Plumb's
Veterinary Drug Handbook

Eighth Edition

Donald C. Plumb, Pharm.D.

DISTRIBUTED BY
John Wiley & Sons, Inc.

PUBLISHED BY

PharmaVet Inc.

Stockholm, Wisconsin

WORLDWIDE PRINT DISTRIBUTION BY:

Wiley-Blackwell

1606 Golden Aspen Drive

Suite 104

Ames, Iowa 50010

(877) 762-2974

www.wiley.com/wiley-blackwell

Wiley-Blackwell is an imprint of John Wiley & Sons, formed by the merger of Wiley's global scientific, technical and medical business with Blackwell Publishing.

DESIGN AND TYPESETTING

Judy Gilats

Peregrine Graphics Services

St. Paul, Minnesota

ISBN: 978-1-1189-1193-8

2015 1

For Benjamin M. Plumb

* * *

Consulting Editors

Gigi Davidson, DICVP
North Carolina State University
Raleigh, NC
Ophthalmology Products, Topical
Principles of Compounding Ophthalmic Products

Lisa Powell, DVM, DACVECC
University of Minnesota Veterinary Medical Center
St. Paul, MN
Small Animal Critical Care Drugs

Contributors to this Edition

Camille DeClementi, VMD, DABVT, DABT, CVJ
ASPCA Animal Poison Control Center
Urbana, IL
Overdose and Toxin Exposure Decontamination
Guidelines

Tina Wismer, DVM, DABVT, DABT
ASPCA Animal Poison Control Center
Urbana, IL
ASPCA Animal Poison Control Center Data for Drug
Monographs

Dinah Jordan, PharmD, DICVP
Mississippi State University
Mississippi State, MS
Insulin Monograph

Katrina L. Mealey, DVM, PhD, DACVIM, DACVCP
Washington State University
Pullman, WA
Multidrug Sensitivity in Dogs

Trishna Patel, PharmD
University of California-Davis
Davis, CA
"Drug Store Toxins"

Tina Wismer, DVM, DABVT, DABT
ASPCA Animal Poison Control Center
Urbana, IL
ASPCA Animal Poison Control Center Data for Drug
Monographs

For errata, updates, and information on other Plumb's resources, follow us at:

Twitter: @PlumbsVetDrug
Facebook: Plumb's Veterinary Drugs
Web: www.vetdruginfo.com

Preface to the Eighth Edition

In this 8th edition of *Plumb's Veterinary Drug Handbook* we continue to strive to provide quality information in a single volume reference to assist veterinarians, other health professionals, and animal caretakers in providing the best possible drug therapy for veterinary patients.

In this edition, in addition to updating all the monographs, 40+ new systemic drug full monographs have been added (see below). A major effort has been to reduce the number of dosage entries for a given indication, primarily by consolidating anecdotal dosage recommendations to reflect the scope of clinical opinions, while giving the prescribing clinician clearer guidance in selecting a dosage for their patient. Dosages in this edition are also identified per their USA label status (i.e. "labeled dose; FDA-approved" or "extra-label") for a given indication and species.

Two new appendices are added to this edition. The first is information on multidrug sensitivity in dogs (MDR1, *ABCB*1) and the second is information on OTC drugs, drug ingredients, products, etc. that can be found in human pharmacies or retail settings that can be toxic to small animals, entitled "Drug Store Toxins". Additionally, the ophthalmology drug monographs have been expanded and are now listed alphabetically by generic name.

New Systemic Monographs: Afoxolaner, Benzonatate, Bumetanide, Calcium Carbonate, Candesartan, Citrate (potassium), Epirubicin, Esomeprazole, Estriol (*Incurin*®), Fenoldopam, Fentanyl Transdermal Solution, Fexofenadine, Fluralaner, Gamithromycin, Hydroxychloroquine, Imepitoin, Imidapril, Iodixanol, L-Theanine, Lithium, Loratadine, Losartan, Masitinib, Nalbuphine, Norepinephrine, Oclacitinib, Osaterone, Paclitaxel, Polyethylene Glycol (PEG) 3350, Pioglitazone, Posaconazole, Pradofloxacin, Rufinamide, Saline Cathartics, Sorbitol, Spinetoram, Tamsulosin, Telmisartan, Theophylline, Thyrotropin-Releasing Hormone, Tildipirosin, Vitamin A, & Zinc Gluconate (neutering agent).

Deleted Monographs: Acemannan, Dichlorphenamide, Dichlorvos, Diethylcarbamazine, Difloxacin, Gold Salts (injectable), Halothane, Ibafloxacin, Inamrinone, Piperacillin (Piperacillin/Tazobactam still listed).

Donald Plumb
September 2014

About the Author

Donald C. Plumb, PharmD was formerly Director of Pharmacy Services and Hospital Director at the University of Minnesota's Veterinary Medical Center. Now retired from the University of Minnesota, he focuses full-time on providing veterinary drug information to veterinarians, other health professionals, and animal caretakers.

Notes and Cautions

Dosages and Extra-Label Use of Medications

Dosages for the various species for the drugs listed in this reference come from a variety of sources and are referenced to their source in the appendix. While a sincere effort has been made to assure that the dosages and information included in this book are accurate and reflect the original source's information, errors can occur; it is recommended that the reader refer to the original reference or the approved labeling information of the product for additional information and verification of all dosages.

Except for labeled dosages for veterinary-approved products (for a given species and indication,) dosages listed in this reference should be considered "extra-label" and are not necessarily endorsed by the manufacturer, the Food and Drug Administration (FDA) or this author. Veterinarians are responsible as per the Animal Medical Drug Use Clarification Act (AMDUCA) for the appropriate use of medications. The Animal Medicinal Drug Use Clarification Act of 1994 (AMDUCA) allows veterinarians to prescribe extra-label uses of certain approved animal drugs and approved human drugs for animals under certain conditions. Extra-label (or extralabel) use refers to the use of an approved drug in a manner that is not in accordance with the approved label directions. The key constraints of AMDUCA are that any extra-label use must be by or on the order of a veterinarian within the context of a veterinarian-client-patient relationship, must not result in violative residues in food-producing animals, and the use must be in conformance with the implementing regulations published at 21 CFR Part 530. A list of drugs specifically prohibited from extra-label use appears in the Code of Federal Regulations. For additional information go to the FDA-Center for Veterinary Medicine Website at: http://www.fda.gov/cvm/

Abbreviations: OTC & Rx

In addition to the abbreviations used in writing prescriptions (*e.g., tid*, q8h, etc.—see the abbreviation list in the appendix), the terms OTC or Rx are found in parentheses after a listed dosage form. If Rx, the drug is considered to be a prescription or legend product, and requires a prescription. OTC denotes that the item is available "over-the-counter" and does not legally require a prescription for purchase.

Trade and Proprietary Names

The notation used to signify trade names or proprietary names is an italicized, capitalized name followed by a ® (*e.g., Amoxi-Tabs*®). This notation may not accurately represent the drug's official registered copyright, trademark, or licensed status (*e.g.*, ™, etc.). For clarity, no use of ® or *italics* are used in the index.

Drug Interactions

Drug interaction identification and evaluation is in its infancy in veterinary medicine, as relatively little specific information is known on the subject for the variety of species treated. While drug interactions can be clinically significant and potentially life-threatening in veterinary patients, most of the interactions listed in the monographs are derived from human medicine (which is only slightly more informed than veterinary medicine on this topic) and are often included primarily to serve as cautions to the prescriber to be alert for unforeseen outcomes, or to enhance monitoring associated with the drug therapy. Additionally, it is likely there are potentially many other clinically significant interactions between drugs that are not listed; prescribers are reminded that the risk for adverse drug interactions occurring increases with the number of different drugs given to an individual patient.

DISCLAIMER

The author/publisher/distributor assume no responsibility for and make no warranty with respect to results that may be obtained from the uses, procedures, or dosages listed, and do not necessarily endorse such uses, procedures, or dosages. The author/publisher shall not be liable to any person whatsoever for any damages, or equivalencies, or by reason of any misstatement or error, negligent or otherwise obtained in this work. Should the purchaser not wish to be bound by the above, he/she may return the reference to the distributor for a full refund.

Contents

SYSTEMIC MONOGRAPHS

Acarbose **1**

Acepromazine Maleate **2**

Acetaminophen **6**

Acetazolamide **7**

Acetic Acid **9**

Acetohydroxamic Acid **10**

Acetylcysteine **11**

Acitretin **13**

Acyclovir **14**

Afoxolaner **16**

Aglepristone **17**

Albendazole **19**

Albumin, Human/Canine **20**

Albuterol Sulfate **23**

Alendronate Sodium **25**

Alfaxalone **26**

Alfentanil HCl **30**

Allopurinol **31**

Alprazolam **33**

Altrenogest **35**

Aluminum Hydroxide **37**

Amantadine HCl **38**

Amikacin Sulfate, Systemic **40**

Aminocaproic Acid **43**

Aminopentamide Hydrogen Sulfate **45**

Aminophylline **46**

Amiodarone HCl **48**

Amitriptyline HCl **50**

Amlodipine Besylate **52**

Ammonium Chloride **54**

Ammonium Molybdate **56**

Ammonium Tetrathiomolybdate **56**

Amoxicillin **56**

Amoxicillin/Clavulanate **59**

Amphotericin B **62**

Ampicillin **67**

Ampicillin Sodium + Sulbactam Sodium **69**

Amprolium HCl **71**

Antivenin (Crotalidae) Polyvalent (Equine Origin) **73**

Antivenin (Crotalidae) Polyvalent Immune Fab (Ovine Origin) **73**

Antivenin (Micrurus fulvias) Eastern and Texas Coral Snake **75**

Antivenin (Latrodectus Mactans) Black Widow Spider **76**

Apomorphine HCl **77**

Apramycin Sulfate **78**

Ascorbic Acid (Vitamin C) **79**

Asparaginase **81**

Aspirin **83**

Atenolol **86**

Atipamezole HCl **88**

Atovaquone **90**

Atracurium Besylate **91**

Atropine Sulfate **93**

Auranofin **96**

Azaperone **97**

Azathioprine **99**

Azithromycin **102**

Aztreonam **104**

Baclofen **106**

Benazepril HCl **107**

Benzonatate **109**

Betamethasone (Systemic) **110**

Bethanechol Chloride **112**

Bisacodyl **114**

Bismuth Subsalicylate **115**

Bleomycin Sulfate **117**

Boldenone Undecylenate **118**

Bromides: Potassium Bromide; Sodium Bromide **120**

Bromocriptine Mesylate **122**

Budesonide **124**

Bumetanide **125**

Buprenorphine HCl **127**

Buspirone HCl **131**

Busulfan **132**

Butaphosphan w/Cyanocobalamin **134**

Butorphanol Tartrate **135**

Cabergoline **140**

Calcitonin Salmon **141**

Calcitriol **143**

Calcium Acetate **145**

Calcium Carbonate **146**

Calcium (Borogluconate, Chloride, Gluconate), Injectable **147**

Candesartan Cilexetil **151**

Captopril **152**

Carbamazepine 154

Carbimazole 156

Carboplatin 158

Carnitine 159

Levocarnitine (L-Carnitine) 159

Carprofen 161

Carvedilol 163

Caspofungin Acetate 165

Cefaclor 167

Cefadroxil 168

Cefazolin Sodium 170

Cefepime HCl 172

Cefixime 173

Cefotaxime Sodium 174

Cefotetan Disodium 176

Cefovecin Sodium 178

Cefoxitin Sodium 180

Cefpodoxime Proxetil 182

Ceftazidime 183

Ceftiofur Crystalline Free Acid 185

Ceftiofur HCl 188

Ceftiofur Sodium 190

Ceftriaxone Sodium 193

Cefuroxime Axetil 195

Cefuroxime Sodium 195

Cephalexin 196

Cephapirin 199

Cetirizine HCl 200

Charcoal, Activated 202

Chlorambucil 204

Chloramphenicol 206

Chlordiazepoxide ± Clidinium Br 209

Chlorothiazide 211

Chlorpheniramine Maleate 213

Chlorpromazine HCl 215

Chlorpropamide 217

Chlortetracycline 218

Chorionic Gonadotropin (HCG) 220

Chromium, Chromium Picolinate 221

Cimetidine 222

Ciprofloxacin 224

Cisapride 226

Cisplatin 228

Citrate, Potassium 230

Clarithromycin 232

Clemastine Fumarate 234

Clenbuterol HCl 236

Clindamycin 237

Clodronate 240

Clofazimine 242

Clomipramine HCl 243

Clonazepam 246

Clonidine 247

Clopidogrel Bisulfate 249

Cloprostenol Sodium 251

Clorazepate Dipotassium 253

Clorsulon 254

Cloxacillin 255

Codeine 256

Colchicine 258

Corticotropin (ACTH) 260

Cortisone Acetate 261

Cosyntropin 263

Cromolyn Sodium (Inhaled) 264

Cyanocobalamin (Vitamin B12) 265

Cyclophosphamide 266

Cyclosporine (Systemic) 269

Cyproheptadine HCl 273

Cytarabine 274

Dacarbazine (DTIC) 276

Dactinomycin 278

Dalteparin Sodium 279

Danazol 281

Danofloxacin Mesylate 282

Dantrolene Sodium 283

Dapsone 285

Darbepoetin Alfa 287

Decoquinate 288

Deferoxamine Mesylate 289

Deracoxib 291

Desflurane 293

Deslorelin Acetate 294

Desmopressin Acetate 295

Desoxycorticosterone Pivalate (DOCP) 297

Detomidine HCl 299

Dexamethasone 301

Dexmedetomidine 306

Dexpanthenol 308

D-Panthenol 308

Dexrazoxane 309

Dextran 70 311

Diazepam 312

Diazoxide, Oral 316

Dichlorphenamide 317

Dichlorvos 318

Diclazuril 319

Diclofenac Sodium, Topical **321**

Dicloxacillin Sodium **322**

Diethylstilbestrol **323**

Digoxin **325**

Dihydrotachysterol **328**

DHT **328**

Diltiazem HCl **330**

Dimenhydrinate **332**

Dimercaprol (BAL) **334**

Dimethyl Sulfoxide (DMSO) **335**

Diminazene Aceturate **337**

Dinoprost Tromethamine **339**

Prostaglandin F2alpha Tromethamine **339**

Diphenhydramine HCl **342**

Diphenoxylate HCl + Atropine Sulfate **344**

Dirlotapide **345**

Disopyramide Phosphate **347**

Dobutamine HCl **349**

Docusate **351**

Dolasetron Mesylate **352**

Domperidone **353**

Dopamine HCl **355**

Doramectin **357**

Doxapram HCl **359**

Doxepin HCl **361**

Doxorubicin HCl **362**

Doxycycline **365**

Edetate Calcium Disodium **370**

Edrophonium Chloride **371**

Emodepside + Praziquantel **373**

Enalapril; Enalaprilat **374**

Enoxaparin Sodium **377**

Enrofloxacin **379**

Ephedrine Sulfate **383**

Epinephrine **385**

Epirubicin HCl **388**

Epoetin Alfa (Erythropoietin) **390**

Eprinomectin **392**

Epsiprantel **394**

Ergocalciferol **394**

Ertapenem Sodium **396**

Erythromycin **397**

Esmolol HCl **400**

Esomeprazole **402**

Estradiol Cypionate **404**

Estriol **406**

Ethambutol HCl **407**

Ethanol **409**

Alcohol, Ethyl **409**

Etidronate Disodium **411**

Etodolac **412**

Etomidate **414**

Euthanasia Agents w/Pentobarbital **415**

Famciclovir **416**

Famotidine **418**

Fat Emulsion, Intravenous **420**

Fatty Acids, Essential/Omega (Oral) **422**

Felbamate **424**

Fenbendazole **425**

Fenoldopam **428**

Fentanyl Citrate, Injection **430**

Fentanyl, Transdermal Patch **432**

Fentanyl Transdermal Solution **436**

Ferrous Sulfate **438**

Fexofenadine HCl **440**

Filgrastim (GCSF) **442**

Finasteride **443**

Firocoxib **444**

Flavoxate HCl **447**

Florfenicol **447**

Fluconazole **449**

Flucytosine **451**

Fludrocortisone Acetate **453**

Flumazenil **454**

Flumethasone **455**

Flunixin Meglumine **458**

Fluorouracil (5-FU) **461**

Fluoxetine HCl **462**

Fluralaner **464**

Fluticasone Propionate **465**

Fluvoxamine Maleate **467**

Folic Acid **469**

Fomepizole **471**

4-Methylpyrazole (4-MP) **471**

Fosfomycin Tromethamine **472**

Furazolidone **474**

Furosemide **475**

Gabapentin **478**

Gamithromycin **481**

Gemcitabine HCl **482**

Gemfibrozil **484**

Gentamicin Sulfate, Systemic **485**

Glimepiride **488**

Glipizide **490**

Glucagon **491**

Glucocorticoid Agents, General Information **493**

Glucosamine/Chondroitin Sulfate **495**

Glutamine **497**

Glyburide **498**

Glycerin, Oral **499**

Glycopyrrolate **500**

Gonadorelin **503**

Granisetron HCl **505**

Griseofulvin **506**

Guaifenesin, Intravenous **507**

Hemoglobin Glutamer-200 (Bovine) **510**

Heparin Sodium **512**

Hyaluronate Sodium **515**

Sodium Hyaluronate **515**

Hyaluronan **515**

Hydralazine HCl **516**

Hydrochlorothiazide **518**

Hydrocodone Bitartrate **521**

Hydrocortisone **522**

Hydrocortisone Sodium Succinate **522**

Hydrogen Peroxide 3% (oral) **525**

Hydromorphone **526**

Hydroxychloroquine Sulfate **529**

Hydroxyethyl Starch Colloids (HES) **530**

Hydroxyurea **533**

Hydroxyzine **534**

Hyoscyamine Sulfate **536**

Hypertonic Saline (7% –7.5%) **537**

Ifosfamide **539**

Imepitoin **541**

Imidapril **543**

Imidocarb Dipropionate **544**

Imipenem-Cilastatin Sodium **546**

Imipramine **548**

Immune Globulin (Human), Intravenous **550**

Insulin **552**

Interferon Alfa, Human Recombinant **558**

Interferon-ω (omega), Feline Origin **560**

Iodide **561**

Iodixanol **563**

Iohexol **564**

Ipodate **566**

Ipratropium Bromide **567**

Irbesartan **568**

Iron Dextran **570**

Isoflupredone Acetate **571**

Isoflurane **573**

Isoniazid (INH) **575**

Isoproterenol HCl **577**

Isosorbide **579**

Isotretinoin **580**

Isoxsuprine HCl **582**

Itraconazole **583**

Ivermectin **586**

Kaolin/Pectin **591**

Ketamine HCl **592**

Ketoconazole, Systemic **599**

Ketoprofen **603**

Ketorolac Tromethamine **605**

L-Theanine **607**

Lactulose **608**

Lanthanum Carbonate **609**

Leflunomide **610**

Leucovorin Calcium **612**

Leuprolide **613**

Levamisole **615**

Levetiracetam **617**

Levothyroxine Sodium **619**

Lidocaine HCl (I.V.; Systemic) **623**

Lincomycin HCl **626**

Liothyronine Sodium **628**

Lisinopril **630**

Lithium **632**

Lomustine (CCNU) **634**

Loperamide HCl **636**

Loratadine **638**

Lorazepam **639**

Losartan Potassium **641**

Lufenuron **643**

Lysine **644**

L-Lysine **644**

Magnesium Hydroxide **645**

Magnesium/Aluminum Antacids **645**

Magnesium, Intravenous **647**

Mannitol **650**

Marbofloxacin **652**

Maropitant Citrate **654**

Masitinib Mesylate **656**

Mavacoxib **658**

Mechlorethamine HCl **660**

Meclizine HCl **662**

Medetomidine HCl **663**

Medium Chain Triglycerides (MCT Oil) **665**

Medroxyprogesterone Acetate **666**

Megestrol Acetate **668**

Meglumine Antimoniate **670**

Melarsomine **671**

Melatonin **673**

Meloxicam **675**

Melphalan **678**

Meperidine HCl **680**

Mercaptopurine **682**

Meropenem **684**

Metergoline **685**

Metformin HCl **686**

Methadone HCl **688**

Methazolamide **690**

Methenamine **692**

Methimazole **693**

Methionine (dl-Methionine) **695**

Methocarbamol **697**

Methohexital Sodium **698**

Methotrexate **700**

Methylene Blue **702**

Methylphenidate **704**

Methylprednisolone **705**

Methyltestosterone **709**

Metoclopramide HCl **710**

Metoprolol **713**

Metronidazole **715**

Metyrapone **718**

Mexiletine HCl **720**

Mibolerone **721**

Midazolam HCl **722**

Milbemycin Oxime **726**

Miltefosine **727**

Mineral Oil **728**

Minocycline HCl **730**

Mirtazapine **732**

Misoprostol **734**

Mitotane **737**

Mitoxantrone HCl **739**

Montelukast Sodium **741**

Morantel Tartrate **742**

Morphine Sulfate **743**

Moxidectin **747**

Mycobacterial Cell Wall Fraction Immunomodulator **751**

Mycophenolate Mofetil **752**

N-Butylscopolammonium Bromide (Hyoscine Butylbromide) **754**

Nalbuphine HCl **756**

Naloxone HCl **757**

Naltrexone HCl **759**

Nandrolone **761**

Naproxen **762**

Narcotic (Opiate) Agonist Analgesics, Pharmacology of **764**

Neomycin Sulfate **764**

Neostigmine **766**

Niacinamide **768**

Nitazoxanide **769**

Nitenpyram **770**

Nitrofurantoin **771**

Nitroglycerin, Transdermal **773**

Nitroprusside Sodium **774**

Nizatidine **776**

Norepinephrine Bitartrate **777**

Novobiocin Sodium **779**

Nystatin (Oral) **780**

Oclacitinib **782**

Octreotide Acetate **783**

Olsalazine Sodium **784**

Omeprazole **785**

Ondansetron HCl **787**

Orbifloxacin **788**

Osaterone Acetate **790**

Oseltamivir Phosphate **791**

Oxacillin Sodium **793**

Oxazepam **795**

Oxfendazole **796**

Oxibendazole **797**

Oxybutynin Chloride **798**

Oxymorphone HCl **799**

Oxytetracycline **802**

Oxytocin **806**

Paclitaxel **809**

Pamidronate Disodium **811**

Pancrelipase **812**

Pancuronium Bromide **813**

Pantoprazole **815**

Parapox Ovis Virus Immunomodulator **816**

Paregoric **817**

Paromomycin Sulfate **819**

Paroxetine HCl **820**

Penicillamine **822**

Penicillins, General Information **823**

Penicillin G **825**

Penicillin V Potassium **829**

Pentazocine **830**

Pentobarbital Sodium **832**

Pentosan Polysulfate Sodium **835**

Pentoxifylline **836**

Pergolide Mesylate **838**

Phenobarbital **840**

Phenoxybenzamine HCl **843**

Phenylbutazone **845**

Phenylephrine HCl, Parenteral **847**

Phenylpropanolamine HCl **849**

Phenytoin Sodium **850**

Pheromones **852**

Phosphate, Parenteral **854**

Physostigmine Salicylate **855**

Phytonadione (Vitamin K**1**) **857**

Pimobendan **858**

Piperacillin Sodium + Tazobactam **861**

Piperazine **863**

Pirlimycin HCl **864**

Piroxicam **865**

Polyethylene Glycol 3350 (PEG 3350) **867**

Polysulfated Glycosaminoglycan (PSGAG) **868**

Ponazuril **869**

Posaconazole **871**

Potassium **872**

Pradofloxacin **875**

Pralidoxime Chloride (2-PAM) **877**

Praziquantel **879**

Prazosin HCl **882**

Prednisolone **883**

Prednisone **883**

Prednisolone Sodium Succinate **883**

Pregabalin **887**

Primaquine Phosphate **889**

Primidone **890**

Probenecid **892**

Procainamide HCl **894**

Procarbazine HCl **896**

Prochlorperazine **898**

Promethazine HCl **899**

Propantheline Bromide **901**

Propionibacterium acnes Injection **903**

Propofol **904**

Propranolol HCl **908**

Protamine Sulfate **910**

Pseudoephedrine HCl **911**

Psyllium Hydrophilic Mucilloid **913**

Pyrantel Pamoate **914**

Pyridostigmine Bromide **916**

Pyridoxine HCl (Vitamin B-6) **918**

Pyrilamine Maleate **919**

Pyrimethamine **920**

Pyrimethamine + Sulfadiazine **922**

Quinacrine HCl **923**

Quinidine **925**

Ramipril **927**

Ranitidine HCl **929**

Remifentanil HCl **931**

Rifampin **933**

Robenacoxib **935**

Rocuronium Bromide **938**

Romifidine HCl **940**

Ronidazole **942**

Rufinamide **944**

S-Adenosyl-Methionine **945**

Saline Cathartics **947**

Selamectin **949**

Selegiline HCl **951**

Sertraline HCl **953**

Sevelamer **954**

Sevoflurane **955**

Sildenafil Citrate **957**

Silymarin **959**

Sodium Bicarbonate **960**

Sodium Polystyrene Sulfonate **963**

Sodium Stibogluconate **964**

Sodium Thiosulfate **965**

Somatotropin (Growth Hormone) **966**

Sorbitol **967**

Sotalol HCl **969**

Spectinomycin **970**

Spinosad **972**

Spironolactone **974**

Stanozolol **976**

Staphylococcal Phage Lysate **978**

Streptozocin **979**

Succimer **981**

Succinylcholine Chloride **982**

Sucralfate **983**

Sufentanil Citrate **985**

Sulfachlorpyridazine Sodium **986**

Sulfadiazine/Trimethoprim **988**

Sulfamethoxazole/Trimethoprim **988**

Sulfadimethoxine **992**

Sulfadimethoxine/Ormetoprim **994**

Sulfasalazine **995**

Tadalafil **997**

Tamsulosin **998**

Taurine **1000**

Telmisartan **1001**

Tepoxalin **1002**

Terbinafine HCl **1004**

Terbutaline Sulfate **1006**

Testosterone **1008**

Tetracycline HCl **1010**

Theophylline **1013**

Thiamine HCl **1015**

Thioguanine **1017**

Thiopental Sodium **1018**

Thiotepa **1020**

Thyrotropin Alfa (RHTSH) **1022**

Thyrotropin-Releasing Hormone **1023**

Tiamulin **1024**

Ticarcillin Disodium + Clavulanate Potassium **1025**

Tildipirosin **1028**

Tiletamine HCl/Zolazepam HCl **1030**

Tilmicosin **1033**

Tiludronate Disodium **1034**

Tinidazole **1036**

Tiopronin **1038**

Tobramycin Sulfate **1039**

Toceranib Phosphate **1042**

Tolazoline HCl **1044**

Tolfenamic Acid **1046**

Toltrazuril **1047**

Topiramate **1049**

Torsemide **1051**

Tramadol HCl **1052**

Trazodone HCl **1055**

Triamcinolone Acetonide **1057**

Triamterene **1061**

Trientine HCl **1062**

Trilostane **1063**

Trimeprazine Tartrate with Prednisolone **1066**

Tripelennamine HCl **1067**

Trypan Blue **1068**

Tulathromycin **1069**

Tylosin **1071**

Ursodiol **1073**

Valproic Acid; (Valproate Divalproex) **1075**

Vanadium (Vanadyl Sulfate) **1076**

Vancomycin HCl **1077**

Vasopressin **1079**

Vecuronium Bromide **1081**

Verapamil HCl **1083**

Vinblastine Sulfate **1085**

Vincristine Sulfate **1087**

Vitamin A **1090**

Vitamin E ± Selenium **1092**

Voriconazole **1094**

Warfarin Sodium **1097**

Xylazine HCl **1099**

Yohimbine HCl **1104**

Zafirlukast **1106**

Zidovudine **1107**

Zinc (Systemic) **1108**

Zinc Gluconate (Neutering Agent) **1110**

Zonisamide **1111**

Ophthalmic Products, Topical 1114

Routes of Administration For Ophthalmic Drugs **1114**

Ophthalmic Agents Listed by Class/Indication **1115**

Acetylcysteine Ophthalmic **1116**

Acyclovir Ophthalmic **1116**

Alcaftadine Ophthalmic **1117**

Amikacin Sulfate Ophthalmic **1117**

Aminocaproic Acid Ophthalmic **1118**

Amphotericin B Ophthalmic **1118**

Apraclonidine Ophthalmic **1119**

Artificial Tears/Ocular Lubricants **1120**

Atropine Sulfate Ophthalmic **1121**

Azelastine Ophthalmic **1122**

Azithromycin Ophthalmic **1123**

Bacitracin Ophthalmic **1123**

Benoxinate Ophthalmic **1124**

Bepotastine Ophthalmic **1125**

Besifloxacin Ophthalmic **1125**

Betamethasone Ophthalmic **1126**

Betaxolol Ophthalmic **1126**

Bimatoprost Ophthalmic **1127**

Brimonidine Ophthalmic **1127**

Brinzolamide Ophthalmic **1128**

Bromfenac Ophthalmic **1129**

Carteolol Ophthalmic **1129**

Chloramphenicol Ophthalmic **1130**

Cidofovir Ophthalmic **1130**

Ciprofloxacin Ophthalmic **1131**

Cromolyn Sodium Ophthalmic **1132**

Cyclopentolate Ophthalmic **1132**

Cyclosporine Ophthalmic **1133**

Demecarium Bromide Ophthalmic **1134**

Dexamethasone Ophthalmic **1135**

Diclofenac Ophthalmic **1136**

Difluprednate Ophthalmic **1136**

Dorzolamide Ophthalmic **1137**

Echothiophate Iodide Ophthalmic **1138**

Edetate Disodium Ophthalmic **1138**

Emedastine Ophthalmic **1139**

Epinastine Ophthalmic **1140**

Erythromycin Ophthalmic **1140**

Fluorometholone Ophthalmic **1141**

Fluorouracil Ophthalmic **1142**

Fluorescein Sodium Ophthalmic **1142**

Flurbiprofen Ophthalmic **1143**

Ganciclovir Ophthalmic **1144**

Gatifloxacin Ophthalmic **1144**

Gentamicin Sulfate Ophthalmic **1145**

Hydrocortisone Ophthalmic **1146**

Idoxuridine Ophthalmic **1147**

Irrigating Solutions, Ophthalmic **1147**

Itraconazole Ophthalmic **1148**

Ketorolac Ophthalmic **1149**

Ketotifen Ophthalmic **1150**

Latanoprost Ophthalmic **1150**

Levobunolol Ophthalmic **1151**

Levofloxacin Ophthalmic **1151**

Lissamine Green Ophthalmic **1152**

Loteprednol Ophthalmic **1153**

Metipranolol Ophthalmic **1153**

Miconazole Ophthalmic **1154**

Mitomycin Ophthalmic **1154**

Morphine Sulfate Ophthalmic **1155**

Moxifloxacin Ophthalmic **1156**

Nalbuphine Ophthalmic **1157**

Natamycin Ophthalmic **1157**

Nedocromil Ophthalmic **1158**

Neomycin Sulfate Ophthalmic **1158**

Nepafenac Ophthalmic **1159**

Ofloxacin Ophthalmic **1160**

Olopatadine Ophthalmic **1161**

Oxytetracycline/Polymyxin B Ophthalmic **1161**

Phenylephrine Ophthalmic **1162**

Pilocarpine Ophthalmic **1163**

Pimecrolimus Ophthalmic **1163**

Polysulfated Glycosaminoglycan Ophthalmic **1164**

Povidone Iodine Ophthalmic **1165**

Prednisolone Ophthalmic **1165**

Proparacaine Ophthalmic **1166**

Rimexolone Ophthalmic **1167**

Rose Bengal Ophthalmic **1168**

Schirmer Tear Test Ophthalmic **1169**

Silver Sulfadiazine Ophthalmic **1169**

Sodium Chloride (Hypertonic) Ophthalmic **1170**

Sulfacetamide Ophthalmic **1171**

Suprofen Ophthalmic **1172**

Tacrolimus Ophthalmic **1172**

Tafluprost Ophthalmic **1173**

Tetracaine Ophthalmic **1174**

Timolol Maleate Ophthalmic **1174**

Tissue Plasminogen Activator (Alteplase) Ophthalmic **1175**

Tobramycin Sulfate Ophthalmic **1176**

Trifluridine Ophthalmic **1177**

Triple Antibiotic Ophthalmic **1177**

Tropicamide Ophthalmic **1178**

Vancomycin Sulfate Ophthalmic **1179**

Voriconazole Ophthalmic **1180**

Principles of Compounding Ophthalmic Products **1180**

Dermatological Agents, Topical 1184

Antipruritics/Antiinflammatories, Topical **1184**

    Non-Corticosteroids **1184**

        Aluminum Acetate Solution (Burow's Solution) **1184**

        Colloidal Oatmeal **1185**

        Essential Fatty Acids, Topical **1185**

        Diphenhydramine HCl, Topical **1186**

        Lidocaine, Topical **1186**

        Lidocaine/Prilocaine (EMLA Cream) **1186**

        Phytosphingosine **1187**

        Pramoxine HCl **1188**

        Phenol/Menthol/Camphor **1189**

        Zinc Gluconate (Neutralized), Topical **1189**

    Corticosteroids, Topical **1190**

        Betamethasone Dipropionate, Topical **1190**

        Hydrocortisone, Topical **1191**

        Isoflupredone Acetate, Topical **1192**

        Mometasone Furoate **1193**

        Triamcinolone Acetonide, Topical **1194**

    Antimicrobials, Topical **1195**

        Antibacterial Agents **1195**

        Bacitracin, Topical **1195**

        Benzoyl Peroxide **1196**

        Clindamycin, Topical **1196**

        Gentamicin Sulfate, Topical **1197**

        Mupirocin (Pseudomonic Acid A) **1198**

        Nitrofurazone, Topical **1199**

        Silver Sulfadiazine (SSD) **1199**

    Antiseptics **1200**

        Acetic Acid/Boric Acid **1200**

        Chlorhexidine **1201**

        Chloroxylenol (PCMX) **1202**

        Enzymes, Topical (Lactoperoxidase, Lysozyme, Lactoferrin) **1203**

        Ethyl Lactate **1204**

        Hypochlorous Acid **1204**

Povidone Iodine **1205**

Triclosan **1206**

Antifungals **1206**

Clotrimazole, Topical **1206**

Enilconazole **1207**

Ketoconazole, Topical **1208**

Lime Sulfur (Sulfurated Lime Solution) **1209**

Miconazole, Topical **1210**

Nystatin & Nystatin Combinations **1211**

Selenium Sulfide **1212**

Terbinafine HCl, Topical **1212**

Keratolytic Agents **1213**

Salicylic Acid **1213**

Sulfur, Precipitated **1214**

Coal Tar & Coal Tar Combinations **1215**

Antiseborrheic Products **1216**

Immunomodulators, Topical **1216**

Imiquimod, Topical **1216**

Pimecrolimus, Topical **1216**

Tacrolimus, Topical **1217**

Retinoids, Topical **1218**

Tretinoin (trans-Retinoic Acid; Vitamin A Acid) **1218**

Antiparasitic Agents, Topical **1218**

Amitraz & Amitraz Combinations **1218**

Crotamiton **1220**

Deltamethrin **1220**

Dinotefuran + Pyriproxyfen (± Permethrin) **1220**

Fipronil & Fipronil Combinations **1221**

Imidacloprid & Imidacloprid Combinations **1223**

Indoxacarb ± Permethrin **1224**

Isopropyl Myristate **1225**

(s)-Methoprene Combinations **1225**

Permethrin & Permethrin Combinations **1227**

Pyrethrins & Pyrethrin Combinations **1228**

Pyriproxyfen & Pyriproxyfen Combinations **1229**

Spinetoram **1230**

Otic Preparations 1231

Ceruminolytic Agents **1231**

Cleaning/Drying Agents **1231**

Antiseptic Agents **1233**

Corticosteroid Preparations **1234**

Antibacterials **1234**

Antibiotic Potentiating Agents **1234**

Antifungals **1235**

Corticosteroid + Antimicrobial Preparations **1235**

Antiparasitic Preparations **1236**

APPENDIX 1238

Multidrug Sensitivity in Dogs **1238**

Overdose and Toxin Exposure Decontamination Guidelines **1239**

"Drug Store" Toxins in Small Animals **1241**

Importation of Unapproved New Animal Drugs into the USA **1245**

ARCI UCGFS Classifications **1245**

Conversion Tables for Weight in Kilograms to Body Surface Area (m2) **1245**

Tables of Parenteral Fluids **1246**

Abbreviations Used in Prescription Writing **1247**

Solubility Definitions **1248**

Conversion: Weights; Temperature; Liquids **1248**

Milliequivalents & Molecular Weights **1248**

"Normal" Vital Signs **1248**

Estrus and Gestation Periods: Dogs & Cats **1249**

Conversion of Conventional Chemistry Units to SI Units **1249**

Reference Laboratory Ranges **1250**

Chemistry: Companion/Small Animals **1250**

Hematology: Companion/Small Animals **1251**

Chemistry: Equine, Food, & Fiber Animals **1251**

Hematology: Equine, Food, & Fiber Animals **1252**

Coagulation: Bovine, Canine, Equine, Feline **1253**

Urinalysis: Canine, Feline **1253**

Cerebral Spinal Fluid: Canine, Feline **1254**

Phone Numbers And Websites 1255

Governmental Veterinary Drug-Related Websites **1255**

Drug Shortage Websites **1255**

Animal Poison Control Centers **1255**

Animal Blood Banks **1255**

Dog/Cat Food Companies **1256**

Veterinary Pharmaceutical Manufacturers & Suppliers **1256**

Systemic Drugs Sorted by Therapeutic Class or Major Indication 1260

Index 1264

Acarbose

(ay-**kar**-bose)   Precose®

Oral Antidiabetic

Prescriber Highlights

▶ Antihyperglycemic agent that reduces the rate & amount of glucose absorbed from the gut after a meal; may be useful for mild reductions in blood glucose in dogs or cats. Unlikely to be effective when used as sole therapy.

▶ Contraindications: Underweight animals, known hypersensitivity, diabetic ketoacidosis, inflammatory bowel disease, colonic ulceration, partial intestinal obstruction or predisposition to obstruction, chronic intestinal disease with marked disorders of digestion or absorption & when excessive gas formation would be detrimental.

▶ Dose–dependent loose stools, diarrhea & flatulence are the adverse effects most likely to be noted.

▶ Give with meals (preferably right before); drug is not very useful if feeding *ad libitum*.

Uses/Indications

May be useful for mild reductions in blood glucose concentrations (250-350 mg/dL range) in dogs and cats with non-insulin-dependent diabetes mellitus and as adjunctive treatment of insulin dependent diabetes mellitus.

Acarbose apparently is most effective in cats that will not eat a low carbohydrate diet and that consume their food within a short time after acarbose is given. Acarbose is usually not effective in cats with advanced renal failure with reduced appetites that are being fed low protein diets *ad libitum. In dogs, acarbose may be considered when glycemic control is poor and the cause is not determined. Acarbose is unlikely to give adequate glucose control when used alone and most recommend dietary therapy and other antihyperglycemic agents (e.g., insulin) instead.*

Pharmacology/Actions

Acarbose competitively inhibits pancreatic alpha-amylase and alpha-glucosidases found in the small intestine. This delays the digestion of complex carbohydrates and disaccharides to glucose and other monosaccharides. Glucose is absorbed lower in the GI tract in lesser amounts than is normal thereby reducing insulin requirements during the postprandial hyperglycemic phase. Acarbose has no effect on lactase.

Pharmacokinetics

In dogs about 4% of an oral dose is absorbed; in humans only about 2% of an oral dose is absorbed from the gut that is then excreted by the kidneys. Practically all the remaining drug in the gut is metabolized in the GI tract by intestinal bacteria. Patients with severe renal dysfunction attain serum levels approximately 5 times those of normal subjects.

Contraindications/Precautions/Warnings

Acarbose is contraindicated in patients with known hypersensitivity to the drug, diabetic ketoacidosis, inflammatory bowel disease, colonic ulceration, partial intestinal obstruction or predisposition to obstruction, chronic intestinal disease with marked disorders of digestion or absorption, and when excessive gas formation would be detrimental. Acarbose is not indicated in patients with low body weight (some say normal body weight as well) as it may have deleterious effects on nutrition status. Use caution in patients with renal dysfunction or severe liver disease.

Adverse Effects

Adverse effects reported in cats include flatulence, soft stools and diarrhea; in dogs, diarrhea and weight loss. Adverse effects are more likely at higher doses.

While acarbose alone does not cause hypoglycemia, it may contribute to it by reducing the rate and amount of glucose absorbed when the patient is receiving other hypoglycemic agents (insulin, oral hypoglycemics).

Reproductive/Nursing Safety

Safety in pregnancy has not been established; weigh any potential risks versus benefits in pregnant animals. In humans, the FDA categorizes this drug as category *B* for use during pregnancy (*Animal studies have not yet demonstrated risk to the fetus, but there are no adequate studies in pregnant women; or animal studies have shown an adverse effect, but adequate studies in pregnant women have not demonstrated a risk to the fetus in the first trimester of pregnancy, and there is no evidence of risk in later trimesters.*)

Overdosage/Acute Toxicity

Acute overdosages are likely to cause only diarrhea and flatulence; no treatment should be necessary. Should acute hypoglycemia occur secondary to other antihypoglycemics, parenteral glucose should be administered. If treating orally, use glucose (do not use sucrose).

Drug Interactions

The following drug interactions with acarbose have either been reported or are theoretical in humans or animals and may be of significance in veterinary patients. Unless otherwise noted, use together is not necessarily contraindicated, but weigh the potential risks and perform additional monitoring when appropriate.

- **CHARCOAL**: Intestinal adsorbents may reduce the efficacy of acarbose.
- **DIGOXIN**: Acarbose may reduce digoxin blood concentrations.
- **HYPERGLYCEMIC AGENTS** (*e.g.*, corticosteroids, thiazides, estrogens, phenothiazines, thyroid hormones, and calcium channel blockers): May reduce or negate the effects of acarbose.
- **HYPOGLYCEMIC AGENTs** (*e.g.*, insulin, sulfonylureas): May increase the risk for hypoglycemia.
- **PANCREATIN, PANCRELIPASE, OR AMYLASE**: Exogenous enzyme formulations may reduce the efficacy of acarbose.

Laboratory Considerations

- Increased **serum aminotransferase levels** have been noted in some humans taking high dosages for a long period.

Doses

- **DOGS:**

  For mild reductions of blood glucose (extra-label): Initial Dosage: 12.5 – 25 mg per dog PO with each meal (usually twice a day). Give only at time of feeding (right before). If response is inadequate after 2 weeks, may titrate dosage up to 50 mg PO twice a day. For dogs weighing >10-25 kg, a further increase up to 100 mg twice daily may be considered if response has been inadequate. Frequency and severity of side effects such as diarrhea and weight loss increase with higher dosages.

- **CATS:**

  For mild reductions of blood glucose (extra-label): 12.5 – 25 mg (per cat) PO with each meal (usually 2 times a day).

Monitoring

- Serum glucose.
- Adverse effects (diarrhea, flatulence).

Client Information

- Give right before feeding for best results.
- Diarrhea and/or gas most likely side effects.
- Acarbose does not cause low blood sugar, but it may add to it if the animal is getting other drugs that lower blood sugar (including insulin); watch for signs of low blood sugar: seizures (convulsions), collapse, rear leg weakness or paralysis, muscle twitching, unsteadiness, tiredness, or depression. If these occur, call veterinarian immediately.
- May take up to two weeks for the drug to work at its peak effect.

Chemistry/Synonyms

A complex oligosaccharide antihyperglycemic agent, acarbose occurs as white to off-white powder, is soluble in water and has a pKa of 5.1.

Acarbose may also be known as: Bay-g-5421, *Precose®*, *Asucrose®*, *Glicobase®*, *Glucobay®*, *Glucor®*, *Glumida®*, or *Prandase®*.

Storage/Stability

Do not store tablets above 25°C (77°F); protect from moisture.

Compatibility/Compounding Considerations

Tablets may be split or crushed and mixed with food just prior to administration.

Dosage Forms/Regulatory Status

VETERINARY-LABELED PRODUCTS: NONE.

HUMAN-LABELED PRODUCTS:

Acarbose Oral Tablets: 25 mg, 50 mg & 100 mg; *Precose®*, generic; (Rx)

Revisions/References

Monograph revised/updated August 2013.

Acepromazine Maleate

(ase-**pro**-ma-zeen)

Acetylpromazine, ACE, ACP, PromAce®

Phenothiazine Sedative/Tranquilizer

Prescriber Highlights

▶ Dosages used are usually much lower than those listed on the approved label. Relatively long duration of action.

▶ Negligible analgesic effects by itself, but can potentiate effects of opiates; little effect on respiratory function.

▶ Dosage may need to be reduced in debilitated or geriatric animals, those with hepatic or cardiac disease, or when combined with other agents. Certain dog breeds (*e.g.*, giant breeds, sight hounds) and dogs with the ABCB1-1Δ (also called MDR1) mutation may be overly sensitive to effects and require dosage reduction.

▶ Inject IV slowly; do not inject into arteries. Requires up to 30 minutes (even after IV injection) to show full effect.

▶ May cause significant hypotension, cardiac rate abnormalities, hypo- or hyperthermia.

▶ May cause penis protrusion (prolapse) in large animals (esp. horses), but associated permanent penile dysfunction is very rare.

Uses/Indications

Acepromazine is FDA-approved for use in dogs, cats, and horses. Labeled indications for dogs and cats include: "...as an aid in controlling intractable animals...alleviate itching as a result of skin irritation; as an antiemetic to control vomiting associated with motion sickness" and as a preanesthetic agent. Because acepromazine has minimal effect on respiratory function, it can be a useful tranquilizer/sedative in small animals with upper airway obstruction (*e.g.*, laryngeal paralysis). Newer, effective agents that have fewer adverse effects have largely supplanted the use of acepromazine as a sedative/tranquilizer in the treatment of adverse behaviors in dogs and cats. Its use for sedation during travel is controversial and many no longer recommend drug therapy for this purpose. In combination with analgesics (*e.g.*, opioids), acepromazine can potentiate their analgesic effect (neuroleptanalgesia).

In horses, acepromazine is labeled "...as an aid in controlling fractious animals," and in conjunction with local anesthesia for various procedures and treatments. It is also commonly used in horses as a pre-anesthetic agent at very small doses to help control behavior.

Although not FDA-approved, it is used as a tranquilizer (see doses) in other species such as swine, cattle, rabbits, sheep and goats. Acepromazine has also been shown to reduce the incidence of halothane-induced malignant hyperthermia in susceptible pigs.

Pharmacology/Actions

Acepromazine is a phenothiazine neuroleptic agent. While the exact mechanisms of action are not fully understood, the phenothiazines block post-synaptic dopamine receptors in the CNS and may also inhibit the release of, and increase the turnover rate of dopamine. They are thought to depress portions of the reticular activating system that assists in the control of body temperature, basal metabolic rate, emesis, vasomotor tone, hormonal balance, and alertness. Additionally, phenothiazines have varying degrees of anticholinergic, antihistaminic, antispasmodic, and alpha-adrenergic blocking effects.

The primary desired effect for the use of acepromazine in veterinary medicine is its tranquilizing/sedating action. Additional pharmacologic actions that acepromazine possesses include antiemetic, antispasmodic, and hypothermic actions.

Acepromazine use has historically been avoided in epileptic animals or in those susceptible to seizures (*e.g.*, post-myelography) secondary to the concern that phenothiazines may lower the seizure threshold and/or precipitate seizures. However, there is no apparent published evidence to support this idea and some research has shown that acepromazine has some anticonvulsant activity.

Acepromazine may decrease respiratory rates, but studies have demonstrated that little or no effect occurs with regard to the blood gas picture, pH or oxyhemoglobin saturation. A dose dependent decrease in hematocrit is seen within 30 minutes after dosing in horses and dogs. Hematocrit values in horses may decrease up to 50% of pre-dose values; this is probably due to increased splenic sequestration of red cells.

Besides lowering arterial blood pressure in dogs, acepromazine causes increases in central venous pressure, a vagally induced bradycardic effect and transient sinoatrial arrest. The bradycardia may be negated by a reflex tachycardic effect secondary to decreases in blood pressure. Acepromazine also has antidysrhythmic effects. Acepromazine has been demonstrated to inhibit the arrhythmias induced by ultra-short acting barbiturates, and protect against the ventricular fibrillatory actions of halothane and epinephrine. Other pharmacologic actions are discussed in the adverse effects section below.

Pharmacokinetics

In dogs, oral bioavailability is about 20% and elimination half-lives are approximately 7.1 hours (IV) and 16 hours (PO) (Hashem et al. 1992). The pharmacokinetics of acepromazine has been studied in the horse (Ballard et al. 1982). The drug has a fairly high volume of distribution (6.6 L/kg), and is more than 99% protein bound. The onset of action is fairly slow, requiring up to 15 minutes following IV administration, with peak effects seen in 30–60 minutes. The elimination half-life in horses is approximately 3 hours.

Acepromazine is metabolized in the liver with both conjugated and unconjugated metabolites eliminated in the urine. Metabolites may be found in equine urine up to 96 hours after dosing.

Contraindications/Precautions/Warnings

Animals may require lower dosages of general anesthetics following acepromazine. Use cautiously and in smaller doses in animals with hepatic dysfunction, mild cardiac disease, or general debilitation. Because of its hypotensive effects, acepromazine is relatively contraindicated in patients with significant cardiac disease, hypovolemia, hypotension or shock. Acepromazine has been said to decrease platelet aggregation and its use avoided in patients with coagulopathies or thrombocytopenia, but a study in 6 healthy dogs showed no platelet inhibition (Conner et al. 2009; Conner et al. 2012). Phenothiazines are usually not recommended in patients with tetanus or strychnine intoxication due to effects on the extrapyramidal system, however the drug is commonly recommended for adjunctive treatment of tetanus in horses.

Intravenous injections should be made slowly. Do not administer intra-arterially in horses since it may cause severe CNS excitement/depression, seizures and death. Because of its effects on thermoregulation, use cautiously in very young or debilitated animals.

In horses, acepromazine's vasodilation effects may be deleterious in acute colic, Cantharidin toxicosis, dehydration/hypovolemia, or hypotension/shock.

Two retrospective studies in dogs (McConnell et al. 2007), (Tobias et al. 2006) did not show any increase in seizure activity after administration of acepromazine.

When used alone, acepromazine has no analgesic effects; treat animals with appropriate analgesics to control pain. The tranquilization effects of acepromazine can be overridden and it cannot always be counted upon when used as a restraining agent.

Do not administer to racing animals within 4 days of a race.

In dogs, acepromazine's effects may be individually variable and breed dependent. Dogs with MDR1 mutations (many Collies, Australian shepherds, etc.) may develop a more pronounced sedation that persists longer than normal. The Veterinary Clinical Pharmacology Lab at Washington State recommends reducing the dose by 25% in dogs heterozygous for the MDR1 mutation (mutant/normal) and by 30-50% in dogs homozygous for the *ABCB1-1Δ* (also called MDR1) mutation (mutant/mutant) (WSU-VetClinPharmLab 2009). Boxer dogs have been reported to be more sensitive to the effects of acepromazine, but published documentation of this was not located. Acepromazine should be used very cautiously as a restraining agent in aggressive dogs as it may make the animal more prone to startle and react to noises or other sensory inputs. In geriatric patients, very low doses have been associated with prolonged effects of the drug. Giant breeds and greyhounds may be extremely sensitive to the drug while terrier breeds are somewhat resistant to its effects. Atropine may be used with acepromazine to help negate its bradycardic effects.

In addition to the legal aspects (not FDA-approved) of using acepromazine in cattle, the drug may cause regurgitation of ruminal contents when inducing general anesthesia.

Adverse Effects

Acepromazine's effect on blood pressure (hypotension) is well described and an important consideration in therapy. This effect is thought mediated by both central mechanisms and through the alpha-adrenergic actions of the drug. Cardiovascular collapse (secondary to bradycardia and hypotension) has been described in all major species. Dogs may be more sensitive to these effects than other animals.

Acepromazine has been shown to decrease tear production in cats (Ghaffari et al. 2010).

In male large animals acepromazine may cause protrusion of the penis; in horses, this effect may last 2 hours. Permanent penile dysfunction in male horses and ponies is possible, but a retrospective study found the risk extremely low (≤1 in 10,000) (Driessen et al. 2011). Other clinical signs that have been reported in horses include excitement, restlessness, sweating, trembling, tachypnea, tachycardia and, rarely, seizures and recumbency.

Acepromazine's effects of causing penis extension in horses and prolapse of the membrana nictitans in horses and dogs may make its use unsuitable for show animals. There are also ethical considerations regarding the use of tranquilizers prior to showing an animal or having an animal examined before sale.

Occasionally an animal may develop the contradictory clinical signs of aggressiveness and generalized CNS stimulation after receiving acepromazine. IM injections may cause transient pain at the injection site.

Reproductive/Nursing Safety

In humans, the FDA categorizes phenothiazines as category *C* for use during pregnancy (*Animal studies have shown an adverse effect on the fetus, but there are no adequate studies in humans; or there are no animal reproduction studies and no adequate studies in humans.*) In a separate system evaluating the safety of drugs in canine and feline pregnancy (Papich 1989), this drug is categorized as class: *B* (*Safe for use if used cautiously. Studies in laboratory animals may have uncovered some risk, but these drugs appear to be safe in dogs and cats or these drugs are safe if they are not administered when the animal is near term.*)

Overdosage/Acute Toxicity

The LD$_{50}$ in mice is 61 mg/kg after IV dosage and 257 mg/kg after oral dose. While a toxicity study in dogs reported no adverse effects in dogs receiving 20 – 40 mg/kg over 6 weeks, since 2004 the ASPCA Animal Poison center has documented adverse effects in dogs receiving single doses between 20 – 42 mg/kg. Dogs have survived oral dosages up to 220 mg/kg, but overdoses can cause serious hypotension, CNS depression, pulmonary edema and hyperemia.

There were 196 single agent exposures to acepromazine reported to the ASPCA Animal Poison Control Center (APCC) during 2009-2013. Of the 156 dogs, 118 were symptomatic with 79% being sedated/lethargic, 42% ataxic, 9% bradycardic and 8% with protrusion of the third eyelids. Of the 39 cats, 32 were symptomatic with 72% being sedated/lethargic, 28% were ataxic and had elevation of third eyelids.

Because of the apparent relatively low toxicity of acepromazine, most overdoses can be handled by monitoring the animal and treating clinical signs as they occur; massive oral overdoses should definitely be treated by emptying the gut if possible. Hypotension should be treated initially with fluids; alpha-adrenergic pressor agents (epinephrine, phenylephrine) can be considered if fluids do not maintain adequate blood pressure. **Note:** The U.K. label (ACP Tablets; Novartis U.K.) states "Epinephrine (adrenaline) is contraindicated in the treatment of acute hypotension produced by overdosage of acepromazine maleate, since further depression of systemic blood pressure can result."

Seizures may be controlled with barbiturates or diazepam. Doxapram has been suggested as an antagonist to the CNS depressant effects of acepromazine and one study in dogs found that 1.25 mg/kg doxapram IV significantly reduced sedation scores and did not induce panting (Zapata et al. 2013).

Drug Interactions

The following drug interactions with acepromazine or other phenothiazines have either been reported or are theoretical in humans or animals and may be of significance in veterinary patients. Unless otherwise noted, use together is not necessarily contraindicated, but weigh the potential risks and perform additional monitoring when appropriate.

- **ACETAMINOPHEN:** Possible increased risk for hypothermia.
- **ANTACIDS:** May cause reduced GI absorption of oral phenothiazines.
- **ANTIDIARRHEAL MIXTURES** (*e.g.,* Kaolin/pectin, bismuth subsalicylate mixtures): May reduce GI absorption of oral phenothiazines.
- **CNS DEPRESSANT AGENTS** (barbiturates, narcotics, anesthetics, etc.): May cause additive CNS depression if used with acepromazine.
- **DOPAMINE:** Acepromazine may impair the vasopressive action of dopamine.
- **EMETICS:** Acepromazine may reduce the effectiveness of emetics.
- **METOCLOPRAMIDE:** May increase risks for extrapyramidal adverse effects.
- **OPIATES:** May enhance the hypotensive effects of acepromazine; dosages of acepromazine are generally reduced when used with an opiate.
- **ORGANOPHOSPHATE AGENTS:** Acepromazine should not be given within one month of worming with these agents as their effects may be potentiated.
- **PHENYTOIN:** Metabolism may be decreased if given concurrently with phenothiazines.
- **PROCAINE:** Activity may be enhanced by phenothiazines.
- **PROPRANOLOL:** Increased blood levels of both drugs may result if administered with phenothiazines.
- **QUINIDINE:** Phenothiazines may cause additive cardiac depression.

Laboratory Considerations

- Acepromazine does not appear to alter the results of glucose tolerance testing in dogs (Ionut et al. 2004).

Doses

- **DOGS/CATS:**

  Labeled Dose (FDA-Approved): As an aid in controlling intractable animals… alleviate itching as a result of skin irritation; as an antiemetic to control vomiting associated with motion sickness and as a preanesthetic agent: 0.55 – 2.2 mg/kg PO or 0.55 – 1.1 mg/kg IV, IM or SC. Give IV doses slowly; allow at least 15 minutes for onset of action (Package Insert; PromAce® —Fort Dodge). **Note:** The labeled dose is considered by most clinicians to be 10 times (or more) greater than is necessary for most indications; consider using dosages below.

  For sedation, tranquilization, premed, or restraint (extra-label): Injectable: 0.01 – 0.2 mg/kg IV (slowly), IM, or SQ once. Total dose should not exceed more than 3 mg (1 mg in cats). "Common" dosages usually are 0.02 – 0.03 mg/kg. Oral: Anecdotal dosage recommendations vary widely, but generally are similar to the labeled dosage range of 0.55 – 2.2 mg/kg, although some think that dosages at the higher end of this range are too high. If oral dosages require repeating, it is usually given every 6-12 hours.

  For anesthetic premedication (extra-label in USA): 0.03 – 0.125 mg/kg IM, SQ, or slow IV. Following acepromazine administration, the amount of anesthetic necessary to induce anesthesia is considerably reduced (by approximately 1/3 of a suitable induction agent). For other uses (tranquilization/sedation): 0.0625 – 0.125 mg/kg IM, SQ or slow IV. Use lower doses for tranquilization, higher doses for sedation. Maximum dose is 4 mg per animal. Normally, single doses are administered; long-term use is not recommended. (Adapted from label information; ACP 2 mg/mL Injection; Novartis U.K.)

- **FERRETS:**

  All doses are extra-label.
  a) **As a tranquilizer:** 0.25 – 0.75 mg/kg IM or SC. Has been used safely in pregnant jills; use with caution in dehydrated animals. (Finkler 1999)
  b) 0.1 – 0.25 mg/kg IM or SC; may cause hypotension/hypothermia. (Williams 2000)

- **RABBITS/RODENTS/SMALL MAMMALS:**

  All doses are extra-label.
  a) **Rabbits: As a tranquilizer:** 1 mg/kg IM, effect should begin in 10 minutes and last for 1–2 hours. (Booth 1988)
  b) **Rabbits: As a premed:** 0.1 – 0.5 mg/kg SC; 0.25 – 2 mg/kg IV, IM, SC 15 minutes prior to induction. No analgesia; may cause hypotension/hypothermia. (Ivey et al. 2000)
  c) **Mice, Rats, Hamsters, Guinea pigs, Chinchillas:** 0.5 mg/kg IM. Do <u>not</u> use in Gerbils. (Adamcak et al. 2000)

- **CATTLE:**

  All doses are extra-label.
  a) **Sedation:** 0.01 – 0.02 mg/kg IV or 0.03 – 0.1 mg/kg IM (Booth 1988).
  b) 0.05 – 0.1 mg/kg IV, IM or SC (Howard 1986).
  c) **Sedative one hour prior to local anesthesia:** 0.1 mg/kg IM (Hall et al. 1983).

- **HORSES:** (NOTE: ARCI UCGFS CLASS 3 DRUG)

  Labeled Dose (FDA-Approved): **As an aid in controlling fractious animals, and in conjunction with local anesthesia for various procedures and treatments:** 0.044 – 0.088 mg/kg (2 – 4 mg/100 lbs. body weight) IV, IM or SC (Package Insert; PromAce® —Fort Dodge)

  For sedation, tranquilization, premed, vasodilator (laminitis); (extra-label): When used alone, acepromazine is usually dosed similarly to the label: 0.02 – 0.1 mg/kg IM, IV or SQ. When used in combination with drugs such as butorphanol as a pre-med or to increase blood flow in the treatment of laminitis, recommended dosages are usually on the low end of this range. Repeat dosages should be limited and ideally given no more often than every 36 hours.

  For anesthetic premedication, tranquilization, or sedation (extra-label in USA): 0.03 – 0.1 mg/kg IM or slow IV. Following acepromazine administration, the amount of anesthetic necessary to induce anesthesia is considerably reduced (by approximately 1/3 of a suitable induction agent). Normally, single doses of acepromazine are administered; long-term use is not recommended. On rare occasions when repeat dosing is required, the dosing interval should be 36-48 hours. Lower dosages may reduce anxiety and be beneficial prior to shoeing or transportation; higher dosages may be effective sedative as an adjunct to, or replacement for, physical restraint (*e.g.,* dentistry, handling and shoeing). (Adapted from label information; ACP 10 mg/mL Injection; Novartis U.K.)

- **SWINE:**

  All doses are extra-label.

  a) 0.1 – 0.2 mg/kg IV, IM, or SC. (Howard 1986)

  b) 0.03 – 0.1 mg/kg. (Hall et al. 1983)

  c) **For brief periods of immobilization:** acepromazine 0.5 mg/kg IM followed in 30 minutes by ketamine 15 mg/kg IM. Atropine (0.044 mg/kg IM) will reduce salivation and bronchial secretions. (Lumb et al. 1984)

- **SHEEP & GOATS:**

  Extra-label: 0.05 – 0.1 mg/kg IM. (Hall et al. 1983)

- **ZOO, EXOTIC, WILDLIFE SPECIES:**

  For use of acepromazine in zoo, exotic and wildlife medicine refer to specific references, including:

  a) *Zoo Animal and Wildlife Immobilization and Anesthesia.* West, G., Heard, D., Caulkett, N. (eds.). Blackwell Publishing, 2007.

  b) *Handbook of Wildlife Chemical Immobilization, 3rd Ed.* Kreeger, T.J. and J.M. Arnemo. 2007.

  c) *Fowler's Zoo and Wild Animal Medicine Current Therapy, Volume 7,* Miller, R.E., Fowler, M.E., Saunders. 2011.

  d) *Exotic Animal Formulary, 4th Ed.* Carpenter, J.W., Saunders. 2012.

  e) *The 2009 American Association of Zoo Veterinarian Proceedings* by D. K. Fontenot also has several dosages listed for restraint, anesthesia, and analgesia for a variety of drugs for carnivores and primates. VIN members can access them at: http://goo.gl/NNIWQ or http://goo.gl/9UJse

Monitoring

- Cardiac rate/rhythm/blood pressure if indicated and possible to measure.
- Degree of tranquilization.
- Male horses should be checked to make sure penis retracts and is not injured.
- Body temperature (especially if ambient temperature is very hot or cold).

Client Information

- When giving by mouth, give dose 45-60 minutes before the procedure or trip for best effect. Your veterinarian may recommend a trial dose a few days before travel to see how the drug will affect your animal.
- Sedative/tranquilizing effects and side effects may last 6-8 hours.
- Keep treated animal in a quiet, comfortable temperature environment.
- This drug may give urine a pinkish to red-brown color; this is nothing to be worried about.
- Unless your veterinarian instructs, don't give other medicines with this drug to tranquilize or sedate your animal.

Chemistry/Synonyms

Acepromazine maleate (formerly acetylpromazine) is a phenothiazine derivative that occurs as a yellow, odorless, bitter tasting powder. One gram is soluble in 27 mL of water, 13 mL of alcohol, or 3 mL of chloroform.

Acepromazine maleate may also be known as: acetylpromazine maleate, "ACE", ACP, *Aceproject®, Aceprotabs®, PromAce®, Plegicil®, Notensil®,* and *Atravet®*.

Storage/Stability

Store protected from light. Tablets should be stored in tight containers. Acepromazine injection should be kept from freezing.

Although controlled studies have not documented the compatibility of these combinations, acepromazine has been mixed with atropine, buprenorphine, chloral hydrate, ketamine, meperidine, oxymorphone, and xylazine. Both glycopyrrolate and diazepam have been reported to be physically **incompatible** with phenothiazines, however glycopyrrolate has been demonstrated to be **compatible** with promazine HCl for injection.

Compatibility/Compounding Considerations

A study (Taylor et al. 2009) evaluating the stability, sterility, pH, particulate formation and efficacy in laboratory rodents of compounded ketamine, acepromazine and xylazine (KAX) supported the finding that the drugs are stable and efficacious for at least 180 days after mixing if stored at room temperature in the dark.

Combinations of acepromazine mixed with atropine, buprenorphine, chloral hydrate, meperidine, and oxymorphone have been commonly used, but studies documenting their compatibility and stability were not located. Both glycopyrrolate and diazepam have been reported to be physically **incompatible** with phenothiazines, however glycopyrrolate has been demonstrated to be **compatible** with promazine HCl for injection.

Dosage Forms/Regulatory Status

VETERINARY-LABELED PRODUCTS:

Acepromazine Maleate for Injection: 10 mg/mL for injection in 50 mL vials; PromAce®; generic; (Rx). FDA-approved forms available for use in dogs, cats and horses not intended for food.

Acepromazine Maleate Tablets: 5 mg, 10 mg & 25 mg in bottles of 100 and 500 tablets; PromAce®; generic; (Rx). FDA-approved forms available for use in dogs, cats and horses not intended for food.

There is a website (dailymed.nlm.nih.gov) with FDA-approved veterinary product labels.

When used in an extra-label manner in food animals, it is recommended to use the withdrawal periods used in Canada: Meat: 7 days; Milk: 48 hours. Contact FARAD (see appendix) for further guidance.

The ARCI (Racing Commissioners International) has designated this drug as a class 3 substance. See the appendix for more information.

HUMAN-LABELED PRODUCTS: NONE.

Revisions/References

Monograph revised/updated August 2013.

Adamcak, A. & B. Otten (2000). Rodent Therapeutics. *Vet Clin NA: Exotic Anim Pract* 3:1(Jan): 221-40.

Booth, N. H. (1988). Drugs Acting on the Central Nervous System. Veterinary *Pharmacology and Therapeutics - 6th Ed.* N. H. Booth and L. E. McDonald. Ames, Iowa State University Press: 153-408.

Conner, B., et al. (2009). The effects of acepromazine upon adenosine diphosphate- and arachidonic acid- mediated platelet activation in healthy dogs. Proceedings: IVECCS. accessed via Veterinary Information Network; vin.com

Conner, B. J., et al. (2012). Effects of acepromazine maleate on platelet function assessed by use of adenosine diphosphate activated- and arachidonic acid-activated modified thromboelastography in healthy dogs. *American Journal of Veterinary Research* 73(5): 595-601.

Driessen, B., et al. (2011). Contemporary use of acepromazine in the anaesthetic management of male horses and ponies: A retrospective study and opinion poll. *Equine Veterinary Journal* 43(1): 88-98.

Finkler, M. (1999). *Anesthesia in Ferrets.* Proceedings: Central Veterinary Conference, Kansas City. accessed via Veterinary Information Network; vin.com

Ghaffari, M. S., et al. (2010). Effect of acepromazine or xylazine on tear production as measured by Schirmer tear test in normal cats. *Vet. Ophthalmol.* 13(1): 1-3.

Hall, L. W. & K. W. Clarke (1983). *Veterinary Anesthesia 8th Ed.,* Bailliere Tindall. London.

Hashem, A., et al. (1992). Pharmacokinetics and Bioavailability of Acepromazine in Plasma of the Dog. *Deutsche Tierarztliche Wochenschrift* 99(10): 396-8.

Howard, J. L., Ed. (1986). *Current Veterinary Therapy 2, Food Animal Practice.* Philadelphia, W.B. Saunders.

Ionut, V., et al. (2004). Investigation of the effect of acepromazine on intravenous glucose tolerance tests in dogs. *American Journal of Veterinary Research* 65(8): 1124-7.

Ivey, E. & J. Morrisey (2000). Therapeutics for Rabbits. *Vet Clin NA: Exotic Anim Pract* 3:1(Jan): 183-216.

Lumb, W. V. & E. W. Jones (1984). *Veterinary Anesthesia, 2nd Ed.,* Lea & Febiger. Philadelphia.

McConnell, J., et al. (2007). Administration of acepromazine maleate to 31 dogs with a history of seizures. *J. Vet. Emerg. Crit. Care* 17(3): 262-7.

Taylor, B. J., et al. (2009). Beyond-Use Dating of Extemporaneously Compounded Ketamine, Acepromazine, and Xylazine: Safety, Stability, and Efficacy over Time. *Journal of the American Association for Laboratory Animal Science* 48(6): 718-26.

Tobias, K. M. & K. Marioni-Henry (2006). A retrospective study on the use of acepromazine maleate in dogs with seizures. *J. Am. Anim. Hosp. Assoc.* 42(4): 283-9.

Williams, B. (2000). Therapeutics in Ferrets. *Vet Clin NA: Exotic Anim Pract* 3:1(Jan): 131-53.

WSU-VetClinPharmLab (2009). "Problem Drugs." http://goo.gl/aIGlM.

Zapata, M. & E. Hofmeister (2013). Refinement of the dose of doxapram to counteract the sedative effects of acepromazine in dogs. J Small Anim Pract 54(8): 405-8.

Acetaminophen

(ah-seet-a-min-a-fen)   Tylenol®, APAP, Paracetamol

Oral Analgesic, Antipyretic

Prescriber Highlights

► *Contraindicated in cats* at any dosage; ferrets may be as sensitive to acetaminophen as cats.

► At recommended dosages, not overly toxic to dogs, rodents, or rabbits. Dogs are more susceptible to red blood cell toxicity than are humans, so dose carefully.

► Often used in combined dosage forms with codeine, tramadol or hydrocodone; see the codeine, tramadol or hydrocodone monographs for more information.

Uses/Indications

Acetaminophen is occasionally used as an oral analgesic in dogs and small mammals. It may be particularly beneficial in dogs with renal dysfunction for the treatment of chronic pain conditions. In situations where moderate pain occurs, it may be used in combination products containing codeine, hydrocodone, or tramadol. See the codeine, hydrocodone and tramadol monographs for more information on the use of acetaminophen combination preparations.

A case report of adjunctive treatment for pain using oral acetaminophen in a pony has been published (West et al. 2011).

Pharmacology/Actions

Acetaminophen's exact mechanisms of action are not completely understood; it produces analgesia and antipyresis via a weak, reversible, isoform-nonspecific inhibition of cyclooxygenase (COX-3; Cox-1-v1). Unlike aspirin, it does not possess significant antiinflammatory activity nor inhibit platelet function when given at clinically recommended dosages.

Pharmacokinetics

Acetaminophen's pharmacokinetics have been evaluated after single oral doses (mean dose = 10.46 mg/kg) in 6 greyhounds (Ku-Kanich 2010). Oral absorption is rapid and peak levels of about 6.8 mcg/mL occurred 51 minutes (mean) after a dose. Terminal half-life was also fast and was approximately 1 hour.

In humans, acetaminophen is rapidly and nearly completely absorbed from the gut and is rapidly distributed into most tissues. Approximately 25% is plasma protein bound.

Contraindications/Precautions/Warnings

Acetaminophen is contraindicated in cats at any dosage. Severe methemoglobinemia, hematuria, and icterus can be seen. Cats are unable to significantly glucuronidate acetaminophen leading to toxic metabolites being formed and resultant toxicity. Presently, acetaminophen should not be used in ferrets as *in vitro* studies indicate they may be as sensitive to acetaminophen as cats. At this time, acetaminophen should not be used in Sugar Gliders or Hedgehogs, as its safety has not been determined.

Dogs do not metabolize acetaminophen as well as humans and its use must be judicious. While dogs are not as sensitive to acetaminophen as cats, they may also be susceptible to methemoglobinemia when given high dosages. In dogs, it is generally not recommended to use acetaminophen during the immediate post-operative phase (first 24 hours) due to an increased risk of hepatotoxicity.

Adverse Effects

Because acetaminophen is not routinely used in veterinary medicine, experience on its adverse effect profile is limited. At suggested dosages in dogs, there is some potential for renal, hepatic, GI, and hematologic effects occurring. Higher dosages (3X) can cause keratoconjunctivitis sicca.

Reproductive/Nursing Safety

Absolute reproductive safety has not been established, but acetaminophen is apparently relatively safe for occasional use in pregnancy (no documented problems in humans). Animal data was not located. In humans, the FDA categorizes this drug as category *B* for use during pregnancy *(Animal studies have not yet demonstrated risk to the fetus, but there are no adequate studies in pregnant women; or animal studies have shown an adverse effect, but adequate studies in pregnant women have not demonstrated a risk to the fetus in the first trimester of pregnancy, and there is no evidence of risk in later trimesters.)* In a separate system evaluating the safety of drugs in canine and feline pregnancy (Papich 1989), this drug is categorized as class: *C (These drugs may have potential risks. Studies in people or laboratory animals have uncovered risks, and these drugs should be used cautiously as a last resort when the benefit of therapy clearly outweighs the risks.)*

Acetaminophen is excreted in milk in low concentrations with reported milk:plasma ratios of 0.91 to 1.42 at 1 and 12 hours, respectively. In nursing human infants, no adverse effects have been reported.

Overdosage/Acute Toxicity

Because of the potentially severe toxicity associated with acetaminophen, consultation with an animal poison control center is highly recommended (see appendix). Effects can include methemoglobinemia, liver necrosis, renal effects, facial and paw swelling, and keratoconjunctivitis sicca (KCS). Liver effects are more common in dogs; facial and paw swelling and methemoglobinemia are more common in cats. Dosages above 100 mg/kg in dogs have been associated with severe toxicosis.

There were 6194 single agent exposures to acetaminophen only products reported to the ASPCA Animal Poison Control Center (APCC) during 2009-2013. Of the 5698 dogs exposed, 1206 were symptomatic. The common signs in the dogs included vomiting (31%), lethargy (24%), ataxia (8%), facial edema (5%), and 3% with elevated liver enzymes and/or methemoglobinemia. Of the 473 cats, 214 were symptomatic with 28% reporting vomiting, 21% hypersalivating, 15% lethargic, 9% tachypneic, 8% had methemoglobinemia, and 6% had elevated liver enzymes. For overdosage in dogs or cats, standard gut emptying techniques and supportive care should be administered when applicable. Further treatment with acetylcysteine, s-adenosyl methionine (SAMe), oxygen, and blood transfusions may be warranted (Richardson 2000, Aronson et al. 1996, Mariani et al. 2001, Steenbergen 2003).

Drug Interactions

The following drug interactions with acetaminophen have either been reported or are theoretical in humans or animals and may be of significance in veterinary patients. Unless otherwise noted, use together is not necessarily contraindicated, but weigh the potential risks and perform additional monitoring when appropriate.

- **BARBITURATES:** Increased conversion of acetaminophen to hepatotoxic metabolites; potentially increased risk for hepatotoxicity.

- **DOXORUBICIN:** May deplete hepatic glutathione, thereby leading to increased hepatic toxicity.

- **FENBENDAZOLE:** May increase the risk for hepatotoxicity (study done in mice; Gardner et al. 2012).
- **ISONIAZID:** Possible increased risk of hepatotoxicity.
- **PHENOTHIAZINES:** Possible increased risk for hypothermia.
- **PROPYLENE GLYCOL:** Foods containing propylene glycol (often found in wet cat foods) may increase the severity of acetaminophen-induced methemoglobinemia or Heinz body formation.
- **WARFARIN:** While acetaminophen is relatively safe to use, large doses may potentiate anticoagulant effects.

Laboratory Considerations
- False positive results may occur for urinary **5-hydroxyindoleacetic acid.**

Doses
Note: For dosages of acetaminophen/codeine, and acetaminophen/hydrocodone combination products refer to the codeine and hydrocodone monographs.

- **DOGS:**
  As an analgesic (extra-label): 10 – 15 mg/kg PO q8h; if using long-term (>5 days) consider giving q12h at the lower end of dosing range.

- **RABBITS/RODENTS/SMALL MAMMALS:**
  As an analgesic (extra-label):
  a) Using Children's *Tylenol®*: 1 – 2 mg/mL in drinking water. Effective for controlling low-grade nociception. (Huerkamp 2000)
  b) **Mice, Rats, Gerbils, Hamsters, Guinea pigs, Chinchillas:** 1 – 2 mg/mL in drinking water. (Adamcak et al. 2000)

Monitoring
- When used at recommended doses for pain control in otherwise healthy patients, little monitoring should be necessary. However, with chronic therapy, occasional liver, renal and hematologic monitoring may be warranted, particularly when clinical signs occur.

Client Information
- Must **NEVER BE USED IN CATS.** Do not use in ferrets.
- Not commonly used in dogs; watch for adverse effects and contact veterinarian if dog stops eating, if the whites of the eyes become yellowish, continues vomiting or having diarrhea, or blood is seen in vomit or stool.
- Do NOT give more than veterinarian prescribes. Unless veterinarian instructs, do NOT give other pain or fever medicines.
- Keep out of reach of children.

Chemistry/Synonyms
A synthetic non-opiate analgesic, acetaminophen (also known as paracetamol)) occurs as a crystalline, white powder with a slightly bitter taste. It is soluble in boiling water and freely soluble in alcohol. Acetaminophen is known in the U.K. as paracetamol.

Acetaminophen may also be known as: paracetamol, N-acetyl-p-aminophenol, MAPAP or APAP; many trade names are available.

Storage/Stability
Acetaminophen products should be stored at temperatures less than 40°C. Do not freeze the oral solution or suspension.

Compatibility/Compounding Considerations
Non-extended release tablets may be split or crushed and mixed with food just prior to administration.

Dosage Forms/Regulatory Status
VETERINARY-LABELED PRODUCTS: NONE.

The ARCI (Racing Commissioners International) has designated this drug as a class 4 substance. See the appendix for more information.

HUMAN-LABELED PRODUCTS:
There are many different trade names and products of acetaminophen available commercially. The most commonly known trade name is *Tylenol®*. Acetaminophen is available in 160 mg, 325 mg and 500 mg tablets, capsules or caplets; 80 mg chewable tablets; 650 mg extended release tablets; oral liquids in several different concentrations and 80 mg, 120 mg, 125 mg, 300 mg, 325 mg and 650 mg rectal suppositories. Combinations with other analgesics (aspirin, codeine phosphate, hydrocodone, tramadol, or oxycodone) or antihistamines (diphenhydramine) are also available.

Revisions/References
Monograph revised/updated August 2013.

Adamcak, A. & B. Otten (2000). Rodent Therapeutics. *Vet Clin NA: Exotic Anim Pract* 3:1(Jan): 221-40.
Aronson, L. & K. J. Drobatz (1996). Acetaminophen Toxicosis in 17 Cats. *Vet Emerg Crit Care* 6: 65-9.
Gardner, C., et al. (2012). Exacerbation of acetaminophen hepatotoxicity by the anthelmintic drug fenbendazole. *Toxicol Sci.* 125(2): 607-12.
Huerkamp, M. (2000). The use of analgesics in rodents and rabbits. Emory University, Division of Animal Resources.
KuKanich, B. (2010). Pharmacokinetics of acetaminophen, codeine, and the codeine metabolites morphine and codeine-6-glucuronide in healthy Greyhound dogs. *J. Vet. Pharmacol. Ther.* 33(1): 15-21.
Mariani, C. & R. Fulton (2001). Atypical Reaction to Acetaminophen Intoxication in a Dog. *Vet Emerg Crit Care* 10: 123-6.
Richardson, J. (2000). Management of Acetaminophen and Ibuprofen Toxicosis in Dogs and Cats. *Vet Emerg Crit Care* 10: 285-91.
Steenbergen, V. (2003). Acetaminophen and Cats A Dangerous Combination. *Vet Tech:* 43-5.
West, E., et al. (2011). Use of acetaminophen (paracetamol) as a short-term adjunctive analgesic in a laminitic pony. Veterinary Anaesthesia and Analgesia 38: 521-2.

Acetazolamide
Acetazolamide Sodium

(ah-seet-a-**zole**-a-mide)   Diamox®, Dazamide®

Carbonic Anhydrase Inhibitor Diuretic; Antiglaucoma Agent

Prescriber Highlights
▶ Used sometimes for metabolic alkalosis or glaucoma in small animals; HYPP in horses.
▶ Contraindicated in patients with significant hepatic, renal, pulmonary or adrenocortical insufficiency, hyponatremia, hypokalemia, hyperchloremic acidosis, or electrolyte imbalance.
▶ Give oral doses with food if GI upset occurs.
▶ Electrolytes & acid/base status should be monitored with chronic or high dose therapy.
▶ Monitor with tonometry if using for glaucoma.

Uses/Indications
Acetazolamide has been used principally in veterinary medicine for its effects on aqueous humor production in the treatment of glaucoma, metabolic alkalosis, and for its diuretic action. It may be useful as an adjunctive treatment for syringomyelia in dogs. Acetazolamide's use in small animals is complicated by a relatively high occurrence of adverse effects.

In horses, acetazolamide is used as an adjunctive treatment for hyperkalemic periodic paralysis (HYPP).

In humans, the drug has been used as adjunctive therapy for epilepsy and for acute high-altitude sickness.

Pharmacology/Actions
The carbonic anhydrase inhibitors act by a noncompetitive, reversible inhibition of the enzyme carbonic anhydrase. This reduces the formation of hydrogen and bicarbonate ions from carbon dioxide thereby reducing the availability of these ions for active transport into body secretions.

Pharmacologic effects of the carbonic anhydrase inhibitors include: decreased formation of aqueous humor, thus reducing intraocular pressure, increased renal tubular secretion of sodium and potassium and, to a greater extent, bicarbonate, leading to increased urine alkalinity and volume. Acetazolamide has some anticonvulsant activity, which is independent of its diuretic effects (mechanism is not fully understood, but may be due to carbonic anhydrase or a metabolic acidosis effect).

In anesthetized cats, methazolamide did not, but acetazolamide did, reduce the hypoxic ventilatory response. The authors believe this is not as a result of carbonic anhydrase inhibition, but due to acetazolamide's effects on carotid bodies or type I cells (Teppema et al. 2006).

Pharmacokinetics

The pharmacokinetics of this agent have apparently not been studied in domestic animals. One report (Roberts 1985) states that after a dose of 22 mg/kg, the onset of action is 30 minutes; maximal effects occur in 2-4 hours; duration of action is about 4-6 hours in small animals.

In humans, the drug is well absorbed after oral administration with peak levels occurring within 1-3 hours. It is distributed throughout the body with highest levels found in the kidneys, plasma and erythrocytes. Acetazolamide has been detected in the milk of lactating dogs and it crosses the placenta (in unknown quantities). Within 24 hours of administration, an average of 90% of the drug is excreted unchanged into the urine by tubular secretion and passive reabsorption processes.

Contraindications/Precautions/Warnings

Carbonic anhydrase inhibitors are contraindicated in patients with significant hepatic disease (may precipitate hepatic coma), renal or adrenocortical insufficiency, hyponatremia, hypokalemia, hyperchloremic acidosis, or electrolyte imbalance. They should not be used in patients with severe pulmonary obstruction that are unable to increase alveolar ventilation or in those who are hypersensitive to them. Long-term use of carbonic anhydrase inhibitors is contraindicated in patients with chronic, noncongestive, angle-closure glaucoma as angle closure may occur and the drug may mask the condition by lowering intraocular pressures.

Acetazolamide should be used with caution in patients with severe respiratory acidosis or having preexisting hematologic abnormalities. Cross sensitivity between acetazolamide and antibacterial sulfonamides or furosemide may occur.

Adverse Effects

Potential adverse effects that may be encountered include: GI disturbances, CNS effects (sedation, depression, weakness, excitement, etc.), hematologic effects (bone marrow depression), renal effects (crystalluria, dysuria, renal colic, polyuria), hypokalemia, hyperchloremia, hyperglycemia, hyponatremia, hyperuricemia, hepatic insufficiency, dermatologic effects (rash, etc.), and hypersensitivity reactions.

At the dosages used for HYPP in horses adverse effects are reportedly uncommon.

Reproductive/Nursing Safety

Acetazolamide has been implicated in fetal abnormalities in mice and rats when used at high (10X) dosages and fetal toxicity has been noted when the drug has been used in pregnant humans. In humans, the FDA categorizes this drug as category *C* for use during pregnancy (*Animal studies have shown an adverse effect on the fetus, but there are no adequate studies in humans; or there are no animal reproduction studies and no adequate studies in humans.*)

In humans, the manufacturer states that either nursing or the drug must be discontinued if the mother is receiving acetazolamide. Veterinary significance is not clear.

Overdosage/Acute Toxicity

Information regarding overdosage of this drug was not located. In the event of an overdose, it is recommended to contact an animal poison control center. Monitor serum electrolytes, blood gases, volume status, and CNS status during an acute overdose; treat symptomatically and supportively.

Drug Interactions

The following drug interactions with acetazolamide have either been reported or are theoretical in humans or animals and may be of significance in veterinary patients. Unless otherwise noted, use together is not necessarily contraindicated, but weigh the potential risks and perform additional monitoring when appropriate.

- **ALKALINE URINE:** Drugs where acetazolamide-caused alkaline urine may affect their excretion rate: Decreased urinary excretion of **quinidine, procainamide, tricyclic antidepressants**; Increased urinary excretion of **salicylates, phenobarbital**.
- **ASPIRIN (or other salicylates):** Increased risk of acetazolamide accumulation and toxicity; increased risk for metabolic acidosis.
- **CYCLOSPORINE:** Acetazolamide may increase levels.
- **DIGOXIN:** As acetazolamide may cause hypokalemia, increased risk for toxicity.
- **INSULIN:** Rarely, carbonic anhydrase inhibitors interfere with the hypoglycemic effects of insulin.
- **METHENAMINE COMPOUNDS:** Acetazolamide may negate methenamine effects in the urine.
- **DRUGS AFFECTING POTASSIUM** (*e.g.*, **corticosteroids, amphotericin B, corticotropin, or other diuretics**): Concomitant use may exacerbate potassium depletion.

Laboratory Considerations

- **Urine Protein.** By alkalinizing the urine, carbonic anhydrase inhibitors may cause false positive results in determining urine protein when using bromphenol blue reagent (Albustix®, Albutest®, Labstix®), sulfosalicylic acid (Bumintest®, Exton's® Test Reagent), nitric acid ring test, or heat and acetic acid test methods.
- **Thyroid function.** Carbonic anhydrase inhibitors may **decrease iodine uptake** by the thyroid gland in hyperthyroid or euthyroid patients.
- **Theophylline concentrations.** May interfere with HPLC determination of theophylline.

Doses

Directions for reconstitution of injection: Reconstitute 500 mg vial with at least 5 mL of Sterile Water for Injection; use within 24 hours after reconstitution.

- **DOGS:**

  For adjunctive therapy of glaucoma, hydrocephalus or metabolic acidosis (extra-label): 4 – 10 mg/kg PO two to three times daily; or IV once.

- **CATS:**

  For adjunctive therapy of glaucoma (extra-label): 6 – 8 mg/kg PO two to three times a day.

- **HORSES:** (NOTE: ARCI UCGFS CLASS 4 DRUG)

  For adjunctive therapy of hyperkalemic periodic paralysis (HYPP) (extra-label): 2 – 3 mg/kg PO q8-12h when diet adjustment does not control episodes. (Valberg 2008)

Monitoring

- Intraocular pressure tonometry (if used for glaucoma).
- Blood gases if used for alkalosis.
- Serum electrolytes.
- Baseline CBC with differential and periodic retests if using chronically.
- Other adverse effects.

Client Information

- Most common side effect is stomach upset; giving with food may help reduce this effect.
- Contact veterinarian immediately if unusual panting or rapid breathing, weakness, staggering, behavior changes, tremors or seizures (convulsions) are seen.
- Horses must have access to water and food while taking this medication.
- Patients will need ongoing lab tests while on this medicine.

Chemistry/Synonyms

A carbonic anhydrase inhibitor, acetazolamide occurs as a white to faintly yellowish-white, odorless, crystalline powder with pK_as of 7.4 and 9.1. It is very slightly soluble in water, sparingly soluble in hot water (90-100°C) and alcohol. Acetazolamide sodium occurs as a white lyophilized solid and is freely soluble in water. The injection has a pH of 9.2 after reconstitution with Sterile Water for Injection.

Acetazolamide may also known as: acetazolam, acetazolamidum, or sodium acetazolamide; many trade names are available.

Storage/Stability

Acetazolamide products should be stored at room temperature.

To prepare parenteral solution: reconstitute with at least 5 mL of Sterile Water for Injection. After reconstitution, the injection is stable for one week when refrigerated, but as it contains no preservatives, it should be used within 24-hours.

Compatibility/Compounding Considerations

Acetazolamide sodium for injection is reportedly physically **compatible** with all commonly used IV solutions and cimetidine HCl for injection.

Compounded preparation stability: Acetazolamide oral suspension compounded from commercially available tablets has been published (Allen et al. 1996). Triturating twelve (12) 250 mg tablets with 60 mL of *Ora-Plus®* and *qs ad* to 120 mL with *Ora-Sweet®* (or *Ora-Sweet® SF*) yields a 25 mg/mL suspension that retains >90% potency for 60 days stored at both 5°C and 25°C. The stability of acetazolamide aqueous liquids decreases at pH values above 9. The optimal stability is reported to be between 3 and 5. Compounded preparations of acetazolamide should be protected from light.

Dosage Forms/Regulatory Status

VETERINARY-LABELED PRODUCTS: NONE.

The ARCI (Racing Commissioners International) has designated this drug as a class 4 substance. See the appendix for more information.

HUMAN-LABELED PRODUCTS:

Acetazolamide Oral Tablets: 125 mg, 250 mg; generic; (Rx)

Acetazolamide Extended-Release Oral Capsules: 500 mg; *Diamox Sequels®*, generic; (Rx)

Acetazolamide Injection (lyophilized powder for solution): 500 mg; generic; (Rx)

Revisions/References

Monograph revised/updated August 2013.

Allen, L. V. & M. A. Erickson (1996). Stability of acetazolamide, allopurinol, azathioprine, clonazepam, and flucytosine in extemporaneously compounded oral liquids. *Am J Health Syst Pharm* 53(16): 1944-9.

Roberts, S. E. (1985). Assessment and management of the ophthalmic emergency. *Comp CE* 7(9): 739-52.

Teppema, L. J., et al. (2006). The carbonic anhydrase inhibitors methazolamide and acetazolamide have different effects on the hypoxic ventilatory response in the anaesthetized cat. *Journal of Physiology-London* 574(2): 565-72.

Valberg, S. (2008). *Muscle Tremors in Horses.* Proceedings: Western Veterinary Conference. accessed via Veterinary Information Network; vin.com

Acetic Acid

(ah-**see**-tick **ass**-id)   Vinegar

GI Acidifier

Prescriber Highlights

▶ Used primarily for treatment of non-protein nitrogen-induced ammonia toxicosis (secondary to urea poisoning, etc.) in ruminants or enterolith prevention in horses.
▶ Contraindicated if potential lactic acidosis (grain overload, rumen acidosis) is possible.
▶ Given via stomach tube.

Uses/Indications

Acetic acid is used via its acidifying qualities in ruminants to treat non-protein nitrogen-induced (*e.g.,* urea poisoning) ammonia toxicosis. It is also used as a potential treatment to prevent enterolith formation in horses by reducing colonic pH.

Pharmacology/Actions

Acetic acid in the rumen lowers pH due to shifting ammonia to ammonium ions and reducing absorption. It may also slow the hydrolysis of urea.

Pharmacokinetics

No information was noted.

Contraindications/Precautions/Warnings

Should not be administered to ruminants until potential lactic acidosis (grain overload, rumen acidosis) is ruled out.

Do NOT use concentrated forms of acetic acid.

Adverse Effects

Because of the unpleasant taste and potential for causing mucous membrane irritation, acetic acid is generally recommended for administration via stomach tube.

Overdosage/Acute Toxicity

When used for appropriate indications there is little likelihood of serious toxicity occurring after minor overdoses. Due to its potential corrosiveness, the greatest concern would occur if a concentrated form of acetic acid is mistakenly used. However, one human patient who had glacial acetic acid used instead of 5% acetic acid during colposcopy (cervix) demonstrated no detectable harm.

Drug Interactions

There are no documented drug interactions with oral acetic acid, but because of its acidic qualities it could, potentially, affect the degradation of several drugs in the gut.

Doses

- **CATTLE/RUMINANTS:**

  For treatment of urea poisoning (non-protein nitrogen-induced ammonia toxicosis); (extra-label): Cattle: Using 5% acetic acid (vinegar) infuse 4 – 10 liters (for cattle) or 250 mL – 1 liter (sheep/goats) into rumen. Follow with cold water to reduce rumen temperature and reduce formation of urea (up to 20 liters in cattle; 2 – 8 liters in sheep/goats). Repeat treatment as required if clinical signs reoccur.

- **HORSES:**

  For enterolith prevention (extra-label): Using vinegar: 250 mL/450 kg body weight PO once daily (Robinson 1992).

Chemistry/Synonyms

Glacial acetic acid is $C_2H_4O_2$. Acetic acid has a distinctive odor and a sharp acid taste. It is miscible with water, alcohol or glycerin. Much confusion can occur with the percentages of $C_2H_4O_2$ contained in various acetic acid solutions. Acetic Acid USP is defined as having a concentration of 36-37% $C_2H_4O_2$. Diluted Acetic Acid NF contains 5.7-6.3% w/v of $C_2H_4O_2$. Solutions containing approximately 3-5% w/v of $C_2H_4O_2$ are commonly known as vinegar. Be certain of the concentration of the product you are using and your dilutions.

Acetic acid may also be known as: E260, eisessig (glacial acetic acid), essigsaure, etanoico, or ethanoic acid.

Storage/Stability

Acetic acid solutions should be stored in airtight containers.

Compatibility/Compounding Considerations

If diluting more concentrated forms of acetic acid to concentrations equivalent to vinegar (3-5%), use safety precautions to protect eyes and skin. It is strongly recommended to have someone check your calculations to prevent potentially serious consequences.

Dosage Forms/Regulatory Status

VETERINARY-LABELED PRODUCTS: NONE.

HUMAN-LABELED PRODUCTS: NONE.

There are no systemic products commercially available. Acetic acid (in various concentrations) may be purchased from chemical supply houses. Distilled white vinegar is available in gallon sizes from grocery stores.

Revisions/References

Monograph revised/updated August 2013.

Acetohydroxamic Acid

(ah-seet-oh-**hy**-drox-am-ik)   Lithostat®, AHA

Urease Inhibitor

Prescriber Highlights

▶ Used occasionally in dogs for persistent struvite uroliths & persistent urease-producing bacteriuria.

▶ Contraindicated in patients with renal impairment & during pregnancy; do not use in cats.

▶ Adverse effects are common & can include GI effects (anorexia, vomiting, mouth/esophageal ulcers), hemolytic anemia, hyperbilirubinemia & bilirubinuria.

▶ Monitor renal function (including urinalysis), CBC's, & bilirubin levels.

Uses/Indications

Acetohydroxamic acid can be used in dogs as adjunctive therapy in some cases of recurrent urolithiasis or in the treatment of persistent urinary tract infections caused by the following bacteria: *E. coli, Klebsiella, Morganella morganii, Staphylococci spp.,* and *Pseudomonas aeruginosa*. Adverse effects limit its usefulness.

Pharmacology/Actions

AHA inhibits urease thereby reducing production of urea and subsequent urinary concentrations of ammonia, bicarbonate and carbonate. While the drug does not directly reduce urine pH, by reducing ammonia and bicarbonate production by urease-producing bacteria, it prevents increases in urine pH. The drug may act synergistically with several antimicrobial agents (*e.g.,* carbenicillin, gentamicin, clindamycin, trimethoprim-sulfa or chloramphenicol) in treating some urinary tract infections. The drug's effects on urinary pH and infection also indirectly inhibit the formation of urinary calculi (struvite, carbonate-apatite).

Pharmacokinetics

No canine specific data was located. In humans, the drug is rapidly absorbed after PO administration. Absolute bioavailability "in animals" is reported to be 50-60%. AHA is well distributed throughout body fluids. It is partially metabolized to acetamide, which is active; 36-65% of a dose is excreted in the urine unchanged, and 9-14%

excreted in the urine as acetamide. The remainder is reportedly excreted as CO_2 via the respiratory tract.

Contraindications/Precautions/Warnings

AHA is contraindicated in patients with poor renal function (*e.g.,* serum creatinine >2.5 mg/dL) or when it is not specifically indicated (see Indications).

Acetohydroxamic acid is reportedly very toxic in cats and should not be used in felines.

Adverse Effects

In dogs, GI effects (anorexia, vomiting, mouth/esophageal ulcers), hemolytic anemia, hyperbilirubinemia and bilirubinuria have been reported. Other potential adverse effects include: CNS disturbances (anxiety, depression, tremulousness), hematologic effects (reticulocytosis, bone marrow depression), phlebitis, and skin rashes/alopecia. Effects on bilirubin metabolism have also been reported.

Reproductive/Nursing Safety

AHA use is considered contraindicated during pregnancy. In pregnant beagles, doses of 25 mg/kg/day caused cardiac, coccygeal, and abdominal wall abnormalities in puppies. At high doses (>750 mg/kg) leg deformities have been noted in test animals. Higher doses (1500 mg/kg) caused significant encephalopathologies. In humans, the FDA categorizes this drug as category **X** for use during pregnancy *(Studies in animals or humans demonstrate fetal abnormalities or adverse reaction; reports indicate evidence of fetal risk. The risk of use in pregnant women clearly outweighs any possible benefit.)*

Overdosage/Acute Toxicity

In humans, mild overdoses have resulted in hemolysis after several weeks of treatment, particularly in patients with reduced renal function. Acute overdoses are expected to cause clinical signs such as anorexia, tremors, lethargy, vomiting and anxiety. Increased reticulocyte counts and a severe hemolytic reaction are laboratory findings that would be expected. Treatment for an acute overdose may include intensive hematologic monitoring with adjunctive supportive therapy, including possible transfusions.

Drug Interactions

The following drug interactions with acetohydroxamic acid (AHA) have either been reported or are theoretical in humans or animals and may be of significance in veterinary patients. Unless otherwise noted, use together is not necessarily contraindicated, but weigh the potential risks and perform additional monitoring when appropriate.

▪ **IRON:** AHA may chelate iron salts in the gut if given concomitantly.

▪ **METHENAMINE:** AHA may have a synergistic effect with methenamine in inhibiting the urine pH increases caused by urease-producing *Proteus* spp.; AHA may also potentiate the antibacterial effect of methenamine against these bacteria.

▪ **ALCOHOL:** In humans, AHA with alcohol has resulted in rashes.

Laboratory Considerations

▪ Although AHA is a true urease inhibitor, it apparently does not interfere with urea nitrogen determination using one of the following: urease-Berthelot, urease-glutamate dehydrogenase or diacetyl monoxime methods.

Doses

▪ **DOGS:**

For adjunctive therapy of persistent struvite uroliths and persistent urease-producing bacteria after treating with antibiotics and calculolytic diets (extra-label): 12.5 mg/kg twice daily PO. (Osborne et al. 1993), (Lulich et al. 2000)

Monitoring
- CBC.
- Renal/Hepatic (bilirubin) function.
- Efficacy.

Client Information
- This medication can cause several adverse effects in dogs; contact veterinarian if dog develops persistent or severe vomiting, has a lack of appetite, a change in urine color, develops yellowing of the whites of the eyes, or has decreased energy/activity.

Chemistry/Synonyms
An inhibitor of urease, acetohydroxamic acid occurs as a white crystal having a pKa of 9.32-9.4 and a pH of about 9.4. 850 mg are soluble in one mL of water, and 400 mg are soluble in one mL of alcohol.

Acetohydroxamic acid may also be known as: AHA, Acetic acid oxime, N-Acetylhydroxylamide, N-Hydroxyacetamide, *Lithostat*® or *Uronefrex*®.

Storage/Stability
Tablets should be stored in tight containers.

Compatibility/Compounding Considerations
No specific information noted.

Dosage Forms/Regulatory Status
VETERINARY-LABELED PRODUCTS: NONE.

HUMAN-LABELED PRODUCTS:
Acetohydroxamic Acid Oral Tablets: 250 mg; *Lithostat*®; (Rx)

Revisions/References
Monograph revised/updated August 2013.

Lulich, J., et al. (2000). Canine Lower Urinary Tract Disorders. *Textbook of Veterinary Internal Medicine: Diseases of the Dog and Cat.* S. Ettinger and E. Feldman. Philadelphia, WB Saunders. 2: 1747-81.

Osborne, C., et al. (1993). Canine and feline urolithiasis: Relationship and etiopathogenesis with treatment and prevention. *Disease mechanisms in small animal surgery.* M. Bojrab. Philadelphia, Lea & Febiger: 464-511.

Acetylcysteine

(assah-**teel**-sis-tay-een)   N-acetylcysteine, NAC, ACC, Mucomyst®

Antidote; Mucolytic

Prescriber Highlights
▶ Used primarily as a treatment for acetaminophen toxicity or other hepatotoxic conditions where glutathione synthesis is inhibited or oxidative stress occurs.

▶ When used as an antidote, if possible give first dosage IV; oral doses should be given on an empty stomach and via gastric- or duodenal tube.

▶ Also has been used as an inhaled solution for its mucolytic effect and, anecdotally, for treating degenerative myelopathy.

▶ Has caused hypersensitivity & bronchospasm when used in pulmonary tree.

Uses/Indications
Acetylcysteine (N-acetylcysteine, NAC) is used in veterinary medicine as both a mucolytic agent in the pulmonary tree and as a treatment for acetaminophen, xylitol, or phenol toxicity in small animals. It potentially could be useful in the adjunctive treatment of sulfonamide hypersensitivity, mushroom hepatotoxicity, doxorubicin-induced hepatotoxicity or phenazopyridine toxicity (Bulucu et al. 2009; Holahan et al. 2010; Puschner et al. 2012). Acetylcysteine is used investigatively as an antiinflammatory for chronic upper respiratory disease in cats, as an adjunct in heavy metal removal, and

topically in the eye to halt the melting effect of collagenases and proteinases on the cornea.

It has been used anecdotally with aminocaproic acid to treat degenerative myelopathy in dogs, but data is lacking showing efficacy.

In horses with strangles, acetylcysteine instilled into the gutteral pouch has been used to help break up chondroids and avoid the need for surgical removal. Acetylcysteine enemas have been used in neonatal foals to break up meconium refractory to repeated enemas. In estrous mares, intrauterine NAC instillation could potentially be useful as an adjunctive treatment of endometritis as it appears to have antiinflammatory effects on equine endometrial cells and improve pregnancy rates (Gores-Lindholm et al. 2013; Melkus et al. 2013).

Pharmacology/Actions
When administered into the pulmonary tree, acetylcysteine (NAC) reduces the viscosity of both purulent and nonpurulent secretions and expedites the removal of these secretions via coughing, suction, or postural drainage. The free sulfhydryl group on the drug is believed to reduce disulfide linkages in mucoproteins; this effect is most pronounced at a pH from 7–9. The drug has no effect on living tissue or fibrin.

Acetylcysteine can reduce the extent of liver injury or methemoglobinemia after ingestion of acetaminophen or phenol, by providing an alternate substrate for conjugation with the reactive metabolite of acetaminophen, thus maintaining or restoring glutathione levels.

When administered to ill dogs (N=30) during the first 48 hours of hospitalization, NAC stabilized erythrocyte glutathione concentrations, but when compared with the placebo group, illness severity scores and survival rates were unchanged (Viviano et al. 2013).

Pharmacokinetics
When given orally, some acetylcysteine is absorbed from the GI tract. Oral bioavailability in healthy cats has been reported as approximately 20% (Buur et al. 2013). When administered via nebulization or intratracheally into the pulmonary tract, most of the drug is involved in the sulfhydryl-disulfide reaction and the remainder is absorbed. Absorbed drug is converted (deacetylated) into cysteine in the liver and then further metabolized. Elimination half-lives in cats are approximately 0.8 hours (IV) and 1.3 hours (PO). The authors postulated that oral doses of 100 mg/kg may be effective in cats when treating chronic diseases, but that additional studies are required to confirm safety and efficacy (Buur et al. 2013).

Contraindications/Precautions/Warnings
Acetylcysteine is contraindicated (for pulmonary indications) in animals hypersensitive to it. There are no contraindications for its use as an antidote.

Because acetylcysteine may cause bronchospasm in some patients when used in the pulmonary system, animals with bronchospastic diseases should be monitored carefully when using this agent.

Adverse Effects
When given orally for acetaminophen toxicity, acetylcysteine can cause GI effects (nausea, vomiting) and rarely, urticaria. Because the taste of the solution is very bad, taste-masking agents (*e.g.*, colas, juices) have been used. Since oral dosing of these drugs may be very difficult in animals, gastric or duodenal tubes may be necessary.

Intravenous administration appears to be very well tolerated in veterinary patients. IV boluses in humans have caused changes in blood pressure (hyper-, hypo-tension), GI effects and allergic reactions.

Adverse effects reported when acetylcysteine is administered into the pulmonary tract include: hypersensitivity, chest tightness, bronchoconstriction, and bronchial or tracheal irritation. A study done in cats with experimentally induced asthma demonstrated that endotracheal nebulization with acetylcysteine increased airway resistance and caused other adverse effects in some cats, including increased airway secretions, cough, and unilateral strabismus (Reinero et al. 2011).

Reproductive/Nursing Safety

Reproduction studies in rabbits and rats have not demonstrated any evidence of teratogenic or embryotoxic effects when used in doses up to 17 times normal. In humans, the FDA categorizes this drug as category *B* for use during pregnancy *(Animal studies have not yet demonstrated risk to the fetus, but there are no adequate studies in pregnant women; or animal studies have shown an adverse effect, but adequate studies in pregnant women have not demonstrated a risk to the fetus in the first trimester of pregnancy, and there is no evidence of risk in later trimesters.)*

It is unknown if acetylcysteine enters milk. Use caution when administering to a nursing dam.

Overdosage/Acute Toxicity

The LD_{50} of acetylcysteine in dogs is 1 gram/kg (PO) and 700 mg/kg (IV). It is believed that acetylcysteine is quite safe (with the exception of the adverse effects listed above) in most overdose situations.

Drug Interactions

- **ACTIVATED CHARCOAL:** The use of activated charcoal as a gut adsorbent of acetaminophen is controversial, as charcoal may also adsorb acetylcysteine. Because cats can develop methemoglobinemia very rapidly after ingestion of acetaminophen, do not delay acetylcysteine treatment and preferably give the first dose intravenously. If using the solution (not labeled for injectable use), it is preferable to use a 0.2 micron in-line filter.
- **NITROGLYCERIN (IV):** May enhance hypotension.

Doses

- **DOGS/CATS:**

  To maintain or restore glutathione levels for the adjunctive treatment of acetaminophen, phenol, or xylitol toxicity, sulfonamide hypersensitivity, mushroom hepatotoxicity, or doxorubicin-induced hepatotoxicity; (extra-label): Initial dose 140 – 180 mg/kg IV (dilute to 5% and give via slow IV over 15-20 minutes) or 280 mg/kg PO (via gastric- or duodenal-tube), followed by 70 mg/kg PO or IV q6h for a minimum of 7 treatments. Large overdoses may require up to 17 doses. Because oral bioavailability may only be 20% (in cats) and fluid/electrolytes may need ongoing adjustment, IV administration is preferred in serious intoxications.

  For degenerative myelopathy (Dogs); (extra-label): 25 mg/kg PO q8h for 2 weeks, then q8h every other day. The 20% solution should be diluted to 5% with chicken broth or suitable diluent. Used in conjunction with aminocaproic acid (500 mg per dog PO q8h indefinitely). Other treatments may include prednisone (0.25 – 0.5 mg/kg PO daily for 10 days then every other day), Vitamin C (1000 mg PO q12h) and Vitamin E (1000 Units PO q12h). **Note:** No treatment has been shown to be effective in published trials. (Shell 2003)

  For adjunctive treatment of hepatic lipidosis (see also Carnitine); (extra-label): Identify underlying cause of anorexia and provide a protein replete feline diet, give acetylcysteine (NAC) at 140 mg/kg IV over 20 minutes, then 70 mg/kg IV q12h; dilute 10% NAC with saline 1:4 and administer IV using a 0.25 micron filter; correct hypokalemia and hypophosphatemia, beware of

electrolyte changes with re-feeding phenomenon (Center 2006).

- **HORSES:**

  To help break up chondroids in the gutteral pouch (extra-label): Instill 20% solution (Foreman 1999).

  In neonatal foals to break up meconium refractory to repeated enemas (extra-label): 8 grams in 20 g sodium bicarbonate in 200 mL water (pH of 7.6), give as enema as needed to effect (Freeman 1999) or with foal in lateral recumbency, insert a 30 french foley catheter with a 30 cc bulb for a retention enema. Using gravity flow, infuse slowly 100–200 mL of 4% acetylcysteine solution and retain for 30–45 minutes. IV fluids and pain medication should be considered. Monitor for possible bladder distention. (Pusterla et al. 2003)

Monitoring

When used for acetaminophen, etc. poisoning:
- Hepatic enzymes (particularly in dogs).
- Acetaminophen level, if available (particularly in dogs).
- Hemogram, with methemoglobin value (particularly in cats).
- Serum electrolytes, hydration status.

Client Information

- This agent should be used in a clinically supervised setting only.

Chemistry/Synonyms

The N-acetyl derivative of L-cysteine, acetylcysteine occurs as a white, crystalline powder with a slight acetic odor. It is freely soluble in water or alcohol.

Acetylcysteine may also be known as: N-acetylcysteine or N-acetyl-L-cysteine, NAC, 5052 acetylcysteinum, NSC-111180, *Acetadote®*, *Mucomyst®* or *ACC®*.

Storage/Stability

When unopened, vials of sodium acetylcysteine should be stored at room temperature (15–30°C). When used for IV infusion, vials should be kept refrigerated and used within 96 hours after opening. The product labeled for IV use states to use within 24 hours. The color may turn from essentially colorless to a slight pink or purple once the stopper is punctured, but color change does not affect quality or concentration.

When stored at room temperature (under fluorescent lighting) or under refrigeration, 20% injection repackaged in 3 mL oral syringes (600 mg/3 mL; for oral use) is physically and chemically stable for 6 months (Kiser et al. 2007).

Compatibility/Compounding Considerations

Acetylcysteine injection (20%) is hyperosmolar and must be diluted before IV administration. It is **compatible** with dextrose 5% (D5W), sodium chloride 0.45% injection (half-normal saline), and water for injection. Acetylcysteine is **incompatible** with oxidizing agents; solutions can become discolored and liberate hydrogen sulfide when exposed to rubber, copper, iron, and during autoclaving. It does not react to aluminum, stainless steel, glass or plastic. If the solution becomes light purple in color, potency is not appreciably affected, but it is best to use non-reactive materials when giving the drug via nebulization. Acetylcysteine solutions are **incompatible** with amphotericin B, ampicillin sodium, erythromycin lactobionate, tetracycline, oxytetracycline, iodized oil, hydrogen peroxide and trypsin.

In veterinary medicine, acetylcysteine 20% is usually diluted to a concentration of 5% (final concentration of 50 mg/mL). This concentration can be obtained by adding one part injection (20%) to 3 parts of diluent. Dextrose 5% is most commonly employed as the diluent.

Dosage Forms/Regulatory Status

VETERINARY-LABELED PRODUCTS: NONE.

HUMAN-LABELED PRODUCTS:

Acetylcysteine injection: 20% (200 mg/mL), EDTA in 30 mL single-dose vials, preservative free; *Acetadote®*, generic; (Rx)

Acetylcysteine Oral Capsules: 600 mg; (Rx and OTC). May be labeled as a nutritional product.

Acetylcysteine Inhalation Solution: 10% & 20% (as sodium) in 4 mL, 10 mL & 30 mL vials; generic; (Rx) **Note:** If using this product for dilution and then intravenous dosing, it is preferable to use a 0.2 micron in-line filter.

Revisions/References

Monograph revised/updated August 2013.

Bulucu, F., et al. (2009). Effects of N-Acetylcysteine, Deferoxamine and Selenium on Doxorubicin-Induced Hepatotoxicity. *Biological Trace Element Research* 132(1-3): 184-96.

Buur, J. L., et al. (2013). Pharmacokinetics of N-acetylcysteine after oral and intravenous administration to healthy cats. *American Journal of Veterinary Research* 74(2): 290-3.

Center, S. (2006). *Treatment for Severe Feline Hepatic Lipidosis.* Proceedings: WSAVA. accessed via Veterinary Information Network; vin.com

Foreman, J. (1999). Equine respiratory pharmacology. *The Veterinary Clinics of North America: Equine Practice* 15:3(December).

Freeman, D. (1999). Gastrointestinal Pharmacology. *The Veterinary Clinics of North America: Equine Practice* 15:3(December): 535-59.

Gores-Lindholm, A., et al. (2013). Relationships between intrauterine infusion of N-acetylcysteine, equine endometrial pathology, neutrophil function, post-breeding therapy, and reproductive performance. *Theriogenology* 80.

Holahan, M. L., et al. (2010). Presumptive hepatotoxicity and rhabdomyolysis secondary to phenazopyridine toxicity in a dog. *J. Vet. Emerg. Crit. Care* 20(3): 352-8.

Kiser, T., et al. (2007). Stability of acetylcysteine solution repackaged in oral syringes and associated cost savings. *Am J Health-Syst Pharm* 64(7): 762-6.

Melkus, E., et al. (2013). Investigations on the Endometrial Response to Intrauterine Administration of N-Acetylcysteine in Oestrous Mares. *Reprod Dom Anim* 48: 591-7.

Puschner, B. & C. Wegenast (2012). Mushroom Poisoning Cases in Dogs and Cats: Diagnosis and Treatment of Hepatotoxic, Neurotoxic, Gastroenterotoxic, Nephrotoxic, and Muscarinic Mushrooms. *Vet Clin Small Anim* 42: 375-87.

Pusterla, N., et al. (2003). *Evaluation and use of acetylcysteine retention enemas in the treatment of meconium impaction in foals.* Proceedings: ACVIM Forum. accessed via Veterinary Information Network; vin.com

Reinero, C. R., et al. (2011). Endotracheal nebulization of N-acetylcysteine increases airway resistance in cats with experimental asthma. *Journal of Feline Medicine & Surgery* 13(2): 69-73.

Shell, L. (2003). "Degenerative Myelopathy (Degenerative Radiculomyelopathy)." *Associates Database.*

Viviano, K. R. & B. VanderWielen (2013). Effect of N-Acetylcysteine Supplementation on Intracellular Glutathione, Urine Isoprostanes, Clinical Score, and Survival in Hospitalized Ill Dogs. *Journal of Veterinary Internal Medicine* 27(2): 250-8.

Acetylsalicylic Acid — See Aspirin

Acitretin

(ase-a-**tre**-tin)   Soriatane®

Retinoid

Prescriber Highlights

▶ Retinoid that may be useful for certain dermatologic conditions in small animals.

▶ Contraindications: Pregnancy; Caution: Cardiovascular disease, hypertriglyceridemia or sensitivity to retinoids.

▶ Adverse Effects: Limited experience; appears to be fairly well tolerated in small animals. Potentially: anorexia/vomiting/diarrhea, cracking of foot pads, pruritus, ventral abdominal erythema, polydipsia, lassitude, joint pain/stiffness, eyelid abnormalities & conjunctivitis (KCS), swollen tongue, & behavioral changes.

▶ Known teratogen; do not use in households with pregnant women present (Plumb's recommendation).

▶ May be very expensive; may need to compound smaller capsules for small dogs or cats.

▶ Drug-drug; drug-lab interactions.

Uses/Indications

Acitretin may be useful in dogs for a variety of dermatologic conditions, including follicular dysplasias (*e.g.*, color dilution alopecia), schnauzer comedo syndrome, lamellar ichthyosis, solar-induced precancerous lesions in Dalmatians or bull Terriers, actinic keratoses, squamous cell carcinomas, epitheliotropic lymphomas, and intracutaneous cornifying epitheliomas (multiple keratoacanthomas). While the drug has provided effective treatment of idiopathic seborrhea (particularly in cocker spaniels), it is not effective in treating the ceruminous otitis that may also be present. Results have been disappointing in treating idiopathic seborrheas seen in basset hounds and West Highland terriers.

Acitretin's usage in cats is very limited, but it may have some usefulness in treating paraneoplastic actinic keratosis, solar-induced squamous cell carcinoma, sebaceous adenitis, feline acne, and Bowen's Disease.

Pharmacology/Actions

Acitretin is a synthetic retinoid agent potentially useful in the treatment of several disorders related to abnormal keratinization and/or sebaceous gland abnormalities in small animals. The drug has some antiinflammatory activity, but its exact mechanism of action is not known.

Pharmacokinetics

Acitretin absorption is enhanced by food in the gut and is highly bound to plasma proteins. The drug is metabolized to conjugate forms that are excreted in the bile and urine. Terminal half-life averages 50 hours in humans.

Contraindications/Precautions/Warnings

Acitretin use should not be considered when the following conditions exist: cardiovascular disease, hypertriglyceridemia or known sensitivity to acitretin. Use with caution in patients with renal or hepatic failure.

Adverse Effects

Veterinary experience with this medication is limited, but the incidence of adverse effects appears to be less in companion animals than in people. Potential adverse effects include: anorexia/vomiting/diarrhea, cracking of foot pads, pruritus, ventral abdominal erythema, polydipsia, lassitude, joint pain/stiffness, eyelid abnormalities and conjunctivitis (KCS), swollen tongue, and behavioral changes.

The most common adverse effect seen in cats is anorexia with resultant weight loss. If cats develop adverse effects, the time between doses may be prolonged (*e.g.*, every other week give every other day) to reduce the total dose given.

Reproductive/Nursing Safety

Acitretin is a known teratogen. Major anomalies have been reported in children of women receiving acitretin. It should not be handled by pregnant women nor used in a household where women are pregnant or planning to become pregnant. It should be considered absolutely contraindicated in pregnant veterinary patients. In humans, the FDA categorizes this drug as category *X* for use during pregnancy (*Studies in animals or humans demonstrate fetal abnormalities or adverse reaction; reports indicate evidence of fetal risk. The risk of use in pregnant women clearly outweighs any possible benefit.*)

Acitretin is excreted in rat milk. At this time, it cannot be recommended for use in nursing dams.

Overdosage/Acute Toxicity

Information on overdoses with this agent remains limited. One oral overdose (525 mg) in a human patient resulted only in vomiting. The oral LD50 in rats and mice is >4 grams/kg.

Drug Interactions

The following drug interactions with acitretin have either been reported or are theoretical in humans or animals and may be of significance in veterinary patients. Unless otherwise noted, use together is not necessarily contraindicated, but weigh the potential risks and perform additional monitoring when appropriate.

- **ALCOHOL:** Acitretin can form etretinate in the presence of alcohol; etretinate is a teratogen with an extremely long terminal half-life and (can persist in adipose tissue for years).
- **CYCLOSPORINE:** Retinoids may increase cyclosporine levels.
- **HEPATOTOXIC DRUGS** (especially **methotrexate**—contraindicated, and potentially **anabolic steroids, androgens, asparaginase, erythromycins, estrogens, fluconazole, halothane, ketoconazole, sulfonamides** or **valproic acid**): May be increased potential for hepatotoxicity.
- **OTHER RETINOIDS** (*e.g.*, **isotretinoin, tretinoin,** or **vitamin A**): May cause additive toxic effects.
- **TETRACYCLINES:** Acitretin with tetracyclines may increase the potential for the occurrence of pseudotumor cerebri (cerebral edema and increased CSF pressure).

Laboratory Considerations

- In humans, acitretin may cause significant increases in **plasma triglycerides, serum cholesterol, serum ALT (SGPT), serum AST (SGOT),** and **serum LDH concentrations. Serum HDL** (high density lipoprotein) concentrations may be decreased. Veterinary significance of these effects is unclear.

Doses

- **DOGS:**

  For dermatologic conditions where retinoids may be useful (see Indications); (extra-label): 0.5 – 3 mg/kg PO once daily. The lower end of this dosing range is generally used for color dilution alopecia and upper end of the dosing range for conditions such as Bowenoid-carcinoma and epitheliotropic lymphoma. Some dogs with sebaceous adenitis can be controlled with every other day dosing.

- **CATS:**

  For dermatologic conditions where retinoids may be useful (see Indications); (extra-label): 3 mg/kg or one 10 mg capsule (per cat) once daily.

Monitoring

- Efficacy.
- Liver function tests (baseline and if clinical signs appear).
- Schirmer tear tests (monthly—especially in older dogs).

Client Information

- Pregnant women must not handle acitretin; veterinarians must take responsibility to educate clients of the potential risk of ingestion by pregnant females.
- Food will increase the absorption of acitretin. To reduce variability of absorption, either have clients consistently give with meals or when fasted.
- Long-term therapy can be quite expensive.

Chemistry/Synonyms

Acitretin, a synthetic retinoid occurs as a yellow to greenish-yellow powder.

Acitretin may also be known as: acitretinum, etretin, Ro-10-1670, Ro-10-1670/000, *Soriatane®, Acetrizoic Acid®,* or *Iodophil Viscous®.*

Storage/Stability

Store at room temperature and protected from light. After bottle is opened, protect from high temperature and humidity.

Compatibility/Compounding Considerations

No specific information noted.

Dosage Forms/Regulatory Status

VETERINARY-LABELED PRODUCTS: NONE.

HUMAN-LABELED PRODUCTS:

Acitretin Capsules: 10 mg, 17.5 mg, 22.5 mg & 25 mg; *Soriatane®*; (Rx)

Revisions/References

Monograph revised/updated August 2013.

ACTH — See Corticotropin

Activated Charcoal — See Charcoal, Activated

Acyclovir

(ay-**sye**-kloe-vir)   Zovirax®

Antiviral (Herpes)

Prescriber Highlights

▶ Used primarily in birds for Pacheco's disease.
▶ If given rapidly IV, may be nephrotoxic. Can cause tissue necrosis in birds when given IM.
▶ Oral use may cause GI distress.
▶ Reduce dosage with renal insufficiency.
▶ May be fetotoxic at high dosages.

Uses/Indications

Acyclovir may be useful in treating herpes infections in a variety of avian species. When used for Pacheco's disease, it appears to be somewhat effective but only when given very early in the disease (before clinical symptoms occur). Acyclovir (systemic) has also been used in cats with corneal or conjunctival herpes infections, but its relatively mild activity against *Feline Herpesvirus-1* when compared to some of the newer antiviral agents (*e.g.*, ganciclovir, cidofovir, or penciclovir), low bioavailability, and potential for toxicity make its use problematic.

Acyclovir is being investigated in horses as a treatment for equine herpes virus type-5 (EHV-5) lymphoma, and equine herpes virus type-1 (EHV-1) myeloencephalopathy, but clinical efficacy has not yet been proven and the drug's poor oral bioavailability is an issue. There continues to be interest in finding a dosing regimen that can achieve therapeutic levels and be economically viable, particularly since the drug's use during a recent outbreak appeared to have some efficacy in reducing morbidity and mortality (not statistically proven). Also, intravenous acyclovir may be economically feasible to treat some neonatal foals.

Pharmacology/Actions

Acyclovir has antiviral activity against a variety of viruses including herpes simplex (types I and II), cytomegalovirus, *Epstein-Barr,* and *varicella-Zoster.* It is preferentially taken up by these viruses, and converted into the active triphosphate form where it inhibits viral DNA replication.

Pharmacokinetics

In dogs, acyclovir bioavailability varies with the dose. At doses of 20 mg/kg and below, bioavailability is about 80%, but declines to about 50% at 50 mg/kg.

Bioavailability in horses after oral administration is very low (<4%) and oral doses of up to 20 mg/kg may not yield sufficient levels to treat equine herpes virus, but some accumulation may occur with prolonged oral dosing. Elimination half-lives in dogs, cats and horses are approximately 3 hours, 2.6 hours, and 10 hours, respectively.

In humans, acyclovir is poorly absorbed after oral administration (approx. 20%) and absorption is not significantly affected by the presence of food. It is widely distributed throughout body tissues and fluids including the brain, semen, and CSF. It has low protein binding and crosses the placenta. Acyclovir is primarily hepatically metabolized and has a half-life of about 3 hours in humans. Renal disease does not significantly alter half-life unless anuria is present.

Contraindications/Precautions/Warnings

Acyclovir is potentially contraindicated (assess risk vs. benefit) during dehydrated states, pre-existing renal function impairment, hypersensitivity to it or other related antivirals, neurologic deficits, or previous neurologic reactions to other cytotoxic drugs.

Adverse Effects

With parenteral therapy potential adverse effects include thrombophlebitis, acute renal failure, and ecephalopathologic changes (rare). GI disturbances may occur with either oral or parenteral therapy.

Reproductive/Nursing Safety

Acyclovir crosses the placenta, but rodent studies have not demonstrated any teratogenic effects thus far. Acyclovir crosses into maternal milk but associated adverse effects have not been noted. In humans, the FDA categorizes this drug as category *C* for use during pregnancy (*Animal studies have shown an adverse effect on the fetus, but there are no adequate studies in humans; or there are no animal reproduction studies and no adequate studies in humans.*)

Acyclovir concentrations in milk of women following oral administration have ranged from 0.6 to 4.1 times those found in plasma. These concentrations would potentially expose the breastfeeding infant to a dose of acyclovir up to 0.3 mg/kg/day. Data for animals was not located. Use caution when administering to a nursing patient.

Overdosage/Acute Toxicity

Acute oral overdosage is unlikely to cause significant toxicity. GI signs predominate although renal failure is possible with higher doses. Crystalluria and elevated renal values occurred at 188.7 mg/kg in a dog. There were 85 exposures to acyclovir reported to the ASPCA Animal Poison Control Center (APCC) during 2008-2009. In these cases 75 were dogs with 9 showing clinical signs. The remaining 10 cases were cats with 4 showing clinical signs. Common findings in dogs (recorded in decreasing frequency) include vomiting, diarrhea, and lethargy. Vomiting was a common finding in cats.

Consider decontamination at 150 mg/kg or higher. Below 150 mg/kg, GI signs will likely predominate.

Drug Interactions

The following drug interactions with acyclovir have either been reported or are theoretical in humans or animals and may be of significance in veterinary patients. Unless otherwise noted, use together is not necessarily contraindicated, but weigh the potential risks and perform additional monitoring when appropriate.

- **NEPHROTOXIC MEDICATIONS:** Concomitant administration of IV acyclovir with nephrotoxic medications may increase the potential for nephrotoxicity occurring. Amphotericin B may potentiate the antiviral effects of acyclovir but it also increases chances for development of nephrotoxicity.
- **ZIDOVUDINE:** Concomitant use with zidovudine may cause additional CNS depression.

Doses

- **BIRDS:**

  For treatment/prophylaxis of Pacheco's Disease (extra-label): Treatment: 80 mg/kg PO (oral gavage) or IM (one time; can cause tissue necrosis) q8h for 7-14 days; For prophylaxis: After an initial dose of 25 mg/kg IM, may be added to drinking water at 1 mg/mL or to food at 400 mg/quart of seed for at least 7 days.

- **HORSES:**

  For equine herpes infections (extra-label): Although efficacy is undetermined and oral bioavailability is very low, 20 mg/kg PO q8h (for months) has been used. In foals it can be used at 10 mg/kg IV (over one hour) q12h.

Monitoring

- Renal function tests (BUN, Serum Creatinine) with prolonged or IV therapy.

Client Information

- Side effects are usually limited gastrointestinal problems (diarrhea, vomiting, lack of appetite).
- For birds it usually given in water or mixed with seed or peanut butter.
- Patients will need ongoing lab tests while taking this medication.

Chemistry/Synonyms

An antiviral agent, acyclovir (also known as ACV or acycloguanosine), occurs as a white, crystalline powder. 1.3 mg is soluble in one mL of water. Acyclovir sodium has a solubility of greater than 100 mg/mL in water. However, at a pH of 7.4 at 37°C it is practically all unionized and has a solubility of only 2.5 mg/mL in water. There is 4.2 mEq of sodium in each gram of acyclovir sodium.

Acyclovir may be known as: aciclovirum, acycloguanosine, acyclovir, BW-248U, *Zovirax®, Acic®, Aciclobene®, Aciclotyrol®, Acivir®, Acyrax®, Cicloviral®, Geavir®, Geavir®, Herpotern®, Isavir®, Nycovir®, Supraviran®, Viclovir®, Virherpes®, Viroxy®, Xorox®,* or *Zovirax®.*

Storage/Stability

Acyclovir capsules and tablets should be stored in tight, light resistant containers at room temperature. Acyclovir suspension and sodium sterile powder should be stored at room temperature.

Compatibility/Compounding Considerations

When reconstituting acyclovir sodium do not use bacteriostatic water with parabens as precipitation may occur. The manufacturer does not recommend using bacteriostatic water for injection with benzyl alcohol because of the potential toxicity in neonates. After reconstitution with 50 – 100 mL of a standard electrolyte or dextrose solution, the resulting solution is stable at 25°C for 24 hours.

Acyclovir is reportedly **incompatible** with biologic or colloidal products (*e.g.,* blood products or protein containing solutions). It is also **incompatible** with dopamine HCl, dobutamine, foscarnet sodium, meperidine and morphine sulfate. Many other drugs have been shown to be **compatible** in specific situations. Compatibility is dependent upon factors such as pH, concentration, temperature and diluent used; consult specialized references or a hospital pharmacist for more specific information.

Dosage Forms/Regulatory Status
VETERINARY-LABELED PRODUCTS: NONE

HUMAN-LABELED PRODUCTS:

Acyclovir Oral Tablets: 400 mg & 800 mg; *Zovirax*®, generic; (Rx)

Acyclovir Oral Capsules: 200 mg; *Zovirax*®; generic; (Rx)

Acyclovir Oral Suspension: 200 mg/5 mL in 473 mL; *Zovirax*®, generic; (Rx)

Acyclovir Sodium; Injection (for IV infusion only): 50 mg/mL (as sodium); generic; (Rx)

Acyclovir Powder for Injection: 500 mg/vial (as sodium) in 10 mL vials; 1000 mg/vial (as sodium) in 20 mL vials; generic; (Rx)

Topical 5% creams and ointments are also available.

Revisions/References
Monograph revised/updated August 2013.

Afoxolaner

(ah-**fox**-ah-lan-er)   NexGard®

Oral insecticide/acaracide

Prescriber Highlights
▶ Chewable oral tablet for treatment and control of flea and American Dog tick infestations in dogs.

▶ New agent with little clinical experience, but thus far, adverse effects appear unlikely (possible vomiting after a dose).

Uses/Indications
Afoxolaner chewable tablets (*NexGard*®) is approved by FDA for the treatment and prevention of flea infestations (*Ctenocephalides felis*), and the treatment and control of American dog tick (*Dermacentor variabilis*) infestations in dogs and puppies 8 weeks of age and older, weighing 4 pounds of body weight or greater, for 1 month.

Pharmacology/Actions
Afoxolaner is in the isoxazoline family of insecticides and acaracides. In the CNS, they block pre- and post-synaptic transfer of chloride ions across cell membranes, by inhibiting gamma-aminobutyric acid (GABA)-mediated ligand-gated chloride channels. Prolonged neuronal hyperexcitation results in death of susceptible insects and acarines. A difference between GABA receptor sensitivities of insects/acarines in comparison to mammals is believed the reason for differential toxicity.

Pharmacokinetics
In dogs, afoxolaner is reported to be rapidly absorbed with a bioavailability of about 75% and peak levels occurring between 2-6 hours. Food does not impair absorption. Protein binding is very high (>99%). Elimination is via biliary excretion of free afoxolaner and renal excretion of hepatically biotransformed metabolites. Terminal elimination half-life is about 15 days.

Contraindications/Precautions/Warnings
There no labeled contraindications when used as indicated. Safe use in breeding, pregnant or lactating dogs has not been evaluated. Use with caution in dogs with a history of seizures or epilepsy. The drug is not labeled for use in puppies less than 8 weeks old or in dogs that weigh less than 4 lbs. (1.8 kg).

Adverse Effects
While experience is very limited at the time of writing (2013), in pre-approval field studies (415 dogs over 90 days) serious adverse effects were not noted, although two dogs with a history of seizures had a seizure during the study (causation could not be determined), hence the caution above. The most prevalent adverse effect noted was vomiting (4.1%). Other adverse effects reported (>1%) included dry flaky skin (3.1%), diarrhea (3.1%), lethargy (1.7%) and anorexia (1.2%).

Reproductive/Nursing Safety
No specific information located. The label states that safe use in breeding, pregnant or lactating dogs has not been evaluated.

Overdosage/Acute Toxicity
No information was located for acute toxicity in dogs. Oral doses up to 1,000 mg/kg in rats and 2,000 mg/kg in mice did not cause lethality. Dogs receiving dosages of 5X (6.3 mg/kg) for three treatments every 28 days, followed by three treatments every 14 days, for a total of six treatments did not show clinically-relevant effects related to treatment on physical examination, body weight, food consumption, clinical pathology (hematology, clinical chemistries, or coagulation tests), gross pathology, histopathology or organ weights. Vomiting occurred throughout the study, with a similar incidence in the treated and control groups, including one dog in the 5X group that vomited four hours after treatment.

Drug Interactions
None have been reported.

Laboratory Considerations
None were noted.

Doses
- **DOGS:**

  For labeled indications of the treatment and control of flea (*Ctenocephalides felis*), American Dog tick (*Dermacentor variabilis*) infestations (FDA-approved): Minimum dosage is 2.5 mg/kg PO once per month. The package insert has a dosing table for the various tablet sizes: 11.3 mg tablet for dogs weighing 4-10 lbs. (1.8-4.6 kg); 28.3 mg tablet for dogs weighing 10.1-24 lbs. (4.7-10.9 kg); 68 mg tablet for dogs weighing 24.1-60 lbs. (11-27.3 kg); 136 mg tablet for dogs weighing 60.1-120 lbs. (27.4-54.6 kg). Dogs that weigh more than 120 lbs. would receive the appropriate combination of chewables. (Label Information; *NexGard*®)

Monitoring
- Clinical efficacy and any adverse effects.

Client Information
- Can be administered with or without food.
- Be sure dog consumes the complete dose. Watch your dog for a minutes after giving to be sure they don't spit out any part of the dose
- If your dog vomits within two hours of dosing, give another full dose. If a dose is missed, give it when you remember and start a new a monthly dosing schedule.
- Treatment may start at any time of the year. In areas where fleas are common year-round, monthly treatment should continue the entire year without stopping.
- To minimize the likelihood of flea reinfestation, treat all animals within a household with an approved flea control product.

Chemistry/Synonyms
Afoxolaner is lipophilic, hydrophobic, and non-ionizable. Its ATCvet code is QP53BX04.

Storage/Stability
Chewable tablets should be stored at or below 30°C (86°F) with excursions permitted up to 40°C (104°F).

Compatibility/Compounding Considerations
No specific information noted.

Dosage Forms/Regulatory Status
VETERINARY-LABELED PRODUCTS:
Afoxolaner Chewable (Beef-flavored) Tablets: 11.3 mg, 28.3 mg, 68 mg, & 136 mg; *NexGard*®; (Rx). FDA-approved (NADA 141-406) for use in dogs.

HUMAN-LABELED PRODUCTS: NONE.

Revisions/References
Monograph written 12/2013.

Aglepristone

(a-gle-**pris**-tone)   Alizin®, Alizine®

Injectable Progesterone Blocker

Prescriber Highlights

▶ Injectable progesterone blocker indicated for pregnancy termination in bitches; may also be of benefit in inducing parturition or in treating pyometra complex in dogs & progesterone-dependent mammary hyperplasia in cats.

▶ Not currently available in USA; marketed for use in dogs in Europe, South America, etc.

▶ Localized injection site reactions are the most commonly noted adverse effect; other adverse effects reported in >5% of patients include: anorexia (25%), excitation (23%), depression (21%), & diarrhea (13%).

Uses/Indications

Aglepristone is labeled (in the U.K. and elsewhere) for pregnancy termination in bitches up to 45 days after mating.

In dogs, aglepristone may prove useful in inducing parturition or treating pyometra complex (often in combination with a prostaglandin F analog such as cloprostenol).

In cats, it may be of benefit for pregnancy termination (one study documented 87% efficacy when administered at the recommended dog dose at day 25) or in treating mammary hyperplasias or pyometras.

Pharmacology/Actions

Aglepristone is a synthetic steroid that binds to the progesterone (P4) receptors thereby preventing biological effects from progesterone. In dogs, it has an affinity for uterine progesterone receptors approximately three times that of progesterone. In queens, affinity is approximately nine times greater than the endogenous hormone. As progesterone is necessary for maintaining pregnancy, pregnancy can be terminated or parturition induced. Abortion occurs within 7 days of administration.

Benign feline mammary hyperplasias (fibroadenomatous hyperplasia; FAHs) are usually under the influence of progesterone and aglepristone can be used to medically treat this condition.

Aglepristone has been shown to have inhibitory effects on progesterone-receptor positive canine mammary carcinoma cells (Guil-Luna et al. 2011).

When used for treating pyometra in dogs, aglepristone can cause opening of the cervix and resumption of miometral contractility.

Within 24 hours of administration, aglepristone does not appreciably affect circulating plasma levels of progesterone, cortisol, prostaglandins or oxytocin. Plasma levels of prolactin are increased within 12 hours when used in dogs during mid-pregnancy which is probably the cause of mammary gland congestion often seen in these dogs.

Aglepristone also binds to glucocorticoid receptors but has no glucocorticoid activity; it can prevent endogenous or exogenously administered glucocorticoids from binding and acting at these sites.

Pharmacokinetics

In dogs, after injecting two doses of 10mg/kg 24 hours apart, peak serum levels occur about 2.5 days later and mean residence time is about 6 days. The majority (90%) of the drug is excreted via the feces.

Contraindications/Precautions/Warnings

Aglepristone is contraindicated in patients who have documented hypersensitivity to it and during pregnancy, unless used for pregnancy termination or inducing parturition.

When being considered for use in treating pyometra in bitches, peritonitis must be ruled out before using.

Because of its antagonistic effects on glucocorticoid receptors, the drug should not be used in patients with hypoadrenocorticism or in dogs with a genetic predisposition to hypoadrenocorticism.

The manufacturer does not recommend using the product in patients in poor health, with diabetes, or with impaired hepatic or renal function, as there is no data documenting its safety with these conditions.

Adverse Effects

As the product is in an oil-alcohol base, localized pain and inflammatory reactions (edema, skin thickening, ulceration, and localized lymph node enlargement) can be noted at the injection site. Resolution of pain generally occurs shortly after injection; other injection site reactions usually resolve within 2–4 weeks. The manufacturer recommends light massage of the injection site after administration. Larger dogs should not receive more than 5 mL at any one subcutaneous injection site. One source states that severe injection reactions can be avoided if the drug is administered into the scruff of the neck.

Systemic adverse effects reported from field trials include: anorexia (25%), excitation (23%), depression (21%), vomiting (2%), diarrhea (13%) and uterine infections (3.4%). Transient changes in hematologic (RBC, WBC indices) or biochemical (BUN, creatinine, chloride, potassium, sodium, liver enzymes) laboratory parameters were seen in <5% of dogs treated.

When used for pregnancy termination, a brown mucoid vaginal discharge can be seen approximately 24 hours before fetal expulsion. This discharge can persist for an additional 3–5 days. If used in bitches after the 20th day of gestation, abortion may be accompanied with other signs associated with parturition (*e.g.,* inappetence, restlessness, mammary congestion).

Bitches may return to estrus in as little as 45 days after pregnancy termination.

Reproductive/Nursing Safety

Unless used for pregnancy termination or at term to induce parturition, aglepristone is contraindicated during pregnancy.

One study (Baan et al. 2005) using aglepristone to induce parturition (day 58) demonstrated no significant differences in weight gain between those puppies in the treatment group versus the control group suggesting that aglepristone did not have effect on milk production of treated bitches.

Overdosage/Acute Toxicity

When administered at 3X (30mg/kg) recommended doses, bitches demonstrated no untoward systemic effects. Localized reactions were noted at the injection site, presumably due to the larger volumes injected.

Drug Interactions

No documented drug interactions were noted. Theoretically, the following interactions may occur with aglepristone:

- **PROGESTINS (natural or synthetic):** Could reduce the efficacy of aglepristone.
- **GLUCOCORTICOIDS:** Aglepristone could reduce the efficacy of glucocorticoid treatment.
- **KETOCONAZOLE, ITRACONAZOLE, ERYTHROMYCIN:** The manufacturer states that although there is no data, these drugs may interact with aglepristone.

Laboratory Considerations

None were noted.

Doses

Warning: As accidental injection of this product can induce abortion; it should not be administered or handled by pregnant women. Accidental injection can also cause severe pain, intense swelling and ischemic necrosis that can lead to serious sequelae, including loss of a digit. In cases of accidental injection, prompt medical attention must be sought.

- **DOGS:**

  To induce parturition: At day 60 (not before day 58; post-estimated LH surge); (extra-label): 15 mg/kg subcutaneously and another dose 9-24 hours later. Use standard protocols to assist with birth (including oxytocin to assist in pup expulsion if necessary) or to intervene if parturition does not proceed.

  To terminate pregnancy (up to day 45) (extra-label in USA): 10 mg/kg (0.33 mL/kg) subcutaneous injection (into the scruff of the neck) only. Repeat one time, 24 hours after the first injection. A maximum of 5 mL should be injected at any one site. Light massage of the injection site is recommended after administration. (Label information; *Alizin*®—Virbac U.K.)

  As an adjunct to treating pyometra/metritis (extra-label):

  a) **When attempting to preserve fertility (mating should occur in the first or second estrus post-treatment) in bitches up to 5 years old with a lack of detectable ovarian cysts:** Treatment begun at week 2-4 of diestrus with a single SC injection of aglepristone at 10 mg/kg. Doses are repeated at days 2, 7, and 14. During first 7 days, daily injections of amoxicillin/clavulanic acid were also given. (Jurka et al. 2010)

  b) **For metritis:** 10 mg/kg subcutaneously once daily on days 1, 2 and 8. For open or closed pyometra: aglepristone 10 mg/kg subcutaneously once daily on days 1, 2 and 8 and cloprostenol 1 microgram/kg subcutaneously on days 3 to 7. Bitches with closed pyometra or with elevated temperature or dehydration should also receive intravenous fluids and antibiotics (*e.g.*, amoxicillin/clavulanate at 24 mg/kg/day on days 1–5). If pyometra has not resolved, additional aglepristone doses should be given on days 14 and 28. (Fieni 2006)

- **CATS:**

  For treating mammary fibroadenomatous hyperplasia (extra-label): 10 – 15 mg/kg subcutaneously on days 1, 2 and 7. Weekly treatment should be made until resolution of signs and may be required for several weeks. Relapses can occur especially in cats that have been treated with a long-acting progestin (*e.g.*, medroxyprogesterone acetate).

  To terminate pregnancy (up to day 45); (extra-label): 10 – 15 mg/kg subcutaneously twice 24 hours apart.

Monitoring

- Clinical efficacy.
- For pregnancy termination: ultrasound 10 days after treatment and at least 30 days after mating.
- Adverse effects (see above).

Client Information

- Only veterinary professionals should handle and administer this product.
- When used for pregnancy termination in the bitch, clients should understand that aglepristone might only be 95% effective in terminating pregnancy when used between days 26–45.
- A brown mucoid vaginal discharge can be seen approximately 24 hours before fetal expulsion.
- Bitch may exhibit the following after treatment: lack of appetite, excitement, restlessness or depression, vomiting, or diarrhea.
- Clients should be instructed to contact veterinarian if bitch exhibits a purulent or hemorrhagic discharge after treatment or if vaginal discharge persists 3 weeks after treatment.
- When used for pyometra, there is a substantial risk of treatment failure and ovariohysterectomy may be required.

Chemistry/Synonyms

Aglepristone is a synthetic steroid. The manufactured injectable dosage form is in a clear, yellow, oily, non-aqueous vehicle that contains arachis oil and ethanol. No additional antimicrobial agent is added to the injection.

Aglepristone may also be known as RU-534, *Alizine*®, or *Alizin*®.

Storage/Stability

Aglepristone injection should be stored below 25°C and protected from light. The manufacturer recommends using the product within 28 days of withdrawing the first dose.

Compatibility/Compounding Considerations

Although no incompatibilities have been reported, due to the product's oil/alcohol vehicle formulation it should not be mixed with any other medication.

Dosage Forms/Regulatory Status

VETERINARY-LABELED PRODUCTS:

Note: Not presently available or approved for use in the USA. In several countries: Aglepristone Injection: 30 mg/mL in 5 mL & 10 mL vials; *Alizine*® or *Alizin*®; (Rx)

HUMAN-LABELED PRODUCTS: NONE.

Revisions/References

Monograph revised/updated August 2013.

Baan, M., et al. (2005). Induction of parturition in the bitch with the progesterone-receptor blocker aglepristone. *Theriogenology* 63(17): 1958-72.

Fieni, F. (2006). Clinical evaluation of the use of aglepristone, with or without cloprostenol, to treat cystic endometrial hyperplasia-pyometra complex. *Theriogenology* 66(6-7): 1550-6.

Guil-Luna, S., et al. (2011). Aglepristone Decreases Proliferation in Progesterone Receptor-Positive Canine Mammary Carcinomas. *Journal of Veterinary Internal Medicine* 25(3): 518-23.

Jurka, P., et al. (2010). Age-Related Pregnancy Results and Further Examination of Bitches after Aglepristone Treatment of Pyometra. *Reproduction in Domestic Animals* 45(3): 525-9.

Albendazole

(al-**ben**-da-zole)   Albenza®, Valbazen®

Antiparasitic

Prescriber Highlights

▶ Broad spectrum against a variety of nematodes, cestodes & protozoa; labeled for cattle & sheep (suspension only).

▶ Contraindicated with hepatic failure, pregnancy, lactating dairy cattle.

▶ Not recommended for use in dogs or cats. While it may be effective, there is an increased risk for bone marrow toxicity in these species.

▶ May cause GI effects (including hepatic dysfunction) & rarely blood dyscrasias (aplastic anemia).

▶ Do not use in pigeons, doves or crias.

Uses/Indications

Albendazole is labeled for the following endoparasites of cattle (not lactating): *Ostertagia ostertagi, Haemonchus* spp., *Trichostrongylus* spp., *Nematodius* spp., *Cooperia* spp., *Bunostomum phlebotomum, Oesphagostomum* spp., *Dictacaulus vivaparus (adult and 4th stage larva), Fasciola hepatica (adults),* and *Moniezia* spp.

In sheep, albendazole is FDA-approved for treating the following endoparasites: *Ostertagia circumcincta, Marshallagia marshalli, Haemonchus contortus, Trichostrongylus* spp., *Nematodius* spp., *Cooperia* spp., *Oesphagostomum* spp., *Chibertia ovina, Dictacaulus filaria, Fasciola hepatica, Fascioides magna, Moniezia expansa,* and *Thysanosoma actinoides.*

Albendazole is also used (extra-label) in small mammals, goats and swine for endoparasite control.

In cats, albendazole has been used to treat Paragonimus kellicotti infections. In dogs and cats, albendazole has been used to treat capillariasis. In dogs, albendazole has been used to treat Filaroides infections. It has been used for treating giardia infections in small animals, but concerns about bone marrow toxicity have diminished enthusiasm for the drug's use.

Pharmacology/Actions

Benzimidazole antiparasitic agents have a broad spectrum of activity against a variety of pathogenic internal parasites. In susceptible parasites, their mechanism of action is believed due to disrupting intracellular microtubular transport systems by binding selectively and damaging tubulin, preventing tubulin polymerization, and inhibiting microtubule formation. Benzimidazoles also act at higher concentrations to disrupt metabolic pathways within the helminth, and inhibit metabolic enzymes, including malate dehydrogenase and fumarate reductase.

Pharmacokinetics

Pharmacokinetic data for albendazole in cattle, dogs and cats was not located.

After oral dosing in sheep, the parent compound was either not detectable or only transiently detectable in plasma due to a very rapid first-pass effect. The active metabolites, albendazole sulphoxide and albendazole sulfone, reached peak plasma concentrations 20 hours after dosing.

Contraindications/Precautions/Warnings

The drug is not FDA-approved for use in lactating dairy cattle. The manufacturer recommends not administering to female cattle during the first 45 days of pregnancy or for 45 days after removal of bulls. In sheep or goats, it should not be administered to ewes or does during the first 30 days of pregnancy or for 30 days after removal of rams or bucks.

Pigeons and doves may be susceptible to albendazole and fenbendazole toxicity (intestinal crypt epithelial necrosis and bone marrow hypoplasia).

Nine alpaca crias receiving albendazole at dosages from 33 – 100 mg/kg/day once daily for 4 consecutive days developed neutropenia and severe watery diarrhea. All required treatment and 7 of 9 animals treated died or were euthanized secondary to sepsis or multiple organ failure (Gruntman et al. 2006).

In humans, caution is recommended for use in patients with liver or hematologic diseases.

Albendazole was implicated as being an oncogen in 1984, but subsequent studies were unable to demonstrate any oncogenic or carcinogenic activity of the drug.

Adverse Effects

Albendazole is tolerated without significant adverse effects when dosed in cattle or sheep at recommended dosages.

Dogs treated at 50 mg/kg twice daily may develop anorexia. Cats may exhibit clinical signs of mild lethargy, depression, anorexia, and resistance to receiving the medication when albendazole is used to treat Paragonimus. Albendazole has been implicated in causing aplastic anemia in dogs, cats, and humans.

Reproductive/Nursing Safety

Albendazole has been associated with teratogenic and embryotoxic effects in rats, rabbits and sheep when given early in pregnancy. The manufacturer recommends not administering to female cattle during the first 45 days of pregnancy or for 45 days after removal of bulls. In sheep, it should not be administered to ewes or does during the first 30 days of pregnancy or for 30 days after removal of rams or bucks.

In humans, the FDA categorizes this drug as category *C* for use during pregnancy (*Animal studies have shown an adverse effect on the fetus, but there are no adequate studies in humans; or there are no animal reproduction studies and no adequate studies in humans.*)

Safety during nursing has not been established.

Overdosage/Toxicity

Doses of 300 mg/kg (30X recommended) and 200 mg/kg (20X) have caused death in cattle and sheep, respectively. Doses of 45 mg/kg (4.5X those recommended) did not cause any adverse effects in cattle tested. Cats receiving 100 mg/kg/day for 14-21 days showed signs of weight loss, neutropenia and mental dullness.

Drug Interactions

The following drug interactions with albendazole have either been reported or are theoretical in humans or animals and may be of significance in veterinary patients. Unless otherwise noted, use together is not necessarily contraindicated, but weigh the potential risks and perform additional monitoring when appropriate.

▪ **CIMETIDINE**: Increased albendazole levels in bile and cystic fluid.

▪ **DEXAMETHASONE**: May increase albendazole serum levels.

▪ **PRAZIQUANTEL**: May increase albendazole serum levels.

▪ **THEOPHYLLINE**: May decrease theophylline levels.

Doses

▪ **DOGS/CATS:**

For Giardia (extra-label): 25 mg/kg PO q12h for 3-5 days. **Note:** Because of the potential for bone marrow toxicity in small animals, albendazole is rarely used in, or recommended for dogs or cats.

▪ **CATTLE:**

For removal and control of liver flukes, tapeworms, stomach worms (including 4th stage inhibited larvae of Ostertagia ostertagi), intestinal worms, and lungworms (FDA-approved label): 10 mg/kg PO (4 mL/100 lbs. of body weight). **Note:** Not approved for use in female dairy cattle of breeding age. (Adapted from *Valbazen®* label information)

- **SHEEP:**

  For removal and control of liver flukes, tapeworms, stomach worms (including 4th stage inhibited larvae of *Ostertagia ostertagi*), intestinal worms, and lungworms (FDA-approved label): 7.5 mg/kg PO (0.75 mL/25 lbs. of body weight). (Adapted from *Valbazen®* label information)

- **GOATS:**

  For the treatment of adult liver flukes in nonlactating goats (FDA-approved label): 10 mg/kg PO (4 mL/100 lbs. of body weight). (Adapted from *Valbazen®* label information)

- **RABBITS/RODENTS/SMALL MAMMALS:**

  All are extra-label.

  a) **Rabbits: For Encephalitozoon phacoclastic uveitis:** 30 mg/kg PO once daily for 30 days, then 15 mg/kg PO once daily for 30 days. (Ivey et al. 2000)

  b) **Rabbits: For *E. cuniculi*:** 20 mg/kg PO once daily for 10 days. (Bryan 2009)

  c) **Chinchillas: For Giardia:** 50 – 100 mg/kg PO once a day for 3 days. (Hayes 2000)

Monitoring

- Efficacy.
- Adverse effects; particularly if used in non-FDA-approved species or at dosages higher than recommended.
- Consider monitoring CBC's and liver enzymes (q4-6 weeks) if treating long-term (>1 month).

Client Information

- Shake well before administering.
- Contact veterinarian if adverse effects occur (*e.g.,* vomiting, diarrhea, yellowish sclera/mucous membranes or skin).

Chemistry/Synonyms

A benzimidazole anthelmintic structurally related to mebendazole, albendazole has a molecular weight of 265. It is insoluble in water and soluble in alcohol.

Albendazole may also be known as albendazolum, SKF-62979, *Valbazen®* or *Albenza®*; many other trade names are available.

Storage/Stability

Albendazole suspension should be stored at room temperature (15-30°C); protect from freezing. Shake well before using. Albendazole tablets should be stored at 20-30°C.

Compatibility/Compounding Considerations

No specific information noted.

Dosage Forms/ Regulatory Status

VETERINARY-LABELED PRODUCTS:

Albendazole Suspension: 113.6 mg/mL (11.36%) in 500 mL, 1 liter, 5 liters; *Valbazen® Suspension*; (OTC). FDA-approved for use in cattle (not female cattle during first 45 days of pregnancy or for 45 days after removal of bulls, or of breeding age) and sheep (do not administer to ewes during the first 30 days of pregnancy or for 30 days after removal of rams). Slaughter withdrawal for cattle = 27 days at labeled doses. Slaughter withdrawal for sheep = 7 days at labeled dose. Since milk withdrawal time has not been established, do not use in female dairy cattle of breeding age. A milk withdrawal time of 7 milkings has been proposed for sheep (Athanasiou et al. 2009).

There is a website (dailymed.nlm.nih.gov) with the FDA-approved veterinary product label: *Valbazen®*

HUMAN-LABELED PRODUCTS:

Albendazole Oral Tablets: 200 mg; *Albenza®*; (Rx)

Revisions/References

Monograph revised/updated August 2013.

Athanasiou, L. V., et al. (2009). Proposals for withdrawal period of sheep milk for some commonly used veterinary medicinal products: A review. *Small Ruminant Research* 86(1-3): 2-5.

Bryan, J. (2009). *E. Cuniculi: Past, Present, and Future.* Proceedings: Western Veterinary Conference. accessed via Veterinary Information Network; vin.com

Gruntman, A. & R. Nolen-Walston (2006). *Albendazole toxicity in nine alpaca crias.* Proceedings: ACVIM Forum 2006. accessed via Veterinary Information Network; vin.com

Hayes, P. (2000). Diseases of Chinchillas. *Kirk's Current Veterinary Therapy: XIII Small Animal Practice.* J. Bonagura. Philadelphia, WB Saunders: 1152-7.

Ivey, E. & J. Morrisey (2000). Therapeutics for Rabbits. *Vet Clin NA: Exotic Anim Pract* 3:1(Jan): 183-216.

Albumin, Human / Albumin, Canine

(al-**byoo**-min)

Natural Protein Colloid

Prescriber Highlights

▶ Natural colloid that may be useful in increasing intravascular oncotic pressure and organ perfusion and decreasing edema secondary to crystalloid fluid replacement, particularly in critically ill animals with reversible diseases/conditions when hypoalbuminemia is present.

▶ Significant concerns with adverse effects, especially immune-mediated reactions when using xeno-albumin products (*i.e.,* human albumin in dogs).

▶ Canine albumin product (lyophilized) available commercially in USA, but little data available on its safety and efficacy.

▶ Treatment can be relatively expensive, but may be cheaper than plasma and may reduce intensive care unit stays.

Uses/Indications

Human serum albumin (HSA) or canine serum albumin (CSA) may be useful as colloid fluid replacement therapy in critically ill small animals. Conditions where albumin therapy may be considered include times when the patient is severely hypoalbuminemic (albumin <2.0 g/dL), severely edematous, or has systemic inflammatory response syndrome/sepsis or increased vascular leak. Because of availability, human albumin is usually used in small animals, but this "xeno-albumin" can pose considerable risks. There is little information available on the use of human albumin in cats.

A recent review article on fluid therapy in emergent small animals recommended that the use of HSA be reserved for critically ill veterinary patients with a life-threateningly low albumin (*e.g.,* septic peritonitis) and not be routinely used for patients with a low colloid osmotic pressure (COP). In those cases, a safer synthetic colloid, such as a hydroxyethyl starch product could be used. In dogs, CSA seems to be a safer option than HSA, but it is not known if these products decrease hospitalization time or improve survival time when compared with dogs with similar conditions not receiving albumin. The authors concluded that to more fully answer these questions, a comparative, prospective study is necessary (Mazzaferro et al. 2013).

Pharmacology/Actions

Albumin provides 75-80% of the oncotic pressure of plasma. When replacing endogenous albumin that has been lost, albumin helps prevent additional crystalloid fluids from leaking from capillaries by reducing hydrostatic pressure. This can allow less volume of crystalloids to be used and increase perfusion, with less risk for edema. Albumin (for its species) also has other actions, including binding and transport of drugs, ions, hormones, lipids, and metals (including iron), maintenance of endothelial integrity and permeability control, antioxidant properties, metabolic and acid–base functions, decreasing platelet aggregation, augmenting antithrombin and serving as a thiol-group. It is unknown what effect, if any, xeno-albumin has on these actions.

Pharmacokinetics

Endogenous circulating albumin represents 30-40% of total body albumin. Elimination of exogenously administered canine albumin is estimated to be between 20-24 days with a half-life of 8-10 days. The kinetics of human albumin in dogs or cats is not well described.

Contraindications/Precautions/Warnings

A history of hypersensitivity to albumin (human or canine) is a specific contraindication for use. Because of the risk for hypersensitivity, repeat administration of xeno-albumin is relatively contraindicated and in otherwise healthy animals that are only volume depleted, its use should be avoided.

The label for the canine albumin products states: Dogs with a pre-existing condition resulting in volume overload should be monitored carefully during administration of hyperosmolar products like canine albumin. Dogs with anemia or extreme dehydration should not receive canine albumin unless concurrent red blood cell products or appropriate fluid therapy is first administered.

Adverse Effects

The incidence of adverse effects reported in retrospective studies in dogs and cats with human albumin (HSA) vary widely, but they can be serious. Hypersensitivity, both immediate (anaphylactoid, anaphylactic) and delayed (type III hypersensitivity; serum sickness), is an issue when using human albumin in dogs and cats; these effects can be serious and deaths have occurred. Immediate adverse effects reported include facial edema, vomiting, urticaria, hyperthermia, and shock. Should facial edema occur, diphenhydramine should be given at 1 – 2 mg/kg IM and repeated every 8 hours as required (Mathews 2008). Delayed adverse effects can include lethargy, lameness, edema, cutaneous lesions/vasculitis, vomiting, inappetence, renal failure and coagulopathies.

A retrospective study evaluating 25% albumin (human) in critically ill dogs and cats, found that it could be safely administered, and it increased albumin levels and systemic blood pressure (Mathews et al. 2005). However, another retrospective study (Trow et al. 2008) evaluating albumin (human) use in 73 critically ill dogs, found that while albumin increased serum albumin, total protein, and colloid osmotic pressure, 23% of treated dogs developed at least one adverse effect that could potentially have been caused by albumin. The authors caution that given the risks for complications and uncertain positive influence, thoughtful consideration and extreme care must be taken when deciding whether to administer human albumin transfusions to critically ill dogs; these concerns should be discussed with clients and frequent monitoring should always be used.

An Italian retrospective study evaluating 5% human albumin in 418 dogs and 170 cats with critical illnesses, severe hypersensitivity reactions such as anaphylaxis, angioedema, or urticaria were not noted in any patient record. In no case was it necessary to discontinue or interrupt the albumin infusion due to adverse effects. Diarrhea, hyperthermia, or tremors were noted in 43% of dogs and 36% of cats treated. A combination of these adverse reactions was seen in 32% of dogs and 34% of cats treated. Adverse reactions that developed one day or more after treatment were noted in 28% of dogs and 11% of cats treated. Reactions beyond Day 3 were not recorded. Perivascular inflammation at catheter sites following albumin were seen in 17% of dogs and 34% of cats. This study did not measure changes in total protein, colloid oncotic pressure or albumin (Viganó et al. 2010).

The incidence of adverse effects in dogs associated with human albumin appears to be higher in healthy dogs than in critically ill dogs possibly due to the blunted immune response that can be seen in critically ill patients. In a study in 6 healthy dogs given 2 mL/kg of 25% human albumin during a 1-hour period an immediate hypersensitivity reaction (vomiting, facial edema) was seen in 1 dog and delayed adverse reactions were seen 5 to 13 days after albumin in all 6 dogs and included lethargy, lameness, peripheral edema, ecchymoses, vomiting, and anorexia. Delayed complications in 2 of these dogs resulted in death due to renal failure and coagulopathy and were suspected to have occurred because of serum sickness secondary to type III hypersensitivity reactions. Another dog had shock and sepsis secondary to a multi-drug resistant *E. coli* infection (Francis et al. 2007). In another study in 9 healthy dogs that were given one or two infusions of human albumin (25% at an initial infusion rate of 0.5 mL/kg/hour that was increased incrementally to a maximum of 4 mL/kg/hour) adverse effects were seen after the first or second infusion in 3 dogs. Anaphylactoid reactions were observed in 1 of 9 dogs during the first infusion and in the 2 dogs that were administered a second infusion. Two dogs developed severe edema and urticaria 6 or 7 days after the initial infusion. All dogs developed anti-HSA antibodies (Cohn et al. 2007).

The adverse effect profile for canine specific albumin (CSA) use in dogs is not well described. One study of 14 dogs with septic peritonitis demonstrated minimal adverse effects (one dog developed tachypnea) that could have been attributable to albumin administration (Craft et al. 2012). Safety studies in healthy normovolemic beagles where canine albumin was administered once weekly for four weeks did not show any evidence of adverse effects or antibody formation.

While the risk appears low, transmission of infectious agents from albumin products is possible. Rash, nausea, vomiting, tachycardia and hypotension have been reported in humans, but hypersensitivity reactions are very rare.

Reproductive/Nursing Safety

In humans, the FDA categorizes this drug as category **C** for use during pregnancy (*Animal studies have shown an adverse effect on the fetus, but there are no adequate studies in humans; or there are no animal reproduction studies and no adequate studies in humans.*) However, it is unlikely to pose much risk to the fetus, particularly when used appropriately. Albumin excretion into maternal milk is not known, but is unlikely to be harmful.

Overdosage/Acute Toxicity

To avoid the effects of hyperalbuminemia/hyperproteinemia, albumin levels should be followed. Most believe that serum albumin should not exceed 2.5 grams/dL (some say 2 grams/dL) when used clinically.

Drug Interactions

While the administration of exogenous albumin could bind drugs that are highly bound to plasma proteins and affect the amount of free drug circulating, this does not appear to be of significance when albumin is used clinically.

Laboratory Considerations

- Exogenous administration of albumin may temporarily decrease serum concentrations of calcium.

Doses

- **DOGS/CATS**

  Human Albumin Dogs: In a review of albumin (human) 25% (HSA) use in small animals the author describes when he considers using 25% human albumin: Patients with: **1)** refractory hypotension; **2)** Severe hypoalbuminemic patients (albumin <1.5 g/dL or <1.8 g/dL) during dehydration and hypovolemia) with ongoing losses (*e.g.*, peritonitis, pleural effusion); **3)** Combined with FFP in hypoalbuminemic septic patients; **4)** Patients that have protein-losing enteropathy before surgical biopsy; **5)** Markedly hypoalbuminemic patients that continue to vomit (likely attributable to bowel edema); **6)** Refractory hypotension associated with gastric dilation-volvulus. The following is an edited dosage protocol (see the reference for more detailed information on use, etc.): When time permits (non-emergent situation), a test dose of 0.25 mL/kg/h is given over 15 minutes while monitoring heart rate, respiratory rate, and temperature (baseline before transfusion and at end of test dose). Discontinue infusion if adverse signs (facial swelling, or other signs of anaphylaxis or anaphylactoid reaction) develop. The maximum volume administered to any dog by the author is 25 mL/kg (6.25 g/kg) administered continuously over 72 hours; the mean volume administered to any dog overall is 5 mL/kg (1.25 g/kg). The maximum volume given as a slow push or bolus to treat hypotension is 4 mL/kg (1 g/kg), with a mean volume of 2 mL/kg (0.5 g/kg). The range for a continuous rate infusion (CRI) after a bolus administration is 0.1 – 1.7 mL/kg/h (0.025 – 0.425 g/kg) over 4 to 72 hours. Infusions are empirically selected to meet low normal values. The shorter infusion times are most commonly used for refractory hypotension. (Mathews 2008)

Human Albumin Dogs: The administration of 10% human albumin may be useful in dogs with reversible disease and clinically affected by marked hypoalbuminemia (serum albumin, <1.5 g/dL) and low colloid osmotic pressure (colloid osmotic pressure, <14 mm Hg), but given the risks for complications and uncertain positive influence, thoughtful consideration and extreme care must be taken when deciding whether to administer human albumin transfusions to critically ill dogs, and these concerns should be discussed with clients and frequent monitoring performed. Reasonable goals for human albumin administration may be to increase serum albumin to 2 – 2.5 g/dL and colloid osmotic pressure to 14 – 20 mm Hg. Dogs with surgical diseases and septic peritonitis should be especially considered because of the role of albumin in wound healing. The protocol most often used for calculating the dosage of human albumin in the study was: albumin deficit (g) = 10X (serum albumin desired – serum albumin of patient) X body weight (kg) X 0.3. Alternatively, some dogs received 0.5 – 1.25 g/kg. In the authors' institution, the calculated dosage of human albumin was aseptically diluted to a 10% solution with saline (0.9% NaCl) solution and administered over a 12-hour period with a transfusion filter. Because of the antigenicity of human albumin in dogs, no dog was eligible for receiving additional human albumin after 7 days following initial human albumin administration. (Trow et al. 2008)

Canine Albumin Dogs: Using the canine albumin lyophilized product (5 gram) for the treatment of septic peritonitis or hypoalbuminemia: Using either a 5% or 16% reconstituted solution give 800 – 844 mg/kg IV over 6 hours. (Product label; Canine Albumin 5gm lyophilized— Animal Blood Resources)

Canine Albumin Dogs: Using the canine albumin lyophilized product (5 gram): 800 mg/kg (reconstituted in 0.9% NaCl to yield a 5% CSA solution) administered intravenously over 6 hours. **Note:** Study was done in hypoalbuminemic dogs following surgical source control for septic peritonitis. (Craft et al. 2012)

Monitoring

- Pre and post serum albumin. Depending on the source, most suggest a target for serum albumin concentrations of 2 – 2.5 g/dL.
- Pre and post colloid osmotic pressure (if possible).

- Adverse effects: body temperature, respiratory rate, blood pressure and heart rate.
- Signs of volume overload.
- Monitor for delayed reactions, which can occur weeks after administration.

Client Information

- The medication must be given in an inpatient setting.
- Clients should understand and accept the risks, costs, and monitoring associated with albumin's use.

Chemistry/Synonyms

Human albumin is a highly soluble, globular protein with a molecular weight of 66,500. The 5% solution has a colloid osmotic pressure (COP) similar to that of normal plasma. Amino acid homology of human and canine albumin is about 79%, but the canine albumin molecule is 2 kDalton larger and has a different relative charge and isoelectric point.

Albumin (human) may also be known as Alb, albumine, HSA, or albuminum. "Salt-poor" albumin is a misnomer, but still occasionally used as a designation for 25% albumin. There are a variety of trade name products.

Storage/Stability

5% solution: Albumin (human) 5% solution is stable for 3 years, providing storage temperature does not exceed 30°C (89°F). Protect from freezing. 25% and 20% solutions: Store at room temperature not exceeding 30°C (86°F). Do not freeze. Do not use after expiration date.

Do not use solutions of they appear turbid or if sediment is noted. Solutions should not be used if more than 4 hours have passed since the container was entered, as it contains no preservatives. Do not use solutions that have been frozen.

The lyophilized canine albumin product should be stored at 4-6°C (refrigerated) until use. Product is stable for 15 months as labeled. After rehydration, it should be used within 6 hours.

Compatibility/Compounding Considerations

Human albumin may be administered either in conjunction with or combined with other parenteral products such as whole blood, plasma, saline, glucose, or sodium lactate. It is reportedly **compatible** with usual carbohydrate or electrolyte solutions, diltiazem or midazolam at a Y-site. The canine specific product label warns not to add supplementary medication or mix with other medicinal products including whole blood or plasma, but that it can be given in conjunction with saline.

Do not mix albumin with protein hydrolysates, amino acid solutions or solutions containing alcohol.

When preparing human albumin for administration use only 16-gauge needles or dispensing pins with 20 mL vial sizes and larger. Needles or dispensing pins should only be inserted within the stopper area delineated by the raised ring. The stopper should be penetrated perpendicular to the plane of the stopper within the ring.

Canine albumin 5 gram lyophilized should be rehydrated with 0.9% sterile saline (sodium chloride 0.9%) as the diluent. Adding 30 mL of sterile saline will yield a 16% (166 mg/mL) solution and 100 mL will yield a 5% (50 mg/mL) solution. DO NOT use sterile water to rehydrate the product. The diluent may be gently warmed before addition to speed rehydration. Do not exceed 90°F (32°C) for the temperature of the warmed diluent. After addition of the diluent, gently swirl the solution intermittently to avoid foaming until all the powder is rehydrated. Do not aggressively agitate the bottle as foaming may occur. Rehydration may take 15-30 minutes with gentle swirling.

Dosage Forms/Regulatory Status

VETERINARY-LABELED PRODUCTS:

Albumin, Canine, lyophilized 5 g, without preservatives or plasma byproducts; (Animal Blood Resources Intl.). Product labeled for intravenous use in dogs and only to be used by or on the order of licensed veterinarian. **Note:** This is not an FDA-approved product. More information can be found at: abrint.net.

HUMAN-LABELED PRODUCTS:

Albumin, Human 5% in 50 mL, 100 mL, 250 mL & 500 mL glass containers, and 25% in 20 mL, 50 mL & 100 mL vials or flex containers; *Albuminar*®, *Albutein*®, *AlbuRX*®, *Albuminate*®, *Flexbumin*®, *Albuked*®, *Kedbumin*®, *Plasbumin*®, generic; (Rx). These are FDA-approved products (human).

Revisions/References

Monograph revised/updated August 2013.

Cohn, L. A., et al. (2007). Response of healthy dogs to infusions of human serum albumin. *American Journal of Veterinary Research* 68(6): 657-63.

Craft, E. M. & L. L. Powell (2012). The use of canine-specific albumin in dogs with septic peritonitis. *J. Vet. Emerg. Crit. Care* 22(6): 631-9.

Francis, A. H., et al. (2007). Adverse reactions suggestive of type III hypersensitivity in six healthy dogs given human albumin. *Javma-Journal of the American Veterinary Medical Association* 230(6): 873-9.

Mathews, K. A. (2008). The therapeutic use of 25% human serum albumin in critically ill dogs and cats. *Veterinary Clinics of North America-Small Animal Practice* 38(3): 595-+.

Mathews, K. A. & M. Barry (2005). The use of 25% human serum albumin: outcome and efficacy in raising serum albumin and systemic blood pressure in critically ill dogs and cats. *J. Vet. Emerg. Crit. Care* 15(2): 110-8.

Mazzaferro, E. & L. L. Powell (2013). Fluid Therapy for the Emergent Small Animal Patient: Crystalloids, Colloids, and Albumin Products. *Veterinary Clinics of North America: Small Animal Practice* 43(4): 721-34.

Trow, A. V., et al. (2008). Evaluation of use of human albumin in critically ill dogs: 73 cases (2003-2006). *Javma-Journal of the American Veterinary Medical Association* 233(4): 607-12.

Viganó, F., et al. (2010). Administration of 5% human serum albumin in critically ill small animal patients with hypoalbuminemia: 418 dogs and 170 cats (1994–2008). *J. Vet. Emerg. Crit. Care* 20(2): 237-43.

Albuterol Sulfate

(al-**byoo**-ter-ole)   Salbutamol, Proventil®, Ventolin®

Beta-Adrenergic Agonist

Prescriber Highlights

▶ Used primarily as a bronchodilator after PO or inhaled dosing.

▶ Use with caution in patients with cardiac dysrhythmias or dysfunction, seizure disorders, hypertension or hyperthyroidism.

▶ May be teratogenic (high doses) or delay labor.

Uses/Indications

Albuterol is used principally in cats and horses for its effects on bronchial smooth muscle to alleviate bronchospasm or cough. True bronchoconstriction is rare in dogs, but when present, albuterol may be useful.

Pharmacology/Actions

Like other beta-agonists, albuterol is believed to act by stimulating production of cyclic AMP through activation of adenyl cyclase. Albuterol is considered to be predominantly a beta2 agonist (relaxation of bronchial, uterine, and vascular smooth muscles). At usual doses, albuterol possesses minimal beta1 agonist (heart) activity. Beta-adrenergics can promote a shift of potassium away from the serum and into the cell, perhaps via stimulation of Na⁺-K⁺-ATPase. Temporary decreases in either normal or high serum potassium levels are possible.

Pharmacokinetics

The specific pharmacokinetics of this agent have apparently not been thoroughly studied in domestic animals. In general, albuterol is absorbed rapidly and well after oral administration. Effects occur within 5 minutes after oral inhalation; 30 minutes after oral administration (*e.g.,* tablets). It does not cross the blood-brain barrier but does cross the placenta. Duration of effect generally persists for 3-6 hours after inhalation and up to 12 hours (depending on dosage form) after oral administration. The drug is extensively metabolized in the liver principally to the inactive metabolite, albuterol 4'-O-sulfate. After oral administration the serum half-life in humans has been reported as 2.7-5 hours.

Contraindications/Precautions/Warnings

Albuterol is contraindicated in patients hypersensitive to it. It should be used with caution in patients with diabetes, hyperthyroidism, hypertension, seizure disorders, or cardiac disease (especially with concurrent arrhythmias).

Use during the late stages of pregnancy may inhibit uterine contractions.

Adverse Effects

Most adverse effects are dose-related and those that would be expected with sympathomimetic agents including increased heart rate, tremors, CNS excitement (nervousness) and dizziness. These effects are generally transient and mild and usually do not require discontinuation of therapy. Decreased serum potassium values may be noted; rarely is potassium supplementation required.

The S-form of albuterol may potentially increase airway inflammation in cats. As "regular" albuterol is the racemic form (R,S-albuterol) it may also increase airway inflammation and its use in cats should probably be limited to acute, rescue treatment only and not for chronic treatment (Reinero 2008), (Reinero 2009). Additionally, cats don't like the "hiss" occurring during actuation of the metered-dose inhaler or the taste of the drug/vehicle.

Reproductive/Nursing Safety

In very large doses, albuterol is teratogenic in rodents. It should be used (particularly the oral dosage forms) during pregnancy only when the potential benefits outweigh the risks. Like some other beta agonists, it may delay pre-term labor after oral administration. In humans, the FDA categorizes this drug as category *C* for use during pregnancy (*Animal studies have shown an adverse effect on the fetus, but there are no adequate studies in humans; or there are no animal reproduction studies and no adequate studies in humans.*)

Overdosage/Acute Toxicity

The oral LD50 of albuterol in rats is reported to be greater than 2 g/kg, but significant toxicity can occur in small animals after oral overdoses or when dogs bite into the metered dose inhalers. Clinical signs of significant overdose after systemic administration (including when dogs bite into an aerosol canister) may include: arrhythmias (tachycardia and extrasystole), hypertension, fever, vomiting, mydriasis, tremors, and CNS stimulation. Hypokalemia and hypophosphatemia may occur.

There were 1703 single agent exposures to albuterol reported to the ASPCA Animal Poison Control Center (APCC) during 2009-2013. Of the 1695 dogs, 1594 were symptomatic with 83% being tachycardic, 31% lethargic, 28% vomiting, 22% panting/tachypneic, 18% hypokalemic, and 15% agitated.

If there is a recent ingestion of tablets, and if the animal does not have significant cardiac or CNS effects, it should be handled like other overdoses (decontamination procedures). For inhalation exposure (when a dog bites into an aerosol canister) decontamination is generally not effective. If cardiac arrhythmias require treatment, a beta-blocking agent (*e.g.,* atenolol, metoprolol) can be used. Diazepam can be used for tremors. Potassium supplementation may be required, but be alert for rebound hyperkalemia. Contact an animal poison control center for further information.

Drug Interactions

The following drug interactions with albuterol (primarily when albuterol is given orally and not via inhalation) have either been reported or are theoretical in humans or animals and may be of significance in veterinary patients. Unless otherwise noted, use together is not necessarily contraindicated, but weigh the potential risks and perform additional monitoring when appropriate.

- **BETA-ADRENERGIC BLOCKING AGENTS** (*e.g.*, **propranolol**): May antagonize the actions of albuterol.
- **DIGOXIN**: Albuterol may increase the risk of cardiac arrhythmias.
- **INHALATION ANESTHETICS** (*e.g.*, **isoflurane**): Albuterol may predispose the patient to ventricular arrhythmias, particularly in patients with preexisting cardiac disease—use cautiously.
- **OTHER SYMPATHOMIMETIC AMINES**: Use with albuterol may increase the risk of developing adverse cardiovascular effects.
- **TRICYCLIC ANTIDEPRESSANTS OR MONOAMINE OXIDASE INHIBITORS**: May potentiate the vascular effects of albuterol.

Doses

- **DOGS:**

  As a bronchodilator for bronchoconstriction (oral); (extra-label): 0.02 – 0.05 mg/kg (20 – 50 micrograms/kg) PO q8-12h, start at low end of dosing range and assess for efficacy and side effects. Increase dosage and/or frequency if response not adequate and side effects are acceptable.

- **CATS:**

  As a bronchodilator (inhaled) for intermittent, short-term treatment of feline asthma (extra-label): Use with an appropriate spacer and mask (*e.g.*, *Aerokat®*) and administer one puff. May repeat every 30 minutes for up to 4 to 6 hours in emergencies. Generally, albuterol should not be used on a chronic basis as tolerance can develop and inhaled corticosteroids (*e.g.*, fluticasone) are usually recommended, but some state that albuterol can be used in cats up to once daily prior to administering fluticasone.

- **HORSES:** (NOTE: ARCI UCGFS CLASS 3 DRUG)

  As a bronchodilator (inhaled) for acute (rescue) treatment of recurrent airway obstruction (RAO); (extra-label): Use a hand-held device (*e.g.*, *AeroHippus®*, *Equine Haler®*): 2 - 3 puffs initially; may repeat up to 3 times every 5-15 minutes. Consider using inhaled corticosteroids (*e.g.*, fluticasone 5 minutes after albuterol) as tolerance to albuterol alone can develop rapidly. Primary therapy for RAO is managing and controlling environment.

Monitoring

- Clinical symptom improvement; auscultation, blood gases (if indicated).
- Cardiac rate, rhythm (if warranted).
- Serum potassium, early in therapy if animal is susceptible to hypokalemia.

Client Information

- Contact veterinarian if animal's condition deteriorates or it becomes acutely ill.
- If using the aerosol, shake well before using and then attach to the spacer/mask. Be certain how to appropriately administer the product to maximize effectiveness. Do not puncture or use near an open flame; do not allow exposure to temperatures greater than 120°F. Keep out of reach of children and pets.
- When using inhaled albuterol with an appropriate spacer/facemask (*e.g.*, *Aerokat®*) in cats, the following tips have been recommended (Scherk 2010): Allow cat to get used to the device over several days letting it investigate it (*e.g.*, leaving it by food bowl). Reward (praise, food, catnip, stroking) fearless approaches to device and start placing it near cat's face. Practice with the mask over the cats face without anything in the chamber. Preload the chamber with a puff of albuterol (in addition to the dose required). Make sure the mask is placed snugly over the muzzle for 4–6 breaths.

Chemistry/Synonyms

A synthetic sympathomimetic amine, albuterol sulfate occurs as a white, almost tasteless crystalline powder. It is soluble in water and slightly soluble in alcohol. One mg of albuterol is equivalent to 1.2 mg of albuterol sulfate.

Albuterol sulfate may also be known as: salbutamol hemisulphate, salbutamol sulphate, or salbutamoli sulfas; many trade names are available.

Storage/Stability

Oral albuterol sulfate products should be stored at 2-30°C. The inhaled aerosol should be stored at room temperature; do not allow exposure to temperatures above 120°F or the canister may burst. The 0.5% nebs should be stored at room temperature; the 0.083% nebs should be stored in the refrigerator. Discard solutions if they become colored.

Compatibility/Compounding Considerations

No specific information noted.

Dosage Forms/Regulatory Status

VETERINARY-LABELED PRODUCTS: NONE.

HUMAN-LABELED PRODUCTS:

Albuterol Oral Tablets: 2 mg & 4 mg; generic; (Rx)

Albuterol Extended Release Oral Tablets: 4 mg & 8 mg; *VoSpire®* ER, generic; (Rx)

Albuterol Oral Syrup: 2 mg (as sulfate)/5 mL in 473 mL; generic; (Rx)

Albuterol Aerosol for Inhalation: Each actualization (puff) delivers 90 micrograms—now labeled as 108 mcg albuterol in 6.7 g, 8 g, 8.5 g and 18 g. Some canisters have 60 actuations and some have 200 actuations; *Proventil HFA®, Ventolin HFA®, ProAir HFA®*; (Rx).

Albuterol Solution for Inhalation ("Nebs"): 0.083% (2.5 mg/3 mL) in 3 mL UD vials; 0.5% (5 mg/mL) in 0.5 mL vials & 20 mL with dropper; 0.021% preservative-free (0.63 mg/3mL) & 0.042% preservative-free (1.25 mg/3 mL), in 3 mL UD vials; *AccuNeb®*, generic; (Rx)

Also available: 14.7 g aerosol metered dose inhaler containing 18 mcg ipratropium bromide (an inhaled anticholinergic) and 103 mcg albuterol sulfate per puff; *Combivent®* (B-I); (Rx) and 3 mL unit dose solution for inhalation (neb) containing 0.5 mg ipratropium bromide and 3 mg albuterol, *DuoNeb®*; generic; (Rx)

Revisions/References

Monograph revised/updated August 2013.

Reinero, C. R. (2008). *The Beta-agonist Paradox: Is Albuterol Detrimental for Asthma?* Proceedings: American College of Veterinary Internal Medicine. accessed via Veterinary Information Network; vin.com

Reinero, C. R. (2009). *Dispelling the myths about diagnosis and treatment of feline asthma.* Proceedings: ACVIM. accessed via Veterinary Information Network; vin.com

Scherk, M. (2010). *Bronchopulmonary Disease in Cats - Is It Really Asthma?* Wild West Veterinary Conference, Vancouver. accessed via Veterinary Information Network; vin.com

Alendronate Sodium

(a-**len**-droe-nate)   Fosamax®

Oral Bisphosphonate Bone Resorption Inhibitor

Prescriber Highlights

▶ Orally dosed bisphosphonate that reduces osteoclastic bone resorption. Potentially useful for refractory hypercalcemia, FORLs, bone pain, osteosarcoma.

▶ Very limited clinical experience with use of this drug in animals; adverse effect profile, dosages, etc. may significantly change with more experience & clinical research.

▶ Potentially can cause esophageal erosions; risks are not clear for dogs or cats.

▶ Accurate dosing may be difficult & bioavailability is adversely affected by food, etc.

▶ Cost may be an issue, but generic forms are now available.

Uses/Indications

Alendronate use in small animals has been limited, but it may prove useful for treating refractory hypercalcemia in dogs or cats, to reduce pain associated with bone tumors and as an osteosarcoma treatment adjuvant.

Pharmacology/Actions

Alendronate, like other bisphosphonates, inhibits osteoclastic bone resorption by inhibiting osteoclast function after binding to bone hydroxyapatite. Secondary actions that may contribute to therapeutic usefulness in osteogenic neoplasms include promoting apoptosis and inhibiting osteoclastogenesis, angiogenesis and cancer cell proliferation.

Pharmacokinetics

Specific pharmacokinetic values are limited for dogs and apparently unavailable for cats. Oral bioavailability in all species studied is less than 2%. In humans, alendronate sodium has very low oral bioavailability (<1%) and the presence of food can reduce bioavailability further to negligible amounts. In women, taking the medication with coffee or orange juice reduced bioavailability by 60% when compared to plain water.

Absorbed drug is rapidly distributed to bone or excreted into the urine. The drug is reportedly not highly plasma protein bound in dogs, but it is in rats. Alendronate apparently accumulates on subgingival tooth surfaces and bordering alveolar bone. Plasma concentrations are virtually undetectable after therapeutic dosing.

Alendronate is not metabolized and drug taken up by bone is very slowly eliminated. It is estimated that the terminal elimination half-life in dogs is approximately 1000 days and, in humans, approximately 10 years, however once incorporated into bone, alendronate is no longer active.

Contraindications/Precautions/Warnings

Alendronate is contraindicated in human patients with esophageal abnormalities (*e.g.,* strictures, achalasia) that cause delayed esophageal emptying and those who cannot stand or sit upright for 30 minutes after administration. At present, it is not believed that small animal patients need to remain upright after administration. Because of a lack of experience, the drug is not recommended for use in human patients with severe renal dysfunction (CrCl <35 mL/minute). Alendronate should not be used in patients who have demonstrated hypersensitivity reactions to it.

Alendronate use in small animals should be considered investigational at this point. Limited research and experience, dosing questions, risks of esophageal irritation or ulcers, and medication expense all are potential hindrances to its therapeutic usefulness.

Adverse Effects

Little information on the specific adverse effect profile for dogs or cats is published. In humans, alendronate can cause upper GI irritation and erosions. Anecdotal reports of GI upset, vomiting and inappetence have been reported in dogs receiving the drug. It has been suggested that after administration, walking or playing with the dog for 30 minutes may reduce the incidence of esophageal problems. In cats, buttering the lips after administration to induce salivation and reduce esophageal transit time has been suggested.

Other potential adverse effects of concern include jaw osteonecrosis and musculoskeletal pain.

Reproductive/Nursing Safety

Alendronate at dosages of 2 mg/kg in rats caused decreased post-implantation survival rates and at 1 mg/kg caused decreased weight gain in healthy pups. Higher dosages (10 mg/kg) caused incomplete fetal ossification of several bone types. In humans, the FDA categorizes alendronate as category **C** for use during pregnancy (*Animal studies have shown an adverse effect on the fetus, but there are no adequate studies in humans; or there are no animal reproduction studies and no adequate studies in humans.*)

While it is unknown if alendronate enters maternal milk, it would be unexpected that measurable quantities would be found in milk or enough would be absorbed in clinically significant amounts in nursing offspring.

Overdosage/Acute Toxicity

No lethality was observed in dogs receiving doses of up to 200 mg/kg. Lethality in mice and rats was seen at dosages starting at 966 mg/kg and 552 mg/kg, respectively. Observed adverse effects associated with overdoses included hypocalcemia, hypophosphatemia, and upper GI reactions.

A recently ingested overdose should be treated with orally administered antacids or milk to bind the drug and reduce absorption. Do not induce vomiting. Monitor serum calcium and phosphorus and treat supportively.

Drug Interactions

The following drug interactions with alendronate have either been reported or are theoretical in humans or animals and may be of significance in veterinary patients. Unless otherwise noted, use together is not necessarily contraindicated, but weigh the potential risks and perform additional monitoring when appropriate.

■ **ASPIRIN:** Increased risk of upper GI adverse effects.

■ **CALCIUM-CONTAINING ORAL PRODUCTS or FOOD:** Likely to significantly decrease oral bioavailability of alendronate.

Laboratory Considerations

■ No specific laboratory concerns or interactions have been noted.

Doses

■ **DOGS:**

For refractory hypercalcemia or to reduce pain associated with bone tumors (extra-label): 0.5 – 1 mg/kg PO once daily on an empty stomach (**Note:** There is little experience using this drug in dogs).

■ **CATS:**

For treatment of idiopathic hypercalcemia (extra-label): Initially 10 mg per cat PO (on an empty stomach) once per week. After dosing, administer at least 6 mL of water and then butter the lips to increase salivation and enhance esophageal transit. May take 3-4 weeks to show effect. Can increase dosage up to 30 mg per cat once per week. If GI side effects are problematic, can split weekly dose and give every 3-4 days.

Monitoring

- Serum calcium (ionized). Usually repeated monthly.
- GI adverse effects. **Note:** Depending on diagnosis (*e.g.,* hypercalcemia, adjunctive treatment of osteogenic sarcomas, or FORLs) other monitoring of serum electrolytes (total calcium, phosphorus, potassium sodium) or disease-associated signs may be required.

Client Information

- Inform clients of the "investigational" nature with using this drug in small animals.
- Must be given with water on an empty stomach. Food can prevent the drug from being absorbed and make it useless; do not offer food for at least 30 minutes after a dose is given. Try to have animal drink some water after dosing to reduce the chances of throat or esophagus problems.
- If animal vomits or acts sick after getting the drug, try walking, exercising or playing with your animal after dosing, encouraging them to drink water, or "buttering" lips.
- Alendronate has not been used in many animals, but possible side effects include: vomiting, lack of appetite, throat or esophagus ulcers or sores, or bone pain.

Chemistry/Synonyms

Alendronate sodium is a synthetic analog of pyrophosphonate with the chemical name: (4-amino-1-hydroxy-1-phosphono-butyl) phosphonic acid. One mg is soluble in one liter of water.

Alendronate may also be known as: alendronic acid, acide alendronique, acido alendronico, acidum alendronicum, *Adronat®, Alendros®, Arendal®, Onclast®* or *Fosamax®*.

Storage/Stability

Alendronate tablets should be stored in well-closed containers at room temperature. The oral solution should be stored at room temperature; do not freeze.

Compatibility/Compounding Considerations

No specific information noted.

Dosage Forms/Regulatory Status

VETERINARY-LABELED PRODUCTS: NONE.

HUMAN-LABELED PRODUCTS:

Alendronate Sodium Oral Tablets: 5 mg, 10 mg, 35 mg, 40 mg, & 70 mg (also effervescent tablet); *Fosamax®*; generic; (Rx)

Alendronate Oral Solution: 70 mg (as base) in 75 mL; raspberry flavor; *Fosamax®*; (Rx)

Revisions/References

Monograph revised/updated August 2013.

Reinero, C. R. (2008). *The Beta-agonist Paradox: Is Albuterol Detrimental for Asthma?* Proceedings: American College of Veterinary Internal Medicine.

Reinero, C. R. (2009). Dispelling the myths about diagnosis and treatment of feline asthma. Proceedings: ACVIM.

Scherk, M. (2010). *Bronchopulmonary Disease in Cats - Is It Really Asthma?* Wild West Veterinary Conference, Vancouver.

Alfaxalone

(al-**fax**-ah-lone)   Alfaxan®

Intravenous Anesthetic

Prescriber Highlights

- ▶ Injectable (IV) anesthetic for dogs and cats. At time of writing (February 2014), not available in USA but marketing is anticipated.
- ▶ Negligible analgesic effects.
- ▶ Respiratory depression/apnea can occur, particularly if administered rapidly IV.
- ▶ Use with premeds allows lower dose (and cost) and may make recoveries smoother.

Uses/Indications

Alfaxalone is FDA-approved (USA) for the induction and maintenance of anesthesia and for induction of anesthesia followed by maintenance with an inhalant anesthetic, in cats and dogs.

Alfaxalone has also been administered deep IM (extra-label in USA) to cats as a deep sedative/light anesthetic which may make it particularly useful in feral or fractious cats.

Because of its short duration of effect and relatively high safety margin, alfaxalone may be considered for use in high-risk patients or in sighthounds (Pasloske et al. 2009; Nieuwendijk 2011; Psatha et al. 2011).

Although not presently approved for use in horses, alfaxalone may prove useful as an injectable induction agent or part of a total intravenous anesthesia (TIVA) protocol for short-term field anesthesia procedures (Leece et al. 2009; Kloppel et al. 2011; Keates et al. 2012; Goodwin et al. 2013).

Alfaxalone has been used clinically in an extra-label manner in a variety of species including small mammals, rabbits, sheep, fish, amphibians and reptiles (Roan 2009; Bertelsen et al. 2011; McMillan et al. 2011; Gil et al. 2012; Jones 2012; Gonzalez et al. 2013; Hansen et al. 2013; Kischinovsky et al. 2013; Knotek et al. 2013; Moll et al. 2013; Tutunaru et al. 2013; Navarrete-Calvo et al. 2014).

Pharmacology/Actions

Alfaxalone is a neuroactive steroid molecule with properties of a general anesthetic. The primary mechanism for the anesthetic action of alfaxalone is the modulation of neuronal cell membrane chloride ion transport, induced by binding of alfaxalone to GABA cell surface receptors. Alfaxalone has negligible analgesic properties at clinical doses.

In dogs, recumbency is usually produced within 60 seconds after the start of injection, and permits intubation within 1-2 minutes. Duration of anesthesia from a single induction dose is approximately 5-10 minutes in dogs not receiving a preanesthetic and may be longer in dogs that received preanesthetic agents. In cats, anesthesia is usually observed within 60 seconds after the start of injection, and permits intubation within 1-2 minutes. Anesthesia duration after a single induction dose ranges between 15-30 minutes in cats that did not receive a preanesthetic and may be longer in cats that received a preanesthetic agent. In pre-approval field studies, recovery times (extubation to head lift) following *Alfaxan®* maintenance anesthesia averaged 22 minutes in dogs and 15 minutes in cats that did not receive a preanesthetic, and 15 minutes in dogs and 17 minutes in cats that did receive preanesthetics. At usual dosages, dogs or cats are expected to recover to sternal recumbency in 60-80 minutes.

Pharmacokinetics

In dogs, alfaxalone's volume of distribution after a single injection of clinical doses (2 mg/kg) is approximately 2.5 L/kg. At this dose, clearance is about 54 mL/kg/minute and elimination terminal half-life around 27 minutes (Ferre et al. 2006). A study done in Greyhounds showed similar results when dogs were not premedicated; however, premedicated (acepromazine/morphine) Greyhounds had substantially longer (5X) anesthetic durations and elimination half-life was approximately 19% longer and clearance about 24% lower then when they were not premedicated (Pasloske et al. 2009).

In cats, the volume of distribution of alfaxalone is approximately 2 L/kg. Clearance is dosage dependent with doses of 5 mg/kg (clinical dose) averaging 25.1 mL/kg/minute and doses of 25 mg/kg (supra-clinical dose) averaging 14.8 mL/kg/minute. The elimination half-lives at these doses were 45.2 and 76.6 minutes respectively. Alfaxalone has nonlinear pharmacokinetics in the cat, but with multiple doses there was no clinically relevant accumulation (Whittem et al. 2008).

Cat and dog hepatocyte (*in vitro*) studies show that alfaxalone undergoes both Phase I (cytochrome P450 dependent) and Phase II (conjugation dependent) metabolism in both species. Both cats and dogs form the same five Phase I metabolites. Phase II metabolites in cats are alfaxalone sulfate and alfaxalone glucuronide, while only alfaxalone glucuronide is found in dogs. Alfaxalone metabolites are likely to be eliminated from both the dog and cat by the hepatic/fecal and renal routes, similarly to other species studied.

In adult horses after receiving a premed of acepromazine, xylazine and guaifenesin, alfaxalone had a plasma elimination half-life of about 33 minutes, volume of distribution of 1.6 L/kg, and a plasma clearance of 33 mL/minute/kg (Goodwin et al. 2011). In neonatal foals receiving a butorphanol premed, alfaxalone had a plasma elimination half-life of about 23 minutes, volume of distribution of 0.6 L/kg, and a plasma clearance of 20 mL/minute/kg (Goodwin et al. 2012).

Contraindications/Precautions/Warnings

Alfaxalone is contraindicated in patients with known hypersensitivity to alfaxalone or its components, or when general anesthesia and/or sedation are contraindicated. It should not be used with other injectable general anesthetic agents (*e.g.,* propofol). As post-induction apnea can occur, alfaxalone should only be used in facilities where patients can be continuously monitored and maintenance of a patent airway, artificial ventilation, and oxygen supplementation can be immediately provided.

Use with caution in patients with significant hepatic dysfunction as they may require lower dosages or increased dosing intervals to maintain anesthesia. Use with caution in elderly, critically ill or debilitated animals.

Patients should be in appropriate facilities and under sufficient supervision during the post-anesthesia recovery period. During recovery, it is preferable that animals are not handled or disturbed as psychomotor excitement may occur. Premedication with only a benzodiazepine may increase this likelihood.

As alfaxalone does not provide analgesia, appropriate pain control should be provided.

Intramuscular administration to dogs or subcutaneous administration to dogs or cats is not recommended by the manufacturer. IM use in cats or dogs is extra-label in USA, but IM use in cats is approved in some countries.

Must be given slow IV (see Dosages); too rapid IV administration or overdosage can cause severe cardiorespiratory depression.

Label information (USA) states that safety of alfaxalone has not been evaluated in cats less than 4 weeks of age or in dogs less than 10 weeks of age. A study done in kittens (est. ages of 6-11 weeks old) concluded that it was a suitable anesthetic induction agent for premedicated kittens less than 12 weeks of age and that anesthetic maintenance with supplemental doses of alfaxalone may be a suit-able alternative in kittens when inhalant maintenance is not feasible (O'Hagan et al. 2012a). The same group did a similar study in 25 puppies (est. ages of 6-11 weeks old) and concluded that alfaxalone was a suitable induction agent for premedicated puppies less than 12 weeks of age requiring anesthesia for surgical or diagnostic procedures. However, two of the dogs had excited recoveries and one dog had an unacceptable anesthetic maintenance period (O'Hagan et al. 2012b).

Adverse Effects

Alfaxalone has a high therapeutic index and for a general anesthetic agent it is relatively safe; respiratory depression and apnea are the biggest concerns and can be exacerbated depending on which premed is used. In clinical studies, 44% of dogs and 19% of cats experienced post-induction apnea (defined as the cessation of breathing for 30 seconds or more). The mean duration of apnea in these animals was 100 seconds in dogs and 60 seconds in cats. Give the drug IV slowly while closely monitoring the patient, stopping administration and placing an endotracheal tube when the patient is sufficiently anesthetized. Supplemental oxygen supply is advisable. Cardiac arrhythmias may occur, but are thought to occur primarily due to hypoxemia/hypercapnia; O2 therapy is recommended as the primary treatment, followed by appropriate cardiotherapy if required.

Alfaxalone's cardiodepressant effects in conjunction with inhalant anesthetics' vasodilatory effects can cause hypotension. Transient hypertension can also be noted possibly due to increased sympathetic activity.

Hypothermia during and post anesthesia is likely. External heat sources and monitoring of patient core body temperature is recommended.

Excitement during recovery can occur (disorientation, nervousness, paddling, muscle twitching, violent movements). Sedative drugs used in combination with alfaxalone can improve recovery (Quandt 2009) and especially in cats, recovery should preferably be in a quiet, darkened room (Nieuwendijk 2011).

Reproductive/Nursing Safety

The safety of alfaxalone has not been established in pregnancy or during lactation, but it is used routinely for Cesarean sections in dogs and cats. Studies in pregnant mice, rats and rabbits have not demonstrated deleterious effects on gestation of the treated animals or on the reproductive performance of their offspring. Alfaxalone's effects upon fertility have not been evaluated.

Overdosage/Acute Toxicity

Hypoventilation, apnea, and hypotension are the most likely consequences of overdoses up to 25 mg/kg (>10X overdose in dogs and 5X overdose in cats). Cardiac arrhythmias are possible. Extended monitoring with appropriate cardiopulmonary support may be required.

Drug Interactions

The USA label states that alfaxalone is compatible (**Note:** *This is therapeutic compatibility, not pharmaceutical compatibility*) with benzodiazepines, opioids, alpha2-agonists, and phenothiazines as commonly used in surgical practice. The Australia/N.Z. (ANZ) label states that alfaxalone has been safely used in combination with the premeds acepromazine, atropine, methadone, butorphanol, diazepam and xylazine. The concomitant use with other CNS depressants is expected to potentiate the depressant effects of either drug, and appropriate dose adjustments should be made. A study evaluating the effects that medetomidine (4 micrograms/kg) and/or butorphanol (0.1 mg/kg) had on the induction doses required for alfaxalone in dogs found that when either was used alone average induction dose was 1.2 mg/kg and when used together average alfaxalone induction dose was 0.8 mg/kg (Maddern et al. 2010).

- **PROPOFOL, THIOPENTAL:** The label (U.K.) states that alfaxalone <u>should not</u> be used with other injectable anesthetics.

Laboratory Considerations
None noted.

Doses
- **DOGS/CATS:**

Note: Refer to actual product information (label) for more specific information.

USA labeled-dose (FDA-approved): **For induction and maintenance of anesthesia and for induction of anesthesia followed by maintenance with an inhalant anesthetic:** Administer IV only. For induction, administer over approximately 60 seconds or until clinical signs show the onset of anesthesia, titrating administration against the response of the patient. Rapid administration may be associated with an increased incidence of cardiorespiratory depression or apnea. Apnea can occur following induction or after the administration of maintenance boluses. The use of preanesthetics may reduce the alfaxalone induction dose. The choice and the amount of phenothiazine, alpha2-adrenoreceptor agonist, benzodiazepine or opioid will influence the response of the patient to an induction dose of alfaxalone.

Dogs: Induction of general anesthesia: From a field study: In dogs that did not receive a preanesthetic, induction doses averaged 2.2 mg/kg IV (range 1.5 – 4.5 mg/kg). In dogs that received preanesthetics induction doses were reduced by 23-50%, depending on the combination of preanesthetics. Average induction doses ranged from 1.1 mg/kg in dogs that received an alpha2-adrenergic agonist to 1.7 mg/kg in dogs that received a benzodiazepine+opioid+acepromazine. Use of a preanesthetic appeared to decrease the occurrence of apnea following alfaxalone induction in dogs. The dose sparing of alfaxalone depends on the potency, dose, and time of administration of the preanesthetics used prior to induction. To avoid anesthetic overdose, titrate the administration of alfaxalone against the response of the patient. See the package insert (label) for more information. Additional doses of alfaxalone similar to those used for maintenance (1.2 – 2.2 mg/kg) may be administered to facilitate intubation.

Dogs: Maintenance of anesthesia: Following induction of anesthesia with alfaxalone and intubation, anesthesia may be maintained using intermittent intravenous boluses or an inhalant anesthetic agent. A maintenance bolus of 1.2 - 1.4 mg/kg provides an additional 6-8 minutes of anesthesia in preanesthetized dogs. A dose of 1.5 – 2.2 mg/kg provides an additional 6-8 minutes anesthesia in unpreanesthetized dogs. Clinical response may vary, and is determined by the dose, rate of administration, and frequency of maintenance injections. Additional low doses, similar to a maintenance dose, may be required to facilitate the transition to inhalant maintenance anesthesia.

Cats: Induction of general anesthesia: From a field study: In cats that did not receive a preanesthetic, induction doses averaged 4 mg/kg IV (range 2.2 – 9.7 mg/kg). In cats that received preanesthetics induction doses were reduced by 10-43%, depending on the combination of preanesthetics. Average induction doses ranged from 2.3 mg/kg in cats that received a benzodiazepine+opioid+phenothiazine to 3.6 mg/kg in cats that received benzodiazepine+phenothiazine, or alpha2-adrenergic agonist with/without a phenothiazine. The dose sparing of alfaxalone depends on the potency, dose, and time of administration of the preanesthetics used prior to induction. To avoid anesthetic overdose, titrate the administration of alfaxalone against the response of the patient. See the package insert (label) for more information. Additional doses of alfaxalone similar to those used for maintenance (1.1 – 1.5 mg/kg) may be administered to facilitate intubation.

Cats: Maintenance of anesthesia: Following induction of anesthesia with alfaxalone and intubation, anesthesia may be maintained using intermittent intravenous boluses or an inhalant anesthetic agent. A maintenance bolus of 1.1 – 1.3 mg/kg provides an additional 7-8 minutes of anesthesia in preanesthetized cats. A dose of 1.4 – 1.5 mg/kg provides an additional 3-5 minutes anesthesia in unpreanesthetized cats. Clinical response may vary, and is determined by the dose, rate of administration, and frequency of maintenance injections. Additional low doses, similar to a maintenance dose, may be required to facilitate the transition to inhalant maintenance anesthesia. (Adapted from label— *Alfaxan*®)

Cats (extra-label dose): For sedation for short procedures (subcutaneous dosing): Study was done in hyperthyroid cats. Alfaxalone at 3 mg/kg and butorphanol 0.2 mg/kg drawn up in the same syringe and administered as a single subcutaneous injection in the region dorsal to the right hip. 45 minutes post injection maximum sedation occurs. Blood pressure, heart rate and respiration rate all were significantly decreased. Monitoring BP is recommended. Further studies are required to determine whether the sedative, respiratory and cardiovascular effects are similar in euthyroid cats (Ramoo et al. 2013).

U.K. Label (extra-label in USA):

Induction: Dogs: Not premedicated: 3 mg/kg IV; Premedicated: 2 mg/kg IV. Cats: Premedicated or not premedicated: 5 mg/kg IV. The rate of administration should be that, if required, the total dose is given over the first 60 seconds. After that, if intubation is still not possible, one further similar dose may be administered to effect. Administration should continue until the clinician is satisfied that the depth of anesthesia is sufficient for endotracheal intubation or until the entire dose has been administered.

Maintenance: Following induction, the animal may be intubated and maintained on alfaxalone or an inhalation anesthetic agent. Maintenance doses of alfaxalone may be given as supplemental boluses or as constant-rate infusion. Alfaxalone has been used safely and effectively in both dogs and cats for procedures lasting for up to one hour. The following doses suggested for maintenance of anesthesia are based on data taken from controlled laboratory and field studies and represent the average amount of drug required to provide maintenance anesthesia for a dog or cat; however, the actual dose will be based on the response of the individual patient.

	DOGS		CATS	
	Unpremedicated	Premedicated	Unpremedicated	Premedicated
Dose for constant rate infusion (CRI)				
mg/kg/hour	8 – 9	6 – 7	10 – 11	7 – 8
mg/kg/minute	0.13 – 0.15	0.1 – 0.12	0.16 – 0.18	0.11 – 0.13
mL/kg/minute	0.013 – 0.015	0.01 – 0.012	0.016 – 0.018	0.011 – 0.013
Bolus dose for each 10 minutes maintenance				
mg/kg	1.3 – 1.5	1 – 1.2	1.6 – 1.8	1.1 – 1.3
mL/kg	0.13 – 0.15	0.1 – 0.12	0.16 – 0.18	0.11 – 0.13

Where maintenance of anesthesia is with alfaxalone for procedures lasting more than 5-10 minutes, a butterfly needle or catheter can be left in the vein, and small amounts of alfaxalone injected subsequently to maintain the required level and duration of anesthesia. In most cases the average duration of recovery when using alfaxalone for maintenance will be longer than if using an inhalant gas as a maintenance agent. (Adapted from label; *Alfaxan®*—Jurox U.K.)

Australia/New Zealand Label (extra-label in USA):

Induction: Dogs: Not premedicated: 3 mg/kg IV; Premedicated: 2 mg/kg IV. Cats: Premedicated or not premedicated: 5 mg/kg IV. IV (Dogs and Cats): Give the total induction dose, if required, IV over the first 60 seconds. If, 60 seconds after complete delivery of this first induction dose, intubation is still not possible, one further similar dose may be administered to effect by administering 25% (1/4) of the calculated dose every 15 seconds and continued until the clinician is satisfied that the depth of anesthesia is sufficient for endotracheal intubation, or until the entire dose has been administered.

Deep sedation/light anesthesia (Cats only): IM for 5 – 10 mg/kg (0.5 mL – 1 mL/kg). Variability in response may be minimized by giving deep IM in the quadriceps muscle mass. (Adapted from label; *Alfaxan®*—Jurox)

- **SMALL MAMMALS, RABBITS, EXOTICS, WILDLIFE SPECIES:**

A therapeutic review of alfaxalone use in a variety of species, including referenced dosages for certain amphibians, reptiles, fish, lagomorphs, rodents, ferrets, marsupials, etc. can be found in the *Journal of Exotic Pet Medicine* 21 (2012), pp. 347-353 (Jones 2012).

Monitoring

- Level of anesthesia/CNS effects.
- Respiratory depression.
- Cardiovascular status (cardiac rate/rhythm; blood pressure).

Chemistry/Synonyms

Alfaxalone is 3-alpha-hydroxy-5-alpha-pregnane-11,20-dione and has a molecular weight of 332.5. It occurs as a white to creamy white powder. It is practically insoluble in water or mineral spirits, soluble in alcohol, and freely soluble in chloroform.

The commercial injection occurs as a clear, colorless sterile solution without preservatives. It is a water-soluble formulation containing 2-hydroxypropyl-beta-cyclodextrin (HPCD) as the solubilizing agent. Another product containing alfaxalone, *Saffan®*, was marketed in the 1970s as an intravenous anesthetic agent for cats, but contained a polyethoxylated castor oil as the solubilizing agent which caused significant histamine release via mast cell degranulation. This product was subsequently removed from the market.

Alfaxalone may also be known as alfaksaloni, alfaxalon, alfaxalona, alfaxalonum, alphaxalone, or GR-2/234. A common trade name is *Alfaxan®*.

Storage/Stability

Alfaxalone solution for injection should be stored at room temperature (<30°C) and protected from light. Do not freeze. The USA label states to store the product at controlled room temperature 20°-25°C (68°-77°F) with excursions permitted between 15°-30°C (59°-86°F).

Stability recommendations vary depending the labeling for respective countries. As there is no preservative, most labels including the USA label states that once the vial has been opened, vial contents should be drawn into sterile syringes with each syringe prepared for single patient use only. Unused product should be discarded within 6 hours. However the ANZ label states: "…contains no preservatives. Solution should be removed from the vial using aseptic technique. Contents of broached vials should preferably be used within 24 hours, but may be stored if necessary at 4°C for up to 7 days provided contamination is avoided. Do not use broached vials if the solution is not clear, colorless and free from particulate matter." A study comparing bacterial growth in propofol, alfaxalone, and thiopental found that while alfaxalone injection supports the growth of some microorganisms (i.e., *E.coli),* this occurred less readily than with propofol and generally after 24 hours

of inoculation. The authors concluded that alfaxalone may be safe to use for a longer period after opening, but further investigation using a wider range of microorganisms and larger sample numbers would be required to state this definitively (Strachan et al. 2008).

Compatibility/Compounding Considerations

Although published stability data was not located, one source (Nieuwendijk 2011) states that alfaxalone injection can be diluted with an equal volume of lactated Ringers solution or 0.9% NaCl to obtain a concentration of 5 mg/mL. Similar dilutions were also done some clinical studies (Zaki et al. 2009; Maddern et al. 2010). The product label (USA) states it should not be mixed with other therapeutic agents prior to administration.

Dosage Forms/Regulatory Status

VETERINARY-LABELED PRODUCTS:

Alfaxalone 10 mg/mL in 10 mL single-use vials; *Alfaxan®*; (Rx). Approved by FDA (NADA 141-342) for use in cats and dogs. **Note:** At time of writing (March 2014) not presently marketed, but release is expected. The drug is a controlled substance (C-IV).

Alfaxalone is available in several other countries, including Australia, New Zealand, U.K. and 6 other European countries, Canada, and Japan. It requires a veterinary prescription.

HUMAN-LABELED PRODUCTS: NONE.

Revisions/References
Monograph revised/updated March 2014.

Bertelsen, M. F. & C. D. Sauer (2011). Alfaxalone anaesthesia in the green iguana (Iguana iguana). *Veterinary Anaesthesia and Analgesia* 38(5): 461-6.

Ferre, P. J., et al. (2006). Plasma pharmacokinetics of alfaxalone in dogs after an intravenous bolus of Alfaxan-CD RTU. *Veterinary Anaesthesia and Analgesia* 33(4): 229-36.

Gil, A. G., et al. (2012). Corticoadrenal Response and Heart and Respiratory Rates after Propofol or Alfaxalone Anesthesia in Rabbits. *Journal of the American Association for Laboratory Animal Science* 51(5): 694-5.

Gonzalez, M. S., et al. (2013). Effects of intramuscular alfaxalone alone or in combination with diazepam in swine. *Veterinary Anaesthesia and Analgesia* 40(4): 399-402.

Goodwin, W., et al. (2012). Plasma pharmacokinetics and pharmacodynamics of alfaxalone in neonatal foals after an intravenous bolus of alfaxalone following premedication with butorphanol tartrate. *Veterinary Anaesthesia and Analgesia* 39(5): 503-10.

Goodwin, W. A., et al. (2011). The pharmacokinetics and pharmacodynamics of the injectable anaesthetic alfaxalone in the horse. *Veterinary Anaesthesia and Analgesia* 38: 431-8.

Goodwin, W. A., et al. (2013). Alfaxalone and medetomidine intravenous infusion to maintain anaesthesia in colts undergoing field castration. *Equine Veterinary Journal* 45(3): 315-9.

Hansen, L. L. & M. F. Bertelsen (2013). Assessment of the effects of intramuscular administration of alfaxalone with and without medetomidine in Horsfield's tortoises (Agrionemys horsfieldii). *Veterinary Anaesthesia and Analgesia* 40(6): E68-E75.

Jones, K. L. (2012). Therapeutic Review: Alfaxalone. *Journal of Exotic Pet Medicine* 21(4): 347-53.

Keates, H. L., et al. (2012). Alfaxalone compared with ketamine for induction of anaesthesia in horses following xylazine and guaifenesin. *Veterinary Anaesthesia and Analgesia* 39(6): 591-8.

Kischinovsky, M., et al. (2013). Intramuscular administration of alfaxalone in red-eared sliders (Trachemys scripta elegans) - effects of dose and body temperature. *Veterinary Anaesthesia and Analgesia* 40(1): 13-20.

Kloppel, H. & E. A. Leece (2011). Comparison of ketamine and alfaxalone for induction and maintenance of anaesthesia in ponies undergoing castration. *Veterinary Anaesthesia and Analgesia* 38(1): 37-43.

Knotek, Z., et al. (2013). Alfaxalone anaesthesia in the green iguana (Iguana iguana). *Acta Veterinaria Brno* 82(1): 109-14.

Leece, E. A., et al. (2009). Alfaxalone in cyclodextrin for induction and maintenance of anaesthesia in ponies undergoing field castration. *Veterinary Anaesthesia and Analgesia* 36(5): 480-4.

Maddern, K., et al. (2010). Alfaxalone induction dose following administration of medetomidine and butorphanol in the dog. *Veterinary Anaesthesia and Analgesia* 37(1): 7-13.

McMillan, M. W. & E. A. Leece (2011). Immersion and branchial/transcutaneous irrigation anaesthesia with alfaxalone in a Mexican axolotl. *Veterinary Anaesthesia and Analgesia* 38(6): 619-23.

Moll, X., et al. (2013). The effects on cardio-respiratory and acid-base variables of a constant rate infusion of alfaxalone-HPCD in sheep. *Veterinary Journal* 196(2): 209-12.

Navarrete-Calvo, R., et al. (2014). Cardiorespiratory, anaesthetic and recovery effects of morphine combined with medetomidine and alfaxalone in rabbits. *Veterinary Record* 174(4).

Nieuwendijk, H. Alfaxalone; Alfaxan®. Veterinary Anesthesia & Analgesia Support Group (VASG.org)

O'Hagan, B. J., et al. (2012a). Clinical evaluation of alfaxalone as an anaesthetic induction agent in cats less than 12 weeks of age. *Australian Veterinary Journal* 90(10): 395-401.

O'Hagan, B. J., et al. (2012b). Clinical evaluation of alfaxalone as an anaesthetic induction agent in dogs less than 12 weeks of age. *Australian Veterinary Journal* 90(9): 346-50.

Pasloske, K., et al. (2009). Plasma pharmacokinetics of alfaxalone in both premedicated and unpremedicated Greyhound dogs after single, intravenous administration of Alfaxan (R) at a clinical dose. *J. Vet. Pharmacol. Ther.* 32(5): 510-3.

Psatha, E., et al. (2011). Clinical efficacy and cardiorespiratory effects of alfaxalone, or diazepam/fentanyl for induction of anaesthesia in dogs that are a poor anaesthetic risk. *Veterinary Anaesthesia and Analgesia* 38(1): 24-36.

Quandt, J. (2009). *Sedation and analgesia for the critically ill patient: Comprehensive review.* Proceedings; ACVIM. accessed via Veterinary Information Network; vin.com

Ramoo, S., et al. (2013). Sedation of hyperthyroid cats with subcutaneous administration of a combination of alfaxalone and butorphanol. *Australian Veterinary Journal* 91(4): 131-6.

Roan, R. (2009). Use of alfaxalone in rabbits. *Veterinary Record* 164(6): 188-.

Strachan, F. A., et al. (2008). A comparison of microbial growth in alfaxalone, propofol and thiopental. *Journal of Small Animal Practice* 49(4): 186-90.

Tutunaru, A. C., et al. (2013). Anaesthetic induction with alfaxalone may produce hypoxemia in rabbits premedicated with fentanyl/droperidol. *Veterinary Anaesthesia and Analgesia* 40(6): 657-9.

Whittem, T., et al. (2008). The pharmacokinetics and pharmacodynamics of alfaxalone in cats after single and multiple intravenous administration of Alfaxan((R)) at clinical and supraclinical doses. *J. Vet. Pharmacol. Ther.* 31(6): 571-9.

Zaki, S., et al. (2009). Clinical evaluation of Alfaxan-CD (R) as an intravenous anaesthetic in young cats. *Australian Veterinary Journal* 87(3): 82-7.

Alfentanil HCl

(al-**fen**-ta-nil)   Alfenta®

Opiate Anesthetic Adjunct

Prescriber Highlights

▶ Injectable, potent opiate that may be useful for adjunctive anesthesia.

▶ Marginal veterinary experience & little published data available to draw conclusions on appropriate usage in veterinary species.

▶ Dose-related respiratory & CNS depression are the most likely adverse effects seen.

▶ Dose may need adjustment in geriatric patients & those with liver disease.

▶ Class-II controlled substance; relatively expensive.

Uses/Indications

An opioid analgesic, alfentanil may be useful for anesthesia, analgesia, or sedation similar to fentanyl; fentanyl is generally preferred because of the additional experience with its use in veterinary patients and cost.

Pharmacology/Actions

Alfentanil is a potent *mu* opioid with the expected sedative, analgesic, and anesthetic properties. When comparing analgesic potencies after IM injection, 0.4 – 0.8 mg of alfentanil is equivalent to 0.1 – 0.2 mg of fentanyl and approximately 10 mg of morphine.

Pharmacokinetics

The pharmacokinetics of alfentanil have been studied in dogs and cats. In dogs, the drug's steady state volume of distribution is about 0.56 L/kg, clearance is approximately 30 mL/kg/minute, and the terminal half-life is approximately 20 minutes. In cats, alfentanil's elimination half-life is approximately 2-3 hours, volume of distribution (steady state) about 0.9 L/kg and clearance 17mL/minute/kg.

In humans, onset of anesthetic action occurs within 2 minutes after intravenous dosing, and within 5 minutes of intramuscular injection. Peak effects occur approximately 15 minutes after IM injection. The drug has a volume of distribution of 0.4 – 1 L/kg. About 90% of the drug is bound to plasma proteins. Alfentanil is primarily metabolized in the liver to inactive metabolites that are excreted by the kidneys into the urine; only about 1% of the drug is excreted unchanged into the urine. Total body clearance in humans ranges from 1.6 – 17.6 mL/minute/kg. Clearance is decreased by about 50% in patients with alcoholic cirrhosis or in those that are obese. Clearance is reduced by approximately 30% in geriatric patients. Elimination half–life in humans is about 100 minutes.

Contraindications/Precautions/Warnings

Alfentanil is contraindicated in patients hypersensitive to opioids. Because of the drug's potency and potential for significant adverse effects, it should only be used in situations where patient vital signs can be continuously monitored. Initial dosage reduction may be required in geriatric or debilitated patients, particularly those with diminished cardiopulmonary function.

Adverse Effects

Adverse effects are generally dose related and consistent with other opiate agonists. In conscious cats, excitement after an IV bolus has been noted. Respiratory depression, bradycardia, and CNS depression are most likely to be encountered. Bradycardia is usually responsive to anticholinergic agents. Dose-related skeletal muscle rigidity is not uncommon and neuromuscular blockers are routinely used. Alfentanil has rarely been associated with asystole, hypercarbia and hypersensitivity reactions.

Respiratory or CNS depression may be exacerbated if alfentanil is given with other drugs that cause those effects.

Reproductive/Nursing Safety

In humans, the FDA categorizes alfentanil as a category *C* drug for use during pregnancy (*Animal studies have shown an adverse effect on the fetus, but there are no adequate studies in humans; or there are no animal reproduction studies and no adequate studies in humans*). If alfentanil is administered systemically to the mother close to giving birth, offspring may show behavioral alterations (hypotonia, depression) associated with opioids. Although high dosages given for 10-30 days to laboratory animals have been associated with embryotoxicity, it is unclear if this is a result of direct effects of the drug or as a result of maternal toxicity secondary to reduced food and water intake.

The effects of alfentanil on lactation or its safety for nursing offspring is not well defined, but it is unlikely to cause significant effects when used during anesthetic procedures in the mother.

Overdosage/Acute Toxicity

Intravenous, severe overdosages may cause circulatory collapse, pulmonary edema, seizures, cardiac arrest and death. Less severe overdoses may cause CNS and respiratory depression, coma, hypotension, muscle flaccidity and miosis. Treatment is a combination of supportive therapy, as necessary, and the administration of an opiate antagonist such as naloxone. Although alfentanil has a relatively rapid half-life, multiple doses of naloxone may be necessary. Because of the drug's potency, the use of a tuberculin syringe to measure dosages less than 1 mL with a dosage calculation and measurement double-check system, are recommended.

Drug Interactions

The following drug interactions with alfentanil have either been reported or are theoretical in humans or animals and may be of significance in veterinary patients. Unless otherwise noted, use together is not necessarily contraindicated, but weigh the potential risks and perform additional monitoring when appropriate.

▪ **DRUGS THAT INHIBIT HEPATIC ISOENZYME CYP3A4,** such as **erythromycin, cimetidine, ketoconazole, itraconazole, fluconazole or diltiazem:** May increase the half-life and decrease the clearance of alfentanil leading to prolonged effect and an increased risk of respiratory depression.

▪ **DRUGS THAT DEPRESS CARDIAC FUNCTION OR REDUCE VAGAL TONE,** such as **beta-blockers** or **other anesthetic agents:** May produce bradycardia or hypotension if used concurrently with alfentanil.

Laboratory Considerations

- Patients receiving opiates may have increased plasma levels of **amylase** or **lipase** secondary to increased biliary tract pressure. Values may be unreliable for 24 hours after administration of alfentanil.

Doses

Note: In very obese patients, figure dosages based upon lean body weight. All dosages below are extra-label.

- **DOGS:**

  As a premed: 5 micrograms/kg alfentanil with 0.3 – 0.6 mg of atropine IV 30 seconds before injecting propofol can reduce the dose of propofol needed to induce anesthesia to 2 mg/kg, but apnea may still occur. (Hall et al. 2001b)

  As a constant rate infusion for pain: Loading dose of 0.5–1 micrograms/kg, then a CRI of 0.5–1 micrograms/kg/minute. (Grint 2008)

  As an analgesic supplement to anesthesia:

  a) 2 – 5 micrograms/kg IV q20 minutes (Hall et al. 2001b), (Hall et al. 2001a)

  b) **For intra-operative analgesia in patients with intracranial disease:** 0.2 micrograms/kg/minute. (Raisis 2005)

- **CATS:**

  As an analgesic supplement to anesthesia (extra-label): Study was done in cats undergoing ovariohysterectomy using propofol CRI general anesthesia. Five minutes after induction of anesthesia, alfentanil IV bolus at 10 mg/kg followed by a CRI of 0.8 micrograms/kg/minute. In the study, if heart rate (HR) or systolic arterial pressure (SAP) increased or decreased by 20% from the previously recorded values, infusion rate was adjusted upward or downwards by 10% and 3 minutes allowed before continuing surgery. (Padilha et al. 2011)

Monitoring

- Anesthetic and/or analgesic efficacy.
- Cardiac and respiratory rate.
- Pulse oximetry or other methods to measure blood oxygenation when used for anesthesia.

Client Information

- Alfentanil is a potent opiate that should only be used by professionals in a setting where adequate patient monitoring is available.

Chemistry/Synonyms

A phenylpiperidine opioid anesthetic-analgesic related to fentanyl, alfentanil HCl occurs as a white to almost white powder. It is freely soluble in alcohol, water, chloroform or methanol. The commercially available injection has a pH of 4–6 and contains sodium chloride for isotonicity. Alfentanil is more lipid soluble than morphine, but less so than fentanyl.

Alfentanil may also be known as: alfentanyl, *Alfenta®*, *Alfast®*, *Fanaxal®*, *Fentalim®*, *Limifen®*, or *Rapifen®*.

Storage/Stability

Alfentanil injection should be stored protected from light at room temperature.

Compatibility/Compounding Considerations

In concentrations of up to 80 micrograms/mL, alfentanil injection has been shown to be **compatible with normal saline, D**5 in normal saline, D5W, and lactated Ringers.

Dosage Forms/Regulatory Status

VETERINARY-LABELED PRODUCTS: NONE.

The ARCI (Racing Commissioners International) has designated this drug as a class 1 substance. See the appendix for more information.

HUMAN-LABELED PRODUCTS:

Alfentanil HCl for injection: 500 micrograms (as base)/mL in 2, 5 mL, 10 mL & 20 mL amps; preservative-free; *Alfenta®*, generic; (Rx, C-II).

Revisions/References

Monograph revised/updated August 2013.

Grint, N. (2008). *Constant Rate Infusions (CRIS) in Pain Management.* Proceedings: BSAVA. accessed via Veterinary Information Network; vin.com

Hall, L., et al. (2001a). Anesthesia of the dog. *Veterinary Anesthesia,* 10th Ed. London, Saunders: 385-440.

Hall, L., et al. (2001b). Principles of sedation, analgesia, and premedication. *Veterinary Anesthesia,* 10th Ed. London, Saunders: 75-112.

Padilha, S. T., et al. (2011). A clinical comparison of remifentanil or alfentanil in propofol-anesthetized cats undergoing ovariohysterectomy. *Journal of Feline Medicine and Surgery* 13(10): 738-43.

Raisis, A. (2005). *Techniques for anesthetizing animals with intracranial disease.* Proceedings: ACVSc2005. accessed via Veterinary Information Network; vin.com

Allopurinol

(al-oh-**pyoor**-i-nol)   Zyloprim®

Xanthine Oxidase Inhibitor; Purine Analog

Prescriber Highlights

- ▶ Used as a uric acid reducer in dogs, cats, reptiles & birds & as an alternative treatment Leishmaniasis & Trypanosomiasis in dogs.
- ▶ Use with caution (dosage adjustment may be required) in patients with renal or hepatic dysfunction.
- ▶ Contraindicated in red-tailed hawks & should be used with caution, if at all, in other raptors.
- ▶ Diet may need to be adjusted to lower purine.
- ▶ GI effects are most likely adverse effects, but hypersensitivity, hepatic & renal effects can occur.
- ▶ Many potential drug interactions.

Uses/Indications

The primary veterinary uses for allopurinol are for the prophylactic treatment of recurrent uric acid uroliths and hyperuricosuric calcium oxalate uroliths in dogs, particularly Dalmatians. It has also been used in an attempt to treat gout in pet birds and reptiles.

Allopurinol has been recommended as an alternative treatment for canine Leishmaniasis. Although it appears to have clinical efficacy, it must be used for many months of treatment and does not apparently clear the parasite in most dogs at usual dosages. Allopurinol may also be useful for American Trypanosomiasis.

Pharmacology/Actions

Allopurinol and its metabolite, oxypurinol, inhibit the enzyme xanthine oxidase. Xanthine oxidase is responsible for the conversion of oxypurines (*e.g.,* hypoxanthine, xanthine) to uric acid. Hepatic microsomal enzymes may also be inhibited by allopurinol. It does not increase the renal excretion of uric acid nor does it possess any antiinflammatory or analgesic activity.

Allopurinol is metabolized by *Leishmania* into an inactive form of inosine that is incorporated into the organism's RNA leading to faulty protein and RNA synthesis.

Allopurinol, by inhibiting xanthine oxidase, can inhibit the formation of superoxide anion radicals, thereby providing protection against hemorrhagic shock and myocardial ischemia in laboratory conditions. The clinical use of the drug for these indications requires further study.

Pharmacokinetics

In Dalmatians, absorption rates were variable between subjects. Peak levels occur within 1-3 hours after oral dosing. Elimination half-life is about 2.7 hours. In dogs (not necessarily Dalmatians), the serum half-life of allopurinol is approximately 2 hours and for oxipurinol, 4 hours. Food does not appear to alter the absorption of allopurinol in dogs.

In horses, oral bioavailability of allopurinol is low (approximately 15%). Allopurinol is rapidly converted to oxypurinol in horses; the elimination half-life of allopurinol is approximately 5-6 minutes. Oxypurinol has an elimination half-life of about 1.1 hours in the horse.

In humans, allopurinol is approximately 90% absorbed from the GI tract after oral dosing. Peak levels after oral allopurinol administration occur 1.5 and 4.5 hours later, for allopurinol and oxypurinol, respectively.

Allopurinol is distributed in total body tissue water but levels in the CNS are only about 50% of those found elsewhere. Neither allopurinol nor oxypurinol are bound to plasma proteins, but both drugs are excreted into milk.

Xanthine oxidase metabolizes allopurinol to oxypurinol. In humans, the serum half-life for allopurinol is 1-3 hours and for oxypurinol, 18-30 hours. Half-lives are increased in patients with diminished renal function. Both allopurinol and oxypurinol are dialyzable.

Contraindications/Precautions/Warnings

Allopurinol is contraindicated in patients that are hypersensitive to it or have previously developed a severe reaction to it. It should be used cautiously and with intensified monitoring in patients with impaired hepatic or renal function. When used in patients with renal insufficiency, dosage reductions and increased monitoring are usually warranted.

Allopurinol does not appear to be effective in dissolving urate uroliths in dogs with portovascular anomalies.

Red-tailed hawks appear to be sensitive to the effects of allopurinol. Doses of 50 mg/kg PO once daily caused clinical signs of vomiting and hyperuricemia with renal dysfunction. Doses of 25 mg/kg PO once daily were safe but not effective in reducing plasma uric acid.

Adverse Effects

Adverse effects in dogs are apparently uncommon with allopurinol when fed low purine diets. There has been one report of a dog developing hemolytic anemia and trigeminal neuropathy while receiving allopurinol. Xanthine coatings have formed around ammonium urate uroliths in dogs that have been fed diets containing purine. If the drug is required for chronic therapy, reduction of purine precursors in the diet with dosage reduction should be considered.

Several adverse effects have been reported in humans including GI distress, bone marrow suppression, skin rashes, hepatitis, and vasculitis. Human patients with renal dysfunction are at risk for further decreases in renal function and other severe adverse effects unless dosages are reduced. Until further studies are performed in dogs with decreased renal function, the drug should be used with caution and at reduced dosages.

Reproductive/Nursing Safety

While the safe use of allopurinol during pregnancy has not been established, dosages of up to 20 times normal in rodents have not demonstrated decreases in fertility. Infertility in males (humans) has been reported with the drug, but a causal effect has not been firmly established. In humans, the FDA categorizes this drug as category **C** for use during pregnancy (*Animal studies have shown an adverse effect on the fetus, but there are no adequate studies in humans; or there are no animal reproduction studies and no adequate studies in humans.*)

Allopurinol and oxypurinol may be excreted into milk; use caution when allopurinol is administered to a nursing dam.

Overdosage/Acute Toxicity

Vomiting has been seen in dogs at doses >44 mg/kg per the APCC database. A human ingesting 22.5 grams did not develop serious toxicity. The oral LD 50 in mice is 78 mg/kg.

There were 52 exposures to allopurinol reported to the ASPCA Animal Poison Control Center (APCC) during 2008-2009. In these cases, 51 were dogs with 6 showing clinical signs. The remaining 1 reported case was a cat that showed no symptoms. Common findings (recorded in decreasing frequency) include vomiting and trembling.

Drug Interactions

The following drug interactions with allopurinol have either been reported or are theoretical in humans or animals and may be of significance in veterinary patients. Unless otherwise noted, use together is not necessarily contraindicated, but weigh the potential risks and perform additional monitoring when appropriate.

- **AMINOPHYLLINE** or **THEOPHYLLINE**: Large doses of allopurinol may decrease metabolism thereby increasing their serum levels.
- **AMOXICILLIN** or **AMPICILLIN**: In humans, concomitant use with allopurinol has been implicated in increased occurrences of skin rashes; the veterinary significance of this interaction is unknown.
- **AZATHIOPRINE** or **MERCAPTOPURINE**: Allopurinol may inhibit metabolism and increase toxicity; if concurrent use is necessary, dosages of the antineoplastic/immunosuppressive agent should be reduced initially to 25-33% of their usual dose and then adjusted, dependent upon patient's response.
- **CHLORPROPAMIDE**: Allopurinol may increase risks for hypoglycemia and hepato-renal reactions.
- **CYCLOPHOSPHAMIDE**: Increased bone marrow depression may occur in patients receiving both allopurinol and cyclophosphamide.
- **CYCLOSPORINE**: Allopurinol may increase cyclosporine levels.
- **DIURETICS** (*e.g.*, **furosemide, thiazides, diazoxide, and alcohol**): Can increase uric acid levels.
- **ORAL ANTICOAGULANTS** (*e.g.*, **warfarin**): Allopurinol may reduce the metabolism of warfarin thereby increasing effect.
- **TRIMETHOPRIM/SULFAMETHOXAZOLE**: In a few human patients, thrombocytopenia has occurred when used with allopurinol.
- **URICOSURIC AGENTS** (*e.g.*, **probenecid, sulfinpyrazone**): May increase the renal excretion of oxypurinol and thereby reduce xanthine oxidase inhibition; in treating hyperuricemia the additive effects on blood uric acid may, in fact, be beneficial to the patient.
- **URINARY ACIDIFIERS** (*e.g.*, **methionine, ammonium chloride**) May reduce the solubility of uric acid in the urine and induce urolithiasis.

Doses

- **DOGS:**

  For urate uroliths (extra-label): Underline: For dissolution: 10 mg/kg PO q8h or 15 mg/kg q12h for up to 4 weeks. Use only in conjunction with low purine foods. Goal is to reduce urate:creatinine ratio by 50%. For prevention: 10 – 15 mg/kg PO once daily. **Note:** Prolonged high doses of allopurinol may result in xanthine uroliths; optimize dietary therapy to reduce recurrences and lessen need to use intermittent higher dose dissolution protocols.

  For Leishmaniasis (extra-label): Best used with an antimonial drug. Meglumine antimoniate (N-methylglucamine antimoniate) 75 – 100 mg/kg once daily for 4-8 weeks plus allopurinol 10 – 15 mg/kg PO twice daily for 6-12 months. Alternatively, miltefosine 2 mg/kg PO once daily for 4 weeks plus allopurinol 10 – 15 mg/kg PO twice daily for 6-12 months. When an antimonial cannot be used, allopurinol can be used alone at 10 – 20 mg/kg PO q12h for 1-4 months or longer. **Note:** If dog has renal insufficiency, allopurinol 5 mg/kg PO twice daily.

- **BIRDS:**

   For gout (extra-label):
   a) **In budgies and cockatiels:** Crush one 100 mg tablet into 10 mL of water. Add 20 drops of this solution to one ounce of drinking water. (McDonald 1989)
   b) **For parakeets:** Crush one 100 mg tablet into 10 mL of water. Add 20 drops of this solution to one ounce of drinking water or give 1 drop 4 times daily. (Clubb 1986)

- **REPTILES:**

   For gout in lizards or iguanas (extra-label): 20 – 25 mg/kg PO once daily.

Monitoring
- Urine uric acid (for urolithiasis).
- Adverse effects.
- Periodic CBC, liver and renal function tests (*e.g.*, BUN, Creatinine, liver enzymes); especially early in therapy.

Client Information
- May be given with or without food. Give with food if vomiting occurs.
- When used long-term in dogs, low-purine diets usually used.
- Usually does not cause many side effects, but contact veterinarian immediately if rash, unusual tiredness or yellowing of the whites of the eyes is seen.
- If using in drinking water for birds or reptiles, make a fresh solution every day.

Chemistry/Synonyms
A xanthine oxidase inhibitor, allopurinol occurs as a tasteless, fluffy white to off-white powder with a slight odor. It melts above 300° with decomposition and has an apparent pK_a of 9.4. Oxypurinol (aka oxipurinol, alloxanthine), its active metabolite, has a pK_a of 7.7. Allopurinol is only very slightly soluble in both water and alcohol.

Allopurinol may also be known as: allopurinolum, BW-56-158, HPP, or NSC-1390; many trade names are available but a common one is *Zyloprim®*.

Storage/Stability
Allopurinol tablets should be stored at room temperature in well-closed containers. The drug is stated to be stable in both light and air.

Compatibility/Compounding Considerations
Compounded preparation stability: Allopurinol oral suspension compounded from commercially available tablets has been published (Allen et al. 1996). Triturating eight (8) 300 mg tablets with 60 mL of *Ora-Plus®* and *qs ad* to 120 mL with *Ora-Sweet®* (or *Ora-Sweet®* SF) yields a 20 mg/mL suspension that retains >95% potency for 60 days stored at both 5°C and 25°C. The optimal stability of allopurinol liquids is reported to be between 3.1 and 3.4. Compounded preparations of allopurinol should be protected from light.

Another extemporaneously prepared suspension containing 20 mg/mL allopurinol for oral use can be prepared from the commercially available tablets. Tablets are crushed and mixed with an amount of *Cologel®* suspending agent equal to 1/3 the final volume. A mixture of simple syrup and wild cherry syrup at a ratio of 2:1 is added to produce the final volume. This preparation has been re-

ported to be stable for at least 14 days when stored in an amber bottle at either room temperature or when refrigerated.

Dosage Forms/Regulatory Status
VETERINARY-LABELED PRODUCTS: NONE.

HUMAN-LABELED PRODUCTS:
Allopurinol Oral Tablets: 100 mg & 300 mg; *Zyloprim®*, generic; (Rx)

Revisions/References
Monograph revised/updated August 2013.

Allen, L. V. & M. A. Erickson (1996). Stability of acetazolamide, allopurinol, azathioprine, clonazepam, and flucytosine in extemporaneously compounded oral liquids. *Am J Health Syst Pharm* **53**(16): 1944-9.
Clubb, S. L. (1986). Therapeutics: Individual and Flock Treatment Regimens. *Clinical Avian Medicine and Surgery.* G. J. Harrison and L. R. Harrison. Philadelphia, W.B. Saunders: 327-55.
McDonald, S. E. (1989). Summary of medications for use in psittacine birds. *JAAV* **3**(3): 120-7.

Alprazolam
(al-**prah**-zoe-lam)   Xanax®

Benzodiazepine Sedative/Tranquilizer

Prescriber Highlights
▶ Oral benzodiazepine that may be useful for adjunctive behavioral treatment in dogs and cats, especially for prophylaxis for storm phobias, etc.
▶ Contraindications: Aggressive animals (controversial), benzodiazepine hypersensitivity.
▶ Caution: Hepatic or renal disease.
▶ Adverse Effects: Sedation, behavior changes, & contradictory responses; physical dependence is a possibility; may impede training.
▶ C-IV controlled substance.

Uses/Indications
Alprazolam may be useful for adjunctive therapy in anxious, aggressive dogs or in those demonstrating panic reactions. It is most effective when used in advance of a triggering event. (**Note:** Some clinicians believe that benzodiazepines are contraindicated in aggressive dogs as anxiety may actually restrain the animal from aggressive tendencies). It may be useful in cats to treat anxiety disorders and unlike oral diazepam in cats, has not been implicated in causing liver failure.

Alprazolam may have less effect on motor function at low doses than does diazepam.

Pharmacology/Actions
Alprazolam and other benzodiazepines depress subcortical levels (primarily limbic, thalamic, and hypothalamic) of the CNS thus producing the anxiolytic, sedative, skeletal muscle relaxant, and anticonvulsant effects seen. The exact mechanism of action is unknown, but postulated mechanisms include: antagonism of serotonin, increased release of and/or facilitation of gamma-aminobutyric acid (GABA) activity, and diminished release or turnover of acetylcholine in the CNS. Benzodiazepine specific receptors have been located in the mammalian brain, kidney, liver, lung, and heart. In all species studied, receptors are lacking in the white matter.

Pharmacokinetics
The pharmacokinetics of alprazolam have not been described for either dogs or cats. In humans, alprazolam is well absorbed and is characterized as having an intermediate onset of action. Peak plasma levels occur in 1-2 hours.

Alprazolam is highly lipid soluble and widely distributed throughout the body. It readily crosses the blood-brain barrier and is somewhat bound to plasma proteins (80%).

Alprazolam is metabolized in the liver to at least two metabolites, including alpha-hydroxy-alprazolam, which is pharmacologically active. Elimination half-lives range from 6-27 hours in humans.

Contraindications/Precautions/Warnings

Some clinicians believe that benzodiazepines are contraindicated in aggressive dogs as anxiety may actually restrain the animal from aggressive tendencies. This remains controversial. Alprazolam is contraindicated in patients with known hypersensitivity to the drug. Use cautiously in patients with hepatic or renal disease, narrow angle glaucoma and debilitated or geriatric patients. Benzodiazepines may impair the abilities of working animals.

Alprazolam, like other benzodiazepines, has human abuse and drug diversion potential; prescribe cautiously.

Adverse Effects

Benzodiazepines can cause sedation, increased appetite, and transient ataxia. Cats may exhibit changes in behavior (irritability, increased affection, depression, aberrant demeanor) after receiving benzodiazepines.

Dogs may rarely exhibit a contradictory response (CNS excitement) following administration of benzodiazepines.

Chronic usage of benzodiazepines may induce physical dependence. Animals appear to be less likely than humans to develop physical dependence at doses normally administered.

Benzodiazepines may impede the ability of the animal to learn and may retard training.

Reproductive/Nursing Safety

Diazepam and other benzodiazepines have been implicated in causing congenital abnormalities in humans if administered during the first trimester of pregnancy. Infants born of mothers receiving large doses of benzodiazepines shortly before delivery have been reported to suffer from apnea, impaired metabolic response to cold stress, difficulty in feeding, hyperbilirubinemia, hypotonia, etc. Withdrawal symptoms have occurred in infants whose mothers chronically took benzodiazepines during pregnancy. The veterinary significance of these effects is unclear, but the use of these agents during the first trimester of pregnancy should only occur when the benefits clearly outweigh the risks associated with their use. In humans, the FDA categorizes this drug as category *D* for use during pregnancy (*There is evidence of human fetal risk, but the potential benefits from the use of the drug in pregnant women may be acceptable despite its potential risks.*)

Overdosage/Acute Toxicity

Alprazolam overdoses are generally limited to CNS signs. CNS depression can be seen and the severity is generally dose dependent. Hypotension, respiratory depression, and cardiac arrest have been reported in human patients but apparently are quite rare. The reported LD_{50} in rats for alprazolam is >330 mg/kg, but cardiac arrest occurred at doses as low as 195 mg/kg. Life threatening signs in small animals are rare. Some animals may present with a paradoxical type reaction (disorientation, vocalization, agitation, etc.). At times, those signs may be followed by CNS depression.

There were 1452 single agent exposures to alprazolam reported to the ASPCA Animal Poison Control Center (APCC) during 2009-2013. Of the 1324 dogs exposed, 725 were symptomatic. The common signs in the dogs included ataxia (73%), hyperactivity/agitation (24%), lethargy/sedation (21%), and vomiting (11%). Of the 118 cats, 80 were symptomatic with 79% ataxic, 24% vocalizing or agitated, 14% polyphagic, and 13% lethargic.

Treatment of acute toxicity consists of standard protocols for decontamination. The decision to give activated charcoal should be weighed carefully, as in some cases the risk of activated charcoal may outweigh the benefit. Flumazenil (see separate monograph) may be used to reverse the sedative effects of benzodiazepines, but

only if the CNS depression is significant, resulting in respiratory depression.

Drug Interactions

The following drug interactions with alprazolam have either been reported or are theoretical in humans or animals and may be of significance in veterinary patients. Unless otherwise noted, use together is not necessarily contraindicated, but weigh the potential risks and perform additional monitoring when appropriate.

- **ANTACIDS**: May slow the rate, but not the extent of oral absorption of alprazolam; administer 2 hours apart to avoid this potential interaction.
- **CNS DEPRESSANT AGENTS** (*e.g.,* **barbiturates, narcotics, anesthetics**, etc.): Additive effects may occur.
- **DIGOXIN**: Serum levels may be increased; monitor serum digoxin levels or clinical signs of toxicity.
- **FLUOXETINE, FLUVOXAMINE**: Increased alprazolam levels.
- **HEPATICALLY METABOLIZED DRUGS** (*e.g.,* **cimetidine, erythromycin, isoniazid, ketoconazole, itraconazole**): Metabolism of alprazolam may be decreased and excessive sedation may occur.
- **RIFAMPIN**: May induce hepatic microsomal enzymes and decrease the pharmacologic effects of benzodiazepines.
- **TRICYCLIC ANTIDEPRESSANTS** (*e.g.,* **amitriptyline, clomipramine, imipramine**): Alprazolam may increase levels of these drugs; clinical significance is not known and some state that clomipramine and alprazolam together may improve efficacy for phobias (*e.g.,* thunderstorm phobia).

Doses

- **DOGS:**

  For adjunctive treatment of canine anxiety disorders or phobias (extra-label): 0.02 – 0.1 mg/kg (usually 0.02 – 0.05 mg/kg initially) PO 2-4 times daily as needed. If used for acute phobias (fireworks, thunderstorms) it should be given in advance (30-60 minutes) of the expected trigger.

- **CATS:**

  For adjunctive treatment of feline anxiety disorders, phobias, or house soiling/marking (extra-label): 0.125 – 0.25 mg per cat 1-3 times a day. If used for phobias, attempt to dose 30-60 minutes before triggering event.

Monitoring

- Efficacy.
- Adverse Effects.
- Consider monitoring hepatic enzymes particularly when treating cats chronically.

Client Information

- When using for thunderstorm phobias or other triggers for phobia, try to give it 30 minutes to an hour before the event or trigger.
- Sleepiness is most common side effect, but sometimes the drug can change behavior or work in the opposite way. It may increase appetite, especially in cats.
- If difficulty with pilling the medication occurs, consider using the orally-disintegrating tablets; hands must be dry before handling.
- If yellowing of the whites of the eyes are seen or the gums have a yellowish tint, contact veterinarian immediately.

Chemistry/Synonyms

A benzodiazepine, alprazolam occurs as a white to off-white, crystalline powder. It is soluble in alcohol and insoluble in water.

Alprazolam may also be known as D65 MT, U 31889, or alprazolamum; many trade names available internationally.

Storage/Stability

Alprazolam tablets should be stored at room temperature in tight, light-resistant containers. The orally disintegrating tablets should be stored at room temperature and protected from moisture.

Compatibility/Compounding Considerations

Compounded preparation stability: Alprazolam oral suspension compounded from commercially available tablets has been published (Allen et al. 1998). Triturating sixty (60) alprazolam 2 mg tablets with 60 mL of *Ora-Plus*® and *qs ad* to 120 mL with *Ora-Sweet*® (or *Ora-Sweet*® SF) yields a 1 mg/mL oral suspension that retains >90% potency for 60 days stored at both 5°C and 25°C. Compounded preparations of alprazolam should be protected from light.

Dosage Forms/Regulatory Status

VETERINARY-LABELED PRODUCTS: NONE.

The ARCI (Racing Commissioners International) has designated this drug as a class 2 substance.

HUMAN-LABELED PRODUCTS:

Alprazolam Oral Tablets: 0.25 mg, 0.5 mg, 1 mg & 2 mg; *Xanax*®, generic; (Rx; C-IV)

Alprazolam Extended-release Oral Tablets: 0.5 mg, 1 mg, 2 mg, & 3 mg; *Xanax XR*®, generic; (Rx; C-IV)

Alprazolam Orally Disintegrating Tablets: 0.25 mg, 0.5 mg, 1 mg, & 2 mg; *Niravam*®, generic; (Rx; C-IV)

Alprazolam Oral Solution: 1 mg/mL in 30 mL; *Alprazolam Intensol*®; (Rx; C-IV)

Revisions/References

Monograph revised/updated August 2013.

Allen, L. V. & M. A. Erickson (1998). Stability of alprazolam, chloroquine phosphate, cisapride, enalapril maleate, and hydralazine hydrochloride in extemporaneously compounded oral liquids. *Am J Health Syst Pharm* **55**(18): 1915-20.

Altrenogest

(al-tre-**noe**-jest)   Regu-Mate®, Matrix®

Oral Progestin

Prescriber Highlights

▶ Progestational drug used in horses to suppress estrus or maintain pregnancy when progestin deficient; used in swine to synchronize estrus.

▶ May be used in dogs for luteal deficiency or as a treatment to prevent premature delivery.

▶ Many "handling" warnings for humans (see below).

▶ Very sensitive to light.

Uses/Indications

Altrenogest (*Regu-Mate*®) is indicated (labeled) to suppress estrus in mares to allow a more predictable occurrence of estrus following withdrawal of the drug. It is used clinically to assist mares to establish normal cycles during the transitional period from anestrus to the normal breeding season often in conjunction with an artificial photoperiod. It is more effective in assisting in pregnancy attainment later in the transition period. Some authors (Squires et al. 1983) suggest selecting mares with considerable follicular activity (mares with one or more follicles 20 mm or greater in size) for treatment during the transitional phase. Mares that have been in estrus for 10 days or more and have active ovaries are also considered excellent candidates for progestin treatment.

Altrenogest is effective in normally cycling mares for minimizing

the necessity for estrus detection, for the synchronization of estrus, and permitting scheduled breeding. Estrus will ensue 2-5 days after treatment is completed and most mares ovulate between 8-15 days after withdrawal. Altrenogest is also effective in suppressing estrus expression in show mares or mares to be raced. Although the drug is labeled as contraindicated during pregnancy, it has been demonstrated to maintain pregnancy in oophorectomized mares and may be of benefit in mares that abort due to sub-therapeutic progestin levels.

The product *Matrix*® is labeled for synchronization of estrus in sexually mature gilts that have had at least one estrous cycle. Treatment with altrenogest results in estrus (standing heat) 4-9 days after completion of the 14-day treatment period.

Altrenogest has been used in dogs for luteal insufficiency and as a treatment to prevent premature delivery.

Pharmacology/Actions

Progestins are primarily produced endogenously by the corpus luteum. They transform proliferative endometrium to secretory endometrium, enhance myometrium hypertrophy and inhibit spontaneous uterine contraction. Progestins have a dose-dependent inhibitory effect on the secretion of pituitary gonadotropins and have some degree of estrogenic, anabolic and androgenic activity.

Pharmacokinetics

In horses, the pharmacokinetics of altrenogest have been studied (Machnik et al. 2007). After oral dosing of 44 mg/kg PO, peak levels usually occur within 15-30 minutes post-dose; 24 hours post-dose, levels were below the level of quantification. Elimination half-lives are approximately 2.5-4 hours. Altrenogest appears to be primarily eliminated in the urine. Peak urine levels occur 3-6 hours after oral dosing. Urine levels were detectable up to 12 days post-administration.

Contraindications/Precautions/Warnings

The label (*Regu-Mate*®) lists pregnancy as a contraindication to the use of altrenogest, however it has been used clinically to maintain pregnancy in certain mares (see Dosages below). When used to maintain pregnancy it should be discontinued within 24 hours of the due date (Baker et al. 2012). Pregnant mares with gastrointestinal diseases may not absorb altrenogest adequately and injectable progesterone is preferred (Volkmann 2010). Altrenogest should not be used in horses intended for food purposes.

Adverse Effects

Adverse effects of altrenogest appear to be minimal when used at labeled dosages. One study (Shideler et al. 1983) found negligible changes in hematologic and most "standard" laboratory tests after administering altrenogest to 4 groups of horses (3 dosages, 1 control) over 86 days. Occasionally, slight changes in Ca^{++}, K^+, alkaline phosphatase and AST were noted in the treatment group, but values were only slightly elevated and only noted sporadically. No pattern or definite changes could be attributed to altrenogest. No outward adverse effects were noted in the treatment group during the trial.

Use of progestational agents in mares with chronic uterine infections should be avoided as the infection process may be enhanced.

Overdosage/Acute Toxicity

The LD_{50} of altrenogest is 175-177 mg/kg in rats. No information was located regarding the effects of an accidental acute overdose in horses or other species.

Drug Interactions

The following drug interaction with altrenogest has either been reported or is theoretical in humans or animals and may be of significance in veterinary patients. Unless otherwise noted, use together is not necessarily contraindicated, but weigh the potential risks and perform additional monitoring when appropriate.

- **RIFAMPIN**: May decrease progestin activity if administered concomitantly. This is presumably due to microsomal enzyme induction with resultant increase in progestin metabolism. The clinical significance of this potential interaction is unknown.

Laboratory Considerations
- Unlike exogenously administered progesterone, altrenogest does not interfere or cross-react with progesterone assays.

Doses
- **DOGS:**

For luteal insufficiency (extra-label):
a) Document luteal insufficiency and rule out infectious causes of pregnancy loss. Best to avoid during first trimester. Give equine product (*Regumate®*) at 2 mL per 100 lbs. of body weight PO once daily. Monitor pregnancy with ultrasound. Remember that exogenous progesterone is the experimental model for pyometra in the bitch, so monitor carefully. (Purswell 1999)
b) For luteal insufficiency, pre-term labor: 0.1 mL per 10 lb. body weight PO once daily. (Barber 2006)
c) To maintain pregnancy if tocolytics (*e.g.,* terbutaline) do not control myometrial contractility: 0.088 mg/kg once daily (q24h). Must be withdrawn 2-3 days prior to predicted whelp date. (Davidson 2006)

- **HORSES:**

To suppress estrus for synchronization (labeled dosage; FDA-approved): Administer 1 mL per 110 pounds body weight (0.044 mg/kg) PO once daily for 15 consecutive days. May administer directly on tongue using a dose syringe or on the usual grain ration. (Package insert; *Regu-Mate®*)

For prevention of abortion/pregnancy loss (all are extra-label):
a) 0.088 mg/kg PO once daily. (Dascanio 2009)
b) To maintain pregnancy in mares with deficient progesterone levels: 0.044 mg/kg PO once daily. Three options for treatment: 1) treatment until day 60 of pregnancy or greater AND measurement of endogenous progesterone level of >4 ng/mL; 2) treatment until day 120 of pregnancy; or 3) treatment until end of pregnancy. (McCue 2003)
c) To maintain pregnancy in mares with placentitis: 22 – 44 mg (total dose; 10 – 20 mL) PO daily. (Valla 2003)

To suppress estrus (long-term) (extra-label): 0.044 mg/kg PO daily. (Squires et al. 1983)

- **SWINE:**

For synchronization of estrous in sexually mature gilts that have had at least one estrous cycle (labeled dosage; FDA-approved): Follow label directions for safe use. Administer 6.8 mL (15 mg) per gilt for 14 consecutive days. Apply as a top-dressing on a portion of gilt's daily feed allowance. Estrous should occur 4–9 days after completing treatment. (Package insert; *Matrix®*)

Client Information
The manufacturer (*Regu-Mate®, Matrix®*) lists the following people as those who should not handle the product:
1. Women who are or suspect that they are pregnant.
2. Anyone with thrombophlebitis or thromboembolic disorders or with a history of these events.
3. Anyone having cerebrovascular or coronary artery disease.
4. Women with known or suspected carcinoma of the breast.
5. People with known or suspected estrogen-dependent neoplasias.
6. Women with undiagnosed vaginal bleeding.
7. People with benign or malignant tumor that developed during the use of oral contraceptives or other estrogen containing products.

- Altrenogest can be absorbed after skin contact and absorption can be enhanced if the drug is covered by occlusive materials (*e.g.,* under latex gloves, etc.). If exposed to the skin, wash off immediately with soap and water. If the eyes are exposed, flush with water for 15 minutes and get medical attention. If the product is swallowed, do not induce vomiting and contact a physician or poison control center.
- This medication is prohibited from use in an extra-label manner to enhance food and/or fiber production in animals.

Chemistry/Synonyms
An orally administered synthetic progestational agent, altrenogest has a chemical name of 17 alpha-Allyl-17beta-hydroxyestra-4,9,11-trien-3-one.

Altrenogest may also be known as: allyl trenbolone, A-35957, A-41300, RH-2267, or RU-2267, *Regu-Mate®*, or *Matrix®*.

Storage/Stability
Altrenogest oral solution should be stored at room temperature. Altrenogest is extremely sensitive to light; dispense in light-resistant containers.

Compatibility/Compounding Considerations
No specific information noted.

Dosage Forms/Regulatory Status
VETERINARY-LABELED PRODUCTS:

Altrenogest 0.22% (2.2 mg/mL) in oil solution in 150 mL and 1000 mL bottles; *Regu-Mate®*; (Rx). FDA-approved for use in horses not intended for food. This medication is banned in racing animals in some countries.

Altrenogest 0.22% (2.2 mg/mL) in 1000 mL bottles; *Matrix®*; (OTC, but extra-label use prohibited). FDA-approved for use in sexually mature gilts that have had at least one estrous cycle. Gilts must not be slaughtered for human consumption for 21 days after the last treatment. The FDA prohibits the extra-label use of this medication to enhance food and/or fiber production in animals.

HUMAN-LABELED PRODUCTS: NONE.

Revisions/References
Monograph revised/updated August 2013.

Baker, T. W. & A. F. Davidson (2012). *Obstetrical Emergencies I.* Western Veterinary Conference 2012. accessed via Veterinary Information Network; vin.com
Barber, J. (2006). *Whelping management in the bitch.* Proceedings: Western Veterinary Conference. accessed via Veterinary Information Network; vin.com
Dascanio, J. (2009). *Hormonal Control of Reproduction.* Proceedings: ABVP. accessed via Veterinary Information Network; vin.com
Davidson, A. (2006). *Myths in small animal reproduction.* Proceedings: Canine Medicine Symposium. accessed via Veterinary Information Network; vin.com
Machnik, M., et al. (2007). Pharmacokinetics of altrenogest in horses. *J Vet Phamacol Ther* **30**: 86-90.
McCue, P. (2003). *Ovarian problems in the non-pregnant mare.* Proceedings: Western Veterinary Conference. accessed via Veterinary Information Network; vin.com
Purswell, B. (1999). *Pharmaceuticals used in canine theriogenology - Part 1 & 2.* Proceedings: Central Veterinary Conference, Kansas City. accessed via Veterinary Information Network; vin.com
Squires, E. L., et al. (1983). Clinical Applications of Progestins in Mares. *Comp CE* **5**(1): S16-S22.
Valla, W. (2003). *Medical management of mares with complicated pregnancies.* Proceedings: ACVIM Forum. accessed via Veterinary Information Network; vin.com
Volkmann, D. (2010). *Rational Use of Progestagen Therapy During Pregnancy.* Western Veterinary Conference 2010. accessed via Veterinary Information Network; vin.com

Aluminum Hydroxide

(ah-**loo**-min-um hye-**droks**-ide)
Aluminium Hydroxide, Amphogel®

Oral Antacid/Phosphate Binder

Prescriber Highlights

▶ Used to treat hyperphosphatemia in small animal patients &
   sometimes as a gastric antacid for ulcers.
▶ Chronic use may lead to electrolyte abnormalities; possible
   aluminum toxicity.
▶ Many potential drug interactions.
▶ Bulk, dried powder available from several sources.

Uses/Indications

Orally administered aluminum hydroxide is used to reduce hyperphosphatemia in patients with renal failure when dietary phosphorus restriction fails to maintain serum phosphorus concentrations
in the normal range. Occasionally, it has been used as an oral antacid in veterinary patients.

Pharmacology/Actions

Aluminum salts reduce the amount of phosphorus absorbed from
the intestine by physically binding to dietary phosphorus. When
used as an antacid the hydroxyl ion interacts with hydrogen ions
in the gut.

Contraindications/Precautions/Warnings

Aluminum-containing antacids may inhibit gastric emptying; use
cautiously in patients with gastric outlet obstruction. Also, use with
caution in patients prone to developing constipation.

Adverse Effects

In small animals, the most likely side effect of aluminum hydroxide
is constipation. If the patient is receiving a low phosphate diet and
the patient chronically receives aluminum antacids, hypophosphatemia can develop.

Potentially, aluminum toxicity could occur with prolonged use.
While previously believed unlikely to occur in small animal patients, at least 2 dogs in renal failure have been documented to have
developed aluminum toxicity after receiving aluminum-containing
phosphate binders (Segev et al. 2008). Aluminum-containing and
calcium-containing phosphate binders may be used in combination
to reduce the dose of each to reduce the risk of aluminum toxicity
or hypercalcemia.

Reproductive/Nursing Safety

In a system evaluating the safety of drugs in canine and feline pregnancy (Papich 1989), these drugs are categorized as class: **A** (*Probably safe. Although specific studies may not have proved the safety of
all drugs in dogs and cats, there are no reports of adverse effects in
laboratory animals or women.*)

Overdosage/Acute Toxicity

Acute toxicity is unlikely with an oral overdose. If necessary, GI and
electrolyte imbalances that occur with chronic or acute overdose
should be treated symptomatically.

Drug Interactions

The following drug interactions with oral aluminum salts have either been reported or are theoretical in humans or animals and may
be of significance in veterinary patients. Unless otherwise noted,
use together is not necessarily contraindicated, but weigh the potential risks and perform additional monitoring when appropriate.

Aluminum salts can **decrease** the amount absorbed or the pharmacologic effect of the drugs listed below; separate oral doses of
aluminum hydroxide and these drugs by two hours to help reduce
he potential for this interaction.

- **ALLOPURINOL**
- **CHLOROQUINE**
- **CORTICOSTEROIDS**
- **DIGOXIN**
- **ETHAMBUTOL**
- **FLUOROQUINOLONES**
- **GABAPENTIN**
- **H-2 ANTAGONISTS** (*e.g.,* **ranitidine, famotidine,** etc.)
- **IRON SALTS**
- **ISONIAZID**
- **PENICILLAMINE**
- **PHENOTHIAZINES**
- **TETRACYCLINES**
- **THYROID HORMONES**

Doses

Note: All dosages are extra-label.

- **DOGS/CATS:**

  For hyperphosphatemia: Aluminum hydroxide gel powder,
  USP is preferred as it can be mixed with food and is tasteless:
  30 – 100 mg/kg per day. Dose is divided and mixed with food.
  Start at low end of dosage range and adjust upward every 2-4
  weeks until desired serum phosphorus attained. Then re-check
  phosphorus and re-adjust dose if necessary every 4-6 weeks. If
  a reduced-phosphorus diet and higher dosages of aluminum hydroxide do not adequately control serum phosphorus, consider
  adding a lanthanum- or calcium-based (*e.g.,* calcium acetate,
  calcium carbonate) phosphate binder to reduce the chances for
  aluminum toxicity.

- **RABBITS/RODENTS/SMALL MAMMALS:**

  Chinchillas: Aluminum hydroxide gel: 1 mL/animal PO as needed. Guinea pigs: 0.5 – 1 mL/animal PO as needed. (Adamcak et
  al. 2000)

- **CATTLE:**

  As an antacid: Aluminum hydroxide: 30 grams/animal. (Jenkins
  1988)

- **HORSES:**

  For adjunctive gastroduodenal ulcer therapy in foals: Alu-
  minum/magnesium hydroxide suspension: 15 mL (total dose)
  4 times a day. (Clark and Becht 1987)

Monitoring

- Serum phosphorus (after a 12-hour fast), initially at 10-14 day
  intervals (some say 5 days); once "stable" at 4-6 week intervals.
  Most recommend maintaining below 6 mg/dL (1.6 mmol/L) with
  a target range (depending on stage of chronic kidney disease) of
  3.5-5.5 mg/dL (1.13-1.78 mmol/L).

- For aluminum toxicity: neuromuscular effects, progressive decreases in mean cell volume (MCV) and microcytosis.

Client Information

- Oral aluminum hydroxide products are available without prescription (OTC), but should be used under the supervision of the
  veterinarian.

- Bulk powder, or compounded capsules are easier to administer
  than liquids or suspensions.

- Give either just before feeding or mixed in food.

- Can cause constipation or decrease appetite.

- Report any unusual neuromuscular signs such as weakness, difficulty walking, or stumbling to veterinarian.

Chemistry/Synonyms

Dried Aluminum Hydroxide Gel (CAS Registry: 21645-51-2) occurs as a white, odorless, tasteless, amorphous powder. It is insoluble in water or alcohol. The USP 36 standard allows varying amounts of basic aluminum carbonate and bicarbonate, but it can contain not less than 76.5% of Al(OH)3.

Aluminum hydroxide may also be known as aluminium hydroxide.

Storage/Stability

Store powder forms in airtight containers. Liquid formulations should not be allowed to freeze.

Compatibility/Compounding Considerations

Because aluminum hydroxide powder USP can vary in the concentration of aluminum hydroxide (must be 76.5% or greater) and powders can vary in density, volume measurements can only approximate actual weight. However, ¼ teaspoonful (1.25 mL) of the dried USP powder has been reported to contain approximately 300 mg of aluminum hydroxide.

Dosage Forms/Regulatory Status

VETERINARY-LABELED PRODUCTS: NONE.

HUMAN-LABELED PRODUCTS:

Aluminum Hydroxide Concentrated Gel Suspension/Liquid (**Note:** These products are usually flavored (mint) and not well accepted by dogs or cats.): 320 mg/5 mL in 360 mL & 480 mL, UD 15 mL & 30 mL; generic; (OTC)

Aluminum Hydroxide Gel, Dried Powder, USP; bulk powder is available from a variety of sources including many compounding pharmacies. See: http://goo.gl/1lYJk for additional source information.

Note: There are also many products available that have aluminum hydroxide and a magnesium or calcium salt (*e.g., Maalox®*, etc.) that are used as antacids. All oral aluminum and magnesium hydroxide preparations are OTC.

Revisions/References

Monograph revised/updated August 2013.

Adamcak, A. & B. Otten (2000). Rodent Therapeutics. *Vet Clin NA: Exotic Anim Pract* **3:1**(Jan): 221-40.

Jenkins, W. L. (1988). Drugs affecting gastrointestinal functions. *Veterinary Pharmacology and Therapeutics 6th Ed.* N. H. Booth and L. E. McDonald. Ames, Iowas Stae Univ. Press: 657- 71.

Segev, G., et al. (2008). Aluminum Toxicity Following Administration of Aluminum-based Phosphate Binders in 2 Dogs with Renal Failure. *J Vet Intern Med* **22**(6): 1432-5.

Amantadine HCl

(a-**man**-ta-deen)   Symmetrel®

Antiviral (Influenza A); NMDA Antagonist

Prescriber Highlights

▶ Antiviral drug with NMDA antagonist properties; may be useful in adjunctive therapy of chronic pain in small animals.

▶ Very limited clinical experience; dogs may exhibit agitation & GI effects, especially early in therapy.

▶ Large interpatient variations of pharmacokinetics in horses limit its therapeutic usefulness.

▶ Overdoses are potentially very serious; fairly narrow therapeutic index in dogs & cats; may need to be compounded to accurately dose small animals.

▶ Extra-label use prohibited (by FDA) in chickens, turkeys & ducks.

Uses/Indications

While amantadine may have efficacy and clinical usefulness against some veterinary viral diseases, presently the greatest interest for its use in small animals is as a NMDA antagonist in the adjunctive treatment of chronic pain, often in those tolerant to opioids. It is generally used in combination with an NSAID, opioid, or gabapentin/pregabalin. It is also used as an adjunct drug for treating neuropathic pain. It has been suggested for use as an early intervention in the treatment of pain associated with osteosarcomas (Gaynor 2008).

Amantadine has also been investigated for treatment of equine-2 influenza virus in the horse. However, because of expense, interpatient variability in oral absorption and other pharmacokinetic parameters, and the potential for causing seizures after intravenous dosing, it is not commonly used for treatment.

In humans, amantadine is used for treatment and prophylaxis of influenza A, parkinsonian syndrome, and drug-induced extrapyramidal effects. As in veterinary medicine, amantadine's effect on NMDA receptors in humans are of active interest, particularly its use as a co-analgesic with opiates and in the reduction of opiate tolerance development.

Pharmacology/Actions

Like ketamine, dextromethorphan and memantine, amantadine antagonizes the N-methyl-D-aspartate (NMDA) receptor. Within the central nervous system, chronic pain can be maintained or exacerbated when glutamate or aspartate bind to this receptor. It is believed that this receptor is particularly important in allodynia (sensation of pain resulting from a normally non-noxious stimulus). Amantadine alone is not a particularly good analgesic, but in combination with other analgesics (*e.g.*, opiates, NSAIDs), it is thought that it may help alleviate chronic pain. However, one small experimental study in cats did not show that amantadine potentiated the antinociceptive effect of oxymorphone in response to thermal stimulus (Siao et al. 2012). But because amantadine is expected to produce effects when pain or CNS sensitization is already present (and not in response to noxious stimuli) these results may not be clinically relevant to naturally occurring pain states (KuKanich 2013).

Amantadine's antiviral activity is primarily limited to strains of influenza A. While its complete mechanism of action is unknown, it does inhibit viral replication by interfering with influenza A virus M2 protein.

Amantadine's antiparkinsonian activity is not well understood, but it apparently increases dopamine levels in the brain. The drug does appear to have potentiating effects on dopaminergic neurotransmission in the CNS and anticholinergic activity. Amantadine is being studied for adjunctive treatment of traumatic brain injury in humans.

Pharmacokinetics

In dogs, oral bioavailability of amantadine is reportedly very high and some of the drug is metabolized; elimination half-life is around 5 hours.

In cats, after oral administration bioavailability is very high and peak levels occur about 2 hours after dosing. After IV administration volume of distribution (VDss) is about 4.3 L/kg, clearance (mean) was 8.2 mL/minute/kg. Elimination half-life is approximately 6 hours (Siao et al. 2011).

In horses, amantadine has a very wide interpatient variability of absorption after oral dosing; bioavailability ranges from 40-60%. The elimination half-life in horses is about 3.5 hours and the steady state volume of distribution is approximately 5 L/kg.

In humans, the drug is well absorbed after oral administration with peak plasma concentrations occurring about 3 hours after dosing. Volume of distribution is 3 – 8 L/kg. Amantadine is primarily eliminated via renal mechanisms. Oral clearance is approximately 0.28 L/hr/kg; half-life is around 9-17 hours.

Contraindications/Precautions/Warnings

In humans, amantadine is contraindicated in patients with known hypersensitivity to it or rimantadine, and those with untreated angle-closure glaucoma. It should be used with caution in patients with liver disease, renal disease (dosage adjustment may be required), congestive heart failure, active psychoses, eczematoid dermatitis or seizure disorders. In veterinary patients with similar conditions, it is advised to use the drug with caution until more information on its safety becomes available.

In 2006, the FDA banned the use of amantadine and other influenza antivirals in chickens, turkeys and ducks.

Adverse Effects

There is very limited experience in domestic animals with amantadine and its adverse effect profile is not well described. It has been reported that dogs given amantadine occasionally develop agitation, loose stools, flatulence or diarrhea, particularly early in therapy. Experience in cats is limited and an adverse effect profile has yet to be fully elucidated, but some report that gastrointestinal effects are more likely than in dogs. Possible signs indicating toxicity include: anxiety, restlessness, and dry mouth.

Reproductive/Nursing Safety

In humans, the FDA categorizes amantadine as a category **C** drug for use during pregnancy (*Animal studies have shown an adverse effect on the fetus, but there are no adequate studies in humans; or there are no animal reproduction studies and no adequate studies in humans*). High dosages in rats demonstrated some teratogenic effects.

Amantadine does enter maternal milk. The manufacturer does not recommend its use in women who are nursing. Veterinary significance is unclear.

Overdosage/Acute Toxicity

Toxic dose reported for cats is 30 mg/kg and behavioral effects may be noted at 15 mg/kg in dogs and cats.

In humans, overdoses as low as 2 grams have been associated with fatalities. Cardiac dysfunction (arrhythmias, hypertension, tachycardia), pulmonary edema, CNS toxicity (tremors, seizures, psychosis, agitation, coma), hyperthermia, renal dysfunction and respiratory distress syndrome have all been documented. There is no known specific antidote for amantadine overdose. Treatment should consist of gut emptying, if possible, intensive monitoring and supportive therapy. Forced urine acidifying diuresis may increase renal excretion of amantadine. Physostigmine has been suggested for cautious use in treating CNS effects.

There were 36 single agent exposures to amantadine reported to the ASPCA Animal Poison Control Center (APCC) during 2009-2013. Of these animals, 31 were dogs, with 11 being symptomatic. Common signs in these dogs included 45% with tremors, and 18% having anxiety, ataxia, hypersalivation and/or vomiting.

Drug Interactions

The following drug interactions with amantadine have either been reported or are theoretical in humans or animals and may be of significance in veterinary patients. Unless otherwise noted, use together is not necessarily contraindicated, but weigh the potential risks and perform additional monitoring when appropriate.

- **ANTICHOLINERGIC DRUGS**: May enhance the anticholinergic effects of amantadine.
- **CNS STIMULANTS** (including **selegiline**): Concomitant use with amantadine may increase the drug's CNS stimulatory effects.
- **TRIMETHOPRIM/SULFA, QUINIDINE, QUININE, THIAZIDE DIURETICS or TRIAMTERENE**: May decrease the excretion of amantadine, yielding higher blood levels.

- **URINARY ACIDIFIERS** (*e.g.*, **methionine, ammonium chloride, ascorbic acid**): May increase the excretion of amantadine.

Laboratory Considerations

- No laboratory interactions identified.

Doses

- **DOGS/CATS:**

  As adjunctive therapy (with another analgesic) for chronic pain, neuropathic pain or to prevent "wind-up" (extra-label): 2 – 5 mg/kg PO once daily; start at lower end of dosing range and increase slowly if needed. Because amantadine has a significantly shorter half-life in dogs and cats when compared to humans, twice daily dosing may be more effective.

Monitoring

- Adverse effects (GI, anxiety, restlessness, and dry mouth).
- Efficacy.

Client Information

- When used in small animals, the drug must be given as prescribed to be effective and may take a week or more to show effect.
- Gastrointestinal effects (loose stools, gas, diarrhea) or some agitation may occur, particularly early in treatment. Contact the veterinarian if these become serious or persist.
- Overdoses with this medication can be serious; keep well out of reach of children and pets.

Chemistry/Synonyms

An adamantane-class antiviral agent with NMDA antagonist properties, amantadine HCl occurs as a white to practically white, bitter tasting, crystalline powder with a pKa of 9. Approximately 400 mg are soluble in 1 mL of water; 200 mg are soluble in 1 mL of alcohol.

Amantadine HCl may also be known as: adamantanamine HCl, *Adekin®, Amanta®, Amantagamma®, Amantan®, Amantrel®, Amixx®, Antadine®, Antiflu-DES®, Atarin®, Atenegine®, Cerebramed®, Endantadine®, Infectoflu®, Influ-A®, Lysovir®, Mantadine®, Mantadix®, Mantidan®, Padiken®, Symadine®, Symmetrel®, Viroifral®* and *Virucid®*.

Storage/Stability

Tablets, capsules and the oral solution should be stored in tight containers at room temperature. Limited exposures to temperatures as low as 15°C and as high as 30°C are permitted. Avoid freezing the liquid.

Compatibility/Compounding Considerations

No specific information noted.

Dosage Forms/Regulatory Status

VETERINARY-LABELED PRODUCTS: NONE.

HUMAN-LABELED PRODUCTS:

Amantadine HCl Oral Tablets & Capsules: 100 mg; generic; (Rx)

Amantadine HCl Oral Syrup: 50 mg/5mL (10 mg/mL) in 480 mL; generic; (Rx). **Note:** It is reported that the oral liquid has a very bad taste and may not be accepted by animal patients.

In 2006, the FDA banned the extra-label use of amantadine and other influenza antivirals in chickens, turkeys and ducks.

Revisions/References

Monograph revised/updated August 2013.

Gaynor, J. S. (2008). Control of Cancer Pain in Veterinary Patients. *Veterinary Clinics of North America-Small Animal Practice* **38**(6): 1429-+.

KuKanich, B. (2013). Outpatient Oral Analgesics in Dogs and Cats Beyond Nonsteroidal Antiinflammatory Drugs: An Evidence-based Approach. *Vet Clin Small Anim* **43**: 1109-25.

Siao, K. T., et al. (2012). Effect of amantadine on oxymorphone-induced thermal antinociception in cats. *J. Vet. Pharmacol. Ther.* **35**(2): 169-74.

Siao, K. T., et al. (2011). Pharmacokinetics of amantadine in cats. *J. Vet. Pharmacol. Ther.* **34**(6): 599-604.

Amikacin Sulfate, Systemic

(am-i-**kay**-sin) Amikin®, Amiglyde-V®

Aminoglycoside Antibiotic

Prescriber Highlights

► Parenteral aminoglycoside antibiotic that has good activity against a variety of bacteria, predominantly gram-negative aerobic bacilli.

► Adverse Effects: Nephrotoxicity, ototoxicity, neuromuscular blockade.

► Cats may be more sensitive to toxic effects.

► Risk factors for toxicity: Preexisting renal disease, age (both neonatal & geriatric), fever, sepsis & dehydration.

► Now usually dosed once daily when used systemically.

Uses/Indications

While parenteral use is only FDA-approved for use in dogs, amikacin is used clinically to treat serious gram-negative infections in most species. It is often used in settings where gentamicin-resistant bacteria are a clinical problem. The inherent toxicity of the aminoglycosides limit their systemic use to serious infections when there is either a documented lack of susceptibility to other, less toxic antibiotics or when the clinical situation dictates immediate treatment of a presumed gram-negative infection before culture and susceptibility results are reported.

Amikacin is also FDA-approved for intrauterine infusion in mares. It is used with intra-articular injection in foals to treat gram-negative septic arthritis. Intravenous regional limb perfusion (IVRLP) using amikacin in horses for the treatment of septic arthritis is actively being researched (Alkabes et al. 2011; Beccar-Verela et al. 2011; Kelmer et al. 2013).

Pharmacology/Actions

Amikacin, like the other aminoglycoside antibiotics, act on susceptible bacteria presumably by irreversibly binding to the 30S ribosomal subunit thereby inhibiting protein synthesis. It is considered a bactericidal concentration-dependent antibiotic.

Amikacin's spectrum of activity includes: coverage against many aerobic gram-negative and some aerobic gram-positive bacteria, including most species of *E. coli*, Klebsiella, Proteus, Pseudomonas, Salmonella, Enterobacter, Serratia, and Shigella, Mycoplasma, and Staphylococcus. Several strains of *Pseudomonas aeruginosa*, Proteus, and Serratia that are resistant to gentamicin will still be killed by amikacin.

Antimicrobial activity of the aminoglycosides is enhanced in an alkaline environment.

The aminoglycoside antibiotics are inactive against fungi, viruses and most anaerobic bacteria.

Pharmacokinetics

Amikacin, like the other aminoglycosides is not appreciably absorbed after oral or intrauterine administration, but is absorbed from topical administration (not from skin or the urinary bladder) when used in irrigations during surgical procedures. Patients receiving oral aminoglycosides with hemorrhagic or necrotic enteritises may absorb appreciable quantities of the drug. After IM administration to dogs and cats, peak levels occur from 1/2-1 hour later. Subcutaneous injection results in slightly delayed peak levels and with more variability than after IM injection. Bioavailability from extravascular injection (IM or SC) is greater than 90%.

After absorption, aminoglycosides are distributed primarily in the extracellular fluid. They are found in ascitic, pleural, pericardial, peritoneal, synovial and abscess fluids; high levels are found in sputum, bronchial secretions and bile. Aminoglycosides are mini-

mally protein bound (<20%, streptomycin 35%) to plasma proteins. Aminoglycosides do not readily cross the blood-brain barrier nor penetrate ocular tissue. CSF levels are unpredictable and range from 0-50% of those found in the serum. Therapeutic levels are found in bone, heart, gallbladder and lung tissues after parenteral dosing. Aminoglycosides tend to accumulate in certain tissues such as the inner ear and kidneys, which may help explain their toxicity. Volumes of distribution have been reported to be 0.15-0.3 L/kg in adult cats and dogs, and 0.26 – 0.58 L/kg in horses. Volumes of distribution may be significantly larger in neonates and juvenile animals due to their higher extracellular fluid fractions. Aminoglycosides cross the placenta; fetal concentrations range from 15-50% of those found in maternal serum.

Elimination of aminoglycosides after parenteral administration occurs almost entirely by glomerular filtration. The approximate elimination half-lives for amikacin have been reported to be 5 hours in foals, 1.14-2.3 hours in adult horses, 2.2-2.7 hours in calves, 1 hour in cows, 1.5 hours in sheep, and 0.5-2 hours in dogs and cats. Patients with decreased renal function can have significantly prolonged half-lives. In humans with normal renal function, elimination rates can be highly variable with the aminoglycoside antibiotics.

Contraindications/Precautions/Warnings

Aminoglycosides are contraindicated in patients who are hypersensitive to them. Because these drugs are often the only effective agents in severe gram-negative infections, there are no other absolute contraindications to their use. However, they should be used with extreme caution in patients with preexisting renal disease with concomitant monitoring and dosage interval adjustments made. Other risk factors for the development of toxicity include age (both neonatal and geriatric patients), fever, sepsis and dehydration.

Because aminoglycosides can cause irreversible ototoxicity, they should be used with caution in "working" dogs (*e.g.*, "seeing-eye," herding, dogs for the hearing impaired, etc.).

Aminoglycosides should be used with caution in patients with neuromuscular disorders (*e.g.*, myasthenia gravis) due to their neuromuscular blocking activity.

Sighthounds may require reduced dosages of aminoglycosides as they have significantly smaller volumes of distribution.

Because aminoglycosides are eliminated primarily through renal mechanisms, they should be used cautiously, preferably with serum monitoring and dosage adjustment in neonatal or geriatric animals.

Aminoglycosides are generally considered contraindicated in rabbits/hares as they adversely affect the GI flora balance in these animals.

Adverse Effects

Aminoglycosides can be nephrotoxic and ototoxic. The nephrotoxic (tubular necrosis) mechanisms of these drugs are not completely understood, but are probably related to interference with phospholipid metabolism in the lysosomes of proximal renal tubular cells, resulting in leakage of proteolytic enzymes into the cytoplasm. Nephrotoxicity risks increase with prolonged therapy. Nephrotoxicity is usually manifested by: increases in BUN, creatinine, nonprotein nitrogen in the serum, and decreases in urine specific gravity and creatinine clearance. Proteinuria and cells or casts may be seen in the urine. Nephrotoxicity is usually reversible once the drug is discontinued. While gentamicin may be more nephrotoxic and amikacin less nephrotoxic than the other aminoglycosides, the incidences of nephrotoxicity with all of these agents require caution and monitoring.

Ototoxicity (8th cranial nerve toxicity) of the aminoglycosides can manifest by either auditory and/or vestibular clinical signs and may be irreversible. Vestibular clinical signs are more frequent with streptomycin, gentamicin, or tobramycin. Auditory clinical signs are more frequent with amikacin or neomycin but either form can occur with any of these drugs. Cats are apparently very sensitive to the vestibular effects of the aminoglycosides.

Aminoglycosides can also cause neuromuscular blockade, facial edema, pain/inflammation at injection site, peripheral neuropathy and hypersensitivity reactions. Rarely, GI clinical signs, hematologic and hepatic effects have been reported.

Reproductive/Nursing Safety

Aminoglycosides can cross the placenta and while rare, may cause 8th cranial nerve toxicity or nephrotoxicity in fetuses. Because the drug should only be used in serious infections, the benefits of therapy may exceed the potential risks. In humans, the FDA categorizes this drug as category **C** for use during pregnancy (*Animal studies have shown an adverse effect on the fetus, but there are no adequate studies in humans; or there are no animal reproduction studies and no adequate studies in humans.*) In a separate system evaluating the safety of drugs in canine and feline pregnancy (Papich 1989), this drug is categorized as class: **C** (*These drugs may have potential risks. Studies in people or laboratory animals have uncovered risks, and these drugs should be used cautiously as a last resort when the benefit of therapy clearly outweighs the risks.*)

Aminoglycosides are excreted in milk. While potentially, amikacin ingested with milk could alter GI flora and cause diarrhea, amikacin in milk is unlikely to be of significant concern after the first few days of life (colostrum period).

Overdosage/Acute Toxicity

Should an inadvertent overdosage be administered, three treatments have been recommended. Hemodialysis is very effective in reducing serum levels of the drug but is not a viable option for most veterinary patients. Peritoneal dialysis also will reduce serum levels but is much less efficacious. Complexation of drug with ticarcillin (12 – 20 g/day in humans) is reportedly nearly as effective as hemodialysis. Amikacin is less affected by this effect than either tobramycin or gentamicin, and it is assumed that reduction in serum levels will also be minimized.

Drug Interactions

The following drug interactions with amikacin have either been reported or are theoretical in humans or animals and may be of significance in veterinary patients. Unless otherwise noted, use together is not necessarily contraindicated, but weigh the potential risks and perform additional monitoring when appropriate.

- **BETA-LACTAM ANTIBIOTICS** (*e.g.*, **penicillins, cephalosporins**): May have synergistic effects against some bacteria; some potential for physical inactivation of aminoglycosides *in vitro* (do not mix together) and *in vivo* (patients in renal failure).
- **CEPHALOSPORINS**: The concurrent use of aminoglycosides with cephalosporins is somewhat controversial. Potentially, cephalosporins could cause additive nephrotoxicity when used with aminoglycosides, but this interaction has only been well documented with cephaloridine and cephalothin (both no longer marketed).
- **DIURETICS, LOOP** (*e.g.*, **furosemide, torsemide**) or **OSMOTIC** (*e.g.,* **mannitol**): Concurrent use with loop or osmotic diuretics may increase the nephrotoxic or ototoxic potential of the aminoglycosides.
- **NSAIDS:** Because NSAIDs may cause nephrotoxic effects; some believe that concurrent use with aminoglycosides should be avoided.

- **NEPHROTOXIC DRUGS, OTHER** (*e.g.*, **cisplatin, amphotericin B, polymyxin B**, or **vancomycin**): Potential for increased risk for nephrotoxicity.
- **NEUROMUSCULAR BLOCKING AGENTS & ANESTHETICS, GENERAL**: Concomitant use with general anesthetics or neuromuscular blocking agents could potentiate neuromuscular blockade.

Laboratory Considerations

- Amikacin serum concentrations may be falsely decreased if the patient is also receiving **beta-lactam antibiotics** and the serum is stored prior to analysis. It is recommended that if assay is delayed, samples be frozen and, if possible, drawn at times when the beta-lactam antibiotic is at a trough.

Doses

Note: There is an FDA-approved dosage for systemic use in dogs, but most infectious disease clinicians now agree that aminoglycosides should be dosed once a day in most patients (mammals). This dosing regimen yields higher peak levels with resultant greater bacterial kill, and as aminoglycosides exhibit a "post-antibiotic effect", surviving susceptible bacteria generally do not replicate as rapidly even when antibiotic concentrations are below MIC. Periods where levels are low may also decrease the "adaptive resistance" (bacteria take up less drug in the presence of continuous exposure) that can occur. Once daily dosing may decrease the toxicity of aminoglycosides as lower urinary concentrations may mean reduced uptake into renal tubular cells. However, patients that are neutropenic (or otherwise immunosuppressed) may benefit from more frequent dosing (q8h). Patients with significantly diminished renal function that must receive aminoglycosides may need to be dosed at longer intervals than once daily. Clinical drug monitoring is strongly suggested for these patients. Except where noted all dosages are extra-label.

- **DOGS:**

  For labeled indications [Genitourinary tract infections (cystitis) caused by susceptible strains of *Escherichia coli* and *Proteus* sp. Skin and soft tissue infections caused by susceptible strains of *Pseudomonas* sp. and *Escherichia coli*.]; (FDA-approved; See the Note above regarding this dosage.): 10 mg/kg SC or IM twice daily. Dogs with skin and soft tissue infections should be treated for a minimum of 7 days and those with genitourinary infections should be treated for 7 to 21 days or until culture negative and asymptomatic. If no response is observed after three days of treatment, therapy should be discontinued and the case re-evaluated. Maximum duration of therapy should not exceed 30 days. (Adapted from label; *Amiglyde-V*®)

  For susceptible infections and empirical therapy (extra-label): 15 – 30 mg/kg IV, IM, SC once daily. **Note:** In Greyhounds (and potentially other sighthounds) a reduction in dose to 10 mg/kg IV q24h or 15 mg/kg SC/IM q24h has been recommended (KuKanich 2008). Neutropenic or immunocompromised patients may need to be dosed q8h (above dose divided) (Trepanier 1999). Septic patients may be started at 20 – 30 mg/kg IV once daily. **Note:** Dosage should be adjusted based on kidney function and serum levels when possible.

- **CATS:**

  For susceptible infections and empirical therapy (extra-label): 10 – 15 mg/kg IV, IM, SC once daily. Neutropenic or immunocompromised patients may still need to be dosed q8h (above dose divided). Septic patients may be started at 20 mg/kg IV once daily. **Note:** Dosage should be adjusted based on kidney function and serum levels when possible. When renal function is significantly decreased (*e.g.* IRS stage II or II) if less nephrotoxic drugs cannot be used, dosage amount remains the same but dosing interval is increased.

■ **FERRETS:**

For susceptible infections (extra-label):

a) 8 – 16 mg/kg IM or IV once daily. (Williams 2000)

b) 8 – 16 mg/kg/day SC, IM, IV divided q8–24h. (Morrisey et al. 2004)

■ **RABBITS/RODENTS/SMALL MAMMALS:**

All are extra-label.

a) **Rabbits:** 8 – 16 mg/kg daily dose (may divide into q8h-q24h) SC, IM or IV. Increased efficacy and decreased toxicity if given once daily. If given IV, dilute into 4 mL/kg of saline and give over 20 minutes. (Ivey et al. 2000)

b) **Rabbits:** 5 – 10 mg/kg SC, IM, IV divided q8–24h. **Guinea pigs:** 10 – 15 mg/kg SC, IM, IV divided q8–24h. **Chinchillas:** 10 – 15 mg/kg SC, IM, IV divided q8–24h. **Hamsters, rats, mice:** 10 mg/kg SC, IM q12h. **Prairie Dogs:** 5 mg/kg SC, IM q12h. (Morrisey et al. 2004)

c) **Chinchillas:** 2 – 5 mg/kg SC, IM q8–12h. (Hayes 2000)

■ **HORSES:**

For uterine infusion (labeled dosage; FDA-approved): 2 grams mixed with 200 mL sterile normal saline (0.9% sodium chloride for injection) and aseptically infused into uterus daily for 3 consecutive days (Package insert; Amiglyde-V®).

For susceptible infections and empirical therapy (extra-label): Adults: 10 mg/kg IV or IM once daily. For neonatal foals: 20 – 25 mg/kg IV or IM once daily. It is strongly recommended to individualize dosage based upon therapeutic drug monitoring.

For treatment of septic joints (extra-label): 20 mg/kg IV once daily. For regional intravenous limb perfusion (RILP) administration in standing horses: Usual dosages range from 500 mg – 2 grams; dosage must be greater than 250 mg when a cephalic vein is used for perfusion and careful placement of tourniquets must be performed (Parra-Sanchez et al. 2006).

■ **BIRDS:**

For susceptible infections (all are extra-label):

a) For sunken eyes/sinusitis in macaws caused by susceptible bacteria: 40 mg/kg IM once or twice daily. Must also flush sinuses with saline mixed with appropriate antibiotic (10 – 30 mL per nostril). May require 2 weeks of treatment. (Karpinski et al. 1986)

b) 15 mg/kg IM or SC q12h. (Hoeffer 1995).

c) For gram-negative infections resistant to gentamicin: Dilute commercial solution and administer 15 – 20 mg/kg (0.015 mg/g) IM once a day or twice a day. (Clubb 1986)

d) **Ratites:** 7.6 – 11 mg/kg IM twice daily; air cell: 10 – 25 mg/egg; egg dip: 2000 mg/gallon of distilled water pH of 6. (Jenson 1998)

■ **REPTILES:**

For susceptible infections (all are extra-label):

a) **For snakes:** 5 mg/kg IM (forebody) loading dose, then 2.5 mg/kg q72h for 7-9 treatments. Commonly used in respiratory infections. Use a lower dose for Python curtus. (Gauvin 1993)

b) Study done in gopher snakes: 5 mg/kg IM loading dose, then 2.5 mg/kg q72h. House snakes at high end of their preferred optimum ambient temperature. (Mader et al. 1985)

c) **For bacterial shell diseases in turtles:** 10 mg/kg daily in water turtles, every other day in land turtles and tortoises for 7-10 days. Used commonly with a beta-lactam antibiotic.

Recommended to begin therapy with 20 mL/kg fluid injection. Maintain hydration and monitor uric acid levels when possible. (Rosskopf 1986)

d) **For Crocodilians:** 2.25 mg/kg IM q 72-96h. (Jacobson 2000)

e) **For gram-negative respiratory disease:** 3.5 mg/kg IM, SC or via lung catheter every 3–10 days for 30 days. (Klaphake 2005)

■ **FISH:**

For susceptible infections (extra-label): 5 mg/kg IM loading dose, then 2.5 mg/kg every 72 hours for 5 treatments. (Lewbart 2006)

Monitoring

■ Efficacy (cultures, clinical signs, WBC's and clinical signs associated with infection). Therapeutic drug monitoring is highly recommended when using this drug systemically. Attempt to draw samples at 1, 2, and 4 hours post dose. Peak level should be at least 40 micrograms/mL and the 4-hour sample less than 10 micrograms/mL.

■ Adverse effect monitoring is essential. Pre-therapy renal function tests and urinalysis (repeated during therapy) are recommended. Casts in the urine are often the initial sign of impending nephrotoxicity.

■ Gross monitoring of vestibular or auditory toxicity is recommended.

Client Information

■ With appropriate training, owners may give subcutaneous injections at home, but routine monitoring of therapy for efficacy and toxicity must still be done.

■ Clients should also understand that the potential exists for severe toxicity (nephrotoxicity, ototoxicity) developing from this medication.

■ Use in food producing animals is controversial as drug residues may persist for long periods.

Chemistry/Synonyms

A semi-synthetic aminoglycoside derived from kanamycin, amikacin occurs as a white, crystalline powder that is sparingly soluble in water. The sulfate salt is formed during the manufacturing process. 1.3 grams of amikacin sulfate is equivalent to 1 gram of amikacin. Amikacin may also be expressed in terms of units. 50,600 Units are equal to 50.9 mg of base. The commercial injection is a clear to straw-colored solution and the pH is adjusted to 3.5-5.5 with sulfuric acid.

Amikacin sulfate may also be known as: amikacin sulphate, amikacini sulfas, or BB-K8; many trade names are available.

Storage/Stability

Amikacin sulfate for injection should be stored at room temperature (15-30°C); freezing or temperatures above 40°C should be avoided. Solutions may become very pale yellow with time but this does not indicate a loss of potency.

Amikacin is stable for at least 2 years at room temperature. Autoclaving commercially available solutions at 15 pounds of pressure at 120°C for 60 minutes did not result in any loss of potency.

Compatibility/Compounding Considerations

When given intravenously, amikacin should be diluted into suitable IV diluent such as normal saline, D5W or LRS and administered over at least 30 minutes.

Amikacin sulfate is reportedly **compatible** and stable in all commonly used intravenous solutions and with the following drugs: ascorbic acid injection, bleomycin sulfate, calcium chloride/gluconate, cefoxitin sodium, chloramphenicol sodium succinate, chlorpheniramine maleate, cimetidine HCl, clindamycin phosphate, dimenhydrinate, diphenhydramine HCl, epinephrine HCl, hyaluronidase, hydrocortisone sodium phosphate/succinate, lincomycin HCl, metronidazole (with or without sodium bicarbonate), norepinephrine bitartrate, pentobarbital sodium, phenobarbital sodium, phytonadione, prochlorperazine edisylate, promethazine HCl, sodium bicarbonate, succinylcholine chloride, vancomycin HCl and verapamil HCl.

The following drugs or solutions are reportedly **incompatible** or only **compatible in specific situations** with amikacin: amphotericin B, ampicillin sodium, cefazolin sodium, chlorothiazide sodium, dexamethasone sodium phosphate, erythromycin glucceptate, heparin sodium, oxytetracycline HCl, penicillin G potassium, phenytoin sodium, potassium chloride (in dextran 6% in sodium chloride 0.9%; stable with potassium chloride in "standard" solutions), vitamin B-complex with C and warfarin sodium. Compatibility is dependent upon factors such as pH, concentration, temperature and diluent used; consult specialized references or a hospital pharmacist for more specific information.

In vitro inactivation of aminoglycoside antibiotics by beta-lactam antibiotics is well documented. While amikacin is less susceptible to this effect, it is usually recommended to avoid mixing these compounds together in the same syringe or IV bag unless administration occurs promptly. See also the information in the Drug Interaction and Drug/Lab Interaction sections.

Dosage Forms/Regulatory Status

VETERINARY-LABELED PRODUCTS:

Amikacin Sulfate, Injection: 50 mg (of amikacin base) per mL in 50 mL vials (Rx). FDA-approved for use in dogs. While this drug is still listed in the FDA's Green Book of approved animal drugs, it may not be commercially available.

Amikacin Sulfate Intrauterine Solution: 250 mg (of amikacin base) per mL in 48 mL vials; (Rx). FDA-approved for use in horses not intended for food. While this drug is still listed in the FDA's Green Book of approved animal drugs, it may not be commercially available.

Warning: Amikacin is not FDA-approved for use in cattle or other food-producing animals in the USA. Drug residues may persist for long periods, particularly in renal tissue. For guidance with determining use and withdrawal times, contact FARAD (see Phone Numbers & Websites in the appendix for contact information).

HUMAN-LABELED PRODUCTS:

Amikacin Injection: 50 mg/mL & 250 mg/mL in 2 mL & 4 mL; generic; (Rx)

Revisions/References

Monograph revised/updated August 2013.

Alkabes, S. B., et al. (2011). Comparison of two tourniquets and determination of amikacin sulfate concentrations after metacarpophalangeal joint lavage performed simultaneously with intravenous regional limb perfusion in horses. *American Journal of Veterinary Research* 72(5): 613-9.

Beccar-Verela, A., et al. (2011). Effect of Experimentally Induced Synovitis on Amikacin Concentrations after Intravenous Regional Limb Perfusion. *Veterinary Surgery* 40: 891-7.

Clubb, S. L. (1986). Therapeutics: Individual and Flock Treatment Regimens. *Clinical Avian Medicine and Surgery*. G. J. Harrison and L. R. Harrison. Philadelphia, W.B. Saunders: 327-55.

Gauvin, J. (1993). Drug therapy in reptiles. *Seminars in Avian & Exotic Med* 2(1): 48-59.

Hayes, P. (2000). Diseases of Chinchillas. *Kirk's Current Veterinary Therapy: XIII Small Animal Practice*. J. Bonagura. Philadelphia, WB Saunders: 1152-7.

Hoeffer, H. (1995). Antimicrobials in pet birds. *Kirk's Current Veterinary Therapy:XII*. J. Bonagura. Philadelphia, W.B. Saunders: 1278-83.

Ivey, E. & J. Morrisey (2000). Therapeutics for Rabbits. *Vet Clin NA: Exotic Anim Pract* 3:1(Jan): 183-216.

Jacobson, E. (2000). Antibiotic Therapy for Reptiles. *Kirk's Current Veterinary Therapy: XIII Small Animal Practice*. J. Bonagura. Philadelphia, WB Saunders: 1168-69.

Jenson, J. (1998). Current ratite therapy. *The Veterinary Clinics of North America: Food Animal Practice* 16:3(November).

Karpinski, L. G. & S. L. Clubb (1986). Clinical aspects of ophthalmology in caged birds. *Current Veterinary Therapy IX: Small Animal Practice*. R. W. Kirk. Philadelphia, W.B. Saunders: 616-21.

Kelmer, G., et al. (2013). Evaluation of regional limb perfusion with amikacin using the saphenous, cephalic, and palmar digital veins in standing horses. *J. Vet. Pharmacol. Ther.* 36(3): 236-40.

Klaphake, E. (2005). *Sneezing turtles and wheezing snakes*. Proceedings: Western Vet Conf. accessed via Veterinary Information Network; vin.com

KuKanich, B. (2008). *Canine breed specific differences in clinical pharmacology*. Proceedings: WVC. accessed via Veterinary Information Network; vin.com

Lewbart, G. (2006). *Medicating the pet fish patient*. Proceedings: Western Vet Conf. accessed via Veterinary Information Network; vin.com

Mader, D. R., et al. (1985). Effects of ambient temperature on the half-life and dosage regimen of amikacin in the gopher snake. *JAVMA* 187(11): 1134-6.

Morrisey, J. & J. Carpenter (2004). Formulary. *Ferrets, Rabbits, and Rodents Clinical Medicine and Surgery 2nd ed.* K. Quesenberry and J. Carpenter. St Louis, Saunders.

Parra-Sanchez, A., et al. (2006). Pharmacokinetics and pharmacodynamics of enrofloxacin and a low dose of amikacin administered via regional intravenous limb perfusion in standing horses. *AJVR* 67(10): 1687-95.

Rosskopf, W. J. (1986). Shell diseases in turtles and tortoises. *Current Veterinary Therapy (CVT) IX Small Animal Practice*. R. W. Kirk. Philadelphia, WB Saunders: 751-9.

Trepanier, L. (1999). *Management of resistant infections in small animal patients*. Proceedings: American Veterinary Medical Association: 16th Annual Convention, New Orleans. accessed via Veterinary Information Network; vin.com

Williams, B. (2000). Therapeutics in Ferrets. *Vet Clin NA: Exotic Anim Pract* 3:1(Jan): 131-53.

Aminocaproic Acid

(a-**mee**-noe-ka-**proe**-ik)   Epsilon Aminocaproic Acid, Amicar®

Fibrinolysis Inhibitor/Antiprotease

Prescriber Highlights

▶ May be useful for treating degenerative myelopathies in dogs; efficacy questionable.

▶ Treatment may be very expensive, especially with large dogs.

▶ Contraindicated in DIC.

▶ Infrequently causes GI distress.

Uses/Indications

Aminocaproic acid is potentially useful to treat conditions of hyperfibrinolysis and prophylactically to prevent post-operative bleeding, especially in Greyhounds or other sighthounds. It has also been used for this purpose to help stabilize the clot or slow bleeding in horses with guttural pouch hemorrhage. A study in horses found that aminocaproic acid was not effective in preventing or reducing the severity of exercise-induced pulmonary hemorrhage (EIPH) (Buchholz et al. 2010).

Aminocaproic acid has been used as a treatment to degenerative myelopathy (seen primarily in German shepherds), but no controlled studies documenting its efficacy were located. One study (Polizopoulou et al. 2008) in 12 dogs where aminocaproic acid was used with acetylcysteine and vitamins B, C, and E, no improvement was noted with treatment and all dogs' neurological signs worsened with time.

There is some interest in evaluating aminocaproic acid for adjunctive treatment of immune-mediated thrombocytopenia in dogs, but efficacy and safety for this purpose remains to be investigated. In humans, it is primarily used for treating hyperfibrinolysis-induced hemorrhage.

Pharmacology/Actions

Aminocaproic acid inhibits fibrinolysis via its inhibitory effects on plasminogen activator substances and via some antiplasmin action.

Aminocaproic acid is thought to affect degenerative myelopathy by its antiprotease activity thereby reducing the activation of inflammatory enzymes that damage myelin.

Pharmacokinetics

No pharmacokinetic data was located for dogs.

In a study where 70 mg/kg doses were given IV to horses over 20 minutes, the drug was distributed rapidly and plasma levels remained above the proposed therapeutic level of 130 mcg/mL for one hour after the end of the infusion. Elimination half-life was

2.3 hours. The authors proposed that a constant rate infusion of 15 mg/kg/hr after the original infusion would maintain more prolonged therapeutic levels (Ross et al. 2006).

In humans, the drug is rapidly and completely absorbed after oral administration. The drug is well distributed in both intravascular and extravascular compartments and penetrates cells (including red blood cells). It is unknown if the drug enters maternal milk. It does not bind to plasma proteins. Terminal half-life is about 2 hours in humans and the drug is primarily renally excreted as unchanged drug.

Contraindications/Precautions/Warnings

Aminocaproic acid is contraindicated in patients with active intravascular clotting. It should only be used when the benefits outweigh the risks in patients with preexisting cardiac, renal or hepatic disease.

Adverse Effects

Aminocaproic acid appears to be well tolerated. In dogs treated with oral aminocaproic acid, about 1% exhibit clinical signs of GI irritation. It potentially can cause hyperkalemia particularly in renal impaired patients.

Reproductive/Nursing Safety

Some, but not all, animal studies have demonstrated teratogenicity; use when risk to benefit ratio merits. In humans, the FDA categorizes this drug as category **C** for use during pregnancy (*Animal studies have shown an adverse effect on the fetus, but there are no adequate studies in humans; or there are no animal reproduction studies and no adequate studies in humans.*)

Overdosage/Acute Toxicity

There is very limited information on overdoses with aminocaproic acid. The IV lethal dose in dogs is reportedly 2.3 g/kg. At lower IV overdosages, tonic-clonic seizures were noted in some dogs. There is no known antidote, but the drug is dialyzable.

Drug Interactions

The following drug interactions with aminocaproic acid have either been reported or are theoretical in humans or animals and may be of significance in veterinary patients. Unless otherwise noted, use together is not necessarily contraindicated, but weigh the potential risks and perform additional monitoring when appropriate.

- **ESTROGENS**: Hypercoagulation states may occur in patients receiving aminocaproic acid and estrogens.

Laboratory Considerations

- Serum **potassium** may be elevated by aminocaproic acid, especially in patients with preexisting renal failure.

Doses

- **DOGS:**

  As an antifibrinolytic to reduce delayed-onset bleeding after surgery in Greyhounds (extra-label): 500 mg (approx. 15.6 – 17.5 mg/kg) PO q8h for 5 days beginning the night of surgery (Marin et al. 2012).

  For adjunctive treatment of degenerative myelopathy (seen primarily in German shepherds); (extra-label): Aminocaproic acid 500 mg/dog PO q8h indefinitely. Used in conjunction with acetylcysteine at 25 mg/kg PO q8h for 2 weeks, then q8h every other day. The 20% solution should be diluted to 5% with chicken broth or suitable diluent. Other treatments may include prednisone (0.25 – 0.5 mg/kg PO daily for 10 days then every other day), Vitamin C (1000 mg PO q12h) and Vitamin E (1000 Int. Units PO q12). **Note:** No treatment has been shown to be effective in published trials. (Shell 2003)

- **HORSES:**

  As an antifibrinolytic for guttural pouch hemorrhage (extra-label): 40 mg/kg intravenous bolus, followed by 10 – 20 mg/kg q6h. (Mudge 2012)

Client Information

- Drug costs to treat a German shepherd-sized dog can be substantial.
- As no well-controlled studies have documented that this drug is effective for treating degenerative myelopathy, its use should be considered investigational.

Chemistry/Synonyms

An inhibitor of fibrinolysis, aminocaproic acid is a synthetic monamino carboxylic acid occurring as a fine, white crystalline powder. It is slightly soluble in alcohol and freely soluble in water and has pKa's of 4.43 and 10.75. The injectable product has its pH adjusted to approximately 6.8.

Aminocaproic acid may also be known as: acidum aminocaproicum, CL-10304 CY-116, EACA, epsilon aminocaproic acid, 6-aminohexanoic acid, JD-177, NSC-26154, *Amicar®, Capracid®, Capramol®, Caproamin®, Caprolisin®, Epsicaprom®, Hemocaprol®, Hemocid®, Hexalense®,* or *Ipsilon®*.

Storage/Stability

Products should be stored at room temperature. Avoid freezing liquid preparations. Discoloration will occur if aldehydes or aldehydic sugars are present.

Compatibility/Compounding Considerations

When given as an intravenous infusion, normal saline, D5W and Ringer's Injection have been recommended for use as the infusion diluent.

Dosage Forms/Regulatory Status

VETERINARY-LABELED PRODUCTS: None

The ARCI (Racing Commissioners International) has designated this drug as a class 4 substance. See the appendix for more information.

HUMAN-LABELED PRODUCTS:

Aminocaproic Acid; Oral Tablets: 500 mg & 1000 mg; *Amicar®*, generic; (Rx)

Aminocaproic Oral Solution: 250 mg/mL in 237 mL & 473 mL; *Amicar®*, generic; (Rx)

Aminocaproic Acid Injection: 250 mg/mL in 20 mL vials; generic; (Rx)

Revisions/References

Monograph revised/updated August 2013.

Buchholz, B. M., et al. (2010). Effects of intravenous aminocaproic acid on exercise-induced pulmonary haemorrhage (EIPH). *Equine Veterinary Journal* **42**: 256-60.
Marin, L. M., et al. (2012). Epsilon Aminocaproic Acid for the Prevention of Delayed Postoperative Bleeding in Retired Racing Greyhounds Undergoing Gonadectomy. *Veterinary Surgery* **41**(5): 594-603.
Mudge, M. (2012). *Guttural Pouch Hemorrhage: Stabilization and Resuscitation.* International Veterinary Emergency and Critical Care Symposium accessed via Veterinary Information Network; vin.com
Polizopoulou, Z. S., et al. (2008). Evaluation of a proposed therapeutic protocol in 12 dogs with tentative degenerative myelopathy. *Acta Veterinaria Hungarica* **56**(3): 293-301.
Ross, J., et al. (2006). *Pharmacokinetics and pharmacodynamics of aminocaproic acid in horses.* Proceedings: IVECC. accessed via Veterinary Information Network; vin.com
Shell, L. (2003). "Degenerative Myelopathy (Degenerative Radiculomyelopathy)." *Associates Database.*

Aminopentamide Hydrogen Sulfate

(a-**mee**-noe-**pent**-a-mide)   Centrine®

Anticholinergic/Antispasmodic

Prescriber Highlights

▶ Anticholinergic/antispasmodic labeled for GI indications in small animals. Today, use is rarely recommended except for vestibular induced vomiting.

▶ Typical adverse effect profile ("dry, hot, red"); potentially could cause tachycardia.

▶ Contraindicated in glaucoma; relatively contraindicated in tachycardias, heart disease, GI obstruction, etc.

Uses/Indications

The manufacturer states that the drug is indicated "in the treatment of acute abdominal visceral spasm, pylorospasm or hypertrophic gastritis and associated nausea, vomiting and/or diarrhea" for use in dogs and cats.

Pharmacology/Actions

Aminopentamide is an anticholinergic agent that when compared to atropine has been described as having a greater effect on reducing colonic contractions and less mydriatic and salivary effects. It reportedly may also reduce gastric acid secretion.

Pharmacokinetics

No information was located.

Contraindications/Precautions/Warnings

The manufacturer lists glaucoma as an absolute contraindication to therapy and to use the drug cautiously, if at all, in patients with pyloric obstruction. Additionally, aminopentamide should not be used if the patient has a history of hypersensitivity to anticholinergic drugs, tachycardias secondary to thyrotoxicosis or cardiac insufficiency, myocardial ischemia, unstable cardiac status during acute hemorrhage, GI obstructive disease, paralytic ileus, severe ulcerative colitis, obstructive uropathy or myasthenia gravis (unless used to reverse adverse muscarinic effects secondary to therapy).

Antimuscarinic agents should be avoided or used with extreme caution in patients with known or suspected GI infections (*e.g.*, parvovirus enteritis), or with autonomic neuropathy. Atropine or other antimuscarinic agents can decrease GI motility and prolong retention of the causative agent(s) or toxin(s) resulting in prolonged clinical signs.

Antimuscarinic agents should be used with caution in patients with hepatic disease, renal disease, hyperthyroidism, hypertension, CHF, tachyarrhythmias, prostatic hypertrophy, esophageal reflux, and in geriatric or pediatric patients.

Adverse Effects

Adverse effects resulting from aminopentamide therapy may include dry mouth, dry eyes, blurred vision, and urinary hesitancy. Urinary retention is a symptom of too high a dose and the drug should be withdrawn until resolved.

Overdosage/Acute Toxicity

No specific information was located regarding acute overdosage clinical signs or treatment for this agent. The following discussion is from the atropine monograph that could be used as a guideline for treating overdoses:

If a recent oral ingestion, emptying of gut contents and administration of activated charcoal and saline cathartics may be warranted. Treat clinical signs supportively and symptomatically. Do not use phenothiazines as they may contribute to the anticholinergic effects. Fluid therapy and standard treatments for shock may be instituted.

The use of physostigmine is controversial and should probably be reserved for cases where the patient exhibits either extreme agitation and is at risk for injuring themselves or others, or for cases where supraventricular tachycardias and sinus tachycardias are severe or life threatening. The usual dose for physostigmine (human) is: 2 mg IV slowly (for average sized adult), if no response, may repeat every 20 minutes until reversal of toxic antimuscarinic effects or cholinergic effects takes place. The human pediatric dose is 0.02 mg/kg slow IV (repeat q10 minutes as above) and may be a reasonable choice for treatment of small animals. Physostigmine adverse effects (*e.g.*, bronchoconstriction, bradycardia, seizures) may be treated with small doses of IV atropine.

Drug Interactions

No specific interactions were noted for this product. The following drug interactions with atropine, a similar drug have either been reported or are theoretical in humans or animals and may be of significance in veterinary patients. Unless otherwise noted, use together is not necessarily contraindicated, but weigh the potential risks and perform additional monitoring when appropriate.

- **ANTIHISTAMINES, PROCAINAMIDE, QUINIDINE, MEPERIDINE, BENZODIAZEPINES, PHENOTHIAZINES**: May enhance the activity of atropine and its derivatives.
- **PRIMIDONE, DISOPYRAMIDE, NITRATES**: May potentiate the adverse effects of atropine and its derivatives.
- **CORTICOSTEROIDS** (**long-term use**): May increase intraocular pressure.
- **NITROFURANTOIN, THIAZIDE DIURETICS, SYMPATHOMIMETICS**: Atropine and its derivatives may enhance actions.
- **METOCLOPRAMIDE**: Atropine and its derivatives may antagonize metoclopramide actions.

Doses

- **DOGS/CATS:**

  For labeled indications (FDA-approved): May be administered every 8-12 hours via IM, SC or oral routes. If the desired effect is not attained, the dosage may be gradually increased up to 5 times those listed below: Animals weighing: 10 lbs. or less: 0.1 mg; 11-20 lbs.: 0.2 mg; 21-50 lbs.: 0.3 mg; 51-100 lbs.: 0.4 mg; over 100 lbs.: 0.5 mg (Package Insert; *Centrine*®)

Monitoring

- Clinical efficacy.
- Adverse effects (see above).

Client Information

- Oral tablets may be given with or without food.
- Side effects can include dry mouth or eyes, difficulty urinating.

Chemistry/Synonyms

An antispasmodic, anticholinergic agent, aminopentamide hydrogen sulfate has a chemical name of 4-(dimethylamino)-2,2-diphenylvaleramide.

Aminopentamide hydrogen sulfate may also be known as dimevamid or *Centrine*®.

Storage/Stability

Store aminopentamide tablets and injection at controlled room temperature (15–30°C; 59–86°F).

Compatibility/Compounding Considerations

No specific information noted.

Dosage Forms/Regulatory Status

VETERINARY-LABELED PRODUCTS:

Aminopentamide Hydrogen Sulfate Tablets: 0.2 mg; *Centrine*®; (Rx). FDA-approved for use in dogs and cats only.

Aminopentamide Hydrogen Sulfate Injection: 0.5 mg/mL in 10 mL vials; *Centrine*®; (Rx). FDA-approved for use in dogs and cats only.

HUMAN-LABELED PRODUCTS: NONE.

Revisions/References
Monograph revised/updated August 2013.

Aminophylline
(am-in-**off**-i-lin)
Phosphodiesterase Inhibitor Bronchodilator

Prescriber Highlights
► Parenteral form of theophylline; bronchodilator drug with diuretic activity. Used short-term for bronchospasm & cardiogenic pulmonary edema. For oral use—see the Theophylline monograph.
► Narrow therapeutic index in humans, but dogs appear to be less susceptible to toxic effects at higher plasma levels.
► Many drug interactions.

Uses/Indications
Aminophylline is the parenteral form for administering theophylline. The theophyllines (aminophylline and theophylline) are used primarily for their bronchodilatory effects. While once used routinely in patients with myocardial failure and/or pulmonary edema, aminophylline is rarely recommended today for this purpose. While theophyllines are still used, especially in animals with 'cough', they must be used cautiously due to their adverse effects and toxicity.

Pharmacology/Actions
The theophyllines competitively inhibit phosphodiesterase thereby increasing amounts of cyclic AMP that then increase the release of endogenous epinephrine. The elevated levels of cAMP may also inhibit the release of histamine and slow reacting substance of anaphylaxis (SRS-A). The myocardial and neuromuscular transmission effects that the theophyllines possess may be a result of translocating intracellular ionized calcium.

The theophyllines directly relax smooth muscles in the bronchi and pulmonary vasculature, induce diuresis, increase gastric acid secretion and inhibit uterine contractions. They have weak chronotropic and inotropic action, stimulate the CNS and can cause respiratory stimulation (centrally-mediated).

Pharmacokinetics
Theophylline is distributed throughout the extracellular fluids and body tissues. It crosses the placenta and is distributed into milk (70% of serum levels). In dogs, at therapeutic serum levels only about 7-14% is bound to plasma proteins. The volume of distribution of theophylline for dogs has been reported to be 0.82 L/kg. The volume of distribution in cats is reported to be 0.46 L/kg, and in horses, 0.85-1.02 L/kg. Because of the low volumes of distribution and theophylline's low lipid solubility, obese patients should be dosed on a lean body weight basis.

Theophylline is metabolized primarily in the liver (in humans) to 3-methylxanthine, which has weak bronchodilator activity. Renal clearance contributes only about 10% to the overall plasma clearance of theophylline. The reported elimination half-lives (mean values) in various species are: dogs ≈ 5.7 hours; cats ≈ 7.8 hours, pigs ≈ 11 hours; and horses ≈ 11.9-17 hours. In humans, there are very wide interpatient variations in serum half-lives and resultant serum levels. It could be expected that similar variability exists in veterinary patients, particularly those with concurrent illnesses.

Contraindications/Precautions/Warnings
Aminophylline is contraindicated in patients who are hypersensitive to any of the xanthines, including theobromine or caffeine. Patients who are hypersensitive to ethylenediamine should not take aminophylline.

The theophyllines should be administered with caution in patients with severe cardiac disease, seizure disorders, gastric ulcers, hyperthyroidism, renal or hepatic disease, severe hypoxia, or severe hypertension. Because it may cause or worsen preexisting arrhythmias, patients with cardiac arrhythmias should receive theophylline only with caution and enhanced monitoring. Neonatal and geriatric patients may have decreased clearances of theophylline and be more sensitive to its toxic effects. Patients with CHF may have prolonged serum half-lives of theophylline.

Adverse Effects
The theophyllines can produce CNS stimulation and gastrointestinal irritation after administration by any route. Most adverse effects are related to the serum level of the drug and may be symptomatic of toxic blood levels; dogs appear to tolerate levels that may be very toxic to humans. Some mild CNS excitement and GI disturbances are not uncommon when starting therapy and generally resolve with chronic administration in conjunction with monitoring and dosage adjustments.

Dogs and cats can exhibit clinical signs of nausea and vomiting, insomnia, increased gastric acid secretion, diarrhea, polyphagia, polydipsia, and polyuria. Side effects in horses are generally dose related and may include: nervousness, excitability (auditory, tactile, and visual), tremors, diaphoresis, tachycardia, and ataxia. Seizures or cardiac dysrhythmias may occur in severe intoxications.

Reproductive/Nursing Safety
In humans, the FDA categorizes this drug as category ***C*** for use during pregnancy (*Animal studies have shown an adverse effect on the fetus, but there are no adequate studies in humans; or there are no animal reproduction studies and no adequate studies in humans.*)

Overdosage/Acute Toxicity
Clinical signs of toxicity (see above) are usually associated with levels greater than 20 micrograms/mL in humans and become more severe as the serum level exceeds that value. Tachycardias, arrhythmias, and CNS effects (seizures, hyperthermia) are considered the most life-threatening aspects of toxicity. Dogs appear to tolerate serum levels higher than 20 micrograms/mL.

Treatment of theophylline toxicity is supportive. Patients suffering from seizures should have an adequate airway maintained and treated with IV diazepam. The patient should be constantly monitored for cardiac arrhythmias and tachycardia. Fluid and electrolytes should be monitored and corrected as necessary. Hyperthermia may be treated with phenothiazines and tachycardia treated with propranolol if either condition is considered life threatening.

Drug Interactions
The following drug interactions with aminophylline or theophylline have either been reported or are theoretical in humans or animals and may be of significance in veterinary patients. Unless otherwise noted, use together is not necessarily contraindicated, but weigh the potential risks and perform additional monitoring when appropriate.

The following drugs can **decrease** theophylline levels:
- **BARBITURATES** (*e.g.,* **phenobarbital**)
- **CARBAMAZEPINE**: May increase or decrease levels.
- **CHARCOAL**
- **HYDANTOINS** (*e.g.,* **phenytoin**)
- **ISONIAZID**: May increase or decrease levels.
- **KETOCONAZOLE**

- **LOOP DIURETICS** (*e.g.,* **furosemide**): May increase or decrease levels.
- **RIFAMPIN**
- **SYMPATHOMIMETICS** (*e.g.,* **beta-agonists**)

The following drugs can **increase** theophylline levels:
- **ALLOPURINOL**
- **BETA-BLOCKERS** (**non-selective such as propranolol**)
- **CALCIUM CHANNEL BLOCKERS** (*e.g.,* **diltiazem, verapamil**)
- **CIMETIDINE**
- **CORTICOSTEROIDS**
- **FLUOROQUINOLONES** (*e.g.,* **enrofloxacin, ciprofloxacin**): If adding either, consider reducing the dose of theophylline by 30%. Monitor for toxicity/efficacy. Marbofloxacin reduces clearance of theophylline in dogs, but not with clinical significance. In animals with renal impairment, marbofloxacin may interfere with theophylline metabolism in a clinically relevant manner.
- **MACROLIDES** (*e.g.,* **erythromycin; clindamycin, lincomycin**)
- **THIABENDAZOLE**
- **THYROID HORMONES** (in hypothyroid patients)

Theophylline may decrease the effects of following drugs:
- **BENZODIAZEPINES**
- **LITHIUM**
- **PANCURONIUM**
- **PROPOFOL**

- **EPHEDRINE, ISOPROTERENOL**: Toxic synergism (arrhythmias) can occur if theophylline is used concurrently with sympathomimetics (especially ephedrine) or possibly isoproterenol.
- **KETAMINE**: Theophylline with ketamine can cause an increased incidence of seizures.

Laboratory Considerations

- Theophylline can cause falsely elevated values of serum **uric acid** if measured by the Bittner or colorimetric methods. Values are not affected if using the uricase method.
- Theophylline serum levels can be falsely elevated by **furosemide, phenylbutazone, probenecid, theobromine, caffeine, sulfathiazole, chocolate, or acetaminophen** if using a spectrophotometric method of assay.

Doses

Note: Theophyllines have a relatively low therapeutic index; determine dosage carefully. Because of aminophylline/theophylline's pharmacokinetic characteristics, it should be dosed on a lean body weight basis in obese patients. Dosage conversions between aminophylline and theophylline can be made using the information found in the Chemistry section below. Aminophylline causes intense local pain when administered IM and is rarely used or recommended via this route.

- **DOGS/CATS:**

  For adjunctive therapy of severe, acute pulmonary edema (rarely used today), **cough or bronchoconstriction** (extra-label): 3 – 11 mg/kg IV or IM (can cause pain) every 6-12 hours. Dogs may require the higher end of the dosage range and dosed every 6-8 hours and for cats the low end of the dosing range is used a given every 12 hours. If effective switch to oral therapy (theophylline) as soon as possible. When giving IV, do not push. Preferably administer over at least several minutes or as an infusion.

- **HORSES:**

  For adjunctive treatment of pulmonary edema or recurrent airway **obstruction (RAO)**; (extra-label): 5 – 11 mg/kg IV q8-12h. IV infusion should be in approximately 1 liter of IV fluids and given over 20-60 minutes. Rarely recommended for use today. Consider monitoring serum levels.

Monitoring

- Therapeutic efficacy and clinical signs of toxicity.
- Serum levels at steady state. The therapeutic serum levels of theophylline in humans are generally described to be between 10 – 20 micrograms/mL. In small animals, one recommendation for monitoring serum levels is to measure trough concentration; level should be at least above 8 – 10 micrograms/mL (**Note:** Some recommend not exceeding 15 micrograms/mL in horses).

Client Information

- Injectable aminophylline should be used in an inpatient setting or under the direct supervision of a veterinarian only.

Chemistry/Synonyms

Aminophylline occurs as bitter-tasting, white or slightly yellow granules or powder with a slight ammoniacal odor and a pK_a of 5. Aminophylline is soluble in water and insoluble in alcohol. 1 mg of aminophylline (hydrous) contains approximately 0.79 mg of theophylline (anhydrous). Conversely, 1 mg of theophylline (anhydrous) is equivalent to 1.27 mg aminophylline (hydrous).

Aminophylline may also be known as: aminofilina, aminophyllinum, euphyllinum, metaphyllin, theophyllaminum, theophylline and ethylenediamine, theophylline ethylenediamine compound, or theophyllinum ethylenediaminum; many trade names are available.

Storage/Stability

Aminophylline for injection should be stored in single-use containers in which carbon dioxide has been removed. It should also be stored at temperatures below 30°C and protected from freezing and light. Upon exposure to air (carbon dioxide), aminophylline will absorb carbon dioxide, lose ethylenediamine and liberate free theophylline that can precipitate out of solution. Do not inject aminophylline solutions that contain either a precipitate or visible crystals.

Compatibility/Compounding Considerations

Aminophylline for injection is reportedly **compatible** when mixed with all commonly used IV solutions, but may be **incompatible** with 10% fructose or invert sugar solutions.

Aminophylline is reportedly **compatible** when mixed with the following drugs: calcium gluconate, chloramphenicol sodium succinate, dexamethasone sodium phosphate, dopamine HCl, erythromycin lactobionate, heparin sodium, hydrocortisone sodium succinate, lidocaine HCl, metronidazole with sodium bicarbonate, phenobarbital sodium, potassium chloride, sodium bicarbonate, sodium iodide, terbutaline sulfate, and verapamil HCl.

Aminophylline is reportedly **incompatible** (or data conflicts) with the following drugs: amikacin sulfate, ascorbic acid injection, bleomycin sulfate, clindamycin phosphate, corticotropin, dimenhydrinate, dobutamine HCl, doxorubicin HCl, epinephrine HCl, erythromycin gluceptate, hydralazine HCl, hydroxyzine HCl, insulin (regular), isoproterenol HCl, meperidine HCl, methadone HCl, methylprednisolone sodium succinate, morphine sulfate, norepinephrine bitartrate, oxytetracycline, penicillin G potassium, pentazocine lactate, procaine HCl, prochlorperazine, promazine HCl, promethazine HCl, vancomycin HCl, and vitamin B complex with C. Compatibility is dependent upon factors such as pH, concentration, temperature, and diluent used and it is suggested to consult specialized references for more specific information.

Dosage Forms/Regulatory Status

VETERINARY-LABELED PRODUCTS: NONE.

The ARCI (Racing Commissioners International) has designated this drug as a class 3 substance.

HUMAN-LABELED PRODUCTS:

Aminophylline Injection: 25 mg/mL (equiv. to 19.7 mg/mL of theophylline) in 10 mL & 20 mL vials or amps; generic; (Rx)

At the time of update (Sept 2013), oral aminophylline tablets have been discontinued for the US market. See the Theophylline monograph for information on using oral products.

Revisions/References

Monograph revised/updated August 2013.

Amiodarone HCl

(a-mee-oh-**da**-rone)   Cordarone®, Pacerone®

Class III Antiarrhythmic

Prescriber Highlights

▶ Antidysrhythmic agent that can be used in dogs for arrhythmias associated with left ventricular dysfunction or to convert atrial fibrillation into sinus rhythm; very limited experience warrants cautious use. May take several days to weeks to have an effect.

▶ May be useful in horses to convert atrial fibrillation or ventricular tachycardia into sinus rhythm.

▶ Contraindicated in 2nd, 3rd degree heart block, bradyarrhythmias. Use caution in patients with thyroid dysfunction.

▶ In *Dogs*: GI disturbances (vomiting, anorexia) most likely adverse effect, but corneal deposits, neutropenia, thrombocytopenia, bradycardia, hepatotoxicity, positive Coombs' test reported. Generic IV forms can cause serious histaminergic effects in dogs.

▶ In *Horses*: Limited use (full adverse effect profile to be determined): Hind limb weakness, increased bilirubin reported when used IV to convert atrial fibrillation.

▶ Many potential drug interactions.

Uses/Indications

Because of its potential toxicity and lack of experience with use in canine and equine patients, amiodarone is usually used when other less toxic or commonly used drugs are ineffective. It may be useful in dogs and horses to convert atrial fib into sinus rhythm and in dogs for arrhythmias associated with left ventricular dysfunction. Using amiodarone to convert a horse with ventricular tachycardia into sinus rhythm has been reported.

As the risk of sudden death is high in Doberman pinschers exhibiting rapid, wide-complex ventricular tachycardia or syncope with recurrent VPC's, amiodarone may be useful when other drug therapies are ineffective.

Pharmacology/Actions

Amiodarone's mechanism of action is not fully understood; it apparently is a potassium channel blocker that possesses unique pharmacology from other antiarrhythmic agents. It can be best classified a Class III antiarrhythmic agent that also blocks sodium and calcium channels, and beta-adrenergic receptors. Major properties include prolongation of myocardial cell action-potential duration and refractory period.

Pharmacokinetics

Amiodarone may be administered parenterally or orally. Amiodarone is widely distributed throughout the body and can accumulate and persist in adipose tissue. Levels in myocardial cells are significantly higher than in plasma. Amiodarone is metabolized by the liver into desethylamiodarone, which is active. After oral administration of a single dose in normal dogs, amiodarone's plasma half-life averaged 7.5 hours, but repeated dosing increased its half-life from 11 hours to 3.2 days.

In horses, amiodarone has a low oral bioavailability (range from 6-34%) and peak levels of amiodarone and desethylamiodarone occur about 7-8 hours after an oral dose. After IV administration amiodarone is rapidly distributed with a high apparent volume of distribution of 31 L/kg. In horses, amiodarone is relatively highly bound to plasma proteins (96%). Clearance was 0.35 L/kg/hr and median elimination half-lives for amiodarone and desethylamiodarone were approximately 51 and 75 hours, respectively (De Clercq, Baert, et al. 2006).

In humans, oral absorption is slow and variable, with bioavailabilities ranging from 22-86%. Elimination half-lives for amiodarone and desethylamiodarone range from 2.5-10 days after a single dose, but with chronic dosing, average 53 days and 60 days, respectively.

Contraindications/Precautions/Warnings

Amiodarone is considered contraindicated in patients (humans) hypersensitive to it, having severe sinus-node dysfunction with severe sinus bradycardia, 2nd or 3rd degree heart block, or bradycardial syncope. Amiodarone should be used with caution in patients with thyroid dysfunction.

Clinical experience in veterinary patients is limited. Until further safety and efficacy data are available, consider use carefully.

Adverse Effects

Gastrointestinal effects (*e.g.*, anorexia, vomiting) are apparently the most likely adverse effects seen in the limited number of canine patients treated. Hepatopathy (bilirubinemia, increased hepatic enzymes) has been reported in dogs on amiodarone. Because hepatic effects can occur before clinical signs are noted, routine serial evaluation of liver enzymes and bilirubin is recommended. Other adverse effects reported in dogs include bradycardia, neutropenia, thrombocytopenia, or positive Coombs' test. A case series of 5 dogs administered IV amiodarone reported pruritus, erythema, subcutaneous edema, hives, agitation, tachypnea, and hypotension (Cober et al. 2009). The authors postulated that the solvent polysorbate 80 found in the IV solutions could be the cause. A newer IV formulation, *Nexterone®*, does not contain polysorbate 80 or benzyl alcohol. Corneal deposits may be seen in dogs treated with amiodarone, but this affect apparently occurs less frequently in dogs than in humans.

Horses treated with IV amiodarone for 36 hours or longer have developed short-term hind limb weakness and diarrhea.

In human patients, adverse effects are very common while on amiodarone therapy. Those that most commonly cause discontinuation of the drug include: pulmonary infiltrates or pulmonary fibrosis (sometimes fatal), liver enzyme elevations, congestive heart failure, paroxysmal ventricular tachycardia, and thyroid dysfunction (hypo- or hyperthyroidism). An odd effect seen in some individuals is a bluish cast to their skin. Reversible corneal deposits are seen in a majority of humans treated with amiodarone.

Reproductive/Nursing Safety

In laboratory animals, amiodarone has been embryotoxic at high doses and congenital thyroid abnormalities have been detected in offspring. Use during pregnancy only when the potential benefits outweigh the risks of the drug. In humans, the FDA categorizes this drug as category *D* for use during pregnancy (*There is evidence of human fetal risk, but the potential benefits from the use of the drug in pregnant women may be acceptable despite its potential risks.*)

Overdosage/Acute Toxicity

Clinical overdosage experience is limited; most likely adverse effects seen are hypotension, bradycardia, cardiogenic shock, AV block, and hepatotoxicity. Treatment is supportive. Bradycardia may be managed with a pacemaker or beta-1 agonists (*e.g.*, isoproterenol); hypotension managed with positive inotropic agents or vasopressors. Neither amiodarone nor its active metabolite are dialyzable.

Drug Interactions

Several potentially significant interactions can occur with amiodarone. The following is a partial list of interactions that have either been reported or are theoretical in humans or animals and may be of significance in veterinary patients. Unless otherwise noted, use together is not necessarily contraindicated, but weigh the potential risks and perform additional monitoring when appropriate.

Amiodarone may significantly **increase** the serum levels and/or pharmacologic or toxic effects of:

- **ANTICOAGULANTS (warfarin)**
- **DIGOXIN**
- **CYCLOSPORINE**
- **LIDOCAINE**
- **METHOTREXATE (with prolonged amiodarone administration)**
- **PHENYTOIN**
- **PROCAINAMIDE**
- **QUINIDINE**

Amiodarone may have **additive effects on QTc interval**; possible serious arrhythmias may result:

- **AZOLE ANTIFUNGALS** (*e.g.*, **ketoconazole, itraconazole, etc.**)
- **CISAPRIDE**
- **DISOPYRAMIDE**
- **DOLASETRON**
- **FLUOROQUINOLONE ANTIBIOTICS** (some, such as **moxifloxacin, pradofloxacin(?), but not enrofloxacin, marbofloxacin,** etc.)
- **MACROLIDE ANTIBIOTICS** (*e.g.*, **erythromycin**)
- **ONDANSETRON**

Other amiodarone drug interactions:

- **ANESTHETICS, GENERAL**: Increased risks for hypotension or arrhythmias.
- **BETA-ADRENERGIC BLOCKERS**: Possible potentiation of bradycardia, AV block or sinus arrest.
- **CALCIUM-CHANNEL BLOCKERS** (*e.g.*, **diltiazem, verapamil**): Possible potentiation of bradycardia, AV block or sinus arrest.
- **CIMETIDINE**: Increased amiodarone levels.
- **CYCLOSPORINE**: Increased cyclosporine levels; may increase creatinine.
- **FENTANYL**: Possible hypotension, bradycardia.
- **RIFAMPIN**: Decreased amiodarone levels.

Laboratory Considerations

- While most human patients remain euthyroid while receiving amiodarone, it may cause an increase in **serum T$_4$** and serum reverse T$_3$ levels, and a reduction in **serum T$_3$** levels.
- The human therapeutic serum concentrations of 1 – 2.5 micrograms/mL are believed to apply to dogs as well.
- Amiodarone may cause a **positive Coombs'** test result.

Doses

Note: Some human references state that because of the potential for drug interactions with previous drug therapies, the life-threatening nature of the arrhythmias being treated, and the unpredictability of response from amiodarone, the drug should be initially given (loaded) over several days in an inpatient setting where adequate monitoring can occur.

- **DOGS:**

  For atrial fibrillation or ventricular arrhythmias (primarily in ambulatory patients); (extra-label): Dosages for oral amiodarone are not well established and significant variation in recommendations can be found. At present, no well-controlled, prospective studies evaluating dosage regimens in clinically ill dogs could be located. A recently published retrospective study concluded that amiodarone might be a safe and effective alternative drug for the treatment of arrhythmias with myocardial dysfunction and not controlled with commonly used anti-arrhythmic drugs at dosages or 5 – 7.5 mg/kg per day PO with careful monitoring (Pedro et al. 2012). Others suggest that due to its unique pharmacokinetics that an initial loading dosage of 8 – 10 mg/kg PO twice daily be given for one week and then reduced to 5 – 10 mg/kg PO once daily thereafter. Adapted from: (Meurs 2005; Kittleson 2006; Saunders, Miller and Gordon 2006; Saunders, Miller, Gordon, et al. 2006; Mucha 2009)

- **HORSES:**

  For conversion of atrial fibrillation or ventricular tachycardia (extra-label): 5 mg/kg/hour for one hour, followed by 0.83 mg/kg/hour for 23 hours and then 1.9 mg/kg/hour for the following 30 hours. In the study (atrial fib), infusion was discontinued when conversion occurred or when any side effects were noted. 4 of 6 horses converted from atrial fib; one horse from ventricular tachycardia. In order to increase success rate and decrease adverse effects, regimen should be further adapted based upon PK/PD studies in horses. (De Clercq, van Loon, et al. 2006a), (De Clercq, van Loon, et al. 2006b)

Monitoring

- Efficacy (ECG).
- Toxicity (GI effects; CBC, serial liver enzymes; thyroid function tests; blood pressure; pulmonary radiographs if clinical signs such as dyspnea/cough occur). One reference recommends that liver enzymes be monitored monthly during therapy and if they become abnormal the dosage is reduced or discontinued (Twedt 2011).

Client Information

- Because relatively few canine/equine patients have received this agent and the drug's potential for toxicity, clients should give informed consent before the drug is prescribed or administered.

Chemistry/Synonyms

An iodinated benzofuran, amiodarone is unique structurally and pharmacologically from other antiarrhythmic agents. It occurs as a white to cream colored lipophilic powder having a pKa of approximately 6.6. Amiodarone 200 mg tablets each contain approximately 75 mg of iodine. Generic forms of the injectable solution contain polysorbate 80 and benzyl alcohol. *Nexterone*® pre-filled IV bags contain dextrose 42.1 mg/mL dextrose, but do not contain benzyl alcohol or polysorbate 80.

Amiodarone HCl may also be known as: amiodaroni hydrochloridum, L-3428, 51087N, or SKF-33134-A; many trade names are available.

Storage/Stability

Tablets should be stored in tight containers, at room temperature and protected from light. A 3-year expiration date is assigned from the date of manufacture.

Injection should be stored at room temperature and protected from light or excessive heat. While administering, light protection is not necessary.

Compatibility/Compounding Considerations

Use D5W as the IV diluent. Amiodarone is reportedly compatible with dobutamine, lidocaine, potassium chloride, procainamide, propafenone, and verapamil. Variable compatibility is reported with furosemide and quinidine gluconate.

Compounded preparation stability: Amiodarone oral suspension compounded from commercially available tablets has been published (Nahata 1997). Triturating one (1) tablet of amiodarone 200 mg with 20 mL of *Ora-Plus®* and *qs ad* to 40 mL with *Ora-Sweet®* (or *Ora-Sweet®SF*) yields a 5 mg/mL oral suspension that retains >90% potency for 91 days stored at 5°C. Compounded preparations of amiodarone should be protected from light. Amiodarone suspensions may be stored at room temperature during short periods (such as travel).

Dosage Forms/Regulatory Status

VETERINARY-LABELED PRODUCTS: NONE.

The ARCI (Racing Commissioners International) has designated this drug as a class 4 substance. See the appendix for more information.

HUMAN-LABELED PRODUCTS:

Amiodarone Oral Tablets: 100 mg, 200 mg & 400 mg; *Cordarone®*; *Pacerone®*; generic; (Rx)

Amiodarone Injection Solution: 50 mg/mL in 3 mL, 10 mL & 30 mL single-dose vials, & 3 mL prefilled syringes; generic; (Rx)

Amiodarone Injection Solution: 150 mg/100 mL & 360 mg/200 mL prefilled IV bags (contains 42.1 mg/mL dextrose as diluent); *Nexterone®*; (Rx)

Revisions/References

Monograph revised/updated August 2013.

Cober, R. E., et al. (2009). Adverse Effects of Intravenous Amiodarone in 5 Dogs. *Journal of Veterinary Internal Medicine* 23(3): 657-61.

De Clercq, D., et al. (2006). Evaluation of the pharmacokinetics and bioavailability of intravenously and orally administered amiodarone in horses. *Am J Vet Res* 67(3): 448-54.

De Clercq, D., et al. (2006a). Intravenous amiodarone treatment in horses with chronic atrial fibrillation. *Vet J* 172(1): 129-34.

De Clercq, D., et al. (2006b). Treatment with amiodarone of refractory ventricular tachycardia in a horse. *J Vet Intern Med* 21(4): 878-80.

Kittleson, M. (2006). "Chapt 29: Drugs used in the treatment of cardiac arrhythmias." *Small Animal Cardiology, 2nd Ed.*

Meurs, K. (2005). Primary Myocardial Disease in the Dog. *Textbook of Veterinary Internal Medicine, 6th Ed.* S. Ettinger and E. Feldman, Elsevier: 1077-82.

Mucha, C. (2009). *Therapeutics in Heart Disease.* Proceedings: WSAVA. accessed via Veterinary Information Network; vin.com

Nahata, M. C. (1997). Stability of amiodarone in an oral suspension stored under refrigeration and at room temperature. *Ann Pharmacother* 31(7-8): 851-2.

Pedro, B., et al. (2012). Retrospective evaluation of the use of amiodarone in dogs with arrhythmias (from 2003 to 2010). *Journal of Small Animal Practice* 53(1): 19-26.

Saunders, A., et al. (2006). Oral amiodarone therapy in dogs with atrial fibrillation. *J Vet Intern Med* 20: 921-6.

Saunders, A. B., et al. (2006). Oral amiodarone therapy in dogs with atrial fibrillation. *Journal of Veterinary Internal Medicine* 20(4): 921-6.

Twedt, D. (2011). *Canine Contemporary Hepatotoxins: Drugs CCNU, Mitotane, Amiodarone and Sulfonamides.* ACVIM 2011. accessed via Veterinary Information Network; vin.com

Amitraz – See the Topical Dermatologic Agents section in the appendix

---

Amitriptyline HCl

(a-mih-**trip**-ti-leen)   Elavil®

Tricyclic Behavior Modifier; Antipruritic; Neuropathic Pain Modifier

Prescriber Highlights

▶ Tricyclic "antidepressant" used primarily for behavior disorders & neuropathic pain/pruritus in small animals.

▶ May reduce seizure thresholds in epileptic animals.

▶ Sedation & anticholinergic effects most likely adverse effects. When discontinuing, taper off medication.

▶ Overdoses can be very serious in both animals & humans.

Uses/Indications

Amitriptyline has been used for behavioral conditions such as separation anxiety or generalized anxiety in dogs, and excessive grooming, spraying and anxiety in cats. Because it is FDA-approved for dogs, clomipramine (*Clomicalm®*) is often chosen over amitriptyline for use in dogs when a tricyclic is to be tried for behavioral indications. Amitriptyline may be useful for adjunctive treatment of pruritus, or chronic pain of neuropathic origin in dogs and cats. In cats, it potentially could be useful for adjunctive treatment of lower urinary tract disease. Amitriptyline has been tried to reduce feather plucking in birds.

Pharmacology/Actions

Amitriptyline (and its active metabolite, nortriptyline) is a tricyclic antidepressant (TCA) and has a complicated pharmacologic profile. From a slightly oversimplified viewpoint, it has 3 main characteristics: blockage of the amine pump, thereby increasing neurotransmitter levels (principally serotonin, but also norepinephrine), sedation, and central and peripheral anticholinergic activity. Other pharmacologic effects include stabilizing mast cells via H-1 receptor antagonism, and antagonism of glutamate receptors and sodium channels. In animals, tricyclic antidepressants are similar to the actions of phenothiazines in altering avoidance behaviors.

Pharmacokinetics

Amitriptyline is rapidly absorbed from both the GI tract and from parenteral injection sites, but transdermal (PLO-gel based) absorption in cats is poor (Mealey et al. 2004). Peak levels occur in 1-2 hours after oral administration in cats and other species within 2-12 hours. Amitriptyline is highly bound to plasma proteins, enters the CNS, and enters maternal milk in levels at, or greater than those found in maternal serum. The drug is metabolized in the liver to several metabolites, including nortriptyline, which is active. In humans, the terminal half-life is approximately 30 hours. Half-life in dogs has been reported to be 6–8 hours. Because TCAs are metabolized through glucuronidation, cats may more sensitive to TCAs than dogs.

Contraindications/Precautions/Warnings

These agents are contraindicated if prior sensitivity has been noted with any other tricyclic. Concomitant use with monoamine oxidase inhibitors is generally contraindicated. Use with extreme caution in patients with seizure disorders as tricyclic agents may reduce seizure thresholds. Use with caution in patients with thyroid disorders, urinary retention, hepatic disorders, KCS, glaucoma, cardiac rhythm disorders, diabetes, or adrenal tumors.

Adverse Effects

The most predominant adverse effects seen with the tricyclics are related to their sedating and anticholinergic (constipation, urinary retention) properties. Occasionally, dogs exhibit hyperexcitability and, rarely, develop seizures. However, adverse effects can run the entire gamut of systems, including cardiac (dysrhythmias), hematologic (bone marrow suppression), GI (diarrhea, vomiting), endocrine, etc. Cats may be more sensitive to amitriptyline than dogs as it is metabolized via glucuronidation, and can develop the following adverse effects: sedation, hypersalivation, urinary retention, anorexia, thrombocytopenia, neutropenia, unkempt hair coat, vomiting/nausea, ataxia, disorientation and cardiac conductivity disturbances.

Reproductive/Nursing Safety

Isolated reports of limb reduction abnormalities have been noted; restrict use to pregnant animals only when the benefits clearly outweigh the risks. In humans, the FDA categorizes this drug as category **D** for use during pregnancy (*There is evidence of human fetal risk, but the potential benefits from the use of the drug in pregnant women may be acceptable despite its potential risks.*)

Overdosage/Acute Toxicity

Overdosage with tricyclics can be life-threatening (arrhythmias, cardiorespiratory collapse). Because the toxicities and therapies for treatment are complicated and controversial, it is recommended to contact an animal poison control center for further information in any potential overdose situation. Intravenous fat emulsion (*Intralipid®*) therapy did not affect amitriptyline mortality rates in rats (Bania et al. 2006).

There were 405 single agent exposures to amitriptyline reported to the ASPCA Animal Poison Control Center (APCC) during 2009-2013. There were 272 dogs, 64 that were symptomatic. Of these dogs, 25% were lethargic, 19% were tachycardic, 16% were ataxic and 11% were vomiting and/or hyperthermic. Of the 133 exposed cats, 81 were symptomatic. Of these cats, 51% were vocalizing, 40% had mydriasis and/or tachycardia, 35% were ataxic, 26% were lethargic, 22% were disoriented and 12% were vomiting.

Drug Interactions

The following drug interactions with amitriptyline have either been reported or are theoretical in humans or animals and may be of significance in veterinary patients. Unless otherwise noted, use together is not necessarily contraindicated, but weigh the potential risks and perform additional monitoring when appropriate.perform additional monitoring when appropriate.

- **ANTICHOLINERGIC AGENTS:** Increased effects; hyperthermia and ileus possible.
- **CIMETIDINE:** May inhibit tricyclic antidepressant metabolism and increase the risk of toxicity.
- **CISAPRIDE:** May have additive effects on QTc interval; possible serious arrhythmias may result.
- **CNS DEPRESSANTS:** Increased effects.
- **CYPROHEPTADINE:** May antagonize the effects of antagonize the effects of SSRIs (*e.g.*, fluoxetine, paroxetine, etc.), tricyclic antidepressants (*e.g.*, clomipramine, amitriptyline, etc.) and tramadol.
- **DIAZEPAM:** Possible increased amitriptyline levels.
- **ITRACONAZOLE, KETOCONAZOLE:** Increased levels of amitriptylin.
- **MONOAMINE OXIDASE INHIBITORS** (including **selegilene, amitraz**): Potential life threatening serotonin syndrome; use together not recommended.
- **QUINIDINE:** Increased risk for QTc interval prolongation and tricyclic adverse effects.
- **SELECTIVE-SEROTONIN RE-UPTAKE INHIBITORS** (*e.g.*, **SSRIs, fluoxetine**, etc.): Potential increased amitriptyline levels, increased risk for serotonin syndrome; **Note:** SSRI's and TCA's such as amitriptyline are often used together in veterinary behavior medicine, but enhanced monitoring for adverse effects is suggested.

- **SYMPATHOMIMETIC AGENTS:** May increase the risk of cardiac effects (arrhythmias, hypertension, hyperpyrexia).
- **THYROID AGENTS:** Increased risk for arrhythmias; monitor.
- **TRAMADOL:** Increased risk for serotonin syndrome; veterinary clinical significance is not known, but one source states that monoamine oxidase inhibitors (selegiline), tricyclic antidepressants (*e.g.*, amitriptyline, clomipramine), selective serotonin reuptake inhibitors (*e.g.*, fluoxetine, paroxetine), and SNRIs (venlafaxine) should not be administered concurrently with tramadol (KuKanich 2013).

Laboratory Considerations

- **ECG:** Tricyclics can widen QRS complexes, prolong PR intervals and invert or flatten T-waves on ECG.
- **Metapyrone:** The response to metapyrone may be decreased by amitriptyline.
- **Blood glucose:** Tricyclics may alter (increase or decrease) blood glucose levels.

Doses

- **DOGS:**

  For adjunctive treatment (with behavior modification and anxiolytics if required) of behavior disorders amenable to tricyclics (extra-label): Initially, 1 – 2 mg/kg PO q12h for 2-4 weeks. May gradually increase by 1 mg/kg as tolerated to a maximum of 4 mg/kg PO twice daily. If discontinuing, taper off slowly.

  For adjunctive treatment of pruritus (extra-label): 1 – 2.2 mg/kg PO q12h. To determine efficacy, treat for 3-4 weeks and assess response. If discontinuing, taper off slowly.

  For adjunctive treatment of chronic (especially neuropathic) pain (extra-label): 1 – 2 mg/kg PO q12-24h. If discontinuing, taper off slowly.

- **CATS:**

  For adjunctive treatment of behavior disorders amenable to tricyclics (extra-label): 0.5 – 1 mg/kg PO once daily (or divided twice daily). Practically, 2.5 mg – 12.5 mg per cat once daily. Start at lower end of dosing range and gradually increase as tolerated. If discontinuing, gradually taper off dosage.

  For adjunctive treatment of pruritus (after other more conventional therapies have failed (extra-label): 2.5 – 12.5 mg per cat PO once daily or 2.5 – 7.5 mg per cat twice daily. To minimize adverse effects start at low end of dosing range (2.5 mg per cat once daily) and gradually increase as tolerated. May need to have compounded to accurately dose and to improve palatability (fish or cod liver oil).

  For symptomatic therapy of idiopathic cystitis, idiopathic feline lower urinary tract disease (FLUTD); (extra-label): 2.5 – 12.5 mg per cat PO once daily at night. Taper off drug when discontinuing.

  For adjunctive treatment of chronic (especially neuropathic) pain (extra-label): 2.5 – 12.5 mg per cat PO once daily.

- **BIRDS:**

  For adjunctive treatment of feather plucking (extra-label): 1 – 2 mg/kg PO q12–24 hours. Anecdotal reports indicate some usefulness. Barring side effects, may be worth a more prolonged course of therapy to determine efficacy. (Lightfoot 2001)

Monitoring

- Efficacy.
- Adverse effects; it is recommended to perform a cardiac evaluation, CBC and serum chemistry panel prior to therapy.
- For cats, some clinicians recommend that liver enzymes be measured prior to therapy, one month after initial therapy, and yearly, thereafter.

Client Information

- May take several days to weeks to determine if the drug is effective.
- Most common side effects are: drowsiness/sleepiness, dry mouth and constipation; be sure your animal has access to water.
- Rare side effects that can be serious (contact veterinarian immediately): abnormal bleeding or fever, seizures, very fast or irregular heart rate.
- Overdoses can be very serious; keep out of the reach of animals and children.
- If your animal wore a flea collar containing amitraz in the past two weeks, let your veterinarian know.

Chemistry/Synonyms

A tricyclic dibenzocycloheptene-derivative antidepressant, amitriptyline HCl occurs as a white or practically white, odorless or practically odorless crystalline powder that is freely soluble in water or alcohol. It has a bitter, burning taste and a pK_a of 9.4.

Amitriptyline may also be known as amitriptylini hydrochloridum; many trade names are available.

Storage/Stability

Amitriptyline tablets should be stored at room temperature.

Compatibility/Compounding Considerations

No specific information noted.

Dosage Forms/Regulatory Status

VETERINARY-LABELED PRODUCTS: NONE.

The ARCI (Racing Commissioners International) has designated this drug as a class 2 substance. See the appendix for more information.

HUMAN-LABELED PRODUCTS:

Amitriptyline HCl Tablets: 10 mg, 25 mg, 50 mg, 75 mg, 100 mg, & 150 mg; generic; (Rx)

Revisions/References

Monograph revised/updated August 2013.

Bania, T. & J. Chu (2006). Hemodynamic effect of intralipid in amitriptyline toxicity. *Acad Emerg Med* **13**: S177.

KuKanich, B. (2013). Outpatient Oral Analgesics in Dogs and Cats Beyond Nonsteroidal Antiinflammatory Drugs: An Evidence-based Approach. *Vet Clin Small Anim* **43**: 1109-25.

Lightfoot, T. (2001). *Feather "Plucking"*. Proceedings: Atlantic Coast Veterinary Conference. accessed via Veterinary Information Network; vin.com

Mealey, K. L., et al. (2004). Systemic absorption of amitriptyline and buspirone after oral and transdermal administration to healthy cats. *Journal of Veterinary Internal Medicine* **18**(1): 43-6.

Amlodipine Besylate

(am-loe-di-peen)   Norvasc®, Istin®

Calcium Channel Blocker

Prescriber Highlights

▶ Calcium channel blocker used most often for treating hypertension, especially in cats.

▶ Slight negative inotrope; use with caution in patients with heart disease, hepatic dysfunction.

▶ Potentially may cause anorexia & hypotension in cats early in therapy; gingival hyperplasia seen in some dogs.

▶ Hypertension may rapidly reoccur if dosages are missed.

Uses/Indications

Oral amlodipine can be a useful agent in the treatment of hypertension in cats and most consider it the drug of choice for this indication. In pharmacokinetic studies, amlodipine has decreased blood pressure in dogs with chronic renal disease, but evidence for its efficacy in dogs as an afterload reducer or in treating hypertensive dogs has not been well established. When used alone in healthy dogs in higher dosages, amlodipine has been shown to activate the renin-angiotensin-aldosterone system (RAAS). Use with an ACE inhibitor (enalapril) at least partially blocks this effect (Atkins et al. 2007).

Hypertension in cats is usually secondary to other diseases (often renal failure or cardiac causes such as thyrotoxic cardiomyopathy or primary hypertrophic cardiomyopathy, etc.) and is most often seen in middle-aged or geriatric cats. These animals often present with acute clinical signs such as blindness, seizures, collapse or paresis. A cat is generally considered hypertensive if systolic blood pressure is >160 mmHg. Early reports indicate that if antihypertensive therapy is begun acutely, some vision may be restored in about 50% of cases of blindness secondary to hypertension.

Pharmacology/Actions

Amlodipine inhibits calcium influx across cell membranes in both cardiac and vascular smooth muscle. It has a greater effect on vascular smooth muscle, thereby acting as a peripheral arteriolar vasodilator and reducing afterload. Amlodipine also depresses impulse formation (automaticity) and conduction velocity in cardiac muscle. After an initial dose in dogs, amlodipine has a mild diuretic action.

Pharmacokinetics

No feline-specific data on the drug's pharmacokinetics was located. In humans, amlodipine's bioavailability does not appear to be altered by the presence of food in the gut. The drug is slowly but almost completely absorbed after oral administration and is reported to be absorbed after rectal administration. In humans, peak plasma concentrations occur between 6-9 hours post-dose and effects on blood pressure are correspondingly delayed. In cats, effects on systemic blood pressure are usually seen within 4 hours of dosing and may persist for approximately 30 hours post dose (Brown 2009). The drug has very high plasma protein binding characteristics (approximately 93%). However, drug interactions associated with potential displacement from these sites have not been elucidated. Amlodipine is slowly, but extensively metabolized to inactive compounds in the liver. Terminal plasma half-life is approximately 30 hours in dogs and 35 hours in healthy humans, but is prolonged in the elderly and in those patients with hypertension or hepatic dysfunction.

Contraindications/Precautions/Warnings

Because amlodipine may have slight negative inotropic effects, it should be used cautiously in patients with heart failure or cardiogenic shock. It should also be used cautiously in patients with hepatic disease or at risk for developing hypotension. A relative contraindication for amlodipine exists for humans with advanced aortic stenosis. Amlodipine use for pulmonary hypertension in dogs is not recommended as systemic hypotension can occur (Kellihan et al. 2010).

There is concern that using amlodipine alone for treating hypertension in cats with renal disease may expose glomeruli to higher pressures secondary to efferent arteriolar constriction. This is caused by localized increases in renin-angiotensin-aldosterone (RAAS) axis activity thereby allowing progressive damage to glomeruli. It is postulated that using an ACE inhibitor with amlodipine may help prevent this occurrence (Stepien 2006). Whether routine use of ACE inhibitors with amlodipine is necessary and beneficial in animals with chronic kidney disease and hypertension is somewhat controversial, particularly in cats.

Adverse Effects

Because of amlodipine's relatively slow onset of action, hypotension and inappetence is usually absent in cats. Infrequently, cats may develop azotemia, lethargy, hypokalemia, reflex tachycardia, and weight loss. In humans taking amlodipine, headache (7.3% incidence) is the most frequent problem reported.

In dogs, reversible gingival hyperplasia has been reported when amlodipine has been used long term; incidence in the retrospective study was 8.5% (Thomason et al. 2009). Gingival hyperplasia could also occur in cats, but is apparently quite rare.

Reproductive/Nursing Safety

While no evidence of impaired fertility was noted in rats given 8X overdoses, amlodipine has been shown to be fetotoxic (intrauterine death rates increased 5 fold) in laboratory animals (rats, rabbits) at very high dosages. No evidence of teratogenicity or mutagenicity was observed in lab animal studies. In rats, amlodipine prolonged labor. It is unknown whether amlodipine enters maternal milk. In humans, the FDA categorizes this drug as category **C** for use during pregnancy (*Animal studies have shown an adverse effect on the fetus, but there are no adequate studies in humans; or there are no animal reproduction studies and no adequate studies in humans.*)

Overdosage/Acute Toxicity

Limited experience with other calcium channel blockers in humans has shown that profound hypotension and bradycardia may result. There were 719 single agent exposures to amlodipine reported to the ASPCA Animal Poison Control Center (APCC) during 2009-2013. Of the 578 dogs, 108 were symptomatic with 39% tachycardic, 32% hypotensive, 26% lethargic, 18% vomiting and 13% hypertensive. Of the 140 cats, 31 were symptomatic. The most common clinical signs included: hypertension (23%), hypotension (23%), tachycardia (23%) and lethargy (13%).

Risk in animals with overdoses is for hypotension and reflex tachycardia (possibly bradycardia). When possible, massive overdoses should be managed with gut emptying and supportive treatment. Beta-agonists, intravenous lipid therapy, and intravenous calcium may be beneficial.

Drug Interactions

The following drug interactions with amlodipine have either been reported or are theoretical in humans or animals and may be of significance in veterinary patients. Unless otherwise noted, use together is not necessarily contraindicated, but weigh the potential risks and perform additional monitoring when appropriate.

- **CYCLOSPORINE**: Amlodipine may increase levels.
- **CYP3A4 STRONG INHIBITORS** (*e.g.*, ketoconazole, itraconazole, grapefruit juice, etc.): Amlodipine levels may be increased.
- **CYP3A4 INDUCERS** (*e.g.*, rifampin, etc.): Amlodipine levels may be decreased.
- **OTHER DRUGS THAT CAN REDUCE BLOOD PRESSURE**: May have additive effects on when used with amlodipine.

Laboratory Considerations
- No specific concerns noted.

Doses
- **DOGS:**

  For adjunctive therapy treatment of systemic hypertension as an afterload reducer for refractory heart failure (extra-label): 0.1 – 0.5 mg/kg PO once daily, start at low end of dosing range. In dogs, amlodipine is generally added after ACE-Inhibitor (*e.g.*, benazepril) therapy has been used.

- **CATS:**

  For treatment of systemic hypertension (extra-label; reasonable evidence to support): 0.625 – 1.25 mg per cat (¼ - ½ of a 1.25 mg tablet per cat) once daily. Cats weighing less than 4 kg generally receive 0.625 mg (¼ of a 2.5 mg tablet) initially and those >4 kg receive 1.25 mg (½ of a 2.5 mg tablet) initially. Some recommend that higher dosages (up to 2.5 mg per cat) can be used if blood pressure is not controlled. In cats that are proteinuric, an ACE inhibitor (*e.g.*, benazepril) is added.

Monitoring
- Blood pressure. A general guideline for treating hypertension in cats is to maintain systolic blood pressure (Doppler forelimb) below 160 mmHg.
- Ophthalmic exam.
- Potassium, especially in cats with chronic kidney disease.
- Adverse effects.

Client Information
- May give with or without food.
- Very important to not skip dosages as high blood pressure can quickly return.
- Side effects are not common in cats but include reduced appetite and low blood pressure, especially early in treatment. In dogs, overgrowth of the gums can occur.
- Patient will need to be seen regularly by veterinarian to check to see if the medication is working properly.

Chemistry/Synonyms

Amlodipine besylate, a dihydropyridine calcium channel-blocking agent, occurs as a white crystalline powder that is slightly soluble in water and sparingly soluble in alcohol.

Amlodipine Besylate may also as: amlodipini besilas, UK-48340-26, or UK-48340-11 (amlodipine maleate); many trade names are available.

Storage/Stability

Store amlodipine tablets at room temperature, in tight, light resistant containers.

Compatibility/Compounding Considerations

Compounded preparation stability: Amlodipine oral suspension compounded from commercially available tablets has been published (Nahata et al. 1999). Triturating six (6) amlodipine 5 mg tablets with 15 mL of *Ora-Plus®* and *qs ad* to 30 mL with *Ora-Sweet®* yields a 1 mg/mL oral suspension that retains >90% potency for 91 days stored at both 5°C and 25°C. Compounded preparations of amlodipine should be protected from light.

Dosage Forms/Regulatory Status

VETERINARY-LABELED PRODUCTS: NONE.

The ARCI (Racing Commissioners International) has designated this drug as a class 4 substance. See the appendix for more information.

HUMAN-LABELED PRODUCTS:

Amlodipine Oral Tablets: 2.5 mg, 5 mg & 10 mg; *Norvasc®*, generic; (Rx)

Fixed-dose combination products with benazepril (*Lotrel®*) or atorvastatin (*Caduet®*) are available.

Revisions/References

Monograph revised/updated August 2013.

Atkins, C. E., et al. (2007). The effect of amlodipine and the combination of amlodipine and enalapril on the renin-angiotensin-aldosterone system in the dog. *J. Vet. Pharmacol. Ther.* **30**(5): 394-400.

Brown, S. (2009). *Amlodipine and Hypertensive Nephropathy in Cats*. Proceedings: ECVIM. accessed via Veterinary Information Network; vin.com

Kellihan, H. B. & R. L. Stepien (2010). Pulmonary Hypertension in Dogs: Diagnosis and Therapy. *Veterinary Clinics of North America-Small Animal Practice* **40**(4): 623-+.

Nahata, M. C., et al. (1999). Stability of amlodipine besylate in two liquid dosage forms. *J Am Pharm Assoc (Wash)* **39**(3): 375-7.

Stepien, R. (2006). *Diagnosis and treatment of systemic hypertension*. Proceedings: ACVIM Forum. accessed via Veterinary Information Network; vin.com

Thomason, J. D., et al. (2009). Gingival Hyperplasia Associated with the Administration of Amlodipine to Dogs with Degenerative Valvular Disease (2004-2008). *Journal of Veterinary Internal Medicine* **23**(1): 39-42.

Ammonium Chloride

(ah-**moe**-nee-um)   Uroeze®

Acidifying Agent

Prescriber Highlights

▶ Urinary acidifier; treatment of metabolic alkalosis.

▶ Contraindicated in patients with hepatic failure or uremia.

▶ Potential adverse effects are primarily GI distress; IV use may lead to metabolic acidosis.

▶ Very unpalatable; addition of sugar (not molasses) may improve palatability to goats and sheep.

▶ May increase excretion of quinidine; decrease efficacy of erythromycin or aminoglycosides in urine.

Uses/Indications

Although rarely recommended for use in small animals today, the veterinary indications for ammonium chloride are as a urinary acidifying agent to help prevent and dissolve certain types of uroliths (*e.g.*, struvite), to enhance renal excretion of some types of toxins (*e.g.*, strontium, strychnine) or drugs (*e.g.*, quinidine), or to enhance the efficacy of certain antimicrobials (*e.g.*, chlortetracycline, methenamine mandelate, nitrofurantoin, oxytetracycline, penicillin G or tetracycline) when treating urinary tract infections. Ammonium chloride has also been used intravenously for the rapid correction of metabolic alkalosis.

Because of changes in feline diets to restrict struvite and as struvite therapeutic diets (*e.g.*, s/d) cause aciduria, ammonium chloride is not commonly recommended for struvite uroliths in cats.

Ammonium chloride is still recommended to help prevent uroliths in small ruminants, but dietary changes can significantly affect its efficacy for this purpose. When used continually, renal compensatory mechanisms may negate its urinary pH lowering effects and pulse therapy may be more effective (Sprake et al. 2012).

Pharmacology/Actions

The acidification properties of ammonium chloride are caused by its dissociation into chloride and ammonium ions *in vivo*. The ammonium cation is converted by the liver to urea with the release of a hydrogen ion. This ion combines with bicarbonate to form water and carbon dioxide. In the extracellular fluid, chloride ions combine with fixed bases and decrease the alkaline reserves in the body. The net effects are decreased serum bicarbonate levels and a decrease in blood and urine pH.

Excess chloride ions presented to the kidney are not completely reabsorbed by the tubules and are excreted with cations (principally sodium) and water. This diuretic effect is usually compensated for in the kidneys after a few days of therapy.

Pharmacokinetics

No information was located on the pharmacokinetics of this agent in veterinary species. In humans, ammonium chloride is rapidly absorbed from the GI.

Contraindications/Precautions/Warnings

Ammonium chloride is contraindicated in patients with severe hepatic disease as ammonia may accumulate and cause toxicity. In general, ammonium chloride should not be administered to uremic patients since it can intensify the metabolic acidosis already existing in some of these patients. As sodium depletion can occur, ammonium chloride should not be used alone in patients with severe renal insufficiency and metabolic alkalosis secondary to vomiting hydrochloric acid. In these cases, sodium chloride repletion with or without ammonium chloride administration should be performed to correct both sodium and chloride deficits. Ammonium chloride is contraindicated in patients with urate calculi or respiratory acidosis with high total CO_2 and buffer base. Ammonium chloride alone cannot correct hypochloremia with secondary metabolic alkalosis due to intracellular potassium chloride depletion; potassium chloride must be administered to these patients.

Do not administer subcutaneously, rectally or intraperitoneally.

Use ammonium chloride with caution in patients with pulmonary insufficiency or cardiac edema.

A high roughage/concentrate ratio diet can decrease the urine pH lowering effect of ammonium chloride in horses (Kienzle et al. 2006).

Adverse Effects

Development of metabolic acidosis (sometimes severe) can occur unless adequate monitoring is performed. When used intravenously, pain at the injection site can develop; slow administration lessens this effect. Gastric irritation, nausea and vomiting may be associated with oral dosing of the drug. Urinary acidification is associated with an increased risk for calcium oxalate urolith formation in cats.

Overdosage/Acute Toxicity

Clinical signs of overdosage may include: nausea, vomiting, excessive thirst, hyperventilation, bradycardias or other arrhythmias, and progressive CNS depression. Profound acidosis and hypokalemia may be noted on laboratory results.

Treatment should consist of correcting the acidosis by administering sodium bicarbonate or sodium acetate intravenously. Hypokalemia should be treated by using a suitable oral (if possible) potassium product. Intense acid-base and electrolyte monitoring should be performed on an ongoing basis until the patient is stable.

Reproductive/Nursing Safety

In humans, the FDA categorizes this drug as category **B** for use during pregnancy (*Animal studies have not yet demonstrated risk to the fetus, but there are no adequate studies in pregnant women; or animal studies have shown an adverse effect, but adequate studies in pregnant women have not demonstrated a risk to the fetus in the first trimester of pregnancy, and there is no evidence of risk in later trimesters.*) In a separate system evaluating the safety of drugs in canine and feline pregnancy (Papich 1989), this drug is categorized as class: **B** (*Safe for use if used cautiously. Studies in laboratory animals may have uncovered some risk, but these drugs appear to be safe in dogs and cats or these drugs are safe if they are not administered when the animal is near term.*)

Drug Interactions

The following drug interactions with ammonium chloride or other urinary acidifying agents have either been reported or are theoretical in humans or animals and may be of significance in veterinary patients. Unless otherwise noted, use together is not necessarily contraindicated, but weigh the potential risks and perform additional monitoring when appropriate.

▪ **AMINOGLYCOSIDES** (*e.g.*, **gentamicin**) and **ERYTHROMYCIN**: Are more effective in an alkaline medium; urine acidification may diminish these drugs effectiveness in treating bacterial urinary tract infections.

▪ **QUINIDINE**: Urine acidification may increase renal excretion.

Doses

▪ **DOGS:**

For urine acidification (extra-label):

a) **As adjunctive therapy for struvite uroliths:** 20 mg/kg PO three times daily. (Labato 2002)

b) **To enhance the renal elimination of certain toxins/drugs:** 200 mg/kg/day divided four times daily. (Grauer et al. 1988)

c) **To enhance elimination of strontium:** 0.2 – 0.5 grams PO 3–4 times a day (used with calcium salts). (Bailey 1986)

For ATT (ammonia tolerance testing); (extra-label):

a) 2 mL/kg of a 5% solution of ammonium chloride deep in the rectum, blood sampled at 20 minutes and 40 minutes; or oral challenge with ammonium chloride 100 mg/kg (maximum dose = 3 grams) either in solution: dissolved in 20 – 50 mL warm water or in gelatin capsules, blood sampled at 30 and 60 minutes. Test may also be done by comparing fasting and 6–hour postprandial samples without giving exogenous ammonium chloride. (Center 2004)

■ **CATS:**

For urine acidification (extra-label):

a) **In struvite dissolution therapy if diet and antimicrobials do not result in acid urine or to help prevent idiopathic FUS in a non-obstructed cat:** 20 mg/kg PO twice daily. (Lage et al. 1988)

b) **As adjunctive therapy for struvite uroliths:** 20 mg/kg PO twice daily. (Labato 2002)

■ **HORSES:**

For urine acidification (extra-label):

a) **Ammonium chloride as a urinary acidifier:** 60 – 520 mg/kg PO daily. Ammonium salts are unpalatable and will have to be dosed via stomach tube or dosing syringe. Alternatively, ammonium sulfate at 165 mg/kg PO per day is more palatable and may be accepted when mixed with grain or hay. (Jose-Cunilleras and Hinchcliff 1999)

b) **As a urinary acidifier to enhance renal excretion of strychnine:** 132 mg/kg PO. (Schmitz 2004)

■ **SHEEP & GOATS:**

For urolithiasis prevention (extra-label):

a) 200 – 300 mg/kg (dosage titrated to the individual in the study) PO twice daily for 3 days and then off for 4 days. 4/10 goats achieved urine pH <6.5 for all treatment cycles. (Sprake et al. 2012)

b) 450 mg/kg (2.25% of dry matter intake) PO per day maintained urine pH <6.5 in study goats. Animals were fed orchard grass diet. Further studies to evaluate the relative risks of urolith formation in goats fed specific diets with and without supplemental ammonium chloride are necessary. (Mavangira et al. 2010)

c) 0.5 – 1% of the daily dry matter will acidify urine, but can be very unpalatable. Table sugar may improve palatability. (Snyder 2009), (Van Metre 2009)

Monitoring

■ Urine pH (Urine pH's of ≤6.5 are recommended as goals of therapy).

■ Blood pH if there are clinical signs of toxicity or treating metabolic alkalosis.

■ Serum electrolytes, if using chronically or if treating metabolic acidosis.

■ Prior to IV use, it is recommended that the carbon dioxide combining power of the patient's serum be measured to insure that serious acidosis is prevented.

Client Information

■ Contact veterinarian if animal exhibits signs of nausea, vomiting, excessive thirst, hyperventilation, or progressive lethargy.

■ Multiple daily dosing is usually necessary.

■ Granules have bitter taste, mix well in food for dogs and cats; usually sprinkled over food for horses.

■ When used as a urinary acidifier, monitoring of urine pH often done by owner.

Chemistry/Synonyms

An acid-forming salt, ammonium chloride occurs as colorless crystals or as white, fine or course, crystalline powder. It is somewhat hygroscopic, and has a cool, saline taste. When dissolved in water, the temperature of the solution is decreased. One gram is soluble in approximately 3 mL of water at room temperature; 1.4 mL at 100°C. One gram is soluble in approximately 100 mL of alcohol.

One gram of ammonium chloride contains 18.7 mEq of ammonium and chloride ions. The commercially available concentrate for injection (26.75%) contains 5 mEq of each ion per mL and contains disodium edetate as a stabilizing agent. The pH of the concentrate for injection is approximately 5.

Ammonium chloride may also be known as muriate of ammonia and sal ammoniac.

Storage/Stability

Ammonium chloride for injection should be stored at room temperature; avoid freezing. At low temperatures, crystallization may occur; it may be resolubolized by warming to room temperature in a water bath.

Compatibility/Compounding Considerations

Ammonium chloride should not be titrated with strong oxidizing agents (*e.g.*, potassium chlorate) as explosive compounds may result.

Ammonium chloride is reported to be physically **compatible** with all commonly used IV replacement fluids and potassium chloride. It is **incompatible** with codeine phosphate, dimenhydrinate, methadone HCl, and warfarin sodium. It is also reportedly **incompatible** with alkalis and their hydroxides.

Dosage Forms/Regulatory Status

VETERINARY-LABELED PRODUCTS:

Note: The following may not be FDA-approved products as they are not located in FDA's "Green Book".

Ammonium Chloride Tablets: 200 mg, 400 mg; *UriKare® 200, 400 Tablets*; (Rx). Labeled for use in cats and dogs.

Ammonium Chloride Granules: 200 mg per 1/4 teaspoonful powder; *Uroeze® 200, UriKare® 200*; (Rx). Labeled for cats and dogs.

Ammonium Chloride Granules: 400 mg per 1/4 teaspoonful powder; *Uroeze®, UriKare® 400*; (Rx). Labeled for cats and dogs.

Ammonium chloride is also found in some veterinary labeled cough preparations, *e.g.*, *Spect-Aid® Expectorant Granules* (7% guaifenesin, 75% ammonium chloride, potassium iodide 2%), and in some cough syrups (also containing guaifenesin, pyrilamine and phenylephrine).

When used in large animals, feed grade ammonium chloride can be obtained from feed mills.

HUMAN-LABELED PRODUCTS:

Ammonium Chloride Injection: 26.75% (5 mEq/mL) in 20 mL (100 mEq) vials; generic; (Rx). Preparation of solution for IV administration: Dilute 1 or 2 vials (100–200 mEq) in either 500 or 1000 mL of sodium chloride 0.9% for injection. Do not administer at a rate greater than 5 mL/minute (human adult).

Revisions/References

Monograph revised/updated August 2013.

Bailey, E. M. (1986). Emergency and general treatment of poisonings. *Current Veterinary Therapy (CVT) IX Small Animal Practice*. R. W. Kirk. Philadelphia, W.B. Saunders: 135-44.

Center, S. (2004). *Current recommendations for liver function testing*. Proceedings: ACVIM Forum. accessed via Veterinary Information Network; vin.com

Grauer, G. F. & J. J. Hjelle (1988). Household Toxins. *Handbook of Small Animal Practice*. R. V. Morgan. New York, Churchill Livingstone: 1109-14.

Kienzle, E., et al. (2006). A high roughage/concentrate ratio decreases the effect of ammonium chloride on acid-base balance in horses. *Journal of Nutrition* **136**(7): 2048S-9S.

Labato, M. (2002). *Those troublesome uroliths I and II.* Proceedings: Tufts Animal Expo. accessed via Veterinary Information Network; vin.com

Lage, A. L., et al. (1988). Diseases of the Bladder. *Handbook of Small Animal Practice.* R. V. Morgan. New York, Churchill Livingstone: 605-20.

Mavangira, V., et al. (2010). Effect of ammonium chloride supplementation on urine pH and urinary fractional excretion of electrolytes in goats. *Journal of the American Veterinary Medical Association* **237**(11): 1299-304.

Schmitz, D. (2004). Toxicologic problems. *Equine Internal Medicine 2nd Ed.* S. Reed, W. Bayly and D. Sellon. Philadelphia, Saunders: 1441-512.

Snyder, J. (2009). *Small Ruminant Medicine & Surgery for Equine and Small Animal Practitioners I & II.* Proceedings: WVC. accessed via Veterinary Information Network; vin.com

Sprake, P., et al. (2012). The Effect of Ammonium Chloride Treatment as a Long Term Preventative Approach for Urolithiasis in Goats and a Comparison of Continuous and Pulse Dosing Regimes. Journal of Veterinary Internal Medicine. accessed via Veterinary Information Network; vin.com

Van Metre, D. (2009). *Urolithiasis in ruminants.* Proceedings: Western Veterinary Conference. accessed via Veterinary Information Network; vin.com

Ammonium Molybdate
Ammonium Tetrathiomolybdate

(ah-**moe**-nee-um moe-**lib**-date; tet-ra-**thye**-oh-moe-**lib**-date) TTM, Molypen®

Copper Poisoning Treatment

Prescriber Highlights

▶ Used primarily to treat copper poisoning in food animals (esp. sheep).

▶ Consider contacting FDA for guidance in treating food animals.

Uses/Indications

Ammonium molybdate and ammonium tetrathiomolybdate (TTM) are used for the investigational or compassionate treatment of copper poisoning in food animals, primarily sheep.

Adverse Effects

After apparent successful treatment for copper poisoning with ammonium tetrathiomolybdate (TTM), a flock of sheep became infertile, progressively unthrifty, and died 2-3 years later. The authors concluded the TTM was retained in the CNS, pituitary and adrenal glands and caused a toxic endocrinopathy (Haywood et al. 2004).

Reproductive/Nursing Safety

In humans, the FDA categorizes this drug as category **C** for use during pregnancy (*Animal studies have shown an adverse effect on the fetus, but there are no adequate studies in humans; or there are no animal reproduction studies and no adequate studies in humans.*)

Doses

Note: In food animals, FARAD recommends a minimum 10-day preslaughter withdrawal time and a minimum 5-day milk withholding interval (Haskell et al. 2005).

Ammonium tetrathiomolybdate does not go into solution readily and ammonium molybdate administered orally is often preferred.

■ **SHEEP:**

For treatment of copper poisoning (extra-label):

a) **Sheep:** Tetrathiomolybdate (TTM): Until more is known about the significance of TTM cuproenzyme inhibition it is recommended that it be used conservatively: 1 mg/kg IV once. Dose could be repeated if there is recurrence of pre-hemolytic copper poisoning. Reduction in available copper in dietary supply is necessary. Zinc (150 mg/kg) may be useful along with the antagonists, molybdate and sulfate. (Suttle 2012)

b) **Food animals:** Ammonium molybdate: 200 mg per head PO once daily for 3 weeks. Ammonium tetrathiomolybdate: 1.7 – 3.4 mg per head IV or SC every other day for 3 treatments (Post et al. 2000).

c) **Ammonium tetrathiomolybdate:** 1.7 mg/kg IV or 3.4 mg/kg SC every other day for 3 treatments. Alternatively, ammonium molybdate 50 – 500 mg PO once daily and sodium thiosulfate 300 – 1000 mg PO once daily for 3 weeks. (Plumlee 1996)

d) **Ammonium tetrathiomolybdate:** 2 – 15 mg/kg IV q24h (once daily) for 3-6 days. (Boileau 2009)

Dosage Forms/Regulatory Status

VETERINARY-LABELED PRODUCTS: NONE.

Note: Ammonium molybdate or ammonium tetrathiomolybdate can be obtained from various chemical supply houses. There are no veterinary FDA-approved products, but the FDA has historically used discretion in enforcement when molybdate is used for copper poisoning in animals. However, it is recommended to contact the FDA-CVM before treating for guidance.

HUMAN-LABELED PRODUCTS:

Ammonium Molybdate Injection: 25 micrograms/mL (as 46 micrograms/mL ammonium molybdate tetrahydrate) in 10 mL vial; generic; (Rx). Approved for use in TPN solutions to help prevent depletion of endogenous molybdenum stores and subsequent deficiency syndromes.

Ammonium molybdate may also be known as: *Molybdene Injectable®*, or *Molypen®*. Ammonium tetrathiomolybdate may also be known as TTM.

Revisions/References

Monograph revised/updated August 2013.

Boileau, M. (2009). *Challenging cases in small ruminant medicine.* Proceedings: ACVIM. accessed via Veterinary Information Network; vin.com

Haskell, S., et al. (2005). Farad Digest: Antidotes in Food Animal Practice. *JAVMA* **226**(6): 884-7.

Haywood, S., et al. (2004). Molybdenum-associated pituitary endocrinopathy in sheep associated with ammonium tetrathiomolybdate. *J Comparative Path* **130**(1): 21-31.

Plumlee, K. (1996). Disorders caused by toxicants: Metals and other inorganic compounds. *Large Animal Internal Medicine 2nd Ed.* B. Smith, Mosby: 1902-8.

Post, L. & W. Keller (2000). Current status of food animal antidotes. *The Veterinary Clinics of North America: Food Animal Practice* **16**:3(November).

Suttle, N. F. (2012). Responsiveness of prehaemolytic copper poisoning in sheep from a specific pathogen-free environment to a relatively high dose of tetrathiomolybdate. *Veterinary Record* **171**(10): 246-+.

Amoxicillin

(a-mox-i-**sill**-in)   Amoxil®, Amoxi-Tabs®

Aminopenicillin

Prescriber Highlights

▶ Bactericidal aminopenicillin with same spectrum as ampicillin (ineffective against bacteria that produce beta-lactamase).

▶ Most likely adverse effects are GI-related, but hypersensitivity & other adverse effects occur rarely.

Uses/Indications

The aminopenicillins have been used for a wide range of infections in various species. FDA-approved indications/species, as well as non-approved uses, are listed in the Dosages section below. Because of its enhanced efficacy against many lactamase-producing bacteria, potentiated amoxicillin (with clavulanate) is often chosen for use in small animals, but amoxicillin (alone) can be effectively and more inexpensively used particularly for treatment of urinary tract infections and Lyme disease (Borelliosis).

According to one reference (Trepanier 2009), amoxicillin (alone) is a reasonable first choice for empiric treatment (before culture and susceptibility results are back) of abscesses in cats. Quadruple therapy (amoxicillin in combination with clarithromycin, metronidazole and a proton pump inhibitor) did not eradicate *H. pylori* in

4/13 treated cats, and may only cause transient suppression (Khosh-negah et al. 2011).

Pharmacology/Actions

Like other penicillins, amoxicillin is a time-dependent, bactericidal (usually) agent that acts by inhibiting cell wall synthesis. Although there may be some slight differences in activity against certain organisms, amoxicillin generally shares the same spectrum of activity and uses as ampicillin. Because it is better absorbed orally (in non-ruminants), higher serum levels may be attained than with ampicillin. Urinary tract-specific breakpoint for amoxicillin in dogs is ≤ 8 mcg/mL.

Penicillins are usually bactericidal against susceptible bacteria and act by inhibiting mucopeptide synthesis in the cell wall resulting in a defective barrier and an osmotically unstable spheroplast. The exact mechanism for this effect has not been definitively determined, but beta-lactam antibiotics have been shown to bind to several enzymes (carboxypeptidases, transpeptidases, endopeptidases) within the bacterial cytoplasmic membrane that are involved with cell wall synthesis. The different affinities that various beta-lactam antibiotics have for these enzymes (also known as penicillin-binding proteins; PBPs) help explain the differences in spectrums of activity the drugs have that are not explained by the influence of beta-lactamases. Like other beta-lactam antibiotics, penicillins are generally considered more effective against actively growing bacteria.

The aminopenicillins, also called the "broad-spectrum" or ampicillin penicillins, have increased activity against many strains of gram-negative aerobes not covered by either the natural penicillins or penicillinase-resistant penicillins, including some strains of E. coli, Klebsiella, and Haemophilus. Like the natural penicillins, they are susceptible to inactivation by beta-lactamase-producing bacteria (e.g., Staph aureus). Although not as active as the natural penicillins, they do have activity against many anaerobic bacteria, including Clostridial organisms. Organisms that are generally not susceptible include Pseudomonas aeruginosa, Serratia, Indole-positive Proteus (Proteus mirabilis is susceptible), Enterobacter, Citrobacter, and Acinetobacter. The aminopenicillins also are inactive against Rickettsia, mycobacteria, fungi, Mycoplasma, and viruses.

In order to reduce the inactivation of penicillins by beta-lactamases, potassium clavulanate and sulbactam have been developed to inactivate these enzymes and thus extend the spectrum of those penicillins. When used with a penicillin, these combinations are often effective againta-lactamase-producing strains of otherwise resistant E. coli, Pasteurella spp., Staphylococcus spp., Klebsiella, and Proteus. Type I beta-lactamases that are often associated with E. coli, Enterobacter, and Pseudomonas are not generally inhibited by clavulanic acid.

Pharmacokinetics

Amoxicillin trihydrate is relatively stable in the presence of gastric acid. After oral administration, it is about 74-92% absorbed in humans and monogastric animals. Food will decrease the rate, but not the extent of oral absorption and many clinicians suggest giving the drug with food, particularly if there is concomitant associated GI distress. Amoxicillin serum levels will generally be 1.5-3 times greater than those of ampicillin after equivalent oral doses.

After absorption, the volume of distribution for amoxicillin is approximately 0.3 L/kg in humans and 0.2 L/kg in dogs. The drug is widely distributed to many tissues, including liver, lungs, prostate (human), muscle, bile, and ascitic, pleural and synovial fluids. Amoxicillin will cross into the CSF when meninges are inflamed in concentrations that may range from 10-60% of those found in serum. Very low levels of the drug are found in the aqueous humor, and low levels found in tears, sweat and saliva. Amoxicillin cross-es the placenta, but it is thought to be relatively safe to use during pregnancy. It is approximately 17-20% bound to human plasma proteins, primarily albumin. Protein binding in dogs is approximately 13%. Milk levels of amoxicillin are considered low.

Amoxicillin is eliminated primarily through renal mechanisms, principally by tubular secretion, but some of the drug is metabolized by hydrolysis to penicilloic acids (inactive) and then excreted in the urine. Elimination half-lives of amoxicillin have been reported as 45-90 minutes in dogs and cats, and 90 minutes in cattle. Clearance is reportedly 1.9 mL/kg/minute in dogs.

Contraindications/Precautions/Warnings

Penicillins are contraindicated in patients with a history of hypersensitivity to them. Because there may be cross-reactivity, use penicillins cautiously in patients who are documented hypersensitive to other beta-lactam antibiotics (e.g., cephalosporins, cefamycins, carbapenems).

Do not administer penicillins, cephalosporins, or macrolides to rabbits, guinea pigs, chinchillas, hamsters, etc. or serious enteritis and clostridial enterotoxemia may occur.

Do not administer systemic antibiotics orally in patients with septicemia, shock, or other grave illnesses as absorption of the medication from the GI tract may be significantly delayed or diminished. Parenteral (preferably IV) routes should be used for these cases.

Adverse Effects

Adverse effects with the penicillins are usually not serious and have a relatively low frequency of occurrence.

Hypersensitivity reactions unrelated to dose can occur with these agents and can manifest as rashes (including serious cutaneous reactions), fever, eosinophilia, neutropenia, agranulocytosis, thrombocytopenia, leukopenia, anemia, lymphadenopathy, or full-blown anaphylaxis.

When given orally, penicillins may cause GI effects (anorexia, vomiting, diarrhea). Because the penicillins may alter gut flora, antibiotic-associated diarrhea can occur and allow the proliferation of resistant bacteria in the colon (superinfections). Healthy dogs given oral amoxicillin had their gut flora altered with a shift in balance toward gram-negative bacteria that included resistant Enterobacteriaceae species (Gronvold et al. 2010).

High doses or very prolonged use have been associated with neurotoxicity (e.g., ataxia in dogs). Although the penicillins are not considered hepatotoxic, elevated liver enzymes have been reported. Other effects reported in dogs include tachypnea, dyspnea, edema and tachycardia.

Reproductive/Nursing Safety

Penicillins have been shown to cross the placenta; safe use during pregnancy has not been firmly established, but neither has there been any documented teratogenic problems associated with these drugs. However, use only when the potential benefits outweigh the risks. In humans, the FDA categorizes this drug as category **B** for use during pregnancy (Animal studies have not yet demonstrated risk to the fetus, but there are no adequate studies in pregnant women; or animal studies have shown an adverse effect, but adequate studies in pregnant women have not demonstrated a risk to the fetus in the first trimester of pregnancy, and there is no evidence of risk in later trimesters.) In a separate system evaluating the safety of drugs in canine and feline pregnancy (Papich 1989), this drug is categorized as class: **A** (Probably safe. Although specific studies may not have proved the safety of all drugs in dogs and cats, there are no reports of adverse effects in laboratory animals or women.)

Overdosage/Acute Toxicity

Acute oral penicillin overdoses are unlikely to cause significant problems other than GI distress but other effects are possible (see Adverse Effects). In humans, very high dosages of parenteral penicillins, especially in patients with renal disease, have induced CNS effects.

Drug Interactions

The following drug interactions with amoxicillin have either been reported or are theoretical in humans or animals and may be of significance in veterinary patients. Unless otherwise noted, use together is not necessarily contraindicated, but weigh the potential risks and perform additional monitoring when appropriate.

- **BACTERIOSTATIC ANTIMICROBIALS** (*e.g.,* **chloramphenicol, erythromycin** and other **macrolides, tetracyclines, sulfonamides,** etc.): Because there is evidence of *in vitro* antagonism between beta-lactam antibiotics and bacteriostatic antibiotics, use together has been generally not recommended in the past, but the actual clinical importance is not clear and in doubt.
- **METHOTREXATE**: Amoxicillin may decrease the renal excretion of MTX causing increased levels and potential MTX toxic effects.
- **PROBENECID**: Competitively blocks the tubular secretion of most penicillins, thereby increasing serum levels and serum half-lives.

Laboratory Considerations

- Amoxicillin may cause false-positive **urine glucose determinations** when using cupric sulfate solution (Benedict's Solution, *Clinitest®*). Tests utilizing glucose oxidase (*Tes-Tape®, Clinistix®*) are not affected by amoxicillin.
- As penicillins and other beta-lactams can inactivate **aminoglycosides** *in vitro* (and *in vivo* in patients in renal failure), serum concentrations of aminoglycosides may be falsely decreased if the patient is also receiving beta-lactam antibiotics particularly when the serum is stored prior to analysis. It is recommended that if the assay is delayed, samples be frozen and if possible, drawn at times when the beta-lactam antibiotic is at a trough.

Doses

- **DOGS:**

  Labeled Dosage (FDA-approved); (**Note:** While the following indications and dosages are on the FDA-approved label, they are not accepted by most today as being consistently efficacious. Indications: Respiratory tract infections (tonsillitis, tracheobronchitis) due to *Staphylococcus aureus, Streptococcus* spp., *E. coli,* and *Proteus mirabilis*. Genitourinary tract infections (cystitis) due to *Staphylococcus aureus, Streptococcus* spp., *E. coli,* and *Proteus mirabilis*. Gastrointestinal tract infections (bacterial gastroenteritis) due to *Staphylococcus aureus, Streptococcus* spp., *E. coli,* and *Proteus mirabilis*. Bacterial dermatitis due to *Staphylococcus aureus, Streptococcus* spp., and *Proteus mirabilis*. Dosage: 11 mg/kg PO twice a day.

  For urinary tract infections (UTI); (extra-label):
  a) Empirically (when waiting for culture/susceptibility results) or after urine culture shows susceptibility: 11 – 15 mg/kg PO q8h. Typically, uncomplicated UTIs are treated for 7-14 days, however shorter treatment time (≤7 days) may be effective, but until objective data is available, 7 days is reasonable. For complicated UTI: Evidence is lacking to support a given duration of treatment but typically, 4 weeks has been recommended and is reasonable until further evidence is forthcoming. Although evidence is lacking, animals with a non-recurrent but deemed complicated (due to a comorbidity) UTI, shorter-term therapy may be reasonable. Urine cul-

  ture should be considered 5-7 days after initiation of therapy, particularly in patients with a history of relapsing or refractory infection, or those considered at high risk for ascending or systemic infection. Adapted from Antimicrobial Use Guidelines for Treatment of Urinary Tract Disease in Dogs and Cats: Antimicrobial Guidelines Working Group of the International Society for Companion Animal Infectious Diseases. (Weese et al. 2011)

  b) For preventative therapy for recurrent (>2 per 6 months) urinary tract gram-positive bacterial infections: 20 mg/kg PO once daily before bedtime after the dog has urinated. Use only after effective treatment completed using full therapeutic doses. (Adams 2009; Adams 2013)

  For Lyme borreliosis (*B. burgdorferi*) infections (extra-label): 20 mg/kg PO three times daily for 30 days. (Krupka et al. 2010)

- **CATS:**

  Labeled Dosage (FDA-approved); (**Note:** While the following indications and dosages are on the FDA-approved label, they are not accepted by most today as being consistently efficacious. Upper respiratory tract infections due to *Staphylococcus aureus, Streptococcus* spp., and *E. coli*. Genitourinary tract infections (cystitis) due to *Staphylococcus aureus, Streptococcus* spp., *E. coli,* and *Proteus mirabilis*. Gastrointestinal tract infections due to *E. coli*. Skin and soft tissue infections (abscesses, lacerations, and wounds) due to *Staphylococcus aureus, Streptococcus* spp., *E. coli,* and *Pasteurella multocida*. As with all antibiotics, appropriate *in vitro* culturing and susceptibility testing of samples taken before treatment should be conducted. Dosage: 50 mg per cat (11 – 22 mg/kg) once a day. Dosage should be continued for 5-7 days or 48 hours after all symptoms have subsided. If no improvement is seen in 5 days, review diagnosis and change therapy. (Label Information; *Amoxi-Tabs®*)

  For urinary tract infections (UTI); (extra-label): Empirically (when waiting for culture/susceptibility results) or after urine culture shows susceptibility: 11 – 15 mg/kg PO q8h. Typically, uncomplicated UTIs are treated for 7-14 days, however shorter treatment time (≤7 days) may be effective, but until objective data is available, 7 days is reasonable. For complicated UTI: Evidence is lacking to support a given duration of treatment but typically, 4 weeks has been recommended and is reasonable until further evidence is forthcoming. Although evidence is lacking, animals with a non-recurrent but deemed complicated (due to a comorbidity) UTI, shorter-term therapy may be reasonable. Urine culture should be considered 5-7 days after initiation of therapy, particularly in patients with a history of relapsing or refractory infection, or those considered at high risk for ascending or systemic infection. Adapted from Antimicrobial Use Guidelines for Treatment of Urinary Tract Disease in Dogs and Cats: Antimicrobial Guidelines Working Group of the International Society for Companion Animal Infectious Diseases. (Weese et al. 2011)

  For treating *H. pylori* infections using quadruple therapy (extra-label): amoxicillin 20 mg/kg PO twice daily, metronidazole 20 mg/kg PO twice daily, clarithromycin 7.5 mg/kg PO twice daily, and omeprazole 0.7 mg/kg q8h for 14 days. Treatment did not eradicate organism in 4 of 13 cats in study. (Khoshnegah et al. 2011)

- **FERRETS:**

  For treating Helicobacter gastritis infections (extra-label): Using triple therapy: Metronidazole 20 mg/kg PO q12h, amoxicillin 20 mg/kg PO q12h and bismuth subsalicylate 17.5 mg/kg PO q8h. Give 21 days. Sucralfate (25 mg/kg PO q8h) and famotidine (0.5 mg/kg PO once daily) are also used. Fluids and assisted feeding should be continued while the primary cause of disease is investigated. (Johnson 2006)

■ **RABBITS/RODENTS/SMALL MAMMALS:**

Note: See warning above in Contraindications; extra-label.

a) **Hedgehogs:** 15 mg/kg IM or PO q12h. (Smith 2000)

■ **BIRDS:**

For susceptible infections (extra-label):

a) 125 mg/kg q12h PO. Mix oral solution to double strength to a final concentration of 125 mg/mL. (Antinoff 2009)

b) 100 mg/kg q8h, IM, SC, PO. (Hoeffer 1995)

■ **REPTILES:**

For susceptible infections (extra-label): For all species: 22 mg/kg PO q12-24h; not very useful unless used in combination with aminoglycosides. (Gauvin 1993)

Monitoring

■ Because penicillins usually have minimal toxicity associated with their use, monitoring for efficacy is usually all that is required unless toxic signs develop. Serum levels and therapeutic drug monitoring are not routinely done with these agents.

Client Information

■ The oral suspension should preferably be refrigerated, but refrigeration is not absolutely necessary; any unused oral suspension should be discarded after 14 days.

■ Can be given with or without food, but gastrointestinal side effects might be prevented if given with food.

■ Most common side effects are diarrhea, vomiting and loss of appetite.

■ Be sure to give as long as veterinarian has prescribed, even if animal seems better.

■ Do not give to rabbits, guinea pigs, chinchillas, hamsters, rodents or other pocket pets since life-threatening diarrhea may occur.

Chemistry/Synonyms

An aminopenicillin, amoxicillin is commercially available as the trihydrate. It occurs as a practically odorless, white, crystalline powder that is sparingly soluble in water. Amoxicillin differs structurally from ampicillin only by having an additional hydroxyl group on the phenyl ring.

Amoxicillin may also be known as: amoxycillin, p-hydroxyampicillin, or BRL 2333; many trade names are available.

Storage/Stability

Amoxicillin capsules, tablets, and powder for oral suspension should be stored at room temperature (15-30°C) in tight containers. After reconstitution, the oral suspension should preferably be refrigerated (refrigeration not absolutely necessary) and any unused product discarded after 14 days.

Compatibility/Compounding Considerations

No specific information noted.

Dosage Forms/Regulatory Status

VETERINARY-LABELED PRODUCTS:

Amoxicillin Oral Tablets: 50 mg, 100 mg, 150 mg, 200 mg, & 400 mg; *Amoxi-Tabs®*, generic; (Rx). FDA-approved for use in dogs and cats.

Amoxicillin Powder for Oral Suspension 50 mg/mL (after reconstitution) in 15 mL or 30 mL bottles; *Amoxi-Drop®*, generic; (Rx). FDA-approved for use in dogs and cats.

HUMAN-LABELED PRODUCTS:

Amoxicillin Oral Tablets (chewable): 125 mg, 200 mg, 250 mg, & 400 mg; *Amoxil®*, generic; (Rx)

Amoxicillin Oral Tablets: 500 mg & 875 mg; *Amoxil®*, generic; (Rx)

Amoxicillin Oral Capsules: 250 mg, & 500 mg; *Amoxil®*, generic; (Rx)

Amoxicillin Powder for Oral Suspension: 200 mg/5 mL in 50 mL, 75 mL & 100 mL; 250 mg/5 mL in 80 mL, 100 mL & 150 mL; 400 mg/5 mL in 50 mL, 75 mL & 100 mL; *Amoxil®*, *Trimox®*, generic; (Rx)

Amoxicillin Oral Extended-Release Tablets: 775 mg in 30s & UD 10s; *Moxatag®*; (Rx)

Revisions/References

Monograph revised/updated August 2013.

Adams, L. (2009). *Recurrent Urinary Tract Infections: Bad Bugs That Won't Go Away*. Proceedings: WVC. accessed via Veterinary Information Network; vin.com

Adams, L. G. (2013). *Recurrent Urinary Tract Infections*. World Small Animal Veterinary Association World Congress. accessed via Veterinary Information Network; vin.com

Antinoff, N. (2009). *Avian Critical Care: What's Old, What's New*. Proceedings: IVECCS. accessed via Veterinary Information Network; vin.com

Gauvin, J. (1993). Drug therapy in reptiles. *Seminars in Avian & Exotic Med* 2(1): 48-59.

Gronvold, A. M. R., et al. (2010). Changes in fecal microbiota of healthy dogs administered amoxicillin. *Fems Microbiology Ecology* 71(2): 313-26.

Hoeffer, H. (1995). Antimicrobials in pet birds. *Kirk's Current Veterinary Therapy:XII*. J. Bonagura. Philadelphia, W.B. Saunders: 1278-83.

Johnson, D. (2006). *Ferrets: the other companion animal*. Proceedings: ACVC. accessed via Veterinary Information Network; vin.com

Khoshnegah, J., et al. (2011). The efficacy and safety of long-term Helicobacter species quadruple therapy in asymptomatic cats with naturally acquired infection. *Journal of Feline Medicine & Surgery* 13(2): 88-93.

Krupka, I. & R. K. Straubinger (2010). Lyme Borreliosis in Dogs and Cats: Background, Diagnosis, Treatment and Prevention of Infections with Borrelia burgdorferi sensu stricto. *Veterinary Clinics of North America-Small Animal Practice* 40(6): 1103-+.

Smith, A. (2000). General husbandry and medical care of hedgehogs. *Kirk's Current Veterinary Therapy: XIII Small Animal Practice*. J. Bonagura. Philadelphia, WB Saunders: 1128-33.

Trepanier, L. (2009). *Appropriate empirical antimicrobial therapy: Making decisions without a culture*. Proceedings: ACVIM. accessed via Veterinary Information Network; vin.com

Weese, J. S., et al. (2011). Antimicrobial Use Guidelines for Treatment of Urinary Tract Disease in Dogs and Cats: Antimicrobial Guidelines Working Group of the International Society for Companion Animal Infectious Diseases. *Veterinary Medicine International*.

Amoxicillin/Clavulanate Potassium; Amoxicillin/Clavulanic Acid

(a-mox-i-**sill**-in clav-yue-**lan**-ate)

Clavamox®, Augmentin®

Potentiated Aminopenicillin

Prescriber Highlights

▶ Bactericidal aminopenicillin with beta-lactamase inhibitor that expands its spectrum. Not effective against Pseudomonas or Enterobacter.

▶ Most likely adverse effects are GI related, but hypersensitivity & other adverse effects occur rarely.

▶ If writing prescriptions to be filled at human pharmacies: Note that when compared to veterinary-labeled products, human-labeled products contain differing ratios of amoxicillin:clavulanate and are expressed in terms of amoxicillin (only) while veterinary products are expressed in terms of both compounds.

Uses/Indications

Amoxicillin/potassium clavulanate tablets and oral suspension products are FDA-approved for use in dogs and cats for the treatment of urinary tract, skin and soft tissue infections caused by susceptible organisms. It is also indicated for canine periodontal disease due to susceptible strains of bacteria. According to one reference (Trepanier 2009), amoxicillin + clavulanate is a reasonable first choice for empiric treatment (before culture and susceptibility results are back) of bacterial cystitis in female dogs, and hepatobiliary infections (with a fluoroquinolone) in dogs or cats.

Pharmacology/Actions

For information on the pharmacology/actions of amoxicillin, refer that monograph.

Clavulanic acid has only weak antibacterial activity when used alone and presently it is only available in fixed-dose combinations with either amoxicillin (oral) or ticarcillin (parenteral). Clavulanic acid acts by competitively and irreversibly binding to beta-lactamases, including types II, III, IV, and V, and penicillinases produced by staphylococci. Staphylococci that are resistant to penicillinase-resistant penicillins (*e.g.*, oxacillin) are considered resistant to amoxicillin/potassium clavulanate, although susceptibility testing may indicate otherwise. Amoxicillin/potassium clavulanate is usually ineffective against type I cephalosporinases. Members of the family Enterobacteriaceae, particularly Pseudomonas aeruginosa, often produce these plasmid-mediated cephalosporinases. When combined with amoxicillin, there is little if any synergistic activity against organisms already susceptible to amoxicillin, but amoxicillin-resistant strains (due to beta-lactamase inactivation) may be covered.

When performing Kirby-Bauer susceptibility testing, the *Augmentin®* (human-product trade name) disk is often used. Because the amoxicillin:clavulanic acid ratio of 2:1 in the susceptibility tests may not correspond to *in vivo* drug levels, susceptibility testing may not always accurately predict efficacy for this combination. A urinary tract-specific breakpoint in dogs and cats for amoxicillin-clavulanate is reported as <8/4 mcg/mL.

Pharmacokinetics

The pharmacokinetics of amoxicillin are presented in that drug's monograph. There is no evidence to suggest that the addition of clavulanic acid significantly alters amoxicillin pharmacokinetics.

Clavulanate potassium is relatively stable in the presence of gastric acid and is readily absorbed. In dogs, the absorption half-life is reportedly 0.39 hours with peak levels occurring about 1 hour after dosing. Specific bioavailability data for dogs or cats was not located.

Clavulanic acid has an apparent volume of distribution of 0.32 L/kg in dogs and is distributed (with amoxicillin) into the lungs, pleural fluid and peritoneal fluid. Low concentrations of both drugs are found in the saliva, sputum and CSF (uninflamed meninges). Higher concentrations in the CSF are expected when meninges are inflamed, but it is questionable whether therapeutic levels are attainable. Clavulanic acid is 13% bound to proteins in dog serum. The drug readily crosses the placenta but is not believed to be teratogenic. Clavulanic acid and amoxicillin are both found in milk in low concentrations.

Clavulanic acid is apparently extensively metabolized in the dog (and rat) primarily to 1-amino-4-hydroxybutan-2-one. It is not known if this compound possesses any beta-lactamase inhibiting activity. The drug is also excreted unchanged in the urine via glomerular filtration. In dogs, 34-52% of a dose is excreted in the urine as unchanged drug and metabolites, 25-27% eliminated in the feces, and 16-33% into respired air. Urine levels of active drug are considered high, but may be only 1/5th of those of amoxicillin.

Contraindications/Precautions/Warnings

Penicillins are contraindicated in patients with a history of hypersensitivity to them. Because there may be cross-reactivity, use penicillins cautiously in patients who are documented hypersensitive to other beta-lactam antibiotics (*e.g.*, cephalosporins, cefamycins, carbapenems).

Do not administer systemic antibiotics orally in patients with septicemia, shock, or other grave illnesses as absorption of the medication from the GI tract may be significantly delayed or diminished.

Do not administer penicillins, cephalosporins, or macrolides to rabbits, guinea pigs, chinchillas, hamsters, etc. or serious enteritis and clostridial enterotoxemia may occur.

Adverse Effects

Adverse effects with the penicillins are usually not serious and have a relatively low frequency of occurrence.

Hypersensitivity reactions unrelated to dose can occur with these agents and can manifest as rashes (including serious cutaneous reactions), fever, eosinophilia, neutropenia, agranulocytosis, thrombocytopenia, leukopenia, anemia, lymphadenopathy, or full-blown anaphylaxis.

When given orally, penicillins may cause GI effects (anorexia, vomiting, diarrhea). Because the penicillins may alter gut flora, antibiotic-associated diarrhea can occur and allow the proliferation of resistant bacteria in the colon (superinfections).

Neurotoxicity (*e.g.*, ataxia in dogs) has been associated with very high doses or very prolonged use. Although the penicillins are not considered hepatotoxic, elevated liver enzymes have been reported. Other effects reported in dogs include tachypnea, dyspnea, edema and tachycardia.

Reproductive/Nursing Safety

In humans, the FDA categorizes this drug as category **B** for use during pregnancy (*Animal studies have not yet demonstrated risk to the fetus, but there are no adequate studies in pregnant women; or animal studies have shown an adverse effect, but adequate studies in pregnant women have not demonstrated a risk to the fetus in the first trimester of pregnancy, and there is no evidence of risk in later trimesters.*) In a separate system evaluating the safety of drugs in canine and feline pregnancy (Papich 1989), this drug is categorized as class: **A** (*Probably safe. Although specific studies may not have proved the safety of all drugs in dogs and cats, there are no reports of adverse effects in laboratory animals or women.*)

Overdosage/Acute Toxicity

Acute oral penicillin overdoses are unlikely to cause significant problems other than GI distress, but other effects are possible (see Adverse Effects). In humans, very high dosages of parenteral penicillins, especially in patients with renal disease, have induced CNS effects.

Drug Interactions

The following drug interactions with amoxicillin-clavulanate have either been reported or are theoretical in humans or animals and may be of significance in veterinary patients. Unless otherwise noted, use together is not necessarily contraindicated, but weigh the potential risks and perform additional monitoring when appropriate.

- **BACTERIOSTATIC ANTIMICROBIALS** (*e.g.*, **chloramphenicol, erythromycin** and other **macrolides, tetracyclines, sulfonamides,** etc.): Because there is evidence of *in vitro* antagonism between beta-lactam antibiotics and bacteriostatic antibiotics, use together has been generally not recommended in the past, but actual clinical importance is not clear and currently in doubt.
- **METHOTREXATE:** Amoxicillin may decrease the renal excretion of MTX causing increased levels and potential MTX toxic effects.
- **PROBENECID:** Competitively blocks the tubular secretion of most penicillins, thereby increasing serum levels and serum half-lives.

Laboratory Considerations

- Amoxicillin may cause false-positive **urine glucose determinations** when using cupric sulfate solution (Benedict's Solution, *Clinitest®*). Tests utilizing glucose oxidase (*Tes-Tape®, Clinistix®*) are not affected by amoxicillin.
- As penicillins and other beta-lactams can inactivate **aminogly-**

cosides *in vitro* (and *in vivo* in patients in renal failure), serum concentrations of aminoglycosides may be falsely decreased if the patient is also receiving beta-lactam antibiotics particularly when the serum is stored prior to analysis. It is recommended that if the assay is delayed, samples be frozen and if possible, drawn at times when the beta-lactam antibiotic is at a trough.

Doses

Note: All doses are for combined quantities of both drugs (unless noted otherwise).

- **DOGS:**

  Labeled Dosage (FDA-approved); Indications: Skin and soft tissue infections such as wounds, abscesses, cellulitis, superficial/juvenile and deep pyoderma due to susceptible strains of the following organisms: β-lactamase-producing *Staphylococcus aureus* non-β-lactamase-producing *Staphylococcus aureus*, *Staphylococcus* spp., *Streptococcus* spp., and *E. coli*. Periodontal infections due to susceptible strains of both aerobic and anaerobic bacteria. Dosage: 13.75 mg/kg PO twice a day. Skin and soft tissue infections such as abscesses, cellulitis, wounds, superficial/juvenile pyoderma, and periodontal infections should be treated for 5-7 days or for 48 hours after all symptoms have subsided. If no response is seen after 5 days of treatment, therapy should be discontinued and the case reevaluated. Deep pyoderma may require treatment for 21 days; the maximum duration of treatment should not exceed 30 days.

  For urinary tract infections (UTI); (extra-label): Empirically (when waiting for culture/susceptibility results) or if organism is susceptible: 12.5 – 25 mg/kg PO q8h is an acceptable option but is not recommended initially because of the lack of evidence for requiring clavulanic acid and the desire to use the narrowest spectrum that is possible while maintaining optimal efficacy (amoxicillin alone or trimethoprim/sulfa are preferred for empirical treatment). Typically, uncomplicated UTIs are treated for 7-14 days, however shorter treatment time (≤7 days) may be effective, but until objective data is available, 7 days is reasonable. For complicated UTI: Evidence is lacking to support a given duration of treatment but typically, 4 weeks has been recommended and is reasonable until further evidence is forthcoming. Although evidence is lacking, animals with a non-recurrent but deemed complicated (due to a comorbidity) UTI, shorter-term therapy may be reasonable. Urine culture should be considered 5-7 days after initiation of therapy, particularly in patients with a history of relapsing or refractory infection, or those considered at high risk for ascending or systemic infection. Adapted from Antimicrobial Use Guidelines for Treatment of Urinary Tract Disease in Dogs and Cats: Antimicrobial Guidelines Working Group of the International Society for Companion Animal Infectious Diseases (ISCAID) (Weese et al. 2011).

  For pyoderma (extra-label): Superficial: 12.5 mg/kg PO twice daily for 21-28 days. Fair evidence available to support moderate to high efficacy. Deep: 12.5 mg/kg PO for at least 28 days. Good level of evidence for high efficacy. (Summers et al. 2012)

  For treatment of endocarditis (chronic therapy) secondary to a susceptible strain of Staphylococcus (extra-label): 20 mg/kg PO three times daily for 6-8 weeks. (MacDonald 2010)

- **CATS:**

  Labeled Dosage (FDA-approved); Indications: Skin and soft tissue infections such as wounds, abscesses, and cellulitis/dermatitis due to susceptible strains of the following organisms: β-lactamase-producing Staphylococcus aureus, non-βeta-lactamase-producing Staphylococcus aureus, Staphylococcus spp., Streptococcus spp., E. coli, Pasteurella multocida, and Pasteurella spp. Urinary tract infections (cystitis) due to susceptible

strains of E. coli. Therapy may be initiated prior to obtaining results from bacteriological and susceptibility studies. A culture should be obtained prior to treatment to determine susceptibility of the organisms to this drug. Following determination of susceptibility results and clinical response to medication, therapy may be reevaluated. Dosage: 62.5 mg per cat twice a day. Skin and soft tissue infections such as abscesses and cellulitis/dermatitis should be treated for 5-7 days or 48 hours after all symptoms have subsided, not to exceed 30 days. If no response is seen after 3 days of treatment, therapy should be discontinued and the case reevaluated. Urinary tract infections may require treatment for 10-14 days or longer. The maximum duration of treatment should not exceed 30 days.

For urinary tract infections (UTI); (extra-label): Empirically (when waiting for culture/susceptibility results) or if organism is susceptible: 12.5 – 25 mg/kg PO q8h is an acceptable option but is not recommended initially because of the lack of evidence for requiring clavulanic acid and the desire to use the narrowest spectrum that is possible while maintaining optimal efficacy (amoxicillin alone or trimethoprim/sulfa are preferred for empirical treatment). Typically, uncomplicated UTIs are treated for 7-14 days, however shorter treatment time (≤7 days) may be effective, but until objective data is available, 7 days is reasonable. For complicated UTI: Evidence is lacking to support a given duration of treatment but typically, 4 weeks has been recommended and is reasonable until further evidence is forthcoming. Although evidence is lacking, animals with a non-recurrent but deemed complicated (due to a comorbidity) UTI, shorter-term therapy may be reasonable. Urine culture should be considered 5-7 days after initiation of therapy, particularly in patients with a history of relapsing or refractory infection, or those considered at high risk for ascending or systemic infection. Adapted from Antimicrobial Use Guidelines for Treatment of Urinary Tract Disease in Dogs and Cats: Antimicrobial Guidelines Working Group of the International Society for Companion Animal Infectious Diseases (ISCAID) (Weese et al. 2011).

For upper respiratory tract disease (URTD) with a bacterial component (extra-label): 12.5 mg/kg PO q12h for 14 days. Study done in shelter cats. (Litster et al. 2012)

- **FERRETS:**

  For susceptible infections (extra-label): 10 – 20 mg/kg PO 2–3 times daily. (Williams 2000)

- **BIRDS:**

  For susceptible infections (extra-label): 50 – 100 mg/kg PO q6–8h. (Hoeffer 1995)

Client Information

- The oral suspension should preferably be refrigerated, but refrigeration is not absolutely necessary; any unused oral suspension should be discarded after 10 days.
- Can be given with or without food, but gastrointestinal side effects might be prevented if given with food.
- Most common side effects are diarrhea, vomiting and loss of appetite.
- Be sure to give as long as veterinarian has prescribed, even if animal seems better.
- Do **not** give to rabbits, guinea pigs, chinchillas, hamsters, rodents or other pocket pets since life-threatening diarrhea may occur.

Monitoring

- Because penicillins usually have minimal toxicity associated with their use, monitoring for efficacy is usually all that is required unless toxic signs or symptoms develop. Serum levels and therapeutic drug monitoring are not routinely performed with these agents.

Chemistry/Synonyms

A beta-lactamase inhibitor, clavulanate potassium occurs as an off-white, crystalline powder that has a pK_a of 2.7 (as the acid) and is very soluble in water and slightly soluble in alcohol at room temperatures. Although available in commercially available preparations as the potassium salt, potency is expressed in terms of clavulanic acid.

Amoxicillin may also be known as: amoxycillin, p-hydroxyampicillin, or BRL 2333; many trade names are available. Clavulanate potassium may also be known as: clavulanic acid, BRL-14151K, or kalii clavulanas.

Storage/Stability

Clavulanate products should be stored at temperatures less than 24°C (75°F) in tight containers. Potassium clavulanate is reportedly very susceptible to moisture and should be protected from excessive humidity.

After reconstitution, oral suspensions are stable for 10 days when refrigerated. Unused portions should be discarded after that time. If kept at room temperature, suspensions are reportedly stable for 48 hours. The veterinary oral suspension should be reconstituted by adding 14 mL of water and shaking vigorously; refrigerate and discard any unused portion after 10 days.

Compatibility/Compounding Considerations

No specific information noted.

Dosage Forms/Regulatory Status

VETERINARY-LABELED PRODUCTS:

Oral Tablets (4:1 ratio):

62.5 mg: Amoxicillin 50 mg/12.5 mg clavulanic acid (as the potassium salt); 125 mg: Amoxicillin 100 mg/25 mg clavulanic acid (as the potassium salt); 250 mg: Amoxicillin 200 mg/50 mg clavulanic acid (as the potassium salt); 375 mg: Amoxicillin 300 mg/75 mg clavulanic acid (as the potassium salt); *Clavamox Tablets®*; (Rx). FDA-approved for use in dogs and cats.

Powder for Oral Suspension:

Amoxicillin 50 mg/12.5 mg clavulanic acid (as the potassium salt) per mL in 15 mL dropper bottles; *Clavamox® Drops*; (Rx). FDA-approved for use in dogs and cats.

HUMAN-LABELED PRODUCTS:

Note: Human-labeled amoxicillin/clavulanate products have varying ratios of amoxicillin:clavulanate ranging from 2:1 to 7:1. Additionally, human products are generally expressed in potency only as the amoxicillin component (*e.g.*, *Augmentin®* 875 contains 875 mg of amoxicillin and 125 mg of clavulanic acid), while the veterinary products are expressed as the total of both drugs.

Amoxicillin (as trihydrate)/Clavulanic Acid (as potassium salt) Tablets: Amoxicillin 250 mg/125 mg clavulanic acid; Amoxicillin 500 mg/125 mg clavulanic acid; Amoxicillin 875 mg/125 mg clavulanic acid; *Augmentin®*, generic (Rx)

Chewable Tablets: Amoxicillin 125 mg/31.25 mg clavulanic acid; Amoxicillin 200 mg/28.5 mg clavulanic acid; 250 mg/62.5 mg clavulanic acid & 400 mg/57 mg clavulanic acid; *Augmentin®*, generic; (Rx)

Powder for Oral Suspension—Amoxicillin/Clavulanic Acid (as potassium salt) after reconstitution: Amoxicillin 125 mg/31.25 mg clavulanic acid per 5 mL in 75 mL, 100 mL & 150 mL; Amoxicillin 200 mg/28.5 mg clavulanic acid per 5 mL in 50 mL, 75 mL &100 mL; Amoxicillin 250 mg/62.5 mg clavulanic acid per 5 mL in 75 mL, 100 mL & 150 mL; Amoxicillin 400 mg/57 mg clavulanic acid per 5 mL in 50 mL, 75 mL & 100 mL; 600 mg/42.9 mg clavulanic acid per 5 mL in 75 mL, 100 mL, 125 mL & 200 mL; *Augmentin®* & *Augmentin ES-600®*, *Amoclan®*, generic; (Rx)

Revisions/References

Monograph revised/updated August 2013.

Hoeffer, H. (1995). Antimicrobials in pet birds. *Kirk's Current Veterinary Therapy:XII*. J. Bonagura. Philadelphia, W.B. Saunders: 1278-83.

Litster, A. L., et al. (2012). Comparison of the efficacy of amoxicillin-clavulanic acid, cefovecin, and doxycycline in the treatment of upper respiratory tract disease in cats housed in an animal shelter. *Javma-Journal of the American Veterinary Medical Association* **241**(2): 218-26.

MacDonald, K. (2010). Infective Endocarditis in Dogs: Diagnosis and Therapy. *Veterinary Clinics of North America-Small Animal Practice* **40**(4): 665-+.

Summers, J. F., et al. (2012). The effectiveness of systemic antimicrobial treatment in canine superficial and deep pyoderma: a systematic review. *Veterinary Dermatology* **23**(4): 305-E61.

Trepanier, L. (2009). *Appropriate empirical antimicrobial therapy: Making decisions without a culture.* Proceedings: ACVIM. accessed via Veterinary Information Network; vin.com

Weese, J. S., et al. (2011). Antimicrobial Use Guidelines for Treatment of Urinary Tract Disease in Dogs and Cats: Antimicrobial Guidelines Working Group of the International Society for Companion Animal Infectious Diseases. *Veterinary Medicine International*.

Williams, B. (2000). Therapeutics in Ferrets. *Vet Clin NA: Exotic Anim Pract* **3**:1(Jan): 131-53.

Amphotericin B

(am-foe-ter-i-sin bee)   Abelcet®, Fungizone®

Antifungal

Prescriber Highlights

▶ Systemic antifungal used for serious mycotic infections. Must be parenterally administered (IV or SC infusion) for systemic infections.

▶ Four different forms available on US market: conventional, formulated with sodium desoxycholate–generic; cholesteryl sulfate complex–*Amphotec®*; lipid complex–*Abelcet®*; liposomal–*AmBisome®*. Each form may have different reconstitution, dilution, stability, storage, and dosage recommendations.

▶ Nephrotoxicity is biggest concern (not in birds), particularly with the deoxycholate form; newer products (lipid-complex, liposome, cholesterol) are less nephrotoxic & penetrate into tissues better, but are more expensive.

▶ Renal function monitoring essential.

▶ Many potential drug interactions.

Uses/Indications

Amphotericin B has activity against most serious fungal pathogens, but because the potential exists for severe toxicity its use should only be considered for progressive, potentially fatal fungal infections.

The liposomal form of amphotericin B can be used to treat Leishmaniasis, and while it can be clinically effective, relapses inevitably occur. Additionally, worries about the development of amphotericin B-resistant Leishmania strains in human Leishmaniasis has prompted the World Health Organization (WHO) to discourage its use in the treatment of dogs with Leishmaniasis (Oliva et al. 2010).

Pharmacology/Actions

Amphotericin B is usually fungistatic, but can be fungicidal against some organisms depending on drug concentration. It acts by binding to sterols (primarily ergosterol) in the cell membrane and alters the permeability of the membrane allowing intracellular potassium and other cellular constituents to "leak out." Because bacteria and rickettsia do not contain sterols, amphotericin B has no activity against those organisms. Mammalian cell membranes do contain sterols (primarily cholesterol) and the drug's toxicity may be a result of a similar mechanism of action, although amphotericin binds less strongly to cholesterol than ergosterol.

Amphotericin B has *in vitro* activity against a variety of fungal organisms, including Blastomyces, Aspergillus, Paracoccidioides,

Coccidioides, Histoplasma, Cryptococcus, Mucor, and Sporothrix. While outright resistance to amphotericin B is apparently very rare, some strains of Aspergillus and Sporothrix species have high MIC values. Additionally, amphotericin B has *in vivo* activity against some protozoa species, including *Leishmania* spp. and *Naegleria* spp. Leishmania species have ergostane-based sterols in their cell membranes, which may explain amphotericin's efficacy for treating Leishmaniasis.

Pharmacokinetics

In humans (and presumably animals), amphotericin B is poorly absorbed from the GI tract and must be given parenterally to achieve sufficient concentrations to treat systemic fungal infections. After intravenous injection, the drug reportedly penetrates well into most tissues but does not penetrate well into the pancreas, muscle, bone, aqueous humor, or pleural, pericardial, synovial, and peritoneal fluids. The drug does enter the pleural cavity and joints when inflamed. CSF levels are approximately 3% of those found in the serum. Approximately 90-95% of amphotericin in the vascular compartment is bound to serum proteins. The newer "lipid" forms of amphotericin B have higher penetration into the lungs, liver and spleen than the conventional form.

The metabolic pathways of amphotericin are not known, but it exhibits biphasic elimination. An initial serum half-life of 24-48 hours, and a longer terminal half-life of about 15 days have been described. Seven weeks after therapy has stopped, amphotericin can still be detected in the urine. Approximately 2-5% of the drug is recovered in the urine in unchanged (biologically active) form.

Contraindications/Precautions/Warnings

Amphotericin is contraindicated in patients who are hypersensitive to it, unless no other alternative therapies are available for treating life-threatening infections.

Because of the serious nature of the diseases treated with systemic amphotericin, it is not contraindicated in patients with renal disease, but it should be used cautiously with adequate monitoring. A recent recommendation for use of amphotericin B in cats with varying stages of renal disease includes using the liposomal formulation only in cats with IRIS stage II & III renal disease, and not using amphotericin B in cats with IRIS stage IV renal disease (Trepanier 2013).

Adverse Effects

Amphotericin B is known for its nephrotoxic effects; most mammalian patients will show some degree of renal toxicity after receiving the drug. The proposed mechanism of nephrotoxicity is via renal vasoconstriction with a subsequent reduction in glomerular filtration rate. The drug may directly act as a toxin to renal epithelial cells. Renal damage may be more common, irreversible and severe in patients who receive higher individual doses or have preexisting renal disease. Renal tubular acidosis, nephrogenic diabetes insipidus, hypokalemia and hypomagnesemia can be associated with nephrotoxicity. Usually, renal function will return to normal after treatment is halted, but may require several months to do so. When compared to dogs, cats may be more sensitive to nephrotoxic effects. Newer forms of lipid-complexed and liposome-encapsulated amphotericin B are more hydrophobic than the deoxycholate form and significantly reduce the nephrotoxic qualities of the drug. Because higher dosages may then be used, these forms may also have enhanced effectiveness. A study in dogs showed that amphotericin B lipid complex was 8-10 times less nephrotoxic than the conventional form. However, newer forms may be associated with more infusion related reactions such as phlebitis.

The patient's renal function should be aggressively monitored during therapy. A pre-treatment serum creatinine, BUN (serum urea nitrogen/SUN), serum electrolytes (including magnesium if possible), total plasma protein (TPP), packed cell volume (PCV), body weight, and urinalysis should be done prior to starting therapy. BUN, creatinine, PCV, TPP, and body weight must be rechecked before each dose is administered. Electrolytes and urinalysis should be monitored at least weekly during the course of treatment. Several different recommendations regarding the stoppage of therapy when a certain BUN is reached have been made. Most clinicians recommend stopping, at least temporarily, amphotericin treatment if the BUN reaches 30 – 40 mg/dL, serum creatinine >3 mg/dL or if other clinical signs of systemic toxicity develop such as serious depression or vomiting.

Several dosing regimens have been used in the attempt to reduce nephrotoxicity in dogs and cats treated with amphotericin desoxycholate (conventional amphotericin) including pre-treatment with sodium and/or mannitol, but mannitol is not commonly used in veterinary medicine for this purpose. A tubuloglomerular feedback mechanism that induces vasoconstriction and decreased GFR has been postulated for amphotericin B toxicity and increasing sodium load at the glomerulus may help prevent that feedback. Slow intravenous infusion with large volumes of fluid may also decrease nephrotoxicity. A diluted subcutaneous infusion technique (see Dosages) that may mimic slow IV infusion has been employed in dogs and cats to potentially reduce nephrotoxic potential and allow outpatient administration. None of these techniques have been proven in animals to be superior over another.

Other adverse effects that have been reported with amphotericin B use in mammals include: anorexia, vomiting, hypokalemia, distal renal tubular acidosis, hypomagnesemia, phlebitis, cardiac arrhythmias, bronchospasm, hypotension, non-regenerative anemia and fever (may be reduced with pretreatment with NSAIDs or a low dosage of steroids). Calcinosis cutis has been reported in dogs treated with amphotericin B. Amphotericin B can increase creatine kinase levels.

Cats with cryptococcosis (CNS involvement) may have increased neurologic signs within the first 3 days of treatment. This is possibly due to an inflammatory response to dying organisms. When administered as a subcutaneous infusion especially in concentrations of 20 mg/kg or greater is used in dogs and cats, sterile abscesses have been reported but do not occur commonly when using this administration technique at lower concentrations (such as 5 mg/mL) (O'Brien, Krockenberger and Martin 2006).

In horses, additional adverse effects reported include: tachycardia, tachypnea, lethargy, fever, restlessness, anorexia, anemia, phlebitis, polyuria and collapse.

In birds, nephrotoxicity does not appear to be an issue with amphotericin B use. It has been postulated that the shorter half-life of the drug noted in birds may be responsible for the lack of nephrotoxicity.

Reproductive/Nursing Safety

The safety of amphotericin B during pregnancy has not been established, but there are apparently no reports of teratogenicity associated with the drug. The risks of therapy should be weighed against the potential benefits. In humans, the FDA categorizes this drug as category ***B*** for use during pregnancy (*Animal studies have not yet demonstrated risk to the fetus, but there are no adequate studies in pregnant women; or animal studies have shown an adverse effect, but adequate studies in pregnant women have not demonstrated a risk to the fetus in the first trimester of pregnancy, and there is no evidence of risk in later trimesters.*) In a separate system evaluating the safety of drugs in canine and feline pregnancy (Papich 1989), this drug is categorized as class: ***A*** (*Probably safe. Although specific studies may not have proved the safety of all drugs in dogs and cats, there are no reports of adverse effects in laboratory animals or women.*)

Overdosage/Acute Toxicity

No case reports were located regarding acute intravenous over-dose of amphotericin B. Because of the toxicity of the drug, dosage calculations and solution preparation procedures should be dou-ble-checked. If an accidental overdose is administered, administer-ing fluids and mannitol may minimize renal toxicity.

Drug Interactions

The following drug interactions with amphotericin B have either been reported or are theoretical in humans or animals and may be of significance in veterinary patients. Unless otherwise noted, use together is not necessarily contraindicated, but weigh the potential risks and perform additional monitoring when appropriate.

- **CORTICOSTEROIDS**: May exacerbate the potassium-losing effects of amphotericin.
- **DIGOXIN**: Amphotericin B-induced hypokalemia may exacer-bate digoxin toxicity.
- **FLUCYTOSINE**: Synergy (*in vitro*) between amphotericin and flucytosine may occur against strains of Cryptococcus and Can-dida, but increased flucytosine toxicity may also occur.
- **NEPHROTOXIC DRUGS** (*e.g.,* **aminoglycosides, cisplatin, cyclosporine,** or **vancomycin**): Since the renal effects of other nephrotoxic drugs may be additive with amphotericin B, avoid, if possible the concurrent or sequential use of these agents.
- **POTASSIUM-DEPLETING DRUGS** (*e.g.,* **thiazide** or **loop di-uretics**): Increase risk for hypokalemia.
- **SKELETAL MUSCLE RELAXANTS** (*e.g.,* **tubocurarine**): Am-photericin B-induced hypokalemia may enhance curariform ef-fects.
- **ZIDOVUDINE (AZT)**: Potential for increased myelotoxicity or nephrotoxicity.

Doses

Note: Amphotericin B (AMB) is not approved by the FDA for use in animals and all use in the USA is considered extra-label. Because of the potential toxicity, expense (drug, and associated administration costs & laboratory tests), and the necessity for parenteral admin-istration, Amphotericin B treatment is generally reserved only for treating serious fungal infections. Dosage (initial dosages, frequen-cy of administration, and cumulative dosage) recommendations can vary widely depending on the disease/organism treated, formu-lation used, and route of administration. Solid evidence supporting any specific dosage is lacking.

- **DOGS:**

For life-threatening fungal infections:

Desoxycholate (conventional AMB), slow IV: Initially, 0.5 mg/kg IV every other day (q48h); practically, 3 times per week (Mon.-Wed.-Fri). Drug should be diluted in D5W and giv-en IV slowly over 4-6 hours. Cumulative dose recommendations vary and are dependent on patient response and drug toxicity; most recommendations are in the 9 – 12 mg/kg range. Patients must be kept well hydrated before and during treatment, but care must be taken to avoid fluid overload.

Desoxycholate (conventional AMB), Subcutaneous Infusion: Generally, the slow intravenous route is more commonly rec-ommended for dogs, but for those clients unable to afford the costs associated with intravenous administration or using lip-id-formulations, SC administration can be an option. Initially, 0.5 mg/kg 2-3 times per week. Drug should initially be diluted to a concentration of 5 mg/mL and then proper dosage for the patient is further diluted into 350-500 mL of sodium chloride 0.45%/Dextrose 2.5% and injected subcutaneously between the scapulae. Alternatively, the subcutaneous fluid (without AMB) can be injected first and the AMB dosage can then be injected

into the "lump" formed by the SC fluid. Cumulative dose rec-ommendations vary and are dependent on patient response and drug toxicity; most recommendations are in the 10 – 15 mg/kg range. Dosage adapted from: (Malik et al. 1996)(Taboada 2000; O'Brien, Krockenberger, Martin, et al. 2006; Barr 2013). Some sources recommending this dosage method state that heating the stock solution to 60°C for 5 minutes prior to administration will decrease nephrotoxicity, but a review article on antifungal treatment in small animals (Foy et al. 2010) states "…no exper-imental or clinical studies exist to warrant this additional step."

Lipid Formulations [most recommend using amphotericin B lipid complex (ABLC; *Abelcet®*)]; especially in animals with pre-existing renal disease or that have developed renal toxicity with the desoxycholate form: 1 – 3.3 mg/kg IV over 2 hours. Cu-mulative dosage recommendations vary and are dependent on patient response and drug toxicity; most recommendations are in the 24 – 30 mg/kg range. One specific dosage protocol pub-lished for treating blastomycosis dogs follows (Foy et al. 2010): Reconstitute ABLC to a concentration of 5 mg/mL with sterile water. Calculate the patient's dosage (1 mg/kg) and dilute the ap-propriate volume of reconstituted ABLC to a concentration of 1 mg/mL in 5% dextrose in water (D5W). Consider pretreat-ment with antiinflammatory dosages of dexamethasone (about 0.1 mg/kg IV) and metoclopramide (0.2 – 0.4 mg/kg IV) approx-imately 30 minutes before ABLC administration. For 30 minutes before ABLC administration, begin an LRS infusion at 2.5 times the maintenance rate. Immediately before ABLC administra-tion, discontinue LRS, and flush the line with D5W. Infuse the ABLC dose in D5W over 2 hours. Once the ABLC infusion is complete, flush the line with D5W and restart LRS at 2.5 times the maintenance rate and continue for 120 minutes after ABLC treatment.

- **CATS:**

For life-threatening fungal infections:

Desoxycholate (conventional AMB), Slow IV: Initially, 0.25 mg/kg IV every other day (q48h); practically, 3 times per week (Mon.-Wed.-Fri). Drug should be diluted in D5W and giv-en IV slowly over 4-6 hours. Cumulative dose recommendations vary and are dependent on patient response and drug toxicity; most recommendations are in the 6 – 9 mg/kg range, but recom-mendations as low as 4 mg/kg to as high as 16 mg/kg have been noted. Patients must be kept well hydrated before and during treatment, but care must be taken to avoid fluid overload.

Desoxycholate (conventional AMB), Subcutaneous Infusion: Initially, 0.5 mg/kg 2-3 times per week. Drug should initially be diluted to a concentration of 5 mg/mL and then proper dosage for the patient is further diluted into 350 mL of sodium chloride 0.45%/Dextrose 2.5% and injected subcutaneously between the scapulae. Alternatively, the subcutaneous fluid (without AMB) can be injected first and the AMB dosage can then be injected into the "lump" formed by the SC fluid. Cumulative dose rec-ommendations vary and are dependent on patient response and drug toxicity; most recommendations are in the 10 – 15 mg/kg range. Dosage adapted from: (Malik et al. 1996)(Taboada 2000; O'Brien, Krockenberger, Martin, et al. 2006; Barr 2013). Some sources recommending this dosage method state that heating the stock solution to 60°C for 5 minutes prior to administration will decrease nephrotoxicity, but a review article on antifungal treatment in small animals (Foy et al. 2010) states "…no exper-imental or clinical studies exist to warrant this additional step."

Lipid Formulations [most recommend using amphotericin B lip-id complex (ABLC; *Abelcet®*)]; especially in animals with pre-ex-isting renal disease or that have developed renal toxicity with the desoxycholate form: 1 mg/kg IV over 1-2 hours. Cumulative dosage recommendations vary and are dependent on patient response and drug toxicity; most recommendations are in the 12 mg/kg range. See the Dog dosage protocol above (Foy et al. 2010) for additional information; however if an antiemetic is used, an alternative antiemetic (*e.g.*, ondansetron, maropitant) that may be more efficacious in cats should be considered.

- **RABBITS/RODENTS/SMALL MAMMALS:**
  a) **Rabbits:** 1 mg/kg/day IV. (Ivey et al. 2000)
- **HORSES:**

  Note: All dosages are extra-label. Using amphotericin B systemically in adult equids can be inordinately expensive and there is little consensus on dosage regimens.

  For treatment of serious susceptible systemic fungal infections: Using deoxycholate (conventional): Starting at 0.3 mg/kg IV (in 1 L of D5W) over at least an hour. and increasing dosage by 0.1 mg per day and giving for 3 days straight. Then give every 2-3 days (practically 3 times per week). Continue increasing dosage by 0.1 mg/kg/dose to 0.6 – 0.9 mg/kg until clinical improvement or toxicity occurs. Oral sodium chloride has been suggested to reduce nephrotoxicity. If toxicity occurs, a dose may be skipped, dosage reduced or dosage interval lengthened. Treatment duration is dependent on response, budget, toxicity, etc. but may be required for a month or more. Cumulative dosage limits are not well described. One source suggests a 6.75 mg/kg cumulative dose for foals (Foreman 1999).

  For pythiosis using regional limb perfusion (IRLP): After surgical excision of granulation tissue and thermocautery, after a catheter was placed in a superficial vein of the affected limb next to the lesion and a tourniquet above the injection site, 50 mg amphotericin B (diluted with 50 mL LRS) was administered over 5 minutes. The catheter was removed 10 minutes post administration, and firm manual pressure applied over injection site. Tourniquet was released 45 minutes after administration and debrided area bandaged. A 2nd administration of amphotericin B was performed if kunkers and/or dark red or black exuberant granulation tissue (necrotic areas) still observed 14 days after surgery. 92% of treated horses had complete lesion resolution after 1 or 2 IRLP treatments 35 or 60 days, respectively. Adverse effects included limb edema/pain on palpation (42%) and inflammation at injection site (33%). Adverse signs resolved after 14 days. (Doria et al. 2012)

  For intrauterine infusion: 200 – 250 mg. Little science is available for recommending doses, volume infused, frequency, diluents, etc. Most intrauterine treatments are commonly performed every day or every other day for 3-7 days. (Perkins 1999)
- **LLAMAS:**

  For treatment of susceptible systemic fungal infections (extra-label; from a single case report). Llama with coccidioidomycosis received 1 mg test dose, then initially at 0.3 mg/kg IV over 4 hours, followed by 3 L of LRS with 1.5 mL of B-Complex and 20 mEq of KCl added. Subsequent doses were increased by 10 mg and given every 48 hours until reaching 1 mg/kg q48h IV for 6 weeks. Animal tolerated therapy well, but treatment was ultimately unsuccessful. (Fowler 1989)
- **BIRDS:**

  For treatment of susceptible systemic fungal infections (all are extra-label):
  a) **For raptors and psittacines with aspergillosis:** 1.5 mg/kg IV three times daily for 3 days with flucytosine or follow with flucytosine. May also use intratracheally at 1 mg/kg diluted in sterile water 1-3 times daily for 3 days in conjunction with flucytosine or nebulized (1 mg/mL of saline) for 15 minutes twice daily. Potentially nephrotoxic and may cause bone marrow suppression. (Clubb 1986)
  b) 1.5 mg/kg IV q12h for 3–5 days; topically in the trachea at 1 mg/kg q12h; 0.3 – 1 mg/mL nebulized for 15 minutes 2–4 times daily. (Flammer 2003)
  c) For treatment of Macrorhabdiasis (*Microrhabdus ornithogaster*): Amphotericin B at 100 – 150 mg/kg <u>PO</u> q12h for 30 days; treatment failures are common especially with shorter durations of treatment. (Flammer 2008)
- **REPTILES:**

  For susceptible fungal respiratory infections (extra-label, anecdotal): For most species: 1 mg/kg diluted in saline and given intra-tracheally once daily for 14-28 treatments. (Gauvin 1993)

Monitoring

Also see the *Adverse Effects* section.
- BUN and serum creatinine every other day while dosage is being increased, and at least weekly thereafter during therapy. Some suggest that before every dose the BUN and urine sediment is checked.
- Serum electrolytes (sodium, potassium and magnesium) weekly.
- Liver function tests weekly.
- CBC weekly.
- Urinalysis weekly.
- TPP at least weekly.
- Animal's weight.

Client Information

- Clients should be informed of the potential seriousness of toxic effects and costs associated with amphotericin B therapy.

Chemistry/Synonyms

A polyene macrolide antifungal agent produced by *Streptomyces nodosus*, amphotericin B occurs as a yellow to orange, odorless or practically odorless powder. It is insoluble in water and anhydrous alcohol. Amphotericin B is amphoteric and can form salts in acidic or basic media. These salts are more water-soluble but possess less antifungal activity than the parent compound. Each mg of amphotericin B must contain not less than 750 micrograms of anhydrous drug. Amphotericin A may be found as a contaminant in concentrations not exceeding 5%. The commercially available powder for injection contains sodium desoxycholate as a solubilizing agent.

These include amphotericin B cholesteryl sulfate complex (amphotericin B colloidal dispersion, ABCD, *Amphotec®*), amphotericin B lipid complex (ABLC, *Abelcet®*), and amphotericin B liposomal (ABL, L-AMB, *Ambisome®*).

Amphotericin B desoxycholate may also be known as: amphotericin generic, AMB, conventional amphotericin B, or *Fungizone®*. Amphotericin B cholesteryl sulfate complex may also be known as amphotericin colloidal dispersion, ABCD, or *Amphotec®*. Amphotericin B lipid complex may also be known as ABLC or *Abelcet®*. Amphoteric B liposome may also be known as liposomal amphotericin B, lip-AmB or *Ambisome®*.

Storage/Stability

The following information is for the conventional (deoxycholate; generic) and lipid complex (ABLC; Abelcet®) forms of Amphotericin B. If using cholesteryl sulfate complex–Amphotec® or liposomal–AmBisome® forms, refer to the appropriate package insert for detailed information.

Vials of amphotericin B deoxycholate powder for injection (conventional; generic) should be stored in the refrigerator (2-8°C), protected from light and moisture. Reconstitution of the powder must be done with sterile water for injection (no preservatives—see directions for preparation in the Dosage Form section below). After reconstitution, if protected from light, the solution is stable for 24 hours at room temperature and for 1 week if kept refrigerated. After diluting with D_5W (must have pH >4.3) for IV use, the manufacturer recommends continuing to protect the solution from light during administration. Additional studies however, have shown that potency remains largely unaffected if the solution is exposed to light for 8-24 hours.

One reference (Orosz 2000) states that for avian use, the conventional amphotericin B can be diluted with sterile water, divided into 10mL aliquots using aseptic technique, and stored at -20°C for approximately 1 month. However, no published data was located documenting the stability of the drug for this practice.

Amphotericin B lipid complex vials should be stored under refrigeration and protected from light and or freezing. The manufacturer recommends keeping the vials in their original cartons until use. When diluted in dextrose 5% for administration, the manufacturer states that it can be stored for 48 hours when refrigerated and then an additional 6 hours at room temperature. However, other sources have stated that at a concentration of 1 mg/mL in dextrose 5% it is stable for 10 days when refrigerated.

Compatibility/Compounding Considerations

The following information is for the conventional (deoxycholate; generic) and lipid complex (ABLC; *Abelcet*®) forms of Amphotericin B. If using cholesteryl sulfate complex–*Amphotec*® or liposomal–*AmBisome*® forms, refer to the appropriate package insert for detailed information.

Amphotericin B deoxycholate (conventional; generic) is reportedly **compatible** with the following solutions and drugs: D_5W, D_5W in sodium chloride 0.2%, heparin sodium, heparin sodium with hydrocortisone sodium phosphate, hydrocortisone sodium phosphate/succinate and sodium bicarbonate.

Amphotericin B (conventional; generic) is reportedly **incompatible** with the following solutions and drugs: normal saline, lactated Ringer's, D_5-normal saline, D_5-lactated Ringer's, amino acids 4.25%-dextrose 25%, amikacin, calcium chloride/gluconate, chlorpromazine HCl, cimetidine HCl, diphenhydramine HCl, dopamine HCl, edetate calcium disodium (CaEDTA), gentamicin sulfate, oxytetracycline HCl, penicillin G potassium/sodium, polymyxin B sulfate, potassium chloride, prochlorperazine mesylate, tetracycline HCl, and verapamil HCl. Compatibility is dependent upon factors such as pH, concentration, temperature and diluent used; consult specialized references or a hospital pharmacist for more specific information.

Directions for reconstitution/administration: Using strict aseptic technique and a 20 gauge or larger needle, rapidly inject 10 mL of sterile water for injection (without a bacteriostatic agent) directly into the lyophilized cake; immediately shake well until solution is clear. A 5 mg/mL colloidal solution results. Further dilute (1:50) for administration to a concentration of 0.1 mg/mL with 5% dextrose in water (pH >4.2). An in-line filter may be used during administration, but must have a pore diameter >1 micron.

Amphotericin B lipid complex is **compatible** with D_5W, but it is **incompatible** with normal saline or other electrolyte solutions.

Directions for Dilution/Administration: The suspension must be diluted in dextrose 5% for administration. Shake the vial gently so that no sediment remains on the vial bottom. Withdraw the dose using a syringe and needle. Attach the 5-micron filter needle that is supplied with the vial, and add the drug suspension into a bag of dextrose 5%. One filter needle may be used for up to four vials of drug. The final concentration is usually 1 mg/mL, although 2 mg/mL may be used in some cases. The bag is shaken just prior to infusion; it should not be used if foreign matter is present. If de-livery proceeds over more than 2 hours, the bag should be shaken every 2 hours. Use a separate infusion line or flush an existing line with dextrose 5% prior to administration.

Dosage Forms/Regulatory Status

VETERINARY-LABELED PRODUCTS: NONE.

HUMAN-LABELED PRODUCTS:

Amphotericin B (conventional; desoxycholate) Powder for Injection: 50 mg in vials; generic; (Rx)

Amphotericin B Lipid-complex Suspension for Injection: 100 mg/20 mL (as lipid complex) in vials with 5 micron filter needles: *Abelcet*®; (Rx)

Amphotericin B Cholesteryl Sulfate Complex for Injection: 50 mg & 100 mg (as cholesteryl) in single-use vials; *Amphotec*®; (Rx)

Amphotericin B Liposomal for Injection: 50 mg in single-dose vials with 5-micron filter; *AmBisome*®; (Rx)

Revisions/References

Monograph revised/updated August 2013.

Barr, V. (2013). *Invasive Fungal Infections.* World Small Animal Veterinary Association World Congress Proceedings. accessed via Veterinary Information Network; vin.com

Clubb, S. L. (1986). Therapeutics: Individual and Flock Treatment Regimens. *Clinical Avian Medicine and Surgery.* G. J. Harrison and L. R. Harrison. Philadelphia, W.B. Saunders: 327-55.

Doria, R. G. S., et al. (2012). Treatment of Pythiosis in Equine Limbs Using Intravenous Regional Perfusion of Amphotericin B. *Veterinary Surgery* 41(6): 759-65.

Flammer, K. (2003). *Antifungal therapy in avian medicine.* Proceedings: Western Veterinary Conference. accessed via Veterinary Information Network; vin.com

Flammer, K. (2008). *Avian Mycoses: Managing those difficult cases.* Proceedings: AAV. accessed via Veterinary Information Network; vin.com

Foreman, J. (1999). Equine respiratory pharmacology. *The Veterinary Clinics of North America: Equine Practice* 15:3(December): 665-86.

Fowler, M. E. (1989). *Medicine and Surgery of South American Camelids,* Iowa State University Press. Ames.

Foy, D. S. & L. A. Trepanier (2010). Antifungal Treatment of Small Animal Veterinary Patients. *Veterinary Clinics of North America-Small Animal Practice* 40(6): 1171-+.

Gauvin, J. (1993). Drug therapy in reptiles. *Seminars in Avian & Exotic Med* 2(1): 48-59.

Ivey, E. & J. Morrisey (2000). Therapeutics for Rabbits. *Vet Clin NA: Exotic Anim Pract* 3:1(Jan): 183-216.

Malik, R., et al. (1996). Combination chemotherapy of canine and feline cryptococcosis using subcutaneously administered amphotericin B. *Australian Veterinary Journal* 73(7): 124-8.

O'Brien, C., et al. (2006). Long-term outcome of therapy for 59 cats and 11 dogs with cryptococcosis. *Australian Veterinary Journal* 84: 384-92.

O'Brien, C. R., et al. (2006). Long-term outcome of therapy for 59 cats and 11 dogs with cryptococcosis. *Australian Veterinary Journal* 84(11): 384-92.

Oliva, G., et al. (2010). Guidelines for treatment of leishmaniasis in dogs. *Journal of the American Veterinary Medical Association* 236(11): 1192-8.

Orosz, S. E. (2000). Overview of aspergillosis: Pathogenesis and treatment options. *Seminars in Avian and Exotic Pet Medicine* 9(2): 59-65.

Perkins, N. (1999). Equine reproductive pharmacology. *The Veterinary Clinics of North America: Equine Practice* 15:3(December): 687-704.

Taboada, J. (2000). Systemic Mycoses. *Textbook of Veterinary Internal Medicine: Diseases of the Dog and Cat.* S. Ettinger and E. Feldman. Philadelphia, WB Saunders. 1: 453-76.

Trepanier, L. (2013). *Feline Therapeutics.* World Small Animal Veterinary Association World Congress Proceedings. accessed via Veterinary Information Network; vin.com

Ampicillin

(am-pi-**sill**-in)   Polyflex®

Aminopenicillin

Prescriber Highlights

▶ Bactericidal aminopenicillin with same spectrum as amoxicillin (ineffective against bacteria that produce beta-lactamase).

▶ Poor oral absorption in dogs and cats; amoxicillin is generally preferred.

▶ Ampicillin trihydrate (Polyflex®) <u>must not</u> be given IV.

▶ Most likely adverse effects are GI-related, but hypersensitivity & other adverse effects occur rarely; may cause more GI effects than amoxicillin when used orally.

▶ Available in both parenteral & oral forms.

Uses/Indications

In dogs and cats, ampicillin is not as well absorbed after oral administration as amoxicillin and its oral use has largely been supplanted by amoxicillin. It is used commonly in parenteral dosage forms when an aminopenicillin is indicated in all species. Ampicillin at high dosages, is still an effective drug for treating penicillin-sensitive enterococci, particularly *E. faecium* and its poor oral absorption may be an advantage when treating *Clostridium perfringens* enteritis. An aminoglycoside (*e.g.*, gentamicin) is often added to treat serious enterococcus infections caused by penicillin-sensitive organisms.

The aminopenicillins, also called the "broad-spectrum" or ampicillin penicillins, have increased activity against many strains of gram-negative aerobes not covered by either the natural penicillins or penicillinase-resistant penicillins, including some strains of *E. coli*, Klebsiella, and Haemophilus.

Pharmacology/Actions

Like other penicillins, ampicillin is a time-dependent, bactericidal (usually) agent that acts via inhibiting cell wall synthesis. Ampicillin and the other aminopenicillins have increased activity against many strains of gram-negative aerobes not covered by either the natural penicillins or penicillinase-resistant penicillins, including some strains of *E. coli*, Klebsiella and Haemophilus. Like the natural penicillins, they are susceptible to inactivation by beta-lactamase-producing bacteria (*e.g.*, Staph aureus).

Although not as active as the natural penicillins, they do have activity against many anaerobic bacteria, including Clostridial organisms. Organisms that are generally not susceptible include *Pseudomonas aeruginosa*, Serratia, Indole-positive Proteus (*Proteus mirabilis* is susceptible), Enterobacter, Citrobacter, and Acinetobacter. The aminopenicillins also are inactive against Rickettsia, mycobacteria, fungi, Mycoplasma, and viruses.

In order to reduce the inactivation of penicillins by beta-lactamases, potassium clavulanate and sulbactam have been developed to inactivate these enzymes and extend the spectrum of those penicillins. See the ampicillin/sulbactam or amoxicillin/clavulanate monographs for more information.

Pharmacokinetics

Ampicillin anhydrous and trihydrate are relatively stable in the presence of gastric acid. After oral administration, ampicillin is about 30-55% absorbed in humans (empty stomach) and monogastric animals. Food will decrease the rate and extent of oral absorption.

When administered parenterally (IM, SC) the trihydrate salt will achieve serum levels of approximately 1/2 those of a comparable dose of the sodium salt. The trihydrate parenteral dosage form should not be used where higher MIC's are required for treating systemic infections.

After absorption, the volume of distribution for ampicillin is approximately 0.3 L/kg in humans and dogs, 0.167 L/kg in cats, and 0.16 – 0.5 L/kg in cattle. The drug is widely distributed to many tissues, including liver, lungs, prostate (human), muscle, bile, and ascitic, pleural and synovial fluids. Ampicillin will cross into the CSF when meninges are inflamed in concentrations that may range from 10-60% those found in serum. Very low levels of the drug are found in the aqueous humor; low levels are found in tears, sweat and saliva. Ampicillin crosses the placenta, but is thought to be relatively safe to use during pregnancy. Ampicillin is approximately 20% bound to plasma proteins, primarily albumin. Milk levels of ampicillin are considered low. In lactating dairy cattle, the milk to plasma ratio is about 0.3.

Ampicillin is eliminated primarily through renal mechanisms, principally by tubular secretion, but some of the drug is metabolized by hydrolysis to penicilloic acids (inactive) and then excreted in the urine. Elimination half-lives of ampicillin have been reported as 45-80 minutes in dogs and cats, and 60 minutes in swine.

Contraindications/Precautions/Warnings

Penicillins are contraindicated in patients with a history of hypersensitivity to them. Because there may be cross-reactivity, use penicillins cautiously in patients who are documented hypersensitive to other beta-lactam antibiotics (*e.g.*, cephalosporins, cefamycins, carbapenems).

The trihydrate form (*Polyflex*®, etc.) must not be given IV as there is a high risk for anaphylaxis and sudden death. Ampicillin sodium for injection is the only form of ampicillin that may be administered intravenously.

Do not administer systemic antibiotics orally in patients with septicemia, shock, or other grave illnesses as absorption of the medication from the GI tract may be significantly delayed or diminished. Parenteral (preferably IV) routes should be used for these cases.

Do not administer penicillins, cephalosporins, or macrolides to rabbits, guinea pigs, chinchillas, hamsters, etc., or serious enteritis and clostridial enterotoxemia may occur.

Adverse Effects

Adverse effects with the penicillins are usually not serious and have a relatively low frequency of occurrence.

Hypersensitivity reactions unrelated to dose can occur with these agents and manifest as rashes, fever, eosinophilia, neutropenia, agranulocytosis, thrombocytopenia, leukopenia, anemia, lymphadenopathy, or full-blown anaphylaxis. In humans, it is estimated that up to 15% of patients hypersensitive to cephalosporins will also be hypersensitive to penicillins. The incidence of cross-reactivity in veterinary patients is unknown.

When given orally, penicillins may cause GI effects (anorexia, vomiting, diarrhea). Because the penicillins may also alter gut flora, antibiotic-associated diarrhea can occur and allow the proliferation of resistant bacteria in the colon (superinfections).

Neurotoxicity (*e.g.*, ataxia in dogs) has been associated with very high doses or very prolonged use. Although the penicillins are not considered hepatotoxic, elevated liver enzymes have been reported. Other effects reported in dogs include tachypnea, dyspnea, edema and tachycardia.

Reproductive/Nursing Safety

Penicillins have been shown to cross the placenta; safe use during pregnancy has not been firmly established, but neither has there been any documented teratogenic problem associated with these drugs. However, use only when the potential benefits outweigh the risks. In humans, the FDA categorizes ampicillin as category ***B*** for use during pregnancy (*Animal studies have not yet demonstrated* *risk to the fetus, but there are no adequate studies in pregnant women; or animal studies have shown an adverse effect, but adequate studies in pregnant women have not demonstrated a risk to the fetus in the first trimester of pregnancy, and there is no evidence of risk in later trimesters.*) In a separate system evaluating the safety of drugs in canine and feline pregnancy (Papich 1989), this drug is categorized as class: *A* (*Probably safe. Although specific studies may not have proved the safety of all drugs in dogs and cats, there are no reports of adverse effects in laboratory animals or women.*)

Overdosage/Acute Toxicity

Acute oral penicillin overdoses are unlikely to cause significant problems other than GI distress, but other effects are possible (see Adverse Effects). In humans, very high dosages of parenteral penicillins, particularly in patients with renal disease, have induced CNS effects.

Drug Interactions

The following drug interactions with ampicillin have either been reported or are theoretical in humans or animals and may be of significance in veterinary patients. Unless otherwise noted, use together is not necessarily contraindicated, but weigh the potential risks and perform additional monitoring when appropriate.

- **BACTERIOSTATIC ANTIMICROBIALS** (*e.g.*, **chloramphenicol, erythromycin** and **other macrolides, tetracyclines, sulfonamides,** etc.): Because there is evidence of *in vitro* antagonism between beta-lactam antibiotics and bacteriostatic antibiotics, use together has not been generally recommended in the past, but actual clinical importance is not clear and currently in doubt.
- **METHOTREXATE**: Ampicillin may decrease the renal excretion of MTX causing increased levels and potential toxic effects.
- **PROBENECID**: Competitively blocks the tubular secretion of most penicillins thereby increasing serum levels and serum half-lives.

Laboratory Considerations

- Ampicillin may cause false-positive **urine glucose determinations** when using cupric sulfate solution (Benedict's Solution, *Clinitest®*). Tests utilizing glucose oxidase (*Tes-Tape®, Clinistix®*) are not affected by ampicillin.
- As penicillins and other beta-lactams can inactivate **aminoglycosides** *in vitro* (and *in vivo* in patients in renal failure), serum concentrations of aminoglycosides may be falsely decreased if the patient is also receiving beta-lactam antibiotics, particularly when the serum is stored prior to analysis. It is recommended that if the assay is delayed, samples be frozen and, if possible, drawn at times when the beta-lactam antibiotic is at a trough.

Doses

- **DOGS/CATS:**

Ampicillin Trihydrate Injection Labeled Dosage (FDA-approved); **Note:** While the following indications and dosages are on the FDA-approved label, the labeled dosages are not accepted by most today as being consistently efficacious. Indications: Respiratory Tract Infections: Upper respiratory infections, tonsillitis and bronchopneumonia due to hemolytic streptococci, *Staphylococcus aureus, Escherichia coli, Proteus mirabilis* and *Pasteurella* spp. Urinary Tract Infections due to *Proteus mirabilis, Escherichia coli, Staphylococcus* spp., hemolytic streptococci and *Enterococcus* spp. Gastrointestinal Infections due to *Enterococcus* spp., *Staphylococcus* spp. and *Escherichia coli.* Skin, Soft Tissue and Post-Surgical Infections: Abscesses, pustular dermatitis, cellulitis and infections of the anal gland, due to *Escherichia coli, Proteus mirabilis,* hemolytic streptococci, *Staphylococcus* spp. and *Pasteurella* spp. Dosage: 6.6 mg/kg SC, or IM twice a day. The dosage will vary according to the animal being treated, the severity of the infection and the animal's response. In all species, 3 days treatment is usually adequate, but treatment should be continued for 48-72 hours after the animal has become afebrile or asymptomatic. (Label Information—*Polyflex®*)

For adjunctive antibiotic therapy for sepsis (empiric therapy) or susceptible systemic infections (extra-label): Ampicillin sodium: 20 – 40 mg/kg IV q6-8h; usually used in combination with an antibiotic that would enhance coverage for gram-negative organisms (*e.g.* an aminoglycoside or fluoroquinolone). Enterococci infections may require much higher (40 – 100 mg/kg) dosages.

For leptospirosis in dogs (extra-label): If vomiting or other adverse reactions preclude doxycycline administration, ampicillin sodium at 20 mg/kg IV q6h. Reduce dosage in azotemic dogs. (Sykes et al. 2011)

For acute treatment in dogs of endocarditis secondary to a susceptible strain of *Streptococcus canis* (extra-label): Ampicillin sodium: 20 – 40 mg/kg IV q6-8h. (MacDonald 2010)

- **CATTLE**

Ampicillin Trihydrate Injection Labeled Dosage (FDA-approved): Respiratory Tract Infections: Bacterial pneumonia (shipping fever, calf pneumonia and bovine pneumonia) caused by *Aerobacter* spp., *Klebsiella* spp., *Staphylococcus* spp., *Streptococcus* spp., *Pasteurella multocida* and *E. coli* susceptible to ampicillin trihydrate. Dosage: From 4.4 – 11 mg/kg once daily IM. Do not treat for more than 7 days. In all species, 3 days treatment is usually adequate, but treatment should be continued for 48-72 hours after the animal has become afebrile or asymptomatic. Withdrawal times at labeled doses: Milk = 48 hours; Slaughter = 6 days (144 hours). (Label Information—*Polyflex®*)

For respiratory **infections:** (extra-label): Ampicillin trihydrate (*Polyflex®*) 22 mg/kg SC q12h (60 day slaughter withdrawal suggested). (Hjerpe 1986)

- **HORSES:**

For streptococcal lower airway infections (extra-label): Ampicillin sodium: 15 mg/kg IV q12h. Ampicillin concentrations in pulmonary epithelial lining fluid (PELF) are above MIC values for at least 12 hours. Treatment of other bacterial pathogens requires susceptibility testing and possibly more frequent dosing, depending on minimum inhibitory concentrations (MIC). (Winther et al. 2012)

Foals (extra-label): Ampicillin sodium 15 – 30 mg/kg IV or IM q6–8h. (Brumbaugh 1999)

- **FERRETS:**

For susceptible infections (extra-label): 5 – 10 mg/kg IM, SC or IV twice daily. (Williams 2000)

- **RABBITS/RODENTS/SMALL MAMMALS:**

Note: All are extra-label.

a) **Rabbits:** Not recommended as it can cause a fatal enteritis. (Ivey et al. 2000)

b) **Gerbils, Mice, Rats:** 20 – 100 mg/kg PO, SC, IM q8–12h. **Guinea pigs, Chinchillas, Hamsters:** Do NOT use as it may cause enterocolitis. (Adamcak et al. 2000)

c) **Hedgehogs:** 10 mg/kg IM or PO once daily. (Smith 2000)

- **REPTILES:**

For respiratory tract infections (extra-label): 50 mg/kg SC or IM q12h. (Schumacher 2011)

Monitoring

- Because penicillins usually have minimal toxicity associated with their use, monitoring for efficacy is usually all that is required unless toxic signs or symptoms develop. Serum levels and therapeutic drug monitoring are not routinely done with these agents.

Client Information

- Unless otherwise instructed by the veterinarian, this drug should be given orally on an empty stomach, at least 1 hour before feeding or 2 hours after.
- Keep oral suspension in the refrigerator and discard any unused suspension after 14 days. If stored at room temperature, discard unused suspension after 7 days.

Chemistry/Synonyms

A semi-synthetic aminopenicillin, ampicillin anhydrous and trihydrate occur as practically odorless, white, crystalline powders that are slightly soluble in water. At usual temperatures (<42°C), ampicillin anhydrous is more soluble in water than the trihydrate (13 mg/mL vs. 6 mg/mL at 20°C). Ampicillin anhydrous or trihydrate oral suspensions have a pH of 5-7.5 after reconstitution with water.

Ampicillin sodium occurs as an odorless or practically odorless, white to off-white, crystalline hygroscopic powder. It is very soluble in water or other aqueous solutions. After reconstitution, ampicillin sodium has a pH of 8-10 at a concentration of 10 mg/mL. Commercially available ampicillin sodium for injection has approximately 3 mEq of sodium per gram of ampicillin.

Potency of the ampicillin salts is expressed in terms of ampicillin anhydrous.

Ampicillin may also be known as: aminobenzylpenicillin, ampicillinum, ampicillinum anhydricum, anhydrous ampicillin, AY-6108, BRL-1341, NSC-528986, or P-50; many trade names are available.

Storage/Stability

Ampicillin trihydrate for injection (*Polyflex®*) was labeled as stable for 12 months when refrigerated (2-8°C) and 3 months when kept at room temperature. Its new labeling states that after reconstitution it is stable for 3 months when refrigerated. It is not clear if this change is a result of more recent scientific stability studies.

Ampicillin anhydrous or trihydrate capsules and powder for oral suspension should be stored at room temperature (15-30°C). After reconstitution, the oral suspension is stable for 14 days if refrigerated (2-8°C); 7 days when kept at room temperature.

Ampicillin sodium for injection is relatively unstable after reconstitution and should generally be used within 1 hour of reconstitution. As the concentration of the drug in solution increases, the stability of the drug decreases. Dextrose may also speed the destruction of the drug by acting as a catalyst in the hydrolysis of ampicillin.

While most sources recommend using solutions of ampicillin sodium immediately, studies have demonstrated that at concentrations of 30 mg/mL, ampicillin sodium solutions are stable up to 48 hours at 4°C in sterile water for injection or 0.9% sodium chloride (72 hours if concentrations are 20 mg/mL or less). Solutions with a concentration of 30 mg/mL or less have been shown to be stable up to 24 hours in solutions of lactated Ringer's solution if kept at 4°C. Solutions of 20 mg/mL or less are reportedly stable up to 4 hours in D5W if refrigerated.

Compatibility/Compounding Considerations

Ampicillin sodium is reportedly **compatible** with the following additives (see the above paragraph for more information): heparin sodium, chloramphenicol sodium succinate, procaine HCl and verapamil HCl.

Ampicillin sodium is reportedly **incompatible** with the following additives: amikacin sulfate, chlorpromazine HCl, dopamine HCl, erythromycin lactobionate, gentamicin HCl, hydralazine HCl,

hydrocortisone sodium succinate, oxytetracycline HCl, polymyxin B sulfate, prochlorperazine edisylate, sodium bicarbonate and tetracycline HCl. Compatibility is dependent upon factors such as pH, concentration, temperature and diluent used; consult specialized references or a hospital pharmacist for more specific information.

Dosage Forms/Regulatory Status

VETERINARY-LABELED PRODUCTS:

Ampicillin Trihydrate Injection Powder for Suspension: 10 g and 25 g (of ampicillin) vials; *Polyflex®*; (Rx). FDA-approved for use in dogs, cats, and cattle. Withdrawal times at labeled doses (cattle; do not treat for more than 7 days): Milk = 48 hours; Slaughter = 6 days (144 hours).

HUMAN-LABELED PRODUCTS:

Ampicillin Sodium Powder for Injection: 125 mg, 250 mg, 500 mg, 1 g, 2 g, & 10 g in vials; generic; (Rx)

Ampicillin Oral Capsules (as trihydrate): 250 mg & 500 mg; generic; (Rx)

Ampicillin (as trihydrate) Powder for Oral Suspension: 125 mg/5 mL & 250 mg/5 mL (as trihydrate) when reconstituted; generic; (Rx)

Revisions/References

Monograph revised/updated August 2013.

Adamcak, A. & B. Otten (2000). Rodent Therapeutics. *Vet Clin NA: Exotic Anim Pract* **3:1**(Jan): 221-40.

Brumbaugh, G. (1999). *Clinical Pharmacology and the Pediatric Patient.* 45th Annual AAEP Convention, Albuquerque. accessed via Veterinary Information Network; vin.com

Hjerpe, C. A. (1986). The bovine respiratory disease complex. *Current Veterinary Therapy: Food Animal Practice 2.* J. L. Howard. Philadelphia, W.B. Saunders: 670-81.

Ivey, E. & J. Morrisey (2000). Therapeutics for Rabbits. *Vet Clin NA: Exotic Anim Pract* **3:1**(Jan): 183-216.

MacDonald, K. (2010). Infective Endocarditis in Dogs: Diagnosis and Therapy. *Veterinary Clinics of North America-Small Animal Practice* **40**(4): 665-+.

Schumacher, J. (2011). Respiratory Medicine of Reptiles. *Vet Clin Exot Anim* **14**: 207-24.

Smith, A. (2000). General husbandry and medical care of hedgehogs. *Kirk's Current Veterinary Therapy: XIII Small Animal Practice.* J. Bonagura. Philadelphia, WB Saunders: 1128-33.

Sykes, J. E., et al. (2011). 2010 ACVIM Small Animal Consensus Statement on Leptospirosis: Diagnosis, Epidemiology, Treatment, and Prevention. *Journal of Veterinary Internal Medicine* **25**(1): 1-13.

Williams, B. (2000). Therapeutics in Ferrets. *Vet Clin NA: Exotic Anim Pract* **3:1**(Jan): 131-53.

Winther, L., et al. (2012). Pharmacokinetics in pulmonary epithelial lining fluid and plasma of ampicillin and pivampicillin administered to horses. *Research in Veterinary Science* **92**: 111-5.

Ampicillin Sodium + Sulbactam Sodium

(am-pi-**sill**-in; sul-**bak**-tam)   Unasyn®

Injectable Potentiated Aminopenicillin

Prescriber Highlights

► Parenteral potentiated aminopenicillin that may be used for infections where amoxicillin/clavulanate would be appropriate but when an injectable antibiotic is required.

► Hypersensitivity reactions possible; contraindicated in patients with documented severe hypersensitivity to penicillins.

► Usually dosed IM or IV q6-8h.

Uses/Indications

Ampicillin sodium/sulbactam sodium in a 2:1 ratio is effective when used parenterally for severa infections caused by many beta-lactamase-producing bacterial strains of otherwise resistant *E. coli, Pasteurella* spp., *Staphylococcus* spp., *Klebsiella*, and *Proteus*. Other aerobic bacteria commonlye to this combination include *Streptococcus, Listeria monocytogenes, Bacillus anthracis, Salmonella, Pasteurella,* and *Acinetobacter*. Anaerobic bacterial infections caused by *Clostridium, Bacteroides, Fusobacterium, Peptostrepto-*

coccus or *Propionibacterium* may be effectively treated with ampicillin/sulbactam.

Type I beta-lactamases that may be associated with *Citrobacter, Enterobacter, Serratia* and *Pseudomonas* are not generally inhibited by sulbactam or clavulanic acid. Ampicillin/sulbactam is ineffective against practically all strains of *Pseudomonas aeruginosa.*

In dogs and cats, ampicillin/sulbactam therapy may be considered when oral amoxicillin/clavulanate treatment is not viable (patient NPO, critically ill) or when large parenteral doses would be desirable for treatment (sepsis, pneumonia, other severe infections) or surgical prophylaxis.

Ampicillin/sulbactam has been used successfully to treat experimentally induced Klebsiella pneumonia in foals.

Pharmacology/Actions

When sulbactam is combined with ampicillin it extends its spectrum of activity to those bacteria that produce beta-lactamases of Richmond-Sykes types II-VI that would otherwise render ampicillin ineffective. Sulbactam binds to beta-lactamases thereby "protecting" the beta-lactam ring of ampicillin from hydrolysis.

Sulbactam has some intrinsic antibacterial activity against some bacteria (*Neisseria, Moraxella, Bacteroides*) at achievable levels. Sulbactam binding to certain penicillin-binding proteins (PBPs) may explain its activity. For most bacteria, sulbactam alone does not achieve levels sufficient to act as an antibacterial but when used in combination with ampicillin, synergistic effects may result.

On a mg for mg basis, clavulanic acid is a more potent beta-lactamase inhibitor than is sulbactam, but sulbactam has advantages of reduced likelihood of inducing chromosomal beta-lactamases, greater tissue penetration and stability.

For further information on the pharmacology of ampicillin, refer to that monograph.

Pharmacokinetics

As sulbactam sodium is not appreciably absorbed from the GI tract, this medication must be given parenterally. A covalently linked double ester form of ampicillin/sulbactam (sultamicillin) is orally absorbed, but this combination is not commercially available in the USA. When administered parenterally (IV/IM), sulbactam's pharmacokinetic profile closely mirrors that of ampicillin in most species studied. During the elimination phase in calves, plasma concentrations of sulbactam were consistently higher than those of ampicillin, leading the authors of the study to propose using a higher ratio (greater than 2:1 ampicillin/sulbactam) if the combination is used in calves.

Contraindications/Precautions/Warnings

Penicillins are contraindicated in patients with a history of severe hypersensitivity (*e.g.,* anaphylaxis) to them. Because there may be cross-reactivity, use penicillins cautiously in patients who are documented hypersensitive to other beta-lactam antibiotics (*e.g.,* cephalosporins, cefamycins, carbapenems).

Patients with severe renal dysfunction may require increased periods of time between doses.

Adverse Effects

Intramuscular injections may be painful. Intravenous injections may cause thrombophlebitis. Hypersensitivity reactions to penicillins occur infrequently in animals, but can be severe (anaphylaxis), particularly after IV administration.

High doses or very prolonged use of penicillins have been associated with neurotoxicity (*e.g.,* ataxia in dogs). Although the penicillins are not considered hepatotoxic, elevated liver enzymes have been reported. Other effects reported in dogs include tachypnea, dyspnea, edema and tachycardia.

Reproductive/Nursing Safety

Penicillins have been shown to cross the placenta and safe use during pregnancy has not been firmly established, but neither has there been any documented teratogenic problems associated with these drugs; however, use only when the potential benefits outweigh the risks. In humans, the FDA categorizes ampicillin as category *B* for use during pregnancy (*Animal studies have not yet demonstrated risk to the fetus, but there are no adequate studies in pregnant women; or animal studies have shown an adverse effect, but adequate studies in pregnant women have not demonstrated a risk to the fetus in the first trimester of pregnancy, and there is no evidence of risk in later trimesters.*) In a separate system evaluating the safety of drugs in canine and feline pregnancy (Papich 1989), ampicillin is categorized as in class: *A* (*Probably safe. Although specific studies may not have proved the safety of all drugs in dogs and cats, there are no reports of adverse effects in laboratory animals or women.*)

It is unknown if sulbactam crosses the placenta and safe use during pregnancy has not been established.

Both ampicillin and sulbactam are distributed into human breast milk in low concentrations. For humans, the World Health Organization (WHO) rates ampicillin as being compatible with breastfeeding and the American Academy of Pediatrics lists sulbactam as compatible with breastfeeding.

Overdosage/Acute Toxicity

Neurological effects (ataxia) have rarely been reported in dogs receiving very high dosages of penicillins; should these develop, weigh the risks of continued use versus those of dosage reduction or using a different antibiotic. In humans, especially those with renal disease, very high dosages of parenteral penicillins have induced CNS effects.

Drug Interactions

The following drug interactions with ampicillin/sulbactam have either been reported or are theoretical in humans or animals and may be of significance in veterinary patients. Unless otherwise noted, use together is not necessarily contraindicated, but weigh the potential risks and perform additional monitoring when appropriate.

- **AMINOGLYCOSIDES** (*e.g.,* **amikacin, gentamicin, tobramycin**): *In vitro* studies have demonstrated that penicillins can have synergistic or additive activity against certain bacteria when used with aminoglycosides. However, beta-lactam antibiotics can inactivate aminoglycosides *in vitro* and *in vivo* in patients in renal failure or when penicillins are used in massive dosages. Amikacin is considered the most resistant aminoglycoside to this inactivation.

- **BACTERIOSTATIC ANTIMICROBIALS** (*e.g.,* **chloramphenicol, erythromycin** and **other macrolides, tetracyclines, sulfonamides,** etc.): Because there is evidence of *in vitro* antagonism between beta-lactam antibiotics and bacteriostatic antibiotics, use together has been generally not recommended in the past, but actual clinical importance is not clear and in doubt.

- **PROBENECID**: Can reduce the renal tubular secretion of both ampicillin and sulbactam, thereby maintaining higher systemic levels for a longer period of time. This potential "beneficial" interaction requires further investigation before dosing recommendations can be made for veterinary patients.

Laboratory Considerations

- Ampicillin may cause false-positive **urine glucose** determinations when using cupric sulfate solution (Benedict's Solution, *Clinitest*®). Tests utilizing glucose oxidase (*Tes-Tape*®, *Clinistix*®) are not affected by ampicillin.

- As penicillins and other beta-lactams can inactivate **aminoglycosides** *in vitro* (and *in vivo* in patients in renal failure or when penicillins are used in massive dosages), serum concentrations of aminoglycosides may be falsely decreased particularly when the serum is stored prior to analysis. It is recommended that if the aminoglycoside assay is delayed, samples be frozen and, if possible, drawn at times when the beta-lactam antibiotic is at a trough.

Doses

- **DOGS/CATS:**

  Note: Dosages are for combined amounts (ampicillin + sulbactam) unless otherwise noted:

  For pre-surgery prophylaxis for colorectal procedures (extra-label): 150 mg (toy breed dogs, cats) – 3 grams (giant breed dogs) IV once within 60 minutes prior to incision. (Extrapolated from human recommendations.)

  For empiric therapy in critically ill animals (extra-label): 15 – 30 mg/kg IV q6-8h; used in combination with a parenteral drug with gram-negative activity (*e.g.*, an aminoglycoside or fluoroquinolone).

Monitoring

- Because penicillins usually have minimal toxicity associated with their use, monitoring for efficacy is usually all that is required unless toxic signs or symptoms develop.
- Serum levels and therapeutic drug monitoring are not routinely performed with these agents.

Client Information

- Because of the dosing intervals required this drug is best administered to inpatients only.

Chemistry/Synonyms

Ampicillin sodium and sulbactam sodium for injection occurs as a white to off-white powder that is freely soluble in water or other aqueous solutions.

Ampicillin/Sulbactam may also be known as: *Ampibactan®, Bacimex®, Begalin-P®, Bethacil®, Comabactan®, Galotam®, Loricin®, Sulam®, Sulperazon®, Synergistin®, Unacid®, Unacim®, Unasyn®* or *Unasyna®*.

Storage/Stability

The unreconstituted powder should be stored at temperatures at, or below 30°C.

Compatibility/Compounding Considerations

Diluents for reconstituting the powder for injection for IV use that are reported **compatible** with ampicillin/sulbactam include sterile water for injection, and 0.9% sodium chloride. If reconstituted to a concentration of 45 mg/mL (30/15), the resulting solution is stable for 8 hours at room temperature and for 48 hours at 4°C. If reconstituted to a concentration of 30 mg/mL (20/10), the resulting solution is stable for 72 hours at 4°C. After reconstitution and before administering, the solution should be further diluted into a 50 mL or 100 mL bag of 0.9% sodium chloride and administered IV over 15-30 minutes. Diluted solutions for IV administration are stable at room temperature for 8 hours.

When reconstituting for IM use, sterile water for injection or 0.5% or 2% lidocaine HCl injection may be used. 3.2 mL of diluent is added to the 1.5 g vial; 6.4 mL of diluent to the 3 g vial. After reconstituting, the solution should be administered within 1 hour.

Ampicillin/sulbactam injection is **not compatible** with aminoglycoside antibiotics (*e.g.*, gentamicin, amikacin) and should not be mixed with these agents.

Ampicillin/sulbactam is **compatible** with vancomycin when mixed at concentrations of 50/25 mg/mL of ampicillin/sulbactam and 20 mg/mL or less of vancomycin.

Dosage Forms/Regulatory Status

VETERINARY-LABELED PRODUCTS: NONE.

HUMAN-LABELED PRODUCTS:

Ampicillin Sodium/Sulbactam Sodium Powder (injection): 1.5 g (1 g ampicillin sodium/0.5 g sulbactam sodium), 3 g (2 g ampicillin sodium/1 g sulbactam sodium) in vials and 15 g (10 g ampicillin sodium/5 g sulbactam sodium) in bulk; *Unasyn®*, generic; (Rx)

Revisions/References

Monograph revised/updated August 2013.

Papich, M. (1989). Effects of drugs on pregnancy. *Current Veterinary Therapy X: Small Animal Practice.* R. Kirk. Philadelphia, Saunders: 1291-9.

Amprolium HCl

(am-proe-**lee**-um)   Corid®

Anticoccidial

Prescriber Highlights

▶ Thiamine analog antiprotozoal (coccidia).
▶ Prolonged high dosages may cause thiamine deficiency; treatment is usually no longer than 14 days.
▶ Occasionally may cause GI or neurologic effects.
▶ May be unpalatable.

Uses/Indications

Amprolium has good activity against *Eimeria tenella* and *E. acervulina* in poultry and can be used as a therapeutic agent for these organisms. It only has marginal activity or weak activity against *E. maxima, E. mivati, E. necatrix,* or *E. brunetti.* It is often used in combination with other agents (*e.g.*, ethopabate) to improve control against those organisms.

In cattle, amprolium has FDA-approval for the treatment and prevention of *E. bovis* and *E. zurnii* in cattle and calves.

Amprolium has been used in dogs, swine, sheep, and goats for the control of coccidiosis, although there are no FDA-approved products in the USA for these species.

Pharmacology/Actions

By mimicking its structure, amprolium competitively inhibits thiamine utilization by the parasite. Prolonged high dosages can cause thiamine deficiency in the host; excessive thiamine in the diet can reduce or reverse the anticoccidial activity of the drug.

Amprolium is thought to act primarily upon the first generation schizont in the cells of the intestinal wall, preventing differentiation of the metrozoites. It may suppress the sexual stages and sporulation of the oocysts.

Pharmacokinetics

No information was located for this agent.

Contraindications/Precautions/Warnings

Not recommended to be used for more than 12 days in puppies.

Adverse Effects

In dogs, neurologic disturbances, depression, anorexia, and diarrhea have been reported but are rare and are probably dose-related. See Overdosage section below for treatment recommendations. The undiluted liquid or pastes are reportedly unpalatable.

High dosages or long-term use of amprolium may induce neurologic signs (polioencephalomalacia—PEM; cerebrocortical necrosis). Parenteral thiamine (vitamin B-1) can be used for treatment.

Overdosage/Acute Toxicity

Amprolium has induced polioencephalomalacia (PEM) in sheep when administered at 880 mg/kg PO for 4-6 weeks and at 1 gram/kg for 3-5 weeks. Erythrocyte production also ceased in lambs receiving these high dosages.

It is reported that overdoses of amprolium can produce neurologic clinical signs in dogs. Treatment should consist of stopping amprolium therapy and administering parenteral thiamine (1 – 10 mg/day IM or IV).

Drug Interactions
The following drug interactions have either been reported or are theoretical in animals receiving amprolium and may be of significance in veterinary patients:

- **THIAMINE:** Exogenously administered thiamine in high doses may reverse or reduce the efficacy of amprolium.

Doses
- **DOGS:**

For coccidiosis (All are extra-label):

a) **Small Pups** (< 10 kg adult weight): 100 mg (total dose) (using the 20% powder) in a gelatin capsule PO once daily for 7-12 days. **Large pups** (>10 kg adult weight): 200 mg (total dose) (using the 20% powder) in a gelatin capsule PO once daily for 7-12 days. In food, for pups or bitches: 250 – 300 mg total dose using the 20% powder on food once daily for 7-12 days. In water, for pups or bitches: 30 mL of the 9.6% solution in one gallon of water (no other water provided) for 7-10 days. (Greene et al. 2006)

b) 150 mg/kg of amprolium and 25 mg/kg of sulfadimethoxine for 14 days. (Blagburn 2003)

c) **For control of coccidiosis:** 1.5 tablespoonsful (22.5 mL) of the 9.6% solution per one gallon of water to be used as the sole drinking water source, not to exceed 10 days. Monitor water consumption both for treatment and hydration assurance; rarely some dogs may not drink the amprolium water due to its bitter taste. In situations where dogs are co-habitants, it is necessary to place enough water for all to have access. (Blagburn 2005), (Blagburn 2007)

- **CATS:**

For coccidiosis (all are extra-label):

a) For *Cystoisospora* spp.: 60 – 100 mg total dose PO once daily for 7 days. (Lappin 2000)

b) On food: 300 – 400 mg/kg on food once daily for 5 days or 110 – 220 mg/kg on food once daily for 7-12 days. In water: 1.5 teaspoonsful (7.5 mL) of the 9.6% solution in one gallon of water per day for 10 days. In combination: amprolium at 150 mg/kg PO once daily with sulfadimethoxine (25 mg/kg PO once daily) for 14 days. (Greene et al. 2006)

- **FERRETS:**

For coccidiosis (extra-label): 19 mg/kg PO once daily. (Lennox 2006)

- **RABBITS/RODENTS/SMALL MAMMALS:**

For coccidiosis (all are extra-label):

a) **Rabbits:** Using 9.6% solution: 1 mL/7 kg BW PO once daily for 5 days; in drinking water: 0.5 mL/500 mL for 10 days. (Ivey et al. 2000)

b) **Gerbils, Mice, Rats, Hamsters:** 10 – 20 mg/kg total daily dose divided q8-24h SC or IM. **Chinchillas:** 10 – 15 mg/kg per day divided q8–24h SC, IM or IV. (Adamcak et al. 2000)

- **CATTLE:**

As an aid in the treatment and prevention of coccidiosis caused by *Eimeria bovis* and *E. zuernii* in calves (FDA-Approved; see restrictions in *Dosage Form* section): 1) 5 day treatment protocol: 10 mg/kg PO for 5 days. 2) PO 21-day prevention protocol: 5 mg/kg PO for 21 days. Can be administered either as an oral drench or mixed into the sole source of fresh drinking water. See product labels for additional information. (Adapted From product label; AmproMed® for Calves)

- **SWINE:**

For coccidiosis (extra-label): Treatment: 25 – 65 mg/kg PO once or twice daily for 3–4 days. (Todd et al. 1986)

- **SHEEP & GOATS:**

For coccidiosis:

a) **Lambs** (extra-label): 55 mg/kg daily PO for 19 days. (Todd et al. 1986)

b) **Goat kids** (extra-label): 50 mg/kg daily PO for 5 days will effectively reduce the fecal shedding of Eimeria oocysts without inducing neurologic disease. The Food Animal Residue Avoidance and Depletion program (FARAD; USA) recommends a minimum slaughter withdrawal interval of 6 days for goats that receive amprolium at doses higher than 40 mg/kg. (Young et al. 2011)

- **CAMELIDS (NEW WORLD):**

For *Eimeria macusaniensis* (E.mac); (extra-label): 10 mg/kg PO as a 1.5% solution PO once daily. Treat for 10-15 days and give thiamine at 10 mg/kg SC once daily every 5 days during treatment. (Cebra et al. 2007)

- **BIRDS:**

For coccidiosis in pet birds (extra-label): 2 mL (using the 9.6% solution) per gallon of water for 5 days or longer. Cages should be steam cleaned to prevent reinfection. Supplement diet with B vitamins. Some strains resistant in Toucans and Mynahs. (Clubb 1986)

Monitoring
- Clinical efficacy.
- If using in high dosages (extra-label) watch for neurological signs such as "stargazing", opisthotonos, central blindness, circling, or ataxia.

Chemistry/Synonyms
A structural analogue of thiamine (vitamin B_1), amprolium hydrochloride occurs as a white or almost white, odorless or nearly odorless powder. One gram is soluble in 2 mL of water and is slightly soluble in alcohol.

Amprolium may also be known as amprocidi, *Amprol®*, *Corid®*, *Coxoid®*, *Coxiprol®* or *Ampromed®*.

Storage/Stability
Unless otherwise instructed by the manufacturer, amprolium products should be stored at room temperature (15–30°C).

Compatibility/Compounding Considerations
No specific information noted.

Dosage Forms/Regulatory Status/Withdrawal Times
VETERINARY-LABELED PRODUCTS:

Amprolium 9.6% (96 mg/mL) Oral Solution in 1 gal jugs; *Ampromed®*, *Corid®*, *generic*; (OTC). FDA-approved for use in calves (not veal calves). Slaughter withdrawal (when used as labeled) = 24 hours; a withdrawal period has not been established for pre-ruminating calves.

Amprolium 20% Soluble Powder; *Corid®*, *Ampromed®*; (OTC). FDA-approved for use in calves (not veal calves). Slaughter withdrawal (when used as labeled) = 24 hours. A withdrawal period has not been established for pre-ruminating calves.

There are also available medicated feeds (amprolium alone) and combination products (medicated feeds, feed additives) containing amprolium with other therapeutic agents. These products may be labeled for use in calves, chickens and/or turkeys.

HUMAN-LABELED PRODUCTS: NONE.

Revisions/References

Monograph revised/updated August 2013.

Adamcak, A. & B. Otten (2000). Rodent Therapeutics. *Vet Clin NA: Exotic Anim Pract* **3:1**(Jan): 221-40.

Blagburn, B. (2003). *Giardiasis and coccidiosis updates.* Proceedings: Western Veterinary Conference. accessed via Veterinary Information Network; vin.com

Blagburn, B. (2005). *Treatment and control of tick borne diseases and other important parasites of companion animals.* Proceedings: ACVC2005. accessed via Veterinary Information Network; vin.com

Blagburn, B. (2007). Personal communication.

Cebra, C. K., et al. (2007). Eimeria macusaniensis infection in 15 llamas and 34 alpacas. *Javma-Journal of the American Veterinary Medical Association* **230**(1): 94-100.

Clubb, S. L. (1986). Therapeutics: Individual and Flock Treatment Regimens. *Clinical Avian Medicine and Surgery.* G. J. Harrison and L. R. Harrison. Philadelphia, W.B. Saunders: 327-55.

Greene, C., et al. (2006). Appendix 8: Antimicrobial Drug Formulary. *Infectious Disease of the Dog and Cat.* C. Greene, Elsevier: 1186-333.

Ivey, E. & J. Morrisey (2000). Therapeutics for Rabbits. *Vet Clin NA: Exotic Anim Pract* **3:1**(Jan): 183-216.

Lappin, M. (2000). Protozoal and Miscellaneous Infections. *Textbook of Veterinary Internal Medicine: Diseases of the Dog and Cat.* S. Ettinger and E. Feldman. Philadelphia, WB Saunders. **1**: 408-17.

Lennox, A. (2006). *Working up gastrointestinal disease in the ferret.* Proceedings: West Vet Conf. accessed via Veterinary Information Network; vin.com

Todd, K. S., et al. (1986). Coccidiosis. *Current Veterinary Therapy 2: Food Animal Practice.* J. L. Howard. Philadelphia, WB Saunders: 632-6.

Young, G., et al. (2011). Efficacy of amprolium for the treatment of pathogenic Eimeria species in Boer goat kids. *Veterinary Parasitology* **178**(3-4): 346-9.

Antacids, Oral – See Aluminum Hydroxide; or Magnesium Hydroxide

Antivenin (Crotalidae) Polyvalent (Equine Origin)
Antivenin (Crotalidae) Polyvalent Immune Fab (Ovine Origin)

(an-tie-ven-nin)   Antivenom; Pit Viper Antivenin; CroFab®

Antidote

Note: The products, availability, and clinical use of antivenins are subject to change. Sources for current information include: The Arizona Poison and Drug Information Center (800-222-1222), ASPCA Animal Poison Control Center (888-426-4435), and Pet Poison HELPLINE (800-213-6680). Consultation fees may apply.

Prescriber Highlights

► May cause hypersensitivity reactions (both acute and delayed). More likely to occur with the Antivenin (Crotalidae) Polyvalent Equine Origin (ACP) product.
► Treatment can be extremely expensive.

Uses/Indications

The equine-derived product is indicated for the treatment of envenomation from most venomous snake bites (pit vipers) in North America and those caused by several species found in Central and South America (fer-de-lance, Central and South American Rattlesnake). The ovine-derived product is indicated for North American Crotalid snake envenomation in humans, but has been used in dogs. There is a fair amount of controversy or unknowns with regard to use of these products in domestic animals and many factors contribute to the potential for toxicity (victim's size and general health, bite site(s), number of bites, age, species and size of snake, etc.). Antivenin treatment is considered the mainstay treatment for moderate to severe pit viper envenomation although use in animals can be dictated by availability and affordability. At the time of writing (2013) there are two antivenin products commercially available in the Unites States: Veterinary-Approved (Dogs): Antivenin (Crotalidae) Polyvalent Equine Origin (ACP) and Human-approved: Antivenin (Crotalidae) Polyvalent Immune Fab (Ovine Origin)(OPCA; *Crofab®*). Additionally, a polyvalent equine-origin F(ab')2 antivenin (*Antivipmyn®*; Bioclon Institute–Mexico) and a polyspecific equine-origin IgG antivenin (*Polyvet-ICP®*, Instituto Clodomiro Picado–Costa Rica) have been successfully used in treating North American Pit Viper envenomation.

Pharmacology/Actions

Antivenins act by neutralizing the venoms (complex proteins) in patients via passive immunization of globulins or antibody fragments obtained from horses or sheep immunized with venom(s). Antivenin can be very effective in reversing venom-related coagulation abnormalities or neurotoxicity (depending on the antivenin), but Timber Rattlesnake venom-induced thrombocytopenia may be resistant to treatment.

Pharmacokinetics

Specific detailed information was not located. It is reported that Fab2 antibody fragment antivenom (*Antivipmyn®*) is cleared from the body faster than IgG (ACP, or *Polyvet-ICP®*), but slower than the Fab1 antibody fragment (*CroFab®*) (Armentano et al. 2011).

Contraindications/Precautions/Warnings

Up to 50% of the veterinary-labeled product contains equine albumin and other equine proteins.

The canine-approved product reads: "Attempts should be made to immobilize the patient until treatment is initiated. The use of excessive heat or cold is contraindicated. Antihistamines and tranquilizers are also contraindicated, and may potentiate the effect of snake venom. Sedatives and analgesics should also be employed with discretion, because large doses may mask important clinical signs."

Adverse Effects

Up to 50% of the veterinary-labeled product (ACP) contains equine albumin and other equine proteins and anaphylaxis or anaphylactoid reactions have been reported in 2-7% of treated dogs (McCown et al. 2009). A 1:10 dilution of the antivenin given intracutaneously at a dose of 0.02 – 0.03 mL has been suggested as a test for hypersensitivity, but this is no longer commonly recommended. A pre-treatment dose of diphenhydramine is often recommended before administering antivenin primarily to sedate the patient and, theoretically, reduce any possible allergic reactions to the antivenin but this too, is somewhat controversial. Epinephrine (0.01 mg/kg intramuscularly and repeated at 15-20-minute intervals until the patient stable) has been recommended if early signs of anaphylaxis (vomiting, salivation, restlessness, urticaria, and facial pruritus) are noted (Armentano et al. 2011). Stopping the infusion, giving an additional dose of diphenhydramine and restarting the infusion 5 minutes later at a slower rate allowing the dose to be administered without further problems has also been suggested. One case of a dog developing antivenin-associated serum sickness has been reported after treatment using Crotilidae antivenin (ACP) (Berdoulay et al. 2005) and a retrospective study of 218 dogs reported signs of delayed hypersensitivity/serum sickness in 2/218 dogs (McCown et al. 2009). While it is believed that the fractionated antibody products would have less antigenic potential than ACP, hypersensitivity reactions are still possible especially if multiple vials are required.

Other potential adverse effects can include hypocalcemia, gastrointestinal effects, cardiac rhythm changes (tachycardia, bradycardia), changes in blood pressure, and agitation/trembling.

Reproductive/Nursing Safety

In humans, the FDA categorizes this drug as category **C** for use during pregnancy (*Animal studies have shown an adverse effect on the fetus, but there are no adequate studies in humans; or there are no animal reproduction studies and no adequate studies in humans*).

Safety during nursing has not been established but it would unlikely pose much risk.

Drug Interactions

The following drug interactions with antivenin have either been reported or are theoretical in humans or animals and may be of significance in veterinary patients. Unless otherwise noted, use together is not necessarily contraindicated, but weigh the potential risks and perform additional monitoring when appropriate.

- **ANALGESICS/SEDATIVES**: Although reducing excessive movement and other supportive therapy are important parts of treating envenomation, drugs that can mask the clinical signs associated with the venom (*e.g.*, analgesics and sedatives) should initially be used with caution.
- **ANTIHISTAMINES**: It has been stated that antihistamines may potentiate the venom; however, documentation of this interaction was not located and diphenhydramine is routinely used by many clinicians to treat snakebite in dogs.
- **BETA-BLOCKERS**: May mask the early signs associated with anaphylaxis.
- **CORTICOSTEROID** use has fallen out of favor in the treatment of snakebite envenomation and is usually not employed, but controversy remains regarding their use. Corticosteroids may be useful to treat anaphylaxis, however.
- **HEPARIN**: Is reportedly not effective in treating the thrombin-like enzymes found in rattlesnake venom.

Doses

Note: The treatment of pit viper snakebite involves significant supportive treatment and monitoring beyond administration of antivenin. It is highly recommended to refer to specialized references (*e.g.*, *Overview and controversies in the medical management of pit viper envenomation in the dog*) (Armentano et al. 2011) or to contact an animal poison control center for guidance beyond what is listed below.

- **DOGS/CATS:**

    Crotilidae antivenin (ACP; equine origin):

    FDA-Approved Label: Dogs: Administer 1 – 5 rehydrated vials (10 – 50 mL) IV depending on severity of symptoms, duration of time after the bite, snake size, patient size (the smaller the victim, the larger the dose). Additional doses may be given every 2 hours as required. If unable to give IV, may administer IM as close to bite as practical. Give supportive therapy (*e.g.*, corticosteroids, antibiotics, fluid therapy, blood products, and tetanus prophylaxis) as required. (Adapted from label; *Antivenin*®—BIVI)

    Dogs/Cats (extra-label): Dose necessary is calculated relative to the amount of venom injected, body mass of patient and the bite site. Average dose required for dogs or cats is 1 – 2 vials of antivenin. The earlier the antivenin is administered the more effective it is. Intravascular bites or bites to the torso or tongue are serious and require prompt, aggressive antivenin administration. Smaller patients may require higher doses (as venom amount/kg body weight is higher), and multiple vials may be necessary. Initially, give one vial, by diluting to 100 – 250 mL of crystalloid fluids and administering by slow IV (if there are no problems, may increase rate and administer volume over 30 minutes). In smaller patients, adjust infusion volume to prevent fluid overload. (Peterson 2006)

- **HORSES:**

    Crotilidae Antivenin (extra-label): Use only if necessary to treat systemic effects, otherwise, avoid use. Administer 1 – 2 vials slowly IV diluted in 250 – 500 mL saline or lactated Ringer's. Administer antihistamines; corticosteroids are contraindicated. (Bailey et al. 1992)

Monitoring

- Signs associated with an allergic response to the antivenin (*e.g.*, anaphylaxis, anaphylactoid-reactions, serum sickness).
- CBC with platelets; coagulation parameters.
- Biochem profile; hydration status.
- ECG.

Client Information

- Clients must be made aware of the potential for anaphylaxis as well as the expenses associated with treatment, monitoring and hospitalization.

Chemistry

Antivenin products are concentrated serum globulins obtained from horses immunized with the venoms of several types of snakes. They are provided as refined, lyophilized product with a suitable diluent. Up to 50% of the proteins contained in the veterinary product may be equine-specific proteins.

Storage/Stability

Do not store above 98°F (37°C); avoid freezing and excessive heat. Reconstitute the vial with the diluent provided; gently swirl the vial (may require several minutes; do not shake) to prevent excessive foaming. Warming the vial to body temperature may speed up reconstitution. Once reconstituted the vial contents are often added to a crystalloid intravenous solution (D5W, normal saline often recommended) for infusion. Depending on dog size, one vial in 100 – 250 mL has been suggested for infusion (Peterson 2006).

The package insert for the veterinary-labeled product states that after rehydration the vial should be used immediately. One reference (anon 2007a) states that the human-labeled equine origin product can be used within 4 hours of reconstitution if refrigerated, but another (anon 2007b) states that it can be used within 48 hours after reconstitution and within 12 hours after further dilution into IV fluids.

The polyvalent immune fab (ovine) product should be stored in the refrigerator and used within 4 hours of reconstitution.

Compatibility/Compounding Considerations

No specific information noted.

Dosage Forms/Regulatory Status

Note: The availability status of antivenins in the USA is in flux. It is highly recommended to contact a poison control center (see phone numbers at the top of this monograph) to get current recommendations on availability and treatment options.

VETERINARY-LABELED PRODUCTS:

Antivenin (Crotalidae) Polyvalent Equine Origin single dose vial lyophilized; 10 mL vials with diluent. *Antivenin*®; (Rx). Approved for use in dogs. Not returnable for credit or exchange.

HUMAN-LABELED PRODUCTS:

Antivenin (Crotalidae) Polyvalent Immune Fab (Ovine Origin) Powder for Injection (lyophilized): 1 g total protein per single use vial; *CroFab*®; (Rx)

The following products are not (at the time of writing; 2013) approved by FDA or USDA for use in the Untied States, but have been used in animals: Polyvalent equine-origin F(ab')2 antivenin (*Antivipmyn*®; Bioclon Institute–Mexico) and Polyspecific equine-origin IgG antivenin (*Polyvet-ICP*®, Instituto Clodomiro Picado–Costa Rica). It is reported that a special importer's permit acquired from the USDA and the approval from the state veterinarian is required to legally import these products into the USA (Armentano et al. 2011).

Revisions/References

Monograph revised/updated August 2013.
anon (2007a). "Facts and Comparisons Online Edition."
anon (2007b). "USP DI® Drug Information for the Health Professional Online Edition."
Armentano, R. A. & M. Schaer (2011). Overview and controversies in the medical management of pit viper envenomation in the dog. *J. Vet. Emerg. Crit. Care* 21(5): 461-70.
Bailey, E. & T. Garland (1992). Management of Toxicoses. *Current Therapy in Equine Medicine 3*. N. Robinson. Philadelphia, W.B. Saunders Co.: 346-53.
Berdoulay, P., et al. (2005). Serum sickness on a dog associated with antivenin therapy for a snake bite caused by Crotalus adamanteus. *J Vet Emerg Crit Care* 15(3): 206-12.
McCown, J. L., et al. (2009). Effect of antivenin dose on outcome from crotalid envenomation: 218 dogs (1988-2006). *J. Vet. Emerg. Crit. Care* 19(6): 603-10.
Peterson, M. (2006). Snake Bite: North American Pit Vipers. *Small Animal Toxicology, 2nd Ed.* M. Peterson and P. Talcott, Elsevier: 1017-38.

Antivenin (Micrurus fulvias) Eastern and Texas Coral Snake

(an-tie-**ven**-nin)   North American Coral Snake Antivenin

Antidote

Note: The products, availability, and clinical use of antivenins are subject to change. Sources for current information include: The Arizona Poison and Drug Information Center (800-222-1222), ASPCA Animal Poison Control Center (888-426-4435), and Pet Poison HELPLINE (800-213-6680). Consultation fees may apply.

Prescriber Highlights

▶ May cause hypersensitivity reactions.

▶ Treatment can be very expensive.

Uses/Indications

This product is indicated for the treatment of envenomation from the Eastern coral snake (*Micrurus fulvius fulvius*) and the Texas coral snake (*Micrurus fulvius tenere*). It will not neutralize the venom from the Sonoran or Arizona coral snake (*Micruroides euryxanthus*) or the Brazilian giant coral snake (*Micrurus frontalis*). Coral snake envenomation is quite rare in the United States and approximately 60% of coral snake bites do not result in envenomation. Unlike pit viper venom, coral snake venom primarily causes neurotoxicity and clinical signs may be delayed. It has been recommended that animals suspected of a coral snake envenomation be hospitalized with close observation for 24-48 hours post-bite.

Pharmacology/Actions

Antivenins act by neutralizing the venoms (complex proteins) in patients via passive immunization of globulins obtained from horses immunized with the venom. Each vial of antivenin will neutralize approximately 2 mg of *M. fulvius fulvius* venom.

Contraindications/Precautions/Warnings

The coral snake antivenin will not neutralize *M. euryxanthus* (Sonoran or Arizona Coral Snake) venom. Because there is a risk of anaphylaxis occurring secondary to the horse serum, many recommend performing sensitivity testing before administration.

Adverse Effects

The most significant adverse effect associated with the use of these products is anaphylaxis secondary to the equine serum source of this product. An incidence rate of less than 2% has been reported. A 1:10 dilution of the antivenin given intracutaneously at a dose of 0.02 – 0.03 mL may be useful as a test for hypersensitivity. Wheal formation and erythema indicate a positive reaction and are generally seen within 30 minutes of administration. A negative response does not insure that anaphylaxis will not occur, however. A pre-treatment dose of diphenhydramine is often recommended before administering antivenin. Should an anaphylactoid reaction be detected, stopping the infusion, giving an additional dose of diphenhydramine and restarting the infusion 5 minutes later at a slower rate may allow the dose to be administered without further problems.

Reproductive/Nursing Safety

In humans, the FDA categorizes this drug as category *C* for use during pregnancy (*Animal studies have shown an adverse effect on the fetus, but there are no adequate studies in humans; or there are no animal reproduction studies and no adequate studies in humans*).

Drug Interactions

The following drug interactions with antivenin have either been reported or are theoretical in humans or animals and may be of significance in veterinary patients. Unless otherwise noted, use together is not necessarily contraindicated, but weigh the potential risks and perform additional monitoring when appropriate.

- **ANALGESICS/SEDATIVES**: Although reducing excessive movement and other supportive therapy are important parts of treating envenomation, drugs that can mask the clinical signs associated with the venom (*e.g.*, analgesics and sedatives) should initially be used with caution.

- **ANTIHISTAMINES**: It has been stated that antihistamines may potentiate the venom; however, documentation of this interaction was not located and diphenhydramine is routinely used by many clinicians to treat snakebite in dogs.

- **BETA-BLOCKERS**: May mask the early signs associated with anaphylaxis.

- **CORTICOSTEROID** use has fallen out of favor in the treatment of snakebite envenomation and is usually considered contraindicated. Corticosteroids may be useful to treat anaphylaxis, however.

Doses

Note: The treatment of Coral snakebite involves significant treatment and monitoring beyond administration of antivenin. It is highly recommended to refer to specialized references *e.g., A retrospective evaluation of coral snake envenomation in dogs and cats: 20 cases (1996–2011)* (Perez et al. 2012) or to contact an animal poison control center for guidance beyond what is listed below.

- **DOGS/CATS:**

  Coral Snake antivenin (not Sonoran or Arizona variety); (extra-label): Dose necessary is calculated relative to the amount of venom injected and the body mass of patient. Average dose required for dogs or cats is 1 – 2 vials of antivenin. The earlier the antivenin is administered the more effective it is. Smaller patients may require higher doses (as venom amount/kg body weight is higher), and multiple vials may be necessary. Initially give one vial, by diluting to 100 – 250 mL of crystalloid fluids and administering by slow IV. In smaller patients, adjust infusion volume to prevent fluid overload. Give additional vials as indicated by the progression of the syndrome. (Peterson 2006)

- **HORSES:**

  Coral Snake Antivenin (extra-label): Use only if necessary to treat systemic effects, otherwise, avoid use. Administer 1 – 2 vials slowly IV diluted in 250 – 500 mL saline or lactated Ringer's. Administer antihistamines; corticosteroids are contraindicated. May be used with Crotalidae antivenin. (Bailey and Garland 1992)

Monitoring

- Signs associated with an allergic response to the antivenin (*e.g.*, anaphylaxis, anaphylactoid-reactions, serum sickness).

- Cardiorespiratory monitoring; mechanical ventilation may be necessary.

- Pulse oximetry.

Client Information

- Clients must be made aware of the potential for anaphylaxis as well as the expenses associated with treatment, monitoring and hospitalization.

Chemistry

These products are concentrated serum globulins obtained from horses immunized with the venoms of several types of snakes. They are provided as refined, lyophilized product with a suitable diluent.

Storage/Stability

Product should be stored in the refrigerator. Avoid freezing and excessive heat. Reconstitute vial with 10 mL of the supplied diluent. Gentle agitation may be used to hasten dissolution of the lyophilized powder. Reconstituted vials should be used within 48 hours (keep refrigerated) and within 12 hours once added to IV solutions.

Compatibility/Compounding Considerations

No specific information noted.

Dosage Forms/Regulatory Status

Note: The availability status of antivenins in the USA is in flux. It is highly recommended to contact a poison control center (see phone numbers at the top of this monograph) to get current recommendations on availability and treatment options.

VETERINARY-LABELED PRODUCTS: NONE.

HUMAN-LABELED PRODUCTS:

Antivenin (*Micrurus fulvius*) Powder for Injection lyophilized: in single-use vials with 1 vial diluent (10 mL water for injection); *Antivenin* (*Micrurus fulvius*); (Rx). **Note:** The manufacturer has discontinued producing this product and availability may an issue. A coral snake antivenin (*Coralmyn*®) is being developed by Bioclon Institute (Mexico), but at the time of writing (2013) was not approved for us in the USA.

Revisions/References

Monograph revised/updated August 2013.

Perez, M. L., et al. (2012). A retrospective evaluation of coral snake envenomation in dogs and cats: 20 cases (1996-2011). *J. Vet. Emerg. Crit. Care* **22**(6): 682-9.

Peterson, M. (2006). Snake Bite: North American Pit Vipers. *Small Animal Toxicology, 2nd Ed.* M. Peterson and P. Talcott, Elsevier: 1017-38.

Antivenin (Latrodectus Mactans) Black Widow Spider

(an-tie-ven-nin)   Black Widow Spider Antivenin

Antidote

Note: The products, availability, and clinical use of antivenins are subject to change. Sources for current information include: The Arizona Poison and Drug Information Center (800-222-1222), ASPCA Animal Poison Control Center (888-426-4435), and Pet Poison HELPLINE (800-213-6680). Consultation fees may apply.

Prescriber Highlights

▶ May cause hypersensitivity reactions.
▶ May be difficult for veterinarians to obtain.

Uses/Indications

Black widow spider antivenin is used to treat envenomation caused by this spider. Cats, camels and horses are considered to be extremely sensitive to the venom. Primary toxic signs are due to neurotoxins in the venom.

Pharmacology/Actions

Antivenins act by neutralizing the venoms (complex proteins) in patients via passive immunization of globulins obtained from horses immunized with the venom. In humans, symptoms begin to subside in 1-2 hours after administration.

Contraindications/Precautions/Warnings

Because there is a risk of anaphylaxis occurring secondary to the horse serum, many recommend performing sensitivity testing before administration.

Adverse Effects

The most significant adverse effect associated with the use of the equine origin product is anaphylaxis secondary to its equine serum source; an incidence rate of less than 2% has been reported. A 1:10 dilution of the antivenin given intracutaneously at a dose of 0.02 – 0.03 mL has been suggested as a test for hypersensitivity. Wheal formation and erythema indicate a positive reaction and are generally seen within 30 minutes of administration. However, a negative response does not insure that anaphylaxis will be avoided and slow intravenous administration is usually sufficient to identify animals that will react to the product. A pre-treatment dose of diphenhydramine is often recommended before administering antivenin primarily to sedate the patient and, theoretically, to reduce any possible allergic reactions to the antivenin. Should an anaphylactoid reaction be detected (nausea, pruritus, hyperemia of the inner pinna), stopping the infusion, giving an additional dose of diphenhydramine and restarting the infusion 5 minutes later at a slower rate may allow the dose to be administered without further problems.

Reproductive/Nursing Safety

In humans, the FDA categorizes this drug as category **C** for use during pregnancy (*Animal studies have shown an adverse effect on the fetus, but there are no adequate studies in humans; or there are no animal reproduction studies and no adequate studies in humans*).

Drug Interactions

The following drug interactions with black widow spider antivenin have either been reported or are theoretical in humans or animals and may be of significance in veterinary patients. Unless otherwise noted, use together is not necessarily contraindicated, but weigh the potential risks and perform additional monitoring when appropriate.

- **BETA-BLOCKERS:** May mask the early signs associated with anaphylaxis.

Doses

- **DOGS/CATS:**

  Note: All are extra-label.

  a) After reconstituting the antivenin, add to 100 mL of normal saline and administer via slow IV over 30 minutes. Pretreatment with 2 – 4 mg/kg of diphenhydramine SC may help calm the patient and may possibly protect against allergic reactions from the antivenin. Monitor inner pinna during infusion for signs of anaphylaxis (hyperemia). If hyperemia occurs, discontinue infusion and give a second dose of diphenhydramine. If allergic reactions abate, may restart infusion at a slower rate; if they recur, stop infusion and seek consultation. Use care with administration of IV fluids as envenomation can cause significant hypertension. Benzodiazepines may alleviate muscle cramping. (Peterson et al. 2006)

  b) Dissolve contents of one vial and add to 100 – 200 mL of warm 0.9% NaCl and infuse over 2–6 hours. Administer diphenhydramine at 0.5 – 1 mg/kg prior to infusion. (Atkins 2006)

Client Information
- Clients must be made aware of the potential for anaphylaxis as well as the expenses associated with treatment, monitoring and hospitalization.

Monitoring
- Signs associated with an allergic response to the antivenin (*e.g.*, anaphylaxis, anaphylactoid-reactions, serum sickness).
- Respiratory/cardiac rate.
- Blood pressure.
- Serum chemistry (blood glucose mandatory).
- CBC.
- Urine output; urinalysis.

Chemistry
This product is concentrated serum globulins obtained from horses immunized with the venom of the black widow spider. It is provided as refined, lyophilized product with a suitable diluent.

Storage/Stability
Product should be stored in the refrigerator (2-8°C). It is reconstituted by adding 2.5 mL of the diluent provided; shake the vial to completely dissolve the contents. Do not freeze the reconstituted solution. For IV use, further dilute the solution in 10 – 100 mL of normal saline injection.

Compatibility/Compounding Considerations
No specific information noted.

Dosage Forms/Regulatory Status
Note: The availability status of antivenins in the USA is in flux. It is highly recommended to contact a poison control center (see phone numbers at the top of this monograph) to get current recommendations on availability and treatment options.

VETERINARY-LABELED PRODUCTS: NONE.

HUMAN-LABELED PRODUCTS:

Antivenin (*Latrodectus mactans*) Powder for Injection: greater than or equal to 6000 antivenin Units/vial in single-use vials with 1 vial diluent (2.5 mL vial of sterile water for injection) and 1 mL vial of normal horse serum (1:10 dilution) for sensitivity testing; Antivenin (Lactrodectus mactans); (Rx)

A Black widow spider antivenin (*Aracmyn Plus®*) is being developed by Bioclon Institute (Mexico), but at the time of writing (2013) was not approved for us in the USA.

Revisions/References
Monograph revised/updated August 2013.
Atkins, L. (2006). *Spiders and Snakes--Envenomation*. Proceedings: IVECCS. accessed via Veterinary Information Network; vin.com
Peterson, M. & J. McNalley (2006). Spider Envenomation: Black Widow. *Small Animal Toxicology, 2nd Ed.* M. Peterson and P. Talcott, Elsevier: 1017-38.

Apomorphine HCl

(a-poe-**mor**-feen)   Apokyn®

Emetic

Prescriber Highlights
▶ Rapid acting, centrally-mediated emetic used in dogs & rarely in cats (as it is often ineffective).
▶ Contraindicated in certain species (*e.g.*, rodents, rabbits) & when vomiting may be deleterious (*e.g.*, impending coma, aspiration).
▶ Can cause protracted vomiting; naloxone should reverse CNS effects or cardio-respiratory depression, but not vomiting.
▶ Availability & expense may be an issue.

Uses/Indications
Apomorphine is used primarily as an emetic in dogs, and is considered the emetic of choice for dogs by most clinicians. It is rarely used in cats; and if emesis is indicated, xylazine is generally preferred in feline patients.

Pharmacology/Actions
Apomorphine stimulates dopamine receptors in the chemoreceptor trigger zone, thus inducing vomiting. It can cause both CNS depression and stimulation, but tends to cause more stimulatory effects. Medullary centers can be depressed with resultant respiratory depression.

Pharmacokinetics
Apomorphine is slowly absorbed after oral administration and has unpredictable efficacy when given by this route, therefore, it is usually administered parenterally or topically to the eye. An evaluative study in dogs reported the mean time to emesis was 18-19 minutes and a mean duration of about 29 minutes (Khan et al. 2012).

Apomorphine is primarily conjugated in the liver and then excreted in the urine.

Contraindications/Precautions/Warnings
Emetics can be an important aspect in the treatment of orally ingested toxins, but they must not be used injudiciously. Emetics should not be used in rodents or rabbits, because they are either unable to vomit or do not have stomach walls strong enough to tolerate the act of emesis. Emetics are also contraindicated in patients that are: hypoxic, dyspneic, in shock, lack normal pharyngeal reflexes, seizuring, comatose, severely CNS depressed or where CNS function is deteriorating, or extremely physically weak. Emetics should also be withheld in patients who have previously vomited repeatedly. Because of the risk for additional esophageal or gastric injury with emesis, emetics are contraindicated in patients who have ingested a sharp object, strong acids, alkalis, or other caustic agents. Because of the risks of aspiration, emetics are usually contraindicated after petroleum distillate ingestion, but may be employed when the risks of toxicity of the compound are greater than the risks of aspiration. Use of emetics after ingestion of strychnine or other CNS stimulants may precipitate seizures.

Emetics generally do not remove more than 80% of the material in the stomach (usually 40-60%) and successful induction of emesis does not signal the end of appropriate monitoring or therapy. In addition to the contraindications outlined in the general statement, apomorphine should not be used in cases of oral opiate or other CNS depressant (*e.g.*, barbiturates) toxicity, or in patients hypersensitive to morphine.

The use of apomorphine in cats is controversial, and several clinicians state that it should not be used in this species as it is much less effective than xylazine and, possibly, less safe.

If vomiting does not occur within the expected time after apomorphine administration, repeated doses are unlikely to induce emesis and may cause clinical signs of toxicity.

Adverse Effects
At usual doses, the principal adverse effect that may be seen with apomorphine is protracted nausea/vomiting. Protracted vomiting after ophthalmic administration may be averted by washing the conjunctival sac with sterile saline or ophthalmic rinsing solution. Lethargy, hypersalivation, and eye redness/irritation are possible. CNS or respiratory depression are usually only associated with overdoses of the drug. Anecdotal reports of corneal ulcers have been noted after conjunctival administration.

Reproductive/Nursing Safety
The reproductive safety of this drug has not been established; weigh the risks of use versus the potential benefits.

Overdosage/Acute Toxicity

Excessive doses of apomorphine may result in respiratory and/or cardiac depression, CNS stimulation (excitement, seizures) or depression and protracted vomiting. Naloxone may reverse the CNS and respiratory effects of the drug but cannot be expected to halt the vomiting. Atropine has been suggested to treat severe bradycardias.

Drug Interactions

The following drug interactions with apomorphine have either been reported or are theoretical in humans or animals and may be of significance in veterinary patients. Unless otherwise noted, use together is not necessarily contraindicated, but weigh the potential risks and perform additional monitoring when appropriate.

- **ANTIDOPAMINERGIC DRUGS** (*e.g.*, **phenothiazines**) may negate the emetic effects of apomorphine.
- **ONDANSETRON:** A human patient that received ondansetron and apomorphine developed severe hypotension. In humans, use together is contraindicated.
- **OPIATES or OTHER CNS or RESPIRATORY DEPRESSANTS** (*e.g.*, **barbiturates**): Additive CNS, or respiratory depression may occur when apomorphine is used with these agents.

Doses

- **DOGS:**

  For induction of emesis (extra-label):
  a) 0.03 mg/kg IV; 0.04 mg/kg IM; or a crushed tablet (typically 6.25 mg) subconjunctivally. (Lee 2013)
  b) 0.03 mg/kg IV, once, or a crushed tablet dissolved in saline (0.9% NaCl) solution, instilled in the conjunctival sac, and rinsed away with water or saline solution after emesis (resulting in a dose to effect). (Khan et al. 2012)

Monitoring

- CNS, respiratory, and cardiac systems should be monitored.
- Vomitus should be quantified, examined for contents and saved for possible later analysis.

Client Information

- This agent must be used in a professionally supervised setting only.

Chemistry/Synonyms

A centrally-acting emetic, apomorphine occurs as a white powder or minute, white or grayish-white crystals and is sparingly soluble in water or alcohol.

Apomorphine HCl may also be known as: apomorphini hydrochloridum, *APO-go®*, *APO-go Pen®*, *Apofin®*, *Apokinon®*, *Apokyn®*, *Apomine®*, *Britaject®*, *Ixense®*, *Taluvian®*, or *Uprima®*.

Storage/Stability

Apomorphine soluble tablets should be stored in tight containers at room temperature (15-30°C) and protected from light.

Upon exposure to light and air, apomorphine gradually darkens in color. Discolored tablets or discolored solutions (green to turquoise) should not be used. Apomorphine solutions are more stable in acidic than in alkaline solutions. A 0.3% solution of apomorphine has a pH of about 3-4.

Compatibility/Compounding Considerations

Solutions of apomorphine can be made by solubilizing tablets in at least 1 – 2 mL of either sterile water for injection or 0.9% sodium chloride for injection. After being sterilized by filtration, the solution is stable for 2 days if protected from light and air and stored in the refrigerator. Do not use solutions that are discolored or form a precipitate after filtering.

Compounded preparation stability: Apomorphine injectable solution compounded from the active pharmaceutical ingredient (API) has been published (Jaeger et al. 1976). Dissolving 10 mg apomorphine to a final volume of 10 mL with 0.1% sodium metabisulfite in sterile water and filtering through a 0.22 micron sterilizing filter yields a 2.5 mg/mL sterile solution that retains potency for two months stored at 25°C. Compounded preparations of apomorphine should be protected from light. Solutions of apomorphine should be cold sterilized and not be autoclaved as autoclaving results in the development of a green color.

Dosage Forms/Regulatory Status

VETERINARY-LABELED PRODUCTS:

Pharmaceutical dosage forms of apomorphine can be difficult to obtain and compounding pharmacies may be required to obtain the drug.

HUMAN-LABELED PRODUCTS:

Apomorphine HCl Injection: 10 mg/mL in 3 mL cartridges; *Apokyn®*; (Rx)

Revisions/References

Monograph revised/updated August 2013.

Jaeger, R. W. & F. J. de Castro (1976). Apomorphine: a stable solution. *Clin Toxicol* **9**(2): 199-202.

Khan, S. A., et al. (2012). Effectiveness and adverse effects of the use of apomorphine and 3% hydrogen peroxide solution to induce emesis in dogs. *Javma-Journal of the American Veterinary Medical Association* **241**(9): 1179-84.

Lee, J. A. (2013). Emergency Management and Treatment of the Poisoned Small Animal Patient. *Veterinary Clinics of North America: Small Animal Practice* **43**(4): 757-71.

Apramycin Sulfate

(a-pra-**mye**-sin)   Apralan®

Aminoglycoside Antibiotic

Prescriber Highlights

▶ Orally administered aminocyclitol antibiotic for porcine *E. coli* bacillosis in swine (sometimes used in calves—not FDA-approved).

▶ Products no longer available in USA, but products labeled for use in pigs, calves and poultry are still available in some other countries.

▶ May be partially absorbed in neonates; potentially nephro- & ototoxic if absorbed systemically.

Uses/Indications

Apramycin is no longer commercially available in the USA, but it is used in some countries for the treatment of bacterial enteritis, colibacillosis, salmonellosis, etc. in pigs, calves and poultry.

Pharmacology/Actions

Apramycminoglycoside that is bactericidal against many gram-negative bacteria (*E. coli, Pseudomonas, Salmonella, Klebsiella, Proteus, Pasteurella, Treponema hyodysenteriae, Bordetella bronchiseptica*), Staphylococcus and Mycoplasma. It prevents protein synthesis by susceptible bacteria, presumably by binding to the 30S ribosomal subunit.

There are human public health concerns about widespread use of apramycin in animals as resistance caused by the aac(3)-IV gene, also confers resistance towards gentamicin. A Danish national surveillance study of antimicrobial resistance of *E. coli* isolates from pigs concluded that: "The present study suggests that the occurrence of the aac(3)- IV gene in diseased and healthy pigs may be an increasing problem, which pleads for the prudent use of antimicrobials in pigs, considering the human health risk associated with apramycin/gentamicin cross-resistance." (Jensen et al. 2006)

Pharmacokinetics

After oral administration, apramycin is partially absorbed, particularly in neonates. Absorption is dose related and decreases substantially with the age of the animal. Absorbed drug is eliminated via the kidneys unchanged.

After IV administration to goats, apramycin had a volume of distribution (steady-state) of 0.26 L/kg, clearance of 2.8 mL/minute/kg and an elimination half-life of 1.3 hours (Dinev et al. 2009).

Contraindications/Precautions/Warnings

Do not use in known cases of apramycin hypersensitivity. The drug apparently has a wide margin of safety when used orally and is safe to use in breeding swine. Apramycin is contraindicated in cats and in patients with myasthenia gravis.

Adverse Effects

When used as labeled, the manufacturer does not list any adverse reactions. Should substantial amounts of the drug be absorbed, both ototoxicity and nephrotoxicity are a distinct possibility.

Drug Interactions/Laboratory Considerations

None were noted. May have similar interaction potential as neomycin; refer to that monograph for more information.

Doses

Note: All dosages are extra-label in the USA.

- **SWINE:**

  For bacterial enteritis in pigs caused by susceptible organisms: To be administered via the drinking water. Add 1 small measure (4.4 mL) or 1 sachet of soluble powder per 20 L of drinking water. (Label information; *Apralan Soluble Powder*®—Elanco U.K.)

- **CATTLE:**

  Calves: For the treatment of colibacillosis or salmonellosis: 1 – 2 sachets to be administered in the drinking water, milk, or milk replacer to provide 20 – 40 mg of apramycin activity per kg of bodyweight daily according to the severity of the disease. Continue treatment for 5 days. (Label information; *Apralan Soluble Powder*®—Elanco U.K.)

- **POULTRY:**

  For the treatment of *Escherichia coli* septicemia in young chickens: To be administered via drinking water to provide 250 – 500 mg of apramycin activity per liter for 5 days. This may be achieved by adding 50 g apramycin per 100 – 200 liters of water. (Label information; *Apralan Soluble Powder*®—Elanco U.K.)

Monitoring

- Clinical efficacy.

Chemistry/Synonyms

Apramycin is an aminocyclitol antibiotic produced from *Streptomyces tenebrarius*; it is soluble in water.

Apramycin may also be known as nebramycin factor 2, nebramcyin II, apramycine, apramicina, AIDS166733, *Apralan*®, *Actavis*® or *Abylan*®.

Storage/Stability

Apramycin powder should be stored in a cool dry place, in tightly closed containers, protected from moisture. Store at temperatures less than 25°C. If exposed to rust, as in a rusty waterer, the drug can be inactivated. Shelf life of the powder is 24 months.

The following information is adapted from: (Label information; *Apralan Soluble Powder*®—Elanco U.K.):

Add the appropriate quantity of soluble powder to five to ten times its own volume of water. Stir well and allow solution to stand for a few minutes then stir again. When completely dissolved, add to the full volume of drinking water, milk or reconstituted milk replacer and stir well.

Any medicated water not consumed within 24 hours, should be discarded.

Solutions in milk and reconstituted milk replacer should be prepared immediately before use. Any medicated milk or milk replacer not consumed within one hour, should be discarded.

Compatibility/Compounding Considerations

No specific information noted.

Dosage Forms/Regulatory Status

VETERINARY-LABELED PRODUCTS:

None at present in the USA. A swine product: Apramycin Sulfate Soluble Powder 37.5 g & 48 g (base) bottle; *Apralan*®; (OTC), was formerly marketed in the USA and is still available in several countries.

In the UK: Apramycin Soluble Powder: 1 gram sachets and 50 g (apramycin activity) in 220 mL; *Apralan Soluble Powder*®; (POM-V). In the UK when used as labeled: Slaughter withdrawal: Pigs = 14 days, Calves = 28 days, Poultry = 7 days. Not for use in laying hens where eggs are for human consumption.

HUMAN-LABELED PRODUCTS: NONE.

Revisions/References

Monograph revised/updated August 2013.

Dinev, T., et al. (2009). Comparative pharmacokinetics and PK/PD parameters of five aminoglycosides in goats. *Turkish Journal of Veterinary & Animal Sciences* 33(3): 223-8.

Jensen, V. F., et al. (2006). Correlation between apramycin and gentamicin use in pigs and an increasing reservoir of gentamicin-resistant Escherichia coli. *Journal of Antimicrobial Chemotherapy* 58(1): 101-7.

ASA – see Aspirin

Ascorbic Acid / Vitamin C

(a-**skor**-bik)

Vitamin/Urinary Acidifier

Prescriber Highlights

▶ Prevention/treatment of scurvy in Guinea pigs most accepted use. Sometimes used in dogs and cats as an antioxidant for treating certain toxicants.

▶ At usual dosages, little downside to use; may exacerbate liver injury in copper toxicosis.

▶ Some drug interactions, primarily due to its urinary acidification qualities.

▶ May alter some lab results (urine glucose, occult blood in stool, serum bilirubin).

Uses/Indications

Ascorbic acid is used to prevent and treat scurvy in guinea pigs. Vitamin C requirements for an adult, non-breeding guinea pig is 10 mg/kg/day; for breeding and growing animals it is 30 mg/kg/day (Johnson 2012).

Ascorbic acid is sometimes recommended as an antioxidant as part of a treatment protocol in treating toxicants that can cause methemoglobinemia (*e.g.* acetaminophen, phenazopyridine, monomethylhydrazine-containing mushrooms) or hepatotoxicity.

Ascorbic acid has been used as a urinary acidifier in small animals, but its efficacy is in question and it is rarely recommended for use. In the past, it was used to treat copper-induced hepatopathy in dogs but this use has fallen into disfavor (see Contraindications below). Supplementation to dogs undergoing stress (*e.g.*, intensive care) does not appear warranted (Groth et al. 2012).

Pharmacology/Actions

Exogenously supplied ascorbic acid is a dietary requirement in some exotic species (including rainbow trout, Coho salmon), guinea pigs, and primates. The other domestic species are able to synthesize *in vivo* enough Vitamin C to meet their nutritional needs. Vitamin C is used for tissue repair and collagen formation. It may be involved with some oxidation-reduction reactions, and with the metabolism of many substances (iron, folic acid, norepinephrine, histamine, phenylalanine, tyrosine, some drug enzyme systems). Vitamin C is believed to play a role in protein, lipid and carnitine synthesis, maintaining blood vessel integrity and immune function. When used as an antioxidant for the adjunctive treatment of intoxicants causing methemoglobinemia and/or hepatotoxicity, it is serves as a reducing agent that neutralizes reactive oxygen compounds (*e.g.,* hydrogen peroxide), can increase conversion of methemoglobin to oxyhemoglobin and act as a substrate for the antioxidant enzyme ascorbate peroxidase.

Pharmacokinetics

Vitamin C is generally well absorbed in the jejunum (human data) after oral administration, but absorption may be reduced with high doses as an active process is involved with absorption. Ascorbic acid is widely distributed and only about 25% is bound to plasma proteins. Vitamin C is biotransformed in the liver. When the body is saturated with vitamin C and blood concentrations exceed the renal threshold, the drug is more readily excreted unchanged into the urine.

Contraindications/Precautions/Warnings

Vitamin C (high doses) should be used with caution in patients with diabetes mellitus due to the laboratory interactions (see below), or in patients susceptible to urolithiasis as it can promote hyperoxaluria.

Because there is some evidence that it may increase copper's oxidative damage to the liver, avoid vitamin C's use in animals with copper-associated hepatopathy.

Adverse Effects

At usual doses vitamin C has minimal adverse effects. Occasionally GI disturbances have been noted in humans. At higher dosages there is an increased potential for urate, oxalate or cystine stone formation, particularly in susceptible patients.

Reproductive/Nursing Safety

The reproductive safety of vitamin C has not been studied, but it is generally considered safe at moderate dosages. In humans, the FDA categorizes this drug as category *A* for use during pregnancy (*Adequate studies in pregnant women have not demonstrated a risk to the fetus in the first trimester of pregnancy, and there is no evidence of risk in later trimesters.*) But in dosages greater than the RDA, the FDA categorizes vitamin C as category *C* for use during pregnancy (*Animal studies have shown an adverse effect on the fetus, but there are no adequate studies in humans; or there are no animal reproduction studies and no adequate studies in humans.*)

Overdosage/Acute Toxicity

Very large doses may result in diarrhea and potentially urolithiasis. Generally, treatment should consist of monitoring and keeping the patient well hydrated.

Drug Interactions

The following drug interactions with ascorbic acid (high dosages) have either been reported or are theoretical in humans or animals and may be of significance in veterinary patients. Unless otherwise noted, use together is not necessarily contraindicated, but weigh the potential risks and perform additional monitoring when appropriate.

- **AMINOGLYCOSIDES:** (*e.g.,* **gentamicin**) and **ERYTHROMYCIN**: Are more effective in an alkaline medium; urine acidification may diminish these drugs' effectiveness in treating bacterial urinary tract infections.
- **QUINIDINE:** Urine acidification may increase renal excretion.

- **DEFEROXAMINE:** While vitamin C may be synergistic with deferoxamine in removing iron, it may lead to increased iron tissue toxicity, especially in cardiac muscle. It should be used with caution, particularly in patients with preexisting cardiac disease.
- **IRON SALTS:** Presence of vitamin C may enhance the oral absorption of iron salts.

Laboratory Considerations

- **Urine Glucose:** Large doses of vitamin C may cause false-negative values.
- **Stool occult blood:** False-negative results may occur if vitamin C is administered within 48-72 hours of an amine-dependent test.
- **Bilirubin, serum:** Vitamin C may decrease concentrations.

Doses

- **DOGS/CATS:**

  As an antioxidant for adjunctive treatment of toxic (*e.g.,* acetaminophen, phenazopyridine, etc.) methemoglobinemia (extra-label): 30 – 33 mg/kg PO q6h.

- **RABBITS:**

  For soft stools (may reduce cecal absorption of clostridial endotoxins); (extra-label): 100 mg/kg PO q12h. (Ivey et al. 2000)

- **GUINEA PIGS:**

  For prevention/treatment of scurvy (extra-label):
  a) Maintenance dose is 25 mg/kg/day and 100 mg/kg/day during pregnancy, and stress, and illness. (Hoefer 2010)
  b) Add 200 mg vitamin C to one liter of dechlorinated water and add to water bottle. 10 – 30 mg/kg PO, SC or IM. (Adamcak et al. 2000)

- **HORSES:**

  For adjunctive treatment of erythrocyte oxidative injury (*e.g.,* red maple toxicity); (extra-label): 10 – 20 grams PO once daily (Davis et al. 2003); 30 – 50 mg/kg IV twice daily diluted in 5 – 10 L of crystalloid fluids. (Alward 2008).

  As a urinary acidifier (extra-label): 1 – 2 g/kg PO daily. (Jose-Cunilleras et al. 1999)

  As adjunctive therapy for perinatal asphyxia syndrome in foals (extra-label): 100 mg/kg per day IV. (Slovis 2003)

- **CATTLE:**

  For vitamin C-responsive dermatitis in calves (extra-label): 3 grams SC once or twice (Miller 1993)

Chemistry/Synonyms

A water-soluble vitamin, ascorbic acid occurs as white to slightly yellow crystal or powder. It is freely soluble in water and sparingly soluble in alcohol. The parenteral solution has a pH of 5.5-7.

Ascorbic acid may also be known as: acidum ascorbicum, L-ascorbic acid, cevitamic acid, E300, or vitamin C; many trade names are available.

Storage/Stability

Protect from air and light. Ascorbic acid will slowly darken upon light exposure; slight discoloration does not affect potency. Because with time ascorbic acid will decompose with the production of CO_2, open ampules carefully. To reduce the potential for excessive pressure within ampules, store in refrigerator and open while still cold.

Compatibility/Compounding Considerations

Ascorbic acid for injection is **compatible** with most commonly used IV solutions, but is **incompatible** with many drugs when mixed in syringes or IV bags. Compatibility is dependent upon factors such as pH, concentration, temperature and diluent used; consult specialized references or a hospital pharmacist for more specific information.

Dosage Forms/Regulatory Status

VETERINARY-LABELED PRODUCTS:

Parenteral Injection: 250 mg/mL (as sodium ascorbate) in 100 mL and 250 mL vials; generic; (Rx or OTC depending on labeling)

Ascorbic Acid Powder: Concentrations vary. (OTC)

HUMAN-LABELED PRODUCTS:

Vitamin C or Ascorbic Acid Oral Tablets & Capsules: 250 mg, 500 mg, 1000 mg & 1500 mg; generic; (OTC)

Ascorbic Acid Oral Extended-release Tablets: 500 mg & 1000 mg; generic; (OTC)

Ascorbic Acid Oral Crystals or Powder: Concentrations vary; (OTC)

Ascorbic Acid Oral Liquid/Solution: 100 mg/mL in 50 mL & 500 mg/5 mL; *Cecon®*, generic; (OTC)

Ascorbic Acid Injection: 500 mg/mL in 50 mL vials; *Ascor L 500®* (0.025% EDTA, preservative-free), generic; (Rx)

Revisions/References

Monograph revised/updated August 2013.

Adamcak, A. & B. Otten (2000). Rodent Therapeutics. *Vet Clin NA: Exotic Anim Pract* **3:1**(Jan): 221-40.

Alward, A. (2008). *Red Maple Leaf Toxicosis in Horses.* Proceedings: ACVIM. accessed via Veterinary Information Network; vin.com

Davis, E. & M. Wilkerson (2003). Hemolytic anemia. *Current Therapy in Equine Medicine: 5.* N. Robinson, Saunders: 344-8.

Groth, E., et al. (2012). Hyperascorbaemia in dogs admitted to a teaching hospital intensive care unit. *Journal of Small Animal Practice* **53**(11): 652-6.

Hoefer, H. (2010). *Common Problems in Guinea Pigs.* Atlantic Coast Veterinary Conference Proceedings. accessed via Veterinary Information Network; vin.com

Ivey, E. & J. Morrisey (2000). Therapeutics for Rabbits. *Vet Clin NA: Exotic Anim Pract* **3:1**(Jan): 183-216.

Johnson, D. (2012). *The Gastrointestinal Tract of the Guinea Pig: Health and Disease.* ABVP Proceedings. accessed via Veterinary Information Network; vin.com

Jose-Cunilleras, E. & K. Hinchcliff (1999). Renal pharmacology. *The Veterinary Clinics of North America: Equine Practice* **15:3**(December): 647-64.

Miller, W. (1993). Nutritional, Endocrine, and Keratinization Abnormalities. *Current Veterinary Therapy 3: Food Animal Practice.* J. Howard. Philadelphia, W.B. Saunders Co.: 911-3.

Slovis, N. (2003). *Perinatal asphyxia syndrome (Hypoxic ischemic encephalopathy).* Proceedings: ACVIM Forum. accessed via Veterinary Information Network; vin.com

Asparaginase

(a-**spar**-a-gin-ase)   L-Asparaginase, Elspar®

Antineoplastic

Prescriber Highlights

▶ Antineoplastic used as part of some protocols for treating lymphomas and leukemias in dogs/cats. Availability a significant issue.

▶ Two primary adverse effects: hypersensitivity & effects on protein synthesis (usually manifested by GI effects, hemorrhagic pancreatitis, hepatotoxicity or coagulation disorders).

▶ Bone marrow suppression is rare and it does not have significant GI mucosal toxicity.

▶ Usually given IM or SC as IV administration may increase risk for anaphylaxis.

Uses/Indications

Asparaginase has been used in combination with other agents in the treatment of lymphoid malignancies. The drug is thought most useful in inducing remission of disease but is also used in maintenance or rescue protocols. It may also have benefit in treating leukemia, particularly ALL.

Use of asparaginase as part of an initial treatment lymphosarcoma protocol is now clouded due to unavailability of commercially-produced drug products and a retrospective study (MacDonald et al. 2005) in dogs that showed no statistical difference for response rates, remission or survival rate, remission or survival duration, or prevalence of toxicity and treatment delay in dogs treated with or without asparaginase as part of a standard CHOP protocol.

Pharmacology/Actions

Some malignant cells are unable to synthesize asparagine and are dependent on exogenous asparagine for DNA and protein synthesis. Asparaginase catalyzes asparagine into ammonia and aspartic acid. The antineoplastic activity of asparaginase is greatest during the post mitotic (G_1) cell phase. While normal cells are able to synthesize asparagine intracellularly, some normal cells, having a high rate of protein synthesis, require some exogenous asparagine and may be adversely affected by asparaginase.

Resistance to asparaginase can develop rapidly, but apparently, there is no cross-resistance between asparaginase and other antineoplastic agents.

Asparaginase possesses antiviral activity, but its toxicity prevents it from being clinically useful in this regard.

Pharmacokinetics

Asparaginase is not absorbed from the GI tract and must be given either IV or IM. After IM injection, serum levels of asparaginase are approximately 1/2 of those after IV injection. Because of its high molecular weight, asparaginase does not diffuse readily out of the capillaries and about 80% of the drug remains within the intravascular space.

In humans after IV dosing, serum levels of asparagine fall almost immediately to zero and remain that way as long as therapy continues. Once therapy is halted, serum levels of asparagine do not recover for at least 23 days.

The metabolic fate of asparaginase is not known. In humans, the plasma half-life is highly variable and ranges from 8-30 hours.

Contraindications/Precautions/Warnings

Asparaginase is contraindicated in patients who have exhibited anaphylaxis to it, or those with pancreatitis or a history of pancreatitis. Asparaginase should be used with caution in patients with preexisting hepatic, renal, hematologic, gastrointestinal, or CNS dysfunction.

No special precautions are required for handling asparaginase, but any inadvertent skin contact should be washed off, as the drug can be a contact irritant.

Adverse Effects

Asparaginase adverse reactions are classified in two main categories, hypersensitivity reactions and effects on protein synthesis. Hypersensitivity reactions can occur with clinical signs of vomiting, diarrhea, urticaria, pruritus, dyspnea, restlessness, hypotension and collapse. The likelihood of hypersensitivity reactions occurring increases with subsequent doses and intravenous administration. Some clinicians recommend giving a test dose before the full dose to test for local hypersensitivity. Many oncologists now recommend administering antihistamines (*e.g.*, diphenhydramine at 2 mg/kg in dogs and 1 mg/kg in cats SC 30 minutes prior to administration) prior to dosing. If a hypersensitivity reaction occurs, diphenhydramine (0.2 – 0.5 mg/kg slow IV), dexamethasone sodium phosphate (1 – 2 mg/kg IV), intravenous fluids and, if severe, epinephrine (0.1 – 0.3 mL of a 1:1000 solution IV) have been suggested (O'Keefe et al. 1990).

The other broad category of toxicity is associated with asparaginase's effects on protein synthesis. Hemorrhagic pancreatitis or other gastrointestinal disturbances, hepatotoxicity and coagulation defects may be noted. Large doses may be associated with hyperglycemia secondary to altered insulin synthesis. A case report of acute hyperammonemia in dogs has been reported (Lyles et al. 2011) and the author's recommended that any animal showing unexplained neurologic symptoms should have serum ammonia levels determined.

Bone marrow depression is an uncommon consequence of asparaginase therapy, but leukopenia has been reported.

Reproductive/Nursing Safety

In humans, the FDA categorizes this drug as category *C* for use during pregnancy (*Animal studies have shown an adverse effect on the fetus, but there are no adequate studies in humans; or there are no animal reproduction studies and no adequate studies in humans.*)

Overdosage/Acute Toxicity

Little information was located regarding overdosages with this agent. It would be expected that toxicity secondary to the protein synthesis altering effects of the drug would be encountered. In dogs, it has been reported that the maximally tolerated dose of asparaginase is 10,000 IU/kg and the lethal dose is 50,000 IU/kg.

It is recommended to treat supportively if an overdose occurs.

Drug Interactions

The following drug interactions with asparaginase have either been reported or are theoretical in humans or animals and may be of significance in veterinary patients. Unless otherwise noted, use together is not necessarily contraindicated, but weigh the potential risks and perform additional monitoring when appropriate.

- **METHOTREXATE**: Asparaginase may reduce methotrexate effectiveness against tumor cells until serum asparagine levels return to normal.
- **PREDNISONE**: Use with asparaginase may increase risk for hyperglycemia; in humans, asparaginase is usually administered after prednisone.
- **VINCRISTINE**: In humans, increased toxicity (neuropathy and erythropoiesis disruption) may occur when asparaginase (IV) is given concurrently with or before vincristine. Myelosuppression reportedly occurs in a minority of dogs treated with vincristine/asparaginase; some veterinary oncologists separate the dosing by a few days to a week, but others do not feel this is beneficial.

Laboratory Considerations

- **Serum ammonia and urea nitrogen**: levels may be increased by the action of the drug.
- **Thyroxine-binding globulin**: Asparaginase may cause rapid (within 2 days) and profound decreases in circulating TBG, which may alter interpretation of thyroid function studies; values may return to normal after approximately 4 weeks.

Doses

Note: Because of the potential toxicity of this drug to patients, veterinary personnel and clients, and since chemotherapy indications, treatment protocols, monitoring and safety guidelines often change, the following dosages should be used only as a general guide. Consultation with a veterinary oncologist and referral to current veterinary oncology references [*e.g.*, (Withrow et al. 2012); (Dobson et al. 2011); (Henry et al. 2009); (North et al. 2009); (Argyle et al. 2008)] are <u>strongly recommended</u>.

- **DOGS/CATS:**
  The following is a usual dose or dose range for asparaginase and should be used only as a general guide (extra-label): Asparaginase is usually dosed in dogs and cats at 400 Units/kg or 10,000 Units/m^2 (NOT Units/kg) IM or SC, with a maximum dose of 10,000 Units per patient. **Note**: Many oncologists recommend administering antihistamines such as diphenhydramine at 2 mg/kg for dogs and 1 mg/kg for cats SC 30 minutes prior to administration.

Monitoring

- Animals should have hepatic, renal, pancreatic (blood glucose, amylase) and hematopoietic function determined prior to initiating therapy and regularly monitored during therapy.

Client Information

- Clients must be briefed on the possibilities of severe toxicity developing from this drug, including drug-related mortality.
- Clients should contact the veterinarian if the patient exhibits any symptoms of profound depression, severe diarrhea, abnormal bleeding (including bloody diarrhea) and/or bruising.

Chemistry/Synonyms

Asparaginase is an enzyme derived from *E. coli* and occurs as a white or almost white, slightly hygroscopic powder that is soluble in water. The commercially available product is a lyophilized powder that also contains mannitol that after reconstituting has a pH of about 7.4. Activity of asparaginase is expressed in terms of International Units (I.U.), or Units.

Asparaginase may also be known as: coloaspase, A-ase, ASN-ase, L-asparaginase, L-asparagine amidohydrolase, MK-965 NSC-109229, Re-82-TAD-15, *Crasnitin®*, *Crasnitine®*, *Elspar®*, *Erwinase®*, *Kidrolase®*, *L-Asp®*, *Laspar®*, *Leucogen®*, *Leunase®*, *Paronal®*, or *Serasa®*.

Storage/Stability

Asparaginase powder for injection should be stored at temperatures less than 8°C, but it is stable for at least 48 hours at room temperature. After reconstituting, the manufacturer states that the drug is stable when refrigerated for up to 8 hours, but other sources state that it is stable for up to 14 days.

Solutions should be used only if clear; turbid solutions should be discarded. Upon standing, gelatinous fibers may be noted in the solution occasionally. These may be removed without loss of potency with a 5 micron filter. Some loss of potency may occur if a 0.2 micron filter is used.

The solution may be gently shaken while reconstituting, but vigorous shaking should be avoided as the solution may become foamy and difficult to withdraw from the vial and some loss of potency can occur. Recommended intravenous diluents for asparaginase include D5W and sodium chloride 0.9%.

Compatibility/Compounding Considerations

No specific information noted.

Dosage Forms/Regulatory Status

VETERINARY-LABELED PRODUCTS: NONE.

HUMAN-LABELED PRODUCTS:

Asparaginase Powder for Injection, lyophilized: 10,000 Units in 10 mL vials (with 80 mg mannitol, preservative-free); Reconstitute vial with 5 mL Sodium Chloride Injection or Sterile Water for Injection for IV use. For IM use, add 2 mL Sodium Chloride Injection. See Storage/Stability section for more information. *Elspar®*; (Rx).

Note: As of December 2012 this product has been discontinued in the USA. Some compounding pharmacies may be able to provide it, however.

Revisions/References

Monograph revised/updated August 2013.

Argyle, D., et al. (2008). *Decision Making in Small Animal Oncology*, Wiley-Blackwell.

Dobson, J. & D. Lascelles (2011). *BSAVA Manual of Canine and Feline Oncology*, BSAVA.

Henry, C. & M. Higginbotham (2009). *Cancer Management in Small Animal Practice*, Saunders.

Lyles, S. E., et al. (2011). Acute hyperammonemia after L-asparaginase administration in a dog. *J. Vet. Emerg. Crit. Care* 21(6): 673-8.

MacDonald, V., et al. (2005). Does L-asparaginase influence efficacy or toxicity when added to a standard CHOP protocol for dogs with lymphoma? *J Vet Intern Med* 19: 732-6.

North, S. & T. Banks (2009). *Small Animal Oncology: An Introduction*, Saunders.

O'Keefe, D. A. & C. L. Harris (1990). Toxicology of Oncologic Drugs. *Vet Clinics of North America: Small Animal Pract* 20(2): 483-504.

Withrow, S., et al. (2012). Withrow and MacEwen's Small Animal Clinical Oncology, 5th Ed., Saunders.

Aspirin

(ass-pir-in)   ASA, Acetylsalicylic Acid

Analgesic; Antipyretic; Platelet Aggregation Reducer;
   Antiinflammatory

Prescriber Highlights

▶ NSAID used for analgesic, antiinflammatory & antiplatelet effects in a variety of species.

▶ Contraindicated in patients hypersensitive to it or with active GI bleeds; Relatively contraindicated in patients with bleeding disorders, asthma, or renal insufficiency (but has been used to treat glomerular disease).

▶ Aspirin has a very long half-life in cats (approx. 30 hours; dose carefully); dogs are relatively sensitive to GI effects (bleeding).

▶ Low grade teratogen & may delay labor; avoid use in pregnancy.

▶ Many drug & lab interactions.

Uses/Indications

Aspirin is used for its analgesic, antipyretic, and antiplatelet effects.

Pharmacology/Actions

Aspirin inhibits cyclooxygenase (COX-1, prostaglandin synthetase) thereby reducing the synthesis of prostaglandins and thromboxanes (TXA2). These effects are thought to be how aspirin produces analgesia, antipyrexia, and reduces platelet aggregation and inflammation.

Most cells can synthesize new cyclooxygenase, but platelets cannot. Therefore, aspirin can cause an irreversible effect on platelet aggregation. A study in dogs investigating the platelet function effects of various aspirin doses, showed that doses <1 mg/kg/day or at 10 mg/kg/day PO did not have any statistically significant effect on platelet aggregation. Doses of 12 mg/kg/day inhibited platelet function and aggregation (Shearer et al. 2009).

Aspirin has been shown to decrease the clinical signs of experimentally induced anaphylaxis in calves and ponies.

While aspirin does not directly inhibit COX-2, it can modify it to produce, with lipoxygenase (LOX), a compound known as aspirin-triggered lipoxin (ATL), which appears to have gastric mucosal protective actions. This may explain why aspirin tends to have reduced gastric damaging effects when used over time.

Pharmacokinetics

Aspirin is rapidly absorbed from the stomach and proximal small intestine in monogastric animals. The rate of absorption is dependent upon factors as stomach content, gastric emptying times, tablet disintegration rates and gastric pH. In cattle, oral dosages of 50 mg/kg did not achieve therapeutic concentrations (Coetzee 2013).

During absorption, aspirin is partially hydrolyzed to salicylic acid where it is distributed widely throughout the body. Highest levels may be found in the liver, heart, lungs, renal cortex, and plasma. The amount of plasma protein binding is variable depending on species, serum salicylate and albumin concentrations. At lower salicylate concentrations it is 90% protein bound, but only 70% protein bound at higher concentrations. Salicylate is excreted into milk but levels appear to be very low. Salicylate will cross the placenta and fetal levels may actually exceed those found in the mother.

Salicylate is metabolized in the liver primarily by conjugation with glycine and glucuronic acid via glucuronyl transferase. Because cats are deficient in this enzymatic pathway, they have prolonged half-lives (27-45 hours) and are susceptible to accumulating the drug. Minor metabolites formed include gentisic acid, 2,3-dihydroxybenzoic acid, and 2,3,5-trihydroxybenzoic acid. Gentisic acid appears to be the only active metabolite, but because of its low concentrations appears to play an insignificant role therapeutically. The rate of metabolism is determined by both first order kinetics and dose-dependent kinetics depending on the metabolic pathway. Serum half-life in dogs is approximately 8 hours, in cats, approximately 38 hours, while in humans it averages 1.5 hours. Generally, steady-state serum levels will increase to levels higher (proportionally) than expected with dosage increases. These effects have not been well studied in domestic animals, however.

The kidneys rapidly excrete salicylate and its metabolites by both filtration and renal tubular secretion. Significant tubular reabsorption occurs which is highly pH dependent. Raising urine pH to 5-8 can significantly increase salicylate excretion. Salicylate and metabolites may be removed using peritoneal dialysis or more rapidly using hemodialysis.

Contraindications/Precautions/Warnings

Aspirin is contraindicated in patients demonstrating previous hypersensitivity reactions to it or with bleeding ulcers. It is relatively contraindicated in patients with hemorrhagic disorders, asthma, or renal insufficiency.

Because aspirin is highly protein bound to plasma albumin, patients with hypoalbuminemia may require lower dosages to prevent clinical signs of toxicity. Aspirin should be used cautiously with enhanced monitoring in patients with severe hepatic failure or diminished renal function. Because of its effects on platelets, aspirin therapy should be halted, if possible, one week prior to surgical procedures.

Aspirin must be used cautiously in cats because of their inability to rapidly metabolize and excrete salicylates. Clinical signs of toxicity may occur if dosed recklessly or without stringent monitoring. Aspirin should be used cautiously in neonatal animals; adult doses may lead to toxicity.

Adverse Effects

The most common adverse effect of aspirin at therapeutic doses is gastric (nausea, anorexia, vomiting) or intestinal irritation with varying degrees of occult GI blood loss occurring. The resultant irritation may result in vomiting and/or anorexia. Severe blood loss may result in a secondary anemia or hypoproteinemia. In dogs, plain uncoated aspirin may be more irritating to the gastric mucosa than either buffered aspirin or enteric-coated tablets. Misoprostol has been shown to reduce GI bleeding and vomiting in dogs receiving aspirin. Hypersensitivity reactions have been reported in dogs although they are thought to occur rarely. Cats may develop acidosis from aspirin therapy.

Reproductive/Nursing Safety

Salicylates are possible teratogens and have been shown to delay parturition; their use should be avoided during pregnancy, particularly during the later stages. In humans, the FDA categorizes this drug as category **D** for use during pregnancy (*There is evidence of human fetal risk, but the potential benefits from the use of the drug in pregnant women may be acceptable despite its potential risks.*) In a separate system evaluating the safety of drugs in canine and feline pregnancy (Papich 1989), this drug is categorized as class: **C** (*These drugs may have potential risks. Studies in people or laboratory animals have uncovered risks, and these drugs should be used cautiously as a last resort when the benefit of therapy clearly outweighs the risks.*)

Overdosage/Acute Toxicity

Clinical signs of acute overdosage in dogs and cats include: depression, vomiting (may be blood tinged), anorexia, hyperthermia, and increased respiratory rate. Initially, a respiratory alkalosis occurs with a compensatory hyperventilation response. A profound metabolic acidosis follows. If treatment is not provided, muscular weakness, pulmonary and cerebral edema, hypernatremia, hypokalemia, ataxia, and seizures may all develop with eventual coma and death.

There were 1939 single agent exposures to aspirin reported to the ASPCA Animal Poison Control Center (APCC) during 2009-2013. There were 1749 dogs exposed, 712 of which were symptomatic. The most common signs included: vomiting (75%), lethargy (21%), panting (9%), hyperthermia (8%), and bloody vomiting (7%). Of the 177 cats, 54 were symptomatic with 56% vomiting, 22% anorexic, 13% lethargic and 6% with bloody vomiting.

Treatment of acute overdosage initially consists of emptying the gut if ingestion has occurred within 12 hours, giving activated charcoal and an oral cathartic, placing an intravenous line, beginning fluids and drawing appropriate lab work (*e.g.*, blood gases). Some clinicians suggest performing gastric lavage with a 3-5% solution of sodium bicarbonate to delay the absorption of aspirin. A reasonable choice for an intravenous solution to correct dehydration would be dextrose 5% in water. Acidosis treatment and forced alkaline diuresis with sodium bicarbonate should be performed for serious ingestions, but should only be attempted if acid-base status can be monitored. Diuresis may be enhanced by the administration of mannitol (1 – 2 grams/kg/hour). GI protectant medications should also be administered. Seizures may be controlled with IV diazepam. Treatment of hypoprothrombinemia may be attempted by using phytonadione (2.5 mg/kg divided q8-12h) and ascorbic acid (25 mg parenterally) but ascorbic acid may negate some of the urinary alkalinization effects of bicarbonate. Peritoneal dialysis or exchange transfusions may be attempted in very severe ingestions when heroic measures are desired.

Drug Interactions

The following drug interactions with aspirin have either been reported or are theoretical in humans or animals and may be of significance in veterinary patients. Unless otherwise noted, use together is not necessarily contraindicated, but weigh the potential risks and perform additional monitoring when appropriate.

- **AMINOGLYCOSIDES**: Some clinicians feel that aspirin should not be given concomitantly with aminoglycoside antibiotics because of an increased likelihood of nephrotoxicity developing. The actual clinical significance of this interaction is not clear, and the risks versus benefits should be weighed when contemplating therapy.
- **CORTICOSTEROIDS**: May increase the clearance of salicylates, decrease serum levels and increase the risks for GI bleeding. One dog study showed no significant difference in gastric mucosal injury when ultra-low dose (0.5 mg/kg/day) aspirin was added to prednisone therapy. Addition of aspirin did increase the incidence of mild, self-limiting diarrhea (Graham et al. 2009).
- **DIGOXIN**: In dogs, aspirin has been demonstrated to increase plasma levels of digoxin by decreasing the clearance of the drug.
- **FUROSEMIDE**: May compete with the renal excretion of aspirin and delay its excretion; this may cause clinical signs of toxicity in animals receiving high aspirin doses. Furosemide diuretic effect may be diminished.
- **HEPARIN or ORAL ANTICOAGULANTS**: Aspirin may increase the risks for bleeding.
- **METHOTREXATE**: Aspirin may displace MTX from plasma proteins increasing the risk for toxicity.
- **NSAIDS**: Increased chances of developing GI ulceration exist. Animals that have been on aspirin therapy that will be replaced with a COX-2 NSAID, should probably have a "wash out" period of 3-10 days between stopping aspirin and starting the NSAID (Bill 2008). Another recommendation for cats is a "washout period" of approximately 7-10 days when switching from aspirin to another NSAID (Sparkes et al. 2010).

- **PHENOBARBITAL**: May increase the rate of metabolism of aspirin by inducing hepatic enzymes.
- **PROBENECID, SULFINPYRAZONE**: At usual doses, aspirin may antagonize the uricosuric effects of probenecid or sulfinpyrazone.
- **SPIRONOLACTONE**: Aspirin may inhibit the diuretic activity of spironolactone.
- **TETRACYCLINE**: The antacids in buffered aspirin may chelate tetracycline products if given simultaneously; space doses apart by at least one hour.
- **URINARY ACIDIFYING DRUGS** (*e.g.,* **methionine, ammonium chloride, ascorbic acid**): Can decrease the urinary excretion of salicylates.
- **URINARY ALKALINIZING DRUGS:** (*e.g.,* **acetazolamide, sodium bicarbonate**) significantly increase the renal excretion of salicylates; because carbonic anhydrase inhibitors (*e.g.,* **acetazolamide, dichlorphenamide**) may cause systemic acidosis and increase CNS levels of salicylates; toxicity may occur.

Laboratory Considerations

- At high doses, aspirin may cause false-positive results for **urinary glucose** if using the cupric sulfate method (*Clinitest*®, Benedict's solution) and false-negative results if using the glucose oxidase method (*Clinistix*® or *Tes-Tape*®).
- **Urinary ketones** measured by the ferric chloride method (Gerhardt) may be affected if salicylates are in the urine (reddish-color produced). Salicylates may interfere with fluorescent methods for determining urine **5-HIAA**. Falsely elevated **VMA** (vanillylmandelic acid) may be seen with most methods used if salicylates are in the urine. Falsely lowered **VMA** levels may be seen if using the Pisano method.
- Urinary excretion of **xylose** may be decreased if aspirin is given concurrently. Falsely elevated **serum uric acid** values may be measured if using colorimetric methods.
- Aspirin can decrease serum concentrations of **total T4**.

Doses

Note: There are no approved FDA-Products/Dosages; all dosages are extra-label.

- **DOGS:**

  To decrease platelet aggregation; as an antithrombotic (extra-label): The ideal aspirin dosage, if any, for prevention of thromboembolism in dogs is unknown (data conflicts, study limitations, etc.) (Smith 2012). Commonly, dosages of 0.5 – 1 mg/kg PO once a day are recommended, but some recommend up to 10 mg/kg PO once a day. A preliminary report demonstrated that platelet activity is increased in dogs with IMHA as compared to normal dogs and that neither low dose aspirin (0.5 mg/kg/day PO) nor individually dosed heparin suppresses platelet thromboxane release *in vivo* (Stiller et al. 2013).

  As an analgesic/antipyretic/antiinflammatory (extra-label): Anecdotal dosages usually range from 10 – 20 mg/kg of buffered aspirin PO twice daily. Anecdotal antiinflammatory dosages are slightly higher (20 – 30 mg/kg q8-12h), but canine-approved NSAIDs generally have significantly fewer gastrointestinal effects and are usually preferred.

- **CATS:**

  For analgesia/antipyrexia/antiinflammatory (extra-label): Anecdotal dosage recommendation is usually 10 mg/kg PO every 2-3 days; practically: ½ to one 81 mg tablet ("baby aspirin") Monday, Wednesday, Friday of each week.

  As an antithrombotic agent (extra-label): Two basic dosage regimens have been recommended, "high dose" and "low dose"; it is unknown if one is superior to the other with regard to efficacy, but "high dose" appears to have a significantly higher risk for causing GI effects. High-dose: As above (10 mg/kg PO q2-3 days; ½ – 1 "baby aspirin" every 2-3 days (M-W-F). Low-dose: 5 mg per cat PO every 3rd day.

- **FERRETS:**

  As an analgesic (extra-label): 10 – 20 mg/kg PO once daily (has short duration of activity). (Williams 2000)

- **RABBITS/RODENTS/SMALL MAMMALS:**

  All are extra-label.

  1) **Rabbits:** 5 – 20 mg/kg PO once daily for low-grade analgesia. (Ivey et al. 2000)
  2) **Mice, Rats, Gerbils, Hamsters:** 100 – 150 mg/kg PO q4h. **Guinea pigs:** 87 mg/kg PO. (Adamcak et al. 2000)

- **HORSES:** (NOTE: ARCI UCGFS CLASS 4 DRUG)

  For anti-platelet activity as an adjunctive treatment of laminitis (extra-label): 5 – 10 mg/kg PO q24–48 hours or 20 mg/kg PO every 4–5 days. (Brumbaugh et al. 1999)

Monitoring

- Analgesic effect &/or antipyretic effect.
- Bleeding times if indicated.
- PCV and stool guaiac tests if indicated.

Client Information

- Contact veterinarian if symptoms of GI bleeding or distress occur (*e.g.,* black, tarry feces; anorexia or vomiting, etc.).
- Because aspirin is a very old drug, formal approvals from the FDA for its use in animals have not been required. There is no listed meat or milk withdrawal times listed for food-producing animals but because there are salicylate-sensitive people, in the interest of public health, this author suggests a minimum of 1 day withdrawal time for either milk or meat.

Chemistry/Synonyms

Aspirin, sometimes known as acetylsalicylic acid or ASA, is the salicylate ester of acetic acid. The compound occurs as a white, crystalline powder or tabular or needle-like crystals. It is a weak acid with a pK$_a$ of 3.5. Aspirin is slightly soluble in water and is freely soluble in alcohol. Each gram of aspirin contains approximately 760 mg of salicylate.

Aspirin may also be known as: ASA, acetylsal acid, acetylsalicylic acid, acidum acetylsalicylicum, polopiryna, or salicylic acid acetate; many trade names are available.

Storage/Stability

Aspirin tablets should be stored in tight, moisture resistant containers. Do not use products past the expiration date or if a strong vinegar-like odor is noted emitting from the bottle.

Aspirin is stable in dry air, but readily hydrolyzes to acetate and salicylate when exposed to water or moist air; it will then exude a strong vinegar-like odor. The addition of heat will speed the rate of hydrolysis. In aqueous solutions, aspirin is most stable at pH's of 2-3 and least stable at pH's <2 or >8. Should an aqueous solution be desirable as a dosage form, the commercial product *Alka-Seltzer*® will remain stable for 10 hours at room temperature in solution.

Compatibility/Compounding Considerations

Compounded preparation stability: Aspirin is hydrolyzed by water to degradative byproducts, acetic acid and salicylic acid.

Effervescent buffered aspirin tablets (*Alka-Seltzer*®) dissolved in water are demonstrated to be stable for 10 hours at room temperature and for 90 hours if refrigerated (McEvoy 2008). Although pharmacists compound aspirin suspensions in fixed oils, the long-term stability of these preparations has not been determined.

Dosage Forms/Regulatory Status

VETERINARY-LABELED PRODUCTS:

Note: No known products are FDA-approved for use in animals.

Aspirin Tablets (Enteric-Coated): 81 mg; (OTC). Labeled for use in dogs.

Aspirin Tablets (Buffered, Microencapsulated, Chewable for dogs): 150 mg & 450 mg; *Canine Aspirin Chewable Tablets for Small & Medium* (150 mg) or *Large Dogs*® (450 mg); (OTC). Labeled for use in dogs.

Aspirin Tablets 60 grain (3.9 g): Aspirin 60 Grain (OTC & Rx); Rx is labeled for use in horses, cattle, sheep and swine; not for use in horses intended for food or in lactating dairy animals.

Aspirin Boluses 240 grain (15.6 g): Labeled for use in horses, foals, cattle and calves; not for use in lactating animals. Aspirin 240 Grain Boluses, Aspirin Bolus (various); (OTC)

Aspirin Boluses 480 grain (31.2 g). Labeled for use in mature horses, & cattle. Aspirin 480 Grain Boluses (various); (OTC)

Oral Aspirin Gel: 250 mg/mL in 30 mL: *Aspir-Flex*® *Aspirin Gel for Small and Medium Dogs*; 500 mg/1 mL in 30 mL: *Aspir-Flex*® *Aspirin Gel for Large Dogs*; (OTC). Labeled for use in dogs.

Aspirin Powder: 1 lb. (various); (OTC); Aspirin Powder Molasses-Flavored 50% acetylsalicylic acid in base; Aspirin USP 204 g/lb. (apple flavored); Acetylsalicylic acid; (OTC)

Aspirin Granules: 2.5 gram per 39 mL scoop (apple and molasses flavor); *Arthri-Eze Aspirin Granules*®; (OTC); Labeled for use in horses

Aspirin Liquid Concentrate (equiv. to 12% aspirin) for Dilution in Drinking Water in 32 oz. btls.; (OTC). Labeled for addition to drinking water for swine, poultry, beef and dairy cattle

There are no listed meat or milk withdrawal times listed for food-producing animals, but because there are salicylate-sensitive people, in the interest of public health, this author suggests a minimum of 1 day withdrawal time for either milk or meat. For further guidance with determining use and withdrawal times, contact FARAD (see Phone Numbers & Websites in the appendix for contact information).

The ARCI (Racing Commissioners International) has designated this drug as a class 4 substance. See the appendix for more information.

HUMAN-LABELED PRODUCTS:

Aspirin, Chewable Tablets: 81 mg (1.25 grains); many trade names, generic; (OTC)

Aspirin, Tablets; plain uncoated; 325 mg (5 grain), & 500 mg (7.8 grain); many trade names, generic; (OTC)

Aspirin Tablets, enteric coated: 81 mg, 165 mg, 325 mg, 500 mg, 650 mg, & 800 mg; many trade names, generic; (OTC)

Aspirin Extended-controlled Release Tablets: 81 mg, 650 mg, 800 mg & 975 mg; many trade names, generic; (OTC)

Aspirin, Tablets; buffered uncoated; 325 mg (5 grain), with aluminum &/or magnesium salts; many trade names, generic; (OTC)

Aspirin Tablets: buffered coated: 325 mg & 500 mg; many trade names, generic; (OTC)

Rectal suppositories, chewing gum and effervescent oral dosage forms are also available commercially for human use.

Revisions/References
Monograph revised/updated August 2013.

Adamcak, A. & B. Otten (2000). Rodent Therapeutics. *Vet Clin NA: Exotic Anim Pract* **3:1**(Jan): 221-40.

Bill, R. (2008). NSAIDs--Keeping up with all the changes. *Proceedings: ACVC.*

Brumbaugh, G., et al. (1999). The pharmacologic basis for the treatment of laminitis. *The Veterinary Clinics of North America: Equine Practice* **15:2**(August).

Coetzee, J. F. (2013). Assessment and Management of Pain Associated with Castration in Cattle. *Veterinary Clinics of North America-Food Animal Practice* **29**(1): 75-+.

Graham, A. H. & M. S. Leib (2009). Effects of Prednisone Alone or Prednisone with Ultralow-Dose Aspirin on the Gastroduodenal Mucosa of Healthy Dogs. *Journal of Veterinary Internal Medicine* 23(3): 482-7.

Ivey, E. & J. Morrisey (2000). Therapeutics for Rabbits. *Vet Clin NA: Exotic Anim Pract* **3:1**(Jan): 183-216.

McEvoy, J., Ed. (2008). *AHFS Drug Information*. Bethesda, American Society of Health System Pharmacists.

Shearer, L., et al. (2009). *Effects of aspirin and clopidogrel on platelet function in healthy dogs*. Proceedings: ECVIM. accessed via Veterinary Information Network; vin.com

Smith, S. A. (2012). Antithrombotic Therapy. *Topics in Companion Animal Medicine* 27(2): 88-94.

Sparkes, A. H., et al. (2010). ISFM AND AAFP CONSENSUS GUIDELINES Long-term use of NSAIDs in cats. *Journal of Feline Medicine and Surgery* **12**(7): 521-38.

Stiller, A., et al. (2013). Effect of Low-Dose Aspirin or Heparin on Platelet-Derived Urinary Thromboxane Metabolite in Dogs with Immune-Mediated Hemolytic Anemia (IMHA). ACVIM Proceedings. accessed via Veterinary Information Network; vin.com

Williams, B. (2000). Therapeutics in Ferrets. *Vet Clin NA: Exotic Anim Pract* **3:1**(Jan): 131-53.

Atenolol
(a-**ten**-oh-lol)   Tenormin®

Beta-Adrenergic Blocker

Prescriber Highlights

▶ Beta-blocker that is used primarily for hypertension & tachyarrhythmias in small animals; use in cats with preclinical hypertrophic cardiomyopathy is controversial.

▶ Has minimal beta$_2$ blocking activity at usual doses; comparatively safe to use in asthmatic patients.

▶ Contraindicated in patients with bradycardic arrhythmias or that are hypersensitive to it.

▶ Negative inotrope so must be used with caution in patients with CHF; use with caution in renal failure patients & those with sinus node dysfunction.

▶ Higher dosages may mask clinical signs of hyperthyroidism or hypoglycemia; may cause hyper- or hypoglycemia—use with caution in brittle diabetics.

▶ Primary adverse effects are lethargy, hypotension, or diarrhea but usually well tolerated.

▶ If discontinuing, recommend withdrawing gradually.

Uses/Indications

Atenolol may be useful in the treatment of supraventricular tachyarrhythmias, premature ventricular contractions (PVC's, VPC's), and systemic hypertension. A study evaluating atenolol as monotherapy for treating systemic hypertension in hyperthyroid cats, found that most cats had their heart rates decrease, but 70% of cases were not controlled (SBP<160 mmHg) and that additional drug therapy (*e.g.*, amlodipine or an ACE inhibitor) is required (Henik et al. 2008).

While atenolol has been used in cats with preclinical hypertrophic cardiomyopathy its use is controversial and a study (prospective, observational, open-label, clinical cohort) found no significant difference in mortality between cats treated or untreated with atenolol (Schober et al. 2013).

Atenolol is relatively safe to use in animals with bronchospastic disease.

Pharmacology/Actions

Atenolol is a relatively specific beta$_1$-blocker. At higher dosages, this specificity may be lost and Beta$_2$ blockade can occur. Atenolol does not possess any intrinsic sympathomimetic activity like pindolol nor does it possess membrane-stabilizing activity like pindolol or propranolol. Cardiovascular effects secondary to atenolol's negative inotropic and chronotropic actions include: decreased sinus heart rate, slowed AV conduction, diminished cardiac output at rest and during exercise, decreased myocardial oxygen demand, reduced blood pressure, and inhibition of isoproterenol-induced tachycardia.

Pharmacokinetics

Only about 50-60% of an oral dose is absorbed in humans, but it is absorbed rapidly. In cats, it is reported to have a bioavailability of approximately 90%. The drug has very low protein binding characteristics (5-15%) and is distributed well into most tissues. Atenolol has low lipid solubility and unlike propranolol, only small amounts of atenolol are distributed into the CNS. Atenolol crosses the placenta and levels in milk are higher than those found in plasma. Atenolol is minimally biotransformed in the liver; 40-50% is excreted unchanged in the urine and the bulk of the remainder is excreted in the feces unchanged (unabsorbed drug). Reported half-lives: dogs = 3.2 hours; cats = 3.7 hours; humans = 6-7 hours. Duration of beta blockade effect in cats persists for about 12 hours.

Contraindications/Precautions/Warnings

Atenolol is contraindicated in patients with overt heart failure, hypersensitivity to this class of agents, greater than first-degree heart block, or sinus bradycardia. Non-specific beta-blockers are generally contraindicated in patients with CHF unless secondary to a tachyarrhythmia responsive to beta-blocker therapy. They are also relatively contraindicated in patients with bronchospastic lung disease. Atenolol may cause increased morbidity in cats with hypertrophic cardiomyopathy with accompanying left-sided CHF.

Atenolol should be used cautiously in patients with significant renal insufficiency or sinus node dysfunction.

Atenolol (at high dosages) can mask the clinical signs associated with hypoglycemia. It can also cause hypoglycemia or hyperglycemia and, therefore, should be used cautiously in labile diabetic patients.

Atenolol can mask the clinical signs associated with thyrotoxicosis, however, it may be used clinically to treat the clinical signs associated with this condition.

Adverse Effects

It is reported that adverse effects most commonly occur in geriatric animals or those that have acute decompensating heart disease. Adverse effects considered clinically relevant include: bradycardia, inappetence, lethargy and depression, impaired AV conduction, CHF or worsening of heart failure, hypotension, hypoglycemia, and bronchoconstriction (less so with Beta$_1$ specific drugs like atenolol). Syncope and diarrhea have also been reported in canine patients with beta-blockers. Lethargy and hypotension may be noted within 1 hour of administration.

Exacerbation of symptoms has been reported following abrupt cessation of beta-blockers in humans. It is recommended to withdraw therapy gradually in patients who have been receiving the drug chronically.

Reproductive/Nursing Safety

In humans, the FDA categorizes this drug as category *C* for use during pregnancy (*Animal studies have shown an adverse effect on the fetus, but there are no adequate studies in humans; or there are no animal reproduction studies and no adequate studies in humans.*)

Overdosage/Acute Toxicity

There were 509 single agent exposures to atenolol reported to the ASPCA Animal Poison Control Center (APCC) during 2009-2013. Of the 362 dogs, 53 were symptomatic with 28% bradycardic, 25% lethargic, 13% vomiting, 11% tachycardic and 9% hypotensive. Of the 145 cats, 20 were symptomatic with 25% experiencing hypotension, 20% bradycardic, 20% tachycardic, 15% hypertensive, 15% lethargic, and 15% vomiting.

Humans have apparently survived dosages of up to 5 grams. The most predominant clinical signs expected would be extensions of the drug's pharmacologic effects: hypotension, bradycardia, bronchospasm, cardiac failure, hypoglycemia, and hyperkalemia.

If overdose is secondary to a recent oral ingestion, emptying the gut and charcoal administration may be considered. Monitor ECG, blood glucose and potassium, and if possible, blood pressure. Treatment of the cardiovascular effects is symptomatic. Use fluids and pressor agents (dopamine or norepinephrine) to treat hypotension. Bradycardia may be treated with atropine. If atropine fails, isoproterenol given cautiously has been recommended. Insulin and dextrose may be needed for hyperkalemia and hypoglycemia. Use of a transvenous pacemaker may be necessary. Cardiac failure can be treated with a digitalis glycoside, diuretics and oxygen. Glucagon (5 – 10 mg IV; human dose) may increase heart rate and blood pressure and reduce the cardiodepressant effects of atenolol.

Drug Interactions

The following drug interactions with atenolol have either been reported or are theoretical in humans or animals and may be of significance in veterinary patients. Unless otherwise noted, use together is not necessarily contraindicated, but weigh the potential risks and perform additional monitoring when appropriate.

- **ANESTHETICS (myocardial depressant):** Additive myocardial depression may occur with the concurrent use of atenolol and myocardial depressant anesthetic agents.
- **CALCIUM-CHANNEL BLOCKERS** (*e.g.,* **diltiazem, verapamil, amlodipine**): Concurrent use of beta-blockers with calcium channel blockers (or other negative inotropics) should be done with caution, particularly in patients with preexisting cardiomyopathy or CHF.
- **CLONIDINE:** Atenolol may exacerbate rebound hypertension after stopping clonidine therapy.
- **FUROSEMIDE, HYDRALAZINE** or **OTHER HYPOTENSIVE DRUGS:** May increase the hypotensive effects of atenolol.
- **PHENOTHIAZINES:** With atenolol may exhibit enhanced hypotensive effects.
- **RESERPINE:** Potential for additive effects (*e.g.,* hypotension, bradycardia).
- **SYMPATHOMIMETICS** (*e.g.,* **metaproterenol, terbutaline, beta-effects of epinephrine, phenylpropanolamine,** etc.): May have their actions blocked by atenolol and they may, in turn, reduce the efficacy of atenolol.

Doses

- **DOGS:**

  For indications where beta-blockade may be indicated (tachyarrhythmias, obstructive heart disease, etc.); (extra-label): Recommended dosages generally are 0.25 – 1 mg/kg PO q12h; practically 6.25 mg (1/4 of a 25 mg tablet) to 50 mg per dog twice daily. In atrial fibrillation, dosage is often started at the low end and titrated upward. In dogs with sub-valvular aortic stenosis, dosage recommendations are on the high end of the dosing range.

- **CATS:**

  For treatment of hypertension (usually with other drugs) or cardiac conditions (e.g., hypertrophic cardiomyopathy) where beta blockade may be indicated (extra-label): Initially 6.25 mg per cat (1/4 of a 25 mg tablet) PO q12h. Dosage may be titrated upwards (*e.g.,* 12.5 mg AM & 6.25 mg PM, etc.). Dosages as high as 25 mg per cat twice daily have been reported. In cats with

renal dysfunction, the following dosage adjustments have been recommended (Trepanier 2013): IRIS Stage II: 0.19 mg/kg PO q12-24h; IRIS Stage III: 0.125 mg/kg PO q12-24h; IRIS stage IV: 0.06 mg/kg PO q24h.

- **FERRETS:**

  For hypertrophic cardiomyopathy (extra-label):
  a) 6.25 mg (total dose per ferret) PO once daily. (Williams 2000)
  b) 3.13 – 6.25 mg (total dose per ferret) PO once daily. (Johnson-Delaney 2005)

Monitoring

- Cardiac function, pulse rate, ECG if necessary, BP if indicated.
- Toxicity (see Adverse Effects/Overdosage).

Client Information

- To be effective, the animal must receive all doses as prescribed. Notify veterinarian if animal becomes lethargic or becomes exercise intolerant; develops shortness of breath or cough; or develops a change in behavior or attitude. Do not stop therapy without first conferring with veterinarian.

Chemistry/Synonyms

A beta$_1$-adrenergic blocking agent, atenolol occurs as a white, crystalline powder. At 37°C, 26.5 mg are soluble in 1 mL of water. The pH of the commercially available injection is adjusted to 5.5-6.5.

Atenolol may also be known as atenololum, or ICI-66082; many trade names are available.

Storage/Stability

Tablets should be stored at room temperature and protected from heat, light and moisture.

Compatibility/Compounding Considerations

Atenolol tablets may be crushed or split/cut into quarters or halves for appropriate dosing.

Compounded preparation/stability:

1) Atenolol oral suspensions should not be compounded with sugar-containing vehicles. Atenolol oral suspension compounded from either active pharmaceutical ingredient (API) or commercially available tablets has been published (Patel et al. 1997). Triturating an appropriate amount of API or tablets with equal volumes of *Ora-Plus®* and *Ora-Sweet® SF* yields a 2 mg/mL oral suspension that retains >90% potency for 90 days stored at both 5°C and 25°C. This investigation also reveals that the presence of sugars (*Ora-Sweet®* and simple syrup) reduces the potency of compounded atenolol suspensions to <90% in 7-14 days after compounding. Atenolol preparations are most stable at pH 4. Atenolol should be stored protected from light as exposure to ultraviolet light results in drug decomposition at all pH ranges.

2) Atenolol suspension (flavored) 25 mg/mL. In the study, 150 mL batches were prepared by adding atenolol powder (3.75 g), PEG 4500 (51 g), processed beef and pork flavor powder (15 g), sodium saccharin (1.8 g) and 50 mL of distilled water in and shaken vigorously. Distilled water was added to volume (150 mL) and shaken again. Stored in refrigerator. Stability is still to be established, but pharmacokinetics in cats was comparable to tablets (Khor et al. 2012).

Dosage Forms/Regulatory Status

VETERINARY-LABELED PRODUCTS: NONE.

The ARCI (Racing Commissioners International) has designated this drug as a class 3 substance. See the appendix for more information.

HUMAN-LABELED PRODUCTS:

Atenolol Oral Tablets: 25 mg, 50 mg, & 100 mg; *Tenormin®*, generic; (Rx)

Revisions/References

Monograph revised/updated August 2013.
Henik, R. A., et al. (2008). Efficacy of atenolol as a single antihypertensive agent in hyperthyroid cats. *Journal of Feline Medicine and Surgery* **10**(6): 577-82.
Johnson-Delaney, C. (2005). *Ferret Cardiology.* Proceedings: Atlantic Coast Veterinary Conference. accessed via Veterinary Information Network; vin.com
Khor, K. H., et al. (2012). Acceptability and compliance of atenolol tablet, compounded paste and compounded suspension prescribed to healthy cats. *Journal of Feline Medicine and Surgery* **14**(2): 99-106.
Patel, D., et al. (1997). Short-term stability of atenolol in oral liquid formulations. *Int J Pharm Compound* **1**: 437-9.
Schober, K. E., et al. (2013). Effect of treatment with atenolol on 5-year survival in cats with preclinical (asymptomatic) hypertrophic cardiomyopathy. *Journal of Veterinary Cardiology* **15**: 93-104.
Trepanier, L. (2013). *Feline Therapeutics.* World Small Animal Veterinary Association World Congress Proceedings. accessed via Veterinary Information Network; vin.com
Williams, B. (2000). Therapeutics in Ferrets. *Vet Clin NA: Exotic Anim Pract* **3**:**1**(Jan): 131-53.

Atipamezole HCl

(at-i-**pam**-a-zole)   Antisedan®

Alpha-2 Adrenergic Antagonist

Prescriber Highlights

▶ Alpha2-adrenergic antagonist; antagonizes agonists such as medetomidine or xylazine.

▶ No safety data on use in pregnant or lactating animals.

▶ May reverse effects rapidly, including analgesia; animals should be observed & protected from self-harm or causing harm to others.

▶ Adverse Effects may include vomiting, diarrhea, hypersalivation, tremors, or excitation.

Uses/Indications

Atipamezole is labeled for use as a reversal agent for medetomidine and dexmedetomidine. It potentially could be useful for reversal of other alpha2-adrenergic agonists as well (*e.g.,* amitraz, xylazine, clonidine, tizanidine, brimonidine).

Pharmacology/Actions

Atipamezole competitively inhibits alpha2-adrenergic receptors, thereby acting as a reversal agent for alpha2-adrenergic agonists (*e.g.,* medetomidine). Net pharmacologic effects are to reduce sedation, decrease blood pressure, increase heart and respiratory rates, and reduce the analgesic effects of alpha2-adrenergic agonists. Atipamezole will antagonize the diuretic action of xylazine in dogs (Talukder et al. 2009).

Pharmacokinetics

After IM administration in the dog, peak plasma levels occur in about 10 minutes. Atipamezole is apparently metabolized in the liver to compounds that are eliminated in the urine. The drug has an average plasma elimination half-life of about 2-3 hours.

Contraindications/Precautions/Warnings

While the manufacturer lists no absolute contraindications to the use of atipamezole, the drug is not recommended in pregnant or lactating animals due to the lack of data establishing safety. Caution should be used in administration of anesthetic agents to elderly or debilitated animals.

When used as a reversal agent (antidote) for alpha2-agonist toxicity, atipamezole's effects may subside before non-toxic levels of the offending agent are reached; repeat dosing may be necessary.

Do not give IV to reptiles as profound hypotension can occur.

Adverse Effects

Potential adverse effects include occasional vomiting, diarrhea, hypersalivation, tremors, and brief excitation or apprehensiveness.

Because reversal can occur rapidly, care should be exercised as animals emerging from sedation and analgesia may exhibit apprehensive or aggressive behaviors. After reversal, animals should be protected from falling. Additional analgesia (*e.g.,* butorphanol) should be considered, particularly after painful procedures.

In reptiles, intravenous administration reportedly can cause profound hypotension.

Reproductive/Nursing Safety

The manufacturer states that the drug is not recommended in pregnant or lactating animals, or in animals intended for breeding due to lack of data establishing safety in these animals. No other data was noted.

Overdosage/Acute Toxicity

Dogs receiving up to 10X the listed dosage apparently tolerated the drug without major effects. When overdosed, dose related effects seen included panting, excitement, trembling, vomiting, soft or liquid feces, vasodilatation of sclera and some muscle injury at the IM injection site. Specific overdose therapy should generally not be necessary.

Drug Interactions

The manufacturer states that information on the use of atipamezole with other drugs is lacking, therefore, caution should be taken when using with other drugs (other than medetomidine). The following drug interactions with atipamezole have either been reported or are theoretical in humans or animals and may be of significance in veterinary patients. Unless otherwise noted, use together is not necessarily contraindicated, but weigh the potential risks and perform additional monitoring when appropriate.

■ **ALPHA₁-ADRENERGIC BLOCKERS** (*e.g.,* **prazosin**): Atipamezole is a relatively specific alpha2 blocker; it can also partially block alpha1 receptors and reduce the effects of prazosin.

■ **ALPHA₂-ADRENERGIC AGONISTS** (*e.g.,* **detomidine, clonidine, brimonidine, xylazine, amitraz,** etc.): Atipamezole can reduce the effects (toxic or therapeutic) of these agents.

Doses

■ **DOGS:**

For reversal of dexmedetomidine or medetomidine (labeled dosage; FDA-approved): 3750 micrograms/m2 IM regardless of the route used for dexmedetomidine or medetomidine. Formulated so that the volume of injection is the same (mL for mL) as the recommended (labeled) dose of dexmedetomidine or medetomidine. The product label (package insert) has a detailed dosage chart that converts dog's weight (in lbs.) to dosage in micrograms/kg and mLs. (Adapted from label; Antisedan®)

For reversal of dexmedetomidine or medetomidine (extra-label): 100 micrograms/kg IV or IO (intraosseous) as part of CPR to reverse alpha2 agonists. Dosage is based on a 10 microgram/kg dexmedetomidine dose. If a higher dose of dexmedetomidine was administered, increase this dose accordingly. (Fletcher et al. 2012)

For treatment of amitraz toxicity (extra-label): 50 mcg/kg IM; doses may need to be repeated every 4-6 hours as the half-life of amitraz is longer than atipamezole in dogs. (Hugnet, Buronrosse et al. 1996), (Papich 2009)

■ **CATS:**

As a reversal agent (extra-label):

a) For reversal of medetomidine as part of a medetomidine/butorphanol or buprenorphine/ketamine/carprofen or meloxicam anesthesia/analgesia injectable combination: Use an equal volume IM of atipamezole as medetomidine was used in the combination. (Ko 2005)

b) 100 micrograms/kg IV or IO as part of CPR to reverse alpha2 agonists. Dosage is based on a 10 microgram/kg dexmedetomidine dose. If a higher dose of dexmedetomidine was administered, increase this dose accordingly. (Fletcher et al. 2012)

c) For reversal of xylazine sedation (when xylazine used as an emetic): 25 – 50 micrograms/kg IM or IV (slowly). (Wells 2012)

- **RABBITS/RODENTS/SMALL MAMMALS:**

a) **Rabbits:** For medetomidine reversal (extra-label): 0.5 mg/kg IM or SC; 0.25 mg/kg IV. (Vella 2009)

b) **Mice, Rats, Gerbils, Hamsters, Guinea pigs:** To reverse xylazine or medetomidine (extra-label): 0.1 – 1 mg/kg IM, IP, IV or SC. (Adamcak et al. 2000)

- **HORSES:**

For reversal of alpha2-adrenergic agonist (such as amitraz, xylazine) toxicity (extra-label): 0.1 mg/kg IV has been suggested. (Dowling 2008)

- **RUMINANTS:**

As a reversal agent for alpha2-adrenergic agonists (e.g., xylazine, detomidine, etc.); (extra-label):

a) For reversal of alpha2-adrenergic agonists in bovine, new world camelids, ovine and caprine species: 0.02 – 0.1 mg/kg IV to effect. (Haskell 2005)

b) **Small ruminants, camelids:** 0.1 – 0.2 mg/kg slow IV or IM; as a rule of thumb, if induction included ketamine or *Telazol®* do not reverse alpha2 sooner than 30 and ideally 60 minutes after induction. This will allow enough of the ketamine or tiletamine to be metabolized. (Snyder 2009), (Wolff 2009)

- **BIRDS:**

As a reversal agent for alpha2-adrenergic agonists (e.g., xylazine, detomidine, etc.); (extra-label): 0.5 mg/kg IM. (Clyde et al. 2000)

- **REPTILES:**

As a reversal agent for alpha2-adrenergic agonists (extra-label): Reversal of all dosages ketamine/medetomidine combination (see ketamine or medetomidine monographs) with atipamezole is 4-5 times the medetomidine dose (Heard 1999). Reversal may take longer (up to one hour) in reptiles than in other species; Do NOT give IV as profound hypotension can occur (Mehler 2009).

- **ZOO, EXOTIC, WILDLIFE SPECIES:**

For use in zoo, exotic and wildlife medicine refer to specific references, including:

a) *Zoo Animal and Wildlife Immobilization and Anesthesia.* West, G., Heard, D., Caulkett, N. (eds.). Blackwell Publishing, 2007.

b) Handbook of Wildlife Chemical Immobilization, 3rd Ed. Kreeger, T.J. and J.M. Arnemo. 2007.

c) Fowler's Zoo and Wild Animal Medicine Current Therapy, Volume 7, Miller, R.E., Fowler, M.E., Saunders. 2011.

d) *Exotic Animal Formulary, 4th Ed.* Carpenter, J.W., Saunders. 2012.

e) The 2009 American Association of Zoo Veterinarian Proceedings by D. K. Fontenot also has several dosages listed for restraint, anesthesia, and analgesia for a variety of drugs for carnivores and primates. VIN members can access them at: http://goo.gl/NNIWQ or http://goo.gl/9UJse

Monitoring
- Level of sedation and analgesia.
- Heart rate.
- Body temperature.

Client Information
- Atipamezole should be administered by veterinary professionals only. Clients should be informed that occasionally vomiting, diarrhea, hypersalivation, excitation and tremors may be seen after atipamezole administration. Should these be severe or persist after leaving the clinic, clients should contact the veterinarian.

Chemistry/Synonyms
Atipamezole is an imidazole alpha2-adrenergic antagonist. The injection is a clear, colorless solution.
Atipamezole HCl may also be known as MPV-1248 or *Antisedan®*.

Storage/Stability
Atipamezole HCl injection should be stored at room temperature (15-30°C) and protected from light.

Compatibility/Compounding Considerations
No specific information noted.

Dosage Forms/Regulatory Status
VETERINARY-LABELED PRODUCTS:
Atipamezole HCl for Injection: 5 mg/mL in 10 mL multidose vials; *Antisedan®*; (Rx). FDA-approved for use in dogs. There is a website (dailymed.nlm.nih.gov) with FDA-approved veterinary product labels.

HUMAN-LABELED PRODUCTS: NONE.

Revisions/References
Monograph revised/updated August 2013.
Adamcak, A. & B. Otten (2000). Rodent Therapeutics. *Vet Clin NA: Exotic Anim Pract* **3:1**(Jan): 221-40.
Clyde, V. & J. Paul-Murphy (2000). Avian Analgesia. *Kirk's Current Veterinary Therapy: XIII Small Animal Practice.* J. Bonagura. Philadelphia, WB Saunders: 1126-8.
Dowling, P. M. (2008). Amitraz Toxicosis. *Blackwell's Five-Minute Veterinary Consult: Equine.* J.-P. Lavoie and K. V. Hinchcliff, Wiley-Blackwell: 55.
Fletcher, D. J., et al. (2012). RECOVER evidence and knowledge gap analysis on veterinary CPR. Part 7: Clinical guidelines. *J. Vet. Emerg. Crit. Care* **22**.
Haskell, R. (2005). *Development of a Small Ruminant Formulary.* Proceedings: WVC. accessed via Veterinary Information Network; vin.com
Heard, D. (1999). *Advances in Reptile Anesthesia.* The North American Veterinary Conference, Orlando. accessed via Veterinary Information Network; vin.com
Ko, J. (2005). *New anesthesia-analgesia injectable combinations in dogs and cats.* Proceedings: ACVC. accessed via Veterinary Information Network; vin.com
Mehler, S. (2009). *Anaesthesia and care of the reptile.* Proceedings: BSAVA. accessed via Veterinary Information Network; vin.com
Papich, M. (2009). *Medication precautions for the neurologic patient.* Proceedings: ACVIM. accessed via Veterinary Information Network; vin.com
Snyder, J. (2009). *Small Ruminant Medicine & Surgery for Equine and Small Animal Practitioners I & II.* Proceedings: WVC. accessed via Veterinary Information Network; vin.com
Talukder, M. H., et al. (2009). Antagonistic Effects of Atipamezole and Yohimbine on Xylazine-Induced Diuresis in Healthy Dogs. *Journal of Veterinary Medical Science* **71**(5): 539-48.
Vella, D. (2009). *Rabbit General Anesthesia.* Proceedings: AAVAC-UEP. accessed via Veterinary Information Network; vin.com
Wells, R. (2012). *Toxins and Poisons.* Western Veterinary Conference Proceedings. accessed via Veterinary Information Network; vin.com
Wolff, P. (2009). *Camelid Medicine.* Proceedings: AAZV. accessed via Veterinary Information Network; vin.com

Atovaquone

(ah-**toe**-va-kwone)   Mepron®

Oral Antiprotozoal Agent

Prescriber Highlights

▶ Atovaquone (with azithromycin) appears effective in treating dogs with *Babesia gibsoni* infections. Alone, it is a second-line agent (after trimethoprim/sulfa) for pneumocystosis in dogs.

▶ In combination with azithromycin, used to treat cytauxzoonosis in cats.

▶ Limited use thus far; appears well tolerated by dogs.

▶ Treatment may be quite expensive.

Uses/Indications

Atovaquone (with azithromycin) appears effective in treating dogs with *Babesia gibsoni* (Asian genotype) infections, particularly in dogs not immunosuppressed or splenectomized. A prospective, unmasked study in dogs comparing atovaquone/azithromycin (AA) with a protocol using clindamycin, diminazene and imidocarb (CDI) found that CDI had higher recovery and lower relapse rates, albeit longer therapy duration and slower reduction in parasite numbers than AA. The authors concluded that CDI was effective for initial therapy and when the M121I gene in *B. gibsoni* had mutated (Lin et al. 2012). Atovaquone (alone) may be of benefit for treating pneumocystosis in dogs, but it is considered second line therapy after potentiated sulfonamides.

Atovaquone (with azithromycin) may be of benefit in treating *Cytauxzoon felis* infections in cats.

Pharmacology/Actions

Atovaquone's antiprotozoal mechanism of action is not completely understood. It is believed that the hydroxynaphthoquinones, like atovaquone, selectively inhibit protozoan mitochondrial electron transport causing inhibition of *de novo* pyrimidine synthesis. Unlike mammalian cells, certain protozoa cannot salvage preformed pyrimidines. The M121I mutation in the *Babesia gibsoni* CYTb gene apparently confers resistance to atovaquone (Lin et al. 2012).

Pharmacokinetics

Pharmacokinetic data for dogs or cats was not located. In humans after oral administration, bioavailability ranges from 23-47%. The presence of food, particularly high in fat, can increase bioavailability significantly (2+ fold over fasted administration). The drug is highly bound to human plasma proteins (99.9%) and levels in the CSF are approximately 1% of those found in plasma. Elimination half-life in people is about 70 hours presumably due to enterohepatic recycling. There may be limited hepatic metabolism, but the bulk of absorbed drug is eventually eliminated unchanged in the feces.

Contraindications/Precautions/Warnings

No absolute contraindications for using atovaquone in dogs or cats have been documented. Animals with malabsorption syndromes or that cannot take the drug with food should have alternate therapies considered.

The drug is contraindicated in human patients that develop or have a prior history of hypersensitivity reactions to the drug.

Reproductive/Nursing Safety

Studies in pregnant rats with atovaquone plasma levels approximately 2-3 times those found in humans receiving therapeutic dosages revealed no increase in teratogenicity. Similar studies in rabbits showed increased maternal and fetal toxicity (decreased fetal growth and increased early fetal resorption). In humans, the FDA categorizes atovaquone as category *C* for use during pregnancy (*Animal studies have shown an adverse effect on the fetus, but there are no adequate studies in humans; or there are no animal reproduc-*

tion studies and no adequate studies in humans.)

Little information is available on the safety of this drug during lactation. In rats, milk levels were approximately 1/3 those found in maternal plasma. It is unlikely atovaquone in milk poses much risk to nursing puppies.

Adverse Effects

Atovaquone use in dogs and cats has been limited and the adverse effect profile is not well known. One study (Birkenheuer et al. 2004) using atovaquone and azithromycin for treating *Babesia gibsoni* infections in 10 dogs reported that no adverse effects were noted. The combination product containing atovaquone and proguanil (*Malarone®*) reportedly causes severe gastrointestinal effects in dogs.

In humans treated with atovaquone, rashes (up to 39% of treated patients) and gastrointestinal effects (nausea, vomiting, diarrhea) are the most frequently reported adverse effects. Rashes or diarrhea may necessitate discontinuation of therapy. Other adverse effects reported in humans include hypersensitivity reactions, increased liver enzymes, CNS effects (headache, dizziness, insomnia), hyperglycemia, hyponatremia, fever, neutropenia, and anemia.

Overdosage/Acute Toxicity

Limited information is available for any species. Minimum toxic doses have not been established; laboratory animals have tolerated doses up to 31.5 grams. The current recommendation for treating overdoses is basically symptomatic and supportive.

Drug Interactions

The following drug interactions with atovaquone have either been reported or are theoretical in humans or animals and may be of significance in veterinary patients. Unless otherwise noted, use together is not necessarily contraindicated, but weigh the potential risks and perform additional monitoring when appropriate.

■ **METOCLOPRAMIDE**: Can decrease atovaquone plasma concentrations.

■ **TETRACYCLINE**: Can decrease atovaquone plasma concentrations.

■ **RIFAMPIN**: Can decrease atovaquone plasma concentrations.

Laboratory Considerations

■ No specific issues; see Monitoring for recommendations for testing for efficacy.

Doses

■ **DOGS:**

For *Babesia gibsoni* (Asian genotype) or *B. microti* infections (extra-label): Atovaquone 13.3 mg/kg PO q8h with a fatty meal and Azithromycin 10 mg/kg PO once daily. Give both drugs for 10 days. Reserve immunosuppressive therapy for cases that are not rapidly responding (3-5 days) to anti-protozoal therapy. (Birkenheuer et al. 2004), (Birkenheuer 2006; Ayoob et al. 2010; Birkenheuer 2012)

For pneumocystosis (extra-label): 15 mg/kg PO once daily for 3 weeks. (Greene et al. 2006)

■ **CATS:**

For cytauxzoonosis (*Cytauxzoon felis*); (extra-label): Atovaquone 15 mg/kg PO q8h with azithromycin 10 mg/kg PO q24h. All cases were treated with IV fluids and most received heparin. (Birkenheuer et al. 2008)

Monitoring

■ Monitoring for therapy for *Babesia gibsoni* in dogs should include surveillance for potential adverse effects and signs for clinical efficacy, including monitoring serial CBCs.

■ Severe cases may have elevated BUN or liver enzymes, and hypokalemia.

- Current recommendation for determining "clearing" of the organism (*B. gibsoni*) is to perform a PCR test at 60 days and 90 days post-therapy.

Client Information

- Store medication at room temperature and away from bright light.
- Before using, shake bottle gently.
- To increase the absorption from the GI tract, give with food high in fat (*e.g.*, ice cream, tuna oil, butter, meat fat).
- Adverse effect profile in dogs and cats for this medication is not well known.
- Report any significant effects such as rash, or severe or persistent vomiting or diarrhea, to the veterinarian.

Chemistry/Synonyms

Atovaquone is a synthetic, hydroxy-1,4-naphthoquinone antiprotozoal agent. It occurs as a yellow powder that is highly lipid soluble, insoluble in water and slightly soluble in alcohol.

Atovaquone may also be known as: BW-556C, Atovacuona, Atovakvon, Atovakvoni, Atovaquonnum, *Malanil®, Mepron®*, or *Wellvone®*.

Storage/Stability

The commercially available oral suspension should be stored at room temperature (15-25°C) in tight containers and protected from bright light; do not freeze.

Compatibility/Compounding Considerations

No specific information noted.

Dosage Forms/Regulatory Status

VETERINARY-LABELED PRODUCTS: NONE.

HUMAN-LABELED PRODUCTS:

Atovaquone Oral Suspension: 150 mg/mL (750 mg/5mL) in 210 mL bottles; citrus flavor; *Mepron®*; (Rx)

A tablet dosage form was previously available, but was discontinued when the oral suspension was approved by FDA; the suspension has much better oral bioavailability in humans. A combination tablet product containing atovaquone and proguanil HCl (*Malarone®*) is available that has labeled indications (human) for malaria prophylaxis and treatment. This combination has reportedly caused significant GI adverse effects in some dogs.

Revisions/References

Monograph revised/updated August 2013.

Ayoob, A. L., et al. (2010). Clinical management of canine babesiosis. *J. Vet. Emerg. Crit. Care* **20**(1): 77-89.

Birkenheuer, A. (2006). *Infectious Hemolytic Anemias.* ACVIM Proceedings. accessed via Veterinary Information Network; vin.com

Birkenheuer, A. (2012). *Canine Babesiosis: What's New?* Second International Society for Companion Animal Infectious Diseases Symposium Proceedings. accessed via Veterinary Information Network; vin.com

Birkenheuer, A., et al. (2008). *Atovaquone and azithromycin for the treatment of Cytauxzoon felis.* Proceedings: ACVIM. accessed via Veterinary Information Network; vin.com

Birkenheuer, A., et al. (2004). Efficacy of combined atovaquone and azithromycin for therapy of chronic Babesia gibsoni (Asian genotype) infections in dogs. *J Vet Intern Med* **18**: 494-8.

Greene, C., et al. (2006). Pneumocystosis. *Infectious Diseases of the Dogs and Cat.* C. Greene, Elsevier: 651-8.

Lin, E. C. Y., et al. (2012). The therapeutic efficacy of two antibabesial strategies against Babesia gibsoni. *Veterinary Parasitology* **186**(3-4): 159-64.

Atracurium Besylate

(a-tra-**cure**-ee-um)   Tracrium®

Nondepolarizing Neuromuscular Blocker

Prescriber Highlights

▶ Non-depolarizing neuromuscular blocking agent; minimal cardiovascular effects; valuable in critically ill patients who cannot receive standard inhalant anesthesia concentrations. Should never be given as a sole agent; has no sedative or analgesic effects.

▶ Intraurethral administration in male cats may assist in urethral plug removal.

▶ More potent in horses than other species.

▶ Relatively contraindicated in patients with myasthenia gravis, hypersensitivity to it.

▶ Less incidence of histamine release than tubocurarine or metocurine.

▶ Potential drug interactions.

Uses/Indications

Atracurium is indicated as an adjunct to general anesthesia to produce muscle relaxation during surgical procedures or mechanical ventilation and also to facilitate endotracheal intubation. Atracurium can be used in patients with significant renal or hepatic disease. It is valuable to paralyze critically ill patients when very low settings, or no inhalant anesthesia can be used.

Intraurethral administration of atracurium in male cats with urethral plugs has been shown to increase the proportion (64% vs. 15% control) of obstruction removal with the first attempt (Galluzzi et al. 2012).

Pharmacology/Actions

Atracurium is a nondepolarizing neuromuscular blocking agent and acts by competitively binding at cholinergic receptor sites at the motor end-plate thereby inhibiting the effects of acetylcholine. Atracurium is considered 1/4 to 1/3 as potent as pancuronium. In horses, atracurium is more potent than in other species tested and more potent than other nondepolarizing muscle relaxants studied.

Atracurium does not provide any analgesia or sedation.

Neuromuscular blockade (NMB) can be variably potentiated when used with different general anesthetics. A study in dogs, demonstrated that when compared with propofol, sevoflurane prolonged atracurium-induced NMB by about 15 minutes (Kastrup et al. 2005).

At usual doses, atracurium exhibits minimal cardiovascular effects, unlike most other nondepolarizing neuromuscular blockers. A related compound, cis-atracurium (*Nimbex®*) has even less cardiovascular effects in cats than does atracurium. While atracurium can stimulate histamine release, it is considered to cause less histamine release than either tubocurarine or metocurine. In humans, less than one percent of patients receiving atracurium exhibit clinically significant adverse reactions or histamine release.

Pharmacokinetics

After IV injection, maximal neuromuscular blockade generally occurs within 3-5 minutes. The duration of maximal blockade increases as the dosage increases. Systemic alkalosis may diminish the degree and duration of blockade; acidosis potentiates it. In conjunction with balanced anesthesia, the duration of blockade generally persists for 20-35 minutes. Recovery times do not appreciably change after giving maintenance doses, so predictable blocking effects can be attained when the drug is administered at regular intervals.

Atracurium is metabolized by ester hydrolysis and Hofmann elimination that occur independently of renal or hepatic function.

Physiologic pH and temperature can affect elimination of atracurium. Increased body temperature can enhance the elimination of the drug. Ester hydrolysis is enhanced by decreases in pH, while Hofmann elimination is reduced by decreases in pH.

Contraindications/Precautions/Warnings

Atracurium is contraindicated in patients who are hypersensitive to it. Because it may rarely cause significant release of histamine, it should be used with caution in patients where this would be hazardous (*e.g.*, severe cardiovascular disease, asthma, etc.). Atracurium has minimal cardiac effects and will not counteract the bradycardia or vagal stimulation induced by other agents. Use of neuromuscular blocking agents must be done with extreme caution in patients suffering from myasthenia gravis (MG). It has been reported that atracurium can be safely used in dogs with MG if dosed at 16-20% of the normal dose and if neuromuscular transmission is monitored throughout the procedure (Jones 2012). Atracurium has no analgesic or sedative/anesthetic actions. To provide amnesia in critically ill patients, when no inhalant anesthesia can be used, midazolam should be considered. Either intermittent boluses (0.1 mg/kg IV every 20-30 minutes) or a continuous IV infusion (0.1 mg/kg/hr) of midazolam has been recommended (Spelts 2009).

It is not known whether this drug is excreted in milk. Safety for use in the nursing mother has not been established.

Adverse Effects

Clinically significant adverse effects are apparently quite rare in patients (<1% in humans) receiving recommended doses of atracurium and usually are secondary to histamine release. They can include: allergic reactions, inadequate or prolonged block, hypotension vasodilatation, bradycardia, tachycardia, dyspnea, broncho-, laryngo-spasm, rash, urticaria, and a reaction at the injection site. Patients developing hypotension usually have preexisting severe cardiovascular disease. Large dosages or rapid administration can release histamine.

Overdosage/Acute Toxicity

Monitoring muscle twitch responses to peripheral nerve stimulation can minimize overdosage possibilities. Increased risks of hypotension and histamine release occur with overdoses, as well as prolonged duration of muscle blockade.

Besides treating conservatively (mechanical ventilation, O_2, fluids, etc.), reversal of blockade may be accomplished by administering an anticholinesterase agent such as edrophonium (0.5 mg/kg IV), or neostigmine (0.02 – 0.04 mg/kg IV) with an anticholinergic (atropine or glycopyrrolate). Reversal is usually attempted (in humans) approximately 20-35 minutes after the initial dose, or 10-30 minutes after the last maintenance dose. Reversal is usually complete within 8-10 minutes. Because the duration of action of atracurium may be longer than the reversal agent, careful observation and monitoring is required. Readministration of the reversal agent may be necessary.

Drug Interactions

The following drug interactions with atracurium have either been reported or are theoretical in humans or animals and may be of significance in veterinary patients. Unless otherwise noted, use together is not necessarily contraindicated, but weigh the potential risks and perform additional monitoring when appropriate.

The following drugs may enhance the neuromuscular blocking activity of atracurium:

- **AMINOGLYCOSIDE ANTIBIOTICS** (*e.g.*, **gentamicin**, etc.)
- **ANESTHETICS, GENERAL** (*e.g.*, **enflurane, isoflurane, halothane**)
- **BACITRACIN, POLYMYXIN B (systemic)**
- **PROCAINAMIDE**
- **QUINIDINE**
- **LITHIUM**
- **MAGNESIUM SALTS**

ANTICONVULSANTS (*e.g.*, **phenytoin, carbamazepine**): Have been reported to both decrease the effects and duration of neuromuscular blockade.

- **OTHER MUSCLE RELAXANT DRUGS:** May cause a synergistic or antagonistic effect.
- **SUCCINYLCHOLINE:** May speed the onset of action and enhance the neuromuscular blocking actions of atracurium. Do not give atracurium until succinylcholine effects have diminished.

Doses

- **DOGS:**

For surgical muscle relaxation (extra-label):

a) **For use in critically ill patients when low concentrations of, or no inhalant anesthesia can be used:** 0.2 mg/kg IV initial dose; subsequent doses 0.1 mg/kg IV. Do not dose more frequently than every 20-30 minutes in critical patients unless a peripheral nerve stimulator is applied, or voluntary movement is observed. Positive pressure ventilation, preferably mechanical, is required. (Spelts 2009)

b) **As a muscle relaxant to facilitate intubation in patients with severe blunt trauma:** IV started and acepromazine 0.01 mg/kg plus butorphanol 0.1 mg/kg plus ketamine 1 mg/kg is infused. If patient requires intubation, give atracurium at 0.25 mg/kg IV push. (Crowe 2004)

c) **For induction of respiratory muscle paralysis during mechanical ventilation:** Loading dose: 0.2 – 0.5 mg/kg IV, then a constant rate infusion 5 minutes later of 3 – 9 micrograms/kg/minute. Use D5W or 0.9% sodium chloride for diluent; do not mix with other drugs. Respiratory and cardiovascular monitoring should be provided. (Dhupa 2005)

- **CATS:**

For surgical muscle relaxation (extra-label):

a) **For induction of respiratory muscle paralysis during mechanical ventilation:** Loading dose: 0.2 – 0.5 mg/kg IV, then a constant rate infusion 5 minutes later of 0.37 micrograms/kg/minute. Use D5W or 0.9% sodium chloride for diluent; do not mix with other drugs. Respiratory and cardiovascular monitoring should be provided. (Dhupa 2005)

b) **For use in critically ill patients when low concentrations of, or no inhalant anesthesia can be used:** 0.2 mg/kg IV initial dose; subsequent doses 0.1 mg/kg IV. Do not dose more frequently than every 20-30 minutes in critical patients unless a peripheral nerve stimulator is applied, or voluntary movement is observed. Positive pressure ventilation, preferably mechanical, is required. (Spelts 2009)

For removal of urethral plugs in male cats (extra-label): 0.2 mL of 10 mg/mL injection diluted in 3.8 mL of normal saline; final concentration 0.5 mg/mL. Then instilled via catheter with steady, gentle pressure over 5 minutes while urethra pressed with two fingers to prevent leakage. Retrograde flushing with saline performed for a maximum of 20 seconds. If obstruction not removed with first attempt, procedure repeated. (Galluzzi et al. 2012)

- **RABBITS/RODENTS/SMALL MAMMALS:**

Rabbits: For paralysis for periophthalmic surgery (extra-label): 0.1 mg/kg. (Ivey et al. 2000)

■ **HORSES:** (NOTE: ARCI UCGFS CLASS 2 DRUG)

For surgical muscle relation (extra-label): Has been extensively used at doses ranging between 0.07 and 0.2 mg/kg without any major complications being reported. (Martin-Flores 2013)

Monitoring

■ Level of neuromuscular blockade; recommend use of a peripheral nerve stimulator to evaluate "train of 4" twitches. If not available, watch for spontaneous ventilation and voluntary muscle movement.

■ Cardiac rate.

Client Information

■ This drug should only be used by professionals familiar with its use.

Chemistry/Synonyms

A synthetic, non-depolarizing neuromuscular blocking agent, atracurium, is a bisquaternary, non-choline diester structurally similar to metocurine and tubocurarine. It occurs as white to pale yellow powder; 50 mg are soluble in 1 mL of water, 200 mg are soluble in 1 mL of alcohol, and 35 mg are soluble in 1 mL of normal saline.

Atracurium besylate may also be known as: 33A74, atracurium besilate, BW-33A, *Abbottracurium®*, *Atracur®*, *Faulcurium®*, *Ifacur®*, *Laurak®*, *Mycurium®*, *Relatrac®*, *Sitrac®*, *Trablok®*, *Tracrium®*, or *Tracur®*.

Storage/Stability

The commercially available injection occurs as clear, colorless solution and is a sterile solution of the drug in sterile water for injection. The pH of this solution is 3.25- 3.65. Atracurium injection should be stored in the refrigerator and protected against freezing. At room temperature, approximately 5% potency loss occurs each month; when refrigerated, a 6% potency loss occurs over a year's time.

Compatibility/Compounding Considerations

Atracurium is **compatible** with the standard IV solutions, but while stable in lactated Ringer's for 8 hours, degradation occurs more rapidly. It should not be mixed in the same IV bag or syringe, or given through the same needle with alkaline drugs (*e.g.*, barbiturates) or solutions (sodium bicarbonate) as precipitation may occur. It is **incompatible** when mixed with propofol, diazepam, thiopental, aminophylline, cefazolin, heparin, ranitidine, and sodium nitroprusside.

Dosage Forms/Regulatory Status

VETERINARY-LABELED PRODUCTS: NONE.

The ARCI (Racing Commissioners International) has designated this drug as a class 2 substance. See the appendix for more information.

HUMAN-LABELED PRODUCTS:

Atracurium Besylate Injection: 10 mg/mL in 5 mL single-use & 10 mL multi-use vials; *Tracrium®*, generic; (Rx)

Revisions/References

Monograph revised/updated August 2013.

Crowe, D. (2004). *Severe blunt trauma: Surgical intervention into the unknown.* Proceedings: IVECCS. accessed via Veterinary Information Network; vin.com

Dhupa, N. (2005). Constant rate infusions. *Textbook of Veterinary Internal Medicine, 6th Ed.* S. Ettinger and E. Feldman, Elsevier: 544-50.

Galluzzi, F., et al. (2012). Effect of intraurethral administration of atracurium besylate in male cats with urethral plugs. *Journal of Small Animal Practice* **53**(7): 411-5.

Ivey, E. & J. Morrisey (2000). Therapeutics for Rabbits. *Vet Clin NA: Exotic Anim Pract* **3**:1(Jan): 183-216.

Jones, R. S. (2012). The use of neuromuscular blocking agents for thymectomy in myasthenia gravis. *Veterinary Anaesthesia and Analgesia* **39**(2): 220-.

Kastrup, M. R., et al. (2005). Neuromuscular blocking properties of atracurium during sevoflurane or propofol anaesthesia in dogs. *Veterinary Anaesthesia and Analgesia* **32**(4): 222-7.

Martin-Flores, M. (2013). Neuromuscular Blocking Agents and Monitoring in the Equine Patient. *Veterinary Clinics of North America-Equine Practice* **29**(1): 131-+.

Spelts, K. (2009). *Anesthesia for the critically ill patient.* Proceedings: WVC. accessed via Veterinary Information Network; vin.com

Atropine Sulfate

(a-troe-peen)

Anticholinergic

Prescriber Highlights

▶ Prototype antimuscarinic agent used for a variety of indications (*e.g.*, bradycardia, premed, antidote, etc.).

▶ Contraindicated in conditions where anticholinergic effects would be detrimental (*e.g.*, narrow angle glaucoma, tachycardias, ileus, urinary obstruction, etc.).

▶ Adverse effects are dose related & anticholinergic in nature: 1) dry secretions, 2) initial bradycardia, then tachycardia, 3) slowed gut & urinary tract, 4) mydriasis/cycloplegia.

▶ Drug interactions.

Uses/Indications

The principal veterinary indications for systemic atropine include:

■ Preanesthetic to prevent or reduce secretions of the respiratory tract.

■ Treat sinus bradycardia, sinoatrial arrest, and incomplete AV block.

■ Differentiate vagally-mediated bradycardia for other causes.

■ As an antidote for overdoses of cholinergic agents (*e.g.*, physostigmine, etc.).

■ As an antidote for organophosphate, carbamate, muscarinic mushroom, blue-green algae intoxication.

■ Hypersialism; reduce secretions.

■ Treatment (adjunctive) of bronchoconstrictive disease.

Pharmacology/Actions

Atropine, like other antimuscarinic agents, competitively inhibits acetylcholine or other cholinergic stimulants at postganglionic parasympathetic neuroeffector sites. High doses may block nicotinic receptors at the autonomic ganglia and at the neuromuscular junction. Pharmacologic effects are dose related. At low doses salivation, bronchial secretions, and sweating (not horses) are inhibited. At moderate systemic doses, atropine dilates and inhibits accommodation of the pupil, and increases heart rate. High doses will decrease GI and urinary tract motility. Very high doses will inhibit gastric secretion.

Pharmacokinetics

Atropine sulfate is well absorbed after oral administration, IM injection, inhalation, or endotracheal administration. After IV administration peak effects in heart rates occur within 3-4 minutes.

Atropine is well distributed throughout the body and crosses into the CNS, across the placenta, and can distribute into the milk in small quantities.

Atropine is metabolized in the liver and excreted into the urine. Approximately 30-50% of a dose is excreted unchanged into the urine. The plasma half-life in humans has been reported to be between 2-3 hours.

Contraindications/Precautions/Warnings

Atropine is contraindicated in patients with narrow-angle glaucoma, synechiae (adhesions) between the iris and lens, hypersensitivity to anticholinergic drugs, tachycardias secondary to thyrotoxicosis or cardiac insufficiency, myocardial ischemia, unstable cardiac status during acute hemorrhage, GI obstructive disease, paralytic ileus, severe ulcerative colitis, obstructive uropathy, and myasthenia gravis (unless used to reverse adverse muscarinic effects secondary to therapy). Atropine may aggravate some signs seen with amitraz toxicity, leading to hypertension and further inhibition of peristalsis.

Atropine is not recommended for treating bradycardias secondary to dexmedetomidine.

Antimuscarinic agents should be used with extreme caution in patients with known or suspected GI infections. Atropine or other antimuscarinic agents can decrease GI motility and prolong retention of the causative agent(s) or toxin(s) resulting in prolonged clinical signs. Antimuscarinic agents must also be used with extreme caution in patients with autonomic neuropathy.

Atropine reportedly is not effective in treating bradycardias in puppies before 14 days of age or kittens younger than 11 days old. It may also damage hypoxic myocardia in neonates (Trass 2009).

Glycopyrrolate is usually the anticholinergic of choice when treating rabbits as a large percentage (40%?) have endogenous atropinesterase present.

Antimuscarinic agents should be used with caution in patients with hepatic or renal disease, geriatric or pediatric patients, hyperthyroidism, hypertension, CHF, tachyarrhythmias, prostatic hypertrophy, or esophageal reflux. Systemic atropine should be used cautiously in horses as it may decrease gut motility and induce colic in susceptible animals. It may also reduce the arrhythmogenic doses of epinephrine. Use of atropine in cattle may result in inappetence and rumen stasis that may persist for several days.

When used in food animals at doses up to 0.2 mg/kg, FARAD recommends a 28-day meat and 6-day milk withdrawal time. (Haskell et al. 2005)

Adverse Effects

Adverse effects are basically extensions of the drug's pharmacologic effects and are generally dose related. At usual doses, effects tend to be mild in relatively healthy patients. The more severe effects listed tend to occur with high or toxic doses. GI effects can include dry mouth (xerostomia), increased viscosity of secretions, dysphagia, constipation, vomiting, and thirst. GU effects may include urinary retention or hesitancy. CNS effects may include stimulation, drowsiness, ataxia, seizures, respiratory depression, etc. Ophthalmic effects include blurred vision, pupil dilation, cycloplegia, and photophobia. Cardiovascular effects include sinus tachycardia (at higher doses), increased myocardial work and oxygen consumption, bradycardia (initially, or at very low doses), hypertension, hypotension, arrhythmias (ectopic complexes), and circulatory failure.

Reproductive/Nursing Safety

In humans, the FDA categorizes this drug as category **C** for use during pregnancy (*Animal studies have shown an adverse effect on the fetus, but there are no adequate studies in humans; or there are no animal reproduction studies and no adequate studies in humans.*) In a separate system evaluating the safety of drugs in canine and feline pregnancy (Papich 1989), this drug is categorized as class: **B** (*Safe for use if used cautiously. Studies in laboratory animals may have uncovered some risk, but these drugs appear to be safe in dogs and cats or these drugs are safe if they are not administered when the animal is near term.*) Atropine use in pregnancy may cause fetal tachycardia.

Overdosage/Acute Toxicity

For signs and symptoms of atropine toxicity see adverse effects above. If a recent oral ingestion, emptying of gut contents and administration of activated charcoal and saline cathartics may be warranted. Treat clinical signs supportively and symptomatically. Do not use phenothiazines as they may contribute to the anticholinergic effects. Fluid therapy and standard treatments for shock may be instituted.

The use of physostigmine is controversial and should probably be reserved for cases where the patient exhibits either extreme agitation and is at risk for injuring themselves or others, or for cas-

es where supraventricular tachycardias and sinus tachycardias are severe or life threatening. The usual dose for physostigmine (human) is: 2 mg IV slowly (for average sized adult). If no response, may repeat every 20 minutes until reversal of toxic antimuscarinic effects or cholinergic effects takes place. The human pediatric dose is 0.02 mg/kg slow IV (repeat q10 minutes as above) and may be a reasonable choice for initial treatment of small animals. Physostigmine adverse effects (bronchoconstriction, bradycardia, seizures) may be treated with small doses of IV atropine.

Drug Interactions

The following drug interactions with atropine have either been reported or are theoretical in humans or animals and may be of significance in veterinary patients. Unless otherwise noted, use together is not necessarily contraindicated, but weigh the potential risks and perform additional monitoring when appropriate.

The following drugs may enhance the activity or toxicity of atropine and its derivatives:

- **AMANTADINE**
- **ANTICHOLINERGIC AGENTS (other)**
- **ANTICHOLINERGIC MUSCLE RELAXANTS**
- **ANTIHISTAMINES** (*e.g.,* **diphenhydramine**)
- **MEPERIDINE**
- **PHENOTHIAZINES**
- **PROCAINAMIDE**
- **PRIMIDONE**
- **TRICYCLIC ANTIDEPRESSANTS** (*e.g.,* **amitriptyline, clomipramine**)

- **ALPHA-2 AGONISTS** (*e.g.,* **dexmedetomidine, medetomidine**): Use of atropine with alpha-2 blockers may significantly increase arterial blood pressure, heart rates and the incidence of arrhythmias (Congdon et al. 2009). Clinical use of atropine or glycopyrrolate to prevent or treat medetomidine- or dexmedetomidine-caused bradycardia is controversial and many discourage using together. This may be particularly important when using higher dosages of the alpha-2 agonist.
- **AMITRAZ**: Atropine may aggravate some signs seen with amitraz toxicity; leading to hypertension and further inhibition of peristalsis.
- **ANTACIDS**: May decrease PO atropine absorption; give oral atropine at least 1 hour prior to oral antacids.
- **CORTICOSTEROIDS** (**long-term use**): May increase intraocular pressure.
- **DIGOXIN** (**slow-dissolving**): Atropine may increase serum digoxin levels; use regular digoxin tablets or oral liquid.
- **KETOCONAZOLE**: Increased gastric pH may decrease GI absorption; administer oral atropine 2 hours after ketoconazole.
- **METOCLOPRAMIDE**: Atropine and its derivatives may antagonize the actions of metoclopramide.

Doses

Note: As FDA-approval has not been required for atropine products in animals all dosages should be considered extra-label.

- **DOGS/CATS:**

  As a preanesthetic adjuvant: Generally, 0.02 mg/kg IM or IV. Consider smaller dosages (0.01 mg/kg) in geriatric or debilitated patients. The veterinary label lists 0.074 mg/kg IV, IM, or SC, but this is usually not recommended today.

  During cardiopulmonary cerebral resuscitation (CPCR) efforts for adjunctive treatment of bradycardias, incomplete AV block, etc.: Atropine at 0.04 mg/kg IV or IO (intraosseous) is most likely to be useful (although not strongly supported in the literature) in dogs/cats with asystole or pulseless electrical activity (PEA) that is associated with high vagal tone. Due to a lack of any clear detrimental effect routine use of atropine (0.04 mg/kg IV or IO; may repeat every other BLS cycle) during CPR can be considered. Intratracheal administration at 0.15 – 0.2 mg/kg can be considered when intravenous or intraosseous access is not possible. (Fletcher et al. 2012)

To differentiate vagally-mediated bradyarrhythmias from non-vagal bradyarrhythmias in dogs (Atropine Response Test):

Rishniw Preference: 1) Record ECG at baseline; 2) Administer 0.04 mg/kg atropine IV; 3) Wait 15 minutes; 4) Record ECG for at least 2 minutes (use slow paper speed). If the response is incomplete, repeat steps 2 through 4. Persistent sinus tachycardia at >140 bpm is expected in most dogs with vagally-mediated bradycardia.

Kittleson Preference: 1) Record ECG at baseline; 2) Administer 0.04 mg/kg atropine SQ; 3) Wait 30 minutes; 4) Record ECG for at least 2 minutes (use slow paper speed). Persistent sinus tachycardia at >140 bpm is expected in most dogs with vagally-mediated bradycardia. (Rishniw et al. 2007)

For treatment of organophosphate/carbamate poisoning: If poisoning/OD is suspected: Get baseline heart rate. Give test dose of atropine (0.02 mg/kg) IV. If heart rate increases and the pupils dilate, likely not organophosphate/OP; look for other causes for signs as it generally requires 10 times (0.2 mg/kg) the test dose to resolve muscarinic signs of OP/carbamate poisoning. If signs do not resolve, consider decontamination procedures when appropriate, supportive care and seizure control if necessary. Muscarinic signs (salivation, lacrimation, urination, defecation, dyspnea, emesis; SLUDDE), miosis and bradycardia can be treated with atropine at 0.2 mg/kg (1/4th of the dose IV, remainder IM or SC). Repeat as required. Atropine will not reverse nicotinic (muscular weakness, etc.) or CNS (seizures) effects. (Wismer et al. 2012)

For treatment of muscarinic mushroom toxicity: Initial dosage of 0.04 mg/kg (1/4th of the dose IV, remainder IM or SC). Can titrate dosage upwards and repeat if required to control severe signs, but avoid over treating. Muscarinic signs usually resolve in 30 minutes. Give supportive care (e.g., IV fluids) as needed. (Puschner et al. 2012)

- **FERRETS:**

  As a premed: 0.05 mg/kg SC or IM. (Williams 2000)

- **RABBITS/RODENTS/SMALL MAMMALS:**

  To treat organophosphate toxicity: 10 mg/kg SC q20 minutes. (Ivey et al. 2000)

- **CATTLE:**

  Note: When used in food animals at doses of 0.1 mg/kg or 0.2 mg/kg, FARAD recommends a 14 or 28 day meat and 3 or 6 day milk withdrawal times, respectively. (Haskell et al. 2005)

  For treatment of cholinergic toxicity (organophosphates): 0.5 mg/kg (average dose); give 1/4th of the dose IV and the remainder SC or IM; repeat and titrate dosages as required.

- **HORSES:** (NOTE: ARCI UCGFS CLASS 3 DRUG)

  For treatment of bradyarrhythmias due to increased parasympathetic tone: 0.01 – 0.02 mg/kg IV. (Mogg 1999)

  As a bronchodilator: 5 – 7 mg IV per horse (450 kg) can serve as a rescue medication in cases with severe airway obstruction, but it has an abbreviated duration of action (0.5-2 hours) and adverse effects (ileus, CNS toxicity, tachycardia, increased mucus secretion, and impaired mucociliary clearance) limit its use to a single rescue dose. (Rush 2006)

For organophosphate poisoning: Most recommendations are similar to the small animal dosage: 0.2 mg/kg (1/4th IV and remainder IM or SC); repeat every 1.5-6 hours as necessary. Mydriasis and absence of salivation can be used as therapy endpoints. Do not over use as gut stasis is a concern.

- **SWINE:**

  For organophosphate poisoning: The equine dose (above) may be used to initially treat.

  As an adjunctive preanesthetic agent: 0.04 mg/kg IM. (Thurmon et al. 1986)

- **SHEEP, GOATS:**

  For treating organophosphate toxicity: Use the dose for cattle (above).

- **BIRDS:**

  For organophosphate poisoning: 0.2 mg/kg IM every 3-4 hours as needed; 1/4th the initial dose is administered. Use with pralidoxime (not in raptors) at 10 – 20 mg/kg IM q8-12h as needed. Do not use pralidoxime in carbamate poisonings. To assist in diagnosing organophosphate poisoning (with history, clinical signs, etc.) in birds presenting with bradycardia: May administer atropine at 0.02 mg/kg IV. If bradycardia does not reverse, may consider organophosphate toxicity. (LaBonde 2006)

  As a preanesthetic: 0.04 – 0.1 mg/kg IM or SC once. (Clubb 1986)

  For adjunctive treatment of cardiac arrest (CPR): 0.2 mg/kg IV with ventilation and epinephrine (0.1 mg/kg diluted in saline and into the trachea). (O'Malley 2011)

- **REPTILES:**

  For organophosphate toxicity in most species: 0.1 – 0.2 mg/kg SC or IM as needed. (Gauvin 1993)

  For ptyalism in tortoises: 0.05 mg/kg (50 micrograms/kg) SC or IM once daily. (Gauvin 1993)

Monitoring

Dependent on dose and indication:
- Heart rate and rhythm.
- Thirst/appetite; urination/defecation capability.
- Mouth/secretions dryness.

Client Information

- Parenteral atropine administration is best performed by professional staff and where adequate cardiac monitoring is available.
- If animal is receiving atropine systemically, allow animal free access to water and encourage drinking if dry mouth is a problem.

Chemistry/Synonyms

The prototype tertiary amine antimuscarinic agent, atropine sulfate is derived from the naturally occurring atropine. It is a racemic mixture of d-hyoscyamine and l-hyoscyamine. The l- form of the drug is active, while the d- form has practically no antimuscarinic activity. Atropine sulfate occurs as colorless and odorless crystals, or white, crystalline powder. One gram of atropine sulfate is soluble in approximately 0.5 mL of water, 5 mL of alcohol, or 2.5 mL of glycerin. Aqueous solutions are practically neutral or only slightly acidic. Commercially available injections may have the pH adjusted to 3.0-6.5.

Atropine may also be known as dl-hyoscyamine. Atropine sulfate may also be known as: atrop. sulph., atropine sulphate, or atropini sulfas; many trade names are available.

Storage/Stability

Atropine sulfate tablets or soluble tablets should be stored in well-closed containers at room temperature (15-30°C). Atropine sulfate for injection should be stored at room temperature; avoid freezing.

Compatibility/Compounding Considerations

Atropine sulfate for injection is reportedly **compatible** with the following agents: benzquinamide HCl, butorphanol tartrate, chlorpromazine HCl, cimetidine HCl (not with pentobarbital), dimenhydrinate, diphenhydramine HCl, dobutamine HCl, fentanyl citrate, glycopyrrolate, hydromorphone HCl, hydroxyzine HCl (also with meperidine), meperidine HCl, morphine sulfate, nalbuphine HCl, pentazocine lactate, pentobarbital sodium (OK for 5 minutes, not 24 hours), perphenazine, prochlorperazine edisylate, promazine HCl, promethazine HCl (also with meperidine), and scopolamine HBr.

Atropine sulfate is reported physically **incompatible** with norepinephrine bitartrate, metaraminol bitartrate, methohexital sodium, and sodium bicarbonate. Compatibility is dependent upon factors such as pH, concentration, temperature, and diluent used; consult specialized references for more specific information.

Dosage Forms/Regulatory Status

VETERINARY-LABELED PRODUCTS:

Atropine Sulfate for Injection: 0.54 mg/mL (1/120 grain); (Rx)

Atropine Sulfate for Injection: 15 mg/mL (organophosphate treatment) 100 mL vial; (Rx)

Atropine is labeled for use in dogs, cats, horses, cattle, sheep, and swine in the USA, but actual FDA-approval has not been required. No withdrawal times are mandated when used in food animals in the USA, but FARAD recommends a 28 day meat and 6 day milk withdrawal time (Haskell et al. 2005). In the UK, slaughter withdrawal for cattle, sheep, and pigs is 14 days when used as an antimuscarinic and 28 days when used as an antidote; milk withdrawal is 3 days when used as an antimuscarinic and 6 days when used as an antidote. For guidance with determining use associated withdrawal times, contact FARAD (see Phone Numbers & Websites in the appendix).

The ARCI (Racing Commissioners International) has designated this drug as a class 3 substance. See the appendix for more information.

HUMAN-LABELED PRODUCTS:

Atropine Sulfate for Injection:

0.05 mg/mL in 5 mL syringes; (Rx)

0.1 mg/mL in 5 mL and 10 mL syringes; (Rx)

0.3 mg/mL in 1 mL and 30 mL vials; (Rx)

0.4 mg/mL in 1 mL amps and 1 mL, 20 mL, and 30 mL vials; (Rx)

0.5mg/mL in 1mL and 30 mL vials & 5 mL syringes; (Rx)

0.8 mg/mL in 0.5 mL and 1 mL amps and 0.5 mL syringes; (Rx)

1 mg/mL in 1 mL amps and vials and 10 mL syringes; (Rx)

0.5 mg, 1 mg & 2 mg pre-filled, auto-injectors; *AtroPen®*; (Rx)

Atropine Sulfate Tablets: 0.4 mg; *Sal-Tropine®*; (Rx)

See also the monograph for atropine sulfate for ophthalmic use in the appendix. Atropine sulfate ophthalmic drops have been used buccally to decrease excessive oral secretions in human patients.

Revisions/References

Monograph revised/updated August 2013.

Clubb, S. L. (1986). Therapeutics: Individual and Flock Treatment Regimens. *Clinical Avian Medicine and Surgery.* G. J. Harrison and L. R. Harrison. Philadelphia, W.B. Saunders: 327-55.

Congdon, J., et al. (2009). *Cardiovascular and sedation paramerters during dexmedetomidine and atropine administration.* Prtoceedings: IVECCS. accessed via Veterinary Information Network; vin.com

Fletcher, D. J., et al. (2012). RECOVER evidence and knowledge gap analysis on veterinary CPR. Part 7: Clinical guidelines. *J. Vet. Emerg. Crit. Care* **22**.

Gauvin, J. (1993). Drug therapy in reptiles. *Seminars in Avian & Exotic Med* **2**(1): 48-59.

Haskell, S., et al. (2005). Farad Digest: Antidotes in Food Animal Practice. *JAVMA* **226**(6): 884-7.

Ivey, E. & J. Morrisey (2000). Therapeutics for Rabbits. *Vet Clin NA: Exotic Anim Pract* **3:1**(Jan): 183-216.

LaBonde, J. (2006). *Avian Toxicology.* Proceedings: AAV. accessed via Veterinary Information Network; vin.com

Mogg, T. (1999). Equine Cardiac Disease: Clinical pharmacology and therapeutics. *The Veterinary Clinics of North America: Equine Practice* **15**:3(December).

O'Malley, B. (2011). *Avian Emergencies.* World Small Animal Veterinary Association World Congress Proceedings. accessed via Veterinary Information Network; vin.com

Puschner, B. & C. Wegenast (2012). Mushroom Poisoning Cases in Dogs and Cats: Diagnosis and Treatment of Hepatotoxic, Neurotoxic, Gastroenterotoxic, Nephrotoxic, and Muscarinic Mushrooms. *Vet Clin Small Anim* **42**: 375-87.

Rishniw, M. & M. Kittleson (2007). "Atropine Response Test."

Rush, B. (2006). *Use of inhalation therapy in management of recurrent airway obstruction.* Proceedings: ACVIM. accessed via Veterinary Information Network; vin.com

Thurmon, J. C. & G. J. Benson (1986). Anesthesia in ruminants and swine. *Current Veterinary Therapy 2: Food Animal Practice.* J. L. Howard. Philadelphia, WB Saunders: 51-71.

Trass, A. (2009). *Pediatric Emergencies.* Proceedings: IVECCS. accessed via Veterinary Information Network; vin.com

Williams, B. (2000). Therapeutics in Ferrets. *Vet Clin NA: Exotic Anim Pract* **3:1**(Jan): 131-53.

Wismer, T. & C. Means (2012). Toxicology of Newer Insecticides in Small Animals. *Veterinary Clinics of North America-Small Animal Practice* **42**(2): 335-+.

Auranofin

(au-**rane**-oh-fin)   Ridaura®

Oral Gold Immunosuppressive

Prescriber Highlights

▶ Orally administered gold; can be tried for pemphigus & idiopathic polyarthritis in dogs or cats.

▶ Can be quite toxic & expensive, intensive ongoing monitoring required; dosages must be compounded from 3 mg capsules.

▶ Considered contraindicated in SLE (exacerbates).

▶ Renal, hepatic & GI toxicity possible; dose dependmediated thrombocytopenia, hemolytic anemia or leukopenias have been seen.

Uses/Indications

Auranofin has been used to treat idiopathic polyarthritis and pemphigus complex in dogs and cats. Several clinicians report that while auranofin may be less toxic, it also less efficacious than injectable gold (aurothioglucose; no longer marketed). There is very limited information published on the safety and efficacy of this drug in dogs and cats.

Pharmacology/Actions

Auranofin is an orally available gold salt. Gold has antiinflammatory, antirheumatic, immunomodulating, and antimicrobial (*in vitro*) effects. The exact mechanisms for these actions are not well understood. Gold is taken up by macrophages where it inhibits phagocytosis and may inhibit lysosomal enzyme activity. Gold also inhibits the release of histamine, and the production of prostaglandins. While gold does have antimicrobial effects *in vitro*, it is not clinically useful for this purpose. Auranofin suppresses helper T-cells, without affecting suppressor T-cell populations.

Pharmacokinetics

Unlike other available gold salts, auranofin is absorbed when given by mouth (20-25% of the gold) primarily in the small and large intestines. In contrast to the other gold salts, auranofin is only moderately bound to plasma proteins (the others are highly bound). Auranofin crosses the placenta and is distributed into maternal milk. Tissues with the highest levels of gold are kidneys, spleen, lungs, adrenals and liver. Accumulation of gold does not appear to occur, unlike the parenteral gold salts. About 15% of an administered dose (60% of the absorbed dose) is excreted by the kidneys, the remainder in the feces.

Contraindications/Precautions/Warnings

Auranofin should only be administered to animals where other less expensive and toxic therapies are ineffective and the veterinarian and owner are aware of the potential pitfalls of auranofin therapy and willing to accept the associated risks and expenses. Gold salts are contraindicated in SLE as they may exacerbate the signs associated with this disease.

Adverse Effects
A dose dependent immune-mediated thrombocytopenia, hemolytic anemia or leukopenias have been noted in dogs. Discontinuation of the drug and administration of steroids has been recommended. Auranofin has a higher incidence of dose dependent GI disturbances (particularly diarrhea) in dogs than with the injectable products. Discontinuation of the drug or a lowered dose will generally resolve the problem. Renal toxicity manifested by proteinuria is possible as is hepatotoxicity (increased liver enzymes). These effects are less likely than either the GI or hematologic effects. Dermatoses including toxic epidermal necrolysis, and corneal ulcers have been associated with auranofin therapy.

Reproductive/Nursing Safety
Auranofin has been demonstrated to be teratogenic and maternotoxic in laboratory animals; it should not be used during pregnancy unless the owner accepts the potential risks of use. In humans, the FDA categorizes this drug as category **C** for use during pregnancy (*Animal studies have shown an adverse effect on the fetus, but there are no adequate studies in humans; or there are no animal reproduction studies and no adequate studies in humans.*)

Following auranofin administration, gold is excreted in the milk of rodents. Trace amounts appear in the serum and red blood cells of nursing offspring. As this may cause adverse effects in nursing offspring, switching to milk replacer is recommended if auranofin is to be continued in the dam. Because gold is slowly excreted, persistence in milk will occur even after the drug is discontinued.

Overdosage/Acute Toxicity
Very limited data is available. The minimum lethal oral dose in rats is 30 mg/kg. It is recommended that gut-emptying protocols be employed after an acute overdose when applicable. Chelating agents (*e.g.*, penicillamine, dimercaprol) for severe toxicities have been used, but are controversial. One human patient who took an overdose over 10 days developed various neurologic sequelae, but eventually (after 3 months) recovered completely after discontinuation of the drug and chelation therapy.

Drug Interactions
The following drug interactions with auranofin have either been reported or are theoretical in humans or animals and may be of significance in veterinary patients. Unless otherwise noted, use together is not necessarily contraindicated, but weigh the potential risks and perform additional monitoring when appropriate.
- **CYTOTOXIC AGENTS** (including **high dose corticosteroids**): Auranofin's safety when used with these agents has not been established; use with caution.
- **PENICILLAMINE or ANTIMALARIAL DRUGS**: Use with gold salts is not recommended due to the increased potential for hematologic or renal toxicity.

Laboratory Considerations
- In humans, response to **tuberculin skin tests** may be enhanced; veterinary significance is unclear.

Doses
- **DOGS:**

  For immune-mediated skin diseases in patients unresponsive to, or that cannot tolerate more conventional therapy (*e.g.*, glucocorticoids or azathioprine); (extra-label): 0.05 – 0.2 mg/kg (up to 9 mg/day total dose per dog) PO two times a day; often in conjunction with glucocorticoids. Allow a 4-week "wash out" before starting therapy after azathioprine discontinued. A lag phase of 6-12 weeks can occur before response can be seen. If remission is

achieved, pulse therapy 1 – 2 mg/kg PO every other week for one month and then once monthly can be attempted. If remission is maintained for 6 months, can attempt discontinuation.
- **CATS:**

  For immune-mediated skin diseases (*e.g.*, feline pemphigus, eosinophilic granuloma complex and plasma cell pododermatitis and stomatitis); (extra-label): 0.2 – 0.3 mg/kg twice daily; must be reformulated for accurate dosing. (Morris 2004)

Monitoring
The following should be performed prior to therapy, then once monthly for 2-3 months, then every other month:
- Hepatic and renal function tests (including urinalysis).
- CBC, with platelet counts; **Note**: eosinophilia may denote impending reaction.

Client Information
- Clients must understand that several months may be required before a positive response may be seen.
- Commitment to the twice daily dosing schedule, the costs associated with therapy, and the potential adverse effects should be discussed before initiating therapy.

Chemistry/Synonyms
An orally administered gold compound, auranofin occurs as a white, odorless, crystalline powder. It is very slightly soluble in water and soluble in alcohol. Auranofin contains 29% gold.

Auranofin may also be known as: SKF-39162, SKF-D-39162, *Crisinor*®, *Crisofin*®, *Goldar*®, *Ridaura*® or *Ridauran*®.

Storage/Stability
Store capsules in tight, light resistant containers at room temperature. After manufacture, expiration dates of 4 years are assigned to the capsules.

Compatibility/Compounding Considerations
No specific information noted.

Dosage Forms/Regulatory Status
VETERINARY-LABELED PRODUCTS: NONE.

HUMAN-LABELED PRODUCTS:
Auranofin Capsules: 3 mg; *Ridaura*®; (Rx)

Revisions/References
Monograph revised/updated August 2013.
Morris, D. (2004). *Immunomodulatory drugs in veterinary dermatology.* Proceedings: Western Veterinary Conf 2004. accessed via Veterinary Information Network; vin.com

---

Azaperone

(a-zap-**peer**-ohne)   Stresnil®

Butyrophenone Tranquilizer

Prescriber Highlights
▶ Butyrophenone tranquilizer for swine; also used in wildlife.
▶ FDA-approved product no longer on US market; compounded dosage forms available.
▶ Do not give IV; allow pigs to be undisturbed for 20 minutes after injecting.
▶ No analgesic activity. May cause transient piling, salivation & shivering.

Uses/Indications
Azaperone is officially indicated for the "control of aggressiveness when mixing or regrouping weanling or feeder pigs weighing up to 36.4 kg" (Package Insert, *Stresnil*®—P/M; Mallinckrodt). It is also used clinically as a general tranquilizer for swine, to allow piglets to be accepted by aggressive sows, and as a preoperative agent prior to general anesthesia or cesarean section with local anesthesia.

Azaperone has been used as a neuroleptic in horses, but some horses develop adverse reactions (sweating, muscle tremors, panic reaction, CNS excitement) and IV administration has resulted in significant arterial hypotension. Because of these effects, most clinicians avoid the use of this drug in equines.

Azaperone, has been used alone as a sedative and in combination with butorphanol and medetomidine (BAM) as an immobilization combination in cervids.

Pharmacology/Actions

The butyrophenones as a class cause tranquilization and sedation (sedation may be less than with the phenothiazines), anti-emetic activity, reduced motor activity, and inhibition of CNS catecholamines (dopamine, norepinephrine). Azaperone appears to have minimal effects on respiration and may inhibit some of the respiratory depressant actions of general anesthetics. A slight reduction of arterial blood pressure has been measured in pigs after IM injections of azaperone, apparently due to slight alpha-adrenergic blockade. Azaperone has been demonstrated to prevent the development of halothane-induced malignant hyperthermia in susceptible pigs. Preliminary studies have suggested that the effects of butyrophenones may be antagonized by 4-aminopyridine.

Pharmacokinetics

Minimal information was located regarding actual pharmacokinetic parameters, but the drug is considered to have a fairly rapid onset of action following IM injections in pigs (5-10 minutes) with a peak effect at approximately 30 minutes post injection. It has a duration of action of 2-3 hours in young pigs and 3-4 hours in older swine. The drug is metabolized in the liver with 13% of it excreted in the feces. At 16 hours post-dose, practically all the drug is eliminated from the body; however in the UK a 10-day slaughter withdrawal has been assigned.

Contraindications/Precautions/Warnings

When used as directed, the manufacturer reports no contraindications (other than for slaughter withdrawal) for the drug. It should not be given IV as a significant excitatory phase may be seen in pigs. Avoid use in very cold conditions as cardiovascular collapse may occur secondary to peripheral vasodilation.

Do not exceed dosing recommendation in boars as the drug may cause the penis to be extruded.

Because Vietnamese Pot Bellied pigs may have delayed absorption due to sequestration of the drug in body fat, re-dose with extreme caution; deaths have resulted after repeat dosing.

Adverse Effects

Transient salivation, piling, panting and shivering have been reported in pigs. Pigs should be left undisturbed after injection (for approximately 20 minutes) until the drug's full effects have been expressed; disturbances during this period may trigger excitement. Azaperone has minimal analgesic effects and is not a substitute for appropriate anesthesia or analgesia. Doses above 1 mg/kg may cause the penis to be extruded in boars.

In wildlife species, azaperone can cause hypersalivation, hypotension and increased heart rates. Equids may show signs of excitement.

Overdosage/Acute Toxicity

Azaperone overdoses can cause hypotension; doses >1 mg/kg in boars may cause penis extrusion leading to damage. There is no reversal agent for azaperone; treat supportively.

Drug Interactions

No specific drug interactions have been reported for azaperone. The following interactions have been reported for the closely related compounds, haloperidol or droperidol:

- **CNS DEPRESSANT AGENTS** (*e.g.,* **barbiturates, narcotics,**

anesthetics, etc.) may cause additive CNS depression if used with butyrophenones.

Doses

- **SWINE:**

For (the formerly) FDA-approved indication of mixing feeder or weanling pigs: 2.2 mg/kg deeply IM (see client information below). (Package Insert—Stresnil®; **Note:** No longer on US market)

For labeled indications (U.K.; adapted from *Stresnil®* label—Elanco U.K.): **Note:** all doses are to be given IM directly behind the ear using a long hypodermic needle and given as closely behind the ear as possible and perpendicular to the skin.

a) **Aggression (prevention and cure of fighting; including regrouping of piglets, porkers, fattening pigs):** 2 mg/kg (1 mL/20 kg); all animals should be treated; will not prevent aggressiveness in non-castrated adult boars.

b) **Treatment of aggression in sows:** 2 mg/kg (1 mL/20 kg); ½ to 1 hour after administration sow will accept piglets including piglets from other litters.

c) **Stress (restlessness, anxiety, etc.):** 1 – 2 mg/kg (0.5 – 1 mL/20 kg); if animal is very nervous, may be given in divided doses at 15 minute intervals.

d) **Transport of boars:** 1 mg/kg (0.5 mL/20 kg); should be left alone in a quiet environment during the induction period (approximately 30 minutes). Do not exceed dose of 1 mg/kg as a higher dose may cause the penis to be extruded, which may then be damaged.

e) **Transport of weaners:** 0.4 – 2 mg/kg (0.4 – 1 mL/20 kg). Administer 15-30 minutes before transport. Dose can be increased up to 2 mg/kg to prevent fighting during transport. Assure that transport is adequately ventilated and that there is space for animals to lie down.

f) **Obstetrics:** 1 mg/kg (0.5 mL/20 kg).

g) **As a premed:** 1 – 2 mg/kg (0.5 – 1 mL/20 kg).

- **ZOO, EXOTIC, WILDLIFE SPECIES:**

For use in zoo, exotic and wildlife medicine refer to specific references, including:

a) *Zoo Animal and Wildlife Immobilization and Anesthesia.* West, G., Heard, D., Caulkett, N. (eds.). Blackwell Publishing, 2007.

b) *Handbook of Wildlife Chemical Immobilization, 3rd Ed.* Kreeger, T.J. and J.M. Arnemo. 2007.

c) *Fowler's Zoo and Wild Animal Medicine Current Therapy, Volume 7,* Miller, R.E., Fowler, M.E., Saunders. 2011.

d) *Exotic Animal Formulary, 4th Ed.* Carpenter, J.W., Saunders. 2012.

e) The 2009 American Association of Zoo Veterinarian Proceedings by D. K. Fontenot also has several dosages listed for restraint, anesthesia, and analgesia for a variety of drugs for carnivores and primates. VIN members can access them at: http://goo.gl/NNIWQ or http://goo.gl/9UJse

Monitoring

- Level of sedation.

Client Information

- Must be injected IM deeply, either behind the ear and perpendicular to the skin or in the back of the ham. All animals in groups to be mixed must be treated.

Chemistry/Synonyms

A butyrophenone neuroleptic, azaperone occurs as a white to yellowish-white macrocrystalline powder with a melting point between 90-95°C. It is practically insoluble in water; 1 gram is soluble in 29 mL of alcohol.

Azaperone may also be known as azaperonum, R-1929, *Stresnil®*, or *Suicalm®*.

Storage/Stability

Azaperone injection should be stored at controlled room temperature (15–25°C) and away from light. Do not store above 25°C. Once the vial is opened it should be used within 28 days.

Compatibility/Compounding Considerations

No published information was located regarding mixing azaperone with other compounds. A compounded product that combines butorphanol, azaperone and medetomidine (BAM) is reportedly available.

Dosage Forms/Regulatory Status

VETERINARY-LABELED PRODUCTS: NONE IN USA.

Note: No FDA-approved azaperone products are currently marketed in the USA. Compounded azaperone injection and a combination injection containing butorphanol, azaperone, and medetomidine (BAM) can be obtained from zoopharm.net.

In the UK: Azaperone 40 mg/mL for Injection in 100 mL vials; *Stresnil®* (Elanco—UK); (POM-V). Pigs may be slaughtered for human consumption only after 10 days from the last treatment.

The ARCI (Racing Commissioners International) has designated this drug as a class 2 substance. See the appendix for more information.

HUMAN-LABELED PRODUCTS: NONE.

Revisions/References

Monograph revised/updated August 2013.

Azathioprine

(ay-za-**thye**-oh-preen)   Imuran®

Immunosuppressant

Prescriber Highlights

▶ Purine antagonist immunosuppressive used for a variety of autoimmune diseases. Usually not used in cats as they are very sensitive to bone marrow effects.

▶ May take several weeks for immunosuppression to occur.

▶ Often used in combination with corticosteroids to reduce doses and dosing frequency of each drug.

▶ Known mutagen & teratogen; use with caution in patients with hepatic disease.

▶ Bone marrow depression principal adverse effect; GI effects (including GI distress, anorexia, pancreatitis & hepatotoxicity) also seen.

Uses/Indications

In veterinary medicine, azathioprine is used primarily as an immunosuppressive agent in the treatment of immune-mediated diseases in dogs, but no large, controlled, prospective studies documenting its efficacy were located. For auto-agglutinizing immune mediated hemolytic anemia, azathioprine is often recommended to start at the time of diagnosis. When used in combination with cyclosporine, azathioprine has been used to prevent rejection of MHC-matched renal allografts in dogs.

Azathioprine is often used in combination with corticosteroids, such as prednisolone, in the hope for synergy and to reduce the incidence of adverse effects of each drug by allowing dosage reductions and eventually, every other day dosing of each drug.

Although the drug can be very toxic to bone marrow in cats, it is sometimes used to treat feline autoimmune skin diseases.

Pharmacology/Actions

While the exact mechanism how azathioprine exerts its immunosuppressive action has not been determined, it is probably dependent on several factors. Azathioprine antagonizes purine metabolism thereby inhibiting RNA, DNA synthesis and mitosis. It may also cause chromosome breaks secondary to incorporation into nucleic acids and cellular metabolism may become disrupted by the drug's ability to inhibit coenzyme formation. Azathioprine has greater activity on delayed hypersensitivity and cellular immunity than on humoral antibody responses. Clinical response to azathioprine may require up to 6 weeks.

Pharmacokinetics

Azathioprine is poorly absorbed from the GI tract and is rapidly metabolized to mercaptopurine. Mercaptopurine is rapidly taken up by lymphocytes and erythrocytes. Mercaptopurine remaining in the plasma is then further metabolized to several other compounds that are excreted by the kidneys. Only minimal amounts of either azathioprine or mercaptopurine are excreted unchanged. Cats have low activity of thiopurine methyltransferase (TPMT), one of the routes used to metabolize azathioprine. Approximately 11% of humans have low thiopurine methyltransferase activity, and these individuals have a greater incidence of bone marrow suppression, but also greater azathioprine efficacy. Dogs have variable TMPT activity levels similar to that seen in humans, which may explain why some canine breeds/patients respond better and/or develop more myelotoxicity than others. TPMT activity is lower in giant schnauzers and much higher in Alaskan malamutes than in other breeds. One study, however in dogs did not show significant correlation between TMPT activity in red blood cells and drug toxicity (Rodriguez et al. 2004).

Contraindications/Precautions/Warnings

Azathioprine is contraindicated in patients hypersensitive to it. The drug should be used cautiously in patients with hepatic dysfunction. Use of azathioprine in cats is rarely recommended as they seem to be more susceptible to azathioprine's bone marrow suppressive effects.

Prescription/order errors have occurred when azithromycin and azathioprine have been confused. The use of "tall man" letters (writing part of a drug's name in upper case) on prescription/orders may reduce the risk for errors: aZITHROmycin; azaTHIOprine.

Adverse Effects

The principal adverse effects associated with azathioprine in dogs are bone marrow suppression, gastrointestinal effects (vomiting, anorexia, diarrhea), pancreatitis, and hepatotoxicity, and poor hair growth. Cats are more prone to develop myelotoxic effects than dogs and the drug is generally not recommended for use in this species. Leukopenia is the most prevalent consequence, but anemia and thrombocytopenia may also be seen. GI upset/anorexia, poor hair growth, acute pancreatitis and hepatotoxicity have been associated with azathioprine therapy in dogs.

Because azathioprine depresses the immune system, animals may be susceptible to infections or neoplastic illnesses with long-term use.

In dogs recovering from immune-mediated hemolytic anemia, taper the withdrawal of the drug slowly over several months and monitor for early signs of relapse. Rapid withdrawal can lead to a rebound hyperimmune response.

Reproductive/Nursing Safety

Azathioprine is mutagenic and teratogenic in lab animals. In humans, the FDA categorizes this drug as category *D* for use during pregnancy (*There is evidence of human fetal risk, but the potential benefits from the use of the drug in pregnant women may be acceptable despite its potential risks.*) In a separate system evaluating the safety of drugs in canine and feline pregnancy (Papich 1989), this drug is categorized as class: **C** (*These drugs may have potential risks. Studies in people or laboratory animals have uncovered risks, and these drugs should be used cautiously as a last resort when the benefit of therapy clearly outweighs the risks.*)

Azathioprine is distributed into milk; it is recommended to use milk replacer while the dam is receiving azathioprine.

Overdosage/Acute Toxicity

There were 122 single agent exposures to azathioprine reported to the ASPCA Animal Poison Control Center (APCC) during 2009-2013. Of the 104 dogs, 38 were symptomatic with 42% vomiting, 21% had elevated liver enzymes, 18% were anorexia, and 13% were thrombocytopenic.

Drug Interactions

The following drug interactions with azathioprine have either been reported or are theoretical in humans or animals and may be of significance in veterinary patients. Unless otherwise noted, use together is not necessarily contraindicated, but weigh the potential risks and perform additional monitoring when appropriate.

- **ACE INHIBITORS** (*e.g.,* benazepril, enalapril, etc.): Increased potential for hematologic toxicity.
- **ALLOPURINOL**: The hepatic metabolism of azathioprine may be decreased by concomitant administration of allopurinol; in humans, it is recommended to reduce the azathioprine dose to 1/4–1/3 usual if both drugs are to be used together.
- **AMINOSALICYLATES** (*e.g.,* **sulfasalazine, mesalamine, olsalazine**): Increased risk for azathioprine toxicity.
- **NON-DEPOLARIZING MUSCLE RELAXANTS** (*e.g.,* **pancuronium, tubocurarine**): The neuromuscular blocking activity of these drugs may be inhibited or reversed by azathioprine.
- **CORTICOSTEROIDS**: Although azathioprine is often used with corticosteroids, there is greater potential risk for toxicity development.
- **DRUGS AFFECTING MYELOPOIESIS** (*e.g.,* **trimethoprim/sulfa, cyclophosphamide,** etc.): Increased potential for hematologic toxicity.
- **WARFARIN**: Potential for reduced anticoagulant effect.

Doses

Note: All dosages are extra-label.

- **DOGS:**

  As an immunosuppressive (no prospective studies supporting any dosage protocol were noted): There are many anecdotal protocols for use of azathioprine; general recommendations are: Initially, 2 mg/kg PO once daily for 1-4 weeks. Then the dosage is reduced to 0.5 – 2 mg/kg PO every other day. After treatment is begun, a lag period of at least a week and often as long as 3-5 weeks is required before there is significant clinical immunosuppressive efficacy. Some protocols include glucocorticoids. During the maintenance phase of treatment (every other day dosing), glucocorticoids are often given on days when azathioprine is not given. Sample dosage protocols follow:

  a) **For inflammatory bowel disease:** Initially 2 mg/kg PO once daily for 2 weeks, then tapered to 2 mg/kg PO every other day for 2-4 weeks, then 1 mg/kg PO every other day. May take 2-6 weeks before beneficial effects are seen. (Moore 2004)

  b) **For immune-mediated anemia, colitis, immune-mediated skin disease, and acquired myasthenia gravis**: 2 mg/kg PO once daily (q24h); long-term therapy 0.5 – 1 mg/kg PO every other day, with prednisolone administered on the alternate days. (Papich 2001)

  c) **For adjunctive therapy in myasthenia gravis in non-re-**

sponsive patients: Initially, 1 mg/kg PO once daily. CBC is evaluated every 1-2 weeks. If neutrophil and platelet counts are normal after 2 weeks, dose is increased to 2 mg/kg PO once daily. CBC is repeated every week for the first month and then monthly thereafter. Recommend to discontinue azathioprine if WBC falls below 4,000 cells/mcL or neutrophil count is less than 1,000 cells/mcL. Serum ACHR antibody concentrations reevaluated q4–6 weeks. Azathioprine dose is tapered to every other day when clinical remission occurs and serum ACHR antibody concentrations are normalized. (Coates 2000)

d) **For lymphoplasmacytic enteritis if clinical response to prednisolone is poor or the adverse effects (of prednisolone) predominate**: azathioprine 2 mg/kg PO once daily for 5 days, then on alternate days to prednisolone. (Simpson 2003)

e) **For severe cases (autoagglutination, hemolytic crisis with rapid decline of hematocrit, intravascular hemolysis, Cocker Spaniels) of immune-mediated hemolytic anemia**: 2.2 mg/kg PO once daily (q24h) in addition to prednisone (initially at 2.2 mg/kg PO q12h until hematocrit reaches 25-30%; then dose is gradually tapered by approximately 25% q2-3 weeks until a dose of 0.5 mg/kg PO q48h is reached). (Macintire 2006)

f) **For use with glucocorticoids in acute immune-mediated hemolytic anemia (IMHA):** Author starts all patients with IMHA with adjunctive immunosuppressants (usually azathioprine) at 1 – 2 mg/kg PO once daily. Often used for long-term maintenance as steroid side effects quickly become intolerable to many pet owners. Generally well tolerated in dogs but may cause bone marrow suppression and hepatotoxicity. (Noonan 2009)

g) **For perianal fistulas (anal furunculosis):** In the study, initially 2 mg/kg PO once daily (q24h) until a reduction in the size, number or inflammation of the fistulas was seen or total WBC <5000 cells/mcL or neutrophil count was <3500 cells/mcL or platelet count <160,000 cells/mcL. Then reduce to 2 mg/kg PO every other day (q48h) and continued for 12 weeks as long as myelosuppression doesn't develop. After 12 weeks, reduce dose to 1 mg/kg PO every other day (q48h) with a planned therapy duration of 12 months. Prednisone was given at 2 mg/kg PO once daily for the first two weeks of therapy; then at 1 mg/kg PO once daily for another 2 weeks and then discontinued. All dogs were placed on a limited antigen diet. No correlation with efficacy and lymphocyte blastogenesis effect. Complete or partial remission in 64% of treated dogs, which is less than systemic cyclosporine or topical tacrolimus treatment, but azathioprine treatment is less expensive. (Harkin et al. 2007)

h) **To reduce inflammation in dogs with chronic hepatitis:** 2.2 mg/kg PO once daily in combination with corticosteroids (Prednis(ol)one initially at 1 – 2 mg/kg/day PO; dose is gradually tapered with clinical improvement). Azathioprine dose is given every other day after 1-2 weeks. (Twedt 2010b), (Twedt 2010a)

- **CATS:**

Warning: Most do not recommend azathioprine for use in cats because the difficulty in accurately dosing and the potential for development of fatal myelotoxicity.

As an immunosuppressive: For severe and refractory inflammatory bowel disease: Must be used with caution; myelotoxicity with severe neutropenia is possible. Azathioprine at 0.3 mg/kg

PO once every other day; may take 3-5 weeks before any beneficial effects. Administration can be enhanced by crushing one 50 mg tablet and suspending it in 15 mL of syrup resulting in a concentration of 3.3 mg/mL. Must be shaken well before each use. If cat becomes ill, rectal temperature and WBC should be determined immediately. (Willard 2002)

- **FERRETS:**

  As an immunosuppressive: For treating inflammatory bowel disease: Treatments include prednisone (1 mg/kg PO q12-24h), azathioprine (0.9 mg/kg PO q24-72h), and dietary management. (Johnson 2006)

- **HORSES:**

  As an immunosuppressive: 3 mg/kg PO q24h. Although clinical experiences are still limited, azathioprine appears to be a relatively safe immunosuppressive treatment in the horse and its cost is relatively low. (Divers 2010)

Monitoring

- Hemograms (including platelets) should be monitored closely; initially every 1-2 weeks and every 1-2 months (some recommend every 2 weeks) once on maintenance therapy. It is recommended by some clinicians that if the WBC count drops to between 5,000–7,000 cells/mm^3 the dose be reduced by 25%. If WBC count drops below 5,000 cells/mm^3 treatment should be discontinued until leukopenia resolves.
- Liver function tests; serum amylase, if indicated.
- Efficacy.

Client Information

- There is the possibility of severe toxicity developing from this drug including drug-related neoplasms or mortality; routine testing to detect toxic effects are necessary.
- May give with or without food.
- May take up to 6 weeks to see positive effects.
- Pregnant women should avoid handling; everyone should wash hands or wear disposable gloves when handling this drug.
- Do not stop the drug unless your veterinarian tells you to.
- Watch for signs of infection, liver or blood problems: fever, reduced activity, bruising, bleeding, vomiting, lack of appetite, yellowing of whites of eyes.

Chemistry/Synonyms

Related structurally to adenine, guanine and hypoxanthine, azathioprine is a purine antagonist antimetabolite that is used primarily for its immunosuppressive properties. Azathioprine occurs as an odorless, pale yellow powder that is insoluble in water and slightly soluble in alcohol. Azathioprine sodium powder for injection occurs as a bright yellow, amorphous mass. After reconstituting with sterile water for injection to a concentration of 10 mg/mL, it has an approximate pH of 9.6.

Azathioprine/Azathioprine sodium may also be known as: azathioprinum, BW-57322, or NSC-39084; many trade names are available.

Storage/Stability

Azathioprine tablets should be stored at room temperature in well-closed containers and protected from light.

The sodium powder for injection should be stored at room temperature and protected from light. It is reportedly stable at neutral or acidic pH, but will hydrolyze to mercaptopurine in alkaline solutions. This conversion is enhanced upon warming or in the presence of sulfhydryl-containing compounds (*e.g.*, cysteine). After reconstituting, the injection should be used within 24-hours as no preservative is present.

Compatibility/Compounding Considerations

Azathioprine sodium is reportedly **compatible** with the following intravenous solutions: dextrose 5% in water, and sodium chloride 0.45% or 0.9%. Compatibility is dependent upon factors such as pH, concentration, temperature and diluent used; consult specialized references or a hospital pharmacist for more specific information.

Compounded preparation stability: Azathioprine oral suspension compounded from commercially available tablets has been published (Allen et al. 1996). Triturating one-hundred twenty (120) azathioprine 50 mg tablets with 60 mL of *Ora-Plus®* and *qs ad* to 120 mL with *Ora-Sweet®* (or *Ora-Sweet® SF*) yields a 50 mg/mL suspension that retains >90% potency for 60 days stored at both 5°C and 25°C. The stability of azathioprine aqueous liquids decreases in the presence of alkaline pH. The optimal stability is reported to be between 5.5-6.5. Compounded preparations of azathioprine should be protected from light.

Dosage Forms/Regulatory Status

VETERINARY-LABELED PRODUCTS: NONE.

HUMAN-LABELED PRODUCTS:

Azathioprine Tablets: 50 mg, 75 mg & 100 mg; *Azasan®*; *Imuran®*; generic; (Rx)

Azathioprine Sodium Injection: 100 mg (as sodium)/vial in 20 mL vials; generic; (Rx) **Note:** At the time of monograph update (Sept 2013), the injection was unavailable (long-term backorder) on the US market.

Revisions/References

Monograph revised/updated August 2013.

Allen, L. V. & M. A. Erickson (1996). Stability of acetazolamide, allopurinol, azathioprine, clonazepam, and flucytosine in extemporaneously compounded oral liquids. *Am J Health Syst Pharm* **53**(16): 1944-9.

Coates, J. (2000). *Use of azathioprine in the myasthenia gravis patient.* Proceedings: The North American Veterinary Conference, Orlando. accessed via Veterinary Information Network; vin.com

Divers, T. J. (2010). Azathioprine - a useful treatment for immune-mediated disorders in the horse? *Equine Veterinary Education* **22**(10): 501-2.

Harkin, K., et al. (2007). Evaluation of azathioprine on lesion severity and lymphocyte blastogenesis in dogs with perianal fistulas. *J Am Anim Hosp Assoc* **43**(21-26).

Johnson, D. (2006). *Ferrets: the other companion animal.* Proceedings: ACVC. accessed via Veterinary Information Network; vin.com

Macintire, D. (2006). *New therapies for immune-mediated hemolytic anemia.* Proceedings: ACVIM 2006. accessed via Veterinary Information Network; vin.com

Moore, L. (2004). *Beyond corticosteroids for therapy of inflammatory bowel disease in dogs and cats.* Proceedings: ACVIM Forum. accessed via Veterinary Information Network; vin.com

Noonan, M. (2009). *Immune Mediated Hemolytic Anemia.* Proceedings: IVECC. accessed via Veterinary Information Network; vin.com

Papich, M. (2001). *Immunosuppressive Drug Therapy.* Proceedings: World Small Animal Veterinary Association World Congress. accessed via Veterinary Information Network; vin.com

Rodriguez, D., et al. (2004). Relationship between red blood cell thiopurine methyltransferase activity and myelotoxicity in dogs receiving azathioprine. *J Vet Intern Med* **18**(3): 339-45.

Simpson, K. (2003). *Chronic enteropathies: How should I treat them.* Proceedings: ACVIM Forum. accessed via Veterinary Information Network; vin.com

Twedt, D. (2010a). *How I treat chronic hepatitis.* Proceedings: WSAVA. accessed via Veterinary Information Network; vin.com

Twedt, D. (2010b). *Update on Medical therapy for hepatobiliary disease.* Proceedings: WSAVA. accessed via Veterinary Information Network; vin.com

Willard, M. (2002). *Stopping "unstoppable" diarrhea-How to stop the flood.* Proceedings: Atlantic Coast Veterinary Conference. accessed via Veterinary Information Network; vin.com

Azithromycin

(ay-zith-roe-**my**-sin)   Zithromax®

Macrolide Antibiotic

Prescriber Highlights

▶ Oral & parenteral human macrolide antibiotic; potentially useful for a variety of infections in veterinary patients; not effective for clearing *Chlamydophila felis* or *Mycoplasma Haemofelis* in cats.

▶ Very long tissue half-lives in dogs & cats.

▶ Contraindications: Hypersensitivity to macrolides. Caution: Hepatic disease.

▶ Adverse Effects: Potentially GI effects (anorexia, vomiting, diarrhea), but less so than with erythromycin.

Uses/Indications

Azithromycin with its relative broad spectrum and favorable pharmacokinetic profile may be useful for a variety of bacterial, rickettsial and parasitic infections in veterinary species.

Azithromycin combined with atovaquone appears effective in treating dogs with *Babesia gibsoni* (Asian genotype) infections, particularly in dogs not immunosuppressed or splenectomized. A prospective, unmasked study in dogs comparing atovaquone/azithromycin (AA) with a protocol using clindamycin, diminazene and imidocarb (CDI) found that CDI had higher recovery and lower relapse rates, albeit longer therapy duration and slower reduction in parasite numbers than AA. The authors concluded that CDI was effective for initial therapy and when the M121I gene in *B. gibsoni* had mutated (Lin et al. 2012).

In dogs, both oral (10 mg/kg/day) and a toothpaste form (8.5%) of azithromycin have been used to treat cyclosporine-induced gingival hyperplasia, but one study found only limited efficacy (Rosenberg et al. 2013).

Azithromycin has been shown to be ineffective in the treatment of *Mycoplasma haemofelis* or eliminating *Chlamydophila felis* in cats.

Azithromycin may be potentially useful for treating Rhodococcus infections in foals. While azithromycin's pharmacokinetics support oral dosing in adult horses, concerns for potential antimicrobial-associated enterocolitis require further studies (Leclere et al. 2012).

Pharmacology/Actions

Like other macrolide antibiotics, azithromycin inhibits protein synthesis by penetrating the cell wall and binding to the 50S ribosomal subunits in susceptible bacteria. It is considered a bacteriostatic antibiotic. It can accumulate and persist in macrophages, neutrophils and in pulmonary epithelial lining fluid (PELF).

Azithromycin has a relatively broad spectrum. It has *in vitro* activity (does not necessarily indicate clinical efficacy) against gram-positive organisms such as *Streptococcus pneumoniae, Staph aureus*; gram-negative organisms such as *Haemophilus influenzae; Bartonella* spp., *Bordetella* spp.; and *Mycoplasma pneumoniae, Borrelia burgdorferi* and *Toxoplasma* spp.

Pharmacokinetics

The pharmacokinetics of azithromycin have been described in cats and dogs. In dogs, the drug has excellent bioavailability after oral administration (97%). Tissue concentrations apparently do not mirror those in the serum after multiple doses and tissue half-lives in the dogs may be up to 90 hours. Greater than 50% of an oral dose is excreted unchanged in the bile. In cats, oral bioavailability is 58%. Tissue half-lives are less than in dogs, and range from 13 hours in adipose tissue to 72 hours in cardiac muscle. As with dogs, cats excrete the majority of a given dose in the bile.

In foals, azithromycin is variably absorbed after oral administration with a mean systemic bioavailability ranging from 40-60%. The affect of food, if any, on absorption is not clear. It has a very high volume of distribution (11.6-18.6 L/kg). Elimination half-life is approximately 20-26 hours. The drug concentrates in bronchoalveolar cells and pulmonary epithelial fluid. Elimination half-life in PMN's is about 2 days. In adult horses after intragastric administration (tablets suspended in 500 mL of water), oral bioavailability averaged 45% with peak levels occurring about an hour after dosing. Plasma elimination half-life after IV dosing was approximately 18 hours. Plasma concentrations after a single intragastric dose remained above the MIC90 for 6-12 hours for beta-hemolytic streptococci, *Pasteurella* spp., and *Staphylococcus* spp. For these bacteria, intracellular concentrations of azithromycin in alveolar macrophages were above MIC90 for at least 48 hours and in neutrophils for at least 120 hours after a dose (Leclere et al. 2012).

When compared to erythromycin, azithromycin has better absorption characteristics, longer tissue half-lives, and higher concentrations in tissues and white blood cells. Azithromycin achieves high concentrations in bronchial secretions and has excellent ocular penetration.

Goats have an elimination half-life of 32.5 hours (IV), 45 hours (IM), an apparent volume of distribution (steady-state) of 34.5 L/kg and a clearance of 0.85 L/kg/hr.

Rabbits have an elimination half-life of 24.1 hours (IV), and 25.1 hours (IM). IM injection has a high bioavailability, but causes some degree of muscle damage at the injection site.

Sheep have an elimination half-life average of 48 hours (IV), 61 hours (IM), an apparent volume of distribution (steady-state) of 34.5 L/kg and a clearance of 0.52 L/kg/hr.

Contraindications/Precautions/Warnings

Azithromycin is contraindicated in animals hypersensitive to any of the macrolides. It should be used with caution in patients with impaired hepatic function.

Prescription/order errors have occurred when azithromycin and azathioprine have been confused. The use of "tall man" letters (writing part of a drug's name in upper case) on prescription/orders may reduce the risk for errors: aZITHROmycin; azaTHIOprine.

Adverse Effects

Azithromycin can cause vomiting, reduced appetite, and diarrhea in small animals, but compared to erythromycin, it has significantly fewer GI adverse effects. Local IV site reactions have occurred in patients receiving IV azithromycin.

A small preliminary study where horses were given 10 mg/kg PO once daily for 5 days, no life-threatening adverse effects were seen, but some GI effects (self-limiting decrease in appetite and change in fecal consistency), raising concerns of the potential for serious antimicrobial-associated enterocolitis (Leclere et al. 2012).

Reproductive/Nursing Safety

Safety during pregnancy has not been fully established; use only when clearly necessary. In humans, the FDA categorizes this drug as category **B** for use during pregnancy (*Animal studies have not yet demonstrated risk to the fetus, but there are no adequate studies in pregnant women; or animal studies have shown an adverse effect, but adequate studies in pregnant women have not demonstrated a risk to the fetus in the first trimester of pregnancy, and there is no evidence of risk in later trimesters.*)

Overdosage/Acute Toxicity

Acute oral overdoses are unlikely to cause significant morbidity other than vomiting, diarrhea and GI cramping.

Drug Interactions

The following drug interactions with azithromycin have either been reported or are theoretical in humans or animals and may be of significance in veterinary patients. Unless otherwise noted, use together is not necessarily contraindicated, but weigh the potential risks and perform additional monitoring when appropriate.

- **ANTACIDS (oral; magnesium-** and **aluminum-containing):** May reduce the rate of absorption of azithromycin; suggest separating dosages by 2 hours.
- **CISAPRIDE:** No data on azithromycin, but other macrolides (*e.g.*, clarithromycin) contraindicated with cisapride; use with caution.
- **CYCLOSPORINE:** Azithromycin may potentially increase cyclosporine blood levels; monitor carefully.
- **DIGOXIN:** No data on azithromycin, but other macrolides (*e.g.*, erythromycin, clarithromycin) can increase digoxin levels; monitor carefully.
- **PIMOZIDE:** Azithromycin use is contraindicated in patients taking pimozide (unlikely to be used in vet med—used for Tourette's disorder in humans). Acute deaths have occurred.

Doses

Note: All dosages are extra-label.

- **DOGS:**

  For susceptible infections: There is significant variability in anecdotal dosing recommendations. Most recommendations are 5 – 10 mg/kg PO once daily for 3-7 days, with skin infections at the higher end of dosage range and duration. Because of the drug's pharmacokinetics, after a few days of once a day dosing, some recommend every other day dosing or giving higher dosages (*e.g.*, 10 – 15 mg/kg) twice per week; these dosing regimens may be effective for longer-term treatment of some infections.

  For *Babesia gibsoni* (Asian genotype) **or *B. microti* infections:** Atovaquone 13.3 mg/kg PO q8h with a fatty meal and azithromycin 10 mg/kg PO once daily. Give both drugs for 10 days. Reserve immunosuppressive therapy for cases that are not rapidly responding (3-5 days) to anti-protozoal therapy. (Birkenheuer et al. 2004), (Birkenheuer 2006; Ayoob et al. 2010; Birkenheuer 2012)

- **CATS:**

  For susceptible infections: There is significant variability in dosing recommendations. Most recommendations are 5 – 10 mg/kg PO once daily for 3-7 days, but for some infections, treatment durations are far longer (see below). Because of the drug's pharmacokinetics, after a few days of once a day dosing, some recommend every other day dosing or giving higher dosages (*e.g.*, 10 – 15 mg/kg) twice per week; these dosing regimens may be effective for longer-term treatment of some infections. Sample indications and treatment recommendations follow:

  a) **For upper respiratory infections:** 5 – 10 mg/kg PO once daily for 5 days, then q72h (every 3rd day) long-term. If there is an initial positive response to the antibiotic, therapy should be continued for 6-8 weeks without changing the antibiotic. (Scherk 2006)

  b) **For bartonellosis:** 10 mg/kg PO once daily for 21 days. Response to therapy is rapid; most cats with anterior uveitis will show significant improvement in less than one week. Recurrence after 21 days of treatment, followed by good flea control, is low. Failure of Bartonella positive cats to respond indicates that Bartonella is part of a polymicrobial disease syndrome. (Ketring 2009)

  c) **For cryptosporidiosis** (particularly in cats that are intolerant or nonresponsive to tylosin): 10 mg/kg PO once daily;

optimal duration of therapy is unknown but is usually several weeks. (Shahiduzzamana et al. 2012)

  d) **For toxoplasmosis:** 10mg/kg PO once daily for a minimum of 4 weeks. (Barrs 2013)

- **HORSES:**

  For treatment of *R. equi* infections in foals: 10 mg/kg PO once daily. Because of persistence of high levels in bronchoalveolar cells and pulmonary epithelial lining fluid, after 5 days of once daily treatment, every other day (q48h) dosing can be considered in foals responding to treatment. Some protocols combine therapy with rifampin (5 mg/kg PO q12h).

- **RODENTS/SMALL MAMMALS:**

  a) **Rabbits:** For Staphylococcus osteomyelitis: 50 mg/kg PO once daily with 40 mg/kg of rifampin q12h PO. (Ivey et al. 2000)

  b) **Rabbits:** For jaw abscesses: 15 – 30 mg/kg PO once daily (q24h). Systemic antibiotic treatment is continued for 2-4 weeks post-operatively. Advise owners to discontinue treatment if anorexia or diarrhea occurs. (Johnson 2006b)

  c) **Guinea pigs:** For Pneumonia: 15 – 30 mg/kg PO once daily (q24h). Advise owners to discontinue treatment if soft stools develop. (Johnson 2006a)

- **BIRDS:**

  For chlamydiosis (study done in experimentally infected cockatiels): Azithromycin 40 mg/kg PO once every other day (q48h) for 21 days (as effective as a 21 or 45 day treatment with doxycycline). Birds were dosed via metallic feeding tube into crop using the commercially available (*Zithromax®*) human oral suspension. (Guzman et al. 2010)

Monitoring

- Clinical efficacy.
- Adverse effects.

Client Information

- Give medication as prescribed. Do not refrigerate oral suspension and shake well before each use. If using the suspension, preferably give to an animal with an empty stomach. Discard any unused oral suspension after 14 days.
- Contact veterinarian if animal develops severe diarrhea or vomiting, or if condition deteriorates after beginning therapy.

Chemistry/Synonyms

A semisynthetic azalide macrolide antibiotic, azithromycin dihydrate occurs as a white crystalline powder. In one mL of water at neutral pH and at 37° C, 39 mg are soluble. Although commercial preparations are available as the dihydrate, potency is noted as the anhydrous form.

Azithromycin may also be known as: azithromycinum, acitromicina, CP-62993, or XZ-450; many trade names are available.

Storage/Stability

The commercially available tablets should be stored at temperatures less than 30°C. Products for reconstitution for oral suspension should be stored between 5-30°C before reconstitution with water. After reconstitution the multiple dose product may be stored between 5-30°C for up to ten days and then discarded. The single dose packets should be given immediately after reconstitution.

The injectable product should be stored below 30°C. After reconstitution with sterile water for injection, solutions containing 100 mg/mL are stable for 24 hours if stored below 30°C.

Compatibility/Compounding Considerations

Azithromycin injection is physically and chemically **compatible** with several intravenous solutions, including: half-normal and normal saline, D5W, LRS, D5 with 0.3% or 0.45% sodium chloride, and D5 in LRS. When azithromycin injection is diluted into 250-500 mL of one of the above solutions, it remains physically and chemically stable for 24 hours at room temperature and up to 7 days if kept refrigerated at 5°C.

Dosage Forms/Regulatory Status

VETERINARY-LABELED PRODUCTS: NONE.

Preparations compounded for dogs and cats may be available from compounding pharmacies.

HUMAN-LABELED PRODUCTS:

Azithromycin Oral Tablets: 250 mg, 500 mg & 600 mg (as dihydrate); *Zithromax®*; generic; (Rx)

Azithromycin Powder for Oral Suspension: After reconstitution: 100 mg/5 mL (20 mg/mL) in 15 mL bottles; 200 mg/5 mL (40 mg/mL) in 15, 22.5 & 30 mL bottles; 1 g/packet in single-dose packets; *Zithromax®*, generic; (Rx)

Azithromycin Powder for Injection (lyophilized): 500 mg in 10 mL vials; *Zithromax®*; generic; (Rx)

Azithromycin Hydrogencitrate for Injection Solution: 2.5 grams/100 mL (bulk package); generic (Rx)

Revisions/References

Monograph revised/updated August 2013.

Ayoob, A. L., et al. (2010). Clinical management of canine babesiosis. *J. Vet. Emerg. Crit. Care* 20(1): 77-89.

Barrs, V. (2013). *Feline Toxoplasmosis*. World Small Animal Veterinary Association World Congress Proceedings. accessed via Veterinary Information Network; vin.com

Birkenheuer, A. (2006). *Infectious Hemolytic Anemias*. ACVIM Proceedings. accessed via Veterinary Information Network; vin.com

Birkenheuer, A. (2012). *Canine Babesiosis: What's New?* Second International Society for Companion Animal Infectious Diseases Symposium Proceedings. accessed via Veterinary Information Network; vin.com

Birkenheuer, A., et al. (2004). Efficacy of combined atovaquone and azithromycin for therapy of chronic Babesia gibsoni (Asian genotype) infections in dogs. *J Vet Intern Med* 18: 494-8.

Guzman, D. S. M., et al. (2010). Evaluating 21-day Doxycycline and Azithromycin Treatments for Experimental Chlamydophila psittaci Infection in Cockatiels (Nymphicus hollandicus). *Journal of Avian Medicine and Surgery* 24(1): 35-45.

Ivey, E. & J. Morrisey (2000). Therapeutics for Rabbits. *Vet Clin NA: Exotic Anim Pract* 3:1(Jan): 183-216.

Johnson, D. (2006a). *Guinea Pig Medicine Primer*. Proceedings: ACVC. accessed via Veterinary Information Network; vin.com

Johnson, D. (2006b). *Treating jaw abscesses in rabbits*. Proceedings: ACVC. accessed via Veterinary Information Network; vin.com

Ketring, K. (2009). Feline Bartonellosis: The naysayers are wrong! It is the most under diagnosed feline ocular disease. Proceedings: WVC. accessed via Veterinary Information Network; vin.com

Leclere, M., et al. (2012). Pharmacokinetics and preliminary safety evaluation of azithromycin in adult horses. *J. Vet. Pharmacol. Ther.* 35(6): 541-9.

Lin, E. C. Y., et al. (2012). The therapeutic efficacy of two antibabesial strategies against Babesia gibsoni. *Veterinary Parasitology* 186(3-4): 159-64.

Rosenberg, A., et al. (2013). Evaluation of azithromycin in systemic and toothpaste forms for the treatment of ciclosporin-associated gingival overgrowth in dogs. *Veterinary Dermatology* 24(3): 337-+.

Scherk, M. (2006). *Snots and Snuffles: Chronic Feline Upper Respiratory Syndrome*. Proceedings: ACVIM. accessed via Veterinary Information Network; vin.com

Shahiduzzamana, M. & A. Daugschiesb (2012). Therapy and prevention of cryptosporidiosis in animals. *Veterinary Parasitology* 188: 203-14.

Aztreonam

(az-tree-oh-nam)   Azactam®

Injectable Monobactam Antibacterial

Prescriber Highlights

► Monobactam injectable antibiotic with good activity against a variety of gram-negative aerobic bacteria.
► May be considered for use for treating serious infections, when aminoglycosides or fluoroquinolones are ineffective or relatively contraindicated.
► Very limited information available regarding dosing & adverse effect profile.

Uses/Indications

Aztreonam is a monobactam antibiotic that may be considered for use in small animals for treating serious infections caused by a variety of aerobic and facultative gram-negative bacteria, including strains of *Citrobacter, Enterobacter, E. coli, Klebsiella, Proteus, Pseudomonas* and *Serratia*. The drug exhibits good penetration into most tissues and low toxic potential and may be of benefit in treating infections when an aminoglycoside or a fluoroquinolone are either ineffective or are relatively contraindicated. Any consideration for using aztreonam must be tempered with the knowledge that little clinical experience or research findings have been published with regard to target species.

Aztreonam has also been used to treat pet fish (koi) infected with *Aeromonas salmonocida*.

Pharmacology/Actions

Aztreonam is a bactericidal antibiotic that binds to penicillin-binding protein-3 thereby inhibiting bacterial cell wall synthesis resulting in cell lyses and death of susceptible bacteria. Aztreonam is relatively stable to the effects of bacterial beta-lactamases and unlike many other beta-lactam antibiotics, it does not induce the activity of beta-lactamases.

Aztreonam has activity against many species and most strains of the following gram-negative bacteria: *Aeromonas, Citrobacter, Enterobacter, E. coli, Klebsiella, Pasteurella, Proteus, Pseudomonas* and *Serratia*. It is not clinically efficacious against gram-positive or anaerobic bacteria.

Aztreonam can be synergistic against *Pseudomonas aeruginosa* and other gram-negative bacilli when used with aminoglycosides.

Pharmacokinetics

There is limited information published on the pharmacokinetic parameters of aztreonam in dogs and none was located for cats.

In dogs, after a 20mg/kg dose was administered IM, peak plasma levels of approximately 40 micrograms/mL occurred in about 20 minutes. Serum protein binding is about 20-30%, compared to 65% in humans. High tissue levels are found in the kidney (approx. 2.5X that of plasma). Liver concentrations approximate those found in plasma and lower levels are found in the lung and spleen. The drug is primarily (80%) excreted unchanged in the dog. Elimination half-lives are approximately 0.7 hours after IV administration and 0.9 hours after IM administration. These values are approximately twice as short as those reported in humans (ages 1 yr. to adult) with normal renal function.

Contraindications/Precaution/Warnings

Aztreonam should not be used in patients with documented severe hypersensitivity to the compound. Patients with serious renal dysfunction may need dosage adjustment. Use cautiously in patients with serious liver dysfunction.

Adverse Effects

Adverse effect profiles for aztreonam specific to target species were not located. Aztreonam's adverse effects in humans are similar to those of other beta-lactam antibiotics: hypersensitivity, gastrointestinal effects including GI bacterial overgrowth/Pseudomembranous colitis, pain and/or swelling after IM injection, and phlebitis after IV administration. Transient increases in liver enzymes, serum creatinine, and coagulation indices have been noted.

In a single-dose IV pharmacokinetic study in foals, watery diarrhea lasting 12-24 hours was noted 6-8 hours post-dose in two of the five treated animals (Paxson et al. 2011).

Reproductive/Nursing Safety

Aztreonam crosses that placenta and can be detected in fetal circulation. However, no evidence of teratogenicity or fetal toxicity have been reported after doses of up to 5 times normal were given to pregnant rats and rabbits. In humans, the FDA categorizes this drug as category **B** for use during pregnancy (*Animal studies have not yet demonstrated risk to the fetus, but there are no adequate studies in pregnant women; or animal studies have shown an adverse effect, but adequate studies in pregnant women have not demonstrated a risk to the fetus in the first trimester of pregnancy, and there is no evidence of risk in later trimesters.*)

Aztreonam has been detected in human breast milk at levels approximately 1% of those found in serum. As the drug is not absorbed orally, it is likely safe to use in nursing animals although antibiotic-associated diarrhea is possible.

Overdosage/Acute Toxicity

There is little reason for concern in patients with adequate renal function. The IV LD50 for mice is 3.3 g/kg. Hemodialysis or peritoneal dialysis may be used to clear aztreonam from the circulation.

Drug Interactions

The following drug interactions with aztreonam have either been reported or are theoretical in humans or animals and may be of significance in veterinary patients. Unless otherwise noted, use together is not necessarily contraindicated, but weigh the potential risks and perform additional monitoring when appropriate.

- **PROBENECID**: Can reduce the renal tubular secretion of aztreonam, thereby maintaining higher systemic levels for a longer period of time; this potential "beneficial" interaction requires further investigation before dosing recommendations can be made for veterinary patients.

For *in vitro* interactions, see the Storage-Stability and Compatibility sections.

Laboratory Considerations

- Aztreonam may cause false-positive **urine glucose determinations** when using cupric sulfate solution (Benedict's Solution, *Clinitest*®). Tests utilizing glucose oxidase (*Tes-Tape*®, *Clinistix*®) are not affected by aztreonam.

Doses

Note: Dosages for this medication are not well established for use in veterinary patients; all are extra-label.

- **DOGS:**

  An anecdotal dosing suggestion is to use the human pediatric dose of 30 mg/kg IM or IV q6-8h. When compared to humans, aztreonam in dogs has a shorter half-life, but is about half as bound to plasma proteins; the human pediatric dose may be a reasonable choice until more data becomes available.

- **HORSES:**

  Foals: Additional multi-dose trials should be completed before aztreonam is recommended for foals with gram-negative infections, but based on pharmacokinetics and reported microbial susceptibility (humans), a possible dosing regimen could be:

For susceptible (<2-4 micrograms/mL) Enterobacteriaceae (*e.g.* *E. coli*): 30 mg/kg IV q6h; for susceptible (<8 micrograms/mL) *P. aeruginosa*: 30 mg/kg IV q4h. Not recommended for Actinobacter. Development of diarrhea and frequent dosing may limit any clinical usefulness. (Paxson et al. 2011)

- **FISH:**

  For treating *Aeromonas salmonicida* in koi: 100 mg/kg IM or ICe (intracoelemic) every 48 hours for 7 treatments. (Lewbart 2005)

Monitoring

- Because monobactams usually have minimal toxicity associated with their use, monitoring for efficacy is usually all that is required unless toxic signs develop.
- Serum levels and therapeutic drug monitoring are not routinely performed with this agent.

Client Information

- Veterinary professionals only should administer this medication.
- Because of the dosing intervals required, this drug is best administered to inpatients only.

Chemistry/Synonyms

Aztreonam is a synthetic monobactam antimicrobial. It occurs as a white, odorless crystalline powder.

Aztreonam may also be know as: Aztreonamum, Azthreonam, Atstreonaami, SQ-26776, *Monobac*®, *Azactam*®, *Aztreotic*®, *Azenam*®, *Primbactam*®, *Trezam*®, or *Urobactam*®.

Storage/Stability

Commercially available powder for reconstitution should be stored at room temperature (15-30°C).

For IM use, add at least 3 mL of diluent (sterile water for injection, bacteriostatic sterile water for injection, NS, or bacteriostatic sodium chloride injection.) Solutions are stable for 48 hours at room temperature, 7 days if refrigerated.

For direct IV use, add 6-10 mL of sterile water for injection to each 15 or 30 mL vial. If the medication is to be given as an infusion, add at least 3 mL of sterile water for injection for each gram of aztreonam powder; then add the resulting solution to a suitable IV diluent (NS, LRS, D5W, etc.) so that the final concentration does not exceed 20 mg/mL. Inspect all solutions for visible particulate matter. Solutions may be colorless or a light, straw yellow color; upon standing, a light pink color may develop which does not affect the drug's potency. Intravenous solutions not exceeding concentrations of 20 mg/mL are stable for 48 hours at room temperature, 7 days if refrigerated. The package insert has specific directions for freezing solutions after dilution.

Compatibility/Compounding Considerations

Intravenous admixtures containing aztreonam are **compatible** with clindamycin, amikacin, gentamicin, tobramycin, ampicillin-sulbactam, imipenem-cilastatin, morphine, propofol, piperacillin-tazobactam, ticarcillin-clavulanate, ranitidine, sodium bicarbonate, potassium chloride, butorphanol, furosemide, hydromorphone, cefotaxime, cefuroxime, ceftriaxone and cefazolin. It is **not compatible** with metronidazole, amphotericin B, or vancomycin.

Dosage Forms/Regulatory Status

VETERINARY-LABELED PRODUCTS: NONE.

HUMAN-LABELED PRODUCTS:

Aztreonam Injection (lyophilized cake or powder for solution): 500 mg, 1 g, 2 g single-dose vials; 1 g in single-dose vials, & single-dose 100 mL infusion bottles; & 2 g in single-dose vials, 30 mL single-dose vials and single-dose 100 mL infusion bottles; *Azactam*®; generic (Rx)

Aztreonam Powder (lyophilized); for inhalation solution: 75 mg preservative free, arginine free (lysine 46.7 mg) in 2 mL single-dose vials with 1 mL amp of sodium chloride 0.17% diluent; *Cayston®*; (Rx)

Revisions/References
Monograph revised/updated August 2013.
Lewbart, G. (2005). Antimicrobial and antifungal agents used in fish. *Exotic Animal Formulary 3rd Ed.* J. Carpenter, Elsevier: 5-12.
Paxson, J. A. & M. R. Paradis (2011). Pharmacokinetics of aztreonam after intravenous administration in foals. *J. Vet. Pharmacol. Ther.* **34**(1): 92-4.

Baclofen
(bak-loe-fen)   Lioresal®

GABA-Derivative Muscle Relaxant

Prescriber Highlights
▶ Muscle relaxant that is used for treating urinary retention in dogs.
▶ Do not use in cats.
▶ Adverse Effects: sedation, weakness, pruritus, & gastrointestinal distress.
▶ Do not stop therapy abruptly.
▶ Overdoses potentially serious.

Uses/Indications
Baclofen is a centrally acting skeletal muscle relaxant that may be useful to decrease urethral resistance in dogs to treat urinary retention. It is not commonly used in dogs and is not recommended for use in cats.

In humans, baclofen is most commonly used for preventing and treating spasticity associated with conditions such as multiple sclerosis, spinal disorders and cerebral palsy.

Pharmacology/Actions
Considered a skeletal muscle relaxant, baclofen's mechanism of action is not well understood, but it acts at the spinal cord level and decreases the frequency and amplitude of muscle spasm. It apparently decreases muscle spasticity by reducing gamma efferent neuronal activity. In the urethra, it reduces striated sphincter tone.

Pharmacokinetics
After oral administration, baclofen is rapidly and well absorbed but at least in humans, there is wide interpatient variation. The drug is widely distributed with only a small percentage crossing the blood-brain barrier. Baclofen is eliminated primarily by the kidneys; less than 15% of a dose is metabolized by the liver. Elimination half-life in humans ranges from 2.5-4 hours.

Baclofen crosses the placenta. It is unknown if it enters maternal milk in quantities sufficient to cause effects in offspring.

Contraindications/Precautions/Warnings
Baclofen is contraindicated in patients hypersensitive to it and is not recommended for use in cats. It should be used with caution in patients that have seizure disorders and working dogs that must be alert. Do not give the intrathecal medication by any other route.

Adverse Effects
Adverse effects reported in dogs include sedation, weakness, pruritus, salivation, and gastrointestinal distress (nausea, abdominal cramping).

Discontinue this medication gradually as hallucinations and seizures have been reported in human patients that have abruptly stopped the medication.

Reproductive/Nursing Safety
Very high doses caused fetal abnormalities in rodents. It is unknown if normal dosages affect fetuses; use during pregnancy with care. In humans, the FDA categorizes this drug as category C for use during pregnancy (*Animal studies have shown an adverse effect on the fetus, but there are no adequate studies in humans; or there are no animal reproduction studies and no adequate studies in humans.*)

Overdosage/Acute Toxicity
Deaths in dogs have been reported with baclofen doses as low as 8 mg/kg. Oral overdoses as low as 1.3 mg/kg may cause vomiting, depression, ataxia, hypersalivation and vocalization. Other signs that may be noted include hypotonia or muscle twitching. Massive overdoses may cause respiratory depression, coma, or seizures. Onset of clinical signs after overdoses in dogs can occur from 15 minutes to 7 hours after ingestion and persist for hours up to days.

There were 743 single agent exposures to baclofen reported to the ASPCA Animal Poison Control Center (APCC) during 2009-2013. Of the 696 dogs, 610 were symptomatic. The most common clinical signs included: vocalization (57%), hypersalivation (46%), vomiting (44%), ataxia (36%), recumbency (29%), lethargy (28%), hypothermia (16%), disorientation (13%), tachycardia (11%), bradycardia (10%), and seizures (10%). Of the 43 cats, 36 were symptomatic with 36% being ataxic, 36% vomiting, 31% hyperthermic, 27% hypersalivating, 27% lethargic, 27% vocalizing and 17% recumbent.

Because of the potential serious consequences of baclofen overdoses and evolving treatment guidelines, it is recommended to contact an animal poison control center for further information and guidance. In alert patients, consider standard decontamination protocols. Avoid the use of magnesium containing saline cathartics as they may compound CNS depression. Forced fluid diuresis may enhance baclofen excretion. Obtunded patients with respiratory depression may need oxygen and mechanical ventilation. Monitor ECG and treat arrhythmias if needed. For patients that are vocalizing or disoriented, cyproheptadine (1.1 mg/kg orally or rectally) may be effective in alleviating the signs. Atropine has been suggested to improve ventilation, heart rate, BP, and body temperature. Diazepam at the lowest effective dose may be useful for treating seizures, tremors or dysphoria/agitation. Intravenous lipids may potentially be useful as baclofen is lipid soluble. (Khorzad et al. 2012; Bates et al. 2013; Lee 2013)

Drug Interactions
The following drug interactions have either been reported or are theoretical in humans or animals receiving baclofen and may be of significance in veterinary patients. Unless otherwise noted, use together is not necessarily contraindicated, but weigh the potential risks and perform additional monitoring when appropriate.
■ **CNS DEPRESSANTS, OTHER:** May cause additive CNS depression.

Laboratory Considerations
■ Increased AST, **alkaline phosphate** and **blood glucose** have been reported in humans.

Doses
■ **DOGS:**

To treat urinary retention by decreasing urethral resistance (extra-label): Baclofen has a very narrow therapeutic index and significant side effects can occur at higher dosages (see Overdosage): Anecdotal dosage recommendations generally have been 1 – 2 mg/kg PO q8h or 5 – 10 mg (per dog) q8h. It is recommended to start at a low dosage and gradually increase if necessary while determining efficacy and adverse effects/toxicity.

Monitoring
■ Efficacy.
■ Adverse effects.

Client Information

- Used in dogs that have difficulty urinating; not used in cats.
- Overdoses can be extremely serious.
- Drowsiness/tiredness is the most common side effect.
- Do not stop the drug abruptly. Hallucinations and seizures have been reported in humans that have stopped the drug suddenly.

Chemistry/Synonyms

A skeletal muscle relaxant that acts at the spinal cord level, baclofen occurs as white to off-white crystals. It is slightly soluble in water and has pKa values of 5.4 and 9.5.

Baclofen may also be known as: aminomethyl chlorohydrocinnamic acid, Ba-34647, baclofenum, *Baclo®, Baclohexal®, Baclon®, Baclopar®, Baclosal®, Baclospas®, Balgifen®, Clinispas®, Clofen®, Kemstro®, Lebic®, Lioresal®, Liotec®, Miorel®, Neurospas®, Nu-Baclo®, Pacifen®,* or *Vioridon®.*

Storage/Stability

Do not store tablets above 30°C (86°F). Intrathecal product should be stored at room temperature; do not freeze or heat sterilize.

Compatibility/Compounding Considerations

Compounded preparation stability: Baclofen oral suspension compounded from commercially available tablets has been published (Allen et al. 1996). Triturating one-hundred twenty (120) baclofen 10 mg tablets with 60 mL of *Ora-Plus®* and *qs ad* to 120 mL with *Ora-Sweet®* (or *Ora-Sweet® SF*) yields a 10 mg/mL oral suspension that retains >90% potency for 60 days stored at both 5°C and 25°C. Compounded preparations of baclofen should be protected from light.

Another oral liquid compounding recipe has been described (Olin 2000): To prepare a 5 mg/mL liquid (35 day expiration date). Grind fifteen 20 mg tablets in a glass mortar to fine powder. Wet the powder with 10 mL of glycerin and form a fine paste. Slowly add 15 mL of simple syrup to the paste and transfer to a glass amber bottle. Rinse the mortar and pestle with another 15 mL of simple syrup and transfer to the bottle. Repeat until final volume is 60 mL. Shake well before each use and store in the refrigerator.

Dosage Forms/Regulatory Status

VETERINARY-LABELED PRODUCTS: NONE.
The ARCI (Racing Commissioners International) has designated this drug as a class 4 substance. See the appendix for more information.

HUMAN-LABELED PRODUCTS:
Baclofen Tablets: 10 mg & 20 mg; generic; (Rx)

Baclofen Intrathecal Injection: 0.05 mg/mL (50 micrograms/mL) preservative-free in single-use amps, 10 mg/20 mL (500 mg/mL) preservative-free in single-use amps (1 amp refill kit) & 10 mg/5 mL (2000 micrograms/mL) preservative-free in single-use amps (2 or 4 amp refill kits); *Lioresal® Intrathecal, Gablofen®*; (Rx)

Revisions/References

Monograph revised/updated September 2013.

Allen, L. V. & M. A. Erickson (1996). Stability of baclofen, captopril, diltiazem hydrochloride, dipyridamole, and flecainide acetate in extemporaneously compounded oral liquids. *Am J Health Syst Pharm* 53(18): 2179-84.

Bates, N., et al. (2013). Lipid infusion in the management of poisoning: a report of 6 canine cases. *Veterinary Record* 172(13).

Khorzad, R., et al. (2012). Baclofen toxicosis in dogs and cats: 145 cases (2004-2010). *Javma-Journal of the American Veterinary Medical Association* 241(8): 1059-64.

Lee, J. A. (2013). Emergency Management and Treatment of the Poisoned Small Animal Patient. *Veterinary Clinics of North America: Small Animal Practice* 43(4): 757-71.

Olin, B. (2000). *Drug Facts and Comparisons: 2000*, Facts and Comparisons. St. Louis.

BAL in Oil — see Dimercaprol

Benazepril HCl

(ben-**a**-za-pril)   Fortekor®, Lotensin®

Angiotensin Converting Enzyme (ACE) Inhibitor

Prescriber Highlights

▶ ACE inhibitor that may be useful for treating heart failure, hypertension, chronic renal failure & protein-losing glomerulonephropathies in dogs & cats; particularly useful in patients with hypertension and proteinuria.

▶ Not recommended for acute kidney injury. Caution in patients with increased serum creatinine, hyponatremia, coronary or cerebrovascular insufficiency, SLE, hematologic disorders.

▶ GI disturbances most likely adverse effects, but hypotension, renal dysfunction, hyperkalemia possible.

▶ Mildly fetotoxic at high dosages.

Uses/Indications

Benazepril may be useful as a vasodilator in the treatment of heart failure and as an antihypertensive agent, particularly in dogs. Reasonable evidence exists that ACE-inhibitors increase survival (when compared to placebo) in dogs with dilated cardiomyopathy and mitral valve disease. Benazepril may be of benefit in treating the clinical signs associated with valvular heart disease and left to right shunts. Use of ACE inhibitors in dogs with ACVIM Class B2 heart disease (myxomatous mitral valve disease, mitral regurgitation, and cardiomegaly but without clinical signs) remains somewhat controversial and the ACVIM Consensus group did not reach consensus on any potential medical therapies. ACE inhibitors may also be of benefit in the adjunctive treatment of chronic renal failure and for protein losing nephropathies. Benazepril is cleared via both renal and hepatic routes in contrast to enalapril (primarily renal), potentially allowing it to be more safely dosed in patients with decreased renal function. Benazepril may be an effective treatment for idiopathic renal hemorrhage in dogs.

In cats, benazepril may be useful for treating hypertension, adjunctive treatment of hypertrophic cardiomyopathy, and reducing protein loss associated with chronic renal failure.

Pharmacology/Actions

Benazepril is a prodrug and has little pharmacologic activity of its own. After being hydrolyzed in the liver to benazeprilat, the drug inhibits the conversion of angiotensin-I to angiotensin-II by inhibiting angiotensin-converting enzyme (ACE). Angiotensin-II acts both as a vasoconstrictor and stimulates production of aldosterone in the adrenal cortex. By blocking angiotensin-II formation, ACE inhibitors generally reduce blood pressure in hypertensive patients and vascular resistance in patients with congestive heart failure. There is no evidence that ACE inhibitors reduce abnormal cardiac hypertrophy in cats.

When administered to dogs with heart failure at low dosages (0.1 mg/kg q12h), benazepril improved clinical signs, but did not significantly affect blood pressure (Wu et al. 2006).

In cats with chronic renal failure, benazepril has been shown to reduce systemic arterial pressure and glomerular capillary pressure while increasing renal plasma flow and glomerular filtration rates. It may also help improve appetite.

ACE inhibitors' proteinuric reducing effects are most likely a result of reducing intraglomerular hypertension by a vasodilating effect on postglomerular arterioles.

Like enalapril and lisinopril, but not captopril, benazepril does not contain a sulfhydryl group. ACE inhibitors containing sulfhydryl groups (*e.g.,* captopril) may have a greater tendency of causing immune-mediated reactions.

Pharmacokinetics

After oral dosing in healthy dogs, benazepril is rapidly absorbed and converted into the active metabolite benazeprilat with peak levels of benazeprilat occurring approximately 75 minutes after dosing. The elimination half-life of benazeprilat is approximately 3.5 hours in healthy dogs. Unlike enalaprilat, which is approximately 95% cleared in dogs via renal mechanisms, benazeprilat is cleared via both renal (45%) and hepatic (55%) routes.

In cats, inhibition of ACE is long-lasting (half-life of 16–23 hours), despite relatively quick elimination of free benazeprilat, due to high affinity of benazeprilat to ACE. Because benazeprilat exhibits non-linear binding to ACE, doses greater than 0.25 mg/kg PO produced only small incremental increases in peak effect or duration of ACE inhibition. (King et al. 2003)

In humans, approximately 37% of an oral dose is absorbed after oral dosing and food apparently does not affect the extent of absorption. About 95% of the parent drug and active metabolite are bound to serum proteins. Benazepril and benazeprilat are primarily eliminated via the kidneys and mild to moderate renal dysfunction apparently does not significantly alter elimination as biliary clearance may compensate somewhat for reductions in renal clearances. Hepatic dysfunction or age does not appreciably alter benazeprilat levels.

Contraindications/Precautions/Warnings

Benazepril is contraindicated in patients that have demonstrated hypersensitivity to the ACE inhibitors.

ACE inhibitors should be used with caution in patients with hyponatremia or sodium depletion, coronary or cerebrovascular insufficiency, preexisting hematologic abnormalities or a collagen vascular disease (e.g., SLE). Patients with severe CHF should be monitored very closely upon initiation of therapy.

Because ACE inhibitors may decrease glomerular filtration rate (GFR) and worsen azotemia, they are generally avoided in critically ill acute kidney injury patients.

Benazepril can potentially be confused with *Benadryl*® on written prescriptions and written or verbal orders.

Adverse Effects

Benazepril's adverse effect profile in dogs is not well described, but other ACE inhibitors effects in dogs usually center around GI distress (e.g., anorexia, vomiting, diarrhea, etc.). Potentially, hypotension, renal dysfunction and hyperkalemia could occur. Because it lacks a sulfhydryl group (unlike captopril), there is less likelihood that immune-mediated reactions will occur, but rashes, neutropenia and agranulocytosis have been reported in humans.

In healthy cats given mild overdoses (2 mg/kg PO once daily for 52 weeks), only increased food consumption and weight were noted.

Reproductive/Nursing Safety

Benazepril apparently crosses the placenta. High doses of ACE inhibitors in rodents have caused decreased fetal weights and increases in fetal and maternal death rates; no teratogenic effects have been reported to date, but use during pregnancy should occur only when the potential benefits of therapy outweigh the risks to the offspring. In humans, the FDA categorizes this drug as category *C* for use during the first trimester of pregnancy (*Animal studies have shown an adverse effect on the fetus, but there are no adequate studies in humans; or there are no animal reproduction studies and no adequate studies in humans.*) During the second and third trimesters, the FDA categorizes this drug as category *D* for use during pregnancy (*There is evidence of human fetal risk, but the potential benefits from the use of the drug in pregnant women may be acceptable despite its potential risks.*)

Benazepril is distributed into milk in very small amounts.

Overdosage/Acute Toxicity

In overdose situations, the primary concern is hypotension; supportive treatment with volume expansion with normal saline is recommended to correct blood pressure. Because of the drug's long duration of action, prolonged monitoring and treatment may be required. Recent massive overdoses should be managed using standard decontamination protocols as appropriate. There were 298 single agent exposures to benazepril reported to the ASPCA Animal Poison Control Center (APCC) during 2009-2013. Of the 256 dogs, 30 were symptomatic with 33% vomiting, 27% lethargic, 27% tachycardic and 17% hypotensive.

Drug Interactions

The following drug interactions have either been reported or are theoretical in humans or animals receiving benazepril and may be of significance in veterinary patients:

- **ASPIRIN**: Aspirin may potentially negate the decrease in systemic vascular resistance induced by ACE inhibitors; however, one study in dogs using low-dose aspirin, the hemodynamic effects of enalaprilat (active metabolite of enalapril, a related drug) were not affected.
- **ANTIDIABETIC AGENTS (insulin, oral agents)**: Possible increased risk for hypoglycemia; enhanced monitoring recommended.
- **DIURETICS** (*e.g.,* **furosemide, hydrochlorothiazide**, etc.): Potential for increased hypotensive effects.
- **DIURETICS, POTASSIUM-SPARING** (*e.g.,* **spironolactone, triamterene**, etc.): Increased hyperkalemic effects, enhanced monitoring of serum potassium.
- **LITHIUM**: Increased serum lithium levels possible; increased monitoring required.
- **NON-STEROIDAL ANTIINFLAMMATORY DRUGS (NSAIDS)**: Potentially could increase the risk for nephrotoxicity and/or reducing efficacy of the ACE inhibitor; monitoring is advised.
- **POTASSIUM SUPPLEMENTS**: Increased risk for hyperkalemia.

Laboratory Considerations

- When using **iodohippurate sodium I^{123}/I^{134} or Technetium Tc^{99} pententate renal imaging** in patients with renal artery stenosis, ACE inhibitors may cause a reversible decrease in localization and excretion of these agents in the affected kidney that may lead to confusion in test interpretation.

Doses

- **DOGS:**

  For adjunctive treatment of heart failure (extra-label in USA): 0.25 – 0.5 mg/kg PO once daily.

  For adjunctive treatment of hypertension and/or proteinuria (extra-label): 0.25 – 0.5 mg/kg PO q12-24h.

- **CATS:**

  For adjunctive treatment of hypertrophic heart failure (extra-label): While definitive evidence for efficacy is lacking, some recommend 0.25 – 0.5 mg/kg PO once to twice daily.

  For adjunctive treatment of hypertension (extra-label): Most recommend using amlodipine as the first-line agent, but in cats that do not have BP controlled with amlodipine alone or in those with concurrent proteinuria, benazepril at 0.5 – 1 mg/kg PO q12-24h has been recommended. Monitor renal function.

  For reduction of proteinuria associated with chronic kidney disease (extra-label in USA): Most recommend 0.5 – 1 mg/kg PO once daily (U.K. labeled dosage). Some anecdotal dosage recommendations state that some cats may require the drug twice daily, but that higher dosages may worsen preexisting azotemia; caution is advised.

Monitoring

- Clinical signs of CHF.
- Serum electrolytes, creatinine, BUN, urine protein.
- Blood pressure (if treating hypertension or clinical signs associated with hypotension arise).

Client Information

- Usually well tolerated, but vomiting and diarrhea can occur. Give with food if vomiting or lack of appetite becomes a problem. If a rash or signs of infection occur (*e.g.*, fever) contact your veterinarian immediately.
- Very important to give benazepril as prescribed. Do not stop or reduce dosage without veterinarian's guidance.
- Your animal will likely need to have blood pressure and lab tests performed while receiving benazepril.

Chemistry/Synonyms

Benazepril HCl, an angiotensin converting enzyme inhibitor, occurs as white to off-white crystalline powder. It is soluble in water and ethanol. Benazepril does not contain a sulfhydryl group in its structure.

Benazepril may also be known as: CGS-14824A (benazepril or benazepril hydrochloride), *Benace®, Boncordin®, Briem®, Cibace®, Cibacen®, Cibacen®, Cibacene®, Fortekor®, Labopal®, Lotensin®, Lotrel®, Tensanil®,* or *Zinadril®*.

Storage/Stability

Benazepril tablets (and combination products) should be stored at temperatures less than 86°F (30°C) and protected from moisture. They should be dispensed in tight containers.

Compatibility/Compounding Considerations

No specific information noted.

Dosage Forms/Regulatory Status

VETERINARY-LABELED PRODUCTS: NONE IN THE USA.

In the UK (and elsewhere): Benazepril Tablets: 2.5 mg, 5 mg, & 20 mg; *Fortekor®*; (POM-V). Labeled for use in cats for chronic renal insufficiency and for heart failure in dogs.

The ARCI (Racing Commissioners International) has designated this drug as a class 3 substance. See the appendix for more information.

HUMAN-LABELED PRODUCTS:

Benazepril HCl Oral Tablets: 5 mg, 10 mg, 20 mg, & 40 mg; *Lotensin®*, generic; (Rx)

Also available in fixed dose combination products containing amlodipine (*Lotrel®*) or hydrochlorothiazide (*Lotensin HCT®*)

Revisions/References

Monograph revised/updated September 2013.

King, J., et al. (2003). Pharmacokinetic/pharmacodynamic modeling of the disposition and effect of benazepril and benazeprilat in cats. *J Vet Phamacol Ther* 26: 213-24.
Wu, S. & H. Juany (2006). *Effect of benazepril on systemic blood pressure in dogs with heart failure*. Proceedings: WSAVA. accessed via Veterinary Information Network; vin.com

Benzonatate

(ben-**zoe**-na-tate)   *Tessalon®, Zonatuss®*

Antitussive

Prescriber Highlights

▶ Cough suppressant (antitussive) that may be useful in veterinary medicine. Very little clinical experience or published data on animal use. Dosages not well established; use with caution.

▶ Possible side effects include: GI (vomiting/nausea) and CNS effects (sedation/depression to agitation/seizures). Cardiovascular effects possible if overdosed.

▶ Possible toxicity and the human dosage form (100 mg round-shaped liquid-filled gelatin capsule) limits potential usefulness in dogs. Potentially could be compounded into smaller dosage forms, but local anesthetic effect of drug makes this challenging.

▶ Must be kept in secure areas in child-resistant packaging to limit possibility of overdoses in children or animals.

Uses/Indications

Benzonatate may be useful in dogs for treating cough secondary to collapsing trachea or other respiratory conditions. Its use in veterinary medicine has been extremely limited and little published information specific to animal patients is available. The drug is potentially very toxic to animals or humans when overdosed.

Pharmacology/Actions

Benzonatate is thought to reduce the cough reflex via its anesthetic effects on stretch receptors of vagal afferent fibers in bronchi, alveoli, and pleura. Cough reflex may also be suppressed in the medulla where afferent impulses are transmitted to motor nerves. In humans, usual dosages do not depress respiration.

Pharmacokinetics

No animal pharmacokinetic data for benzonatate was located. In humans, pharmacokinetic data is not well described but benzonatate's onset of activity usually occurs within 20 minutes of oral dosing and activity lasts for 3-8 hours post-dose. It is believed that plasma esterases hydrolyze it to para-aminobenzoic acid (PABA).

Contraindications/Precautions/Warnings

Benzonatate is contraindicated in human patients with known hypersensitivity to it. It should be used with caution in dogs with seizure disorders or with aggressive behavioral conditions.

Adverse Effects

An adverse effect profile for animal use has not been established. In dogs, the most likely adverse effect expected would be nausea/vomiting. CNS effects ranging from depression/sedation to agitation and seizures, and cardiovascular effects (heart rate changes, hypotension) are possible and more likely associated with higher or toxic dosages. Hypersensitivity reactions have been reported in humans.

Benzonatate has a local anesthetic effect. If direct contact with oral mucosa occurs, swallowing difficulty, choking and aspiration are possible.

Reproductive/Nursing Safety

Safe use of benzonatate during pregnancy or nursing has not been established. For humans, the FDA has classified this drug as category **C** (*Animal studies have shown an adverse effect and there are no adequate studies in pregnant women or no animal studies have been conducted and there are no adequate studies in pregnant women*).

Overdosage/Acute Toxicity

Benzonatate is potentially very toxic to animals and humans when overdosed, but very limited data are available with respect to animal ingestions. Severe intoxication in humans has led to death and, reportedly, one or two capsules can be lethal in human infants. Severe toxicity can include cardiac arrest, arrhythmias, hypotension, and seizures.

There were 176 single agent exposures to benzonatate reported to the ASPCA Animal Poison Control Center (APCC) during 2009-2013. Of the 163 dogs, 58 were symptomatic with 53% vomiting, 14% lethargic, 12% hypersalivating, 12% tachycardic, 9% retching, and 7% ataxic. Of the 12 cats, 7 were symptomatic with 57% lethargic, 43% hypersalivating, 29% anorexic and 29% vomiting.

Due to the potential for toxicity, evaluation and management of benzonatate overdoses are best guided by an animal poison control center.

Drug Interactions

No clinically significant drug interactions for animal or human patients were located. Potentially, other local anesthetic drugs (e.g., procaine, tetracaine) could have an additive effect.

Laboratory Considerations

None noted.

Dosages

- **DOGS:**

  For adjunctive treatment of cough (extra-label): There is very little clinical experience using this drug in animal patients and dosages referenced to supporting scientific data for animal patients were not located. Use with caution. Dosages of 1 – 2 mg/kg PO two to three times daily or one 100 mg capsule (in dogs weighing more than 10 lbs./4.5 kg) PO twice daily have been noted. Dosage form must be given whole (do not give capsule contents directly into mouth, crush, or allow animal to chew on capsule).

Monitoring

- Clinical efficacy to reduce cough.
- Adverse effects, especially CNS/behavior-related.

Client Information

- Not commonly used in veterinary medicine; report unusual effects to veterinarian. Benzonatate may cause nausea/vomiting and behavioral changes (depression/sedation to agitation).
- Benzonatate can be very toxic if overdosed. Never exceed your veterinarian's dosage instructions. Benzonatate overdoses have caused death in children with as few as one or two capsules. The capsules can look like "candy" to children and the FDA has warned that they should be stored in child-resistant containers out of reach of children and pets.
- Capsules or compounded dosage forms must be given whole— do not break, or split capsules. The animal must not be allowed to chew them or let them dissolve in their mouth or choking may occur.

Chemistry/Synonyms

Benzonatate (CAS Registry: 0000104-31-4; ATC: R05DB01) is chemically related to tetracaine and procaine. It occurs as a clear, pale yellow, viscous liquid having a faint, characteristic odor. Benzonatate is miscible in water and freely soluble in alcohol. The commercially available liquid-filled, soft-gelatin capsules contain benzoate in a vehicle of glycerin.

Storage/Stability

Commercially available liquid filled capsules should be stored in tight, light-resistant containers at 15-30°C (59-86°F).

Compatibility/Compounding Considerations

Because of the potential toxicity, local anesthetic activity, and drug form (viscous liquid), compounding an acceptable dosage form for use in animals is challenging. Any compounded preparation must protect oral mucosa from direct contact with the drug.

Dosage Forms/Regulatory Status

VETERINARY-LABELED PRODUCTS: NONE.

HUMAN-LABELED PRODUCTS:

Oral Capsules, liquid filled: 100 mg & 200 mg capsules (round); *Tessalon® Perles*, generic; (Rx) There is a website (dailymed.nim.hih.gov) listing FDA-approved (human drug) labels for benzonatate. Benzonatate is not commercially available in Canada.

Revisions/References

Monograph written July 2013.

Betamethasone (Systemic)

(bet-ta-meth-a-sone)   Celestone®

Glucocorticoid

Note: For more information on the pharmacology of glucocorticoids refer to the monograph: Glucocorticoids, General information. For topical or otic use, see the Topical Dermatology & Otic sections in the appendix.

Prescriber Highlights

- ▶ Injectable glucocorticoid. Long acting; 25-40X more potent than hydrocortisone; no mineralocorticoid activity.
- ▶ Primary use is intraarticular administration in horses.
- ▶ When used systemically goal is to use as much as is required & as little as possible for as short an amount of time as possible.
- ▶ Primary adverse effects are "Cushingoid" in nature with sustained systemic use.
- ▶ Many potential drug & lab interactions when used systemically (IM).

Uses/Indications

In veterinary medicine, betamethasone for systemic or articular effects is usually administered as the injection combining betamethasone sodium phosphate (prompt effect) and betamethasone acetate (sustained effect). It can be used when an injectable glucocorticoid having both rapid- and long-acting glucocorticoid is desired.

In horses, intraarticular injection of betamethasone sodium phosphate/acetate can be useful for treating pain and inflamed joints. Duration of pain relief can be up to 4 weeks after injection (Edwards 2011).

Betamethasone injection (0.5 mg on day 55) has been shown in pregnant dogs to induce premature labor. No long-term negative clinical effects in preterm puppies (delivered by C-section on day 58) were detected and appeared to enhance vital organ maturation (Vannucchi et al. 2012). Comparing IV or PO glucocorticoid potency: A dosage of 0.75 mg of betamethasone is approximately equivalent to 5 mg of prednisone, 4 mg of methylprednisolone or 20 mg of hydrocortisone (intraarticular or IM may be different).

Contraindications/Precautions/Warnings

For the product *Betasone®* (Schering), the manufacturer states that the drug is "contraindicated in animals with acute or chronic bacterial infections unless therapeutic doses of an effective antimicrobial agent are used." Systemic use of glucocorticoids is generally considered contraindicated in systemic fungal infections (unless used for replacement therapy in Addison's), when administered IM in patients with idiopathic thrombocytopenia and in patients hypersensitive to a particular compound. Use of sustained-release injectable glucocorticoids is contraindicated for chronic corticosteroid therapy of systemic diseases.

Animals that have received glucocorticoids systemically, other than with "burst" therapy, should be tapered off the drugs. Patients that have received the drugs chronically should be tapered off slowly as endogenous ACTH and corticosteroid function may return slowly. Should the animal undergo a "stressor" (*e.g.*, surgery, trauma, illness, etc.) during the tapering process or until normal adrenal and pituitary function resume, additional glucocorticoids should be administered.

Corticosteroid therapy may induce parturition in large animal species during the latter stages of pregnancy.

Adverse Effects
When used systemically in horses, betamethasone, like other glucocorticoids, may potentially increase the risk for laminitis. When used as an intraarticular (IA) injection in adult horses, betamethasone sodium phosphate/acetate does not appear to have deleterious effects (McIlwraith 2010). However, there is a slight risk for infection (septic arthritis) and post-corticosteroid reactive synovitis after IA injection.

Adverse effects are generally associated with long-term systemic administration of these drugs, especially if given at high dosages or not on an alternate day regimen. Effects generally manifest as clinical signs of hyperadrenocorticism. When administered to young, growing animals, glucocorticoids can retard growth. Many of the potential effects, adverse and otherwise, are outlined in the Pharmacology section of the Glucocorticoids, General information monograph.

In dogs, polydipsia (PD), polyphagia (PP) and polyuria (PU), may all be seen with short-term "burst" therapy as well as with alternate-day maintenance therapy on days when given the drug. Adverse effects in dogs associated with long-term use can include: dull, dry haircoat, weight gain, panting, vomiting, diarrhea, elevated liver enzymes, pancreatitis, GI ulceration, lipidemias, activation or worsening of diabetes mellitus, muscle wasting and behavioral changes (*e.g.*, depression, lethargy, viciousness, etc.). Discontinuation of the drug may be necessary; changing to an alternate steroid may also alleviate the problem. With the exception of PU/PD/PP, adverse effects associated with antiinflammatory therapy are relatively uncommon. Adverse effects associated with immunosuppressive doses are more common and potentially more severe.

Cats generally require higher dosages than dogs for clinical effect but tend to develop fewer adverse effects. Occasionally, polydipsia, polyuria, polyphagia with weight gain, diarrhea, or depression can be seen. Long-term, high dose therapy can lead to "Cushingoid" effects.

Reproductive/Nursing Safety
In addition to the contraindications, precautions and adverse effects outlined above, betamethasone has been demonstrated to cause decreased sperm output and semen volume and increased percentages of abnormal sperm in dogs.

Use with caution in nursing dams. Corticosteroids appear in milk and could suppress growth, interfere with endogenous corticosteroid production or cause other unwanted effects in the nursing offspring. However, in humans, several studies suggest that amounts excreted in breast milk are negligible when prednisone or prednisolone doses in the mother are less than or equal to 20 mg/day or methylprednisolone doses are less than or equal to 8 mg/day. Larger doses for short periods may not harm the infant.

Overdosage/Acute Toxicity
Acute overdoses of glucocorticoids rarely cause serious problems, but in large overdoses contact an animal poison control center for further guidance. One incidence of a dog developing acute CNS effects after accidental ingestion of glucocorticoids has been reported. Should clinical signs occur, use supportive treatment if required.

Chronic usage of glucocorticoids can lead to serious adverse effects. Refer to Adverse Effects above for more information.

Drug Interactions
The following drug interactions have either been reported or are theoretical in humans or animals receiving betamethasone systemically and may be of significance in veterinary patients. Unless otherwise noted, use together is not necessarily contraindicated, but weigh the potential risks and perform additional monitoring when appropriate.

- **AMPHOTERICIN B:** When administered concomitantly with glucocorticoids may cause hypokalemia.
- **ANTICHOLINESTERASE AGENTS** (*e.g.*, **pyridostigmine, neostigmine**, etc.): In patients with myasthenia gravis, concomitant glucocorticoid and anticholinesterase agent administration may lead to profound muscle weakness; if possible, discontinue anticholinesterase medication at least 24 hours prior to corticosteroid administration.
- **ASPIRIN and OTHER SALICYLATES:** Glucocorticoids may reduce salicylate blood levels.
- **BARBITURATES:** May increase the metabolism of glucocorticoids.
- **CYCLOPHOSPHAMIDE:** Glucocorticoids may inhibit the hepatic metabolism of cyclophosphamide; dosage adjustments may be required.
- **CYCLOSPORINE:** Concomitant administration of glucocorticoids and cyclosporine may increase the blood levels of each by mutually inhibiting hepatic metabolism; clinical significance is not clear.
- **DIGOXIN:** When glucocorticoids are used concurrently with digitalis glycosides, an increased chance of digitalis toxicity may occur should hypokalemia develop; diligent monitoring of potassium and digitalis glycoside levels is recommended.
- **DIURETICS, POTASSIUM-DEPLETING** (*e.g.*, **furosemide, thiazides**, etc.): When administered concomitantly with glucocorticoids may cause hypokalemia.
- **ESTROGENS:** May decrease corticosteroid clearance.
- **INSULIN** Requirements may increase in patients receiving glucocorticoids.
- **ISONIAZID:** May have serum levels decreased by corticosteroids.
- **KETOCONAZOLE:** Corticosteroid clearance may be reduced and the AUC increased.
- **MITOTANE:** May alter the metabolism of steroids; higher than usual doses of steroids may be necessary to treat mitotane-induced adrenal insufficiency.
- **RIFAMPIN:** May increase the metabolism of glucocorticoids.
- **THEOPHYLLINES:** Alterations of pharmacologic effects of either drug can occur.
- **ULCEROGENIC DRUGS** (*e.g.*, NSAIDs): Use with glucocorticoids may increase the risk of gastrointestinal ulceration.
- **VACCINES:** Patients receiving corticosteroids at immunosuppressive dosages should generally not receive live attenuated-virus vaccines as virus replication may be augmented; diminished immune response may occur after vaccine, toxoid, or bacterin administration in patients receiving glucocorticoids.

Laboratory Considerations
- Glucocorticoids may increase **serum cholesterol** and **urine glucose** levels.
- Glucocorticoids may decrease **serum potassium.**
- Glucocorticoids can suppress the release of thyroid stimulating hormone (TSH) and reduce T_3 & T_4 values; thyroid gland atrophy has been reported after chronic glucocorticoid administration.

- Uptake of I^{131} by the thyroid may be decreased by glucocorticoids.
- Reactions to **skin tests** may be suppressed by glucocorticoids.
- False-negative results of the **nitroblue tetrazolium test** for systemic bacterial infections may be induced by glucocorticoids.
- Betamethasone does not cross-react with the cortisol assay.

Doses

- **DOGS:**

  For the control of pruritus: 0.25 – 0.5 mL per 20 pounds body weight IM. Dose dependent on severity of condition. May repeat when necessary. Relief averages 3 weeks in duration. Do not exceed more than 4 injections. (Package Insert; *Betasone®*—Schering) **Note:** Product no longer marketed in the USA.

- **HORSES: (NOTE: ARCI UCGFS CLASS 4 DRUG)**

  For intraarticular administration (extra-label): Most dosage recommendations range from 3 – 18 mg per joint intra-articularly. Repeat dosages should be limited to the minimum required to achieve soundness.

Monitoring

Monitoring of glucocorticoid therapy is dependent on its reason for use, dosage, agent used (amount of mineralocorticoid activity), dosage schedule (daily versus alternate day therapy), duration of therapy, and the animal's age and condition. The following list may not be appropriate or complete for all animals; use clinical assessment and judgment should adverse effects be noted:

- Weight, appetite, signs of edema.
- Serum and/or urine electrolytes.
- Total plasma proteins, albumin.
- Blood glucose.
- Growth and development in young animals.
- ACTH stimulation test, if necessary.

Client Information

- Clients should carefully follow the dosage instructions and should not discontinue the drug abruptly without consulting veterinarian beforehand.
- Clients should be briefed on the potential adverse effects that can be seen with these drugs and instructed to contact the veterinarian should these effects become severe or progress.

Chemistry/Synonyms

A synthetic glucocorticoid, betamethasone is available as the base and as the dipropionate, acetate and sodium phosphate salts. The base is used for oral dosage forms. The sodium phosphate and acetate salts are used in injectable preparations. The dipropionate salt is used in topical formulations and in combination with the sodium phosphate salt in a veterinary-approved injectable preparation.

Betamethasone occurs as an odorless, white to practically white, crystalline powder. It is insoluble in water and practically insoluble in alcohol. The dipropionate salt occurs as a white or creamy-white, odorless powder. It is practically insoluble in water and sparingly soluble in alcohol. The sodium phosphate salt occurs as an odorless, white to practically white, hygroscopic powder. It is freely soluble in water and slightly soluble in alcohol.

Betamethasone may also be known as flubenisolone or *Celestone®*.

Storage/Stability

The oral solution should be stored in well-closed containers, protected from light and kept at temperatures less than 40°C. The combination injectable product (*Celestone®*) should be stored between 2-30°C and protected from light and freezing. Shake well before using.

Compatibility/Compounding Considerations

If coadministration with a local anesthetic is desired, lidocaine 1% or 2% (without parabens or phenol) mixed with betamethasone sodium phosphate/acetate injection has been suggested. The lidocaine should be drawn into the syringe after the dose of betamethasone is drawn up. Do not add lidocaine to the vial of betamethasone.

Dosage Forms/Regulatory Status

VETERINARY-LABELED PRODUCTS:

The following product is apparently no longer marketed in the USA: Betamethasone Dipropionate Injection equivalent to 5 mg/mL of betamethasone and betamethasone sodium phosphate equivalent to 2 mg/mL betamethasone in 5 mL vials; *Betasone®*; (Rx). FDA-approved for use in dogs.

Betamethasone valerate is also found in *Gentocin® Otic*, *Gentocin® Topical Spray* and *Topagen® Ointment*. There are several other otic and topical products containing betamethasone and gentamicin on the veterinary market.

The ARCI (Racing Commissioners International) has designated this drug as a class 4 substance. See the appendix for more information.

HUMAN-LABELED PRODUCTS:

Betamethasone Oral Solution: 0.6 mg/5 mL in 118 mL; *Celestone®*; (Rx)

Betamethasone Injection: betamethasone (as sodium phosphate) 3 mg/mL and betamethasone acetate 3 mg/mL suspension in 5 mL multi-dose vials; *Celestone Soluspan®*, generic;(Rx)

Revisions/References

Monograph revised/updated September 2013.

Edwards, S. H. R. (2011). Intra-articular drug delivery: The challenge to extend drug residence time within the joint. *The Veterinary Journal* 190(1): 15-21.

McIlwraith, C. W. (2010). The use of intra-articular corticosteroids in the horse: What is known on a scientific basis? *Equine Veterinary Journal* 42(6): 563-71.

Vannucchi, C. I., et al. (2012). Cortisol Profile and Clinical Evaluation of Canine Neonates Exposed Antenatally to Maternal Corticosteroid Treatment. *Reproduction in Domestic Animals* 47: 173-6.

Bethanechol Chloride

(beh-than-e-kole)   Urecholine®

Cholinergic

Prescriber Highlights

▶ Cholinergic agent used primarily to increase bladder contractility; symptomatic treatment of dysautonomia. May be useful for equine gastric ulcer syndrome (EGUS).

▶ Principle contraindications are GI or urinary tract obstructions or if bladder wall integrity is in question.

▶ Adverse Effects: "SLUD" (salivation, lacrimation, urination, defecation).

▶ Cholinergic crisis possible if injecting IV or SC; have atropine at the ready.

Uses/Indications

Bethanechol can be useful to stimulate bladder contractions in small animals. It appears to be most effective in acute and partial detrusor atony secondary to acute bladder overdistension and partial neurogenic lesions. Bethanechol also can be useful as an esophageal prokinetic. While it can be used a general GI prokinetic agent, other agents such as metoclopramide or cisapride have largely supplanted it.

Bethanechol has been shown to increase abomasum and duodenum contractility in both healthy dairy cattle and those with left displacement of the abomasum (LDA) (Niederberger et al. 2010).

In horses, bethanechol has been suggested as an adjunctive prokinetic agent for treatment of equine gastric ulcer syndrome (EGUS) when there is adynamic ileus and gastroduodenal reflux.

Pharmacology/Actions

Bethanechol directly stimulates cholinergic receptors. Its effects are principally muscarinic and at usual doses has negligible nicotinic activity. It is more resistant to hydrolysis than acetylcholine by cholinesterase and, therefore, has an increased duration of activity.

Pharmacologic effects include increased esophageal peristalsis and lower esophageal sphincter tone, increased tone and peristaltic activity of the stomach and intestines, increased gastric and pancreatic secretions, increased tone of the detrusor muscle of the bladder, and decreased bladder capacity. At high doses after parenteral administration, effects such as increased bronchial secretions and constriction, miosis, lacrimation, and salivation can be seen. When administered SC or orally, effects are predominantly on the GI and urinary tracts. A ceiling effect (decreased response after high dosages) can be seen secondary to receptor desensitization and calcium depletion.

Pharmacokinetics

No information was located on the pharmacokinetics of this agent in veterinary species. In humans, bethanechol is poorly absorbed from the GI tract, and the onset of action is usually within 30-90 minutes after oral dosing. After subcutaneous administration, effects begin within 5-15 minutes and usually peak within 30 minutes. The duration of action after oral dosing may persist up to 6 hours after large doses and 2 hours after SC dosing. Subcutaneous administration yields a more enhanced effect on urinary tract stimulation than does oral administration.

Bethanechol does not enter the CNS after usual doses; other distribution aspects of the drug are not known. The metabolic or excretory fate of bethanechol has not been described.

Contraindications/Precautions/Warnings

Contraindications to bethanechol therapy include: bladder neck or other urinary outflow obstruction, when the integrity of the bladder wall is in question (*e.g.*, as after recent bladder surgery), hyperthyroidism, peptic ulcer disease or when other inflammatory GI lesions are present, recent GI surgery with resections/anastomoses, GI obstruction or peritonitis, hypersensitivity to the drug, epilepsy, asthma, coronary artery disease or occlusion, hypotension, severe bradycardia or vagotonia or vasomotor instability. If urinary outflow resistance is increased due to enhanced urethral tone (not mechanical obstruction!), bethanechol should only be used in conjunction with another agent that will sufficiently reduce outflow resistance [*e.g.*, diazepam, dantrolene (striated muscle) or phenoxybenzamine (smooth muscle)].

Adverse Effects

When administered orally to small animals, adverse effects are usually mild with vomiting, diarrhea, salivation, and anorexia being the most likely to occur. Cardiovascular (*e.g.*, bradycardia, arrhythmias, hypotension, etc.) and respiratory effects (*e.g.*, asthma, dyspnea, etc.) are most likely only seen after overdosage situations or with high dose SC therapy.

In horses, salivation, lacrimation and abdominal pain (colic) are potential adverse effects.

IM or IV use is not recommended except in emergencies when the IV route may be used. Severe cholinergic reactions are likely if given IV. If injecting the drug (SC or IV), it is recommended that atropine be immediately available.

Reproductive/Nursing Safety

In humans, the FDA categorizes this drug as category *C* for use during pregnancy (*Animal studies have shown an adverse effect on the fetus, but there are no adequate studies in humans; or there are no animal reproduction studies and no adequate studies in humans.*) It is unknown if bethanechol is distributed into milk.

Overdosage/Acute Toxicity

Clinical signs of overdosage are basically cholinergic in nature. Muscarinic effects (*e.g.*, salivation, urination, defecation, etc.) are usually seen with oral or SC administration. If given IM or IV, a full-blown cholinergic crisis can occur with circulatory collapse, bloody diarrhea, shock and cardiac arrest possible.

Treatment for bethanechol toxicity is atropine. Refer to the atropine monograph for more information on its use. Epinephrine may also be employed to treat clinical signs of bronchospasm.

Drug Interactions

The following drug interactions have either been reported or are theoretical in humans or animals receiving bethanechol and may be of significance in veterinary patients. Unless otherwise noted, use together is not necessarily contraindicated, but weigh the potential risks and perform additional monitoring when appropriate.

- **ANTICHOLINERGIC DRUGS:** (*e.g.*, **atropine, glycopyrrolate, propantheline,** etc.): Can antagonize bethanechol's effects.
- **CHOLINERGIC DRUGS** (*e.g.*, **neostigmine, physostigmine, pyridostigmine,** etc.): Because of additional cholinergic effects, bethanechol should generally not be used concomitantly with other cholinergic drugs.
- **GANGLIONIC BLOCKING DRUGS** (*e.g.*, **mecamylamine,** etc.): Can produce severe GI and hypotensive effects.
- **QUINIDINE, PROCAINAMIDE:** Can antagonize the effects of bethanechol.

Doses

Note: The injectable product is no longer commercially marketed in the USA.

- **DOGS:**

  To increase bladder contractility in detrusor atony or symptomatic treatment of dysautonomia: (extra-label): 2.5 mg – 25 mg per dog PO three times daily. Some dogs may respond to twice daily dosing.

- **CATS:**

  To increase bladder contractility or symptomatic treatment of dysautonomia (extra-label): 1.25 mg (1/4 of a 5 mg tablet) – 7.5 mg per cat PO three times daily. Some cats may respond to twice daily dosing.

- **HORSES: (NOTE: ARCI UCGFS CLASS 4 DRUG)**

  To stimulate detrusor muscle activity (extra-label): 0.025 – 0.075 mg/kg SC q8h for 2-3 doses, then 0.25 – 0.75 mg/kg PO 2-4 times a day. If no response after 5 days, discontinue. **Note:** Oral dose is 10X that of SC dose.

  To adjunctive treatment of equine gastric ulcer syndrome (EGUS); (extra-label): 0.025 – 0.03 mg/kg SC q4-8 hours until no reflux, followed by 0.3 – 0.4 mg/kg PO 3-4 times daily.

- **CATTLE:**

  For adjunctive medical therapy (with fluids, mineral oil, and NSAIDs if needed) of cecal dilation/dislocation (CDD); (extra-label): Only if animal is "normal" or only slightly disturbed, defecation is present, and rectal exam does not reveal torsion or retroflexion. If these criteria are not met, or no improvement within 24 hours of medical therapy, surgical therapy is recommended. Bethanechol at 0.07 mg/kg SC three times daily for 2 days. Withhold feed for 24 hours and then gradually give increasing amounts of hay if defecation is present and CDD is resolved. **Note:** Compounded preparations are required as no commercial products are on the market. (Meylan 2004)

Monitoring

- Clinical efficacy.
- Urination frequency, amount voided, bladder palpation.
- Adverse effects (see above section).

Client Information

- Usually given on an empty stomach, but if animal vomits after getting the drug try giving it with food.
- Side effects in dogs and cats include: vomiting, diarrhea, lack of appetite and increased drooling. Contact veterinarian if these are severe or continue.

Chemistry/Synonyms

A synthetic cholinergic ester, bethanechol occurs as a slightly hygroscopic, white or colorless crystalline powder with a slight, amine-like or "fishy" odor. It exhibits polymorphism, with one form melting at 211° and the other form at 219°. One gram of the drug is soluble in approximately 1 mL of water or 10 mL of alcohol.

Bethanechol Chloride may also be known as: carbamylmethylcholine chloride, *Duvoid®*, *Miotonachol®*, *Muscaran®*, *Myo Hermes®*, *Myocholine®*, *Myotonine®*, *Ucholine®*, *Urecholine®*, *Urocarb®*, or *Urotonine®*.

Storage/Stability

Bethanechol tablets should be stored at room temperature in tight containers.

Compounded preparation stability: Bethanechol oral suspension compounded from commercially available tablets has been published (Allen et al. 1998). Triturating twelve (12) bethanechol 50 mg tablets with 60 mL of *Ora-Plus®* and *qs ad* to 120 mL with *Ora-Sweet®* (or *Ora-Sweet® SF*) yields a 5 mg/mL oral suspension that retains >90% potency for 60 days stored at both 5°C and 25°C. Compounded preparations of bethanechol should be protected from light.

Compatibility/Compounding Considerations

No specific information noted.

Dosage Forms/Regulatory Status

VETERINARY-LABELED PRODUCTS: NONE.

The ARCI (Racing Commissioners International) has designated this drug as a class 4 substance. See the appendix for more information.

HUMAN-LABELED PRODUCTS:

Bethanechol Chloride Oral Tablets: 5 mg, 10 mg, 25 mg & 50 mg; *Urecholine®*, generic; (Rx)

An injectable product was formerly commercially available; a compounding pharmacy may be able to prepare a bethanechol injectable form.

Revisions/References

Monograph revised/updated September 2013.

Allen, L. V. & M. A. Erickson (1998). Stability of bethanechol chloride, pyrazinamide, quinidine sulfate, rifampin, and tetracycline hydrochloride in extemporaneously compounded oral liquids. *Am J Health Syst Pharm* 55(17): 1804-9.

Meylan, M. (2004). *Motility in the bovine large intestine and pathogenesis of cecal dilatation/dislocation.* Proceedings: ACVIM Forum. accessed via Veterinary Information Network; vin.com

Niederberger, M. D., et al. (2010). In vitro effects of bethanechol on abomasal and duodenal smooth muscle preparations from dairy cows with left displacement of the abomasum and from healthy dairy cows. *The Veterinary Journal* 184(1): 88-94.

Bicarbonate — see Sodium Bicarbonate

Bisacodyl

(bis-a-koe-dill)   Dulcolax®

Oral/Rectal Laxative

Prescriber Highlights

▶ Stimulant laxative used in dogs & cats.
▶ Contraindicated in GI obstruction.
▶ GI cramping/diarrhea possible.
▶ Don't give with milk products or antacids; do not crush or split tablets.

Uses/Indications

Bisacodyl oral and rectal products are used as stimulant cathartics in dogs and cats.

Pharmacology/Actions

A stimulant laxative, bisacodyl's exact mechanism is unknown. It is thought to produce catharsis by increasing peristalsis by direct stimulation on the intramural nerve plexuses of intestinal smooth muscle. It has been shown to increase fluid and ion accumulation in the large intestine thereby enhancing catharsis.

Pharmacokinetics

Bisacodyl is minimally absorbed after either oral or rectal administration. Onset of action after oral administration is generally 6-10 hours and 15 minutes to an hour after rectal administration.

Contraindications/Precautions/Warnings

Stimulant cathartics are contraindicated in the following conditions: intestinal obstruction (not constipation), undiagnosed rectal bleeding, or when the patient is susceptible to intestinal perforation.

Bisacodyl should only be used short-term as chronic use can damage myenteric neurons.

Adverse Effects

Bisacodyl has relatively few side effects when used occasionally; cramping, nausea, or diarrhea may be noted after use.

Reproductive/Nursing Safety

In humans, the FDA categorizes this drug as category *B* for use during pregnancy (*Animal studies have not yet demonstrated risk to the fetus, but there are no adequate studies in pregnant women; or animal studies have shown an adverse effect, but adequate studies in pregnant women have not demonstrated a risk to the fetus in the first trimester of pregnancy, and there is no evidence of risk in later trimesters.*)

Bisacodyl may be distributed into milk but at quantities unlikely to cause any problems in nursing offspring.

Overdosage/Acute Toxicity

Overdoses may result in severe cramping, diarrhea, vomiting and, potentially, fluid and electrolyte imbalances. Animals should be monitored and given replacement parenteral fluids and electrolytes as necessary.

Drug Interactions

The following drug interactions have either been reported or are theoretical in humans or animals receiving bisacodyl and may be of significance in veterinary patients. Unless otherwise noted, use together is not necessarily contraindicated, but weigh the potential risks and perform additional monitoring when appropriate.

- **ANTACIDS/MILK:** Do not give milk or antacids within an hour of bisacodyl tablets as it may cause premature disintegration of the enteric coating.
- **ORAL DRUGS:** Stimulant laxatives may potentially decrease GI transit time thereby affecting absorption of other oral drugs. Separate doses by two hours if possible.

Doses

Note: Bisacodyl enema products and pediatric suppositories are no longer available in the USA. Human pediatric suppositories were 5 mg; the 10 mg "adult" suppositories can be cut lengthwise to approximate one pediatric suppository.

- **DOGS/CATS:**

  As a cathartic (extra-label): One 5 mg tablet PO per cat or small dog; one to three 5 mg tablets (5 – 15 mg) per dog for medium to large dogs. Do not break or crush tablets.

Client Information

- Do not crush, split, or allow animals to chew tablets; severe cramping can occur.
- Do not give milk (dairy) products or antacids within one hour of giving the oral tablets as it can dissolve the protective coating on the tablets.
- If you are giving other drugs by mouth to your animal, try to give them two hours apart from the bisacodyl oral dose. Bisacodyl can speed up the movement of these drugs through the intestines and prevent them from being absorbed properly.
- Bisacodyl should only be used on an occasional basis; long-term, regular use can damage the nerves in the intestinal tract.

Chemistry/Synonyms

A diphenylmethane laxative, bisacodyl occurs as white to off-white crystalline powder. It is practically insoluble in water and sparingly soluble in alcohol.

Bisacodyl may also be known as bisacodylum; many trade names are available.

Storage/Stability

Bisacodyl suppositories and enteric-coated tablets should be stored at temperatures less than 30°C.

Compatibility/Compounding Considerations

Do not crush tablets.

Dosage Forms/Regulatory Status

VETERINARY-LABELED PRODUCTS: NONE.

HUMAN-LABELED PRODUCTS:

Bisacodyl Enteric-coated Oral Tablets: 5 mg; Many trade names including *Dulcolax®*, generic; (OTC)

Bisacodyl Rectal Suppositories: 10 mg: *Dulcolax®*, *Bisa-Lax®*, *Bisac-Evac®*, generic; (OTC). Pediatric suppositories (5 mg) are no longer available in the USA; 10 mg "adult" suppositories can be cut lengthwise to approximate a pediatric suppository.

Bisacodyl Rectal Enema: 10 mg/30 mL; (OTC)

Revisions/References

Monograph revised/updated September 2013.

Bismuth Subsalicylate

(biz-mith sub-sal-iss-ih-layt)   *BSS, Pepto-Bismol®*

Antidiarrheal; Gastroprotectant

Prescriber Highlights

▶ Used to treat diarrhea & as a component of "triple/quadruple therapy" for treating Helicobacter GI infections.

▶ High doses may cause salicylism, use with caution in cats.

▶ Constipation/impactions may occur.

▶ Refrigeration may improve palatability.

Uses/Indications

In veterinary medicine, bismuth subsalicylate products are used to treat diarrhea, as a gastroprotectant, and as a component of "triple therapy" for treating Helicobacter GI infections. The drug is also used in humans for other GI symptoms (indigestion, cramps, gas pains) and in the treatment and prophylaxis of traveler's diarrhea.

Pharmacology/Actions

Bismuth subsalicylate is thought to possess protectant, anti-endotoxic and weak antibacterial properties. It is believed that the parent compound is cleaved in the small intestine into bismuth carbonate and salicylate. The protectant, anti-endotoxic and weak antibacterial properties are thought to be because of the bismuth. The salicylate component has antiprostaglandin activity that may contribute to its effectiveness and reduce clinical signs associated with secretory diarrheas.

Pharmacokinetics

No specific veterinary information was located. In humans, the amount of bismuth absorbed is negligible while the salicylate component is rapidly and completely absorbed. Salicylates are highly bound to plasma proteins and are metabolized in the liver to salicylic acid. Salicylic acid, conjugated salicylate metabolites and any absorbed bismuth are all excreted renally.

Contraindications/Precautions/Warnings

Salicylate absorption may occur; use with caution in patients with preexisting bleeding disorders. Because of the potential for adverse effects caused by the salicylate component, this drug should be used cautiously, if at all, in cats.

As bismuth is radiopaque, it may interfere with GI tract radiologic examinations.

Adverse Effects

Antidiarrheal products are not a substitute for adequate fluid and electrolyte therapy when required. May change stool color to a gray-black or greenish-black; do not confuse with melena. In human infants and debilitated individuals, use of this product may cause impactions to occur.

Reproductive/Nursing Safety

The FDA has not, apparently, given bismuth subsalicylate a pregnancy risk category. As it is a form of salicylate, refer to the aspirin monograph for further guidance. Use with caution in pregnant animals.

Use with caution in nursing dams.

Overdosage/Acute Toxicity

Bismuth subsalicylate liquid/suspension contains approximately 8.7 mg/mL salicylate. Two tablespoonsful (30 mL) are approximately equivalent to one 325 mg aspirin tablet. See the Aspirin monograph for more information. There were 63 single agent exposures to bismuth subsalicylate reported to the ASPCA Animal Poison Control Center (APCC) during 2009-2013. Of the 41 exposed dogs, 27 were symptomatic. The most common clinical signs included: diarrhea (26%), lethargy (26%), vomiting (22%), ataxia (19%), hind limb weakness (19%), and panting (15%). Of the 22 cats, 10 were symptomatic with 50% having diarrhea, 40% lethargic, and 20% anorexic.

Drug Interactions

The following drug interactions have either been reported or are theoretical in humans or animals receiving bismuth subsalicylate and may be of significance in veterinary patients. Unless otherwise noted, use together is not necessarily contraindicated, but weigh the potential risks and perform additional monitoring when appropriate.

- **TETRACYCLINE:** Bismuth containing products can decrease the absorption of orally administered tetracycline products. If both agents are to be used, separate drugs by at least 2 hours and administer tetracycline first.

- **ASPIRIN:** Because bismuth subsalicylate contains salicylate, concomitant administration with aspirin may increase salicylate serum levels; monitor appropriately.

Laboratory Considerations

- At high doses, salicylates may cause false-positive results for **urinary glucose** if using the cupric sulfate method (*Clinitest®*, Benedict's solution) and false-negative results if using the glucose oxidase method (*Clinistix®* or *Tes-Tape®*).
- **Urinary ketones** measured by the ferric chloride method (Gerhardt) may be affected if salicylates are in the urine (reddish-color or produced).
- **5-HIAA** determinations by the fluorometric method may be interfered by salicylates in the urine.
- Falsely elevated **VMA** (vanillylmandelic acid) may be seen with most methods used if salicylates are in the urine. Falsely lowered **VMA** levels may be seen if using the Pisano method.
- Urinary excretion of **xylose** may be decreased if salicylates are given concurrently.
- Falsely elevated **serum uric acid** values may be measured if using colorimetric methods.

Doses

Note: Doses of liquids below are for the 17.5 mg/mL (1.75%) liquids (veterinary suspensions; original *Pepto-Bismol®* liquid, etc.) unless otherwise specified.

- **DOGS:**

  For acute diarrhea or as a GI "coating agent" (extra-label): Liquid: 0.25 – 2 mL/mg PO 3-4 times per day.

  For treating Helicobacter gastritis infections (extra-label):

  a) Using triple therapy: Metronidazole 15.4 mg/kg q8h, amoxicillin 11 mg/kg q8h and bismuth subsalicylate (original *Pepto-Bismol®*) 0.22 mL/kg PO q4-6h. Give each for 3 weeks. (Hall 2000)

  b) Using triple therapy: Metronidazole 10 mg/kg PO q12h, amoxicillin 15 mg/kg q12h and bismuth subsalicylate 262 mg tablets given based upon body weight (< 5kg = 0.25 tablet; 5-9.9 kg = 0.5 tablet; 10-24.9kg = 1 tablet; >25kg = 2 tablets) q12h. Give each for 2 weeks. (Leib et al. 2007)

- **CATS:**

  For diarrhea (extra-label): 0.25 – 1 mL/kg PO q6-12h. Use cautiously in cats; recommend not treating for more than a few days.

  For treating Helicobacter gastritis infections (extra-label):

  a) Metronidazole 10 mg/kg PO twice daily, amoxicillin 10 – 20 mg/kg PO three times daily, bismuth subsalicylate (262 mg tablets; *Pepto-Bismol®*) ¼ tablet PO twice daily, ± H2 blocker (*e.g.,* famotidine) or omeprazole. All are given for two weeks. (Leib 2012)

  b) Using triple therapy: Metronidazole 15.4 mg/kg PO q8h, amoxicillin 11 mg/kg PO q8h and bismuth subsalicylate (original *Pepto-Bismol®*) 0.22 mL/kg PO q4-6h. Give each for 3 weeks. (Hall 2000)

- **FERRETS:**

  For treating Helicobacter gastritis infections (extra-label):

  a) Using triple therapy: Metronidazole 20 mg/kg PO, amoxicillin 30 mg/kg PO and bismuth subsalicylate 7.5 mg/kg PO. Give each q8h for 3-4 weeks. (Johnson-Delaney 2009)

  b) Using triple therapy: Metronidazole 20 mg/kg PO q12h, amoxicillin 20 mg/kg PO q12h and bismuth subsalicylate 17.5 mg/kg PO q8h; continue for 21 days. Used with famoti-

dine (0.5 mg/kg PO once daily) and sucralfate (25 mg/kg PO q8h). (Johnson 2006)

- **CATTLE:**

  For diarrhea in calves (extra-label): 60 – 90 mL per calf PO two to four times a day.

- **HORSES:**

  For diarrhea in foals (extra-label): 60 – 120 mL per foal PO two to four times per day.

- **SWINE:**

  For diarrhea in baby pigs (extra-label): 2 – 5 mL PO two to four times a day for 2 days.

Monitoring

- Clinical efficacy.
- Fluid and electrolyte status in severe diarrhea.

Client Information

- Use with caution in cats, as they may be sensitive to the salicylate (aspirin-like compound).
- May cause constipation.
- Don't give other drugs within two hours of this drug unless veterinarian approves.
- Shake suspension well; store in refrigerator to improve palatability. Do not mix with milk.
- May cause stool to change color to a gray-black or greenish-black, this is normal; contact veterinarian if stool becomes tarry black.

Chemistry/Synonyms

Bismuth subsalicylate occurs as white or nearly white, tasteless, odorless powder and contains about 58% bismuth. It is insoluble in water, glycerin and alcohol.

Bismuth subsalicylate may also be known as: BSS, basic bismuth salicylate, bismuth oxysalicylate, bismuth salicylate, bismuthi subsalicylas, *Bismu-kote®*, *Bismukote®*, *Bismupaste®*, *Bismatrol®*, *Bismed®*, *Bismusal®*, *Bismylate®*, *Bisval®*, *Equi-Phar®*, *Gastrocote®*, *Jatrox®*, *Kalbeten®*, *Kaopectate®*, *Katulcin-R®*, *PalaBIS®*, *Peptic Relief®*, *Pink Biscoat®*, *Pink Bismuth Rose®*, or *Ulcolind Wismut®*; many other human trade names are available.

Storage/Stability

Bismuth subsalicylate should be stored protected from light. Unless otherwise labeled store at room temperature; do not freeze.

Compatibility/Compounding Considerations

Bismuth subsalicylate is **incompatible** with mineral acids and iron salts. When exposed to alkali bicarbonates, bismuth subsalicylate decomposes with effervescence.

Dosage Forms/Regulatory Status

VETERINARY-LABELED PRODUCTS:

Note: Veterinary labeling does not imply that the product is FDA-approved.

Bismuth Subsalicylate Paste: 5% (50 mg/mL); 10% (100 mg/mL); (OTC). Depending on product, labeled for use in small, medium and large dogs; 20% (200 mg/mL); (OTC). Labeled for use in horses.

Bismuth subsalicylate Oral Suspension 1.75% (17.5 mg/mL; 262 mg/15 mL). Many trade names available, generic; (OTC). Available in gallons. Labeled for use in cattle, horses, calves, foals, dogs and cats. Each mL contains about 8.7 mg salicylate.

Bismuth Subsalicylate Tablets (each tablet contains 262 mg of bismuth subsalicylate). Labeled for use in dogs; (OTC). One tablet contains about 102 mg salicylate.

HUMAN-LABELED PRODUCTS:

Bismuth Subsalicylate (BSS) Liquid/Suspension: 87 mg/5 mL; 130 mg/15 mL; 262 mg/15 mL; 524 mg/15 mL; 525 mg/15 mL; in

120 mL, 236 mL, 237 mL, 240 mL, 355 mL, 360 mL, or 480 mL; Many trade names including *Pepto-Bismol®*, *Kaopectate®*, *Pink Bismuth*; (OTC). **Note:** Regular strength (262 mg/mL) contains 8.7 mg salicylate per mL; Extra-Strength (525 mg/mL) contains 15.7 mg of salicylate per mL.

Bismuth Subsalicylate Tablets and Caplets: 262 mg (regular & chewable); Many trade names including *Pepto-Bismol®*, *Kaopectate®*; (OTC). One tablet contains about 102 mg salicylate.

Revisions/References

Monograph revised/updated September 2013.

Hall, J. (2000). Diseases of the Stomach. *Textbook of Veterinary Internal Medicine: Diseases of the Dog and Cat.* S. Ettinger and E. Feldman. Philadelphia, WB Saunders. **2:** 1154-82.

Johnson, D. (2006). *Ferrets: the other companion animal.* Proceedings: ACVC. accessed via Veterinary Information Network; vin.com

Johnson-Delaney, C. (2009). *Gastrointestinal physiology and disease of carnivorous exotic companion animals.* Proceedings: ABVP. accessed via Veterinary Information Network; vin.com

Leib, M. S. (2012). *Helicobacter Gastritis: Does it Cause Vomiting in Dogs and Cats?* Western States Veterinary Conference Proceedings. accessed via Veterinary Information Network; vin.com

Leib, M. S., et al. (2007). Triple antimicrobial therapy and acid suppression in dogs with chronic vomiting and gastric Helicobacter spp. *Journal of Veterinary Internal Medicine* 21(6): 1185-92.

Bleomycin Sulfate

(blee-oh-mye-sin)   Blenoxane

Antineoplastic

Prescriber Highlights

▶ Antibiotic antineoplastic agent infrequently used for a variety of neoplasms in dogs & cats; intralesional administration may have promise.

▶ Two main toxicities: acute (fever, anorexia, vomiting, & allergic reactions) & delayed (dermatologic effects, stomatitis, pneumonitis & pulmonary fibrosis).

▶ Do not exceed total dosage recommendations.

▶ Intensive adverse effect monitoring required when used systemically.

Uses/Indications

Bleomycin has occasionally been used as adjunctive treatment of lymphomas, oral squamous cell carcinomas, teratomas, and nonfunctional thyroid tumors in both dogs and cats. Recent research has demonstrated that bleomycin may be promising for intralesional treatment for a variety of localized tumors with or without concomitant electropermeabilization. Intralesional bleomycin has been successfully used to treat dogs with acanthomatous ameloblastoma (Kelly et al. 2010).

Pharmacology/Actions

Bleomycin is an antibiotic that has activity against a variety of gram-negative and gram-positive bacteria as well as some fungi. While its cytotoxicity prevents it from being clinically useful as an antimicrobial, it has activity against a variety of tumors.

Bleomycin has both a DNA binding site and a site that binds to the ferrous form of iron. By accepting an electron from ferrous ion to an oxygen atom in the DNA strand, DNA is cleaved.

Resistance to bleomycin therapy is via reduced cellular uptake of the drug, reduced ability to damage DNA and increased rates of DNA repair by the cell and, probably most importantly, via the enzyme bleomycin hydrolase.

Pharmacokinetics

Bleomycin is not appreciably absorbed from the gut and must be administered parenterally. It is mainly distributed to the lungs, kidneys, skin, lymphatics and peritoneum. In patients with normal renal function, terminal half-life is about 2 hours. In humans, 60-70% of a dose is excreted as active drug in the urine.

Contraindications/Precautions/Warnings

Because bleomycin is a toxic drug with a low therapeutic index, only those with the facilities to actively monitor patients and ability to handle potential complications should use it. Bleomycin is contraindicated in patients with prior hypersensitivity reactions from the drug, preexisting pulmonary disease, or adverse pulmonary effects from prior therapy. The drug should be used very cautiously in patients with significant renal impairment and dosage reduction may be necessary. Bleomycin can be teratogenic; it should only be used in pregnant animals when the owners accept the associated risks.

Adverse Effects

Toxicity falls into two broad categories: acute and delayed. Acute toxicities include fever, anorexia, vomiting (usually mild), and allergic reactions (including anaphylaxis). Delayed toxic effects include dermatologic effects (*e.g.*, alopecia, rashes, etc.), stomatitis, pneumonitis and pulmonary fibrosis. These latter two effects have been associated with drug-induced fatalities. Initial signs associated with pulmonary toxicity include pulmonary interstitial edema with alveolar hyaline membrane formation and hyperplasia of type II alveolar macrophages. Pulmonary toxicity is potentially reversible if treatment is stopped soon enough. Unlike many other antineoplastics, bleomycin does not usually cause bone marrow toxicity but thrombocytopenia, leukopenia and slight decreases in hemoglobin levels are possible. Renal toxicity and hepatotoxicity are potentially possible.

To reduce the likelihood of pulmonary toxicity developing, a total maximum dosage of $125 - 200$ mg/m^2 should not be exceeded.

Reproductive/Nursing Safety

In humans, the FDA categorizes this drug as category *D* for use during pregnancy (*There is evidence of human fetal risk, but the potential benefits from the use of the drug in pregnant women may be acceptable despite its potential risks.*)

It not known if bleomycin enters milk; it is not recommended to nurse while receiving the medication.

Overdosage/Acute Toxicity

No specific information was located. Because of the toxicity of the drug, it is important to determine dosages carefully.

Drug Interactions

The following drug interactions have either been reported or are theoretical in humans or animals receiving bleomycin and may be of significance in veterinary patients. Unless otherwise noted, use together is not necessarily contraindicated, but weigh the potential risks and perform additional monitoring when appropriate.

■ **ANESTHETICS, GENERAL:** Use of general anesthetics in patients treated previously with bleomycin should be exercised with caution. Bleomycin sensitizes lung tissue to oxygen (even to concentrations of inspired oxygen considered to be safe) and rapid deterioration of pulmonary function with post-operative pulmonary fibrosis can occur.

■ **PRIOR OR CONCOMITANT CHEMOTHERAPY WITH OTHER AGENTS OR RADIATION THERAPY:** Can lead to increased hematologic, mucosal and pulmonary toxicities with bleomycin therapy.

Doses

Note: Because of the potential toxicity of this drug to patients, veterinary personnel and clients, and since chemotherapy indications, treatment protocols, monitoring and safety guidelines often change, the following dosages should be used only as a general guide. Consultation with a veterinary oncologist and referral to current veterinary oncology references [*e.g.*, (Withrow et al. 2012); (Dobson et al.

2011); (Henry et al. 2009); (North et al. 2009); (Argyle et al. 2008)] are strongly recommended.

- **SMALL ANIMALS:**

  The following is a usual dosage or dose range for bleomycin and should be used only as a general guide: 10 Units mg/m^2 (**NOT** mg/kg) or 0.3 – 0.5 mg/kg (**Note:** 1 Unit = 1 mg). Some protocols use the drug once daily for a few days and then back off to once weekly; some give the drug once weekly at the start. To reduce the likelihood of pulmonary toxicity, a total maximum dosage of 125 – 200 mg/m^2 should not be exceeded.

Monitoring

- Efficacy.
- Pulmonary Toxicity: Obtain chest films, (baseline and on a regular basis—in humans they are recommended q1-2 weeks); lung auscultation (dyspnea and fine rales may be early signs of toxicity); other initial signs associated with pulmonary toxicity include pulmonary interstitial edema with alveolar hyaline membrane formation and hyperplasia of type II alveolar macrophages.
- Blood chemistry (encompassing renal and hepatic function markers) and hematologic profiles (CBC) may be useful to monitor potential renal, hepatic and hematologic toxicities.
- Total dose accumulation.

Client Information

- Bleomycin is a chemotherapy (cancer) drug. The drug and its byproducts can be hazardous to other animals and people that come in contact with it. On the day your animal gets the drug and then for a few days afterward, all bodily waste (urine, feces, litter), blood, or vomit should only be handled while wearing disposable gloves. Seal the waste in a plastic bag and then place both the bag and gloves in with the regular trash.
- Can have very serious side effects, including fatal lung damage; report any change in breathing (*e.g.*, shortness of breath, wheezing, etc.) immediately.

Chemistry/Synonyms

An antibiotic antineoplastic agent, bleomycin sulfate is obtained from *Streptomyces verticillus*. It occurs as a cream colored, amorphous powder that is very soluble in water and sparingly soluble in alcohol. After reconstitution, the pH of the solution ranges from 4.5-6. Bleomycin is assayed microbiologically. One unit of bleomycin is equivalent to one mg of the reference Bleomycin A$_2$ standard.

Bleomycin sulfate may also be known as: bleomycin sulphate, bleomycini sulfas, *Bileco®*, *Blanoxan®*, *Blenamax®*, *Blenoxane®*, *Bleo®*, *Bleo-S®*, *Bleo-cell®*, *Bleocin®*, *Bleolem®*, *Blio®*, *Blocamicina®*, *Bonar®*, *Oil Bleo®*, or *Tecnomicina®*.

Storage/Stability

Powder for injection should be kept refrigerated. After reconstituting with sterile saline, water, or dextrose, the resulting solution is stable for 24 hours. Bleomycin is less stable in dextrose solutions than in saline. After reconstituting with normal saline, bleomycin is reportedly stable for at least two weeks at room temperature and 4 weeks when refrigerated; however, since there are no preservatives in the resulting solution, the product is recommended for use within 24 hours.

Compatibility/Compounding Considerations

Bleomycin sulfate is reported to be **compatible** with the following drugs: amikacin sulfate, cisplatin, cyclophosphamide, dexamethasone sodium phosphate, diphenhydramine HCl, doxorubicin, heparin sodium, metoclopramide HCl, vinblastine sulfate, and vincristine sulfate. Compatibility is dependent upon factors such as pH, concentration, temperature and diluent used; consult specialized references or a hospital pharmacist for more specific information.

Dosage Forms/Regulatory Status

VETERINARY-LABELED PRODUCTS: NONE.

HUMAN-LABELED PRODUCTS:

Bleomycin Sulfate Lyophilized Powder for Injection after reconstitution: 15 Units & 30 Units per vial; generic; (Rx)

Revisions/References

Monograph revised/updated September 2013.

Argyle, D., et al. (2008). *Decision Making in Small Animal Oncology*, Wiley-Blackwell.
Dobson, J. & D. Lascelles (2011). *BSAVA Manual of Canine and Feline Oncology*, BSAVA.
Henry, C. & M. Higginbotham (2009). *Cancer Management in Small Animal Practice*, Saunders.
Kelly, J. M., et al. (2010). Acanthomatous ameloblastoma in dogs treated with intralesional bleomycin. *Veterinary and Comparative Oncology* **8**(2): 81-6.
North, S. & T. Banks (2009). *Small Animal Oncology: An Introduction*, Saunders.
Withrow, S., et al. (2012). *Withrow and MacEwen's Small Animal Clinical Oncology, 5th Ed.*, Saunders.

Boldenone Undecylenate

(bole-di-nohn un-de-sil-en-ate)   Equipoise®

Anabolic Steroid

Prescriber Highlights

▶ Long-acting anabolic steroid labeled for horses.
▶ Not recommended for use in stallions or pregnant mares.
▶ May cause androgenic effects, including aggressiveness; potentially a hepatotoxin.
▶ Potentially a drug of abuse by humans, watch for diversion scams.

Uses/Indications

Boldenone is labeled for use as adjunctive therapy "… as an aid for treating debilitated horses when an improvement in weight, haircoat, or general physical condition is desired" (Package Insert; *Equipoise®*).

Pharmacology/Actions

In the presence of adequate protein and calories, anabolic steroids promote body tissue building processes and can reverse catabolism. As these agents are either derived from or are closely related to testosterone, the anabolics have varying degrees of androgenic effects. Endogenous testosterone release may be suppressed by inhibiting luteinizing hormone (LH). Large doses can impede spermatogenesis by negative feedback inhibition of FSH.

Anabolic steroids can also stimulate erythropoiesis possibly by stimulation of erythropoietic stimulating factor. Anabolics can cause nitrogen, sodium, potassium and phosphorus retention and decrease the urinary excretion of calcium.

Pharmacokinetics

No specific information was located for this agent. It is considered a long-acting anabolic, with effects persisting up to 8 weeks. It is unknown if the anabolic agents cross into milk.

Contraindications/Precautions/Warnings

The manufacturer (Solvay) recommends not using the drug on stallions or pregnant mares. Other clinicians state that anabolic steroids should not be used in either stallions or non-pregnant mares intended for reproduction. Boldenone should not be administered to horses intended for food purposes.

In humans, anabolic agents are contraindicated in patients with hepatic dysfunction, hypercalcemia, patients with a history of myocardial infarction (can cause hypercholesterolemia), pituitary insufficiency, prostate carcinoma, in selected patients with breast carcinoma, benign prostatic hypertrophy and during the nephrotic stage of nephritis.

Adverse Effects

In the manufacturer's (*Equipoise®*—Solvay) package insert, only androgenic (over aggressiveness) effects are listed. However, in work reported in both stallions and mares (Squires and McKinnon 1987), boldenone caused a detrimental effect in testis size, and sperm production and quality in stallions. In mares, the drug caused fewer total and large follicles, smaller ovaries, increased clitoral size, shortened estrus duration, reduced pregnancy rates and severely altered sexual behavior.

Although not reported in horses, anabolic steroids have the potential to cause hepatic toxicity.

Reproductive/Nursing Safety

The anabolic agents are category X (*Risk of use outweighs any possible benefit*) agents for use in pregnancy and are contraindicated because of possible fetal masculinization.

Overdosage/Acute Toxicity

No information was located for this specific agent. In humans, sodium and water retention can occur after overdosage of anabolic steroids. It is suggested to treat supportively and monitor liver function should an inadvertent overdose be administered.

Drug Interactions

No drug interactions were located for boldenone specifically. The following drug interactions have either been reported or are theoretical in humans or animals receiving anabolic steroids and may be of significance in veterinary patients. Unless otherwise noted, use together is not necessarily contraindicated, but weigh the potential risks and perform additional monitoring when appropriate.

- **ANTICOAGULANTS** (*e.g.*, **warfarin**, etc.): Anabolic agents as a class may potentiate the effects of anticoagulants; monitoring of INR and dosage adjustment of the anticoagulant (if necessary) are recommended.
- **CORTICOSTEROIDS, ACTH:** Anabolics may enhance the edema that can be associated with ACTH or adrenal steroid therapy.
- **INSULIN:** Diabetic patients receiving insulin may need dosage adjustments if anabolic therapy is added or discontinued; anabolics may decrease blood glucose and decrease insulin requirements.

Laboratory Considerations

- Concentrations of **protein bound iodine (PBI)** can be decreased in patients receiving androgen/anabolic therapy, but the clinical significance of this is probably not important.
- Androgen/anabolic agents can decrease amounts of **thyroxine-binding globulin** and decrease **total T4** concentrations and increase **resin uptake of T3 and T4**; free thyroid hormones are unaltered and, clinically, there is no evidence of dysfunction.
- Both **creatinine** and **creatine excretion** can be decreased by anabolic steroids.
- Anabolic steroids can increase the urinary excretion of **17-ketosteroids.**
- Androgenic/anabolic steroids may alter **blood glucose** levels.
- Androgenic/anabolic steroids may suppress **clotting factors II, V, VII, and X.**
- Anabolic agents can affect **liver function tests** (*e.g.*, BSP retention, SGOT, SGPT, bilirubin, and alkaline phosphatase).

Doses

- **HORSES:** (NOTE: ARCI UCGFS CLASS 4 DRUG)

  For labeled indications (as adjunctive therapy "...as an aid for treating debilitated horses when an improvement in weight, haircoat, or general physical condition is desired"): 1.1 mg/kg IM; may repeat in 3 week intervals (most horses will respond with one or two treatments). (Package Insert; *Equipoise®*)

Monitoring

- Androgenic side effects.
- Fluid and electrolyte status, if indicated.
- Liver function tests if indicated.
- Red blood cell count, indices, if indicated.
- Weight, appetite.

Client Information

- Because of the potential for abuse by humans, anabolic steroids are controlled drugs. Boldenone should be kept in a secure area and out of the reach of children.
- Contact veterinarian if patient develops yellowing of whites of the eyes, or develops a decreased appetite or lethargy.

Chemistry/Synonyms

An injectable anabolic steroid derived from testosterone, boldenone undecylenate has a chemical name of 17 beta-hydroxyandrosta-1,4-dien-3-one. The commercially available product is in a sesame oil vehicle.

Boldenone undecylenate may also be known as: Ba-29038, boldenone undecenoate, *Equipoise®*, or *Vebonol®*.

Storage/Stability

Boldenone injection should be stored at room temperature; avoid freezing.

Compatibility/Compounding Considerations

Because boldenone injection is in an oil vehicle, it should not be physically mixed with any other medications.

Dosage Forms/Regulatory Status

VETERINARY-LABELED PRODUCTS:

Boldenone Undecylenate for Injection: 25 mg/mL in 10 mL vials, 50 mg/mL in 10 mL & 50 mL vials; *Equipoise®*; (Rx, C-III). FDA-approved for use in horses not to be used for food.

The ARCI (Racing Commissioners International) has designated this drug as a class 4 substance. See the appendix for more information.

HUMAN-LABELED PRODUCTS: NONE.

Revisions/References

Monograph revised/updated September 2013.

Bromides: Potassium Bromide; Sodium Bromide

(broe-mide)

Anticonvulsant

Prescriber Highlights

▶ Primary or adjunctive therapy for seizure disorders in dogs; rarely used in cats as it can cause eosinophilic bronchitis.

▶ Very long half-life, must give loading dose to see therapeutic levels within a month.

▶ Most prevalent adverse effect in dogs is sedation, especially when used with phenobarbital. Polyphagia with resultant weight gain is also commonly noted, particularly in the first few months of therapy. Polydipsia and polyuria can also be seen.

▶ Therapeutic levels in dogs approximately 1 – 3 mg/mL. Monotherapy with bromide may require higher levels, but risk for toxicity is significantly increased.

▶ Do not feed salty snacks; keep chloride in diet stable.

▶ Toxic effects include profound sedation to stupor, ataxia, tremors, hind limb paresis, or other CNS manifestations.

▶ If using sodium bromide (vs. potassium bromide), dosage adjustments must be made.

Uses/Indications

Bromide is used both as primary therapy and as adjunctive therapy to control seizures in dogs. While historically bromide was only recommended for use as sole therapy in patients suffering from phenobarbital hepatotoxicity, it has been used by some as a drug of first choice in recent years or as an additional treatment in dogs not adequately controlled with phenobarbital alone (when steady state trough phenobarbital levels are >30 micrograms/mL for at least one month). However, as more experience is gained in veterinary medicine with newer human anticonvulsants (*e.g.*, zonisamide, levetiracetem, gabapentin, etc.) and their transition to less expensive generically available products, bromide use in dogs may become less prevalent. A recently published study comparing phenobarbital with bromide as a first-choice antiepileptic drug for treatment of epilepsy in dogs (N=46; 21 phenobarbital, 25 bromide) found that while both were reasonable choices, phenobarbital was more effective (seizure eradication in 85% of phenobarbital treated and 52% of bromide treated) and better tolerated than bromide during the first 6 months of treatment (Boothe et al. 2012).

Although rarely used, bromides may be suitable for use in some cats with chronic seizure disorders, but the high incidence of respiratory adverse effects precludes its routine use in feline patients.

Pharmacology/Actions

Bromide's anti-seizure activity is thought to be the result of its generalized depressant effects on neuronal excitability and activity. Bromide ions compete with chloride transport across cell membranes resulting in membrane hyperpolarization, thereby raising seizure threshold and limiting the spread of epileptic discharges.

Pharmacokinetics

Bromides are well absorbed after oral administration, primarily in the small intestine. Oral bioavailability in dogs averages 46% but there can be wide interpatient variation. The presence of food does not appear to affect absorption. Bromides are also well absorbed after solutions are administered rectally in dogs (bioavailability of 60-100%). Bromide is distributed in the extracellular fluid and mimics the volume of distribution of chloride (0.2-0.4 L/Kg). It is not bound to plasma proteins and readily enters the CSF (in dogs: 87% of serum concentration; in humans: 37%). Bromides enter maternal

milk (see Reproductive Safety below). Bromide is predominantly excreted unchanged via renal mechanisms. The half-life in dogs has been reported to be from 16-46 days; cats, 10 days; and humans, 12 days. Alterations in serum chloride levels or diminished renal function can significantly affect bromide elimination rates.

Contraindications/Precautions/Warnings

Older animals and those with additional disease may be prone to intolerance (see Adverse Effects below) at blood levels that are tolerable by younger, healthier dogs. Patients with renal dysfunction may require dosage adjustments.

Because bromides have been associated with serious pulmonary effects in cats, it should be used with extreme caution. Some state that the drug should not be used in cats.

Adverse Effects

A transient sedation (lasting up to 3 weeks) is commonly seen in dogs receiving bromides, but conversely some dogs show signs of irritability and restlessness. Toxicity is generally associated with higher bromide levels (>2.5 mg/mL), but some dogs appear to be 'sensitive' to bromide's effects and can show toxic signs at lower levels. Additionally, some dogs can tolerate serum levels as high as 4 mg/mL or higher. Toxicity is usually neurotoxic in nature and present as profound sedation to stupor, ataxia, tremors, mydriasis, or other CNS manifestations (*e.g.*, upper and lower motor neuron tetraparesis/paraparesis, megaesophagus, etc.). Pancreatitis has been reported in dogs receiving combination therapy of bromides with phenobarbital; however, since this effect has also been reported with both primidone and phenobarbital alone, its direct relationship with bromide is unknown. Additional potential adverse effects reported include: polyphagia with weight gain, polydipsia, polyuria, anorexia, vomiting, diarrhea and constipation. Gastrointestinal effects may be reduced or avoided by giving with food or dividing the dose. If the patient cannot tolerate the gastrointestinal effects (vomiting) of potassium bromide and divided doses with food do not alleviate the problem, switching to sodium bromide may be tried. Monitoring weight and dietary intake may help prevent weight gain. Pruritic dermatitis and paradoxical hyperactivity are rarely reported.

If administering an oral loading dose of potassium bromide, acute GI upset may occur if given too rapidly. Potentially, large loading doses could affect serum potassium levels in patients receiving potassium bromide.

In cats, lower respiratory effects (*e.g.*, cough, dyspnea, eosinophilic bronchitis, etc.) have been associated with bromide therapy and its use is rarely recommended. Peribronchial infiltrates may be seen on radiographs and dyspnea may be serious or fatal. Signs appear to be reversible in most cats once bromides are discontinued. Other adverse effects in cats include polydipsia, sedation, and weight gain.

Reproductive/Nursing Safety

Reproductive safety has not been established. Human infants have suffered bromide intoxication and growth retardation after maternal ingestion of bromides during pregnancy. Bromide intoxication has also been reported in human infants breastfeeding from mothers taking bromides. Use with caution in pregnancy or lactation.

Overdosage/Acute Toxicity

Toxicity is more likely with chronic overdoses, but acute overdoses are a possibility. In addition to the adverse effects noted above, animals that have developed bromism (whether acute or chronic) may develop signs of muscle pain, conscious proprioceptive deficits, anisocoria, hyperreflexia and other neurologic deficits.

Standard gut removal techniques should be employed after a known acute overdose. Death after an acute oral ingestion is apparently rare as vomiting generally occurs spontaneously. Administration of parenteral (0.9% sodium chloride) or oral sodium chloride, parenteral glucose and diuretics (*e.g.*, furosemide, etc.) may be helpful in reducing bromide loads in either acutely or chronically intoxicated individuals. Contact an animal poison control center for further guidance.

There were 111 single agent exposures to potassium bromide reported to the ASPCA Animal Poison Control Center (APCC) during 2009-2013. Of these cases, 97 were dogs and 35 were symptomatic. The most common signs were ataxia (43%), lethargy/sedation (43%), and vomiting (17%).

Drug Interactions

The following drug interactions have either been reported or are theoretical in humans or animals receiving bromides and may be of significance in veterinary patients. Unless otherwise noted, use together is not necessarily contraindicated, but weigh the potential risks and perform additional monitoring when appropriate.

- **CNS SEDATING DRUGS:** Because bromides can cause sedation, other CNS sedating drugs may cause additive sedation.
- **DIURETICS** (*e.g.,* **furosemide, thiazides, etc.**): May enhance the excretion of bromides thereby affecting seizure control and dosage requirements.
- **INTRAVENOUS FLUIDS CONTAINING SODIUM.** Can reduce serum bromide levels.
- **LOW/HIGH SALT (SODIUM CHLORIDE) DIETS:** Bromide toxicity can occur if chloride ion ingestion is markedly reduced. Patients put on low salt diets may be at risk. Conversely, additional sodium chloride in the diet (including prescription diets high in chloride) could reduce serum bromide levels, affecting seizure control. Keep chloride content of diet relatively constant while bromides are being administered. If chloride content must be altered, monitor bromide levels more frequently.
- **DRUGS THAT CAN LOWER SEIZURE THRESHOLD** (*e.g.,* **xylazine**): May potentially reduce efficacy of antiseizure medications.

Laboratory Considerations

- **Gold Chloride Assay for Serum Bromide.** This assay is considered reliable for bromide levels below 4 mg/mL, but at levels above 4 mg/mL, results can become non-linear and may not be accurate.
- **Chloride, Serum.** See drug interactions above regarding chloride. Bromide may interfere with serum chloride determinations yielding falsely high results.
- **Hypertriglyceridemia, Lipemia.** May interfere with colorimetric assays for serum bromide and give falsely elevated bromide values. A 12-hour fast prior to drawing levels has been recommended (Rusbridge 2013).
- Potassium bromide does not affect canine thyroid function test results.

Doses

- **DOGS:**

  For treatment of epilepsy (extra-label); **Note:** Unless otherwise noted, the following dosages are for potassium bromide. If substituting sodium bromide, reduce dosage by 15%:

  Loading Dose: Because of the long serum elimination half-life (weeks) in dogs, (it may take up to 4-5 months for blood levels to reach steady state concentrations), many dosing recommendations include an initial oral loading dose regimen to reduce the time required to attain therapeutic concentrations. Loading dosage recommendations for potassium bromide are generally in the 500 – 600 mg/kg range, but some recommend 400 mg/kg (or lower). This is divided in multiple doses and given over 1-5 days PO with food. In dogs that are unable to eat, it can be divided and given rectally every 4 hours. Sodium bromide 3% in sterile water

can potentially be administered intravenously as an infusion over at least 8 hours, but this must be done with caution as there is little clinical experience giving the drug IV and are no commercially available intravenous preparations available; an in-line IV filter is required. Potassium bromide must **NOT** be administered IV.

  Maintenance Dose: Initially, most recommend dosages in the 30 – 35 mg/kg range PO once daily with food. Some state that if using bromide as an add-on drug in dogs already on phenobarbital, initial lower dosages (15 – 30 mg/kg PO once daily) should be used. Adjust dosages based upon clinical efficacy, adverse effects and bromide serum levels (see Monitoring). Dosage increases should generally be in less than 5 mg/kg increments particularly at the higher end of the dosing range; a retrospective study found that dosage increases of 5 mg/kg increased by almost 5-fold the risk for toxicity (bromism) (Rossmeisl et al. 2009).

- **CATS:**

  As second line therapy for epilepsy (extra-label): **Note:** Rarely recommended due to adverse effects; 30 mg/kg PO once daily. (Munana 2004)

Monitoring

- Efficacy/Toxicity. One review of the safety of potassium bromide in dogs states: "…the use of clinical signs to judge appropriateness of treatment may be more important than monitoring serum bromide concentration alone." (Baird-Heinz et al. 2012)
- Serum Levels. In dogs, therapeutic bromide concentrations are generally agreed to be 1-3 mg/mL (100-300 mg/dL; 1000-3000 mg/L; 12.5-37.5 mmol/L). Some state that 2 mg/mL is the upper end of the range. Levels in the lower range may be effective for dogs on phenobarbital therapy and the higher range for dogs on bromide alone. Time of day (hours post-dose) for sampling is not critical, but it has been recommended that a 12-hour fast prior to blood draw is desirable (to reduce interference from triglycerides). Actual monitoring recommendations vary and depend on whether the patient received a loading dose or not. One recommendation (Boothe 2004) based upon pharmacokinetic principles is: If no load was given and maintenance dose was used initially, monitor at 3-4 weeks and then at steady-state (2.5-3 months). The first sample indicates about 50% of what will be achieved at steady-state and allows adjustment of the dosage early. If a loading dose was used, an immediate level after the load (day 6 or 7 after a 5 day loading protocol), followed by a sample at 1 month and then 3 months. The immediate sample indicates what was achieved with loading; the 1 month level indicates the success of the maintenance dose, maintains what was achieved with the loading dose and allows dosage adjustment, if required; and the 3 month level establishes the new baseline.

Client Information

- Best given with food. Dosage measurements of bromide solutions should be done with a needle-less syringe or other accurate measuring device. The dose may either be sprinkled on the dog's food (assuming it is consumed entirely) or squirted in the side of the mouth. If mixed with food, elevate the food bowl.
- Dogs that cannot tolerate the gastrointestinal effects (vomiting) of potassium bromide with single daily doses may better tolerate doses divided through the day and given with food. Do not give salty snacks or salty food.
- Most common side effect is drowsiness (usually gets better in a few weeks). Some dogs will consume more water or food than usual.
- Watch for serious side effects that may indicate that the dosage is too high, including behavior changes, difficulty walking, stumbling, incoordination, severe vomiting, difficulty swallowing, etc.

Chemistry

Potassium bromide occurs as white, odorless, cubical crystals or crystalline powder. One gram will dissolve in 1.5 mL of water. Potassium bromide contains 67.2% bromide. Each gram contains 8.4 mEq (mMol) of potassium and bromide.

Sodium bromide occurs as white, odorless, cubic crystals or granular powder. One gram will dissolve in 1.2 mL of water. Sodium bromide contains 77.7% bromide.

Because of the different molecular weights of sodium and potassium, with respect to actual bromide content, sodium bromide solutions of 250 mg/mL contain about 20% more bromide than potassium bromide 250 mg/mL solution. This is generally not clinically significant unless changing from one salt to another in a given patient.

Storage/Stability

Store in tight containers. Solutions may be stored for up to one year in clear or brown, glass or plastic containers at room temperature. Refrigerating the solution may help reduce the chance for microbial growth, but may cause crystals or precipitants to form. Should precipitation occur, warming the solution should resolubolize the bromide.

Compatibility/Compounding Considerations

Bromides can precipitate out alkaloids in solution. Mixing with strong oxidizing agents can liberate bromine. Metal salts can precipitate solutions containing bromides. Sodium bromide is hygroscopic; potassium bromide is not.

To compound a solution with a concentration of 250 mg/mL, 25 grams of potassium bromide are weighed; a sufficient amount of distilled water is added to a final volume of 100 mL; potassium bromide dissolves easily in water, sodium bromide may take longer to dissolve. Flavoring agents are not usually necessary for patient acceptance.

Dosage Forms/Regulatory Status

At the time of writing (September 2013), neither potassium or sodium bromide are available in FDA-approved dosage forms in the USA. Reagent grade or USP grade powder/crystals may be obtained from various chemical supply houses to compound an acceptable oral product (see Compatibility/Compounding above). If purchasing a reagent grade, specify American Chemical Society (ACS) grade.

A licensed product for use in dogs is available in the UK: Potassium Bromide Oral Tablets: 325 mg; *Libromide®*; (POM-V)

Revisions/References

Monograph revised/updated September 2013.

Baird-Heinz, H. E., et al. (2012). A systematic review of the safety of potassium bromide in dogs. *Javma-Journal of the American Veterinary Medical Association* 240(6): 705-15.

Boothe, D. M. (2004). *Bromide: The "old" new anticonvulsant.* Proceedings: WSAVA. accessed via Veterinary Information Network; vin.com

Boothe, D. M., et al. (2012). Comparison of phenobarbital with bromide as a first-choice antiepileptic drug for treatment of epilepsy in dogs. *Javma-Journal of the American Veterinary Medical Association* 240(9): 1073-83.

Munana, K. (2004). *Seizures and cats.* Proceedings: ACVIM Forum, Minneapolis. accessed via Veterinary Information Network; vin.com

Rossmeisl, J. H. & K. D. Inzana (2009). Clinical signs, risk factors, and outcomes associated with bromide toxicosis (bromism) in dogs with idiopathic epilepsy. *Javma-Journal of the American Veterinary Medical Association* 234(11): 1425-31.

Rusbridge, C. (2013). Choosing the right drug 1. Anticonvulsants used for first-line therapy. *In Practice* 35(3): 106-13.

Bromocriptine Mesylate

(broe-moe-krip-teen)   Parlodel®

Dopamine Agonist/Prolactin Inhibitor

Prescriber Highlights

▶ Dopamine agonist & prolactin inhibitor occasionally used in dogs for estrus induction or treatment for pseudocyesis; in horses for pituitary adenomas or inappropriate lactation; in cats for acromegaly or mammary hyperplasia. Cabergoline is generally preferred for use in small animals, but can be more expensive than bromocriptine.

▶ Many adverse effects possible; GI, CNS depression & hypotension are most likely; much more likely to cause emesis in dogs than cabergoline.

▶ Interferes with lactation.

Uses/Indications

Bromocriptine may potentially be of benefit in treating acromegaly/pituitary adenomas in a variety of species. However, because of adverse effects, its potential value for treating hyperadrenocorticism in dogs is low. It has been used in dogs for pregnancy termination and pseudopregnancy, but cabergoline is used more commonly.

Pharmacology/Actions

Bromocriptine exhibits multiple pharmacologic actions. It inhibits prolactin release from the anterior pituitary thereby reducing serum prolactin. The mechanism for this action is by a direct effect on the pituitary and/or stimulating postsynaptic dopamine receptors in the hypothalamus to cause release of prolactin-inhibitory factor. Bromocriptine also activates dopaminergic receptors in the neostriatum of the brain.

Pharmacokinetics

In humans, only about 28% of a bromocriptine dose is absorbed from the gut and, due to a high first-pass effect, only about 6% reaches the systemic circulation. Distribution characteristics are not well described but in humans, it is highly bound (90-96%) to serum albumin. Bromocriptine is metabolized by the liver to inactive and non-toxic metabolites. It has a biphasic half-life; the alpha phase is about 4 hours and the terminal phase is about 15 hours, but one source says 45-50 hours.

Contraindications/Precautions/Warnings

Bromocriptine is generally contraindicated in patients with hypertension. It should be used with caution in patients with hepatic disease as metabolism of the drug may be reduced.

Adverse Effects

Bromocriptine may cause a plethora of adverse effects that are usually dose related and minimized with dosage reduction. Some more likely possibilities include: gastrointestinal effects (*e.g.*, nausea, vomiting, etc.), nervous system effects (*e.g.*, sedation, fatigue, etc.), and hypotension (particularly with the first dose, but it may persist). At dosages used in dogs, it is more likely to cause emesis than cabergoline.

Reproductive/Nursing Safety

Usage during pregnancy is contraindicated in humans, although documented teratogenicity has not been established.

Because bromocriptine interferes with lactation, it should not be used in animals that are nursing.

Overdosage/Acute Toxicity

Overdosage may cause vomiting, severe nausea, and profound hypotension. There were 35 single agent exposures to bromocriptine reported to the ASPCA Animal Poison Control Center (APCC) during 2009-2013. Of the 34 dogs, 29 were symptomatic with vomiting (93%), 17% lethargic and 14% hypothermic or tachycardic. Standardized gut removal techniques should be employed when applicable, but emesis often occurs spontaneously. Institute cardiovascular monitoring (blood pressure, heart rate) and support as needed.

Drug Interactions

The following drug interactions have either been reported or are theoretical in humans or animals receiving bromocriptine and may be of significance in veterinary patients. Unless otherwise noted, use together is not necessarily contraindicated, but weigh the potential risks and perform additional monitoring when appropriate.

- **ALCOHOL:** Use with alcohol may cause a disulfiram-type reaction.
- **BUTYROPHENONES** (*e.g.,* **haloperidol, azaperone,** etc.), **AMITRIPTYLINE, PHENOTHIAZINES,** and **RESERPINE:** May increase prolactin concentrations and bromocriptine doses may need to be increased.
- **CYCLOSPORINE:** May elevate cyclosporine levels.
- **ERYTHROMYCIN, CLARITHROMYCIN:** May increase bromocriptine levels.
- **ESTROGENS** or **PROGESTINS:** May interfere with the effects of bromocriptine.
- **ERGOT ALKALOIDS:** Use of bromocriptine and ergot alkaloids is not recommended; some human patients receiving both have developed severe hypertension and myocardial infarction.
- **HYPOTENSIVE MEDICATIONS:** May cause additive hypotension if used with bromocriptine.
- **MAO INHIBITORS** (including **amitraz,** and maybe **selegiline**): Avoid use of bromocriptine with these compounds.
- **METOCLOPRAMIDE:** May cause prolactin release in dogs, thereby negating the effects of bromocriptine for treating pseudopregnancy.
- **OCTREOTIDE:** May increase bromocriptine levels.
- **SYMPATHOMIMETICS** (*e.g.,* **phenylpropanolamine,** etc.): Enhanced bromocriptine effects have been reported in humans (rare), including ventricular tachycardia and cardiac dysfunction.

Doses

- **DOGS:**

  For treatment of pseudocyesis (extra-label): 10 – 50 micrograms/kg (0.01 – 0.05 mg/kg) PO twice daily until lactation ceases. Vomiting, depression and anorexia are common side effects and often is more problematic than the inappropriate lactation. Reducing dosage and giving after meals may help.

  For inducing estrus (extra-label): Not often recommended, but dosing regimens of 10 micrograms/kg PO 3 times a day with food and 25 micrograms/kg PO twice daily with food have been noted.

  For pregnancy termination (extra-label): Not often recommended, but regimens using bromocriptine at 15 – 30 micrograms/kg PO once to twice daily in conjunction with a prostaglandin (*e.g.,* cloprostenol at 1 microgram/kg SC every other day) starting 25 days after LH surge have been noted.

- **CATS:**

  For adjunctive treatment of acromegaly (extra-label): Initial dose of 0.2 mg per cat PO once daily. May have some effect, especially in reducing insulin requirements. (Jones 2004)

  For adjunctive treatment of mammary fibroadenomatous hyperplasia (extra-label): 0.25 mg per cat; may need to be compounded. (Little 2011)

- **HORSES:** (NOTE: ARCI UCGFS CLASS 2 DRUG)

  For treatment of pituitary adenoma (extra-label):
  a) 0.03 – 0.09 mg/kg (30 – 90 micrograms/kg) twice daily PO or SC, but its use is limited. (Toribio 2004)
  b) 5 mg (per horse) IM q12h. To prepare an injectable formulation for IM use from oral dosage forms: Bromocriptine mesylate 70 mg is added to 7 mL of a solution of 80% normal saline and 20% absolute alcohol (v/v). Final concentration is 1% (10 mg/mL). (Beck 1992)

  For inappropriate lactation (extra-label; based upon a case report): 0.04 mg/kg PO twice daily for 10 days. In conjunction with local hydrotherapy (20 minutes twice daily) and milking restricted to times when the mare was in extreme discomfort. (Meirelles et al. 2012)

Monitoring

- Monitoring is dependent upon the reason for use to evaluate efficacy. However, blood pressures should be evaluated if patients have clinical signs associated with hypotension.

Client Information

- For dogs and cats the drug works best when given with food.
- Vomiting, fatigue and low blood pressure are possible.
- Pregnant or nursing women should take precautions to avoid exposure.

Chemistry/Synonyms

A dopamine agonist and prolactin inhibitor, bromocriptine mesylate is a semisynthetic ergot alkaloid derivative. It occurs as a yellowish-white powder and is slightly soluble in water and sparingly soluble in alcohol.

Bromocriptine mesylate may also be known as: bromocryptine, brom-ergocryptine, 2-bromergocryptine, bromocriptine methanesulphonate, bromocriptini mesilas, 2-bromo-alpha-ergocryptine mesylate, 2-bromoergocryptine monomethanesulfonate, or CB-154 (bromocriptine); many trade names are available.

Storage/Stability

Tablets and capsules should be protected from light and stored in tight containers at temperatures less than 25°C.

Compatibility/Compounding Considerations

No specific information noted.

Dosage Forms/Regulatory Status

VETERINARY-LABELED PRODUCTS: NONE.

The ARCI (Racing Commissioners International) has designated this drug as a class 2 substance. See the appendix for more information.

HUMAN-LABELED PRODUCTS:

Bromocriptine Mesylate Oral Capsules: 5 mg (as base); *Parlodel®,* generic; (Rx)

Bromocriptine Mesylate Oral Tablets: 0.8 mg & 2.5 mg (as base); *Cycloset®, Parlodel®,* generic; (Rx)

Revisions/References

Monograph revised/updated September 2013.

Beck, D. (1992). Effective long-term tratment of a suspected pituitary adenoma in a pony. *Equine Vet Educ* **4**(3): 119-22.
Jones, B. (2004). *Less common feline endocrinopathies.* Proceedings: WSAVA. accessed via Veterinary Information Network; vin.com
Little, S. (2011). Feloine Reproduction: Problems and clinical challenges. *Journal of Feline Medicine and Surgery* **13**: 508-15.
Meirelles, M. G., et al. (2012). Bromocriptine Treatment for Inappropriate Lactation in Mares: A Case Report. *Journal of Equine Veterinary Science* **32**(12): 840-3.
Toribio, R. (2004). Pars intermedia dysfunction (Equine Cushing's Disease). *Equine Internal Medicine 2nd Edition.* M. Reed, W. Bayly and D. Sellon. Phila, Saunders: 1327-40.

Budesonide

(bue-**des**-oh-nide)   Entocort EC®

Glucocorticoid

Prescriber Highlights

▶ Orally administered glucocorticoid with limited systemic glucocorticoid effects; may be useful in treating IBD in small animals that are either refractory to, or intolerant of, systemic steroids.

▶ Hyperadrenocorticism possible, but much less likely then with systemic steroids.

▶ Inhaled (pulmonary) dosage forms may be useful in feline asthma or RAO in horses, but fluticasone has been used more frequently.

▶ Drug interactions (CYP3A inhibitors, antacids).

▶ Expense may be an issue, but generic forms now available; may need to be compounded to smaller dosage strengths.

Uses/Indications

Most veterinary interest is in budesonide's potential oral use to treat inflammatory intestinal diseases in small animals that are either refractory to, or intolerant of, systemic steroids. No prospective studies evaluating the safety or efficacy of budesonide were located.

In humans, oral budesonide is indicated for Crohn's disease and ulcerative colitis. It also used in an extra-label manner for treating eosinophilic esophagitis (as an oral slurry) in children.

There are inhalational human dosage forms for treating asthma or allergic rhinitis and theoretically these could be used in animals. One study comparing ACTH-stimulated cortisol levels in healthy beagles, found that inhaled budesonide (200 mcg twice daily) did not significantly affect cortisol levels while oral prednisolone (1 mg/kg/day) and inhaled fluticasone (250 mcg twice daily) did after 35 days of treatment (Melamies et al. 2012).

Pharmacology/Actions

Budesonide is a potent glucocorticoid (15X more potent than prednisolone) with high topical activity. It has weak mineralocorticoid activity. By delaying dissolution until reaching the duodenum and subsequent controlled release of the drug, the drug can exert its topical antiinflammatory activity in the intestines. While the drug is absorbed from the gut into the portal circulation, it has a high first-pass metabolism effect through the liver that reduces systemic blood levels and resultant glucocorticoid effects of the drug. However, significant suppression of the HPA-axis does occur in patients taking the drug.

Pharmacokinetics

Budesonide's pharmacokinetics have been reported in healthy dogs. The drug has a bioavailability of 10-20%. When dosed at 10 micrograms/kg, half-life is about 2 hours and clearance 2.2 L/hr/kg. At 100 micrograms/kg, half-life is slightly prolonged to 2-3 hours. In dogs with inflammatory bowel disease, budenoside (as the commercial oral product) is apparently rapidly absorbed with peak levels occurring at 1-hour post dose (Pietra et al. 2013).

Upon oral administration of the commercially available product in humans, budesonide is nearly completely absorbed from the gut, but time to achieve peak concentrations are widely variable (30-600 minutes). The presence of food in the gut may delay absorption, but does not impact the amount of drug absorbed. Because of a high first-pass effect, only about 10% of a dose is systemically bioavailable in healthy adults. In patients with Crohn's disease, oral bioavailability may be twice that initially, but with further dosing, reduces to amounts similar to healthy subjects. Budesonide's mean volume of distribution in humans ranges from 2.2 – 3.9 L/kg. The drug is completely metabolized and these metabolites are excreted in the feces and urine. Budesonide's terminal half-life is about 4 hours.

Contraindications/Precautions/Warnings

Budesonide is contraindicated in patients hypersensitive to it. Because budesonide can cause systemic corticosteroid effects, it should be used with caution in any patient where glucocorticoid therapy may be problematic including those with GI ulcers, active infections, diabetes mellitus, or cataracts.

Because budesonide does suppress the HPA-axis, animals undergoing stressful procedures such as surgery, should be considered for exogenous steroid administration.

Adverse Effects

There are limited reports of the clinical use of budesonide in small animals and the determination of the drug's adverse effect profile is ongoing. Budesonide can cause significant hypothalamic-pituitary-adrenal axis (HPAA) suppression, but does not necessarily cause cushingoid effects. Steroid hepatopathy is possible. In humans, oral budesonide is generally well tolerated and glucocorticoid adverse effects occur infrequently when the drug is used for courses of therapy of no more than 8 weeks duration. Patients with moderate to severe hepatic dysfunction may be more likely to develop signs associated with hypercorticism.

Reproductive/Nursing Safety

In humans, the FDA categorizes budesonide as a category C drug for use during pregnancy (*Animal studies have shown an adverse effect on the fetus, but there are no adequate studies in humans; or there are no animal reproduction studies and no adequate studies in humans*). Like other corticosteroids, budesonide has been demonstrated to be embryocidal and teratogenic in rats and rabbits.

Specific data on budesonide levels in maternal milk are not available and the manufacturer warns against use by nursing women; however, because of the drugs high first-pass effect, the amounts are unlikely to be of clinical significance to nursing animal offspring.

Overdosage/Acute Toxicity

Acute, oral overdoses are unlikely to be of much concern although doses of 200 mg/kg were lethal in mice. Decontamination should be considered for massive overdoses.

Drug Interactions

The following drug interactions have either been reported or are theoretical in humans or animals receiving budesonide and may be of significance in veterinary patients. Unless otherwise noted, use together is not necessarily contraindicated, but weigh the potential risks and perform additional monitoring when appropriate.

■ **ERYTHROMYCIN, CIMETIDINE, KETOCONAZOLE, ITRACONAZOLE, FLUCONAZOLE, DILTIAZEM, GRAPEFRUIT JUICE POWDER,** etc.: Because the hepatic enzyme CYP3A extensively metabolizes budesonide, drugs that inhibit this isoenzyme can significantly increase the amount of drug that enters the systemic circulation. Ketoconazole given with budesonide may increase the area under the curve (AUC) of budesonide by eight fold.

■ **ORAL ANTACIDS:** Because the dissolution of the drug's coating is pH dependent, oral antacids should not be given at the same time as the drug. Other drugs that potentially would increase gastric pH (*e.g.*, omeprazole, ranitidine, etc.) apparently do not significantly impact the oral pharmacokinetics of the drug.

Laboratory Considerations

■ **Intradermal skin testing** (IDST) for allergens: Inhaled budesonide (for one month) eliminated skin reactivity in 3/6 cats tested. A 2-week withdrawal is suggested if using IDST, but may not be necessary if using serum IgE testing for allergies (Chang et al. 2011).

- While no other specific laboratory interactions were located, budesonide could potentially alter laboratory test results similarly to other corticosteroids (*e.g.*, serum ALT, ALP in dogs).

Doses

- **DOGS**

  For adjunctive treatment of IBD (extra-label): Initial dosage recommendations vary, but practically: <u>Toy or Small breeds:</u> 1 mg (must be compounded) PO once daily. <u>Medium breeds:</u> 2 mg (must be compounded) PO once daily. <u>Large or Giant breeds:</u> 3 mg (commercially available) PO once daily. Once adequately controlled, gradual reductions in dosage amounts or frequency (every other day) are desirable.

- **CATS:**

  For adjunctive treatment of IBD (extra-label): Most cats tolerate oral glucocorticoids, but in those that cannot and especially in diabetic cats, budesonide can be considered: 1 mg per cat (must be compounded) PO once daily.

Monitoring

- Efficacy.
- Adverse effects.

Client Information

- Do not crush capsules or allow animals to chew them. Do not open capsules unless your veterinarian has instructed you to do so.
- Once your animal has been taking this drug for a while, don't stop giving it unless your veterinarian says it is OK. There can be serious withdrawal effects if the medication is stopped suddenly.
- Side effects are not well documented in animals, but are likely to be associated with steroid effects: Increased appetite/thirst/urination, lethargy, muscle weakness, increased panting (dogs), changes in skin and hair/coat, weight gain, pot belly. Contact your veterinarian if these occur.

Chemistry/Synonyms

Budesonide, a non-halogenated glucocorticoid, occurs as a white to off-white, odorless, tasteless powder. It is practically insoluble in water, freely soluble in chloroform and sparingly soluble in alcohol. The commercially available capsules contain a granulized micronized form of the drug that is coated to protect from dissolution in gastric juice, but will dissolve at pH >5.5. In humans, this pH usually corresponds with the drug reaching the duodenum.

Budesonide may also be known as S 1320, *Entocord®*, *Entocort EC®*, *Pulmicort®*, and *Rhinocort®*.

Storage/Stability

Budesonide oral capsules should be stored in tight containers at room temperature. Exposures to temperatures as low as 15°C (59°F) and as high as 30°C (86°F) are permitted.

Compatibility/Compounding Considerations

If reformulating into smaller capsules, do not alter (damage) the micronized enteric-coated sugar spheres inside of the capsules.

Dosage Forms/Regulatory Status

VETERINARY-LABELED PRODUCTS: NONE.

HUMAN-LABELED PRODUCTS:

Budesonide Extended-Release Capsules: 3 mg & 9 mg (micronized); *Entocort EC®*, *Uceris®*, generic; (Rx)

Human budesonide capsules may need to be compounded into dosage strengths suitable for dogs and cats, but the enteric-coated sugar spheres found inside the capsule should not be altered or damaged.

There are also budesonide products (powder and suspension for oral inhalation, and nasal sprays) for the treatment of asthma or allergic rhinitis. Trade names for these products include *Pulmicort®* and *Rhinocort®*.

Revisions/References

Monograph revised/updated September 2013.

Chang, C. H., et al. (2011). The impact of oral versus inhaled glucocorticoids on allergen specific IgE testing in experimentally asthmatic cats. *Veterinary Immunology and Immunopathology* 144(3-4): 437-41.

Melamies, M., et al. (2012). Endocrine effects of inhaled budesonide compared with inhaled fluticasone propionate and oral prednisolone in healthy Beagle dogs. *Veterinary Journal* 194(3): 349-53.

Pietra, M., et al. (2013). Plasma concentrations and therapeutic effects of budesonide in dogs with inflammatory bowel disease. *American Journal of Veterinary Research* 74(1): 78-83.

Bumetanide

(bue-MET-a-nide)   Bumex®, Burinex®

Loop Diuretic

Prescriber Highlights

▶ Loop diuretic similar to furosemide, but more potent (on a mg/kg basis). Available both in oral and injectable dosage forms.

▶ Limited use and experience in veterinary medicine; primary reason to consider use is if furosemide is unavailable.

▶ The following information is for furosemide but may be applicable to bumetanide. Contraindications: Patients with anuria, hypersensitivity, or seriously depleted electrolytes. Caution: Patients with pre-existing electrolyte or water balance abnormalities, impaired hepatic function, & diabetes mellitus. Adverse Effects: Fluid & electrolyte (esp. hyponatremia) abnormalities; others include: ototoxicity, GI distress, hematologic effects, ototoxicity, weakness, & restlessness. Pre-renal azotemia is possible if dehydration occurs; encourage normal food & water intake.

Uses/Indications

Bumetanide is a sulfonamide loop diuretic similar to furosemide that potentially could be used in place of furosemide. Uses may include congestive cardiomyopathy, pulmonary edema, hypercalciuric nephropathy, uremia, as adjunctive therapy in hyperkalemia, or hypertension. It is unknown if it has efficacy to help prevent or reduce epistaxis (exercise-induced pulmonary hemorrhage; EIPH) in racehorses.

Pharmacology/Actions

Like furosemide, bumetanide reduces the absorption of electrolytes in the ascending section of the loop of Henle, decreases the reabsorption of both sodium and chloride and increases the excretion of potassium in the distal renal tubule, and directly effects electrolyte transport in the proximal tubule. Renal excretion of water, sodium, potassium, chloride, calcium, magnesium, hydrogen, ammonium, and bicarbonate are increased. In dogs, potassium excretion is affected much less than sodium and chloride; hyponatremia may be more of a concern than hypokalemia. Bumetanide, like furosemide, causes some renal venodilation, renal artery dilation (blocked by prostaglandin synthetase inhibitors such as indomethacin) and an increase in renin secretion.

In dogs and humans, bumetanide may be 25-60 times more potent a diuretic than furosemide. This increased potency is likely due to a greater effect on sodium transport in the ascending loop of Henle and increased renal uptake of the drug. In healthy cats when compared to furosemide, bumetanide was 2-3 times more potent on a mg/kg basis when determining a defined standard diuretic dose (SDD; IV dosage given over 2 minutes necessary to produce diuresis of 30 mL/kg over for 4 hours) (Gottl et al. 1985).

Pharmacokinetics

In dogs, bumetanide has a rapid onset of action. After intravenous dosing peak diuresis occurs within 1 hour and diuresis continues up to 4 hours. Oral dosing causes diuresis within one hour and the duration of effect continues for approximately 4-5 hours. About 2/3 of the drug is excreted unchanged in the urine and feces with the majority of the remainder glucuronidated in the liver.

In humans, oral bioavailability is high (85-95%) and peak plasma levels occur in 0.5 to 2 hours. The presence of food may delay absorption but does not alter diuretic efficacy. Plasma protein binding is approximately 95% but may be decreased in patients with renal impairment. After oral administration plasma half-life is 1-1.5 hours. Clearance may be decreased in patients with renal impairment. Unlike dogs, only about 50% of the drug is excreted unchanged in the urine, with the remaining eliminated as metabolites in the urine and feces.

Contraindications/Precautions/Warnings

Bumetanide is contraindicated in patients with anuria or that are hypersensitive to the drug. Like furosemide, it should be used with caution in patients with preexisting electrolyte or water balance abnormalities, impaired hepatic function (may precipitate hepatic coma), and diabetes mellitus. Patients with conditions that may lead to electrolyte or water balance abnormalities (*e.g.*, vomiting, diarrhea, etc.) should be monitored carefully. Patients hypersensitive to sulfonamides may also be hypersensitive to bumetanide (not documented in veterinary species). Cross-sensitivity in human patients allergic to furosemide apparently does not apparently occur.

The human label has a "black box warning" that states: Bumetanide is a potent diuretic that if given in excessive amounts, can lead to a profound diuresis with water and electrolyte depletion. Therefore, careful medical supervision is required; dosage selection and titration should be adjusted to the individual patient's needs.

Adverse Effects

Adverse effect profiles for bumetanide in dogs, cats, and horses are not well described, but would likely mirror those of furosemide, including fluid and electrolyte abnormalities. Patients should be monitored for hydration status and electrolyte imbalances; prerenal azotemia may result if moderate to severe dehydration occurs. Hyponatremia is probably the greatest concern, but hypocalcemia, hypokalemia, and hypomagnesemia may all occur. Animals that have normal food and water intake are much less likely to develop water and electrolyte imbalances than those who do not. Other potential effects include gastrointestinal disturbances, hematologic effects (anemia, leukopenia), weakness, ototoxicity (see below) and restlessness.

In a study (Martinez-Alcaine et al. 2001) in 32 dogs with CHF (stage II) using bumetanide (0.1 mg/kg PO once daily) in conjunction with an ACE-inhibitor (quinapril 0.5 mg/kg PO once daily) and low-sodium diet over 30 days, adverse effects attributable to the drug treatment were not discerned.

Like other loop diuretics, bumetanide has potential for causing ototoxicity (primarily hearing loss) in dogs and cats. For an equivalent diuretic effect in cats, bumetanide has about 3 times the ototoxic potential of furosemide (Gottl et al. 1985), but in dogs, relative ototoxic potential is 0.11-0.16 times that of furosemide. (Brown et al. 1979) However loop diuretic-caused ototoxicity is usually transient.(Oishi et al. 2012)

Reproductive/Nursing Safety

It is not known if bumetanide is safe to use during pregnancy, but only extremely high dosages have caused issues in pregnant laboratory animals. In humans, the FDA categorizes this drug as category **C** for use during pregnancy (*Animal studies have shown an adverse effect on the fetus, but there are no adequate studies in humans; or there are no animal reproduction studies and no adequate studies in humans*).

Safe use during lactation/nursing is not known, but it is likely compatible with nursing. However in humans, the manufacturer cautions against using it when nursing.

Overdosage/Acute Toxicity

The LD_{50} of bumetanide following IV administration is approximately 330 mg/kg in mice. In rabbits, the LD_{50} is reportedly 70 mg/kg (IV) and 350 mg/kg (PO). Bumetanide overdosages can cause acute volume and electrolyte depletion, hypovolemia and circulatory collapse. Standard gut decontamination procedures may be considered if oral overdose was recent. Acute overdoses should be managed with supportive and symptomatic fluid and electrolyte therapy. Serum and urinary electrolytes, urine output, CNS and cardiovascular status should be monitored. Contact an animal poison center for additional advice and support.

Drug Interactions

The following drug interactions have either been reported or are theoretical in humans or animals receiving bumetanide and may be of significance in veterinary patients. Unless otherwise noted, use together is not necessarily contraindicated, but weigh the potential risks and perform additional monitoring when appropriate.

- **ACE INHIBITORS** (*e.g.*, **enalapril, benazepril**): Increased risks for hypotension, particularly in patients who are volume or sodium depleted secondary to diuretics.
- **AMINOGLYCOSIDES** (**gentamicin, amikacin**, etc.): Increased risk for ototoxicity and nephrotoxicity.
- **AMPHOTERICIN B:** Loop diuretics may increase the risk for nephrotoxicity development and hypokalemia.
- **CISPLATIN:** Increased risk for ototoxicity.
- **CORTICOSTEROIDS:** Increased risk for GI ulceration and hypokalemia.
- **DIGOXIN:** Bumetanide-induced hypokalemia may increase the potential for digoxin toxicity.
- **DIURETICS, OTHER:** May result in enhanced effects and depending on species and diuretic, alter electrolyte excretion.
- **INDOMETHACIN:** Reduced effects of bumetanide.
- **INSULIN:** Bumetanide may alter insulin requirements.
- **MUSCLE RELAXANTS, NON-DEPOLARIZING** (*e.g.*, **atracurium, tubocurarine**): Bumetanide may prolong neuromuscular blockade.
- **PROBENECID:** Bumetanide can reduce uricosuric effects.
- **SALICYLATES:** Loop diuretics can reduce the excretion of salicylates.
- **THEOPHYLLINE:** Pharmacologic effects of theophylline may be enhanced when used with bumetanide.

Laboratory Considerations

- **FREE T4:** Furosemide can result in an increased free T4 fraction; furosemide inhibits T4 binding to canine serum *in vitro*. It is unknown if bumetanide may also have this effect.

Dosages

- **DOGS/CATS:**

  As a diuretic for adjunctive therapy of cardiogenic or pulmonary edema, acute oliguric renal failure, or moderate to severe hypercalcemia/hypercalcuric nephropathy (extra-label):

Note: There is very little clinical experience using this drug in animal patients and furosemide would usually be preferred. In dogs, bumetanide may be 25-50 times more potent on a mg/mg basis when compared with furosemide. Initially reducing the "furosemide dose" to reflect this potency difference appears reasonable (divide furosemide dosage by 25 or 50); adjust dosage to achieve desired clinical effect. One study in dogs with CHF (Martinez-Alcaine et al. 2001) gave bumetanide at 0.1 mg/kg PO once daily (with quinapril and a low sodium diet). Anecdotal bumetanide dosages for dogs and cats of 0.02 - 0.1 mg/kg IV or PO q8-24h have been reported. If giving IV, bumetanide may be administered directly, but should be given over at least 2 minutes time.

Monitoring
- Serum electrolytes, BUN, creatinine, glucose.
- Hydration status.
- Blood pressure, if indicated.
- Clinical signs of edema, patient weight, if indicated.
- Evaluation of ototoxicity, particularly with prolonged therapy in cats.

Client Information
- Animal may urinate more frequently than normal. This usually improves after a while.
- May be given with or without food. Allow free access to water at all times; encourage normal food intake.
- Because this drug can change electrolytes (salts) in the blood, your veterinarian will probably want to do more frequent testing.
- Contact veterinarian immediately if excessive thirst, weakness or collapse, head tilt, lack of urination, or a racing heartbeat is noticed.

Chemistry/Synonyms
Bumetanide (Chemical Name: 3-(Aminosulfonyl)-5-(butylamino)-4-phenoxybenzoic acid; CAS Registry: 28395-03-1, ATC: C03CA02) occurs as a white, or practically white powder with a slightly bitter taste. It is structurally related to furosemide but differs by the presence of 4-phenoxy and 5-butylamino substituents. Bumetanide is slightly soluble in water and soluble in alkaline solutions.

Bumetanide may also be known as Ro-10-6338 or by several trade names including *Bumex®* and *Burinex®*.

Storage/Stability
Bumetanide tablets should be stored at 5-30°C (59-86°F) in tight, light resistant containers.

The injection should be stored at 15-30°C; (59-86°F) and protected from light. The injectable product has sodium hydroxide added during the manufacture of the injection to adjust the pH to 6.8-7.8; it reportedly is stable between a pH of 4-10 and does not adsorb to glass or PVC containers. It is compatible with 5% dextrose, 0.9% sodium chloride, or lactated Ringer's solutions. If diluted with an infusion solution, it should be used within 24 hours.

Compatibility/Compounding Considerations
Bumetanide injection is reported to be incompatible when mixed and/or at Y-site with dobutamine, fenoldopam mesylate and midazolam. The injection is physically and chemically compatible in glass or PVC containers.

Dosage Forms/Regulatory Status
VETERINARY-LABELED PRODUCTS: NONE.

HUMAN-LABELED PRODUCTS:
Oral Tablets: 0.5 mg, 1 mg, 2 mg; generic; (Rx)
Injection: 0.25 mg/mL in 2 mL, 4 mL and 10 mL vials; generic; (Rx)

There is a website (dailymed.nim.hih.gov) listing FDA-approved (human drug) labels for bumetanide products.

Revisions/References
Monograph written August 2013.
Brown, R. D., et al. (1979). Comparative Acute Ototoxicity of intravenous Bumetanide and Furosemide in the Pure-Bred Beagle. *Toxicology and Applied Pharmacology* 48(1): 157-69.
Gottl, K. H., et al. (1985). Quantitative-Evaluation of Ototoxic Side-Effects of Furosemide, Piretanide, Bumetanide, Azosemide and Ozolinone in the Cat - A New Approach To the Problem of Ototoxicity. *Naunyn-Schmiedebergs Archives of Pharmacology* 331(2-3): 275-82.
Martinez-Alcaine, M. A., et al. (2001). Effect of short-term treatment with bumetanide, quinapril and low-sodium diet on dogs with moderate congestive heart failure. *Australian Veterinary Journal* 79(2): 102-5.
Oishi, N., et al. (2012). Ototoxicity in Dogs and Cats. *Veterinary Clinics of North America-Small Animal Practice* 42(6): 1259-+.

Buprenorphine HCl
(byoo-pre-nor-feen) Buprenex®, Simbadol®
Opiate Partial Agonist

Prescriber Highlights
▶ Partial *mu* opiate agonist used primarily as an injectable & buccal analgesic in small animals, especially cats; has been used in horses also.
▶ Often used as a component of short-term immobilization "cocktails".
▶ Buccal administration well tolerated & can be effective.
▶ Rarely, may cause respiratory depression.
▶ At standard doses, naloxone may not completely reverse respiratory depressant effects in overdoses.

Uses/Indications
Buprenorphine is most often used as an analgesic for mild to moderate pain or in combination in pre-anesthetic "cocktails" in small animals. In many species, it is not as an effective analgesic as pure *mu*-agonists (*e.g.*, morphine, hydromorphone, etc.), but it generally causes fewer adverse effects.

In cats, buccal (oral transmucosal; OTM) administration can be a practical, effective method for helping to control post-operative pain and it may provide better analgesia in cats than does parenteral morphine or oxymorphone. One study however, found that IV or IM buprenorphine provided better post-operative (OHE) analgesia than when the drug was administered SC or via the oral transmucosal route (Giordano et al. 2010). Multi-dose injectable formulations may be less palatable to cats than the preservative-free formulation (Bortolami et al. 2012). Combining opiates such as buprenorphine with short-term NSAIDs for post-op pain control is being used more commonly.

In the UK, there are licensed products that are labeled as indicated for postoperative analgesia in dogs, cats and horses and potentiation of the sedative effects of centrally acting agents in dogs and horses.

For acute pain control, buprenorphine may have the disadvantage of a longer onset of action than other opiates.

Pharmacology/Actions
Buprenorphine has partial agonist activity at the *mu*-receptor. This is in contrast to pentazocine that acts as an antagonist at the *mu*-receptor. Buprenorphine is considered 30 times as potent as morphine and exhibits many of the same actions as the opiate agonists. It produces a dose-related analgesia but at higher dosages analgesic effects may actually decrease. Buprenorphine appears to have a high affinity for *mu*-receptors in the CNS, which may explain its relatively long duration of action. In dogs, sedative effects are generally present after 15 minutes, but analgesia may not develop fully until 30 minutes post-dose. Analgesia may persist for 12 hours, but usually a 6-8 hour duration of analgesic effect is typical.

The cardiovascular effects of buprenorphine may cause a decrease in both blood pressure and cardiac rate. Rarely, human patients may exhibit increases in blood pressure and cardiac rate. Respiratory depression is a possibility, and decreased respiratory rates have been noted in horses treated with buprenorphine. Gastrointestinal effects appear to be minimal in cats treated with buprenorphine.

Pharmacokinetics

In cats, buprenorphine is rapidly absorbed when given IM, but bioavailability may only be around 50%. Peak levels after subcutaneous injection can vary widely and blood levels are low. Buprenorphine has a volume of distribution [Vd(ss)] of approximately 3-8 L/kg and a clearance of about 8-20 mL/kg/min. Elimination half-life is about 6-7 hours. When administered via oral mucosa (liquid placed into the side of cat's mouth), absorption can be comparable to that seen with IM or IV administration. Human transdermal patch buprenorphine (*Transtac®*—Napp Pharm.; UK) applied to cats has demonstrated widely variable blood levels and without a loading dose does not appear to provide adequate analgesia.

In dogs, oral bioavailability is very low (5%), but oral transmucosal administered buprenorphine is about 35-50% absorbed. Elimination half-life has been reported as various times and wide interpatient variability exists; mean half-life ranges from 5-9 hours in most reports. In a small pilot study, application of topical buprenorphine patches showed that plasma concentrations increased during the first 36 hours and then remained in the 0.7-1 ng/mL range during the study period (Andaluz et al. 2009).

In the horse, onset of action is approximately 15 minutes after IV dosing. The drug is reportedly well absorbed after sublingual administration; IM bioavailability is variable. Volume of distribution is about 2.5-3 L/kg. The peak effect occurs in 30-45 minutes and the duration of action may last up to 8 hours. Elimination half-life after an IV or an IM dose is about 3.5-6 hours. Because acepromazine exhibits a similar onset and duration of action, many equine clinicians favor using this drug in combination with buprenorphine.

In humans, buprenorphine is rapidly absorbed following IM injection, with 40-90% absorbed systemically when tested in humans. The drug is also absorbed sublingually (bioavailability≈55%) in people. Oral doses appear to undergo a high first-pass effect with metabolism occurring in the GI mucosa and liver.

The distribution of the drug has not been well studied. Data from work done in rats reflects that buprenorphine concentrates in the liver, but is also found in the brain, GI tract, and placenta. It is highly bound (96%) to plasma proteins (not albumin), crosses the placenta, and it and its metabolites are found in maternal milk at concentrations equal to or greater than those found in plasma.

Buprenorphine is metabolized in the liver by N-dealkylation and glucuronidation. These metabolites are then eliminated by biliary excretion into the feces (≈70%) and urinary excretion (≈27%).

Contraindications/Precautions/Warnings

All opiates should be used with caution in patients with hypothyroidism, severe renal insufficiency, adrenocortical insufficiency (Addison's), and in geriatric or severely debilitated patients.

Rarely, patients may develop respiratory depression from buprenorphine; it, therefore, should be used cautiously in patients with compromised cardiopulmonary function. Like other opiates, buprenorphine must be used with extreme caution in patients with head trauma, increased CSF pressure or other CNS dysfunction (*e.g.*, coma).

Patients with severe hepatic dysfunction may eliminate the drug more slowly than normal patients. Buprenorphine may increase bile duct pressure and should be used cautiously in patients with biliary tract disease. It should also be used with caution in horses that show signs of diminished GI tract motility.

The drug is contraindicated in patients having known hypersensitivity to it.

The UK label states that it is contraindicated preoperatively for Caesarian section due to concerns for respiratory depression in the offspring. Labeling states that it should not be administered via the intrathecal or peridural routes. Because it does not cause much sedation in horses, when used as a preop an intravenous sedative should be administered prior to, or in conjunction with buprenorphine injection.

Adverse Effects

Although rare, respiratory depression appears to be the major adverse effect to monitor for with buprenorphine; other adverse effects (sedation) may be noted. IM injections may be more painful than other parenteral routes of administration.

In dogs, salivation, bradycardia, hypothermia, agitation, dehydration and miosis have been reported. Tachycardia, vomiting and high blood pressure rarely occur.

In cats, mydriasis and behavioral effects (*e.g.*, excessive purring, pacing, rubbing, etc.) can be seen. Vomiting and hyperthermia occur rarely.

In horses, buprenorphine may cause some excitement and diminished gut sounds, but colic has not been a major concern. Administration with a sedative (*e.g.*, acepromazine, detomidine, etc.) may help decrease excitement, and cardiac and respiratory rates.

The primary side effect seen in humans is sedation with an incidence of approximately 66%. May cause urine retention or difficulty voiding, particularly with high IV doses or epidural administration.

Reproductive/Nursing Safety

Although no controlled studies have been performed in domestic animals or humans, the drug has exhibited no evidence of teratogenicity or causing impaired fertility in laboratory animals. In humans, the FDA categorizes this drug as category *C* for use during pregnancy (*Animal studies have shown an adverse effect on the fetus, but there are no adequate studies in humans; or there are no animal reproduction studies and no adequate studies in humans.*)

Overdosage/Acute Toxicity

The intraperitoneal LD_{50} of buprenorphine has been reported to be 243 mg/kg in rats. The ratio of lethal dose to effective dose is at least 1000:1 in rodents. Because of the apparent high index of safety, life-threatening acute overdoses should be a rare event in veterinary medicine, but most overdoses will cause signs. There were 55 exposures to buprenorphine reported to the ASPCA Animal Poison Control Center (APCC) during 2008-2009. In these cases, 34 were dogs with 25 showing clinical signs, and 20 were cats with 6 showing clinical signs. The 1 remaining case was a lagomorph that showed clinical signs. Common findings in dogs (recorded in decreasing frequency) include vocalization, ataxia, hypersalivation, hypothermia, and lethargy.

Treatment with naloxone and doxapram has been suggested in cases of acute overdoses causing respiratory or cardiac effects. Secondary to buprenorphine's high affinity for the *mu* receptor, high doses of naloxone may be required to treat respiratory depression.

Drug Interactions

The following drug interactions have either been reported or are theoretical in humans or animals receiving buprenorphine and may be of significance in veterinary patients. Unless otherwise noted, use together is not necessarily contraindicated, but weigh the potential risks and perform additional monitoring when appropriate.

- **ANESTHETICS, LOCAL** (*e.g.*, **mepivacaine, bupivacaine, etc.**): May be potentiated by concomitant use of buprenorphine.

- **ANTICONVULSANTS** (*e.g.*, **phenobarbital, phenytoin, etc.**): May decrease plasma buprenorphine levels.
- **BENZODIAZEPINES:** Case reports of humans developing respiratory/cardiovascular/CNS depression; use with caution.
- **CNS DEPRESSANTS** (*e.g.*, **anesthetic agents, antihistamines, phenothiazines, barbiturates, tranquilizers, alcohol**, etc.): May cause increased CNS or respiratory depression when used with buprenorphine.
- **ERYTHROMYCIN:** Can increase plasma buprenorphine levels.
- **FENTANYL** (and other **pure opiate agonists**): Buprenorphine may potentially antagonize some analgesic effects (**Note:** *This is controversial*), but may also reverse some of the sedative and respiratory depressant effects of pure agonists.
- **HALOTHANE:** Potentially can increase buprenorphine effects.
- **KETOCONAZOLE, ITRACONAZOLE, FLUCONAZOLE:** Can increase plasma buprenorphine levels.
- **MONAMINE OXIDASE (MAO) INHIBITORS** (*e.g.*, **selegiline, amitraz**, etc.): Possible additive effects or increased CNS depression.
- **NALOXONE:** May reduce analgesia associated with high dose buprenorphine.
- **PANCURONIUM:** If used with buprenorphine may cause increased conjunctival changes.
- **RIFAMPIN:** Potentially decrease plasma buprenorphine concentrations.

Doses

- **DOGS:**

  For analgesia (all dosages are extra-label in the USA):

  a) 5 – 30 micrograms/kg (0.005 – 0.03 mg/kg) IV, IM or SC q6-12h. Following an IV loading dose of 5 – 10 micrograms/kg (0.005 – 0.01 mg/kg), continuous IV infusions of 2 – 4 micrograms/kg/hr have also been suggested.

  b) **Post-operative Analgesia:** 10 – 20 micrograms/kg (0.01 – 0.02 mg/kg) IV or IM. For further pain relief, repeat if necessary after 3-4 hours with 10 micrograms/kg (0.01 mg/kg) or after 5-6 hours with 20 micrograms/kg (0.02 mg/kg). (Adapted from label; *Vetergesic*® Multi-Dose; UK)

  c) **Buccal (oral transmucosal; OTM) for post-surgical anesthesia:** Based upon the study results the authors concluded that 120 micrograms/kg buccally before OHE was an effective analgesic with minimal intraoperative and postoperative adverse effects. (Ko et al. 2011)

  As a premed before surgery or an anesthetic adjunct (extra-label): **Note:** there are many potential combinations that have been suggested; the following are examples and not inclusive. For additional information refer to other anesthesia-specific references such as *Handbook of Veterinary Anesthesia*, 5th Ed., Muir & Hubbell, Elsevier 2012; *Essentials of Small Animal Anesthesia & Analgesia*, Grimm et al, Wiley-Blackwell 2011 or the website Veterinary Anesthesia & Analgesia Support Group (vasg.org).

  a) In the study, buprenorphine at 20 micrograms/kg (0.02 mg/kg) was combined in the same syringe with either acepromazine (at 0.03 mg/kg) or dexmedetomidine (dosed by body surface area at 250 micrograms/m²) and injected IM. IV catheters were placed 30-45 minutes post premedication and general anesthesia induction was done using propofol or alfaxalone. Meloxicam was given IV (dogs at 0.2 mg/kg) after induction and before surgery started. General anesthesia maintained with isoflurane. Both combinations (buprenorphine with either acepromazine or dexme-

detomidine) resulted in suitable anesthesia and analgesia for dogs and cats undergoing elective procedures; some animals required additional analgesia within 4 hours of the premed. Analgesic effect differences post-surgery were not clinically significant. (Hunt et al. 2013)

  b) In the study, efficacy and cardiorespiratory effects of a combination of dexmedetomidine (15 micrograms/kg), ketamine (3 mg/kg) and either buprenorphine (40 micrograms/kg), butorphanol, or hydromorphone as a single IM injection, (with or without reversal by atipamezole) in dogs undergoing castration. Supplemental isoflurane used when anesthesia was considered inadequate during surgery. Authors concluded that the most suitable combination was with buprenorphine and that atipamezole shortened recovery times. (Barletta et al. 2011)

- **CATS:**

  For analgesia:

  a) **For the control of postoperative pain associated with surgical procedures using the feline-labeled product (*Simbadol*®);** (labeled dose; FDA-approved): 0.24 mg/kg SC once daily, for up to 3 days. Administer the first dose approximately 1 hour prior to surgery. Do not dispense for administration at home by the pet owner. (Adapted from label; Simbadol®—Abbott) Note: This product was approved just as this edition was going to press; refer to the label (package insert) for additional information.

  b) Extra-label dose: 10 – 30 micrograms/kg (0.01 – 0.03 mg/kg) IM, IV, Buccal (oral transmucosal; OTM) q6-8h. Dosages at the high end of the dosing range may be required for more severe pain. If using OTM, suggest using upper end of dosing range.

  As a premed before surgery (extra-label):

  a) In the study, buprenorphine at 20 micrograms/kg (0.02 mg/kg) was combined in the same syringe with either acepromazine (at 0.03 mg/kg) or dexmedetomidine (dosed by body surface area at 250 micrograms/m2) and injected IM. IV catheters were placed 30-45 minutes post premedication and general anesthesia induction was done using propofol or alfaxalone. Meloxicam was given IV (cats at 0.3 mg/kg) after induction and before surgery started. General anesthesia maintained with isoflurane. Both combinations (buprenorphine with either acepromazine or dexmedetomidine) resulted in suitable anesthesia and analgesia for dogs and cats undergoing elective procedures; some animals required additional analgesia within 4 hours of the premed. Dexmedetomidine cats were more sedated than when acepromazine was used. Analgesic effect differences post-surgery were not clinically significant. (Hunt et al. 2013)

  b) In the study (assessing analgesia after OHE), one of the protocols used was: Ten minutes prior to surgery, ketamine 60 mg/m² (~3 mg/kg), midazolam 3 mg/m² (~0.2 mg/kg), medetomidine 600 micrograms/m2 (~30 micrograms/kg), and buprenorphine 180 micrograms/m2 (~9 micrograms/kg) combined and given as a single IM injection in quadriceps muscles. Additionally, either carprofen (4 mg/kg) or meloxicam (0.3 mg/kg) were given subcutaneously. All protocols in the study provided adequate analgesia. (Polson et al. 2012)

- **FERRETS:**

  As an analgesic (extra-label): 0.01 – 0.05 mg/kg SC or IM 2-3 times daily. (Williams 2000)

HORSES: (NOTE: ARCI UCGFS CLASS 2 DRUG)

For neuroleptanalgesia (all are extra-label in USA):

a) 4 – 6 micrograms/kg (0.004 – 0.006 mg/kg) IV (given with a sedative such as acepromazine, detomidine, etc.). IM administration could also be used, but bioavailability may be reduced and onset of action somewhat delayed.

b) **For analgesia:** 10 micrograms/kg (0.01 mg/kg) IV, 5 minutes after administration of an IV sedative. The dose may be repeated if necessary, once, after not less than 1-2 hours. For potentiation of sedation: 5 micrograms/kg (0.005 mg/kg) IV 5 minutes after administration of an IV sedative. The dose may be repeated if necessary after 10 minutes. (Adapted from label; *Vetergesic®* Multi-Dose; UK)

■ **RABBITS/RODENTS/SMALL MAMMALS:**

As an analgesic (for control of acute or chronic visceral pain); (extra-label):

a) **Rabbits:** 0.01 – 0.05 mg/kg SC, IM or IV q6–12h; 0.5 mg/kg rectally q12h. (Ivey et al. 2000)

b) **Guinea pigs:** 0.05 mg/kg SC or IV q8-12h. **Mice:** 0.05 – 0.1 mg/kg SC q12h. **Rats:** 0.01– 0.05 mg/kg SC or IV q8-12h or 0.1 – 0.25 mg/kg PO q8-12h. (Adamcak et al. 2000)

As a premedication (extra-label):

a) **Rabbits: In compromised patients:** 0.05 – 0.1 mg/kg SC alone. (Vella 2009)

b) **Rabbits: In healthy animals before uncomplicated elective procedures:** Buprenorphine 0.02 – 0.06 mg/kg with midazolam (0.25 – 0.5 mg/kg) IM within 20 minutes of procedure along with a local or line incisional block using lidocaine and bupivacaine. Protocols are modified for ill or unstable animals. (Lennox 2009)

■ **ZOO, EXOTIC, WILDLIFE SPECIES:**

For use of buprenorphine in zoo, exotic and wildlife medicine refer to specific references, including:

a) *Zoo Animal and Wildlife Immobilization and Anesthesia.* West, G., Heard, D., Caulkett, N. (eds.), Blackwell Publishing, 2007.

b) *Handbook of Wildlife Chemical Immobilization, 3rd Ed.* Kreeger, T.J. and J.M. Arnemo. 2007.

c) *Fowler's Zoo and Wild Animal Medicine Current Therapy, Volume 7,* Miller, R.E., Fowler, M.E., Saunders. 2011.

d) *Exotic Animal Formulary, 4th Ed.* Carpenter, J.W., Saunders. 2012.

e) The 2009 American Association of Zoo Veterinarian Proceedings by D. K. Fontenot also has several dosages listed for restraint, anesthesia, and analgesia for a variety of drugs for carnivores and primates. VIN members can access them at: http://goo.gl/NNIWQ or http://goo.gl/9UJse

Monitoring

■ Analgesic efficacy.
■ Respiratory status.
■ Cardiac status.

Client Information

■ Opiate analgesic often used for short-term pain relief. Given either by injection or buccally (squirted into the mouth).
■ When given buccally to cats, squirt just under the tongue or in the cheek pouch for the best effect. The doses are very small for this potent drug, so be sure that you are giving the exact amount your veterinarian has prescribed.
■ Sedation is the most common side effect.

Chemistry/Synonyms

A thebaine derivative, buprenorphine is a synthetic partial opiate agonist. It occurs as a white, crystalline powder with a solubility of 17 mg/mL in water and 42 mg/mL in alcohol. The commercially available injectable product (*Buprenex®*) has a pH of 3.5-5 and is a sterile solution of the drug dissolved in D5W. Terms of potency are expressed in terms of buprenorphine. The commercial product contains 0.324 mg/mL of buprenorphine HCl, which is equivalent to 0.3 mg/mL of buprenorphine.

Buprenorphine HCl may also be known as: buprenorphini hydrochloridum, CL-112302, NIH-8805, UM-952; trade names include *Vetergesic®*, *Buprenex®*, *Buprenodale®*, *Suboxone®*, *Subutex®*, and *Temgesic®*.

Storage/Stability

Buprenorphine should be stored at room temperature (15-30° C). Temperatures above 40° C or below freezing should be avoided. Buprenorphine products should be stored away from bright light. Autoclaving may considerably decrease drug potency. The drug is stable between a pH of 3.5-5. The UK labeling states that the injection should not be stored above 25°C; the vial protected from light and to shake well before using.

Compatibility/Compounding Considerations

Buprenorphine is reported to be **compatible** with the following IV solutions and drugs: acepromazine, atropine, diphenhydramine, D5W, D5W and normal saline, droperidol, glycopyrrolate, haloperidol, hydroxyzine, lactated Ringer's, normal saline, scopolamine, and xylazine.

Although no published data could be located to support stability for this combination, buprenorphine injection has been mixed in syringes with detomidine, dexmedetomidine, ketamine, medetomidine, and xylazine.

Buprenorphine is reportedly **incompatible** with diazepam and lorazepam.

Dosage Forms/Regulatory Status

VETERINARY-LABELED PRODUCTS: NONE IN THE USA.

Buprenorphine Injection 1.8 mg/mL in 10 mL multi-dose vials; Simbadol®; (Rx; C-III). FDA-approved (NADA 141-434) for use in cats.

The ARCI (Racing Commissioners International) has designated this drug as a class 2 substance. See the appendix for more information.

HUMAN-LABELED PRODUCTS:

Buprenorphine HCl for Injection: 0.324 mg/mL (equivalent to 0.3 mg/mL buprenorphine); 1 mL amps, vials, & syringes; *Buprenex®*, generic; (Rx, C-III)

Buprenorphine HCl Sublingual Tablets: 2 & 8 mg (as base); generic; (Rx, C-III)

Buprenorphine HCl Transdermal System: 5 mcg/hr, 10 mcg/hr, & 20 mcg/hr; *Butrans®*; (Rx, C-III) **Note:** In the study comparing buprenorphine SC with a topical patch in dogs for surgical pain (Moll et al. 2011), a 70 mcg/hr patch (*Transtec®*, Grünenthal) was used. In the study comparing buprenorphine IV with a topical patch in dogs for its antinociceptive effects (Pieper et al. 2011), a 52.5 mcg/hr patch (*Transtec Pro®*, Grünenthal) was used. At the time of writing (2013), neither of these products are available commercially in the USA.

A combination sublingual product containing buprenorphine and naloxone is also available.

Revisions/References

Monograph revised/updated September 2013.

Adamcak, A. & B. Otten (2000). Rodent Therapeutics. *Vet Clin NA: Exotic Anim Pract* **3:**1(Jan): 221-40.

Andaluz, A., et al. (2009). Plasma buprenorphine concentrations after the application of a 70 mu g/h transdermal patch in dogs. Preliminary report. *J. Vet. Pharmacol. Ther.* **32**(5): 503-5.

Barletta, M., et al. (2011). Evaluation of dexmedetomidine and ketamine in combination with opioids as injectable anesthesia for castration in dogs. *Journal of the American Veterinary Medical Association* **238**(9): 1159-67.

Bortolami, E., et al. (2012). Comparison of two formulations of buprenorphine in cats administered by the oral transmucosal route. *Journal of Feline Medicine and Surgery* **14**(8): 534-9.

Catbagan, D. L., et al. (2011). Comparison of the efficacy and adverse effects of sustained-release buprenorphine hydrochloride following subcutaneous administration and buprenorphine hydrochloride following oral transmucosal administration in cats undergoing ovariohysterectomy. *American Journal of Veterinary Research* **72**(4): 461-6.

Giordano, T., et al. (2010). Postoperative analgesic effects of intravenous, intramuscular, subcutaneous or oral transmucosal buprenorphine administered to cats undergoing ovariohysterectomy. *Veterinary Anaesthesia and Analgesia* **37**(4): 357-66.

Hunt, J. R., et al. (2013). Sedative and analgesic effects of buprenorphine, combined with either acepromazine or dexmedetomidine, for premedication prior to elective surgery in cats and dogs. *Veterinary Anaesthesia and Analgesia* **40**(3): 297-307.

Ivey, E. & J. Morrisey (2000). Therapeutics for Rabbits. *Vet Clin NA: Exotic Anim Pract* **3:**1(Jan): 183-216.

Ko, J. C., et al. (2011). Efficacy of oral transmucosal and intravenous administration of buprenorphine before surgery for postoperative analgesia in dogs undergoing ovariohysterectomy. *Journal of the American Veterinary Medical Association* **238**(3): 318-28.

Lennox, A. (2009). Anaesthesia and analgesia of the rabbit. Proceedings: BSAVA. accessed via Veterinary Information Network; vin.com

Moll, X., et al. (2011). Comparison of subcutaneous and transdermal administration of buprenorphine for pre-emptive analgesia in dogs undergoing elective ovariohysterectomy (vol 187, pg 124, 2011). *Veterinary Journal* **189**(3): 364-.

Pieper, K., et al. (2011). Antinociceptive efficacy and plasma concentrations of transdermal buprenorphine in dogs. *The Veterinary Journal* **187**(3): 335-41.

Polson, S., et al. (2012). Analgesia after feline ovariohysterectomy under midazolam-medetomidine-ketamine anaesthesia with buprenorphine or butorphanol, and carprofen or meloxicam: a prospective, randomised clinical trial. *Journal of Feline Medicine and Surgery* **14**(8): 553-9.

Vella, D. (2009). *Rabbit General Anesthesia*. Proceedings: AAVAC-UEP. accessed via Veterinary Information Network; vin.com

Williams, B. (2000). Therapeutics in Ferrets. *Vet Clin NA: Exotic Anim Pract* **3:**1(Jan): 131-53.

Buspirone HCl

(byoo-spye-rone) BuSpar®

Anxiolytic

Prescriber Highlights

▶ Non-benzodiazepine anxiolytic agent used in dogs & cats. Usually given 2-3 times a day.

▶ May take a week or more to be effective; not appropriate for acute treatment of situational anxieties.

▶ Use with caution in patients with severe hepatic or renal disease.

▶ Adverse Effects relatively uncommon; cats may exhibit behavior changes.

▶ Human generic forms of medication are relatively inexpensive.

Uses/Indications

Buspirone may be effective in treating certain behavior disorders in dogs and cats, principally those that are fear/phobia related and especially those associated with social interactions. Buspirone may also be useful for urine spraying or treatment of motion sickness in cats. Approximately 50% of cats show improvement in urine marking when buspirone is given. Buspirone may be more effective in multi-cat households than in single cat households.

Pharmacology/Actions

Buspirone is an anxioselective agent. Unlike the benzodiazepines, buspirone does not possess any anticonvulsant or muscle relaxant activity and little sedative or psychomotor impairment activity. Buspirone does not share the same mechanisms as the benzodiazepines (does not have significant affinity for benzodiazepine receptors and does not affect GABA binding). It appears to act as a partial agonist at serotonin (5-HT1A) receptors and as an agonist/antagonist of dopamine (D2) receptors in the CNS. In neurons, buspirone slows the neuronal flow depletion of serotonin stores.

Pharmacokinetics

In humans, buspirone is rapidly and completely absorbed but a high first pass effect limits systemic bioavailability to approximately 5%. Binding to plasma proteins is very high (95%). In rats, highest tissue concentrations are found in the lungs, kidneys, and fat. Lower levels are found in the brain, heart, skeletal muscle, plasma and liver. Both buspirone and its metabolites are distributed into maternal milk. The elimination half-life (in humans) is about 2-4 hours. Buspirone is hepatically metabolized to several metabolites (including one that is active: 1-PP). These metabolites are excreted primarily in the urine.

In a limited study done in 6 cats (Mealey et al. 2004), oral administration of buspirone gave peak levels in about 1.4 hours, but oral bioavailability appeared to be significantly lower than in humans. Transdermal administration of buspirone (PLO-base) did not yield detectable levels (ELISA method).

Contraindications/Precautions/Warnings

Buspirone should be used with caution in animals with either significant renal or hepatic disease. Because buspirone may reduce disinhibition, it should be used with caution in aggressive animals. While buspirone has far less sedating properties than many other anxiolytic drugs, it should be used with caution in working or service dogs.

Because buspirone often takes a week or more for effect, it should not be used as the sole therapy for situational anxieties.

Prescription/order errors have occurred when buspirone and bupropion have been confused. The use of "tall man" letters (writing part of a drug's name in upper case) on prescription/orders may reduce the risk for errors: BusPIRone/BuPROPion.

Adverse Effects

Adverse effects are usually minimal in animals treated with buspirone and it is generally well tolerated. Bradycardia, GI disturbances and stereotypic behaviors are possible. Cats may demonstrate increased affection, which may be the desired effect. In multi-cat households, cats that have previously been extremely timid in the face of repeated aggression from other cats may, after receiving buspirone become less anxious, more assertive and begin turning on their attacker.

The most likely adverse effect profile seen with buspirone in humans includes dizziness, headache, nausea/anorexia, and restlessness; other neurologic effects (including sedation) may be noted. Rarely, tachycardias and other cardiovascular clinical signs may be present.

Reproductive/Nursing Safety

While the drug has not been proven safe during pregnancy, doses of up to 30 times the labeled dosage in rabbits and rats demonstrated no teratogenic effects. In humans, the FDA categorizes this drug as category *B* for use during pregnancy (*Animal studies have not yet demonstrated risk to the fetus, but there are no adequate studies in pregnant women; or animal studies have shown an adverse effect, but adequate studies in pregnant women have not demonstrated a risk to the fetus in the first trimester of pregnancy, and there is no evidence of risk in later trimesters.*)

Buspirone and its metabolites have been detected in the milk of lactating rats; avoid use during nursing if possible.

Overdosage/Acute Toxicity

Limited information is available. The oral LD_{50} in dogs is 586 mg/kg. Oral overdoses may produce vomiting, dizziness, drowsiness, miosis and gastric distention. Standard overdose protocols should be followed after ingestion has been determined.

Drug Interactions

Buspirone may be used in combination with tricyclic or SSRI agents, but dosage reductions may be necessary to minimize adverse effects.

The following drug interactions have either been reported or are theoretical in humans or animals receiving buspirone and may be of significance in veterinary patients. Unless otherwise noted, use together is not necessarily contraindicated, but weigh the potential risks and perform additional monitoring when appropriate.

- **CNS DEPRESSANTS**: Potentially could cause increased CNS depression.
- **DILTIAZEM**: May cause increased buspirone plasma levels and adverse effects.
- **ERYTHROMYCIN**: May cause increased buspirone plasma levels and adverse effects.
- **GRAPEFRUIT JUICE (powder)**: May cause increased buspirone plasma levels and adverse effects.
- **KETOCONAZOLE, ITRACONAZOLE**: May cause increased buspirone plasma levels and adverse effects.
- **MONOAMINE OXIDASE INHIBITORS** (*e.g.*, **selegiline, amitraz**): Use with buspirone is not recommended because dangerous hypertension may occur.
- **RIFAMPIN**: May cause decreased buspirone plasma levels.
- **TRAZODONE**: Use with buspirone may cause increased ALT.
- **VERAPAMIL**: May cause increased buspirone plasma levels.

Doses

- **DOGS:**

  For adjunctive treatment of low-grade anxieties and fears (extra-label): Most recommendations fall into a range of 0.5 – 1 mg/kg PO q8-12h, but anecdotal recommendations as high as 2 mg/kg have been noted. Some put upper end maximum dosage limits such as 10 – 15 mg per dog PO q8-12h.

- **CATS:**

  For adjunctive treatment of low-grade anxieties/fears, spraying, overgrooming (extra-label): Most recommend 0.5 – 1 mg/kg PO q8-12h; or practically, using 5 mg tablets: 2.5 – 7.5 mg per cat PO 2-3 times per day.

Monitoring

- Efficacy.
- Adverse effect profiles.

Client Information

- May be given either with food or on an empty stomach. If animal vomits or acts sick after getting it on an empty stomach, give with food or small treat to see if this helps.
- May take a few weeks for the full benefits of this medication to be noticeable. Best used in conjunction with behavioral therapy.
- If your animal wore a flea collar in the past two weeks, let your veterinarian know.
- Buspirone is usually well tolerated by dogs and cats. Cats may show increased friendliness/affection while receiving buspirone.

Chemistry/Synonyms

An arylpiperazine derivative azaspirone anxiolytic agent, buspirone HCl differs structurally from the benzodiazepines. It occurs as a white, crystalline powder with solubility's at 25°C of 865 mg/mL in water and about 20 mg/mL in alcohol.

Buspirone HCl may also be known as MJ-9022; many trade names are available. A common trade name is *BuSpar®*.

Storage/Stability

Buspirone HCl tablets should be stored in tight, light-resistant containers at room temperature. After manufacture, buspirone tablets have an expiration date of 36 months.

Compatibility/Compounding Considerations

No specific information noted.

Dosage Forms/Regulatory Status

VETERINARY-LABELED PRODUCTS: NONE.

The ARCI (Racing Commissioners International) has designated this drug as a class 2 substance. See the appendix for more information.

HUMAN-LABELED PRODUCTS:

Buspirone HCl Oral Tablets: 5 mg (4.6 mg as base), 7.5 mg (6.85 mg as base), 10 mg (9.1 mg as base), 15 mg (13.7 mg as base) and 30 mg (27.4 mg as base); generic; (Rx)

Revisions/References

Monograph revised/updated September 2013.

Mealey, K. L., et al. (2004). Systemic absorption of amitriptyline and buspirone after oral and transdermal administration to healthy cats. *Journal of Veterinary Internal Medicine* 18(1): 43-6.

Busulfan

(byoo-sul-fan)   Myleran®, Busulfex®

Antineoplastic

Prescriber Highlights

- ▶ Antineoplastic sometimes used in treating chronic granulocytic leukemias in small animals.
- ▶ Myelosuppression; may be severe.
- ▶ May increase uric acid levels.

Uses/Indications

Busulfan may be useful in the adjunctive therapy of chronic granulocytic leukemias or polycythemia vera in small animals. Not commonly used in veterinary medicine.

Pharmacology/Actions

Busulfan is a bifunctional alkylating agent antineoplastic and is cell cycle-phase nonspecific. The exact mechanism of action has not been determined but is thought to be due to its alkylating, cross-linking of strands of DNA and myelosuppressive properties. Busulfan's primary activity is against cells of the granulocytic series.

Pharmacokinetics

Busulfan is well absorbed after oral administration. Distribution characteristics are not well described but in humans, drug concentrations in the CSF are nearly equal to those found in plasma. It is unknown whether the drug enters maternal milk. Busulfan is rapidly, hepatically metabolized to at least 12 different metabolites that are slowly excreted into the urine. In humans, serum half-life of busulfan averages about 2.5 hours.

Contraindications/Precautions/Warnings

Busulfan is contraindicated in patients that have shown resistance to the drug in the past or are hypersensitive to it. Only veterinarians with the experience and resources to monitor the toxicity of this agent should administer this drug. The risk versus benefits of therapy must be carefully considered in patients with preexisting bone marrow depression or concurrent infections. Additive bone marrow depression may occur in patients undergoing concomitant radiation therapy.

Adverse Effects

The most commonly associated adverse effect seen with busulfan therapy is myelosuppression. In humans, anemia, leukopenia, and thrombocytopenia may be observed. Onset of leukopenia is generally 10-15 days after initiation of therapy and leukocyte nadirs occurring on average around 11-30 days. Severe bone marrow depression can result in pancytopenia that may take months to years for recovery. In humans, bronchopulmonary dysplasia with pulmonary fibrosis, uric acid nephropathy, and stomatitis have been reported. These effects are uncommon and generally associated with chronic, higher dose therapy.

Reproductive/Nursing Safety

Busulfan's teratogenic potential has not been well documented, but it is mutagenic in mice and may potentially cause a variety of fetal abnormalities. It is generally recommended to avoid the drug during pregnancy, but because of the seriousness of the diseases treated with busulfan, the potential benefits to the mother must be considered. In humans, the FDA categorizes this drug as category **D** for use during pregnancy (*There is evidence of human fetal risk, but the potential benefits from the use of the drug in pregnant women may be acceptable despite its potential risks.*)

It is unknown if busulfan enters milk; avoid nursing if the dam is receiving the drug.

Overdosage/Acute Toxicity

There is limited experience with busulfan overdoses. The LD50 in mice is 120 mg/kg. Chronic overdosage is more likely to cause serious bone marrow suppression than is an acute overdose; however, any overdose, should be treated seriously with standard gut emptying protocols used when appropriate and supportive therapy initiated when required. There is no known specific antidote for busulfan intoxication.

Drug Interactions

The following drug interactions have either been reported or are theoretical in humans or animals receiving busulfan and may be of significance in veterinary patients. Unless otherwise noted, use together is not necessarily contraindicated, but weigh the potential risks and perform additional monitoring when appropriate.

- **ACETAMINOPHEN:** Use within 72 hours prior to busulfan can reduce busulfan clearance by reducing glutathione concentrations in tissues and blood.
- **CYCLOPHOSPHAMIDE:** Can potentially reduce clearance of busulfan, probably by competing for available glutathione.
- **ITRACONAZOLE:** Potential decreased busulfan clearance.
- **MYELOSUPPRESSANT AGENTS:** Concurrent use with other bone marrow depressant medications may result in additive myelosuppression.
- **PHENYTOIN:** Possible increased clearance of busulfan.
- **THIOGUANINE:** Used concomitantly with busulfan may result in hepatotoxicity.

Laboratory Considerations

- Busulfan may raise serum **uric acid** levels. Drugs such as allopurinol may be required to control hyperuricemia.

Doses

Note: Because of the potential toxicity of this drug to patients, veterinary personnel and clients, and since chemotherapy indications, treatment protocols, monitoring and safety guidelines often change, the following dosages should be used only as a general guide. Consultation with a veterinary oncologist and referral to current veterinary oncology references [*e.g.*, (Withrow et al. 2012); (Dobson et al. 2011); (Henry et al. 2009); (North et al. 2009); (Argyle et al. 2008)] are strongly recommended.

- **SMALL ANIMALS:**
  Busulfan is rarely used in veterinary medicine, but when used it is usually dosed in a range of 2 – 4 mg/m^2 (**NOT** mg/kg) PO once daily.

Monitoring

- CBC.
- Serum uric acid.
- Efficacy.

Client Information

- Clients must understand the importance of both administering busulfan as directed and reporting immediately any signs associated with toxicity (*e.g.*, abnormal bleeding, bruising, urination, depression, infection, shortness of breath, etc.).

Chemistry/Synonyms

An alkylsulfonate antineoplastic agent, busulfan occurs as white, crystalline powder. It is slightly soluble in alcohol and very slightly soluble in water.

Busulfan may also be known as: bussulfam, busulfanum, busulphan, CB-2041, GT-41, myelosan, NSC-750, WR-19508, *Bussulfam*®, *Busulfanum*®, *Busulivex*®, *Mielucin*®, *Misulban*®, or *Myleran*®.

Storage/Stability

Busulfan tablets should be stored in well-closed containers at room temperature.

Compatibility/Compounding Considerations

A busulfan 2 mg/mL oral suspension can be prepared by crushing 30 (thirty) 2 mg oral tablets completely and diluting with simple syrup to a total volume of 30 mL.

Dilute with simple syrup for a final total volume of 30 mL. Shake suspension well before dosing. Stable up to 30-days when refrigerated (White et al. 2007).

Dosage Forms/Regulatory Status

VETERINARY-LABELED PRODUCTS: NONE.

HUMAN-LABELED PRODUCTS:

Busulfan Oral Tablets: 2 mg; *Myleran*®; (Rx)

Busulfan Injection Solution: 6 mg/mL in 10 mL single-use amps with syringe filters; *Busulfex*®; (Rx)

Revisions/References

Monograph revised/updated September 2013.

Argyle, D., et al. (2008). *Decision Making in Small Animal Oncology*, Wiley-Blackwell.
Dobson, J. & D. Lascelles (2011). *BSAVA Manual of Canine and Feline Oncology*, BSAVA.
Henry, C. & M. Higginbotham (2009). *Cancer Management in Small Animal Practice*, Saunders.
North, S. & T. Banks (2009). *Small Animal Oncology: An Introduction*, Saunders.
White, R. & V. Bradnam (2007). *Handbook of Drug Administration via Enteral Feeding Tubes*, Pharmaceutical Press.
Withrow, S., et al. (2012). *Withrow and MacEwen's Small Animal Clinical Oncology, 5th Ed.*, Saunders.

Butaphosphan with Cyanocobalamin

(byoo-ta-fos-fan; sye-an-oh-koe-bal-ah-min)   Catosal®

Injectable Phosphate/Vitamin B12

Prescriber Highlights

▶ An injectable organic phosphorous and vitamin B-12 product.

▶ Not an FDA-approved drug.

Because this product has not undergone FDA-approval process as a drug, there is a limited amount of information available; refer to the Cyanocobalamin and Phosphate monographs for more information.

Uses/Indications

The combination product *Catosal®* contains butaphosphan with cyanocobalamin (Vitamin B-12). It is marketed in several countries for a variety of species (sheep, poultry, pigs, horses, goats, dogs, cattle, fur-bearing animals, and cats) when a parenteral source of phosphorous and vitamin B-12 is indicated. In the USA, the label states that it is a source of Vitamin B12 and phosphorus for prevention or treatment of deficiencies of these nutrients in cattle, swine, horses and poultry.

Pharmacology/Actions

For more detail on pharmacology/actions, see the *Cyanocobalamin* and *Phosphate* monographs. A study (Furll et al. 2010) done in dairy cattle where butaphosphan/cyanocobalamin was injected daily one to two weeks before parturition either 0, 3, or 6 times (0.1 mL/kg IV; 10 mg/kg butaphosphan and 5 micrograms/kg cyanocobalamin) showed that multiple daily IV injections before parturition increased serum cyanocobalamin levels, post-partum glucose availability, and decreased peripheral fat mobilization and ketone body formation. Puerperal infection rates in the first 5 days post-partum were decreased in the group receiving 6 injections versus the cows receiving placebo.

Another study done in dairy cattle to determine the effect of butaphosphan/cyanocobalamin on the prevalence of subclinical ketosis in dairy cattle in the early postpartum period has been published (Rollin et al. 2010). Cows received either placebo (25 mL sterile water SC) or butaphosphan/cyanocobalamin injection (25 mL SC) on the day of, and one day after, calving. Only mature cows (3 or more lactations) receiving the drug had a lower rate of hyperketonemia than the non-treated cattle. These mature cows also showed significantly lower increases in serum concentrations of beta-hydroxybutyrate (BHBA) when measured at 3 and 10 days post-calving.

Pharmacokinetics

No specific information located; refer to the phosphate and cyanocobalamin monographs for further information.

Contraindications/Precautions/Warnings

This product should <u>not</u> be used in patients with hyperphosphatemia. Use with caution in patients with chronic renal failure.

Use standard aseptic procedures during administration of injections. Volumes of more than 10 mL should be split and given at separate intramuscular or subcutaneous sites.

Adverse Effects

None noted.

Reproductive/Nursing Safety

No specific information located.

Overdosage/Acute Toxicity

No specific information located.

Drug Interactions

No specific information located. Refer to the phosphate monograph for more information.

Laboratory Considerations

No specific information located.

Doses

- **HORSES:**

  1 – 2 mL per 100 lbs. body weight SC, IM, or IV; repeat daily as needed. Use standard aseptic procedures during administration of injections. Volumes of more than 10 mL should be split and given at separate intramuscular or subcutaneous sites. (*Catosal®*; (USA) label information)

- **CATTLE:**

  1 – 2 mL per 100 lbs. body weight SC, IM, or IV; repeat daily as needed. Volumes of more than 10 mL should be split and given at separate intramuscular or subcutaneous sites. Calves: 2 – 4 mL per 100 lbs. body weight; repeat daily as needed. (*Catosal®*; (USA) label information)

- **SWINE:**

  2 – 5 mL per 100 lbs. body weight SC, IM, or IV repeat daily as needed. Volumes of more than 10 mL should be split and given at separate intramuscular or subcutaneous sites. Piglets: 1 – 2.5 mL (total dose) per animal SC, IM, or IV; repeat daily as needed. (*Catosal®*; (USA) label information)

- **BIRDS:**

  Poultry (turkeys): 1 – 3 mL per liter of drinking water; repeat daily as needed. (*Catosal®*; (USA) label information)

Chemistry/Synonyms

Butaphosphan is 1-(n-Butylamino)-1-methylethyl phosphonous acid. One gram (10 mL of injection) provides 173 mg of phosphorous.

Storage/Stability

The injectable product should be stored at temperatures below 30°C (86°F); avoiding freezing.

Compatibility/Compounding Considerations

No specific information located. Consult the cyanocobalamin and Phosphate monographs for guidance.

Dosage Forms/Regulatory Status

VETERINARY-LABELED PRODUCTS:

Butaphosphan 100 mg/mL and Cyanocobalamin (Vitamin B-12) 0.05 mg/mL in 100 mL & 250 mL multidose (each mL contains 30 mg of n-Butyl alcohol as a preservative); *Catosal®*. This is not an FDA-approved drug product (not listed in Green Book). The USA labeling for the product states that federal law (USA) restricts this drug for use by or on the order of a licensed veterinarian (Rx) and that there is a zero day withdrawal period for meat, milk, and eggs.

HUMAN-LABELED PRODUCTS: NONE.

Revisions/References

Monograph revised/updated September 2013.

Furll, M., et al. (2010). Effect of multiple intravenous injections of butaphosphan and cyanocobalamin on the metabolism of periparturient dairy cows. *Journal of Dairy Science* **93**(9): 4155-64.

Rollin, E., et al. (2010). The effect of injectable butaphosphan and cyanocobalamin on postpartum serum beta-hydroxybutyrate, calcium, and phosphorus concentrations in dairy cattle. *Journal of Dairy Science* **93**(3): 978-87.

Butorphanol Tartrate

(byoo-tor-fa-nol)   Stadol®, Torbutrol®, Torbugesic®

Opiate Partial Agonist

Prescriber Highlights

▶ Partial opiate agonist/antagonist used in a variety of species as an analgesic, premed, antitussive, or antiemetic.

▶ Better choices available for moderate to severe pain in small animals, but a reasonably good analgesic for horses.

▶ Contraindicated or caution in patients with liver disease, hypothyroidism, or renal insufficiency, Addison's, head trauma, increased CSF pressure or other CNS dysfunction (*e.g.*, coma) & in geriatric or severely debilitated patients.

▶ Reduce dose in dogs with MDR1 (ABCB-1) mutation.

▶ Potential adverse effects in **Dogs/Cats:** Sedation, ataxia, anorexia or diarrhea (rarely).

▶ Horses (at usual doses) may include a transient ataxia, reduced gut sounds & sedation, but CNS excitement possible.

▶ Controlled substance (C-IV).

Uses/Indications

FDA-approved indication for dogs is "...for the relief of chronic non-productive cough associated with tracheobronchitis, tracheitis, tonsillitis, laryngitis and pharyngitis originating from inflammatory conditions of the upper respiratory tract" (Package Insert; *Torbugesic SA®*). In cats, it is labeled as indicated for is indicated for the relief of pain in cats caused by major or minor trauma, or pain associated with surgical procedures (Package Insert; *Torbutrol®*). It is also used in practice in both dogs and cats as an adjunctive preanesthetic medication (premed), analgesic, and as an antiemetic prior to cisplatin treatment (although not very effective in cats for this indication). Compared with other opiate analgesics, butorphanol is not very useful in small animals (particularly dogs) for treating pain and has to be dosed frequently. Butorphanol can be a useful reversal agent for the CNS and respiratory depressant effects of *mu*-agonists. Due to its kappa effects, it can reverse CNS and respiratory depression without completely reversing the analgesic effect of the *mu* agonist drugs.

The FDA-approved indication for horses is "...for the relief of pain associated with colic in adult horses and yearlings" (Package Insert; *Torbugesic®*). In horses, it appears that by adding butorphanol to an alpha agonist (*e.g.*, detomidine, xylazine, etc.), analgesia and sedation can be enhanced.

Butorphanol has also been used in cattle, camelids, small ruminants, small mammals, and several wildlife species. Butorphanol use in reptiles is somewhat controversial, but most studies show it has minimal analgesic or anesthetic-sparing efficacy in most species.

Pharmacology/Actions

Butorphanol is considered to be, on a weight basis, 4-7 times as potent an analgesic as morphine, 15-30 times as pentazocine, and 30-50 times as meperidine; however a ceiling effect is reached at higher dosages, where analgesia is no longer enhanced and may be reduced. Its agonist activity is thought to occur primarily at the kappa and sigma receptors and the analgesic actions at sites in the limbic system (sub-cortical level and spinal levels). Its use as an analgesic in small animals has been disappointing, primarily because of its very short duration of action and ability to alleviate only mild to moderate pain.

The antagonist potency of butorphanol is considered to be approximately 30 times that of pentazocine and 1/40th that of naloxone and will antagonize the effect of true agonists (*e.g.*, morphine, meperidine, oxymorphone, etc.).

Besides the analgesic qualities of butorphanol, it possesses significant antitussive activity. In dogs, butorphanol has been shown to elevate CNS respiratory center threshold to CO_2 but, unlike opiate agonists, not depress respiratory center sensitivity. Butorphanol, unlike morphine, apparently does not cause histamine release in dogs. CNS depression may occur in dogs, while CNS excitation has been noted (usually at high doses) in horses and dogs.

Although possessing less cardiovascular effects than the classical opiate agonists, butorphanol can cause a decrease in cardiac rate secondary to increased parasympathetic tone and mild decreases in arterial blood pressures. However, increased heart rates have been noted in horses after intravenous injection (Knych et al. 2013).

The risk of causing physical dependence seems to be minimal when butorphanol is used in veterinary patients.

Pharmacokinetics

Butorphanol is absorbed completely in the gut when administered orally but, because of a high first-pass effect, only about 1/6th of the administered dose reaches the systemic circulation. The drug has also been shown to be completely absorbed following IM administration.

Butorphanol is well distributed, with highest levels (of the parent compound and metabolites) found in the liver, kidneys, and intestine. Concentrations in the lungs, endocrine tissues, spleen, heart, fat tissue and blood cells are also higher than those found in plasma. Approximately 80% of the drug is bound to plasma proteins (human data). Butorphanol will cross the placenta and neonatal plasma levels have been roughly equivalent to maternal levels. The drug is also distributed into maternal milk.

Butorphanol is metabolized in the liver, primarily by hydroxylation. Other methods of metabolism include N-dealkylation and conjugation. The metabolites of butorphanol do not exhibit any analgesic activity. These metabolites and the parent compound are mainly excreted into the urine (only 5% is excreted unchanged), but 11-14% of a dose is excreted into the bile and eliminated with the feces.

Following IV doses in adult horses, the onset of action is approximately 3 minutes with a peak analgesic effect at 15-30 minutes. The duration of action in horses may be up to 4 hours after a single dose. After single 0.1 mg/kg IV doses, volume of distribution is approximately 1.4 L/kg, clearance approximately 12 mL/min/kg, and elimination half-life of 6 hours. In plasma, concentrations below the level of detection (0.1 ng/mL) occurred in 48 hours. In urine (as the conjugate), 7/10 horses had butorphanol urine levels below the level of detection (0.05 ng/mL) at 120 hours post dose (Knych et al. 2013). Bioavailability after IM injections in adult horses is relatively low (approx. 37%) (Sellon et al. 2009). In neonatal foals, IM bioavailability is approximately 67%, and peak levels occurred about 6 minutes after dosing. Terminal half-life was about 2 hours after an IV dose (Arguedas et al. 2008).

Contraindications/Precautions/Warnings

The drug is contraindicated in patients having known hypersensitivity to it. All opiates should be used with caution in patients with hypothyroidism, severe renal insufficiency, adrenocortical insufficiency (Addison's), and in geriatric or severely debilitated patients.

Like other opiates, butorphanol must be used with extreme caution in patients with head trauma, increased CSF pressure or other CNS dysfunction (*e.g.*, coma).

Dogs with MDR1 mutations ('white feet', many Collies, Australian shepherds, etc.) may develop a more pronounced sedation that persists longer than normal. The Washington State University Veterinary Clinical Pharmacology Lab recommends reducing the dose by 25% in dogs heterozygous for the MDR1 mutation and by 30-50% in dogs homozygous (mutant/mutant) for the mutation.

The manufacturer states that butorphanol "should not be used in dogs with a history of liver disease" and, because of its effects on suppressing cough, "it should not be used in conditions of the lower respiratory tract associated with copious mucous production." The drug should be used cautiously in dogs with heartworm disease, as safety for butorphanol has not been established in these cases.

Butorphanol may not be a very good analgesic and may cause respiratory depression in turtles or tortoises (Sladky et al. 2007).

As butorphanol injection is available in different concentrations, be certain which concentration is being used when drawing up dosages. Avoid ordering dosages in mLs only.

Adverse Effects

Adverse effects reported in dogs/cats include sedation, excitement, respiratory depression, ataxia, anorexia or diarrhea (rarely). Adverse effects may be less severe than those seen with pure agonists.

Adverse effects seen in horses (at usual doses) may include a transient ataxia and sedation, but excitement has been noted as well (see below). Although reported to have minimal effects on the GI, butorphanol has the potential to decrease intestinal motility and ileus is possible. Horses may exhibit increased heart rates and CNS excitement (e.g., tossing and jerking of head, increased ambulation, augmented avoidance response to auditory stimuli, etc.) particularly if given high doses (0.2 mg/kg) IV rapidly. Very high doses IV (1 – 2 mg/kg) may lead to the development of nystagmus, salivation, seizures, hyperthermia and decreased GI motility. It has been suggested that when used for analgesia, butorphanol administered as a continuous rate IV infusion can minimize adverse effects and maximize analgesia.

Reproductive/Nursing Safety

Although no controlled studies have been performed in domestic animals or humans, the drug has exhibited no evidence of teratogenicity or of causing impaired fertility in laboratory animals. The manufacturer, however, does not recommend its use in pregnant bitches, foals, weanlings (equine), and breeding horses. In humans, the FDA categorizes this drug as category C for use during pregnancy (*Animal studies have shown an adverse effect on the fetus, but there are no adequate studies in humans; or there are no animal reproduction studies and no adequate studies in humans.*) In a separate system evaluating the safety of drugs in canine and feline pregnancy (Papich, 1989), this drug is categorized as class: B (*Safe for use if used cautiously. Studies in laboratory animals may have uncovered some risk, but these drugs appear to be safe in dogs and cats; or these drugs are safe if they are not administered when the animal is near term.*)

Butorphanol can be distributed into milk, but not in amounts that would cause concern in nursing offspring.

Overdosage/Acute Toxicity

Acute life-threatening overdoses with butorphanol should be unlikely. The LD_{50} in dogs is reportedly 50 mg/kg. However, because butorphanol injection is available in different dosage strengths (0.5 mg/mL, 2 mg/mL and 10 mg/mL) for veterinary use, the possibility exists that inadvertent overdoses may occur in small animals. It has been suggested that animals exhibiting clinical signs of overdose (e.g., CNS effects, cardiovascular changes, and respiratory depression, etc.) be treated immediately with intravenous naloxone. Additional supportive measures (e.g., fluids, O_2, vasopressor agents, and mechanical ventilation) may be required. Should seizures occur and persist, diazepam may be used for control.

Drug Interactions

The following drug interactions have either been reported or are theoretical in humans or animals receiving butorphanol and may be of significance in veterinary patients. Unless otherwise noted, use together is not necessarily contraindicated, but weigh the potential risks and perform additional monitoring when appropriate.

- **OTHER CNS DEPRESSANTS** (*e.g.,* **anesthetic agents, antihistamines, phenothiazines, barbiturates, tranquilizers, alcohol,** etc.): May cause increased CNS or respiratory depression when used with butorphanol; dosage may need to be decreased.
- **ERYTHROMYCIN**: Could potentially decrease metabolism of butorphanol.
- **FENTANYL** (and other **pure opiate agonists**): Butorphanol may potentially antagonize some analgesic effects (**Note**: *this is controversial*), but may also reverse some of the sedative and respiratory depressant effects of pure agonists.
- **PANCURONIUM** If used with butorphanol may cause increased conjunctival changes.
- **THEOPHYLLINE**: Could potentially decrease metabolism of butorphanol.

Doses

Note: All doses are expressed in mg/kg of the <u>base</u> activity. If using the human product (*Stadol®*), 1 mg of tartrate salt = 0.68 mg base.

- **DOGS:**

  As an antitussive (labeled dosage; FDA-approved indication):

  <u>Injection</u>: 0.055 mg/kg SC q6-12h; may be increased to 0.11 mg/kg SC q6-12h. Treatment should not normally be required for longer than 7 days.

  <u>Oral</u>: 0.55 mg/kg PO q6-12h; may increase dose to 1.1 mg/kg PO q6-12h (These oral doses correspond to one 5 mg tablet per 20 lbs. and 10 lbs. of body weight, respectively); treatment should not normally be required for longer than 7 days. (Adapted from Package Insert; *Torbutrol®*)

  As an analgesic (all are extra-label):

  a) 0.1 – 0.5 mg/kg IV, IM, SQ. Commonly 0.2 mg/kg is chosen. Butorphanol provides only mild to moderate analgesia (good visceral analgesia); duration of sedative action 2-4 hours, but analgesic action may be less than one hour.

  b) **As a constant rate infusion** (CRI): 0.1 – 0.4 mg/kg/hr, following a loading dose of 0.2 mg/kg IV.

  c) **As an epidural analgesic:** 0.25 mg/kg diluted with preservative-free saline (0.2 mL) or local anesthetic epidurally. Onset of action less than 30 minutes and duration is 2-4 hours. Has predominantly supraspinal effects. (Valverde 2008)

  In combination as an anesthetic adjunct/immobilizing agent (all are extra-label): **Note**: There are many potential combinations that have been suggested; the following are examples and not inclusive. For additional information refer to other anesthesia-specific references such as *Handbook of Veterinary Anesthesia*, 5th Ed., Muir & Hubbell, Elsevier 2012; *Essentials of Small Animal Anesthesia & Analgesi*a, Grimm et al, Wiley-Blackwell 2011 or the website Veterinary Anesthesia & Analgesia Support Group (vasg.org).

  a) **For difficult dogs and short procedures** (*e.g.,* nail trims, X-rays, etc.): butorphanol 0.2 mg/kg; medetomidine 0.001 – 0.01 mg/kg; midazolam 0.05 – 0.2 mg/kg. All given IM.

  b) **For dogs requiring more sedation:** butorphanol 0.2 mg/kg; medetomidine 0.01 – 0.02 mg/kg; midazolam 0.05 – 0.2 mg/kg; all are given IM. Consider adding tiletamine/zolazepam (*Telazol®*) 1 - 2 mg/kg if insufficient sedation from above. For painful procedures consider adding buprenorphine at 0.02 – 0.04 mg/kg or substituting butorphanol or buprenorphine with either morphine 0.5 – 1 mg/kg or hydromorphone 0.1 – 0.2 mg/kg. More information is available from vasg.org. (Moffat 2008)

  c) Butorphanol (0.4 mg/kg) with acepromazine

(20 micrograms/kg) mixed in same syringe and given IM. Study was done in dogs undergoing OHE. Approx. 30 minutes post-dose, propofol IV used as induction agent and isoflurane used for maintenance anesthesia. Meloxicam used for rescue analgesia if needed post-op. Authors concluded that ace/butorphanol or ace/meperidine (pethidine), produced satisfactory sedation, decreased the amount of anesthetic necessary to induce and maintain anesthesia, and produced similar postoperative analgesia in dogs. (Vettorato et al. 2011)

As reversal agent for the sedative and respiratory depressant effects of *mu***-agonist opiates** (extra-label): 0.05 – 0.1 mg/kg IV; the benefit of using butorphanol over naloxone is that it does not completely reverse analgesic effects. (Quandt 2009)

As an anti-emetic prior to cisplatin treatment (extra-label): 0.4 mg/kg IM 1/2 hour prior to cisplatin infusion; can be repeated in 4-6 hours. (Klausner et al. 1988)

■ **CATS:**

As an analgesic:

a) Labeled dosage (FDA-approved): 0.4 mg/kg SC. The dose may be repeated up to 4 times per day for up to 2 days. (Adapted from label; *Torbugesic SA®*)

The following are extra-label dosages:

b) 0.1 – 0.5 mg/kg IV, IM, SQ; provides only mild to moderate analgesia (good visceral analgesia); duration of sedative action 2-4 hours, but analgesic action may be 1 hour or less. (Perkowski 2006)

c) **As a postoperative CRI** (usually in combination with ketamine) for mild to moderate pain: Loading dose of 0.1 – 0.2 mg/kg IV, then a CRI of 0.1 – 0.2 mg/kg/hr; Ketamine is used at a loading dose of 0.1 mg/kg IV with a CRI of 0.4 mg/kg/hr. When used with an opioid CRI may allow reduction in dosage of both. (Lichtenberger 2006b)

d) **As an epidural analgesic:** 0.25 mg/kg diluted with preservative-free saline (0.2 mL) or local anesthetic epidurally. Onset of action less than 30 minutes and duration is 2-4 hours. Has predominantly supraspinal effects. (Valverde 2008)

In combination as a preop or immobilizing agent (all are extra-label): **Note:** There are many potential combinations that have been suggested; the following are examples and not inclusive. For additional information refer to other anesthesia-specific references such as *Handbook of Veterinary Anesthesia*, 5th Ed., Muir & Hubbell, Elsevier 2012; *Essentials of Small Animal Anesthesia & Analgesi*a, Grimm et al, Wiley-Blackwell 2011 or the website Veterinary Anesthesia & Analgesia Support Group (vasg.org).

a) **Combining butorphanol, ketamine, midazolam and medetomidine:** In the study (assessing analgesia after OHE), one of the protocols used was: Ten minutes prior to surgery, Ketamine 60 mg/m² (~3 mg/kg), midazolam 3 mg/m² (~0.2 mg/kg), medetomidine 600 micrograms/m2 (~30 micrograms/kg), and butorphanol 6 mg/m² (~0.4 micrograms/kg) combined and given as a single IM injection in quadriceps muscles. Additionally, either 4 mg/kg carprofen (4 mg/kg) or meloxicam (0.3 mg/kg) were given subcutaneously. All protocols in the study provided adequate analgesia. (Polson et al. 2012)

b) **Combining butorphanol and dexmedetomidine:** In the study comparing dexmedetomidine alone (20 micrograms/kg IM), or <u>dexmedetomidine (10 micrograms/kg) with</u> either <u>butorphanol (0.4 mg/kg)</u> or meperidine (pethidine; 2.5 mg/kg) combined in same syringe and given IM, the results were similar

for quality of sedation, analgesia, muscle relaxation and possibility of performing some clinical procedures; all were deemed suitable. (Nagore et al. 2013)

c) **Combining butorphanol and midazolam with ketamine or dexmedetomidine:** In a small (N=6) healthy cat crossover study, the combination of butorphanol (0.4 mg/kg), midazolam (0.4 mg/kg) and ketamine (3 mg/kg) combined and given IM, the authors concluded that it provided acceptable sedation and minimal cardiovascular changes. Substituting dexmedetomidine (5 micrograms/kg) for the ketamine produced excellent sedation/recovery, but caused more cardiovascular depression and hematologic changes. (Biermann et al. 2012)

d) **Combining butorphanol and alfaxalone (SC dosing): For sedation for short procedures:** Study was done in hyperthyroid cats. Alfaxalone at 3 mg/kg and butorphanol 0.2 mg/kg drawn up in the same syringe and administered as a single subcutaneous injection in the region dorsal to the right hip. 45 minutes post injection maximum sedation occurs. Blood pressure, heart rate and respiration rate all were significantly decreased. Monitoring BP is recommended. Further studies are required to determine whether the sedative, respiratory and cardiovascular effects are similar in euthyroid cats. (Ramoo et al. 2013)

e) **Combining butorphanol, dexmedetomidine, and ketamine:** The study evaluated efficacy and cardiorespiratory effects of a combination of dexmedetomidine (25 micrograms/kg), ketamine (3 mg/kg) and either butorphanol (0.2 mg/kg), hydromorphone (0.05 mg/kg) or buprenorphine (30 micrograms/kg) as a single IM injection, (with or without reversal by atipamezole) in cats undergoing castration. Cats also received meloxicam (0.2 mg/kg SC) immediately prior to the conclusion of surgery. Supplemental isoflurane used when anesthesia was considered inadequate during surgery. Authors concluded that combinations including butorphanol or hydromorphone were suitable injectable anesthetic protocols for castration in cats commencing at 10 minutes after injection. Atipamezole shortened recovery times. (Ko et al. 2011)

As reversal agent for the sedative and respiratory depressant effects of *mu***-agonist opiates** (extra-label): 0.05 – 0.1 mg/kg IV; the benefit of using butorphanol over naloxone is that it does not completely reverse analgesic effects. (Quandt 2009)

■ **FERRETS:**

As an analgesic (extra-label): Because butorphanol appears to have shorter duration of action, buprenorphine is more commonly recommended for use as an analgesic in ferrets, but a butorphanol CRI of 0.1 – 0.2 mg/kg can be useful. Recommended analgesic dosages generally range from 0.1 – 0.4 mg/kg IM, IV, or SC q2-6h.

As an anesthetic adjunct (extra-label):

a) Butorphanol 0.1 mg/kg, ketamine 5 mg/kg, medetomidine 80 micrograms/kg. Combine in one syringe and give IM. May need to supplement with isoflurane (0.5-1.5%) for abdominal surgery. (Finkler 1999)

b) Xylazine (2 mg/kg) plus butorphanol (0.2 mg/kg) IM; Telazol (1.5 mg/kg) plus xylazine (1.5 mg/kg) plus butorphanol (0.2 mg/kg) IM; may reverse xylazine with yohimbine (0.05 mg/kg IM). (Williams 2000)

■ **RABBITS/RODENTS/SMALL MAMMALS:**

As an analgesic (extra-label):

a) **Rabbits:** Dosage recommendations generally range from 0.1 – 0.5 mg/kg SC, IM or IV q2-4 hours. An IV CRI dosage of 0.1 – 0.2 mg/kg/hr has also been recommended. (Lichtenberger 2006a)

b) **Rodents, Guinea pigs:** 1 – 2 mg/kg SC q4h. **Chinchillas:** 0.2 – 2 mg/kg SC q2-4h. (Miller et al. 2011)

- **BIRDS:**

As an analgesic (extra-label): 1 – 4 mg/kg IM has been suggested in birds but dosing frequencies range from q2-24 hours. Limited pharmacokinetic studies in birds suggests that frequent dosing may be necessary in birds raising issues of the practicality of using this drug. (Hawkins et al. 2011)

- **CATTLE:**

Note: FARAD recommends a 5-day meat withdrawal and 3-day milk withdrawal (Smith 2013).

As an analgesic (extra-label): When used alone in cattle, butorphanol has been recommended anecdotally at dosages such as 0.02 – 0.04 mg/kg IV or SC q4h.

To provide analgesia, sedation/restraint, and disassociation from a noxious procedure in combination as "ketamine stun" (extra-label): A combination of xylazine (0.02 to 0.05 mg/kg), ketamine (0.04 to 0.1 mg/kg) with butorphanol (0.01 – 0.04 mg/kg) IV or IM has been recommended. See the ketamine monograph for further details.

- **HORSES:** (NOTE: ARCI UFGFS CLASS 3 DRUG)

As an analgesic:

a) Labeled dosage; FDA-approved): 0.1 mg/kg IV q3-4h; not to exceed 48 hours. (Package Insert; *Torbugesic®*—Fort Dodge)

The following are extra-label:

b) As a continuous rate IV infusion (CRI; extra-label): There is evidence that giving butorphanol via a CRI may provide better analgesia and reduce the potential for adverse effects. One study (Sellon et al. 2004) that administered butorphanol at 13 micrograms/kg/hr as a CRI (begun at the time surgery ended and continued for 24 hours, along with flunixin at 1.1 mg/kg IV q12h) in horses following celiotomy, showed that butorphanol treated horses had delayed passage of feces following surgery, but pain scores were significantly decreased, less weight was lost, and had improved recovery scores. Treated horses were discharged on average, 3 days sooner than those treated with flunixin alone; cost savings were considerable.

c) Foals: Most recommend dosages of around 0.1 mg/kg IV or IM. One study in pony foals (both neonatal and older) (McGowan et al. 2013), found that 0.1 mg/kg IV, but not 0.05 mg/kg significantly raised thermal nociceptive threshold. However, a pharmacokinetic study done in neonatal foals found that dosages of 0.05 mg/kg IV significantly changed behaviors (increased nursing, sedation). Because elimination half-life in foals is longer than in adults, consider giving repeat dosages q4-6h when needed.

As a sedative/analgesic in combination with other agents (extra-label): Several protocols have been described using butorphanol in conjunction with an alpha agonist (*e.g.*, xylazine, romifidine, detomidine, etc.); often butorphanol is used at a lower dosage than labeled (such as 0.02 – 0.05 mg/kg). One such protocol for field anesthesia follows: Sedate with xylazine (1 mg/kg IV; 2 mg/kg IM) given 5-10 minutes (longer for IM route) before induction of anesthesia with ketamine (2 mg/kg IV). Horse must be adequately sedated (head to the knees) before giving the ketamine (ketamine can cause muscle rigidity and seizures). If adequate sedation does not occur, either 1) Redose xylazine: up to half the original dose, 2) Add butorphanol

(0.02 – 0.04 mg/kg IV). Butorphanol can be given with the original xylazine if you suspect that the horse will be difficult to tranquilize (*e.g.*, high-strung Thoroughbreds, etc.) or added before the ketamine. This combination will improve induction, increase analgesia and increase recumbency time by about 5-10 minutes. 3) Diazepam (0.03 mg/kg IV). Mix the diazepam with the ketamine. This combination will improve induction when sedation is marginal, improve muscle relaxation during anesthesia and prolong anesthesia by about 5-10 minutes. 4) Guaifenesin (5% solution administered IV to effect) can also be used to increase sedation and muscle relaxation. (Mathews 1999)

- **CAMELIDS (LLAMAS AND ALPACAS):**

As an analgesic/sedative (extra-label): Most dosage recommendations fall into the 0.05 – 0.1 mg/kg range either IM or IV and administered every 4-6 hours. In combination, with other sedative/anesthetics several dosing protocols have been suggested, including:

a) **As an anesthetic:** butorphanol 0.07 – 0.1 mg/kg; ketamine 0.2 – 0.3 mg/kg; xylazine 0.2 – 0.3 mg/kg IV or butorphanol 0.05 – 0.1 mg/kg; ketamine 0.2 – 0.5 mg/kg; xylazine 0.2 – 0.5 mg/kg IM. (Wolff 2009)

b) **For procedural pain** (*e.g.*, castrations, etc.) when recumbency (up to 30 minutes) is desired: Alpacas: butorphanol 0.046 mg/kg; xylazine 0.46 mg/kg; ketamine 4.6 mg/kg. Llamas: butorphanol 0.037 mg/kg; xylazine 0.37 mg/kg; ketamine 3.7 mg/kg. All drugs are combined in one syringe and given IM. May administer 50% of original dose of ketamine and xylazine during anesthesia to prolong effect up to 15 minutes. If doing mass castrations on 3 or more animals, can make up bottle of the "cocktail". Add 10 mg (1 mL) of butorphanol and 100 mg (1 mL) xylazine to a 1 gram (10 ml vial) of ketamine. This mixture is dosed at 1 mL/40 lbs. (18 kg) for alpacas, and 1 mL per 50 lbs. (22 kg) for llamas. Handle quietly and allow plenty of time before starting procedure. Expect 20 minutes of surgical time; patient should stand 45 minutes to 1 hour after injection. (Miesner 2009)

- **ZOO, EXOTIC, WILDLIFE SPECIES:**

For use of butorphanol in zoo, exotic and wildlife medicine refer to specific references, including:

a) *Zoo Animal and Wildlife Immobilization and Anesthesia.* West, G., Heard, D., Caulkett, N. (eds.). Blackwell Publishing, 2007.

b) *Handbook of Wildlife Chemical Immobilization, 3rd Ed.* Kreeger, T.J. and J.M. Arnemo. 2007.

c) *Fowler's Zoo and Wild Animal Medicine Current Therapy, Volume 7,* Miller, R.E., Fowler, M.E., Saunders. 2011.

d) *Exotic Animal Formulary, 4th Ed.* Carpenter, J.W., Saunders. 2012.

e) The 2009 American Association of Zoo Veterinarian Proceedings by D. K. Fontenot also has several dosages listed for restraint, anesthesia, and analgesia for a variety of drugs for carnivores and primates. VIN members can access them at: http://goo.gl/NNIWQ or http://goo.gl/9UJse

Monitoring

- Analgesic and/or antitussive efficacy.
- Respiratory rate/depth.
- Appetite and bowel function.
- CNS effects.

Client Information

- Clients should report any significant changes in behavior, appetite, bowel or urinary function in their animals.

Chemistry/Synonyms

A synthetic opiate partial agonist, butorphanol tartrate is related structurally to morphine but exhibits pharmacologic actions similar to other partial agonists such as pentazocine or nalbuphine. The compound occurs as a white, crystalline powder that is sparingly soluble in water and insoluble in alcohol. It has a bitter taste and a pK_a of 8.6. The commercial injection has a pH of 3-5.5. One mg of the tartrate is equivalent to 0.68 mg of butorphanol base.

Butorphanol tartrate may also be known as: levo-BC-2627 (butorphanol), *Dolorex®*, *Equanol®*, *Stadol®*, *Torbutrol®*, *Torbugesic®*, and *Verstadol®*.

Storage/Stability

The injectable product should be stored out of bright light and at room temperature; avoid freezing.

Compatibility/Compounding Considerations

The injectable product is reported to be **compatible** with the following drugs mixed into the same syringe: acepromazine, atropine sulfate, chlorpromazine, diphenhydramine HCl, fentanyl citrate, hydroxyzine HCl, meperidine, metoclopramide, midazolam, morphine sulfate, pentazocine lactate, perphenazine, prochlorperazine, promethazine HCl, and scopolamine HBr, and xylazine. Although studies confirming compatibility were not located, it is reportedly also compatible with alfaxalone, detomidine, dexmedetomidine, ketamine, medetomidine, and xylazine.

The drug is reportedly **incompatible** with the following agents: dimenhydrinate, and pentobarbital sodium. It is unlikely to be compatible with diazepam.

Dosage Forms/Regulatory Status

Note: Butorphanol is a class IV controlled substance. The veterinary products (*Torbutrol®*, *Torbugesic®*) strengths are listed as base activity. The human product (*Stadol®*) strength is labeled as the tartrate salt.

VETERINARY-LABELED PRODUCTS:

Butorphanol Tartrate Injection: 0.5 mg/mL (activity as base) in 10 mL vials; *Torbutrol®-IV*; (Rx, C-IV). FDA-approved for use in dogs. NADA 102-990.

Butorphanol Tartrate Injection: 2 mg/mL (activity as base) in 10 mL vials. *Torbugesic-SA®*; (Rx, C-IV). FDA-approved for use in cats. NADA 141-047.

Butorphanol Tartrate Injection: 10 mg/mL (activity as base) in 10 mL, 50 mL vials; *Torbugesic®*, *Dolorex®*, *Butorphic®*, generic; (Rx, C-IV). FDA-approved for use in horses not intended for food.

Butorphanol Tartrate Tablets: 1 mg, 5 mg, and 10 mg (activity as base) tablets; bottles of 100; *Torbutrol®*; (Rx, C-IV). FDA-approved for use in dogs. NADA 103-390.

The ARCI (Racing Commissioners International) has designated this drug as a class 3 substance. See the appendix for more information.

HUMAN-LABELED PRODUCTS:

Butorphanol Tartrate Injection: 1 mg/mL (as tartrate salt; equivalent to 0.68 mg base) in 1 mL & 2 mL vials; 2 mg/mL (as tartrate salt) in 1 mL, 2 mL & 10 mL vials; generic; (Rx, C-IV)

Butorphanol Nasal Spray: 10 mg/mL in 2.5 mL metered dose; generic; (Rx, C-IV)

Revisions/References

Monograph revised/updated September 2013.

Arguedas, M. G., et al. (2008). Pharmacokinetics of Butorphanol and Evaluation of Physiologic and Behavioral Effects after Intravenous and Intramuscular Administration to Neonatal Foals. *Journal of Veterinary Internal Medicine* 22(6): 1417-26.

Biermann, K., et al. (2012). Sedative, cardiovascular, haematologic and biochemical effects of four different drug combinations administered intramuscularly in cats. *Veterinary Anaesthesia and Analgesia* 39(2): 137-50.

Finkler, M. (1999). *Anesthesia in Ferrets.* Proceedings: Central Veterinary Conference, Kansas City. accessed via Veterinary Information Network; vin.com

Hawkins, M. G. & J. Paul-Murphy (2011). Avian Analgesia. *Vet Clin Exot Anim* 14: 61-80.

Hellyer, P. (2006). *Pain assessment and multimodal analgesic therapy in dogs and cats.* Proceedings: ABVP. accessed via Veterinary Information Network; vin.com

Klausner, J. S. & F. W. Bell (1988). Personal Communication.

Knych, H. K., et al. (2013). Pharmacokinetics and pharmacodynamics of butorphanol following intravenous administration to the horse. *J. Vet. Pharmacol. Ther.* 36(1): 21-30.

Ko, J. C., et al. (2011). Evaluation of dexmedetomidine and ketamine in combination with various opioids as injectable anesthetic combinations for castration in cats. *Javma-Journal of the American Veterinary Medical Association* 239(11): 1453-62.

Lichtenberger, M. (2006a). *Anesthesia Protocols and Pain Management for Exotic Animal Patients.* Proceedings: Western Vet Conf. accessed via Veterinary Information Network; vin.com

Lichtenberger, M. (2006b). *Pain management protocols for the ICU patient.* Proceedings: Western Vet Conf. accessed via Veterinary Information Network; vin.com

Mathews, N. (1999). *Anesthesia in large animals— Injectable (field) anesthesia: How to make it better.* Proceedings: Central Veterinary Conference, Kansas City. accessed via Veterinary Information Network; vin.com

McGowan, K. T., et al. (2013). Effect of butorphanol on thermal nociceptive threshold in healthy pony foals. *Equine Veterinary Journal* 45(4): 503-6.

Miesner, M. (2009). *Field anesthesia techniques in camelids.* Proceedings: WVC. accessed via Veterinary Information Network; vin.com

Miller, A. L. & C. Richardson (2011). Rodent Analgesia. *Vet Clin Exot Anim* 14: 81-92.

Moffat, K. (2008). Addressing canine and feline aggression in the veterinary clinic. *Vet Clin NA: Sm Anim Pract* 38: 983-1003.

Nagore, L., et al. (2013). Sedative effects of dexmedetomidine, dexmedetomidine/pethidine and dexmedetomidine/butorphanol in cats. *J. Vet. Pharmacol. Ther.* 36(3): 222-8.

Perkowski, S. (2006). *Practicing pain management in the acute setting.* Proceedings: ACVIM. accessed via Veterinary Information Network; vin.com

Polson, S., et al. (2012). Analgesia after feline ovariohysterectomy under midazolam-medetomidine-ketamine anaesthesia with buprenorphine or butorphanol, and carprofen or meloxicam: a prospective, randomised clinical trial. *Journal of Feline Medicine and Surgery* 14(8): 553-9.

Quandt, J. (2009). *Sedation and analgesia for the critically ill patient: Comprehensive review.* Proceedings; ACVIM. accessed via Veterinary Information Network; vin.com

Ramoo, S., et al. (2013). Sedation of hyperthyroid cats with subcutaneous administration of a combination of alfaxalone and butorphanol. *Australian Veterinary Journal* 91(4): 131-6.

Sellon, D. C., et al. (2009). Pharmacokinetics of butorphanol in horses after intramuscular injection. *J. Vet. Pharmacol. Ther.* 32(1): 62-5.

Sellon, D. C., et al. (2004). Effects of continuous rate intravenous infusion of butorphanol on physiologic and outcome variables in horses after celiotomy. *Journal of Veterinary Internal Medicine* 18(4): 555-63.

Sladky, K. K., et al. (2007). Analgesic efficacy and respiratory effects of butorphanol and morphine in turtles. *Javma-Journal of the American Veterinary Medical Association* 230(9): 1356-62.

Smith, G. (2013). Extralabel Use of Anesthetic and Analgesic Compounds in Cattle. *Veterinary Clinics of North America-Food Animal Practice* 29(1): 29-+.

Valverde, A. (2008). Epidural analgesia and anesthesia in dogs and cats. *Vet Clin NA: Sm Anim Pract* 38: 1205-30.

Vettorato, E. & S. Bacco (2011). A comparison of the sedative and analgesic properties of pethidine (meperidine) and butorphanol in dogs. *Journal of Small Animal Practice* 52(8): 426-32.

Williams, B. (2000). Therapeutics in Ferrets. *Vet Clin NA: Exotic Anim Pract* 3:1(Jan): 131-53.

Wolff, P. (2009). *Camelid Medicine.* Proceedings: AAZV. accessed via Veterinary Information Network; vin.com

N-Butylscopolammonium Bromide –
See the monograph found in the "N's" before neomycin

Cabergoline

(ka-**ber**-go-leen)   Dostinex®, Galastop®

Prolactin Inhibitor/Dopamine (D2) Agonist

Prescriber Highlights

▶ Ergot derivative used for reducing prolactin levels in bitches and queens. Indications include: inducing/synchronizing estrus, inducing abortion, treating pseudopregnancy, mastitis, and pre-surgery for mammary tumors.

▶ Appears to be well tolerated in dogs & cats; vomiting has been infrequently reported, but adverse effects are much less than with bromocriptine. Can change coat color and texture.

▶ Potentially very expensive particularly in large dogs, but generic tablets now available. Can be difficult to dose small dogs; usually must be compounded for accurate dosing.

Uses/Indications

For dogs and cats, cabergoline may be useful for inducing estrus, treatment of primary or secondary anestrus, mastitis, pseudopregnancy, as a treatment prior to mammary tumor surgery, and pregnancy termination in the second half of pregnancy. Cabergoline may be useful in treating some cases of pituitary-dependent hyperadrenocorticism (Cushing's).

Preliminary work has been done in psittacines (primarily Cockatiels) for adjunctive treatment of reproductive-related disorders, particularly persistent egg laying.

In humans, cabergoline is indicated for the treatment of disorders associated with hyperprolactenemia or the treatment of Parkinson's disease.

Pharmacology/Actions

Cabergoline has a high affinity for dopamine$_2$ (D$_2$) receptors and a long duration of action. It exerts a direct inhibitory effect on the secretion of prolactin from the pituitary. Its effect in inducing estrus is probably due more to its dopamine agonist effects than its effects on prolactin. When compared to bromocriptine it has greater D$_2$ specificity, a longer duration of action, and fewer tendencies to cause vomiting.

Pharmacokinetics

The pharmacokinetics of cabergoline have apparently not been reported for dogs or cats. In humans, the drug is absorbed after oral dosing but its absolute bioavailability is not known. Food does not appear to significantly alter absorption. The drug is only moderately bound to plasma proteins (50%). Cabergoline is extensively metabolized in the liver via hydrolysis; these metabolites and about 4% of unchanged drug are excreted into the urine. Half-life is estimated to be around 60 hours. Duration of pharmacologic action may persist for 48 hours or more. Renal dysfunction does not appear to significantly alter elimination characteristics of the drug.

Contraindications/Precautions/Warnings

Cabergoline is contraindicated in dogs and cats that are pregnant unless abortion is desired (see indications). Cabergoline should not be used in patients that are hypersensitive to ergot derivatives. Patients that do not tolerate bromocriptine may or may not tolerate cabergoline. In humans, cabergoline is contraindicated in patients that have uncontrolled hypertension.

Patients with significantly impaired liver function should receive the drug with caution, and if required, possibly at a lower dosage.

When using to induce estrus, it is recommended to wait at least 4 months after the prior cycle to allow the uterus to recover.

Adverse Effects

Cabergoline is usually well tolerated by animal patients. Vomiting has been reported, but may be alleviated by administering with food. Dogs receiving cabergoline for more than 14 days may exhibit changes in coat color or texture. This is likely reversible.

Human patients have reported postural hypotension, dizziness, headache, nausea and vomiting while receiving cabergoline.

Reproductive/Nursing Safety

This drug can cause spontaneous abortion in pregnant dogs or cats. In pregnant humans, cabergoline is designated by the FDA as a category **B** drug (*Animal studies have not demonstrated risk to the fetus, but there are no adequate studies in pregnant women; or animal studies have shown an adverse effect, but adequate studies in pregnant women have not demonstrated a risk to the fetus during the first trimester of pregnancy, and there is no evidence of risk in later trimesters.*)

Because cabergoline suppresses prolactin, it should not be used in nursing mothers.

Overdosage/Acute Toxicity

Overdose information is not available for dogs or cats, and remains very limited for humans. It is postulated that cabergoline overdoses in people could cause hypotension, nasal congestion, syncope or hallucinations. Treatment is basically supportive and primarily focuses on supporting blood pressure.

Drug Interactions

The following drug interactions have either been reported or are theoretical in humans or animals receiving cabergoline and may be of significance in veterinary patients. Unless otherwise noted, use together is not necessarily contraindicated, but weigh the potential risks and perform additional monitoring when appropriate.

■ **HYPOTENSIVE DRUGS**: Because cabergoline may have hypotensive effects, concomitant use with other hypotensive drugs may cause additive hypotension.

■ **METOCLOPRAMIDE**: Use with cabergoline may reduce the efficacy of both drugs and use together should be avoided.

■ **PHENOTHIAZINES** (*e.g.*, **acepromazine**, **chlorpromazine**, etc.): Use of cabergoline with dopamine (D$_2$) antagonists may reduce the efficacy of both drugs and should be avoided.

Laboratory Considerations

■ No particular laboratory interactions or considerations were located for this drug.

Doses

Because of the dosage differences in animals versus human patients and the strength of the commercially available product in the USA, a compounding pharmacist must usually reformulate this medication.

■ **DOGS:**

For estrus induction (extra-label):

a) Anecdotal: Most commonly recommended at 5 micrograms/kg PO once daily for 25-40 days until proestrus induced.

b) 0.6 micrograms/kg PO once daily. Make a 10 micrograms per mL solution by dissolving commercial tablets in warm distilled water (One 0.5 mg tablet (500 micrograms) per 50 mL of distilled water.) Give the appropriate dose for the patient within 15 minutes of preparation and discard the remaining solution. Continue until day 2 after the onset of the first signs of proestrus, or until day 42 without signs of proestrus. 81% (22 of 27) of dogs treated at this low dose showed proestrus between days 4 and 48. (Cirit et al. 2006)

For pseudocyesis (pseudopregnancy)/suppression of lactation (all are extra-label in USA):

a) Labeled Dose (U.K.): 5 micrograms/kg (if using *Galastop®* equivalent to 0.1 mL/kg) PO (either directly into the mouth or by mixing with food) once daily for 4-6 consecutive days depending on the severity of the clinical condition. For dogs weighing less than 5 kg measure the dosage in drops, 3 drops being equivalent to 0.1 mL. If signs do not resolve after a course of treatment, or if they recur, treatment may be repeated. (Adapted from label; *Galastop®*–Ceva U.K.)

b) Anecdotal dosages: Most recommend treating at 5 micrograms/kg PO once daily for 4-10 days.

For adjunctive treatment of pyometra (extra-label): Cabergoline at 5 micrograms/kg PO and cloprostenol at 1 microgram/kg SC once a day for 7 days with oral antibiotic therapy and supportive hydration. If no response to treatment cloprostenol (without cabergoline) with supportive treatment is continued for another 7 days. (Corrada, Rodriguez, Tortora, et al. 2006; Castillo et al. 2008; Jena et al. 2013)

For pregnancy termination (extra-label): Between days 35-45: Cabergoline 5 micrograms/kg PO once daily for 7 days in food and cloprostenol at 1 microgram/kg SC (after a tenfold dilution with physiologic saline) on days 1 and 3 given at least 8 hours after food. If pregnancy not terminated by day 8, continue cabergoline (at same dose) until day 12. (Corrada, Rodriguez and Tortora 2006)

For pituitary-dependent hyperadrenocorticism (Cushing's Disease) (extra-label): 0.07 mg/kg per week PO. Dose is divided by 3 (0.023 mg/kg; 23.3 micrograms/kg) and given every other day (q48h). 42.5% of treated dogs were considered responders, and 41% of cabergoline treated dogs were still alive 4 years later. (Castillo et al. 2008)

- **CATS:**

For pregnancy termination (extra-label): At 30 days post-coitus, cabergoline at 5 micrograms/kg PO q24h and cloprostenol 5 micrograms/kg SC q48h in 7-13 days was used to induce abortion. (Davidson 2004)

To reduce prolactin production in queens (extra-label): 5 micrograms/kg PO once daily. (Romagnoli 2009)

During the diestrus period to pre-treat mammary tumors prior to surgery (extra-label): 5 micrograms/kg PO 5-7 days before surgery. (Fontbonne 2007)

- **BIRDS:**

For persistent egg laying in psittacines combination with removal of males, altered light cycle (extra-label): Initially 10 – 20 micrograms/kg PO daily; higher dosages were also used. Further work needed to determine the dose rate, etc. (Chitty et al. 2006)

Monitoring
- Efficacy.
- Adverse effects.

Client Information
- Give with food to help prevent vomiting.
- Usually very well tolerated in dogs and cats.
- Pregnant and nursing women should be careful when handling this drug as it can cause serious birth defects and miscarriage.

Chemistry/Synonyms
Cabergoline, a synthetic, ergot-derivative, dopamine agonist similar to bromocriptine, occurs as a white powder that is insoluble in water, and soluble in ethanol or chloroform. The commercially available tablets also contain the inactive ingredients leucine and lactose.

Cabergoline may also be known as FCE-21336, cabergolina, *Cabasar®*, *Actualene®*, *Sostilar®*, *Dostinex®* or *Galastop®*.

Storage/Stability
The commercially available tablets should be stored at controlled room temperature (20°-25°C; 68°-77°F). The veterinary (Europe) oral liquid product *Galastop®* should be stored below 25°C and protected from light. Do not refrigerate. Once opened, it should be used within 28 days.

Compatibility/Compounding Considerations
It has been reported that the drug is unstable or degrades in aqueous suspensions and if compounded into a liquid that will not be used immediately, should be compounded into a lipid-based product. Preparing a fresh aqueous solution for immediate use should be stable (see estrus induction for dogs dose "c" above).

Dosage Forms/Regulatory Status
VETERINARY-LABELED PRODUCTS: None in USA.
Cabergoline is available in Europe as *Galastop®* 50 micrograms/mL oral liquid (miglyol base). An injectable product, *Galastop® Injectable* is available in some countries.

HUMAN-LABELED PRODUCTS:
Cabergoline Oral Tablets: 0.5 mg (500 micrograms); generic; (Rx)

Revisions/References
Monograph revised/updated September 2013.

Castillo, V. A., et al. (2008). Cushing's disease in dogs: Cabergoline treatment. *Research in Veterinary Science* 85(1): 26-34.
Chitty, J., et al. (2006). *Use of cabergoline in companion psittacine birds.* Proceedings: AAV. accessed via Veterinary Information Network; vin.com
Cirit, U., et al. (2006). The effects of low dose cabergoline on induction of estrus and pregnancy rates in anestrus bitches. *Anim Repro Sci* in press.
Corrada, Y., et al. (2006). A combination of oral cabergoline and double cloprostenol injections to produce third-quarter gestation termination in the bitch. *J Am Anim Hosp Assoc* 42(366-370).
Corrada, Y., et al. (2006). A combination of oral cabergoline and double cloprostenol injections to produce third-quarter gestation termination in the bitch. *J. Am. Anim. Hosp. Assoc.* 42(5): 366-70.
Davidson, A. (2004). *Update: Therapeutics for reproductive disorders in small animal practice.* Proceedings: ACVIM Forum. accessed via Veterinary Information Network; vin.com
Fontbonne, A. (2007). *Hormones and antibiotics in canine and feline reproduction.* Proceedings: WSAVA. accessed via Veterinary Information Network; vin.com
Jena, B., et al. (2013). Comparative efficacy of various therapeutic protocols in the treatment of pyometra in bitches. *Veterinarni Medicina* 58(5): 271-6.
Romagnoli, S. (2009). *An update on pseudopregnancy.* Proceedings: WSAVA. accessed via Veterinary Information Network; vin.com

Calcitonin Salmon

(kal-si-toe-nin sam-in)   Miacalcin®, Calcimar®

Osteoclast Inhibiting Hormone

Prescriber Highlights
▶ Hormone used primarily to control hypercalcemia in dogs and reptiles. Very short duration of action in dogs and can be expensive.
▶ Hypersensitivity possible. May cause GI effects.
▶ Young animals may be extremely sensitive to effects.
▶ Do not confuse with calcitriol.

Uses/Indications
In small animals, calcitonin has been used as adjunctive therapy to control hypercalcemia. It potentially may be of use in the adjunctive treatment of pain, particularly when originating from bone. Calcitonin's use in veterinary medicine has been limited by expense, availability, and development of resistance to its effects after several days of treatment.

Pharmacology/Actions
Calcitonin has a multitude of physiologic effects. It principally acts on bone inhibiting osteoclastic bone resorption. By reducing tubular reabsorption of calcium, phosphate, sodium, magnesium, potassium and chloride, it promotes their renal excretion. Calcitonin

also increases jejunal secretion of water, sodium, potassium and chloride (not calcium).

Pharmacokinetics

Calcitonin is destroyed in the gut after oral administration and therefore must be administered parenterally. In humans, the onset of effect after IV administration of calcitonin salmon is immediate. After IM or SC administration, onset occurs within 15 minutes with maximal effects occurring in about 4 hours. Duration of action is 6-12 hours after IM or SC injection. The drug is believed to be rapidly metabolized by the kidneys, and in blood and peripheral tissues.

Contraindications/Precautions/Warnings

Calcitonin is contraindicated in animals hypersensitive to it. Patients with a history of hypersensitivity to other proteins may be at risk. Young animals are reportedly up to 100 times more sensitive to calcitonin than are older animals (adults).

Do not confuse calcitriol with calcitonin. Consider writing orders and prescriptions using tall man letters; calciTONIN and calciTRIOL.

Adverse Effects

There is not a well-documented adverse effect profile for calcitonin in domestic animals. Anorexia and vomiting have been reported in dogs. Overmedicating can lead to hypocalcemia. The following effects are documented in humans and potentially could be seen in animals: diarrhea, anorexia, vomiting, swelling and pain at injection site, redness and peripheral paresthesias. Rarely, allergic reactions may occur. Tachyphylaxis (resistance to drug therapy with time) may occur in some dogs treated.

Reproductive/Nursing Safety

There is little information on the reproductive safety of calcitonin; however, it does not cross the placenta. Very high doses have decreased birth weights in laboratory animals, presumably due to the metabolic effects of the drug. In humans, the FDA categorizes this drug as category *C* for use during pregnancy (*Animal studies have shown an adverse effect on the fetus, but there are no adequate studies in humans; or there are no animal reproduction studies and no adequate studies in humans.*)

Calcitonin has been shown to inhibit lactation. Safe use during nursing has not been established.

Overdosage/Acute Toxicity

Very limited data is available. Nausea and vomiting have been reported after accidental overdose injections. Chronic overdosing can lead to hypocalcemia.

Drug Interactions

The following drug interactions have either been reported or are theoretical in humans or animals receiving calcitonin and may be of significance in veterinary patients. Unless otherwise noted, use together is not necessarily contraindicated, but weigh the potential risks and perform additional monitoring when appropriate.

- **PAMIDRONATE:** While pamidronate and calcitonin are used together in human medicine, this combination is not recommended in veterinary patients. When used together in dogs, studies do not show any benefit and outcomes can potentially worsen. (DeClementi et al. 2012)
- **VITAMIN D ANALOGS** or **CALCIUM** products: May interfere with the efficacy of calcitonin.

Doses

- **DOGS:**

  For hypervitaminosis D (toxicity)/hypercalcemia (extra-label): Calcitonin treatment is not routinely recommended due to expense, frequency of dosing and limited efficacy. In a re-cent review of management of hypercalcemia associated with cholecalciferol and vitamin D analogs (DeClementi et al. 2012), the authors stated that the following protocol using calcitonin could be used, but due to inconsistent results, some patients becoming refractory to treatment, and the potential for greater soft tissue mineralization, they prefer substituting pamidronate (1.3 – 2 mg/kg; diluted in normal saline and administered IV over a 2-hours) for calcitonin: **1)** Normal saline; twice maintenance; forced diuresis; maintain diuresis until calcium levels have dropped; **2)** Furosemide at 2.5 – 4.5 mg/kg PO three to four times a day or 0.5 mg/kg/hour via continuous IV infusion; **3)** Either dexamethasone at 1 mg/kg SQ or IV divided four times a day or prednisone at 2 – 3 mg/kg PO twice daily; Calcitonin at 4 – 6 Units/kg SC two to three times a day.

- **REPTILES:**

  For hypercalcemia: Green iguanas in combination with fluid therapy: 1.5 Units/kg SC q8h for several weeks if necessary. (Gauvin 1993)

  For nutritional secondary hyperparathyroidism (NSHP):

  a) If reptile is not hypocalcemic: 50 Units/kg IM once weekly for 2-3 doses. (Hernandez-Divers 2005)

  b) Correct husbandry problems and correct hypocalcemia with calcium and vitamin D. Once calcium level is normal and patient is on oral calcium supplementation (usually about 7 days after starting therapy) give calcitonin at 50 Units/kg IM weekly for 2-3 doses. Supportive care can be tapered off once patient becomes stable. (Johnson 2004)

Monitoring

- Serum ionized (if possible) calcium. Directly measured serum ionized calcium is a better indicator of calcium status than total calcium, but requires specific collection techniques and/or analyzers. Refer to your laboratory's guidelines or your analyzer's instructions. A more thorough discussion of this topic can be found at the following reference: (Schenck et al. 2008).
- Phosphorus, BUN/creatinine.
- Fluid status.

Chemistry/Synonyms

A polypeptide hormone, calcitonin is a 32-amino acid polypeptide having a molecular weight of about 3600. Calcitonin is available commercially as either calcitonin human or calcitonin salmon, both of which are synthetically prepared. Potency of calcitonin salmon is expressed in international units (IU), in this reference this is expressed as Units. Calcitonin salmon is approximately 50X more potent than calcitonin human on a per weight basis.

Calcitonin salmon may also be known as calcitonin-salmon, calcitoninum salmonis, salmon calcitonin, SCT-1, or *Calcimar®*; many other trade names are available internationally.

Storage/Stability

Calcitonin salmon for injection should be stored in the refrigerator (2-8°C). The nasal solution should be stored in the refrigerator but protected from freezing. Once in use it should be stored at room temperature in an upright position; use within 35 days.

Compatibility/Compounding Considerations

No specific information noted.

Dosage Forms/Regulatory Status

VETERINARY-LABELED PRODUCTS: NONE.

HUMAN-LABELED PRODUCTS:

Calcitonin Salmon for Injection: 200 IU/mL in 2 mL vials; *Miacalcin®*; (Rx)

Calcitonin Salmon Intranasal Spray: 200 Units/activation; *Miacalcin®*; *Fortical®*, generic; (Rx)

Revisions/References

Monograph revised/updated September 2013.

DeClementi, C. & B. R. Sobczak (2012). Common Rodenticide Toxicoses in Small Animals. *Veterinary Clinics of North America-Small Animal Practice* 42(2): 349-+.

Gauvin, J. (1993). Drug therapy in reptiles. *Seminars in Avian & Exotic Med* 2(1): 48-59.

Hernandez-Divers, S. (2005). *Reptile Non-Infectious Diseases.* Proceedings: WSAVA World Congress. accessed via Veterinary Information Network; vin.com

Johnson, D. (2004). *Metabolic bone disease in reptiles.* Proceedings: ACVC. accessed via Veterinary Information Network; vin.com

Schenck, P. A. & D. J. Chew (2008). Calcium: Total or ionized? *Veterinary Clinics of North America-Small Animal Practice* 38(3): 497-+.

Calcitriol

(kal-si-trye-ole)   Rocaltrol®, Calcijex®, Active Vitamin D3

Vitamin D Analog

Prescriber Highlights

▶ Vitamin D analog may be useful in dogs (& possibly cats) for treatment of hypocalcemia, chronic renal disease or idiopathic seborrhea.

▶ Contraindications: Hypercalcemia, hyperphosphatemia, malabsorption syndromes.

▶ Adverse Effects: Hypercalcemia, hypercalcuria or hyperphosphatemia greatest concerns.

▶ May need to have oral dosage forms compounded.

▶ Do not confuse with calcitonin.

Uses/Indications

Calcitriol can be useful when combined with oral calcium therapy for the long-term treatment of hypocalcemia associated with hypoparathyroidism. It may be potentially beneficial in the adjunctive treatment of chronic renal disease in dogs and cats but its use is somewhat controversial, particularly the decision on how soon in the course of chronic renal insufficiency it should be employed. Calcitriol may be a useful adjunctive drug for treating certain neoplasias (*e.g.*, mast cell tumors) as it may potentiate some chemotherapy agents (Malone et al. 2010). It reportedly can improve cats' appetite and general well being. It may also be of benefit in treating some types of dermatopathies (primary idiopathic seborrhea).

Pharmacology/Actions

Calcitriol is a vitamin D analog. Vitamin D is considered a hormone and, in conjunction with parathormone (PTH) and calcitonin, regulates calcium homeostasis in the body. Active analogues (or metabolites) of vitamin D enhance calcium absorption from the GI tract, promote reabsorption of calcium by the renal tubules, and increase the rate of accretion and resorption of minerals in bone. Calcitriol has a rapid onset of action (approximately 1 day) and a short duration of action. Unlike other forms of vitamin D, calcitriol does not require renal activation for it to be effective.

Pharmacokinetics

If fat absorption is normal, vitamin D analogs are readily absorbed from the GI tract (small intestine). Bile is required for adequate absorption and patients with steatorrhea, liver or biliary disease will have diminished absorption. Calcitriol has a rapid onset of biologic action and has a short duration of action (<1 day to 2-3 days). Dogs and cats appear to require much smaller doses of calcitriol than do humans.

Contraindications/Precautions/Warnings

Calcitriol is contraindicated in patients with hypercalcemia, vitamin D toxicity, malabsorption syndrome, or abnormal sensitivity to the effects of vitamin D. It should be used with extreme caution in patients with hyperphosphatemia (many clinicians believe hyperphosphatemia or a combined calcium/phosphorous product of >70 is a contraindication to the use of vitamin D analogs). Using calcitriol in patients with hyperphosphatemia can increase risks for tissue mineralization with additional renal tissue damage and dysfunction. Generally, calcium and phosphorus levels should be in the low normal range before beginning treatment.

As calcitriol can promote hypercalciuria, it should be used with caution in animals susceptible to calcium oxalate uroliths.

Do not confuse calcitriol with calcitonin. Consider writing orders and prescriptions using tall man letters; calciTONIN and calciTRIOL.

Adverse Effects

While hypercalcemia is a definite concern, calcitriol administered in low dosages to dogs with chronic renal disease infrequently causes hypercalcemia, unless it is used with a calcium-containing phosphorus binder, particularly calcium carbonate. Signs of hypercalcemia include polydipsia, polyuria and anorexia. Hyperphosphatemia may also occur and patients' serum phosphate levels should be normalized before therapy is begun. Monitoring of serum calcium levels is mandatory while using this drug.

Reproductive/Nursing Safety

Calcitriol has proven to be teratogenic in laboratory animal when given at doses several times higher than those used therapeutically. In humans, the FDA categorizes this drug as category C for use during pregnancy (*Animal studies have shown an adverse effect on the fetus, but there are no adequate studies in humans; or there are no animal reproduction studies and no adequate studies in humans.*)

Safe use during lactation has not been established.

Overdosage/Acute Toxicity

Overdosage can cause hypercalcemia, hypercalciuria, and hyperphosphatemia. Intake of excessive calcium and phosphate may also cause the same effect. Acute ingestions should be managed using established protocols for removal or prevention of the drug being absorbed from the GI. Orally administered mineral oil may reduce absorption and enhance fecal elimination.

There were 120 single agent exposures to calcitriol reported to the ASPCA Animal Poison Control Center (APCC) during 2009-2013. Of the 106 dogs, 65 were symptomatic with 62% vomiting, 52% hypercalcemic, 49% lethargic, 43% hyperphosphatemic, 34% diarrhea and 20% azotemic.

Hypercalcemia secondary to chronic dosing of the drug should be treated by first temporarily discontinuing (not dose reduction) calcitriol and exogenous calcium therapy. If the hypercalcemia is severe, pamidronate, furosemide, calcium-free IV fluids (*e.g.*, normal saline), urine acidification, and corticosteroids may be employed.

Drug Interactions

The following drug interactions have either been reported or are theoretical in humans or animals receiving calcitriol and may be of significance in veterinary patients. Unless otherwise noted, use together is not necessarily contraindicated, but weigh the potential risks and perform additional monitoring when appropriate.

■ **CALCIUM-CONTAINING PHOSPHORUS BINDING AGENTS** (*e.g.,* **calcium carbonate, calcium acetate,** etc.): Use with calcitriol may induce hypercalcemia.

■ **CORTICOSTEROIDS:** Can nullify the effects of vitamin D analogs.

■ **DIGOXIN** or **VERAPAMIL:** Patients on verapamil or digoxin are sensitive to the effects of hypercalcemia; intensified monitoring is required.

■ **PHENYTOIN, BARBITURATES** or **PRIMIDONE:** May induce hepatic enzyme systems and increase the metabolism of Vitamin D analogs thus decreasing their activity.

■ **THIAZIDE DIURETICS:** May cause hypercalcemia when given in conjunction with Vitamin D analogs.

Laboratory Considerations

- **SERUM CHOLESTEROL** levels may be falsely elevated by vitamin D analogs when using the Zlatkis-Zak reaction for determination.

Doses

- **DOGS:**

To suppress secondary hyperparathyroidism and slow progression of chronic kidney disease (extra-label):

a) There is strong evidence to support use in dogs with IRIS CKD Stages 3 & 4 (and possibly Stage 2). Recommended dose is initially 2 – 2.5 nanograms/kg PO once daily (q24h) preferably in the evening on an empty stomach. Ionized calcium and PTH must be monitored to adjust dosage. Goal is to minimize PTH and avoid hypercalcemia. Do not exceed 5 nanograms/kg per day. If hypercalcemia develops, may try giving double the daily dosage every other day to reduce GI calcium absorption. Life-long treatment is required. (Polzin 2013)

b) **1)** Confirm the diagnosis of chronic renal failure (serum creatinine >2 mg/dL); **2)** Reduce hyperphosphatemia to <6 mg/dL; **3)** If serum creatinine between 2 – 3 mg/dL and serum phosphorus <6 mg/dL, start calcitriol at 2.5 – 3.5 nanograms/kg/day PO (so-called "preventative" dose); if serum creatinine >3 mg/dL and serum phosphorus <6 mg/dL, obtain a baseline PTH level and start calcitriol at 3.5 nanograms/kg/day.

Monitoring of preventative dose: assess serum calcium on days 7 and 14 after starting calcitriol and then every 6 months. Serum creatinine should be measured every 1-3 months. If hypercalcemia occurs, stop calcitriol for one week to determine if the drug is causing the hypercalcemia or if it's due to another cause (*e.g.*, too little calcitriol).

Monitoring patients with elevated PTH: monitor as above, but also determine PTH levels at 4-6 weeks after starting calcitriol. If still elevated increase dose by 1 – 2 nanograms/kg/day, but do not exceed 6.6 nanograms/kg/day unless monitoring ionized calcium. If higher daily doses are required (5 – 7 nanograms/kg/day), a pulsed-dosing strategy may be considered. This is usually about 20 nanograms/kg given twice weekly PO at bedtime on an empty stomach. (Nagode 2005)

For hypocalcemia (extra-label): **For long-term maintenance in animals with hypoparathyroidism:** 0.03 – 0.06 micrograms/kg/day (30 – 60 nanograms/kg/day). Maximal effect is in 1-4 days. Combine with oral calcium to reduce vitamin D dose requirements. Adjust dose by monitoring serum calcium. (Crystal 2007)

For primary idiopathic seborrhea (especially in spaniel breeds) (extra-label): 10 nanograms/kg PO once daily. Give as far away from the main meal as possible. (Kwochka 1999)

- **CATS:**

To suppress secondary hyperparathyroidism in CRF: There is only weak evidence to support use in cats (Polzin 2013).

a) 1.5 – 3.5 nanograms/kg PO daily given separately from meals. Remove oil from capsule, dilute in corn oil, then give the appropriate volume. Store for up to 2 weeks. (Gunn-Moore 2008)

b) 2.5 – 3.5 nanograms/kg PO once daily. (Chew 2003)

c) See the dog dose in "b" above. (Nagode 2005)

For hypocalcemia (extra-label): **For long-term maintenance in animals with hypoparathyroidism:** 0.03 – 0.06 mcg/kg/day (30 – 60 nanograms/kg/day). Maximal effect is in 1-4 days. Combine with oral calcium to reduce vitamin D dose requirements. Adjust dose by monitoring serum calcium. (Crystal 2007)

Monitoring

- Serum ionized (if possible) calcium; baseline and at one week; then every 2-4 weeks thereafter. Directly measured serum ionized calcium is a better indicator of calcium status than total calcium, but requires specific collection techniques and/or analyzers. Refer to your laboratory's or analyzer's instructions. A more thorough discussion of this topic can be found at the following reference: (Schenck et al. 2008).
- Serum phosphate, creatinine. Baseline and at one week; then every 2-4 weeks thereafter.
- Serum PTH levels.
- Clinical efficacy (*e.g.*, improved appetite, activity level, slowed progression of disease, etc.).

Client Information

- Best given on an empty stomach, usually at bedtime.
- Watch for signs of too high blood calcium (*e.g.*, greater thirst and urination, reduced or lack of appetite, etc.) and too low blood calcium (*e.g.*, muscle tremors, twitching, stiffness, weakness, stiff gait, unsteadiness, behavioral changes, seizures, etc.). If any of these are seen, contact veterinarian immediately.
- Don't give calcium supplements or antacids (*e.g.*, *Tums*®, etc.) without veterinarian's approval.

Chemistry/Synonyms

Calcitriol, a vitamin D analog is synthesized for pharmaceutical use. It is a white crystalline compound and insoluble in water.

Calcitriol may also be known as: calcitrolo, calcitriolum, 1,25-dihydroxycholecalciferol, 1-alpha,25 dihydrocholecalciferol, 1alpha, 25-Dihydroxyvitamin D_3 or 1,25-DHCC, 1,25-dihidroxyvitamin D_3, Ro 21-5535, U 49562, or *Rocaltrol*®.

Storage/Stability

Protect from light. Store in tight, light resistant containers at room temperature. The injection does not contain preservatives and remaining drug should be discarded after opening ampule.

Compatibility/Compounding Considerations

No specific information noted.

Dosage Forms/Regulatory Status

VETERINARY-LABELED PRODUCTS: NONE.

HUMAN-LABELED PRODUCTS:

Note: Most doses are expressed in nanograms/kg (ng/kg); to convert micrograms to nanograms: 1 microgram = 1000 ng, 0.25 micrograms = 250 ng, etc. Reformulation by a compounding pharmacy is usually required to assure accurate dosing.

Calcitriol Oral Capsules: 0.25 micrograms & 0.5 micrograms; *Rocaltrol*®, generic; (Rx)

Calcitriol Oral Solution: 1 microgram/mL in 15 mL btls & single-use graduated oral dispensers; *Rocaltrol*®, generic; (Rx)

Calcitriol Injection: 1 microgram/mL in 1 mL amps & vials; generic; (Rx)

Topical calcitriol may also be available.

Revisions/References

Monograph revised/updated September 2013.

Chew, D. (2003). *Chronic Renal Failure Treatment Updates*. Proceedings: Western Veterinary Conf. accessed via Veterinary Information Network; vin.com

Crystal, M. (2007). Hypoparathyroidism. *Backwell's 5-Minute Veterinary Consult: Canine & Feline*. L. Tilley and F. Smith, Blackwell: 720-1.

Gunn-Moore, D. (2008). *The diagnosis and treatment of renal insufficiency in cats*. Proceedings: World Veterinary Congress. accessed via Veterinary Information Network; vin.com

Kwochka, K. (1999). *The Cutting Edge of Dermatologic Therapy.* North American Veterinary Conference, Orlando. accessed via Veterinary Information Network; vin.com

Malone, E. K., et al. (2010). Calcitriol (1,25-dihydroxycholecalciferol) enhances mast cell tumour chemotherapy and receptor tyrosine kinase inhibitor activity in vitro and has single-agent activity against spontaneously occurring canine mast cell tumours. *Veterinary and Comparative Oncology* 8(3): 209-20.

Nagode, L. (2005). "Medical FAQ's: Protocol for calcitriol use in CRF dogs and cats."

Polzin, D. J. (2013). Evidence-based step-wise approach to managing chronic kidney disease in dogs and cats. *J. Vet. Emerg. Crit. Care* 23(2): 205-15.

Schenck, P. A. & D. J. Chew (2008). Calcium: Total or ionized? *Veterinary Clinics of North America-Small Animal Practice* 38(3): 497-+.

Calcium Acetate

(kal-see-um ass-ah-tate)   PhosLo®

Oral Phosphate Binder

Prescriber Highlights

▶ Oral calcium salt used as a phosphorus binding agent in treating hyperphosphatemia associated with chronic renal failure.

▶ Must monitor serum phosphorus & calcium.

Uses/Indications

Calcium acetate can be used for oral administration to treat hyperphosphatemia in patients with chronic renal failure. Secondary to its phosphorus binding efficiency and lower concentration of elemental calcium, calcium acetate is considered the most effective and having the lowest potential for causing hypercalcemia of the calcium-based phosphorus-binding agents. When compared to calcium carbonate, calcium acetate binds approximately twice as much phosphorus per gram of elemental calcium administered. Unlike calcium citrate, calcium acetate does not promote aluminum absorption.

Pharmacology/Actions

When calcium acetate is given with meals it binds to dietary phosphorus and forms calcium phosphate, an insoluble compound that is eliminated in the feces. Calcium acetate is soluble over a range of pH and, therefore, available for binding phosphorus in the stomach and proximal small intestine.

Pharmacokinetics

No information was located on the pharmacokinetics of calcium acetate in dogs and cats. In humans, approximately 30% is absorbed when given with food.

Contraindications/Precautions/Warnings

This agent should not be used when hypercalcemia is present. Because hypercalcemia can result from administering oral calcium products to animals with renal failure, adequate monitoring of serum ionized calcium and phosphorus is required.

Use calcium containing phosphate binders with caution in patients having a serum calcium and phosphorus product greater than 60.

Using calcium-based phosphate binders and calcitriol together is controversial. Some authors state the combination is contraindicated, while others state that intensified monitoring for hypercalcemia is required.

Adverse Effects

Hypercalcemia and extraosseous (soft tissue) calcification are the primary concerns associated with calcium acetate; especially when using high dosages long-term; adequate monitoring is required.

In humans, GI intolerance (nausea) has been reported.

Reproductive/Nursing Safety

No reproductive safety studies were located and the human label states that it is not known whether the drug can cause fetal harm. However, it would be surprising if calcium acetate caused teratogenic effects. In humans, the FDA categorizes calcium acetate as category C for use during pregnancy (*Animal studies have shown an adverse effect on the fetus, but there are no adequate studies in humans; or there are no animal reproduction studies and no adequate studies in humans.*)

It would be expected that calcium acetate would be safe to administer during lactation.

Overdosage/Acute Toxicity

Potentially, acute overdoses could cause hypercalcemia. Patients should be monitored and treated symptomatically. If dosage was massive and recent, consider using standard protocols to empty the gut.

Drug Interactions

The following drug interactions have either been reported or are theoretical in humans or animals receiving calcium acetate and may be of significance in veterinary patients. Unless otherwise noted, use together is not necessarily contraindicated, but weigh the potential risks and perform additional monitoring when appropriate.

- **CALCITRIOL:** If administered with calcium acetate, may lead to hypercalcemia; if calcitriol is used concomitantly, intensified monitoring for hypercalcemia is mandatory.

- **DIGOXIN:** Calcium acetate is not recommended for use in human patients that are on digoxin therapy, as hypercalcemia may cause serious arrhythmias.

- **FLUOROQUINOLONES, TETRACYCLINES:** Oral calcium-containing products can reduce absorption of fluoroquinolones; if both calcium acetate and one of these antibiotics are required, separate dosages by at least two hours.

- **LEVOTHYROXINE:** Oral calcium products may reduce levothyroxine absorption if given at the same time. Separate dosages by at least two hours if possible.

Laboratory Considerations

- No specific concerns noted; see Monitoring.

Doses

- **DOGS/CATS:**

  For hyperphosphatemia associated with chronic renal failure, in conjunction with a low-phosphorus diet (extra-label): 60 – 90 mg/kg/day PO divided and given with food, mixed with food, or just prior to each meal. Dosed "to effect," meaning the dose is adjusted to assure that the serum phosphorus target is achieved. Therapy usually begins at the lower end of the recommended dose range and adjusted upward as needed every 4-6 weeks until the therapeutic target is reached. Monitor ionized calcium; hypercalcemia is possible. Decrease dose if serum calcium exceeds normal limits. (Polzin et al. 2005; Bartges 2012; Polzin 2013)

Monitoring

Initially at 10-14 day intervals; once "stable", then at 4-6 week intervals:

- Serum phosphorus (after a 12-hour fast).

- Serum ionized (if possible) calcium. Directly measured serum ionized calcium is a better indicator of calcium status than total calcium, but requires specific collection techniques and/or analyzers. Refer to your laboratory's guidelines or analyzer's instructions. A more thorough discussion of this topic can be found at the following reference: (Schenck et al. 2008).

Client Information

- Give with meals; either just before feeding or mixed into food. Veterinarian may prescribe additional doses to be administered between meals.

- Use of this medication will require ongoing laboratory monitoring.

Chemistry/Synonyms

Calcium acetate is a white, odorless, hygroscopic powder that is freely soluble in water and slightly soluble in alcohol. Each gram contains approximately 254 mg of elemental calcium.

Calcium acetate may also be known as: calcii acetas, acetato de calcio, kalcio acetates, kalciumacetat, or kalciumasetaatti, *PhosLo®*.

Storage/Stability

The commercially available tablets, capsules and gelcaps should be stored at room temperature (25°C); excursions are permitted to 15-30°C.

Compatibility/Compounding Considerations

No specific information noted.

Dosage Forms/Regulatory Status

VETERINARY-LABELED PRODUCTS: NONE.

HUMAN-LABELED PRODUCTS:

Calcium Acetate Oral Tablets: 667 mg (169 mg elemental calcium); *Calphron®*, *Eliphos®*; (Rx)

Calcium Acetate Oral Capsules & Gelcaps: 667 mg (169 mg elemental calcium); *PhosLo®*; (Rx)

Revisions/References

Monograph revised/updated September 2013.

Bartges, J. W. (2012). Chronic Kidney Disease in Dogs and Cats. *Veterinary Clinics of North America-Small Animal Practice* 42(4): 669-+.

Polzin, D., et al. (2005). Chronic Kidney Disease. *Textbook of Veterinary Internal Medicine: Diseases of the Dog and Cat 6th Ed.* S. Ettinger and E. Feldman, Elsevier: 1756-85.

Polzin, D. J. (2013). Evidence-based step-wise approach to managing chronic kidney disease in dogs and cats. *J. Vet. Emerg. Crit. Care* 23(2): 205-15.

Schenck, P. A. & D. J. Chew (2008). Calcium: Total or ionized? *Veterinary Clinics of North America-Small Animal Practice* 38(3): 497-+.

Calcium Carbonate

(kal-see-um kar-boe-nate)

Oral Phosphate Binder; Antacid

Prescriber Highlights

▶ Oral calcium salt used as a phosphorus binding agent for use in treating hyperphosphatemia associated with chronic renal failure and as a calcium supplement in animals with chronic hypocalcemia. It could also be used as an oral antacid, but is rarely recommended for this use in small animals.

▶ Must monitor serum phosphorus & calcium.

Uses/Indications

Calcium carbonate can be used for oral administration to treat hyperphosphatemia in patients with chronic renal failure and as a calcium supplement in animals with chronic hypocalcemia. Secondary to its phosphorus binding efficiency and lower concentration of elemental calcium, calcium acetate is considered the most effective and having the lowest potential for causing hypercalcemia of the calcium-based phosphorus-binding agents. Unlike calcium citrate, calcium carbonate does not promote aluminum absorption. It could also be used as an oral antacid, but is rarely recommended for this use in small animals.

Pharmacology/Actions

When calcium carbonate is given with meals it binds to dietary phosphorus and forms calcium phosphate, an insoluble compound that is eliminated in the feces. Calcium carbonate binds approximately 50% as much phosphorous as does calcium acetate.

Pharmacokinetics

No information was located on the pharmacokinetics of calcium acetate in dogs and cats. In humans, calcium carbonate is converted to calcium chloride by gastric acid. Approximately 30% is absorbed when given with food.

Contraindications/Precautions/Warnings

This agent should not be used when hypercalcemia is present. Because hypercalcemia can result from administering oral calcium products to animals with renal failure, adequate monitoring of serum ionized calcium and phosphorus is required.

Use calcium containing phosphate binders with caution in patients having a serum calcium and phosphorus product greater than 60.

Using calcium-based phosphate binders and calcitriol together is controversial. Some authors state the combination is contraindicated, while others state that intensified monitoring for hypercalcemia is required.

Adverse Effects

Hypercalcemia and extraosseous (soft tissue) calcification are the primary concerns associated with calcium carbonate; especially when using high dosages long-term; adequate monitoring is required.

In humans, constipation has been reported.

Reproductive/Nursing Safety

No reproductive safety studies were located and the human label states that it is not known whether the drug can cause fetal harm. However, it would be surprising if calcium carbonate caused teratogenic effects. In humans, the FDA categorizes calcium acetate as category C for use during pregnancy (*Animal studies have shown an adverse effect on the fetus, but there are no adequate studies in humans; or there are no animal reproduction studies and no adequate studies in humans.*)

It would be expected that calcium carbonate would be safe to administer during lactation.

Overdosage/Acute Toxicity

Potentially, acute overdoses could cause hypercalcemia in susceptible animals. Patients should be monitored and treated symptomatically. If dosage was massive and recent, consider using standard protocols to empty the gut.

Drug Interactions

The following drug interactions have either been reported or are theoretical in humans or animals receiving calcium carbonate and may be of significance in veterinary patients. Unless otherwise noted, use together is not necessarily contraindicated, but weigh the potential risks and perform additional monitoring when appropriate.

- **CALCITRIOL:** If administered with calcium carbonate, may lead to hypercalcemia; if calcitriol is used concomitantly, intensified monitoring for hypercalcemia is mandatory.
- **DIGOXIN:** Calcium carbonate is not recommended for use in human patients that are on digoxin therapy, as hypercalcemia may cause serious arrhythmias.
- **FLUOROQUINOLONES, TETRACYCLINES:** Oral calcium-containing products can reduce absorption of fluoroquinolones; if both calcium carbonate and one of these antibiotics are required, separate dosages by at least two hours.
- **LEVOTHYROXINE:** Oral calcium products may reduce levothyroxine absorption if given at the same time. Separate dosages by at least two hours if possible.
- **PROTON PUMP INHIBITORS, H2 BLOCKERS:** Reducing stomach acid may lower the phosphorous binding capacity of calcium carbonate.

Laboratory Considerations

When using to treat hypocalcemia:

- **HEMOLYZED BLOOD SAMPLES** or **HYPERLIPIDEMIA:** Can cause falsely elevated total calcium reports.
- **HYPERBILIRUBINEMA:** Can cause falsely low total calcium reports.
- **OXALATE, CITRATE, ETHYLENEDIAMINETETRA-ACETIC ACID (EDTA):** These anticoagulants in blood sample collection tubes can bind calcium and cause falsely low total calcium reports. Heparinized samples are acceptable.

Doses

- **DOGS/CATS:**

    For hyperphosphatemia associated with chronic renal failure, in conjunction with a low-phosphorus diet (extra-label): 90 – 150 mg/kg/day calcium carbonate PO divided and given with food, mixed with food, or just prior to each meal. Dosed "to effect," meaning the dose is adjusted to assure that the serum phosphorus target is achieved. Therapy usually begins at the lower end of the recommended dose range and adjusted upward as needed every 4-6 weeks until the therapeutic target is reached. Monitor ionized calcium; hypercalcemia is possible. Decrease dose if serum calcium exceeds normal limits. (Polzin et al. 2005; Polzin 2013)

    As a calcium supplement for chronic hypocalcemia: Dogs: Approximately 1250 mg (toy breeds) - 10 grams (giant breeds) of calcium carbonate PO per day. This is 0.5 – 4 grams of <u>elemental</u> calcium PO per day. Cats: 1250 mg – 2.5 grams (0.5 – 1 gram of <u>elemental</u> calcium) PO per day.

Monitoring

Initially at 10-14 day intervals; once "stable", then at 4-6 week intervals:

- Serum phosphorus (after a 12-hour fast).
- Serum ionized (if possible) calcium; baseline and at one week. Directly measured serum ionized calcium is a better indicator of calcium status than total calcium, but requires specific collection techniques and/or analyzers. Refer to your laboratory's guidelines or your analyzers instructions. A more thorough discussion of this topic can be found at the following reference: (Schenck et al. 2008).

Client Information

- Give with meals; either just before or mixed into food.
- The veterinarian may prescribe additional doses to be administered between meals if additional calcium is required, give only with meals unless the veterinarian instructs to do so.
- Use of this medication will require ongoing laboratory monitoring.

Chemistry/Synonyms

Calcium carbonate occurs as a fine, white, odorless, microcrystalline powder. It is practically insoluble in water, but water solubility is increased by presence of carbon dioxide or ammonium salts. It dissolves with effervescence in hydrochloric acid. It is insoluble in alcohol.

One gram of calcium carbonate contains 400 mg of elemental calcium (40%).

Calcium carbonate may also be known as calcii carbonas, E170, or precipitate chalk. A common oral dosage form trade name is *Tums®*.

Storage/Stability

The commercially available tablets, capsules and gelcaps should be stored at room temperature (25°C); excursions are permitted to 15-30°C.

Compatibility/Compounding Considerations

No specific information noted.

Dosage Forms/Regulatory Status

VETERINARY-LABELED PRODUCTS: NONE.

There is an oral nutritional supplement (not FDA-approved) product (*Epakitin®*) that contains calcium carbonate 10% (100 mg/gram) and chitosan (8%).

HUMAN-LABELED PRODUCTS:

There are many oral calcium carbonate products available and are all OTC. Dosage forms include:

Chewable and Regular Tablets in strengths ranging from 420 mg to 1250 mg. Common sizes are 500 mg or 750 mg.

Oral Powders 800 mg/2 grams and suspensions 1250 mg/5mL.

Capsules: 200 mg (*Cal-CO3S®*); 1250 mg (*Calci-Mix®*).

Revisions/References

Monograph revised/updated September 2013.

Polzin, D., et al. (2005). Chronic Kidney Disease. *Textbook of Veterinary Internal Medicine: Diseases of the Dog and Cat 6th Ed.* S. Ettinger and E. Feldman, Elsevier: 1756-85.
Polzin, D. J. (2013). Evidence-based step-wise approach to managing chronic kidney disease in dogs and cats. *J. Vet. Emerg. Crit. Care* 23(2): 205-15.
Schenck, P. A. & D. J. Chew (2008). Calcium: Total or ionized? *Veterinary Clinics of North America-Small Animal Practice* 38(3): 497-+.

Calcium EDTA—see Edetate Calcium Disodium

Calcium (Borogluconate, Chloride, Gluconate), Injectable

(kal-**see**-um)

Essential Cation Nutrient

Prescriber Highlights

▶ Used IV to treat or prevent severe hypocalcemia, acute hyperkalemia and hypermagnesemia; SC administration is somewhat controversial.

▶ Contraindicated in V-fib or hypercalcemia.

▶ Determine dosages carefully; can be confusing. Must NOT give IV too rapidly.

▶ Must monitor therapy carefully depending on condition, etc.

▶ Potential drug interactions & physical incompatibilities prevalent.

Uses/Indications

Parenteral calcium is used for treatment of documented ionized hypocalcemia, calcium channel blocker toxicity, hypermagnesemia, or hyperkalemia. Parenteral calcium salts include calcium gluconate, calcium borogluconate, and calcium chloride. Calcium gluconate is generally preferred as it is less irritating to vascular tissues.

Routine administration of intravenous calcium during CPR is not recommended, but it may be considered in cases with documented moderate to severe hypocalcemia (Fletcher et al. 2012).

Pharmacology/Actions

Calcium is an essential element that is required for many functions within the body, including proper nervous and musculoskeletal system function, cell membrane and capillary permeability, and activation of enzymatic reactions.

Pharmacokinetics

After administration or absorption, ionized calcium enters the extracellular fluid and then is rapidly incorporated into skeletal tissue. Calcium administration does not necessarily stimulate bone formation. Approximately 99% of total body calcium is found in bone. Of circulating calcium, approximately 50% is bound to serum proteins or complexed with anions and 50% is in the ionized form. Total serum calcium is dependent on serum protein concentrations. Total serum calcium changes by approximately 0.8 mg/dL for every 1.09 g/dL change in serum albumin. Calcium crosses the placenta and is distributed into milk.

Calcium is eliminated primarily in the feces, contributed by both unabsorbed calcium and calcium excreted into the bile and pancreatic juice. Only small amounts of the drug are excreted in the urine as most of cationic calcium is filtered by the glomeruli and reabsorbed by the tubules and ascending loop of Henle. Vitamin D, parathormone, and thiazide diuretics decrease the amount of calcium excreted by the kidneys. Loop diuretics (*e.g.*, furosemide, etc.), calcitonin, and somatotropin increase calcium renal excretion.

Contraindications/Precautions/Warnings

Calcium is contraindicated in patients with ventricular fibrillation or hypercalcemia. Parenteral calcium should not be administered to patients with above normal serum calcium levels. Calcium should be used very cautiously in patients receiving digitalis glycosides, or having cardiac or renal disease. Calcium chloride, because it can be acidifying, should be used with caution in patients with respiratory failure, respiratory acidosis, or renal disease.

In dogs, calcium gluconate diluted 1:1 (but not calcium chloride) has been generally regarded as safe to administer subcutaneously for the treatment of primary hypoparathyroidism in the past, but there are now several case reports of severe tissue reactions (*e.g.*, pyogranulomatous panniculitis, adipocyte mineralization, etc.) at the injection site. A recent review article on hypocalcemia in critically ill dogs and cats stated that subcutaneous administration of calcium salts is not recommended (Holowaychuk 2013). If considering SC administration use with caution, particularly when using with calcitriol or in smaller dogs.

Adverse Effects

Hypercalcemia can be associated with calcium therapy, particularly in patients with cardiac or renal disease; animals should be adequately monitored. Other effects that may be seen include mild to severe tissue reactions after IM or SC administration of calcium salts and venous irritation after IV administration. Calcium chloride may be more irritating than other parenteral salts and is more likely to cause hypotension. Too rapid intravenous injection of calcium can cause hypotension, cardiac arrhythmias and cardiac arrest. Calcinosis cutis has been observed in animals receiving diluted 10% calcium gluconate subcutaneously. This can be more prevalent in small dogs or cats and those with concurrent hypophosphatemia.

Should calcium salts be infused perivascularly, stop the infusion; treatment then may include: infiltrating the affected area with normal saline, corticosteroids administered locally, applying heat and elevating the area, and infiltrating the affected area with a local anesthetic and hyaluronidase.

Reproductive/Nursing Safety

Although parenteral calcium products have not been proven safe for use during pregnancy, they are often used before, during, and after parturition in cows, ewes, bitches, and queens to treat parturient paresis secondary to hypocalcemia. In humans, the FDA categorizes this drug as category *C* for use during pregnancy (*Animal studies have shown an adverse effect on the fetus, but there are no adequate studies in humans; or there are no animal reproduction studies and no adequate studies in humans.*)

Overdosage/Acute Toxicity

Hypercalcemia can occur with parenteral therapy or oral therapy in combination with vitamin D or increased parathormone levels. Treat hypercalcemia by withholding calcium therapy and other calcium elevating drugs (*e.g.*, vitamin D analogs). Mild hypercalcemia generally will resolve without further intervention when renal function is adequate.

More serious hypercalcemia (>12 mg/dL) should generally be treated by hydrating with IV normal saline and administering a loop diuretic (*e.g.*, furosemide, etc.) to increase both sodium and calcium excretion. Potassium and magnesium must be monitored and replaced as necessary. ECG should also be monitored during treatment. Corticosteroids, and in humans, calcitonin and hemodialysis, have also been employed in treating hypercalcemia.

Drug Interactions

The following drug interactions have either been reported or are theoretical in humans or animals receiving calcium and may be of significance in veterinary patients. Unless otherwise noted, use together is not necessarily contraindicated, but weigh the potential risks and perform additional monitoring when appropriate.

- **CALCIUM CHANNEL BLOCKERS** (*e.g.*, **diltiazem, verapamil**, etc.): Intravenous calcium may antagonize the effects of calcium-channel blocking agents.
- **DIGOXIN**: Patients on digitalis therapy are more apt to develop arrhythmias if receiving IV calcium—use with caution.
- **MAGNESIUM SULFATE**: Parenteral calcium can neutralize the effects of hypermagnesemia or magnesium toxicity secondary to parenteral magnesium sulfate.
- **NEUROMUSCULAR BLOCKERS** (*e.g.*, **tubocurarine, metubine, gallamine, pancuronium, atracurium, and vecuronium**): Parenteral calcium may reverse the effects of nondepolarizing neuromuscular blocking agents; calcium has been reported to prolong or enhance the effects of tubocurarine.
- **POTASSIUM SUPPLEMENTS**: Patients receiving both parenteral calcium and potassium supplementation may have an increased chance of developing cardiac arrhythmias—use cautiously.
- **THIAZIDE DIURETICS**: Used in conjunction with large doses of calcium may cause hypercalcemia.

Laboratory Considerations

- **SERUM and URINARY MAGNESIUM**: Parenteral calcium may cause false-negative results for serum and urinary magnesium when using the Titan yellow method of determination.
- **HEMOLYZED BLOOD SAMPLES or HYPERLIPIDEMIA**: Can cause falsely elevated total calcium reports.
- **HYPERBILIRUBINEMA**: Can cause falsely low total calcium reports.
- **OXALATE, CITRATE, ETHYLENEDIAMINE TETRA ACETIC ACID (EDTA)**: These anticoagulants in blood sample collection tubes can bind calcium and cause falsely low total calcium reports. Heparinized samples are acceptable.

Doses

Warning: Dosing parenteral calcium can be confusing and potentially dangerous. Depending on the reference, dosages can be listed by mL/kg, mEq/kg, mmol/kg or mg/kg. These may be for the calcium salt being used OR for elemental calcium. Calcium chloride 10% (100 mg/mL) injection contains approximately 3 times more **elemental calcium** per mL as calcium gluconate 10% (100 mg/mL). Parenteral treatment using calcium should be considered "High Alert" with dosages double-checked by another person.

- **DOGS/CATS:**

  For emergency treatment of severe hypocalcemia (extra-label): Intravenous dosage for severe hypocalcemia (tetany; seizures) ranges from 5 – 15 mg/kg of elemental calcium IV slowly over 10-30 minutes. This would correspond to:

  If using **calcium gluconate** **10% injection** each mL contains 9.3 mg of **elemental** calcium. Doses of 5 – 15 mg/kg **elemental** calcium would equate to 0.54 – 1.61 **mL/kg** of calcium gluconate 10% injection.

If using **calcium** chloride **10% injection** each mL contains 27.2 mg of **elemental** calcium. Doses of 5 – 15 mg/kg **elemental calcium** would equate to 0.18 – 0.56 **mL/kg** of calcium chloride 10% injection.

If using other concentrations or other salts (*e.g.*, calcium borogluconate) the actual volume to inject will vary depending on the concentration of the solution and which salt is being used.

Patient response determines the final dose of calcium. During the infusion, patients should be continually monitored for heart rate/rhythm with an ECG and respiration rate. If bradycardia, S-T segment elevation or QT interval shortening occurs, temporarily stop the infusion.

For short-term maintenance after tetany has been corrected using a constant-rate intravenous infusion (preferred) or subcutaneous administration: The goal is to maintain calcium within the normal range, but to wean off parenteral calcium as soon as oral calcium and vitamin D take effect and serum calcium concentration remains stable. Parenteral calcium is preferably given by IV constant-rate infusion (calcium gluconate or calcium chloride) or subcutaneous administration (calcium gluconate only).

If giving as a constant-rate infusion (CRI): **2.5 – 3.5 mg/kg/hour of elemental calcium.**

If using **calcium** gluconate **10% injection** each mL contains 9.3 mg of **elemental** calcium. A dosage of **2.5 – 3.5 mg/kg/hour of elemental calcium** would equate to 0.27 – 0.38 mL/hour of calcium gluconate 10% injection.

If using **calcium** chloride **10% injection** each mL contains 27.2 mg of **elemental** calcium. A dosage of **2.5 – 3.5 mg/kg/hour of elemental calcium** would equate to 0.092 – 0.128 mL/kg/hour of calcium chloride 10% injection.

If using the SC route: Use calcium gluconate only. Determine the dosage of calcium gluconate that was required to correct tetany and dilute the corresponding dosage amount in an equal volume of saline and administer SC q4-6 hours. Small dogs and cats may be prone to developing calcinosis cutis. Gradually increase the dosing interval to q12h as oral calcium and vitamin D take effect. [Adapted from (Crystal 2004; Ross 2004; Greco 2012)]

For hyperkalemic cardiotoxicity (extra-label): **Note:** Intravenous calcium treatment can antagonize the cardiotoxic effects of calcium, but does not reduce potassium concentrations. Correct metabolic acidosis, if present, with sodium bicarbonate (bicarbonate may also be beneficial even if acidosis is not present). **Calcium gluconate** (10%) is indicated if serum K+ is >8 mEq/L, or with evident ECG changes (bradycardia, tall/tented T-waves, atrial standstill). Give at an approximate dose of 0.5 – 1 mL/kg of the 10% solution (this corresponds to 50 – 100 mg/kg of calcium gluconate) over 10-20 minutes; monitor ECG. Rapidly corrects arrhythmias but effects are very short (10-15 minutes). IV glucose (0.5 – 1 g/kg body weight with or without regular insulin) can be administered to lower serum K+ concentrations. (Polzin et al. 1985)

- **CATTLE:**

For hypocalcemia (extra-label): **Calcium gluconate injection:** 150 – 250 mg/kg (as the gluconate) IV slowly to effect (intraperitoneal route may also be used). Monitor respirations and cardiac rate and rhythm during administration. (USPC 1990)

- **HORSES:**

For hypocalcemia (extra-label):

a) **Mild hypocalcemia:** As routine therapy, adding 50 mL of 23% calcium borogluconate per 5 L of lactated Ringer's solution (at twice the maintenance rate) is sufficient to restore normocalcemia in horses with mild hypocalcemia. Horses with functional kidneys can eliminate large amounts of calcium; hypercalcemia from excessive calcium administration is rare, especially if the horse is receiving fluid therapy.

Severe hypocalcemia: Higher doses, adding 100 – 150 mL of 23% calcium borogluconate per 5 L of LRS may be required. In animals with chronic or refractory hypocalcemia, oral supplementation with calcium carbonate (limestone; 100 – 300 grams/horse/day) or dicalcium phosphate (100 – 200 grams/horse/day) should be considered. Adding vitamin D treatment is questionable and some horses may develop toxicity (hypervitaminosis D). However, low doses of vitamin D might be of benefit to horses with decreased calcium absorption and reabsorption. Hypocalcemia may not resolve in some animals until they receive magnesium supplementation. (Toribio 2011)

b) **Calcium gluconate injection:** 150 – 250 mg/kg IV slowly to effect (intraperitoneal route may also be used). Monitor respirations and cardiac rate and rhythm during administration. (USPC 1990)

c) **For lactation tetany:** 250 mL per 450 kg body weight of a standard commercially available solution that also contains magnesium and phosphorous IV slowly while auscultating heart. If no improvement after 10 minutes, repeat. Intensity in heart sounds should be noted, with only an infrequent extrasystole. Stop infusion immediately if a pronounced change in rate or rhythm is detected. (Brewer 1987)

- **SHEEP & GOATS:**

For hypocalcemia:

a) Slow IV infusion of calcium should show immediate clinical response. A typical dose using 23% calcium borogluconate is approximately 50 – 75 mL/45 kg (100 lbs.) body weight slow IV. May also give SC.

b) Sheep: Calcium gluconate injection: 150 – 250 mg/kg (as the gluconate) IV slowly to effect (intraperitoneal route may also be used). Monitor respirations and cardiac rate and rhythm during administration. (USPC 1990)

- **SWINE:**

For hypocalcemia: Calcium gluconate injection: 150 – 250 mg/kg IV slowly to effect (intraperitoneal route may also be used). Monitor respirations and cardiac rate and rhythm during administration. (USPC 1990)

- **BIRDS:**

For hypocalcemic tetany: Calcium gluconate: 50 – 100 mg/kg (as gluconate) IV slowly to effect; may be diluted and given IM if a vein cannot be located. (Clubb 1986)

For egg-bound birds: Initially, calcium gluconate 1% solution 0.01 – 0.02 mL/g IM. Provide moist heat (80-85°F) and allow 24 hours for bird to pass egg. (Nye 1986)

- **REPTILES:**

For egg binding in combination with oxytocin (oxytocin: 1 – 10 Units/kg IM): **Calcium glubionate:** 10 – 50 mg/kg IM as needed until calcium levels back to normal or egg binding is resolved. Use care when giving multiple injections. Calcium/oxytocin is not as effective in lizards as in other species. (Gauvin 1993)

Monitoring

- During IV administration: heart rate/rhythm with ECG.
- Serum ionized (if possible) calcium. Directly measured serum ionized calcium is a better indicator of calcium status than total calcium, but requires specific collection techniques and/or analyzers. Refer to your laboratory's or analyzer's instructions. A more thorough discussion of this topic can be found at the following references: (Schenck et al. 2008; Holowaychuk 2013).
- Serum magnesium, phosphate, and potassium when indicated.
- Serum PTH (parathormone) if indicated.
- Renal function tests initially and as required.
- Urine calcium if hypercalcuria develops.

Chemistry

Several different salts of calcium are available in various formulations. Calcium gluceptate and calcium chloride are freely soluble in water; calcium lactate is soluble in water; calcium gluconate and calcium glycerophosphate are sparingly soluble in water, and calcium phosphate and carbonate are insoluble in water. Calcium gluconate for injection has a pH of 6-8.2 and calcium chloride for injection has a pH of 5.5-7.5.

To determine approximate elemental calcium content per gram of various calcium salts:

Calcium Borogluconate: 90 mg (4.6 mEq; 2.3 mmol)
Calcium Chloride: 273 mg (13.6 mEq; 6.8 mmol)
Calcium Glubionate: 66 mg (3.29 mEq; 1.64 mmol)
Calcium Gluceptate: 82 mg (4.08 mEq; 2.04 mmol)
Calcium Gluconate: 93 mg (4.65 mEq; 2.32 mmol)
Calcium Glycerophosphate: 191 mg (9.6 mEq)

Storage/Stability

Calcium gluconate injection, calcium borogluconate injection, calcium gluceptate injection, and calcium chloride injection should be stored at room temperature and protected from freezing.

Compatibility/Compounding Considerations

Calcium chloride for injection is reportedly **compatible** with the following intravenous solutions and drugs: amikacin sulfate, ascorbic acid, chloramphenicol sodium succinate, dopamine HCl, hydrocortisone sodium succinate, isoproterenol HCl, lidocaine HCl, norepinephrine bitartrate, penicillin G potassium/sodium, pentobarbital sodium, phenobarbital sodium, sodium bicarbonate, verapamil HCl, and vitamin B-complex with C.

Calcium chloride for injection **compatibility information conflicts** or is dependent on diluent or concentration factors with the following drugs or solutions: fat emulsion 10%, dobutamine HCl, oxytetracycline HCl, and tetracycline HCl. Compatibility is dependent upon factors such as pH, concentration, temperature and diluent used.

Calcium chloride for injection is reportedly **incompatible** with the following solutions or drugs: amphotericin B and chlorpheniramine maleate.

Calcium gluconate for injection is reportedly **compatible** with the following intravenous solutions and drugs: sodium chloride for injection 0.9%, lactated Ringer's injection, dextrose 5%-20%, dextrose-lactated Ringer's injection, dextrose-saline combinations, amikacin sulfate, aminophylline, ascorbic acid injection, chloramphenicol sodium succinate, corticotropin, dimenhydrinate, erythromycin glucheptate, heparin sodium, hydrocortisone sodium succinate, lidocaine HCl, norepinephrine bitartrate, penicillin G potassium/sodium, phenobarbital sodium, potassium chloride, tobramycin sulfate, vancomycin HCl, verapamil and vitamin B-complex with C.

Calcium gluconate compatibility information conflicts or is dependent on diluent or concentration factors with the follow-ing drugs or solutions: phosphate salts, oxytetracycline HCl, and prochlorperazine edisylate. Compatibility is dependent upon factors such as pH, concentration, temperature and diluent used.

Calcium gluconate is reportedly **incompatible** with the following solutions or drugs: intravenous fat emulsion, amphotericin B, dobutamine HCl, methylprednisolone sodium succinate, and metoclopramide HCl.

Consult specialized references or a hospital pharmacist for more specific information.

Dosage Forms/Regulatory Status

VETERINARY-LABELED PRODUCTS:

Note: Not necessarily a complete list; veterinary-labeled products are apparently not FDA-approved as they do not appear in the Green Book.

Calcium borogluconate 23% [230 mg/mL; equivalent to 20.7 mg (1.06 mEq) elemental calcium per mL], in 500 mL bottles; generic; (OTC). Depending on the product, labeled for use in cattle, horses, swine, sheep, cats, and dogs. No withdrawal times are required and these products may not be FDA-approved.

Products are also available that include calcium, phosphorus, potassium and/or dextrose; refer to the individual product's labeling for specific dosage information. Trade names for these products include: *Norcalciphos*®, and *Cal-Dextro*® *Special, #2, C, and K*; (Rx).

Oral Products: No products containing only calcium (as a salt) are available commercially with veterinary labeling. There are several products (*e.g.*, *Pet-Cal*® and *Osteoform*® *Improved*) that contain calcium with phosphorous and vitamin D (plus other ingredients in some preparations).

HUMAN-APPROVED PRODUCTS: (NOT A COMPLETE LIST)

Calcium Gluconate Injection 10% [100 mg/mL; equivalent to 9.3 mg (0.465 mEq) elemental calcium per mL], preservative-free in 10 mL & 50 mL single-dose vials & 100 mL & 200 mL pharmacy bulk vials; generic; (Rx)

Calcium Chloride Injection 10% [100 mg/mL; equivalent to 27.2 mg (1.36 mEq) elemental calcium per mL] in 10 mL amps, vials, and syringes; generic; (Rx)

Revisions/References

Monograph revised/updated September 2013.

Brewer, B. D. (1987). Disorders of calcium metabolism. *Current Therapy in Equine Medicine.* N. E. Robinson. Philadelphia, WB Saunders: 189-92.

Clubb, S. L. (1986). Therapeutics: Individual and Flock Treatment Regimens. *Clinical Avian Medicine and Surgery.* G. J. Harrison and L. R. Harrison. Philadelphia, W.B. Saunders: 327-55.

Crystal, M. (2004). Hypocalcemia. *The 5-Minute Veterinary Consult: Canine and Feline 3rd Ed.* L. Tilley and F. Smith, Lippincott Williams & Wilkins: 662-3.

Fletcher, D. J., et al. (2012). RECOVER evidence and knowledge gap analysis on veterinary CPR. Part 7: Clinical guidelines. *J. Vet. Emerg. Crit. Care* 22.

Gauvin, J. (1993). Drug therapy in reptiles. *Seminars in Avian & Exotic Med* 2(1): 48-59.

Greco, D. S. (2012). Endocrine Causes of Calcium Disorders. *Topics in Companion Animal Medicine* 27(4): 150-5.

Holowaychuk, M. K. (2013). Hypocalcemia of Critical Illness in Dogs and Cats. *Veterinary Clinics of North America-Small Animal Practice* 43(6): 1299-+.

Nye, R. R. (1986). Dealing with the Egg-bound Bird. *Current Veterinary Therapy (CVT) IX Small Animal Practice.* R. W. Kirk. Philadelphia, W.B. Saunders: 746-7.

Polzin, D. J. & C. A. Osborne (1985). Diseases of the Urinary Tract. *Handbook of Small Animal Therapeutics.* L. E. Davis. New York, Churchill Livingstone: 333-95.

Ross, L. (2004). *Life-Threatening Metabolic Emergencies.* ACVIM Proceedings. accessed via Veterinary Information Network; vin.com

Schenck, P. A. & D. J. Chew (2008). Calcium: Total or ionized? *Veterinary Clinics of North America-Small Animal Practice* 38(3): 497-+.

Toribio, R. E. (2011). Disorders of Calcium and Phosphate Metabolism in Horses. *Veterinary Clinics of North America-Equine Practice* 27(1): 129-+.

USPC (1990). Veterinary Information- Appendix III. *Drug Information for the Health Professional.* Rockville, United States Pharmacopeial Convention. 2: 2811- 60.

Camphorated Tincture of Opium — See Paregoric

Candesartan Cilexetil

(kan-de-sar-tan sye-lex-e-til)   Atacand®

Angiotensin-II Receptor Blocker (ARB)

Prescriber Highlights

▶ ARB that potentially could be useful in dogs and cats for the adjunctive treatment of proteinuria, hypertension secondary to renal insufficiency, or congestive heart failure.

▶ Very limited experience in veterinary medicine; little data on efficacy, safety, adverse effects, etc.

▶ Not safe for use during pregnancy.

Uses/Indications

Candesartan is a human-approved angiotensin-II AT1-receptor blocker that potentially could be useful for the adjunctive treatment of hypertension, proteinuria and cardiomyopathies in dogs and cats, but very little information on its safety and efficacy are known for veterinary species.

One study in Beagles with experimentally-induced pulmonary artery stenosis, candesartan (1 mg/kg PO once daily) prevented right ventricular remodeling (Yamane et al. 2008). It is not yet known if candesartan alone or in combination with a beta-blocker would be effective medical treatment for clinical cases of pulmonary artery stenosis in dogs.

Pharmacology/Actions

Candesartan is an angiotensin-II receptor blocker (ARB). By selectively blocking the AT1-receptor, aldosterone synthesis and secretion is reduced causing vasodilation and decreased potassium and increased sodium excretion. While plasma concentrations of renin and angiotensin-II are increased, this does not counteract the blood pressure lowering effects of candesartan. Candesartan does not interfere with substance P or bradykinin responses.

ARBs potentially can reduce blood pressure, reduce proteinuria, slow the progression of kidney disease, prevent or reverse ventricular hypertrophy, and improve congestive heart failure, but the evaluation of their clinical usefulness, if any, in veterinary medicine is in its very early stages.

Pharmacokinetics

Candesartan cilexetil is a pro-drug and has little activity until it is hydrolyzed to candesartan in the small intestine during absorption. Little pharmacokinetic information is published for veterinary species. In dogs, orally administered radiolabeled candesartan cilexetil had a bioavailability of 5% (of the active compound) and peak levels occurred 1.3 hours post-dose. The elimination half-life was about 4-5 hours.(Kondo et al. 1996)

In humans, candesartan is rapidly absorbed, but oral bioavailability of the tablets is only about 15%. Food does not significantly alter bioavailability. Greater than 99% of the drug is bound to plasma proteins. Candesartan if primarily excreted unchanged in the urine or via bile in the feces. Elimination half-life is about 9 hours.

Contraindications/Precautions/Warnings

Candesartan is contraindicated in patients that are allergic (hypersensitive) to it. In humans, it is also contraindicated in diabetic patients taking aliskiren. Hypotensive patients should not receive the drug. Patients that are volume or electrolyte depleted should not receive the drug until volume/electrolytes have been replenished/corrected.

Candesartan should be used with caution in patients with moderate hepatic impairment; dosage reduction may be warranted.

The human label has the following Black Box Warning: "Fetal toxicity: "When pregnancy is detected, discontinue candesartan as soon as possible. Drugs that act directly on the renin-angiotensin

system can cause injury and even death to the developing fetus." See the Reproductive Safety section for more information.

Adverse Effects

The adverse effect profile for this drug when used clinically in veterinary species is not known. In humans, adverse effects are not common. The most commonly reported adverse effects include headache and orthostatic dizziness/hypotension. Changes in renal function and hyperkalemia are possible. Very rarely in humans, neutropenia, leukopenia, agranulocytosis, and increased liver enzymes have been reported.

Reproductive/Nursing Safety

Candesartan is not considered safe to use during pregnancy. Studies in pregnant rats given high doses of ARBs demonstrated a variety of fetal abnormalities (renal pelvic cavitation, hydroureter, absence of renal papilla). Smaller doses in rabbits caused increased maternal death and spontaneous abortion. In humans, the drug is considered teratogenic, particularly during the 2nd and 3rd trimesters. During this time, the FDA categorizes candesartan as category **D** for use during pregnancy *(There is evidence of human fetal risk, but the potential benefits from the use of the drug in pregnant women may be acceptable despite its potential risks.)* If pregnancy is detected in patients receiving candesartan, the drug should be discontinued as soon as possible.

Because small amounts of candesartan have been detected in rat milk, and there is significant concern about the safety of the drug in neonates, the manufacturer recommends that it not be used in nursing women.

Overdosage/Acute Toxicity

In acute toxicity studies in mice, rats, and dogs single oral doses of up to 2 grams/kg of candesartan cilexetil were not lethal. Likely effects seen in an overdose situation include hypotension and either bradycardia or tachycardia; treatment is supportive. Candesartan is not dialyzable. In the event of an overdose, contact an animal poison control center for further information.

Drug Interactions

The following drug interactions have either been reported or are theoretical in humans or animals receiving candesartan and potentially could be of significance in veterinary patients:

■ **ACE INHIBITORS (benazepril, enalapril**, etc.): Increased risk for adverse effects (*e.g.*; hypotension, hyperkalemia, renal function changes); increased monitoring may be warranted.

■ **ASPIRIN:** Possible reduced antihypertensive effect of candesartan and increased risk for renal impairment; increased monitoring may be warranted.

■ **NSAIDs** (*e.g.,* **carprofen, meloxicam**, etc.): Possible reduced antihypertensive effect of candesartan and increased risk for renal impairment; increased monitoring may be warranted.

■ **POTASSIUM PREPARATIONS, POTASSIUM–SPARING DIURETICS** (*e.g.,* spironolactone): Increased risk for hyperkalemia; increased monitoring of serum potassium may be warranted.

Laboratory Considerations

■ No specific concerns were noted.

Dosages

■ **DOGS:**

As adjunctive treatment for hypertension, heart failure, or proteinuria (extra-label): Note: There is very little clinical experience using this drug in animal patients and nearly nothing published on its clinical usage; consider use at this time as experimental—use with caution. One study done in Beagles with experimentally induced pulmonary artery stenosis, candesartan was dosed at 1 mg/kg PO once daily. (Yamane et al.

2008). Human pediatric (ages 1-6) patients are initially started at 0.2 mg/kg once daily and dosage titrated up to 0.4 mg/kg once daily if needed. Oral bioavailability in dogs appears to be lower than humans, so larger dosages may be required (unconfirmed).

Monitoring

- Depending on reason for use and patient's clinical condition: Renal function, urine protein, blood pressure, serum potassium levels, and volume status.

Client Information

- This medication may be given with or without food.
- Because this medication has not been frequently used in dogs or cats, watch carefully for any side effects and report them to your veterinarian. Possible side effects could include: diarrhea, vomiting, lack of appetite, fatigue, and low blood pressure (fainting, weakness, inability to exercise, etc.).
- This drug has caused birth defects and should not be used in pregnant animals. If a human in the household is pregnant, they should be very careful not to ingest these tablets and should either wear disposable gloves when administering doses or wash hands after touching these tablets.

Chemistry/Synonyms

Candesartan cilexetil (CAS Registry: 145040-37-5; ATC: C09CA06) occurs as a white to off-white powder. It is practically insoluble in water, sparingly soluble in methyl alcohol, and freely soluble in dichlormethane.

Candesartan cilexetil may also be known as CV-11974, H-212/9 or TCV-116. A common trade name is *Atacand®*.

Storage/Stability

Candesartan tablets should be stored in tight containers at room temperature (15-30°C; 59-86°F).

Compatibility/Compounding Considerations

The human-label product has the following information in its package insert: Oral suspension can be prepared with any strength of candesartan tablets in concentrations within the range of 0.1 to 2 mg/mL. Typically, a concentration of 1 mg/mL will be suitable for the prescribed dose. The following steps below will yield 160 mL of a candesartan 1 mg/mL suspension:

Prepare the vehicle by adding equal volumes of *Ora-Plus®* (80 mL) and *Ora-Sweet®* SF (80 mL), or alternatively, use *Ora-Blend SF®* (160 mL).

- Add a small amount of vehicle to the required number of candesartan tablets (five 32 mg tablets) and grind into a smooth paste using a mortar and pestle.
- Add the paste to a preparation vessel of suitable size.
- Rinse the mortar and pestle clean using the vehicle and add this to the vessel. Repeat, if necessary.
- Prepare the final volume by adding the remaining vehicle.
- Mix thoroughly.
- Dispense into suitably sized amber PET bottles.
- Label with an expiry date of 100 days and include the following instructions: Store at room temperature (below 30°C/86°F). Use within 30 days after first opening. Do not use after the expiry date stated on the bottle. Do not freeze. Shake well before each use. (2009)

Dosage Forms/Regulatory Status

VETERINARY-LABELED PRODUCTS: NONE.

HUMAN-LABELED PRODUCTS:

Oral Tablets: 4 mg, 8 mg, 16 mg, 32 mg; *Atacand®*, generic; (Rx).

Combination products containing candesartan and hydrochlorothiazide are also available. There is a website (dailymed.nim.hih.

gov) listing FDA-approved (human drug) labels for candesartan products.

Revisions/References

Monograph written August 2013.

(2009). Atacand® Tablets [Package Insert]. Wilminton, DE, AstraZeneca

Kondo, T., et al. (1996). Disposition of the new angiotensin II receptor antagonist candesartan cilexetil in rats and dogs. *Arzneimittel-Forschung/Drug Research* 46(6): 594-600.

Yamane, T., et al. (2008). Comparison of the effects of candesartan cilexetil and enalapril maleate on right ventricular myocardial remodeling in dogs with experimentally induced pulmonary stenosis. *American Journal of Veterinary Research* 69(12): 1574-9.

Captopril

(kap-toe-pril)   Capoten®

Angiotensin-Converting Enzyme (ACE) Inhibitor

Prescriber Highlights

▶ First available ACE inhibitor; rarely used today as enalapril, benazepril & other newer ACE inhibitors are preferred.

▶ Shorter duration of activity & more adverse effects than other newer ACE inhibitors.

Uses/Indications

The principle use of captopril in veterinary medicine has been as a vasodilator in the treatment of CHF and hypertension. Because of approval status, fewer adverse effects, and longer duration of action, enalapril and benazepril have largely supplanted the use of this drug in veterinary medicine.

Pharmacology/Actions

Captopril prevents the formation of angiotensin-II (a potent vasoconstrictor) by competing with angiotensin-I for the enzyme angiotensin-converting enzyme (ACE). ACE has a much higher affinity for captopril than for angiotensin-I. Because angiotensin-II concentrations are decreased, aldosterone secretion is reduced and plasma renin activity is increased.

The cardiovascular effects of captopril in patients with CHF include decreased total peripheral resistance, pulmonary vascular resistance, mean arterial and right atrial pressures, and pulmonary capillary wedge pressure; no change or decrease in heart rate; and increased cardiac index and output, stroke volume, and exercise tolerance. Renal blood flow can be increased with little change in hepatic blood flow.

Pharmacokinetics

In dogs, approximately 75% of an oral dose is absorbed but food in the GI tract reduces bioavailability by 30-40%. It is distributed to most tissues (not the CNS) and is 40% bound to plasma proteins in dogs. The half-life of captopril is about 2.8 hours in dogs and less than 2 hours in humans. Its duration of effect in dogs may only persist for 4 hours. The drug is metabolized and renally excreted. More than 95% of a dose is excreted renally, both as unchanged (45-50%) drug and as metabolites. Patients with significant renal dysfunction can have significantly prolonged half-lives.

Contraindications/Precautions/Warnings

Captopril is contraindicated in patients that have demonstrated hypersensitivity with ACE inhibitors. It should be used with caution and under close supervision in patients with renal insufficiency; doses may need to be reduced.

Captopril should also be used with caution in patients with hyponatremia or sodium depletion, coronary or cerebrovascular insufficiency, preexisting hematologic abnormalities or a collagen vascular disease (*e.g.*, SLE).

Patients with severe CHF should be monitored very closely upon initiation of therapy.

Adverse Effects

There have been some reports of hypotension, renal failure, hyperkalemia, vomiting and diarrhea developing in dogs after captopril administration. Captopril may have a higher incidence of gastrointestinal effects in dogs than other available ACE inhibitors. Although seen in people, skin rashes (4-7% incidence) and neutropenia/agranulocytosis (rare) have not been reported in dogs.

Reproductive/Nursing Safety

Captopril apparently crosses the placenta. High doses of ACE inhibitors in rodents have caused decreased fetal weights and increases in fetal and maternal death rates; no teratogenic effects have been reported to date, but use during pregnancy should occur only when the potential benefits of therapy outweigh the risks to the offspring. In humans, the FDA categorizes this drug as category *C* for use during the first trimester of pregnancy (*Animal studies have shown an adverse effect on the fetus, but there are no adequate studies in humans; or there are no animal reproduction studies and no adequate studies in humans.*) During the second and third trimesters, the FDA categorizes this drug as category *D* for use during pregnancy (*There is evidence of human fetal risk, but the potential benefits from the use of the drug in pregnant women may be acceptable despite its potential risks.*) In a separate system evaluating the safety of drugs in canine and feline pregnancy (Papich 1989), this drug is categorized as class: *C* (*These drugs may have potential risks. Studies in people or laboratory animals have uncovered risks, and these drugs should be used cautiously as a last resort when the benefit of therapy clearly outweighs the risks.*)

Captopril enters milk in concentrations of about 1% of that found in maternal plasma.

Overdosage/Acute Toxicity

In overdose situations, the primary concern is hypotension; supportive treatment with volume expansion with normal saline is recommended to correct blood pressure. Dogs given 1.5 g/kg orally developed emesis and decreased blood pressure. Dogs receiving doses greater than 6.6 mg/kg q8h may develop renal failure.

Drug Interactions

The following drug interactions have either been reported or are theoretical in humans or animals receiving captopril and may be of significance in veterinary patients. Unless otherwise noted, use together is not necessarily contraindicated, but weigh the potential risks and perform additional monitoring when appropriate.

- **ANTACIDS:** Reduced oral absorption of captopril may occur if given concomitantly with antacids; it is suggested to separate dosing by at least two hours.
- **CIMETIDINE:** Used concomitantly with captopril has caused neurologic dysfunction in two human patients.
- **DIGOXIN:** Levels may increase 15-30% when captopril is added, automatic reduction in dosage is not recommended, but monitoring of serum digoxin levels should be performed.
- **DIURETICS:** Concomitant diuretics may cause hypotension if used with captopril; titrate dosages carefully.
- **NON-STEROIDAL ANTIINFLAMMATORY AGENTS (NSAIDs):** May reduce the clinical efficacy of captopril when it is being used as an antihypertensive agent.
- **POTASSIUM** or **POTASSIUM SPARING DIURETICS** (*e.g.,* **spironolactone**): Hyperkalemia may develop with captopril.
- **PROBENECID:** Can decrease renal excretion of captopril and possibly enhance the clinical and toxic effects of the drug.
- **VASODILATORS** (*e.g.,* **prazosin, hydralazine, nitrates**, etc.): Concomitant vasodilators may cause hypotension if used with captopril; titrate dosages carefully.

Laboratory Considerations

- Captopril may cause a false positive **urine acetone test** (sodium nitroprusside reagent).
- When using **iodohippurate sodium I^{123}/I^{134} or Technetium Tc^{99} pententate renal imaging** in patients with renal artery stenosis, ACE inhibitors may cause a reversible decrease in localization and excretion of these agents in the affected kidney that may lead to confusion in test interpretation.

Doses

Note: Because of fewer adverse effects in dogs, longer duration of activity, and/or veterinary labeling/dosage forms, enalapril and other newer ACE inhibitors have largely supplanted the use of this drug in veterinary medicine. Dosages below are extra-label and anecdotal.

- **DOGS:**
  a) 0.5 – 2 mg/kg PO three times daily. (Atkins 2008)
- **CATS:**
  a) 1/4 to 1/2 of a 12.5 mg tablet PO q8-12h. (Bonagura 1989)

Monitoring

- Clinical signs of CHF.
- Serum electrolytes, creatinine, BUN, urine protein.
- CBC with differential; periodic.
- Blood pressure (if treating hypertension or signs associated with hypotension arise).

Client Information

- Give medication on an empty stomach unless otherwise instructed. Do not abruptly stop or reduce therapy without veterinarian's approval. Contact veterinarian if vomiting or diarrhea persist or are severe, or if animal's condition deteriorates.

Chemistry/Synonyms

Related to a peptide isolated from the venom of a South American pit viper, captopril occurs as a slightly sulfurous smelling, white to off-white, crystalline powder. It is freely soluble in water or alcohol.

Captopril may also be known as: captoprilum, or SQ-14225; many trade names are available.

Storage/Stability

Captopril tablets should be stored in tight containers at temperatures not greater than 30°C.

Compatibility/Compounding Considerations

Compounded preparation stability: Captopril oral suspension compounded from commercially available tablets has been published (Allen et al. 1996). Triturating one (1) captopril 100 mg tablet with 65 mL of *Ora-Plus*® and *qs ad* to 134 mL with *Ora-Sweet*® (or *Ora-Sweet*® SF) yields a 0.75 mg/mL oral suspension that retains >90% potency for 14 days stored at 5°C and for 7 days at 25°C. Compounded preparations of captopril should be protected from light.

Dosage Forms/Regulatory Status

VETERINARY-LABELED PRODUCTS: NONE.

The ARCI (Racing Commissioners International) has designated this drug as a class 3 substance. See the appendix for more information.

HUMAN-LABELED PRODUCTS:

Captopril Oral Tablets: 12.5 mg, 25 mg, 50 mg, & 100 mg; *Capoten*®, generic; (Rx)

Revisions/References

Monograph revised/updated September 2013.
Allen, L. V. & M. A. Erickson (1996). Stability of baclofen, captopril, diltiazem hydrochloride, dipyridamole, and flecainide acetate in extemporaneously compounded oral liquids. *Am J Health Syst Pharm* 53(18): 2179-84.

Atkins, C. (2008). *Therapeutic advances in the management of heart disease: An overview.* Proceedings: World Veterinary Congress. accessed via Veterinary Information Network; vin.com

Bonagura, J. D. (1989). Cardiovascular Diseases. *The Cat: Diseases and Clinical Management.* R. G. Sherding. New York, Churchill Livingstone. 2: 649-86.

Carbamazepine

(Kar-bam-aye-zuh-peen)   Tegretol®

Dibenzazepine Anticonvulsant, Neuropathic Pain & Psychotherapeutic Agent

Prescriber Highlights

▶ Potentially useful for behavior disorders (aggression), neuropathic pain states, or epilepsy in dogs and cats.

▶ Very little information published on use, adverse effects, etc. for veterinary patients.

▶ Pharmacokinetic profile in dogs a serious roadblock for clinical use.

▶ Reportedly can be used successfully for photic head shaking in horses not responding to cyproheptadine.

▶ Many potential drug interactions.

Uses/Indications

Carbamazepine potentially could be useful for treating behavior disorders, neuropathic pain states, or epilepsy in dogs and cats, but its unfavorable pharmacokinetic profile in dogs is problematic. Despite this, there are sporadic case reports that it has had efficacy in dogs (aggression, psychomotor seizures) and it has been proposed that there may be an as of yet unidentified active metabolite in dogs that is more slowly eliminated. There is extremely scant information published on the use of this drug in cats, but it has been stated that it has had some efficacy in reducing aggression.

Until more information is available, carbamazepine should be considered as a 3rd-line agent for use in small animals, but if formulations can be developed to increase absorption and methods developed to reduce hepatic metabolism (*e.g.*, ketoconazole, grapefruit juice powder), its potential is intriguing.

In horses with photic head shaking, cyproheptadine is generally the drug of first choice, but carbamazepine has been used.

Pharmacology/Actions

Carbamazepine has a variety of pharmacological effects similar to drugs such as phenytoin in the central nervous system, including modulation of ion channels (sodium and calcium) and receptor-mediated neurotransmission (GABA, glutamate, monoamines). Its antiseizure effects are due primarily to limiting seizure propagation by reduction of post-tetanic potentiation (PTP) of synaptic transmission. It also has antiarrhythmic, antidiuretic, anticholinergic, antidepressant, sedative, muscle relaxant, and neuromuscular transmission-inhibitory actions, but only mild analgesic effects.

Carbamazepine has been shown to reduce electrical- and chemical-induced seizures in rats and mice. It appears to act by reducing polysynaptic responses and blocking the post-tetanic potentiation. Carbamazepine has been shown in cats and rats to reduce or block pain induced by stimulation of the infraorbital nerve. Also in cats, it depresses thalamic potential and bulbar and polysynaptic reflexes, including the linguomandibular reflex.

The principal metabolite of carbamazepine, carbamazepine-10,11-epoxide, also has anticonvulsant activity.

Pharmacokinetics

When compared to humans, carbamazepine is eliminated much more rapidly in dogs. Humans may eliminate carbamazepine and its active metabolite, carbamazepine-10,11-epoxide, up to 25 times more slowly then dogs.

The pharmacokinetics of carbamazepine were reported in the dog in 1980 (Frey et al. 1980). The drug was better absorbed when given as liquid preparation than from tablets. Elimination half-life was 1.5 hours for carbamazepine and 2.2 hours for carbamazepine-10,11-epoxide. However after dosing for a week, plasma concentrations showed a pronounced and progressive decline from Day 2 and the authors concluded that carbamazepine was not a suitable drug for treating epilepsy in dogs.

A study evaluating the pharmacokinetics of carbamazepine in the dog using a 2-hydroxypropyl-beta-cyclodextrin-based formulation administered orally and intravenously compared with oral commercially available tablets and suspensions was published (Brewster et al. 1997). They found that the oral bioavailability of tablets was low in dogs (around 28%) and that oral suspensions or solutions increased bioavailability. After IV dosing, volume of distribution (steady-state) was 0.58 L/kg, and elimination half-life of carbamazepine was 38 minutes and 110 minutes for the epoxide metabolite. Renal clearance was only 12 mL/min or about 4% of total body clearance. Elimination half-life after tablet administration was 116 minutes. As this was a single-dose study (with a 2-week washout period between doses), no effect of hepatic enzyme induction could be measured.

A study comparing the oral bioavailability of carbamazepine in a beta-cyclodextrin complex with hydroxymethylcellulose matrix tablets (sustained-release; *Tegretol® CR 200*) in 4 Beagles found that the experimentally produced beta-cyclodextrin complexes had higher bioavailability then the commercial product. However, there was significant inter-subject variability. The dose given to these dogs was approximately 20 mg/kg of the commercial sustained release tablets. At this dosage, peak levels occurred at approximately 1 hour after dosing and averaged 0.5 micrograms/mL. Elimination half-life was 46 minutes. No determination of any metabolites was measured in this study.

Contraindications/Precautions/Warnings

There is extremely limited information for carbamazepine's safety in animals; the following pertains to humans and may apply to veterinary patients: Carbamazepine is **contraindicated** in patients with a history of bone marrow depression; concomitant use of an MAO-I, or use within 14 days of discontinuing an MAOI or hypersensitivity to carbamazepine or tricyclic compounds. Use with caution in patients with significant hepatic dysfunction.

Potential drug interactions involving carbamazepine are numerous, but documentation for veterinary patients is very scant. Use with caution when patients are receiving other medications.

Adverse Effects

There is extremely limited information for carbamazepine's adverse effect profile in animals. In humans, adverse effects (dizziness, drowsiness, nausea, and vomiting) are often seen when therapy is begun and the drug is usually started at a low dosage and then increased as the patient tolerates. Serious adverse effects reported in humans are usually associated with the cardiovascular (AV block, CHF) or hematopoietic system (aplastic anemia, agranulocytosis), skin (TEN, Stevens-Johnson Syndrome), and hepatotoxicity.

Reproductive/Nursing Safety

Carbamazepine can cause teratogenic effects. The drug crosses the placenta readily and has been implicated in increased rates of congenital malformations in humans. The FDA lists carbamazepine as a category *D* drug (*There is evidence of human fetal risk, but the potential benefits from the use of the drug in pregnant women may be acceptable despite its potential risks.*)

While carbamazepine is excreted into maternal milk and has the potential for some risks to nursing offspring, it is generally considered compatible with breast-feeding in humans.

Overdosage/Acute Toxicity

Reported oral median lethal dose (LD_{50}) in animals: Mice: 1,100 to 3,750 mg/kg; Rats: 3,850 to 4,025 mg/kg; Rabbits: 1,500 to 2,680 mg/kg; Guinea pigs: 920 mg/kg. Overdose treatment consists of using decontamination protocols when appropriate, and supportive care. In the event of an overdose in a veterinary species, contact a veterinary poison control center for further guidance.

Drug Interactions

The following drug interactions have either been reported or are theoretical in humans or animals receiving carbamazepine and may be of significance in veterinary patients. Unless otherwise noted, use together is not necessarily contraindicated, but weigh the potential risks and perform additional monitoring when appropriate.

The following drugs may increase the plasma levels or effects of carbamazepine:

- ACETAZOLAMIDE
- AZOLE ANTIFUNGALS (*e.g.,* **ketaconazole, itraconazole**)
- CALCIUM CHANNEL BLOCKERS, (*e.g.,* **diltiazem, verapamil**)
- CIMETIDINE
- DANAZOL
- GRAPEFRUIT JUICE
- ISONIAZID
- MACROLIDES (*e.g.,* **erythromycin, clarithromycin**)
- MAO INHIBITORS (including **selegiline**): Contraindicated in humans; discontinue MAOI at least 14 days prior to carbamazepine.
- NIACIN
- SSRI ANTIDEPRESSANTS (**fluoxetine**, etc.)
- TRICYCLIC ANTIDEPRESSANTS (**clomipramine, amitriptyline**, etc.)
- VALPROIC ACID

The following drugs may decrease the plasma levels or effects of carbamazepine:

- BARBITURATES (*e.g.,* **phenobarbital**)
- CISPLATIN
- DOXORUBICIN
- FELBAMATE
- PHENYTOIN
- PRIMIDONE
- RIFAMPIN
- THEOPHYLLINE

Carbamazepine may increase the plasma levels or effects of the following drugs:

- CLOMIPRAMINE
- ISONIAZID

Carbamazepine (particularly after chronic therapy) may decrease the effect of the following drugs/drug classes by lowering their serum concentrations or pharmacological effects:

- ACETAMINOPHEN
- BENZODIAZEPINES
- BUPROPION
- BUSPRIONE
- CALCIUM CHANNEL BLOCKERS
- CYCLOSPORINE
- DOXYCYCLINE
- GLUCOCORTICOIDS
- ITRACONAZOLE
- LAMOTRIGINE
- LEVOTHYROXINE
- METHADONE
- METHOTREXATE
- MIRTAZAPINE
- NON-DEPOLARIZING MUSCLE BLOCKERS (*e.g.,* **atracurium**)
- PRAZIQUANTEL
- TOPIRAMATE
- TRAMADOL
- ZONISAMIDE
- TOPIRAMATE
- TRAZODONE
- TRICYCLIC ANTIDEPRESSANTS
- VALPROIC ACID (may also increase risk for phenobarbital toxicity)
- VERAPAMIL
- WARFARIN

Laboratory Considerations

- In humans, thyroid function tests have been reported to show decreased values and interference with some pregnancy tests has been reported. Veterinary significance is unclear.

Doses

- **DOGS:**

  As a psychotherapeutic agent (extra-label): 4 – 8 mg/kg PO q12h; not commonly used, but may have some utility in dogs that seem to have amygdalar hyperactivity; sometimes used in conjunction with SSRIs to control explosive aggression. (Haug 2008)

- **HORSES:**

  For photic head shaking (extra-label): 10 mg/kg PO q6h or 29 mg/kg PO q12h. May be helpful in some horses that do not respond to cyproheptadine. (Brooks 2008)

Monitoring

- Occasional CBC's and liver function tests are suggested.
- Clinical efficacy.

Client Information

- Many possible drug interactions; don't give other drugs to animal without first checking with your veterinarian.
- May require dosing multiple times per day.
- If using extended-release forms, do not crush.
- Pregnant women should handle this drug cautiously as it may cause birth defects.
- Report any adverse effects seen to the veterinarian.

Chemistry/Synonyms

Carbamazepine is a dibenzoazepine iminostilbene derivative and is chemically related to imipramine. It has the chemical name 5H-Dibenz[b,f]azepine-5-carboxamide and a molecular weight of 236.3. Carbamazepine is a white or off-white powder and is practically insoluble in water, but soluble in alcohol and in acetone.

Carbamazepine may also be known as G-32883, carbamazepine, carbamazepine, carbamazepinum, karbamatsepiini, karbamazepin, karbamazepinas, or karbamazepinum. Trade names include: *Tegretol®* and *Carbatrol®*.

Storage/Stability

Carbamazepine should be stored below 30°C (86°F) in airtight containers as humid conditions can reduce potency by up to one-third. Protect from light.

Compatibility/Compounding Considerations

Compounded preparation stability: Carbamazepine oral suspension compounded from commercially available tablets has been published (Burkart et al. 1981). Triturating one (1) carbamazepine 200 mg tablet with 5 mL simple syrup yields a 40 mg/mL oral suspension that retains >90% potency for 90 days stored at both 5°C and 25°C. Suspensions may separate over the 90 day storage period but can be re-suspended when shaken vigorously. Compounded preparations of carbamazepine should be protected from light.

Dosage Forms/Regulatory Status

VETERINARY-LABELED PRODUCTS: NONE.

HUMAN-LABELED PRODUCTS:

Carbamazepine Oral Tablets: 100 mg (regular and chewable) & 200 mg; *Tegretol®, Epitol®*, generic; (Rx)

Carbamazepine Oral Tablets or Capsules Extended-Release (12-hour): 100 mg, 200 mg, 400 mg; *Tegretol® XR; Carbatrol®, Equetro®*, generic; (Rx)

Carbamazepine Oral Suspension: 100 mg/5 mL (20 mg/mL); *Tegretol®*, generic; (Rx)

Revisions/References

Monograph revised/updated September 2013.

Brewster, M. E., et al. (1997). Intravenous and oral pharmacokinetic evaluation of a 2-hydroxypropyl-beta-cyclodextrin-based formulation of carbamazepine in the dog: Comparison with commercially available tablets and suspensions. *Journal of Pharmaceutical Sciences* **86**(3): 335-9.

Brooks, D. (2008). Photic Head Shaking. *Blackwell's Five-Minute Veterinary Consult: Equine 2nd Edition.* J.-P. Lavoie and K. W. Hinchcliff. Ames, IA, WIley-Blackwell: 590-1.

Burkart, G., et al. (1981). Stability of extemporaneous suspensions of carbamazepine. *Am J Hosp Pharm* **38**: 1929.

Frey, H. H. & W. Loscher (1980). Pharmacokinetics of carbamazepine in the dog. *Archives Internationales De Pharmacodynamie Et De Therapie* **243**(2): 180-91.

Haug, L. (2008). Canine aggression toward unfamiliar people and dogs. *Vet Clin NA: Sm Anim Pract* **38**: 1023-41.

Carbimazole

(kar-bi-ma-zole)   Neo-Carbimazole®, Carbazole®

Anti-Thyroid

Note: *This drug is not available in the USA, but is routinely used in Europe and elsewhere in place of methimazole.*

Prescriber Highlights

▶ Used outside of USA & Canada for medical treatment of feline hyperthyroidism.

▶ Contraindications/Cautions: Hypersensitive to carbimazole; not recommended in cats intolerant to methimazole; history of, or concurrent hematologic abnormalities, liver disease or autoimmune disease.

▶ Adverse Effects: Most occur within first 3 months of treatment; vomiting, anorexia & depression most frequent. Eosinophilia, leukopenia, & lymphocytosis are usually transient. Rare, but serious: self-induced excoriations, bleeding, hepatopathy, thrombocytopenia, agranulocytosis, positive direct antiglobulin test, & acquired myasthenia gravis.

▶ Dosing requirements may change with time.

▶ Place kittens on milk replacer if mother receiving carbimazole.

▶ Unlike methimazole, has no bitter taste. Give with food.

▶ Potentially efficacious when used transdermally in cats.

Uses/Indications

Carbimazole (a pro-drug of methimazole) or methimazole are considered by most clinicians to be the agents of choice when using drugs to treat feline hyperthyroidism. Propylthiouracil has significantly higher incidences of adverse reactions when compared to methimazole.

Methimazole and therefore, carbimazole, may be useful for the prophylactic prevention of cisplatin-induced nephrotoxicity in dogs.

Pharmacology/Actions

Carbimazole is converted almost entirely to methimazole *in vivo*. Methimazole inhibits thyroid peroxidase thereby interfering with iodine incorporation into tyrosyl residues of thyroglobulin and inhibiting the synthesis of thyroid hormones. It also inhibits iodinated tyrosyl residues from coupling to form iodothyronine. Methimazole has no effect on the release or activity of thyroid hormones already formed or in the general circulation.

Pharmacokinetics

Carbimazole is rapidly absorbed from the GI tract and rapidly and nearly totally converted to methimazole. Because of differences in molar weight, to attain an equivalent serum level, carbimazole must be dosed approximately 2 times that of methimazole.

In cats, the volume of distribution of methimazole is variable (0.12 – 0.84 L/kg). Methimazole apparently concentrates in thyroid tissue and biologic effects persist beyond measurable blood levels. After oral dosing, plasma elimination half-life ranges from 2.3-10.2 hours. There is usually a 1-3 week lag time between starting the drug and significant reductions in serum T4. Timed-release formulations of carbimazole can extend methimazole (active metabolite) half-life and allow once daily dosing. Carbimazole may be amenable for use transdermally in cats to control hyperthyroidism.

In dogs, methimazole has a serum half-life of 8-9 hours.

Contraindications/Precautions/Warnings

Carbimazole is contraindicated in patients that are hypersensitive to it or methimazole. It should be used very cautiously in patients with a history of or concurrent hematologic abnormalities, liver disease or autoimmune disease.

Because carbimazole is a prodrug and is converted into methimazole, cats that have had prior serious reactions to methimazole should receive carbimazole with great caution.

Adverse Effects

Adverse effects are reported less often with carbimazole than methimazole. Whether they indeed occur less frequently is debatable. Most adverse effects associated with carbimazole or methimazole use in cats occur within the first three months of therapy with vomiting, anorexia and depression occurring most frequently. The GI effects may be related to the drug's bitter taste and are usually transient. Eosinophilia, leukopenia, and lymphocytosis may be noted in approximately 15% of cats treated within the first 8 weeks of therapy. These hematologic effects usually are also transient and generally do not require drug withdrawal. Other more serious but rare adverse effects include: self-induced excoriations (2.3%), bleeding (2.3%), hepatopathy (1.5%), thrombocytopenia (2.7%), agranulocytosis (1.5%), and positive direct antiglobulin test (1.9%). These effects generally require withdrawal of the drug and adjunctive therapy. Up to 50% of cats receiving methimazole chronically (>6 months), will develop a positive ANA, which requires dosage reduction. Rarely, cats will develop an acquired myasthenia gravis that requires either withdrawal or concomitant glucocorticoid therapy.

Potentially, treatment with methimazole or carbimazole could precipitate renal dysfunction in some cats. The hyperthyroid state may increase GFR and expedite elimination of nitrogenous waste. By treating the hyperthyroidism this effect could be abolished.

High levels of methimazole cross the placenta and may induce hypothyroidism in kittens born of queens receiving the drug. Levels higher than those found in plasma are found in human breast milk. It is suggested that kittens be placed on a milk replacer after receiving colostrum from mothers on methimazole.

Reproductive/Nursing Safety

Carbimazole, like methimazole (carbimazole is converted to methimazole), has been associated with teratogenic effects in humans (scalp defects). It may also affect offspring thyroid development or function. In humans, the FDA categorizes methimazole as category D for use during pregnancy (*There is evidence of human fetal risk, but the potential benefits from the use of the drug in pregnant women may be acceptable despite its potential risks.*)

As methimazole can enter milk and have deleterious effects on offspring, switch to milk replacer if carbimazole or methimazole are required for nursing dams.

Overdosage

Acute toxicity that may be seen with overdosage include those that are listed above under Adverse Effects. Agranulocytosis, hepatopathy, and thrombocytopenias are perhaps the most serious effects that may be seen. Treatment consists of following standard protocols in handling an oral ingestion (empty stomach if not contraindicated, administer charcoal, etc.) and to treat symptomatically and supportively.

Drug Interactions

The following drug interactions have either been reported or are theoretical in humans or animals receiving carbimazole and may be of significance in veterinary patients. Unless otherwise noted, use together is not necessarily contraindicated, but weigh the potential risks and perform additional monitoring when appropriate.

- **BUPROPION**: Potential for increased risk for hepatotoxicity; increased monitoring (LFT's) necessary.
- **DIGOXIN**: Carbimazole may decrease digoxin efficacy.
- **FENBENDAZOLE**: Carbimazole may increase blood levels.
- **PHENOBARBITAL**: May decrease carbimazole efficacy.
- **WARFARIN**: Potential for decreased anticoagulant efficacy if carbimazole added.

Laboratory Considerations

- **FRUCTOSAMINE, SERUM**: Methimazole and carbimazole may affect serum fructosamine levels in diabetic cats; increased serum fructosamine after 6 weeks of treatment has been reported. It has been recommended that serum fructosamine not be used to initially diagnose or assess the adequacy of diabetic control in cats with concurrent hyperthyroidism until hyperthyroidism is controlled for at least six weeks (Bruyette 2012).

Doses

Note: See also Methimazole. Usually, carbimazole dosages are twice that of methimazole.

- **CATS:**

  For hyperthyroidism:

  a) **Regular Tablets** (extra-label): Most dosage recommendations (anecdotal) are initially 5 mg PO 2-3 times a day. Once euthyroid state is established the dosage amount or frequency given is titrated downward. Most cats will require 2.5 – 5 mg PO twice daily, but some can be controlled on once a day dosing.

  b) **Sustained-Release Tablets** (labeled dose U.K.; extra-label in the USA): Using the sustained-release tablets (*Vidalta®*) 15 mg PO once daily at the same time each day; food increase absorption. 10 mg PO once daily can be considered for cats with moderate hyperthyroidism (total T4 between 50-100 nmol/L; 3.9-7.8 mcg/dL). Do not break or crush tabs. Adjust dose upwards or downwards within a range of 10 mg – 25 mg per day in 5 mg increments depending on clinical signs and TT4 (tablets cannot be split, so combinations of 10 mg and 15 mg tablets must be used). If cat requires doses less than 10 mg per day, use alternative treatment. (Adapted from label information; *Vidalta®*— MSD U.K.)

Monitoring

During first 3 months of therapy (baseline values and every 2-3 weeks):
- CBC, platelet counts.
- Serum T4.
- Serum creatine.
- If indicated by clinical signs: liver function tests, ANA.

After stabilized (at least 3 months of therapy):
- T4 at 3-6 month intervals.
- Other diagnostic tests as dictated by adverse effects.

Client Information

- It must be stressed to owners that this drug will decrease excessive thyroid hormones, but does not cure the condition.
- Adherence with the treatment regimen is necessary for success.
- Give with food.
- Watch for lethargy (tiredness), vomiting, lack of appetite, jaundice (yellowing of whites of the eyes), or itching. If any of these occur, stop giving the drug and contact veterinarian.

Chemistry/Synonyms

A thioimidazole-derivative antithyroid drug, carbimazole occurs as a white to creamy white powder having a characteristic odor. It is slightly soluble in water and soluble in alcohol.

Carbimazole may also be known as: carbimazolum, *Basolest®*, *Camazol®*, *Carbimazole®*, *Carbazole®*, *Carbistad®*, *Cazole®*, *Neo Tomizol®*, *Neo-Mercazole®*, *Neo-Thyreostat®*, *Thyrostat®*, *Tyrazol®*, *Vidalta®* or *Neo-morphazole®*.

Storage/Stability

Unless otherwise labeled, carbimazole tablets should be stored at room temperature in well-closed containers.

Compatibility/Compounding Considerations

No specific information noted.

Dosage Forms/Regulatory Status

VETERINARY-LABELED PRODUCTS: NONE IN USA.

In some countries: Carbimazole Oral Sustained-Release Tablets: 10 mg & 15 mg; *Vidalta®*; POM-V in the U.K.

HUMAN-LABELED PRODUCTS:

There are no FDA-approved products in the USA; elsewhere it may be available as: Carbimazole Oral Tablets: 5 mg & 20 mg. Trade names include *Neo-Carbimazole®*, *Carbazole®*, *Neo Mercazole®*, etc.

Revisions/References

Monograph revised/updated September 2013.

Bruyette, D. (2012). *Feline Hyperthyroidism: Diagnosis and Treatment,* Proceedings: Atlantic Coast Veterinary Conference. accessed via Veterinary Information Network; vin.com

Carboplatin

(kar-boe-pla-tin)   Paraplatin®

Antineoplastic

Prescriber Highlights

▶ Platinum antineoplastic agent used for a variety of carcinomas & sarcomas.

▶ Unlike cisplatin, may be used in cats.

▶ Contraindications: History of hypersensitivity to it or other platinum agents; severe bone marrow depression; fetotoxic. Caution: Hepatic/renal disease, hearing impairment, active infection.

▶ Primary adverse effects: GI, Bone marrow depression. Nadir (neutrophils/platelets) in dogs about 14 days; in cats (neutrophils) about 17-21 days.

▶ Must be given IV in D5W.

▶ May adversely affect vaccinations (safety/efficacy).

▶ Treatment may be very expensive.

Uses/Indications

Like cisplatin, carboplatin may be useful in a variety of veterinary neoplastic diseases including squamous cell carcinomas, ovarian carcinomas, mediastinal carcinomas, pleural adenocarcinomas, nasal carcinomas and thyroid adenocarcinomas. Carboplatin's primary use currently in small animal medicine is in the adjunctive treatment (post amputation) of osteogenic sarcomas. Its effectiveness in treating transitional cell carcinoma of the bladder has been disappointing; however, intra-arterial administration with NSAID (*e.g.*, meloxicam, etc.) may prove to enhance efficacy. Intracavitary carboplatin for recurrent idiopathic or malignant pleural effusion after pericardectomy holds promise.

Carboplatin, unlike cisplatin, appears to be relatively safe for use in cats.

Carboplatin may be considered for intralesional use in conditions such as equine sarcoids or in treating adenocarcinoma in birds.

Whether carboplatin is more efficacious than cisplatin for certain cancers does not appear to be decided at this point, but the drug does appear to have fewer adverse effects (less renal toxicity and reduced vomiting) in dogs.

Pharmacology/Actions

Carboplatin's exact mechanism of action is not fully understood. Both carboplatin's and cisplatin's properties are analogous to those of bifunctional alkylating agents producing inter- and intrastrand crosslinks in DNA, thereby inhibiting DNA replication, RNA transcription, and protein synthesis. Carboplatin is cell-cycle nonspecific.

Pharmacokinetics

After IV administration, carboplatin is well distributed throughout the body; highest concentrations are found in the liver, kidney, skin and tumor tissue. The metabolic fate and elimination of carboplatin are complex and the discussion of this aspect of the drug's pharmacokinetics is beyond the scope of this reference. Suffice it to say, the parent drug degrades into platinum and platinum-complexed compounds that are primarily eliminated by kidneys. In dogs, almost one half of the dose is excreted in the urine within 24 hours and approximately 70% of the platinum administered is secreted in the urine after 72 hours.

Contraindications/Precautions/Warnings

Carboplatin is contraindicated in patients hypersensitive to it or other platinum-containing compounds. It is also contraindicated in patients with severe bone marrow suppression. Patients with severe carboplatin-induced myelosuppression should be allowed to recover their counts before additional therapy.

Caution is advised in patients with active infections, hearing impairment or preexisting renal or hepatic disease.

Do not give carboplatin IM or SC.

It has been anecdotally reported that small dogs may be more susceptible to developing adverse effects from carboplatin.

Do not confuse carboplatin with cisplatin. Consider using tall man lettering when writing orders or prescriptions: CARBOplatin; CISplatin.

Adverse Effects

Established adverse effects in dogs include anorexia and/or vomiting and diarrhea that usually occur 2-4 days after a dose, and dose-related bone marrow suppression that is exhibited primarily as thrombocytopenia and/or neutropenia. The nadir of platelet and neutrophil counts generally occur about 14 days post treatment in dogs. Recovery is generally seen by day 21. In cats, thrombocytopenia occurs infrequently, but the neutrophil nadir occurs about 21 days post treatment. Recovery usually occurs by day 28 in cats. In dogs, lithium carbonate did not prevent carboplatin-induced thrombocytopenia (Leclerc et al. 2010). One case of a dog developing a cutaneous delayed hypersensitivity reaction has been reported (Lanore et al. 2010). Nephrotoxicity is uncommon, but can occur in dogs or cats.

Hepatotoxicity (increased serum bilirubin and liver enzymes) is seen in about 15% of human patients treated with carboplatin. Other potential adverse effects include: nephrotoxicity, neuropathies and ototoxicity. These effects occur with carboplatin therapy much less frequently than with cisplatin therapy. Anaphylactoid reactions have been reported rarely in humans that have received platinum-containing compounds (*e.g.*, cisplatin). Hyperuricemia may occur after therapy in a small percentage of patients.

Reproductive/Nursing Safety

Carboplatin is fetotoxic and embryotoxic in rats and the risks of its use during pregnancy should be weighed with its potential benefits. In humans, the FDA categorizes this drug as category *D* for use during pregnancy (*There is evidence of human fetal risk, but the potential benefits from the use of the drug in pregnant women may be acceptable despite its potential risks.*)

It is unknown whether carboplatin enters maternal milk. In humans, it is recommended to discontinue nursing if the mother is receiving the drug.

Overdosage/Acute Toxicity

There is limited information available. An overdose of carboplatin would be expected to cause aggravated effects associated with the drug's bone marrow nephro- and liver toxicity. Monitor for neurotoxicity, ototoxicity, hepatotoxicity and nephrotoxicity.

Treatment is basically supportive; no specific antidote is available. Plasmapheresis or hemodialysis could potentially be of benefit in removing the drug.

Drug Interactions

The following drug interactions have either been reported or are theoretical in humans or animals receiving carboplatin and may be of significance in veterinary patients. Unless otherwise noted, use together is not necessarily contraindicated, but weigh the potential risks and perform additional monitoring when appropriate.

■ **AMINOGLYCOSIDES:** Potential for increased risk of nephrotoxicity or ototoxicity.

■ **CISPLATIN:** Human patients previously treated with cisplatin have an increased risk of developing neurotoxicity or ototoxicity after receiving carboplatin.

- **MYLEOSUPPRESSIVE DRUGS:** The leukopenic or thrombocytopenic effects secondary to carboplatin may be enhanced by other myelosuppressive medications.
- **RADIATION THERAPY:** Potential for increased hematologic toxicity.
- **VACCINES:** Live or killed virus vaccines administered after carboplatin therapy may not be as effective as the immune response to these vaccines may be modified by carboplatin therapy; carboplatin may also potentiate live virus vaccines replication and increase the adverse effects associated with these vaccines.

Doses

Note: Because of the potential toxicity of this drug to patients, veterinary personnel and clients, and since chemotherapy indications, treatment protocols, monitoring and safety guidelines often change, the following dosages should be used only as a general guide. Consultation with a veterinary oncologist and referral to current veterinary oncology references [*e.g.*, (Withrow et al. 2012); (Dobson et al. 2011); (Henry et al. 2009); (North et al. 2009); (Argyle et al. 2008)] are <u>strongly recommended</u>.

Do not confuse cisplatin and carboplatin dosages; cisplatin dosages are much lower.

The following is a usual dosage (dosage may need adjustment in patients with reduced renal function) or dose range for carboplatin and should be used only as a general guide:

Dogs: 300 – 350 mg/m^2 IV every 3 weeks.

Cats and Rabbits: 180 – 260 mg/m^2 IV every 3 weeks. It has also been administered intratumorally in cats for nasal planum carcinomas.

Monitoring

- CBC. Often, if neutrophil count is less than 3,000 per microliter the dose is held.
- Serum electrolytes, uric acid.
- Baseline and ongoing renal and hepatic function tests.

Client Information

- Care should be taken to avoid contact with the administration site.
- Carboplatin is a chemotherapy (cancer) drug. The drug and its byproducts can be hazardous to other animals and people that come in contact with it. On the day your animal gets the drug and then for a few days afterward, all bodily waste (urine, feces), blood, or vomit should only be handled while wearing disposable gloves. Seal the waste in a plastic bag and then place both the bag and gloves in with the regular trash.

Chemistry/Synonyms

Carboplatin, like cisplatin, is a platinum-containing antineoplastic agent. It occurs as white to off-white crystalline powder having a solubility of 14 mg/mL in water and is insoluble in alcohol. The commercially available powder for injection contains equal parts of mannitol and carboplatin. After reconstitution with sterile water for injection, a resulting solution of 10 mg/mL of carboplatin has a pH of 5-7 and an osmolality of 94 mOsm/kg.

Carboplatin may also be known as: cis-Diammine-1,1-cyclobutanedicarboxylato-platinum, carboplatinum; CBDCA; JM-8; or NSC-241240; many trade names are available.

Storage/Stability

The powder for injection should kept stored at room temperature and protected from light.

After reconstitution, solutions containing 10 mg/mL are stable for at least 8 hours. Some sources say that the solution is stable for up to 24 hours and can be refrigerated, but because there are no preservatives in the solution, the manufacturer recommends discarding unused portions after 8 hours. Previous recommendations to avoid the use of solutions to dilute carboplatin containing sodium chloride are no longer warranted as only a minimal amount of carboplatin is converted to cisplatin in these solutions.

Because aluminum can displace platinum from carboplatin, the solution should not be prepared, stored or administered where aluminum-containing items can come into contact with the solution. Should carboplatin come into contact with aluminum, a black precipitate will form and the product should not be used.

Compatibility/Compounding Considerations

Directions for reconstitution for the 50 mg vial: Add 5 mL of either sterile water for injection, normal saline injection or D5W that will provide a solution containing 10 mg/mL. May infuse directly (usually over 15 minutes) or further dilute. Visually inspect after reconstitution/dilution for discoloration or particulate matter.

Dosage Forms/Regulatory Status

VETERINARY-LABELED PRODUCTS: NONE.

HUMAN-LABELED PRODUCTS:

Carboplatin lyophilized Powder for reconstitution and IV Injection: 50 mg, 150 mg, 450 mg & 600 mg in single-dose vials (contains mannitol); generic; (Rx)

Carboplatin Injection: 10 mg/mL in 15 mL single-use vials; generic; (Rx)

Revisions/References

Monograph revised/updated September 2013.

Argyle, D., et al. (2008). *Decision Making in Small Animal Oncology*, Wiley-Blackwell.
Dobson, J. & D. Lascelles (2011). *BSAVA Manual of Canine and Feline Oncology*, BSAVA.
Henry, C. & M. Higginbotham (2009). *Cancer Management in Small Animal Practice*, Saunders.
Lanore, D. & D. Sayag (2010). Probable cutaneous hypersensitivity to carboplatin single-agent chemotherapy in a dog. *Journal of Small Animal Practice* 51(12): 654-6.
Leclerc, A., et al. (2010). Effects of lithium carbonate on carboplatin-induced thrombocytopenia in dogs. *American Journal of Veterinary Research* 71(5): 555-63.
North, S. & T. Banks (2009). *Small Animal Oncology: An Introduction*, Saunders.
Withrow, S., et al. (2012). *Withrow and MacEwen's Small Animal Clinical Oncology, 5th Ed.*, Saunders.

Carnitine
Levocarnitine
L-Carnitine

(kar-ni-teen)   Carnitor®

Nutrient

Prescriber Highlights

▶ Nutrient required for normal fat utilization & energy metabolism.
▶ May be useful in certain cardiomyopathies (including doxorubicin induced) in dogs.
▶ Use only L (levo-) forms. Expense can be an issue.
▶ Preferably give with meals.

Uses/Indications

Levocarnitine may potentially be useful as adjunctive therapy of dilated cardiomyopathy in dogs. Up to 90% of dogs with dilated cardiomyopathy may have a carnitine deficiency. American Cocker spaniels, Boxers, English bulldogs, Dalmatians, dogs with cysteine or urate urolithiasis, and dilated cardiomyopathy may all especially benefit. Any breed with dilated cardiomyopathy may receive a trial of the drug as approximately 5% will respond.

Levocarnitine may also protect against doxorubicin-induced cardiomyopathy and reduce risks of myocardial infarction and may be beneficial in the adjunctive treatment of valproic acid toxicity.

In cats, levocarnitine has been recommended as being useful as an adjunctive therapy in feline hepatic lipidosis by facilitating hepatic lipid metabolism. Its use for this indication is somewhat controversial.

Pharmacology/Actions

Levocarnitine is required for normal fat utilization and energy metabolism in mammalian species. It serves to facilitate entry of long-chain fatty acids into cellular mitochondria where they can be used during oxidation and energy production.

Severe chronic deficiency is generally a result of an inborn genetic defect where levocarnitine utilization is impaired and not the result of dietary insufficiency. Effects seen in levocarnitine deficiency may include hypoglycemia, progressive myasthenia, hepatomegaly, CHF, cardiomegaly, hepatic coma, neurologic disturbances, encephalopathy, hypotonia and lethargy.

Pharmacokinetics

In humans, levocarnitine is absorbed via the GI with a bioavailability of about 15%, but is absorbed rapidly in the intestine via passive and active mechanisms. Highest levels of levocarnitine are found in skeletal muscle. Levocarnitine is distributed in milk. Exogenously administered levocarnitine is eliminated by both renal and fecal routes. Plasma levocarnitine levels may be increased in patients with renal failure.

Contraindications/Precautions/Warnings

Levocarnitine may also be known as carnitine or Vitamin B$_T$. Products labeled as such may have both D and L racemic forms. Use only Levo- (L-) forms as the D- form may competitively inhibit L- uptake with a resulting deficiency.

Adverse Effects

Adverse effect profile is minimal. Gastrointestinal upset is the most likely effect that may be noted and usually associated with high dosages. GI effects are usually mild and limited to loose stools or possibly diarrhea; nausea and vomiting are possible. Human patients have reported increased body odor.

Reproductive/Nursing Safety

Studies done in rats and rabbits have demonstrated no teratogenic effects and it is generally believed that levocarnitine is safe for use in pregnancy though documented safety during pregnancy has not been established. In humans, the FDA categorizes this drug as category *B* for use during pregnancy (*Animal studies have not yet demonstrated risk to the fetus, but there are no adequate studies in pregnant women; or animal studies have shown an adverse effect, but adequate studies in pregnant women have not demonstrated a risk to the fetus in the first trimester of pregnancy, and there is no evidence of risk in later trimesters.*)

Overdosage/Acute Toxicity

Levocarnitine is a relatively safe drug. Minor overdoses need only to be monitored; with massive overdoses consider gut emptying. Refer to a poison control center for more information.

Drug Interactions

The following drug interactions have either been reported or are theoretical in humans or animals receiving levocarnitine and may be of significance in veterinary patients. Unless otherwise noted, use together is not necessarily contraindicated, but weigh the potential risks and perform additional monitoring when appropriate.

- **VALPROIC ACID:** Patients receiving valproic acid may require higher dosages of levocarnitine.

Doses

- **DOGS:**

For myocardial carnitine deficiency associated with dilated cardiomyopathy (extra-label):

a) For boxers with severe myocardial failure: Give 2 – 3 grams carnitine PO q12h for 2-4 months to determine if they respond. (Kittleson 2006)

b) For adjunctive treatment of American cocker spaniels with dilated cardiomyopathy: Carnitine 1 g PO q12h with taurine 500 mg q12h PO. (Kittleson 2006)

c) For cardiac indications (dilated cardiomyopathy) when carnitine supplementation may benefit: American Cocker spaniels: 1 g PO q8h. Boxer dogs with dilated cardiomyopathy: 2 g PO q8h. Documented systemic carnitine deficiency: 50 – 100 mg/kg PO q8h. Myocardial carnitine deficiency only: 200 mg/kg PO q8h. (Smith 2009)

- **CATS:**

As adjunctive dietary therapy in cats with severe hepatic lipidosis (extra-label):

a) 250 mg PO once daily (use *Carnitor®*); also supplement with taurine (250 mg once to twice daily), Vitamin E (10 Units/kg/day), water soluble vitamins and determine B12 status (treat while awaiting data at 1 mg/cat SC). See also Acetylcysteine. (Center 2006)

b) For supplementation in cats with liver disease: 250 – 500 mg/day. (Zoran 2006)

Monitoring

- Efficacy.
- Periodic blood chemistries have been recommended for human patients; their value in veterinary medicine is undetermined.

Client Information

- Usually causes no side effects but when giving larger doses vomiting or diarrhea can occur. Giving it with food may help.
- If using a powder form, mix into food.
- Do NOT use any carnitine product that contains D-carnitine; use only L-carnitine.
- Most dogs that respond to carnitine therapy for dilated cardiomyopathy will require other medication to control clinical signs.

Chemistry/Synonyms

Levocarnitine (the L-isomer of carnitine) is an amino acid derivative, synthesized *in vivo* from methionine and lysine. It is required for energy metabolism and has a molecular weight of 161.

Carnitine may also be known as: vitamin B(T), L-carnitine, or levocarnitinum; many trade names are available.

Storage/Stability

Levocarnitine capsules, tablets and powder should be stored in well-closed containers at room temperature. The oral solution should be kept in tight containers at room temperature. The injection should be stored at room temperature in the original carton; discard any unused portion after opening, as the injection contains no preservative.

Compatibility/Compounding Considerations

No specific information noted.

Dosage Forms/Regulatory Status

VETERINARY-LABELED PRODUCTS: NONE.

HUMAN-LABELED PRODUCTS:

Levocarnitine Oral Tablets: 330 mg & 500 mg; *Carnitor®*, generic; (Rx & OTC)

Levocarnitine or L-Carnitine Oral Capsules: 250 mg; generic; (OTC—as a food supplement)

Levocarnitine Oral Solution: 100 mg/mL in 118 mL; *Carnitor®*, generic; (Rx)

Levocarnitine Injection: 200 mg/mL in single-dose vials & preservative-free in single-dose vials and amps; *Carnitor®*, generic; (Rx)

Note: L-carnitine may also be available in bulk powder form from local health food stores.

Revisions/References

Monograph revised/updated September 2013.

Center, S. (2006). *Treatment for Severe Feline Hepatic Lipidosis*. Proceedings: WSAVA. accessed via Veterinary Information Network; vin.com

Kittleson, M. (2006). "Chapt 10: Management of Heart Failure." *Small Animal Cardiology, 2nd Ed.*

Smith, F. (2009). *Alternative therapies for the cardiac diseases*. Proceedings: WVC. accessed via Veterinary Information Network; vin.com

Zoran, D. (2006). *Inflammatory liver disease in cats*. Proceedings: ABVP 2006. accessed via Veterinary Information Network; vin.com

Carprofen

(kar-pro-fen)   Rimadyl®, quellin®

Non-Steroidal Antiinflammatory Agent

Prescriber Highlights

► NSAID used in dogs & other small animals.
► Contraindicated in dogs with bleeding disorders (*e.g.*, Von Willebrand's), history of serious reactions to it or other propionic-class NSAIDs.
► Caution: Geriatric patients or those with preexisting chronic diseases (*e.g.*, inflammatory bowel disease, renal or hepatic insufficiency).
► GI adverse effects are less likely than with older NSAIDs, but can occur.
► Rarely may cause hepatic failure; monitor liver enzymes.

Uses/Indications

Carprofen is labeled (in the USA) for the relief of pain and inflammation in dogs. An evaluation of the literature, concluded that the current evidence suggests that there is a clinical benefit of longer-term (>28 days) NSAID use for dogs with chronic osteoarthritis and that this is associated with a low risk of serious adverse events (Innes et al. 2010). Carprofen potentially could be useful as an adjunctive treatment of certain neoplasias.

Carprofen may also be of benefit in other species as well, but data is scant to support its safety beyond very short-term use at this time, especially in cats. In Europe, carprofen is registered for use in cattle and single dose use in cats, but there have been reported problems (*e.g.*, vomiting) with cats receiving more than a single dose.

Carprofen is being investigated for antineoplastic effects in dogs and may be a useful adjunctive treatment for some types of tumors with COX-2 overexpression.

Pharmacology/Actions

Like other NSAIDs, carprofen exhibits analgesic, antiinflammatory, and antipyretic activity probably through its inhibition of cyclooxygenase, phospholipase A_2 and inhibition of prostaglandin synthesis. Carprofen appears to be more sparing of COX-1 *in vitro* and in dogs appears to have fewer COX-1 effects (GI distress/ulceration, platelet inhibition, renal damage) when compared to older non-COX-2 specific agents. COX-2 specificity appears to be species, dose, and tissue dependent. Carprofen in horses or cats does not seem to be as COX-2 specific as it is in dogs.

Pharmacokinetics

When administered orally to dogs, carprofen is approximately 90% bioavailable. Peak serum levels occur between 1-3 hours post dosing. The drug is highly bound to plasma proteins (99%) and has a low volume of distribution (0.12 – 0.22 L/kg). Carprofen is extensively metabolized in the liver primarily via glucuronidation and oxidative processes. About 70-80% of a dose is eliminated in the feces; 10-20% eliminated in the urine. Some enterohepatic recycling of the drug occurs.

Elimination half-life of carprofen in the dog is approximately 8 hours with the S form having a longer half-life than the R form. The half-life of carprofen is reportedly 22 hours in horses and averages 20 hours in cats, but interpatient variability is very high in cats (9-49 hours). Half-life is not necessarily a good predictor of duration of effect, as the drug's high affinity for tissue proteins may act as a reservoir for the drug at inflamed tissue.

In cattle, carprofen shows age dependent pharmacokinetics. Calves less than 10 weeks old have an approximate half-life of 50 hours, while half-life is about 30 hours after subcutaneous administration to adult cattle.

Contraindications/Precautions/Warnings

Carprofen is contraindicated in dogs with bleeding disorders (*e.g.*, Von Willebrand's) or those that have had prior serious reactions to it or other propionic-class antiinflammatory agents. It should be used with caution in geriatric patients or those with preexisting chronic diseases (*e.g.*, inflammatory bowel disease, renal or hepatic insufficiency, etc.).

The manufacturer states that the safe use of carprofen in dogs less than 6 weeks of age, pregnant dogs, dogs used for breeding purposes, or lactating bitches has not been established.

Adverse Effects

Although adverse effects appear to be uncommon with carprofen use in dogs, they can occur. Mild gastrointestinal effects (*e.g.*, vomiting, diarrhea, inappetence, etc.) or lethargy are the most likely to appear but incidence is low (<2%). Rarely, serious effects including hepatocellular damage and/or renal disease; hematologic and serious gastrointestinal effects (ulceration) have been reported. Increased risks for the development of renal toxicity include preexisting renal insufficiency, dehydration or sodium depletion.

Reported incidence of hepatopathy is approximately 0.05% or less in dogs. It has been postulated that this adverse effect could be caused by formation of reactive acyl glucuronide metabolites that bind to and form haptites on hepatocytes; an immunological reaction then occurs causing hepatotoxicity. Geriatric dogs or dogs with chronic diseases (*e.g.*, inflammatory bowel disease, renal or hepatic insufficiency, etc.) may be at greater risk for developing hepatic toxicity while receiving this drug, but the effect may be idiosyncratic and unpredictable. Although not proven statistically significant, Labrador Retrievers have been associated with 1/4 of the initially reported cases associated with the reported hepatic syndrome; but it is not believed that this breed has any greater chance of developing this adverse effect than others. Before initiating therapy, pre-treatment patient evaluation and discussion with the owner regarding the potential risks versus benefits of therapy are advised. Rare, case reports of neutrophilic dermatosis (Sweet's syndrome) have been reported.

Carprofen has been used in cats, but as cats have limited ability hepatically to glucuronidate there is a greater potential for drug accumulation with resultant adverse effects. In particular, cats appear to be more susceptible to developing renal adverse effects from NSAIDs. Prolonged administration of carprofen in cats has also caused gastrointestinal effects. Hepatotoxicity does not appear to be a significant concern with NSAID use in cats, perhaps since they do not form significant amounts of glucuronidated metabolites.

Reproductive/Nursing Safety

The manufacturer states that the safe use of carprofen in dogs less than 6 weeks of age, pregnant dogs, dogs used for breeding purposes, or lactating bitches has not been established. Carprofen has been given to pregnant rats at dosages of up to 20 mg/kg during day 7-15 of gestation. While no teratogenic effects were noted in pups, the drug did delay parturition with an increased number of dead pups at birth.

Overdosage/Acute Toxicity

In dog toxicologic studies, repeated doses of up to 10X resulted in little adversity. Some dogs exhibited hypoalbuminemia, melena or slight increases in ALT. However, post-marketing surveillance suggests that there may be significant interpatient variability in response to acute or chronic overdoses. According to the APCC database, vomiting has been reported at doses as low as 5.3 mg/kg in dogs and 3.9 mg/kg in cats. The APCC level of concern for renal damage is 50 mg/kg in dogs and 8 mg/kg in cats.

There were 4341 single agent exposures to carprofen reported to the ASPCA Animal Poison Control Center (APCC) during 2009-2013. Of the 3795 dogs, 757 were symptomatic with 62% vomiting, 14% lethargic, 12% with diarrhea, 8% anorexic, 7% with elevated liver enzymes and 5% with elevated kidney values. Of the 607 cats, 90 were symptomatic with 59% vomiting, 19% anorexic, 18% lethargic, 14% azotemic and 9% with diarrhea.

This medication is a NSAID. As with any NSAID, overdosage can lead to gastrointestinal and renal effects. Decontamination with emetics and/or activated charcoal is appropriate. For doses where GI effects are expected, the use of gastrointestinal protectants is warranted. If renal effects are also expected, fluid diuresis is warranted.

Drug Interactions

Note: Although the manufacturer does not list any specific drug interactions in the package insert, it does caution to avoid or closely monitor carprofen's use with other ulcerogenic drugs (*e.g.,* **corticosteroids** or other **NSAIDs**). While some advocate a multi-day washout period when switching from one NSAID to another (not aspirin—see below), there does not appear to be any credible evidence that this is required. Until so, consider starting the new NSAID when the next dose would be due for the old one.

The following drug interactions have either been reported or are theoretical in humans or animals receiving carprofen and may be of significance in veterinary patients. Unless otherwise noted, use together is not necessarily contraindicated, but weigh the potential risks and perform additional monitoring when appropriate.

- **ACE INHIBITORS** (*e.g.,* **benazepril, enalapril**, etc.): Because ACE inhibitors potentially can reduce renal blood flow, use with NSAIDs could increase the risk for renal injury. However, one study in dogs receiving tepoxalin did not show any adverse effect. It is unknown what effects, if any, occur if other NSAIDs and ACE inhibitors are used together in dogs.
- **ASPIRIN:** When aspirin is used concurrently with carprofen, plasma levels of carprofen could decrease and an increased likelihood of GI adverse effects (blood loss) could occur. Concomitant administration of aspirin with carprofen cannot be recommended. Washout periods of several days is probably warranted when switching from an NSAID to aspirin therapy in dogs.
- **CORTICOSTEROIDS:** Concomitant administration with NSAIDs may significantly increase the risks for GI adverse effects.
- **DIGOXIN:** Carprofen may increase serum levels of digoxin; use with caution in patients with severe cardiac failure.
- **FUROSEMIDE:** Carprofen may reduce the saluretic and diuretic effects of furosemide. After 8 days of use together in dogs, GFR has been shown to decrease (Surdyk et al. 2012).
- **HIGHLY PROTEIN BOUND DRUGS** (*e.g.,* **phenytoin, valproic acid, oral anticoagulants, other antiinflammatory agents, salicylates, sulfonamides, sulfonylurea antidiabetic agents**): Because carprofen is highly bound to plasma proteins (99%), it

potentially could displace other highly bound drugs; increased serum levels and duration of actions may occur. Although these interactions are usually of little concern clinically, use together with caution.

- **METHOTREXATE:** Serious toxicity has occurred when NSAIDs have been used concomitantly with methotrexate; use together with extreme caution.
- **PHENOBARBITAL, RIFAMPIN,** or **OTHER HEPATIC ENZYME INDUCING AGENTS:** As carprofen hepatotoxicity may be mediated by its hepatic metabolites, these drugs should be avoided if carprofen is required. One source states: Patients should not receive phenobarbital or other hepatic drug metabolizing enzyme inducers when receiving this drug (Boothe 2005).
- **PROBENECID:** May cause a significant increase in serum levels and half-life of carprofen.

Laboratory Considerations

- In dogs, carprofen can have no effect or slightly lower **Free T$_4$**, **Total T$_4$** and TSH levels in dogs.

Doses

- **DOGS:**

  As an antiinflammatory/analgesic (Labeled Dose): 4.4 mg/kg PO; may be given once daily or divided and given as 2.2. mg/kg twice daily; round dose to nearest half caplet increment. For postoperative pain, administer approximately 2 hours before the procedure. Injectable is dosed as the oral products, but administered SC. (Package Insert; *Rimadyl®*)

- **CATS:**

  As an antiinflammatory/analgesic:

  Warning: Extreme caution is advised, particularly with continued dosing.

  a) Labeled Dose (U.K.; not approved in USA—extra-label): 4 mg/kg SC or IV once; best given pre-operatively at the time of induction of anesthesia. (Adapted from label; *Rimadyl® Small Animal Solution for Injection* 50 mg/ml; *Zoetis®* U.K.)

  b) Anecdotal; extra-label: 12.5 mg per cat (adult) PO or SC once weekly. (Grubb 2010)

- **HORSES: (NOTE: ARCI UCGFS CLASS 4 DRUG)**

  Labeled Dose (U.K.); (extra-label in USA): 0.7 mg/kg IV, one time; may follow with 0.7 mg/kg PO (granules, mixed with a little feed) for up to 4-9 days according to clinical response (Adapted from label information; *Rimadyl® Large Animal Solution, Rimadyl Granules®*—Pfizer U.K.)

- **CATTLE:**

  Labeled Dose (U.K.); (extra-label in USA): In young cattle (<12 months old) for adjunctive therapy of acute inflammation associated with respiratory disease: 1.4 mg/kg IV or SC once. Slaughter withdrawal = 21 days; not to be used in cows producing milk for human consumption. (Label information; *Rimadyl® Large Animal Solution*—Pfizer U.K.).

- **FERRETS:**

  As an antiinflammatory/analgesic (extra-label): 1 – 4 mg/kg SC q12-24h; 4 mg/kg PO q24h.

- **RABBITS/RODENTS/SMALL MAMMALS:**

  As an antiinflammatory/analgesic (all are extra-label):

  a) **Rabbits:** 2 – 4 mg/kg PO q12-24; 4 mg/kg SC. (Barter 2011)

  b) **Rats & mice:** 5 mg/kg SC q12-24h; **Guinea pigs & Chinchillas:** 4 mg/kg SC q12-24h. (Miller et al. 2011)

- **BIRDS:**

  As an antiinflammatory/analgesic (all are extra-label):

  a) 2 mg/kg PO q8-24 hours. (Clyde et al. 2000)

b) 1 mg/kg SC. Study demonstrated increased walking ability in lame chickens. (Paul-Murphy 2003)

c) 1 – 4 mg/kg IM, IV, PO. (Bays 2006)

■ **REPTILES:**

As an antiinflammatory (extra-label): 1 – 4 mg/kg IV, IM, SC, PO q 24-72h. (Bays 2006)

Monitoring

■ Baseline (especially in geriatric dogs, dogs with chronic diseases, or when prolonged treatment is likely): physical exam, CBC, Serum chemistry panel (including liver and renal function tests), and UA. It is recommended to reassess the liver enzymes at 1, 2, and 4 weeks of therapy and then at 3-6 month intervals. Should elevation occur, recommend discontinuing the drug.

■ Clinical efficacy.

■ Signs of potential adverse reactions: inappetence, diarrhea, vomiting, melena, polyuria/polydipsia, anemia, jaundice, lethargy, behavior changes, ataxia or seizures.

■ Chronic therapy: Consider repeating CBC, UA and serum chemistries on an ongoing basis.

Client Information

■ Read and understand the client information sheet provided with this medication; contact the veterinarian with any questions or concerns.

■ Can give with or without food, but food may reduce the chances for stomach problems.

■ Most dogs usually tolerate very it well, but rarely some will develop ulcers, or serious kidney and liver problems. Watch for these signs: Decreased or increased appetite, vomiting, changes in bowel movements; changes in behavior or activity level (more or less active than normal), muscle weakness (*e.g.*, stumbling, clumsiness, etc.), seizures (convulsions) or aggression; yellowing of gums, skin, or whites of the eyes (jaundice); changes in drinking habits (frequency, amount consumed) or urination habits (frequency, color, or smell).

■ Store chewable tablets well out of reach of animals and children.

■ Periodic lab tests to check for liver and kidney side effects are required.

Chemistry/Synonyms

A propionic acid derivative non-steroidal antiinflammatory agent, carprofen occurs as a white crystalline compound. It is practically insoluble in water and freely soluble in ethanol at room temperature. Carprofen has both an S (+) enantiomer and R (-) enantiomer. The commercial product contains a racemic mixture of both. The S (+) enantiomer has greater antiinflammatory potency than the R (-) form.

Carprofen may also be known as: C-5720; Ro-20-5720/000, *Rimadyl®*, *Zinecarp®*, *Canidryl®*, *Novox®*, *Carprodyl®* or *Norocarp®*.

Storage/Stability

The commercially available caplets or chewable tablets should be stored at room temperature (15-30°C).

The commercially available (in the USA) injection should be stored in the refrigerator (2-8°C; 36-46°F). Once broached, the injection may be stored at temperatures of up to 25°C for 28 days.

Compatibility/Compounding Considerations

Compounded preparation stability: Carprofen oral suspension compounded from commercially available tablets has been published (Hawkins et al. 2006). Triturating one (1) carprofen 100 mg tablet with 10 mL of *Ora-Plus®* and *qs ad* to 20 mL with *Ora-Sweet®* yields a 5 mg/mL suspension that retains 90% potency for 21 days stored at both 5°C and 25°C. Compounded preparations of carprofen should be protected from light.

Dosage Forms/Regulatory Status

VETERINARY-LABELED PRODUCTS:

Carprofen Scored Caplets: 25 mg, 75 mg & 100 mg; *Rimadyl® Caplets*, *Novocox®*, *Vetprofen®*, *Norocarp®*; (Rx). FDA-approved for use in dogs.

Carprofen Chewable Tablets: 25 mg, 75 mg & 100 mg; *quellin®* (soft chewable; scored), *Rimadyl® Chewable Tablets*; (Rx). FDA-approved for use in dogs.

Carprofen Sterile Injectable Solution: 50 mg/mL in 20 mL vials; *Rimadyl®*; (Rx). FDA-approved for use in dogs.

In the U.K., *Rimadyl® Injection* is labeled for use in dogs, cats, horses, ponies and cattle (less than 12 months old; slaughter withdrawal = 21 days; not to be used in cattle producing milk for human consumption). *Rimadyl® Granules* are labeled for use in horses and ponies. See Doses for more information.

The ARCI (Racing Commissioners International) has designated this drug as a class 4 substance. See the appendix for more information.

HUMAN-LABELED PRODUCTS: NONE.

Revisions/References

Monograph revised/updated September 2013.
Barter, L. S. (2011). Rabbit Analgesia. *Vet Clin Exot Anim* 14: 93-104.
Bays, T. (2006). *Recognizing and managing pain in exotic species.* Proceedings: Western Vet Conf. accessed via Veterinary Information Network; vin.com
Boothe, D. M. (2005). *New information on nonsteroidal antiinflammatories: What every criticalist must know.* Proceedings: IVECC. accessed via Veterinary Information Network; vin.com
Clyde, V. & J. Paul-Murphy (2000). Avian Analgesia. *Kirk's Current Veterinary Therapy: XIII Small Animal Practice.* J. Bonagura. Philadelphia, WB Saunders: 1126-8.
Grubb, T. (2010). What Do We Really Know About the Drugs We Use to Treat Chronic Pain? *Topics in Companion Animal Medicine* 25(1): 10-9.
Hawkins, M. G., et al. (2006). Drug distribution and stability in extemporaneous preparations of meloxicam and carprofen after dilution and suspension at two storage temperatures. *J Am Vet Med Assoc* 229(6): 968-74.
Innes, J. F., et al. (2010). Review of the safety and efficacy of long-term NSAID use in the treatment of canine osteoarthritis. *Veterinary Record* 166(8): 226-30.
Miller, A. L. & C. Richardson (2011). Rodent Analgesia. *Vet Clin Exot Anim* 14: 81-92.
Paul-Murphy, J. (2003). *Managing pain in birds.* Proceedings: Pain 2003. accessed via Veterinary Information Network; vin.com
Surdyk, K. K., et al. (2012). Renal effects of carprofen and etodolac in euvolemic and volume-depleted dogs. *American Journal of Veterinary Research* 73(9): 1485-90.

Carvedilol

(kar-vah-da-lol)   Coreg®

Beta & Alpha-1 Adrenergic Blocker

Prescriber Highlights

▶ Non-selective beta-adrenergic blocker with selective alpha₁-adrenergic blocking activity that could be useful for treating heart failure in dogs; use is controversial.

▶ Negative inotrope that may prohibit its use in severely symptomatic patients; potentially could decompensate patient.

▶ Additional adverse effects that may demonstrate intolerance include lassitude, inappetence, & hypotension.

Uses/Indications

Carvedilol may be useful as adjunctive therapy in the treatment of heart failure (dilated cardiomyopathy) in dogs. There is a fair amount of controversy at present among veterinary cardiologists as to whether this drug will find a therapeutic niche as there is no definitive proof that any medication can delay disease progression or improve mortality in dogs with stage B1 or B2 (with or without cardiac remodeling) chronic valvular heart disease. One study (Oyama et al. 2006) done in a small number of dogs with dilated cardiomyopathy showed that carvedilol dosed at 0.3 mg/kg PO q12h for 3 months did not produce any significant improvements in neurohormonal activation, heart size, or owner-perceived quality of life. The authors stated that doses >0.3 mg/kg q12h are likely to be required to effect changes in ventricular remodeling and function. A retrospective study (Gordon et al. 2012) of 38 dogs (33 were Cavalier King Charles Spaniels) with preclinical ACVIM Stage B2 chronic valvular heart disease, found average initial doses of 0.31 mg/kg PO twice daily and average uptitration target dosages of 1.11 mg/kg PO twice daily. In this study, median survival was 48.5 months.

Pharmacology/Actions

Carvedilol is a non-selective, beta-adrenergic blocker with selective alpha$_1$-adrenergic blocking activity. Despite their negative inotropic effects, chronic dosing of beta blockers in human patients with dilated cardiomyopathy can be useful in reducing both morbidity and mortality. Patients in heart failure, chronically activate their sympathetic nervous system, thereby leading to tachycardia, activation of the renin-angiotensin-aldosterone system, down-regulation of beta-receptors, induction of myocyte necrosis and myocyte energy substrate and calcium ion handling. By giving beta-blockers, these negative effects may be reversed or diminished. As carvedilol also inhibits alpha$_1$-adrenergic activity, it can cause vasodilation and reduce afterload. Carvedilol has free-radical scavenging and antidysrhythmic effects that could be beneficial in heart failure patients.

Pharmacokinetics

In dogs, a pilot study (Arsenault et al. 2003) showed carvedilol's bioavailability after oral dosing (standard tablets) averaged about 23% in the 4 dogs studied, but in 3 of the 4, bioavailability ranged from 3-10%. Volume of distribution averaged about 1.4 L/kg; elimination half-life was about 100 minutes. At least 15 different metabolites of carvedilol have been identified after dosing in dogs. Hydroxylation of the carbazolyl ring and glucuronidation of the parent compound are the most predominant processes of metabolism in dogs. No pharmacokinetic data for the extended-release oral capsules (*Coreg CR®*) in dogs was located.

In cats, oral carvedilol has a relatively low mean bioavailability (15.7%) with wide interpatient variation. Peak levels occur about one hour post oral dose. Elimination half-life is about 4.5 hours (Durtschi et al. 2011).

In humans, carvedilol is rapidly and extensively absorbed but due to a high first-pass effect, bioavailability is about 30%. The drug is extensively bound to plasma proteins (98%). It is extensively metabolized and the R(+) enantiomer is metabolized 2–3 times greater than the S(-) form during the first pass. Both the R(+) and S(-) enantiomers have equal potency as non-specific beta- or alpha-adrenergic blockers. CYP2D6 and CYP2C9 are the P450 isoenzymes most responsible for hepatic metabolism. Some of these metabolites have pharmacologic activity. Metabolites are primarily excreted via the bile and feces. Elimination half-life of carvedilol in humans is about 8-9 hours.

Contraindications/Precautions/Warnings

In humans, carvedilol is contraindicated in class IV decompensated heart failure, bronchial asthma, 2nd or 3rd degree AV block, sick sinus syndrome (unless artificially paced), severe bradycardia, cardiogenic shock or hypersensitivity to the drug. Dogs with equivalent conditions should not receive the drug.

Too rapid dose uptitration can cause cardiac decompensation.

Adverse Effects

Veterinary experience is very limited and an accurate portrayal of adverse effects in dogs has yet to be elucidated. Too rapid beta blockade can cause decompensation in patients with heart failure; cautious dosage titration is mandatory. Dogs that do not tolerate the medication may show signs of inappetence, lassitude, or hypotension. Bronchospasm has been reported in humans.

Because the drug is extensively metabolized in the liver, patients with hepatic insufficiency should receive the drug with caution. In humans, carvedilol has on rare occasions, caused mild hepatocellular injury.

Reproductive/Nursing Safety

In humans, the FDA categorizes carvedilol as a category C drug for use during pregnancy (*Animal studies have shown an adverse effect on the fetus, but there are no adequate studies in humans; or there are no animal reproduction studies and no adequate studies in humans*). In rats and rabbits, carvedilol increased post-implantation loss.

It is unknown if carvedilol enters maternal milk in dogs, but it does enter milk in rats. Use with caution in nursing patients.

Overdosage/Acute Toxicity

The acute oral LD$_{50}$ in healthy rats and mice is greater than 8 grams/kg. Clinical signs associated with large overdoses include: severe hypotension, cardiac insufficiency, bradycardia, cardiogenic shock and death due to cardiac arrest. Gut emptying protocols should be considered if ingestion was recent. In humans, bradycardia is treated with atropine, and cardiovascular function supported with glucagon and sympathomimetics (*e.g.*, dobutamine, epinephrine, etc.). Contact an animal poison control center for specific information in the case of overdose.

There were 406 single agent exposures to carvedilol reported to the ASPCA Animal Poison Control Center (APCC) during 2009-2013. Of the 380 dogs, 62 were symptomatic. The clinical signs included: lethargy (42%), bradycardia (21%), hypotension (8%), hypertension (8%) and tachycardia (8%). Of the 25 cats, 4 were symptomatic with 75% being lethargic and 50% vomiting.

Drug Interactions

The following drug interactions have either been reported or are theoretical in humans or animals receiving carvedilol and may be of significance in veterinary patients. Unless otherwise noted, use together is not necessarily contraindicated, but weigh the potential risks and perform additional monitoring when appropriate.

- **BETA-BLOCKERS (other):** Use with carvedilol may cause additive effects.
- **CALCIUM CHANNEL BLOCKERS** (*e.g., diltiazem, verapamil*, etc.): Carvedilol may rarely cause hemodynamic compromise in patients taking diltiazem or verapamil.
- **CIMETIDINE:** May decrease metabolism and increase AUC of carvedilol.
- **CLONIDINE:** Carvedilol may potentiate the cardiovascular effects of clonidine.
- **CYCLOSPORINE:** Carvedilol may increase cyclosporine levels.
- **DIGOXIN:** Carvedilol can increase (in humans) digoxin plasma concentrations by approximately 15%.
- **FLUOXETINE, PAROXETINE, QUINIDINE:** May increase R(+)-carvedilol concentrations and increase alpha$_1$ blocking effects (vasodilation).
- **INSULIN; ORAL ANTIDIABETIC AGENTS:** Carvedilol may enhance the blood glucose lowering effects of insulin or other antidiabetic agents.
- **RIFAMPIN:** Can decrease carvedilol plasma concentrations by as much as 70%.
- **RESERPINE:** Drugs such as reserpine can cause increased bradycardia and hypotension in patients taking carvedilol.

Laboratory Considerations

- No specific laboratory interactions or considerations noted.

Doses

- **DOGS:**

  For adjunctive treatment of chronic valvular heart disease (Stage B); (extra-label): From a retrospective study: Carvedilol at an initial dose of 0.31 mg/kg (mean) PO twice daily and a target dose of 1.11 mg/kg (mean) PO twice daily is safe and well tolerated in dogs with Stage B1 and early Stage B2 if an up titration protocol is used that involves a 50-100% increase in dose every 7-14 days until the target dose is reached. This study suggests that carvedilol at the doses reported is well tolerated in small breed dogs with Stage B CVD. Additional prospective studies to assess efficacy are warranted. (Gordon et al. 2012)

Monitoring

- During the dosage uptitration phase (q1-2 weeks) patients should be assessed for clinical response.
- Clinical efficacy.
- Adverse effects.
- Plasma drug levels potentially could be useful.

Client Information

- This medication is best given with food.
- When starting this drug, your veterinarian may start with a low dose and gradually increase it over time. It is important to be aware of the changing doses and not administer more at one time than your veterinarian prescribes. Do not stop the medication without the approval and guidance of veterinarian.
- If the first doses are too large, it may cause your animal's condition to worsen and show signs of loss of appetite, depression, lack of energy or weakness. If any of these symptoms occur, call your veterinarian immediately.
- Compounded liquids of carvedilol should NOT be stored in the refrigerator.

Chemistry/Synonyms

A non-selective beta-adrenergic blocker with selective alpha$_1$-adrenergic blocking activity, carvedilol occurs as a white to off-white crystalline powder that is practically insoluble in water, dilute acids, and gastric or intestinal fluids. It is sparingly soluble in ethanol. The compound exhibits polymorphism and contains both R(+) and S(-) enantiomers. It is a basic, lipophilic compound.

Carvedilol may also be known as: BM-14190, carvedilolum, *Cardilol®*, *Cardiol®*, *Carloc®*, *Carvil®*, *Carvipress®*, *Coreg®*, *Coritensil®*, *Coropres®*, *Dilatrend®*, *Dilbloc®*, *Dimitone®*, *Divelol®*, *Eucardic®*, *Hybridil®*, *Kredex®*, or *Querto®*.

Storage/Stability

Carvedilol tablets and extended release capsules should be stored below 30°C (86°F) and protected from moisture. They should be dispensed in tight, light-resistant containers.

Compatibility/Compounding Considerations

Compounded preparation stability: Carvedilol oral suspension compounded from commercially available tablets has been published (Yamreudeewong et al. 2006); however, HPLC analysis of drug samples in this study gave erratic and variable results indicating a loss of potency at refrigerated temperatures as compared to room temperature. Results of this study do not necessarily confirm that carvedilol is stable when prepared as an oral liquid.

Another published (Gordon et al. 2006) compounded oral suspension with documented 90 day stability to accurately dose dogs is to powder 25 mg tablets and add enough de-ionized water to make a paste, allowing the tablet coating to dissolve. Then suspend in a commercially available simple syrup to a concentration of either 2 mg/mL or 10 mg/mL. Store in amber bottles at temperatures not exceeding 25°C and protect from light for up to 90 days. Shake well before administering.

Dosage Forms/Regulatory Status

VETERINARY-LABELED PRODUCTS: NONE.

The ARCI (Racing Commissioners International) has designated this drug as a class 3 substance. See the appendix for more information.

HUMAN-LABELED PRODUCTS:

Carvedilol Oral Tablets: 3.125 mg, 6.25 mg, 12.5 mg, & 25 mg; *Coreg®*, generic; (Rx)

Carvedilol Extended-Release Oral Capsules: 10 mg, 20 mg, 40 mg & 80 mg (as phosphate); *Coreg CR*; (Rx)

Revisions/References

Monograph revised/updated September 2013.

Arsenault, W., et al. (2003). *The pharmacokinetics of carvedilol in healthy dogs: A pilot study.* Proceedings ACVIM Forum. accessed via Veterinary Information Network; vin.com

Durtschi, A. L., et al. (2011). *Pharmacokinetics and Bioavailability of Carvedilol in Cats.* ACVIM Proceedings. accessed via Veterinary Information Network; vin.com

Gordon, S., et al. (2006). *Stability of carvedilol in an oral liquid preparation.* Proceedings: ACVIM. accessed via Veterinary Information Network; vin.com

Gordon, S. G., et al. (2012). Retrospective review of carvedilol administration in 38 dogs with preclinical chronic valvular heart disease. *Journal of veterinary cardiology : the official journal of the European Society of Veterinary Cardiology* 14(1).

Oyama, M. & M. Prosek (2006). Acute Conversion of atrial fibrillation in two dogs by intravenous amiodarone administration. *J Vet Intern Med* 20(5): 1224-7.

Yamreudeewong, W., et al. (2006). Stability of two extemporaneously prepared oral metoprolol and carvedilol liquids. *Hosp Pharm* 41: 254-9.

Caspofungin Acetate

(kas-poe-fun-jin)   Cancidas®

Parenteral Antifungal

Prescriber Highlights

▶ Parenteral antifungal that has potential for treating invasive aspergillosis or disseminated candidal infections in companion animals.

▶ Very limited clinical experience in veterinary medicine. Must be given slow IV.

▶ Very expensive.

Uses/Indications

Caspofungin has potential for treating invasive aspergillosis or disseminated candidal infections in companion animals although little, if any, information on its use in dogs or cats is available.

Pharmacology/Actions

Caspofungin represents the echinocandins, a new class of antifungal agent. These drugs inhibit beta-glucan synthase, thereby blocking the synthesis of beta-(1,3)-D-glucan, a component found in cell walls of filamentous fungi. Caspofungin has activity against *Aspergillus* and *Candida* species and is effective in treating pneumonia caused by *Pneumocystis carinii*. Because it contains very little beta-glucan synthase, *Cryptococcus neoformans* infections are not effectively treated with caspofungin. An *in vitro* study found that caspofungin had significant, but only minimal to moderate inhibition of *Pythium insidiosum* and a *Lagenidium* species (Brown et al. 2008).

Pharmacokinetics

No information was located on the pharmacokinetics of caspofungin in dogs or cats.

In humans, the drug is not appreciably absorbed from the gut and must be administered IV. Protein binding (primarily to albumin) is high (97%) and the drug is distributed to tissues over a 36-48 hour period. Caspofungin is slowly metabolized via hydrolysis and N-acetylation. It also spontaneously degrades chemically. Caspofungin exhibits polyphasic elimination, but little drug is excreted or biotransformed during the first 30 hours post-administration. Elimination half-life for the primary phase is about 10 hours; the secondary phase between 40-50 hours. Excretion, consisting mostly as metabolites, is via the feces and urine. Only small amounts (1-2%) are excreted unchanged into the urine.

Contraindications/Precautions/Warnings

No specific information is available for veterinary patients. Caspofungin is contraindicated in human patients hypersensitive to it. Dosage adjustment is recommended in humans with moderate hepatic impairment. No information is available for use in patients with significant hepatic impairment; avoid use.

Reproductive/Nursing Safety

In humans, the FDA categorizes caspofungin as category C for use during pregnancy (*Animal studies have shown an adverse effect on the fetus, but there are no adequate studies in humans; or there are no animal reproduction studies and no adequate studies in humans.*) Studies with caspofungin performed in pregnant rats and rabbits demonstrated changes in fetal ossification. The drug should be avoided during the first trimester of pregnancy unless the benefits associated with treating outweigh the risks.

Although no data is available, because the drug is not appreciably absorbed from the gut, it would be expected that caspofungin would be safe to administer during lactation.

Adverse Effects

An adverse effect profile for animals has not been determined. In humans, caspofungin is generally well tolerated. Histamine-mediated signs have occurred (rash, facial swelling, pruritus) and anaphylaxis has been reported. Intravenous site reactions (pain, redness, phlebitis) have occurred. Hepatic dysfunction has been reported but frequency is unknown.

Overdosage/Acute Toxicity

Limited information is available. Dosages of 210 mg (about 3x) in humans were well tolerated. Some monkeys receiving 5 – 8 mg/kg (approx. 4-6X) over 5 weeks developed sites of microscopic subcapsular necrosis on their livers.

Drug Interactions

The following drug interactions have either been reported or are theoretical in humans or animals receiving caspofungin and may be of significance in veterinary patients. Unless otherwise noted, use together is not necessarily contraindicated, but weigh the potential risks and perform additional monitoring when appropriate.

- **CARBAMAZEPINE:** Reduced caspofungin plasma levels.
- **CYCLOSPORINE:** Increased caspofungin plasma levels and increased risk of hepatic enzyme increases.
- **DEXAMETHASONE:** Reduced caspofungin plasma levels.
- **PHENYTOIN:** Reduced caspofungin plasma levels.
- **RIFAMPIN:** Reduced caspofungin plasma levels.

Laboratory Considerations

- No specific concerns noted; see Monitoring.

Doses

- **DOGS/CATS:**

  No published dosage recommendations for dogs or cats were located and the use of this medication in animal patients must be considered highly investigational. A single case report using caspofungin in a cat with upper respiratory aspergillosis at 1 mg/kg IV once daily (cumulative dose of 22 mg/kg) has been reported. This cat tolerated the treatment well and the authors stated it was "efficacious" (Barrs et al. 2012). Another case where caspofungin showed potential efficacy in a dog with *A. deflectus* has been reported (Brown et al. 2008). This dog received caspo-

fungin at 1 mg/kg IV in 250 mL 0.9% NaCl over 1 hour q24h. Rapid clinical improvement and resolution of lymphadenomegaly was noted 6 weeks after starting therapy, at which time caspofungin was administered 3 times weekly for 2 months, then on 3 consecutive days every 3 weeks for 4 months, then discontinued. One month later, small numbers of *A. deflectus* (sensitive to caspofungin) were noted in urine culture and twice weekly caspofungin treatment was administered for two weeks and urine culture again was negative. Treatment was continued on 3 consecutive days every 3 weeks. One year later, the dog showed clinical signs of disease recurrence and enlarged mesenteric lymph nodes revealed fungal hyphae with marked necrosis.

Monitoring

- Clinical efficacy.
- Periodic liver function tests, CBC, serum electrolytes.

Client Information

- This medication is appropriate for inpatient use only.
- Clients should understand the investigational nature and the associated expense of using this drug on veterinary patients.

Chemistry/Synonyms

Caspofungin acetate is a semisynthetic echinocandin compound produced from a fermentation product of *Glarea lozoyensis*. It occurs as a white to off-white powder that is freely soluble in water and slightly soluble in ethanol. The commercially available lyophilized powder for injection also contains acetic acid, sodium hydroxide, mannitol and sucrose.

Caspofungin may also be known as: caspofungina, caspofungine, caspofungini, kaspofungiinia, kaspofungina, L-743873, MK-0991, or *Cancidas*®.

Storage/Stability

The commercially available product should be stored refrigerated (2-8°C). Refer to the package insert for very specific directions on preparing the solution for intravenous use.

Do not use if the solution is cloudy or has precipitated.

Compatibility/Compounding Considerations

It is recommended to not mix or infuse with any other medications. Do not use with intravenous solutions containing dextrose.

Dosage Forms/Regulatory Status

VETERINARY-LABELED PRODUCTS: NONE.

HUMAN-LABELED PRODUCTS:

Caspofungin Acetate Lyophilized Powder for Injection: 50 mg & 70 mg in single-use vials; *Cancidas*®; (Rx)

Revisions/References

Monograph revised/updated September 2013.

Barrs, V. R., et al. (2012). Sinonasal and sino-orbital aspergillosis in 23 cats: Aetiology, clinicopathological features and treatment outcomes. *Veterinary Journal* 191(1): 58-64.

Brown, T. A., et al. (2008). In vitro susceptibility of Pythium insidiosum and a Lagenidium sp to itraconazole, posaconazole, voriconazole, terbinafine, caspofungin, and mefenoxam. *AJVR* 69(11): 1463-8.

Cefaclor

(sef-a-klor)   Ceclor®

Oral 2nd Generation Cephalosporin

Prescriber Highlights

▶ Oral 2nd generation cephalosporin that is more active against some gram-negative bacteria then first generation (*e.g.*, cephalexin, etc.) cephalosporins.

▶ Potentially useful when an oral cephalosporin is desired to treat bacterial infections that are susceptible to cefaclor, but resistant to first generation cephalosporins.

▶ Very limited clinical experience in veterinary medicine.

▶ Adverse effects most likely seen in small animals would be GI-related.

Uses/Indications

Cefaclor may potentially be useful when an oral cephalosporin is desired to treat infections that are susceptible to it but resistant to first generation cephalosporins such as cephalexin or cefadroxil. Little information is available with regard to its clinical use in small animals, however.

Pharmacology/Actions

Cefaclor, like other cephalosporins, is bactericidal and acts via inhibiting cell wall synthesis. Its spectrum of activity is similar to that of cephalexin, but it is more active against gram-negative bacteria including strains of *E. coli*, *Klebsiella pneumoniae*, and *Proteus mirabilis*.

Pharmacokinetics

Limited information is available on the pharmacokinetics of cefaclor in dogs and none was located for cats. In dogs, about 75% of an oral dose is absorbed, but an apparent first-pass effect reduces bioavailability to about 60%. Cefaclor is distributed to many tissues, but levels are lower in interstitial fluid than those found in serum. Very high levels are excreted into the urine unchanged. Bile levels are higher than those found in serum. Dogs appear to metabolize a greater percentage of cefaclor than do rats, mice, or humans. Approximate elimination half-life is about 2 hours in dogs. Pharmacokinetic information for the extended-release oral tablets in dogs was not located.

In humans, cefaclor is well absorbed after oral administration; food delays, but does not appreciably alter the amount absorbed. The drug is widely distributed, crosses the placenta and enters breast milk. Up to 85% of a dose is excreted unchanged into the urine; elimination half-life is less than 1 hour in patients with normal renal function.

Contraindications/Precautions/Warnings

No specific information is available for veterinary patients. Cefaclor is contraindicated in human patients hypersensitive to it and must be cautiously used in patients with penicillin-allergy. Dosage adjustment is recommended in humans with severe renal impairment.

Reproductive/Nursing Safety

In humans, the FDA categorizes cefaclor as category *B* for use during pregnancy (*Animal studies have not yet demonstrated risk to the fetus, but there are no adequate studies in pregnant women; or animal studies have shown an adverse effect, but adequate studies in pregnant women have not demonstrated a risk to the fetus in the first trimester of pregnancy, and there is no evidence of risk in later trimesters.*) Studies performed in pregnant rats (doses up 12X human dose) and ferrets (doses up to 3X human dose) demonstrated no overt fetal harm.

Cefaclor enters maternal milk in low concentrations. Although probably safe for nursing offspring the potential for adverse effects cannot be ruled out, particularly, alterations to gut flora with resultant diarrhea.

Adverse Effects

As usage of cefaclor in animals has been very limited, a comprehensive adverse effect profile has not been determined. In humans, cefaclor is generally well tolerated but commonly can cause gastrointestinal effects (*e.g.*, nausea, diarrhea, etc.). Hypersensitivity reactions including anaphylaxis are possible; cefaclor appears to cause a higher incidence of serum-sickness-like reactions than other cephalosporins, particularly in children who have received multiple courses of treatment. Rare adverse effects reported include erythema multiforme, rash, increases in liver function tests, and transient increases in BUN and serum creatinine.

Overdosage/Acute Toxicity

Cefaclor appears quite safe in dogs. Dogs given daily PO doses of 200 mg/kg/day for 30 days developed soft stools and occasional emesis. Two dogs in this study group developed transient moderate decreases in hemoglobin. One dog in another study group that was given 400 mg/kg/day for one year developed a reversible thrombocytopenia.

Drug Interactions

The following drug interactions have either been reported or are theoretical in humans or animals receiving cefaclor and may be of significance in veterinary patients. Unless otherwise noted, use together is not necessarily contraindicated, but weigh the potential risks and perform additional monitoring when appropriate.

- **ANTACIDS (magnesium- or aluminum-containing):** Reduces extent of absorption of extended-release cefaclor tablets in humans.

- **PROBENECID:** Reduced renal excretion of cefaclor.

- **WARFARIN:** Rare reports of increased anticoagulant effect.

Laboratory Considerations

- Except for cefotaxime, cephalosporins may cause false-positive **urine glucose determinations** when using the copper reduction method (Benedict's solution, Fehling's solution, *Clinitest*®); tests utilizing glucose oxidase (*Tes-Tape*®, *Clinistix*®) are not affected by cephalosporins.

- When using the Jaffe reaction to measure **serum or urine creatinine**, cephalosporins (not ceftazidime or cefotaxime) given in high dosages may cause falsely elevated values.

- In humans, particularly with azotemia, cephalosporins have caused a false-positive direct **Coombs' test**.

- Cephalosporins may also cause falsely elevated **17-ketosteroid** values in urine.

Doses

- **DOGS/CATS:**

  For susceptible infections (extra-label): 7 – 20 mg/kg PO q8h. Maximum dose is 1 gram.

Monitoring

- Clinical efficacy.

- Patients with renal insufficiency should have renal function monitored.

Client Information

- Preferably should be administered to animal without food; however, if patient vomits or develops a lack of appetite while receiving medication it can be administered with food.

- Most common side effects are diarrhea, vomiting and loss of appetite.

- Be sure to give as long as veterinarian has prescribed, even if animal seems better.
- Cephalosporin antibiotics have an odor that resembles cat urine, but this is normal.

Chemistry/Synonyms

Cefaclor occurs as a white to off-white powder that is slightly soluble in water.

Cefaclor may also be known as: cefaclorum, cefaklor, cefkloras, kefakloori or compound 99638. There are many internationally registered trade names.

Storage/Stability

Capsules, tablets, and powder for suspension should be stored at room temperature (15-30°C). After reconstituting, the oral suspension should be stored in the refrigerator and discarded after 14 days.

Compatibility/Compounding Considerations

No specific information noted.

Dosage Forms/Regulatory Status

VETERINARY-LABELED PRODUCTS: NONE.

HUMAN-LABELED PRODUCTS:

Cefaclor Oral Capsules: 250 mg & 500 mg; generic; (Rx)

Cefaclor Extended-Release Oral Tablets: 500 mg; generic; (Rx)

Cefaclor Powder for Oral Suspension: 125 mg/5 mL, 187 mg/5 mL, 250 mg/5 mL, & 375 mg/5 mL, generic; (Rx)

Revisions/References

Monograph revised/updated September 2013.

Cefadroxil

(sef-a-drox-ill)   Cefa-Drops®, Duricef®

Oral 1st Generation Cephalosporin

Prescriber Highlights

▶ Oral 1st generation cephalosporin.
▶ May be administered with food (especially if GI upset occurs).
▶ Most likely adverse effects are GI in nature.
▶ May need to reduce dose in renal failure.
▶ May be expensive when compared to generic cephalexin.

Uses/Indications

Cefadroxil is FDA-approved for oral therapy in treating susceptible infections of the skin, soft tissue, and genitourinary tract in dogs and cats. The veterinary oral tablets have been discontinued in the USA, but human-labeled oral capsules and tablets are still available. At present, a fair level of evidence exists for moderate to high efficacy using cefadroxil for treating superficial and deep pyodermas in dogs (Summers et al. 2012).

Pharmacology/Actions

A first generation cephalosporin, cefadroxil exhibits activity against the bacteria usually covered by this class. First generation cephalosporins are usually bactericidal and act via inhibition of cell wall synthesis.

While there may be differences in MIC's for individual first generation cephalosporins, their spectrums of activity are quite similar. They generally possess excellent coverage against most gram-positive pathogens; variable to poor coverage against most gram-negative pathogens. These drugs are very active *in vitro* against groups A beta-hemolytic and B Streptococci, non-enterococcal group D Streptococci (*S. bovis*), *Staphylococcus pseudintermedius* and *aureus*, *Proteus mirabilis* and some strains of *E. coli*, *Klebsiella* spp., Actinobacillus, Pasteurella, *Haemophilus equigenitalis*, Shigella and Salmonella. With the exception of *Bacteroides fragilis*, most an-

aerobes are very susceptible to the first generation agents. Most species of Corynebacteria are susceptible, but *C. equi* (*Rhodococcus*) is usually resistant. Strains of *Staphylococcus epidermidis* are usually sensitive to the parenterally administered 1st generation drugs, but may have variable susceptibilities to the oral drugs. The following bacteria are regularly resistant to the 1st generation agents: Group D streptococci/enterococci (*S. faecalis, S. faecium*), Methicillin-resistant Staphylococci, *indole-positive Proteus* spp., *Pseudomonas* spp., *Enterobacter* spp., *Serratia* spp. and *Citrobacter* spp.

Pharmacokinetics

Cefadroxil is reportedly well absorbed after oral administration to dogs without regard to feeding state. After an oral dose of 22 mg/kg, peak serum levels of approximately 18.6 micrograms/mL occur within 1-2 hours of dosing. Only about 20% of the drug is bound to canine plasma proteins. The drug is excreted into the urine and has a half-life of about 2 hours. Over 50% of a dose can be recovered unchanged in the urine within 24 hours of dosing.

In cats, the serum half-life has been reported as approximately 3 hours.

Oral absorption of cefadroxil in adult horses after oral suspension was administered was characterized as poor and erratic. In a study done in foals (Duffee, Christensen, and Craig 1989), oral bioavailability ranged from 36-99.8% (mean=58.2%); mean elimination half-life was 3.75 hours after oral dosing.

Contraindications/Precautions/Warnings

Cephalosporins are contraindicated in patients with a history of hypersensitivity to them. Because there may be cross-reactivity, use cephalosporins cautiously in patients that are documented hypersensitive to other beta-lactam antibiotics (*e.g.*, penicillins, cefamycins, carbapenems, etc.).

Oral systemic antibiotics should not be administered in patients with septicemia, shock or other grave illnesses as absorption of the medication from the GI tract may be significantly delayed or diminished. Parenteral routes (preferably IV) should be used for these cases.

Cefadroxil can be easily confused with other cephalosporins. Consider writing orders and prescriptions using tall man letters: cefaDROXil.

Adverse Effects

Adverse effects with the cephalosporins are usually not serious and have a relatively low frequency of occurrence.

Hypersensitivity reactions unrelated to dose can occur with these agents and can manifest as rashes, fever, eosinophilia, lymphadenopathy, or full-blown anaphylaxis. The use of cephalosporins in patients documented to be hypersensitive to penicillin-class antibiotics is controversial. In humans, it is estimated that up to 15% of patients hypersensitive to penicillins will also be hypersensitive to cephalosporins. The incidence of cross-reactivity in veterinary patients is unknown.

When given orally, cephalosporins may cause GI effects (*e.g.*, anorexia, vomiting, diarrhea, etc.). Administering the drug with a small meal may help alleviate these effects. Because the cephalosporins may alter gut flora, antibiotic-associated diarrhea can occur and allow the proliferation of resistant bacteria in the colon (superinfections).

While cephalosporins (particularly cephalothin) have the potential for causing nephrotoxicity, at clinically used doses in patients with normal renal function, risks for the occurrence of this adverse effect appear minimal.

Cefadroxil or cephalexin may rarely cause tachypnea.

High doses or very prolonged use of cephalosporins have been associated with neurotoxicity, neutropenia, agranulocytosis, thrombocytopenia, hepatitis, positive Comb's test, interstitial nephritis, and tubular necrosis. Except for tubular necrosis and neurotoxicity, these effects have an immunologic component.

Reproductive/Nursing Safety

Cephalosporins have been shown to cross the placenta and safe use of them during pregnancy has not been firmly established, but neither have there been any documented teratogenic problems associated with these drugs. However, use only when the potential benefits outweigh the risks. In humans, the FDA categorizes this drug as category *B* for use during pregnancy (*Animal studies have not yet demonstrated risk to the fetus, but there are no adequate studies in pregnant women; or animal studies have shown an adverse effect, but adequate studies in pregnant women have not demonstrated a risk to the fetus in the first trimester of pregnancy, and there is no evidence of risk in later trimesters.*)

Cephalosporins can be distributed into milk, but are unlikely to pose much risk to nursing offspring; diarrhea is possible.

Overdosage/Acute Toxicity

Acute oral cephalosporin overdoses are unlikely to cause significant problems other than GI distress, but other effects are possible (see Adverse Effects section).

Drug Interactions

The following drug interactions have either been reported or are theoretical in humans or animals receiving cefadroxil and may be of significance in veterinary patients. Unless otherwise noted, use together is not necessarily contraindicated, but weigh the potential risks and perform additional monitoring when appropriate.

- **PROBENECID:** Competitively blocks the tubular secretion of most cephalosporins thereby increasing serum levels and serum half-lives.

Laboratory Considerations

- Except for cefotaxime, cephalosporins may cause false-positive **urine glucose determinations** when using cupric sulfate solution (Benedict's Solution, *Clinitest*®). Tests utilizing glucose oxidase (*Tes-Tape*®, *Clinistix*®) are not affected by cephalosporins.
- When using the Jaffe reaction to measure **serum or urine creatinine**, cephalosporins (not ceftazidime or cefotaxime) in high dosages may cause falsely elevated values.
- In humans, particularly with azotemia, cephalosporins have caused a false-positive direct **Combs' test.**
- Cephalosporins may also cause falsely elevated **17-ketosteroid** values in urine.

Doses -

- **DOGS:**

  For susceptible infections:

  a) **Labeled Dose:** 22 mg/kg PO twice daily. Treat skin and soft tissue infections for at least 3 days, and GU infections for at least 7 days. Treat for at least 48 hours after animal is afebrile and asymptomatic. Reevaluate therapy if no response after 3 days of treatment. Maximum therapy is 30 days. (Package Insert; *Cefa-Drops*®).

  b) **Superficial pyoderma** (extra-label): 22 – 35 mg/kg PO twice daily for 28-42 days. Fair level of evidence for moderate to high efficacy. (Summers et al. 2012)

  c) **Deep pyoderma** (extra-label): Either 20 mg/kg PO twice daily or 40 mg/kg PO once daily for 21 days. Fair level of evidence for moderate to high efficacy. (Summers et al. 2012)

  d) **UTI** (extra-label): Several anecdotal widely ranging (10 – 40 mg/kg PO once to three times daily) dosage recommendations have been published. In the absence of any evidence supporting one or the other, consider using the labeled dosage recommendations (22 mg/kg PO twice daily);

treatment duration is dependent on the infection's etiology, location and chronicity. Chronic urethrocystitis or pyelonephritis may require several weeks of treatment.

- **CATS:**

  For susceptible infections:

  a) **Labeled Dose:** 22 mg/kg PO once daily. Treat for at least 48 hours after animal is afebrile and asymptomatic Reevaluate therapy if no response after 3 days of treatment. Maximum therapy is 21 days. (Package Insert; *Cefa-Drops*®— BIVI).

  b) **Extra-label Dose:** Note some recommend using the above dosage (22 mg/kg) twice daily in cats and treating certain infections (*e.g.*, orthopedic, pyoderma) longer than the 21 day labeled maximum.

- **FERRETS:**

  For susceptible infections (extra-label): 15 – 20 mg/kg PO twice daily. (Williams 2000)

Monitoring

- Because cephalosporins usually have minimal toxicity associated with their use, monitoring for efficacy is usually all that is required.
- Patients with diminished renal function may require intensified renal monitoring. Serum levels and therapeutic drug monitoring are not routinely performed with these agents.

Client Information

- Can be given with or without food, but gastrointestinal side effects might be prevented if given with food.
- Most common side effects are diarrhea, vomiting and loss of appetite.
- Be sure to give as long as veterinarian has prescribed, even if animal seems better.
- Cephalosporin antibiotics have an odor that resembles cat urine, but this is normal.

Chemistry/Synonyms

A semisynthetic cephalosporin antibiotic, cefadroxil occurs as a white to yellowish-white, crystalline powder that is soluble in water and slightly soluble in alcohol. The commercially available product is available as the monohydrate.

Cefadroxil may also be known as: BL-S578; cefadroxilum, cephadroxil, or MJF-11567-3; many trade names are available.

Storage/Stability

Cefadroxil tablets, capsules and powder for oral suspension should be stored at room temperature (15-30°C) in tight containers. After reconstitution, the oral suspension is stable for 14 days when kept refrigerated (2-8°C).

Compatibility/Compounding Considerations

No specific information noted.

Dosage Forms/Regulatory Status

VETERINARY-LABELED PRODUCTS:

Cefadroxil Powder for Oral Suspension: 50 mg/mL in 15 mL and 50 mL btls; *Cefa-Drops*®; (Rx). FDA-approved for use in dogs and cats. NADA: 140684.

HUMAN-LABELED PRODUCTS:

Cefadroxil Oral Tablets: 1 gram; generic; (Rx)

Cefadroxil Oral Capsules: 500 mg; generic; (Rx)

Cefadroxil Powder for Oral Suspension: 250 mg/5 mL & 500 mg/5 mL in 50 mL, 75 mL (500 mg/5 mL only) & 100 mL; generic; (Rx)

Revisions/References
Monograph revised/updated September 2013.
Summers, J. F., et al. (2012). The effectiveness of systemic antimicrobial treatment in canine superficial and deep pyoderma: a systematic review. *Veterinary Dermatology* 23(4): 305-E61.
Williams, B. (2000). Therapeutics in Ferrets. *Vet Clin NA: Exotic Anim Pract* 3:1(Jan): 131-53.

Cefazolin Sodium

(sef-a-zoe-lin)   Ancef®, Kefzol®, Zolicef®

1st Generation Cephalosporin

Prescriber Highlights

▶ 1st generation parenteral cephalosporin. Often used for surgical prophylaxis for gram-positive coverage.

▶ Potentially could cause hypersensitivity reactions.

▶ Can cause pain on IM injection; Give IV over 3-5 minutes (or more).

▶ May need to reduce dose in renal failure.

Uses/Indications

In the United States, there are no cefazolin products FDA-approved for veterinary species but it has been used clinically in several species when an injectable, first generation cephalosporin is indicated. It is used for surgical prophylaxis, and for a variety of systemic infections (including orthopedic, soft tissue, sepsis) caused by susceptible bacteria. Most commonly given every 6-8 hours via parenteral routes. Since cefazolin is a time dependent (above MIC) antibiotic, constant rate intravenous infusion protocols are being developed so that serum/tissue concentrations can remain above MIC.

Pharmacology/Actions

A first generation cephalosporin, cefazolin exhibits activity against the bacteria usually covered by this class. First generation cephalosporins are usually bactericidal and act via inhibition of cell wall synthesis. They are considered time-dependent antibiotics.

While there may be differences in MIC's for individual first generation cephalosporins, their spectrums of activity are quite similar. They possess generally excellent coverage against most gram-positive pathogens; variable to poor coverage against most gram-negative pathogens. These drugs are very active *in vitro* against groups A beta-hemolytic and B Streptococci, non-enterococcal group D Streptococci (*S. bovis*), *Staphylococcus pseudintermedius* and *aureas*, *Proteus mirabilis* and some strains of *E. coli*, *Klebsiella* spp., Actinobacillus, Pasteurella, *Haemophilus equigenitalis*, Shigella and Salmonella. With the exception of *Bacteroides fragilis*, most anaerobes are very susceptible to the first generation agents. Most species of Corynebacteria are susceptible, but *C. equi* (Rhodococcus) is usually resistant. Strains of *Staphylococcus epidermidis* are usually sensitive to the parenterally administered 1st generation drugs, but may have variable susceptibilities to the oral drugs. The following bacteria are regularly resistant to the 1st generation agents: Group D streptococci/enterococci (*S. faecalis, S. faecium*), Methicillin-resistant Staphylococci, *indole-positive Proteus* spp., *Pseudomonas* spp., *Enterobacter* spp., *Serratia* spp. and *Citrobacter* spp.

Pharmacokinetics

Cefazolin is not appreciably absorbed after oral administration and must be given parenterally to achieve therapeutic serum levels. Absorbed drug is excreted unchanged by the kidneys into the urine. Elimination half-lives may be significantly prolonged in patients with severely diminished renal function.

In dogs, peak levels occur in about 30 minutes after IM administration. The apparent volume of distribution at steady state is 700 mL/kg, total body clearance of 10.4 mL/min/kg with a serum elimination half-life of 48 minutes. Approximately 64% of the clearance can be attributed to renal tubular secretion. The drug is approximately 16-28% bound to plasma proteins in dogs. Penetration into pancreatic tissue is poor.

In horses, the apparent volume of distribution at steady state is 190 mL/kg, total body clearance of 5.51 mL/min/kg with a serum elimination half-life of 38 minutes when given IV and 84 minutes after IM injection (gluteal muscles). Cefazolin is about 4-8% bound to equine plasma proteins. Because of the significant tubular secretion of the drug, it would be expected that probenecid administration would alter the kinetics of cefazolin. One study performed in horses (Donecker, Sams, and Ashcroft 1986), did not show any effect, but the authors concluded that the dosage of probenecid may have been sub-therapeutic in this species.

In calves, the volume of distribution is 165 mL/kg, and had a terminal elimination half-life of 49-99 minutes after IM administration.

Contraindications/Precautions/Warnings

Cephalosporins are contraindicated in patients with a history of hypersensitivity to them. Because there may be cross-reactivity, use cephalosporins cautiously in patients that are documented hypersensitive to other beta-lactam antibiotics (*e.g.*, penicillins, cefamycins, carbapenems, etc.). Cephalosporins in small mammals such as Syrian hamsters and guinea pigs may cause antibiotic-induced enterocolitis; 25% mortality was reported in guinea pigs receiving 100 mg IM q6h for 5 days.

Patients in renal failure may need dosage adjustments.

Cefazolin can be easily confused with other cephalosporins. Consider writing orders and prescriptions using tall man letters: ceFAZolin.

Adverse Effects

Adverse effects with the cephalosporins are usually not serious and have a relatively low frequency of occurrence.

Hypersensitivity reactions unrelated to dose can occur with these agents and manifest as rashes, fever, eosinophilia, lymphadenopathy, or full-blown anaphylaxis. The use of cephalosporins in patients documented to be hypersensitive to penicillin-class antibiotics is controversial. In humans, it is estimated 1-15% of patients hypersensitive to penicillins will also be hypersensitive to cephalosporins. The incidence of cross-reactivity in veterinary patients is unknown.

Cephalosporins can cause pain at the injection site when administered intramuscularly, although this effect occurs less with cefazolin than with other agents. Sterile abscesses or other severe local tissue reactions are possible but are much less common. Thrombophlebitis is also possible after IV administration of these drugs.

While cephalosporins (particularly cephalothin) have the potential for causing nephrotoxicity at clinically used doses in patients with normal renal function, risks for the occurrence of this adverse effect appear minimal.

High doses or very prolonged use has been associated with neurotoxicity, neutropenia, agranulocytosis, thrombocytopenia, hepatitis, positive Comb's test, interstitial nephritis, and tubular necrosis. Except for tubular necrosis and neurotoxicity, these effects have an immunologic component. Cefazolin may be more likely than other cephalosporins to cause seizures at very high doses.

Reproductive/Nursing Safety

Cephalosporins have been shown to cross the placenta and safe use of them during pregnancy has not been firmly established, but neither have there been any documented teratogenic problems associated with these drugs. However, use only when the potential benefits outweigh the risks. In humans, the FDA categorizes this drug as category *B* for use during pregnancy (*Animal studies have not yet demonstrated risk to the fetus, but there are no adequate studies in pregnant women; or animal studies have shown an adverse effect, but adequate studies in pregnant women have not demonstrated a risk to the fetus in the first trimester of pregnancy, and there is no evidence of risk in later trimesters.)*

Cefazolin is distributed into milk and could potentially alter neonatal gut flora. Use with caution in nursing dams.

Overdosage/Acute Toxicity

Cephalosporin overdoses are unlikely to cause significant problems, but other effects are possible (see Adverse Effects section). Very high doses given IV rapidly could potentially cause seizures.

Drug Interactions

The following drug interactions have either been reported or are theoretical in humans or animals receiving cefazolin and may be of significance in veterinary patients. Unless otherwise noted, use together is not necessarily contraindicated, but weigh the potential risks and perform additional monitoring when appropriate.

- **NEPHROTOXIC DRUGS:** The concurrent use of parenteral aminoglycosides or other nephrotoxic drugs (*e.g.,* **amphotericin B**, etc.) with cephalosporins is somewhat controversial. Potentially, cephalosporins could cause additive nephrotoxicity when used with these drugs, but this interaction has only been well documented with cephaloridine (no longer marketed). Nevertheless, use caution.
- **PROBENECID:** Competitively blocks the tubular secretion of most cephalosporins thereby increasing serum levels and serum half-lives.

Laboratory Considerations

- Except for cefotaxime, cephalosporins may cause false-positive **urine glucose determinations** when using cupric sulfate solution (Benedict's Solution, *Clinitest®*). Tests utilizing glucose oxidase (*Tes-Tape®, Clinistix®*) are not affected by cephalosporins.
- When using the Jaffe reaction to measure **serum or urine creatinine**, cephalosporins (not ceftazidime or cefotaxime) in high dosages may cause falsely elevated values.
- In humans, particularly with azotemia, cephalosporins have caused a false-positive direct **Coombs' test**.
- Cephalosporins may also cause falsely elevated **17-ketosteroid** values in urine.

Doses

Note: If injecting IM, must be injected into a large muscle mass. IV injections should not be given faster than over 3–5 minutes.

- **DOGS/CATS:**

  For surgical prophylaxis (extra-label): For orthopedic, soft-tissue or colonic (with metronidazole) procedures: Usually given just before incision or within 1 hour before incision (colon surgery): 20 – 22 mg/kg IV followed by 20 – 22 mg/kg IV every 90-120 minutes until wound closure.

  For susceptible infections (extra-label):
  a) **Pulse Treatment:** 15 – 35 mg/kg q6-8h IV, IM (large muscle) or SC. An "average" standard dosage is 20 mg/kg q8h.
  b) **Constant-rate IV infusion:** Loading dose 1.3 mg/kg IV, then 1.2 mg/kg/hour CRI.
  c) **Empirical dosage adjustment for renal failure:** Consider giving standard dosage (20 mg/kg) q12h if CrCl is 0.15 – 0.4 mL/kg/min (roughly a serum creatine between 2.3 – 5.5 mg/dL in cats) and q24h if CrCL is <0.15 mL/kg/min (roughly a serum creatine of 8.5 mg/dl in cats) (Trepanier 2013).
  d) Neonates: 10 – 30 mg/kg IV or intraosseous (IO) q8h.

- **HORSES:**

  For susceptible infections (extra-label):

  a) 25 mg/kg IV or IM q6-8h.
  b) Neonatal foals: 15 – 20 mg/kg q8-12h.

- **REPTILES:**

  For susceptible infections (extra-label): Chelonians: 22 mg/kg IM q24h. (Johnson 2002)

Monitoring

- Because cephalosporins usually have minimal toxicity associated with their use, monitoring for efficacy is usually all that is required.
- Patients with diminished renal function may require intensified renal monitoring. Serum levels and therapeutic drug monitoring are not routinely done with these agents.

Chemistry/Synonyms

An injectable, semi-synthetic cephalosporin antibiotic, cefazolin sodium occurs as a practically odorless or having a faint odor, white to off-white, crystalline powder or lyophilized solid. It is freely soluble in water and very slightly soluble in alcohol. Each gram of the injection contains 2 mEq of sodium. After reconstitution, the solution for injection has a pH of 4.5-6 and a light-yellow to yellow color.

Cefazolin sodium may also be known as: 46083, cefazolinum natricum, cephazolin sodium, or SKF-41558; many trade names are available.

Storage/Stability

Cefazolin sodium powder for injection and solutions for injection should be protected from light. The powder for injection should be stored at room temperature (15-30°C); avoid temperatures above 40°C. The frozen solution for injection should be stored at temperatures no higher than -20°C.

After reconstitution, the solution is stable for 24 hours when kept at room temperature; 96 hours if refrigerated. If after reconstitution, the solution is immediately frozen in the original container, the preparation is stable for at least 12 weeks when stored at -20°C.

Compatibility/Compounding Considerations

The following solutions are reportedly **compatible** with cefazolin: Amino acids 4.25%/dextrose 25%, D5W in Ringer's, D5W in Lactated Ringer's, D5W in sodium chloride 0.2%-0.9%, D5W, D10W, Ringer's Injection, Lactated Ringer's Injection, and normal saline The following drugs are reportedly **compatible with cefazolin when given together at a Y-site:** amiodarone, atracurium, calcium gluconate, famotidine, cyclophosphamide, dexmedetomidine, diltiazem, doxorubicin liposome, heparin, hetastarch, insulin, lidocaine, magnesium sulfate, midazolam, metronidazole, morphine, propofol, ranitidine, vancomycin, vecuronium, verapamil HCl, and vitamin B-complex.

The following drugs or solutions are reportedly **incompatible** or only compatible in specific situations with cefazolin: amikacin sulfate, ascorbic acid injection, bleomycin sulfate, calcium chloride/gluconate, cimetidine HCl, erythromycin glucceptate, lidocaine HCl, oxytetracycline HCl, pentobarbital sodium, polymyxin B sulfate, tetracycline HCl and vitamin B-complex with C injection.

Compatibility is dependent upon factors such as pH, concentration, temperature and diluent used; consult specialized references or a hospital pharmacist for more specific information.

Dosage Forms/Regulatory Status

VETERINARY-LABELED PRODUCTS: NONE.

HUMAN-LABELED PRODUCTS:

Cefazolin Sodium Powder for Injection: 100 mg, 300 mg, 500 mg, 1 g, 2 g, 10 g, & 20 g in vials & piggyback vials; generic; (Rx)

Cefazolin Sodium for Injection (IV infusion): 1 g in 50 mL plastic containers, or duplex bags; generic; (Rx)

Revisions/References

Monograph revised/updated September 2013.
Johnson, J. (2002). *Medical management of ill chelonians.* Proceedings; Western Veterinary Conference. accessed via Veterinary Information Network; vin.com
Trepanier, L. A. (2013). Applying Pharmacokinetics to Veterinary Clinical Practice. *Veterinary Clinics of North America-Small Animal Practice* 43(5): 1013-+.

Cefepime HCl

(sef-eh-pim)   Maxipime®

4th Generation Cephalosporin

Prescriber Highlights

▶ Injectable 4th generation cephalosporin that is more active against some gram-negative & gram-positive bacteria than 3rd generation cephalosporins.

▶ Potentially useful for treating neonatal foals & dogs with serious infections.

▶ Limited clinical experience in veterinary medicine.

▶ Adverse effects most likely seen in small animals or foals would be GI-related (*e.g.*, diarrhea, etc.).

Uses/Indications

Cefepime is a semi-synthetic 4th generation cephalosporin with enhanced activity against many gram-negative and gram-positive pathogens. It potentially may be useful in treating serious infections in dogs or foals particularly when aminoglycosides, fluoroquinolones or other more commonly used beta-lactam drugs are ineffective or contraindicated.

Pharmacology/Actions

Cefepime, like other cephalosporins, is usually bactericidal and acts by inhibiting cell wall synthesis. It is classified as a 4th-generation cephalosporin, implying increased gram-negative activity (particularly against *Pseudomonas*) and better activity against many gram-positive bacteria than would be seen with the 3rd generation agents. It rapidly penetrates into gram-negative bacteria and targets penicillin-binding proteins (PBPs). Cefepime does not readily induce beta-lactamases and is highly resistant to hydrolysis by them.

Cefepime has activity against many gram-positive aerobes including many species and strains of Staphylococci and Streptococci. It is not clinically effective in treating infections caused by enterococci, *L. monocytogenes,* or methicillin-resistant staphylococci.

Cefepime has good activity against many gram-negative bacteria and has better activity than other cephalosporins against many Enterobacteriaceae including *Enterobacter* spp., *E. coli, Proteus* spp. and Klebsiella. Its activity against *Pseudomonas* is similar to, or slightly less than, that of ceftazidime.

Cefepime also has activity against certain atypicals like *Mycobacterium avium-intracellulare* complex.

Some anaerobes are sensitive to cefepime, but *Clostridia* and *Bacteroides* are not.

Pharmacokinetics

Cefepime is not absorbed from the GI tract and must be administered parenterally. In dogs, cefepime's volume of distribution at steady state is approximately 0.14 L/kg, elimination half-life about 1.1 hours and clearance, 0.13 L/kg/hr.

In neonatal foals, cefepime's volume of distribution at steady state is approximately 0.18 L/kg, elimination half-life about 1.65 hours and clearance, 0.08 L/kg/hr.

In humans, volume of distribution is about 18 L in adults; 20% of the drug is bound to plasma proteins. Elimination half-life is about 2 hours. Approximately 85% of a dose is excreted unchanged into the urine; less than 1% is metabolized.

Contraindications/Precautions/Warnings

No specific information is available for veterinary patients. Cefepime is contraindicated in human patients hypersensitive to it or other cephalosporins. Dosage adjustment is recommended in humans with severe renal impairment.

Adverse Effects

As usage of cefepime in animals has been very limited, a comprehensive adverse effect profile has not been determined.

There are some reports of dogs or foals developing loose stools or diarrhea after receiving cefepime. IM injections may be painful (alleviated by using 1% lidocaine as diluent).

Human patients generally tolerate cefepime well. Injection site inflammation and rashes occur in approximately 1% of treated patients. Gastrointestinal effects (*e.g.*, dyspepsia, diarrhea, etc.) occur in less than 1% treated patients. Hypersensitivity reactions including anaphylaxis are possible. Rarely, patients with renal dysfunction who have received cefepime without any dosage adjustment will develop neurologic effects (see Overdosage).

Reproductive/Nursing Safety

Studies performed in pregnant mice, rats, and rabbits demonstrated no overt fetal harm. In humans, the FDA categorizes cefepime as category *B* for use during pregnancy (*Animal studies have not yet demonstrated risk to the fetus, but there are no adequate studies in pregnant women; or animal studies have shown an adverse effect, but adequate studies in pregnant women have not demonstrated a risk to the fetus in the first trimester of pregnancy, and there is no evidence of risk in later trimesters.*)

Cefepime enters maternal milk in very low concentrations. Although probably safe for nursing offspring, the potential for adverse effects cannot be ruled out, particularly alterations to gut flora with resultant diarrhea.

Overdosage/Acute Toxicity

No specific information was located for acute toxicity in veterinary patients.

Humans with impaired renal function receiving inadvertent overdoses have developed encephalopathy, seizures and neuromuscular excitability.

Drug Interactions

The following drug interactions have either been reported or are theoretical in humans or animals receiving cefepime and may be of significance in veterinary patients. Unless otherwise noted, use together is not necessarily contraindicated, but weigh the potential risks and perform additional monitoring when appropriate.

■ **AMINOGLYCOSIDES:** Potential for increased risk of nephrotoxicity; monitor renal function.

Laboratory Considerations

■ Cefepime may cause false-positive **urine glucose determinations** when using the copper reduction method (Benedict's solution, Fehling's solution, *Clinitest®*); tests utilizing glucose oxidase (*Tes-Tape®, Clinistix®*) are not affected by cephalosporins.

■ In humans, particularly with azotemia, cephalosporins have caused a false-positive direct **Coombs' test.**

Doses

■ **DOGS/CATS:**

For susceptible infections (extra-label): Based on a pharmacokinetic, 40 mg/kg IV q6h has been recommended for dogs (Gardner et al. 2001). Other sources (anecdotal) state that it can be given to both dogs and cats at 50 mg/kg q8h IM or IV or that a constant-rate IV infusion can be used: 1.4 mg/kg IV load, then 1.04 mg/kg IV CRI.

HORSES:

For susceptible gram-negative infections in foals: 11 mg/kg IV q8h; use has been limited primarily to neonates with poor aminoglycoside kinetics or documented multi-resistant infections. (Gardner et al. 2001; McKenzie 2005)

Monitoring
- Clinical efficacy.
- Monitor renal function in patients with renal insufficiency.

Client Information
- Veterinary professionals only should administer this medication.
- Because of the dosing intervals required, this drug is best administered to inpatients only.

Chemistry/Synonyms
Cefepime HCl occurs as a white to off-white, non-hygroscopic powder that is freely soluble in water.

Cefepime may also be known as: BMY-28142, cefepimi, or cefepima; internationally registered trade names include: *Axepime®*, *Biopime®*, *Cefepen®*, *Ceficad®*, *Cemax®*, *Cepim®*, *Cepimix®*, *Forpar®*, *Maxcef®*, *Maxipime®* or *Maxil®*.

Storage/Stability
The powder for injection should be stored between (2-25°C) and protected from light. Cefepime can be reconstituted and administered with a variety of diluents including normal saline and D5W. Generally, the solution is stable for up 24 hours at room temperature; up to 7 days if kept refrigerated.

Compatibility/Compounding Considerations
Drugs that may be admixed with cefepime include: amikacin (but not gentamicin or tobramycin), ampicillin, vancomycin, metronidazole and clindamycin. These admixtures have varying times that they remain stable. For more information on dosage preparation, stability and compatibility, refer to the package insert for *Maxipime®* or contact a hospital pharmacist.

Dosage Forms/Regulatory Status
VETERINARY-LABELED PRODUCTS: NONE.

HUMAN-LABELED PRODUCTS:

Cefepime Powder for Injection: 500 mg, 1 g & 2 g in vials, 15 mL & 20 mL vials, ADD-Vantage vials, & 100 mL piggyback bottles; *Maxipime®*, generic; (Rx)

Cefepime Injection Solution: 1 g & 2 g in 50 mL & 100 mL (respectively) single-dose containers; generic; (Rx)

Revisions/References
Monograph revised/updated September 2013.

Gardner, S. & M. Papich (2001). Comparison of cefepime pharmacokinetics in neonatal foals and adult dogs. *J Vet Pharmacol Therap* 24: 187-92.

McKenzie, H. (2005). *Pathophysiology and treatment of pneumonia in foals.* ACVIM 2005 Proceedings. accessed via Veterinary Information Network; vin.com

Cefixime

(sef-ix-eem)   Suprax®

3rd Generation Cephalosporin

Prescriber Highlights
▶ Oral 3rd generation cephalosporin that may be useful in dogs and cats.
▶ Contraindications: Hypersensitivity to it or other cephalosporins.
▶ May need to adjust dose if patient has renal disease.
▶ Adverse Effects: Primarily GI, but hypersensitivity possible.

Uses/Indications
Uses for cefixime are limited in veterinary medicine. Its use should be reserved for those times when infections (systemic or urinary tract) are caused by susceptible gram-negative organisms where oral treatment is indicated or when FDA-approved fluoroquinolones or other 3rd generation cephalosporins (*e.g.*, cefpodoxime, etc.) are either contraindicated or ineffective.

Pharmacology/Actions
Like other cephalosporins, cefixime inhibits bacteria cell wall synthesis. It is considered bactericidal and relatively resistant to bacterial beta-lactamases.

Cefixime's main spectrum of activity is against gram-negative bacteria in the family Enterobacteriaceae (excluding Pseudomonas) including Escherichia, Proteus, and Klebsiella. It is efficacious against Streptococcus, Rhodococcus, and apparently, Borrelia. Efficacy for *E. coli* is rapidly decreasing as significant resistance has developed in recent years.

Cefixime is not efficacious against *Pseudomonas aeruginosa*, Enterococcus, Staphylococcus, Bordetella, Listeria, Enterobacter, Bacteroides, Actinomyces or Clostridium. For other than *Streptococcus* spp., it has limited efficacy against many gram-positive organisms or anaerobes.

Because sensitivity of various bacteria to the 3rd generation cephalosporin antibiotics is unique to a given agent, cefixime specific disks or dilutions must be used to determine susceptibility.

Pharmacokinetics
Cefixime is relatively rapidly absorbed after oral administration. Bioavailability in the dog is about 50%. Food may impede the rate, but not the extent, of absorption. The suspension may have a higher bioavailability than tablets. The drug is fairly highly bound to plasma proteins in the dog (about 90%). It is unknown if the drug penetrates into the CSF.

Elimination of cefixime is by both renal and non-renal means, but serum half-lives are prolonged in patients with decreased renal function. In dogs, elimination half-life is about 7 hours.

Contraindications/Precautions/Warnings
Cefixime is contraindicated in patients hypersensitive to it or other cephalosporins. Because cefixime is excreted by the kidneys dosages and/or dosage frequency may need to be adjusted in patients with significantly diminished renal function. Use with caution in patients with seizure disorders and patients allergic to penicillins.

Adverse Effects
Adverse effects in the dog may include GI distress (*e.g.*, vomiting, etc.) and hypersensitivity reactions (*e.g.*, urticaria and pruritus, possibly fever).

Reproductive/Nursing Safety
Cefixime has not been shown to be teratogenic, but should only be used during pregnancy when clearly indicated. In humans, the FDA categorizes this drug as category *B* for use during pregnancy (*Animal studies have not yet demonstrated risk to the fetus, but there are no adequate studies in pregnant women; or animal studies have shown an adverse effect, but adequate studies in pregnant women have not demonstrated a risk to the fetus in the first trimester of pregnancy, and there is no evidence of risk in later trimesters.*)

Overdosage/Acute Toxicity
Cephalosporin overdoses are unlikely to cause significant problems, but other effects are possible (see Adverse Effects section).

Drug Interactions
The following drug interactions have either been reported or are theoretical in humans or animals receiving cefixime and may be of significance in veterinary patients. Unless otherwise noted, use

together is not necessarily contraindicated, but weigh the potential risks and perform additional monitoring when appropriate.

- **PROBENECID:** Competitively blocks the tubular secretion of most cephalosporins thereby increasing serum levels and serum half-lives.
- **SALICYLATES:** May displace cefixime from plasma protein binding sites; clinical significance is unclear.

Laboratory Considerations

- Cefixime may cause false-positive **urine glucose determinations** when using cupric sulfate solution (Benedict's Solution, *Clinitest®*). Tests utilizing glucose oxidase (*Tes-Tape®*, *Clinistix®*) are not affected by cephalosporins.
- If using the nitroprusside test for determining **urinary ketones,** cefixime may cause false-positive results.

Doses

- **DOGS/CATS:**

    For susceptible infections (extra-label): Dosage recommendations range from 5 mg/kg PO 1-2 times a day for UTI to 10 – 12.5 mg/kg PO twice daily for systemic infections.

Monitoring

- Efficacy.
- Adverse effects.

Client Information

- Can be given with or without food, but gastrointestinal side effects might be prevented if given with food.
- Most common side effects are diarrhea, vomiting and loss of appetite.
- Be sure to give as long as veterinarian has prescribed, even if animal seems better.
- Cephalosporin antibiotics have an odor that resembles cat urine, but this is normal.

Chemistry/Synonyms

An oral 3rd generation semisynthetic cephalosporin antibiotic, cefixime is available commercially as the trihydrate. Cefixime occurs as a white to slightly yellowish white crystalline powder with a characteristic odor and a pKa of 3.73. Solubility in water is pH dependent. At a pH of 3.2, 0.5 mg/mL is soluble and 18 mg/mL at pH 4.2. The oral suspension is strawberry flavored and after reconstitution has pH of 2.5-4.2.

Cefixime may also be known as: cefiximum, CL-284635, FK-027, FR-17027 and *Suprax®*; many internationally registered trade names are available.

Storage/Stability

Cefixime powder for suspension should be stored at room temperature in tight containers. After reconstitution of the oral suspension, refrigeration is not required, but it should be discarded after 14 days whether refrigerated or not.

Compatibility/Compounding Considerations

No specific information noted.

Dosage Forms/Regulatory Status

VETERINARY-LABELED PRODUCTS: NONE.

HUMAN-LABELED PRODUCTS:

Cefixime Oral Tablets or Capsules: 400 mg; *Suprax®*; (Rx)

Cefixime Oral Chewable Tablets: 100 mg & 200 mg; *Suprax®*; (Rx)

Cefixime Powder for Oral Suspension: 100 mg/5 mL in 50 mL, 75 mL & 100 mL, 200 mg/5 mL in 25 mL, 37.5 mL, 50 mL, 75 mL & 100 mL; *Suprax®*; (Rx)

Revisions/References

Monograph revised/updated September 2013.

Cefotaxime Sodium

(sef-oh-taks-eem)   Claforan®

3rd Generation Cephalosporin

Prescriber Highlights

► 3rd generation parenteral cephalosporin.
► Potentially could cause hypersensitivity reactions, granulocytopenia, or diarrhea.
► Causes pain on IM injection; give IV over 3-5 minutes (or more).
► May need to reduce dose in renal failure.

Uses/Indications

In the United States, there are no cefotaxime products FDA-approved for veterinary species but it has been used clinically in several species when an injectable 3rd generation cephalosporin may be indicated.

Pharmacology/Actions

Cefotaxime is a 3rd generation injectable cephalosporin agent and, like other cephalosporins, inhibits bacteria cell wall synthesis. It is usually bactericidal and it is a time-dependent antibiotic. Cefotaxime has a relatively wide spectrum of activity against both gram-positive and gram-negative bacteria. While less active against *Staphylococcus* spp. than the first generation agents, it still has significant activity against those and other gram-positive cocci. Cefotaxime, like the other 3rd generation agents, has extended coverage of gram-negative aerobes particularly in the family *Enterobacteriaceae*, including *Klebsiella* spp., *E. coli, Salmonella, Serratia marcescens, Proteus* spp., and *Enterobacter* spp. Cefotaxime's *in vitro* activity against *Pseudomonas aeruginosa* is variable and results are usually disappointing when the drug is used clinically against this organism. Many anaerobes are also susceptible to cefotaxime including strains of *Bacteroides fragilis, Clostridium* spp., *Fusobacterium* spp., *Peptococcus* spp., and *Peptostreptococcus* spp.

Because 3rd generation cephalosporins exhibit specific activities against bacteria, a 30 microgram cefotaxime disk should be used when performing Kirby-Bauer disk susceptibility tests for this antibiotic.

Pharmacokinetics

Cefotaxime is not appreciably absorbed after oral administration and must be given parenterally to attain therapeutic serum levels. After administration, the drug is widely distributed in body tissues including bone, prostatic fluid (human), aqueous humor, bile, ascitic and pleural fluids. Cefotaxime crosses the placenta and activity in amniotic fluid either equals or exceeds that in maternal serum. Cefotaxime distributes into milk in low concentrations. In humans, approximately 13-40% of the drug is bound to plasma proteins.

Unlike the 1st generation cephalosporins (and most 2nd generation agents), cefotaxime will enter the CSF in therapeutic levels (at high dosages) when the patient's meninges are inflamed.

Cefotaxime is partially metabolized by the liver to desacetylcefotaxime that exhibits some antibacterial activity. Desacetylcefotaxime is partially degraded to inactive metabolites by the liver. Cefotaxime and its metabolites are primarily excreted in the urine. Because tubular secretion is involved in the renal excretion of the drug, in several species probenecid has been demonstrated to prolong the serum half-life of cefotaxime.

Pharmacokinetic parameters in certain veterinary species follow: In dogs, the apparent volume of distribution at steady state is 480 mL/kg, and a total body clearance of 10.5 mL/min/kg after intravenous injection. Serum elimination half-lives of 45 minutes when given IV, 50 minutes after IM injection, and 103 minutes after SC injection have been noted. Bioavailability is about 87% after IM injection and approximately 100% after SC injection.

In cats, total body clearance is approximately 3 mL/min/kg after intravenous injection and the serum elimination half-life is about 1 hour. Bioavailability is about 93-98% after IM injection.

In foals, several pharmacokinetic studies have been performed with reported values for volume of distribution ranging from 0.29 L/kg to 4.2 L/kg. Half-life is around one hour and clearance, approximately 0.32 L/kg/hr.

Contraindications/Precautions/Warnings

Cephalosporins are contraindicated in patients with a history of hypersensitivity to them. Because there may be cross-reactivity, use cephalosporins cautiously in patients that are documented hypersensitive to other beta-lactam antibiotics (*e.g.*, penicillins, cefamycins, carbapenems).

Patients in renal failure may need dosage adjustments.

Cefotaxime can be easily confused with other cephalosporins. Consider writing orders and prescriptions using tall man letters: cefoTAXime.

Adverse Effects

Adverse effects with the cephalosporins are usually not serious and have a relatively low frequency of occurrence.

Hypersensitivity reactions unrelated to dose can occur with these agents and can manifest as rashes, fever, eosinophilia, lymphadenopathy, or full-blown anaphylaxis. The use of cephalosporins in patients documented to be hypersensitive to penicillin-class antibiotics is controversial. In humans, it is estimated 1-15% of patients hypersensitive to penicillins will also be hypersensitive to cephalosporins. The incidence of cross-reactivity in veterinary patients is unknown.

Cephalosporins can cause pain at the injection site when administered intramuscularly. Sterile abscesses or other severe local tissue reactions are also possible but much less common. Thrombophlebitis is also possible after IV administration of these drugs.

Because the cephalosporins may also alter gut flora, antibiotic-associated diarrhea can occur and allow the proliferation of resistant bacteria in the colon (superinfections).

While cephalosporins (particularly cephalothin) have the potential for causing nephrotoxicity at clinically used doses in patients with normal renal function, risks for the occurrence of this adverse effect appear minimal.

High doses or very prolonged use has been associated with neurotoxicity, neutropenia, agranulocytosis, thrombocytopenia, hepatitis, positive Comb's test, interstitial nephritis, and tubular necrosis. Except for tubular necrosis and neurotoxicity, these effects have an immunologic component.

Reproductive/Nursing Safety

Cephalosporins have been shown to cross the placenta and safe use of them during pregnancy has not been firmly established, but neither have there been any documented teratogenic problems associated with these drugs. However, use only when the potential benefits outweigh the risks. In humans, the FDA categorizes this cefotaxime as category *B* for use during pregnancy (*Animal studies have not yet demonstrated risk to the fetus, but there are no adequate studies in pregnant women; or animal studies have shown an adverse effect, but adequate studies in pregnant women have not demonstrated a risk to the fetus in the first trimester of pregnancy, and there is no evidence of risk in later trimesters.*)

Most of these agents (cephalosporins) are excreted in milk in small quantities. Modification/alteration of bowel flora with resultant diarrhea is theoretically possible.

Overdosage/Acute Toxicity

Cephalosporin overdoses are unlikely to cause significant problems, but other effects are possible (see Adverse effects section).

Drug Interactions

The following drug interactions have either been reported or are theoretical in humans or animals receiving cefotaxime and may be of significance in veterinary patients. Unless otherwise noted, use together is not necessarily contraindicated, but weigh the potential risks and perform additional monitoring when appropriate.

- **AMINOGLYCOSIDES/NEPHROTOXIC DRUGS:** The concurrent use of parenteral aminoglycosides or other nephrotoxic drugs (*e.g.*, **amphotericin B**, etc.) with cephalosporins is somewhat controversial. Potentially, cephalosporins could cause additive nephrotoxicity when used with these drugs, but this interaction has only been well documented with cephaloridine (no longer marketed). *In vitro* studies have demonstrated that cephalosporins can have synergistic or additive activity against certain bacteria when used with aminoglycosides, but they should not be mixed together (administer separately).

- **PROBENECID:** Competitively blocks the tubular secretion of most cephalosporins, thereby increasing serum levels and serum half-lives.

Laboratory Considerations

- In humans, particularly with azotemia, cephalosporins have caused a false-positive direct **Coombs' test**.

- Cephalosporins may cause falsely elevated **17-ketosteroid** values in urine.

- Cefotaxime like most other cephalosporins, may cause a **false-positive urine glucose determination** when using the cupric sulfate solution test (*e.g.*, *Clinitest®*), Benedict's solution or Fehling's solution.

Doses

- **DOGS/CATS:**

  For susceptible infections (extra-label): Pulse therapy dosage recommendations vary widely, ranging from 20 – 80 mg/kg IV, SC or IM q6-12h. A "common" anecdotal dose is 40 – 50 mg/kg q8h. Some sources recommend giving as a CRI with an initial IV load of 3.2 mg/kg IV followed by a CRI of 5 mg/kg/hour.

- **HORSES:**

  For susceptible infections (extra-label):

  a) **Neonatal foals:** Based on their pharmacokinetic study: foals were given a bolus IV dose of 40 mg/kg and then a constant rate infusion of 120 mg/kg/24 hours (5 mg/kg/hour) was given the first day. On subsequent days the dose was 160 mg/kg/24 hours (6.66 mg/kg/hour) as a CRI infusion. The authors concluded that to optimize the time that cefotaxime concentrations exceed the MIC of common equine pathogens their results support continuous drug infusion over bolus dosing in the treatment of neonatal foal septicemia. They also stated that a subsequent study was desirable to determine whether a lower dose would still be effective to reduce the cost associated with cefotaxime therapy. (Hewson et al. 2013)

  b) **Foals:** As regional perfusion for adjunctive treatment of septic arthritis: 1 gram cefotaxime in 20 mL of saline. Tourniquet above and below joint. Inject antibiotic solution and leave tourniquet in place for 20 minutes. (Stewart 2008)

- **BIRDS:**

  For susceptible infections (extra-label):

  a) **For bacterial infections, bacterial hepatitis:** 75 – 100 mg/kg IM or IV q4-8h. (Oglesbee 2009a), (Oglesbee 2009b)

b) **Ratites (young birds):** 25 mg/kg IM 3 times daily. (Jenson 1998)

c) 75 – 100 mg/kg IM or IV q4-8h. (Hess 2002)

- **REPTILES:**

  For susceptible infections (extra-label):

  a) 20 – 40 mg/kg IM once daily for 7-14 days. (Gauvin 1993)

  b) Chelonians: 20 – 40 mg/kg IM q24h. (Johnson 2002)

  c) Nebulized antibiotic therapy: 100 mg twice daily. (Raiti 2003)

Monitoring

- Because cephalosporins usually have minimal toxicity associated with their use, monitoring for efficacy is usually all that is required.

- Patients with diminished renal function may require intensified renal monitoring.

Chemistry/Synonyms

A semisynthetic, 3rd generation, aminothiazolyl cephalosporin, cefotaxime sodium occurs as an odorless, white to off-white crystalline powder with a pK_a of 3.4. It is sparingly soluble in water and slightly soluble in alcohol. Potency of cefotaxime sodium is expressed in terms of cefotaxime. One gram of cefotaxime (sodium) contains 2.2 mEq of sodium.

Cefotaxime sodium may also be known as: cefotaximum natricum, CTX, HR-756, RU-24756 and *Claforan®*; many other trade names are available internationally.

Storage/Stability

Cefotaxime sodium sterile powder for injection should be stored at temperatures of less than 30°C; protected from light. The commercially available frozen injection should be stored at temperatures no greater than -20°C. Depending on storage conditions, the powder or solutions may darken which may indicate a loss in potency. Cefotaxime is not stable in solutions with pH >7.5 (sodium bicarbonate).

Compatibility/Compounding Considerations

All commonly used IV fluids and the following drugs are reportedly **compatible** with cefotaxime: clindamycin, metronidazole and verapamil. Compatibility is dependent upon factors such as pH, concentration, temperature, and diluent used; consult specialized references or a hospital pharmacist for more specific information.

Dosage Forms/Regulatory Status

VETERINARY-LABELED PRODUCTS: NONE.

HUMAN-LABELED PRODUCTS:

Cefotaxime Sodium Powder for Injection: 500 mg, 1 g, 2 g, & 10 g in vials, bottles, infusion bottles & *ADD-Vantage* system vials; *Claforan®*, generic; (Rx)

Cefotaxime Sodium for Injection: 1 g & 2 g in infusion bottles & premixed 50 mL; *Claforan®*, generic; (Rx)

Revisions/References

Monograph revised/updated September 2013.

Gauvin, J. (1993). Drug therapy in reptiles. *Seminars in Avian & Exotic Med* 2(1): 48-59.

Hess, L. (2002). *Practical emergency/critical care of pet birds.* Proceedings: Atlantic Coast Veterinary Conference. accessed via Veterinary Information Network; vin.com

Hewson, J., et al. (2013). Comparison of continuous infusion with intermittent bolus administration of cefotaxime on blood and cavity fluid drug concentrations in neonatal foals. *J. Vet. Pharmacol. Ther.* 36(1): 68-77.

Jenson, J. (1998). Current ratite therapy. *The Veterinary Clinics of North America: Food Animal Practice* 16:3(November).

Johnson, J. (2002). *Medical management of ill chelonians.* Proceedings; Western Veterinary Conference. accessed via Veterinary Information Network; vin.com

Oglesbee, B. (2009a). *Liver disease in pet birds.* Proceedings: WVC. accessed via Veterinary Information Network; vin.com

Oglesbee, B. (2009b). *Working up the pet bird with lower respiratory tract disorders.* Proceedings: WVC. accessed via Veterinary Information Network; vin.com

Raiti, P. (2003). *Administration of aerosolized antibiotics to reptiles.* Proceedings: Atlantic Coast Veterinary Conference. accessed via Veterinary Information Network; vin.com

Stewart, A. (2008). *Equine Neonatal Sepsis.* Proceedings: WVC. accessed via Veterinary Information Network; vin.com

Cefotetan Disodium

(sef-oh-tee-tan)   Cefotan®

2nd Generation Cephalosporin (Cephamycin)

Prescriber Highlights

▶ 2nd to 3rd generation parenteral cephalosporin (cephamycin) similar to cefoxitin.

▶ Pharmacokinetic profile better and may be more effective against *E. coli* in dogs than cefoxitin.

▶ Contraindications: Hypersensitivity to it or cephalosporins.

▶ Adverse Effects: Unlikely; potentially could cause bleeding.

▶ If severe renal dysfunction, may need to increase time between doses.

Uses/Indications

Cefotetan may be a reasonable choice for treating serious infections caused by susceptible bacteria, including *E. coli* or anaerobes. It appears to be well tolerated in small animals and may be given less frequently than cefoxitin.

Pharmacology/Actions

Often categorized as a 2nd or 3rd generation cephalosporin, cefotetan is usually bactericidal and acts by inhibiting mucopeptide synthesis in the bacterial cell wall.

Cefotetan's *in vitro* activity against aerobes include *E. coli*, Proteus, Klebsiella, Salmonella, Staphylococcus and most Streptococcus. It has efficacy against most strains of the following anaerobes: Actinomyces, Clostridium, Peptococcus, Peptostreptococcus and Propionibacterium. Many strains of Bacteroides are still sensitive to cefotetan.

Cefotetan is generally ineffective against *Pseudomonas aeruginosa* and Enterococci.

Because 2nd generation cephalosporins exhibit specific activities against bacteria, a 30-microgram cefoxitin disk should be used when performing Kirby-Bauer disk susceptibility tests for this antibiotic.

Pharmacokinetics

Cefotetan is not appreciably absorbed after oral administration and must be given parenterally to achieve therapeutic serum levels. The drug is well distributed into most tissues, but only has limited penetration into the CSF. Cefotetan is primarily excreted unchanged by the kidneys into the urine via both glomerular filtration (primarily) and tubular secretion. Elimination half-lives may be significantly prolonged in patients with severely diminished renal function.

Contraindications/Precautions/Warnings

Cephamycins are contraindicated in patients that have a history of hypersensitivity to them. Because there may be cross-reactivity, use cephalosporins cautiously in patients that are documented to be hypersensitive to other beta-lactam antibiotics (*e.g.*, penicillins, cephalosporins, carbapenems).

Cefotetan can be easily confused with other cephalosporins. Consider writing orders and prescriptions using tall man letters: cefoTEtan.

Adverse Effects

There is little information on the adverse effect profile of this medication in veterinary species, but it appears to be well tolerated. In humans, less than 5% of patients report adverse effects. Because cefotetan contains an N-methylthiotetrazole side chain (like cefoperazone), it may have a greater tendency to cause hematologic effects (*e.g.*, hypoprothrombinemia, etc.) or disulfiram-like reactions (*e.g.*, vomiting, etc.) than other parenteral cephalosporins.

Hypersensitivity reactions unrelated to dose can occur with these agents and can manifest as rashes, fever, eosinophilia, lymphadenopathy, or full-blown anaphylaxis. The use of cephalosporins in patients documented to be hypersensitive to penicillin-class antibiotics is controversial. In humans, it is estimated 1-15% of patients hypersensitive to penicillins will also be hypersensitive to cephalosporins. The incidence of cross-reactivity in veterinary patients is unknown.

Cephalosporins can cause pain at the injection site when administered intramuscularly. Sterile abscesses or other severe local tissue reactions are also possible but are less common. Thrombophlebitis is also possible after IV administration of these drugs.

Even when administered parenterally, cephalosporins may alter gut flora and antibiotic-associated diarrhea or the proliferation of resistant bacteria in the colon (superinfections) can occur.

While cephalosporins (particularly cephalothin) have the potential for causing nephrotoxicity at clinically used doses in patients with normal renal function, risks for the occurrence of this adverse effect appear minimal. High doses or very prolonged use has been associated with neurotoxicity, neutropenia, agranulocytosis, thrombocytopenia, hepatitis, positive Comb's test, interstitial nephritis, and tubular necrosis. Except for tubular necrosis and neurotoxicity, these effects have an immunologic component.

Reproductive/Nursing Safety

Safe use during pregnancy has not been established; use only when justified. In humans, the FDA categorizes this drug as category *B* for use during pregnancy (*Animal studies have not yet demonstrated risk to the fetus, but there are no adequate studies in pregnant women; or animal studies have shown an adverse effect, but adequate studies in pregnant women have not demonstrated a risk to the fetus in the first trimester of pregnancy, and there is no evidence of risk in later trimesters*)

Cefotetan enters maternal milk in small quantities. Alteration of bowel flora with resultant diarrhea is theoretically possible.

Overdosage/Acute Toxicity

Unlikely to cause adverse effects, unless massive or chronically overdosed; seizures possible. Treat symptomatically.

Drug Interactions

The following drug interactions have either been reported or are theoretical in humans or animals receiving cefotetan and may be of significance in veterinary patients. Unless otherwise noted, use together is not necessarily contraindicated, but weigh the potential risks and perform additional monitoring when appropriate.

- **ALCOHOL:** A disulfiram reaction is possible.
- **AMINOGLYCOSIDES/NEPHROTOXIC DRUGS:** The concurrent use of parenteral aminoglycosides or other nephrotoxic drugs (*e.g.*, **amphotericin B**, etc.) with cephalosporins is somewhat controversial. Potentially, cephalosporins could cause additive nephrotoxicity when used with these drugs, but this interaction has only been well documented with cephaloridine (no longer marketed). *In vitro* studies have demonstrated that cephalosporins can have synergistic or additive activity against certain bacteria when used with aminoglycosides, but they should not be mixed together (administer separately).

Laboratory Considerations

- Except for cefotaxime, cephalosporins may cause false-positive **urine glucose determinations** when using cupric sulfate solution (Benedict's Solution, *Clinitest®*). Tests utilizing glucose oxidase (*Tes-Tape®, Clinistix®*) are not affected by cephalosporins.
- When using the Jaffe reaction to measure **serum or urine creatinine**, cephalosporins (not ceftazidime or cefotaxime) in high dosages may cause falsely elevated values.
- In humans, particularly with azotemia, cephalosporins have caused a false-positive direct **Coombs' test**.

- Cephalosporins may also cause falsely elevated **17-ketosteroid** values in urine.

Doses

- **DOGS/CATS:**

  For susceptible infections (extra-label):

  a) 30 mg/kg IV or SC q8h; several references state that q12h can be used when giving SC, but this was based on a very small (N=4) study done in dogs (Petersen et al. 1993).

  b) Empirical dosage adjustment for renal failure: Consider giving q24h if CrCl is 0.15 – 0.4 mL/kg/min (roughly a serum creatine between 2.3 – 5.5 mg/dL in cats) and q48h if CrCL is <0.15 mL/kg/min (roughly a serum creatine of 8.5 mg/dL in cats). (Trepanier 2013)

  For surgical (GI surgery) prophylaxis (extra-label): 30 mg/kg IV 30-60 minutes prior to incision. May repeat one time in 6-12 hours.

Monitoring

- Because cephalosporins usually have minimal toxicity associated with their use, monitoring for efficacy is usually all that is required.
- Patients with diminished renal function may require intensified renal monitoring and decreased dosage frequency. Serum levels and therapeutic drug monitoring are not routinely done with these agents.

Chemistry/Synonyms

A semisynthetic cephamycin similar to cefoxitin, cefotetan disodium occurs as a white to pale yellow, lyophilized powder. It is very soluble in water and alcohol. The injection contains approximately 3.5 mEq of sodium per gram of cefotetan and after reconstitution has a pH of 4-6.5.

Cefotetan Disodium may also be known as: ICI-156834, YM-09330, *Apacef®*, *Apatef®*, *Cefotan®*, Ceftenon®, *Cepan®*, *Darvilen®*, or *Yamatetan®*.

Storage/Stability

The sterile powder for injection should be stored below 22°C and protected from light. A darkening of the powder with time does not indicate lessened potency. After reconstituting with sterile water for injection, the resultant solution is stable for 24 hours if stored at room temperature, 96 hours if refrigerated, and at least one week if frozen at -20°C.

Dosage Forms/Regulatory Status

VETERINARY-LABELED PRODUCTS: NONE.

HUMAN-LABELED PRODUCTS:

Cefotetan Disodium Powder for Solution: 1 g, 2 g, & 10 g in 10 mL & 20 mL vials and 1 g and 2 g premixed bags (with dextrose); generic; (Rx)

Revisions/References

Monograph revised/updated September 2013.

Petersen, S. & E. Rosin (1993). In vitro antibacterial activity of cefoxitin and cefotetan and pharmacokinetics in dogs. *Am J Vet Res* 54(Sep 9): 1496-9.

Trepanier, L. A. (2013). Applying Pharmacokinetics to Veterinary Clinical Practice. *Veterinary Clinics of North America-Small Animal Practice* 43(5): 1013-+.

Cefovecin Sodium

(sef-oh-vee-sin)   Convenia®

Injectable Long-Acting Cephalosporin

Prescriber Highlights

▶ Long-acting injectable cephalosporin labeled for use in dogs and cats.

▶ Primary benefit is for patients whose owners have difficulty adhering to an oral dosing regimen or when oral antibiotics are not tolerated or absorbed.

Uses/Indications

In the USA, cefovecin is FDA-approved for dogs to treat skin infections (secondary superficial pyoderma, abscesses, and wounds) caused by susceptible strains of *Staphylococcus pseudintermedius* and *Streptococcus canis* (Group G) and in cats to treat skin infections (wounds and abscesses) caused by susceptible strains of *Pasteurella multocida*. A recent review of the evidence supporting efficacy of various antibiotics for superficial and deep pyoderma in dogs, found that for SC dosing of cefovecin, there was a good level of evidence for high efficacy for superficial pyoderma and a fair level of evidence for moderate to high efficacy in deep pyoderma. The Working Group of the International Society for Companion Animal Infectious Diseases recommended that cefovecin be used for urinary tract infections in dogs and cats only in situations where oral treatment is problematic; Enterococci are resistant and the long duration of excretion in urine makes it difficult to interpret post-treatment culture results (Weese et al. 2011). A study comparing oral amoxicillin-clavulanic acid, cefovecin, and oral doxycycline in the treatment of upper respiratory tract disease in shelter cats, found that single-dose cefovecin appeared to be less effective than the other two treatments (Litster et al. 2012).

In the UK, cefovecin is also labeled for dogs for skin and soft tissue infections caused by *E. coli* and/or *Pasteurella multocida*, for the treatment of urinary tract infections associated with *E. coli* and/or *Proteus* spp., and as adjunctive treatment to mechanical or surgical periodontal therapy of severe infections of the gingival and periodontal tissues associated with *Porphyromonas* spp. and *Prevotella* spp. Cefovecin is also labeled there for use in cats for skin infections caused by *Fusobacterium* spp., *Bacteroides* spp., *Prevotella oralis*, beta-hemolytic *Streptococci* and/or *Staphylococcus pseudintermedius*, and the treatment of urinary tract infections associated with *E. coli*.

Cefovecin's long half-life in dogs and cats allows a single dose or extended dosing intervals (determined by organism susceptibility and MIC) for treating a variety of infections off-label (in USA).

Pharmacology/Actions

Cefovecin is a cephalosporin antibiotic that described as a 3rd-generation cephalosporin, but it is not as active as cefotaxime or ceftazidime against gram-negative organisms. Its mechanism of action in susceptible bacteria, like other beta-lactams, is to bind to and disrupt the actions of bacterial transpeptidase and carboxypeptidase thereby interfering with bacterial cell wall synthesis.

At present, there are no established CLSI-approved standards for susceptibility testing for cefovecin, but an MIC ≤ 2 mcg/mL should be considered as a susceptible breakpoint (Papich 2013). Cefovecin is not active against *Pseudomonas* spp., methicillin-resistant staphylococci, or enterococci. Its high protein binding does not allow it (at labeled doses) to achieve effective serum levels to treat systemic (non-UTI) *E. coli* or other gram-negative bacilli infections.

Pharmacokinetics

After SC injection in dogs or cats, cefovecin is completely absorbed.

In dogs, peak levels occur about 6 hours after a dose, and in cats, about 2 hours. The drug is highly bound to plasma proteins (98.5% dogs; 99.8% cats) that slowly dissociate giving the drug its long elimination half-life. As cefovecin exhibits non-linear kinetics, an increase in dosage does not proportionally increase the plasma concentration. In the product label the following additional pharmacokinetic values are listed: terminal elimination half-life: 133 ± 16 hours (dog), 166 ± 18 hours (cat), maximum plasma concentration: 121 ± 51 micrograms/mL (dog), 141 ± 12 micrograms/mL (cat); volume of distribution (steady-state): 0.122 ± 0.011 L/kg (dog), 0.09 ± 0.01 L/kg (cat); total body clearance: 0.76 ± 0.13 mL/hr/kg (dog), 0.350 ± 0.40 mL/kg/hr (cat).

Elimination of cefovecin is primarily via renal mechanism and the majority of a dose is excreted unchanged in the urine, but a small amount is excreted unchanged in the bile. Cefovecin is a highly protein-bound molecule in dog plasma (98.5%) and cat plasma (99.8%) and may compete with other highly protein-bound drugs for plasma protein binding sites. Cefovecin may persist in the body for up to 65 days and be excreted in urine at therapeutic concentrations for 14 days in dogs and 21 days in cats.

Contraindications/Precautions/Warnings

Cefovecin is contraindicated in animals with a known allergy to cefovecin or to other beta-lactam antibiotics. Anaphylaxis has been reported with the use of this product. Because cefovecin is primarily eliminated via renal mechanisms, use with caution in animals with severe renal dysfunction.

The UK labeling warns against using in small herbivores (*e.g.*, Guinea pigs, rabbits, etc.).

Safe use in dogs or cats less than 4 months of age has not been established. The UK labeling warns against using in dogs or cats less then 8 weeks old.

Cefovecin can be easily confused with other cephalosporins. Consider writing orders and prescriptions using tall man letters: cefoVEcin.

Adverse Effects

In dogs and cats, cefovecin appears to be well tolerated. Pre-marketing (USA) studies in dogs and cats found no significant increases in adverse effect types or rates when compared with control. However, treated animals did have some changes in laboratory values. Several dogs had mild to moderate increases in liver enzymes (GGT, ALT). In treated cats, 4/147 cats had increases (mild) in ALT concentrations, 24/147 had increases in BUN, and 6/147 had moderately elevated serum creatinine values.

In the FDA's Cumulative Veterinary Adverse Drug Experience (ADE) Reports (through November 2010), the most common adverse effects listed (in decreasing order of frequency) are: Dogs: depression/lethargy, anorexia, and vomiting; Cats: anorexia, depression/lethargy, and vomiting. As more experience is gained with this agent, a clearer adverse drug reaction profile is expected.

Hypersensitivity reactions, anaphylaxis and death associated with this drug are possible and have been reported. The manufacturer also states: Occasionally, cephalosporins and NSAIDs have been associated with myelotoxicity, thereby creating a toxic neutropenia. Other hematological reactions seen with cephalosporins include neutropenia, anemia, hypoprothrombinemia, thrombocytopenia, prolonged prothrombin time (PT) and partial thromboplastin time (PTT), platelet dysfunction and transient increases in serum aminotransferases.

Because the drug can persist in the body for up to 65 days, adverse reactions may occur that require prolonged treatment.

Reproductive/Nursing Safety

The manufacturer states that safe use in breeding or lactating animals has not been determined. However, cephalosporins are generally considered safe for use during pregnancy and lactation and veterinarians and owners can weigh any risks of using the drug versus the benefits to the dam and offspring.

Overdosage/Acute Toxicity

Acute overdoses should be relatively safe. Dogs administered cefovecin SC up to 180 mg/kg (22.5X) showed only site irritation, vocalization, and edema. Edema resolved within 8-24 hours. Cats given the same dose (22.5X) injection showed the same signs but 10 days post had a lower mean white blood cell counts than controls, and one cat had a small amount of bilirubinuria on day 10.

Drug Interactions

As cefovecin is so highly bound to plasma proteins it potentially could displace (or be displaced) from plasma protein binding sites by other highly bound agents. The manufacturer reports that in an experimental *in vitro* system, cefovecin demonstrated that it could increase the free (active) concentrations of other highly protein-bound dugs such as **carprofen, furosemide, doxycycline,** and **ketoconazole.** They caution that concurrent use of these or other drugs that have a high degree of protein binding (*e.g.,* **NSAIDs, propofol, cardiac, anticonvulsant,** and **behavioral medications**) may compete with cefovecin-binding and cause adverse reactions. However, actual clinical significance has not been established and a recent report concluded that a clinically significant drug interaction is unlikely from the concurrent administration of **carprofen** and cefovecin in dogs (Messenger et al. 2013).

Laboratory Considerations

- Cephalosporins may cause false-positive **urine glucose determinations** when using the copper reduction method (Benedict's solution, Fehling's solution, *Clinitest®*); tests utilizing glucose oxidase (*Tes-Tape®, Clinistix®*) are not affected by cephalosporins.

- When using the Jaffe reaction to measure **serum or urine creatinine,** cephalosporins (not ceftazidime or cefotaxime) given in high dosages may cause falsely elevated values.

- Cephalosporins may cause falsely lowered **albumin** levels when certain tests are used to measure albumin.

- In humans, particularly with azotemia, cephalosporins have caused a false-positive direct **Coombs' test.**

- Cephalosporins may also cause falsely elevated **17-ketosteroid** values in urine.

Doses

- **DOGS:**

  For labeled indications:

  a) USA: Skin infections due to susceptible-strains of *Staph. pseudintermedius* or *Strep. canis* (Group G): Administer 8 mg/kg SC once. A second injection (same dose/route) may be administered if response to therapy is not complete 7 days later (for *S. pseudintermedius* infections) and 14 days later for *S. canis* (Group G) infections. Maximum treatment should not exceed 2 injections. (Adapted from label information; *Convenia®*—Zoetis)

  b) UK (for indicated organisms see Uses above): Skin and soft tissue infections: 8 mg/kg SC once. If required, treatment may be repeated at 14 day intervals up to three more times. In accordance with good veterinary practice, treatment of pyoderma should be extended beyond complete resolution of clinical signs.

  Severe infections of the gingival and periodontal tissues: 8 mg/kg SC once.

  UTI: 8 mg/kg SC once. (Adapted from label information; *Convenia®*—Pfizer U.K.)

- **CATS:**

  For labeled indications:

  a) USA: Skin infections (wounds and abscesses) caused by susceptible strains of *Pasteurella multocida*: 8 mg/kg SC as a single, one-time subcutaneous injection. Therapeutic concentrations are maintained for approximately 7 days for *Pasteurella multocida* infections. (Adapted from label information; *Convenia®*—Zoetis USA)

  b) UK (for indicated organisms see Uses above): Skin and soft tissue abscesses and wounds: 8 mg/kg SC once. If required, an additional dose may be administered 14 days after the first injection. UTI: 8 mg/kg SC once. (Adapted from label information; *Convenia®*—Pfizer UK)

Monitoring

- Efficacy. When performing urine cultures after treatment with cefovecin, because of the drug's prolonged excretion optimal timing of sampling is unclear, but testing 3 weeks after the last dose may be reasonable (Weese et al. 2011).
- Adverse effects.

Client Information

- This drug must be injected; it does not work when given by mouth.
- Antibiotic effect is long lasting after a single injection in dogs and cats and side effects can occur up to 2 months after an injection.
- If giving at home, store in refrigerator; throw out any unused liquid after 56 days.
- Do not use in small mammals (*e.g.,* Guinea pigs, rabbits, hamsters, etc.).

Chemistry/Synonyms

Cefovecin sodium is a so-called 3rd-generation cephalosporin antibacterial agent with a molecular weight of 475.5. Each mL of reconstituted lyophilized powder contains cefovecin sodium equivalent to 80 mg of cefovecin; methylparaben 1.8 mg and propylparaben 0.2 mg are added as preservatives, and sodium citrate dihydrate 5.8 mg and citric acid monohydrate 0.1 mg, sodium hydroxide or hydrochloric acid are added to adjust pH.

Cefovecin sodium may also be known as UK-287074-02, cefovecina sodica, céfovécine sodique or natrii cefovecinum. A trade name is *Convenia®*.

Storage/Stability

Store the powder and the reconstituted product in the original carton, refrigerated at 2°-8°C (36°-46°F). Use the entire contents of the vial within 56 days of reconstitution. Cefovecin is light sensitive; protect from light. After each use return the unused portion back to the refrigerator in the original carton. Color of the solution may vary from clear to amber at reconstitution and may darken over time, but if stored as recommended, solution color does not adversely affect potency.

Compatibility/Compounding Considerations

To deliver the appropriate dose, aseptically reconstitute vial with 10 mL sterile water for injection. Shake then allow vial to sit until all material is visually dissolved. The resulting solution contains cefovecin sodium equivalent to 80 mg/mL of cefovecin.

Dosage Forms/Regulatory Status

VETERINARY-LABELED PRODUCTS:

Cefovecin Sodium (lyophilized) 800 mg (of cefovecin) per 10 mL multidose vial (80 mg/mL when reconstituted); *Convenia®*; (Rx). FDA-approved as labeled for use in dogs and cats.

HUMAN-LABELED PRODUCTS: NONE.

Revisions/References
Monograph revised/updated September 2013.

Litster, A. L., et al. (2012). Comparison of the efficacy of amoxicillin-clavulanic acid, cefovecin, and doxycycline in the treatment of upper respiratory tract disease in cats housed in an animal shelter. *Javma-Journal of the American Veterinary Medical Association* 241(2): 218-26.

Messenger, K. M. & M. G. Papich (2013). The Influence of Cefovecin on the Enantioselective Pharmacokinetics of Carprofen in Dogs. *Journal of Veterinary Internal Medicine* 27(3): 749-.

Papich, M. G. (2013). Antibiotic Treatment of Resistant Infections in Small Animals. *Veterinary Clinics of North America-Small Animal Practice* 43(5): 1091-+.

Weese, J. S., et al. (2011). Antimicrobial Use Guidelines for Treatment of Urinary Tract Disease in Dogs and Cats: Antimicrobial Guidelines Working Group of the International Society for Companion Animal Infectious Diseases. *Veterinary Medicine International*.

Cefoxitin Sodium

(se-fox-i-tin)   Mefoxin®

2nd Generation Cephalosporin (Cephamycin)

Prescriber Highlights

▶ 2nd generation parenteral cephalosporin; effective against anaerobes, including Bacteroides.

▶ Potentially could cause hypersensitivity reactions, thrombocytopenia, & diarrhea.

▶ Causes pain on IM injection; Give IV over 3-5 minutes (or more).

▶ May need to reduce dose in renal failure.

Uses/Indications

In the United States, there are no cefoxitin products FDA-approved for veterinary species, but it has been used clinically in several species when an injectable second generation cephalosporin may be indicated.

Pharmacology/Actions

Although not a true cephalosporin, cefoxitin is usually classified as a 2nd generation agent. Cefoxitin has activity against gram-positive cocci, but less so on a per weight basis than the 1st generation agents and methicillin-resistant staphylococci are resistant. Unlike the first generation agents, it has good activity against many strains of *E. coli*, Klebsiella, Campylobacter and Proteus that may be resistant to the first generation agents. However, *E. coli* resistance is an ongoing concern. In human medicine, cefoxitin's activity against many strains of *Bacteroides fragilis* has placed it in a significant therapeutic role. While *Bacteroides fragilis* has been isolated from anaerobic infections in veterinary patients, it may not be as significant a pathogen in veterinary species as in humans.

Because 2nd generation cephalosporins exhibit specific activities against bacteria, a 30-microgram cefoxitin disk should be used when performing Kirby-Bauer disk susceptibility tests for this antibiotic.

Pharmacokinetics

Cefoxitin is not appreciably absorbed after oral administration and must be given parenterally to achieve therapeutic serum levels. The absorbed drug is primarily excreted unchanged by the kidneys into the urine via both tubular secretion and glomerular filtration. In humans, approximately 2% of a dose is metabolized to descarbamylcefoxitin, which is inactive. Elimination half-lives may be significantly prolonged in patients with severely diminished renal function.

In dogs (N=4) after 30 mg/kg doses (IV, SC), plasma cefoxitin concentrations remained above MIC90 (*E. coli*) for 4-6 hours after an IV dose, and about 8 hours after SC administration (Petersen et al. 1993).

In cats after 30 mg/kg doses, peak levels are similar when given IV or IM and IM bioavailability is about 90%. Apparent volume of distribution is 0.32 L/kg, clearance 0.14 L/hr/kg, and elimination

half-life about 1.5 hours. No significant accumulation occurs when dosed at 30 mg/kg every 8 or 12 hours and time of MIC (estimated for cefoxitin) was almost equal after IV or IM administration, 75% for q8h and 50% for q12h. (Albarellos et al. 2010).

In horses, the apparent volume of distribution at steady state is 110 mL/kg, total body clearance of 4.32 mL/min/kg with a serum elimination half-life of 49 minutes.

In calves, the volume of distribution is 318 mL/kg, and it has a terminal elimination half-life of 67 minutes after IV dosing, and 81 minutes after IM administration. Cefoxitin is approximately 50% bound to calf plasma proteins. Probenecid (40 mg/kg) has been demonstrated to significantly prolong elimination half-lives.

Contraindications/Precautions/Warnings

Cephalosporins are contraindicated in patients with a history of hypersensitivity to them. Because there may be cross-reactivity, use cephalosporins cautiously in patients that are documented hypersensitive to other beta-lactam antibiotics (*e.g.*, penicillins, cefamycins, carbapenems).

Patients in renal failure may need dosage adjustments.

Cephalosporins in small mammals such as Syrian hamsters and guinea pigs may cause antibiotic-induced enterocolitis.

Cefoxitin can be easily confused with other cephalosporins. Consider writing orders and prescriptions using tall man letters: CefOXitin.

Adverse Effects

Adverse effects with the cephalosporins are usually not serious and have a relatively low frequency of occurrence.

Hypersensitivity reactions unrelated to dose can occur with these agents and can manifest as rashes, fever, eosinophilia, lymphadenopathy, or full-blown anaphylaxis. The use of cephalosporins in patients documented to be hypersensitive to penicillin-class antibiotics is controversial. In humans, it is estimated 1-15% of patients hypersensitive to penicillins will also be hypersensitive to cephalosporins. The incidence of cross-reactivity in veterinary patients is unknown.

Cephalosporins can cause pain at the injection site when administered intramuscularly. Sterile abscesses or other severe local tissue reactions are also possible but are less common. Thrombophlebitis is also possible after IV administration of these drugs.

Even when administered parenterally, cephalosporins may alter gut flora and antibiotic-associated diarrhea or the proliferation of resistant bacteria in the colon (superinfections) can occur.

While cephalosporins (particularly cephalothin) have the potential for causing nephrotoxicity at clinically used doses in patients with normal renal function, risks for the occurrence of this adverse effect appear minimal. High doses or very prolonged use has been associated with neurotoxicity, neutropenia, agranulocytosis, thrombocytopenia, hepatitis, positive Comb's test, interstitial nephritis, and tubular necrosis. Except for tubular necrosis and neurotoxicity, these effects have an immunologic component.

Reproductive/Nursing Safety

Cephalosporins have been shown to cross the placenta and safe use of them during pregnancy has not been firmly established, but neither has there been any documented teratogenic problems associated with these drugs; however, use only when the potential benefits outweigh the risks. In humans, the FDA categorizes this drug as category *B* for use during pregnancy (*Animal studies have not yet demonstrated risk to the fetus, but there are no adequate studies in pregnant women; or animal studies have shown an adverse effect, but adequate studies in pregnant women have not demonstrated a risk to the fetus in the first trimester of pregnancy, and there is no evidence of risk in later trimesters.*)

Cefoxitin can be distributed into milk in low concentrations. It is unlikely to pose significant risk to nursing offspring.

Overdosage/Acute Toxicity

Acute oral cephalosporin overdoses are unlikely to cause significant problems other than GI distress, but other effects are possible (see Adverse Effects section).

Drug Interactions

The following drug interactions have either been reported or are theoretical in humans or animals receiving cefoxitin and may be of significance in veterinary patients. Unless otherwise noted, use together is not necessarily contraindicated, but weigh the potential risks and perform additional monitoring when appropriate.

- **AMINOGLYCOSIDES/NEPHROTOXIC DRUGS:** The concurrent use of parenteral aminoglycosides or other nephrotoxic drugs (*e.g.*, **amphotericin B**, etc.) with cephalosporins is somewhat controversial. Potentially, cephalosporins could cause additive nephrotoxicity when used with these drugs, but this interaction has only been well documented with cephaloridine (no longer marketed). *In vitro* studies have demonstrated that cephalosporins can have synergistic or additive activity against certain bacteria when used with aminoglycosides, but they should not be mixed together (administer separately).
- **PROBENECID:** Competitively blocks the tubular secretion of most cephalosporins thereby increasing serum levels and serum half-lives.

Laboratory Considerations

- **Methicillin-resistant staphylococci:** Certain strains of methicillin-resistant staphylococci (*e.g.*, *S. pseudintermedius*, etc.) may be falsely identified as methicillin-susceptible if the laboratory uses (lack of) cefoxitin susceptibility as the indicator. At present it is not recommended to use cefoxitin susceptibility as an indicator for staphylococci obtained from animal patients. But one recent study concluded that "With careful measurement of zone diameters and attention to standard testing procedures, it should be possible to increase the sensitivity and specificity of such a screening assay for detection of methicillin resistance" (Bemis et al. 2012).
- Except for cefotaxime, cephalosporins may cause false-positive **urine glucose determinations** when using cupric sulfate solution (Benedict's Solution, *Clinitest®*). Tests utilizing glucose oxidase (*Tes-Tape®*, *Clinistix®*) are not affected by cephalosporins.
- When using the Jaffe reaction to measure **serum or urine creatinine**, cephalosporins (not ceftazidime or cefotaxime) in high dosages may cause falsely elevated values.
- In humans, particularly with azotemia, cephalosporins have caused a false-positive direct **Coombs' test.**
- Cephalosporins may also cause falsely elevated **17-ketosteroid** values in urine.

Doses

- **DOGS/CATS:**

  For susceptible infections (extra-label): 30 mg/kg IV or IM q6-8h.

  For surgical (GI surgery) prophylaxis (extra-label): 20 – 30 mg/kg IV, IM 30-60 minutes prior to incision. May repeat one time in 3-6 hours.

- **HORSES:**

  For susceptible infections (extra-label): Foals: 20 mg/kg IV q4–6h. (Brumbaugh 1999)

Monitoring

- Because cephalosporins usually have minimal toxicity associated with their use, monitoring for efficacy is usually all that is required.
- Patients with diminished renal function may require intensified renal monitoring.

Chemistry/Synonyms

Actually a cephamycin, cefoxitin sodium is a semisynthetic antibiotic that is derived from cephamycin C that is produced by *Streptomyces lactamdurans*. It occurs as a white to off-white, somewhat hygroscopic powder or granules with a faint but characteristic odor. It is very soluble in water and only slightly soluble in alcohol. Each gram of cefoxitin sodium contains 2.3 mEq of sodium.

Cefoxitin may also be known as: MK-306, L-620-388, cefoxitinum, cefoxitina, cefoxitine, *Mefoxin®*, *Mefoxitin®*, *Cefociclin®*, or *Cefoxin®*.

Storage/Stability

Cefoxitin sodium powder for injection should be stored at temperatures less than 30°C and should not be exposed to temperatures greater than 50°C. The frozen solution for injection should be stored at temperatures no higher than -20°C.

After reconstitution, the solution is stable for 24 hours when kept at room temperature and from 48 hours to 1 week if refrigerated. If after reconstitution the solution is immediately frozen in the original container, the preparation is stable up to 30 weeks when stored at -20°C. Stability is dependent on the diluent used and the reader should refer to the package insert or other specialized references for more information. The powder or reconstituted solution may darken but this apparently does not affect the potency of the product.

Compatibility/Compounding Considerations

All commonly used IV fluids and the following drugs are reportedly **compatible** with cefoxitin: amikacin sulfate, cimetidine HCl, gentamicin sulfate, kanamycin sulfate, mannitol, metronidazole, multivitamin infusion concentrate, sodium bicarbonate, tobramycin sulfate and vitamin B-complex with C. Compatibility is dependent upon factors such as pH, concentration, temperature and diluent used; consult specialized references or a hospital pharmacist for more specific information.

Dosage Forms/Regulatory Status

VETERINARY-LABELED PRODUCTS: NONE.

HUMAN-LABELED PRODUCTS:

Cefoxitin Sodium Powder for Injection: 1 g, 2 g, & 10 g in vials; generic; (Rx)

Cefoxitin Sodium Injection Solution (with dextrose): 1 g & 2 g in 50 mL bags; *Mefoxin®*, generic; (Rx)

Revisions/References

Monograph revised/updated September 2013.

Albarellos, G. A., et al. (2010). Pharmacokinetics of cefoxitin after intravenous and intramuscular administration to cats. *J. Vet. Pharmacol. Ther.* 33(6): 619-21.

Bemis, D. A., et al. (2012). Evaluation of cefoxitin disk diffusion breakpoint for detection of methicillin resistance in Staphylococcus pseudintermedius isolates from dogs. *Journal of Veterinary Diagnostic Investigation* 24(5): 964-7.

Brumbaugh, G. (1999). *Clinical Pharmacology and the Pediatric Patient.* 45th Annual AAEP Convention, Albuquerque. accessed via Veterinary Information Network; vin.com

Petersen, S. & E. Rosin (1993). In vitro antibacterial activity of cefoxitin and cefotetan and pharmacokinetics in dogs. *Am J Vet Res* 54(Sep 9): 1496-9.

Cefpodoxime Proxetil

(sef-poe-docks-eem) Simplicef®, Vantin®

3rd Generation Cephalosporin

Prescriber Highlights

▶ Oral 3rd generation cephalosporin that may be useful in dogs or cats.
▶ Contraindications: Hypersensitivity to it or other cephalosporins.
▶ May need to adjust dose if patient has renal disease.
▶ Adverse Effects: Primarily GI, but hypersensitivity possible.

Uses/Indications

In dogs, cefpodoxime is indicated for the treatment of skin infections caused by susceptible strains of *Staphylococcus pseudintermedius, Staphylococcus aureus, Streptococcus canis, E. coli, Proteus mirabilis,* and *Pasteurella multocida.* Although not currently FDA-approved for cats, it may also be useful as well.

Pharmacology/Actions

Like other cephalosporins, cefpodoxime inhibits bacterial cell wall synthesis. It is considered a time-dependent bactericidal antibiotic that is relatively resistant to bacterial beta-lactamases.

Cefpodoxime is sometimes characterized as a so-called 3rd generation cephalosporin. But while it does have activity against many gram-negative bacteria in the family *Enterobacteriaceae,* including may species/strains of Escherichia, Proteus, and Klebsiella, MIC's are often significantly higher than with some other 3rd generation drugs such as cefotaxime or ceftazidime. Cefpodoxime has good activity against methicillin-sensitive staphylococci and many streptococci.

Cefpodoxime is not efficacious against *Pseudomonas aeruginosa,* Enterococcus, anaerobes, and methicillin-resistant Staphylococcus strains. The development of *E. coli* resistant strains to cefpodoxime is an ongoing concern.

Because sensitivity of various bacteria to the 3rd generation cephalosporin antibiotics is unique to a given agent, cefpodoxime specific disks or dilutions must be used to determine susceptibility.

Pharmacokinetics

Cefpodoxime proxetil is not active as an antibiotic. Cefpodoxime is active after the proxetil ester is cleaved *in vivo.* After single oral doses of 5 or 10 mg/kg in dogs, bioavailability is approximately 63%; volume of distribution 150 mL/kg; peak concentrations about 16 mg/mL; time to peak was 2.2 hours; and terminal elimination half-life of approximately 3–6 hours. High levels of drug are found in urine and approximately 70-95% is excreted unchanged (Kumar et al. 2011). Approximately 83% of the drug is bound to plasma proteins (Papich et al. 2010).

In humans, cefpodoxime proxetil is about 40-50% absorbed from the GI tract. Food can alter the rate, but not the extent, of absorption. Cefpodoxime penetrates most tissues well; it is unknown if it penetrates into the CSF. The drug is eliminated in both the urine and feces. Serum half-life may be prolonged in patients with impaired renal function.

In foals after an oral dose (suspension) of 10 mg/kg, peak levels occur in about 100 minutes and peak at about 0.8 micrograms/mL. Elimination half-life is about 7 hours in foals. Levels in synovial and peritoneal fluids were similar to those found in the serum, but no drug was detected in the CSF.

Contraindications/Precautions/Warnings

Cefpodoxime is contraindicated in patients hypersensitive to it or other cephalosporins. Because cefpodoxime is excreted by the kidneys, dosages and/or dosage frequency may need to be adjusted in patients with significantly diminished renal function. Use with caution in patients with seizure disorders.

Adverse Effects

The most likely adverse effects seen in dogs with this medication include inappetence, diarrhea, vomiting, and lethargy. Hypersensitivity and pemphigus-like drug reactions are very rare, but possible.

Cefpodoxime may occasionally induce a positive direct Coombs' test. Rarely, blood dyscrasias may be seen following high doses of cephalosporins.

Reproductive/Nursing Safety

Cefpodoxime has not shown to be teratogenic but should only be used during pregnancy when clearly indicated. The veterinary product is labeled: "The safety of cefpodoxime proxetil in dogs used for breeding, pregnant dogs, or lactating bitches has not been demonstrated." In humans, the FDA categorizes this drug as category *B* for use during pregnancy (*Animal studies have not yet demonstrated risk to the fetus, but there are no adequate studies in pregnant women; or animal studies have shown an adverse effect, but adequate studies in pregnant women have not demonstrated a risk to the fetus in the first trimester of pregnancy, and there is no evidence of risk in later trimesters.*)

The drug enters maternal milk in low concentrations. Modification/alteration of bowel flora with resultant diarrhea is theoretically possible.

Overdosage/Acute Toxicity

Cephalosporin overdoses are unlikely to cause significant problems but other effects are possible (see Adverse effects section).

Drug Interactions

The following drug interactions have either been reported or are theoretical in humans or animals receiving cefpodoxime and may be of significance in veterinary patients. Unless otherwise noted, use together is not necessarily contraindicated, but weigh the potential risks and perform additional monitoring when appropriate.

- **AMINOGLYCOSIDES/NEPHROTOXIC DRUGS:** The concurrent use of parenteral aminoglycosides or other nephrotoxic drugs (*e.g.,* **amphotericin B,** etc.) with cephalosporins is somewhat controversial. Potentially, cephalosporins could cause additive nephrotoxicity when used with these drugs, but this interaction has only been well documented with cephaloridine (no longer marketed). *In vitro* studies have demonstrated that cephalosporins can have synergistic or additive activity against certain bacteria when used with aminoglycosides.
- **ANTACIDS:** Drugs that can increase stomach pH may decrease the absorption of the drug.
- **H-2 ANTAGONISTS** (*e.g.,* **ranitidine, famotidine,** etc.): Drugs that can increase stomach pH may decrease the absorption of the drug.
- **PROBENECID:** Competitively blocks the tubular secretion of most cephalosporins thereby increasing serum levels and serum half-lives.
- **PROTON PUMP INHIBITORS** (*e.g.,* **omeprazole,** etc.): Drugs that can increase stomach pH may decrease the absorption of the drug.

Laboratory Considerations

- Cefpodoxime may cause false-positive **urine glucose determinations** when using cupric sulfate solution (Benedict's Solution, *Clinitest®*). Tests utilizing glucose oxidase (*Tes-Tape®, Clinistix®*) are not affected by cephalosporins.
- If using the nitroprusside test for determining **urinary ketones,** cefpodoxime may cause false-positive results.

Doses

- **DOGS:**

  a) Labeled Dose; FDA-approved: **For susceptible skin infections:** 5 – 10 mg/kg PO once daily. Should be administered for 5-7 days or 2-3 days beyond cessation of clinical signs, up to a maximum of 28 days. Treatment of acute infections should not be continued for more than 3-4 days if no response to therapy is seen. May be given with or without food. (Label information; *Simplicef*®—Zoetis)

  b) From a PK/PD study that included measuring free cefpodoxime in subcutaneous fluid. Authors concluded that: "…cefpodoxime would yield good therapeutic outcome in treating skin infections in dogs for bacteria with MIC50 up to 0.5 mcg / mL with 10 mg/ kg dose while higher doses (or more frequent dosing) may be needed for bacteria with higher MICs. Urinary excretion data suggested that oral administration of cefpodoxime proxetil could be efficacious for UTIs treatment in dogs and further study may be needed to confirm these findings." (Kumar et al. 2011)

- **CATS:**

  For susceptible skin and soft tissue infections (extra-label): 5 mg/kg PO q12h or 10 mg/kg PO once daily (**Note**: Extrapolated from human dosage). (Greene et al. 1998)

- **HORSES:**

  Foals (neonates) with bacterial infections (extra-label): 10 mg/kg PO q6-12 hours. Additional studies required to confirm clinical efficacy and safety. (Carrillo et al. 2005)

Monitoring

- Clinical efficacy, adverse effects.

Client Information

- Can be given with or without food, but gastrointestinal side effects might be prevented if given with food.
- Most common side effects are diarrhea, vomiting and loss of appetite.
- Be sure to give as long as veterinarian has prescribed, even if your animal seems better.
- Cephalosporin antibiotics have an odor that resembles cat urine, but this is normal.

Chemistry/Synonyms

An orally administered semisynthetic 3rd generation cephalosporin, cefpodoxime proxetil is a prodrug that is hydrolyzed *in vivo* to cefpodoxime. The esterified form (proxetil) enhances lipid solubility and oral absorption.

Cefpodoxime proxetil may also be known as: CS-807; R-3763, U-76252, U-76253, *Banan*®, *Biocef*®, *Cefodox*®, *Cepodem*®, *Garia*®, *Instana*®, *Kelbium*®, *Orelox*®, *Otreon*®, *Podomexef*®, *Simplicef*®, or *Vantin*®.

Storage/Stability

Tablets and unreconstituted powder should be stored at 20-25°C in well-closed containers. After reconstitution, the oral suspension should be stored in the refrigerator and discarded after 14 days.

Dosage Forms/Regulatory Status

VETERINARY-LABELED PRODUCTS:

Cefpodoxime Proxetil Tablets: 100 mg & 200 mg; *Simplicef*®, generic; (Rx). FDA-approved for use in dogs.

HUMAN-LABELED PRODUCTS:

Cefpodoxime Proxetil Oral Tablets: 100 mg & 200 mg; *Vantin*®, generic; (Rx)

Cefpodoxime Proxetil Granules for Suspension, Oral: 50 mg/5 mL & 100 mg/5 mL in 50 mL, 75 mL & 100 mL bottles; *Vantin*®, generic; (Rx)

Revisions/References

Monograph revised/updated September 2013.

Carrillo, N. A., et al. (2005). Disposition of orally administered cefpodoxime proxetil in foals and adult horses and minimum inhibitory concentration of the drug against common bacterial pathogens of horses. *American Journal of Veterinary Research* **66**(1): 30-5.

Greene, C. & A. Watson (1998). Antimicrobial Drug Formulary. *Infectious Diseases of the Dog and Cat.* C. Greene. Philadelphia, WB Saunders: 790-919.

Kumar, V., et al. (2011). Pharmacokinetics of cefpodoxime in plasma and subcutaneous fluid following oral administration of cefpodoxime proxetil in male beagle dogs. *J. Vet. Pharmacol. Ther.* **34**(2): 130-5.

Papich, M. G., et al. (2010). Pharmacokinetics, protein binding, and tissue distribution of orally administered cefpodoxime proxetil and cephalexin in dogs. *American Journal of Veterinary Research* **71**(12): 1484-91.

Ceftazidime

(sef-**taz**-i-deem)   Ceptaz®, Fortaz®, Tazicef®

3rd Generation Cephalosporin

Prescriber Highlights

▶ 3rd generation parenteral cephalosporin for gram-negative infections. May be particularly useful in reptiles.

▶ For serious systemic Pseudomonas infections in dogs and cats, constant rate IV infusion or frequent parenteral administration is probably necessary.

▶ Could cause hypersensitivity reactions, granulocytopenia, thrombocytopenia, diarrhea, mild azotemia.

▶ May cause pain on IM injection; SC injection probably less painful.

▶ May need to increase time between dosages in renal failure; use with caution.

▶ Check drug-lab interactions.

Uses/Indications

Ceftazidime is potentially useful in treating serious gram-negative bacterial infections particularly against susceptible Enterobacteriaceae including *Pseudomonas aeruginosa*, that are not susceptible to other, less-expensive agents, or when aminoglycosides are not indicated (due to their potential toxicity). It is of particular interest for treating gram-negative infections in reptiles due to a very long half-life in many species.

Pharmacology/Actions

Ceftazidime is a third generation injectable cephalosporin agent. It is bactericidal and acts via its inhibition of enzymes responsible for bacterial cell wall synthesis. The third generation cephalosporins retain much of the gram-positive activity of the first- and second-generation agents, but have much expanded gram-negative activity. As with the 2nd generation agents, enough variability exists with individual bacterial sensitivities that susceptibility testing is necessary for most bacteria. Ceftazidime is considered an anti-pseudomonal cephalosporin, but resistance development is an issue. A European study (Seol et al. 2002) looking at antibiotic susceptibility of *Pseudomonas aeruginosa* isolates obtained from dogs, demonstrated that 77% of strains tested were sensitive to ceftazidime.

Pharmacokinetics

Ceftazidime is not appreciably absorbed after oral administration. In dogs after SC injection, the terminal half-life of ceftazidime was 0.8 hours; a 30 mg/kg dose was above the MIC for *Pseudomonas aeruginosa* for 4.3 hours. When administered as a 4.1 mg/kg/hr constant rate infusion (after a loading dose of 4.4 mg/kg), mean serum concentration was above 165 micrograms/mL (Moore et al. 2000). Another study done in dogs (Monfrinotti et al. 2010), obtained somewhat different results as the reported average terminal elimination half-lives after IV, IM or SC dosing were between 1-2 hours.

In cats, ceftazidime is about 83% bioavailable after IM administration. It has an apparent volume of distribution of 0.18 L/kg, a clearance of 0.19 L/kg/hr. Elimination half-life is approximately 0.8 hr (IV) to 1 hr (IM) (Albarellos et al. 2008).

Ceftazidime is widely distributed throughout the body, including into bone and CSF and is primarily excreted unchanged by the kidneys via glomerular filtration. As renal tubular excretion does not play a major role in the drug's excretion probenecid does not affect elimination kinetics.

Contraindications/Precautions/Warnings

Only prior allergic reaction to cephalosporins contraindicates ceftazidime's use. In humans documented hypersensitive to penicillin, up to 16% may also be allergic to cephalosporins; veterinary significance is unclear.

Because the drug is primarily excreted via the kidneys, accumulation may result in patients with significantly impaired renal function; use with caution and adjust dose as required.

Ceftazidime can be easily confused with other cephalosporins. Consider writing orders and prescriptions using tall man letters: cefTAZidime.

Adverse Effects

Because veterinary usage of ceftazidime has been very limited, a full adverse effect profile has not been determined for veterinary patients. Gastrointestinal effects have been reported in dogs that have received the drug subcutaneously. When given IM, pain may be noted at the injection site; pain on injection could also occur after SC administration in animals.

Hypersensitivity reactions and gastrointestinal signs have been reported in humans and may not apply to veterinary patients. Pseudomembranous colitis (*C. difficile*) may occur with this antibiotic. Increased serum concentrations of liver enzymes have been described in 1-8% of human patients given ceftazidime.

Reproductive/Nursing Safety

In humans, the FDA categorizes this drug as category *B* for use during pregnancy (*Animal studies have not yet demonstrated risk to the fetus, but there are no adequate studies in pregnant women; or animal studies have shown an adverse effect, but adequate studies in pregnant women have not demonstrated a risk to the fetus in the first trimester of pregnancy, and there is no evidence of risk in later trimesters.*) No teratogenic effects were demonstrated in studies in pregnant mice and rats given up to 40X labeled doses of ceftazidime.

Because of the drug's low absorbability, it is unlikely to be harmful to nursing offspring, but alterations to GI flora of nursing animals could occur.

Overdosage/Acute Toxicity

An acute overdose in patients with normal renal function is unlikely to be of great concern; but in humans with renal failure, overdosage of ceftazidime has caused seizures, encephalopathy, coma, neuromuscular excitability, asterixis, and myoclonia. Treatment of signs associated with overdose is primarily symptomatic and supportive. Hemodialysis could be used to enhance elimination. Ceftazidime is significantly cleared during continuous renal replacement therapies (CRRTs).

Drug Interactions

The following drug interactions have either been reported or are theoretical in humans or animals receiving ceftazidime and may be of significance in veterinary patients. Unless otherwise noted, use together is not necessarily contraindicated, but weigh the potential risks and perform additional monitoring when appropriate.

- **AMINOGLYCOSIDES/NEPHROTOXIC DRUGS:** The concurrent use of parenteral aminoglycosides or other nephrotoxic drugs (*e.g.,* **amphotericin B**, etc.) with cephalosporins is somewhat controversial. Potentially, cephalosporins could cause additive nephrotoxicity when used with these drugs, but this interaction has only been well documented with cephaloridine (no longer marketed). *In vitro* studies have demonstrated that cephalosporins can have synergistic or additive activity against certain bacteria when used with aminoglycosides, but they should not be mixed together (administer separately).

- **CHLORAMPHENICOL:** May be antagonistic to the ceftazidime's effects on gram-negative bacilli; concurrent use is not recommended.

Laboratory Considerations

- Ceftazidime, like most other cephalosporins, may cause a **false-positive urine glucose** determination when using the cupric sulfate solution test (*e.g., Clinitest®*).

- In humans, ceftazidime rarely causes positive direct antiglobulin (**Coombs'**) tests and increased **prothrombin times**.

- When using Kirby-Bauer disk diffusion procedures for testing susceptibility, a specific 30 microgram ceftazidime disk should be used. An inhibition zone of 18 mm or more indicates susceptibility; 15-17 mm, intermediate; and 14 mm or less, resistant. When using a dilution susceptibility procedure, an organism with a MIC of 8 micrograms/mL or less is considered susceptible; 16 micrograms/mL intermediate; and 32 micrograms/mL or greater is resistant. With either method, infections caused by organisms with intermediate susceptibility may be effectively treated if the infection is limited to tissues where the drug concentrates, or when a higher than normal dose is used.

Doses

- **DOGS:**

  For susceptible *P. aeruginosa* infections (extra-label):

  a) Based on a PK/PD study: 30 mg/kg IV, IM, SC q4h or be given as a continuous IV infusion (CRI) with a loading dose of 4.4 mg/kg and a CRI infusion rate of 4.1 mg/kg/hour. The authors recommended that these regimens be tested in clinical trials dogs with *P. aeruginosa* infections and that ceftazidime should be reserved for those dogs with *P. aeruginosa* isolates that are resistant to, or develop adverse effects to aminoglycosides and fluoroquinolones. (Moore et al. 2000)

  b) Based on a PK/PD study: The authors concluded that: when treating *P. aeruginosa* infections in dogs … ceftazidime administered at 20 mg/kg (IV) or 25 mg/kg (IM, SC) q8h should prove a useful alternative to aminoglycosides and fluoroquinolones for the empirical treatment of the majority of the *P. aeruginosa* infections in dogs. However, higher doses may be needed and clinical trials must be conducted to verify these recommendations. (Monfrinotti et al. 2010)

  c) Other recommendations (anecdotal) suggest that the drug could be given at 30 – 50 mg/kg at q8-12h intervals for susceptible infections other than Pseudomonas.

- **CATS:**

  For susceptible infections (extra-label): Based on a PK/PD study: The authors suggest that for organisms with MIC values between 4 mcg/mL to ≤8 mcg/mL, that IM dosages of 30 mg/kg IM q8h should be effective, but for Pseudomonas infections ceftazidime would either need to be dosed much more frequently (q2-4h) or as a continuous infusion similarly to the Moore et al dog dose (see above). (Albarellos et al. 2008)

- **REPTILES:**
  a) **For susceptible infections:** 20 mg/kg IM or SC q72h (every 3 days). (Lewbart 2001)
  b) **For bacterial infections in snakes**, particularly when Enterobacteriaceae or Pseudomonas aeruginosa are confronted: 20 mg/kg IM q72h at 30°C. (Klingenberg 1996), (Johnson 2008)
  c) **For chelonians:** 50 mg/kg IM q24h. (Johnson 2002)

Monitoring
- Efficacy.
- Baseline renal function.

Client Information
- This drug must be injected; it does not work when given by mouth.
- Causes pain when given in the muscle. Usually given at home by injecting under the skin (subcutaneously).
- Once mixed store in refrigerator, do not use mixed liquid after 5 days.

Chemistry/Synonyms
A semi-synthetic, third-generation cephalosporin antibiotic, ceftazidime occurs as a white to cream-colored crystalline powder that is slightly soluble in water (5 mg/mL) and insoluble in alcohol, chloroform and ether. The pH of a 0.5% solution in water is between 3 and 4.

Ceftazidime may also be known as ceftazidimum, GR-20263, or LY-139381, *Fortaz®*, *Ceptaz®*, *Tazicef®*, and *Tazidime®*; there are many international trade names.

Storage/Stability
Commercially available powders for injection should be stored at 15-30°C (59-86°F) and protected from light.

The commercial products containing the sodium carbonate (*Fortaz®*, *Tazicef®*) all release carbon dioxide (effervesce) when reconstituted and are supplied in vials under negative pressure; do not allow pressure to normalize before adding diluent.

Once reconstituted, the solution retains potency for 24 hours (18 hours for arginine formulation) at room temperature and 7 days when refrigerated. Solutions frozen in the original glass vial after reconstitution with sterile water are stable for 3 months when stored at -20°C (-4°F). While no stability data was located, veterinarians have anecdotally reported efficacy when individual dosages are frozen in plastic syringes. Once thawed, they should not be refrozen. Thawed solutions are stable for 8 hours at room temperature and 4 days when refrigerated.

Compatibility/Compounding Considerations
Ceftazidime is **compatible** with the following diluents when being prepared for IM (or SC) injection: sterile or bacteriostatic water for injection, 0.5% or 1% lidocaine. Once reconstituted it is **compatible** with the more commonly used IV fluids, including: D5W, normal saline or half-normal saline, Ringer's, or lactated Ringer's.

Do not use sodium bicarbonate solution for a diluent; it is not recommended to mix with aminoglycosides, vancomycin or metronidazole.

Dosage Forms/Regulatory Status
VETERINARY-LABELED PRODUCTS: NONE.

HUMAN-LABELED PRODUCTS:
Ceftazidime Powder for Injection: 500 mg, 1 g, 2 g, & 6 g in 20 mL & 100 mL vials, infusion packs, *ADD-Vantage* vials & piggyback vials; *Fortaz®*, *Tazicef®*, generic; (Rx)

Revisions/References
Monograph revised/updated October 2013.

Albarellos, G. A., et al. (2008). Pharmacokinetics of ceftazidime after intravenous and intramuscular administration to domestic cats. *Veterinary Journal* 178(2): 238-43.

Johnson, J. (2002). *Medical management of ill chelonians.* Proceedings; Western Veterinary Conference. accessed via Veterinary Information Network; vin.com

Johnson, R. (2008). *Critical care of reptiles.* Procceedings: AAVAC-UEP. accessed via Veterinary Information Network; vin.com

Klingenberg, R. (1996). Therapeutics. *Reptile Medicine and Surgery.* D. Mader. Philadelphia, Saunders: 299-321.

Lewbart (2001). *Reptile Formulary.* Proceedings: Atlantic Coast Veterinary Conference. accessed via Veterinary Information Network; vin.com

Monfrinotti, A., et al. (2010). Pharmacokinetics of ceftazidime after intravenous, intramuscular and subcutaneous administration to dogs. *J. Vet. Pharmacol. Ther.* 33(2): 204-7.

Moore, K., et al. (2000). Pharmacokinetics of ceftazidime in dogs following subcutaneous administration and constant infusion and association with in vitro susceptibility of Pseudomonas aeruginosa. *Am J Vet Res* 61(10): 1204-8.

Seol, N., et al. (2002). In vitro antimicrobial susceptibility of 182 Pseudomonas aeruginosa strains isolated from dogs to selected antipseudomonal agents. *J Vet Med B Infect Dis Vet Public Health* 49(4): 188-92.

Ceftiofur Crystalline Free Acid
(sef **tee** oh fur) Excede®

3rd Generation Cephalosporin

Prescriber Highlights
▶ Veterinary-only 3rd generation cephalosporin labeled for use in cattle, horses & swine.
▶ Potentially could cause hypersensitivity reactions, granulocytopenia, thrombocytopenia, or diarrhea.
▶ Administered SC at the posterior aspect of ear in cattle; administered IM in swine.
▶ Shake well prior to use.

Uses/Indications
In beef and lactating/non-lactating, dairy cattle, ceftiofur crystalline free acid (CCFA) is labeled for the treatment of bovine respiratory disease (BRD, shipping fever, pneumonia) associated with *Mannheimia haemolytica, Pasteurella multocida, and Histophilus somni* and for the treatment of foot rot (interdigital necrobacillosis) associated with *Fusobacterium necrophorum* and *Porphyromonas levii*. In beef and non-lactating dairy cattle it is indicated for the control of respiratory disease at high risk of developing BRD associated with *M. haemolytica, P. multocida*, and *H. somni*.

In swine, ceftiofur CFA is labeled for the treatment of swine respiratory disease (SRD) associated with *Actinobacillus pleuropneumoniae, Pasteurella multocida, Haemophilus parasuis*, and *Streptococcus suis*.

In horses, ceftiofur CFA is FDA-approved for the treatment of lower respiratory tract infections caused by susceptible strains of *Streptococcus equi* ssp. *zooepidemicus*.

Pharmacology/Actions
Ceftiofur is a 3rd generation cephalosporin time-dependent, bactericidal antibiotic active against a variety of gram-positive and gram-negative bacteria and like other cephalosporins, inhibits bacteria cell wall synthesis.

After administration, the parent compound (ceftiofur) is rapidly cleaved into furoic acid and desfuroylceftiofur (active). Desfuroylceftiofur inhibits cell wall synthesis (at stage three) of susceptible multiplying bacteria and exhibits a spectrum of activity similar to that of cefotaxime. Parent ceftiofur and the primary metabolite are equally potent and assays to measure microbial sensitivity (plasma and tissue levels) are based on ceftiofur equivalents referred to as CE. The protein binding activity of ceftiofur creates a "reservoir effect" to maintain active levels at the site of infection.

In cattle, ceftiofur has a broad range of *in vitro* activity against a variety of pathogens including many species of Pasteurella, Streptococcus, Staphylococcus, Salmonella, and *E. coli*.

In swine, ceftiofur CFA at a single IM dosage of 2.27 mg/lb. (5 mg/kg) BW provides concentrations of ceftiofur and desfuroylceftiofur-related metabolites in plasma that are multiples above the MIC90 for an extended period of time for the swine respiratory disease (SRD) label pathogens *Actinobacillus pleuropneumoniae*, *Pasteurella multocida*, *Haemophilus parasuis* and *Streptococcus suis*.

Pharmacokinetics

In cattle, subcutaneous administration of ceftiofur CFA, in the middle third of the posterior aspect of the ear (middle third of the ear) of beef and non-lactating dairy cattle, or in the posterior aspect of the ear where it attaches to the head (base of the ear) of beef, non-lactating dairy, and lactating dairy cattle, provides therapeutic concentrations of ceftiofur and desfuroylceftiofur-related metabolites in plasma above the MIC90 for the bovine respiratory disease (BRD) label pathogens, *Pasteurella multocida*, *Mannheimia haemolytica* and *Histophilus somni* for generally not less than 150 hours after single administration.

Pharmacokinetic studies indicate that base of ear administrations (BOE) in dairy cattle are consistent with middle of ear (MOE) administration in beef cattle with blood levels at therapeutic threshold within 2 hours of administration at labeled doses.

The systemic safety of ceftiofur concentrations resulting from product administration at the base of the ear was established via a pharmacokinetic comparison of the two routes of administration (base of the ear versus middle third of the ear). Based upon the results of this relative bioavailability study, the two routes of administration are therapeutically equivalent.

In swine, therapeutic plasma levels for the parent compound and primary metabolite, desfuroylceftiofur, are reached within 1 hour of treatment. Plasma levels remained above the MIC for nearly 100% of target swine respiratory disease (SRD) pathogens for an average of 8 days.

In horses, ceftiofur CFA at 6.6 mg/kg IM is relatively slowly absorbed and eliminated. After the first dose the time to peak serum level is about 22 hours and after a second dose 96 hours apart from the first, time to peak was about 16 hours. When dosed at this regiment the drug and its active metabolites stay above the determined therapeutic concentration (0.2 micrograms/mL) for susceptible strains of *Streptococcus equi* spp. *zooepidemicus* for 10 days.

Approximate half-lives of ceftiofur/desfurolylceftiofur after ceftiofur CFA administration of 6.6 mg/kg SC in a variety of species include alpacas: 45 hours; goats: 37 hours; & elephants: 84 hours.

Contraindications/Precautions/Warnings

Cephalosporins are contraindicated in patients with a history of hypersensitivity to them. Because there may be cross-reactivity, use cephalosporins cautiously in patients that are documented hypersensitive to other beta-lactam antibiotics (*e.g.*, penicillins, cefamycins, carbapenems).

Hypersensitivity reactions unrelated to dose can occur with these agents and manifest as rashes, fever, eosinophilia, lymphadenopathy, or full-blown anaphylaxis. The use of cephalosporins in patients documented to be hypersensitive to penicillin-class antibiotics is controversial. In humans, it is estimated 1-15% of patients hypersensitive to penicillins will also be hypersensitive to cephalosporins. The incidence of cross-reactivity in veterinary patients is unknown.

Avoid direct contact of the product with the skin, eyes, mouth and clothing. Sensitization of the skin may be avoided by wearing latex gloves. Persons with a known hypersensitivity to penicillin or cephalosporins should avoid exposure to this product.

In cattle, administration of ceftiofur free acid into the ear arteries is likely to result in sudden death.

Following label use as a single treatment in cattle, slaughter withdrawal time = 13 days and zero day (no) milk discard time. Extra-label drug use may result in violative residues. A withdrawal

period has not been established for this product in pre-ruminating calves; do not use in calves to be processed for veal.

In swine, slaughter withdrawal is 14 days. A maximum of 2 mL of formulation should be injected at each injection site. Injection volumes in excess of 2 mL may result in violative residues.

In horses, the manufacturer warns that if acute diarrhea is observed after dosing, additional doses should not be administered and appropriate therapy should be initiated. Use has not been evaluated in horses less than 4 months of age and in breeding, pregnant, or lactating horses. The long-term effects on injection sites have not been evaluated. Additionally the manufacturer warns that due to the extended exposure in horses, based on the drug's pharmacokinetic properties, adverse reactions may require prolonged care. Approximately 17 days are needed to eliminate 97% of the dose from the body. Animals experiencing adverse reactions may need to be monitored for this duration of time.

Ceftiofur can be easily confused with other cephalosporins. Consider writing orders and prescriptions using tall man letters: cefTIOfur. Do not confuse between the three distinct formulations for this drug (HCl, Sodium, and CFA).

Adverse Effects

Adverse effects with the cephalosporins are usually not serious and have a relatively low frequency of occurrence, but cephalosporins can cause allergic reactions in sensitized individuals. Topical exposures to such antimicrobials, including ceftiofur, may elicit mild to severe allergic reactions in some individuals. Repeated or prolonged exposure may lead to sensitization.

In cattle, administration of ceftiofur free acid into the ear arteries is likely to result in sudden death. Following SC injection in the middle third of the posterior aspect of the ear, thickening and swelling (characterized by aseptic cellular infiltrate) of the ear may occur. As with other parenteral injections, localized post-injection bacterial infections may result in abscess formation; attention to hygienic procedures can minimize occurrence. Following SC injections at the posterior aspect of the ear where it attaches to the head (base of the ear), areas of discoloration and signs of inflammation may persist at least 13 days post administration resulting in trim loss of edible tissue at slaughter. Injection of volumes greater than 20 mL in the middle third of the ear may result in open draining lesions in a small percentage of cattle.

In horses, ceftiofur CFA may cause swelling at the injection site and diarrhea, soft or loose stools. When used in an extra-label manner (long-term weekly SC injections), significantly greater swelling occurred at the injection site compared to that observed after IM administration (Fultz et al. 2013).

Reproductive/Nursing Safety

The manufacturer states that the effects of ceftiofur on bovine reproductive performance, pregnancy, and lactation have not been determined and the safety of ceftiofur has not been demonstrated for pregnant swine or swine intended for breeding. However, cephalosporins as a class are relatively safe for use during pregnancy, and teratogenic or embryotoxic effects would not be anticipated.

Target animal safety studies report administration of a single dose of ceftiofur free acid at the base of the ear to high-producing dairy cattle did not adversely affect milk production compared to untreated controls. Ceftiofur in maternal milk would unlikely pose significant risk to offspring.

Overdosage/Acute Toxicity

Cephalosporin overdoses are unlikely to cause significant problems other than GI distress, but other effects are possible (see Adverse Effects section). Use of dosages in excess of 6.6 mg ceftiofur equivalents (CE)/kg or administration by unapproved routes in cattle (subcutaneous injection in the neck or intramuscular injection) may cause violative residues. Dosages in excess of 5 mg ceftiofur equivalents (CE)/kg or administration by an unapproved route in swine may result in illegal residues in edible tissues. Contact FARAD (see appendix) for assistance in determining appropriate withdrawal times in circumstances where the drug has been used at higher than labeled dosages.

Drug Interactions

Although the manufacturer does not list any drug interactions on the label for ceftiofur, the following drug interactions have either been reported or are theoretical in humans or animals receiving injectable 3rd generation cephalosporins and may be of significance in veterinary patients receiving ceftiofur:

- **AMINOGLYCOSIDES/NEPHROTOXIC DRUGS:** The concurrent use of parenteral aminoglycosides or other nephrotoxic drugs (*e.g.*, **amphotericin B**, etc.) with cephalosporins is somewhat controversial. Potentially, cephalosporins could cause additive nephrotoxicity when used with these drugs, but this interaction has only been well documented with cephaloridine (no longer marketed). *In vitro* studies have demonstrated that cephalosporins can have synergistic or additive activity against certain bacteria when used with aminoglycosides, but they should not be mixed together (administer separately).
- **PROBENECID:** Competitively blocks the tubular secretion of most cephalosporins, thereby increasing serum levels and serum half-lives.

Laboratory Considerations

Note: Ceftiofur is structurally similar to cefotaxime and it is not known if these interactions occur with ceftiofur.

- Except for cefotaxime, cephalosporins may cause false-positive **urine glucose determinations** when using cupric sulfate solution (Benedict's Solution, *Clinitest*®). Tests utilizing glucose oxidase (*Tes-Tape*®, *Clinistix*®) are not affected by cephalosporins.
- When using the Jaffe reaction to measure **serum or urine creatinine**, cephalosporins (not ceftazidime or cefotaxime) in high dosages may cause falsely elevated values.
- In humans, particularly with azotemia, cephalosporins have caused a false-positive direct **Coombs' test**.
- Cephalosporins may also cause falsely elevated **17-ketosteroid** values in urine.

Doses

- **CATTLE:**

  Treatment of BRD and bovine foot rot (labeled-dose): Shake well before using. Administer as a single subcutaneous (SC) injection in the posterior aspect of the ear where it attaches to the head (base of the ear) at a dosage of 6.6 mg/kg (3 mg/lb.) ceftiofur equivalents (1.5 mL sterile suspension per 100 lb. BW). In beef and non-lactating dairy cattle, it may also be administered as a single SC injection in the middle third of the posterior aspect of the ear at the same dosage. Most animals will respond to treatment within three to five days. If no improvement is observed, the diagnosis should be reevaluated. (Adapted from *Excede*® *Sterile Suspension*; Package Insert—Zoetis)

  Control of BRD (labeled for beef and non-lactating dairy cattle only): Shake well before using. Give at the same dosage as above (6.6 mg/kg) either in the middle third of the posterior aspect of the ear or in the posterior aspect of the ear where it attaches to the head (base of the ear). (Adapted from *Excede*® *Sterile Suspension*; Package Insert—Zoetis)

- **SWINE:**

  Labeled-Dose: Shake well before using. Administer by IM injection in the post-auricular region of the neck as a single dosage of 2.27 mg ceftiofur equivalents (CE)/lb. (5 mg CE/kg) body

weight (BW). This is equivalent to 1 mL sterile suspension per 44 lb. (20 kg) BW. No more than 2 mL should be injected in a single injection site. Injection volumes in excess of 2 mL may result in violative residues. Pigs heavier than 88 lb. (40 kg) will require more than one injection. Most animals will respond to treatment within 3-5 days. If no improvement is observed, the diagnosis should be reevaluated. (*Excede*® *For Swine*; Package Insert—Zoetis)

- **HORSES:**

  Labeled Dose: Shake well before using. 6.6 mg/kg IM; repeat in 4 days. A maximum of 20 mL per injection site may be administered. Shake well before using. (*Excede*® *Sterile Suspension*; Package Insert—Zoetis)

Monitoring

Because cephalosporins usually have minimal toxicity associated with their use, monitoring for efficacy is usually all that is required. Some clinicians recommend weekly CBC monitoring of small animals receiving ceftiofur. Patients with diminished renal function may require intensified renal monitoring. Serum levels and therapeutic drug monitoring are not routinely done with these agents.

Client Information

- This drug must be injected; it does not work when given by mouth.
- In cattle, pigs, and horses the antibiotic effect is long lasting after a single injection under the skin.
- In cattle, it is injected under the skin in the ear; do not give in ear veins or arteries. In swine, it is given in the neck. In horses, it is given into the muscle.
- Observe recommended withholding times when using in an animal that will be used for human food.

Chemistry/Synonyms

Ceftiofur CFA has a molecular weight of 523.58.

Ceftiofur may also be known as CM-31916, ceftiofuri, or *Excede*®.

Storage/Stability

Ceftiofur CFA cattle and swine products should be stored at controlled room temperature 20-25 °C (68-77°F). Shake well before using. Contents should be used within 12 weeks after the first dose is removed.

Compatibility/Compounding Considerations

No specific information noted.

Dosage Forms/Regulatory Status

VETERINARY-LABELED PRODUCTS:

Ceftiofur Crystalline Free Acid equivalent to 200 mg/mL ceftiofur (in a *Miglyol*® cottonseed oil based suspension) in 100 mL vials; *Excede*®. FDA-approved for use in horses, beef, lactating and non-lactating cattle. Following label use as either a single-dose or 2-dose regimen, no milk discard period is required, but a 13-day pre-slaughter withdrawal period is required after the last treatment. Use of dosages in excess of 6.6 mg/kg or administration by unapproved routes (subcutaneous injection in the neck or intramuscular injection) may cause violative residues. A withdrawal period has not been established for this product in preruminating calves. Do not use in calves to be processed for veal. If used in an extra-label manner, contact FARAD (see appendix) for guidance in determining withdrawal times for milk or meat. Approved label information for *Excede*® can be found at dailymed.nlm.nih.gov or at zoetis.com.

Ceftiofur Crystalline Free Acid equivalent to 100 mg/mL ceftiofur (in a *Miglyol*® cottonseed oil based suspension) in 100 mL vials; *Excede*® *for Swine*; (Rx). Following labeled use as a single treatment, a 14-day pre-slaughter withdrawal period is required.

HUMAN-LABELED PRODUCTS: NONE.
Revisions/References
Monograph revised/updated October 2013.
Fultz, L., et al. (2013). Concentrations of desfuroylceftiofur acetamide after weekly administration of ceftiofur crystalline free acid to adult horses and comparative pharmacokinetics of the drug after intramuscular versus subcutaneous administration. *Journal of Veterinary Internal Medicine* 27(3): 667-.

Ceftiofur HCl

(sef-tee-oh-fur)   Excenel® RTU, Spectramast®

3rd Generation Cephalosporin

Prescriber Highlights

▶ A veterinary-only 3rd generation cephalosporin approved as intramammary tubes for dairy cattle and as an injection (given daily) for swine and cattle.
▶ Potentially could cause hypersensitivity reactions, granulocytopenia, thrombocytopenia, or diarrhea.
▶ Causes pain on IM injection to small animals.
▶ May need to reduce dose in renal failure.

Uses/Indications

In swine, ceftiofur HCl injection is labeled for the treatment and control of swine bacterial respiratory disease (swine bacterial pneumonia) associated with *Actinobacillus (Haemophilus) pleuropneumoniae*, *Pasteurella multocida*, *Salmonella choleraesuis* and *Streptococcus suis*.

In cattle, ceftiofur HCl is labeled for the treatment of the following bacterial diseases: Bovine respiratory diseases (*e.g.*, BRD, shipping fever, pneumonia) associated with *Mannheimia haemolytica*, *Pasteurella multocida*, and *Histophilus somni*; Acute bovine interdigital necrobacillosis (foot rot, pododermatitis) associated with *Fusobacterium necrophorum* and *Bacteroides melaninogenicus*; and acute metritis (0-14 days post-partum) associated with bacterial organisms susceptible to ceftiofur.

The intramammary syringe for dry dairy cattle (*Spectramast DC®*) is labeled for the treatment of subclinical mastitis in dairy cattle at the time of dry off associated with *Staphylococcus aureus*, *Streptococcus dysgalactiae*, and *Streptococcus uberis*. The intramammary syringe for lactating dairy cattle (*Spectramast LC®*) is labeled for the treatment of clinical mastitis in lactating dairy cattle associated with coagulase-negative staphylococci, *Streptococcus dysgalactiae*, and *Escherichia coli*.

Pharmacology

Ceftiofur is a 3rd generation time-dependent, bactericidal cephalosporin antibiotic active against a variety of gram-positive and gram-negative bacteria and like other cephalosporins inhibits bacteria cell wall synthesis.

After administration, the parent compound (ceftiofur) is rapidly cleaved into furoic acid and desfuroylceftiofur (active). Desfuroylceftiofur inhibits cell wall synthesis (at stage three) of susceptible multiplying bacteria and exhibits a spectrum of activity similar to that of cefotaxime. Parent ceftiofur and the primary metabolite are equally potent and assays to measure microbial sensitivity (plasma and tissue levels) are based on ceftiofur equivalents referred to as CE. The protein binding activity of ceftiofur creates a "reservoir effect" to maintain active levels at the site of infection.

In cattle, ceftiofur has a broad range of *in vitro* activity against a variety of pathogens, including many species of Pasteurella, Streptococcus, Staphylococcus, Salmonella, and *E. coli*.

In swine, ceftiofur HCl has activity against the pathogens *Actinobacillus pleuropneumoniae*, *Pasteurella multocida*, *Haemophilus parasuis* and *Streptococcus suis* for an extended period of time.

Pharmacokinetics

In cattle and swine, ceftiofur is rapidly metabolized to desfuroylceftiofur, the primary metabolite. In cattle, ceftiofur sodium and HCl have practically equivalent pharmacokinetic parameters. The following pharmacokinetic values for cattle are for the active metabolite desfuroylceftiofur. The volume of distribution in cattle is about 0.3 L/kg. Peak levels are about 7 micrograms/mL after IM injection of ceftiofur sodium (*Naxcel®*), but areas under the curve are practically equal as well as elimination half-lives (approx. 8-12 hours).

The elimination kinetics of ceftiofur HCl in milk when used in an extra-label manner to treat coliform mastitis has been studied. Milk samples were tested after two, 300 mg doses (6 mL), administered 12 hours apart into the affected mammary quarters. The samples tested at less than the tolerance level for this drug set by FDA by 7 hours after the last intramammary administration. However, the authors noted considerable variability in the time required for samples from individual cows and mammary gland quarters to consistently have drug residues less than the tolerance level and reported that elimination rates of the drug may be related to milk production. Therefore, cows producing smaller volumes of milk many have prolonged withdrawal times (Smith et al. 2004).

In lactating dairy cattle, active ceftiofur concentrations were measured after the administration of 1 mg/kg SC in healthy dairy cattle within 24 hours of calving. Drug concentrations were found to exceed MIC in uterine tissues and lochial fluid for common pathogens (Okker et al. 2002).

In swine, a study measuring tissue distribution following IM injection of varying doses revealed the highest concentration were detected in the kidneys, followed by lungs, liver and muscle tissue (Beconi-Barker et al. 1996). In swine, the intramuscular bioavailability of the ceftiofur sodium salt and the hydrochloride salt at doses of 3mg/kg or 5mg/kg were compared. The study reported similar therapeutic efficacy for both salt forms (Brown et al. 1999).

Contraindications/Precautions/Warnings

Cephalosporins are contraindicated in patients with a history of hypersensitivity to them. Because there may be cross-reactivity, use cephalosporins cautiously in patients that are documented hypersensitive to other beta-lactam antibiotics (*e.g.*, penicillins, cefamycins, carbapenems).

In swine, areas of discoloration associated with the injection site at time periods of 11 days or less may result in trim-out of edible tissues at slaughter.

In cattle, after intramuscular or subcutaneous administration in the neck, areas of discoloration at the site may persist beyond 11 days resulting in trim loss of edible tissues at slaughter. Following intramuscular administration in the rear leg, areas of discoloration at the injection site may persist beyond 28 days resulting in trim loss of edible tissues at slaughter.

Swine treated with ceftiofur HCl (*Excenel® RTU*) must not be slaughtered for 4 days following the last treatment.

Cattle treated with ceftiofur HCl (*Excenel® RTU*) must not be slaughtered for 3 days following the last treatment. There is no required milk discard time.

Cattle treated with *Spectramast DC®*, must not be slaughtered for 16 days following the last treatment. Milk taken from cows completing a 30-day dry cow period may be used with no milk discard. Following label use, no slaughter withdrawal period is required for neonatal calves born from treated cows regardless of colostrum consumption.

Cattle treated with *Spectramast LC®*, must not be slaughtered for 2 days following the last treatment. Milk taken from cows during treatment and for 72 hours after the last treatment must be discarded.

Patients in renal failure may need dosage adjustments.

Ceftiofur can be easily confused with other cephalosporins. Consider writing orders and prescriptions using tall man letters: cefT-IOfur. Do not confuse between the three distinct formulations for this drug (HCl, Sodium, and CFA).

Adverse Effects

Adverse effects with the cephalosporins are usually not serious and have a relatively low frequency of occurrence.

Hypersensitivity reactions unrelated to dose can occur with these agents and manifest as rashes, fever, eosinophilia, lymphadenopathy, or full-blown anaphylaxis. The use of cephalosporins in patients documented to be hypersensitive to penicillin-class antibiotics is controversial. In humans, it is estimated 1-15% of patients hypersensitive to penicillins will also be hypersensitive to cephalosporins. The incidence of cross-reactivity in veterinary patients is unknown.

Swine safety data: results from a five-day tolerance study in normal feeder pigs indicated that ceftiofur sodium was well tolerated when administered at 125 mg ceftiofur equivalents/kg BW (more than 25 times the highest recommended daily dosage) for five consecutive days. Ceftiofur administered intramuscularly to pigs produced no overt adverse signs of toxicity.

Cattle safety data: results from a five-day tolerance study in feeder calves indicated that ceftiofur sodium was well tolerated at 55 mg ceftiofur equivalents/kg BW (25 times the highest recommended dose) for five consecutive days. Ceftiofur administered intramuscularly had no adverse systemic effects.

Reproductive/Nursing Safety

The effects of ceftiofur on cattle and swine reproductive performance, pregnancy, and lactation have not been determined. However, cephalosporins as a class are relatively safe for use during pregnancy, and teratogenic or embryotoxic effects would not be anticipated.

Overdosage/Acute Toxicity

Cephalosporin overdoses are unlikely to cause significant problems other than GI distress, but other effects are possible (see Adverse Effects section). Use of dosages in excess of those labeled or by unapproved routes of administration may cause violative residues. Contact FARAD (see appendix) for assistance in determining appropriate withdrawal times in circumstances where the drug has been used at higher than labeled dosages.

Drug Interactions

Although the manufacturer does not list any drug interactions on the label for ceftiofur, the following drug interactions have either been reported or are theoretical in humans or animals receiving injectable 3rd generation cephalosporins and may be of significance in veterinary patients receiving injectable ceftiofur:

- **AMINOGLYCOSIDES/NEPHROTOXIC DRUGS:** The concurrent use of parenteral aminoglycosides or other nephrotoxic drugs (*e.g.*, **amphotericin B**, etc.) with cephalosporins is somewhat controversial. Potentially, cephalosporins could cause additive nephrotoxicity when used with these drugs, but this interaction has only been well documented with cephaloridine (no longer marketed). *In vitro* studies have demonstrated that cephalosporins can have synergistic or additive activity against certain bacteria when used with aminoglycosides, but they should not be mixed together (administer separately).
- **PROBENECID:** Competitively blocks the tubular secretion of most cephalosporins thereby increasing serum levels and serum half-lives.

Laboratory Considerations

Note: Ceftiofur is structurally similar to cefotaxime and it is not known if these interactions occur with ceftiofur.

- Except for cefotaxime, cephalosporins may cause false-positive **urine glucose determinations** when using cupric sulfate solution (Benedict's Solution, *Clinitest®*). Tests utilizing glucose oxidase (*Tes-Tape®*, *Clinistix®*) are not affected by cephalosporins.
- When using the Jaffe reaction to measure **serum or urine creatinine**, cephalosporins (not ceftazidime or cefotaxime) in high dosages may cause falsely elevated values.
- In humans, particularly with azotemia, cephalosporins have caused a false-positive direct **Coombs' test**.
- Cephalosporins may also cause falsely elevated **17-ketosteroid** values in urine.

Doses

- **SWINE:**

  For labeled indications (FDA-approved labeled dose): Administer IM at 3 to 5 mg/kg body weight (1 mL of sterile suspension per 22 to 37 lb. body weight). Treatment should be repeated at 24-hour intervals for a total of three consecutive days. Shake well before using. (*Excenel® RTU*; Package Insert)

- **CATTLE:**

  For bovine respiratory disease and acute bovine interdigital necrobacillosis (FDA-approved labeled dose): Administer IM or SC at 1.1 – 2.2 mg/kg (1 – 2 mL sterile suspension per 100 lb.) daily for a total of three consecutive days. Additional treatments may be administered on Days 4 and 5 for animals that do not show a satisfactory response. For or BRD only: based on an assessment of the severity of disease, pathogen susceptibility and clinical response, can administer IM or SC 2.2 mg/kg every other day on Days 1 and 3 (48h interval). Do not inject more than 15 mL per injection site. Shake well before using. (*Excenel® RTU*; Package Insert)

  For acute post-partum metritis (FDA-approved labeled dose): Administer by IM or SC 2.2 mg/kg (2 mL sterile suspension per 100 lb.) daily for five consecutive days. Do not inject more than 15 mL per injection site. Shake well before using. (*Excenel® RTU*; Package Insert)

  For neonatal salmonellosis (extra-label): Ceftiofur HCl 5 mg/kg IM once daily for 5 days. (Fecteau et al. 2002)

  For the treatment of subclinical mastitis in dairy cattle at time of dry off associated with *Staphylococcal aureus*, *Streptococcus dysgalactiae* or *Streptococcus uberis* (FDA-approved labeled dose): Infuse one syringe of *Spectramast® DC* into each affected quarter at the time of dry off. (*Spectramast® DC*; Package Insert)

  For the treatment of clinical mastitis in lactating dairy cattle associated with coagulase-negative staphylococci *Streptococcus dysgalactiae* or *E. coli* (FDA-approved labeled dose): Infuse one syringe of *Spectromast® LC* into each affected quarter. Repeat this treatment in 24 hours. For extended duration therapy, once daily treatment may be repeated for up to 8 consecutive days. (*Spectramast® LC*; Package Insert)

Monitoring

Because cephalosporins usually have minimal toxicity associated with their use, monitoring for efficacy is usually all that is required. Some clinicians recommend weekly CBC monitoring of small animals receiving ceftiofur. Patients with diminished renal function may require intensified renal monitoring. Serum levels and therapeutic drug monitoring are not routinely performed with these agents.

Client Information

For the injectable product:

- This drug must be injected; it does not work when given by mouth.
- Do not give more than 15 mL at one site.
- May cause discoloration of the skin at the injection site.
- Do not give in a vein or artery.
- Observe recommended withholding times if injecting an animal that will be used for human food.

Chemistry/Synonyms

Ceftiofur HCl is a semisynthetic 3rd generation cephalosporin. Ceftiofur HCl is a weak acid and acid stable and water-soluble with a molecular weight of 560. The injectable sterile suspension in a ready-to-use formulation that contains ceftiofur hydrochloride equivalent to 50 mg ceftiofur, 0.50 mg phospholipon, 1.5 mg sorbitan monooleate, 2.25 mg sterile water for injection, and cottonseed oil. Both *Spectramast*® products are sterile, oil based suspensions of ceftiofur HCl.

Ceftiofur HCl may also be known as U-64279A, ceftiofuri hydrochloridium or *Excenel RTU*®.

Storage/Stability

The ready-to-use injectable product should be stored at controlled room temperature 20-25 °C (68-77 °F). Shake well before using; protect from freezing.

The intramammary syringes should be stored at controlled room temperature 20-25 °C (68- 77 °F). Protect from light. Store plastets in carton until used.

Compatibility/Compounding Considerations

No specific information noted.

Dosage Forms/Regulatory Status

VETERINARY-LABELED PRODUCTS:

Ceftiofur HCL Sterile Suspension for injection, 50 mg/mL in 100 mL vials; *Excenel RTU*®; (Rx). FDA-approved for use in cattle and swine. Slaughter withdrawal = 3 days in cattle, and 4 days in swine. There is no required milk discard time.

Ceftiofur HCl Sterile Suspension for Intramammary Infusion in Dry Cows 500 mg ceftiofur equivalents (as the HCl) per 10 mL syringe (plastets) in packages of 12 syringes with 70% isopropyl alcohol pads; *Spectramast*® DC; (Rx) Slaughter withdrawal for cattle = 16 days (no slaughter withdrawal required for neonatal calves born from treated cows)

Ceftiofur HCl Sterile Suspension for Intramammary Infusion in Lactating Cows 125 mg ceftiofur equivalents (as the HCl) per 10 mL syringe (plastets) in packages of 12 syringes with 70% isopropyl alcohol pads; *Spectramast*® LC; (Rx) Cattle slaughter withdrawal = 2 days; milk discard = 72 hours

HUMAN-LABELED PRODUCTS: NONE.

Revisions/References

Monograph revised/updated October 2013.

Beconi-Barker, M., et al. (1996). Ceftiofur hydrochloride: plasma and tissue distribution in swine following intramuscular administration at various doses. *J Vet Phamacol Ther* 19(3): 192-9.

Brown, S., et al. (1999). Comparison of plasma pharmacokinetics and bioavailability of ceftiofur sodium and ceftiofur hydrochloride in pigs after a single intramuscular injection. *J Vet Phamacol Ther* 22: 35-40.

Fecteau, M.-E., et al. (2002). *Efficacy of ceftiofur for treatment of bovine neonatal salmonellosis.* Proceedings: ACVIM Forum. accessed via Veterinary Information Network; vin.com

Okker, H., et al. (2002). Pharmacokinetics of ceftiofur in plasma and uterine secretions and tissues after subcutaneous postpartum administration in lactating dairy cows. *J Vet Phamacol Ther* 25: 33-8.

Smith, G., et al. (2004). Elimination kinetics of ceftiofur hydrochloride after intramammary administration in lactating dairy cows. *JAVMA* 224(11).

Ceftiofur Sodium

(sef-tee-oh-fur)   Naxcel®, Ceftiflex®

3rd Generation Cephalosporin

Prescriber Highlights

- ▶ A veterinary-only 3rd generation cephalosporin approved for use in cattle, sheep/goats, swine, horses, dogs, and poultry. Also used in an extra-label manner in a variety of other species.
- ▶ Potentially could cause hypersensitivity reactions, granulocytopenia, thrombocytopenia, or diarrhea.
- ▶ Causes pain on IM injection to small animals.
- ▶ May need to reduce dose in patients with renal failure.

Uses/Indications

Labeled indications for ceftiofur sodium include:

In cattle for treatment of bovine respiratory disease (shipping fever, pneumonia) associated with *Mannheimia haemolytica, Pasteurella multocida* and *Histophilus somni*. It is also indicated for treatment of acute bovine interdigital necrobacillosis (foot rot, pododermatitis) associated with *Fusobacterium necrophorum* and *Bacteroides melaninogenicus*.

In swine for treatment/control of swine bacterial respiratory disease (swine bacterial pneumonia) associated with *Actinobacillus (Haemophilus) pleuropneumoniae, Pasteurella multocida, Salmonella choleraesuis* and *Streptococcus suis*.

In sheep/goats for treatment of sheep/caprine respiratory disease (sheep/goat pneumonia) associated with *Mannheimia haemolytica* and *Pasteurella multocida*.

In horses for treatment of respiratory infections in horses associated with *Streptococcus* ssp. *zooepidemicus*.

In dogs for the treatment of canine urinary tract infections associated with *E. coli* and *Proteus mirabilis*.

In day old chicks/poults for the control of early mortality, associated with *E. coli* organisms susceptible to ceftiofur.

Ceftiofur sodium has also been used in an extra-label manner in a variety of veterinary species (see Doses) to treat infections that likely to be susceptible to a 3rd generation cephalosporin.

Pharmacology/Actions

Ceftiofur is a 3rd generation cephalosporin time-dependent, bactericidal antibiotic active against a variety of gram-positive and gram-negative bacteria and like other cephalosporins inhibits bacteria cell wall synthesis.

Ceftiofur is rapidly cleaved into furoic acid and desfuroylceftiofur, which is active. Desfuroylceftiofur inhibits cell wall synthesis (at stage three) of susceptible multiplying bacteria and exhibits a spectrum of activity similar to that of cefotaxime. It has a broad range of *in vitro* activity against a variety of pathogens, including many species of Pasteurella, Streptococcus, Staphylococcus, Salmonella, and *E. coli*. Enterococcus is resistant to ceftiofur.

Pharmacokinetics

In cattle, ceftiofur sodium and HCl have practically equivalent pharmacokinetic parameters. The following pharmacokinetic values for cattle are for the active metabolite desfuroylceftiofur. The volume of distribution in cattle is about 0.3 L/kg. Peak levels are about 7 mcgs/mL after IM injection of *Naxcel*®, but areas under the curve are practically equal as well as elimination half-lives (approx. 8-12 hours). Peak levels occur 30-45 minutes after IM dosing. Pharmacokinetic parameters of ceftiofur sodium are very similar for either SC or IM injection in cattle.

In dairy goats, dosing at 1.1 mg/kg or 2.2 mg/kg, administered IV or IM, demonstrated 100% bioavailability via the IM route. After 5 daily IM doses of the drug, serum concentrations were found to be dose-proportional (Courtin et al. 1997).

In horses, 2 grams of ceftiofur were administered via regional IV perfusion or systemic IV to determine radiocarpal joint synovial fluid and plasma concentrations. Mean synovial fluid concentrations were higher for the regional IV perfusion than systemic IV administration. The study concluded regional IV perfusion induced significantly higher intraarticular antibiotic concentrations in the radiocarpal joint compared to systemic IV administration. Additionally, synovial fluid drug concentrations remained above the MIC for common pathogens for more than 24 hours (Pille et al. 2005).

In dogs, ceftiofur sodium only attains effective concentrations in urine (Papich 2013).

Contraindications/Precautions/Warnings

Cephalosporins are contraindicated in patients with a history of hypersensitivity to the drug. Because there may be cross-reactivity, use cephalosporins cautiously in patients that are documented hypersensitive to other beta-lactam antibiotics (*e.g.*, penicillins, cefamycins, carbapenems).

Hypersensitivity reactions unrelated to dose can occur with these agents and manifest as rashes, fever, eosinophilia, lymphadenopathy, or full-blown anaphylaxis. The use of cephalosporins in patients documented to be hypersensitive to penicillin-class antibiotics is controversial. In humans, it is estimated 1-15% of patients hypersensitive to penicillins will also be hypersensitive to cephalosporins. The incidence of cross-reactivity in veterinary patients is unknown.

Withdrawal times: Cattle: 4-day slaughter withdrawal time is required. No milk discard time is required. Swine: A 4-day slaughter withdrawal time is required. Sheep/Goats: No slaughter withdrawal time or milk discard time is required. Not to be used in horses intended for human consumption.

Patients in renal failure may need dosage adjustments.

Ceftiofur can be easily confused with other cephalosporins. Consider writing orders and prescriptions using tall man letters: cefT-IOfur. Do not confuse between the three distinct formulations for this drug (HCl, Sodium, and CFA).

Adverse Effects

Adverse effects with the cephalosporins are usually not serious and have a relatively low frequency of occurrence when used at recommended dosages. The use of ceftiofur may result in some signs of immediate and transient local pain to the animal. Following subcutaneous administration of ceftiofur sodium in the neck, small areas of discoloration at the site may persist beyond five days, potentially resulting in trim loss of edible tissues at slaughter. Localized post-injection bacterial infections may result in abscess formation in cattle. Attention to hygienic procedures can minimize their occurrence.

The administration of antimicrobials to horses under conditions of stress may be associated with acute diarrhea that could be fatal. If acute diarrhea is observed, discontinue use of this antimicrobial and initiate appropriate therapy. One report however, found that ceftiofur administered to horses (4 mg/kg IM) had minimal effects on fecal flora (Clark et al. 2005).

Hypersensitivity reactions unrelated to dose can occur with these agents and manifest as rashes, fever, eosinophilia, lymphadenopathy, or full-blown anaphylaxis. The use of cephalosporins in patients documented to be hypersensitive to penicillin-class antibiotics is controversial. In humans, it is estimated 1-15% of patients hypersensitive to penicillins will also be hypersensitive to cephalosporins. The incidence of cross-reactivity in veterinary patients is unknown.

Reproductive/Nursing Safety

The effects of ceftiofur on the reproductive performance, pregnancy, and lactation of cattle, dogs, horses, swine, sheep, and goats have not been determined.

Cephalosporins have been shown to cross the placenta and safe use of them during pregnancy have not been firmly established, but neither have there been any documented teratogenic problems associated with these drugs. However, use only when the potential benefits outweigh the risks.

Most of these agents (cephalosporins) are excreted in milk in small quantities. Modification/alteration of bowel flora with resultant diarrhea is theoretically possible. When dosed as labeled, there are no milk withdrawal times necessary for ceftiofur products in dairy cattle.

Overdosage/Acute Toxicity

Cephalosporin overdoses are unlikely to cause significant problems other than GI distress, but other effects are possible (see Adverse Effects section). However, overdoses in food animals may result in significantly extended withdrawal times; contact FARAD (see appendix) for assistance.

Drug Interactions

Although the manufacturer does not list any drug interactions on the label for ceftiofur, the following drug interactions have either been reported or are theoretical in humans or animals receiving injectable 3rd generation cephalosporins and may be of significance in veterinary patients receiving ceftiofur:

- **AMINOGLYCOSIDES/NEPHROTOXIC DRUGS:** The concurrent use of parenteral aminoglycosides or other nephrotoxic drugs (*e.g.*, **amphotericin B**, etc.) with cephalosporins is somewhat controversial. Potentially, cephalosporins could cause additive nephrotoxicity when used with these drugs, but this interaction has only been well documented with cephaloridine (no longer marketed). *In vitro* studies have demonstrated that cephalosporins can have synergistic or additive activity against certain bacteria when used with aminoglycosides, but they should not be mixed together (administer separately).
- **PROBENECID:** Competitively blocks the tubular secretion of most cephalosporins thereby increasing serum levels and serum half-lives.

Laboratory Considerations

Note: Ceftiofur is structurally similar to cefotaxime and it is not known if these interactions occur with ceftiofur.

- Except for cefotaxime, cephalosporins may cause false-positive **urine glucose determinations** when using cupric sulfate solution (Benedict's Solution, *Clinitest®*). Tests utilizing glucose oxidase (*Tes-Tape®*, *Clinistix®*) are not affected by cephalosporins.
- When using the Jaffe reaction to measure **serum or urine creatinine**, cephalosporins (not ceftazidime or cefotaxime) in high dosages may cause falsely elevated values.
- In humans, particularly with azotemia, cephalosporins have caused a false-positive direct **Coombs' test**.
- Cephalosporins may also cause falsely elevated **17-ketosteroid** values in urine.

Doses

- **CATTLE:**

  For labeled indications (FDA-approved labeled dose): Administer to cattle by IM or SC injection at 1.1 to 2.2 mg/kg of body weight (1 – 2 mL reconstituted sterile solution per 100 lbs. body weight). Treatment should be repeated at 24-hour intervals for a total of three consecutive days. Additional treatments may be given on days four and five for animals that do not show a satisfactory response (not recovered) after the initial three treatments. (Package Insert; *Naxcel®*)

- **SWINE:**

For labeled indications (FDA-approved labeled dose): Administer to swine by IM injection at 3 to 5 mg/kg of body weight (1 mL of reconstituted sterile solution per 22-37 lbs. body weight). Treatment should be repeated at 24-hour intervals for a total of three consecutive days. (Package Insert; *Naxcel®*)

- **SHEEP/GOATS:**

For labeled indications (FDA-approved labeled dose): Administer to sheep/goats by IM injection at 1.1 to 2.2 mg/kg of body weight (1 – 2 mL reconstituted sterile solution per 100 lbs. body weight). Treatment should be repeated at 24-hour intervals for a total of three consecutive days. Additional treatments may be given on days four and five for animals that do not show a satisfactory response (not recovered) after the initial three treatments. When used in lactating does, the high end of the dosage is recommended. (Package Insert; *Naxcel®*)

- **HORSES:**

For labeled indications (FDA-approved labeled dose): Administer to horses by IM injection at the dosage of 1 to 2 mg ceftiofur per pound (2.2 – 4.4 mg/kg) of body weight (2 – 4 mL reconstituted sterile solution per 100 lbs. body weight). A maximum of 10 mL may be administered per injection site. Repeat treatment at 24-hour intervals, continued for 48 hours after symptoms have disappeared. Do not exceed 10 days of treatment. (Package Insert; *Naxcel®*)

Extra-label doses:

a) **Foals:** Based upon a PK study: a bolus loading dose of 1.26 mg/kg followed immediately by a continuous IV infusion of 2.86 micrograms/kg/min should be administered. Approximate daily dose is 5.4 mg/kg. This dosage could presumably be used to treat bacterial with an MIC of ≤ 4 mcg/mL. Once foal's clinical condition improves, dosing can be switched to from CRI to q12h IM dosing. (Wearn et al. 2013)

b) **Foals:** 2.2 – 5 mg/kg IM q12h. (Giguere 2003)

c) **For intrauterine infusion:** 1 gram. Little science is available for recommending doses, volume infused, frequency, diluents, etc. Most treatments are commonly performed every day or every other day for 3-7 days. (Perkins 1999)

- **DOGS:**

For labeled indications; UTI (FDA-approved labeled dose): **For susceptible UTI's:** 2.2 mg/kg SC once daily for 5-14 days Administer to dogs by subcutaneous injection at the dosage of 1 mg ceftiofur per pound (2.2 mg/kg) of body weight (0.1 mL reconstituted sterile solution per 5 lbs. body weight). Treatment should be repeated at 24-hour intervals for 5-14 days. (Package Insert; *Naxcel®*)

Extra-label doses:

a) **For UTI:** 2 mg/kg SC q12-24h. (Weese et al. 2011)

b) **For neonatal septicemia:** 2.5 mg/kg SC q12h for no longer than 5 days; presumptive therapy with vitamin K1 (0.01 – 1 mg per neonate SC) may be used in puppies and kittens less than 48 hours old. (Davidson 2004), (Davidson 2009)

- **CATS:**

Extra-label doses: For UTI: 2 mg/kg SC q12-24h. (Weese et al. 2011)

- **BIRDS:**

For labeled indications (FDA-approved labeled dose): **Day-Old Turkey Poults:** Administer by SC injection in the neck region of day-old turkey poults at the dosage of 0.17 to 0.5 mg ceftiofur/poult. One mL of the 50 mg/mL reconstituted solution will treat approximately 100-294 day-old poults. **Day Old Chicks:** Administer by SC injection in the neck region of day-old chicks at the dosage of 0.08 to 0.20 mg ceftiofur/chick. One mL of the 50 mg/mL reconstituted solution will treat approximately 250-625 day-old chicks. A sterile 26-gauge needle and syringe or properly cleaned automatic injection machine should be used. (Package Insert; *Naxcel®*—Pfizer)

- **REPTILES:**

Extra-label doses:

a) **For chelonians:** 4 mg/kg IM once daily for 2 weeks. Commonly used in respiratory infections. (Gauvin 1993)

b) Based on PK study in Green iguanas: for microbes susceptible at > 2 µg/mL, 5 mg/kg, IM or SC, every 24 hours. (Bensen et al. 2003)

c) **For bacterial pneumonia:** 2.2 mg/kg IM q24-48h; keep patient at upper end of ideal temperature range. (Johnson 2004)

Monitoring

Because cephalosporins usually have minimal toxicity associated with their use, monitoring for efficacy is usually all that is required. Some clinicians recommend weekly CBC monitoring of small animals receiving ceftiofur. Patients with diminished renal function may require intensified renal monitoring. Serum levels and therapeutic drug monitoring are not routinely done with these agents.

Client Information

- This drug must be injected; it does not work when given by mouth.
- Causes pain when given in the muscle. If given at home to small animals it usually is given by injecting under the skin (subcutaneously).
- Observe recommended withholding times if injecting an animal that will be used for human food.

Chemistry/Synonyms

Ceftiofur sodium is a semisynthetic 3rd generation cephalosporin. Ceftiofur sodium is a weak acid and acid stable and water-soluble.

Ceftiofur sodium may also be known as CM 31-916, U 64279E, ceftiofen sodium, *Excenel®* (not *Excenel® RTU*), *Naxcel®*, *Ceftiflex®*, or *Accent®*.

Storage/Stability

Unreconstituted ceftiofur sodium powder for reconstitution should be stored at room temperature. Protect from light. Color of the cake may vary from off-white to tan, but this does not affect potency.

After reconstitution with bacteriostatic water for injection or sterile water for injection, the solution is stable up to 7 days when refrigerated and for 12 hours at room temperature (15-30°C). According to the manufacturer, if a precipitate should form while being stored refrigerated during this time, the product may be used if it goes back into solution after warming. If not, contact the manufacturer. Frozen reconstituted solutions are stable up to 8 weeks. Thawing may be done at room temperature or by swirling the vial under running warm or hot water.

One-time salvage procedure for reconstituted product: At the end of the 7-day refrigeration or 12-hour room temperature storage period following reconstitution, any remaining reconstituted product may be frozen up to 8 weeks without loss in potency or other chemical properties. This is a one-time only salvage procedure for the remaining product. To use this salvaged product at any time during the 8-week storage period, hold the vial under warm running water, gently swirling the container to accelerate thawing, or allow the frozen material to thaw at room temperature. Rapid freez-

Revisions/References

Monograph revised/updated October 2013.

Albarellos, G. A., et al. (2007). Pharmacokinetics of ceftriaxone after intravenous, intramuscular and subcutaneous administration to domestic cats. *J. Vet. Pharmacol. Ther.* **30**(4): 345-52.

Krupka, I. & R. K. Straubinger (2010). Lyme Borreliosis in Dogs and Cats: Background, Diagnosis, Treatment and Prevention of Infections with Borrelia burgdorferi sensu stricto. *Veterinary Clinics of North America-Small Animal Practice* **40**(6): 1103-+.

Rebuelto, M., et al. (2002). Pharmacokinetics of ceftriaxone administered by the intravenous, intramuscular and subcutaneous routes to dogs. *J Vet Phamacol Ther* **25**: 73-6.

Stewart, A. (2008). *Equine Neonatal Sepsis.* Proceedings: WVC. accessed via Veterinary Information Network; vin.com

Cefuroxime Axetil
Cefuroxime Sodium

(sef-yoor-oks-eem)   Ceftin®, Zinacef®

2nd Generation Cephalosporin

Prescriber Highlights

▶ Oral & parenterally administered 2nd generation cephalosporin that is more active against some gram-negative bacteria than first generation (*e.g.,* cephalexin, cefazolin) cephalosporins.

▶ Potentially useful in small animals when a cephalosporin is desired to treat bacterial infections susceptible to cefuroxime, but resistant to first generation cephalosporins, when slightly enhanced gram-negative coverage is desired for surgery prophylaxis, or when high CNS levels are necessary.

▶ Limited clinical experience in veterinary medicine.

▶ Adverse effects most likely seen in small animals would be GI-related.

Uses/Indications

Cefuroxime is a semi-synthetic 2nd generation cephalosporin with enhanced activity against some gram-negative pathogens when compared to the first generation agents. Cefuroxime is available in both oral and parenteral dosage forms. It potentially may be useful in small animals when a cephalosporin is desired to treat bacterial infections susceptible to cefuroxime, but resistant to first generation cephalosporins, when slightly enhanced gram-negative coverage is desired for surgery prophylaxis, or when high CNS levels are necessary. Little information is available with regard to its clinical use in small animals, however.

Pharmacology/Actions

Cefuroxime, like other cephalosporins, is a time-dependent, bactericidal antibiotic and acts by inhibiting cell wall synthesis. Its spectrum of activity is similar to that of cephalexin, but it is more active against gram-negative bacteria including strains of *E. coli, Klebsiella pneumoniae,* Salmonella and Enterobacter. It is not effective against methicillin-resistant Staphylococcus, Pseudomonas, Serratia or Enterococcus and has little activity against *Bacteroides fragilis.*

Pharmacokinetics

No information was located for the pharmacokinetics of cefuroxime in dogs, cats or horses.

In goats after 40 mg/kg was administered, IM bioavailability is high and protein binding is low. Volume of distribution is about 0.46 L/kg. Elimination half-life is about 2.1 hours (IM) (El-Sooud et al. 2000).

In humans, cefuroxime axetil is well absorbed after oral administration and is rapidly hydrolyzed in the intestinal mucosa and circulation to the parent compound. Bioavailability ranges on average from 37% (fasted) to 52% (with food). Peak serum levels occur in about 2-3 hours after oral dosing. When the sodium salt is administered IM, peak levels occur within 15 minutes to 1 hour. Cefuroxime is widely distributed after absorption, including to bone, aqueous humor and joint fluid. Therapeutic levels can be attained in the CSF if meninges are inflamed. Binding to human plasma proteins ranges from 35-50%. Cefuroxime is primarily excreted unchanged in the urine; elimination half-life in patients with normal renal function is between 1-2 hours.

Contraindications/Precautions/Warnings

No specific information is available for veterinary patients. In humans, cefuroxime is contraindicated in patients hypersensitive to it or other cephalosporins. Dosage adjustment is recommended in humans with severe renal impairment.

Cefuroxime can be easily confused with other cephalosporins. Consider writing orders and prescriptions using tall man letters: cefUROXime.

Adverse Effects

As usage of cefuroxime in animals has been limited, a comprehensive adverse effect profile has not been determined. A six-month toxicity study of oral cefuroxime axetil given at dosages ranging from 100 mg/kg/day to 1600 mg/kg/day in Beagles demonstrated little adversity associated with cefuroxime. At the highest dosing levels (approximately 80X), some vomiting and slight suppression of body weight gain were noted. Minor reductions in neutrophils and red cells, with increases in prothrombin times were also seen.

When used clinically in dogs, gastrointestinal effects (*e.g.,* inappetence, vomiting, diarrhea, etc.) would be the most likely expected adverse effects, but incidence rates are not known.

Cefuroxime is generally well tolerated in human patients. Injection site inflammation can occur when cefuroxime is used intravenously. Gastrointestinal effects (*e.g.,* nausea, diarrhea, etc.) may occur, but are not frequently reported. Eosinophilia and hypersensitivity reactions (including anaphylaxis) are possible. Neurologic effects (*e.g.,* hearing loss, seizures), pseudomembranous colitis, serious dermatologic reactions (*e.g.,* TEN, Stevens-Johnson syndrome, etc.), hematologic effects (*e.g.,* pancytopenia, thrombocytopenia), and interstitial nephritis have all been reported rarely in humans.

Reproductive/Nursing Safety

Studies performed in pregnant mice at dosages of up to 6400 mg/kg and rabbits at 400 mg/kg demonstrated no adverse fetal effects. In humans, the FDA categorizes cefuroxime as category *B* for use during pregnancy (*Animal studies have not yet demonstrated risk to the fetus, but there are no adequate studies in pregnant women; or animal studies have shown an adverse effect, but adequate studies in pregnant women have not demonstrated a risk to the fetus in the first trimester of pregnancy, and there is no evidence of risk in later trimesters.*)

Cefuroxime enters maternal milk in low concentrations. Although probably safe for nursing offspring the potential for adverse effects cannot be ruled out, particularly alterations to gut flora with resultant diarrhea.

Overdosage/Acute Toxicity

Beagles receiving daily dosages of up to 1600 mg/kg/day orally tolerated cefuroxime well (see Adverse Effects).

Cerebral irritation with seizures has been reported with large overdoses in humans. Plasma levels of cefuroxime can be reduced with hemodialysis or peritoneal dialysis.

Drug Interactions

The following drug interactions have either been reported or are theoretical in humans or animals receiving cefuroxime and may be of significance in veterinary patients. Unless otherwise noted, use together is not necessarily contraindicated, but weigh the potential risks and perform additional monitoring when appropriate.

▪ **AMINOGLYCOSIDES:** Potential for increased risk of nephrotoxicity—monitor renal function; however, aminoglycosides and cephalosporins may have synergistic or additive actions against some gram-negative bacteria (Enterobacteriaceae).

- **FUROSEMIDE, TORSEMIDE:** Possible increased risk of nephrotoxicity.
- **PROBENECID:** Reduced renal excretion of cefuroxime.

Laboratory Considerations

- Cefuroxime may cause false-positive **urine glucose determinations** when using the copper reduction method (Benedict's solution, Fehling's solution, *Clinitest®*); tests utilizing glucose oxidase (*Tes-Tape®*, *Clinistix®*) are not affected by cephalosporins.
- In humans, particularly with azotemia, cephalosporins have caused a false-positive direct **Coombs' test.**

Doses

- **DOGS/CATS:**

  For susceptible infections (extra-label): 10 – 15 mg/kg IV q8-12h. Oral dosages are not established. An anecdotal dosage of 62.5 mg (per cat or toy breed dog) – 500 mg (giant breed dogs) PO twice daily could be considered.

  For surgery prophylaxis (extra-label): 20 – 50 mg/kg IV slowly (over at least 3-5 minutes) approximately 30 minutes prior to surgery (often at time of induction) and every 1.5-3 hours during surgery.

- **GOATS:**

  For susceptible infections (extra-label) for organisms with MIC ≤ 1 mcg/mL: Based on their PK study, the authors recommend 40 mg/kg IM q12h. (El-Sooud et al. 2000)

Monitoring

- Clinical efficacy.
- Monitor renal function in patients with renal insufficiency.

Client Information

- Give with food.
- Don't crush tablets; the drug is very bitter so this would make it more difficult to dose the animal.
- Most common side effects are diarrhea, vomiting and loss of appetite. Contact veterinarian if animal develops severe vomiting/diarrhea or rash/itching.
- Be sure to give as long as veterinarian has prescribed, even if your animal seems better.
- Cephalosporin antibiotics have an odor that resembles cat urine, but this is normal.

Chemistry/Synonyms

Cefuroxime axetil occurs as a white or almost white, powder that is insoluble in water and slightly soluble in dehydrated alcohol.

Cefuroxime sodium occurs as a white or almost white, hygroscopic powder that is freely soluble in water.

Cefuroxime may also be known as: CCI-15641, cefuroxim, cefuroxima, cefuroximum, cefuroksiimi, or cefuroksimas; many internationally registered trade names are available.

Storage/Stability

Cefuroxime axetil tablets should be stored in tight containers at room temperature (15-30°C); protect from excessive moisture.

The powder for suspension should be stored at 2-30°C. Once reconstituted, it should be kept refrigerated (2-8°C) and any unused suspension discarded after 10 days.

The powder for injection of infusion should be stored at room temperature (15-30°C). The powder may darken, but this does not indicate any loss of potency. When reconstituted with sterile water to a concentration of 90 mg/mL, the resulting solution is stable for 24 hours at room temperature; 48 hours if refrigerated. If further

diluted into a **compatible** IV solution such as D5W, normal saline or Ringer's, the resulting solution is stable for 24 hours at room temperature; up to 7 days if refrigerated.

Compatibility/Compounding Considerations

Drugs that are reportedly **compatible** when mixed with cefuroxime for IV use include, clindamycin, furosemide and metronidazole. Drugs that may be given at a Y-site with a cefuroxime infusion running include, morphine, hydromorphone, and propofol. Aminoglycosides, ciprofloxacin, or ranitidine should not be admixed with cefuroxime.

Dosage Forms/Regulatory Status

VETERINARY-LABELED PRODUCTS: NONE.

HUMAN-LABELED PRODUCTS:

Cefuroxime Axetil Oral Tablets (film coated): 125 mg, 250 mg, & 500 mg; *Ceftin®*, generic; (Rx)

Cefuroxime Axetil Oral Suspension: 25 mg/mL & 50 mg/mL (125 mg/5 mL & 250 mg/5 mL; as base) when reconstituted in 50 mL &100 mL; generic; (Rx)

Cefuroxime Sodium for Injection: 750 mg, 1.5 g, 7.5 g, & 225 g (as sodium); *Zinacef®*, generic; (Rx)

Revisions/References

Monograph revised/updated October 2013.

El-Sooud, K. A., et al. (2000). Pharmacokinetics and intramuscular bioavailability of cefuroxime sodium in goats. *Research in Veterinary Science* **69**(3): 219-24.

Cephalexin

(sef-a-**lex**-in)   Cefalexin, Rilexine®

1st Generation Cephalosporin

Prescriber Highlights

- ▶ 1st generation oral cephalosporin. Some countries may have an injectable form.
- ▶ May be administered with food (especially if GI upset occurs).
- ▶ Most likely adverse effects are GI in nature; hypersensitivity reactions possible.
- ▶ May need to reduce dose in patients with renal failure.

Uses/Indications

In the USA an FDA-approved oral product for dogs is available (*Rilexine®*). It is labeled as indicated for the treatment of secondary superficial bacterial pyoderma in dogs caused by susceptible strains of *Staphylococcus pseudintermedius*. Cephalexin has also been used clinically in cats, horses, rabbits, ferrets, and birds, particularly for susceptible Staphylococcal infections.

Pharmacology/Actions

A first generation cephalosporin, cephalexin exhibits activity against the bacteria usually covered by this class. Cephalosporins are considered time-dependent and bactericidal against susceptible bacteria and act by inhibiting mucopeptide synthesis in the cell wall resulting in a defective barrier and an osmotically unstable spheroplast. The exact mechanism for this effect has not been definitively determined, but beta-lactam antibiotics have been shown to bind to several enzymes (carboxypeptidases, transpeptidases, endopeptidases) within the bacterial cytoplasmic membrane that are involved with cell wall synthesis. The different affinities that various beta-lactam antibiotics have for these enzymes (also known as penicillin-binding proteins; PBPs) help explain the differences in spectrums of activity of these drugs that are not explained by the influence of beta-lactamases. Like other beta-lactam antibiotics, cephalosporins are generally considered to be more effective against actively growing bacteria.

While there may be differences in MIC's for individual first generation cephalosporins, their spectrums of activity are quite similar. They possess generally excellent coverage against most gram-positive pathogens and variable to poor coverage against most gram-negative pathogens. These drugs are very active *in vitro* against groups A beta-hemolytic and B Streptococci, non-entero-coccal group D Streptococci (*S. bovis*), *Staphylococcus pseudinter-medius* and *aureus*, *Proteus mirabilis* and some strains of *E. coli*, *Klebsiella* spp., Actinobacillus, Pasteurella, *Haemophilus equigen-italis*, Shigella and Salmonella. With the exception of *Bacteroides fragilis*, most anaerobes are very susceptible to the first generation agents. Most species of Corynebacteria are susceptible, but *C. equi* (Rhodococcus) is usually resistant. Strains of *Staphylococcus epidermidis* are usually sensitive to the parenterally administered 1st generation drugs, but may have variable susceptibilities to the oral drugs. The following bacteria are regularly resistant to the 1st generation agents: Group D streptococci/enterococci (*S. faecalis*, *S. faecium*), Methicillin-resistant Staphylococci, *indole-positive Proteus* spp., *Pseudomonas* spp., *Enterobacter* spp., *Serratia* spp. and Citrobacter. *E. coli* resistance is an ongoing concern.

Pharmacokinetics

After oral administration, cephalexin is rapidly and completely absorbed in humans. Cephalexin (base) must be converted to the HCl before absorption can occur and, therefore, absorption can be delayed. There is a form of cephalexin HCl commercially available for oral use that apparently is absorbed more rapidly, but the clinical significance of this is in question. Food apparently has little impact on absorption.

In a study done in dogs and cats (Silley et al. 1988), peak serum levels reached 18.6 micrograms/mL about 1.8 hours after a mean oral dose of 12.7 mg/kg in dogs, and 18.7 micrograms/mL, 2.6 hours after an oral dose of 22.9 mg/kg in cats. Elimination half-lives ranged from 1-2 hours in both species. Bioavailability was about 75% in both species after oral administration. A different study (Papich et al. 2010), found that protein binding of cephalexin in dogs is low (15-26%) and elimination half-life in interstitial fluid (protein unbound) is approximately 3.2 hours, compared to 4.7 hours in total plasma.

Oral bioavailability in adult horses is low.

There may be temporal differences in pharmacokinetics depending on the time of day the drug is administered. Six beagles given cephalexin orally at 10:00 and 22:00 had significantly lower peak levels (77%) after the 22:00 dose versus the 10:00 dose. Additionally, the elimination half-life was approximately 50% longer with the evening dose versus the morning dose. Clinical significance is not clear as times above an MIC of 0.5 micrograms/mL were not different (Prados et al. 2007).

In horses, oral cephalexin has low bioavailability (approx. 5%) and a short plasma half-life (about 2 hours), but at doses of 30 mg/kg PO q8h sufficient plasma and interstitial levels were achieved to treat gram-positive bacteria (MIC ≤5 micrograms/mL) (Davis et al. 2005).

Outside the USA, an oily suspension of the sodium salt (*Ceporex® Injection*—Glaxovet; Cefalexina Injection 20%—Labatorino Burnet) is available in several countries for IM or SC injection in animals. In calves, the sodium salt had a 74% bioavailability after IM injection and a serum half-life of about 90 minutes. When 7.5 mg/kg was injected either SC or IM in adult cattle, the 20% suspension had longer durations of time above MIC90 for common gram positive pathogens when injected SC versus IM (11-14 hours vs. 8-9 hours) (Dova et al. 2008).

Contraindications/Precautions/Warnings

Cephalosporins are contraindicated in patients with a history of hypersensitivity to them. Because there may be cross-reactivity, use cephalosporins cautiously in patients that are documented hypersensitive to other beta-lactam antibiotics (*e.g.*, penicillins, cefamycins, carbapenems).

Oral systemic antibiotics should not be administered in patients with septicemia, shock or other grave illnesses as absorption of the medication from the GI tract may be significantly delayed or diminished. Parenteral routes (preferably IV) should be used for these cases.

Although cephalexin has been used in some small mammal species, a product (*Ceporex Vet®*) licensed in the UK states: "Do not use in rabbits, guinea pigs, hamsters and gerbils and other small rodents"; potentially serious enterocolitis can result.

Cephalexin can be easily confused with other cephalosporins. Consider writing orders and prescriptions using tall man letters: cephaLEXin.

Adverse Effects

Adverse effects with the cephalosporins are usually not serious and have a relatively low frequency of occurrence.

In addition to the adverse effects listed below, cephalexin has reportedly caused salivation, tachypnea and excitability in dogs, and emesis and fever in cats. Nephrotoxicity occurs rarely during therapy with cephalexin, but patients with renal dysfunction, receiving other nephrotoxic drugs or that are geriatric may be more susceptible. Interstitial nephritis, a hypersensitivity reaction, has been reported with many of the cephalosporins including cephalexin. The incidence of these effects is not known.

Hypersensitivity reactions unrelated to dose can occur with these agents and can manifest as rashes, fever, eosinophilia, lymphadenopathy, or full-blown anaphylaxis. The use of cephalosporins in patients documented to be hypersensitive to penicillin-class antibiotics is controversial. In humans, it is estimated 1-15% of patients hypersensitive to penicillins will also be hypersensitive to cephalosporins. The incidence of cross-reactivity in veterinary patients is unknown.

When given orally, cephalosporins may cause GI effects (*e.g.*, anorexia, vomiting, diarrhea, etc.). Administering the drug with a small meal may help alleviate these effects. Because the cephalosporins may also alter gut flora, antibiotic-associated diarrhea or proliferation of resistant bacteria in the colon can occur.

Rarely, cephalexin has been implicated in causing serious skin reactions (*e.g.*, erythema multiforme, cutaneous vasculitis, toxic epidermal necrolysis, etc.) in small animals.

While cephalosporins (particularly cephalothin) have the potential for causing nephrotoxicity at clinically used doses in patients with normal renal function, risks for the occurrence of this adverse effect appear minimal.

High doses or very prolonged use has been associated with neurotoxicity, neutropenia, agranulocytosis, thrombocytopenia, hepatitis, positive Coomb's test, interstitial nephritis, and tubular necrosis. Except for tubular necrosis and neurotoxicity, these effects have an immunologic component.

Reproductive/Nursing Safety

Cephalosporins have been shown to cross the placenta and safe use of them during pregnancy has not been firmly established, but neither have there been any documented teratogenic problems associated with these drugs. However, use only when the potential benefits outweigh the risks. The veterinary-labeled (USA) product's (*Rilexine®*) label states "Safe use in dogs intended for breeding and in pregnant or lactating bitches has not been evaluated."

In humans, the FDA categorizes cephalexin as category *B* for use during pregnancy (*Animal studies have not yet demonstrated risk to the fetus, but there are no adequate studies in pregnant women; or animal studies have shown an adverse effect, but adequate studies in pregnant women have not demonstrated a risk to the fetus in the first trimester of pregnancy, and there is no evidence of risk in later trimesters.*)

Small amounts of cephalexin may be distributed into maternal milk; it could potentially affect gut flora in neonates.

Overdosage/Acute Toxicity

Acute oral cephalosporin overdoses are unlikely to cause significant problems other than GI distress, but other effects are possible (see Adverse Effects section).

Drug Interactions

The following drug interactions have either been reported or are theoretical in humans or animals receiving cephalexin and may be of significance in veterinary patients. Unless otherwise noted, use together is not necessarily contraindicated, but weigh the potential risks and perform additional monitoring when appropriate.

- **PROBENECID:** Competitively blocks the tubular secretion of most cephalosporins thereby increasing serum levels and serum half-lives.

Laboratory Considerations

- Except for cefotaxime, cephalosporins may cause false-positive **urine glucose determinations** when using cupric sulfate solution (Benedict's Solution, *Clinitest®*). Tests utilizing glucose oxidase (*Tes-Tape®, Clinistix®*) are not affected by cephalosporins.

- When using the Jaffe reaction to measure **serum or urine creatinine**, cephalosporins (not ceftazidime or cefotaxime) in high dosages may cause falsely elevated values.

- In humans, particularly with azotemia, cephalosporins have caused a false-positive direct **Coombs' test**. Cephalosporins may also cause falsely elevated **17-ketosteroid** values in urine.

Doses

- **DOGS:**

For susceptible skin infections:

a) Labeled-dose; FDA-approved: 22 mg/kg (10 mg/lb.) of body weight PO twice daily for 28 days. (Label; *Rilexine®*)

b) Extra-label: 22 – 30 mg/kg PO twice daily is often recommended; some suggest that 30 – 40 mg/kg PO once daily can be used. Good evidence to support treatment duration is lacking, but continuing treatment for 7 days (superficial pyoderma) or 14 days (deep pyoderma) after clinical signs have resolved is commonly recommended.

c) Extra-label in USA: One product licensed in the UK for this indication (*Cefaseptin®*) has a labeled dose of 25 mg/kg PO twice daily for up to 3 weeks. The treatment should be re-assessed if no improvement is seen after 14 days. (Adapted from label; *Cefaseptin®*—Vetoquinol UK). Another product (*Therios®*) has a labeled dose of 15 mg/kg PO twice daily. Treat for at least 15 days in cases of superficial infectious dermatitis and at least 28 days in cases of deep infectious dermatitis. (Adapted from label; *Therios®*—Sogeval UK)

For susceptible urinary tract infections (extra-label): 12 – 25 mg/kg PO q12h. Enterococci are resistant and resistance may be common in Enterobacteriaceae in some regions. (Weese et al. 2011)

For other susceptible infections:

a) Extra-label; anecdotal: 10 – 40 mg/kg PO q8-12h.

b) Extra-label in USA: 10 – 15 mg/kg PO twice daily. (Labeled dose; *Ceporex® Vet*—MSD UK)

- **CATS:**

For susceptible skin infections:

a) Extra-label: 22 – 30 mg/kg PO twice daily is often recommended. Good evidence to support treatment duration is lacking, but continuing treatment for 7 days (superficial pyoderma) or 14 days (deep pyoderma) after clinical signs have resolved is commonly recommended.

b) Extra-label in USA: One product licensed in the UK for this indication (*Therios®*) has a labeled dose of 15 mg/kg PO twice daily. Treat for 5 days for wounds and abscesses and 14 days at least in case of pyoderma. The treatment must be continued for 10 days once the lesions have disappeared. (Adapted from label; *Therios®*—Sogeval UK)

For susceptible urinary tract infections (extra-label): 12 – 25 mg/kg PO q12h. Enterococci are resistant and resistance may be common in Enterobacteriaceae in some regions. (Weese et al. 2011)

For other susceptible infections:

a) Extra-label; anecdotal: 10 – 40 mg/kg PO q8-12h.

b) Extra-label in USA: 10 – 15 mg/kg PO twice daily. (Labeled dose; *Ceporex® Vet*—MSD UK)

- **RABBITS/RODENTS/SMALL MAMMALS:**

For susceptible infections (extra-label); **Note:** Use with caution in small mammals. See Contraindications/Warnings.

a) **Rabbits:** 11 – 22 mg/kg PO q8h. (Ivey et al. 2000)

b) **Guinea pigs:** 50 mg/kg IM q24h. (Adamcak et al. 2000)

- **FERRETS:**

For susceptible infections (extra-label): 15 – 25 mg/kg PO 2-3 times daily. (Williams 2000)

- **HORSES:**

For susceptible infections (extra-label): **Foals:** 30 mg/kg PO q12h.

- **REPTILES:**

For susceptible infections respiratory infections (extra-label): 20 – 40 mg/kg PO q12-24h. (Schumacher 2011)

- **BIRDS:**

For susceptible infections (extra-label):

a) 35 – 50 mg/kg PO four times daily (using suspension); most preps are well accepted. (Clubb 1986)

b) 40 – 100 mg/kg q6h PO. (Hoeffer 1995)

Monitoring

- Because cephalosporins usually have minimal toxicity associated with their use, monitoring for efficacy is usually all that is required.

- Patients with diminished renal function may require intensified renal monitoring. Serum levels and therapeutic drug monitoring are not routinely done with these agents.

Client Information

- Can be given with or without food, but gastrointestinal side effects might be prevented if given with food.

- Most common side effects are diarrhea, vomiting and loss of appetite. Contact veterinarian if animal develops severe vomiting/diarrhea or rash/itching.

- Be sure to give as long as veterinarian has prescribed, even if your animal seems better.

- Cephalosporin antibiotics have an odor that resembles cat urine, but this is normal.

Chemistry/Synonyms

A semi-synthetic oral cephalosporin, cephalexin (as the monohydrate) occurs as a white to off-white crystalline powder. It is slightly soluble in water and practically insoluble in alcohol.

Cephalexin may also be known as: cefalexin, 66873, or cefalexinum; many trade names are available.

Storage/Stability

Cephalexin tablets, chewable tablets, capsules, and powder for oral suspension should be stored at room temperature (15-30°C) in tight containers. After reconstitution, the oral suspension is stable for 2 weeks.

Compatibility/Compounding Considerations

No specific information noted.

Dosage Forms/Regulatory Status

VETERINARY-LABELED PRODUCTS:

Cephalexin Chewable Tablets: 75 mg, 150 mg, 300 mg, & 600 mg; *Rilexine®*; (Rx). Approved for use in dogs. The FDA-approved label information for *Rilexine®* may be found on the dailymed.nlm.nih.gov website.

In the UK and some other countries, there are other oral dosage forms licensed for dogs and cats. Trade names include *Cefaceptin®*, *Ceporex®*, *Cephorum®*, and *Therios®*.

HUMAN-LABELED PRODUCTS:

Cephalexin Oral Capsules: 250 mg, 333 mg, 500 mg & 750 mg; Oral Tablets: 250 mg & 500 mg; generic; (Rx)

Cephalexin Powder for Oral Suspension: 125 mg/5 mL & 250 mg/5 mL (after reconstitution) in 100 mL & 200 mL; *Keflex®*, generic; (Rx)

Revisions/References

Monograph revised/updated October 2013.

Adamcak, A. & B. Otten (2000). Rodent Therapeutics. *Vet Clin NA: Exotic Anim Pract* 3:1(Jan): 221-40.
Clubb, S. L. (1986). Therapeutics: Individual and Flock Treatment Regimens. *Clinical Avian Medicine and Surgery.* G. J. Harrison and L. R. Harrison. Philadelphia, W.B. Saunders: 327-55.
Davis, J., et al. (2005). *The pharmacokinetics and tissue distribution of cephalexin in the horse.* Proceedings: ACVIM 2005. accessed via Veterinary Information Network; vin.com
Dova, S. W., et al. (2008). Comparative pharmacokinetics of an injectable cephalexin suspension in beef cattle. *Research in Veterinary Science* 85(3): 570-4.
Hoeffer, H. (1995). Antimicrobials in pet birds. *Kirk's Current Veterinary Therapy:XII.* J. Bonagura. Philadelphia, W.B. Saunders: 1278-83.
Ivey, E. & J. Morrisey (2000). Therapeutics for Rabbits. *Vet Clin NA: Exotic Anim Pract* 3:1(Jan): 183-216.
Papich, M. G., et al. (2010). Pharmacokinetics, protein binding, and tissue distribution of orally administered cefpodoxime proxetil and cephalexin in dogs. *American Journal of Veterinary Research* 71(12): 1484-91.
Prados, A. P., et al. (2007). Chronopharmacological study of cephalexin in dogs. *Chronobiology International* 24(1): 161-70.
Schumacher, J. (2011). Respiratory Medicine of Reptiles. *Vet Clin Exot Anim* 14: 207-24.
Weese, J. S., et al. (2011). Antimicrobial Use Guidelines for Treatment of Urinary Tract Disease in Dogs and Cats: Antimicrobial Guidelines Working Group of the International Society for Companion Animal Infectious Diseases. *Veterinary Medicine International.*
Williams, B. (2000). Therapeutics in Ferrets. *Vet Clin NA: Exotic Anim Pract* 3:1(Jan): 131-53.

Cephapirin Sodium
Cephapirin Benzathine

(sef-a-pye-rin)   Cefapirin, Cefa-Lak®, Cefa-Dri®

1st Generation Cephalosporin

Prescriber Highlights

► 1st generation intramammary cephalosporin; also used via intrauterine infusions for endometritis.
► Potentially could cause hypersensitivity reactions.
► Watch withdrawal times.

Uses/Indications

In the USA, there are no longer parenterally administered cephapirin products available. A 500 mg intrauterine suspension (*Metricure®*) is available in many countries worldwide.

An intramammary cephapirin sodium product is FDA-approved in the USA for use in the treatment of mastitis in lactating dairy cows and cephapirin benzathine is FDA-approved in dry cows.

Pharmacology/Actions

A first generation cephalosporin, cephapirin exhibits activity against the bacteria usually covered by this class. A cephalothin disk is usually used to determine bacterial susceptibility to this antibiotic when using the Kirby-Bauer method. Cephalosporins are usually bactericidal against susceptible bacteria and act by inhibiting mucopeptide synthesis in the cell wall resulting in a defective barrier and an osmotically unstable spheroplast. The exact mechanism for this effect has not been definitively determined, but beta-lactam antibiotics have been shown to bind to several enzymes (*e.g.*, carboxypeptidases, transpeptidases, endopeptidases) within the bacterial cytoplasmic membrane that are involved with cell wall synthesis. The different affinities that various beta-lactam antibiotics have for these enzymes (also known as penicillin-binding proteins; PBPs) help explain the differences in these drugs' spectrums of activity that are not explained by the influence of beta-lactamases. Like other beta-lactam antibiotics, cephalosporins are generally considered more effective against actively growing bacteria.

Pharmacokinetics

In cattle when used systemically, the apparent volume of distribution has been reported as 0.335 – 0.399 L/kg; total body clearance is 12.66 mL/min/kg and serum elimination half-life is about 64-70 minutes.

When cephapirin sodium (*Cefa-Lak®*) was administered to healthy (no mastitis) dairy cattle via intramammary infusion it was rapidly metabolized to the active metabolite desacetylcephapirin in milk. Times above MIC$_{90}$ for common mastitis pathogens and time to reach FDA tolerance concentrations is similar whether the cow was milked two or three times daily. Additionally, giving the second dose 16 hours later (rather then 12 hours as labeled) to cows that are milked three times daily caused no significant effect on withdrawal times or times above MIC. Cows with low daily milk production (<25 kg) appear to absorb more cephalothin systemically and had longer mean residence times than those with high milk production. The authors caution that extended withdrawal times would be prudent in cows with very low milk production and that more studies are required to determine the pharmacokinetics in animals with mastitis (Stockler et al. 2009).

Contraindications/Precautions/Warnings

Cephalosporins are contraindicated in patients with a history of hypersensitivity to them. Because there may be cross-reactivity, use cephalosporins cautiously in patients that are documented hypersensitive to other beta-lactam antibiotics (*e.g.*, penicillins, cefamycins, carbapenems).

Adverse Effects

Adverse effects with the cephalosporins are usually not serious and have a relatively low frequency of occurrence.

Potentially, hypersensitivity reactions could occur with intramammary infusion. Hypersensitivity reactions unrelated to dose can occur with these agents and can manifest as rashes, fever, eosinophilia, lymphadenopathy, or full-blown anaphylaxis. The use of cephalosporins in patients documented to be hypersensitive to penicillin-class antibiotics is controversial. In humans, it is estimated 1-15% of patients hypersensitive to penicillins will also be hypersensitive to cephalosporins. The incidence of cross-reactivity in veterinary patients is unknown.

Reproductive/Nursing Safety

Cephalosporins have been shown to cross the placenta and safe use of them during pregnancy has not been firmly established, but neither have there been any documented teratogenic problems associated with these drugs. See label information for more information.

Overdosage/Acute Toxicity

No clinical effects would be expected but if used at doses or rates higher than labeled, withdrawal times may be prolonged.

Drug Interactions

No significant concerns when used via the intramammary or intrauterine routes.

Laboratory Considerations

- No significant concerns when used via the intramammary route or intrauterine routes.

Doses

- **CATTLE:**

  For mastitis:

  a) **Lactating cow** (*Cefa-Lak®, ToDAY®*): After milking out udder, clean and dry teat area. Swab teat tip with alcohol wipe and allow to dry. Insert tip of syringe into teat canal; push plunger to instill entire contents. Massage quarter and do not milk out for 12 hours. May repeat dose q12h. (Label directions; *Cefa-Lak®*—BIVI)

  b) **Dry Cow** (*Cefa-Dri®, ToMorrow®*): Same basic directions as above, but should be done at the time of drying off and not later than 30 days prior to calving. (Label directions; *Cefa-Dri®*—BIVI)

  For subacute and chronic endometritis (at least 14 days after parturition) caused by cephapirin sensitive bacteria (extra-label in USA): Using the Intrauterine suspension: Contents of syringe (500 mg) instilled through the cervix into the lumen of the uterus; depending on response may re-treat in 7-14 days if signs persist. May be used one day after insemination. If pyometra, pretreatment with a prostaglandin is recommended. (From label information; *Metricure®*—Intervet U.K.)

Monitoring

- Because cephalosporins usually have minimal toxicity associated with their use, monitoring for efficacy is usually all that is required.
- Patients with diminished renal function may require intensified renal monitoring. Serum levels and therapeutic drug monitoring are not routinely done with these agents.

Client Information

- Follow all label information and milk and slaughter withdrawal times.

Chemistry/Synonyms

A semi-synthetic cephalosporin antibiotic, cephapirin sodium occurs as a white to off-white, crystalline powder having a faint odor. It is very soluble in water and slightly soluble in alcohol. Each gram of the injection contains 2.36 mEq of sodium. After reconstitution, the solution for injection has a pH of 6.5-8.5.

Cephapirin sodium may also be known as: BL-P-1322, cefapirin, cefapirinum natricum, *Brisfirina®, Cefa-Dri®, Cefa-Lak®, Cefaloject®, Cefatrex®, Lopitrex®, Metricure®, Piricef®, ToDAY®* or *ToMORROW®*.

Storage/Stability

Cephapirin intramammary syringes should be stored at controlled room temperature (15-30°C); avoid excessive heat.

Compatibility/Compounding Considerations

No specific information noted.

Dosage Forms/Regulatory Status

VETERINARY-LABELED PRODUCTS:

Cephapirin Sodium Mastitis Tube: 200 mg cephapirin per 10 mL tube; *ToDAY®, Cefa-Lak®*; (OTC). FDA-approved for use in lactating dairy cattle. Milk withdrawal = 96 hours; Slaughter withdrawal = 4 days.

Cephapirin Benzathine Mastitis Tube: 300 mg cephapirin per 10 mL tube; *ToMORROW®, Cefa-Dri®*; (OTC). FDA-approved for use in dry dairy cattle. Milk withdrawal = 72 hours after calving and must not be administered within 30 days of calving; Slaughter withdrawal = 42 days.

In many countries, including Canada, Australia and the UK, 500 mg cephapirin benzathine intrauterine infusion syringes are available for treating endometritis in dairy or beef cattle. *Metricure®*; (Rx). Milk and meat withdrawal times may vary with each country; refer to the label, but usually: milk withdrawal = 0 hours and meat withdrawal = 48 hours.

HUMAN-LABELED PRODUCTS: NONE.

Revisions/References

Monograph revised/updated October 2013.

Stockler, R. M., et al. (2009). Effect of milking frequency and dosing interval on the pharmacokinetics of cephapirin after intramammary infusion in lactating dairy cows. *Journal of Dairy Science* 92(9): 4262-75.

Cetirizine HCl

(she-tih-ra-zeen)   Zyrtec®

2nd Generation Antihistamine

Prescriber Highlights

- ▶ Oral, relatively non-sedating antihistamine.
- ▶ Limited clinical experience in veterinary medicine; recommended dosages for dogs & cats vary widely but the drug appears well tolerated.
- ▶ Potentially may cause vomiting, hypersalivation, or somnolence in small animals.

Uses/Indications

Cetirizine is an H1 receptor blocking antihistamine agent that may be useful for the adjunctive treatment of histamine-mediated pruritic conditions in dogs or cats. It may also find a role in treating horses.

Pharmacology/Actions

Cetirizine, a human metabolite of hydroxyzine, is a piperazine-class non-sedating (when compared to first generation drugs) antihistamine. It selectively inhibits peripheral H1 receptors. Also, cetirizine appears to decrease histamine release from basophils in some species, but in cats, cetirizine or cyproheptadine do not reduce eosinophilic airway inflammation (experimentally produced) (Schooley et al. 2007). Cetirizine does not possess significant anticholinergic or anti-serotonergic effects. Tolerance to its antihistaminic effects is thought not to occur.

Pharmacokinetics

No specific information was located for the pharmacokinetics of cetirizine in dogs. In a study performed in cats (Papich et al. 2006) after an oral dose of 5 mg, volume of distribution was 0.26 L/kg and clearance about 0.3 mL/L/minute. Terminal elimination half-life was approximately 11 hours. The mean plasma concentrations remained above 0.85 micrograms/mL (a concentration reported to be effective for humans) for 24 hours after dosing. In horses, the terminal elimination half-life is reported to be around 6 hours (Olsen et al. 2008). After oral administration to humans, cetirizine peak concentrations occur in about one hour. Food can delay, but not affect the extent of, absorption. It is 93% bound to human plasma proteins and brain levels are approximately 10% of those found in plasma. Approximately 80% is excreted in the urine, primarily as unchanged drug. Terminal elimination half-life is around 8 hours; antihistaminic effect generally persists for 24 hours after a dose.

Contraindications/Precautions/Warnings

No specific information is available for veterinary patients. In humans, cetirizine is contraindicated in patients hypersensitive to it or hydroxyzine. Dosage adjustment is recommended in humans with severe renal or hepatic impairment, or older than 76 years of age.

The combination product containing pseudoephedrine is not appropriate for use in dogs or cats.

Adverse Effects

Cetirizine appears well tolerated in dogs and cats. Vomiting or hypersalivation after dosing have been reported in some dogs. Drowsiness has been reported in small dogs at higher dosages.

A pharmacokinetic/pharmacodynamic study performed in a small number of horses yielded no visible adverse effects.

In humans, the primary adverse effects reported have been drowsiness (13%) and dry mouth (5%). Rarely, hypersensitivity reactions or hepatitis have been reported.

Reproductive/Nursing Safety

In pregnant mice, rats, and rabbits, dosages of approximately 40X, 180X, and 220X respectively, of the human dose when compared on mg/m² basis, caused no teratogenic effects. In humans, the FDA categorizes cetirizine as category *B* for use during pregnancy (*Animal studies have not yet demonstrated risk to the fetus, but there are no adequate studies in pregnant women; or animal studies have shown an adverse effect, but adequate studies in pregnant women have not demonstrated a risk to the fetus in the first trimester of pregnancy, and there is no evidence of risk in later trimesters.*)

In Beagles, approximately 3% of a dose was excreted into milk. The manufacturer does not recommend that nursing women use cetirizine although it is probably safe for use in nursing veterinary patients.

Overdosage/Acute Toxicity

Limited information is available. Reported minimum lethal oral doses for mice and rats are 237 mg/kg (95X human adult dose on a mg/m² basis) and 562 mg/kg (460X human adult dose on a mg/m² basis), respectively. Cetirizine may cross into the CNS in overdose situations and cause neurologic signs. Unlike the earlier non-sedating antihistamines, terfenadine and astemizole (both no longer available in the USA), cetirizine does not appreciably prolong the QT interval on ECG at high serum levels.

There were 591 single agent exposures to cetirizine reported to the ASPCA Animal Poison Control Center (APCC) during 2009-2013. Of the 563 dogs, 120 were symptomatic. The most common clinical signs included: hyperactivity (58%), lethargy (17%), vomiting (14%), panting (12%), mydriasis (12%), and tachycardia (11%).

Overdoses of cetirizine products that also contain pseudoephedrine (*e.g., Zyrtec-D 12 Hour®*) may be serious. It is advised to contact an animal poison control center in this event.

Drug Interactions

The following drug interactions have either been reported or are theoretical in humans or animals receiving cetirizine and may be of significance in veterinary patients. Unless otherwise noted, use together is not necessarily contraindicated, but weigh the potential risks and perform additional monitoring when appropriate.

- **CNS DEPRESSANTS:** Additive CNS depression if used with cetirizine.

Laboratory Considerations

- Discontinue medication well in advance of any **hypersensitivity skin testing**. Usually a 2-week period is suggested before intradermal skin testing is performed.

Doses

- **DOGS:**

  For pruritus associated with atopic dermatitis (extra-label):
  a) Based on a single-blinded (owners), placebo-controlled study: 1 mg/kg PO once daily with or without food. Satisfactory control of pruritus occurred in 18% of dogs evaluated in the study. (Cook et al. 2004)

  b) Anecdotal: 1 mg/kg or 10 – 20 mg/dog PO q12-24h.

- **CATS:**

  For adjunctive treatment of pruritus (extra-label):
  a) Based on an open trial: 5 mg per cat once daily (q24h); 41% of cats had pruritus reduced. (Griffin et al. 2012)

  b) Anecdotal: 0.5 – 1 mg/kg or 2.5 – 5 mg/per cat PO q12-24h.

- **HORSES:**
  a) Extra-label: Based on pharmacokinetic and pharmacodynamic data, cetirizine at 0.2 – 0.4 mg/kg PO q12h may be a useful antihistamine in horses. (Olsen et al. 2008)

Monitoring

- Clinical efficacy.
- Adverse effects (*e.g.*, vomiting, somnolence, etc.).

Client Information

- Antihistamines should be used on a regular, ongoing basis in animals that respond to them. They work better if used before exposure to an allergen.
- May cause less drowsiness/sleepiness than some other antihistamines, but this can still happen.
- Can be given on an empty stomach, but if your animal vomits or drools, try giving with food.

Chemistry/Synonyms

Cetirizine HCl occurs as a white to almost white, crystalline powder that is freely soluble in water. A 5% solution has a pH of 1.2-1.8.

Cetirizine may also be known as: UCB-P071, P-071, cetirizina, cetirizini, cetirizin, ceterizino, or *Zyrtec®*; many internationally registered trade names are available.

Storage/Stability

Tablets should be stored at 20-25°C; excursions are permitted to 15-30°C. The oral syrup may be stored at room temperature or in the refrigerator.

Compatibility/Compounding Considerations

No specific information noted.

Dosage Forms/Regulatory Status

VETERINARY-LABELED PRODUCTS: NONE.

The ARCI (Racing Commissioners International) has designated this drug as a class 4 substance.

HUMAN-LABELED PRODUCTS:

Cetirizine HCl Oral Tablets (film-coated): 5 mg & 10 mg; *Zyrtec®*, generic; (Rx)

Cetirizine HCl Chewable Tablets (grape flavor): 5 mg & 10 mg; *Zyrtec®*; (Rx)

Cetirizine HCl Oral Syrup: 1 mg/mL (grape flavor) in 118 & 473 mL; *Zyrtec®*, generic; (Rx)

Revisions/References

Monograph revised/updated October 2013.

Cook, C., et al. (2004). Treatment of canine atopic dermatitis with cetirizine, a second-generation antihistamine: a single-blinded, placebo-controlled study. *Can Vet J* 45: 414-7.

Griffin, J. S., et al. (2012). An open clinical trial on the efficacy of cetirizine hydrochloride in the management of allergic pruritus in cats. *Canadian Veterinary Journal-Revue Veterinaire Canadienne* 53(1): 47-50.

Olsen, L., et al. (2008). Cetirizine in horses: Pharmacokinetics and pharmacodynamics following repeated oral administration. *Veterinary Journal* 177(2): 242-9.

Papich, M., et al. (2006). *Cetirizine (Zyrtec®) pharmacokinetics in healthy cats.* Proceedings: ACVIM 2006. accessed via Veterinary Information Network; vin.com

Schooley, E. K., et al. (2007). Effects of cyproheptadine and cetirizine on eosinophilic airway inflammation in cats with experimentally induced asthma. *American Journal of Veterinary Research* 68(11): 1265-71.

Charcoal, Activated

(char-kole)

Oral Adsorbent

Prescriber Highlights

▶ Orally administered adsorbent for GI tract toxins/drug overdoses; recommend consulting with an animal poison control center before use.

▶ Not effective for mineral acids/alkalis.

▶ Too rapid administration may induce emesis/aspiration.

▶ In small dogs & cats, monitor for hypernatremia.

▶ Handle with care as charcoal stains clothing very easily; dry powder "floats".

Uses/Indications

Activated charcoal is administered orally to adsorb certain drugs or toxins to prevent or reduce their systemic absorption.

Pharmacology/Actions

Activated charcoal has a large surface area and adsorbs many chemicals and drugs via ion-ion, hydrogen bonding, dipole and Van der Walle forces in the upper GI tract thereby preventing or reducing their absorption. Efficiency of adsorption increases with the molecular size of the toxin and poorly water-soluble organic substances are better adsorbed than small, polar, water-soluble organic compounds.

While activated charcoal also adsorbs various nutrients and enzymes from the gut, when used for acute poisonings, generally no nutritional significance results. Activated charcoal reportedly is not effective in adsorbing cyanide, but this has been disputed in a recent study. It is not very effective in adsorbing alcohols, ferrous sulfate, lithium, caustic alkalies, nitrates, sodium chloride/chlorate, petroleum distillates or mineral acids. Activated charcoal slurries are more effective in adsorbing most toxins than are tablets.

Pharmacokinetics

Activated charcoal is not absorbed nor metabolized in the gut. As activated charcoal slurries can slow GI transit times, an osmotic cathartic is often given concurrently that can enhance expulsion of the toxin-charcoal moiety. A study demonstrated that the presence of food can reduce the adsorptive capacity of activated charcoal of acetaminophen in dogs, but the authors concluded that charcoal was likely to remain efficacious (Wilson et al. 2013).

Contraindications/Precautions/Warnings

Charcoal should not be used for mineral acids, salt toxicosis (including paintballs, homemade play dough), hydrocarbons or caustic alkalies, as it is either ineffective or dangerous (*e.g.*, gut perforation). Although not contraindicated for ethanol, methanol, ethylene glycol, xylitol, heavy metals or iron salts, activated charcoal is ineffective in adsorbing these products and may obscure GI lesions during endoscopy. Patients with a decreased gag reflex or otherwise at risk for aspiration pneumonia (*e.g.*, megaesophagus, CNS depression)

should not be given charcoal/cathartics by mouth. Other potential contraindications to charcoal therapy include: GI obstruction or ileus, hypernatremia, hyperosmolar states, or imminent GI surgery/endoscopy.

To enhance elimination of the charcoal-toxin moiety, an osmotic cathartic (*e.g.*, sorbitol) is often given with activated charcoal. If multiple doses of activated charcoal are administered, it has been recommended that only the first dose contain the cathartic to prevent diarrhea, dehydration, and potentially, hypernatremia (Jutkowitz et al. 2009).

Adverse Effects

Very rapid GI administration of charcoal can induce emesis. If aspiration occurs after activated charcoal is administered, pneumonitis/aspiration pneumonia may result. Charcoal can cause either constipation or diarrhea and feces will be black. Products containing sorbitol may cause loose stools and vomiting.

There have been reports of hypernatremia occurring in small dogs and cats after charcoal (with or without sorbitol) administration, presumably due an osmotic effect pulling water into the GI tract. Reduced sodium fluids (*e.g.*, D5W, 1/2 normal saline/D2.5W) with warm water enemas can be administered to alleviate the condition.

Charcoal powder is very staining and the dry powder tends to "float" covering wide areas.

Overdosage/Acute Toxicity

Potentially could cause electrolyte abnormalities; see Adverse Effects for more information.

Drug Interactions

The following drug interactions have either been reported or are theoretical in humans or animals receiving charcoal and may be of significance in veterinary patients. Unless otherwise noted, use together is not necessarily contraindicated, but weigh the potential risks and perform additional monitoring when appropriate.

- **OTHER ORALLY ADMINISTERED THERAPEUTIC AGENTS:** Separate by at least 3 hours the administration of any other orally administered therapeutic agents from the charcoal dose.
- **DAIRY PRODUCTS:** May reduce the adsorptive capacity of activated charcoal.
- **MINERAL OIL:** May reduce the adsorptive capacity of activated charcoal.
- **POLYETHYLENE GLYCOL ELECTROLYTE SOLUTIONS** (*e.g.*, *Go-Lytely®*): May reduce the adsorptive capacity of activated charcoal.

Laboratory Considerations

- When used with sorbitol, a false-positive **ethylene glycol test** may result.

Doses

- **DOGS & CATS:**

  As an adjunctive treatment for toxin ingestions (extra-label): Note: Depending on the toxin exposure, recommendations for using activated charcoal can vary. It is highly recommended to contact an animal poison control center for specific guidance on using activated charcoal in veterinary patients.

  Current recommended dosage for single-dose activated charcoal is 1 – 5 grams/kg PO. A "standard dose" is 2 g/kg PO. When a cathartic is not contraindicated, charcoal w/sorbitol is commonly employed to reduce GI transit time. For drugs/toxins that are enterohepatically recirculated (*e.g.*, caffeine, phenobarbital, theobromine, theophylline, bromethalin, pyrethrins, organophosphate insecticides, ivermectin, antidepressants), multiple doses of activated charcoal WITHOUT sorbitol at 1 – 2 grams/kg PO q4-8 hours for 24 hours is suggested. Dogs and cats with no clinical signs may freely drink the charcoal suspension if administered via syringe. A small amount of food may be added to the solution to enhance palatability. In animals exhibiting clinical signs, administration of activated charcoal slurries/suspensions may be administered via an orogastric tube with a cuffed endotracheal tube in place to help prevent aspiration. Administration via a nasogastric tube may be useful, particularly in cats. (Adapted from: (Jutkowitz et al. 2009; Talcott 2012; Lee 2013)

■ **RUMINANTS:**

For plant intoxications (extra-label): Activated charcoal (AC) slurry dosage range of 1 – 5 g/kg (~1 g of activated charcoal per 5 ml of water). Multi-dose activated charcoal is beneficial for a number of plant intoxications, including oleander. Administration of a cathartic mixed in the AC slurry helps to hasten elimination of contents from the gastrointestinal tract. Commonly used cathartics include sodium sulfate (Glauber's salts), magnesium sulfate (Epsom salts), and sorbitol. Sodium or magnesium sulfate can be administered at 250 – 500 mg/kg mixed in the AC slurry. Sorbitol (70%), also mixed in the AC slurry, can be administered at 3 mL/kg. There is little need to administer a cathartic if significant diarrhea is already present. (Puschner 2010)

■ **HORSES:**

As an adjunctive treatment for toxin ingestions (extra-label):

a) **Foals:** 250 grams (minimum). **Adult horses:** up to 750 grams. Make a slurry by mixing with up to 4 L (depending on animal's size) of warm water and administer via stomach tube. Leave in stomach for 20-30 minutes and then give a laxative to hasten removal of toxicants. (Oehme 1987)

b) See the reference by Puschner in the Ruminants section above.

Monitoring

■ Monitoring for efficacy of charcoal is usually dependent upon the toxin/drug that it is being used for and could include the drug/toxin's serum level, clinical signs, etc.

■ Serum sodium, particularly if patient develops neurologic signs associated with hypernatremia (*e.g.,* tremors, ataxia, seizures, etc.).

Client Information

■ This agent should generally be used with professional supervision; if used on an outpatient basis animals must be observed for at least 4 hours after administration for signs associated with too much sodium in the blood (*e.g.,* weakness, unsteadiness, tremors, convulsions, etc.). Should these occur, animals must be seen immediately by a veterinarian.

■ Charcoal can permanently stain fabrics.

Chemistry/Synonyms

Activated charcoal occurs as a fine, black, odorless, tasteless powder that is insoluble in water or alcohol. Commercially available activated charcoal products may differ in their adsorptive properties, but one gram must adsorb 100 mg of strychnine sulfate in 50 mL of water to meet USP standards.

Activated charcoal may also be known as: active carbon, activated carbon, carbo activatus, adsorbent charcoal, decolorizing carbon, or medicinal charcoal. There are many trade names available.

Storage/Stability

Store activated charcoal in well-closed glass or metal containers or in the manufacturer's supplied container.

Compatibility/Compounding Considerations

No specific information noted.

Dosage Forms/Regulatory Status

VETERINARY-LABELED PRODUCTS:

In the USA, the following products are labeled for veterinary use, but there are no oral activated charcoal products listed as FDA-approved on the FDA's "Green Book" website.

Activated charcoal 47.5%, Kaolin 10% granules (free flowing and wettable) in 1 lb. bottles, and 5 kg pails; *Toxiban® Granules* ; (OTC). Labeled for use in both large and small animals.

Activated charcoal 10.4%, Kaolin 6.25% suspension in 240 mL bottles; *Toxiban® Suspension* ; (OTC). Labeled for use in both large and small animals.

Activated charcoal 10%, Kaolin 6.25%, sorbitol 10% suspension in 240 mL bottles; *Toxiban® Suspension* with *Sorbitol*; (OTC). Labeled for use in small animals.

Activated Charcoal 10%, Attapulgite 20%, sodium chloride 35 mg/mL, potassium chloride 35 mg/mL Gel/Paste in 80 mL & 300 mL; *D-Tox-Besc®*; *Activated Charcoal Gel with Electrolytes®* & *DVM Formula®*, *Activated Charcoal Paste®*; (OTC). Labeled for use in small and large animals.

Activated Hardwood Charcoal and thermally activated attapulgite clay (concentrations not labeled) in an aqueous gel suspension in 8 fl oz. bottle, 60 mL tube and 300 mL tube with easy dose syringe; *UAA®* (*Universal Animal Antidote) Gel*; (OTC). Labeled for use in dogs, cats and grain overload in ruminants.

HUMAN-LABELED PRODUCTS:

Activated Charcoal Oral Powder: 15 g, 30 g, 40 g, 120 g, 240 g and UD 30 g; generic; (OTC)

Activated Charcoal Oral Liquid/Suspension with sorbitol: 15 g & 30 g in 150 mL & 50 g in 240 mL; *CharcoAid®*; 25 g in 120 mL & 50 g in 240 mL; *Actidose®* with *Sorbitol*; (OTC)

Activated Charcoal Liquid/Suspension without sorbitol: 15 g & 50 g in 120 mL & 240 mL; *CharcoAid® 2000*; (OTC); 208 mg/mL — 12.5 g in 60 mL & 25 g in 120 mL; 12.5 g in 60 mL, 15 g in 75 mL, 25 g in 120 mL, 30 g in 120 mL, 50 g in 240 mL; *Actidose-Aqua®*, generic; (OTC)

Activated Charcoal Oral Granules: 15 g in 120 mL; *CharcoAid® 2000*; (OTC)

Revisions/References

Monograph revised/updated October 2013.

Jutkowitz, L. & J. Schildt (2009). *Management of common household toxins.* Proceedings: WVC. accessed via Veterinary Information Network; vin.com

Lee, J. A. (2013). Emergency Management and Treatment of the Poisoned Small Animal Patient. *Veterinary Clinics of North America: Small Animal Practice* 43(4): 757-71.

Oehme, F. W. (1987). General Principles in Treatment of Poisoning. *Current Therapy in Equine Medicine 2.* N. E. Robinson. Philadelphia, W.B. Saunders: 653-6.

Puschner, B. (2010). *Diagnostic and therapeutic approach to plant poisonings in large animals.* accessed via Veterinary Information Network; vin.com

Talcott, P. A. (2012). *Decontamination Procedures in Poisoned Companion Animals - Facts & Fiction.* Western Veterinary Conference. accessed via Veterinary Information Network; vin.com

Wilson, H. E. & K. R. Humm (2013). In vitro study of the effect of dog food on the adsorptive capacity of activated charcoal. *J. Vet. Emerg. Crit. Care* 23(3): 263-7.

Chlorambucil

(klor-am-byoo-sil)   Leukeran®

Immunosuppressant/Antineoplastic

Prescriber Highlights

▶ Nitrogen mustard derivative immunosuppressant & antineoplastic in dogs, cats and horses.

▶ Caution: Preexisting bone marrow depression, infection.

▶ Potential teratogen.

▶ Adverse Effects primarily myelosuppression & GI toxicity.

Uses/Indications

Chlorambucil may be useful as part of multi-drug protocols or as a solo metronomic agent (Leach et al. 2012; Schrempp et al. 2013) in a variety of neoplastic diseases, including lymphocytic leukemia, multiple myeloma, polycythemia vera, macroglobulinemia, and ovarian adenocarcinoma. It may also be useful as adjunctive therapy for some immune-mediated conditions (*e.g.,* inflammatory bowel disease, non-erosive arthritis, or immune-mediated skin disease).

Pharmacology/Actions

Chlorambucil is a cell-cycle nonspecific alkylating antineoplastic/immunosuppressive agent. Its cytotoxic activity stems from cross-linking with cellular DNA. Immunosuppressive effects may not be noted until 2-4 weeks after starting the drug.

Pharmacokinetics

Chlorambucil is rapidly and nearly completely absorbed after oral administration; peak levels occur in about one hour. It is highly bound to plasma proteins. While it is not known whether it crosses the blood-brain barrier, neurological side effects have been reported. Chlorambucil crosses the placenta, but it is not known whether it enters maternal milk. Chlorambucil is extensively metabolized in the liver, primarily to phenylacetic acid mustard, which is active. Phenylacetic acid mustard is further metabolized to other metabolites that are excreted in the urine.

Contraindications/Precautions/Warnings

Chlorambucil is contraindicated in patients that are hypersensitive to it or have demonstrated resistance to its effects. It should be used with caution in patients with preexisting bone marrow depression or infection, or susceptible to bone marrow depression or infection.

Adverse Effects

The most commonly associated major adverse effects seen with chlorambucil therapy is myelosuppression manifested by anemia, leukopenia, and thrombocytopenia and gastrointestinal toxicity (*e.g.,* vomiting, diarrhea, etc.). A greater likelihood of toxicity occurs with higher dosages. This may occur gradually with nadirs occurring usually within 7-14 days of the start of therapy. Recovery generally takes from 7-14 days. Severe bone marrow depression can result in pancytopenia that may take months to years for recovery. Alopecia and delayed regrowth of shaven fur have been reported in dogs; Poodles or Kerry blues are reportedly more likely to be affected than other breeds. Lower dose metronomic therapy (4 mg/m² once daily) in dogs, is associated with a lower incidence of adverse effects.

One case report in cat of neurotoxicity (*e.g.,* facial twitching, myoclonus, agitation, seizures) after chlorambucil therapy has been reported (Benitah et al. 2003). In another report in a dog, chlorambucil was suspected of causing seizures (Giuliano 2013).

In humans, bronchopulmonary dysplasia with pulmonary fibrosis, neurotoxicity, and uric acid nephropathy have been reported. These effects are uncommon and generally associated with chronic, higher dose therapy. Hepatotoxicity has been reported rarely in humans.

Reproductive/Nursing Safety

Chlorambucil's teratogenic potential remains poorly documented, but it may potentially cause a variety of fetal abnormalities. It is generally recommended to avoid the drug during pregnancy, but because of the seriousness of the diseases treated with chlorambucil, the potential benefits to the mother must be considered. Chlorambucil has been documented to cause irreversible infertility in male humans, particularly when given during pre-puberty and puberty. In humans, the FDA categorizes this drug as category *D* for use during pregnancy (*There is evidence of human fetal risk, but the potential benefits from the use of the drug in pregnant women may be acceptable despite its potential risks.*) In a separate system evaluating the safety of drugs in canine and feline pregnancy (Papich 1989), this drug is categorized as class: *C* (*These drugs may have potential risks. Studies in people or laboratory animals have uncovered risks, and these drugs should be used cautiously as a last resort when the benefit of therapy clearly outweighs the risks.*)

Overdosage/Acute Toxicity

The oral LD_{50} in mice is 123 mg/kg. There have been limited experiences with acute overdoses in humans. Doses of up to 5 mg/kg resulted in neurologic (seizures) toxicity and pancytopenia (nadirs at 1-6 weeks post ingestion). All patients recovered without long-term sequelae. Treatment should consist of gut emptying when appropriate (beware of rapidly changing neurologic status if inducing vomiting). Monitoring of CBC's several times a week for several weeks should be performed after overdoses and blood component therapy may be necessary.

Drug Interactions

The following drug interactions have either been reported or are theoretical in humans or animals receiving chlorambucil and may be of significance in veterinary patients. Unless otherwise noted, use together is not necessarily contraindicated, but weigh the potential risks and perform additional monitoring when appropriate.

■ **MYELOSUPPRESSIVE DRUGS** (*e.g.,* **other antineoplastics, chloramphenicol, flucytosine, amphotericin B, or colchicine**): Bone marrow depression may be additive.

■ **IMMUNOSUPPRESSIVE DRUGS** (*e.g.,* **azathioprine, cyclophosphamide, cyclosporine, corticosteroids**): Use with other immunosuppressant drugs may increase the risk of infection.

Laboratory Considerations

■ Chlorambucil may raise serum **uric acid** levels. Drugs such as **allopurinol** may be required to control hyperuricemia in some patients.

Doses

Note: Because of the potential toxicity of this drug to patients, veterinary personnel and clients, and since chemotherapy indications, treatment protocols, monitoring and safety guidelines often change, the following dosages should be used only as a general guide. Consultation with a veterinary oncologist and referral to current veterinary oncology references [*e.g.,* (Withrow et al. 2012); (Dobson et al. 2011); (Henry et al. 2009); (North et al. 2009); (Argyle et al. 2008)] are strongly recommended.

Dosages are commonly listed as mg/m². Do not confuse with mg/kg dosages.

■ **DOGS:**

As an immunosuppressant (extra-label): Dosage recommendations vary. Commonly dosed at 0.1 – 0.2 mg/kg (corresponds approximately to 2 – 6 mg/m²) once daily initially. Dosages are generally rounded to the nearest 2 mg. When remission occurs, attempt to dose every other day; use lowest dosage that will control condition. Often used in conjunction with prednisolone.

For adjunctive therapy of lymphoreticular neoplasms, macroglobulinemia, and polycythemia vera (extra-label): For first level treatment of dogs of canine lymphoma where clients cannot afford, or will not accept combination chemotherapy due to risks of toxicity: Prednisone alone 40 mg/m² (NOT mg/kg) PO daily for 7 days then every other day or in combination with chlorambucil at 6 – 8 mg/m² (NOT mg/kg) PO every other day. Perform a CBC every 2-3 weeks. (Ogilvie 2006)

For metronomic treatment of cancer (extra-label): 4 mg/m² (NOT mg/kg) PO once daily. For dogs weighing >8 kg, the dose is rounded to the nearest 2 mg; dogs weighing ≤8 kg, dose is compounded to 4 mg/m² (Leach et al. 2012; Schrempp et al. 2013). **Note:** In the second reference (Schrempp et al. 2013), dogs enrolled in the study had bladder transitional cell carcinoma. 70% of dogs either had a partial remission (1/30) or stable disease (20/30).

- **CATS:**

As an immunosuppressant (extra-label): Chlorambucil is generally considered a second-line immunosuppressant (after glucocorticoids) in cats and often used in conjunction with prednisolone. Anecdotal chlorambucil dosing recommendations vary and the commercial tablet size (2 mg) may make precise dosing difficult without compounding. For immune-mediated conditions it is commonly dosed initially at 0.1 – 0.2 mg/kg (approximately 1.5 – 4 mg/m²; ½ of a 2 mg tablet for larger cats or a compounded dosage form) PO once daily. If using the whole 2 mg tablets, it is dosed in a practical manner every 48 hours for cats weighing more than 4 kg, and every 72 hours for cats weighing less than 4 kg. Once remission occurs the dosage is reduced or the dosage interval (often every 3-4 days) is extended to where the condition is still controlled.

For low-grade gastrointestinal lymphosarcoma (extra-label): Several protocols using chlorambucil with prednisolone have had a relatively high degree of efficacy, including:

a) Chlorambucil 15 mg/m² PO once daily for 4 days; repeated every 3 weeks and prednisolone initially at 3 mg/kg PO once daily. (Lingard et al. 2009)

b) Chlorambucil 20 mg/m² (rounded to nearest 2 mg) PO once every 2 weeks and prednisolone 2 mg/kg PO once daily. (Stein et al. 2010)

c) Chlorambucil 2 mg per cat PO every 2-3 days (q48-72h) and prednisolone 5 – 10 mg per cat PO q12-24h. (Kiselow et al. 2008)

- **HORSES:**

For adjunctive therapy in treating lymphoma using the LAP protocol (extra-label): Cytarabine 200 – 300 mg/m² (NOT mg/kg) SC or IM once every 1-2 weeks; Chlorambucil 20 mg/m² (NOT mg/kg) PO every 2 weeks (alternating with cytarabine) and Prednisone 1.1 – 2.2 mg/kg PO every other day. If this protocol is not effective (no response seen in 2-4 weeks) add vincristine at 0.5 mg/m² (NOT mg/kg) IV once a week. Side effects are rare. (Couto 1994)

Monitoring

- Efficacy.
- CBC, Platelets once weekly (or once stable, every other week) during therapy; once stable, dogs may require only monthly monitoring. If neutrophils are <3,000/microL hold drug until recovered and reduce dose by 25% or increase dosing interval. Other references recommend CBCs at 0, 1, 2, 4, 8, & 12 weeks and then every 3-6 months (Mueller 2000) or in cats, CBCs at 2

to 3 weeks after starting therapy and every 3-6 months thereafter (Ashley 2009).
- Uric acid, liver enzymes; if warranted.

Client Information

- Give this drug with food.
- Chlorambucil is a chemotherapy (cancer) drug. The drug and its byproducts can be hazardous to other animals and people that come in contact with it. On the day your animal gets the drug and then for a few days afterward, all bodily waste (urine, feces, litter), blood, or vomit should only be handled while wearing disposable gloves. Seal the waste in a plastic bag and then place both the bag and gloves in with the regular trash.
- Chlorambucil can be very toxic to the gastrointestinal tract and cause vomiting and gastrointestinal upset.
- Contact your veterinarian immediately if you notice abnormal bleeding, bruising, depression, infection, shortness of breath, bloody diarrhea, etc.

Chemistry/Synonyms

A nitrogen mustard derivative antineoplastic agent, chlorambucil occurs as an off-white, slightly granular powder. It is very slightly soluble in water.

Chlorambucil may also be known as: CB-1348, NSC-3088, WR-139013, chlorambucilum, chloraminophene, chlorbutinum, *Chloraminophene®*, *Leukeran®*, or *Linfolysin®*.

Storage/Stability

Chlorambucil tablets should be stored in light-resistant, well-closed containers under refrigeration (2-8°C; 36-46°F). Tablets can be stored at a maximum of 30°C (86°F) up to one week. An expiration date of one year after manufacture is assigned to the commercially available tablets.

Compatibility/Compounding Considerations

Compounded preparation stability: Chlorambucil oral suspension compounded from commercially available tablets has been published (Dressman et al. 1983). Triturating six (6) chlorambucil 2 mg tablets with 2 mL *Cologel®* and *qs ad* to 6 mL with simple syrup yields a 2 mg/mL oral suspension that retains 90% potency for 7 days at 5°C. Suspensions of chlorambucil stored at room temperature rapidly decompose with losses >15% in one day. Chlorambucil is rapidly hydrolyzed independently of pH, but minimal hydrolysis occurs at pH 2. Refrigeration also slows hydrolysis.

Dosage Forms/Regulatory Status

VETERINARY-LABELED PRODUCTS: NONE.

HUMAN-LABELED PRODUCTS:

Chlorambucil Oral Tablets (film-coated): 2 mg; *Leukeran®*; (Rx)

Revisions/References

Monograph revised/updated October 2013.

Argyle, D., et al. (2008). *Decision Making in Small Animal Oncology*, Wiley-Blackwell.
Ashley, P. (2009). *Thinking outside the box of DepoMedrol: Dermatology drug choices for cats.* Proceedings: WVC. accessed via Veterinary Information Network; vin.com
Benitah, N., et al. (2003). Chlorambucil-induced myoclonus in a cat with lymphoma. *J. Am. Anim. Hosp. Assoc.* 39(3): 283-7.
Couto, C. (1994). *Lymphoma in the Horse.* Proceedings of the Twelfth Annual Veterinary Medical Forum, San Francisco, American College of Veterinary Internal Medicine. accessed via Veterinary Information Network; vin.com
Dobson, J. & D. Lascelles (2011). *BSAVA Manual of Canine and Feline Oncology*, BSAVA.
Dressman, J. & R. Poust (1983). Stability of allopurinol and of five antineoplastics in suspension. *Am J Hosp Pharm* 40(4): 616-8.

Giuliano, A. (2013). Suspected chlorambucil-related neurotoxicity with seizures in a dog. *Journal of Small Animal Practice* **54**(8): 437-.

Henry, C. & M. Higginbotham (2009). *Cancer Management in Small Animal Practice*, Saunders.

Kiselow, M. A., et al. (2008). Outcome of cats with low-grade lymphocytic lymphoma: 41 cases (1995-2005). *Javma-Journal of the American Veterinary Medical Association* **232**(3): 405-10.

Leach, T. N., et al. (2012). Prospective trial of metronomic chlorambucil chemotherapy in dogs with naturally occurring cancer. *Veterinary and Comparative Oncology* **10**(2): 102-12.

Lingard, A. E., et al. (2009). Low-grade alimentary lymphoma: clinicopathological findings and response to treatment in 17 cases. *Journal of Feline Medicine and Surgery* **11**(8): 692-700.

Mueller, R. (2000). *Dermatology for the Small Animal Practitioner*, Teton New Media.

North, S. & T. Banks (2009). *Small Animal Oncology: An Introduction*, Saunders.

Ogilvie, G. (2006). *Canine Lymphoma*. Proceedings WSAVA. accessed via Veterinary Information Network; vin.com

Schrempp, D. R., et al. (2013). Metronomic administration of chlorambucil for treatment of dogs with urinary bladder transitional cell carcinoma. *Javma-Journal of the American Veterinary Medical Association* **242**(11): 1534-8.

Stein, T. J., et al. (2010). Treatment of Feline Gastrointestinal Small-Cell Lymphoma With Chlorambucil and Glucocorticoids. *J. Am. Anim. Hosp. Assoc.* **46**(6): 413-7.

Withrow, S., et al. (2012). *Withrow and MacEwen's Small Animal Clinical Oncology, 5th Ed.*, Saunders.

Chloramphenicol

(klor-am-fen-i-kole)　Chloromycetin®

Broad-Spectrum Antibacterial

Prescriber Highlights

▶ Broad-spectrum antibiotic.

▶ Contraindications: Banned in food animals. Extreme caution/avoid use: Preexisting hematologic disorders, pregnancy, neonates, hepatic failure, and in cats, renal failure; IV use in animals with cardiac failure; use long-term (>14 days) in cats with caution.

▶ May need to reduce dose in animals with hepatic or renal insufficiency.

▶ Adverse Effects: GI; potentially myelosuppressive, especially with high dose, long-term treatment.

▶ Potentially toxic to humans; have dosage-giver avoid direct contact with medication.

Uses/Indications

Chloramphenicol is used for a variety of infections in small animals and horses, particularly those caused by anaerobic bacteria. In dogs, it is a potentially useful drug in treating methicillin-resistant staphylococcal infections or treating bacterial prostatic infections. Chloramphenicol appears to pose a low risk for serious enteropathies to hindgut-fermenting species (*e.g.*, rabbits, Guinea pigs, etc.) and it may be useful in those species. The FDA has prohibited the use of chloramphenicol in animals used for food production because of the human public health implications.

Pharmacology/Actions

Chloramphenicol usually acts as a time-dependent, bacteriostatic antibiotic, but at higher concentrations or against some very susceptible organisms it can be bactericidal. Chloramphenicol acts by binding to the 50S ribosomal subunit of susceptible bacteria, thereby preventing bacterial protein synthesis. Erythromycin, clindamycin, lincomycin, tylosin, etc., also bind to the same site, but unlike these drugs, chloramphenicol appears to also have an affinity for mitochondrial ribosomes of rapidly proliferating mammalian cells (*e.g.*, bone marrow) that may result in reversible bone marrow suppression.

Chloramphenicol has a wide spectrum of activity against many gram-positive and gram-negative organisms. Gram-positive aerobic organisms that are generally susceptible to chloramphenicol include many streptococci and staphylococci. It is also effective against some gram-negative aerobes including Neisseria, Brucella, Salmonella, Shigella, and Haemophilus. Many anaerobic bacteria are sensitive to chloramphenicol including Clostridium, Bacteroides (including *B. fragilis*), Fusobacterium, and Veillonella. Chloramphenicol also has activity against Nocardia, Chlamydia, Mycoplasma, and Rickettsia. In dogs, most isolates of *Enterococcus faecalis* are resistant to chloramphenicol.

Pharmacokinetics

Chloramphenicol is rapidly absorbed after oral administration with peak serum levels occurring approximately 30 minutes after dosing. The palmitate oral suspension produces significantly lower peak serum levels when administered to fasted cats. The sodium succinate salt is rapidly and well absorbed after IM or SC administration in animals and, contrary to some recommendations, need not be administered only intravenously. The palmitate and sodium succinate is hydrolyzed in the GI tract and liver to the base.

Chloramphenicol is widely distributed throughout the body. Highest levels are found in the liver and kidney, but the drug attains therapeutic levels in most tissues and fluids, including the aqueous and vitreous humor, and synovial fluid. CSF concentrations may be up to 50% of those in the serum when meninges are uninflamed and higher when meninges are inflamed. A 4-6 hour lag time before CSF peak levels occur may be seen. Chloramphenicol concentrations in the prostate are approximately 50% of those in the serum. Because only a small amount of the drug is excreted unchanged into the urine in dogs, chloramphenicol may not be the best choice for lower urinary tract infections in that species. The volume of distribution of chloramphenicol has been reported as 1.6-1.8 L/kg in the dog, 2.4 L/kg in the cat, and 1.41 L/kg in horses. Chloramphenicol is about 30-60% bound to plasma proteins, enters milk and crosses the placenta.

In most species, chloramphenicol is eliminated primarily by hepatic metabolism via glucuronidative mechanisms. Only about 5-15% of the drug is excreted unchanged in the urine. The cat, having little ability to glucuronidate drugs, excretes 25% or more of a dose as unchanged drug in the urine.

The elimination half-life has been reported as 1.1-5 hours in dogs but it appears to average around 2.4 hours, <1 hour in foals and ponies, and 4-8 hours in cats. The elimination half-life of chloramphenicol in birds is highly species variable, ranging from 26 minutes in pigeons to nearly 5 hours in bald eagles and peafowl.

Contraindications/Precautions/Warnings

Chloramphenicol is prohibited by the FDA for use in food animals.

Chloramphenicol is contraindicated in patients hypersensitive to it. Because of the potential for hematopoietic toxicity, the drug should be used with extreme caution, if at all, in patients with preexisting hematologic abnormalities, especially a preexisting non-regenerative anemia. The drug should only be used in patients in hepatic failure when no other effective antibiotics are available and then only with prolonged dosing intervals. Chloramphenicol should be used with caution in patients with impaired hepatic or renal function as drug accumulation can occur. Those patients may need dosing adjustment, and monitoring of blood levels should be considered.

Use with caution in cats. Dosages for dogs and cats are very different.

Chloramphenicol should be used with caution in neonatal animals, particularly in young kittens. In neonates (humans), circulatory collapse (so-called "Gray-baby syndrome") has occurred with chloramphenicol, probably due to toxic levels accumulating secondary to an inability to conjugate the drug or excrete the conjugate effectively.

Adverse Effects

While the toxicity of chloramphenicol in humans has been greatly discussed, the drug is generally considered to have a low order of toxicity in adult companion animals when appropriately dosed. However, a recent retrospective review found that 53% of 51 dogs treated with chloramphenicol at usual dosages (approx. 50 mg/kg) for methicillin-resistant *Staphylococcus pseudintermedius* (MRSP) pyoderma developed adverse effects that included: GI signs (47%), lethargy (14%), shaking (8%), increased liver enzymes (6%). Anemia, panting, and aggression were reported in individual dogs (Bryan et al. 2012).

Development of aplastic anemia reported in humans, does not appear to be a significant problem for veterinary patients; however, a dose-related bone marrow suppression (reversible) is seen in all species, primarily with long-term therapy. Early signs of bone marrow toxicity can include vacuolation of many of the early cells of the myeloid and erythroid series, lymphocytopenia, and neutropenia. Thrombocytopenia associated with chloramphenicol use in cats has been reported.

Other adverse effects that may be noted include anorexia, vomiting, diarrhea, and depression.

It has been said that cats tend to be more sensitive to developing adverse reactions to chloramphenicol than dogs, but this is probably more as a result of the drug's longer half-life in the cat. Cats dosed at high dosages for prolonged periods (*e.g.*, 50 mg/kg q12h for 2-3 weeks) do develop a high incidence of adverse effects, including bone marrow hypoplasia and should be closely monitored.

Reproductive/Nursing Safety

Chloramphenicol has not been determined to be safe for use during pregnancy. The drug may decrease protein synthesis in the fetus, particularly in the bone marrow. It should only be used when the benefits of therapy clearly outweigh the risks. In humans, the FDA categorizes this drug as category *C* for use during pregnancy (*Animal studies have shown an adverse effect on the fetus, but there are no adequate studies in humans; or there are no animal reproduction studies and no adequate studies in humans.*) In a separate system evaluating the safety of drugs in canine and feline pregnancy (Papich 1989), this drug is categorized as class: *C* (*These drugs may have potential risks. Studies in people or laboratory animals have uncovered risks, and these drugs should be used cautiously as a last resort when the benefit of therapy clearly outweighs the risks.*)

Because chloramphenicol is found in milk in humans at 50% of serum levels, the drug should be given with caution to nursing bitches or queens, particularly within the first week after giving birth.

Overdosage/Acute Toxicity

Because of the potential for serious bone marrow toxicity, large overdoses of chloramphenicol should be handled by emptying the gut using standard protocols. For more information on the toxicity of chloramphenicol, refer to the Adverse Effects section above.

Drug Interactions

Chloramphenicol is a cytochrome P450 CYP2B11 inhibitor in dogs, and may possibly inhibit other CYP isoenzymes in dogs or other veterinary species. The following drug interactions have either been reported or are theoretical in humans or animals receiving chloramphenicol and may be of significance in veterinary patients (**Note:** Cats may be particularly susceptible to chloramphenicol's effects on the hepatic metabolism of other drugs):

- **ANTI-ANEMIA DRUGS** (*e.g.*, **Iron, Vitamin B12, folic acid**): Chloramphenicol may delay hematopoietic response.
- **ASPIRIN** (and other **SALICYLATES**): Chloramphenicol may delay hepatic metabolism.

- **BETA-LACTAM ANTIBIOTICS** (*e.g.*, **penicillins, cephalosporins, aminoglycosides**): Potential for antagonism; clinical significance, if any, is not clear.
- **CIMETIDINE:** May reduce the metabolism of chloramphenicol increasing the risks for toxicity.
- **KETAMINE:** Chloramphenicol may prolong effects. Chloramphenicol did not prolong anesthesia in dogs receiving xylazine/ketamine in one study.
- **LIDOCAINE:** Chloramphenicol may delay hepatic metabolism.
- **MIDAZOLAM:** Chloramphenicol may prolong effects.
- **MYELOSUPPRESSIVE DRUGS** (*e.g.*, **cyclophosphamide**): Potential for additive bone marrow depression.
- **OPIATES:** Chloramphenicol can significantly inhibit metabolism and prolong opiate effects.
- **PENTOBARBITAL:** Chloramphenicol has been demonstrated to prolong the duration of pentobarbital anesthesia by 120% in dogs, and 260% in cats.
- **PHENOBARBITAL:** Chloramphenicol may inhibit hepatic metabolism and phenobarbital may decrease chloramphenicol concentrations.
- **PROPOFOL:** Chloramphenicol may prolong anesthesia.
- **RIFAMPIN:** May decrease serum chloramphenicol levels.

Laboratory Considerations

False-positive **glucosuria** has been reported, but the incidence is unknown.

Doses

- **DOGS:**

  For susceptible infections (extra-label): Most current recommendations, based on pharmacokinetic and bacterial susceptibility data recommend 40 – 50 mg/kg PO, IV, SC, IM q8h. Some suggest that dosages up to 60 mg/kg PO q8h may be necessary for some infections.

- **CATS:**

  For susceptible infections (extra-label): Most current recommendations are 10 – 20 mg/kg q12h PO, IV, IM or SC. Practically, it is often administered at 50 mg per cat PO twice a day.

- **RABBITS/RODENTS/SMALL MAMMALS:**

  All dosages are extra-label.

  a) **Rabbits:** 30 – 50 mg/kg PO, SC, IM, IV q8–24h. (Ivey et al. 2000)

  b) **Hedgehogs:** 50 mg/kg PO q12h; 30 – 50 mg/kg SC, IM, IV or IO q12h. (Smith 2000)

  c) **Chinchillas:** 30 – 50 mg/kg PO, SC, IM q12h. (Hayes 2000)

  d) **Gerbils, Guinea Pigs, Hamsters, Mice, Rats:** 20 – 50 mg/kg (succinate salt) SC q6–12h. (Adamcak et al. 2000)

  e) **Guinea pigs for pneumonia:** 30 – 50 mg/kg PO q12h. (Johnson 2006)

- **FERRETS:**

  For susceptible infections (extra-label): 50 mg/kg PO, SC, IV q12h.

- **HORSES:**

  All dosages are extra-label.

  For susceptible infections (extra-label):

  a) 45 – 60 mg/kg PO q8h; 45 – 60 mg/kg IM, SC or IV q6–8h. (USPC 1990)

  b) **Foals:** 20 mg/kg PO or IV q4h. (Furr 1999)

  c) **Foals:** Chloramphenicol sodium succinate: 25 – 50 mg/kg IV q4–8h; chloramphenicol base or palmitate: 40 – 50 mg/kg PO q6–8h. (Brumbaugh 1999)

■ **BIRDS:**

For susceptible infections (extra-label):

a) Chloramphenicol sodium succinate: 80 mg/kg IM two to three times daily, 50 mg/kg IV three to four times daily.

b) Succinate: 50 mg/kg IM or IV q8h. (Hoeffer 1995)

■ **REPTILES:**

For susceptible infections (extra-label):

a) For most species using the sodium succinate salt: 20 – 50 mg/kg IM or SC for up to 3 weeks. Chloramphenicol is often a good initial choice until sensitivity results are available. (Gauvin 1993)

b) 30 – 50 mg/kg/day IV, or IM for 7-14 days. (Lewbart 2001)

Monitoring

- Clinical efficacy.
- Adverse effects; chronic therapy should be associated with routine CBC monitoring.

Client Information

- Rarely, this drug can be very toxic to humans. Wear gloves when handling this medication.
- Usually given three times daily. Missing dosages can cause the drug not to work properly for your animal.
- Best given with food. Extremely bitter taste can make oral administration of the tablets difficult.
- Most common adverse effects are stomach upset, vomiting and diarrhea. Cats may be more likely to get serious adverse effects of this drug.
- Banned for use in animals that are used for food (including egg laying chickens and dairy animals).

Chemistry/Synonyms

Originally isolated from *Streptomyces venezuelae*, chloramphenicol is now produced synthetically. It occurs as fine, white to grayish, yellow white, elongated plates or needle-like crystals with a pK_a of 5.5. It is freely soluble in alcohol and about 2.5 mg are soluble in 1 mL of water at 25°C.

Chloramphenicol sodium succinate occurs as a white to light yellow powder. It is freely soluble in both water and alcohol. Commercially available chloramphenicol sodium succinate for injection contains 2.3 mEq of sodium per gram of chloramphenicol.

Chloramphenicol may also be known as: chloramphenicolum, chloranfenicol, cloranfenicol, kloramfenikol, or laevomycetinum; many trade names are available.

Storage/Stability

Chloramphenicol capsules and tablets should be stored in tight containers at room temperature (15-30°C). The palmitate oral suspension should be stored in tight containers at room temperature and protected from light or freezing.

The sodium succinate powder for injection should be stored at temperatures less than 40°C, preferably between 15-30°C. After reconstituting the sodium succinate injection with sterile water, the solution is stable for 30 days at room temperature and 6 months if frozen. The solution should be discarded if it becomes cloudy.

Compatibility/Compounding Considerations

The following drugs and solutions are reportedly **compatible** with chloramphenicol sodium succinate injection: all commonly used intravenous fluids, amikacin sulfate, aminophylline, ampicillin sodium (in syringe for 1 hr.) ascorbic acid, calcium chloride/gluconate, corticotropin, cyanocobalamin, dimenhydrinate, dopamine HCl, ephedrine sulfate, heparin sodium, hydrocortisone sodium succinate, hydroxyzine HCl, lidocaine HCl, magnesium sulfate, methylprednisolone sodium succinate, metronidazole with or without sodium bicarbonate, oxytocin, penicillin G potassium/sodium, pentobarbital sodium, phenylephrine HCl with or without sodium bicarbonate, phytonadione, plasma protein fraction, potassium chloride, promazine HCl, ranitidine HCl, sodium bicarbonate, verapamil HCl, and vitamin B-complex with C.

The following drugs and solutions are reportedly **incompatible** (or compatibility data conflicts) with chloramphenicol sodium succinate injection: chlorpromazine HCl, glycopyrrolate, metoclopramide HCl, oxytetracycline HCl, prochlorperazine edislyate/mesylate, promethazine HCl, tetracycline HCl, and vancomycin HCl.

Compatibility is dependent upon factors such as pH, concentration, temperature and diluent used; consult specialized references or a hospital pharmacist for more specific information.

Dosage Forms/Regulatory Status

VETERINARY-LABELED PRODUCTS:

Chloramphenicol Oral Tablets and Capsules: 50 mg, 100 mg, 250 mg, 500 mg, & 1 g; FDA-approved for use in dogs only. Trade names and manufacturers/sponsors vary. (Rx)

Chloramphenicol Injection: 100 mg/mL; (Rx). FDA-approved for use in dogs, but availability and marketing status unknown.

Chloramphenicol (as palmitate) Oral Suspension: 30 mg/mL; *Chloromycetin®*; (Rx). FDA-approved for use in dogs, but availability and marketing status unknown.

HUMAN-LABELED PRODUCTS:

Chloramphenicol Powder for Injection: 1 gram (100 mg/mL as sodium succinate when reconstituted); generic; (Rx)

Revisions/References

Monograph revised/updated October 2013.

Adamcak, A. & B. Otten (2000). Rodent Therapeutics. *Vet Clin NA: Exotic Anim Pract* 3:1(Jan): 221-40.

Brumbaugh, G. (1999). *Clinical Pharmacology and the Pediatric Patient.* 45th Annual AAEP Convention, Albuquerque. accessed via Veterinary Information Network; vin.com

Bryan, J., et al. (2012). Treatment outcome of dogs with meticillin-resistant and meticillin-susceptible Staphylococcus pseudintermedius pyoderma. *Veterinary Dermatology* 23(4): 361-E65.

Furr, M. (1999). *Antimicrobial treatments for the septic foal.* Proceedings: The North American Veterinary Conference, Orlando. accessed via Veterinary Information Network; vin.com

Gauvin, J. (1993). Drug therapy in reptiles. *Seminars in Avian & Exotic Med* 2(1): 48-59.

Hayes, P. (2000). Diseases of Chinchillas. *Kirk's Current Veterinary Therapy: XIII Small Animal Practice.* J. Bonagura. Philadelphia, WB Saunders: 1152-7.

Hoeffer, H. (1995). Antimicrobials in pet birds. *Kirk's Current Veterinary Therapy:XII.* J. Bonagura. Philadelphia, W.B. Saunders: 1278-83.

Ivey, E. & J. Morrisey (2000). Therapeutics for Rabbits. *Vet Clin NA: Exotic Anim Pract* 3:1(Jan): 183-216.

Johnson, D. (2006). *Guinea Pig Medicine Primer.* Proceedings: ACVC. accessed via Veterinary Information Network; vin.com

Lewbart (2001). *Reptile Formulary.* Proceedings: Atlantic Coast Veterinary Conference. accessed via Veterinary Information Network; vin.com

Smith, A. (2000). General husbandry and medical care of hedgehogs. *Kirk's Current Veterinary Therapy: XIII Small Animal Practice.* J. Bonagura. Philadelphia, WB Saunders: 1128-33.

USPC (1990). Veterinary Information- Appendix III. *Drug Information for the Health Professional.* Rockville, United States Pharmacopeial Convention. 2: 2811- 60.

Chlordiazepoxide ± Clidinium Br

(klor-dye-az-e-pox-ide) ± (kli-din-ee-um)   Librium®, Librax®

Benzodiazepine ± Antimuscarinic

Prescriber Highlights

▶ Benzodiazepine for behavior problems (*e.g.*, phobias, etc.) & with an antimuscarinic (clidinium) for irritable bowel syndrome in dogs.

▶ Not commonly used, so little has been published on adverse effects (similar to diazepam +/- atropine).

▶ Potentially teratogenic.

Uses/Indications

Chlordiazepoxide alone may be a useful adjunct in treating certain behaviors where benzodiazepines may be useful including noise phobias in dogs, and inter-cat aggression and urine spraying in cats. When combined with clidinium, it may be useful symptomatic therapy for dogs with irritable bowel syndrome.

Pharmacology/Actions

The subcortical levels (primarily limbic, thalamic, and hypothalamic) of the CNS are depressed by chlordiazepoxide and other benzodiazepines thus producing the anxiolytic, sedative, skeletal muscle relaxant and anticonvulsant effects seen. The exact mechanism of action is unknown but postulated mechanisms include: antagonism of serotonin, increased release of and/or facilitation of gamma-aminobutyric acid (GABA) activity, and diminished release or turnover of acetylcholine in the CNS. Benzodiazepine specific receptors have been located in the mammalian brain, kidney, liver, lung, and heart. In all species studied, receptors are lacking in the white matter.

Clidinium bromide is an antimuscarinic with its main action to reduce GI motility and secretion similarly to atropine. Clidinium is a quaternary ammonium compound and, unlike atropine, does not cross appreciably into the CNS or the eye and should not exhibit the same extent of CNS or ocular adverse effects that atropine possesses. For further information, refer to the atropine monograph.

Pharmacokinetics

Chlordiazepoxide is rapidly absorbed following oral administration. It is highly lipid soluble and is widely distributed throughout the body. It readily crosses the blood-brain barrier and is fairly highly bound to plasma proteins. Chlordiazepoxide is metabolized in the liver to several metabolites, including: desmethyldiazepam (nordiazepam), desmethylchlordiazepoxide and oxazepam, all of which are pharmacologically active and can have considerable half lives. These are eventually conjugated with glucuronide and eliminated primarily in the urine. Because of the active metabolites, serum values of chlordiazepoxide are not useful in predicting efficacy.

Little pharmacokinetic data for clidinium is available. The drug is incompletely absorbed from the gut (small intestine). Effects in humans are seen in about an hour; duration of effect is about 3 hours. As the compound is completely ionized *in vivo*, it does not enter the CNS or the eye and therefore unlike atropine does not have effects on those systems. The drug is metabolized principally in the liver, but is also excreted unchanged in the urine.

Contraindications/Precautions/Warnings

Use benzodiazepines cautiously in patients with hepatic or renal disease and in debilitated or geriatric patients. Chlordiazepoxide should only be administered very cautiously to patients in coma, shock or with significant respiratory depression. It is contraindicated in patients with known hypersensitivity to the drug. Chlordiazepoxide should be used very cautiously, if at all, in aggressive patients as it may disinhibit the anxiety that may help prevent these animals from aggressive behavior. Benzodiazepines may impair the abilities of working animals. If administering the drug IV (rarely warranted), be prepared to administer cardiovascular or respiratory support. Give IV slowly.

Clidinium, like other antimuscarinic agents should not be used in patients with tachycardias secondary to thyrotoxicosis or cardiac insufficiency, myocardial ischemia, unstable cardiac status during acute hemorrhage, GI obstructive disease, paralytic ileus, severe ulcerative colitis, obstructive uropathy, or myasthenia gravis.

Antimuscarinic agents should be used with extreme caution in patients with known or suspected GI infections. Antimuscarinic agents can decrease GI motility and prolong retention of the causative agent(s) or toxin(s) resulting in prolonged effects of the toxin. Antimuscarinic agents must also be used with extreme caution in patients with autonomic neuropathy.

Antimuscarinic agents should be used with caution in geriatric or pediatric patients, and in patients with hepatic or renal disease, hyperthyroidism, hypertension, CHF, tachyarrhythmias, prostatic hypertrophy, or esophageal reflux.

Adverse Effects

Chlordiazepoxide's adverse effects are similar to other benzodiazepines, especially diazepam (they share several active metabolites). As there is much more information with respect to diazepam in dogs or cats than chlordiazepoxide, the following is extrapolated from diazepam information: Dogs could exhibit a contradictory response (CNS excitement) following administration of chlordiazepoxide. The effects with regard to sedation and tranquilization are extremely variable with each dog. Cats could exhibit changes in behavior (*e.g.*, irritability, depression, aberrant demeanor, etc.) after receiving chlordiazepoxide. There have been reports of cats developing hepatic failure after receiving oral diazepam for several days. It is unknown if chlordiazepoxide also shares this effect. Clinical signs have been reported to occur 5-11 days after beginning oral therapy. Cats that receive diazepam should have baseline liver function tests. These should be repeated and the drug discontinued if emesis, lethargy, inappetence, or ataxia develops.

Clidinium's adverse effects are basically extensions of the drug's pharmacologic effects and are generally dose related. At usual doses, effects tend to be mild in relatively healthy patients; more severe effects tend to occur with high or toxic doses. GI effects can include dry mouth (xerostomia), dysphagia, constipation, vomiting, and thirst. GU effects may include urinary retention or hesitancy. Cardiovascular effects include sinus tachycardia (at higher doses), bradycardia (initially or at very low doses), hypertension, hypotension, arrhythmias (ectopic complexes), and circulatory failure.

Reproductive/Nursing Safety

Benzodiazepines have been implicated in causing congenital abnormalities in humans if administered during the first trimester of pregnancy. Infants born of mothers receiving large doses of benzodiazepines shortly before delivery have been reported to suffer from apnea, impaired metabolic response to cold stress, difficulty in feeding, hyperbilirubinemia, hypotonia, etc. Withdrawal symptoms have occurred in infants whose mothers chronically took benzodiazepines during pregnancy. The veterinary significance of these effects is unclear, but the use of these agents during the first trimester of pregnancy should only occur when the benefits clearly outweigh the risks associated with their use. In humans, the FDA categorizes chlordiazepoxide as category *D* for use during pregnancy (*There is evidence of human fetal risk, but the potential benefits from the use of the drug in pregnant women may be acceptable despite its potential risks.*)

Benzodiazepines and their metabolites are distributed into milk and may cause CNS effects in nursing neonates.

Overdosage/Acute Toxicity

When administered alone, chlordiazepoxide overdoses are generally limited to significant CNS depression (*e.g.,* confusion, coma, decreased reflexes, etc.). Hypotension, respiratory depression, and cardiac arrest have been reported in human patients but apparently are quite rare.

Treatment of acute toxicity consists of standard protocols for removing and/or binding the drug in the gut if taken orally, and supportive systemic measures. The use of analeptic agents (CNS stimulants such as caffeine) is generally not recommended. Flumazenil may be considered for adjunctive treatment of overdoses of benzodiazepines.

Drug Interactions

The following drug interactions have either been reported or are theoretical in humans or animals receiving chlordiazepoxide or other benzodiazepines and may be of significance in veterinary patients. Unless otherwise noted, use together is not necessarily contraindicated, but weigh the potential risks and perform additional monitoring when appropriate.

- **DIGOXIN:** The pharmacologic effects of digoxin may be increased; monitor serum digoxin levels or signs of toxicity.
- **OTHER CNS DEPRESSANT DRUGS** (*e.g.,* **barbiturates, opiates, anesthetics**): Additive effects may occur.
- **PROBENECID:** May interfere with benzodiazepine metabolism in the liver, causing increased or prolonged effects.
- **RIFAMPIN:** May induce hepatic microsomal enzymes and decrease the pharmacologic effects of benzodiazepines.

The following drugs may decrease the metabolism of chlordiazepoxide and excessive sedation may occur:

- **CIMETIDINE**
- **ERYTHROMYCIN**
- **FLUOXETINE**
- **ISONIAZID**
- **KETOCONAZOLE**
- **METOPROLOL**
- **PROPRANOLOL**

When using the product containing clidinium the following potential interactions noted with atropine may apply and the following drugs may enhance the activity or toxicity of clidinium:

- **AMANTADINE**
- **ANTICHOLINERGIC AGENTS, OTHER**
- **ANTICHOLINERGIC MUSCLE RELAXANTS**
- **ANTIHISTAMINES** (*e.g.,* **diphenhydramine,** *etc.*)
- **DISOPYRAMIDE**
- **MEPERIDINE**
- **PHENOTHIAZINES**
- **PROCAINAMIDE**
- **PRIMIDONE**
- **TRICYCLIC ANTIDEPRESSANTS** (*e.g.,* **amitriptyline, clomipramine, etc.**)

- **AMITRAZ:** Atropine may aggravate some signs seen with amitraz toxicity; hypertension and further inhibition of peristalsis are possible.
- **ANTACIDS:** May decrease PO atropine absorption; give oral atropine at least 1 hour prior to oral antacids.
- **CORTICOSTEROIDS** (long-term use): may increase intraocular pressure.
- **DIGOXIN** (slow-dissolving): Atropine may increase serum digoxin levels; use regular digoxin tablets or oral liquid.

- **KETOCONAZOLE:** Increased gastric pH may decrease GI absorption; administer atropine 2 hours after ketoconazole.
- **METOCLOPRAMIDE:** Atropine and its derivatives may antagonize the actions of metoclopramide.

Laboratory Considerations

- Chlordiazepoxide can cause interference with the Zimmerman reaction for **17-ketosteroids**, resulting in false results.
- It can also cause a false-positive result in the *Gravindex®* **pregnancy test**.

Doses

- **DOGS:**

  Chlordiazepoxide (alone) for behavior indications (*e.g.,* thunderstorm/noise phobias, etc.); (extra-label): 2.2 – 6.6 mg/kg PO as needed (start low). (Overall 2000)

  Chlordiazepoxide with clidinium or symptomatic treatment of irritable bowel syndrome (extra-label):

  a) Using the combination product (*e.g.,* *Librax®*), give 0.1 – 0.25 mg/kg of clidinium or 1-2 capsules PO 2-3 times a day. Owner may give when abdominal pain or diarrhea first noticed or if stressful conditions are encountered. Drug can usually be discontinued in a few days. (Leib 2004)

  b) Using the combination product (*e.g.,* *Librax®*), give 0.44 – 1.1 mg/kg of clidinium PO 2-3 times a day. Use at first signs of cramping or abdominal pain. Most dogs only require treatment for a day to 2 weeks. Some require long-term treatment at 1-2 doses per day. (Tams 2000)

- **CATS:**

  As an anxiolytic (extra-label): Chlordiazepoxide: 0.5 – 1 mg/kg PO q12–24h. (Virga 2002)

Monitoring

- Clinical efficacy.
- Adverse effects.

Client Information

- When using for thunderstorm phobias or other triggers (*e.g.,* owners separation anxiety, etc.) that upset your animal, try to give it about an hour before the event or trigger. Notify veterinarian if animal's behavior worsens.
- If you see yellowing of the whites of the eyes or the gums have a yellowish tint, contact your veterinarian immediately.
- Sleepiness is most common side effect, but sometimes the drug can change behavior or work opposite from what is expected.
- This drug may increase appetite, especially in cats.

Chemistry/Synonyms

A benzodiazepine, chlordiazepoxide HCl occurs as an odorless, white crystalline powder. It is soluble in water and alcohol, but is unstable in aqueous solutions.

A synthetic quaternary antimuscarinic agent similar to glycopyrrolate, clidinium bromide occurs as a white to nearly white, crystalline powder. It is soluble in alcohol and water.

Chlordiazepoxide HCl may also be known as: chlordiazepoxidi hydrochloridum, methamino-diazepoxide hydrochloride, NSC-115748, or Ro-5-0690; many trade names are available.

Storage/Stability

Chlordiazepoxide HCl capsules or tablets should be stored protected from light. The chlordiazepoxide HCl injection should be prepared immediately prior to use and any unused portions discarded. The diluent should be stored in the refrigerator before use.

Clidinium bromide with chlordiazepoxide capsules should be stored at room temperature in tight, light-resistant containers.

Compatibility/Compounding Considerations
No specific information noted.

Dosage Forms/Regulatory Status
VETERINARY-LABELED PRODUCTS: NONE.
The ARCI (Racing Commissioners International) has designated this drug as a class 2 substance. See the appendix for more information.

HUMAN-LABELED PRODUCTS:

Chlordiazepoxide HCl Oral Capsules: 5 mg, 10 mg & 25 mg; generic; (Rx, C-IV)

Chlordiazepoxide HCl 5 mg and Clidinium Br 2.5 mg Capsules; *Librax® Capsules*, generic; (Rx, C-IV)

Revisions/References
Monograph revised/updated October 2013.

Leib, M. (2004). *Chronic idiopathic large bowel diarrhea in dogs.* Proceedings: ACVIM Forum. accessed via Veterinary Information Network; vin.com

Overall, K. (2000). *Behavioral Pharmacology.* Proceedings: American Animal Hospital Association 67th Annual Meeting, Toronto. accessed via Veterinary Information Network; vin.com

Tams, T. (2000). *Diagnosis and Management of Large Intestinal Disorders in Dogs.* Proceedings: American Animal Hospital Association 67th Annual Meeting, Toronto. accessed via Veterinary Information Network; vin.com

Virga, V. (2002). *Which drug and why: An update on psychopharmacology.* Proceedings: Atlantic Coast Veterinary Conference. accessed via Veterinary Information Network; vin.com

Chlorothiazide
(klor-oh-thye-a-zide)   Diuril®

Thiazide Diuretic

Prescriber Highlights
▶ Thiazide diuretic used for nephrogenic diabetes insipidus; udder edema in dairy cattle (cattle product now discontinued in USA).
▶ Contraindications: Hypersensitivity; pregnancy (relative contraindication).
▶ Extreme caution/avoid: Severe renal disease, preexisting electrolyte/water balance abnormalities, impaired hepatic function, hyperuricemia, SLE, diabetes mellitus.
▶ Adverse Effects: Hypokalemia, hypochloremic alkalosis, other electrolyte imbalances, hyperuricemia, GI effects.
▶ Many drug-drug & laboratory test interactions.

Uses/Indications
In veterinary medicine, furosemide has largely supplanted the use of thiazides as a general diuretic (edema treatment). Thiazides are still used for the treatment of nephrogenic diabetes insipidus and to help prevent the recurrence of calcium oxalate uroliths in dogs.

Chlorothiazide was FDA-approved for use in dairy cattle for the treatment of post parturient udder edema, but the veterinary-labeled product has been discontinued in the USA.

Pharmacology/Actions
Thiazide diuretics act by interfering with the transport of sodium ions across renal tubular epithelium possibly by altering the metabolism of tubular cells. The principle site of action is at the cortical diluting segment of the nephron; enhanced excretion of sodium, chloride, and water results. Thiazides also increase the excretion of potassium, magnesium, phosphate, iodide, and bromide and decrease the glomerular filtration rate (GFR). Plasma renin and resulting aldosterone levels are increased which contributes to the hypokalemic effects of the thiazides. Bicarbonate excretion is increased, but effects on urine pH are usually minimal. Thiazides usually initially have a hypercalciuric effect but with continued therapy, calcium excretion is significantly decreased. But in dogs,

hydrochlorothiazide, but not chlorothiazide, has been shown to decrease urinary calcium excretion. Uric acid excretion is also decreased by the thiazides. Thiazides can cause, or exacerbate, hyperglycemia in diabetic patients, or induce diabetes mellitus in prediabetic patients.

The antihypertensive effects of thiazides are well known, and these agents are used extensively in human medicine for treating essential hypertension. The exact mechanism of this effect has not been established.

Thiazides paradoxically reduce urine output in patients with diabetes insipidus (DI). They have been used as adjunctive therapy in patients with neurogenic DI and are the only drug therapy for nephrogenic DI.

Pharmacokinetics
The pharmacokinetics of the thiazides have apparently not been studied in domestic animals. In humans, chlorothiazide is only 10-21% absorbed after oral administration. The onset of diuretic activity occurs in 1-2 hours and peaks at about 4 hours. The serum half-life is approximately 1-2 hours and the duration of activity is from 6-12 hours. Like all thiazides, the antihypertensive effects of chlorothiazide can take several days to transpire.

Thiazides are found in the milk of lactating humans. Because of the chance of idiosyncratic or hypersensitive reactions, it is recommended that these drugs not be used in lactating females or nursing mothers.

Contraindications/Precautions/Warnings
Thiazides are contraindicated in patients with anuria or that are hypersensitive to any one of these agents. Although many sources state that thiazides are contraindicated in patients that are hypersensitive to sulfonamides, clear evidence for cross-reactivity has not been established in humans or animals. They are also contraindicated in pregnant females who are otherwise healthy and have only mild edema; newborn human infants have developed thrombocytopenia when their mothers received thiazides.

Thiazides should be used with extreme caution, if at all, in patients with severe renal disease or with preexisting electrolyte or water balance abnormalities, impaired hepatic function (may precipitate hepatic coma), hyperuricemia, lupus (SLE); or diabetes mellitus. Patients with conditions that may lead to electrolyte or water balance abnormalities (*e.g.*, vomiting, diarrhea, etc.) should be monitored carefully.

Adverse Effects
Hypokalemia is one of the most common adverse effects associated with the thiazides but rarely causes clinical signs or progresses further; however, monitoring of potassium is recommended with chronic therapy.

Hypochloremic alkalosis (with hypokalemia) may develop, especially if there are other causes of potassium and chloride loss (*e.g.*, vomiting, diarrhea, potassium-losing nephropathies, etc.) or if the patient has cirrhotic liver disease. Dilutional hyponatremia and hypomagnesemia may also occur. Hyperparathyroid-like effects of hypercalcemia and hypophosphatemia have been reported in humans, but have not led to effects such as nephrolithiasis, bone resorption, or peptic ulceration.

Hyperuricemia can occur but is usually asymptomatic.

Other possible adverse effects include GI reactions (*e.g.*, vomiting, diarrhea, etc.), pancreatitis, hypersensitivity/dermatologic reactions, GU reactions (polyuria), hematologic toxicity, hyperglycemia, hyperlipidemias, and orthostatic hypotension.

Reproductive/Nursing Safety
In humans, the FDA categorizes this drug as category *B* for use during pregnancy (*Animal studies have not yet demonstrated risk*

to the fetus, but there are no adequate studies in pregnant women; or animal studies have shown an adverse effect, but adequate studies in pregnant women have not demonstrated a risk to the fetus in the first trimester of pregnancy, and there is no evidence of risk in later trimesters.)

Chlorothiazide enters maternal milk and can reduce milk volume and suppress lactation. Generally, either discontinuation of the drug or nursing is recommended in humans.

Overdosage

Acute overdosage may cause electrolyte and water balance problems, CNS effects (lethargy to coma and seizures), and GI effects (*e.g.*, hypermotility, GI distress, etc.). Transient increases in BUN have also been reported.

Treatment consists of emptying the gut after recent oral ingestion using standard protocols. Avoid giving concomitant cathartics as they may exacerbate the fluid and electrolyte imbalances that may ensue. Monitor and treat electrolyte and water balance abnormalities supportively. Additionally, monitor respiratory, CNS and cardiovascular status; treat supportively and symptomatically, if required.

Drug Interactions

The following drug interactions have either been reported or are theoretical in humans or animals receiving chlorothiazide and may be of significance in veterinary patients. Unless otherwise noted, use together is not necessarily contraindicated, but weigh the potential risks and perform additional monitoring when appropriate.

- **AMPHOTERICIN B:** Use with thiazides can lead to an increased risk for severe hypokalemia.
- **CORTICOSTEROIDS, CORTICOTROPIN:** Use with thiazides can lead to an increased risk for severe hypokalemia.
- **DIAZOXIDE:** Increased risk for hyperglycemia, hyperuricemia, and hypotension may occur.
- **DIGITALIS, DIGOXIN:** Thiazide-induced hypokalemia, hypomagnesemia, and/or hypercalcemia may increase the likelihood of digitalis toxicity.
- **INSULIN:** Thiazides may increase insulin requirements.
- **LITHIUM:** Thiazides can increase serum lithium concentrations.
- **METHENAMINE:** Thiazides can alkalinize urine and reduce methenamine effectiveness.
- **NSAIDS:** Thiazides may increase risk for renal toxicity and NSAIDs may reduce diuretic actions of thiazides.
- **NEUROMUSCULAR BLOCKING AGENTS:** Tubocurarine or other nondepolarizing neuromuscular blocking agents response or duration may be increased in patients taking thiazide diuretics.
- **PROBENECID:** Blocks thiazide-induced uric acid retention (used to therapeutic advantage).
- **QUINIDINE:** Half-life may be prolonged by thiazides (thiazides can alkalinize the urine).
- **VITAMIN D** or **CALCIUM SALTS:** Hypercalcemia may be exacerbated if thiazides are concurrently administered with Vitamin D or calcium salts.

Laboratory Considerations

- **AMYLASE:** Thiazides can increase serum amylase values in asymptomatic patients and those in the developmental stages of acute pancreatitis (humans).
- **CORTISOL:** Thiazides can decrease the renal excretion of cortisol.
- **ESTROGEN, URINARY:** Hydrochlorothiazide may falsely decrease total urinary estrogen when using a spectrophotometric assay.
- **HISTAMINE:** Thiazides may cause false-negative results when testing for pheochromocytoma.
- **PARATHYROID-FUNCTION TESTS:** Thiazides may elevate serum calcium; recommend discontinuing thiazides prior to testing.
- **PHENOLSULFONPHTHALEIN (PSP):** Thiazides can compete for secretion at proximal renal tubules.
- **PHENTOLAMINE TEST:** Thiazides may give false-negative results.
- **PROTEIN-BOUND IODINE:** Thiazides may decrease values.
- **TRIIODOTHYRONINE RESIN UPTAKE TEST:** Thiazides may slightly reduce uptake.
- **TYRAMINE:** Thiazides can cause false-negative results.

Doses

- **DOGS/CATS:**

    For treatment of nephrogenic diabetes insipidus or as a diuretic (extra-label): 20 – 40 mg/kg PO q12h.

Monitoring

- Serum electrolytes, BUN, creatinine, glucose.
- Hydration status.
- Blood pressure, if indicated.
- Hemograms, if indicated.

Client Information

- When beginning this medicine your animal may urinate more frequently than normal.
- May be given with or without food. Allow access to water at all times and encourage normal food intake.
- Because this drug can change electrolytes (salts) in the blood, your veterinarian will probably want to do more frequent testing.
- Contact your veterinarian immediately if excessive thirst, weakness or collapse, head tilt, lack of urination, or a racing heartbeat is noticed.

Chemistry/Synonyms

Chlorothiazide is a thiazide diuretic and occurs as a white to practically white, odorless, crystalline powder having a slightly bitter taste. It is very slightly soluble in water and slightly soluble in alcohol.

Chlorothiazide may also be known as: chlorothiazidum, clorotiazida, *Azide®*, *Diuril®*, or *Saluric®*.

Storage/Stability

Tablets should be stored at room temperature. The oral suspension should be protected from freezing. The injectable preparation is stable for 24 hours after reconstitution. If the pH of the reconstituted solution is less than 7.4, precipitation will occur in less than 24 hours.

Compatibility/Compounding Considerations

Chlorothiazide sodium for injection is reportedly **compatible** with the following IV solutions: dextrose and/or saline products for IV infusion (with the exception of many Ionosol and Normosol products), Ringer's injection and Lactated Ringer's, 1/6 M sodium lactate, Dextran 6% with dextrose or sodium chloride, and fructose 10%. It is also reportedly **compatible** with the following drugs: cimetidine HCl, lidocaine HCl, and sodium bicarbonate.

Chlorothiazide sodium is reportedly **incompatible** with the following drugs: amikacin sulfate, chlorpromazine HCl, codeine phosphate, hydralazine HCl, insulin (regular), morphine sulfate, norepinephrine bitartrate, procaine HCl, prochlorperazine edisylate and mesylate, promazine HCl, promethazine HCl, tetracycline HCl, and vancomycin HCl.

Dosage Forms/Regulatory Status

VETERINARY-LABELED PRODUCTS: NONE.

The ARCI (Racing Commissioners International) has designated this drug as a class 4 substance. See the appendix for more information.

HUMAN-LABELED PRODUCTS:

Chlorothiazide Tablets: 250 mg & 500 mg; generic; (Rx)

Chlorothiazide Oral Suspension: 50 mg/mL in 237 mL; *Diuril®*; (Rx)

Chlorothiazide Sodium Powder for Injection (lyophilized): 500 mg (0.25 g mannitol) in 20 mL vials; *Diuril®*; (Rx)

Revisions/References

Monograph revised/updated October 2013.

Chlorpheniramine Maleate

(klor-fen-ir-a-meen)   Chlor-Trimetron®

Antihistamine

Prescriber Highlights

▶ An alkylamine antihistamine used primarily for its antihistamine/antipruritic effects; occasionally used for CNS depressant (sedative) effects.

▶ Contraindications: Hypersensitivity. Caution: narrow angle glaucoma, hypertension, GI or urinary obstruction, hypertension, hyperthyroidism, cardiovascular disease.

▶ Adverse Effects: Sedation, anticholinergic effects, GI effects.

Uses/Indications

Chlorpheniramine is an orally administered, type-1 antihistamine. Antihistamines are used in veterinary medicine to reduce or help prevent histamine mediated adverse effects. In dogs with pruritic atopic dermatitis (AD), there is no conclusive evidence of efficacy of oral type-1 antihistamines for treatment of active AD and whether these drugs would be of benefit in dogs with mild AD or prevent the recurrence of flares has not been determined (Olivry et al. 2010). The response to chlorpheniramine, as with other antihistamines in dogs and cats, is individualized and not predictable. One patient may respond to one and not another. Potentially, better results could be obtained if chlorpheniramine is combined with hydroxyzine as this has been reported to be efficacious in reducing the clinical signs of canine atopic dermatitis in about 1 in 3 treated dogs (Ewert et al. 2001). In small animals, type-1 antihistamines are best given as preventative therapy and on a regular basis to keep the histamine receptors blocked before histamine is released. Because of its CNS depressant effects, chlorpheniramine may also be of benefit as a mild sedative in small animals.

Pharmacology/Actions

Antihistamines (H_1-receptor antagonists) competitively inhibit histamine at H_1 receptor sites. They do not inactivate or prevent the release of histamine, but can prevent histamine's action on the cell. Besides their antihistaminic activity, these agents all have varying degrees of anticholinergic and CNS activity (sedation).

Pharmacokinetics

Chlorpheniramine pharmacokinetics have not been described in domestic species. In humans, the drug is well absorbed after oral administration, but because of a relatively high degree of metabolism in the GI mucosa and the liver, only about 25-60% of the drug is available to the systemic circulation.

Chlorpheniramine is well distributed after IV injection; the highest distribution of the drug (in rabbits) occurs in the lungs, heart, kidneys, brain, small intestine, and spleen. In humans, the apparent steady-state volume of distribution is 2.5 – 3.2 L/kg and about 70% is bound to plasma proteins. It is unknown if chlorpheniramine is excreted into the milk.

Chlorpheniramine is metabolized in the liver and practically all the drug (as metabolites and unchanged drug) is excreted in the urine. In human patients with normal renal and hepatic function, the terminal serum half-life the drug ranges from 13.2-43 hours.

Contraindications/Precautions/Warnings

Chlorpheniramine is contraindicated in patients that are hypersensitive to it or other antihistamines in its class. Because of their anticholinergic activity, antihistamines should be used with caution in patients with angle closure glaucoma, prostatic hypertrophy, pyloroduodenal or bladder neck obstruction, and COPD if mucosal secretions are a problem. Additionally, they should be cautiously used in patients with hyperthyroidism, cardiovascular disease or hypertension.

Adverse Effects

Most commonly seen adverse effects are CNS depression (*e.g.,* lethargy, somnolence) and GI effects (*e.g.,* diarrhea, vomiting, anorexia, etc.). The sedative effects of antihistamines may diminish with time. Anticholinergic effects (*e.g.,* dry mouth, urinary retention, etc.) are a possibility.

The sedative effects of antihistamines may adversely affect the performance of working dogs.

Chlorpheniramine may cause paradoxical excitement in cats. Palatability of this drug is also an issue in felines.

Reproductive/Nursing Safety

In humans, the FDA categorizes this drug as category *B* for use during pregnancy (*Animal studies have not yet demonstrated risk to the fetus, but there are no adequate studies in pregnant women; or animal studies have shown an adverse effect, but adequate studies in pregnant women have not demonstrated a risk to the fetus in the first trimester of pregnancy, and there is no evidence of risk in later trimesters.*)

It is unknown if chlorpheniramine is excreted into milk; use with caution in dams nursing neonates.

Overdosage/Acute Toxicity

Overdosage may cause CNS stimulation (excitement to seizures) or depression (lethargy to coma), anticholinergic effects, respiratory depression, and death. A 9-month-old dachshund ingesting 25 mg/kg showed signs of ataxia, tremors, bradycardia, coma, & cardiac arrest and died within 11 hours of ingestion (Murphy 2001). Another source states not to use dosages greater than 1.1 mg/kg/day in dogs as sudden death has occurred (Bloom 2013).

Treatment consists of emptying the gut (if the ingestion was oral) using standard protocols. Induce emesis if the patient is alert and CNS status is stable. Administration of a saline cathartic and/or activated charcoal may be given after emesis or gastric lavage. Treatment of other clinical signs should be performed using symptomatic and supportive therapies. Phenytoin (IV) is recommended in the treatment of seizures caused by antihistamine overdoses in humans; barbiturates and diazepam should be avoided.

Drug Interactions

The following drug interactions have either been reported or are theoretical in humans or animals receiving chlorpheniramine and may be of significance in veterinary patients. Unless otherwise noted, use together is not necessarily contraindicated, but weigh the potential risks and perform additional monitoring when appropriate.

- ANTICOAGULANTS (*e.g.,* **heparin, warfarin**): Antihistamines may partially counteract the anticoagulation effects of heparin or warfarin.
- MAO INHIBITORS (including **amitraz**, and possibly **selegiline**): May prolong and exacerbate anticholinergic effects.
- OTHER CNS DEPRESSANT DRUGS: Increased sedation can occur.

Laboratory Considerations

- Antihistamines can decrease the wheal and flare response to **antigen skin testing**. In humans, it is suggested that antihistamines be discontinued at least 2 weeks before testing.

Doses

- **DOGS:**

  For the adjunctive treatment (prevention) of histamine-related pruritic conditions or as a mild sedative (extra-label): Most recommendations range from 0.2 – 0.5 (maximum) mg/kg PO q8-12h. Using commercially available oral tablets, this is usually rounded off to the nearest 2 mg with doses ranging from 2 – 8 mg per dog 2-3 times a day. If using sustained-release capsules, the capsule contents may be placed on food, but should not be allowed to dissolve before ingestion. Trial periods to determine an individual antihistamine's efficacy are usually 1-2 weeks long.

- **CATS:**

  For the adjunctive treatment (prevention) of histamine-related pruritic conditions or as a mild sedative (extra-label): Most recommended dosages from 1 – 4 mg per cat PO 2-3 times per day. Commonly dosed at 2 mg per cat twice daily. Some cats may be controlled with once daily dosing. Palatability/acceptance may be enhanced by dipping the split tablet into tuna fish "juice", butter or petrolatum, or by placing split tablets into empty gelatin capsules. If using sustained-release capsules, the capsule contents may be placed on food, but should not be allowed to dissolve before ingestion.

- **FERRETS:**

  For the adjunctive treatment (prevention) of histamine-related pruritic conditions or as a mild sedative (extra-label): 1 – 2 mg/kg PO 2–3 times a day. (Williams 2000)

- **BIRDS:**

  For the adjunctive treatment (prevention) of histamine-related pruritic conditions or as a mild sedative (extra-label): One 4 mg tablet in one cup (240 mL; 8 oz.) of bottled water to be used as drinking water; changed daily. (Clubb 2009)

Monitoring

- Clinical efficacy.
- Adverse effects.

Client Information

- Antihistamines should be used on a regular, ongoing basis in animals that respond to them. They work better if used before exposure to an allergen.
- Drowsiness/sleepiness can occur with this medication, but usually this will lessen with time. Cats sometimes become excited after getting it.
- If using a sustained-release product, do not split or crush the tablets. If using a long-acting capsule, you may empty the contents of the capsule over food, but do not allow the beads to dissolve before the pet eats the food.
- May be difficult to give to cats as it has a bitter taste.

Chemistry/Synonyms

A propylamine (alkylamine) antihistaminic agent, chlorpheniramine maleate occurs as an odorless, white, crystalline powder with a melting point between 130-135° C and a pK_a of 9.2. One gram is soluble in about 4 mL of water or 10 mL of alcohol.

Chlorpheniramine maleate may also be known as chlorphenamini maleas; many trade names are available; a commonly known brand is *Chlor-Trimeton®*.

Storage/Stability

Chlorpheniramine tablets and sustained-release tablets should be stored in tight containers. The sustained-release capsules should be stored in well-closed containers. The oral solution should be stored in light-resistant containers; avoid freezing. All chlorpheniramine products should be stored at room temperature (15-30°C).

Compatibility/Compounding Considerations

Timed-release forms of the drug should not be crushed or allowed to dissolve in liquids.

Dosage Forms/Regulatory Status

VETERINARY-LABELED PRODUCTS: NONE.

The ARCI (Racing Commissioners International) has designated this drug as a class 4 substance. See the appendix for more information.

HUMAN-LABELED PRODUCTS:

Chlorpheniramine Maleate Oral Tablets: 2 mg (chewable) & 4 mg tablets; (OTC)

Chlorpheniramine Maleate Extended-Release Tablets & Capsules: 8 mg, 12 mg & 16 mg; (Rx & OTC)

Chlorpheniramine Maleate Oral Syrup: 2 mg/5 mL in 118 mL; (OTC)

Oral Suspension: 4 mg/5 mL in 118 mL; (Rx)

Many combination products are available that combine chlorpheniramine with decongestants, analgesics, and/or antitussives, but these are generally inappropriate for use in animal patients.

Revisions/References

Monograph revised/updated October 2013.

Bloom, P. (2013). Nonsteroidal, Nonimmunosuppressive Therapies for Pruritus. *Veterinary Clinics of North America-Small Animal Practice* 43(1): 173-+.

Clubb, S. (2009). *Feather damaging behavior.* Proceedings; WVC. accessed via Veterinary Information Network; vin.com

Ewert, G. & T. Daems (2001). Treatment of canine atopic dermatitis by a fatty acid copolymer: comparative double blind study. *Pratique Medicale Et Chirurgicale De L Animal De Compagnie* 36(4): 401-8.

Murphy, L. (2001). Antihistamine Toxicosis. *Veterinary Medicine*(October 2001).

Olivry, T., et al. (2010). Treatment of canine atopic dermatitis: 2010 clinical practice guidelines from the International Task Force on Canine Atopic Dermatitis. *Veterinary Dermatology* 21(3): 233-48.

Williams, B. (2000). Therapeutics in Ferrets. *Vet Clin NA: Exotic Anim Pract* 3:1(Jan): 131-53.

Chlorpromazine HCl

(klor-proe-ma-zeen)   Thorazine®

Phenothiazine Sedative/Antiemetic

Prescriber Highlights

▶ Prototype phenothiazine used primarily as an antiemetic, may be particularly useful to treat motion sickness in cats.

▶ Generally contraindicated in horses.

▶ Negligible analgesic effects.

▶ Dosage may need to be reduced in debilitated/geriatric animals, those with hepatic or cardiac disease or when combined with other agents.

▶ Use with caution in dehydrated patients because phenothiazines can cause vasodilation & reduce perfusion; rehydrate before use.

▶ Inject diluted solution IV slowly; do not inject into arteries; do not inject IM in rabbits.

▶ May cause significant hypotension, cardiac rate abnormalities, hypo- or hyperthermia; may cause extrapyramidal effects at high doses in cats.

Uses/Indications

The clinical use of chlorpromazine as a neuroleptic agent has diminished, but the drug is still used for its antiemetic effects in small animals and occasionally as a preoperative medication and sedative/tranquilizer. Once the principle phenothiazine used in veterinary medicine, chlorpromazine has been largely supplanted by acepromazine.

In patients exhibiting severe anxiety, tachycardia, or hypertension secondary to a toxin/overdose of amphetamine-like ADD/ADHD medications, SSRI antidepressants, (or other agents that can cause "serotonin syndrome"), or the paradoxical CNS stimulation that can be seen with overdoses of human sleep aids (*e.g.*, zolpidem, *Ambien*®, *Lunesta*®, etc.), acepromazine or chlorpromazine can be useful (Lee 2013). As an antiemetic, chlorpromazine use is limited to normotensive or hypertensive patients as it can potentiate hypotension. It will inhibit apomorphine-induced emesis in the dog but not the cat. It will also inhibit the emetic effects of morphine in the dog. It does not inhibit emesis caused by copper sulfate, or digitalis glycosides.

Pharmacology/Actions

Chlorpromazine has similar pharmacologic activities as acepromazine, but is less potent and has a longer duration of action. For further information, refer to the acepromazine monograph.

Pharmacokinetics

Chlorpromazine is absorbed rapidly after oral administration, but undergoes extensive first pass metabolism in the liver. The drug is also well absorbed after IM injection, but onsets of action are slower than after IV administration.

Chlorpromazine is distributed throughout the body and brain concentrations are higher than those in plasma. Approximately 95% of chlorpromazine in plasma is bound to plasma proteins (primarily albumin).

The drug is extensively metabolized principally in the liver and kidneys, but little specific information is available regarding its excretion in dogs and cats.

Contraindications/Precautions/Warnings

Chlorpromazine causes severe muscle discomfort and swelling when injected IM into rabbits; use IV only in this species.

Animals may require lower dosages of general anesthetics following phenothiazines. Use cautiously and in smaller doses in animals with hepatic dysfunction, cardiac disease, or general debilitation.

Because of its hypotensive effects, phenothiazines are relatively contraindicated in patients with hypovolemia or shock, and those with tetanus or strychnine intoxication due to effects on the extrapyramidal system.

Intravenous injections must be diluted with saline to concentrations of no more than 1 mg/mL and administered slowly. Chlorpromazine has no analgesic effects; treat animals with appropriate analgesics to control pain.

Dogs with MDR1 (ABCB1) mutations may develop a more pronounced sedation that persists longer than normal with this agent. It may be prudent to reduce initial doses by 25% to determine the reaction of a patient identified or suspect of having this mutation.

Phenothiazines should be used very cautiously as restraining agents in aggressive dogs: it may make the animal more prone to startle and react to noises or other sensory inputs.

Adverse Effects

In addition to the possible effects listed in the acepromazine monograph (*e.g.*, hypotension, contradictory effects such as CNS stimulation, bradycardia), chlorpromazine may cause extrapyramidal signs cats when used at high dosages. These can include tremors, shivering, rigidity and loss of the righting reflexes. Lethargy, diarrhea, and loss of anal sphincter tone may also be seen.

Horses may develop an ataxic reaction with resultant excitation and violent consequences. These ataxic periods may cycle with periods of sedation. Because of this effect, chlorpromazine is rarely used in equine medicine today.

Reproductive/Nursing Safety

In humans, the FDA categorizes this drug as category *C* for use during pregnancy (*Animal studies have shown an adverse effect on the fetus, but there are no adequate studies in humans; or there are no animal reproduction studies and no adequate studies in humans.*)

Chlorpromazine is thought to be excreted into maternal milk and safety to nursing offspring cannot be assured.

Overdosage/Acute Toxicity

Most small overdoses cause only somnolence; larger overdoses can cause serious effects including coma, agitation/seizures, ECG changes/arrhythmias, hypotension and extrapyramidal effects. Contact an animal poison control center in the event of a suspected large overdose or if multiple drugs are involved.

Most overdoses can be handled by monitoring the patient and treating signs as they occur; massive oral overdoses should definitely be treated by emptying the gut if possible. Hypotension should not be treated with epinephrine; use either phenylephrine or norepinephrine (levarterenol). Seizures may be controlled with barbiturates or diazepam.

Drug Interactions

The following drug interactions have either been reported or are theoretical in humans or animals receiving chlorpromazine or other phenothiazines and may be of significance in veterinary patients. Unless otherwise noted, use together is not necessarily contraindicated, but weigh the potential risks and perform additional monitoring when appropriate.

- **ACETAMINOPHEN**: Possible increased risk for hypothermia.

- **ANTACIDS**: May cause reduced GI absorption of oral phenothiazines.

- **ANTIDIARRHEAL MIXTURES** (*e.g.*, **kaolin/pectin, bismuth subsalicylate mixtures**, etc.): May cause reduced GI absorption of oral phenothiazines.

- **CNS DEPRESSANT AGENTS** (*e.g.*, **barbiturates, narcotics, anesthetics**, etc.): May cause additive CNS depression if used with phenothiazines.

- **DIPYRONE**: May cause serious hypothermia.

- **EPINEPHRINE:** Phenothiazines block alpha-adrenergic receptors and concomitant epinephrine can lead to unopposed beta-activity causing vasodilation and increased cardiac rate.
- **OPIATES:** May enhance the hypotensive effects of the phenothiazines; dosages of chlorpromazine may need to be reduced when used with an opiate.
- **ORGANOPHOSPHATE AGENTS:** Phenothiazines should not be given within one month of worming with these agents as their effects may be potentiated.
- **PARAQUAT:** Toxicity may be increased by chlorpromazine.
- **PHENYTOIN:** Metabolism may be decreased if given concurrently with phenothiazines.
- **PHYSOSTIGMINE:** Toxicity may be enhanced by chlorpromazine.
- **PROCAINE:** Activity may be enhanced by phenothiazines.
- **PROPRANOLOL:** Increased blood levels of both drugs may result if administered with phenothiazines.
- **QUINIDINE:** With phenothiazines may cause additive cardiac depression.

Doses

- **DOGS/CATS:**

  As an antiemetic or sedative (extra-label): Most recommendations range from 0.2 – 0.5 mg/kg IM or SC q6-8h. Intravenous dosage recommendations can vary widely from 0.05 – 0.5 mg/kg (dogs); 0.025 – 0.5 mg/kg (cats) IV q6-8h. It is advised when giving the drug IV to start at the lower end of the dosage range and increase dosage as necessary (to effect) while monitoring blood pressure.

- **CATTLE:**

  Premedication for cattle undergoing standing procedures (extra-label): Up to 1 mg/kg IM (may cause regurgitation if animal undergoes general anesthesia). (Hall et al. 1983)

- **HORSES: (NOTE: ARCI UCGFS CLASS 2 DRUG)**

  Note: Because of side effects (*e.g.,* ataxia, panic reaction, etc.) this drug is not recommended for use in horses; use acepromazine or promazine if phenothiazine therapy is desired.

- **SWINE:**

  All are extra-label.
  a) Premedication: 1 mg/kg IM. (Hall et al. 1983)
  b) 0.55 – 3.3 mg/kg IV; 2 – 4 mg/kg IM.
  c) Restraint: 1.1 mg/kg IM (effects are at peak in 45-60 minutes); Prior to barbiturate anesthesia: 2 – 4 mg/kg IM. (Booth 1988)

- **SHEEP & GOATS:**

  All are extra-label.
  a) 0.55 – 4.4 mg/kg IV, 2.2 – 6.6 mg/kg IM. (Lumb et al. 1984)
  b) **Goats:** 2 – 3.5 mg/kg IV q5-6h. (Booth 1988)

Monitoring

- Cardiac rate/rhythm/blood pressure if indicated and possible to measure.
- Degree of tranquilization/anti-emetic activity if indicated.
- Body temperature (especially if ambient temperature is very hot or cold).

Client Information

- Avoid getting solutions on hands or clothing; contact dermatitis may develop.
- May discolor the urine to a pink or red-brown color; this is not abnormal.

Chemistry/Synonyms

A propylamino-phenothiazine derivative, chlorpromazine is the prototypic phenothiazine agent. It occurs as a white to slightly creamy white, odorless, bitter tasting, crystalline powder. One g is soluble in 1 mL of water and 1.5 mL of alcohol. The commercially available injection is a solution of chlorpromazine HCl in sterile water at a pH of 3-5.

Chlorpromazine HCl may also be known as aminazine, or chlorpromazini hydrochloridum; many trade names are available.

Storage/Stability

Protect from light and store at room temperature; avoid freezing the oral solution and injection. Dispense oral solution in amber bottles. Store oral tablets in tight containers. Do not store in plastic syringes or IV bags for prolonged periods as the drug may adsorb to plastic.

Chlorpromazine will darken upon prolonged exposure to light; do not use solutions that are darkly colored or if precipitates have formed. A slight yellowish color will not affect potency or efficacy.

Compatibility/Compounding Considerations

Alkaline solutions will cause the drug to oxidize.

The following products have been reported to be **compatible** when mixed with chlorpromazine HCl injection: all usual intravenous fluids, ascorbic acid, atropine sulfate, butorphanol tartrate, diphenhydramine, fentanyl citrate, glycopyrrolate, heparin sodium, hydromorphone HCl, hydroxyzine HCl, lidocaine HCl, meperidine, metoclopramide, metaraminol bitartrate, morphine sulfate, pentazocine lactate, promazine HCl, promethazine, scopolamine HBr, and tetracycline HCl.

The following products have been reported as being **incompatible** when mixed with chlorpromazine: aminophylline, amphotericin B, chloramphenicol sodium succinate, chlorothiazide sodium, dimenhydrinate, methohexital sodium, penicillin g potassium, pentobarbital sodium, phenobarbital sodium, and thiopental sodium. Compatibility is dependent upon factors such as pH, concentration, temperature, and diluent used; consult specialized references or a hospital pharmacist for more specific information.

Dosage Forms/Regulatory Status

VETERINARY-LABELED PRODUCTS: NONE.

The ARCI (Racing Commissioners International) has designated this drug as a class 2 substance. See the appendix for more information.

HUMAN-LABELED PRODUCTS:

Chlorpromazine Oral Tablets: 10 mg, 25 mg, 50 mg, 100 mg & 200 mg; generic; (Rx)

Chlorpromazine Injection: 25 mg/mL in 1 & 2 mL amps; generic; (Rx)

Revisions/References

Monograph revised/updated October 2013.

Booth, N. H. (1988). Drugs Acting on the Central Nervous System. *Veterinary Pharmacology and Therapeutics - 6th Ed.* N. H. Booth and L. E. McDonald. Ames, Iowa State University Press: 153-408.

Hall, L. W. & K. W. Clarke (1983). *Veterinary Anesthesia 8th Ed.*, Bailliere Tindall. London.

Lee, J. A. (2013). Emergency Management and Treatment of the Poisoned Small Animal Patient. *Veterinary Clinics of North America: Small Animal Practice* 43(4): 757-71.

Lumb, W. V. & E. W. Jones (1984). *Veterinary Anesthesia, 2nd Ed.*, Lea & Febiger. Philadelphia.

Chlorpropamide

(klor-**proe**-pa-mide)   Diabenese®

Sulfonylurea Antidiabetic

Prescriber Highlights

▶ Oral sulfonylurea antidiabetic agent sometimes used in dogs or cats for diabetes insipidus; potentially for diabetes mellitus. Not commonly used in veterinary medicine.

▶ Many contraindications/cautions.

▶ Most likely adverse effects are hypoglycemia or GI distress.

Uses/Indications

While chlorpropamide could potentially be of benefit in the adjunctive treatment of diabetes mellitus in small animals, its use has been primarily for adjunctive therapy in diabetes insipidus in dogs and cats.

Pharmacology/Actions

Sulfonylureas lower blood glucose concentrations in both diabetic and non-diabetic patients. The exact mechanism of action is not known, but these agents are thought to exert the effect primarily by stimulating the beta cells in the pancreas to secrete additional endogenous insulin. Ongoing use of the sulfonylureas appears to enhance peripheral sensitivity to insulin and reduce the production of hepatic basal glucose. The mechanisms causing these effects are yet to be fully explained. Chlorpropamide has antidiuretic activity, presumably by potentiating vasopressin's effects on the renal tubules. It may also stimulate secretion of vasopressin.

Pharmacokinetics

Chlorpropamide is absorbed well from the GI tract. Its distribution characteristics have not been well described, but it is highly bound to plasma proteins and is excreted into milk. Elimination half-lives have not been described in domestic animals, but in humans the elimination half-life is about 36 hours. The drug is both metabolized in the liver and excreted unchanged. Elimination of chlorpropamide is enhanced in alkaline urine; decreased in acidic urine.

Contraindications/Precautions/Warnings

Oral antidiabetic agents are considered contraindicated with the following conditions: severe burns, severe trauma, severe infection, diabetic coma or other hypoglycemic conditions, major surgery, ketosis, ketoacidosis, or other significant acidotic conditions. Chlorpropamide should only be used when its potential benefits outweigh its risks during untreated adrenal or pituitary insufficiency, thyroid, cardiac, renal or hepatic function impairment, prolonged vomiting, high fever, malnourishment or debilitated condition, or when fluid retention is present.

Adverse Effects

Hypoglycemia and GI disturbances are the most common adverse effects noted with this agent. Syndrome of inappropriate antidiuretic hormone (SIADH), anorexia, diarrhea, hepatotoxicity, skin eruptions, lassitude or other CNS effects, and hematologic toxicity are all potentially possible.

Reproductive/Nursing Safety

Safe use during pregnancy has not been established. In humans, the FDA categorizes this drug as category *C* for use during pregnancy (*Animal studies have shown an adverse effect on the fetus, but there are no adequate studies in humans; or there are no animal reproduction studies and no adequate studies in humans.*)

Chlorpropamide enters maternal milk; in humans it is not recommended for use during nursing.

Overdosage/Acute Toxicity

Profound hypoglycemia is the greatest concern after an overdose. Gut emptying protocols should be employed when warranted. Because of its long half-life, blood glucose monitoring and treatment with parenteral glucose may be required for several days. Overdoses may require additional monitoring (blood gases, serum electrolytes) and supportive therapy.

Drug Interactions

The following drug interactions have either been reported or are theoretical in humans or animals receiving chlorpropamide and may be of significance in veterinary patients. Unless otherwise noted, use together is not necessarily contraindicated, but weigh the potential risks and perform additional monitoring when appropriate.

- **ALCOHOL:** A disulfiram-like reaction (*e.g.,* anorexia, nausea, vomiting, etc.) has been reported in humans who have ingested alcohol within 48-72 hours of receiving chlorpropamide.

- **BARBITURATES:** Barbiturate duration of action may be prolonged.

The following drugs may potentiate hypoglycemia if administered with chlorpropamide, or be displaced by chlorpropamide from plasma proteins thereby causing enhanced pharmacologic effects of the two drugs involved:

- **CHLORAMPHENICOL**
- **BETA-BLOCKERS**
- **MAOI'S** (including **amitraz** and possibly, **selegiline**)
- **NSAIDS**
- **PROBENECID**
- **SALICYLATES**
- **SULFONAMIDES**
- **WARFARIN**

The following drugs may potentiate hyperglycemia if administered with chlorpropamide:

- **CALCIUM CHANNEL BLOCKERS** (*e.g.,* **diltiazem, amlodipine,** etc.)
- **CORTICOSTEROIDS**
- **ESTROGENS**
- **ISONIAZID**
- **PHENOTHIAZINES**
- **PHENYTOIN**
- **THIAZIDES**
- **THYROID MEDICATIONS**

Laboratory Considerations

- Chlorpropamide may mildly increase values of **liver enzymes, BUN,** or **serum creatinine.**

Doses

- **DOGS & CATS:**

  For adjunctive treatment of diabetes insipidus in animals with partial ADH deficiency (extra-label): 10 – 40 mg/kg PO once daily (or dose divided twice daily). Using the commercially available tablets (100 mg or 250 mg), it is practically dosed at 50 mg per cat (1/2 of a 100 mg tablet) or 50 – 250 mg (in 50 mg increments) per dog PO once daily. Beneficial effects may be seen in less than 50% of animals treated. A trial period of at least one week of therapy should be given before assessing effect.

Monitoring

- Serum electrolytes, plasma and urine osmolarity, urine output; if used for DI.

- Blood Glucose.

Client Information

- Usually given once a day with or without food. If stomach upset occurs, giving half the dose twice a day with food may be suggested by your veterinarian.
- May take up to a week to see if it is working.
- Low blood sugar or GI disturbances are the most common side effects.

Chemistry/Synonyms

An oral sulfonylurea antidiabetic agent, chlorpropamide occurs as a white, crystalline powder having a slight odor. It is practically insoluble in water.

Chlorpropamide may also be known as: chlorpropamidum, or *Diabenese®*.

Storage/Stability

Chlorpropamide tablets should be stored in well-closed containers at room temperature.

Compatibility/Compounding Considerations

No specific information noted.

Dosage Forms/Regulatory Status

VETERINARY-LABELED PRODUCTS: NONE.

HUMAN-LABELED PRODUCTS:

Chlorpropamide Oral Tablets: 100 mg & 250 mg; generic; (Rx)

Revisions/References

Monograph revised/updated October 2013.

Chlortetracycline

(klor-te-tra-sye-kleen)   Aureomycin®

Tetracycline Antibiotic

Prescriber Highlights

▶ Tetracycline antibiotic used primarily in water or feed treatments or topically for ophthalmic use.

▶ Many bacteria are now resistant; may still be very useful to treat mycoplasma, rickettsia, spirochetes, & Chlamydia.

▶ Contraindications: Hypersensitivity. Extreme caution: Pregnancy. Caution: liver, renal insufficiency.

▶ Adverse Effects: GI distress, staining of developing teeth & bones, superinfections, photosensitivity.

▶ Drug-drug; drug-lab interactions.

Uses/Indications

There are a variety of FDA-approved chlortetracycline products for use in food animals. It may also be useful in treating susceptible infections in dogs, cats, birds and small mammals (not Guinea pigs). For more information, refer to the Doses section below.

Pharmacology/Actions

Tetracyclines generally act as bacteriostatic antibiotics inhibiting protein synthesis by reversibly binding to 30S ribosomal subunits of susceptible organisms thereby preventing binding to those ribosomes of aminoacyl transfer-RNA. Tetracyclines are believed to reversibly bind to 50S ribosomes and additionally alter cytoplasmic membrane permeability in susceptible organisms. In high concentrations, tetracyclines can inhibit protein synthesis by mammalian cells.

As a class, the tetracyclines have activity against most mycoplasma, spirochetes (including the Lyme disease organism), Chlamydia, and Rickettsia. Against gram-positive bacteria, the tetracyclines have activity against some strains of staphylococcus and streptococci, but resistance of these organisms is increasing. Gram-positive bacteria that are usually covered by tetracyclines include: *Actinomyces* spp., *Bacillus anthracis*, *Clostridium perfringens* and *tetani*, *Listeria monocytogenes*, and Nocardia. Among gram-negative bacteria that tetracyclines usually have *in vitro* and *in vivo* activity include *Bordetella* spp., *Brucella*, Bartonella, *Haemophilus* spp., *Pasteurella multocida*, Shigella, and *Yersinia pestis*. Many or most strains of *E. coli*, Klebsiella, Bacteroides, Enterobacter, Proteus and *Pseudomonas aeruginosa* are resistant to the tetracyclines. While most strains of *Pseudomonas aeruginosa* show *in vitro* resistance to tetracyclines, those compounds attaining high urine levels (*e.g.*, tetracycline, oxytetracycline) have been associated with clinical cures in dogs with UTI secondary to this organism.

Oxytetracycline, chlortetracycline, and tetracycline share nearly identical spectrums of activity and patterns of cross-resistance and a tetracycline susceptibility disk is usually used for *in vitro* testing for chlortetracycline susceptibility.

Pharmacokinetics

Refer to the oxytetracycline monograph for general information on the pharmacokinetics of tetracyclines.

Contraindications/Precautions/Warnings

Chlortetracycline is contraindicated in patients hypersensitive to it or other tetracyclines. Because tetracyclines can retard fetal skeletal development and discolor deciduous teeth, they should only be used in the last half of pregnancy when the benefits outweigh the fetal risks. Oxytetracycline, chlortetracycline and tetracycline are considered more likely to cause these abnormalities than either doxycycline or minocycline.

In patients with renal insufficiency or hepatic impairment, chlortetracycline must be used cautiously. Lower than normal dosages are recommended with enhanced monitoring of renal and hepatic function. Avoid concurrent administration of other nephrotoxic or hepatotoxic drugs.

Because it may cause clostridial enterotoxemia in guinea pigs, chlortetracycline should not be used this species.

Adverse Effects

Chlortetracycline given to young animals can cause discoloration of bones and teeth to a yellow, brown, or gray color. High dosages or chronic administration may delay bone growth and healing.

Tetracyclines in high levels can exert an antianabolic effect that can cause an increase in BUN and/or hepatotoxicity, particularly in patients with preexisting renal dysfunction. As renal function deteriorates secondary to drug accumulation, this effect may be exacerbated.

In ruminants, high oral doses can cause ruminal microflora depression and ruminoreticular stasis. Rapid intravenous injection of undiluted propylene glycol-based products can cause intravascular hemolysis with resultant hemoglobinuria. Propylene glycol based products have also caused cardiodepressant effects when administered to calves.

In small animals, tetracyclines can cause nausea, vomiting, anorexia, and diarrhea. Cats do not tolerate oral tetracycline or oxytetracycline very well; signs of colic, fever, hair loss, and depression may be seen. There are reports that long-term tetracycline use may cause urolith formation in dogs.

Horses that are stressed by surgery, anesthesia, trauma, etc., may break with severe diarrheas after receiving tetracyclines (especially with oral administration).

Tetracycline therapy (especially long-term) may result in overgrowth (superinfections) of non-susceptible bacteria or fungi.

Tetracyclines have been associated with photosensitivity reactions and, rarely, hepatotoxicity or blood dyscrasias.

Reproductive/Nursing Safety

In humans, the FDA categorizes this drug as category *D* (tetracyclines-general) for use during pregnancy (*There is evidence of hu-*

man fetal risk, but the potential benefits from the use of the drug in pregnant women may be acceptable despite its potential risks.)

Tetracyclines are excreted in milk, but because much of the drug will be bound to calcium in milk, it is unlikely to be of significant risk to nursing animals.

Overdosage/Acute Toxicity

Tetracyclines are generally well tolerated after acute overdoses. Dogs given more than 400 mg/kg/day orally or 100 mg/kg/day IM of oxytetracycline did not demonstrate any toxicity. Oral overdoses would most likely be associated with GI disturbances (vomiting, anorexia, and/or diarrhea). Should the patient develop severe emesis or diarrhea, fluids and electrolytes should be monitored and replaced if necessary. Chronic overdoses may lead to drug accumulation and nephrotoxicity.

High oral doses given to ruminants, can cause ruminal microflora depression and ruminoreticular stasis. Rapid intravenous injection of undiluted propylene glycol-based products can cause intravascular hemolysis with resultant hemoglobinuria.

Rapid intravenous injection of tetracyclines has induced transient collapse and cardiac arrhythmias in several species, presumably due to chelation with intravascular calcium ions. Overdose quantities of drug could exacerbate this effect if given too rapidly IV. If the drug must be given rapidly IV (less than 5 minutes), some clinicians recommend pre-treating the animal with intravenous calcium gluconate.

Drug Interactions

The following drug interactions have either been reported or are theoretical in humans or animals receiving chlortetracycline and may be of significance in veterinary patients. Unless otherwise noted, use together is not necessarily contraindicated, but weigh the potential risks and perform additional monitoring when appropriate.

- **BETA-LACTAM OR AMINOGLYCOSIDE ANTIBIOTICS:** Bacteriostatic drugs, like the tetracyclines, may interfere with bactericidal activity of the penicillins, cephalosporins, and aminoglycosides; there is some controversy regarding the actual clinical significance of this interaction, however.
- **DIGOXIN:** Tetracyclines may increase the bioavailability of digoxin in a small percentage of patients (human) and lead to digoxin toxicity. These effects may persist for months after discontinuation of the tetracycline.
- **DIVALENT OR TRIVALENT CATIONS (oral antacids, saline cathartics** or other **GI products containing aluminum, calcium, iron, magnesium, zinc,** or **bismuth cations**): When orally administered, tetracyclines can chelate divalent or trivalent cations that can decrease the absorption of the tetracycline or the other drug if it contains these cations; it is recommended that all oral tetracyclines be given at least 1-2 hours before or after the cation-containing products.
- **WARFARIN:** Tetracyclines may depress plasma prothrombin activity and patients on anticoagulant (*e.g.,* warfarin) therapy may need dosage adjustment.

Laboratory Considerations

- Tetracyclines (not minocycline) may cause falsely elevated values of **urine catecholamines** when using fluorometric methods of determination.
- Tetracyclines reportedly can cause false-positive **urine glucose** results if using the cupric sulfate method of determination (Benedict's reagent, *Clinitest®*), but this may be the result of ascorbic acid that is found in some parenteral formulations of tetracyclines. Tetracyclines have also reportedly caused false-negative results in determining urine glucose when using the glucose oxidase method (*Clinistix®, Tes-Tape®*).

Doses

- **CATS:**

  To prevent recurrence of mycoplasma or chlamydial conjunctivitis in large catteries where topical therapy is impractical (extra-label): Soluble chlortetracycline powder in food at a dose of 50 mg per day per cat for 1 month. (Carro 1994)

- **RABBITS/RODENTS/SMALL MAMMALS:**

  Note: Not recommended for use in guinea pigs. All dosages are extra-label.

  a) **Rabbits:** 50 mg/kg PO q12-24h. (Ivey et al. 2000)

  b) **Chinchillas:** 50 mg/kg PO q12h. (Hayes 2000)

  c) **Hamsters:** 20 mg/kg IM or SC q12h; **Mice:** 25 mg/kg SC or IM q12h; **Rats:** 6 – 10 mg/kg SC or IM q12h. (Adamcak et al. 2000)

- **BIRDS:**

  All dosages are extra-label. Refer to actual product labels for FDA- approved dosing rates in poultry and withdrawal times.

  a) **For the treatment of chlamydiosis:** In small birds add chlortetracycline to food in a concentration of 0.05%; larger psittacines require 1% CTC. (Flammer 1992)

  b) **Pigeons:** 50 mg/kg PO q6-8h; or 1000 – 1500 mg/gallon drinking water; in warm weather mix fresh every 12 hours. Best used in combination with tylosin for ornithosis complex; calcium inhibits absorption therefore grit and layer pellets should be withheld during treatment. (Harlin 2006)

Monitoring

- Adverse effects.
- Clinical efficacy.
- Long-term use or in susceptible patients: periodic renal, hepatic, hematologic evaluations.

Client Information

- Avoid giving this drug orally within 1–2 hours of feeding, milk, or other dairy products.
- If used in food animals, follow labeled doses and withdrawal times.

Chemistry/Synonyms

A tetracycline antibiotic, chlortetracycline occurs as yellow, odorless crystals. It is slightly soluble in water.

Chlortetracycline may also be known as clortetraciclina, A-377, NRRL-2209, SF-66, *Aureomycin®* is a common trade name.

Storage/Stability

Chlortetracycline should be stored in tight containers and protected from light.

Compatibility/Compounding Considerations

No specific information noted.

Dosage Forms/Regulatory Status

VETERINARY-LABELED PRODUCTS:

There are several feed additive/water mix preparations available containing chlortetracycline. There are also combination products containing chlortetracycline and sulfamethazine (*Aureomycin Sulmet®, Aureo S 700®*), chlortetracycline, sulfamethazine and penicillin (*Aureomix 500®, Pennclor SP 250®* & *500®*), chlortetracycline, sulfathiazole, and penicillin (*Aureozol 500®*)

See individual labels for more information. Chlortetracycline-containing product labels may be found at dailymed.nlm.nih.gov

HUMAN-LABELED PRODUCTS: NONE.

Revisions/References

Monograph revised/updated October 2013.

Adamcak, A. & B. Otten (2000). Rodent Therapeutics. *Vet Clin NA: Exotic Anim Pract* 3:1(Jan): 221-40.

Carro, T. (1994). L-forms and mycoplasmal infections. *Consultations in Feline Internal Medicine: 2.* J. August. Philadelphia, W.B. Saunders Company: 13-20.

Flammer, K. (1992). An update on the diagnosis and treatment of avian chlamydiosis. *Current Veterinary Therapy XI: Small Animal Practice.* R. Kirk and J. Bonagura. Philadelphia, W.B. Saunders Company: 1150-3.

Harlin, R. (2006). *Practical pigeon medicine.* Proceedings: AAV 2006. accessed via Veterinary Information Network; vin.com

Hayes, P. (2000). Diseases of Chinchillas. *Kirk's Current Veterinary Therapy: XIII Small Animal Practice.* J. Bonagura. Philadelphia, WB Saunders: 1152-7.

Ivey, E. & J. Morrisey (2000). Therapeutics for Rabbits. *Vet Clin NA: Exotic Anim Pract* 3:1(Jan): 183-216.

Chondroitin Sulfate – See Glucosamine/Chondroitin

Chorionic Gonadotropin (HCG)

(kor-ee-on-ic goe-nad-oh-troe-pin)   Chorulon®

Reproductive Hormone

Prescriber Highlights

▶ Human hormone that mimics luteinizing hormone & some FSH activity; used for a variety of theriogenology conditions in many species.

▶ Only administered parenterally.

▶ Contraindications: Androgen responsive neoplasias, hypersensitivity.

▶ Adverse Effects: Antibodies/hypersensitivity, pain on injection.

Uses/Indications

The veterinary product's labeled indication is for "parenteral use in cows for the treatment of nymphomania (frequent or constant heat) due to cystic ovaries." It has been used for other purposes in several species; refer to the Dosage section for more information.

Pharmacology/Actions

HCG mimics quite closely the effects of luteinizing hormone (LH) but also has some FSH-like activity. In males, HCG can stimulate the differentiation of, and androgen production by, testicular interstitial (Leydig) cells. It may also stimulate testicular descent when no anatomical abnormality is present.

In females, HCG will stimulate the corpus luteum to produce progesterone and can induce ovulation (possibly also in patients with cystic ovaries). In the bitch HCG will induce estrogen secretion.

Pharmacokinetics

HCG is destroyed in the GI tract after oral administration, so it must be given parenterally. After IM injection, peak plasma levels occur in about 6 hours.

HCG is distributed primarily to the ovaries in females and to the testes in males, but some may also be distributed to the proximal tubules in the renal cortex.

HCG is eliminated from the blood in biphasic manner. The initial elimination half-life is about 11 hours and the terminal half-life is approximately 23 hours.

Contraindications/Precautions/Warnings

In humans, HCG is contraindicated in patients with prostatic carcinoma or other androgen-dependent neoplasias, precocious puberty or having a previous hypersensitivity reaction to HCG. No labeled contraindications for veterinary patients were noted, but the above human contraindications should be used as guidelines.

Antibody production to this hormone has been reported after repetitive use, resulting in diminished effect.

Adverse Effects

Potentially, hypersensitivity reactions are possible with this agent. HCG may cause abortion in mares prior to the 35th day of pregnancy possibly due to increased estrogen levels.

Problems associated with using the combined equine and human chorionic gonadotrophin product labeled for swine (*PG600®*) in dogs for estrus induction, include unpredictability of response, potential for allergic reactions and premature luteal failure (Kustritz 2012).

In humans, HCG has caused pain at the injection site, gynecomastia, headache, depression, irritability, and edema.

Reproductive/Nursing Safety

In humans, the FDA categorizes this drug as category *X* for use during pregnancy (*Studies in animals or humans demonstrate fetal abnormalities or adverse reaction; reports indicate evidence of fetal risk. The risk of use in pregnant women clearly outweighs any possible benefit.*)

It is unknown if HCG enters maternal milk.

Overdosage/Acute Toxicity

No overdosage cases have been reported with HCG.

Drug/Lab Interactions

No interactions have apparently been reported with HCG.

Doses

■ **DOGS:**

For treatment of cryptorchidism or increase libido in male dogs (extra-label): 25 – 500 Units IM two times per week for 4-6 weeks.

For HCG Challenge test to determine if testicular tissue remains in castrated male dogs (extra-label): **Note:** Contact your laboratory for specific recommendations for testing. Various protocols exist including: Take sample for resting testosterone level. Administer 44 micrograms/kg HCG IM and take a 4-hour post sample.

To produce luteinization of a persistent follicular cyst (extra-label): 500 – 1000 Units IM; repeat in 48 hours or once daily for 3 days.

■ **CATS:**

For HCG Challenge test (to determine if testicular tissue remains in castrated male cats) (extra-label): **Note:** Contact your laboratory for specific recommendations for testing. Various protocols exist including: Take baseline serum testosterone sample, administer 250 Units IM; take second sample 4-hours later.

For infertility, reduced libido, testis descent in male cats (extra-label): 50 – 100 Units repeated if necessary. (Verstegen 2000)

■ **BIRDS:**

To reduce feather plucking (especially in female birds); (extra-label): Dosage is empirical; 500 – 1,000 Units/kg IM. If no response in 3 days, repeat. If no response after second injection, unlikely to be of benefit at any dose. If reduces feather plucking, will need to repeat after 4-6 weeks. Major drawback is that with repeated usage, time between treatments is reduced. (Lightfoot 2001)

■ **CATTLE:**

For treatment of ovarian cysts (labeled dose): The reconstituted contents of one vial (10,000 Units; 10 mL) should be administered as a single deep intramuscular injection. Dosage may be repeated in 14 days if the animal's behavior or rectal examination of the ovaries indicates the necessity for retreatment. (Adapted from package insert; *Chorlulon®*)

■ **SWINE:**

For induction of fertile estrus (heat) in healthy prepuberal (non-cycling) gilts over five and one-half months of age and weighing at least 85 kg (187 lb.) or in healthy sows at weaning experiencing delayed return to estrus (labeled dose): One dose (5 mL) of reconstituted *P.G. 600®* injected into the gilt or sow's neck behind the ear. Prepuberal gilts should be injected when they are selected for addition to the breeding herd. Sows should be injected at weaning during periods of delayed return to estrus. (adapted from label; *P.G. 600®*)

Chemistry/Synonyms

A gonad-stimulating polypeptide secreted by the placenta, chorionic gonadotropin is obtained from the urine of pregnant women. It occurs as a white or practically white, amorphous, lyophilized powder. It is soluble in water and practically insoluble in alcohol. One International Unit (called Units in this reference) of HCG is equal to one USP unit. There are at least 1500 USP Units per mg.

Chorionic gonadotropin may also be known as: human chorionic gonadotropin, HCG, hCG, LH 500, CG, chorionic gonadotrophin, dynatropin, gonadotropine chorionique, gonadotrophinum chorionicum, choriogonadotrophin, chorionogonadotropin, pregnancy-urine hormone, or PU; there are many trade names internationally.

Storage/Stability

Chorionic gonadotropin powder for injection should be stored at room temperature (15-30°C) and protected from light. After reconstitution, the resultant solution is stable for 30-90 days (depending on the product) when stored at 2-15°C. The labels for the veterinary products, *Chorulon®* and *P.G. 600®* state to use the vial immediately after reconstituting with the supplied diluent.

Compatibility/Compounding Considerations

No specific information noted.

Dosage Forms/Regulatory Status

VETERINARY-LABELED PRODUCTS:

Chorionic Gonadotropin (HCG) Injection: 10,000 Units per 10 mL double vial packs containing 10,000 USP Units per vial with bacteriostatic water for injection; single dose 10 mL vials of freeze-dried powder and five 10 mL vials of sterile diluent; *Chorulon®*; (Rx). FDA-approved for use in cows and finfish. No withdrawal time is required when used as labeled.

Chorionic Gonadotropin freeze-dried powder: Single dose 5 mL vials when reconstituted contains pregnant mare serum gonadotropin (equine chorionic gonadotrophin, eCG, PMSG) 400 Units and human chorionic gonadotropin (hCG) 200 Units; five dose 25 mL vials that when reconstituted contains pregnant mare serum gonadotropin (PMSG) 2,000 Units and human chorionic gonadotropin (hCG) 1,000 Units; *P.G. 600®* ; (OTC). FDA-approved for use in swine (prepuberal gilts and sows at weaning); no meat withdrawal time is required when used as labeled.

HUMAN-LABELED PRODUCTS:

Chorionic Gonadotropin (Human) Powder for Injection: 5,000 Units/vial with 10 mL diluent (to make 500 Units/mL); 10,000 Units/vial with 10 mL diluent (to make 1,000 Units/mL); 20,000 Units/vial with 10 mL diluent (to make 2,000 Units/mL) in 10 mL vials; *Novarel®*, *Pregnyl®*, generic; (Rx)

Revisions/References

Monograph revised/updated October 2013.

Kustritz, M. V. R. (2012). Managing the Reproductive Cycle in the Bitch. *Veterinary Clinics of North America-Small Animal Practice* **42**(3): 423-37.

Lightfoot, T. (2001). *Feather "Plucking"*. Proceedings: Atlantic Coast Veterinary Conference. accessed via Veterinary Information Network; vin.com

Verstegen, J. (2000). Feline Reproduction. *Textbook of Veterinary Internal Medicine: Diseases of the Dog and Cat*. S. Ettinger and E. Feldman. Philadelphia, WB Saunders. 2: 1585-98.

Chromium / Chromium Picolinate

(kroe-mee-um pik-oh-lin-ate)

Transition Trace Metal

Prescriber Highlights

▶ Trace metal "nutraceutical" that may be useful as an adjunctive treatment for diabetes mellitus & obesity in cats.

▶ Efficacy in question, but probably safe.

Uses/Indications

Chromium supplementation may be useful in the adjunctive treatment of diabetes mellitus or obesity, particularly in cats; there is controversy whether this treatment is beneficial. It does not appear to be useful in dogs with diabetes mellitus.

Pharmacology/Actions

Metallic chromium has no pharmacologic activity, but other valence states have activity. Chromium VI (hexavalent form) is used in the welding and chemical industries and is considered a carcinogen. Chromium III (trivalent) is the form used in supplements and found naturally in foods. Chromium is thought to play a role in insulin function. It is an active component of so-called glucose tolerance factor (GTF). GTF is a complex of molecules that includes glycine, glutamic acid, cysteine and nicotinic acid. Chromium's exact role in carbohydrate and nitrogen metabolism is not clear. It does not lower blood glucose levels in normal patients. In humans, chromium deficiency can cause impaired tolerance to glucose and insulin function, increased serum cholesterol and triglyceride levels, neuropathy, weight loss, impaired nitrogen metabolism, and decreased respiratory function.

Pharmacokinetics

Chromium is not absorbed very well from the GI tract and most of a dose is excreted in the feces. When given as a salt (picolinate, chloride, nicotinate), lipophilicity and solubility are increased and absorption is enhanced. Absorbed chromium is eliminated via the kidneys.

Contraindications/Precautions/Warnings

Chromium supplements could, potentially, exacerbate renal insufficiency; use with caution in these patients. Because the picolinate salt can potentially alter behavior, consider using chromium chloride, or chromium nicotinate in patients receiving SSRI's or other behavioral therapies.

Adverse Effects

Chromium supplements (Cr III) at usual dosages appear to be well tolerated. Some human patients have complained of cognitive, perceptual, and motor dysfunction after receiving the picolinate salt.

Reproductive/Nursing Safety

In humans, chromium (up to 8 micrograms/kg) is probably safe for use in pregnancy but information remains sketchy. Because cats may receive much higher dosages than the human dosages for treating diabetes, use cautiously in pregnant animals.

Chromium supplements are likely to be safe for use in lactating animals.

Overdosage/Acute Toxicity

Little information on acute overdoses was located. There are at least two case reports of women developing renal failure after taking excessive doses of chromium picolinate.

Drug Interactions

The following drug interactions have either been reported or are theoretical in humans or animals receiving chromium and may be of significance in veterinary patients. Unless otherwise noted, use

together is not necessarily contraindicated, but weigh the potential risks and perform additional monitoring when appropriate.

- **CORTICOSTEROIDS**: May increase the urinary excretion of chromium.
- **H$_2$ BLOCKERS** (*e.g.,* **cimetidine, ranitidine, famotidine**, etc.) or **PROTON PUMP INHIBITORS** (*e.g.,* **PPI's, omeprazole**, etc.): May decrease chromium levels by inhibiting their absorption; clinical significance is unclear.
- **NSAIDs**: May increase the absorption and retention of chromium; clinical significance is unlikely.
- **ZINC**: Theoretically, co-administration of zinc with chromium could decrease the oral absorption of both.

Laboratory Considerations

- No specific laboratory interactions or considerations noted.

Doses -

- **CATS:**

  For use as an oral hypoglycemic agent (extra-label): Chromium picolinate 200 micrograms (per cat) PO once a day.

Monitoring

- As there is no reliable way to measure chromium in the body, a clinical trial is the only way to determine whether chromium is effective in helping to control blood glucose. Standard methods of monitoring diabetes treatment efficacy should be followed (*e.g.,* fasting blood glucose, appetite, attitude, body condition/weight, PU/PD resolution and, perhaps, serum fructosamine and/or glycosylated hemoglobin levels).

Client Information

- Clients should give the medication only as prescribed and not change brands without their veterinarian's approval.

Chemistry/Synonyms

A trace element (Cr; atomic number 24), oral chromium supplements are usually given as the picolinate salt (also known as chromium tripicolinate).

Storage/Stability

Chromium picolinate should be stored in tight containers. For storage recommendations, refer to the label for each product used.

Compatibility/Compounding Considerations

No specific information noted.

Dosage Forms/Regulatory Status

VETERINARY-LABELED PRODUCTS: NONE.

HUMAN-LABELED PRODUCTS:

No oral products FDA-approved as pharmaceuticals.

Injectable chromium: (as chromic chloride hexahydrate): 4 micrograms/mL (as 20.5 micrograms chromic chloride hexahydrate) and 20 micrograms/mL (as 102.5 micrograms chromic chloride hexahydrate) in 5 mL (20 micrograms/mL only), 10 mL & 30 mL; Chromic Chloride (various); *Chroma-Pak*®; generic; (Rx). Oral chromium products are considered to be nutritional supplements by the FDA. No standards have been accepted for potency, purity, safety or efficacy by regulatory bodies.

Supplements are available from a wide variety of sources. Most veterinary use in small animals is with chromium picolinate dosage forms. Common tablet sizes include 200 micrograms, 400 micrograms, 500 micrograms and 800 micrograms. Bioequivalence between products cannot be assumed.

Revisions/References

Monograph revised/updated October 2013.

Cimetidine

(sye-met-i-deen)   Tagamet®

Histamine$_2$ Blocker

Prescriber Highlights

▶ Prototype histamine$_2$-blocker primarily used to reduce GI acid production. Newer H$_2$-blockers (*e.g.,* ranitidine, famotidine) & other agents (*e.g.,* omeprazole) may be more effective, have longer duration of activity, & fewer drug interactions.

▶ Caution: Geriatric patients, hepatic or renal insufficiency.

▶ Compared with newer H$_2$ blockers, there are many drug interactions.

Uses/Indications

In veterinary medicine, cimetidine has been used for the treatment and/or prophylaxis of gastric, abomasal and duodenal ulcers, uremic gastritis, stress-related or drug-induced erosive gastritis, esophagitis, duodenal gastric reflux, and esophageal reflux. It has also been employed to treat hypersecretory conditions associated with gastrinomas and systemic mastocytosis. Cimetidine has also been used investigationally as an immunomodulating agent (see doses) in dogs. Cimetidine has been used for the treatment of melanomas in horses, but efficacy is unproven. Its use in veterinary and human medicine has been largely supplanted by newer agents that compared to cimetidine are more effective, need less frequent dosing, and do not have as many drug interaction issues.

Pharmacology/Actions

At the H$_2$ receptors of the parietal cells, cimetidine competitively inhibits histamine thereby reducing gastric acid output both during basal conditions and when stimulated by food, pentagastrin, histamine, or insulin. Gastric emptying time, pancreatic or biliary secretion, and lower esophageal pressures are not altered by cimetidine. By decreasing the amount of gastric juice produced, cimetidine also decreases the amount of pepsin secreted.

Cimetidine has an apparent immunomodulating effect as it has been demonstrated to reverse suppressor T-cell-mediated immune suppression. It also possesses weak anti-androgenic activity.

Pharmacokinetics

In dogs, the oral bioavailability is reported to be approximately 75-95%; food can significantly reduce oral bioavailability. Serum half-life is 1.3-1.6 hours and volume of distribution is 1.2 L/kg.

In horses, after intragastric administration oral bioavailability is only about 14%, steady-state volume of distribution 0.77 L/kg, median plasma clearance 8.2 mL/min/kg, and terminal elimination half-life is approximately 90 minutes.

In humans, cimetidine is rapidly and well absorbed after oral administration, but a small amount is metabolized in the liver before entering the systemic circulation (first-pass effect). The oral bioavailability is 70-80%. Food may delay absorption and slightly decrease the amount absorbed, but when given with food, peak levels occur when the stomach is not protected by the buffering capabilities of the ingesta.

Cimetidine is well distributed in body tissues and only 15-20% is bound to plasma proteins. The drug enters milk and crosses the placenta.

Cimetidine is both metabolized in the liver and excreted unchanged by the kidneys. More of the drug is excreted by the kidneys when administered parenterally (75%) than when given orally (48%). The average serum half-life is 2 hours in humans, but can be prolonged in elderly patients and those with renal or hepatic disease. Peritoneal dialysis does not appreciably enhance the removal of cimetidine from the body.

Contraindications/Precautions/Warnings

Cimetidine is contraindicated in patients with known hypersensitivity to the drug.

Cimetidine should be used cautiously in geriatric patients and patients with significantly impaired hepatic or renal function. In humans meeting these criteria, increased risk of CNS effects (confusion) may occur; dosage reductions may be necessary.

Cimetidine has been used in the past as an adjunctive treatment for acetaminophen toxicity in cats, but as it does not appear to be efficacious and could complicate therapy, it is generally not used.

Adverse Effects

Adverse effects appear to be very rare in animals at the dosages generally used. Potential adverse effects (documented in humans) that could be seen include mental confusion, headache (upon discontinuation of the drug), gynecomastia, and decreased libido. Rarely, agranulocytosis may develop and, if given rapidly IV, transient cardiac arrhythmias may be seen. Pain at the injection site may occur after IM administration.

Cimetidine does inhibit microsomal enzymes in the liver and may alter the metabolic rates of other drugs (see Drug Interactions below).

Reproductive/Nursing Safety

In humans, the FDA categorizes this drug as category *B* for use during pregnancy (*Animal studies have not yet demonstrated risk to the fetus, but there are no adequate studies in pregnant women; or animal studies have shown an adverse effect, but adequate studies in pregnant women have not demonstrated a risk to the fetus in the first trimester of pregnancy, and there is no evidence of risk in later trimesters.*) In a separate system evaluating the safety of drugs in canine and feline pregnancy (Papich 1989), this drug is categorized as class: *B* (*Safe for use if used cautiously. Studies in laboratory animals may have uncovered some risk, but these drugs appear to be safe in dogs and cats or these drugs are safe if they are not administered when the animal is near term.*)

Cimetidine is distributed into milk; while safety during nursing is not assured, it is usually considered compatible with nursing in humans.

Overdosage/Acute Toxicity

Clinical experience with cimetidine overdosage is limited. In laboratory animals, very high dosages have been associated with tachycardia and respiratory failure; respiratory support and beta-adrenergic blockers have been suggested for use should these signs occur.

Drug Interactions

The following drug interactions have either been reported or are theoretical in humans or animals receiving cimetidine and may be of significance in veterinary patients. Unless otherwise noted, use together is not necessarily contraindicated, but weigh the potential risks and perform additional monitoring when appropriate.

Cimetidine may inhibit the hepatic microsomal enzyme system and thereby reduce the metabolism, prolong serum half-lives, and increase the serum levels of several drugs and/or reduce the hepatic blood flow and reduce the amount of hepatic extraction of drugs that have a high first-pass effect, including:

- **BENZODIAZEPINES** (*e.g.,* **diazepam**, etc.)
- **BETA-BLOCKERS** (*e.g.,* **propranolol**, etc.)
- **CALCIUM CHANNEL BLOCKERS** (*e.g.,* **verapamil**, etc.)
- **CHLORAMPHENICOL**
- **LIDOCAINE**
- **METRONIDAZOLE**
- **PHENYTOIN**
- **PROCAINAMIDE**
- **THEOPHYLLINE**

- **TRIAMTERENE**
- **TRICYCLIC ANTIDEPRESSANTS**
- **WARFARIN**
- **ANTACIDS:** May decrease the absorption of cimetidine; stagger doses (separate by 2 hours if possible).
- **KETOCONAZOLE, ITRACONAZOLE,** etc.: Cimetidine may decrease the absorption of these drugs; give these medications at least two hours before cimetidine.
- **MYELOSUPPRESSIVE DRUGS:** Cimetidine may exacerbate leukopenias when used with myelosuppressive agents.

Laboratory Considerations

- **Creatinine:** Cimetidine may cause small increases in plasma creatinine concentrations early in therapy; these increases are generally mild, non-progressive, and have disappeared when therapy is discontinued.
- **Gastric Acid Secretion Tests:** Histamine$_2$ blockers may antagonize the effects of histamine and pentagastrin in the evaluation of gastric acid secretion; it is recommended that histamine$_2$ blockers be discontinued at least 24 hours before performing this test.
- **Allergen Extract Skin Tests:** Histamine$_2$ antagonists may inhibit histamine responses; it is recommended that histamine$_2$ blockers be discontinued at least 24 hours before performing this test.

Doses

- **DOGS/CATS:**
  For GI indications (extra-label): 5 – 10 mg/kg PO q6-8h.
- **FERRETS:**
  For stress induced ulcers (extra-label): 5 – 10 mg/kg PO 3 times daily. (Williams 2000)
- **RABBITS/RODENTS/SMALL MAMMALS:**
  All are extra-label.
  a) **Rabbits:** For GI ulcers: 5 – 10 mg/kg PO q8–12h. (Ivey et al. 2000)
  b) **Mice, Rats, Gerbils, Hamsters, Guinea pigs, Chinchillas:** 5 – 10 mg/kg PO q6-12h. (Adamcak et al. 2000)
- **HORSES:** (NOTE: ARCI UCGFS CLASS 5 DRUG)
  For GI indications in foals (extra-label): 300 – 600 mg per foal PO 3-4 times daily.
  For adjunctive treatment of melanomas (extra-label): 2.5 – 5 mg/kg PO once to twice a day.

Monitoring

- Clinical efficacy (dependent on reason for use); monitored by decrease in symptomatology, endoscopic examination, blood in feces, etc.
- Adverse effects if noted.

Client Information

- Used to treat or prevent stomach ulcers.
- Doses often need to be given 2-4 times per day; signs may reoccur if dosages are missed.
- Cimetidine interacts with many other medications. Don't give new medicines without your veterinarian's approval.
- Cimetidine is available OTC (over the counter; without a prescription), but only give it to your animal if your veterinarian recommends it.

Chemistry/Synonyms

An H$_2$-receptor antagonist, cimetidine occurs as a white to off-white, crystalline powder. It has what is described as an "unpleasant" odor and a pK$_a$ of 6.8. Cimetidine is sparingly soluble in water and soluble in alcohol. Cimetidine HCl occurs as white, crystalline powder and is very soluble in water and soluble in alcohol. It has a pK$_a$ of 7.11 and the commercial injection has a pH of 3.8-6.

Cimetidine may also be known as: cimetidinum, or SKF-92334; many trade names are available.

Storage/Stability

Cimetidine products should be stored protected from light and kept at room temperature. Do not refrigerate the injectable product as precipitation may occur. Oral dosage forms should be stored in tight containers.

Compatibility/Compounding Considerations

Compounded preparation stability: Cimetidine oral suspension compounded from commercially available tablets has been published (Tortorici 1979). Triturating twenty-four (24) cimetidine 300 mg tablets with 10 mL of glycerin and *qs ad* to 120 mL with simple syrup yields a 60 mg/mL oral suspension that retains >90% potency for 17 days stored at 4°C.

Dosage Forms/Regulatory Status

VETERINARY-LABELED PRODUCTS: NONE.

The ARCI (Racing Commissioners International) has designated this drug as a class 5 substance. See the appendix for more information.

HUMAN-LABELED PRODUCTS:

Cimetidine Oral Tablets: 200 mg, 300 mg, 400 mg, & 800 mg; *Tagamet*®, generic; (Rx, OTC)

Cimetidine HCl Oral Solution: 300 mg (as HCl)/5 mL in 240 mL, 480 mL & UD 5 mL; generic; (Rx)

A parenteral solution was formerly available, but has been withdrawn.

Revisions/References

Monograph revised/updated October 2013.

Adamcak, A. & B. Otten (2000). Rodent Therapeutics. *Vet Clin NA: Exotic Anim Pract* **3:**1(Jan): 221-40.

Ivey, E. & J. Morrisey (2000). Therapeutics for Rabbits. *Vet Clin NA: Exotic Anim Pract* **3:**1(Jan): 183-216.

Tortorici, M. (1979). Formulation of a cimetidine oral suspension. *Am J Hosp Pharm* **36**(1): 22.

Williams, B. (2000). Therapeutics in Ferrets. *Vet Clin NA: Exotic Anim Pract* **3:**1(Jan): 131-53.

Ciprofloxacin

(sip-roe-flox-a-sin)   Cipro®

Fluoroquinolone Antibiotic

Prescriber Highlights

▶ Human-label fluoroquinolone antibiotic. In dogs and cats oral bioavailability can be very low.

▶ Available as a true IV product.

▶ Contraindications: Food animals. History of hypersensitivity. Relatively contraindicated for young, growing animals due to cartilage abnormalities. Caution: Hepatic or renal insufficiency, dehydration.

▶ Adverse Effects: GI distress, CNS stimulation, crystalluria/urolithiasis, & hypersensitivity.

▶ Many potential drug interactions.

Uses/Indications

Because of its similar spectrum of activity, ciprofloxacin could be used as an alternative to enrofloxacin when a larger oral dosage form or intravenous product is desired. But the two compounds cannot be considered equivalent because of pharmacokinetic differences (see below). Because there are approved fluoroquinolones for some species, ciprofloxacin use in animals should be reserved for when it is clearly indicated.

Pharmacology/Actions

Ciprofloxacin is a bactericidal and a concentration dependent agent, with susceptible bacteria cell death occurring within 20-30 minutes of exposure. Ciprofloxacin has demonstrated a significant post-antibiotic effect for both gram-negative and gram-positive bacteria and is active in both stationary and growth phases of bacterial replication. Its mechanism of action is not thoroughly understood, but it is believed to act by inhibiting bacterial DNA-gyrase (a type-II topoisomerase), thereby preventing DNA supercoiling and DNA synthesis.

Both enrofloxacin and ciprofloxacin have similar spectrums of activity. These agents have good activity against many gram-negative bacilli and cocci, including most species and strains of *Pseudomonas aeruginosa*, *Klebsiella* spp., *E. coli*, Enterobacter, Campylobacter, Shigella, Salmonella, Aeromonas, Haemophilus, Proteus, Yersinia, Serratia, and Vibrio species. Of the currently commercially available quinolones, ciprofloxacin and enrofloxacin have the lowest MIC values for the majority of these pathogens treated. Other organisms that are generally susceptible include *Brucella* spp. *Chlamydia trachomatis*, Staphylococci (including penicillinase-producing and methicillin-resistant strains), Mycoplasma, and *Mycobacterium* spp. (not the etiologic agent for Johne's disease). When combined with either ceftazidime or cefepime, fluoroquinolones may have an additive or synergistic effect against certain bacteria.

The fluoroquinolones have variable activity against most Streptococci and are not usually recommended for use in treating these infections. These drugs have weak activity against most anaerobes and are ineffective in treating anaerobic infections.

Resistance does occur by mutation, particularly with *Pseudomonas aeruginosa*, *Klebsiella pneumonia*, Acinetobacter, and enterococci, but plasmid-mediated resistance does not seem to occur.

Pharmacokinetics

In dogs, ciprofloxacin's bioavailability can be variable and significantly less than enrofloxacin. In one study after oral tablets (250 mg/dog) were administered to beagles, bioavailability ranged from 32-80% (mean of 58%) (Papich 2012). Elimination half-life is reported to be about 2.5-2.6 hours (PO) and about 3.7 hours (IV).

Oral bioavailability in cats can be very low. A study (Albarellos et al. 2004) found that the oral bioavailability average is only about 33% in cats. After intravenous dosing, volume of distribution (steady state) is about 3.9 L/kg, clearance is approximately 0.64 L/hr/kg and elimination half-life averaged about 4.5 hours.

Studies of the oral bioavailability in ponies have shown that ciprofloxacin is poorly absorbed (2-12%) while enrofloxacin in foals apparently is well absorbed.

In humans, the oral bioavailability of ciprofloxacin has been reported to be between 50-85%.

In humans, the volume of distribution in adults for ciprofloxacin is about 2-3.5 L/kg and it is approximately 20-40% bound to serum proteins.

Ciprofloxacin is one of the metabolites of enrofloxacin. Approximately 15-50% of the drugs are eliminated unchanged into the urine by both tubular secretion and glomerular filtration. Enrofloxacin/ciprofloxacin are metabolized to various metabolites that are less active than the parent compounds. Approximately 10-40% of circulating enrofloxacin is metabolized to ciprofloxacin in most species. These metabolites are eliminated in both the urine and feces. Because of the dual (renal and hepatic) means of elimination, patients with severely impaired renal function may have slightly prolonged half-lives and higher serum levels but may not require dosage adjustment.

Contraindications/Precautions/Warnings

The extra-label use of ciprofloxacin (and other fluoroquinolones) is banned from use in food animals by the FDA.

Ciprofloxacin, as is enrofloxacin, should be considered relatively contraindicated in small and medium breed dogs from 2-8 months of age. Bubble-like changes in articular cartilage have been noted when the drug was given at 2-5 times recommended doses for 30 days, although clinical signs have only been seen at the 5X dose. To avoid cartilage damage, large and giant breed dogs may need to wait longer than the recommended 8 months since they may be in the rapid-growth phase past 8 months of age. Quinolones are also contraindicated in patients hypersensitive to them.

Because ciprofloxacin has occasionally been reported to cause crystalluria, animals should not be allowed to become dehydrated during therapy. In humans, ciprofloxacin has been associated with CNS stimulation and should be used with caution in patients with seizure disorders. Patients with severe renal or hepatic impairment may require dosage adjustments to prevent drug accumulation.

Use high dose ciprofloxacin in cats with caution. No reports of retinal toxicity (as can be seen with high dose enrofloxacin) secondary to ciprofloxacin in cats were located and retinal toxicity appears to be less likely since it is less lipophilic than enrofloxacin.

Adverse Effects

Potential adverse effects include cartilage abnormalities in young, growing animals (see Contraindications above), GI distress (*e.g.,* vomiting, anorexia, diarrhea, etc.), crystalluria/urolithiasis (dogs), CNS stimulation, and hypersensitivity reactions (dogs).

Reproductive/Nursing Safety

In humans, the FDA categorizes this drug as category *C* for use during pregnancy (*Animal studies have shown an adverse effect on the fetus, but there are no adequate studies in humans; or there are no animal reproduction studies and no adequate studies in humans.*)

Ciprofloxacin is distributed into milk, but oral absorption should be negligible. No adverse effects have been reported in nursing human infants of mothers receiving ciprofloxacin.

Overdosage

Little specific information is available. See the enrofloxacin monograph for more information.

Drug Interactions

The following drug interactions have either been reported or are theoretical in humans or animals receiving ciprofloxacin and may be of significance in veterinary patients. Unless otherwise noted, use together is not necessarily contraindicated, but weigh the potential risks and perform additional monitoring when appropriate.

- **ANTACIDS/DAIRY PRODUCTS** containing cations (Mg^{++}, Al^{+++}, Ca^{++}) may bind to ciprofloxacin and prevent its absorption; separate doses of these products by at least 2 hours from ciprofloxacin.
- **ANTIBIOTICS, OTHER (aminoglycosides, 3rd-generation cephalosporins, penicillins—extended-spectrum):** Synergism may occur, but is not predictable, against some bacteria (particularly *Pseudomonas aeruginosa*) with these compounds. Although enrofloxacin/ciprofloxacin has minimal activity against anaerobes, *in vitro* synergy has been reported when used with **clindamycin** against strains of Peptostreptococcus, Lactobacillus and *Bacteroides fragilis*.
- **CYCLOSPORINE:** Fluoroquinolones may exacerbate the nephrotoxicity, and reduce the metabolism of, cyclosporine (used systemically).
- **GLYBURIDE:** Severe hypoglycemia possible.
- **IRON, ZINC (oral):** Decreased ciprofloxacin absorption; separate doses by at least two hours.

- **METHOTREXATE:** Increased MTX levels possible with resultant toxicity
- **NITROFURANTOIN:** May antagonize the antimicrobial activity of the fluoroquinolones; concomitant use is not recommended.
- **PHENYTOIN:** Ciprofloxacin may alter phenytoin levels.
- **PROBENECID:** Blocks tubular secretion of ciprofloxacin and may increase its blood level and half-life.
- **QUINIDINE:** Increased risk for cardiotoxicity.
- **SUCRALFATE:** May inhibit absorption of ciprofloxacin; separate doses of these drugs by at least 2 hours.
- **THEOPHYLLINE:** Ciprofloxacin may increase theophylline blood levels.
- **WARFARIN:** Potential for increased warfarin effects.

Laboratory Considerations

- In some human patients, the fluoroquinolones have caused increases in **liver enzymes, BUN,** and **creatinine** and decreases in **hematocrit**. The clinical relevance of these mild changes is not known at this time.

Doses

- **DOGS:**

  For susceptible infections (extra-label): 20 – 25 mg/kg PO or IV once daily; some recommend dividing the dosage and giving q12h. **Note:** Dosage recommendations vary considerably. Because of the drug's variable oral bioavailability in dogs and the availability of other approved fluoroquinolone drugs for oral administration, ciprofloxacin is best reserved for use when an intravenous fluoroquinolone is indicated.

- **CATS:**

  For susceptible infections (extra-label): 20 – 25 mg/kg PO or IV once daily; some recommend dividing the dosage and giving q12h. **Note:** Because of the drug's relatively low oral bioavailability in cats and the availability of other approved fluoroquinolone drugs for oral administration, ciprofloxacin is best reserved for use when an intravenous fluoroquinolone is indicated.

- **FERRETS:**

  For susceptible infections (extra-label): 5 – 15 mg/kg PO twice daily. (Williams 2000)

- **RABBITS/RODENTS/SMALL MAMMALS:**

  All are extra-label.
  a) **Rabbits:** 5 – 20 mg/kg PO q12h. (Ivey et al. 2000)
  b) **Chinchillas, Gerbils, Guinea Pigs, Hamsters, Mice, Rats:** 7 – 20 mg/kg PO q12h. (Adamcak et al. 2000)
  c) **For treating pasteurellosis in rabbits:** ciprofloxacin or enrofloxacin 15 – 20 mg/kg PO twice daily for a minimum of 14 days in mild cases and up to several months in chronic infections. (Antinoff 2008)

- **BIRDS:**

  For susceptible gram-negative infections (extra-label):
  a) Using ciprofloxacin 500 mg tablets: 20 – 40 mg/kg PO twice daily. Crushed tablet goes into suspension well, but must be shaken well before administering. (McDonald 1989)
  b) Using crushed tablets: 20 mg/kg PO q12h. (Bauck et al. 1993)
  c) Using crushed tablets or compounded suspension: 10 – 15 mg/kg PO q12h. (Hoeffer 1995)

Monitoring

- Clinical efficacy.
- Adverse effects.

Client Information

- This drug is best given without food on an empty stomach, but if your animal vomits or acts sick after getting it, give with food or small treat (no dairy products, antacids or anything containing iron) to see if this helps. If vomiting continues, contact your veterinarian.
- Do not give at the same time with other drugs or vitamins that contain calcium, iron, or aluminum (including sucralfate) as these can reduce the amount of drug absorbed.
- May stunt bone growth or cause joint abnormalities if used in young animals, during pregnancy or while nursing.
- Most common side effects are vomiting, nausea, or diarrhea.

Chemistry/Synonyms

A fluoroquinolone antibiotic, ciprofloxacin HCl occurs as a faintly yellowish to yellow, crystalline powder. It is slightly soluble in water. Ciprofloxacin is related structurally to the veterinary-FDA-approved drug enrofloxacin (enrofloxacin has an additional ethyl group on the piperazinyl ring).

Ciprofloxacin may also be known as ciprofloxacine, ciprofloxacinum, ciprofloxacino, Bay-q-3939, or *Cipro®*.

Storage/Stability

Unless otherwise directed by the manufacturer, ciprofloxacin tablets should be stored in tight containers at temperatures less than 30°C. Protect from strong UV light. The injection should be stored at 5°-25°C and protected from light and freezing.

Compatibility/Compounding Considerations

The manufacturer recommends administering IV ciprofloxacin alone (temporarily discontinuing other solutions or drugs while ciprofloxacin running). However, other sources state that ciprofloxacin injection is reportedly **compatible** with the following IV solutions and drugs: Dextrose 5%, D5 and 1/4 or 1/2 NaCl, Ringer's, LRS, normal saline; **Y-site compatible with** amikacin sulfate, aztreonam, ceftazidime, cimetidine, cyclosporine, dexmedetomidine, dobutamine, dopamine, fluconazole, gentamicin, lidocaine, midazolam, KCl, ranitidine, tobramycin, and vitamin B complex.

Ciprofloxacin injection is reportedly **incompatible** with aminophylline, amphotericin B, azithromycin, cefuroxime, clindamycin, heparin sodium, sodium bicarbonate, and ticarcillin.

Compatibility is dependent upon factors such as pH, concentration, temperature and diluent used; consult specialized references or a hospital pharmacist for more specific information.

Dosage Forms/Regulatory Status

VETERINARY-LABELED PRODUCTS: NONE.

HUMAN-LABELED PRODUCTS:

Ciprofloxacin Oral Tablets: 100 mg, 250 mg, 500 mg & 750 mg; *Cipro®*, generic; (Rx)

Ciprofloxacin Extended-Release Oral Tablets: 500 mg & 1000 mg; *Cipro XR®*, generic; (Rx)

Ciprofloxacin Solution for Injection: 200 mg & 400 mg in 100 mL & 200 mL (respectively) in 5% dextrose flexible containers (0.2%); *Cipro® I.V.*, generic; (Rx)

The extra-label use of ciprofloxacin (and other fluoroquinolones) is banned from use in food animals by the FDA.

Revisions/References

Monograph revised/updated October 2013.

Adamcak, A. & B. Otten (2000). Rodent Therapeutics. *Vet Clin NA: Exotic Anim Pract* 3:1(Jan): 221-40.

Albarellos, G. A., et al. (2004). Pharmacokinetics of ciprofloxacin after single intravenous and repeat oral administration to cats. *J. Vet. Pharmacol. Ther.* 27(3): 155-62.

Antinoff, N. (2008). *Respiratory diseases of ferrets, rabbits, and rodents.* Proceedings: IVECCS. accessed via Veterinary Information Network; vin.com

Bauck, L. & H. Hoefer (1993). Avian antimicrobial therapy. *Seminars in Avian & Exotic Med* 2(1): 17-22.

Hoeffer, H. (1995). Antimicrobials in pet birds. *Kirk's Current Veterinary Therapy:XII.* J. Bonagura. Philadelphia, W.B. Saunders: 1278-83.

Ivey, E. & J. Morrisey (2000). Therapeutics for Rabbits. *Vet Clin NA: Exotic Anim Pract* 3:1(Jan): 183-216.

McDonald, S. E. (1989). Summary of medications for use in psittacine birds. *JAAV* 3(3): 120-7.

Papich, M. G. (2012). Ciprofloxacin pharmacokinetics and oral absorption of generic ciprofloxacin tablets in dogs. *American Journal of Veterinary Research* 73(7): 1085-91.

Williams, B. (2000). Therapeutics in Ferrets. *Vet Clin NA: Exotic Anim Pract* 3:1(Jan): 131-53.

Cisapride

(sis-a-pride)

Pro-motility Agent

Prescriber Highlights

▶ Oral GI prokinetic agent, used in several species for GI stasis, reflux esophagitis, & constipation/megacolon (cats).

▶ No longer commercially available, must be obtained from a compounding pharmacy.

▶ Contraindications: Hypersensitivity, GI perforation or obstruction, hemorrhage.

▶ Adverse effects appear to be minimal in veterinary patients; vomiting, diarrhea, and abdominal discomfort can occur.

▶ Drug interactions are possible.

Uses/Indications

Proposed uses for cisapride in small animals include esophageal reflux including during surgery, esophagitis and treatment of primary gastric stasis disorders. Cisapride has been found to be useful in the treatment of constipation and megacolon in cats. It has also been proposed to enhance detrusor contractility in dogs with micturition disorders, but it is not commonly used for this purpose.

Pharmacology/Actions

Cisapride increases lower esophageal peristalsis and sphincter pressure and accelerates gastric emptying. The drug's proposed mechanism of action enhances the release of acetylcholine at the myenteric plexus, but does not induce nicotinic or muscarinic receptor stimulation. Acetylcholinesterase activity is not inhibited. Cisapride blocks dopaminergic receptors to a lesser extent than does metoclopramide and does not increase gastric acid secretion.

Pharmacokinetics

In cats, oral bioavailability is variable but averages 30% and elimination half-life is about 5-6 hours (LeGrange et al. 1997). A study evaluating lower esophageal pressure in dogs after cisapride administration (0.5 mg/kg PO) found that effects were lacking after 7 hours (Kempf et al. 2013).

Human data: After oral administration, cisapride is rapidly absorbed with an absolute bioavailability of 35-40%. The drug is highly bound to plasma proteins and apparently extensively distributed throughout the body. Cisapride is extensively metabolized and its elimination half-life is about 8-10 hours.

Contraindications/Precautions/Warnings

Cisapride is contraindicated in patients where increased gastrointestinal motility could be harmful (*e.g.*, perforation, obstruction, GI hemorrhage, etc.) or those who are hypersensitive to the drug.

Adverse Effects

Cisapride appears to be safe in small animals at the dosages recommended. Occasionally vomiting, diarrhea, and abdominal discomfort may be noted. Although no reports have been noted in dogs or cats, prolonged QT intervals or other cardiac arrhythmias are possible but unlikely.

In humans, the primary adverse effects are gastrointestinal related with diarrhea and abdominal pain most commonly reported, but the drug was removed from the market due to concerns with QT-interval prolongation.

Dosage may need to be decreased in patients with severe hepatic impairment.

Reproductive/Nursing Safety

Cisapride at high dosages (>40 mg/kg/day) caused fertility impairment in female rats. At doses 12 to 100 times the maximum recommended, cisapride caused embryotoxicity and fetotoxicity in rabbits and rats. Its use during pregnancy should occur only when the benefits outweigh the risks. Cisapride is excreted in maternal milk in low levels; use with caution in nursing mothers.

Overdosage/Acute Toxicity

LD_{50} doses in various lab animals range from 160 – 4000 mg/kg. The reported oral lethal dose in dogs is 640 mg/kg. In one reported human overdose of 540 mg, the patient developed GI distress and urinary frequency. There were 29 exposures to cisapride reported to the ASPCA Animal Poison Control Center (APCC) during 2008-2009. In these cases, 21 were cats with 6 showing clinical signs, and 8 were dogs with 5 showing clinical signs. Most common adverse effects seen in dogs and cats are diarrhea, lethargy, ataxia, hypersalivation, muscle fasciculations, agitation, abnormal behavior, hyperthermia, and possibly seizures (dogs) (APCC unpublished data).

Significant overdoses should be handled using standard gut emptying protocols when appropriate; supportive therapy should be initiated when required. Activated charcoal is effective in binding unabsorbed cisapride (Volmer 1996).

Drug Interactions

The following drug interactions have either been reported or are theoretical in humans or animals receiving cisapride and may be of significance in veterinary patients. Unless otherwise noted, use together is not necessarily contraindicated, but weigh the potential risks and perform additional monitoring when appropriate.

- **ANTICHOLINERGIC AGENTS:** Use of anticholinergic agents may diminish the effects of cisapride.
- **BENZODIAZEPINES:** Cisapride may enhance the sedative effects of alcohol or benzodiazepines.
- **WARFARIN:** Cisapride may enhance anticoagulant effects; additional monitoring and anticoagulant dosage adjustments may be required.
- **ORAL DRUGS WITH A NARROW THERAPEUTIC INDEX:** May need serum levels monitored more closely when adding or discontinuing cisapride as cisapride can decrease GI transit times and potentially affect the absorption of other oral drugs.

As cisapride is metabolized via cytochrome P450 (3A4 in humans), the following medications/foods that can inhibit this enzyme may lead to increased cisapride levels with an increased risk for cisapride cardiotoxicity:

- **AMIODARONE**
- **ANTIFUNGALS** (*e.g.*, ketoconazole, itraconazole, fluconazole, etc.)
- **CHLORAMPHENICOL**
- **CIMETIDINE**
- **FLUVOXAMINE**
- **GRAPEFRUIT JUICE/POWDER**
- **MACROLIDE ANTIBIOTICS (except azithromycin) Note:** Erythromycin did not alter cisapride pharmacodynamics in one study in dogs.

The following drugs may increase QT interval and use with cisapride may increase this risk:

- **AMIODARONE**
- **CLARITHROMYCIN**

- **MOXIFLOXACIN**
- **PROCAINAMIDE**
- **QUINIDINE**
- **SOTALOL**
- **TRICYCLIC ANTIDEPRESSANTS** (*e.g.*, amitriptyline, imipramine, etc.)

Doses

- **DOGS:**

  As a promotility agent (extra-label): Most recommend initially dosing between 0.1 – 0.5 mg/kg PO q8-12h and some gastroenterologists recommend giving 30 minutes before feeding. Some sources state that dosages (gradually increased) up to 1 mg/kg PO q8h may be required (if tolerated).

- **CATS:**

  As a promotility agent (extra-label): Initially, 2.5 mg per cat PO twice daily preferably 15-30 minutes before food. Dosages may be titrated upwards, if tolerated, to as high as 7.5 mg per cat PO three times daily in large cats. Cats with hepatic insufficiency may need dosage interval extensions.

- **RABBITS/RODENTS/SMALL MAMMALS:**

  As a promotility agent (extra-label):

  a) **Mice, Rats, Gerbils, Hamsters, Guinea pigs, Chinchillas:** 0.1 – 0.5 mg/kg PO q12h (Adamcak et al. 2000).

  b) **Rabbits for GI stasis:** 0.5 mg/kg PO q6-12h. With IV or SC fluids, depending on amount of dehydration, feeding a high fiber slurry, with or without metoclopramide (0.2 – 1 mg/kg PO, SC q6–8h). (Hess 2002)

  c) **For ileus if GI tract not obstructed in Guinea pigs, chinchillas:** 0.5 mg/kg q8–12h (*Route not specified; assume PO*). (Orcutt 2005)

  d) **For gastric stasis in rabbits:** Usually started at 0.5 mg/kg PO (via NG tube) q8h after first stools were produced or no intestinal obstruction appreciated. May be synergistic if used with ranitidine (0.5 mg/kg IV q24h). (Lichtenberger 2008)

- **HORSES:**

  As a promotility agent in foals with periparturient asphyxia (extra-label): 10 mg (total dose) PO q6-8h. Adequate time for healing of damaged bowel before using prokinetic agents is essential. (Vaala 2003)

Monitoring

- Efficacy.
- Adverse effects profile.

Client Information

- Must be obtained from a compounding pharmacy; commercially available dosage forms are unavailable.
- Adverse effects appear to be minimal in veterinary patients; vomiting, diarrhea, and abdominal discomfort can occur.
- May give with or without food. Give with food if animal vomits after a dose.
- Many possible drug interactions; don't give any new drugs without checking with your veterinarian.

Chemistry/Synonyms

An oral GI prokinetic agent, cisapride is a substituted piperidinyl benzamide and is structurally, but not pharmacologically, related to procainamide. It is available commercially as a monohydrate, but potency is expressed in terms of the anhydrate.

Cisapride may also be known as: cisapridum, or R-51619; many trade names are registered.

Storage/Stability

Unless otherwise instructed by the manufacturer, store cisapride tablets in tight, light-resistant containers at room temperature.

Compatibility/Compounding Considerations

Compounded preparation stability: Cisapride oral suspension compounded from commercially available tablets has been published (Allen et al. 1998). Triturating twelve (12) cisapride 10 mg tablets with 60 mL of *Ora-Plus®* and *qs ad* to 120 mL with *Ora-Sweet®* with pH finally adjusted to 7 with sodium bicarbonate yields a 1 mg/mL oral suspension that retains >90% potency for 60 days stored at both 5°C and 25°C. Although cisapride tablets are no longer commercially available, the active pharmaceutical ingredient powder may be used to compound suitable oral suspensions of cisapride. Compounded preparations of cisapride should be protected from light.

Dosage Forms/Regulatory Status

VETERINARY-LABELED PRODUCTS: NONE.

HUMAN-LABELED PRODUCTS: NONE.

Because of adverse effects in humans, cisapride has been removed from the US market. It may be available from compounding pharmacies.

Revisions/References

Monograph revised/updated October 2013.

Adamcak, A. & B. Otten (2000). Rodent Therapeutics. *Vet Clin NA: Exotic Anim Pract* 3:1(Jan): 221-40.

Allen, L. V. & M. A. Erickson (1998). Stability of alprazolam, chloroquine phosphate, cisapride, enalapril maleate, and hydralazine hydrochloride in extemporaneously compounded oral liquids. *Am J Health Syst Pharm* 55(18): 1915-20.

Hess, L. (2002). *Practical Emergency/Critical Care of the Pet Rabbit.* Proceedings: Atlantic Coast Veterinary Conference. accessed via Veterinary Information Network; vin.com

Kempf, J., et al. (2013). Evaluation of the Effect of Oral Cisapride On Lower Esophageal Sphincter Pressure in Awake Dogs Using High-Resolution Manometry. *Journal of Veterinary Internal Medicine* 27(3): 697-.

LeGrange, S. N., et al. (1997). Pharmacokinetics and suggested oral dosing regimen of cisapride: A study in healthy cats. *J. Am. Anim. Hosp. Assoc.* 33(6): 517-23.

Lichtenberger, M. (2008). *What's new in small mammal critical care.* Proceedings: AAV. accessed via Veterinary Information Network; vin.com

Orcutt, C. (2005). *Chinchilla and Guinea pig diseases.* Proceedings: Western Veterinary Conf. accessed via Veterinary Information Network; vin.com

Vaala, W. (2003). Perinatal asphyxia syndrome in foals. *Current Therapy in Equine Medicine* 5. N. Robinson and E. Carr. Phila., Saunders: 644-9.

Volmer, P. A. (1996). Cisapride toxicosis in dogs. *Veterinary and Human Toxicology* 38(2): 118-20.

Cisplatin

(sis-pla-tin)   CDDP, Platinol-AQ®

Antineoplastic

Prescriber Highlights

▶ Platinum antineoplastic agent used for a variety of carcinomas & sarcomas; palliative control of neoplastic pulmonary effusions with intracavitary administration; intralesional injection for skin tumors in horses.

▶ Contraindications: Cats; preexisting significant renal impairment or myelosuppression.

▶ Drug-related deaths possible. Primary adverse effects: Vomiting (pretreat with antiemetic); nephrotoxicity (use forced saline diuresis); ototoxicity (permanent hearing loss), myelosuppression; many other adverse effects possible.

▶ Teratogenic, fetotoxic; may cause azoospermia.

▶ Must be handled with care by dosage preparer/administerer.

▶ Must be given as slow IV infusion; fast administration (<5 minutes) may increase toxicity.

Uses/Indications

In veterinary medicine, the systemic use of cisplatin is presently limited to use in dogs. The drug has been, or may be, useful in a variety of neoplastic diseases including squamous cell carcinomas, transitional cell carcinomas, ovarian carcinomas, mediastinal carcinomas, osteosarcomas, pleural adenocarcinomas, nasal carcinomas, and thyroid adenocarcinomas. There is some evidence that efficacy for transitional cell carcinoma can be enhanced with concurrent NSAIDs (firocoxib) (Knapp et al. 2013).

Cisplatin may be useful for the palliative control of neoplastic pulmonary effusions after intracavitary administration.

Intralesional injections of compounded cisplatin suspension in oil or as cisplatin-impregnated beads have been used for intralesional injection for skin tumors (sarcoids) in horses. Cisplatin also shows some promise as an electrochemotherapy agent for treating incompletely excised mast cell tumors in dogs (Spugnini et al. 2011) or sarcoids in horses.

Pharmacology/Actions

While the exact mechanism of action of cisplatin has not been determined, its properties are analogous to those of bifunctional alkylating agents producing inter- and intrastrand crosslinks in DNA. Cisplatin is cell cycle nonspecific.

Pharmacokinetics

After administration, the drug concentrates in the liver, intestines and kidneys. Platinum will accumulate in the body and may be detected 6 months after a course of therapy has been completed. Cisplatin is highly bound (90%) to serum proteins.

In dogs, cisplatin exhibits a biphasic elimination profile. The initial plasma half-life is short (approximately 20-50 minutes), but the terminal phase is very long (about 60-80 hours). Approximately 80% of a dose can be recovered as free platinum in the urine within 48 hours of dosing in dogs.

Contraindications/Precautions/Warnings

Cisplatin is <u>contraindicated in cats</u> because of severe dose-related primary pulmonary toxicoses (dyspnea, hydrothorax, pulmonary edema, mediastinal edema, and death). Death can occur within 2-4 days of administration. Cisplatin is also contraindicated in patients with preexisting significant renal impairment, myelosuppression, or a history of hypersensitivity to platinum-containing compounds. Because of the fluid loading required prior to dosing, it should be used with caution in patients with congestive heart failure.

When preparing the product for injection, wear gloves and protective clothing as local reactions may occur with skin or mucous membrane contact. Should accidental exposure occur, wash the area thoroughly with soap and water.

Do not confuse cisplatin with carboplatin. Consider using tall man lettering when writing orders or prescriptions: CISplatin; CARBOplatin.

Adverse Effects

In dogs, the most frequent adverse effect seen after cisplatin treatment is vomiting, which usually occurs within 6 hours after dosing and persists for 1-6 hours. This is because of direct effects on the chemoreceptor trigger zone (CTZ). Maropitant, ondansetron, dolasetron, metoclopramide and butorphanol have all been used successfully as antiemetics when given before cisplatin administration.

Nephrotoxicity may occur unless the animal is adequately diuresed with sodium chloride prior to, and after therapy; diuresis will generally significantly reduce the incidence and severity of nephrotoxicity in the majority of dogs. Intravenous methimazole (40 mg/kg) has been demonstrated to protect cisplatin-induced nephrotoxicity in dogs in experimental models.

Ototoxicity (high-frequency permanent hearing loss and tinnitus) has been reported, but incidence in dogs is not known. In human patients, up to 100% of treated patients develop some degree of hearing loss. Co-administered antioxidants (*e.g.*, vitamins A & E, glutathione, etc.) have been proposed to help protect against cisplatin-induced ototoxicity. This is somewhat controversial as potentially these could also reduce cisplatin's antitumor efficacy (Oishi et al. 2012).

Other adverse effects that have been reported include hematologic abnormalities (thrombocytopenia and/or granulocytopenia), anorexia, diarrhea (including hemorrhagic diarrhea), seizures, peripheral neuropathies, electrolyte abnormalities, hyperuricemia, increased hepatic enzymes, anaphylactoid reactions, and death.

Direct IV infusion over 1-5 minutes should be avoided as it may cause increased nephrotoxicity or ototoxicity.

Reproductive/Nursing Safety

Cisplatin's safe use in pregnancy has not been established. It is teratogenic and embryotoxic in mice. In human males, the drug may cause azoospermia and impaired spermatogenesis. In humans, the FDA categorizes this drug as category *D* for use during pregnancy (*There is evidence of human fetal risk, but the potential benefits from the use of the drug in pregnant women may be acceptable despite its potential risks.*) In a separate system evaluating the safety of drugs in canine and feline pregnancy (Papich 1989), this drug is categorized as class: *C* (*These drugs may have potential risks. Studies in people or laboratory animals have uncovered risks, and these drugs should be used cautiously as a last resort when the benefit of therapy clearly outweighs the risks.*)

Overdosage/Acute Toxicity

The minimum lethal dose of cisplatin in dogs is reportedly 2.5 mg/kg ($\approx$80 mg/m^2). Because of the potential for serious toxicity associated with this agent, dosage calculations should be checked thoroughly to avoid overdosing. See Adverse Effects above for more information.

Drug Interactions

The following drug interactions have either been reported or are theoretical in humans or animals receiving cisplatin and may be of significance in veterinary patients. Unless otherwise noted, use together is not necessarily contraindicated, but weigh the potential risks and perform additional monitoring when appropriate.

- **AMINOGLYCOSIDES**: Potential for increased risk for nephrotoxicity and/or nephrotoxicity; if possible, delay aminoglycoside administration by at least two weeks after cisplatin.

- **AMPHOTERICIN B**: Potential for increased risk for nephrotoxicity; if possible, delay amphotericin B administration by at least two weeks after cisplatin.

- **FUROSEMIDE** (and other **loop diuretics**): Potential for increased ototoxicity.

- **PHENYTOIN**: Cisplatin may reduce serum levels of phenytoin.

Doses

Note: Because of the potential toxicity of this drug to patients, veterinary personnel and clients, and since chemotherapy indications, treatment protocols, monitoring and safety guidelines often change, the following dosages should be used only as a general guide. Consultation with a veterinary oncologist and referral to current veterinary oncology references [*e.g.,* (Withrow et al. 2012); (Dobson et al. 2011); (Henry et al. 2009); (North et al. 2009); (Argyle et al. 2008)] are strongly recommended.

Dosages are commonly listed as mg/m^2. Do not confuse them as mg/kg.

- **DOGS:**

  For potentially susceptible carcinomas and sarcomas (extra-label): The following is a usual dosage or dose range for cisplatin and should be used only as a general guide: Dogs: 30 – 70 mg/m^2 (NOT mg/kg) IV over 20 minutes to several hours every 3-5 weeks. **Warning:** Do not confuse cisplatin and carboplatin dosages; cisplatin dosages are much lower. Dogs must un-

dergo saline diuresis before and after cisplatin therapy to reduce the potential for nephrotoxicity development. Some clinicians also recommend using either mannitol or furosemide with saline, but this is somewhat controversial.

Intracavitary administration for palliative control of neoplastic pulmonary effusions (extra-label): Give dog IV normal saline at 10 mL/kg/hr for 4 hours prior to treating. Dose cisplatin at 50 mg/m^2 (NOT mg/kg) (diluted in normal saline to a total volume of 250 mL/m^2). Warm solution to body temperature; place a 16-gauge over-the-needle catheter into the pleural space using sterile technique. Remove as much pleural fluid as possible and then slowly infuse cisplatin solution through same catheter. Once completed, remove catheter. May repeat every 3-4 weeks as needed to control effusion. If resolves completely, discontinue therapy after the 4th treatment. Reinstitute if effusion recurs. (Hawkins et al. 2000)

- **HORSES:**

  For intralesional injection of skin tumors (extra-label): Add 10 mg of cisplatin powder (if available) to 1 mL of water and 2 mL of medical-grade sesame oil. Resultant solution contains 3.3 mg of cisplatin per mL. Inject 1 mg per cm^3 of tumor/tumor bed intralesionally with a small gauge needle (22-25 gauge) attached to an extension set with Luer-lock connections. Inject in multiple planes no further than 0.6 to 1 cm apart. Because the volume of tumor is difficult to measure, the rule of thumb is to discontinue injection when fluid is extruded from the skin surface. Because recurrence at the periphery of the treated area is the primary cause of treatment failure, injection into 1-2 cm of normal tissue surrounding the tumor has been recommended. Intralesional injection is generally repeated at 2-week intervals for 4 total treatments. (Moll 2002)

Monitoring

- Toxicity. Baseline laboratory data: urinalysis, hemogram, platelet count, serum biochemical and electrolyte determination. Repeat tests before each dose if animal is receiving high-dose therapy (monthly) or as needed if signs of toxicity develop. Animals receiving frequent small doses should be monitored at least weekly. Not recommended to use cisplatin if WBC is <3200/mcl, platelets <100,000, creatinine clearance is <1.4 mL/min/kg, or uremia, electrolyte or acid-base imbalance is present. Reduce dose if rapid decreases occur with either WBC or platelets, changes in urine specific gravity or serum electrolytes, elevated serum creatinine or BUN, or if creatinine clearance is >1.4 but <2.9 mL/min/kg.

- Efficacy. Tumor measurement and radiography at least monthly. In one study (Knapp et al. 1988), the authors state that dogs should be evaluated at 42 days into therapy. Dogs demonstrating complete or partial remission or stable disease should receive additional therapy. Dogs whose disease has progressed should have cisplatin therapy stopped and receive alternate therapies if warranted.

Client Information

- Cisplatin is a chemotherapy (cancer) drug. The drug and its byproducts can be hazardous to other animals and people that come in contact with it. On the day your animal gets the drug and then for 2 days afterward, all bodily waste (urine, feces, litter), blood, or vomit should only be handled while wearing disposable gloves. Seal the waste in a plastic bag and then place both the bag and gloves in with the regular trash.

- Not to be used in cats.

- Care should be taken to avoid contact with the administration site if your veterinarian injected cisplatin directly into a tumor (sarcoid) on your animal.

Chemistry/Synonyms

An inorganic platinum-containing antineoplastic, cisplatin occurs as white powder. One mg is soluble in 1 mL of water or normal saline. The drug is available commercially as a solution for injection. Cisplatin injection (premixed solution) has a pH of 3.7-6.

Cisplatin may also be known as: cis-Platinum II, cis-DDP, CDDP, cis-diamminedichloroplatinum, cisplatina, cisplatinum, cis-platinum, DDP, NSC-119875, Peyrone's salt, or platinum diamminodichloride; many trade names are available.

Storage/Stability

The injection should be stored at room temperature and away from light; do not refrigerate as a precipitate may form. During use, the injection should be protected from direct bright sunlight, but does not need to be protected from normal room incandescent or fluorescent lights.

Do not use aluminum hub needles or aluminum containing IV sets as aluminum may displace platinum from the cisplatin molecule with the resulting formation of a black precipitate. Should a precipitate form from either cold temperatures or aluminum contact, discard the solution.

Compatibility/Compounding Considerations

Cisplatin is reportedly **compatible** with the following intravenous solutions and drugs: dextrose/saline combinations, sodium chloride 0.225%-0.9%, magnesium sulfate, and mannitol. It is also **compatible** in syringes or at Y-sites with: bleomycin sulfate, cyclophosphamide, doxorubicin HCl, fluorouracil, furosemide, heparin sodium, leucovorin calcium, methotrexate, vinblastine sulfate, and vincristine sulfate.

Cisplatin **compatibility information conflicts** or is dependent on diluent or concentration factors with the following drugs or solutions: dextrose/saline combinations, dextrose 5% in water, and metoclopramide. Compatibility is dependent upon factors such as pH, concentration, temperature and diluent used; consult specialized references or a hospital pharmacist for more specific information.

Cisplatin is reportedly **incompatible** with the following solutions or drugs: sodium chloride 0.1% and sodium bicarbonate 5%.

Dosage Forms/Regulatory Status

VETERINARY-LABELED PRODUCTS: NONE.

HUMAN-LABELED PRODUCTS:

Cisplatin Injection: 1 mg/mL in 50 mL, 100 mL & 200 mL multidose vials; generic; (Rx)

Cisplatin powder or compounded formulations appropriate for intralesional injection may be available from compounding pharmacies.

Revisions/References

Monograph revised/updated October 2013.

Argyle, D., et al. (2008). *Decision Making in Small Animal Oncology*, Wiley-Blackwell.

Dobson, J. & D. Lascelles (2011). *BSAVA Manual of Canine and Feline Oncology*, BSAVA.

Hawkins, E. & T. Fossum (2000). Medical and Surgical Management of Pleural Effusion. *Kirk's Current Veterinary Therapy: XIII Small Animal Practice*. J. Bonagura. Philadelphia, WB Saunders: 819-25.

Henry, C. & M. Higginbotham (2009). *Cancer Management in Small Animal Practice*, Saunders.

Knapp, D. W., et al. (2013). Randomized Trial of Cisplatin versus Firocoxib versus Cisplatin/Firocoxib in Dogs with Transitional Cell Carcinoma of the Urinary Bladder. *Journal of Veterinary Internal Medicine* 27(1): 126-33.

Moll, H. (2002). *Skin tumor management*. Proceedings: Western Veterinary Conference. accessed via Veterinary Information Network; vin.com

North, S. & T. Banks (2009). *Small Animal Oncology: An Introduction*, Saunders.

Oishi, N., et al. (2012). Ototoxicity in Dogs and Cats. *Veterinary Clinics of North America-Small Animal Practice* 42(6): 1259-+.

Spugnini, E. P., et al. (2011). Evaluation of Cisplatin as an Electrochemotherapy Agent for the Treatment of Incompletely Excised Mast Cell Tumors in Dogs. *Journal of Veterinary Internal Medicine* 25(2): 407-11.

Withrow, S., et al. (2012). *Withrow and MacEwen's Small Animal Clinical Oncology, 5th Ed.*, Saunders.

Citrate, Potassium

(si-trate)   Urocit-K®

Urinary Alkalinizer

Prescriber Highlights

▶ Oral administered precursor to bicarbonate; used for urinary alkalization & treatment of chronic metabolic acidosis; may be useful to prevent calcium oxalate urolith formation.

▶ Potassium citrate is also used to treat hypokalemia.

▶ Many contraindications to therapy, including heart failure, severe renal impairment, UTI with calcium or struvite stones.

▶ Contraindications for potassium citrate alone include hyperkalemia, ulcer disease; tablets in patients with delayed gastric emptying conditions, esophageal compression, or intestinal obstruction.

▶ Most prevalent adverse effect is GI distress but, potentially, hyperkalemia, fluid retention & metabolic alkalosis possible.

▶ Adequate lab monitoring mandatory.

Uses/Indications

Potassium citrate alone (*Uracit-K*®) has been used for the prevention of calcium oxalate uroliths. The citrate can complex with calcium thereby decreasing urinary concentrations of calcium oxalate. The urinary alkalinizing effects of the citrate also increase the solubility of calcium oxalate.

Citrate salts serve as source of bicarbonate; but are usually more palatable than bicarbonate preparations. They are used as urinary alkalinizers and in the management of chronic metabolic acidosis accompanied with conditions such as renal tubular acidosis or chronic renal insufficiency. Compounds containing potassium citrate can also serve to treat hypokalemia.

Pharmacology/Actions

Citrate salts are oxidized in the body to bicarbonate thereby acting as alkalinizing agents. The citric acid component of multi-component products is converted only to carbon dioxide and water and has only a temporary effect on systemic acid-base status.

Pharmacokinetics

Absorption and oxidation are nearly complete after oral administration; less than 5% of a dose is excreted unchanged.

Contraindications/Precautions/Warnings

Contraindications for products containing potassium citrate: aluminum toxicity, heart failure, severe renal impairment (with azotemia or oliguria), UTI associated with calcium, or struvite stones. Additional contraindications for potassium citrate alone include hyperkalemia (or conditions that predispose to hyperkalemia such as adrenal insufficiency, acute dehydration, renal failure, uncontrolled diabetes mellitus), or peptic ulcer (particularly with the tablets). The potassium citrate tablets are contraindicated in patients with delayed gastric emptying conditions, esophageal compression, or intestinal obstruction or stricture. These products should be used with caution (weigh risks vs. benefit) in severe renal tubular acidosis or chronic diarrheal syndromes as they may be ineffective. Products containing sodium citrate should be used with caution in patients with congestive heart disease.

Adverse Effects

The primary adverse effects noted with these agents are gastrointestinal in nature, however, most dogs receiving these products tolerate them well. Potassium citrate products have the potential of causing hyperkalemia, especially in susceptible patients.

The oral liquids containing potassium citrate can be bitter making patient acceptance more difficult.

Reproductive/Nursing Safety

In humans, the FDA categorizes potassium citrate as a category *C* drug for use during pregnancy (*Animal studies have shown an adverse effect on the fetus, but there are no adequate studies in humans; or there are no animal reproduction studies and no adequate studies in humans*). In dosages not resulting in hypernatremia, hyperkalemia or metabolic alkalosis, these products should not cause fetal harm.

No specific data is available on the safety of citrates during nursing, but no documented adverse effects have been reported.

Overdosage/Acute Toxicity

Overdosage and acute toxicity would generally fall into three categories: gastrointestinal distress and ulceration, metabolic alkalosis, and hyperkalemia (potassium citrate). Should an overdose occur and there are reasonable expectations of preventing absorption (especially with the tablets), gut-emptying protocols should be employed if not contraindicated. Otherwise, treat GI effects, if necessary, with intravenous fluids or other supportive care. Hyperkalemia, hypernatremia, and metabolic alkalosis should be treated if warranted. It is suggested to refer to an animal poison control center, an internal medicine text or other references for additional information for specific treatment modalities for these conditions.

Drug Interactions

The following drug interactions have either been reported or are theoretical in humans or animals receiving citrates and may be of significance in veterinary patients. Unless otherwise noted, use together is not necessarily contraindicated, but weigh the potential risks and perform additional monitoring when appropriate.

- **ALUMINUM-CONTAINING PHOSPHATE BINDERS:** Increased risk for aluminum toxicity and systemic alkalosis particularly in patients with renal insufficiency.
- **AMPHETAMINES; PSEUDOEPHEDRINE; EPHEDRINE:** Alkalinized urine can decrease excretion.
- **ANTACIDS:** Citrate alkalinizers used with antacids (particularly those containing bicarbonate or aluminum salts) may cause systemic alkalosis, and aluminum toxicity (aluminum antacids only) particularly in patients with renal insufficiency. Sodium citrate combined with sodium bicarbonate may cause hypernatremia, and may cause the development of calcium stones in patients with preexisting uric acid stones.
- **ASPIRIN:** Alkalinized urine can increase the excretion of salicylates.
- **FLUOROQUINOLONES:** The solubility of ciprofloxacin & enrofloxacin is decreased in an alkaline environment. Patients with alkaline urine should be monitored for signs of crystalluria.
- **LITHIUM:** Alkalinized urine can decrease excretion.
- **METHENAMINE:** Concurrent use with methenamine is not recommended as it requires an acidic urine for efficacy.
- **PHENOBARBITAL:** Alkalinized urine can increase phenobarbital excretion (Fukunaga et al. 2008).
- **QUINIDINE:** Alkalinized urine can decrease excretion.
- **TETRACYCLINES:** Alkalinized urine can decrease excretion.

With potassium citrate products, the following agents may lead to increases in serum potassium levels (including severe hyperkalemia), particularly in patients with renal insufficiency:

- **ACE INHIBITORS** (*e.g.,* **enalapril, lisinopril**)
- **CYCLOSPORINE**
- **DIGOXIN**
- **HEPARIN**
- **NONSTEROIDAL ANTIINFLAMMATORY DRUGS (NSAIDS)**
- **POTASSIUM-CONTAINING DRUGS/FOODS**
- **SPIRONOLACTONE; TRIAMTERENE**

Doses

- **DOGS:**

  For adjunctive therapy to inhibit calcium oxalate crystal formation in dogs with hypocitraturia (extra-label): Potassium citrate: 50 – 75 mg/kg PO twice daily. If urine pH is already above 7.5, do not use potassium citrate. Usually used with dietary therapy; some recommend hydrochlorothiazide also.

  For adjunctive therapy of chronic renal failure as a potassium supplement and alkalinizing agent (extra-label): Potassium citrate: Initially, 60 – 75 mg/kg PO twice daily.

- **CATS:**

  For adjunctive therapy to inhibit calcium oxalate formation (extra-label): Potassium Citrate: Initial dosage recommendations range from 50 – 75 mg/kg PO twice daily. Efficacy is not well established for cats.

  For adjunctive therapy of chronic renal failure as a potassium supplement and alkalinizing agent (extra-label): Potassium citrate initial dosage 50 – 75 mg/kg PO twice daily. Monitor serum potassium every 7-14 days to establish the final maintenance dosage.

Monitoring

Depending on patient's condition, product chosen and reason for use:

- Serum potassium, sodium, bicarbonate, chloride.
- Acid/base status.
- Urine pH, Urinalysis.
- Serum creatinine, CBC, particularly in chronic renal failure.

Client Information

- Can be used to help prevent the formation of calcium oxalate bladder/kidney stones. In animals with chronic renal failure (chronic kidney disease) it can be used to increase blood potassium levels and make the urine and blood (temporarily) more alkaline.
- Usually given with or mixed into food.
- Use of this medication will require ongoing laboratory monitoring.

Chemistry/Synonyms

Potassium citrate occurs as odorless, transparent crystals or a white, granular powder having a cooling, saline taste. It is freely soluble in water. 108 mg of potassium citrate contains approximately 1 mEq of potassium.

Potassium citrate may also be known as citrate of potash, or citric acid tripotassium salt monohydrate. Sodium citrate and citric acid solutions may also be known as Shohl's solution.

Storage/Stability

Store solutions and potassium citrate tablets in tight containers at room temperature unless otherwise recommended by manufacturer.

Compatibility/Compounding Considerations

No specific information noted.

Dosage Forms/Regulatory Status

VETERINARY-LABELED PRODUCTS:

Potassium Citrate Tablets: 675 mg (6.25 mEq potassium); *CitraVet®* (also contains liver flavoring); (OTC). Labeled for dogs and cats, but does not appear to be an FDA-approved product.

Potassium Citrate and Fatty Acids Granules: each 5 g (one scoop) contains 300 mg potassium citrate (approximately 2.8 mEq of potassium) and 423 mg total fatty acids; also contains several amino acids—quantities not labeled; *Nutrived® Potassium Citrate Granules for Cats and Dogs*; (OTC). This does not appear to be an FDA-approved product.

HUMAN-LABELED PRODUCTS:

Potassium Citrate Extended-Release Oral Tablets: 5 mEq (540 mg), 10 mEq (1080 mg) & 15 mEq (1620 mg); *Urocit-K®*, generic; (Rx)

Potassium Citrate/Sodium Citrate Combinations:

Tablets: 50 mg potassium citrate and 950 mg sodium citrate. *Citrolith®*; (Rx)

Syrup: 550 mg potassium citrate, 500 mg sodium citrate, 334 mg citric acid/5 mL (1mEq K, 1 mEq Na per mL equivalent to 2 mEq bicarbonate); in 120 and 480 mL; *Polycitra®*; (Rx)

Solution: 550 mg K citrate, 500 mg sodium citrate, 334 mg citric acid/5 mL (1 mEq K, 1 mEq Na per mL; equiv. to 2 mEq bicarbonate) in 120 and 480 mL; *Polycitra-LC®*; (Rx)

1100 mg potassium citrate, 334 mg citric acid/5 mL, (2 mEq K/mL; equiv. to 2 mEq bicarbonate) in 120 and 480 mL; *Polycitra-K®*; (Rx)

Crystals for Reconstitution: 3300 mg potassium citrate, 1002 mg citric acid per UD packet (equiv. To 30 mEq bicarbonate) in single dose packets; *Polycitra-K®*; (Rx)

Potassium Citrate, Sodium Citrate/Citric Acid Solutions:

550 mg potassium citrate monohydrate, 500 mg sodium citrate dihydrate, 334 mg citric acid monohydrate per 5 mL (1 mEq potassium and 1 mEq sodium per mL and is equivalent to 2 mEq bicarbonate in 60 oz. bottles; *Cytra-LC®*; (Rx)

1100 mg potassium citrate monohydrate and 334 mg citric acid monohydrate per 5 mL (2 mEq potassium per mL and is equivalent to 2 mEq bicarbonate) in 473 mL; *Cytra-K®*; (Rx)

20 mEq potassium, 30 mEq citrate (20 g dextrose, 5 g fructose, 35 mEq chloride, 45 mEq sodium)/L in 1 liter; *Naturalyte® Oral Electrolyte Solution*; (OTC)

Revisions/References

Monograph revised/updated October 2013.

Fukunaga, K., et al. (2008). Effects of urine pH modification on pharmacokinetics of phenobarbital in healthy dogs. *J. Vet. Pharmacol. Ther.* 31(5): 431-6.

Clarithromycin

(klar-ith-ro-my-sin)   Biaxin®

Macrolide Antibiotic

Prescriber Highlights

▶ Macrolide antibiotic that may useful for treating atypical mycobacterial infections or treatment of *Helicobacter* spp. infections in dogs, cats, & ferrets; *Rhodococcus equi* infections in foals.

▶ Appears to be well tolerated by domestic animals, but clinical experience is limited.

▶ Many potential drug interactions. Rifampin appears to negate its usefulness in foals.

▶ Expense may be an issue, but generics now available.

Uses/Indications

In small animal medicine, clarithromycin is primarily of interest in treating atypical mycobacterial infections or treatment of *Helicobacter* spp. infections in cats and ferrets. However one recent study using quadruple therapy (amoxicillin, clarithromycin, metronida-

zole and a proton pump inhibitor) demonstrated it did not eradicate *H. pylori* in 4/13 treated cats, and may only cause transient suppression (Khoshnegah et al. 2011). In equine medicine, clarithromycin may be useful in treating *Rhodococcus equi* infections in foals, but drug interactions with rifampin raise questions for its usefulness.

Pharmacology/Actions

Clarithromycin, like other macrolide antibiotics, penetrate susceptible bacterial cell walls and bind to the 50S ribosomal subunit inhibiting protein synthesis. The drug is usually bacteriostatic, but may be bactericidal at high concentrations in very susceptible organisms.

Clarithromycin's spectrum of activity is similar to that of erythromycin, but it also has activity against a variety of bacteria that are not easily treated with other antibiotics (*e.g.*, atypical mycobacteria). Activity against gram-positive aerobic cocci is similar to that of erythromycin, but lower concentrations are required to be effective against susceptible organisms. The drug is typically not effective against oxacillin-resistant Staph or coagulase-negative Staph. Clarithromycin also has activity against *Rhodococcus equi*. Activity against gram-negative aerobic bacteria includes *Haemophilus influenzae, Pasteurella multocida, Legionella pneumophilia, Bordetella pertussis* and *Campylobacter* spp. Clarithromycin has inhibitory activity against a variety of atypical mycobacteria, including *M. avium complex* and *M. leprae*. Clarithromycin has good activity against *Mycoplasma pneumoniae* and *Ureaplasma ureatlyticum*. Other organisms where clarithromycin may have therapeutic usefulness include: *Nocardia* spp. *Toxoplasma gondii, Helicobacter pylori, Borrelia burgdorferi,* and *Cryptosporidium parvum*.

Pharmacokinetics

In horses (foals), the drug is apparently well absorbed (approx. 50-60%) after intragastric administration with peak serum concentrations occurring about 1.6 hours after dosing. Elimination half-life is about 5.4 hours (Womble et al. 2006). However, when used with chronic rifampin treatment, oral bioavailability can be reduced by 90% (Peters et al. 2011).

In dogs, clarithromycin bioavailability ranges from 60-83% with the higher values obtained when given to fasted animals.

Contraindications/Precautions/Warnings

In humans, clarithromycin is contraindicated in patients hypersensitive to it or other macrolide antibiotics (*e.g.*, erythromycin, azithromycin, etc.).

Adverse Effects

The adverse effect profile for clarithromycin in domestic animals is not well described. With limited clinical experience, it appears to be relatively well tolerated in dogs, cats, ferrets, and foals. Like all orally administered antibiotics, GI disturbances are possible. The incidence of diarrhea in foals may be higher than with other macrolides. Pinnal or generalized erythema may be associated with this drug when used in cats. Orange staining of skin is possible.

Adverse effects in humans include gastrointestinal adverse effects (primarily nausea, vomiting, abdominal pain, abnormal taste, diarrhea) that, when compared with erythromycin, are milder and occur less frequently. Approximately 4% of treated humans develop transient, mildly elevated BUN levels. Rarely, prolonged QT interval (torsades de pointes), hepatotoxicity, thrombocytopenia, or hypersensitivity reactions have been reported. Pseudomembranous colitis secondary to *Clostridium difficile* has been reported after clarithromycin use.

Reproductive/Nursing Safety

In humans, the FDA categorizes clarithromycin as a category *C* drug for use during pregnancy (*Animal studies have shown an adverse effect on the fetus, but there are no adequate studies in humans;*

or there are no animal reproduction studies and no adequate studies in humans). Teratogenic studies in rats and rabbits failed to document any teratogenic effects in some studies, but, at high dosages (yielding plasma levels 2-17 times achieved in humans with maximum recommended dosages) in pregnant rats, rabbits and monkeys, some effects (cleft palate, cardiovascular abnormalities, fetal growth retardation) were noted.

Clarithromycin is excreted into milk of lactating animals and levels may be higher in milk than in the dam's plasma, but this is unlikely to be of clinical significance.

Overdosage/Acute Toxicity

Generally, overdoses of clarithromycin are usually not serious with only gastrointestinal effects seen. Patients ingesting large overdoses may be given activated charcoal/cathartic to remove any unabsorbed drug. Forced diuresis, peritoneal dialysis, or hemodialysis does not appear to be effective in removing the drug from the body.

Drug Interactions

The following drug interactions have either been reported or are theoretical in humans or animals receiving clarithromycin and may be of significance in veterinary patients. Unless otherwise noted, use together is not necessarily contraindicated, but weigh the potential risks and perform additional monitoring when appropriate.

- **CISAPRIDE:** Clarithromycin can inhibit the metabolism of cisapride and the manufacturer states that use of these drugs together (in humans) is contraindicated.
- **CYCLOSPORINE:** Clarithromycin can significantly increase oral bioavailability in cats and reduce dosage requirements by 35% (Katayama et al. 2012).
- **FLUCONAZOLE:** Possible increased clarithromycin levels.
- **DIGOXIN:** Clarithromycin may increase the serum levels of digoxin.
- **OMEPRAZOLE:** Clarithromycin and omeprazole can increase the plasma levels of one another.
- **RIFAMPIN:** Can significantly decrease the oral bioavailability of clarithromycin in foals and can negate its efficacy (Peters et al. 2011; Peters et al. 2012).
- **WARFARIN:** Clarithromycin may potentiate the effects of oral anticoagulant drugs.
- **ZIDOVUDINE:** Clarithromycin may decrease serum concentrations of zidovudine.

Clarithromycin, like erythromycin, can inhibit the metabolism of other drugs that use the CYP3A subfamily of the cytochrome P450 enzyme system. Depending on the therapeutic index of the drug(s) involved, therapeutic drug monitoring and/or dosage reduction may be required if the drugs must be used together. These drugs include:

- **ALFENTANIL**
- **BROMOCRIPTINE**
- **BUSPIRONE**
- **CARBAMAZEPINE**
- **DISOPYRAMIDE** (also risk of increased QT interval)
- **METHYLPREDNISOLONE**
- **MIDAZOLAM, ALPRAZOLAM, TRIAZOLAM**
- **QUINIDINE** (also risk of increased QT interval)
- **RIFABUTIN**
- **TACROLIMUS** (systemic)
- **THEOPHYLLINE**

Laboratory Considerations

- No clarithromycin-related laboratory interactions noted.

Doses

- **DOGS:**

  For treatment of severe or refractory cases of canine leproid granuloma syndrome (extra-label): Using a combination of clarithromycin 15 – 25 mg/kg total daily dose PO given divided q8-12h; and rifampin 10 – 15 mg/kg PO once daily. Usually treatment should be continued for 4-8 weeks until lesions are at least substantially reduced in size and ideally have resolved completely. (Malik et al. 2001)

  For susceptible infections (extra-label): 5 – 10 mg/kg PO twice daily.

- **CATS:**

  Susceptible infections (extra-label): 7.5 mg/kg PO q12h.

  For treatment of feline leprosy syndrome or other opportunist mycobacteria (extra-label):

  Note: Combination therapy using two or more antibiotics has been recommended and appears to be more efficacious than single antibiotic therapy. Long treatment courses are often needed (2-14 months) and should be continued for at least 2 months beyond resolution of the lesions. Several treatment protocols have been suggested (see below). No evidence was located that clearly supports one over the other.

  a) Combination of clarithromycin 7.5 – 15 mg/kg PO twice daily with pradofloxacin (3 mg/kg PO q24h) and either rifampin (10 – 15 mg/kg PO q24h) or clofazimine (4 – 10 mg/kg PO q24h or 25 – 50 mg/cat/day q24-48h). (Malik et al. 2013)

  b) Clarithromycin 62.5 mg per cat q12h combined with doxycycline 5 mg/kg PO q12h, or enrofloxacin/marbofloxacin 5 mg/kg PO q24h, or clofazimine 8 – 12 mg/kg PO q24h, and/or rifampin at 10 – 15 mg/kg PO q24h. (Koch et al. 2011)

  For treatment of *Nocardia* (*N. nova*) infections (extra-label): Combination therapy with: amoxicillin 20 mg/kg PO twice daily with clarithromycin 62.5 – 125 mg (total dose per cat) PO twice daily and/or doxycycline 5 mg/kg or higher PO twice daily. (Malik 2006)

  For treating *H. pylori* infections (extra-label):

  a) Using quadruple therapy: Amoxicillin 20 mg/kg PO twice daily, metronidazole 20 mg/kg PO twice daily, clarithromycin 7.5 mg/kg PO twice daily, and omeprazole 0.7 mg/kg q8h for 14 days. Treatment did not eradicate organism in 4 of 13 cats in study. (Khoshnegah et al. 2011)

  b) Using triple therapy (anecdotal): Amoxicillin (20 mg/kg PO twice daily), clarithromycin (7.5 mg/kg PO twice daily) and metronidazole (10 mg/kg PO twice daily) for 14-21 days. Further studies are required before clear guidelines can be made. The author recommends treating only symptomatic patients that have biopsy-confirmed *Helicobacter* spp. infection and gastritis. (Simpson 2012)

- **FERRETS:**

  For treatment of *Helicobacter mustelae* infections (extra-label):

  a) Clarithromycin 12.5 mg/kg PO q12h with ranitidine bismuth citrate (**Note:** not currently available in the USA, but may be available from compounding pharmacies) 24 mg/kg PO q12h. Treat for 14 days. Same regimen, but given q8h is also published. (Johnson-Delaney 2009)

  b) 12.5 – 50 mg/kg q8-24h with omeprazole at 0.7 mg/kg PO once daily (q24h). (Fisher 2005)

■ **HORSES:**

For treatment of *Rhodococcus equi* infection in foals (extra-label): Based on a retrospective study, 7.5 mg/kg PO twice daily in combination with rifampin (Giguere et al. 2004). **Note:** It is unclear at the time of this writing (2103) whether the recently published drug interaction studies will impact this dosage recommendation.

For treatment of *Lawsonia intracellularis* infections in foals (extra-label): Chloramphenicol (50 mg/kg PO q6-8h) and oxytetracycline (10 mg/kg IV q24h) followed by doxycycline (10 mg/kg PO q12h), erythromycin (25 mg/kg PO q12h) or clarithromycin (7.5 mg/kg PO q12h). Treatment length determined by clinical response, but 3 weeks minimum is likely indicated. (Mallicote et al. 2012)

Monitoring

■ Antibacterial efficacy.
■ Adverse effects.

Client Information

■ May give with or without food. Give with food if stomach upset or vomiting occurs.
■ May cause stomach and intestinal pain and cramping when given by mouth.
■ Cats may experience reddening of the skin (especially the ears) while taking this drug.
■ Do not give to rabbits, gerbils, guinea pigs, hamsters, or to adult horses/ponies.
■ Many possible drug interactions. Tell your veterinarian and pharmacist what other drugs your animal is receiving.
■ If using the oral suspension, do <u>not</u> refrigerate; keep at room temperature and discard after 14 days.

Chemistry/Synonyms

Clarithromycin is a semi-synthetic macrolide antibiotic related to erythromycin. It differs from erythromycin by the methylation of position 6 in the lactone ring. Clarithromycin occurs as a white to off-white crystalline powder. It is practically insoluble in water, slightly soluble in ethanol, and soluble in acetone. It is slightly soluble in a phosphate buffer at pH's of 2-5.

Clarithromycin may also be known as: 6-O-methylerythromycin, TE-031, A-56268. *Biaxin®* is a common trade name.

Storage/Stability

The conventional 250 mg tablets should be protected from light and stored in well-closed containers at 15-30°C (59-86°F). The conventional or extended-release 500 mg tablets should be stored in well-closed containers at controlled room temperature (20-25°C; 68-77°F). The granules for reconstitution into an oral suspension should be stored in well-closed containers at 15-30°C. After reconstitution, it should be stored at room temperature (do not refrigerate) and any unused drug discarded after 14 days.

Compatibility/Compounding Considerations

No specific information noted.

Dosage Forms/Regulatory Status

VETERINARY-LABELED PRODUCTS: NONE.

HUMAN-LABELED PRODUCTS:

Clarithromycin Regular & Film-coated Oral Tablets: 250 mg & 500 mg; Extended-release Tablets: 500 mg; *Biaxin® & Biaxin XL®*, generic; (Rx)

Clarithromycin Granules for Oral Suspension: 125 mg/5 mL & 250 mg/5 mL (after reconstitution) in 50 mL & 100 mL; *Biaxin®*, generic; (Rx)

A pre-packaged combination containing lansoprazole, amoxicillin and clarithromycin for *H. pylori* in humans marketed as *Prevpak®*; (Rx)

Revisions/References

Monograph revised/updated October 2013.

Fisher, P. (2005). *Ferret Medicine I.* Proceedings: Western Vet Conf. accessed via Veterinary Information Network; vin.com
Giguere, S., et al. (2004). Retrospective comparison of azithromycin, clarithromycin, and erythromycin for the treatment of foals with Rhodococcus equi pneumonia. *Journal of Veterinary Internal Medicine* 18(4): 568-73.
Johnson-Delaney, C. (2009). *Gastrointestinal physiology and disease of carnivorous exotic companion animals.* Proceedings: ABVP. accessed via Veterinary Information Network; vin.com
Katayama, M., et al. (2012). Interaction of clarithromycin with cyclosporine in cats: pharmacokinetic study and case report. *Journal of Feline Medicine and Surgery* 14(4): 257-61.
Khoshnegah, J., et al. (2011). The efficacy and safety of long-term Helicobacter species quadruple therapy in asymptomatic cats with naturally acquired infection. *Journal of Feline Medicine & Surgery* 13(2): 88-93.
Koch, S., et al. (2011). *Small Animal Dermatology Drug Handbook*, Wiley-Blackwell. Ames.
Malik, R. (2006). *Nocardia infections in cats.* Proceedings Western Vet Conf. accessed via Veterinary Information Network; vin.com
Malik, R., et al. (2001). Treatment of canine leproid granuloma syndrome: preliminary findings in dogs. *Aust Vet J* 79(Jan): 30-6.
Malik, R., et al. (2013). Ulcerated and nonulcerated nontuberculous cutaneous mycobacterial granulomas in cats and dogs. *Veterinary Dermatology* 24(1): 146-+.
Mallicote, M., et al. (2012). A review of foal diarrhoea from birth to weaning. *Equine Veterinary Education* 24(4): 206-14.
Peters, J., et al. (2011). Oral Absorption of Clarithromycin Is Nearly Abolished by Chronic Comedication of Rifampicin in Foals. *Drug Metabolism and Disposition* 39(9): 1643-9.
Peters, J., et al. (2012). Clarithromycin Is Absorbed by an Intestinal Uptake Mechanism That Is Sensitive to Major Inhibition by Rifampicin: Results of a Short-Term Drug Interaction Study in Foals. *Drug Metabolism and Disposition* 40(3): 522-8.
Simpson, K. W. (2012). *Managing Persistent Vomiting.* Western Veterinary Conference Proceedings. accessed via Veterinary Information Network; vin.com
Womble, A. Y., et al. (2006). Pharmacokinetics of clarithromycin and concentrations in body fluids and bronchoalveolar cells of foals. *American Journal of Veterinary Research* 67(10): 1681-6.

Clavulanate/Amoxicillin — See Amoxicillin/Clavulanate

Clavulanate/Ticarcillin — See Ticarcillin /Clavulanate

Clemastine Fumarate

(klem-as-teen)   Tavist®

Antihistamine

Prescriber Highlights

▶ Oral antihistamine with greater anticholinergic, but less sedative activity.
▶ Poor pharmacokinetic profile for oral administration in dogs or horses.
▶ Caution: Prostatic hypertrophy, bladder neck obstruction, severe cardiac failure, angle-closure glaucoma, or pyeloduodenal obstruction.
▶ Most likely adverse effects: <u>Dogs:</u> Sedation, paradoxical hyperactivity & anticholinergic effects (dryness of mucous membranes, etc.). <u>Cats:</u> Diarrhea.

Uses/Indications

Clemastine may be used for symptomatic relief of histamine$_1$-related allergic conditions.

Pharmacology/Actions

Like other H$_1$-receptor antihistamines, clemastine acts by competing with histamine for sites on H$_1$-receptor sites on effector cells. They do not block histamine release, but can antagonize its effects. Clemastine has greater anticholinergic activity, but less sedation than average.

Pharmacokinetics

In dogs, oral bioavailability is very low (3%). Clemastine has a high volume of distribution (13.4 L/kg; 98% protein bound) and clearance (2.1 L/hr/kg). After IV administration, clarithromycin completely inhibited wheal formation for 7 hours; elimination half-life was about 4 hours. Oral administration of 0.5 mg/kg only yielded minor inhibition of wheal formation. The authors of the study concluded that most oral dosage regimens in the literature are likely to give too low a systemic exposure of the drug to allow effective therapy (Hansson et al. 2004).

In horses, clemastine has poor oral bioavailability (3-4%), a volume of distribution at steady-state of 3.8 L/kg, a clearance (TBC) of 0.79 L/hr/Kg and a terminal half-life of about 5.4 hours. The authors concluded that the drug is not appropriate for oral administration in the horse and must be dosed at least 3-4 times a day intravenously to maintain therapeutic plasma concentrations (Torneke et al. 2003).

In humans, clemastine has a variable bioavailability (20-70%); its distribution is not well characterized, but it does distribute into milk. Metabolic fate has not been clearly determined, but it appears to be extensively metabolized with metabolites eliminated in the urine. In humans, its duration of action is about 12 hours.

Contraindications/Precautions/Warnings

Clemastine is contraindicated in patients hypersensitive to it. It should be used with caution in patients with prostatic hypertrophy, bladder neck obstruction, severe cardiac failure, angle-closure glaucoma, or pyeloduodenal obstruction.

Adverse Effects

The most likely adverse effects seen in dogs receiving clemastine are sedation, paradoxical hyperactivity, and anticholinergic effects (dryness of mucous membranes, etc.). In cats, diarrhea has been noted most commonly; one cat reportedly developed a fixed drug reaction while on this medication.

Reproductive/Nursing Safety

Clemastine has been tested in pregnant lab animals in doses up to 312 times labeled without evidence of harm to fetuses. However, because safety has not been established in other species, its use during pregnancy should be weighed carefully. In humans, the FDA categorizes this drug as category *B* for use during pregnancy (*Animal studies have not yet demonstrated risk to the fetus, but there are no adequate studies in pregnant women; or animal studies have shown an adverse effect, but adequate studies in pregnant women have not demonstrated a risk to the fetus in the first trimester of pregnancy, and there is no evidence of risk in later trimesters.*)

Clemastine enters maternal milk and may potentially cause adverse effects in offspring. Use with caution, especially with newborns.

Overdosage/Acute Toxicity

There are no specific antidotes available. Significant overdoses should be handled using standard gut emptying protocols, when appropriate, and supportive therapy initiated when required. The adverse effects seen with overdoses are an extension of the drug's side effects; principally CNS depression (although CNS stimulation may be seen), anticholinergic effects (severe drying of mucous membranes, tachycardia, urinary retention, hyperthermia, etc.), and possibly hypotension. Physostigmine may be considered to treat serious CNS anticholinergic effects and diazepam employed to treat seizures, if necessary.

Drug Interactions

The following drug interactions have either been reported or are theoretical in humans or animals receiving clemastine and may be of significance in veterinary patients. Unless otherwise noted, use together is not necessarily contraindicated, but weigh the potential risks and perform additional monitoring when appropriate.

- **CNS DEPRESSANT MEDICATIONS:** Additive CNS depression may be seen if combining clemastine with other CNS depressant medications such as barbiturates, tranquilizers, etc.

- **MONOAMINE OXIDASE INHIBITORS** (including **furazolidone, amitraz,** and possibly **selegiline**) may intensify the anticholinergic effects of clemastine.

Laboratory Considerations

Because antihistamines can decrease the wheal and flair response to **skin allergen testing**, antihistamines should be discontinued 3-14 days (depending on the antihistamine used and the reference) before intradermal skin tests.

Doses

- **DOGS:**

Note: Relatively recent published information (Hansson et al. 2004) on the pharmacokinetics of clemastine in dogs puts the efficacy of previously published doses for this drug in doubt, but some veterinary dermatologists still recommend its use. Usual doses published are approximately 0.05 – 0.1 mg/kg PO q12h; however oral bioavailability (see Pharmacokinetics above) in dogs is less than 5% versus approximately 20-70% in humans. An oral dose of 0.5 mg/kg (10X most published doses) in dogs only inhibited histamine-induced wheal formation to a slight degree, while IV administration inhibited it for 7 hours. Further dosing studies must be performed before this drug can be recommended for therapeutic use in the dog.

- **CATS:**

As an antihistamine (extra-label): 0.34 – 0.68 mg per cat PO twice a day.

Monitoring

- Efficacy.
- Adverse Effects.

Client Information

- Antihistamines are used on a regular, ongoing basis in animals that respond to them. They work better if used before exposure to an allergen.
- Drowsiness/sleepiness can occur with this medication, but usually this lessens with time.
- Cats can develop diarrhea.

Chemistry/Synonyms

Also known as meclastine fumarate or mecloprodin fumarate, clemastine fumarate is an ethanolamine antihistamine. It occurs as an odorless, faintly yellow, crystalline powder. It is very slightly soluble in water and sparingly soluble in alcohol.

Clemastine fumarate may also be known by the following synonyms and internationally registered trade names: clemastini fumaras, or HS-592; a common trade name is *Tavist®*.

Storage/Stability

Oral tablets and solution should be stored in tight, light resistant containers at room temperature.

Compatibility/Compounding Considerations

No specific information noted.

Dosage Forms/Regulatory Status

VETERINARY-LABELED PRODUCTS: NONE.

The ARCI (Racing Commissioners International) has designated this drug as a class 3 substance. See the appendix for more information.

HUMAN-LABELED PRODUCTS:

Clemastine Fumarate Oral Tablets: 1.34 mg as fumarate (equivalent to 1 mg clemastine), 2.68 mg (equivalent to 2 mg clemastine); *Dayhist-1®*, *Tavist® Allergy*, generic; (Rx & OTC)

Clemastine Oral Syrup: 0.67 mg/5 mL (equivalent to 0.5 mg clemastine) in 118 mL & 120 mL; generic; (Rx)

Revisions/References

Monograph revised/updated October 2013.

Hansson, H., et al. (2004). Clinical pharmacology of clemastine in healthy dogs. *Vet Derm* 15: 152-8.

Torneke, K., et al. (2003). Pharmacokinetics and pharmacodynamics of clemastine in healthy horses. *J Vet Phamacol Ther* 26(2): 151-7.

Clenbuterol HCl

(klen-byoo-ter-ol)   Ventipulmin®

Beta-2 Agonist

Prescriber Highlights

▶ Beta$_2$-adrenergic agonist used in horses as a short-term bronchodilator in the management of airway obstruction and for dystocia as a uterine relaxant.

▶ Banned in food animals in USA and several other countries.

▶ In pregnancy, antagonizes the effects of dinoprost (prostaglandin F$_2$alpha) & oxytocin & can diminish normal uterine contractility.

▶ Acute adverse effects include tachycardia, muscle tremors, sweating, restlessness, & urticaria.

▶ Tachyphylaxis can occur with chronic administration and potentially cause deleterious effects on endocrine, immune and reproductive functions.

Uses/Indications

Clenbuterol is FDA-approved for use in horses as a bronchodilator in the management of airway obstruction, such as recurrent airway obstruction (RAO; formerly COPD). It has been used both parenterally and orally as a uterine relaxant for the adjunctive treatment of dystocia.

It has been used as a partitioning agent in food producing animals, but its use for this purpose is banned in the USA as relay toxicity in humans has been documented.

Pharmacology/Actions

Like other beta-2 agonists, clenbuterol is believed to act by stimulating production of cyclic AMP through the activation of adenyl cyclase. By definition, beta-2 agonists have more smooth muscle relaxation activity (bronchial, vascular, and uterine smooth muscle) versus its cardiac effects (beta-1). Clenbuterol appears to have secondary modes of action in horses as it can inhibit the release from macrophages of pro-inflammatory cytokines such as interleukin–1(beta) and tumor necrosis factor (alpha), increase ciliary beat frequency to enhance mucous clearance, and reduce mucous production.

Tachyphylaxis has been observed for tracheal mucociliary clearance rate after 12 days (Barr et al. 2013) or histamine-induced airway reactivity after 21 days (Read et al. 2012).

Clenbuterol has anabolic action in humans and cattle. In horses it can increase muscle mass, but any performance increases are offset by a negative ergonomic effect.

Compared to control, when clenbuterol was administered IV to healthy horses, aerobic capacity was not improved, insulin levels were increased, and treadmill velocities for defined heart rates were reduced (Ferraz et al. 2007).

Chronic administration of clenbuterol to horses can cause decreased aerobic performance which may be due effects on thermoregulation. It can induce cardiac hypertrophy and infiltration of collagen in cardiac muscle, and suppress cortisol response to exercise. Chronic clenbuterol administration in combination with exercise training can alter immune function (reduced killer and CD8+ cells).

In pregnant mares, clenbuterol can inhibit uterine tone and contractility, but these effects are not considered detrimental. In non-pregnant mares, clenbuterol's effects on uterine contractility may potentially increase risks for mating-induced endometritis. Some studies have shown that clenbuterol can impair reproductive function in males. (Kearns et al. 2009)

Pharmacokinetics

After oral administration to horses, peak plasma levels of clenbuterol occur 2 hours after administration and the average half-life is about 10-13 hours. Oral bioavailability is approximately 84%. The manufacturer states the duration of effect varies from 6-8 hours. After multiple oral doses, the drug's volume of distribution is approximately 1.6 L/kg and clearance was 94 mL/kg/hr. Urinary concentrations of clenbuterol are approximately 100X those found in plasma and can persist at quantifiable levels for 288 hours (12 days) in urine after the last oral dose (Soma et al. 2004).

Contraindications/Precautions/Warnings

The drug is contraindicated in food producing animals (legal ramifications). The label states that the drug should not be used in horses suspected of having cardiovascular impairment as tachycardia may occur.

Adverse Effects

Muscle tremors, sweating, restlessness, urticaria, and tachycardia may be noted, particularly early in the course of therapy. Creatine kinase elevations have been noted in some horses and, rarely, ataxia can occur. Clenbuterol is reported to induce abortion in pregnant animals.

Clenbuterol has been touted in some body building circles as an alternative to anabolic steroids for muscle development and body fat reduction; however, its safe use for this purpose is in serious question. Be alert for scams to divert legitimately obtained clenbuterol for this purpose.

Reproductive/Nursing Safety

Clenbuterol's safety in breeding stallions and brood mares has not been established. Clenbuterol should not be used in pregnant mares near full-term as it antagonizes the effects of dinoprost (prostaglandin F2alpha) and oxytocin and can diminish normal uterine contractility.

Overdosage/Acute Toxicity

Some case reports of clenbuterol overdoses have been reported in various species. In recent years, clenbuterol has been used as an adulterant in illicit heroin. Depending on dosage and species, emptying gut may be appropriate, otherwise supportive therapy and administration of parenteral beta-blockers to control heart rate and rhythm and elevated blood pressure may be considered.

Drug Interactions

The following drug interactions have either been reported or are theoretical in humans or animals receiving clenbuterol and may be of significance in veterinary patients. Unless otherwise noted, use together is not necessarily contraindicated, but weigh the potential risks and perform additional monitoring when appropriate.

- **ANESTHETICS, INHALANT:** Use with inhalation anesthetics (*e.g.,* **isoflurane**), may predispose the patient to ventricular arrhythmias, particularly in patients with preexisting cardiac disease—use cautiously.

- **BETA-BLOCKERS** (*e.g.,* **propranolol**): May antagonize clenbuterol's effects.

- **DIGOXIN:** Use with digitalis glycosides may increase the risk of cardiac arrhythmias.

- **DINOPROST:** Clenbuterol may antagonize the effects of dinoprost (prostaglandin F2alpha).

- **OXYTOCIN:** Clenbuterol may antagonize the effects of oxytocin.

- SYMPATHOMIMETIC AMINES, OTHER (*e.g.*, **terbutaline, albuterol**): Concomitant administration with other sympathomimetic amines may enhance the adverse effects of clenbuterol.
- TRICYCLIC ANTIDEPRESSANTS or MONOAMINE OXIDASE INHIBITORS: May potentiate the vascular effects of clenbuterol.

Doses

- **HORSES:** (NOTE: ARCI UCGFS CLASS 3 DRUG)

As a bronchodilator (FDA-approved label): Initially, 0.8 micrograms/kg (practically: 0.5 mL of the commercially available syrup/100 lb. BW) twice daily for 3 days; if no improvement increase to 1.6 micrograms/kg (practically: 1 mL of the commercially available syrup/100 lb. BW) twice daily for 3 days; if no improvement increase to 2.4 micrograms/kg (practically: 1.5 mL of the commercially available syrup/100 lb. BW) twice daily for 3 days; if no improvement increase to 3.2 micrograms/kg (practically: 2 mL of the commercially available syrup/100 lb. BW) twice daily for 3 days; if no improvement discontinue therapy. Recommended duration of therapy is 30 days; then withdraw therapy and reevaluate. If signs return, reinitiate therapy as above. (Package Insert; *Ventipulmin®*)

As adjunctive treatment for dystocia emergencies (extra-label):

a) IV administration (Not available in USA): 300 micrograms per 500 kg mare IV slowly (**Note:** parenteral formulation not available commercially in the USA). The drug's fast onset of action when given IV allows veterinarian to decide quickly if uterine relaxation will correct the problem. Clenbuterol is particularly useful when repelling the equine fetus to allow manipulation of the head and limbs. May be used in combination with sedatives, analgesics and tranquilizers. Xylazine or detomidine may potentiate uterine relaxant effects of clenbuterol. (Card 2002)

b) Oral administration: At the author's hospital: Upon arrival of a dystocia, on the clinician's orders the nurse administers 10 mLs of clenbuterol syrup orally as the mare walks in the door. (McCafferty 2007)

Monitoring

- Clinical efficacy.
- Adverse effects.

Client Information

- Usually used in horses with airway obstruction to relax muscles to improve breathing. Also used by veterinarians to treat dystocia (difficult delivery) emergencies in mares.
- Use with caution in pregnancy; can possibly induce abortion or prevent labor.
- Drug has been abused by humans; keep secure and dispose of unused drug appropriately.
- Illegal to use in food animals (USA and other countries). Use may be prohibited in show or racing horses.

Chemistry/Synonyms

A beta-2-adrenergic agonist, clenbuterol HCl's chemical name is 1-(4-Amino-3,5-dichlorophenyl)-2-tert-butyl aminoethanol HCl.

Clenbuterol HCl may also be known as: NAB-365, *Aeropulmin®, Broncodil®, Broncoterol®, Bronq-C®, Cesbron®, Clembumar®, Clenasma®, Clenbutol®, Contrasmina®, Contraspasmin®, Monores®, Novegam®, Oxibron®, Oxyflux®, Prontovent®, Spiropent®, Ventilan®, Ventipulmin®* or *Ventolase®*.

Storage/Stability

The commercially available syrup is colorless and should be stored at room temperature (avoid freezing). The manufacturer warns to replace the safety cap on the bottle when not in use.

Compatibility/Compounding Considerations

No specific information noted.

Dosage Forms/Regulatory Status

VETERINARY-LABELED PRODUCTS:

Clenbuterol HCl Oral Syrup: 72.5 micrograms/mL in 100 mL, 330 mL, 460 mL bottles; *Ventipulmin® Syrup, Aeropulmin® Syrup*; (Rx). FDA-approved for use in horses not intended for use as food.

Extra-label clenbuterol use in food animals is prohibited by federal (USA) law.

The ARCI (Racing Commissioners International) has designated this drug as a class 3 substance. See the appendix for more information.

HUMAN-LABELED PRODUCTS: NONE.

Revisions/References

Monograph revised/updated October 2013.

Barr, C. A., et al. (2013). The effect of chronic clenbuterol administration on mucociliary clearance and repartitioning in adult horses. *Journal of Veterinary Internal Medicine* 27(3): 668-9.
Card, C. (2002). Dystocia in mares. *Large Animal Veterinary Rounds* 2(4).
Ferraz, G. C., et al. (2007). Effect of acute administration of Clenbuterol on athletic performance in horses. *Journal of Equine Veterinary Science* 27(10): 446-9.
Kearns, C. F. & K. H. McKeever (2009). Clenbuterol and the horse revisited. *Veterinary Journal* 182(3): 384-91.
McCafferty, K. (2007). *Nursing's role in equine dystocia*. Proceedings: IVECCS. accessed via Veterinary Information Network; vin.com
Read, J. R., et al. (2012). Effect of prolonged administration of clenbuterol on airway reactivity and sweating in horses with inflammatory airway disease. *American Journal of Veterinary Research* 73(1): 140-5.
Soma, L., et al. (2004). Pharmacokinetics and disposition of clenbuterol in the horse. *J Vet Phamacol Ther* 27: 71-7.

Clindamycin

(klin-da-mye-sin)   Antirobe®, Cleocin®

Lincosamide Antibiotic

Prescriber Highlights

- Lincosamide antibiotic, broad spectrum against many anaerobes, gram-positive aerobic cocci, Toxoplasma, etc.
- Contraindications: Horses, rodents, ruminants, lagomorphs; patients hypersensitive to lincosamides.
- Caution: Liver or renal dysfunction; consider reducing dosage if severe.
- Adverse Effects: gastroenteritis, esophageal injuries possible if "dry pilled", pain at injection site if given IM.

Uses/Indications

There are clindamycin products FDA-approved for use in dogs and cats. The labeled indications for dogs include wounds, abscesses and osteomyelitis caused by *Staphylococcus aureus*. Because clindamycin has excellent activity against most pathogenic anaerobic organisms, it is also used extensively for those infections. Clindamycin is used for a variety of protozoal infections, including toxoplasmosis but CNS and eye levels do not reach effective concentrations. For further information, refer to the Dosage or Pharmacology sections.

Pharmacology/Actions

The lincosamide antibiotics, lincomycin and clindamycin, share mechanisms of action and have similar spectrums of activity, although lincomycin is usually less active against susceptible organisms. Complete cross-resistance occurs between the two drugs; at least partial cross-resistance occurs between the lincosamides and erythromycin. They may act as bacteriostatic or bactericidal agents, depending on the concentration of the drug at the infection site and the susceptibility of the organism. The lincosamides are believed to act by binding to the 50S ribosomal subunit of susceptible bacteria, thereby inhibiting peptide bond formation.

Most aerobic gram-positive cocci are susceptible to the lincosamides (*Strep. faecalis* is not) including Staphylococcus and Streptococci. Clindamycin's use in recurrent pyoderma can be limited by development of resistance; methicillin-resistant staphylococci are usually resistant to clindamycin. Other organisms that are generally susceptible include: *Corynebacterium diphtheriae, Nocardia asteroides,* Erysepelothrix, Toxoplasma, and *Mycoplasma* spp. Anaerobic bacteria that are generally susceptible to the lincosamides include: *Clostridium perfringens, C. tetani* (not *C. difficile*), Bacteroides (including many strains of *B. fragilis*), Fusobacterium, Peptostreptococcus, Actinomyces, and Peptococcus.

Clindamycin has activity against a variety of protozoal organisms, but it may be more suppressive than curative for *Toxoplasma gondii* infections. It can have a delayed onset of action (1-3 days) and drug concentrations may not be high enough to achieve complete efficacy. Clindamycin is not effective against extracellular tachyzoites.

Pharmacokinetics

In dogs, oral bioavailability is about 73%, elimination half-life is reportedly 2-5 hours after oral administration and 10-13 hours after subcutaneous administration. Volume of distribution is about 0.9 L/kg. Half-life may be longer with higher dosages. One study in dogs found a mean half-life of about 4 hours after 5.5 mg/kg PO versus 7-10 hours for 11 mg/kg (Saridomichelakis et al. 2011).

In cats, clindamycin half-life after a dose of 11 mg/kg is about 16 hours (capsules) and 8 hours (liquid). Volume of distribution is approximately 1.6-3 L/kg. Highest levels are found in lungs, liver, spleen, jejunum and colon.

In humans, the drug is rapidly absorbed from the gut and about 90% of the total dose is absorbed. Food decreases the rate of absorption, but not the extent. Peak serum levels are attained about 45-60 minutes after oral dosing. IM administration gives peak levels about 1-3 hours post injection.

Clindamycin is distributed into most tissues. Therapeutic levels are achieved in bone, synovial fluid, bile, pleural fluid, peritoneal fluid, skin, and heart muscle. Clindamycin also penetrates well into abscesses, scar tissue, and white blood cells. CNS levels may only reach 40% of those found in serum if meninges are inflamed. It does not penetrate into the eye at levels required to treat infections. Clindamycin is about 93% bound to plasma proteins. The drug crosses the placenta and can be distributed into milk at concentrations equal to those in plasma.

Clindamycin is partially metabolized in the liver to both active and inactive metabolites. Unchanged drug and metabolites are excreted in the urine, feces, and bile. Half-lives can be prolonged in patients with severe renal or hepatic dysfunction.

Contraindications/Precautions/Warnings

Although there have been case reports of parenteral administration of lincosamides to horses, cattle, and sheep, the lincosamides are considered to be contraindicated for use in rabbits, hamsters, chinchillas, guinea pigs, horses, and ruminants because of serious gastrointestinal effects that may occur, including death. Clindamycin is contraindicated in patients with known hypersensitivity to it or lincomycin.

Clindamycin has been implicated in causing esophagitis and potentially, esophageal strictures in small animals. Avoid dry "pilling" when administering this drug.

Patients with very severe renal and/or hepatic disease should receive the drug with caution and the manufacturer suggests monitoring serum clindamycin levels during high-dose therapy; consider dosage reduction.

Clindamycin use is generally avoided in neonatal small animals.

Adverse Effects

Adverse effects after oral administration reported in dogs and cats include gastroenteritis (emesis, loose stools, and infrequently bloody diarrhea in dogs). There have been case reports of esophageal injuries (esophagitis, strictures) occurring in cats when solid dosage forms were given without food or a water bolus. Cats may occasionally show signs of hypersalivation or lip smacking after oral administration. IM injections reportedly cause pain at the injection site.

C. difficile–associated pseudomembranous colitis has been reported in some species, but does not appear to be a significant risk when clindamycin is used in dogs or cats.

Reproductive/Nursing Safety

Clindamycin crosses the placenta, and cord blood concentrations are approximately 46% of those found in maternal serum. Safe use during pregnancy has not been established, but neither has the drug been implicated in causing teratogenic effects. In humans, the FDA categorizes this drug as category *B* for use during pregnancy (*Animal studies have not yet demonstrated risk to the fetus, but there are no adequate studies in pregnant women; or animal studies have shown an adverse effect, but adequate studies in pregnant women have not demonstrated a risk to the fetus in the first trimester of pregnancy, and there is no evidence of risk in later trimesters.*) In a separate system evaluating the safety of drugs in canine and feline pregnancy (Papich 1989), this drug is categorized as class: *A* (*Probably safe. Although specific studies may not have proved the safety of all drugs in dogs and cats, there are no reports of adverse effects in laboratory animals or women.*)

Because clindamycin is distributed into milk, nursing puppies or kittens of mothers receiving clindamycin may develop diarrhea. However, in humans, the American Academy of Pediatrics considers clindamycin compatible with breastfeeding.

Overdosage/Acute Toxicity

There is little information available regarding overdoses of this drug. In dogs, oral doses of up to 300 mg/kg/day for up to one year did not result in toxicity. Dogs receiving 600 mg/kg/day, developed anorexia, vomiting, and weight loss.

Drug Interactions

The following drug interactions have either been reported or are theoretical in humans or animals receiving clindamycin and may be of significance in veterinary patients. Unless otherwise noted, use together is not necessarily contraindicated, but weigh the potential risks and perform additional monitoring when appropriate.

- **CYCLOSPORINE:** Clindamycin has been reported to reduce levels in humans, but this apparently does not occur in dogs.
- **ERYTHROMYCIN:** *in vitro* antagonism when used with clindamycin; concomitant use should probably be avoided.
- **NEUROMUSCULAR BLOCKING AGENTS** (*e.g.,* **pancuronium**): Clindamycin possesses intrinsic neuromuscular blocking activity and should be used cautiously with other neuromuscular blocking agents.

Laboratory Considerations

- Slight increases in **liver function tests** (AST, ALT, Alk. Phosph.) can occur. There is apparently not any clinical significance associated with these increases.

Doses

- **DOGS:**

  For skin infections (wounds, abscesses), osteomyelitis and dental infections (FDA-approved dosage): 5.5 – 33 mg/kg PO q12h; for osteomyelitis: 11 – 33 mg/kg PO q12h. Treatment may continue for up to 28 days. If no response after 3-4 days, discontinue. (Adapted from label; *Antirobe*®)

Pyoderma, superficial (extra-label): 5.5 mg/ kg PO twice daily or 11 mg/kg PO once daily for 21 days. Fair level of evidence for moderate to high efficacy (Summers et al. 2012). A recently published study evaluated levels in skin homogenates of normal dogs concluded that 11 mg/kg once daily doses were at least equal, if not better, than when given at 5.5. mg/kg twice daily (Saridomi-chelakis et al. 2013).

Pyoderma, deep (extra-label): 11 mg/kg PO q12-24h.

For serious systemic infections (*e.g.,* sepsis); (extra-label): 10 – 15 mg/kg IV q12h. **Note:** Empirical treatment would require an additional antibiotic (*e.g.,* an aminoglycoside, 3rd generation cephalosporin, a carbapenem, etc.) for gram-negative coverage.

For surgical prophylaxis for gram-positive aerobes and anaerobic coverage (extra-label): 5 – 11 mg/kg PO 16-60 minutes preoperatively. (Greene et al. 2006) Additionally, parenteral clindamycin at 10 mg/kg could be given IM 15-30 minutes prior to incision or IV slowly (over 10-30 minutes) so that infusion is completed prior to incision.

For susceptible protozoal infections (anecdotal): Most recommendations for adjunctive treatment for Neospora, Hepatozoon, Babesia or Toxoplasma infections are 12.5 mg PO twice daily for at least two weeks or longer. Often additional drugs are used (*e.g.,* TMP/sulfa, pyrimethamine). However the Companion Animal Parasite Council (CAPC) (www.capcvet.org) recommends dogs with American canine hepatozoonosis be treated with either a triple combination of trimethoprim-sulfadiazine (15 mg/kg PO twice daily), clindamycin (10 mg/kg PO three times daily) and pyrimethamine (0.25 mg/kg PO once daily), or ponazuril (10 mg/kg twice daily) for 14 days followed by 2 years of twice-daily decoquinate administration (10 – 20 mg/kg) (Allen et al. 2011).

■ **CATS:**

For skin infections (wounds, abscesses) and dental infections (FDA-approved dosage): 11 – 33 mg/kg PO once a day (q24h). Do not treat acute infections for more than 3-4 days if no clinical response is seen. Maximum labeled treatment period = 14 days. (Adapted from label; *Antirobe® Aquadrops*)

For refractory infections (extra-label): Up to 33 mg/kg PO q12h.

For serious systemic infections (*e.g.,* sepsis); (extra-label): 10 – 15 mg/kg IV q12h. **Note:** Empirical treatment would require an additional antibiotic (*e.g.,* an aminoglycoside, 3rd generation cephalosporin, a carbapenem, etc.) for gram-negative coverage.

For surgical prophylaxis for gram-positive aerobes and anaerobic coverage (extra-label): 5 – 11 mg/kg PO 16-60 minutes preoperatively (Greene et al. 2006). Additionally, parenteral clindamycin at 10 mg/kg could be given IM 15-30 minutes prior to incision or IV slowly (over 10-30 minutes) so that infusion is completed prior to incision.

For Toxoplasmosis (extra-label): **Note:** Treatment of toxoplasmosis in cats is somewhat controversial and there is presently no strong evidence supporting one treatment regimen over another. The following have been recommended:

a) Clindamycin 12.5 mg/kg PO or IV q12h, or trimethoprim/sulfa 15 mg/kg PO q12h, or azithromycin 10 mg/kg PO q24h for a minimum of 4 weeks. Pyrimethamine 0.25 – 0.5 mg/kg PO q12h is synergistic when combined with sulfonamides. A 5 mL water swallow should be administered after giving clindamycin since esophagitis and esophageal strictures can occur. A CBC should be performed every 2 weeks for detection of myelosuppression in cats treated with sulfonamides or pyrimethamine. (Barrs 2013)

b) To decrease zoonotic risk to susceptible humans by reducing shedding period in cats suspected of toxoplasmosis after fecal exam: Clindamycin 25 – 50 mg/kg PO daily; alternative medications include sulfonamides at 100 mg/kg PO daily, or pyrimethamine at 2 mg/kg daily PO.

For treatment of clinical toxoplasmosis: Clindamycin at 10 mg/kg PO q12h, trimethoprim-sulfonamide combination at 15 mg/kg PO q12h, and azithromycin at 10 mg/kg once daily for at least 28 days. Institute supportive care as needed. Patients with uveitis should receive topical, oral or parenteral glucocorticoids to reduce risk for secondary glaucoma and lens luxations. (Lappin 2004)

■ **FERRETS:**

For susceptible infections (extra-label): 5 – 10 mg/kg PO twice daily. (Williams 2000)

■ **BIRDS:**

For susceptible infections (extra-label):

a) 25 mg/kg PO q8h. (Tully 2002)

b) For mild spore-forming enteric bacterial infections: 50 mg/kg PO q12h for 5-10 days. (Flammer 2006)

■ **REPTILES:**

For susceptible infections (anaerobes); (extra-label):

a) 5 mg/kg PO once daily. (Lewbart 2001)

b) For respiratory infections (anaerobes, mycoplasma): 5 mg/kg PO once daily for 14 days. (Klaphake 2005)

Monitoring

■ Clinical efficacy.

■ Adverse effects; particularly severe diarrhea.

■ Manufacturer recommends doing periodic liver and kidney function tests and blood counts if therapy persists for more than 30 days.

Client Information

■ Used for infections of skin, wounds, and bone, but also useful for Toxoplasmosis.

■ Do not give to horses, rabbits, mice, rats, hamsters, guinea pigs, cattle, sheep, goats or deer as it may cause fatal diarrhea.

■ May give with or without food, but do not "dry pill" or it may cause throat burns. Give a small amount of food or a small bit of water (little over a teaspoonful) after pilling.

■ Very bitter taste; may require disguising in food to get animal to take it.

■ Report any severe, prolonged, or bloody diarrhea to the veterinarian

Chemistry/Synonyms

A semisynthetic derivative of lincomycin, clindamycin is available as the hydrochloride hydrate, phosphate ester, and palmitate hydrochloride. Potency of all three salts is expressed as milligrams of clindamycin. The hydrochloride occurs as a white to practically white, crystalline powder. The phosphate occurs as a white to off-white, hygroscopic crystalline powder. The palmitate HCl occurs as a white to off-white amorphous powder. All may have a faint characteristic odor and are freely soluble in water. With the phosphate, about 400 mg are soluble in one mL of water. Clindamycin has a pK$_a$ of 7.45. The commercially available injection has a pH of 5.5-7.

Clindamycin HCl may also be known as: chlorodeoxylincomycin hydrochloride, (7S)-chloro-7-deoxy-lincomycin hydrochloride, clindamycini hydrochloridum, U-28508, or U-25179E; many trade names are available.

Storage/Stability

Clindamycin capsules and the palmitate powder for oral solution should be stored at room temperature (15-30°C). After reconstitution, the palmitate oral solution (human-product) should not be refrigerated or thickening may occur. It is stable for 2 weeks at room temperature. The veterinary oral solution should be stored at room temperature and has an extended shelf life.

Clindamycin phosphate injection should be stored at room temperature. If refrigerated or frozen, crystals may form which re-solubolize upon warming.

Compatibility/Compounding Considerations

Clindamycin for injection is reportedly **compatible** for at least 24 hours in the following IV infusion solutions: D5W, Dextrose combinations with Ringer's, lactated Ringer's, sodium chloride, D10W, sodium chloride 0.9%, Ringer's injection, and lactated Ringer's injection. Clindamycin for injection is reportedly **compatible** with the following drugs: amikacin sulfate, ampicillin sodium, aztreonam, cefazolin sodium, cefonicid sodium, cefoperazone sodium, cefotaxime sodium, ceftazidime sodium, cefuroxime sodium, cimetidine HCl, gentamicin sulfate, heparin sodium, hydrocortisone sodium succinate, methylprednisolone sodium succinate, magnesium sulfate, meperidine HCl, metoclopramide HCl, metronidazole, morphine sulfate, penicillin G potassium/sodium, piperacillin sodium, potassium chloride, sodium bicarbonate, tobramycin HCl (not in syringes), verapamil HCl, and vitamin B-complex with C.

Drugs that are reportedly **incompatible** with clindamycin include: aminophylline, ciprofloxacin, ranitidine HCl, and ceftriaxone sodium. Compatibility is dependent upon factors such as pH, concentration, temperature, and diluent used; consult specialized references or a hospital pharmacist for more specific information.

Dosage Forms/Regulatory Status

VETERINARY-LABELED PRODUCTS:

Clindamycin (as the HCl) Oral Capsules: 25 mg, 75 mg, 150 mg, 300 mg; *Antirobe*®, generic; (Rx). Depending on label, FDA-approved for use in dogs (only) or dogs and cats. Approved label information for *Antirobe*® can be found at dailymed.nlm.nih.gov

Clindamycin (as the HCl) Oral Tablets: 25 mg, 75 mg, 150 mg; *Clintabs*®; (Rx). FDA-approved for use in dogs.

Clindamycin (as the HCl) Oral Solution 25 mg/mL in 30 mL bottles; *Antirobe*® *Aquadrops*, *Clinsol*®; generic; (Rx). FDA-approved for use in dogs and cats.

HUMAN-LABELED PRODUCTS:

Clindamycin (as the HCl) Oral Capsules: 75 mg, 150 mg, & 300 mg; *Cleocin*®, generic; (Rx)

Clindamycin (as the palmitate HCl) Granules for Oral Solution: 75 mg/5 mL in 100 mL; *Cleocin*® *Pediatric*, generic; (Rx)

Clindamycin (as the Phosphate) Solution Concentrate for Injection: 150 mg/mL in 2 mL, 4 mL, 6 mL & 2 mL, 4 mL and 6 mL vials and 150 mg, 300 mg, 600 mg, and 900 mg in 50 mL with dextrose flexible bags; *Cleocin*®, generic; (Rx)

Also available in topical and vaginal preparations.

Revisions/References

Monograph revised/updated October 2013.

Allen, K. E., et al. (2011). Hepatozoon spp Infections in the United States. *Veterinary Clinics of North America-Small Animal Practice* 41(6): 1221-+.

Barrs, V. (2013). *Feline Toxoplasmosis*. World Small Animal Veterinary Association World Congress Proceedings. accessed via Veterinary Information Network; vin.com

Flammer, K. (2006). *Managing Avian Bacterial Diseases II*. Proceedings: WVC2006. accessed via Veterinary Information Network; vin.com

Greene, C. & S. Jang (2006). Surgical and traumatic wound infections. *Infectious Diseases of the Dog and Cat, 3rd Ed.* C. Greene, Elsevier: 524-31.

Klaphake, E. (2005). *Sneezing turtles and wheezing snakes*. Proceedings: Western Vet Conf. accessed via Veterinary Information Network; vin.com

Lappin, M. (2004). *Toxoplasmosis*. Proceedings: WSAVA World Congress. accessed via Veterinary Information Network; vin.com

Lewbart (2001). *Reptile Formulary*. Proceedings: Atlantic Coast Veterinary Conference. accessed via Veterinary Information Network; vin.com

Saridomichelakis, M. N., et al. (2013). Concentrations of clindamycin hydrochloride in homogenates of normal dog skin when administered at two oral dosage regimens. *Veterinary Quarterly* 33(1): 8-14.

Saridomichelakis, M. N., et al. (2011). Serum pharmacokinetics of clindamycin hydrochloride in normal dogs when administered at two dosage regimens. *Veterinary Dermatology* 22(5): 429-35.

Summers, J. F., et al. (2012). The effectiveness of systemic antimicrobial treatment in canine superficial and deep pyoderma: a systematic review. *Veterinary Dermatology* 23(4): 305-E61.

Tully, T. (2002). *Avian Therapeutic Options*. Proceedings: Western Veterinary Conference. accessed via Veterinary Information Network; vin.com

Williams, B. (2000). Therapeutics in Ferrets. *Vet Clin NA: Exotic Anim Pract* 3:1(Jan): 131-53.

Clodronate

(kloe-**dron**-ayte)   OSPHOS®, Clodronic Acid

Bisphosphonate

Prescriber Highlights

▶ Bisphosphonate approved for clinical signs associated with navicular syndrome in horses.

▶ Adverse effect profile not well established (new drug); most adverse effects noted in field studies occurred within 2 hours of the dose; highest incidence (9%) were discomfort or agitation-related.

▶ Given IM; dose is divided into 3 equal injections. Single-use vial; discard unused drug.

▶ May be re-administered every 3-6 months if initially effective.

Uses/Indications

In horses, clodronate disodium is indicated for the control of clinical signs associated with navicular syndrome in horses (Anon 2014b). Based on a pre-approval study, 75% of treated horses were deemed a treatment success (if the lameness grade in the primarily affected limb improved by at least 1 AAEP grade and there was no worsening of lameness grade in the other forelimb on Day 56). Clinical improvement was most evident at 2 months post-treatment; approximately 65% of horses that responded to initial treatment, maintained their level of improvement through the 6 month evaluation.

A human-labeled (E.U.) intravenous form was used in a study to determine the effects of clodronate (4 mg/kg in 150 mL 0.9% NaCl IV infusion 24-hours post vitamin D3 administration; administration rate not reported) on vitamin D3-induced hypercalcemia in dogs. The authors concluded that clodronate may be useful within the first 24 hours to treat vitamin D3-induced hypercalcemia in dogs, but that further studies are necessary to define toxicity and appropriate dosing. (Ulutas *et al.* 2006)

Liposome-encapsulated clodronate (LCP) is preferentially phagocytosed by macrophages and dendritic cells, which then undergo apoptosis and therefore LCP may be clinically useful for treating certain autoimmune diseases. Research is ongoing to evaluate LCP for the management of immune-mediated hemolytic anemia and malignant histiocytosis in dogs (Whitley *et al.* 2011).

Pharmacology/Actions

Clodronate is a bisphosphonate that inhibits bone resorption by binding to calcium phosphate crystals thereby inhibiting their formation and dissolution, and by directly inhibiting osteoclast cell function. Clodronate's mechanism of action for treating navicular disease is not well understood.

Pharmacokinetics

After IM injection in horses, clodronate disodium is rapidly absorbed and cleared from the plasma. Plasma half-life of the parent compound is relatively fast ($\approx$ 2-3 hours). Like other bisphosphonates, a percentage of bioavailable clodronate is taken up by bone and then slowly excreted over a sustained period of time (months to years). The actual residence time in equine bone has not been established.

Contraindications/Precautions/Warnings

Clodronate is contraindicated in animals with a known hypersensitivity to clodronate or clodronic acid, in pregnant or lactating mares (USA label; see Reproductive/Nursing Safety), or horses to be used for human consumption.

Use with caution in horses <4 years of age as the drug has not been evaluated in this age group. Since bisphosphonates can affect bone, they may affect bone growth in young, growing horses.

As a class, bisphosphonates are renally excreted and may be associated with gastrointestinal and renal toxicity. Use clodronate with caution in patients with existing renal dysfunction or if using with other potentially nephrotoxic drugs (e.g., gentamicin, amikacin, etc.). The equine label states: "Use of bisphosphonates in patients with conditions or diseases affecting renal function is not recommended."

Use with caution in horses with conditions affecting mineral or electrolyte homeostasis (e.g. hyperkalemic periodic paralysis, hypocalcemia, etc.) as bisphosphonates can affect plasma concentrations of electrolytes (e.g., calcium, magnesium and potassium) immediately post-treatment, with effects lasting up to several hours.

Adverse Effects

In pre-approval field studies the following adverse reactions in horses were reported: Within 2 hours of injection: discomfort, agitation, pawing, or signs of colic (reported together; incidence rate 9%); lip licking (5.4%); yawning (4.5%); head shaking (2.7%); and injection site swelling (1.8%). One horse (of 111) develop colic that required treatment and another, hives and pruritus.

Increased bone fragility is possible, especially with long-term use.

Reproductive/Nursing Safety

The equine product label (USA) states: "Bisphosphonates should not be used in pregnant or lactating mares, or mares intended for breeding. The safe use…has not been evaluated in breeding horses or pregnant or lactating mares." Bisphosphonates have been shown to cause fetal developmental abnormalities in laboratory animals and uptake into fetal bone may be greater than into maternal bone creating a possible risk for fetal skeletal or other abnormalities. However, the U.K. label states: "Use only accordingly to the benefit-risk assessment by the responsible veterinarian. Laboratory studies in rats and rabbits have not produced any evidence of teratogenic, fetotoxic or maternotoxic effects." (Anon 2014a)

Although oral bioavailability is likely very low, bisphosphonates may be excreted in milk and absorbed by nursing animals.

Overdosage/Acute Toxicity

Six horses given single doses of 9 mg/kg (5X) IM divided evenly into 5 separate injection sites caused 5 of 6 to show changes in attitude (e.g., agitation, nervousness, pawing, circling, and tail twitching) within 6 minutes of the dose. Four of 6 also showed excessive yawning, flehmen, tongue rolling, head shaking, and head bobbing. All horses developed mild to moderate muscle fasciculations between 2 and 30 minutes post-treatment. By 30 minutes post-treatment, 4 of 6 also developed signs of discomfort and possible abdominal pain including full body stretching, repetitive lying down and rising, and kicking at the abdomen. At approximately 1-hour post-treatment, 1 horse exhibited agitation and clinical signs of colic requiring medical therapy. This horse responded to medical therapy and

was clinically normal at 7-hours post-treatment. Three of 6 developed temporary gait abnormalities that included mild to moderate hypermetria, spasticity, or mild ataxia. Four of 6 developed mildly elevated BUN concentrations by 48-hours post-treatment and one had a creatinine concentration slightly above the reference range (2.0 mg/dL; reference range 0.9-1.9 mg/dL) for 12 hours post-treatment.

Drug Interactions

The following drug interactions have either been reported or are theoretical in humans or animals receiving clodronate and may be of significance in veterinary patients. Unless otherwise noted, use together is not necessarily contraindicated, but weigh the potential risks and perform additional monitoring when appropriate.

- **AMINOGLYCOSIDES:** Potential for additive effect in lowering serum calcium concentrations and increasing risk for nephrotoxicity. UK label states; "…should not be given for 72 hours after administration with clodronic acid (clodronate)."
- **DIGOXIN:** May increase digoxin levels. Use together with caution.
- **FUROSEMIDE (or other loop diuretics):** Increased risk of hypocalcemia. Use together with caution.
- **PHENYLBUTAZONE:** In a pre-approval pilot study, 3 of 6 horses had post-treatment elevations in BUN above the reference range. Clinical significance, if any is unclear.
- **TETRACYCLINES:** UK label states: "medications such as tetracyclines that can reduce serum calcium should not be given for 72 hours after administration with clodronic acid (clodronate)."

Laboratory Considerations

- No specific information noted.

Doses

- **HORSES:**

  For the control of clinical signs associated with navicular syndrome (labeled dose; FDA-approved): 1.8 mg/kg IM (up to a maximum dose of 900 mg per horse). Divide the total volume equally and administer into three separate injection sites. If no response to initial therapy, re-evaluate patient. In horses that initially respond, but do not maintain clinical improvement for 6 months it may be re-administered at 3-6 month intervals based on recurrence of clinical signs. In horses that respond initially and maintain clinical improvement for 6 months, re-administer after clinical signs recur. (Adapted from label—OSPHOS®)

Monitoring

- Efficacy.
- Adverse effects.

Client Information

- Watch horse for at least two hours after treatment for agitation, signs of colic, and other abnormal behavior, such as head shaking and lip licking. If horse seems uncomfortable or nervous, or experiences cramping, hand-walk the horse for 15 minutes. Contact veterinarian if signs don't resolve or if the horse displays other abnormal symptoms.

Chemistry/Synonyms

Clodronate disodium, a non-amino, chloro-containing bisphosphonate occurs as a white or almost white, crystalline powder. It is freely soluble in water, practically insoluble in alcohol, and slightly soluble in methyl alcohol. A 5% solution in water has a pH of 3-4.5. Sodium hydroxide is used in the equine product to adjust pH. Clodronic acid is also used to describe the active entity in some research or products. 60 mg of clodronate disodium is equivalent to 51 mg of clodronic acid.

Clodronate disodium may also be known as 177501, BM-06.011,

ZK-00091106, clodronate sodium, sodium clodronate, dichloromethane diphosphonate, or dichloromethylene diphosphonate disodium.

Storage/Stability

Store at controlled room temperature 25°C (77°F) with excursions between 15°-30°C (59°-86°F) permitted. Discard unused vial contents; single use vial and does not contain a preservative.

Compatibility/Compounding Considerations

Do not mix the IM injection with other medications or solutions.

Dosage Forms/Regulatory Status

VETERINARY-LABELED PRODUCTS:

Clodronate Disodium Injection 60 mg/mL, 15 mL/single-use vial; OSPHOS®; (Rx). FDA-approved (NADA 141-427) for use in horses not intended for human consumption. The UK label states: "Treated horses may never be slaughtered for human consumption."

HUMAN-LABELED PRODUCTS:

None in the USA; both injectable and oral products may be available elsewhere.

Revisions/References

Monograph written July 2014.

Anon (2014a). OSPHOS® Label Information (U.K.), Dechra Veterinary Products Limited.

Anon (2014b). OSPHOS® Label Information (USA), Dechra Veterinary Products.

Ulutas, B., et al. (2006). Clodronate treatment of vitamin D-induced hypercalcemia in dogs. *J. Vet. Emerg. Crit. Care* 16(2): 141-5.

Whitley, N. T. & M. J. Day (2011). Immunomodulatory drugs and their application to the management of canine immune-mediated disease. *Journal of Small Animal Practice* 52(2): 70-85.

Clofazimine

(kloe-fa-zi-meen)   Lamprene®

Antimycobacterial Antibiotic

Prescriber Highlights

▶ May be difficult for veterinarians to obtain & accurately dose.

▶ Antimycobacterial antibiotic that may be used as part of multi-drug therapy for leprosy-like or M. avium-related diseases in small animals.

▶ Very limited clinical experience & documentation supporting its use in veterinary patients.

▶ Stains skin, eyes, bodily fluids and excreta. Dose limiting gastrointestinal adverse effects.

▶ Treatment usually must continue for weeks to months.

Uses/Indications

In small animals, clofazimine is sometimes used as part of multi-drug therapy against mycobacterial diseases, primarily leprosy-like or *M. avium*-related disease states.

In humans, clofazimine is used primarily as part of a multi-drug regimen in the treatment of all forms of leprosy (with rifampin and dapsone), or the treatment of Mycobacterium avium complex (MAC) (with at least two of the following agents: clarithromycin or azithromycin, rifampin or rifabutin, and ethambutol). It has also been used in some treatment regimens for Crohn's disease, pyoderma gangrenosum, etc.

Pharmacology/Actions

Clofazimine binds to mycobacterial DNA and inhibits growth. It is considered to be slowly bactericidal against susceptible organisms. Clofazimine has activity against a variety of mycobacteria including: *M. leprae, M. tuberculosis, M. avium* complex (MAC), *M. bovis*, and *M. chelonei*. Resistance is thought to occur only rarely; cross-resistance with dapsone or rifampin apparently does not occur. Clofazimine may have some antileishmanial activity. Clofazimine has antiinflammatory and immunosuppressive effects, but the mechanisms of action for these effects are not understood.

Pharmacokinetics

Clofazimine's pharmacokinetics have apparently not been determined in domestic animals. In humans, the microcrystalline form of the drug is variably absorbed after oral administration; bioavailability ranges from 45-70%. Food enhances absorption but increasing the dosage decreases the percentage absorbed. Clofazimine is highly lipid soluble and is distributed primarily to lipid tissue and the reticuloendothelial system. Throughout the body macrophages take up clofazimine. The drug crosses the placenta and is distributed into milk, but does not apparently cross into the CNS or CSF. Clofazimine is retained in the body for a long period; its elimination half-life is at least 70 days long. Bile excretion may be responsible for the majority of the drug's excretion, but excretion in sputum, sebum, and sweat may also contribute.

Contraindications/Precautions/Warnings

It is suggested that clofazimine be used with caution in patients with pre-existing gastrointestinal conditions such as diarrhea or abdominal pain.

Adverse Effects

There is very limited clinical experience with this medication in domestic animals and its adverse effect profile is not well documented. Apparently, the skin, eye, and excretion discoloration (described below) also occurs in animals. Gastrointestinal effects have been reported. One case of a dog receiving clofazimine and rifampin to treat canine leproid granuloma resulted in hepatotoxicity. There is a report of one cat treated with clofazimine developing a photosensitization reaction (Bennett 2007).

In humans, clofazimine is usually well tolerated, particularly at dosages of 100 mg/day or less. The most troubling adverse effect in many human patients is the dose-related discoloration (pink to brownish-black) of skin, eyes, and body fluids, which occurs in most patients. This discoloration can persist for months to years after clofazimine has been discontinued. In dosages greater than 100 mg/day, gastrointestinal effects (pain, nausea, vomiting, diarrhea) become more likely and often limit the dosage that can be administered. Other adverse effects (CNS, increased liver enzymes, etc.) are reported in less than 1% of patients receiving the drug.

Reproductive/Nursing Safety

In humans, the FDA categorizes clofazimine as a category *C* drug for use during pregnancy (*Animal studies have shown an adverse effect on the fetus, but there are no adequate studies in humans; or there are no animal reproduction studies and no adequate studies in humans*). Very large doses (12-25X) demonstrated no teratogenic effects in rats or rabbits, but some effects were noted in mice. The World Health Organization (WHO) states that the drug is safe for use during pregnancy when used as part of one of their treatment protocols for leprosy.

Clofazimine does enter maternal milk and skin discoloration of nursing offspring can occur.

Overdosage/Acute Toxicity

Very limited data is available; the LD_{50} for rabbits is 3.3 g/kg and is greater than 5 g/kg in mice, rats, and guinea pigs. Treatment, if required, would include gut emptying and supportive care. Contact an animal poison control center for additional guidance.

Drug Interactions

The following drug interactions have either been reported or are theoretical in humans or animals receiving clofazimine and may be of significance in veterinary patients. Unless otherwise noted, use together is not necessarily contraindicated, but weigh the potential risks and perform additional monitoring when appropriate.

▪ **ISONIAZID:** May reduce the clofazimine levels in the skin and increase the amounts in plasma and urine; clinical significance is unclear.

- **DAPSONE:** There is sketchy evidence that suggests dapsone may reduce the antiinflammatory effects of clofazimine; clinical significance is unclear.

Laboratory Considerations
- No clofazimine-related laboratory interactions noted.

Doses
- **DOGS:**

  For *M. avium intracellularae* complex infections, or opportunistic mycobacteriosis (extra-label): 4 – 8 mg/kg PO once a day for 4 weeks usually as part of a multi-drug protocol. (Greene et al. 1998)

- **CATS:**

  For *M. avium intracellularae* complex infections, feline leprosy or opportunistic mycobacteriosis (extra-label): 4 – 8 mg/kg PO once a day or 25 – 50 mg per cat once a day for 4 weeks usually as part of a multi-drug protocol.

- **BIRDS:**

  For avian mycobacteriosis (extra-label): Treatment protocols include: 1) rifampin 45 mg/kg, ethambutol 30 mg/kg and clofazimine 6 mg/kg PO once daily; or 2) ethambutol 20 mg/kg q12h, cycloserine 5 mg/kg q12h, enrofloxacin 15 mg/kg q12h, and clofazimine 1.5 mg/kg PO q24h (recommended regime for raptors). Regular monitoring of fecal samples is needed; antifungal medication may be required. Surgery for discrete nodules may be curative. (Turner 2008)

Monitoring
- Efficacy against mycobacterial disease.
- Adverse effects (primarily GI, but consider monitoring hepatic function in dogs).

Client Information
- Unless otherwise instructed give this medication with food.
- This medication may cause your animal's skin to turn color (usually pink, but from red to orange to brown). It may also cause discoloring of tears, urine, feces, and other body fluids to a brownish-black color. This discoloration may persist for many months after therapy is concluded.

Chemistry/Synonyms
Clofazimine, a phenazine dye antimycobacterial agent, occurs as an odorless or nearly odorless, reddish-brown powder that is highly insoluble in water. In room temperature alcohol, clofazimine's solubility is 1 mg/mL.

Clofazimine may also be known as: B-663, G-30320, NSC-141046, Chlofazimine, *Clofozine*®, *Hansepran*®, *Lamcoin*®, *Lamprene*®, or *Lampren*®.

Storage/Stability
Clofazimine oral capsules should be stored in tight containers, protected from moisture at temperatures less than 30°C.

Compatibility/Compounding Considerations
The commercially available capsules are a micronized form of the drug in a wax matrix base; it may be difficult to obtain an accurate dosage for small animals. It is suggested to contact a compounding pharmacist for advice.

Dosage Forms/Regulatory Status
VETERINARY-LABELED PRODUCTS: NONE.

HUMAN-LABELED PRODUCTS: NONE.

In November 2004, clofazimine (*Lamprene*®) became available in the USA only on a limited basis. The FDA now restricts its use to physicians enrolled as investigators under an Investigational New Drug (IND) for treating Hansen's Disease (Leprosy) or multi-drug resistant tuberculosis. Its status for use in veterinary patients is uncertain at the time of writing (2013); contact the FDA Center for Veterinary Medicine (see appendix) for more information.

Revisions/References
Monograph revised/updated October 2013.
Bennett, S. L. (2007). Photosensitisation induced by clofazimine in a cat. *Australian Veterinary Journal* 85(9): 375-80.
Greene, C. & A. Watson (1998). Antimicrobial Drug Formulary. *Infectious Diseases of the Dog and Cat.* C. Greene. Philadelphia, WB Saunders: 790-919.
Turner, K. (2008). *A review of avian mycobacteriosis.* Proceedings: AAVAC-UEP. accessed via Veterinary Information Network; vin.com

Clomipramine HCl

(kloe-mi-pra-meen)   Clomicalm®, Anafranil®

Tricyclic Antidepressant

Prescriber Highlights
▶ Tricyclic antidepressant used in dogs & cats for obsessive-compulsive disorders, but may be useful for other behavior disorders.
▶ Used in birds to treat feather picking.
▶ Caution: Seizure disorders, liver disease, cardiac rate/rhythm disorders, urinary retention or reduced GI motility.
▶ Not a teratogen, but may affect testicular size/function.
▶ Adverse Effects: Emesis, diarrhea, sedation, anticholinergic effects (dry mouth, tachycardia, etc.); cats may be more sensitive than dogs.

Uses/Indications
In veterinary medicine, clomipramine is used primarily in dogs as a treatment for obsessive-compulsive disorders (ritualistic stereotypical behaviors) and may be useful for dominance aggression and anxiety (separation).

Clomipramine may also be useful in cats, particularly for behaviors such as urine spraying. One prospective, double-blinded controlled study in cats with psychogenic alopecia comparing clomipramine (0.5 mg/kg PO daily) versus placebo showed no statistic differences in study parameters (Mertens et al. 2006).

In small animals, clomipramine may be useful as adjunctive treatment for neuropathic pain, but evidence documenting efficacy is currently lacking.

Clomipramine has been used to treat feather picking in birds.

Pharmacology/Actions
While the exact mechanism of action of tricyclic antidepressants is not completely understood, it is believed that their most significant effects result from their action in preventing the reuptake of norepinephrine and serotonin at the neuronal membrane. Clomipramine is predominantly an inhibitor of serotonin (5-HT) reuptake, but it also has effects on other neurotransmitters. Clomipramine's active metabolite, desmethylclomipramine has primarily noradrenergic activity and, at least in humans, may be responsible for the majority of the drug's adverse effects.

Pharmacokinetics
In dogs, after absorption, clomipramine is rapidly converted in the liver to its active metabolite desmethylclomipramine. Both the parent drug and the active metabolite are highly bound to plasma proteins (96%). Repeated oral dosing increases clomipramine concentrations but not desmethylclomipramine. The presence of food decreases the area under the curve for the parent compound by about 25% but not the metabolite. Giving without food probably is not necessary for efficacy. After a single dose in dogs, the elimination half-life of clomipramine averages 7 hours and desmethylclomipramine averages about 2 hours, but a wide variability can be seen between patients. When dosed for 28 days, half-life averaged

5.7 hours (range from 1.5-9 hours) for clomipramine and 2.1 hours (1.4-4.3 hours) for the active metabolite (Hewson et al. 1998).

Cats appear to metabolize clomipramine more slowly than dogs and wide interpatient variability in pharmacokinetic parameters have been shown after single oral doses. Male cats may metabolize clomipramine more slowly than female cats. In a limited (6 subject) pharmacokinetic study, oral bioavailability averaged 90%.

In humans, the drug is well absorbed from the GI tract but a substantial first pass effect reduces its systemic bioavailability to approximately 50%. The presence of food in the gut apparently does not significantly alter its absorption. Clomipramine is highly lipophilic and widely distributed throughout the body with an apparent volume of distribution of 17 L/kg. The drug crosses the placenta and into maternal milk. Plasma levels have been detected in nursing babies of mothers taking the drug. Both clomipramine and its active metabolite (desmethylclomipramine) cross the blood-brain barrier and significant levels are found in the brain. It should be noted that although therapeutic effects may take several weeks to be seen, adverse effects can occur early on in treatment. Clomipramine is metabolized principally in the liver to several metabolites including desmethylclomipramine, which is active. About two-thirds of these metabolites are eliminated in the urine and the rest in the feces. After a single dose, the elimination half-life of clomipramine averages 32 hours and desmethylclomipramine averages 69 hours, but there remains wide interpatient variation.

Contraindications/Precautions/Warnings

These agents are contraindicated if prior sensitivity has been noted with any other tricyclic. Concomitant use with monoamine oxidase inhibitors is generally contraindicated. As aged cheeses can contain high levels of tyramine, avoid giving to animals receiving clomipramine.

In humans, tricyclic antidepressants may lower seizure threshold. Use with caution in animals with preexisting seizure disorders. Because of their anticholinergic effects, use with caution in patients with decreased GI motility, urinary retention, cardiac rhythm disturbances, or increased intraocular pressure. One study in dogs however, showed little effect on intra-ocular pressure or cardiac rhythm. In humans, tricyclic antidepressants have caused hepatic abnormalities. Baseline and annual monitoring of liver enzymes is suggested for animals receiving clomipramine long-term. Tricyclics should be used cautiously in patients with hyperthyroidism or those that are receiving thyroid supplementation as there may be an increased risk of cardiac rhythm abnormalities developing.

Adverse Effects

The primary adverse effects reported thus far with the use of clomipramine in dogs are anorexia, emesis, diarrhea, dry mouth, elevation of liver enzymes, and sedation/lethargy/depression. Cardiac effects such as tachycardia secondary to the drugs anticholinergic activity may also result. One case of a dog developing pancreatitis after receiving clomipramine has been published (Kook et al. 2009).

Cats have been reported to be more susceptible than dogs to development of adverse effects including anticholinergic effects (dry mouth, mydriasis, urine retention, constipation), sedation, and diarrhea. This may be the result of slower elimination of the desmethyl metabolite in cats.

Adverse effects reported in birds include ataxia, drowsiness and regurgitation.

Reproductive/Nursing Safety

No teratogenic effects were noted in mice and rats given clomipramine at dosages of up 20X usual maximum human dosage. Data in other domestic species appear to be lacking. The manufacturer warns not to use in breeding male dogs as high dose (12.5X) toxicity studies demonstrated testicular atrophy.

In humans, the FDA categorizes this drug as category *C* for use during pregnancy (*Animal studies have shown an adverse effect on the fetus, but there are no adequate studies in humans; or there are no animal reproduction studies and no adequate studies in humans.*)

Overdosage/Acute Toxicity

Clomipramine has a narrow margin of safety; significant clinical signs can be seen at or slightly above therapeutic range (at 2 – 3 mg/kg, APCC database). Overdosage with tricyclics can be life-threatening (arrhythmias, seizures, cardiorespiratory collapse). In dogs, lethal doses are approximately between 50 – 100 mg/kg/day PO (12.5-25X recommended dose).

There were 344 single agent exposures to clomipramine reported to the ASPCA Animal Poison Control Center (APCC) during 2009-2013. Of the 276 dogs, 110 were symptomatic with lethargy/sedation (61%), tachycardia (21%), vomiting (16%), vocalization (15%) and ataxia (13%) being the most common clinical signs. Of the 66 cats, 29 were symptomatic with 52% mydriatic, 34% lethargic, 34% tachycardic, 24% ataxic, 24% vocalizing, 17% vocalizing and 14% agitated.

Clomipramine toxicity may potentially be amenable to treatment with intravenous lipid emulsion "lipid rescue"; it is strongly recommended to contact an animal poison control center for further treatment information and guidance.

Drug Interactions

The following drug interactions have either been reported or are theoretical in humans or animals receiving clomipramine and may be of significance in veterinary patients. Unless otherwise noted, use together is not necessarily contraindicated, but weigh the potential risks and perform additional monitoring when appropriate.

- **ANTICHOLINERGIC AGENTS:** Because of additive effects, use with clomipramine cautiously.
- **BUTYREPHENONE ANTIPSYCHOTIC AGENTS** (*e.g.,* **haloperidol**): There is a case report (Starkey et al. 2008) of a macaw developing extrapyramidal side effects after it had received a long acting haloperidol injection and then subsequently received clomipramine.
- **CIMETIDINE:** May inhibit tricyclic antidepressant metabolism and increase the risk of toxicity.
- **CISAPRIDE:** Increased risk for prolonged QT interval.
- **CLONIDINE:** May cause increased blood pressure.
- **CNS DEPRESSANTS:** Because of additive effects, use with clomipramine cautiously.
- **CYPROHEPTADINE:** May antagonize the effects of antagonize the effects of SSRIs (*e.g.,* fluoxetine, paroxetine, etc.), tricyclic antidepressants (*e.g.,* clomipramine, amitriptyline, etc.) and tramadol.
- **MEPERIDINE, PENTAZOCINE, DEXTROMETHORPHAN:** Increased risk for serotonin syndrome.
- **MONOAMINE OXIDASE INHIBITORS** (including **amitraz** and possibly, **selegiline**): Concomitant use (within 14 days) with monoamine oxidase inhibitors is generally contraindicated (serotonin syndrome).
- **QUINIDINE:** Increased risk for QTc interval prolongation and tricyclic adverse effects.
- **RIFAMPIN:** May decrease tricyclic blood levels.
- **SSRIs** (*e.g.,* **fluoxetine, paroxetine, sertraline**, etc.): Increased risk for serotonin syndrome. In dogs, if switching from clomipramine to an SSRI, a 3-4 day washout period has been recommended (Trepanier 2013).
- **SYMPATHOMIMETIC AGENTS:** Use in combination with sympathomimetic agents may increase the risk of cardiac effects (arrhythmias, hypertension, hyperpyrexia).

- **TRAMADOL:** Increased risk for serotonin syndrome. Veterinary clinical significance is not known, but one source states that monoamine oxidase inhibitors (selegiline), tricyclic antidepressants (*e.g.*, amitriptyline, clomipramine), selective serotonin reuptake inhibitors (*e.g.*, fluoxetine, paroxetine), and SNRIs (venlafaxine) should not be administered concurrently with tramadol (KuKanich 2013).

Laboratory Considerations

- **ECG:** Tricyclics can widen QRS complexes, prolong PR intervals and invert or flatten T-waves on ECG.
- **METAPYRONE TEST:** The response to metapyrone may be decreased by clomipramine.
- **GLUCOSE, BLOOD:** Tricyclics may alter (increase or decrease) blood glucose levels.
- **THYROID TESTS:** Clomipramine may decrease T3, T4 and free T4 levels in dogs and cats.

Doses

- **DOGS:**

  For adjunctive treatment of behavioral conditions:

  a) Labeled Dose (FDA-approved): 2 – 4 mg/kg once daily or divided twice daily PO. (Label directions; *Clomicalm®*)

  b) Extra-label Dosage: Recommendations vary somewhat, most range from 1 – 2 mg/kg PO twice daily initially and eventually up to 3 mg/kg PO once to twice daily. Dosages are generally started at the low end and are increased gradually (i.e., every 2 weeks) until efficacy is noted or limited by adverse effects. Up to 8 weeks of treatment are required to determine efficacy. When being used for situational anxiety/phobias, many recommend using in conjunction with a *prn* benzodiazepine (*e.g.*, alprazolam). When behavioral modification treatment efficacy is established, dosages may be reduced in many patients. Discontinuation of the drug should be done gradually, preferably over several weeks.

- **CATS:**

  For adjunctive treatment of behavioral conditions (extra-label): Dosage recommendations range from 0.25 – 1 mg/kg PO once daily. This often translates into a dose of 2.5 – 5 mg per cat PO once daily. As per dogs, dosages are gradually increased and gradually discontinued.

- **BIRDS:**

  For adjunctive treatment of feather picking (extra-label): Reported dosages range from 0.5 – 9 mg/kg PO q12-24h. (Siebert 2007)

Monitoring

- Clinical efficacy.
- Adverse Effects: Baseline liver function tests; EKG.

Client Information

- May be given with or without food; if patient vomits from the medication, give with food.
- Works best when used with behavior therapy. May take several days to weeks to determine if the drug is effective.
- Most common side effects are: drowsiness/sleepiness, dry mouth and constipation; be sure your animal has access to water.
- Rare side effects that can be serious: abnormal bleeding or fever, seizures, very fast or irregular heartbeat. Contact your veterinarian immediately if you see any of these.
- Overdoses can be very serious; keep out of the reach of animals and children.
- If your animal wore a flea collar in the past two weeks, let your veterinarian know and don't use a new flea collar without your veterinarian's OK.

Chemistry/Synonyms

A dibenzazepine-derivative tricyclic antidepressant, clomipramine HCl occurs as a white to off-white crystalline powder and is freely soluble in water.

Clomipramine HCl may also be known as: chlorimipramine hydrochloride, clomipramini hydrochloridum, G-34586, monochlorimipramine hydrochloride, *Clofranil®*, *Clomicalm®*, *Clopram®*, *Clopress®*, *Equinorm®*, *Hydiphen®*, *Maronil®*, *Novo-Clopamine®*, *Placil®*, *Tranquax®*, or *Zoiral®*.

Storage/Stability

The commercially available veterinary tablets should be stored in a dry place at controlled room temperature (15-30°C) in the original closed container. The (human label) capsules should be stored at temperatures less than 30°C in tight containers and protected from moisture. An expiration date of 3 years from the date of manufacture is assigned to the commercially available capsules.

Compatibility/Compounding Considerations

No specific information noted.

Dosage Forms/Regulatory Status

VETERINARY-LABELED PRODUCTS:

Clomipramine HCl Oral Tablets: 5 mg, 20 mg, 40 mg, & 80 mg; FDA-approved for dogs. *Clomicalm®*; (Rx)

The ARCI (Racing Commissioners International) has designated this drug as a class 2 substance. See the appendix for more information.

HUMAN-LABELED PRODUCTS:

Clomipramine Oral Capsules: 25 mg, 50 mg, & 75 mg; *Anafranil®*; generic; (Rx)

Revisions/References

Monograph revised/updated October 2013.

Hewson, C. J., et al. (1998). The pharmacokinetics of clomipramine and desmethylclomipramine in dogs: parameter estimates following a single oral dose and 28 consecutive daily oral doses of clomipramine. *J. Vet. Pharmacol. Ther.* 21(3): 214-22.

Kook, P. H., et al. (2009). Pancreatitis associated with clomipramine administration in a dog. *Journal of Small Animal Practice* 50(2): 95-8.

KuKanich, B. (2013). Outpatient Oral Analgesics in Dogs and Cats Beyond Nonsteroidal Antiinflammatory Drugs: An Evidence-based Approach. *Vet Clin Small Anim* 43: 1109-25.

Mertens, P., et al. (2006). The effects of clomipramine hydrochloride in cats with psychogenic alopecia: a prospective study. *J Am Anim Hosp Assoc* 42.

Siebert, L. (2007). Pharmacotherapy for behavioral disorders in pet birds. *Journal of Exotic Pet Medicine* 16(1): 30-7.

Starkey, S. R., et al. (2008). Extrapyramidal Side Effects in a Blue and Gold Macaw (Ara ararauna) Treated With Haloperidol and Clomipramine. *Journal of Avian Medicine and Surgery* 22(3): 234-9.

Trepanier, L. A. (2013). Applying Pharmacokinetics to Veterinary Clinical Practice. *Veterinary Clinics of North America-Small Animal Practice* 43(5): 1013-+.

Clonazepam

(kloe-na-ze-pam)   Klonopin®

Benzodiazepine

Prescriber Highlights

▶ Benzodiazepine anticonvulsant, used primarily as adjunctive therapy for short-term treatment of epilepsy in dogs & for longer-term adjunctive treatment of epilepsy in cats; may also be used as an anxiolytic particularly when a longer-acting benzodiazepine is desired.

▶ Contraindications: Hypersensitivity to benzodiazepines, narrow angle glaucoma, significant liver disease. May exacerbate myasthenia gravis.

▶ If using for seizures, discontinue gradually.

▶ Adverse Effects: Sedation & ataxia most prevalent; Cats: Possible hepatic necrosis, but thought less likely to occur than with diazepam.

▶ Dogs: Tolerance to efficacy may occur (over a few weeks.)

▶ Controlled substance (C-IV).

Uses/Indications

Clonazepam is used primarily as a short-term adjunctive anticonvulsant for the treatment of epilepsy in dogs. It has been considered as long-term adjunctive therapy in dogs not controlled with other, more standard therapies, but like diazepam, tolerance tends to develop in a few weeks of treatment. It can also be used as an anxiolytic agent or as a muscle relaxant.

Clonazepam has been used as an anxiolytic and in the treatment of epilepsy in cats. The availability of oral dispersible tablets (ODT) in strengths from 0.125 mg may make dosing in cats easier than with other dosage forms.

Pharmacology/Actions

The subcortical levels (primarily limbic, thalamic, and hypothalamic) of the CNS are depressed by diazepam and other benzodiazepines thereby producing the anxiolytic, sedative, skeletal muscle relaxant, and anticonvulsant effects that are seen. The exact mechanism of action is unknown, but postulated mechanisms include: antagonism of serotonin, increased release of and/or facilitation of gamma-aminobutyric acid (GABA) activity, and diminished release or turnover of acetylcholine in the CNS. Benzodiazepine specific receptors have been located in the mammalian brain, kidney, liver, lung, and heart. In all species studied, receptors are lacking in the white matter.

Pharmacokinetics

In dogs, clonazepam's oral bioavailability is variable (20-60%) but absorption is rapid. Protein binding is about 82% and the drug rapidly crosses into the CNS. Clonazepam exhibits saturation kinetics in dogs as elimination rates are dose dependent.

In humans, the drug is well absorbed from the GI tract, crosses the blood-brain barrier and placenta and is metabolized in the liver to several metabolites that are excreted in the urine. Peak serum levels occur about 3 hours after oral dosing. Half-lives range from 19-40 hours.

Contraindications/Precautions/Warnings

Clonazepam is contraindicated in patients that are hypersensitive to it or other benzodiazepines, have significant liver dysfunction, or acute narrow angle glaucoma. Benzodiazepines have been reported to exacerbate myasthenia gravis.

Clonazepam orally dispersible tablets (ODT) that contain xylitol (unknown quantity) should be used with caution in dogs.

Do not confuse clonazepam with clonidine, or other benzodiaz-epines (*e.g.*, clorazepate). Consider writing orders and prescriptions using tall man letters; clonazePAM.

Adverse Effects

There is very limited information on the adverse effect profile of this drug in domestic animals. Sedation (or excitement) and ataxia may occur. Clonazepam has been reported to cause a multitude of various adverse effects in humans. Some of the more significant effects include increased salivation, hypersecretion in upper respiratory passages, GI effects (vomiting, constipation, diarrhea, etc.), transient elevations of liver enzymes, and hematologic effects (anemia, leukopenia, thrombocytopenia, etc.). Tolerance (usually noted after several weeks) to the anticonvulsant effects has been reported in dogs.

In cats, clonazepam may cause sedation, ataxia and possibly, acute hepatic necrosis.

Patients discontinuing clonazepam, particularly those who have been on the drug chronically at high dosages, should be tapered off or status epilepticus may be precipitated. Vomiting and diarrhea may occur during this process.

Reproductive/Nursing Safety

Safe use during pregnancy has not been established; adverse teratogenic effects have been seen in rabbits and rats. In humans, the FDA categorizes this drug as category *D* for use during pregnancy (*There is evidence of human fetal risk, but the potential benefits from the use of the drug in pregnant women may be acceptable despite its potential risks.*)

It is not known if clonazepam drug is excreted into milk, but several other benzodiazepines have been documented to enter milk. Theoretically, accumulation of the drug and its metabolites to toxic levels are possible; use with caution in nursing dams.

Overdosage/Acute Toxicity

Overdoses commonly cause sedation, depression, and ataxia. Some animals will exhibit paradoxical signs, such as hyperactivity, disorientation, and vocalization. Emesis is generally not indicated. With mild to moderate overdoses, animals can often be monitored at home, as long as the animal is rousable and does not show paradoxical signs. Animals should be confined and stimulation kept to a minimum. Paradoxical excitation can be treated with a mild sedative, such as diphenhydramine.

There were 1335 single agent exposures to clonazepam reported to the ASPCA Animal Poison Control Center (APCC) during 2009-2013. Of the 1214 dogs, 725 were symptomatic with 74% being ataxic, 33% sedated, 21% agitated and 11% vomiting. Of the 119 cats, 85 were symptomatic with 85% being ataxic, 27% agitated and 27% sedated.

Massive overdoses can lead to respiratory depression or hypotension. Flumazenil can be used to reverse respiratory depression or severe depression. The half-life of flumazenil is short and the animal may require multiple doses.

Drug Interactions

The following drug interactions have either been reported or are theoretical in humans or animals receiving clonazepam and may be of significance in veterinary patients. Unless otherwise noted, use together is not necessarily contraindicated, but weigh the potential risks and perform additional monitoring when appropriate.

■ **ANTIFUNGALS, AZOLE (itraconazole, ketoconazole, etc.):** May increase clonazepam levels.

■ **CIMETIDINE:** May decrease metabolism of benzodiazepines.

■ **CNS DEPRESSANT DRUGS:** If clonazepam administered with other CNS depressant agents (**barbiturates, narcotics, anesthetics,** etc.) additive effects may occur.

■ **ERYTHROMYCIN:** May decrease the metabolism of benzodiazepines.

- **PHENOBARBITAL:** May decrease clonazepam concentrations.
- **PHENYTOIN:** May decrease clonazepam concentrations.
- **PROPANTHELINE:** May decrease clonazepam concentrations.
- **RIFAMPIN:** May induce hepatic microsomal enzymes and decrease the pharmacologic effects of benzodiazepines.

Laboratory Considerations

- Benzodiazepines may decrease the thyroidal uptake of I^{123} or I^{131}.

Doses

- **DOGS:**

  As an anxiolytic (extra-label): Dosage recommendations vary considerably. Most range from 0.1 – 1 mg/kg PO up to 2-3 times per day, but some recommend up to q6h dosing or dosages up to 2 mg/kg PO q12h. Generally dosages are started near the low end and increased if necessary. If discontinuing after long-term use, do so gradually.

  As an adjunctive medication in the treatment of seizures or sleep disorders (extra-label): Most dosage recommendations range from 0.5 – 1 mg/kg PO 2-3 times per day, but some recommend up to q6h dosing or dosages up to 2 mg/kg PO q12h. Generally dosages are started near the low end and increased if necessary. If discontinuing after long-term use, do so gradually.

- **CATS:**

  As an anxiolytic (extra-label): Dosage recommendations vary considerably. Most range from 0.02 – 0.25 mg/kg PO up to 2 times per day. A 4 kg cat receiving one 0.125 mg oral dispersible tablet would receive a dosage of approximately 0.03 mg/kg. Generally dosages are started near the low end and increased if necessary. If discontinuing after long-term use, do so gradually.

  As an adjunctive medication in the treatment of seizures (extra-label): Dosage recommendations vary considerably. Most range from 0.02 – 0.5 mg/kg PO up to 2 times per day. A 4 kg cat receiving one 0.125 mg oral dispersible tablet would receive a dosage of approximately 0.03 mg/kg. Generally dosages are started near the low end and increased if necessary. If discontinuing after long-term use, do so gradually.

Monitoring

- Efficacy.
- Adverse effects.
- The therapeutic blood level has been reported as 0.015 – 0.07 micrograms/mL but is not routinely monitored in veterinary patients.
- Cats: Liver function tests.

Client Information

- Used both for epilepsy and as a tranquilizer.
- When using for thunderstorm phobias or other triggers (*e.g.*, owner separation, etc.) that upset your animal try to give it about an hour before the event or trigger. Works best along with behavior therapy.
- When used for epilepsy it is very important to give doses regularly.
- If you see yellowing of the whites of the eyes or the gums have a yellowish tint, contact veterinarian immediately.
- Sleepiness is most common side effect, but sometimes the drug can change behavior or work in a way that's opposite from what is expected.
- This drug may increase appetite, especially in cats.

Chemistry/Synonyms

A benzodiazepine anticonvulsant, clonazepam occurs as an off-white to light yellow, crystalline powder having a faint odor. It is insoluble in water and slightly soluble in alcohol.

Clonazepam may also be known as: clonazepamum, Ro-5-4023, *Antelepsin®*, *Clonagin®*, *Clonapam®*, *Clonax®*, *Clonex®*, *Diocam®*, *Epitril®*, *Iktorivil®*, *Kenoket®*, *Klonopin®*, *Kriadex®*, *Neuryl®*, *Paxam®*, *Rivatril®*, *Rivotril®*, or *Solfidin®*.

Storage/Stability

Tablets should be stored in airtight, light resistant containers at room temperature. After manufacture, a 5-year expiration date is assigned.

Compatibility/Compounding Considerations

Compounded preparation stability: Clonazepam oral suspension compounded from commercially available tablets has been published (Allen et al. 1996). Triturating six (6) clonazepam 2 mg tablets with 60 mL of *Ora-Plus®* and *qs ad* to 120 mL with *Ora-Sweet®* (or *Ora-Sweet® SF*) yields a 0.1 mg/mL suspension that retains >90% potency for 60 days stored at both 5°C and 25°C. Compounded preparations of clonazepam should be protected from light.

Dosage Forms/Regulatory Status

VETERINARY-LABELED PRODUCTS: NONE.
The ARCI (Racing Commissioners International) has designated this drug as a class 2 substance. See the appendix for more information.

HUMAN-LABELED PRODUCTS:

Clonazepam Oral Tablets: 0.5 mg, 1 mg, & 2 mg; *KlonoPIN®*, generic; (Rx, C-IV)

Clonazepam Orally Dispersible (Disintegrating) Tablets: 0.125 mg, 0.25 mg, 0.5 mg, 1 mg & 2 mg (with mannitol); generic; (Rx, C-IV). **Note:** May contain xylitol.

Revisions/References

Monograph revised/updated October 2013.

Allen, L. V. & M. A. Erickson (1996). Stability of acetazolamide, allopurinol, azathioprine, clonazepam, and flucytosine in extemporaneously compounded oral liquids. *Am J Health Syst Pharm* 53(16): 1944-9.

Clonidine

(kloe-ni-deen)   Duraclon®, Catapres®

Central Alpha-2 Agonist

Prescriber Highlights

▶ Centrally acting alpha-adrenergic agonist used as a diagnostic for growth hormone deficiency or pheochromocytoma in dogs, adjunctive treatment for behavioral conditions and IBD, & potentially, epidurally as an adjunct for pain &/or anesthesia or a premed prior to surgery.

▶ Limited experience in veterinary species for therapeutic purposes.

▶ Potential adverse effects include: Transient hyperglycemia, dry mouth, constipation, sedation, aggressive behavior, hypotension, collapse, & bradycardia.

Uses/Indications

Clonidine potentially could be useful as a diagnostic agent to determine growth hormone deficiency or pheochromocytoma in dogs, and as an adjunctive treatment for refractory inflammatory bowel disease. It is being investigated as a premed in dogs and a variety of species as an epidural adjunct with or without opiates in the treatment of severe pain or for surgical procedures using epidural anesthesia.

In recent years, clonidine's use as an adjunctive treatment for certain behavioral conditions in dogs has been of interest but little information or evidence supporting its use is available. An open trial using clonidine on a *prn* basis for fear-based behavioral problems suggested that clonidine reduced phobic signs and aggression in most treated dogs (Ogata et al. 2011).

Pharmacology/Actions

Clonidine acts centrally (brain stem), stimulating alpha-adreno-receptors, thereby reducing sympathetic outflow from the CNS; decreased renal vascular resistance, peripheral resistance, cardiac rate, and blood pressure result. Renal blood flow and glomerular filtration rates are not affected. Clonidine stimulates growth hormone release by stimulating release of GHRH, but this effect does not persist with continued dosing. Clonidine possesses centrally acting analgesic effects probably at presynaptic and postjunctional alpha$_2$-adrenoreceptors in the spinal cord thereby blocking pain signal transmission to the brain. It may also increase seizure threshold but the clinical significance for this effect is unclear.

Pharmacokinetics

Limited information is available on the pharmacokinetics of clonidine in domestic animals. In cats, clonidine exhibits a two-compartment open model and penetrates into tissues rapidly.

In humans, the drug is well absorbed after oral administration. Peak plasma concentrations occur approximately 3-5 hours after oral administration. After epidural administration, maximal analgesia occurs within 30-60 minutes. Clonidine is apparently widely distributed into body tissues; tissue concentrations are higher than in plasma. Clonidine does enter into the CSF, but brain concentrations are low compared with other tissues. In humans with normal renal function, clonidine's half-life is 6-20 hours. Elimination may be prolonged with higher dosages (dose-dependent elimination kinetics) or in patients with renal dysfunction. Up to 60% of a dose is eliminated unchanged in the urine, but the remainder is metabolized in the liver; one active metabolite (p-hydroxyclonidine) has been identified.

Contraindications/Precautions/Warnings

Clonidine is contraindicated in patients known to be hypersensitive to it. It should be used with caution in patients with severe cardiovascular disease, including conduction disturbances or heart failure; it should be used very cautiously in patients with renal failure.

Do not confuse clonidine with other drugs including *Klonipin*® or clonazepam; consider writing orders or prescriptions using tall man lettering: cloNIDine.

Adverse Effects

Reported adverse effects most likely to occur include: vomiting, transient hyperglycemia, dry mouth, constipation, sedation, aggressive behavior, hypotension, collapse, and bradycardia (responsive to atropine). Tolerance to its therapeutic effects has been reported in humans.

Reproductive/Nursing Safety

At reasonable dosages no significant teratogenic effects have been described in laboratory animals, but at very high dosages some effects (increased perinatal mortality, growth retardation, cleft palates) have been seen. In humans, the FDA categorizes clonidine as a category *C* drug for use during pregnancy (*Animal studies have shown an adverse effect on the fetus, but there are no adequate studies in humans; or there are no animal reproduction studies and no adequate studies in humans*).

Clonidine does enter maternal milk at concentrations of about 20% of those found in plasma; clinical significance to nursing offspring is unknown, but clonidine was undetectable in plasma of an infant one hour after nursing from a mother taking clonidine.

Overdosage/Acute Toxicity

Clonidine has a narrow margin of safety. Common signs include hypotension, bradycardia, vomiting, weakness, and depression. Rarely, seizures or respiratory depression is seen. The LD$_{50}$ val-

ues reported for oral clonidine in rats are 465 mg/kg and mice, 206 mg/kg.

There were 344 single agent exposures to clonidine reported to the ASPCA Animal Poison Control Center (APCC) during 2009-2013. There were 307 exposed dogs, of which 132 became symptomatic. The most common clinical signs included: lethargy/sedation (64%), bradycardia (28%), ataxia (18%), pale mucus membranes (14%), vomiting (14%), and hypotension (9%). Of the 37 cats, 22 became symptomatic with vomiting (45%), ataxia (36%), lethargy (32%), bradycardia (18%) and hypotension (14%) being the most common.

Fluids and dopamine can be used to treat hypotension.

Treatment for large overdoses includes gut evacuation using standard protocols. Use of emetics should be carefully considered, as level of consciousness may deteriorate rapidly. Treatment of systemic effects is primarily symptomatic and supportive. Hypotensive effects may be treated, if necessary, using fluids or pressors (*e.g.*, dopamine); bradycardia may be treated with IV atropine, if required. Atipamezole or yohimbine may also be used to help reverse the cardiovascular effects, but multiple doses may be required as clinical signs can last up to 48 hours, depending on clonidine dosage.

Drug Interactions

The following drug interactions have either been reported or are theoretical in humans or animals receiving clonidine and may be of significance in veterinary patients. Unless otherwise noted, use together is not necessarily contraindicated, but weigh the potential risks and perform additional monitoring when appropriate.

- **ANTIHYPERTENSIVE DRUGS, OTHER:** Possible additive hypotensive effects.
- **BETA-ADRENERGIC BLOCKING AGENTS** (*i.e.*, **propranolol**) may enhance bradycardia when given with clonidine. In patients receiving clonidine and beta-adrenergic blocking agents together: if clonidine is to be discontinued, the beta-blocker should be discontinued prior to clonidine and clonidine gradually discontinued, otherwise rebound hypertension may occur.
- **CNS DEPRESSANT DRUGS** (**opiates, barbiturates**, etc.): Clonidine may exacerbate the actions of other CNS depressant drugs.
- **DIGOXIN:** Possible additive bradycardia.
- **PRAZOSIN:** May decrease the antihypertensive effects of clonidine.
- **TRICYCLIC ANTIDEPRESSANTS** (*e.g.*, **amitriptyline, clomipramine**): May block the antihypertensive effects of clonidine.

Laboratory Considerations

- No specific laboratory interactions were noted for clonidine.

Doses

- **DOGS:**

  As an adjunctive treatment (with other medications and behavioral therapy) **for situational use for fears, phobias, and separation anxiety** (extra-label): 0.01 – 0.05 mg/kg PO approximately 1.5-2 hours prior to the triggering event. A 0.1 mg tablet given to a 10 kg (22 lb.) dog would be a dose of 0.01 mg/kg.

  For diagnosing hyposomatotropism (extra-label): Dosage may be variable depending on the laboratory's protocol. Contact lab prior to test to determine protocol and sample handling instructions. Usual dose is 10 micrograms/kg IV. Obtain plasma for growth hormone (GH) levels, prior to clonidine dosing and at 15, 30, 45, 60, and 120 minutes. Larger dosages may cause a more pronounced and prolonged hyperglycemia and a higher incidence of other adverse reactions that may include sedation, aggressive behavior, hypotension, collapse, and bradycardia (responsive to atropine). Adverse effects may persist for 15-60 minutes post dose. Healthy dogs should demonstrate GH levels of

10 ng/mL after clonidine administration. (Feldman et al. 1996)

For adjunctive antidiarrheal therapy for refractory cases of inflammatory bowel disease (extra-label): 5 – 10 micrograms/kg PO or SC two to three times a day; can activate alpha$_2$-receptors in the CRT and cause vomiting. (Washabau 2009)

- **CATS:**

  For adjunctive antidiarrheal therapy for refractory cases of inflammatory bowel disease (extra-label): As fourth line therapy after prostaglandin synthetase inhibitors (*i.e.*, sulfasalazine, bismuth subsalicylate), opioid agonists (*i.e.*, loperamide), and 5-HT3 serotonergic antagonists (*i.e.*, ondansetron) are being used: clonidine 5 – 10 micrograms/kg two to three times a day, SC or PO. (Washabau 2000)

- **CATTLE:**

  For epidural analgesia/analgesia (extra label): 2 – 3 micrograms/kg diluted to 8 mL with sterile normal saline epidurally; onset/duration of analgesia = 19 minutes/192 minutes with a 2 microgram/kg dose, and = 9 minutes/311 minutes with a 3 microgram/kg dose; peak effects from 60-180 minutes. (De Rossi et al. 2003)

Monitoring

- Dependent upon purpose for use. When used for determining GH levels, adverse effects (noted in dosage section) should be evaluated.
- Blood pressure and cardiac rate are most likely to be affected, but effects usually only persist for an hour after dose.
- When used for ongoing diarrhea treatment, evaluation of efficacy and adverse effect profile should be monitored.

Client Information

- May be given with or without food.
- Not very much experience with this drug in dogs or cats. Sedation and lowered blood pressure are the most likely side effects. Report unusual effects to veterinarian.
- When used to treat fear-based behavioral problems, usually given 90 minutes to 2 hours before the event. Dosages are started low and then gradually raised, depending on side effects and effectiveness. Sometimes used longer term on a regular basis (up to twice daily).
- Best used with behavioral modification training for fear-based problems.
- When used on a daily basis, don't change dosages or discontinue treatment without veterinarian's advice.

Chemistry/Synonyms

An imidazoline derivative centrally acting alpha-adrenergic agonist, clonidine HCl occurs as an odorless, bitter, white or almost white crystalline powder. It is soluble in water and alcohol. It is also considered highly lipid soluble. The commercially available injection for epidural use has its pH adjusted to between 5-7.

Clonidine may also be known as: ST-155 or clonidini hydrochloridum; *Catapres®* and *Duraclon®* are common trade names.

Storage/Stability

Clonidine tablets should be stored in tight, light-resistant containers at room temperature; excursions permitted to 15-30°C (59-86°F). The preservative-free injection for epidural use should be stored at controlled room temperature (25°C). Because it contains no preservative, unused portions of the injection should be discarded.

Compatibility/Compounding Considerations

No specific information noted.

Dosage Forms/Regulatory Status

VETERINARY-LABELED PRODUCTS: NONE.

The ARCI (Racing Commissioners International) has designated this drug as a class 3 substance. See the appendix for more information.

HUMAN-LABELED PRODUCTS:

Clonidine HCl Injection for epidural use: 100 micrograms/mL, & 500 micrograms/mL (must be diluted before use) preservative-free in 10 mL vials; *Duraclon®*, generic; (Rx)

Clonidine HCl Oral Tablets: 0.1 mg, 0.2 mg & 0.3 mg; *Catapres®*, generic; (Rx)

Clonidine HCl Oral Modified-release (12-hour for humans) Tablets: 0.1 mg (equivalent to 0.087 mg of base); *Kapvay®*; (Rx)

Clonidine HCl Transdermal: 0.1 mg/24hrs (2.5 mg total clonidine content), 0.2 mg/24hrs (5 mg total clonidine content), & 0.3 mg/24hrs (7.5 mg total clonidine content); *Catapres-TTS-1®*, *2®* or *3®*, generic; (Rx)

Revisions/References

Monograph revised/updated October 2013.

De Rossi, R., et al. (2003). Perineal analgesic actions of epidural clonidine in cattle. *Vet Anaesth Analg* 30: 63-70.

Feldman, E. & R. Nelson (1996). *Canine and Feline Endocrinology and Reproduction*, Saunders. Philadelphia.

Ogata, N. & N. H. Dodman (2011). The use of clonidine in the treatment of fear-based behavior problems in dogs: An open trial. *Journal of Veterinary Behavior-Clinical Applications and Research* 6(2): 130-7.

Washabau, R. (2000). *Intestinal Diseases/IBD*. Proceedings: American Association of Feline Practitioners. accessed via Veterinary Information Network; vin.com

Washabau, R. (2009). *Principles in the therapy of canine inflammatory bowel disease*. Proceedings: WSAVA. accessed via Veterinary Information Network; vin.com

Clopidogrel Bisulfate

(kloe-pid-oh-grel) Plavix®

Platelet Aggregation Inhibitor

Prescriber Highlights

▶ Oral, once-daily platelet aggregation inhibitor that may be useful in hypercoagulable states in dogs and preventing thromboembolic disease in cats.

▶ Limited clinical experience in feline medicine; but appears well tolerated.

▶ Potentially may cause vomiting or bleeding.

Uses/Indications

Clopidogrel, a platelet aggregation inhibitor, may be useful for preventing thrombi in susceptible cats. A report from the multi-center study (FAT CAT) comparing clopidogrel at 18.75 mg/cat/day with aspirin (81 mg/cat every 3 days) demonstrated that at 1 year and for the total study period clopidogrel was associated with a significant improvement in survival compared to aspirin (Hogan et al. 2013). Some clinicians use aspirin and clopidogrel together, but there does not appear to be any evidence published that supports combining these drugs. Clopidogrel may also improve pelvic limb circulation in cats after a cardiogenic embolic event via a vasomodulating effect secondary to inhibition of serotonin release from platelets. It may also prove to be of benefit in treating hypercoagulable states in dogs although studies to date have not found significant benefits for its use in dogs with IMHA (Mellett et al. 2011; Smith 2012).

Pharmacology/Actions

Clopidogrel is metabolized to an active, highly unstable thiol compound (not yet identified) that is responsible for its inhibitory platelet-aggregation (both primary and secondary aggregation) activity. This compound binds selectively to platelet surface low-affinity ADP-receptors and inhibits ADP binding to the site thereby reducing platelet aggregation. Clopidogrel's active metabolite irreversibly alters the ADP receptor; the platelet is affected for its lifespan.

Clopidogrel's mechanism of action on platelet aggregation is different than aspirin's effects. Aspirin acetylates and inactivates COX-1 in platelets, thereby preventing formation of thromboxane A2.

Pharmacokinetics

No specific information was located for the pharmacokinetics of clopidogrel in cats. In a pharmacodynamic study in cats (Hogan et al. 2004), doses as low as 18.75 mg were as effective as higher dosages in reducing platelet aggregation; maximal effects were seen after 3 days of therapy and platelet function returned to normal 7 days after stopping treatment. While lower dosages may be effective in cats, they have not been evaluated and are not practical to administer with the presently available 75 mg human-labeled dosage form (tablets).

In dogs, clopidogrel's pharmacokinetics have not been fully elucidated, but in a pharmacodynamic study done in healthy dogs, most subjects had significant inhibition of platelet function within 3 hours after the initial PO dose; inhibition lasted at least 24 hours (Brainard et al. 2010). Others have reported that the onset of clinical effects on platelets may require two days.

In horses, clopidogrel did decrease adenosine diphosphate-induced platelet aggregation in the horse, but the time to onset and total required dose in horses was greater than in other species (Brainard et al. 2011).

In humans, clopidogrel is rapidly absorbed with a bioavailability of about 50%. Food does not alter its absorption. Clopidogrel is highly bound to plasma proteins in humans and rapidly hydrolyzed to a carboxylic acid derivative inactive metabolite (SR 26334) that is excreted via the urine and feces. The 2% of drug that is covalently bound to platelets has an approximate elimination half-life of 11 days.

Contraindications/Precautions/Warnings

No specific information is available for cats. In humans, clopidogrel is contraindicated in patients with active pathologic bleeding or known hypersensitivity to the drug.

Adverse Effects

Clopidogrel appears well tolerated by cats, but numbers treated have been relatively few. Some cats may vomit, or develop anorexia or diarrhea; giving the drug with food may alleviate these effects. Non-regenerative anemia has been reported in some cats receiving long-term clopidogrel therapy.

In humans, the primary adverse effects reported have been bleeding related. In a major pre-clinical study, major bleeding occurred in approximately 2% of patients treated. Use of aspirin with clopidogrel may increase this incidence. Rashes and gastrointestinal effects (diarrhea) have also been reported. Rarely, thrombotic thrombocytopenic purpura (TTP) has been noted; onset can occur after a short period of treatment (<2 weeks). Aplastic anemia is reported very rarely.

Reproductive/Nursing Safety

In pregnant rats and rabbits, dosages of approximately 65X and 78X respectively, of the human dose when compared on mg/m² basis, caused no teratogenic effects. In humans, the FDA categorizes clopidogrel as category *B* for use during pregnancy (*Animal studies have not yet demonstrated risk to the fetus, but there are no adequate studies in pregnant women; or animal studies have shown an adverse effect, but adequate studies in pregnant women have not demonstrated a risk to the fetus in the first trimester of pregnancy, and there is no evidence of risk in later trimesters.*)

In rats, clopidogrel or its metabolites are distributed into milk. Although probably safe for use in nursing veterinary patients, weigh the potential risks to nursing offspring before allowing patients receiving the drug to nurse their young, or use a milk replacer.

Overdosage/Acute Toxicity

Limited information is available. Reported lethal oral doses for mice and rats were 1500 mg/kg and 2000 mg/kg (460X human adult dose on a mg/m² basis), respectively. Acute toxic signs may include bleeding or vomiting. Platelet transfusions have been suggested if rapid reversal is required.

Drug Interactions

The following drug interactions have either been reported or are theoretical in humans or animals receiving clopidogrel and may be of significance in veterinary patients. Unless otherwise noted, use together is not necessarily contraindicated, but weigh the potential risks and perform additional monitoring when appropriate.

- **ASPIRIN:** Increased risk for bleeding, however many human patients take both medications.
- **CIMETIDINE:** May decrease the effects of clopidogrel.
- **CYCLOSPORINE:** A study in dogs showed that clopidogrel can increase cyclosporine peak levels, but areas under the curve were the same when cyclosporine was used alone (Lee et al. 2012).
- **HEPARIN; LOW MOLECULAR WEIGHT HEPARINS:** Clopidogrel appears safe to use with heparin (both unfractionated and LMW).
- **NSAIDS:** Increased risk for bleeding; clopidogrel may interfere with metabolism.
- **PHENYTOIN:** Clopidogrel may interfere with metabolism.
- **PROTON PUMP INHIBITORS** (*e.g.*, **omeprazole**): Proton pump inhibitors may decrease the efficacy of clopidogrel.
- **RIFAMPIN:** May increase the effects of clopidogrel.
- **TORSEMIDE:** Clopidogrel may interfere with metabolism.
- **WARFARIN:** Increased risk for bleeding; clopidogrel may interfere with metabolism.

Laboratory Considerations

- None noted. No washout period is required before performing intradermal skin testing (allergy) or IgE serological testing.

Doses

- **DOGS:**

  As an antiplatelet agent (extra-label): 1 – 5 mg/kg PO once daily. A "standard" dosage recommendation is 1 mg/kg PO once daily. Some have suggested that if aspirin is also being used the clopidogrel dosage be reduced to 0.5 mg/kg PO once daily. At the time of writing (2013), there is no substantial evidence supporting clopidogrel use in dogs.

- **CATS:**

  To prevent thrombus formation; antiplatelet agent (extra-label). **Note:** There is little scientific evidence and no general consensus as to the ideal treatment of arterial thromboembolism (ATE):

  a) Based on the FAT CAT trial (Hogan et al. 2013): 18.75 mg (practically, 1/4 of a 75 mg tablet) per cat PO once daily; cats under 3 kg may need dosages to be compounded.

  b) Anecdotal: Clopidogrel 18.75 mg (practically, 1/4 of a 75 mg tablet) per cat PO once daily AND aspirin either at 5 mg per cat PO every 2-3 days or 81 mg per cat PO every 3 days. **Note:** there may be a higher risk for bleeding when combining therapy especially with the high dose aspirin regimen. See the Aspirin monograph for using aspirin alone.

Monitoring

- Clinical efficacy.
- Adverse effects (vomiting, bleeding).

Client Information

- Bleeding is not likely, but can occur. If your pet shows any signs of bleeding, bruising, or black, tarry stools, please consult your veterinarian immediately.
- This medication may be given with or without food, but if vomiting occurs, give with food.

Chemistry/Synonyms

Clopidogrel bisulfate, a thienopyridine, occurs as a white to off-white powder that is practically insoluble in water at a pH of 7, but freely soluble at a pH of 1.

Clopidogrel may also be known as: SR-259990C, PCR-4099, or clopedogreli. A common trade name is *Plavix®*.

Storage/Stability

Clopidogrel tablets should be stored at 25°C; excursions are permitted to 15-30°C.

Compatibility/Compounding Considerations

Compounded preparation stability: Clopidogrel oral suspension compounded from commercially available tablets has been published (Skillman et al. 2010). Triturating four (4) clopidogrel 75 mg tablets with 30 mL of *Ora-Plus®* and *qs ad* to 60 mL with *Ora-Sweet®* (or *Ora-Sweet® SF*) yields a 5 mg/mL oral suspension that retains >90% potency for 60 days stored at both 5°C and 25°C. Compounded preparations of clopidogrel should be protected from light.

Dosage Forms/Regulatory Status

VETERINARY-LABELED PRODUCTS: NONE.

HUMAN-LABELED PRODUCTS:

Clopidogrel Bisulfate Tablets: 75 mg & 300 mg; *Plavix®*, generic; (Rx)

Revisions/References

Monograph revised/updated October 2013.

Brainard, B. M., et al. (2011). Effects of Clopidogrel and Aspirin on Platelet Aggregation, Thromboxane Production, and Serotonin Secretion in Horses. *Journal of Veterinary Internal Medicine* 25(1): 116-22.

Brainard, B. M., et al. (2010). Pharmacodynamic and pharmacokinetic evaluation of clopidogrel and the carboxylic acid metabolite SR 26334 in healthy dogs. *American Journal of Veterinary Research* 71(7): 822-30.

Hogan, D., et al. (2004). Antiplatelet effects and pharmacodynamics of clopidogrel in cats. *JAVMA* 225(9): 1406-11.

Hogan, D., et al. (2013). *Analysis of the Feline Arterial Thromboembolism: Clopidogrel vs. Aspirin Trial (Fat Cat).* Proceedings ACVIM accessed via Veterinary Information Network; vin.com

Lee, J. H., et al. (2012). Pharmacokinetic interactions of clopidogrel with quercetin, telmisartan, and cyclosporine A in rats and dogs. *Archives of Pharmacal Research* 35(10): 1831-7.

Mellett, A. M., et al. (2011). A Prospective Study of Clopidogrel Therapy in Dogs with Primary Immune-Mediated Hemolytic Anemia. *Journal of Veterinary Internal Medicine* 25(1): 71-5.

Skillman, K. L., et al. (2010). Stability of an extemporaneously prepared clopidogrel oral suspension. *Am J Health Syst Pharm* 67(7): 559-61.

Smith, S. A. (2012). Antithrombotic Therapy. *Topics in Companion Animal Medicine* 27(2): 88-94.

Cloprostenol Sodium

(kloe-**pros**-te-nol)   Estrumate®

Prostaglandin (F-Class)

Prescriber Highlights

▶ Synthetic F-class prostaglandin used in cattle to induce luteolysis, induce abortion, treat pyometra, endometritis, etc.

▶ Contraindications: Pregnancy (when abortion or induced parturition are not desired).

▶ Can cause cholinergic-like adverse effects in dogs.

▶ Do not give IV.

▶ Pregnant women should not handle; caution handling in humans with asthma & women of childbearing age.

Uses/Indications

Cloprostenol is FDA-approved for use in beef or dairy cattle to induce luteolysis. Labeled uses include: for unobserved or undetected estrus in cows cycling normally, pyometra or chronic endometritis, expulsion of mummified fetus, luteal cysts, induced abortions after mismating, and to schedule estrus and ovulation for controlled breeding.

Cloprostenol has been used in dogs for pregnancy termination and treatment of open pyometra. The use of cloprostenol for pyometra is controversial as some believe dinoprost (PGF$_2$alpha) is more effective and has fewer adverse effects than cloprostenol.

In horses, cloprostenol has been used for luteolysis, inducing abortion, and stimulating uterine contractions.

Pharmacology/Actions

Prostaglandin F$_2$alpha and its analogues cloprostenol and fluprostenol are powerful luteolytic agents. They cause rapid regression of the corpus luteum and arrest its secretory activity. These prostaglandins also have direct stimulating effect on uterine smooth muscle causing contraction and a relaxant effect on the cervix.

In normally cycling animals, estrus will generally occur 2-5 days after treatment. In pregnant cattle treated between 10-150 days of gestation, abortion will usually occur 2-3 days after injection.

Pharmacokinetics

No information was located on the pharmacokinetics of cloprostenol. It is reported to have a longer duration of action than dinoprost tromethamine.

Contraindications/Precautions/Warnings

Should not be administered to pregnant animals when abortion is not desired.

Women of child-bearing age, persons with asthma or other respiratory diseases should use extreme caution when handling cloprostenol as the drug may induce abortion or acute bronchoconstriction. Cloprostenol is readily absorbed through the skin and must be washed off immediately with soap and water.

Do not administer IV.

Adverse Effects

The manufacturer does not list any adverse effects for this product when used as labeled. If used after the 5th month of gestation, increased risk of dystocia and decreased efficacy occur.

In dogs, cloprostenol can cause increased salivation, tachycardia, increased urination and defecation, gagging, vomiting, ataxia, and mild depression. Pretreatment with an anticholinergic drug (such as atropine) may reduce the severity of these effects.

At higher doses in horses, cloprostenol can cause sweating, cramping and loose stools, but incidence of adverse effects is less than with dinoprost tromethamine. In horses, uterine contractions are stimulated for approximately 5 hours post-dose.

Reproductive/Nursing Safety

Cloprostenol is contraindicated in pregnant animals when abortion or induced parturition is not desired.

Overdosage/Acute Toxicity

The manufacturer states that at doses of 50X and 100X's those recommended, cattle may show signs of uneasiness, slight frothing, and milk let-down.

Overdoses of cloprostenol or other synthetic prostaglandin F$_2$alpha analogs in small animals reportedly can result in shock and death.

Drug Interactions

The following drug interactions have either been reported or are theoretical in humans or animals receiving cloprostenol and may be of significance in veterinary patients. Unless otherwise noted, use together is not necessarily contraindicated, but weigh the potential risks and perform additional monitoring when appropriate.

- **OXYTOCIC AGENTS, OTHER:** Activity may be enhanced by cloprostenol.

Doses

- **DOGS:**

For adjunctive treatment of pyometra (extra-label): Cabergoline at 5 micrograms/kg PO and cloprostenol at 1 microgram/kg SC once a day for 7 days with oral antibiotic therapy and supportive hydration. If no response to treatment, cloprostenol (without cabergoline) with supportive treatment continued for another 7 days. (Corrada et al. 2006; Castillo et al. 2008; Jena et al. 2013)

For pregnancy termination (extra-label):

a) 1 – 2.5 micrograms/kg SC once daily for 4-7 days has been successful in terminating pregnancy in dogs after 30 days gestation. (Davidson 2004)

b) 1 – 2.5 micrograms/kg SC every 48 hours for three doses. At higher dose (2.5 mcg/kg), appears very effective starting at 30 days of pregnancy. Anticholinergic drug administration (*e.g.*, atropine) 15 minutes prior to dosing appears to lessen adverse effects. (Romagnoli 2006)

- **CATTLE:**

For all labeled (see Indications) uses (FDA-approved): 500 micrograms IM once.

As part of a controlled breeding program there are two labeled methods:

Single injection method: Use only animals with mature corpus luteum. Examine rectally to determine corpus luteum maturity, anatomic normality, and lack of pregnancy. Give 500 micrograms cloprostenol IM. Estrus should occur in 2-5 days. Inseminate at usual time after detecting estrus, or inseminate once at 72 hours post injection, or twice at 72 and 96 hours post injection.

Double injection method: Examine rectally to determine if animal is anatomically normal, not pregnant, and cycling normally. Give 500 micrograms IM. Repeat dose 11 days later. Estrus should occur in 2-5 days after second injection. Inseminate at usual time after detecting estrus, or inseminate once at 72 hours post second injection, or twice at 72 and 96 hours post second injection.

Animals that come into estrus after first injection may be inseminated at the usual time after detecting estrus.

Any controlled breeding program should be completed by either observing animals and re-inseminating or hand mating after returning to estrus, or turning in clean-up bull(s) five to seven days after the last injection of cloprostenol to cover any animals returning to estrus. (Adapted for Package Insert; *Estrumate®*)

- **HORSES:**

All are extra-label.

For pregnancy termination: To cause abortion prior to the twelfth day of gestation: 100 micrograms IM, most effective day 7 or 8 post estrus. Mare will usually return to estrus within 5 days. (Lofstedt 1986)

For luteolysis and to stimulate uterine contractions:

a) 250 micrograms (per horse) IM once. Research has shown that 1/10th of a dose (25 micrograms) can still cause luteolysis and if this is given once or on two consecutive days, side effects can be avoided. (Dascanio 2009)

b) For luteolysis: 25 – 250 micrograms per horse (0.1 – 1 mL) IM once. As an ecbolic: 250 micrograms (1 mL) IM q24h. Clo-

prostenol should not be used more than one day after ovulation because it can damage the corpus luteum and reduce progesterone. (Foss 2009)

- **SWINE:**

To induce parturition in sows (extra-label): 175 micrograms IM; give 2 days or less before anticipated date of farrowing. Farrowing generally occurs in approximately 36 hours after injection. (Pugh 1982)

- **SHEEP/GOATS:**

All are extra-label.

For estrus synchronization (extra-label): During the breeding period 125 micrograms IM or SC twice 9-10 days apart. Males (female:male ratio of 10:1) can be reintroduced 48 hours after the second injection. (Abecia et al. 2011)

To induce parturition in does:

a) 62.5 – 125 micrograms IM at 144 days of gestation in early morning. Deliveries will peak at 30-35 hours after injection. Maintain goat in usual surroundings and minimize outside disturbances. (Williams 1986)

b) For adjunctive treatment of toxemia in does: If there is only a partial response to medical therapy induction of parturition with 250 micrograms IM cloprostenol can be attempted. Kidding or abortion typically occurs in 30-36 hours. A caesarian section may be needed if the animal does not respond quickly to medical therapy. (Smith 2011)

To treat pseudopregnancy (hydrometra/mucometra): 125 micrograms IM once. (Tibary 2009)

- **CAMELIDS:**

As a luteolytic (extra-label): **Alpacas:** 100 micrograms IM once. **Llamas:** 250 micrograms IM once. Not to be given more than 4 days after ovulation. Luteolysis and abortion can be induced at any stage of pregnancy with 2-4 injections of cloprostenol. (Adams 2008)

Client Information

- Cloprostenol should be used by individuals familiar with its use and precautions.
- Pregnant women, asthmatics or other persons with bronchial diseases should handle this product with extreme caution.
- Wear disposable gloves when handling and any accidental exposure to skin should be washed off immediately.

Chemistry/Synonyms

A synthetic prostaglandin of the F class, cloprostenol sodium occurs as a white or almost white, amorphous, hygroscopic powder. It is freely soluble in water and alcohol. Potency of the commercially available product is expressed in terms of cloprostenol.

Cloprostenol sodium may also be known as ICI-80996, *Estrumate®*, or *estroPLAN®*.

Storage/Stability

Cloprostenol sodium should be stored at room temperature (15-30°C); protect from light.

Compatibility/Compounding Considerations

No specific information noted.

Dosage Forms/Regulatory Status

VETERINARY-LABELED PRODUCTS:

Cloprostenol Sodium Injection equivalent to 250 micrograms/mL cloprostenol in 20 mL vials; *Estrumate®*, estroPLAN® *Injection*; (Rx). FDA-approved for use in beef and dairy cattle. No pre-slaughter or milk withdrawal is required; no specific tolerances for cloprostenol residues have been published.

HUMAN-LABELED PRODUCTS: NONE.

Revisions/References

Monograph revised/updated October 2013.

Abecia, J., et al. (2011). Pharmaceutical Control of Reproduction in Sheep and Goats. *Vet Clin Food Anim* 27: 67-79.

Adams, G. (2008). *Breeding management of llamas and alpacas.* Proceedings: WVC. accessed via Veterinary Information Network; vin.com

Castillo, V. A., et al. (2008). Cushing's disease in dogs: Cabergoline treatment. *Research in Veterinary Science* 85(1): 26-34.

Corrada, Y., et al. (2006). A combination of oral cabergoline and double cloprostenol injections to produce third-quarter gestation termination in the bitch. *J. Am. Anim. Hosp. Assoc.* 42(5): 366-70.

Dascanio, J. (2009). *Hormonal Control of Reproduction.* Proceedings: ABVP. accessed via Veterinary Information Network; vin.com

Davidson, A. (2004). *Update: Therapeutics for reproductive disorders in small animal practice.* Proceedings: ACVIM Forum. accessed via Veterinary Information Network; vin.com

Foss, R. (2009). *Breeding the Problem Mare.* Proceedings: WVC. accessed via Veterinary Information Network; vin.com

Jena, B., et al. (2013). Comparative efficacy of various therapeutic protocols in the treatment of pyometra in bitches. *Veterinarni Medicina* 58(5): 271-6.

Lofstedt, R. M. (1986). Termination of unwanted pregnancy in the mare. *Current Therapy in Theriogenology 2: Diagnosis, Treatment and Prevention of Reproductive Diseases in Small and Large Animals.* D. A. Morrow, WB Saunders: 715-8.

Pugh, D. M. (1982). The Hormones II: Control of reprductive function. *Veterinary Applied Pharmacolgy and Therapeutics.* London, Baillière Tindall: 181-201.

Romagnoli, S. (2006). *Control of reproduction in dogs and cats: Use and misuse of hormones.* Proceedings: WSAVA World Congress. accessed via Veterinary Information Network; vin.com

Smith, M. (2011). *Dystocia in Small Ruminants: Management & Prevention.* Western Veterinary Conference. accessed via Veterinary Information Network; vin.com

Tibary, A. (2009). *Infertility in goats: Individual & herd approach.* Proceedings: WVC. accessed via Veterinary Information Network; vin.com

Williams, C. S. F. (1986). Practical management of induced parturition. *Current Therapy in Theriogenology 2: Diagnosis, Treatment and Prevention of Reproductive Diseases in Small and Large Animals.* D. A. Morrow. Philadelphia, WB Saunders: 588-9.

Clorazepate Dipotassium

(klor-az-e-pate)   Tranxene-SD®, Gen-Xene®

Benzodiazepine

Prescriber Highlights

▶ Benzodiazepine anxiolytic, sedative-hypnotic, & anticonvulsant used in dogs & cats.

▶ Contraindications: Hypersensitivity to benzodiazepines, narrow angle glaucoma, or significant liver disease.

▶ Use extreme caution in aggressive animals (especially fear induced).

▶ May exacerbate myasthenia gravis.

▶ Can interact with phenobarbital.

▶ Adverse Effects: Sedation & ataxia most prevalent.

Uses/Indications

Clorazepate has been used in dogs both as an adjunctive anticonvulsant (usually in conjunction with phenobarbital) and in the treatment of behavior disorders, primarily those that are anxiety or phobia-related. In dogs, clorazepate has been reported to develop tolerance to its anticonvulsant effects less rapidly than clonazepam.

Clorazepate may be useful as an anxiolytic agent in cats.

Pharmacology/Actions

The subcortical levels (primarily limbic, thalamic, and hypothalamic) of the CNS are depressed by clorazepate and other benzodiazepines thus producing the anxiolytic, sedative, skeletal muscle relaxant and anticonvulsant effects seen. The exact mechanism of action is unknown, but postulated mechanisms include: antagonism of serotonin, increased release of and/or facilitation of gamma-aminobutyric acid (GABA) activity and diminished release or turnover of acetylcholine in the CNS. Benzodiazepine specific receptors have been located in the mammalian brain, kidney, liver, lung and heart. In all species studied, receptors are lacking in the white matter. Clorazepate is considered an intermediate-action benzodiazepine.

Pharmacokinetics

In dogs, clorazepate peak serum levels generally occur within 1-2 hours. Volume of distribution is about 1.8 L/kg after multiple dosing. Clorazepate is metabolized to nordiazepam and other metabolites. Nordiazepam is active and has a very long half-life (in humans up to 100 hours). In dogs, the sustained release preparation apparently offers no pharmacokinetic advantage over the non-sustained preparations (Brown et al. 1989).

Contraindications/Precautions/Warnings

Clorazepate is contraindicated in patients that are hypersensitive to it or other benzodiazepines, have significant liver dysfunction or acute narrow angle glaucoma. Clorazepate should be used very cautiously, if at all, in aggressive patients as it may disinhibit the anxiety that may help prevent these animals from aggressive behavior. Benzodiazepines have been reported to exacerbate myasthenia gravis.

Use with caution in dogs displaying fear-induced aggression; these drugs may actually provoke dogs to attack.

Do not confuse clorazepate with clonazepam. Consider writing orders and prescriptions using tall man letters; clorazePATE.

Adverse Effects

In dogs, the most likely adverse effects seen include sedation and ataxia. These effects apparently occur infrequently, are mild and usually transient. Physical dependence may occur and abrupt withdrawal of clorazepate may precipitate seizures.

In cats, clorazepate may cause sedation, ataxia and, potentially, acute hepatic necrosis.

Reproductive/Nursing Safety

Safe use during pregnancy has not been established; teratogenic effects of similar benzodiazepines have been noted in rabbits and rats. In humans, the FDA categorizes this drug as category *D* for use during pregnancy (*There is evidence of human fetal risk, but the potential benefits from the use of the drug in pregnant women may be acceptable despite its potential risks.*)

Nordiazepam is distributed into milk and may affect nursing neonates.

Overdosage/Acute Toxicity

When used alone, clorazepate overdoses are generally limited to significant CNS depression (confusion, coma, decreased reflexes, etc.). Treatment of significant oral overdoses consists of standard protocols for removing and/or binding the drug in the gut and supportive systemic measures. The use of analeptic agents (CNS stimulants such as caffeine, amphetamines, etc.) is generally not recommended. Flumazenil may be considered for very serious overdoses.

Drug Interactions

The following drug interactions have either been reported or are theoretical in humans or animals receiving clorazepate and may be of significance in veterinary patients. Unless otherwise noted, use together is not necessarily contraindicated, but weigh the potential risks and perform additional monitoring when appropriate.

▪ **ANTIFUNGALS, AZOLE (itraconazole, ketoconazole,** etc.): May increase levels.

▪ **CIMETIDINE:** May decrease metabolism of benzodiazepines.

▪ **CNS DEPRESSANT DRUGS:** If clorazepate is administered with other CNS depressant agents (**barbiturates, narcotics, anesthetics,** etc.) additive effects may occur.

▪ **ERYTHROMYCIN:** May decrease the metabolism of benzodiazepines.

▪ **PHENOBARBITAL:** While used together in the treatment of seizures in dogs, can interact with one another. Clorazepate (especially high serum concentrations), may increase the serum levels of phenobarbital, particularly if added to patients that received phenobarbital long-term. In time, clorazepate levels may decrease, leading to decreased phenobarbital levels.

- **PHENYTOIN:** May decrease clorazepate concentrations.
- **RIFAMPIN:** May induce hepatic microsomal enzymes and decrease the pharmacologic effects of benzodiazepines.

Laboratory Considerations

- Benzodiazepines may decrease the thyroidal uptake of I^{123} or I^{131}.
- Clorazepate may increase **serum alkaline phosphatase** and **serum cholesterol** levels; clinical significance is unclear.

Doses

- **DOGS:**

   As an adjunctive medication in the treatment of epilepsy (extra-label): Clorazepate is generally used in conjunction with phenobarbital (see Drug Interactions above). Dosing recommendations vary, but consider: 0.5 – 1.5 mg/kg PO q8h or 1 – 2.5 mg/kg PO q12h. Tolerance can occur with continued use.

   As adjunctive therapy for the treatment of fears and phobias (extra-label): 0.55 – 2.2 mg/kg PO up to q8h.

- **CATS:**

   As an anxiolytic or for compulsive behaviors: 0.2 – 0.5 mg/kg PO q12–24h. (Virga 2002)

   As an alternative drug to phenobarbital for seizures: 3.75 – 7.5 mg (total dose per cat) PO once to twice daily. Similar precautions are necessary as described for diazepam use in cats. (Podell 2008)

Monitoring

- Efficacy.
- Adverse effects.

Client Information

- Used for epilepsy or as a tranquilizer.
- When using for thunderstorm phobias or other triggers (*e.g.*, owner separation, etc.) that upset your animal try to give it about an hour before the event or trigger. Works best along with behavior therapy.
- When used for epilepsy it is very important to give doses regularly.
- If you see yellowing of the whites of the eyes or the gums have a yellowish tint, contact veterinarian immediately.
- Sleepiness is most common side effect, but sometimes the drug can change behavior or work in a way that's opposite from what is expected.
- This drug may increase appetite, especially in cats.

Chemistry/Synonyms

A benzodiazepine anxiolytic, sedative-hypnotic, and anticonvulsant, clorazepate dipotassium occurs as a light yellow, fine powder that is very soluble in water and slightly soluble in alcohol.

Clorazepate dipotassium may also be known as Abbott-35616, AH-3232, 4306-CB, clorazepic acid, dipotassium clorazepate, dikalii clorazepas, or potassium clorazepate; many trade names are available.

Storage/Stability

Clorazepate dipotassium is unstable in the presence of water. It has been recommended to keep the desiccant packets in with the original container of the capsules and tablets and to consider adding a desiccant packet to the prescription vial when dispensing large quantities of tablets or capsules to the client.

Compatibility/Compounding Considerations

No specific information noted.

Dosage Forms/Regulatory Status

VETERINARY-LABELED PRODUCTS: NONE.

The ARCI (Racing Commissioners International) has designated this drug as a class 2 substance. See the appendix for more information.

HUMAN-LABELED PRODUCTS:

Clorazepate Dipotassium Tablets: 3.75 mg, 7.5 mg, & 15 mg; *Tranxene® T-tab*, generic; (Rx, C-IV)

Revisions/References

Monograph revised/updated October 2013.

Brown, S. & S. Forrester (1989). Serum disposition of oral clorazepate from regular-release and sustained-release tablets in dogs. *J Vet Int Med* 3(2): 116.

Podell, M. (2008). *Novel approaches to feline epilepsy.* Proceedings: ACVIM. accessed via Veterinary Information Network; vin.com

Virga, V. (2002). *Which drug and why: An update on psychopharmacology.* Proceedings: Atlantic Coast Veterinary Conference. accessed via Veterinary Information Network; vin.com

Clorsulon

(klor-su-lon)   Curatrem®, Ivomec Plus®

Antiparasitic (Flukicide)

Prescriber Highlights

▶ Adult flukicide (*Fasciola hepatica*).

▶ Not for female dairy cattle.

▶ Slaughter withdrawal: 8 days at labeled doses for *Curatrem®*, 49 days for *Ivomec Plus®*.

Uses/Indications

Clorsulon is FDA-approved for use in the treatment of immature and adult forms of *Fasciola hepatica* (Liver fluke) in cattle. It is not effective against immature flukes less than 8 weeks old. It also has activity against *Fasciola gigantica*. Although not FDA-approved, the drug has been used in practice in various other species (*e.g.*, sheep, goats, llamas). It has activity against *F. magna* in sheep, but is not completely effective in eradicating the organism after a single dose, thus severely limiting its clinical usefulness against this parasite. Clorsulon is also not effective against the rumen fluke (Paramphistomum).

Pharmacology/Actions

In susceptible flukes, clorsulon inhibits the glycolytic enzymes 3-phosphoglycerate kinase and phosphoglyceromutase, thereby blocking the Emden-Myerhof glycolytic pathway; the fluke is deprived of its main metabolic energy source and dies. Clorsulon at 7 mg/kg is effective against migrating *F. hepatica* 8 weeks post-infection, but at 2 mg/kg is effective only against adult flukes (14 weeks post infection).

Pharmacokinetics

After oral administration to cattle, the drug is absorbed rapidly with peak levels occurring in about 4 hours. Approximately 75% of the circulating drug is found in plasma and 25% in erythrocytes. At 8-12 hours after administration, clorsulon levels peak in the fluke.

Contraindications/Precautions/Warnings

No milk withdrawal time has been determined, and the drug is labeled not for use in female dairy cattle of breeding age.

The combination injectable product (*Ivomec Plus®*) must be administered subcutaneously only; do not give IV or IM. The manufacturer warns to use this product only in cattle as severe reactions, including fatalities in dogs, may occur.

Adverse Effects

When used as directed adverse effects are unlikely to occur with the oral suspension (*Curatrem®*). Local swelling may occur at injection sites with *Ivomec Plus®*.

Reproductive/Nursing Safety

Clorsulon is considered safe for use in pregnant or breeding animals.

Overdosage/Acute Toxicity

Clorsulon is very safe when administered orally to cattle or sheep. Doses of up to 400 mg/kg have not produced toxicity in sheep. A dose that is toxic in cattle has also not been determined.

Drug Interactions/Laboratory Considerations

- None identified.

Doses

- **CATTLE:**

    For *Fasciola hepatica* infections (Labeled Dose; FDA-approved): 7 mg/kg PO; deposit suspension over the back of the tongue (Label directions; *Curatrem®*)

    For *Fasciola hepatica* infections, **round worms, lungworms, cattle grubs, sucking lice, mange mites** (see Ivermectin monograph or product label for more information on species covered) (Labeled Dose; FDA-approved): Inject 1mL per 110 lb. body weight SC behind the shoulder. (Label directions; *Ivomec Plus®*)

- **SHEEP:**

    For *Fasciola hepatica* infections (extra-label): 7 mg/kg PO.

- **CAMELIDS:**

    For *Fasciola hepatica* infections (extra-label): 7 mg/kg PO.

Monitoring

- Clinical efficacy.

Client Information

- Shake well before using (*Curatrem®*).
- Follow withdrawal times for slaughter (8 days for *Curatrem®*, 49 days for *Ivomec Plus®*).
- Do not use in female dairy cattle of breeding age.

Chemistry/Synonyms

A benzenesulfonamide, clorsulon has a chemical name of 4-amino-6-trichloroethenyl-1,3-benzenedisulfonamide. Clorsulon may also be known as MK-401, *Curatrem®*, or *Ivomec®*.

Storage/Stability

Unless otherwise instructed by the manufacturer, clorsulon should be stored at room temperature (15-30°C).

Compatibility/Compounding Considerations

No specific information noted.

Dosage Forms/Regulatory Status

VETERINARY APPROVED PRODUCTS:

Clorsulon 8.5% (85 mg/mL) Oral Drench in quarts or gallons; *Curatrem®*; (OTC). FDA-approved for use in cattle. Slaughter withdrawal = 8 days (when used as labeled); Because a withdrawal time in milk has not been established, do not use in female dairy cattle of breeding age.

Clorsulon 10% (100 mg/mL) and Ivermectin 1% (10 mg/mL) Injection in 50 mL, 200 mL, 500 mL, & 1000 mL; *Ivomec® Plus, Alverin Plus®, Noromectin® Plus*; (OTC). FDA-approved for subcutaneous injection use in cattle. Do not use within 49 days of slaughter; do not use in female dairy cattle of breeding age.

HUMAN APPROVED PRODUCTS: NONE.

Revisions/References

Monograph revised/updated October 2013.

Cloxacillin Sodium
Cloxacillin Benzathine

(klox-a-sill-in)

Anti-Staphylococcal Penicillin

Prescriber Highlights

▶ Intramammary isoxazolyal (anti-staphylococcal) penicillin.
▶ Contraindicated: Hypersensitivity to penicillins.
▶ Oral dosage forms (human) no longer marketed in USA.

Uses/Indications

Cloxacillin is used via intramammary infusion in dry and lactating dairy cattle.

Pharmacology/Actions

Cloxacillin, dicloxacillin and oxacillin have nearly identical spectrums of activity and can be considered therapeutically equivalent when comparing *in vitro* activity. These penicillinase-resistant penicillins have a narrower spectrum of activity than the natural penicillins. Their antimicrobial efficacy is aimed directly against penicillinase-producing strains of gram-positive cocci, particularly Staphylococcal species. They are sometimes called anti-staphylococcal penicillins. There are documented strains of Staphylococci that are resistant to these drugs (so-called methicillin-resistant Staph), but these strains have not yet become a major problem in veterinary species. While this class of penicillins does have activity against some other gram-positive and gram-negative aerobes and anaerobes, other antibiotics (penicillins and otherwise) are usually better choices. The penicillinase-resistant penicillins are inactive against *Rickettsia*, mycobacteria, fungi, Mycoplasma, and viruses.

Pharmacokinetics

Cloxacillin is only available in intramammary dosage forms in the USA.

Contraindications/Precautions/Warnings

Penicillins are contraindicated in patients with a history of hypersensitivity to them. Because there may be cross-reactivity, use penicillins cautiously in patients that are documented hypersensitive to other beta-lactam antibiotics (*e.g.*, cephalosporins, cefamycins, carbapenems).

Adverse Effects

Adverse effects with the penicillins are usually not serious and have a relatively low frequency of occurrence.

Hypersensitivity reactions unrelated to dose can occur with these agents and can manifest as rashes, fever, eosinophilia, neutropenia, agranulocytosis, thrombocytopenia, leukopenia, anemias, lymphadenopathy, or full-blown anaphylaxis. In humans, it is estimated that 1-15% of patients hypersensitive to cephalosporins will also be hypersensitive to penicillins. The incidence of cross-reactivity in veterinary patients is unknown.

Reproductive/Nursing Safety

Penicillins have been shown to cross the placenta and safe use of them during pregnancy has not been firmly established, but neither have there been any documented teratogenic problems associated with these drugs. However, use only when the potential benefits outweigh the risks. In humans, the FDA categorizes this drug as category *B* for use during pregnancy (*Animal studies have not yet demonstrated risk to the fetus, but there are no adequate studies in pregnant women; or animal studies have shown an adverse effect, but adequate studies in pregnant women have not demonstrated a risk to the fetus in the first trimester of pregnancy, and there is no evidence of risk in later trimesters.*) In a separate system evaluating the safety of drugs in canine and feline pregnancy (Papich 1989), this drug is categorized as class: *A* (*Probably safe. Although specific studies may not have proved the safety of all drugs in dogs and cats, there are no reports of adverse effects in laboratory animals or women.*)

Overdosage/Acute Toxicity

Overdosage of intramammary infusions is unlikely to pose much risk to the patient, but may prolong withdrawal times.

Drug Interactions

- No significant interactions are likely when intramammary dosage forms are used as labeled.

Laboratory Considerations

- No specific concerns noted

Doses

- **CATTLE:**

  For mastitis (treatment or prophylaxis) caused by susceptible organisms (Labeled dose; FDA-approved):

  Lactating cow (using lactating cow formula; *Dari-Clox®*): After milking out and disinfecting teat, instill contents of syringe; massage. Repeat q12h for 3 total doses.

  Dry (non-lactating) cows (using dry cow formula; benzathine): After last milking (or early in the dry period), instill contents of syringe and massage into each quarter. (Package inserts; *Dari-Clox®*, *Orbenin-DC®*; *Dri-Clox®*)

Monitoring

- Because penicillins usually have minimal toxicity associated with their use, monitoring for efficacy is usually all that is required unless toxic signs develop. Serum levels and therapeutic drug monitoring are not routinely done with these agents.

Client Information

- Dry cow products (benzathine; *Orbenin-DC®*, *Dry-Clox®*) slaughter withdrawal = 28-30 days (depending on product used).
- Lactating cow product (*Dariclox®*) withdrawal times when used as labeled; milk withdrawal = 48 hours; slaughter withdrawal = 10 days.

Chemistry/Synonyms

An isoxazolyl-penicillin, cloxacillin sodium is a semisynthetic, penicillinase-resistant penicillin. It is available commercially as the monohydrate sodium salt that occurs as an odorless, bitter-tasting, white, crystalline powder. It is freely soluble in water and soluble in alcohol and has a pK_a of 2.7. One mg of cloxacillin sodium contains not less than 825 micrograms of cloxacillin.

Cloxacillin benzathine occurs as white or almost white powder that is slightly soluble in water and alcohol. A 1% (10 mg/mL) suspension has a pH from 3-6.5.

Cloxacillin sodium may also be known as: BRL-1621, sodium cloxacillin, chlorphenylmethyl isoxazolyl penicillin sodium, methylchlorophenyl isoxazolyl penicillin sodium, cloxacilina sodica, cloxacillinum natricum, or P-25; many trade names are available.

Storage/Stability

Unless otherwise instructed by the manufacturer, cloxacillin benzathine or cloxacillin sodium mastitis syringes should be stored at temperatures less than 25°C in tight containers.

Compatibility/Compounding Considerations

No specific information noted.

Dosage Forms/Regulatory Status

VETERINARY-LABELED PRODUCTS:

Cloxacillin Benzathine 500 mg (of cloxacillin) in a peanut-oil gel; 10 mL syringe for intramammary infusion: *Orbenin-DC®*, *Dry-Clox®*, *Boviclox®*; (Rx). FDA-approved for use in dairy cows during the dry period (immediately after last milking or early in the dry period). Do not use *Dry-Clox®* or *Boviclox®* within 30 days prior to calving;

(28 days for *Orbenin-DC®*). Slaughter withdrawal for Dry-Clox® = 30 days; *Orbenin®-DC* = 28 days; *Boviclox®* = 72 hours for milk and meat. A tolerance of 0.01 ppm has been established for negligible residues in uncooked edible meat and milk from cattle.

Cloxacillin Sodium 200 mg (of cloxacillin) in vegetable oils; 10 mL syringe for intramammary infusion: *Dariclox®*; (Rx). FDA-approved for use in lactating dairy cows. When used as labeled, Milk withdrawal = 48 hours; Slaughter withdrawal = 10 days.

HUMAN-LABELED PRODUCTS: NONE.

Revisions/References

Monograph revised/updated October 2013.

Codeine

(koe-deen)

Opiate

Prescriber Highlights

▶ Opiate used for analgesia, cough, & sometimes diarrhea in dogs & cats. Oral bioavailability in dogs is very low (high first pass effect) and it is unknown how much, if any analgesic efficacy it has.

▶ Often used in combination products with acetaminophen (NOT for cats).

▶ Adverse Effects most likely noted include: Sedation, constipation, high doses may cause respiratory depression. Cats may also show CNS stimulation.

▶ Controlled Substance (Class-II when used as a sole agent).

Uses/Indications

In small animal medicine, codeine is potentially useful as an oral analgesic (mild pain), antitussive or an antidiarrheal. Its pharmacokinetic profile raises questions of utility in dogs.

Pharmacology/Actions

Codeine possesses activity similar to other opiate agonists, but its pharmacokinetics and metabolic fate can vary widely in differing species. It is an effective antitussive and a mild analgesic. It produces similar respiratory depression, as does morphine at equianalgesic dosages.

Pharmacokinetics

In dogs, oral codeine is well absorbed, but its bioavailability is very low (approx. 4% systemically as codeine) as it appears to undergo high first-pass metabolism primarily to codeine-6-glucuronide. Codeine-6-glucuronide has opiate activity, but it is not clear how much antinociceptive, antitussive or antidiarrheal activity it has in dogs. The author of this kinetics study concluded that future studies are needed to assess the antinociceptive effects of oral codeine in dogs to determine if it can be effectively used (KuKanich 2010).

The following information is human data unless otherwise noted. After oral administration, codeine salts are rapidly absorbed. Codeine is about 2/3's as effective after oral administration when compared with parenteral administration. After oral dosing, onset of action is usually within 30 minutes and analgesic effects persist for 4-6 hours. Codeine is metabolized in the liver and then excreted into the urine.

Contraindications/Precautions/Warnings

Do not use the combination product containing acetaminophen in cats. All opiates should be used with caution in patients with hypothyroidism, severe renal insufficiency, adrenocortical insufficiency (Addison's disease), and in geriatric or severely debilitated patients. Codeine is contraindicated in cases where the patient is hypersensitive to narcotic analgesics, or taking monoamine oxidase inhibitors (MAOIs). It is also contraindicated in patients with diarrhea caused by a toxic ingestion (until the toxin is eliminated from the GI tract) or when used repeatedly in patients with severe inflammatory bowel disease.

Codeine should be used with caution in patients with head injuries or increased intracranial pressure, and in those with acute abdominal conditions (*e.g.*, colic) as it may obscure the diagnosis or clinical course of these conditions. Use with extreme caution in patients suffering from respiratory disease or from acute respiratory dysfunction (*e.g.*, pulmonary edema secondary to smoke inhalation).

Opiate analgesics are contraindicated in patients that have been stung by the scorpion species *Centuroides sculpturatus Ewing* and *C. gertschi Stahnke* as they may potentiate these venoms.

Codeine, like other opioids can have immunosuppressive effects. It is not clear if this is clinically significant.

Codeine has a high human abuse potential; be alert to drug seeking clients and maintain security for in-house stock.

Adverse Effects

Codeine generally is well tolerated, but adverse effects are possible, particularly at higher dosages or with repeated use. Sedation is the most likely effect seen. Potential gastrointestinal effects include anorexia, vomiting, constipation, ileus, and biliary and pancreatic duct spasms. Respiratory depression is generally not noted unless the patient receives high doses or is at risk (see contraindications above).

In cats, opiates may cause CNS stimulation with hyperexcitability, tremors, and seizures.

Reproductive/Nursing Safety

Opiates cross the placenta. Very high doses in mice have caused delayed ossification. Use during pregnancy only when the benefits outweigh the risks, particularly with chronic use. In humans, the FDA categorizes this drug as category *C* for use during pregnancy (*Animal studies have shown an adverse effect on the fetus, but there are no adequate studies in humans; or there are no animal reproduction studies and no adequate studies in humans.*) In a separate system evaluating the safety of drugs in canine and feline pregnancy (Papich 1989), this drug is categorized as class: *B* (*Safe for use if used cautiously. Studies in laboratory animals may have uncovered some risk, but these drugs appear to be safe in dogs and cats or these drugs are safe if they are not administered when the animal is near term.*)

Although codeine enters maternal milk, no documented problems have been associated with its use in nursing mothers.

Overdosage/Acute Toxicity

Opiate overdosage may produce profound respiratory and/or CNS depression in most species. Other effects can include cardiovascular collapse, hypothermia, and skeletal muscle hypotonia. Oral ingestions of codeine should be removed when possible using standard gut removal protocols. Because rapid changes in CNS status may occur, inducing vomiting should be attempted with caution. Naloxone is the agent of choice in treating respiratory depression. In massive overdoses, naloxone doses may need to be repeated and animals should be closely observed because naloxone's effects may diminish before subtoxic levels of codeine are attained. Mechanical respiratory support should also be considered in cases of severe respiratory depression. Serious overdoses involving any of the opiates should be closely monitored; it is suggested to contact an animal poison control center for further information.

Drug Interactions

The following drug interactions have either been reported or are theoretical in humans or animals receiving codeine and may be of significance in veterinary patients. Unless otherwise noted, use together is not necessarily contraindicated, but weigh the potential risks and perform additional monitoring when appropriate.

- **ANTICHOLINERGIC DRUGS:** Use with codeine may increase the chances of constipation developing.
- **ANTIDEPRESSANTS (tricyclic/monoamine oxidase inhibitors):** May potentiate CNS depressant effects.
- **CNS DEPRESSANTS, OTHER** (*e.g.*, **anesthetic agents, antihistamines, phenothiazines, barbiturates, tranquilizers, alcohol,** etc.) May cause increased CNS or respiratory depression when used with codeine.

Laboratory Considerations

- As they may increase biliary tract pressure, opiates can increase plasma amylase and lipase values up to 24 hours following their administration.

Doses

- **DOGS:**

  As an antitussive (extra-label): 1 – 2 mg/kg PO q6-12h.

  As an analgesic (extra-label):

  a) When used alone, anecdotal analgesic dosages for codeine are usually 1 – 2 mg/kg q4-6h, but some have suggested that dosages up to 4 mg/kg may required. Codeine's pharmacokinetics in dogs may be problematic as it undergoes a high first-pass effect and it is not clear how much analgesic efficacy the primary metabolite possesses.

  b) When used with the acetaminophen combination products (*e.g.*, Tylenol #3 etc.): Most recommend using either the #3 (30 mg of codeine) or the #4 (60 mg codeine) combination tablets, and dosing as per the acetaminophen component at 10 – 15 mg/kg (of acetaminophen) PO q8h. For example, if using one tablet PO every 8 hours the "Tylenol #4" (acetaminophen 300 mg/codeine 60 mg) product in a 20 kg dog, the dose for each would be acetaminophen 15 mg/kg and codeine 3 mg/kg. The codeine dose would be 1.5 mg/kg if using the "#3" (acetaminophen 300 mg/codeine 30 mg) product in the same dog.

- **CATS:**

  Note: Do **NOT** use the combination product containing acetaminophen in cats.

  As an analgesic (extra-label): 0.5 – 2 mg/kg PO q6-8h.

- **RABBITS:**

  Using acetaminophen and codeine elixir (extra-label): 1 mL in 10 – 20 mL of drinking water (add dextrose to enhance palatability). (Ivey et al. 2000)

Monitoring

- Efficacy.
- Adverse effects (see above).

Client Information

- May give with food or on an empty stomach.
- Sedation and constipation are the most common side effects. Cats may also show CNS stimulation (overly excited).
- Combination with acetaminophen (*e.g.*, Tylenol #3) **must not be used in cats or ferrets**.
- Codeine (alone) is a controlled drug (C-II); requires a new written prescription each time.
- Keep out of reach of children.
- Report any significant changes in behavior or activity level, or GI effects (constipation, lack of appetite, vomiting) to veterinarian.

Chemistry/Synonyms

A phenanthrene-derivative opiate agonist, codeine is available as the base and three separate salts. Codeine base is slightly soluble in water and freely soluble in alcohol. Codeine phosphate occurs as fine, white, needle-like crystals or white, crystalline powder. It is freely soluble in water. Codeine sulfate's appearance resembles codeine phosphate, but it is soluble in water.

Codeine may also be known as: codeini or codeinii; many trade names are available.

Storage/Stability

Codeine sulfate tablets should be stored in light-resistant, well-closed containers at room temperature. Codeine phosphate injection should be stored at room temperature (avoid freezing) and protected from light. Do not use the injection if it is discolored or contains a precipitate.

Compatibility/Compounding Considerations

Codeine phosphate injection is reportedly **compatible** with glycopyrrolate or hydroxyzine HCl. It is reportedly **incompatible** with aminophylline, ammonium chloride, heparin sodium, pentobarbital sodium, phenobarbital sodium, phenytoin sodium, sodium bicarbonate, and sodium iodide.

Dosage Forms/Regulatory Status

VETERINARY-LABELED PRODUCTS: NONE.
The ARCI (Racing Commissioners International) has designated this drug as a class 1 substance. See the appendix for more information.

HUMAN-LABELED PRODUCTS:
There are many products available containing codeine. The following is a partial listing:

Codeine Sulfate Oral Solution: 30 mg/5 mL (6 mg/mL); generic; (Rx, C-II)

Codeine Sulfate Tablets: 15 mg, 30 mg & 60 mg; generic; (Rx, C-II)

Codeine Phosphate Parenteral Injection: 15 mg/mL & 30 mg/mL in 2 mL *Carpuject* syringe; generic; (Rx, C-II)

Codeine Phosphate 7.5 mg (#1), 15 mg (#2), 30 mg (#3), 60 mg (#4) with Acetaminophen 300 mg tablets; *Tylenol® with Codeine #'s 1, 2, 3, 4* (McNeil); generic; (Rx, C-III) **Warning:** Do not use in cats.

Note: Codeine-only products are Class-II controlled substances. Combination products with aspirin or acetaminophen are Class-III. Codeine containing cough syrups are either Class-V or Class-III, depending on the state.

Revisions/References

Monograph revised/updated October 2013.

Ivey, E. & J. Morrisey (2000). Therapeutics for Rabbits. *Vet Clin NA: Exotic Anim Pract* 3:1(Jan): 183-216.
KuKanich, B. (2010). Pharmacokinetics of acetaminophen, codeine, and the codeine metabolites morphine and codeine-6-glucuronide in healthy Greyhound dogs. *J. Vet. Pharmacol. Ther.* 33(1): 15-21.

Colchicine

(kol-chi-seen)   Colcrys®

Antiinflammatory

Prescriber Highlights

► Unique antiinflammatory has been used for Shar-Pei fever; occasionally used in dogs for hepatic cirrhosis/fibrosis; relatively experimental.
► Contraindications: Serious renal, GI, or cardiac dysfunction.
► Caution: Geriatric or debilitated patients.
► Teratogenic, reduces spermatogenesis.
► Most likely adverse effects are GI distress (diarrhea, vomiting; may be an early sign of toxicity), but several serious effects are possible including bone marrow suppression.

Uses/Indications

In veterinary medicine, colchicine has been proposed as a treatment in small animals for amyloidosis or Shar Pei fever. For colchicine to be effective, however, it must be given early in the course of the disease and it is ineffective once renal failure has occurred. At the time of writing (2013), no conclusive evidence exists for its efficacy for these or any other indication in dogs.

Colchicine has also been proposed for treating chronic hepatic fibrosis presumably by decreasing the formation and increasing the breakdown of collagen, but its efficacy is in question.

A case report (Brown et al. 2008) using colchicine to treat endotracheal stent granulation stenosis in a dog has been published and the drug may find a place in therapy for this indication after further investigation.

Colchicine possibly may be benefit in reducing hyperuricemia in birds with renal disease, amyloidosis or to reduce renal or hepatic fibrosis. No controlled studies were located to document efficacy for any of these potential uses.

Pharmacology/Actions

Colchicine inhibits cell division during metaphase by interfering with sol-gel formation and the mitotic spindle. The mechanism for its antifibrotic activity is believed secondary to collagenases activity stimulation.

Colchicine apparently blocks the synthesis and secretion of serum amyloid A (SAA; an acute-phase reactant protein) by hepatocytes thereby preventing the formation of amyloid-enhancing factor and preventing amyloid disposition.

Colchicine is best known in human medicine for its anti-gout activity. The mechanism for this effect is not fully understood, but it probably is related to the drug's ability to reduce the inflammatory response to the disposition of monosodium urate crystals.

Pharmacokinetics

No information was located specifically for domestic animals; the following information is human/lab animal data unless otherwise noted. After oral administration, colchicine is absorbed from the GI tract. Some of the absorbed drug is metabolized in the liver (first-pass effect). These metabolites and unchanged drug are re-secreted into the GI tract via biliary secretions where it is reabsorbed. This "recycling" phenomena may explain the intestinal manifestations noted with colchicine toxicity. Colchicine is distributed into several tissues, but is concentrated in leukocytes. Plasma half-life is about 20 minutes, but leukocyte half-life is approximately 60 hours. Colchicine is deacetylated in the liver and metabolized in other tissues. While most of a dose (as colchicine and metabolites) is excreted in the feces, some is excreted in the urine. More may be excreted in the urine in patients with hepatic disease. Patients with severe renal disease may have prolonged half-lives.

Contraindications/Precautions/Warnings

Colchicine is contraindicated in patients with serious renal, GI, or cardiac dysfunction and should be used with caution in patients in early stages of these disorders. It should also be used with caution in geriatric or debilitated patients.

Colchicine use in veterinary medicine is somewhat controversial, as safety and efficacy have not been well documented.

Adverse Effects

There has been only marginal experience with colchicine in domestic animals. Colchicine can cause nausea, vomiting, and diarrhea in dogs, particularly at higher dosages. Rarely, bone marrow depression (neutropenia), renal toxicity and peripheral neuropathy can occur.

In humans, GI effects have been noted (abdominal pain, anorexia, vomiting, diarrhea) and can be an early indication of toxicity; it is recommended to discontinue therapy (in humans) should these occur. Prolonged administration has caused bone marrow depression.

Reproductive/Nursing Safety

Because colchicine has been demonstrated to be teratogenic in laboratory animals (mice and hamsters) it should be used during pregnancy only when its potential benefits outweigh its risks. Colchicine may decrease spermatogenesis. In humans, the FDA categorizes this drug as category *C* (ORAL) for use during pregnancy (*Animal studies have shown an adverse effect on the fetus, but there are no adequate studies in humans; or there are no animal reproduction studies and no adequate studies in humans.*) In humans, the FDA categorizes this drug as category *D* (PARENTERAL) for use during pregnancy (*There is evidence of human fetal risk, but the potential benefits from the use of the drug in pregnant women may be acceptable despite its potential risks.*)

It is unknown if colchicine enters maternal milk; use cautiously in nursing mothers.

Overdosage/Acute Toxicity

Colchicine can be a very toxic drug after relatively small overdoses. Deaths in humans have been reported with a single oral ingestion of as little as 7 mg, but 65 mg is considered the lethal dose in an adult human. GI manifestations are usually the presenting signs seen. These can range from anorexia and vomiting to bloody diarrhea or paralytic ileus. Renal failure, hepatotoxicity, pancytopenia, paralysis, shock, and vascular collapse may also occur.

There is no specific antidote to colchicine. Gut removal techniques should be employed when applicable. Because of the extensive GI "recycling" of the drug, repeated doses of activated charcoal and a saline cathartic may reduce systemic absorption. Other treatment is symptomatic and supportive. Dialysis (peritoneal) may be of benefit.

Drug Interactions

The following drug interactions have either been reported or are theoretical in humans or animals receiving colchicine and may be of significance in veterinary patients. Unless otherwise noted, use together is not necessarily contraindicated, but weigh the potential risks and perform additional monitoring when appropriate.

- **AMPHOTERICIN B:** Potentially, increased risk for nephrotoxicity.
- **ANTINEOPLASTICS, IMMUNOSUPPRESSANTS, CHLORAMPHENICOL:** May cause additive myelosuppression or GI effects when used with colchicine.
- **CYCLOSPORINE:** Potentially, increased risk for nephrotoxicity or bone marrow depression.

Laboratory Considerations

- Colchicine may cause false-positive results when testing for **erythrocytes or hemoglobin in urine**.
- Colchicine may interfere with **17-hydroxycorticosteroid** determinations in urine if using the Reddy, Jenkins, and Thorn procedure.
- Colchicine may cause increased serum values of **alkaline phosphatase**.

Doses

- **DOGS:**

  For the adjunctive treatment of hepatic cirrhosis/fibrosis; 'Shar Pei fever', amyloidosis (extra-label): Most recommend a dosage of 0.03 mg/kg PO once daily. Some suggest starting at a lower initial dosage to determine if dog will tolerate (GI effects). For adult Shar Pei dogs, if using the commercially available 0.6 mg tablets, it has been suggested to start with ½ tablet (0.3 mg) PO once daily and increase dosage in 0.3 increments every 4-5 days as tolerated until a "target" dose of up to 0.6 mg/dog PO twice daily is reached. In dogs that cannot tolerate a given dosage, the dosage is reduced or the drug is temporarily discontinued and restarted at a lower dose.

- **BIRDS:**

  For the adjunctive treatment of hepatic fibrosis, amyloidosis, or hyperuricemia (extra-label): Recommended anecdotal doses can vary widely, from 0.01 mg/kg PO q12h to 0.2 mg/kg PO twice daily. It is recommended to start at the lower end of the dosage range and increase dosage gradually.

Monitoring

- Efficacy.
- Adverse effects (see above).
- CBC.
- Cobalamin levels. Consider when using long-term.

Client Information

- Little experience using this drug in animals; side effects are not well known. Report any side effects to your veterinarian.
- May give with or without food.
- Pregnant women should avoid exposure to the drug or urine of animals being treated.

Chemistry/Synonyms

An antigout drug possessing many other pharmacologic effects, colchicine occurs as a pale yellow, amorphous powder or scales. It is soluble in water and freely soluble in alcohol.

Colchicine may also be known as: colchicinum, or *Colcrys®*.

Storage/Stability

Colchicine tablets should be stored in tight, light resistant containers.

Compatibility/Compounding Considerations

No specific information noted.

Dosage Forms/Regulatory Status

VETERINARY-LABELED PRODUCTS: NONE.

The ARCI (Racing Commissioners International) has designated this drug as a class 4 substance. See the appendix for more information.

HUMAN-LABELED PRODUCTS:

Colchicine Oral Tablets: 0.6 mg (1/100 gr); *Colcrys®*; (Rx). **Note:** At the time of writing (2103) there is only one commercially available FDA-approved product and expense may be considerable. However, it has been reported that the manufacturer may offer a reduced cost program when this drug is used in animal patients. More information may be found at colcrys.com or the direct link. Compounding pharmacies may also be able to provide colchicine preparations.

Revisions/References

Monograph revised/updated October 2013.

Brown, S. A., et al. (2008). Endotracheal stent granulation stenosis resolution after colchicine therapy in a dog. *Journal of Veterinary Internal Medicine* 22(4): 1052-5.

Co-Trimoxazole; Co-trimazine — See Sulfa/Trimethoprim

Corticotropin (ACTH)

(kor-ti-koe-troe-pin)   Acthar®

Hormonal Diagnostic Agent

Prescriber Highlights

▶ Stimulates cortisol release; used primarily to test for hyper- or hypoadrenocorticism (ACTH-stimulation test); use as a screening test for naturally occurring "Cushing's" is becoming less popular than in the past. Also used to test for iatrogenic Cushing's and to monitor therapy when treating with anti-adrenal drugs.

▶ Adverse Effects: Unlikely unless using chronically.

▶ Do not administer gel form IV.

▶ Issues include availability & expense; may need to obtain via a compounding pharmacy. Most have switched to using cosyntropin.

Uses/Indications

Availability of corticotropin in FDA-approved products is an issue as no commercially products were commercially available for veterinary use at the time of this writing. Either cosyntropin (see monograph) or compounded ACTH products are potential substitutes.

In veterinary medicine, an ACTH product (*Adrenomone®*) was FDA-approved for use in dogs, cats, and beef or dairy cattle for stimulation of the adrenal cortex when there is a deficiency of ACTH and as a therapeutic agent in primary bovine ketosis, but apparently is no longer commercially available.

In practice, ACTH tends to be used most often in the diagnosis of hypoadrenocorticism (ACTH-stimulation test), iatrogenic Cushing's syndrome, and to monitor the response to mitotane or trilostane therapy in Cushing's syndrome. It is less often recommended as a screening test for naturally occurring "Cushing's" syndrome in dogs as the test is relatively insensitive. One reference (Behrend 2003) recommends using the ACTH stimulation test if the dog has non-adrenal illness, received any form of exogenous glucocorticoids (including topicals) or phenobarbital. If the dog has no known non-adrenal illness and moderate to severe clinical signs of hyperadrenocorticism, use the low-dose dexamethasone suppression test. If using the ACTH-stim test, the author states that cosyntropin is the agent of choice (see that monograph).

Pharmacology/Actions

ACTH stimulates the adrenal cortex (principally the zona fasciculata) to stimulate the production and release of glucocorticoids (primarily cortisol in mammals and corticosterone in birds). ACTH release is controlled by corticotropin-releasing factor (CRF) activated in the central nervous system and via a negative feedback pathway, whereby either endogenous or exogenous glucocorticoids suppresses ACTH release.

Pharmacokinetics

Because it is rapidly degraded by proteolytic enzymes in the gut, ACTH cannot be administered PO. It is not effective if administered topically to the skin or eye.

After IM injection in humans, repository corticotropin injection is absorbed over 8-16 hours. The elimination half-life of circulating ACTH is about 15 minutes but because of the slow absorption after IM injection of the gel, effects may persist up to 24 hours.

Contraindications/Precautions/Warnings

When used for diagnostic purposes, it is unlikely that increases in serum cortisol levels induced by ACTH will have significant deleterious effects on conditions where increased cortisol levels are contraindicated (*e.g.*, systemic fungal infections, osteoporosis, peptic ulcer disease, etc.). ACTH gel should not be used in patients hypersensitive to porcine proteins.

Adverse Effects

Prolonged use may result in fluid and electrolyte disturbances and other adverse effects; if using on a chronic basis, refer to the human literature for an extensive listing of potential adverse reactions. The veterinary manufacturer suggests giving potassium supplementation with chronic therapy.

Do not administer the repository form (gel) IV.

Reproductive/Nursing Safety

ACTH should only be used during pregnancy when the potential benefits outweigh the risks. It may be embryocidal. Neonates born from mothers receiving ACTH should be observed for signs of adrenocortical insufficiency. In humans, the FDA categorizes this drug as category *C* for use during pregnancy (*Animal studies have shown an adverse effect on the fetus, but there are no adequate studies in humans; or there are no animal reproduction studies and no adequate studies in humans.*)

Overdosage/Acute Toxicity

When used for diagnostic purposes, acute inadvertent overdoses are unlikely to cause any significant adverse effects. Monitor as required and treat symptomatically if necessary.

Drug Interactions

The following drug interactions have either been reported or are theoretical in humans or animals receiving corticotropin for diagnostic purposes and may be of significance in veterinary patients. Unless otherwise noted, use together is not necessarily contraindicated, but weigh the potential risks and perform additional monitoring when appropriate.

- **ANTICHOLINESTERASES** (*e.g.*, **pyridostigmine**): ACTH may antagonize effects in patients with myasthenia gravis.
- **DIURETICS**: ACTH may increase electrolyte loss.

Laboratory Considerations

- Patients should not receive **hydrocortisone** or **cortisone** on test day.
- ACTH may decrease ^{131}I uptake by the thyroid gland.
- ACTH may suppress **skin test reactions.**
- ACTH may interfere with **urinary estrogen** determinations.
- Obtain specific information from the laboratory on sample handling and laboratory normals for cortisol when doing ACTH stimulation tests.

Doses

Note: When using compounded ACTH products, it is recommended to get several post-ACTH samples, at a minimum one and two hours following injection. (Behrend 2005)

- **DOGS:**

  ACTH Stimulation Test (extra-label): Draw baseline blood sample for cortisol determination and administer 2.2 Units/kg of ACTH gel IM. Draw sample 120 minutes after injection. (Feldman et al. 1984), (Kemppainen et al. 1989)

- **CATS:**

  ACTH Stimulation Test (extra-label): Draw baseline blood sample for cortisol determination and administer 2.2 Units/kg of ACTH gel IM. Draw samples at 60 minutes and 120 minutes after injection. (Kemppainen et al. 1989)

- **HORSES:**

  ACTH Stimulation Test (extra-label): Obtain pre-dose level. Administer 1 Unit/kg IM of ACTH gel between 8 and 10 AM; take post ACTH cortisol levels at 2 and 4 hours post dose. Horses with a functional adrenal gland should have a 2- to 3-fold increase in plasma cortisol when compared with baseline. (Toribio 2004)

- **BIRDS:**

ACTH Stimulation Test (extra-label): Draw baseline blood sample for corticosterone (not cortisol) determination and administer 16 – 25 Units IM. Draw second sample 1-2 hours later. Normal baseline corticosterone levels vary with regard to species, but generally range from 1.5 – 7 ng/mL. After ACTH, corticosterone levels generally increase by 5-10X's those of baseline. Specific values are listed in the reference. (Lothrop et al. 1986)

Chemistry/Synonyms

A 39 amino acid polypeptide, corticotropin is secreted from the anterior pituitary. The first 24 amino acids (from the N-terminal end of the chain) define its biologic activity. While human, sheep, cattle and swine corticotropin have different structures, the first 24 amino acids are the same and, therefore, biologic activity is thought to be identical. Commercial sources of ACTH have generally been obtained from porcine pituitaries. One USP unit of corticotropin is equivalent to 1 mg of the international standard.

Corticotropin may also be known as: ACTH, adrenocorticotrophic hormone, adrenocorticotrophin, corticotrophin, corticotropinum, *Acethropan®, Acortan simplex®, Actharn®, Acthelea®, Acton prolongatum®, H.P. Acthar®* or *Cortrophin-Zinc®.*

Storage/Stability

Corticotropin in the past has been available commercially as corticotropin for injection, repository corticotropin for injection, and corticotropin zinc hydroxide suspension. Corticotropin is commonly called ACTH (abbreviated from adrenocorticotropic hormone). Repository corticotropin is often called ACTH gel and was the most commonly used ACTH product in veterinary medicine.

Corticotropin for injection (aqueous) can be stored at room temperature (15-30°C) before reconstitution. After reconstitution, it should be refrigerated and used within 24 hours. Repository corticotropin injection should be stored in the refrigerator (2-8°C). To allow ease in withdrawing the gel into a syringe, the vial may be warmed with warm water prior to use.

Compatibility/Compounding Considerations

No specific information noted.

Dosage Forms/Regulatory Status

VETERINARY-LABELED PRODUCTS: NONE.

Compounded ACTH products may be available from compounding pharmacies.

HUMAN-LABELED PRODUCTS:

Corticotropin Repository Injection: 80 Units/mL in 5 mL multidose vials; *H.P. Acthar® Gel* ; (Rx) **Note:** This product is only available through a specialty pharmacy distribution system and is not available via regular retail pharmacies or drug wholesalers.

Revisions/References

Monograph revised/updated October 2013.

Behrend, E. (2003). *Common questions in endocrine diagnostic testing.* Proceedings: Western Veterinary Conference. accessed via Veterinary Information Network; vin.com

Behrend, E. (2005). *Use of compounded ACTH for adrenal function testing in dogs.* Proceedings: ACVIM. accessed via Veterinary Information Network; vin.com

Feldman, E. C. & M. E. Peterson (1984). Hypoadrenocorticism. *Vet Clin of North America: Small Anim Prac* **14**(4): 751-66.

Kemppainen, R. J. & C. A. Zerbe (1989). Common Endocrine Diagnostic Tests: Normal Values and Interpretation. *Current Veterinary Therapy X: Small Animal Practice.* R. W. Kirk. Philadelphia, WB Saunders: 961-8.

Lothrop, C. D. & G. J. Harrison (1986). Miscellaneous diagnostic tests. *Clinical Avian Medicine and Surgery.* G. J. Harrison and L. R. Harrison. Philadelphia, W.B. Saunders: 293-7.

Toribio, R. (2004). The adrenal glands. *Equine Internal Medicine 2nd Edition.* M. Reed, W. Bayly and D. Sellon. Phila, Saunders: 1357-61.

Cortisone Acetate

(kor-ti-zone ass-*ah-tate*)

Adrenal Corticosteroid

Prescriber Highlights

► Oral glucocorticoid with both glucocorticoid and mineralocorticoid effects; may be a lower drug cost way to manage Addison's by reducing dosage requirements for mineralocorticoid drugs.

► Not commonly used in veterinary medicine; whether it has any clinically significant benefit in dogs over oral prednis(ol)one is controversial.

► Typical cautions and adverse effects associated with other corticosteroid drugs if used at supra-physiologic replacement doses; otherwise should be very well tolerated.

► Relatively inexpensive.

Uses/Indications

Cortisone acetate potentially could be an alternative to predniso(lo)ne for the oral treatment of hypoadrenocorticism in dogs. *In vivo* it is rapidly converted to cortisol and thereby could serve as a total replacement for both glucocorticoid and mineralocorticoid effects. Whether cortisone acetate is any more effective then prednis(ol)one for long-term treatment in dogs is controversial as some believe that any benefit the increased mineralocorticoid activity cortisone acetate has is clinically insignificant.

Pharmacology/Actions

Cortisone/cortisol has effects on practically every body system. For a more complete description refer to the Hydrocortisone monograph.

Pharmacokinetics

Like other glucocorticoids, cortisone acetate's pharmacokinetics do not correlate with its pharmacodynamic activity. Cortisol acetate is absorbed and converted to cortisol (hydrocortisone) *in vivo*. Oral bioavailability in humans ranges widely, but is approximately 50%.

Contraindications/Precautions/Warnings

When used for physiologic replacement in dogs with hypoadrenocorticism, cortisone acetate is contraindicated if the patient is hypersensitive to it. If used at supra-physiologic dosages, the typical contraindications and warnings for drugs like prednisone should be followed. See that monograph for more information.

Adverse Effects

When used for physiologic replacement in dogs with hypoadrenocorticism, cortisone acetate should be very well tolerated. Potentially, GI effects (vomiting, inappetence, diarrhea) could occur and hypersensitivity reactions are theoretically possible. If used at supra-physiologic dosages, the typical adverse effect profile for drugs like prednisone is possible. See the prednisone monograph for more information.

Reproductive/Nursing Safety

Glucocorticoids are probably necessary for normal fetal development. They may be required for adequate surfactant production, myelin, retinal, pancreatic, and mammary development. However, excessive dosages early in pregnancy may lead to teratogenic effects. In humans, the FDA categorizes this drug as category *C* for use during pregnancy (*Animal studies have shown an adverse effect on the fetus, but there are no adequate studies in humans; or there are no animal reproduction studies and no adequate studies in humans.*)

Glucocorticoids unbound to plasma proteins will enter milk. High dosages or prolonged administration to mothers may potentially inhibit the growth of nursing newborns.

Overdosage/Acute Toxicity

Acute ingestion is rarely a clinical problem and clinical effects are unlikely with acute overdose. However, neuropsychiatric effects can occur; cardiac arrhythmias and anaphylaxis are possible, but very rare.

Drug Interactions

The following drug interactions have either been reported or are theoretical in humans or animals receiving cortisone and may be of significance in veterinary patients. Unless otherwise noted, use together is not necessarily contraindicated, but weigh the potential risks and perform additional monitoring when appropriate.

- **AMPHOTERICIN B**: Administered concomitantly with glucocorticoids may cause hypokalemia; in humans, there have been cases of CHF and cardiac enlargement reported after using hydrocortisone to treat Amphotericin B adverse effects.
- **ASPIRIN**: Glucocorticoids may reduce salicylate blood levels and increase risk for GI ulceration/bleeding.
- **DIURETICS, POTASSIUM-DEPLETING** (*e.g.*, **spironolactone, triamterene**): Administered concomitantly with glucocorticoids may cause hypokalemia.
- **ESTROGENS**: The effects of hydrocortisone and, possibly other glucocorticoids, may be potentiated by concomitant administration with estrogens.
- **INSULIN; ANTIDIABETIC AGENTS**: Insulin requirements may increase in patients receiving glucocorticoids.
- **MITOTANE**: May alter the metabolism of steroids; higher than usual doses of steroids may be necessary to treat mitotane-induced adrenal insufficiency.
- **NSAIDs**: Administration of ulcerogenic drugs with glucocorticoids may increase the risk of gastrointestinal ulceration.
- **POTASSIUM-DEPLETING DRUGS** (*e.g.*, **amphotericin B, furosemide, thiazides**): Administered concomitantly with glucocorticoids may cause hypokalemia.
- **VACCINES**: Patients receiving corticosteroids at immunosuppressive dosages should generally not receive live attenuated-virus vaccines as virus replication may be augmented; a diminished immune response may occur after vaccine, toxoid, or bacterin administration in patients receiving glucocorticoids.
- **WARFARIN**: Hydrocortisone may affect INR's; monitor.

Laboratory Considerations

- Cortisone can cross react with cortisol in ACTH response test. This test must be performed before cortisone is administered. (**Note**: Dexamethasone does not cross react).
- Glucocorticoids may increase **serum cholesterol**.
- Glucocorticoids may increase **urine glucose** levels.
- Glucocorticoids may decrease **serum potassium**.
- Glucocorticoids can suppress the release of **thyroid stimulating hormone** (TSH) and reduce T_3 & T_4 values. Thyroid gland atrophy has been reported after chronic glucocorticoid administration. Uptake of I^{131} by the thyroid may be decreased by glucocorticoids.
- Reactions to **skin tests** may be suppressed by glucocorticoids.
- False-negative results of the **nitroblue tetrazolium** test for systemic bacterial infections may be induced by glucocorticoids.
- Glucocorticoids may cause **neutrophilia** within 4-8 hours after dosing and return to baseline within 24-48 hours after drug discontinuation.
- Glucocorticoids can cause **lymphopenia** that can persist for weeks after drug discontinuation in dogs.

Doses

- **DOGS:**

  For long-term treatment of hypoadrenocorticism (extra-label): In the changeover period as animals recover from an acute crisis, start eating and drinking and are changed from parenteral to oral medication, traditionally a semi-selective mineralocorticoid (fludrocortisone) and a semi-selective glucocorticoid (cortisone acetate or prednisolone) are initially used together. The former is discontinued in a proportion of patients after one to two months. When using cortisone acetate most hypoadrenocorticoid dogs are started on a dose of 0.5 – 1 mg/kg PO q12-24h. Once stable, generally a dose of 0.5 mg/kg PO q12-24h provides adequate additional glucocorticoid supplementation. Some clinicians advocate prednisolone use as a glucocorticoid supplement in the long-term management of hypoadrenocorticism, but in the author's (Church) opinion cortisone acetate is a more effective alternative. (Church 2008), (Church 2009)

Client Information

- Not commonly used, but may be effective for long-term treatment of Addison's disease (hypoadrenocorticism) in dogs.
- May allow using lower (or no) doses of mineralocorticoid drugs (*e.g.*, desoxycorticosterone—DOCP, fludrocortisone).
- Side effects not likely, but if dose is too high (long-term) "Cushingoid" effects could occur; if too low, Addison's effects could occur.
- Surgery or stress (*e.g.*, trauma, illness) may require additional glucocorticoids (*e.g.*, methylprednisolone, etc.).
- Do not stop drug abruptly.

Monitoring

Monitoring of cortisone therapy is dependent on its reason for use, dosage, adjunctive mineralocorticoid therapy, dosage schedule (daily versus alternate day therapy), duration of therapy, and the animal's age and condition. The following list may not be appropriate or complete for all animals; use clinical assessment and judgment should adverse effects be noted:

- Weight, appetite, signs of edema.
- Serum and/or urine electrolytes.
- Total plasma proteins, albumin.
- Blood glucose.
- Growth and development in young animals.
- ACTH stimulation test, if necessary.

Chemistry/Synonyms

Cortisone acetate is synthetic acetate ester of cortisone. It occurs as a white or practically white, odorless, crystalline powder. It is insoluble in water and slightly soluble in alcohol.

Cortisone acetate may also be known as acetato de cortisona, compound E acetate, acétate de cortisone, cortisoni acetas, or 11-dehydro-17-hydroxycorticosterone acetate.

Storage/Stability

Cortisone acetate tablets should be stored in well-closed containers at a temperature less than 40°C, preferably at 15-30°C.

Compatibility/Compounding Considerations

No specific information noted.

Dosage Forms/Regulatory Status

VETERINARY-LABELED PRODUCTS: NONE.

HUMAN-LABELED PRODUCTS:

Cortisone Acetate Oral Tablets: 25 mg; generic; (Rx)

Revisions/References

Monograph revised/updated October 2013.

Church, D. B. (2008). *Addison's Disease: What's The Best Treatment?* Proceedings: WSAVA. accessed via Veterinary Information Network; vin.com

Church, D. B. (2009). *Management of Hypoadrenocorticism.* Proceedings: WSAVA. accessed via Veterinary Information Network; vin.com

Cosyntropin

(koh-sin-troh-pin)   Tetracosactide, Cortrosyn®

Hormonal Diagnostic Agent

Prescriber Highlights

▶ Alternative to ACTH for adrenal function tests. Should be given IV. Low doses have been shown to be useful for screening tests.

▶ Drug-lab interactions.

Uses/Indications

Cosyntropin is used primarily as an alternative to ACTH to test for adrenocortical insufficiency (Addison's), or hyperadrenocorticism. Additionally, it is used to help diagnose iatrogenic Cushing's syndrome, and monitor the response to mitotane or trilostane therapy in Cushing's syndrome.

Pharmacology/Actions

Like endogenous corticotropin, cosyntropin stimulates the adrenal cortex (in normal patients) to secrete cortisol, corticosterone, etc. Because of its structure, corticotropin is not as immunogenic as endogenous corticotropin. Apparently, the bulk of immunogenicity resides in the C-terminal portion of corticotropin (22–39 amino acids) and cosyntropin ends after amino acid #24.

Pharmacokinetics

Cosyntropin must be given parenterally because it is inactivated by gut enzymes. The two commercially available parenteral forms in the USA appear to be bioequivalent in dogs when given IV (Cohen et al. 2012). In humans, it is rapidly absorbed after being given IM. After giving IM or rapid IV, plasma cortisol levels reach their peak within an hour, but this can be variable and dosage dependent in some veterinary species. It is unknown how cosyntropin is inactivated or eliminated.

Contraindications/Precautions/Warnings

Contraindicated in patients with known hypersensitivity to cosyntropin. Use caution in patients that have shown hypersensitive reactions to ACTH in the past; there is a possibility that cross-reactivity could occur.

Adverse Effects

When used short-term, the only real concern is hypersensitivity reactions.

Reproductive/Nursing Safety

In humans, the FDA categorizes this drug as category *C* for use during pregnancy (*Animal studies have shown an adverse effect on the fetus, but there are no adequate studies in humans; or there are no animal reproduction studies and no adequate studies in humans.*)

Overdosage/Acute Toxicity

Unlikely to be of clinical consequence if used one-time.

Drug Interactions

The following drug interactions have either been reported or are theoretical in humans or animals receiving corticotropin for diagnostic purposes and may be of significance in veterinary patients receiving cosyntropin:

- **ANTICHOLINESTERASES** (*e.g.*, **pyridostigmine**): ACTH may antagonize effects in patients with myasthenia gravis.
- **DIURETICS**: ACTH may increase electrolyte loss.

Laboratory Considerations

- Patients should not receive **hydrocortisone** or **cortisone** on test day; dexamethasone sodium phosphate does not interfere with cortisol assays.
- If using a fluorometric analysis: Falsely high values may be observed if the patient is taking **spironolactone.**
- Falsely high values may be observed in patients with high **bilirubin** or if free plasma hemoglobin is present.

Doses

Note: The following dosages are for the cosyntropin aqueous (either liquid or lyophilized) products available commercially in the USA. There is also depot injectable cosyntropin zinc hydroxide (*Synacthen® Depot*) available in some countries. That product should only be used IM and not given IV. Contact your laboratory for specific dosing protocols if using the depot form.

- **DOGS:**

  For testing (screening) adrenal function using low dose "ACTH" stimulation test (extra-label): From a prospective study. Draw pre-level. Give 5 micrograms/kg IV; peak concentrations at 60 minutes after dose. (Lathan et al. 2008)

- **CATS:**

  For testing (screening) adrenal function using low dose "ACTH" stimulation test (extra-label): From a study in healthy cats. Draw pre-level. Give 5 micrograms/kg IV followed by blood sample collection at 60 to 75 minutes. Serum cortisol and aldosterone concentrations were equivalent to those achieved following administration of cosyntropin at 125 mcg/cat. (DeClue et al. 2011)

- **HORSES:**

  For testing (screening) adrenal function (extra-label): A study done in healthy adult horses showed that 0.1 micrograms/kg IV resulted in maximum adrenal stimulation, with peak cortisol concentration 30 minutes after cosyntropin administration. In healthy neonatal foals, the lowest dose of cosyntropin to result in significant adrenal gland stimulation was 0.25 micrograms/kg IV, with peak cortisol concentration 20 minutes after cosyntropin administration. (Stewart et al. 2011; Stewart 2013; Stewart et al. 2013)

Monitoring

- See specific protocols for test procedures.

Chemistry/Synonyms

A synthetic polypeptide that mimics the effects of corticotropin (ACTH), cosyntropin is commercially available as a lyophilized white to off-white powder containing mannitol. Cosyntropin's structure is identical to the first 24 (of 39) amino acids in natural corticotropin. 0.25 mg of cosyntropin is equivalent to 25 Units of corticotropin.

Cosyntropin may also be known as: tetracosactide, alpha(1–24)-corticotrophin, beta(1–24)-corticotrophin, tetracosactido, tetracosactidum, tetracosactrin, tetracosapeptide, *Cortrosina®*, *Cortrosyn®*, *Nuvacthen Depot®*, *Synacthen®*, *Synacthen Depot®*, *Synacthen Retard®*, or *Synacthene®*.

Storage/Stability

After reconstituting the lyophilized product with sterile normal saline, the solution is stable for 24 hours at room temperature; 21 days if refrigerated. Anecdotally it has been reported that when stored in plastic vials it remains stable up to 4 months when refrigerated. Do not add the drug to blood or plasma infusions. The commercially available injectable solution is labeled to be stored refrigerated between 2-8°C (36-46°F); protect from light and freezing.

One study (Frank and Oliver 1998) showed that cosyntropin can be reconstituted and stored frozen (-20°C) in plastic syringes for up to 6 months and still show biologic activity in the dog. It is recommended to freeze in small aliquots as it is unknown what effect thawing and refreezing has on potency. At present it is recommended to store in plastic containers (*e.g.*, tuberculin syringes) as it may bind to glass.

Compatibility/Compounding Considerations

No specific information noted.

Dosage Forms/Regulatory Status

VETERINARY-LABELED PRODUCTS: NONE.

HUMAN-LABELED PRODUCTS:

Cosyntropin Powder for Injection: 0.25 mg lyophilized (250 mcg) in single-dose vials with diluent; *Cortrosyn®*, generic; (Rx)

Cosyntropin Solution for Injection: 0.25 mg/mL, preservative free in 1 mL single-dose vials; generic; (Rx)

Revisions/References

Monograph revised/updated October 2013.

Cohen, T. A. & E. C. Feldman (2012). Comparison of IV and IM Formulations of Synthetic ACTH for ACTH Stimulation Tests in Healthy Dogs. *Journal of Veterinary Internal Medicine* 26(2): 412-4.

DeClue, A. E., et al. (2011). Cortisol and aldosterone response to various doses of cosyntropin in healthy cats. *Journal of the American Veterinary Medical Association* 238(2): 176-82.

Lathan, P., et al. (2008). Use of a low-dose ACTH stimulation test for diagnosis of hypoadrenocorticism in dogs. *Journal of Veterinary Internal Medicine* 22(4): 1070-3.

Stewart, A. (2013). *Understanding Testing for Equine Endocrinopathies.* ACVIM. accessed via Veterinary Information Network; vin.com

Stewart, A. J., et al. (2011). Validation of a low-dose ACTH stimulation test in healthy adult horses. *Javma-Journal of the American Veterinary Medical Association* 239(6): 834-41.

Stewart, A. J., et al. (2013). Validation of a low-dose adrenocorticotropic hormone stimulation test in healthy neonatal foals. *Javma-Journal of the American Veterinary Medical Association* 243(3): 399-405.

Cromolyn Sodium (Inhaled)

(kroh-mah-lin)

Disodium Cromoglycate, Sodium Cromoglicate, Intal®
Mast Cell Stabilizer

For ophthalmic use, see the monograph in the Ophthalmic Drug Appendix

Prescriber Highlights

▶ Inhaled mast cell stabilizer that may be useful adjunctive treatment in preventing airway hyper-reactivity in horses with type 2 (high mast cell count in BAL) IAD or with RAO (heaves).

▶ Not for treatment of acute bronchoconstriction; used as a preventative agent.

▶ May take several days or weeks for efficacy.

Uses/Indications

Cromolyn sodium is a mast cell stabilizer that may be useful in reducing airway hyper-reactivity in horses with type 2 (high mast cell count in bronchoalveolar lavage fluid; mast cells of >2% of the total cell count) inflammatory airway disease (IAD) or with recurrent airway obstruction (RAO; heaves). Use of this agent is somewhat controversial; studies have yielded conflicting efficacy results and it is not widely used clinically.

Pharmacology/Actions

Cromolyn inhibits the release of histamine and leukotrienes from sensitized mast cells found in lung mucosa, nasal mucosa and eyes. Its exact mechanism of activity is not understood, but it is thought to be a result from blocking indirect entry of calcium ions into cells. Other effects of cromolyn include inhibiting neuronal reflexes in the lung, inhibiting bronchospasm secondary to tachykins, inhibiting the movement of other inflammatory cells (neutrophils, monocytes, eosinophils), and preventing the down-regulation of beta-2

adrenergic receptors on lymphocytes. Cromolyn does not possess antihistaminic, anticholinergic, antiserotonin, corticosteroid-like, or antiinflammatory actions.

Pharmacokinetics

Limited information is available for horses. The amount of cromolyn reaching the distal airways is probably variable and dependent on the type of nebulizer used and the amount of concurrent bronchoconstriction present. Absorbed cromolyn is eliminated in the urine and via the bile into the feces.

In humans, less than 2% is absorbed from the GI tract after oral dosing. Approximately 8% is absorbed when inhaled into the lung. Absorbed drug is eliminated via the feces and urine as unchanged drug.

Contraindications/Precautions/Warnings

Do not use in patients with documented hypersensitivity to cromolyn.

Unlikely to be of benefit in treating horses with types 1 and 3 IAD. Cromolyn has no efficacy in treating acute bronchospasm.

Adverse Effects

Adverse effects associated with inhaled cromolyn use in horses are not well documented. Cough and treatment avoidance (secondary to bad taste?) have been reported. It has been proposed that pretreatment with albuterol may reduce the incidence of cough.

Humans can occasionally develop cough, throat irritation or complain of unpleasant taste. Rarely, bronchoconstriction and anaphylaxis (<0.0001%) have been reported.

Reproductive/Nursing Safety

Laboratory animal studies have shown no effect on fertility. Teratogenicity studies in mice, rats and rabbits have not demonstrated any teratogenic effects and it is likely safe for use during pregnancy. Extremely low (or undetectable) levels have been detected in milk; cromolyn is most likely safe for use during nursing.

Overdosage/Acute Toxicity

Because of the drug's low systemic bioavailability after inhalation or oral administration, acute overdoses are unlikely to cause significant morbidity.

Drug Interactions

No notable drug interactions have been reported.

Laboratory Considerations

No notable laboratory interactions or alterations have been reported.

Doses

- **HORSES:**

  For adjunctive treatment of type-2 inflammatory airway disease (extra-label): Using a jet nebulizer: 200 mg (total dose) q12 hours; using an ultrasonic nebulizer 80 mg once daily (q24h). (Couetil 2002)

Monitoring

- Clinical efficacy.
- For horses with type 2 IAD, reductions in mast cell counts in bronchoalveolar lavage fluid could help confirm efficacy.

Client Information

- This medication does not treat airway constriction but is used to prevent airway constriction by reducing the release of substances from cells that can cause it; it should not be used to treat acute bronchoconstriction (difficulty breathing).
- This medicine must be must be dosed once to twice daily and it may take several days or weeks before it can be determined if it is working.
- Proper use of the drug delivery device is very important; if any questions arise regarding proper use, contact the veterinarian.

Chemistry/Synonyms

Cromolyn sodium occurs as a white, odorless, hygroscopic, crystalline powder that is soluble in water and insoluble in alcohol.

Cromolyn sodium may also be known as cromoglicic acid, cromoglycic acid, sodium cromoglicate, disodium cromoglycate, sodium cromoglycate, DSCG, SCG, FPL–670, or DNSG; there are many international trade names.

Storage/Stability/Compatibility

Cromolyn sodium solution for inhalation should be stored below 40°C (104°F); preferably between 15-30°C. Protect from freezing, light and humidity. Store in foil pouch until ready for use. Do not use solution if it is cloudy or contains a precipitate. Solution remaining in nebulizers after use should be discarded.

Compatibility/Compounding Considerations

Cromolyn solution is reportedly **compatible** with acetylcysteine, albuterol, epinephrine, isoetherine, isoproterenol, metaproterenol, or terbutaline solutions for up to 60 minutes. It is **not compatible** with bitolterol.

Dosage Forms/Regulatory Status

VETERINARY-LABELED PRODUCTS: NONE IN THE USA.

HUMAN-LABELED PRODUCTS:

Cromolyn Sodium Solution for Inhalation: 20 mg/2 mL vials or amps; generic; (Rx)

There is also an OTC nasal solution (*Nasalcrom®*), and an oral concentrate (*Gastrocrom®*) indicated for mastocystosis available, but these dosage forms are unlikely to be of use in veterinary medicine.

Revisions/References

Monograph revised/updated October 2013.

Couetil, L. (2002). *Aerosol medications for the management of inflammatory airway disease (IAD)*. Proceedings: ACVIM 2002. accessed via Veterinary Information Network; vin.com

Cyanocobalamin (Vitamin B12)

(sye-an-oh-koe-bal-ah-min)

Vitamin/Nutritional

Prescriber Highlights

▶ Used for parenteral treatment of vitamin B12 deficiency.
▶ Very safe.

Uses/Indications

Cyanocobalamin is used for treating deficiencies of vitamin B12 secondary to gastrointestinal tract disease or exocrine pancreatic insufficiency, or dietary chromium deficiencies (in ruminants) that can be associated with dietary deficiencies of vitamin B12. As there appears to be a high percentage of cats with exocrine pancreatic insufficiency or gastrointestinal disease that are deficient in cobalamin, there is considerable interest in evaluating serum cobalamin (vitamin B12) in these patients. Giant schnauzers, Beagles, Border Collies, Australian Shepherds, and Chinese Shar-Peis may have a genetic defect affecting the location of the cobalamin-intrinsic factor, causing cobalamin deficiency. Dogs with inflammatory bowel disease may also develop cobalamin deficiency.

Pharmacology/Actions

Vitamin B12 (cobalamin), a cobalt-containing water-soluble vitamin, serves as an important cofactor for many enzymatic reactions in mammals that are required for normal cell growth, function and reproduction, nucleoprotein and myelin synthesis, amino acid metabolism, and erythropoiesis. Cobalamin is required for folate utilization; B12 deficiency can cause functional folate deficiency. Unlike humans, macrocytic anemias do not appear to be a significant component to cobalamin deficiency in dogs or cats.

Clinical signs associated with cobalamin deficiency in cats may include weight loss, poor haircoat, vomiting, or diarrhea. Increases in serum methionine and methylmalonic acid, and decreased serum cystathionine and cysteine values may be noted. Homocysteine levels do not appear to be affected.

In dogs, cobalamin deficiency may cause or contribute to inappetence, diarrhea, weight loss, leukopenia, or methylmalonylaciduria.

In ruminants, vitamin B12 appears to be synthesized by rumen microflora and requires dietary cobalt to be present for its formation. Clinical signs seen with cobalamin deficiency states associated with cobalt deficiency in cattle and sheep include inappetence, lassitude, poor haircoat/fleece, poor milk production, weight loss, or failure to grow.

Pharmacokinetics

After food is consumed in monogastric mammals, cobalamin in food is bound to a protein (haptocorrin) in the stomach. Haptocorrin/cobalamin is degraded by pancreatic proteases in the duodenum, but cobalamin is then bound by Intrinsic factor (IF), a protein produced in the stomach and pancreas in dogs, in the pancreas (only) in cats, and in the stomach (only) in humans. The cobalamin-IF complex is absorbed in the small intestine where it binds to cubulin, which facilitates its entry into the portal circulation. A protein called transcobalamin 2 (TCII) then binds to cobalamin allowing its entry into target cells. Some cobalamin is rapidly excreted into the bile where entero-hepatic recirculation occurs. Dogs and cats, unlike humans, do not possess cobalamin-binding protein TC1. This means that dogs and cats with B12 dietary deficiency or malabsorption can rapidly deplete their stores of B12 in 1-2 months, whereas in humans it may require 1-2 years.

In normal cats, circulating half-life of cobalamin is approximately 13 days, but in two cats with inflammatory bowel disease, it was only 5 days (Simpson et al. 2001).

Contraindications/Precautions/Warnings

For injectable use, no contraindications are documented for domestic animals. In humans, cyanocobalamin is contraindicated in patients hypersensitive to it or hydroxocobalamin.

Adverse Effects

Cyanocobalamin appears very well tolerated when used parenterally in animals. In humans, anaphylaxis has been reported rarely after parenteral use. Some human patients complain of pain at the injection site, but this is uncommon.

Reproductive/Nursing Safety

Studies documenting safety during pregnancy have apparently not been done in humans or animals, but it is likely safe to use. Vitamin B12 deficiency states are thought to cause teratogenic effects.

While vitamin B12 can be excreted into milk, it is safe for use while nursing.

Overdosage/Acute Toxicity

No overdose information was located, but an inadvertent overdose of cyanocobalamin given via SC or IM injection is unlikely to cause significant morbidity.

Drug Interactions

No significant drug interactions have been identified when cyanocobalamin is administered parenterally.

Laboratory Considerations

- Serum samples to be analyzed for cobalamin and/or folate should be protected from bright light and excessive heat.
- If a microbiologic method assay is used to determine cobalamin values, concurrent use of antibiotics can cause falsely low serum or red blood cell values.

Doses

- **DOGS:**

  For cobalamin deficiency (extra-label): Injectable cyanocobalamin at 25 micrograms/kg, or practically, 250 – 1200 micrograms per dog (based on dog's size) SC once per week for 4-6 weeks, then every 14 days for 4-6 weeks, then monthly thereafter to maintain normal serum levels. May take as long as 3-4 weeks to see a response and lifelong therapy may be required depending on the status of underlying cause (disease).

- **CATS:**

  For cobalamin deficiency (extra-label): 250 micrograms (per cat) SC once per week for 6 weeks, then every 1-2 months based on cobalamin levels.

- **HORSES:**

  For vitamin B12 deficiency: 1 – 2 mL of a 1000 micrograms/mL injection (1000 – 2000 micrograms per horse) injected IM or SC; dosage may be repeated once or twice weekly, as indicated by condition or response.

- **CATTLE, SHEEP:**

  For treatment of vitamin B12 deficiency associated with cobalt deficiency (extra-label): Cattle: 2000 micrograms per head IM or SC weekly as needed; **Lambs:** 100 micrograms per head; **Adult sheep:** 300 – 1000 micrograms per head injected IM or SC once weekly as needed.

- **SWINE:**

  For vitamin B12 deficiency (extra-label): 500 – 2000 micrograms injected IM or SC; dosage may be repeated in weekly intervals if necessary.

Monitoring

- Cobalamin levels.
- In small animals: folate status, both before and after treatment with cyanocobalamin.
- Clinical signs associated with deficiency.
- CBC, baseline and ongoing if abnormal.

Client Information

- Vitamin injected under the skin (subcutaneously) to treat vitamin B-12 (cobalamin) deficiency. May be needed for the life of the animal.
- May take several weeks before improvement is seen.
- Very safe. Injections may sting.
- Dispose of needles and syringes safely in a "sharps" container.

Chemistry/Synonyms

Cyanocobalamin occurs as dark red crystals or crystalline powder. It is sparingly soluble in water (1 in 80) and soluble in alcohol. When in the anhydrous form, it is very hygroscopic and can absorb substantial amounts of water from the air.

Vitamin B12 may also be known as cobalamins. Cyanocobalamin may also be known as: cyanocobalamine, cyanocobalaminum, cobamin, cianokobalaminas, cianocobalamina, or cycobemin; many internationally registered trade names.

Storage/Stability

Cyanocobalamin injection should be stored below 40°C; protect from light and freezing.

Compatibility/Compounding Considerations

Cyanocobalamin injection is reportedly **compatible** with all commonly used intravenous fluids.

Dosage Forms

VETERINARY-LABELED PRODUCTS:

Cyanocobalamin (Vitamin B12) Injection: 1000, 3000 and 5000 micrograms/mL in 100 mL, 250 mL and 500 mL multi-dose vials depending on source; generic; (Rx). Products may be labeled as cyanocobalamin or vitamin B12, and be labeled for use in cattle, horses, dogs, cats, sheep, or swine.

There are many combination products, both oral and injectable containing cyanocobalamin as one of the ingredients. These are not recommended for use when cobalamin deficiency states exist.

HUMAN-LABELED PRODUCTS:

Cyanocobalamin (crystalline, Vitamin B12) Injection 100 micrograms (0.1 mg) per mL and 1000 micrograms (1 mg) per mL, vial sizes range from 1 mL single-use to 10 mL and 30 mL multi-dose; generic; (Rx). Besides generically labeled products there are several products available with a variety of trade names including *Cyanoject®*, *Rubesol®*, *Crysti®*, or *Crystamine®*.

Oral tablet dosage forms are also available, but have not been shown to be appropriate for therapy of cobalamin deficient states in small animal medicine. A nasally administered product and an oral sub lingual tablet are marketed, but there is no information on their use in dogs or cats.

Revisions/References

Monograph revised/updated October 2013.

Simpson, K., et al. (2001). Subnormal concentrations of serum cobalamin (vitamin B12) in cats with gastrointestinal disease. *J Vet Intern Med* 15: 26-32.

Cyclophosphamide

(sye-kloe-foss-fa-mide)   Cytoxan®, Neosar®

Immunosuppressive/Antineoplastic

Prescriber Highlights

► Antineoplastic/immunosuppressive used in dogs & cats for a variety of conditions.

► Low dose metronomic (continuous) therapy with piroxicam shows promise for preventing sarcoma recurrence in dogs with fewer adverse effects then high dose treatment.

► Contraindications: Prior anaphylaxis. Caution in patients with leukopenia, thrombocytopenia, previous radiotherapy, impaired hepatic or renal function, or in those for whom immunosuppression may be dangerous (*e.g.*, infection).

► Potentially teratogenic, fetotoxic.

► Primary adverse effects are myelosuppression, GI effects, alopecia (especially Poodles, Old English Sheepdogs, etc.), & hemorrhagic cystitis.

► Adequate monitoring essential.

Uses/Indications

In veterinary medicine, cyclophosphamide is used primarily in small animals (dogs and cats) in combination with other agents both as an antineoplastic agent (lymphomas, leukemias, carcinomas, and sarcomas) and as an immunosuppressant (SLE, ITP, pemphigus, rheumatoid arthritis, proliferative urethritis, etc.). Its use in treating acute immune-mediated hemolytic anemia is controversial and it is rarely used for this indication today, as there is evidence it does not produce additional beneficial effects when used with prednisone. A recent review article on immunomodulating drugs for dogs states: "It has been proposed that the primary indication for cyclophosphamide therapy in the dog should now be for cancer therapy. As for most other immunosuppressive agents, there is a lack of published efficacy data, but studies suggesting increased morbidity and the increased incidence of serious adverse effects of cyclophosphamide (*e.g.*, hemorrhagic cystitis and myelosuppression) do not justify its use as an immunosuppressive agent." (Whitley et al. 2011)

Cyclophosphamide has historically been used as a chemical shearing agent in sheep, but this use is discouraged.

Pharmacology/Actions

While commonly categorized as an alkylating agent, the parent compound (cyclophosphamide) is a prodrug and one of cyclophosphamide's primary metabolites, 4-hydroxycyclophosphamide (4-OHCP) is thought to be responsible for most of the drug's pharmacologic activity. 4-OHCP enters cells where it rapidly decomposes to phosphoramide mustard and acrolein, thereby acting as an alkylating agent interfering with DNA replication, RNA transcription and replication, and ultimately disrupting nucleic acid function. The cytotoxic properties of cyclophosphamide are also enhanced by the phosphorylating activity the drug possesses.

Cyclophosphamide has marked immunosuppressive activity and both white cells and antibody production are decreased, but the exact mechanisms for this activity have not been fully elucidated.

Pharmacokinetics

The pharmacokinetics of cyclophosphamide after PO or IV dosing in dogs with lymphomas has been reported. After oral administration, peak levels of cyclophosphamide occurred about 45 minutes later. Elimination half-life was between 30-60 minutes. Pharmacokinetics of 4-OHCP (active metabolite) in plasma, were similar to cyclophosphamide after IV or PO dosing, but there were significant differences in peak levels (IV was about twice as high as PO) and time to reach peak levels (IV about 13 minutes and PO about 75 minutes). The authors concluded that it is likely that oral and intravenous cyclophosphamide can be used interchangeably with the same exposure of active metabolite being achieved in dogs with lymphoma (Warry et al. 2011).

The pharmacokinetics of cyclophosphamide apparently have not been detailed in cats and it is presumed that the drug is handled in a manner similar to humans.

In horses, preliminary reports indicate that higher dosages may be necessary to obtain clinically useful levels of 4-OHCP (Duran 2014).

In humans, cyclophosphamide is well absorbed after oral administration with peak levels occurring about 1 hour after dosing. Cyclophosphamide and its metabolites are distributed throughout the body, including the CSF (albeit in subtherapeutic levels). Cyclophosphamide is metabolized in the liver to several metabolites. The active metabolite, 4-hydroxycyclophosphamide (4-OHCP) is believed responsible for its primary cytotoxic effect. The drug is only minimally protein bound and is distributed into milk and presumed to cross the placenta. After IV injection, the serum half-life of cyclophosphamide is approximately 4-12 hours, but drug/metabolites can be detected up to 72 hours after administration. The majority of the drug is excreted as metabolites and unchanged drug in the urine.

Contraindications/Precautions/Warnings

Cyclophosphamide should not be used in patients with prior anaphylactic reactions to the drug, otherwise there are no absolute contraindications to the use of cyclophosphamide. It must be used with caution, however in patients with leukopenia, thrombocytopenia, previous radiotherapy, impaired hepatic or renal function, or in those for which immunosuppression may be dangerous (e.g., infected patients). Patients that develop myelosuppression should have subsequent doses delayed until adequate recovery occurs.

Because of the potential for development of serious adverse effects, cyclophosphamide should only be used in patients that can be adequately and regularly monitored.

Do not confuse cyclophosphamide with cyclosporine (ciclosporin) or *Cytoxan*® with *Cytotec*®. Consider writing orders using tall man lettering: cycloPHOSphamide. Additionally, do not write prescriptions for this drug using the abbreviation "SID". Many "human" pharmacists are not aware of this abbreviation and could interpret it as another abbreviation (e.g., QID).

Adverse Effects

Primary adverse effects in animals associated with cyclophosphamide are myelosuppression, gastroenterocolitis (anorexia—especially in cats, nausea, vomiting, diarrhea), alopecia (especially in breeds where hair coat continually grows, e.g., Poodles, Old English Sheepdogs), and hemorrhagic cystitis.

Cyclophosphamide's myelosuppressant effects primarily impact the white cells lines, but may also affect red cell and platelet production. The nadir for leukocytes generally occurs between 5-14 days after dosing and may require up to 4 weeks for recovery. When used with other drugs causing myelosuppression, toxic effects may be exacerbated. A study in dogs using recombinant-canine granulocyte colony-stimulating factor (rcG-SCF) at 2.5 mcg/kg 3 times a day for 2-5 days after cyclophosphamide accelerated recovery and reduced the severity of neutropenia (Yamamoto et al. 2011). Thrombocytopenia occurs only rarely.

Sterile hemorrhagic cystitis induced by cyclophosphamide is thought to be caused by the metabolite acrolein. Up to 30% of dogs receiving long-term (>2 months) cyclophosphamide can develop this problem. Furosemide administered with cyclophosphamide may reduce the occurrence of this adverse effect.

In cats, cyclophosphamide-induced-cystitis (CIC) is rare. Initial signs may present as hematuria and dysuria. Because bacterial cystitis is not uncommon in immunosuppressed patients, it must be ruled out by taking urine cultures. Diagnosis of CIC is made by a negative urine culture and inflammatory urine sediment found during urinalysis. Because bladder fibrosis and/or transitional cell carcinoma of the bladder is also associated with cyclophosphamide use, these may need to be ruled out by contrast radiography. It is believed that the incidence of CIC may be minimized by increasing urine production and frequent voiding. The drug should be given in the morning and animals should be encouraged to drink/urinate whenever possible. Recommendation for treatment of CIC includes discontinuing cyclophosphamide, furosemide, and corticosteroids. Refractory cases have been treated by surgical debridement, 1% formalin or 25% DMSO instillation in the bladder.

Other adverse effects that may be noted with cyclophosphamide therapy include pulmonary infiltrates and fibrosis, depression, immune-suppression with hyponatremia, leukemia, and increased risks for future neoplastic disease.

In recovering dogs with immune-mediated hemolytic anemia, taper the withdrawal of the drug slowly over several months and monitor for early signs of relapse. Rapid withdrawal can lead to a rebound hyperimmune response.

Reproductive/Nursing Safety

Cyclophosphamide's safe use in pregnancy has not been established and it is potentially teratogenic and embryotoxic. Cyclophosphamide may induce sterility (may be temporary) in male animals. In humans, the FDA categorizes this drug as category *D* for use during pregnancy (*There is evidence of human fetal risk, but the potential benefits from the use of the drug in pregnant women may be acceptable despite its potential risks.*) In a separate system evaluating the safety of drugs in canine and feline pregnancy (Papich 1989), this drug is categorized as class: *C* (*These drugs may have potential risks. Studies in people or laboratory animals have uncovered risks, and these drugs should be used cautiously as a last resort when the benefit of therapy clearly outweighs the risks.*)

Cyclophosphamide is distributed in milk and nursing is generally not recommended when dams are receiving the drug.

Overdosage/Acute Toxicity

There is only limited information on acute overdoses of this drug. The lethal dose in the dogs has been reported as 40 mg/kg IV. If an oral overdose occurs, gut emptying should proceed if indicated and the animal should be hospitalized for supportive care.

There were 22 single agent exposures to cyclophosphamide reported to the ASPCA Animal Poison Control Center (APCC) during 2009-2013. Of the 18 dogs, only 3 were symptomatic with 67% having neutrophilia. Other signs included anorexia, hematuria, hyperchloremia, hypernatremia, polydipsia, nystagmus, seizures, tremors, and vomiting.

Drug Interactions

The following drug interactions have either been reported or are theoretical in humans or animals receiving cyclophosphamide and may be of significance in veterinary patients. Unless otherwise noted, use together is not necessarily contraindicated, but weigh the potential risks and perform additional monitoring when appropriate.

- **ALLOPURINOL**: May increase the myelosuppression caused by cyclophosphamide.
- **CARDIOTOXIC DRUGS** (*e.g.*, **doxorubicin**): Use caution when using cyclophosphamide with other cardiotoxic agents as potentiation of cardiotoxicity may occur.
- **CHLORAMPHENICOL**: May reduce cyclophosphamide efficacy.
- **CYCLOSPORINE**: May cause decreased cyclosporine levels.
- **DIGOXIN**: May decrease digoxin's efficacy.
- **HYDROCHLOROTHIAZIDE**: May result in increased cyclophosphamide exposure and enhanced myelosuppression.
- **ONDANSETRON**: May reduce cyclophosphamide efficacy.
- **PHENOBARBITAL** (or other **barbiturates**) given chronically may increase the rate of metabolism of cyclophosphamide to active metabolites via microsomal enzyme induction and increase the likelihood of toxicity development.
- **PHENOTHIAZINES**: May inhibit cyclophosphamide metabolism.
- **POTASSIUM IODIDE**: May inhibit cyclophosphamide metabolism.
- **SUCCINYLCHOLINE**: Metabolism may be slowed with resulting prolongation of effects, as cyclophosphamide may decrease the levels of circulating pseudocholinesterases.
- **VACCINES, LIVE**: Increased risk for infection by live vaccine.
- **WARFARIN**: May result in increased risk for bleeding.

Laboratory Considerations

- **Uric acid** levels (blood and urine) may be increased after cyclophosphamide use.
- The immunosuppressant properties of cyclophosphamide may cause false negative **antigenic skin test** results to a variety of antigens, including tuberculin, Candida, and Trichophyton.

Doses

Note: In oral tablets, the active ingredient may be contained within an inner tablet surrounded by an inert flecked outer tablet. Accurate dosing may be difficult if splitting or crushing tablets. When dosing in cats or very small dogs, or if using low-dose therapy, compounding pharmacies may be able to compound oral dosage forms containing less than 25 mg. Another method has been suggested (Mackin 2009) to allow use of whole 25 mg tablets when used as an immunosuppressant: Convert daily (or every other day) doses into a weekly total dose and then administer whole tablets at a suitable interval to allow using whole tablets.

- **DOGS:**

  As an antineoplastic; often used as part of a multi-drug chemotherapy protocols (*e.g.*, COP, CHOP, etc.); (extra-label): **Note** Because of the potential toxicity of this drug to patients, veterinary personnel and clients, and since chemotherapy indications treatment protocols, monitoring and safety guidelines often change, the following dosages should be used only as a general guide. Consultation with a veterinary oncologist and referral to current veterinary oncology references [*e.g.*, (Withrow et al. 2012); (Dobson et al. 2011); (Henry et al. 2009); (North et al 2009); (Argyle et al. 2008)] are strongly recommended.

  Dosages and dosage frequency vary considerably depending on the protocol used and it is most often dosed by body surface area (mg/m^2). Dosages can range from 10 – 15 mg/m^2 as a daily metronomic dose to 50 mg/m^2 PO once a day for 3-4 days each week to larger dosages of 250 – 300 mg/m^2 once very 3 weeks.

  As an immunosuppressant (usually for short-term use and with glucocorticoids); (extra-label): 50 mg/m^2 (not mg/kg) PO every other day or as a pulse therapy 4 days on, 3 days off. 50 mg/m^2 is approximately 1.5 mg/kg for dogs over 30 kg, 2 mg/kg for dogs 15–30 kg, and 2.5 mg/kg for dogs for dogs under 15 kg. Because of adverse effects, most clinicians prefer using other immunosuppressives (*e.g.*, cyclosporine, azathioprine).

- **CATS:**

  As an antineoplastic (extra-label): See the **Note** as per dogs above. Dosages range as per dogs depending on the protocol used.

  As an immunosuppressant (extra-label): 2 – 2.5 mg/kg PO once daily; some suggest dosing 4 days per week. Not commonly used as many clinicians prefer cyclosporine or chlorambucil.

- **HORSES:**

  Note: Recently performed research in horses found that cyclophosphamide administered at doses of 400 mg/m^2 (IV) and 600 mg/m^2 (PO) did not achieve therapeutic concentrations of 4-OHCP at levels proven for the treatment of malignancies in other species. Additional research is ongoing in the attempt to define a clinically useful dosage for cyclophosphamide (Duran 2014).

  For neoplastic diseases; consultation with a veterinary oncologist is encouraged before use (extra-label): Doses historically used in horses have been 200 mg/m^2 (usually 1 gram per horse per dose) IV every 1-2 weeks. For generalized lymphoma the CAP protocol was used at the time of publication by one of the authors. See the reference or the vincristine monograph for more information (Mair et al. 2006).

- **RABBITS:**

  As an antineoplastic (lymphoma) agent (extra-label): 50 mg/m^2 (NOT mg/kg) PO daily for 3 days each week or 100 – 200 mg/m^2 IV (cephalic or saphenous veins) every 7 days. Consider using a fully implantable vascular access device for multiple IV chemo administration. (Bryan 2009)

Monitoring

- Efficacy; See the Protocol section or refer to the references from the Dosage section above for more information.
- Toxicity, see Adverse Effects above. Regular hemograms and urinalyses are mandatory.

Client Information

- Cyclophosphamide is a chemotherapy (cancer) and immune suppressive drug. The drug and its byproducts can be hazardous to other animals and people that come in contact with it. On the day your animal gets the drug and then for a few days afterward, all bodily waste (urine, feces, litter), blood, or vomit should only be handled while wearing disposable gloves. Seal the waste in a plastic bag and then place both the bag and gloves in with the regular trash.

- Cyclophosphamide can be very toxic to the gastrointestinal tract and cause vomiting and gastrointestinal upset. Give with food.
- Watch for bleeding, bruising, infection/fever, blood in urine.
- After dosing in dogs, frequent walks to encourage urination is suggested to attempt to lessen the risk for bladder toxicity.

Chemistry/Synonyms

A nitrogen-mustard derivative, cyclophosphamide occurs as a white, crystalline powder that is soluble in water and alcohol. The commercially available injection has pH of 3 to 7.5.

Cyclophosphamide may also be known as: CPM, CTX, CYT, B-518, ciclofosfamida, cyclophosphamidum, cyclophosphanum, NSC-26271, or WR-138719. *Cytoxan®* is a common trade name.

Storage/Stability

Cyclophosphamide tablets and powder for injection should be stored at temperatures less than 25°C. They may be exposed to temperatures up to 30°C for brief periods, but should not be exposed to temperatures above 30°C. Tablets should be stored in tight containers. The commercially available tablets (*Cytoxan®*) are manufactured in a bi-level manner with a white tablet containing the cyclophosphamide found within a surrounding flecked outer tablet. Therefore, the person administering the drug need not protect their hands from cyclophosphamide exposure unless the tablets are crushed. Because of their construction, accurately splitting tablets is problematic and cannot be recommended.

After reconstituting the powder for injection with either sterile water for injection or bacteriostatic water for injection, the product should be used within 24 hours if stored at room temperature; 6 days if refrigerated.

Compatibility/Compounding Considerations

Commercially available cyclophosphamide tablets may not have the active ingredient dispersed evenly throughout the tablet. To assure accurate oral dosing, it is recommended to obtain dosing forms from an experienced compounding pharmacist.

Cyclophosphamide injection may be dissolved in aromatic elixir to be used as an oral solution. When refrigerated, it is stable for 14 days.

Cyclophosphamide is reportedly **compatible** with the following intravenous solutions and drugs: Amino acids 4.25%/dextrose 25%, D5 in normal saline, D5W, sodium chloride 0.9%. It is also **compatible** in syringes or at Y-sites for brief periods with the following: bleomycin sulfate, cefazolin, cisplatin, doxorubicin HCl, droperidol, fluorouracil, furosemide, heparin sodium, leucovorin calcium, methotrexate sodium, metoclopramide HCl, mitomycin, vinblastine sulfate, and vincristine sulfate. Compatibility is dependent upon factors such as pH, concentration, temperature and diluent used; consult specialized references or a hospital pharmacist for more specific information.

Dosage Forms/Regulatory Status

VETERINARY-LABELED PRODUCTS: NONE.

HUMAN-LABELED PRODUCTS:

Cyclophosphamide Tablets: 25 mg & 50 mg; generic; (Rx)

Cyclophosphamide Powder for Solution for Injection: 500 mg, 1 g & 2 g in vials; generic (Rx)

Revisions/References

Monograph revised/updated October 2013.

Argyle, D., et al. (2008). *Decision Making in Small Animal Oncology*, Wiley-Blackwell.
Bryan, J. (2009). *Neoplasia in rabbits: Therapy*. Proceedings: WVC. accessed via Veterinary Information Network; vin.com
Dobson, J. & D. Lascelles (2011). *BSAVA Manual of Canine and Feline Oncology*, BSAVA.
Duran, S. (2014). Personal Communication.
Henry, C. & M. Higginbotham (2009). *Cancer Management in Small Animal Practice*, Saunders.
Mackin, A. (2009). *Chronic management of the immune-mediated blood disorders*. Proceedings: World Veterinary Congress. accessed via Veterinary Information Network; vin.com
Mair, T. S. & C. G. Couto (2006). The use of cytotoxic drugs in equine practice. *Equine Veterinary Education* 18(3): 149-56.
North, S. & T. Banks (2009). *Small Animal Oncology: An Introduction*, Saunders.
Warry, E., et al. (2011). Pharmacokinetics of Cyclophosphamide after Oral and Intravenous Administration to Dogs with Lymphoma. *Journal of Veterinary Internal Medicine* 25(4): 903-8.
Whitley, N. T. & M. J. Day (2011). Immunomodulatory drugs and their application to the management of canine immune-mediated disease. *Journal of Small Animal Practice* 52(2): 70-85.
Withrow, S., et al. (2012). *Withrow and MacEwen's Small Animal Clinical Oncology, 5th Ed.*, Saunders.
Yamamoto, A., et al. (2011). Recombinant canine granulocyte colony-stimulating factor accelerates recovery from cyclophosphamide-induced neutropenia in dogs. *Veterinary Immunology and Immunopathology* 142(3-4): 271-5.

Cyclosporine (Systemic)

(sye-kloe-spor-een)   Ciclosporin, Cyclosporine A, Atopica®, Neoral®, Sandimmune®

Immunosuppressive

Note: Cyclosporine topical ophthalmic information is found in the ophthalmology section in the appendix.

Prescriber Highlights

- ▶ Immunosuppressant (primarily cellular immunity). FDA-approved products available for dogs (control of atopic dermatitis) and cats (allergic dermatitis as manifested by excoriations–including facial and neck, miliary dermatitis, eosinophilic plaques, and self-induced alopecia). Good evidence to support use in treating perianal fistulas in dogs.
- ▶ Adverse Effects: Primarily GI related, but uncommon in dogs at usual dosages. Cats may be more susceptible to GI effects.
- ▶ If using human-labeled products, don't confuse *Sandimmune®* with *Atopica®/Neoral®/Gengraf®* dosages; they are not bioequivalent.
- ▶ Consider measuring serum levels to assure efficacy & minimize adverse effect potential.
- ▶ Cost may be an issue. Ketoconazole has been used to lower dosages in dogs.
- ▶ Many potential drug-drug interactions. Variation between species' susceptibility to a given interaction exist.

Note: Cyclosporine topical ophthalmic information is found in the ophthalmology section in the appendix.

Uses/Indications

The FDA-approved indication for dogs is for the control of atopic dermatitis. The FDA-approved indication for cats is for the control of feline allergic dermatitis as manifested by excoriations (including facial and neck), miliary dermatitis, eosinophilic plaques, and self-induced alopecia in cats at least 6 months of age and at least 3 lbs. (1.4 kg) in body weight.

In dogs, reasonable evidence exists for cyclosporine efficacy in treating anal furunculosis and in dogs and cats for treating atopic dermatitis and reducing allograft transplant rejection. While cyclosporine may also be useful in dogs and cats as a treatment for other immune-mediated diseases or keratinization disorders, evidence supporting efficacy is either weak or not currently available.

Pharmacology/Actions

Cyclosporine is an immunosuppressant that focuses on cell-mediated immune responses (but it has some humoral immunosuppressive action). Cyclosporine binds to T-cell cyclophilin and blocks calcineurin-mediated T-cell activation. T-helper lymphocytes are the primary target, but T-suppressor cells are also affected. Cyclosporine can also inhibit cytokine production and release (including IL-2, IL-3, IL-4, and tissue necrosis factor-alpha) thereby affecting function of eosinophils, mast cells, granulocytes and macrophages.

Pharmacokinetics

Cyclosporine is relatively poorly absorbed after oral administration and bioavailability can vary widely between patients. The emulsion form oral products (*Atopica*®, *Neoral*®) reportedly achieve much higher blood levels in dogs and cats for a given dosage. **Note:** *Neoral*®/*Atopica*® and *Sandimmune*® are **NOT** bioequivalent.

In dogs, the veterinary-labeled oral product (*Atopica*®) is rapidly absorbed, but bioavailability is variable and can range from 23-45%. Food in the GI increases variability of bioavailability and reduces it by about 20%. Cyclosporine is distributed in high levels into the liver, fat and blood cells (RBC's lymphocytes). It does not appreciably enter the CNS. The drug is primarily metabolized in the liver via the cytochrome P450 system (probably CYP3A) and excreted into the bile. Less than 1% of a dose is excreted unchanged into the urine. Elimination half-life in the dog is approximately 5-12 hours.

In cats, oral cyclosporine bioavailability is highly variable but drug absorption is not significantly altered when administered with/without food or mixed in with food. However the product label recommends giving on a consistent schedule with regard to meals and time of day. Elimination half-life in cats also varies considerably with estimates as short as 6.8 hours to longer than 40 hours in some normal healthy cats.

Contraindications/Precautions/Warnings

Cyclosporine is contraindicated in patients hypersensitive to it or any component (*e.g.*, polyoxyethylated castor oil) in the injectable micro-emulsion products. It is labeled as being contraindicated in dogs with a history of malignant neoplasia. Cyclosporine should be used with caution in patients with hepatic or renal disease. Killed vaccines are recommended for dogs receiving cyclosporine as the drug's impact on the immune response to modified live vaccines is not known.

Cyclosporine is pumped by P-glycoprotein, but the Washington State University Clinical Pharmacology Lab reports that it has not seen any increased sensitivity to cyclosporine and does not recommend any dose reductions in dogs with MDR1 (ABCB1) mutations. They do however, recommend therapeutic drug monitoring (WSU-VetClinPharmLab 2009).

In cats, the approved product is labeled as contraindicated in cats with a history of cyclosporine hypersensitivity, malignant disorders or suspected malignancy, infected with feline leukemia virus (FeLV), feline immunodeficiency virus (FIV), clinical toxoplasmosis or other serious systemic illness. Use may increase susceptibility to infection and development of neoplasia. It is also labeled that safe use has not been established in cats less than 6 months of age or less than 3 lbs. (1.4 kg) body weight. It is not for use in breeding cats, pregnant or lactating queens and cats should be tested and found to be negative for FeLV and FIV infections before treatment.

Diminished immune response to vaccinations can occur. As it may cause elevated levels of serum glucose, creatinine, and urea nitrogen, it should be used with caution in cases with diabetes mellitus or renal insufficiency.

Do not confuse cyclosporine (ciclosporin) with cyclophosphamide. Consider writing orders using tall man lettering: cycloSPORine. Additionally, do not write prescriptions for this drug using the abbreviation "SID". Many "human" pharmacists are not aware of this abbreviation and could interpret it as another abbreviation (*e.g.*, QID).

Adverse Effects

In dogs, vomiting, anorexia, and diarrhea are the most commonly adverse effects seen. Dogs quite commonly will vomit when start-

ing therapy, but this generally abates with time. GI effects rarely require drug discontinuation. Giving the drug with a small amount of food or freezing the capsule for 30-60 minutes before administration have anecdotally been suggested to alleviate vomiting when it is a problem. Gingival hyperplasia, hypertrichosis, altered glucose metabolism/diabetes mellitus, excessive shedding, and papillomatosis have been reported. Gingival hyperplasia has been treated with oral and toothpaste-forms of azithromycin with limited efficacy (Rosenberg et al. 2013). Hepatotoxicity or thromboembolic events have been reported, but are believed rare. Because of its immunosuppressive effects, patients may be more susceptible to opportunistic infections (*e.g.*, nocardiosis, etc.) or neoplastic disease.

In order to reduce the incidence of vomiting in dogs when starting therapy, some clinicians will start at a low dose, give with food and gradually increase oral doses over the first week or so. One protocol (Bloom 2006) is: 1 – 2 mg/kg PO once daily for 2 days, 2 – 3 mg/kg PO once daily for 2 days, 3 – 4 mg/kg PO once daily for 3 days, and then 5 mg/kg PO once daily for 30 days. For the first 10 days metoclopramide is given 30 minutes prior to cyclosporine. For the first 14 days cyclosporine is given with a meal and after that, 2 hours prior to a meal.

In cats, gastrointestinal effects including vomiting, diarrhea, hypersalivation, decreased appetite/anorexia are often reported during the first month of therapy. Resultant weight loss may rarely lead to hepatic lipidosis. Lethargy, malaise, behavior changes, increased hair growth, gingival hyperplasia, and flares of latent viral infections have also been noted in feline patients on cyclosporine. A case of a cat developing fatal systemic toxoplasmosis while on cyclosporine therapy has been reported. Anaphylaxis is very rare, but possible.

While nephrotoxicity and hepatotoxicity are potentially an issue in dogs and cats, it appears that extremely high blood levels (>3,000 ng/mL) are necessary before this is a significant problem.

Long-term use, particularly in combination with other immunosuppressants (steroids), may predispose the patient to develop neoplastic diseases.

Because the drug has an unpleasant taste, it has been suggested that compounded dosages be placed in gelatin capsules or used with taste-masking flavoring agents.

Reproductive/Nursing Safety

Cyclosporine has been shown to be fetotoxic and embryotoxic in rats and rabbits at dosages 2-5 times normal. Use during pregnancy only when the risks outweigh the benefits. In humans, the FDA categorizes this drug as category C for use during pregnancy (*Animal studies have shown an adverse effect on the fetus, but there are no adequate studies in humans; or there are no animal reproduction studies and no adequate studies in humans.*)

Cyclosporine is distributed into milk and safety cannot be assured for nursing offspring. In humans, it is not recommended that women nurse while taking cyclosporine.

Overdosage/Acute Toxicity

Acute overdoses may cause transient renal- or hepato-toxicity. Overdoses may be treated with gut evacuation (emesis is apparently effective in humans if used within 2 hours of ingestion); otherwise, treat supportively and symptomatically.

There were 276 single agent exposures to cyclosporine reported to the ASPCA Animal Poison Control Center (APCC) during 2009-2013. Of the 259 dogs, 61 were symptomatic with vomiting (67%), diarrhea, (34%) and lethargy (18%) being the most common. In the 18 exposed cats, 4 were symptomatic with 100% vomiting.

Drug Interactions

The following drug interactions have either been reported or are theoretical in humans or animals receiving cyclosporine and may be of significance in veterinary patients. Unless indicated, a listed potential drug interaction does not imply that using the drugs together are contraindicated, but does mean they should be used cautiously with enhanced awareness and monitoring.

The following drugs may **increase** cyclosporine blood levels and **increase** the risk for cyclosporine toxicity:

- **ACETAZOLAMIDE**
- **ALLOPURINOL**
- **AMLODIPINE**
- **AZITHROMYCIN**
- **AZOLE ANTIFUNGALS** (*e.g.,* **ketoconazole, itraconazole, fluconazole**): Ketoconazole and fluconazole have been shown to significantly alter the pharmacokinetics of cyclosporine in dogs. Itraconazole appears to affect cyclosporine pharmacokinetics in cats, but not in dogs. Many clinicians concurrently use ketoconazole in dogs to reduce the dose and resultant cost of cyclosporine treatment. Attempt this with caution only, and with the realization that monitoring of cyclosporine levels may be required.
- **BROMOCRIPTINE**
- **CALCIUM CHANNEL BLOCKERS** (*e.g.,* **verapamil, diltiazem**)
- **CARVEDILOL**
- **CIMETIDINE**: This interaction does not appear to occur in dogs.
- **CHLORAMPHENICOL**
- **CIPROFLOXACIN/ENROFLOXACIN**
- **CISAPRIDE**
- **CLARITHROMYCIN**
- **CLOPIDOGREL**: A study in dogs showed that clopidogrel can increase cyclosporine peak levels, but areas under the curve were the same when cyclosporine was used alone (Lee et al. 2012).
- **COLCHICINE** (colchicine levels may also increase)
- **CORTICOSTEROIDS**: Methylprednisolone does not appear to affect cyclosporine levels in dogs.
- **DANAZOL**
- **DIGOXIN**
- **ESTROGENS**
- **FLUVOXAMINE**
- **GLIPIZIDE/GLYBURIDE**
- **GRAPEFRUIT JUICE/GRAPEFRUIT JUICE POWDER**
- **IMIPENEM**
- **LOSARTAN, VALSARTAN**
- **MEDROXYPROGESTERONE**
- **METOCLOPRAMIDE**: A study in dogs demonstrated that metoclopramide did not significantly alter cyclosporine pharmacokinetics (Radwanski et al. 2011).
- **METRONIDAZOLE**
- **OMEPRAZOLE**
- **SERTRALINE**
- **TINIDAZOLE**

The following drugs may **decrease** the blood levels of cyclosporine:

- **AZATHIOPRINE**
- **CARBAMAZEPINE**
- **CLINDAMYCIN** (may decrease cyclosporine bioavailability): This interaction does not appear to occur in dogs.
- **CYCLOPHOSPHAMIDE**
- **FAMOTIDINE**
- **GRISEOFULVIN**

- **OCTREOTIDE**
- **RIFAMPIN**
- **PHENOBARBITAL**
- **PHENYTOIN**
- **St. JOHN'S WORT**: This interaction appears to be of significance in dogs.
- **SULFADIAZINE/SULFAMETHOXAZOLE**
- **SULFASALAZINE**
- **TERBINAFINE**
- **TRIMETHOPRIM** (may also increase risk for nephrotoxicity)
- **WARFARIN** (may also reduce efficacy of warfarin)

Additional interactions/notes:

- **ACE INHIBITORS** (**benazepril, enalapril**, etc.): Have been case reports in humans where renal function declined.
- **DIGOXIN**: Cyclosporine can cause increased digoxin levels with possible toxicity.
- **DOXORUBICIN**: Cyclosporine can increase doxorubicin and doxorubicinol (active metabolite) levels.
- **MELPHALAN**: Increased risk for renal failure.
- **METHOTREXATE**: Cyclosporine may increase MTX levels.
- **MYCOPHENOLATE**: Reduced levels of mycophenolate.
- **NEPHROTOXIC DRUGS, OTHER** (*e.g.,* **acyclovir, amphotericin B, aminoglycosides, colchicine, vancomycin, NSAIDs, tacrolimus**): Possible additive nephrotoxicity.
- **SPIRONOLACTONE** and other **potassium sparing diuretics**: Increased risk for hyperkalemia.
- **VACCINATIONS**: May be less effective while patients are receiving cyclosporine; avoid the use of live attenuated vaccines.

Doses

Note: Dosages are for cyclosporine (modified), *Atopica*®, *Neoral*®, or equivalent; they are not interchangeable with *Sandimmune*® (or equivalent) dosages.

- **DOGS:**

    For control of atopic dermatitis:

    a) **Labeled dosage; FDA-approved**: In dogs weighing at least 1.8 kg: 5 mg/kg (3.3 – 6.7 mg/kg) PO once daily for 30 days. Following this initial treatment period, dosage may be tapered to every other day, and then 2 times per week, until a minimum frequency is reached that will maintain the desired therapeutic effect. Give at least one hour before, or two hours after meals. If a dose is missed, the next dose should be administered (without doubling) as soon as possible, but dosing should be no more frequent than once daily. (Adapted from label information; *Atopica*®)

    b) **Extra-label using cyclosporine (modified); (*e.g., Atopica*®) with ketoconazole**: Ideally should be given on an empty stomach, but if causes GI upset, administration with food may help. In larger dogs, administration of cyclosporine at 2.5 – 3 mg/kg PO once daily with ketoconazole (2.5 – 5 mg/kg/day) may be effective and reduce costs. One study found similar cyclosporine levels in dogs treated with either 5 mg/kg cyclosporine (alone) PO once daily or cyclosporine 2.5 mg/kg PO once daily with ketoconazole 2.5 mg/kg PO once daily (Gray et al. 2013). Once control of pruritus is achieved, the clinician may be able to reduce the daily dosage or switch to every second or third day therapy.

    For perianal fistulas (anal furunculosis); (extra-label): Dosed similarly as for atopic dermatitis although some give q12h. Cyclosporine (alone) 5 – 7.5 mg PO once daily or 2.5 – 3 mg/kg PO once daily with ketoconazole (2.5 – 5 mg/kg/day). Once controlled, dosing interval is increased to the lowest frequency that controls symptoms.

As an immunosuppressant (extra-label): Reasonable evidence supports use for transplant rejection, but despite widespread clinical use, retrospective studies, case reports, etc., the evidence supporting cyclosporine efficacy for other immune-mediated diseases or keratinization disorders is either weak or not currently available. Empirical dosages generally range from 3 – 6 mg/kg PO twice daily or 5 – 7.5 mg/kg once daily. As with other uses (above), ketoconazole or grapefruit juice powder have been used to lower cyclosporine dosage requirements. When used to reduce transplant rejection twice daily administration is generally used and blood levels are monitored.

■ **CATS:**

For allergic dermatitis as manifested by excoriations (including facial and neck), miliary dermatitis, eosinophilic plaques, and self-induced alopecia (labeled dosage; FDA-approved): Initial dose: 7 mg/kg/day PO once daily for a minimum of 4-6 weeks or until resolution of clinical signs. Following this initial daily treatment period, the dose may be tapered by decreasing the frequency of dosing to every other day or twice weekly to maintain the desired therapeutic effect. Administer directly on a small amount of food or orally just after feeding. Whenever possible, administer on a consistent schedule with regard to meals and time of day. If a dose is missed, the next dose should be administered (without doubling) as soon as possible, but dosing should be no more frequent than once daily. (Adapted from label; *Atopica® for Cats*)

As an immunosuppressant (usually as part of an immunosuppressive protocol); (extra-label): 3 – 4 mg/kg PO q12h; 5 – 7 mg/kg PO once daily. When used to reduce transplant rejection twice daily administration is generally used and blood levels are monitored.

Monitoring
■ Therapeutic efficacy.
■ Adverse effects.
■ Consider therapeutic drug monitoring, particularly when response is poor or adverse effects occur; ideally no sooner than 60 hours after starting therapy. Trough whole-blood levels (12 hours after last dose) have been suggested to be between 400-600 ng/mL, but may not reliably predict clinical response for immunosuppression. Because different methodologies may yield different results; contact your laboratory for recommendations on the evaluation of levels.
■ CBC and biochem profile: baseline and then monthly to every 3 months has been suggested; others believe this is not warranted.

Client Information
■ Provide a client information sheet when dispensing this medication.
■ Preferably dogs should receive the drug on an empty stomach and cats should get it with food. If dog vomits after getting the drug, try giving with food.
■ May take up to two weeks to see if the drug is working. Cyclosporine blood level tests may be done.
■ Vomiting, reduced appetite, & diarrhea are the most common side effects. These usually get better on their own, but if they are severe or continue, contact your veterinarian.
■ Watch for signs of infection; if seen, contact veterinarian immediately.

Chemistry/Synonyms
Also known as Cyclosporin A, ciclosporin, or cyclosporin, cyclosporine is a naturally produced immunosuppressant agent. It is a non-polar, cyclic, polypeptide antibiotic consisting of 11 amino acids and occurs as a white, fine crystalline powder. It is relatively insoluble in water, but generally soluble in organic solvents and oils.

Commercially cyclosporine is available in several dosage forms, including an oral liquid, capsules, and a concentrate for injection. To increase oral absorption, a micro emulsion forming preparation (*Neoral®*) is also available in capsules and oral liquid. The veterinary product, *Atopica®*, is a micro-emulsion product equivalent to *Neoral®*.

Cyclosporine may also be known as: ciclosporin, 27-400, ciclosporinum, cyclosporine, cyclosporine A, OL-27-400, *Atopica®*, *Gengraf®*, *Neoral®*, *Sandimmune®*, or *Sigmasporin®*.

Storage/Stability
The veterinary product (*Atopica®*) for dogs should be stored and dispensed in the original unit-dose container at controlled room temperature (15-35°C; 59-77°C). The oral solution for cats is labeled to only be dispensed in the original container and stored at controlled room temperature between 59-77°F (15-25°C). Once opened, use contents within two months for the 5 mL container and within 11 weeks for the 17 mL container.

The oral liquid and oral capsules (*Sandimmune®*) should be stored in their original containers at temperatures less than 30°C; protect from freezing and do not refrigerate. After opening the oral liquid, use within 2 months.

The oral liquid and capsules for emulsion (*Neoral®*) should be stored in their original containers at 25°C. Temperatures below 20°C may cause the solution to gel or flocculate. Rewarming to 25°C can reverse this process without harm.

The injection should be stored at temperatures less than 30°C and be protected from light. After diluting to a concentration of approximately 2 mg/mL, the resultant solution is stable for 24 hours in D5W or normal saline; if diluting with normal saline it would be wise to use the solution within 12 hours. It does not need to be protected from light after diluting.

Compatibility/Compounding Considerations
Cyclosporine for injection is compatible with sodium chloride 0.9%, or dextrose 5% intravenous solutions.

Because there are approved oral dosage forms for both dogs and cats, routine compounding for use in these species is discouraged. A recent study evaluating the accuracy and precision of compounded cyclosporine preparations found some compounded solutions deviated by more than 10% from the labeled concentration (Umstead et al. 2012).

Dosage Forms/Regulatory Status
VETERINARY-LABELED PRODUCTS:

Cyclosporine (Modified) Capsules: 10 mg, 25 mg, 50 mg, & 100 mg; *Atopica®*; (Rx). FDA-approved for use in dogs. The FDA-approved label information for *Atopica®* may be found on the dailymed.nlm. nih.gov website.

Cyclosporine (Modified) Oral Solution 100 mg/mL in 5 & 17 mL bottles; *Atopica for Cats®*; (Rx). FDA-approved for use in cats. The FDA-approved label information for *Atopica® for Cats* may be found on the dailymed.nlm.nih.gov website.

See the appendix for more information on the topical ophthalmic preparation.

HUMAN-LABELED PRODUCTS:

Cyclosporine Modified (Microemulsion) Oral Capsules (Soft-gelatin): 25 mg, & 100 mg; *Neoral®*, *Gengraf®*, generic; (Rx) These products may be bioequivalent with veterinary-approved products (*Atopica®*).

Cyclosporine Modified Oral Solution (Microemulsion): 100 mg/mL in 50 mL btls; *Neoral®*, generic; (Rx). This product is may be bioequivalent with the veterinary-approved product (*Atopica® for Cats*).

Cyclosporine Oral Solution: 100 mg/mL in 50 mL btls with syringe; *Sandimmune®*; (Rx). This product is not bioequivalent with the veterinary-approved product (*Atopica® for Cats*).

Cyclosporine Oral Capsules (Soft-gelatin): 25 mg, 50 mg & 100 mg; *Sandimmune®*; generic; (Rx). These products are not bioequivalent with veterinary-approved products (*Atopica®*).

Cyclosporine Concentrated Solution for Injection: 50 mg/mL in 5 mL single-use vials & amps; *Sandimmune®*, generic; (Rx)

Revisions/References

Monograph revised/updated October 2013.

Bloom, P. (2006). *Cyclosporine and emesis.* Proceedings: Western Vet Conf. accessed via Veterinary Information Network; vin.com

Gray, L. L., et al. (2013). The effect of ketoconazole on whole blood and skin ciclosporin concentrations in dogs. *Veterinary Dermatology* 24(1): 118-+.

Lee, J. H., et al. (2012). Pharmacokinetic interactions of clopidogrel with quercetin, telmisartan, and cyclosporine A in rats and dogs. *Archives of Pharmacal Research* 35(10): 1831-7.

Radwanski, N. E., et al. (2011). Effects of powdered whole grapefruit and metoclopramide on the pharmacokinetics of cyclosporine in dogs. *American Journal of Veterinary Research* 72(5): 687-93.

Rosenberg, A., et al. (2013). Evaluation of azithromycin in systemic and toothpaste forms for the treatment of ciclosporin-associated gingival overgrowth in dogs. *Veterinary Dermatology* 24(3): 337-+.

Umstead, M. E., et al. (2012). Accuracy and precision of compounded ciclosporin capsules and solution. *Veterinary Dermatology* 23(5).

WSU-VetClinPharmLab (2009). "Problem Drugs." http://goo.gl/aIGlM.

Cyproheptadine HCl

(sip-roe-hep-ta-deen)   Periactin®

Antihistamine

Prescriber Highlights

▶ Serotonin antagonist antihistamine used as an appetite stimulant, primarily in cats: can be useful in management of serotonin-syndrome in small animals. Has also been tried as an antipruritic/antihistamine in dogs & cats and for photic head shaking or treatment of equine Cushing's (PPID) in horses.

▶ Caution: Urinary or GI obstruction, severe CHF, narrow angle glaucoma.

▶ Adverse Effects: Sedation (cats may demonstrate paradoxical hyperexcitability) & anticholinergic effects; some reports of hemolytic anemia in cats.

Uses/Indications

Cyproheptadine may be useful in cats as an appetite stimulant, but it apparently is not effective in the management of hepatic lipidosis. It potentially may be of benefit in the treatment of feline asthma or pruritus in cats, but clinical efficacy is marginal for these indications. Cyproheptadine use as monotherapy for eosinophilic airway inflammation in cats is not recommended (Schooley et al. 2007).

Cyproheptadine is an antihistamine but its efficacy is questionable for this indication in dogs. The drug may be useful as adjunctive therapy for Cushing's syndrome probably as result of its anti-serotonin activity, however one study demonstrated efficacy in less than 10% of dogs treated for pituitary dependent hyperadrenocorticism.

Cyproheptadine may be useful as adjunctive treatment in dogs or cats with serotonin syndrome or to reduce dysphoria (vocalization, disorientation) associated with baclofen, carisoprodol, SSRI, or ephedra/ma huang toxicosis.

In horses, cyproheptadine has been used for treating photic head shaking and pituitary pars intermedia dysfunction (PPID, Equine Cushing's Disease). Pergolide is generally considered to be superior to cyproheptadine for treating PPID. However, cyproheptadine combined with pergolide may increase efficacy in refractory cases that do not respond to pergolide alone.

Pharmacology/Actions

Like other H_1-receptor antihistamines, cyproheptadine acts by competing with histamine for sites on H_1-receptor sites on effector cells. Antihistamines do not block histamine release, but can antagonize its effects. Cyproheptadine also possesses potent antiserotonin activity and, reportedly, has calcium channel blocking action as well.

Pharmacokinetics

Limited data is available. Cyproheptadine is well absorbed after oral administration. Its distribution characteristics are not well described. Cyproheptadine is apparently nearly completely metabolized in the liver and these metabolites are then excreted in the urine; elimination is reduced in renal failure. Elimination half-life in cats averages about 13 hours, but there is wide interpatient variability.

Contraindications/Precautions/Warnings

Cyproheptadine is contraindicated in patients hypersensitive to it. It should be used with caution in patients with prostatic hypertrophy, bladder neck obstruction, severe cardiac failure, epilepsy, angle-closure glaucoma, or pyeloduodenal obstruction.

Adverse Effects

The most likely adverse effects seen with cyproheptadine are related to its CNS depressant (sedation) and anticholinergic effects (dryness of mucous membranes, etc.). Cats can develop a paradoxical agitated state that resolves upon dose reduction or discontinuation. There have been reports of cyproheptadine-induced hemolytic anemia in cats. Horses may show mild depression, anorexia, or lethargy.

At higher dosages, cyproheptadine has caused significant polyphagia in dogs.

Reproductive/Nursing Safety

Cyproheptadine has been tested in pregnant lab animals in doses up to 32X labeled dose without evidence of harm to fetuses. Nevertheless, because safety has not been established in other species, its use during pregnancy should be weighed carefully. In humans, the FDA categorizes this drug as category *B* for use during pregnancy (*Animal studies have not yet demonstrated risk to the fetus, but there are no adequate studies in pregnant women; or animal studies have shown an adverse effect, but adequate studies in pregnant women have not demonstrated a risk to the fetus in the first trimester of pregnancy, and there is no evidence of risk in later trimesters.*)

It is not known if cyproheptadine is distributed into milk.

Overdosage/Acute Toxicity

There are no specific antidotes available. Significant overdoses should be handled using standard gut emptying protocols when appropriate and supportive therapy when required. The adverse effects seen with overdoses are an extension of the drug's side effects, principally CNS depression (although CNS stimulation may be seen), anticholinergic effects (severe drying of mucous membranes, tachycardia, urinary retention, hyperthermia, etc.) and possibly hypotension. Physostigmine may be considered to treat serious CNS anticholinergic effects, and diazepam employed to treat seizures, if necessary.

Horses that have received doses 2 times greater than recommended apparently showed no untoward effects.

Drug Interactions

The following drug interactions have either been reported or are theoretical in humans or animals receiving cyproheptadine and may be of significance in veterinary patients. Unless otherwise noted, use together is not necessarily contraindicated, but weigh the potential risks and perform additional monitoring when appropriate.

- **CNS DEPRESSANT MEDICATIONS:** Additive CNS depression may be seen if combining cyproheptadine with other CNS depressant medications, such as barbiturates, tranquilizers, etc.
- **MIRTAZAPINE:** Although no supporting published documentation was located, it has been anecdotally reported that cyproheptadine and mirtazapine should not be given together.
- **SSRIs** (including **sertraline, fluoxetine, paroxetine,** etc.); **TRICYCLIC ANTIDEPRESSANTS** (**clomipramine, amitriptyline,** etc.): Cyproheptadine may decrease the efficacy of the SSRI or TCA.
- **TRAMADOL:** Cyproheptadine may decrease the efficacy.

Laboratory Considerations

- Because antihistamines can decrease the wheal and flair response to **skin allergen testing**, antihistamines should be discontinued from 7-14 days (depending on the antihistamine used and the reference) before intradermal skin tests.
- Cyproheptadine may increase amylase and prolactin serum levels when administered with **thyrotropin-releasing hormone**.

Doses

- **DOGS:**

  As an appetite stimulant (extra-label): 0.2 mg/kg PO q12h. May be dosed less frequently if inappetence is mild.

  For adjunctive treatment of dysphoria associated with serotonin syndrome; toxicoses of SSRIs, TCAs, ephedra, amphetamines, baclofen, etc.; (extra-label): 1.1 mg/kg PO; doses may be repeated q4-6h as needed until signs have resolved. In cases where PO dosing not possible (severe vomiting), may crush tablets and mix with saline and give rectally.

  As an antihistamine (extra-label): 0.3 – 2 mg/kg PO twice daily. Can be very expensive at higher dosage range and there is little evidence to support dose recommendation or efficacy.

- **CATS:**

  As an appetite stimulant (extra-label): 1 – 2 mg per cat PO q12-24h. Most cats require twice daily dosing and it may take 3 days to see effect. Before starting treatment, adequate antiemetic and/or analgesic therapy is necessary. If discontinuing, taper off drug to prevent rebound anorexia.

  As an antihistamine/antipruritic/anti-asthma (extra-label): 2 mg per cat PO q12h. Little evidence to support use.

  For adjunctive treatment of serotonin syndrome (extra-label): 2 – 4 mg (total dose) PO; doses may be repeated q4-6h as needed until signs have resolved. In cases where PO dosing not possible (severe vomiting), may crush tablets and mix with saline and give rectally. (Wismer 2006)

- **HORSES: (NOTE: ARCI UCGFS CLASS 4 DRUG)**

  For photic head shaking (extra-label): 0.3 – 0.6 mg/kg PO q12h.

  For treatment of equine Cushing's (PPID); (extra-label): Pergolide therapy is preferred, but cyproheptadine at 0.25 mg/kg PO once to twice daily can be added in refractory cases. May require 4-8 weeks to determine efficacy and can be very expensive.

Monitoring

- Efficacy (weight if used for anorexia).
- Adverse effects, if any.

- With long-term use, should occasionally monitor serum BUN in cats.

Client Information

- When used as an antihistamine it should be given on a regular, ongoing basis. Antihistamines work better if used before exposure to an allergen. It may take several weeks to see if the drug is working.
- Drowsiness/sleepiness can occur with this medication, but usually will lessen with time. Cats can become excited when receiving this medication; if cat becomes very lethargic, weak or develops pale mucous membranes contact veterinarian immediately.

Chemistry/Synonyms

An antihistamine that also possesses serotonin antagonist properties, cyproheptadine HCl occurs as a white to slightly yellow crystalline powder. Approximately 3.64 mg are soluble in one mL of water and 28.6 mg in one mL of alcohol.

Cyproheptadine HCl may also be known as: cyproheptadini hydrochloridum, *Ciplactin*®, *Cyheptine*®, *Cyprogin*®, *Cyprono*®, *Cyprosian*®, *Klarivitina*®, *Nuran*®, *Periactine*®, *Periactinol*®, *Periatin*®, *Peritol*®, *Polytab*®, *Practin*®, *Preptin*®, *Supersan*®, or *Trimetabol*®.

Storage/Stability

Cyproheptadine HCl tablets and oral solution should be stored at room temperature and freezing should be avoided.

Compatibility/Compounding Considerations

No specific information noted.

Dosage Forms/Regulatory Status

VETERINARY-LABELED PRODUCTS: NONE.

The ARCI (Racing Commissioners International) has designated this drug as a class 4 substance. See the appendix for more information.

HUMAN-LABELED PRODUCTS:

Cyproheptadine HCl Oral Tablets: 4 mg; generic; (Rx)

Cyproheptadine HCl Oral Syrup: 2 mg/5 mL in 473 mL; generic; (Rx)

Revisions/References

Monograph revised/updated October 2013.

Schooley, E. K., et al. (2007). Effects of cyproheptadine and cetirizine on eosinophilic airway inflammation in cats with experimentally induced asthma. *American Journal of Veterinary Research* 68(11): 1265-71.

Wismer, T. (2006). *Serotonin Syndrome*. Proceedings: IVECC Symposium. accessed via Veterinary Information Network; vin.com

Cytarabine

(sye-tare-a-bean) Cytosine arabinoside, Cytosar-U®

Antineoplastic

Prescriber Highlights

▶ Parenteral immunosuppressant/antineoplastic for meningoencephalomyelitis of unknown origin in dogs and for lymphoreticular neoplasms & leukemias in dogs & cats.

▶ Contraindications: Hypersensitivity; potentially, embryotoxic & teratogenic.

▶ Adverse Effects: Primarily myelosuppression, but GI & other toxicities can occur.

▶ Adequate monitoring essential.

Uses/Indications

In veterinary medicine, cytarabine is used primarily in small animals as an antineoplastic agent for lymphoreticular neoplasms, myeloproliferative disease (leukemias), and CNS lymphoma. Cytarabine appears to be efficacious (with glucocorticoids) for treating meningoencephalomyelitis of unknown origin in dogs.

Pharmacology/Actions

Cytarabine is converted intracellularly into cytarabine triphosphate that apparently competes with deoxycytidine triphosphate, thereby inhibiting DNA polymerase with resulting inhibition of DNA synthesis. Cytarabine is cell phase specific, and acts principally during the S-phase (DNA synthesis). It may also, under certain conditions, block cells from the G_1 phase to the S phase.

Pharmacokinetics

Cytarabine has very poor systemic availability after oral administration and is only used parenterally. The pharmacokinetics of cytarabine have been described in dogs following 50 mg/m² SC injections and an 8-hour IV constant rate infusion (CRI) of 25 mg/m² per hour. Volume of distribution was about 0.67 L/kg. Elimination half-lives were similar (1.35 hours SC; 1.15 hours CRI) as were peak concentrations. Rate of absorption after SC was very rapid with peak levels occurring under an hour after the dose. Dose corrected area under the curve was greater with the CRI (Crook et al. 2012).

Cytarabine is distributed widely throughout the body, but crosses into the CNS in only a limited manner. If given via continuous IV infusion, CSF levels are higher than with IV bolus injection and can reach 20-60% of those levels found in plasma. Elimination half-life in the CSF is significantly longer than that of serum. In humans, cytarabine is only about 13% bound to plasma proteins. The drug apparently crosses the placenta, but it is not known if it enters milk.

Circulating cytarabine is rapidly metabolized by the enzyme cytidine deaminase, principally in the liver but also in the kidneys, intestinal mucosa, and granulocytes, to the inactive metabolite ara-U (uracil arabinoside). About 80% of a dose is excreted in the urine within 24 hours as both ara-U (≈90%) and unchanged cytarabine (≈10%).

Contraindications/Precautions/Warnings

Cytarabine is contraindicated in patients hypersensitive to it. Because of the potential for development of serious adverse reactions, cytarabine should only be used in patients that can be adequately and regularly monitored.

The person preparing or administering cytarabine for injection, need not observe any special handling precautions other than wearing gloves, however, should any contamination occur, thoroughly wash the drug from skin or mucous membranes.

Adverse Effects

The principal adverse effect of cytarabine is myelosuppression (with leukopenia being most prevalent), but anemia and thrombocytopenia can also be seen. Myelosuppressive effects are more pronounced with IV administration and reach a nadir at 5-7 days, and generally recover at 7-14 days.

GI disturbances (anorexia, nausea, vomiting, diarrhea), conjunctivitis, oral ulceration, neurotoxicity, hepatotoxicity and fever may also be noted with cytarabine therapy, but occur rarely in veterinary patients. Anaphylaxis has been reported, but is believed to occur very rarely. Calcinosis cutis at cytarabine injection sites was reported in 3 dogs that also were receiving prednisolone (Volk et al. 2012).

Cytarabine is a mutagenic and, potentially, carcinogenic agent.

Reproductive/Nursing Safety

Cytarabine's safe use in pregnancy has not been established and it is potentially teratogenic and embryotoxic. In humans, the FDA categorizes this drug as category *D* for use during pregnancy (*There is evidence of human fetal risk, but the potential benefits from the use of the drug in pregnant women may be acceptable despite its potential risks.*)

It is unknown if cytarabine enters milk; safe use during nursing cannot be assured.

Overdosage/Acute Toxicity

Cytarabine efficacy and toxicity (see Adverse Effects) are dependent not only on the dose, but also the rate the drug is given. In dogs, the IV LD_{50} is 384 mg/kg when given over 12 hours and 48 mg/kg when infused IV over 120 hours. Should an inadvertent overdose occur, supportive therapy should be instituted.

Drug Interactions

The following drug interactions have either been reported or are theoretical in humans or animals receiving cytarabine and may be of significance in veterinary patients. Unless otherwise noted, use together is not necessarily contraindicated, but weigh the potential risks and perform additional monitoring when appropriate.

- **DIGOXIN:** Presumably due to causing alterations in the intestinal mucosa, cytarabine may decrease the amount of digoxin (tablets only) absorbed after oral dosing; this effect may persist for several days after cytarabine has been discontinued.
- **FLUCYTOSINE (5-FC):** Limited studies have indicated that cytarabine may antagonize the anti-infective activity of flucytosine; monitor for decreased efficacy.
- **GENTAMICIN:** Limited studies have indicated that cytarabine may antagonize the anti-infective activity of gentamicin; monitor for decreased efficacy.

Laboratory Considerations

- None noted.

Doses

Note: Because of the potential toxicity of this drug to patients, veterinary personnel and clients, and since chemotherapy indications, treatment protocols, monitoring and safety guidelines often change, the following dosages should be used only as a general guide. Consultation with a veterinary oncologist or referral to current veterinary oncology references [*e.g.,* (Withrow et al. 2012); (Dobson et al. 2011); (Henry et al. 2009); (North et al. 2009); (Argyle et al. 2008)] are strongly recommended. All dosages below are extra-label uses.

- **DOGS:**

    For susceptible neoplastic diseases: The following is a usual dosage or dose range for cytarabine in dogs and should be used only as a general guide: Usually, cytarabine is dosed at 100 mg/m² (**NOT** mg/kg) IV either as a continuous infusion over 2-3 days or divided and given IV or SC for 2-4 days.

    For adjunctive treatment (with glucocorticoid therapy) of inflammatory brain disease (*e.g.,* meningoencephalomyelitis of unknown etiology; MUE); (empirical): At present, recommendations for dosage amounts and route of administration vary. Both 50 mg/m² (**NOT** mg/kg) SC twice daily for 2 consecutive days or 25 mg/m² per hour for an 8 hour CRI have each been recommended. May be repeated every 3-4 weeks. A recent pharmacokinetic study (Crook et al. 2012), suggests that the CRI may produce a more prolonged exposure of cytarabine at cytotoxic levels in plasma, but it is not known if this correlates with differences in efficacy or toxicity.

- **CATS:**

    For susceptible neoplastic diseases: The following is a usual dosage or dose range for cytarabine in cats and should be used only as a general guide: Usually, cytarabine is dosed at 100 mg/m² (**NOT** mg/kg) IV either as a continuous infusion over 2-3 days or divided and given IV or SC for 2-4 days. Cats are generally dosed similarly as dogs.

- **HORSES:**

    For neoplastic diseases; consultation with a veterinary oncologist is encouraged before use: Usual doses used in horses are: 200 – 300 mg/m² (usually 1 – 1.5 grams per horse per dose) SC, IM or

IV every 1-2 weeks. For generalized lymphoma the CAP protocol was used at the time of publication by one of the authors. See the reference or the vincristine monograph for more information. (Mair et al. 2006)

Monitoring

- Efficacy; refer to the references from the Dosage section above for more information.
- Toxicity; see Adverse Effects above. Regular hemograms are mandatory. Periodic liver and kidney function tests are suggested.

Client Information

- Clients must be briefed on the possibilities of severe toxicity developing from this drug, including drug-related mortality.
- Clients should contact the veterinarian should the patient exhibit any signs of profound depression, abnormal bleeding and/or bruising.

Chemistry/Synonyms

A synthetic pyrimidine nucleoside antimetabolite, cytarabine occurs as an odorless, white to off-white, crystalline powder with a pK_a of 4.35. It is freely soluble in water and slightly soluble in alcohol.

Cytarabine may also be known as: 1-beta-D-arabinofuranosylcytosine, arabinosylcytosine, ara-C, cytarabine liposome, cytarabinum, cytosine arabinoside, liposomal cytarabine, NSC-63878, U-19920, U-19920A, WR-28453, ARA-cell®, *Alexan®, Arabine®, Aracytin®, Aracytine®, Citab®, Citagenin®, Citaloxan®, Cylocide Cytarbel®, Cytarine®, DepoCyt®, DepoCyte®, Erpalfa®, Ifarab®, Laracit®, Medsara®, Novutrax®, Serotabir®, Starasid®, Tabine®, Tarabine®* or *Udicil®*.

Storage/Stability

Cytarabine sterile powder for injection should be stored at room temperature (15-30°C). After reconstituting with bacteriostatic water for injection, solutions are stable for at least 48 hours when stored at room temperature. One study, however, demonstrated that the reconstituted solution retains 90% of its potency for up to 17 days when stored at room temperature. If the solution develops a slight haze, the drug should be discarded.

Compatibility/Compounding Considerations

Cytarabine is reportedly **compatible** with the following intravenous solutions and drugs: amino acids 4.25%/dextrose 25%, dextrose containing solutions, dextrose-saline combinations, dextrose-lactated Ringer's injection combinations, Ringer's injection, lactated Ringer's injection, sodium chloride 0.9%, sodium lactate 1/6 M, corticotropin, lincomycin HCl, methotrexate sodium, metoclopramide HCl, potassium chloride, prednisolone sodium phosphate, sodium bicarbonate, and vincristine sulfate.

Cytarabine **compatibility information conflicts** or is dependent on diluent or concentration factors with the following drugs or solutions: gentamicin sulfate, hydrocortisone sodium succinate, and methylprednisolone sodium succinate. Compatibility is dependent upon factors such as pH, concentration, temperature and diluent used; consult specialized references or a hospital pharmacist for more specific information.

Cytarabine is reportedly **incompatible** with the following solutions or drugs: fluorouracil, regular insulin, and penicillin G sodium.

Dosage Forms/Regulatory Status

VETERINARY-LABELED PRODUCTS: NONE.

HUMAN-LABELED PRODUCTS:

Cytarabine Powder for Injection: 100 mg, 500 mg, 1 g & 2 g in vials; generic; (Rx)

Cytarabine Injection: 20 mg/mL in 5 mL single- & multi-dose vials

& preservative free 50 mL bulk package vials, & 100 mg/mL in 20 mL single-dose vials, generic; (Rx)

Cytarabine Injection: 10 mg/mL (liposomal) preservative free (for intrathecal use) in 5 mL vials; *DepoCyt®*; (Rx)

Revisions/References

Monograph revised/updated October 2013.

Argyle, D., et al. (2008). *Decision Making in Small Animal Oncology*, Wiley-Blackwell.
Crook, K. I., et al. (2012). The pharmacokinetics of cytarabine in dogs when administered via subcutaneous and continuous intravenous infusion routes. *J. Vet. Pharmacol. Ther.* 36(4): 408-11.
Dobson, J. & D. Lascelles (2011). *BSAVA Manual of Canine and Feline Oncology*, BSAVA.
Henry, C. & M. Higginbotham (2009). *Cancer Management in Small Animal Practice*, Saunders.
Mair, T. S. & C. G. Couto (2006). The use of cytotoxic drugs in equine practice. *Equine Veterinary Education* 18(3): 149-56.
North, S. & T. Banks (2009). *Small Animal Oncology: An Introduction*, Saunders.
Volk, A. V., et al. (2012). Calcinosis cutis at cytarabine injection site in three dogs receiving prednisolone. *Veterinary Record* 171(13).
Withrow, S., et al. (2012). *Withrow and MacEwen's Small Animal Clinical Oncology*, 5th Ed., Saunders.

d-Panthenol —see Dexpanthenol

Dacarbazine (DTIC)

(da-kar-ba-zeen)

Antineoplastic

Prescriber Highlights

- ▶ Parenteral antineoplastic used in dogs for relapsed lymphomas, soft tissue sarcomas, & melanoma.
- ▶ Not recommended for use in cats.
- ▶ Contraindications: Hypersensitivity; potentially teratogenic.
- ▶ Primary adverse effects are GI (can be severe & dose limiting) & bone marrow suppression; adequate monitoring essential.
- ▶ Must give diluted IV; extravasation injuries can be serious.

Uses/Indications

Dacarbazine has been used to treat relapsed canine lymphoma, soft tissue sarcomas and melanoma in dogs. In combination with doxorubicin, dacarbazine has been used to treat dogs with relapsed lymphosarcoma. Ongoing studies evaluating various protocols are ongoing for this indication.

Pharmacology/Actions

The mechanism for dacarbazine's antineoplastic activity has not been precisely determined, but it is believed the drug acts as an alkylating agent through the formation of reactive carbonium ions. Dacarbazine also possesses antimetabolic activity by inhibiting DNA's of purine nucleoside. It possesses minimal immunosuppressant activity and is probably not a cell cycle-phase specific drug.

Pharmacokinetics

Dacarbazine (DTIC) is poorly absorbed from the GI tract and is administered intravenously. It is converted into an active form of the drug in the liver. The drug's distribution characteristics are not well known, but it is only slightly bound to plasma proteins and probably concentrates in the liver. Only limited amounts cross the blood-brain barrier; it probably crosses the placenta, but it is unknown if it is distributed into milk. Dacarbazine is extensively metabolized in the liver and is excreted in the urine via tubular secretion. Elimination half-life is about 5 hours.

Contraindications/Precautions/Warnings

Dacarbazine is not recommended for use in cats as it is unknown whether the feline liver can adequately metabolize it.

Dacarbazine (DTIC) is contraindicated in patients that are hypersensitive to it. DTIC can cause life-threatening toxicity. It should only be used where adequate monitoring and support can be administered. It should be used with caution in patients with preexisting bone marrow depression, hepatic or renal dysfunction, or infection.

Adverse Effects

Gastrointestinal toxicity (including vomiting, anorexia, diarrhea) can commonly be seen after administration and is dose limiting. Some oncologists pretreat with an antiemetic (*e.g.*, dolasetron, ondansetron).

Bone marrow toxicity is usually asymptomatic with leukocyte and platelet nadirs seen several weeks after therapy. Occasionally severe hematopoietic toxicity can occur with fatal consequences. Other delayed toxic effects can include, alopecia, severe hepatotoxicity, renal impairment, and photosensitivity reactions. These delayed reactions appear rarely.

Because DTIC can cause extensive pain and tissue damage, avoid extravasation injuries. Venous spasm and phlebitis may occur during IV administration. Pretreatment with dexamethasone and/or butorphanol has been suggested to reduce vasospasm, phlebitis and pain. Severe pain at the injection site can occur if giving the concentrated drug; dilution and administration by IV infusion is recommended. If signs of extravasation occur, the following has been recommended: Stop the infusion immediately and if possible, withdraw 3-5 mL of blood to remove some of the drug. Remove the infusion needle. Delineate the infiltrated area on the patient's skin with a felt tip marker. Elevate for 48 hours above heart level using a sling or stockinette dressing with an observation window cut in the dressing. Avoid pressure or friction; do not rub the area. Observe for signs of increased erythema, pain, or skin necrosis. Ensure that no medication is given distally to the extravasation site. After 48 hours, encourage the patient to use the extremity normally to promote full range of motion (Beckwith et al. 2008).

There is increasing evidence that chronic exposure by health care givers to antineoplastic drugs increases the mutagenic, teratogenic, and carcinogenic risks associated with these agents. Proper precautions in the handing, preparation, administration, and disposal of these drugs and supplies associated with their use are strongly recommended.

Reproductive/Nursing Safety

DTIC is teratogenic in rats at higher than clinically used dosages. It should be used during pregnancy only when the potential benefits outweigh its risks. In humans, the FDA categorizes this drug as category **C** for use during pregnancy (*Animal studies have shown an adverse effect on the fetus, but there are no adequate studies in humans; or there are no animal reproduction studies and no adequate studies in humans.*)

While it is unknown if DTIC enters milk, the potential carcinogenicity of the drug warrants using extreme caution in allowing the mother to continue nursing while receiving DTIC.

Overdosage/Acute Toxicity

Because of the toxic potential of this agent, iatrogenic overdoses must be avoided. Recheck dosage calculations. See Adverse Effects above for additional information on toxicity.

Drug Interactions

The following drug interactions have either been reported or are theoretical in humans or animals receiving dacarbazine and may be of significance in veterinary patients. Unless otherwise noted, use together is not necessarily contraindicated, but weigh the potential risks and perform additional monitoring when appropriate.

- **MYELOSUPPRESSIVE DRUGS, OTHER** (*e.g.*, **other antineoplastics, immunosuppressives, chloramphenicol, flucytosine, colchicine**, etc.): May cause additive myelosuppression when used with DTIC.

- **RIFAMPIN**: May increase the metabolism of DTIC.
- **PHENOBARBITAL**: May increase the metabolism of DTIC.
- **PHENYTOIN**: May increase the metabolism of DTIC.

Doses

Note: Because of the potential toxicity of this drug to patients, veterinary personnel and clients, and since chemotherapy indications, treatment protocols, monitoring and safety guidelines often change, the following dosages should be used only as a general guide. Consultation with a veterinary oncologist and referral to current veterinary oncology Revisions/References [*e.g.*, (Withrow et al. 2012); (Dobson et al. 2011); (Henry et al. 2009); (North et al. 2009); (Argyle et al. 2008)] are recommended.

- **DOGS:**

  Usual doses for DTIC in dogs (depending on the protocol used) are either: 800 – 1000 mg/m² (NOT mg/kg) IV over 4-8 hours every 2-3 weeks OR at a lower dosage such as 200 – 250 mg/m² once daily IV (as a bolus in a freely running IV solution) for 5 days with the treatment cycle repeated every 3-4 weeks.

Monitoring

- Efficacy.
- Toxicity, including CBC with differential and platelets; renal and hepatic function tests.

Client Information

- Dacarbazine is a chemotherapy (cancer) drug. The drug and its byproducts can be hazardous to other animals and people that come in contact with it. On the day your animal gets the drug and then for a few days afterward, all bodily waste (urine, feces, litter), blood, or vomit should only be handled while wearing disposable gloves. Seal the waste in a plastic bag and then place both the bag and gloves in with the regular trash.
- GI toxicity (*e.g.*, ulcers, diarrhea, etc.) can occur. If diarrhea is severe or continues, contact your veterinarian.
- Bone marrow depression can occur. The greatest effects on bone marrow usually occur within a few weeks after treatment. Your veterinarian will do blood tests to watch for this, but if you see bleeding, bruising, fever (indicating an infection), or if your animal becomes very tired easily, contact your veterinarian right away.

Chemistry/Synonyms

An antineoplastic agent, dacarbazine occurs as a colorless to ivory colored crystalline solid. It is slightly soluble in water or alcohol. After reconstituting with sterile water, the injection has a pH of 3-4.

Dacarbazine may also be known as: dacarbazinum, DIC, DTIC, imidazole carboxamide, diemthyl triazeno imadazol carboxamide, NSC-45388, WR-139007, *Asercit®*, *DTI®*, *DTIC-Dome®*, *Dacarb®*, *Dacarbaziba®*, *Dacatic®*, *Deticene®*, *Detilem®*, *Detimedac®*, *Fauldetic®*, *Ifadac®*, or *Oncocarbil®*.

Storage/Stability

The powder for injection should be protected from light and kept refrigerated. If exposed to heat, the powder may change color from ivory to pink indicating some decomposition.

After reconstituting with sterile water for injection the resultant solution is stable for up to 72 hours if kept refrigerated; up to 8 hours at room temperature. If further diluted (up to 500 mL) with either D5W or normal saline, the solution is stable for at least 24 hours when refrigerated; 8 hours at room temperature under normal room lighting.

Compatibility/Compounding Considerations

Drug additives that are reported to be **compatible** with dacarbazine include: bleomycin, cyclophosphamide, cytarabine, dactinomycin, doxorubicin, ondansetron and vinblastine. **Y-site compatibility** includes: doxorubicin liposome, granisetron, and ondansetron.

Compatibility is dependent upon factors such as pH, concentration, temperature and diluent used; consult specialized references or a hospital pharmacist for more specific information.

Dosage Forms/Regulatory Status
VETERINARY-LABELED PRODUCTS: NONE.

HUMAN-LABELED PRODUCTS:
Dacarbazine Powder for Injection: 100 mg & 200 mg (may contain mannitol) vials; generic; (Rx)

Revisions/References
Monograph revised/updated January 2014.

Argyle, D., et al. (2008). *Decision Making in Small Animal Oncology*, Wiley-Blackwell.
Beckwith, M. & L. Tyler (2008). Summary of extravasation management for antineoplastic agents. *Cancer Chemotherapy Manual [loose-leaf information service].* St Louis, Walters Kluwer Health.
Dobson, J. & D. Lascelles (2011). *BSAVA Manual of Canine and Feline Oncology*, BSAVA.
Henry, C. & M. Higginbotham (2009). *Cancer Management in Small Animal Practice*, Saunders.
North, S. & T. Banks (2009). *Small Animal Oncology: An Introduction*, Saunders.
Withrow, S., et al. (2012). Withrow and MacEwen's Small Animal Clinical Oncology, 5th Ed., Saunders.

Dactinomycin

(dak-ti-noe-mye-sin)   Actinomycin D, Cosmegen®

Antineoplastic

Prescriber Highlights
▶ Parenteral antibiotic antineoplastic used in dogs & cats.
▶ Contraindications: Hypersensitivity. Caution: Preexisting bone marrow depression, hepatic dysfunction, or infection.
▶ Teratogenic.
▶ Primary adverse effects are GI & bone marrow depression (may be life threatening); adequate monitoring essential.
▶ Specific administration techniques required, avoid extravasation injuries.

Uses/Indications
Dactinomycin has been used as adjunctive treatment of lymphoreticular neoplasms, bone and soft tissue sarcomas, and carcinomas in small animals. It appears to have low efficacy against most carcinomas and sarcomas. A study in dogs demonstrated that doxorubicin was superior to dactinomycin when used as part of a 'CHOP' protocol to treat lymphoma (Khanna et al. 1998).

Pharmacology/Actions
Dactinomycin is an antibiotic antineoplastic. While it has activity against gram-positive bacteria, the drug's toxicity precludes its use for this purpose. Dactinomycin's exact mechanism of action for its antineoplastic activity has not been determined, but it apparently inhibits DNA-dependent RNA synthesis. Dactinomycin forms a complex with DNA and interferes with DNA's template activity. Dactinomycin also possesses immunosuppressing and some hypocalcemic activity.

Pharmacokinetics
Because dactinomycin is poorly absorbed it must be given IV. It is rapidly distributed and high concentrations may be found in bone marrow and nucleated cells. Dactinomycin crosses the placenta, but it is unknown whether it enters maternal milk. The majority of the drug is excreted unchanged in the bile and urine.

Contraindications/Precautions/Warnings
Dactinomycin can cause life-threatening toxicity. It should only be used where adequate monitoring and support can be administered. Dactinomycin is contraindicated in patients that are hypersensitive to it. It should be used with caution in patients with preexisting bone marrow depression, hepatic dysfunction, or infection.

The p-glycoprotein pump actively transports dactinomycin and certain breeds susceptible to MDR1-allele mutation (*e.g.*, Collies, Australian Shepherds, Shelties, Long-haired Whippets) are at higher risk for toxicity. It is suggested to test susceptible breeds prior to treating (test available at Washington State Univ. Vet. School).

Consider using tall man lettering when writing orders for dactinomycin: DACTINomycin.

Adverse Effects
Adverse effects that may be seen more frequently include: anemia, leukopenia, thrombocytopenia (or other signs of bone marrow depression), diarrhea, and ulcerative stomatitis or other GI ulceration. Because dactinomycin may cause increased serum uric acid levels, allopurinol may be required to prevent urate stone formation in susceptible patients. Hepatotoxicity is potentially possible with this agent.

Because dactinomycin can cause extensive pain and tissue damage, avoid extravasation injuries. Dilution and administration by IV infusion is recommended or to administer slowly into a running IV line. If signs of extravasation occur, the following has been recommended: Stop the infusion immediately and if possible, withdraw 3-5 mL of blood to remove some of the drug. Remove the infusion needle. Delineate the infiltrated area on the patient's skin with a felt tip marker. Elevate for 48 hours above heart level using a sling or stockinette dressing with an observation window cut in the dressing. Avoid pressure or friction; do not rub the area. Observe for signs of increased erythema, pain, or skin necrosis. Ensure that no medication is given distally to the extravasation site. After 48 hours, encourage the patient to use the extremity normally to promote full range of motion (Beckwith et al. 2008).

There is increasing evidence that chronic exposure by health care givers to antineoplastic drugs increases the mutagenic, teratogenic and carcinogenic risks associated with these agents. Proper precautions in the handing, preparation, administration, and disposal of these drugs and supplies associated with their use are strongly recommended.

Reproductive/Nursing Safety
Dactinomycin has been demonstrated to be embryotoxic and teratogenic in rats, rabbits, and hamsters at higher than clinically used dosages. It should be used during pregnancy only when the potential benefits outweigh its risks. In humans, the FDA categorizes this drug as category *C* for use during pregnancy (*Animal studies have shown an adverse effect on the fetus, but there are no adequate studies in humans; or there are no animal reproduction studies and no adequate studies in humans.*)

While it is unknown if dactinomycin enters maternal milk, the potential mutagenicity and carcinogenicity of the drug warrants using extreme caution in allowing the mother to continue nursing while receiving dactinomycin.

Overdosage/Acute Toxicity
Because of the toxic potential of this agent, iatrogenic overdoses must be avoided; recheck dosage calculations. See Adverse Effects above for additional information on toxicity.

Drug Interactions
The following drug interactions have either been reported or are theoretical in humans or animals receiving dactinomycin and may be of significance in veterinary patients. Unless otherwise noted, use together is not necessarily contraindicated, but weigh the potential risks and perform additional monitoring when appropriate.

■ **DOXORUBICIN:** Additive cardiotoxicity may occur if used concurrently or sequentially with doxorubicin.

■ **MYELOSUPPRESSIVE DRUGS, OTHER** (*e.g.*, other **antineoplastics, chloramphenicol, flucytosine, colchicine,** etc.): May cause additive myelosuppression when used with dactinomycin.

- VITAMIN K: Patients requiring vitamin K may require higher dosages when receiving dactinomycin.

Laboratory Considerations

- Dactinomycin may interfere with determination of antibacterial **drug levels** if using bioassay techniques.

Doses

Note: Because of the potential toxicity of this drug to patients, veterinary personnel and clients, and since chemotherapy indications, treatment protocols, monitoring and safety guidelines often change, the following dosages should be used only as a general guide. Consultation with a veterinary oncologist and referral to current veterinary oncology references [*e.g.*, (Withrow et al. 2012); (Dobson et al. 2011); (Henry et al. 2009); (North et al. 2009); (Argyle et al. 2008)] are <u>strongly recommended</u>.

- **DOGS:**

Depending on the protocol, usual doses for dactinomycin in dogs range from 0.5 – 1 mg/m^2 (NOT mg/kg) IV over 20 minutes; doses may be repeated (depending on the protocol) at 1-3 week intervals.

Monitoring

- Efficacy.
- Toxicity: including CBC with differential and platelets; hepatic function tests; check inside patient's mouth for ulceration.

Client Information

- Dactinomycin is a chemotherapy (cancer) drug. The drug and its byproducts can be hazardous to other animals and people that come in contact with it. On the day your animal gets the drug and then for a few days afterward, all bodily waste (urine, feces, litter), blood, or vomit should only be handled while wearing disposable gloves. Seal the waste in a plastic bag and then place both the bag and gloves in with the regular trash.
- GI toxicity (*e.g.*, ulcers, diarrhea, etc.) can occur. If diarrhea is severe or continues, contact your veterinarian.
- Bone marrow depression can occur. The greatest effects on bone marrow usually occur within a few weeks after treatment. Your veterinarian will do blood tests to watch for this, but if you see bleeding, bruising, fever (indicating an infection), or if your animal becomes very tired easily, contact your veterinarian right away.

Chemistry/Synonyms

An antibiotic antineoplastic agent, dactinomycin (also known as actinomycin D;) occurs as a bright red, crystalline powder. It is somewhat hygroscopic and soluble in water at 10°C and slightly soluble at 37°C. The commercially available preparation is a yellow lyophilized mixture of dactinomycin and mannitol.

Dactinomycin may also be known as: DTIC, ACT, actinomycin C(1), actinomycin D, meractinomycin, NSC-3053, *Ac-De®*, *Bioact-D®*, or *Dacmozen®*.

Storage/Stability

The commercially available powder should be stored at room temperature and protected from light. When reconstituting, sterile water for injection without preservatives must be used as preservatives may cause precipitation. After reconstituting, the manufacturer recommends using the solution immediately and discarding any unused portion (no preservatives). When stored in the refrigerator, reconstituted solution loses 2-3% potency over 6 hours. The reconstituted solution may be added to D5W or normal saline IV infusions. IV fluid sterilizing filters (cellulose ester membrane) may partially remove dactinomycin.

Compatibility/Compounding Considerations

A precipitate may form when dactinomycin is added to sterile water that contains preservatives. Dextrose 5% or saline intravenous solutions are compatible with reconstituted solutions of dactinomycin.

Drugs that reported to be **compatible with dactinomycin when injected at a Y-site** include: granisetron and ondansetron. Compatibility is dependent upon factors such as pH, concentration, temperature and diluent used; consult specialized references or a hospital pharmacist for more specific information

Dosage Forms/Regulatory Status

VETERINARY-LABELED PRODUCTS: NONE.

HUMAN-LABELED PRODUCTS:

Dactinomycin Powder for Injection, lyophilized: 500 micrograms (0.5 mg) with mannitol 20 mg in vials; *Cosmegen®*, generic; (Rx)

Revisions/References

Monograph revised/updated January 2014.

Argyle, D., et al. (2008). *Decision Making in Small Animal Oncology*, Wiley-Blackwell.

Beckwith, M. & L. Tyler (2008). Summary of extravasation management for antineoplastic agents. *Cancer Chemotherapy Manual [loose-leaf information service].* St Louis, Walters Kluwer Health.

Dobson, J. & D. Lascelles (2011). *BSAVA Manual of Canine and Feline Oncology*, BSAVA.

Henry, C. & M. Higginbotham (2009). *Cancer Management in Small Animal Practice*, Saunders.

Khanna, C., et al. (1998). Randomized controlled trial of doxorubicin versus dactinomycin in a multiagent protocol for treatment of dogs with malignant lymphoma. JAVMA **213**(7): 985-90.

North, S. & T. Banks (2009). *Small Animal Oncology: An Introduction*, Saunders.

Withrow, S., et al. (2012). Withrow and MacEwen's Small Animal Clinical Oncology, 5th Ed., Saunders.

Dalteparin Sodium

(dahl-tep-ah-rin)   Fragmin®

Anticoagulant

Prescriber Highlights

▶ Low molecular weight (fractionated) heparin that may be useful for treatment or prophylaxis of thromboembolic disease.

▶ Preferentially inhibits factor Xa & usually only minimally impacts thrombin & clotting time (TT or aPTT).

▶ Hemorrhage unlikely, but possible.

▶ Must be given subcutaneously.

▶ Cats & dogs may require very frequent dosing making outpatient administration unfeasible.

▶ Expense may be an issue, particularly in large dogs/horses.

Uses/Indications

Dalteparin may be useful for prophylaxis or treatment of deep vein thrombosis or pulmonary embolus. Recent pharmacokinetic work in dogs and cats raises questions whether the drug can be effectively and practically administered long-term. In humans, it is also indicated for prevention of ischemic complications associated with unstable angina/non Q-wave MI.

Pharmacology/Actions

By binding to and accelerating antithrombin III, low molecular weight heparins (LMWHs) enhance the inhibition of factor Xa and thrombin. The potential advantage to using these products over standard (unfractionated) heparin is that they preferentially inhibit factor Xa and only minimally impact thrombin and clotting time (TT or aPTT).

Pharmacokinetics

In dogs, dalteparin is completely absorbed after SC injection. It has a volume of distribution of 50-70 mL/kg and a half-life of about 2 hours. Dalteparin half-life in dogs is shorter than in humans.

After SC administration to cats, dalteparin is completely absorbed, but half-life is quite short (around two hours) (Mischke et al. 2012). Cats appear to have a much shorter duration of activity (anti-Xa) associated with LMWHs than do humans and to maintain a therapeutic target of anti-XA activity of 0.5-1 IU/mL requires 150 Units/kg SC q4h dosing of dalteparin (Alwood et al. 2007).

In horses, dalteparin's pharmacokinetics are similar to humans, but a pharmacodynamic study where 50 Units/kg SC were used showed that twice daily (q12h) dosing kept anti-factor Xa activity above the thromboprophylactic range, but that once daily administration did not (Whelchel et al. 2013).

In humans, after subcutaneous injection, dalteparin is absorbed rapidly with a bioavailability of about 87%; peak plasma levels (activity) occur in about 4 hours. Anti-factor Xa activity persists for up to 24 hours and doses are usually given once to twice a day. Dalteparin is excreted via the kidneys in the urine; elimination half-life is about 3-5 hours. Half-life may be prolonged in patients with renal dysfunction.

Contraindications/Precautions/Warnings

Dalteparin is contraindicated in patients that are hypersensitive to it, heparin, or pork products. It is also contraindicated in patients with major bleeding, or thrombocytopenia associated with positive *in vitro* tests for anti-platelets in the presence of dalteparin. Use dalteparin cautiously in patients with significant renal dysfunction as drug accumulation could result. It should be used with extreme caution in patients with heparin-induced thrombocytopenia or increased risk of hemorrhage.

Adverse Effects

In humans, adverse effects do not routinely occur but hemorrhage is a possibility. Injection site hematomas or pain, allergic reactions, and neurologic sequelae secondary to epidural or spinal hematomas have been reported.

Do not administer via IM or IV routes; dalteparin must be given via subcutaneous injection only. Dalteparin cannot be used interchangeably with other LMWHs or heparin sodium, as dosages differ for each.

Reproductive/Nursing Safety

In humans, dalteparin is designated by the FDA as a category *B* drug (*Animal studies have not demonstrated risk to the fetus, but there are no adequate studies in pregnant women; or animal studies have shown an adverse effect, but adequate studies in pregnant women have not demonstrated a risk to the fetus during the first trimester of pregnancy, and there is no evidence of risk in later trimesters.*)

Dalteparin is likely safe to use during nursing.

Overdosage/Acute Toxicity

Overdosage may lead to hemorrhagic complications. If treatment is necessary, protamine sulfate via slow IV may be administered. 1 mg of protamine sulfate can inhibit the effects of 100 units of administered anti-Xa dalteparin. Avoid overdoses of protamine.

Drug Interactions

The following drug interactions have either been reported or are theoretical in humans or animals receiving dalteparin and may be of significance in veterinary patients:

- **ANTICOAGULANTS, ORAL (warfarin)**: Increased risk for hemorrhage.
- **PLATELET-AGGREGATION INHIBITORS (aspirin, clopidogrel)**: Increased risk for hemorrhage.
- **THROMBOLYTIC AGENTS**: Increased risk for hemorrhage.

Laboratory Considerations

- Low molecular weight heparins may cause asymptomatic, fully-reversible increases in **AST** or **ALT**; **bilirubin** is only rarely increased in these patients, therefore, interpret these tests with caution, as increases do not necessarily indicate hepatic damage or dysfunction.

Doses

- **DOGS:**

  For thromboprophylaxis (extra-label): 150 Units/kg SC q8h daily; twice daily dosing may be effective.

- **CATS:**

  For thromboprophylaxis (extra-label): There appears to be no consensus as to an appropriate dosage or efficacy of LMWHs in cats. Dosage recommendations range from 100 Units/kg SC once daily to 180 Units/kg SC q4-6h. A dosage of 100 – 175 Units/kg SC q8-12h could be considered until further data are available.

- **HORSES:**

  For thromboprophylaxis (extra-label; based on a pharmacodynamic study): 50 Units/kg SC twice daily (q12h). There was considerable variability in anti-factor Xa activity between horses, which may indicate the need for more frequent monitoring. Maintaining higher anti-factor Xa activity might increase the risk of bleeding complications although this was not evident in the study; further investigation of dosing regimens are warranted particularly in critically ill horses. (Whelchel et al. 2013)

Monitoring

- Baseline and ongoing during therapy CBC (with platelet count).
- Urinalysis.
- Stool occult blood test.
- Routine coagulation tests (aPTT, PT) are usually insensitive measures of activity and normally not warranted.
- Factor Xa activity (available at Cornell Coagulation Laboratory) may be useful, particularly if bleeding occurs or patient has renal dysfunction. **Note:** To measure peak anti-Xa activity in cats, sample at 2 hours post-dose.

Client Information

- Must be injected subcutaneously (SC, under the skin); be sure you understand how to properly give the shots. Several shots a day may be required and treatment may be very expensive. Shots may be painful.
- Bleeding is not likely, but can occur. Contact your veterinarian immediately if it happens.
- If your animal is very listless (lacking energy or interest in things), appears to be having trouble breathing, trouble walking or loses the use of its rear legs, contact your veterinarian immediately as it may mean clots have formed.

Chemistry/Synonyms

A low molecular weight heparin (LMWH), dalteparin sodium is obtained by nitrous acid depolymerization of heparin derived from pork intestinal mucosa. The average molecular weight is about 5000 and 90% ranges from 2000-9000 daltons (heparin sodium has a molecular weight around 12000). 1 mg of dalteparin is equivalent to not less than 110 Units and not more than 210 Units of anti-factor Xa.

Dalteparin sodium may also be known as: Daltaparinum natricum, Kabi-2165, *Boxol®*, *Fragmine®*, *Ligofragmin®*, or *Low Liquemine®*.

Storage/Stability

The manufacturer of the commercially available injection states the product should be stored at controlled room temperature (20-25°C, 68-77°F). Do not use if particulate matter or discoloration occur. Once the multi-dose vial is punctured, store at room temperature; discard any unused solution after 2 weeks.

A study showed that commercially available dalteparin solution was stable when drawn into syringes for up to 30 days when stored at room temperature or refrigerated (Laposata et al. 2003).

Compatibility/Compounding Considerations

Do not mix with other compounds.

Dosage Forms/Regulatory Status

VETERINARY-LABELED PRODUCTS: NONE.

HUMAN-LABELED PRODUCTS:

Dalteparin Sodium Injection (Anti-factor Xa International Units): Available in a variety of preservative-free single dose syringes that range from 2500 Units (16 mg/0.2 mL) to 18,000 Units per 0.72 mL (115.2 mg/0.72 mL); these are less likely to be of clinical use in veterinary medicine. A multi-dose vial containing 25,000 Units/mL in a 3.8 mL/vial is available; also contains benzyl alcohol; *Fragmin*®; (Rx)

Revisions/References

Monograph revised/updated January 2014.

Alwood, A., et al. (2007). Anticoagulant effects of low -molecular weight heparins in healthy cats. J Vet Intern Med 21(3): 378-87.

Laposata, M. & S. Johnson (2003). Assessment of the stability of dalteparin sodium in prepared syringes for up to thirty days: an in vitro study. Clin Ther 25(4): 1219-25.

Mischke, R., et al. (2012). Pharmacokinetics of the low molecular weight heparin dalteparin in cats. Veterinary Journal 192(3): 299-303.

Whelchel, D. D., et al. (2013). Pharmacodynamics of Multi-Dose Low Molecular Weight Heparin in Healthy Horses. Veterinary Surgery 42(4): 448-54.

Danazol

(da-na-zole)   Danocrine®

Androgen

Prescriber Highlights

▶ Synthetic androgen; suppresses the pituitary-ovarian axis. Sometimes used for adjunctive treatment of autoimmune hemolytic anemia/thrombocytopenia in dogs & cats. Efficacy is unpredictable and slow.

▶ Caution: Severe cardiac, renal or hepatic function impairment, or undiagnosed abnormal vaginal bleeding.

▶ Teratogenic; contraindicated in pregnancy.

▶ Can cause dramatic weight gain; rare hepatotoxicity in dogs.

▶ Expense may be an issue.

Uses/Indications

Because of expense and unpredictable efficacy, danazol is not commonly used in veterinary medicine, but has been used as adjunctive therapy (with corticosteroids) in the treatment of canine immune-mediated thrombocytopenia and hemolytic anemia, particularly if the patient becomes refractory to glucocorticoids and other immunosuppressive therapy. There may be synergism when danazol is combined with corticosteroids for these indications. Once remission is attained, some dogs may have their dosage reduced or other medications may be eliminated and controlled with danazol alone. In humans, danazol has been used for the treatment of endometriosis, fibrocystic breast disease, idiopathic thrombocytopenic purpura and a variety of other conditions.

Pharmacology/Actions

Danazol is a synthetic androgen with weak androgenic effects. It suppresses the pituitary-ovarian axis. Danazol probably directly inhibits the synthesis of sex steroids and binds to sex steroid receptors in tissues where it may express anabolic, weak androgenic, and antiestrogenic effects. Danazol appears to reduce affinity of antibodies with the mononuclear phagocytic system Fc receptor. It also may compete with glucocorticoids on steroid-binding globulin, thereby allowing greater free glucocorticoid to act.

Pharmacokinetics

There is very limited data available. Danazol is absorbed from the GI tract, but appears to be a rate limited process as increasing the dosage does not yield a corresponding increase in serum level. Distribution information is practically nonexistent; the drug apparently crosses the placenta. Danazol is thought metabolized primarily in the liver. In humans, half-lives average about 4-5 hours.

Contraindications/Precautions/Warnings

Danazol should be used in patients with severe cardiac, renal, or hepatic function impairment, or undiagnosed abnormal vaginal bleeding only when its benefits outweigh its risks. It is contraindicated in pregnancy.

Adverse Effects

Hepatotoxicity (incidence is rare) is the most significant of the adverse effects that have been reported thus far in dogs. Otherwise virilization in females is the most likely other effect that may be seen. Danazol may cause weight gain or lethargy. Human patients have developed vaginitis. Other potential adverse effects include edema, testicular atrophy, hirsutism, or alopecia.

Reproductive/Nursing Safety

Because of documented teratogenic effects, danazol is contraindicated during pregnancy. In humans, the FDA categorizes this drug as category *X* for use during pregnancy (*Studies in animals or humans demonstrate fetal abnormalities or adverse reaction; reports indicate evidence of fetal risk. The risk of use in pregnant women clearly outweighs any possible benefit.*)

While it is unknown if danazol enters milk, the potential adverse effects associated with androgens in young animals warrants caution. In humans, breastfeeding is contraindicated in patients taking danazol.

Overdosage/Acute Toxicity

No information was located. Significant overdoses should initially be handled by contacting an animal poison control center and initiate gut emptying protocols when applicable.

Drug Interactions

The following drug interactions have either been reported or are theoretical in humans or animals receiving danazol and may be of significance in veterinary patients. Unless otherwise noted, use together is not necessarily contraindicated, but weigh the potential risks and perform additional monitoring when appropriate.

- **CYCLOSPORINE:** Danazol may significantly increase cyclosporine levels.
- **INSULIN:** By affecting carbohydrate metabolism, danazol may affect insulin requirements (doses may need to be increased) in diabetic patients.
- **WARFARIN:** Concomitant use of danazol with anticoagulants may enhance the anticoagulant effect as danazol may decrease the synthesis of procoagulant factors in the liver.

Laboratory Considerations

- Danazol may decrease **total serum thyroxine** (T4) and increase T3 uptake; because thyroid-binding globulin is decreased, free T4 and TSH remain normal.
- **ALT** (SGPT) and **AST** (SGOT) may increase early in therapy but decrease towards baseline later in therapy. After discontinuation of danazol, levels usually return to baseline.

Doses

- **DOGS:**

  For **adjunctive treatment of immune-mediated hemolytic anemia or thrombocytopenia** (extra-label): 5 mg/kg PO 2-3 times a day (in addition to glucocorticoids) has been anecdotally recommended, particularly in dogs that are refractory to glucocorticoid treatment. Potentially could allow the reduction of gluco-corticoid dosage, but there is little evidence to support efficacy.

- **CATS:**

    For adjunctive treatment of immune-mediated hemolytic anemia (extra-label): There is very little data published to support using this drug in cats; 5 mg/kg PO twice daily has been suggested as a dosage.

Monitoring

For autoimmune hematologic disorders:

- Efficacy (CBC, platelets, etc.).
- Hepatic function, baseline and at regular intervals while on therapy.

Client Information

- May be given with or without food. If your animal vomits or acts sick after getting it on an empty stomach, give with food or small treat to see if this helps. If vomiting continues, contact your veterinarian.
- May take 2-3 months to see if the drug is working.
- Watch for liver toxicity (rare): jaundice (yellowing), severe vomiting, lack of appetite, or lack of energy. If any of these occur, contact your veterinarian immediately.
- Can cause birth defects; pregnant women should not handle this drug.

Chemistry/Synonyms

A synthetic derivative of ethisterone (ethinyl testosterone), danazol occurs as a white to pale yellow, crystalline powder. It is practically insoluble in water and sparingly soluble in alcohol.

Danazol may also be known as: Win-17757, *Anargil®, Azol®, Cyclomen®, D-Zol®, Danalem®, Danatrol®, Danazant®, Danogen®, Danocrine®, Danokrin®, Danol®, Ectopal®, Gonablok®, Kendazol®, Ladazol®, Ladogal®, Lisigon®, Mastodanatrol®, Norciden®, Vabon®, Winobanin®, Zendol®,* or *Zoldan-A®.*

Storage/Stability

Danazol capsules should be stored in well-closed containers at room temperature.

Compatibility/Compounding Considerations

No specific information noted.

Dosage Forms/Regulatory Status

VETERINARY-LABELED PRODUCTS: NONE.

The ARCI (Racing Commissioners International) has designated this drug as a class 4 substance. See the appendix for more information.

HUMAN-LABELED PRODUCTS:

Danazol Capsules: 50 mg, 100 mg, & 200 mg; generic; (Rx)

Revisions/References

Monograph revised/updated January 2014.

Danofloxacin Mesylate

(dan-oh-floks-a-sin)   A180®, Advocin®

Injectable Fluoroquinolone

Prescriber Highlights

▶ Parenteral fluoroquinolone antibiotic labeled for use in cattle (not dairy or veal) to treat BRD associated with *Mannheimia* (Pasteurella) *hemolytica* & *P. multocida*; may also be of benefit in treating fluoroquinolone-susceptible infections in non-food producing species (horses, camelids, exotics).

▶ Labeled in cattle for two SC injections 48 hours apart.

▶ FDA prohibits extra-label use in food animals.

Uses/Indications

Danofloxacin mesylate injection is indicated for the treatment of Bovine Respiratory Disease (BRD) associated with *Mannheimia* (*Pasteurella*) *hemolytica* and *P. multocida* in cattle (not dairy or veal). Because of the drug's spectrum of activity, it may also be of benefit in the treatment of infections caused by *Histophilus somni* (*Haemophilus somnus*) or *M. bovis,* but the drug is not labeled (at the time of writing) for treating these pathogens. In other countries, danofloxacin may be labeled for use in swine and chickens (non-laying), but in the USA it is illegal to use the drug in an extra-label manner in food-producing species.

Danofloxacin may be of benefit in treating susceptible infections in adult horses, camelids and other non-food producing species.

Pharmacology/Actions

Danofloxacin is a fluoroquinolone bactericidal antibiotic that inhibits bacterial DNA-gyrase, preventing DNA supercoiling and DNA synthesis. Fluoroquinolones have good activity against many gram-negative bacilli and some gram-positive cocci (*Staphylococcus aureus* and *Staphylococcus pseudintermedius).* In general, fluoroquinolones have a dose or concentration dependent effect rather than a time-dependent bactericidal effect.

MIC90 values for *Mannheimia* (*Pasteurella*) *hemolytica* and *Pasteurella multocida* average 0.06 micrograms/mL and 0.015 micrograms/mL, respectively.

Pharmacokinetics

After subcutaneous injection in the neck in cattle, danofloxacin is reportedly rapidly absorbed with high bioavailability (≈90%). Peak serum levels occur about 2-3 hours after dosing. Steady-state volume of distribution is approximately 2.7 L/kg; lung levels exceed those in plasma. Terminal elimination half-life ranges from 3-6 hours. In cattle, elimination is primarily unchanged drug into the urine. Other species may metabolize greater percentages of the drug into a desmethyl metabolite (desmethyldanofloxacin).

In horses, a research study on the pharmacokinetics of IM, IV and IG (intragastric) administration of danofloxacin at 1.25 mg/kg to healthy mature horses revealed favorable bioavailability with the IM route at 89% and poor bioavailability of the IG route at 22%. The authors reported good tolerability of the IG route (Fernandez-Varon et al. 2006).

In sheep, the drug quickly reaches high tissue concentrations. One hour after IM administration, the concentration peaks in lung tissue and interdigital skin. A study dosing sheep at 1.25 mg/kg IV and IM resulted in similar levels for serum, exudates and transudates (Aliabadi, Landoni, et al. 2003).

In goats, a study of danofloxacin administered at 1.25 mg/kg IV or IM, revealed similar half-lives of 4.67 and 4.41 hours after IV and IM, respectively. Volume of distribution was high via either route with 100% bioavailability reported after IM administration. The drug's penetration into both exudates and transudates were slightly slower after IM administration (Aliabadi et al. 2001). Another study found that goats challenged with *E. coli* endotoxin receiving danofloxacin at 1.25 mg/kg IV or IM had an altered clearance of the drug with significant increases in plasma concentrations and AUC (Ismail 2006).

In camels, IV administration of the drug at 1.25mg/kg results in a high volume of distribution, a half-life of 5.37 hours and rapid clearance. The IM administration of the drug at the same dose resulted in rapid and near complete absorption, with a half life of 5.71 hours (Aliabadi, Badrelin, et al. 2003).

In pigs, the drug has been shown to reach a high concentration in lung tissue and gastrointestinal tissue, including mucosa. In the first 24-hours after an intramuscular dose of 2 mg/kg, 43% of the dose is eliminated in the urine. Elimination half-life in swine is about 7 hours.

Contraindications/Precautions/Warnings

The FDA prohibits extra-label usage of this drug in food animals. The manufacturer cautions use of danofloxacin in animals with known or suspected CNS disorders as quinolones have rarely caused CNS stimulation.

Adverse Effects

Hypersensitivity reactions and lameness have been reported after administration to calves at labeled dosages. Incidence rates are not known, but they are believed to occur uncommonly. In cattle, subcutaneous injections can cause a local tissue reaction that may result in trim loss.

Reproductive/Nursing Safety

Studies documenting safety during pregnancy in cattle are not available. In studies performed in rats (100 mg/kg/day), mice (50 mg/kg/day) and rabbits (15 mg/kg/day), no teratogenic effects were observed.

Danofloxacin safety during nursing is not known, but it is prohibited from use in lactating dairy cattle where the milk is for human consumption.

Overdosage/Acute Toxicity

Limited information is available for cattle. High dosages, 18 – 60 mg/kg for 3-6 days in feeder calves reportedly can cause arthropathies/lameness (consistent with other fluoroquinolones), CNS stimulation (ataxia, nystagmus, tremors), inappetence, recumbency, depression, and exophthalmos. Some (3/6) 21-day-old calves receiving 18 mg/kg twice 48 hours apart developed nasal pad erythema.

Studies performed in adult dogs given 2.4 mg/kg/day PO for 90 days developed no observable effects.

Drug Interactions

No specific interactions have been reported when danofloxacin is used in cattle. In humans:

- **THEOPHYLLINE (aminophylline):** Some injectable fluoroquinolones (*e.g.*, ciprofloxacin) can potentially increase serum concentrations; increased monitoring of theophylline concentrations is recommended.

Laboratory Considerations

- No issues identified.

Doses

- **CATTLE (NOT DAIRY CATTLE OR VEAL CALVES):**

  For labeled indications (FDA-approved): Either 8 mg/kg SC (2 mL/100 lb. B.W.) as a one-time injection, or 6 mg/kg SC (1.5 mL/100 lb. B.W.) repeated once approximately 48 hours following the first injection. Administered dose volume should not exceed 15 mL per injection site. (Adapted from label, *Advocin*—Zoetis)

- **REPTILES:**

  For mycoplasma infections in desert tortoises (extra-label): 6 mg/kg SC (vary injection site) q48h (every other day) for 3-6 weeks. (Boyer 2011)

Monitoring

- Clinical efficacy.

Client Information

- If clients are to administer this product to food animals, they should be advised on proper injection technique and the importance of using the product per the label only.

Chemistry/Synonyms

Danofloxacin mesylate is a synthetic fluoroquinolone that occurs as a white to off-white crystalline powder. Approximately 180 grams are soluble in 1 liter of water.

Danofloxacin may also be known by the following synonyms: CP-76136-27, danofloxacine or danofloxacino. Internationally registered trade names include: *Advocin®, Advocine®, Danocin®, Advocid®,* and *Advovet®.*

Storage/Stability

Danofloxacin mesylate for injection should be stored at or below 30° C and protected from light and freezing. The color of the injectable solution is yellow to amber and does not affect potency.

Compatibility/Compounding Considerations

Danofloxacin injection for SC use should not be mixed with other medications or diluents. Fluoroquinolone injectable products can be very sensitive to pH changes or chelation with cationic substances (calcium, magnesium, zinc, etc.).

Dosage Forms/Regulatory Status

VETERINARY-LABELED PRODUCTS:

Danofloxacin Mesylate: 180 mg/mL (of danofloxacin) in 100 mL & 250 mL multi-dose vials; *Advocin®;* (Rx). FDA-approved for use in cattle only. Not for use in cattle intended for dairy production or calves to be processed for veal. When administered per the label directions, slaughter withdrawal is 4 days from the time of the last treatment. Approved label information for *Advocin®* can be found at dailymed.nlm.nih.gov

HUMAN-LABELED PRODUCTS: NONE.

Revisions/References

Monograph revised/updated January 2014.

Aliabadi, F., et al. (2003). Pharmacokinetics and PH-PD modeling of danofloxacin in camel serum and tissue fluid cages. *Vet J* 165(2): 104-8.

Aliabadi, F., et al. (2003). Pharmacokinetics (PK), pharmacodynamics (PD) and PK-PD integration of danofloxacin in sheep biological fluids. Antimicrob. Agents Chemother. Feb:47(2): 626-635. 2003. Antimicrob. Agents Chemotherap. 47(2): 626-35.

Aliabadi, F. & P. Lees (2001). Pharmacokinetics and pharmacodynamics of danofloxacin in serum and tissue fluids of goats following intravenous and intramuscular administration. AJVR 62(12): Dec 2001.

Boyer, T. H. (2011). Common Problems of Tortoises. Western Veterinary Conference. accessed via Veterinary Information Network; vin.com

Fernandez-Varon, E., et al. (2006). Pharmacokinetics of danofloxacin in horses after intravenous, intramuscular and intragastric administration. *Equine Vet J* 38(4): 342-6.

Ismail, M. (2006). A pharmacokinetic study of danofloxacin in febrile goats following repeated administration of endotoxin. *J Vet Phamacol Ther* 29: 313-6.

Dantrolene Sodium

(dan-troe-leen)   Dantrium®

Skeletal Muscle Relaxant

Prescriber Highlights

- ▶ Direct acting muscle relaxant.
- ▶ Primary indications: **Horses:** post-anesthesia myositis/acute rhabdomyolysis; **Dogs & Cats:** functional urethral obstruction, potentially rhabdomyolysis.
- ▶ Extreme caution: Animals with hepatic dysfunction. Caution: Severe cardiac dysfunction or pulmonary disease.
- ▶ Adverse Effects: Weakness, sedation, increased urinary frequency, GI effects; hepatotoxicity possible especially with chronic use.
- ▶ Injectable is very expensive.

Uses/Indications

In humans, oral dantrolene is indicated primarily for the treatment associated with upper motor neuron disorders (*e.g.*, multiple sclerosis, cerebral palsy, spinal cord injuries, etc.). In veterinary medicine, its proposed indications include: the prevention and treatment of malignant hyperthermia syndrome in various species, the treatment of functional urethral obstruction due to increased external urethral tone in dogs and cats, the prevention and treatment of equine post-anesthetic myositis (PAM), and equine exertional rhabdomyolysis. It has also been recommended for use in the treatment of bites from Black Widow Spiders in small animals and for the treatment of porcine stress syndrome.

Pharmacology/Actions

Dantrolene exhibits muscle relaxation activity by direct action on muscle. While the exact mechanism is not well understood, it probably acts on skeletal muscle by interfering with the release of calcium from the sarcoplasmic reticulum. It has no discernible effects on the respiratory or cardiovascular systems, but can cause drowsiness and dizziness. The reasons for these CNS effects are not known.

Pharmacokinetics

After intragastric administration to horses, bioavailability is approximately 39%. The drug is fairly slowly absorbed, with peak levels occurring in about 1.5 hours in horses. Oral dantrolene absorption can be affected by food. Although there was considerable interpatient variation in the results, a study concluded that where possible, feed restriction before nasogastric dantrolene administration should be avoided or should not exceed 4 hours (McKenzie et al. 2010). Oral dantrolene is has an approximate half-life of 3-4 hours in horses.

In humans, bioavailability of dantrolene after oral administration in humans is only about 35%. Peak levels occur about 5 hours after oral administration. The drug is substantially bound to plasma proteins (principally albumin), and many drugs can displace it (see Drug Interactions). The elimination half-life in humans is approximately 8 hours. Dantrolene is metabolized in the liver and metabolites are excreted in the urine. Only about 1% of the parent drug is excreted unchanged in the urine and bile.

Contraindications/Precautions/Warnings

Because dantrolene can cause hepatotoxicity, it should be used with extreme caution in patients with preexisting liver disease and with caution in patients with severe cardiac dysfunction or pulmonary disease.

In horses, dantrolene is an ARCI class 4 drug. Analysis of urine samples show that parent and metabolites (5-hydroxydantrolene) are below the limit of detection by 168 hours post oral dantrolene administration; a 48 hour (blood) and 168 hour (urine) withdrawal guideline should be adopted after oral administration (Knych et al. 2011).

Adverse Effects

The most significant adverse reaction with dantrolene therapy is hepatotoxicity. In humans, it is most commonly associated with high dose chronic therapy, but may also be seen after short high dose therapy. The incidence of this reaction is unknown in veterinary medicine, but monitor for its occurrence.

More common, but less significant, are the CNS associated signs of weakness, sedation, dizziness, headache, and GI effects (nausea, vomiting, constipation). Also seen are increased urinary frequency and, possibly, hypotension.

Reproductive/Nursing Safety

The safe use of dantrolene during pregnancy has not been determined. In humans, the FDA categorizes this drug as category *C* for use during pregnancy (*Animal studies have shown an adverse effect on the fetus, but there are no adequate studies in humans; or there are no animal reproduction studies and no adequate studies in humans.*) In a separate system evaluating the safety of drugs in canine and feline pregnancy (Papich 1989), this drug is categorized

as class: *C* (*These drugs may have potential risks. Studies in people or laboratory animals have uncovered risks, and these drugs should be used cautiously as a last resort when the benefit of therapy clearly outweighs the risks.*)

Dantrolene is distributed into milk; safe use cannot be assured during nursing.

Overdosage/Acute Toxicity

There is no specific antidotal therapy to dantrolene overdoses, therefore, remove the drug from the gut if possible and treat supportively.

Drug Interactions

The following drug interactions have either been reported or are theoretical in humans or animals receiving dantrolene and may be of significance in veterinary patients. Unless otherwise noted, use together is not necessarily contraindicated, but weigh the potential risks and perform additional monitoring when appropriate.

- **BENZODIAZEPINES & OTHER CNS DEPRESSANTS:** Increased sedation may be seen if tranquilizing agents are used concomitantly with dantrolene.
- **CALCIUM-CHANNEL BLOCKERS:** Rare reports of cardiovascular collapse in humans; concomitant use with dantrolene during malignant hyperthermia crises not recommended.
- **ESTROGENS:** Increased risks of hepatotoxicity from dantrolene have been seen in women >35 years of age that are also receiving estrogen therapy; veterinary significance is unknown.
- **VECURONIUM:** Dantrolene may potentiate neuromuscular blockade.
- **WARFARIN:** Dantrolene may be displaced from plasma proteins by warfarin with increased effects or adverse reactions resulting.

Doses

- **DOGS:**

  For treatment of functional urethral obstruction due to increased external urethral tone (extra-label): 1 – 5 mg/kg PO q8-12h; limited evidence to support this dosage.

  For canine stress syndrome (CSS)/Malignant Hyperthermia (MH); (extra-label):

  a) To treat an acute attack: 0.2 – 3 mg/kg IV. (Axlund 2004)

  b) For MH-like syndrome associated with hops (*Humulus lupulus*) ingestion: 2 – 3 mg/kg IV or 3.5 mg/kg PO as soon as possible after ingestion. (Wismer 2004)

  For adjunctive treatment of rhabdomyolysis (extra-label): 1.5 mg/kg PO q8h (from a case report; very intensive drug and supportive therapy used in this case). (Wells et al. 2009)

- **CATS:**

  For treatment of functional urethral obstruction due to increased external urethral tone (extra-label): 0.5 – 2 mg/kg PO q12h; limited evidence to support this dosage.

- **HORSES:** (NOTE: ARCI CLASS 4 DRUG; SEE CONTRAINDICATIONS ABOVE)

  For prevention of rhabdomyolysis (all are extra-label):

  a) In Thoroughbreds: 4 mg/kg PO or via NG tube. Feed restriction before nasogastric dantrolene administration should be avoided or should not exceed 4 hours. (McKenzie et al. 2010)

  b) Several dosage regimens have been recommended, but use caution as use and efficacy are uncertain: 2 mg/kg PO once daily for 3-5 days and then every 3rd day for a month has been recommended. Drug is diluted in normal saline and given via stomach tube. Another dosage recommendation is 300 mg (total dose) PO once daily (may be preferable because the drug is hepatotoxic). Another recommendation is 500 mg (total dose) PO for 3-5 days and then 300 mg PO every third day. Monitor hepatic function and status. (MacLeay 2004)

c) 800 mg (total dose); within 30 minutes prior to administration contents of capsules mixed with 9 mL tap water to make a suspension and given PO one hour before exercise. (Edwards et al. 2003)

For prevention of post-anesthetic myositis (PAM); (extra-label): To prevent muscle damage in horses undergoing hypotensive anesthesia: 6 mg/kg enterally (in 2 L of water given via NG tube) 60-90 minutes prior to general anesthesia. Dantrolene reduces muscle damage in horses undergoing general anesthesia without inhibiting anesthetic recovery, but decreases cardiac output and can precipitate hyperkalemia and arrhythmias. (McKenzie et al. 2009), (McKenzie et al. 2012)

Monitoring
Depending on the reason for use:
- Baseline and periodic liver function tests (ALT, AST, Alk Phos, etc.) if projecting to be used chronically or using high dosages.
- Body temperature (malignant hyperthermia).
- Urine volume, frequency, continence.

Client Information
- Drowsiness, vomiting, constipation, and a greater need to urinate are the most likely side effects.
- Liver toxicity can rarely occur. If animal shows signs of extreme lack of energy, frequent vomiting (small animals), not eating, bleeding, or yellow discoloration of the whites of the eyes, contact your veterinarian right away.

Chemistry/Synonyms
A hydantoin derivative that is dissimilar structurally and pharmacologically from other skeletal muscle relaxant drugs, dantrolene sodium is a weak acid with a pK_a of 7.5. It occurs as an odorless, tasteless, orange, fine powder that is slightly soluble in water. It rapidly hydrolyzes in aqueous solutions to the free acid form that precipitates out of solution.

Dantrolene Sodium may also be known by the following synonyms and internationally registered trade names: F-440, F-368, *Danlene*®, *Dantamacrin*®, *Dantralen*®, or *Dantrolen*®.

Storage/Stability
Dantrolene capsules should be stored in well-closed containers at room temperature. Dantrolene powder for injection should be stored at temperatures less than 30°C and protected from prolonged exposure to light. After reconstitution, the powder for injection should be used within 6 hours when stored at room temperature and should be protected from direct light. It is **not compatible** with either normal saline or D5W injection.

Compatibility/Compounding Considerations
To dose in small dogs or cats, it has been suggested to re-encapsulate 1/8th to ¼ of the contents of a 25 mg capsule and place into a size 2 or 4 gelatin capsule (Gunn-Moore 2008).

Dosage Forms/Regulatory Status
VETERINARY-LABELED PRODUCTS: NONE.

HUMAN-LABELED PRODUCTS:

Dantrolene Sodium Oral Capsules: 25 mg, 50 mg, & 100 mg; *Dantrium*®, generic; (Rx)

Dantrolene Sodium Powder for Injection Solution: 20 mg/vial (approx. 0.32 mg/mL dantrolene after reconstitution; with mannitol 3 g/vial) in 70 mL vials; *Dantrium*® *Intravenous*, *Revonto*®; (Rx). **Note:** Because of the expense, minimum order quantity, and non-returnable nature of the commercially available intravenous product, it may not be practical for veterinary use.

Revisions/References
Monograph revised/updated January 2014.

Axlund, T. (2004). Exercise induced collapse and hyperthermic myopathy: What every clinician should know. Proceedings: ACVC. accessed via Veterinary Information Network; vin.com

Edwards, J. G. T., et al. (2003). The efficacy of dantrolene sodium in controlling exertional rhabdomyolysis in the Thoroughbred racehorse. *Equine Veterinary Journal* 35(7): 707-11.

Gunn-Moore, D. (2008). Feline lower urinary tract disease (FLUTD)--Cystitis in cats. Proceedings: World Veterinary Congress. accessed via Veterinary Information Network; vin.com

Knych, H. K. D., et al. (2011). Pharmacokinetics and metabolism of dantrolene in horses. *J. Vet. Pharmacol. Ther.* 34(3): 238-46.

MacLeay, J. (2004). Diseases of the musculoskeletal system. *Equine Internal Medicine 2nd Ed.* S. Reed, W. Bayly and D. Sellon. Philadelphia, Saunders: 461-521.

McKenzie, E., et al. (2012). Reduced Cardiac Output in Horses Anesthetized After Dantrolene Administration. ACVIM Proceedings. accessed via Veterinary Information Network; vin.com

McKenzie, E. & C. Mosley (2009). Dantrolene sodium prevents myopathy in horses undergoing hypotensive anesthesia. Proceedings: IVECCS. accessed via Veterinary Information Network; vin.com

McKenzie, E. C., et al. (2010). Effect of feed restriction on plasma dantrolene concentrations in horses. *Equine Veterinary Journal* 42: 613-7.

Wells, R. J., et al. (2009). Successful management of a dog that had severe rhabdomyolysis with myocardial and respiratory failure. *Javma-Journal of the American Veterinary Medical Association* 234(8): 1049-54.

Wismer, T. (2004). Newer antidotal therapies. Proceedings: IVECC Symposium. accessed via Veterinary Information Network; vin.com

Dapsone

(dap-sone) DDS

Antimycobacterial Antibiotic

Prescriber Highlights
▶ Rarely used due to potential for severe adverse effects. Potentially useful for treating mycobacterial & some protozoal (Pneumocystis) infections, Brown Recluse spider bites, & cutaneous vasculitis.

▶ Relatively contraindicated in cats.

▶ Adverse effects: hepatotoxicity, methemoglobinemia, anemia, thrombocytopenia, neutropenia, gastrointestinal effects, neuropathies, & cutaneous drug eruptions; photosensitivity reactions are possible.

Uses/Indications
Dapsone may be useful as a second-line agent in the treatment of mycobacterial diseases in dogs and, possibly, cats. It potentially may be a useful treatment for *Pneumocystis jiroveci* (formerly *Pneumocystis carinii*) infections.

Because of its leukocyte inhibitory characteristics, dapsone may be useful for adjunctive treatment of Brown recluse spider (*Loxosceles rectusa recluse*) bites, or when an underlying etiology causing cutaneous vasculitis cannot be determined. In humans, dapsone has been used as a second-line treatment for immune-mediated thrombocytopenia.

Pharmacology/Actions
Dapsone's antimicrobial actions are thought due to inhibition of the synthesis of dihydrofolic acid via competition with para-aminobenzoate for the active site of dihydropteroate synthetase. Dapsone also decreases neutrophil chemotaxis, complement activation, antibody production and lysosomal enzyme synthesis. The mechanisms for these actions are not well understood.

Pharmacokinetics
After oral administration to dogs, dapsone is rapidly and completely absorbed. Elimination half-life ranges from about 6-10 hours. In humans, the monoacetyl metabolite is almost completely bound to plasma proteins, but in dogs, it is only about 60% bound. Dapsone is primarily eliminated via the kidneys as conjugates and unidentified metabolites. Half-life in humans is widely variable and ranges from about 10-50 hours.

Contraindications/Precautions/Warnings

Because of increased incidences of neurotoxicity and hemolytic anemia, dapsone is generally not recommended for use in cats. Dapsone in contraindicated in patients hypersensitive to it or other sulfone drugs. It should not be used in patients with severe anemias or other preexisting blood dyscrasias. Because of its potential for causing hepatic toxicity, dapsone should be used with caution in animals with preexisting hepatic dysfunction.

Adverse Effects

Adverse effects include hepatotoxicity, dose-dependent methemoglobinemia, hemolytic anemia, thrombocytopenia, neutropenia, gastrointestinal effects, neuropathies, and cutaneous drug eruptions. Photosensitivity is possible. Dapsone is a potential carcinogen.

Reproductive/Nursing Safety

In pregnant animals, dapsone should be used with caution. In humans, the FDA categorizes dapsone as a category *C* drug for use during pregnancy (*Animal studies have shown an adverse effect on the fetus, but there are no adequate studies in humans; or there are no animal reproduction studies and no adequate studies in humans*). Animal studies have apparently not been performed with dapsone to determine its effects in pregnancy.

Dapsone is excreted into milk in concentrations equivalent to those found in plasma; and hemolytic reactions have been seen in human neonates. Consider switching to milk replacer if dapsone is required in a nursing dam.

Overdosage/Acute Toxicity

Because of its toxicity potential, specific species differences in sensitivity, and pharmacokinetics, it is recommended to contact an animal poison control center in cases of dapsone overdoses. In humans, dapsone overdoses generally cause nausea, vomiting, and hyperexcitability that can occur within minutes of an overdose. Methemoglobinemia with associated depression, seizures, and cyanosis can occur. Hemolysis may be delayed, occurring from 7-14 days after the overdose. Treatment in humans includes removal of drug from the gut, methylene blue for methemoglobinemia and, sometimes, hemodialysis to enhance removal of the drug and the monoacetyl metabolite.

Drug Interactions

The following drug interactions have either been reported or are theoretical in humans or animals receiving dapsone and may be of significance in veterinary patients. Unless otherwise noted, use together is not necessarily contraindicated, but weigh the potential risks and perform additional monitoring when appropriate.

- **PROBENECID:** May decrease the renal excretion of active metabolites of dapsone.
- **PYRIMETHAMINE:** May increase risk of hematologic reactions occurring with dapsone.
- **RIFAMPIN:** May decrease plasma dapsone concentrations (7-10 fold).
- **TRIMETHOPRIM:** May increase plasma dapsone concentrations (and vice versa) and potentially increase each other's toxicity.

Laboratory Considerations

- No specific laboratory interactions or considerations noted.

Doses

- **DOGS:**

  As an alternative immunomodulatory for cutaneous conditions (e.g., cutaneous vasculitis); (extra-label): 1 – 1.1 mg/kg PO q8h initially. Has been used in combination with other immunomodulating drugs (*e.g.*, prednisone). Once remission occurs, taper to lowest effective dosage frequency (*e.g.*, once daily). Evidence is relatively weak to support use.

  For adjunctive treatment of Brown Recluse spider (*Loxosceles* spp.) bite (extra-label): 1 mg/kg PO 3 times daily for 10 days. (Peterson 2006)

- **CATS:**

  Caution: Dapsone can potentially cause serious side effects in cats (*e.g.*, blood dyscrasias, and hepatic or neuro-toxicities); many consider its use relatively contraindicated in cats. If this drug is to be used, clients must accept the risks associated with its use; intensive monitoring for adverse effects must be performed.

  For feline leprosy or oral chondritis (extra-label): Anecdotal dosage suggestion is 1 mg/kg PO once daily.

- **HORSES:**

  As an alternative treatment for *Pneumocystis carinii* pneumonia (extra-label): 3 mg/kg PO once daily (q24h). **Note:** From one case report of treatment of a foal treatment period was 56 days. (Clark-Price et al. 2004)

Monitoring

- CBC with platelets every 2-3 weeks during first 4 months of treatment and then every 3-4 months.
- Liver function tests.
- Other adverse effects (GI, drug eruptions, neurotoxicity, etc.).
- Efficacy.

Client Information

- Clients should understand that limited experience has occurred with dapsone in domestic animals and that serious toxicity may occur.
- Because photosensitivity can occur, exposed skin should be protected from prolonged exposure to sunlight.

Chemistry/Synonyms

A sulfone antimycobacterial/antiprotozoan, dapsone occurs as a white or creamy-white, odorless, crystalline powder. It is very slightly soluble in water, freely soluble in alcohol, and insoluble in fixed or vegetable oils.

Dapsone may also be known as: DADPS, dapsonum, DDS, diaminodiphenylsulfone, NSC-6091, diaphenylsulfone, disulone, sulfonyldianiline, *Avlosulfone®, Daps®, Dapsoderm-X®, Dopsan®, Novasulfone®, Servidapsone®*, and *Sulfona®*.

Storage/Stability

Dapsone tablets should be stored protected from light at controlled room temperature (20-25°C, 68-77°F).

Compatibility/Compounding Considerations

Dapsone tablets may be compounded into a stable liquid dosage form. The simplest method is to use a 1:1 ratio of *Ora-Plus®*: *Ora-Sweet®* and use crushed tablets to make a concentration of 2 mg/mL. This preparation is stable either stored refrigerated or at room temperature for 90 days (Nahata et al. 2000).

Dosage Forms/Regulatory Status

VETERINARY-LABELED PRODUCTS: NONE.

HUMAN-LABELED PRODUCTS:

Dapsone Oral Tablets: 25 mg & 100 mg (scored); generic; (Rx)

Revisions/References

Monograph revised/updated January 2014.

Clark-Price, S., et al. (2004). Use of dapsone on the treatment of Pneumocystis carinii pneumonia in a foal. JAVMA **224**(3): 407-10.
Nahata, M. C., et al. (2000). Stability of dapsone in two oral liquid dosage forms. Ann Pharmacother **34**(7-8): 848-50.
Peterson, M. (2006). Venomous arthropods. Proceedings: Western Vet Conf. accessed via Veterinary Information Network; vin.com

Darbepoetin Alfa

(dar-beh-poe-eh-tin al-fah)   Aranesp®

Erythropoietic Agent

Prescriber Highlights

▶ Biosynthetic erythropoietic agent potentially useful for treating anemia of chronic kidney disease in dogs & cats.

▶ May be less immunogenic (not proven) in dogs and cats than epoetin alfa (rHuEPO).

▶ Longer duration of effect, initially only dosed once per week.

▶ Considerably more expensive than rHuEPO and treatment expense may be formidable.

Uses/Indications

Darbepoetin may potentially be useful in treating anemia of chronic kidney disease in dogs and cats. It may be less immunogenic than epoetin, but this has not been fully documented in dogs or cats. Another advantage is that doses may be administered less often to maintain PCV. Treatment costs may be higher than using epoetin, however. One group with experience treating over 70 cats with epoetin or darbepoetin report only that about 60-65% had an adequate response (Chalhoub et al. 2011). Because of concerns associated with expense and adverse effects (red cell aplasia), most do not recommend starting therapy in cats until PCV is less than 20%.

Pharmacology/Actions

Darbepoetin is a recombinant DNA-produced protein related to erythropoietin. It stimulates erythropoiesis using the same mechanism as endogenous erythropoietin by interacting with progenitor stem cells to increase RBC production. Darbepoetin may be less immunogenic in animals than epoetin secondary to its formulation utilizing carbohydrates as part of its structure. Theoretically, carbohydrates may "shield" the sites on the drug of greatest antigenic potential from immune cell detection. Carbohydrates also increase the solubility and stability of the compound causing less aggregate formation and, therefore, potentially less immunogenicity.

Pharmacokinetics

In dogs, darbepoetin has an elimination half-life of about 25 hours, which is approximately 3X that of epoetin. Clearance was also correspondingly reduced. No information was noted for cats. In humans with chronic renal failure after subcutaneous injection, bioavailability is about 37% and the drug is absorbed slowly with a distribution half-life of about 1.4 hours. It is extensively metabolized and terminal elimination half-life averages 21 hours. Terminal half-life is about 3 times greater than that of epoetin alfa.

Contraindications/Precautions/Warnings

Darbepoetin should not be used in dogs or cats with documented anti-rHuEPO antibodies. Antibody formation diagnosis is based upon high myeloid:erythroid ratio on bone marrow cytology and exclusion of other causes of anemia. In humans, darbepoetin is contraindicated in patients hypersensitive to it or excipients in the formulation and in those with uncontrolled hypertension.

Adequate iron stores are necessary for efficacy. Most clinicians prefer using injectable iron dextran rather than oral iron products for this purpose.

Adverse Effects

The adverse effect profile for darbepoetin is unknown, but adverse effects reported with rHuEPO (epoetin) therapy in animals include: anti-rHuEPO antibody formation with resultant pure red blood cell aplasia (PRCA), injection site reactions, polycythemia, hypertension, seizures, or iron deficiency.

Anecdotally, PRCA is reported to occur less often than with epoetin. One source states that incidence of PRCA is about 25-30% in dogs and cats receiving epoetin and less than 10% with darbepoetin (Chalhoub et al. 2011). PRCA can be difficult to treat, but immediate discontinuation of epoetin or darbepoetin is required. Immunosuppressive therapy and blood transfusions can potentially help, but long-term prognosis is often grave.

Hypertension is reported to occur in up to 50% of dogs and cats treated. Hypertension may be a result of increased blood viscosity and cardiac output, and decreased anemia-mediated vasodilation. Seizures may be in response to hypertension.

Reproductive/Nursing Safety

Studies performed in pregnant rats and rabbits demonstrated no overt teratogenicity at IV dosages of up to 20 mg/kg/day. Decreased body weights were noted in some rat pups.

It is unknown if darbepoetin is distributed into milk, but it is unlikely to pose much risk to animals nursing.

Overdosage/Acute Toxicity

Little information is available. Humans have received therapeutic dosages of up to 8 micrograms/kg every week for 12 weeks. Polycythemia is possible and therapeutic phlebotomy may be required.

Drug Interactions

None have been identified. For epoetin (a related compound) and theoretically for darbepoetin:

- **ANDROGENS:** May increase the sensitivity of erythroid progenitors and this interaction has been used for therapeutic effect.
- **DESMOPRESSIN:** With EPO can decrease bleeding times.

Laboratory Considerations

- No specific lab issues were identified; see Contraindications and Monitoring for more information.

Doses

- **DOGS/CATS:**

  To stimulate erythropoiesis (extra-label): There are several dosage recommendations for using darbepoetin in dogs and cats; no conclusive evidence exists to choose one over the other. Adequate iron stores are required. Most suggest using injectable iron dextran (e.g.; 50 mg per cat IM or 50 – 300 mg per dog IM once, or every month while on darbepoetin). An "average" initial dose for the induction phase of darbepoetin is 1 microgram/kg SC once weekly, but other recommendations have ranged from 0.25 micrograms/kg SC per week (cats) to 1.5 micrograms per week SC until the target PCV is attained. PCV target goals vary by author, with most falling into a 25-35% range, but some suggest that 35-40% is preferred. Ideally an increase in PCV of no more than 3% per week is suggested as greater increases may increase the risks for hypertension (in cats). Once target range is met, most recommend increasing the dosing interval to once every 2-3 weeks and continuing to titrate dosage to maintain PCV in the target range. Based on: (Chalhoub et al. 2011; Bartges 2012; Chalhoub et al. 2012; DiBartola 2012; Adams 2013; Polzin 2013)

Monitoring

- Before re-dosing check PCV each time or at least until stable and then once monthly. Consider performing reticulocyte counts during the induction phase, but it has been reported that reticulocyte counts in cats receiving darbepoetin may not reflect efficacy (Chalhoub et al. 2011).
- Monitor patient's iron stores or supplement with iron.
- Blood pressure.

Client Information

- Injectable (subcutaneous; under the skin) drug used to treat anemia (too few red blood cells) from chronic renal failure. May take several weeks before it works.
- Biggest concern is the development of antibodies after using it

awhile. Watch for skin reactions at the site of the shot. Also, if seizures (convulsions), fever, joint pain, mouth ulcers are seen, or animal has no appetite, contact veterinarian right away.

- Ongoing lab tests are necessary and treatment can be very expensive.

Chemistry/Synonyms

Darbepoetin alfa is a 165-amino acid protein that is produced using recombinant DNA technology in Chinese hamster ovary cells. Two additional N-linked oligosaccharide chains are added to human erythropoietin yielding a glycoprotein with an approximate molecular weight of 37,000 daltons.

Darbepoetin may also be known by the following synonyms: NESP, novel erythropoiesis stimulating protein, darbepoetina or darbepoetinum. Internationally registered trade names include: *Aranesp®* and *Nespo®*.

Storage/Stability

The commercially available injection solutions (polysorbate-based) should be stored refrigerated at 2-8°C and protected from light. Do not freeze or shake.

Compatibility/Compounding Considerations

No specific information noted. Do not mix with other compounds.

Dosage Forms/Regulatory Status

VETERINARY-LABELED PRODUCTS: NONE.

The ARCI (Racing Commissioners International) has designated this drug as a class 2 substance. It is also prohibited on the premises of a racing facility.

HUMAN-LABELED PRODUCTS:

Darbepoetin Alfa Solution for Injection (preservative free; albumin-free); *Aranesp®*; (Rx)

25 micrograms/0.42 mL in single-dose prefilled syringes
25 micrograms/mL in 1 mL single-dose vials
40 micrograms/0.4 mL in single-dose prefilled syringes
40 micrograms/mL in 1 mL single-dose vials
60 micrograms/0.3 mL in single-dose prefilled syringes
60 micrograms/mL in single-dose vials
100 micrograms/0.5 mL single-dose prefilled syringes
100 micrograms/mL in 1 mL single-dose vials
150 micrograms/0.3 mL single-dose prefilled syringes
150 micrograms/0.75 mL in 1 mL single-dose vials
200 micrograms/0.4 mL single-dose prefilled syringes
200 micrograms/mL in 1 mL single-dose vials
300 micrograms/0.6 mL single-dose prefilled syringes
300 micrograms/mL in 1 mL single-dose vials
500 micrograms/mL single-dose vials and prefilled syringes

Revisions/References

Monograph revised/updated January 2014.

Adams, L. G. (2013). Managing Chronic Kidney Disease in Cats. British Small Animal Veterinary Conference. accessed via Veterinary Information Network; vin.com

Bartges, J. W. (2012). Chronic Kidney Disease in Dogs and Cats. Veterinary Clinics of North America-Small Animal Practice 42(4): 669-+.

Chalhoub, S., et al. (2011). Anemia of Chronic Renal Disease What it is, what to do and what's new. Journal of Feline Medicine and Surgery 13(9): 629-40.

Chalhoub, S., et al. (2012). The Use of Darbepoetin to Stimulate Erythropoiesis in Anemia of Chronic Kidney Disease in Cats: 25 Cases. Journal of Veterinary Internal Medicine 26(2): 363-9.

DiBartola, S. P. (2012). Medical Management of Chronic Renal Failure in Cats. Atlantic Coast Veterinary Conference accessed via Veterinary Information Network; vin.com

Polzin, D. J. (2013). Evidence-based step-wise approach to managing chronic kidney disease in dogs and cats. J. Vet. Emerg. Crit. Care 23(2): 205-15.

Decoquinate

(de-koe-kwin-ate)   Deccox®

Antiprotozoal/Coccidiostat

Prescriber Highlights

▶ Coccidiostat.

▶ Not FDA-approved for lactating dairy animals, laying chickens.

▶ Not effective against adult coccidia; no effect on clinical coccidiosis; results in treating calves with cryptosporidiosis have been disappointing.

Uses/Indications

Decoquinate is labeled for use in cattle for the prevention of coccidiosis in either ruminating or non-ruminating calves, cattle or young goats caused by the species *E. christenseni* or *E. ninakohlyakimoviae*. It is used for prevention of coccidiosis in broilers caused by *E. tenella*, *E. necatrix*, *E. acervulina*, *E. mivati*, *E. maxima* or *E. burnetti*.

It may be useful in dogs as prophylactic treatment for coccidiosis and hepatozoonosis.

Pharmacology/Actions

Decoquinate is 4-hydroxy quinolone agent that has anticoccidial activity. Decoquinate acts on the sporozoite stage of the life cycle. The sporozoite apparently can still penetrate the host intestinal cell, but further development is prevented. The mechanism of action for decoquinate is to disrupt electron transport in the mitochondrial cytochrome system of coccidia.

Pharmacokinetics

No information was located.

Contraindications/Precautions/Warnings

Decoquinate is not effective for treating clinical coccidiosis and has no efficacy against adult coccidia. Decoquinate is not FDA-approved for use in animals producing milk for food or in laying chickens.

Adverse Effects

No adverse effects listed when given as directed.

Overdosage/Acute Toxicity

No specific information located. Decoquinate is considered to have a wide safety margin.

Drug Interactions/Laboratory Considerations

- None noted.

Doses

- **DOGS:**

For canine hepatozoonosis (*Hepatozoon americanum*) (extra-label): **Note:** When using decoquinate for this indication, obtain the decoquinate 6% (27.2 gram/lb.) powder. An approximate conversion is 1/4 teaspoonful is equivalent to approximately 45 mg decoquinate and 1 teaspoonful (5 mL) is equivalent to approximately 180 mg decoquinate. Currently, the Companion Animal Parasite Council (CAPC) (www.capcvet. org) recommends presenting ACH patients be treated with either a triple combination (TCP) of trimethoprim-sulfadiazine (15 mg/kg twice daily), clindamycin (10 mg/kg 3 times daily), and pyrimethamine (0.25 mg/kg once daily) or ponazuril (10 mg/kg twice daily) for 14 days followed by 2 years of twice-daily decoquinate administration (10 – 20 mg/kg). Supplemental nonsteroidal anti-inflammatory drugs (NSAIDs) may be given for fever and pain control. Although this treatment regimen is not curative, it does extend life expectancy and improve quality of life for many ACH patients. Should clinical relapse occur, repeat TCP or ponazuril treatments and again follow with long-term decoquinate. (Allen et al. 2011)

For canine sarcocystosis myositis (extra-label; from a case report) (extra-label): Appeared to be effective in the one dog treated with decoquinate at 10 – 20 mg/kg PO q12h. Dog also received clindamycin initially (discontinued after 3 months on decoquinate) and tramadol. Authors concluded that additional research is required to evaluate decoquinate efficacy, but the clinical improvement seen in Dog 2 suggests it may be of value. (Sykes et al. 2011)

- **CATTLE:**

For the prevention of coccidiosis in ruminating and non-ruminating calves (including veal calves) and cattle caused by *Eimeria bovis* **and** *E. zuerni* **(labeled dosage; FDA-approved):** 0.5 mg/kg PO per day. Feed for at least 28 days during periods of coccidiosis exposure or when experience indicates that coccidiosis is likely to be a hazard. Coccidiostats are not indicated for use in adult animals due to continuous previous exposure. (Adapted from label; *Deccox®* Granules)

For treatment of coccidiosis in calves (extra-label): 1 mg/kg in feed PO daily for at least 28 days. (Taylor et al. 2012)

For cryptosporidium in calves (extra-label): 2 mg/kg PO twice daily for 21 days. (Shahiduzzamana et al. 2012)

- **SHEEP/GOATS:**

Sheep (labeled dosage; FDA-approved): **For the prevention of coccidiosis in young sheep caused by** *Eimeria ovinoidalis*, *E. crandallis*, *E. parva*, **and** *E. bakuensis*: 0.5 mg/kg PO per day. Feed for at least 28 days during periods of coccidiosis exposure or when experience indicates that coccidiosis is likely to be a hazard. (Adapted from label; *Deccox®* Granules)

Lambs: **For prevention or treatment of coccidiosis (extra-label):** 1 mg/kg in feed PO daily for at least 28 days. (Taylor et al. 2012)

Ewes (extra-label): **To aid in the prevention of abortions and perinatal losses caused by toxoplasmosis:** 2 mg/kg daily in feed continuously for 14 weeks prior to lambing. (Taylor et al. 2012)

Goats (labeled dosage; FDA-approved): **For the prevention of coccidiosis in young goats caused by** *Eimeria christenseni* **and** *E. ninakohlyakimovae*: Thoroughly mix *Deccox®* into the feed ration at a rate to provide decoquinate at a daily dose of 22.7 mg/100 lbs. (0.5 mg/kg) of body weight. Feed for at least 28 days during periods of coccidiosis exposure or when experience indicates that coccidiosis is likely to be a hazard. (Adapted from label; *Deccox®* Granules)

- **CAMELIDS:**

Llamas (extra-label): **For prophylaxis of coccidiosis:** Using the 6% premix: 0.5 mg/kg per day in feed for at least 28 days. (Johnson 1993)

Client Information

- Decoquinate should be used for at least 4 weeks when used for preventing coccidiosis outbreaks.
- When used in dogs for Hepatozoonosis treatment may continue for up to two years.
- Mix well into food.

Chemistry/Synonyms

A coccidiostat, decoquinate occurs as a cream to buff-colored fine amorphous powder having a slight odor. It is insoluble in water.

Decoquinate may also be known as HC-1528, M&B-15497, or *Deccox®*.

Storage/Stability

Follow label storage directions; store in a cool, dry place, preferably in airtight containers.

Compatibility/Compounding Considerations

Decoquinate is reportedly **incompatible** with strong bases or oxidizing material. *Deccox®* is labeled as being **compatible** (and cleared for use) with bacitracin zinc (with or without roxarsone), chlortetracycline, and lincomycin.

Dosage Forms/Regulatory Status

VETERINARY-LABELED PRODUCTS:

Decoquinate 6% (27.2 gram/lb.) Feed Additive (with corn meal, soybean oil, lecithin and silicon dioxide) in 50 lb. bags; *Deccox®*; (OTC). FDA-approved for use in cattle, sheep, goats (**DO NOT** feed to cows, goats or sheep producing milk for food) and chickens (NOT laying chickens). Approved label information for *Deccox®* can be found at dailymed.nlm.nih.gov

Decoquinate 0.5% (2.271 grams/lb.) Feed Additive in 50 lb. bags; *Doccox®-L*; (OTC). FDA-approved for use in ruminating and non-ruminating calves and cattle. **DO NOT** feed to cows producing milk for food.

Decoquinate 0.8% (3.632 grams/lb.) in 5 lb. and 50 lb. bags; *Deccox®-M*; (OTC). FDA-approved for use in ruminating and non-ruminating calves including veal calves.

Also available are calf milk replacers that contain 22.7 mg decoquinate per pound for the prevention of coccidiosis in non-ruminating and calves and cattle. *Advance® Calvita® Supreme 20/21* (and *18/21*) *Medicated with Decoquinate*; (OTC)

HUMAN-LABELED PRODUCTS: NONE.

Revisions/References

Monograph revised/updated January 2014.

Allen, K. E., et al. (2011). Hepatozoon spp Infections in the United States. Veterinary Clinics of North America-Small Animal Practice 41(6): 1221-+.
Johnson, L. (1993). Llama Herd health management. *Current Veterinary Therapy 3: Food Animal Practice.* J. Howard. Philadelphia, W.B. Saunders Co.: 172-7.
Shahiduzzamana, M. & A. Daugschiesb (2012). Therapy and prevention of cryptosporidiosis in animals. Veterinary Parasitology 188: 203-14.
Sykes, J. E., et al. (2011). Severe Myositis Associated with Sarcocystis spp. Infection in 2 Dogs. Journal of Veterinary Internal Medicine 25(6): 1277-83.
Taylor, M. A. & D. J. Bartram (2012). The history of decoquinate in the control of coccidial infections in ruminants. J. Vet. Pharmacol. Ther. 35(5): 417-27.

Deferoxamine Mesylate

(de-fer-**ox**-a-meen)   Desferal®, DFO

Chelating Agent

Prescriber Highlights

▶ Parental iron chelating agent used primarily for treatment of iron or aluminum intoxication in dogs/cats; has been used as a ferric ion chelator in cardiac arrest/GDV.
▶ Contraindications: Severe renal failure unless dialysis used.
▶ Caution: Pregnancy.
▶ Adverse Effects: Allergic reactions, auditory neurotoxicity, pain or swelling at injection sites, GI distress.
▶ When used IV, must be given slowly.

Uses/Indications

Deferoxamine is used for the treatment of either acute or chronic iron toxicity. It is being evaluated as an iron chelator for adjunctive treatment of acute cardiac ischemia and chelator for aluminum toxicity. Its efficacy in treating reperfusion injuries has been disappointing.

Pharmacology/Actions

Deferoxamine (DFO) binds ferric (Fe^{+++}) ions to its three hydroxamic groups forming ferrioxamine a stable, water-soluble compound that is readily excreted by the kidneys. DFO does not appear to chelate other trace metals (except aluminum) or electrolytes in clinically significant quantities.

Pharmacokinetics

DFO is poorly absorbed from the GI and is usually given parenterally. The drug is widely distributed in the body. DFO and ferrioxamine are excreted primarily in the urine.

Contraindications/Precautions/Warnings

DFO is contraindicated in patients with severe renal failure unless dialysis is used to remove ferrioxamine.

Adverse Effects

There is little veterinary experience with this drug. Potential adverse effects include, allergic reactions, auditory neurotoxicity (particularly with chronic, high-dose therapy), pain or swelling at injection sites, and GI distress. Too rapid IV injection may cause rapid heart rates, convulsions, hypotension, hives, and wheezing. Ferrioxamine will give the urine a reddish color ("vin rosé"), which is innocuous and indicates iron removal.

Oral administration of DFO is controversial. Some have recommended oral administration after oral iron ingestions, but DFO may actually increase the amount of iron absorbed from the gut. At present, oral sodium bicarbonate solution 5% given as a gastric lavage is probably a better treatment in reducing oral absorption of iron.

Reproductive/Nursing Safety

Because deferoxamine has caused skeletal abnormalities in animals at dosages just above those recommended for iron toxicity, it should be used during pregnancy only when its benefits outweigh it risks. In humans, the FDA categorizes this drug as category *C* for use during pregnancy (*Animal studies have shown an adverse effect on the fetus, but there are no adequate studies in humans; or there are no animal reproduction studies and no adequate studies in humans.*)

Overdosage/Acute Toxicity

See Adverse Effects above. Chronic high dose use may also lead to hypocalcemia and thrombocytopenia.

Drug Interactions

The following drug interactions have either been reported or are theoretical in humans or animals receiving deferoxamine and may be of significance in veterinary patients. Unless otherwise noted, use together is not necessarily contraindicated, but weigh the potential risks and perform additional monitoring when appropriate.

- **PROCHLORPERAZINE:** Use with deferoxamine may cause temporary impairment of consciousness.
- **VITAMIN C:** May be synergistic with deferoxamine in removing iron, but could lead to increased tissue iron toxicity especially in cardiac muscle; it should be used with caution, particularly in patients with preexisting cardiac disease.

Laboratory Considerations

- DFO may interfere (falsely low values) with colorimetric **iron** assays.
- DFO may cause falsely high total iron binding capacity (**TIBC**) measurements.

Doses

- **DOGS & CATS:**

In animals at risk for, or exhibiting signs of severe iron toxicosis (extra-label):

a) Most effective within the first 24 hours. Extrapolated animal dose is 40 mg/kg IM q4-8 hours. IM route is preferred as too rapid IV administration can cause hypotension and pulmonary edema. Giving ascorbic acid after the gut has been cleared of iron can increase efficacy. Deferoxamine-iron complex gives a salmon pink ("vin rose") color to urine. Continue to chelate until urine clears or serum iron levels return to normal. (Wismer 2004)

b) Initiate ASAP or at least within 12 hours of ingestion; give as a constant rate infusion at 15 mg/kg/hour. More rapid infusion may precipitate arrhythmias or aggravate hypotension. If constant rate infusion is not possible or are unable to monitor patient during infusion, give 40 mg/kg IM q4-8h, depending on clinical status. Continue therapy until serum iron levels are below 300 microliters/dL or decrease below the TIBC, whichever is lower. Chelation therapy may require 2-3 days of therapy. Following recovery, monitor for signs of GI obstruction, which may develop 4-6 weeks post-ingestion. (Greentree et al. 1995)

Experimentally, as a ferric ion chelator during treatment of cardiac arrest (extra-label):

a) 5 – 15 mg/kg IV, IM or SC. (Muir 1994)

b) 10 mg/kg IV, IM q2h for two doses, then 3 times daily for 24 hours. (Hackett et al. 1995)

- **HORSES:**

Foals: To reduce iron overload after transfusion (extra-label): In the study healthy foals were treated with 1 gram (in 5 mL) SC twice daily for 14 days beginning immediately before transfusion. Results suggest that deferoxamine increases urinary iron elimination after blood transfusion and may help prevent hepatotoxic iron overload. Additional studies needed to evaluate the effects of deferoxamine on iron elimination in foals with neonatal isoerythrolysis that require multiple transfusions. (Elfenbein et al. 2010)

Client Information

Deferoxamine should only used in an inpatient setting.

Monitoring

For iron overload:

- Efficacy (serum ferritin, serum iron, TIBC are recommended to monitor iron overload).
- Treatment is continued until serum iron levels decrease below total iron-binding capacity or until urine loses its "vin rosé" color.
- Adverse effects (see above). Additionally, if chronic iron overload: eye examinations (iron toxicity and its subsequent removal may adversely affect vision).

Chemistry/Synonyms

An iron-chelating agent, deferoxamine mesylate occurs as a white to off-white powder that is freely soluble in alcohol or water.

Deferoxamine mesylate may also be known as: desferoxamine mesylate, DFO, Ba-33112, Ba-29837, deferoxamini mesilas, desferrioxamine mesylate, desferrioxamine methanesulphonate, NSC-527604, *Desferal®* or *Desferin®*.

Storage/Stability

Store at room temperature. After aseptic reconstitution (2 – 5 mL for 500 mg vial; 8 – 20 mL for 2 gram vial) with sterile water for injection, the solution may be stored for up 24 hours at room temperature and protected from light.

Compatibility/Compounding Considerations

It is recommended not to mix this agent with other drugs; do not use if solution is turbid. Dilution in normal saline, lactated Ringer's or dextrose 5% has been recommended when administering as an intravenous infusion.

Dosage Forms/Regulatory Status

VETERINARY-LABELED PRODUCTS: NONE.

HUMAN-LABELED PRODUCTS:

Deferoxamine Mesylate Powder for Injection (lyophilized): 500 mg & 2 g in vials; *Desferal®*, generic; (Rx)

Revisions/References

Monograph revised/updated January 2014.

Elfenbein, J. R., et al. (2010). The Effects of Deferoxamine Mesylate on Iron Elimination after Blood Transfusion in Neonatal Foals. *Journal of Veterinary Internal Medicine* **24**(6): 1475-82.

Greentree, W. & J. Hall (1995). Iron Toxicosis. *Kirk's Current Veterinary Therapy:XII.* J. Bonagura. Philadelphia, W.B. Saunders: 240-2.

Hackett, T. & D. Van Pelt (1995). Cardiopulmonary resuscitation. *Kirk's Current Veterinary Therapy:XII.* J. Bonagura. Philadelphia, W.B. Saunders: 167-75.

Muir, W. (1994). Cardiopulmonary cerebral resuscitation. *Saunders Manual of Small Animal Practice.* S. Birchard and R. Sherding. Philadelphia, W.B. Saunders Company: 513-24.

Wismer, T. (2004). Newer antidotal therapies. Proceedings: IVECC Symposium. accessed via Veterinary Information Network; vin.com

---

Deracoxib

(dare-a-cox-ib)   Deramaxx®

Non-Steroidal Antiinflammatory Agent

Prescriber Highlights

▶ Coxib-class NSAID FDA-approved for use in dogs for treatment of post-operative pain (higher dose, 7 day maximum) & for treatment of pain & inflammation associated with osteoarthritis (lower dose, ongoing dosing).

▶ May be useful alternative to piroxicam in adjunctive treatment of transitional cell carcinoma of bladder.

▶ At lower doses, appears to cause predominantly COX-2 inhibition.

▶ Adverse effect profile still being fully determined, but GI & renal effects are possible.

Uses/Indications

Deracoxib is indicated for the treatment of post-operative pain (higher dose, 7 day maximum), and for the treatment of pain and inflammation associated with osteoarthritis (lower dose, ongoing dosing) in dogs.

Like piroxicam, deracoxib is of interest in adjunctive treatment of transitional cell carcinoma of the bladder; investigations into this use are ongoing (McMillan et al. 2011).

Pharmacology/Actions

Deracoxib is a coxib-class, nonsteroidal antiinflammatory drug (NSAID). It is believed to predominantly inhibit cyclooxygenase-2 (COX-2) and spare COX-1 at therapeutic dosages. This, theoretically, would inhibit production of the prostaglandins that contribute to pain and inflammation (COX-2) and spare those that maintain normal gastrointestinal and renal function (COX-1). However, COX-1 and COX-2 inhibition studies are done *in vitro* and do not necessarily correlate perfectly with clinical effects seen in actual patients.

Deracoxib's effect on platelet function in dogs is not entirely understood. In one study, healthy dogs given 2 mg/kg PO once daily for 7 days had a decrease in platelet aggregation induced by 50µM ADP, but deracoxib did not affect results of other platelet function tests; clinical significance is not known (Blois et al. 2010). Another study concluded that all of the COX-2 selective NSAIDs evaluated (meloxicam, deracoxib, carprofen) caused significantly prolonged PFA-100 closure times as measured using collagen/EPI cartridges, suggesting NSAID-induced alterations in platelet function (Mullins et al. 2012).

Pharmacokinetics

After oral administration to dogs, bioavailability is greater than 90%; the time to peak serum concentration occurs at approximately 2 hours. The presence of food in the gut can enhance bioavailability. The drug has an apparent volume of distribution of 1.5 L/kg in dogs and is at least 90% bound to canine plasma proteins. Deracoxib is hepatically metabolized to four primary metabolites. These metabolites and unchanged drug are principally eliminated in the feces. Some excretion of metabolites occurs via renal mechanisms. Terminal elimination half-life in the dog is dependent upon dose. In dosages up to approximately 8 mg/kg, half-life is about 3 hours (clearance ≈ 5 mL/min/kg). Half-life at a dose of 20 mg/kg is approximately 19 hours (clearance ≈ 1.7 mL/min/kg). Drug accumulation can occur with higher dosages, leading to increased toxic effects as increased COX-1 inhibition can occur at higher concentrations. Serum half-life is not necessarily a good predictor of duration of efficacy, possibly due to the drug's high protein binding.

In cats, after 1 mg oral doses of deracoxib, peak levels (0.28 micrograms/mL) occurred about 3.6 hours after administration. Elimination half-life was about 8 hours (Gassel et al. 2006).

In horses, deracoxib has a long half-life of about 13 hours. Based on dosage simulations and plasma levels, the authors suggested that dosages of 2 mg/kg PO q12-24h be further studied for safety and efficacy (Davis et al. 2011).

Contraindications/Precautions/Warnings

Deracoxib is contraindicated in patients known to be hypersensitive to it. It should be used with caution in patients with concurrent GI ulcerative diseases, renal or hepatic dysfunction, those in hypoproteinemic states, or with conditions that may predispose them to hypercoagulability. Deracoxib is not approved or recommended for use in cats.

Adverse Effects

In the majority of dogs treated, deracoxib appears to be well tolerated, particularly when dosed as labeled and not in conjunction with other NSAIDs or corticosteroids. However, like other NSAIDs used in dogs, many adverse effects associated with deracoxib have been reported and include: gastrointestinal (vomiting, anorexia/weight loss, diarrhea, melena, hematemesis, hematochezia, GI ulceration/perforation); urinary (azotemia, polydipsia, polyuria, UTI, hematuria, incontinence, renal failure); hematologic (anemia, thrombocytopenia); hepatic (increased hepatic enzymes, changes in total protein, etc.); neurologic (lethargy/weakness, seizures, etc.); cardiovascular/respiratory (tachypnea, bradycardia, cough); and dermatologic/immunologic (fever, facial/muzzle edema, urticaria, dermatitis). Rare occurrences of death associated with these effects are possible. As additional clinical experience is gained with this agent, relative instances of these effects and the potential risk for them to occur in a given patient population should be clarified.

Reproductive/Nursing Safety

No information on the drug's safety in pregnancy or in nursing pups was located. Use with caution in these animals.

Overdosage/Acute Toxicity

There is little data available regarding this drug's acute toxicity. A 14-day study in dogs demonstrated no clinically observable adverse effects in the dogs that received 10 mg/kg. Dogs that received 25 mg/kg, 50 mg/kg or 100 mg/kg per day for 10-11 days survived, but showed vomiting and melena; no hepatic or renal lesions were demonstrated in these dogs.

In safety studies performed by the drug manufacturer (Roberts et al. 2009), oral deracoxib was well tolerated by dogs when administered for up to six months at a variety of doses. Some dogs receiving ≥ 6 mg/kg/day (1.5-5X) showed signs of focal tubular degeneration/regeneration on histopathology. Focal tubular necrosis was seen in 4 dogs (of a total of 20) when dosed at 8 mg/kg/day (1 of 10 dogs) or 10 mg/kg/day (3 of 10 dogs) in the 6-month safety study.

There were 979 exposures to deracoxib reported to the ASPCA Animal Poison Control Center (APCC) during 2008-2009. In these cases 948 were dogs with 96 showing clinical signs and the remaining 31 cases were cats with 1 showing clinical signs. Common findings in dogs (recorded in decreasing frequency) include vomiting, diarrhea, lethargy, and elevated creatinine.

Because non-linear elimination occurs in dogs at dosages of 10 mg/kg and above, dogs acutely ingesting dosages above this amount should be observed for gastrointestinal erosion or ulceration and treated symptomatically for vomiting and GI bleeding.

This medication is a NSAID. As with any NSAID, overdosage can lead to gastrointestinal and renal effects. Decontamination with emetics and/or activated charcoal is appropriate. For doses where GI effects are expected, the use of gastrointestinal protectants is warranted. The ASPCA APCC recommends GI protectants at acute dosages of 15 mg/kg and above and IV fluid diuresis at dosages of 30 mg/kg and above in healthy dogs.

Drug Interactions

No specific drug interactions were noted, but the manufacturer warns that use in conjunction with other **NSAIDs** or **corticosteroids** be avoided. A 5-7 day washout period between other NSAIDs, aspirin or a glucocorticoid is recommended.

It is also possible deracoxib may cause increased renal dysfunction if used with other drugs that can cause or contribute to **renal dysfunction** (*e.g.*, **diuretics, aminoglycosides**), but the clinical significance of this potential interaction is unclear.

The following drug interactions have either been reported or are theoretical in humans or animals receiving coxib-class NSAIDs and may be of significance in veterinary patients. Unless otherwise noted, use together is not necessarily contraindicated, but weigh the potential risks and perform additional monitoring when appropriate.

- **ACE INHIBITORS** (*e.g.*, **enalapril, benazepril,** etc.): Some NSAIDs can reduce effects on blood pressure. Because ACE inhibitors potentially can reduce renal blood flow, use with NSAIDs could increase the risk for renal injury. However, one study in dogs receiving tepoxalin did not show any adverse effect. It is unknown what effects, if any, occur if other NSAIDs and ACE inhibitors are used together in dogs.
- **ASPIRIN:** May increase the risk of gastrointestinal toxicity (*e.g.*, ulceration, bleeding, vomiting, diarrhea, etc.). Washout periods several days long are warranted when switching from an NSAID to aspirin therapy in dogs.
- **CORTICOSTEROIDS** (*e.g., prednisone,* etc.): May increase the risk of gastrointestinal toxicity (*e.g.*, ulceration, GI perforation, bleeding, vomiting, diarrhea, etc.). Not recommended to use corticosteroids in conjunction with an NSAID.
- **DIGOXIN:** NSAIDS may increase serum levels.
- **FLUCONAZOLE:** Administration has increased plasma levels of celecoxib in humans and potentially could also affect deracoxib levels in dogs.
- **FUROSEMIDE:** NSAIDs may reduce saluretic and diuretic effects.
- **METHOTREXATE:** Serious toxicity has occurred when NSAIDs have been used concomitantly with methotrexate; use together with extreme caution.
- **NEPHROTOXIC DRUGS** (*e.g.*, **furosemide, aminoglycosides, amphotericin B,** etc.): May enhance the risk of nephrotoxicity development.
- **NSAIDS, OTHER:** May increase the risk of gastrointestinal toxicity (*e.g.*, ulceration, bleeding, vomiting, diarrhea, etc.). A 5-7 day washout period between NSAIDs is strongly recommended.
- **TRAMADOL:** May increase the risk of gastrointestinal toxicity. From a case report (Case et al. 2010).

Laboratory Considerations

- No specific laboratory interactions were noted for deracoxib. Deracoxib does not appear to affect thyroid function tests in dogs.

Doses

- **DOGS:**

  Labeled Doses (FDA-approved):

  For the control of pain and inflammation associated with osteoarthritis: 1 – 2 mg/kg PO once a day as needed.

  For treatment of post-operative pain: 3 – 4 mg/kg PO once a day as needed, not to exceed 7 days of therapy at this dosage. (Package insert; *Deramaxx®*)

Monitoring

- Baseline and periodic CBC and serum chemistry (including BUN/serum creatinine, and liver function assessment).
- Baseline history and physical.
- Efficacy of therapy.
- Adverse effect monitoring via client.

Client Information

Note: The manufacturer provides a client information sheet they recommend be given with every prescription for this medication.

- NSAID used in dogs for pain and inflammation. Can give with or without food, but food may reduce the chances for stomach problems. If your animal vomits or acts sick after getting it on an empty stomach, give with food or small treat to see if this helps. If vomiting continues, contact your veterinarian. Fresh water should always be available.
- Most dogs tolerate it very well, but rarely some will develop ulcers or serious kidney and liver problems. Watch for these signs: Decreased or increased appetite (eating less or more than normal), vomiting, changes in bowel movements, changes in behavior or activity levels (more or less active than normal), incoordination/weakness (*e.g.*, stumbling, clumsiness, etc.), seizures (convulsions) or aggression, yellowing of gums, skin, or whites of the eyes (jaundice), changes in drinking habits (frequency, amount consumed) or urination habits (frequency, color, or smell).
- Store chewable tablets well out of reach of animals and children.
- Periodic lab tests to check for liver and kidney side effects are required.
- Other drugs for pain or inflammation should not be used with this medication without the approval of the veterinarian.
- Do not increase or alter the dose of this medication without the approval of the veterinarian.

Chemistry/Synonyms

Deracoxib is a diaryl-substituted pyrazole that is chemically related to other coxib-class NSAIDs such as celecoxib. Its molecular weight is 397.38.

Storage/Stability

The commercially available chewable tablets for dogs should be stored at room temperature between 15-30°C (59-86°F).

Compatibility/Compounding Considerations

No specific information noted.

Dosage Forms/Regulatory Status

VETERINARY-LABELED PRODUCTS:

Deracoxib Chewable (scored) Tablets: 25 mg, 50 mg, 75 mg, & 100 mg in bottles of 7, 30 and 90 tablets; *Deramaxx®*; (Rx). FDA-approved for use in dogs.

The ARCI (Racing Commissioners International) has designated this drug as a class 4 substance. See the appendix for more information.

HUMAN-LABELED PRODUCTS: NONE.

Revisions/References
Monograph revised/updated January 2014.

Blois, S. L., et al. (2010). Effects of aspirin, carprofen, deracoxib, and meloxicam on platelet function and systemic prostaglandin concentrations in healthy dogs. American Journal of Veterinary Research 71(3): 349-58.

Case, J., et al. (2010). Proximal duodenal perforation in three dogs following deracoxib administration. J Am Anim Hosp Assoc 46: 255-8.

Davis, J. L., et al. (2011). The pharmacokinetics and in vitro cyclooxygenase selectivity of deracoxib in horses. J. Vet. Pharmacol. Ther. 34(1): 12-6.

Gassel, A. D., et al. (2006). Disposition of deracoxib in cats after oral administration. J. Am. Anim. Hosp. Assoc. 42(3): 212-7.

McMillan, S. K., et al. (2011). Antitumor effects of deracoxib treatment in 26 dogs with transitional cell carcinoma of the urinary bladder. Javma-Journal of the American Veterinary Medical Association 239(8): 1084-9.

Mullins, K. B., et al. (2012). Effects of carprofen, meloxicam and deracoxib on platelet function in dogs. Veterinary Anaesthesia and Analgesia 39(2): 206-17.

Roberts, E. S., et al. (2009). Safety and tolerability of 3-week and 6-month dosing of Deramaxx® (Deracoxib) chewable tablets in dogs. J. Vet. Pharmacol. Ther. 32(4): 329-37.

Dermcaps® — see Fatty Acids

DES — see Diethylstilbestrol

Desflurane
(dez-floor-ane)   Suprane®

Inhalant Anesthetic

Prescriber Highlights
▶ Primary benefit is when very rapid recoveries are desired.
▶ Similar effects on CNS, respiratory and cardiovascular systems as isoflurane.
▶ Requires desflurane-specific vaporizer (electric, heated, pressurized, expensive).

Uses/Indications
Desflurane is a volatile anesthetic with a chemical structure identical to isoflurane except for substitution of a fluorine atom for chlorine at the alpha-ethyl carbon. Desflurane may be of particular use when rapid recoveries are desired.

Pharmacology/Actions
Desflurane is a halogenated inhalant anesthetic. It is structurally related to isoflurane (has a fluorine atom substituted for chlorine at the alpha-ethyl carbon). While the precise mechanism that inhalant anesthetics exert their general anesthetic effect is not precisely known, they may interfere with functioning of nerve cells in the brain by acting at the lipid matrix of the membrane. Like sevoflurane, desflurane has a very low blood/gas partition coefficient (0.42). Minimal Alveolar Concentration (MAC; %) in oxygen reported for desflurane: dogs = 7; cats = 9.8; horse = 7.23; rabbit = 8.9, alpacas/llamas = 7.8-8.

Some key pharmacologic effects noted with desflurane include: rapid inductions and recoveries; rapid recoveries may be a benefit, but could also be detrimental particularly if perioperative analgesics are not used. It is relatively resistant to biodegradation that may minimize risk for nephrotoxicity.

Like sevoflurane, desflurane does not potentiate catecholamine-induced arrhythmias, and like all the inhalant anesthetics it does decrease arterial blood pressure and depress ventilation in a dose-dependent manner. Unlike sevoflurane, it is a respiratory irritant, has a pungent odor and is not well suited for mask inductions.

Pharmacokinetics
Onset of action is very rapid after inhalation; some have described as "one breath" induction. At body temperature (37°C) desflurane has a blood/gas coefficient (predicts rate of recovery) of 0.47, an oil/gas coefficient (indicates potency) of 19 and a brain/blood coefficient of 1.3.

Very little of desflurane is eliminated via hepatic routes as only 0.02% is recovered as metabolites. In humans, elimination half-life is 2.5 minutes (isoflurane about 9.5 minutes).

Contraindications/Precautions/Warnings
Desflurane is contraindicated in patients that are hypersensitive to it or other halogenated agents or that have a history or predilection towards malignant hyperthermia. It should be used with caution (benefits vs. risks) in patients with increased CSF pressure or head injury.

Because of its rapid action, use caution not to overdose during the induction phase. Because of the rapid recovery associated with desflurane, use caution (and appropriate analgesia and sedation during the recovery phase) particularly with large animals.

Geriatric or critically ill animals may require less inhalation anesthetic.

The National Institute for Occupational Safety and Health Administration has recommended that no worker should be exposed at ceiling concentrations greater than 2 ppm of any halogenated anesthetic agent over a sampling period not to exceed 1 hour.

Adverse Effects
Desflurane is usually very well tolerated. Hypotension and respiratory depression may occur and are considered dose-dependent. Like all halogenated anesthetics, desflurane can cause malignant hyperthermia in susceptible individuals (usually humans or pigs). Desflurane may have a lower incidence rate of this effect than other halogenated anesthetics.

When used for mask inductions, desflurane can cause respiratory irritation and cause salivation in dogs and cats. Rapid changes in desflurane concentrations may result in a sympathetic response and temporarily increase cardiac work.

Reproductive/Nursing Safety
Desflurane appears to be relatively safe to use during pregnancy, but data is limited. Because of its low blood solubility, desflurane may be one of the safest inhalant anesthetics for use during pregnancy. In rats and rabbits, no overt teratogenic effects were observed when exposed at 1 MAC-hour/day during organogenesis (10-13 days exposure). For humans, desflurane is categorized by the FDA as a category *B* drug (*Animal studies have not demonstrated risk to the fetus, but there are no adequate studies in pregnant women; or animal studies have shown an adverse effect, but adequate studies in pregnant women have not demonstrated a risk to the fetus during the first trimester of pregnancy, and there is no evidence of risk in later trimesters.*)

Desflurane is likely compatible with nursing as levels are low in milk and rapidly washout within 24 hours of use. However, safety during nursing has not been established.

Overdosage/Acute Toxicity
In the event of an overdosage, discontinue desflurane; maintain airway and support respiratory and cardiac function as necessary.

Drug Interactions
The following drug interactions have either been reported or are theoretical in humans or animals receiving desflurane and may be of significance in veterinary patients. Unless otherwise noted, use together is not necessarily contraindicated, but weigh the potential risks and perform additional monitoring when appropriate.

▪ **ACE INHIBITORS OR OTHER HYPOTENSIVE AGENTS:** Concomitant use may increase risks for hypotension. Enalapril caused significant decreases in systolic blood pressure in cats and dogs undergoing isoflurane anesthesia (Ishikawa et al. 2007). Similar effects may be expected with desflurane.

▪ **NON-DEPOLARIZING NEUROMUSCULAR BLOCKING AGENTS:** Additive neuromuscular blockade may occur.

▪ **SUCCINYLCHOLINE:** With inhalation anesthetics, may induce increased incidences of cardiac effects (bradycardia, arrhythmias, sinus arrest and apnea) and, in susceptible patients, malignant hyperthermia.

Laboratory Considerations

- Like other halogenated anesthetics, desflurane can cause transient increases in **glucose** and white blood cell count.

Doses

For general anesthesia (all are extra-label):

a) Clinically useful concentrations: Induction = 8 – 15%; Maintenance = 5 – 9%. (Grubb 2004)

b) Approximate MAC for emergency patients: 6%. (Gaynor 2010)

c) Following intravenous induction: the author usually starts with a vaporizer setting of about 8% (around MAC in most animals), increasing the concentration as required. (Clarke 2008)

Monitoring

- Respiratory, ventilatory status.
- Cardiac rate/rhythm; blood pressure.
- Level of anesthesia.
- Body temperature.
- Neuromuscular function.

Client Information

- Desflurane is only used in an inpatient setting.

Chemistry/Synonyms

Desflurane has the chemical name: (±)-2-Difluoromethyl 1,2,2,2-tetrafluoroethyl ether and has molecular weight of 168. It is a clear, colorless, heavy liquid. It is non-flammable and non-explosive. At one atmosphere it has a boiling point of 22-23°C, a vapor pressure of 669mm Hg at 20°C, specific gravity is 1.465 at 20°C. Desflurane is practically insoluble in water, but miscible with anhydrous alcohol. Desflurane has a very low blood:gas solubility ratio of 0.42 (at 37°C).

Desflurane may also be known as I-653, desfluraani, desflurano, or desfluranum. A common trade name is *Suprane®*.

Storage/Stability

Desflurane solution should be stored in its original container at 15°-30°C (59°-86°F). Secure cap on bottle tightly after use. Protect from light.

Before opening, the contents of the bottle should be cooled to below 10°C (48°F). Desflurane is relatively stable in soda lime at room temperature, but can produce carbon monoxide and formaldehyde. At 80°C, rate of degradation per hour is 0.44%.

Compatibility/Compounding Considerations

No specific information noted.

Dosage Forms/Regulatory Status

VETERINARY-LABELED PRODUCTS: NONE.

HUMAN-LABELED PRODUCTS:

Desflurane Solution for Inhalation Anesthesia in 240 mL btls; *Suprane®*; (Rx)

Revisions/References

Monograph revised/updated January 2014.

Clarke, K. W. (2008). Options for inhalation anaesthesia. In Practice **30**(9): 513-8.

Gaynor, J. S. (2010). Critical Anesthesia: Not All Patients Are Created Equal. Proceedings: WVC. accessed via Veterinary Information Network; vin.com

Grubb, T. (2004). Gas Anesthetics: Where Are We Now? Proceedings: IVECCS. accessed via Veterinary Information Network; vin.com

Ishikawa, Y., et al. (2007). Effect of Isoflurane Anesthesia on Hemodynamics Following Administration of an Angiotensin-Converting Enzyme Inhibitor in Cats. Proceedings: ACVIM. accessed via Veterinary Information Network; vin.com

Deslorelin Acetate

(dess-lor-a-lin)   SucroMate®, Suprelorin® F

Hormonal Agent

Prescriber Highlights

- ▶ Synthetic GnRH analog for estrual mares to induce & time ovulation; implants may also be effective to control reproduction in the bitch or as a contraceptive in male dogs.
- ▶ May be useful for treating ferrets with adrenal gland disease.
- ▶ No labeled contraindications.
- ▶ Adverse Effects: May cause some local swelling, pain, etc.; interovulatory period may be prolonged if implant not removed.

Uses/Indications

Deslorelin is FDA-approved for inducing ovulation in estrual mares. There is also interest in developing dosages and dosage forms as a long-term, reversible contraceptive in a variety of animal species, a treatment for prostatic disease in male dogs, and incontinence in ovariectomized dogs. An implant is "unapproved", but deemed legal to market by the FDA for management of adrenal disease in ferrets.

In humans, deslorelin has been investigated for treating children with precocious puberty, and in adults for prostate carcinoma, dysmenorrhea, fibroids, and endometriosis.

Pharmacology/Actions

Deslorelin increases the levels of endogenous luteinizing hormone (LH), thereby inducing ovulation. When developing follicles are greater than 30 mm in diameter, deslorelin induces ovulation in approximately 78% of mares within 48 hours of administration.

Pharmacokinetics

In horses after implantation of a 2.1 mg pellet, concentrations of LH and FSH peak about 12 hours after implant and return to pretreatment levels approximately 3-4 days after implantation. Oral dosing of 100 micrograms/kg to Beagles, demonstrated no increase in LF or FSH.

Contraindications/Precautions/Warnings

Deslorelin acetate is contraindicated in horses known to be hypersensitive to it. Do not use in horses intended for human consumption. Do not administer IV.

Adverse Effects

The IM gel can cause swelling at the site of injection, which generally subsides within 5 days. With the implants, minor local swelling, sensitivity to touch, and elevated skin temperature at injection site may occur; these effects should resolve within 5 days of implantation.

There is some evidence that deslorelin implants can suppress pituitary FSH secretion and decrease follicular development in subsequent diestrus, leading to a prolonged interovulatory period. Some clinicians (see the dose recommendation by McCue 2003, below) recommend removing the implant to negate this possibility.

Reproductive/Nursing Safety

Abnormalities in foal viability or behavior related to the use of deslorelin have not been observed in foals born to treated mares.

Overdosage/Acute Toxicity

In 8 mares that received a single IM injection at 10X the recommended of 1.8 mg dose, one exhibited moderate tremors and hives 6 hours after injection. If inadvertent administration of additional implant is done, it should be removed upon detection if within 96 hours of implant.

Drug Interactions

- No specific interactions noted.

Laboratory Considerations
- None noted.

Doses
- **DOGS:**

  Note: There are several deslorelin products licensed/approved for various species; see the specific labels for more information.

  As a contraceptive in male dogs (extra-label in USA): Using the licensed (not in USA) 4.7 mg implant (*Suprelorin-6®*—Virbac/Peptech): Implant SC every 6 months. Using the 9.4 mg implant (*Suprelorin-12®*—Peptech): Implant SC every 12 months. Implant in loose skin between lower neck and lumbar area; avoid implanting into fat. Pregnant women should not administer the implant. (Adapted from label information; see full label for further dosing instructions, precautions and adverse effects)

  To induce estrus in bitches (extra-label): Estrus induction more successful in bitches with serum progesterone concentrations of <5 ng/mL. Implant most commonly described for use in dogs is the equine product containing 2.1 mg (*Ovuplant®*; may not be commercially available in USA). A 2.1-mg implant is placed in the subcutaneous space, often in the vestibular mucosa just within the vulvar lips. Placement of the implant in an area from which it can be removed may be desirable. Compounded products may have significantly more variable success rates. (Kustritz 2012)

- **FERRETS:**

  For the management of adrenal gland cortical disease in the male and female domestic ferret (labeled dose; *Suprelorin F®*; USA): One 4.7 mg implant per ferret every 12 months. Appropriate clinical monitoring is suggested to determine that the symptoms of adrenal gland disease are being adequately controlled. See label for specific administration instructions. (Adapted from label; *Suprelorin F®*)

- **HORSES:**

  For inducing ovulation within 48 hours in cyclic estrous mares with an ovarian follicle between 30 and 40 mL in diameter (labeled dose; FDA-approved): Shake vial well before drawing into syringe. Administer 1.8 mg (1 mL) by intramuscular injection in the neck. (Label Information—*SucroMate® Equine*)

Monitoring
- None required.

Client Information
- Administered only by a veterinarian.
- Swelling or inflammation can occur at injection site; if this gets worse contact veterinarian.

Chemistry/Synonyms
Deslorelin acetate is a synthetic gonadotropin-releasing hormone (GnRH, gonadorelin) analog. It is a nonapeptide and has chemical modifications in the amino aide composition at positions 6 and 9/10.

Storage/Stability
Deslorelin implants or injectable suspension should be stored refrigerated (2-8°C, 36-46°F).

Compatibility/Compounding Considerations
No specific information noted.

Dosage Forms/Regulatory Status
VETERINARY-LABELED PRODUCTS:

Deslorelin Suspension for Injection 1.8 mg/mL in 10 mL multi-dose vials; *SucroMate® Equine*; (Rx). FDA-approved for horses (not intended for food); (NADA 141-319).

Deslorelin 2.1 mg cylindrical implant with implanter; 5 per box

Ovuplant®; (Rx). FDA-approved for ovulation induction in mares. Not for use in horses intended for food. This product is FDA-approved in the USA (per the FDA's Green Book), but it may not be currently marketed.

Deslorelin Implants 4.7 mg; *Suprelorin-F®*; Not approved by FDA, but legally marketed for use in ferrets only as an FDA Indexed Product under MIF 900-013. Extra-label use is prohibited. This product is not to be used in animals intended for use as food for humans or other animals. A link to the label information for *Suprelorin-F®* can be found at dailymed.nlm.nih.gov

Other deslorelin products may be licensed for animal use in other countries and compounded preparations may be available.

HUMAN-LABELED PRODUCTS: NONE.

Revisions/References
Monograph revised/updated January 2014.

Kustritz, M. V. R. (2012). Managing the Reproductive Cycle in the Bitch. Veterinary Clinics of North America-Small Animal Practice **42**(3): 423-37.

Desmopressin Acetate

(des-moe-press-in)   Stimate®, DDAVP®

Hormonal Agent

Prescriber Highlights

▶ Synthetic vasopressin analogue used to treat diabetes insipidus & von Willebrand's disease (limited usefulness).

▶ Contraindications: Hypersensitivity to desmopressin, type IIB or platelet-type (pseudo) Von Willebrand's (German shorthair pointers?).

▶ Use caution in patients susceptible to thrombosis.

▶ Adverse Effects: Eye irritation after conjunctival administration; hypersensitivity possible.

▶ Overdoses can cause fluid retention/hyponatremia.

Uses/Indications

Desmopressin has been found to be useful in the treatment of central diabetes insipidus in small animals. It may be useful in treating von Willebrand's disease, but its short duration of activity (2-4 hours) in this condition, resistance development, and expense limit its usefulness for this disorder. Desmopressin, secondary to its hemostatic effects may be useful as a surgical adjuvant perioperatively to reduce lymph node involvement and metastatic disease in canine mammary carcinoma or other aggressive tumors.

Pharmacology/Actions

Desmopressin is related structurally to arginine vasopressin, but it has more antidiuretic activity and less vasopressor properties on a per weight basis. Desmopressin increases water reabsorption by the collecting ducts in the kidneys, thereby increasing urine osmolality and decreasing net urine production. Therapeutic doses do not directly affect either urinary sodium or potassium excretion.

Desmopressin causes a dose-dependent increase in plasma factor VIII and plasminogen factor and also causes smaller increases in factor VIII-related antigen and ristocetin cofactor activities.

Pharmacokinetics

Because desmopressin is destroyed in the GI tract, it usually is given parenterally or topically. Oral tablets have been used in those dogs that cannot tolerate ophthalmic administration, but bioavailability is very low. In humans, intranasal administration is commonly used, while in veterinary medicine topical administration to the conjunctiva is preferred. The onset of antidiuretic action in dogs usually occurs within one hour of administration, peaks in 2-8 hours, and may persist for up to 24 hours. Distribution characteristics of desmopressin are not well described, but it does enter maternal milk. The metabolic fate is also not well understood. Terminal half lives in humans after IV administration are from 0.4-4 hours.

Contraindications/Precautions/Warnings

Desmopressin is contraindicated in patients hypersensitive to it. It should not be used for treatment of type IIB or platelet-type (pseudo) von Willebrand's disease as platelet-aggregation and thrombocytopenia may occur. German shorthair pointers apparently can have this type of vWD. Desmopressin should be used with caution in patients susceptible to thrombotic events.

When desmopressin is used to stimulate von Willebrand factor, with repeated administration tachyphylaxis (increasing lack of efficacy) will occur to a variable extent within 24 hours.

Adverse Effects

Side effects in small animals apparently are uncommon. Occasionally eye irritation may occur after conjunctival administration. Hypersensitivity reactions are possible. Humans using the drug have complained about increased headache frequency.

Reproductive/Nursing Safety

Safe use during pregnancy has not been established; however safe doses of up to 125X the average human antidiuretic dose have been given to rats and rabbits without demonstration of fetal harm. In humans, the FDA categorizes this drug as category *B* for use during pregnancy (*Animal studies have not yet demonstrated risk to the fetus, but there are no adequate studies in pregnant women; or animal studies have shown an adverse effect, but adequate studies in pregnant women have not demonstrated a risk to the fetus in the first trimester of pregnancy, and there is no evidence of risk in later trimesters.*)

Desmopressin is likely safe to use during nursing.

Overdosage/Acute Toxicity

Oral doses of 0.2 mg/kg/day have been administered to dogs for 6 months without any significant drug-related toxicity reported. Dosages that are too high may lead to fluid retention and hyponatremia; dosage reduction and fluid restriction may be employed to treat. Adequate monitoring should be performed.

Drug Interactions

The following drug interactions have either been reported or are theoretical in humans or animals receiving desmopressin and may be of significance in veterinary patients. Unless otherwise noted, use together is not necessarily contraindicated, but weigh the potential risks and perform additional monitoring when appropriate.

- CHLORPROPAMIDE, FLUDROCORTISONE, UREA: May enhance the antidiuretic effects of desmopressin.

Laboratory Considerations

- See Monitoring Parameters.

Doses

Note: When doses listed below use "drops" of the nasal solution they are referencing the 0.1 mg/mL product and **NOT** the 1.5 mg/mL product (*Stimate®*). **Do not** confuse the two.

- **DOGS:**

  For treatment of central diabetes insipidus (extra-label): In dogs, using the 0.1 mg/mL (0.01%) human intranasal product is most commonly employed. Initially, one drop is placed into the conjunctival sac once to twice daily. Up to 4 drops per dose may be required in some patients.

  As a trial in place of water deprivation test (extra-label): one-half to one 0.1 or 0.2 mg DDAVP tablet PO q8h or 1 – 4 drops of nasal spray from an eye dropper into the conjunctival sac every 12 hours for 5-7 days. If central DI, owners should notice a decrease in PU/PD by the end of treatment period. Increase in

urine specific gravity by 50% or more, compared with pre-treatment values, also support diagnosis of central DI. (Nelson 2002)

To improve hemostatic function (all are extra-label):

a) **For pre-surgery prophylaxis or treatment of von Willebrand's Disease** (not Types 2 or 3 vWD): 1 microgram/kg SC 30-minutes hour before surgery. It has been suggested that the intranasal solution can be used subcutaneously. Duration of activity is approximately 2 hours. Have transfusion capability ready.

b) **For aspirin-induced coagulopathy** (extra-label; based on a 3 dog case report): Desmopressin at 0.3 – 1 micrograms/kg IV over 15-30 minutes dramatically shortened buccal mucosal bleeding time measured 15-120 minutes later and reduced the risk of intraoperative hemorrhage during surgery (Di Mauro et al. 2013). Subcutaneous dosages of 1 – 4 micrograms prior to surgery have also been suggested.

c) **For hemorrhage secondary to canine monocytic ehrlichiosis** (extra-label; based on a 3 dog case report): 1 microgram/kg SC once daily (q24h) for 3 days. (Giudice et al. 2010)

- **CATS:**

To help differentiate central diabetes insipidus from the nephrogenic form: 1 drop into the conjunctival sac twice daily for 2-3 days; a dramatic reduction in water intake or a 50% or greater increase in urine concentration gives strong evidence for a deficit in ADH production. For treatment of central DI: 1 – 2 drops into the conjunctival sac once or twice a day; duration of activity is 8-24 hours. (Bruyette 1991)

For treatment of diabetes insipidus (central): 1 – 4 drops of the intranasal solution in the conjunctival sac once to twice daily; may use intranasal solution parenterally at 2 – 5 micrograms per cat SC once to twice daily (Nichols 2000). For PO use in cats whose owners find the intranasal or conjunctival application inconvenient: 25 – 50 micrograms (per cat; 1/4th to 1/2 of a 100 microgram tablet) PO q12h. Dose and response may be variable. (Aroch et al. 2005)

- **HORSES:**

For diagnosis of diabetes insipidus (extra-label):

a) 20 micrograms per horse IV. (Barnes et al. 2002)

b) Dilute the nasal spray formulation (0.1 mg/ml) in sterile water and administer 0.05 micrograms/kg IV. Urine specific gravity (SG) should be measured every 2 hours. An increase in SG to 1.025 or greater within 2-7 hours is consistent with central DI. No change in urine SG is consistent with nephrogenic DI if medullary washout has been accounted for. (McKenzie 2009)

Monitoring

For Central DI:
- Serum electrolytes.
- Urine osmolality and/or urine volume.

For von Willebrand's disease, other coagulopathies:
- Bleeding times.

Client Information

- In dogs and cats, human nasal spray is usually prescribed, but it is given by putting drops into the conjunctival sac (just below the eye).
- Usually tolerated very well as an eye drop though sometimes eye irritation occurs.
- Store in refrigerator; discard open bottles after 30 days.

Chemistry/Synonyms

A synthetic polypeptide related to arginine vasopressin (antidiuretic hormone), desmopressin acetate occurs as a fluffy white powder with a bitter taste. The commercially available nasal solution has HCl added and the pH is approximately 4. This preparation also contains chlorobutanol 0.5% as a preservative.

Desmopressin Acetate may also be known as: 1-Deamino-8-D-Arginine Vasopressin, *DFDAVP®*, *Concentraid®*, *D-Void®*, *Defirin®*, *Desmogalen®*, *Desmospray®*, *Desmotabs®*, *Emosint®*, *Minirin®*, *Minirin/DDAVP®*, *Minrin®*, *Minurin®*, *Nocutil®*, *Octim®*, *Octostim®*, *Presinex®*, or *Stimate®*.

Storage/Stability

The nasal solution should be refrigerated (2-8°C). It has an expiration date of one year after manufacture. While the nasal solution should be stored in the refrigerator, it is stable at room temperature for 3 weeks in the unopened bottle. The product for injection should be stored refrigerated (4°C); do not freeze.

Compatibility/Compounding Considerations

Parenteral drug products should be inspected visually for particulate matter and discoloration prior to administration. In humans it is recommended that for IV infusion, the appropriate dose of desmopressin acetate be diluted in 10 or 50 mL of 0.9% sodium chloride injection for administration in children weighing 10 kg or less or in adults and children weighing more than 10 kg, respectively; the solution is then infused IV slowly over 15-30 minutes. It has been anecdotally suggested that the intranasal solution can be administered SC or diluted and given IV to veterinary patients. However, no specific published safety or stability data was located.

Dosage Forms/Regulatory Status

VETERINARY-LABELED PRODUCTS: NONE.

HUMAN-LABELED PRODUCTS:

Desmopressin Acetate Intranasal Spray Solution: 0.1 mg/mL (0.01%; 10 micrograms/spray) in 5 mL bottle or 2.5 mL rhinal tube delivery system; *DDAVP®*; generic; (Rx)

Desmopressin Acetate Intranasal Spray Solution: 1.5 mg/mL (0.15%; 150 micrograms/spray) in 2.5 mL bottle; *Stimate®*; (Rx)

Desmopressin Acetate Injection Solution: 4 micrograms/mL in 1 mL single-dose amps & 10 mL multiple dose vials; *DDAVP®*; generic; (Rx)

Desmopressin Acetate Oral Tablets: 0.1 mg & 0.2 mg; *DDAVP®*; generic; (Rx)

Revisions/References

Monograph revised/updated January 2014.

Aroch, I., et al. (2005). Central diabetes insipidus in five cats: clinical presentation, diagnosis and oral desmopressin therapy. Journal of Feline Medicine and Surgery 7(6): 333-9.

Barnes, D., et al. (2002). Antidiuretic response to horses to DDAVP (desmopressin acetate). Proceedings ACVIM Forum. accessed via Veterinary Information Network; vin.com

Bruyette, D. (1991). Polyuria and polydipsia. *Consultations in Feline Internal Medicine*. J. August. Philadelphia, W.B. Saunders Company: 227-35.

Di Mauro, F. M. & M. K. Holowaychuk (2013). Intravenous administration of desmopressin acetate to reverse acetylsalicylic acid-induced coagulopathy in three dogs. J. Vet. Emerg. Crit. Care 23(4): 455-8.

Giudice, E., et al. (2010). Effect of desmopressin on immune-mediated haemorrhagic disorders due to canine monocytic ehrlichiosis: a preliminary study. J. Vet. Pharmacol. Ther. 33(6): 610-4.

McKenzie, E. (2009). Polyuria/polydipsia in Horses. Proceedings: Western Veterinary Conference. accessed via Veterinary Information Network; vin.com

Nelson, R. (2002). Polyuria, polydipsia, and diabetes insipidus. Proceedings: World Small Animal Veterinary Asssoc. World Congress. accessed via Veterinary Information Network; vin.com

Nichols, R. (2000). Clinical use of DDAVP for the diagnosis and treatment of diabetes insipidus. *Kirk's Current Veterinary Therapy: XIII Small Animal Practice*. J. Bonagura. Philadelphia, WB Saunders: 325-6.

Desoxycorticosterone Pivalate (DOCP)

(de-sox-ee-kor-ti-kost-er-ohn pih-vah-late)   Percorten-V®

Mineralocorticoid

Prescriber Highlights

▶ Parenteral mineralocorticoid used to treat Addison's in dogs/cats.

▶ Relative contraindications: congestive heart failure, severe renal disease, or edema; Caution: pregnancy.

▶ Addison's patients must receive glucocorticoid supplementation in periods of high stress/illness.

▶ May cause irritation at injection site.

▶ Adjust dosage based upon monitoring parameters.

Uses/Indications

DOCP is indicated for the parenteral treatment of adrenocortical insufficiency in dogs. It is also used in an extra-label manner in cats.

Pharmacology/Actions

Desoxycorticosterone pivalate (DOCP) is a long-acting mineralocorticoid agent. The site of action of mineralocorticoids is at the renal distal tubule where it increases the absorption of sodium. Mineralocorticoids also enhance potassium and hydrogen ion excretion. To be effective, mineralocorticoids require a functioning kidney.

Pharmacokinetics

Little information is available. It is injected IM (or subcutaneously) as a microcrystalline depot for slow dissolution into the circulation. Duration of action after injection is usually 21-30 days.

Contraindications/Precautions/Warnings

The drug is labeled as contraindicated in dogs suffering from congestive heart failure, severe renal disease, or edema.

Because some animals may be more (or less) sensitive to the effects of the drug, "cookbook" dosing without ongoing monitoring is inappropriate. Some animals may require additional supplementation with a glucocorticoid agent on an ongoing basis. If glucocorticoid dosages are too high, polydipsia, polyuria, or polyphagia can occur. All animals with hypoadrenocorticism should receive additional glucocorticoids (2-10 times basal) during periods of stress or acute illness.

Do not administer DOCP IV; acute collapse and shock may result. If given IV, treat immediately for shock with IV fluids and glucocorticoids.

Adverse Effects

Occasionally, irritation at the site of injection may occur. Post-approval reported adverse effects in dogs include (in decreasing frequency): depression/lethargy, vomiting, anorexia, polydipsia, polyuria, diarrhea, facial/muzzle edema, weakness, urticaria and anaphylaxis. Anemia has been reported following DOCP administration.

Reproductive/Nursing Safety

The manufacturer states that the drug should not be used in pregnant dogs as safe use during pregnancy has not been established. Use in pregnant animals only when the potential benefits outweigh the risks.

DOCP should be safe for offspring when administered to nursing dams.

Overdosage/Acute Toxicity

Overdosage may cause polyuria, polydipsia, hypernatremia, hypertension, edema, and hypokalemia. Cardiac enlargement is possible with prolonged overdoses. Excessive weight gain may be indicative of fluid retention secondary to sodium retention. Electrolytes should be aggressively monitored and potassium may need to be supplemented. Discontinue the drug in patients until clinical signs associated with overdosage have resolved and then restart the drug at a lower dosage.

Drug Interactions
The following drug interactions have either been reported or are theoretical in humans or animals receiving DOCP and may be of significance in veterinary patients. Unless otherwise noted, use together is not necessarily contraindicated, but weigh the potential risks and perform additional monitoring when appropriate.
- **AMPHOTERICIN B:** Patients may develop hypokalemia if mineralocorticoids are administered concomitantly with amphotericin B.
- **ASPIRIN:** DOCP may reduce salicylate levels.
- **DIGOXIN:** Because DOCP may cause hypokalemia it should be used with caution and increased monitoring in patients receiving digitalis glycosides.
- **INSULIN:** Potentially, DOCP could increase the insulin requirements of diabetic patients.
- **POTASSIUM-DEPLETING DIURETICS** (*e.g.,* **furosemide, thiazides**): Patients may develop hypokalemia if mineralocorticoids are administered concomitantly with potassium-depleting diuretics; as diuretics can cause a loss of sodium, they may counteract the effects DOCP.

Doses
- **DOGS:**

  For maintenance of hypoadrenocorticism (labeled dose; FDA-approved): Dosage requirements are variable and must be individualized on the basis of the response of the patient to therapy. Begin treatment at a dose of 2.2 mg/kg IM (**Note:** *Some administer the drug SC in an extra-label manner—Plumb*) every 25 days. In some patients the dose may be reduced. Serum sodium and potassium levels should be monitored. Most patients are well controlled with a dose range of 1.65 – 2.2 mg/kg every 21-30 days. Well-controlled patients have normal electrolytes at 14 days after administration or may exhibit slight hyponatremia and hyperkalemia. This needs no additional therapy as long as the patient is active and eating normally. Monitor for depression, lethargy, vomiting or diarrhea, which indicate a probable glucocorticoid deficiency. At the end of the 25-day dosing interval, the patient should be clinically normal and have normal serum electrolytes; may have slight hyponatremia and slight hyperkalemia. This indicates that the dosage and dosage interval should not be altered. If the dog is not clinically normal or serum electrolytes are abnormal, then the dosage interval should be decreased 2-3 days.

  Note: DOCP replaces the mineralocorticoid hormones only. Glucocorticoid replacement must be supplied by small daily doses of glucocorticoid hormones (e.g., prednisone or prednisolone) (0.2 – 0.4 mg/kg/day). Failure to administer glucocorticoids is the most common reason for treatment failure. Signs of glucocorticoid deficiency include depression, lethargy, vomiting and diarrhea. Such signs should be treated with high doses of injectable glucocorticoids (prednisolone or dexamethasone), followed by continued oral therapy 0.2 – 0.4 mg/kg/day. Polyuria and polydipsia (PU/PD) usually indicate excess glucocorticoid, but may also indicate DOCP excess. Begin by decreasing the glucocorticoid dose first. If the PU/PD persists, then decrease the dose without changing the interval between doses.

Oral supplementation with salt (NaCl) is not necessary with animals receiving DOCP. (Adapted from label; *Percorten®-V*)

- **CATS:**

  For maintenance therapy of hypoadrenocorticism (all are extra-label):
  a) 2.2 mg/kg IM every 25 days plus prednisolone (0.25 – 1 mg/cat PO twice daily; if daily oral dosing not feasible, may give 10 mg of methylprednisolone acetate once a month IM). (Reusch 2000)
  b) 10 – 12.5 mg (per cat) IM per month. Adjust dose based-upon follow-up serum electrolyte concentrations monitored every 1-2 weeks during initial maintenance period. Normal electrolyte values 2 weeks following injection, suggests adequate dosing, but does not provide information regarding duration of action. Prednisone at 1.25 mg PO once a day or IM methylprednisolone acetate 10 mg once a month can provide long-term glucocorticoid supplementation. (Bruyette 2002)

Monitoring
- Serum electrolytes, BUN, creatinine; initially every 1-2 weeks, then once stabilized, every 3-4 months. See Dosage above.
- Weight, PE for edema.

Client Information
- Most commonly injected into the muscle (IM) every 20-30 days; sometimes veterinarians will have you inject it under the skin (subcutaneously). Your veterinarian will adjust the dose and times between doses depending on your animal's response.
- Shake vial vigorously before drawing up into syringe.
- Must not be given IV (into the vein).
- Watch for symptoms of the dose being too high: greater thirst and need to urinate, swelling/edema, weight gain, pot belly; or the dose being too low: muscle weakness, lethargy (lack of energy), shaking, collapsing/fainting, loss of appetite/weight loss, vomiting, diarrhea, slower heartbeat, or painful abdomen. If any of these are seen, contact veterinarian right away.

Chemistry/Synonyms
A mineralocorticoid, desoxycorticosterone pivalate (DOCP) occurs as a white or creamy white powder that is odorless and stable in air. It is practically insoluble in water, slightly soluble in alcohol and vegetable oils. The injectable product is a white aqueous suspension and has a pH between 5-8.5. The commercially available injection (*Percorten-V®*) contains (per mL): 25 mg desoxycorticosterone pivalate, 10.5 mg methylcellulose, 3 mg sodium carboxymethylcellulose, 1 mg polysorbate 80, and 8 mg sodium chloride with 0.002% thimerosal added as preservative in water for injection.

Desoxycorticosterone pivalate may also be known as: deoxycorticosterone pivalate, deoxycorticosterone trimethyl-acetate, deoxycortone pivalate, deoxycortone trimethylacetate, desoxycorticosterone pivalate, desoxycorticosterone trimethyl-acetate, *Cortiron®,* or *Percorten-V®*.

Storage/Stability
Store the injectable suspension at room temperature and protect from light or freezing. The label states that once the vial is broached, product should be used within 4 months.

Compatibility/Compounding Considerations
Do not mix with any other agent.

Dosage Forms/Regulatory Status
VETERINARY-LABELED PRODUCTS:
Desoxycorticosterone Pivalate Injectable Suspension: 25 mg/mL in 4 mL vials; *Percorten-V®*; (Rx). FDA-approved for use in dogs; NADA # 141-029. A link to the label information for *Percorten-V®* can be found at dailymed.nlm.nih.gov

The ARCI (Racing Commissioners International) has designated this drug as a class 4 substance. See the appendix for more information.

HUMAN-LABELED PRODUCTS: NONE.

Revisions/References
Monograph revised/updated January 2014.
Bruyette, D. (2002). Feline adrenal disease. Proceedings: Atlantic Coast Veterinary Conference. accessed via Veterinary Information Network; vin.com
Reusch, C. (2000). Hypoadrenocorticism. *Textbook of Veterinary Internal Medicine: Diseases of the Dog and Cat.* S. Ettinger and E. Feldman. Philadelphia, WB Saunders. 2: 1488-99.

Detomidine HCl

(de-toe-ma-deen)   Dormosedan®

Alpha-2 Adrenergic Agonist

Prescriber Highlights

▶ Alpha₂ sedative analgesic used primarily in horses.
▶ Contraindications: Heart block, severe coronary, cerebrovascular, or respiratory disease, chronic renal failure.
▶ Caution: Horses with endotoxic or traumatic shock or approaching shock, advanced hepatic or renal disease; stress due to temperature extremes, fatigue, or high altitude; patients treated for intestinal impactions; with suspected colic as it may mask abdominal pain or changes in respiratory & cardiac rates.
▶ May respond (*i.e.*, kick) to external stimuli even after fully sedated; use caution, opioids may temper.
▶ Adverse Effects: Initial blood pressure increase, then bradycardia/heart block; piloerection.

Uses/Indications
At present, detomidine is only FDA-approved for use as a sedative analgesic in horses, but it has been used clinically in other species.

Pharmacology/Actions
Detomidine, like xylazine, is an alpha₂-adrenergic agonist that produces a dose-dependent sedative and analgesic effect, but it also has cardiac and respiratory effects. For more information, refer to the xylazine monograph or the adverse effects section below. Detomidine is approximately 50-100X as potent as xylazine.

Pharmacokinetics
Detomidine is well absorbed after oral administration, but due to a high first-pass effect, little drug is available systemically. The drug is apparently rapidly distributed into tissues, including the brain after parenteral administration and extensively metabolized then excreted primarily into the urine. Peak sedative actions can range from 5-20 minutes post IM injection in horses. After 40 mcg/kg of the sublingual (SL) gel, - peak effects times in various measurements were: heart rate 40 minutes, head height and ataxia 60 minutes, and response to stimuli 100 minutes (l'Ami et al. 2013). Published mean or median pharmacokinetic values for detomidine in horses include: Volume of distribution: 0.47-0.59 L/kg (at rest), 1.3 L/kg (after exercise). Times to reach maximum blood level concentration were approximately 2 minutes (IV), 77 minutes (IM), and 1.83 hours (SL). Clearance is about12-16 mL/min/kg. Elimination half-lives are 24-26 minutes (IV, at rest), 46 minutes (IV, after exercise), and 51 minutes (IM, at rest) (Hubbell et al. 2009), (Mama et al. 2009). The oromucosal gel product bioavailability is lower than IM (22% vs. 38%) (Kaukinen et al. 2009); the product label states that the peak concentrations observed after administration of the gel are approximately 40% of those observed after IM injection.

After exercise, the volume of distribution of detomidine is higher then at rest. Initial dose requirements may be higher and subsequent doses lower after exercise (Hubbell et al. 2009).

Contraindications/Precautions/Warnings
Detomidine is contraindicated in horses with preexisting AV or SA heart block, severe coronary insufficiency, cerebrovascular disease, respiratory disease or chronic renal failure. Use cautiously in animals with endotoxic or traumatic shock or approaching shock, and advanced hepatic or renal disease. Horses that are stressed due to temperature extremes, fatigue, or high altitude should be given the drug carefully. Because this drug may inhibit gastrointestinal motility, use with prudence in patients treated for intestinal impactions. In horses with suspected colic, the use of detomidine analgesia should be used cautiously as it may mask abdominal pain and conceal changes in respiratory and cardiac rates, thereby making diagnosis more difficult.

Although animals may appear to be deeply sedated, some may respond (kick, etc.) to external stimuli; use appropriate caution. The addition of opioids (*e.g.*, butorphanol, etc.) may help temper this effect. The manufacturer recommends allowing the horse to stand quietly for 5 minutes prior to injection and for 10-15 minutes after injection to improve the effect of the drug. After administering detomidine, protect the animal from temperature extremes.

During times of ambient temperature extremes, especially summer heat, consider using dosages in the lower range to reduce chances for toxicity.

When using the gel, wear impermeable gloves during drug administration or doing procedures that require contact with the horse's mouth.

In cattle, use of alpha-2 agonists under emergency conditions is discouraged as the risk of profound cardiovascular instability or recumbency exceeds the benefits observed with the use of these drugs (Anderson et al. 2013).

Adverse Effects
Detomidine can cause an initial rise in blood pressure that is then followed by bradycardia and heart block. Atropine at 0.02 mg/kg IV has been successfully used to prevent or correct the bradycardia that may be seen when the detomidine is used at labeled dosages. However, routine use of anticholinergics is generally not recommended due to the potential for GI motility reduction and hypertension. In addition detomidine can cause piloerection, sweating, ataxia, salivation, slight muscle tremors, and penile prolapse after injection.

When compared to xylazine, detomidine causes more pronounced bradycardia and bradyarrhythmias. Because the sedative and muscle-relaxing effects of detomidine in horses can persist for up to 90 minutes, it may influence the quality of recovery and contribute to post-anesthesia ataxia.

Reproductive/Nursing Safety
The manufacturer states that "Information on the possible effects of detomidine HCl in breeding horses is limited to uncontrolled clinical reports; therefore, this drug is not recommended for use in breeding animals." In pregnant ruminants however, at recommended doses detomidine is considered less likely than xylazine to induce premature parturition.

Overdosage/Acute Toxicity
The manufacturer states that detomidine is tolerated by horses at doses 5X (0.2 mg/kg) the high dose level (0.04 mg/kg). Doses of 0.4 mg/kg given daily for 3 consecutive days produced microscopic foci of myocardial necrosis in 1 of 8 horses tested. Doses of 10-40X recommended may cause severe respiratory and cardiovascular changes that can become irreversible and cause death. Yohimbine or atipamezole could be used to reverse some or all of the effects of the drug. Atipamezole at a dose of 50 – 100 micrograms/kg has

been successfully used to treat inadvertent overdoses of detomidine in horses.

Drug Interactions

The following drug interactions have either been reported or are theoretical in humans or animals receiving detomidine and may be of significance in veterinary patients. Unless otherwise noted, use together is not necessarily contraindicated, but weigh the potential risks and perform additional monitoring when appropriate.

- **ALPHA-2 AGONISTS, OTHER** (*e.g.*, **xylazine, medetomidine, romifidine, clonidine** and including **epinephrine**): Not recommended to be used together with detomidine as effects may be additive.

- **ANESTHETICS, OPIATES, SEDATIVE/HYPNOTICS**: Effects may be additive; dosage reduction of one or both agents may be required; potential for increased risk for arrhythmias when used in combination with thiopental, ketamine or halothane.

- **EPINEPHRINE**: As epinephrine possesses alpha agonist effects, do not use to treat cardiac effects caused by detomidine.

- **PHENOTHIAZINES** (*e.g.*, **acepromazine**): Severe hypotension can result.

- **SEDATIVES OR ANALGESICS, OTHER**: The manufacturer warns to use with extreme caution in combination with other sedative or analgesic drugs.

- **SULFONAMIDES, POTENTIATED** (*e.g.*, **trimethoprim/sulfa**): The manufacturer warns against using this agent with intravenous potentiated sulfonamides as fatal dysrhythmias may occur.

- **YOHIMBINE**: IV yohimbine has been shown in horses to effectively reverse detomidine-induced sedation, bradycardia, AV block and hyperglycemia (Knych, Covarrubias, et al. 2012), but a study done in horses demonstrated that yohimbine's clearance and volume of distribution decreased and plasma concentrations were higher when it was given after detomidine. Any clinical significance is not yet clear, and further study is warranted. (Knych, Steffey, et al. 2012)

Doses

CAUTION: Do not confuse <u>microgram/kg</u> with <u>mg/kg</u> doses.

- **DOGS:**

  As a sedative/anxiolytic (extra-label; from a study in 6 dogs): Using the equine oromucosal gel; 0.35 mg/m² administered via the OTM route. For 4 dogs, maximal global sedation (GS) scores occurred at 45 minutes post-treatment, and duration of maximal GS scores was 30 minutes. Five of 6 dogs achieved adequate GS scores. Ease of handling scores were significantly higher during time points of adequate GS scores as compared with time points when adequate GS scores were not achieved. 5 of 6 dogs developed transient bradycardia and one dog developed intermittent second-degree atrioventricular block. Further evaluation is warranted for use in client-owned dogs. (Hopfensperger et al. 2013)

- **HORSES:** (NOTE: ARCI UCGFS CLASS 3 DRUG)

  For sedation/analgesia (labeled doses; FDA-approved):

  Injection: 20 – 40 micrograms/kg (0.02 – 0.04 mg/kg) IV or IM (IV only for analgesia). Effects generally occur within 2-5 minutes. Lower dose will generally provide 30-90 minutes of sedation and 30-45 minutes of analgesia. The higher dose will generally provide 90-120 minutes of sedation and 45-75 minutes of analgesia. Allow animal to rest quietly prior to and after injection.

  Sublingual Gel: 0.04 mg/kg (0.018 mg/lb.) placed beneath the tongue of the horse; not meant to be swallowed. The dosing syringe delivers the product in 0.25 mL increments. The package insert provides a dosing table to determine correct amount of gel

to administer for the weight of the horse. (Adapted from label; *Dormosedan®*; *Dormosedan Gel®*—Pfizer)

For sedation, chemical restraint, analgesia (extra-label doses):

As a premedicant: 0.005 – 0.03 mg/kg IV. (Lerche 2013)

For caudal epidural analgesia: 0.06 mg/kg, given between S4-S5; duration of analgesia is 2-3 hours <u>or</u> detomidine 0.03 mg/kg with morphine (0.2 mg mg/kg) given between S1-L6; duration of analgesia is >6 hours. (Muir 2004)

As a CRI for total intravenous anesthesia (TIVA): Using the GKD triple-drip protocol: Add 10 mg detomidine and 500 – 1000 mg of ketamine to 500 mL of 5% guaifenesin. This will yield concentrations of: 50 mg/mL of guaifenesin; 1 – 2 mg/mL of ketamine and 20 micrograms/mL of detomidine. The CRI infusion rate is: 1.2 – 1.6 mL/kg/hour. **Note:** If using 500mL of 10% guaifenesin as the base, amounts of the other drugs added should be doubled, leading to final concentrations that are doubled, and infusion rate will be halved. (Lerche 2013)

As a CRI for sedation or partial intravenous anesthesia (PIVA): Sedation: 22 micrograms/kg/hour. **PIVA:** 13 – 38 micrograms/kg/hour seem appropriate to obtain a significant MAC reduction, because lower doses were not associated with a MAC-sparing effect. (Valverde 2013)

- **CATTLE:**

  To produce standing sedation with a low incidence of recumbency (extra-label): <u>Tractable cattle</u>: 0.002 – 0.005 mg/kg (IV), 0.006 – 0.01 mg/kg (IM); <u>Anxious cattle</u>: 0.005 – 0.0075 mg/kg (IV), 0.01 – 0.015 mg/kg IM; <u>Extremely anxious or unruly cattle</u>: 0.01 – 0.015 mg/kg (IV), 0.0015 – 0.02 mg/kg (IM). Information regarding the use of detomidine in ruminants is limited. The dose ranges provided are estimates and should be adjusted based on experience. Administering the IV dose IM further reduces the possibility of recumbency. (Abrahamsen 2013)

  For analgesia (extra-label): 0.01 mg/kg IV; short (1/2 hour) duration of action. Appropriate withdrawal times are: Milk = 72 hours; Slaughter = 7 days. (Walz 2006)

- **SHEEP, GOATS:**

  Extra-label: For anesthesia: Detomidine at 0.01 mg/kg IM, followed by propofol at 3 – 5 mg/kg IV. **For analgesia:** 0.005 – 0.05 mg/kg IV or IM q3-6 hours (once). (Haskell 2005)

- **LLAMAS, ALPACAS:**

  For analgesia (extra-label): 0.005 – 0.05 mg/kg IV or IM q3-6 hours (once). (Haskell 2005)

- **BIRDS:**

  For sedation/analgesia (extra-label): 0.3 mg/kg IM; limited data available on duration of effect, adverse effects, etc. (Clyde et al. 2000)

Monitoring

- Level of sedation, analgesia.
- Cardiac rate/rhythm; blood pressure if indicated.

Client Information

- When used parenterally (by injection), detomidine should be used in a professionally supervised setting by individuals familiar with its properties.
- When handling the oromucosal gel wear disposable gloves; avoid skin contact.
- If dispensing gel for client administration, give client the **Client Information Sheet For Owner/Handler Use and Safety.**

Chemistry/Synonyms

An imidazoline derivative alpha$_2$-adrenergic agonist, detomidine HCl occurs as a white crystalline substance that is soluble in water.

Detomidine HCl may also be known as: demotidini hydrochloridum, MPV-253-AII, or *Dormosedan®*.

Storage/Stability

Detomidine HCl for injection should be stored at room temperature (59-85°F; 15-30°C) and protected from light.

Detomidine gel for SL administration should be stored at controlled room temperature (68-77°F; 20-25°C); excursions are permitted to 59-85°F (15-30°C).

Dosage Forms/Regulatory Status

VETERINARY-LABELED PRODUCTS:

Detomidine HCl for Injection: 10 mg/mL in 5 mL and 20 mL vials; *Dormosedan®*; (Rx). FDA-approved for use in mature horses and yearlings. In ruminants, the reported FARAD-suggested withdrawal time for single doses of detomidine of up to 0.08 mg/kg IM or IV are 3 days for meat and 72 hours for milk (Lin 2012).

Detomidine HCL Oromucosal Gel for Sublingual Administration: 7.8 mg/mL in 3 mL graduated dosing syringes; *Dormosedan Gel®*; (Rx). FDA-approved (NADA #141-306) for use in horses not intended for human consumption. Based upon the times when detomidine was not detectable in blood and urine, one study recommended a 72-hour wait time after a single 40 mcg/kg SL dose for horses (l'Ami et al. 2013). A link to the label information for *Dormosedan Gel®* can be found at dailymed.nlm.nih.gov

The ARCI (Racing Commissioners International) has designated this drug as a class 3 substance.

HUMAN-LABELED PRODUCTS: NONE.

Revisions/References

Monograph revised/updated January 2014.

Abrahamsen, E. J. (2013). Chemical Restraint and Injectable Anesthesia of Ruminants. Veterinary Clinics of North America-Food Animal Practice 29(1): 209-+.

Anderson, D. E. & M. A. Edmondson (2013). Prevention and Management of Surgical Pain in Cattle. Veterinary Clinics of North America-Food Animal Practice 29(1): 157-+.

Clyde, V. & J. Paul-Murphy (2000). Avian Analgesia. *Kirk's Current Veterinary Therapy: XIII Small Animal Practice.* J. Bonagura. Philadelphia, WB Saunders: 1126-8.

Haskell, R. (2005). Development of a Small Ruminant Formulary. Proceedings: WVC. accessed via Veterinary Information Network; vin.com

Hopfensperger, M. J., et al. (2013). The use of oral transmucosal detomidine hydrochloride gel to facilitate handling in dogs. Journal of Veterinary Behavior-Clinical Applications and Research 8(3): 114-23.

Hubbell, J. A. E., et al. (2009). Pharmacokinetics of detomidine administered to horses at rest and after maximal exercise. Equine Veterinary Journal 41(5): 419-22.

Kaukinen, H., et al. (2009). Bioavailability of Detomidine Administered to Horses as an Oromucosal (Sublingual) Gel and Comparison of Absorption of Detomidine by the Sublingual and Intramuscular Routes. Proceedings: ACVIM. accessed via Veterinary Information Network; vin.com

Knych, H., et al. (2012). Effect of yohimbine on detomidine induced changes in behavior, cardiac and blood parameters in the horse. Vet Anaesth Analg 39(6): 574-83.

Knych, H. K., et al. (2012). The effects of yohimbine on the pharmacokinetic parameters of detomidine in the horse. Veterinary Anaesthesia and Analgesia 39(3): 221-9.

l'Ami, J. J., et al. (2013). Sublingual administration of detomidine in horses: Sedative effect, analgesia and detection time. Veterinary Journal 196(2): 253-9.

Lerche, P. (2013). Total Intravenous Anesthesia in Horses. Veterinary Clinics of North America-Equine Practice 29(1): 123-+.

Lin, H.-C. (2012). Large Ruminants Anesthesia: Review and Update. Western Veterinary Conference. accessed via Veterinary Information Network; vin.com

Mama, K. R., et al. (2009). Plasma concentrations, behavioural and physiological effects following intravenous and intramuscular detomidine in horses. Equine Veterinary Journal 41(8): 772-7.

Muir, W. (2004). Recognizing and treating pain in horses. *Equine Internal Medicine, 2nd Ed.* S. Reed, W. Bayly and D. Sellon. Philadelphia, Saunders: 1529-42.

Valverde, A. (2013). Balanced Anesthesia and Constant-Rate Infusions in Horses. Veterinary Clinics of North America-Equine Practice 29(1): 89-+.

Walz, P. (2006). Practical management of pain in cattle. Proceedings: ABVP. accessed via Veterinary Information Network; vin.com

---

Dexamethasone
Dexamethasone Sodium Phosphate

(dex-a-meth-a-zone)   Azium®, Dexasone®

Glucocorticoid

Prescriber Highlights

▶ Injectable, oral & ophthalmic glucocorticoid.

▶ Long acting; 30X more potent than hydrocortisone; no mineralocorticoid activity.

▶ If using for therapy, goal is to use as much as is required, but as little and for as short an amount of time as possible.

▶ Primary adverse effects are "Cushingoid" in nature with sustained use, but acute effects (primarily GI, colon perforation in dogs after high doses) can be seen.

▶ Many potential drug & lab interactions.

Uses/Indications

Glucocorticoids have been used in an attempt to treat practically every malady that afflicts man or animal, but there are three broad uses and dosage ranges for use of these agents: 1) Replacement of glucocorticoid activity in patients with adrenal insufficiency, 2) as an antiinflammatory agent, and 3) as an immunosuppressive. Glucocorticoids are used in the treatment of endocrine conditions (*e.g.*, adrenal insufficiency), rheumatic diseases (*e.g.*, rheumatoid arthritis), collagen diseases (*e.g.*, systemic lupus), allergic states/anaphylaxis, envenomation, inducing fetal maturation, respiratory diseases (*e.g.*, asthma), dermatologic diseases (*e.g.*, pemphigus, allergic dermatoses), hematologic disorders (*e.g.*, thrombocytopenias, autoimmune hemolytic anemia), neoplasias, nervous system disorders (increased CSF pressure), GI diseases (*e.g.*, ulcerative colitis exacerbations), and renal diseases (*e.g.*, nephrotic syndrome). Some glucocorticoids are used topically in the eye and skin for various conditions or are injected intra-articularly or intra-lesionally. This listing is certainly not complete. High dose fast-acting corticosteroids are no longer recommended for use in shock or CNS trauma; recent studies have not demonstrated significant benefit and it actually may cause increased deleterious effects.

Pharmacology/Actions

Glucocorticoids have effects on virtually every cell type and system in mammals. An overview of the effects of these agents follows:

Cardiovascular System: Glucocorticoids can reduce capillary permeability and enhance vasoconstriction. A relatively clinically insignificant positive inotropic effect can occur after glucocorticoid administration. Increased blood pressure can result from both the drugs' vasoconstrictive properties and increased blood volume that may be produced.

Cells: Glucocorticoids inhibit fibroblast proliferation, macrophage response to migration inhibiting factor, sensitization of lymphocytes and the cellular response to mediators of inflammation. Glucocorticoids stabilize lysosomal membranes.

CNS/Autonomic Nervous System: Glucocorticoids can lower seizure threshold, alter mood and behavior, diminish the response to pyrogens, stimulate appetite and maintain alpha rhythm. Glucocorticoids are necessary for normal adrenergic receptor sensitivity.

Endocrine System: When animals are not stressed, glucocorticoids will suppress the release of ACTH from the anterior pituitary, thereby reducing or preventing the release of endogenous corticosteroids. Stress factors (*e.g.*, renal disease, liver disease, diabetes) may sometimes nullify the suppressing aspects of exogenously administered steroids. Release of thyroid-stimulating hormone (TSH), follicle-stimulating hormone (FSH), prolactin, and luteinizing hormone (LH) may all be reduced when glucocorticoids are administered at pharmacological doses. Conversion of thyroxine (T$_4$) to triiodothyronine (T$_3$) may be reduced by glucocorticoids; plasma levels of parathyroid hormone increased. Glucocorticoids may inhibit osteoblast function. Vasopressin (ADH) activity is reduced at the renal tubules and diuresis may occur. Glucocorticoids inhibit insulin binding to insulin-receptors and the post-receptor effects of insulin.

Hematopoietic System: Glucocorticoids can increase the numbers of circulating platelets, neutrophils and red blood cells, but platelet aggregation is inhibited. Decreased amounts of lymphocytes (peripheral), monocytes and eosinophils are seen as glucocorticoids can sequester these cells into the lungs and spleen and prompt decreased release from the bone marrow. Removal of old red blood cells becomes diminished. Glucocorticoids can cause involution of lymphoid tissue.

GI Tract and Hepatic System: Glucocorticoids increase the secretion of gastric acid, pepsin, and trypsin. They alter the structure of mucin and decrease mucosal cell proliferation. Iron salts and calcium absorption are decreased while fat absorption is increased. Hepatic changes can include increased fat and glycogen deposits within hepatocytes, increased serum levels of alanine aminotransferase (ALT), and gamma-glutamyl transpeptidase (GGT). Significant increases can be seen in serum alkaline phosphatase levels. Glucocorticoids can cause minor increases in BSP (bromosulfophthalein) retention time.

Immune System (also see Cells and Hematopoietic System): Glucocorticoids can decrease circulating levels of T-lymphocytes; inhibit lymphokines; inhibit neutrophil, macrophage, and monocyte migration; reduce production of interferon; inhibit phagocytosis and chemotaxis; antigen processing; and diminish intracellular killing. Specific acquired immunity is affected less than nonspecific immune responses. Glucocorticoids can also antagonize the complement cascade and mask the clinical signs of infection. Mast cells are decreased in number and histamine synthesis is suppressed. Many of these effects only occur at high or very high doses and there are species differences in response.

Metabolic effects: Glucocorticoids stimulate gluconeogenesis. Lipogenesis is enhanced in certain areas of the body (*e.g.*, abdomen) and adipose tissue can be redistributed away from the extremities to the trunk. Fatty acids are mobilized from tissues and their oxidation is increased. Plasma levels of triglycerides, cholesterol, and glycerol are increased. Protein is mobilized from most areas of the body (not the liver).

Musculoskeletal: Glucocorticoids may cause muscular weakness (also caused if there is a lack of glucocorticoids), atrophy, and osteoporosis. Bone growth can be inhibited via growth hormone and somatomedin inhibition, increased calcium excretion and inhibition of vitamin D activation. Resorption of bone can be enhanced. Fibrocartilage growth is also inhibited.

Ophthalmic: Prolonged corticosteroid use (both systemic or topically to the eye) can cause increased intraocular pressure and glaucoma, cataracts, and exophthalmos.

Renal, Fluid, & Electrolytes: Glucocorticoids can increase potassium and calcium excretion, sodium and chloride reabsorption, and extracellular fluid volume. Hypokalemia and/or hypocalcemia rarely occur. Diuresis may develop following glucocorticoid administration.

Skin: Thinning of dermal tissue and skin atrophy can be seen with glucocorticoid therapy. Hair follicles can become distended and alopecia may occur.

Pharmacokinetics

The pharmacokinetics of dexamethasone does not translate into pharmacologic effect. The half-life of dexamethasone in dogs is about 2-5 hours, but biologic activity can persist for 48 hours or more. In horses, after dosages of 0.05 mg/kg PO, IV, IM, or IA, endogenous cortisol levels did not return to baseline until between 96-120 hours (IV, IM, IA) and 72 hours (PO) (Soma et al. 2013).

Contraindications/Precautions/Warnings

Because dexamethasone has negligible mineralocorticoid effect, it should generally not be used alone in the treatment of adrenal insufficiency.

Do not administer the propylene glycol base injectable product rapidly intravenously; hypotension, collapse, and hemolytic anemia can occur. Many clinicians only use dexamethasone sodium phosphate when giving the drug intravenously.

In dogs, dexamethasone can cause more gastrointestinal complications and bleeding than prednisone, so careful attention to the minimum dosing necessary is required. There is a high incidence of gastrointestinal bleeding and colonic perforation in canine neurosurgical patients treated with dexamethasone (also seen with methylprednisolone sodium succinate); the dose and duration of therapy should be limited to as short a time as possible, and prednisone or prednisolone used when possible instead of dexamethasone (Wilson 2011). Animals with significantly diminished renal function may be more susceptible to GI adverse effects.

Rabbits reportedly can develop serious adverse effects to dexamethasone, even after single doses.

Systemic use of glucocorticoids is generally considered contraindicated in systemic fungal infections (unless used for replacement therapy in Addison's), when administered IM in patients with idiopathic thrombocytopenia and those hypersensitive to a particular drug. Use of sustained-release injectable glucocorticoids is considered contraindicated for chronic corticosteroid therapy of systemic diseases.

Unless very short-term burst therapy is used, patients that have received systemic glucocorticoids systemically should be tapered off the drug. Tapers should be slow if the patient has been receiving a glucocorticoid chronically as endogenous ACTH and corticosteroid function may return slowly. Should the animal undergo a "stressor" (*e.g.*, surgery, trauma, illness, etc.) during the tapering process and/or until normal adrenal and pituitary function resume, additional glucocorticoids should be administered.

Animals, particularly cats, at risk for diabetes mellitus or with concurrent cardiovascular disease should receive glucocorticoids with caution due to these agents' potent hyperglycemic effect.

Adverse Effects

Serious adverse effects are generally associated with long-term administration of these drugs, especially if given at high dosages or not on an alternate day regimen though acute use at high dosages, especially in dogs, can produce serious effects including GI ulceration/perforation and bleeding. Effects associated with chronic therapy generally are manifested as clinical signs of hyperadrenocorticism. Glucocorticoids can retard growth in young animals. Many of the potential effects, adverse and otherwise, are outlined above in the Pharmacology section.

In dogs, polydipsia (PD), polyphagia (PP) and polyuria (PU), may all be seen with short-term "burst" therapy as well as with alternate-day maintenance therapy on days when giving the drug. Very high doses in dogs with spinal chord injuries have caused fatal colon perforations. Other adverse effects in dogs can include: dull, dry haircoat, weight gain, panting, vomiting, diarrhea, elevated liver enzymes, pancreatitis, GI ulceration, lipidemias, activation or worsening of diabetes mellitus, muscle wasting, and behavioral changes (depression, lethargy, viciousness). Discontinuation of the drug may be necessary; changing to an alternate steroid may also alleviate the problem. With the exception of PU/PD/PP, adverse effects associated with antiinflammatory therapy are relatively uncommon. Adverse effects associated with immunosuppressive doses are more common and, potentially, more severe.

Cats generally require higher dosages than dogs for clinical effect, but tend to develop fewer adverse effects. Glucocorticoids appear to have a greater hyperglycemic effect in cats than other species. Occasionally, polydipsia, polyuria, polyphagia with weight gain, diarrhea, or depression can be seen. Long-term, high dose therapy can lead to "Cushingoid" effects, however.

Administration of dexamethasone or triamcinolone may play a role in the development of laminitis in horses, but this is thought to occur only rarely.

Reproductive/Nursing Safety

Corticosteroid therapy may induce parturition in large animal species during the latter stages of pregnancy. In humans, the FDA categorizes this drug as category *C* for use during pregnancy (*Animal studies have shown an adverse effect on the fetus, but there are no adequate studies in humans; or there are no animal reproduction studies and no adequate studies in humans.*) In a separate system evaluating the safety of drugs in canine and feline pregnancy (Papich 1989), this drug is categorized as class: C (*These drugs may have potential risks. Studies in people or laboratory animals have uncovered risks, and these drugs should be used cautiously as a last resort when the benefit of therapy clearly outweighs the risks.*)

Overdosage/Acute Toxicity

Glucocorticoids when given short-term are unlikely to cause significant harmful effects, but dogs may be susceptible to GI ulceration/perforation. One incidence of a dog developing acute CNS effects after accidental ingestion of glucocorticoids has been reported. Should clinical signs occur, use supportive treatment if necessary.

Chronic usage of glucocorticoids can lead to serious adverse effects. Refer to Adverse Effects above for more information.

Drug Interactions

The following drug interactions have either been reported or are theoretical in humans or animals receiving dexamethasone and may be of significance in veterinary patients. Unless otherwise noted, use together is not necessarily contraindicated, but weigh the potential risks and perform additional monitoring when appropriate.

- **AMPHOTERICIN B:** Administered concomitantly with glucocorticoids may cause hypokalemia.
- **ANTICHOLINESTERASE AGENTS** (*e.g.,* **pyridostigmine, neostigmine,** etc.): In patients with myasthenia gravis, concomitant glucocorticoid and anticholinesterase agent administration may lead to profound muscle weakness. If possible, discontinue anticholinesterase medication at least 24 hours prior to corticosteroid administration
- **ASPIRIN:** Glucocorticoids may reduce salicylate blood levels.
- **BARBITURATES:** May increase the metabolism of glucocorticoids and decrease dexamethasone blood levels.
- **CYCLOPHOSPHAMIDE:** Glucocorticoids may also inhibit the hepatic metabolism of cyclophosphamide; dosage adjustments may be required.
- **CYCLOSPORINE:** Concomitant administration of glucocorticoids and cyclosporine may increase the blood levels of each, by mutually inhibiting the hepatic metabolism of each other; the clinical significance of this interaction is not clear.
- **DIAZEPAM:** Dexamethasone may decrease diazepam levels.
- **DIURETICS, POTASSIUM-DEPLETING** (*e.g.,* **spironolactone, triamterene**): Administered concomitantly with glucocorticoids may cause hypokalemia.

- **EPHEDRINE:** May reduce dexamethasone blood levels and interfere with dexamethasone suppression tests.
- **INDOMETHACIN:** Can cause false negative test results in the dexamethasone suppression test.
- **INSULIN:** Insulin requirements may increase in patients receiving glucocorticoids.
- **KETOCONAZOLE** and other **AZOLE ANTIFUNGALS:** May decrease the metabolism of glucocorticoids and increase dexamethasone blood levels; ketoconazole may induce adrenal insufficiency when glucocorticoids are withdrawn by inhibiting adrenal corticosteroid synthesis.
- **MACROLIDE ANTIBIOTICS** (*e.g.,* **erythromycin, clarithromycin**): May decrease the metabolism of glucocorticoids and increase dexamethasone blood levels.
- **MITOTANE:** May alter the metabolism of steroids; higher than usual doses of steroids may be necessary to treat mitotane-induced adrenal insufficiency.
- **NSAIDS:** Administration of ulcerogenic drugs with glucocorticoids may increase the risk of gastrointestinal ulceration.
- **PHENYTOIN:** May increase the metabolism of glucocorticoids and decrease dexamethasone blood levels.
- **RIFAMPIN:** May increase the metabolism of glucocorticoids and decrease dexamethasone blood levels.
- **DEXAMETHASONE:** In dogs, dexamethasone increased quinidine volume of distribution (49-78%) and elimination half-life (1.5-2.3X). (Zhang et al. 2006)
- **VACCINES:** Patients receiving corticosteroids at immunosuppressive dosages should generally not receive live attenuated-virus vaccines as virus replication may be augmented; a diminished immune response may occur after vaccine, toxoid, or bacterin administration in patients receiving glucocorticoids.

Laboratory Considerations

- While dexamethasone does not interfere with the cortisol assay, over a few days it will suppress the HPA axis and suppress endogenous release of cortisol, so if using it to diagnose hypoadrenocorticism, **ACTH stimulation tests** should be performed as soon as possible.
- Glucocorticoids may increase **serum cholesterol.**
- Glucocorticoids may increase **urine glucose** levels.
- Glucocorticoids may decrease **serum potassium.**
- Glucocorticoids can suppress the release of thyroid stimulating hormone (TSH) and reduce T3 & T4 values. Thyroid gland atrophy has been reported after chronic glucocorticoid administration. Uptake of I¹³¹ by the thyroid may be decreased by glucocorticoids.
- Reactions to **skin tests** may be suppressed by glucocorticoids.
- False-negative results of the **nitroblue tetrazolium** test for systemic bacterial infections may be induced by glucocorticoids.
- Glucocorticoids may cause **neutrophilia** within 4-8 hours after dosing and return to baseline within 24-48 hours after drug discontinuation.
- Glucocorticoids can cause **lymphopenia** in dogs that can persist for weeks after drug discontinuation.

Doses

- **DOGS:**

Note: Generally, most veterinarians use prednisone or prednisolone when a glucocorticoid is administered as an antiinflammatory agent or immunosuppressive orally to dogs. Despite a short circulating half-life, dexamethasone has a long biologic duration of effect (thought to be >48 hours, whereas the biologic duration of effect of prednisone is 12-36 hours). Thus, it is difficult to spare normal adrenal function, even when dexamethasone is given every other day. (Wilson 2011)

For labeled indications (antiinflammatory; glucocorticoid agent): Note: The labeled dose for dogs does not represent what is generally used by most veterinarians today. Injection: 0.5 – 1 mg IV or IM; may be repeated for 3-5 days; Tablets: 0.25 – 1.25 mg PO daily in single or two divided doses. (Package Insert; *Azium®*)

Replacement of glucocorticoid activity in patients with adrenal insufficiency (Note: Dexamethasone has no mineralocorticoid activity):

a) **For Addisonian crises:** give 0.1 – 0.2 mg/kg dexamethasone sodium phosphate IV as the initial dose. Dexamethasone is not measured on the cortisol assay, so the ACTH stimulation test will be valid after dexamethasone is used. If the dog is vomiting/inappetent, dexamethasone may be continued at a dose of 0.05 – 0.1 mg/kg q12h until able to switch to oral prednisone as the glucocorticoid replacement (see Prednisone monograph for more information). (Wilson 2011)

b) **For Addisonian crisis:** Dexamethasone sodium phosphate at 0.2 – 0.5 mg/kg IV once; maintenance therapy with prednisone. Dexamethasone, unlike prednisone will not interfere with cortisol assays. (Jutkowitz 2009)

c) **For adjunctive acute treatment** (including correction of hypotension/hypovolemia, electrolyte imbalances, acidosis, hypoglycemia, and hypercalcemia): Immediately place IV catheter in cephalic or jugular vein, and collect a blood sample for measurement of electrolytes and cortisol. Cosyntropin (synthetic ACTH) is then administered IV, and a second blood sample for measurement of cortisol collected 1 hour later. Fluid therapy (0.9% saline IV, 30 – 80 mL/kg/24 hours plus correction for dehydration) should be started immediately. After the second blood sample is collected, give prednisolone sodium succinate (4 – 20 mg/kg IV), or hydrocortisone hemisuccinate or hydrocortisone phosphate (2 – 4 mg/kg IV) or dexamethasone sodium phosphate at 0.5 – 2 mg/kg as an initial dose. Then add dexamethasone at a dose of 0.05 – 0.1 mg/kg q12 hours into fluids until able to switch to oral glucocorticoids. If animal is in shock, administration of steroids should be at shock doses and this should take precedence over establishing an immediate diagnosis. For dogs with hyperkalemia consider IV glucose and insulin to rapidly lower serum potassium, and calcium gluconate to protect the heart from the cardiosuppressive effects of hyperkalemia. (Scott-Moncrieff 2010)

As an IV alternative to PO prednisone for immune-suppression (e.g., immune-mediated thrombocytopenia); (extra-label): Dexamethasone sodium phosphate 0.35 mg/kg IV q24h.

For use a diagnostic agent:

Low-Dose Dexamethasone Suppression (LDDS) Test (extra-label): Obtain plasma samples for cortisol before and 4 and 8 hours after IV administration of 0.01 mg/kg dexamethasone. The 8-hour plasma cortisol is used as a screening test for hyperadrenocorticism, with concentrations >1.4 micrograms/dL being consistent with (not confirming) the diagnosis of Cushing's syndrome. Test is relatively sensitive and specific, but not perfect. Approximately 90% of dogs with Cushing's syndrome have an 8 hour post-dexamethasone plasma cortisol concentration >1.4 micrograms/dL and another 6-8% have values of 0.9-1.3 micrograms/dL. The results of a low dose test can also aid in discriminating pituitary-dependent hyperadrenocorticism (PDH) from adrenocortical tumor (ACT), using 3 criteria: 1) an 8 hour plasma cortisol >1.4 micrograms/dL but <50% of the basal value; 2) a 4 hour plasma cortisol concentration <1.0 micrograms/dL; and 3) a 4 hour plasma cortisol concentration <50% of the basal value. If a dog has Cushing's and it meets any of these 3 criteria, it most likely has PDH. Approximately 65% of dogs with naturally occurring PDH demonstrate suppression, as defined by these 3 criteria. A dog with Cushing's that fails to meet any of these 3 criteria could have either PDH or ACT. However, if two relatively equal sized adrenals on abdominal ultrasonography, it most likely has PDH. (Feldman 2009)

Oral Dexamethasone Suppression Test (extra-label): An alternative 'at home' oral dexamethasone suppression test relies on results of urine cortisol/creatinine ratio (UCCR) to establish the diagnosis of hyperadrenocorticism and identify pituitary-dependent hyperadrenocorticism (PDH). The owner collects 2 urine samples from the dog on 2 consecutive mornings and stores them in the refrigerator. After collection of the second urine sample, the owner administers 3 doses of dexamethasone (0.1 mg/kg/dose) at 8-hour intervals. Urine is collected on the morning of the third day and UCCR is determined on all 3 samples. The first 2 urine samples establish the diagnosis of hyperadrenocorticism; both results must be abnormal. If both values are abnormal, then the average of the 2 values are used as the 'baseline' value and compared with the third value obtained after dexamethasone. A diagnosis of PDH is established if the UCCR result from the third urine sample is less than 50% of the 'baseline' value. Dogs failing to meet these criteria could have either cortisol secreting adrenocortical tumor (ADH) or PDH. (Nelson 2013)

High-Dose Dexamethasone Suppression (HDDS) Test (extra-label): Relatively easy to perform (plasma obtained before and 4 or 8 hours after IV administration of 0.1 mg/kg dexamethasone), readily available and inexpensive. If a dog has Cushing's syndrome and the plasma cortisol, 8 hours post-dexamethasone, is <50% of the basal value, the dog has pituitary-dependent hyperadrenocorticism (PDH). However, our experience with the LDDS and abdominal ultrasonography has limited the need and use of HDDS. Approximately 75% of dogs with PDH demonstrate suppression with the HDDS. Realizing that approximately 65% of PDH dogs demonstrate "suppression" consistent with PDH on the LDDS limits the value of this test by only identifying an additional 10% of afflicted dogs. (Feldman 2009)

- **CATS:**

Note: Generally, most veterinarians use prednisolone when a glucocorticoid is administered orally to cats. If using dexamethasone, figure the dose for prednisolone and administer 10-20% of that dose as dexamethasone. Approximately 0.75 mg of dexamethasone is equivalent to 5 mg prednisone.

For labeled indications (antiinflammatory; glucocorticoid agent): Injection: 0.125 – 0.5 mg IV or IM; may be repeated for 3-5 days; Tablets: 0.125 – 0.5 mg daily in single or divided doses. (Package Insert; *Azium®*)

Low-Dose Dexamethasone Suppression (LDDS) Test (extra-label): Test of choice for diagnosis of feline hyperadrenocorticism; uses a higher dose of dexamethasone (0.1 mg/kg IV) than in dogs. A base-line blood sample is collected, and additional samples are collected at 4 and 8 hours after dexamethasone administration. Cortisol concentration will be suppressed (<1.5 micrograms/dL) at 8 hours in normal cats but not in cats with hyperadrenocorticism. A few cats with HAC will suppress normally on the LDDS. If the index of suspicion for hyperadrenocorticism is high, a second test using the lower dose of dexamethasone (0.01 mg/kg) can be performed, but some normal cats will fail to suppress at this dose. (Scott-Moncrieff 2010)

- **RABBITS/RODENTS/SMALL MAMMALS:**

  Extra-label: Mice, Rats, Gerbils, Hamsters, Guinea pigs, Chinchillas: 0.6 mg/kg IM (as an antiinflammatory). (Adamcak et al. 2000)

- **CATTLE:**

  For adjunctive therapy of insect bites or stings (extra-label): 2 mg/kg IM or IV q4h (use epinephrine if anaphylaxis develops). (Fowler 1993)

  For primary bovine ketosis (labeled-dose): 5 – 20 mg IV or IM. (Package Insert; *Azium®*)

- **HORSES:** (NOTE: ARCI UCGFS CLASS 4 DRUG)

  For labeled indications (antiinflammatory; glucocorticoid agent): Dexamethasone Injection: 2.5 – 5 mg IV or IM. (Package Insert; *Azium®*—Schering); Dexamethasone sodium phosphate injection: 2.5 – 5 mg IV. (Package Insert; *Azium® SP*)

  For adjunctive treatment of recurrent airway obstruction (extra-label):

  a) For a 500 kg horse give 40 mg IM once every other day for 3 treatments, followed by 35 mg IM once every other day for 3 treatments, followed by 30 mg IM once every other day for 3 treatments, etc., until horse is weaned off dexamethasone. Corticosteroid use may be contraindicated in horses predisposed to laminitis or exhibiting endocrinopathies. (Ainsworth et al. 2004)

  b) For short term treatment with environmental control: In the study, dexamethasone sodium phosphate was dosed at 0.1 mg/kg IM once daily for 4 days, 0.075 mg/kg IM once daily for 4 days, and 0.05 mg/kg IM for 4 days. Except for bronchoalveolar lavage cytology, oral prednisolone (1 mg/kg PO X 4d, 0.75 mg/kg PO x 4d, 0.5 mg/kg PO x 4d) was as effective as IM dexamethasone. (Courouce-Malblanc et al. 2008)

  c) In this study, horses were under continuous antigen exposure: Dexamethasone was given at 0.05 mg/kg PO once daily for 7 days or prednisolone (2 mg/kg PO once daily for 7 days). Both were effective, but dexamethasone more so. (Leclere et al. 2010)

  Dexamethasone suppression test (extra-label): 20 mg IM. Normal values: Cortisol levels decrease 50% in 2 hours, 70% in 4 hours, and 80% at 6 hours. At 24 hours, levels are still depressed about 30% of original value. (Beech 1987)

Monitoring

Monitoring of glucocorticoid therapy is dependent on its reason for use, dosage, agent used (amount of mineralocorticoid activity), dosage schedule (daily versus alternate day therapy), duration of therapy, and the animal's age and condition. The following list may not be appropriate or complete for all animals; use clinical assessment and judgment should adverse effects be noted:

- Weight, appetite, signs of edema.
- Serum and/or urine electrolytes.
- Total plasma proteins, albumin.
- Blood glucose.
- Growth and development in young animals
- ACTH stimulation test if necessary.

Client Information

- Long acting glucocorticoid. Goal is to find the lowest dose possible and use for the shortest period of time, but do not discontinue the drug on your own without first talking with your veterinarian.
- May be given with food (preferred way) or without food. If your animal vomits or acts sick after getting it on an empty stomach, give with food or small treat to see if this helps. If vomiting continues, contact your veterinarian.
- Many side effects, especially when used long term.
- In dogs, stomach or intestinal ulcers, perforation or bleeding can occur. If your dog stops eating, or you notice a high fever, black tarry stools or bloody vomit, contact your veterinarian right away.

Chemistry/Synonyms

A synthetic glucocorticoid, dexamethasone occurs as an odorless, white to practically white, crystalline powder that melts with some decomposition at about 250°C. It is practically insoluble in water and sparingly soluble in alcohol. Dexamethasone sodium phosphate occurs as an odorless or having a slight odor, white to slightly yellow, hygroscopic powder. One gram is soluble in about 2 mL of water; it is slightly soluble in alcohol.

1.3 mg of dexamethasone sodium phosphate is equivalent to 1 mg of dexamethasone; 4 mg/mL of dexamethasone sodium phosphate injection is approximately equivalent to 3 mg/mL of dexamethasone.

Dexamethasone may also be known as: desamethasone, dexametasone, dexamethasonum, 9alpha-Fluoro-16alpha-methylprednisolone; hexadecadrol; many trade names are available.

Storage/Stability

Dexamethasone is heat labile and should be stored at room temperature (15-30°C) unless otherwise directed by the manufacturer. Dexamethasone sodium phosphate injection should be protected from light. Dexamethasone tablets should be stored in well-closed containers.

Compatibility/Compounding Considerations

Dexamethasone sodium phosphate for injection is reportedly **compatible** with the following drugs: amikacin sulfate, aminophylline, bleomycin sulfate, cimetidine HCl, glycopyrrolate, lidocaine HCl, prochlorperazine edisylate and verapamil.

Dexamethasone sodium phosphate is reportedly **incompatible** with: daunorubicin HCl, doxorubicin HCl, metaraminol bitartrate, and vancomycin. Compatibility is dependent upon factors such as pH, concentration, temperature and diluent used; consult specialized references or a hospital pharmacist for more specific information.

Dosage Forms/Regulatory Status

VETERINARY-LABELED PRODUCTS:

Dexamethasone Injection: 2 mg/mL; *Azium® Solution*, generic; (Rx). FDA-approved for use in dogs, cats, horses (those not intended for food) and cattle. There are no withdrawal times required when used in cattle. A withdrawal period has not been established for this product in preruminal calves; do not use in veal calves.

Dexamethasone Oral Powder: 10 mg crystalline in 10 mg packets; *Azium® Powder*; (Rx). FDA-approved for use in cattle and horses (not horses intended for food).

Dexamethasone Sodium Phosphate Injection: 4 mg/mL (equivalent to 3 mg/mL dexamethasone), generic; (Rx). FDA-approved for use in horses.

Dexamethasone 5 mg and trichlormethiazide 200 mg oral bolus: in boxes of 30 and 100 boluses; *Naquasone® Bolus*; (Rx). FDA-approved for use in cattle. Milk withdrawal = 72 hours.

The ARCI (Racing Commissioners International) has designated dexamethasone as a class 4 substance. See the appendix for more information.

HUMAN-LABELED PRODUCTS:

Dexamethasone Oral Tablets: 0.25 mg, 0.5 mg, 0.75 mg, 1 mg, 1.5 mg, 2 mg, 4 mg, & 6 mg; *Decadron®*, generic; (Rx)

Dexamethasone Oral Elixir/Solution: 0.5 mg/5 mL in 100 mL, 237 mL, 500 mL and UD 5 & UD 20 mL; 1 mg/mL (concentrate) in 30 mL with dropper; *Dexamethasone Intensol®*, generic; (Rx)

Dexamethasone Sodium Phosphate Injection: 4 mg/mL (as sodium phosphate solution) in 1 mL, 5 mL, 10 mL & 30 mL vials, 1 mL syringe & 1 mL fill in 2 mL vials; generic; (Rx); 10 mg/mL (as sodium phosphate solution) in 1 mL and 10 mL vials & 1 mL syringes; generic; (Rx); 20 mg/mL (as sodium phosphate solution) in 5 mL vials (IV); *Hexadrol® Phosphate*; (Rx)

Dexamethasone is also available in topical ophthalmic (see ophthalmic products in the appendix) and inhaled aerosol dosage forms.

Revisions/References

Monograph revised/updated January 2014.

Adamcak, A. & B. Otten (2000). Rodent Therapeutics. Vet Clin NA: Exotic Anim Pract **3**:1(Jan): 221-40.

Ainsworth, D. & R. Hackett (2004). Disorders of the Respiratory System. *Equine Internal Medicine 2nd Ed*. M. Reed, W. Bayly and D. Sellon. Phila., Saunders: 289-354.

Beech, J. (1987). Respiratory Tract—Horse, Cow. *The Bristol Handbook of Antimicrobial Therapy*. D. E. Johnston. Evansville, Veterinary Learning Systems: 88-109.

Courouce-Malblanc, A., et al. (2008). Comparison of prednisolone and dexamethasone effects in the presence of environmental control in heaves-affected horses. Veterinary Journal **175**(2): 227-33.

Feldman, E. C. (2009). Diagnosis & Treatment of Canine Cushing's I: Diagnosis of Hyperadrenocorticism (Cushing's Syndrome) in Dogs--Which Tests are Best? Proceedings: Western Veterinary Conference. accessed via Veterinary Information Network; vin.com

Fowler, M. E. (1993). Zootoxins. *Current Veterinary Therapy: Food Animal Practice 3*. J. L. Howard. Philadelphia, W.B. Saunders: 411-3.

Jutkowitz, L. (2009). Diagnosis and Management of the Addisonian Crisis. Proceedings: WVC. accessed via Veterinary Information Network; vin.com

Leclere, M., et al. (2010). Efficacy of oral prednisolone and dexamethasone in horses with recurrent airway obstruction in the presence of continuous antigen exposure. Equine Veterinary Journal **42**(4): 316-21.

Nelson, R. (2013). Diagnosing Hyperadrenocorticism. World Small Animal Veterinary Association World Congress Proceedings. accessed via Veterinary Information Network; vin.com

Scott-Moncrieff, J. C. (2010). Hypoadrenocorticism in dogs and cats: Update on diagnosis & treatment. Proceedings: ACVIM Forum. accessed via Veterinary Information Network; vin.com

Soma, L. R., et al. (2013). Pharmacokinetics of dexamethasone following intra-articular, intravenous, intramuscular, and oral administration in horses and its effects on endogenous hydrocortisone. J. Vet. Pharmacol. Ther. **36**(2): 181-91.

Wilson, S. (2011). Personal Communication.

Zhang, K. W., et al. (2006). Clinical oral doses of dexamethasone decreases intrinsic clearance of quinidine, a cytochrome P450 3A substrate in dogs. Journal of Veterinary Medical Science **68**(9): 903-7.

Dexmedetomidine

(deks-mee-deh-**toe**-mih-deen)   Dexdomitor®

Alpha-2 Adrenergic Agonist

Prescriber Highlights

▶ Alpha-2 agonist similar to medetomidine used as a preanesthetic & for sedation, analgesia in dogs & cats.

▶ Contraindications: cardiac disease, liver or kidney diseases, shock, severe debilitation, or animals stressed due to heat, cold or fatigue; caution in very old or young animals, animals with seizure disorders, respiratory, renal or kidney disorders.

▶ Adverse Effects: Bradycardia, occasional AV blocks, decreased respiration, hypothermia, urination, vomiting, hyperglycemia, & pain on injection (IM). Rarely: prolonged sedation, paradoxical excitation, hypersensitivity, apnea & death from circulatory failure.

▶ Dosed in dogs based upon body surface area, not weight.

▶ Effects may be reversed with atipamezole.

Uses/Indications

In the USA, dexmedetomidine is FDA-approved for dogs and cats for use as a sedative and analgesic to facilitate clinical examinations, clinical procedures, minor surgical procedures, and minor dental procedures, and as a preanesthetic to general anesthesia.

Pharmacology/Actions

Dexmedetomidine is the dextrorotatory enantiomer of the alpha$_2$-adrenergic agonist, medetomidine. The other enantiomer, levomedetomidine is thought to be pharmacologically inactive so dexmedetomidine is about 2X more potent than medetomidine.

Dexmedetomidine is much more specific than xylazine for alpha$_2$-receptors versus alpha$_1$-receptors. The pharmacologic effects of dexmedetomidine include: depression of CNS (sedation, anxiolysis), analgesia, GI (decreased secretions, varying affects on intestinal muscle tone) and endocrine functions, peripheral and cardiac vasoconstriction, bradycardia, respiratory depression, diuresis, hypothermia, analgesia (somatic and visceral), muscle relaxation (but not enough for intubation), and blanched or cyanotic mucous membranes. Effects on blood pressure are variable, but dexmedetomidine can cause hypertension for a longer time than xylazine.

Pharmacokinetics

In dogs after IM administration, dexmedetomidine is absorbed (bioavailability 60%) and reaches peak plasma levels in about 35 minutes. Volume of distribution is 0.9 L/kg and elimination half-life is approximately 40-50 minutes. The drug is primarily metabolized in the liver via glucuronidation and N-methylation. No metabolites are active and they are eliminated primarily in the urine and, to lesser extent, the feces.

In cats after IM administration, dexmedetomidine is absorbed and reaches peak plasma levels of about 17 ng/mL occur in about 15 minutes. Oral transmucosal (OTM, buccal) administration of dexmedetomidine (40 micrograms/kg) appears to give similar levels (extrapolated from clinical effects) as IM administration in cats (Slingsby et al. 2009). But in comparing OTM versus IM dexmedetomidine (20 micrograms/kg combined with buprenorphine 20 micrograms/kg, another report found that cats in the IM group were more sedated than in the OTM group, but that OTM administration allowed placement of an IV catheter in 75% of the cats (Santos et al. 2009). Volume of distribution is 2.2 L/kg and elimination half-life is approximately 1 hour. Metabolites are eliminated primarily in the urine and to lesser extent, the feces.

In humans after IV administration, dexmedetomidine is rapidly distributed, undergoes almost complete biotransformation via both glucuronidation and CY-450 enzymes systems and has a terminal elimination half-life of about 2 hours. Metabolites are eliminated in the urine and feces.

Contraindications/Precautions/Warnings

The US labeling states not to use in dogs or cats with cardiovascular disease, respiratory disorders, liver or kidney diseases, or in conditions of shock, severe debilitation, or stress due to extreme heat, cold or fatigue. It is not recommended in cats with respiratory disease. Due to the pronounced cardiovascular effects of dexmedetomidine, only clinically healthy dogs and cats should be treated. While not contraindicated in pediatric or geriatric dogs or cats in the US label, it states that the drug has not been evaluated in dogs younger than 16 weeks of age or in cats younger than 12 weeks of age, or in geriatric dogs and cats.

The UK labeling states not to use in puppies less than 6 months old or kittens less than 5 months old; in animals with cardiovascular disorders, or severe systemic disease or that are moribund, or animals known to be hypersensitive to the active substance or any of the excipients.

Use with caution in animals with, or prone to developing, seizures. Dexmedetomidine lowered the seizure threshold in cats undergoing anesthesia with enflurane.

Because blinking may be impaired in cats during sedation and dexmedetomidine/butorphanol has been shown to reduce tear production in dogs (Jalornaki et al. 2007), eye lubricants should be used when using dexmedetomidine.

Adverse Effects

The adverse effects reported with medetomidine or dexmedetomidine are essentially extensions of their pharmacologic effects including bradycardia, vasoconstriction, muscle tremors, transient hypertension, reduced tear production, occasional AV blocks, decreased respiration, hypothermia, urination, vomiting, hyperglycemia, and pain on injection (IM). Rare effects that have been reported include: prolonged sedation, paradoxical excitation, hypersensitivity, pulmonary edema, apnea, and death from circulatory failure. Adverse effects that require treatment can generally be alleviated with atipamezole, however analgesic effects will also be reversed.

Reproductive/Nursing Safety

The drug is not recommended for use in pregnant dogs or those used for breeding purposes because safety data for use during pregnancy is insufficient; therefore use only when the benefits clearly outweigh the drug's risks. However, no teratogenic effects were observed when rats were given up to 200 micrograms/kg SC from days 5-16 of gestation or when rabbits were given up 96 micrograms/kg IV from days 6-18 of gestation. In humans, the FDA categorizes this drug as category C for use during pregnancy (*Animal studies have shown an adverse effect on the fetus, but there are no adequate studies in humans; or there are no animal reproduction studies and no adequate studies in humans.*)

Dexmedetomidine is distributed into the milk of lactating rats; safe use during nursing has not been established.

Overdosage/Acute Toxicity

Single doses of up to 5X (IV) and 10X (IM) were tolerated in dogs, but adverse effects can occur (see above). Because of the potential of additional adverse effects occurring (heart block, PVC's, or tachycardia), treatment of dexmedetomidine-induced bradycardia with anticholinergic agents (atropine or glycopyrrolate) is usually not recommended. Atipamezole is probably a safer choice to treat any dexmedetomidine-induced effect.

Drug Interactions

Note: Before attempting combination therapy with dexmedetomidine, it is strongly advised to access references from veterinary anesthesiologists familiar with the use of this drug. The following drug interactions have either been reported or are theoretical in humans or animals receiving dexmedetomidine or medetomidine (a related compound) and may be of significance in veterinary patients. Unless otherwise noted, use together is not necessarily contraindicated, but weigh the potential risks and perform additional monitoring when appropriate.

- **ANESTHETICS, OPIATES, SEDATIVE/HYPNOTICS:** Effects may be additive; dosage reduction of one or both agents may be required. General anesthetic requirements may be reduced between 30-60%.

- **ATROPINE, GLYCOPYRROLATE:** The use of atropine (or glycopyrrolate) with dexmedetomidine can significantly increase arterial blood pressure and heart rate; use together is not recommended in dogs (and probably other species) (Congdon et al. 2009).

- **EPINEPHRINE:** As epinephrine possesses alpha agonist effects, do not use to treat cardiac effects caused by dexmedetomidine.

- **YOHIMBINE:** May reverse the effects of medetomidine; but atipamezole is preferred for clinical use to reverse the drug's effects.

Laboratory Considerations

- Medetomidine (and presumably dexmedetomidine) can inhibit ADP-induced **platelet aggregation** in cats.

Doses

Note: there are many potential extra-label combinations that have been suggested; the following are examples and not inclusive. For additional information refer to other anesthesia-specific references such as *Handbook of Veterinary Anesthesia*, 5th Ed., Muir & Hubbell, Elsevier 2012; *Essentials of Small Animal Anesthesia & Analgesia*, Grimm et al, Wiley-Blackwell 2011 or the website Veterinary Anesthesia & Analgesia Support Group (vasg.org). See also the doses listed in the buprenorphine and butorphanol monographs.

- **DOGS:**

Labeled dose (FDA-approved):

For sedation and analgesia: 375 micrograms/m² body surface area (BSA) IV; 500 micrograms/m² BSA IM. The microgram/kg dosage decreases as body weight increases.

As a preanesthetic: Depending on duration and severity of the procedure and anesthetic regimen: 125 – 375 micrograms/m² IM. The microgram/kg dosage decreases as body weight increases. Accurate dosing is not possible with dogs weighing less than 2 kg. An extensive dosing table using patient weights is available in the package insert. It is recommended that patients be fasted for 12 hours prior to use. After injection allow animal to rest quietly for 15 minutes, sedation/analgesia occur within 5-15 minutes, with peak effects at 30 minutes post dose. (Label Information; *Dexdomitor®*—Pfizer)

Extra-label doses:

a) For use in combination with an opioid and ketamine (so-called "doggie magic") to provide anesthesia and pain management (Note: reference has dosing tables for conversion of patient weight to various microgram/m² doses of dexmedetomidine; opioid concentrations used in the reference are: Butorphanol 10 mg/mL, Hydromorphone 2 mg/mL, Morphine 15 mg/mL, & Buprenorphine 0.3 mg/mL. Ketamine concentration is 100 mg/mL. As these drugs may be available in other concentrations, only use those products with the above concentrations if using this protocol.)

For geriatric dogs, dogs with renal or liver dysfunction as a premed prior to propofol or face mask induction, followed by maintenance on isoflurane or sevoflurane: dexmedetomidine at 62.5 micrograms/m². Combine with equal volumes of one of the opioids noted above and ketamine. May administer IM or IV.

For slightly heavier sedation in ASA class II or II dogs requiring sedation for radiographic procedures: Dexmedetomidine at 125 micrograms/m². Combine with equal volumes of one of the opioids noted above and ketamine. May administer IM or IV.

For dogs undergoing minor surgery, Penn hip or OFA-types of radiographic procedures that require significant muscle relaxation: Dexmedetomidine at 250 micrograms/m². Combine with equal volumes of one of the opioids noted above and ketamine. May administer IM or IV.

To induce a surgical plane of anesthesia for OHE, castration, or other abdominal surgery: Dexmedetomidine at 375 micrograms/m². Combine with equal volumes of one of the opioids noted above and ketamine. May administer IM or IV. Provides rapid immobilization; lateral recumbency in 5-8 minutes. Dogs can be intubated and maintained on oxygen. Supplemental low doses of isoflurane (0.5%) or sevoflurane (1%) can be used.

For immobilizing extremely fractious dogs and wolf-hybrid dogs: Dexmedetomidine at 500 micrograms/m². Combine with equal volumes of one of the opioids noted above and ketamine. Administer IM. This dose is rarely required.

To reverse above, atipamezole IM at the same volume as the dexmedetomidine. (Ko 2009)

b) **As a constant rate infusion for post-operative pain management in critically ill dogs:** After surgery a loading dose of 25 micrograms/m² IV, followed by a constant rate infusion for 24 hours at 25 micrograms/m²/hr. In study, morphine at 0.2 mg/kg IV was used when rescue analgesia required (about half the dogs in the study). In this study, dexmedetomidine was as effective as morphine CRI (2.5 mg/m² load, and 2.5 mg/m²/hour CRI). Authors concluded that CRI's of dexmedetomidine have potential to provide postoperative analgesia in critically ill patients, but additional studies required to determine appropriate doses and/or use with other analgesics to provide maximal and safe post-surgical analgesia. (Valtolina et al. 2009)

■ **CATS:**

For sedation and analgesia (Labeled dose; FDA-approved): 40 micrograms/kg IM. A dosing table is available in the package insert. Recommended that patients be fasted for 12 hours prior to use. Apply an eye lubricant. After injection allow animal to rest quietly for 15 minutes, sedation/analgesia occurs within 5-15 minutes, with peak effects at 30 minutes post dose. When used as a preanesthetic it can markedly reduce anesthetic requirements. The anesthetic dose should always be titrated against the response of the patient. (Adapted from label information; *Dexdomitor*—Zoetis)

For use in combination with an opioid and ketamine (so-called "kitty magic", "DKT" or "Triple Combination") to provide sedation and analgesia (extra-label): **Note:** Opioid concentrations used in the reference are: Butorphanol 10 mg/mL, Hydromorphone 2 mg/mL, Morphine 15 mg/mL, & Buprenorphine 0.3 mg/mL. Ketamine concentration is 100 mg/mL. Dexmedetomidine concentration is 0.5 mg/mL. As these drugs may be available in other concentrations, only use those products with the above concentrations if using this protocol.

For the chart below: MILD = For sedation or as a premed prior to propofol or face mask induction; MODERATE = For castration or minor surgical procedures; PROFOUND = Invasive surgical procedures including OHE and declaws. Cats can be reversed immediately with an equal volume (of the dexmedetomidine dose) of atipamezole.

Cat Weight		Volume (of each) of: Dexmedetomidine-Opioid-Ketamine		IM Route
Lbs.	Kg	MILD	MODERATE	PROFOUND
4-7	2-3	0.025 mL	0.05 mL	0.1 – 0.15 mL
7-9	3-4	0.05 mL	0.1 mL	0.2 – 0.25 mL
9-13	4-6	0.1 mL	0.2 mL	0.3 – 0.35 mL
14-15	6-7	0.2 mL	0.3 mL	0.4 – 0.45 mL
15-18	7-8	0.3 mL	0.4 mL	0.5 – 0.55 mL

(Ko 2009)

Monitoring

■ Level of sedation and analgesia; heart rate; body temperature.

■ Heart rhythm, blood pressure, respiration rate, and pulse oximetry should be considered, particularly in higher risk patients.

Client Information

■ This drug should be administered and monitored by veterinary professionals only.

■ Clients should be made aware of the potential adverse effects associated with its use, particularly in dogs at risk (older, preexisting conditions).

Chemistry/Synonyms

Dexmedetomidine is the dextrorotatory enantiomer of medetomidine.

Dexmedetomidine HCl may also be known as (S)-medetomidine, (+)-medetomidine, MPV 1440, MPV 295, or MPV 785. Trade names include: *Precedex®* or *Dexdomitor®*.

Storage/Stability

Store the injection at room temperature (15-30°C); do not freeze.

Compatibility/Compounding Considerations

Information "on file" with the manufacturer states that dexmedetomidine 0.5 mg/mL solution for injection can be mixed with butorphanol 2 mg/mL or with ketamine 50 mg/ml solution, or with butorphanol 2 mg/mL solution and ketamine 50 mg/mL solution, in the same syringe and possesses no pharmacological risk. Anecdotal comments have been noted that buprenorphine, hydromorphone, morphine can also be mixed with dexmedetomidine.

Dosage Forms/Regulatory Status

VETERINARY-LABELED PRODUCTS:

Dexmedetomidine HCl 0.5 mg/mL (500 micrograms/mL) in 10 mL multidose vials; *Dexdomitor®*; (Rx).

HUMAN-LABELED PRODUCTS:

Dexmedetomidine HCl Concentrated Solution for Injection: 100 micrograms/mL (equiv. to dexmedetomidine hydrochloride 118 mcg), preservative free, sodium chloride 9 mg in 2 mL vials; *Precedex®*; (Rx)

Revisions/References

Monograph revised/updated January 2014.

Congdon, J., et al. (2009). Cardiovascular and sedation paramerters during dexmedetomidine and atropine administration. Prtoceedings: IVECCS. accessed via Veterinary Information Network; vin.com

Jalornaki, S. & E. Eskelinen (2007). Effect of dexmedetomidine-butorphanol combination on Schirmer 1 tear test (STT1) readings in dogs. Proceedings: ACVO. accessed via Veterinary Information Network; vin.com

Ko, J. (2009). Dexmedetomidine and its injectable anesthetic-pain management combinations. Proceedings: ACVC. accessed via Veterinary Information Network; vin.com

Santos, L., et al. (2009). Sedative and Cardiorespiratory Effects of Dexmedetomidine and Buprenorphine Administered to Cats via Oral Trans-Mucosal or Intramuscular Routes. Proceedings: IVECCS. accessed via Veterinary Information Network; vin.com

Slingsby, L., et al. (2009). Thermal antinociception after dexmedetomidine administration in cats: a comparison between intramuscular and oral transmucosal administration. Journal of Feline Medicine and Surgery 11(829-834).

Valtolina, C., et al. (2009). Clinical evaluation of the efficacy and safety of a constant rate infusion of dexmedetomidine for postoperative pain management in dogs. Veterinary Anaesthesia and Analgesia 36(4): 369-83.

Dexpanthenol
D-Panthenol

(dex-pan-the-nole)   Ilopan®

Pantothenic Acid Precursor

Prescriber Highlights

▶ Precursor to Coenzyme A that ostensibly aids in production of acetylcholine.

▶ Potentially may be useful in the prevention of post-surgical ileus, but efficacy is in doubt.

▶ Contraindications: Ileus secondary to mechanical obstruction or in cases of colic caused by the treatment of cholinergic anthelmintics.

Uses/Indications

Dexpanthenol has been suggested for use in intestinal atony or distension, postoperative retention of flatus and feces, prophylaxis and treatment of paralytic ileus after abdominal surgery or traumatic injuries, equine colic (not due to mechanical obstruction) and any other condition when there is an impairment of smooth muscle function. Controlled studies are lacking with regard to proving the efficacy of the drug for any of these indications.

Pharmacology/Actions

A precursor to pantothenic acid, dexpanthenol acts as a precursor to coenzyme A that is necessary for acetylation reactions to occur during gluconeogenesis and in the production of acetylcholine. It has been postulated that giving high doses of dexpanthenol, thereby assuring adequate levels of acetylcholine, can prevent post-surgical ileus. However, one study in normal horses (Adams, Lamar, and Masty 1984) failed to demonstrate any effect of dexpanthenol on peristalsis.

Pharmacokinetics

Dexpanthenol is rapidly converted to pantothenic acid *in vivo*, which is widely distributed throughout the body, primarily as coenzyme A.

Contraindications/Precautions/Warnings

Dexpanthenol is contraindicated in ileus secondary to mechanical obstruction, or in cases of colic caused by the treatment of cholinergic anthelmintics. It is also contraindicated in humans with hemophilia as it may exacerbate bleeding.

Adverse Effects

Adverse reactions are reportedly rare. Hypersensitivity reactions have been reported in humans, but may have been due to the preservative agents found in the injectable product. Potentially, GI cramping and diarrhea are possible.

Reproductive/Nursing Safety

Safety in use during pregnancy has not been established. In humans, the FDA categorizes this drug as category *C* for use during pregnancy (*Animal studies have shown an adverse effect on the fetus, but there are no adequate studies in humans; or there are no animal reproduction studies and no adequate studies in humans.*)

Overdosage/Acute Toxicity

The drug is considered non-toxic even when administered in high doses.

Drug Interactions

The following drug interactions have either been reported or are theoretical in humans or animals receiving dexpanthenol and may be of significance in veterinary patients. Unless otherwise noted, use together is not necessarily contraindicated, but weigh the potential risks and perform additional monitoring when appropriate.

- **NEOSTIGMINE; SUCCINYLCHOLINE:** The manufacturers have recommended that dexpanthenol not be administered within 12 hours of neostigmine or other parasympathomimetic agents or within 1 hour of receiving succinylcholine. The clinical significance of these potential interactions has not been documented, however.

Doses

- **DOGS & CATS:**

  For GI indications: 11 mg/kg IM; may be repeated in 2 hours after initial injection and followed every 6-8 hours until condition is alleviated. The time interval and duration of therapy will depend upon the degree of severity that the animal is exhibiting from the clinical standpoint. (Label Instructions; *d-Panthenol® Injectable*—Vedco)

- **HORSES:**

  For GI Indications: 2.5 grams IV or IM; repeat if indicated at 4-6 hour intervals. (Rossoff 1974), (Label Instructions; *d-Panthenol® Injectable*—Vedco)

Monitoring

- Clinical efficacy.

Client Information

- Should be used in a professionally monitored situation where gastrointestinal motility can be monitored.

Chemistry/Synonyms

The alcohol of D-pantothenic acid, dexpanthenol occurs as a slightly bitter-tasting, clear, viscous, somewhat hygroscopic liquid. It is freely soluble in water or alcohol.

Dexpanthenol may also be known as: D-panthenol, dexpanthenolum, dextro-pantothenyl alcohol, panthenol; many trade names are available.

Storage/Stability

Dexpanthenol should be protected from both freezing and excessive heat. It is incompatible with strong acids and alkalis.

Dosage Forms/Regulatory Status

VETERINARY-LABELED PRODUCTS:

Dexpanthenol Injection: 250 mg/mL in 100 mL vials; *D-Panthenol Injectable*, generic; (Rx). Labeled for use in dogs, cats, and horses, but it does not appear to be an FDA-approved product.

HUMAN-LABELED PRODUCTS:

Dexpanthenol Injection: 250 mg/mL; generic; (Rx). Not an FDA-approved drug.

Revisions/References

Monograph revised/updated January 2014.
Rossoff, I. S. (1974). *Handbook of Veterinary Drugs*, Springer Publishing. New York.

Dextrose — see the Tables of Parenteral Fluids in the Appendix

Dexrazoxane

(dex-ra-**zox**-ane)   Zinecard®

Antidote

Prescriber Highlights

▶ May be useful in attenuating the cardiotoxic effects of doxorubicin in patients (dogs) showing signs of anthracycline cardiotoxicity, that have cardiac disease, or are at maximum cumulative dosages of doxorubicin; also used to treat extravasation injuries associated with doxorubicin.

▶ Potentially may reduce efficacy of doxorubicin & increase myelosuppression.

▶ For extravasation treatment, must be administered within hours of injury.

▶ Very expensive.

Uses/Indications

Dexrazoxane may be useful to attenuate the cardiotoxic effects of doxorubicin in patients that are showing signs of anthracycline cardiotoxicity, have cardiac disease, or are at maximum cumulative dosages of doxorubicin. It is also used to treat extravasation injuries associated with doxorubicin. In a published retrospective study in 4 dogs, it was recommended that because of the importance of timely administration (within 6 hours), veterinarians treating patients with doxorubicin should have dexrazoxane readily available (Venable et al. 2012).

While dexrazoxane has been shown to be cardioprotective when given at dosages of 10X the doxorubicin dose, there is evidence that it may also partially protect the cancer cells being treated.

Pharmacology/Actions

Dexrazoxane is hydrolyzed to an active metabolite that chelates intracellular iron that is believed to prevent the formation of a anthracycline-iron complex free radicals thought to be the primary cause of anthracycline-induced cardiomyopathy and extravasation injury.

Pharmacokinetics

In dogs, dexrazoxane's pharmacokinetics fit a two compartment open model. Steady-state volume of distribution is 0.67 L/kg; terminal half life is about 1.2 hours and clearance, about 11 mL/min/kg. Clearance was dose-independent and the drug showed low tissue and protein binding. Dexrazoxane is primarily excreted in the urine as unchanged drug and metabolites.

Contraindications/Precautions/Warnings

Dexrazoxane should not be used unless an anthracycline antineoplastic agent is being used.

Efficacy and safety for use in cats is not known.

Adverse Effects

Dexrazoxane may cause additive myelosuppression when used with other myelosuppressive agents. There is some evidence in humans, that dexrazoxane may reduce the efficacy of anthracycline antitumor agents. Clinical significance in veterinary patients is unknown.

Wear gloves when handling and use normal procedures for handling and disposing of anti-cancer medications. If unreconstituted powder contacts skin or mucous membranes, thoroughly wash the exposed area with soap and water.

Reproductive/Nursing Safety

Dexrazoxane has been shown to cause testicular atrophy in dogs when administered at usual doses for 13 weeks. In humans, the FDA categorizes dexrazoxane as a category C drug for use during pregnancy (*Animal studies have shown an adverse effect on the fetus, but there are no adequate studies in humans; or there are no animal reproduction studies and no adequate studies in humans*). In rats and rabbits, dexrazoxane was teratogenic at doses lower than those administered to humans.

It is unknown if dexrazoxane enters maternal milk; human mothers are advised to discontinue nursing if given the drug.

Overdosage/Acute Toxicity

Because of the method of administration and drug expense, overdoses are unlikely in veterinary medicine. As there is no known antidote, treatment would be supportive. Potentially, the drug could be removed via hemodialysis.

Drug Interactions

Dexrazoxane does not influence the pharmacokinetics of doxorubicin.

The following drug interactions have either been reported or are theoretical in humans or animals receiving dexrazoxane and may be of significance in veterinary patients. Unless otherwise noted, use together is not necessarily contraindicated, but weigh the potential risks and perform additional monitoring when appropriate.

- MYELOSUPPRESSIVE AGENTS, OTHER: Additive myelo-suppression may occur when used with other myelosuppressive agents.

Laboratory Considerations

- No specific laboratory interactions or considerations were noted.

Doses

- **DOGS:**

  For treatment of anthracycline (doxorubicin, epirubicin, etc.) **extravasation** (extra-label): **Note:** In a retrospective study of 4 dogs, the authors concluded that the most effective dosage and timing of administration are unknown, however, there is evidence to suggest that administration within 6 hours after the event is warranted; further studies are needed (Venable et al. 2012).

  a) Terminate doxorubicin infusion immediately, and infuse intravenously 1000 mg/m² of dexrazoxane in a separate infusion within 6 hours and again on day 2. Infuse 500 mg/m² on day 3. Acute surgical evaluation is performed. **Note:** Dosage recommendations are for human patients, but may apply to veterinary patients. (Langer et al. 2000)

  b) Anecdotally: IV administration of dexrazoxane at 10X the doxorubicin dose within 3 hours and again at 24 and 48 hours after extravasation significantly reduces local tissue injury. (Vail 2006)

  For prevention of doxorubicin-induced cardiomyopathy (extra-label; from a retrospective study in 25 dogs): In the study, dogs had to meet at least one of the following criteria: pre-existing diagnosed clinical heart disease; onset of impaired systolic function during the course of doxorubicin therapy; cumulative dose of doxorubicin of 180 mg/m² or cardiac disease as determined by echocardiographic evaluation. Ten minutes prior to doxorubicin infusion, dexrazoxane was administered for 5-10 min IV at a level of 10X the administered milligram dose of doxorubicin. While no information regarding efficacy of cardioprotection could be gleaned, it appears that 1-2 doses of dexrazoxane administered with doxorubicin are safe and well tolerated (FitzPatrick et al. 2010).

Monitoring

- CBC.
- If used for cardioprotection: echocardiogram, ECG, etc.

Client Information

- Clients should understand and accept the potential costs associated with this drug and that when used for extravasation injuries, may not be fully effective.

Chemistry/Synonyms

A derivative of EDTA, dexrazoxane occurs as a white crystalline powder that is soluble in water and slightly soluble in ethanol and practically insoluble in nonpolar organic solvents. It has a pKa of 2.1 and degrades rapidly at pH above 7.

Dexrazoxane may also be known as: 2,6-Piperazinedione, ADR-529, ICRF-187, NSC-169780, *Zinecard®, Cardioxane®* or *Eucardion®*.

Storage/Stability

Unreconstituted dexrazoxane vials should be stored at 25°C (77°F); excursions permitted to 15-30°C (59-86°F). Once reconstituted with the supplied diluent, it is stable for 6 hours at room temperature or refrigerated. Unused solutions after that time should be discarded. After reconstitution, the resulting solution may be diluted with either 0.9% sodium chloride injection or D₅W in concentrations of 1.3-5 mg/mL. Inspect visually for particulate matter and discoloration prior to administering.

Compatibility/Compounding Considerations

The manufacturer states that dexrazoxane should not be mixed with any other drug.

Dosage Forms/Regulatory Status

VETERINARY-LABELED PRODUCTS: NONE.

HUMAN-LABELED PRODUCTS:

Dexrazoxane Lyophilized Powder for Injection Solution: 250 mg in single-use vials with 25 mL vial of sodium lactate injection; and 500 mg regular & preservative free (equiv. to dexrazoxane hydrochloride 589 mg) in single-use vials with 50 mL vial of sodium lactate injection; *Zinecard®, Totect®*, generic; (Rx)

Revisions/References

Monograph revised/updated January 2014.

FitzPatrick, W. M., et al. (2010). Safety of concurrent administration of dexrazoxane and doxorubicin in the canine cancer patient. Veterinary and Comparative Oncology **8**(4): 273-82.

Langer, S., et al. (2000). Treatment of anthracycline extravasation with dexrazoxane. Clin Cancer Res **6**(Sept): 3680-6.

Vail, D. (2006). New supportive therapies for cancer patients. Proceedings: ACVIM. accessed via Veterinary Information Network; vin.com

Venable, R. O., et al. (2012). Dexrazoxane treatment of doxorubicin extravasation injury in four dogs. Javma-Journal of the American Veterinary Medical Association **240**(3): 304-7.

Dextran 70

(dex-tran)

Plasma Volume Expander

Synthetic Colloid

Note: Dextran is also available as Dextran 40. As Dextran 70 has been the most commonly used version in veterinary medicine, the following monograph is limited to it alone.

Prescriber Highlights

▶ Branched polysaccharide plasma volume expander. Other colloids (*e.g.*, hetastarch) have largely supplanted use.

▶ Contraindications: Preexisting coagulopathies. Caution: Patients susceptible to circulatory overload (severe heart or renal failure), thrombocytopenia.

▶ Adverse Effects: Quite rare in dogs. Increased bleeding times, acute renal failure & anaphylaxis possible (but very rare).

▶ Must monitor for fluid overload.

Uses/Indications

Dextran 70 is a relatively low cost colloid for the adjunctive treatment of hypovolemic shock. Hydroxyethyl starches are the more commonly employed synthetic colloids in use today.

Pharmacology/Actions

Dextran 70 has osmotic effects similar to albumin. Dextran's colloidal osmotic effect draws fluid into the vascular system from the interstitial spaces, resulting in increased circulating blood volume.

Pharmacokinetics

After IV infusion, circulating blood volume is increased maximally within one hour and effects can persist for 24 hours or more. Approximately 20-30% of a given dose remains in the intravascular compartment at 24 hours and it may be detected in the blood 4-6 weeks after dosing. Dextran 70 is slowly degraded to glucose by dextranase in the spleen and then metabolized to carbon dioxide and water. A small amount may be excreted directly into the gut and eliminated in the feces.

Contraindications/Precautions/Warnings

Patients overly susceptible to circulatory overload (severe heart or renal failure) should receive dextran 70 with great caution. Dextran 70 is contraindicated in patients with severe coagulopathies and should be used with caution in patients with thrombocytopenia as it can interfere with platelet function. Do not give dextran IM. Patients on strict sodium restriction should receive dextran cautiously as a 500 mL bag contains 77 mEq of sodium.

Adverse Effects

Dextran 70 may increase bleeding time and decrease von Willebrand's factor antigen and factor VIII activity. This does not usually cause clinical bleeding in dogs.

While anaphylactoid reactions are not rare in humans, they do occur rarely in dogs, but at a higher rate than with hetastarch. Unlike dextran 40, dextran 70 has rarely been associated with acute renal failure. In humans, GI effects (abdominal pain, nausea/vomiting) have been reported with use of dextran 70.

Reproductive/Nursing Safety

In humans, the FDA categorizes this drug as category *C* for use during pregnancy (*Animal studies have shown an adverse effect on the fetus, but there are no adequate studies in humans; or there are no animal reproduction studies and no adequate studies in humans.*).

Overdosage/Acute Toxicity

The drug should be dosed and monitored carefully as volume overload may result.

Drug Interactions

Dextran reportedly has no drug interactions that are clinically significant.

Laboratory Considerations

▪ Dextran 70 may interfere with **blood cross-matching** as it can cross-link with red blood cells and appear as rouleaux formation. Isotonic saline may be used to negate this effect.

▪ **Blood glucose** levels may be increased as dextran is degraded.

▪ Falsely elevated **bilirubin** levels may be noted; reason unknown.

Doses

▪ **DOGS:**

For volume resuscitation (extra-label):

a) Small volume resuscitation techniques are recommended in any dog with closed cavity hemorrhage, head injury, pulmonary contusions or edema, cardiogenic shock, or oliguric renal failure. An initial dose of balanced isotonic crystalloids (10 – 15 mL/kg) for dogs is given. Either a hydroxyethyl starch or dextran-70 is then administered (5 mL/kg in dogs) over 1-5 minutes. The perfusion parameters are reassessed and the initial mL/kg bolus repeated as needed until the end-point of resuscitation is reached. (Kirby 2008)

b) 20 mL/kg/day; when acute resuscitation is required, may be given as a slow bolus over 30 minutes to an hour. May also be given as a constant rate infusion over a longer period to augment colloid oncotic pressure or decrease the volume of crystalloids infused, thereby reducing hemodilution. (Martin 2004)

▪ **CATS:**

For volume resuscitation (extra-label):

a) Small volume resuscitation techniques are recommended in the hypovolemic cat with closed cavity hemorrhage, head injury, pulmonary contusions or edema, cardiogenic shock, or oliguric renal failure. An initial dose of balanced isotonic crystalloids (5 – 10 mL/kg for cats) is given. Either hetastarch or dextran-70 is then administered (2 – 5 mL/kg in cats) over 1-5 minutes. The perfusion parameters are reassessed and the initial mL/kg bolus repeated as needed until the end-point of resuscitation is reached. (Kirby 2008)

b) 10 mL/kg/day; when acute resuscitation is required. May be given as a slow bolus over 30 minutes to an hour. May also be given as a constant rate infusion over a longer period to augment colloid oncotic pressure or decrease the volume of crystalloids infused, thereby reducing hemodilution. (Martin 2004)

▪ **CATTLE:**

For dehydrated (secondary to diarrhea) calves given as 6% Dextran 70 in 7.2% sodium chloride: To prepare solution, add 31.6 g sodium chloride into the barrel of a 60 mL syringe. Draw 60 mL of 6% dextran 70 in 0.9% NaCl from the bag/bottle to dilute the NaCl crystals. Re-inject the dissolved solution into the bag/bottle through a 0.22 micron filter giving a 6% dextran 70 in 7.2% NaCl solution. Resultant solution may be refrigerated for up to 3 months. Inject IV 4 – 5 mL/kg of this solution over 4-5 minutes, followed immediately by oral administration of isotonic electrolyte solution. Give dextran 70 solution one time only or hypernatremia may result and follow-up with isotonic fluids (oral or IV) is critical. (Sweeney 2003)

Monitoring

- Other than the regular monitoring performed in patients that would require volume expansion therapy, there is no inordinate monitoring required specific to dextran therapy.

Chemistry/Synonyms

A branched polysaccharide used intravenously as a plasma volume expander, dextran 70 occurs as a white to light yellow amorphous powder. It is freely soluble in water and insoluble in alcohol. Dextran 70 contains (on average) molecules of 70,000 daltons. Each 500 mL of the commercially available 6% dextran 70 in normal saline provides 77 mEq of sodium. Dextran 70 in normal saline has a viscosity of 3.68 centipose (blood is 3 centipose) and a colloid osmotic pressure of 62 mmHg (canine plasma is approximately 20 mmHg).

Dextran 70 may also be known as: dextranum 70, polyglucin, *Dextran 70®*, *Fisiodex 70®*, *Gentran 70®*, *Hyskon®*, *Lomodex 70®*, *Longasteril 70®*, *Macrodex®*, *Macrohorm 70®*, *Neodextril 70®*, *Plander®*, *RescueFlow®*, or *Solplex 70®*.

Storage/Stability

Dextran 70 injection should be stored at room temperature, preferably in an area with little temperature variability. While only clear solutions should be used, dextran flakes can form but may be resolubolized by heating the solution in a boiling water bath until clear, or autoclaving at 110°C for 15 minutes.

Compatibility/Compounding Considerations

Dextran 70 is **compatible** with many other solutions and drugs; refer to specialized references or a hospital pharmacist for more information.

Dosage Forms/Regulatory Status

VETERINARY-LABELED PRODUCTS: NONE.

HUMAN-LABELED PRODUCTS:

Dextran 70: 6% in 5% dextrose in 500 mL; generic; (Rx)

Revisions/References

Monograph revised/updated January 2014.

Kirby, R. (2008). Shock and Resuscitation: Parts 1 & 2. "Be a Shock Buster...!". Proceedings: World Veterinary Congress. accessed via Veterinary Information Network; vin.com

Martin, L. (2004). Plasma vs Synthetic Colloids: Do you know which to use? Proceedings: ACVIM Forum. accessed via Veterinary Information Network; vin.com

Sweeney, R. (2003). When salt water isn't enough: TPN, colloid, and blood product therapy in cattle. Proceedings: ACVIM Forum. accessed via Veterinary Information Network; vin.com

Diazepam

(dye-az-e-pam)   Valium®, Diastat®

Benzodiazepine

Prescriber Highlights

▶ Benzodiazepine used for a variety of indications (anxiolytic, muscle relaxant, hypnotic, appetite stimulant, & anticonvulsant) in several species; use in cats is controversial secondary to potential hepatotoxicity.

▶ In dogs, tolerance to anticonvulsant effects occurs with long-term use making it less useful to treat status epilepticus.

▶ Contraindications: Hypersensitivity to benzodiazepines, significant liver disease (especially in cats), cats exposed to chlorpyrifos. Caution: hepatic or renal disease, aggressive, debilitated or geriatric patients, patients in coma, shock or with significant respiratory depression. May be teratogenic.

▶ Adverse Effects: Sedation & ataxia most prevalent. **Dogs:** CNS excitement, increased appetite; **Cats:** Hepatic failure or behavior changes; **Horses:** Muscle fasciculations.

▶ Inject IV slowly. IV form incompatible with many other drugs.

▶ Many potential drug interactions.

▶ Controlled substance (C-IV).

Uses/Indications

Diazepam is used clinically for its anxiolytic, muscle relaxant, hypnotic, appetite stimulant, and anticonvulsant activities. It is also used in preanesthetic protocols for neuroleptanalgesia.

While diazepam is a drug of choice for treating status epilepticus and cluster seizures in dogs, it is relatively short acting (15-30 minutes). Long-term administration usually causes tolerance to its anticonvulsant effects. Additionally, long-term use in dogs may prevent effective use of diazepam for the emergency treatment of seizures. In cats, diazepam has a longer elimination half-life and tolerance does not appear to be a major concern, but many neurologists avoid its use because of the risk for serious hepatotoxicity.

Pharmacology/Actions

Diazepam and other benzodiazepines depress CNS subcortical levels (primarily limbic, thalamic, and hypothalamic) thereby producing the anxiolytic, sedative, skeletal muscle relaxant, and anticonvulsant effects seen. The exact mechanism of action is unknown, but postulated mechanisms include: antagonism of serotonin, increased release of and/or facilitation of gamma-aminobutyric acid (GABA) activity, and diminished release or turnover of acetylcholine in the CNS. Benzodiazepine specific receptors have been located in the mammalian brain, kidney, liver, lung, and heart. In all species studied, receptors are lacking in the white matter.

Pharmacokinetics

Diazepam is rapidly absorbed following oral administration. Peak plasma levels occur within 30 minutes to 2 hours after oral dosing. The drug is slowly (slower than oral) and incompletely absorbed following IM administration. In dogs, rectally administered diazepam has a bioavailability of <10%, but when factoring in diazepam plus the active (20-50% of the anticonvulsant activity of diazepam) metabolites desmethyldiazepam and oxazepam, bioavailability is closer to 80%. When administered intranasally to dogs, bioavailability is about 80%.

Diazepam is highly lipid soluble and is widely distributed throughout the body. It readily crosses the blood-brain barrier and is fairly highly bound to plasma proteins. In the horse at a serum concentration of 75 ng/mL, 87% of the drug is bound to plasma proteins. In humans, this value has been reported to be 98-99%.

Diazepam is metabolized in the liver to several metabolites including desmethyldiazepam (nordiazepam), temazepam, and oxazepam, all of which are pharmacologically active. These are eventually conjugated with glucuronide and eliminated primarily in the urine. Because of the active metabolites, serum values of diazepam are not useful in predicting efficacy. Serum half-lives (approximated) have been reported for diazepam and metabolites in dogs, cats, and horses:

	Dogs	Cats	Horses	Humans
Diazepam	1-3.2 hrs.	5.5 hrs.	7-22 hrs.	20-50 hrs.
Nordiazepam	2-3 hrs.	21.3 hrs.		30-200 hrs.

Contraindications/Precautions/Warnings

Inject intravenously slowly. This is particularly true when using a small vein for access or in small animals; diazepam may cause significant thrombophlebitis. Rapid injection of intravenous diazepam in small animals or neonates may cause hypotension/cardiotoxicity secondary to the propylene glycol in the formulation. Intra-carotid artery injections must be avoided.

Use of diazepam in cats is controversial, primarily because of case reports of serious hepatotoxicity. Some are of the opinion that the drug should not be used chronically in cats.

Use cautiously in patients with hepatic or renal disease and debilitated or geriatric patients. The drug should be administered very cautiously to patients in coma, shock, or with significant respiratory depression. It is contraindicated in patients with known hypersensitivity to the drug. Diazepam should be used very cautiously, if at all, in aggressive patients as it may disinhibit the anxiety that may help prevent these animals from aggressive behavior. Diazepam may impair the abilities of working or service animals. If administering the drug IV, be prepared to administer cardiovascular or respiratory support.

It is recommended to not use diazepam for seizure control in cats exposed to chlorpyrifos as organophosphate toxicity may be potentiated.

Animals that have toxicity from ingesting human sleep aids such as zolpidem (*Ambien®*) or eszopiclone (*Lunesta®*) should not receive diazepam or other benzodiazepines to treat paradoxical CNS stimulation as these drugs also increase GABA activity; IV phenothiazines such as acepromazine or chlorpromazine or phenobarbital are recommended instead.

Rapid IV bolus administration can potentially cause hypotension; administer over 1-3 minutes depending on dose and patient size.

Adverse Effects

Rapid IV administration of diazepam can potentially cause hypotension; give IV slowly and flush IV catheter with fluids after administration to help prevent phlebitis.

Adverse effects reported in dogs include sedation, increased appetite, agitation, ataxia, and aggression. Additionally, dogs may exhibit a contradictory response (CNS excitement) following administration of diazepam. Doses of 0.8 mg/kg or higher are more likely to cause this effect. Diazepam's effects with regard to sedation and tranquilization in dogs can be variable and some feel that this makes it less than an ideal inpatient sedating agent, particularly when used alone.

Cats may exhibit changes in behavior (irritability, depression, aberrant demeanor) after receiving diazepam. There have been sporadic reports of cats developing idiosyncratic hepatic failure after receiving oral diazepam (not dose dependent) for several days. Clinical signs (anorexia, lethargy, increased ALT/AST, hyperbilirubinemia) have been reported to occur 5-11 days after beginning oral therapy. Cats that receive diazepam should have baseline liver function tests. These should be repeated and the drug discontinued if emesis, lethargy, inappetence or ataxia develops.

In horses, diazepam may cause muscle fasciculations, weakness and ataxia at doses sufficient to cause sedation. Doses greater than 0.2 mg/kg may induce recumbency as a result of its muscle relaxant properties and general CNS depressant effects.

Reproductive/Nursing Safety

Diazepam has been implicated in causing congenital abnormalities in humans if administered during the first trimester of pregnancy. Infants born of mothers receiving large doses of benzodiazepines shortly before delivery have been reported to suffer from apnea, impaired metabolic response to cold stress, difficulty in feeding, hyperbilirubinemia, hypotonia, etc. Withdrawal symptoms have occurred in infants whose mothers chronically took benzodiazepines during pregnancy. The veterinary significance of these effects is unclear, but the use of these agents during the first trimester of pregnancy should only occur when the benefits clearly outweigh the risks associated with their use. In humans, the FDA categorizes this drug as category *D* for use during pregnancy (*There is evidence of human fetal risk, but the potential benefits from the use of the drug in pregnant women may be acceptable despite its potential risks.*) In a separate system evaluating the safety of drugs in canine and feline pregnancy (Papich 1989), this drug is categorized as class: *C* (*These drugs may have potential risks. Studies in people or laboratory animals have uncovered risks, and these drugs should be used cautiously as a last resort when the benefit of therapy clearly outweighs the risks.*)

Benzodiazepines and their metabolites are distributed into milk and may cause CNS effects in nursing neonates.

Overdosage/Acute Toxicity

When administered alone, diazepam overdoses are generally limited to significant CNS depression (confusion, coma, decreased reflexes, etc.). Hypotension, respiratory depression, and cardiac arrest have been reported in human patients, but apparently are quite rare.

Treatment of acute toxicity consists of standard protocols for removing and/or binding the drug in the gut if taken orally, and supportive systemic measures. The use of analeptic agents (CNS stimulants such as caffeine) is generally not recommended. Flumazenil may be considered for adjunctive treatment of overdoses of benzodiazepines.

Drug Interactions

The following drug interactions have either been reported or are theoretical in humans or animals receiving diazepam and may be of significance in veterinary patients. Unless otherwise noted, use together is not necessarily contraindicated, but weigh the potential risks and perform additional monitoring when appropriate.

- **AMITRIPTYLINE:** Diazepam may increase levels.
- **ANTACIDS:** May decrease oral diazepam absorption.
- **ANTIFUNGALS, AZOLE (itraconazole, ketoconazole,** etc.): May increase diazepam levels.
- **CIMETIDINE:** May decrease metabolism of benzodiazepines.
- **CNS DEPRESSANT DRUGS (barbiturates, narcotics, anesthetics,** etc.): If diazepam administered with other CNS depressant agents, additive effects may occur.
- **DEXAMETHASONE:** May decrease diazepam levels.
- **DIGOXIN:** Diazepam may increase digoxin levels.
- **ERYTHROMYCIN:** May decrease the metabolism of benzodiazepines.
- **MINERAL OIL:** May decrease oral diazepam absorption.
- **OMEPRAZOLE:** May inhibit the metabolism of diazepam and increase levels.
- **PHENOBARBITAL:** May decrease diazepam concentrations.

- **PHENYTOIN**: May decrease diazepam concentrations.
- **QUINIDINE**: May increase diazepam levels.
- **RIFAMPIN**: May induce hepatic microsomal enzymes and decrease the pharmacologic effects of benzodiazepines.

Laboratory Considerations

- Patients receiving diazepam, may show false negative **urine glucose** results if using *Diastix®* or *Clinistix®* tests.
- Secondary to propylene glycol in IV diazepam, patients may show a false-positive **ethylene glycol** test.

Doses

- **DOGS:**

For treatment of cluster seizures or status epilepticus (all are extra-label):

Rectal: 0.5 – 1 mg/kg rectally; if on phenobarbital, use diazepam at 2 mg/kg (using diazepam parenteral solution) rectally. Administer at the onset of seizure and up to 3 times in a 24-hour period, but should not be given within 10 minutes of the prior dose. If client administered, they should stay with dog for one hour after administration. Because diazepam is inactivated by light and adheres to plastic, it is best to dispense the drug in the original glass vial and instruct the owner to draw the required amount into a syringe when needed. A rubber catheter or teat cannula is then placed on the syringe for rectal administration (Podell 2009), (Munana 2010), (Mariani 2010b). A study found that compounded 2 mg rectal suppositories did not achieve plasma levels of diazepam/nordiazepam levels sufficient for emergency treatment of seizures in dogs (Probst et al. 2013).

Intranasal: Based on a pharmacokinetic study (Musulin et al. 2011), diazepam may be also be given intranasally (at home or in the clinic) at 0.5 mg/kg. Dogs that are on chronic phenobarbital therapy may require higher doses (1 – 2 mg/kg).

Intravenous (bolus): 0.5 – 1 mg/kg IV. Rule out hypoglycemia, electrolyte abnormalities as primary cause.

Intravenous (CRI): For refractory status epilepticus using constant rate IV infusion: 0.1 – 2 mg/kg/hour. Use with caution as diazepam can crystallize in solution and adsorb to PVC tubing. (see Compatibility and Storage/Stability sections below)

For functional urethral obstruction/urethral sphincter hypertonus (extra-label): 2 – 10 mg per dog PO 3 times a day.

As a psychotherapeutic agent (*e.g.*, situational anxiety); (extra-label): 0.5 – 2 mg/kg PO prn; preferably 30 minutes to one hour in advance of anticipated event. **Note:** Compared to human dosages, diazepam dosages for dogs are very high; 'human' pharmacists may be unaware that these are appropriate.

For adjunctive treatment of metronidazole toxicity (CNS); (extra-label): Doses of diazepam averaged 0.43 mg/kg in the study and were given as an IV bolus once, and then PO q8h for 3 days. (Evans et al. 2002)

- **CATS:**

Note: because of concerns associated with oral diazepam and rare idiosyncratic hepatic failure in cats, many clinicians avoid diazepam use in cats.

As a psychotherapeutic agent (extra-label): 0.2 – 0.5 mg/kg PO 1-3 times a day.

For treatment of seizure disorders: For maintenance therapy: 0.2 – 1 mg/kg PO q12h. Use with caution; associated with fatal hepatic necrosis. Phenobarbital is preferred as a maintenance drug in cats. (Mariani 2010a)

Functional urethral obstruction/urethral sphincter hypertonus: 1 – 5 mg per cat PO q8-12h.

- **FERRETS:**

For premedication/sedation (extra-label): 0.5 mg/kg IM or IV (IV preferred); 0.2 mg/kg if using with ketamine (2 – 5 mg/kg). (Kaiser-Klingler 2009)

- **RABBITS/RODENTS/SMALL MAMMALS:**

Note: All are extra-label.

Rabbits: For sedation: 0.5 – 2 mg/kg IV or IM (IV preferred). For anesthesia: Diazepam at 0.5 – 1 mg/kg with ketamine (20 – 35 mg/kg) IM or IV. (Kaiser-Klingler 2009)

Hedgehogs: For long anesthesia: Diazepam at 0.5 – 2 mg/kg with ketamine at 5 – 20 mg/kg IM. (Kaiser-Klingler 2009)

Hamsters, Gerbils, Mice, Rats: 3 – 5 mg/kg IM. **Guinea pigs:** 0.5 – 3 mg/kg IM. (Adamcak et al. 2000)

- **HORSES:** (NOTE: ARCI UCGFS CLASS 2 DRUG)

For field anesthesia (extra-label):

Sedate with xylazine (1 mg/kg IV; 2 mg/kg IM) given 5-10 minutes (longer for IM route) before induction of anesthesia with ketamine (2 mg/kg IV). Horse must be adequately sedated (head to the knees) before giving the ketamine as ketamine can cause muscle rigidity and seizures.

If adequate sedation does not occur, either 1) Re-dose xylazine: up to half the original dose; or 2) Add butorphanol (0.02 – 0.04 mg/kg IV). Butorphanol can be given with the original xylazine if you suspect that the horse will be difficult to tranquilize (*e.g.*, high-strung Thoroughbreds) or added before the ketamine. This combination will improve induction, increase analgesia and increase recumbency time by about 5-10 minutes; or 3) Give Diazepam (0.03 mg/kg IV) with the ketamine Mix the diazepam with the ketamine. This combination will improve induction when sedation is marginal, improve muscle relaxation during anesthesia and prolong anesthesia by about 5-10 minutes; 4) Guaifenesin (5% solution administered IV to effect) can also be used to increase sedation and muscle relaxation. (Mathews 1999)

- **BIRDS:**

For adjunctive therapy of pain control (with analgesics); (extra-label): 0.5 – 2 mg/kg IV or IM. (Clyde et al. 2000)

For sedation/induction (extra-label): 0.5 – 2 mg/kg IV or IM. Doses apply to pet birds to the medium parrots. Adjustments would need to be made for large parrots or wild species such as raptors. (Kaiser-Klingler 2009)

ZOO, EXOTIC, WILDLIFE SPECIES:

For use in zoo, exotic and wildlife medicine refer to specific references, including:

a) *Zoo Animal and Wildlife Immobilization and Anesthesia.* West, G., Heard, D., Caulkett, N. (eds.). Blackwell Publishing, 2007.

b) *Handbook of Wildlife Chemical Immobilization, 3rd Ed.* Kreeger, T.J. and J.M. Arnemo. 2007.

c) *Fowler's Zoo and Wild Animal Medicine Current Therapy, Volume 7*, Miller, R.E., Fowler, M.E., Saunders. 2011.

d) *Exotic Animal Formulary, 4th Ed.* Carpenter, J.W., Saunders. 2012.

e) The 2009 American Association of Zoo Veterinarian Proceedings by D. K. Fontenot also has several dosages listed for restraint, anesthesia, and analgesia for a variety of drugs for carnivores and primates. VIN members can access them at: http://goo.gl/NNIWQ or http://goo.gl/9UJse

Monitoring

- Horses should be observed carefully after receiving this drug.
- Cats receiving diazepam should have baseline liver function tests. Repeat and discontinue drug if emesis, lethargy, inappetence, or ataxia develop. When used for seizure control in cats, one source (Quesnel 2000) recommends obtaining serum level 5 days after beginning therapy. Therapeutic serum concentration goals for seizure control in cats ranges from 2500 – 700 nmol/L (200 – 700 ng/mL), depending on the source.

Client Information

- When using for thunderstorm phobias or other triggers (*e.g.*, owner separation anxiety, etc.) that upset your animal, try to give it about an hour before the event or trigger.
- May be given with or without food. If your animal vomits or acts sick after getting it on an empty stomach, give with food or small treat to see if this helps. If vomiting continues, contact your veterinarian.
- If you see yellowing of the whites of the eyes or the gums have a yellowish tint, contact veterinarian immediately.
- Sleepiness is most common side effect, but sometimes the drug can change behavior or work in the opposite way from what is expected.
- This drug may increase appetite, especially in cats.
- Contact your veterinarian immediately if your cat stops eating or seems depressed.

Chemistry/Synonyms

A benzodiazepine, diazepam is a white to yellow, practically odorless crystalline powder with a melting point between 131°-135°C and pK$_a$ of 3.4. Diazepam is tasteless initially, but develops a bitter after-taste. One g is soluble in 333 mL of water, 25 mL of alcohol, and is sparingly soluble in propylene glycol. The pH of the commercially prepared injectable solution is adjusted with benzoic acid/sodium benzoate to 6.2-6.9. It consists of a 5 mg/mL solution with 40% propylene glycol, 10% ethanol, 5% sodium benzoate/benzoic acid buffer, and 1.5% benzyl alcohol as a preservative.

Diazepam may also be known as: diazepamum, LA-III, NSC-77518, or Ro-5-2807; many trade names are available.

Storage/Stability

All diazepam products should be stored at room temperature (15°-30°C). The injection should be kept from freezing and protected from light. The oral dosage forms (tablets/capsules) should be stored in tight containers and protected from light.

Because diazepam may adsorb to plastic, it should not be stored drawn up into plastic syringes. The drug may also significantly adsorb to IV solution plastic (PVC) bags and infusion tubing. This adsorption appears to be dependent on several factors (temperature, concentration, flow rates, line length, etc.).

The following are recommended to minimize the adsorption of diazepam: glass or polyolefin containers should be used; if PVC bags are used, the lowest possible surface-to-volume ratio should be selected and storage time should be minimized. The use of non-PVC administration sets will reduce loss. If PVC tubing is used, it should be the shortest possible length with a small diameter, and the set should not contain a burette chamber. More rapid flow rates (consistent with safe clinical use) will also reduce the loss of diazepam (Trissel 2013).

Compatibility/Compounding Considerations

The manufacturers of injectable diazepam do not recommend the drug be mixed with any other medication or IV diluent and diluting for infusion cannot be recommended. While some studies have shown that dilution in some IV solutions at low concentrations may not exhibit visible precipitates, microcrystal formation could not be ruled out. Because there is continued interest in IV infusions of diazepam, some studies indicate that diazepam injection may be compatible with various drugs and IV fluids (e.g., diluted to a concentration of 5 mg/50 mL to 5 mg/100 mL with 0.9% sodium chloride, 5% dextrose, Ringer's, or lactated Ringer's injection), compatibility may depend on several factors (e.g., the concentration of the drugs, resulting pH, temperature). Specialized references (e.g., (Trissel 2013)) or a hospital pharmacist should be consulted for the most current specific compatibility information.

Mixing ketamine with diazepam in the same syringe or IV bag has been suggested, but is not recommended as precipitation may occur. Although there are many anecdotal reports of mixing ketamine with diazepam in the same syringe just prior to injection, there does not appear to be any published information documenting the stability of the drugs after mixing. Do not use if a visible precipitate forms.

Dosage Forms/Regulatory Status

VETERINARY-LABELED PRODUCTS: NONE.

The ARCI (Racing Commissioners International) has designated this drug as a class 2 substance. See the appendix for more information.

HUMAN-LABELED PRODUCTS:

Diazepam Oral Tablets: 2 mg, 5 mg, & 10 mg; *Valium®*, generic; (Rx, C-IV)

Diazepam Oral Solution: 1 mg/mL in 500 mL, and 5 mg & 10 mg patient cups; generic; (Rx, C-IV); Concentrated oral solution: 5 mg/mL in 30 mL with dropper; *Diazepam Intensol®*; (Rx, C-IV)

Diazepam Injection: 5 mg/mL in 2 mL *Carpuject* cartridges; generic; (Rx, C-IV)

Diazepam Rectal Gel: 2.5 mg, 10 mg, & 20 mg; *Diastat®*, generic; (Rx, C-IV)

Revisions/References

Monograph revised/updated January 2014.

Adamcak, A. & B. Otten (2000). Rodent Therapeutics. Vet Clin NA: Exotic Anim Pract 3:1(Jan): 221-40.

Clyde, V. & J. Paul-Murphy (2000). Avian Analgesia. *Kirk's Current Veterinary Therapy: XIII Small Animal Practice*. J. Bonagura. Philadelphia, WB Saunders: 1126-8.

Evans, J., et al. (2002). The use of diazepam in the treatment of metronidazole toxicosis in the dog. Proceedings: ACVIM Forum. accessed via Veterinary Information Network; vin.com

Kaiser-Klingler, S. (2009). Exotic animal anesthesia for the small animal practice. Proceedings: World Veterinary Congress. accessed via Veterinary Information Network; vin.com

Mariani, C. (2010a). Maintenance therapy for the routine & difficult to control epileptic patient. Proceedings: ACVIM Forum. accessed via Veterinary Information Network; vin.com

Mariani, C. (2010b). Treatment of cluster seizures and stauts epilepticus. Proceedings: ACVIM Forum. accessed via Veterinary Information Network; vin.com

Mathews, N. (1999). Anesthesia in large animals— Injectable (field) anesthesia: How to make it better. Proceedings: Central Veterinary Conference, Kansas City. accessed via Veterinary Information Network; vin.com

Munana, K. (2010). Current Approaches to Seizure Management. Proceedings: ACVIM Forum. accessed via Veterinary Information Network; vin.com

Musulin, S. E., et al. (2011). Diazepam pharmacokinetics after nasal drop and atomized nasal administration in dogs. J. Vet. Pharmacol. Ther. 34(1): 17-24.

Podell, M. (2009). Status epilepticus: Stopping seizures from home to hospital. Proceedings: IVECCS. accessed via Veterinary Information Network; vin.com

Probst, C. W., et al. (2013). Evaluation of plasma diazepam and nordiazepam concentrations following administration of diazepam intravenously or via suppository per rectum in dogs. American Journal of Veterinary Research 74(4): 611-5.

Quesnel, A. (2000). Seizures. *Textbook of Veterinary Internal Medicine: Diseases of the Dog and Cat*. S. Ettinger and E. Feldman. Philadelphia, WB Saunders. 1: 148-52.

Trissel, L. 2013. Handbook on Injectable Drugs - 17th Edition. Accessed via STAT!Ref; Teton Data Systems

Diazoxide, Oral

(di-az-ok-side) Proglycem®, Hyperstat IV®

Direct Vasodilator/Hyperglycemic

Prescriber Highlights

▶ Orally administered drug used to treat insulinomas in small animals.

▶ Contraindications/Cautions: Functional hypoglycemia or hypoglycemia secondary to insulin overdosage (diabetics); hypersensitive to thiazide diuretics; CHF or renal disease.

▶ Adverse Effects: Most likely are anorexia, vomiting &/or diarrhea (may be reduced by giving with food). Less likely: tachycardia, hematologic abnormalities, diabetes mellitus, cataracts, & sodium & water retention. Adverse effects are more likely in dogs with hepatic disease.

▶ Availability and expense may be issues. May need to be compounded.

Uses/Indications

In veterinary medicine, oral diazoxide has been used for the treatment of hypoglycemia secondary to hyperinsulin secretion (*e.g.,* insulinoma) in patients refractory to glucocorticoid and dietary therapy. In cats, there is little experience using diazoxide, as insulinomas are apparently very rare.

Pharmacology/Actions

Although related structurally to the thiazide diuretics, diazoxide does not possess any appreciable diuretic activity. By directly causing a vasodilatory effect on the smooth muscle in peripheral arterioles, diazoxide reduces peripheral resistance and blood pressure. To treat malignant hypertension, intravenous diazoxide is generally required for maximal response.

Diazoxide exhibits hyperglycemic activity by directly inhibiting pancreatic insulin secretion. This action may be a result of the drug's capability to decrease the intracellular release of ionized calcium, thereby preventing the release of insulin from the insulin granules. Diazoxide does not apparently affect the synthesis of insulin, nor does it possess any antineoplastic activity. Diazoxide also enhances hyperglycemia by stimulating the beta-adrenergic system thereby stimulating epinephrine release and inhibiting the uptake of glucose by cells.

Pharmacokinetics

The serum half-life of diazoxide has been reported to be about 5 hours in the dog; other pharmacokinetic parameters in the dog appear to be unavailable. In humans, serum diazoxide levels (at 10 mg/kg PO) peaked at about 12 hours after dosing with capsules. It is unknown what blood levels are required to obtain hyperglycemic effects. Highest concentrations of diazoxide are found in the kidneys with high levels also found in the liver and adrenal glands. Approximately 90% of the drug is bound to plasma proteins and it crosses the placenta and into the CNS. It is not known if diazoxide is distributed into milk. Diazoxide is partially metabolized in the liver and is excreted as both metabolites and unchanged drug by the kidneys. Serum half-life of the drug is prolonged in patients with renal impairment.

Contraindications/Precautions/Warnings

Diazoxide should not be used in patients with functional hypoglycemia or for treating hypoglycemia secondary to insulin overdosage in diabetic patients. Unless the potential advantages outweigh the risks, do not use in patients hypersensitive to thiazide diuretics.

Because diazoxide can cause sodium and water retention, use cautiously in patients with congestive heart failure or renal disease.

Adverse Effects

When used to treat insulinomas in dogs, the most commonly seen adverse reactions include hypersalivation, anorexia, vomiting and/or diarrhea; administering the drug with food may lessen these effects. Other effects that may be seen include: tachycardia, hematologic abnormalities (agranulocytosis, aplastic anemia, thrombocytopenia), diabetes mellitus, cataracts (secondary to hyperglycemia?), and sodium and water retention.

Administering the drug with meals or temporarily reducing the dose may alleviate the gastrointestinal side effects. Adverse effects may be more readily noted in dogs with concurrent hepatic disease.

Adverse effects reported with diazoxide use in ferrets include: inappetence, vomiting, diarrhea, malaise, and bone marrow suppression.

The drug is reportedly very bitter.

Reproductive/Nursing Safety

In humans, the FDA categorizes this drug as category *C* for use during pregnancy (*Animal studies have shown an adverse effect on the fetus, but there are no adequate studies in humans; or there are no animal reproduction studies and no adequate studies in humans.*)

It is unknown if diazoxide enters milk.

Overdosage/Acute Toxicity

Acute overdosage may result in severe hyperglycemia and ketoacidosis. Treatment should include insulin (see insulin monograph), fluids and electrolytes. Intensive and prolonged monitoring is recommended.

Drug Interactions

The following drug interactions have either been reported or are theoretical in humans or animals receiving diazoxide and may be of significance in veterinary patients. Unless otherwise noted, use together is not necessarily contraindicated, but weigh the potential risks and perform additional monitoring when appropriate.

- **ALPHA-ADRENERGIC AGENTS** (*e.g.,* **phenoxybenzamine**): May decrease the effectiveness of diazoxide by increasing glucose levels.
- **HYPOTENSIVE AGENTS, OTHER** (*e.g.,* **hydralazine**, **prazosin**, etc.): Diazoxide may enhance the hypotensive actions of other hypotensive agents.
- **PHENOTHIAZINES** (*e.g.,* **acepromazine**, **chlorpromazine**): May enhance the hyperglycemic effects of diazoxide.
- **PHENYTOIN**: Diazoxide may increase the metabolism, or decrease the protein binding of phenytoin.
- **THIAZIDE DIURETICS**: May potentiate the hyperglycemic effects of oral diazoxide. Some clinicians have recommended using hydrochlorothiazide (2 – 4 mg/kg/day PO) in combination with diazoxide, if diazoxide is ineffective alone to increase blood glucose levels; Caution: hypotension may occur.

Laboratory Considerations

- Diazoxide will cause a false-negative insulin response to the **glucagon-stimulation** test.
- Diazoxide may displace **bilirubin** from plasma proteins.

Doses

- **DOGS/CATS:**

  For adjunctive treatment of hypoglycemia secondary to insulin-secreting islet cell or non-islet cell tumors (extra-label): Initially 5 mg/kg PO twice daily. May gradually increase to 30 mg/kg PO twice daily.

- **FERRETS:**

  For hypoglycemia secondary to insulin-secreting islet cell tumors (extra-label): After surgical resection of pancreatic nodules or partial pancreatectomy: Prednisone at 0.5 – 2 mg/kg PO q12h will usually control mild to moderate clinical signs. Begin at lowest dose and gradually increase as needed. Add diazoxide when clinical signs cannot be controlled with prednisone alone. Begin at 5 – 10 mg/kg PO q12h. At same time prednisone dosage may be lowered. (Johnson 2006)

- **SMALL MAMMALS:**

Guinea pigs; for hypoglycemia secondary to insulin-secreting islet cell tumors (extra-label): Based on a single case report: Initially at 5 mg/kg PO every 12 hours. Based blood glucose curve dosage was gradually increased to 25mg/kg (PO every 12 hours. (Hess et al. 2013)

Monitoring

- Blood (serum) glucose.
- CBC (at least every 3-4 months).
- Physical exam (monitor for clinical signs of other adverse effects—see above).

Client Information

- Used to raise blood sugar.
- Give with food to reduce the gastrointestinal side effects of the drug.
- Can be very bitter tasting; taste masking agents are often used to get animals to take the drug. Shake suspensions well.
- Watch for signs of blood sugar that's too high (hyperglycemia) such as drinking more than normal or not drinking much, needing to urinate more, dehydration (not urinating), no appetite, lack of energy, muscle weakness, depression, or severe vomiting, and signs of blood sugar that is or too low (hypoglycemia) such as seizures, muscle weakness, collapse, muscle twitching, depression, or unsteadiness.

Chemistry/Synonyms

Related structurally to the thiazide diuretics, diazoxide occurs as an odorless, white to creamy-white, crystalline powder with a melting point of about 330°F. It is practically insoluble to sparingly soluble in water and slightly soluble in alcohol.

Diazoxide may also be known as: diazoxidum, NSC-64198, Sch-6783, SRG-95213, *Eudemine®*, *Glicemin®*, *Hypertonalum®*, *Hyperstat IV®*, *Proglicem®*, *Sefulken®*, or *Tensuril®*.

Storage/Stability

Diazoxide capsules and oral suspensions should be stored at 2-30°C and protected from light. Protect solutions/suspensions from freezing. Do not use darkened solutions/suspensions, as they may be subpotent.

Compatibility/Compounding Considerations

Diazoxide has a very bitter taste and taste-masking agents (preferably sugar free) may be useful in increasing patient acceptance of this medication.

Dosage Forms/Regulatory Status

VETERINARY-LABELED PRODUCTS: NONE.

The ARCI (Racing Commissioners International) has designated this drug as a class 3 substance. See the appendix for more information.

HUMAN-LABELED PRODUCTS:

Diazoxide Oral Suspension: 50 mg; with sorbitol in 30 mL calibrated dropper; *Proglycem®*; (Rx)

Revisions/References

Monograph revised/updated January 2014.

Hess, L. R., et al. (2013). Diagnosis and treatment of an insulinoma in a guinea pig (Cavia porcellus). Javma-Journal of the American Veterinary Medical Association **242**(4): 522-6.

Johnson, D. (2006). Ferrets: the other companion animal. Proceedings: ACVC. accessed via Veterinary Information Network; vin.com

Dichlorphenamide

(dye-klor-fen-a-mide)   Daranide®

Carbonic Anhydrase Inhibitor

Prescriber Highlights

▶ Used primarily for open angle glaucoma.

▶ Contraindicated in patients with significant hepatic, renal, pulmonary or adrenocortical insufficiency, hyponatremia, hypokalemia, hyperchloremic acidosis, or electrolyte imbalance.

▶ Give oral doses with food if GI upset occurs.

▶ Monitor with tonometry for glaucoma; check electrolytes.

▶ Availability issues; may need to be obtained from a compounding pharmacy.

Uses/Indications

Dichlorphenamide is used for the medical treatment of glaucoma. Because of availability issues and toxic effects associated with systemic therapy, human (and many veterinary) ophthalmologists are using topical carbonic anhydrase inhibitors (*e.g.,* dorzolamide or brinzolamide) in place of acetazolamide, dichlorphenamide or methazolamide.

Pharmacology/Actions

The carbonic anhydrase inhibitors act by a noncompetitive, reversible inhibition of the enzyme carbonic anhydrase. This reduces the formation of hydrogen and bicarbonate ions from carbon dioxide and reduces the availability of these ions for active transport into body secretions.

Pharmacologic effects of the carbonic anhydrase inhibitors include decreased formation of aqueous humor, thereby reducing intraocular pressure; increased renal tubular secretion of sodium and potassium and, to a greater extent, bicarbonate, leading to increased urine alkalinity and volume; and anticonvulsant activity, which is independent of its diuretic effects (mechanism not fully understood, but may be due to carbonic anhydrase or a metabolic acidosis effect).

Pharmacokinetics

The pharmacokinetics of this agent have apparently not been studied in domestic animals. In small animals, onset of action is 30 minutes, maximal effect in 2-4 hours, and duration of action is 8-12 hours.

Contraindications/Precautions/Warnings

Carbonic anhydrase inhibitors are contraindicated in patients with significant hepatic disease (may precipitate hepatic coma), renal or adrenocortical insufficiency, hyponatremia, hypokalemia, hyperchloremic acidosis, or electrolyte imbalance. They should not be used in patients with severe pulmonary obstruction unable to increase alveolar ventilation or those that are hypersensitive to them. Long-term use of carbonic anhydrase inhibitors is contraindicated in patients with chronic, noncongestive, angle-closure glaucoma as angle closure may occur and the drug may mask the condition by lowering intra-ocular pressures.

Adverse Effects

Potential adverse effects that may be encountered include panting, GI disturbances (inappetence, vomiting, diarrhea), CNS effects (sedation, depression, excitement, etc.), hematologic effects (bone marrow depression), renal effects (crystalluria, dysuria, renal colic, polyuria), metabolic acidosis, hypokalemia, hyperglycemia, hyponatremia, hyperuricemia, hepatic insufficiency, dermatologic effects (rash, etc.), and hypersensitivity reactions.

Reproductive/Nursing Safety

In humans, the FDA categorizes this drug as category *C* for use during pregnancy (*Animal studies have shown an adverse effect on the fetus, but there are no adequate studies in humans; or there are no animal reproduction studies and no adequate studies in humans.*)

Overdosage/Acute Toxicity

Information regarding overdosage of this drug is not readily available. It is suggested to monitor serum electrolytes, blood gases, volume status, and CNS status during an acute overdose. Treat symptomatically and supportively.

Drug Interactions

The following drug interactions have either been reported or are theoretical in humans or animals receiving dichlorphenamide and may be of significance in veterinary patients. Unless otherwise noted, use together is not necessarily contraindicated, but weigh the potential risks and perform additional monitoring when appropriate.

- **ANTIDEPRESSANTS, TRICYCLIC:** Alkaline urine cause by dichlorphenamide may decrease excretion.
- **ASPIRIN** (or other **salicylates**): Increased risk of dichlorphenamide accumulation and toxicity; increased risk for metabolic acidosis; dichlorphenamide increases salicylate excretion.
- **DIGOXIN:** As dichlorphenamide may cause hypokalemia, increased risk for toxicity.
- **INSULIN:** Rarely, carbonic anhydrase inhibitors interfere with the hypoglycemic effects of insulin.
- **METHENAMINE COMPOUNDS:** Dichlorphenamide may negate effects in the urine.
- **POTASSIUM, DRUGS AFFECTING** (**corticosteroids, amphotericin B, corticotropin,** or other **diuretics**): Concomitant use may exacerbate potassium depletion.
- **PHENOBARBITAL:** Increased urinary excretion, may reduce phenobarbital levels.
- **PRIMIDONE:** Decreased primidone concentrations
- **QUINIDINE:** Alkaline urine cause by dichlorphenamide may decrease excretion.

Laboratory Considerations

- By alkalinizing the urine, carbonic anhydrase inhibitors may cause false positive results in determining **urine protein** using bromphenol blue reagent (*Albustix®, Albutest®, Labstix®*), sulfosalicylic acid (*Bumintest®,* Exton's Test Reagent), nitric acid ring test, or heat and acetic acid test methods.
- Carbonic anhydrase inhibitors may decrease **iodine uptake** by the thyroid gland in hyperthyroid or euthyroid patients.

Doses

- **DOGS:**
  For adjunctive treatment of glaucoma (extra-label):
  a) 2.2 – 4.4 mg/kg PO 2-3 times daily (q8-12h). (Nasisse 2005), (Miller 2005)
  b) 10 – 15 mg/kg per day divided 2-3 times daily. (Brooks 2002)
  c) 2 – 5 mg/kg PO q8-12h. (Wilkie 2003)
- **CATS:**
  For adjunctive treatment of glaucoma (extra-label):
  a) 0.5 – 1.5 mg/kg PO 2-3 times daily. (Powell 2003)
  b) 1 – 2 mg/kg PO q8-12h. (Miller 2005)

Monitoring

- Intraocular pressure/tonometry.
- Serum electrolytes; may need to supplement potassium.

- Baseline CBC with differential and periodic retests if using chronically.
- Other adverse effects.

Client Information

- If GI upset occurs, give with food.
- Notify veterinarian if abnormal bleeding or bruising occurs or if animal develops tremors or a rash.

Chemistry/Synonyms

A carbonic anhydrase inhibitor, dichlorphenamide occurs as a white or nearly white, crystalline powder with a melting range of 235-240°C, and pK$_a$s of 7.4 and 8.6. It is very slightly soluble in water and soluble in alcohol.

Dichlorphenamide may also be known as: dichlorphenamide, diclofenamidum, *Antidrasi®, Fenamide®, Glaucol®, Glauconide®, Glaumid®, Oralcon®, Oratrol®,* or *Tensodilen®.*

Storage/Stability

Store tablets in well-closed containers and at room temperature. An expiration date of 5 years after the date of manufacture is assigned to the commercially available tablets.

Compatibility/Compounding Considerations

No specific information noted.

Dosage Forms/Regulatory Status

VETERINARY-LABELED PRODUCTS: NONE.

HUMAN-LABELED PRODUCTS: NONE.

Dichlorphenamide availability has been an issue and it may not be available commercially; if not, contact a compounding pharmacy for information.

Revisions/References

Monograph revised/updated January 2014.

Brooks, D. E. (2002). Glaucoma-Medical and Surgical Treatment. Proceedings: Western Veterinary Conference. accessed via Veterinary Information Network; vin.com
Miller, P. (2005). New drugs for glaucoma. Proceedings: Western Vet Conf. accessed via Veterinary Information Network; vin.com
Nasisse, M. (2005). Treatment of canine glaucoma, Proceedings: ACVIM. accessed via Veterinary Information Network; vin.com
Powell, C. (2003). Feline Glaucoma. Proceedings: Western Veterinary Conference. accessed via Veterinary Information Network; vin.com
Wilkie, D. (2003). Glaucoma. Proceedings: Atlantic Coast Veterinary Conference. accessed via Veterinary Information Network; vin.com

Dichlorvos

(dye-klor-vose)   Atgard®

Organophosphate Antiparasitic

Prescriber Highlights

▶ Organophosphate used orally as a wormer (primarily roundworms) in pigs & as ectoparasiticide ("No Pest Strip") for small mammals, etc.

▶ Contraindications: Anticholinesterase drugs; do not allow fowl access to medicated feed or manure from treated animals.

▶ Adverse Effects (dose related): Vomiting, tremors, bradycardia, respiratory distress, hyperexcitability, salivation, & diarrhea.

▶ Drug Interactions.

Uses/Indications

Dichlorvos is effective in swine against Ascaris, Trichuris, *Ascarops strongylina* and *Oesophagostomum* spp.

Dichlorvos as a "No Pest Strip" is used as an ectoparasiticide for small mammals. It is also used as a premise spray to keep fly populations controlled.

In horses, dichlorvos is labeled as being effective for the treatment and control of bots, pinworms, large and small bloodworms, and large roundworms, but no systemic equine products are currently being marketed in the USA.

Dichlorvos was available for use internally in dogs and cats for the treatment of roundworms and hookworms, but no products are currently being marketed since newer, safer and more effective anthelmintics have replaced dichlorvos.

Pharmacology/Actions

Like other organophosphate agents, dichlorvos inhibits acetylcholinesterase interfering with neuromuscular transmission in susceptible parasites.

Pharmacokinetics

Specific information was not located for this agent.

Contraindications/Precautions/Warnings

For the product (*Atgard®*) for use in swine, no absolute contraindications are labeled, but it should not be used within a few days of any other cholinesterase inhibiting drug, pesticide or chemical.

Do not allow fowl access to medicated feed or manure from treated animals.

Unused medication or medicated feed should be buried 18 inches below the ground and covered so that it is unavailable to any other animal.

Avoid contact with the skin and keep out of reach of children.

Adverse Effects

When used as labeled, there are no listed adverse effects in swine. Adverse effects are generally dose-related and may include those listed below in the Overdosage/Acute Toxicity section.

Reproductive/Nursing Safety

Studies performed in target species have demonstrated no teratogenic effects at usual doses. In pigs, no effects have been noted on reproductive capability, performance or litter survivability.

Overdosage/Acute Toxicity

If overdoses occur, vomiting, tremors, bradycardia, respiratory distress, hyperexcitability, salivation, and diarrhea may occur. Atropine (see atropine and pralidoxime monographs for more information) may be antidotal. Use of succinylcholine, theophylline, aminophylline, reserpine, or respiratory depressant drugs (*e.g.*, narcotics, phenothiazines) should be avoided in patients with organophosphate toxicity. If ingestion occurs by a human, contact a poison control center, physician, or hospital emergency room.

Drug Interactions

The following drug interactions have either been reported or are theoretical in humans or animals receiving dichlorvos and may be of significance in veterinary patients. Unless otherwise noted, use together is not necessarily contraindicated, but weigh the potential risks and perform additional monitoring when appropriate.

- **ACEPROMAZINE** or other **phenothiazines**: Should not be given within one month of worming with an organophosphate agent as their effects may be potentiated.
- **ANTICHOLINESTERASE DRUGS** (*e.g.*, **neostigmine**, **physostigmine**, and **pyridostigmine**): Avoid use when using organophosphates as they can inhibit cholinesterase.
- **DMSO**: Because of its anticholinesterase activity, avoid the use of organophosphates with DMSO.
- **MORPHINE**: Avoid use when using organophosphates as it can inhibit cholinesterase.
- **PYRANTEL PAMOATE** (or **tartrate**): Adverse effects could be intensified if used concomitantly with an organophosphate.
- **SUCCINYLCHOLINE**: Patients receiving organophosphate anthelmintics should not receive succinylcholine or other depolarizing muscle relaxants for at least 48 hours.

Doses

- **RABBITS/RODENTS/SMALL MAMMALS:**

  Mice, Rats, Gerbils, Hamsters, Guinea pigs, Chinchillas: Hang

5 cm of a dichlorvos strip (*e.g., Vapona® No Pest Strip*) 6 inches above cage for 24 hours, twice weekly for 3 weeks (Anderson 1994); (Adamcak et al. 2000) or hang in room for 24 hours once a week for 6 weeks or a 1 inch square laid on cage for 24 hours once a week for 6 weeks (Adamcak et al. 2000)

- **SWINE:**

  For *Atgard® Swine Wormer*: Dosing for pigs is accomplished by adding to feed (crumble-type or dry meal). Specific amounts of feed per packet are dependent on pig weight. See the label for specific recommendations.

Monitoring

- Efficacy.
- Adverse effects.

Client Information

- Keep out of reach of children. Handling of dichlorvos liquid preparations (*e.g.*, premise spray) must be done with extreme care; follow all label directions!
- Oral pellets are non-digestible and may be seen in the animals' feces.

Chemistry/Synonyms

An organophosphate insecticide, dichlorvos may also known as: 2,2,-dichlorovinyl dimethyl phosphate DDVP, NSC-6738, OMS-14, SD-1750, *Atgard®*, or *Ravap E.C.®*.

Storage/Stability

Store *Atgard®* swine wormer at less than 80°F. Dichlorvos feed additives should not be stored at temperatures below freezing. Dichlorvos is sensitive to hydrolysis if exposed to moisture or oxidizing agents.

Compatibility/Compounding Considerations

No specific information noted.

Dosage Forms/Regulatory Status

VETERINARY-LABELED PRODUCTS:

Dichlorvos Feed Additives: *Atgard® C*; *Atgard® Swine Wormer*; (OTC). When used as labeled there are no slaughter withdrawal times required in swine.

Dichlorvos with Tetrachlorvinphos (*Rabon®*) Premise and Topical Insecticide: *Ravap E.C.®*; (OTC)

Dichlorvos may also be found in premise insecticidal products.

HUMAN-LABELED PRODUCTS: NONE.

Revisions/References

Monograph revised/updated January 2014.

Adamcak, A. & B. Otten (2000). Rodent Therapeutics. Vet Clin NA: Exotic Anim Pract 3:1(Jan): 221-40.
Anderson, N. (1994). Basic husbandry and medicine of pocket pets. *Saunders Manual of Small Animal Practice*. S. Birchard and R. Sherding. Philadelphia, W.B. Saunders Company: 1363-89.

Diclazuril

(dye-klaz-yoor-il)   Protazil®, Clinicox®

Antiprotozoal

Prescriber Highlights

▶ FDA-approved (in USA) for equine protozoal myeloencephalitis (EPM) in horses & as a coccidiostat in broiler chickens.
▶ Adverse effect profile not well known.

Uses/Indications

In the USA, diclazuril is FDA-approved for the treatment of equine protozoal myeloencephalitis (EPM) caused by *Sarcocystis neurona* and as a coccidiostat in broiler chickens.

In the U.K., oral diclazuril suspension is approved for the treatment and prevention of coccidial infections in lambs caused, in particular, by the more pathogenic *Eimeria* species *E. crandallis* and *E. ovinoidalis* and to aid in the control of coccidiosis in calves caused by *Eimeria bovis* and *Eimeria zuernii*. Recent studies, comparing diclazuril and toltrazuril have shown that toltrazuril is more effective in reducing oocyte shedding in lambs and calves than is diclazuril (Le Sueur et al. 2009), (Mundt et al. 2009), (Mundt et al. 2007).

Diclazuril could potentially be useful in treating coccidiosis, *Neospora caninum* and Toxoplasma infections in dogs or cats.

Pharmacology/Actions

The triazine class of antiprotozoals is believed to target the "plastid" body, an organelle found in the members of the Apicomplexa phylum, including *Sarcocystis neurona*. The actual mechanism of action is not well described. *In vitro* levels required to inhibit (95%) *Sarcocystis neurona* are about 1 ng/mL.

Pharmacokinetics

In horses, oral bioavailability is about 5%. CSF levels are approximately 1-5% of those found in plasma. Elimination half-life is prolonged (43-65 hours). Doses of 1 mg/kg/day should give mean steady-state plasma levels of about 2 – 2.5 mg/mL with corresponding CSF levels of 20 – 70 ng/mL which is in excess of the *in vitro* IC_{95} (1 ng/mL).

Contraindications/Precautions/Warnings

The drug is contraindicated in patients known to be hypersensitive to diclazuril.

The safe use of *Protazil®* in horses used for breeding purposes, during pregnancy, in lactation, or with other therapies has not been evaluated.

Adverse Effects

The adverse effect profile in horses is not well known. In field trials, no adverse effects could be ascribed to the drug.

On rare occasions, highly susceptible lambs may develop severe diarrhea (scour) after dosing; fluid therapy is required and antibiotics may be necessary.

Reproductive/Nursing Safety

The manufacturer states that the safe use of *Protazil®* in horses used for breeding purposes, during pregnancy, or in lactation has not been evaluated.

Overdosage/Acute Toxicity

Limited information is available, but the drug appears to have a large safety margin in animals. Normal horses dosed up to 50 mg/kg/day (50X) for 42 days developed only marginal effects (decreased weight gain, increased creatinine, BUN). Doses of up to 60X in lambs and calves did not cause any demonstrable side effects.

Drug Interactions

- None were noted. The manufacturer states that the safety of *Protazil®* with concomitant therapies in horses has not been evaluated.

Laboratory Considerations

- None were noted.

Doses

- **HORSES:**

  For treatment of equine protozoal myeloencephalitis (*S. neurona*): Using the oral pellets and the provided cup: Top dress at the rate of 1 mg/kg bodyweight for 28 days. If horse's bodyweight is in between two graduations on the dosing cup, fill the cup to the higher of the two marks. (Label information; *Protazil®*)

- **DOGS/CATS:**

  For coccidiosis (extra-label): 25 mg/kg PO once. (Greene et al.

2006)

For coccidiosis in kittens (extra-label): 1 mL (2.5 mg) PO of the sheep solution per 4 kg body mass. (Miller 2007)

For *Isospora* spp. infections in cats (extra-label): 25 mg/kg PO once. (Dubey et al. 2009)

- **SHEEP (LAMBS):**

  Therapeutic use (extra-label in USA): 1 mg/kg (1 mL of the 2.5mg/mL suspension per 2.5 kg bodyweight) PO once. **For preventative use** (extra-label in USA): 1 mg/kg PO at about 4-6 weeks of age at the time that coccidiosis can normally be expected on the farm. Under conditions of high infection pressure, a second treatment may be indicated about 3 weeks after the first dosing. Recommended to treat all lambs in flock. (Label Information; *Vecoxan®*—Janssen U.K.)

- **CATTLE (CALVES):**

  As an aid to control coccidiosis (extra-label in USA): 1 mg/kg (1 mL of the 2.5 mg/mL suspension per 2.5 kg bodyweight) PO as a single dose, 14 days after moving into a potentially high risk environment. If a satisfactory response is not observed, then further advice should be sought from your veterinary surgeon and the cause of the condition reviewed. It is good practice to ensure the cleanliness of calf housing. Recommended to treat all calves in pen. (Label Information; *Vecoxan®*—Janssen U.K.)

Monitoring

- Clinical efficacy (neuro exams).

Client Information

- Antiprotozoal drug used for treating equine protozoal myeloencephalitis (EPM) in horses. Also used to treat coccidiosis in dogs, cats, chickens and other species.

- In small animals may be given with or without food. If your animal vomits or acts sick after getting it on an empty stomach, give with food or small treat to see if this helps. If vomiting continues, contact your veterinarian.

- Used as a "top-dress" over feed in horses. Must be dosed daily; be sure horse eats the entire dose.

- Appears to be tolerated well, but report any side effects to veterinarian.

Chemistry/Synonyms

Diclazuril occurs as a white to light yellow powder. It is practically insoluble in water and alcohol.

Diclazuril may also be known as diclazurilo, diclazurilum, R 64433 and by the trade names, *Clinicox®*, *Protazil®*, and *Vecoxan®*.

Compatibility/Compounding Considerations

No specific information noted.

Storage/Stability

Diclazuril pellets should be stored at room temperature (15-30°C).

Dosage Forms/Regulatory Status

VETERINARY-LABELED PRODUCTS:

Diclazuril Oral Pellets 1.56% in 2 lb. and 10 lb. containers: *Protazil®*; (Rx). FDA-approved for use in horses not intended for food. One 2 lb. bucket will treat a 1100 lb. horse for 28 days.

Diclazuril 0.2% Type A Medicated Feed Article in 50 lb. containers; *Clinicox®*; (OTC). FDA-approved for use in broiler chickens.

In the UK and other countries, diclazuril may be available as an oral suspension containing 2.5 mg/mL diclazuril. One trade name is *Vecoxan®* (Janssen). When used as labeled, no withdrawal time is required in the U.K.

HUMAN-LABELED PRODUCTS: NONE.

Revisions/References

Monograph revised/updated January 2014.

Dubey, J., et al. (2009). Toxoplasmosis and other intestinal coccidial infections in cats and dogs. Vet Clin Small Anim **39**: 1009-34.

Greene, C., et al. (2006). Appendix 8: Antimicrobial Drug Formulary. *Infectious Disease of the Dog and Cat.* C. Greene, Elsevier: 1186-333.

Le Sueur, C., et al. (2009). Efficacy of toltrazuril (BaycoxA (R) 5% suspension) in natural infections with pathogenic Eimeria spp. in housed lambs. Parasitology Research **104**(5): 1157-62.

Miller, D. (2007). Kitten Diarrhoea. Proceedings: World Small Animal Association. accessed via Veterinary Information Network; vin.com

Mundt, H. C., et al. (2009). Study of the Comparative Efficacy of Toltrazuril and Diclazuril against Ovine Coccidiosis in Housed Lambs. Parasitology Research **105**: S141-S50.

Mundt, H. C., et al. (2007). Control of coccidiosis due to Eimeria bovis and Eimeria zuernii in calves with toltrazuril under field conditions in comparison with diclazuril and untreated controls. Parasitology Research **101**: S93-S104.

Diclofenac Sodium, Topical

(dye-kloe-fen-ak)   Surpass®

Non-Steroidal Antiinflammatory Agent (NSAID)

Prescriber Highlights

▶ NSAID FDA-approved for topical use in horses for local control of joint pain & inflammation.

▶ Appears well-tolerated at recommended dosage.

Uses/Indications

The equine topical cream (*Surpass®*) is labeled for the control of pain and inflammation associated with osteoarthritis in tarsal, carpal, metacarpophalangeal, metarsophalangeal, and proximal interphalangeal (hock, knee, fetlock, pastern) joints for use up to 10 days duration. While, theoretically, diclofenac could be used systemically (orally) in other veterinary species, there are other FDA-approved and safer alternatives.

Pharmacology/Actions

Diclofenac is a non-specific inhibitor of cyclooxygenase (both COX-1 and COX-2). It may also have some inhibitory effects on lipooxygenase. By inhibiting COX-2 enzymes, diclofenac reduces the production of prostaglandins associated with pain, hyperpyrexia, and inflammation.

Pharmacokinetics

When diclofenac is administered topically to horses via the 1% liposomal cream, it is absorbed locally, but specific bioavailability data was not located. Peak levels in transudate obtained from tissue cages were about 80 ng/mL; levels stay increased from 6 hours to at least 18 hours after administration. At the dosages recommended for the topical cream, most of the drug remains in the tissues local to the administration point, but detectable levels in the systemic circulation may occur. In humans, diclofenac is more than 99% bound to plasma proteins. It is metabolized in the liver and the metabolites are excreted primarily into the urine.

Contraindications/Precautions/Warnings

Topical diclofenac should not be used in horses hypersensitive to it or any component of the cream. It has not been evaluated in horses less than one year old.

Exceeding the recommended dosage or treating multiple joints may cause adverse effects.

Do not use diclofenac in birds as it has been implicated in causing death in vultures.

Adverse Effects

The topical cream in horses appears to be well tolerated. One case of a horse developing colic during therapy has been reported. Other adverse effects that may be seen include weight loss, gastric ulcers, diarrhea, or uterine discharge. In the FDA's adverse reaction database local reactions (inflammation, swelling, alopecia) have been reported.

Reproductive/Nursing Safety

Reproductive safety for topical diclofenac has not been investigated in breeding, pregnant or lactating horses.

Overdosage/Acute Toxicity

When overdoses are administered topically to horses, adverse effects may occur including weight loss, gastric ulcers, colic, diarrhea, and uterine discharge. Treatment is supportive.

In small animals, there were 140 exposures to diclofenac sodium reported to the ASPCA Animal Poison Control Center (APCC) during 2008-2009. In these cases 131 were dogs with 37 showing clinical signs and the remaining 9 cases were cat exposures with 3 showing clinical signs. Common findings in dogs (recorded in decreasing frequency) include vomiting, diarrhea, bloody diarrhea, melena and polydipsia.

This medication is a NSAID. As with any NSAID, overdosage can lead to gastrointestinal and renal effects. Decontamination with emetics and/or activated charcoal is appropriate. For doses where GI effects are expected, the use of gastrointestinal protectants is warranted. If renal effects are also expected, fluid diuresis is warranted.

Diclofenac ingestion has caused death in vultures eating dead carcasses of animals that received diclofenac.

Drug Interactions

When used topically at recommended dosages, there are no reported drug interactions in horses.

Laboratory Considerations

■ No specific laboratory interactions or considerations were noted.

Doses

■ **HORSES:**

For the control of pain and inflammation associated with osteoarthritis in tarsal, carpal, metacarpophalangeal, metarsophalangeal, and proximal interphalangeal (hock, knee, fetlock, pastern) joints (labeled-dose): Using *Surpass®* topical cream apply a five inch ribbon twice daily over the affected joint for up to 10 days. Wear rubber gloves and rub cream thoroughly into the hair covering the joint until cream disappears. (Label information; *Surpass®*—Idexx)

Monitoring

■ Efficacy.

■ Adverse effects.

Client Information

■ A client information sheet is supplied with the medication and should be given to the client.

■ Topical NSAID cream used on horses for joint pain and inflammation. Approved for use for up to 10 days.

■ Horses usually tolerate very well; loss of hair or mild swelling at application site is possible.

■ Manufacturer warns against using on more than one joint or using more than a 5-inch ribbon as this may cause adverse effects. Do not use more than veterinarian prescribes.

■ Wear rubber or other disposable non-permeable gloves and rub cream thoroughly into the hair covering the joint until cream disappears.

Chemistry/Synonyms

A phenyl-acetic acid derivative non-steroidal antiinflammatory agent, diclofenac sodium occurs as a white to off-white, hygroscopic, crystalline powder. It is sparingly soluble in water, soluble in alcohol and practically insoluble in chloroform and ether.

Diclofenac may also be known as: GP-45840, diclofenacum or diclophenac; many trade names are available for diclofenac products outside of the USA.

Storage/Stability

Unless otherwise labeled, diclofenac sodium products should be stored in airtight containers and protected from light. The commercially available 1% cream (*Surpass®*) should be stored at temperatures up to 25°C (77°F); protect from freezing.

Compatibility/Compounding Considerations

No specific information noted.

Dosage Forms/Regulatory Status

VETERINARY-LABELED PRODUCTS:

Diclofenac sodium (liposomal) 1% topical cream in 124 gram tubes, *Surpass®*; (Rx). FDA-approved for use in horses.

Injectable forms of this medication are available in some countries.

HUMAN-LABELED PRODUCTS:

Diclofenac Tablets: 50 mg (as potassium); *Cataflam®*, generic; (Rx)

Diclofenac Delayed-release Tablets: 25 mg, 50 mg, 75 mg & 100 mg (as sodium); *Voltaren-XR®*, generic; (Rx)

Diclofenac Sodium Gel: 3% (1 g contains 30 mg diclofenac sodium) with benzyl alcohol in 25 g & 50 g; *Solaraze®*; (Rx)

Diclofenac Sodium/Misoprostol Tablets: (each tablet consists of an enteric-coated core containing diclofenac sodium surrounded by an outer mantle containing misoprostol) 50 mg/misoprostol 200 mcg & 75 mg/misoprostol 200 mcg; *Arthrotec®*; (Rx)

Diclofenac sodium is also FDA-approved as a topical ophthalmic agent (see the ophthalmology drug appendix).

Revisions/References

Monograph revised/updated January 2014.

Dicloxacillin Sodium

(di-klox-a-**sill**-in)   Dynapen®

Anti-Staphylococcal Penicillin

Prescriber Highlights

▶ Oral isoxazolyl (anti-staphylococcal) penicillin.

▶ Contraindications: hypersensitivity to penicillins; do not use oral medications in critically ill patients.

▶ Most predominant adverse effects are GI in nature.

▶ Must dose orally quite often (q6-8h); expense, efficacy & owner compliance may be issues.

Uses/Indications

The veterinary use of dicloxacillin has been primarily in the PO treatment of bone, skin, and other soft tissue infections in small animals when penicillinase-producing Staphylococcus species have been isolated. Because of its low oral bioavailability and short half-life, other drugs with good staph coverage are usually employed.

Pharmacology/Actions

Cloxacillin, dicloxacillin and oxacillin have nearly identical spectrums of activity and can be considered therapeutically equivalent when comparing *in vitro* activity. These penicillinase-resistant penicillins have a narrower spectrum of activity than the natural penicillins. Their antimicrobial efficacy is aimed directly against penicillinase-producing strains of gram-positive cocci, particularly Staphylococcal species. They are sometimes called anti-staphylococcal penicillins. There are documented strains of Staphylococcus that are resistant to these drugs (so-called methicillin-resistant Staph, MRSA), but these strains have not yet been a major problem in veterinary species. While this class of penicillins does have activity against some other gram-positive and gram-negative aerobes and anaerobes, other antibiotics (penicillins and others) are usually

better choices. The penicillinase-resistant penicillins are inactive against Rickettsia, mycobacteria, fungi, Mycoplasma and viruses.

Pharmacokinetics

Dicloxacillin is only available in oral dosage forms. Dicloxacillin sodium is resistant to acid inactivation in the gut but is only partially absorbed. The bioavailability after oral administration in dogs is only about 23% and in humans has been reported to range from 35-76%. If given with food, both the rate and extent of absorption is decreased.

The drug is distributed to the liver, kidneys, bone, bile, pleural, synovial and ascitic fluids. However, one manufacturer states that levels of the drug that are achieved in ascitic fluid are not clinically therapeutic. As with the other penicillins, only minimal amounts are distributed into the CSF. In humans, approximately 95-99% of the drug is bound to plasma proteins.

Dicloxacillin is partially metabolized to both active and inactive metabolites. These metabolites and the parent compound are rapidly excreted in the urine via both glomerular filtration and tubular secretion mechanisms. A small amount of the drug is also excreted in the feces via biliary elimination. The serum half-life in humans with normal renal function ranges from about 24-48 minutes. In dogs, 20-40 minutes to 2.6 hours have been reported as the elimination half-life.

Contraindications/Precautions/Warnings

Penicillins are contraindicated in patients with a history of hypersensitivity to them. Because there may be cross-reactivity, use penicillins cautiously in patients that are documented hypersensitive to other beta-lactam antibiotics (*e.g.*, cephalosporins, cefamycins, carbapenems).

Do not administer systemic antibiotics orally in patients with septicemia, shock, or other grave illnesses as absorption of the medication from the GI tract may be significantly delayed or diminished. Parenteral (preferably IV) routes should be used for these cases.

Adverse Effects

Adverse effects with the penicillins are usually not serious and have a relatively low frequency of occurrence.

Hypersensitivity reactions unrelated to dose can occur with these agents and can manifest as rashes, fever, eosinophilia, neutropenia, agranulocytosis, thrombocytopenia, leukopenia, anemias, lymphadenopathy, or full-blown anaphylaxis. In humans, it is estimated that 1-15% of patients hypersensitive to cephalosporins will also be hypersensitive to penicillins. The incidence of cross-reactivity in veterinary patients is unknown.

When given orally, penicillins may cause GI effects (anorexia, vomiting, diarrhea). Because the penicillins may also alter gut flora, antibiotic-associated diarrhea can occur and allow the proliferation of resistant bacteria in the colon (superinfections).

Neurotoxicity (*e.g.*, ataxia in dogs) has been associated with very high doses or very prolonged use. Although the penicillins are not considered hepatotoxic, elevated liver enzymes have been reported. Other effects reported in dogs include tachypnea, dyspnea, edema, and tachycardia.

Reproductive/Nursing Safety

Penicillins have been shown to cross the placenta and safe use of them during pregnancy has not been firmly established, but neither have there been any documented teratogenic problems associated with these drugs. However, use only when the potential benefits outweigh the risks. In humans, the FDA categorizes this drug as category *B* for use during pregnancy (*Animal studies have not yet demonstrated risk to the fetus, but there are no adequate studies in pregnant women; or animal studies have shown an adverse effect, but adequate studies in pregnant women have not demonstrated a risk to the fetus in the first trimester of pregnancy, and there is no evidence of risk in later trimesters.*) In a separate system evaluating the safety of drugs in canine and feline pregnancy (Papich 1989), this drug is categorized as class: A (*Probably safe. Although specific studies may not have proved the safety of all drugs in dogs and cats, there are no reports of adverse effects in laboratory animals or women.*)

Dicloxacillin is distributed into milk. While safety cannot be assured (may alter neonatal gut flora or cause hypersensitivity), it is unlikely to pose much risk to nursing offspring.

Overdosage/Acute Toxicity

Acute oral penicillin overdoses are unlikely to cause significant problems other than GI distress, but other effects are possible (see Adverse Effects). In humans, very high dosages of parenteral penicillins, especially in patients with renal disease, have induced CNS effects.

Drug Interactions

The following drug interactions have either been reported or are theoretical in humans or animals receiving dicloxacillin and may be of significance in veterinary patients. Unless otherwise noted, use together is not necessarily contraindicated, but weigh the potential risks and perform additional monitoring when appropriate.

- **AMINOGLYCOSIDES:** *In vitro* evidence of synergism with dicloxacillin against *S. aureus* strains.
- **CYCLOSPORINE:** Dicloxacillin may reduce levels.
- **PROBENECID:** Competitively blocks the tubular secretion of dicloxacillin, thereby increasing serum levels and serum half-lives.
- **TETRACYCLINES:** Theoretical antagonism; use together usually not recommended.
- **WARFARIN:** Dicloxacillin may cause decreased warfarin efficacy.

Laboratory Considerations

- As penicillins and other beta-lactams can inactivate aminoglycosides *in vitro* (and *in vivo* in patients in renal failure), serum concentrations of aminoglycosides may be falsely decreased if the patient is also receiving beta-lactam antibiotics and the serum is stored prior to analysis. It is recommended that if the assay is delayed, samples be frozen and, if possible, drawn at times when the beta-lactam antibiotic is at a trough.

Doses

- **DOGS/CATS:**

  For susceptible infections (extra-label): 20 – 30 mg/kg PO q6-8h.

Monitoring

- Because penicillins usually have minimal toxicity associated with their use, monitoring for efficacy is usually all that is required unless toxic clinical signs develop. Serum levels and therapeutic drug monitoring are not routinely done with these agents.

Client Information

- Owners should be instructed to give oral penicillins to animals with an empty stomach, unless using amoxicillin or if GI effects (anorexia, vomiting) occur.
- Compliance with the therapeutic regimen should be stressed.
- Reconstituted oral suspensions should be kept refrigerated and discarded after 14 days.

Chemistry/Synonyms

An isoxazolyl-penicillin, dicloxacillin sodium is a semisynthetic, penicillinase-resistant penicillin. It is available commercially as the monohydrate sodium salt that occurs as a white to off-white, crystalline powder that is freely soluble in water and has a pK$_a$ of

2.7-2.8. One mg of dicloxacillin sodium contains not less than 850 micrograms of dicloxacillin.

Dicloxacillin Sodium may also be known as: sodium dicloxacillin, dichlorphenylmethyl isoxazolyl penicillin sodium, methyldichlorophenyl isoxazolyl penicillin sodium, dicloxacilina sodica, dicloxacillinum natricum, or P-1011; many trade names are available.

Storage/Stability

Dicloxacillin sodium capsules should be stored at temperatures less than 40°C and preferably at room temperature (15-30°C).

Compatibility/Compounding Considerations

No specific information noted.

Dosage Forms/Regulatory Status

VETERINARY-LABELED PRODUCTS:

No products are apparently being currently marketed in the USA. The FDA's "Green Book" still lists 100 mg and 500 mg capsules; *Dicloxin®* as approved for use in dogs.

HUMAN-LABELED PRODUCTS:

Dicloxacillin Sodium Capsules: 250 mg & 500 mg; generic; (Rx)

Revisions/References

Monograph revised/updated January 2014.

Diethylstilbestrol

(dye-ethel-stil-bes-tral)   DES

Hormonal Agent

Prescriber Highlights

- ► Synthetic estrogen used in dogs primarily for estrogen responsive incontinence & other estrogen indications (prostatic hypertrophy, estrus induction, etc.). With the FDA-approval of estriol for dogs, using DES now is controversial, particularly in dogs starting estrogen therapy for urinary incontinence.
- ► Prohibited for use in food animals (potential carcinogen).
- ► Teratogen.
- ► Many potential adverse effects: blood dyscrasias, GI effects, cystic endometrial hyperplasia & pyometra (non-spayed females), feminization (males), neoplasia.
- ► Availability issues; must be obtained via a compounding pharmacy.

Uses/Indications

DES has been used in estrogen responsive incontinence in spayed female dogs and the medical treatment of benign prostatic hypertrophy in male dogs. It has also been used for the prevention of pregnancy after mismating in female dogs and cats, but is typically no longer recommended because of serious side effects.

Pharmacology/Actions

Estrogens are necessary for the normal growth and development of the female sex organs and in some species contribute to the development and maintenance of secondary female sex characteristics. Estrogens cause increased cell height and secretions of the cervical mucosa, thickening of the vaginal mucosa, endometrial proliferation, and increased uterine tone.

Estrogens have effects on the skeletal system. They increase calcium deposition, accelerate epiphyseal closure and increase bone formation. Estrogens have a slight anabolic effect and can increase sodium and water retention.

Estrogens affect the release of gonadotropins from the pituitary gland, which can cause inhibition of lactation, inhibition of ovulation, and inhibition of androgen secretion.

Excessive estrogen will delay the transport of the ovum and prevent it from reaching the uterus at the appropriate time for implantation. DES also possesses antineoplastic activity against some types of neoplasias (perianal gland adenoma and prostatic hyperplasia). It affects mRNA and protein synthesis in the cell nucleus and is cell cycle nonspecific.

The mechanism of action for estrogen-responsive urinary incontinence is thought due to increasing sphincter sensitivity to norepinephrine.

Pharmacokinetics

DES is well absorbed from the GI tract of monogastric animals. It is slowly metabolized by the liver, primarily to a glucuronide form and then excreted in the urine and feces.

Contraindications/Precautions/Warnings

DES is prohibited by the FDA for use in food animals.

Because of potential effects on bone marrow, DES should be used with extreme caution in patients with preexisting anemias or leukopenias. DES is contraindicated in females with estrogen-sensitive neoplasms.

Adverse Effects

While adverse effects with estrogen therapy can be serious (see below) in small animals, when used for estrogen-responsive incontinence at the lowest effective dose, it is usually well-tolerated.

In cats and dogs, estrogens are considered toxic to the bone marrow and can cause blood dyscrasias. Blood dyscrasias are more prevalent in older animals and if higher dosages are used. Initially, a thrombocytosis and/or leukocytosis may be noted, but thrombocytopenia/leukopenias will gradually develop. Changes in a peripheral blood smear may be apparent within two weeks after estrogen administration. Chronic estrogen toxicity may be characterized by a normochromic, normocytic anemia, thrombocytopenia, and neutropenia. Bone marrow depression may be transient and begin to resolve within 30-40 days or may persist or progress to a fatal aplastic anemia. Doses of 2.2 mg/kg per day have caused death in cats secondary to bone marrow toxicity.

Estrogens may induce mammary neoplasias.

In cats, daily administration of DES has resulted in pancreatic, hepatic, and cardiac lesions.

Estrogens may cause cystic endometrial hyperplasia and pyometra. After therapy is initiated, an open-cervix pyometra may be noted 1-6 weeks after therapy.

When used chronically in male animals, feminization may occur. In females, signs of estrus may occur and persist for 7-10 days.

Experimental administration of DES to female dogs as young as 8 months of age have induced malignant ovarian adenocarcinomas. Doses ranging from 60-495 mg given over 1 month to 4 years were implicated in causing these tumors.

Reproductive/Nursing Safety

DES is contraindicated during pregnancy, as it can cause fetal malformations of the genitourinary system.

Estrogens have been documented to be carcinogenic at low levels in some laboratory animals. Because of the potential for danger to the public health, DES must not be used in animals to be used for human consumption.

Overdosage/Acute Toxicity

Acute overdosage in humans with estrogens has resulted in nausea, vomiting and withdrawal bleeding in females. No information was located regarding acute overdose in veterinary patients, however, the reader is referred to the warnings and adverse effects listed above.

Drug Interactions

The following drug interactions have either been reported or are theoretical in humans or animals receiving DES and may be of significance in veterinary patients. Unless otherwise noted, use together is not necessarily contraindicated, but weigh the potential risks and perform additional monitoring when appropriate.

- **ANTIFUNGALS, AZOLE (itraconazole, ketoconazole**, etc.): May increase estrogen levels.
- **CIMETIDINE:** May decrease metabolism of estrogens.
- **CORTICOSTEROIDS:** Enhanced glucocorticoid effects may result if estrogens are used concomitantly with corticosteroid agents. It has been postulated that estrogens may either alter the protein binding of corticosteroids and/or decrease their metabolism. Corticosteroid dosage adjustment may be necessary when estrogen therapy is either started or discontinued.
- **ERYTHROMYCIN, CLARITHROMYCIN:** May decrease the metabolism of estrogens.
- **PHENOBARBITAL:** May decrease estrogen concentrations.
- **PHENYTOIN:** May decrease estrogen concentrations.
- **RIFAMPIN:** May induce hepatic microsomal enzymes and decrease estrogen levels.
- **WARFARIN:** Oral anticoagulant activity may be decreased if estrogens are administered concurrently; increases in anticoagulant dosage may be necessary if adding estrogens.

Laboratory Considerations

- Estrogens in combination with progestins (*e.g.*, oral contraceptives) have been demonstrated in humans to increase thyroxine-binding globulin (TBG) with resultant increases in total circulating thyroid hormone. Decreased T3 resin uptake also occurs, but free T4 levels are unaltered.

Doses

- **DOGS:**

  For treatment of primary sphincter mechanism incompetence (idiopathic incontinence, hormone-responsive incontinence); (extra-label): 0.5 – 1 mg (0.02 mg/kg; maximum dose of 1 mg) for 3-5 days as an induction dose and then periodically decreased to every other day and then to the lowest dose that will maintain continence. In difficult cases, may be used with phenylpropanolamine. (Chew et al. 2006)

Monitoring

When therapy is either at high dosages or chronic; see Adverse Effects for more information.

Perform at least monthly:
- Packed Cell Volumes (PCV).
- White blood cell counts.
- Platelet counts.
- Perform liver function tests at baseline, and one month after therapy begins, repeat in 2 months after cessation of therapy if abnormal.

Client Information

- Contact veterinarian if signs of lethargy, diarrhea, vomiting, abnormal discharge from vulva, excessive water consumption and urination or abnormal bleeding occur.

Chemistry/Synonym

A synthetic nonsteroidal estrogen agent, diethylstilbestrol occurs as an odorless, white, crystalline powder with a melting range of 169°–175°C. It is practically insoluble in water and soluble in alcohol or fatty oils.

Diethylstilbestrol may also be known as: DES, diethylstilbestrolum, diethylstilboestrol, NSC-3070, stilbestrol, stilboestrol, *Apstil®*, *Boestrol®*, *Destilbenol®*, or *Distilbene®*.

Storage/Stability

All commercially available DES tablets (plain tablets, enteric-coated tablets) should be stored at room temperature (15-30°C) in well-closed containers.

Compatibility/Compounding Considerations

No specific information noted. It is recommended that when compounding DES it be treated as a cytotoxic agent with appropriate safety precautions toprevent exposure to humans.

Dosage Forms/Regulatory Status

VETERINARY-LABELED PRODUCTS: NONE.

HUMAN-LABELED PRODUCTS: NONE.

No commercially available regular oral DES products are available in the USA. Compounded preparations may be available from compounding pharmacies.

Revisions/References

Monograph revised/updated January 2014.

Chew, D. & S. DiBartola (2006). Tips for managing lower urinary tract disorders: Urinary incontinence. Proceedings: ACVIM. accessed via Veterinary Information Network; vin.com

Digoxin

(di-jox-in) Lanoxin®

Cardiac Glycoside

Prescriber Highlights

▶ Oral & parenteral cardiac glycoside used primarily for SVT's.
▶ Contraindications: V-fib, digitalis intoxication; many veterinarians feel that digoxin is relatively contraindicated in cats with hypertrophic cardiomyopathy. Extreme Caution: Patients with glomerulonephritis & heart failure or with idiopathic hypertrophic subaortic stenosis (IHSS).
▶ Adverse Effects usually associated with high or toxic blood levels: Cardiac effects may include almost every type of cardiac arrhythmia described with a resultant worsening of heart failure clinical signs. Extracardiac: mild GI upset, anorexia, weight loss & diarrhea.
▶ Drug Interactions.
▶ Monitoring of blood levels highly suggested.

Uses/Indications

The labeled veterinary indications for digoxin include treatment of congestive heart failure (CHF), atrial fibrillation or flutter, and supraventricular tachycardias. Presently, digoxin use (often combined with diltiazem) is generally limited to dogs in the management of rapid atrial fibrillation with concurrent CHF caused by either dilated cardiomyopathy or mitral valve disease (MVD) without evidence of renal insufficiency. Digoxin therapy is more controversial for treating heart failure without accompanying supraventricular arrhythmias and its use for this has diminished. Today, most cardiologists no longer feel that digoxin is first line therapy for heart failure in dogs and cats. In a review of the pharmacologic management of myxomatous mitral valve disease in dogs (Atkins et al. 2012), the authors state: "digoxin has little role in veterinary cardiology other than for heart rate control in atrial fibrillation or as an inotrope in patients whose owners have financial constraints."

Pharmacology/Actions

The pharmacology of the digitalis glycosides has been extensively studied, but a thorough discussion is beyond the scope of this reference. Digitalis glycosides cause the following effects in patients with a failing heart: increased myocardial contractility (inotropism) with increased cardiac output; increased diuresis with reduction of edema secondary to a decrease in sympathetic tone;

reduction in heart size, heart rate, blood volume, and pulmonary and venous pressures; and (usually) no net change in myocardial oxygen demand.

The digitalis glycosides have several electrocardiac effects, including: decreased conduction velocity through the AV node, and prolonged effective refractory period (ERP). They may increase the PR interval, decrease the QT interval and cause ST segment depression.

The exact mechanism of action of these agents has not been fully described, but their ability to increase the availability of Ca^{++} to myocardial fibers and to inhibit Na^+-K^+-ATPase with resultant increased intracellular Na^+ and reduced K^+ probably explains their actions.

Pharmacokinetics

Absorption following oral administration occurs in the small intestine and is variable dependent upon the oral dosage form used (see Dosage Forms below). Food may delay, but not alter, the extent of absorption in most species studied. Food reportedly decreases the amount absorbed by 50% in cats after tablet administration. Peak serum levels generally occur within 45-60 minutes after oral elixir and about 90 minutes after oral tablet administration. In patients receiving an initial oral dose of digoxin, peak effects may occur in 6-8 hours after the dose.

The drug is distributed widely throughout the body with highest levels found in kidneys, heart, intestine, stomach, liver and skeletal muscle. Lowest concentrations are found in the brain and plasma. Digoxin does not significantly enter ascitic fluid, so dosage adjustments may be required in animals with ascites. At therapeutic levels, approximately 20-30% of the drug is bound to plasma proteins. Because only small amounts are found in fat, obese patients may receive dosages too high if dosing is based on total body weight versus lean body weight.

Digoxin is metabolized slightly, but the primary method of elimination is renal excretion both by glomerular filtration and tubular secretion. As a result, dosage adjustments must be made in patients with significant renal disease. Values reported for the elimination half-life of digoxin in dogs and cats have been highly variable, with values reported from 14.4-56 hours for dogs; 30-173 hours for cats. Approximate elimination half-lives reported in other species include: sheep 7 hours; horses 17-29 hours; cattle 8 hours.

Contraindications/Precautions/Warnings

Many cardiologists feel that digoxin is relatively contraindicated in cats with hypertrophic cardiomyopathy as it may increase myocardial oxygen demand and lead to dynamic outflow obstruction.

The p-glycoprotein pump actively transports digoxin, but the Washington State University Clinical Pharmacology Lab reports that it has not documented any increased sensitivity to digoxin and does not recommend any dose reductions in dogs with MDR1 mutations. They do however, recommend therapeutic drug monitoring (WSU-VetClinPharmLab 2009).

Digitalis cardioglycosides are contraindicated in patients with ventricular fibrillation or in digitalis intoxication. They should be used with extreme caution in patients with glomerulonephritis and heart failure or with idiopathic hypertrophic subaortic stenosis (IHSS). They should be used with caution in patients with severe pulmonary disease, hypoxia, acute myocarditis, myxedema, or acute myocardial infarction, frequent ventricular premature contractions, ventricular tachycardias, chronic constrictive pericarditis or incomplete AV block. They may be used in patients with stable, complete AV block or severe bradycardia with heart failure if the block was not caused by the cardiac glycoside.

When used to treat atrial fibrillation or flutter prior to administration with an antiarrhythmic agent that has anticholinergic activity (*e.g.*, quinidine, procainamide, disopyramide), digitalis glycosides will reduce, but not eliminate, the increased ventricular rates that may be produced by those agents. Since digitalis glycosides may cause increased vagal tone, they should be used with caution in patients with increased carotid sinus sensitivity.

Elective cardioversion of patients with atrial fibrillation should be postponed until digitalis glycosides have been withheld for 1-2 days, and should not be attempted in patients with signs of digitalis toxicity.

Principally eliminated by the kidneys, digoxin should be used with caution and serum levels monitored in patients with renal disease. Animals that are hypernatremic, hypokalemic, hypercalcemic, hyper- or hypothyroid may require smaller dosages; monitor carefully.

As digoxin does not distribute well into ascitic fluid or fat, dosing is generally based upon lean body weight.

Adverse Effects

Adverse effects of digoxin are usually associated with high or toxic serum levels and are categorized into cardiac and extracardiac clinical signs. There are species differences with regard to the sensitivity to digoxin's toxic effects also. Cats are relatively sensitive to digoxin while dogs tend to be more tolerant of high serum levels.

Cardiac effects may be seen before other extra-cardiac clinical signs and include almost every type of cardiac arrhythmia described with a resultant worsening of heart failure clinical signs. More common arrhythmias or ECG changes observed include: complete or incomplete heart block, bigeminy, ST segment changes, paroxysmal ventricular or atrial tachycardias with block, and multifocal premature ventricular contractions. Because these effects can also be caused by worsening heart disease, it may be difficult to determine if they are a result of the disease process or digitalis intoxication. If in doubt, monitor serum levels or stop digoxin therapy temporarily.

Extracardiac clinical signs most commonly seen in veterinary medicine include mild GI upset, anorexia, weight loss, and diarrhea. Vomiting has been associated with IV injections and should not cause anxiety or alarm. Ocular and neurologic effects are routinely seen in humans, but are not prevalent in animals or are not detected.

Reproductive/Nursing Safety

In humans, the FDA categorizes this drug as category *C* for use during pregnancy (*Animal studies have shown an adverse effect on the fetus, but there are no adequate studies in humans; or there are no animal reproduction studies and no adequate studies in humans.*) In a separate system evaluating the safety of drugs in canine and feline pregnancy (Papich 1989), this drug is categorized as class: *A* (*Probably safe. Although specific studies may not have proved the safety of all drugs in dogs and cats, there are no reports of adverse effects in laboratory animals or women.*)

Studies have shown that digoxin concentrations in mother's serum and milk are similar; however, it is unlikely to have any pharmacological effect in nursing offspring.

Overdosage/Acute Toxicity

Clinical signs of chronic toxicity are discussed above. In dogs the acute toxic dose after IV administration has been reported to be 0.177 mg/kg.

Treatment of chronic digoxin toxicity is dictated by the severity of the clinical signs associated with it. Many patients will do well after temporarily stopping the drug and reevaluating the dosage regimen.

If an acute ingestion has recently occurred and no present cardiotoxic or neurologic signs (coma, seizures, etc.) have manifested,

emptying the stomach may be indicated followed with activated charcoal administration. Because digoxin can be slowly absorbed and there is some enterohepatic recirculation of the drug, repeated charcoal administration may be beneficial even if the ingestion occurred well before treatment. Anion-exchange resins such as colestipol or cholestyramine have been suggested to reduce the absorption and enterohepatic circulation of digoxin, but are not readily available in most veterinary practices.

Dependent on the type of cardiotoxicity, supportive and symptomatic therapy should be implemented. Serum electrolyte concentrations, drug level if available on a "stat" basis, arterial blood gases if available, and continuous ECG monitoring should be instituted. Acid-base, hypoxia, and fluid and electrolyte imbalances should be corrected. The use of potassium in normokalemic patients is very controversial and should only be attempted with constant monitoring and clinical expertise.

The use of specific antiarrhythmic agents in treating life-threatening digitalis-induced arrhythmias may be necessary. Lidocaine and phenytoin are most commonly employed for these arrhythmias. Atropine may be used to treat sinus bradycardia, SA arrest, or 2nd or 3rd degree AV block.

Digoxin immune Fab is a potential treatment for digoxin life-threatening toxicity. It is produced from specific digoxin antibodies from sheep and will bind directly to the drug, inactivating it. It is very expensive and veterinary experience with it is extremely limited.

Drug Interactions

There are many potential drug interactions associated with digoxin and the following list is not necessarily all-inclusive. Because of the narrow therapeutic index associated with the drug, consider enhanced monitoring when these drugs (are those in the same class) are added to patients stabilized on digoxin.

The following drug interactions have either been reported or are theoretical in humans or animals receiving digoxin and may be of significance in veterinary patients. Unless otherwise noted, use together is not necessarily contraindicated, but weigh the potential risks and perform additional monitoring when appropriate.

The following drugs may **reduce digoxin serum levels**:

- **AMINOSALICYLIC ACID**
- **ALUMINUM HYDROXIDE**
- **ANTACIDS, ORAL**
- **CHLORAMPHENICOL** (dogs) (Pedersoli 1980)
- **CHOLESTYRAMINE**
- **CIMETIDINE**
- **METOCLOPRAMIDE**
- **NEOMYCIN (oral)**
- **PHENOBARBITAL**
- **ST. JOHN'S WORT**
- **SUCRALFATE**
- **SULFASALAZINE**

The following drugs or herbs may **increase serum levels**, **decrease** the **elimination rate**, or **enhance** the **toxic effects** of digoxin:

- **AMIODARONE**
- **ANTICHOLINERGICS**
- **CAPTOPRIL** (or other **ACEIs**)
- **COLEUS**
- **CYCLOSPORINE**
- **DIAZEPAM**
- **DILTIAZEM** (data conflicts); See Doses
- **ERYTHROMYCIN**

- FUROSEMIDE (not significantly altered in cats receiving furosemide and aspirin)
- HAWTHORN
- KETOCONAZOLE/ITRACONAZOLE
- OMEPRAZOLE (or other PPIs)
- QUINIDINE (if used together the rule of thumb is to decrease digoxin dose by 50%).
- RESERPINE
- SUCCINYLCHOLINE
- TETRACYCLINE
- VERAPAMIL

Other potential drug interactions:

- BETA-BLOCKERS: Can have additive negative effects on AV conduction, complete heart block possible.
- CALCIUM-CHANNEL BLOCKERS (diltiazem, etc.): Can have additive negative effects on AV conduction.
- PENICILLAMINE: May decrease serum levels of digoxin independent of route of digoxin dosing.
- POTASSIUM/ELECTROLYTE BALANCE, DRUGS AFFECTING (e.g., diuretics, amphotericin B, glucocorticoids, laxatives, sodium polystyrene sulfonate, glucagon, high dose IV dextrose, dextrose/insulin infusions, furosemide, thiazides): May predispose the patient to digitalis toxicity.
- SPIRONOLACTONE: May enhance or decrease the toxic effects of digoxin.
- THYROID SUPPLEMENTS: Patients on digoxin that receive thyroid replacement therapy may need their digoxin dosage adjusted.

Laboratory Considerations

- No specific laboratory test concerns.
- Digoxin can cause prolonged PR interval and ST segment depression, and false-positive changes on EKG ST-T in human patients during exercise testing.

Doses

NOTE: Do not confuse microgram/kg, mg/kg, and microgram/m^2 doses.

- **DOGS:**

  For atrial fibrillation and CHF in dogs with normal renal function (extra-label): Initially, 0.0025 – 0.003 mg/kg PO q12h (alternatively in dogs weighing more than 20 kg using body surface area digoxin at 0.22 mg/m^2.) Do not exceed 0.25 mg per dog (regardless of size) twice daily. Monitor for signs of toxicity and efficacy and measure serum levels to adjust dosage (See Monitoring). One study (Gelzer et al. 2009) demonstrated that digoxin and diltiazem used together had a more effective ventricular rate reduction in dogs with secondary atrial fibrillation than when either was given alone, but it still remains unknown if this translates into decreased morbidity or mortality.

- **CATS:**

  For dilated cardiomyopathy or advanced atrioventricular valve insufficiency (Note: digoxin is generally contraindicated for feline hypertrophic cardiomyopathy); (extra-label): The starting dose for normal cats is 1/4th of a 0.125 mg tablet administered every other day for cats weighing less than 3 kg; 1/4th of a tablet every day for cats weighing 3 to 6 kg; and 1/4th of a tablet every day to q12h for cats weighing more than 6 kg. Tablets are better tolerated than the alcohol-based elixir. (Kittleson 2010)

- **FERRETS:**

  For adjunctive therapy for heart failure associated with dilated cardiomyopathy (extra-label): 0.005 – 0.01 mg/kg PO once daily initially (use oral liquid). May increase to twice daily if necessary. Monitor as per dogs and cats. Furosemide, and an ACE-inhibitor are also commonly employed.

- **HORSES:** (NOTE: ARCI UCGFS CLASS 4 DRUG)
  For SVTs (extra-label):

  a) Loading dose: 11 micrograms/kg IV given slowly or in divided doses, or 44 micrograms/kg PO; Maintenance Dose: 2.2 micrograms/kg IV every 12h or 11 micrograms/kg PO every 12 hours. Maintain plasma concentrations between 0.5 – 2 ng/mL. (Mogg 1999)

  b) 2.2 micrograms/kg IV. If unsuccessful, propranolol (0.03 mg/kg IV) may be tried. (van Loon 2013)

Monitoring

- Serum levels: Because of the significant interpatient pharmacokinetic variation seen with this drug, and its narrow therapeutic index, it is strongly recommended to monitor serum levels to help guide therapy. Unless the patient received an initial loading dose, at least 6 days should pass after beginning therapy to monitor serum levels to allow levels to approach steady-state. Historically, suggested therapeutic serum levels in the dog have ranged widely (0.8 – 3 ng/mL), but most now believe that levels above 1.2 ng/mL are potentially "toxic". A recent reference (Luis Fuentes 2009) states that trough serum levels should be in the 0.9 – 1.2 ng/mL, a range that is lower than previously recommended; other sources list the therapeutic range as 0.8 – 1.2 ng/mL (Trepanier 2013) or 0.5 – 1 ng/mL (Ferasin 2013). Therapeutic levels in cats are reported to be between 0.9 – 2 ng/mL (Lainesse 2009). For other species, values from 0.5 – 2 ng/mL can be used as guidelines. Levels at the higher end of the suggested range may be necessary to treat some atrial arrhythmias, but may also result in greater incidences of adverse effects. Usually a trough level (just before next dose or at least 6-8 hours after the last dose) is recommended.
- Appetite/weight.
- Cardiac rate, ECG changes.
- Serum electrolytes.
- Renal Function Tests.
- Clinical efficacy for CHF (improved perfusion, decreased edema, increased venous (or arterial) O2 levels).

Client Information

- Can be given with or without food. If your animal vomits or acts sick after getting it on an empty stomach, give with food or small treat to see if this helps. If vomiting continues, contact your veterinarian.
- Usually side effects of digoxin occur when there is too much drug in the bloodstream and can include mild gastrointestinal effects (e.g., lack of appetite, vomiting, diarrhea, etc.), lethargy (lacking energy), behavior changes and serious heart rhythm abnormalities. Because digoxin toxicity can be very serious, contact your veterinarian immediately if your animal develops any of these signs to make sure it is not becoming toxic to your animal.
- Monitoring of digoxin levels and blood electrolytes will be necessary.

Chemistry/Synonyms

A cardiac glycoside, digoxin occurs as bitter tasting, clear to white crystals or as white, crystalline powder. It is practically insoluble in water, slightly soluble in diluted alcohol, and very slightly soluble in 40% propylene glycol solution. Above 235°C, it melts with decomposition.

Digoxin may also be known as: digoxinum or digoxosidum; many trade names are available. Occasionally, digoxin is described as digitalis.

Storage/Stability

The commercial injection consists of a 40% propylene glycol, 10% alcohol solution having a pH of 6.6-7.4.

Digoxin tablets, capsules, elixir and injection should be stored at room temperature (15-30°C) and protected from light.

At pH's from 5-8, digoxin is stable, but in solutions with a pH of less than 3, it is hydrolyzed.

Compatibility/Compounding Considerations

The injectable product is **compatible** with most commercially available IV solutions, including lactated Ringer's, D5W, and normal saline. To prevent the possibility of precipitation occurring, one manufacturer recommends that the injection be diluted by a volume at least 4 times; with either sterile water, D5W, or normal saline. Digoxin injection has been demonstrated to be **compatible** with bretylium tosylate, cimetidine HCl, lidocaine HCl, and verapamil HCl.

Digoxin is **incompatible** with dobutamine HCl, acids, and alkalies. The manufacturer does not recommend mixing digoxin injection with other medications. Compatibility is dependent upon factors such as pH, concentration, temperature and diluent used; consult specialized references or a hospital pharmacist for more specific information.

Dosage Forms/Regulatory Status

There are bioavailability differences between dosage forms and in tablets produced by different manufacturers. It is recommended that tablets be used from a manufacturer that the clinician has confidence in and that brands not be routinely interchanged. Should a change in dosage forms be desired, the following bioavailability differences can be used as guidelines in altering the dose: Intravenous = 100%, IM ≈ 80%, Oral tablets ≈ 60%, Oral elixir ≈ 75%, Oral capsules ≈ 90-100%. The bioavailability of digoxin in veterinary species has only been studied in a limited manner. One study in dogs yielded similar values as those above for oral tablets and elixir, but in horses only about 20% of an intragastric dose was bioavailable.

VETERINARY-LABELED PRODUCTS:

The veterinary-labeled products are no longer available commercially in the USA.

The ARCI (Racing Commissioners International) has designated this drug as a class 4 substance. See the appendix for more information.

HUMAN-LABELED PRODUCTS:

Digoxin Solution for Injection: 250 micrograms/mL (0.25 mg/mL), Pediatric solution for Injection: 100 micrograms/mL (0.1 mg/mL) in 1 mL amps; *Lanoxin*®, generic, (Rx)

Digoxin Oral Tablets: 125 micrograms (0.125 mg), and 250 micrograms (0.25 mg); *Lanoxin*®, generic; (Rx)

Digoxin Oral Solution: 50 micrograms/mL (0.05 mg/mL) & 100 micrograms/mL (0.1 mg/mL); generic; (Rx)

Revisions/References

Monograph revised/updated January 2014.

Atkins, C. E. & J. Haggstrom (2012). Pharmacologic management of myxomatous mitral valve disease in dogs. Journal of veterinary cardiology : the official journal of the European Society of Veterinary Cardiology **14**(1).

Ferasin, L. (2013). Diagnosing and treating arrhythmias. Britsih Small Animal Veterinary Congress. accessed via Veterinary Information Network; vin.com

Gelzer, A. R. M., et al. (2009). Combination Therapy with Digoxin and Diltiazem Controls Ventricular Rate in Chronic Atrial Fibrillation in Dogs Better than Digoxin or Diltiazem Monotherapy: A Randomized Crossover Study in 18 Dogs. Journal of Veterinary Internal Medicine **23**(3): 499-508.

Kittleson, M. (2010). Management of Heart Failure - Pharmacokinetics. *Small Animal Cardiovascular Medicine, 2nd Ed.* M. Kittleson and R. Kienle, Accessed Online via the Veterinary Drug Information Network.

Lainesse, C. (2009). TDM: Basic Pharmacokinetics for Dosage Adjustements! Proceedings: WVC. accessed via Veterinary Information Network; vin.com

Luis Fuentes, V. (2009). Treatment of Canine Heart Failure. Proceedings: WSAVA World Congress. accessed via Veterinary Information Network; vin.com

Mogg, T. (1999). Equine Cardiac Disease: Clinical pharmacology and therapeutics. The Veterinary Clinics of North America: Equine Practice **15**:3(December).

Pedersoli, W. M. (1980). Serum Digoxin Concentrations in Dogs Before and After Concomitant Treatment with Chloramphenicol. J. Am. Anim. Hosp. Assoc. **16**(6): 839-44.

Trepanier, L. A. (2013). Applying Pharmacokinetics to Veterinary Clinical Practice. Veterinary Clinics of North America-Small Animal Practice **43**(5): 1013-+.

van Loon, G. (2013). Treatment of Common Arrhythmias: How and When to Treat. ACVIM. accessed via Veterinary Information Network; vin.com

WSU-VetClinPharmLab (2009). "Problem Drugs." Veterinary Clinical Pharmacology Lab, College of Vet Med, Washington State University http://goo.gl/aIGlM.

Dihydrotachysterol DHT

(dye-hye-droe-tak-ee-ster-ole)   DHT®, Hytakerol®

Vitamin D Analog

Prescriber Highlights

▶ Commercial dosage forms discontinued; may be available from compounding pharmacies.

▶ Vitamin D analog for hypocalcemia secondary to hypoparathyroidism or renal disease; calcitriol more often recommended.

▶ Raises calcium faster than ergocalciferol & effects dissipate more rapidly after the drug is stopped.

▶ Contraindications: Hypercalcemia, vitamin D toxicity, malabsorption syndrome, or abnormal sensitivity to the effects of vitamin D. Extreme caution: Hyperphosphatemia, renal dysfunction (when receiving the drug for non-renal indications).

▶ Adverse Effects: Hypercalcemia (may present as polydipsia, polyuria & anorexia), nephrocalcinosis, & hyperphosphatemia.

▶ Some animals are resistant to therapy.

▶ Monitoring serum calcium mandatory.

Uses/Indications

DHT is used in small animals to treat hypocalcemia secondary to hypoparathyroidism or severe renal disease. Because of availability issues and time to resolve hypercalcemia secondary to DHT toxicity, most are now recommending calcitriol.

Pharmacology/Actions

DHT is hydroxylated in the liver to 25-hydroxy-dihydrotachysterol that is the active form of the drug and is an analog of 1,25-dihydroxyvitamin D. Vitamin D is considered a hormone and, in conjunction with parathormone (PTH) and calcitonin, regulates calcium homeostasis in the body. Active analogues (or metabolites) of vitamin D enhance calcium absorption from the GI tract, promote reabsorption of calcium by the renal tubules, and increase the rate of accretion and resorption of minerals in bone.

Pharmacokinetics

If fat absorption is normal, vitamin D analogs are readily absorbed from the GI tract (small intestine). There are anecdotal reports of dogs and cats not responding to the oral tablets or capsule forms of the drug, but responding to the oral liquid dosage forms. Bile is required for adequate absorption and patients with steatorrhea, liver or biliary disease will have diminished absorption. DHT is hydroxylated in the liver to 25-hydroxy-dihydrotachysterol that is the active form of the drug. Unlike some other forms of vitamin D, DHT does not require parathormone activation in the kidneys. The time required for maximal therapeutic effect is usually seen within the first week of treatment. Unlike some other forms of vitamin D, DHT offloads relatively rapidly (1-3 weeks).

Contraindications/Precautions/Warnings

DHT is contraindicated in patients with hypercalcemia, vitamin D toxicity, malabsorption syndrome, or abnormal sensitivity to the effects of vitamin D. It should be used with extreme caution in patients with hyperphosphatemia (many clinicians believe hyperphosphatemia or a combined calcium/phosphorous product of >70 mg/dL is a contraindication to its use), or in patients with renal dysfunction (when receiving the drug for non-renal indications).

Adverse Effects

Hypercalcemia, nephrocalcinosis, and hyperphosphatemia are potential complications of DHT therapy. Clinical signs of hypercalcemia include polydipsia, polyuria, and anorexia. Monitoring of serum calcium levels is mandatory while using this drug.

Reproductive/Nursing Safety

Hypervitaminosis D has caused fetal abnormalities in a variety of species. In humans, the FDA categorizes this drug as category *C* for use during pregnancy (*Animal studies have shown an adverse effect on the fetus, but there are no adequate studies in humans; or there are no animal reproduction studies and no adequate studies in humans.*) Weigh the risks versus benefits of treating animal patients with this drug during pregnancy.

Vitamin D is excreted in breast milk in limited amounts; use with caution.

Overdosage/Acute Toxicity

Acute ingestions should be managed using established protocols for removal or prevention of the drug being absorbed from the GI. Orally administered mineral oil may reduce absorption and enhance fecal elimination.

Hypercalcemia secondary to chronic dosing of the drug should be treated by first temporarily discontinuing DHT and exogenous calcium therapy. If the hypercalcemia

is severe, furosemide, calcium-free IV fluids (*e.g.*, normal saline), urine acidification, and corticosteroids may be employed. Because of the long duration of action of DHT (usually one week and potentially up to 3 weeks), hypercalcemia may persist. Restart DHT/calcium therapy at a reduced dosage with diligent monitoring when calcium serum levels return to the normal range.

Drug Interactions

The following drug interactions have either been reported or are theoretical in humans or animals receiving DHT and may be of significance in veterinary patients. Unless otherwise noted, use together is not necessarily contraindicated, but weigh the potential risks and perform additional monitoring when appropriate.

- **CALCIUM-CONTAINING PHOSPHORUS BINDING AGENTS** (*e.g.,* calcium carbonate): Use with vitamin D analogs may induce hypercalcemia.
- **CORTICOSTEROIDS:** Can nullify the effects of vitamin D analogs.
- **DIGOXIN** or **VERAPAMIL:** Patients on verapamil or digoxin are sensitive to the effects of hypercalcemia; intensified monitoring is required.
- **MINERAL OIL, SUCRALFATE, CHOLESTYRAMINE:** May reduce the amount of drug absorbed.
- **PHENYTOIN, BARBITURATES** or **PRIMIDONE:** May induce hepatic enzyme systems and increase the metabolism of Vitamin D analogs thus decreasing their activity.
- **THIAZIDE DIURETICS:** May cause hypercalcemia when given in conjunction with Vitamin D analogs.

Laboratory Considerations

- **Serum cholesterol** levels may be falsely elevated by vitamin D analogs when using the Zlatkis-Zak reaction for determination.

Doses

Vitamin D therapy for hypocalcemic conditions is often used with exogenously administered calcium products. Refer to the calcium monograph for further information.

- **DOGS/CATS:**

For hypocalcemia secondary to hypoparathyroidism (extra-label): Initially give 0.03 mg/kg PO for several days or until effect is demonstrated, then give 0.02 mg/kg for 2 days, then 0.01 mg/kg per day. Pet should remain hospitalized until serum calcium concentration remains stable between 8-9.5 mg/dL. Recheck serum calcium on a weekly basis during early stages of treatment; recheck every 2-3 months long-term. Some dogs and cats that appear to be resistant to treatment on tablets or capsules may respond to the liquid form. (Feldman 2005)

Monitoring

- Serum calcium levels should be monitored closely (some clinicians recommend twice daily) during the initial treatment period. When the animal is stabilized, frequency may be reduced but never discontinued. All animals receiving DHT therapy should have calcium levels determined at least 2-4 times yearly.
- Serum phosphorous (particularly in renal failure patients).

Client Information

- Clients should be briefed on the clinical signs of hypercalcemia (polydipsia, polyuria, anorexia) and hypocalcemia (muscle tremors, twitching, tetany, weakness, stiff gait, ataxia, behavioral changes, and seizures) and instructed to report these symptoms to the veterinarian.

Chemistry/Synonyms

A vitamin D analog, dihydrotachysterol (DHT) occurs as odorless, colorless or white crystals, or crystalline white powder. It is practically insoluble in water, sparingly soluble in vegetable oils, and soluble in alcohol.

Dihydrotachysterol may also be known as: DHT, dichysterol, or dihydrotachysterol$_2$, AT 10, Atiten, *DHT®*, *Dihydral®*, *Dygratyl®*, *Tachyrol®*, or *Tachystin®*.

Storage/Stability

All DHT products should be stored at room temperature (15-30°C). Capsules or tablets should be stored in well-closed, light-resistant containers and the oral concentrate should be stored in tight, light-resistant containers.

Compatibility/Compounding Considerations

No specific information noted.

Dosage Forms/Regulatory Status

VETERINARY-LABELED PRODUCTS: NONE.

HUMAN-LABELED PRODUCTS: NONE.

Note: Dosage forms may be available from compounding pharmacies.

Revisions/References

Monograph revised/updated January 2014.

Feldman, E. (2005). Disorders of the parathyroid glands. *Textbook of Veterinary Internal Medicine, 6th Ed.* S. Ettinger and E. Feldman, Elsevier: 1508-35.

Diltiazem HCl

(dil-tye-a-zem)   Cardizem®, Dilacor XR®

Calcium Channel Blocker

Prescriber Highlights

▶ Calcium channel blocker used in dogs, cats, & ferrets for SVT's, pulmonary hypertension, systemic hypertension, or hypertrophic cardiomyopathy; may prove useful in horses in combination with quinidine to treat atrial fibrillation.

▶ Contraindications: Severe hypotension, sick sinus syndrome or 2nd or 3rd degree AV block, acute MI, radiographically documented pulmonary congestion, hypersensitivity.

▶ Caution: Geriatric patients or those with heart failure (particularly if also receiving beta blockers), or hepatic or renal impairment.

▶ Potential teratogen (high doses).

Uses/Indications

Diltiazem may be useful in dogs for supraventricular tachycardia or decreasing the ventricular rate associated with atrial fibrillation. One study (Gelzer et al. 2009) demonstrated that digoxin and diltiazem used together had more effective ventricular rate reduction in dogs with secondary atrial fibrillation than when either was given alone. However, it still remains unknown if this translates into decreased morbidity or mortality. In cats, diltiazem is used for the treatment of feline hypertrophic cardiomyopathy, but enthusiasm for its use for this indication has cooled somewhat in recent years. It potentially could be used for hypertension, pulmonary artery hypertension, adjunctive treatment of acute kidney injury and the treatment of supraventricular tachycardia.

Pharmacology/Actions

Diltiazem is a calcium-channel blocker similar in action to drugs such as verapamil or nifedipine. While the exact mechanism remains unknown, diltiazem inhibits the transmembrane influx of extracellular calcium ions in myocardial cells and vascular smooth muscle, but does not alter serum calcium concentrations. The net effect of this action is to inhibit the cardiac and vascular smooth muscle contractility, thereby dilating main systemic and coronary arteries. Total peripheral resistance, blood pressure, and cardiac afterload are all reduced.

Diltiazem has effects on cardiac conduction. It slows AV node conduction and prolongs refractory times. Diltiazem rarely affects SA node conduction, but in patients with Sick Sinus Syndrome, resting heart rates may be reduced.

Although diltiazem can cause negative inotropic effects, it is rarely of clinical importance (unlike verapamil or nifedipine). Diltiazem apparently does not affect plasma renin, aldosterone, glucose, or insulin concentrations.

Pharmacokinetics

In dogs, bioavailability of tablet forms may only be around 25%. Volume of distribution is approximately 8 L/kg and elimination half-life is about 2-4 hours.

Bioavailability in cats is reported to range from 50-80% with peak levels occurring about 45 minutes after oral dosing. Pharmacokinetics of a long acting product (*Cardizem® CD*) given at 10 mg/kg once daily to healthy cats were: bioavailability 22-59%; half-life 411 +/-59 minutes; peak levels achieved in 340 +/-140 minutes. A different sustained-release product (*Dilacor XR*) has a bioavailability of about 94% in cats and doses of 1 mg/kg PO q8h maintained the serum concentration within the suspected therapeutic range for 8 hours. Serum half-life in cats is about 2 hours.

In horses, elimination half-life is about 90 minutes.

Approximately 70-75% of the drug is bound to serum proteins. Diltiazem enters milk in concentrations approximating those found in plasma. Diltiazem is rapidly and almost completely metabolized by the liver into several metabolites, including two that are active. Renal impairment may only slightly increase half-lives.

In humans after an oral dose, about 80% of the dose is absorbed rapidly from the gut, but because of a high first pass effect, only about half of the absorbed drug reaches the systemic circulation; elimination half-life ranges from 3.5-10 hours.

Contraindications/Precautions/Warnings

Diltiazem is contraindicated in patients with severe hypotension (<90 mm Hg systolic), sick sinus syndrome or 2nd or 3rd degree AV block (unless a functioning pacemaker is in place), acute MI, radiographically documented pulmonary congestion, or when the patient is hypersensitive to it.

Diltiazem should be used with caution in geriatric patients or those with heart failure (particularly if also receiving beta blockers), or hepatic or renal impairment.

If giving direct IV administration (push), give over at least two minutes.

Adverse Effects

At usual doses, bradycardia is the most prominent side effect reported in dogs. In cats, vomiting is reportedly the most common side effect. One study done in cats, found that the 60 mg sustained-release "pellet" (9.3 – 14.8 mg/kg) was associated with lethargy, gastrointestinal disturbances, and weight loss in 36% of treated cats. Gastrointestinal disturbances were recognized within 1 week, and weight loss was detected after 2-6 months of treatment (Wall et al. 2005). Potentially, lethargy, GI distress (anorexia), hypotension, heart block or other rhythm disturbances, CNS effects, rashes, or elevations in liver function tests could occur in any species.

Reproductive/Nursing Safety

High doses in rodents have resulted in increased fetal deaths and skeletal abnormalities. Use during pregnancy only when the benefits outweigh the potential risks. In humans, the FDA categorizes this drug as category C for use during pregnancy (*Animal studies have shown an adverse effect on the fetus, but there are no adequate studies in humans; or there are no animal reproduction studies and no adequate studies in humans.*)

Diltiazem is excreted in milk and concentrations may approximate those found in the serum; use during nursing with caution.

Overdosage/Acute Toxicity

The oral LD_{50} in dogs has been reported as >50 mg/kg. Clinical signs noted after overdosage may include GI signs, heart block, bradycardia, hypotension, and heart failure. A dog that ingested approximately 100 mg/kg PO of a sustained release product developed bradycardia, hypotension, CNS depression, 2nd degree AV block with ventricular escape, and gastrointestinal effects. Ultimately the dog required a transvenous pacemaker for 19 hours, but recovered (Syring et al. 2008).

Treatment for calcium-channel blocker intoxication can be complicated and treatment modalities are evolving; consultation with a veterinary poison control center is advised. Gut decontamination should be considered when warranted, along with supportive and symptomatic treatment. Atropine may be used to treat bradycardias or 2nd or 3rd degree AV block. If these do not respond to vagal blockade, isoproterenol may be tried (with caution). Fixed block may require cardiac pacing. Inotropics (*e.g.*, dobutamine, dopamine, isoproterenol) and pressors (*e.g.*, dopamine, norepinephrine) may be required to treat heart failure and hypotension. A slow intravenous calcium infusion (1 mL/10 kg body weight of 10% calcium gluconate) may also be useful for severe acute toxicity. Intravenous lipid emulsion (ILE) and high-dose insulin have been suggested as potential therapies for severe diltiazem toxicity. A case report of successful treatment in a 4-year old Pomeranian has been published (Maton et al. 2013).

Drug Interactions

The following drug interactions have either been reported or are theoretical in humans or animals receiving diltiazem and may be of significance in veterinary patients. Unless otherwise noted, use together is not necessarily contraindicated, but weigh the potential risks and perform additional monitoring when appropriate.

- **ANESTHETICS, GENERAL**: May increase cardiac depressant effects of diltiazem.
- **BENZODIAZEPINES**: Diltiazem may increase benzodiazepine levels.
- **BETA-BLOCKERS**: Diltiazem may increase the likelihood of bradycardia, AV block or CHF developing in patients also receiving beta-blockers (including **ophthalmic beta-blockers**); additionally, diltiazem may substantially increase the bioavailability of propranolol.
- **BUSPIRONE**: Diltiazem may increase buspirone levels.
- **CISAPRIDE**: Diltiazem could potentially increase risk for increased QT intervals.
- **DIGOXIN**: While data conflicts regarding whether diltiazem affects digoxin pharmacokinetics, diligent monitoring of digoxin serum concentrations should be performed.
- **CIMETIDINE/RANITIDINE**: Cimetidine may increase plasma diltiazem concentrations; increased monitoring of diltiazem's effects is warranted. Ranitidine may also affect diltiazem concentrations, but to a lesser extent.
- **CYCLOSPORINE**: Diltiazem may increase cyclosporine serum concentrations; increased monitoring and dosage adjustments may be required.
- **RIFAMPIN**: May decrease diltiazem levels.
- **QUINIDINE**: Diltiazem may increase quinidine serum concentrations; increased monitoring and dosage adjustments may be required.

Doses

Note: Oral diltiazem is available in numerous human dosage forms, including several different types of sustained-release products; there is only limited information available on their pharmacokinetics in dogs or cats (Johnson et al. 1996; Wall et al. 2005; Leach et al. 2011). There are multiple trade names and strengths, and four basic technologies: Standard release tablets, sustained-release capsules containing coated beads, sustained-release compressed tablets containing coated beads, and sustained-release capsules containing multiples of 60 mg pellets. Sustained-release products for use in small animals are most commonly reformulated (compounded) capsules using the coated beads or pellets.

- **DOGS:**

For treatment of supraventricular tachyarrhythmias (extra-label): **Note:** Dosage recommendations can vary significantly and evidence supporting any dosage recommendation is not strong. The following are adapted from, among other sources: (Ware 2000; Rush 2005; Kittleson 2010)

For acute treatment of supraventricular tachycardia: Initially, 0.05 mg/kg IV administered over 1-2 minutes. May repeat this dose up to two times, with 5 minutes between doses. Some cardiologists use a dose of 0.25 mg/kg administered over 2-5 minutes; if required, dosage may be carefully increased up to a total dose of 0.75 mg/kg. Oral dosage suggestions include 0.5 mg/kg PO followed by 0.25 mg/kg PO every hour until conversion or a total

oral dose of 1.5 – 2 mg/kg has been given. (Ware 2000; Rush 2005; Kittleson 2010)

For chronic treatment of supraventricular tachycardia: Initially, 1 mg/kg PO q8h and titrated upward to a maximum of 4 mg/kg PO q8h. Doses from 2 – 4 mg/kg q8h should probably not be given to dogs that have moderate to severe myocardial failure or with significant cardiac compromise due to any reason. Dosages required for this indication are generally higher than those needed in atrial fibrillation to control ventricular rate.

For decreasing ventricular rate associated with atrial fibrillation (extra-label):

a) Using regular tablets, initially at 0.5 – 1.5 mg/kg PO 3 times daily. Titrate upward if necessary. Using a sustained-release product initially at 3 – 5 mg/kg PO twice daily. Dosage may carefully be titrated upward if required.

b) One prospective, randomized crossover, clinical trial study in 18 dogs (Gelzer et al. 2009), demonstrated that digoxin and diltiazem used together had a more effective ventricular rate reduction in dogs with secondary atrial fibrillation than when either was given alone, but it still remains unknown if this translates into decreased morbidity or mortality. Dosages used in the study were digoxin at approximately 0.005 mg/kg PO q12h, and diltiazem (extended-release; Dilt-XR®) at approximately 3 mg/kg PO q12h.

- **CATS:**

For adjunctive treatment of hypertrophic cardiomyopathy; supraventricular arrhythmias (extra-label): Dosage recommendations vary and evidence is not strong supporting any dosage. Diltiazem is usually dosed orally. If using the regular tablets at 7.5 – 15 mg per cat PO 2-3 times a day. If using a sustained-release product 30 – 45 mg per cat PO once daily is employed. (**Note:** Using compounded capsules made from the pelleted beads or ½ of a 60 mg pellet is preferred over the sustained-release tablets.)

If emergency IV treatment is required: 0.125 – 0.25 mg/kg IV over 2 minutes; with subsequent boluses at 15 minute intervals until conversion or to a total dose of 0.75 mg/kg has been recommended. (Rush 2005)

- **FERRETS:**

For hypertrophic cardiomyopathy (extra-label): 2 – 7.5 mg/kg PO twice daily; adjust as necessary. May result in heart block. (Williams 2000)

Monitoring

- ECG/Heart rate.
- Blood pressure.
- Adverse effects.

Client Information

- Used in dogs and cats to treat high blood pressure, heart rhythm problems and in cats only, heart failure.
- Very important to not skip dosages.
- May be given with or without food. If your animal vomits or acts sick after getting it on an empty stomach, give with food or small treat to see if this helps. If vomiting continues, contact your veterinarian.
- Common side effects include vomiting (cats), and slowed heart rate.
- Patient will need to be seen regularly by veterinarian to check to see if the medication is working properly.

Chemistry/Synonyms

A benzothiazepine calcium channel blocker, diltiazem HCl occurs as a white to off-white crystalline powder having a bitter taste. It is soluble in water and alcohol. Potencies may be expressed in terms of base (active moiety) and the salt. Dosages are generally expressed in terms of the salt.

Diltiazem may also be known as: CRD-401, diltiazemi hydrochloridum, latiazem hydrochloride, and MK-793; many trade names are available.

Storage/Stability

Diltiazem oral products should be stored at room temperature in tight, light resistant containers.

The powder for injection should be stored between 15-30°C. Discard 24 hours after reconstituting.

Compatibility/Compounding Considerations

Diltiazem is **compatible** with D5W and sodium chloride 0.9% digoxin, bumetanide, dobutamine, dopamine, epinephrine, lidocaine, morphine, nitroglycerin, potassium chloride, sodium nitroprusside, and vasopressin. It is **incompatible** with diazepam, furosemide, phenytoin and thiopental.

Dosage Forms/Regulatory Status

VETERINARY-LABELED PRODUCTS: NONE.

The ARCI (Racing Commissioners International) has designated this drug as a class 4 substance. See the appendix for more information.

HUMAN-LABELED PRODUCTS:

Diltiazem Oral Tablets: 30 mg, 60 mg, 90 mg, & 120 mg; *Cardizem®*, generic; (Rx)

Diltiazem Tablet & Capsules Extended/Sustained Release: 120 mg, 180 mg, 240 mg, 300 mg, 360 mg and 420 mg; *Cardizem CD®* & *LA®*, *Cartia XT®*, *Dilacor XR®*, *Tiazac®*, *Diltia XT®* & *Taztia XT®*, *Dilt-CD®* & *XR®*, generic; (Rx) **Note:** Products are labeled (for humans) as either q12h or q24h administration.

Diltiazem Injection: 5 mg/mL in 5 mL, 10 mL and 25 mL vials; Powder for Injection: 25 mg in single-use containers (carton of 6 Lyo-Ject syringes with diluent); *Cardizem®*, generic; (Rx)

Revisions/References

Monograph revised/updated January 2014.

Gelzer, A. R. M., et al. (2009). Combination Therapy with Digoxin and Diltiazem Controls Ventricular Rate in Chronic Atrial Fibrillation in Dogs Better than Digoxin or Diltiazem Monotherapy: A Randomized Crossover Study in 18 Dogs. Journal of Veterinary Internal Medicine 23(3): 499-508.

Johnson, L. M., et al. (1996). Pharmacokinetic and pharmacodynamic properties of conventional and CD-formulated diltiazem in cats. Journal of Veterinary Internal Medicine 10(5): 316-20.

Kittleson, M. (2010). "Chapt 29: Drugs used in treatment of cardiac arrhythmias- Drugs used to treat tachyarrhythmias - part 6." Small Animal Cardiovascular Medicine, 2nd Ed Veterinary Information Network http://goo.gl/FXvDZ.

Leach, S. B., et al. (2011). Single-dose and apparent steady state pharmacokinetics and pharmacodynamics of an extended release diltiazem formulation in the dog-a pilot study. Journal of Veterinary Internal Medicine 25(3): 646-.

Maton, B. L., et al. (2013). The use of high-dose insulin therapy and intravenous lipid emulsion to treat severe, refractory diltiazem toxicosis in a dog. J. Vet. Emerg. Crit. Care 23(3): 321-7.

Rush, J. (2005). Treatment of life-threatening arrhythmias. Proceedings: IVECCS. accessed via Veterinary Information Network; vin.com

Syring, R. S., et al. (2008). Temporary transvenous cardiac pacing in a dog with diltiazem intoxication. J. Vet. Emerg. Crit. Care 18(1): 75-80.

Wall, M., et al. (2005). Evaluation of extended-release diltiazem once daily for cats with hypertrophic cardiomyopathy. J. Am. Anim. Hosp. Assoc. 41(2): 98-103.

Ware, W. (2000). Therapy for Critical Arrhythmias: New Advances. Proceedings: The North American Veterinary Conference, Orlando. accessed via Veterinary Information Network; vin.com

Williams, B. (2000). Therapeutics in Ferrets. Vet Clin NA: Exotic Anim Pract 3:1(Jan): 131-53.

Dimenhydrinate

(dye-men-**hye**-dri-nate)   Dramamine®, Gravol®

Antihistamine

Prescriber Highlights

▶ Antihistamine used primarily for prevention of motion sickness in dogs & less so in cats; may be useful as an adjunctive treatment for feline pancreatitis.

▶ Contraindications: Hypersensitivity to it or others in its class. Caution: Angle closure glaucoma, GI or urinary obstruction, COPD, hyperthyroidism, seizure disorders, cardiovascular disease or hypertension; may mask clinical signs of ototoxicity.

▶ Adverse Effects: CNS depression & anticholinergic effects. GI effects (diarrhea, vomiting, anorexia) are less common.

Uses/Indications

In veterinary medicine, dimenhydrinate is used primarily for its antiemetic effects for vomiting and in the prophylactic treatment of motion sickness in dogs and cats. Because histamine is thought not to be an important mediator of vomiting in cats, other choices such as NK-1 antagonists (*e.g.,* maropitant) or M_1-cholinergic antagonists (*e.g.,* prochlorperazine, chlorpromazine) may be better choices for treating motion sickness or vomiting in cats. As dimenhydrinate is often thought of as "half-strength diphenhydramine" it can be employed whenever a histamine-1 blocker is desired.

Pharmacology/Actions

Dimenhydrinate has antihistaminic (H1), antiemetic, anticholinergic, CNS depressant and local anesthetic effects. These principle pharmacologic actions are thought to be a result of only the diphenhydramine moiety. Used most commonly for its antiemetic/motion sickness effects, dimenhydrinate's exact mechanism of action for this indication is unknown, but the drug does inhibit vestibular stimulation. The anticholinergic actions of dimenhydrinate may play a role in blocking acetylcholine stimulation of the vestibular and reticular systems. Tolerance to the CNS depressant effects can ensue after a few days of therapy and antiemetic effectiveness may also diminish with prolonged use.

Theoretically, histamine-1 (diphenhydramine, dimenhydrinate, etc.) and histamine-2 (ranitidine, famotidine, etc.) blockers may reduce histamine-mediated increases in microvasculature permeability that is associated with the development of hemorrhagic necrosis in feline pancreatitis.

Pharmacokinetics

The pharmacokinetics of this agent have apparently not been studied in veterinary species. In humans, the drug is well absorbed after oral administration with antiemetic effects occurring within 30 minutes of administration. Antiemetic effects occur almost immediately after IV injection. The duration of effect is usually 3-6 hours.

Diphenhydramine is metabolized in the liver, and the majority of the drug is excreted as metabolites into the urine. The terminal elimination half-life in adult humans ranges from 2.4-9.3 hours.

Contraindications/Precautions/Warnings

Dimenhydrinate is contraindicated in patients that are hypersensitive to it or to other antihistamines in its class. Because of their anticholinergic activity, antihistamines should be used with caution in patients with angle closure glaucoma, prostatic hypertrophy, pyloroduodenal or bladder neck obstruction, and COPD if mucosal secretions are a problem. Additionally, they should be used with caution in patients with hyperthyroidism, seizure disorders, cardiovascular disease or hypertension. It may mask the clinical signs of ototoxicity and should therefore be used with this knowledge when concomitantly administering with ototoxic drugs.

The sedative effects of antihistamines, may adversely affect the performance of working dogs.

Adverse Effects

Most common adverse reactions seen are CNS depression (lethargy, somnolence) and anticholinergic effects (dry mouth, urinary retention). GI effects (diarrhea, vomiting, anorexia) are less common, but have been noted. The sedative effects of antihistamines may diminish with time.

Do not confuse diphenhydrAMINE with dimenhyDRINATE.

Reproductive/Nursing Safety

In humans, the FDA categorizes this drug as category *B* for use during pregnancy (*Animal studies have not yet demonstrated risk to the fetus, but there are no adequate studies in pregnant women; or animal studies have shown an adverse effect, but adequate studies in pregnant women have not demonstrated a risk to the fetus in the first trimester of pregnancy, and there is no evidence of risk in later trimesters.*) In a separate system evaluating the safety of drugs in canine and feline pregnancy (Papich 1989), this drug is categorized as class: *B* (*Safe for use if used cautiously. Studies in laboratory animals may have uncovered some risk, but these drugs appear to be safe in dogs and cats or these drugs are safe if they are not administered when the animal is near term.*)

Small amounts of dimenhydrinate are excreted in milk; this is unlikely to pose much risk to nursing offspring.

Overdosage/Acute Toxicity

Overdosage may cause CNS stimulation (excitement to seizures) or depression (lethargy to coma), anticholinergic effects, respiratory depression and death. Treatment consists of emptying the gut if the ingestion was oral. Induce emesis if the patient is alert and CNS status is stable. Administration of a saline cathartic and/or activated charcoal may be given after emesis or gastric lavage. Treatment of other clinical signs should be performed using symptomatic and supportive therapies. Phenytoin (IV) is recommended in the treatment of seizures caused by antihistamine overdose in humans; use of barbiturates and diazepam are avoided.

Drug Interactions

Dimenhydrinate has been demonstrated to induce hepatic microsomal enzymes in animals (species not specified); the clinical implications of this effect are unclear.

The following drug interactions have either been reported or are theoretical in humans or animals receiving dimenhydrinate and may be of significance in veterinary patients. Unless otherwise noted, use together is not necessarily contraindicated, but weigh the potential risks and perform additional monitoring when appropriate.

- **ANTICHOLINERGIC DRUGS** (including **tricyclic antidepressants**): Dimenhydrinate may potentiate the anticholinergic effects of other anticholinergic drugs.
- **CNS DEPRESSANT DRUGS:** Increased sedation can occur if dimenhydrinate (diphenhydramine) is combined with other CNS depressant drugs.

Laboratory Considerations

- Antihistamines can decrease the wheal and flare response to **antigen skin testing**. In humans, it is suggested that antihistamines be discontinued at least 4 days before testing.

Doses

- **DOGS/CATS:**

  As an antiemetic (particularly for prevention and treatment of motion sickness) or antihistamine (extra-label): 4 – 8 mg/kg PO q8h.

Monitoring

- Clinical efficacy.
- Adverse effects (sedation, anticholinergic signs, etc.).

Client Information

- Antihistamine related to diphenhydramine (*Benadryl®*); is usually used for prevention of motion sickness in dogs and cats, but also may be tried for treating vomiting in cats.
- May cause drowsiness/sleepiness, which is usually useful.
- Can be given on an empty stomach, but if animal vomits or drools, try giving with food. If vomiting continues, contact your veterinarian.

Chemistry/Synonyms

An ethanolamine derivative antihistamine, dimenhydrinate contains approximately 54% diphenhydramine and 46% 8-chlorotheophylline. Hence, it is sometimes called "½ strength diphenhydramine." It occurs as an odorless, bitter-tasting and numbing, white crystalline powder with a melting range of 102°-107°C. Dimenhydrinate is slightly soluble in water and is freely soluble in propylene glycol or alcohol. The pH of the commercially available injection ranges from 6.4-7.2.

Dimenhydrinate may also be known as: chloranautine, dimenhydrinatum, diphenhydramine teoclate, and diphenhydramine theoclate; many trade names are available.

Storage/Stability

Dimenhydrinate products should be stored at room temperature; avoid freezing and injectable products. Store tablets in well-closed containers.

Compatibility/Compounding Considerations

Dimenhydrinate injection is reportedly physically **compatible** with all commonly used intravenous replenishment solutions and the following drugs: amikacin sulfate, atropine sulfate, calcium gluconate, chloramphenicol sodium succinate, corticotropin, diatrizoate meglumine and sodium, diphenhydramine HCl, droperidol, fentanyl citrate, heparin sodium, iothalamate meglumine and sodium, meperidine HCl, metoclopramide, morphine sulfate, norepinephrine bitartrate, oxytetracycline HCl, penicillin G potassium, pentazocine lactate, phenobarbital sodium, potassium chloride, scopolamine HBr, vancomycin HCl and vitamin B-complex with vitamin C.

The following drugs are either physically **incompatible** or **compatible only in certain concentrations** with dimenhydrinate: aminophylline, ammonium chloride, butorphanol tartrate, glycopyrrolate, hydrocortisone sodium succinate, hydroxyzine, iodipamide meglumine, pentobarbital sodium, prochlorperazine edisylate, promazine HCl, promethazine HCl, and tetracycline HCl. Compatibility is dependent upon factors such as pH, concentration, temperature, and diluent used; consult a hospital pharmacist or specialized references for more specific information.

Dosage Forms/Regulatory Status

VETERINARY-LABELED PRODUCTS: NONE.

HUMAN-LABELED PRODUCTS:

Dimenhydrinate Oral Tablets: 50 mg (regular & chewable); *Dramamine®, Travtabs®, Driminate®, Triptone®*, generic; (OTC)

Dimenhydrinate Injection: 50 mg/mL in 1 mL and 10 mL vials; generic; (Rx)

Revisions/References

Monograph revised/updated January 2014.

Dimercaprol (BAL)

(dye-mer-kap-role)   BAL in Oil®

Antidote

Prescriber Highlights

▶ Chelating agent for arsenicals; sometimes used for lead, mercury, & gold compounds.

▶ Contraindications: Patients with impaired hepatic function, unless secondary to acute arsenic toxicity, & in iron, cadmium, & selenium poisoning. Caution: Patients with impaired renal function.

▶ Alkalinize urine and administer deep IM (still painful).

▶ Adverse Effects: Usually transient & can include vomiting & seizures with higher dosages; increased blood pressure with tachycardia possible.

Uses/Indications

The principal use of dimercaprol in veterinary medicine is treating intoxications caused by arsenical compounds, although succimer in small animals and sodium thiosulfate in large animals, are usually preferred. It is occasionally used for lead (with CaEDTA), mercury and gold intoxication.

Pharmacology/Actions

The sulfhydryl groups found on dimercaprol form heterocyclic ring complexes with heavy metals, principally arsenic, lead, mercury and gold. This binding helps prevent or reduce heavy metal binding to sulfhydryl-dependent enzymes. Different metals have differing affinities for both dimercaprol and sulfhydryl-dependent enzymes and the drug is relatively ineffective in chelating some metals (*e.g.*, selenium). Chelation to dimercaprol is not irreversible and metals can dissociate from the complex as dimercaprol concentrations decrease, in an acidic environment, or if oxidized. The dimercaprol-metal complex is excreted via renal and fecal routes.

Pharmacokinetics

After IM injection, peak blood levels occur in 30-60 minutes. The drug is slowly absorbed through the skin after topical administration.

Dimercaprol is distributed throughout the body, including the brain. Highest tissue levels are found in the liver and kidneys.

Non-metal bound drug is rapidly metabolized to inactive compounds and excreted in the urine, bile and feces. In humans, the duration of action is thought to be about 4 hours with the drug completely eliminated within 6-24 hours.

Contraindications/Precautions/Warnings

Dimercaprol is contraindicated in patients with impaired hepatic function, unless secondary to acute arsenic toxicity. The drug is also contraindicated in iron, cadmium, and selenium poisoning, as the chelated complex can be more toxic than the metal alone.

Because dimercaprol is potentially nephrotoxic, it should be used cautiously in patients with impaired renal function. In order to protect the kidneys, the urine should be alkalinized to prevent the chelated drug from dissociating in the urine. Animals with diminished renal function or that develop renal dysfunction while on therapy should either have the dosage adjusted or discontinue therapy dependent on the clinical situation.

Adverse Effects

IM injections are necessary with this compound but can be very painful, particularly if the drug is not administered deeply. Vomiting and seizures can occur with higher dosages. Transient increases in blood pressure with concomitant tachycardia have been reported. Most adverse effects are transient in nature as the drug is eliminated rapidly.

Dimercaprol is potentially nephrotoxic.

Reproductive/Nursing Safety

In humans, the FDA categorizes this drug as category *C* for use during pregnancy (*Animal studies have shown an adverse effect on the fetus, but there are no adequate studies in humans; or there are no animal reproduction studies and no adequate studies in humans.*).

It is not known if dimercaprol is excreted in milk.

Overdosage/Acute Toxicity

Clinical signs of dimercaprol overdosage in animals include vomiting, seizures, tremors, coma, and death. No specific doses were located to correspond with these clinical signs, however.

Drug Interactions

The following drug interactions have either been reported or are theoretical in humans or animals receiving dimercaprol and may be of significance in veterinary patients. Unless otherwise noted, use together is not necessarily contraindicated, but weigh the potential risks and perform additional monitoring when appropriate.

▪ **IRON** or **SELENIUM**: Because dimercaprol can form a toxic complex with certain metals (**cadmium, selenium, uranium** and **iron**), do not administer with iron or selenium salts. At least 24 hours should pass after the last dimercaprol dose, before iron or selenium therapy can begin.

Laboratory Considerations

▪ Iodine I^{131} thyroidal uptake values may be decreased during or immediately following dimercaprol therapy as it interferes with normal iodine accumulation by the thyroid. (Osweiler 2007)

Doses

▪ **DOGS & CATS:**

Note: It is highly recommended to contact an animal poison center before treating heavy metal poisonings.

For adjunctive treatment of arsenic toxicity (extra-label; evidence is scant to support any dosage regimen): Most recommended dosages are between 2.5 – 5 mg/kg IM q4h for the first two days of treatment (some recommend that 5 mg/kg dosages be given only on the first day of treatment and then for acute cases only); then q12h until recovery. Aggressive supportive therapy is likely required.

▪ **RUMINANTS:**

For treatment for arsenic, lead or mercury poisonings (extra-label): 2.5 – 5 mg/kg IM q4h for 2 days. Withdrawal information is not available in food animals. Efficacy questionable unless dimercaprol is given before signs appear or very early in the clinical course. FDA has not exempted this drug for compounding from bulk supplies. (Osweiler 2007)

▪ **HORSES:**

For arsenic toxicity (extra-label):

a) Dimercaprol therapy in horses is difficult because of the amounts of dimercaprol that are required, the necessity to inject the drug IM, that it must be used acutely, and any substantial delays in treatment significantly decrease its effectiveness. If available, the dose is: 5 mg/kg IM initially, followed by 3 mg/kg IM q6h for the remainder of the first day, then 1 mg/kg IM q6h for two or more additional days, as needed. (Oehme 1987)

b) Wash off topically absorbable arsenic and empty the digestive tract with laxatives. Administer sodium thiosulfate at 50 – 75 grams PO every 6-8 hours to bind unabsorbed arsenic. IV thiosulfate (25 – 30 grams as a 20% solution in distilled water) may counter-absorb arsenic. Dimercaprol is effective if administered within hours of ingestion. Initial treatment is: 5 mg/kg IM, followed by 3 mg/kg IM q6h for the remainder of the first day, then 1 mg/kg IM q6h for the next 48 hours. IM injections are painful; identify source of arsenic and eliminate it. (Rees 2004)

Monitoring
- Liver function.
- Renal function.
- Hemogram.
- Hydration and perfusion status.
- Electrolytes and acid/base status.
- Urinary pH.

Client Information
- Because of the potential toxicity of this agent and the seriousness of most heavy metal intoxications, this drug should be used with close professional supervision only.
- Dimercaprol can impart a strong, unpleasant mercaptan-like odor to the animal's breath.

Chemistry/Synonyms
A dithiol chelating agent, dimercaprol occurs as a colorless or nearly colorless, viscous liquid that is soluble in alcohol, vegetable oils, and water, but is unstable in aqueous solutions. It has a very disagreeable mercaptan-like odor. The commercially available injection is a peanut oil and benzyl benzoate solution. Although the solution may be turbid or contain small amounts of flocculent material or sediment, this does not mean that the solution is deteriorating.

Dimercaprol may also be known as: BAL, British Anti-Lewisite, dimercaptopropanol, dithioglycerol dimercaprolum, *BAL® in Oil* or *Sulfactin Homburg®*.

Storage/Stability
Dimercaprol injection should be stored below 40°C; preferably at room temperature (15-30°C).

Compatibility/Compounding Considerations:
Dimercaprol is not on the FDA's CPG 608.400 list of drugs allowed to be compounded from bulk supplies.

Dosage Forms/Regulatory Status
VETERINARY-LABELED PRODUCTS: NONE.

HUMAN-LABELED PRODUCTS:

Dimercaprol Injection: 100 mg/mL (10%) (for IM use only) in 3 mL amps; *BAL® in Oil*; (Rx)

Revisions/References
Monograph revised/updated January 2014.

Oehme, F. W. (1987). Arsenic. *Current Therapy in Equine Medicine.* N. E. Robinson. Philadelphia, WB Saunders: 668-70.
Osweiler, G. (2007). Detoxification and Antidotes for Ruminant Poisoning. Proceedings: ACVIM. accessed via Veterinary Information Network; vin.com
Rees, C. (2004). Disorders of the skin. *Equine Internal Medicine 2nd Ed.* S. Reed, W. Bayly and D. Sellon. Philadelphia, Saunders: 667-720.

Dimethyl Sulfoxide (DMSO)

(dye-meth-el sul-fox-ide) Domoso®

Free Radical Scavenger

Prescriber Highlights
▶ Free radical scavenger that has antiinflammatory, cryopreservative, anti-ischemic, & radioprotective effects.
▶ Caution: Mastocytomas, dehydration/shock; may mask existing pathology.
▶ Handle cautiously; will be absorbed through skin & can carry toxic compounds across skin.
▶ May cause localized "burning" when administered topically.
▶ Administer IV to horses slowly & at concentrations of 20% or preferably, less (10%); may occasionally cause diarrhea, tremors, & colic.
▶ Odor may be an issue.

Uses/Indications
Purported uses for DMSO are rampant, but the only FDA-approved veterinary indication for DMSO is: "...as a topical application to reduce acute swelling due to trauma" (Package Insert; *Domoso®*—Syntex). Other possible indications for DMSO include: adjunctive treatment in transient ischemic conditions, CNS trauma and cerebral edema, calcinosis cutis, endometritis, skin ulcers/wounds/burns, adjunctive therapy in intestinal surgeries, and analgesia for post-operative or intractable pain, amyloidosis in dogs, reduction of mammary engorgement in the nursing bitch, enhancement of antibiotic penetration in mastitis in cattle, and limitation of tissue damage following extravasation injuries secondary to chemotherapeutic agents.

DMSO's effect on alcohol dehydrogenase, may make it useful in the treatment of ethylene glycol poisoning, but this has not been sufficiently studied as of yet. DMSO's attributes as a potential carrier of therapeutic agents across the skin and into the systemic circulation and its synergistic effects with other agents are potentially exciting, but require much more study before they can be routinely recommended.

While the potential indications for DMSO are many, unfortunately, the lack of well-controlled studies leaves many more questions than answers regarding this drug.

Pharmacology/Actions
The pharmacologic effects of DMSO are diverse. DMSO traps free radical hydroxide and its metabolite, dimethyl sulfide (DMS), traps free radical oxygen. It appears that these actions help to explain some of the antiinflammatory, cryopreservative, antiischemic, and radioprotective qualities of DMSO.

DMSO will easily penetrate the skin. It serves as a carrier agent in promoting the percutaneous absorption of other compounds (including drugs and toxins) that normally would not penetrate. Drugs such as insulin, heparin, phenylbutazone, and sulfonamides may all be absorbed systemically when mixed with DMSO and applied to the skin. DMSO has been shown to increase the rate of oral absorption of the triazine antiprotozoal drugs, diclazuril and toltrazuril in horses (Dirikolu et al. 2013).

DMSO has weak antibacterial activity and possibly has some clinical efficacy as an antifungal when used topically. The mechanism for these antimicrobial effects has not been elucidated.

The antiinflammatory/analgesic properties of DMSO have been thoroughly investigated. DMSO appears to be more effective as an antiinflammatory agent when used for acute inflammation versus chronic inflammatory conditions. The analgesic effects of DMSO have been compared to that produced by narcotic analgesics. It can be efficacious for both acute and chronic musculoskeletal pain.

DMSO decreases platelet aggregation but reports of its effect on coagulability have been conflicting, as has its effect on the myocardium. DMSO has diuretic activity independent of the method of administration. It provokes histamine release from mast cells, which probably contributes to the local vasodilatory effects seen after topical administration.

DMSO also apparently has some anticholinesterase activity and enhances prostaglandin E, but blocks the synthesis of prostaglandins E_2, F_2-alpha, H_2, and G_2. DMSO inhibits the enzyme alcohol dehydrogenase, which not only is responsible for the metabolism of alcohol, but also the metabolism of ethylene glycol into toxic metabolites.

Pharmacokinetics

DMSO is well absorbed after topical administration, especially at concentrations between 80-100%. It is extensively and rapidly distributed to virtually every area of the body. After IV administration to horses, the serum half-life was approximately 9 hours. In dogs, the elimination half-life is approximately 1.5 days. DMSO is metabolized to dimethyl sulfide (DMS) and primarily excreted by the kidneys, although biliary and respiratory excretion also takes place.

In cattle, the drug is eliminated quite rapidly and after 20 days no detectable drug or metabolites are found in milk, urine, blood, or tissues.

Contraindications/Precautions/Warnings

Wear rubber gloves when applying topically, and apply with clean or sterile cotton to minimize the chances for contaminating with potentially harmful substances. Apply only to clean, dry areas to avoid carrying other chemicals into the systemic circulation. Do not apply topically mixed with compounds (heavy metals, etc.) that could be toxic if absorbed systemically.

DMSO may mask existing pathology with its antiinflammatory and analgesic activity.

Because DMSO may degranulate mast cells, animals with mastocytomas should only receive DMSO with extreme caution. DMSO should be used cautiously in animals suffering from dehydration or shock as its diuretic and peripheral vasodilatory effects may exacerbate these conditions.

Adverse Effects

When used as labeled, DMSO appears to be an extremely safe drug. Local effects ("burning", erythema, vesiculation, dry skin, local allergic reactions) and garlic or oyster-like breath odor are the most likely adverse effects. They are transient and quickly resolve when therapy is discontinued. Lenticular changes, which may result in myopia, have been noted primarily in dogs and rabbits when DMSO is used chronically and at high doses. These effects are slowly reversible after the drug is discontinued.

When DMSO is administered intravenously to horses it may cause hemolysis and hemoglobinuria. While older dosage references often recommended concentrations of 20% or less for IV use in horses, 10% solutions, which are probably safer, are more commonly recommended today. Slow IV administration may reduce adverse effects. Other adverse effects can include diarrhea, muscle tremors and colic.

Reports of hepatotoxicity and renal toxicity have been reported for various species and dosages. These occur fairly rarely and some clinicians actually believe DMSO has a protective effect on ischemically insulted renal tissue.

Reproductive/Nursing Safety

At high doses, DMSO has been shown to be teratogenic in hamsters and chicks, but not mice, rats, or rabbits; weigh the risks versus benefits when using in pregnant animals. In humans, the FDA cat-egorizes this drug as category *C* for use during pregnancy (*Animal studies have shown an adverse effect on the fetus, but there are no adequate studies in humans; or there are no animal reproduction studies and no adequate studies in humans.*). In a separate system evaluating the safety of drugs in canine and feline pregnancy (Papich 1989), this drug is categorized as class: *C* (*These drugs may have potential risks. Studies in people or laboratory animals have uncovered risks, and these drugs should be used cautiously as a last resort when the benefit of therapy clearly outweighs the risks.*)

It is not known whether this drug is excreted in milk; use in nursing dams with caution.

Overdosage/Acute Toxicity

The reported LD_{50}'s following IV dosage in dogs and cats are: Cats ≈ 4 g/kg, and Dogs ≈ 2.5 g/kg. Signs of toxicity include: sedation and hematuria at non-lethal doses; coma, seizures, opisthotonus, dyspnea and pulmonary edema at higher dosages. Should an acute overdosage be encountered, treat supportively.

Drug Interactions

The following drug interactions have either been reported or are theoretical in humans or animals receiving DMSO and may be of significance in veterinary patients. Unless otherwise noted, use together is not necessarily contraindicated, but weigh the potential risks and perform additional monitoring when appropriate.

- **ALCOHOL**: Effects may be potentiated by DMSO.
- **ATROPINE**: Effects may be potentiated by DMSO.
- **CORTICOSTEROIDS**: Effects may be potentiated by DMSO.
- **INSULIN**: Effects may be potentiated by DMSO.
- **ORGANOPHOSPHATES** (or other cholinesterase inhibitors): Avoid use with DMSO.

Doses

- **DOGS:**

  To reduce acute swelling due to trauma (labeled dose; FDA-approved): Liberal application should be administered topically to the skin over the affected area 3-4 times daily. Total daily dosage should not exceed 20 grams (or mL of liquid) and therapy should not exceed 14 days. (Package Insert; *Domoso*®)

  For calcinosis cutis (extra-label): Treatment recommendations generally are to treat each lesion with topical DMSO (gel is preferred if available) once daily. If there are many sites or a large area is involved, treat 1/3 of the lesions (or 1/3 of the affected areas) each day. There are differing recommendations to: 1) either rotate these sites each day, or 2) add new treatment areas as the treated sites improve. Dogs reportedly "feel bad" if large areas are treated initially, but usually do not become hypercalcemic. Wear non-permeable gloves when applying. Treatment may require several weeks and not all cases resolve. Most recommend monitoring serum calcium levels occasionally.

  For bladder instillation to treat persistent cases of hemorrhagic cystitis (secondary to cyclophosphamide treatment): 10 mL of DMSO medical grade 50% solution is diluted with 10 mL of water and instilled into bladder and removed after 20 minutes. (Blackwood 2008)

  For doxorubicin extravasation—see the doxorubicin monograph for more information.

- **HORSES:** (NOTE: ARCI UCGFS CLASS 5 DRUG)

  To reduce acute swelling due to trauma; topical application (labeled dose; FDA-approved): Liberal application should be administered topically to the skin over the affected area 2-3 times daily. Total daily dosage should not exceed 100 grams (or mL of liquid) and therapy should not exceed 30 days. (Package Insert; *Domoso*®)

As an antiinflammatory/hydroxyl radical scavenger (IV administration); (extra-label): Note: While DMSO has been used intravenously for many years in horses for a variety of purposes, actual evidence demonstrating its efficacy is very slim. Older dosage references often recommended concentrations of 20% or less for IV use in horses, but 10% solutions are probably safer and are more commonly recommended today. Some recent references state unequivocally "do not exceed 10% concentrations". It is most commonly dosed at 1 g/kg via slow IV infusion and can be repeated q12h.

For chronic endometritis; abnormal mucous; (extra-label): 30% solution as an intrauterine infusion daily; up to 5 days during estrus. In order to prepare a 30% solution using 90% DMSO, 33 mL of a 90% DMSO solution is added to 64 mL of sterile saline. (Lyle 2013)

Monitoring

- Efficacy.
- Hemoglobinuria/hematocrit if indicated.
- Ophthalmic exams with high doses or chronic use in the dog.

Client Information

- Do not use non-medical grades of DMSO as they may contain harmful impurities.
- Wear rubber gloves when applying topically. Use in well-ventilated area; avoid inhalation and contact with eyes.
- Apply with clean or sterile cotton to reduce chances for contaminating DMSO with other substances. Apply only to clean, dry skin.
- Do not mix DMSO with other drugs or chemicals without veterinarian's approval. Keep lid tightly on container when not in use.
- Can cause a "garlic- or oyster-like" breath odor or local skin reactions.
- If used on dogs for large areas for calcinosis cutis, can make dog feel "bad" for a while.

Chemistry/Synonyms

DMSO is a clear, colorless to straw-yellow liquid. It is dipolar, aprotic (acts as a Lewis base) and extremely hygroscopic. It has a melting/freezing point of 18.5°C, boiling point of 189°C, and a molecular weight of 78.1. It is miscible with water (heat is produced), alcohol, acetone, chloroform, ether and many organic solvents. A 2.15% solution in water is isotonic with serum.

Dimethylsulfoxide may also be known as: dimethyl sulphoxide, dimethylis sulfoxidum, DMSO, methyl sulphoxide, NSC-763, SQ-9453, sulphinylbismethane, *Domoso®*, *Kemsol®*, *Rheumabene®*, *Rimso®*, or *Synotic®*.

Storage/Stability

Must be stored in airtight containers away from light. As DMSO may react with some plastics, it should be stored in glass or in the container provided by the manufacturer. If DMSO is allowed to contact room air it will self-dilute to a concentration of 66-67%.

Compatibility/Compounding Considerations

DMSO is apparently compatible with many compounds, but because of the chances for accidental percutaneous absorption of potentially toxic compounds, the admixing of DMSO with other compounds is not to be done casually.

Dosage Forms/Regulatory Status

VETERINARY APPROVED PRODUCTS:
Dimethyl Sulfoxide Veterinary Gel 90%: *Domoso® Gel* 90% (medical grade) in 60 g, and 120 g tubes, and 425 g containers. FDA-approved (NADA 47-925) for use in dogs and horses. Do not administer to horses that are to be used for food.

Dimethyl Sulfoxide Veterinary Solution 90%: *Domoso® Solution* 90% (medical grade) in 1 pint and 1 gallon bottles. FDA-approved (NADA 32-168) for use in canines and equines. Do not administer to horses that are to be used for food.

The ARCI (Racing Commissioners International) has designated this drug as a class 5 substance. See the appendix for more information.

Note: A topical otic product, *Synotic®* that contains: DMSO 60% and fluocinolone acetonide 0.01% is also available for veterinary use. Supplied in 8 mL and 60 mL dropper bottles.

HUMAN APPROVED PRODUCTS:
Dimethylsulfoxide Solution: 50% aqueous solution in 50 mL; *Rimso-50®*; (Rx)

Revisions/References
Monograph revised/updated January 2014.

Blackwood, L. (2008). Problems with Chemotherapy of Lymphoma--How to Cope. Proceedings: World Small Afnimal Assoc World Congress. accessed via Veterinary Information Network; vin.com
Dirikolu, L., et al. (2013). Current therapeutic approaches to equine protozoal myeloencephalitis. Javma-Journal of the American Veterinary Medical Association 242(4): 482-91.
Lyle, S. K. (2013). Incorporating Non-Antibiotic Anti-Infective Agents into the Treatment of Equine Endometritis. SAVMA Symposium. accessed via Veterinary Information Network; vin.com

Diminazene Aceturate

(dye-min-ah-zeen ass-ah-**toor**-ate)   Berenil®

Antiprotozoal

Prescriber Highlights

▶ Antiprotozoal agent used in several species for trypanosomiasis, babesiosis, or cytauxzoonosis.
▶ Usually administered once; repeat dosages may increase risk for toxicity.
▶ Available in several countries, but not in USA.

Uses/Indications

Diminazene is used to treat trypanosomiasis in dogs and livestock (sheep, goats, cattle), Babesia infections in dogs and horses, cytauxzoonosis and babesiosis in cats, and leishmaniasis in humans. A prospective, unmasked study in dogs comparing atovaquone/azithromycin (AA) with a protocol using clindamycin, diminazene and imidocarb (CDI) found that CDI had higher recovery and lower relapse rates, albeit longer therapy duration and slower reduction in parasite numbers than AA. The authors concluded that CDI was effective for initial therapy and when the M121I gene in *B. gibsoni* had mutated (Lin et al. 2012). A recent study in naturally infected cats with chronic *Cytauxzoon felis* parasitemia, found no difference in parasite burden between diminazene (3 mg/kg IM; 2 doses 7 days apart) and placebo-treated cats (Lewis, Cohn, Marr, et al. 2012).

The drug is not commercially available in the USA, but available and used in many countries.

Pharmacology/Actions

Diminazene's exact mechanism of action is not well understood. With Babesia, it is thought to interfere with aerobic glycolysis and DNA synthesis.

Diminazene may not completely eradicate the organism but because it is slowly metabolized, suppression of recurrence of clinical signs or prophylaxis can be attained for several weeks after a single dose.

Pharmacokinetics

Diminazene's pharmacokinetics have been investigated in several species. The drug is rapidly absorbed after IM administration in target species studied and distributed rapidly. High levels can be found in the liver and kidney. The drug appears to enter the CSF, but at levels significantly lower than that found in plasma in healthy animals. CSF levels are higher in infected dogs with African trypanosomiasis, probably due to meningeal inflammation. Diminazene apparently is metabolized somewhat in the liver, but identification of, these metabolites and whether they possess anti-protozoal activity is not known.

Reported elimination half-lives are widely variable. Values range from 5-30 hours in dogs, goats, and sheep, to over 200 hours in one study for cattle. Elimination half-life in cats is quite short with an average of about 1.7 hours (Lewis, Cohn, Birkenheuer, et al. 2012). Differences in assay methodology and study design may account for some of this variation, but even within one individual study in dogs using a modern assay (HPLC), wide inter-patient variability was noted.

Contraindications/Precautions/Warnings

Camels appear highly susceptible to the toxic effects of diminazene, and product labels may state the drug is contraindicated in camelids.

CNS toxic effects in dogs may be associated with cumulative dosages of diminazene, and repeated dosing must be carefully considered. One reference states "the dose cannot be repeated with this or another diaminidine-derivative within a 6-week period" (Ayoob et al. 2010).

Adverse Effects

At usual dosages in domestic livestock, diminazene is reportedly relatively free of adverse effects. Adverse effects associated with therapeutic dosages of diminazene in dogs may include vomiting and diarrhea, pain and swelling at the injection site, and transient decreases in blood pressure. Very rarely (<0.1%) ataxia, seizures, or death have been reported.

Reproductive/Nursing Safety

Little information is available. Rats given up to 1 g/kg PO on days 8-15 demonstrated no teratogenic effects, but decreased body weights and increased resorptions were noted at the highest dose.

Diminazene is distributed into milk; safety for nursing offspring has not been established.

Overdosage/Acute Toxicity

Little information is available. Diminazene appears most toxic in dogs and camels. Dosages greater than 7 mg/kg can be very toxic to camels; dosages above 10 mg/kg IM in dogs can cause severe gastrointestinal, respiratory, nervous system, or musculoskeletal effects.

Drug Interactions

- No significant drug interactions were identified.

Laboratory Considerations

- No issues were noted.

Doses

Note: There is a multitude of protozoal diseases worldwide that may respond to diminazene. Depending on the species/strain (protozoan) and species of the patient treated, there may be local specific recommendations for chemotherapy treatment or prevention. The following should be used as general guidelines only.

- **DOGS:**

  For treatment of Babesia (extra-label):

  a) For large or small Babesia (extra-label): 3.5 mg/kg IM once. Variable efficacy and unpredictable toxicity (CNS signs may be severe). (Irwin 2010)

  b) For babesiosis when the M121I gene in *B. gibsoni* has mutated (based on a prospective, unmasked study): clindamycin 30 mg/kg PO q12h; diminazene aceturate 3.5 mg/kg IM once on

the day of presentation; imidocarb diproprionate 6 mg/kg SC once on the day after the diminazene was administered. (Lin et al. 2012)

For treatment of African trypanosomiasis (extra-label): 3.6 – 7 mg/kg IM every 2 weeks as needed to control relapse or reinfection. (Barr 2006)

- **HORSES, CATTLE, SHEEP, GOATS:**

  For treatment of susceptible protozoal (Trypanosomes, Babesia) infections (West Africa); (extra-label in USA): In general, 3.5 mg/kg IM one time. Depending on susceptibility, dose can be increased to 8 mg/kg. Do not exceed 4 grams total dose per animal. (Label directions; *Berenil*®—Intervet West Africa)

Monitoring

- For Babesia infections in dogs monitoring would include surveillance for potential adverse effects of diminazene and signs for clinical efficacy, including monitoring serial CBCs. Severe cases may have elevated BUN or liver enzymes and hypokalemia.
- Current recommendation for determining "clearing" of the organism (*Babesia gibsoni*) is to perform a PCR test at 60 and 90 days post-therapy.

Client Information

- Clients should understand that depending on the species treated, parasites may not be completely eradicated and that retreatment may be required.

Chemistry/Synonyms

Diminazene aceturate is an aromatic diamidine derivative chemically related to pentamidine. One gram of diminazene is soluble in approximately 14 mL of water and it is slightly soluble in alcohol.

Diminazene aceturate may also be known as: diminazene diaceturate, or diminazeno; many international trade names are available.

Storage/Stability

Read and follow label directions for storage and preparation of each product used; diminazene powder, granules, or packets for reconstitution for injection should generally be stored in a dry, cool place out of direct sunlight. Once reconstituted, the solution's stability is temperature dependent; up to 14 days when refrigerated, up to 5 days at 20°C and only for 24 hours at temperatures above 50°C.

Compatibility/Compounding Considerations

No specific information noted.

Dosage Forms/Regulatory Status

VETERINARY-LABELED PRODUCTS: NONE.

Diminazene aceturate is available in many countries either alone, or in combination products (*e.g.,* with antipyrine), with the following trade names: *Azidine*®, *Azidin*®, *Babezeen*®, *Crede-Bab-Minazene*®, *Berenil*®, *Dimisol*®, *Dizine*®, *Ganaseng*®, *Ganasegur*®, *Pirocide*®, or *Veriben*®.

Withdrawal times may vary depending on the product, dosage, and the country where it is used. In South Africa, *Berenil*® (Intervet), has an animal slaughter withdrawal period of 21 days.

The JECFA of FAO/WHO has established the following maximum residue limit recommendations for diminazene in cattle: muscle (500 micrograms/kg), liver (12000 micrograms/kg), kidney (6000 micrograms/kg), and milk (150 micrograms/L).

HUMAN-LABELED PRODUCTS: NONE.

Revisions/References

Monograph revised/updated January 2014.

Ayoob, A. L., et al. (2010). Clinical management of canine babesiosis. J. Vet. Emerg. Crit. Care **20**(1): 77-89.
Barr, S. (2006). Trypanosomiasis. *Infectious Diseases of the Dog and Cat.* C. Greene, Elsevier: 676-85.

Irwin, P. J. (2010). Canine Babesiosis. Veterinary Clinics of North America-Small Animal Practice **40**(6): 1141-+.

Lewis, K. M., et al. (2012). Pharmacokinetics of diminazene diaceturate in healthy cats. J. Vet. Pharmacol. Ther. **35**(6): 608-10.

Lewis, K. M., et al. (2012). Diminazene Diaceturate for Treatment of Chronic Cytauxzoon felis Parasitemia in Naturally Infected Cats. Journal of Veterinary Internal Medicine **26**(6): 1490-3.

Lin, E. C. Y., et al. (2012). The therapeutic efficacy of two antibabesial strategies against Babesia gibsoni. Veterinary Parasitology **186**(3-4): 159-64.

Dinoprost Tromethamine
Prostaglandin F$_2$alpha Tromethamine

(dye-noe-prost)   Lutalyse®

Prostaglandin

Prescriber Highlights

▶ (THAM) salt of the naturally occurring prostaglandin F$_2$alpha used as a luteolytic agent for estrous synchronization, pyometra treatment, & as an abortifacient.

▶ Contraindications: Pregnancy (when abortion or induced parturition not wanted); manufacturer lists several contraindications for horses; has been associated with serious toxicity and death in camelids.

▶ Do NOT administer IV; extreme caution in elderly or debilitated animals.

▶ Pregnant women should not handle; humans with asthma & women of childbearing age should handle with caution.

▶ Adverse effects (**Dogs/Cats**): Abdominal pain, emesis, defecation, urination, pupillary dilation followed by constriction, tachycardias, restlessness & anxiety, fever, hypersalivation, dyspnea & panting; fatalities possible (esp. dogs).

▶ Adverse Effects: (**Cattle**): Infection at injection site, salivation, & hyperthermia possible.

▶ Adverse Effects (**Swine**): Erythema & pruritus, urination, defecation, slight ataxia, hyperpnea, dyspnea, nesting behavior, abdominal muscle spasms, tail movements, increased vocalization & salivation.

▶ Adverse Effects (**Horses**): Body temperature changes/sweating; seen less frequently: increased respiratory & heart rates, ataxia, abdominal pain, & lying down; usually has more side effects then cloprostenol.

Uses/Indications

Dinoprost (prostaglandin-F$_2$alpha; PGF2; *Lutalyse®*) is labeled for use in cattle as a luteolytic agent for estrous synchronization, unobserved (silent) estrous in lactating dairy cattle, pyometra, and as an abortifacient in feedlot and non-lactating dairy cattle. It is labeled in swine to act as a parturient inducing agent. The product is labeled for use in cycling mares as a luteolytic agent to control the time of estrus and to assist in inducing estrus in "difficult to breed mares."

Unlabeled uses of dinoprost include its use in small animals as an abortifacient agent and adjunctive medical therapy in pyometra, but newer regimens for pyometra that combine aglepristone with cloprostenol or misoprostol appear to be effective without the side effects of dinoprost. Although not FDA-approved, dinoprost is used also in sheep and goat reproductive medicine.

A recent review of the evidence for the therapeutic efficiency of antibiotics and dinoprost in postpartum dairy cows with clinical endometritis, concluded that no scientific evidence supports the effectiveness of dinoprost as a treatment for clinical endometritis in postpartum dairy cows (Lefebvre et al. 2012).

Pharmacology/Actions

Dinoprost has several pharmacologic effects on the female reproductive system, including stimulation of myometrial activity, relaxation of the cervix, and inhibition of steroidogenesis by corpora lutea. It can potentially lyse corpora lutea.

Pharmacokinetics

In studies done in rodents, dinoprost was demonstrated to distribute very rapidly to tissues after injection. In cattle, the serum half-life of dinoprost has been stated to be only "minutes" long.

Contraindications/Precautions/Warnings

Unless being used as an abortifacient or parturition inducer, dinoprost should not be used in any species during pregnancy. Dinoprost is contraindicated in animals with bronchoconstrictive respiratory disease (*e.g.*, asthma, RAO in horses). It should not be administered intravenously.

According to the manufacturer, dinoprost is contraindicated in mares with acute or subacute disorders of the vascular system, GI tract, respiratory system, or reproductive tract.

Dinoprost should be used with extreme caution, if at all, in dogs or cats greater than 8 years old, or with preexisting cardiopulmonary or other serious disease (liver, kidney, etc.). Some clinicians regard closed-cervix pyometra as a relative contraindication to the use of dinoprost.

Dinoprost has been associated with acute toxicity and death in camelids.

Adverse Effects

In cattle, increased temperature has been reported when administered in overdose (5-10X recommended doses) quantities. Limited salivation and bacterial infections at the injection site have been reported. If administered intravenously, increased heart rates have been noted.

In mares, transient decreased body (rectal) temperature and sweating have been reported most often. Less frequently, increased respiratory and heart rates, ataxia, abdominal pain, and lying down have also been noted. These effects are generally seen within 15 minutes of administration and resolve within an hour.

In swine, dinoprost has caused erythema and pruritus, urination, defecation, slight ataxia, hyperpnea, dyspnea, nesting behavior, abdominal muscle spasms, tail movements, increased vocalization and salivation. These effects may last up to 3 hours. At doses of 10X recommended, vomiting may be seen.

In dogs and cats, dinoprost can cause abdominal pain, emesis, defecation, urination, and pupillary dilation followed by constriction, tachycardias, restlessness and anxiety, fever, hypersalivation, dyspnea, and panting. Cats may also exhibit increased vocalization and intense grooming behavior. Severity of effects is generally dose dependent. Defecation can be seen even with very low dosages. Reactions generally appear in 5-120 minutes after administration and may persist for 20-30 minutes. Fatalities have occurred (especially in dogs) after use. Dogs and cats should be monitored for cardiorespiratory effects, especially after receiving higher dosages.

When used as an abortifacient in humans, dinoprost causes nausea, vomiting, or diarrhea in about 50% of patients.

Reproductive/Nursing Safety

Unless being used as an abortifacient or parturition inducer, dinoprost should not be used in any species during pregnancy. In swine, dinoprost should not be administered prior to 3 days of normal predicted farrowing as increased neonatal mortality may result.

Overdosage/Acute Toxicity

Dogs are apparently more sensitive to the toxic effects of dinoprost than other species. The LD$_{50}$ in the bitch has been reported to be

5.13 mg/kg after SC injection, which may be only 5X greater than the recommended dose by some clinicians.

In cattle, swine, and horses, dinoprost's effects when administered in overdose quantities are outlined above in the Adverse Effects section. In any species, if clinical signs are severe and require treatment, supportive therapy is recommended.

Drug Interactions

The following drug interactions have either been reported or are theoretical in humans or animals receiving dinoprost and may be of significance in veterinary patients. Unless otherwise noted, use together is not necessarily contraindicated, but weigh the potential risks and perform additional monitoring when appropriate.

- **OTHER OXYTOCIC AGENTS**: Activity may be enhanced by dinoprost. Reduced effect of dinoprost would be expected with concomitant administration of a progestin.

Doses

- **DOGS:**

For treatment of pyometra (extra-label): Use is restricted to bitches 6 years of age or younger that are not critically ill, do not have significant concurrent illness, do have an open cervix, and an owner who is adamant about saving the animal's reproductive potential. After making definitive diagnosis; use natural prostaglandin F2alpha (*Lutalyse®*): Day 1: 0.1 mg/kg SC once; Day 2: 0.2 mg/kg SC once; Days 3-7: 0.25 mg/kg SC once daily. Use antibiotics (effective against *E. coli*) concurrent with prostaglandin treatment and for 14 days after completion. Reevaluate at 7 and 14 days after treating with prostaglandin. Re-treat at 14 days if purulent discharge persists or fever, increased WBC and fluid filled uterus persist. (Feldman 2000)

As an abortifacient (extra-label):

a) After day 25 or 30: SC injections must be given at least twice a day, using a maximum dosage of 80 – 100 micrograms/kg, starting with half the dose for the first day (or first two administrations). Treatment must initially be done under the supervision of a clinician, after which the bitch can be sent home (with owner administration) once side effects have been carefully (monitored) after the first injection. Side effects include: emesis, salivation, defecation, urination and slight tachypnea. Treatment must continue (for 6 days or longer) until verification with ultrasound or palpation. (Romagnoli 2006)

b) As an adjunctive therapy for the termination of mid-term pregnancy in the bitch: Pregnancy is confirmed with ultrasound and begun no sooner than 30 days after breeding. 1 – 3 micrograms/kg misoprostol given intravaginally once daily concurrently with prostaglandin F2alpha (*Lutalyse®*) at 0.1 mg/kg SC 3 times daily for 3 days and then 0.2 mg/kg SC 3 times daily to effect. Monitor efficacy with ultrasound. (Cain 1999)

- **CATS:**

For treatment of pyometra (extra-label): Initially 0.1 mg/kg SC, then 0.25 mg/kg SC once a day for 5 days. Give bactericidal antibiotics concurrently. Not recommended in animals >8 yrs. old or if severely ill. Closed-cervix pyometra is a relative contraindication. Reevaluate in 2 weeks; retreat for 5 more days if necessary. (Nelson et al. 1988), (Feldman et al. 1989)

As an abortifacient (extra-label): 2 mg (total dose) per cat IM once a day beginning at day 33. Side effects include prostration, vomiting and diarrhea. (Romagnoli 2006)

- **CATTLE:**

For labeled (FDA-approved) indications as a luteolytic agent: Dinoprost is effective only in those cattle having a corpus lute-

um, i.e., those that ovulated at least five days prior to treatment. Future reproductive performance of animals that are not cycling will be unaffected by injection of dinoprost.

For Use for Estrus Synchronization in Beef Cattle and Non-Lactating Dairy Heifers: Dinoprost is used to control the timing of estrus and ovulation in estrous cycling cattle that have a corpus luteum. Inject a dose of 25 mg dinoprost IM either once or twice at a 10-12 day interval. With the single injection, cattle should be bred at the usual time relative to estrus. If receiving two injections of dinoprost, cattle can be bred after the second injection either at the usual time relative to detected estrus or at about 80 hours after the second injection. Estrus is expected to occur 1-5 days after injection if a corpus luteum was present. Cattle that do not become pregnant to breeding at estrus on days 1-5 after injection will be expected to return to estrus in about 18-24 days.

For Use for Unobserved (Silent) Estrus in Lactating Dairy Cows with a Corpus Luteum: Inject a dose of 25 mg dinoprost IM. If the cow returns to estrus, breed at the usual time relative to estrus. If estrus has not been observed by 80 hours after injection, breed at 80 hours.

Management Considerations: Many factors contribute to success and failure of reproduction management and these factors are important also when time of breeding is to be regulated with dinoprost sterile solution. Some of these factors are: a) cattle must be ready to breed—they must have a corpus luteum and be healthy; b) nutritional status must be adequate as this has a direct effect on conception and the initiation of estrus in heifers or return of estrous cycles in cows following calving; c) physical facilities must be adequate to allow cattle handling without being detrimental to the animal; d) estrus must be detected accurately if timed AI is not employed; and e) semen of high fertility must be used and inseminated properly. A successful breeding program can employ dinoprost effectively, but a poorly managed breeding program will continue to be poor when dinoprost is employed unless other management deficiencies are remedied first. Cattle expressing estrus following dinoprost are receptive to breeding by a bull. Using bulls to breed large numbers of cattle in heat following dinoprost will require proper management of bulls and cattle.

For Treatment of Pyometra (chronic endometritis): Inject a dose of 5 mL dinoprost (25 mg PGF2α) intramuscularly.

For Use for Abortion of Feedlot and Other Non-Lactating Cattle: Dinoprost is indicated for its abortifacient effect in feedlot and other non-lactating cattle during the first 100 days of gestation. Inject a dose of 25 mg intramuscularly. Cattle that abort will do so within 35 days of injection. (Adapted from label; *Lutalyse®*)

To induce parturition (extra-label): 25 – 30 mg IM; delivery will occur in about 72 hours. (Drost 1986)

- **HORSES:**

For labeled (FDA-approved) indications; as a luteolytic agent to control the timing of estrus in estrous cycling and clinically anestrous difficult to breed mares that have a corpus luteum: Evaluate the reproductive status of the mare. Administer a single IM injection of 1 mg per 45 kg bodyweight. Observe for signs of estrus by means of daily teasing with a stallion, and evaluate follicular changes on the ovary by palpation of the ovary *per rectum*. Some clinically anestrous mares will not express estrus but will develop a follicle that will ovulate. These mares may become pregnant if inseminated at the appropriate time relative to rupture of the follicle. Breed mares in estrus in a manner consistent with normal management. (Adapted from label; *Lutalyse®*)

For estrus synchronization in normally cycling mares (extra-label): Three different methods can be considered:

1) Two injection method: On day 1 give 5 mg dinoprost and again on day 16. Most mares (60%) will begin estrus 4 days after the second injection and about 90% will show estrous behavior by the 6th day after the second injection. Breed using AI every second day during estrus or inseminate at pre-determined times without estrus detection. Alternatively, an IM injection of HCG (2500 – 3300 Units) can be added on the first or second day (usually day 21) of estrus to hasten ovulation. Breed using AI on days: 20, 22, 24, and 26. This may be of more benefit when used early in the breeding season.

2) Progestagen/Prostaglandin method: Give altrenogest (0.44 mg/kg) for 8-12 days PO. On last day of altrenogest therapy (usually day 10) give dinoprost (dose not noted, but suggest using same dose as "1" above). Majority of mares will show estrus 2-5 days after last treatment. Inseminate every 2 days after detection of estrus. Synchronization may be improved by giving 2500 Units of HCG IM on first or second day of estrus or 5-7 days after altrenogest is withdrawn.

3) On day 1, inject 150 mg progesterone and 10 mg estradiol-17beta daily for 10 days. On last day, also give dinoprost (dose not noted, but suggest using same dose as "1" above). Perform AI on alternate days after estrus detection or on days 19, 21, and 23. (Bristol 1987)

As an abortifacient (extra-label):

a) Prior to the 12th day of pregnancy: 5 mg IM. After the 4th month of pregnancy: 1 mg per 45 kg body weight (1 mg per 100 pounds) daily until abortion takes place. (Lofstedt 1986)

b) From day 80-300: 2.5 mg q12h; approximately 4 injections required on average to induce abortion. (Roberts 1986)

- **SWINE:**

For parturition induction in swine when injected within 3 days of normal predicted farrowing (labeled dose; FDA-approved): 10 mg (2 mL) IM. (Adapted from label; *Lutalyse®*)

For estrus synchronization (grouping); (extra-label): At 15-55 days of gestation: 15 mg dinoprost IM followed in 12 hours by 10 mg IM. Animals will abort and return to estrus in 4-5 days. Close observation of estrus over several days is needed. (Carson 1986)

- **SHEEP & GOATS:**

For estrus synchronization in cycling ewes and does (extra-label): **Ewes:** Give 8 mg IM on day 5 of estrous cycle and repeat in 11 days. Estrus will begin approximately 2 days after last injection. **Does:** Give 8 mg IM on day 4 of estrous cycle and repeat in 11 days. Estrus will begin approximately 2 days after last injection. (Carson 1986)

To treat pseudopregnancy (hydrometra/mucometra) in goats (extra-label): 5 mg IM once. (Tibary 2009)

As an abortifacient (extra-label): **Does:** 5 – 10 mg IM throughout entire pregnancy; abortion takes place in 4-5 days. **Ewes** (during first two months of pregnancy): 10 – 15 mg IM; abortion takes place within 72 hours. (Drost 1986)

To induce parturition (extra-label): **Does:** 2.5 – 20 mg on days 144-149. Higher dosage (20 mg) yields more predictable interval from injection to delivery (≈32 hours). (Ott 1986)

Monitoring

- Depending on use, see above. Monitoring for adverse effects is especially important in small animals.

Client Information

- Dinoprost should be used by individuals familiar with its use and precautions.
- Pregnant women, asthmatics, or other persons with bronchial diseases should handle this product with extreme caution. Any accidental exposure to skin should be washed off immediately.

Chemistry/Synonyms

The tromethamine (THAM) salt of the naturally occurring prostaglandin F2alpha, dinoprost tromethamine occurs as a white to off-white, very hygroscopic, crystalline powder with a melting point of about 100°C. One gram is soluble in about 5 mL of water. 1.3 micrograms of dinoprost tromethamine is equivalent to 1 microgram of dinoprost.

Dinoprost and dinoprost tromethamine may also be known as: PGF(2alpha), prostaglandin F(2alpha), idinoprostum trometamoli, PGF(2alpha) THAM, prostaglandin F(2alpha) trometamol, U-14583E, U-14583, *Amtech Prostamate®, Lutalyse®, Enzaprost®, In-Synch®, Minprostin F(2)alpha®, Prostamate®, Prostin®, Prostin F2®, Prostin F2 Alpha®, Prostin F2 Alpha®, and Prostine F(2) Alpha®, Oriprost®, Glandin®, Noroprost®, Dinolytic®,* and *Prostarmon F®.*

Storage/Stability

Dinoprost for injection should be stored at room temperature (15-30°C) in airtight containers. The human FDA-approved product is recommended to be stored under refrigeration. Dinoprost is considered to be relatively insensitive to heat, light, and alkalis.

Compatibility/Compounding Considerations

No specific information noted. Should not be compounded by pregnant humans.

Dosage Forms/Regulatory Status

VETERINARY-LABELED PRODUCTS:

Dinoprost Tromethamine for injection, equivalent to 5 mg/mL of dinoprost in 10 mL and 30 mL vials; *Lutalyse® Sterile Solution, Prostamate®;* (Rx). FDA-approved for use in beef and non-lactating dairy cattle, swine and mares. No preslaughter withdrawal or milk withdrawal is required when used as labeled; no specific tolerance for dinoprost residues has been published. It is not for use in horses intended for food.

HUMAN-LABELED PRODUCTS: NONE.

Revisions/References

Monograph revised/updated January 2014.

Bristol, F. (1987). Synchronization of estrus. *Current Therapy in Equine Medicine: 2.* N. E. Robinson. Phialdelphia, WB Saunders: 495-8.

Cain, J. (1999). Canine reproduction: Commonly referred problems. Proceedings: American College of Veterinary Internal Medicine: 17th Annual Veterinary Medical Forum, Chicago. accessed via Veterinary Information Network; vin.com

Carson, R. L. (1986). Synchronization of estrus. *Current Veterinary Therapy: Food Animal Practice 2.* J. L. Howard. Philadelphia, W.B. Saunders: 781-3.

Drost, M. (1986). Elective termination of pregnancy. *Current Veterinary Therapy 2: Food Animal Practice.* J. L. Howard. Philadelphia, WB Saunders: 797-8.

Feldman, E. (2000). The cystic endometrial hyperplasia/pyometra complex and infertility in female dogs. *Textbook of Veterinary Internal Medicine: Diseases of the Dog and Cat.* S. Ettinger and E. Feldman. Philadelphia, WB Saunders. 2: 1549-65.

Feldman, E. C. & R. W. Nelson (1989). Diagnosis and treatment alternatives for pyometra in dogs and cats. *Current Veterinary Therapy X: Small Animal Practice.* R. W. Kirk. Philadelphia, WB Saunders: 1305-10.

Lefebvre, R. C. & A. E. Stock (2012). Therapeutic Efficiency of Antibiotics and Prostaglandin F-2 alpha in Postpartum Dairy Cows with Clinical Endometritis: An Evidence-Based Evaluation. *Veterinary Clinics of North America-Food Animal Practice* **28**(1): 79-+.

Lofstedt, R. M. (1986). Termination of unwanted pregnancy in the mare. Current Therapy in Theriogenology 2: Diagnosis, Treatment and Prevention of Reproductive Diseases in Small and Large Animals. D. A. Morrow. Philadelphia, WB Saunders: 715-8.

Nelson, R. W. & E. C. Feldman (1988). Diseases of the Endocrine Pancreas. *Handbook of Small Animal Practice.* R. V. Morgan. New York, Churchill Livingstone: 527-35.

Ott, R. S. (1986). Prostaglandins for induction of estrous, estrous synchronization, abortion and induction of parturition. *Current Therapy in Theriogenology 2: Diagnosis, Treatment and Prevention of Reproductive Diseases in Small and Large Animals.* D. A. Morrow. Philadelphia, WB Saunders: 583-5.

Roberts, S. J. (1986). Abortion and other gestational diseases in mares. *Current Therapy in Theriogenology 2: Diagnosis, Treatment and Prevention of Reproductive Diseases in Small and Large Animals*. D. A. Morrow. Philadelphia, WB Saunders: 705-10.

Romagnoli, S. (2006). Control of reproduction in dogs and cats: Use and misuse of hormones. Proceedings: WSAVA World Congress. accessed via Veterinary Information Network; vin.com

Tibary, A. (2009). Infertility in goats: Individual & herd approach. Proceedings: WVC. accessed via Veterinary Information Network; vin.com

Diphenhydramine HCl

(dye-fen-**hye**-dra-meen)   Benadryl®

Antihistamine

Prescriber Highlights

▶ Antihistamine used primarily for its antihistaminic effects, but with various indications (prevention of motion sickness, sedative, antiemetic, etc.).

▶ Caution: Angle closure glaucoma, GI or urinary obstruction, COPD, hyperthyroidism, seizure disorders, cardiovascular disease or hypertension. May mask clinical signs of ototoxicity.

▶ Adverse Effects: CNS depression & anticholinergic effects; GI effects (diarrhea, vomiting, anorexia) are less common.

Uses/Indications

In veterinary medicine, diphenhydramine is used principally for its antihistaminic effects, but also for other pharmacologic actions. Its sedative effects can be of benefit in treating the agitation (pruritus, etc.) associated with allergic responses. It has also been used for treatment and prevention of motion sickness and as an antiemetic in small animals. Because histamine is thought not to be an important mediator of vomiting in cats, other choices such as NK-1 antagonists (*e.g.,* maropitant) or M_1-cholinergic antagonists (*e.g.,* prochlorperazine, chlorpromazine) may be better choices for treating motion sickness or vomiting in cats. It has been suggested for use as adjunctive treatment of aseptic laminitis in cattle and it may be useful as an adjunctive treatment for feline pancreatitis. For other suggested uses, refer to the Dosage section below.

Pharmacology/Actions

Like other first generation type-1 antihistamines, diphenhydramine competitively inhibits histamine at H_1 receptors. In addition, it possesses substantial sedative, anticholinergic, antitussive, and antiemetic effects.

Pharmacokinetics

The pharmacokinetics of this agent have apparently not been studied in domestic animals. In humans, diphenhydramine is well absorbed after oral administration, but because of a relatively high first-pass effect, only about 40-60% reaches the systemic circulation.

Following IV administration in rats, diphenhydramine reaches its highest levels in the spleen, lungs and brain. The drug is distributed into milk, but has not been measured quantitatively. In humans, diphenhydramine crosses the placenta and is approximately 80% bound to plasma proteins.

Diphenhydramine is metabolized in the liver and the majority of the drug is excreted as metabolites into the urine. The terminal elimination half-life in adult humans ranges from 2.4-9.3 hours.

Contraindications/Precautions/Warnings

Diphenhydramine is contraindicated in patients that are hypersensitive to it or other antihistamines in its class. Because of their anticholinergic activity, antihistamines should be used with caution in patients with angle closure glaucoma, prostatic hypertrophy, pyloroduodenal or bladder neck obstruction, and COPD if mucosal secretions are a problem. Additionally, they should be used with caution in patients with hyperthyroidism, cardiovascular disease or hypertension.

Do not confuse diphenhydrAMINE with dimenhyDRINATE.

Adverse Effects

The most commonly seen adverse effects are CNS depression (lethargy, somnolence), and anticholinergic effects (dry mouth, urinary retention). The sedative effects of antihistamines may diminish with time and dogs may tolerate the sedative effects without much clinical effect, however sedative effects of antihistamines may adversely affect the performance of working or service dogs. GI effects (diarrhea, vomiting, anorexia) are a possibility.

Diphenhydramine may cause paradoxical excitement in cats.

The liquid formulation is distasteful and may not be accepted by animal patients.

Reproductive/Nursing Safety

In humans, the FDA categorizes this drug as category *B* for use during pregnancy (*Animal studies have not yet demonstrated risk to the fetus, but there are no adequate studies in pregnant women; or animal studies have shown an adverse effect, but adequate studies in pregnant women have not demonstrated a risk to the fetus in the first trimester of pregnancy, and there is no evidence of risk in later trimesters.*) In a separate system evaluating the safety of drugs in canine and feline pregnancy (Papich 1989), this drug is categorized as class: *B* (*Safe for use if used cautiously. Studies in laboratory animals may have uncovered some risk, but these drugs appear to be safe in dogs and cats or these drugs are safe if they are not administered when the animal is near term.*)

Diphenhydramine is excreted milk. Use with caution, particularly in neonates.

Overdosage/Acute Toxicity

Overdosage can cause CNS stimulation (excitement to seizures) or depression (lethargy to coma), anticholinergic effects, respiratory depression and death. Treatment consists of emptying the gut after oral ingestion using standard protocols. Induce emesis if the patient is alert and CNS status is stable. Administration of a saline cathartic and/or activated charcoal may be given after emesis or gastric lavage. Treatment of other clinical signs should be performed using symptomatic and supportive therapies. Phenytoin (IV) is recommended in the treatment of seizures caused by antihistamine overdose in humans; barbiturates and diazepam should be avoided.

Drug Interactions

The following drug interactions have either been reported or are theoretical in humans or animals receiving diphenhydramine and may be of significance in veterinary patients. Unless otherwise noted, use together is not necessarily contraindicated, but weigh the potential risks and perform additional monitoring when appropriate.

■ **ANTICHOLINERGIC DRUGS** (including **tricyclic antidepressants**): Diphenhydramine may potentiate anticholinergic effects.

■ **CNS DEPRESSANT DRUGS**: Increased sedation can occur.

Laboratory Considerations

■ Antihistamines can decrease the wheal and flare response to antigen **skin testing**. In humans, it is suggested that antihistamines be discontinued at least 4 days before testing.

Doses

■ **DOGS/CATS:**

As an antihistamine (adjunctive treatment of atopic dermatitis, anaphylaxis, mast cell tumors, transfusion reactions, etc.); (extra-label): Despite its long-time use, evidence for efficacy is primarily anecdotal. Most commonly dosed at 2 – 4 mg/kg PO 2-3 times a day; 0.5 – 2 mg/kg IM, SC or IV.

Prevention of motion sickness/antiemetic (extra-label): 2 – 4 mg/kg PO, IM q8h. Usually not very effective in cats.

- **FERRETS:**

  Prevaccination (extra-label): 2 mg/kg PO, IM or IV 10 minutes prior to vaccination. (Williams 2000)

  Pretreatment before doxorubicin (extra-label): 5 mg (total dose) IM. (Johnson 2006)

- **RABBITS/RODENTS/SMALL MAMMALS:**

  Guinea pigs: 7.5 mg/kg PO. (Adamcak et al. 2000)

  Rabbits: 1 – 2 mg/kg PO twice daily as an antihistamine. (Morrisey et al. 2003), (Antinoff 2008)

- **BIRDS:**

  For adjunctive treatment of pruritus causing feather picking in Psittacines: 2 mg/kg PO q12h. (Siebert 2003)

- **HORSES:** (NOTE: ARCI UCGFS CLASS 3 DRUG)

  As an antihistamine (extra-label): 1 – 2 mg/kg PO 2-3 times a day; 0.5 – 1 mg/kg IV or IM.

- **CATTLE:**

  a) **For adjunctive therapy of anaphylaxis** (extra-label): 0.5 – 1 mg/kg IM or IV (used with epinephrine and steroids). (Clark 1986)

  b) **For adjunctive therapy of aseptic laminitis** (extra-label): During the acute phase (with corticosteroids): 55 – 110 mg/100 kg body weight (0.55 – 1.1 mg/kg) IV or IM. (Berg 1986)

Monitoring

- Clinical efficacy.
- Adverse effects.

Client Information

- Antihistamines should be used on a regular, ongoing basis in animals that respond to them. They work better if used before exposure to an allergen.
- May cause drowsiness/sleepiness; this may lessen with time.
- Rarely, cats may become excited when given this medication.
- Can be given either with or without food, but if animal vomits or drools after getting the medication on an empty stomach, try giving with food. If vomiting continues, contact your veterinarian.

Chemistry/Synonyms

An ethanolamine-derivative antihistamine, diphenhydramine HCl occurs as an odorless, white, crystalline powder which will slowly darken upon exposure to light. It has a melting range of 167-172°C. One gram is soluble in about 1 mL of water or 2 mL of alcohol. Diphenhydramine HCl has a pK_a of about 9; the commercially available injection has its pH adjusted to 5-6.

Diphenhydramine HCl may also be known as: chloranautine, dimenhydrinatum, diphenhydramine teoclate, and diphenhydramine theoclate; many trade names are available.

Storage/Stability

Preparations containing diphenhydramine should be stored at room temperature (15-30°C) and solutions should be protected from freezing. Tablets and oral solutions should be kept in well-closed containers. Capsules and the elixir should be stored in tight containers.

Compatibility/Compounding Considerations

Diphenhydramine for injection is reportedly physically **compatible** with all commonly used IV solutions and the following drugs: amikacin sulfate, aminophylline, ascorbic acid injection, atropine sulfate, bleomycin sulfate, butorphanol tartrate, cephapirin sodium, chlorpromazine HCl, diatrizoate meglumine/sodium, dimenhydrinate, erythromycin lactobionate, fentanyl citrate, glycopyrrolate, hydromorphone HCl, hydroxyzine HCl, iothalamate meglumine/sodium, lidocaine HCl, meperidine HCl, metoclopramide, morphine sulfate, penicillin G potassium/sodium, pentazocine lactate, perphenazine, prochlorperazine edisylate, promazine HCl, promethazine HCl, scopolamine tetracycline HCl, and vitamin B complex with C. Compatibility is dependent upon factors such as pH, concentration, temperature, and diluent used; consult specialized references or a hospital pharmacist for more specific information.

Diphenhydramine is reportedly physically **incompatible** with the following drugs: amphotericin B, hydrocortisone sodium succinate, iodipamide meglumine, and pentobarbital sodium.

Dosage Forms/Regulatory Status

VETERINARY-LABELED PRODUCTS:

No systemic products. A shampoo, topical spray and topical liquid are available. See the topical dermatology section in the appendix for more information.

The ARCI (Racing Commissioners International) has designated this drug as a class 3 substance. See the appendix for more information.

HUMAN-LABELED PRODUCTS:

Diphenhydramine HCl Capsules and Tablets: 12.5 mg (as hydrochloride, chewable), 25 mg (as either hydrochloride or tannate, chewable), 50 mg (as hydrochloride); There are many trade name products that contain diphenhydramine. *Benadryl®*, *Banophen®* & *Diphenhist®* are commonly seen; generic; (OTC and Rx)

Diphenhydramine HCl Orally Disintegrating Tablets: 25 mg; *Unisom SleepMelts®*; (OTC)

Diphenhydramine Orally Disintegrating Strips: 12.5 mg (as hydrochloride); *Triaminic® Dissolve Strips*; (OTC)

Diphenhydramine HCl Oral Liquid, Solution, Suspension, Elixir or Syrup: 12.5 mg/5 mL (as hydrochloride) in 30 mL, 118 mL, 120 mL, 236 mL, 237 mL, 473 mL, and 3.8 L; 25 mg/5 mL (as tannate) in 118 mL; There are many trade name products including: *Benadryl®*, *Diphenhist®*, *Banophen®*, *Hydramine Cough* (various), generic; (OTC and Rx)

Diphenhydramine Injection: 50 mg/mL (as hydrochloride); generic; (Rx)

Revisions/References

Monograph revised/updated January 2014.

Adamcak, A. & B. Otten (2000). Rodent Therapeutics. Vet Clin NA: Exotic Anim Pract 3:1(Jan): 221-40.
Antinoff, N. (2008). Respiratory diseases of ferrets, rabbits, and rodents. Proceedings: IVECCS. accessed via Veterinary Information Network; vin.com
Berg, J. N. (1986). Aseptic laminitis in cattle. *Current Veterinary Therapy: Food Animal Practice 2.* J. L. Howard. Philadelphia, W.B. Saunders: 896-8.
Clark, D. R. (1986). Diseases of the general circulation. *Current Veterinary Therapy: Food Animal Practice 2.* J. L. Howard. Phialdelphia, W.B. Saunders: 694-6.
Johnson, D. (2006). Ferrets: the other companion animal. Proceedings: ACVC. accessed via Veterinary Information Network; vin.com
Morrisey, J. & N. Antinoff (2003). Respiratory diseases of rabbits, ferrets, and rodents. Proceedings: IVECCS. accessed via Veterinary Information Network; vin.com
Siebert, L. (2003). Psittacine feather picking. Proceedings: Western Veterinary Conference. accessed via Veterinary Information Network; vin.com
Williams, B. (2000). Therapeutics in Ferrets. Vet Clin NA: Exotic Anim Pract 3:1(Jan): 131-53.

Diphenoxylate HCl + Atropine Sulfate

(dye-fen-**ox**-i-late/at-roe-peen) Lomotil®

Opiate Agonist/Anticholinergic

Prescriber Highlights

▶ Opiate GI motility modifier with antitussive properties used primarily in dogs.

▶ Contraindications: Known hypersensitivity to narcotic analgesics, patients receiving monoamine oxidase inhibitors (MAOIs), diarrhea caused by a toxic ingestion until the toxin is eliminated from the GI tract, intestinal obstruction.

▶ Caution: Respiratory disease, hepatic encephalopathy, hypothyroidism, severe renal insufficiency, adrenocortical insufficiency (Addison's), head injuries, or increased intracranial pressure, acute abdominal conditions, & in geriatric or severely debilitated patients.

▶ Adverse Effects: Constipation, bloat, & sedation. Potential for: paralytic ileus, toxic megacolon, pancreatitis, & CNS effects.

▶ Dose carefully in small dogs; not advisable to use in very young kittens.

▶ Diphenoxylate is a class-V controlled substance in USA.

Uses/Indications

Diphenoxylate is an opiate and commercially available in a fixed-dose combination with atropine. It is used primarily in dogs for its antidiarrheal and antitussive properties. Use in cats is controversial and many clinicians do not recommend its use in this species.

Pharmacology/Actions

Among their other actions, opiates inhibit GI motility and excessive GI propulsion. They decrease intestinal secretion induced by cholera toxin, prostaglandin E_2 and diarrheas caused by factors where calcium is the second messenger (non-cyclic AMP/GMP mediated). Opiates may also enhance mucosal absorption.

Pharmacokinetics

In humans, diphenoxylate is rapidly absorbed after administration of either the tablets or oral solution; bioavailability of the tablets is approximately 90% that of the solution. Generally, onset of action occurs within 45-60 minutes after dosing and is sustained for 3-4 hours. Diphenoxylate is metabolized into diphenoxylic acid, an active metabolite. The serum half-lives of diphenoxylate and diphenoxylic acid are approximately 2.5 hours and 3-14 hours, respectively.

Contraindications/Precautions/Warnings

All opiates should be used with caution in patients with hypothyroidism, severe renal insufficiency, adrenocortical insufficiency, (Addison's), and in geriatric or severely debilitated patients. Opiate antidiarrheals are contraindicated in cases where the patient is hypersensitive to narcotic analgesics, in patients receiving monoamine oxidase inhibitors (MAOIs), and patients with diarrhea caused by a toxic ingestion (until the toxin is eliminated from the GI tract).

Opiate antidiarrheals should be used with caution in patients with head injuries or increased intracranial pressure and acute abdominal conditions (*e.g.,* colic), as it may obscure the diagnosis or clinical course of these conditions. It should be used with extreme caution in patients suffering from respiratory disease or from acute respiratory dysfunction (*e.g.,* pulmonary edema secondary to smoke inhalation). Opiate antidiarrheals should be used with extreme caution in patients with hepatic disease with CNS clinical signs of hepatic encephalopathy; hepatic coma may result.

Many clinicians recommend not using diphenoxylate or loperamide in dogs weighing less than 10 kg, but this is probably a result of the potency of the tablet or capsule forms of the drugs. Dosage titration using the liquid forms of these agents should allow their safe use in dogs when indicated.

Adverse Effects

In dogs, constipation, bloat, and sedation are the most likely adverse reactions encountered when usual doses are given. Potentially, paralytic ileus, toxic megacolon, pancreatitis, and CNS effects could be seen.

Use of antidiarrheal opiates in cats is controversial; this species may react with excitatory behavior.

Opiates used in horses with acute diarrhea (or in any animal with a potentially bacterial-induced diarrhea) may have a detrimental effect. Opiates may enhance bacterial proliferation, delay the disappearance of the microbe from the feces, and prolong the febrile state.

Reproductive/Nursing Safety

Diphenoxylate/atropine is classified as category C for use during pregnancy (*Animal studies have shown an adverse effect on the fetus, but there are no adequate studies in humans; or there are no animal reproduction studies and no adequate studies in humans.*)

Exercise caution when administering diphenoxylate HCl with atropine to nursing patients. Diphenoxylic acid may be, and atropine is, excreted in maternal milk but effects on the infant may not be significant.

Overdosage/Acute Toxicity

Acute overdosage of the opiate antidiarrheals could result in CNS, cardiovascular, GI, or respiratory toxicity. Because opiates may significantly reduce GI motility, absorption from the GI tract may be delayed and prolonged. For more information, refer to the morphine monograph. Naloxone may be necessary to reverse the opiate effects.

Massive overdoses of diphenoxylate/atropine sulfate may induce atropine toxicity. Refer to the atropine monograph for more information.

Drug Interactions

The following drug interactions have either been reported or are theoretical in humans or animals receiving opiate antidiarrheals and may be of significance in veterinary patients. Unless otherwise noted, use together is not necessarily contraindicated, but weigh the potential risks and perform additional monitoring when appropriate.

▪ **CNS DEPRESSANT DRUGS:** Other CNS depressants (*e.g.,* **anesthetic agents, antihistamines, phenothiazines, barbiturates, tranquilizers, alcohol,** etc.) may cause increased CNS or respiratory depression when used with opiate antidiarrheal agents.

▪ **MONOAMINE OXIDASE INHIBITORS** (including **amitraz,** and possibly **selegiline**): Opiate antidiarrheal agents are contraindicated in human patients receiving systemic monoamine oxidase (MAO) inhibitors for at least 14 days after receiving MAO inhibitors.

Laboratory Considerations

▪ Plasma **amylase** and **lipase** values may be increased for up to 24 hours following administration of opiates.

Doses

▪ **DOGS:**

As an antidiarrheal (extra-label): Dosage is per the diphenoxylate component: 0.05 – 0.1 mg/kg (some recommend up to 0.2 mg/kg) PO q8-12h. Use with caution, if at all, when diarrhea is suspected caused by an enteric infection.

As an **antitussive** (extra-label): 0.2 – 0.4 mg/kg PO q8-12h. If constipation develops, stool softeners may alleviate.

- **CATS:**

As an **antidiarrheal** (extra-label; not usually recommended for cats): 0.08 – 0.1 mg/kg PO q12h. (Marks 2008)

Monitoring
- Clinical efficacy.
- Fluid and electrolyte status in severe diarrhea.
- CNS effects, if using high dosages.

Client Information
- If diarrhea persists or if animal appears listless or develops a high fever, contact veterinarian.
- When used for cough watch for constipation; contact veterinarian if this is a problem.
- May be given with or without food. If your animal vomits or acts sick after getting it on an empty stomach, give with food or small treat to see if this helps. If vomiting continues, contact your veterinarian.
- Constipation and sedation (sleepiness/fatigue) are the most common side effects in dogs.
- Must use very cautiously in cats; can get overly excited.
- Controlled drug in USA. It is against federal law to use, give away or sell this medication to others than for whom it was prescribed.

Chemistry/Synonyms
Structurally related to meperidine, diphenoxylate HCl is a synthetic phenylpiperidine-derivative opiate agonist. It occurs as an odorless, white, crystalline powder that is slightly soluble in water and sparingly soluble in alcohol. Commercially available preparations also contain a small amount of atropine sulfate to discourage the abuse of the drug for its narcotic effects. At therapeutic doses, the atropine has no clinical effect.

This combination may be known as co-phenotrope in the U.K. and elsewhere. Other synonyms include: R 1132, NIH 7562 or difenoxilato. A commonly used trade name is *Lomotil®*.

Compatibility/Compounding Considerations
No specific information noted.

Storage/Stability
Diphenoxylate/atropine tablets should be stored at room temperature in well-closed, light-resistant containers. Diphenoxylate/atropine oral solution should be stored at room temperature in tight, light-resistant containers; avoid freezing.

Dosage Forms/Regulatory Status
VETERINARY-LABELED PRODUCTS: NONE.

HUMAN-LABELED PRODUCTS:

Diphenoxylate HCl Tablets: 2.5 mg with 0.025 mg Atropine Sulfate; *Lofene®*, *Lomotil®*, *Lonox®*, generic; (Rx, C-V)

Diphenoxylate HCl Liquid: 2.5 mg with 0.025 mg Atropine Sulfate per 5 ml; generic; (Rx, C-V)

Revisions/References
Monograph revised/updated January 2014.
Marks, S. (2008). GI Therapeutics: Which Ones and When? Proceedings; IVECCS. accessed via Veterinary Information Network; vin.com

Diphenylhydantoin – see Phenytoin Sodium

Dirlotapide
(dir-loe-ta-pyde)   Slentrol®
Gut Microsomal Triglyceride Transfer Protein (gMTP) Inhibitor

Prescriber Highlights
▶ Indicated for the management of obesity in dogs; not for use in cats.
▶ Not recommended for dogs with liver disease, unmanaged Cushing's, or receiving corticosteroids.
▶ Primary adverse effects are GI (vomiting, diarrhea); increased liver enzymes possible.
▶ Safe use not established for treatment beyond one year.
▶ Fairly complex dosing guidelines; regular monitoring & dosage adjustment required.

Uses/Indications
Dirlotapide oral solution is indicated for the management of obesity in dogs.

Pharmacology/Actions
Dirlotapide is a selective microsomal triglyceride transfer protein inhibitor that blocks the formation and release of lipoproteins into the systemic circulation. The mechanism of action for weight reduction is not completely understood, but it seems to result from reduced fat absorption and a satiety signal (Peptide YY) from lipid-filled enterocytes.

Dirlotapide primarily acts locally in the gut to reduce appetite, increase fecal fat and produce weight loss in the management of obesity in dogs. Although systemic blood levels do not directly correlate with efficacy, they seem to correlate with the drug's systemic toxicity.

Pharmacokinetics
In dogs, dirlotapide is available systemically, but absorption is highly variable (22-41%). Presence of food in the gut apparently increases bioavailability. Dirlotapide in the circulation is highly protein bound and the volume of distribution is 1.3 L/kg. Systemically absorbed dirlotapide is metabolized in the liver. Dirlotapide and its metabolites are excreted in the bile and may undergo enterohepatic circulation. Non-linear pharmacokinetics with less-than-proportional exposure, drug accumulation (at higher doses), and large inter-patient variability have been observed in multiple studies and at various doses. The mean elimination half-life in dogs ranged between 5 and 18 hours, and may increase with dosage and after repeated dosing. The fecal and biliary routes are the predominant routes of elimination. Renal excretion accounts for less than 1% of the drug administered.

Contraindications/Precautions/Warnings
The manufacturer states that dirlotapide is not recommended for use in dogs currently receiving long-term corticosteroid therapy. Do not use in dogs with liver disease. Pre-existing endocrine disease, including hyperadrenocorticism (Cushing's disease), should be managed prior to use of dirlotapide.

Dirlotapide should not be used in cats; increases risk of hepatic lipidosis during weight loss in obese cats.

Safe use for longer than one year has not been evaluated.

Adverse Effects
Adverse effects most likely seen with dirlotapide in dogs include (in decreasing order of frequency): vomiting (especially during the first month of treatment and 3-4 hours after dosing), diarrhea, lethargy, anorexia, salivation, constipation and dehydration. As additional patients receive this medication, this profile could change.

During field trials, some dogs developed mild to moderate elevation in serum hepatic transaminase activity early in treatment that decreased over time while treatment continued.

Reproductive/Nursing Safety

Safety in breeding, pregnant, or lactating dogs has not been established.

Overdosage/Acute Toxicity

Oral doses of 0.5, 1 and 2 mL/kg (2.5X, 5X, 10X of maximum labeled dose) were administered to normal weight Beagles for two weeks. The drug was tolerated but vomiting, diarrhea, anorexia, lethargy, transient elevations in liver enzymes (transaminase) were noted. No histopathologic evidence of hepatic necrosis was seen.

Drug Interactions

Drug interactions with dirlotapide have not been reported at the time of writing, but the drug could potentially alter the oral absorption (rate and extent) of many drugs. Until safe concomitant use is determined with oral drugs with narrow therapeutic indexes, it is suggested to dose these drugs at least two hours prior to administering dirlotapide; additional monitoring may be required.

- **FAT SOLUBLE VITAMINS (A, E, K):** During the first 6 months of treatment, plasma vitamin A and E concentrations of treated dogs were significantly below the vitamin A and E concentrations of the control dogs. Plasma vitamin A concentration was low after one month and the median values did not decline any further. Plasma vitamin E concentrations were lowest after 6 months of treatment but adipose tissue levels of vitamin E appeared to be increased compared to control dogs after 12 months of treatment. Plasma vitamin A and E concentrations appeared to increase during the weight stabilization phase (second 6 months of treatment) and returned to concentrations similar to the control dogs when treatment was discontinued. Prothrombin times were similar in the treated and the control dogs and there were no clinical signs of abnormal hemostasis observed during the 12-month study.

Laboratory Considerations

- No specific alterations to laboratory tests have been noted; the drug can increase **serum transaminase** in some patients.

Doses

- **DOGS:**

  WEIGHT LOSS PHASE:

  Initial assessment and dosing in first month: Assess the dog prior to initiation of therapy to determine the desired weight and to assess the animal's general health (See Precautions). The initial dosage is 0.01 mL/kg (0.05 mg/kg) body weight, administered once daily, orally, for the first 14 days. After the first 14 days of treatment, the dose volume should be doubled to 0.02 mL/kg (0.1 mg/kg) of body weight, administered once daily for the next 14 days (days 15 to 28 of treatment).

  Subsequent Monthly Dose Adjustments for Weight Loss: Dogs should be weighed monthly and the dose volume adjusted every month, as necessary, to maintain a target percent weight loss of ≥ 0.7% per week. To determine if a dose adjustment is necessary, compare the Actual % weight loss to the Target % weight loss and use the following guidelines. **Note:** All dose adjustments are based solely on volume (mL).

  First (or Subsequent) Dose Adjustment Section: <u>If the dog has lost weight</u>, determine if an adjustment in dose is required using the following calculations: (Number of weeks between visits) X 0.7 % per week = Target % weight loss. Example – in 4 weeks (28 days) the Target weight loss would be 4 X 0.7% per week, or at least 2.8% of the total body weight. Compare the Target % weight loss (of ≥ 0.7% per week) with the Actual % weight loss for that dog.

  Monthly weight loss rate achieved. If the Actual % weight loss is the same or greater than the Target % weight loss, the dose volume (number of mL administered each day) should remain the same for the next month of dosing until the next scheduled assessment.

  Monthly weight loss not achieved. If the Actual % weekly weight loss is less than the Target % weight loss of 0.7% weekly, the following dose adjustment instructions apply:

  First dose adjustment: The dose volume (number of mL administered each day) should be increased by 100%, resulting in an increase of the dose volume to 2X the dose administered during the previous month of dosing. Only perform a 100% dose increase once during treatment after day 14.

  Subsequent dose adjustments: If additional dose increases are necessary in the following months, the dose volume (number of mL administered each day) should be increased by 50%, resulting in an increase of the dose volume to 1.5X the dose administered the previous month of dosing. Based on the dog's current body weight a daily dose of 0.2 mL/kg (0.09 mL/lb.) should not be exceeded.

  If a dog's food consumption is greatly reduced for several consecutive days, the dose may be withdrawn until the appetite returns (usually 1–2 days) and then resume dosing at the same volume.

  The monthly adjustments should continue in this way until the desired weight determined at the start of therapy is reached. When the desired weight is reached, begin the weight management phase.

  WEIGHT MANAGEMENT PHASE

  A 3-month weight management phase is recommended to successfully maintain the weight loss achieved with treatment. During the weight management phase, the veterinarian and the pet owner should establish the optimal level of food intake and physical activity needed. Dirlotapide administration should be continued during the weight management phase until the dog owner can establish the food intake and physical activity needed to stabilize body weight at the dog's desired weight. To dose for weight management, body weight should continue to be assessed at monthly intervals.

  First dose adjustment:

  <u>If the dog lost ≥1% body weight per week</u> in the last month of the weight loss phase, the dose volume (number of mL administered each day) should be decreased by 50% resulting in a decrease of the dose volume to 0.5 times the dose administered the previous month.

  <u>If the dog lost between 0 and 1%</u> the dose should remain the same.

  <u>If the dog gained weight,</u> the dose should be increased by 50% resulting in an increase of the dose volume to 1.5 times the dose administered the previous month.

  Subsequent dose adjustments:

  In subsequent months the dose volume should be increased or decreased by 25% to maintain a constant weight.

  If the dog is within -5% to +5% of the body weight at the end of the weight loss phase, the dose volume (number of mL administered each day) should remain unchanged.

  If the dog lost >5% body weight, then the dose should be decreased by 25%.

If the dog gained > 5% body weight, then the dose should be increased by 25%. Based on the dog's current body weight a daily dose of 0.2 mL/kg (0.09 mL/lb.) should not be exceeded.

When dirlotapide is discontinued, the daily amount of food offered and physical activity should be continued as established during the weight management phase. Reverting to previous food intake or physical activity levels at this point can contribute to a re-gain of some or all of the weight loss that has been achieved.

(Package Insert; *Slentrol®*)

Monitoring

- Patient weight (see dosing).
- Adverse effects.
- Liver enzymes (baseline, and occasional).

Client Information

- Not a cure for obesity, dirlotapide decreases the food intake of the dog by decreasing appetite and associated begging behavior. Decreased appetite seen in treated dogs is only temporary and lasts no longer than 1-2 days beyond the cessation of therapy. Weight gain will occur if the amount of food offered is not limited at the time the drug is discontinued.
- Successful, long-term weight management requires changes that extend beyond the period of drug therapy. To maintain weight loss; adjustments in dietary management and physical activity that were begun as part of the overall weight loss program must be continued.
- If total lack of appetite (inappetence or anorexia) is observed for more than one day, contact veterinarian.
- Almost 1 in 4 of dogs placed on therapy experienced occasional episodes of vomiting and diarrhea. In most cases these episodes lasted for one or two days. Vomiting occurred most often during the first month of treatment or within a week of a dose increase. If vomiting occurs it is recommended to continue dosing at the same dose volume, however, the time of day or method of administration (with or without food) may be changed. If vomiting is severe or lasts longer than 2 days, consult veterinarian.
- To prepare for oral administration, remove the bottle cap and insert the supplied oral dosing syringe through the membrane into the bottle. Invert the bottle and withdraw the appropriate volume required using the graduation marks on the side of the oral dosing syringe.
- Can be administered directly into the dog's mouth or on a small amount of food; can be given with a meal or at a different time of day.
- Wipe the oral dosing syringe clean after each use with a clean dry cloth or disposable towel; do not introduce water into the oral dosing syringe or the solution.
- Not for use in humans. Keep this and all drugs out of reach of children.
- If accidental eye exposure occurs, flush the eyes immediately with clean water.

Chemistry/Synonyms

Dirlotapide has the chemical name 5-[(4'-trifluoromethyl-biphenyl-2-carbonyl)-amino]-1H-indole-2-carboxylic acid benzylmethyl carbamoylamide. It has a molecular weight of 674.7. The commercial product is a liquid formulation containing 5 mg/mL of dirlotapide in medium chain triglyceride (MCT) oil.

Dirlotapide may also be known as CP-742,033 or by its trade name *Slentrol®*.

Storage/Stability

Dirlotapide liquid should be stored in the original container at room temperature 15-30°C (59-86°F).

Compatibility/Compounding Considerations

No specific information noted.

Dosage Forms/Regulatory Status

VETERINARY-LABELED PRODUCTS:

Dirlotapide Oral Solution 5 mg/mL in 20 mL, 50 mL and 150 mL bottles; *Slentrol®*; (Rx). Labeled for use in dogs.

HUMAN-LABELED PRODUCTS: NONE.

Revisions/References

Monograph revised/updated January 2014.

Disopyramide Phosphate

(dye-soe-peer-a-mide)   Norpace®

Antiarrhythmic Agent

Prescriber Highlights

▶ Rarely used 3rd line antiarrhythmic for use in dogs; negative inotrope & can prolong QT interval.

▶ Contraindications: Hypersensitivity to the drug, 2nd or 3rd degree AV block, cardiogenic shock, severe uncompensated or poorly compensated cardiac failure or hypotension, glaucoma (closed-angle), urinary retention, or myasthenia gravis.

▶ Caution: Sick sinus syndrome, bundle branch block, or Wolff-Parkinson-White (WPW) syndrome, hepatic or renal disease.

▶ Adverse effects most likely noted: Anticholinergic effects (dry mouth, eyes, nose; constipation; urinary hesitancy or retention) & cardiovascular effects including edema, hypotension, dyspnea, syncope, & conduction disturbances (AV block); can reduce serum glucose.

▶ Drug interactions.

Uses/Indications

Disopyramide potentially could be used for the oral treatment or prevention of ventricular tachyarrhythmias in dogs. Because of its negative inotropic effects and short half-life, disopyramide is generally considered to be a 3rd line agent for veterinary (canine) use. An oral controlled-release product is available that could prove useful, but it has not been extensively evaluated in dogs.

Pharmacology/Actions

Considered to be a class 1A (membrane-stabilizing) antiarrhythmic with actions similar to either quinidine or procainamide, disopyramide reduces myocardial excitability and conduction velocity and also possesses anticholinergic activity (150 mg of disopyramide ≈ 0.09 mg of atropine) that may contribute to the effects of the drug.

The drug's exact mechanism of action has not been established. Disopyramide's cardiac electrophysiologic effects include: 1) shortened sinus node recovery time; 2) increased atrial and ventricular refractory times; 3) decreased conduction velocity through the atria and ventricles; 4) decreased automaticity of ectopic atrial or ventricular pacemakers.

Disopyramide has direct negative inotropic effects. It generally has minimal effects on resting heart rates or blood pressure. Systemic peripheral resistance may increase by 20%.

Pharmacokinetics

The half-life of the disopyramide is approximately 7 hours in humans with normal renal function, but only 2-3 hours in the dog. Oral bioavailability in dogs is about 70% and it is rapidly absorbed. In humans, disopyramide is rapidly absorbed following oral administration with peak levels occurring within 2-3 hours after the conventional capsules are administered. Peak levels occur at about 6 hours post dose with the controlled-release capsules.

Disopyramide is distributed throughout the body in the extracellular water and is not extensively bound to tissues. Binding to plasma proteins is variable and dependent on the drug's concentration. At therapeutic levels it is approximately 50-65% plasma protein bound (human data). Disopyramide crosses the placenta and milk concentrations may exceed those found in plasma.

Disopyramide is metabolized in the liver, but 40-65% of it is excreted unchanged in the urine. Patients with renal disease may need dosage adjustments made to prevent drug accumulation.

Contraindications/Precautions/Warnings

Disopyramide usually should not be used in patients with glaucoma (closed-angle), urinary retention, or myasthenia gravis because of its anticholinergic effects.

Disopyramide is contraindicated in 2nd or 3rd degree AV block (unless pacemaker inserted), cardiogenic shock, or if the patient is hypersensitive to the drug.

Disopyramide should not be used in patients with severe uncompensated or poorly compensated cardiac failure or hypotension because of its negative inotropic effects. Patients with atrial fibrillation or flutter must be digitalized before disopyramide therapy to negate increased ventricular response (beyond acceptable). Disopyramide should be used with caution in patients with sick sinus syndrome, bundle branch block, or Wolff-Parkinson-White (WPW) syndrome.

Use of disopyramide with other class 1A antiarrhythmics or propranolol may cause additive negative inotropic effects (see Drug Interactions).

Disopyramide should be used with caution (and possibly at a reduced dosage) in patients with hepatic or renal disease.

Adverse Effects

Most common adverse reactions are secondary to disopyramide's anticholinergic effects (*e.g.*, dry mouth, eyes, or nose; constipation; urinary hesitancy or retention) and cardiovascular effects (edema, hypotension, dyspnea, syncope, or conduction disturbances such as AV block). Other adverse effects that have been reported in humans include: GI effects (vomiting, diarrhea, etc.), intrahepatic cholestasis, hypoglycemia, fatigue, headache, muscle weakness and pain. In contrast to the urinary hesitancy effects, disopyramide can also cause urinary frequency and urgency.

Doses of 15 mg/kg q8h in dogs prolong the QT interval and doses above 30 mg/kg widen the QRS complex.

Reproductive/Nursing Safety

In humans, the FDA categorizes this drug as category *C* for use during pregnancy (*Animal studies have shown an adverse effect on the fetus, but there are no adequate studies in humans; or there are no animal reproduction studies and no adequate studies in humans.*)

Disopyramide has been detected in milk at a concentration not exceeding that found in maternal plasma. Use with caution in nursing animals.

Overdosage/Acute Toxicity

Clinical signs of overdosage/toxicity include: anticholinergic effects, apnea, loss of consciousness, hypotension, cardiac conduction disturbances and arrhythmias, widening of the QRS complex and QT interval, bradycardia, congestive heart failure, seizures, asystole, and death.

Treatment consists initially of prompt gastric emptying, charcoal, and cathartics. Followed by vigorous symptomatic therapy using, if necessary, cardiac glycosides, vasopressors and sympathomimetics, diuretics, mechanically assisted respiration, and endocardial pacing. Disopyramide can be removed with hemodialysis.

Drug Interactions

The following drug interactions have either been reported or are theoretical in humans or animals receiving disopyramide and may be of significance in veterinary patients. Unless otherwise noted, use together is not necessarily contraindicated, but weigh the potential risks and perform additional monitoring when appropriate.

- **ANTICHOLINERGIC DRUGS:** Additive anticholinergic effects may be encountered if disopyramide is used concomitantly with other anticholinergics (*e.g.*, atropine, glycopyrrolate).
- **CISAPRIDE:** Additional prolongation of QT interval.
- **MACROLIDE ANTIBIOTICS** (*e.g.*, **erythromycin, clarithromycin**): Increased disopyramide levels; prolongation of QT interval may occur. A study done in dogs with complete AV block indicated that a potentially fatal interaction could occur between disopyramide and erythromycin administered in clinically relevant doses (Watanabe et al. 2011).
- **PHENOBARBITAL:** May increase disopyramide's metabolism, thereby reducing disopyramidi levels.
- **PROCAINAMIDE, LIDOCAINE:** May be used with disopyramide, but widening of QRS and prolongation of QT interval may occur.
- **QUINIDINE:** May increase disopyramide levels; disopyramide may decrease quinidine levels.
- **RIFAMPIN:** May increase disopyramide's metabolism and reduce serum levels.
- **VERAPAMIL:** Because of additional negative inotropic effects, use of disopyramide within 48 hours of using verapamil is not recommended.

Doses

- **DOGS:**

  As an antiarrhythmic (almost never used); (extra-label): 7 – 30 mg/kg PO q4h. (Kittleson 2006)

Monitoring

- ECG.
- Blood pressure.
- Clinical signs of adverse effects (see above); liver function tests if chronic therapy.
- Serum levels if indicated (lack of efficacy, toxicity).
- Therapeutic levels in humans have been reported to be between 2-7 micrograms/mL and toxic levels are considered to be above 9 micrograms/mL. Levels of up to 7 micrograms/mL may be necessary to treat and prevent the recurrence of refractory ventricular tachycardias.

Client Information

- Contact veterinarian if animal has persistent problems with difficult urination, dry mouth, vomiting, constipation, becomes lethargic or depressed, or has difficulty breathing.

Chemistry/Synonyms

Structurally dissimilar from other available antiarrhythmic agents, disopyramide phosphate occurs as a white or practically white crystalline powder with a pK_a of 10.4. It is freely soluble in water and slightly soluble in alcohol.

Disopyramide Phosphate may also be known as: disopyramidi phosphas, SC-13957, *Norpace*®, *Dicorantil*®, *Dirythmin*®, *Dirytmin*®, *Diso-Duriles*®, *Disomet*®, *Disonorm*®, *Durbis*®, *Durbis*®, *Isomide*®, *Isorythm*®, *Ritmodan*®, *Ritmoforine*®, *Rythmical*®, *Rythmodan*®, and *Rythmodul*®.

Storage/Stability

Disopyramide capsules should be stored at room temperature (15-30°C) in well-closed containers. An extemporaneously prepared suspension of 1 – 10 mg/mL of disopyramide (from capsules) in cherry syrup has been shown to be stable for one month if stored in amber bottles and refrigerated (2-8°C).

Compatibility/Compounding Considerations

No specific information noted.

Dosage Forms/Regulatory Status

VETERINARY-LABELED PRODUCTS: NONE.

The ARCI (Racing Commissioners International) has designated this drug as a class 4 substance. See the appendix for more information.

HUMAN-LABELED PRODUCTS:

Disopyramide Phosphate Capsules: 100 mg & 150 mg; *Norpace®*, generic; (Rx)

Disopyramide Phosphate Capsules Extended-Release: 100 mg & 150 mg; *Norpace CR®*, generic; (Rx)

Revisions/References

Monograph revised/updated January 2014.

Kittleson, M. (2006). "Chapt 29: Drugs used in the treatment of cardiac arrhythmias." *Small Animal Cardiology, 2nd Ed* Veterinary Information Network.

Watanabe, I., et al. (2011). Combined effect of disopyramide and erythromycin on ventricular repolarization in dogs with complete atrioventricular block. Int Heart J 52(6): 393-7.

dl-Methionine – see Methionine

DMSO – see Dimethyl Sulfoxide

Dobutamine HCl

(doe-byoo-ta-meen)   Dobutrex®

Parenteral Beta-Adrenergic Inotropic

Prescriber Highlights

▶ Parenteral, rapid acting inotropic agent. Use only in an "ICU" setting.

▶ Contraindications: Known hypersensitivity to the drug or to the preservative (sodium bisulfite); patients with idiopathic hypertropic subaortic stenosis (IHSS). Caution: Post myocardial infarction (MI).

▶ Animals with atrial fibrillation should be digitalized prior to receiving dobutamine.

▶ Most common adverse effects: facial twitching in dogs, tachycardia; higher doses can cause CNS effects (especially in cats).

Uses/Indications

Dobutamine is used as a rapid-acting injectable positive inotropic agent for short-term treatment (usually less than 72 hours) of heart failure. It is also useful in shock patients when fluid therapy alone has not restored acceptable arterial blood pressure, cardiac output, or tissue perfusion.

Pharmacology/Actions

Dobutamine is considered a direct beta₁-adrenergic agonist. It also has mild beta₂- and alpha₁-adrenergic effects at therapeutic doses. These effects tend to balance one another and cause little direct effect on the systemic vasculature. In contrast to dopamine, dobutamine does not cause the release of norepinephrine. It has relatively mild chronotropic, arrhythmogenic, and vasodilative effects, but higher dosages can cause tachycardia.

Increased myocardial contractility and stroke volumes result in increased cardiac output. Decreases in left ventricular filling pressures (wedge pressures) and total peripheral resistance occur in patients with a failing heart. Blood pressure and cardiac rate generally are unaltered or slightly increased because of increased cardiac output. Increased myocardial contractility may increase myocardial oxygen demand and coronary blood flow.

Pharmacokinetics

Because it is rapidly metabolized in the GI tract and is not available after oral administration, dobutamine is only administered intravenously (as a constant infusion). After intravenous administration, the onset of action generally occurs within 2 minutes and peaks after 10 minutes.

Dobutamine is metabolized rapidly in the liver and other tissues and has a plasma half-life of approximately 2 minutes in humans. The drug's effects diminish rapidly after cessation of therapy.

Pharmacokinetic data for domestic animals is apparently unavailable. It is unknown if dobutamine crosses the placenta or into milk.

Contraindications/Precautions/Warnings

Dobutamine is contraindicated in patients with known hypersensitivity to the drug or with idiopathic hypertropic subaortic stenosis (IHSS). The injectable formulation contains sodium bisulfite as a preservative that has been documented to cause allergic-type reactions in some human patients. Hypovolemic states must be corrected before administering dobutamine. Because it may increase myocardial oxygen demand and increase infarct size, dobutamine should be used very cautiously after myocardial infarction.

Adequate vascular volume is required for dobutamine use.

Use with extreme caution in patients with ventricular tachyarrhythmias or atrial fibrillation. Dobutamine can enhance atrioventricular conduction. In animals with atrial fibrillation, rapid IV digitalization with digoxin is recommended before dobutamine administration to slow AV nodal conduction. In horses that will receive electrocardioversion for atrial fibrillation, it has been recommended to stop dobutamine for at least 5 minutes before shock delivery (McGurrin 2010).

Do not confuse DOBUTamine with DOPamine.

Adverse Effects

Adverse effects reported in dogs include: tachycardia, facial twitching, seizures and tachyphylaxis (increased dosages required over time). Tachyphylaxis can become apparent within 48-72 hours in dogs. In cats, doses greater than 5 micrograms/kg/min may cause CNS effects such as tremors or seizures.

The most commonly reported adverse effects in humans are: ectopic beats, increased heart rate, increased blood pressure, chest pain, and palpitations. At usual doses these effects are generally mild and will not necessitate halting therapy, but dosage reductions should be performed. Other, more rare, adverse effects reported include: nausea, headache, vomiting, leg cramps, paresthesias, and dyspnea.

Reproductive/Nursing Safety

In humans, the FDA categorizes this drug as category *B* for use during pregnancy (*Animal studies have not yet demonstrated risk to the fetus, but there are no adequate studies in pregnant women; or animal studies have shown an adverse effect, but adequate studies in pregnant women have not demonstrated a risk to the fetus in the first trimester of pregnancy, and there is no evidence of risk in later trimesters.*)

No specific information on lactation safety for dobutamine was found.

Overdosage/Acute Toxicity

Clinical signs reported with excessive dosage include tachycardias, increased blood pressure, nervousness, and fatigue. Because of the drug's short duration of action, temporarily halting therapy is usually all that is required to reverse these effects.

Drug Interactions

The following drug interactions have either been reported or are theoretical in humans or animals receiving dobutamine and may be of significance in veterinary patients. Unless otherwise noted, use together is not necessarily contraindicated, but weigh the potential risks and perform additional monitoring when appropriate.

- **ATROPINE; GLYCOPYROLATE:** May increase the risk for tachyarrhythmias in horses; use with caution.
- **BETA-BLOCKERS** (*e.g.*, **metoprolol, propranolol**): May antagonize the cardiac effects of dobutamine, and result in a preponderance of alpha-adrenergic effects and increased total peripheral resistance.
- **NITROPRUSSIDE:** Synergistic effects (increased cardiac output and reduced wedge pressure) can result if dobutamine is used with nitroprusside.
- **OXYTOCIC DRUGS:** May induce severe hypertension when used with dobutamine in obstetric patients.

Doses

Dobutamine is administered as a constant rate intravenous infusion (CRI) only. An online drip rate table generator can be found at: http://www.globalrph.com/drip.htm

- **DOGS:**

  For short-term treatment of low cardiac output and acute heart failure (extra-label): Dosages are usually started on the low end and titrated upward. Most recommendations fall in the 1 – 20 micrograms/kg/minute range, but suggested lower end dosages ranging from 1 – 5 micrograms/kg/minute and upper end dosages of up to 40 micrograms/kg/minute can be found. Infusions greater than 20 micrograms/kg/minute may cause tachycardia. Tachyphylaxis (reduced response over time to a given dosage) and arrhythmias can occur.

- **CATS:**

  For short-term treatment of low cardiac output and acute heart failure (extra-label): Dosage suggestions tend to be lower for cats (than dogs) with 1 – 5 micrograms/kg/minute noted. Dosages are usually started on the low end and titrated upward. Some have suggested that maximum infusion rates of up to 15 micrograms/kg/minute may be used, however others caution that doses above 5 mcg/kg/min in cats can cause seizures.

- **HORSES:** (NOTE: ARCI UCGFS CLASS 2 DRUG)

  For cardiovascular support in anesthetized horses (extra-label): At IV infusion rates below 1 – 1.5 micrograms/kg/min, arterial blood pressure increases, but cardiac output is marginally affected. At higher rates, both cardiac output and arterial blood pressure are increased, but there also is an increased risk for arrhythmias. Dobutamine is a weaker proarrhythmic than most other catecholamines, and arrhythmias observed at 3 – 5 micrograms/kg/min in horses are usually limited to bradyarrhythmias, second-degree atrioventricular blocks, premature atrial contractions, and isorhythmic atrioventricular dissociation. Use parasympatholytics (e.g., atropine) with caution, as there is an increased risk for tachyarrhythmias. (Schauvliege et al. 2013)

  Foals (after volume repletion); (extra-label): 2 – 20 micrograms/kg per minute CRI (**Note:** another section of this reference states the dose is 3 – 40 micrograms/kg/minute). Follow the rule of "6": 6 times the weight of foal (in kg) = the number of mg to add to 100 mL of saline (1 mL/hr. = 1 microgram/kg/minute). (Wilkins 2004)

- **BIRDS:**

  For isoflurane-induced severe hypotension in Hispaniolan Amazon parrots (extra-label): In the study, dobutamine CRI at a rate of 15 micrograms/kg/min caused the greatest increases in arterial blood pressure of the three tested dobutamine infusions (5, 10, or 15 mcg/kg/min.). (Schnellbacher et al. 2012)

Monitoring

- Heart rate and rhythm, blood pressure.
- Mucous membrane color.
- Urine flow.
- Ideally, measurement of central venous or pulmonary wedge pressures and cardiac output.

Client Information

- This drug should only be used by professionals familiar with its use and in a setting where adequate patient monitoring can be performed.

Chemistry/Synonyms

Dobutamine HCl is a synthetic inotropic agent related structurally to dopamine. It occurs as a white, to off-white, crystalline powder with a pK_a of 9.4. Dobutamine is sparingly soluble in water and alcohol.

Dobutamine HCl may also be known as: 46236, compound 81929, dobutamini hydrochloridum, and LY-174008; many trade names are available.

Storage/Stability

Dobutamine injection should be stored at room temperature (15-30°C); diluted solutions should be used within 24 hours.

Compatibility/Compounding Considerations

Preparation for Injection: The solution for injection must be further diluted to a concentration no greater than 5 mg/mL (total of at least 50 mL of diluent) before administering.

Generally, dobutamine is added to D5W, normal saline (if animal not severely sodium restricted) or other compatible IV solution. The following approximate concentrations will result if 1 vial (250 mg) is added either 250, 500, or 1000 mL IV solutions: 1 vial (250 mg) in: 250 mL ≈ 1000 micrograms/mL; 500 mL ≈ 500 micrograms/mL; 1000 mL ≈ 250 micrograms/mL.

A mechanical fluid administration control device should be used, if available, to administer dobutamine. When using a mini-drip IV administration set (60 drops ≈ 1 mL), 1 drop contains approximately 8.3 micrograms at the 500 micrograms/mL concentration (one 250 mg vial in 500 mL IV fluids).

A formula for calculating dobutamine or dopamine CRI's has been published (Plunkett et al. 2008): 6 x body weight (in kg) = the number of milligrams of dobutamine or dopamine added to a sufficient quantity of 0.9% NaCl to obtain a total volume of 100 mL. When delivered at a rate of 1 mL/hour IV, 1 microgram/kg/min is administered.

Dobutamine is physically **compatible** with the usually used IV solutions (D5W, sodium chloride 0.45% and 0.9%, dextrose-saline combinations, lactated Ringer's) and is reported to be physically **compatible** with the following drugs: amiodarone HCl, atropine sulfate, dopamine HCl, epinephrine HCl, hydralazine HCl, isoproterenol HCl, lidocaine HCl, meperidine HCl, morphine sulfate, nitroglycerin, norepinephrine (levarterenol) bitartrate, phentolamine mesylate, phenylephrine HCl, procainamide HCl, propranolol HCl, and verapamil HCl.

Dobutamine may be physically **incompatible** with the following agents: aminophylline, bumetanide, calcium chloride or gluconate, diazepam, digoxin, furosemide, heparin (inconsistent results), regular insulin, magnesium sulfate, phenytoin sodium, potassium chloride (at high concentrations only – 160 mEq/L), potassium phosphate, and sodium bicarbonate.

Dosage Forms/Regulatory Status

VETERINARY-LABELED PRODUCTS: NONE.

The ARCI (Racing Commissioners International) has designated this drug as a class 2 substance. See the appendix for more information.

Dobutamine HCl Injection Concentrated Solution: 12.5 mg/mL in 20 mL & 40 mL single-use vials & 100 mL pharmacy bulk packages; generic; (Rx)

Dobutamine HCL Solution for Injection: 250 mg/250 mL (1 mg/mL) preservative free in 250 mL single use containers; 500 mg/500 mL (1 mg/mL) preservative free in 500 mg single-use containers; 500 mg/250 mL (2 mg/mL) preservative free in 250 mL single-use containers & 1,000 mg/250 mL (4 mg/mL) preservative free in 250 mL single-use containers; Dobutamine Hydrochloride in 5% Dextrose Injection; (Rx)

Revisions/References

Monograph revised/updated January 2014.
McGurrin, M. (2010). Therapeutic Options in Atrial Fibrillation. Proceedings: ACVIM. accessed via Veterinary Information Network; vin.com
Plunkett, S. J. & M. McMichael (2008). Cardiopulmonary resuscitation in small animal medicine: An update. Journal of Veterinary Internal Medicine 22(1): 9-25.
Schauvliege, S. & F. Gasthuys (2013). Drugs for Cardiovascular. Support in Anesthetized Horses. Veterinary Clinics of North America-Equine Practice 29(1): 19-+.
Schnellbacher, R. W., et al. (2012). Effects of dopamine and dobutamine on isoflurane-induced hypotension in Hispaniolan Amazon parrots (Amazona ventralis). American Journal of Veterinary Research 73(7): 952-8.
Wilkins, P. (2004). Disorders of foals. *Equine Internal Medicine, 2nd Ed.* S. Reed, W. Bayly and D. Sellon. Philadelphia, Saunders: 1381-431.

Docusate

(dok-yoo-sate)   Colace®

Surfactant; Stool Softener

Prescriber Highlights

▶ Surfactant stool softener.
▶ Caution: Fluid/electrolyte abnormalities.
▶ Adverse Effects: Cramping, diarrhea, & GI mucosal damage.

Uses/Indications

Docusate is used in small animals when feces are hard or dry, or with anorectal conditions when passing firm feces would be painful or detrimental. Docusate is used alone and in combination with mineral oil in treating fecal impactions in horses.

Pharmacology/Actions

Docusate salts reduce surface tension and allow water and fat to penetrate the ingesta and formed feces thereby softening the stool. Recent *in vivo* studies have demonstrated that docusate also increases cAMP concentrations in colonic mucosal cells that may increase both ion secretion and fluid permeability from these cells into the colon lumen.

Pharmacokinetics

It is unknown how much docusate is absorbed after oral administration, but it is believed that some is absorbed from the small intestine and then excreted into the bile.

Contraindications/Precautions/Warnings

Use with caution in patients with pre-existing fluid or electrolyte abnormalities; monitor.

Adverse Effects

At usual doses, clinically significant adverse effects should be very rare. Cramping, diarrhea, and intestinal mucosal damage are possible. The liquid preparations may cause throat irritation if administered by mouth. Docusate sodium is very bitter tasting.

Overdoses in horses may be serious.

Reproductive/Nursing Safety

In humans, the FDA categorizes this drug as category C for use during pregnancy (*Animal studies have shown an adverse effect on the fetus, but there are no adequate studies in humans; or there are no animal reproduction studies and no adequate studies in humans.*)

It is not known whether docusate calcium, docusate potassium, or docusate sodium are excreted in milk, but it is unlikely to be of concern.

Overdosage/Acute Toxicity

In horses, single doses of 0.65 – 1 g/kg have caused dehydration, intestinal mucosal damage, and death. Maximum therapeutic dosages of up to 0.2 g/kg have been reported. Signs of overdoses in horses can begin in 1-2 hours after dosing with initial signs including restlessness and increased intestinal sounds; increases in respiratory and cardiac rates can follow. Abdominal pain, watery diarrhea, and dehydration can occur with horses deteriorating over hours to several days to lateral recumbency and death. Because high dose docusate can cause secretory effects, hydration and electrolyte status should be monitored and treated if necessary. Treatment is supportive; GI protectants, bicarbonate, corticosteroids, and antiendotoxemic agents (NSAIDs) have been suggested as being potentially helpful.

Drug Interactions

The following drug interactions have either been reported or are theoretical in humans or animals receiving docusate and may be of significance in veterinary patients. Unless otherwise noted, use together is not necessarily contraindicated, but weigh the potential risks and perform additional monitoring when appropriate.

- **MINERAL OIL:** Theoretically, mineral oil should not be given with docusate (DSS) as enhanced mineral oil absorption could occur, however this interaction does not appear to be of significant clinical concern with large animals. It is less clear whether this could be of significance with small animals, therefore the concurrent use of these agents together in dogs or cats cannot be recommended. If it is deemed necessary to use both docusate and mineral oil in small animals, separate doses by at least two hours.

Doses

- **DOGS:**

  As a stool softener (extra-label): 25 – 100 mg per dog (depending dog size) PO once to twice daily. May give 240 mg or 250 mg once daily to very large dogs.

- **CATS:**

  As a stool softener (extra-label): 50 mg per cat PO once daily.

- **HORSES:**

  For large colon impaction (to soften); (extra-label): 6 – 12 g/500 kg diluted in 2-4 liters of water by nasogastric tube q12-24h. (Blikslager et al. 2004)

Monitoring

- Clinical efficacy.
- Hydration and electrolyte status, if indicated.

Client Information

- Used to treat constipation caused by hard or dry stools.
- Generally well tolerated with few side effects.
- Should be given on an empty stomach: one hour before or two hours after a meal.
- Docusate is available OTC (over-the-counter; without a prescription), but don't give it (or any other laxatives or medications) to your animal without first consulting a veterinarian.

Chemistry/Synonyms

Docusate is available in sodium and calcium salts. They are anionic, surface-active agents and possess wetting and emulsifying properties.

Docusate sodium (also known as dioctyl sodium succinate, DSS, or DOSS) occurs as a white, wax-like plastic solid with a characteristic odor. One g is soluble in approximately 70 mL of water and it is freely soluble in alcohol and glycerin. Solutions are clear and have a bitter taste.

Docusate calcium (also known as dioctyl calcium succinate) occurs as a white, amorphous solid with a characteristic odor (octyl alcohol). It is very slightly soluble in water, but freely soluble in alcohol.

Docusate sodium may also be known as: dioctyl sodium sulphosuccinate, dioctyl sodium sulfosuccinate, docusatum natricum, DSS, and sodium dioctyl sulphosuccinate; many trade names are available; Colace® is the most commonly known sodium salt product and Surfak® the most commonly known calcium salt product.

Storage/Stability

Capsules of salts of docusate should be stored in tight containers at room temperature. Temperatures above 86°F can soften or melt soft gelatin capsules. Docusate sodium solutions should be stored in tight containers and the syrup should be stored in tight, light-resistant containers.

Compatibility/Compounding Considerations

No specific information noted.

Dosage Forms/Regulatory Status

VETERINARY APPROVED PRODUCTS:

There are several docusate products marketed for veterinary use; their FDA-approval status is unknown and no entries were found in the FDA "green book". Docusate products are available without prescription (OTC). Commercially available products may include:

Docusate Sodium Bloat Preparation: 240 mg/30 mL in 360 mL containers; (OTC). Labeled milk withdrawal = 96 hours; slaughter withdrawal = 3 days.

Docusate Sodium Enema: 5% water miscible solution in 1 gal containers; *Dioctynate®*; (OTC).

Docusate Sodium Enema: 250 mg in 12 mL syringes; *Pet-Enema®*, *Enema SA®*, *Docu-Soft® Enema*; (OTC or RX)

Docusate sodium oral liquid 5% in gallons; various; generic. May also be called Veterinary Surfactant. (OTC)

HUMAN-LABELED PRODUCTS:

There are many trade name products for docusate. The two most commonly known are *Colace®* (sodium salt) and *Surfak®* (calcium salt).

Docusate Sodium Oral Tablets: 100 mg; (OTC)

Docusate Sodium Oral Capsules & Soft-gel Capsules: 50 mg, 100 mg, & 250 mg; generic; (OTC)

Docusate Sodium Oral Syrup/Liquid: 50 mg/5 mL (10 mg/mL); (OTC)

Docusate Calcium Capsules: 240 mg (regular and soft gel); (OTC).

Revisions/References

Monograph revised/updated January 2014.

Blikslager, A. & S. Jones (2004). Obstructive disorders of the gastrointestinal tract. *Equine Internal Medicine 2nd Ed.* S. Reed, W. Bayly and D. Sellon. Philadelphia, Saunders: 623-936.

Dolasetron Mesylate

(doe-laz-e-tron)   Anzemet®

Antiemetic Agent

Prescriber Highlights

▶ 5-HT₃ receptor antagonist antiemetic particularly useful for chemo-related nausea & vomiting in small animals.

▶ Once daily administration for IV or PO doses.

▶ Usually well tolerated; may cause dose-related ECG changes.

▶ Oral human tablets not easily dosed in small animals (strength); must be reformulated for PO use in cats.

▶ Expense may be an issue.

Uses/Indications

Dolasetron may be effective in treating severe nausea and vomiting in dogs and cats, particularly if caused by cancer chemotherapy drugs. Because it is given once a day, the injectable form of dolasetron is often preferred over ondansetron, a similarly effective antiemetic. However, for oral use in small animals, dolasetron tablets are too large (50 and 100 mg) to be practically administered.

Pharmacology/Actions

Dolasetron exerts its anti-nausea and antiemetic actions by selectively antagonizing 5-hydroxytryptamine₃ (5-HT₃) receptors. These receptors are found primarily in the CNS chemoreceptor trigger zone, on vagal nerve terminals and enteric neurons in the GI tract. Chemotherapy induced vomiting is believed to be caused principally by serotonin release from the mucosal enterochromaffin cells in the small intestine. Dolasetron does not have prokinetic activity.

Pharmacokinetics

After dolasetron is administered IV to dogs, its half-life is only minutes long as it is rapidly reduced via carbonyl reductase to hydrodolasetron (also called reduced dolasetron or red-dolasetron). Hydrodolasetron is primarily responsible for the drug's pharmacologic effect. Oral dolasetron is also rapidly absorbed and converted to hydrodolasetron. Hydrodolasetron's volume of distribution in dogs is 8.5 L/kg; total body clearance is 25 mL/min/kg and half-life about 4 hours.

In humans, dolasetron is rapidly absorbed and converted to hydrodolasetron. Oral bioavailability is about 75%. Hydrodolasetron's half-life in humans is about 7-8 hours. The drug is partially metabolized in the liver, but 50-60% is excreted unchanged into the urine. Clearance may be reduced in patients with severe renal or hepatic impairment.

Contraindications/Precautions/Warnings

Dolasetron is contraindicated in patients hypersensitive to it, with atrioventricular block II to III, or with markedly prolonged QT$_c$. It should be given with caution to patients with, or susceptible to, developing prolongation of cardiac conduction intervals. This includes patients with hypokalemia, hypomagnesemia, receiving anti-arrhythmic drugs or diuretics that may induce electrolyte abnormalities, congenital QT syndrome, or a cumulative high dose of anthracycline chemotherapy.

These agents are generally ineffective when used for vomiting associated with feline hepatic lipidosis or GI obstruction.

Adverse Effects

Dolasetron appears to be well tolerated in the limited numbers of small animal patients that have received it. In humans, it has been associated with dose-related ECG interval prolongation (PR, QT$_c$, JT prolongation and QRS widening). Other adverse effects that have been reported in humans using the drug during chemotherapy include headache and dizziness.

Reproductive/Nursing Safety

In pregnant humans, dolasetron is designated by the FDA as a category *B* drug (*Animal studies have not demonstrated risk to the fetus, but there are no adequate studies in pregnant women; or animal studies have shown an adverse effect, but adequate studies in pregnant women have not demonstrated a risk to the fetus during the first trimester of pregnancy, and there is no evidence of risk in later trimesters.*) Teratogenicity studies in laboratory animals failed to demonstrate any teratogenic effects.

It is unknown if the drug enters milk; the manufacturer urges caution.

Overdosage/Acute Toxicity

There is very limited data available. One human patient who received 13 mg/kg of dolasetron developed severe hypotension and dizziness and was treated with pressors and fluids. The patient's blood pressure returned to baseline 3 hours after the dose was administered. It is suggested to manage overdoses with supportive therapy. The lethal intravenous doses in mice and rats were 160 mg/kg and 140 mg/kg respectively. This is equivalent to 6-12X the human recommended dose when comparing equivalent body surface areas.

Drug Interactions

The following drug interactions have either been reported or are theoretical in humans or animals receiving dolasetron and may be of significance in veterinary patients. Unless otherwise noted, use together is not necessarily contraindicated, but weigh the potential risks and perform additional monitoring when appropriate.

- **APOMORPHINE:** 5HT3 antagonists may enhance the hypotensive effect of apomorphine. In humans it is recommended to avoid this combination.
- **ATENOLOL:** May reduce the clearance and increase blood levels of hydrodolasetron.
- **CIMETIDINE:** May reduce the clearance and increase blood levels of hydrodolasetron.
- **KETOCONAZOLE:** May reduce the clearance and increase blood levels of hydrodolasetron.
- **PHENOBARBITAL:** Can reduce hydrodolasetron blood levels.
- **RIFAMPIN:** Can reduce hydrodolasetron blood levels.
- **TRAMADOL:** 5HT3 antagonists may reduce the analgesic effects of tramadol.

Laboratory Considerations

- No dolasetron-related laboratory interactions were noted.

Doses

In humans, the injection can be given as rapidly as 100 mg over 30 seconds or diluted into 50 mL of a compatible IV solution and infused over a period of up to 15 minutes.

- **DOGS/CATS:**

  As an anti-emetic (extra-label): To prevent or treat vomiting 0.6 mg/kg PO, IV or SC q24h. Some recommend giving higher dosages up to 1 mg/kg to treat active vomiting disorders. May give IV push undiluted or diluted in up to 50 mL of an IV solution and infused over a period of up to 15 minutes.

Monitoring

- Efficacy.
- Heart rhythm in at-risk patients.

Client Information

- The injectable form of this drug is most appropriately administered at the veterinary clinic/hospital. Oral forms of the drug will most likely need to be compounded to lesser strengths; maropitant or ondansetron tablets may be more practical for oral dosing in small animal patients.

Chemistry/Synonyms

A 5-HT$_3$ receptor antagonist antiemetic, dolasetron mesylate occurs as a white to off-white powder. It is freely soluble in water or propylene glycol, and slightly soluble in 0.9% sodium chloride solution or alcohol.

Dolasetron may also be known as *Anzemet®*, *Anemet®* or *Zamanon®*.

Storage/Stability

The commercially available tablets should be stored at room temperature 20-25°C (68-77°F) and protected from light. The commercially available injection should be stored at room temperature (20-25°C; 68-77°F) with excursions permitted to 15-30°C (59-86°F); protect from light.

Compatibility/Compounding Considerations

Dolasetron injection is reportedly **compatible** with the following injectable solutions: sodium chloride 0.9%, 5% dextrose, sodium chloride 0.45% with 5% dextrose, 5% dextrose and lactated Ringer's, lactated Ringer's, and mannitol 10% injection. After dilution, the injectable is stable under normal lighting at room temperatures for 24 hours; 48 hours if refrigerated. The manufacturer does not recommend mixing with other injectable drugs and states to flush the infusion line before and after administering dolasetron.

Dosage Forms/Regulatory Status

VETERINARY-LABELED PRODUCTS: NONE.

HUMAN-LABELED PRODUCTS:

Dolasetron Tablets: 50 mg & 100 mg; *Anzemet®*; (Rx)

Dolasetron Injection: 20 mg/mL with 38.2 mg/mL mannitol in single use 0.625 mL ampules, 0.625 mL fill in 2 mL *Carpuject*, single-use 5 mL vials & 25 mL multi-dose vials; *Anzemet®*; (Rx)

Revisions/References

Monograph revised/updated January 2014.

Domperidone

(dohm-pare-i-dohne)   Equidone®, Motilium®

Dopamine-2 Agonist

Prescriber Highlights

- ▶ Dopamine-2 antagonist.
- ▶ Used in horses for treatment of tall fescue toxicity and as a diagnostic agent for PPID. Potential treatment for Leishmaniasis in dogs.
- ▶ Galactorrhea or gynecomastia most likely adverse effects.

Uses/Indications

Domperidone is FDA-approved in the USA for prevention of fescue toxicosis in periparturient mares. Domperidone has been shown to increase plasma ACTH in horses with equine pituitary pars intermedia dysfunction (PPID, Equine Cushing's) and may be useful in helping diagnose this condition.

It has been tried as a GI prokinetic or antiemetic agent in small animals, but efficacy appears poor. A study and a follow-up report in dogs showed that domperidone may have some efficacy in treating mild to moderate Canine leishmaniasis (Gomez-Ochoa et al. 2009; Gomez-Ochoa et al. 2011).

Pharmacology/Actions

Domperidone's apparent efficacy for the treatment of fescue toxicosis in pregnant mares is related to the fact that tall fescue toxicosis causes decreased prolactin levels. Dopamine is involved in the reduction of prolactin production and it is postulated that the alkaloids found in tall fescue act as dopamine-mimetic agents. Domperidone ostensibly blocks this effect.

Domperidone is a dopamine antagonist (D2-receptors) with similar actions as metoclopramide. It has been stated that the drug does not cross the blood brain barrier and thus does not have CNS effects as does metoclopramide, but it may be more accurate to say that it does not readily cross into the CNS, as extrapyramidal adverse effects have been reported in some human patients. In dogs and cats, metoclopramide appears to have more prokinetic effects on gastric emptying than domperidone. Domperidone does not appreciably affect small intestinal transit time.

Domperidone antagonizes dopamine in the GI tract and chemoreceptor trigger zone, which is thought to be the primary cause for its prokinetic and antiemetic effects. It also is an antagonist for alpha$_2$- and beta$_2$-adrenergic receptors in the stomach, which may contribute to the drug's pharmacological actions.

Domperidone may have effects on cell-mediated immunity possibly due to its stimulation of prolactin. Prolactin has been classified as a pro-inflammatory lymphocyte-derived cytokine and a study done in healthy dogs found that domperidone induced a statistically significant increase in the percentages of activated phagocytes in the treated group during and for up to one month after treatment (Gomez-Ochoa et al. 2012).

Pharmacokinetics

Domperidone is absorbed from the GI tract, but its bioavailability in dogs is only about 20%, presumably due to a high first pass effect. Peak serum levels occur about 2 hours after oral dosing and the drug is highly bound (93%) to serum proteins. Domperidone is primarily metabolized and metabolites are excreted in the feces and urine.

Contraindications/Precautions/Warnings

Domperidone should not be used in animals with known hypersensitivity to it or when GI obstructions are present or suspected. Do not use in pregnant mares >15 days prior to the expected foaling date (see Reproductive Safety below). In horses, domperidone failure of passive transfer of immunoglobulins (IgG) may occur even in the absence of leakage of colostrum or milk. All foals born to mares treated with domperidone should be tested for serum IgG concentrations. Do not use in horses intended for human consumption.

Because domperidone is potentially a neurotoxic substrate of P-glycoprotein, it should be used with caution in those herding breeds (e.g., Collies, etc.) that may have the gene mutation (MDR1) that causes a nonfunctional protein. Also see Drug Interactions.

Adverse Effects

Because plasma prolactin levels may be increased, galactorrhea or gynecomastia may result. In horses the most commonly reported adverse effects are premature lactation (dripping of milk prior foaling) and failure of passive transfer. Injectable products (now withdrawn) have been associated with arrhythmias in human patients with heart disease or hypokalemia. Rarely, somnolence or dystonic reactions have occurred in people.

Reproductive/Nursing Safety

The equine product label states: *Equidone® Gel* may lead to premature birth, low birth weight foals or foal morbidity if administered >15 days prior to the expected foaling date. Accurate breeding date(s) and an expected foaling date are needed for the safe use of *Equidone® Gel*. The safety of *Equidone® Gel* has not been evaluated in breeding, pregnant and lactating mares other than in the last 45 days of pregnancy and the first 15 days of lactation (see Animal Safety). The safety in stallions has not been evaluated. The long-term effects on foals born to mares treated with *Equidone® Gel* have not been evaluated.

Domperidone has been shown to have teratogenic effects when used at high doses in mice, rats and rabbits. The drug's effect of causing prolactin release may impact fertility in both females and males.

Domperidone has been used to increase milk supply in women. In rats, it enters milk in small amounts with approximately 1/500th of the adult dose reaching the pups.

Overdosage/Acute Toxicity

There is no specific antidote for domperidone overdose. Use standard decontamination procedures and treat supportively.

Drug Interactions

The following drug interactions have either been reported or are theoretical in humans or animals receiving domperidone and may be of significance in veterinary patients. Unless otherwise noted, use together is not necessarily contraindicated, but weigh the potential risks and perform additional monitoring when appropriate.

- **AZOLE ANTIFUNGALS** (*e.g.*, **ketoconazole**, etc.): May increase domperidone levels.
- **ANTICHOLINERGIC DRUGS**: May reduce the efficacy of domperidone.
- **BROMOCRIPTINE/CABERGOLINE**: Domperidone may antagonize effects on prolactin.
- **MACROLIDE ANTIBIOTICS** (*e.g.*, **erythromycin, clarithromycin**): May increase domperidone levels.
- **OPIOIDS**: May reduce the efficacy of domperidone.
- **SUSTAINED-RELEASE** or **ENTERIC-COATED ORAL MEDICATIONS**: Domperidone may alter the absorptive characteristics of these drugs by decreasing GI transit times.

Laboratory Considerations

- Domperidone may increase **serum prolactin** levels.
- Domperidone may increase **ALT** and **AST**.
- Domperidone may cause a false positive result on the **milk calcium** test used to predict foaling.

Doses

- **DOGS:**

  As a prokinetic agent (extra-label): Domperidone is rarely recommended for use in dogs, as it does not appear to be very useful as a prokinetic. It has been tried at 0.05 – 0.1 mg/kg PO 1-3 times a day.

  As an alternative treatment for Leishmaniasis in dogs with mild to moderate clinical signs (extra-label: Based on a preliminary clinical study in dogs. In the initial study dogs received 1 mg/kg PO twice daily for 30 days. In the short-term follow-up report dosages reported were 0.5 mg/kg PO q24h for 30 days (Gomez-Ochoa et al. 2009; Gomez-Ochoa et al. 2011). (**Note:** *At the time of writing it is not known if combination therapies using domperidone are effective or safe—Plumb*)

- **CATS:**

  As a prokinetic agent (extra-label): Domperidone is rarely recommended for use in cats as there is little information published or clinical experience with it. Dog dose (above) has been suggested.

- **HORSES:**

  For fescue toxicity (labeled dose; FDA-approved): 1.1 mg/kg PO once daily starting 10-15 days prior to Expected Foaling Date (EFD). Treatment may be continued for up to 5 days after foaling if mares are not producing adequate milk after foaling. (Label information—*Equidone Gel®*; Dechra)

  For assisting in the diagnosis of pituitary par intermedia dysfunction (PPID)–Domperidone Response Test (extra-label): Collect EDTA plasma (1 mL) at 8 AM. Administer domperidone at 3.3 mg/kg PO. Collect EDTA plasma at 2- and 4-hours after domperidone administration. A 2-fold increase in plasma ACTH concentration suggests PPID. Higher doses (5 mg/kg PO) may improve response. The 2-hour sample is more diagnostic in the summer and autumn, and the 4-hour sample is best in the winter and spring. (McFarlane 2011)

Monitoring

- Clinical efficacy.

Client Information

- Equine gel: Owners should be directed on the proper use of the multi-dose dosing syringe, including how to set the dial ring for accurate dosing after the first dose.

- Should not be given to mares more than 15 days before expected foaling date as premature birth can occur.

- In mares, premature lactation (dripping of milk prior to foaling) and failure of the mare's milk to pass on immunoglobulins to the foal are the most common side effects.

- In small animals, may be given with or without food. Do not give antacids or other drugs that reduce stomach acidity to your animal while it's receiving this medication. If your animal vomits or acts sick after getting it on an empty stomach, give with food or small treat to see if this helps. If vomiting continues, contact your veterinarian.

- Pregnant or nursing women should use caution when handling this medication.

Chemistry/Synonyms

Domperidone maleate occurs as a white or almost white powder that exhibits polymorphism. It is very slightly soluble in water or alcohol.

Domperidone may also be known as domperidonum and R-33812. Common trade names include *Motilium®* or *Equidone®*, but many trade names are available internationally.

Storage/Stability

Domperidone gel should be stored at controlled room temperature 25°C (77°F) with excursions between 15°-30°C (59°-86°F) permitted. Recap after each use. Domperidone tablets should be stored at room temperature and protected from light and moisture.

Compatibility/Compounding Considerations

No specific information noted.

Dosage Forms/Regulatory Status

VETERINARY-LABELED PRODUCTS: NONE.

Domperidone Oral Gel 11% (110 mg/mL) in 25 mL multi-dose oral syringes; *Equidone® Gel*; (Rx). FDA-approved for use in horses (NADA #141-314). A link to the product label can be found at dailymed.nlm.nih.gov

HUMAN-LABELED PRODUCTS: NONE IN THE USA.

In Canada (10 mg tablet only) and in Europe, human oral tablets of 10 mg, suppositories and oral suspension may be available.

Revisions/References

Monograph revised/updated January 2014.

Gomez-Ochoa, P., et al. (2009). Use of domperidone in the treatment of canine visceral leishmaniasis: A clinical trial. Veterinary Journal 179(2): 259-63.

Gomez-Ochoa, P., et al. (2011). Efficacy of Domperidone for the Treatment of Mild and Moderate Cases of Canine Leishmaniosis: Clinical and Immunological Short-Term Follow-Up. 21st ECVIM-CA Congress. accessed via Veterinary Information Network; vin.com

Gomez-Ochoa, P., et al. (2012). Use of the nitroblue tetrazolium reduction test for the evaluation of Domperidone effects on the neutrophilic function of healthy dogs. Veterinary Immunology and Immunopathology 146(1): 97-9.

McFarlane, D. (2011). Equine Pituitary Pars Intermedia Dysfunction. Vet Clin Equine 27: 93-113.

Dopamine HCl

(doe-pa-meen)   Intropin®

Adrenergic/Dopaminergic Inotropic Agent

Prescriber Highlights

▶ Catecholamine that (in most species) at lower doses dilates the renal mesenteric, coronary, & intracerebral vascular beds; at higher doses, systemic peripheral resistance is increased & hypotension treated.

▶ Use in an "ICU" setting.

▶ Contraindications: Pheochromocytoma, ventricular fibrillation, & uncorrected tachyarrhythmia.

▶ Not a substitute for adequate reperfusion therapy.

▶ Adverse Effects: Nausea/vomiting, ectopic beats, tachycardia, hypotension, hypertension, dyspnea, headache & vasoconstriction.

▶ Avoid extravasation injuries.

Uses/Indications

Dopamine should be used only in critical care settings where adequate monitoring can be provided. It is used to correct the hemodynamic imbalances present in shock after adequate fluid volume replacement and as adjunctive therapy for the treatment of acute heart failure.

It has now been shown that low-dose dopamine for the treatment of oliguric renal failure is not efficacious in improving GFR in humans; its use for this purpose in dogs is unproven and somewhat controversial. In cats, low dose dopamine reportedly does not cause renal vasodilatation.

Pharmacology/Actions

Dopamine is a precursor to norepinephrine and acts directly and indirectly (by releasing norepinephrine) on both alpha- and beta$_1$-receptors. Dopamine also has dopaminergic effects.

While there are species differences, in general at very low IV doses, 0.5 – 2 micrograms/kg/min, dopamine acts predominantly on dopaminergic receptors and dilates the renal, mesenteric, coronary, and intracerebral vascular beds. At doses from 2 – 10 micrograms/kg/min, dopamine also stimulates alpha$_1$- and beta$_1$-adrenergic receptors. The net effect at this dosage range is to exert positive cardiac inotropic activity, increase organ perfusion, renal blood flow and urine production, but GFR does not appreciably improve. At these lower doses, systemic vascular resistance increases with the dose. At higher doses, >10 – 12 micrograms/kg/min, the dopaminergic effects are overridden by alpha effects. Systemic peripheral resistance is increased and hypotension may be corrected in cases where systemic vascular resistance is diminished; renal and peripheral blood flows are thus decreased. One study in cats showed that dopamine at 15 micrograms/kg/min did not increase systemic vascular resistance (Pascoe et al. 2006).

Pharmacokinetics

Dopamine is not administered orally as it is rapidly metabolized in the GI tract. After IV administration, the onset of action is usually within 5 minutes and persists for less than 10 minutes after the infusion has stopped.

Dopamine is widely distributed in the body but does not cross the blood-brain barrier in appreciable quantities. It is unknown if dopamine crosses the placenta.

The plasma half-life of dopamine is approximately 2 minutes. It is metabolized in the kidney, liver, and plasma by monoamine oxidase (MAO) and catechol-O-methyltransferase (COMT) to inactive compounds. Up to 25% of a dose of dopamine is metabolized to norepinephrine in the adrenergic nerve terminals. In human patients receiving monoamine oxidase inhibitors, dopamine's duration of activity can be as long as one hour.

Contraindications/Precautions/Warnings

Dopamine is contraindicated in patients with pheochromocytoma, ventricular fibrillation, and uncorrected tachyarrhythmias. It is not a substitute for adequate fluid, electrolyte or blood product replacement therapy. Dopamine should be used with caution in patients with ischemic heart disease or an occlusive vascular disease. Decrease dose or discontinue the drug should clinical signs occur implicating dopamine as the cause of reduced circulation to the extremities or the heart. The drug should be discontinued or dosage reduced should arrhythmias (PVC's) occur.

Cats are unlikely to benefit (and it may be detrimental) from low dose dopamine therapy for oliguric renal failure.

Do not confuse DOBUTamine with DOPamine.

Adverse Effects

Most frequent adverse effects seen include: nausea and vomiting, ectopic beats, tachycardia, palpitation, hypotension, hypertension, dyspnea, headache, and vasoconstriction.

Extravasation injuries with dopamine can be very serious with necrosis and sloughing of surrounding tissue. Patient's IV sites should be routinely monitored. Should extravasation occur, infiltrate the site (ischemic areas) with a solution of 5 – 10 mg phentolamine (*Regitine*®) in 10 – 15 mL of normal saline. A syringe with a fine needle should be used to infiltrate the site with many injections.

Reproductive/Nursing Safety

In humans, the FDA categorizes this drug as category *C* for use during pregnancy (*Animal studies have shown an adverse effect on the fetus, but there are no adequate studies in humans; or there are no animal reproduction studies and no adequate studies in humans.*) In a separate system evaluating the safety of drugs in canine and feline pregnancy (Papich 1989), this drug is categorized as class: *B* (*Safe for use if used cautiously. Studies in laboratory animals may have uncovered some risk, but these drugs appear to be safe in dogs and cats or these drugs are safe if they are not administered when the animal is near term.*)

It is not known whether dopamine is excreted in breast milk.

Overdosage/Acute Toxicity

Accidental overdosage is manifested by excessive blood pressure elevation (see adverse effects above). Treatment consists only of temporarily discontinuing therapy since dopamine's duration of activity is so brief. Should the patient's condition fail to stabilize, phentolamine has been suggested for use.

Drug Interactions

The following drug interactions have either been reported or are theoretical in humans or animals receiving dopamine and may be of significance in veterinary patients. Unless otherwise noted, use together is not necessarily contraindicated, but weigh the potential risks and perform additional monitoring when appropriate.

- **ALPHA-ADRENERGIC BLOCKERS** (*e.g.*, **prazosin**): May antagonize the vasoconstrictive properties of dopamine (high-dose).
- **ANESTHETICS, GENERAL HALOGENATED HYDRO-CARBON**: Use of halothane with dopamine may result in increased incidences of ventricular arrhythmias.
- **ANTIDEPRESSANTS, TRICYCLIC**: May potentiate adverse cardiovascular effects.
- **BETA-BLOCKERS** (*e.g.*, **metoprolol, propranolol**): May antagonize the cardiac effects of dopamine.
- **DIURETICS**: May potentiate urine production effects of low-dose dopamine.
- **MONOAMINE OXIDASE INHIBITORS**: Monoamine oxidase inhibitors can significantly prolong and enhance the effects on dopamine.
- **OXYTOCIC DRUGS**: May cause severe hypertension when used with dopamine.
- **PHENOTHIAZINES**: In animals (species not specified), the renal and mesenteric vasodilatation effects of dopamine have been antagonized by phenothiazines.
- **VASOPRESSORS/VASOCONSTRICTORS**: Use with dopamine may cause severe hypertension.

Laboratory Considerations

Dopamine may:
- Suppress **serum prolactin** secretion from the pituitary.
- Suppress **thyrotropin** secretion from the pituitary.
- Suppress **growth hormone** secretion from the pituitary.

Doses

The dosage of dopamine is determined by its indication (for more information refer to the pharmacology section above). Dopamine is administered as a constant rate intravenous infusion (CRI) only. Use an IV pump or other flow-controlling device to increase precision in dosing. An online drip rate table generator can be found at: http://www.globalrph.com/drip.htm

- **DOGS/CATS:**

  For severe hypotension/shock due to poor cardiac contractility and/or vasodilation (extra-label): In general, constant rate infusion (CRI) rates are titrated to effect. Adequate volume replacement is required before use. Commonly, initial rates of 2 – 2.5 micrograms/kg/minute are recommended and then titrated upward. In dogs and cats a CRI of 5 – 10 micrograms/kg per minute will have predominantly beta-1 effects and from 10 – 15 micrograms/kg /minute will have both beta-1 and alpha-1 effects. Adapted from: (Plunkett et al. 2008; Scroggin et al. 2009; Butler 2011; Fletcher et al. 2012)

Monitoring

- Urine flow.
- Cardiac rate/rhythm.
- Blood pressure.
- IV site.

Client Information

- Dopamine should be used only in an intensive care setting or where adequate monitoring is possible.

Chemistry/Synonyms

An endogenous catecholamine that is the immediate precursor to norepinephrine, dopamine (as the HCl salt) occurs as a white to off-white crystalline powder. It is freely soluble in water and soluble in alcohol. The injectable concentrated solution has a pH of 2.5-5.5 and may contain an antioxidant (sodium bisulfate). The pH of the ready-to-use injectable products in dextrose range from 3-5.

Dopamine HCl may also be known as: ASL-279, dopamini hydrochloridum, and 3-hydroxytyramine hydrochloride; many trade names are available.

Storage/Stability

Dopamine injectable products should be protected from light. Solutions that are pink, yellow, brown, or purple indicate decomposition of the drug. Solutions that are darker than a light yellow should be discarded. Dopamine solutions should be stored at room temperature (15-30°C).

After dilution in a common IV solution (not 5% bicarbonate), dopamine is stable for at least 24 hours at room temperature, but it is recommended to dilute the drug just prior to use. Dopamine is stable in solutions with a pH of less than 6.4, and most stable at a pH less than 5. It is oxidized at alkaline pH.

Compatibility/Compounding Considerations

To prepare solution: Add contents of vial to either 250 mL, 500 mL, or 1000 mL of normal saline, D5W, lactated Ringer's injection, or other compatible IV fluid. If adding a 200 mg vial (5 mL @ 40 mg/mL) to a one-liter bag, the resultant solution will contain an approximate concentration of 200 micrograms/mL. If using a mini-drip IV set (60 drops/mL), each drop will contain approximately 3.3 micrograms. In small dogs and cats, it may be necessary to use less dopamine so the final concentration will be less; in large animals, a higher concentration may be necessary.

A formula for calculating dobutamine or dopamine CRI's has been published (Plunkett et al. 2008): 6 x body weight (in kg) = the number of milligrams of dobutamine or dopamine added to a sufficient quantity of 0.9% NaCl to obtain a total volume of 100 mL. When delivered at a rate of 1 mL/hour IV, 1 microgram/kg/min is administered. When delivered at a rate of 1 mL/hour IV, 1 microgram/kg/min is administered.

Dopamine is reported to be physically **compatible** with the following IV fluids: D5 in LRS, D5 in half-normal saline, D5 in normal saline, D5W, mannitol 20% in water, lactated Ringer's, normal saline, and 1/6M sodium lactate. Dopamine is reported to be physically **compatible** with the following drugs: aminophylline, calcium chloride, chloramphenicol sodium succinate, dobutamine HCl, gentamicin sulfate (gentamicin potency retained for only 6 hours), heparin sodium, hydrocortisone sodium succinate, lidocaine HCl, methylprednisolone sodium succinate, potassium chloride, tetracycline HCl, and verapamil HCl.

Dopamine is reported to be physically **incompatible** with: amphotericin B, ampicillin sodium, iron salts, metronidazole with sodium bicarbonate, penicillin G potassium, and sodium bicarbonate. Compatibility is dependent upon factors such as pH, concentration, temperature, and diluent used; it is suggested to consult specialized references for more specific information.

Dosage Forms/Regulatory Status

VETERINARY-LABELED PRODUCTS: NONE.

The ARCI (Racing Commissioners International) has designated this drug as a class 2 substance. See the appendix for more information.

HUMAN-LABELED PRODUCTS:

Dopamine HCl for Concentrated Solution for Injection: 40 mg/mL, 80 mg/mL and 160 mg/mL in 5 mL & 10 mL vials; generic; (Rx)

Dopamine HCl in Dextrose 5% Injection Solution: 200 mg/250 mL (0.8 mg/mL); 400 mg/500 mL (0.8 mg/mL); 400 mg/250 mL (1.6 mg/mL); 800 mg/500 mL (1.6 mg/mL); & 800 mg/250 mL (3.2 mg/mL) in 250 mL premixed single-use containers; generic; (Rx)

Revisions/References

Monograph revised/updated January 2014.

Butler, A. L. (2011). Goal-Directed Therapy in Small Animal Critical Illness. Veterinary Clinics of North America-Small Animal Practice 41(4): 817-+.

Fletcher, D. J., et al. (2012). RECOVER evidence and knowledge gap analysis on veterinary CPR. Part 7: Clinical guidelines. J. Vet. Emerg. Crit. Care 22.

Pascoe, P. J., et al. (2006). Effects of increasing infusion rates of dopamine, dobutamine, epinephrine, and phenylephrine in healthy anesthetized cats. American Journal of Veterinary Research 67(9): 1491-9.

Plunkett, S. J. & M. McMichael (2008). Cardiopulmonary resuscitation in small animal medicine: An update. Journal of Veterinary Internal Medicine 22(1): 9-25.

Scroggin, R. D. & J. Quandt (2009). The use of vasopressin for treating vasodilatory shock and cardiopulmonary arrest. J. Vet. Emerg. Crit. Care 19(2): 145-57.

Doramectin

(dor-a-mek-tin)   Dectomax®

Avermectin Antiparasitic

Prescriber Highlights

▶ Injectable (cattle, swine) & topical (cattle only) avermectin antiparasiticide.
▶ Potentially useful for generalized demodicosis in small animals.
▶ Manufacturer warns about using in other species.
▶ IM injections may cause muscle blemishes.
▶ Not labeled for female dairy cattle (20 months or older).
▶ Relatively long slaughter withdrawal times.

Uses/Indications

Doramectin injection is indicated for the treatment and control of the following endo- and ectoparasites in cattle: roundworms (adults and some fourth stage larvae)—*Ostertagia ostertagi* (including inhibited larvae), *O. lyrata, Haemonchus placei, Trichostrongylus axei, T. colubriformis, T. longispicularis, Cooperia oncophora, C. pectinata, C. punctata, C. surnabada* (syn. *mcmasteri*), *Bunostomum phlebotomum, Strongyloides papillosus, Oesophagostomum radiatum, Trichuris* spp.; lungworms (adults and fourth stage larvae)—*Dictyocaulus viviparus*; eyeworms (adults)—*Thelazia* spp.; grubs (parasitic stages)—*Hypoderma bovis, H. lineatum*; lice—*Haematopinus eurysternus, Linognathus vituli, Solenopotes capillatus*; and mange mites—*Psoroptes bovis, Sarcoptes scabiei*.

In swine the injection is labeled for the treatment and control gastrointestinal roundworms (adults and 4th stage *Ascaris suum*, adults and 4th stage *Oesophagostomum dentatum, Oesophagostomum quadrispinolatum* adults, *Strongyloides ransomi* adults, and *Hydrostrongylus rubidus* adults), lungworms (*Stephanurus dentatus* adults), mange mites (adults and immature stages *Sarcoptes scabeii var. suis*), and sucking lice (adults and immature stages *Haematopinus suis*)

The manufacturer states the doramectin protects cattle against infection or reinfection with *Ostertagia ostertagi* for up to 21 days.

Doramectin topical (pour-on) is FDA-approved for use in cattle and has a similar spectrum of action against a variety of endo- and ectoparasites, including biting lice.

Injectable doramectin has been used in an extra-label manner orally or as a SC injection for treating a variety of nematode and arthropod parasites in companion animals, including generalized demodicosis in dogs and cats. No controlled, long-term studies were noted confirming its safety and efficacy in dogs, cats, or rabbits.

Pharmacology/Actions

The primary mode of action of avermectins like doramectin is to affect chloride ion channel activity in the nervous system of nematodes and arthropods. Doramectin binds to receptors that increase membrane permeability to chloride ions. This inhibits the electrical activity of nerve cells in nematodes and muscle cells in arthropods and causes paralysis and death of the parasites. Avermectins also enhance the release of gamma amino butyric acid (GABA) at presynaptic neurons. GABA acts as an inhibitory neurotransmitter and blocks the post-synaptic stimulation of the adjacent neuron in nematodes or the muscle fiber in arthropods. Avermectins are generally not toxic to mammals as they do not have glutamate-gated chloride channels and these compounds do not readily cross the blood-brain barrier where mammalian GABA receptors occur.

Pharmacokinetics

After subcutaneous injection, the time to peak plasma concentration in cattle is about 5 days. Bioavailability is, for practical purposes, equal with SC and IM injections in cattle.

Contraindications/Precautions/Warnings

The manufacturer warns to not use in other animal species as severe adverse reactions, including fatalities in dogs, may result.

If using in an extra-label manner in small animals, it is recommended to test all dogs for the MDR-1 (*ABCB*1) mutation before treating. If this not possible: 1) Use alternative treatments in untested dogs of breeds susceptible to MDR1-allele mutation (Collies, Australian Shepherds, Shelties, Long-haired Whippet, etc.) as they are at higher risk for toxicity; 2) Obtain informed consent from owner; 3) Use only in dogs tested negative for heartworm microfilaria or heartworm disease.

Adverse Effects

No listed adverse effects. Intramuscular injections may have a higher incidence of injection site blemishes at slaughter than do subcutaneous injections.

When used for demodicosis in dogs, adverse effects are uncommon but may include pupil dilation, lethargy, blindness, or coma.

Reproductive/Nursing Safety

In studies performed in breeding animals (bulls and cows in early and late pregnancy), at a dose of 3X recommended had no effect on breeding performance.

Overdosage/Acute Toxicity

In field trials, no toxic signs were seen in cattle given up to 25X the recommended dose. In breeding animals (bulls, and cows in early and late pregnancy), a dose 3X the recommended dose had no effect on breeding performance.

Doramectin toxicity may be alleviated with the use of intravenous lipid emulsions; for more information contact an animal poison center.

Drug Interactions

- None noted.

Doses

- **DOGS:**

  For adjunctive treatment of generalized demodicosis (extra-label): Based on an open, clinical study in 38 dogs: Initial dose of 300 micrograms/kg PO was given as a precaution because of the possibility of adverse reactions, then 600 micrograms/kg (0.6 mg/kg) PO once weekly. Re-examination was carried out every 2-4 weeks. Treatment with doramectin was terminated after remission of clinical signs and no evidence of demodectic mites. Each dog was confirmed as cured if there were no signs of relapse during follow-up over the next 12 months. 72% with generalized demodicosis and 89% with localized demodicosis showed remission after a mean of 11.4 weeks (generalized) and 7.8 weeks (localized). Caution is warranted when administering doramectin to dog breeds at the highest-risk breed for *ABCB*1 mutation. A double-blind control study will be needed to confirm the evidence from this study (Murayama et al. 2010). Another source suggests that alternatively to the above, giving 300 micrograms/kg PO twice a week may decrease adverse effects and that treatment should continue for 4 weeks past two consecutive negative skin scrapings 4-6 weeks apart (Koch et al. 2011). A review of published evidence for treatment of demodicosis in dogs concluded that based on the two studies published (at the time of the review) there is evidence that doramectin at a dose of 0.6 mg/kg PO or SC weekly may be used for the treatment of demodicosis (COE III) (Mueller et al. 2012).

  For sarcoptic mange (extra-label): 200–400 mcg/kg (0.2–0.3 mg/kg) SC once weekly for 3–4 treatments. (Koch et al. 2011)

- **CATS:**

  For feline follicular demodicosis (*D. cati*) (extra-label): 400 – 600 mcg/kg (0.4 – 0.6 mg/kg) SC once weekly for 4 weeks past two consecutive negative skin scrapings 4-6 weeks apart. (Koch et al. 2011)

  For notoedric mange (*Notoedris cati*) (extra-label): 200 – 300 mcg/kg (0.2 – 0.3 mg/kg) SC single dose or once weekly for 2-3 treatments. (Koch et al. 2011)

- **CATTLE:**

  For labeled indications (Injectable) (FDA-approved): 200 micrograms/kg (1 mL per 110 lb. body weight) SC or IM. Injections should be made using 16-18 gauge needles. Subcutaneous injections should be administered under the loose skin in front of or behind the shoulder. Intramuscular injections should be administered into the muscular region of the neck. Beef Quality Assurance guidelines recommend subcutaneous administration as the preferred route. (Label Directions; *Dectomax®*—Pfizer)

  For labeled indications (Pour-on) (FDA-approved): Topically at a dosage of 500 micrograms/kg (1 mL per 22 lb. body weight). Administer topically along the mid-line of the back in a narrow strip between the withers and tailhead. (Label Directions; *Dectomax® Pour-On*—Pfizer)

- **SWINE:**

  For labeled indications (FDA-approved): 300 micrograms/kg (1 mL per 75 lb. body weight) IM. Injections should be made using 16 g x 1.5 inch needles for sows and boars and 18 g x 1 inch needles for young animals. Use a tuberculin syringe and a 20 g x 1 inch needle for piglets. Intramuscular injections should be administered into the muscular region of the neck. See the label for recommended treatment program for sows, gilts, boars, feeder pigs, weaners, growers and finishers. (Label Directions; *Dectomax®*—Pfizer)

- **RABBITS:**

  For *P. cuniculi* infestations (extra-label): 200 micrograms/kg IM once. (Kanbur et al. 2008)

Monitoring

- Efficacy.

Client Information

- As an anti-parasite drug in cattle in and swine: Read and follow all labeled instructions and drug residue withdrawal times carefully.
- Should not be used in dog breeds ("white feet" *e.g.*, collies, shelties, etc.) untested for MDR-1 (ABCB-1) gene mutation.
- If using in small animals, have veterinarian or pharmacist draw up the correct dosage into syringe.

Chemistry/Synonyms

An avermectin antiparasitic compound, doramectin is isolated from fermentations from the soil organism *Streptomyces avermitilis*.

Doramectin may also be known as UK-67994, or *Dectomax®*.

Storage/Stability

The commercially available injectable solution is a colorless to pale yellow, sterile solution. The injectable solution should be stored below 86°F (30°C). The topical pour-on solution should be stored below 30°C (86°F) and protected from light.

Compatibility/Compounding Considerations

No specific information noted.

Dosage Forms/Regulatory Status

VETERINARY-LABELED PRODUCTS:

Doramectin Injectable Solution: 10 mg/mL in 100 mL, 250 mL,

and 500 mL multi-dose vials; *Dectomax®*; (OTC). FDA-approved for use in cattle and swine. When used at labeled doses: Slaughter withdrawal: cattle = 45 days, swine = 24 days. Do not use in female dairy cattle 20 months of age or older or in calves to be used for veal. A withdrawal period has not been established in preruminating calves.

Doramectin Pour-On Solution: 5 mg/mL in 250 mL, 1 L, 2.5 L and 5 L multi-dose containers; *Dectomax® Pour-On*; (OTC). FDA-approved for use in cattle. Slaughter withdrawal = 45 days. Not for use in female dairy cattle 20 months of age or older. A withdrawal period has not been established in preruminating calves. Do not use in calves to be used for veal.

HUMAN-LABELED PRODUCTS: NONE.

Revisions/References
Monograph revised/updated January 2014.

Kanbur, M., et al. (2008). The curative and antioxidative efficiency of doramectin and doramectin plus vitamin AD(3)E treatment on Psoroptes cuniculi infestation in rabbits. Research in Veterinary Science 85(2): 291-3.

Koch, S., et al. (2011). *Small Animal Dermatology Drug Handbook*, Wiley-Blackwell. Ames.

Mueller, R. S., et al. (2012). Treatment of demodicosis in dogs: 2011 clinical practice guidelines. Veterinary Dermatology 23(2): 86-+.

Murayama, N., et al. (2010). Efficacy of weekly oral doramectin treatment in canine demodicosis. Veterinary Record 167(2): 63-4.

Doxapram HCl

(docks-a-pram)   Dopram-V®

CNS/Respiratory Stimulant

Prescriber Highlights

▶ CNS stimulant usually used to stimulate respirations in newborns or after anesthesia; also used for assessment of laryngeal function in small animals; use in small animal neonates is controversial.

▶ Not a substitute for aggressive artificial (mechanical) respiratory support when required.

▶ Possible contraindications: Receiving mechanical ventilation, hypersensitivity, seizure disorders, head trauma/CVA, uncompensated heart failure, severe hypertension, respiratory failure secondary to neuromuscular disorders, airway obstruction, pulmonary embolism, pneumothorax, acute asthma, dyspnea, or whenever hypoxia is not associated with hypercapnia.

▶ Caution: History of asthma, arrhythmias, or tachycardias. Use extreme caution in patients with cerebral edema or increased CSF pressure, pheochromocytoma, or hyperthyroidism.

▶ Avoid IV extravasation or using a single injection site for a prolonged period.

▶ Adverse Effects: Hypertension, arrhythmias, seizures, & hyperventilation leading to respiratory alkalosis.

Uses/Indications

The manufacturer of *Dopram®-V* lists the following indications: For dogs, cats, and horses: To stimulate respiration during and after general anesthesia and/or to speed awakening and reflexes after anesthesia. For neonatal dogs and cats: stimulate respirations following dystocia or cesarean section.

It is reported that in small animals doxapram is most likely to be beneficial in increasing respiratory efforts in neonates with low-frequency, gasping, erratic pattern of breathing after receiving oxygen therapy (Traas 2009).

Doxapram has been used for treatment of CNS depression in food animals (not FDA-approved) and has been suggested as a treatment of respiratory depression in small animals caused by reactions to radiopaque contrast media or for barbiturate overdosage (see precautions below).

The use of doxapram to initiate and stimulate respirations in newborns is controversial, as the drug has been shown in experimental animals to increase myocardial oxygen demand and reduce cerebral blood flow. Many no longer recommend its use for this purpose and some state that the drug is contraindicated in situations of respiratory arrest.

Doxapram has been shown to be useful to offset suppression of general anesthetic agents when laryngeal function is being assessed.

Pharmacology/Actions

Doxapram is a general CNS stimulant, with all levels of the CNS affected. The effects of respiratory stimulation are a result of direct stimulation of the medullary respiratory centers and, possibly, through the reflex activation of carotid and aortic chemoreceptors. Transient increases in respiratory rate and volume occur, but increases in arterial oxygenation usually do not ensue. This is because doxapram usually increases the work associated with respirations with resultant increased oxygen consumption and carbon dioxide production.

Pharmacokinetics

Little published pharmacokinetic data appears for domestic animals. Onset of effect in humans and animals after IV injection usually occurs within 2 minutes. The drug is well distributed into tissues. In dogs, doxapram is rapidly metabolized and most is excreted as metabolites in the urine within 24-48 hours after administration. Small quantities of metabolites may be excreted up to 120 hours after dosing.

Contraindications/Precautions/Warnings

Doxapram should not be used as a substitute for aggressive artificial (mechanical) respiratory support in instances of severe respiratory depression. Use to stimulate respiration in newborns is controversial and some state it is contraindicated in apnea.

In calves, doxapram has been reported as contraindicated in premature calves or other patients with clinical signs indicative of lung immaturity as effects are only minimal and use could lead to increased pulmonary blood pressure with fetal circulation persisting resulting from a right-to-left shunt via the patent ductus and foramen ovale (Bleul et al. 2010).

Contraindications from the human literature include: seizure disorders, head trauma, uncompensated heart failure, severe hypertension, cardiovascular accidents, respiratory failure secondary to neuromuscular disorders, airway obstruction, pulmonary embolism, pneumothorax, acute asthma, dyspnea, or whenever hypoxia is not associated with hypercapnia. Doxapram should be used with caution in patients with a history of asthma, arrhythmias, or tachycardias. It should be used with extreme caution in patients with cerebral edema or increased CSF pressure, pheochromocytoma or hyperthyroidism. Patients with a history of hypersensitivity to the drug or that are receiving mechanical ventilation should not receive doxapram. The above contraindications/precautions are not listed in the veterinary product literature provided by the manufacturer.

Avoid the use of a single injection site for a prolonged period of time or extravasation when administering intravenously.

Repeated IV doses in neonates should be done with caution as the product contains benzyl alcohol.

Adverse Effects

Hypertension, arrhythmias, seizures, and hyperventilation leading to respiratory alkalosis have been reported. These effects appear most probable with repeated or high doses. The drug reportedly has a narrow margin of safety when used in humans.

Doxapram has been shown in experimental animals to increase myocardial oxygen demand and reduce cerebral blood flow.

Reproductive/Nursing Safety

Safety of doxapram has not been established in pregnant animals. The potential risks versus benefits should be weighed before using. In humans, the FDA categorizes this drug as category *B* for use during pregnancy (*Animal studies have not yet demonstrated risk to the fetus, but there are no adequate studies in pregnant women; or animal studies have shown an adverse effect, but adequate studies in pregnant women have not demonstrated a risk to the fetus in the first trimester of pregnancy, and there is no evidence of risk in later trimesters.*)

It is not known whether this drug is excreted in milk.

Overdosage/Acute Toxicity

Reported LD_{50} for IV administration in neonatal dogs and cats is approximately 75 mg/kg. Clinical signs of overdosage include: respiratory alkalosis, hypertension, skeletal muscle hyperactivity, tachycardia, and generalized CNS excitation including seizures. Treatment is supportive. Drugs such as short acting IV barbiturates may be used to help decrease CNS hyperactivity. Oxygen therapy may be necessary.

Drug Interactions

The following drug interactions have either been reported or are theoretical in humans or animals receiving doxapram and may be of significance in veterinary patients. Unless otherwise noted, use together is not necessarily contraindicated, but weigh the potential risks and perform additional monitoring when appropriate.

- **ANESTHETICS, GENERAL:** Doxapram may increase epinephrine release; therefore, use should be delayed for approximately 10 minutes after discontinuation of anesthetic agents (*e.g.,* **halothane, enflurane**) that have been demonstrated to sensitize the myocardium to catecholamines.
- **MUSCLE RELAXANTS:** Doxapram may mask the effects of muscle relaxant drugs.
- **SYMPATHOMIMETIC AGENTS:** Additive pressor effects may occur with sympathomimetic agents.

Doses

- **DOGS/CATS:**

  For labeled indications (FDA-approved): 1.1 mg/kg (for gas anesthesia) or 5.5 – 11 mg/kg (for barbiturate anesthesia) IV; adjust dosage for depth of anesthesia, respiratory volume and rate. Dosage may be repeated in 15-20 minutes if necessary. **To initiate or stimulate respirations in neonates** after caesarian section or dystocia: May be administered either SC, sublingually, or via the umbilical vein in doses of 1-5 drops (1 – 5 mg) depending on size of neonate and degree of respiratory crisis. (Package Insert; *Dopram*®-*V*)

  To stimulate respiratory function in neonates (extra-label): 0.1 mL (2 mg) IV (IM or SL also possible); most likely to be beneficial to increase efforts in neonates with low-frequency, gasping, erratic pattern of breathing after receiving oxygen therapy. (Traas 2009)

  To assess laryngeal function (extra-label): 2.2 mg/kg IV to stimulate respiration and increase intrinsic laryngeal motion. Onset of effect occurs within 15-30 seconds and persists for approximately 2 minutes. Anesthetic depth may lighten substantially. Prepare for immediate intubation should airway obstruction or laryngeal paralysis occur. (McKiernan 2007)

  To reduce the sedation associated with acepromazine (extra-label; from a study done in 10 dogs): When given 30 minutes after acepromazine (0.05 mg/kg IM), doxapram at 1.25 mg/kg IV significantly reduced acepromazine sedation without causing panting. (Zapata et al. 2013)

- **FERRETS/RABBITS/RODENTS/SMALL MAMMALS:**

  For the emergency treatment of respiratory depression (extra-label): Suggested anecdotal dosages range from 1 – 10 mg/kg. Suggested routes of administration include IV, SL, IO, IP, SC and intratracheally.

- **BIRDS:**

  For the emergency treatment of respiratory depression (extra-label): 5 – 10 mg/kg IM or IV (Harris 2003). Another source suggests 5 – 20 mg/kg IM, IV, IO or IT (Korbel 2012).

- **REPTILES:**

  To stimulate respiration after general anesthesia (extra-label): 5 mg/kg IV. (Wilson 2002)

- **CATTLE & SWINE:**

  For primary apnea in asphyxic calves when intubation and mechanical ventilation are not feasible (extra-label): 2 mg/kg IV. Contraindicated in premature calves or other patients with clinical signs indicative of lung immaturity. (Bleul et al. 2010), (Constable 2006)

- **HORSES:** (NOTE: ARCI UCGFS CLASS 2 DRUG)

  For labeled indications (FDA-approved): 0.44 mg/kg (for halothane, methoxyflurane anesthesia) or 0.55 mg/kg (for chloral hydrate ± magnesium sulfate anesthesia) IV; adjust dosage for depth of anesthesia, respiratory volume and rate. Dosage may be repeated in 15-20 minutes if necessary. (Package Insert; *Dopram*®-*V*)

  For adjunctive treatment to stimulate respirations in foals with sepsis or hypoxic-ischemic encephalopathy (extra-label): 0.02 – 0.05 mg/kg/hour IV CRI; foals with significant hypercapnia and hypoxia despite O_2 treatment require positive pressure ventilation. (Giguere et al. 2008), (McKenzie 2009)

Monitoring

- Respiratory rate.
- Cardiac rate and rhythm.
- Blood gases if available and indicated.
- CNS level of excitation; reflexes.
- Blood pressure if indicated.

Client Information

- This agent should be used in an inpatient setting or with direct professional supervision.

Chemistry/Synonyms

Doxapram HCl is a white to off-white, odorless, crystalline powder that is stable in light and air. It is soluble in water, sparingly soluble in alcohol and practically insoluble in ether. Injectable products have a pH from 3.5-5. Benzyl alcohol or chlorobutanol is added as a preservative agent in the commercially available injections.

Doxapram HCl may also be known as: AHR-619, doxaprami hydrochloridum, *Docatone*®, *Dopram*®, *Doxapril*®, or *Respiram*®.

Storage/Stability

Store at room temperature and avoid freezing solution.

Compatibility/Compounding Considerations

Doxapram is physically **compatible** with D5W or normal saline. Do not mix with alkaline solutions (*e.g.,* thiopental, aminophylline, sodium bicarbonate).

Dosage Forms/Regulatory Status

VETERINARY-LABELED PRODUCTS:

Doxapram HCl for Injection: 20 mg/mL; 20 mL multi-dose vial; *Dopram-V*®, *Respiram*®; (Rx). FDA-approved for use in dogs, cats and horses.

The ARCI (Racing Commissioners International) has designated this drug as a class 2 substance. See the appendix for more information.

HUMAN-LABELED PRODUCTS:

Doxapram HCl for Injection: 20 mg/mL in 20 mL multi-dose vials; *Dopram*®, generic; (Rx)

Revisions/References

Monograph revised/updated January 2014.

Bleul, U., et al. (2010). Respiratory and cardiovascular effects of doxapram and theophylline for the treatment of asphyxia in neonatal calves. Theriogenology 73(5): 612-9.

Constable, P. (2006). Resuscitation of calves after dystocia. Proceedings: ACVIM. accessed via Veterinary Information Network; vin.com

Giguere, S., et al. (2008). Retrospective comparison of caffeine and doxapram for the treatment of hypercapnia in foals with hypoxic-ischemic encephalopathy. Journal of Veterinary Internal Medicine 22(2): 401-5.

Harris, D. (2003). Emergency management of acute illness and trauma in avian patients. Proceedings: Atlantic Coast Veterinary Conference. accessed via Veterinary Information Network; vin.com

Korbel, R. (2012). Avian Anaesthesia and Critical Care. WSAVA/FECCAVA/BSAVA World Congress. accessed via Veterinary Information Network; vin.com

McKenzie, E. (2009). Management of the Septic Foal. Proceedings: WVC. accessed via Veterinary Information Network; vin.com

McKiernan, B. (2007). Laryngeal function and doxapram HCl (Dopram). Proceedings: Veterinary Information Network MEDFAQ. accessed via Veterinary Information Network; vin.com

Traas, A. (2009). Pediatric Emergencies. Peroceedings: IVECCS. accessed via Veterinary Information Network; vin.com

Wilson, H. (2002). Reptile anesthesia and surgery. Proceedings: Atlantic Coast Veterinary Conference. accessed via Veterinary Information Network; vin.com

Zapata, M. & E. Hofmeister (2013). Refinement of the dose of doxapram to counteract the sedative effects of acepromazine in dogs. J Small Anim Pract 54(8): 405-8.

Doxepin HCl

(dox-e-pin)   Sinequan®

Trycyclic Antidepressant/Antihistamine

Prescriber Highlights

▶ Tricyclic antidepressant used primarily in small animals for adjunctive therapy of psychogenic dermatoses, particularly those that have an anxiety component; also has antihistaminic (H-1) properties.

▶ Contraindications: Prior sensitivity to tricyclics; concomitant use with MAOIs (selegiline?); probably contraindicated in dogs with urinary retention or glaucoma.

▶ Most likely adverse effects: Hyperexcitability, GI distress, or lethargy; ventricular arrhythmias after overdoses possible.

Uses/Indications

The primary use for doxepin in veterinary medicine is the adjunctive therapy of psychogenic dermatoses, particularly those that have an anxiety component. Its efficacy as an antihistamine for atopic dermatoses is in question.

Pharmacology/Actions

Doxepin is a tricyclic agent that has antihistaminic, anticholinergic, and alpha1-adrenergic blocking activity. In the CNS, doxepin inhibits the reuptake of norepinephrine and serotonin (5-HT) by the presynaptic neuronal membrane, thereby increasing their synaptic concentrations. Doxepin is considered a moderate inhibitor of norepinephrine and weak inhibitor of serotonin.

Pharmacokinetics

Doxepin appears to be well absorbed after oral administration. The drug is extensively metabolized in the liver.

Contraindications/Precautions/Warnings

These agents are contraindicated if prior sensitivity has been noted with any other tricyclic. Concomitant use with monoamine oxidase inhibitors is generally contraindicated. Doxepin is probably contraindicated in dogs with urinary retention or glaucoma.

Adverse Effects

While doxepin has less potential for cardiac adverse effects than many other tricyclics, it can cause ventricular arrhythmias, particularly after overdoses. In dogs, it may also cause hyperexcitability, GI distress, or lethargy. However, potential adverse effects can run the entire gamut of systems. Refer to other human drug references for additional information.

Reproductive/Nursing Safety

Rodent studies have demonstrated no teratogenic effects, but safety during pregnancy has not been established. In humans, the FDA categorizes this drug as category C for use during pregnancy (*Animal studies have shown an adverse effect on the fetus, but there are no adequate studies in humans; or there are no animal reproduction studies and no adequate studies in humans.*)

Doxepin and its N-demethylated active metabolite are distributed into milk. One case report of sedation and respiratory depression in a human infant has been reported. Exercise caution when using in a nursing patient.

Overdosage/Acute Toxicity

Overdosage with tricyclics can be life-threatening (arrhythmias, cardiorespiratory collapse). Because the toxicities and therapies for treatment are complicated and controversial, it is recommended to contact an animal poison control center for further information in any potential overdose situation. Doxepin toxicity may be amenable to intravenous lipid emulsion (ILE) treatment.

Drug Interactions

The following drug interactions have either been reported or are theoretical in humans or animals receiving doxepin and may be of significance in veterinary patients. Unless otherwise noted, use together is not necessarily contraindicated, but weigh the potential risks and perform additional monitoring when appropriate.

- **ANTICHOLINERGIC AGENTS:** Because of additive effects, use with doxepin cautiously.
- **CIMETIDINE:** May inhibit tricyclic antidepressant metabolism and increase the risk of toxicity.
- **CNS DEPRESSANTS:** Because of additive effects, use with doxepin cautiously.
- **MEPERIDINE, PENTAZOCINE, DEXTROMETHORPHAN:** Increased risk for serotonin syndrome.
- **MONOAMINE OXIDASE INHIBITORS** (including **amitraz**, and possibly **selegiline**): Concomitant use (within 14 days) of tricyclics with monoamine oxidase inhibitors is generally contraindicated (serotonin syndrome).
- **QUINIDINE:** Increased risk for QTc interval prolongation and tricyclic adverse effects.
- **SSRIs** (*e.g.,* **fluoxetine, paroxetine, sertraline,** etc.): Increased risk for serotonin syndrome.
- **SYMPATHOMIMETIC AGENTS:** Use in combination with tricyclic agents may increase the risk of cardiac effects (arrhythmias, hypertension, hyperpyrexia).

Laboratory Considerations

- Tricyclics can widen QRS complexes, prolong PR intervals and invert or flatten T-waves on ECG.
- Tricyclics may alter (increase or decrease) **blood glucose** levels.
- It is unknown how long to delay **intradermal allergy skin testing** after stopping therapy. One source recommends waiting for at least two weeks (Koch et al. 2011).

Doses

- **DOGS:**

   For treatment of psychogenic dermatoses (extra-label): Little evidence to support any dosage recommendation, but most recommend dosages of 3 – 5 mg/kg PO q12h, although some put limits on a the maximum dose per dog (50 mg and 150 mg per dog have been noted). Generally start at the low end of the dosing range and increase in 1 mg/kg q12h increments every two weeks to the maximum. If after 4 weeks no effect, wean off in 1 mg/kg q12h increments every two weeks to the starting dosage before discontinuing.

For antihistaminic effects in treatment of atopy (extra-label): Little evidence to support any dosage recommendation, but most recommend dosages initial dosages of 0.5 – 1 mg/kg PO q12h and then titrating upwards to maximum as for psychogenic dermatoses (above).

- **CATS:**

  For treatment of psychogenic dermatoses (extra-label): Little evidence to support any dosage recommendation, but most recommend initial dosages of 0.5 mg/kg PO q12-24h. May titrate slowly upwards if cat tolerates, but many will become profoundly sedated and ataxic at higher dosages.

- **HORSES:**

  As an antihistamine (extra-label): 0.5 – 0.75 mg/kg PO q12h.

- **BIRDS:**

  For treatment of anxiety, pruritus caused feather plucking in psittacines (extra-label): 0.5 – 2 mg/kg PO q12h.

Monitoring

- Efficacy.
- Adverse effects.

Client Information

- When used as an antihistamine it should be used on a regular, ongoing basis. It works better if used before exposure to an allergen. May take several days to weeks to determine if the drug is effective.
- May be given with or without food. If your animal vomits or acts sick after getting it on an empty stomach, give with food or small treat to see if this helps. If vomiting continues, contact your veterinarian.
- Most common side effects are: drowsiness/sleepiness, dry mouth and constipation; be sure your animal has access to water.
- Rare side effects that can be serious (contact veterinarian immediately): abnormal bleeding or fever, seizures, very fast or irregular heartbeat.
- Overdoses (in animals and in humans) can be very serious; keep out of the reach of animals and children.
- If your animal wore a flea collar in the past two weeks, let your veterinarian know. Do not use a flea collar on your animal during the time it's getting this drug without first talking to your veterinarian.

Chemistry/Synonyms

A dibenzoxazepine derivative tricyclic antidepressant, doxepin HCl occurs as a white powder that is freely soluble in alcohol.

Doxepin may also be known as: doxepini hydrochloridum, NSC-108160, P-3693A, *Adapin®, Anten®, Aponal®, Deptran®, Desidoxepin®, Doneurin®, Doxal®, Doxepia®, Gilex®, Mareen®, Quitaxon®, Sinequan®, Triadapin®, Xepin®,* and *Zonalon®.*

Compatibility/Compounding Considerations

No specific information noted.

Storage/Stability

Store hydroxyzine products protected from direct sunlight in tight, light-resistant containers at room temperature.

Dosage Forms/Regulatory Status

VETERINARY-LABELED PRODUCTS: NONE.

The ARCI (Racing Commissioners International) has designated this drug as a class 2 substance. See the appendix for more information.

HUMAN-LABELED PRODUCTS:

Doxepin Capsules: 10 mg, 25 mg, 50 mg, 75 mg, 100 mg & 150 mg; generic; (Rx)

Doxepin Tablets: 3 mg, & 6 mg; *Silenor®*; (Rx)

Doxepin Oral Concentrate: 10 mg/mL in 120 mL; generic; (Rx)

Revisions/References

Monograph revised/updated January 2014.

Koch, S., et al. (2011). *Small Animal Dermatology Drug Handbook*, Wiley-Blackwell. Ames.

Doxorubicin HCl

(dox-oh-**roo**-bi-sin)   Adriamycin®, Doxil®

Antineoplastic

Prescriber Highlights

▶ Injectable antibiotic antineoplastic widely used alone or in combination protocols for small animals.

▶ Relatively contraindicated in patients with myelosuppression, impaired cardiac function, or that have reached the total cumulative dose level of doxorubicin &/or daunorubicin.

▶ Caution: Patients with hyperuricemia/hyperuricuria, or impaired hepatic function (dosage adjustments necessary).

▶ Breeds predisposed to developing cardiomyopathy (Doberman pinchers, Great Danes, Rottweilers, Boxers); monitor carefully.

▶ Handle very carefully.

▶ Teratogenic & embryotoxic.

▶ Adverse Effects include bone marrow suppression, cardiac toxicity, nephrotoxicity (esp. cats), alopecia, gastroenteritis (vomiting, diarrhea), & stomatitis.

▶ Immediate-hypersensitivity reported (primarily in dogs); potentially brand specific.

▶ Extravasation injuries can be serious.

Uses/Indications

Doxorubicin is perhaps the most widely used antineoplastic agent at present in small animal medicine. It may be useful in the treatment of a variety of lymphomas, carcinomas, leukemias, and sarcomas in both the dog and cat, either alone or in combination protocols.

Pharmacology/Actions

Although possessing antimicrobial properties, doxorubicin's cytotoxic effects preclude its use as an anti-infective agent. The drug causes inhibition of DNA synthesis, DNA-dependent RNA synthesis and protein synthesis, but the precise mechanisms for these effects are not well understood. The drug acts throughout the cell cycle and also possesses some immunosuppressant activity.

Doxorubicin is most cytotoxic to cardiac cells, followed by melanoma, sarcoma cells, and normal muscle and skin fibroblasts. Other rapidly proliferating "normal" cells, (such as bone marrow, hair follicles, GI mucosa), may also be affected by the drug.

Pharmacokinetics

Doxorubicin must be administered IV as it is not absorbed from the GI tract and is extremely irritating to tissues if administered SC or IM. After IV injection, the drug is rapidly and widely distributed, but does not appreciably enter the CSF. It is highly bound to tissue and plasma proteins, probably crosses the placenta and is distributed into milk.

Via aldo-keto reductase, doxorubicin is extensively metabolized by the liver and other tissues primarily to doxorubicinol (active) and other inactive metabolites. Doxorubicin and metabolites are excreted mostly in bile and feces. Only about 5% of the drug is excreted in the urine within 5 days of dosing. Doxorubicin is eliminated in a triphasic manner. During the first phase (half-life $\approx$ 0.6 hours) doxorubicin is rapidly metabolized, via the "first pass" effect followed by a second phase (half-life $\approx$ 3.3 hours). The third phase has a much slower elimination half-life (17 hours for doxorubicin; 32 hours for metabolites), presumably due to the slow release of the drug from tissue proteins.

Contraindications/Precautions/Warnings

Doxorubicin is contraindicated or relatively contraindicated (measure risk vs. benefit) in patients with myelosuppression, impaired cardiac function, or that have reached the total cumulative dose level of doxorubicin and/or daunorubicin. It is also contraindicated in cats with preexisting renal insufficiency. It should be used with caution in patients with hyperuricemia/hyperuricuria, or impaired hepatic function. Dosage adjustments are necessary in patients with hepatic impairment.

Doxorubicin should be administered IV slowly, over at least 10 minutes in a free flowing line. Extreme care must be taken to avoid perivascular infusion (extravasation).

Breeds predisposed to developing cardiomyopathy (Doberman pinchers, Great Danes, Rottweilers, Boxers, etc.) should be monitored carefully while receiving doxorubicin therapy.

Doxorubicin is actively transported by the p-glycoprotein pump and certain breeds susceptible to *ABCB1* (MDR1)-allele mutation (Collies, Australian Shepherds, Shelties, Long-haired Whippet, etc.) may be at higher risk for toxicity. Bone marrow suppression (decreased blood cell counts, particularly neutrophils) and GI toxicity (anorexia, vomiting, diarrhea) are more likely to occur at normal doses in dogs with the *ABCB1* mutation. To reduce the likelihood of severe toxicity in these dogs (mutant/normal or mutant/mutant), the Veterinary Clinical Pharmacology Laboratory at Washington State University recommends reducing the dose by 25-30% and carefully monitoring these patients (WSU-VetClinPharm-Lab 2009).

Because doxorubicin can be very irritating to skin, gloves should be worn when administering or preparing the drug. Ideally, doxorubicin injection should be prepared in a biological safety cabinet. Should accidental skin or mucous membrane contact occur, wash the area immediately using soap and copious amounts of water.

Do not confuse DOXOrubicin with DAUNOrubicin or EPIrubicin.

Adverse Effects

Doxorubicin may cause several adverse effects including bone marrow suppression, cardiac toxicity, alopecia, gastroenteritis (vomiting, diarrhea), and stomatitis. After administration, nausea and vomiting most commonly occur within the first 72-hours; diarrhea can occur in approximately 4-5 days; myelosuppression nadirs are generally 7-10 days after treatment.

An immediate histamine-mediated hypersensitivity reaction may be seen (particularly in dogs) characterized by urticaria, facial swelling, vomiting, arrhythmias (see below), and/or hypotension. The rate of infusion can have a direct impact on this effect; generally IV infusions should be administered no faster than over 10-20 minutes. Pretreatment with a histamine$_1$ blocker such as diphenhydramine (IV prior to treatment at 10 mg for dogs up to 9 kg; 20 mg for dogs 9-27 kg; and 30 mg for dogs over 27 kg) or an intravenous glucocorticoid may also reduce or eliminate histamine-me-

diated effects. There is some evidence to suggest that a given brand of doxorubicin may be more allergenic than another. Patients that have developed hypersensitive reactions to one brand may not react if switched to another.

Cardiac toxicity of doxorubicin falls into two categories, acute and cumulative. Acute cardiac toxicity may occur during IV administration or several hours after receiving the drug, and is manifested by cardiac arrest preceded by ECG changes (T-wave flattening, S-T depression, voltage reduction, arrhythmias). Rarely, an acute hypertensive crisis has been noted after infusion. Acute cardiac toxicity does not preclude further use of the drug but additional treatment should be delayed. The administration of diphenhydramine and/or glucocorticoids before doxorubicin administration may prevent these effects.

Anthracycline-iron complex free radicals are thought the primary cause of anthracycline-induced cardiomyopathy and extravasation injury. Cumulative cardiotoxicity can be extremely serious and necessitates halting any further therapy. Diffuse cardiomyopathy with severe congestive heart failure refractory to traditional therapies is generally noted. It is believed the risk for cardiac toxicity is greatly increased in dogs when the cumulative dose exceeds 240 mg/m^2. However it may be seen at cumulative doses as low as 90 mg/m^2, particularly in dog breeds predisposed to dilative cardiomyopathy. Therefore in dogs, it is not recommended to exceed 240 mg/m^2 total cumulative dose.

In cats, doxorubicin is a potential nephrotoxin and feline patients should have their renal function monitored both before and during therapy. It is unknown what the incidence of cardiotoxicity or the dosage ceiling for doxorubicin is in cats. Most clinicians believe that 180-240 mg/m^2 should be used as the upper limit cumulative dose.

Extravasation injuries secondary to perivascular administration of doxorubicin can be quite serious, with severe tissue ulceration and necrosis possible. Prevention of extravasation should be a priority and animals frequently checked during the infusion. Should extravasation occur, it is suggested to treat as per recommendations for human patients. There are currently two treatments recommended for doxorubicin extravasation injuries. Both have been shown to be effective but no comparative trials have been published. 1) Apply dimethyl sulfoxide (DMSO) 99% by saturating a gauze pad and painting on an area twice the size of the extravasation. Allow the site to air dry and repeat the application every 6 hours for 14 days. Do not cover the area with dressing. 2) Dexrazoxane is FDA-approved for the treatment of extravasation resulting from anthracycline IV therapy, refer to the dexrazoxane monograph for more information. Additionally, ice compresses applied to the affected area for 15 minutes every 6 hours for 48 hours may be useful.

Reproductive/Nursing Safety

Doxorubicin is teratogenic and embryotoxic in laboratory animals. It is unknown if it affects male fertility. In humans, the FDA categorizes this drug as category *D* for use during pregnancy (*There is evidence of human fetal risk, but the potential benefits from the use of the drug in pregnant women may be acceptable despite its potential risks.*). In a separate system evaluating the safety of drugs in canine and feline pregnancy (Papich 1989), this drug is categorized as class: *C* (*These drugs may have potential risks. Studies in people or laboratory animals have uncovered risks, and these drugs should be used cautiously as a last resort when the benefit of therapy clearly outweighs the risks.*)

Doxorubicin is excreted in milk in concentrations that may exceed those found in plasma. Because of risks to nursing offspring, consider using milk replacer if the dam is receiving doxorubicin.

Overdosage/Acute Toxicity

Acute overdoses may manifest by exacerbations of the adverse effects outlined above. A lethal dose for dogs has been reported as 72 mg/m^2 (O'Keefe and Harris 1990). Supportive and symptomatic therapy is suggested should an overdose occur. Dexrazoxane may be useful to help prevent cardiac toxicity.

Drug Interactions

The following drug interactions have either been reported or are theoretical in humans or animals receiving doxorubicin and may be of significance in veterinary patients. Unless otherwise noted, use together is not necessarily contraindicated, but weigh the potential risks and perform additional monitoring when appropriate.

- **ANTINEOPLASTIC AGENTS (other):** May potentiate the toxic effects of doxorubicin.
- **CALCIUM-CHANNEL BLOCKERS:** Potentially could increase risk for cardiotoxicity associated with doxorubicin.
- **CISPLATIN:** Increased risk of toxicity for both agents; carefully weigh risks versus benefits.
- **CYCLOPHOSPHAMIDE:** May increase doxorubicin blood levels (AUC) and prolong hematologic toxicity; coma and seizures have been reported in human patients. A study in dogs where one of the treatment protocols combined doxorubicin and cyclophosphamide, did not find a significant difference in the prevalence of toxicity (Lori et al. 2010).
- **CYCLOSPORINE:** Cyclosporine can increase doxorubicin and doxorubicinol (active metabolite) levels. Avoid use together.
- **GLUCOSAMINE:** May reduce doxorubicin effectiveness; use together not recommended in humans.
- **KETOCONAZOLE:** Can increase doxorubicin and doxorubicinol (active metabolite) levels and lead to toxicity. Avoid use together.
- **PHENYTOIN:** Doxorubicin may decrease phenytoin levels.
- **PHENOBARBITAL:** May increase elimination and reduce blood levels of doxorubicin.
- **SPINOSAD:** Can increase doxorubicin and doxorubicinol (active metabolite) levels and lead to toxicity. Avoid use together.
- **STREPTOZOCIN:** May inhibit doxorubicin metabolism.
- **VACCINES.** Live or live-attenuated vaccines may result in active infections in immunocompromised patients.
- **VERAPAMIL:** May increase doxorubicin levels.
- **WARFARIN:** Increased risk for bleeding.
- **ZIDOVUDINE:** Increased risk for neutropenia.

Laboratory Considerations

- Doxorubicin may significantly increase both blood and urine concentrations of **uric acid.**
- Handling of blood samples should pose no health hazard after 7 days (Knobloch, Mohring, Eberle, Nolte, et al. 2010).

Doses

NOTE: Because of the potential toxicity of this drug to patients, veterinary personnel and clients, and since chemotherapy indications, treatment protocols, monitoring and safety guidelines often change, the following dosages should be used only as a general guide. Consultation with a veterinary oncologist and referral to current veterinary oncology references [*e.g.*, (Withrow et al. 2012); (Dobson et al. 2011); (Henry et al. 2009); (North et al. 2009); (Argyle et al. 2008)] are strongly recommended.

- **DOGS:**
  Depending on the protocol used, doxorubicin is usually dosed at 30 mg/m^2 (**NOT** mg/kg) IV every 2-3 weeks. Maximum cumulative dose = 240 mg/m^2.

- **CATS:**
  Depending on the protocol used, doxorubicin is usually dosed at 20 – 30 mg/m^2 (**NOT** mg/kg) IV every 2-4 weeks. Maximum cumulative dose is usually 240 mg/m^2.

- **FERRETS:**
  Depending on the protocol used, doxorubicin is usually dosed at 30 mg/m^2 (**NOT** mg/kg) IV every 3 weeks.

Monitoring

- Efficacy.
- Toxicity:
  a) CBC with platelets. Neutrophil counts of <3000/mcL (some say <2000/mcL) generally require delay in dosing.
  b) Dogs with pre-existing heart disease should be monitored with regular ECG's (insensitive to early toxic changes caused doxorubicin) and/or echocardiogram.
  c) Evaluate hepatic function prior to therapy.
  d) Urinalyses and serum creatinine/BUN in cats.

Client Information

- Doxorubicin is a chemotherapy (cancer) drug. The drug and its byproducts can be hazardous to other animals and people that come in contact with it. After treatment, doxorubicin drug residues may be found in treated dog's urine up to 21 days and in feces for several days. (Knobloch, Mohring, Eberle and Nolte 2010). On the day your animal gets the drug and then for a few days afterward, all bodily waste (urine, feces, litter), blood, or vomit should only be handled while wearing disposable gloves. Seal the waste in a plastic bag and then place both the bag and gloves in with the regular trash.
- GI toxicity (*e.g.,* vomiting, lack of appetite, diarrhea, etc.): Doxorubicin can cause severe vomiting after it is given; veterinarians often will prescribe medication to help lessen this. Mild loss of appetite (eating less) and occasional vomiting 2-5 days after a dose are not unusual. If you see severe vomiting or bloody diarrhea, call your veterinarian immediately.
- Bone marrow suppression is also a problem that will occur about 10-14 days after doxorubicin is given, so watch your pet for signs of this (muscle weakness, fever, bruising and bleeding). If you see any of these, you should contact your veterinarian immediately.
- Although it is unknown how much drug is found in the saliva of treated animals, do not allow treated animals to lick human skin while receiving chemotherapy treatment.

Chemistry/Synonyms

An anthracycline glycoside antibiotic antineoplastic, doxorubicin HCl occurs as a lyophilized, red-orange powder that is freely soluble in water, slightly soluble in normal saline, and very slightly soluble in alcohol. The commercially available powder for injection also contains lactose and methylparaben to aid dissolution. After reconstituting, the solution has a pH from 3.8-6.5. The commercially available solution for injection has a pH of approximately 3.

Doxorubicin HCl may also be known as: cloridrato de doxorrubicina, doxorubicin hydrochloride liposome, doxorubicini hydrochloridum, liposomal doxorubicin hydrochloride, NSC-123127, *Adriamycin RDF*®, *Adriblastin*®, *Adriblastina*®, *Adriblastine*®, *Adrim*®, *Adrimedac*®, *Biorrub*®, *Caelyx*®, *DOXO-cell*®, *Doxolem*®, *Doxorbin*®, *Doxorubin*®, *Doxotec*®, *Doxtie*®, *Farmiblastina*®, *Fauldoxo*®, *Flavicina*®, *Ifadox*®, *Myocet*®, *Neoxan*®, *Ranxas*®, *Ribodoxo-L*®, and *Rubex*®.

Storage/Stability

Lyophilized powder for injection should be stored away from direct sunlight in a dry place. After reconstituting with sodium chloride 0.9%, the single-use lyophilized powder product is reportedly stable for 24 hours at room temperature and 48 hours when refrigerated. The manufacturer recommends protecting from sunlight, not freezing the product and discarding any unused portion. However, one study found that powder reconstituted with sterile water to a concentration of 2 mg/mL lost only about 1.5% of its potency per month over 6 months when stored in the refrigerator. When frozen at -20°C, no potency loss after 30 days was detected and sterility was maintained by filtering the drug through a 0.22-micron filter before injection.

The commercially available solution for injection is stable for 18 months when stored in the refrigerator (2-8°C) and protected from light.

The manufacturer states that after reconstitution, the multi-dose vials may be stored for up to 7 days at room temperature in normal room light, and for up to 15 days in the refrigerator.

Compatibility/Compounding Considerations

Doxorubicin HCl is reportedly physically **compatible** with the following intravenous solutions and drugs: dextrose 3.3% in sodium chloride 3%, D5W, *Normosol® R* (pH 7.4), lactated Ringer's injection, and sodium chloride 0.9%. In syringes with: bleomycin sulfate, cisplatin, cyclophosphamide, droperidol, fluorouracil, leucovorin calcium, methotrexate sodium, metoclopramide HCl, mitomycin, and vincristine sulfate. The drug is physically **compatible during Y-site injection** with bleomycin sulfate, cisplatin, cyclophosphamide, droperidol, fluorouracil, leucovorin calcium, methotrexate sodium, metoclopramide HCl, mitomycin, and vincristine sulfate.

Doxorubicin HCl **compatibility information conflicts** or is dependent on diluent or concentration factors with the following drugs or solutions: vinblastine sulfate (in syringes and as an IV additive). Compatibility is dependent upon factors such as pH, concentration, temperature and diluent used; consult specialized references or a hospital pharmacist for more specific information

Doxorubicin HCl is reportedly physically **incompatible** with the following solutions or drugs: aminophylline, dexamethasone sodium phosphate, diazepam, fluorouracil (as an IV additive only), furosemide, heparin sodium, and hydrocortisone sodium succinate. Do not flush IV catheters with heparin; use sterile saline.

Dosage Forms/Regulatory Status

VETERINARY-LABELED PRODUCTS: NONE.

HUMAN-LABELED PRODUCTS:

Doxorubicin HCl (Conventional) Lyophilized Powder for Injection, (conventional): 10 mg, 20 mg, 50 mg, and 150 mg vials; *Adriamycin RDF®*, generic; (Rx). Reconstitute with appropriate amount of 0.9% sodium chloride for final concentration of 2 mg/mL.

Doxorubicin HCl (Conventional) Injection (aqueous): 2 mg/mL in 5 mL, 10 mL, 25 mL, and 100 mL; *Adriamycin PFS®*, generic; (Rx)

Doxorubicin, Liposomal Injection: 20 mg in 10 mL & 50 mg in 30 mL single-use vials; *Doxil®*; (Rx)

Revisions/References

Monograph revised/updated January 2014.

Argyle, D., et al. (2008). *Decision Making in Small Animal Oncology*, Wiley-Blackwell.
Dobson, J. & D. Lascelles (2011). *BSAVA Manual of Canine and Feline Oncology*, BSAVA.
Henry, C. & M. Higginbotham (2009). *Cancer Management in Small Animal Practice*, Saunders.
Knobloch, A., et al. (2010). Cytotoxic Drug Residues in Urine of Dogs Receiving Anticancer Chemotherapy. J Vet Intern Med **24**: 384-90.
Knobloch, A., et al. (2010). Drug Residues in Serum of Dogs Receiving Anticancer Chemotherapy. Journal of Veterinary Internal Medicine 24(2): 379-83.
Lori, J. C., et al. (2010). Doxorubicin and cyclophosphamide for the treatment of canine lymphoma: a randomized, placebo-controlled study. Veterinary and Comparative Oncology 8(3): 188-95.
North, S. & T. Banks (2009). *Small Animal Oncology: An Introduction*, Saunders.
Withrow, S., et al. (2012). Withrow and MacEwen's Small Animal Clinical Oncology, 5th Ed., Saunders.
WSU-VetClinPharmLab (2009). "Problem Drugs." Veterinary Clinical Pharmacology Lab, College of Vet Med, Washington State University http://goo.gl/aIGlM.

Doxycycline

(dox-i-sye-kleen)   Vibramycin®
Tetracycline Antibiotic

Prescriber Highlights

▶ Oral & parenteral tetracycline antibiotic.
▶ Bone & teeth abnormalities are much less likely than with other tetracyclines, but use with caution in pregnant & young animals.
▶ May be used in patients with renal insufficiency.
▶ Not for IV injection in horses; do not give IM or SC to any species.
▶ Most common adverse effects are GI, but increased liver enzymes can occur.
▶ Esophagitis and strictures possible; must follow oral doses with sufficient fluid to get medication into stomach.
▶ Drug Interactions.

Uses/Indications

Although there are no veterinary FDA-approved doxycycline products available, its favorable pharmacokinetic parameters (longer half-life, higher CNS penetration) when compared to either tetracycline HCl or oxytetracycline HCl make it a reasonable choice to use in small animals when a tetracycline is indicated, particularly when a tetracycline is indicated in an azotemic patient. It is commonly used in small animals to treat a variety of infections caused by several different microorganisms that include Borrelia, Leptospira, Rickettsiae, Chlamydia, Mycoplasma, Bartonella, and Bordetella.

Doxycycline therapy is part of the recommended canine heartworm treatment protocol of The American Heartworm Society and it states "Doxycycline is administered at 10 mg/kg twice daily for 4 weeks…and has been shown to eliminate over 95% of the *Wolbachia* organisms in the filarial nematode *Wuchereria bancrofti* resulting in amicrofilaremia for 12 months. This data suggests that the absence or at least very low *Wolbachia* numbers are present as the organism is necessary for embryogenesis. Preliminary data indicate *Wolbachia* numbers remain low in *D. immitis* following doxycycline administration for at least 3 months." (The-American-Heartworm-Society 2012)

In avian species, some clinicians feel that doxycycline is the drug of choice in the oral treatment of chlamydiosis, particularly when treating only a few birds.

Pharmacology/Actions

Tetracyclines are time-dependent, bacteriostatic antibiotics that inhibit protein synthesis by reversibly binding to 30S ribosomal subunits of susceptible organisms, thereby preventing aminoacyl transfer-RNA binding to those ribosomes. Tetracyclines also alter cytoplasmic membrane permeability in susceptible organisms. In high concentrations, tetracyclines can also inhibit protein synthesis by mammalian cells.

As a class, the tetracyclines have activity against most mycoplasma, spirochetes (including the Lyme disease organism), Chlamydia and Rickettsia. Against gram-positive bacteria, the tetracyclines have activity against some strains of staphylococcus and streptococci but resistance by these organisms is increasing.

Staphylococcal resistance to tetracyclines is via the *tet*(K) and *tet*(M) genes. *tet*(K) is the primary MRSP clone found in Europe and *tet*(M) in North America. *tet*(K) confers resistance to tetracycline, but not doxycycline or minocycline, while *tet*(M) confers resistance to all three. Use of doxycycline for treating methicillin-resistant *Staphylococcus pseudintermedius* (MRSP) in dogs is somewhat controversial. One review states that "To date, the North American MRSP isolates all contain *tet*(M), making doxycycline or any tetracycline a poor choice to treat MRSP in this region" (Bryan et al. 2012). In another review of this subject, the author states "Susceptibility testing of doxycycline for methicillin-resistant staphylococci is generally not advised as doxycycline-resistance of MRSA (MRSP is not known) can be induced by pre-incubation with tetracycline or doxycycline and it is recommended that all tetracycline-resistant strains be treated as resistant to doxycycline regardless of susceptibility testing results. In order to determine whether minocycline is a valid choice for treating MRSP, minocycline susceptibility should be performed. Resistance to minocycline should indicate the presence of *tet*(M), while susceptibility to minocycline but resistance to tetracycline should indicate the presence of *tet*(K) (Frank et al. 2012).

Other gram-positive bacteria that are usually covered by tetracyclines include: *Actinomyces* spp., *Bacillus anthracis*, *Clostridium perfringens* and *tetani*, *Listeria monocytogenes* and Nocardia. Among gram-negative bacteria that tetracyclines usually have *in vitro* and *in vivo* activity against, include *Bordetella* spp., Brucella, Bartonella, *Haemophilus* spp., *Pasteurella multocida*, Shigella, and *Yersinia pestis*. Many or most strains of *E. coli*, Klebsiella, Bacteroides, Enterobacter, Proteus and *Pseudomonas aeruginosa* are resistant to the tetracyclines (Bryan et al. 2012).

Doxycycline generally has very similar activity as other tetracyclines against susceptible organisms, but some strains of bacteria may be more susceptible to doxycycline or minocycline and additional *in vitro* testing may be required.

Minocycline and doxycycline have significant inhibitory properties against the activity of matrix metalloproteinases (collagenase, gelatinase) and can act as a disease-modifying agent for osteoarthritis.

Pharmacokinetics

In most species, doxycycline is well absorbed after oral administration. Bioavailability is 90-100% in humans and it is thought that the drug is readily absorbed in most monogastric animals. Unlike tetracycline HCl or oxytetracycline, doxycycline absorption in humans may only be reduced by 20% by either food or dairy products in the gut. But in horses, giving doxycycline orally in the fed state may reduce bioavailability to less than 5%, possibly due to the high fiber content in most equine diets.

Tetracyclines as a class, are widely distributed to the heart, kidney, lungs, muscle, pleural fluid, bronchial secretions, sputum, bile, saliva, synovial fluid, ascitic fluid, and aqueous and vitreous humor. When doxycycline was dosed to horses at 10 mg/kg PO q12h, it did not yield appreciable levels in the aqueous or vitreous humor (Gilmour et al. 2005). In horses, doxycycline has been shown to penetrate into the synovial fluid with an AUC synovial fluid:plasma factor of 4.6 and is eliminated from synovial fluid more slowly than plasma (Schnabel et al. 2010).

Doxycycline is more lipid-soluble and penetrates body tissues and fluids better than tetracycline HCl or oxytetracycline, including into the CSF, prostate, and eye. While CSF levels are generally insufficient to treat most bacterial infections, doxycycline has been shown to be efficacious in the treatment of the CNS effects associated with Lyme disease in humans. The volume of distribution at steady-state in dogs is approximately 1.5 L/kg. Doxycycline is bound to plasma proteins in varying amounts dependent upon species. The drug is approximately 25-93% bound to plasma proteins in humans, 75-86% in dogs, 82% in horses, and about 93% in cattle and pigs. Cats have higher binding to plasma proteins than

dogs. Doxycycline accumulates intracellularly and concentrates in equine PMNs (Davis et al. 2006).

Doxycycline's elimination from the body is relatively unique. The drug is primarily excreted into the feces via non-biliary routes in an inactive form. It is thought that the drug is partially inactivated in the intestine by chelate formation and then excreted into the intestinal lumen. In dogs, about 75% of a given dose is handled in this manner. Renal excretion of doxycycline can only account for about 25% of a dose in dogs, and biliary excretion less than 5%. The serum half-life of doxycycline in dogs is approximately 10-12 hours and a clearance of about 1.7 mL/kg/min. In calves, the drug has similar pharmacokinetic values. In horses, elimination half-life is about 12 hours and clearance is approximately 0.7 mL/kg/min. Doxycycline does not accumulate in patients with renal dysfunction.

Contraindications/Precautions/Warnings

Doxycycline is contraindicated in patients hypersensitive to the drug. Because tetracyclines can retard fetal skeletal development and discolor deciduous teeth, they should only be used in the last half of pregnancy when the benefits outweigh the fetal risks, but doxycycline is much less likely to cause these abnormalities than other more water-soluble tetracyclines (*e.g.*, tetracycline, oxytetracycline). Unlike either oxytetracycline or tetracycline, doxycycline can be used in patients with renal insufficiency. Since increases in hepatic enzymes have been documented in some dogs after doxycycline treatment, use with caution in dogs with significant liver dysfunction.

If using oral tablets "pilling" should be followed by at least 6 mL of water or food. Do not dry pill. It has been suggested that oral doxycycline monohydrate may not have the same esophageal issues as the hyclate salt as it is much less acidic and slower to dissolve in neutral solutions (German et al. 2005), however, it is recommended that each dose be followed by a water or food swallow regardless of the salt used. Another source states that the incidence of gastrointestinal upset may be greater with doxycycline monohydrate however (Boothe 2013).Tetracycline therapy (especially long-term) may result in overgrowth (superinfections) of non-susceptible bacteria or fungi.

Until further studies documenting the safety of intravenous doxycycline in horses are done, the parenteral route of administering this drug in horses should be considered contraindicated.

Doxycycline is pumped by P-glycoprotein, but the Washington State University Clinical Pharmacology Lab reports that it has not seen any increased sensitivity to doxycycline and does not recommend any dose alterations in dogs with MDR-1 mutations. (WSU-VetClinPharmLab 2009)

Adverse Effects

The most commonly reported side effects of oral doxycycline therapy in dogs and cats are vomiting, diarrhea and anorexia. Giving the drug with food may help alleviate these GI effects without significantly reducing drug absorption. Increased liver enzymes (ALT, ALP) have been reported in up to 40% of dogs and 19% of cats treated. The clinical significance of increased liver enzymes has not been determined.

Oral doxycycline has been implicated in causing esophagitis and esophageal strictures in cats. See Warnings for more information.

In humans, doxycycline (or other tetracyclines) has also been associated with photosensitivity reactions and, rarely, hepatotoxicity or blood dyscrasias.

Intravenous injection of even relatively low doses of doxycycline has been associated with cardiac arrhythmias, collapse, and death in horses.

Reproductive/Nursing Safety

In humans, the FDA categorizes this drug as category *D* for use during pregnancy (*There is evidence of human fetal risk, but the potential benefits from the use of the drug in pregnant women may be acceptable despite its potential risks.*) In a separate system evaluating the safety of drugs in canine and feline pregnancy (Papich 1989), this drug is categorized as class: *D* (*Contraindicated. These drugs have been shown to cause congenital malformations or embryotoxicity.*)

Tetracyclines are excreted in milk. Milk:plasma ratios vary between 0.25 and 1.5. Avoid nursing if the dam requires doxycycline.

Overdosage/Acute Toxicity

With the exception of intravenous dosing in horses (see above), doxycycline is apparently quite safe in most mild overdose situations. Oral overdoses would most likely be associated with GI disturbances (vomiting, anorexia, and/or diarrhea). Although doxycycline is less vulnerable to chelation with cations than other tetracyclines, oral administration of divalent or trivalent cation antacids may bind some of the drug and reduce GI distress. Should the patient develop severe emesis or diarrhea, fluids and electrolytes should be monitored and replaced if necessary.

Rapid intravenous injection of doxycycline has induced transient collapse and cardiac arrhythmias in several species, presumably due to chelation with intravascular calcium ions. If overdose quantities are inadvertently administered, these effects may be more pronounced.

Drug Interactions

The following drug interactions have either been reported or are theoretical in humans or animals receiving doxycycline and may be of significance in veterinary patients. Unless otherwise noted, use together is not necessarily contraindicated, but weigh the potential risks and perform additional monitoring when appropriate.

- **ANTACIDS, ORAL:** When orally administered, tetracyclines can chelate divalent or trivalent cations that can decrease the absorption of the tetracycline or the other drug if it contains these cations. Oral antacids, saline cathartics, or other GI products containing aluminum, calcium, magnesium, zinc, or bismuth cations are most commonly associated with this interaction. Doxycycline has a relatively low affinity for calcium ions, but it is recommended that all oral tetracyclines be given at least 1-2 hours before or after the cation-containing product.
- **BISMUTH SUBSALICYLATE, KAOLIN, PECTIN:** May reduce absorption
- **IRON, ORAL:** Oral iron products are associated with decreased tetracycline absorption, and administration of iron salts should preferably be given 3 hours before or 2 hours after the tetracycline dose.
- **PENICILLINS:** Bacteriostatic drugs like the tetracyclines may interfere with bactericidal activity of the penicillins, cephalosporins, and aminoglycosides. The actual clinical significance, if any, of this interaction has probably been overstated.
- **PHENOBARBITAL:** May decrease doxycycline half-life and reduce levels.
- **WARFARIN:** Tetracyclines may depress plasma prothrombin activity and patients on anticoagulant (*e.g.*, warfarin) therapy may need dosage adjustment.

Laboratory Considerations

- Tetracyclines (not minocycline) may cause falsely elevated values of **urine catecholamines** when using fluorometric methods of determination.
- Tetracyclines reportedly can cause false-positive **urine glucose** results if using the cupric sulfate method of determination (Benedict's reagent, *Clinitest®*), but this may be the result of ascorbic acid that is found in some parenteral formulations of tetracyclines. Tetracyclines have also reportedly caused false-negative results in determining urine glucose when using the glucose oxidase method (*Clinistix®*, *Tes-Tape®*).

Doses

- **DOGS:**

For susceptible bacterial infections (extra-label): 5 mg/kg PO q12h. Treatment durations vary, but 7-14 days are commonly recommended.

For adjunctive treatment of canine heartworm disease (extra-label): On days 1-28 doxycycline 10 mg/kg PO twice daily for 4 weeks. Give prior to melarsomine treatment. If after melarsomine therapy (day 120) microfilaria positive, treat with another 30-day regimen of doxycycline and re-test in 4 weeks. When used in the alternative treatment protocol in cases where arsenical therapy is not possible or is contraindicated, the use of a monthly heartworm preventive along with doxycycline might be considered. Doxycycline at 10 mg/kg PO twice daily for a 4-week period every 3-4 months should eliminate most *Wolbachia* organisms and not allow them to repopulate. (The-American-Heartworm-Society 2012)

For leptospirosis (extra-label): Thee consensus panel recommends doxycycline 5mg/kg PO or IV q12h for 2 weeks, but the optimal duration of antimicrobial therapy requires further investigation. Dogs should receive doxycycline for 2 weeks after gastrointestinal signs abate in order to eliminate organisms from the renal tubules. (Sykes et al. 2011)

For granulocytic anaplasmosis (*Anaplasma phagocytotophilum*); (extra-label): 5 mg/kg PO q12h for 14 days; most dogs show clinical improvement in 24-48 hours. (Carrade et al. 2009)

For Lyme disease (extra-label): 10 mg/kg PO q12-24h PO for 30 days. (Krupka et al. 2010)

For Ehrlichiosis (extra-label): The AVCIM consensus statement recommends that doxycycline be administered at a dose of 10 mg/kg by mouth every 24 hours for 28 days. (Neer et al. 2002)

For rickettsial diseases such as Rocky Mountain Spotted-Fever (*Rickettsia rickettsii*); (extra-label): 5 mg/kg PO q12h. (Breitschwerdt 2000)

For periodontitis (subantimicrobial regimen); (extra-label): 2 mg/kg PO daily appeared to be an appropriate dose and may be suitable for long-term treatment of gelatinolytic inflammatory diseases such as periodontitis. (Kim et al. 2013)

- **CATS:**

Warning: Do not dry pill cats with oral doxycycline; follow with at least 6 mL of water or use a compounded slurry (e.g., "triple fish" or similar) to administer.

For susceptible infections (extra-label): 5 mg/kg PO twice daily or 10 mg/kg PO once daily is generally recommended. The following are sample treatment protocols and recommendations for a variety of conditions.

a) For *Mycoplasma felis* upper respiratory tract infections (extra-label; study done in shelter cats): Cats were either given 10 mg/kg (as oral liquid) once daily for 7 or 14 days. Authors concluded that the 14-day course produced superior microbiological, but not clinical results. (Kompare et al. 2013)

b) For Hemotropic mycoplasmosis: 10 mg/kg PO once daily for a minimum of 2 weeks. (Sykes 2010)

c) For Ehrlichiosis or Anaplasmosis: 5 – 10 mg/kg PO q12h for 21 days. (Greene et al. 2006)

d) For hemoplasmosis or bartonellosis: 10 mg/kg PO q12–24h. (Lappin 2006)

e) For clinical *Toxoplasma gondii*: 5 – 10 mg/kg PO q12h for 4 weeks. (Lappin 2000)

f) For susceptible mycobacterial, L-Forms, or mycoplasma infections: 5 – 10 mg/kg PO q12h. (Bonenberger 2009)

g) For treatment of *Nocardia* (*N. nova*) infections: Combination therapy with: amoxicillin 20 mg/kg PO twice daily with clarithromycin 62.5 – 125 mg (total dose per cat) PO twice daily and/or doxycycline 5 mg/kg or higher PO twice daily. (Malik 2006)

h) For feline chlamydial infections (*C. felis*): 10 mg/kg PO once daily for a minimum of 3-4 weeks; additional topical ocular treatment may reduce ocular discomfort. (Gruffyd-Jones 2009)

- **HORSES:**

Warning: Doxycycline intravenously in horses has been associated with fatalities. Until further work is done demonstrating the safety of this drug, it cannot be recommended for parenteral use in this species. Commercially available PO doxycycline hyclate or monohydrate has low bioavailability in horses and successfully treating Lyme disease or anaplasmosis may be problematic.

For Lyme disease (extra-label): A common intensive treatment scenario has been to give IV tetracycline, 6.6 mg/kg q12h for 7-10 days, followed by PO doxycycline at 10 mg/kg q12h for 1-2 months.

For equine granulocytic ehrlichiosis (anaplasmosis; EGE) as an alternative to oxytetracycline (extra-label): 10 mg/kg PO q12h for 10-14 days. (Lewis et al. 2009)

For organisms with an MIC ≤ 0.25 micrograms/mL including many susceptible *Streptococcus* spp, *Staphylococcus* spp, *Pasteurella* spp, *Rhodococcus equi*, *Actinobacillus equuli*, and most ehrlichial organisms; (extra-label): 20 mg/kg PO q24h; preferably food should be withheld for at least 8 hours before and 2 hours after dosing. For bacteria with an MIC of 0.5 – 1 micrograms/mL, 20 mg/kg PO q12h is necessary to maintain adequate trough levels. Feeding should ideally be withheld as above, but may not be practically possible. One horse in the study developed a severe, acute colitis and the authors recommended that further clinical and safety studies be performed before using this regimen. (Davis et al. 2006)

- **RABBITS/RODENTS/SMALL MAMMALS:**

Mice, Rats (extra-label): For mycoplasmal pneumonia: 5 mg/kg PO twice daily with enrofloxacin (10 mg/kg PO twice daily). (Burke 1999)

Chinchillas, Gerbils, Guinea Pigs, Hamsters, Mice, Rats (extra-label): 2.5 – 5 mg/kg PO q12h. Do not use in young or pregnant animals. (Adamcak et al. 2000)

- **BIRDS:**

For Psittacosis (Chlamydiosis); (extra-label):

a) Study done in experimentally infected cockatiels: Doxycycline 35 mg/kg PO once daily for 21 days (as effective as a 45-day treatment). Birds were dosed via metallic feeding tube into crop using the commercially available (*Vibramycin®*) human oral suspension. (Guzman et al. 2010)

b) Routes of treatment include intramuscular injections, oral dosage with a suspension, medicated mash (approximately 1000 mg per kg of feed), and water-soluble approaches. IM: 75 – 100 mg/kg IM every 5-7 days for the first 4 weeks and subsequently every 5 days for the duration of a 45 day treatment. PO: 40 – 50 mg/kg PO once daily for cockatiels, Senegal parrots, Blue fronted and Orange winged amazons, 25 mg/kg PO once daily for African Grey parrots, Goffin's cockatoos, Blue and gold macaws and Green winged macaws. Empirically: 25 – 50 mg/kg PO once a day is the recommended starting dosage for unstudied avian species. (Speer 1999)

c) Using the oral liquid/suspension: 50 mg/kg PO every 24 hours, or divided every 12 hours (use less for macaws). Using the hyclate salt on corn, beans, rice and oatmeal: 1 gram per kg of feed. Using the injectable product (*Vibaravenos®*—may not be available commercially in the USA): 100 mg/kg IM once weekly (75 mg/kg IM once weekly in macaws and lovebirds). (Bauck et al. 1993)

- **REPTILES:**

For susceptible infections (extra-label):

For chelonians: 10 mg/kg PO once daily for 4 weeks. Useful for bacterial respiratory infections in tortoises having suspected Mycoplasma infections.

In most species: 10 mg/kg PO once daily for 10-45 days. (Gauvin 1993)

Monitoring

- Clinical efficacy.
- Adverse effects.

Client Information

- Do not give as a "dry pill." Give with a moist treat or small amount of liquid to be sure that it reaches the stomach; this is especially important for cats. Doxycycline can cause ulcers in the throat and esophagus if it gets stuck there before it reaches the stomach. If your animal has trouble swallowing or eating, contact your veterinarian immediately.
- May upset stomach. Give with a small amount of food that does not contain iron or dairy products.
- Do not give multivitamins, calcium supplements, antacids, or laxatives within 2 hours before or after giving doxycycline. These products can reduce the drug's effectiveness.
- This drug may make your animal's skin more sensitive to sunlight and increase the risk of sunburn on hairless areas such as the nose and around the eyelids and ears. Tell your veterinarian if you notice any reddening/sunburning of the skin while your animal is on this medication.

Chemistry/Synonyms

A semi-synthetic tetracycline that is derived from oxytetracycline, doxycycline is available as hyclate, calcium and monohydrate salts. The hyclate salt is used in the injectable dosage form and oral tablets and capsules. It occurs as a yellow, crystalline powder that is soluble in water and slightly soluble in alcohol. After reconstitution with sterile water, the hyclate injection has a pH of 1.8-3.3. Doxycycline hyclate may also be known as doxycycline hydrochloride.

The monohydrate salt is found in the oral powder for reconstitution. It occurs as a yellow, crystalline powder that is very slightly soluble in water and sparingly soluble in alcohol. The calcium salt is formed *in situ* during manufacturing. It is found in the commercially available oral syrup and other oral dosage forms.

Doxycycline may also be known as: doxycycline monohydrate, doxycyclinum, and GS-3065; many trade names are available.

Storage/Stability

Doxycycline hyclate tablets and capsules should be stored in tight, light-resistant containers at temperatures less than 30°C, and preferably at room temperature (15-30°C). After reconstituting with water, the monohydrate oral suspension is stable for 14 days when stored at room temperature.

The hyclate injection when reconstituted with a suitable diluent (*e.g.*, D5W, Ringer's injection, Sodium Chloride 0.9%, or Plasma-Lyte 56 in D5W) to a concentration of 0.1 – 1 mg/mL may be stored for 72 hours if refrigerated. Frozen reconstituted solutions (10 mg/mL in sterile water) are stable for at least 8 weeks if kept at -20°C, but should not be refrozen once thawed. If solutions are stored at room temperature, different manufacturers give different recommendations regarding stability, ranging from 12-48 hours. Infusions should generally be completed within 12 hours of administration.

Compatibility/Compounding Considerations

Doxycycline hyclate for injection is reportedly physically **compatible** with the following IV infusion solutions and drugs: D5W, Ringer's injection, sodium chloride 0.9%, or Plasma-Lyte 56 in D5W, Plasma-Lyte 148 in D5W, Normosol M in D5W, Normosol R in D5W, invert sugar 10%, acyclovir sodium, hydromorphone HCl, magnesium sulfate, meperidine HCl, morphine sulfate, and ranitidine HCl. Compatibility is dependent upon factors such as pH, concentration, temperature, and diluent used; consult specialized references or a hospital pharmacist for more specific information.

One study examining doxycycline blood levels in birds following injection of commercially available (not in USA) intramuscular formulation (*Vibravenös*®; Pfizer Switz.) and two concentrations of a pharmacist compounded product, showed variable blood levels and a high incidence of localized tissue reactions, including necrosis, with the compounded products (Flammer et al. 2005).

Doxycycline administered to budgerigars at 250 – 300 ppm in a hulled seed diet has been shown to maintain doxycycline levels sufficient to treat chlamydiosis.

Doxycycline oral suspensions should be stored in the refrigerator, protected from light and used within 7 days. Although some compounding pharmacies claim stability of 6 months for compounded doxycycline suspensions, others have demonstrated that compounded doxycycline suspensions degrade rapidly between 7 and 14 days even if refrigerated. A study evaluating compounded oral suspensions made from 100 mg doxycycline tablets at concentrations of 33.3 and 166.7 mg/mL concluded that stability cannot be assured beyond 7 days (Papich et al. 2013). Another study (Sadrieh et al. 2005) demonstrated that doxycycline tablets mixed with water or foods (*e.g.*, milk, pudding, yogurt, apple sauce, jellies) lose more than 10% potency after 24 hours.

Dosage Forms/Regulatory Status

VETERINARY-LABELED PRODUCTS:

None for systemic use.

Doxycycline gel: 8.5% activity once mixed. (2 syringe system); *Doxirobe*®; (Rx). FDA-approved for oral application for the prevention and treatment of periodontal disease in dogs;.

HUMAN-LABELED PRODUCTS:

Doxycycline (as the hyclate) Tablets & Capsules: 20 mg, 50 mg, & 100 mg; *Periostat*®, *Alodox Convenience Kit*®, *Vibramycin*® & *Vibra-Tabs*®, *Oraxyl*®, generic; (Rx)

Doxycycline (as the hyclate) Delayed-Release Tablets & Capsules: 75 mg, 100 mg & 150 mg, & 40 mg (30 mg immediate release & 10 mg delayed release); *Doryx*®; *Oracea*®; (Rx)

Doxycycline (as monohydrate) Tablets and Capsules: 50 mg, 75 mg, 100 mg & 150 mg; *Monodox*®, *Adoxa*®, generic; (Rx)

Doxycycline Capsules (coated-pellets) (as hyclate): 75 mg & 100 mg; *Doryx*®, generic; (Rx)

Doxycycline (as the monohydrate) Powder for Oral Suspension: 5 mg/mL after reconstitution in 60 mL; *Vibramycin*®, generic; (Rx)

Doxycycline (as the calcium salt) Oral Syrup: 10 mg/mL in 473 mL; *Vibramycin*®; (Rx)

Doxycycline Injection: 42.5 mg (as hyclate, 10%) in vials; *Atridox*®; (Rx)

Doxycycline (as the hyclate) Lyophilized Powder for Injection: 100 mg & 200 mg with 300 mg & 600 mg mannitol respectively in vials; *Doxy*®-100 & -200; generic; (Rx)

Revisions/References

Monograph revised/updated January 2014.

Adamcak, A. & B. Otten (2000). Rodent Therapeutics. Vet Clin NA: Exotic Anim Pract 3:1(Jan): 221-40.

Bauck, L. & H. Hoefer (1993). Avian antimicrobial therapy. Seminars in Avian & Exotic Med 2(1): 17-22.

Bonenberger, T. (2009). Typical Cat Bite Abscess, or Not: Chronic Draining Tracts & Nodules. Proceedings: WVC. accessed via Veterinary Information Network; vin.com

Boothe, D. M. (2013). Doxycycline for veterinary use during shortage. Javma-Journal of the American Veterinary Medical Association 242(10): 1340-.

Breitschwerdt, E. (2000). Rocky Mountain Spotted Fever. Proceedings: American Animal Hospital Association 67th Annual Meeting, Toronto. accessed via Veterinary Information Network; vin.com

Bryan, J., et al. (2012). Treatment outcome of dogs with meticillin-resistant and meticillin-susceptible Staphylococcus pseudintermedius pyoderma. Veterinary Dermatology 23(4): 361-E65.

Burke, T. (1999). Husbandry and Medicine of Rodents and Lagomorphs. Proceedings: Central Veterinary Conference, Kansas City. accessed via Veterinary Information Network; vin.com

Carrade, D. D., et al. (2009). Canine Granulocytic Anaplasmosis: A Review. Journal of Veterinary Internal Medicine 23(6): 1129-41.

Davis, J. L., et al. (2006). Pharmacokinetics and tissue distribution of doxycycline after oral administration of single and multiple doses in horses. American Journal of Veterinary Research 67(2): 310-6.

Flammer, K. & M. Papich (2005). Assessment of plasma concentrations and effects of injectable doxycycline in three psittacine species. Journal of Avian Medicine and Surgery 19(3): 216-24.

Frank, L. A. & A. Loeffler (2012). Meticillin-resistant Staphylococcus pseudintermedius: clinical challenge and treatment options. Veterinary Dermatology 23(4): 283-E56.

Gauvin, J. (1993). Drug therapy in reptiles. Seminars in Avian & Exotic Med 2(1): 48-59.

German, A. J., et al. (2005). Oesophageal strictures in cats associated with doxycycline therapy. Journal of Feline Medicine and Surgery 7(1): 33-41.

Gilmour, M. A., et al. (2005). Ocular penetration of oral doxycycline in the horse. Vet. Ophthalmol. 8(5): 331-5.

Greene, C., et al. (2006). Appendix 8: Antimicrobial Drug Formulary. *Infectious Disease of the Dog and Cat.* C. Greene, Elsevier: 1186-333.

Gruffyd-Jones, T. (2009). Chlamydial infections of cats. Proceedings: WSAVA. accessed via Veterinary Information Network; vin.com

Guzman, D. S. M., et al. (2010). Evaluating 21-day Doxycycline and Azithromycin Treatments for Experimental Chlamydophila psittaci Infection in Cockatiels (Nymphicus hollandicus). Journal of Avian Medicine and Surgery 24(1): 35-45.

Kim, S. E., et al. (2013). Experimental determination of a subantimicrobial dosage of doxycycline hyclate for treatment of periodontitis in Beagles. American Journal of Veterinary Research 74(1): 130-5.

Kompare, B., et al. (2013). Randomized masked controlled clinical trial to compare 7-day and 14-day course length of doxycycline in the treatment of Mycoplasma felis infection in shelter cats. Comparative Immunology Microbiology and Infectious Diseases 36(2): 129-35.

Krupka, I. & R. K. Straubinger (2010). Lyme Borreliosis in Dogs and Cats: Background, Diagnosis, Treatment and Prevention of Infections with Borrelia burgdorferi sensu stricto. Veterinary Clinics of North America-Small Animal Practice 40(6): 1103-+.

Lappin, M. (2000). Protozoal and Miscellaneous Infections. *Textbook of Veterinary Internal Medicine: Diseases of the Dog and Cat.* S. Ettinger and E. Feldman. Philadelphia, WB Saunders. 1: 408-17.

Lappin, M. (2006). Chronic feline infectious disease. Proceedings: Western Vet Conf. accessed via Veterinary Information Network; vin.com

Lewis, S. R., et al. (2009). Equine Granulocytic Anaplasmosis: A Case Report and Review. Journal of Equine Veterinary Science 29(3): 160-6.

Malik, R. (2006). Nocardia infections in cats. Proceedings Western Vet Conf. accessed via Veterinary Information Network; vin.com

Neer, T., et al. (2002). Consensus statement on ehrlichial disease of small animals from the infectious disease study group of the ACVIM. J Vet Intern Med 16(3): 309-15.

Papich, M. G., et al. (2013). Doxycycline concentration over time after storage in a compounded veterinary preparation. Javma-Journal of the American Veterinary Medical Association 242(12): 1674-8.

Sadrieh, N., et al. (2005). Stability, dose uniformity, and palatability of three counterterrorism drugs - Human subject and electronic tongue studies. Pharmaceutical Research 22(10): 1747-56.

Schnabel, L. V., et al. (2010). Orally administered doxycycline accumulates in synovial fluid compared to plasma. Equine Veterinary Journal 42(3): 208-12.

Speer, B. (1999). An update on avian chlamydiosis. Proceedings: Central Veterinary Conference, Kansas City. accessed via Veterinary Information Network; vin.com

Sykes, J. E. (2010). Feline Hemotropic Mycoplasmas. Veterinary Clinics of North America-Small Animal Practice 40(6): 1157-+.

Sykes, J. E., et al. (2011). 2010 ACVIM Small Animal Consensus Statement on Leptospirosis: Diagnosis, Epidemiology, Treatment, and Prevention. Journal of Veterinary Internal Medicine 25(1): 1-13.

The-American-Heartworm-Society (2012). "Current Canine Guidelines for the Diagnosis, Prevention, and Management of Heartworm (*Dirofilaria immitis*) Infection in Dogs (revised January, 2012)." http://www.heartwormsociety.org/veterinary-resources/canine-guidelines.html.

WSU-VetClinPharmLab (2009). "Problem Drugs." Veterinary Clinical Pharmacology Lab, College of Vet Med, Washington State University http://goo.gl/aIGlM.

Edetate Calcium Disodium

(ed-a-tayt)   Calcium EDTA, Calcium Disodium Versenate®

Antidote

Prescriber Highlights

▶ Heavy metal chelator used primarily for lead or zinc toxicity.

▶ Contraindications: Patients with anuria or lead still in gut; Extreme Caution: Patients with decreased renal function.

▶ Recommend using SC route when treating small animals; do not give PO.

▶ Adverse Effects: Painful on injection, renal toxicity (renal tubular necrosis); may cause depression & GI clinical signs in dogs.

Uses/Indications

Edetate calcium disodium also known as calcium disodium EDTA (CaEDTA) is used as a chelating agent in the treatment of lead or zinc poisoning. Succimer is more commonly recommended today for treating lead poisoning in dogs and cats.

CaEDTA may be used in combination with dimercaprol treatment.

Pharmacology/Actions

The calcium in CaEDTA can be displaced by divalent or trivalent metals to form a stable, water-soluble complex that can be excreted in the urine. One gram of CaEDTA can theoretically bind 620 mg of lead, but in reality only about 5 mg per gram is actually excreted into the urine in lead poisoned patients. In addition to chelating lead, CaEDTA chelates and eliminates zinc from the body. CaEDTA also binds cadmium, copper, iron, and manganese, but to a much lesser extent than either lead or zinc. CaEDTA is relatively ineffective for use in treating mercury, gold, or arsenic poisoning.

There is some evidence that thiamine supplementation may increase the clinical efficacy of CaEDTA in treating acute lead poisoning in cattle.

Pharmacokinetics

CaEDTA is well absorbed after either IM or SC administration. It is distributed primarily in the extracellular fluid. Unlike dimercaprol, CaEDTA does not penetrate erythrocytes or enter the CNS in appreciable amounts. The drug is rapidly excreted renally, either as unchanged drug or chelated with metals. Changes in urine pH or urine flow do not significantly alter the rate of excretion. Decreased renal function can cause accumulation of the drug and can increase its nephrotoxic potential. In humans with normal renal function, the average elimination half-life of CaEDTA is 20-60 minutes after IV administration, and 1.5 hours after IM administration.

Contraindications/Precautions/Warnings

CaEDTA is contraindicated in patients with anuria. It should be used with extreme caution and dosage adjustment in patients with diminished renal function.

Most small animal clinicians recommend using the SC route when treating small animals as IV administration of CaEDTA has been associated with abrupt increases in CSF pressure and death in children with lead-induced cerebral edema.

Lead should be removed from the GI tract before using CaEDTA. Do not administer CaEDTA orally as it may increase the amount of lead absorbed from the GI tract.

Animals with clinical signs of cerebral edema should not be over-hydrated.

Adverse Effects

The most serious adverse effect associated with this compound is renal toxicity (renal tubular necrosis), but in dogs CaEDTA can cause depression, vomiting, and diarrhea. GI clinical signs may be alleviated by zinc supplementation. Pain can occur at the site of injection.

Chronic therapy may lead to zinc deficiency; zinc supplementation should be considered in these animals.

Reproductive/Nursing Safety

In humans, the FDA categorizes this drug as category *B* for use during pregnancy (*Animal studies have not yet demonstrated risk to the fetus, but there are no adequate studies in pregnant women; or animal studies have shown an adverse effect, but adequate studies in pregnant women have not demonstrated a risk to the fetus in the first trimester of pregnancy, and there is no evidence of risk in later trimesters*).

It is not known whether this drug is excreted in milk.

Overdosage/Acute Toxicity

Doses greater than 12 g/kg are lethal in dogs; refer to Adverse Effects for more information.

Drug Interactions

The following drug interactions have either been reported or are theoretical in humans or animals receiving CaEDTA and may be of significance in veterinary patients. Unless otherwise noted, use together is not necessarily contraindicated, but weigh the potential risks and perform additional monitoring when appropriate.

- **GLUCOCORTICOIDS:** The renal toxicity of CaEDTA may be enhanced by the concomitant administration of glucocorticoids.
- **INSULIN (NPH, PZI):** Concurrent administration of CaEDTA with zinc insulin preparations (NPH, PZI) will decrease the sustained action of the insulin preparation.
- **NEPHROTOXIC DRUGS, OTHER:** Use with caution with other nephrotoxic compounds (*e.g.*, **aminoglycosides, amphotericin B**).

Laboratory Considerations

- CaEDTA may cause increased urine glucose values and/or cause inverted T-waves on ECG.

Doses

The manufacturer of the injectable (human) product recommends diluting the injection to a concentration of 2 – 4 mg/mL with either normal saline or 5% dextrose when used for intravenous use. Because the injection is painful when given IM, it is recommended to add 1 mL of lidocaine HCl 1% to each mL of injection before administering IM.

- **DOGS & CATS:**

  As an alternative to succimer for lead or zinc poisoning (extra-label): 25 mg/kg (diluted in dextrose 5% to a concentration of 10 mg/mL) SC 4 times a day for 5 days. Some sources say not to exceed 2 grams per animal per day. Recheck lead or zinc in approximately 1-2 weeks and repeat course of treatment if required. Maintain adequate hydration throughout treatment.

- **HORSES:**

  For lead poisoning (extra-label): Remove animal from source of lead. If severely affected give CaEDTA at 75 mg/kg IV slowly in D5W or saline daily for 4-5 days (may divide daily dose into 2-3 administrations per day). Stop therapy for 2 days and repeat for another 4-5 days. Give adequate supportive and nutritional therapy. (Oehme 1987)

- **FOOD ANIMALS:**

  For lead poisoning (extra-label): **Note:** FARAD recommends a 2-day meat and milk withdrawal time after use in food animals (Haskell et al. 2005).

  a) 110 mg/kg per day in 3-4 divided doses; dilute to 1 gram/mL in D5W; first dose IV, then subcutaneously. (Post et al. 2000)

  b) Cattle: 67 mg/kg slow IV twice daily for 2 days; withhold dose for 2 days and then give again for 2 days. Cattle may require 10-14 days to recover and may require several series of treatments. (Bailey 1986)

- **BIRDS:**

  For lead or zinc poisoning (extra-label):

  a) For lead or zinc poisoning: 30 – 35 mg/kg IM q12h x 3-5 days, off 3-5 days, may repeat and/or use another chelator. Maintain hydration. Do not give orally as this may increase lead absorption from the GI tract. Can be used IV short-term (48 hrs.) at 20 – 35 mg/kg diluted in saline. Many published regimens. (Johnson-Delaney et al. 2009)

  b) In raptors (falcons): In this study, 25% CaEDTA was given undiluted IM at a dose of 100 mg/kg q12h for 5-25 consecutive days. Falcons were treated if blood lead was >65 micrograms/dL for 5 day courses, until blood lead was <20 micrograms/dL. No evidence of muscle damage, nephrotoxicity or hepatotoxicity seen. (Samour et al. 2004)

Monitoring

- Blood lead or zinc (serial), and/or urine d-ALA.
- Renal function tests, urinalyses, hydration status.
- Serum phosphorus and calcium values.
- Zinc, iron, copper stores in the body may be affected; consider monitoring when treating long-term for lead intoxication.
- Periodic cardiac rate/rhythm monitoring may be warranted during administration.

Client Information

- Because of the potential toxicity of this agent and the seriousness of most heavy metal intoxications, this drug should only be used with close professional supervision.

Chemistry/Synonyms

A heavy metal chelating agent, edetate calcium disodium (CaEDTA) occurs as an odorless, white, crystalline powder or granules and is a mixture of dihydrate and trihydrate forms. It has a slight saline taste and is slightly hygroscopic. CaEDTA is freely soluble in water and very slightly soluble in alcohol. The commercially available injection (human) has a pH of 6.5-8 and has approximately 5.3 mEq of sodium per gram of CaEDTA.

Edetate calcium disodium may also be known as: sodium calcium edetate, calcium disodium edathamil, calcium disodium edetate, calcium disodium ethylenediaminetetra-acetate, calcium disodium versenate, calcium EDTA, disodium calcium tetracemate, E385, natrii calcii edetas, sodium calciumedetate, *Calcium Disodium Versenate®*, *Calcium Vitis®*, *Calciumedetat-Heyl®*, *Chelante®*, *Chelintox®*, or *Ledclair®*.

Storage/Stability

CaEDTA should be stored at temperatures less than 40°, and preferably at room temperature (15-30°C). The injection can be diluted with either normal saline or 5% dextrose.

Compatibility/Compounding Considerations

Commercially available CaEDTA injection is usually diluted to a 1% solution with 5% dextrose for SC administration in small animals. To minimize pain from intramuscular injection, it can be mixed in equal quantities with lidocaine hydrochloride 1% (e.g., 1 mL of lidocaine 1% for each mL of edetate calcium disodium).

Dosage Forms/Regulatory Status

Note: Do not confuse with Edetate Disodium, which should **not** be used for lead poisoning as it may cause severe hypocalcemia.

VETERINARY-LABELED PRODUCTS:
None in the USA; may be available from compounding pharmacies.

HUMAN-LABELED PRODUCTS:
Edetate Calcium Disodium Injection Solution: 200 mg/mL in 5 mL amps (1 gram/amp); *Calcium Disodium Versenate®*; (Rx)

Revisions/References

Monograph revised/updated January 2014.

Bailey, E. M. (1986). Management and treatment of toxicosis in cattle. *Current Veterinary Therapy 2: Food Animal Practice*. J. L. Howard. Philadelphia, WB Saunders: 341-54.

Haskell, S., et al. (2005). Farad Digest: Antidotes in Food Animal Practice. JAVMA **226**(6): 884-7.

Johnson-Delaney, C. & D. Reavill (2009). Toxicoses in Birds: Ante- and Postmortem Findings for Practitioners. Proceedings: AAV. accessed via Veterinary Information Network; vin.com

Oehme, F. W. (1987). LEad. *Current Therapy in Equine Medicine*. N. E. Robinson. Philadelphia, WB Saunders: 667-8.

Post, L. & W. Keller (2000). Current status of food animal antidotes. The Veterinary Clinics of North America: Food Animal Practice **16**:3(November).

Samour, J. & J. Naldo (2004). The use of Ca Na2 EDTA in the treatment of lead toxicosis in falcons. Proceedings: AAV. accessed via Veterinary Information Network; vin.com

Edrophonium Chloride

(ed-roe-foe-nee-um)   Tensilon®, Enlon®

Cholinergic (Anticholinesterase) Agent

Prescriber Highlights

▶ Short-acting parenteral quaternary ammonium cholinergic used primarily to test for myasthenia gravis.

▶ Secondary indications are to reverse nondepolarizing agents and to treat some SVT's.

▶ Relatively contraindicated: Asthma or mechanical urinary or intestinal tract obstruction.

▶ Caution: Bradycardias or atrioventricular block.

▶ Overdoses can cause cholinergic crisis.

Uses/Indications

The primary use for edrophonium is in the presumptive diagnosis of myasthenia gravis (MG). The so-called "Tensilon Test" for MG is not specific or sensitive and has limitations, but a dramatic positive response is suggestive of MG. Both false-positive and false-negative results can occur, therefore it is best to use while awaiting results from a more specific, sensitive test such as the acetylcholine receptor antibody test.

Edrophonium can also be used for the reversal of nondepolarizing agents (*e.g.*, pancuronium, metocurine, atracurium, rocuronium or tubocurarine). Because of its short duration of action, its clinical usefulness for this indication is questionable as longer acting drugs such as neostigmine or pyridostigmine may be more useful. Edrophonium does not appear to reverse vecuronium-induced neuromuscular blockade very efficiently (Martin-Flores et al. 2011).

Edrophonium, in a controlled intensive care-type setting, may also be useful in the diagnosis and treatment of some supraventricular arrhythmias, particularly when other more traditional treatments are ineffective.

Pharmacology/Actions

Edrophonium is an anticholinesterase agent that is very short acting. It briefly attaches to acetylcholinesterase thereby inhibiting its hydrolytic activity on acetylcholine. As acetylcholine accumulates, the following clinical signs may be noted: miosis, increased skeletal and intestinal muscle tone, bronchoconstriction, ureter constriction, salivation, sweating (in animals with sweat glands), and bradycardia.

Pharmacokinetics

Edrophonium is only effective when given parenterally. After IV administration, it begins to have effects on skeletal muscle within one minute and effects may persist for up to 10 minutes. Myasthenic patients may have effects persisting longer after the first dose. Edrophonium's exact metabolic fate and excretion characteristics have not been well described.

Contraindications/Precautions/Warnings

Edrophonium is considered relatively contraindicated in patients with bronchial asthma, or mechanical urinary or intestinal tract obstruction. It should be used with caution (with adequate monitoring and treatment available) in patients with bradycardias or atrioventricular block. Some human patients are documented to be hypersensitive to the drug and exhibit severe cholinergic reactions.

It is recommended to have IV atropine and an endotracheal tube readily available before administering edrophonium.

Adverse Effects

Adverse effects associated with edrophonium are generally dose related and cholinergic in nature (urination, lacrimation, vomiting, defecation, bradycardia, bronchospasm). Although usually mild and easily treated with a "tincture of time", pre-treatment or treatment with an anticholinergic drug (e.g., atropine) can help prevent or alleviate these effects. Severe adverse effects are possible with large overdoses (see below).

Reproductive/Nursing Safety

Edrophonium's safety profile during pregnancy is not established; use only when necessary. While no problems have been documented in nursing humans or animals, its safety has not been established. In humans, the FDA categorizes this drug as category *C* for use during pregnancy (*Animal studies have shown an adverse effect on the fetus, but there are no adequate studies in humans; or there are no animal reproduction studies and no adequate studies in humans.*)

It is unknown whether edrophonium enters maternal milk.

Overdosage/Acute Toxicity

Overdosage of edrophonium may induce a cholinergic crisis. Clinical signs of cholinergic toxicity can include: GI effects (nausea, vomiting, diarrhea), salivation, sweating (in animals able to do so), respiratory effects (increased bronchial secretions, bronchospasm, pulmonary edema, respiratory paralysis), ophthalmic effects (miosis, blurred vision, lacrimation), cardiovascular effects (bradycardia or tachycardia, cardiospasm, hypotension, cardiac arrest), muscle cramps and weakness.

Treatment of edrophonium overdose consists of both respiratory and cardiac supportive therapy and, atropine, if necessary. Refer to the atropine monograph for more information on its use for cholinergic toxicity.

Drug Interactions

The following drug interactions have either been reported or are theoretical in humans or animals receiving edrophonium and may be of significance in veterinary patients. Unless otherwise noted, use together is not necessarily contraindicated, but weigh the potential risks and perform additional monitoring when appropriate.

- **ATROPINE:** Atropine will antagonize the muscarinic effects of edrophonium. While some clinicians routinely use the two together, caution is advised as atropine can mask the early clinical signs of cholinergic crisis.
- **DEXPANTHENOL:** Theoretically, dexpanthenol may have additive effects when used with edrophonium.
- **DIGOXIN:** Edrophonium's cardiac effects may be increased in patients receiving digoxin; excessive slowing of heart rate may occur.

- **MUSCLE RELAXANTS:** Edrophonium may prolong the Phase I block of depolarizing muscle relaxants (*e.g.*, **succinylcholine, decamethonium**) and edrophonium antagonizes the actions of non-depolarizing neuromuscular blocking agents (*e.g.*, **pancuronium, tubocurarine, gallamine, vecuronium, atracurium**, etc.).

Doses

- **DOGS:**

  For presumptive diagnosis of myasthenia gravis (MG); see limitations in Uses/Indications; (extra-label): This test is easiest to assess in patients with the generalized form of MG; those that tire with exercise. The patient is gently exercised until fatigued. Place indwelling catheter. Edrophonium dose is 0.1 – 0.2 mg/kg IV. (Have atropine drawn up so that if cholinergic signs (SLUD) develop, it can be given at 0.02 – 0.04 mg/kg IV). The catheter is flushed with sterile saline, and then the patient is immediately lightly exercised, or if non-ambulatory, encouraged to rise. In patients with focal MG such as facial muscle weakness, the palpebral reflex may be assessed after IV edrophonium. Patients are assessed as having a positive or negative "Tensilon Test". (Vernau 2009); (Khorzad et al. 2011)

- **CATS:**

  For presumptive diagnosis of myasthenia gravis (MG); (extra-label): This test is easiest to assess in patients with the generalized form of MG; those that tire with exercise. The patient is gently exercised until fatigued. Place indwelling catheter. Edrophonium dose is 0.25 – 0.5 mg (per cat) IV. (Have atropine drawn up so that if cholinergic signs (SLUD) develop, it can be given at 0.02 – 0.04 mg/kg IV). The catheter is flushed with sterile saline and then the patient is immediately lightly exercised, or if non-ambulatory, encouraged to rise. In patients with focal MG such as facial muscle weakness, the palpebral reflex may be assessed after IV edrophonium. Patients are assessed as having a positive or negative "Tensilon Test". (Vernau 2009)

- **HORSES:**

  To help reverse neuromuscular block from atracurium or rocuronium (extra-label): Doses of edrophonium ranging between 0.1 – 0.5 mg/kg have been commonly used in horses, but because edrophonium (and neostigmine) can increase the levels of acetylcholine, parasympathetic tone may increase; bradycardia and bronchospasm and increased salivation can occur. Slow administration and low doses help to prevent this problem. (Martin-Flores 2013)

Monitoring

- Cholinergic adverse effects.
- Improvement (for 1-15 minutes) of paresis for presumptive diagnosis of MG.

Client Information

- Edrophonium is a drug that should be used in a controlled clinical setting.
- Clients should be briefed on the side effects that can occur with its use. It is used only in an inpatient setting.

Chemistry/Synonyms

A synthetic quaternary ammonium cholinergic (parasympathomimetic) agent, edrophonium chloride occurs as a white crystalline powder having a bitter taste. Approximately 2 grams are soluble in 1 mL of water. The injection has a pH of approximately 5.4.

Edrophonium chloride may also be known as: edrophonii chloridum, *Anticude®*, *Camsilon®*, *Enlon®*, *Reversol®*, or *Tensilon®*.

Storage/Stability

Edrophonium chloride injection should be stored at room temperature.

Compatibility/Compounding Considerations

Edrophonium is reportedly physically **compatible** at Y-site injections with heparin sodium, hydrocortisone sodium succinate, potassium chloride and vitamin B complex with C. Compatibility is dependent upon factors such as pH, concentration, temperature and diluent used; consult specialized references or a hospital pharmacist for more specific information.

Dosage Forms/Regulatory Status

VETERINARY-LABELED PRODUCTS: NONE.

HUMAN-LABELED PRODUCTS:

Edrophonium Chloride Solution for Injection: 10 mg/mL in 10 mL & 15 mL vials; *Enlon®*; (Rx)

Edrophonium Chloride/Atropine Sulfate for Injection: 10 mg/mL with 0.14 mg/mL atropine sulfate in 5 mL single-dose amps & 15 mL multi-dose vials; *Enlon-Plus®*; (Rx)

Revisions/References

Monograph revised/updated January 2014.

Khorzad, R., et al. (2011). Myasthenia gravis in dogs with an emphasis on treatment and critical care management. J. Vet. Emerg. Crit. Care **21**(3): 193-208.

Martin-Flores, M. (2013). Neuromuscular Blocking Agents and Monitoring in the Equine Patient. Veterinary Clinics of North America-Equine Practice **29**(1): 131-+.

Martin-Flores, M., et al. (2011). Failure to Reverse Prolonged Vecuronium-Induced Neuromuscular Blockade with Edrophonium in an Anesthetized Dog. J. Am. Anim. Hosp. Assoc. **47**(4): 294-8.

Vernau, K. (2009). Beyond Tensilon and Titers: Myasthenia Gravis. Veterinary Neurology Symposium; Univ. of Calif.-Davis. accessed via Veterinary Information Network; vin.com

EFA-Caps® – see Fatty Acids

Emodepside + Praziquantel

(ee-moe-dep-side + pra-zi-kwon-tel)   Profender®

Topical Antiparasitic (Nematocide; Cestocide)

Prescriber Highlights

▶ Topical cestocide & nematocide labeled for cats (in USA). Oral products for dogs may be available in other countries.

▶ Appears safe in cats >1 kg & at least 8 weeks old.

▶ Applied to back of cat's neck; do not allow patient or other cats to lick area of application for at least one hour.

Uses/Indications

Emodepside/Praziquantel topical solution (*Profender®*) is indicated for the treatment and control of hookworm infections caused by *Ancylostoma tubaeforme* (adults, immature adults, and fourth stage larvae), roundworm infections caused by *Toxocara cati* (adults and fourth stage larvae), and tapeworm infections caused by *Dipylidium caninum* (adults) and *Taenia taeniaeformis* (adults) in cats.

Topical *Profender®* may also be of use in an extra-label manner for treating other species (*e.g.*, reptiles) where oral dosing may be overly stressful.

There are also oral products available (not in USA at the time of writing) for use in dogs.

Pharmacology/Actions

Emodepside has a unique mode of action in comparison to other antiparasitic compounds. The drug attaches pre-synaptically at the neuromuscular junction to a latrophilin-like receptor, resulting in an increase in intracellular calcium and diacylglycerol levels. At the end of the signal transduction cascade, vesicles containing inhibitory neuropeptide fuse with pre-synaptic membranes. Inhibitory neuropeptides such as PF1- and/or PF2-like receptor are then released into the synaptic cleft, stimulating postsynaptic receptors and resulting in an inhibition of pharyngeal pumping and locomotion of the nematode. The end result is flaccid paralysis and death of the parasite.

Praziquantel's exact mechanism of action against cestodes has not been determined, but it may be the result of interacting with phospholipids in the integument causing ion fluxes of sodium, potassium and calcium. At low concentrations *in vitro*, the drug appears to impair the function of their suckers and stimulates the worm's motility. At higher concentrations *in vitro*, praziquantel increases the contraction (irreversibly at very high concentrations) of the worm's strobilla (chain of proglottids). In addition, praziquantel causes irreversible focal vacuolization with subsequent cestodal disintegration at specific sites of the cestodal integument.

Pharmacokinetics

Following dermal application of the product (*Profender®*) to cats, emodepside and praziquantel are absorbed through the skin and into the systemic circulation. Absorption of both active ingredients through the skin is relatively rapid, with serum concentrations detectable within 2 hours for emodepside and 1 hour for praziquantel. Peak concentrations occur within 6 hours for praziquantel and 2 days for emodepside. After a single application, both emodepside and praziquantel were detectable for up to 28 days following treatment.

A study looking at topical absorption in a variety of reptiles found variability in blood levels that was associated with skin thickness (Schilliger et al. 2009).

Contraindications/Precautions/Warnings

There are no absolute contraindications for use of this product on cats noted on the label. However, safe use has not been evaluated in cats: less than 8 weeks of age or weighing less than 2.2 lb. (1 kg), used for breeding, during pregnancy or in lactating queens. Use with caution in sick, debilitated, or heartworm positive cats.

Dogs with the *ABCB1* (MDR1) mutation (mutant/mutant) may be susceptible to emodepside toxicity (vomiting, mydriasis, ataxia, muscle tremors and seizures was reported) and it is advisable to test susceptible breeds before using emodepside-containing products (Hugnet 2012).

Adverse Effects

In pre-approval efficacy studies, the most common side effects observed were dermal- and gastrointestinal-related. In a field study, adverse reactions reported by cat owners included licking/excessive grooming (3%), scratching treatment site (2.5%), salivation (1.7%), lethargy (1.7%), alopecia (1.3%), agitation/nervousness (1.2%), vomiting (1%), diarrhea (0.5%), eye irritation in 3 cats (0.5%), respiratory irritation (0.2%) and shaking/tremors (0.2%). All adverse reactions were self-limiting. The following adverse events were reported voluntarily during post-approval use of the product in foreign markets: application site reaction (hair loss, dermatitis, pyoderma, edema, and erythema), salivation, pruritus, lethargy, vomiting, diarrhea, dehydration, ataxia, loss of appetite, facial swelling, rear leg paralysis, seizures, hyperesthesia, twitching, and death. A case report of one cat developing a morphea-like (scleroderma) lesion after application has been reported (Seixas et al. 2009).

Reproductive/Nursing Safety

Safe use has not been evaluated in cats used for breeding, during pregnancy, or in lactating queens. Studies performed in laboratory animals (rats, rabbits) suggest that emodepside may interfere with fetal development in those species.

Overdosage/Acute Toxicity

Oral doses of emodepside of 200 mg/kg were tolerated by rats without mortalities. The oral LD50 in rats is >500 mg/kg; in mice >2,500 mg/kg. The acute dermal toxicity dose of emodepside in rats is high; a dose of 2,000 mg/kg was tolerated without mortality.

Praziquantel has a wide margin of safety. In rats and mice, the oral LD50 is at least 2 g/kg. An oral LD50 could not be determined in dogs, as at doses greater than 200 mg/kg, the drug induced vomiting. Parenteral doses of 50 – 100 mg/kg in cats caused transient ataxia and depression. Injected doses at 200 mg/kg were lethal in cats.

Kittens approximately 8 weeks of age were treated topically with the combination product up to 5X at 2-week intervals for treatments. Clinical signs of transient salivation and/or tremors were seen in a few animals in the 5X group, all of which were self-limiting.

Seven- to eight-month-old cats treated topically with the topical solution at 10X the labeled dose developed transient salivation, tremor, and lethargy.

Studies where the product was administered orally in cats have caused salivation, vomiting, anorexia, tremors, abnormal respirations, and ataxia. Adverse effects in all animals treated in these studies resolved without treatment.

Drug Interactions

No drug interactions have been documented for this product, but emodepside is reportedly a substrate for P-glycoprotein. Use with other drugs that are P-glycoprotein substrates or inhibitors (*e.g.*, **ivermectin, erythromycin, prednisolone, cyclosporine**) could cause pharmacokinetic drug interactions.

Doses

- **CATS:**

    For labeled indications (**certain species of hookworms, tapeworms, roundworms**); (FDA-approved): Minimum dose is 3 mg/kg emodepside & 12 mg/kg praziquantel applied to the skin on the back of the neck as a single topical dose. A second treatment should not be necessary. If re-infection occurs, the product can be re-applied after 30 days. (Label information; *Profender®*—Bayer)

- **DOGS:**

    For certain species of ascarids, whipworms, hookworms and tapeworms (extra-label in USA): 1 mg emodepside and 5 mg praziquantel/kg PO on an empty stomach once. (*Trichuris vulpis* being the dose-limiting species). In certain countries oral tablets are available for use in dogs. (Epe et al. 2013)

- **REPTILES:**

    Extra-label: Serum levels vary between species, but a dose of 4 drops/100 g body weight appears to be effective. Aquatic species must be kept in a dry place for 48 hours after treatment. Caution is advised until further studies verify safety and efficacy, particularly in sick animals. (Schilliger et al. 2009)

Monitoring

- Clinical efficacy.

Client Information

- Topical (spot-on) for treating hookworms, roundworms and tapeworms in cats. Applied once. May re-treat in 30 days if re-infected.
- Very well tolerated.
- Do not apply to broken skin or if hair coat is wet.
- Do not get in the cat's mouth or eyes or allow the cat to lick the application site for one hour. Oral exposure can cause salivation and vomiting; treatment at the base of the head will minimize the opportunity for ingestion while grooming.
- In households with multiple pets, keep animals separated to prevent licking of the application site.
- Not for human use. Keep out of reach of children. To prevent accidental ingestion of the product, children should not come in contact with the application site for 24 hours while the product is being absorbed. Pregnant women or women who may become pregnant should avoid direct contact with, or wear disposable gloves when applying, this product.

Chemistry/Synonyms

Emodepside is an N-methylated 24-membered cyclooctadepsipeptide, consisting of four alternating residues of N-methyl-L-leucine, two residues of D-lactate, and two residues of D-phenylacetate.

Praziquantel occurs as a white to practically white, hygroscopic, bitter tasting, crystalline powder, either odorless or having a faint odor. It is very slightly soluble in water and freely soluble in alcohol.

Praziquantel may also be known as: EMBAY-8440, or praziquantelum.

Storage/Stability

Store product at or below 25°C (77°F); do not allow to freeze.

Compatibility/Compounding Considerations

No specific information noted.

Dosage Forms/Regulatory Status

VETERINARY-LABELED PRODUCTS:

Emodepside (1.98% w/w; 21.4 mg/mL) and Praziquantel (7.94% w/w; 85.8 mg/mL) Topical Solution in 0.35 mL (cats 2.2-5.5 lb.), 0.7 mL (cats >5.5-11 lb.) & 1.12 mL (cats >11-17.6 lb.) tubes: *Profender®*, (Rx). FDA-approved for use on cats.

An oral product for dogs, *Profender® for Dogs* is available in many countries, but is not currently FDA-approved in the USA. A combination oral suspension for dogs and cats containing emodepside and toltrazuril (*Procox®*) is also available in some markets. (Petry et al. 2013)

HUMAN-LABELED PRODUCTS: NONE.

Revisions/References

Monograph revised/updated January 2014.

Epe, C. & R. Kaminsky (2013). New advancement in anthelmintic drugs in veterinary medicine. Trends in Parasitology 29(3): 129-34.

Hugnet, C. (2012). Emodepside Sensitivity in German Shepherd Dog is Associated with Deletion Mutation of the MDR1 Gene. 22nd ECVIM-CA Congress. accessed via Veterinary Information Network; vin.com

Petry, G., et al. (2013). Efficacy of Emodepside plus Toltrazuril Oral Suspension for Dogs (Procox(A (R)), Bayer) against Trichuris vulpis in Naturally Infected Dogs. Parasitology Research 112(1): 133-8.

Schilliger, L., et al. (2009). Absorption and efficacy of a spot-on combination containing emodepside plus praziquantel in reptiles. Revue De Medecine Veterinaire 160(12): 557-61.

Seixas, G. & P. Taboada (2009). Morphea-Like Lesion Following Topical Application of an Endectocide in a Cat. Proceedings: WSAVA. accessed via Veterinary Information Network; vin.com

Enalapril Maleate
Enalaprilat

(e-nal-a-pril)   Enacard®, Vasotec®

Angiotensin-Converting Enzyme (ACE) Inhibitor

Prescriber Highlights

▶ Veterinary & human ACE inhibitor used in the treatment of heart failure, proteinuria or hypertension; may also be of benefit in the treatment of chronic renal failure

▶ Caution: pregnancy, renal insufficiency (doses may need to be reduced), patients with hyponatremia, coronary or cerebrovascular insufficiency, preexisting hematologic abnormalities or a collagen vascular disease (*e.g.*, SLE).

▶ Adverse Effects: GI distress (anorexia, vomiting, diarrhea); Potentially: weakness, hypotension, renal dysfunction & hyperkalemia.

Uses/Indications

Use of enalapril in the adjunctive treatment of heart failure (CHF) in dogs and cats is somewhat controversial. While a product was approved for use in dogs and published studies have found benefits in dogs with CHF, concerns about those studies, coupled with a lack of prospective, controlled studies in cats have raised questions of enalapril's actual value in small animals with CHF. Despite these valid concerns and ongoing debate, ACE inhibitors continue to be used by many veterinary cardiologists for CHF in cats and in dogs with CHF secondary to both dilated cardiomyopathy and myxomatous mitral valve disease (MMVD).

ACE inhibitors can decrease efferent glomerular resistance, reduce proteinuria and have renoprotective effects. They are used for adjunctive treatment in idiopathic glomerulonephritis, chronic renal failure and protein losing nephropathies in small animals. There is stronger evidence for efficacy in dogs with protein-losing nephropathy (PLN) compared to animals with chronic kidney disease without severe PLN.

While ACE inhibitors are a mainstay for treating hypertension in humans, they have not been particularly useful when used alone in treating hypertension in cats, but can be effective in treating hypertension in dogs that have accompanying chronic kidney disease.

Pharmacology/Actions

Enalapril is converted in the liver to the active compound enalaprilat. Enalaprilat prevents the formation of angiotensin-II (a potent vasoconstrictor) by competing with angiotensin-I for the enzyme angiotensin-converting enzyme (ACE). ACE has a much higher affinity for enalaprilat than for angiotensin-I. Because angiotensin-II concentrations are decreased, aldosterone secretion is reduced and plasma renin activity is increased.

The cardiovascular effects of enalaprilat in patients with CHF include: decreased total peripheral resistance, pulmonary vascular resistance, mean arterial and right atrial pressures, and pulmonary capillary wedge pressure, no change or decrease in heart rate, and increased cardiac index and output, stroke volume, and exercise tolerance.

ACE inhibitors increase renal blood flow and decrease glomerular efferent arteriole resistance. In animals with glomerular disease, ACE inhibitors decrease proteinuria and may help to preserve renal function. Enalapril, at least partially blocks amlodipine's activation of the renin-angiotensin-aldosterone system (RAAS) in dogs (Atkins et al. 2007).

Pharmacokinetics

Enalapril/enalaprilat has different pharmacokinetic properties than captopril in dogs. It has a slower onset of action (4-6 hours) but a longer duration of action (12-14 hours). In dogs, approximately 95% of enalaprilat is cleared via renal routes and reduced renal function can impact elimination rates.

In humans, enalapril is well absorbed after oral administration, but enalaprilat is not. Approximately 60% of an oral dose is bioavailable. Both enalapril and enalaprilat are distributed poorly into the CNS and are distributed into milk in trace amounts. Enalaprilat crosses the placenta. In humans, the half-life of enalapril is about 2 hours; enalaprilat about 11 hours. Half-lives are increased in patients with renal failure or severe CHF.

Contraindications/Precautions/Warnings

Enalaprilat is contraindicated in patients that have demonstrated hypersensitivity to the ACE inhibitors. It should be used with caution and close supervision in patients with renal insufficiency and doses may need to be reduced. One recommendation for an empiric reduction of dosage in dogs and cats with renal failure is to start the daily dosage at 50% of the usual total daily dose of 0.5 mg/kg q12h when creatinine clearance is >0.4 mL/kg/min (roughly a serum creatine of >2.3 mg/dL in cats) (Trepanier 2013). Use of ACE inhibitors in critically ill patients in acute kidney injury (AKI) is generally not recommended because of their potential negative effects on glomerular filtration rate (GFR); patients should be stable after recovery from AKI before receiving them.

Enalaprilat should also be used with caution in patients with hyponatremia or sodium depletion, coronary or cerebrovascular insufficiency, preexisting hematologic abnormalities, or a collagen vascular disease (e.g., SLE). Patients with severe CHF should be monitored very closely upon initiation of therapy.

Adverse Effects

Enalapril/enalaprilat's adverse effect profile in dogs is principally GI distress (anorexia, vomiting, diarrhea). Potentially, weakness, hypotension, renal dysfunction and hyperkalemia could occur. Because it lacks a sulfhydryl group (unlike captopril), there is less likelihood that immune-mediated reactions will occur, but rashes, neutropenia, and agranulocytosis have been reported in humans. In humans, ACE inhibitors commonly cause coughs, but this occurs rarely in dogs or cats.

Adverse effects associated with enalapril in cats include lethargy and inappetence.

Reproductive/Nursing Safety

Enalapril crosses the placenta and the human label has a "black box" warning to discontinue enalapril as soon as possible when pregnancy is detected. High doses in rodents have caused decreased fetal weights and increases in fetal and maternal death rates; teratogenic effects have not been reported. In humans, the FDA categorizes this drug as category C for use during pregnancy in the first trimester (*Animal studies have shown an adverse effect on the fetus, but there are no adequate studies in humans; or there are no animal reproduction studies and no adequate studies in humans.*) In humans, the FDA categorizes this drug as category D for use during pregnancy in second and third trimesters (*There is evidence of human fetal risk, but the potential benefits from the use of the drug in pregnant women may be acceptable despite its potential risks.*) as ACE inhibitors may cause abnormal fetal and postnatal kidney development.

Enalapril/enalaprilat is excreted into milk. Safe use during nursing cannot be assumed.

Overdosage/Acute Toxicity

In dogs, a dose of 200 mg/kg was lethal, but 100 mg/kg was not. In overdose situations, the primary concern is hypotension; supportive treatment with volume expansion with normal saline is recommended to correct blood pressure. Because of the drug's long duration of action, prolonged monitoring and treatment may be required. Recent overdoses should be managed by using gut emptying protocols when warranted.

Drug Interactions

The following drug interactions have either been reported or are theoretical in humans or animals receiving enalaprilat and may be of significance in veterinary patients. Unless otherwise noted, use together is not necessarily contraindicated, but weigh the potential risks and perform additional monitoring when appropriate.

- **ANTIDIABETIC AGENTS (insulin, oral agents):** Possible increased risk for hypoglycemia; enhanced monitoring recommended.
- **DIURETICS** (e.g., **furosemide, hydrochlorothiazide**): Potential for increased hypotensive effects; some veterinary clinicians recommend reducing furosemide doses (by 25-50%) when adding enalapril or benazepril to therapy in CHF.
- **DIURETICS, POTASSIUM-SPARING** (e.g., **spironolactone, triamterene**): Increased hyperkalemic effects, enhanced monitoring of serum potassium recommended.

- **HYPOTENSIVE AGENTS, OTHER:** Potential for increased hypotensive effect.
- **LITHIUM:** Increased serum lithium levels possible; increased monitoring required.
- **NSAIDS:** May reduce the anti-hypertensive or positive hemodynamic effects of enalapril; may increase risk for reduced renal function, but clinical significance has not been demonstrated in dogs receiving enalapril and an NSAID.
- **POTASSIUM SUPPLEMENTS:** Increased risk for hyperkalemia.

Laboratory Considerations

- When using iodohippurate sodium I^{123}/I^{134} or Technetium Tc^{99} pententate **renal imaging** in patients with renal artery stenosis, ACE inhibitors may cause a reversible decrease in localization and excretion of these agents in the affected kidney that may lead to confusion in test interpretation.

Doses

- **DOGS:**

For adjunctive treatment of heart failure: Most cardiologists recommend 0.5 mg/kg PO twice daily. However, labeled dosage is 0.5 mg/kg once daily initially with or without food; if response is inadequate, increase to 0.5 mg/kg twice daily (Package Insert; *Enacard®*).

For adjunctive treatment of proteinuria (extra-label): The therapeutic goal is to reduce the urine protein:creatinine ratio by at least half or ideally, into the normal range. Dosages vary somewhat but usually fall into a range from 0.25 – 1 mg/kg PO q12-24h. Most initially will treat at approximately 0.5 mg/kg PO q12h if cat is not azotemic. Laboratory guidelines for serum creatinine "cut-offs" for an initial lower dosage (0.25 mg/kg PO q12h) vary by the reference but a rough guide is approximately 3 mg/dL. If azotemia has not worsened after 7 days, dosage is then increased with continued monitoring. Regardless of initial dosage serum creatinine should be measured before and 1-2 weeks after initiating therapy. Large or progressive increases in serum creatinine should prompt reassessment of therapy. One recommendation is that if serum creatinine increases by more than 0.2 mg/dL, a decrease in dosage should be made. Dosage of ACE inhibitors should be cautiously increased to maximize impact on proteinuria. Serum potassium should be monitored as hyperkalemia or anorexia may limit dosage increases. Higher dosages (*e.g.*, 2 mg/kg/day) may reduce progression of chronic kidney disease in dogs. Adapted from: (Polzin 2013), (Bartges 2012), (Littman 2011)

For systemic hypertension in dogs with chronic kidney disease (extra-label): Initially 0.5 mg/kg PO q12h. If not effective, dosage is increased as tolerated to 1 mg/kg PO q12h if necessary.

- **CATS:**

For adjunctive treatment of heart failure due to hypertrophic cardiomyopathy (extra-label): 0.25 – 0.5 mg/kg PO once daily. This is practically given as 1.25 – 2.5 mg per cat PO once a day.

For adjunctive treatment of proteinuria (extra-label): The therapeutic goal is to reduce the urine protein:creatinine ratio by at least half or, ideally, into the normal range. Dosages vary somewhat but usually fall into a range from 0.25 – 0.5 mg/kg PO q12-24h. Most initially will treat at approximately 0.25 mg/kg PO q12h if cat is not azotemic. Laboratory guidelines for serum creatinine "cut-offs" for an initial lower dosage (0.25 mg/kg PO q24h) vary by the reference but a rough guide is approximately 2.5 – 3 mg/dL. If azotemia has not worsened after 7 days, dosage is then increased with continued monitoring. Regardless of initial dosage serum creatinine should be measured before and 1-2

weeks after initiating therapy. Large or progressive increases in serum creatinine should prompt reassessment of therapy. One recommendation is that if serum creatinine increases by more than 0.2 mg/dL, a decrease in dosage should be made. Dosage of ACE inhibitors should be cautiously increased to maximize impact on proteinuria. Serum potassium should be monitored as hyperkalemia or anorexia may limit dosage increases. Adapted from: (Polzin 2013), (Bartges 2012), (Littman 2011)

For systemic hypertension (extra-label): Most recommend using amlodipine as the first-line agent, but in cats that do not have BP controlled with amlodipine alone or in those with concurrent proteinuria, then enalapril can be added at 0.25 – 0.5 mg/kg PO q12-24h; this may practically be administered as 0.625 mg per cat PO q24h (if cat is greater than 6 kg, then 1.25 mg/cat q24h). Monitor renal function.

- **FERRETS:**

For adjunctive therapy for heart failure (extra-label):

a) 0.5 mg/kg PO once every other day (q48h) initially and may be increased to once a day if tolerated. Dissolve tablet(s) in distilled water and add a methylcellulose suspending agent (*e.g.*, *Ora-Plus®*) and cherry syrup for flavor. (Hoeffer 2000)

b) For dilative cardiomyopathy: 0.25 – 0.5 mg/kg PO once a day to every other day. (Williams 2000)

- **BIRDS:**

For adjunctive therapy for heart failure (extra-label):

a) 1.25 mg/kg PO 2-3 times daily. (Pees et al. 2006)

b) 0.25 – 0.5 mg/kg PO q24-48h with furosemide. (Oglesbee 2009)

Monitoring

- Clinical signs of CHF.
- Serum electrolytes, creatinine, BUN, urine protein.
- CBC with differential, periodic.
- Blood pressure (if treating hypertension or clinical signs associated with hypotension arise).

Client Information

- Enalapril is used to treat heart failure, high blood pressure and some forms of kidney disease in dogs and cats.
- Usually well tolerated, but vomiting and diarrhea can occur. May be given with or without food. If your animal vomits, stops eating, or acts sick after getting it on an empty stomach, give with food or small treat to see if this helps. If vomiting continues, contact your veterinarian.
- If a rash or signs of infection occur (*e.g.*, fever) contact your veterinarian immediately.
- Very important to give as prescribed. Do not stop or reduce dosage without veterinarian's guidance.
- Your animal will likely need to have blood pressure and lab tests performed.

Chemistry/Synonyms

Angiotensin-converting enzyme (ACE) inhibitors, enalapril maleate and enalaprilat are structurally related to captopril. Enalapril is a prodrug and is converted *in vivo* by the liver to enalaprilat. Enalapril maleate occurs as a white to off white crystalline powder. 25 mg are soluble in one mL of water. Enalaprilat occurs as a white to off white crystalline powder and is slightly soluble in water.

Enalapril maleate may also be known as: enalaprili maleas, and MK-421; many trade names are available. Enalaprilat may also be known as: enalaprilic acid, MK-422, *Enacard®*, *Glioten®*, *Lotrial®*, *Pres®*, *Renitec®*, *Reniten®*, *Vasotec®*, and *Xanef®*.

Storage/Stability

The commercially available tablets should be stored at temperatures less than 30°C in tight containers. When stored properly, the tablets have an expiration date of 30 months after manufacture.

Enalaprilat injection should be stored at temperatures less than 30°C. After dilution with D5W, normal saline, or D5 in lactated Ringer's it is stable for up to 24 hours at room temperature.

Compatibility/Compounding Considerations

Enalaprilat has been documented to be physically **incompatible** with amphotericin B or phenytoin sodium. Many other medications have been noted to be compatible with enalaprilat at various concentrations. Compatibility is dependent upon factors such as pH, concentration, temperature and diluent used; consult specialized references or a hospital pharmacist for more specific information.

Compounded preparation stability: Enalapril oral suspension compounded from commercially available tablets has been published (Allen et al. 1998). Triturating six (6) enalapril 20 mg tablets with 60 mL of *Ora-Plus®* and *qs ad* to 120 mL with *Ora-Sweet®* (or *Ora-Sweet® SF*) yields a 1 mg/mL oral suspension that retains >90% potency for 60 days stored at both 5°C and 25°C. Degradation of enalapril is pH dependent with maximum stability at pH 3 and increased decomposition above pH 5. Compounded preparations of enalapril should be protected from light.

Dosage Forms/Regulatory Status

VETERINARY-LABELED PRODUCTS:

Enalapril Maleate Tablets: 1 mg, 2.5 mg, 5 mg, 10 mg, & 20 mg; *Enacard®*; (Rx). FDA-approved for use in dogs. While this product is still listed as approved on FDA's "Green book", it may no longer be marketed in the USA.

The ARCI (Racing Commissioners International) has designated this drug as a class 3 substance. See the appendix for more information.

HUMAN-LABELED PRODUCTS:

Enalapril Maleate Tablets: 2.5 mg, 5 mg, 10 mg & 20 mg; *Vasotec®*, generic; (Rx).

Enalaprilat Injection: (for IV use) equivalent to 1.25 mg/mL in 1 mL & 2 mL vials; generic; (Rx)

Revisions/References

Monograph revised/updated January 2014.

Allen, L. V. & M. A. Erickson (1998). Stability of alprazolam, chloroquine phosphate, cisapride, enalapril maleate, and hydralazine hydrochloride in extemporaneously compounded oral liquids. Am J Health Syst Pharm 55(18): 1915-20.

Atkins, C. E., et al. (2007). The effect of amlodipine and the combination of amlodipine and enalapril on the renin-angiotensin-aldosterone system in the dog. J. Vet. Pharmacol. Ther. 30(5): 394-400.

Bartges, J. W. (2012). Chronic Kidney Disease in Dogs and Cats. Veterinary Clinics of North America-Small Animal Practice 42(4): 669-+.

Hoeffer, H. (2000). Heart Disease in Ferrets. *Kirk's Current Veterinary Therapy: XIII Small Animal Practice*. J. Bonagura. Philadelphia, WB Saunders: 1144-8.

Littman, M. P. (2011). Protein-losing Nephropathy in Small Animals. Veterinary Clinics of North America-Small Animal Practice 41(1): 31-+.

Oglesbee, B. (2009). Working up the pet bird with lower respiratory tract disorders. Proceedings: WVC. accessed via Veterinary Information Network; vin.com

Pees, M., et al. (2006). Bioavailability and compatibility of enalapril in birds. Proceedings: AAV. accessed via Veterinary Information Network; vin.com

Polzin, D. J. (2013). Evidence-based step-wise approach to managing chronic kidney disease in dogs and cats. J. Vet. Emerg. Crit. Care 23(2): 205-15.

Trepanier, L. A. (2013). Applying Pharmacokinetics to Veterinary Clinical Practice. Veterinary Clinics of North America-Small Animal Practice 43(5): 1013-+.

Williams, B. (2000). Therapeutics in Ferrets. Vet Clin NA: Exotic Anim Pract 3:1(Jan): 131-53.

Enoxaparin Sodium

(en-ocks-a-par-in)   Lovenox®

Anticoagulant

Prescriber Highlights

▶ Low molecular weight (fractionated) heparin that may be useful for treatment or prophylaxis of thromboembolic disease.

▶ Preferentially inhibits factor Xa & only minimally impacts thrombin & clotting time (TT or aPTT).

▶ Hemorrhage unlikely, but possible.

▶ Must be given subcutaneously; fair amount of uncertainty about effective dosing requirements for dogs or cats.

▶ Expense may be a significant issue, particularly in large dogs or horses. Generic forms are now available.

Uses/Indications

Enoxaparin may be useful for prophylaxis or treatment of thromboembolic disease, including in dogs with primary immune-mediate hemolytic anemia. However for dogs and cats, at the time of writing (January 2014) there is very little published science to support its use and it is still not known if it is safe, effective, and can be practically and economically administered. In humans, enoxaparin is also indicated for prevention of ischemic complications associated with unstable angina/non Q-wave MI.

Pharmacology/Actions

By binding to and accelerating antithrombin III, low molecular weight heparins (LMWHs) enhance the inhibition of factor Xa and thrombin. The potential advantage to using these products over standard (unfractionated) heparin is that they preferentially inhibit factor Xa and only minimally impact thrombin and clotting times (TT or aPTT). Recent work in cats (Van De Wiele et al. 2010), has suggested that anti-Xa activity may not be an accurate determiner for predicting antithrombotic activity and there may not be an association between the pharmacokinetics and pharmacodynamics *in vivo*.

Pharmacokinetics

It is unclear if enoxaparin's pharmacokinetics directly relate to its antithrombotic actions in animals. In dogs after SC administration, enoxaparin has a shorter duration of anti-Xa activity than in humans and probably must be dosed more frequently. A study examining enoxaparin dose response (anti-Xa activity) in dogs, showed that an enoxaparin dose of 0.8 mg/kg SC q6h would be required to effectively and consistently inhibit factor Xa activity in dogs (Lunsford et al. 2009).

Cats appear to have a much shorter duration of activity (anti-Xa) associated with LMWHs than do humans and to maintain a therapeutic target of anti-XA activity of 0.5 – 1 IU/mL requires 1.5 mg/kg SC q6h dosing of enoxaparin (Alwood et al. 2007). However, a recently published study (Van De Wiele et al. 2010) has suggested that anti-Xa activity may not be an accurate determiner for antithrombotic activity of enoxaparin in cats. In their venous stasis model, antithrombotic activity persisted well beyond the time after anti-Xa levels were below what are thought to be therapeutic.

After subcutaneous injection in humans, enoxaparin is absorbed rapidly, with a bioavailability of about 92%; peak plasma levels (activity) occur in 3-5 hours. Anti-factor Xa activity persists for up to 24 hours; doses are usually given once to twice a day. Enoxaparin is metabolized in the liver and excreted in the urine as both unchanged drug and metabolites; elimination half-life is about 4-5 hours.

Contraindications/Precautions/Warnings

Enoxaparin is contraindicated in patients that are hypersensitive to it, other LMWHs, heparin, or porcine products. Use enoxaparin cautiously in patients with significant renal dysfunction as drug accumulation could result.

Do **not** administer via IM or IV routes; enoxaparin must be given via deep subcutaneous injection only. Enoxaparin cannot be used interchangeably with other LMWHs or heparin sodium because the dosages differ for each.

Adverse Effects

In humans, adverse effects do not routinely occur; hemorrhage is a possibility and has been reported in up to 13% of patients in one study. Injection site hematoma, anemia, thrombocytopenia, nausea, and fever have also been reported.

Reproductive/Nursing Safety

In humans, enoxaparin is designated by the FDA as a category *B* drug (*Animal studies have not demonstrated risk to the fetus, but there are no adequate studies in pregnant women; or animal studies have shown an adverse effect, but adequate studies in pregnant women have not demonstrated a risk to the fetus during the first trimester of pregnancy, and there is no evidence of risk in later trimesters.*)

Overdosage/Acute Toxicity

Overdosage may lead to hemorrhagic complications. If treatment is necessary, protamine sulfate may be administered via slow IV. One mg of protamine sulfate can inhibit the effects of one mg of enoxaparin.

Drug Interactions

The following drug interactions have either been reported or are theoretical in humans or animals receiving enoxaparin and may be of significance in veterinary patients. Unless otherwise noted, use together is not necessarily contraindicated, but weigh the potential risks and perform additional monitoring when appropriate.

- **ANTICOAGULANTS, ORAL (warfarin):** Increased risk for hemorrhage.
- **PLATELET-AGGREGATION INHIBITORS (aspirin, clopidogrel):** Increased risk for hemorrhage.
- **THROMBOLYTIC AGENTS:** Increased risk for hemorrhage.

Laboratory Considerations

Low molecular weight heparins may cause asymptomatic, fully reversible increases in **AST** or **ALT**; bilirubin is only rarely increased in these patients. Therefore, interpret these tests with caution; increased values do not necessarily indicate hepatic damage or dysfunction.

Doses

- **DOGS:**

  As an antithrombotic agent (extra-label): At present, there is no substantial evidence to support any dosage, but based upon pharmacokinetic and anti-Xa activity in dogs, doses of 0.8 – 1 mg/kg SC q6-8h have been noted.

- **CATS:**

  As an antithrombotic (extra-label): An effective dose is not known at present. Some maintain that the previous recommendation of 1.25 mg/kg SC q6h is not necessary and that 1 mg/kg SC q12h for treatment and 1.5 mg/kg q24h for prophylaxis is sufficient. At the time of writing (January 2014) there is not does not appear to be convincing evidence to support any dosage.

- **HORSES:**

  As an antithrombotic (extra-label): No published dosage recommendations were located and the drug's expense is problematic. A study (Schwarzwald et al. 2002) investigating the pharmacokinetic variables of enoxaparin in horses demonstrated that the drug has similar activity (effect, duration) as in humans and the once daily SC injections may be useful for anticoagulant therapy.

Monitoring

- CBC (with platelet count); baseline and ongoing during therapy.
- Urinalysis.
- Stool occult blood test.
- Routine coagulation tests (aPTT, PT) are usually insensitive measures of activity and usually not warranted.
- Factor Xa activity (available at Cornell Coagulation Laboratory) may be useful, particularly if bleeding occurs or patient has renal dysfunction.

Client Information

- Must be injected subcutaneously (SC, under the skin); be sure you understand how to properly give the shots. Several shots a day may be required and treatment may be very expensive. Shots may be painful.
- Bleeding is not likely, but can occur. Contact your veterinarian immediately if it happens.
- If your animal is very listless (lacking energy or interest in things), appears to be having trouble breathing, trouble walking or loses the use of its rear legs, contact your veterinarian immediately as it may mean clots have formed.

Chemistry/Synonyms

A low molecular weight heparin (LMWH), enoxaparin sodium is obtained by alkaline depolymerization of heparin derived from pork intestinal mucosa. The average molecular weight is about 4500 and ranges from 3500-5500 (heparin sodium has a molecular weight around 12,000). 1 mg of enoxaparin is equivalent to 100 Units of anti-factor Xa.

Enoxaparin sodium may also be known as: Enoxaparinum natricum, PK-10169, RP-54563, *Clexane®*, *Decipar®*, *Klexane®*, *Lovenox®*, *Plaucina®*, and *Trombenox®*.

Storage/Stability

The commercially available injection should be stored at room temperature (25°C, 77°F); excursions permitted to 15-30°C (59-86°F).

One study showed that diluting 100 mg/mL commercially available solution with sterile water to 20 mg/mL was stable for 4 weeks when stored in a glass vial or in plastic syringes at room temperature or refrigerated. (Dager et al. 2004)

Compatibility/Compounding Considerations

No specific information noted.

Dosage Forms/Regulatory Status

VETERINARY-LABELED PRODUCTS: NONE.

HUMAN-LABELED PRODUCTS:

Enoxaparin Sodium for Injection: 30 mg/0.3 mL, 40 mg/0.4 mL, 60 mg/0.6 mL, 80 mg/0.8 mL, 100 mg/1 mL, 120 mg/0.8 mL, & 150 mg/1 mL preservative free in single-dose prefilled syringes; 300 mg/3 mL containing 15 mg/mL benzyl alcohol in 3 mL multi-dose vials; *Lovenox®*, generic; (Rx)

Revisions/References

Monograph revised/updated January 2014.

Alwood, A., et al. (2007). Anticoagulant effects of low -molecular weight heparins in healthy cats. J Vet Intern Med **21**(3): 378-87.

Dager, W., et al. (2004). AntiXa stability of enoxaparin for use in pediatrics. Ann Pharmacother **38**(4): 569-73.

Lunsford, K. V., et al. (2009). Pharmacokinetics of Subcutaneous Low Molecular Weight Heparin (Enoxaparin) in Dogs. J. Am. Anim. Hosp. Assoc. **45**(6): 261-7.

Schwarzwald, C., et al. (2002). Comparison of pharmacokinetic variables for two low-molecular-weight heparins after subcutaneous administration of a single dose to horses. Am J Vet Res **63**(Jun): 868-73.

Van De Wiele, C. M., et al. (2010). Antithrombotic Effect of Enoxaparin in Clinically Healthy Cats: A Venous Stasis Model. Journal of Veterinary Internal Medicine **24**(1): 185-91.

Enrofloxacin

(en-roe-flox-a-sin)   Baytril®

Fluoroquinolone Antibiotic

Prescriber Highlights

▶ Veterinary oral & injectable fluoroquinolone antibiotic effective against a variety of pathogens; not effective against anaerobes. In dogs, oral bioavailability is better than ciprofloxacin.

▶ Relatively contraindicated for young, growing animals due to cartilage abnormalities.

▶ Caution: Hepatic or renal insufficiency, dehydration.

▶ Higher doses (>5 mg/kg/day) not recommended in cats; may cause blindness.

▶ Adverse Effects: GI distress, CNS stimulation, crystalluria, or hypersensitivity; IV administration can potentially be very risky in small animals.

▶ Administer PO to dogs/cats preferably on an empty stomach (unless vomiting occurs).

▶ Drug interactions.

▶ FDA prohibits extra-label use in food animals. Should not be used in humans (CNS effects).

Uses/Indications

Enrofloxacin is FDA-approved for use in dogs and cats (oral only) for the management of diseases associated with bacteria susceptible to enrofloxacin. Because of the dosage restriction (5 mg/kg) for cats, enrofloxacin is generally used in this species only for the most susceptible bacterial infections. It is also FDA-approved for use in cattle (not dairy cattle or veal calves) and pigs, but extra-label use is prohibited in food animals.

Pharmacology/Actions

Enrofloxacin is a bactericidal agent. The bactericidal activity of enrofloxacin is concentration dependent, with susceptible bacteria cell death occurring within 20-30 minutes of exposure. Enrofloxacin has demonstrated a significant post-antibiotic effect for both gram-negative and -positive bacteria and is active in both stationary and growth phases of bacterial replication. In evaluating *in vitro* kill assays for enrofloxacin and its active metabolite, ciprofloxacin in dog and cat isolates of *Escherichia coli, Staphylococcus pseudintermedius* and *Pseudomonas aeruginosa*, an additive response (effect equal to the combined action of each of the drugs used separately) was observed (Blondeau et al. 2012).

Its mechanism of action is believed to act by inhibiting bacterial DNA-gyrase (a type-II topoisomerase), thereby preventing DNA supercoiling and DNA synthesis.

Both enrofloxacin and ciprofloxacin have similar spectrums of activity. These agents have good activity against many gram-negative bacilli and cocci, including most species and strains of *Pseudomonas aeruginosa, Klebsiella* spp., *E. coli,* Enterobacter, Campylobacter, Shigella, Salmonella, Aeromonas, Haemophilus, Proteus, Yersinia, Serratia, and Vibrio species. Other organisms that are generally susceptible include *Brucella* spp., *Chlamydia trachomatis,* Staphylococci (including penicillinase-producing and methicillin-resistant strains), Mycoplasma, and *Mycobacterium* spp. (not the etiologic agent for Johne's Disease).

The fluoroquinolones have variable activity against most streptococci and are not usually recommended for use in these infections. These drugs have weak activity against most anaerobes and are ineffective in treating anaerobic infections.

Bacterial resistance development is an ongoing concern, as many isolates of *Pseudomonas aeruginosa* are now resistant to enrofloxacin. *E. coli* resistance is becoming more prevalent. Resistance occurs by mutation, particularly with *Pseudomonas aeruginosa, Klebsiella pneumonia,* Acinetobacter and enterococci, but plasmid-mediated resistance is not thought to commonly occur.

Pharmacokinetics

Enrofloxacin is well absorbed after oral administration in most species. In dogs, enrofloxacin's bioavailability (approximately 80%) is about twice that of ciprofloxacin after oral dosing. Oral bioavailability in horses is between 60-80%. 50% of Cmax is reportedly attained within 15 minutes of dosing and peak levels (Cmax) occur within one hour of dosing. In sheep, enrofloxacin administered orally is about 65-75% bioavailable. The presence of food in the stomach generally delays the rate, but not the extent of absorption, but foods with increased divalent or trivalent cation concentrations such as milk, can reduce bioavailability.

Enrofloxacin is distributed throughout the body. Volume of distribution in dogs is approximately 3-4 L/kg. Only about 27% is bound to canine plasma proteins. Highest concentrations are found in the bile, kidney, liver, lungs, and reproductive system (including prostatic fluid and tissue). Enrofloxacin reportedly concentrates in macrophages. Therapeutic levels are also attained in bone, synovial fluid, skin, muscle, aqueous humor and pleural fluid. In hospitalized horses, volume of distribution was about 1.25 L/kg. After mechanical disruption of the blood-aqueous humor barrier (BAB) in horses, 7.5 mg/kg IV produced levels in the aqueous humor sufficient to treat *Leptospira pomona* (Divers et al. 2008). Low concentrations are found in the CSF; levels may only reach 6-10% of those found in the serum. In cattle, the volume of distribution is about 1.5 L/kg and in sheep, 0.4 L/kg.

Enrofloxacin is eliminated via both renal and non-renal mechanisms. Approximately 15-50% of the drug is eliminated unchanged into the urine, by both tubular secretion and glomerular filtration. Enrofloxacin is metabolized to various metabolites, most of which are less active than the parent compounds. Approximately 10-40% of circulating enrofloxacin is metabolized to ciprofloxacin in most species including humans, dogs, cats, adult horses, cattle, turtles, and snakes. Foals, pigs, and some lizards apparently do not convert much enrofloxacin, if any, to ciprofloxacin. These metabolites are eliminated both in the urine and feces. Because of the dual means of elimination (renal & hepatic), dogs with moderately impaired renal function may have slightly prolonged half-lives and higher serum levels, but not require any dosage adjustment. The approximate elimination half-lives in various species are: dogs 4-5 hours; cats 6 hours; sheep 1.5-4.5 hours; horses 5-10 hours, turtles 18 hours; and alligators 55 hours.

Contraindications/Precautions/Warnings

Enrofloxacin is labeled as contraindicated in small and medium breed dogs from 2-8 months of age. Bubble-like changes in articular cartilage have been noted when the drug was given at 2-5X recommend doses for 30 days, although clinical signs have only been seen at the 5X dose. To avoid cartilage damage, large and giant breed dogs may need to wait longer than the recommended 8 months before treatment since they may be in the rapid-growth phase past 8 months of age. Quinolones are contraindicated in patients hypersensitive to them.

Because ciprofloxacin has occasionally been reported to cause crystalluria in humans, animals should not be allowed to become dehydrated during therapy with either ciprofloxacin or enrofloxacin. Enrofloxacin may cause CNS stimulation and should be used with caution in patients with seizure disorders. Patients with severe renal or hepatic impairment may require dosage interval adjustments to prevent drug accumulation. Enrofloxacin is not recommended in cats with impaired renal function, secondary to an increased risk for retinotoxicity.

Use of the canine or bovine injectable products in cats or administered to dogs via other non-FDA-approved parenteral routes (IV, SC) is controversial and may result in significant adverse effects. Parenteral administration in cats at doses less than 5 mg/kg have reportedly caused ophthalmic toxicity (blindness). Because of the high pH (approx. 11) of the solution, subcutaneous administration in any species may cause pain and tissue damage. If administered rapidly or undiluted IV to dogs, there is an increased risk for cardiac arrhythmias, hypotension, vomiting, and mast cell degranulation (histamine and other mediator release).

The extra-label use in dogs of the IM 22.7 mg/mL (2.27%) product diluted 1:1 to 1:10 with sodium chloride 0.9% for slow IV administration (over at least 10 minutes; some give over 30-45 minutes) has anecdotally been described. However, the rapid absorption of enrofloxacin after IM administration in dogs (peak levels in about 30 minutes) questions the necessity of using this non-approved route (IV) of administration. Injectable enrofloxacin must not be mixed with, or come into contact with any IV solution containing magnesium (e.g., Normosol-R, Plasmalyte-R, -A, or –56); morbidity and mortality secondary to micro-precipitants lodging in patients' lungs have been reported. Dilution and extra-label use in small animals of the large animal product (100 mg/mL; 10%) via any route is discouraged.

Do not use in foals as they appear to be highly susceptible to the fluoroquinolone's arthropathic effects. Do not give rapidly IV to horses as ataxia and other neurologic effects may occur. IM injections are not recommended in horses as localized tissue reactions can occur. Intrauterine infusion of enrofloxacin is not suitable as it can cause serious tissue changes (endometrial ulceration, necrosis, fibrosis, inflammation and hemorrhage) (Rodriguez et al. 2012).

Extra-label use of fluoroquinolones is prohibited in animals to be used for food.

Enrofloxacin should not be used by humans; it may cause hallucinations, vivid dreams, and headache.

Adverse Effects

When used as labeled, the adverse effect profile of enrofloxacin is usually limited to GI distress (vomiting, anorexia). In dogs, rare incidences of elevated hepatic enzymes, ataxia, seizures, depression, lethargy, and nervousness have also been reported. Hypersensitivity reactions or crystalluria could potentially occur.

In cats, rare incidences of ocular toxicity have been reported characterized by mydriasis, retinal degeneration, and blindness. These effects were generally seen at higher dosage ranges (>15 mg/kg) and have necessitated a reduction in dosage recommendations in cats to a maximum of 5 mg/kg/day. Other rare adverse effects seen in cats can include: vomiting, anorexia, elevated hepatic enzymes, diarrhea, ataxia, seizures, depression/lethargy, vocalization, and aggression.

Articular cartilage abnormalities have been noted in young, rapidly growing animals (see Contraindications above).

While enrofloxacin has been implicated in causing antibiotic-associated diarrhea/enterocolitis in horses, due its poor activity against anaerobes, oral or parenterally administered enrofloxacin appears to carry a low risk of causing antibiotic-associated diarrhea.

Reproductive/Nursing Safety

The safety of enrofloxacin in pregnant dogs has been investigated. Breeding, pregnant, and lactating dogs receiving up to 15 mg/kg day demonstrated no treatment related effects. However, because of the risks of cartilage abnormalities in young animals, the fluoroquinolones are not generally recommended for use during pregnancy unless the benefits of therapy clearly outweigh the risks.

Limited studies in male dogs at various dosages have indicated no effects on male breeding performance.

Safety in breeding, pregnant, or lactating cats has not been established.

Overdosage/Acute Toxicity

It is unlikely an acute overdose in dogs with enrofloxacin would result in clinical signs more serious than either anorexia or vomiting, but the adverse effects noted above could occur. Dogs receiving 10X the labeled dosage rate of enrofloxacin for at least 14 days developed only vomiting and anorexia. Death occurred in some dogs when fed 25X the labeled rate for 11 days, however.

In cats overdoses can be serious (blindness, seizures); 20 mg/kg or more can cause retinopathy and blindness which can be irreversible.

There were 322 exposures to enrofloxacin reported to the ASPCA Animal Poison Control Center (APCC) during 2008-2009. In these cases 301 were dogs with 85 showing clinical signs and the remaining 21 cases were cats with 6 showing clinical signs. Common findings in dogs (recorded in decreasing frequency) include vomiting, lethargy, seizures, anorexia, depression, and diarrhea. Findings in cats (recorded in decreasing frequency) include seizures and recumbency.

Drug Interactions

The following drug interactions have either been reported or are theoretical in humans or animals receiving ciprofloxacin or enrofloxacin and may be of significance in veterinary patients. Unless otherwise noted, use together is not necessarily contraindicated, but weigh the potential risks and perform additional monitoring when appropriate.

- **ANTACIDS/DAIRY PRODUCTS**: Containing cations (Mg⁺⁺, Al⁺⁺⁺, Ca⁺⁺) may bind to enrofloxacin and prevent its absorption; separate doses of these products by at least 2 hours.
- **ANTIBIOTICS, OTHER (aminoglycosides, 3rd-generation cephalosporins, penicillins—extended-spectrum)**: Synergism may occur, but is not predictable against some bacteria (particularly Pseudomonas aeruginosa) with these compounds. Although enrofloxacin/ciprofloxacin has minimal activity against anaerobes, in vitro synergy has been reported when used with **clindamycin** against strains of Peptostreptococcus, Lactobacillus and Bacteroides fragilis.
- **CYCLOSPORINE**: Fluoroquinolones may exacerbate the nephrotoxicity and reduce the metabolism of cyclosporine (used systemically).
- **FLUNIXIN**: Has been shown in dogs to increase the AUC and elimination half-life of enrofloxacin and enrofloxacin increases the AUC and elimination half-life of flunixin; it is unknown if other NSAIDs interact with enrofloxacin in dogs.
- **GLYBURIDE**: Severe hypoglycemia possible.
- **IRON, ZINC (oral)**: Decreased enrofloxacin/ciprofloxacin absorption; separate doses by at least two hours.
- **METHOTREXATE**: Increased MTX levels possible with resultant toxicity.
- **NITROFURANTOIN**: May antagonize the antimicrobial activity of the fluoroquinolones and their concomitant use is not recommended.
- **PHENYTOIN**: Enrofloxacin/ciprofloxacin may alter phenytoin levels.
- **PROBENECID**: Blocks tubular secretion of ciprofloxacin and may increase its blood level and half-life.
- **QUINIDINE**: Increased risk for cardiotoxicity.
- **SUCRALFATE**: May inhibit absorption of enrofloxacin; separate doses of these drugs by at least 2 hours.

- **THEOPHYLLINE:** Enrofloxacin/ciprofloxacin may increase theophylline blood levels; in dogs theophylline levels may be increased by about 30-50% (Trepanier 2008).
- **WARFARIN:** Potential for increased warfarin effects.

Laboratory Considerations

- Enrofloxacin may cause false-positive **urine glucose** determinations when using cupric sulfate solution (Benedict's Solution, *Clinitest*®). Tests utilizing glucose oxidase (*Tes-Tape*®, *Clinistix*®) are not affected by enrofloxacin.
- In some human patients, the fluoroquinolones have caused increases in **liver enzymes, BUN,** and **creatinine** and decreases in **hematocrit.** The clinical relevance of these mild changes is not known at this time.

Doses

- **DOGS:**

For susceptible infections (labeled-dose; FDA-approved): 5 – 20 mg/kg per day PO, may be given once daily or divided and given twice daily (q12h). Treatment should continue for at least 2-3 days beyond cessation of clinical signs, to a maximum duration of therapy is 30 days. The injectable 22.7 mg/mL product dosage is labeled as 2.5 mg/kg IM once, followed by oral therapy (Adapted from label; *Baytril*®; *Baytril*® *Injection*).

Extra-label use of the 22.7 mg/mL injection: Has also been given at higher dosages 2.5 – 10 mg/kg q12h or 10 – 20 mg/kg q24h IM, SC (must be diluted in saline) or IV depending on the susceptibility and site of the infection. If using IV, the 22.7% injection is first diluted into sterile saline (0.9% sodium chloride) at approximately 10X of the volume of the enrofloxacin. It then is infused slowly IV (over at least 10 minutes and preferably over 30-45 minutes). Dogs may vomit after receiving the drug IV. Do not mix with other drugs or with other IV fluids containing calcium, magnesium, etc. The 100 mg/mL large animal injectable product is not recommended (see Contraindications/Warnings) for use in small animals.

For urinary tract infections (extra-label):

a) 10 – 20 mg/kg PO q24h. Excreted in urine predominantly in active form. Reserve for documented resistant UTIs but good first-line choice for pyelonephritis at 20 mg/kg PO q24h. Limited efficacy against enterococci. From the Antimicrobial Guidelines Working Group of the International Society for Companion Animal Infectious Diseases. (Weese et al. 2011)

b) In dogs with uncomplicated UTI: A high-dose short duration treatment with oral enrofloxacin at 18 – 20 mg/kg PO once daily for 3 days was shown to be non-inferior to conventional 14-day treatment with amoxicillin/clavulanate. (Westropp et al. 2012)

For enteric infections (extra-label):

a) For enrofloxacin-sensitive *E. coli* in granulomatous colitis of Boxer dogs (extra-label): 5 mg/kg PO q12h for 8 weeks. (Craven et al. 2011)

b) For campylobacteriosis: 5 mg/kg PO q12h. Resistance can develop during treatment. Avoid in young, growing animals. (Weese 2011)

For bacterial skin infections (extra-label): Most consider enrofloxacin to be a second-line drug for the treatment of deep pyoderma in dogs (used when culture evidence is that first-line drugs will not be effective). Usual dosage is 5 mg/kg PO once daily. Prolonged treatment may be required, and higher dosages (*e.g.,* 10 mg/kg PO q12h or 20 mg/kg PO q24h may be required for *Pseudomonas* infections.

- **CATS:**

For susceptible infections (labeled dose; FDA-approved): 5 mg/kg per day PO, may be given once daily or divided and given twice daily (q12h). Treatment should continue for at least 2-3 days beyond cessation of clinical signs, to a maximum duration of therapy is 30 days (Package insert; *Baytril*®—Bayer). In an extra-label manner, the canine injectable product (22.7 mg/mL) has also been used in cats at 5 mg/kg or less per day IM. IV use is not recommended for cats.

- **HORSES:**

Note: Usage of enrofloxacin in horses remains somewhat controversial and there are no FDA-approved enrofloxacin products for horses. While there has been much discussion regarding the potential for cartilage abnormalities or other arthropathies in horses, objective data is lacking. At present however, enrofloxacin probably should only be used in adult horses when other antibiotics are inappropriate.

If using *Baytril*® injection orally in horses, it can be very irritating to the mouth. This may be alleviated by coating the liquid with molasses or preparing a gel (see Compounding Considerations below) and rinsing the horse's mouth with water after administration. All of the following are extra-label:

a) 5 mg/kg IV q24h; 5 – 7.5 mg/kg PO q24h. (Haggett et al. 2008)

b) 7.5 mg/kg PO or IV once daily for susceptible respiratory infections. (Ainsworth et al. 2004)

c) Using the compounded gel as described below (Compatibility/Compounding Considerations): 7.5 mg/kg PO once daily. Horses should be fasted for 11-14 hours prior to dosing and for 1-2 hours after dosing, but should have access to water. Rinse horse's mouth with water after dosing to reduce risks for oral ulceration. (Epstein et al. 2004)

- **CATTLE:**

For the treatment of bovine respiratory disease associated with *Pasteurella haemolytica,* *Pasteurella multocida,* **and** *Haemophilus sommus* (Labeled-dose; FDA-approved): 2.5 – 5 mg/kg SC once daily for 3-5 days or 7.5 – 12.5 mg/kg SC once; not for use in cattle intended for dairy production or in veal calves. Animals intended for human consumption must not be slaughtered within 28 days from the last treatment. Extra-label use of fluoroquinolones in food animals is prohibited by the FDA.

- **SWINE:**

For the treatment and control of swine respiratory disease (SRD) associated with *Actinobacillus pleuropneumoniae,* *Pasteurella multocida,* *Haemophilus parasuis,* **and** *Streptococcus suis* (Labeled-dose; FDA-approved): 7.5 mg/kg (3.4 mL/100 lbs.) SC (behind the ear) once. Administered dose volume should not exceed 5 mL per injection site. (Adapted from label; *Baytril*®100)

- **FERRETS:**

For susceptible infections (extra-label): 10 – 20 mg/kg PO, IM, SC (must be diluted) twice daily. (Williams 2000)

- **RABBITS/RODENTS/SMALL MAMMALS:**

Note: All are extra-label.

a) **Rabbits:** For Pasteurella upper respiratory infections: 15 – 20 mg/kg PO twice daily for a minimum of 14 days in mild cases and up to several months for chronic infections; first dose may be made by SC injection (do **NOT** give subsequent doses SC or severe tissue reactions can occur). (Antinoff 2008)

b) **Rabbits:** 5 mg/kg PO, SC, IM or IV q12h for 14 days. Drug of choice for Pasteurella. If giving SC, dilute or skin may slough. Do not give injectable product PO because it is very unpalatable. (Ivey et al. 2000)

c) **Hedgehogs:** 5 – 10 mg/kg PO or SC q12h. (Smith 2000)

d) **Chinchillas:** 5 – 10 mg/kg PO, IM q12h. (Hayes 2000)

e) **Mice** and **Rats:** For mycoplasmal pneumonia: 10 mg/kg PO twice daily with doxycycline (5 mg/kg PO twice daily). (Burke 1999)

f) **Chinchillas, Gerbils, Guinea Pigs, Hamsters, Mice, Rats:** 5 – 10 mg/kg PO or IM q12h or 5 – 20 mg/kg PO or SC q24h. In drinking water: 50 – 200 mg/liter for 14 days. Do not use in young animals. (Adamcak et al. 2000)

g) **Rats:** Chronic respiratory disease: 10 – 25 mg/kg PO twice daily. If using theophylline concurrently, reduce theophylline dose by 30%. (Monks et al. 2009)

- **CAMELIDS:**

For susceptible infections in alpacas (extra-label): 5 mg/kg SC or 10 mg/kg PO once daily. (Gandolf et al. 2005)

- **BIRDS:**

For susceptible gram-negative infections (extra-label):

Psittacines: For empirical treatment: For stable, immune competent birds: 20 mg/kg PO once daily. For debilitated immune competent birds: 15 – 20 mg/kg SC in fluid pocket once daily. For debilitated, immunocompromised birds: 15 – 20 mg/kg SC in fluid pocket twice daily. When used orally, compounding the liver-flavored tablets grape syrup (*Syrpalta*®; Humco Labs) may improve acceptance. (Flammer 2006)

- **REPTILES:**

For susceptible respiratory infections for most species (extra-label): 5 mg/kg IM every 5 days for 25 days; for chronic respiratory infections in tortoises: 15 mg/kg IM every 72 hours for 5-7 treatments. (Gauvin 1993)

Monitoring

- Clinical efficacy.
- Adverse effects.
- In cats, monitor for mydriasis and/or retinal changes.

Client Information

- This drug is best given on an empty stomach without food, but if your animal vomits or acts sick after getting it, give with food or small treat (no dairy products, antacids or anything containing iron) to see if this helps. If vomiting continues, contact your veterinarian.
- Do not crush film-coated tablets as the drug is very bitter tasting and it will be more difficult to get your animal to take it.
- Do not give at the same time with other drugs or vitamins that contain calcium, iron, or aluminum (including sucralfate) as these can reduce the amount of drug absorbed.
- May stunt bone growth or cause joint abnormalities if used in young animals, during pregnancy or while nursing.
- Most common side effects are vomiting, nausea, or diarrhea.
- Do not exceed dosing recommendations in cats, as blindness can result.

Chemistry/Synonyms

A fluoroquinolone antibiotic, enrofloxacin occurs as a pale yellow, crystalline powder. It is slightly soluble in water. Enrofloxacin is related structurally to the human-FDA-approved drug ciprofloxacin (enrofloxacin has an additional ethyl group on the piperazinyl ring).

Enrofloxacin may also be known as: Bay-Vp-2674 or *Baytril*®.

Storage/Stability

Unless otherwise directed by the manufacturer, enrofloxacin tablets should be stored in tight containers at temperatures less than 30°C. Protect from strong UV light. Enrofloxacin has been reported to be soluble and stable in water, but solubility is pH dependent and altering the pH of the commercially available injections can cause precipitation.

The canine FDA-approved product (2.27%) for IM injection should be stored protected from light; do not freeze.

The cattle FDA-approved product (10%) injectable solution should be stored protected from sunlight. It should not be refrigerated, frozen or stored above 40°C (104°F). If exposed to cold temperatures, precipitation may occur; to redissolve, warm and then shake the vial.

Compatibility/Compounding Considerations

Injectable enrofloxacin must not be mixed with, or come into contact with any IV solution containing calcium or magnesium (*e.g.*, *Normosol*®-R, *Plasmalyte*®-R, -A, or -56); morbidity and mortality secondary to micro-precipitants lodging in patients' lungs have been reported.

For horses, an oral gel formulated from the bovine injectable product has been described (Epstein et al. 2004). 100 mL of the 100 mg/mL bovine injection (*Baytril*®100) is used. Stevia (0.35 g) is mixed with approximately 15 mL of liquid enrofloxacin until dissolved. Apple flavoring 0.6 mL is added until dissolved. Sodium carboxymethylcellulose (2 g) is sprinkled over the mixture and stirred until incorporated. Immediately begin gradually adding the remaining enrofloxacin (85 mL) before the mixture solidifies. Approximate concentration is 100 mg/mL. Stable for up to 84 days if kept in the refrigerator and protected from light.

For exotic animals, the following three compounded oral suspension preparations were shown to be stable for up to 56 days when stored at room temperature in amber-colored containers (Petritz et al. 2013):

1) Formulation A: 40 ml of corn syrup and 40 ml of distilled water were mixed together. 30 mL of this solution was placed in a small mortar. 27 film-coated tablets of 68 mg commercially available enrofloxacin 68 mg product were then added to the mortar and allowed to sit for 15 minutes. Once the film-coating was dissolved, tablets film-coated tablets were pulverized in the mortar with a pestle until a homogeneous paste was formed. The mixture was then carefully transferred into a plastic amber colored 8-oz (240 mL) dispensing vial (bottle). Another 30 mL of the corn syrup–distilled water mixture was poured into the mortar and carefully stirred to facilitate the transfer of any remaining enrofloxacin residue in the mortar to the vial. A sufficient quantity of the corn syrup-distilled water vehicle was then added to the vial to bring the final volume of the suspension to 80 mL resulting in a final concentration of 22.95 mg/mL.

2) Formulation B made in the way as Formulation A, but a 50:30 mixture of cherry syrup (50 mL) and distilled water (30 mL) was used resulting in a final concentration of 22.95 mg/mL.

3) Formulation C was made using 40 mL of the 2.27% (22.7 mg/mL) injectable product and 40 mL of a liquid sweetener (*Ora-Sweet*®–Paddock Labs) resulting in a final concentration of 11.35 mg/mL.

The authors concluded that while all three compounds were stable as described above, subjectively the cheery syrup mixture (Formulation B) was the best at masking the smell and taste of enrofloxacin.

Dosage Forms/Regulatory Status

VETERINARY-LABELED PRODUCTS:

Enrofloxacin Tablets (Film-Coated) & Oral Flavored Tablets: 22.7 mg, 68 mg, 136 mg; *Baytril®*, Enrofloxacin Flavored Tablets (generic); (Rx). FDA-approved for use in dogs and cats.

Enrofloxacin Injection: 22.7 mg/mL (2.27%) in 20 mL vials; *Baytril®*; (Rx). FDA-approved for use in dogs.

Enrofloxacin Injection: 100 mg/mL in 100 mL and 250 mL bottles; *Baytril 100®, Enroflox®*; (Rx). FDA-approved for use in cattle only. Not for use in cattle intended for dairy production or in calves to be processed for veal. Any extra-label use in food animals is banned by the FDA. Slaughter withdrawal cattle = 28 days when used as labeled. A withdrawal period has not been established in pre-ruminating calves. Slaughter withdrawal swine = 5 days when used as labeled.

HUMAN-LABELED PRODUCTS: NONE.

Note: Use of enrofloxacin by humans cannot be recommended due to a high degree of CNS effects.

Revisions/References

Monograph revised/updated January 2014.

Adamcak, A. & B. Otten (2000). Rodent Therapeutics. Vet Clin NA: Exotic Anim Pract **3**:1(Jan): 221-40.

Ainsworth, D. & R. Hackett (2004). Disorders of the Respiratory System. *Equine Internal Medicine 2nd Ed.* M. Reed, W. Bayly and D. Sellon. Phila., Saunders: 289-354.

Antinoff, N. (2008). Respiratory diseases of ferrets, rabbits, and rodents. Proceedings: IVECCS. accessed via Veterinary Information Network; vin.com

Blondeau, J. M., et al. (2012). In vitro killing of Escherichia coli, Staphylococcus pseudintermedius and Pseudomonas aeruginosa by enrofloxacin in combination with its active metabolite ciprofloxacin using clinically relevant drug concentrations in the dog and cat. Veterinary Microbiology **155**(2-4): 284-90.

Burke, T. (1999). Husbandry and Medicine of Rodents and Lagomorphs. Proceedings: Central Veterinary Conference, Kansas City. accessed via Veterinary Information Network; vin.com

Craven, M., et al. (2011). Granulomatous Colitis of Boxer Dogs. Vet Clin Small Anim **41**: 433-45.

Divers, T. J., et al. (2008). Ocular penetration of intravenously administered enrofloxacin in the horse. Equine Veterinary Journal **40**(2): 167-70.

Epstein, K., et al. (2004). Pharmacokinetics, stability, and retrospective analysis of use of an oral gel formulation of the bovine injectable enrofloxacin in horses. Vet Therapeutics **5**(2): 155-67.

Flammer, K. (2006). Antibiotic drug selection in companion birds. Journal of Exotic Pet Medicine **15**(3): 166-76.

Gandolf, A., et al. (2005). Pharmacokinetics after intravenous, subcutaneous and oral administration of enrofloxacin to alpacas. AJVR **66**(5): 767-71.

Gauvin, J. (1993). Drug therapy in reptiles. Seminars in Avian & Exotic Med **2**(1): 48-59.

Haggett, E. F. & W. D. Wilson (2008). Overview of the use of antimicrobials for the treatment of bacterial infections in horses. Equine Veterinary Education **20**(8): 433-48.

Hayes, P. (2000). Diseases of Chinchillas. *Kirk's Current Veterinary Therapy: XIII Small Animal Practice.* J. Bonagura. Philadelphia, WB Saunders: 1152-7.

Ivey, E. & J. Morrisey (2000). Therapeutics for Rabbits. Vet Clin NA: Exotic Anim Pract **3**:1(Jan): 183-216.

Monks, D. & M. Cowan (2009). Chronic respiratory disease in rats. Proceedings: AAVC-UEP. accessed via Veterinary Information Network; vin.com

Petritz, O. A., et al. (2013). Stability of three commonly compounded extemporaneous enrofloxacin suspensions for oral administration to exotic animals. Javma-Journal of the American Veterinary Medical Association **243**(1): 85-90.

Rodriguez, J. S., et al. (2012). Consequences of Intrauterine Enrofloxacin Infusion on Mare Endometrium. Journal of Equine Veterinary Science **32**(2): 106-11.

Smith, A. (2000). General husbandry and medical care of hedgehogs. *Kirk's Current Veterinary Therapy: XIII Small Animal Practice.* J. Bonagura. Philadelphia, WB Saunders: 1128-33.

Trepanier, L. (2008). Top Ten Potential Drug Interactions in Dogs and Cats. Proceedings: WSAVA. accessed via Veterinary Information Network; vin.com

Weese, J. S. (2011). Bacterial Enteritis in Dogs and Cats: Diagnosis, Therapy, and Zoonotic Potential. Veterinary Clinics of North America-Small Animal Practice **41**(2): 287-+.

Weese, J. S., et al. (2011). Antimicrobial Use Guidelines for Treatment of Urinary Tract Disease in Dogs and Cats: Antimicrobial Guidelines Working Group of the International Society for Companion Animal Infectious Diseases. Veterinary Medicine International.

Westropp, J. L., et al. (2012). Evaluation of the Efficacy and Safety of High Dose Short Duration Enrofloxacin Treatment Regimen for Uncomplicated Urinary Tract Infections in Dogs. Journal of Veterinary Internal Medicine **26**(3): 506-12.

Williams, B. (2000). Therapeutics in Ferrets. Vet Clin NA: Exotic Anim Pract **3**:1(Jan): 131-53.

Ephedrine Sulfate

(e-fed-rin)

Sympathomimetic Bronchodilator/Vasopressor

Prescriber Highlights

▶ Sympathomimetic used primarily for oral treatment of urinary incontinence, topically for nasal uses and parenterally as an indirect acting catecholamine pressor agent.

▶ Contraindications: Severe CV disease, especially with arrhythmias.

▶ Caution: Patients with glaucoma, prostatic hypertrophy, hyperthyroidism, diabetes mellitus, cardiovascular disorders or hypertension.

▶ Adverse Effects: CNS stimulation, tachycardia, hypertension, or anorexia.

▶ Excreted into milk, may affect neonates.

Uses/Indications

Ephedrine is used chiefly for the treatment of urethral sphincter hypotonus with resulting incontinence in dogs and cats. In a single oral dose study in incontinent female dogs, both ephedrine (2 mg/kg PO) and phenylpropanolamine (1.5 mg/kg PO) increased urethral pressure and functional length. During micturition, bladder capacity increased with both drugs but a decrease in detrusor pressure was observed only after ephedrine administration (Noel et al. 2012).

Ephedrine has also been used in an attempt to treat nasal congestion and/or bronchoconstriction in small animals. It can be used parenterally as a pressor agent in the treatment of shock or anesthesia-associated hypotension. In a study in horses with isoflurane-induced hypotension, ephedrine increased mean arterial pressure by increasing the cardiac index and systemic vascular resistance. The authors concluded that ephedrine would be preferable to phenylephrine for this indication since it increases both blood flow and blood pressure (Fantoni et al. 2013).

Pharmacology/Actions

While the exact mechanism of ephedrine's actions is undetermined, it is believed that it indirectly stimulates alpha-, beta1-, and beta2-adrenergic receptors by causing the release of norepinephrine. Prolonged use or excessive dosing frequency can deplete norepinephrine from its storage sites and tachyphylaxis (decreased response) may ensue. Tachyphylaxis has not been documented in dogs or cats when used for urethral sphincter hypotonus.

Pharmacologic effects of ephedrine include: increased vasoconstriction, heart rate, coronary blood flow, blood pressure, mild CNS stimulation, and decreased bronchoconstriction, nasal congestion and appetite. Ephedrine can also increase urethral sphincter tone and produce closure of the bladder neck; its principle veterinary indications are as a result of these effects.

Pharmacokinetics

Ephedrine is rapidly absorbed after oral or parenteral administration. Although not confirmed, ephedrine is thought to cross both the blood-brain barrier and the placenta. Ephedrine is metabolized in the liver and excreted unchanged in the urine. Urine pH may significantly alter excretion characteristics. In humans: at urine pH of 5, half-life is about 3 hours; at urine pH of 6.3, half-life is about 6 hours.

Contraindications/Precautions/Warnings

Ephedrine is contraindicated in patients with severe cardiovascular disease, particularly with arrhythmias. Ephedrine should be used with caution in patients with glaucoma, prostatic hypertrophy, hyperthyroidism, diabetes mellitus, cardiovascular disorders or hypertension.

When administered IV, administration rate should not exceed 10 mg/minute (in humans); it is suggested to scale the infusion rate similarly for veterinary patients.

Do not confuse ePHEDrine with EPINEPHrine.

Adverse Effects

Most likely side effects include restlessness, irritability, tachycardia, or hypertension. Anorexia may be a problem in some animals.

Tachyphylaxis (decreased response to subsequent doses) secondary to depleted stores of endogenous norepinephrine can occur with repeated doses.

Reproductive/Nursing Safety

Ephedrine's effects on fertility, pregnancy or fetal safety are not known. Use with caution during pregnancy. The drug is excreted in milk and may have deleterious effects on nursing animals. In humans, the FDA categorizes this drug as category C for use during pregnancy (*Animal studies have shown an adverse effect on the fetus, but there are no adequate studies in humans; or there are no animal reproduction studies and no adequate studies in humans.*)

Ephedrine is excreted in milk. If ephedrine is absolutely necessary for the dam, consider using milk replacer.

Overdosage/Acute Toxicity

Clinical signs of overdosage may consist of an exacerbation of the adverse effects listed above or, if a very large overdose, severe cardiovascular (hypertension to rebound hypotension, bradycardias to tachycardias, and cardiovascular collapse) or CNS effects (stimulation to coma) can be seen.

If the overdose was recent, empty the stomach using the usual precautions and administer charcoal and a cathartic. Treat clinical signs supportively as they occur.

Drug Interactions

The following drug interactions have either been reported or are theoretical in humans or animals receiving ephedrine and may be of significance in veterinary patients. Unless otherwise noted, use together is not necessarily contraindicated, but weigh the potential risks and perform additional monitoring when appropriate.

- **ACEPROMAZINE (and other PHENOTHIAZINES):** A study in dogs with acepromazine/isoflurane-induced hypotension found that ephedrine (initially at 0.1 mg/kg IV, followed by 10 micrograms/kg/min IV infusion) effectively countered cardiovascular depression by significantly increasing arterial blood pressure, cardiac output, and hemoglobin oxygen content and delivery. However, extremes in arterial blood pressure associated with initial vasoconstriction and a trend towards tachycardia prevented their recommendation at this dose (Sinclair et al. 2012).
- **ALPHA-BLOCKERS** (*e.g.,* **phentolamine, prazosin**): May negate the therapeutic effects of ephedrine.
- **BETA-BLOCKERS:** Concomitant use of ephedrine with beta-blockers may diminish the effects of both drugs.
- **DIGOXIN:** An increased risk of arrhythmias may occur if ephedrine is used concurrently with digitalis glycosides.
- **MONAMINE OXIDASE INHIBITORS** (including **amitraz**): Ephedrine should not be given within two weeks of a patient receiving monoamine oxidase inhibitors; severe hypertension, hyperpyrexia possible.
- **SYMPATHOMIMETIC AGENTS** (other, *e.g.* **phenylpropanolamine**): Ephedrine should not be administered with other sympathomimetic agents as increased toxicity may result.
- **RESERPINE:** May reverse the pressor effects of ephedrine.

- **THEOPHYLLINE:** Ephedrine may increase the risk for theophylline toxicity.
- **TRICYCLIC ANTIDEPRESSANTS:** May decrease the pressor effects of ephedrine.
- **URINARY ALKALINIZERS** (*e.g.,* **sodium bicarbonate, citrates, carbonic anhydrase inhibitors**): May reduce the urinary excretion of ephedrine and prolong its duration of activity. Dosage adjustments may be required to avoid toxic clinical signs.

Laboratory Considerations

- Beta-adrenergic agonists may decrease **serum potassium** concentrations. Clinical relevance is unknown.

Doses

- **DOGS:**

  For treatment of urinary incontinence responsive to adrenergic drugs (extra-label): Dosage recommendations vary considerably and there appears to be little evidence to support any dosage regimen. Most recommend around 1 – 1.2 mg/kg PO q8h, but dosages ranging from 1 – 4 mg/kg PO q8-12h have been noted. One formulary states that 2.5 mg/kg PO q12h is the maximum dosage.

  For treatment of hypotension associated with anesthesia (extra-label):
  a) For relatively short procedures in ASA I or II patients when hypotension is not responsive to 1 or 2 crystalloid boluses: 0.1 – 0.2 mg/kg IV bolus; duration of action is approximately 15-60 minutes after a single bolus. (Teixereia Neto 2009)
  b) Can give 0.15 – 0.25 mg/kg diluted into 5 mL of a balanced electrolyte solution or saline and give small increment IV boluses until desirable blood pressure achieved. Can also give as a CRI at 5 – 10 micrograms/kg/minute. (Ko 2009)

- **CATS:**

  For treatment of urinary incontinence responsive to adrenergic drugs (extra-label): Not commonly recommended; anecdotal dosages have generally been 2 – 4 mg per cat PO q8-12h.

  For treatment of hypotension associated with anesthesia (extra-label): Can give 0.15 – 0.25 mg/kg diluted into 5 mL of a balanced electrolyte solution or saline and give small increment IV boluses until desirable blood pressure achieved. Can also give as a CRI at 5 – 10 micrograms/kg/minute. (Ko 2009)

- **HORSES:**

  For adjunctive treatment of isoflurane-induced hypotension (extra-label): In the study, ephedrine CRI was given at 0.02 mg/kg/minute when mean arterial pressure (MAP) was <60 mmHg and was ended when the target MAP (50% higher than baseline) was achieved. (Fantoni et al. 2013)

Monitoring

- Clinical effectiveness.
- Adverse effects (see above).

Client Information

- In order for this drug to be effective, it must be administered as directed by the veterinarian; missed doses will negate its effect. It may take several days for the full benefit of the drug to take place.
- Contact veterinarian if the animal demonstrates ongoing changes in behavior (restlessness, irritability) or if incontinence persists or increases.

Chemistry/Synonyms

A sympathomimetic alkaloid, ephedrine sulfate occurs as fine, odorless, white crystals or powder. Approximately 770 mg are soluble in one mL of water. The commercially available injection has a pH of 4.5-7.

Ephedrine sulfate may also be known as ephedrine sulphate.

Storage/Stability

Store ephedrine sulfate products in tight, light resistant containers at room temperature unless otherwise directed.

Compatibility/Compounding Considerations

When used parenterally, ephedrine sulfate is usually administered directly and not diluted.

Dosage Forms/Regulatory Status

VETERINARY-LABELED PRODUCTS: NONE.

The ARCI (Racing Commissioners International) has designated this drug as a class 2 substance. See the appendix for more information.

HUMAN-LABELED PRODUCTS:

Ephedrine Sulfate Capsules: 25 mg; generic; (OTC)

Ephedrine Sulfate Injection: 50 mg/mL in 1 mL single-dose vials & preservative free in 1 mL single-dose amps; generic; (Rx)

In the USA, ephedrine sulfate is classified as a list 1 chemical (drugs that can be used as precursors to manufacture methamphetamine) and in some states it may be a controlled substance or have other restrictions placed upon its sale. Be alert to persons desiring to purchase this medication.

Revisions/References

Monograph revised/updated January 2014.

Fantoni, D. T., et al. (2013). Effect of ephedrine and phenylephrine on cardiopulmonary parameters in horses undergoing elective surgery. Veterinary Anaesthesia and Analgesia 40(4): 367-74.

Ko, J. (2009). Anesthesia monitoring techniques and management. Proceedings: ACVC. accessed via Veterinary Information Network; vin.com

Noel, S., et al. (2012). Urodynamic and haemodynamic effects of a single oral administration of ephedrine or phenylpropanolamine in continent female dogs. Veterinary Journal 192(1): 89-95.

Sinclair, M. D. & D. H. Dyson (2012). The impact of acepromazine on the efficacy of crystalloid, dextran or ephedrine treatment in hypotensive dogs under isoflurane anesthesia. Veterinary Anaesthesia and Analgesia 39(6): 563-73.

Teixereia Neto, F. (2009). Intraoperative hypotension: a stepwise approach to treatment. Proceedings: WSAVA. accessed via Veterinary Information Network; vin.com

Epinephrine

(ep-i-nef-rin)   Adrenalin®

Alpha- & Beta-Adrenergic Agonist

Prescriber Highlights

▶ Alpha- & beta-adrenergic agonist agent used systemically for treating anaphylaxis & cardiac resuscitation.

▶ Contraindications: Narrow-angle glaucoma, hypersensitivity to epinephrine, shock due to non-anaphylactoid causes, during general anesthesia with halogenated hydrocarbons, during labor (may delay the second stage), cardiac dilatation or coronary insufficiency; cases where vasopressor drugs are contraindicated (*e.g.,* thyrotoxicosis, diabetes, hypertension, toxemia of pregnancy).

▶ Use extreme caution patients with a prefibrillatory cardiac rhythm. Caution: Hypovolemia (not a substitute for adequate volume replacement).

▶ Do not inject with local anesthetics into small appendages of the body (*e.g.,* toes, ears, etc.); may cause necrosis/sloughing.

▶ Adverse Effects: Anxiety, tremor, excitability, vomiting, hypertension (overdosage), arrhythmias, hyperuricemia, & lactic acidosis (prolonged use or overdosage).

▶ Concentrations must not be confused.

▶ Drug interactions possible.

Uses/Indications

Epinephrine is employed primarily in veterinary medicine as a treatment for anaphylaxis or cardiac resuscitation. Because of its vasoconstrictive properties, epinephrine is added to local anesthetics to retard systemic absorption and prolong effect.

Pharmacology/Actions

Epinephrine is an endogenous adrenergic agent that has both alpha and beta activity. It relaxes smooth muscle in the bronchi and iris, antagonizes the effects of histamine, increases glycogenolysis, and raises blood sugar. If given by rapid IV injection, it causes direct stimulation of the heart (increased heart rate and contractility) and increases systolic blood pressure. If given slowly IV, epinephrine usually produces a modest rise in systolic pressure and a decrease in diastolic blood pressure. Total peripheral resistance is decreased because of beta effects.

Pharmacokinetics

Epinephrine is well-absorbed following IM or SC administration. IM injections are absorbed slightly faster than after SC administration; absorption can be expedited by massaging the injection site. Epinephrine is rapidly metabolized in the GI tract and liver after oral administration and is not effective via this route. Following SC injection, the onset of action is generally within 5-10 minutes. The onset of action following IV administration is immediate and intensified.

Epinephrine does not cross the blood-brain barrier, but does cross the placenta and is distributed into milk.

Epinephrine's actions are ended primarily by the uptake and metabolism of the drug into sympathetic nerve endings. Metabolism takes place in both the liver and other tissues by monoamine oxidase (MAO) and catechol-O-methyltransferase (COMT) to inactive metabolites.

Contraindications/Precautions/Warnings

Epinephrine is contraindicated in patients with narrow-angle glaucoma, hypersensitivity to epinephrine, shock due to non-anaphylactoid causes, during general anesthesia with halogenated hydrocarbons, during labor (may delay the second stage), and cardiac dilatation or coronary insufficiency. Epinephrine should not be used in cases where vasopressor drugs are contraindicated (*e.g.,* thyrotoxicosis, diabetes, hypertension, toxemia of pregnancy). It should not be injected with local anesthetics into small appendages of the body (*e.g.,* toes, ears, etc.) because of the chance of necrosis and sloughing.

Use epinephrine with caution in cases of hypovolemia; it is not a substitute for adequate fluid replacement therapy. It should be used with extreme caution in patients with a prefibrillatory cardiac rhythm, because of its excitatory effects on the heart. While epinephrine's usefulness in asystole is well documented, it can cause ventricular fibrillation; use cautiously in cases of ventricular fibrillation.

Do not confuse EPINEPHrine with ePHEDrine or the two concentrations of commercially available epinephrine injection: 1 mg/mL (1:1000) and 0.1 mg/mL (1:10,000).

Adverse Effects

Epinephrine can induce feelings of fear or anxiety, tremor, excitability, vomiting, hypertension (overdosage), arrhythmias (especially if patient has organic heart disease or has received another drug that sensitizes the heart to arrhythmias), hyperuricemia, and lactic acidosis (prolonged use or overdosage). Repeated injections can cause necrosis at the injection site.

Reproductive/Nursing Safety

In humans, the FDA categorizes this drug as category *C* for use during pregnancy (*Animal studies have shown an adverse effect on*

the fetus, but there are no adequate studies in humans; or there are no animal reproduction studies and no adequate studies in humans.)
It is not known if this drug is excreted in milk.

Overdosage/Acute Toxicity

Clinical signs seen with overdosage or inadvertent IV administration of SC or IM dosages can include: sharp rises in systolic, diastolic, and venous blood pressures, cardiac arrhythmias, pulmonary edema and dyspnea, vomiting, headache, and chest pain. Cerebral hemorrhages may result because of the increased blood pressures. Renal failure, metabolic acidosis and cold skin may also result.

Because epinephrine has a relatively short duration of effect, treatment is mainly supportive. If necessary, the use an alpha-adrenergic blocker (*e.g.*, phentolamine) or a beta-adrenergic blocker (*e.g.*, propranolol) can be considered to treat severe hypertension and cardiac arrhythmias. Prolonged periods of hypotension may follow, which may require treatment with norepinephrine.

Drug Interactions

The following drug interactions have either been reported or are theoretical in humans or animals receiving epinephrine and may be of significance in veterinary patients. Unless otherwise noted, use together is not necessarily contraindicated, but weigh the potential risks and perform additional monitoring when appropriate.

- **ALPHA-BLOCKERS** (*e.g.*, **phentolamine, phenoxybenzamine, prazosin**): May negate the therapeutic effects of epinephrine.
- **ALPHA-2 AGONISTS** (*e.g.*, **detomidine, dexmedetomidine, medetomidine, xylazine**): As epinephrine possesses alpha agonist effects, do **NOT** use to treat cardiac effects caused by alpha2 agonists.
- **ANESTHETICS, GENERAL**: An increased risk of arrhythmias developing can occur if epinephrine is administered to patients that have received a halogenated hydrocarbon anesthetic agent. Propranolol may be administered should these occur.
- **ANTIHISTAMINES**: Certain antihistamines (**diphenhydramine, chlorpheniramine**, etc.) may potentiate the effects of epinephrine.
- **BETA-BLOCKERS**: Propranolol (or other beta-blockers) may potentiate hypertension, and antagonize epinephrine's cardiac and bronchodilating effects by blocking the beta effects of epinephrine.
- **DIGOXIN**: An increased risk of arrhythmias may occur if epinephrine is used concurrently with digitalis glycosides.
- **NITRATES**: May reverse the pressor effects of epinephrine.
- **LEVOTHYROXINE**: May potentiate the effects of epinephrine.
- **OXYTOCIC AGENTS**: Hypertension may result if epinephrine is used with oxytocic agents.
- **SYMPATHOMIMETIC AGENTS, OTHER**: Epinephrine should not be administered with other sympathomimetic agents (*e.g.*, **isoproterenol**) as increased toxicity may result.
- **PHENOTHIAZINES**: May reverse the pressor effects of epinephrine.
- **RESERPINE**: May potentiate the pressor effects of epinephrine.
- **TRICYCLIC ANTIDEPRESSANTS**: May potentiate the effects of epinephrine.

Doses

Note: Be certain when preparing injection that you do not confuse 1:1000 (1 mg/mL) with 1:10,000 (0.1 mg/mL) concentrations. To convert a 1:1000 solution to a 1:10,000 solution for IV or intratracheal use, dilute each mL with 9 mL of normal saline for injection. Epinephrine is only one aspect of treating cardiac arrest; refer to specialized references or protocols for more information.

- **DOGS/CATS:**

Cardiac resuscitation (asystole); (extra-label): **Note:** Veterinarians are highly encouraged to obtain the *RECOVER evidence and knowledge gap analysis on veterinary CPR* available for free download via the Veterinary Emergency & Critical Care Society website: veccs.org. Part 7 of this document (summarized in "a" below) includes treatment algorithms and drug dosage tables.

a) Use of low-dose (0.01 mg/kg IV/IO) epinephrine administered every 3-5 minutes early in CPR is recommended, but high-dose (0.1 mg/kg IV/IO) epinephrine may be considered after prolonged CPR. In order to minimize underdosing or overdosing during CPR, this drug should be administered during every other cycle of basic life support (BLS; one cycle is 2 minutes long of uninterrupted compression/ventilation). In animals where intravenous or intraosseous access is not possible, the intratracheal (IT) route may be considered. Dilute with saline or sterile water (1:1) and administered via a catheter longer than the endotracheal tube. Optimal doses are not known, but IT dosages up to 10X of standard dosages have been recommended. (In a subsequent reference, one of the authors lists the IT dose as 0.02 mg/kg low dose; 0.2 mg/kg high dose. (Fletcher et al. 2013), (Fletcher et al. 2012)

b) Using the epinephrine first protocol: After the "ABC's" (airway, breathing, compressions) give epinephrine 0.01 mg/kg IV, continue ABCs for 3-5 minutes. If no response (return to spontaneous circulation; ROSC), vasopressin at 0.2 – 0.8 Units/kg IV, continue ABC's for 3-5 minutes. If no ROSC, epinephrine 0.01 mg/kg IV, continue ABC's for 3-5 minutes.

Using the vasopressin first protocol: After the "ABC's" (airway, breathing, compressions) give vasopressin 0.2 – 0.8 Units/kg IV, continue ABCs for 3-5 minutes. If no response (return to spontaneous circulation; ROSC), epinephrine 0.01 mg/kg IV, continue ABC's for 3-5 minutes. If no ROSC, repeat epinephrine 0.01 mg/kg IV, continue ABC's for 3-5 minutes.

For either protocol, the authors suggest trying atropine 0.04 mg/kg IV and/or naloxone 0.02 – 0.04 mg/kg IV. (Scroggin et al. 2009)

For anaphylaxis (extra-label): Initially, 0.01 mg/kg IM using a 1 mg/mL (1:1,000 solution); maximum dose of 0.3 mg in patients <40 kg and 0.5 mg in patients >40 kg. Depending on the severity of the episode and the response to the initial injection, the dose can be repeated every 5-15 minutes, as needed. However, if shock has already developed, epinephrine should be given by slow IV infusion at 0.05 micrograms/kg/min, ideally with the dose titrated to clinical response. The SC route should be avoided. No randomized controlled trials that meet optimal standards have been published, however, strong evidence for epinephrine supports its use as a first line drug. (Shmuel et al. 2013)

For treatment of hypotension associated with anesthesia (extra-label): **Note:** Because it can cause increased tissue oxygen demand and severe splanchnic vasoconstriction, epinephrine is considered a second- or third-line agent for this indication. Two very different dosage strategies have been noted:

a) As a last line of defense: 1 – 10 micrograms/kg/minute CRI. (Ko 2009)

b) 0.05 – 0.4 micrograms/kg/min IV. (Dodam 2005), (Mazzaferro 2005)

- **SMALL MAMMALS**

  For CPR in small herbivores (guinea pigs, chinchillas, and rabbits); (extra-label): 0.2 – 0.4 mg/kg IM, IV (bolus), or IT. (Schnellbacher et al. 2012)

- **BIRDS:**

  For CPR (extra-label):

  a) 0.1 mg/kg IV or intracardiac. (Harris 2003)

  b) 0.01mg.kg diluted in saline via a catheter down the trachea. If there is tracheal obstruction then a sterile endotracheal tube needs to be inserted and stitched into the left abdominal air sac. (O'Malley 2011)

- **HORSES:** (NOTE: ARCI UCGFS CLASS 2 DRUG)

  For anaphylaxis (extra-label): 3 – 5 mL of 1:1,000 per 450 kg of body weight either IM or SC. **For foal resuscitation**: 0.1 mL/kg of 1:1,000 IV (preferably diluted with saline). (Robinson 1987)

  For cardiopulmonary resuscitation of newborn foals (extra-label): 0.01 – 0.02 mg/kg (0.5 – 1 mL of a 1:1000 solution for a 50 kg foal) IV every 3 minutes until return of spontaneous circulation. If given intratracheally (IT), dose is 0.1 – 0.2 mL/kg. (Corley 2003)

- **RUMINANTS, SWINE:**

  For treatment of anaphylaxis (extra-label): 0.5 – 1 mL/100 lbs. body weight of 1:1,000 SC or IM; dilute to 1:10,000 if using IV; may be repeated at 15-minute intervals. Often used in conjunction with corticosteroids and diphenhydramine. (Clark 1986)

Monitoring

- Cardiac rate/rhythm.
- Respiratory rate/auscultation during anaphylaxis.
- Urine flow, if possible.
- Blood pressure and blood gases, if indicated and possible.

Client Information

- Note to pharmacist or veterinarian: Anaphylaxis clinical signs (depending on species) should be discussed. Review proper use of using the injector including determining dosage (if required) and injection technique using manufacturer's patient insert.
- Always have medication easily accessible (consider attaching it to leash, crate or something that always travels with animal).
- Absorption can be sped up by gently massaging the site of the shot.
- Store in carrier tube at room temperature; do not refrigerate. Do not use if liquid is discolored (pinkish or dark yellow) or particles are seen floating in it.
- Check expiration date and refill before medicine expires.

Chemistry/Synonyms

An endogenous catecholamine, epinephrine occurs as white to nearly white, microcrystalline powder or granules. It is only very slightly soluble in water, but it readily forms water-soluble salts (*e.g.*, HCl) when combined with acids. Both the commercial products and endogenous epinephrine are in the levo- form, which is about 15X more active than the dextro-isomer. The pH of the commercial injection range from 2.5-5.

Epinephrine is commonly called adrenalin.

Storage/Stability

Epinephrine HCl for injection should be stored in tight containers protected from light. Epinephrine will darken (oxidation) upon exposure to light and air. Do not use the injection if it is pink, brown, or contains a precipitate. The stability of the injection is dependent on the form and the preservatives present and may vary from one manufacturer to another. Epinephrine is rapidly destroyed by alkalies, or oxidizing agents.

Compatibility/Compounding Considerations

Epinephrine HCl is reported to be physically **compatible** with the following intravenous solutions and drugs: Dextran 6% in dextrose 5%, Dextran 6% in normal saline, dextrose-Ringer's combinations, dextrose-lactated Ringer's combinations, dextrose-saline combinations, dextrose 2.5%, dextrose 5% (becomes unstable at a pH >5.5), dextrose 10%, Ringer's injection, lactated Ringer's injection, normal saline, and sodium lactate 1/6 M, amikacin sulfate, cimetidine HCl, dobutamine HCl, and verapamil HCl.

Epinephrine HCl is reported to be physically **incompatible** with the following intravenous solutions and drugs: Ionosol-D-CM, Ionosol-PSL (Darrow's), Ionosol-T with dextrose 5% (**Note:** other Ionosol products are compatible), sodium chloride 5%, and sodium bicarbonate 5%, aminophylline, hyaluronidase, sodium bicarbonate, and warfarin sodium. Compatibility is dependent upon factors such as pH, concentration, temperature, and diluent used; consult specialized references or a hospital pharmacist for more specific information.

Dosage Forms/Regulatory Status

VETERINARY-LABELED PRODUCTS:

Epinephrine HCl for Injection 1 mg/mL (1:1,000) in 1 mL amps and syringes and 10 mL, 30 mL and 100 mL vials; *Epinject®*, generic; (Rx). Labeled for dogs, cats, cattle, horses, sheep and swine.

The ARCI (Racing Commissioners International) has designated this drug as a class 2 substance. See the appendix for more information.

HUMAN-LABELED PRODUCTS:

Epinephrine HCl Solution for Injection: 1 mg/mL (1:1,000) in 1 mL amps & 30 mL vials; *Adrenalin Chloride®*, generic; (Rx)

Epinephrine HCl Solution for Injection: 0.1 mg/mL (1:10,000) 10 mL syringes & vials; generic; (Rx)

Epinephrine HCl Solution for Injection: 0.3 mg/0.3 mL; in prefilled single-dose syringes or in dual-dose auto-injectors; *EpiPen®*, *Twinject®*, *Adrenaclick®*, *Auvi-Q®*; generic; (Rx)

Epinephrine HCl Solution for Injection: 0.15 mg/0.15 mL in single dose or dual-dose auto-injectors with chlorobutanol & sodium bisulfite; *Twinject®*, *Adrenaclick®*, *Auvi-Q®*; (Rx)

Epinephrine HCl Solution for Injection: 0.15 mg/0.3 mL; *EpiPen Jr®*; (Rx)

Epinephrine bitartrate is available as a powder form (aerosol) for inhalation, topical solution and a solution for nebulization; ophthalmic preparations are available.

Revisions/References

Monograph revised/updated January 2014.

Clark, D. R. (1986). Diseases of the general circulation. *Current Veterinary Therapy: Food Animal Practice 2.* J. L. Howard. Philadelphia, W.B. Saunders: 694-6.

Corley, K. (2003). Cardiopulmonary resuscitation of the newborn foal. Proceedings: ACVIM Forum. accessed via Veterinary Information Network; vin.com

Dodam, J. (2005). Recognizing and treating hypotension. Proceedings: Western Vet Conf. accessed via Veterinary Information Network; vin.com

Fletcher, D. J. & M. Boller (2013). Updates in Small Animal Cardiopulmonary Resuscitation. Vet Clin Small Anim 43: 971-87.

Fletcher, D. J., et al. (2012). RECOVER evidence and knowledge gap analysis on veterinary CPR. Part 7: Clinical guidelines. J. Vet. Emerg. Crit. Care 22.

Harris, D. (2003). Emergency management of acute illness and trauma in avian patients. Proceedings: Atlantic Coast Veterinary Conference. accessed via Veterinary Information Network; vin.com

Ko, J. (2009). Anesthesia monitoring techniques and management. Proceedings: ACVC. accessed via Veterinary Information Network; vin.com

Mazzaferro, E. (2005). Anesthesia in critically ill patients. Proceedings: Western Vet Conf. accessed via Veterinary Information Network; vin.com

O'Malley, B. (2011). Avian Emergencies. World Small Animal Veterinary Association World Congress Proceedings. accessed via Veterinary Information Network; vin.com

Robinson, N. E. (1987). Table of Common Drugs: Approximate Doses. *Current Therapy in Equine Medicine, 2.* N. E. Robinson. Philadelphia, W.B. Saunders: 761.

Schnellbacher, R., et al. (2012). Emergency presentations associated with cardiovascular disease in exotic herbivores. Journal of Exotic Pet Medicine 21(4): 316-27.

Scroggin, R. D. & J. Quandt (2009). The use of vasopressin for treating vasodilatory shock and cardiopulmonary arrest. J. Vet. Emerg. Crit. Care 19(2): 145-57.

Shmuel, D. L. & Y. Cortes (2013). Anaphylaxis in dogs and cats. J. Vet. Emerg. Crit. Care 23(4): 377-94.

Epirubicin HCl

(ep-ee- roo-bi-sin)   Ellence®

Antineoplastic

Prescriber Highlights

▶ Injectable anthracycline antineoplastic that potentially could be used in place of doxorubicin in dogs.

▶ Very little experience or published information available for use in animal patients.

▶ Adverse effect profile for animals not well documented, but it may have less cardiotoxicity potential, but more gastrointestinal adverse effects. Otherwise, similar cautions and caveats as doxorubicin apply.

Uses/Indications

Epirubicin could potentially be used as a replacement for doxorubicin in dogs and cats, but there is much less published on it for veterinary use. At the time of writing, three retrospective studies in dogs are available: in the adjuvant treatment of splenic hemangiosarcoma (Kim et al. 2007), as part of a multi-agent protocol for lymphoma (Elliott et al. 2013), and a third looking specifically at toxicity (Marrington et al. 2012). From this work it appears that epirubicin has similar efficacy as doxorubicin and the potential for less cardiotoxicity, but may have a higher incidence of adverse gastrointestinal effects.

Pharmacology/Actions

Epirubicin has a similar mode of action as doxorubicin. It causes inhibition of DNA synthesis, DNA-dependent RNA synthesis and protein synthesis, but the precise mechanisms for these effects are not well understood. The drug acts throughout the cell cycle and also possesses some immunosuppressant activity.

Pharmacokinetics

No published data on the epirubicin pharmacokinetics or pharmacodynamics in dogs or cats was located. Epirubicin, like doxorubicin must be administered IV as it is not absorbed from the GI tract and is extremely irritating to tissues if administered SC or IM.

In humans after IV injection, epirubicin is rapidly and widely distributed but does not appreciably enter the CSF. It is marginally bound (77%) to tissue and plasma proteins and concentrates into red blood cells.

Epirubicin is metabolized extensively by the liver and other tissues via aldo-keto reductase primarily to epirubicinol, which is active but only at 10% of the parent compound's activity; other inactive metabolites are also formed. Epirubicin and its metabolites are primarily excreted in the bile and feces with lesser amounts excreted into urine. Epirubicin is eliminated in a triphasic manner. Average half-lives for the three elimination phases are: first phase (3 minutes), second phase (2.5 hours), and third phase (33 hours).

Contraindications/Precautions/Warnings

In humans, and likely in dogs as well, epirubicin is contraindicated or relatively contraindicated (measure risk vs. benefit) in patients with myelosuppression (baseline neutrophil count less than 1,500 cells/mm3); severe myocardial insufficiency, cardiomyopathy and/or heart failure, recent myocardial infarction, severe arrhythmias, or with previous treatment with anthracyclines (e.g. doxorubicin) that have received maximum cumulative dose. It should be used with caution in patients with hyperuricemia/hyperuricuria, or impaired hepatic function. Dosage adjustments may be necessary in patients with hepatic impairment.

Epirubicin, like doxorubicin should be administered IV slowly, over at least 3-5 minutes in a free flowing IV line. Extreme care must be taken to avoid perivascular infusion (extravasation). IM or SC dosages are contraindicated.

Breeds predisposed to developing cardiomyopathy (e.g., Doberman pinchers, Great Danes, Rottweilers, Boxers) should be monitored carefully while receiving epirubicin therapy.

The p-glycoprotein pump, actively transports doxorubicin and possibly epirubicin, and certain breeds susceptible to *ABCB1* (MDR1)-allele mutation (e.g., Collies, Australian Shepherds, Shelties, Long-haired Whippet) may be at higher risk for toxicity. Bone marrow suppression (decreased blood cell counts, particularly neutrophils) and GI toxicity (anorexia, vomiting, diarrhea) are more likely to occur at normal doses of doxorubicin in dogs with the *ABCB1* mutation. To reduce the likelihood of severe toxicity in these dogs (mutant/normal or mutant/mutant), the Veterinary Clinical Pharmacology Laboratory at Washington State University recommends reducing doxorubicin doses by 25-30% and carefully monitoring these patients (WSU-VetClinPharmLab 2009).

Because epirubicin can be very irritating to skin, gloves should be worn when administering or preparing the drug. Ideally, doxorubicin injection should be prepared in a biological safety cabinet using standard chemo preparation procedures. If accidental skin or mucous membrane contact occurs, wash the area immediately using soap and copious amounts of water. Spills or leakage of epirubicin solutions should be diluted with sodium hypochlorite solutions (with 1% available chlorine), preferably by soaking, and then diluted further with water.

Do not confuse EPIrubicin with DOXOrubicin or DAUNOrubicin.

Adverse Effects

Epirubicin can potentially cause several adverse effects similarly to doxorubicin, including bone marrow suppression, cardiac toxicity, alopecia, gastroenteritis (vomiting, diarrhea), and stomatitis. Cardiotoxic effects may be less likely to occur than with doxorubicin. After administration of doxorubicin in dogs (and probably with epirubicin), nausea and vomiting commonly occur within the first 72-hour; diarrhea can occur within approximately 4-5 days and myelosuppression nadirs are generally seen 7-10 days after treatment.

An immediate histamine-mediated hypersensitivity reaction may be seen characterized by urticaria, facial swelling, vomiting, arrhythmias (see below), and/or hypotension. The rate of infusion can have a direct impact on this effect and generally IV infusions should be administered no faster than over 10-20 minutes. Pretreatment with a histamine₁ blocker such as diphenhydramine (IV prior to treatment at 10 mg for dogs up to 9 kg; 20 mg for dogs 9-27 kg; and 30 mg for dogs over 27 kg) or an intravenous glucocorticoid may also reduce or eliminate these effects.

For more information on cardiac toxicity of anthracycline antineoplastics, refer to the doxorubicin monograph.

In cats, doxorubicin (and potentially epirubicin) is a potential nephrotoxin and renal function should be monitored both before and during therapy.

Extravasation injuries secondary to perivascular administration of epirubicin can be quite serious, with severe tissue ulceration and necrosis possible. Prevention of extravasation should be a priority and animals should be frequently checked during the infusion. Should extravasation occur, it is suggested to treat as per the recommendations for humans. There are currently two treatments recommended for doxorubicin (and epirubicin) extravasation injuries. Both have been shown to be effective, but no comparative trials have been published. 1) Apply dimethyl sulfoxide (DMSO) 99% by saturating a gauze pad and painting on an area twice the size of the extravasation. Allow the site to air dry and repeat the application every 6 hours for 14 days. Do not cover the area with dressing. 2) Dexrazoxane is FDA-approved for the treatment of extravasation resulting from anthracycline IV therapy, Refer to the dexrazoxane monograph for more information. Additionally, ice compresses applied to the affected area for 15 minutes every 6 hours for 48 hours may be useful.

Reproductive/Nursing Safety

Epirubicin is teratogenic and embryotoxic in laboratory animals. It is unknown if it affects male fertility. In humans, the FDA categorizes this drug as category *D* for use during pregnancy (*There is evidence of human fetal risk, but the potential benefits from the use of the drug in pregnant women may be acceptable despite its potential risks.*) In a separate system evaluating the safety of drugs in canine and feline pregnancy (Papich 1989), this drug is categorized as class: *C* (*These drugs may have potential risks. Studies in people or laboratory animals have uncovered risks, and these drugs should be used cautiously as a last resort when the benefit of therapy clearly outweighs the risks.*)

Epirubicin is excreted in milk in concentrations that may exceed those found in plasma. Because of risks to nursing offspring, consider using milk replacer if the dam is receiving doxorubicin. In humans, nursing is contraindicated in patients receiving the drug.

Overdosage/Acute Toxicity

Inadvertent acute overdosage may be manifested by exacerbations of the adverse effects outlined above. A lethal dose for dogs of doxorubicin has been reported as 72 mg/m^2 (O'Keefe and Harris 1990). Supportive and symptomatic therapy is suggested should an overdose occur. Dexrazoxane may be useful to help prevent cardiac toxicity.

Drug Interactions

The following drug interactions have either been reported or are theoretical in humans or animals receiving doxorubicin or epirubicin and may be of significance in veterinary patients. Unless otherwise noted, use together is not necessarily contraindicated, but weigh the potential risks and perform additional monitoring when appropriate.

- **ANTINEOPLASTIC AGENTS, OTHER:** May potentiate the toxic effects of doxorubicin.
- **CIMETIDINE:** Can increase epirubicin levels; avoid using together.
- **CYCLOSPORINE:** Cyclosporine can increase doxorubicin and doxorubicinol (active metabolite) levels. Avoid using together.
- **GLUCOSAMINE:** May reduce doxorubicin effectiveness; use together not recommended in humans.
- **IMMUNOSUPPRESIVE AGENTS, OTHER** (*e.g.,* **leflunomide, tacrolimus**). Immunosuppressant effects may be enhanced.
- **KETOCONAZOLE:** Can increase doxorubicin and doxorubicinol (active metabolite) levels and lead to toxicity. Avoid using together.
- **PHENYTOIN:** Doxorubicin may decrease phenytoin levels.
- **PHENOBARBITAL:** May increase elimination and reduce blood levels of doxorubicin.
- **SPINOSAD:** Can increase doxorubicin and doxorubicinol (active metabolite) levels and lead to toxicity. Avoid using together.
- **STREPTOZOCIN:** May inhibit doxorubicin metabolism.
- **VACCINES:** Live or live-attenuated vaccines may result in active infections in immunocompromised patients.
- **VERAPAMIL:** May increase doxorubicin levels.

- **WARFARIN:** Increased risk for bleeding.
- **ZIDOVUDINE:** Increased risk for neutropenia.

Laboratory Considerations

- Epirubicin may significantly increase both blood and urine concentrations of **uric acid**.
- Handling of blood samples should pose no health hazard after 7 days (Knobloch, Mohring, Eberle, Nolte, et al. 2010). **Note:** Reference pertains to doxorubicin; epirubicin not determined.

Doses

NOTE: Because of the potential toxicity of this drug to patients, veterinary personnel and clients, and since chemotherapy indications, treatment protocols, monitoring and safety guidelines often change, the following dosages should be used only as a general guide. Consultation with a veterinary oncologist and referral to current veterinary oncology references [*e.g.,* (Withrow et al. 2012); (Dobson et al. 2011); (Henry et al. 2009); (North et al. 2009); (Argyle et al. 2008)] are strongly recommended.

- **DOGS:**

Depending on the protocol used, epirubicin is usually dosed similarly as doxorubicin at 30 mg/m^2 (**NOT** mg/kg) IV in free-flowing line over at least 3-5 minutes. Maximum cumulative dose is probably similar to doxorubicin at 240 mg/m2.

For lymphoma (extra-label): In the retrospective study, either a modified Wisconsin-Madison continuous chemotherapy protocol (CEOP-C; vincristine, prednisolone, cyclophosphamide, asparaginase and epirubicin) at 30 mg/m^2 or 1 mg/kg IV on weeks 4 and 9; followed by vincristine, chlorambucil and methotrexate weeks 11-17; OR a modified Wisconsin-Madison discontinuous chemotherapy protocol (CEOP-25) used; same epirubicin dosage and frequency. (Elliott et al. 2013)

For splenic hemangiosarcoma (extra-label): In the retrospective study, after splenectomy treated dogs received epirubicin at 30 mg/m^2 IV every 3 weeks for up to 4 to 6 treatments. (Kim et al. 2007)

Monitoring

- Efficacy.
- Toxicity:
  a) CBC with platelets. Neutrophil counts of <3000/mcL (some say <2000/mcL) generally require delay in dosing.
  b) Dogs with pre-existing heart disease should be monitored with regular ECG's (insensitive to early toxic changes) and/or echocardiogram.
  c) Evaluate hepatic function prior to therapy.
  d) Urinalyses and serum creatinine/BUN in cats.

Client Information

- Clients must be briefed on the possibilities of severe toxicity developing from this drug, including drug-related mortality. Clients should contact the veterinarian should the animal exhibit any clinical signs of profound depression, abnormal bleeding (including bloody diarrhea) and/or bruising.
- Epirubicin may cause urine to be colored orange to red for 1-2 days after dosing; although uncommon in veterinary patients, it is not harmful should it occur.
- Mild anorexia and occasional vomiting are commonly seen 2-5 days post-therapy.
- Avoid skin contact with urine or feces of treated animals. After treatment, doxorubicin drug residues may be found in treated dog's urine up to 21 days and feces for several days. (Knobloch, Mohring, Eberle and Nolte 2010).
- Although it is unknown how much drug is found in the saliva of

treated animals, do not allow treated animals to lick human skin while receiving chemotherapy treatment.

Chemistry/Synonyms

Epirubicin (4-epidoxorubicin) is a semisynthetic stereoisomer of the anthracycline doxorubicin antibiotic antineoplastic and occurs as a red-orange powder soluble in water and methyl alcohol, slightly soluble in alcohol, and practically insoluble in acetone. The commercially available solution for injection has a pH of approximately 3. CAS Registry: 56420-45-2 (epirubicin); 56390-09-1 (epirubicin hydrochloride); ATC: L01DB03.

Epirubicin HCl may also be known as: 4-epidoxorubicin, 4-epi-adriamycin HCl, IMI-28, or pidorubicin HCl. A common trade name is *Ellence®*.

Storage/Stability

Lyophilized powder for injection should be stored at 25°C (77°F); excursions are permitted to 15°-30°C (59°-86°F). Reconstituted solutions are stable for 24 hours when stored at 2°-8°C (36°-46°F) and protected from light, or 25°C (77°F) in normal lighting conditions. Discard any unused portion.

The commercially available solution should be stored in a refrigerator between 2°-8°C (36°-46°F). Do not freeze. Store protected from light, but no light protection is needed when administering the drug. The manufacturer recommends using solution within 24 hours of removal from the refrigerator or first penetration of the rubber stopper and to discard any unused solution. When reconstituted the solution should be clear and red in color. Do not use the solution if precipitation or significant discoloration is present.

Studies have shown that 2 mg/mL concentrations in sterile water for injection are stable for at least 43 days at 4°C in plastic syringes.

Compatibility/Compounding Considerations

To reconstitute the lyophilized powder: Reconstitute 50 mg vial with 25 mL sterile water for injection, to a final concentration of 2 mg/mL. Shake vigorously; it may take up to 4 minutes for the mixture to completely dissolve. Epirubicin can be further diluted with sterile water for injection.

Epirubicin can be used in combination with other antitumor agents, but do not mix with other drugs in the same syringe. Prolonged contact with any solution of an alkaline pH should be avoided as hydrolysis can occur. Epirubicin should not be mixed with heparin or fluorouracil due to chemical incompatibility that may lead to precipitation.

Epirubicin HCl is reportedly physically **compatible** with the following intravenous solutions and drugs: dextrose 3.3% in sodium chloride 3%, D_5W, lactated Ringer's injection, sodium chloride 0.9% and ifosfamide.

Dosage Forms/Regulatory Status

VETERINARY-LABELED PRODUCTS: NONE.

HUMAN-LABELED PRODUCTS:

Epirubicin HCl for Injection: 50 mg/ 25 mL & 200 mg/100 mL; *Ellence®*, generic; (Rx).

Revisions/References

Monograph revised/updated January 2014.
Argyle, D., et al. (2008). *Decision Making in Small Animal Oncology*, Wiley-Blackwell.
Dobson, J. & D. Lascelles (2011). *BSAVA Manual of Canine and Feline Oncology*, BSAVA.
Elliott, J. W., et al. (2013). Epirubicin as part of a multi-agent chemotherapy protocol for canine lymphoma. Veterinary and Comparative Oncology 11(3): 185-98.
Henry, C. & M. Higginbotham (2009). *Cancer Management in Small Animal Practice*, Saunders.
Kim, S. E., et al. (2007). Epirubicin in the adjuvant treatment of splenic hemangiosarcoma in dogs: 59 cases (1997-2004). Javma-Journal of the American Veterinary Medical Association 231(10): 1550-7.
Knobloch, A., et al. (2010). Cytotoxic Drug Residues in Urine of Dogs Receiving Anticancer Chemotherapy. J Vet Intern Med 24: 384-90.

Knobloch, A., et al. (2010). Drug Residues in Serum of Dogs Receiving Anticancer Chemotherapy. Journal of Veterinary Internal Medicine 24(2): 379-83.
Marrington, A. M., et al. (2012). Toxicity associated with epirubicin treatments in a large case series of dogs. Veterinary and Comparative Oncology 10(2): 113-23.
North, S. & T. Banks (2009). *Small Animal Oncology: An Introduction*, Saunders.
Withrow, S., et al. (2012). Withrow and MacEwen's Small Animal Clinical Oncology, 5th Ed., Saunders.
WSU-VetClinPharmLab (2009). "Problem Drugs." Veterinary Clinical Pharmacology Lab, College of Vet Med, Washington State University http://goo.gl/aIGlM.

Epoetin Alfa (Erythropoietin)

(eh-poe-ee-tin al-fah)   EPO, rHuEPO, Epogen®, Procrit®

Erythropoietic Agent

Prescriber Highlights

▶ Hormone that regulates erythropoiesis; used for anemia associated with chronic renal failure.

▶ Contraindications: Patients with uncontrolled hypertension or in those that are hypersensitive to it; formation of significant autoantibodies with prior treatment.

▶ Adverse Effects: Autoantibodies with resultant resistance to treatment, vomiting, hypertension, seizures, uveitis, iron depletion (iron supplementation often used), local reactions at injection sites, fever, arthralgia, & mucocutaneous ulcers.

▶ Adequate monitoring vital.

Uses/Indications

Epoetin alfa or rHuEPO (human recombinant erythropoietin) has been used to treat dogs and cats for anemia associated with chronic renal failure. One group with experience treating over 70 cats with epoetin or darbepoetin report only that about 60-65% had an adequate response (Chalhoub et al. 2011). Because of concerns associated expense and adverse effects (red cell aplasia), most do not recommend starting therapy in dogs or cats until PCV is less than 20-22%. It is hoped that canine and feline recombinant products will become available commercially in the future to reduce the risks for autoantibody formation.

Despite increased cost versus epoetin, many clinicians opt for darbepoetin. Darbepoetin may be less immunogenic than epoetin, however this has not been fully documented in dogs or cats. Another advantage of darbepoetin is that doses may be administered less often to maintain PCV.

Pharmacology/Actions

Erythropoietin is a naturally occurring substance produced in the kidney and considered a hormone as it regulates erythropoiesis. It stimulates erythrocyte production by stimulating the differentiation and proliferation of committed red cell precursors. EPO also stimulates the release of reticulocytes.

Recombinant Human EPO alfa (r-HuEPO-alpha) serves as a substitute for endogenous EPO, primarily in patients with renal disease. Various uremic toxins may be responsible for the decreased production of EPO by the kidney.

Pharmacokinetics

EPO is only absorbed after parenteral administration. It is unclear whether the drug crosses the placenta or enters milk. The drug's metabolic fate is unknown. In patients with chronic renal failure, half-lives are prolonged approximately 20% over those with normal renal function. In dogs, epoetin has an elimination half-life of about 8-10 hours, which is approximately 3X shorter than darbepoetin. Depending on initial hematocrit and dose, correction of hematocrit may require 2-8 weeks.

Contraindications/Precautions/Warnings

EPO is contraindicated in patients with uncontrolled hypertension or those that are hypersensitive to it (see Adverse Effects below). EPO cannot be recommended for use in equines. In animals with moderate to severe hypertension or iron deficiency, therapy should be started with caution or withheld until hypertension or deficiency is corrected.

In patients receiving EPO, adequate iron stores are necessary for efficacy. Most clinicians prefer using injectable iron dextran rather than oral iron products for this purpose.

Adverse Effects

In dogs and cats, the most troublesome aspect of EPO therapy is the development of anti-rHuEPO antibody formation in up to 70% of patients. Perhaps up to 30% of all patients will develop antibodies significant enough to cause pure red blood cell aplasia (PRCA) with resultant profound anemia, arrestment of erythropoiesis, and transfusion dependency. Should a patient develop refractory anemia while receiving adequate EPO doses and have normal iron metabolism, a bone marrow aspirate should be considered. A myeloid:erythroid ratio of greater than 6 predicts significant autoantibody formation and contraindicates further EPO therapy. Some clinicians believe that the drug (EPO) should be withdrawn if PCV starts to drop while on therapy. Commercially available epoetin contains 2.5 mg/mL human albumin and anecdotally, PRCA is reported to occur less often than with darbepoetin (does not contain human albumin). One source states that incidence of PRCA is about 25-30% in dogs and cats receiving epoetin and less than 10% with darbepoetin (Chalhoub et al. 2011). PRCA can be difficult to treat, but immediate discontinuation of epoetin or darbepoetin is required. Immunosuppressive therapy and blood transfusions can potentially help but long-term prognosis is often grave.

Other adverse effects reported include: systemic hypertension, high blood viscosity/polycythemia, seizures, and iron depletion. Hypertension may be a result of increased blood viscosity and cardiac output, and decreased anemia-mediated vasodilation. Seizures may be in response to hypertension. Local reactions at injection sites (which may be a predictor of antibody formation), fever, arthralgia, and mucocutaneous ulcers are also possible. Additionally, cardiac disease has been noted that may be a result of, or compounded by, the animal's chronic kidney disease and hypertension.

Therapy should be discontinued if any of the following are recognized: polycythemia, fever, anorexia, joint pain, cellulitis, cutaneous or mucosal ulceration (Cowgill 2002).

Reproductive/Nursing Safety

Some teratogenic effects (decrease in body weight gain, delayed ossification, etc.) have been noted in pregnant rats given high dosages. Rabbits receiving 500 mg/kg during days 6-18 of gestation showed no untoward effects on offspring; however, use during pregnancy only when benefits outweigh the potential risks. In humans, the FDA categorizes this drug as category C for use during pregnancy (*Animal studies have shown an adverse effect on the fetus, but there are no adequate studies in humans; or there are no animal reproduction studies and no adequate studies in humans.*)

It is not known whether epoetin alfa is excreted in milk, but it is unlikely to pose much risk to nursing offspring.

Overdosage/Acute Toxicity

Acute overdoses appear to be relatively free of adverse effects. Single doses of up to 1600 Units/kg in humans demonstrated no signs of toxicity. Chronic overdoses may lead to polycythemia or other adverse effects. Cautious phlebotomy may be employed should polycythemia occur.

Drug Interactions

The following drug interactions have either been reported or are theoretical in humans or animals receiving EPO and may be of significance in veterinary patients. Unless otherwise noted, use together is not necessarily contraindicated, but weigh the potential risks and perform additional monitoring when appropriate.

- **ANDROGENS:** May increase the sensitivity of erythroid progenitors; this interaction has been used for therapeutic effect; **Note:** This effect has not been confirmed in well-controlled studies nor has the safety of this combination been determined.
- **DESMOPRESSIN:** Using with EPO can decrease bleeding times.
- **PROBENECID:** Probenecid has been demonstrated to reduce the renal tubular excretion of EPO; clinical significance remains unclear at this time.

Laboratory Considerations

- No laboratory interactions of major clinical importance have been described.

Doses

- **DOGS/CATS:**

  As adjunctive therapy for the treatment of anemia associated with end-stage renal disease (extra-label): Most recommend an initial dose of 100 Units/kg SC 3 times per week until the low-end of the target hematocrit range of 37-45% for dogs and 30-40% for cats is attained. Then reduce dosage frequency to twice weekly. An initial response is usually seen within 3-4 weeks. If adequate control is not achieved within 8-12 weeks, dosage can be increased by an additional 25 – 50 Units/kg every 3-4 weeks while maintaining dosing interval at 3 times a week. Continue monitoring (PCV, blood pressure) and adjusting dose and frequency as necessary, but take lag phase into account and do not adjust more often than once every three weeks. Iron supplementation is required. If animal requires >145 Units/kg 3 times a week, evaluate for epoetin resistance. Adapted from: (Cowgill 2002) (Chalhoub et al. 2011; Bartges 2012; Chalhoub et al. 2012; DiBartola 2012; Adams 2013; Polzin 2013)

- **FERRETS:**

  For adjunctive treatment of anemia (extra-label): 50 – 150 Units/kg IM 3 times weekly; may decrease to once weekly if RBC indices are significantly improved. (Williams 2000)

- **RABBITS/RODENTS/SMALL MAMMALS:**

  Rabbits; for adjunctive treatment of anemia (extra-label): 50 – 150 Units/kg SC every 2-3 days until PVC is normal; then once weekly (q7 days) for at least 4 weeks. (Ivey et al. 2000)

Monitoring

- Hematocrit; PCV; (Initially weekly to every other week for 2-4 months, then when dose and Hct are stable, at 1-2 month intervals).
- Blood Pressure (initially, at least monthly then every 1-2 months thereafter).
- Renal Function Status.
- Iron status (serum iron, TIBC), RBC indices (initially and regularly during therapy to insure adequate iron availability).

Client Information

- Injectable (subcutaneous; under the skin) drug used to treat anemia (too few red blood cells) from chronic renal failure. If you are giving this at home be sure you understand how and where to administer the shots. May take several weeks before it works.
- Biggest concern is the development of antibodies after using it awhile. Watch for skin reactions at the site of the shot. Also, if seizures (convulsions), fever, joint pain, mouth ulcers are seen or animal has no appetite, contact veterinarian right away.
- Ongoing lab tests are necessary and treatment can be very expensive.

Chemistry/Synonyms

A biosynthetic form of the glycoprotein human hormone erythropoietin, epoetin alfa (EPO) has a molecular weight of approximately 30,000. It is commercially available as a sterile, preservative-free, colorless solution. Sodium chloride solution is added to adjust tonicity and is buffered with sodium citrate or citric acid. Human albumin (2.5 mg/mL) is also added to the solution.

Epoetins may also be known as: erythropoietin, r-HuEPO, BI-71.052 (epoetin gamma), BM-06.019 (epoetin beta), EPO (epoetin alfa), EPOCH (epoetin beta), *Epogen®*, or *Procrit®*.

Storage/Stability

The injectable solution should be stored in the refrigerator (2-8°C); do not freeze. Do not shake the solution as denaturation of the protein with resultant loss of activity may occur. If light exposure is limited to 24 hours or less, no effects on potency should occur. When stored as directed, the solution has an expiration date of 2 years after manufacture. Do not mix with other drugs or use the same IV tubing with other drugs running. Because the solution contains no preservatives, the manufacturer recommends using each vial only as a single use.

Compatibility/Compounding Considerations

A method of diluting the Amgen product to facilitate giving very small dosages has been described (Grodsky 1994). Using a 1:20 dilution (1 part *Epogen®* to 19 parts bacteriostatic normal saline does not require any additional albumin to prevent binding of the drug to container). No data is available commenting on this dilution's stability.

Dosage Forms/Regulatory Status

VETERINARY-LABELED PRODUCTS: NONE.

The ARCI (Racing Commissioners International) has designated this drug as a class 2 substance. It is also prohibited on the premises of a racing facility.

HUMAN-LABELED PRODUCTS:

Epoetin Alfa, Solution for Injection: 2000 Units/mL, 3000 Units/mL, 4000 Units/mL, 10,000 Units/mL, 20,000 Units/mL and 40,000 Units/mL in 1 mL single-dose and 2 mL (10,000 Unit only) multi-dose (contains benzyl alcohol) vials; *Epogen®*, *Procrit®*; (Rx). **Note:** All products contain human albumin 2.5 mg/mL.

Revisions/References

Monograph revised/updated January 2014.

Adams, L. G. (2013). Managing Chronic Kidney Disease in Cats. British Small Animal Veterinary Conference. accessed via Veterinary Information Network; vin.com

Bartges, J. W. (2012). Chronic Kidney Disease in Dogs and Cats. Veterinary Clinics of North America-Small Animal Practice 42(4): 669-+.

Chalhoub, S., et al. (2011). Anemia of Chronic Renal Disease What it is, what to do and what's new. Journal of Feline Medicine and Surgery 13(9): 629-40.

Chalhoub, S., et al. (2012). The Use of Darbepoetin to Stimulate Erythropoiesis in Anemia of Chronic Kidney Disease in Cats: 25 Cases. Journal of Veterinary Internal Medicine 26(2): 363-9.

Cowgill, L. (2002). Anemia and hypertension: The ignored consequences of chronic renal failure, Proceedings: Tufts Animal Expo. accessed via Veterinary Information Network; vin.com

DiBartola, S. P. (2012). Medical Management of Chronic Renal Failure in Cats. Atlantic Coast Veterinary Conference accessed via Veterinary Information Network; vin.com

Grodsky, B. (1994). Personal Communication.

Ivey, E. & J. Morrisey (2000). Therapeutics for Rabbits. Vet Clin NA: Exotic Anim Pract 3:1(Jan): 183-216.

Polzin, D. J. (2013). Evidence-based step-wise approach to managing chronic kidney disease in dogs and cats. J. Vet. Emerg. Crit. Care 23(2): 205-15.

Williams, B. (2000). Therapeutics in Ferrets. Vet Clin NA: Exotic Anim Pract 3:1(Jan): 131-53.

Eprinomectin

(e-pri-no-mek-tin) Ivomec®   Eprinex®; LongRange®

Topical Avermectin Antiparasitic Agent

Prescriber Highlights

► Topically applied (pour-on) or extended-release injection (for cattle on pasture only) avermectin antiparasiticide for cattle.

► When pour-on is used as labeled there are no milk or meat withdrawal times required.

► Injectable has a 48-day slaughter withdrawal and specific syringe compatibilities. Must be administered SC in front of shoulder.

Uses/Indications

In cattle, eprinomectin topical (*Ivomec® Eprinex®*) is indicated for a variety gastrointestinal roundworms including adult and L4 stages of *Haemonchus placei*, *Ostertagia ostertagi*, *Trichostrongylus axei* and *colubriformis*, *Cooperia oncophora/punctata/surnabada*, *Nematodirus helvetianus*, *Oesophagostomum radiatum*, *Bunostomum phlebotomum*, and *Trichuris* spp. (adults only); cattle grubs; lice; mange mites; horn flies (for 7 days after treatment), and lungworms (*Dictyocaulus vivaparus*—for 21 days after treatment).

The extended-release 5% injection (*LongRange®*) is indicated for the treatment and control of internal and external parasites (susceptible GI roundworms, grubs, lungworms, mites) in cattle on pasture with persistent effectiveness. It is not approved for use in female dairy cattle 20 months of age or older, including dry dairy cows; calves to be processed for veal; breeding bulls; calves less than 3 months of age; or cattle managed in feedlots or under intensive rotational grazing. Topical eprinomectin may be useful in an extra-label manner for the topical treatment of psoroptic mange (*P. equi*) in horses or ear mites (*Psoroptes cuniculi*) in rabbits. One small study (6 subjects) showed partial response when rabbits were dosed at 5 mg/kg topically, twice at 14-day intervals. (Ulutas et al. 2005)

Pharmacology/Actions

Eprinomectin binds selectively to glutamate-gated chloride ion channels that occur in invertebrate nerve and muscle cells. This leads to an increase in cell membrane permeability to chloride ions, leading to paralysis and death of the parasite. Like ivermectin, eprinomectin enhances the release of gamma amino butyric acid (GABA) at presynaptic neurons. GABA acts as an inhibitory neurotransmitter and blocks the post-synaptic stimulation of the adjacent neuron in nematodes or the muscle fiber in arthropods. These compounds are generally not toxic to mammals as they do not have glutamate-gated chloride channels and do not readily cross the blood-brain barrier.

Pharmacokinetics

No information noted for the pour-on product. When the injectable product is injected as labeled, a polymeric PLGA matrix is formed allowing a gradual release of eprinomectin into the systemic circulation. Effective plasma levels may persist for at least 100 days.

Contraindications/Precautions/Warnings

Do not give the pour-on orally or intravenously.

The injectable product's label states that: "this product should not be used in other animal species" and is "not for intravenous or intramuscular use." Underdosing and/or subtherapeutic concentrations of extended-release anthelmintic products may encourage the development of parasite resistance.

Adverse Effects

For the pour-on, no adverse reactions are listed on the product label. On the FDA's Cumulative Adverse Drug Experience database for topical administration on cattle, the three most common adverse experiences reported are: ineffectiveness for parasite control, anorexia, and udder hypogalactia (Anon 2009). It must be noted that incidence rates are not listed and causal effect is not established for listings on this database.

For the injection, the label states that it "is likely to cause tissue damage at the site of injection, including possible granulomas and necrosis. These reactions have disappeared without treatment. Local tissue reaction may result in trim loss of edible tissue at slaughter."

Reproductive/Nursing Safety

The label states that the injection is not for use in bulls, as reproductive safety testing has not been conducted in males intended for breeding or actively breeding. Not for use in calves less than 3 months of age because safety testing has not been conducted in calves less than 3 months of age. Administration at 3X the recommended therapeutic dose had no adverse reproductive effects on beef cows at all stages of breeding or pregnancy or on their calves.

It is likely safe to use in nursing cattle, but it is not approved for use in lactating dairy cattle.

Overdosage/Acute Toxicity

For the pour-on, calves given up to 5X dosage showed no signs of adverse effects. One subject (of 6) showed signs of mydriasis when given a 10X dose. The sustained-release injectable at 3-5X the recommended dose resulted in a statistically significant reduction in average weight gain when compared to the group tested at label dose. Treatment-related lesions observed in most cattle administered the product included swelling, hyperemia, or necrosis in the subcutaneous tissue of the skin.

Drug Interactions

- No interactions noted.

Doses

- **CATTLE:**

  For labeled indications (pour-on; FDA-approved): 1 mL per 10 kg (22 lb.) body weight applied topically along backline in a narrow strip from the withers to the tailhead. (Package Insert; *Ivomec® Eprinex®*—Merial)

  For labeled indications (extended-release injection; FDA-approved): 1 mg/kg (1 mL per 110 lb. body weight) SC under the loose skin in front of the shoulder. Divide doses greater than 10 mL between two injection sites to reduce discomfort or site reaction. Animals should be appropriately restrained to achieve the proper route of administration. Inject using a 16 or 18 gauge, ½ to ¾ inch needle. Sanitize the injection site by applying a suitable disinfectant. Clean, properly disinfected needles should be used to reduce the potential for injection site infections. See additional information on syringe compatibility and automatic syringes in the Compatibility/Compounding Considerations section below. (Adapted from label; *LongRange®*)

- **HORSES:**

  For treatment of psoroptic (*P. equi*) mange (extra-label): 500 micrograms/kg (0.5 mg/kg) topically once weekly for 4 treatments. Authors suggest getting informed consent before use. (Ural et al. 2008)

Client Information

For the pour-on:

- When used as labeled, there are no milk or meat withdrawal times required.

- Weather conditions (including rainfall) during administration do not affect efficacy.
- Do not apply to backline if covered with mud or manure.
- Dispose of containers in an approved landfill or by incineration; do not contaminate water as eprinomectin may adversely affect fish and aquatic organisms.

For the injectable:

- 48-day withdrawal time.
- Several restrictions on use. Not approved for bulls, veal calves, dairy cattle, etc.
- Specific syringes required. Must be administered SC in front of shoulder.
- Observe for injection site reactions. If suspected, consult your veterinarian.

Chemistry/Synonyms

A member of the avermectin-class of antiparasitic agents, eprinomectin is also known as MK-397 or 4-epi-acetylamino-4-deoxy-avermectin B1.

Storage/Stability

The commercially available pour-on product should be stored protected from light and kept at 86°F (30°C) or less. Storage up to 104°F (40°C) is permitted for a short period.

The injectable should be stored at 77° F (25° C) with excursions permitted between 59°-86° F (15°-30° C). Protect from light. Do not be store in automatic syringe equipment.

Compatibility/Compounding Considerations

For the injectable: 50 mL bottle: Use only polypropylene syringes with the 50 mL bottle size. Not for use with polycarbonate syringe material. If syringe material is not known, contact the syringe manufacturer prior to use for identification. Do not use beyond 3 months after stopper has been punctured. Discard bottle after 15 stopper punctures.

250 ml & 500 mL bottle sizes: Use only automatic syringe equipment provided by Merial. To obtain compatible equipment, contact Merial at 1-888-637-4251 or your veterinarian; should not be stored in automatic syringe equipment. Automatic syringe equipment should be thoroughly cleaned after each use. Discard bottle after one stopper puncture with draw-off spike. No special handling or protective clothing is necessary.

Dosage Forms/Regulatory Status

VETERINARY-LABELED PRODUCTS:

Eprinomectin Topical (Pour-On) Solution: 5 mg/mL in 250 mL/8.5 fl. oz. and 1 L/33.8 fl. oz. bottle with a squeeze-measure-pour-system, or a 2.5 L/84.5 fl. oz. and 5 L/169 fl. oz. collapsible pack for use with appropriate automatic dosing equipment; *Ivomec®*, *Eprinex®*; (OTC). FDA-approved for use in beef or dairy cattle.

Eprinomectin 5% (50 mg/mL) Sustained-release Injectable: In 50, 250, and 500 mL bottles; *LongRange®*; (Rx). FDA-approved (NADA 141-327) for use in cattle on pasture with persistent effectiveness. It is not approved for use in female dairy cattle 20 months of age or older, including dry dairy cows; calves to be processed for veal; breeding bulls; calves less than 3 months of age; or cattle managed in feedlots or under intensive rotational grazing. Animals intended for human consumption must not be slaughtered within 48 days of the last treatment. The product label *LongRange®* may be found at dailymed.nlm.nih.gov.

HUMAN-LABELED PRODUCTS: NONE.

Revisions/References

Monograph revised/updated December 2013.

Anon (2009). "Cumulative Veterinary Adverse Drug Experience (ADE) Reports." U.S. Food and Drug Administration http://www.fda.gov/AnimalVeterinary/SafetyHealth/ProductSafetyInformation/ucm055394.htm.

Ulutas, B., et al. (2005). Efficacy of topical administration of eprinomectin for treatment of ear mite infestation in six rabbits. Vet Derm **16**: 334-7.

Ural, K., et al. (2008). Eprinomectin treatment of psoroptic mange in hunter jumper and dressage horses: A prospective, randomized, double-blinded, placebo-controlled clinical trial. Veterinary Parasitology 156(3-4): 353-7.

Epsom Salts – see Magnesium Sulfate

Epsiprantel

(ep-si-pran-tel)   Cestex®

Cestocidal Antiparasitic Agent

Prescriber Highlights

▶ Oral cestocide for dogs & cats.
▶ Not appreciably absorbed when given orally.
▶ Not FDA-approved in puppies or kittens less than 7 weeks old.
▶ Adverse Effects: GI (vomiting, diarrhea) possible.

Uses/Indications

Epsiprantel is indicated for the treatment (removal) of *Dipylidium caninum* and *Taenia pisiformis* in dogs, and *Dipylidium caninum* and *Taenia taeniaeformis* in cats. For *D. caninum*, adequate flea/louse control is mandatory or re-infestation is likely.

Pharmacology/Actions

Epsiprantel's exact mechanism of action against cestodes has not been determined. The tapeworm's ability to regulate calcium is apparently affected, causing tetany and disruption of attachment to the host. Alteration to the integument makes the worm vulnerable to digestion by the host animal.

Pharmacokinetics

Unlike praziquantel, epsiprantel is absorbed very poorly after oral administration and the bulk of the drug is eliminated in the feces. Less than 0.1% of the drug is recovered in the urine after dosing. No metabolites have thus far been detected.

Contraindications/Precautions/Warnings

There are no labeled contraindications to this drug, but the manufacturer states not to use it in puppies or kittens less than 7 weeks of age.

Adverse Effects

Adverse effects would be unexpected with this agent, although vomiting and/or diarrhea could potentially occur.

Reproductive/Nursing Safety

Safety for use in pregnant or breeding animals has not been determined, but teratogenic effects would be highly unlikely since the drug is so poorly absorbed.

Overdosage/Acute Toxicity

Acute toxicity resulting from an inadvertent overdose is highly unlikely. Doses as high as 36X the recommended dose resulted in vomiting in some of the kittens tested. Single doses of 36X those recommended in dogs caused no adverse effects.

Drug Interactions

■ None reported; theoretically, prokinetic agents or fast acting laxatives may reduce the drug's efficacy.

Laboratory Considerations

■ None reported.

Doses

■ **DOGS:**

For the treatment (removal) of tapeworms (*Dipylidium caninum* and *Taenia pisiformis*); (Labeled-dose; FDA-approved): 5.5 mg/kg (2.5 mg/lb.) PO once; round up to the next larger tablet size. (Package insert; *Cestex®*—Pfizer)

■ **CATS:**

For the treatment (removal) of tapeworms (*Dipylidium caninum* and *Taenia taeniaeformis*); (Labeled-dose; FDA-approved): 2.75 mg/kg PO once. Cats up to 10 lb. should receive one 12.5 mg tablet; cats 11-20 lb. should receive one 25 mg tablet (Package insert; *Cestex®*—Pfizer)

Monitoring

■ Clinical efficacy.

Client Information

■ Oral drug for treating tapeworms in dogs & cats. Not much drug is absorbed when given orally (by mouth), but it is still effective for killing tapeworms.
■ Give with food.
■ Adverse Effects: GI effects (*e.g.*, vomiting, diarrhea, etc.) are possible, but not likely.
■ Because the worm may be partially or completely digested, worm fragments may not be seen in the feces after treatment.
■ A single dose is usually effective, but measures should be taken to prevent reinfection, particularly against *D. caninum*.

Chemistry/Synonyms

A pyrazino-benzazepine oral cestocide, epsiprantel occurs as a white powder that is sparingly soluble in water.

Epsiprantel may also be known as BRL-38705 or *Cestex®*.

Storage/Stability

Tablets should be stored at room temperature.

Compatibility/Compounding Considerations

No specific information noted.

Dosage Forms/Regulatory Status

VETERINARY-LABELED PRODUCTS:

Epsiprantel Oral Tablets (Film-coated): 12.5 mg, 25 mg, 50 mg & 100 mg; *Cestex®*; (Rx). FDA-approved (NADA 140-893) for use in dogs and cats. A link to the Cestex® label may be found at dailymed. nlm.nih.gov

HUMAN-APPROVED PRODUCTS: NONE.

Revisions/References

Monograph revised/updated January 2014.

Ergocalciferol

(er-goh-kal-sif-er-ole)   Vitamin D2, Calciferol, Drisdol®

Form Of Vitamin D

Prescriber Highlights

▶ May be used to treat hypocalcemia associated with hypoparathyroidism, but calcitriol usually recommended first.
▶ Less expensive than DHT or calcitriol, but takes large initial doses for effect, effects take longer to be seen, & if hypercalcemia develops, takes longer (up to 18 weeks) for toxicity relief.

Uses/Indications

Ergocalciferol is sometimes used in dogs or cats to treat hypocalcemia secondary to parathyroid gland failure, particularly when dihydrotachysterol or calcitriol are too expensive for the owner. When compared to those agents, ergocalciferol takes longer to have a maximal effect on serum calcium. Additionally, if hypercalcemia should develop, ergocalciferol's effects persist longer than either calcitriol or dihydrotachysterol.

Pharmacology/Actions

Ergocalciferol is first hydroxylated in the liver to 25-hydroxyvitamin D (has some activity) and then activated in the kidneys to 1,25-dihydroxyvitamin D, the primary active form of the drug. Vitamin D is considered a hormone and, in conjunction with parathormone (PTH) and calcitonin, regulates calcium homeostasis in the body. Active analogues (or metabolites) of vitamin D enhance calcium and phosphate absorption from the GI tract, promote reabsorption of calcium by the renal tubules, and increase the rate of accretion and resorption of minerals in bone.

Pharmacokinetics

Specific pharmacokinetic values for dogs and cats were not located. But the following information (human-based) generally applies: In the presence of bile salts, ergocalciferol is absorbed from the small intestine; after conversion to its 25-hydroxylated form in the liver and kidneys, it is stored in the liver and fat. Cats do not appear to convert ergocalciferol to its 25-hydroxylate form as well as cholecalciferol. Several days of therapy may be required until distribution steady state is achieved. In dogs and cats, maximal effect on calcium homeostasis is usually noted from 5-21 days after treatment was begun; effects may persist for up to 18 weeks once treatment is discontinued (Feldman 2005).

Contraindications/Precautions/Warnings

Ergocalciferol, at therapeutic dosages, is contraindicated in patients with hypercalcemia, vitamin D toxicity, malabsorption syndrome, or abnormal sensitivity to the effects of vitamin D. It should be used with extreme caution in patients with hyperphosphatemia. As patients with kidney dysfunction may not convert ergocalciferol into the primary active metabolite, calcitriol or DHT would be preferred since they do not require activation by the kidney. Chronic therapy should not be initiated unless owners are willing to commit to ongoing patient monitoring.

Adverse Effects

The primary concern with using ergocalciferol is "overshooting" the dosage with resultant hypercalcemia and, potentially, hyperphosphatemia or nephrocalcinosis. Hypercalcemia can persist for weeks to months.

Reproductive/Nursing Safety

Hypervitaminosis D in pregnant females has been implicated in causing teratogenic effects in animals and infants. Potential benefits of therapy must be weighed against the risks if considering use in pregnant dogs or cats.

As large doses of vitamin D can be excreted into milk, consider using milk replacer in offspring of dams receiving therapeutic dosages of ergocalciferol.

Overdosage/Acute Toxicity

Because of the potential serious ramifications of overdoses, contacting an animal poison control center is strongly recommended. The toxic acute oral dose of ergocalciferol in dogs is reported as 4 mg/kg (160,000 Units/kg).

Acute ingestions should be managed using established protocols for removal or prevention of the drug being absorbed from the GI. Orally administered mineral oil may reduce absorption and enhance fecal elimination.

Hypercalcemia secondary to chronic dosing of the drug should be treated by first temporarily discontinuing it and exogenous calcium therapy. If the hypercalcemia is severe, furosemide, calcium-free IV fluids (e.g., normal saline), urine acidification, and corticosteroids may be employed. Because of the long duration of

action of ergocalciferol (potentially up to 18 weeks), hypercalcemia may persist. Restart therapy (if desired) at a reduced dosage only when calcium serum levels return to the normal range. Diligent monitoring is required.

Drug Interactions

The following drug interactions have either been reported or are theoretical in humans or animals receiving ergocalciferol and may be of significance in veterinary patients. Unless otherwise noted, use together is not necessarily contraindicated, but weigh the potential risks and perform additional monitoring when appropriate.
- **CORTICOSTEROIDS**: Can reduce the effects of vitamin D.
- **DIGOXIN** or **VERAPAMIL**: Patients on these drugs are sensitive to the effects of hypercalcemia; intensified monitoring is required.
- **MINERAL OIL**: May reduce the amount of ergocalciferol absorbed.
- **THIAZIDE DIURETICS**: May cause hypercalcemia when given in conjunction with Vitamin D.

Laboratory Considerations
- Serum cholesterol levels may be falsely elevated by vitamin D analogs when using the Zlatkis-Zak reaction for determination.

Doses
- **DOGS/CATS:**

  For maintenance therapy of parathyroid failure after using parenteral calcium to control hypocalcemic tetany (extra-label): Calcitriol is generally preferred due to the concerns with ergocalciferol of "overshooting" the dosage leading to persistent hypercalcemia, but ergocalciferol can be less expensive. Doses used are relative high 4000 – 6000 Units/kg PO once daily. Effect is usually seen between 5-14 days after initiation of treatment. After 1-5 days, parenteral calcium can usually be discontinued. Patient should remain hospitalized until serum calcium concentration remains between 8 – 10 mg/dL without parenteral calcium support, then patient can be discharged. Continue ergocalciferol, but administer every other day. Weekly serum calcium concentrations should be performed and ergocalciferol dosage adjusted to maintain serum calcium concentrations between 8 – 9.5 mg/dL. Maintenance doses usually range from 1000 – 2000 Units/kg PO once daily to once weekly. Goal is to prevent hypocalcemic tetany, but not induce hypercalcemia (Schoeman 2011). Once animal is stable, monthly rechecks for 6 months are strongly advised; then every 2-3 months thereafter. Adapted from (Feldman 2005), (Schoeman 2011).

Monitoring
- See dosage information above.

Client Information
- While ergocalciferol is less expensive than DHT or calcitriol, it takes longer to have an effect and can persist in the body much longer than DHT or calcitriol. Do not give more than is prescribed.
- Using vitamin D products may require lifelong treatment and regular laboratory monitoring.
- While this agent can treat low calcium, it can cause calcium levels in the blood to become too high; this effect can last for many weeks, even after the medication is discontinued.

Chemistry/Synonyms

Ergocalciferol is obtained by irradiating (with ultraviolet light) ergosterol, a sterol present in fungi and yeasts. It occurs as white or almost white crystals or yellowish crystalline powder and is practically insoluble in water, but is soluble in fatty oils. One mg of ergocalciferol provides 40,000 Units of vitamin D activity.

Ergocalciferol may be known as calciferol, vitamin D2, viosterol, activated ergosterol, or irradiated ergosterol; there are many international trade names.

Storage/Stability

Ergocalciferol is sensitive to light, heat and air. Store capsules or liquid at room temperature (15-30°C) and protect from light.

Compatibility/Compounding Considerations

No specific information noted.

Dosage Forms/Regulatory Status

VETERINARY-LABELED PRODUCTS: NONE.

HUMAN-LABELED PRODUCTS:

Ergocalciferol Oral Liquid (Drops): 8,000 Units/mL (200 micrograms/mL) in 60 mL; *Drisdol® Drops, Calcidol®, Calciferol® Drops*, generic; (OTC)

Ergocalciferol Oral Capsules: 50,000 Units (1.25 mg); *Drisdol®*, generic; (Rx)

Revisions/References

Monograph revised/updated January 2014.

Feldman, E. (2005). Disorders of the parathyroid glands. *Textbook of Veterinary Internal Medicine, 6th Ed.* S. Ettinger and E. Feldman, Elsevier: 1508-35.
Schoeman, J. P. (2011). Endocrine Emergencies. WSAVA World Congress Proceedings. accessed via Veterinary Information Network; vin.com

Ertapenem Sodium

(er-ta-pen-um)   Invanz®

Carbapenem Antibiotic

Prescriber Highlights

► Carbapenem antibiotic similar to imipenem & meropenem, but has a narrower spectrum of activity.

► Not effective against Pseudomonas or Acinetobacter.

► May only need to be dosed once daily.

► Rarely used in veterinary medicine and very limited information available for use in dogs or cats; must be considered investigational. Currently no generic forms available and relatively expensive.

Uses/Indications

Ertapenem may be useful in treating resistant gram-negative bacterial infections, particularly when aminoglycoside use would be risky (*i.e.*, renal failure) or not effective (*i.e.*, resistance or CNS infections), and when meropenem is not available. While ertapenem has a broad spectrum, it is not active against *Pseudomonas aeruginosa*. It potentially could be useful against mixed anaerobic/gram-negative aerobic infections when *Pseudomonas* is not considered a likely pathogen.

Pharmacology/Actions

Ertapenem is a carbapenem antibiotic similar to imipenem and meropenem. Like other beta-lactams, it inhibits bacterial cell wall synthesis and is usually bactericidal.

Ertapenem has a broad antibacterial spectrum similar to that of imipenem, but it is more active against *Enterobacteriaceae* and anaerobes, has equivalent activity against gram-positive bacteria, and minimal activity against *Pseudomonas aeruginosa* and *Acinetobacter*. Methicillin-resistant *Staphylococci* and *Enterococcus* are usually resistant to ertapenem. Because ertapenem, like meropenem, is more stable than imipenem to renal dehydropeptidase I, it does not require the addition of cilastatin to inhibit that enzyme.

Pharmacokinetics

At the time of writing, no pharmacokinetic data was available for dogs or cats.

In humans, the drug must be administered parenterally as it is not appreciably absorbed after oral administration. Intramuscular bioavailability is about 90% and peak plasma levels occur in approximately 2.3 hours. Ertapenem exhibits concentration-dependent binding to human plasma proteins. At plasma concentrations of <100 micrograms/mL it is 95% bound; at 300 micrograms/mL, 85% bound. Ertapenem biotransformation is not dependent on hepatic mechanisms as the major metabolite (inactive) is formed by hydrolysis of the beta-lactam ring. Approximately 80% of an IV dose is excreted in the urine, evenly split between inactive metabolites and unchanged drug. Approximately 10% is excreted in the feces. In young, healthy adults, elimination half-life is about 4 hours; about 2.5 hours in pediatric patients.

Contraindications/Precautions/Warnings

Ertapenem is contraindicated in patients hypersensitive to it or other carbapenems and those that have developed anaphylaxis after receiving any beta-lactam antibiotic. It is contraindicated in patients hypersensitive to lidocaine or other amide-type local anesthetics (if used IM with 1% lidocaine as the diluent).

As ertapenem has not been widely used clinically in veterinary medicine and little information for use in dogs or cats is published, consider its use investigational.

Adverse Effects

The adverse effect profile for ertapenem in dogs or cats is unknown. In humans, intravenous injection site reactions are the most common adverse reaction. Gastrointestinal effects (nausea, vomiting, diarrhea), headache, or tachycardia have occasionally been reported. Rarely, hypersensitivity or CNS effects (hallucinations, agitation, seizures, etc.) have been seen.

Reproductive/Nursing Safety

Ertapenem has been shown to cross the placenta in rats, but no teratogenic effects have been reported. In humans, ertapenem is designated by the FDA as a category **B** drug (*Animal studies have not demonstrated risk to the fetus, but there are no adequate studies in pregnant women; or animal studies have shown an adverse effect, but adequate studies in pregnant women have not demonstrated a risk to the fetus during the first trimester of pregnancy, and there is no evidence of risk in later trimesters.*)

Although risk cannot be ruled out, it is likely that ertapenem is safe to use while nursing.

Overdosage/Acute Toxicity

Inadvertent overdoses are unlikely. Humans receiving 3 grams intravenously had an increased incidence of nausea and diarrhea. Should an overdose occur and adverse effects noted, treat supportively.

Drug Interactions

The following drug interactions have either been reported or are theoretical in humans or animals receiving ertapenem and may be of significance in veterinary patients. Unless otherwise noted, use together is not necessarily contraindicated, but weigh the potential risks and perform additional monitoring when appropriate.

▪ **PROBENECID:** In humans, coadministration of ertapenem with probenecid can increase ertapenem AUC by 25% and elimination half-life by about 20%. Because of these relatively small effects, the manufacturer does not recommend using probenecid to extend the half-life of ertapenem.

Laboratory Considerations

▪ No specific laboratory interactions or concerns were noted.

Doses

▪ **DOGS/CATS:**

Note: There is very little information available regarding ertapenem use in dogs or cats and, therefore use must be considered investigational. If the drug is to be administered, it is suggested to use the human pediatric dose of 15 mg/kg IV or IM every 12 hours (not to exceed a daily dosage of 1 gram). Monitor the literature for additional data and recommendations.

Monitoring

- Clinical efficacy (WBC, fever, etc.).
- Adverse effects (potentially: GI, neurotoxicity, hypersensitivity); in humans receiving ertapenem for a prolonged period, hepatic, hematopoietic, and renal function tests are suggested for periodic assessment.

Client Information

- Must be injected into a muscle (IM) or under the skin (SC; subcutaneously).
- The time between doses must be longer in patients with kidney damage.

Chemistry/Synonyms

Ertapenem sodium is a synthetic 1-(beta) methyl carbapenem antibiotic that occurs as a white to off-white, hygroscopic, crystalline powder. It is soluble in water and normal saline.

Ertapenem may also be known as L-749345, ML-0826, ZD-4433, ertapenemum or *Invanz®*.

Storage/Stability

The 1 gram injectable product contains approximately 6 mEq of sodium and 175 mg of sodium bicarbonate (as an excipient). It should be stored at temperatures at, or below, 25°C.

Compatibility/Compounding Considerations

For intravenous use, vial contents can be reconstituted with 10 mL of water for injection, bacteriostatic water for injection, or 0.9% sodium chloride injection. After shaking to dissolve the powder, immediately transfer to a 50 mL bag of 0.9% sodium chloride. Do not use diluents containing dextrose. Once reconstituted and diluted in normal saline for IV use, ertapenem is stable at room temperature for 6 hours. If refrigerated, it can be stored for 24 hours and used within 4 hours after removal from the refrigerator. Do not freeze reconstituted solutions.

If ertapenem is to be given IM, dilute the vial with 3.2 mL of 1% lidocaine HCl injection (<u>without epinephrine</u>). Use within one hour. Do not give IV.

Do not mix ertapenem with other medications or use IV solutions containing dextrose.

Dosage Forms/Regulatory Status

VETERINARY-LABELED PRODUCTS: NONE.

HUMAN-LABELED PRODUCTS:

Ertapenem Sodium Lyophilized Powder for Injection: 1 g (as 1.045 g ertapenem) in single-dose vials; *Invanz®*; (Rx)

Revisions/References

Monograph revised/updated January 2014.

Erythromycin

(er-ith-roe-mye-sin)   Gallimycin®

Macrolide Antibiotic

Prescriber Highlights

▶ Macrolide antibiotic; also used as a prokinetic agent. Most commonly used (with rifampin) in foals; uncommonly used in dogs and cats.

▶ Contraindicated in rabbits, gerbils, guinea pigs, & hamsters; oral use in ruminants, adult horses(?), hypersensitivity.

▶ Adverse Effects: GI distress (oral), pain on IM injection; thrombophlebitis (IV), hyperthermia (foals). May cause neurological signs in dogs with MDR1 mutation.

▶ Many drug interactions possible.

Uses/Indications

An injectable erythromycin product is approved is for use to treat infections caused by susceptible organisms in cats, dogs, and cattle, but it is no longer commonly used for this purpose in these species.

Erythromycin is still one of the treatments (with rifampin) for the treatment of C. (*Rhodococcus*) *equi* infections in foals, but many now use other macrolides (clarithromycin or azithromycin ± rifampin/rifampicin). Erythromycin estolate and microencapsulated base appear to be the most efficacious forms of the drug in foals due to better absorption and less frequent adverse effects.

Erythromycin may be used as a prokinetic agent to increase gastric emptying in dogs and cats. It may also be beneficial in treating reflux esophagitis, especially in cats and for treating colonic motility disorders in dogs (not cats).

Pharmacology/Actions

Erythromycin is usually a bacteriostatic agent, but in high concentrations or against highly susceptible organisms (*e.g.,* streptococci) it may be bactericidal (time-dependent). The macrolides (erythromycin, tylosin, etc.) are believed to act by binding to the 50S ribosomal subunit of susceptible bacteria, thereby inhibiting peptide bond formation.

Erythromycin has *in vitro* activity against gram-positive cocci (staphylococci, streptococci), gram-positive bacilli [*Bacillus anthracis*, Corynebacterium, *Clostridium* spp., (not *C. difficile*), Listeria, Erysipelothrix], and some strains of gram-negative bacilli, including Haemophilus, Pasteurella, and Brucella. Some strains of Actinomyces, Mycoplasma, Chlamydia, Ureaplasma, and Rickettsia are also inhibited by erythromycin. Most strains of the family Enterobacteriaceae (Pseudomonas, *E. coli*, Klebsiella, etc.) and methicillin-resistant staphylococci are resistant to erythromycin. Tolerance (increasing MICs) by *R. equi* to both erythromycin and rifampin is troubling, and resistance has been documented in some isolates.

Like other macrolides, antimicrobial activity is reduced at lower pH, in abscesses, or necrotic tissues. When used to treat bacterial UTI, alkalinizing the urine is sometimes suggested.

At sub-antimicrobial doses, erythromycin mimics the effects of motilin (in cats, humans, rabbits) or 5-hydroxytryptophan3 (5-HT3) and can stimulate migrating motility complexes and antegrade peristalsis. By inducing antral contractions, gastric emptying is enhanced. Erythromycin also increases lower esophageal pressure and could be useful in treating cats (and dogs possibly) with gastroesophageal reflux and reflux esophagitis. Erythromycin is reported to stimulate colonic activity in dogs, but not in cats. Erythromycin's prokinetic mechanism of action in dogs is not completely understood, but probably is via activation of 5-HT3 receptors. Prokinetic activity may diminish with chronic use (tachyphylaxis).

It has been suggested that combining erythromycin with metoclopramide could lessen tachyphylaxis.

Pharmacokinetics

Erythromycin is absorbed after oral administration in the upper small intestine. Several factors can influence the bioavailability of erythromycin, including salt form, dosage form, GI acidity, food in the stomach, and stomach emptying time. Both erythromycin base and stearate are susceptible to acid degradation; enteric coatings are often used to alleviate this. In most species, ethylsuccinate and estolate forms are dissociated in the upper small intestine and then absorbed. But a study in cats found that oral administration of erythromycin ethylsuccinate tablets or suspension did not result in measureable serum concentrations (Albarellos et al. 2011). After IM or SC injection of the polyethylene-based veterinary product (*Erythro*®-200; *Gallimycin*®-200) in cattle, absorption is very slow. Bioavailabilities are only about 40% after SC injection and 65% after IM injection.

Erythromycin is distributed throughout the body into most fluids and tissues including the prostate, macrophages, and leukocytes. CSF levels are poor. In foals, erythromycin levels in bronchiolar lavage cells are equivalent to those found in the serum, but concentrations in pulmonary epithelial lining fluid are lower. Erythromycin may be 73-81% bound to serum proteins and the estolate salt, 96% bound. Erythromycin will cross the placenta; fetal serum levels are 5-20% of maternal levels. Erythromycin levels of about 50% of those found in the serum can be detected in milk. The volume of distribution for erythromycin in dogs is reportedly 2 L/kg; 3.7 – 7.2 L/kg in foals; 2.3 L/kg in mares; 2.34 L/kg in cats, and 0.8 – 1.6 L/kg in cattle. In lactating dairy cattle, the milk:plasma ratio is 6:7.

Erythromycin is primarily excreted unchanged in the bile, but is also partly metabolized by the liver via N-demethylation to inactive metabolites. Some of the drug is reabsorbed after biliary excretion. Only about 2-5% of a dose is excreted unchanged in the urine.

The reported elimination half-life of erythromycin in various species is: 60-90 minutes in dogs and cats, 60-70 minutes in foals and mares, and 190 minutes in cattle.

Contraindications/Precautions/Warnings

Erythromycin is contraindicated in patients hypersensitive to it. In humans, the estolate form has been associated rarely with the development of cholestatic hepatitis. This effect has not apparently been reported in veterinary species, but the estolate should probably be avoided in patients with preexisting liver dysfunction.

As it may induce a toxic enterocolitis, erythromycin (and other macrolides) is contraindicated in rabbits, gerbils, guinea pigs, and hamsters.

Many clinicians believe that erythromycin is contraindicated in adult horses (see Adverse Effects below), and oral erythromycin should not be used in ruminants as severe diarrhea may result. Unless *R. equi* is confirmed, erythromycin should be used with caution in horses greater than 4 months old (Divers 2009). In foals with *R. equi* infections, prolonged monotherapy could potentially induce *R. equi* resistance; treating without concomitant rifampin is best avoided.

Because erythromycin is implicated in causing hyperthermia/fatal respiratory distress in foals treated during hot weather, provision of shade and close observation is advised.

Adverse Effects

Adverse effects are relatively infrequent with erythromycin when used in small animals, swine, sheep, or cattle. When injected IM, local reactions and pain at the injection site may occur. Oral erythromycin may occasionally cause GI disturbances such as diarrhea, anorexia, and vomiting. Rectal edema and partial anal prolapse have been associated with erythromycin in swine. Intravenous injections must be given very slowly, as they can readily cause thrombophlebitis. Allergic reactions can occur but are thought to be rare.

A case of a dog with the MDR1 mutation developing neurological signs after receiving erythromycin has been reported.

Oral erythromycin should not be used in ruminants as severe diarrheas may result.

In foals treated with erythromycin, partial anorexia, bruxism, and a mild, self-limiting diarrhea can occur; these generally resolve after temporarily stopping treatment. However, severe enterocolitis is possible. Erythromycin may alter temperature homeostasis in foals. Foals between the ages of 2-4 months old have reportedly developed hyperthermia with associated respiratory distress and tachypnea. Physically cooling off these animals has been successful in controlling this effect. Mares of treated foals can develop clostridial enterocolitis, presumably via coprophagia of the foal's feces.

Adult horses may develop severe, sometimes fatal, diarrheas from erythromycin making the use of the drug in adults very controversial. Mares of foals treated with erythromycin have, on occasion, developed severe diarrhea/fatal colitis, possibly through contamination of feeders, water buckets, or via coprophagia.

When used as prokinetic agent, erythromycin may actually increase clinical signs of intestinal distress as it can stimulate emptying of larger food particles into the intestine than is normal.

Reproductive/Nursing Safety

While erythromycin has not demonstrated teratogenic effects in rats, and the drug is not thought to possess serious teratogenic potential, it should only be used during pregnancy when the benefits outweigh the risks. In humans, the FDA categorizes erythromycin and its salts, except ethylsuccinate, as category *B* for use during pregnancy (*Animal studies have not yet demonstrated risk to the fetus, but there are no adequate studies in pregnant women; or animal studies have shown an adverse effect, but adequate studies in pregnant women have not demonstrated a risk to the fetus in the first trimester of pregnancy, and there is no evidence of risk in later trimesters.*) In a separate system evaluating the safety of drugs in canine and feline pregnancy (Papich 1989), this drug is categorized as class: *A* (*Probably safe. Although specific studies may not have proved the safety of all drugs in dogs and cats, there are no reports of adverse effects in laboratory animals or women.*)

In humans, the FDA categorizes erythromycin ethylsuccinate as category *C* for use during pregnancy (*Animal studies have shown an adverse effect on the fetus, but there are no adequate studies in humans; or there are no animal reproduction studies and no adequate studies in humans.*)

Erythromycin is excreted in milk and may concentrate (observed milk:plasma ratio of 0.5). Erythromycin is considered compatible with breastfeeding by the American Academy of Pediatrics.

Overdosage/Acute Toxicity

With the exception of the adverse effects outlined above, erythromycin is relatively non-toxic; however, shock reactions have been reported in baby pigs receiving erythromycin overdosages.

Drug Interactions

The following drug interactions have either been reported or are theoretical in humans or animals receiving erythromycin and may be of significance in veterinary patients. Unless otherwise noted, use together is not necessarily contraindicated, but weigh the potential risks and perform additional monitoring when appropriate.

- **AZOLE ANTIFUNGALS (ketoconazole, fluconazole, itraconazole**, etc.): Possible increased erythromycin levels.
- **CISAPRIDE:** Erythromycin can inhibit the metabolism of cisapride and the manufacturer states that use of these drugs together (in humans) is contraindicated; however it has been re-

ported that in one study in dogs, erythromycin did not alter the pharmacodynamics of cisapride (Trepanier 2008).

- **CHLORAMPHENICOL:** *in vitro* evidence of antagonism.
- **CLINDAMYCIN, LINCOMYCIN:** *in vitro* evidence of antagonism.
- **DIGOXIN:** Erythromycin may increase the serum level of digoxin.
- **DILTIAZEM, VERAPAMIL:** May increase erythromycin levels.
- **OMEPRAZOLE:** Erythromycin and omeprazole can increase the plasma levels of one another.
- **SUCRALFATE:** May reduce the absorption of erythromycin; separate doses by two hours if possible.
- **WARFARIN:** Erythromycin may potentiate the effects of oral anticoagulant drugs.

Erythromycin can inhibit the metabolism of other drugs that use the CYP3A subfamily of the cytochrome P450 enzyme system. Depending on the therapeutic index of the drug(s) involved, therapeutic drug monitoring and/or dosage reduction may be required if the drugs must be used together. These drugs include:

- **ALFENTANIL**
- **BROMOCRIPTINE**
- **BUSPIRONE**
- **CARBAMAZEPINE**
- **CYCLOSPORINE**
- **DISOPYRAMIDE** (also risk of increased QT interval)
- **METHYLPREDNISOLONE**
- **MIDAZOLAM, ALPRAZOLAM, TRIAZOLAM**
- **QUINIDINE** (also risk of increased QT interval)
- **SILDENAFIL**
- **TACROLIMUS (SYSTEMIC)**
- **THEOPHYLLINE**

Laboratory Considerations
- Erythromycin may cause falsely elevated values of **AST** (SGOT), and **ALT** (SGPT) when using colorimetric assays.
- Fluorometric determinations of **urinary catecholamines** can be altered by concomitant erythromycin administration.

Doses
- **DOGS:**

  For susceptible infections (extra-label): Not commonly used in dogs. Erythromycin has a short half-life, oral bioavailability can be very low, and it can cause significant GI side effects; 10 – 20 mg/kg PO q8-12h has been suggested. One reference states that oral erythromycin at 10 – 15 mg/kg PO q8h is the drug of choice for treating enteric campylobacteriosis (Weese 2011).

  As a prokinetic agent (extra-label): 0.5 – 1 mg/kg PO q8h. (Hall et al. 2000), (Twedt 2008)

- **CATS:**

  For susceptible infections (extra-label): Not commonly used in cats; has a short half-life and oral bioavailability can be very low: 10 – 20 mg/kg PO q8-12h has been suggested.

  As a prokinetic agent (extra-label): 0.5 – 1 mg/kg PO q8h. (Hall et al. 2000) Does not appear to have colonic motility stimulating effects in cats.

- **FERRETS:**

  For susceptible infections (extra-label): 10 mg/kg PO 4 times daily. (Williams 2000)

- **BIRDS:**

  For susceptible infections (extra-label): Oral suspension: 60 mg/kg PO q12h. (Hoeffer 1995)

- **CATTLE:**

  For treatment of bovine respiratory disease (shipping fever complex and bacterial pneumonia) associated with *Pasteurella multocida* organisms susceptible to erythromycin (Label dosage; FDA-approved for use in beef cattle): Administer 4 mL/100 lbs. body weight (4 mg/lb.; 8.8 mg/kg) once daily for up to 5 days as needed. Administer via deep intramuscular injection (no more than 10 mL per site) into the heavy neck muscles, or if necessary for alternating injection sites, into the heavy muscular portion of the leg muscle (round). In calves less than 200 lbs., no more than 4 mL/site deep intramuscular injection into the heavy muscles of the leg only. Use a 1-inch to 2-inch, 16 or 18 gauge needle depending on the animal's size. Do not use in female dairy cattle greater than 20 months of age or in calves to be processed for veal. (Adapted from label; *Gallimycin®*-100)

- **HORSES:**

  For treatment of *C.* (*Rhodococcus*) *equi* infections in foals (extra-label): Most recommend using the estolate or enteric-coated (base) forms of erythromycin at 20 – 25 mg/kg orally q8h (although some say q6-8h or q8-12h) and rifampin (at 5 mg/kg PO q12h or 10 mg/kg PO q24h). Treatment may be required for 1-3 months. Early diagnosis and treatment may reduce treatment duration.

  For treatment of proliferative enteropathy caused by *L. intracellularis* infections in foals: Erythromycin estolate at 25 mg/kg PO q6-8h, with rifampin: 10 mg/kg PO q12h for a minimum of 21 days. (Lavoie et al. 2003)

Monitoring
- Clinical efficacy.
- Adverse effects (periodic liver function tests if patient receiving erythromycin estolate long-term; may not be necessary for foals receiving erythromycin and rifampin for Rhodococcus infections).

Client Information
- The intramuscular 100 mg/mL (*Erythro-100®*) product has quite specific instructions on where and how to inject the drug. Refer to the label directions or package insert for more information before using.
- When administering orally to small animals, give on an empty stomach unless gastrointestinal signs (vomiting, lack of appetite, diarrhea) occur, then give with food. The estolate, ethylsuccinate or enteric-coated forms of erythromycin may be given with or without food.
- If gastrointestinal adverse effects are severe or persist, contact veterinarian.

Chemistry/Synonyms
A macrolide antibiotic, produced from *Streptomyces erythreus*, erythromycin is a weak base that is available commercially in several salts and esters. It has a pK$_a$ of 8.9.

Erythromycin base occurs as a bitter tasting, odorless or practically odorless, white to slight yellow, crystalline powder. Approximately 1 mg is soluble in 1 mL of water; it is soluble in alcohol.

Erythromycin estolate occurs as a practically tasteless and odorless, white, crystalline powder. It is practically insoluble in water and approximately 50 mg are soluble in 1 mL of alcohol. Erythromycin estolate may also be known as erythromycin propionate lauryl sulfate.

Erythromycin ethylsuccinate occurs as a practically tasteless and odorless, white to slight yellow, crystalline powder. It is very slightly soluble in water and freely soluble in alcohol.

Erythromycin lactobionate occurs as white to slightly yellow crystals or powder. It may have a faint odor and is freely soluble in water and alcohol.

Erythromycin may also be known as: eritromicina, and erythromycinum; many trade names are available.

Storage/Stability

Erythromycin (base) capsules and tablets should be stored in tight containers at room temperature (15-30°C). Erythromycin estolate preparations should be protected from light. To retain palatability, the oral suspensions should be refrigerated.

Erythromycin ethylsuccinate tablets and powder for oral suspension should be stored in tight containers at room temperature. The commercially available oral suspension should be stored in the refrigerator to preserve palatability. After dispensing, the oral suspensions are stable for at least 14 days at room temperature, but individual products may have longer labeled stabilities.

Erythromycin lactobionate powder for injection should be stored at room temperature. For initial reconstitution (vials), only sterile water for injection should be used. After reconstitution, the drug is stable for 24 hours at room temperature and 2 weeks if refrigerated. To prepare for administration via continuous or intermittent infusion, the drug is further diluted in 0.9% sodium chloride, Lactated Ringer's, or Normosol-R. Other infusion solutions may be used, but first must be buffered with 4% sodium bicarbonate injection (1 mL per 100 mL of solution). At pH's of <5.5, the drug is unstable and loses potency rapidly.

Compatibility/Compounding Considerations

Many drugs are physically **incompatible** with erythromycin lactobionate; it is suggested to consult specialized references or a hospital pharmacist for more specific information.

Dosage Forms/Regulatory Status

VETERINARY-LABELED PRODUCTS:

Erythromycin 100 mg/mL for IM Injection (with 2% butyl aminobenzoate as a local anesthetic) in 100 mL vials; *Gallimycin®-100*; (OTC). FDA-approved (NADA 012-123) for use in cattle, dogs, and cats. Slaughter withdrawal (when used as labeled) for cattle = 21 days. A link to the *Gallimycin®-100* label may be found at dailymed. nlm.nih.gov

There may also be erythromycin premixes alone and in combination with other drugs for use in swine and/or poultry.

HUMAN-LABELED PRODUCTS:

Erythromycin Base Delayed-release Oral Tablets enteric-coated: 250 mg, 333 mg & 500 mg; *Ery-Tab®*; (Rx)

Erythromycin Base Tablets Film-coated: 250 mg, & 500 mg; generic; (Rx)

Erythromycin Base Delayed-release Oral Capsules enteric-coated pellets: 250 mg; *Erythrocin Stearate®*; (Rx)

Erythromycin Stearate Film-coated tablets: 250 mg; generic; (Rx)

Erythromycin Ethylsuccinate Tablets: 400 mg; *E.E.S. 400®*, generic; (Rx)

Erythromycin Ethylsuccinate Powder for Oral Suspension: 200 mg/5 mL when reconstituted 100 mL & 200; *EryPed® 200 & 400, E.E.S. Granules®*; (Rx)

Erythromycin Ethylsuccinate Granules for Oral Suspension: 200 mg/5 mL in 100 & 200 mL; *E.E.S. Granules®*; (Rx)

Erythromycin Ethylsuccinate Powder for Oral Suspension: 400 mg/5 mL in 100, 200, & UD 5 mL; *EryPed 400®*; (Rx)

Erythromycin Ethylsuccinate Powder for Oral Suspension: 100 mg/2.5 mL in 50 mL *EryPed Drops®*; (Rx)

Erythromycin Lactobionate Lyophilized Powder for Injection Solution: 500 mg & 1 g (as lactobionate) in vials; *Eythrocin®*; (Rx)

Erythromycin & Sulfisoxazole Granules for Oral Suspension: erythromycin ethylsuccinate (equivalent to 200 mg erythromycin activity) and sulfisoxazole acetyl (equivalent to 600 mg sulfisoxazole) per 5 mL when reconstituted in 100 mL, 150 mL & 200 mL; *Eryzole®*; *Pediazole®*; generic; (Rx)

Topical and ophthalmic preparations are also available.

Revisions/References

Monograph revised/updated January 2014.

Albarellos, G. A., et al. (2011). Pharmacokinetics of erythromycin after intravenous, intramuscular and oral administration to cats. Veterinary Journal **187**(1): 129-32.

Divers, T. J. (2009). Diagnosing, treating and preventing Rhodococcus equi. Proceedings: WVC. accessed via Veterinary Information Network; vin.com

Hall, J. & R. Washabau (2000). Gastric Prokinetic Agents. *Kirk's Current Veterinary Therapy: XIII Small Animal Practice*. J. Bonagura. Philadelphia, WB Saunders: 609-17.

Hoeffer, H. (1995). Antimicrobials in pet birds. *Kirk's Current Veterinary Therapy:XII.* J. Bonagura. Philadelphia, W.B. Saunders: 1278-83.

Lavoie, J.-P. & R. Drolet (2003). Proliferative enteropathy in foals. Proceedings: ACVIM Forum. accessed via Veterinary Information Network; vin.com

Trepanier, L. (2008). Top Ten Potential Drug Interactions in Dogs and Cats. Proceedings: WSAVA. accessed via Veterinary Information Network; vin.com

Twedt, D. (2008). Antiemetics, prokinetics & antacids. Proceedings: ACVIM. accessed via Veterinary Information Network; vin.com

Weese, J. S. (2011). Bacterial Enteritis in Dogs and Cats: Diagnosis, Therapy, and Zoonotic Potential. Veterinary Clinics of North America-Small Animal Practice **41**(2): 287-+.

Williams, B. (2000). Therapeutics in Ferrets. Vet Clin NA: Exotic Anim Pract 3:**1**(Jan): 131-53.

Esmolol HCl

(ess-moe-lol)   Brevibloc®

Beta-1 Blocker

Prescriber Highlights

▶ Ultra-short acting beta₁-blocker used IV for short-term treatment of SVT's or to determine if beta-blockers are effective for controlling arrhythmias.

▶ Contraindications: Patients with overt cardiac failure, 2nd or 3rd degree AV block, sinus bradycardia, or in cardiogenic shock.

▶ Caution: Patients with CHF, bronchoconstrictive lung disease, or diabetes mellitus.

▶ Adverse Effects: Hypotension & bradycardia are the effects most likely seen.

Uses/Indications

Esmolol may be used as a test drug to indicate whether beta-blocker therapy is warranted, as an antiarrhythmic agent particularly in cats with hypertrophic cardiomyopathy, or as an infusion in the short-term treatment of supraventricular tachyarrhythmias (*e.g.*, atrial fibrillation/flutter, sinus tachycardia).

Pharmacology/Actions

Esmolol primarily blocks both beta₁-adrenergic receptors in the myocardium. At clinically used doses, esmolol does not have any intrinsic sympathomimetic activity (ISA) and unlike propranolol, does not possess membrane-stabilizing effects (quinidine-like) or bronchoconstrictive effects. Cardiovascular effects secondary to esmolol include negative inotropic and chronotropic activity that can lead to reduced myocardial oxygen demand. Systolic and diastolic blood pressures are reduced at rest and during exercise. Esmolol's antiarrhythmic effect is thought to be due to its blockade of adrenergic stimulation of cardiac pacemaker potentials. Esmolol increases sinus cycle length, slows AV node conduction, and prolongs sinus node recovery time.

Pharmacokinetics

After IV injection esmolol is rapidly and widely distributed but not appreciably to the CNS, spleen or testes. The distribution half-life is about 2 minutes. Steady-state blood levels occur in about 5 minutes if a loading dose was given or about 30 minutes if no load was given. It is unknown whether the drug crosses the placenta or enters milk. Esmolol is rapidly metabolized in the blood by esterases to a practically inactive metabolite. Renal or hepatic dysfunction does not appreciably alter elimination characteristics. Terminal half-life is about 10 minutes and duration of action after discontinuing IV infusion is usually about 20 minutes post-infusion in dogs.

Contraindications/Precautions/Warnings

Esmolol is contraindicated in patients with overt cardiac failure, 2nd or 3rd degree AV block, sinus bradycardia, or in cardiogenic shock. It should be used with caution (weigh benefit vs. risk) in patients with CHF, bronchoconstrictive lung disease, or diabetes mellitus.

In patients with tachycardia secondary to pheochromocytoma, esmolol should be given in combination with (or after) an alpha-blocker, or a paradoxical increase in blood pressure can occur secondary to attenuation of beta-mediated vasodilation in skeletal muscle.

Adverse Effects

At usual doses adverse effects are uncommon and generally an extension of the drug's pharmacologic effects. Hypotension (with resultant clinical signs) and bradycardia are the most likely adverse effects seen. These usually prove mild and transient in nature. Esmolol may mask certain clinical signs of developing hypoglycemia (such as increased heart rate or blood pressure).

Reproductive/Nursing Safety

Studies done in rats and rabbits demonstrated no teratogenic effects at doses up to 3X the maximum human maintenance dose (MHMD). Higher doses (8X or more MHMD) demonstrated some maternal death and fetal resorption.

It is unknown if esmolol is excreted in milk.

Overdosage/Acute Toxicity

The IV LD$_{50}$ in dogs is approximately 32 mg/kg. Dogs receiving 2 mg/kg per minute for one hour showed no adverse effects; doses of 3 mg/kg/minute for one hour produced ataxia and salivation and 4 mg/kg/minute for one hour caused muscular rigidity, tremors, seizures, ptosis, vomiting, hyperpnea, vocalizations, and prostration. These effects all resolved within 90 minutes of the end of infusion. Because of the short duration of action of the drug, discontinuation or dosage reduction may be all that is required; otherwise, symptomatic and supportive treatment may be initiated.

Drug Interactions

The following drug interactions have either been reported or are theoretical in humans or animals receiving esmolol and may be of significance in veterinary patients. Unless otherwise noted, use together is not necessarily contraindicated, but weigh the potential risks and perform additional monitoring when appropriate.

- **CALCIUM CHANNEL BLOCKERS** (*e.g.*, **diltiazem, verapamil**): Pharmacologic effects of both classes of agents may be potentiated. IV administration in close proximity is contraindicated. Monitor cardiac function and adjust therapy as needed. Generally, drugs such as diltiazem can be safely administered 30 minutes after esmolol administration has been discontinued.
- **DIGOXIN**: Esmolol may increase serum digoxin levels up to 20%, but these drugs have been used together safely and effectively.

- **MONOAMINE OXIDASE INHIBITORS**: Concurrent use of monoamine oxidase inhibitors with esmolol is not recommended due to potential risk of hypertension.
- **MORPHINE**: Titrate esmolol dosage carefully in patients also receiving morphine as it may increase steady-state esmolol serum concentrations up to 50%.
- **RESERPINE**: May see additive effects (hypotension, bradycardia) if used with esmolol.
- **VASOCONSTRICTORS/INOTROPES** (*e.g.*, **dopamine, epinephrine, norepinephrine**): If systemic vascular resistance is high, there is an increase risk for blocked cardiac contractility; esmolol is not recommended to control SVT's in patients receiving these drugs.

Doses

- **DOGS/CATS:**

   For ultra-short acting beta blockade (for treating or assisting in treatment of ventricular arrhythmias) (extra-label): Dosage recommendations vary somewhat and there does not appear to be clear evidence supporting any dosage. Often an initial IV loading dose of 0.25 – 0.5 mg/kg (250 – 500 micrograms/kg) is administered IV over 2-5 minutes and then a CRI of 10 – 200 micrograms/kg/minute IV is started. Some recommend initial dosages as low as 0.05 – 0.1 mg/kg (50 – 100 micrograms/kg) with intermittent IV bolus doses of 0.05 – 0.1 mg/kg (50 – 100 micrograms/kg) administered every 5 minutes up to a maximum dose of 0.5 mg/kg (500 micrograms/kg). If esmolol is to be used in animals with severe heart failure or mitral regurgitation, it is best dosed without an initial bolus and at the lower end of the CRI rates. CRI can be adjusted upwards every 10 minutes while patient is continuously monitored.

Monitoring

- Blood Pressure.
- ECG.
- Heart Rate.

Client Information

- Esmolol should only be used in an in-patient setting where appropriate monitoring is available.

Chemistry/Synonyms

A short acting beta$_1$-adrenergic blocker, esmolol occurs as white or off white crystalline powder. It is not as lipophilic as either labetalol or propranolol, but is comparable to acebutolol. 650 mg are soluble in one mL of water and 350 mg are soluble in one mL of alcohol.

Esmolol HCl may also be known as ASL-8052, *Brevibloc®* or *Miniblock®*.

Storage/Stability

The concentrate for injection should be stored at room temperature; do not freeze and protect from excessive heat. It is a clear, colorless to light yellow solution. Expiration dates of 3 years are assigned after manufacture.

After diluted to a concentration of 10 mg/mL esmolol HCl is stable (at refrigeration temperatures or room temperature) for at least 24 hours in commonly used IV solutions.

Compatibility/Compounding Considerations

Esmolol may be diluted in standard D5, LRS or saline (or combinations thereof) IV fluids. At this concentration it is reportedly physically **compatible** with digoxin, dopamine, fentanyl, lidocaine, morphine sulfate, nitroglycerin, and nitroprusside. Compatibility is dependent upon factors such as pH, concentration, temperature, and diluent used; consult specialized references or a hospital pharmacist for more specific information.

Dosage Forms/Regulatory Status

VETERINARY-LABELED PRODUCTS: NONE.

The ARCI (Racing Commissioners International) has designated this drug as a class 3 substance. See the appendix for more information.

HUMAN-LABELED PRODUCTS:

Esmolol HCl Injection: 10 mg/mL regular & preservative free in 10 mL vials; 20 mg/mL preservative free in 5 mL vials & 100 mL bags; and 250 mg/mL in 10 mL amps; *Brevibloc®*; generic; (Rx)

Revisions/References

Monograph revised/updated January 2014.

Esomeprazole

(ess-oh-meh-prah-zahl)   NexIUM®

Proton Pump Inhibitor

Prescriber Highlights

▶ Proton pump inhibitor (PPI) used for GI ulcers & erosions; little information on its use in veterinary species is published. Available in oral capsules/suspensions and IV forms.

▶ PO doses should be given on an empty stomach (preferably one hour before food).

▶ Adverse Effects: **Horses:** Unlikely; potentially, hypersensitivity. **Small Animals:** Likely to be well tolerated. Potentially: GI distress (anorexia, colic, nausea, vomiting, flatulence, diarrhea), hematologic abnormalities, urinary tract infections, proteinuria, or CNS disturbances are possible.

▶ Human generic forms expected in 2014 in USA.

Uses/Indications

Esomeprazole is a proton pump inhibitor (PPI) potentially useful in treating both gastroduodenal ulcer disease and to prevent or treat gastric erosions caused by ulcerogenic drugs (*e.g.*, aspirin). It is unclear how esomeprazole's efficacy compares with other PPI's in veterinary species as little information has been published. A study to determine whether preanesthetic IV administration of esomeprazole alone or esomeprazole with cisapride increased esophageal pH and decreased frequency of gastrointestinal reflux (GER) in anesthetized dogs found that while esomeprazole alone increased gastric and esophageal pH, it did not alter the incidence of GER when compared to the control group. Subjects that received both esomeprazole and cisapride had significantly reduced numbers of reflux events (Zacuto et al. 2012). Two studies in horses (PO/NGT and IV) found that it caused significant increases in gastric pH (Pereira et al. 2009; Videla et al. 2011). At present, the greatest potential attribute for this agent are the multiple dosage forms (oral capsules, oral suspensions, intravenous) and strengths that are commercially available. At the time of writing (12/2013), the drug is comparatively more expensive than other PPI's available as generic products, but approved generic forms are expected sometime in 2014.

Pharmacology/Actions

Esomeprazole is a substituted benzimidazole gastric acid (proton) pump inhibitor. It binds irreversibly at the secretory surface of parietal cells to the enzyme, H^+/K^+ ATPase. There it inhibits the transport of hydrogen ions into the stomach. Esomeprazole reduces acid secretion during both basal and stimulated conditions. There is a lag time between administration and efficacy in most species, but it appears that in both dogs and horses effects can be rapid. Esomeprazole may also inhibit some hepatic cytochrome P-450 oxidase system isoenzymes (see Drug Interactions below).

Pharmacokinetics

Specific pharmacokinetic information for esomeprazole in veterinary species was not located.

In humans oral esomeprazole is well absorbed when taken on an empty stomach, but the presence of food can reduce bioavailability from approximately 90% to about 50%. Peak levels occur about 1.5 hours after dosing. Esomeprazole is 97% bound to human plasma proteins and in healthy human adults the apparent volume of distribution at steady state is approximately 16 L. Esomeprazole is predominantly metabolized in the liver by the cytochrome P450 (CYP-450) enzyme system with the isoenzyme CYP2C19 forming the majority of metabolites (hydroxy and desmethyl forms) and to a lesser extent the CYP3A4 isoenzyme forming the sulphone metabolite. Plasma elimination half-life of esomeprazole in humans is approximately 1-1.5 hours. Less than 1% of parent drug is excreted in the urine unchanged with about 80% of the dose excreted into the urine as metabolites. The remainder is excreted in the feces as unabsorbed drug or as metabolites.

Contraindications/Precautions/Warnings

Esomeprazole is contraindicated in patients hypersensitive to it. In patients with severe hepatic disease, the drug's half-life may be prolonged and dosage adjustment may be necessary.

Do not confuse ESOmeprazole with Omeprazole or other similar sounding proton pump inhibitors.

Adverse Effects

There is little clinical experience or published data on the safety of this drug in animal patients, but it is likely to be well tolerated similarly to other PPIs. Potentially, GI distress (anorexia, colic, nausea, vomiting, flatulence, diarrhea; *C. difficile* infection) could occur, as well as hematologic abnormalities (rare in humans), urinary tract infections, proteinuria, or CNS disturbances.

Reproductive/Nursing Safety

Esomeprazole's safety during pregnancy has not been established, but it is not considered a significant teratogen. In humans, the FDA categorizes this drug as category *B* for use during human pregnancy (*Animal studies have not yet demonstrated risk to the fetus, but there are no adequate studies in pregnant women; or animal studies have shown an adverse effect, but adequate studies in pregnant women have not demonstrated a risk to the fetus in the first trimester of pregnancy, and there is no evidence of risk in later trimesters.*)

It is not known whether esomeprazole is excreted in maternal milk. For humans, because of the potential for serious adverse reactions in nursing infants, and the potential for tumorigenicity shown in rat carcinogenicity studies, nursing is discouraged if the drug is required.

Overdosage/Acute Toxicity

Little information on acute toxicity is available. The LD_{50} of esomeprazole in rats after oral administration is reportedly >4 grams/kg. Humans have tolerated oral dosages of 360 mg/day of esomeprazole without significant toxicity. Should a massive overdose occur, treat symptomatically and supportively.

Drug Interactions

The following drug interactions have either been reported or are theoretical in humans or animals receiving esomeprazole and may be of significance in veterinary patients. Unless otherwise noted, use together is not necessarily contraindicated, but weigh the potential risks and perform additional monitoring when appropriate.

- **AZOLE ANTIFUNGALS (ketoconazole, itraconazole**, etc.): Esomeprazole can reduce absorption, and azoles potentially can increase esomeprazole exposure.

- **BENZODIAZEPINES** (*e.g.*, **diazepam**): Esomeprazole may potentially alter benzodiazepine metabolism and prolong CNS effects.

- **CLARITHROMYCIN:** Increased levels of esomeprazole, clarithromycin and 14-hydroxyclarithromycin are possible.
- **CYANOCOBALAMIN (oral):** Esomeprazole may decrease oral absorption.
- **CYCLOSPORINE:** Esomeprazole may reduce cyclosporine metabolism.
- **DIGOXIN:** Esomeprazole may increase digoxin levels.
- **DIURETICS (LOOP or THIAZIDES):** Increased risk for hypomagnesemia; increased monitoring suggested particularly in susceptible patients.
- **IRON, ORAL:** Esomeprazole may decrease iron absorption.
- **METHOTREXATE:** Esomeprazole may increase and prolong methotrexate (and its metabolite) levels.
- **MYCOPHENOLATE:** Esomeprazole may reduce mycophenolic acid (MPA; active metabolite) levels.
- **SUCRALFATE:** May inhibit absorption of esomeprazole; stagger dosages.
- **WARFARIN:** Esomeprazole may increase anticoagulant effect.

Laboratory Considerations
- Esomeprazole may cause increased **liver enzymes.**
- Esomeprazole will increase **serum gastrin** levels early in therapy.

Doses
- **DOGS:**

  As a PPI to reduce gastric acid production (extra-label):

  IV: In the study (measuring gastric/esophageal pH and gastric reflux in anesthetized dogs): 12-18 hours and again 1-1.5 hours before induction, esomeprazole sodium (1 mg/kg IV over 3 minutes); and cisapride (1 mg/kg IV diluted with sterile saline (0.9%) to a total volume of 100 mL and administered over 15 minutes) significantly increased pH and reduced reflux events. (Zacuto et al. 2012)

  Oral: There is little published supporting any oral esomeprazole dosage in dogs, anecdotally it could be used at similarly dosage rates as oral omeprazole (0.5 – 1.5 mg/kg PO once daily on an empty stomach).

- **CATS:**

  As a PPI to reduce gastric acid production (extra-label): Although there is little published supporting any oral esomeprazole dosage in cats, anecdotally it could be used at similarly dosage rates as oral omeprazole (0.5 – 1.5 mg/kg PO once daily on an empty stomach).

- **HORSES:**

  As a PPI to reduce gastric acid production (extra-label):

  PO/NG: A study done in 15 adult thoroughbred horses (5 control, 5 each for esomeprazole at 40 mg per horse & 80 mg per horse via NG tube before feeding for 5 days) found that both the 40 mg and 80 mg dosages (no significant differences between the two) increased gastric pH >5 when measured (90 minutes-6 hours after a dose. Effects occurred after the first dose. It is not known from the study how long (after 6 hours) pH effects persist so dosage frequency is not clear. (Pereira et al. 2009)

  IV: A study done in 12 quarter horses (4 control, 8 treatment group) found that esomeprazole (0.5 mg/kg IV once a day for 13 consecutive days) found on day 14 average gastric juice pH in treated animals was significantly higher than prior to treatment (6.43 vs. 4.24) and also when compared to control subjects. The authors concluded that IV esomeprazole caused a rapid and sustained increase in gastric juice pH in horses after the 1st and 5th daily doses and that it shows promise for treatment of gastric ulcers in horses with signs of dysphagia, gastric reflux, or other

conditions when the approved oral omeprazole paste cannot be used. (Videla et al. 2011)

Monitoring
- Efficacy.
- Adverse effects.

Client Information
- Should be given on an empty stomach (preferably in the morning one hour before food).

Chemistry/Synonyms
A substituted benzimidazole proton pump inhibitor, esomeprazole is the S-isomer of omeprazole and is available commercially as two primary salts: magnesium (PO use) and sodium (IV use). Esomeprazole magnesium (CAS Registry: 217087-09-7; ATC: A02BC05) occurs as a white to slightly colored powder. It is slightly soluble in water, soluble in methyl alcohol and practically insoluble in heptane. Esomeprazole sodium (CAS Registry: 161796-78-7; ATC: A02BC05) commercially available injection is a lyophilized powder with edetate disodium 1.5 mg and sodium hydroxide added to adjust pH (9-11) during manufacturing.

Nexium® 20 and 40 mg capsules contain sugar spheres. *Nexium®* 2.5, 5, 10, 20, and 40 mg powder for oral suspension also contains dextrose.

Esomeprazole may also be known as: (S)-omeprazole, H199/18I or perprazole. A common trade name is *Nexium*.

Storage/Stability
Oral capsules should be stored at 25°C (may be exposed to 15-30°C) in tightly closed containers.

Intact vials of esomeprazole sodium for injection should be stored at controlled room temperature and protected from light. After reconstitution and dilution with sodium chloride 0.9% or lactated Ringer's injection are used, it should be administered within 12 hours when stored at room temperature. If dextrose 5% is used for reconstitution and dilution, use within six hours at room temperature. The manufacturer states that refrigeration is not required. Stability of esomeprazole sodium in solution is strongly dependent on pH; stability of the drug decreases with decreasing pH.

Compatibility/Compounding Considerations
Esomeprazole sodium for injection should be reconstituted only with sterile 0.9% sodium chloride, lactated Ringer's injection or dextrose 5% (see stability above). Flushing the administration line with sodium chloride 0.9%, Ringer's injection, lactated, or dextrose 5% is required both before and after administering the drug. Mixing or giving with other drugs is not recommended.

For humans: If mixing capsule contents with food, only cold or room temperature applesauce is recommended and administration should occur immediately after mixing.

The human label (*Nexium®*) has the following directions for using the delayed oral suspension packets: Empty the contents of a 2.5 or 5 mg packet into a container with 5 mL of water; empty the contents of a 10, 20, or 40 mg packet into a container with 15 mL of water. Stir, then leave 2-3 minutes to thicken. Stir and drink within 30 minutes. If any material remains after drinking, add more water, stir, and drink immediately. In cases where there is a need to use 2 packets, they may be mixed in a similar way by adding twice the required amount of water, or follow the mixing instructions provided by the health care provider or pharmacist.

Nasogastric/Gastric tube administration: Add 5 mL of water to a catheter-tipped syringe and then add the contents of a 2.5 or 5 mg packet; for the 10, 20, or 40 mg packet, the volume of water in the syringe should be 15 mL. It is important to only use a catheter-tipped syringe when administering esomeprazole through a nasogastric or gastric tube. Immediately shake the syringe and leave

2-3 minutes to thicken. Shake the syringe and inject through the nasogastric or gastric tube (French size 6 or larger) into the stomach within 30 minutes. Refill the syringe with an equal amount of water (5 or 15 mL). Shake and flush any remaining contents from the nasogastric or gastric tube into the stomach.

Dosage Forms/Regulatory Status

VETERINARY-LABELED PRODUCTS: NONE.

HUMAN-LABELED PRODUCTS:

Esomeprazole Magnesium Oral Delayed-Release Capsules (containing enteric-coated granules): 20 mg & 40 mg; *NexIUM®*; generic; (Rx)

Esomeprazole Magnesium Powder for Oral Delayed-Release Suspension (containing enteric-coated granules): 2.5, 5, 10, 20, and 40 mg packets. NexIUM®; (Rx)

Esomeprazole Sodium for Injection: 20 & 40 mg; *NexIUM I.V.®*; (Rx)

There is also an oral product combined with naproxen but this would not be appropriate for veterinary use.

Revisions/References

Monograph written December 2013.

Pereira, M. C., et al. (2009). Preliminary Study of the Gastric Acidity in Thoroughbred Horses at Rest after Enteral Administration of Esomeprazole Magnesium (Nexium). Journal of Equine Veterinary Science 29(11): 791-4.

Videla, R., et al. (2011). Effects of Intravenously Administered Esomeprazole Sodium on Gastric Juice pH in Adult Female Horses. Journal of Veterinary Internal Medicine 25(3): 558-62.

Zacuto, A. C., et al. (2012). The Influence of Esomeprazole and Cisapride on Gastroesophageal Reflux During Anesthesia in Dogs. Journal of Veterinary Internal Medicine 26(3): 518-25.

Estradiol Cypionate

(ess-tra-dye-ole)   ECP®

Hormonal Agent (Estrogen)

Prescriber Highlights

▶ Natural estrogen salt used primarily to induce estrus; has been used as an abortifacient (but rarely recommended today).

▶ Contraindications: Pregnancy (abortifacient, teratogen); the FDA has stated that the use of ECP in food animals is illegal.

▶ Adverse Effects: In **cats & dogs**: Bone marrow toxicity, cystic endometrial hyperplasia, and pyometra.

▶ In male animals, feminization may occur; in females, signs of estrus may occur.

▶ Drug Interactions.

Uses/Indications

For mares, indications for the use of estradiol include enhancing estrus behavior and receptivity in ovariectomized mares and to treat estrogen-responsive incontinence. Historically, estradiol cypionate has been used as an abortifacient agent in cattle, cats and dogs, but estrogens are no longer recommended by most theriogenologists for use as an abortifacient in small animals and the FDA stated (April 5, 2006): "The use of ECP in food-producing animals is illegal, and manufacturing and compounding of ECP for such use is illegal."

Pharmacology/Actions

The most active endogenous estrogen, estradiol possesses the pharmacologic profile expected of the estrogen class. Estrogens are necessary for the normal growth and development of the female sex organs and in some species contribute to the development and maintenance of secondary female sex characteristics. Estrogens cause increased cell height and secretions of the cervical mucosa, thickening of the vaginal mucosa, endometrial proliferation, and increased uterine tone.

Estrogens have effects on the skeletal system. They increase calcium deposition, accelerate epiphyseal closure, and increase bone formation. Estrogens have a slight anabolic effect and can increase sodium and water retention.

Estrogens affect the release of gonadotropins from the pituitary gland. This can cause inhibition of lactation, ovulation, and androgen secretion.

Pharmacokinetics

No specific information was located regarding the pharmacokinetics of estradiol in veterinary species. In humans, estrogen in oil solutions after IM administration are absorbed promptly and absorption continues over several days. Esterified estrogens (*e.g.*, estradiol cypionate) have delayed absorption after IM administration. Estrogens are distributed throughout the body and accumulate in adipose tissue. Elimination of the steroidal estrogens occurs principally by hepatic metabolism. Estrogens and their metabolites are primarily excreted in the urine, but are also excreted into the bile where most are reabsorbed from the GI.

Contraindications/Precautions/Warnings

Estradiol is contraindicated during pregnancy as it can cause fetal malformations of the genitourinary system and induce bone marrow depression in the fetus.

Estradiol cypionate should not be used to treat estrogen–responsive incontinence in small animals; other estrogens (DES, conjugated estrogens) are less toxic.

In cases of prolonged corpus luteum in cows, a thorough uterine exam should be completed to determine if endometritis or a fetus is present.

In ferrets, estradiol is reportedly very toxic to bone marrow.

Adverse Effects

Estrogens have been associated with severe adverse reactions in small animals. In cats and dogs, estrogens are considered toxic to the bone marrow and can cause blood dyscrasias. Blood dyscrasias are more prevalent in older animals and if higher dosages are used. Initially, a thrombocytosis and/or leukocytosis may be noted but thrombocytopenia and leukopenia will gradually develop. Changes in a peripheral blood smear may be apparent within two weeks after estrogen administration. Chronic estrogen toxicity may be characterized by a normochromic, normocytic anemia, thrombocytopenia, and neutropenia. Bone marrow depression may be transient and begin to resolve within 30-40 days or may persist or progress to a fatal aplastic anemia.

Estrogens may cause cystic endometrial hyperplasia and pyometra. After therapy is initiated, an open-cervix pyometra may be noted 1-6 weeks after therapy.

Estrogens may induce mammary neoplasia.

When used chronically in male animals, feminization may occur. In females, signs of estrus may occur and persist for 7-10 days.

In cattle, prolonged estrus, genital irritation, decreased milkflow, precocious development, and follicular cysts may develop after estrogen therapy. These effects may be secondary to overdosage and dosage adjustment may reduce or eliminate them.

Reproductive/Nursing Safety

Estradiol is contraindicated during pregnancy. In humans, the FDA categorizes this drug as category *X* for use during pregnancy (*Studies in animals or humans demonstrate fetal abnormalities or adverse reaction; reports indicate evidence of fetal risk. The risk of use in pregnant women clearly outweighs any possible benefit.*) In a separate system evaluating the safety of drugs in canine and feline pregnancy (Papich 1989), this drug is categorized as class: *D* (*Contraindicated. These drugs have been shown to cause congenital malformations or embryotoxicity.*)

Estrogens have been shown to decrease the quantity and quality of maternal milk.

Overdosage/Acute Toxicity

No reports of inadvertent acute overdosage in veterinary patients were located; see Adverse Effects above.

Drug Interactions

The following drug interactions have either been reported or are theoretical in humans or animals receiving estradiol and may be of significance in veterinary patients. Unless otherwise noted, use together is not necessarily contraindicated, but weigh the potential risks and perform additional monitoring when appropriate.

- **AZOLE ANTIFUNGALS (fluconazole, itraconazole, keto-conazole, etc.):** May increase estrogen levels.
- **CORTICOSTEROIDS:** Enhanced glucocorticoid effects may result if estrogens are used concomitantly with corticosteroid agents. It has been postulated that estrogens may either alter the protein binding of corticosteroids and/or decrease their metabolism; corticosteroid dosage adjustment may be necessary when estrogen therapy is either started or discontinued.
- **MACROLIDE ANTIBIOTICS (erythromycin, clarithromycin, etc.):** May increase estrogen levels.
- **PHENOBARBITAL:** May decrease estrogen activity if administered concomitantly.
- **RIFAMPIN:** May decrease estrogen activity if administered concomitantly.
- **ST. JOHN'S WORT:** May decrease estrogen activity if administered concomitantly.
- **WARFARIN:** Oral anticoagulant activity may be decreased if estrogens are administered concurrently; increases in anticoagulant dosage may be necessary if adding estrogens.

Laboratory Considerations

- Estrogens in combination with progestins (*e.g.*, oral contraceptives) have been demonstrated in humans to increase **thyroxine-binding globulin (TBG)** with resultant increases in total circulating thyroid hormone. Decreased T_3 resin uptake also occurs, but free T_4 levels are unaltered. It is unclear if estradiol affects these laboratory tests in veterinary patients.

Doses

- **DOGS:**

  For pregnancy avoidance after mismating (extra-label): **Note:** This drug is rarely used or recommended for this indication today as there are safer, more effective treatments. 44 mcg/kg (0.044 mg/kg) IM once; during day 4 estrus to day 2 of diestrus, toxic at ≥100 micrograms/kg. (Wiebe et al. 2009)

- **CATS:**

  For pregnancy avoidance after mismating (extra-label): **Note:** This drug is rarely used or recommended for this indication today as there are safer, more effective treatments. 250 micrograms/kg (0.25 mg/kg) IM once 6 days after coitus; or 0.25 mg/cat IM at 40 hours after coitus. (Wiebe et al. 2009)

- **CATTLE:**

  The FDA has stated that the use of ECP in food-producing animals is <u>illegal</u>.

- **HORSES:**

  To enhance estrus behavior and receptivity in ovariectomized mares (extra-label): 5 – 10 mg (total dose) IM once. (Dascanio 2009)

  For treatment of mares with estrogen-responsive incontinence (extra-label): 4 – 10 micrograms/kg estradiol cypionate IM daily for three days and then every other day. Some mares will improve, but does not "cure." (Schott II et al. 2003)

Monitoring

When therapy is either at high dosages or chronic, see adverse effects for more information. Done at least monthly:

- Packed Cell Volumes (PCV).
- White blood cell counts (CBC).
- Platelet counts; Baseline, one month after therapy, and repeated two months after cessation of therapy if abnormal.
- Liver function tests.

Client Information

Injectable estrogen that should only be given by veterinarians.

Chemistry/Synonyms

Estradiol is a naturally occurring steroidal estrogen. Estradiol cypionate is produced by esterifying estradiol with cyclopentanepropionic acid, and occurs as a white to practically white, crystalline powder. It is either odorless or may have a slight odor and has a melting range of 149-153°C. Less than 0.1 mg/mL is soluble in water and 25 mg/mL is soluble in alcohol. Estradiol cypionate is sparingly soluble in vegetable oils.

Estradiol may also be known as: beta-oestradiol, dihydrofolliculin, dihydrotheelin, dihydroxyoestrin, estradiolum, NSC-9895, NSC-20293 (alpha-estradiol), and oestradiol; many trade names are available.

Estradiol Cypionate may also be known as: oestradiol cyclopentylpropionate, oestradiol cypionate, *Delestrogen®*, *Depo-Estradiol®*, *Depogen®*, *Dura-Estrin®*, *ECP®*, *E-Cypionate®*, *Estra-D®*, *Estrace®*, *Estro-Cyp®*, *Estroject®*, *depGynogen®*, *Femtrace®*, or *Gynodiol®*.

Storage/Stability

Estradiol cypionate should be stored in light-resistant containers at temperatures of less than 40°C, preferably at room temperature (15-30°C); avoid freezing.

Commercially available injectable solutions of estradiol cypionate are sterile solutions in a vegetable oil (usually cottonseed oil); they may contain chlorobutanol as a preservative.

Compatibility/Compounding Considerations

It is not recommended to mix estradiol cypionate with other medications.

In the USA it is illegal to compound estradiol for use in food producing animals.

Dosage Forms/Regulatory Status

VETERINARY-LABELED PRODUCTS:

There are several estradiol-containing implants for use in beef cattle.

HUMAN-LABELED PRODUCTS:

Estradiol Cypionate in Oil for Injection: 5 mg/mL in 5 mL vials; *Depo-Estradiol®*; (Rx)

Estradiol Valerate in Oil for Injection: 10 mg/mL, 20 mg/mL & 40 mg/mL in 5 mL multi-dose vials; *Delestrogen®*, generic; (Rx)

Estradiol Tablets: 0.5 mg, 1 mg, 1.5 mg, & 2 mg micronized estradiol; *Estrace®*, generic; (Rx)

Revisions/References

Monograph revised/updated January 2014.

Dascanio, J. (2009). Hormonal Control of Reproduction. Proceedings: ABVP. accessed via Veterinary Information Network; vin.com
Schott II, H. & E. Carr (2003). Urinary incontinence in horses. Proceedings: ACVIM Forum. accessed via Veterinary Information Network; vin.com
Wiebe, V. J. & J. P. Howard (2009). Pharmacologic Advances in Canine and Feline Reproduction. Topics in Companion Animal Medicine **24**(2): 71-99.

Estriol

(ess-TRYE-ole) Oestriol, Incurin®, E3

Estrogen

Prescriber Highlights

▶ Short-acting estrogen approved for treating estrogen-responsive urinary incontinence in ovariohysterectomized female dogs.

▶ Not dosed by animal's weight. Dosage tapered to lowest effective dose.

▶ Most likely side effects are gastrointestinal and estrogen-related; bone marrow depression risk appears to be low.

Uses/Indications

The FDA (USA) has approved estriol tablets for the control of estrogen-responsive urinary incontinence (urethral sphincter mechanism incompetence; USMI) in ovariohysterectomized female dogs. At present, estriol is the only estrogen approved in the USA for this use.

No clinical studies in female dogs with urethral sphincter mechanism incompetence (USMI) comparing efficacy or adverse effects of estriol with other estrogens (*e.g.*, diethylstilbestrol) or alpha-adrenergic drugs (*e.g.*, phenylpropanolamine) were found. Some have proposed that using an estrogen with an alpha-adrenergic may be effective and allow dosage reductions for both drugs.

Pharmacology/Actions

Estriol is short acting estrogenic drug. By binding to estrogen receptors found in the female canine lower urinary tract estriol can, in ovariohysterectomized dogs, improve urinary continence via several possible mechanisms, including enhancing urethral sphincter tone via increased sensitivity of urethral smooth muscle receptors to norepinephrine with resultant increased smooth muscle contractility. In comparison to estradiol-17beta or diethylstilbestrol, estradiol binds to estrogen receptors for a much shorter period, yet can still yield therapeutic effects but apparently reduces the risk for tumorigenic effects or bone marrow toxicity.

Pharmacokinetics

After oral administration estriol is nearly completely absorbed from gastrointestinal tract and peak plasma levels occur in about one hour. Absorbed estriol is highly but weakly bound to plasma proteins, which partly explains its short acting character. In dogs, it is not known how the drug is biotransformed, but in other species it is oxidated, sulfated, and glucuronidated in the liver. Enterohepatic circulation and urinary excretion of conjugated forms occur.

Contraindications/Precautions/Warnings

Estriol is labeled (depending on the country) as not for use in male dogs, intact females, female dogs less than one year old, pregnant or lactating dogs, or dogs with signs of polyuria-polydipsia.

Estriol should be used with caution in dogs with liver disease or with glucocorticoids (*Incurin*® Label; USA).

Adverse Effects

Reduced appetite/anorexia and/or vomiting are the most likely adverse effects seen in dogs. Estrogenic effects such as swollen vulva, vulvovaginitis, mammary hyperplasia, behavioral changes, enhanced attractiveness to male dogs, etc. are also possible. Rarely, alopecia has been reported. Very rarely, blood dyscrasias, vaginal bleeding, and an increased incidence of seizures have been noted.

Estrogens have been implicated as being potentially tumorigenic or having bone marrow toxic potential in dogs; the risk for these effects in dogs at recommended dosages of estriol appears thus far to be very low, probably due its relatively short duration of action.

Reproductive/Nursing Safety

Exogenously administered estrogens are contraindicated for use during pregnancy. Some estrogens (*e.g.*, diethylstilbestrol) have been associated with significant fetal malformations or tumorigenic effects in humans.

Exogenous estrogen administration during nursing is generally not recommended due to the potential for milk transmission and reduction in milk quality and quantity.

Overdosage/Acute Toxicity

Acute oral overdoses may cause emesis or other gastrointestinal effects. Estrogenic effects (see adverse effects) are possible in both male and female animals. One time overdoses are unlikely to pose much risk unless they are massive. For further information or guidance, contact an animal poison control center.

Long-term (26 weeks) overdoses of 6-10 mg (3-5X) demonstrated redness and swelling of the vulva, vulvar discharges, mammary hyperplasia, and higher white blood cell counts.

Drug Interactions

The following drug interactions have either been reported or are theoretical in humans or animals receiving oral estrogens and potentially could be of significance in veterinary patients:

▪ **CYP-3A4 INHIBITORS:** (*e.g.*, **cimetidine, clarithromycin, ketoconazole**, etc.): Possible decreased estrogen metabolism and increased estrogen levels.

▪ **CYP-3A4 INDUCERS:** (*e.g.*, **phenobarbital, rifampin**, etc.): Possible increased estrogen metabolism and decreased estrogen levels.

▪ **ESTROGENS, OTHER** (*e.g.*, **diethylstilbestrol**): Possible additive effects. The USA label states: Do not use with other estrogens; concomitant use with other estrogens has not been evaluated.

▪ **THYROID HORMONES:** Possible alteration of thyroxine and thyrotropin serum concentrations.

Dosages

▪ **DOGS:**

For the control of estrogen-responsive urinary incontinence in ovariohysterectomized female dogs (labeled dose; FDA approved): The dose of is not dependent upon body weight. All dogs should receive an initial dose of 2 mg (2 tablets) orally once per day for a minimum of 14 days. After urinary incontinence is controlled, the lowest effective daily dose of should be determined by decreasing the dose in a step-wise manner from 2 mg once daily (2 tablets) to 1 mg once daily (1 tablet), then 0.5 mg once daily (1/2 tablet) depending upon the response of the individual dog. There should be a minimum of 7 days between each dose adjustment. After the lowest daily dose that controls urinary incontinence is identified, the dose may be decreased further by administering once every two days. Dogs should not receive more than 2 mg per day (2 tablets). If the dog does not respond to 2 mg per day, the diagnosis should be re-assessed. (Adapted from product label, *Incurin*®; Merck Animal Health)

For the treatment of hormone-dependent urinary incontinence due to sphincter mechanism incompetence in ovariohysterectomized bitches (extra-label in USA, labeled dose, U.K.): For oral administration. A relationship between final effective dose and body weight has not been established and therefore the dose has to be determined for each dog on an individual basis. The following dosing schedule is advised: start treatment with 1 tablet (1 mg estriol) every day. If treatment is successful, lower the dose to half a tablet a day. If treatment is not successful, increase the dose to 2 tablets a day to be given in one dose. Some dogs do not need daily treatment; treatment every other day may be tried once the effective daily dose has been established. The minimum dose given should not be less than 0.5 mg per dog per day. Ensure the dose used to achieve the therapeutic effect is as low as possible. Do not use more than 2 tablets per dog per day. If no response to treatment is obtained the diagnosis should be reconsidered in order to investigate other causes for the incontinence such as neurological disorders, bladder neoplasia, etc. Animals should be re-examined every 6 months during treatment. (Product Label, *Incurin*®; MSD Animal Health—U.K.)

For the treatment of hormone-responsive urinary incontinence due to sphincter mechanism incompetence in female dogs (extra-label in USA, labeled dose, Aus/NZ): For oral administration. A relationship between final effective dose and body weight has not been established and therefore the dose for each dog has to be determined on an individual basis. Ensure the dose used to achieve the therapeutic effect is as low as possible. Effectiveness of treatment is defined as no signs of incontinence for 7 consecutive days. An improvement will usually be noticed within a few days. However, adjustment of the initial dose will often be necessary, so at least 7 days should be allowed before judging the full effect of a dose rate. The minimum dose given should not be less than half a tablet (0.5 mg) per dog per day. The maximum dose should not exceed 2 tablets (2 mg) per dog per day. If no response to treatment is obtained the diagnosis should be reconsidered in order to investigate other causes of urinary incontinence such as neurological disorders, bladder neoplasia, etc. Treatment will continue for the remainder of the life of the dog. Animals should be re-examined every 6 months during treatment. The following dosing schedule is advised: Initial dose: 1 tablet (1 mg) per day for 7-14 days. (**a**) If treatment with 1 tablet (1 mg) daily is effective, then the dose should be reduced to the minimum possible with 7 days of treatment as follows: Half a tablet (0.5 mg) per day.Ÿ If treatment is ineffective at the lower dose, titrate back to the previous effective dose. (**b**) If treatment with 1 tablet (1 mg) daily is ineffective, increase the dose to 2 tablets (2 mg) daily for 7 days. (Maximum dose should not exceed 2 tablets per day). If effective, reduce dose to 2 tablets on (2 mg) on alternate days. If treatment with 2 tablets (2 mg) daily is ineffective, reassess case to confirm diagnosis. (Product Label, *Incurin*®; MSD Animal Health—N.Z.)

Monitoring
- Clinical efficacy, adverse effects.

Client Information
- Estrogen used in dogs to treat estrogen-responsive urinary incontinence.
- Most common side effects include lack of appetite, vomiting, greater thirst, and swollen vulva.
- May give with or without food. If your animal vomits or acts sick after getting it on an empty stomach, give with food or small treat to see if this helps. If vomiting continues, contact your veterinarian.
- Pregnant women and those who are breastfeeding should use caution when handling. Wash hands with soap and water thoroughly after administration to avoid exposure to the drug.

Chemistry/Synonyms
Estriol (CAS registry: 50-27-1; ATCvet: QG03CA04; ATC: G03CA04) is an estrogenic sex hormone that occurs as a white or practically white, odorless, crystalline powder. It is insoluble in water; sparingly soluble in alcohol; soluble in acetone, chloroform, dioxan, ether, and vegetable oils. The commercially available veterinary tablets contain amylopectin, magnesium stearate, potato starch and anhydrous lactose.

Estriol may also be known as oestriol, follicular hormone hydrate, or theelol. A veterinary product trade name is *Incurin*®.

Storage/Stability
Store estriol tablets at or below 25°C (77°F) with excursions permitted to 40°C (104°F). Shelf life is generally labeled as 3 years post manufacture.

Compatibility/Compounding Considerations
No specific information noted.

Dosage Forms/Regulatory Status
VETERINARY-LABELED PRODUCTS:
Oral Tablets: (scored) 1 mg; *Incurin*®; (Rx). Approved by FDA (NADA 141-325) for oral use in dogs.

There is a website (dailymed.nlm.nih.gov) with the FDA-approved veterinary product's label: *Incurin*®.
HUMAN-LABELED PRODUCTS: NONE.

Revisions/References
Monograph written July 2013.

Ethambutol HCl
(e-tham-byoo-tole)   Myambutol®

Oral Antimycobacterial

Prescriber Highlights
▶ Can be used as an ingredient in an antimycobacterial "cocktail" for dogs, cats, and birds.
▶ Treating these infections is controversial because of potential public health risks associated with the infections.
▶ Optic- or neuro- toxicity greatest concern.

Uses/Indications
In combination with other antimycobacterial drugs, ethambutol may be useful in treating mycobacterial infections caused by *M. bovis*, *M. tuberculosis*, *M. genavense*, *M. avium-intracellulare* complex (MAC) in dogs or cats, particularly when the organism is resistant to treatment with other drug combinations (*e.g.*, rifampin, enrofloxacin, azithromycin). In birds, ethambutol has been used in combination with other agents for treating mycobacterial (*e.g.*, *M. avium*) infections.

Because of public health risks, particularly in the face of increased populations of immunocompromised people, treatment of mycobacterial (*M. bovis*, *M. tuberculosis*, etc.) infections in domestic or captive animals is controversial.

Pharmacology/Actions
A synthetic, bacteriostatic, antimycobacterial agent, ethambutol is only active against actively dividing mycobacteria. It enters mycobacterial cells and interferes with RNA synthesis and appears to interfere with the incorporation of mycolic acid into cell walls, allowing other antimycobacterial agents to penetrate the cell wall. Ethambutol does not have appreciable activity against other bacteria or fungi. Resistance can occur and is thought to develop in a step-wise manner. Cross-resistance with other antimycobacterial agents has not been reported.

Pharmacokinetics
Pharmacokinetic values for cats or birds were not located. In dogs, ethambutol is reported to have a volume of distribution of 3.8 L/kg, a total body clearance of 13.2 mL/min/kg, and an elimination half-life of 4.1 hours. Nephrectomized dogs had an elimination half-life of 5 hours.

In humans, ethambutol is rapidly absorbed after PO administration and bioavailability is around 75%. The drug is distributed widely in the body, but CSF levels only range from 10-50% of those found in serum. Erythrocyte concentrations are about twice that of the serum and can serve as a depot for the drug. About 15% of absorbed drug is hepatically metabolized to inactive metabolites. The majority of the drug is eliminated both by tubular secretion and glomerular filtration as unchanged drug in the urine. Elimination half-life in humans with normal renal function is about 3-4 hours; up to 8 hours if renal function is impaired.

Contraindications/Precautions/Warnings

Ethambutol should not be used in patients with a history of prior hypersensitivity reactions to it.

Patients with markedly reduced renal function may need dosage adjustment.

To help ensure human health, it is recommended to contact local public health authorities and obtain their recommendations before treating mycobacterial infections in companion animals.

Adverse Effects

Well-described adverse effect profiles for ethambutol in dogs, cats or birds are not available. Because ethambutol is used in combination with other medications, adverse effects associated with treatment may not be a result of ethambutol. In pre-clinical studies, some dogs receiving ethambutol over prolonged periods developed non-dose related degenerative changes in the central nervous system. In toxicology studies, dogs receiving large, prolonged doses developed signs of myocardial toxicity and depigmentation of the tapetum lucidum of the eyes. However, doses as large as 400 mg/kg/day for 4 weeks in dogs demonstrated no significant abnormalities in electroretinogram or visual evoked potential. In humans, optic neuritis (usually reversible after drug discontinuation) causing decreased visual acuity has been reported; routine ophthalmologic exams are recommended for humans taking this medication long-term.

Because antimycobacterial therapy involves multiple drugs for extended periods of time, bacterial or fungal overgrowth infections can occur. Antifungal medications may be required.

Reproductive/Nursing Safety

Ethambutol crosses the placenta; fetal levels are reported to range from 30-75% of that found in maternal serum. Teratogenic effects associated with ethambutol have not been reported in humans, but studies in mice, rats, and rabbits given high doses yielded a variety of abnormalities in offspring. Although risks exist, most believe that ethambutol is relatively safe to use during human pregnancy and untreated tuberculosis poses a much greater risk to the fetus.

Ethambutol is excreted into milk in levels approximating those found in maternal serum. While no problems have been documented and it is most likely safe, risk to offspring cannot be ruled out.

Overdosage/Acute Toxicity

Very limited information exists. Acute overdoses of greater than 10 grams in humans have caused optic neuritis. Other adverse effects noted with human overdoses can include: CNS effects (confusion, visual hallucinations), abdominal pain, nausea, fever and headache; treatment is supportive.

Drug Interactions

The following drug interactions have either been reported or are theoretical in humans or animals receiving ethambutol and may be of significance in veterinary patients. Unless otherwise noted, use together is not necessarily contraindicated, but weigh the potential risks and perform additional monitoring when appropriate.

- **ALUMINUM-CONTAINING ANTACIDS:** In humans, it has been documented that co-administration can reduce oral absorption of ethambutol; it is suggested to separate dosing by at least 4 hours if both drugs are necessary.

Laboratory Considerations

- No specific concerns; in humans, increased **serum uric acid** levels have been noted.

Doses

- **DOGS:**

  For treatment of disseminated *M. tuberculosis*: Ethambutol: 10 – 25 mg/kg PO once daily, in combination with rifampin (5 – 10 mg/kg PO q12-24h; maximum of 600 mg/day) and isoniazid (10 – 20 mg/kg PO once daily; maximum of 300 mg/day). May also add pyrazinamide at 15 – 40 mg/kg PO once daily. **Note:** pyrizinamide is ineffective for *M. bovis*. Treatment must continue for more than 9 months. (Greene et al. 2006)

- **CATS:**

  For treatment of feline tuberculosis: Initial treatment phase with rifampin (10 – 20 mg/kg PO q12-24h); enrofloxacin (5 mg/kg PO q12-24h); azithromycin (5 – 10 mg/kg PO q12-24h) for the first two months, then continuation phase (for approximately another 4 months) with rifampin and either enrofloxacin or azithromycin. If resistance develops, rifampin, isoniazid (10 – 20 mg/kg PO once daily) and ethambutol (15 mg/kg PO once daily) may be considered. If only two drugs are required, suggest using only rifampin and isoniazid. (Hartmannn et al. 2005)

- **BIRDS:**

  For treatment of *M. avium* **infections in caged birds:** Several protocols have been used, but controlled trials have not been performed. Combination therapy and treatment for 6-12 months is required.

  Protocol 1: Ciprofloxacin 20 mg/kg PO q12h or Enrofloxacin 15 mg/kg PO or IM (**Note:** repeated IM injections can cause muscle necrosis) for 10 days; Clofazimine 1.5 mg/kg PO once daily; Cycloserine 5 mg/kg PO q12h; and Ethambutol 20 mg/kg PO q12h.

  Protocol 2: Clofazimine 6 mg/kg PO once daily; Ethambutol 30 mg/kg PO once daily; Rifampin 45 mg/kg PO once daily.

  Protocol 3: Ciprofloxacin 80 mg/kg PO once daily or Enrofloxacin 30 mg/kg PO once daily; Ethambutol 30 mg/kg PO once daily; Rifampin 45 mg/kg PO once daily or Rifabutin 15 mg/kg PO once daily. (Phalen 2006)

  For Avian mycobacteriosis: All are dosed PO once daily for 9-12 months: Rifabutin 45 – 55 mg/kg; Clarithromycin 60 – 85 mg/kg; Ethambutol 30 – 85 mg/kg; Enrofloxacin 20 mg/kg. (Flammer 2006)

Monitoring

- Clinical efficacy.
- With long-term therapy, consider periodic monitoring of visual, liver, and renal function; CBC.
- Monitor for fungal or bacterial overgrowth infections.

Client Information

- Clients must be informed of the potential public health issues associated with mycobacterium infections and should be encouraged to contact a physician, preferably an infectious disease specialist for guidance.
- Treatment can be very prolonged (many months) and expensive.
- May be administered with or without food.
- Report any changes noted with patient's eyes or vision to the veterinarian.

Chemistry/Synonyms

Ethambutol HCl occurs as a white, crystalline powder that is freely soluble in water and soluble in alcohol.

Ethambutol may also be known as: CL-40882, etambutol, or ethambutoli; there are many trade names for international products.

Storage/Stability
Ethambutol tablets should be stored below 40°C and preferably, between 15-30°C in well-closed containers.

Compatibility/Compounding Considerations
No specific information noted.

Dosage Forms/Regulatory Status
VETERINARY-LABELED PRODUCTS: NONE.

HUMAN-LABELED PRODUCTS:

Ethambutol HCl Tablets: 100 mg, & 400 mg (scored); *Myambutol®*, generic; (Rx)

Revisions/References
Monograph revised/updated January 2014.

Flammer, K. (2006). Managing Avian Bacterial Diseases II. Proceedings: WVC2006. accessed via Veterinary Information Network; vin.com

Greene, C. & D. Gunn-Moore (2006). Mycobacterial Infections: Infections caused by slow-growing mycobacteria. *Infectious Diseases of the Dog and Cat, 3rd Ed.* C. Greene, Elsevier: 462-77.

Hartmannn, K. & C. Greene (2005). Diseases caused by systemic bacterial infections. *Textbook of Veterinary Internal Medicine, 6th Ed.* S. Ettinger and E. Feldman, Elsevier: 616-31.

Phalen, D. (2006). Selected Infectious Diseases: A Review for the ABVP V. Proceedings: ABVP 2006. accessed via Veterinary Information Network; vin.com

Ethanol
Alcohol, Ethyl

(eth-a-nol)   *Alcohol*

Antidote

Prescriber Highlights
▶ Used for treatment of ethylene glycol (EG) or methanol toxicity; for EG toxicity most now recommend fomepizole (4-MP) for dogs and cats.
▶ Adverse Effects: CNS/respiratory depression, hypoglycemia, diuresis, pain/infection at the injection site.
▶ Avoid extravasation. Monitor fluid & electrolyte and respiratory status, alcohol & toxin levels (if possible).
▶ Usually must be compounded.

Uses/Indications
The principal use of ethanol in veterinary medicine is for the treatment of ethylene glycol or methanol toxicity. While fomepizole (4-methyl pyrazole) is now the treatment of choice for ethylene glycol poisoning, alcohol is a readily available and an economical alternative when patients present within a few hours after ingestion.

Percutaneous injection of ethanol 95% has been used successfully to treat feline hyperthyroidism.

In horses, ethanol has also been used in aerosol form as a mucokinetic agent and for intraarticular administration to promote distal tarsal joint ankylosis with osteoarthritis.

Pharmacology/Actions
By competitively inhibiting alcohol dehydrogenase, alcohol can prevent the formation of ethylene glycol to its toxic metabolites (glycoaldehyde, glycolate, glyoxalate, and oxalic acid). This allows the ethylene glycol to be principally excreted in the urine unchanged. A similar scenario exists for the treatment of methanol poisoning. For alcohol to be effective, however, it must be given very early after ingestion; it is seldom useful if started 8 hours after a significant ingestion.

Pharmacokinetics
Alcohol is well absorbed orally, but is administered intravenously for toxicity treatment. It rapidly distributes throughout the body and crosses the blood-brain barrier. Alcohol crosses the placenta.

Contraindications/Precautions/Warnings
Because ethylene glycol and methanol intoxications are life threatening, there are no absolute contraindications to ethanol's use for these indications.

Use of ethanol with fomepizole is usually contraindicated; see drug interactions for more information.

Adverse Effects
The systemic adverse effects of alcohol are quite well known. The CNS depression and respiratory depression associated with the high levels used to treat ethylene glycol and methanol toxicity can confuse the clinical monitoring of these toxicities. A high risk for respiratory arrest is associated with high blood levels. Ethanol's affects on antidiuretic hormone (vasopressin) may enhance diuresis. As both ethylene glycol and methanol may also cause diuresis, fluid and electrolyte therapy requirements need to be monitored and managed. Hypoglycemia, hypocalcemia and metabolic acidosis may be seen and pulmonary edema can occur. Other adverse affects include pain and infection at the injection site, phlebitis and intravascular hemolysis. Extravasation should be watched for and avoided. When aerosolized in horses, irritation and bronchoconstriction may result. With intraarticular administration in horses mild swelling at the injection site can occur; severe swelling with secondary cellulitis and fibrosis occur rarely.

Reproductive/Nursing Safety
Alcohol's safety during pregnancy has not been established for short-term use. Use only when necessary. In humans, the FDA categorizes this drug as category C for use during pregnancy (*Animal studies have shown an adverse effect on the fetus, but there are no adequate studies in humans; or there are no animal reproduction studies and no adequate studies in humans.*)

Alcohol passes freely into milk in levels that approximate maternal serum levels, but it is unlikely to have negative effects on nursing offspring.

Overdosage/Acute Toxicity
If clinical signs of overdosage occur (lateral nystagmus, respiratory depression, profound obtundation), either slow the infusion or discontinue temporarily. Alcohol blood levels may be used to monitor both efficacy and toxicity of alcohol.

Drug Interactions
The following drug interactions have either been reported or are theoretical in humans or animals receiving ethanol and may be of significance in veterinary patients. Unless otherwise noted, use together is not necessarily contraindicated, but weigh the potential risks and perform additional monitoring when appropriate.

- **BROMOCRIPTINE:** Alcohol may increase the severity of side effects seen with bromocriptine.
- **CHARCOAL, ACTIVATED:** Will inhibit absorption of orally administered ethanol; do not use activated charcoal if administering ethanol orally for methanol or ethylene glycol intoxication.
- **CNS DEPRESSANT DRUGS** (*e.g.,* **barbiturates, benzodiazepines, phenothiazines,** etc.): Alcohol may cause additive CNS depression when used with other CNS depressant drugs.
- **FOMEPIZOLE (4-MP):** Inhibits alcohol dehydrogenase; ethanol metabolism is reduced significantly and alcohol poisoning (CNS depression, coma, death) can occur. Use together is generally not recommended but if both drugs are used, monitoring of ethanol blood levels is mandatory.
- **INSULIN and other antidiabetic drugs:** Alcohol may affect glucose metabolism and the actions of insulin or oral antidiabetic agents.
- **CHLORPROPAMIDE, METRONIDAZOLE:** A disulfiram

reaction (increased acetaldehyde with tachycardia, vomiting, weakness) may occur if alcohol is used concomitantly with these drugs.

Laboratory Considerations

Ethylene Glycol Testing Kits: Ethanol may cause false positive reports on ethylene glycol screening tests. Refer to the label of the product used for more information.

Doses

- **DOGS:**

  For ethylene glycol poisoning (extra-label): **Note:** Fomepizole is generally preferred.

  a) As a 20% solution, give 5.5 mL/kg IV q4h for 5 treatments, then q6h for four additional treatments; dosed as a CRI over 1 hour. (Forrester et al. 1994), (Hall 2009)

  b) Make a 7% ethanol solution (see Compatibility/Compounding Considerations below) and give 8.6 mL/kg slowly IV followed by a CRI of 1.43 mL/kg/hour for at least 36 hours although 48 hours is probably better. If the EG test was positive initially, then check it before stopping treatment; discontinue treatment if it reverts to negative. (Shell 2006)

- **CATS:**

  For ethylene glycol poisoning (extra-label): **Note:** High dose fomepizole is generally preferred.

  a) As a 20% solution, give 5 mL/kg IV q6h for 5 treatments, then q8h for four additional treatments; dosed as a CRI over 1 hour. (Forrester et al. 1994), (Hall 2009)

  b) Make a 7% ethanol solution (see Compatibility/Compounding Considerations below) and give 8.6 mL/kg slowly IV followed by a CRI of 1.43 mL/kg/hour for at least 36 hours although 48 hours is probably better. If the EG test was positive initially, then check it before stopping treatment; discontinue treatment if it reverts to negative. (Shell 2006)

- **HORSES:**

  To promote ankylosis in horses with distal tarsal joint osteoarthritis (extra-label): In the study, joints were treated if there was no contrast-mediated radiographic evidence of communication with the proximal intertarsal joint (PITJ). The same needle was kept in the joint space and either 70% ethanol solution in sterile water or 100% ethanol was injected until minor resistance was felt (2-4 mL). In their conclusion, the authors stated: "...findings of this study support the use of 70% ethanol solution for treatment of distal tarsal joint OA in cases that do not respond to corticosteroid medication. Careful case selection and accurate contrast-facilitated injection technique are mandatory to minimize potential complications of this treatment." (Lamas et al. 2012)

Monitoring

- Alcohol blood levels (and ethylene glycol or methanol levels). **Note:** In humans, blood ethanol levels should be maintained at 100 – 130 mg/deciliter (21.7 – 28.2 milliMoles/liter). It is safer to maintain a blood ethanol concentration greater than 130 mg/deciliter than to have it fall below 100 mg/deciliter. (*POISINDEX® Managements*, Thompson; *MICROMEDEX®* Healthcare Series, 2007)
- Degree of CNS and respiratory effects.
- Fluid/electrolyte, blood glucose status.

Client Information

- Systemically administered alcohol should be given in a controlled clinical environment.

Chemistry/Synonyms

A transparent, colorless, volatile liquid having a characteristic odor and a burning taste, ethyl alcohol is miscible with water and many other solvents.

"Proof" is considered 2X the percentage of ethanol. For example, a 100 proof vodka is 50% ethanol; an 80 proof vodka is 40% ethanol. In some states, pure grain alcohol (often called "Everclear") can be purchased which is a 95% ethanol (190 proof) product.

Ethanol may also be known as aethanolum, alcool, grain alcohol, ethanolum, and ethyl alcohol.

Storage/Stability/Preparation

Alcohol should be protected from extreme heat or freezing. Do not use unless the solution is clear. Alcohol may precipitate many drugs; do not administer other medications in the alcohol infusion solution unless compatibility is documented (consult specialized references or a hospital pharmacist for more specific information).

Compatibility/Compounding Considerations

Note: Since alcohol infusions are generally only used in veterinary medicine for the treatment of ethylene glycol/methanol toxicity and obtaining medical or laboratory grade alcohol or pharmaceutical grade products can be very difficult in an emergency, veterinarians have often had to improvise. One method that has been successful, albeit not pharmaceutically elegant, is to use commercially available vodka (40%-80 proof; 50%-100 proof) or grain alcohol ("Everclear"; 95%-190 proof) diluted in an appropriate IV solution (*e.g.*, LRS, D5W, etc.).

- To make an ethanol solution of a lesser concentration than the stock solution:
- Choose the percentage you want (5%-20%) to administer.
- Divide this number by the % (**NOT** proof) of ethanol of the stock solution.
- Multiply this amount by the total volume of the IV bag that will be used (250 mL-1000 mL) to determine the mLs of stock solution to use.
- Remove this amount from the fluid bag and add the appropriate amount of alcohol solution to make a solution of the desired alcohol percentage.
- Examples:
- To make a 20% ethanol solution using 80 proof (40% ethanol) vodka in a one liter bag of fluids: 20% ÷ 40% = 0.5; multiply by 1000 = 500 mL. Remove 500 mL of fluids from the bag and add 500 mL of 80 proof vodka = 1000 mL of a 20% ethanol solution.
- To make a 5% solution using 100 proof (50% ethanol) vodka in a 500 mL bag of fluids: 5% ÷ 50% = 0.1; multiply by 500 = 50 mL. Remove 50 mL of fluids from the bag and add 50 mL of 100 proof vodka = 500 mL of a 5% ethanol solution.
- To make a 7% ethanol solution from 190 proof (95% ethanol) "Everclear" in a 250 mL bag of fluids: 7% ÷ 95% = 0.074; multiply by 250 = 18.5 mL. Remove 18.5 mL of fluids from the bag and add 18.5 mL of 190 proof (95%) grain alcohol = 250 mL of a 7% ethanol solution.

Regardless of the product used, it is recommended that an in-line filter be used for the IV and the client give informed consent for the use of this non-pharmaceutical product.

Dosage Forms/Regulatory Status

VETERINARY-LABELED PRODUCTS: NONE.

HUMAN-LABELED PRODUCTS:

Alcohol (Ethanol) in Dextrose Infusions: 5% and 10% alcohol (ethanol) in dextrose 5% IV solutions were available commercially, but apparently are no longer marketed in the USA.

For information on obtaining tax-free alcohol for medicinal purposes, contact a regional office of the Bureau of Alcohol, Tobacco, and Firearms.

Revisions/References

Monograph revised/updated January 2014.

Forrester, S. & G. Lees (1994). Disease of the Kidney and Ureter. *Saunders Manual of Small Animal Practice.* S. Birchard and R. Sherding. Philadelphia, W.B. Saunders Company: 799-820.

Hall, K. (2009). Toxicosis Treatments. *Kirk's Current Veterinary Therapy XIV.* J. Bonagura and D. Twedt. 112-116, Saunders Elsevier: 112-6.

Lamas, L. P., et al. (2012). Use of ethanol in the treatment of distal tarsal joint osteoarthritis: 24 cases. Equine Veterinary Journal 44(4): 399-403.

Shell, L. (2006). "Ethylene Glycol Toxicity." *Associate Database* Veterinary Information Network http://goo.gl/qHd1h.

Etidronate Disodium

(e-ti-droe-nate)   Didronel®

Oral Bisphosphonate Bone Resorption Inhibitor

Prescriber Highlights

▶ Bisphosphonate that reduces calcium resorption from bone; occasionally used to treat hypercalcemia associated with malignancy.

▶ Contraindications: Treatment of hypercalcemia in patients with severe renal function impairment. Caution in patients with bone fractures, enterocolitis, cardiac failure, or moderate renal function impairment.

▶ Adverse Effects: Potentially, diarrhea, nausea, or bone pain/tenderness.

▶ Do not confuse etidronate with etretinate or etomidate.

▶ Expense may be an issue.

Uses/Indications

Etidronate is a first generation bisphosphonate that may be useful for the treatment of severe hypercalcemia associated with neoplastic disease. Its use in human medicine has been largely replaced with newer, more potent bisphosphonates that can be dosed less often or have fewer adverse effects. Etidronate is also indicated in humans for the treatment of Paget's disease and heterotopic ossification (*e.g.*, after total hip replacement).

Pharmacology/Actions

Etidronate's primary site of action is bone. It reduces normal and abnormal bone resorption. This effect can reduce hypercalcemia associated with malignant neoplasms. Etidronate can also increase serum phosphate concentrations, presumably by increasing the renal tubular reabsorption of phosphate. Some early studies in lab animals suggest that etidronate may inhibit the formation of bone metastases with some tumor types.

Pharmacokinetics

Oral absorption is poor and dose dependent. As little as 1% of a dose (smaller doses) may be absorbed; with higher doses, up to 20% may be absorbed. Food substantially reduces the amount absorbed. After oral dosing, the drug is rapidly cleared from blood and 50% of the drug absorbed goes into bone. At usual doses, it appears that etidronate does not cross the placenta. Duration of effect may be very prolonged. In humans, effects have persisted for up to one year after discontinuation in patients with Paget's disease. Effects for hypercalcemia may last for 11 days. Absorbed etidronate is excreted unchanged by the kidneys. Approximately 50% of the absorbed dose is excreted within 24 hours; the remainder is chemisorbed to bone and then slowly eliminated.

Contraindications/Precautions/Warnings

Etidronate is considered contraindicated for the treatment of hypercalcemia in patients with renal function impairment (serum creatinines >5 mg/dL). Risk vs. benefit should be carefully considered in patients with bone fractures (delays healing), enterocolitis (higher risk of diarrhea), cardiac failure (especially with parenteral etidronate as patients may not tolerate the extra fluid load), or those with renal function impairment (serum creatinines 2.5-5 mg/dL).

Do not confuse ETIDROnate with ETRETInate or ETOMIdate.

Adverse Effects

Adverse effects are not well described in small animals. In humans, diarrhea, nausea (with higher oral doses), and bone pain/tenderness are most the likely adverse effects reported. Increases in serum creatinine are possible.

A syndrome called "frozen bone" has been reported in dogs on moderately high doses of etidronate or other non-amino bisphosphonates (clodronate). Bone remodeling and repair are inhibited enough that bones can weaken and fracture. Newer bisphosphonates appear to be much safer with respect to this syndrome.

Reproductive/Nursing Safety

Etidronate's safety during pregnancy has not been established. Rabbits given oral doses 5X those recommended in humans, demonstrated no overt problems with offspring. Rats, given very large doses IV, showed skeletal malformations. In humans, the FDA categorizes this drug as category C for use during pregnancy (*Animal studies have shown an adverse effect on the fetus, but there are no adequate studies in humans; or there are no animal reproduction studies and no adequate studies in humans.*)

It is unknown if the drug enters milk.

Overdosage/Acute Toxicity

Very little information is available at this time. Overdoses may result in hypocalcemia (ECG changes may occur), bleeding problems (secondary to rapid chelation of calcium) and proximal renal tubule damage.

Use standard gut emptying protocols after oral ingestion when warranted. IV calcium administration (*e.g.*, calcium gluconate) may be used to reverse hypocalcemia. Intensive monitoring is suggested.

Drug Interactions

The following drug interactions have either been reported or are theoretical in humans or animals receiving etidronate and may be of significance in veterinary patients. Unless otherwise noted, use together is not necessarily contraindicated, but weigh the potential risks and perform additional monitoring when appropriate.

▪ **ANTACIDS, DIARY PRODUCTS, MINERAL SUPPLEMENTS**, and medications containing **iron, magnesium, calcium** or **aluminum**: Absorption of oral etidronate may be inhibited; separate etidronate doses from these substances by at least two hours.

Laboratory Considerations

▪ Etidronate may interfere with bone uptake of technetium Tc 99m medronate or technetium Tc 99m oxidronate.

Doses

▪ **DOGS/CATS:**

For severe hypercalcemia associated with neoplastic disease (extra-label): 5 – 20 mg/kg PO once daily (or divided into two daily doses); unlikely to restore serum calcium to "normal", but may prolong survival and animals may "feel" better.

Monitoring

▪ Serum calcium.

▪ Serum protein.

Client Information

▪ Recommended to give dose to animal that has an empty stomach.

▪ If anorexia or vomiting occurs, notify veterinarian.

Chemistry/Synonyms

An analog of pyrophosphate, etidronate disodium (also known as EHDP, Na2EHDP, or sodium etidronate) is a bisphosphonate agent that occurs as a white powder and is freely soluble in water. Unlike pyrophosphate, etidronate is resistant to enzymatic degradation in the gut.

Etidronate disodium may also be known as: EHDP, disodium etidronate, etidronate disodium, or *Didronel®*.

Storage/Stability

Store tablets in tight containers at room temperature.

Compatibility/Compounding Considerations

No specific information noted.

Dosage Forms/Regulatory Status

VETERINARY-LABELED PRODUCTS: NONE.

HUMAN-LABELED PRODUCTS:

Etidronate Disodium Tablets: 200 mg & 400 mg; generic; (Rx)

Revisions/References

Monograph revised/updated January 2014.

Etodolac

(ee-toe-doe-lak)   EtoGesic®, Lodine®

Non-Steroidal Antiinflammatory Agent

▶ 2nd generation NSAID used in dogs; uncommonly used today. Veterinary-approved dosage forms may no longer be commercially available.

▶ Contraindications: Hypersensitivity. Caution: Patients with preexisting or occult GI, hepatic, renal, cardiovascular, or hematologic abnormalities.

▶ Safe use not established for dogs less than 12 months of age or in breeding, pregnant, or lactating dogs.

▶ Adverse Effects: Vomiting, diarrhea, lethargy, surgical bleeding, hypoproteinemia; keratoconjunctivitis sicca possible; localized pain or tissue reactions at injection site.

▶ Drug interactions.

Uses/Indications

Etodolac is labeled for the management of pain and inflammation associated with osteoarthritis in dogs.

Pharmacology/Actions

Like other NSAIDs, etodolac has analgesic, antiinflammatory, and antipyretic activity. Etodolac appears to be more selective for inhibition of cyclooxygenase-2 than cyclooxygenase-1, but studies conflict and a definitive answer is not presently agreed upon. It may be better to describe etodolac as a COX-1 sparing drug, rather than a COX-2 selective drug. In dogs, etodolac dose also affects whether the drug causes gastrointestinal adverse effects. Doses as little as 2.7X can produce gastrointestinal lesions. Etodolac is also thought to inhibit macrophage chemotaxis, which may explain some of its antiinflammatory activity.

In horses, etodolac does not exhibit much COX-2 selectivity.

Pharmacokinetics

The S(+) enantiomer is thought to provide the bulk of the pharmacologic activity, but the drug is supplied as a racemic mixture. Pharmacokinetic studies that measure both forms as one are not very relevant clinically. After oral administration to healthy dogs, etodolac is rapidly and nearly completely absorbed. The presence of food may alter the rate, but not the extent, of absorption. Peak serum levels occur about 2 hours post dosing. Etodolac is highly bound to serum proteins. The drug is primarily excreted via the bile into the feces. Glucuronide conjugates have been detected in the

bile but not the urine. Elimination half-life in dogs varies depending whether food is present in the gut, which may affect the rate of enterohepatic circulation of the drug. These values range from about 8 hours (fasted) to 12 hours (non-fasted). Serum half-life is not necessarily a good predictor for duration of efficacy, possibly due the drug's high protein binding.

In horses, etodolac has an oral bioavailability of about 77%. After IV dosing, volume of distribution was 0.29 L/kg and the clearance was 235 mL/hr/kg. Elimination half-life (after IV dosing) was approximately 2.5-3 hours.

Contraindications/Precautions/Warnings

Etodolac is contraindicated in dogs previously found to be hypersensitive to it. It should be used with caution in dogs with preexisting or occult GI, hepatic, cardiovascular, or hematologic abnormalities (*e.g.*, von Willebrand's disease or on anticoagulants) as NSAIDs may exacerbate these conditions. Patients may be more susceptible to renal injury from etodolac if they are dehydrated, on diuretics, or have preexisting renal, hepatic, or cardiovascular dysfunction.

Safety of etodolac has not been established in dogs less than 12 months of age.

Adverse Effects

In clinical field studies, etodolac's primary adverse effect was vomiting/regurgitation, reported in about 5% of dogs tested. Diarrhea, lethargy, and hypoproteinemia have also been reported in dogs. Urticaria, behavioral changes, and inappetence were reported in less than 1% of dogs treated. Potentially, hepatotoxicity and/or nephrotoxicity are possible but are not well-documented problems in dogs.

Etodolac injection may cause localized pain or tissue reactions at injection site.

Etodolac may decrease total serum T4 in some dogs. Clinical significance is unclear.

Etodolac appears to have less impact on clotting times than some other canine-FDA-approved NSAIDs, but bleeding during surgery has been reported.

Cases have been reported of dogs developing keratoconjunctivitis sicca (KCS) after receiving etodolac treatment. Incidence rate is unknown at this time.

The manufacturer warns to terminate therapy if inappetence, vomiting, fecal abnormalities, or anemia are observed.

Reproductive/Nursing Safety

Safe use has not been established in breeding, pregnant, or lactating dogs; use only when the benefits clearly outweigh the potential risks in these animals. In humans, the FDA categorizes this drug as category *C* for use during pregnancy (*Animal studies have shown an adverse effect on the fetus, but there are no adequate studies in humans; or there are no animal reproduction studies and no adequate studies in humans.*)

Most NSAIDs are excreted in milk; use with caution.

Overdosage/Acute Toxicity

Limited information is available, but in a safety study where dogs were given 40 mg/kg/day (2.7X) GI ulcers, weight loss, emesis and local occult blood were noted. Doses of 80 mg/kg/day (5.3X) caused 6 of 8 dogs to either die or become moribund secondary to GI ulceration. It should be noted that these were not single dose overdoses. However, they demonstrate that there is a relatively narrow therapeutic window for the drug in dogs and that doses should be carefully determined (*i.e.*, do not confuse mg/kg dosages with mg/lb.).

There were 39 exposures to etodolac reported to the ASPCA Animal Poison Control Center (APCC) during 2006-2009. In these cases 4 were cats with 2 showing clinical signs and the remaining 35 cases were dogs with 5 showing clinical signs. Common findings in theses cats (recorded in decreasing frequency) included acute renal failure, anorexia, collapse, hyperkalemia and hypersalivation. As with any NSAID, overdosage can lead to gastrointestinal and renal effects. Decontamination with emetics and/or activated charcoal may be appropriate. For doses where GI effects are expected, the use of gastrointestinal protectants is warranted. If renal effects are also expected, fluid diuresis is warranted.

Drug Interactions

Note: Although the manufacturer does not list any specific drug interactions in the package insert, it does caution to avoid or closely monitor etodolac's use with other drugs, especially those that are also highly protein bound. It also recommends close monitoring, or to **avoid using etodolac with any other ulcerogenic drugs** (*e.g.*, **corticosteroids, other NSAIDs**). While some advocate a multi-day washout period when switching from one NSAID to another (not aspirin—see below), there does not appear to be any substantial evidence that this is required. Until there is more evidence, consider starting the new NSAID when the next dose would be due for the old one.

The following drug interactions have either been reported or are theoretical in humans or animals receiving etodolac and may be of significance in veterinary patients. Unless otherwise noted, use together is not necessarily contraindicated, but weigh the potential risks and perform additional monitoring when appropriate.

- **ACE INHIBITORS (enalapril, benazepril**, etc.): Etodolac may reduce the antihypertensive effects of ACE inhibitors. Because ACE inhibitors potentially can reduce renal blood flow, use with NSAIDs could increase the risk for renal injury. However, one study in dogs receiving tepoxalin did not show any adverse effects. It is unknown what effects, if any, occur if other NSAIDs and ACE inhibitors are used together in dogs.
- **ASPIRIN:** When aspirin is used concurrently with etodolac, plasma levels of etodolac could decrease and an increased likelihood of GI adverse effects (blood loss) could occur; concomitant administration of aspirin with etodolac cannot be recommended. Washout periods of several days is probably warranted when switching from an NSAID to aspirin therapy in dogs.
- **CYCLOSPORINE:** Etodolac may increase cyclosporine blood levels and increase the risk for nephrotoxicity.
- **DIGOXIN:** Etodolac may increase serum levels of digoxin. Use with caution in patients with severe cardiac failure.
- **FUROSEMIDE & OTHER DIURETICS:** Etodolac with diuretics may reduce the saluretic and diuretic effects of furosemide and transiently decrease glomerular filtration rate (GFR).
- **METHOTREXATE:** Serious toxicity has occurred when NSAIDs have been used concomitantly with methotrexate; use together with caution.
- **NEPHROTOXIC AGENTS** (*e.g.*, **amphotericin B, aminoglycosides, cisplatin**, etc.): Potential for increased risk of nephrotoxicity if used with NSAIDs.
- **PHENOBARBITAL:** May increase the metabolism of etodolac in dogs.
- **PROBENECID:** May cause a significant increase in serum levels and half-life of etodolac.
- **WARFARIN:** Etodolac may increase the risk for bleeding.

Laboratory Considerations

- Etodolac may cause false-positive determinations of **urine bilirubin.**
- Etodolac therapy may alter **thyroid function tests** and their interpretation; falsely low values may occur in dogs receiving etodolac.

Doses

- **DOGS:**

For treatment of pain and inflammation associated with osteoarthritis (labeled-dose; FDA-approved):

Oral Tablets: 10 – 15 mg/kg PO once daily. Dogs less than 5 kg cannot be accurately dosed with *EtoGesic®* tablets. Adjust dose to obtain satisfactory response, but do not exceed 15 mg/kg. For long-term therapy, reduce dose level to minimum effective dosage.

Injection: 10 – 15 mg/kg as a dorsoscapular subcutaneous (SC) injection. If needed, daily doses of tablets may begin 24 hours after the last injectable treatment. Use alternate injection sites. The likelihood of injection site reactions increases when administered near previous injection sites. (Package Insert; *EtoGesic® Tablets; Injection*—BIVI)

Monitoring

- Baseline (especially in geriatric dogs or dogs with chronic diseases or those where prolonged treatment is likely): physical exam, CBC, Serum chemistry panel (including liver and renal function tests), UA. It is recommended to reassess liver enzymes at one week of therapy. Should elevation occur, recommend discontinuing the drug.
- Tear production prior to, and during therapy.
- Clinical efficacy.
- Signs of potential adverse reactions: inappetence, diarrhea, mucoid feces, vomiting, melena, polyuria/polydipsia, anemia, jaundice, lethargy, behavior changes, ataxia, or seizures.
- Chronic therapy: Consider repeating CBC, UA, and serum chemistries on an ongoing basis.

Client information

- Can give with or without food, but food may reduce the chances for stomach problems. If your animal vomits or acts sick after getting it on an empty stomach, give with food or small treat to see if this helps. If vomiting continues, contact your veterinarian.
- Most dogs usually tolerate very it well, but rarely some will develop ulcers, or serious kidney and liver problems. Watch for these: Not eating normally (more or less), vomiting, changes in bowel movements; changes in behavior or activity levels (more or less active than normal), incoordination (*e.g.*, stumbling, clumsiness, etc.), seizure (convulsions) or aggression; yellowing of gums, skin, or whites of the eyes (jaundice); changes in drinking (frequency, amount consumed) or urination habits (frequency, color, or smell).
- Periodic lab tests to check for liver and kidney side effects are required.

Chemistry/Synonyms

An indole acetic acid derivative non-steroidal antiinflammatory agent (NSAID), etodolac occurs as a white, crystalline compound that is insoluble in water, but soluble in alcohol or DMSO. Etodolac has a chirally active center with a corresponding S (+) enantiomer and an R (-) enantiomer. The commercially available product is supplied as a racemic mixture of the forms.

Etodolac may also be known as: AY-24236, etodolacum, etodolic acid, *Acudor®, Articulan®, Dualgan®, Eccoxolac®, Edolan®, Elderin®, EtoGesic®, Etonox®, Etopan®, Flancox®, Hypen®, Lodot®, Lonine®, Metazin®, Sodolac®, Todolac®, Ultradol®*, and *Zedolac®*.

Storage/Stability

The commercially available veterinary tablets should be stored at controlled room temperature (15-30°C).

The commercially available injection should be stored at or below 77°F (25°C).

Compatibility/Compounding Considerations

No specific information noted.

Dosage Forms/Regulatory Status

VETERINARY-LABELED PRODUCTS:

Note: Both of the following veterinary products are still listed (as of Dec 2013) on FGA's "green book" as approved, but may not be currently marketed.

Etodolac Scored Tablets: 150 mg & 300 mg; *EtoGesic®*; (Rx). FDA-approved for use in dogs. Do not use in cats.

Etodolac Injection 10% (100 mg/mL); *EtoGesic® Injectable*; (Rx). FDA-approved for use in dogs. The ARCI (Racing Commissioners International) has designated this drug as a class 4 substance. See the appendix for more information.

HUMAN-LABELED PRODUCTS:

Etodolac Tablets: 400 mg & 500 mg; Extended-release Tablets: 400 mg, 500 mg, 600 mg; Capsules: 200 mg & 300 mg; and 400 mg, 500 mg & 600 mg extended-release tablets; generic; (Rx)

Revisions/References

Monograph revised/updated January 2014.

Etomidate

(ee-toe-mi-date)   Amidate®

Injectable Anesthetic

Prescriber Highlights

▶ Injectable non-barbiturate anesthetic agent that may be useful as an alternative to thiopental or propofol for induction, particularly in patients with preexisting cardiac dysfunction, head trauma, or that are critically ill.

▶ Can inhibit cortisol production; may need to supplement corticosteroids in critically ill patients.

▶ Not a controlled substance.

▶ Relatively expensive, especially in large dogs.

Uses/Indications

Etomidate may be useful as an alternative to thiopental or propofol for anesthetic induction in small animals, particularly in patients with preexisting cardiac dysfunction, head trauma, or that are critically ill.

Pharmacology/Actions

The exact mechanism of action of etomidate is not well defined. Etomidate causes minimal hemodynamic changes and little effect on the cardiovascular system when compared to other injectable anesthetic agents. At usual doses, etomidate has little effect on respiratory rate or rhythm. Etomidate decreases cerebral blood flow and oxygen consumption. It usually lowers intraocular pressure and causes slight decreases in intracranial pressure. Etomidate reportedly does not induce malignant hyperthermia, but can speed its onset in susceptible patients secondary to a triggering agent.

The reported therapeutic index (toxic dose/therapeutic dose) for etomidate is 16. Therapeutic indexes for propofol and thiopental are 3 and 5 respectively.

In comparing etomidate with propofol when used for inductions in dogs, patients receiving etomidate had higher systolic arterial pressures and mean arterial pressures, but it caused longer and poorer recoveries than propofol (Sams et al. 2008).

Pharmacokinetics

No specific information on the pharmacokinetics of etomidate in domesticated animals was located. In humans, after intravenous injection etomidate is rapidly distributed into the CNS and then rapidly cleared from the brain back into systemic tissues. Duration of hypnosis is short (3-5 minutes) and dependent upon dose. Recovery from anesthesia appears to be as fast as with thiopental, but slower than propofol. Etomidate is 75% bound to plasma proteins. The drug is rapidly metabolized in the liver primarily via hydrolysis or glucuronidation to inactive metabolites. The majority of the drug and metabolites are excreted into the urine with the remainder into the bile and feces. Elimination half-life ranges from 1.25-5 hours.

Contraindications/Precautions/Warnings

Etomidate is contraindicated in patients known to be hypersensitive to it.

Etomidate can inhibit adrenocortical function; it should not be used for purposes other than induction. Although somewhat controversial in veterinary medicine, use with caution in patients with impaired adrenocortical function, particularly those with septic shock. Exogenous glucocorticoid administration may be considered in severely compromised animals.

Etomidate does not provide significant analgesia.

Limited studies in patients with impaired hepatic or renal function have shown that elimination half-lives may be significantly increased in these patients and the propylene glycol carrier in the injection may be problematic in patients with liver dysfunction.

A study in dogs concluded that midazolam/etomidate anesthesia be used with caution in dogs undergoing ocular surgery as it caused clinically relevant miosis, significant increases in intraocular pressure, and commonly caused ptyalism, gagging, and abdominal heaving (Gunderson et al. 2013).

Adverse Effects

Common adverse effects include pain at intravenous injection site/phlebitis, vomiting, skeletal muscle movements (myoclonus), eye movements, and post-operative retching. Preanesthetic medications and a benzodiazepine (*e.g.,* diazepam, midazolam) just prior to etomidate can minimize these effects.

Some hemolysis may occur due to the propylene glycol content of the injection, especially in cats. Some anesthesiologists recommend injecting etomidate into a running IV line to decrease the pain associated with injection and, potentially, reduce hemolysis.

While etomidate causes minimal cardiopulmonary depression, a brief period of hypoventilation and decreased arterial blood pressure can occur after administration.

Apnea, laryngospasm, hiccups, hyperventilation, hypoventilation, hypertension, hypotension, lactic acidosis, arrhythmias, and postoperative vomiting have all been reported in human patients that have received the drug. Seizures have been reported in a few human patients receiving etomidate; this adverse effect may be reduced if an opiate premed is first administered.

Reproductive/Nursing Safety

In humans, the FDA categorizes etomidate as a category *C* drug for use during pregnancy (*Animal studies have shown an adverse effect on the fetus, but there are no adequate studies in humans; or there are no animal reproduction studies and no adequate studies in humans*). Etomidate has caused embryocidal effects in rats and maternal toxicity in rabbits and rats.

Some etomidate is excreted into maternal milk; use with caution in nursing patients.

Overdosage/Acute Toxicity

Acute overdoses would be expected to cause enhanced pharmacologic effects of the drug. Treatment would be supportive (*i.e.*, mechanical ventilation), until the effects of the medication are diminished.

Drug Interactions

The following drug interactions have either been reported or are theoretical in humans or animals receiving etomidate and may be of significance in veterinary patients. Unless otherwise noted, use together is not necessarily contraindicated, but weigh the potential risks and perform additional monitoring when appropriate.

- **CNS/RESPIRATORY DEPRESSANTS** (*e.g.*, **barbiturates, opiates, anesthetics,** etc.): Additive pharmacological effects can occur if etomidate is used concurrently with other drugs that can depress CNS or respiratory function.
- **VERAPAMIL**: Has been associated with potentiating the anesthetic and respiratory depressant effects of etomidate.

Laboratory Considerations

- Etomidate's effects on inhibiting cortisol may invalidate **ACTH stimulation** and **glucose tolerance** tests. Cortisol function may be affected for 2-6 hours in dogs, and up to 5.5 hours in cats after etomidate.

Doses

- **DOGS & CATS:**

As an induction agent (extra-label): Dosing recommendations vary somewhat but range generally from 0.5 – 2 mg/kg IV, although dosages up to 4 mg/kg IV have been noted. A suitable premed is required and can help reduce the incidence and severity of vomiting and myoclonus/tremors. A benzodiazepine (*e.g.*, midazolam ± low dose ketamine) just prior to use can further reduce adverse effects and potentially allow lower induction dosages (0.25 – 1 mg/kg) of etomidate. Some also recommend giving a short-acting intravenous glucocorticoid to help offset etomidate's effects on cortisol production.

- **FERRETS:**

As an induction agent in the cardiovascular unstable patient (extra-label): etomidate 1 – 2 mg/kg IV after diazepam (0.5 mg/kg IV). (Lichtenberger 2006)

- **SMALL MAMMALS:**

As an induction agent (extra-label):

a) **Rabbits:** As an induction agent in the cardiovascular unstable patient: etomidate 1 – 2 mg/kg IV after diazepam (0.5 mg/kg IV). (Lichtenberger 2006)

b) 1 – 2 mg/kg IV; must use with a benzodiazepine to prevent seizures. (Lennox 2013)

Monitoring

As per any anesthetic agent:

- Level of consciousness.
- Respiration rate and depth.
- Cardiovascular function.

Client Information

- Etomidate is a potent sedative-hypnotic that should only be used by professionals in a setting where adequate patient monitoring is available.

Chemistry/Synonyms

An injectable, carboxylic imidazole anesthetic, etomidate occurs as a white or almost white powder. It is very slightly soluble in water and freely soluble in alcohol. The commercially available injection has a pH of 8.1, contains 35% propylene glycol, and is hyperosmolar (4640 mosm/L).

Etomidate may also be known as: R-16659, *Amidate*®, *Hypnomidate*®, *Radenarcon*®, or *Sibul*®.

Storage/Stability

Unless otherwise labeled, store etomidate injection at room temperature and protected from light.

Compatibility/Compounding Considerations

No specific information noted.

Dosage Forms/Regulatory Status

VETERINARY-LABELED PRODUCTS: NONE.

HUMAN-LABELED PRODUCTS:

Etomidate Injection: 2 mg/mL in 10 mL & 20 mL single-dose vials, 10 mL & 20 mL amps and 20 mL *Abboject* syringes; *Amidate*®; generic; (Rx)

Revisions/References

Monograph revised/updated January 2014.

Gunderson, E. G., et al. (2013). Effects of anesthetic induction with midazolam-propofol and midazolam-etomidate on selected ocular and cardiorespiratory variables in clinically normal dogs. American Journal of Veterinary Research 74(4): 629-35.

Lennox, A. (2013). Sedation and Local Analgesia as an Alternative to General Anaesthesia in Exotic Companion Mammals. British Small Animal Veterinary Congress accessed via Veterinary Information Network; vin.com

Lichtenberger, M. (2006). Anesthesia Protocols and Pain Management for Exotic Animal Patients. Proceedings: Western Vet Conf. accessed via Veterinary Information Network; vin.com

Sams, L., et al. (2008). A comparison of the effects of propofol and etomidate on the induction of anesthesia and on cardiopulmonary parameters in dogs. Veterinary Anaesthesia and Analgesia 35(6): 488-94.

Etretinate – see Acitretin

Euthanasia Agents with Pentobarbital

(yoo-thon-ayzh-ya; pen-toe-barb-i-tal)

For therapeutic uses (other than euthanasia) of pentobarbital, see the main pentobarbital monograph for this agent. The sections on chemistry, storage, pharmacokinetics, overdosage, drug interactions, and monitoring parameters can be found in the main pentobarbital monograph.

Prescriber Highlights

▶ Used for humane euthanasia for animals not to be used for food.

▶ Store so that it will not be confused with therapeutic agents; keep out of reach of children.

▶ Use care in handling filled syringes & dispose of used injection equipment properly.

▶ Avoid any contact with open wounds or accidental injection.

▶ Tranquilizing agent may be necessary when the animal is in pain or agitated.

▶ Renderers may not accept carcasses euthanized with pentobarbital.

Uses/Indications

For rapid, humane euthanasia in animals not intended for food purposes. Individual products may be labeled for use in specific species.

The AVMA Guidelines for the Euthanasia of Animals: 2013 Edition states that "All barbituric acid derivatives used for anesthesia are acceptable for euthanasia when administered IV. There is a rapid onset of action, and loss of consciousness induced by barbiturates results in minimal or transient pain associated with venipuncture. Desirable barbiturates are those that are potent, nonirritating, long acting, stable in solution, and inexpensive. Sodium pentobarbital best fits these criteria and is most widely used, although others such as secobarbital are also acceptable...the advantages of using barbiturates for euthanasia in dogs and cats far outweigh the disadvantages. Intravenous injection of a barbituric acid derivative is the preferred method for euthanasia of dogs, cats, other small animals, and horses. Barbiturates are also acceptable for all other species of animals if circumstances permit their use. Intraperitoneal or intracoelomic injection may be used in situations when an IV injection would be distressful, dangerous, or difficult due to small patient size. Intracardiac (in mammals and birds), intrasplenic, intrahepatic, and intrarenal injections must only be used if the animal is unconscious or anesthetized (with the exception of intrahepatic injections in cats as discussed in the Companion Animals section of the text)." (Leary et al. 2013)

Pharmacology/Actions

Pentobarbital causes death by severely depressing the medullary respiratory and vasomotor centers when administered at high doses. Cardiac activity may persist for several minutes following administration.

Phenytoin is added to *Beuthanasia®-D Special* for its added cardiac depressant effects and to denature the compounds from a Class-II controlled substance to Class-III drugs.

Contraindications/Precautions/Warnings

Must not be used in animals to be used for food purposes (human or animal consumption); care must be taken to prevent scavenging wildlife from consuming carcasses. Contact the US Fish and Wildlife Service for additional advice for prevention of relay pentobarbital toxicity in wildlife. Should be stored in such a manner that these products will not be confused with therapeutic agents. Extreme care in handling filled syringes and proper disposal of used injection equipment must be undertaken. Avoid any contact with open wounds or accidental injection. Keep out of reach of children.

Prior use of a tranquilizing agent may be necessary when the animal is in pain or agitated.

Adverse Effects

Minor muscle twitching may occur after injection. Death may be delayed or not accomplished if injection given perivascularly.

Doses

For a through discussion of the use of pentobarbital (and other methods) for humane euthanasia in a variety of species, all veterinarians are urged to download and refer to AVMA Guidelines for the Euthanasia of Animals: 2013 Edition available on the AVMA. org website. Additionally, because products may have differing concentrations of pentobarbital, refer to the information provided with the product in use.

- **DOGS:**
  a) Pentobarbital sodium (as a single agent): Approximately 120 mg/kg for the first 4.5 kg of body weight, and 60 mg/kg for every 4.5 kg of body weight thereafter. Preferably administer IV.

  b) Pentobarbital sodium with phenytoin (*Beuthanasia®-D Special*): 1 mL for each 4.5 kg of body weight.

- **CATS:**
  a) Pentobarbital sodium (as a single agent): Approximately 120 mg/kg for the first 4.5 kg of body weight, and 60 mg/kg for every 4.5 kg of body weight thereafter. Administer IV.

  b) Pentobarbital sodium with phenytoin: (*Beuthanasia®-D Special*): 1 mL for each 4.5 kg of body weight (not FDA-approved for use in this species)

- **LARGE ANIMALS:**
  Depending on product concentration, most animals require 10 – 15 mLs per 100 lbs. of body weight IV. **Note:** must not be used in animals to be consumed by either humans or other animals.

Monitoring
- Respiratory rate.
- Cardiac rate.
- Corneal reflex.

Client Information
- Must be administered by an individual familiar with its use.
- Animals must be restrained during administration.
- Inform clients observing euthanasia that animal may give a terminal gasp after becoming unconscious.

Compatibility/Compounding Considerations
No specific information noted.

Dosage Forms/Regulatory Status
See other pentobarbital dosage forms under the main pentobarbital monograph for lower concentration products that are used therapeutically.

VETERINARY-LABELED PRODUCTS:
Pentobarbital Sodium 390 mg/mL & Phenytoin Sodium 50 mg/mL for Injection (Euthanasia) in 100 mL vials; *Beuthanasia®-D Special, Euthasol®, Euthanasia-III® Solution, Somnasol®*; (Rx, C-III). Approved for use in dogs.

Pentobarbital Sodium Powder for reconstitution and injection: 392 mg/mL when constituted with 250 mL of water. *Fatal-Plus® Powder, Pentasol® Powder*; (Rx, C-II). Labeled for use in animals regardless of species.

Pentobarbital Sodium for Injection (Euthanasia): 260 mg/mL: *Sleepaway®* 26%: in 100 mL bottles; (Rx, C-II). Labeled for use in dogs and cats. 324 mg/mL: *SP5®* in 100 mL vials; (Rx, C-II). Labeled for use in dogs and cats. 389 mg/mL: *Socumb-6gr®, Somlethol®, SP6®*; 100 mL & 250 mL vials; (Rx, C-II). Labeled for use in dogs and cats. 390 mg/mL: *Fatal-Plus®* Solution in 250 mL vials (Rx, C-II). Labeled for use in animals regardless of species.

HUMAN-LABELED PRODUCTS: NONE.

Revisions/References
Monograph revised/updated January 2014.

Leary, S., et al. (2013). AVMA Guidelines for the Euthanasia of Animals: 2013 Edition. Javma-Journal of the American Veterinary Medical Association **242**(6): 715-6.

Famciclovir

(fam-sye-klow-veer)   Famvir®

Antiviral (Herpes)

Prescriber Highlights

▶ May be effective in treating feline herpes (FHV-1) infections. Dosage recommendations still in flux, but currently recommended to be given 3 times daily.

▶ Appears to be well tolerated when used short-term (2-3 weeks).

▶ Relatively expensive, but prices may decrease now that generics are available.

Uses/Indications

Famciclovir may be of benefit in treating feline herpes (FHV) infections. Experimentally infected cats with FHV-1 dosed at 90 mg/kg 3 times daily had improved clinical outcomes (Thomasy et al. 2011). It may also prove beneficial in horses with equine herpes virus-1 (EHV-1) infections, but additional research is needed before it can be confidently recommended.

Pharmacology/Actions

In most species, famciclovir is rapidly converted *in vivo* to penciclovir. In cells infected with susceptible Herpes virus or varicella zoster virus, viral thymidine kinase phosphorylates penciclovir to penciclovir monophosphate. Cellular kinases further convert this compound to penciclovir triphosphate, which inhibits herpes virus DNA polymerase via competition with deoxyguanosine triphosphate, thereby selectively inhibiting herpes viral DNA synthesis. It is considered a virostatic agent and therefore does not affect latent virus or necessarily clear the virus.

Viral resistance can occur by mutation.

Pharmacokinetics

Famciclovir is deacetylated (primarily in the blood) and then oxidized via aldehyde oxidase in the liver to the active compound, penciclovir. Cats are deficient in aldehyde oxidase complicating the pharmacokinetics of famciclovir. Extrapolating kinetics data from other species to cats is not reliable. Pharmacokinetics are non-linear in cats probably due to saturation of biotransformation enzymatic systems. Oral administration of 40 mg/kg or 90 mg/kg famciclovir demonstrated variable famciclovir absorption and low bioavailability of penciclovir (7-13%). Food may reduce oral bioavailability. Both dosages had similar peak levels of penciclovir (approx. 1.3 mcg/mL) and peak times (3 hours). Penciclovir elimination half-life was between 4-5 hours at both dosages. IV penciclovir demonstrated a volume of distribution that approximated the total body water of cats (Thomasy, Whittem, et al. 2012). Penciclovir concentrations in cats' tears approximates that found in plasma.

In horses, after oral famciclovir doses of 20 mg/kg, peak plasma penciclovir levels occurred about one hour after dosing with peaks concentrations of about 3 mcg/mL. Elimination was bi-phasic with a slow terminal half-life of about 33 hours (Tsujimura et al. 2010).

In humans, famciclovir is well absorbed after oral administration, but undergoes extensive first pass metabolism (not by CYP enzymes). Food can decrease peak levels but does not significantly impact clinical efficacy. Penciclovir (active metabolite) is only marginally bound to plasma proteins. In humans, penciclovir elimination half-life is about 2-3 hours; excretion is primarily via renal mechanisms. Intracellular half-lives of penciclovir in infected cells are significantly longer.

Contraindications/Precautions/Warnings

Famciclovir is contraindicated in patients known to be hypersensitive to it or penciclovir.

It should be used with caution (and dosage adjustment) in patients with renal dysfunction. In humans patients with CrCl <40 mL/min, dosage adjustments are recommended.

Adverse Effects

Adverse effects in cats are not well documented, but the drug appears to be tolerated quite well when used for up to 3 weeks. At doses of 90 mg/kg PO q8h, anorexia and polydipsia have been noted in some cats.

In humans, famciclovir can cause nausea, vomiting, diarrhea, and headache. Neutropenia has been reported and renal failure can occur particularly when doses are not adjusted in patients with renal dysfunction.

Reproductive/Nursing Safety

In laboratory animals, doses of up to 1,000 mg/kg/day did not cause any observed effects on developing embryos or fetuses. In humans, the FDA categorizes this drug as category *B* for use during pregnancy (*Animal studies have not yet demonstrated risk to the fetus, but there are no adequate studies in pregnant women; or animal studies have shown an adverse effect, but adequate studies in pregnant women have not demonstrated a risk to the fetus in the first trimester of pregnancy, and there is no evidence of risk in later trimesters.*)

Famciclovir (as penciclovir) is excreted in the milk of rats. It is unclear if there is any clinical significance for nursing offspring.

Overdosage/Acute Toxicity

Little information is available. Supportive treatment has been recommended. Penciclovir can be removed by hemodialysis.

Drug Interactions

The following drug interactions have either been reported or are theoretical in humans or animals receiving famciclovir and may be of significance in veterinary patients. Unless otherwise noted, use together is not necessarily contraindicated, but weigh the potential risks and perform additional monitoring when appropriate.

- **PROBENECID:** Can reduce the amount of penciclovir excreted by the kidneys and increase penciclovir plasma levels.

Laboratory Considerations

- No concerns noted.

Doses

- **CATS:**

  For feline herpes virus (FHV-1); (extra-label): At time of writing (12/2013), based upon pharmacokinetic studies in plasma and tears (Thomasy, Covert, et al. 2012; Thomasy, Whittem, et al. 2012) a dosage of approximately 40 mg/kg PO 3 times a day is reasonable, although lower dosages or dosing frequency may yet prove efficacious. Topical antiviral treatment may not be required, but other topical drugs such as an antibacterial agent or mucinomimetic artificial tear replacement may be critical (Maggs 2013). Treatment duration recommendations can vary somewhat with 2-4 week durations often suggested. Kittens (at least 5 days old) may only require treatment for 2 weeks. Available human oral dosage forms of 125 mg or 250 mg tablets may be split to achieve a dose that can be practically administered.

Monitoring

- Clinical efficacy.
- Adverse effects (most likely GI).
- Consider occasional CBC's and creatinine to monitor for neutropenia or renal dysfunction if using the drug chronically.

Client Information

- Try giving without food, but if cat vomits or acts sick after receiving the medication, give with a small amount of food.
- There is limited experience with this drug in cats, report any unusual effects to the veterinarian.
- FHV-1 infections are controlled, not cured, and recurrence may occur even if the cat is treated life-long.

Chemistry/Synonyms

A prodrug, famciclovir is a purine-derived, synthetic, acyclic purine nucleoside analog.

Famciclovir may also be known as AV 42810, BRL 42810, famciclovirum, or by the trade name *Famvir®*.

Storage/Stability

Famciclovir tablets should be stored at room temperature (15-30°C).

Compatibility/Compounding Considerations

The film-coated tablets may be split.

Dosage Forms/Regulatory Status

VETERINARY-LABELED PRODUCTS: NONE.

HUMAN-LABELED PRODUCTS:

Famciclovir Oral Tablets (film-coated): 125 mg, 250 mg, & 500 mg; *Famvir®*, generic; (Rx)

Revisions/References

Monograph revised/updated January 2014.

Maggs, D. J. (2013). Feline Herpesvirus-1: Antiviral Drugs From Bench-Top to Clinic. ACVIM 2013. accessed via Veterinary Information Network; vin.com

Thomasy, S. M., et al. (2012). Pharmacokinetics of famciclovir and penciclovir in tears following oral administration of famciclovir to cats: a pilot study. Vet. Ophthalmol. 15(5): 299-306.

Thomasy, S. M., et al. (2011). Evaluation of orally administered famciclovir in cats experimentally infected with feline herpesvirus type-1. American Journal of Veterinary Research 72(1): 85-95.

Thomasy, S. M., et al. (2012). Pharmacokinetics of penciclovir in healthy cats following oral administration of famciclovir or intravenous infusion of penciclovir. *American Journal of Veterinary Research* 73(7): 1092-9.

Tsujimura, K., et al. (2010). Pharmacokinetics of Penciclovir after Oral Administration of its Prodrug Famciclovir to Horses. *Journal of Veterinary Medical Science* 72(3): 357-61.

Famotidine

(fa-moe-ti-deen)   Pepcid®

H2-Receptor Antagonist

Prescriber Highlights

▶ H$_2$-receptor antagonist used to reduce GI acid production. Recent studies in dogs suggest that omeprazole is superior to famotidine for increasing gastric pH.

▶ Longer duration of action & fewer drug interactions than cimetidine.

▶ Caution: Patients with severe cardiac disease, significantly impaired hepatic or renal function; consider dosage reduction.

▶ Adverse Effects: Too rapid IV infusion may cause bradycardia. Potentially: GI effects, headache, or dry mouth or skin; rare idiopathic intravascular hemolysis anecdotally reported when given IV to cats.

Uses/Indications

In veterinary medicine, famotidine may be useful for the treatment and/or prophylaxis of gastric, abomasal and duodenal ulcers, uremic gastritis, stress-related or drug-induced erosive gastritis, esophagitis, duodenal gastric reflux, and esophageal reflux. It has been recommended in dogs as an "…excellent drug for routine prophylaxis where cost is a concern and where an injectable drug is preferred or… in dogs requiring extended therapy (a minimum of one week), since its effects will improve with time and become comparable to the more expensive PPIs" (Bersenas 2007). However, in a recent study comparing oral omeprazole and oral famotidine in 6 dogs, oral famotidine at 1 – 1.3 mg/kg PO q12h did not significantly increase intragastric pH levels above those of placebo and the authors concluded that oral omeprazole provided superior gastric acid suppression when compared to famotidine (Tolbert et al. 2011). Omeprazole was also deemed superior to famotidine when used to prevent exercise-induced gastritis in racing Alaskan sled dogs (Williamson et al. 2010).

Famotidine has significantly fewer drug interactions than cimetidine and activity may persist longer.

In dogs, famotidine did not improve outcomes (eradication) of Helicobacter infections when added to triple antibiotic therapy (Leib et al. 2007).

Pharmacology/Actions

At the H$_2$-receptors of the parietal cells, famotidine competitively inhibits histamine, thereby reducing gastric acid output both during basal conditions and when stimulated by food, pentagastrin, histamine or insulin. Gastric emptying time, pancreatic or biliary secretion, and lower esophageal pressures are not altered by famotidine. By decreasing the amount of gastric juice produced, H$_2$-blockers reduce the amount of pepsin secreted.

Pharmacokinetics

Famotidine is not completely absorbed after oral administration, but undergoes only minimal first-pass metabolism. In humans, systemic bioavailability is about 40-50%. Distribution characteristics are not well described. In rats, the drug concentrates in the liver, pancreas, kidney and submandibular gland. Only about 15-20% is bound to plasma proteins. In rats, the drug does not cross the blood brain barrier or the placenta. It is distributed into milk. When the drug is administered orally, about 1/3 is excreted unchanged in the urine and the remainder is primarily metabolized in the liver and then excreted in the urine. After intravenous dosing, about 2/3's of a dose is excreted unchanged.

The pharmacokinetics of famotidine, ranitidine, and cimetidine have been investigated in horses (Duran et al. 1993). After a single IV dosage, elimination half-lives of cimetidine, ranitidine, and famotidine all were in the 2-3 hour range and were not significantly different. Of the three drugs tested, famotidine had a larger volume of distribution (4.28 L/kg) than either cimetidine (1.14 L/kg) or ranitidine (2.04 L/kg). Bioavailability of each of the drugs was low; famotidine (13%), ranitidine (13.5%) and cimetidine (30%).

Contraindications/Precautions/Warnings

Famotidine is contraindicated in patients with known hypersensitivity to the drug.

Famotidine should be used cautiously in geriatric patients and patients with significantly impaired hepatic or renal function. Consider dosage reduction in patients with significant renal dysfunction. One recommendation is to give the drug (1 mg/kg) every 24 hours instead of every 12 hours in these patients (Trepanier 2013). Famotidine may have slight negative inotropic effects and some cardioarrhythmogenic properties. Use with caution in patients with severe cardiac disease.

Adverse Effects

Too rapid IV infusion may cause bradycardia. Other H$_2$-blockers have demonstrated to be relatively safe and exhibit minimal adverse effects. Potential adverse effects (documented in humans) that could be seen include GI effects (anorexia, vomiting, diarrhea), headache, or dry mouth or skin. Rarely, agranulocytosis may develop particularly when famotidine is used concomitantly with other drugs that can cause bone marrow depression.

There have been rare anecdotal reports of famotidine causing intravascular hemolysis when given intravenously to cats. It is believed this is probably an idiosyncratic reaction that occurs in a very small percentage of cats treated. A retrospective study evaluating IV famotidine in 56 hospitalized cats did not show any evidence of hemolysis. The authors concluded that the IV route appeared safe in cats when famotidine was administered over 5 minutes (Galvao et al. 2008).

Reproductive/Nursing Safety

In lab animal studies, famotidine demonstrated no detectable harm to offspring. Large doses could affect the mother's food intake and weight gain during pregnancy that could indirectly be harmful. Use in pregnancy when potential benefits outweigh the risks. In rats, nursing from mothers receiving very high doses of famotidine, transient decreases in weight gain occurred. In humans, the FDA categorizes this drug as category *B* for use during pregnancy (*Animal studies have not yet demonstrated risk to the fetus, but there are no adequate studies in pregnant women; or animal studies have shown an adverse effect, but adequate studies in pregnant women have not demonstrated a risk to the fetus in the first trimester of pregnancy, and there is no evidence of risk in later trimesters.*)

Famotidine is excreted in the milk of rats. It is unclear if there is any clinical significance for nursing offspring.

Overdosage/Acute Toxicity

The minimum acute lethal dose in dogs is reported to be >2 g/kg for oral doses and approximately 300 mg/kg for intravenous doses. IV doses in dogs ranging from 5 – 200 mg/kg IV caused: vomiting, restlessness, mucous membrane pallor and redness of the mouth and ears. Higher doses caused hypotension, tachycardia and collapse.

Because of this wide margin of safety associated with the drug, most overdoses should require only monitoring. In massive oral overdoses, gut-emptying protocols should be considered and supportive therapy initiated when warranted.

Drug Interactions

The following drug interactions have either been reported or are theoretical in humans or animals receiving famotidine and may be of significance in veterinary patients. Unless otherwise noted, use together is not necessarily contraindicated, but weigh the potential risks and perform additional monitoring when appropriate.

- **AZOLE ANTIFUNGALS** (*e.g.*, **ketoconazole, itraconazole, fluconazole**): By raising gastric pH, famotidine may decrease the absorption of these agents; if both drugs are required, administer the azole one hour prior to famotidine.
- **CEFPODOXIME, CEFUROXIME**: Famotidine may decrease the absorption of these cephalosporins; giving with food may alleviate this effect.
- **IRON SALTS (ORAL)**: Famotidine may decrease the absorption of oral iron; administer iron at least one hour prior to famotidine.

Unlike cimetidine or ranitidine, famotidine does not appear to inhibit hepatic cytochrome P-450 enzyme systems and dosage adjustments of other drugs (*e.g.*, warfarin, theophylline, diazepam, procainamide, phenytoin) that are metabolized by this metabolic pathway should usually not be required.

Laboratory Considerations

- Histamine$_2$-blockers may antagonize the effects of **histamine** and **pentagastrin** in the evaluation gastric acid secretion.
- A study in dogs showed that famotidine only had transient effects on **serum gastrin** levels. Authors concluded that in dogs with clinical features consistent with gastrinomas, chronic famotidine administration would not likely contribute to increases in serum gastrin concentration (Mordecai et al. 2011).
- After using allergen extract **skin tests**, histamine$_2$ antagonists may inhibit histamine responses. It is recommended that histamine$_2$ blockers be discontinued at least 24 hours before performing either of these tests.

Doses

- **DOGS:**

  To reduce gastric acid production (extra-label): Dosage recommendations vary and there is no compelling evidence to support any specific dosage. Recommended dosages generally are 0.5 – 1.1 mg/kg PO q12-24 hours. Rounding doses to the nearest 5 mg increment (*e.g.*, 5 mg per cat) is reasonable. Once daily administration is most often recommended in patients with significantly diminished renal function. Recommended doses for parenteral use are generally 0.5 mg/kg IV (slowly), IM or SC q12-24h.

- **FERRETS:**

  For stress induced ulcers (extra-label): 0.25 – 0.5 mg/kg PO, IV once daily. (Williams 2000)

  In combination with antibiotics for Helicobacter treatment (extra-label): 0.25 – 0.5 mg/kg PO, IV q24h. (Fisher 2005)

- **SMALL MAMMALS:**

  Rabbits: For stress induced ulcer prevention once critically ill animal has stabilized (extra-label): 1 mg/kg IV once daily (q24h). (Johnston 2006)

- **HORSES:** (NOTE: ARCI UCGFS CLASS 5 DRUG)

  As an adjunct in ulcer treatment: IV doses (extra-label): 0.23 mg/kg, IV q8h or 0.35 mg/kg IV q12h. Oral doses: 1.88 mg/kg, PO q8h or 2.8 mg/kg PO q12h. (Duran et al. 1993)

Monitoring

- Clinical efficacy (dependent on reason for use); monitored by decrease in symptomatology, endoscopic examination, blood in feces, etc.
- Adverse effects, if noted.

Client Information

- Used to treat or prevent stomach ulcers. Doses often are given 1-2 times per day. Clinical signs may reoccur if dosages are missed.
- Works best if given before the first meal of the day. If your animal vomits or acts sick after getting it on an empty stomach, give with food or small treat to see if this helps. If vomiting continues, contact your veterinarian.
- Famotidine is available OTC (over the counter; without a prescription), but only give it to your animal if your veterinarian recommends.

Chemistry/Synonyms

An H$_2$-receptor antagonist, famotidine occurs as a white to pale yellow, crystalline powder. It is odorless, but has a bitter taste. 740 micrograms are soluble in one mL of water.

Famotidine may also be known as: famotidinum, L-643341, MK-208, and YM-11170; many trade names are available.

Storage/Stability

Tablets should be stored in well-closed, light-resistant containers at room temperature. Tablets are assigned an expiration date of 30 months after date of manufacture.

The powder for oral suspension should be stored in tight containers at temperatures less than 40°C. After reconstitution, the resultant suspension is stable for 30 days when stored at temperatures less than 30°C; do not freeze.

Famotidine injection should be stored in the refrigerator (2-8°C).

Compatibility/Compounding Considerations

Commercially available famotidine tablets can be split or crushed but have a bitter taste.

Famotidine for injection is physically **compatible** with most commonly used IV infusion solutions and is stable for 48 hours at room temperature when diluted in these solutions.

Compounded preparation stability: Famotidine oral suspension compounded from commercially available tablets has been published (Dentinger et al. 2000). Triturating twenty-four (24) famotidine 40 mg tablets with 60 mL of *Ora-Plus*® and *qs ad* to 120 mL with *Ora-Sweet*® (or *Ora-Sweet*® *SF*) brought to a favorable pH of 5.8 yields an 8 mg/mL oral suspension that retains >90% potency for 95 days stored at 25°C. Famotidine is stable in buffered solutions at pH 4-6, but rapid and extensive drug degradation occurs at pH less than 2.

Another "recipe" to make a 4 mg/mL flavored, oral aqueous-based suspension from 10 mg tablets: To make a 30 mL suspension: Pulverize twelve 10 mg tabs (0.12 g) to a fine powder in a mortar and pestle. Wet with glycerin (1 – 2 mL) to make a thick paste. Add up to 1 mL of a water-soluble flavoring agent. Add enough oral suspending vehicle—OSV (*e.g.*, *Ora-Plus*®, *Ora-Sweet*®, etc.) and mix to allow transfer to an amber prescription bottle. May need to repeat this process several times to "wash" the mortar. "qs ad" to 30 mL with additional OSV. Shake well before use, store in the refrigerator and dispose any unused amount after 30 days.

Dosage Forms/Regulatory Status

VETERINARY-LABELED PRODUCTS: NONE.

The ARCI (Racing Commissioners International) has designated this drug as a class 5 substance. See the appendix for more information.

HUMAN-LABELED PRODUCTS:

Famotidine Oral Tablets (plain, film-coated, chewable) & Gelcaps: 10 mg & 20 mg, & 40 mg; *Pepcid*®, *Pepcid AC*® & *Pepcid RPD*®, generic; (Rx & OTC)

Famotidine Powder for Oral Suspension: 8 mg/mL when reconstituted in 400 mg bottles; *Pepcid*®, generic; (Rx)

Famotidine Injection: 10 mg/mL in 1 & 2 mL single dose vials and 4 mL, 20 mL & 50 mL multi-dose vials (may contain mannitol or benzyl alcohol); 20 mg/50 mL premixed in 50 mL single-dose containers; generic; (Rx)

Revisions/References

Monograph revised/updated January 2014.

Bersenas, A. (2007). Antacids: What is the evidence? Proceedings: IVECCS. accessed via Veterinary Information Network; vin.com

Dentinger, P. J., et al. (2000). Stability of famotidine in an extemporaneously compounded oral liquid. Am J Health Syst Pharm 57(14): 1340-2.

Duran, S. & W. Ravis (1993). Comparative pharmacokinetics of H2 antagonists in horses. Proceedings of the Eleventh Annual Veterinary Medical Forum, Washington D.C., American College of Veterinary Internal Medicine. accessed via Veterinary Information Network; vin.com

Fisher, P. (2005). Ferret Medicine I. Proceedings: Western Vet Conf. accessed via Veterinary Information Network; vin.com

Galvao, J. & L. A. Trepanier (2008). Risk of hemolytic anemia with intravenous administration of famotidine to hospitalized cats. Journal of Veterinary Internal Medicine 22(2): 325-9.

Johnston, M. (2006). Clinical monitoring of the critically ill rabbit. Proceedings: IVECCS. accessed via Veterinary Information Network; vin.com

Leib, M. S., et al. (2007). Triple antimicrobial therapy and acid suppression in dogs with chronic vomiting and gastric Helicobacter spp. Journal of Veterinary Internal Medicine 21(6): 1185-92.

Mordecai, A., et al. (2011). Normal Dogs Treated with Famotidine for 14 days Have Only Transient Increases in Serum Gastrin Concentrations. Journal of Veterinary Internal Medicine 25(6): 1248-52.

Tolbert, K., et al. (2011). Efficacy of Oral Famotidine and 2 Omeprazole Formulations for the Control of Intragastric pH in Dogs. J Vet Intern Med 25(1): 47-54.

Trepanier, L. A. (2013). Applying Pharmacokinetics to Veterinary Clinical Practice. Veterinary Clinics of North America-Small Animal Practice 43(5): 1013-+.

Williams, B. (2000). Therapeutics in Ferrets. Vet Clin NA: Exotic Anim Pract 3:1(Jan): 131-53.

Williamson, K. K., et al. (2010). Efficacy of Omeprazole versus High-Dose Famotidine for Prevention of Exercise-Induced Gastritis in Racing Alaskan Sled Dogs. Journal of Veterinary Internal Medicine 24(2): 285-8.

Fat Emulsion, Intravenous

Parenteral Nutritional Agent; Antidote

Intralipid®, Intravenous Lipid Emulsion, ILE, IFE

Prescriber Highlights

▶ Parenteral calorie and fatty acid source.

▶ Can be useful in overdoses or poisonings to reduce free-drug blood levels of fat-soluble drugs or toxins. Not a substitute for standard supportive measures in intoxicated patients.

▶ Potentially serious adverse effects can occur (hypersensitivity, lipemia/fat overload, etc.)

▶ When used for parenteral nutrition, use in critically ill veterinary patients is controversial.

Uses/Indications

Intravenous fat emulsions (IFE; intravenous lipid emulsion; ILE) can be used as a source of calories or essential fatty acids when parenteral feeding is required.

IFE can be considered as a rescue treatment for intoxications caused by fat-soluble drugs/toxins when traditional treatments are not effective (Fernandez, Lee and Rahilly 2011). At present, this use is extra-label and solid evidence supporting routine clinical use in veterinary medicine is sparse. Evidence exists that IFE could be useful for reducing free-drug levels for drugs or drug classes such as local anesthetics (bupivacaine, mepivacaine, ropivacaine, lidocaine) macrocyclic lactones (e.g., ivermectin, moxidectin), calcium channel blockers (e.g., diltiazem, verapamil, amlodipine) beta-blockers (e.g., propranolol, carvedilol), antidepressants (e.g., bupropion, doxepin, sertraline, clomipramine), antipsychotics (e.g., chlorpromazine, quetiapine), antiepileptics (e.g., carbamazepine, lamotrigine), and muscle relaxants (e.g., baclofen, cyclobenzaprine) (Crandell et al. 2009), (O'Brien et al. 2010), (Maton et al. 2013). As certain treatments available for humans (*e.g.*, hemoperfusion, hemodialysis, long-term ventilator or intensive care) are either unavailable or cost prohibitive in veterinary medicine, early intervention with IFE for fat-soluble intoxications in patients with severe clinical signs may be a relatively low cost and safe method to effectively treat veterinary patients.

Pharmacology/Actions

Intravenously administered lipid emulsions can provide an efficient method (1 mL of a 20% emulsion provides approximately 2 kCal) of providing calories, and serve as a source of essential fatty acids. In addition, intravenous lipids can have immunosuppressive effects, increase pro-inflammatory cytokines, and affect pulmonary function.

When used for toxicologic indications, IFE's exact mechanism of action is unknown, but it may serve as a "lipid sink" for fat-soluble compounds, reducing the amount of free drug in the circulation thereby reducing the drug's toxic effects. Other hypotheses include: improving cardiac performance/function by increasing intracellular calcium and/or providing myocytes an energy substrate, and increasing the pool of fatty acids thus overcoming the inhibition of mitochondrial fatty acid metabolism by drugs such as bupivacaine.

Pharmacokinetics

IFE appears to be removed from the blood stream about as rapidly as chylomicrons, but the rate of removal requires prior lipolysis of IFE into free fatty acids and seems to be increased with heparin activated lipoprotein. In humans, elimination half-life is about 30 minutes.

Contraindications/Precautions/Warnings

Intravenous lipids are contraindicated in patients with severe egg yolk allergies or abnormal fat metabolism.

Strict aseptic technique and good IV catheter care are imperative when using IFE with or without amino acids and dextrose. When used alone, IFE may be administered via a peripheral line but when combined with amino acids/dextrose as total parenteral nutrition (TPN), a dedicated central line is required due to the solution's hypertonicity.

Use with caution in neonates as there is an increased risk for lipid emboli.

When managing poisoned patients, IFE is not a substitute for standard supportive and symptomatic care.

Use of IFE in critically ill animals is somewhat controversial. While there are no studies specifically addressing the role or safety of lipids in critically ill animals, human data suggests that lipid administration may be associated with significant immunosuppression, exacerbation of pre-existing pulmonary pathology, and increasing infection rates. Data also supports that withholding lipids for moderate periods of time is not associated with an increase in morbidity or mortality administration (Crandell 2005).In humans, intravenous lipids are used with caution in premature and low-birth weight infants (Black Box Warning; lipemia), patients with blood coagulation disorders, pulmonary disease, renal impairment, severe liver damage, and those at risk for fat emboli.

Adverse Effects

While IFE's adverse effect profile/incidence rates in veterinary patients have not been thoroughly reported, they are likely similar to those seen in human patients.

In humans, adverse effects associated with IFE are infrequent and usually associated with IFE use for nutritional support. Most commonly reported are sepsis or thrombophlebitis secondary to IV administration, but these can occur whether or not intravenous lipids are used in parenteral nutrition therapy. Fat overload syndrome (hyperlipidemia, hepatomegaly, icterus, splenomegaly, fat embolism, thrombocytopenia, hemolysis, and prolonged clotting times) can occur, particularly if doses are too high or administration is too fast. More rarely (<1%), IFE can cause pulmonary toxicity, GI effects, somnolence, headache, flushing, fat emboli, hyperlipemia, pancreatitis, hypercoagulability, and hypersensitivity. IFE effects on pulmonary function and oxygenation are temporary and resolve after discontinuation.

Reproductive/Nursing Safety

When used when clearly needed, the benefits of using intravenous lipids during pregnancy would likely outweigh the risks. However, the FDA has placed them in category *C* (*Animal studies have shown an adverse effect on the fetus, but there are no adequate studies in humans; or there are no animal reproduction studies and no adequate studies in humans.*). No data regarding the safe use of IFE during lactation is available, and while IFE is likely safe, nursing may not be appropriate for mothers that require IFE.

Overdosage/Acute Toxicity

In the case of an inadvertent overdose, stop the infusion until the lipid has cleared. This can be evaluated in a gross manner by visually inspecting the plasma (hematocrit tubes), or by laboratory methods (triglyceride concentrations, plasma light-scattering activity by nephelometry).

When using IFE for drug toxicity and in cases where severe hyperlipidemia is present, heparin therapy (75 – 250 Units/kg SC q6h) can be considered. Heparin may increase lipid clearance (not proven) and the use of heparin may potentially affect the mechanism of action of IFE for fat-soluble toxicosis. Some advocate using heparin when hyperlipemia occurs in dog breeds susceptible to pancreatitis (*e.g.*, Shetland sheepdog, miniature schnauzer, Yorkshire terrier, obese animals, etc.), although there is no direct proof that hyperlipidemia secondary to IFE increases the risk for pancreatitis. Otherwise, heparin therapy is not recommended unless clinical signs or advanced diagnostics indicate otherwise. Monitor partial thromboplastin time (PTT) prior to use of heparin to ensure the patient is not already coagulopathic. If PTT exceeds 2-2.5X normal, the dose of heparin should be either reduced (75 Units/kg SC q6-8h) or discontinued (Lee 2010).

Drug Interactions

The following drug interactions have either been reported or are theoretical in humans or animals receiving IFE and may be of significance in veterinary patients. Unless otherwise noted, use together is not necessarily contraindicated, but weigh the potential risks and perform additional monitoring when appropriate.

- **LIPID SOLUBLE DRUGS:** Intravenous lipids (IFE) may affect the pharmacokinetics of lipid soluble drugs by serving as a "lipid sink" for free drug in the circulation. At present, clinical significance is not clear. However, when IFE is used (as a nutritional agent) concurrently with a fat-soluble drug, monitor for decreased efficacy of the drug.

Laboratory Considerations

- Blood samples for diagnostics should be collected prior to administration of IFE to minimize affects from hyperlipidemia.
- Falsely high **hemoglobin, MCH and MCHC** values can occur if samples are drawn during or shortly after fat emulsion infusion.
- Some analyzers (*e.g.*, *Hemocue®*) may report falsely high **blood glucose** values.
- **Serum bilirubin** values may be affected by IFE.

Doses

As a nutritional agent for parenteral nutrition (PN); (extra-label): Note: If using IFE for parenteral nutrition, the reader is advised to consult with a veterinary nutritionist and refer to more detailed references on the subject including: Small Animals: (Thomovsky, Backus, et al. 2007), (Thomovsky, Reniker, et al. 2007), (Chandler et al. 2008), (Campbell et al. 2006), (Freeman et al. 2006), Horses: (Magdesian 2010). The following are examples:

a) Most recommendations are to consider intravenous lipids as energy substrates, and to administer them at 30-40% of total calories. In veterinary medicine, lipid administration ranges from 25-60% of calories administered (Crandell 2005). Traditionally, IFE administration is not recommended at >2 g/kg/day for TPN therapy (Lee 2011).

b) There are two strategies employed by nutritionists to supply calories. One approach is to provide daily resting energy requirements (RER) with a mixture of all three nutrients (protein, dextrose, lipids) starting with provision of adequate protein (4 – 6 grams/100 kcal). Other nutritionists advocate supplying the daily RER in dextrose and lipids and adding protein "on top." This approach asserts that proteins not catabolized for energy can be used to maintain protein synthesis. Hyperalimentation may be more frequent with the second approach. Generally, either approach can be used for total parenteral nutrition (TPN), but with partial parenteral nutrition (PPN) care should be taken with the second approach to keep the solution below 600 mOsm/L. Some nutritionists will supplement lipids alone for up to 3 days at RER. For example, a 10 kg dog with RER of 370 kcal/day. *Intralipid®* 20% solution (2 kcal/mL) could supply RER peripherally at 8 mL/hr. The lipid component of PN is controversial and some nutritionists do not include lipids in PN for critically ill patients because of concerns of increases in infection complications, immunosuppression, free radical generation and inflammation. Use caution when using imbalanced strategies. (Waldrop 2009)

As a rescue agent for fat-soluble drug/toxin intoxication (extra-label): Note: For additional guidance it is highly recommended to contact an animal poison center. Currently, 20% ILE is recommended for all suggested treatment protocols in small animal medicine. Additional information on using IFE for this purpose may also be found at: (Jamaty et al. 2010; Fernandez, Lee, et al. 2011b; Gwaltney-Brant et al. 2012; Bates et al. 2013). Several suggested treatment protocols exist, but at the time of writing (Dec 2013) not enough controlled experimental evidence exists to fully establish any one protocol. The following are examples:

a) Based on available information, suggest an IV bolus of 20% ILE between 1.5 – 4 mL/kg over 1 minute, followed by a CRI of 0.25 mL/kg/minute (15 mL/kg/hour) over 30-60 minutes in dogs. In animals nonresponsive after this traditional dosing protocol, additional individual bolus doses can be administered slowly at up to 7 mL/kg IV. Authors have recommended intermittent IV boluses of 1.5 mL/kg every 4-6 hours for the initial 24 hours with anecdotal success. In addition, it is likely safe to assume that follow-up CRI doses of 0.05 mL/kg/hour can be continued until clinical signs improve (not to exceed 24 hours). That said, there have been no safety studies evaluating the use of ILE in the clinically poisoned veterinary patient, and careful monitoring and risk assessment is important. (Fernandez, Lee, et al. 2011a)

b) The "standard" protocol is: using the 20% ILE is 1.5 mL/kg IV over 5-15 minutes followed by a 0.25 mL/kg/minute CRI over 1-2 hours. This dose can be repeated in several hours if clinical signs of toxicity return. Prior to repeating the dose, a peripheral blood sample should be evaluated for evidence of lipemia; additional doses should not be given if serum is lipemic. (Johnson 2011)

Monitoring

- When used for toxicology indications: **drug levels (serum or plasma)** to evaluate the response to IFE therapy. This will aid in data collection for future retrospective study analysis. While blood sampling times should be based on the pharmacokinetics of the drug, general recommended sample times for drug levels are: time 0 (at the time of presentation), 30 minutes after administration of IFE, 1 hour post, 6, hours post, 12 hours post, and 24 hours post (Lee 2010). Another recommendation is to monitor serum every 2 hours and consider additional infusions if the patient is still symptomatic and the serum clear of **lipemia**. Do not repeat ILE if the serum is very orange or yellow. If no improvement is noted after 3 doses (bolus and CRI), discontinue ILE therapy (Gwaltney-Brant et al. 2012).

- When used for nutritional support; monitoring can be very involved and include: blood glucose, serum triglycerides/lipemia, PCV, total protein, catheter and catheter site status, hydration status, vital signs (temperature, respiration rate, cardiac rate), serum electrolytes (including phosphorous), renal and liver function tests, CBC, etc. It is recommended to consult with a veterinary nutritionist and refer to a more detailed reference (see references) for more information.

Client Information

- Intravenous fat emulsion products should only be used by professionals in a setting where adequate patient monitoring is available.

Chemistry/Synonyms

Fat Emulsion, intravenous are emulsified soybean (*Intralipid®*, *Liposyn® III*), or soybean and safflower (*Liposyn® II*) oils that provide the fatty acids: linoleic, stearic, linolenic, oleic and palmitic acids. Egg yolk phospholipids serve as the primary emulsifying agent and glycerol is used to adjust tonicity. Osmolarity varies with product, but range from 200-293 mOsm/L. The pH of IFE is between 6-9. Initially the pH is around 9, but secondary to hydrolysis of triglycerides into free fatty acids (FFA), the pH decreases to 6 at the end of the product's shelf-life.

Storage/Stability

Unopened IFE products should be stored at room temperature (not above 25°C, 77°F) and not allowed to freeze. If accidentally frozen, it should be discarded. If a partial amount of a bag or bottle is used, the remaining product should be stored protected in the refrigerator (2-8°C), and discarded 24 hours after opening. A new bag or vial must be used every 24 hours.

Compatibility/Compounding Considerations

IFE is **compatible** when mixed with the usual components used in parenteral nutrition (dextrose, amino acids, parenteral multivitamins and trace elements), but as concentrations and mixing order can affect compatibility it is advisable to contact a hospital pharmacist or refer to a drug compatibility reference for more information. This is particularly important as the opaque nature of IFE makes detection of precipitates very difficult.

Admixtures must be prepared with strict aseptic technique. Do not add additives directly to IFE, and in no case add fat emulsion to the total parenteral nutrition container first. The proper order of mixing: 1) transfer dextrose to the admixture container; 2) transfer amino acid solution; then 3) transfer fat emulsion. Alternatively, amino acids, dextrose, and fat emulsion may be simultaneously transferred to the admixture container; gently agitate the mixture. Use these admixtures promptly; store under refrigeration (2°-8°C; 36°-46°F) for 24 hours or less and use within 24 hours after removal from refrigeration.

Dosage Forms/Regulatory Status

VETERINARY-LABELED PRODUCTS: NONE.

HUMAN-LABELED PRODUCTS:

Fat Emulsion, Intravenous 10%, 20%, 30%; depending on product, in 50 mL, 100 mL, 200 mL, 250 mL, & 500 mL bottles or bags; *Intralipid®*, Liposyn® II & *Liposyn® III*; (Rx)

Revisions/References

Monograph revised/updated January 2014.

Bates, N., et al. (2013). Lipid infusion in the management of poisoning: a report of 6 canine cases. Veterinary Record 172(13).

Campbell, S., et al. (2006). Central and peripheral parenteral nutrition. Waltham Focus 16(3): 22-30.

Chandler, M., et al. (2008). Parenteral Nutrition. *Small Animal Critical Care Medicine*. D. Silverstein and K. Hopper. St Louis, Elsevier: 58-62.

Crandell, D. (2005). Use of Lipids in Parenteral Nutrition. Proceedings: IVECCS. accessed via Veterinary Information Network; vin.com

Crandell, D. E. & G. L. Weinberg (2009). Moxidectin toxicosis in a puppy successfully treated with intravenous lipids. J. Vet. Emerg. Crit. Care 19(2): 181-6.

Fernandez, A., et al. (2011). The Use of Intravenous Lipid Emulsion as an Antidote in Toxicology: A Review. J Vet Emerg Crit Care **Pending Publication**.

Fernandez, A. L., et al. (2011a). The use of intravenous lipid emulsion as an antidote in veterinary toxicology. J. Vet. Emerg. Crit. Care 21(5): 570-.

Fernandez, A. L., et al. (2011b). The use of intravenous lipid emulsion as an antidote in veterinary toxicology. J. Vet. Emerg. Crit. Care 21(4): 309-20.

Freeman, L. & D. Chan (2006). Total parenteral nutrition. *Fluid, Electrolyte, and Acid-base Disorders in Small Animal Practice*. S. P. DiBartola. St Louis, Elsevier: 584-600.

Gwaltney-Brant, S. & I. Meadows (2012). Use of Intravenous Lipid Emulsions for Treating Certain Poisoning Cases in Small Animals. Veterinary Clinics of North America-Small Animal Practice 42(2): 251-+.

Jamaty, C., et al. (2010). Lipid emulsions in the treatment of acute poisoning: a systematic review of human and animal studies. Clinical Toxicology 48(1): 1-27.

Johnson, T. (2011). Intravenous Lipid Emulsion (IVLE) Therapy for Selected Toxicoses. International Veterinary Emergency and Critical Care Symposium. accessed via Veterinary Information Network; vin.com

Lee, J. A. (2010). Advances in Toxicology: The Use of Intra-Lipid Therapy & High-Dextrose Insulin Therapy. Proceedings: ACVIM. accessed via Veterinary Information Network; vin.com

Lee, J. A. (2011). Personal Communication.

Magdesian, K. G. (2010). Parenteral nutrition in the mature horse. Equine Veterinary Education 22(7): 364-71.

Maton, B. L., et al. (2013). The use of high-dose insulin therapy and intravenous lipid emulsion to treat severe, refractory diltiazem toxicosis in a dog. J. Vet. Emerg. Crit. Care 23(3): 321-7.

O'Brien, T. Q., et al. (2010). Infusion of a lipid emulsion to treat lidocaine intoxication in a cat. Javma-Journal of the American Veterinary Medical Association 237(12): 1455-8.

Thomovsky, E., et al. (2007). Parenteral nutrition: Formulation, monitoring, and complications. Compendium on Continuing Education for the Practicing Veterinarian 29(2): 88-103.

Thomovsky, E., et al. (2007). Parenteral nutrition: Uses, indications, and compounding. Compendium on Continuing Education for the Practicing Veterinarian 29(2): 76-+.

Waldrop, J. (2009). Parenteral Nutrition in Real Practice. Proceedings: IVECCS. accessed via Veterinary Information Network; vin.com

Fatty Acids, Essential/Omega (Oral)

Nutritional   Fish Oil; Vegetable Oil

Prescriber Highlights

▶ Orally used for treatment of pruritus in dogs and cats; may be useful in cats with heart failure. Injectable forms (not available in USA) may be beneficial for parenteral nutrition use. May also be useful in other species & for other disease states

▶ Safety in pregnancy not established; use **caution** in patients with coagulopathies.

▶ Adverse Effects: High doses may cause GI distress; rarely some dogs may become lethargic or more pruritic.

Uses/Indications

These products are usually used for the treatment of pruritus associated with atopy, idiopathic seborrhea, miliary dermatitis and eosinophilic granuloma complex. In cats, omega-3 (n-3) fatty acids may be helpful to reduce cytokines and improve appetite in cats with heart failure. Fatty acids may improve coat quality and be helpful for adjunctive therapy for arthropathies such as hip dysplasia. Generally, products containing the polyunsaturated fatty acids (PUFA n-3s) eicosapentaenoic acid (EPA) and docosahexaenoic acid (DHA) are recommended in dogs. Omega-3's are added to some commercial diets.

When used for pruritus, significant therapeutic effects may be noted in only 25-50% of treated patients and 2-3 months of treatment is required before evaluating efficacy. Antihistamine and fatty acid therapy may be synergistic for treatment of pruritus.

Polyunsaturated fatty acids, particularly the omega-3's with their antiinflammatory properties, may prove to be useful for a variety of conditions including renal failure, arthritis (both degenerative and autoimmune), cardiovascular disease (hypercoagulable states, heart failure, dysrhythmias), inflammatory bowel disease, hepatic fibrosis and steatosis, and some neoplastic diseases.

One study in dogs with chronic osteoarthritis fed a diet supplemented with fish oil omega-3 fatty acids suggested that carprofen dosage reductions could be possible (Fritsch et al. 2010). In another, dogs with osteoarthritis fed a diet with a very high omega-3 to omega-6 ratio (compared with the control diet, omega-3 levels were 31X greater, and omega-6 levels were 34X lower) had significantly lower serum levels of arachadonic acid and owners reported subjective improvement in arthritic condition (Roush et al. 2010).

The ACVIM consensus statement on proteinuria in dogs and cats (Lees et al. 2005), states: "The treatment strategies to be considered are to feed an appropriate diet (one with reduced quantity but high-quality protein with omega-3 fatty acid supplementation), to administer an angiotensin-converting-enzyme inhibitor drug or both."

Fish oil (but not Flax oil) significantly reduced VPCs in Boxer dogs with arrhythmogenic right ventricular cardiomyopathy (Smith et al. 2007).

Pharmacology/Actions

The exact pharmacologic actions of these products are not well described; particularly in light of the combination nature of the commercial products being marketed, it is difficult to ascertain which compounds may be responsible for their proposed efficacy. The particular therapeutic benefits and ratios of omega-3 versus omega-6 fatty acids are still being debated.

Fish oils affect arachadonic acid levels in plasma lipids and platelet membranes. They may affect production of inflammatory prostaglandins in the body, thereby reducing inflammation and pruritus. Essential fatty acids are necessary for normal skin and haircoat; linolenic or linoleic acids may be used as sources.

Contraindications/Precautions/Warnings

Most commercial pet foods contain a source of omega-3 fatty acids, administering additional omega-3's may cause adverse effects. Before supplementation determine the amount of omega-3's in the diet to determine appropriate dosing.

Because of potential affects on bleeding times, use with caution in patients with coagulation disorders or those receiving anticoagulant medications. Use with caution in patients with non-insulin dependent diabetes as omega-3 fatty acids have impaired insulin secretion with resultant increased glucose levels in humans with type-2 diabetes. Fatty acids should be used with caution in dogs that have had previous bouts of pancreatitis or protracted diarrhea.

Adverse Effects

At high dosages, GI disturbances (*e.g.*, vomiting, diarrhea) may be seen. Rarely, some dogs become lethargic, have reduced wound healing, or become more pruritic. Alterations in platelet function (aggregation) can occur, particularly in cats. Omega 3's may alter immune function, but any clinical significance of these effects is not clearly known (Lenox et al. 2013).

Reproductive/Nursing Safety

Safe use in pregnancy has not been established; these products are not recommended for use in pregnant human patients. Use cautiously in veterinary patients.

Overdosage/Acute Toxicity

With products containing vitamin A, acute toxicosis may result after accidental overdoses. Contact a poison control center for additional information.

Drug Interactions

The following drug interactions have either been reported or are theoretical in humans or animals receiving fatty acids/fish oils and may be of significance in veterinary patients. Unless otherwise noted, use together is not necessarily contraindicated, but weigh the potential risks and perform additional monitoring when appropriate.

- **ANTICOAGULANTS** (*e.g.,* **aspirin, warfarin, heparin**): Because of potential affects on bleeding times, use with caution in patients receiving anticoagulant medications.

Laboratory Considerations

Omega 3's may affect **clotting times.**

Doses

- **DOGS:**

  As a source of Omega-3's (extra-label):
  NRC recommended daily allowances/safe upper limits and suggested dosages for therapeutic use are determined using "metabolic weight" (not actual body weight) and the combined weight of eicosapentaenoic acid (EPA) and docosahexaenoic acid (DHA). To first convert the dog's body weight in kg to the metabolic body weight take the actual weight in kg and raise it to the 0.75 power. For example, a dog weighing 10 kg would convert to 5.62. (*Plumb's note: Those not adept at using a scientific calculator for this purpose can use a calculator that has a square root function key. In the example above of a dog weighing 10 kg; cube the bodyweight in kg (10x10x10=1000); then take the square root of 1000 twice=5.62.*) This value is then multiplied by the recommended dosage for a particular condition. Consider the amount of EPA/DHA consumed in the diet when determining daily dose. The following are suggested daily dosages of combined EPA/DHA per metabolic weight:

  NRC recommended daily allowance: 30 mg/kg$^{0.75}$

  NRC safe upper limit: 370 mg/kg$^{0.75}$

  Idiopathic hyperlipidemia: 120 mg/kg$^{0.75}$

  Kidney Disease: 140 mg/kg$^{0.75}$; may be increased to the NRC safe upper limit.

  Cardiovascular Disorders: 115 mg/kg$^{0.75}$

  Osteoarthritis: 310 mg/kg$^{0.75}$; may be increased to the NRC safe upper limit.

  Inflammatory or Immunologic Disorders (*e.g.* inflammatory bowel disease, atopy): 125 mg/kg$^{0.75}$

  Adapted from: (Bauer 2011, 2012)

  For adjunctive treatment of glomerular disease (extra-label): The IRIS Canine GN Study Group Standard Therapy Subgroup recommends that dogs with glomerular disease be fed a diet with a reduced omega-6/omega-3 polyunsaturated fatty acids (PUFA) ratio, approximating 5:1. Where dietary supplementation with an omega-3 PUFA by the owner is used to alter this ratio, a dosage of 0.25 – 0.50 g/kg of an omega-3 containing eicosapentaenoic acid and docosahexaenoic acid is appropriate for a typical canine diet. (Brown et al. 2013)

- **CATS:**

  To find the metabolic weight for cats; weight in kg is raised to the 0.67 power (kg$^{0.67}$). There is less evidence supporting safety and efficacy use of omega-3's in cats than in dogs and dosages > 75 mg of EPA and DHA/kg$^{0.67}$ per day should be used with caution and under veterinary supervision until further evaluations of long-term safety are performed. (Bauer 2011)

For adjunctive treatment in cats with CHF: Optimal dose of omega-3 fatty acids for cats is not yet known, author currently recommends 40 mg/kg EPA and 25 mg/kg DHA in cats. Fish oil supplements vary widely in the amount of EPA and DHA they contain so know the exact amount in supplements recommended. Capsules that contain approximately 180 mg EPA and 120 mg DHA can be purchased OTC at human pharmacies and administered at a dose of 1 capsule per 10 pounds body weight. Fish oil should contain vitamin E as an antioxidant, but supplements that contain other nutrients are not recommended to avoid toxicities. Cod liver oil and flax oil should not be used. (Freeman 2010)

Monitoring
- Efficacy.
- Adverse effects.

Client Information
- When used for itching, may require treatment for 2-3 months to see if it will be effective.
- Give with or without food.
- Usually tolerated very well. GI effects (*e.g.*, vomiting, diarrhea, etc.) are possible with higher dosages. Bleeding or lethargy (lack of energy) are very rare.

Chemistry/Synonyms
The commercially available veterinary products generally contain a combination of fish oil (eicosapentanoic and docosahexanoic acids) and vegetable oil (gamma linolenic acid) that serve as essential fatty acids. They may also contain vitamin E (d-alpha tocopherol) and vitamin A.

Storage/Stability
The oral capsules should be stored in tight containers and protected from heat (cool, dry place).

Compatibility/Compounding Considerations
No specific information noted.

Dosage Forms/Regulatory Status
VETERINARY-LABELED PRODUCTS:
There are many combination products available without prescription having various trade names, including (partial listing): *Dermapet Eicosderm®, Dermapet OFA plus EZ-C Caps®, F.A. Caps®, F.A. Caps ES®, Omega EFA® Capsules, Omega EFA® Capsules XS, Performer® OFA Gel Capsules Extra Strength, etc.*

HUMAN-LABELED PRODUCTS:
There are many fish oil capsules available without prescription having various trade names.

Revisions/References
Monograph revised/updated January 2014.
Bauer, J. E. (2011). Therapeutic use of fish oils in companion animals. Javma-Journal of the American Veterinary Medical Association 239(11): 1441-51.

Bauer, J. E. (2012). Question about fish oil dosages Response. Javma-Journal of the American Veterinary Medical Association 240(3): 262-.

Brown, S., et al. (2013). Consensus Recommendations for Standard Therapy of Glomerular Disease in Dogs. Journal of Veterinary Internal Medicine 27: S27-S43.

Freeman, L. (2010). Optimal Nutrition for Feline Cardiac Patients. Proceedings: ACVIM. accessed via Veterinary Information Network; vin.com

Fritsch, D. A., et al. (2010). A multicenter study of the effect of dietary supplementation with fish oil omega-3 fatty acids on carprofen dosage in dogs with osteoarthritis. Javma-Journal of the American Veterinary Medical Association 236(5): 535-9.

Lees, G., et al. (2005). Assessment and Management of Proteinuria in Dogs and Cats: 2004 ACVIM Forum Consensus Statement (Small Animal). J Vet Intern Med 19: 377-85.

Lenox, C. E. & J. E. Bauer (2013). Potential Adverse Effects of Omega-3 Fatty Acids in Dogs and Cats. J Vet Intern Med 274(3): 217-26.

Roush, J. K., et al. (2010). Multicenter veterinary practice assessment of the effects of omega-3 fatty acids on osteoarthritis in dogs. Javma-Journal of the American Veterinary Medical Association 236(1): 59-66.

Smith, C. E., et al. (2007). Omega-3 fatty acids in boxer dogs with arrhythmogenic right ventricular cardiomyopathy. Journal of Veterinary Internal Medicine 21(2): 265-73.

Febantel – See the product *Drontal® Plus* listed in the Praziquantel and Pyrantel monographs

Felbamate
(fell-ba-mate)   Felbatol®

Anticonvulsant

Prescriber Highlights
▶ 2nd or 3rd line antiseizure medication for dogs.
▶ Appears relatively safe to use in dogs, but because of limited use, adverse effect profile may be incomplete.
▶ Cost & accessibility may be issues.

Uses/Indications
Felbamate is an anticonvulsant agent that may useful for treating seizure disorders (generalized seizures, but especially complex partial seizures) in dogs. A potential advantage of felbamate therapy is that when used alone or in combination with phenobarbital and/or bromides, it does not appear to cause additive sedation.

Pharmacology/Actions
Felbamate's anticonvulsant activity is thought to be due its ability to reduce excitatory neurotransmission; its exact mechanism is unknown, but it is believed to increase activation of sodium channels thereby decreasing sustained high-frequency firing of action potentials.

Pharmacokinetics
Felbamate is well absorbed after oral administration in dogs. Felbamate is both excreted unchanged and as metabolites in the urine (about 50:50). The half-life in dogs may range from 5-14 hours, but averages around 6 hours. Because the drug can induce liver enzyme induction, half-lives may decrease with time and dosages may need adjustment.

Contraindications/Precautions/Warnings
Felbamate is contraindicated in patients hypersensitive to it or other carbamates (meprobamate). In humans, felbamate should not be used in patients with a history of blood dyscrasias or hepatic dysfunction. Use with caution in dogs with hepatic impairment. Dogs that require felbamate are often close to euthanasia and there is a lack of evidence that felbamate causes liver toxicity in dogs.

Adverse Effects
Adverse reactions in the dog include keratoconjunctivitis sicca (KCS), liver enzyme induction, tremor, limb rigidity, salivation, restlessness and agitation (at high doses). In humans, aplastic anemia and hepatic necrosis have been noted and could be a factor in canine medicine. There apparently have not been any case reports yet of aplastic anemia in dogs, but blood dyscrasias (thrombocytopenia, lymphopenia, and leukopenia) have been reported. Additionally, sedation, and vomiting/nausea have been reported in dogs, but usually in those receiving other anticonvulsants as well.

Reproductive/Nursing Safety
Although no overt teratogenicity has been documented, felbamate should only be used during pregnancy when its potential benefits outweigh its potential risks. In humans, the FDA categorizes this drug as category *C* for use during pregnancy (*Animal studies have shown an adverse effect on the fetus, but there are no adequate studies in humans; or there are no animal reproduction studies and no adequate studies in humans.*)

The drug is excreted into maternal milk, but adverse consequences to nursing puppies appear remote.

Overdosage/Acute Toxicity

Limited information is available. One human subject taking 12 grams over 12 hours only developed mild gastric distress and a slightly increased heart rate.

Drug Interactions

The following drug interactions have either been reported or are theoretical in humans or animals receiving felbamate and may be of significance in veterinary patients. Unless otherwise noted, use together is not necessarily contraindicated, but weigh the potential risks and perform additional monitoring when appropriate.

- **PHENOBARBITAL:** When felbamate is added to patients taking phenobarbital it may cause increases in phenobarbital levels. When phenobarbital is added to patients taking felbamate, felbamate levels may decrease. The same effect can occur with **phenytoin.**
- **VALPROATE:** Felbamate can cause increases in valproic acid levels.

Doses

- **DOGS:**

  For seizures; 2nd to 3rd line agent; (extra-label): Felbamate is not commonly used, but it can be considered as an add-on drug when acceptable seizure control is not attained or adverse effects are not tolerated with other standard treatments. Evidence supporting any dosage regimen was not located. Most recommend using initially at 15 – 20 mg/kg PO q8h, with gradual dosage increases of approx. 15 mg/kg every 2 weeks, if required and tolerated. Some start at lower dosages 5 – 10 mg/kg q12h and titrate to q8h. Upper limits of 60 – 70 mg/kg q8h have been noted.

Monitoring

- There is some controversy about monitoring felbamate use in dogs, probably due to limited experience. Some clinicians state that liver function tests and CBC's should be regularly assessed (q2-3 months). Others state that the drug is very safe in dogs and monitoring does not appear to be necessary. If the dog is receiving other drugs (especially phenobarbital), monitoring is essential.
- Therapeutic drug levels for felbamate in dogs are not truly known, but appear to be in the 25 – 100 micrograms/mL range. The usefulness of monitoring serum levels is questionable at this point.

Client Information

- Human anticonvulsant that may be useful to treat seizure disorders (e.g., epilepsy, etc.) in dogs. Not very much experience using it in veterinary medicine. It usually does not cause sleepiness/sedation.
- May be given with or without food. If your animal vomits or acts sick after getting it on an empty stomach, give with food or small treat to see if this helps. If vomiting continues, contact your veterinarian.
- Appears to be relatively safe in dogs, but report anything out of the ordinary to veterinarian. Possible side effects include: Tremors/shaking, stiff legs, salivation/drooling, restlessness/agitation, dry eyes or increases in liver enzymes.
- May require dosing several times a day. It will not be effective if dosages are missed.

Chemistry/Synonyms

Felbamate is a unique dicarbamate anticonvulsant agent that is slightly soluble in water.

Felbamate may also be known by as: AD-03055, W-554, *Felbamyl®, Felbatol®, Taloxa®,* and *Taloxa®.*

Storage/Stability

Felbamate preparations should be stored at room temperature. The suspension should be shaken well before use.

Compatibility/Compounding Considerations

No specific information noted.

Dosage Forms/Regulatory Status

VETERINARY-LABELED PRODUCTS: NONE.

The ARCI (Racing Commissioners International) has designated this drug as a class 3 substance. See the appendix for more information.

HUMAN-LABELED PRODUCTS:

Felbamate Tablets: 400 mg & 600 mg; *Felbatol®,* generic; (Rx)

Felbamate Suspension: 120 mg/mL in 240 & 960 mL; *Felbatol®,* generic; (Rx)

Revisions/References

Monograph revised/updated January 2014.

Fenbendazole

(fen-ben-da-zole)   Panacur®, Safe-Guard®

Antiparasitic Agent

Prescriber Highlights

▶ Anthelmintic useful for a variety of parasites in dogs, cats, cattle, horses, swine, etc.
▶ Adverse Effects: Antigen release by dying parasites may occur, particularly at high dosages; vomiting may occur infrequently in dogs or cats.
▶ In dogs, give with food.

Uses/Indications

Fenbendazole is indicated (labeled) for the removal of the following parasites in dogs: ascarids (*Toxocara canis, T. leonina*), Hookworms (*Ancylostoma caninum, Uncinaria stenocephala*), whipworms (*Trichuris vulpis*), and tapeworms (*Taenia pisiformis*). It is not effective against *Dipylidium caninum*. Fenbendazole has also been used clinically to treat *Capillaria aerophilia, Filaroides hirthi,* and *Paragonimus kellicotti* infections in dogs.

Fenbendazole is indicated (labeled) for the removal of the following adult forms of parasites in cattle: *Haemonchus contortus, Ostertagia ostertagi, Trichostrongylus axei, Bunostomum phlebotomum, Nematodirus helvetianus, Cooperia* spp., *Trichostrongylus colubriformis, Oesophagostomum radiatum,* and *Dictyocaulus vivaparus.* It is also effective against most immature stages of the above listed parasites. Although not FDA-approved, it has good activity against *Moniezia* spp., and arrested 4th stage forms of *Ostertagia ostertagi.*

Fenbendazole is indicated (labeled) for the removal of the following parasites in horses: large strongyles (*S. edentatus, S. equinus, S. vulgaris*), small strongyles (*Cyathostomum* spp., *Cylicocylus* spp., *Cylicostephanus* spp., *Triodontophorus* spp.), and pinworms (*Oxyuris equi*).

Fenbendazole is indicated (labeled) for the removal of the following parasites in swine: large roundworms (*Ascaris suum*), lungworms (*Metastrongylus pair*), nodular worms (*Oesphagostomum dentatum, O. quadrispinolatum*), small stomach worms (*Hyostrongylus rubidus*), whipworms (*Trichuris suis*), and kidney worms (*Stephanurus dentatus*; both mature and immature).

Although not FDA-approved, fenbendazole has been used in cats, small mammals, reptiles, sheep, goats, pet birds, and llamas. See Dosage section for more information.

Pharmacology/Actions

Fenbendazole is a methylcarbamate benzimidazole antiparasitic agent and has a broad spectrum of activity against a variety of pathogenic internal parasites. In susceptible parasites, benzimidazole mechanism of action is believed due to disrupting intracellular microtubular transport systems by binding selectively and damaging tubulin, preventing tubulin polymerization, and inhibiting microtubule formation. Benzimidazoles also act at higher concentrations to disrupt metabolic pathways within the helminth, and inhibit metabolic enzymes, including malate dehydrogenase and fumarate reductase. Benzimidazoles may be considered time-dependent antiparasitic agents.

Pharmacokinetics

Fenbendazole is only marginally absorbed after oral administration. The amount absorbed from the gut is apparently more associated with the solubility of the drug and not the dose given. In dogs, when doses ranging from 25 – 100 mg/kg were administered, the area-under-the-curves were similar. Bioavailability is increased in dogs when fenbendazole is administered with food. Fat content of food does not significantly alter bioavailability (McKellar et al. 1993).

After oral dosing in calves and horses, peak blood levels of 0.11 micrograms/mL and 0.07 micrograms/mL, respectively, were measured. Absorbed fenbendazole is metabolized (and vice-versa) to the active compound, oxfendazole (sulfoxide) and the sulfone. In sheep, cattle, and pigs, 44-50% of a dose of fenbendazole is excreted unchanged in the feces, and <1% in the urine.

Contraindications/Precautions/Warnings

Fenbendazole is not FDA-approved for use in horses intended for food purposes.

Adverse Effects

At usual doses, fenbendazole generally does not cause any adverse effects. Hypersensitivity reactions secondary to antigen release by dying parasites may occur, particularly at high dosages. Salivation, vomiting, and diarrhea may infrequently occur in dogs or cats receiving fenbendazole. Pancytopenia has been reported in one dog (Gary et al. 2004).

Reproductive/Nursing Safety

Fenbendazole is considered safe to use in pregnant bitches and generally considered safe to use in pregnancy for all species. It is the drug of choice for treating giardia in pregnant animals (Tams 2007). In a system evaluating the safety of drugs in canine and feline pregnancy (Papich 1989), this drug is categorized as class: *A (Probably safe. Although specific studies may not have proved the safety of all drugs in dogs and cats, there are no reports of adverse effects in laboratory animals or women.)*

Overdosage/Toxicity

Fenbendazole is apparently well tolerated at doses up to 100X recommended. The LD_{50} in laboratory animals exceeds 10 grams/kg when administered PO. It is unlikely an acute overdosage would lead to clinical signs.

Drug Interactions

- **BROMSALAN FLUKICIDES (dibromsalan, tribromsalan**; not available in the USA): Oxfendazole or fenbendazole should not be given concurrently with the bromsalan flukicides; abortions in cattle and death in sheep have been reported after using these compounds together.

Doses

- **DOGS:**

  Labeled Indications/Dosages:

  For the treatment and control of Roundworms (Toxocara canis, *Toxascaris leonina*), Hookworms (*Ancylostoma caninum, Uncinaria stenocephala*), Whipworms (*Trichuris vulpis*), and Tapeworms (*Taenia pisiformis*); (labeled dose; FDA-approved): 50 mg/kg PO for 3 consecutive days. (Package insert; *Panacur®*)

  Extra-Label Indications/Dosages:
  a) **For the above labeled indications:** Some suggest re-treating in 2 weeks and then 3 months later. One-time dosages of 100 mg/kg PO have been suggested for dogs older than 6 months.
  b) **For a variety of other parasites:** 50 mg/kg PO once daily is generally used but treatment duration may be extended: **Oslerus (Filaroides):** twice daily for 10-14 days, repeat in 3 weeks; **Capillaria:** 10 days, repeat every 3 months; **Giardia, Balantidium, Entamoeba:** 3-10 days; **Crenosoma:** 10-14 days; **Angiostrongylus:** 7 days; **Paragonimus:** 10-14 days.
  c) **To prevent transplacental and transmammary transmission of somatic** *T. canis* **and** *A. caninum*: 50 mg/kg PO once daily from the 40th day of gestation to the 14th day of lactation. (Kazacos 2002)
  d) **For** *Mesocestoides* **spp.:** 100 mg/kg PO twice daily for at least 4 weeks and up to 3 months.

- **CATS, DOMESTIC:**

  Note: All dosages are extra-label in the USA.

  For susceptible ascarids, hookworms, strongyloides, giardia, lungworms (Capillaria and *Aelurostrongylus)* **and tapeworms (***Taenia* **spp. only):** 50 mg/kg PO for 3-5 days. Longer treatments may be required for lungworms (10-14 days). Some recommend giving 25 – 50 mg/kg PO twice daily for 10+ days in cats with *Paragonimus kellicotti, Capillaria feliscati*, or *Eucoleus aerophilus* (formerly *Capillaria aerophilia*) infections.

  In the U.K. there is additional labeling for *Ascarid* spp. *(Toxocara), Ancylostoma* spp., *Trichuris* spp., *Uncinaria* spp. and *Taenia* spp.: Adult cats (>6 mos. old), and pregnant cats: 100 mg PO once. For kittens (<6 mos. old): 50 mg/kg PO once a day for 3 days. For control of *Aelurostrongylus abstrusus*: 50 mg/kg PO once a day for 3 days. (Label information; *Panacur® Small Animal*; U.K.)

  For *Eurytrema procyonis* **(pancreatic fluke):** 30 mg/kg, PO daily for 6 days. (Steiner et al. 2000)

- **CATS, LARGE (EXOTIC):**

  For labeled parasites: 10 mg/kg PO once daily for 3 consecutive days. (Label information; *Panacur® 22.25 Granules*—Intervet)

- **BEARS (URSIDAE):**

  For labeled parasites: 10 mg/kg PO once daily for 3 consecutive days. (Label information; *Panacur® 22.25 Granules*—Intervet)

- **SMALL MAMMALS/RODENTS:**

  a) **Mice, Rats, Gerbils, Hamsters, Guinea pigs, Chinchillas** (extra-label): 20 – 50 mg/kg PO once daily for 5 days. (Higher dose is for Giardia). (Adamcak et al. 2000)
  b) **For Giardia in Chinchillas** (extra-label): 25 mg/kg PO once a day for 3 days. (Hayes 2000)
  c) **Rabbits: For Treatment/prevention of** *E. cuniculi* (extra-label in USA): 20 mg/kg PO once daily for 28 days. Routine dosing of rabbits is recommended 2-4 times yearly. (Label information; *Panacur Rabbit®*; U.K.)
  d) **Rabbits: For routine worming** (extra-label in USA): 20 mg/kg PO once daily for 5 days; repeat every 3 months. (Label information; *Zerofen®*; U.K.)

- **FERRETS:**

  For routine worming (extra-label in USA): 20 mg/kg PO once daily for 5 days; repeat every 3 months. (Label information; *Zerofen®*; U.K.)

- **CATTLE:**

For the removal and control of lungworm (*Dictyocaulus vi-viparus*); stomach worm (adults) brown stomach worm (*Ostertagia ostertagi*); stomach worms (adults and 4th-stage larvae); barberpole worm (*Haemonchus contortus* and *H. placei*) and small stomach worm (*Trichostrongylus axei*); intestinal worms (adults and 4th-stage larvae); hookworm (*Bunostomum phlebotomum*), threadnecked intestinal worm (*Nematodirus helvetianus*), small intestinal worm (*Cooperia punctata* and *C. oncophora*), bankrupt worm (*Trichostrongylus colubriformis*), and nodular worm (*Oesophagostomum radiatum*); (Labeled dose; FDA-approved): 5 mg/kg PO. Retreatment may be needed after 4 to 6 weeks. Cattle must not be slaughtered within 8 days following last treatment. Do not use in dairy cattle of breeding age. (Adapted from label; *Panacur® Suspension 10%*)

For giardiasis in calves (extra-label): 15 mg/kg PO for 3 successive days and then moved to a pen that was thoroughly cleaned and disinfected with 10% ammonia. (Claerebout 2006)

- **HORSES:**

For control of large strongyles (*Strongylus edentatus, S. equinus, S. vulgaris*), small strongyles, pinworms (*Oxyuris equi*), and ascarids (*Parascaris equorum*); (labeled dose; FDA-approved): Adult horses: 5 mg/kg PO; regular deworming at intervals of 6-8 weeks may be required due to the possibility of reinfection. For foals and weanlings (less than 18 months of age) where ascarids are a common problem: 10 mg/kg PO; regular deworming at intervals of 6-8 weeks may be required due to the possibility of reinfection. (Adapted from label information; *Panacur® Paste*)

For treatment of encysted early 3rd stage, late 3rd stage and 4th stage cyathostome larvae and 4th stage *Strongylus vulgaris* larvae: (labeled dose; FDA-approved): 10 mg/kg PO for 5 consecutive days. In the case of 4th stage larvae of *Strongylus vulgaris*, treatment and retreatment should be based on the life cycle and the epidemiology. Treatment should be initiated in the spring and repeated in the fall after a six-month interval. (Adapted from label information; *Panacur® Paste*)

- **SWINE:**

For whipworms in potbellied pigs (extra-label): 9 mg/kg PO for days. (Braun 1995) **Note:** There are medicated feed/premix products labeled for use in swine.

- **SHEEP & GOATS:**

For the removal and control of stomach worms (adults) *Haemonchus contortus* and *Teladorsagia circumcincta* in non-lactating goats (labeled-dose; FDA-approved): 5 mg/kg PO: Retreatment may be needed after 4-6 weeks. Goats must not be slaughtered within 6 days of last treatment. Do not use in lactating goats. (Adapted from label; *Panacur® 10% Suspension*)

- **CAMELIDS:**

For susceptible parasites in new world camelids (extra-label): 10 – 20 mg/kg PO for 3-5 days. (Wolff 2009)

For adjunctive treatment of meningeal worm infestation (*Parelaphostrongylus tenius*); (extra-label): Fenbendazole 50 mg/kg PO for 5 days with ivermectin 0.3 mg/kg SC for 5 days. Also use prophylactic treatment for stress ulcers (*e.g.,* ranitidine, omeprazole), anti-inflammatories (*e.g.,* flunixin, dexamethasone, DMSO), fluids, nutritional support, etc. (Edmondson 2009)

- **BIRDS:**

For routine worming (extra-label in USA): 20 mg/kg PO once daily for 5 days. (Label information; *Zerofen®*; U.K.)

- **REPTILES:**

For routine worming (extra-label in USA): 50 mg/kg PO once every 7 days. (Label information; *Zerofen®*; U.K.)

For nematodes (extra-label): 50 – 100 mg/ PO repeated in 2 weeks. If fecal exam is positive 14 days later, another dose is administered and repeated until cleared. For trematodes (extra-label): 100 mg/kg repeated in 2 weeks. (de la Navarre 2012)

Monitoring
- Efficacy.

Client Information
- Oral wormer used in many species.
- Must be given for several days to be effective. Do not stop early or miss dosages.
- Best given with food in small animals.
- Usually no side effects, but GI effects (*e.g.,* vomiting, drooling, diarrhea, etc.) can occur. Rarely, allergic reactions can occur when many parasites die in the body.

Chemistry/Synonyms
A benzimidazole anthelmintic, fenbendazole occurs as a white, crystalline powder. It is only slightly soluble in water.

Fenbendazole may also be known as: Hoe-881V, *Panacur®* and *Safe-Guard®*.

Storage/Stability
Fenbendazole products should be stored at room temperature.

Compatibility/Compounding Considerations
No specific information noted.

Dosage Forms/Regulatory Status
VETERINARY-LABELED PRODUCTS:

Fenbendazole Granules: 222 mg/gram (22.2%) in 0.18 oz and 1 g, 2 g, 4 g packets and 1 lb. jars; *Panacur C® Granules 22.2%, Safeguard® Canine Dewormer*, (OTC). FDA-approved for use in dogs, horses, large exotic cats (lions, etc.), and bears (black bears, polar bears, etc.)

Fenbendazole Granules: 222 mg/gram (22.2%); *Panacur® C Granules 22.2%*; (OTC). FDA-approved for use in horses not intended for food.

Fenbendazole Suspension: 100 mg/mL (10%); There are products labeled for use horses, cattle, and goats: *Panacur® Suspension*; (Rx). FDA-approved for use in horses (not intended for food) and cattle. Slaughter withdrawal = 8 days (cattle). *Safe-Guard® Suspension*; (OTC). FDA-approved for use in beef and dairy cattle, and goats. Cattle must not be slaughtered within 8-days following treatment. A withdrawal period has not been established for this product in pre-ruminating calves. Do not use in calves to be processed for veal. Goats must not be slaughtered for food within 6-days following treatment. Because a withdrawal time in milk has not been established, do not use in lactating goats. For dairy cattle, there is no milk withdrawal period.

Fenbendazole Paste: 100 mg/gram (10%); available in both equine and bovine labeled products and sizes. *Panacur® Paste; Safe Guard® Paste;* (OTC). FDA-approved for use in horses not intended for food and cattle. Slaughter withdrawal at labeled doses = 8 days; no milk withdrawal time at labeled doses. A link to the label for *Panacur® Paste* may be found at dailymed.nlm.nih.gov

Fenbendazole Pellets: *Safe-Guard® 0.5% Cattle Top Dress* and *Safe-Guard® 1.96% Scoop Dewormer Mini Pellets;* (OTC). FDA-approved for use in beef and dairy cattle. No milk withdrawal time at labeled doses; slaughter withdrawal time at labeled doses = 13 days.

Fenbendazole Premix 20% Type A (200 mg/gram): *Safe-Guard® Pre-*

mix; (OTC). FDA-approved for use in swine, growing turkeys, dairy and beef cattle, zoo and wildlife animals. Slaughter withdrawal for cattle = 13 days; no milk withdrawal time. Slaughter withdrawal for swine at labeled doses = none. Wildlife animal slaughter (hunting) withdrawal = 14 days at labeled doses.

There may also be Type B and C medicated feeds available.

Combination Products: Fenbendazole 454 mg, Ivermectin 27 mcg, & Praziquantel 23 mg (2.16 g small chews) Chewable Tablets; *Panacur Plus® Soft Chews*; (Rx). FDA-approved for use in adult dogs. Fenbendazole 1.134 g, Ivermectin 68 mcg, & Praziquantel 57 mg (5.4 g large chews) Chewable Tablet; *Panacur Plus® Soft Chews*; (Rx). FDA-approved (NADA 141-286) for use in adult dogs. At the time of writing (1/2014) this product is still listed in the FDA "green book", but it may not be marketed.

HUMAN-LABELED PRODUCTS: NONE.

Revisions/References

Monograph revised/updated January 2014.

Adamcak, A. & B. Otten (2000). Rodent Therapeutics. Vet Clin NA: Exotic Anim Pract **3**:1(Jan): 221-40.
Braun, W. (1995). Potbellied pigs: General medical care. *Kirk's Current Veterinary Therapy:XII*. J. Bonagura. Philadelphia, W.B. Saunders: 1388-9.
Claerebout, E. (2006). New therapeutic approaches to Cryptosporidiosis and Giardiasis. Proceedings: ACVIM. accessed via Veterinary Information Network; vin.com
de la Navarre, B. (2012). Identification and Treatment of Parasites in Reptiles and Amphibians. Atlantic Coast Veterinary Conf. accessed via Veterinary Information Network; vin.com
Edmondson, M. (2009). Internal parasites of goats, sheep, and camelids. ABVP. accessed via Veterinary Information Network; vin.com
Gary, A. T., et al. (2004). Bone marrow hypoplasia associated with fenbendazole administration in a dog. J. Am. Anim. Hosp. Assoc. **40**(3): 224-9.
Hayes, P. (2000). Diseases of Chinchillas. *Kirk's Current Veterinary Therapy: XIII Small Animal Practice*. J. Bonagura. Philadelphia, WB Saunders: 1152-7.
Kazacos, K. (2002). Treatment and control of gastrointestinal helminths. Proceedings: Western Veterinary Conference. accessed via Veterinary Information Network; vin.com
McKellar, Q. A., et al. (1993). Oral Absorption and Bioavailability of Fenbendazole in the Dog and the Effect of Concurrent Ingestion of Food. J. Vet. Pharmacol. Ther. **16**(2): 189-98.
Steiner, J. & D. Williams (2000). Feline Exocrine Pancreatic Disease. *Kirk's Current Veterinary Therapy: XIII Small Animal Practice*. J. Bonagura. Philadelphia, WB Saunders: 701-5.
Tams, T. (2007). Acute diarrhea in dogs and cats. Proceedings: ACVC. accessed via Veterinary Information Network; vin.com
Wolff, P. (2009). Camelid Medicine. Proceedings: AAZV. accessed via Veterinary Information Network; vin.com

Fenoldopam

(fe-NOL-doe-pam)   *Corlopam®*

Dopamine Agonist (DA1); Antihypertensive

Prescriber Highlights

▶ Injectable (CRI) dopamine (DA1) agonist that may be useful in treating nonpolyuric, acute kidney injury in dogs, cats, and foals. Little information known about efficacy and safety in animal patients.

▶ No known contraindications; can cause tachycardia and hypokalemia.

▶ Blood pressure, heart rate, urine output, and serum electrolytes should be monitored closely.

▶ Must be administered with an accurate infusion pump; must not be given as IV bolus.

Uses/Indications

Fenoldopam is a selective DA1-receptor agonist and may be useful in the adjunctive treatment of nonpolyuric, acute kidney injury in dogs, cats, and foals. However, little published research and clinical experience has occurred with this drug in animal patients and at present, its use should be considered 'investigational' in clinically ill animals.

In human patients, fenoldopam is labeled for treatment of severe hypertension, but it is also used as a renoprotectant after cardiovascular surgery, to improve gastrointestinal oxygen flow in hypovolemic patients, and because of its selectivity and lower risk for adverse effects, fenoldopam has largely replaced dopamine use for adjunctive treatment of acute kidney injury. No beneficial effect on renal function has been noted in human patients with severe renal disease, heart failure, or hepatic disease.

Pharmacology/Actions

Fenoldopam is a selective agonist at postsynaptic dopamine DA1-receptors. It causes peripheral arterial vasodilation, increased mesenteric and renal blood flow, diuresis, and reduces total peripheral resistance and systemic blood pressure. In humans, it has shown to be renoprotective after cardiovascular surgery. Heart rates can increase secondary to a reflex-response to vasodilation.

Fenoldopam causes dose-related increases in renal plasma flow, decreases in renal vascular resistance and produces diuresis, natriuresis, and kaliuresis without significantly affecting glomerular filtration rate.

Fenoldopam antagonizes alpha-receptors (alpha2>alpha1) at dosages higher than those that activate DA1-receptors. It has no affinity for DA2-receptors, beta-adrenergic receptors, serotonin receptors, or muscarinic receptors.

While clinical studies are lacking for dogs, cats or horses there has been some experimental research performed. In anesthetized, healthy dogs with experimentally-induced hypovolemia, fenoldopam was shown to be renoprotective during hypovolemia and helped to maintain renal blood flow, glomerular filtration rate, and natriuresis without causing hypotension (Halpenny et al. 2001). Fenoldopam demonstrated dose-dependent increased oxygenation of gastric mucosa in dogs, while dopamine did not (Schwarte et al. 2003). Renal function in dogs did not significantly change after renal bisection nephrotomy (15-minute renal artery occlusion) and fenoldopam had no affect on renal function (Zimmerman-Pope et al. 2003).

In an experimental study in young, healthy cats a 2-hour infusion of 0.5 micrograms/kg/minute induced diuresis (delayed effect) and natriuresis. Creatinine clearance significantly increased 6 hours after the infusion was stopped (Simmons et al. 2006).

In normotensive neonatal foals, low-dosage fenoldopam (0.04 micrograms/kg/min) had no significant effects on systemic hemodynamics, creatinine clearance, sodium, chloride or potassium excretion, but did significantly increase urine output. High-dosage fenoldopam (0.4 micrograms/kg/min) increased heart rate, decreased systemic arterial blood pressure and had no significant affects on renal function. The authors concluded that low-dose fenoldopam had potential clinical application for the prophylaxis or treatment of acute renal failure in neonatal foals and that additional study was warranted (Hollis et al. 2006).

Pharmacokinetics

A pharmacokinetic/hemodynamic effect study done in six, healthy beagles given a 3-hour fenoldopam constant rate infusion at 0.8 microgram/kg/min showed highly variable interpatient values of plasma concentrations and clearance, but the drug achieves steady-state plasma levels within 10 minutes of the infusion start and is rapidly eliminated with the drug becoming undetectable within 10 minutes of discontinuation. The authors suspected that in dogs, fenoldopam undergoes complete first-pass hepatic elimination and may undergo additional extra-hepatic clearance including metabolism and/or renal excretion of unchanged drug (Bloom et al. 2012).

In humans, fenoldopam has a rapid onset of action with most antihypertensive effect occurring within 15 minutes. It is about 88% bound to plasma proteins and almost no drug crosses the blood-brain barrier. Elimination half-life is 5-10 minutes but the duration of effect can persist for 48 hours. Fenoldopam is metabolized in the liver to glucuronide, and methyl and sulfate metabolites. The majority of a dose is excreted into urine, primarily as the glucuronide metabolite (inactive). Only 4% is excreted unchanged. Clearance is not appreciably affected by renal function.

Contraindications/Precautions/Warnings

Manufacturer states that there are no known contraindications to the use of fenoldopam. The drug should be used with caution in patients with glaucoma as increased intraocular pressure has been reported.

Adverse Effects

The adverse effect profile for fenoldopam is not well documented in animals. Experimental studies in dogs and cats did not show any overt adverse effects. Foals administered "high-dosage" fenoldopam (0.4 micrograms/kg/min) had significantly high heart rates compared to low-dose fenoldopam or baseline values and 3/6 foals showed signs of 'restlessness' (Hollis et al. 2006).

In humans, fenoldopam has caused tachycardia (dose-related), headache, flushing, nausea, vomiting, hypotension and hypokalemia.

Reproductive/Nursing Safety

In humans, the FDA categorizes this drug as category *B* for use during pregnancy (*Animal studies have not yet demonstrated risk to the fetus, but there are no adequate studies in pregnant women; or animal studies have shown an adverse effect, but adequate studies in pregnant women have not demonstrated a risk to the fetus in the first trimester of pregnancy, and there is no evidence of risk in later trimesters.*)

It is not known if fenoldopam is excreted in milk.

Overdosage/Acute Toxicity

Overdosages of fenoldopam would likely increase the incidence and severity of adverse effects, including tachycardia. Diligent monitoring heart rate, blood pressure and electrolytes are mandatory. The drug must not be given as an IV bolus.

Drug Interactions

The following drug interactions have either been reported or are theoretical in humans or animals receiving fenoldopam and may be of significance in veterinary patients. Unless otherwise noted, use together is not necessarily contraindicated, but weigh the potential risks and perform additional monitoring when appropriate.

- **BETA-ADRENERGIC BLOCKERS** (e.g., **propranolol**, etc.): Can inhibit sympathetic reflex response to fenoldopam; concomitant use is not recommended.

- **HYPOTENSIVE DRUGS (OTHER):** Fenoldopam's hypotensive effects may be enhanced.

Laboratory Considerations

No concerns noted.

Dosages

Note: Fenoldopam is administered as a constant rate intravenous infusion (CRI) only. An online drip rate table generator can be found at: http://www.globalrph.com/drip.htm

- **DOGS:**

  For adjunctive treatment of acute, nonpolyuric kidney injury (extra-label): The clinical use of fenoldopam in veterinary medicine is still in the 'investigational' stage and its role (if any) in the treatment of acute kidney injury is yet to be determined (Ross 2011). Based upon a pharmacokinetic study in healthy Beagles a constant rate IV infusion of 0.8 micrograms/kg/min has been suggested (Balakrishnan et al. 2013). Duration of infusion for clinical use in dogs is not fully described, but for severe hyper-

tension in human patients the drug is labeled that infusions should continue for no longer than 4 hours in pediatric patients and for 48 hours in adults. Fenoldopam should be administered as an intravenous constant rate infusion using a calibrated, mechanical infusion pump. Fenoldopam infusions—in humans and likely in animal patients—can be discontinued abruptly or slowly withdrawn.

- **CATS:**

  For adjunctive treatment of acute kidney injury (oliguric, anuric); (extra-label): The clinical use of fenoldopam in veterinary medicine is still in the 'investigational' stage and its role (if any) in the treatment of acute kidney injury is yet to be determined. A dosage range of 0.1 – 1 micrograms/kg/min as a constant rate infusion for two hours has been recommended (Simmons et al. 2006; Monaghan et al. 2012). Fenoldopam should be administered as a constant rate infusion intravenously using a calibrated, mechanical infusion pump. Fenoldopam infusions—in humans and likely in animal patients—can be discontinued abruptly or slowly withdrawn.

Monitoring

- Blood pressure, heart rate, urine output.

- Serum electrolytes, especially potassium. Infusions of fenoldopam have caused hypokalemia in human patients with infusions lasting less than 6 hours; every 6-hours monitoring of serum electrolytes is recommended while this drug is being used (in human patients).

Client Information

Fenoldopam should only be used in an inpatient setting.

Chemistry/Synonyms

Fenoldopam mesylate (CAS Registry: 67227-56-9 fenoldopam, 67227-57-0 fenoldopam mesylate; ATC: C01CA190) occurs as a white to off-white powder and is soluble in water. Dosages are expressed as fenoldopam. The injectable solution contains propylene glycol and sodium metabisulfite. Unlike nitroprusside, fenoldopam is not degraded by light nor does it cause thiocyanate toxicity.

Fenoldopam mesylate may also be known as fenoldopam mesilate or SKF-82526-j. A trade name for it is *Corlopam®*.

Storage/Stability

Ampules or vials should be stored between 2-30°C (37-86°F). Ampules and vials of fenoldopam injection concentrate are for single use only; discard unused portion.

Diluted solutions are stable under normal ambient light and temperature conditions for at least 24 hours but should be discarded after 24 hours.

Compatibility/Compounding Considerations

Drugs (partial listing) that have been reported as **incompatible** with fenoldopam infusions at Y-sites, include: ampicillin sodium, bumetanide, dexamethasone sodium phosphate, diazepam, fosphenytoin, furosemide, methylprednisolone sodium succinate, and sodium bicarbonate (Trissel 2013).

Drugs (partial listing) that have been reported to be **compatible** with fenoldopam infusions at Y-sites, include: alfentanil, amikacin, atracurium, atropine, butorphanol, calcium gluconate, dexmedetomidine, diltiazem, diphenhydramine, dolasetron, epinephrine, fentanyl, heparin, hydrocortisone sodium succinate, hydromorphone, mannitol, naloxone, ondansetron, potassium chloride, and propofol (Trissel 2013).

Before administration, the 10 mg/mL injectable concentrate should be diluted in 0.9% sodium chloride injection (NS) or 5% dextrose (D5W) injection. The following directions are for diluting to 60 micrograms/mL, which is the usual dilution guideline for human pediatric patients and is recommended for small animal patients to reduce the risk for volume overload: To obtain a final concentration of 60 mcg/mL: add 30 mg of fenoldopam (3 ml of concentrate) to 500 mL NS or D5W; or add 15 mg of fenoldopam (1.5 mL of concentrate) to 250 mL NS or D5W. The diluted solution is stable under normal ambient light and temperature for at least 24 hours. Diluted solution not used within 24 hours should be discarded. Fenoldopam should be administered as a constant rate infusion intravenously using a calibrated, mechanical infusion pump.

Dosage Forms/Regulatory Status

VETERINARY-LABELED PRODUCTS: NONE.

HUMAN-LABELED PRODUCTS:

Injection, IV (for dilution): 10 mg/mL in 1 & 2 mL ampules or vials; *Corlopam®*, generic; (Rx)

Revisions/References

Monograph written August 2013.

Balakrishnan, A. & K. J. Drobatz (2013). Management of Urinary Tract Emergencies in Small Animals. Veterinary Clinics of North America: Small Animal Practice 43(4): 843-67.

Bloom, C. A., et al. (2012). Preliminary pharmacokinetics and cardiovascular effects of fenoldopam continuous rate infusion in six healthy dogs. J. Vet. Pharmacol. Ther. 35(3): 224-30.

Halpenny, M., et al. (2001). Effects of prophylactic fenoldopam infusion on renal blood flow and venal tubular function during acute hypovolemia in anesthetized dogs. Critical Care Medicine 29(4): 855-60.

Hollis, A. R., et al. (2006). Effects of fenoldopam mesylate on systemic hemodynamics and indices of renal function in normotensive neonatal foals. Journal of Veterinary Internal Medicine 20(3): 595-600.

Monaghan, K., et al. (2012). Feline Acute Kidney Injury: Approach to diagnosis, treatment and prognosis. Journal of Feline Medicine and Surgery 14(11): 785-93.

Ross, L. (2011). Acute Kidney Injury in Dogs and Cats. Veterinary Clinics of North America-Small Animal Practice 41(1): 1-+.

Schwarte, L. A., et al. (2003). Fenoldopam - but not dopamine - selectively increases gastric mucosal oxygenation in dogs. Critical Care Medicine 31(7): 1999-2005.

Simmons, J. P., et al. (2006). Diuretic effects of fenoldopam in healthy cats. J. Vet. Emerg. Crit. Care 16(2): 96-103.

Trissel, L. 2013. Handbook on Injectable Drugs - 17th Edition. Accessed via STAT!Ref; Teton Data Systems

Zimmerman-Pope, N., et al. (2003). Effect of fenoldopam on renal function after nephrotomy in normal dogs. Veterinary Surgery 32(6): 566-73.

Fentanyl Citrate, Injection

(fen-ta-nil)   Sublimaze®

Opioid

Prescriber Highlights

▶ Class-II opiate analgesic used parenterally in small animals; potentially useful as a CRI in horses.

▶ Contraindications: Use extreme caution when additional respiratory, or CNS depression would be deleterious.

▶ Use caution in geriatric, very ill or debilitated patients & those with a preexisting respiratory problem.

▶ Adverse Effects: Dose related respiratory, CNS & circulatory depression (bradycardia); also urine retention, constipation, dysphoria, or agitation. Dogs may become dysphoric when used as a post-op CRI.

▶ Lab values (amylase, lipase) may be altered.

▶ *See also the Fentanyl, Transdermal Patch and Fentanyl, Transdermal Solution monographs.*

Uses/Indications

In veterinary medicine, fentanyl injection is used primarily in dogs and cats and has been shown to be useful for the adjunctive control of postoperative pain and in the control of severe pain associated with chronic pain, dull pain, and non-specific, widespread pain (*e.g.*, associated with cancer, pancreatitis, aortic thromboemboli, peritonitis, etc.). Perioperative injectable fentanyl may also reduce the requirements for inhalational anesthetics during surgery, which could be particularly advantageous in patients with compromised cardiac function. Because of its short duration of action, fentanyl CRI's are particularly useful in critically ill or post-surgical patients as it can be adjusted to meet the analgesia needs of the patient, minimize adverse effects and temporarily halted to assess neurologic status. Injectable fentanyl may be particularly useful in cats for perioperative pain control, especially when higher analgesic doses are required, as it appears to have fewer adverse effects than either hydromorphone or morphine.

In horses, fentanyl CRI's may be useful as part of a partial intravenous anesthesia (PIVA) protocol.

Pharmacology/Actions

Fentanyl is a *mu* opiate agonist that is very short acting and approximately 80-100X more potent than morphine. *Mu* receptors are found primarily in the pain regulating areas of the brain. They are thought to contribute to the analgesia, euphoria, respiratory depression, physical dependence, miosis, and hypothermic actions of opiates. Receptors for opiate analgesics are found in high concentrations in the limbic system, spinal cord, thalamus, hypothalamus, striatum, and midbrain. They are also found in tissues such as the gastrointestinal tract, urinary tract, and other smooth muscle.

The pharmacology of the opiate agonists is discussed in more detail in the monograph Narcotic (opiate) Agonist Analgesics.

Pharmacokinetics

When used via a single dose IV injection, fentanyl has a relatively short duration of effect in most species studied.

When administered to dogs as 10 micrograms/kg IV bolus, fentanyl rapidly distributes and exhibits a large volume of distribution (5 L/kg). The terminal elimination half-life is about 45 minutes; total clearance is 78 mL/min/kg. After a 10 micrograms/kg bolus, dogs administered a constant rate intravenous infusion of 10 micrograms/kg/hour were able to maintain blood levels around 1 ng/mL (the assumed, but not verified therapeutic analgesic level) (Sano et al. 2006).

Half-life after IV administration in cats is approximately 2.5 hours and in horses about 49 minutes

Contraindications/Precautions/Warnings

Fentanyl is contraindicated in patients with known hypersensitivity to it or any component within the product.

Because of its potency, fentanyl injection should be used only by professionals familiar with its use and in circumstances where patients can be adequately monitored and supported.

Use cautiously and with adequate monitoring when using with other CNS, respiratory or cardio- depressant agents.

Because opioids may cause mydriasis in cats, approach slowly so as not to startle, and keep animal out of very bright light or sunlight while pupils are dilated.

Adverse Effects

Dose-related respiratory, CNS and circulatory depression (bradycardia) are the primary adverse effects with fentanyl injection. Hypothermia is possible in dogs. When fentanyl is used intraoperatively, anticholinergic agents may be required to treat bradycardia. Dogs and cats appear less prone than humans but are not immune to opiate-induced respiratory depression. In a study done in normal dogs, concurrent administration of fentanyl and isoflurane resulted in significant decreases in mean arterial blood pressure, heart rate, and cardiac index and a significant increase in P_aCO_2. All except P_aCO_2 retuned to pre-treatment levels with time (Keating et al. 2013). Dysphoria has been reported in approximately 25% of dogs treated with fentanyl (IV CRI) post-operatively (Becker et al. 2013).

In horses, fentanyl, like morphine, can initially stimulate then inhibit cecocolic activity.

Reproductive/Nursing Safety

Safe use in pregnancy has not been established. In humans, the FDA categorizes fentanyl as category *C* for use during pregnancy

(*Animal studies have shown an adverse effect on the fetus, but there are no adequate studies in humans; or there are no animal reproduction studies and no adequate studies in humans.*) In a separate system evaluating the safety of drugs in canine and feline pregnancy (Papich 1989), this drug is categorized as class: *B* (*Safe for use if used cautiously. Studies in laboratory animals may have uncovered some risk, but these drugs appear to be safe in dogs and cats or these drugs are safe if they are not administered when the animal is near term.*)

Most narcotic agonist analgesics are excreted into milk, but effects on nursing offspring may not be significant.

Overdosage/Acute Toxicity

Overdosage may produce profound respiratory and/or CNS depression in most species. Newborns may be more susceptible to these effects than adult animals. Other toxic effects may include cardiovascular collapse, tremors, neck rigidity, and seizures. There were 679 single agent exposures to fentanyl reported to the ASPCA Animal Poison Control Center (APCC) during 2009-2013. Of the 652 dogs, 548 were symptomatic. The most common clinical signs included: lethargy/sedation (60%), hypersalivation (37%), hypothermia (24%), ataxia (24%), and bradycardia (20%). Of the 27 cats, 19 were symptomatic with 42% being mydriatic, 26% lethargic, and 11% agitated.

Naloxone is the agent of choice in treating respiratory depression. In massive overdoses, naloxone doses may need to be repeated; animals should be closely observed as naloxone's effects sometimes diminish before sub-toxic levels of fentanyl are attained. Mechanical respiratory support should also be considered in cases of severe respiratory depression.

Drug Interactions

The following drug interactions have either been reported or are theoretical in humans or animals receiving fentanyl and may be of significance in veterinary patients. Unless otherwise noted, use together is not necessarily contraindicated, but weigh the potential risks and perform additional monitoring when appropriate.

- **AZOLE ANTIFUNGALS** (*e.g.,* **ketoconazole, itraconazole, fluconazole**): May inhibit fentanyl metabolism. A study in dogs however, showed that ketoconazole did not significantly alter the elimination of fentanyl (KuKanich et al. 2010).
- **CNS DEPRESSANTS, OTHER**: Additive CNS effects possible.
- **DEXMEDETOMIDINE**: When used post-operatively in dogs <u>after</u> fentanyl/isoflurane general anesthesia, the study findings suggest that postanesthetic treatment with dexmedetomidine causes significantly greater cardiovascular and respiratory compromise than treatment with fentanyl alone or with fentanyl/acepromazine (Holahan et al. 2010; Keating et al. 2013).
- **DIURETICS**: Opiates may decrease efficacy in CHF patients.
- **MACROLIDE ANTIBIOTICS** (*e.g.,* **erythromycin, clarithromycin**): May inhibit fentanyl metabolism.
- **ISOFLURANE (and other inhalant anesthetics)**: Perioperative fentanyl can reduce the anesthetic-requirements for isoflurane, but can also enhance respiratory- and cardio- depressant effects; adequate monitoring required when used together.
- **MONOAMINE OXIDASE INHIBITORS** (*e.g.,* **amitraz,** and possibly **selegiline**): Severe and unpredictable opiate potentiation may be seen; not recommended (in humans) if MAO inhibitor has been used within 14 days.
- **MUSCLE RELAXANTS, SKELETAL**: Fentanyl may enhance neuromuscular blockade.
- **NITROUS OXIDE**: High fentanyl doses may cause cardiovascular depression.
- **PHENOBARBITAL, PHENYTOIN**: May increase the metabolism of fentanyl.
- **RIFAMPIN**: May increase the metabolism of fentanyl.
- **TRICYCLIC ANTIDEPRESSANTS** (*e.g.,* **clomipramine, amitriptyline,** etc.): Fentanyl may exacerbate the effects of tricyclic antidepressants.
- **WARFARIN**: Opiates may potentiate anticoagulant activity.

Laboratory Considerations

- As they may increase biliary tract pressure, opiates can increase plasma amylase and lipase values up to 24 hours following their administration.

Doses

WARNING: Do not confuse dosages reported as micrograms/kg versus mg/kg; CRI dosages may be reported as mg/kg/hour, micrograms/kg/<u>hour</u>, or micrograms/kg/<u>minute</u>. Always double-check dosages and resulting volumes when using injectable fentanyl. Adequate patient monitoring is essential. Have naloxone readily available. If using as a CRI an online drip rate table generator can be found at: http://www.globalrph.com/drip.htm

- **DOGS/CATS:**

For perioperative pain (extra-label): The combination of a 10 microgram/kg loading dose IV followed by a CRI of 10 micrograms/kg/hour investigated in this study might be a guideline for a CRI dose of fentanyl during general anesthesia to provide analgesia in dogs (Sano et al. 2006). Others have recommended loading doses ranging from 2 – 10 micrograms/kg IV, followed by a CRI at 2 – 10 micrograms/kg/hour for pain management in dogs; cat dosages are generally recommended at the low ends of these dosage ranges. If bolus IV, IM or SC doses (usually 5 – 8 micrograms/kg) are administered without a follow-up CRI, duration of action is very short and re-dosing may need to be repeated at 1-2 hour intervals.

For severe to excruciating pain in the emergent patient (extra-label): Fentanyl at 10 – 50 micrograms/kg, administered IV titrated to effect; use the effective dose as an hourly CRI. NSAIDs when not contraindicated. Ketamine at 4 mg/kg as a bolus can be used with fentanyl. Lidocaine at 2 – 4 mg/kg bolus, followed by 2 – 4mg/kg/hour CRI; caution with respect to overdosing if local anesthetics have been administered by means of a different route. Tachycardia may persist and it may be impossible to control the pain. Consider combining these analgesics with epidurally placed analgesics or local blocks, or anesthetize the patient while attempting to find or treat the inciting cause. Remove the inciting cause immediately. This degree of pain can cause death. (Dyson 2008)

As an epidural for pain control (extra-label) 0.004 mg/kg (4 micrograms/kg), diluted with 0.2 mL with preservative-free saline or local anesthetic. Has predominantly supraspinal effects, onset in less than 10 minutes and duration of ½ hour. (Valverde 2008)

As an anesthetic (extra-label): Dosages are generally higher than those used for analgesia but like all anesthetic agents, vary depending on the patient, patient response and other co-administered drugs/anesthetics. As a sole agent, dosages have been noted of 20 – 40 micrograms/kg as an IV bolus (or SC, IM); lower if using with other cardio- or respiratory depressant agents. To reduce MAC and provide intraoperative pain control this may then be administered as a CRI. CRI dosage recommendations vary considerably, but usually are in the 5 – 20 micrograms/kg/hour (up to 40 mcg/kg/hour in dogs) range.

- **FERRETS:**

  As a perioperative analgesic/anesthetic adjunct (extra-label): Pre-op dose: 5 – 10 micrograms/kg IV; Intra-operatively: CRI at 10 – 20 micrograms/kg/hour with a ketamine CRI (0.3 – 0.4 mg/kg/hour); Post-operatively: 2 – 5 micrograms/kg/hour with a ketamine CRI. (Lichtenberger 2006)

- **RABBITS/RODENTS/SMALL MAMMALS:**

  For perioperative pain (extra-label): 5 – 20 micrograms/kg IV bolus; 30-60 minute duration; causes sedation and respiratory depression. (Ivey et al. 2000)

- **HORSES:**

  As part of a partial intravenous anesthesia (PIVA) protocol (extra-label): Effects of a CRI of fentanyl have not been determined in horses. If plasma concentrations of at least 1 ng/mL are in fact analgesic in horses, the pharmacokinetic data generated by one study would indicate that a loading dose of 0.7 mg/kg IV followed by a CRI of 0.36 mg/kg/hour would be necessary. If using another pharmacokinetic study's data, then a loading dose of 0.8 mg/kg and a CRI of 0.96 mg/kg/hour would be necessary. (Valverde 2013)

Monitoring

- Analgesic efficacy.
- Heart rate and respiratory rate.

Client Information

- Fentanyl injection should be used only by professionals familiar with its use and in a setting where adequate monitoring can occur.

Chemistry/Synonyms

Fentanyl citrate, a very potent opiate agonist, occurs as a white, crystalline powder. It is sparingly soluble in water and soluble in alcohol. It is odorless and tasteless (not recommended for taste test because of extreme potency) with a pK_a of 8.3 and a melting point between 147-152°C.

Fentanyl and fentanyl citrate may also be known as: fentanylum, fentanyli citras, McN-JR-4263-49, phentanyl citrate, R-4263, or *Sublimaze®*.

Storage/Stability

Fentanyl injection should be stored protected from light. It is hydrolyzed in an acidic solution.

Compatibility/Compounding Considerations

The injection is **compatible** with normal saline and D5W. Fentanyl citrate injection is reported **compatible** with clonidine, bupivacaine, ropivacaine, and ketamine.

Dosage Forms/Regulatory Status

VETERINARY-LABELED PRODUCTS: NONE.

The ARCI (Racing Commissioners International) has designated this drug as a class 1 substance. See the appendix for more information.

HUMAN-LABELED PRODUCTS:

Fentanyl Injectable: 0.05 mg/mL (50 micrograms/mL) in 2 mL, 5 mL, 10 mL, & 20 mL amps; 30 mL and 50 mL vials; preservative free in 2 mL, 5 mL, 10 mL, & 20 mL amps; *Sublimaze®*, generic; (Rx, C-II)

All fentanyl products are Class-II controlled substances.

Revisions/References

Monograph revised/updated January 2014.

Becker, W. M., et al. (2013). Prevalence of Dysphoria after Fentanyl in Dogs Undergoing Stifle Surgery. Veterinary Surgery 42(3): 302-7.
Dyson, D. (2008). Analgesia and Chemical Restraint for the Emergent Veterinary Patient. Vet Clin Small Anim 38: 1329-52.
Holahan, M. L., et al. (2010). Presumptive hepatotoxicity and rhabdomyolysis secondary to phenazopyridine toxicity in a dog. J. Vet. Emerg. Crit. Care 20(3): 352-8.
Ivey, E. & J. Morrisey (2000). Therapeutics for Rabbits. Vet Clin NA: Exotic Anim Pract 3:1(Jan): 183-216.
Keating, S. C. J., et al. (2013). Cardiopulmonary effects of intravenous fentanyl infusion in dogs during isoflurane anesthesia and with concurrent acepromazine or dexmedetomidine administration during anesthetic recovery. American Journal of Veterinary Research 74(5): 672-82.
KuKanich, B. & M. Hubin (2010). The pharmacokinetics of ketoconazole and its effects on the pharmacokinetics of midazolam and fentanyl in dogs. J. Vet. Pharmacol. Ther. 33(1): 42-9.
Lichtenberger, M. (2006). Clinical monitoring of the critically ill ferret. Proceedings: IVECCS. accessed via Veterinary Information Network; vin.com
Sano, T., et al. (2006). Pharmacokinetics of fentanyl after single intravenous injection and constant rate infusions in dogs. Vet Anaesth Analg 33: 266-73.
Valverde, A. (2008). Epidural analgesia and anesthesia in dogs and cats. Vet Clin NA: Sm Anim Pract 38: 1205-30.
Valverde, A. (2013). Balanced Anesthesia and Constant-Rate Infusions in Horses. Veterinary Clinics of North America-Equine Practice 29(1): 89-+.

Fentanyl, Transdermal Patch

(fen-ta-nil)   Duragesic®

Opioid

Prescriber Highlights

▶ Human Class-II opiate analgesic used in an extra-label manner transdermally in small animals. A transdermal solution product (*Recuvyra®*) is approved for use in dogs; see Fentanyl, Transdermal Solution monograph for more information.

▶ Contraindications: Use extreme caution when additional respiratory or CNS depression would be deleterious. Use caution in geriatric, very ill or debilitated patients & those with a preexisting respiratory problem.

▶ Adverse Effects: Dose related respiratory, CNS & circulatory depression (bradycardia); also, rashes at the patch site, urine retention, constipation, dysphoria, or agitation.

▶ Lag time before effective analgesia; dispose of properly.

▶ *See also the Fentanyl Citrate, Injection and Fentanyl, Transdermal Solution monographs.*

Uses/Indications

In veterinary medicine, transdermal patches are used primarily in dogs and cats and have been shown to be useful for the adjunctive control of postoperative pain, severe pain associated with chronic pain, dull pain, and non-specific, widespread pain (*e.g.*, associated with cancer, pancreatitis, aortic thromboemboli, peritonitis, etc.).

Overall, transdermal fentanyl is thought clinically effective and not demonstrated substantial adverse effects. A non-controlled study in 10 dogs following spinal surgery that measured plasma fentanyl concentrations of fentanyl after transdermal patch (mean patch concentration 4.1 ± 0.8 mcg/kg/hour) concluded that fentanyl patches could represent a valid aid in pain therapy in small animals and contribute to the postoperative well-being of patients undergoing major surgery (Bellei et al. 2011). However, one study in dogs comparing transdermal (patch) fentanyl versus IM morphine for pain control during the first 24 hours post-orthopedic surgery did not show any significant pain control benefit from the patch and was considerably more expensive then IM morphine (Egger et al. 2007).

In humans, significant respiratory depression with use of the patches after surgery has precluded post-operative use, but this has not been a significant problem in veterinary medicine.

Pharmacology/Actions

Fentanyl is a *mu* opiate agonist that is very short acting and approximately 100X more potent than morphine. *Mu* receptors are found primarily in the pain regulating areas of the brain. They are thought to contribute to the analgesia, euphoria, respiratory depression, physical dependence, miosis, and hypothermic actions of opiates. Receptors for opiate analgesics are found in high concentrations in the limbic system, spinal cord, thalamus, hypothalamus, striatum, and midbrain. They are also found in tissues such as the gastrointestinal tract, urinary tract, and other smooth muscles.

The pharmacology of the opiate agonists is discussed in more detail in the monograph Narcotic (opiate) Agonist Analgesics.

Pharmacokinetics

There have been limited pharmacokinetic studies performed with transdermal fentanyl patches in dogs, cats, horses, and sheep. While therapeutic levels of fentanyl are usually attained, there is a significant interpatient variability with both the time to achieve therapeutic levels and the levels themselves. Some animals may not achieve serum levels thought to be therapeutic (0.6-1 ng/mL). In an *in vitro* study of canine skin, fentanyl penetrated skin from the groin region of dogs more rapidly and with a shorter lag time, compared to skin from the neck and thorax (Mills et al. 2004). Cats tend to achieve therapeutic levels faster than dogs. In dogs, the patch should be applied 24 hours in advance of need if possible; minimum of 12 hours pre-need. Most cats attain therapeutic benefit in about 6 hours after application. While applied, duration of action persists for at least 72 hours (usually for at least 104 hours). Duration of action is generally longer in cats than in dogs. For continued use, patches may need to be changed every 48 hours in dogs or horses.

In horses, fentanyl from patches is rapidly absorbed with therapeutic levels (thought to be 0.6-1 ng/mL) achieved in about 6 hours after application and persists for 48+ hours. However, in about one-third of the horses in the study, plasma levels never reached ≥ 1 ng/mL (Orsini et al. 2006).

In sheep, patches applied at a mean dose of 2.05 mcg/kg/hour had an average Tmax of 12 hours (range 4-24 hours) and a Cmax of 1.3 ng/mL (range of 0.62-2.73 ng/mL); concentrations remained above 0.5 ng/mL for 40 hours after application (Ahern et al. 2010).

Contraindications/Precautions/Warnings

Fentanyl is contraindicated in patients with known hypersensitivity to it or any component of the product (including the adhesive for the patch).

When transdermal patches are used, absorption and efficacy can be highly patient variable; injectable rescue analgesia should be available.

Use cautiously with other CNS depressants. Dosages of other opiates may need to be reduced when given with fentanyl transdermal, particularly several hours after application of the patch. Transdermal fentanyl should be used cautiously in geriatric, very ill or debilitated patients and those with a preexisting respiratory problem. Febrile patients may have increased absorption of fentanyl and will require increased monitoring.

Because opioids may cause mydriasis in cats, approach slowly so as not to startle, and keep animal out of very bright light or sunlight while pupils are dilated.

In the past, fentanyl patches were only available in a gel-matrix form that could not be cut. Brands are now available that potentially can be cut, but with the availability of 12 mg patches there is little therapeutic reason to do so. It is advised to obtain a pharmacist's advice before cutting patches. Do not allow applied fentanyl patch to be exposed to exogenous heat sources (heating pads, etc.). Increased drug release and absorption have occurred with fatal results.

Used fentanyl patches must be disposed of safely as they can contain significant amounts of residual drug and can pose a risk for intoxication of exposed humans, especially children (Reed et al. 2011). Human abusers of opiates have also used them and the FDA recommends that used patches be flushed down the toilet.

Adverse Effects

Respiratory depression and bradycardia associated with fentanyl patches are the most concerning adverse effects, but incidence of these effects have not been widespread thus far when used alone (without other opiates or other respiratory and cardiodepressant medications). Rashes at the patch site have been reported and should they occur, the patch should be removed; if an additional patch is warranted, a different site should be chosen. Urine retention and constipation may occur. Consider removing patch in patients developing a fever after application as fentanyl absorption may increase. Some patients exhibit dysphoria or agitation after application; acepromazine or other mild tranquilizers may alleviate dysphoria.

Reproductive/Nursing Safety

Safe use in pregnancy has not been established. In humans, the FDA categorizes fentanyl as category *C* for use during pregnancy (*Animal studies have shown an adverse effect on the fetus, but there are no adequate studies in humans; or there are no animal reproduction studies and no adequate studies in humans.*) In a separate system evaluating the safety of drugs in canine and feline pregnancy (Papich 1989), this drug is categorized as class: *B* (*Safe for use if used cautiously. Studies in laboratory animals may have uncovered some risk, but these drugs appear to be safe in dogs and cats or these drugs are safe if they are not administered when the animal is near term.*)

Most narcotic agonist analgesics are excreted into milk, but effects on nursing offspring may not be significant.

Overdosage/Acute Toxicity

Overdosage may produce profound respiratory and/or CNS depression in most species. Newborns may be more susceptible to these effects than adult animals. Other toxic effects may include cardiovascular collapse, tremors, neck rigidity, and seizures. There were 374 exposures to fentanyl reported to the ASPCA Animal Poison Control Center (APCC) during 2008-2009. In these cases, 362 were dogs with 295 showing clinical signs, and 12 were cats with 5 showing clinical signs. Common findings in dogs (recorded in decreasing frequency) include lethargy, hypersalivation, ataxia, bradycardia, hypothermia, depression, and diarrhea.

Naloxone is the agent of choice in treating respiratory depression. In massive overdoses, naloxone doses may need to be repeated; animals should be closely observed as naloxone's effects sometimes diminish before sub-toxic levels of fentanyl are attained. Mechanical respiratory support should also be considered in cases of severe respiratory depression.

Drug Interactions

The following drug interactions have either been reported or are theoretical in humans or animals receiving fentanyl and may be of significance in veterinary patients. Unless otherwise noted, use together is not necessarily contraindicated, but weigh the potential risks and perform additional monitoring when appropriate.

- **AZOLE ANTIFUNGALS** (*e.g.*, **ketoconazole, itraconazole, fluconazole**): May inhibit fentanyl metabolism. A study in dogs however, showed that ketoconazole did not significantly alter the elimination of fentanyl (KuKanich et al. 2010).
- **CNS DEPRESSANTS, OTHER**: Additive CNS effects possible.
- **DIURETICS**: Opiates may decrease efficacy in CHF patients.
- **MACROLIDE ANTIBIOTICS** (*e.g.*, **erythromycin, clarithromycin**): May inhibit fentanyl metabolism.
- **MONOAMINE OXIDASE INHIBITORS** (*e.g.*, **amitraz**, and possibly **selegiline**): Severe and unpredictable opiate potentiation may be seen; not recommended (in humans) if MAO inhibitor has been used within 14 days.
- **MUSCLE RELAXANTS, SKELETAL**: Fentanyl may enhance

neuromuscular blockade.

- **NITROUS OXIDE:** High fentanyl doses may cause cardiovascular depression.
- **PHENOBARBITAL, PHENYTOIN:** May increase the metabolism of fentanyl.
- **RIFAMPIN:** May increase the metabolism of fentanyl.
- **TRICYCLIC ANTIDEPRESSANTS** (*e.g.,* **clomipramine, amitriptyline,** etc.): Fentanyl may exacerbate the effects of tricyclic antidepressants.
- **WARFARIN:** Opiates may potentiate anticoagulant activity.

Laboratory Considerations

- As they may increase biliary tract pressure, opiates can increase plasma amylase and lipase values up to 24 hours following their administration.

Doses

WARNING: Do not confuse doses listed as micrograms/kg/hour or mg/kg/hour in this, and other references. Always double-check dosages when using fentanyl. Human-labeled fentanyl patches are used in an extra-label manner in all species.

Fentanyl Transdermal Patch for post-operative pain control or palliative short-term control of cancer pain (extra-label in all species):

- Choose your patient carefully, realizing that the fentanyl patch alone may not provide sufficient analgesia. Fentanyl patches are effective for relief of chronic pain, dull pain and non-specific, widespread pain (peritonitis, pancreatitis, cancer, aortic thromboemboli, declaws, etc.) In the face of acute surgical pain or severe traumatic pain (fractures, thoracotomies, HBC/traumatic injuries/head trauma), analgesia provided by a fentanyl patch tends to be inadequate. Therefore, the patch should be used as an adjunctive measure for pain relief in these patients. If the patient is febrile, do not use fentanyl patch.
- There is significant interspecies and interpatient variability on the response of the transdermal product. When used as the primary analgesic for post-operative pain, application prior to surgery is advised as many hours may be required for "therapeutic" levels to be achieved. Generally in dogs = 12-24 hours may be necessary; cats = 6-24 hours; and horses = 6+ hours. When used for short-term cancer pain control, patches generally are replaced every 4-5 days in dogs or cats.
- To transition to a fentanyl patch in cats: Adjust CRI infusion rate to reach optimal effect before patch is applied; after patch applied, the infusion is then tapered and discontinued over the next 8-24 hours while observing patient response. If the patient does well on the infusion, but poorly on the patch, then failure of the patch is suspected. In cats, fentanyl delivery from the patch is highly variable. A 25 microgram patch provides approximately 10 micrograms/hour. 12 mg patches are available for very small cats. (Hansen 2008)

Dosage range recommendations vary somewhat and range from 1 – 5 micrograms/kg/hour; higher dosage rates may induce sedation and dysphoria. The following table can be used as a general guide:

Patient	Dose (Patch Size)
Small Dogs (<5kg) and Cats	12 mcg/hr (some recommend that a 25 mcg/kg/hr patch can be used in larger cats)
Dogs: 5–10 kg	25 mcg/hr
Dogs: 10–20 kg	50 mcg/hr
Dogs: 20–30 kg	75 mcg/hr
Dogs: >30 kg	100 mcg/hr
Horses: 350–500 kg	2 x 100 mcg/hr
Pigs: 17–25 kg	50 – 100 mcg/hr
Sheep	50 – 100 mcg/hr
Goats	50 mcg/hr
Rabbits	12 – 25 mcg/hr

Choose your location:

- **Dog:** Thorax, inguinal area, metatarsal/carpal areas, base of tail (dorsal or lateral cervical area has been used, but leashes must not be placed around the neck if fentanyl patches are in place)
- **Cat:** Lateral thorax, inguinal area, metatarsal/carpal areas; base of tail (the cervical area is NOT recommended, as the patch tends not to remain on)
- **Horse:** Neck, antebrachium (foals)
- **Pig; Rabbit:** Lateral thorax
- **Sheep, Goat:** Abdomen, cervical area

Note: Direct patch contact with heating pads can significantly increase fentanyl absorption and risk toxicity. The patch should be kept dry; be aware of potential surgical clip sites.

1) Clip close, but don't shave the site. DO NOT use depilatory agents in preparation of the site. Clip at least a 1 cm margin around the patch.

2) Wipe the site with a damp cloth and allow the skin to dry. This step is absolutely necessary, or patch will not stick to the skin. DO NOT wipe the area with alcohol or surgical scrub solution. Alcohol and surgical scrubs may "de-fat" the skin and alter drug absorption.

3) Place the patch on the skin and hold it in place with the palm of your hand for 2-3 minutes. The heat of your hand will help the adhesive bond to the skin. Failure to perform this step will allow the patch to fall off. If patch is not fully adhered to the skin, fentanyl will not be absorbed properly.

4) Cover the patch with a light bandage or clear adhesive bandage (*e.g., Bioclusive®*). If you choose to use *Bioclusive®*, apply the fentanyl patch as described above. Spray around the perimeter and over the patch with medical adhesive spray (*e.g., Medical Adhesive®*). Place the *Bioclusive®* over the site and press it down firmly. Be sure to clip an area large enough so that the *Bioclusive®* can adhere to the patch and the skin. If the *Bioclusive®* only adheres to the patch and fur without good adherence to skin, the patch will tend to peel up and dislodge.

5) Label the site with the size of patch (25, 50, 75 or 100 mcg/hr) and the date and time the patch was placed. Patches have shown to release effective fentanyl levels for up to five days in cats, three days in dogs and two days in horses. Potentially, the patches could be left longer, especially in dogs.

6) Potential side effects include bradycardia, respiratory depression, urinary retention, and constipation. All patients with

fentanyl patches should be monitored accordingly. If a patient with a patch develops a fever, consider patch removal. If the patch is left in place, the patient must be closely monitored since the rate of fentanyl absorption may increase.

7) Person applying or removing the patch must gently, but thoroughly rinse their hands with water to remove any drug residue. Soap, cleansers or solvents should not be used. Surgical gloves may be worn to place or remove patches, as skin contact does occur when handling the adhesive edges.

8) Dispose of used patches by flushing down toilet.

Monitoring
- Analgesic efficacy.
- Heart rate and respiratory rate.
- CNS effects (sedation; dysphoria; excitement)

Client Information
- Narcotic pain reliever topical patch. May take several hours before it starts working. May provide pain relief for 3-5 days in dogs and cats.
- Explain carefully to clients how to apply (if applicable), remove and dispose of patches. Consider making application, removal, and disposal an outpatient procedure, thereby bypassing concerns with clients.
- Usually tolerated very well by animals. High doses can cause sedation, dysphoria (howling, whining), slowed heart rate, and reduced breathing (respiration). Skin rash is the most likely side effect when doses are not too high.
- Patches (new, on the animal, or used) must be kept away from children; use cautiously in households where young children or animals could remove and ingest or be exposed to patches. Should accidental human skin contact occur with the patch, wash with water only (no soap, etc.).
- Dispose by flushing patch down toilet.

Chemistry/Synonyms
Fentanyl citrate, a very potent opiate agonist, occurs as a white, crystalline powder. It is sparingly soluble in water and soluble in alcohol. It is odorless and tasteless (not recommended for taste test because of extreme potency) with a pK_a of 8.3 and a melting point between 147-152°C.

Fentanyl and fentanyl citrate may also be known as: fentanylum, fentanyli citras, McN-JR-4263-49, phentanyl citrate, R-4263, *Actiq®*, *Fenodid®*, *Fenta-Hameln®*, *Fentabbott®*, *Fentanest®*, *Fentax®*, *Fentora®*, *Haldid®*, *Ionsys®*, *Leptanal®*, *Nafluvent®*, *Sintenyl®*, *Sublimaze®*, *Tanyl®*, and *Trofentyl®*.

Storage/Stability
Fentanyl transdermal patches should be stored at temperatures less than 25°C and applied immediately after removing from the individually sealed package. Do not cut patches.

Compatibility/Compounding Considerations
Most modern transdermal fentanyl patches can be cut, but it is advised to obtain the opinion of a pharmacist before doing so.

Dosage Forms/Regulatory Status
VETERINARY-LABELED PRODUCTS: NONE.
The ARCI (Racing Commissioners International) has designated this drug as a class 1 substance. See the appendix for more information.

HUMAN-LABELED PRODUCTS:
Fentanyl Transdermal System (Patch):

1.25 (5 cm2; **12 mcg/hr**);

2.5 to 2.75 (6.25 – 10 cm2; **25 mcg/hr**);

2.5 to 5.5 (12.5 – 20 cm2; **50 mcg/hr**);

7.5 to 8.25 (18.75 – 30 cm2; **75 mcg/hr**);

10 to 11 (25 – 40 cm2; **100 mcg/hr**);

Duragesic®-12, -25, -50, -75 and -100, generic; (Rx, C-II)

The following human products are available, but no information on their clinical usefulness or safety in animal patients was located:

Fentanyl Iontophoretic Transdermal System: 40 mcg/dose fentanyl hydrochloride (equivalent to 44.4 mcg of fentanyl) delivered over a 10-minute period upon each activation of the dose button; Each system contains fentanyl hydrochloride 10.8 mg; *Ionsys®*; (Rx; C-II)

All fentanyl products are Class-II controlled substances.

Revisions/References
Monograph revised/updated January 2014.

Ahern, B. J., et al. (2010). Pharmacokinetics of fentanyl administered transdermally and intravenously in sheep. American Journal of Veterinary Research 71(10): 1127-32.

Bellei, E., et al. (2011). The use of fentanyl-patch in dogs undergoing spinal surgery: plasma concentration and analgesic efficacy. J. Vet. Pharmacol. Ther. 34(5): 437-41.

Egger, C. M., et al. (2007). Efficacy and cost-effectiveness of transdermal fentanyl patches for the relief of post-operative pain in dogs after anterior cruciate ligament and pelvic limb repair. Veterinary Anaesthesia and Analgesia 34(3): 200-8.

Hansen, B. (2008). Analgesia for the critically ill dog or cat: An update. Vet Clin NA: Sm Anim Pract 38: 1353-63.

KuKanich, B. & M. Hubin (2010). The pharmacokinetics of ketoconazole and its effects on the pharmacokinetics of midazolam and fentanyl in dogs. J. Vet. Pharmacol. Ther. 33(1): 42-9.

Mills, P. C., et al. (2004). Investigation of in vitro transdermal absorption of fentanyl from patches placed on skin samples obtained from various anatomic regions of dogs. American Journal of Veterinary Research 65(12): 1697-700.

Orsini, J. A., et al. (2006). Pharmacokinetics of fentanyl delivered transdermally in healthy adult horses - variability among horses and its clinical implications. J. Vet. Pharmacol. Ther. 29(6): 539-46.

Reed, F., et al. (2011). Evaluation of transdermal fentanyl patch attachment in dogs and analysis of residual fentanyl content following removal. Veterinary Anaesthesia and Analgesia 38(4): 407-12.

Fentanyl Transdermal Solution

(fen-ta-nil)   Recuvyra®

Opiate

Prescriber Highlights

WARNING: Because there are very specific and important instructions, safeguards/controls, and restrictions for the use of this product (Recuvyra') that are beyond the scope of this reference, the information in this monograph is a brief synopsis and not meant as a substitute for FDA-approved information. The reader MUST refer to, and follow the FDA-approved information and Risk Minimization Action Plan (RiskMAP) before use.

► Class-II opiate analgesic approved for transdermal application in an **inpatient setting** for **dogs only**. Not for injection.

► Adequate training mandatory for use of the transdermal solution; can only be received and administered by veterinarians through the restricted distribution program because of the potential for human abuse and safety risks associated with its use in dogs. The Risk Minimization Action Plan (RiskMAP) for *Recuvyra®* must be followed; the drug can only be applied to the patient by two trained hospital staff after the dog owner has read and understood the materials (by signing the client information sheet).

► Veterinarian must report serious adverse effects to manufacturer.

► Adverse Effects: Dose related hypothermia, respiratory, CNS & circulatory depression (bradycardia); GI effects (vomiting, diarrhea, anorexia) can occur.

► See also the Fentanyl Citrate, Injection and Fentanyl, Transdermal Patch monographs.

Uses/Indications

In veterinary medicine, fentanyl transdermal solution (*Recuvyra®*) is approved for the control of postoperative pain associated with surgical procedures in dogs.

Pharmacology/Actions

Fentanyl is a *mu* opiate agonist that is very short acting when administered parenterally and approximately 80-100X more potent than morphine. The transdermal solution once applied to the skin, rapidly dries with fast dermal absorption and sequestration of fentanyl in the stratum corneum. It then slowly releases (up to one week) into the systemic circulation,

Mu receptors are found primarily in the pain regulating areas of the brain. They are thought to contribute to the analgesia, euphoria, respiratory depression, physical dependence, miosis, and hypothermic actions of opiates. Receptors for opiate analgesics are found in high concentrations in the limbic system, spinal cord, thalamus, hypothalamus, striatum, and midbrain. They are also found in tissues such as the gastrointestinal tract, urinary tract, and other smooth muscles.

The pharmacology of the opiate agonists is discussed in more detail in the monograph: Narcotic (opiate) Agonist Analgesics.

Pharmacokinetics

When transdermal fentanyl solution (*Recuvyra®*) is applied to canine skin, solvent evaporation results in super-saturation of both a penetration enhancer and fentanyl. At the moment of drying (approximately 2-5 minutes following application), rapid dermal absorption and sequestration of fentanyl into the stratum corneum occurs. From the stratum corneum, fentanyl is then slowly absorbed (up to one week) into the bloodstream. Pharmacokinetic values in individual dogs can vary considerably, but in a "typical"

dog the time to reach a plasma level of 0.6 ng/mL (thought to be the minimum therapeutic analgesic plasma concentration in dogs) is 1.85 hours and to reach 1 ng/mL, 3.08 hours; absorption lag-time averaged around 33 minutes. Peak levels of 1.83 ng/mL occurred about 13.6 hours after administration. Terminal half-life was about 3 days. Mean plasma concentrations from days 0-4 were 1.32 ng/mL (Freise, Linton, et al. 2012).

Contraindications/Precautions/Warnings

Fentanyl is contraindicated in patients with known hypersensitivity to it or any component of the product. Do not use in an extra-label manner in dogs or in other species; safety in cats, horses, or other species has not been evaluated. Fentanyl transdermal solution has not been evaluated in dogs with respiratory disorders, cardiovascular disease, renal disease, hepatic disease, dogs younger than 6 months of age, geriatric dogs, or breeding, pregnant, or lactating dogs.

Do not apply to skin that is diseased or injured or to anatomic areas other than the dorsal scapular area because absorption characteristics may be different.

Do not administer to dogs where postoperative pain is expected to be mild or absent, that have, or are suspected of having paralytic ileus, and that are hypovolemic or debilitated.

Do not administer a second dose; accumulation of fentanyl following repeated administration could result in severe adverse reactions, including death.

Use cautiously with other CNS depressants (sedatives, hypnotics, general anesthetics, phenothiazines, and skeletal muscle relaxants) as respiratory depression, hypothermia, bradycardia, hypotension, and profound sedation may occur. If concomitant therapy is used, the doses of these agents should be reduced. The product's label states "To prevent potential overdose and severe adverse reactions, do not administer other opioids within 7 days of *Recuvyra®* administration."

Dogs must not be discharged to owners until post-operative sedation is mild or absent and are drinking water and eating on their own at an appropriate level for the condition that required surgery.

Abuse Potential: *Recuvyra®* is a very potent, concentrated *mu*-agonist opioid and a Class-II controlled substance (in the USA) with high potential for abuse and drug diversion similar to other opioids. Class II opioid substances have the highest potential for human abuse and criminal diversion. Safe, secure storage and accurate recordkeeping are mandatory.

Risk Minimization and Action Plan: This product is distributed under a Risk Minimization Action Plan (RiskMAP) and its use is limited to certified veterinarians.

Human Safety: *Secondary Exposure To Fentanyl In Children And Adults*: Strict adherence to the requirements of the RiskMAP and the *Instructions For Use* provided in this product insert is imperative in order to reduce the potential of secondary exposure to fentanyl from *Recuvyra®* treated skin.

■ The dog should be isolated from children for 72 hours (3 days) from the time of *Recuvyra®* application to the dog.

■ If a child comes in direct contact with the application site within 72 hours (3 days) from the time of *Recuvyra®* application to the dog, the exposed area should not contact the child's mouth or eyes, and the exposed area should be washed with soap and water.

■ If a child's tongue comes in contact with the dog, or another part of the child's body comes in contact with the dog and is then placed in the mouth, it is possible for fentanyl to enter the bloodstream; this is a medical emergency and the child should be seen immediately by a physician.

■ Adults should avoid contact with the application site for 72 hours (3 days) following the application of *Recuvyra®* to the dog. Within this period, any part of the body that directly contacts the application site should be washed with soap and not inserted into the mouth.

- The antidote for human exposure to *Recuvyra®* transdermal solution is an opioid reversal agent such as naltrexone or naloxone.

Adverse Effects

Dose related hypothermia, respiratory, CNS (sedation) and circulatory depression (bradycardia) are the primary adverse effects with fentanyl. Anticholinergic agents may be required to treat bradycardia when fentanyl is used intraoperatively. Dogs and cats appear less prone than humans but are not immune to opiate-induced respiratory depression. Moderate to severe sedation may persist up to 2 days after dosing. Gastrointestinal effects (diarrhea, vomiting, and anorexia) can occur. To report adverse drug reactions, contact *Elanco Animal Health* at 1-888-545-5973; they may also be reported to the FDA-CVM at 1-888-FDA-VETS or http://www.fda.gov/AnimalVeterinary/SafetyHealth.

Reproductive/Nursing Safety

Safe use in pregnancy has not been established. In humans, the FDA categorizes fentanyl as category *C* for use during pregnancy (*Animal studies have shown an adverse effect on the fetus, but there are no adequate studies in humans; or there are no animal reproduction studies and no adequate studies in humans.*) In a separate system evaluating the safety of drugs in canine and feline pregnancy (Papich 1989), this drug is categorized as class: *B* (*Safe for use if used cautiously. Studies in laboratory animals may have uncovered some risk, but these drugs appear to be safe in dogs and cats or these drugs are safe if they are not administered when the animal is near term.*)

Most narcotic agonist analgesics are excreted into milk, but effects on nursing offspring may not be significant.

Overdosage/Acute Toxicity

Overdosage may produce profound respiratory and/or CNS depression in most species.

Naloxone is the agent of choice in treating respiratory depression. The product label states: "Emergency administration of naloxone at 0.04 mg/kg may be used to reverse serious adverse reactions associated with *Recuvyra®*. Administer the reversal agent slowly to avoid abrupt increases in blood pressure and catecholamine levels. Reversal should occur rapidly (1-2 minutes); however, the duration of action of naloxone is variable (1-3 hours). The effects of *Recuvyra®* could last longer than the effects of the opioid reversal agent." Mechanical respiratory support should also be considered in cases of severe respiratory depression.

Drug Interactions

The following drug interactions have either been reported or are theoretical in humans or animals receiving fentanyl and may be of significance in veterinary patients. Unless otherwise noted, use together is not necessarily contraindicated, but weigh the potential risks and perform additional monitoring when appropriate.

- **AZOLE ANTIFUNGALS** (*e.g.,* **ketoconazole, itraconazole, fluconazole**): May inhibit fentanyl metabolism. A study in dogs however, showed that ketoconazole did not significantly alter the elimination of fentanyl (KuKanich et al. 2010).
- **CNS DEPRESSANTS, OTHER:** Additive CNS effects possible; see Warnings above.
- **DIURETICS:** Opiates may decrease efficacy in CHF patients.
- **MACROLIDE ANTIBIOTICS** (*e.g.,* **erythromycin, clarithromycin**): May inhibit fentanyl metabolism.
- **MONOAMINE OXIDASE INHIBITORS** (*e.g.,* **amitraz,** and possibly **selegiline**): Severe and unpredictable opiate potentiation may be seen; not recommended (in humans) if MAO inhib-

itor has been used within 14 days.

- **MUSCLE RELAXANTS, SKELETAL:** Fentanyl may enhance neuromuscular blockade.
- **NITROUS OXIDE:** High fentanyl doses may cause cardiovascular depression.
- **OPIOIDS, OTHER:** The product's label states "To prevent potential overdose and severe adverse reactions, do not administer other opioids within 7 days of *Recuvyra®* administration."
- **PHENOBARBITAL, PHENYTOIN:** May increase the metabolism of fentanyl.
- **RIFAMPIN:** May increase the metabolism of fentanyl.
- **TRICYCLIC ANTIDEPRESSANTS** (*e.g.,* **clomipramine, amitriptyline,** etc.): Fentanyl may exacerbate the effects of tricyclic antidepressants.
- **WARFARIN:** Opiates may potentiate anticoagulant activity.

Laboratory Considerations

- As they may increase biliary tract pressure, opiates can increase plasma amylase and lipase values up to 24 hours following their administration.

Doses

- **DOGS:**

Warning: The following is a synopsis of the dosage administration instructions for this product. Refer to the actual product information for specific and required information (including RiskMAP and printed Instructions for Use). While handling and applying the product specific safety measures include:

- *At least two trained staff present required for handling and administration; must not be dispensed for home administration by dog owner.*
- *Protective covering must be used by wearing non-permeable gloves, protective glasses and laboratory coat; remove and dispose of protective garments after a minimum drying time of 5 minutes.*
- *If accidental eye, oral or other mucous membrane contact occurs to humans, patient or other animals during administration, flush the area with water and seek immediate medical attention. If human skin contact occurs during administration, wash the exposed area with soap and water and seek medical attention immediately. Physician information: The antidote for human exposure to Recuvyra® (fentanyl transdermal solution) is an opioid reversal agent such as naltrexone or naloxone. In the case of an emergency, provide the physician with the package insert and Client Information Sheet.*
- Not for injection.

For the control of postoperative pain associated with surgical procedures in dogs (labeled dose; FDA-approved): 2.7 mg/kg (1.2 mg/lb.) using only the syringes/applicator provided and applied topically per the instructions to the dorsal scapular area 2-4 hours prior to surgery. Applied one time only; a single application provides analgesia for 4 days. Do not store the product in the syringes. Not for injection. Cannot be safely dosed in dogs weighing less than 2.7 kg (6 lbs.). (Adapted from label information; *Recuvyra®*)

Monitoring

During anesthesia:

- Rectal temperature, heart rate/rhythm, blood pressure, respiratory rate, and O_2 saturation. During general anesthesia following administration, dogs should be continuously monitored and facilities should be available for the maintenance of a patent airway, artificial ventilation, IV fluids, and oxygen supplementation.

Post-surgery:

- Analgesic efficacy.
- Heart and respiratory rate.
- CNS status (sedation).
- Body temperature. Hypothermia may be severe and prolonged (greater than 24 hours) necessitating the use of an external heat source during surgery, throughout recovery, and after recovery from anesthesia.
- Hydration & GI function status.

Client Information

- Prior to administration, dog owners should understand the safety outcomes that could affect them, their family, and their dog. A client information sheet should be discussed and sent home with every dog treated. The *Recuvyra®* RiskMAP program considers the client information sheet as an informed consent form for the dog owner and contains a signature line which should be signed prior to use to document that the dog owner has read and understood the client information sheet.
- The owner should be able to isolate the dog from family members, especially children, for several days after discharge.
- This product must not he used (applied) at home.
- Owners should be advised to contact veterinarian immediately if adverse effects (e.g. excessive sedation, decreased appetite or water intake, vomiting, diarrhea) occur.
- *Adult exposure*: Adults should avoid contact with the application site for 72 hours (3 days) following the application of *Recuvyra®* to the dog. Within this period, any part of the body that directly contacts the application site should be washed with soap and water and not placed in the mouth.
- **Contact or suspected contact in children should be treated as a medical emergency.** *Child exposure*: The dog should be isolated from children for 72 hours (3 days) from the time of *Recuvyra®* application to the dog. If a child comes in direct contact (or if you suspect that contact has happened) with the dog within 72 hours (3 days) from the time of *Recuvyra®* application to the dog, the exposed part of the child's body should not contact the child's mouth or eyes, and the area should be washed with soap and water. If a child's tongue comes in contact with the dog, or another part of the child's body comes in contact with the dog and is then placed in the mouth, it is possible for fentanyl to enter the bloodstream; this is a medical emergency and the child should be seen immediately by a physician.

Chemistry/Synonyms

The transdermal solution (*Recuvyra®*) is a clear, colorless to light yellow, volatile solution that contains 5% w/v (50 mg/mL) fentanyl as the active pharmaceutical ingredient in alcohol and octyl salicylate.

Fentanyl and fentanyl citrate may also be known as: fentanylum, fentanyli citras, McN-JR-4263-49, phentanyl citrate, R-4263, and *Recuvyra®*.

Storage/Stability

Fentanyl transdermal solution (*Recuvyra®*) should be stored in a locked, substantially constructed cabinet according to DEA and local controlled substance guidelines. Once broached with the needleless adaptor, store the vial upright at controlled room temperature, 20-25°C (68-77°F), with the needleless adaptor attached. Discard broached vials after 30 days. Any unused or expired vials must be destroyed by a DEA registered reverse distributor; for further information call 1-888-545-5973.

Compatibility/Compounding Considerations

This product must not be mixed or diluted with any other compound.

Dosage Forms/Regulatory Status

VETERINARY-LABELED PRODUCTS:

Fentanyl Transdermal Solution 50 mg/mL in 10 mL vials (not for injection); *Recuvyra®*; (Rx; C-II). FDA-approved (NADA 141-337) for use in dogs. All fentanyl products are Class-II controlled substances.

HUMAN-LABELED PRODUCTS: NONE.

Revisions/References

Monograph written January 2014.

Refer to the package insert, instructions for use and RiskMAP documents; these may be found at Recuvyra.com. Additional references include:

Freise, K. J., et al. (2012). Population pharmacokinetics of transdermal fentanyl solution following a single dose administered prior to soft tissue and orthopedic surgery in dogs. J. Vet. Pharmacol. Ther. 35: 65-72.

Freise, K. J., et al. (2012a). Naloxone reversal of an overdose of a novel, long-acting transdermal fentanyl solution in laboratory Beagles. J. Vet. Pharmacol. Ther. 35: 45-51.

Freise, K. J., et al. (2012b). Pharmacokinetics and the effect of application site on a novel, long-acting transdermal fentanyl solution in healthy laboratory Beagles. J. Vet. Pharmacol. Ther. 35: 27-33.

Freise, K. J., et al. (2012). Pharmacokinetics and dose selection of a novel, long-acting transdermal fentanyl solution in healthy laboratory Beagles. J. Vet. Pharmacol. Ther. 35: 21-6.

Kukanich, B. & T. P. Clark (2012). The history and pharmacology of fentanyl: relevance to a novel, long-acting transdermal fentanyl solution newly approved for use in dogs. J. Vet. Pharmacol. Ther. 35: 3-19.

KuKanich, B. & M. Hubin (2010). The pharmacokinetics of ketoconazole and its effects on the pharmacokinetics of midazolam and fentanyl in dogs. J. Vet. Pharmacol. Ther. 33(1): 42-9.

Linton, D. D., et al. (2012). The effectiveness of a long-acting transdermal fentanyl solution compared to buprenorphine for the control of postoperative pain in dogs in a randomized, multicentered clinical study. J. Vet. Pharmacol. Ther. 35: 53-64.

Savides, M. C., et al. (2012). The margin of safety of a single application of transdermal fentanyl solution when administered at multiples of the therapeutic dose to laboratory dogs. J. Vet. Pharmacol. Ther. 35: 35-43.

Ferrous Sulfate

(fer-us sul-fayte)   Fer-In-Sol®, Feosol®

Nutritional/Hematinic

Prescriber Highlights

▶ Oral iron supplement for the treatment of iron-deficiency anemia or as an iron supplement when epoetin or darbepoetin is used.

▶ Contraindications: Patients with hemosiderosis, hemochromatosis, hemolytic anemia, or known hypersensitivity; some consider it contraindicated with GI ulcers.

▶ Adverse Effects: With non-toxic doses, gastrointestinal upset. Dogs and cats may not tolerate oral iron products.

▶ May be very toxic (life threatening) if overdosed.

Uses/Indications

While iron is a necessary trace element in all hemoglobin-utilizing animals, the use of therapeutic dosages of ferrous sulfate (or other oral iron) preparations in veterinary medicine is limited primarily to the treatment of iron-deficiency anemia in dogs (usually due to chronic blood loss) and as adjunctive therapy in dogs or cats when receiving epoetin (erythropoietin) or darbepoetin therapy. Injectable iron products are usually used in the treatment of iron deficiency anemia associated with newborn animals.

Pharmacology/Actions

Iron is necessary for myoglobin and hemoglobin in the transport and utilization of oxygen. While neither stimulating erythropoiesis nor correcting hemoglobin abnormalities not caused by iron deficiency, iron administration does correct both physical signs and decreased hemoglobin levels secondary to iron deficiency.

Ionized iron is a component in the enzymes cytochrome oxidase, succinic dehydrogenase, and xanthine oxidase.

Pharmacokinetics

Oral absorption of iron salts is complex and determined by a variety of factors including diet, iron stores present, degree of erythropoiesis, and dose. Iron is thought to be absorbed throughout the GI tract but is most absorbed in the duodenum and proximal jejunum. Food in the GI tract may reduce the amount absorbed.

After absorption, the ferrous iron is immediately bound to transferrin, transported to the bone marrow and eventually incorporated into hemoglobin. Iron metabolism occurs in a nearly closed system. Because iron liberated by the destruction of hemoglobin is reused by the body and only small amounts are lost by the body via hair and nail growth, normal skin desquamation and GI tract sloughing, normal dietary intake usually is sufficient to maintain iron homeostasis.

Contraindications/Precautions/Warnings

Ferrous sulfate (or other oral iron products) are considered contraindicated in patients with hemosiderosis, hemochromatosis, hemolytic anemias, or known hypersensitivity to any component of the product. Because of the GI irritating properties of the drugs, oral iron products are considered contraindicated by some clinicians in patients with GI ulcerative diseases.

Adverse Effects

Adverse effects associated with non-toxic doses are usually limited to mild gastrointestinal upset. Division of the daily dosage may reduce this effect, but dosage reduction may also be necessary in some animals.

Reproductive/Nursing Safety

In humans, the FDA categorizes this drug as category A for use during pregnancy (*Adequate studies in pregnant women have not demonstrated a risk to the fetus in the first trimester of pregnancy, and there is no evidence of risk in later trimesters.*)

Overdosage/Acute Toxicity

Ingestion of iron containing products may result in serious toxicity and acute intoxication should be considered an emergency. It is recommended to consult with an animal poison center for diagnostic and management guidance. While lethal doses are not readily available in domestic species, as little as 400 mg (of elemental iron) is potentially fatal in a child. Initial clinical signs of acute iron poisoning usually present with an acute onset of gastrointestinal irritation and distress (vomiting—possibly hemorrhagic, abdominal pain, diarrhea). The onset of these effects may be seen within 30 minutes of ingestion, but can be delayed for several hours. Peripheral vascular collapse may rapidly follow with clinical signs of depression, weak and/or rapid pulse, hypotension, cyanosis, ataxia, and coma possible. Some patients do not exhibit this phase of toxicity and may be asymptomatic for 12-48 hours after ingestion, when another critical phase may occur. This phase may be exhibited by pulmonary edema, vasomotor collapse, cyanosis, pulmonary edema, fulminant hepatic failure, coma and death. Animals that survive this phase may exhibit long-term sequelae, including gastric scarring and contraction and have persistent digestive disturbances.

Because an acute onset of gastroenteritis may be associated with a multitude of causes, diagnosis of iron intoxication may be difficult unless the animal has been observed ingesting the product or physical evidence suggests ingestion. Ferrous sulfate (and gluconate) tablets are radiopaque and often can be observed on abdominal radiographs. Serum iron levels and total iron binding capacity (TIBC) may also be helpful in determining the diagnosis, but must be done on an emergency basis to have any clinical benefit.

Deferoxamine is useful in chelating iron that has been absorbed. See that monograph for further information.

In addition to chelation therapy, other supportive measures may be necessary including treatment of acidosis, prophylactic antibiotics, oxygen, treatment for shock, coagulation abnormalities, seizures, and/or hyperthermia. After the acute phases have resolved, dietary evaluation and management may be required.

Drug Interactions

The following drug interactions have either been reported or are theoretical in humans or animals receiving ferrous sulfate and may be of significance in veterinary patients. Unless otherwise noted, use together is not necessarily contraindicated, but weigh the potential risks and perform additional monitoring when appropriate.

- **ANTACIDS:** May bind to iron and decrease oral absorption; administer at least two hours apart.
- **CALCIUM (ORAL):** May bind to iron and decrease oral absorption; administer at least two hours apart.
- **CHLORAMPHENICOL:** Because chloramphenicol may delay the response to iron administration, avoid using chloramphenicol in patients with iron deficiency anemia.
- **FLUOROQUINOLONES** (*e.g.,* **enrofloxacin**, etc.): Iron may reduce the absorption of oral fluoroquinolones; administer at least two hours apart.
- **H2-RECEPTOR ANTAGONISTS** (*e.g.,* **ranitidine, famotidine**, etc.): Increased gastric pH may decrease iron absorption.
- **PENICILLAMINE:** Iron can decrease the efficacy of penicillamine, probably by decreasing its absorption; if both drugs are required, space doses of the two drugs as far apart as possible.
- **PROTON-PUMP INHIBITORS** (*e.g.,* **omeprazole**): Increased gastric pH may decrease iron absorption.
- **TETRACYCLINES:** Oral iron preparations can bind to orally administered tetracyclines, thereby decreasing the absorption of both compounds.
- **THYROXINE:** Iron may reduce the absorption of oral thyroxine; administer at least two hours apart.
- **VITAMIN C:** May enhance the absorption of iron.

Laboratory Considerations

- Large doses of oral iron can color the feces black and cause false-positives with the guaiac test for occult blood in the feces.
- Iron does not usually affect the benzidine test for occult blood.

Doses

Caution: Unless otherwise noted, doses are for ferrous sulfate (regular—not dried). Dosing of oral iron products can be confusing; some authors state doses in terms of the iron salt and some state doses in terms of elemental iron. For the doses below, assume that the doses are for ferrous sulfate and not elemental iron unless specified.

- **DOGS:**

  For iron deficiency anemia or patients to be treated with epoetin or darbepoetin: More commonly injectable iron dextran is used, but oral ferrous sulfate may be considered. Usual recommended dosages are 100 – 300 mg per dog PO once daily. If underlying blood loss is the cause for iron deficiency, it must be corrected before treatment.

- **CATS:**

  For iron deficiency anemia or patients treated with epoetin or darbepoetin: More commonly injectable iron dextran is used as cats usually do not tolerate oral iron products, but oral ferrous sulfate may be considered. Usual recommended dosages are 50 – 100 mg per cat PO once daily. If underlying blood loss is the cause for iron deficiency, it must be corrected before treatment.

Monitoring

Efficacy; adverse effects:

- Hemograms.
- Serum iron and total iron binding capacity, if necessary.

Normal serum iron values for dogs and cats are reported as 80-180 micrograms/dL and 70-140 micrograms/dL, respectively. Total iron binding for dogs and cats are reported as 280-340 micrograms/dL and 270-400 micrograms/dL, respectively. (Morgan 1988).

- Serum transferrin saturation can be estimated by dividing serum iron by total iron binding capacity.

Client Information

- Oral iron supplement for the treatment of iron-deficiency anemia or when animals are receiving epoetin or darbepoetin.
- Best given with food to avoid stomach upset, but do not give with dairy products (including cheese).
- Side effects can include vomiting or nausea. If black tarry stools or bloody vomit are seen, contact veterinarian immediately.
- Overdoses can be very toxic to animals or children; keep well out of reach.

Chemistry/Synonyms

An orally available iron supplement, ferrous sulfate occurs as odorless, pale-bluish-green, crystals or granules having a saline, styptic taste. In dry air the drug is efflorescent.

If exposed to moisture or moist air, the drug is rapidly oxidized to a brownish-yellow ferric compound that should not be used medicinally. Exposure to light or an alkaline medium will enhance the conversion from the ferrous to ferric state.

Ferrous sulfate is available commercially in two forms, a "regular" and a "dried" form. Regular ferrous sulfate contains 7 molecules of water of hydration and is freely soluble in water and insoluble in alcohol. Ferrous sulfate contains approximately 200 mg of elemental iron per gram. Dried ferrous sulfate consists primarily of the monohydrate with some tetrahydrate. It is slowly soluble in water and insoluble in water. Dried ferrous sulfate contains 300 mg of elemental iron per gram. Ferrous sulfate, dried may also be known as ferrous sulfate, exsiccated.

Ferrous sulfate may also be known as: eisen(II)-sulfat, ferreux (sulfate), ferrosi sulfas heptahydricus, ferrous sulphate, ferrum sulfuricum oxydulatum, iron (II) sulphate heptahydrate, iron sulphate; many trade names are available.

Storage/Stability

Unless otherwise instructed, store ferrous sulfate preparations in tight, light-resistant containers.

Compatibility/Compounding Considerations

No specific information noted.

Dosage Forms/Regulatory Status

VETERINARY-LABELED PRODUCTS:

No veterinary-FDA-approved products containing only ferrous sulfate could be located, but there are many multivitamin with iron containing products available.

HUMAN-LABELED PRODUCTS:

Ferrous Sulfate Oral Tablets: 325 mg (65 mg iron); *Feosol*®, *Fero-Sul*®, generic; (OTC)

Ferrous Sulfate Oral Elixir/Liquid: 220 mg/5 mL (44 mg iron/5 mL) in 473 mL, 300 mg/5 mL (60 mg iron/5 mL) in 5 mL; generic; (OTC)

Ferrous Sulfate Oral Drops: 15 mg iron/mL & 75 mg/0.6 mL (15 mg iron/0.6 mL) in 50 mL; *Enfamil Fer-In-Sol*®, *Fer-Gen-Sol*®, generic; (OTC)

Revisions/References

Monograph revised/updated January 2014.

Morgan, R. V., Ed. (1988). *Handbook of Small Animal Practice*. New York, Churchill Livingstone.

Fexofenadine HCl

(fex-oh-FEN-ah-deen) *Allegra*®, *Telfast*®

Antihistamine (2nd Generation)

Prescriber Highlights

▶ Second-generation (non-sedating, non-anticholinergic) antihistamine that may be useful in treating or preventing allergic-related conditions. Little experience in veterinary medicine and little published data to support use.

▶ Side effect incidence appears minimal, but sedation/depression and gastrointestinal effects are possible.

▶ Do not confuse with, or use combination products containing pseudoephedrine (*Allegra-D*®); human fexofenadine oral suspension contains xylitol (may be toxic in dogs).

Uses/Indications

Fexofenadine, is a second-generation (non-sedating) antihistamine that may be useful in small animals for controlling clinical signs associated with histamine-mediated conditions, including atopic dermatitis and allergic rhinitis. However, little scientific evidence exists to support antihistaminic therapy in animals, or any one antihistamine over another. Antihistamines have anecdotally shown benefit for treating mild pruritus in dogs with atopic dermatitis (without chronic skin lesions) and appear to be more effective if given consistently and before dogs become moderately pruritic (Bloom 2013). One small, random controlled non-inferiority trial suggested consistent benefit from fexofenadine in treated dogs with atopic dermatitis (Plevnik et al. 2006; Plevnik et al. 2009), however this study has been criticized for its design and thus its conclusions (Olivry & Bizikova 2013).

Pharmacology/Actions

Fexofenadine, a second-generation antihistamine, is a selective peripheral histamine1-receptor (H1-receptor) antagonist. Second-generation antihistamines are more lipophobic than those of the first generation (*e.g.*, diphenhydramine, chlorpheniramine), therefore they do not readily cross into the CNS and cause sedation or have substantial anticholinergic effects. Fexofenadine also may have other anti-inflammatory effects, including mast cell stabilization, and effects on leukotrienes and prostaglandins that are associated with allergic responses.

Fexofenadine is an active metabolite of terfenadine (*Seldane*®), which was withdrawn from the market secondary to concerns that it could increase QT intervals (QTc) in humans. Fexofenadine does not have this effect.

Pharmacokinetics

Pharmacokinetic data for fexofenadine was not located for dogs or cats. In humans, fexofenadine is rapidly absorbed following oral administration with peak levels occurring between 2-3 hours after dosing. Tablets or oral suspension yield similar values. Absolute bioavailability has not been established. Administering with a high fat meal can somewhat reduce area under the curve. Elimination half-life is around 14.5 hours when dosed twice daily. Approximately 5% of the total dose is eliminated by hepatic metabolism. The majority of an oral dose is eliminated in the feces, which may be due to low oral absorption or biliary excretion. Moderate to severe renal function impairment can increase plasma concentration by 100% or more and dosing adjustment is recommended.

Fexofenadine is a P-glycoprotein (P-gp) substrate drug and theoretically could have altered bioavailability in dogs with deficient P-gp function (ABCB-1delta mutation), however, it is unclear if fexofenadine pharmacokinetics are altered in these dogs. One study found that plasma concentrations of fexofenadine were significantly higher at 4 and 8 hours post dose in ABCB-1delta dogs (Kitamura et al. 2008), but the results are in question as dogs also received famotidine (another P-gp substrate) one hour before dosing and additional P-gp/CYP-3A substrates (quinidine, loperamide) were administered at the same time as fexofenadine (Mealey et al. 2010).

A pharmacokinetic study done in horses (Olsen et al. 2007) showed low oral bioavailability (median = 2.6% alone; 1.5% when PO ivermectin given 12 hours prior), volume of distribution (steady state) of 0.8 L/kg, plasma clearance of 0.75 mL/hr/kg and a terminal half-life of 5 hours after oral administration. The authors concluded that despite fexofenadine having antihistaminic effects in the horse at low plasma concentrations and that extended studies are needed to determine its therapeutic value, low bioavailability in horses may mean that oral treatment is not suitable.

Contraindications/Precautions/Warnings

Do not use in patients allergic (hypersensitive) to fexofenadine. Dosage adjustment is recommended in humans with severe renal impairment.

Adverse Effects

Although there has been little clinical experience with fexofenadine in animal patients, adverse effects are not common. Sedation/CNS depression and gastrointestinal effects are possible.

Reproductive/Nursing Safety

Teratogenicity from fexofenadine has not been reported in humans or laboratory animals, even at high dosages. In rats, doses of 3X (human equivalent) were associated with decreased pup weights and survival rates. In humans, the FDA categorizes this drug as category C for use during pregnancy (*Animal studies have shown an adverse effect on the fetus, but there are no adequate studies in humans; or there are no animal reproduction studies and no adequate studies in humans.*)

It is unknown if fexofenadine is excreted into milk, but it is unlikely to pose much risk to nursing offspring.

Overdosage/Acute Toxicity

In laboratory studies, dogs receiving oral doses up to 2 grams/kg (300X the maximum recommended adult human daily oral dose) no evidence of toxicity was observed. QT intervals were not prolonged in dogs receiving 30 mg/kg orally twice daily for 5 days; fexofenadine plasma concentrations were approximately 9X those of humans receiving 180 mg per day (maximum recommended human dose). There were 215 single agent exposures to fexofenadine reported to the ASPCA Animal Poison Control Center (APCC) during 2009-2013. Of the 198 dogs, 34 were symptomatic with lethargy (35%), facial edema (21%) and vomiting (21%) being the most common clinical signs. Overdoses may cause CNS depression. Because fexofenadine may be found in combination with other drugs (*e.g.*, pseudoephedrine) determine what product was actually ingested. Contact an animal control center for further advice and clinical management assistance.

Drug Interactions

The following drug interactions have either been reported or are theoretical in humans or animals receiving fexofenadine and may be of significance in veterinary patients. Unless otherwise noted, use together is not necessarily contraindicated, but weigh the potential risks and perform additional monitoring when appropriate.

- **ANTACIDS CONTAINING ALUMINUM or MAGNESIUM:** Oral bioavailability of fexofenadine reduced; separate dosing by at least one hour.
- **ERYTHROMYCIN, KETOCONAZOLE:** Possibly increases fexofenadine levels by enhancing its absorption. Because of the wide margin of safety with this medication and since fexofenadine does not affect QT interval, any clinical significance is doubtful.
- **FRUIT JUICES:** In humans, grapefruit, apple or orange juices

may reduce bioavailability; therefore it is recommended that fexofenadine be taken with water.
- **IVERMECTIN:** In a small pharmacokinetic study in horses, oral ivermectin decreased the oral bioavailability of fexofenadine (Olsen et al. 2007).

Laboratory Considerations

- **Allergy Testing (Allergen-specific intradermal tests):** Most veterinary dermatologists recommend discontinuing oral antihistamines 1-2 weeks prior to intradermal skin tests in dogs or cats, but one PK/PD study with hydroxyzine and cetirizine in dogs (Bizikova et al. 2008) suggests that when tests cannot be delayed, a minimum wait time of 2 days may be acceptable for some drugs in dogs (Olivry, Saridomichelakis, et al. 2013).
- **Allergy Testing (IgE serological tests):** Withdrawal of antihistamines prior to testing is theoretically not necessary, but this has not been proven (Olivry, Saridomichelakis, et al. 2013).

Dosages

- **DOGS:**

  As an antihistamine for treatment of allergic (histamine-mediated) conditions (extra-label): 2 – 5 mg/kg PO q12-24h although some have recommended higher dosages, including one study that used 18 mg/kg PO once daily and reported positive results in dogs with atopic dermatitis (Plevnik et al. 2009). Practically, because of available tablet dosage forms, initial dosages should be rounded to the nearest multiple of 15 mg (smaller dogs) and 30 mg (large dogs). As with other antihistamines, patient response is individualized and not predictable. When evaluating efficacy for any antihistamine a trial of 2-weeks minimum has been recommended (Bloom 2013). In patients exhibiting benefit, response may be improved when used prior to allergen exposure and regular, ongoing use is recommended.

- **CATS:**

  As an antihistamine for treatment of allergic (histamine-mediated) conditions (extra-label): 10 – 15 mg per cat (**NOT** mg/kg) PO q12-24h. There are some that recommend up to 30 mg per cat PO q12h. The oral 30 mg dispersible tablets may be a useful dosage form for use in cats as it rapidly dissolves on the tongue/inside the mouth. When splitting tablets of this dosage form, protect from moisture. As with other antihistamines, patient response is not predictable. In patients exhibiting benefit, response may be improved when used prior to allergen exposure and regular, ongoing use is recommended.

Monitoring

- Clinical efficacy.

Client Information

- Antihistamines should be used on a regular, ongoing basis in animals that respond to them. They work better if used before exposure to an allergen.
- May be given with or without food. If your animal vomits or acts sick after getting it on an empty stomach, give with food or small treat to see if this helps. If vomiting continues, contact your veterinarian.
- May cause less drowsiness/sleepiness than some other antihistamines, but this can still occur.

Chemistry/Synonyms

Fexofenadine HCl (CAS Registry: 138452-21-8; ATC: R06AX26) occurs as a white to off-white powder. It is slightly soluble in water; freely soluble in methyl alcohol; very slightly soluble in acetone.

Fexofenadine may also be known as terfenadine carboxylate hydrochloride or MDL-16455A. A common trade name is *Allegra®* or *Telfast®*.

Storage/Stability

Fexofenadine tablets, orally dispersible (disintegrating) tablets, capsules and oral suspension should be stored at room temperature (20-25°C; 68-77°F).

Orally dispersible tablets should be protected from moisture and are recommended for use immediately after opening individual tablet blisters.

Compatibility/Compounding Considerations

No specific information noted.

Dosage Forms/Regulatory Status

VETERINARY-LABELED PRODUCTS: NONE.

HUMAN-LABELED PRODUCTS:

Oral Tablets: 60 mg & 180 mg; *Allegra Allergy®*, generic; (OTC).

Oral Dispersible Tablets (ODT): 30 mg; *Allegra Allergy Children's®*; (OTC). **Note:** The orally disintegrating tablet is designed to disintegrate on the tongue and may be of use in animals difficult to pill. Some ODT products may contain xylitol.

Oral Suspension: 30 mg/5 mL (6 mg/mL); *Allegra Allergy Children's®*; (OTC). Also contains xylitol; <u>avoid use</u> in dogs.

There are also fexofenadine/pseudoephedrine combination products available (*e.g., Allegra D®*), but they are **NOT** recommended for use in animal patients.

Revisions/References

Monograph revised/updated January 2014.

Bizikova, P., et al. (2008). Hydroxyzine and cetirizine pharmacokinetics and pharmacodynamics after oral and intravenous administration of hydroxyzine to healthy dogs. Veterinary Dermatology 19(6): 348-57.

Bloom, P. (2013). Nonsteroidal, Nonimmunosuppressive Therapies for Pruritus. Veterinary Clinics of North America-Small Animal Practice 43(1): 173-+.

Kitamura, Y., et al. (2008). Modest effect of impaired P-glycoprotein on the plasma concentrations of fexofenadine, quinidine, and loperamide following oral administration in collies. Drug Metabolism and Disposition 36(5): 807-10.

Mealey, K. L., et al. (2010). Oral bioavailability of P-glycoprotein substrate drugs do not differ between ABCB1-1Δ and ABCB1 wild type dogs. J. Vet. Pharmacol. Ther. 33(5): 453-60.

Olivry, T. & P. Bizikova (2013). A systematic review of randomized controlled trials for prevention or treatment of atopic dermatitis in dogs: 2008-2011 update. Veterinary Dermatology 24(1): 97-+.

Olivry, T., et al. (2013). Evidence-based guidelines for anti-allergic drug withdrawal times before allergen-specific intradermal and IgE serological tests in dogs. Veterinary Dermatology 24(2).

Olsen, L., et al. (2007). Cetirizine in horses: pharmacokinetics and effect of ivermectin pretreatment. J. Vet. Pharmacol. Ther. 30(3): 194-200.

Plevnik, A., et al. (2009). The Efficacy of Antihistamine Fexofenadine versus Methylprednisolone in the Treatment of Atopic Dermatitis in Dogs. Slovenian Veterinary Research 46(1): 5-12.

Plevnik, A., et al. (2006). Fexofenadine treatment of atopic dogs: Preliminary clinical results. Acta Veterinaria Brno 75(4): 549-55.

Filgrastim (Granulocyte Colony Stimulating Factor; GCSF)

(fill-grass-stim)   Neupogen®

Cytokine Hematopoietic Agent

Prescriber Highlights

► Cytokine that in the bone marrow primarily increases the proliferation, differentiation, & activation of progenitor cells in the neutrophil-granulocyte line.

► Human origin product; antibodies may form that can cause prolonged neutropenia.

► Treatment is very expensive.

Uses/Indications

Filgrastim may be of benefit in treating neutropenias in dogs, cats or foals. It should be used only when the intrinsic response to endogenously produced cytokines is thought inadequate and there is evidence that there are precursors in the bone marrow available. Because of the drug's cost, potential for antibody development and the lack of good evidence for its efficacy in reducing mortality versus using antibiotic therapy alone, its use in veterinary medicine is controversial.

Pharmacology/Actions

Filgrastim is a hematopoietic agent that primarily affects bone marrow to increase the proliferation, differentiation, and activation of progenitor cells in the neutrophil-granulocyte line. While derived from human DNA, the product is not species specific on its effects on bone marrow.

Pharmacokinetics

After subcutaneous injection, filgrastim is rapidly absorbed and distributed with highest concentrations found in the bone marrow, liver, kidneys and adrenal glands. It is unknown if it crosses the blood-brain barrier, placenta, or enters maternal milk. The elimination pathways of filgrastim are still under investigation.

Contraindications/Precautions/Warnings

Filgrastim is contraindicated in patients hypersensitive to it. Dogs or cats that have developed antibodies to filgrastim with resultant neutropenia should probably not receive it in the future.

Adverse Effects

Because the human DNA origin product can be immunogenic to dogs and cats, some patients may develop severe neutropenia by mounting an immune response against both endogenously produced and exogenously administered G-CSF. Studies in cats have demonstrated that short pulse doses of 3-5 days at the time of neutropenia may be safe and minimize the development of neutrophil neutralizing antibodies. Preliminary studies using canine origin G-CSF have not demonstrated autoantibody formation in either dogs or cats.

Additionally, there are concerns that exogenously administered filgrastim can cause undesirable responses in other tissues, including myelofibrosis and medullary histiocytosis.

Occasionally irritation at the injection site may occur. Bone pain, splenomegaly, and hypotension have been reported in humans.

Reproductive/Nursing Safety

Adverse effects in females and offspring have been demonstrated after filgrastim was administered to pregnant laboratory animals at high dosages. To interpret this data for use in a clinical setting is difficult, but filgrastim should be used in pregnant females only when the benefits of treating outweigh the potential risks. In humans, the FDA categorizes this drug as category *C* for use during pregnancy (*Animal studies have shown an adverse effect on the fetus, but there are no adequate studies in humans; or there are no animal reproduction studies and no adequate studies in humans.*)

It is not known whether filgrastim is excreted in milk, but it is unlikely to pose significant risk to nursing offspring.

Overdosage/Acute Toxicity

Limited information is available. Because of the expense of the drug and its apparent limited acute toxic potential, clinically significant overdoses are unlikely.

Drug Interactions

The following drug interactions have either been reported or are theoretical in humans or animals receiving filgrastim and may be of significance in veterinary patients. Unless otherwise noted, use together is not necessarily contraindicated, but weigh the potential risks and perform additional monitoring when appropriate.

■ **ANTINEOPLASTICS:** While filgrastim was developed primarily to prevent neutropenia associated with some chemotherapeutic agents, some controversy exists about using filgrastim within 24 hours of a dose of antineoplastic agents that target rapidly proliferating cells; generally, in human medicine, use is avoided within 24 hours of such antineoplastics.

Doses

Note: To avoid the development of autoantibody formation, most clinicians that use this agent in dogs or cats recommend a "pulse" therapy of no more than 5 days in duration.

- **DOGS/CATS:**

  For adjunctive therapy of neutropenia (extra-label): No consensus or evidence was located on any dosing strategy for this agent in animals. Most commonly a dosage of 5 micrograms/kg SC daily is recommended. Some have suggested dosages as low as 1 microgram/kg daily and up to 5 micrograms/kg SC twice daily.

- **HORSES:**

  For the treatment of neutropenia in foals (extra-label): From a retrospective study (abstract) of the 13 foals that were dosed at 5 micrograms/kg SC; 8 were discharged, 5 died or were euthanized. From the data the authors concluded that the use of filgrastim in foals was safe; adverse effects were not observed. Leukopenic foals treated with filgrastim that survived to discharge tended to have higher mean WBC, higher percent of neutrophils, and lower percent of band neutrophils than foals that did not survive.

Monitoring

- CBC with platelets, routinely.

Client Information

- Clients should be briefed on the cost of this agent as well as the possibility that it may cause antibodies to form against endogenously produced G-CSF, thereby causing a potentially life threatening neutropenia.

Chemistry/Synonyms

Prepared via recombinant DNA technology from human DNA, filgrastim is a single chain polypeptide containing 175 amino acids with a molecular weight of about 18,800 daltons. The commercially available injection occurs as a clear solution; buffered to a pH of 4.

Filgrastim may also be known as: granulocyte colony-stimulating factor, G-CSF, recombinant methionyl human GCS-F, r-metHuG-CSF, *Filgen*®, *Gran*®, *Granulen*®, *Granulokine*®, *Neulasta*®, *Neupogen*®, and *Neutromax*®.

Storage/Stability

Injection should be stored in the refrigerator (2-8°C). Do not freeze or shake contents of vial.

Compatibility/Compounding Considerations

The drug should never be diluted with saline as a precipitate may form. If necessary it may be diluted into 5% dextrose for injection, but if diluted to concentrations between 5-15 micrograms/mL, it is recommended that albumin be added to the solution to a concentration of 2 mg/mL to reduce adsorption to plastic IV tubing. It is not recommended to dilute to concentrations of less than 5 micrograms/mL.

Dosage Forms/Regulatory Status

VETERINARY-LABELED PRODUCTS: NONE.

HUMAN-LABELED PRODUCTS:

Filgrastim Injection: 300 micrograms/mL preservative free in 1 mL and 1.6 mL single dose vials; 300 micrograms/0.5 mL preservative free in 0.5 mL and 0.8 mL prefilled syringes; *Neupogen*®; (Rx)

Revisions/References

Monograph revised/updated January 2014.

Finasteride

(fin-as-te-ride)   Proscar®, Propecia®

5-Alpha-Reductase Inhibitor

Prescriber Highlights

- ▶ 5-alpha-reductase inhibitor potentially useful for dogs with benign prostatic hypertrophy & ferrets with adrenal disease.
- ▶ Contraindications: Hypersensitivity to finasteride; sexually developing animals.
- ▶ Caution: Patients with significant hepatic impairment.
- ▶ Adverse Effects: Potentially may cause some minor sexual side effects.
- ▶ Expense may be an issue, but generics now available.

Uses/Indications

Finasteride may be useful in treating the benign prostatic hypertrophy in canine patients, particularly those that are used for breeding. Because of the drug's relative expense and the long duration of therapy required to see a response (up to 8 weeks), its usefulness may be limited in veterinary medicine.

It may also be useful in the adjunctive treatment of adrenal disease in ferrets.

Pharmacology/Actions

Finasteride specifically and totally inhibits 5-alpha-reductase. This enzyme is responsible for metabolizing testosterone to dihydrotestosterone (DHT) in the prostate, liver and skin. DHT is a potent androgen and the primary hormone responsible for the development of the prostate. In dogs with BPH, clinical effects may be noted in as little as one week, but full efficacy may require up to 8 weeks of treatment.

Pharmacokinetics

Finasteride is absorbed after oral administration and in humans about 65% is bioavailable. The presence of food does not affect absorption. It is distributed across the blood-brain barrier and is found in seminal fluid. In humans, about 90% is bound to plasma proteins. Finasteride is metabolized in the liver and the half-life is about 6 hours. Metabolites are excreted in the urine and feces. In humans, a single daily dose suppresses DHT concentrations for 24 hours.

Contraindications/Precautions/Warnings

Finasteride is contraindicated in patients hypersensitive to it. It should be used with caution in patients with significant hepatic impairment as metabolism of the drug may be reduced. Finasteride should be used in males only; do not use in sexually developing animals.

Adverse Effects

One study done in dogs reported no adverse effects or irreversibility of effects after treating for 21 weeks at 1 mg/kg. Potentially finasteride may reduce semen volume while maintaining semen quality in breeding dogs. Clinical signs begin to resolve after one week of therapy.

Adverse effects reported in humans have been very limited, mild and transient. Decreased libido, decreased ejaculate volume, and impotence have been reported.

Reproductive/Nursing Safety

In humans, the FDA categorizes this drug as category X for use during pregnancy (*Studies in animals or humans demonstrate fetal abnormalities or adverse reaction; reports indicate evidence of fetal risk. The risk of use in pregnant women clearly outweighs any possible benefit.*)

Finasteride is not indicated for use in females. It is not known whether finasteride is excreted in milk.

Overdosage/Acute Toxicity

Limited information is available; gastrointestinal effects may be noted.

Drug Interactions

The following drug interactions have either been reported or are theoretical in humans or animals receiving finasteride and may be of significance in veterinary patients. Unless otherwise noted, use together is not necessarily contraindicated, but weigh the potential risks and perform additional monitoring when appropriate.

- **ANTICHOLINERGIC DRUGS:** May precipitate or aggravate urinary retention thereby negating the effects of the drug when used for BPH.

Doses

- **DOGS:**

    For benign prostatic hypertrophy (extra-label): Castration is considered the treatment of choice, but finasteride may be tried in dogs that are potentially to be used for breeding. Controlled studies were not located evaluating efficacy, but dosages of 0.1 – 0.5 mg/kg PO once daily are often noted. Because of available commercial dosage forms (1 mg & 5 mg tablets) dosages are often rounded to the nearest full or half tablet. 5 mg is generally the maximum dosage given.

- **FERRETS:**

    For adjunctive treatment of adrenal disease (extra-label): No controlled studies are available for this use, but 5 mg per ferret PO once daily has been noted.

Monitoring

- Efficacy: Prostate exam in dogs.

Client Information

- May be given with or without food. If your animal vomits or acts sick after getting it on an empty stomach, give with food or small treat to see if this helps. If vomiting continues, contact your veterinarian.
- Limited experience in veterinary medicine; could possibly cause GI effects (*e.g.,* vomiting, diarrhea, etc.).
- May take several weeks to determine if the drug is working; do not skip dosages.
- Pregnant women should use caution when handling this medication.

Chemistry/Synonyms

Finasteride is a 4-azasteroid synthetic drug that inhibits 5 alpha-dihydroreductase (DH), and has a molecular weight of 372.55.

Finasteride may also be known as: finasteridum, MK-0906, and MK-906; many trade names are available.

Storage/Stability

Store tablets below 30°C in tight containers and protected from light.

Compatibility/Compounding Considerations

No specific information noted.

Dosage Forms/Regulatory Status

VETERINARY-LABELED PRODUCTS: NONE.

HUMAN-LABELED PRODUCTS:

Finasteride Oral Tablets: 1 mg & 5 mg; *Proscar*®, *Propecia*®, generic; (Rx)

Revisions/References

Monograph revised/updated January 2014.

Fipronil – See the listing in the Dermatological Agents, Topical Appendix

Firocoxib

(feer-oh-koks-ib)   Previcox®, Equioxx®

Oral COX-2 Inhibitor (NSAID)

Prescriber Highlights

- ▶ Oral COX-2 NSAID labeled for the control of pain & inflammation associated with osteoarthritis in dogs & horses.
- ▶ Adverse effects in **dogs**: GI effects (vomiting, anorexia) most likely, but serious effects are possible.
- ▶ Adverse effects in **horses** include mouth ulcers, facial skin lesions, & excitation (rare).

Uses/Indications

Firocoxib is indicated in dogs and horses for the control of pain and inflammation associated with osteoarthritis and in dogs for the control of post-operative pain and inflammation associated with orthopedic surgery. A chewable tablet form for dogs and an oral paste for horses are available.

Like other NSAIDs, firocoxib can be useful for treating fever, pain, and/or inflammation associated with other conditions, post-surgery, trauma, etc.

In dogs with transitional cell carcinoma, firocoxib had antitumor effects and significantly enhanced the antitumor activity of cisplatin. Potentially it could be useful as a palliative treatment (Knapp et al. 2013).

Firocoxib may also be useful in other species, but information is scant regarding its safety and efficacy. One study in cats (McCann et al. 2005) evaluating firocoxib in experimentally induced pyrexia, demonstrated that the drug was effective after a single oral dose in preventing or attenuating pyrexia at all doses studied (0.75 – 3 mg/kg).

Pharmacology/Actions

Firocoxib is a coxib-class, nonsteroidal antiinflammatory drug (NSAID). It is believed to predominantly inhibit cyclooxygenase-2 (COX-2) and spare COX-1 at therapeutic dosages. This theoretically would inhibit production of the prostaglandins that contribute to pain and inflammation (COX-2) and spare those that maintain normal gastrointestinal, platelet and renal function (COX-1). However, COX-1 and COX-2 inhibition studies are done *in vitro* and do not necessarily correlate perfectly with clinical effects seen in actual patients.

Firocoxib also has some anti-tumor activity and it may find a role in treating cancer in animals.

Pharmacokinetics

In dogs, firocoxib absorption after oral dosing varies among individuals. Oral bioavailability with the chewable tablets, on average, is about 38%. Food will delay, but not affect the amount absorbed. Peak levels occur about 1 hour after dosing if fasted, and 5 hours if the patient is fed. Volume of distribution at steady state is about 3 L/kg; it is 96% bound to plasma proteins. Biotransformation occurs predominantly via dealkylation and glucuronidation in the liver; elimination is principally in the bile and feces. Elimination half-life in dogs is approximately 6-8 hours.

In horses, oral availability after administering the paste is approximately 79%. Peak levels occur 4-12 hours after dosing. Volume of distribution at steady state is about 1.7-2.3 L/kg and it is 98% bound to plasma proteins. Biotransformation in horses occurs primarily via decyclopropylmethylation and then glucuronidation. Metabolites are primarily excreted in the urine. Elimination half-life is approximately 30-40 hours. In neonatal foals, firocoxib at 0.1 mg/kg q24h for nine consecutive days, was rapidly absorbed and a maximum plasma concentration was reached in 30 minutes after the first dosage. Estimated terminal elimination half-life was approximately 11 hours after the last dose (Hovanessian et al. 2011).

Pharmacokinetics of firocoxib have only been reported in two cats studied (McCann et al. 2005). Oral bioavailability after administering an oral suspension was about 60% and the volume of distribution, between 2-3 L/kg. Elimination half-life in the two cats studied averaged about 10 hours.

Contraindications/Precautions/Warnings

Firocoxib should not be used in animals hypersensitive to it or other NSAIDs. The drug should be used with caution and enhanced monitoring in patients with preexisting renal, hepatic or cardiovascular dysfunction, and those that are dehydrated, hypovolemic, hypotensive, or on concomitant diuretic therapy. Because geriatric patients have reduced renal function and firocoxib is often used for osteoarthritis in this patient population, ongoing monitoring for adverse effects is mandatory.

The product's label states that it cannot be accurately dosed in dogs less than 12.5 pounds (5.7 kg) body weight.

Because all NSAIDs can potentially cause GI toxicity, firocoxib is relatively contraindicated in dogs with active GI ulcerative conditions. As it may affect platelet function, it is relatively contraindicated in patients with bleeding disorders or thrombocytopenia, but one study done in dogs did not show any changes on platelet aggregation (Roiz Martin et al. 2009).

A chronic dosing (5 mg/kg for 6 months) study performed in puppies 10-13 weeks old, showed subclinical periportal hepatic fatty changes in half the dogs studied. Higher doses (15 – 25 mg/kg; 3-5X) in this age range caused increased rates of hepatic fatty changes; some dogs died or were euthanized due to moribund conditions. The manufacturer states in the package insert: "Use of this product at doses above the recommended 5 mg/kg in puppies less than 7 months old has been associated with serious adverse reactions, including death" and "…this product cannot be accurately dosed in dogs weighing less than seven pounds in body weight." The labeling in the UK states that it should not be used in dogs "less than 10 weeks of age."

If changing from one NSAID to another in dogs for reasons of efficacy, consider a washout period between agents. While the actual length of time between agents is controversial and opinions vary widely, often a 24-hour washout period between COX-2 selective agents is recommended. Recommendations for washout periods before starting a COX-2 selective agent after using a non-selective agent or aspirin are usually much longer (72 hours to 1 week).

For horses, the labeling states that the safety of firocoxib in horses less than one year old, horses used for breeding, or in pregnant or lactating mares has not been established and treatment should be terminated in horses if signs such as inappetence, colic, abnormal feces, or lethargy are observed.

Adverse Effects

Because firocoxib is a relatively new product, its adverse effect profile in dogs is yet to be fully determined. In pre-approval studies (128 dogs treated), vomiting and decreased appetite/anorexia were the most common adverse effects noted with an approximate incidence rate of 4% and 2%, respectively. The drug sponsor has a toll-free overdose hotline in the USA: 877-217-3543.

In the FDA's CVM Cumulative Adverse Drug Experiences (ADE) Summaries Report (through 4/30/2013) for firocoxib in dogs, the most prevalent ADE reported was vomiting followed by anorexia. Other effects on this list included (in decreasing order): increases in BUN, depression/lethargy, alkaline phosphatase and ALT, creatinine,, and diarrhea,. It should be noted that this data reflects voluntary reporting to the FDA and does not reflect actual incidence rates, nor is causation necessarily proven.

In pre-approval studies done in horses treated for 14 days, diarrhea/loose stools were seen in about 2%. Excitation was rarely (<1%) detected. In safety studies, oral lesions/ulcers were seen in some horses after dosages of 1-5X were given.

Reproductive/Nursing Safety

Information on the safety of firocoxib in breeding, pregnant or lactating dogs or horses is not available. Studies performed in pregnant rabbits at dosages approximating those given to dogs, demonstrated maternotoxic and fetotoxic effects.

Overdosage/Acute Toxicity

Limited information is available for acute overdoses in animals. The reported oral LD50 for rats is > 2 grams per kg. Should an overdose occur, contacting an animal poison control center or the manufacturer (1-877-217-3543) is highly recommended. Use of gut emptying protocols and supportive treatment (IV fluids, oral sucralfate, etc.) may be useful in managing the case.

Drug Interactions

In the package insert for *Previcox®*, the manufacturer states the following (**Note**: bold *mine—Plumb*): "As a class, cyclooxygenase inhibitory NSAIDs may be associated with renal and gastrointestinal toxicity. Sensitivity to drug-associated adverse events varies with the individual patient. Patients at greatest risk for renal toxicity are those that are dehydrated, on concomitant **diuretic therapy**, or those with existing renal, cardiovascular, and/or hepatic dysfunction. Concurrent administration of **potentially nephrotoxic drugs** should be carefully approached. NSAIDs may inhibit the prostaglandins that maintain normal homeostatic function. Such antiprostaglandin effects may result in clinically significant disease in patients with underlying or pre-existing disease that has not been previously diagnosed. Since many NSAIDs possess the potential to produce gastrointestinal ulcerations, concomitant use with other antiinflammatory drugs, such as **NSAIDs** or **corticosteroids**, should be avoided or closely monitored. The concomitant use of **protein bound drugs** with *Previcox®* Chewable Tablets has not been studied in dogs. Commonly used **protein-bound drugs** include cardiac, anticonvulsant, and behavioral medications. The influence of concomitant drugs that may inhibit the metabolism of *Previcox®* Chewable Tablets has not been evaluated."

Drug interactions reported in humans taking NSAIDS, that may be of significance in veterinary patients receiving firocoxib include:

- **ACE INHIBITORS** (*e.g., enalapril, benazepril*): Some NSAIDs can reduce effects on blood pressure.
- **ASPIRIN**: May increase the risk of gastrointestinal toxicity (*e.g.*, ulceration, bleeding, vomiting, diarrhea).
- **CORTICOSTEROIDS** (*e.g.,* **prednisone**): May increase the risk of gastrointestinal toxicity (*e.g.*, ulceration, bleeding, vomiting, diarrhea).
- **DIGOXIN**: NSAIDS may increase serum levels.
- **FLUCONAZOLE**: Administration has increased plasma levels of celecoxib in humans and potentially could also affect firocoxib levels in dogs.
- **FUROSEMIDE**: NSAIDs may reduce the saluretic and diuretic effects.
- **HIGHLY PROTEIN BOUND DRUGS** (**phenytoin, valproic acid, oral anticoagulants, other antiinflammatory agents, salicylates, sulfonamides, sulfonylurea antidiabetic agents**): As firocoxib is highly bound to plasma proteins (95-98%), it may displace other highly bound drugs or these agents could displace firocoxib. Increased serum levels, duration of actions and toxicity could occur.
- **METHOTREXATE**: Serious toxicity has occurred when NSAIDs have been used concomitantly with **methotrexate**; use together with extreme caution.

- NEPHROTOXIC DRUGS (*e.g.*, **furosemide, aminoglycosides, amphotericin B**, etc.): May enhance the risk of nephrotoxicity development.

Laboratory Considerations
- No specific laboratory concerns; see Monitoring.

Doses
- **DOGS:**

  For the control of pain and inflammation associated with osteoarthritis and for the control of postoperative pain and inflammation associated with soft-tissue and orthopedic surgery in dogs (labeled indication; FDA-approved): 5 mg/kg (2.27 mg/lb.) PO once daily as needed for osteoarthritis and for 3 days as needed for postoperative pain and inflammation associated with soft-tissue and orthopedic surgery. Dosage should be calculated in half tablet increments and can be administered with or without food. Use the lowest effective dose for the shortest duration consistent with individual response. (Adapted from package insert; *Previcox®*), (Kondo et al. 2012; Davila et al. 2013)

  As an adjunctive treatment for transitional cell carcinoma of the bladder (extra-label): In the study, firocoxib at 5 mg/kg PO q24h was used alone and in combination with cisplatin (60 mg/m² IV q21d). (Knapp et al. 2013)

- **CATS:**

  Caution: While firocoxib may ultimately be shown to be safe for use in cats, FDA approval or supporting evidence is not currently available for it to be recommended.

- **HORSES:**

  For the control of pain and inflammation associated with osteoarthritis (Labeled indication; FDA-approved):

  Oral: 0.1 mg/kg (0.045 mg/lb.) body weight PO with or without food daily for up to 14 days. (Adapted from package insert; *Equioxx*—Merial)

  Parenteral: 0.09 mg/kg (0.04 mg/lb.) IV once daily for up to 5 days. If further treatment is needed, the oral paste can be used at 0.1 mg/kg PO for additional 9 days of treatment. Overall duration of treatment with injection and oral paste will be dependent on the response observed, but should not exceed 14 days. (Adapted from label; *Equioxx® Injection*)

Monitoring
- Baseline and periodic physical exam including clinical efficacy and adverse effect queries.
- Baseline and periodic: CBC, liver function, renal function, and electrolytes; urinalysis.

Client Information
- The manufacturer provides a client handout that is recommended to be distributed each time the drug is dispensed.
- For dogs: Can give with or without food, but food may reduce the chances for stomach problems. If your animal vomits or acts sick after getting it on an empty stomach, give with food or small treat to see if this helps. If vomiting continues, contact your veterinarian.
- Most dogs usually tolerate very it well, but rarely some will develop ulcers or serious kidney and liver problems. Watch for these: Eating more or less than normal, vomiting, changes in bowel movements; changes in behavior or activity levels (more or less active than normal), incoordination (*e.g.*, stumbling, clumsiness, etc.), seizures (convulsions) or aggression, yellowing of gums, skin, or whites of the eyes (jaundice); changes in drinking habits (frequency, amount consumed) or urination habits (frequency, color, or smell).
- Store chewable tablets well out of reach of animals and children.

- For dogs: Periodic lab tests to check for liver and kidney side effects are required.
- For horses, contact veterinarian if patient develops ulcers or sores on tongue or in mouth, sores or lesions on facial skin or lips, diarrhea/loose stools, changes in behavior/activity, changes in feed or water consumption, or yellowing of whites of eyes or mucous membranes. Don't use with other NSAIDs (*e.g.*, flunixin, phenylbutazone, aspirin).

Chemistry/Synonyms
Firocoxib occurs a white crystalline powder. The commercially available injection occurs as a colorless to pale yellow solution.

Firocoxib may also be known as: 3-(cyclopropylmethoxy)-5,5-dimethyl-4-(4-methylsulfonyl) phenylfuran-2(5H)-on or ML-1,785,713, *Equioxx®*, and *Previcox®*.

Storage/Stability
Commercially available tablets and oral paste should be stored at room temperature (15-30°C); brief excursions are permitted up to 40°C (104°F). The injection should be stored at 20-25°C with excursions between 15-30°C permitted.

Compatibility/Compounding Considerations
The injection is a non-aqueous solution and should not be mixed with aqueous solutions. Do not flush through intravenous lines using aqueous flush solutions.

Dosage Forms/Regulatory Status
VETERINARY-LABELED PRODUCTS:

Firocoxib Chewable Tablets (scored): 57 mg, & 227 mg; *Previcox®*; (Rx). FDA-approved (NADA 141-230) for use in dogs. The product label for *Previcox®* can be found at dailymed.nlm.nih.gov

Firocoxib Oral Paste: 0.82% w/w (8.2 mg firocoxib per gram of paste) in a 6.93 gram oral syringe (total of 56.8 mg of firocoxib per syringe); *Equioxx Oral Paste®*; (Rx). Approved (NADA 141-253) for use in horses. The product label for *Equioxx Paste®* can be found at dailymed.nlm.nih.gov

Firocoxib Injection: 20 mg/mL in 25 mL vials; *Equioxx® Injection*; (Rx). FDA-approved (NADA 141-313) for use in horses. Do not use in horses intended for human consumption. The product label for *Equioxx Injection®* can be found at dailymed.nlm.nih.gov

Firocoxib use may be restricted in racing animals; contact local racing authority for additional guidance. The ARCI UCGFS classifies it as a class-4 substance.

HUMAN-LABELED PRODUCTS: NONE.

Revisions/References
Monograph revised/updated January 2014.

Bartges, J. (2006). Broken plumbing: urinary incontinence. Proceedings: ACVC 2006. accessed via Veterinary Information Network; vin.com

Davila, D., et al. (2013). Comparison of the analgesic efficacy of perioperative firocoxib and tramadol administration in dogs undergoing tibial plateau leveling osteotomy. Javma-Journal of the American Veterinary Medical Association 243(2): 225-31.

Hovanessian, N., et al. (2011). Pharmacokinetics of Firocoxib in Neonatal Foals. ACVIM accessed via Veterinary Information Network; vin.com

Knapp, D. W., et al. (2013). Randomized Trial of Cisplatin versus Firocoxib versus Cisplatin/Firocoxib in Dogs with Transitional Cell Carcinoma of the Urinary Bladder. Journal of Veterinary Internal Medicine 27(1): 126-33.

Kondo, Y., et al. (2012). Efficacy and Safety of Firocoxib for the Treatment of Pain Associated with Soft Tissue Surgery in Dogs under Field Conditions in Japan. Journal of Veterinary Medical Science 74(10): 1283-9.

McCann, M., et al. (2005). In vitro effects and in vivo efficacy of a novel cyclooxygenase-2 inhibitor in cats with lipopolysaccharide-induced pyrexia. AJVR 66(7): 1278-84.

Roiz Martin, S., et al. (2009). Evaluation of the Effects of Firocoxib on Platelet Function of Healthy Dogs Studied By PFA-100. Proceedings: ECVIM. accessed via Veterinary Information Network; vin.com

Fish Oil – See Fatty Acids

Flavoxate HCl

(fla-vox-ate)   Urispas®

Parasympathetic Blocker; Urinary Antispasmodic

Prescriber Highlights

▶ Alternative medication to treat detrusor hyperspasticity (hyperactive bladder; urge incontinence) in dogs.

▶ Not commonly used; little information available on veterinary use. Must be dosed frequently (3-4 times per day).

▶ Most likely adverse effect is weakness, but may also cause anticholinergic effects.

Uses/Indications

Flavoxate may be considered for treating dogs with detrusor hyperspasticity (hyperactive bladder, urge incontinence). Flavoxate, propantheline or oxybutynin can be particularly useful in dogs where phenylpropanolamine alone has not resulted in continence.

Pharmacology/Actions

Flavoxate has direct smooth muscle relaxing properties and antimuscarinic effects.

Pharmacokinetics

No information was located for dogs or cats. In humans, the drug's onset of action is within an hour with peak effects at around 2 hours post dose. 57% of a dose is excreted in the urine within 24 hours.

Contraindications/Precautions/Warnings

Flavoxate is contraindicated in human patients with pyloric or duodenal obstruction, obstructive intestinal lesions or ileus, achalasia, GI hemorrhage or obstructive uropathies of the lower urinary tract. It is to be used with caution in patients with suspected glaucoma.

Adverse Effects

Weakness is the most likely adverse effect seen in dogs treated with flavoxate, but it mays also cause anticholinergic effects (dry mouth, constipation, tachycardia, etc.).

Reproductive/Nursing Safety

In laboratory animals, doses of up to 34X (human dose) demonstrated no harm to fetuses or impaired fertility. In humans, flavoxate is designated by the FDA as a category *B* drug (*Animal studies have not demonstrated risk to the fetus, but there are no adequate studies in pregnant women; or animal studies have shown an adverse effect, but adequate studies in pregnant women have not demonstrated a risk to the fetus during the first trimester of pregnancy, and there is no evidence of risk in later trimesters.*)

It is not known whether this drug is excreted into milk; use with caution in nursing mothers.

Overdosage/Acute Toxicity

The approximate oral LD-50 for rats and mice are 4300 mg/kg and 1800 mg/kg respectively.

Drug Interactions

▪ No significant drug interactions with flavoxate were located, however concomitant use with other **anticholinergic drugs** may cause additive effects.

Laboratory Considerations

▪ No concerns noted.

Doses

▪ **DOGS:**

To decrease urinary bladder contractility (extra-label): Not commonly used and no substantial evidence is available to recommend, but may be tried at 100 – 200 mg (per dog) PO q6-8h. (Bartges 2006)

Monitoring

▪ Clinical efficacy.

▪ Adverse effects (most likely GI).

▪ Consider occasional CBC's and creatinine to monitor for neutropenia or renal dysfunction if using the drug chronically.

Client Information

▪ May give with or without food. If your animal vomits or acts sick after getting it on an empty stomach, give with food or small treat to see if this helps. If vomiting continues, contact your veterinarian.

▪ Not much experience with this drug in animals. Most likely side effects are vomiting, diarrhea and muscle weakness.

Chemistry/Synonyms

Flavoxate HCl occurs as a white or almost white crystalline powder. It is slightly soluble in water or alcohol.

Flavoxate may also be known as flavoxato, AK 123, or Rec 7-0040. A common trade name is *Urispas®*.

Storage/Stability

Flavoxate tablets should be stored at room temperature (15-30°C).

Compatibility/Compounding Considerations

No specific information noted.

Dosage Forms/Regulatory Status

VETERINARY-LABELED PRODUCTS: NONE.

HUMAN-LABELED PRODUCTS:

Flavoxate HCl Oral Tablets (film-coated): 100 mg; *Urispas®*, generic; (Rx)

Revisions/References

Monograph revised/updated January 2014.

Florfenicol

(flor-fen-i-col)   NuFlor®

Antibiotic

Prescriber Highlights

▶ Broad spectrum antibiotic FDA-approved for use in cattle, swine, & fish, but may be useful in other species (*e.g.*, dogs, cats).

▶ Contraindications: Do not give IV. Not for use in veal calves or cattle of breeding age (per manufacturer).

▶ Adverse Effects: Cattle: Anorexia, decreased water consumption, diarrhea, injection site reactions (may result in trim loss); IM injection may be painful in small animals.

▶ Slaughter withdrawals depend upon route of administration (IM shorter than SC).

Uses/Indications

The drug is FDA-approved for use in cattle only (in the USA) for the treatment of bovine respiratory disease (BRD) associated with *Mannheimia haemolytica*, *Pasteurella multocida*, *Histophilus somni*, and *Mycoplasma bovis*.

Because florfenicol has activity against a wide range of microorganisms, it may be useful for treating other infections in cattle (or other species) as well, but specific data is limited.

The combination product containing florfenicol and flunixin (*Resflor Gold®*) is FDA-approved for SC use in beef and non-lactating dairy cattle (not veal calves) for treatment of BRD associated with *Mannheimia haemolytica*, *Pasteurella multocida*, *Histophilus somni*, *Mycoplasma bovis* and control BRD-associated pyrexia.

Pharmacology/Actions

Like chloramphenicol, florfenicol is a broad-spectrum antibiotic that has activity against many bacteria. It acts by binding to the 50S ribosome, thereby inhibiting bacterial protein synthesis.

Pharmacokinetics

After IM injection in cattle, approximately 79% of the dose is bioavailable. The drug appears to be well distributed throughout the body, including achievement of therapeutic levels in the CSF. In cattle, the volume of distribution is about 0.7 L/kg and only about 13% is bound to serum proteins. Mean serum half-life is 18 hours, but wide interpatient variation exists. When dosed at 40 mg/kg IM, serum levels are above the MIC_{90} (1 microgram/mL) for *M. haemolytica* for 72 hours and above MIC_{90} (0.5 micrograms/mL) for *P. multocida* and *H. somnus* for 96 hours.

In dogs, florfenicol is absorbed poorly after subcutaneous injection and has an elimination half-life of less than 5 hours. After IV administration, total body clearance is approximately 1 L/kg/hour PO administration results in good bioavailability (95%), but the drug is eliminated rapidly (elimination half-life 1.25 hours) (Park et al. 2008).

Cats have high absorption of a 100 mg/mL solution when either given IM or orally and an elimination half-life of less than 5 hours. Time duration above an MIC of 2 mg/mL were 12 hours (IM) and 18 hours (PO); and above an MIC of 8 mg/mL were 10 hours (IM) and 6 hours (PO), respectively, in cats.

In sheep, florfenicol elimination half-life is about 9 hours and has a mean residence time of approximately 20 hours for its major metabolite (FFC-a). Based upon these values the authors agreed with an earlier study in which a calculated withdrawal time of 42 days was determined (Lane et al. 2007; Palma et al. 2012).

Contraindications/Precautions/Warnings

Not for use in animals intended for breeding purposes. The effects of florfenicol on bovine reproductive performance, pregnancy, and lactation have not been determined. Also see the residue warnings in the Dosage Forms section.

Do not use in female dairy cattle 20 months of age or older. Do not use in calves to be processed for veal.

Note: Do **NOT** give this drug IV.

Adverse Effects

Noted transient adverse reactions in cattle include anorexia, decreased water consumption, or diarrhea. Injection site reactions can occur that may result in trim loss. Reactions may be more severe if injected at sites other than the neck. Anaphylaxis and collapse have been reported in cattle.

When used in other species (mammals), gastrointestinal effects, including severe diarrheas are potentially possible.

Reproductive/Nursing Safety

Safety or adverse effects when used in breeding cattle or swine, during pregnancy, or during lactation are unknown and the manufacturer states that the drug is not for use in cattle of breeding age or swine intended for breeding.

Overdosage/Acute Toxicity

In toxicology studies where feeder calves were injected with up to 10X the recommended dosage, the adverse effects noted above were seen, plus increased serum enzymes. These effects were generally transient in nature. Long-term (43 day) standard dosage studies showed a transient decrease in feed consumption, but no long-term negative effects were noted.

Drug Interactions

No specific drug interactions for florfenicol were located, but the drug may behave similarly to chloramphenicol. If so, florfenicol could antagonize the bactericidal activity of **penicillins** or **aminoglycosides**. This antagonism has not been demonstrated *in vivo*, and these drug combinations have been used successfully many times clinically. Other antibiotics that bind to the 50S ribosomal subunit of susceptible bacteria (**erythromycin, clindamycin, lincomycin, tylosin**, etc.) may potentially antagonize the activity of chloramphenicol or vice versa, but the clinical significance of this potential interaction has not been determined. For other drug interactions that florfenicol may share with chloramphenicol, see the monograph for chloramphenicol or refer to other drug information resources.

Doses

- **CATTLE:**

  Labeled Indications/Dosages (FDA-approved):

  For treatment of BRD: 20 mg/kg IM (in neck muscle only); repeat in 48 hours. Alternatively, a single 40 mg/kg SC dose (in neck) may be used. **Note:** 20 mg/kg equates to 3 mL of the injection per 100 lb. of body weight. Do not exceed 10 mL per injection site. (Package Insert; *Nuflor®*)

  For treatment of bovine respiratory disease (BRD) associated with *Mannheimia haemolytica, Pasteurella multocida, Histophilus somni*, and *Mycoplasma bovis* in beef and non-lactating dairy cattle: 40 mg/kg (6 mL/100 lb. body weight) administered once by SC injection. Do not administer more than 15 mL at each site. The injection should be given only in the neck. Injection sites other than the neck have not been evaluated. (Label Information; *Nuflor Gold®*)

  For the treatment bovine respiratory disease (BRD) associated with *Mannheimia haemolytica, Pasteurella multocida*, and *Histophilus somni*, and control of BRD-associated pyrexia in beef and non-lactating dairy cattle. Using the combination product containing florfenicol and flunixin (*Resflor Gold®*): 40 mg/kg florfenicol and 2.2 mg/kg flunixin (6 mL/100 lb. body weight) SC once. Do not administer more than 10 mL at each site. The injection should be given only in the neck. Injection sites other than the neck have not been evaluated. (Label Information — *Resflor Gold®*)

- **DOGS:**

  For susceptible systemic (bacterial or rickettsial) infections when myelotoxic potential (in humans or animals) of chloramphenicol is to be avoided (extra-label): The half-life of florfenicol is very rapid in dogs and the drug must be dosed fairly often (q6-8h). It has been suggested that the injectable form can be administered orally, but because the drug is very bitter, patient acceptance may be problematic. Published dosage recommendations are scant, variable and range from 20 mg/kg IM or PO q6h to 20 – 50 mg/kg PO, SC or IM q8h.

- **CATS:**

  For susceptible systemic infections (bacterial or rickettsial) infections when myelotoxic potential (in humans or animals) of chloramphenicol is to be avoided (extra-label): The half-life of florfenicol in cats is longer than in dogs, but it still must be dosed fairly frequently (q8-12h). Oral administration (using the injectable) is possible, but the drug's bitterness is problematic. Dosage recommendations are scant, variable and range from 20 – 50 mg/kg PO, SC or IM q8h to 22 mg/kg IM, PO q12h for 3-5 days.

- **SHEEP & GOATS:**

  For respiratory disease complex in kids (extra-label): 20 mg/kg a day (route not specified; assume IM) for 2 days. (de la Concha 2002)

■ **SWINE:**

For swine respiratory disease (labeled-dose; FDA-approved): In water at a concentration of 400 mg/gallon (100 ppm). Use as only source of drinking water for 5 days. For bulk tank add one gallon concentrate to 128 gallons of water; for proportioner set to 1:128 (0.8%). (Label information; *NuFlor® Concentrate Solution*)

Monitoring
- Clinical efficacy.
- Injection site reactions.

Client Information
- Residue Warnings: When administered as labeled, cattle slaughter withdrawal is 28 days post injection if using the IM route; 38 days after the SC route. Swine (in drinking water) = 16 days.
- Not to be used in female dairy cattle 20 months of age or older.
- A withdrawal period has not been established in preruminating calves. Do not use in calves to be processed for veal.
- Do not give IV.

Chemistry/Synonyms
A fluorinated analog of thiamphenicol, florfenicol is commercially available as light yellow to straw-colored injectable solution also containing n-ethyl-2-pyrolidone, propylene glycol, and polyethylene glycol. The commercially available products range from a bright yellow to straw color. Color does not affect potency.

Florfenicol may also be known as Sch-25298 and *NuFlor®*.

Storage/Stability
Florfenicol injection (*Nuflor®, Nuflor Gold®*) should be stored between 2°-30°C (36°-86°F). Use within 28 days of first use.

The oral solution (swine) should be stored between 2°-26°C (36°-77°F).

The combination product with flunixin (*Resflor Gold®*) should not be stored above 30°C (86°F) and used within 28 days. The 500 mL vial should not be punctured more than 10 times.

Compatibility/Compounding Considerations
No specific information noted.

Dosage Forms/Regulatory Status/Withdrawal Times
VETERINARY-LABELED PRODUCTS:
Florfenicol Injection: 300 mg/mL in 100 mL, 250 mL and 500 mL multi-dose vials; *NuFlor®*; (Rx). FDA-approved (NADA 141-063) for use in cattle; see residue warnings above. Slaughter withdrawal (at labeled dosages) = 28 days (IM treatment), 38 days (SC treatment). Do not use in female dairy cattle 20 months of age or older. A withdrawal period has not been established in preruminating calves. Do not use in calves to be processed for veal.

Florfenicol Injection: 300 mg/mL (also contains 300 mg of 2-pyrrolidone, and triacetin) in 100 mL, 250 mL, & 500 mL vials; *NuFlor Gold®*; (Rx). FDA-approved (NADA 141-265) for use in beef and non-lactating dairy cattle. Do not slaughter within 44 days of last treatment. Do not use in female dairy cattle 20 months of age or older. Use may cause milk residues. A withdrawal period has not been established in preruminating calves. The product label for *NuFlor Gold®* can be found at dailymed.nlm.nih.gov

Florfenicol 2.3% (23 mg/mL) Concentrate Solution in 2.2 btls; *NuFlor® Concentrate Solution, Florvio 2.3% Concentrate Solution*; (Rx). FDA-approved (NADA 141-206) for use in swine. Slaughter withdrawal (at labeled dosages) = 16 days.

There are florfenicol products for addition to catfish or salmonid feeds (*Aquaflor®*) and swine feed.

Florfenicol 300 mg/mL with Flunixin 16.5 mg/mL Injection in 100 mL, 250 mL and 500 mL vials; *Resflor Gold®*; (Rx). FDA-approved (NADA 141-299) for use in beef and non-lactating dairy cat-

tle. Do not slaughter within 38 days of last treatment. Not for use in female dairy cattle 20 months of age or older or in calves to be processed for veal. Use may cause milk residues. A withdrawal period has not been established in preruminating calves. The product label for *ResFlor Gold®* can be found at dailymed.nlm.nih.gov

HUMAN-LABELED PRODUCTS: NONE.

Revisions/References
Monograph revised/updated January 2014.
de la Concha, A. (2002). Diseases of kids. Proceedings: Western Veterinary Conference. accessed via Veterinary Information Network; vin.com

Lane, V., et al. (2007). Tissue residues of florfenicol in sheep. J. Vet. Pharmacol. Ther. **31**: 178-80.

Palma, C., et al. (2012). Pharmacokinetics of florfenicol and florfenicol-amine after intravenous administration in sheep. J. Vet. Pharmacol. Ther. **35**(5): 508-11.

Park, B. K., et al. (2008). Pharmacokinetics of florfenicol and its metabolite, florfenicol amine, in dogs. Research in Veterinary Science **84**(1): 85-9.

Fluconazole
(floo-kon-a-zole)   Diflucan®

Antifungal

Prescriber Highlights
▶ Oral or parenteral antifungal particularly useful for CNS infections. Treatment for systemic mycosis may be required for many months.

▶ Similar efficacy as itraconazole, but (at present) considerably less expensive. Unlike itraconazole, does not require an acidic environment for PO absorption. Can be given with or without food.

▶ Caution: Renal failure (dosage adjustment needed), pregnancy (safety not established), hepatic failure.

▶ Adverse Effects: Occasional GI effects (inappetence, vomiting, diarrhea) in cats or dogs; may see increased liver enzymes and rarely, severe hepatotoxicity.

▶ Drug Interactions.

Uses/Indications
Fluconazole can be useful in the treatment of systemic mycoses, including cryptococcal meningitis, blastomycosis, and histoplasmosis. A retrospective study in dogs with blastomycosis, found that there was no significant difference in efficacy between fluconazole and itraconazole and while treatment with fluconazole was required for a longer time than itraconazole (median of 183 days vs. 138 days), treatment costs were about 1/3 less (Mazepa et al. 2011).

Fluconazole may also be useful for superficial candidiasis or dermatophytosis. Because of the drug's unique pharmacokinetic qualities, it is probably more useful in treating CNS infections or fungal urinary tract infections than other azole derivatives. Unlike ketoconazole, fluconazole does not have appreciable effects on hormone synthesis and may have fewer side effects in small animals.

Pharmacology/Actions
Fluconazole is a fungistatic triazole compound. Triazole-derivative agents, like the imidazoles (clotrimazole, ketoconazole, etc.), presumably act by altering the cellular membranes of susceptible fungi, thereby increasing membrane permeability and allowing leakage of cellular contents and impaired uptake of purine and pyrimidine precursors. Fluconazole has efficacy against a variety of pathogenic fungi including yeasts and dermatophytes. *In vivo* studies using laboratory models have shown that fluconazole has fungistatic activity against some strains of Candida, Cryptococcus, Histoplasma, and Blastomyces. *In vivo* studies of efficacy against Aspergillus strains have been conflicting.

Pharmacokinetics

Fluconazole is rapidly and nearly completely absorbed (90%) after oral administration. Gastric pH or the presence of food, do not appreciably alter fluconazole's oral bioavailability. It has low protein binding and is widely distributed throughout the body and penetrates well into the CSF, eye, and peritoneal fluid. Fluconazole is eliminated primarily via the kidneys and achieves high concentrations in the urine. In humans, fluconazole's serum half-life is about 30 hours in patients with normal renal function. Because of it's long half-life, fluconazole does not reach steady state plasma levels for 6–14 days after beginning therapy, unless loading doses are given. Patients with impaired renal function may have half-lives extended significantly and dosage adjustment may be required.

Contraindications/Precautions/Warnings

Fluconazole should not be used in patients hypersensitive to it or other azole antifungal agents. In patients with hepatic impairment it should be used only when the potential benefits outweigh the risks. Fluconazole is eliminated primarily by the kidneys, doses or dosing intervals may need to be adjusted in patients with renal impairment.

Fluconazole is reportedly toxic to budgerigars.

Adverse Effects

Fluconazole is well tolerated in the majority of dogs and cats treated. Occasionally, inappetence, vomiting, or diarrhea has been reported. Hepatotoxicity is possible and approximately 15-20% of dogs treated long-term may have increased ALT concentrations. Occasionally ALT increases will worsen necessitating fluconazole discontinuation.

In humans, side effects have been generally limited to occasional GI effects (vomiting, diarrhea, anorexia/nausea) and headache. Rarely, increased liver enzymes and hepatic toxicity, exfoliative skin disorders, and thrombocytopenia have been reported in humans.

Reproductive/Nursing Safety

Safety during pregnancy has not been established and it is not recommended for use in pregnant animals unless the benefits outweigh the risks. In humans, the FDA categorizes this drug as category *C* for use during pregnancy (*Animal studies have shown an adverse effect on the fetus, but there are no adequate studies in humans; or there are no animal reproduction studies and no adequate studies in humans.*)

Fluconazole is excreted in milk at concentrations similar to plasma. Use with caution in nursing dams.

Overdosage/Acute Toxicity

There is very limited information on the acute toxicity of fluconazole. Rats and mice survived doses of 1 g/kg, but died within several days after receiving 1 – 2 g/kg. Rats and mice receiving very high dosages demonstrated respiratory depression, salivation, lacrimation, urinary incontinence, and cyanosis. If a massive overdose occurs, consider gut emptying and give supportive therapy as required. Fluconazole may be removed by hemodialysis or peritoneal dialysis.

Drug Interactions

The following drug interactions have either been reported or are theoretical in humans or animals receiving fluconazole and may be of significance in veterinary patients. Unless otherwise noted, use together is not necessarily contraindicated, but weigh the potential risks and perform additional monitoring when appropriate.

- **AMPHOTERICIN B**: Lab animal studies have shown that fluconazole used concomitantly with amphotericin B may be antagonistic against Aspergillus or Candida; the clinical importance of these findings is not yet clear.
- **BENZODIAZEPINES**: Increased benzodiazepine levels/effects possible.
- **BUSPIRONE**: Plasma concentrations may be elevated.
- **CIMETIDINE**: May reduce fluconazole levels.
- **CISAPRIDE**: Fluconazole may increase cisapride levels and the possibility for toxicity.
- **COLCHICINE**: Increased colchicine levels and effects possible. Considered contraindicated in human patients with hepatic or renal impairment.
- **CORTICOSTEROIDS**: Fluconazole may inhibit the metabolism of corticosteroid; potential for increased adverse effects.
- **CYCLOPHOSPHAMIDE**: Fluconazole may inhibit the metabolism of cyclophosphamide and its metabolites; potential for increased toxicity.
- **CYCLOSPORINE**: Fluconazole increases cyclosporine levels. In normal dogs, fluconazole at 5 mg/kg once daily decreased cyclosporine dosages by 29%-51% to achieve similar therapeutic trough levels. In renal transplant dogs (also on mycophenolate), fluconazole decreased cyclosporine dose requirements 33% on average (Katayama et al. 2010).
- **DIURETICS, THIAZIDES**: Increased fluconazole concentrations possible.
- **FENTANYL/ALFENTANIL**: Fluconazole may increase fentanyl levels.
- **LOSARTAN**: Increased losartan effects possible; increased monitoring of blood pressure recommended.
- **NSAIDs**: Fluconazole may increase plasma levels of some agents; increased risk for adverse effects.
- **QUINIDINE**: Increased risk for cardiotoxicity.
- **RIFAMPIN**: May decrease fluconazole efficacy; fluconazole may increase rifampin levels.
- **THEOPHYLLINE/AMINOPHYLLINE**: Increased theophylline concentrations possible.
- **TRICYCLIC ANTIDEPRESSANTS (clomipramine, amitriptyline,** etc.): Fluconazole may exacerbate the effects of tricyclic antidepressants.
- **SULFONYLUREA ANTIDIABETIC AGENTS (***e.g.,* **glipizide, glyburide**): Fluconazole may increase levels; hypoglycemia possible.
- **VINCRISTINE/VINBLASTINE**: Fluconazole may inhibit vinca alkaloid metabolism.
- **WARFARIN**: Fluconazole may cause increased prothrombin times in patients receiving warfarin or other coumarin anticoagulants.

Doses

- **DOGS:**

  For systemic mycosis for fluconazole-sensitive organisms (potentially **cryptococcosis, blastomycosis, histoplasmosis, nasal aspergillosis**); (extra-label): The empiric dosage for dogs is 5 mg/kg q12h PO or IV (slowly; over 1-2 hours); some recommend giving twice this dose the first day of treatment. Depending on response the dosage may be increased to 10 mg/kg PO q12h for refractory cases or the frequency of administration reduced 5 – 10 mg/kg PO q24h. Treatment may be required for months and generally should continue for 1-3 months after resolution of clinical signs.

  For urinary candidiasis (extra-label): 5 – 10 mg/kg PO q24h for 3-5 weeks.

  For systemic treatment of *Malassezia* dermatitis, dermatophytosis, onychomycosis (extra-label): 5 mg/kg PO q24h. Continue to treat for at least one week after complete resolution of signs (*Malassezia*) or until two negative skin cultures are obtained (dermatophytosis, onychomycosis).

- **CATS:**

  For systemic mycosis for fluconazole-sensitive organisms (potentially cryptococcosis, blastomycosis, histoplasmosis, nasal aspergillosis); (extra-label): The empiric dosage for cats is 10 mg/kg PO q12h. This is practically administered as one 50 mg tablet per cat PO q12h. Rapidly progressing or severe disseminated infections may require 100 mg/cat PO q12h. Tablets may be crushed. Treatment usually required for several months and should continue for 1-3 months after clinical resolution or antigen test results on serum and CSF are negative.

- **HORSES:**

  For *C. immitis* infection or Candida bacteremia (extra-label): Loading dose of 14 mg/kg PO followed by 5 mg/kg PO once daily. There have been anecdotal reports of successful treatment of fungal keratitis using 1 mg/kg PO q24h. (Stewart et al. 2008)

  For the treatment of infectious endometritis caused by susceptible fungal organisms of *Candida* spp. (extra-label): Based upon plasma and endometrial tissue levels a 14 mg/kg PO loading dose and maintenance dose of 5 mg/kg PO q24h will result in endometrial tissue levels near the accepted MIC values for most *Candida* spp. and surpass the MIC for *Candida albicans* in the reproductive tract of mares. (Scofield et al. 2013)

- **RABBITS/RODENTS/SMALL MAMMALS:**

  Rabbits (extra-label): 25 – 43 mg/kg slow IV q12h. (Ivey et al. 2000)

- **BIRDS:**

  For treating candidiasis (extra-label): A report where fluconazole pharmacokinetics were determined in Goffin's cockatoos, Timneh African grey parrots, and orange-winged Amazon parrots showed that fluconazole dosed at 20 mg/kg PO q24-48h or 10 mg/kg PO q24h would likely be effective for treating *C. albicans*. *C. galabrata* and *C. papasilosis* may have MIC's greater than this dose could effectively treat. (Flammer 2008)

  For treating candidiasis in cockatiels (extra-label): In this report, both a 10 mg/kg fluconazole PO suspension and 100 mg/mL fluconazole treated drinking water maintained plasma levels above the MIC for most strains of *Candida albicans*. (Ratzlaff et al. 2009)

  As an alternate treatment of aspergillosis (extra-label): 5 – 10 mg/kg PO once daily for up to 6 weeks, with or after amphotericin B. (Oglesbee et al. 1994)

- **REPTILES:**

  For dermatophytosis (iguanas); (extra-label): 5 mg/kg PO once daily.

Monitoring

- Clinical Efficacy.
- With long-term therapy, occasional liver function tests are recommended.

Client Information

- May give with or without food. If your animal vomits or acts sick after getting it on an empty stomach, give with food or small treat to see if this helps. If vomiting continues, contact your veterinarian.
- Most likely side effects are gastrointestinal (*e.g.,* vomiting, diarrhea, lack of appetite, etc.). Liver toxicity is possible, but very rare.
- Do not to skip doses.

Chemistry/Synonyms

A synthetic triazole antifungal agent, fluconazole occurs as a white crystalline powder. It is slightly soluble (8 mg/mL) in water.

Fluconazole may also be known as UK-49858; many trade names are available.

Storage/Stability

Fluconazole tablets should be stored at temperatures less than 30°C in tight containers. Fluconazole injection should be stored at temperatures from 5-30°C (5-25°C for the *Viaflex®* bags); avoid freezing.

Compatibility/Compounding Considerations

Do not add additives to the injection.

Dosage Forms/Regulatory Status

VETERINARY-LABELED PRODUCTS: NONE.

HUMAN-LABELED PRODUCTS:

Fluconazole Oral Tablets: 50 mg, 100 mg, 150 mg, & 200 mg; *Diflucan®*, generic; (Rx)

Fluconazole Powder for Oral Suspension: 10 mg/mL & 40 mg/mL (when reconstituted) in 35 mL; *Diflucan®*, generic; (Rx)

Fluconazole Injection: 2 mg/mL in 100 mL or 200 mL bottles or *Viaflex® Plus* (available with sodium chloride or dextrose diluents); *Diflucan®*, generic; (Rx)

Revisions/References

Monograph revised/updated January 2014.

Flammer, K. (2008). Avian Mycoses: Managing those difficult cases. Proceedings: AAV. accessed via Veterinary Information Network; vin.com
Ivey, E. & J. Morrisey (2000). Therapeutics for Rabbits. Vet Clin NA: Exotic Anim Pract **3:1**(Jan): 183-216.
Katayama, M., et al. (2010). Fluconazole decreases cyclosporine dosage in renal transplanted dogs. Research in Veterinary Science **89**(1): 124-5.
Mazepa, A. S. W., et al. (2011). Retrospective Comparison of the Efficacy of Fluconazole or Itraconazole for the Treatment of Systemic Blastomycosis in Dogs. Journal of Veterinary Internal Medicine **25**(3): 440-5.
Oglesbee, B. & C. Bishop (1994). Avian Infectious Diseases. *Saunders Manual of Small Animal Practice.* S. Birchard and R. Sherding. Philadelphia, W.B. Saunders Company: 1257-70.
Ratzlaff, K. & K. Flammer (2009). Fluconazole in cockatiels. Proceedings: AAV. accessed via Veterinary Information Network; vin.com
Scofield, D. B., et al. (2013). Equine Endometrial Tissue Concentration of Fluconazole Following Oral Administration. Journal of Equine Veterinary Science **33**(1): 44-50.
Stewart, A., et al. (2008). Pulmonary and systemic fungal infections. Compendium Equine(-June): 260-72.

Flucytosine

(floo-sye-toe-seen)   Ancobon®

Antifungal

Prescriber Highlights

▶ Infrequently used antifungal used in combination with other drugs (to reduce resistance development). CSF penetration is excellent and high urinary concentrations are attainable. Frequent dosing (q6-12h) and cost may be issues.

▶ Extreme Caution: Patients with renal impairment, preexisting bone marrow depression, hematologic diseases, or receiving other bone marrow suppressant drugs; dogs may not tolerate therapy for more than 10-14 days. Caution: Hepatic disease.

▶ Teratogenic in rats.

▶ Adverse Effects: Most common: GI disturbances; Potentially: dose dependent bone marrow depression, cutaneous eruption & rash primarily seen on the scrotum & nasal planum (in dogs), oral ulceration, increased hepatic enzymes, CNS effects in cats.

Uses/Indications

Flucytosine is principally active against strains of Cryptococcus and Candida. Flucytosine is used in combination with other antifungals (*e.g.,* an azole, amphotericin B). When used alone, resistance can develop rapidly to flucytosine, particularly with Cryptococcus. Because it penetrates relatively well into the CNS, it has been used for the treatment of CNS cryptococcosis. Some cases of subcutaneous and systemic chromoblastosis may also respond to flucytosine.

Pharmacology/Actions

Flucytosine penetrates fungal cells where it is deaminated by cytosine deaminase to fluorouracil. Fluorouracil acts as an antimetabolite by competing with uracil, thereby interfering with pyrimidine metabolism and eventually RNA and protein synthesis. It is thought that flucytosine is converted to fluorodeoxyuredylic acid that inhibits thymidylate synthesis and ultimately DNA synthesis.

In human cells, cytosine deaminase is apparently not present or only has minimal activity. Rats apparently metabolize some of the drug to fluorouracil, which may explain the teratogenic effects seen in this species. It is unclear how much cytosine deaminase activity dog and cat cells possess.

Flucytosine can have synergistic efficacy when used with amphotericin B.

Pharmacokinetics

Flucytosine is well absorbed after oral administration. The rate, but not extent, of absorption will be decreased if given with food.

Flucytosine is distributed widely throughout the body. CSF concentrations may be 60-100% of those found in the serum. In healthy humans, the volume of distribution is about 0.7 L/kg. Only about 2-4% of the drug is bound to plasma proteins. It is unknown if flucytosine is distributed into milk.

Absorbed flucytosine is excreted basically unchanged in the urine via glomerular filtration. In humans, the half-life is about 3-6 hours in patients with normal renal function, but may be significantly prolonged in patients with renal dysfunction.

Contraindications/Precautions/Warnings

Flucytosine is contraindicated in patients hypersensitive to it.

Flucytosine should be used with extreme caution in patients with renal impairment. Some clinicians recommend monitoring serum flucytosine levels in these patients and adjusting dosage (or dosing interval) to maintain serum levels at less than 100 micrograms/mL. One clinician (Macy, 1987) recommends dividing the flucytosine dose by the serum creatinine level if azotemia develops.

Use in dogs with extreme caution, cutaneous drug eruptions can develop rapidly (within 10-14 days).

Use flucytosine with extreme caution in patients with preexisting bone marrow depression, hematologic diseases, or receiving other bone marrow suppressant drugs. Flucytosine should also be used cautiously (with enhanced monitoring) in patients with hepatic disease.

Because resistance can develop rapidly when flucytosine is used alone, it should only be used in combination with other antifungal drugs.

Adverse Effects

Most common adverse effects seen with flucytosine are GI disturbances (nausea, vomiting, diarrhea, etc.). Other potential adverse effects include a dose dependent bone marrow depression (anemia, leukopenia, thrombocytopenia), cutaneous eruption and rash primarily seen on the scrotum and nasal planum (occurring in dogs), oral ulceration and increased levels of hepatic enzymes. Dogs receiving flucytosine often develop a severe drug reaction within 10-14 days of treatment.

Reports of aberrant behavior and seizures in a cat without concurrent CNS infection have been noted after flucytosine use. There are anecdotal reports of toxic epidermal necrolysis occurring in cats treated with flucytosine.

Reproductive/Nursing Safety

Flucytosine has caused teratogenic effects in rats. It should be used in pregnant animals only when the benefits of therapy outweigh the risks. In humans, the FDA categorizes this drug as category C for use during pregnancy (*Animal studies have shown an adverse effect on the fetus, but there are no adequate studies in humans; or there are no animal reproduction studies and no adequate studies in humans.*)

It is not known whether this drug is excreted in milk. Because there are potential serious adverse reactions in nursing offspring, consider using milk replacer.

Overdosage/Acute Toxicity

No specifics regarding flucytosine overdosage were located. It is suggested that a substantial overdose be handled with gut emptying, charcoal and cathartic administration unless contraindicated.

Drug Interactions

The following drug interactions have either been reported or are theoretical in humans or animals receiving flucytosine and may be of significance in veterinary patients. Unless otherwise noted, use together is not necessarily contraindicated, but weigh the potential risks and perform additional monitoring when appropriate.

- **AMPHOTERICIN** B: When used with amphotericin B, synergism against Cryptococcus and Candida has been demonstrated *in vitro*. However, if amphotericin B induces renal dysfunction, toxicity of flucytosine may be enhanced if it accumulates. Should clinically significant renal toxicity develop, flucytosine dosage may need to be adjusted.

Laboratory Considerations

- When determining **serum creatinine** using the *Ektachem*® analyzer, false elevations in levels may be noted if patients are also taking flucytosine.

Doses

- **DOGS:**

  Note: Because of potential serious toxicity, flucytosine is usually **not recommended** for use in dogs.

  For cryptococcosis (extra-label): 50 – 75 mg/kg PO q8h; treatment requires 1-12 months. Must be given with a polyene or azole antifungal agent. (Malik et al. 2006)

- **CATS:**

  For cryptococcosis (extra-label): Must be used with another antifungal (amphotericin B or an azole). Flucytosine at 30 mg/kg PO q6h or 50 mg/kg PO q8h or 75 mg/kg PO q12h. Cats 3.5 kg or greater should receive 250 mg (total) q6-8h. Must be given with a polyene (amphotericin B) or azole antifungal agent. Treatment requires 1-9 months. (Malik et al. 2006)

  For candidiasis (extra-label): 25 – 50 mg/kg PO q6h or 50 – 65 mg/kg PO q8h for 42 days. Must be given with a polyene or azole antifungal agent. (Greene et al. 1998)

Monitoring

- Renal function (at least twice weekly if also receiving amphotericin B).
- CBC with platelets.
- Hepatic enzymes at least monthly.

Client Information

- Clients should report any clinical signs associated with hematologic toxicity (abnormal bleeding, bruising, etc.).
- Pregnant women should take precautions handling this medication. It has caused birth defects in laboratory animals.
- Prolonged treatment times, as well as costs of medication and associated monitoring, require substantial client commitment.

Chemistry/Synonyms

A fluorinated pyrimidine antifungal agent, flucytosine occurs as a white to off-white, crystalline powder that is odorless or has a slight odor with pK_as of 2.9 and 10.71. It is sparingly soluble in water and slightly soluble in alcohol.

Flucytosine may also be known as: 5-FC, 5-fluorocytosine, flucytosinum, Ro-2-9915, *Alcobon®*, and *Ancotil®*.

Storage/Stability

Store flucytosine capsules in tight, light-resistant containers at temperatures less than 40°C, and preferably at room temperature (15-30°C). The commercially available capsules are assigned an expiration date of 5 years from the date of manufacture.

Compatibility/Compounding Considerations

Compounded preparation stability: Flucytosine oral suspension compounded from commercially available capsules has been published (Allen et al. 1996). Triturating four (4) flucytosine 250 mg capsules with 50 mL of *Ora-Plus®* and *qs ad* to 100 mL with *Ora-Sweet®* (or *Ora-Sweet®* SF) yields a 10 mg/mL oral suspension that retains >95% potency for 60 days stored at both 5°C and 25°C.

Dosage Forms/Regulatory Status

VETERINARY-LABELED PRODUCTS: NONE.

HUMAN-LABELED PRODUCTS:

Flucytosine Oral Capsules: 250 mg & 500 mg; *Ancobon®*; (Rx)

Revisions/References

Monograph revised/updated January 2014.

Allen, L. V. & M. A. Erickson (1996). Stability of acetazolamide, allopurinol, azathioprine, clonazepam, and flucytosine in extemporaneously compounded oral liquids. Am J Health Syst Pharm 53(16): 1944-9.

Greene, C. & A. Watson (1998). Antimicrobial Drug Formulary. *Infectious Diseases of the Dog and Cat.* C. Greene. Philadelphia, WB Saunders: 790-919.

Malik, R., et al. (2006). Cryptococcosis. *Infectious Diseases of the Dog and Cat, 3rd Ed.* C. Greene, Elsevier: 584-98.

Fludrocortisone Acetate

(flue-droe-kor-ti-sone)   Florinef®

Mineralocorticoid

Prescriber Highlights

▶ Oral mineralocorticoid alternative to DOCP used to treat adrenal insufficiency in small animals; may be useful to treat hyperkalemia as well.

▶ Also has some glucocorticoid effect that could cause adverse effects.

▶ Adverse Effects: Dosage related; PU/PD, hypertension, edema, & hypokalemia possible.

▶ May be excreted in significant quantities in milk.

▶ Patients may require supplemental glucocorticoids.

▶ Expense may be an issue, especially in larger dogs.

Uses/Indications

Fludrocortisone is used in small animal medicine for the treatment of adrenocortical insufficiency (Addison's disease). It can also be used as adjunctive therapy in hyperkalemia.

In humans, fludrocortisone has also been used for severe postural hypotension, and salt-losing, congenital adrenogenital syndrome.

Pharmacology/Actions

Fludrocortisone acetate is a potent corticosteroid that possesses both glucocorticoid and mineralocorticoid activity. It is approximately 10-15X as potent a glucocorticoid agent as hydrocortisone, but is a much more potent mineralocorticoid (125X that of hydrocortisone). It is only used clinically for its mineralocorticoid effects.

The site of action of mineralocorticoids is at the renal distal tubule where they increase the absorption of sodium. Mineralocorticoids also enhance potassium and hydrogen ion excretion.

Pharmacokinetics

In humans, fludrocortisone is well absorbed from the GI with peak levels occurring in approximately 1.7 hours; plasma half-life is about 3.5 hours, but biologic activity persists for 18-36 hours.

Contraindications/Precautions/Warnings

Fludrocortisone is contraindicated in patients known to be hypersensitive to it.

Some dogs or cats may require additional supplementation with a glucocorticoid agent on an ongoing basis. All animals with hypoadrenocorticism should receive additional glucocorticoids (at least 2X basal) during periods of stress or acute illness.

Adverse Effects

Adverse effects of fludrocortisone are generally a result of chronic, excessive dosage (see Overdosage section below) or if withdrawal is too rapid. Since fludrocortisone also possesses glucocorticoid activity, it theoretically could cause the adverse effects associated with those compounds such as polyuria/polydipsia, which could be a problem for some dogs. (See the monograph on glucocorticoids for more information.)

Reproductive/Nursing Safety

In humans, the FDA categorizes this drug as category C for use during pregnancy (*Animal studies have shown an adverse effect on the fetus, but there are no adequate studies in humans; or there are no animal reproduction studies and no adequate studies in humans.*)

Fludrocortisone may be excreted in clinically significant quantities in milk. Puppies or kittens of mothers receiving fludrocortisone should receive milk replacer after colostrum is consumed.

Overdosage/Acute Toxicity

Overdosage may cause hypertension, edema, and hypokalemia. Electrolytes should be aggressively monitored and potassium may need to be supplemented. Patients should have the drug discontinued until clinical signs associated with overdosage have resolved; then restart the drug at a lower dosage.

Drug Interactions

The following drug interactions have either been reported or are theoretical in humans or animals receiving fludrocortisone and may be of significance in veterinary patients. Unless otherwise noted, use together is not necessarily contraindicated, but weigh the potential risks and perform additional monitoring when appropriate.

■ **AMPHOTERICIN B:** Patients may develop hypokalemia if fludrocortisone is administered concomitantly with amphotericin B.

■ **ASPIRIN:** Fludrocortisone may reduce salicylate levels.

■ **DIURETICS, POTASSIUM-DEPLETING** (*e.g.,* thiazides, furosemide): Patients may develop hypokalemia if fludrocortisone is administered concomitantly with diuretics; diuretics can cause a loss of sodium, and may counteract the effects of fludrocortisone.

■ **INSULIN:** Potentially, fludrocortisone could increase the insulin requirements of diabetic patients.

Doses

■ **DOGS:**

For maintenance therapy of hypoadrenocorticism (extra-label): Initial dosage recommendations vary somewhat but most recommend 0.01 mg/kg PO q12h. Dosages are adjusted in 0.05 – 0.1 mg increments (1/2 to one 0.1 mg tablet) based on monitoring serum electrolyte concentrations every 1-2 weeks until stable; many dogs can be transitioned to once daily dosing. Once stable, recheck every 3-4 months. Most dogs will eventually require 0.02 – 0.03 mg/kg per day. Approximately 50% of dogs will not require supplemental prednisone, but owners should have supplemental prednisone on hand and instructed to use it when animal undergoes stress or illness (*e.g.* veterinary visits, boarding etc.). In dogs that develop signs associated with Cushing's (*e.g.,* polyuria/polydipsia) even when hyponatremia and, less frequently, hyperkalemia persist, the addition of NaCl (0.1 g/kg/day) may be useful to reduce the dose of fludrocortisone, while maintaining normal serum sodium.

- **CATS:**

  For maintenance therapy of hypoadrenocorticism (extra-label): 0.02 mg/kg PO once daily with prednisolone. Practically, one 0.1 mg tablet PO once daily with prednisolone (at 1.25 mg per cat PO once daily; ¼ of a 5 mg tablet).

- **FERRETS:**

  For hypoadrenocorticism (extra-label): For those animals that still exhibit Addisonian signs even with prednisone therapy: 0.05 – 0.1 mg/kg PO q24h or divided q12h. (Johnson 2006)

Monitoring

- Serum electrolytes, BUN, creatinine; initially every 1-2 weeks, then every 3-4 months once stabilized.
- Weight, PE for edema.

Client Information

- May give with or without food. If your animal vomits or acts sick after getting it on an empty stomach, give with food or small treat to see if this helps. If vomiting continues, contact your veterinarian.
- Side effects not likely, but if dose is too high (long-term) "Cushingoid" effects (change in coat, swelling abdomen, etc.) could occur; if too low, Addison's effects (*e.g.,* weakness, depression, lack of appetite, vomiting, diarrhea, etc.) could occur.
- Surgery or stress (*e.g.,* trauma, illness) may require additional glucocorticoids (*e.g.,* prednisolone, etc.).
- Do not stop the drug abruptly ('cold turkey') or serious side effects could occur.

Chemistry/Synonyms

A synthetic glucocorticoid with significant mineralocorticoid activity, fludrocortisone acetate occurs as hygroscopic, fine, white to pale yellow powder or crystals. It is odorless or practically odorless. Fludrocortisone is insoluble in water and slightly soluble in alcohol.

Fludrocortisone acetate may also be known as: fluohydrisone acetate, fluohydrocortisone acetate, 9alpha-fluorohydrocortisone acetate, fludrocortisoni acetas, 9alpha-fluorohydrocortisone 21-acetate, *Astonin*®, *Astonin H*®, *Florinef*®, *Florinefe*®, and *Lonikan*®.

Storage/Stability

Fludrocortisone acetate tablets should be stored at room temperature (15-30°C) in well-closed containers; avoid excessive heat. The drug is relatively stable in light and air.

Compatibility/Compounding Considerations

No specific information noted.

Dosage Forms/Regulatory Status

VETERINARY-LABELED PRODUCTS: NONE.

HUMAN-LABELED PRODUCTS:

Fludrocortisone Acetate Tablets: 0.1 mg; generic; (Rx)

Revisions/References

Monograph revised/updated January 2014.

Johnson, D. (2006). Current Therapies for Ferret Adrenal Disease. Proceedings: ACVC. accessed via Veterinary Information Network; vin.com

Flumazenil

(floo-maz-eh-nill)   Romazicon®

Benzodiazepine Antagonist

Prescriber Highlights

▶ Benzodiazepine antagonist to reverse after overdose (OD)/ toxicity. May also have efficacy in improving neurologic function in patients with hepatic encephalopathy or for OD's of non-benzodiazepine sleep aids ("z" drugs such a zolpidem).

▶ Contraindications: Known hypersensitivity, when benzodiazepines are treating life-threatening conditions (*e.g.*, status epilepticus, increased CSF pressure), & during tricyclic antidepressant OD treatment. Use extreme caution in mixed overdoses.

▶ Adverse Effects: Potentially injection site reactions, vomiting, cutaneous vasodilatation, vertigo, ataxia, & blurred vision; seizures, and cardiac arrhythmias have been reported in humans.

▶ Potentially teratogenic at high dosages.

Uses/Indications

Flumazenil may be useful for the reversal of benzodiazepine effects after overdoses or toxic effects. Flumazenil may be of benefit in the treatment of encephalopathy in patients with severe hepatic failure or in treating overdoses of zolpidem (*Ambien*®) or other imidazopyridine hypnotic agents.

A report of using flumazenil to reverse the anesthetic effects of tiletamine-zolazepam in dogs, demonstrated that analgesia, posture, and auditory effects were reversed, but it had no effect on sedation or muscle relaxation. Recovery times (head up, sternal recumbency, standing, walking) from anesthesia were reduced in the flumazenil treated dogs. Heart rates, glucose levels, body temperature were significantly higher in the flumazenil treated group (Kim et al. 2009).

Pharmacology/Actions

Flumazenil is a competitive blocker of benzodiazepines at benzodiazepine receptors in the CNS. It antagonizes the sedative and amnestic qualities of benzodiazepines.

Pharmacokinetics

Flumazenil is administered by IV injection. Therapeutic effect may occur within 1-2 minutes of administration. It is rapidly distributed and metabolized in the liver. In humans, the average half-life is about one hour.

Contraindications/Precautions/Warnings

Flumazenil is contraindicated in patients hypersensitive to it or other benzodiazepines or in patients where benzodiazepines are being used to treat a potentially life-threatening condition (*e.g.*, status epilepticus, increased CSF pressure). It should not be used in patients with a serious tricyclic antidepressant overdose. Flumazenil should not be used, or used with extreme caution, in patients with mixed overdoses where benzodiazepine reversal may lead to seizures or other complications.

While flumazenil has been tried as treatment for overdoses of baclofen or carisoprodol, it may actually be contraindicated as it can cause worsening of clinical signs (Mazzaferro 2008).

Flumazenil does not alter benzodiazepine pharmacokinetics. Effects of long-acting benzodiazepines may recur after flumazenil's effects subside.

Routine use of flumazenil as a benzodiazepine reversal agent is not advised as adverse reactions, including cardiac arrhythmias, seizures and sudden death have been reported in humans and experimental canine studies.

Adverse Effects

In some human patients (usually having a long history of benzodiazepine use or showing signs of serious tricyclic antidepressant toxicity) and in pre-clinical canine experimental studies, flumazenil has been associated with seizures. Other adverse effects reported in humans include injection site reactions, vomiting, cutaneous vasodilatation, arrhythmias, vertigo, ataxia and blurred vision. Deaths have been associated with its use in humans having serious underlying diseases.

Overdosage/Acute Toxicity

Large IV overdoses have rarely caused symptoms in otherwise healthy humans. Seizures, if precipitated, have been treated with barbiturates, benzodiazepines and phenytoin, usually with prompt responses.

Drug Interactions

The following drug interactions have either been reported or are theoretical in humans or animals receiving flumazenil and may be of significance in veterinary patients. Unless otherwise noted, use together is not necessarily contraindicated, but weigh the potential risks and perform additional monitoring when appropriate.

- **CYCLIC** (tri-, tetra-) **ANTIDEPRESSANTS** (*e.g.*, **clomipramine, amitriptyline**, etc.): Increased risk for seizures; use is contraindicated.
- **NEUROMUSCULAR BLOCKING AGENTS:** Not recommended to use flumazenil until neuromuscular blockade has been fully reversed.

Doses

- **DOGS & CATS:**

  As an antagonist for benzodiazepine toxicity (*e.g.*, **respiratory depression**); toxicity of imidazopyridine sleep-aid drugs (*Ambien*®, etc.); to improve neurologic function in dogs with hepatic encephalopathy; (extra-label): Most sources recommend an initial dose of 0.01 mg/kg IV (or IO) and repeat every hour if needed. Intratracheal administration has been suggested in an emergency situation when venous access is not possible.

  Note: *Dosages of 0.08 – 0.2 mg/kg IV (approximately 10-20X greater) have been noted in some recent veterinary publications, but without published data to support them they are currently not recommended by this author (Plumb). Adult human doses of flumazenil for benzodiazepine overdoses are 0.2 mg (approx. 0.003 mg/kg for a 70kg person) IV over 30 seconds; if the desired level of consciousness is not obtained 30 seconds after the dose, 0.3 mg (approx. 0.004 mg/kg) can be given over another 30 seconds. Further doses of 0.5 mg over 30 seconds can be administered at 1 minute intervals, up to a cumulative dose of 3 mg (approx. 0.04 mg/kg). Most patients will respond to a cumulative dose of 1 mg to 3 mg.*

- **ZOO, EXOTIC, WILDLIFE SPECIES:**

  For use in zoo, exotic and wildlife medicine refer to specific references, including:

  a) *Zoo Animal and Wildlife Immobilization and Anesthesia.* West, G., Heard, D., Caulkett, N. (eds.). Blackwell Publishing, 2007.

  b) Handbook of Wildlife Chemical Immobilization, 3rd Ed. Kreeger, T.J. and J.M. Arnemo. 2007.

  c) *Fowler's Zoo and Wild Animal Medicine Current Therapy*, Volume 7, Miller, R.E., Fowler, M.E., Saunders. 2011.

  d) *Exotic Animal Formulary, 4th Ed.* Carpenter, J.W., Saunders. 2012.

  e) The 2009 American Association of Zoo Veterinarian Proceedings by D. K. Fontenot also has several dosages listed for

restraint, anesthesia, and analgesia for a variety of drugs for carnivores and primates. VIN members can access them at: http://goo.gl/NNIWQ or http://goo.gl/9UJse

Monitoring

- Efficacy.
- Monitor for seizures in susceptible patients.

Client Information

- Flumazenil should only be used in a controlled environment by clinically experienced professionals.

Chemistry/Synonyms

A benzodiazepine antagonist, flumazenil is a 1,4-imidazobenzodiazepine derivative.

Flumazenil may also be known as: flumazenilum, flumazepil, Ro-15-1788, Ro-15-1788/000, *Anexate*®, *Fadaflumaz*®, *Flumage*®, *Flumanovag*®, *Flumazen*®, *Fluxifarm*®, *Lanexat*® and *Romazicon*®.

Storage/Stability

Store flumazenil at 25°C (77°F); excursions are permitted from 15°-30°C (59°-86°F). Once drawn into a syringe or mixed with the above solutions, discard after 24 hours.

Compatibility/Compounding Considerations

Flumazenil is physically **compatible** with lactated Ringer's, D_5W, or normal saline solutions.

Dosage Forms/Regulatory Status

VETERINARY-LABELED PRODUCTS: NONE.

HUMAN-LABELED PRODUCTS:

Flumazenil Injection: 0.1 mg/mL in 5 mL & 10 mL vials; generic; (Rx)

Revisions/References

Monograph revised/updated January 2014.

Kim, M., et al. (2009). Antagonistic Effects of Flumazenil on Tiletamine-Zolazepam Induced Anesthesia in Dogs. Proceedings: WSAVA. accessed via Veterinary Information Network; vin.com

Mazzaferro, E. (2008). Emergency Intoxications. Proceedings: WVC. accessed via Veterinary Information Network; vin.com

Flumethasone

(floo-meth-a-sone)   Flucort®

GLUCOCORTICOID

Prescriber Highlights

▶ Injectable & oral glucocorticoid (oral may not be available commercially in USA).

▶ Long-acting; 15X more potent than hydrocortisone; no appreciable mineralocorticoid activity.

▶ Therapy goal is to use as much as is required & as little as possible for as short an amount of time as possible.

▶ Primary adverse effects are "Cushingoid" in nature with sustained use.

▶ Many potential drug & lab interactions.

Uses/Indications

Flumethasone injection is available commercially as a free steroid alcohol solution. While it does not work quite as rapidly as the corticosteroid phosphate and succinate esters (methylprednisolone sodium succinate, prednisolone sodium succinate, or dexamethasone sodium phosphate), it can be given either IM or IV and is useful for acute reactions such as insect bite hypersensitivity or vaccine reactions (Dowling 2007).

Flumethasone injection (*Flucort*®) is labeled in horses as indicated for: 1) Musculoskeletal conditions due to inflammation, where permanent structural changes do not exist, such as bursitis, carpitis, osselets and myositis. Following therapy an appropriate period of rest should be instituted to allow a more normal return to function of the affected part. 2) In allergic states such as hives, urticaria and insect bites.

Flumethasone injection (*Flucort®*) is labeled in dogs as indicated for: 1) Musculoskeletal conditions due to inflammation of muscles or joints and accessory structures, where permanent structural changes do not exist, such as arthritis, osteoarthritis, the disc syndrome and myositis. In septic arthritis appropriate antibacterial therapy should be concurrently administered. 2) In certain acute and chronic dermatoses of varying etiology to help control the pruritus, irritation and inflammation associated with these conditions. The drug has proven useful in otitis externa in conjunction with topical medication for similar reasons. 3) In allergic states such as hives, urticaria and insect bites. 4) Shock and shock-like states, by intravenous administration.

Flumethasone injection (*Flucort®*) is labeled in cats as indicated for certain acute and chronic dermatoses of varying etiology to help control the pruritus, irritation and inflammation associated with these conditions.

Pharmacology/Actions

Flumethasone is considered a long-acting glucocorticoid agent with duration of effect of 36-48 hours. Flumethasone is about 15X more potent than hydrocortisone; 1.3 mg of flumethasone is approximately equivalent to 5 mg of prednisone. It does not have significant mineralocorticoid activity and it is not suitable for every other day dosing. For more information refer to the Glucocorticoids, General Information monograph.

Pharmacokinetics

No information was located for this agent.

Contraindications/Precautions/Warnings

Flumethasone is contraindicated during the last trimester of pregnancy. Systemic use of glucocorticoids is generally considered contraindicated in systemic fungal infections (unless used for replacement therapy in Addison's), when administered IM in patients with idiopathic thrombocytopenia, and those hypersensitive to a particular compound. Use of sustained-release, injectable glucocorticoids is contraindicated for chronic corticosteroid therapy of systemic diseases.

Animals that have received glucocorticoids systemically, other than with "burst" therapy, should be tapered off the drugs. Patients that have received the drugs chronically should be tapered off slowly as endogenous ACTH and corticosteroid function may return slowly. Should the animal undergo a "stressor" (*e.g.*, surgery, trauma, illness, etc.) during the tapering process or until normal adrenal and pituitary function resume, additional glucocorticoids should be administered.

Adverse Effects

Adverse effects are generally associated with long-term administration of these drugs, especially if given at high dosages or not on an alternate day regimen. Effects generally manifest as clinical signs of hyperadrenocorticism. When administered to young, growing animals, glucocorticoids can retard growth. Many of the potential effects, adverse and otherwise, are outlined above in the Pharmacology section.

In dogs, GI effects (including GI ulceration) can occur with acute dosing. Polydipsia (PD), polyphagia (PP), and polyuria (PU) may be seen with short-term "burst" therapy. Adverse effects in dogs can include: dull, dry haircoat, weight gain, panting, vomiting, diarrhea, elevated liver enzymes, pancreatitis, GI ulceration, lipidemias, activation or worsening of diabetes mellitus, muscle wasting and behavioral changes (depression, lethargy, viciousness). Discontinuation of the drug may be necessary; changing to an alternate-day steroid may also alleviate the problem. With the exception of PU/PD/PP, adverse effects associated with antiinflammatory therapy are relatively uncommon. Adverse effects associated with immunosuppressive doses are more common and potentially more severe.

Cats generally require higher dosages than dogs for clinical effect, but tend to develop fewer adverse effects. Occasionally, polydipsia, polyuria, polyphagia with weight gain, diarrhea, or depression can be seen. Long-term, high dose therapy can lead to "Cushingoid" effects, however.

Reproductive/Nursing Safety

Corticosteroid therapy may induce parturition in large animal species during the latter stages of pregnancy. In a system evaluating the safety of drugs in canine and feline pregnancy (Papich 1989), this drug is categorized as class: C (*These drugs may have potential risks. Studies in people or laboratory animals have uncovered risks, and these drugs should be used cautiously as a last resort when the benefit of therapy clearly outweighs the risks.*)

Overdosage/Acute Toxicity

Glucocorticoids when given short-term are unlikely to cause harmful effects, even in massive dosages. One incidence of a dog developing acute CNS effects after accidental ingestion of glucocorticoids has been reported. Should clinical signs occur, use supportive treatment if required.

Chronic usage of glucocorticoids can lead to serious adverse effects. Refer to Adverse Effects above for more information.

Drug Interactions

The following drug interactions have either been reported or are theoretical in humans or animals receiving flumethasone and may be of significance in veterinary patients. Unless otherwise noted, use together is not necessarily contraindicated, but weigh the potential risks and perform additional monitoring when appropriate.

- **AMPHOTERICIN B:** Administered concomitantly with glucocorticoids may cause hypokalemia.
- **ANTICHOLINESTERASE AGENTS** (*e.g.*, **pyridostigmine**, **neostigmine**, etc.): In patients with myasthenia gravis, concomitant glucocorticoid and anticholinesterase agent administration may lead to profound muscle weakness. If possible, discontinue anticholinesterase medication at least 24 hours prior to corticosteroid administration.
- **ASPIRIN:** Glucocorticoids may reduce salicylate blood levels.
- **BARBITURATES:** May increase the metabolism of glucocorticoids and decrease flumethasone blood levels.
- **CYCLOPHOSPHAMIDE:** Glucocorticoids may inhibit the hepatic metabolism of cyclophosphamide; dosage adjustments may be required.
- **CYCLOSPORINE:** Concomitant administration of glucocorticoids and cyclosporine may increase the blood levels of each by mutually inhibiting the hepatic metabolism of the other; the clinical significance of this interaction is not clear.
- **DIAZEPAM:** Flumethasone may decrease diazepam levels.
- **DIURETICS, POTASSIUM-DEPLETING** (*e.g.*, **spironolactone, triamterene**): Administered concomitantly with glucocorticoids may cause hypokalemia.
- **EPHEDRINE:** May reduce flumethasone blood levels.
- **INSULIN:** Insulin requirements may increase in patients receiving glucocorticoids.
- **KETOCONAZOLE AND OTHER AZOLE ANTIFUNGALS:** May decrease the metabolism of glucocorticoids and increase flumethasone blood levels; ketoconazole may induce adrenal insufficiency when glucocorticoids are withdrawn by inhibiting adrenal corticosteroid synthesis.

- **MACROLIDE ANTIBIOTICS** (*e.g.*, **erythromycin, clarithromycin**): May decrease the metabolism of glucocorticoids and increase flumethasone blood levels.
- **MITOTANE**: May alter the metabolism of steroids; higher than usual doses of steroids may be necessary to treat mitotane-induced adrenal insufficiency.
- **NSAIDS**: Administration of ulcerogenic drugs with glucocorticoids may increase the risk of gastrointestinal ulceration.
- **PHENYTOIN**: May increase the metabolism of glucocorticoids and decrease flumethasone blood levels.
- **RIFAMPIN**: May increase the metabolism of glucocorticoids and decrease flumethasone blood levels.
- **VACCINES**: Patients receiving corticosteroids at immunosuppressive dosages should generally not receive live attenuated-virus vaccines as virus replication may be augmented; a diminished immune response may occur after vaccine, toxoid, or bacterin administration in patients receiving glucocorticoids.

Laboratory Considerations

- Glucocorticoids may increase **serum cholesterol** and **urine glucose levels**
- Glucocorticoids may decrease **serum potassium.**
- Glucocorticoids can suppress the release of thyroid stimulating hormone (TSH) and reduce T_3 & T_4 values. Thyroid gland atrophy has been reported after chronic glucocorticoid administration. Uptake of I^{131} by the thyroid may be decreased by glucocorticoids.
- Reactions to **skin tests** may be suppressed by glucocorticoids.
- False-negative results of the **nitroblue tetrazolium** test for systemic bacterial infections may be induced by glucocorticoids.
- Glucocorticoids may cause **neutrophilia** within 4-8 hours after dosing and return to baseline within 24-48 hours after drug discontinuation.
- Glucocorticoids can cause **lymphopenia**, which can persist for weeks after drug discontinuation in dogs.

Doses

- **DOGS:**

For labeled (FDA-approved) indications; musculoskeletal conditions due to inflammation; certain acute and chronic dermatoses when given orally, and also for allergic states or shock when given intravenously. Treat and adjust dosage on an individual basis: Orally: 0.0625 – 0.25 mg daily in divided doses. Dosage is dependent on size of animal, stage and severity of disease. **Note:** *Tablets no longer marketed in the USA.* Parenterally: 0.0625 – 0.25 mg IV, IM, SC daily; may repeat; Intra-articularly: 0.166 – 1 mg; Intra-lesionally: 0.125 – 1 mg. (Adapted from label; *Flucort®*)

- **CATS:**

For labeled (FDA-approved) indications (**certain acute and chronic dermatoses**); Treat and adjust dosage on an individual basis: Orally: 0.03125 – 0.125 mg daily in divided doses; **Note:** *Tablets no longer marketed in the USA.* Parenterally: 0.03125 – 0.125 mg IV, IM, or SC. If necessary, may repeat. (Adapted from label; *Flucort®*)

- **HORSES:** (NOTE: ARCI UCGFS CLASS 4 DRUG)

For labeled (FDA-approved) indications (**musculoskeletal conditions due to inflammation, where permanent changes do not exist; and also for allergic states such as hives, urticaria and insect bites**): 1.25 – 2.5 mg per horse daily by IV, IM or intra-articular injection. If necessary, the dose may be repeated. (Adapted from label; *Flucort®*)

Monitoring

Monitoring of glucocorticoid therapy is dependent on its reason for use, dosage, agent used (amount of mineralocorticoid activity), dosage schedule (daily versus alternate day therapy), duration of therapy, and the animal's age and condition. The following list may not be appropriate or complete for all animals; use clinical assessment and judgment should adverse effects be noted:

- Weight, appetite, signs of edema.
- Serum and/or urine electrolytes.
- Total plasma proteins, albumin.
- Blood glucose.
- Growth and development in young animals.
- ACTH stimulation test if necessary.

Client Information

- Clients should carefully follow the dosage instructions and should not discontinue the drug abruptly without consulting with veterinarian beforehand.
- Clients should be briefed on the potential adverse effects that can be seen with these drugs and instructed to contact the veterinarian should these effects become severe or progress.

Chemistry/Synonyms

Flumethasone occurs as an odorless, white to creamy white, crystalline powder. Its chemical name is 6alpha, 9alpha-difluoro-16alpha methylprednisolone.

Flumethasone may also be known as: flumetasone, glumetasoni pivalas, NSC-107680, *Cerson®, Flucort®, Locacorten®, Locacortene®, Locorten®, Locortene®,* and *Lorinden®.*

Storage/Stability

Flumethasone injection should be stored at room temperature; avoid freezing.

Dosage Forms/Regulatory Status

VETERINARY-LABELED PRODUCTS:

Flumethasone Injection: 0.5 mg/mL in 100 mL vials; *Flucort® Solution*; (Rx). FDA-approved for use in dogs, cats, and horses.

The ARCI (Racing Commissioners International) has designated this drug as a class 4 substance. See the appendix for more information.

HUMAN-LABELED PRODUCTS: NONE.

Revisions/References

Monograph revised/updated January 2014.

Dowling, P. (2007). Corticosteroids: The wonderful, terrible drugs. Proceedings: AAFP. accessed via Veterinary Information Network; vin.com

Flunixin Meglumine

(floo-nix-in)   Banamine®

Non-Steroidal Antiinflammatory Agent

Prescriber Highlights

▶ Veterinary-only non-steroidal antiinflammatory agent used in a variety of species.

▶ Caution in patients with preexisting GI ulcers, renal, hepatic, or hematologic diseases; in horses with colic, flunixin may mask the behavioral & cardiopulmonary signs associated with endotoxemia or intestinal devitalization.

▶ Use in small animals largely supplanted by FDA-approved agents or those with better adverse effect profile in target species. Still may play a role in ophtho surgery.

▶ If first dose is ineffective for pain control, subsequent doses unlikely to be of benefit.

▶ Adverse Effects in **Horses & Cattle:** Rare anaphylaxis (especially after rapid IV administration); IM injections (extra-label in food animals) may cause pain/swelling; myonecrosis reported in some horses.

Uses/Indications

In the United States, flunixin meglumine is FDA-approved for use in horses, cattle and swine; however, it is approved for use in dogs in other countries. The FDA-approved indications for its use in the horse are for the alleviation of inflammation and pain associated with musculoskeletal disorders and alleviation of visceral pain associated with colic. In cattle it is FDA-approved for the control of pyrexia associated with bovine respiratory disease and endotoxemia, and control of inflammation in endotoxemia. In swine, flunixin is FDA-approved for use to control pyrexia associated with swine respiratory disease. In ruminants, there is some evidence that flunixin is a better analgesic for visceral pain rather than musculoskeletal pain.

Flunixin has been suggested for many other indications in various species, including: Horses: foal diarrheas, shock, colitis, respiratory disease, post-race treatment, and pre- and post-ophthalmic and general surgery; Dogs: disk problems, arthritis, heat stroke, diarrhea, shock, ophthalmic inflammatory conditions, pre- and post-ophthalmic and general surgery, and treatment of parvovirus infection; Cattle: acute respiratory disease, acute coliform mastitis with endotoxic shock, pain (downer cow), and calf diarrheas; Swine: agalactia/hypogalactia, lameness, and piglet diarrhea. It should be noted that the evidence supporting some of these indications is equivocal and flunixin may not be appropriate for every case.

The combination product containing florfenicol and flunixin (*Resflor Gold*®) is FDA-approved for SC use in beef and non-lactating dairy cattle (not veal calves) for treatment of BRD associated with *Mannheimia haemolytica, Pasteurella multocida, Histophilus somni, Mycoplasma bovis* and control BRD-associated pyrexia.

Pharmacology/Actions

Flunixin is a very potent inhibitor of cyclooxygenase and, like other NSAIDs, it exhibits analgesic, antiinflammatory, and antipyretic activity. Flunixin does not appreciably alter GI motility in horses and may improve hemodynamics in animals with septic shock.

Pharmacokinetics

In the horse, flunixin is rapidly absorbed following oral administration with an average bioavailability of 80% and peak serum levels in 30 minutes. Oral bioavailability is good when the injection is mixed with molasses and given orally. The onset of action is generally within 2 hours; peak response occurs between 12-16 hours and the duration of action lasts up to 30 hours. Flunixin is highly bound to plasma proteins (>99% cattle, 92% dogs, 87% horses). Volume of distributions ranges from approximately 0.15 L/kg in horses to 0.78 L/kg in cattle. Elimination is primarily via hepatic routes by biliary excretion. Serum half-lives have been determined in horses ≈ 1.6-4.2 hours, dogs ≈ 3.7 hours; cattle ≈ 3.1-8.1 hours; swine ≈ 6-8 hours. Flunixin is detectable in equine urine for at least 48 hours after a dose.

Contraindications/Precautions/Warnings

The only contraindication the manufacturer lists for flunixin's use in horses is for patients with a history of hypersensitivity reactions to it. It is suggested, however, that flunixin be used cautiously in animals with renal, hepatic, or hematologic diseases. When using to treat colic, flunixin may mask the behavioral and cardiopulmonary signs associated with endotoxemia or intestinal devitalization and must be used with caution.

Do not inject intra-arterially.

In horses with known or suspected EGUS, use should be avoided; single doses of flunixin will probably not result in catastrophic consequences, but repeated doses can exacerbate gastric ulcers (Videla et al. 2009).

In cattle, the drug is contraindicated in animals that have shown prior hypersensitivity reactions. The IM route is extra-label in cattle and should only be used when the IV route is not feasible for use. Longer withdrawal times would be required after IM use. Flunixin should not be used in an attempt to ambulate cattle to be shipped for slaughter.

Flunixin is usually considered contraindicated in cats, but some clinicians have used it short-term. However, FDA-approved (and safer?) NSAIDs are available for cats.

Usage in birds is generally avoided as flunixin can have significant effects on renal function in some species.

Adverse Effects

When used for pain, if the animal does not respond to an initial dose, it is unlikely additional doses will be effective and may increase the chance for toxicity. In horses following IM injection, reports of localized swelling/tissue necrosis, induration, stiffness, and sweating have been reported. Do not inject intra-arterially as it may cause CNS stimulation (hysteria), ataxia, hyperventilation, and muscle weakness. Clinical signs are transient and generally do not require any treatment. Flunixin appears to be a relatively safe agent for use in the horse, but the potential exists for GI intolerance, hypoproteinemia, and hematologic abnormalities to occur. Flunixin is not to be used in horses intended for food.

Horses have developed oral and gastric ulcers, anorexia, and depression when given high doses for prolonged periods (>2 weeks). Although gastric ulceration is frequently observed in adult horses and foals, evidence of an association between this disease and administration of NSAIDs such as flunixin at recommended dosages is lacking. On the basis of current evidence, giving prophylactic anti-ulcer medications to horses receiving therapeutic doses of NSAIDs is probably unnecessary in horses that are otherwise at low risk for gastric ulceration (Fennell et al. 2009).

In horses and cattle, rare anaphylactic-like reactions have been reported, primarily after rapid IV administration. IM injections may rarely be associated with clostridial myonecrosis.

Hematochezia and hematuria have been reported in cattle treated for longer than the 3-day recommendation.

In dogs, GI distress is the most likely adverse reaction. Clinical signs may include, vomiting, diarrhea, and ulceration with very high doses or chronic use. There have been anecdotal reports of flunixin causing renal shutdown in dogs when used at higher dosages pre-operatively.

In birds, flunixin has been shown to cause dose-related, significant renal ischemia and nephrotoxicity.

Reproductive/Nursing Safety

Although reports of teratogenicity, effects on breeding performance, or gestation length have not been noted, flunixin should be used cautiously in pregnant animals. Flunixin is not recommended for use in breeding bulls (lack of reproductive safety data).

In a system evaluating the safety of drugs in canine and feline pregnancy (Papich 1989), this drug is categorized as class: **C** (*These drugs may have potential risks. Studies in people or laboratory animals have uncovered risks, and these drugs should be used cautiously as a last resort when the benefit of therapy clearly outweighs the risks.*)

Overdosage/Acute Toxicity

No clinical case reports of flunixin overdoses were discovered. It is suggested that acute overdosage be handled by using established protocols of emptying the gut (if oral ingestion and practical or possible) and treating the patient supportively.

Gastric ulceration is a distinct possibility in horses that have received overdoses of flunixin. Consider using anti-ulcer medications in overdosed horses.

Drug Interactions

Drug/drug interactions have not been appreciably studied for flunixin and the label does not mention any drug interactions. However, the following drug interactions have either been reported or are theoretical in humans or animals receiving other NSAIDs and may be of significance in veterinary patients receiving flunixin:

- **ASPIRIN:** When aspirin is used concurrently with NSAIDs, plasma levels of the NSAID could decrease and an increased likelihood of GI adverse effects (*e.g.*, blood loss) could occur.
- **CYCLOSPORINE:** NSAIDs may increase cyclosporine blood levels and increase the risk for nephrotoxicity.
- **DIGOXIN:** NSAIDs may increase serum levels of digoxin; use with caution in patients with severe cardiac failure.
- **ENROFLOXACIN:** Has been shown in dogs to increase the AUC and elimination half-life of flunixin and flunixin increases the AUC and elimination half-life of enrofloxacin; it is unknown if other NSAIDs interact with enrofloxacin in dogs. Enrofloxacin and flunixin did not interact in rabbits.
- **FUROSEMIDE & OTHER DIURETICS:** NSAIDs may reduce the saluretic and diuretic effects of furosemide.
- **METHOTREXATE:** Serious toxicity has occurred when NSAIDs have been used concomitantly with methotrexate; use together with caution.
- **NEPHROTOXIC AGENTS** (*e.g.*, **amphotericin B, aminoglycosides, cisplatin,** etc.): Potential for increased risk of nephrotoxicity if used with NSAIDs.
- **PROBENECID:** May cause a significant increase in serum levels and half-life of some NSAIDs.
- **WARFARIN:** Use with NSAIDs may increase the risk for bleeding.

Doses

- **DOGS:**

  As an analgesic/antipyretic (extra-label): **Note:** There are many canine doses published from the time when there were no FDA-approved NSAIDs for dogs; using FDA-approved drugs is recommended. Dosage recommendations vary and there is little evidence to support any suggested dosage. Most recommended dosages are 1 – 1.1 mg/kg IV, IM or SC one time; some say dosages can be repeated once daily for up to 3 days.

  Prior to intraocular surgery (extra-label): In the study a dose of flunixin 0.5 mg/kg IV thirty minutes prior to procedure was more effective than meloxicam or carprofen for minimizing the

PGE2 concentration in the aqueous humor of dogs with experimentally induced uveitis. (Gilmour et al. 2012)

For adjunctive treatment of uveitis (extra-label): 0.25 – 0.5 mg/kg IV once. Some recommended that dosages can be repeated once in 12-24 hours time; others state repeated dosages can be repeated q12-24h for up to 5 treatments however little evidence appears to available to support any specific dosage recommendation.

- **CATS:**

  Prior to intraocular surgery/adjunctive treatment of uveitis (extra-label): Little efficacy/safety evidence to support use in cats, but some suggest that 0.5 – 0.55 mg/kg IV once can be used.

- **FERRETS:**

  As an analgesic/antiinflammatory (extra-label): 0.5 – 2 mg/kg PO or IM one time daily. (Williams 2000)

- **RABBITS/RODENTS/SMALL MAMMALS:**
  a) **Rabbits:** 1.1 mg/kg SC, IM, IV q12–24h. (Ivey et al. 2000)
  b) **Rabbits:** 1.1 mg/kg SC or IM q12h; **Rodents:** 2.5 mg/kg SC or IM q12h. (Huerkamp 1995)
  c) **Chinchillas:** 1 – 3 mg/kg SC q12h; **Guinea pigs:** 2.5 – 5 mg/kg SC q12h; **Gerbils, Mice, Rats, Hamsters:** 2.5 mg/kg SC q12–24h. (Adamcak et al. 2000)

- **CATTLE:**

  Labeled Indication/Dose Flunixin-alone (FDA-approved). **For control of fever associated with respiratory disease or mastitis and fever and inflammation associated with endotoxemia:** 1.1 – 2.2 mg/kg (1 – 2 mL per 100 lbs. body weight) given slow IV either once a day as a single dose or divided into two doses q12h for up to 3 days. Avoid rapid IV administration. (Package Insert; *Banamine®*).

  Labeled Indication/Dose Flunixin/Florfenicol (FDA-approved). **For treatment of bovine respiratory disease (BRD) associated with *Mannheimia haemolytica, Pasteurella multocida,* and *Histophilus somni,* and control of BRD-associated pyrexia in beef and non-lactating dairy cattle:** Using the combination product containing florfenicol/flunixin (*Resflor Gold®*): 40 mg/kg florfenicol/2.2 mg/kg flunixin (6 mL/100 lb. body weight) SC once. Do not administer more than 10 mL at each site. The injection should be given only in the neck. Injection sites other than the neck have not been evaluated. (Label Information — *Resflor Gold®*)

  As an analgesic (extra-label): 1.1 – 2.2 mg/kg IV q6-12 hours; recommend 72-hour milk withdrawal at this dose rate. (Walz 2006)

- **HORSES:** (NOTE: ARCI UCGFS CLASS 4 DRUG)

  For labeled indications (FDA-approved). **For the alleviation of inflammation and pain associated with musculoskeletal disorders and alleviation of visceral pain associated with colic:**

  Injectable: 1.1 mg/kg IV or IM once daily for up to 5 days (**Note:** *IM use has sometimes been associated with muscle necrosis–Plumb*). For colic cases, use IV route and may re-dose when necessary.

  Oral Paste: 1.1 mg/kg PO (see markings on syringe—calibrated in 250 lb. weight increments) once daily. One syringe will treat a 1000 lb. horse for 3 days. Do not exceed 5 days of consecutive therapy.

  Oral Granules: 1.1 mg/kg PO once daily. One packet will treat 500 lbs. of body weight. May apply on feed. Do not exceed 5 consecutive days of therapy. (Package Inserts; *Banamine®*)

  To decrease pain, inflammation, and edema in laminitis (extra-label): 0.5 – 1.1 mg/kg IV or PO q8-12 hours. A dose of

0.25 mg/kg can be administered IV q8h to interrupt eicosanoid production associated with endotoxemia. (Moore 2003)

For adjunctive treatment of uveitis in foals (extra-label): 0.5 – 1 mg/kg (route not noted) twice daily. (Cutler 2003)

- **SHEEP, GOATS:**

As an analgesic (extra-label): 1 – 2 mg/kg IV q24h; oral paste has also been used at 1 – 4 mg/kg PO once daily. (Snyder 2009)

- **SWINE:**

To control pyrexia associated with swine respiratory disease (labeled-dose; FDA-approved): 2.2 mg/kg IM once, only in the neck musculature with a maximum of 10 mL per site. (Label information; *Banamine®-S*—Schering-Plough)

- **ZOO, EXOTIC, WILDLIFE SPECIES:**

For use in zoo, exotic and wildlife medicine refer to specific references, including:

a) *Zoo Animal and Wildlife Immobilization and Anesthesia.* West, G., Heard, D., Caulkett, N. (eds.). Blackwell Publishing, 2007.

b) *Handbook of Wildlife Chemical Immobilization, 3rd Ed.* Kreeger, T.J. and J.M. Arnemo. 2007.

c) *Fowler's Zoo and Wild Animal Medicine Current Therapy, Volume 7,* Miller, R.E., Fowler, M.E., Saunders. 2011.

d) *Exotic Animal Formulary, 4th Ed.* Carpenter, J.W., Saunders. 2012.

e) The 2009 American Association of Zoo Veterinarian Proceedings by D. K. Fontenot also has several dosages listed for restraint, anesthesia, and analgesia for a variety of drugs for carnivores and primates. VIN members can access them at: http://goo.gl/NNIWQ or http://goo.gl/9UJse

Monitoring

- Analgesic/antiinflammatory/antipyretic effects.
- GI effects in dogs.
- CBC's, occult blood in feces with chronic use in horses.

Client Information

- If injecting IM, do not inject into neck muscles.
- The IM route is extra-label in cattle and should only be used when the IV route is not feasible for use. Longer withdrawal times would be required after IM use.
- Flunixin should not be used in an attempt to ambulate cattle to be shipped for slaughter.

Chemistry/Synonyms

Flunixin meglumine, a nonsteroidal antiinflammatory agent is a highly substituted derivative of nicotinic acid, and is unique structurally when compared to other NSAIDs. It occurs as a white to off-white powder that is soluble in water and alcohol. The chemical name for flunixin is 3-pyridine-carboxylic acid.

Flunixin may also be known as 3-pyridine-carboxylic acid, flunixin meglumine, Sch-14714, *Banamine®*, *Flumeglumine®*, and *Finadyne®*, *Flu-Nix®D*, *Flunixamine®*, *Flunixiject®*, *Flunizine®*, *Prevail®*, *Suppressor®*, and *Vedagesic®*.

Storage/Stability

All flunixin products should be stored between 2-30°C (36-86°F).

The combination product with florfenicol (*Resflor Gold®*) should not be stored above 30°C (86°F). Once the vial is entered it should be used within 28 days. The 500 mL vial should not be punctured more than 10 times.

Compatibility/Compounding Considerations

It has been recommended that flunixin meglumine injection not be mixed with other drugs because of unknown compatibilities.

Dosage Forms/Regulatory Status

VETERINARY-LABELED PRODUCTS:

Note: Individual products may be FDA-approved and labeled for different species, lactation status, different routes of administration (IV, IM). Flunixin is also FDA-approved only for use in horses not intended for food. Refer to the specific product label for more information.

Flunixin Meglumine for Injection: 50 mg/mL in 50 mL, 100 mL and 250 mL vials; *Banamine®*, *Flumeglumine®*, *Flunixamine®*, *Flunixiject®*, *Prevail®*, *Suppressor® Dairy*, *Flunizine®*, *Vedagesic®*; *Flu-Nix-®D*, generic; (Rx). Products may be FDA-approved for use in horses and beef and dairy cattle (not for use in dry dairy cows or veal calves). Depending on product, when used as labeled: withdrawal (Cattle): Milk: 36 hours; Slaughter: 4 days (US); 6 days (Canada). The product label for *Banamine Injection®* can be found at dailymed.nlm.nih.gov

Flunixin Meglumine for Injection: 50 mg/mL in 100 mL vials; *Banamine®-S*; (Rx) FDA-approved for IM use in swine; Withdrawal: Slaughter: 12 days.

Flunixin Meglumine for Injection: 50 mg/mL in 100 mL vials; *Suppressor®*; (Rx). FDA-approved for use in horses.

Flunixin Meglumine Oral Paste: 1500 mg/syringe in 30 gram syringes in boxes of 6; *Banamine® Paste*; (Rx). FDA-approved for use in horses.

Flunixin Meglumine Oral Granules: 250 mg in 10 gram sachets in boxes of 50; 20 g sachets containing 500 mg flunixin in boxes of 25; *Banamine® Granules*; (Rx). FDA-approved for use in horses.

Flunixin 16.5 mg/mL with Florfenicol 300 mg/mL Injection in 100 mL, 250 mL and 500 mL vials; *Resflor Gold®*; (Rx). FDA-approved for use in beef and non-lactating dairy cattle. Do not slaughter within 38 days of last treatment. Not for use in female dairy cattle 20 months of age or older or calves to be processed for veal. Use may cause milk residues. A withdrawal period has not been established in preruminating calves. The ARCI (Racing Commissioners International) has designated flunixin/florfenicol as a class 4 substance. See the appendix for more information. The product label for Resflor Gold® can be found at dailymed.nlm.nih.gov

HUMAN-LABELED PRODUCTS: NONE.

Revisions/References

Monograph revised/updated January 2014.

Adamcak, A. & B. Otten (2000). Rodent Therapeutics. Vet Clin NA: Exotic Anim Pract 3:1(Jan): 221-40.

Cutler, T. (2003). Neonatal foals: beyond corneal ulcers. Proceedings: ACVIM Forum. accessed via Veterinary Information Network; vin.com

Fennell, L. C. & R. P. Franklin (2009). Do nonsteroidal anti-inflammatory drugs administered at therapeutic dosages induce gastric ulcers in horses? Equine Veterinary Education 21(12): 660-2.

Gilmour, M. A. & M. E. Payton (2012). Comparison of the effects of IV administration of meloxicam, carprofen, and flunixin meglumine on prostaglandin E-2 concentration in aqueous humor of dogs with aqueocentesis-induced anterior uveitis. American Journal of Veterinary Research 73(5): 698-703.

Huerkamp, M. (1995). Anesthesia and postoperative management of rabbits and pocket pets. *Kirk's Current Veterinary Therapy:XII.* J. Bonagura. Philadelphia, W.B. Saunders: 1322-7.

Ivey, E. & J. Morrisey (2000). Therapeutics for Rabbits. Vet Clin NA: Exotic Anim Pract 3:1(Jan): 183-216.

Moore, R. (2003). New developments in the treatment of reperfusion injury and acute laminitis in horses. Proceedings: ACVIM Forum. accessed via Veterinary Information Network; vin.com

Snyder, J. (2009). Anesthesia and pain management: Minor surgeries. Proceedings: WVC. accessed via Veterinary Information Network; vin.com

Videla, R. & F. M. Andrews (2009). New Perspectives in Equine Gastric Ulcer Syndrome. Veterinary Clinics of North America-Equine Practice 25(2): 283-+.

Walz, P. (2006). Practical management of pain in cattle. Proceedings: ABVP. accessed via Veterinary Information Network; vin.com

Williams, B. (2000). Therapeutics in Ferrets. Vet Clin NA: Exotic Anim Pract 3:1(Jan): 131-53.

5-Fluorocytosine – see Flucytosine

Fluorouracil (5-FU)

(flure-oh-yoor-a-sill)   Adrucil®

Antineoplastic Agent

Prescriber Highlights

▶ Antineoplastic agent used in dogs for susceptible tumors (see doses) & intralesionally in horses for skin tumors.

▶ Contraindications: Do **NOT** use in any form on cats; Patients hypersensitive to it, in poor nutritional states, depressed bone marrow, serious infections.

▶ Known teratogen.

▶ Adverse Effects: Dose-dependent myelosuppression, GI toxicity, & neurotoxicity.

Uses/Indications

Chemotherapeutic agent that has been used for canine mammary carcinoma (in combination with doxorubicin and cyclophosphamide—FAC protocol), dermal squamous cell carcinoma and GI tract tumors. It is also used topically and for intralesional injection with epinephrine into certain skin neoplasms (squamous cell carcinoma, melanoma, sarcoid) in horses.

Pharmacology/Actions

Fluorouracil is converted via intracellular mechanisms to active metabolites (fluoruridine monophosphate—FUMP and fluoruridine triphosphate—FUTP). FUMP inhibits the synthesis of deoxythymidine triphosphate thereby interfering with DNA synthesis. FUTP incorporates into RNA and inhibits cell function.

Pharmacokinetics

Fluorouracil is administered systemically via the IV route. It rapidly disappears from the systemic circulation (plasma half live is about 15 minutes in humans) and is primarily distributed into tumor cells, intestinal mucosa, liver, and bone marrow. While some of the drug is converted to active metabolites, (see Pharmacology above), the majority of it is metabolized by the liver. A small amount (about 15% of dose) is excreted unchanged into the urine.

Contraindications/Precautions/Warnings

Cats develop a severe, potentially fatal neurotoxicity when given fluorouracil. Do **NOT** use in cats in any form (including topical).

5-FU is contraindicated in patients hypersensitive to it, in poor nutritional states, with depressed or reduced bone marrow function or concurrent serious infections.

Adverse Effects

In dogs, 5-FU causes a dose-dependent myelosuppression, GI toxicity (diarrhea, GI ulceration/sloughing, stomatitis), and neurotoxicity (seizures). Fluorouracil has a very narrow therapeutic index and should be used only by clinicians with experience using cancer chemotherapeutic agents.

Reproductive/Nursing Safety

The drug is a known teratogen and its use should be weighed against any risks to offspring. In humans, the FDA categorizes this drug as category *D* for use during pregnancy (*There is evidence of human fetal risk, but the potential benefits from the use of the drug in pregnant women may be acceptable despite its potential risks.*)

It is not known whether fluorouracil is excreted in milk. Because fluorouracil inhibits DNA, RNA and protein synthesis, milk replacer should be considered if the dam requires 5-FU.

Overdosage/Acute Toxicity

While overdoses are possible with IV use, careful checking of dosages and preparation should minimize the risks. Oral ingestions of topical products have occurred with dogs and cats and can be very serious. The prognosis for dogs with ingestion of 5-FU is dependent on the amount consumed, with severe intoxication carrying a poor prognosis. Toxic doses in dogs can be as little as 5 mg/kg, and doses ≥40 mg/kg are reported to be uniformly fatal (Sayre et al. 2012). Signs at lower doses include mild GI irritation and vomiting. Seizures and death have been reported at doses as low as 10.3 mg/kg (APCC database) and survival in dogs may be as low as 25% Very small ingestions can reportedly cause death in cats. Clinical signs may be seen within 30 minutes to 6 hours after ingestion; death has been reported in 7 hours. Clinical signs include acute nausea, vomiting, hemorrhagic diarrhea, abdominal pain, GI sloughing, ataxia, severe and non-responsive seizures, and severe dose-dependent myelosuppression affecting all cell lines. Severe metabolic acidosis and signs of multi-organ failure can be seen (Lee 2010).

There were 190 single agent exposures to fluorouracil reported to the ASPCA Animal Poison Control Center (APCC) during 2009-2013. Of the 186 dogs, 156 were symptomatic with vomiting (73%), seizures (62%), death/euthanasia (24%) and ataxia (16%) being the most commonly reported.

Should an oral ingestion occur, aggressive GI decontamination with GI protection should be done, especially if the ingestion was very recent. However, decontamination may not be effective due to the rapid onset of toxicity. Treatment is primarily supportive and can include antiemetics, anticonvulsants, fluid support, etc. Intensive monitoring is required. Seizure control with diazepam is often unrewarding and a barbiturate or general anesthesia is often required. Pain and body temperature control are important. Use broad-spectrum antibiotics to prevent secondary bacterial infections. If bone marrow suppression develops, filgrastim (*Neupogen*®) can be considered to stimulate bone marrow stem cell proliferation in dogs. Complete blood counts should be routinely performed (every 3-4 days) for at least 18 days, as it may take up to 3 weeks before all cell lines return to normal (Lee 2010).

Patients given an accidental parenteral overdose should undergo intensive hematologic monitoring for at least 4 weeks and be supported as required.

Drug Interactions

The following drug interactions have either been reported or are theoretical in humans or animals receiving fluorouracil and may be of significance in veterinary patients. Unless otherwise noted, use together is not necessarily contraindicated, but weigh the potential risks and perform additional monitoring when appropriate.

■ **LEUCOVORIN:** May increase the GI toxic effects of 5-FU.

Laboratory Considerations

■ Fluorouracil may cause increases in alkaline phosphatase, serum transaminase, serum bilirubin, and lactic dehydrogenase.

Doses

NOTE: Because of the potential toxicity of this drug to patients, veterinary personnel and clients, and since chemotherapy indications, treatment protocols, monitoring and safety guidelines often change, the following dosages should be used only as a general guide. Consultation with a veterinary oncologist and referral to current veterinary oncology references [*e.g.,* (Withrow et al. 2012); (Dobson et al. 2011); (Henry et al. 2009); (North et al. 2009); (Argyle et al. 2008)] are <u>strongly recommended</u>.

■ **DOGS:**

For canine mammary carcinoma (in combination with doxorubicin and cyclophosphamide—FAC protocol), dermal squamous cell carcinoma and GI tract tumors: 150 mg/m² IV weekly, or 5 – 10 mg/kg IV weekly. (Kitchell et al. 2000)

- **CATS:**

  5-FU is CONTRAINDICATED in cats in any form (including topical).

- **HORSES:**

  For intratumoral injection for squamous cell carcinoma (SCC), melanoma, sarcoids (extra-label): 5-FU can be injected intralesionally at doses of 1 – 3 mL per tumor site (depending on size of tumor). Epinephrine is typically added to the injection at a ratio of 1 part epinephrine to 10 parts 5-FU. Can also be mixed with sterile sesame seed oil (1:1) immediately prior to usage then injected. Generally, this can be successful for resolution of small sarcoids and SCC, but is often ineffective for melanoma. Maximum systemic dosage ~750 mg for average horse. (Phillips 2011)

Monitoring

- CBC's (nadirs usually occur between days 9-14 with recovery by day 30; no dog info located).
- GI and CNS adverse effects.
- Efficacy.

Client Information

- Fluorouracil is a chemotherapy (cancer) drug. The drug and its byproducts can be hazardous to other animals and people that come in contact with it. On the day your animal gets the drug and then for a few days afterward, all bodily waste (urine, feces, litter), blood, or vomit should only be handled while wearing disposable gloves. Seal the waste in a plastic bag and then place both the bag and gloves in with the regular trash.
- If applying fluorouracil to the skin of your animal, wear disposable gloves and wash your hands immediately after each use.
- Fluorouracil should NEVER be used in cats.
- Fluorouracil can be very toxic to the nervous system (seizures, convulsions) and to the gastrointestinal tract (vomiting and gastrointestinal upset).

Chemistry/Synonyms

A pyrimidine antagonist antineoplastic agent, fluorouracil (5-FU) occurs as a white, practically odorless, crystalline powder. It is sparingly soluble in water and slightly soluble in alcohol. The commercially available injection has its pH adjusted to 8.6–9.4 and may be colorless or slightly yellow in color.

Fluorouracil may also be known as 5-fluorouracil, fluorouracilo, fluorouracilum, 5-FU, NSC-19893, Ro-2-9757, and WR-69596; many trade names are available.

Storage/Stability

The injection should be stored between 15-30°C; avoid freezing and exposure to light.

Compatibility/Compounding Considerations

Slight color changes in the solution can be ignored. If a precipitate forms, the solution can be heated to 60°C and shaken vigorously to redissolve the drug. Cool to body temperature before administering. If unsuccessful in redissolving the drug, it should not be used.

Dosage Forms/Regulatory Status

VETERINARY-LABELED PRODUCTS: NONE.

HUMAN-LABELED PRODUCTS:

Fluorouracil Injection: 50 mg/mL in 10 mL, 20 mL, 50 mL, & 100 mL vials and 10 mL amps; *Adrucil®*; generic; (Rx)

Also available in topical creams and solutions in concentrations ranging from 0.5%-5%. These are indicated in humans for treating multiple actinic or solar keratoses, and superficial basal cell carcinomas (5%) when other treatments are impractical.

Revisions/References

Monograph revised/updated January 2014.

Argyle, D., et al. (2008). *Decision Making in Small Animal Oncology*, Wiley-Blackwell.

Dobson, J. & D. Lascelles (2011). *BSAVA Manual of Canine and Feline Oncology*, BSAVA.

Henry, C. & M. Higginbotham (2009). *Cancer Management in Small Animal Practice*, Saunders.

Kitchell, B. & R. Dhaliwal (2000). CVT Update: Anticancer Drugs and Protocols Using Traditional Drugs. *Kirk's Current Veterinary Therapy: XIII Small Animal Practice*. J. Bonagura. Philadelphia, WB Saunders: 465-73.

Lee, J. A. (2010). Top Ten Small Animal Toxins: Recognition, Diagnosis, Treatment. Proceedings: ACVIM. accessed via Veterinary Information Network; vin.com

North, S. & T. Banks (2009). *Small Animal Oncology: An Introduction*, Saunders.

Phillips, J. (2011). Standard and Novel Treatments for Solid Tumors in Equids. ACVIM. accessed via Veterinary Information Network; vin.com

Sayre, R. S., et al. (2012). Accidental and experimentally induced 5-fluorouracil toxicity in dogs. J. Vet. Emerg. Crit. Care 22(5).

Withrow, S., et al. (2012). Withrow and MacEwen's Small Animal Clinical Oncology, 5th Ed., Saunders.

Fluoxetine HCl

(floo-ox-e-teen)   Prozac®, Reconcile®

Selective Serotonin-Reuptake Inhibitor (SSRI)

Prescriber Highlights

▶ A selective-serotonin reuptake inhibitor antidepressant used in dogs (approved) & cats (extra-label) for a variety of behavior disorders.

▶ Contraindications: Patients with known hypersensitivity or receiving monoamine oxidase inhibitors.

▶ Caution: Patients with diabetes mellitus or seizure disorders; dosages may need to be reduced in patients with severe hepatic impairment.

▶ Adverse Effects: <u>Dogs:</u> Anorexia, lethargy, GI effects, anxiety, irritability, insomnia/hyperactivity, or panting, & aggressive behavior in previously unaggressive dogs is possible; <u>Cats:</u> May exhibit behavior changes (anxiety, irritability, sleep disturbances), anorexia, & changes in elimination patterns.

▶ Drug Interactions.

Uses/Indications

Fluoxetine may be beneficial for the treatment of canine aggression, stereotypic behaviors (and other obsessive-compulsive behaviors), and anxiety. It may be useful in cats for the aforementioned behaviors and, additionally, for inappropriate elimination.

The veterinary FDA-approved product (*Reconcile®*) is labeled for the treatment of canine separation anxiety in conjunction with a behavior modification plan.

Pharmacology/Actions

Fluoxetine is a highly selective inhibitor of the reuptake of serotonin in the CNS thereby potentiating the pharmacologic activity of serotonin. Fluoxetine apparently has little effect on other neurotransmitters (*e.g.*, dopamine or norepinephrine). In dogs and cats, fluoxetine has anxiolytic and anticompulsive effects, and may also reduce aggressive behaviors.

Pharmacokinetics

Fluoxetine is apparently well absorbed after oral administration. In a study done in beagles, approximately 70% of an oral dose reached the systemic circulation. The presence of food altered the rate, but not the extent, of absorption. The oral capsules and oral liquid apparently are bioequivalent. When applied transdermally (15% in a PLO gel) to cats, bioavailability was approximately 10% of the oral route (Ciribassi et al. 2003).

Fluoxetine and its principal metabolite, norfluoxetine (active), are apparently distributed throughout the body with highest levels found in the lungs and liver. CNS concentrations are detected within one hour of dosing. In humans, fluoxetine is approximately 95% bound to plasma proteins. Fluoxetine crosses the placenta in rats, but it is unknown if it does so in other species. Fluoxetine enters maternal milk in concentrations about 20-30% of those found in plasma.

Fluoxetine is primarily metabolized in the liver to a variety of metabolites, including norfluoxetine (active). Both fluoxetine and norfluoxetine are eliminated slowly. In dogs, elimination half-life average for fluoxetine is about 6+ hours and for norfluoxetine, about 2 days; wide interpatient variation does occur, however. Renal impairment does not apparently affect elimination rates substantially, but liver impairment will decrease clearance rates. In humans, the elimination half-life of fluoxetine is about 2-3 days and norfluoxetine, about 7-9 days.

Contraindications/Precautions/Warnings

The labeling for the veterinary (canine) FDA-approved drug states that fluoxetine should not be used in dogs with epilepsy or a history of seizures and it should not be given with drugs that lower the seizure threshold (*e.g.*, acepromazine, chlorpromazine). Fluoxetine is contraindicated in patients with known hypersensitivity to it, as well as those receiving monoamine oxidase inhibitors (see Drug Interactions below).

Fluoxetine should be used with caution in patients with diabetes mellitus as it may alter blood glucose. Dosages may need to be reduced in patients with severe hepatic impairment.

Because of the long half-life of norfluoxetine, tapering off the drug is probably only necessary when a patient has been on the drug long-term (>8 weeks) (Landsberg 2008).

Do not confuse FLUoxetine with DULoxetine or PARoxetine.

Adverse Effects

In multi-site field trials in dogs, seizures were reported in some of the dogs treated with fluoxetine. Absolute causality and incidence rate has not been determined. Fluoxetine may cause lethargy, GI effects, anxiety, irritability, insomnia/hyperactivity, or panting. Anorexia is a common side-affect in dogs (usually transient and may be negated by temporarily increasing the palatability of food and/or hand feeding). Some dogs have persistent anorexia that precludes further treatment. Aggressive behavior in previously unaggressive dogs has been reported. Post-approval (2010) reported adverse events include (listed in decreasing order of frequency): decreased appetite, depression/lethargy, shaking/shivering/tremor, vomiting, restlessness and anxiety, seizures, aggression, diarrhea, mydriasis, vocalization, weight loss, panting, confusion, incoordination, and hypersalivation.

Cats may exhibit behavior changes (anxiety, irritability, sleep disturbances), anorexia, diarrhea and changes in elimination patterns.

In humans, potential adverse effects are extensive and diverse, but most those most commonly noted include anxiety, nervousness, insomnia, drowsiness, fatigue, dizziness, anorexia, nausea, rash, diarrhea, and sweating; seizures or hepatotoxicity are possible. About 15% of human patients discontinue treatment due to adverse effects.

Reproductive/Nursing Safety

Fluoxetine's safety during pregnancy has not been established. The canine FDA-approved product states that studies to determine the effects of fluoxetine in breeding, pregnant, or lactating dogs or in patients less than 6 months of age have not been conducted. Preliminary studies done in rats demonstrated no overt teratogenic effects. In humans, the FDA categorizes this drug as category *C* for use during pregnancy (*Animal studies have shown an adverse effect on the fetus, but there are no adequate studies in humans; or there are no animal reproduction studies and no adequate studies in humans.*)

The drug is excreted into milk (20-30% of plasma levels), so caution is advised in nursing patients. Clinical implications for nursing offspring are not clear.

Overdosage/Acute Toxicity

The LD$_{50}$ for rats is 452 mg/kg and in dogs >100 mg/kg, but a median dose of 15.9 mg/kg is reported to cause clinical signs of SSRI toxicity in dogs (Thomas et al. 2012). A retrospective study in cats found dosages as low as 3.7 mg/kg caused clinical signs of toxicity (Pugh et al. 2013). In a study, five of six dogs given an oral "toxic" dose developed seizures that immediately stopped after giving IV diazepam. The dog having the lowest plasma level of fluoxetine that developed seizures had a level twice that expected of a human taking 80 mg day (highest recommended dose).

There were 860 single agent exposures to fluoxetine reported to the ASPCA Animal Poison Control Center (APCC) during 2009-2013. Of the 707 dogs, 189 were symptomatic with lethargy (23%), vomiting (21%), mydriasis (16%), tachycardia (12%) and vocalization (11%) being the most common. Of the 154 cats, 50 were symptomatic with 24% vomiting, 20% hypersalivating, 16% mydriatic and 14% vocalizing.

Treatment of fluoxetine overdoses consists of symptomatic and supportive therapy. Gut emptying techniques should be employed when warranted and otherwise not contraindicated. Diazepam should be considered to treat seizures. Cyproheptadine can be used as a serotonin antagonist.

Drug Interactions

The following drug interactions have either been reported or are theoretical in humans or animals receiving fluoxetine and may be of significance in veterinary patients. Unless otherwise noted, use together is not necessarily contraindicated, but weigh the potential risks and perform additional monitoring when appropriate.

- **BUSPIRONE:** Increased risk for serotonin syndrome.
- **CYPROHEPTADINE:** May decrease or reverse the effects of SSRIs.
- **DIAZEPAM, ALPRAZOLAM:** Fluoxetine may increase diazepam levels.
- **DIURETICS:** Increased risk for hyponatremia.
- **INSULIN:** May alter insulin requirements.
- **ISONIAZID:** Increased risk for serotonin syndrome.
- **MAO INHIBITORS** (including **amitraz** and potentially, **selegiline**): High risk for serotonin syndrome; use contraindicated; in humans, a 5 week washout period is required after discontinuing fluoxetine and a 2 week washout period if first discontinuing the MAO inhibitor.
- **NONSTEROIDAL ANTIINFLAMMATORY DRUGS (NSAIDS, ASPIRIN):** SSRI's may increase the risk for GI ulceration.
- **PENTAZOCINE:** Serotonin syndrome-like adverse effects possible.
- **PHENYTOIN:** Increased plasma levels of phenytoin possible.
- **PROPRANOLOL, METOPROLOL:** Fluoxetine may increase these beta-blocker's plasma levels; atenolol may be safer to use if fluoxetine required.
- **ST JOHNS WORT:** Increased risk for serotonin syndrome.
- **TRAMADOL:** SSRI's can inhibit the metabolism of tramadol to the active metabolites decreasing its efficacy and increasing the risk of toxicity (serotonin syndrome, seizures).
- **TRICYCLIC ANTIDEPRESSANTS** (*e.g.*, **clomipramine, amitriptyline**): Fluoxetine may increase TCA blood levels and the risk for serotonin syndrome.
- **TRAZODONE:** Increased plasma levels of trazodone possible.
- **WARFARIN:** Fluoxetine may increase the risk for bleeding.

Doses

- **DOGS:**

  Labeled dose (FDA-approved): **For the treatment of canine separation anxiety in conjunction with a behavior modification plan:** 1 – 2 mg/kg PO once daily. (Label Information; *Reconcile®*)

  Extra-label Doses: For the adjunctive treatment of behavior disorders (noise aversion, compulsive disorder, aggression, etc.): Most recommend the labeled dosage (1 – 2 mg/kg PO once daily), but dosages as high as 3 mg/kg once daily have been noted. May take 4-8 weeks before efficacy can be fully assessed.

- **CATS:**

  For adjunctive treatment of behavior disorders (urine marking, separation anxiety, aggression, etc.); (extra-label): Recommended doses in cats are usually 0.5 – 1 mg/kg PO once daily. Some have recommended up to 1.5 mg/kg PO once daily. Treatment may be required for up to 8 weeks before full determination of efficacy. When using for urine marking, after 8-12 weeks of successful treatment dosage may be reduced gradually (approx. 25%) per week to see if urine marking returns. If so, dosage is increased.

Monitoring

- Efficacy.
- Adverse effects; including appetite (weight).

Client Information

- May be given with or without food. If your animal vomits or acts sick after getting it on an empty stomach, give with food or small treat to see if this helps. If vomiting continues, contact your veterinarian.
- This medication is most effective when used with a behavior modification program. May take several days to weeks to determine if the drug is effective.
- Do not stop this medication abruptly without veterinarian's guidance.
- Most common side effects are: drowsiness/sleepiness, and reduced appetite. Rare side effects that can be serious: seizures, aggression; contact veterinarian immediately.
- Overdoses can be very serious; keep out of the reach of animals and children.
- If your animal wore a flea collar in the past two weeks, let your veterinarian know. Do not use one on your animal while it's getting this medicine without first talking to your veterinarian.

Chemistry/Synonyms

A member of the phenylpropylamine-derivative antidepressant group, fluoxetine differs both structurally and pharmacologically from either the tricyclic or monoamine oxidase inhibitor antidepressants. Fluoxetine HCl occurs as a white to off-white crystalline solid. Approximately 50 mg are soluble in 1 mL of water.

Fluoxetine may also be known as: fluoxetini hydrochloridum, and LY-110140; many trade names are available.

Storage/Stability

Capsules and tablets should be stored in well-closed containers at room temperature. The oral liquid should be stored in tight, light-resistant containers at room temperature.

Compatibility/Compounding Considerations

No specific information noted.

Dosage Forms/Regulatory Status

VETERINARY-LABELED PRODUCTS:

Fluoxetine Chewable Tablets: 8 mg, 16 mg, 32 mg, & 64 mg; *Reconcile®*; (Rx). FDA-approved (NADA 141-272) for use in dogs. The label information for *Reconcile®* can be found at dailymed.nlm.nih.gov

The ARCI (Racing Commissioners International) has designated this drug as a class 2 substance. See the appendix for more information.

HUMAN-LABELED PRODUCTS:

Fluoxetine HCl Oral Tablets: 10 mg, 15 mg & 20 mg; generic; (Rx)

Fluoxetine HCl Oral Capsules: 10 mg, 20 mg, 40 mg & 90 mg (delayed-release only); *Prozac® Pulvules & Prozac® Weekly, Sarafem® Pulvules*, generic; (Rx)

Fluoxetine HCl Oral Solution 20 mg/5 mL (may contain alcohol, sucrose) in 120 mL & 473 mL; *Prozac®*, generic; (Rx)

Revisions/References

Monograph revised/updated January 2014.

Ciribassi, J., et al. (2003). Comparative bioavailability of fluoxetine after transdermal and oral administration to healthy cats. American Journal of Veterinary Research **64**(8): 994-8.

Landsberg, G. (2008). Treating canine and feline anxiety: Drug therapy and pheromones. Proceedings: BSAVA. accessed via Veterinary Information Network; vin.com

Pugh, C. M., et al. (2013). Selective serotonin reuptake inhibitor (SSRI) toxicosis in cats: 33 cases (2004-2010). J. Vet. Emerg. Crit. Care **23**(5): 565-70.

Thomas, D. E., et al. (2012). Retrospective evaluation of toxicosis from selective serotonin reuptake inhibitor antidepressants: 313 dogs (2005-2010). J. Vet. Emerg. Crit. Care **22**(6): 674-81.

Fluralaner

(floor-ah-lan-er)   Bravecto®

Insecticide; Acaricide

Prescriber Highlights

▶ Oral (chewable tablets), long-acting insecticide/acaracide for dogs.

▶ Contraindications: None known at present. Not labeled for use in dogs weighing less than 4.4 lbs. (2 kg) or less than 6 months old.

▶ Adverse Effects: GI effects possible.

Uses/Indications

The veterinary FDA-approved product (*Bravecto®*) is labeled for the for the treatment and prevention of flea infestations (*Ctenocephalides felis*) and the treatment and control of tick infestations [*Ixodes scapularis* (black-legged tick), *Dermacentor variabilis* (American dog tick), and *Rhipicephalus sanguineus* (brown dog tick)] for 12 weeks in dogs and puppies 6 months of age and older, and weighing 4.4 pounds or greater. It also indicated for the treatment and control of *Amblyomma americanum* (Lone Star tick) infestations for 8 weeks in dogs and puppies 6 months of age and older, and weighing 4.4 pounds or greater.

Pharmacology/Actions

Fluralaner inhibits gamma-aminobutyric acid- (GABA-) and glutamate-gated chloride channels with significant selectivity for insect neurons over mammalian neurons (Gassel et al. 2014). Inhibition induces uncontrolled neuronal activity with resultant paralysis and death of fleas and ticks. After feeding onset of action is within 8 hours for fleas and 12 hours for ticks.

Pharmacokinetics

After IV administration (12.5 mg/kg slowly) in dogs, volume of distribution was 3.1 L/kg and mean clearance 0.14 L/kg/day and elimination half-life 15 days. The drug is highly bound to plasma proteins. After oral or IV administration elimination half-life averaged 12-15 days. Giving chewable tablets with food increases bioavailability by approximately 2-2.5X. Because fluralaner is highly bound to plasma proteins, it is assumed the primary route of elimination is hepatic, but the hepatic extraction ratio is estimated to be low (0.3%). (Kilp et al. 2014; Walther, Allan, et al. 2014)

Contraindications/Precautions/Warnings

The labeling for the veterinary (canine) FDA-approved product states: "There are no known contraindications for the use of the product." However, the product is not labeled for use in dogs weighing less than 4.4 lbs. (2 kg) or less than 6 months old.

No adverse effects were noted after 3X doses were administered to Collies homozygous for the MDR1 deletion mutation (Walther, Paul, et al. 2014).

Adverse Effects

At the time of writing (May 2014) fluralaner appears to be quite safe in dogs, however the adverse effect profile should be further clarified after post-approval clinical experience. In pre-approval field trials in dogs, vomiting was the most common adverse effect reported. Decreased appetite, hypersalivation, and diarrhea were also reported.

Reproductive/Nursing Safety

While safe use during pregnancy is not firmly established, the product labeling (USA) has no specific cautions regarding use in breeding, pregnant or lactating dogs. A reproductive safety study in Beagles (doses up to 3X) found no clinically relevant effects on body weight, food consumption, reproductive performance, semen analysis, litter data, gross necropsy (adult dogs) or histopathology findings (adult dogs and puppies). However, abnormalities were noted in 7 pups from 2 of the 10 dams in the treated group: limb deformity (4 pups), enlarged heart (2 pups), enlarged spleen (3 pups), and cleft palate (2 pups). Weigh the potential risks versus benefits in treating pregnant dogs.

No information regarding fluralaner's distribution in maternal milk was located, but concentrations would be expected to be very low.

Overdosage/Acute Toxicity

Some puppies (8-9 week old) receiving up to 5X developed diarrhea, mucoid, and bloody feces. If clinical signs occur after an overdose, treat supportively.

Drug Interactions

None reported at present. In field trials, vaccines, anthelmintics, antibiotics, and steroids were given concurrently to some dogs without observed adverse reactions.

Doses

- **DOGS:**

  For approved indications (see Uses/Indications); (FDA-approved): A minimum dose of 11.4 mg/lb. (25 mg/kg) PO with food every 12 weeks (8 weeks for *Amblyomma americanum* ticks). The product is available in 5 different strengths for dogs weighing between 2-56 kg (4.4-123 lbs.); dogs weighing more than 56 kg (123 lbs.) should receive the appropriate number of tablets. Adapted from label; *Bravecto*®. (Anon 2014)

Monitoring

- Efficacy.
- Adverse effects if any.

Client Information

- Keep this and all drugs out of the reach of children. The label states to keep the product in the original packaging until use to prevent children from getting direct access.
- Do not eat, drink or smoke while handling the product. Wash hands thoroughly with soap and water immediately after use.
- Report any side effects to veterinarian.

Chemistry/Synonyms

Fluralaner is an isoxazoline-substituted benzamide derivative insecticide/acaracide. It has a molecular weight of 556.29 and an octa-nol/water partition coefficient of 5.35. ATCvet code is QP53BX and trade name is *Bravecto*®.

Storage/Stability

Do not store above 86°F (30°C).

Compatibility/Compounding Considerations

No specific information noted.

Dosage Forms/Regulatory Status

VETERINARY-LABELED PRODUCTS:

Fluralaner Chewable Tablets: 112 mg (2-4.5 kg; 4.4-9.9 lbs.), 250 mg (>4.5-10 kg; >9.9-22 lbs.), 500 mg (>10-20 kg; >22-44 lbs.), 1000 mg (>20-40 kg; >44-88 lbs.) & 1400 mg (>40-56 kg; >88-123 lbs.); *Bravecto*®®; (Rx). FDA-approved (NADA 141-426) for use in dogs.

HUMAN-LABELED PRODUCTS: NONE.

Revisions/References

Monograph written May 2014.

Anon (2014). Bravecto® (Fluralaner) [Package Insert]. Secondary Bravecto® (Fluralaner) [Package Insert]. Secondary Anon, Merck Animal Health-USA. Volume

Gassel, M., et al. (2014). The novel isoxazoline ectoparasiticide fluralaner: Selective inhibition of arthropod gamma-aminobutyric acid- and L-glutamate-gated chloride channels and insecticidal/acaricidal activity. Insect Biochemistry and Molecular Biology 45: 111-24.

Kilp, S., et al. (2014). Pharmacokinetics of fluralaner in dogs following a single oral or intravenous administration. Parasites & Vectors 7.

Walther, F. M., et al. (2014). The effect of food on the pharmacokinetics of oral fluralaner in dogs. Parasites & Vectors 7.

Walther, F. M., et al. (2014). Safety of fluralaner, a novel systemic antiparasitic drug, in MDR1(-/-) Collies after oral administration. Parasites & Vectors 7.

Fluticasone Propionate

(floo-ti-ca-sone)   Flovent®

Glucocorticoid, Inhaled

Prescriber Highlights

▶ Glucocorticoid used most commonly in veterinary medicine as an inhaled aerosol.

▶ Has shown efficacy in treating feline asthma, dogs with chronic cough, & in horses for recurrent airway obstruction or inflammatory airway disease.

▶ May be useful as a nasally inhaled treatment for allergy-related rhinosinusitis.

▶ Appears to be well tolerated; suppression of HPA axis possible.

▶ Must be used with a species-appropriate delivery device.

▶ Expense may be an issue.

Uses/Indications

While there are topical forms of fluticasone, most veterinary interests are in the inhaled versions of the drug. The aerosol for pulmonary inhalation appears to be effective in treating feline lower airway disease (FLAD, feline asthma), recurrent airway obstruction (RAO, heaves) or inflammatory airway disease (IAD) in horses, and dogs with chronic tracheobronchial disease. While the majority of small animal use has been with fluticasone, there are several other aerosol corticosteroids for inhalation (beclomethasone dipropionate, flunisolide, and budesonide) that theoretically could be used for the same purpose. The optimal dosing of inhaled corticosteroids is unknown and to date, there have been no studies specifically showing any advantages of inhaled corticosteroids over oral prednisolone in dogs and cats with naturally occurring airway disease (Sumner et al. 2013). In an 8-week study in cats (n=9) with naturally-occurring lower airway disease (FLAD) comparing oral prednisolone vs. 110 mcg fluticasone via inhalation twice daily, the authors concluded that while both treatments were effective in eliminating clinical signs/reducing airway eosinophilia, and fluticasone was well tolerated by all treated cats, oral glucocorticoids were associated with more robust improvement in airway resistance and static compliance (Rozanski et al. 2013).

The nasal inhalation corticosteroid products potentially could be useful for allergy-related chronic rhinosinusitis in cats and dogs.

Pharmacology/Actions

Like other glucocorticoids, fluticasone has potent antiinflammatory activity. Fluticasone has an affinity 18X that of dexamethasone for human glucocorticoid receptors. For a more thorough discussion of glucocorticoid effects, refer to the Glucocorticoids, General Information monograph.

Pharmacokinetics

In humans, when fluticasone aerosol is administered via the lung, about 30% is absorbed into the systemic circulation. In humans, a dose of 880 micrograms (4 puffs of the 220 microgram aerosol) showed peak plasma concentrations of 0.1 to 1 ng/mL. Volume of distribution averages 4.2 L/kg and it is 91% bound to human plasma proteins. Fluticasone is metabolized via cytochrome P450 3A4 isoenzymes to a metabolite with negligible pharmacologic activity. Terminal elimination half-life is about 8 hours. Most of the drug is excreted in the feces as parent drug and metabolites.

Contraindications/Precautions/Warnings

Fluticasone is contraindicated when patients are hypersensitive to it or during acute bronchospasm (status asthmaticus).

When transferring patients from systemic steroid therapy to inhaled steroids, wean slowly off systemic therapy to avoid acute adrenal insufficiency. Prepare to cover patients with additional steroid therapy during periods of acute stress, severe asthma attacks occurring during the withdrawal stage, or after transfer to inhaled steroids. Fluticasone is not useful for acute bronchospasm; cases of fluticasone-induced bronchospasm have been reported in humans.

Adverse Effects

In humans, the most likely adverse effects are pharyngitis and upper respiratory infections. While inhaled steroids generally cause significantly fewer adverse effects than injectable or oral therapy, suppression of the HPA axis can potentially occur. One study comparing ACTH-stimulated cortisol levels in healthy beagles, found that inhaled budesonide (200 mcg twice daily) did not significantly affect cortisol levels while oral prednisolone (1 mg/kg/day) and inhaled fluticasone (250 mcg twice daily) did after 35 days of treatment (Melamies et al. 2012). However, one study in cats using different concentrations of inhaled fluticasone, did not show any significant HPAA suppression at any of the doses used (Cohn et al. 2010). Another study in horses demonstrated that long-term inhaled fluticasone did not cause detectable effects on innate and adaptive (both humoral and cell-mediated) immune parameters studied (Dauvillier et al. 2011).

Reproductive/Nursing Safety

In humans, the FDA categorizes inhaled fluticasone as a category *C* drug for use during pregnancy (*Animal studies have shown an adverse effect on the fetus, but there are no adequate studies in humans; or there are no animal reproduction studies and no adequate studies in humans*). When given subcutaneously to laboratory animals, fluticasone caused a variety of teratogenic effects, including growth retardation, cleft palate, omphalocele and retarded cranial ossification. It should be used during pregnancy only when the benefits clearly outweigh the risks of therapy.

It is not known if the drug enters maternal milk; use with caution in nursing dams.

Overdosage/Acute Toxicity

Acute overdoses of this medication are unlikely, but there have been reported cases of dogs puncturing canisters of albuterol and developing adverse effects. A similar occurrence with fluticasone would unlikely require treatment. Chronic overdoses could result in significant HPA axis suppression and cushingoid effects.

Drug Interactions

While the manufacturer states that due to the low systemic plasma levels associated with inhalational therapy clinically significant drug interactions are unlikely, use caution when used in conjunction with other drugs (such as **ketoconazole**) that can inhibit CYP 3A4 isoenzymes; theoretically, fluticasone levels could be increased.

Laboratory Considerations

- **Intradermal skin testing** (IDST) for allergens: A related inhaled corticosteroid (budesonide) in cats (for one month) eliminated skin reactivity in 3/6 cats tested. The authors suggested a 2-week withdrawal if using IDST, but withdrawal may not be necessary if using serum IgE testing for allergies (Chang et al. 2011).

Doses

- **CATS:**

For treatment of feline "asthma"; feline lower airway disease (FLAD); (extra-label): Use with an aerosol metered dose inhaler, a spacer, and a facemask designed for use on cats (*e.g., Aerokat®*). The optimal dosing of inhaled corticosteroids is unknown and there have been no studies specifically showing any advantages of inhaled glucocorticoids over oral prednisone/prednisolone in dogs or cats with naturally occurring airway disease. Most commonly, oral glucocorticoid therapy is continued for about 10-14 days with a tapering overlap. (Sumner et al. 2013)

a) Initially, try the 44 micrograms/puff MDI: one puff q12h. In the study, all three dosages (44 micrograms, 110 micrograms and 220 micrograms) significantly reduced the proportion of eosinophils in airway lavage fluid. (Cohn et al. 2010)

b) For cats with signs of bronchial disease that occur more than once per week: Give prednisolone at 1 – 2 mg/kg PO twice daily for 5-7 days. Most newly diagnosed cats will have greatly diminished signs; then the dose is slowly tapered over at least 2-3 months. Some cats are effectively managed by low dose, alternate day corticosteroids, but most will continue to wheeze/cough. For those, encourage inhaled corticosteroids such as fluticasone. Use a delivery device (*e.g., AeroKat®*) in combination with a spacer and 110 micrograms fluticasone metered dose inhaler (MDI) and administer one puff twice daily. Cats with more serious disease may require the 220 micrograms MDI. Author has not found the 44 microgram inhaler to provide consistent clinical results. Attach MDI and the facemask to the spacer. Place facemask gently over cats mouth and nose and actuates the MDI to fill the spacer with medication. The cat breathes in and out for 7-10 times with the mask in place. (Padrid 2006), (Padrid 2008)

- **DOGS:**

For adjunctive treatment of chronic tracheobronchial disease; (extra-label):

a) In dogs with excessive side effects associated with oral steroids therapy: Use a delivery device (*e.g., AeroDawg®*) in combination with either fluticasone 220 microgram or 110 microgram (1 puff) twice daily. Ensure a tightly fitting facemask and counting 7-10 respirations after actuating the MDI into the spacer is important for optimizing therapy. (Johnson 2007)

b) Using the 220 micrograms/puff MDI: 2 puffs q12h. (Hawkins 2009)

■ **HORSES:**

For treatment of recurrent airway disease (heaves); (extra-label): Use a delivery device (*e.g., AeroHippus®* or *Equine-haler®*) in combination with a metered dose inhaler: In a year long study of 11 horses (6 horses treated with inhaled fluticasone/antigen avoidance; 5 with antigen avoidance alone). In the treated group fluticasone propionate was administered via inhalation at 2000 micrograms q12h for a month, then dosages were adjusted to control clinical signs (2000 – 3000 micrograms q12-24h). Authors concluded that the benefits of using inhaled corticosteroids in the treatment of heaves include a more rapid effect on lung function and airway smooth muscle remodeling compared to antigen avoidance alone, without inducing detectable side effects with prolonged use. However, antigen avoidance leads to a better control of inflammation and has additional beneficial effects on pulmonary function of inhaled corticosteroids-treated horses, even when clinical signs are apparently controlled by medication. (Leclere et al. 2013)

Monitoring
■ Efficacy.

Client Information
■ Before using, shake well and, if possible, bring canister to room temperature. Do not puncture or incinerate can. Must be used with a spacer device appropriate for the species being treated.
■ When using inhaled fluticasone with an appropriate spacer/facemask (*e.g., Aerokat®*) in cats, the following tips have been recommended (Scherk 2010): Allow cat to get used to the device over several days letting it investigate it (*e.g.,* leaving it by food bowl). Reward (praise, food, catnip, stroking) fearless approaches to device and start placing it near cat's face. Practice with the mask over the cats face without anything in the chamber. Pre-load the chamber with a puff of albuterol (in addition to the dose required). Make sure the mask is placed snugly over the muzzle for 4-6 breaths.
■ Allow animal to breath with the mask on for 7-10 times before removing.
■ One puff twice a day will last approximately 2 months.

Chemistry/Synonyms
A trifluorinated glucocorticoid, fluticasone propionate occurs as a white to off-white powder that is practically insoluble in water and slightly soluble in ethanol.

Fluticasone may also be known as: CCI-18781, fluticasoni propionas, *Advair Diskus®, Cutovate®, Flixotide®, Flixonase®, Flovent®,* and *Flutivate®.*

Storage/Stability
Fluticasone propionate aerosol for inhalation (*Flovent®*) should be stored between 2-30°C (36-86°F); protect from freezing and direct sunlight. Store canister with the mouthpiece down.

Compatibility/Compounding Considerations
No specific information noted.

Dosage Forms/Regulatory Status
VETERINARY-LABELED PRODUCTS: NONE.

HUMAN-LABELED PRODUCTS:

Fluticasone Propionate aerosol for inhalation: 44 micrograms per actuation, 110 micrograms per actuation, 220 micrograms per actuation in 10.6 g & 12 g canisters with actuator. Each canister contains approximately 120-metered inhalations; *Flovent® HFA;* (Rx). **Note:** There is also a breath-activated inhalation powder: *Flovent® Diskus,* and *Advair® Diskus* (with salmeterol), but for veterinary use the HFA aerosol is used (not *Diskus*-aerosol powder).

Fluticasone is also available commercially in combination as:

Fluticasone Propionate/Salmeterol Aerosol for Inhalation: 45 mcg fluticasone propionate/salmeterol 21 mcg per actuation; 115 mcg fluticasone propionate /salmeterol 21 mcg per actuation & 230 mcg fluticasone propionate/salmeterol 21 mcg per actuation equiv. to salmeterol xinafoate 30.45 mcg in 12 g pressurized canisters containing 120 metered inhalations.

Nasal solutions, topical creams and ointments containing fluticasone are also available.

Revisions/References
Monograph revised/updated January 2014.

Chang, C. H., et al. (2011). The impact of oral versus inhaled glucocorticoids on allergen specific IgE testing in experimentally asthmatic cats. Veterinary Immunology and Immunopathology **144**(3-4): 437-41.
Cohn, L. A., et al. (2010). Effects of fluticasone propionate dosage in anexperimental model of feline asthma. Jnl Fel Med Surg **12**: 91-6.
Dauvillier, J., et al. (2011). Effect of Long-Term Fluticasone Treatment on Immune Function in Horses with Heaves. Journal of Veterinary Internal Medicine **25**(3): 549-57.
Hawkins, E. (2009). Treating Canine Chronic Bronchitis: Revisiting the Basics. Proceedings: WVC. accessed via Veterinary Information Network; vin.com
Johnson, L. (2007). The coughing dog. Proceedings: Univ Cal-Davis Canine Medicine Symposium. accessed via Veterinary Information Network; vin.com
Leclere, M., et al. (2013). Inhaled Corticosteroids and Antigen Avoidance in Heaves: A Year-long Study. ACVIM. accessed via Veterinary Information Network; vin.com
Melamies, M., et al. (2012). Endocrine effects of inhaled budesonide compared with inhaled fluticasone propionate and oral prednisolone in healthy Beagle dogs. Veterinary Journal **194**(3): 349-53.
Padrid, P. (2006). Diagnosis and therapy of feline asthma. Proceedings: ACVIM 2006. accessed via Veterinary Information Network; vin.com
Padrid, P. (2008). Inhaled Steroids to Treat Feline Lower Airway Disease: 300 Cases 1995-2007. Proceedings: ACVIM. accessed via Veterinary Information Network; vin.com
Rozanski, E., et al. (2013). Fluticasone or Prednisolone for Treatment of Cats with Naturally-Occurring Lower Airway Disease. ACVIM. accessed via Veterinary Information Network; vin.com
Scherk, M. (2010). Bronchopulmonary Disease in Cats - Is It Really Asthma? Wild West Veterinary Conference, Vancouver. accessed via Veterinary Information Network; vin.com
Sumner, C. & E. Rozanski (2013). Management of Respiratory Emergencies in Small Animals. Veterinary Clinics of North America: Small Animal Practice **43**(4): 799-815.

Fluvoxamine Maleate

(floo-vox-a-meen)   Luvox®

Selective Serotonin-Reuptake Inhibitor (SSRI)

Prescriber Highlights
▶ Uncommonly used selective-serotonin reuptake inhibitor (SSRI) antidepressant similar to fluoxetine; can be used in dogs & cats for a variety of behavior disorders, but little information available to recommend its use in place of more commonly prescribed SSRIs.
▶ Contraindications: Patients with known hypersensitivity or receiving MAOIs. Caution: Patients with severe cardiac, renal or hepatic disease; dosages may need to be reduced in patients with severe renal or hepatic impairment.
▶ Must treat for 6-8 weeks before evaluating efficacy.
▶ Adverse effect profile not well established: Potentially, **Dogs:** Anorexia, lethargy, GI effects, anxiety, irritability, insomnia/hyperactivity, or panting; aggressive behavior in previously non-aggressive dogs possible. **Cats:** May exhibit sedation, decreased appetite/anorexia, vomiting, diarrhea, behavior changes (anxiety, irritability, sleep disturbances), & changes in elimination patterns.
▶ Drug-drug interactions.

Uses/Indications
Fluvoxamine may be considered for use in treating a variety of behavior-related diagnoses in dogs and cats, including aggression and stereotypic behaviors (and other obsessive-compulsive behaviors). Because of a lack of published information documenting its safety and efficacy in animals, it is not commonly prescribed.

Pharmacology/Actions

Fluvoxamine is a highly selective inhibitor of the reuptake of serotonin in the CNS thereby potentiating the pharmacologic activity of serotonin. Fluvoxamine apparently has little effect on dopamine or norepinephrine, and apparently no effect on other neurotransmitters.

Pharmacokinetics

There is limited data on the pharmacokinetics of fluvoxamine in domestic animals. In dogs, fluvoxamine appears to be completely absorbed; only about 10% of a dose is excreted unchanged in the urine. Half-life appears to be similar to humans (15 hours). No pharmacokinetic information for cats was located.

In humans, fluvoxamine is absorbed after oral administration, but bioavailability is only around 50%. Peak plasma concentrations occur between 3-8 hours post-dose. Food does not appear to affect the absorptive characteristics of the drug. Fluvoxamine is widely distributed in the body and about 80% bound to plasma proteins. The drug is extensively metabolized in the liver to non-active metabolites and eliminated in the urine. Plasma half-life is about 15 hours.

Contraindications/Precautions/Warnings

Fluvoxamine is contraindicated in patients hypersensitive to it or any SSRI or if the patient is receiving a monoamine oxidase inhibitor (MAOI) or cisapride. Consider using a lower dosage in patients with hepatic impairment or in geriatric patients.

Adverse Effects

The adverse effect profile of fluvoxamine in dogs or cats has not been well established. In dogs, SSRIs can cause lethargy, GI effects, anxiety, irritability, insomnia/hyperactivity, or panting. Anorexia is a common side effect in dogs (usually transient and may be negated by temporarily increasing the palatability of food and/or hand feeding). Some dogs have persistent anorexia that precludes further treatment. Aggressive behavior in previously non-aggressive dogs has been reported. SSRIs in cats can cause sedation, decreased appetite/anorexia, vomiting, diarrhea, behavior changes (anxiety, irritability, sleep disturbances), and changes in elimination patterns.

In humans, common adverse reactions (>10%) include sexual side effects (abnormal ejaculation, anorgasmia), agitation/nervousness, insomnia, nausea, dry mouth, constipation/diarrhea, dyspepsia, dizziness, headache, and somnolence.

Reproductive/Nursing Safety

In humans, the FDA categorizes fluvoxamine as a category C drug for use during pregnancy (*Animal studies have shown an adverse effect on the fetus, but there are no adequate studies in humans; or there are no animal reproduction studies and no adequate studies in humans*). In rats, fluvoxamine reportedly increased pup mortality at birth and was associated with decreased birth weights.

Fluvoxamine enters maternal milk, although it appears unlikely to be of significant clinical concern.

Overdosage/Acute Toxicity

Limited data exists for animals. Reportedly, any dosage over 10 mg/kg can cause tremors and lethargy. A case of dog developing clinical signs (CNS depression) at 1.5 mg/kg has been reported (Thomas et al. 2012). Other signs associated with overdoses may include vomiting, somnolence/coma, tremors, diarrhea, hypotension, heart rate/rhythm disturbances (bradycardia/tachycardia, ECG changes), seizures, etc.

Cyproheptadine may be useful in the adjunctive treatment of serotonin syndrome.

Fatalities have been reported in human overdoses; the highest reported dose where the patient survived was 10,000 mg. Treatment recommendations include standard protocols for drug adsorption/removal from the GI for potentially dangerous overdoses and symptomatic and supportive therapy. Serotonin effects may be negated somewhat by administration (oral or rectal) with cyproheptadine at a dose of 1.1 mg/kg. Seizures or other neurologic signs may be treated with diazepam. The drug has an elimination half-life of approximately 15 hours in dogs.

Drug Interactions

The following drug interactions have either been reported or are theoretical in humans or animals receiving fluvoxamine and may be of significance in veterinary patients. Unless otherwise noted, use together is not necessarily contraindicated, but weigh the potential risks and perform additional monitoring when appropriate.

- **BUSPIRONE:** Fluvoxamine may paradoxically decrease the clinical efficacy of buspirone.
- **CISAPRIDE:** Fluvoxamine may increase plasma levels of cisapride leading to toxicity.
- **CYPROHEPTADINE:** May decrease or reverse the effects of SSRIs.
- **DIAZEPAM, ALPRAZOLAM, MIDAZOLAM:** Fluvoxamine may increase diazepam levels.
- **DILTIAZEM:** Fluvoxamine may increase the effects of diltiazem; bradycardia has been reported in humans taking this drug combination.
- **MAO INHIBITORS** (including **amitraz** and potentially, **selegiline**): High risk for serotonin syndrome; use contraindicated; in humans, a 5 week washout period is required after discontinuing fluvoxamine and a 2 week washout period if first discontinuing the MAO inhibitor.
- **METHADONE:** Fluvoxamine may increase plasma levels of methadone, leading to toxicity.
- **PHENYTOIN:** Increased plasma levels of phenytoin possible.
- **PROPRANOLOL, METOPROLOL:** Fluvoxamine may increase these beta-blocker's plasma levels; atenolol may be safer to use if fluvoxamine is required.
- **THEOPHYLLINE:** Fluvoxamine may increase plasma levels of theophylline.
- **TRAMADOL:** SSRI's can inhibit the metabolism of tramadol to the active metabolites decreasing its efficacy and increasing the risk of toxicity (serotonin syndrome, seizures).
- **TRICYCLIC ANTIDEPRESSANTS** (*e.g.,* **clomipramine, amitriptyline**): Fluvoxamine may increase TCA blood levels and the risk for serotonin syndrome.
- **WARFARIN:** Fluvoxamine may increase the risk for bleeding.

Laboratory Considerations

- No fluvoxamine-related laboratory interactions noted.

Doses

Note: Fluvoxamine is available commercially as both regular tablets and extended-release capsules. While the contents of the extended-release capsules could be compounded into smaller strengths for use in veterinary patients, there does not appear to be any information available to support this practice.

- **DOGS:**

For adjunctive treatment of behavioral disorders (extra-label): Several dosages have been suggested, but little evidence exists to support any single recommendation. Dosage suggestions range from 0.5 – 2 mg/kg PO twice daily to 1 – 3 mg/kg PO once daily. 3-8 weeks of treatment may be required before assessing efficacy. If discontinuing therapy after this time, wean off over at least 3 weeks time (preferably longer).

■ **CATS:**

For adjunctive treatment of behavioral disorders (extra-label): Several dosages have been suggested, but little evidence exists to support any single recommendation. Dosage suggestions generally range from 0.25 mg/kg PO twice daily to 0.25 – 0.5 mg/kg PO once daily. 3-8 weeks of treatment may be required before assessing efficacy. If discontinuing therapy after this time, wean off over at least 3 weeks time (preferably longer). The smallest practical dosage available (without compounding) is ¼ of a 25 mg tablet (approximately 6 mg), which may be too high for the suggested dosages above.

Monitoring

■ Efficacy.

■ Adverse Effects; including appetite (weight).

■ Consider doing baseline liver function tests and ECG and re-test as needed.

Client Information

■ May be given with or without food. If your animal vomits or acts sick after getting it on an empty stomach, give with food or small treat to see if this helps. If vomiting continues, contact your veterinarian.

■ This medication is most effective when used with a behavior modification program. May take several days to weeks to determine if the drug is effective.

■ Do not stop this medication abruptly without veterinarian's guidance.

■ Most common side effects are: drowsiness/sleepiness, and reduced appetite. Rare side effects that can be serious: seizures, aggression; contact veterinarian immediately.

■ Overdoses can be very serious; keep out of the reach of animals and children.

■ If your animal wore a flea collar in the past two weeks, let your veterinarian know. Do not use one on your animal while it's getting this medicine without first talking to your veterinarian.

Chemistry/Synonyms

A selective serotonin-reuptake inhibitor (SSRI), fluvoxamine maleate occurs as a white to almost white crystalline powder. It is freely soluble in alcohol and sparingly soluble in water.

Fluvoxamine may also be known as DU-23000, desifluvoxamin, and Luvox®.

Storage/Stability

The commercially available tablets should be stored in tight containers at room temperatures of 15-30° C (59-86° F) and protected from high humidity.

Compatibility/Compounding Considerations

No specific information noted.

Dosage Forms/Regulatory Status

VETERINARY-LABELED PRODUCTS: NONE.

The ARCI (Racing Commissioners International) has designated this drug as a class 2 substance. See the appendix for more information.

HUMAN-LABELED PRODUCTS:

Fluvoxamine Oral Tablets: 25 mg, 50 mg, & 100 mg; generic; (Rx)

Fluvoxamine Oral Extended-release (24-hour for humans) Capsules: 100 mg & 150 mg; Luvox CR®, generic; (Rx)

Revisions/References

Monograph revised/updated January 2014.

Thomas, D. E., et al. (2012). Retrospective evaluation of toxicosis from selective serotonin reuptake inhibitor antidepressants: 313 dogs (2005-2010). J. Vet. Emerg. Crit. Care 22(6): 674-81.

Folic Acid

(foe-lik ass-id)   Folate, Folacin, Vitamin B9

Water-Soluble "B" Vitamin

Prescriber Highlights

▶ "B" Vitamin necessary for nucleoprotein synthesis & normal erythropoiesis.

▶ Injectable or oral dosage forms.

▶ Folic acid deficiency may be seen in animals (especially cats) with proximal or diffuse small intestinal inflammatory disease.

▶ May be used when dihydrofolate reductase inhibitor drugs (*e.g.*, trimethoprim, ormetoprim, pyrimethamine) are used for a prolonged period.

▶ Very safe.

Uses/Indications

Folic acid is used to treat folic acid deficiency in dogs, cats, and horses (theoretically in other animal species as well) often due to small intestinal disease. Cats with exocrine pancreatic insufficiency appear to be most at risk for folate and cobalamin deficiencies secondary to malabsorption of folic acid in the diet. Dogs with exocrine pancreatic insufficiency often are noted to have increased folate levels secondary to overgrowths of folate-synthesizing bacteria in the proximal small intestine. Chronic administration of dihydrofolate reductase inhibiting drugs such as pyrimethamine, ormetoprim or trimethoprim can potentially lead to reduced activated folic acid (tetrahydrofolic acid); folic acid supplementation is sometimes prescribed in an attempt to alleviate this situation. Folic acid supplementation during pregnancy has been shown to reduce the occurrence of lip and/or palate cleft (CL/CP) in Pug and Chihuahua puppies (Domoslawska et al. 2013).

Pharmacology/Actions

Folic acid is required for several metabolic processes. It is reduced via dihydrofolate reductase in the body to tetrahydrofolate (5-methyltetrahydrofolate), which acts as a coenzyme in the synthesis of purine and pyrimidine nucleotides that are necessary for DNA synthesis. Folic acid is also required for maintenance of normal erythropoiesis.

Pharmacokinetics

Therapeutically administered folic acid is primarily absorbed in the proximal small intestine via carrier-mediated diffusion. In humans, synthetic folic acid is nearly completely absorbed after oral administration while folate in foodstuffs is about 50% bioavailable. Folic acid is converted to its active form, tetrahydrofolic acid, principally in the liver and plasma. Folate is distributed widely throughout the body and stored in the liver. Erythrocyte and CSF levels can be significantly higher than those found in serum. It can undergo enterohepatic recirculation and is excreted primarily in the urine either as metabolites or unchanged drug (when administered in excess of body requirements).

Contraindications/Precautions/Warnings

Folic acid treatment is contraindicated only when known intolerance to the drug is documented. In humans, cobalamin (B-12) levels may be reduced with megaloblastic anemias; folic acid therapy may mask the signs associated with it. Folic acid doses in people above 0.4 mg/day (except during pregnancy and lactation) are not to be used until pernicious anemia has been ruled out.

As dogs may have increased, normal, or decreased folate levels associated with enteropathies, do not administer therapeutic doses until folate and cobalamin levels have been determined.

Adverse Effects

Folic acid is quite non-toxic and should not cause significant adverse effects. Rarely in humans, folic acid tablets or injection have reportedly caused hypersensitivity reactions or gastrointestinal effects. Very high oral doses in humans (15 mg/day) have occasionally caused CNS effects (*e.g.*, difficulty sleeping, excitement, confusion, etc.).

Reproductive/Nursing Safety

Folic acid is safe to use during pregnancy and in humans it is routinely prescribed as part of prenatal vitamin supplementation as folate deficiency can increase the risk for fetal neural tube defects. In humans, the FDA categorizes this drug as category A for use during pregnancy (*Adequate studies in pregnant women have not demonstrated a risk to the fetus in the first trimester of pregnancy, and there is no evidence of risk in later trimesters.*)

Folic acid is distributed into milk, but is safe. Folic acid requirements may be increased in lactating animals.

Overdosage/Acute Toxicity

Folic acid is relatively non-toxic and no treatment should be required if an inadvertent overdose occurs. Excess drug is metabolized or rapidly excreted unchanged in the urine.

Drug Interactions

The following drug interactions or have been reported in humans and may be of significance in veterinary patients receiving folic acid or may alter patient folic acid requirements:

- **CHLORAMPHENICOL**: May delay response to folic acid.
- **METHOTREXATE, TRIMETHOPRIM, PYRIMETHAMINE (drugs that inhibit dihydrofolate reductase)**: May interfere with folic acid utilization.
- **PHENYTOIN**: May decrease serum folate levels, and phenytoin dosage may need to be increased; increased frequency in seizures can occur.
- **SULFASALAZINE, BARBITURATES, NITROFURANTOIN, PRIMIDONE**: May increase risk for folate deficiency.

Laboratory Considerations

- **Serum samples** to be analyzed for cobalamin and/or folate should be protected from bright light and excessive heat.
- **Hemolysis** can cause falsely elevated serum concentrations of folate.
- Potentially, decreased **cobalamin serum levels** (B-12) can occur in patients receiving prolonged folic acid supplementation.

Doses

- **DOGS/CATS:**

  For folate deficiency associated with inflammatory bowel disease, pancreatic insufficiency (extra-label): Dosage recommendations vary and there is little evidence to support any specific dosage recommendation. Suggested PO dosages for small animals generally range from 400 micrograms – 1 mg per dog or cat once daily although doses of 2 mg & 5 mg per dog PO once daily have been noted. When used for IBD, many recommend also using parenteral cyanocobalamin (B-12).

  For cats on long-term use of high dose trimethoprim/sulfa (for treating *Nocardia*) (extra-label): 2 mg (per cat) PO once daily has been recommended. (Wolf 2006)

- **HORSES:**

  Prolonged therapy with antifolate medications (*e.g.*, trimethoprim, pyrimethamine); (extra-label): Sometimes recommend folic acid at 20 – 40 mg (per horse) PO per day. Pregnant mares should routinely receive folic acid supplementation during treatment with antifolates. (Granstrom et al. 1998)

Monitoring

- Small Animals: folate & cobalamin levels (serum) before and after treatment.
- Clinical signs associated with deficiency.
- CBC, baseline and ongoing if abnormal.

Client Information

- May be given either orally or as a shot. If giving orally, may give with or without food. If your animal vomits or acts sick after getting it on an empty stomach, give with food or small treat to see if this helps. If vomiting continues, contact your veterinarian.
- Usually no side effects.
- When used to treat folate deficiency associated with small intestinal disease or pancreatic insufficiency, lifelong monitoring and periodic replacement therapy may be required.

Chemistry/Synonyms

Folic acid occurs as a yellow, yellow-brownish, or yellowish-orange, odorless crystalline powder. It is very slightly soluble in water and insoluble in alcohol. Commercially available folic acid is obtained synthetically.

Folic acid may also be known as: folate, folacin, vitamin B9, acidum folicum, pteroylglutamic acid, pteroylmonoglutamic acid, *Folvite®* and vitamin B11.

Storage/Stability

Folic acid tablets should be stored in well-closed containers below 40°C (104°F), preferably between 15-30°C; protect from light and moisture. The injection should be stored protected from light below 40°C (104°F), preferably between 15-30°C. Do not allow to freeze.

Compatibility/Compounding Considerations

No specific information noted.

Dosage Forms/Regulatory Status

VETERINARY-LABELED PRODUCTS:

None as sole ingredient products. There are many products available that contain folic acid as one of the ingredients. If using one of these products, be certain it has enough folic acid to treat folate deficiency without overdosing fat soluble vitamins A or D.

HUMAN-LABELED PRODUCTS:

Folic Acid Tablets: 0.4 mg & 0.8 mg; generic (OTC); 1 mg, 7.5 mg, & 15 mg; *Deplin®*; generic; (Rx)

Folic Acid Injection: 5 mg/mL in 10 mL vials; *Folvite®*, generic; (Rx)

Revisions/References

Monograph revised/updated January 2014.

Domoslawska, A., et al. (2013). Oral folic acid supplementation decreases palate and/or lip cleft occurrence in Pug and Chihuahua puppies and elevates folic acid blood levels in pregnant bitches. Polish Journal of Veterinary Sciences 16(1): 33-7.

Granstrom, D. & W. Saville (1998). Equine Protozoal Myeloencephalitis. *Equine Internal Medicine*. S. Reed and W. Bayly, Saunders: 486-91.

Wolf, A. (2006). Chronic draining tracts and nodules in cats. Proceedings: ABVP2006, Accessed from the Veterinary information Network, Jan 2007. accessed via Veterinary Information Network; vin.com

Fomepizole
4-Methylpyrazole (4-MP)

(foe-me-pi-zole)   Antizol-Vet®

Antidote

Prescriber Highlights

▶ Synthetic alcohol dehydrogenase inhibitor used to treat dogs and cats for ethylene glycol poisoning.

▶ Has been shown to be efficacious in cats at high dosages if given within 3 hours of ingestion.

▶ Adverse Effects: Rapid IV infusion may cause vein irritation & phlebosclerosis; anaphylaxis is potentially possible.

▶ Dilute as directed in the commercially available kit.

▶ Monitor & treat acid/base, fluid, electrolyte imbalances.

▶ May inhibit elimination of ethanol (& vice versa).

▶ Expense & timely availability may be issues.

Uses/Indications

Fomepizole (4-methylpyrazole; 4-MP) is used for the treatment of known or suspected ethylene glycol toxicity in dogs (and humans). Fomepizole, at high doses, may be efficacious in treating recent (within 3 hours) ingestion of ethylene glycol in cats. Ethanol treatment has been recommended as the drug of choice for ethylene glycol toxicity in cats, but a recent study demonstrated that high dose fomepizole was more effective (Connally et al. 2010).

Pharmacology/Actions

Ethylene glycol itself is only mildly toxic in dogs, but when it is metabolized to glycoaldehyde, glycolate, glyoxalic acid, and oxalic acid, the resultant metabolic acidosis and renal tubular necrosis can be fatal. Fomepizole is a competitive inhibitor of alcohol dehydrogenase, the primary enzyme that converts ethylene glycol into glycoaldehyde and other toxic metabolites. This allows ethylene glycol to be excreted primarily unchanged in the urine decreasing the morbidity and mortality associated with ethylene glycol ingestion.

Pharmacokinetics

Fomepizole is excreted primarily by the kidneys and apparently exhibits a dose-dependent accumulation of the drug over time; therefore, a reduction in subsequent doses can safely occur.

Contraindications/Precautions/Warnings

There are no labeled contraindications to fomepizole's use. In dogs, fomepizole treatment may be successful as late as 8 hours post-ingestion, but if azotemia is noted, treatment is less successful and the prognosis is poor. If so, treatment should still be considered up to 36 hours post-ingestion, as fomepizole can potentially prevent further renal damage and some dogs may survive with dialysis and supportive therapy.

Fomepizole has been shown to be effective in treating ethylene glycol in cats, but a high dosage is required and treatment should be started within 3 hours of ingestion.

Use of fomepizole alone without adequate monitoring and adjunctive supportive care (*e.g.*, correction of acid/base, fluid, electrolyte imbalances) may lead to therapeutic failure. However, as fomepizole may increase serum bicarbonate (HCO_3) it has been recommended that correction of severe metabolic acidosis in cats (*and presumably dogs as fomepizole has increased bicarb in experimental studies in dogs–Plumb*) be treated with appropriate IV fluid therapy and fomepizole before consideration of HCO_3 administration (Tart et al. 2011). If animal presents within 1-2 hours post ingestion, consider inducing vomiting and/or gastric lavage with activated charcoal to prevent further absorption.

Adverse Effects

Giving concentrated drug rapidly intravenously may cause vein irritation and phlebosclerosis. Dilute as directed in the commercially available kit.

One dog during clinical trials was reported to develop anaphylaxis.

Cats may develop mild sedation when receiving fomepizole.

Fomepizole may increase serum bicarbonate levels in dogs and cats (See Warnings above).

Reproductive/Nursing Safety

Fomepizole's safe use during pregnancy, lactation or in breeding animals has not been established. However, because of the morbidity and mortality associated with ethylene glycol toxicity, the benefits of fomepizole should generally outweigh its risks. In humans, the FDA categorizes this drug as category *C* for use during pregnancy (*Animal studies have shown an adverse effect on the fetus, but there are no adequate studies in humans; or there are no animal reproduction studies and no adequate studies in humans.*)

It is not known whether this drug is excreted in milk.

Overdosage/Acute Toxicity

Overdosage may cause significant CNS depression. No specific treatment is recommended.

Drug Interactions

The following drug interactions have either been reported or are theoretical in humans or animals receiving fomepizole and may be of significance in veterinary patients. Unless otherwise noted, use together is not necessarily contraindicated, but weigh the potential risks and perform additional monitoring when appropriate.

■ **ETHANOL**: Fomepizole inhibits alcohol dehydrogenase; ethanol metabolism is reduced significantly and alcohol poisoning (*e.g.*, CNS depression, coma, death) can occur. Use together is generally not recommended, but if both drugs are used, monitoring of ethanol blood levels is mandatory.

Laboratory Considerations

Ethylene Glycol Testing Kits: Fomepizole may cause false readings on ethylene glycol screening tests. Refer to the product used for more information.

Doses

■ **DOGS:**

For treatment of ethylene glycol toxicity (labeled dose; FDA-approved): Initially load at 20 mg/kg IV; at 12 hours post initial dose give 15 mg/kg IV; at 24 hours post initial dose give another 15 mg/kg IV and at 36 hours after initial dose give 5 mg/kg; may give additional 5 mg/kg doses as necessary (animal has not recovered or has additional ethylene glycol in blood). (Package Insert; *Antizol-Vet*®)

■ **CATS:**

For treatment of ethylene glycol toxicity (extra-label): Evidence from an experimental study and naturally occurring EG intoxication (3 cats). Initially, 125 mg/kg slow IV; at 12, 24, 36 hours give 31.25 mg/kg IV. In addition, treat supportively with supplemental fluids. Cats must be treated within 3 hours of ingestion. Cats whose treatment began 4 hours post ethylene glycol had 100% mortality with either fomepizole or ETOH therapy. (Connally et al. 2010; Tart et al. 2011)

Monitoring

■ Ethylene glycol blood levels; mostly important to document diagnosis if necessary and to determine if therapy can be discontinued after 36 hours of treatment.

■ Blood gases and serum electrolytes.

■ Hydration status.

- Renal function tests (*e.g.*, urine output and urinalysis; BUN or serum creatinine).
- Cats: body temperature.

Client Information

- Clients should be informed that treatment of serious ethylene glycol toxicity is an "intensive care" admission and appropriate monitoring and therapy can be quite expensive, particularly when fomepizole is used in large dogs.
- Because time is critical for therapy, clients will need to make an informed decision rapidly. Dogs treated within 8 hours post ingestion have a significantly better prognosis than those treated after 10-12 hours post ingestion. Cats must be treated within 3 hours of ingestion with high dosages.

Chemistry/Synonyms

A synthetic alcohol dehydrogenase inhibitor, fomepizole is commonly called 4-methylpyrazole (4-MP). Its chemical name is 4-methyl-1H-pyrazole. It has a molecular weight of 81; it is soluble in water and very soluble in ethanol.

Fomepizole may also be known as: 4-methylpyrazole, 4-MP, fomepisol, fomepizolum, and *Antizol®*.

Storage/Stability

Commercially available solutions should be stored at room temperature. The concentrate for injection may solidify at temperatures less than 25°C. Should this occur, resolubolize by running warm water over the vial. Solidification or resolubolization does not affect drug potency or stability. Store reconstituted vial at room temperature and discard after 72 hours.

Compatibility/Compounding Considerations

Preparation: If drug has solidified, run warm water over vial; Add entire contents to 30 mL vial of 0.9% NaCl (in kit), mix well. Resultant solution is: 50 mg/mL. Reconstituted solutions may be further diluted in D5W or normal saline for IV infusion.

If commercial fomepizole products (veterinary- or human-approved) are not available (back-ordered/discontinued), compounded 1 gram/mL fomepizole (4-methylpyrazole) sterile injection may be considered, but should be prepared via USP 797 standards.

Dosage Forms/Regulatory Status

VETERINARY-LABELED PRODUCTS:

Fomepizole 1.5 g Kit for Injection; *Antizol-Vet®*; (Rx). FDA-approved (NADA 141-075) for use in dogs. **Note:** At recommended doses 1 kit will treat a 26 kg dog (up to 58 lb.); larger dogs will require additional kits.

HUMAN-LABELED PRODUCTS:

Fomepizole Injection Concentrate: 1 g/mL & 1.5 g/mL preservative free (must be diluted) in 1.5 mL vials; *Antizol®*, generic; (Rx)

Revisions/References

Monograph revised/updated January 2014.

Connally, H. E., et al. (2010). Safety and efficacy of high-dose fomepizole compared with ethanol as therapy for ethylene glycol intoxication in cats. J. Vet. Emerg. Crit. Care 20(2): 191-206.

Tart, K. M. & L. L. Powell (2011). 4-Methylpyrazole as a treatment in naturally occurring ethylene glycol intoxication in cats. J. Vet. Emerg. Crit. Care 21(3): 268-72.

Fosfomycin Tromethamine

(fos-foe-my-sin)   Monurol®

Phosphonic Acid Antimicrobial

Prescriber Highlights

▶ Human phosphonic acid derivative urinary antibiotic; only oral dose form (granules) available in USA.

▶ Potentially could be useful in dogs for UTI, especially multi-drug resistant *E.coli*; may be useful for systemic infections, but data supporting clinical use is lacking.

▶ Appears to be nephrotoxic in cats; use with extreme caution in this species.

▶ Currently, very expensive.

Uses/Indications

Fosfomycin is an antibacterial agent that may be useful for treating multi-drug resistant urinary tract infections in dogs. Very little information has been published for this agent in veterinary medicine and its use must be considered relatively investigational for treating UTI's, when other antibiotics are not effective.

Pharmacology/Actions

Fosfomycin is a phosphonic acid derivative, synthetic, antibacterial agent. It irreversibly inhibits phosphoenol pyruvate transferase, an enzyme that catalyzes the formation of uridine diphosphate-N-acetylmuramic acid, which is the first step of microbial cell wall peptidoglycan synthesis. Additionally, it reduces adherence of bacteria to uroepithelial cells. Fosfomycin is primarily a time-dependent antibacterial, but it also exhibits some characteristics of a concentration-dependent agent. It is bactericidal in urine (at therapeutic doses) against susceptible bacteria. It has activity (*in vitro*) against a variety of gram-positive and gram-negative bacteria, including multi-drug resistant isolates of *E.coli* and enterococcus. Cross-resistance apparently does not occur with beta-lactams or aminoglycosides. Resistance to fosfomycin, when it occurs, is via hydrolysis secondary to FosX or FosA enzymes that are chromosomally mediated.

Pharmacokinetics

Fosfomycin tromethamine is rapidly converted to the free acid fosfomycin after absorption. Fosfomycin is distributed into the kidneys, bladder wall, and prostate, and crosses the placenta. Primary route of elimination is as unchanged drug in urine (38% of an oral dose in humans). Renal dysfunction can substantially increase half-life and reduce urine levels.

In dogs, fosfomycin (disodium salt) is rapidly absorbed after oral administration; peak levels occur about 2 hours after oral dosing. Bioavailability in dogs is about 29%, which is similar to the values reported for humans (tromethamine salt). Volume of distribution (steady-state) is about 0.7 L/kg and protein binding is very low; clearance is approximately 15 mL/kg/hour, and terminal half-life is approximately 2 hours (Gutierrez et al. 2008).

The commercially available oral product is the tromethamine salt. Dogs receiving 80 mg/kg PO showed high (approx. 100%) oral bioavailability when given with food. Fasted bioavailability was lower and averaged 66%. Elimination half-life was approximately 2.5 hours. Serum concentrations exceeded the MIC90 reported for multidrug resistant (MDR) *E. coli* (1.5 µg/ml) for 12 hours (Boothe 2011).

In horses (using fosfomycin disodium), SC bioavailability is about 85%. Peak levels occur about 3.25 hours after SC dosing. Mean volume of distribution (steady-state) is 0.21 L/kg; clearance 16-24 mL/kg/hour; and terminal half-life about 1.3 hours (Zozaya et al. 2008).

Contraindications/Precautions/Warnings

Because of concerns that fosfomycin may be nephrotoxic in cats, it presently should be considered contraindicated in young cats and used with caution in adult cats. In a study where cats where given 20 mg/kg of fosfomycin (as the calcium or sodium salt) once daily for 3 days, all young cats (actual age not noted) given the drug orally had significant increases in serum creatinine. Tubular necrosis, disappearance of tubular cells and rearrangement of eosinophilic non-structural material were observed in the kidneys of all the young and adult cats (Fukata et al. 2008).

In humans, this drug is used as a one-time dose; multiple doses do not enhance efficacy and increase incidence of adverse events.

Adverse Effects

There is very little information available on this drug's adverse effect profile in animals. Reduced appetite, anorexia and diarrhea have been reported in some dogs receiving the drug. In cats, renal tubular damage is possible (see contraindications above). In humans, the most common adverse effect is diarrhea.

Reproductive/Nursing Safety

In humans, fosfomycin is listed as a category *B* drug (*Animal studies have not demonstrated risk to the fetus, but there are no adequate studies in pregnant women; or animal studies have shown an adverse effect, but adequate studies in pregnant women have not demonstrated a risk to the fetus during the first trimester of pregnancy, and there is no evidence of risk in later trimesters.*)

It is unknown if fosfomycin is distributed into milk; use with caution in nursing dams.

Overdosage/Acute Toxicity

Single overdoses would most likely cause GI effects. Single oral overdoses in dogs of up to 5 g/kg caused diarrhea and anorexia occurring 2-3 days after administration. Overdoses in cats may cause nephrotoxicity.

Drug Interactions

The following drug interactions have either been reported or are theoretical in humans or animals receiving fosfomycin and may be of significance in veterinary patients. Unless otherwise noted, use together is not necessarily contraindicated, but weigh the potential risks and perform additional monitoring when appropriate.

- **METOCLOPRAMIDE:** Can decrease serum concentrations and reduce urine levels. Although no interactions have been reported, other drugs that can increase GI motility (*e.g.,* **bethanechol, cisapride, domperidone, ranitidine, laxatives**) may have a similar effect.

Laboratory Considerations
- No specific concerns noted.

Doses

- **DOGS:**

  For UTI (extra-label): Until scientific evidence defines the most appropriate dose, interval and duration, the use of fosfomycin might be prudently reserved for treatment of MDR-*E. coli* for which no other alternative exists and the risk of not treating the infection presents harm to the patient. Use of fosfomycin should be based on susceptibility testing only. If the decision is made to use fosfomycin, re-culture and supportive care are indicated. A single dose of 40 mg/kg (disodium salt) PO was well tolerated in dogs in a pharmacokinetic study. 80 mg/kg doses of the commercially available tromethamine salt had high oral bioavailability when administered with food and serum levels remained above MIC90 for multi-drug resistant *E. coli* for 12 hours. 5 of 12 treated dogs at this dosage developed diarrhea. Fosfomycin levels and antibacterial effects in urine have not (at time of writing) been reported for dogs. Multi-center randomized clinical trials involving dogs with spontaneous UTI associated with *E. coli* should be preformed to determine efficacy and safety. Adapted from: (Boothe et al. 2010), (Hubka et al. 2010; Boothe 2011)

- **HORSES:**
  Based on their pharmacokinetic study, the authors concluded that clinically effective plasma concentrations might be obtained for up to 10 hours administering 20 mg/kg SC. (Zozaya et al. 2008) (**Note:** In this study, fosfomycin disodium was used. This salt is not currently commercially available in the USA)

Monitoring
- Adverse Effects: GI.
- Standard monitoring for UTI treatment (*i.e.,* before and after culture and susceptibility, clinical signs, urinalysis).
- Cats: Renal function tests.

Client Information
- There is little clinical experience with this drug in animals; report any possible side effects to the veterinarian immediately
- It is likely that this drug will be provided to you as a compounded product; follow the directions for using it exactly as prescribed. For human use, the granules are to be diluted in water (not hot water) just prior to dosing. The drug can be given regardless of feeding status (full or empty stomach).

Chemistry/Synonyms

Fosfomycin tromethamine (also known as fosfomycin trometamol) is an antibacterial isolated from *Streptomyces fradiae*. It occurs as a white or almost white, hygroscopic powder that is very soluble in water, slightly soluble in alcohol or methyl alcohol, and practically insoluble in acetone. A 5% solution in water has a pH of 3.5-5.5.

Fosfomycin may also be known as MK-955, phosphomycin, phosphonomycin, fosfomicina, fosfomycine, fosfomycinum, or fosfomysiini. Its chemical name is cis-1, 2-epoxyphosphonic acid.

Storage/Stability

Fosfomycin tromethamine granules should be stored at room temperature (25°C).

Compatibility/Compounding Considerations

The product's label (for human use) states: Pour the entire contents of a single-dose sachet of fosfomycin into 90-120 mL of water (1/2 cup) and stir to dissolve. Do not use hot water. Fosfomycin should be taken immediately after dissolving in water.

Dosage Forms/Regulatory Status
VETERINARY-LABELED PRODUCTS: NONE.

HUMAN-LABELED PRODUCTS:

Fosfomycin Tromethamine 3 grams per packet (for dilution and oral use); *Monurol®*; (Rx)

Revisions/References

Monograph revised/updated January 2014.

Boothe, D. (2011). Pharmacokinetics and Time Dependent Killing of Fosfomycin in Multi Drug Resistant-Escherichia coli Urinary Tract Infections in Dogs. ACVIM. accessed via Veterinary Information Network; vin.com

Boothe, D. & P. Hubka (2010). Fosfomycin: An Alternative Drug for Treatment of E. coli Urinary Tract Infections? Proceedings: ACVIM. accessed via Veterinary Information Network; vin.com

Fukata, T., et al. (2008). Acute renal insufficiency in cats after fosfomycin administration. Veterinary Record **163**(11): 337-8.

Gutierrez, O. L., et al. (2008). Pharmacokinetics of disodium-fosfomycin in mongrel dogs. Research in Veterinary Science **85**(1): 156-61.

Hubka, P. & D. M. Boothe (2010). In vitro susceptibility of canine and feline Escherichia coli to fosfomycin. Veterinary Microbiology **In Press, Corrected Proof**.

Zozaya, D. H., et al. (2008). Pharmacokinetics of a single bolus intravenous, intramuscular and subcutaneous dose of disodium fosfomycin in horses. J. Vet. Pharmacol. Ther. **31**(4): 321-7.

Furazolidone

(fyoor-a-zoe-li-done)   Furoxone®

Antibacterial/Antiprotozoal

Prescriber Highlights

▶ Antibacterial/antiprotozoal nitrofuran that has been used in dogs & cats; availability is an issue.

▶ Contraindications: Known hypersensitivity; food animals.

▶ Adverse Effects: GI effects (anorexia, vomiting, cramping & diarrhea) possible.

▶ May innocuously discolor urine to a dark yellow to brown color.

▶ Drug Interactions.

Uses/Indications

Furazolidone is usually a drug of second choice in small animals to treat enteric infections caused by the organisms listed below. Because it is no longer commercially available (in the USA), it may be difficult to locate.

Pharmacology/Actions

Furazolidone interferes with susceptible bacterial enzyme systems. Its mechanism against susceptible protozoa is not well determined. Furazolidone has activity against Giardia, *Vibrio cholerae*, Trichomonas, Coccidia, and many strains of *E. coli*, Enterobacter, Campylobacter, Salmonella, and Shigella. Not all strains are sensitive, but resistance is usually limited and develops slowly. Furazolidone also inhibits monoamine oxidase.

Pharmacokinetics

Conflicting information on furazolidone's absorption characteristics are published. As colored metabolites are found in the urine, it is clearly absorbed to some extent. Because furazolidone is used to treat enteric infections, absorption becomes important only when discussing adverse reactions and drug interaction issues. Furazolidone reportedly distributes into the CSF. Absorbed furazolidone is rapidly metabolized in the liver and the majority of absorbed drug is eliminated in the urine.

Contraindications/Precautions/Warnings

Furazolidone is contraindicated in patients hypersensitive to it.

The FDA has prohibited the extra-label use of furazolidone in food animals.

Adverse Effects

Adverse effects noted with furazolidone are usually minimal. Anorexia, vomiting, cramping, and diarrhea may occasionally occur. Some human patients are reported to be hypersensitive to the drug. Because furazolidone also inhibits monoamine oxidase it may, potentially, interact with several other drugs and foods (see Drug Interactions below). The clinical significance of these interactions remains unclear, particularly in light of the drug's poor absorptive characteristics.

Reproductive/Nursing Safety

While the safe use of furazolidone during pregnancy has not been established, neither were there any teratogenic issues located for it. However, one reference (Tams 2003) states that furazolidone should not be used in pregnant queens. In humans, the FDA categorizes this drug as category *C* for use during pregnancy (*Animal studies have shown an adverse effect on the fetus, but there are no adequate studies in humans; or there are no animal reproduction studies and no adequate studies in humans.*)

It is unknown if furazolidone enters maternal milk.

Overdosage/Acute Toxicity

No information was located; but moderate overdoses are unlikely to cause significant toxicity. Gut emptying may be considered for large overdoses.

Drug Interactions

The following drug interactions have either been reported or are theoretical in humans or animals receiving furazolidone and may be of significance in veterinary patients. Unless otherwise noted, use together is not necessarily contraindicated, but weigh the potential risks and perform additional monitoring when appropriate.

▪ **ALCOHOL**: With furazolidone may cause a disulfiram-like reaction.

Because furazolidone inhibits monoamine oxidase, its use concurrently with the following drugs is not recommended because dangerous hypertension could occur:

▪ **AMITRAZ**

▪ **BUSPIRONE**

▪ **SELEGILINE**

▪ **SYMPATHOMIMETIC AMINES** (phenylpropanolamine, ephedrine, etc.)

▪ **TRICYCLIC ANTIDEPRESSANTS**

▪ **FISH OR POULTRY** (high tyramine content)

Laboratory Considerations

▪ Furazolidone may cause a false-positive **urine glucose** determination when using the cupric sulfate solution test (*e.g., Clinitest®*).

Doses

▪ **CATS:**

For treatment of Giardia: 4 mg/kg PO twice daily (q12h) for 7-10 days; if re-treatment is required, elevated dosages or lengthened treatment regimens may provide better results. (Reinemeyer 1992), (Lappin 2000)

Monitoring

▪ Efficacy (stool exams for parasitic infections).

Client Information

▪ Furazolidone may discolor urine to a dark yellow to brown color; this is not significant.

▪ Have clients report prolonged or serious GI effects.

Chemistry/Synonyms

A synthetic nitrofuran-derivative antibacterial/antiprotozoal, furazolidone occurs as a bitter-tasting, yellow, crystalline powder. It is practically insoluble in water.

Furazolidone may also be known as: nifurazolidonum, *Enterolidon®, Exofur®, Furasian®, Furion®, Furoxona®, Fuxol®, Giarcid®, Giardil®, Giarlam®, Neo Furasil®, Nifuran®, Novafur®, Salmocide®,* and *Seforman®*.

Storage/Stability

Store protected from light in tight containers.

Compatibility/Compounding Considerations

No specific information noted.

Dosage Forms/Regulatory Status

VETERINARY-LABELED PRODUCTS:

No systemic products are available; a 4% topical powder/spray is available. The FDA prohibits its use on food producing animals.

HUMAN-LABELED PRODUCTS:

None; the human product *Furoxone®* has apparently been withdrawn from the USA market. Preparations may be available from compounding pharmacies.

Revisions/References

Monograph revised/updated January 2014.

Lappin, M. (2000). Protozoal and Miscellaneous Infections. *Textbook of Veterinary Internal Medicine: Diseases of the Dog and Cat.* S. Ettinger and E. Feldman. Philadelphia, WB Saunders. 1: 408-17.

Reinemeyer, C. (1992). Feline Gastrointestinal Parasites. *Current Veterinary Therapy XI: Small Animal Practice.* R. Kirk and J. Bonagura. Philadelphia, W.B. Saunders Company: 626-30.

Tams, T. (2003). Giardiasis, Clostridium perfringens enterotoxicosis, and cryptosporidiosis. Proceedings: Atlantic Coast Veterinary Conference. accessed via Veterinary Information Network; vin.com

Furosemide

(fur-oh-se-mide)   Lasix®, Frusomide

Loop Diuretic

Prescriber Highlights

▶ A loop diuretic commonly used in many species for treatment of congestive cardiomyopathy, pulmonary edema, udder edema, hypercalcuric nephropathy, uremia, as adjunctive therapy in hyperkalemia &, occasionally, as an antihypertensive agent. Used in racehorses to prevent/reduce EIPH.

▶ Contraindications: Patients with anuria, hypersensitivity, or seriously depleted electrolytes. Caution: Patients with pre-existing electrolyte or water balance abnormalities, impaired hepatic function, & diabetes mellitus.

▶ Adverse Effects: Fluid & electrolyte (esp. hyponatremia) abnormalities; others include: ototoxicity, GI distress, hematologic effects, ototoxicity, weakness, & restlessness. SC injection may cause ulcerative skin lesions in dogs (and potentially in other species).

▶ Pre-renal azotemia possible if dehydration occurs.

▶ Encourage normal food & water intake.

Uses/Indications

Furosemide is used for its diuretic activity in all species. It is used in small animals for the treatment of congestive cardiomyopathy, pulmonary edema, hypercalcuric nephropathy, uremia, as adjunctive therapy in hyperkalemia and, occasionally, as an antihypertensive agent. In cattle, it is FDA-approved for use for the treatment of post-parturient udder edema. It has been used to help prevent or reduce epistaxis (exercise-induced pulmonary hemorrhage; EIPH) in racehorses.

Pharmacology/Actions

Furosemide reduces the absorption of electrolytes in the ascending section of the loop of Henle, decreases the reabsorption of both sodium and chloride and increases the excretion of potassium in the distal renal tubule, and directly effects electrolyte transport in the proximal tubule. The exact mechanisms of furosemide's effects have not been fully established. It has no effect on carbonic anhydrase nor does it antagonize aldosterone.

Furosemide increases renal excretion of water, sodium, potassium, chloride, calcium, magnesium, hydrogen, ammonium, and bicarbonate. In dogs, excretion of potassium is affected much less than sodium; hyponatremia may be more of a concern than hypokalemia. It causes some renal venodilation and transiently increases glomerular filtration rates (GFR). Renal blood flow is increased and decreased peripheral resistance may occur. While furosemide increases renin secretion, due to its effects on the nephron, increases in sodium and water retention do not occur. Furosemide can cause hyperglycemia, but to a lesser extent than the thiazides.

Dosages of 1 – 4 mg/kg IV or PO decreased in a dosage proportional manner, left atrial pressure in dogs with experimentally induced mitral regurgitation (Suzuki et al. 2011). At high doses (10 – 12 mg/kg), thoracic duct lymph flow is increased in dogs. In horses, guinea pigs and humans, furosemide has some bronchodilative effects. Cats are reportedly more sensitive than other species to the diuretic effects of furosemide.

Pharmacokinetics

The pharmacokinetics of furosemide have been studied in a limited fashion in domestic animals. In dogs, the oral bioavailability is approximately 77% and the elimination half-life approximately 1-1.5 hours.

In humans, furosemide is 60-75% absorbed following oral administration. The diuretic effect takes place within 5 minutes after IV administration and within one hour after oral dosing. Peak effects occur approximately 30 minutes after IV dosing, and 1-2 hours after oral dosing. The drug is approximately 95% bound to plasma proteins in both azotemic and normal patients. The serum half-life is about 2 hours, but prolonged in patients with renal failure, uremia, CHF, and in neonates.

Contraindications/Precautions/Warnings

Furosemide is contraindicated in patients with anuria or that are hypersensitive to the drug. The manufacturer states that the drug should be discontinued in patients with progressive renal disease if increasing azotemia and oliguria occur during therapy.

Furosemide should be used with caution in patients with preexisting electrolyte or water balance abnormalities, impaired hepatic function (may precipitate hepatic coma), and diabetes mellitus. Patients with conditions that may lead to electrolyte or water balance abnormalities (*e.g.*, vomiting, diarrhea, etc.) should be monitored carefully. Patients hypersensitive to sulfonamides may also be hypersensitive to furosemide (not documented in veterinary species).

Use very cautiously with other drugs that can cause renal- or ototoxicity as furosemide may potentiate toxic effects.

Adverse Effects

Furosemide may induce fluid and electrolyte abnormalities. Patients should be monitored for hydration status and electrolyte imbalances (especially potassium, calcium, magnesium and sodium). Prerenal azotemia may result if moderate to severe dehydration occurs. Hyponatremia is probably the greatest concern, but hypocalcemia, hypokalemia, and hypomagnesemia may all occur. Animals that have normal food and water intake are much less likely to develop water and electrolyte imbalances than those that do not.

Other potential adverse effects include ototoxicity, especially in cats with high dose IV therapy. Dogs reportedly require dosages greater than 22 mg/kg IV to cause hearing loss. Other effects include gastrointestinal disturbances, hematologic effects (anemia, leukopenia), weakness, and restlessness.

A case of a dermatologic reaction (ulcerative lesions) at the injection sites after subcutaneous administration of furosemide in a dog has been reported (Scruggs et al. 2013). This dog had received injections from two separate manufacturers/formulations. The product suspected of causation had a pH of between 8.66-9.05 in the samples analyzed whereas the product used prior without reaction had pH's between 7.2-7.47 (none of the tested lots were actually used in the patient). The authors concluded that this report suggests that veterinarians should exercise caution when prescribing SC furosemide and consider the potential effects of furosemide formulation (e.g., pH) in their choice when prescribing this route.

Reproductive/Nursing Safety

In humans, the FDA categorizes this drug as category *C* for use during pregnancy (*Animal studies have shown an adverse effect on the fetus, but there are no adequate studies in humans; or there are no animal reproduction studies and no adequate studies in humans.*) In a separate system evaluating the safety of drugs in canine and feline pregnancy (Papich 1989), this drug is categorized as class: *B* (*Safe for use if used cautiously. Studies in laboratory animals may have uncovered some risk, but these drugs appear to be safe in dogs and cats or these drugs are safe if they are not administered when the animal is near term.*)

Furosemide appears in milk; clinical significance to nursing offspring is unknown.

Overdosage/Acute Toxicity

The LD_{50} in dogs after oral administration is >1000 mg/kg; after IV injection >300 mg/kg. Chronic overdosing at 10 mg/kg for six months in dogs led to development of calcification and scarring of the renal parenchyma.

Acute overdosage may cause electrolyte and water balance problems, CNS effects (lethargy to coma and seizures) and cardiovascular collapse.

Treatment consists of emptying the gut after recent oral ingestion, using standard protocols. Avoid giving concomitant cathartics as they may exacerbate the fluid and electrolyte imbalances that can occur. Aggressively monitor and treat electrolyte and water balance abnormalities supportively. Also monitor respiratory, CNS, and cardiovascular status; treat supportively and symptomatically if necessary.

Drug Interactions

The following drug interactions have either been reported or are theoretical in humans or animals receiving furosemide and may be of significance in veterinary patients. Unless otherwise noted, use together is not necessarily contraindicated, but weigh the potential risks and perform additional monitoring when appropriate.

- **ACE INHIBITORS** (*e.g.,* **enalapril, benazepril**): Increased risks for hypotension, particularly in patients that are volume or sodium depleted secondary to diuretics.
- **AMINOGLYCOSIDES** (**gentamicin, amikacin,** etc.): Increased risk for ototoxicity.
- **AMPHOTERICIN B**: Loop diuretics may increase the risk for nephrotoxicity development; hypokalemia.
- **CISPLATIN**: Ototoxic effects may be enhanced.
- **CORTICOSTEROIDS**: Increased risk for GI ulceration; hypokalemia.
- **DIGOXIN**: Furosemide-induced hypokalemia may increase the potential for digoxin toxicity.
- **INSULIN**: Furosemide may alter insulin requirements.
- **MUSCLE RELAXANTS, NON-DEPOLARIZING** (*e.g.,* **atracurium, tubocurarine**): Furosemide may prolong neuromuscular blockade.
- **PROBENECID**: Furosemide can reduce uricosuric effects.
- **SALICYLATES**: Loop diuretics can reduce the excretion of salicylates.
- **SUCCINYLCHOLINE**: Furosemide may potentiate effects.
- **THEOPHYLLINE**: Pharmacologic effects of theophylline may be enhanced when used with furosemide.

Laboratory Considerations

- **Free T4**: Furosemide can result in an increased free T4 fraction; furosemide inhibits T4 binding to canine serum *in vitro*.

Doses

- **DOGS & CATS:**

  Labeled Doses (FDA-approved): **Treatment of edema (pulmonary congestion, ascites) associated with cardiac insufficiency and acute noninflammatory tissue edema** (labeled dose; FDA-approved): Injection: 2.75 – 5.5 mg/kg IV or IM once or twice daily after a 6- to 8-hour interval. The dosage should be adjusted to the individual animal's response. In refractory or severe edematous cases the dosage may be doubled or increased by increments of 2.2 mg/kg of body weight to establish the effective dose. The established effective dose should be administered once

or twice daily on an intermittent daily schedule. Diuretic therapy should be discontinued after reduction of edema, or when necessary, maintained after determining a programmed dosage schedule to prevent recurrence. PO: 0.45 – 0.9 mg/kg PO once or twice daily. (Adapted from label; *Salix®*)

Extra-label Doses:

For acute cardiogenic or pulmonary edema (parenteral dosing): Initially a dosage of 1 – 4 mg/kg IV, IM, or SC—see Adverse Effects—is administered and adjusted/repeated every 1–2 hours until respiratory rate and/or respiratory character improves. A maximum daily dose of 12 mg/kg has been noted in some references; alternately a CRI of furosemide administered at 0.66 – 1 mg/kg/hour may produce greater diuresis, natriuresis and less kaliuresis. Adapted from: (Kittleson 2009; DeFrancesco 2013); (Atkins et al. 2009)

For adjunctive treatment of chronic heart failure (PO dosing): Oral dosage recommendations can vary widely and are tailored for the specific patient. Dogs with mild heart failure signs may initially be controlled with 1 mg/kg PO every other day while dogs with severe heart failure may require doses as high as 6 mg/kg PO q8h. Generally the goal is to give the lowest "effective dose" of furosemide. Many cardiologists counsel clients to maintain a clinical sign (respiration rate) diary and to make minor adjustments to dosage within a given range based upon clinical signs (e.g. "give more for difficulty breathing or rapid respirations, and give less if the animal appears weak, lethargic, anorexic or depressed.") Dogs must have adequate fluid and food intake. Adapted from: (Rush 2008), (Kittleson 2009), (Atkins et al. 2009)

For adjunctive treatment of dogs with glomerular disease and pulmonary edema or hyperkalemia: Furosemide may be administered at an initial dosage of 1 mg/kg q6-12h (*route of administration not listed; assume IV or IM—Plumb*), with incremental increases of 0.5 – 1 mg/kg q6-12h or conversion into continuous IV infusion at a rate of 2 – 15 micrograms/kg/minute after an initial loading dose of 2 mg/kg in animals with insufficient response. (Brown et al. 2013)

For adjunctive treatment of moderate to severe hypercalcemia: Volume expansion is necessary prior to use of furosemide; 2 – 4 mg/kg 2-3 times daily, IV, SC or PO. (Chew et al. 2003)

For acute oliguric renal failure: Furosemide can increase urine output so that IV fluid therapy can correct acid-base and electrolyte imbalances but it does not improve GFR or necessarily affect clinical outcome. Two basic dosing protocols have been recommended:

a) IV CRI of 0.5 – 1 mg/kg/hour. If furosemide administration fails to increase urine production, osmotic diuresis (mannitol) can be attempted.

b) Initial IV bolus of 1 – 2 mg/kg (up to 4 mg/kg in dogs if no response seen within 30-60 minutes) followed by a CRI of 0.1 – 2 mg/kg/hour adjusted depending on patient's response.

- **CATS:**

  Labeled-doses (FDA-approved): For treatment of edema (pulmonary congestion, ascites) associated with cardiac insufficiency and acute noninflammatory tissue edema: Injection: 2.75 mg/kg IV or IM once or twice daily after a 6- to 8-hour interval. The dosage should be adjusted to the individual animal's response. In refractory or severe edematous cases the dosage may be doubled or increased by increments of 2.2 mg/kg of body weight to establish the effective dose. The established effective dose should be administered once or twice daily on an intermittent daily schedule. Diuretic therapy should be discontinued after reduction of edema, or when necessary, maintained after determining a programmed dosage schedule to prevent recurrence. PO: 0.45 – 0.9 mg/kg PO once or twice daily. (Adapted from label; *Salix®*)

<u>Extra-label Doses:</u>

For severe acute cardiogenic or pulmonary edema (parenteral dosing): Up to 4 mg/kg IV, IM, or SC—see Adverse Effects—is administered and adjusted/repeated every 1–2 hours until respiratory rate and/or respiratory character improves. Cats that can tolerate an IV injection may benefit from a faster onset of action (5 minutes IV vs. 30 minutes IM). The dose may be repeated within 1-2 hours. To avoid severe dehydration, dosing must be reduced sharply once respiratory rate starts to decrease. Adapted from: (Kittleson 2009; DeFrancesco 2013)

For adjunctive treatment of chronic heart failure (PO dosing): Oral dosage recommendations can vary widely in cats and range from 1 mg/kg PO every 2 to 3 days to 2 mg/kg PO q8-12h for most cases. But dosages of up to 7 mg/kg q12h have been noted. Practically, many cats are dosed in 6.25 mg increments (½ of a 12.5 mg tablet). Like dogs, dosages are tailored to the patient and in general the goal is to give the lowest "effective dose" of furosemide. Often owners are counseled to adjust dosages within a given range based upon respiratory rates (*e.g.,* more if >35 breaths per minute when not purring, and less furosemide if cat seems weak, lethargic, anorexic, or depressed.) Adapted from: (Kittleson 2009), (Freeman et al. 2013)

For acute oliguric renal failure: Furosemide can increase urine output so that IV fluid therapy can correct acid-base and electrolyte imbalances but it does not improve GFR or necessarily affect clinical outcome. Two basic dosing protocols have been recommended:

a) IV CRI of 0.25 – 1 mg/kg/hour. If furosemide administration fails to increase urine production, osmotic diuresis (mannitol) can be attempted.

b) Bolus of 1 – 2 mg/kg IV and, if an effect is seen, start a continuous rate infusion at 0.25 – 1 mg/kg/hour adjusted depending on patient's response.

■ **FERRETS:**

For adjunctive therapy for heart failure (extra-label): For fulminant CHF, initially at 1 - 4 mg/kg IV or IM every 8-12 hours; repeat after 30 minutes if there is no improvement, then transition to PO at 1 – 2 mg/kg PO q12h. Adapted from (Hoeffer 2000), (Williams 2000), (Watson 2011)

■ **RABBITS/RODENTS/SMALL MAMMALS:**

Note: Dosages are primarily extrapolated (extra-label) from those recommended for dogs and cats with similar disease states. Use caution with SC dosing as local tissue reactions can occur.

Rabbits: For CHF: 2 – 5 mg/kg PO, SC, IM or IV q12h; **For pulmonary edema:** 1 – 4 mg/kg IV or IM q4–6h. (Ivey et al. 2000)

Mice, Rats, Gerbils, Hamsters, Guinea pigs, Chinchillas: 5 – 10 mg/kg q12h. (Adamcak et al. 2000)

■ **CATTLE:**

For the treatment of physiological parturient edema of the mammary gland and associated structures (labeled dose; FDA-approved): The drug is administered at a dosage of 500 mg IM or IV per animal once daily or 250 mg per animal IV or IM q12h; treatment not to exceed 48 hours post-parturition. Milk and slaughter withdrawal = 48 hours after last treatment. (Adapted from label; *Salix®*)

■ **HORSES:**

Note: Refer to state/country guidelines for use of furosemide in racing animals.

<u>Labeled doses</u> (FDA-approved):

For the treatment of edema (pulmonary congestion, ascites) associated with cardiac insufficiency, and acute non-inflammatory tissue edema: 250 – 500 mg per horse IM or IV once or twice daily. Do not use in horses intended for human consumption. (Adapted from label; *Salix®*)

For treatment of acute noninflammatory tissue edema: 1 mg/kg IV or IM; once or twice daily at 6-to 8-hour intervals. (Adapted from label; *Disal®*, *Furos-A-Vet®*)

Extra-label Doses:

For adjunctive therapy for congestive heart failure: Initially, 1 – 2 mg/kg IM or IV q6-12h to control edema. Long-term therapy: 0.5 – 2 mg/kg PO or IM q8–12h. (Mogg 1999)

For adjunctive therapy of acute renal failure: 2 – 4 mg/kg q6h. (Jose-Cunilleras et al. 1999)

For epistaxis/EIPH prevention: 500 mg (per horse) IV 4 hours prior to race (Hinchcliff et al. 2009). There appears to be substantial evidence supporting the efficacy of furosemide for this purpose.

■ **BIRDS:**

For cardiopulmonary disorders (edema, pericardial effusion); (extra-label): Recommended dosages ranging from 0.15 – 2 mg/kg/day PO or IM. (Watson 2011) **Note:** Lories are very sensitive to this agent and can be easily overdosed. (Clubb 1986).

■ **REPTILES:**

For edema/pulmonary congestion (extra-label): The use of furosemide is limited in reptiles as they lack a loop of Henle. It has been suggested that a dose of 5 mg/kg PO, IM, IV every 12-24 hours can be used. (Watson 2011)

Monitoring

■ Serum electrolytes, BUN, creatinine, glucose.

■ Hydration status.

■ Blood pressure, if indicated.

■ Clinical signs of edema, patient weight, if indicated.

■ Evaluation of ototoxicity, particularly with prolonged therapy or in cats.

Client Information

■ Your animal may urinate more often than normal. This usually improves after a while.

■ May be given with or without food. Allow access to water at all times; encourage normal food intake. If your animal vomits or acts sick after getting it on an empty stomach, give with food or small treat to see if this helps. If vomiting continues, contact your veterinarian.

■ Because this drug can change electrolytes (salts) in the blood, your veterinarian will probably want to do more frequent testing.

■ Contact veterinarian immediately if excessive thirst, muscle weakness or collapse, head tilt, lack of urination, or a very fast heartbeat is noticed.

Chemistry/Synonyms

A loop diuretic related structurally to the sulfonamides, furosemide occurs as an odorless, practically tasteless, white to slightly yellow, fine, crystalline powder. Furosemide has a melting point between 203-205°C with decomposition, and a pK_a of 3.9. It is practically insoluble in water, sparingly soluble in alcohol, and freely soluble in alkaline hydroxides. The veterinary injectable products use either the diethanolamine or monoethanolamine salts of furosemide. Diethanolamine salts of have a pH of 7-7.8 and monoethanolamine salts have a pH of 8-9.3. pH may be adjusted with NaOH or HCl.

Furosemide may also be known as: frusemide, furosemidum, and LB-502; many trade names are available.

Storage/Stability

Furosemide tablets should be stored in light-resistant, well-closed containers. The oral solution should be stored at room temperature and protected from light and freezing. Furosemide injection should be stored at room temperature. A precipitate may form if the injection is refrigerated, but will resolubolize when warmed without alteration in potency. The human injection (10 mg/mL) should not be used if it has a yellow color. The veterinary injection (50 mg/mL) normally has a slight yellow color. Furosemide is unstable at an acid pH, but is very stable under alkaline conditions.

Compatibility/Compounding Considerations

Furosemide injection (10 mg/mL) is reportedly physically **compatible** with all commonly used intravenous solutions and the following drugs (depending on concentration): amikacin sulfate, atropine sulfate, dexmedetomidine, digoxin, epinephrine, heparin, mannitol, potassium chloride, ranitidine, sodium nitroprusside, tobramycin sulfate, vasopressin, and verapamil. Refer to a specialized reference or consult a hospital pharmacist for additional information.

It is reportedly physically **incompatible** with the following agents: ascorbic acid solutions, dobutamine HCl, esmolol, gentamicin sulfate, hydralazine and tetracyclines. It should generally not be mixed with antihistamines, local anesthetics, alkaloids, hypnotics, or opiates.

Dosage Forms/Regulatory Status

VETERINARY-LABELED PRODUCTS:

Furosemide Tablets: 12.5 mg, & 50 mg; *Salix®*, *Disal®*, generic; (Rx). Products may be FDA-approved for use in dogs and cats.

Furosemide Oral Solution (Syrup): 10 mg/mL in 60 mL; generic; (Rx). FDA-approved for use in dogs.

Furosemide for Injection: 50 mg/mL (5%) in 50 mL & 100 mL vials; *Disal® Injection*, *Salix® Injection*, generic; (Rx). Products may be FDA-approved for use in dogs, cattle, cats and horses. 48 hour milk/meat withdrawal in cattle.

HUMAN-LABELED PRODUCTS:

Furosemide Oral Tablets: 20 mg, 40 mg, & 80 mg; *Lasix®*, generic; (Rx)

Furosemide Oral Solution: 10 mg/mL & 40 mg/5 mL (8 mg/mL); generic; (Rx)

Furosemide Injection: 10 mg/mL in 2 mL (20 mg), 4 mL (40 mg) & 10 mL (100 mg) single-dose vials; generic; (Rx)

Revisions/References

Monograph revised/updated January 2014.
Adamcak, A. & B. Otten (2000). Rodent Therapeutics. Vet Clin NA: Exotic Anim Pract 3:1(Jan): 221-40.
Atkins, C., et al. (2009). Guidelines for the Diagnosis and Treatment of Canine Chronic Valvular Heart Disease. Journal of Veterinary Internal Medicine 23(6): 1142-50.
Brown, S., et al. (2013). Consensus Recommendations for Standard Therapy of Glomerular Disease in Dogs. Journal of Veterinary Internal Medicine 27: S27-S43.
Chew, D., et al. (2003). Assessment and treatment of clinical cases with elusive disorders of hypercalcemia. Proceedings: ACVIM Forum. accessed via Veterinary Information Network; vin.com
Clubb, S. L. (1986). Therapeutics: Individual and Flock Treatment Regimens. *Clinical Avian Medicine and Surgery.* G. J. Harrison and L. R. Harrison. Philadelphia, W.B. Saunders: 327-55.
DeFrancesco, T. C. (2013). Management of Cardiac Emergencies in Small Animals. Veterinary Clinics of North America: Small Animal Practice 43(4): 817-42.
Freeman, L. A. & J. E. Rush (2013). Top Ten Treatment Tips for Feline Heart Disease: Feeding and Pharmacology. ACVIM. accessed via Veterinary Information Network; vin.com
Hinchcliff, K. W., et al. (2009). Efficacy of furosemide for prevention of exercise-induced pulmonary hemorrhage in Thoroughbred racehorses. Javma-Journal of the American Veterinary Medical Association 235(1): 76-82.
Hoeffer, H. (2000). Heart Disease in Ferrets. *Kirk's Current Veterinary Therapy: XIII Small Animal Practice.* J. Bonagura. Philadelphia, WB Saunders: 1144-8.
Ivey, E. & J. Morrisey (2000). Therapeutics for Rabbits. Vet Clin NA: Exotic Anim Pract 3:1(Jan): 183-216.
Jose-Cunilleras, E. & K. Hinchcliff (1999). Renal pharmacology. The Veterinary Clinics of North America: Equine Practice 15:3(December): 647-64.
Kittleson, M. (2009). Treatment of feline hypertrophic cardiomyopathy (HCM)--Lost Dreams. Proceedings: ACVIM. accessed via Veterinary Information Network; vin.com
Mogg, T. (1999). Equine Cardiac Disease: Clinical pharmacology and therapeutics. The Veterinary Clinics of North America: Equine Practice 15:3(December).
Rush, J. (2008). Heart failure in dogs and cats. Proceedings: IVECCS. accessed via Veterinary Information Network; vin.com
Scruggs, S. M. & M. Rishniw (2013). Dermatologic Adverse Effect of Subcutaneous Furosemide Administration in a Dog. Journal of Veterinary Internal Medicine 27(5): 1248-50.
Suzuki, S., et al. (2011). The Effect of Furosemide on Left Atrial Pressure in Dogs with Mitral Valve Regurgitation. Journal of Veterinary Internal Medicine 25(2): 244-50.
Watson, M. (2011). Furosemide. Journal of Exotic Pet Medicine 20(1): 60-3.
Williams, B. (2000). Therapeutics in Ferrets. Vet Clin NA: Exotic Anim Pract 3:1(Jan): 131-53.
Adamcak, A. & B. Otten (2000). Rodent Therapeutics. Vet Clin NA: Exotic Anim Pract 3:1(Jan): 221-40.
Atkins, C., et al. (2009). Guidelines for the Diagnosis and Treatment of Canine Chronic Valvular Heart Disease. Journal of Veterinary Internal Medicine 23(6): 1142-50.
Brown, S., et al. (2013). Consensus Recommendations for Standard Therapy of Glomerular Disease in Dogs. Journal of Veterinary Internal Medicine 27: S27-S43.
Chew, D., et al. (2003). Assessment and treatment of clinical cases with elusive disorders of hypercalcemia. Proceedings: ACVIM Forum. accessed via Veterinary Information Network; vin.com
Clubb, S. L. (1986). Therapeutics: Individual and Flock Treatment Regimens. *Clinical Avian Medicine and Surgery.* G. J. Harrison and L. R. Harrison. Philadelphia, W.B. Saunders: 327-55.
DeFrancesco, T. C. (2013). Management of Cardiac Emergencies in Small Animals. Veterinary Clinics of North America: Small Animal Practice 43(4): 817-42.
Freeman, L. A. & J. E. Rush (2013). Top Ten Treatment Tips for Feline Heart Disease: Feeding and Pharmacology. ACVIM. accessed via Veterinary Information Network; vin.com
Hinchcliff, K. W., et al. (2009). Efficacy of furosemide for prevention of exercise-induced pulmonary hemorrhage in Thoroughbred racehorses. Javma-Journal of the American Veterinary Medical Association 235(1): 76-82.
Hoeffer, H. (2000). Heart Disease in Ferrets. *Kirk's Current Veterinary Therapy: XIII Small Animal Practice.* J. Bonagura. Philadelphia, WB Saunders: 1144-8.
Ivey, E. & J. Morrisey (2000). Therapeutics for Rabbits. Vet Clin NA: Exotic Anim Pract 3:1(Jan): 183-216.
Jose-Cunilleras, E. & K. Hinchcliff (1999). Renal pharmacology. The Veterinary Clinics of North America: Equine Practice 15:3(December): 647-64.
Kittleson, M. (2009). Treatment of feline hypertrophic cardiomyopathy (HCM)--Lost Dreams. Proceedings: ACVIM. accessed via Veterinary Information Network; vin.com
Mogg, T. (1999). Equine Cardiac Disease: Clinical pharmacology and therapeutics. The Veterinary Clinics of North America: Equine Practice 15:3(December).
Rush, J. (2008). Heart failure in dogs and cats. Proceedings: IVECCS. accessed via Veterinary Information Network; vin.com
Scruggs, S. M. & M. Rishniw (2013). Dermatologic Adverse Effect of Subcutaneous Furosemide Administration in a Dog. Journal of Veterinary Internal Medicine 27(5): 1248-50.
Suzuki, S., et al. (2011). The Effect of Furosemide on Left Atrial Pressure in Dogs with Mitral Valve Regurgitation. Journal of Veterinary Internal Medicine 25(2): 244-50.
Watson, M. (2011). Furosemide. Journal of Exotic Pet Medicine 20(1): 60-3.
Williams, B. (2000). Therapeutics in Ferrets. Vet Clin NA: Exotic Anim Pract 3:1(Jan): 131-53.

Gabapentin

(gab-ah-pen-tin)   Neurontin®

Anticonvulsant; Neuropathic Pain Analgesic

Prescriber Highlights

▶ May be useful in dogs & cats as adjunctive therapy for refractory or complex partial seizures and in many species for the treatment of pain (especially neuropathic pain). Efficacy evidence to support extensive clinical usage is currently weak.

▶ Caution in patients with diminished renal function, but dogs partially (30-40%) metabolize the drug (humans do not).

▶ Avoid use of xylitol-containing oral liquid in dogs.

▶ Sedation or ataxia most likely adverse effects in small animals.

▶ Three times a day dosing in dogs or cats may be problematic.

Uses/Indications

Gabapentin may be useful as adjunctive therapy for refractory or complex partial seizures. As an analgesic, gabapentin has been demonstrated to be most useful in treating chronic pain, particularly neuropathic pain in small animals.

Gabapentin does not appear to be of significant use for treating acute pain, but it may be of benefit when given preemptively for acute pain (*e.g.*, before surgery) when used adjunctively with other analgesics; studies are ongoing to evaluate this indication for small animals. Gabapentin has been proposed for further study in horses to determine its efficacy as an adjunctive treatment for laminitis pain (Terry, McDonnell, van, et al. 2010) and in cattle for treating neuropathic pain (Coetzee et al. 2011).

Pharmacology/Actions

Gabapentin has analgesic effects and can prevent allodynia (sensation of pain resulting from a normally non-noxious stimulus) or hyperalgesia (exaggerated response to painful stimuli). It also has anticonvulsant activity. The mechanism of action of gabapentin, for either its anticonvulsant or analgesic actions is not fully understood, but it appears to bind to CaVa2-d (alpha2-delta subunit of the voltage-gated calcium channels). By decreasing calcium influx, the release of excitatory neurotransmitters (*e.g.*, substance P, glutamate, norepinephrine) is inhibited. While gabapentin is structurally related to GABA, it does not appear to alter GABA binding, reuptake, or degradation, or serve as a GABA agonist *in vivo*.

Pharmacokinetics

In dogs, oral bioavailability is about 80% at a dose of 50 mg/kg. Peak plasma levels occur about 2 hours post dose. Elimination is primarily via renal routes, but gabapentin is partially metabolized to N-methyl-gabapentin in dogs. Elimination half-life is approximately 2-4 hours.

In cats, gabapentin is well absorbed after oral dosing with a bioavailability average of 90%, but there was significant interpatient variation (50%-120%). Peak levels occurred about 100 minutes after dosing. Volume of distribution is relatively low (apparent Vd_{ss} of 0.65 L/kg.) Clearance was about 3 mL/min/kg and mean elimination half-life of 2.8 hours is similar to that of dogs (Siao et al. 2010).

In four horses given single oral doses of 5 mg/kg, gabapentin was rapidly absorbed with peak levels noted within 2 hours (mean 1.4 hours). Plasma elimination half-life was about 3.4 hours (Dirikolu et al. 2008). Another study done in 6 horses showed that oral gabapentin had a low oral bioavailability (about 16%) and peak levels occurred about one hour after oral dosing. Elimination half-life (oral) was about 7-8 hours (Terry, McDonnell, Van Eps, et al. 2010).

In ruminating calves, oral gabapentin (with or without meloxicam) at 10 or 15 mg/kg yielded plasma gabapentin levels of >2 mcg/mL for up to 15 hours and elimination half-life was about 8-10 hours (Coetzee et al. 2011).

In humans, gabapentin bioavailability decreases as dosage increases. At doses of 900 mg/day, 60% of the dose is absorbed. Percentage absorbed is reduced as doses are increased to a minimum of 27% of the dose being absorbed when 4800 mg/day is administered. Presence of food only marginally alters absorption rate and extent of absorption. Gabapentin is only minimally bound to plasma proteins; CSF levels are approximately 20% of those in plasma. The drug is not significantly metabolized and is almost exclusively excreted unchanged into the urine. Elimination half-lives in humans are approximately 5-7 hours.

An extended-release tablet formulation (gabapentin enacarbil) is available for humans, but no pharmacokinetic information for this product was noted for veterinary species.

Contraindications/Precautions/Warnings

Gabapentin is considered contraindicated in patients hypersensitive to it. Because gabapentin is eliminated via renal routes (practically 100% in humans), it should be used with caution in patients with renal insufficiency; if required, dosage adjustment should be considered. In dogs, the drug is also metabolized (30-40% of a dose), so dosage adjustment may not be required in dogs with mild to moderate renal dysfunction. However, one reference recommends that dosages be reduced and/or dosing intervals increased in dogs and cats when creatine clearance is 0.7 mL/kg/min or less (Trepanier 2013).

In general, avoid the use of the commercially available human oral solution (*Neurontin®*) in dogs as it reportedly contains 300 mg/mL xylitol. As the threshold dose that can cause hypoglycemia in dogs is approximately 100 mg/kg, doses of up to 15 mg/kg in dogs using the solution should be safe, but further data is needed to confirm this. Additionally, xylitol may be hepatotoxic in dogs. Doses of 500 mg/kg of xylitol are currently thought to be the threshold for this toxicity, but there have been anecdotal reports of it occurring at much lower doses. In cats, at the dosages used presently, xylitol toxicity does not appear to be a problem with gabapentin oral solution, but use with caution.

Abrupt discontinuation of the drug after chronic use has lead to withdrawal-precipitated seizures. In humans, it is recommended to wean off the drug when it is used for epilepsy treatment and similar advice for animal patients seems prudent.

Adverse Effects

Sedation and ataxia are probably the most likely adverse effects seen in small animals. Starting the dose at the lower end of the range and increasing with time may alleviate these effects. In humans, the most common adverse effects associated with gabapentin therapy are dizziness, somnolence, and peripheral edema.

Gabapentin was associated with an increased rate of pancreatic adenocarcinoma in male rats. It is unknown if this effect occurs in other species.

Reproductive/Nursing Safety

In humans, the FDA categorizes gabapentin as a category *C* drug for use during pregnancy (*Animal studies have shown an adverse effect on the fetus, but there are no adequate studies in humans; or there are no animal reproduction studies and no adequate studies in humans*). At high dosages (at or above human maximum dosages), gabapentin was associated with a variety of fetotoxic and teratogenic effects (*e.g.*, delayed ossification, hydronephrosis, fetal loss) in rats, mice and rabbits.

Gabapentin enters maternal milk. It has been calculated that a nursing human infant could be exposed to a maximum dosage of 1 mg/kg/day. This is 5-10% of the usual pediatric (>3 yrs. old) therapeutic dose. In veterinary patients, this appears unlikely to be of significant clinical concern.

Overdosage/Acute Toxicity

In humans, doses of up to 49 grams have been reported without fatality. Most likely effects include ataxia, lethargy/somnolence, diarrhea, etc.

The commercially available oral solution contains 300 mg/mL of xylitol; doses of 0.33 mL/kg may cause hypoglycemia or liver toxicity in dogs.

There were 568 single agent exposures to gabapentin reported to the ASPCA Animal Poison Control Center (APCC) during 2009-2013. Of the 462 dogs, 90 were symptomatic with 24% ataxic, 22% lethargic, 21% lethargic and 16% vomiting. Of the 103 exposed cats, 47 were symptomatic. The most common signs were lethargy/sedation (55%) and ataxia (49%).

Treatment is basically supportive with general decontamination procedures including emesis, activated charcoal, and cathartics. The drug can be removed with hemodialysis. Should xylitol toxicity be suspected secondary to the human-labeled liquid formulation, contact an animal poison control center for further guidance.

Drug Interactions

The following drug interactions have either been reported or are theoretical in humans or animals receiving gabapentin and may be of in veterinary patients. Unless otherwise noted, use together is not necessarily contraindicated, but weigh the potential risks and perform additional monitoring when appropriate.

- **ANTACIDS:** Oral antacids given concurrently with gabapentin may decrease oral bioavailability by 20%; if antacids are required, separate doses at least 2 hours from gabapentin.
- **HYDROCODONE:** Co-administration of gabapentin and hydrocodone may increase the AUC (area under the curve) of gabapentin and increase the efficacy and/or adverse effects of the drug. Gabapentin can reduce the AUC of hydrocodone, potentially reducing the drug's effectiveness.
- **MORPHINE:** May increase gabapentin levels.

Laboratory Considerations

- There are reports of gabapentin causing false-positive **urinary protein** readings on *Ames N-Multistix SG* dipstick tests. The use of a sulfosalicylic acid precipitation test to determine presence of urine protein is recommended for patients receiving gabapentin.

Doses

- **DOGS:**

  For ancillary therapy of refractory seizures (extra-label):
  a) Evidence to support use is relatively weak, suggested dosages usually fall into the 10 – 20 mg/kg PO q8h range. Some recommend starting therapy at 10 mg/kg PO q8h to reduce potential for over-sedation; some suggest that dosages up to 30 mg/kg PO q8h or administering every 6 hours may be required for efficacy.
  b) Study was done in dogs with uncontrolled seizures (at least 2 per month and at least 6 over the prior 3 months) when phenobarbital and potassium bromide levels were therapeutic or sub-therapeutic but had unacceptable side effects: Dogs were dosed at approximately 10 mg/kg PO q8h for 3 months. Six of eleven dogs had a minimum of 50% reduction in seizures per week. (Platt et al. 2006)

  As an adjunctive analgesic (extra-label): Evidence to support use is weak, but anecdotally it has been reported to be effective in some dogs, particularly for chronic pain conditions with a neuropathic component. Dosage recommendations usually are 5 – 10 mg/kg PO q12h, but dosing similarly as for seizures (10 – 20 mg/kg PO q8h), may be considered.

- **CATS:**

  For ancillary therapy of refractory seizures (extra-label): Evidence to support use is weak, but anecdotal initial dosages of 5 – 10 mg/kg PO q8-12h have been noted. A recently published review article on epilepsy in cats, lists an anecdotal dosage of 5 – 20 mg/kg PO q6-12h (Pakozdy et al. 2014). Some have suggested initially giving the drug once per day and giving more often as necessary.

  As an adjunctive analgesic (extra-label): Evidence to support use is weak, but anecdotally it has been reported to be effective in some cats, particularly for chronic pain conditions with a neuropathic component. There is no strong evidence to support one dosage recommendation over another and suggested initial dosages range from 3 mg/kg PO once daily and titrated upwards to 5 – 10 mg/kg PO q12h (if required). Others start at 5 – 10 mg/kg PO q8-12h.

Monitoring

- **Note:** Gabapentin serum levels are usually not monitored; therapeutic levels are thought to be 4-16 micrograms/mL. In dogs, if monitoring levels, samples should be when peak levels occur (about two hours after a dose). Subsequent levels should be drawn at consistent times after dosing.
- Monitor clinical efficacy and adverse effects.

Client Information

- May be given with or without food. If your animal vomits or acts sick after getting it on an empty stomach, give with food or small treat to see if this helps. If vomiting continues, contact your veterinarian.
- Drowsiness and loss of coordination are the most common side effects.
- Do not use the oral liquid made for humans in dogs. It contains xylitol, which is toxic to dogs.

Chemistry/Synonyms

Gabapentin occurs as white to off-white crystalline solid that is freely soluble in water. It has a pK_{a1} of 3.7 and a pK_{a2} of 10.7. It is structurally related to GABA (gamma-aminobutyric acid).

Gabapentin may also be known as: CI-945, GOE-3450, *Aclonium®*, *Equipax®*, *Gantin®*, *Gabarone®*, *Neurontin®*, *Neurostil®* and *Progresse®*.

Storage/Stability

The commercially available capsules and tablets should be stored at room temperature (25°C, 77°F); excursions permitted to 15-30°C (59-86°F). The oral liquid should be stored in the refrigerator at 2-8°C (36-46°F).

Compatibility/Compounding Considerations

Compounded preparation stability: Commercially available gabapentin solutions contain amounts of xylitol, which may be toxic to canine patients. Gabapentin oral suspension compounded from commercially available tablets has been published (Nahata 1999). Triturating twenty (20) gabapentin 600 mg tablets with 60 mL of *Ora-Plus®* and *qs ad* to 120 mL with *Ora-Sweet®* (or *Ora-Sweet® SF*) yields a 100 mg/mL oral suspension that retains >90% potency for 56 days stored at both 4°C and 25°C. Liquid formulations of gabapentin are most stable in the pH range of 5.5-6.5.

Dosage Forms/Regulatory Status

VETERINARY-LABELED PRODUCTS: NONE.

The ARCI (Racing Commissioners International) has designated this drug as a class 4 substance. See the appendix for more information.

HUMAN-LABELED PRODUCTS:

Gabapentin Oral Capsules & Tablets: 100 mg, 300 mg, 400 mg; 600 mg, & 800 mg (film-coated); *Neurontin®*, generic; (Rx)

Gabapentin Oral Solution: 250 mg/5mL (50 mg/mL) in 470 mL; *Neurontin®*; (Rx). **Note:** Contains xylitol. Use with caution in dogs.

There is also a gabapentin enacarbil 600 mg oral extended-release tablet product (*Horizant®*), but no information on its pharmacokinetics or clinical usage in dogs and cats was noted.

Revisions/Revisions/References

Monograph revised/updated January 2014.

Coetzee, J. F., et al. (2011). Pharmacokinetics of oral gabapentin alone or co-administered with meloxicam in ruminant beef calves. The Veterinary Journal **190**(1): 98-102.

Dirikolu, L., et al. (2008). Pharmacokinetics of gabapentin in horses. J. Vet. Pharmacol. Ther. **31**(2): 175-7.

Nahata, M. C. (1999). Development of two stable oral suspensions for gabapentin. Pediatr Neurol **20**(3): 195-7.

Pakozdy, A., et al. (2014). Epilepsy in cats: Theory and practice. J Vet Intern Med.

Platt, S. R., et al. (2006). Treatment with gabapentin of 11 dogs with refractory idiopathic epilepsy. Veterinary Record **159**(26): 881-4.

Siao, K. T., et al. (2010). Pharmacokinetics of gabapentin in cats. American Journal of Veterinary Research **71**(7): 817-21.

Terry, R. L., et al. (2010). Pharmacokinetics and Pharmacodynamics of Gabapentin in Horses: A Potentially Useful Analgesic Agent for the Treatment of Laminitis. Journal of Equine Veterinary Science **30**(2): 100-1.

Terry, R. L., et al. (2010). Pharmacokinetic profile and behavioral effects of gabapentin in the horse. J. Vet. Pharmacol. Ther. **33**(5): 485-94.

Trepanier, L. A. (2013). Applying Pharmacokinetics to Veterinary Clinical Practice. Veterinary Clinics of North America-Small Animal Practice **43**(5): 1013-+.

Gamithromycin

(gah-mith-roe-my-sin)   Zactran®

Macrolide (Azalide) Antibiotic

Prescriber Highlights

▶ Injectable azalide-class macrolide antibiotic approved for BRD in cattle (not dairy cattle); potentially could be useful in horses, especially foals, but presently little information available on efficacy and safety to support routine use.

▶ Pain/swelling most common adverse effect.

▶ 35 day slaughter withdrawal (63 day in UK).

Uses/Indications

The FDA has approved (see restrictions in the Dosage Form/Regulatory Status section) gamithromycin for the treatment of bovine respiratory disease (BRD) associated with *Mannheimia haemolytica*, *Pasteurella multocida*, *Histophilus somni* and *Mycoplasma bovis* in beef and non-lactating dairy cattle. It is also indicated for the control of respiratory disease in beef and non-lactating dairy cattle at high risk of developing BRD associated with *Mannheimia haemolytica* and *Pasteurella multocida*.

Gamithromycin potentially could be useful in other species as well. One study done in foals showed that IM doses of 6 mg/kg every 7 days would maintain pulmonary epithelial lining fluid (PELF) concentrations above the MIC_{90} for susceptible isolates of *S. zooepidemicus* and phagocytic cell concentrations above the MIC_{90} for susceptible isolates of *R. equi* (Berghaus et al. 2012). Additional studies are ongoing.

Pharmacology/Actions

Like other macrolides, gamithromycin penetrates bacterial cell membranes and binds to the 50s ribosomal subunit thereby inhibiting protein synthesis. It inhibits the translocation process between 30S and 50s ribosomes, causing premature detachment of incomplete peptide chains.

Significant increases in MIC can occur in *P. multocida* and *M. haemolytica* with the *msr*(E)-*mph*(E) gene (Michael et al. 2012).

Pharmacokinetics

In cattle, after a 6 mg/kg subcutaneous injection (in neck), gamithromycin absorption is complete and peak plasma levels occur in about an hour. Volume of distribution is very high (approximately 25 L/kg) and only 26% of drug in plasma is bound to plasma proteins. Clearance is 712 mL/kg/hour and elimination half-life is approximately 51 hours. The primary route of elimination is biliary excretion of unchanged drug. After a single (6 mg/kg) dose, gamithromycin concentrations in pulmonary epithelial lining fluid (PELF), bronchiolar lavage fluid (BAL) cells, and lung tissue can persist above reported MIC_{90} for labeled organisms for 7 days (PELF) to 10-15+ days (BAL cells and lung tissue). (Huang et al. 2010; Giguere et al. 2011; anon 2012b, a)

In foals after a 6 mg/kg IM dose, peak plasma levels occur in about an hour and elimination half-life around 39 hours. Gamithromycin concentrations in PELF were above the MIC_{90} for susceptible isolates of *S. zooepidemicus* and phagocytic cell concentrations above the MIC_{90} for susceptible isolates of *R. equi* for approximately 7 days. (Berghaus et al. 2012)

Contraindications/Precautions/Warnings

Gamithromycin is contraindicated in animals that are hypersensitive to it. Potentially animals hypersensitive to other azalide or macrolide antibiotics could also react to gamithromycin. Subcutaneous injection may cause a temporary local tissue reaction in some animals that may result in trim loss of edible tissues at slaughter.

Cross-resistance may occur with other macrolide/azalide antibiotics (*e.g.*, tulathromycin, tilmicosin).

Adverse Effects

Pain and swelling at the injections site can be seen. Swelling/local inflammation at injection site usually resolves within 3-14 days, but has been reported to persist up to 35 days post injection (anon 2011).

Potentially, hypersensitivity reactions could occur, however no case reports were noted.

Reproductive/Nursing Safety

While the drug is not labeled for use in pregnant animals, the product's material safety data sheet (MSDS) lists: none of the ingredients are considered to be reproductive, teratogenic, or developmental toxin. The UK label reads: "Based on laboratory animal data, gamithromycin has not produced any evidence of selective developmental or reproductive effects. The safety of gamithromycin during pregnancy and lactation has not been evaluated in cattle. Use only according to the risk/benefit assessment by the responsible veterinarian."(anon 2011)

Overdosage/Acute Toxicity

Subcutaneous injections of 18 and 30 mg/kg (3X and 5X label dose) given every 5 days for 3 doses to 6-month old beef cattle caused swelling and pain at the injection site (neck twisting, attempts to scratch or lick the injection site, and pawing at the ground). Other clinically relevant treatment-related effects were not observed.

Drug Interactions

No drug interactions have been reported for this drug when used in cattle.

Laboratory Considerations

Nothing noted.

Dosages

- **CATTLE**

  Note: See restrictions and withdrawal times in the Dosage Forms/Regulatory Status section.

  U.S. labeled dose for the treatment of bovine respiratory disease (BRD) associated with *Mannheimia haemolytica*, *Pasteurella multocida*, *Histophilus somni* and *Mycoplasma bovis* in beef and non-lactating dairy cattle; also indicated for the control of respiratory disease in beef and non-lactating dairy cattle at high risk of developing BRD associated with *Mannheimia haemolytica* and *Pasteurella multocida* (labeled dose; FDA-approved): Administer one time as a subcutaneous injection in the neck at 6 mg/kg (2 mL/110 lb.) body weight (BW). If the total dose exceeds 10 mL, divide the dose so that no more than 10 mL is administered at each injection site. Animals should be appropriately restrained to achieve the proper route of administration. Use sterile equipment. Inject under the skin in front of the shoulder. (Adapted from label information; *Zactran*®—Merial USA)

  U.K. labeled dose (extra-label in USA): For use in cattle for therapeutic and preventative treatment of bovine respiratory disease (BRD) associated with *Mannheimia haemolytica*, *Pasteurella multocida* and *Histophilus somni*. The presence of the disease in the herd should be established before preventative treatment: A single subcutaneous injection of 6 mg gamithromycin/kg bodyweight (equivalent to 1 mL/25 kg bodyweight) in the neck. For treatment of cattle over 250 kg bodyweight, divide the dose so that no more than 10 mL are injected at one site. To ensure correct dosage, bodyweight should be determined as accurately as possible to avoid under dosing. (Adapted from label information; *Zactran*®—Merial U.K.)

Monitoring

- Clinical response. In field trials, animals that responded to therapy did so within 24 hours of injection.

Client Information

- Understand and follow use restrictions and withdrawal times for food animals.
- Humans with known hypersensitivity (drug allergy) to macrolide antibiotics (e.g. erythromycin, clarithromycin) should avoid contact with the medication.
- In case of skin or eye exposure, wash/flush with clean water. If accidental self-injection, seek medical advice immediately and show the package leaflet or label to the physician.

Chemistry/Synonyms

Gamithromycin is a 7a-azalide macrolide antibiotic (CAS Registry: 145435-72-9). It differs structurally from other macrolides by having a 15-membered semisynthetic lactone ring with an alkylated nitrogen at the 7a-position. The commercially available injectable solution contains per mL: 150 mg of gamithromycin as the free base, 1 mg of monothioglycerol and 40 mg of succinic acid in a glycerol formal vehicle.

Gamithromycin may also be known as ML-1,709,460 or UNII-ZE856183S0. A trade name is *Zactran®*.

Storage/Stability

The injection should be stored at or below 77°F (25°C) with excursions between 59-86°F (15-30°C). Use within 18 months of first puncture (USA label); once opened, use within 28 days (U.K. label). Viscosity of the injectable solution may increase at sub-freezing temperatures, but should not affect syringability. (anon 2012b)

Compatibility/Compounding Considerations

No information was noted on the label (USA) or in other references, but the U.K. label states: Do not mix with any other veterinary medicinal product.

Dosage Forms/Regulatory Status

VETERINARY-LABELED PRODUCTS:

Solution for Injection: 150 mg/mL in 100 mL, 250 mL & 500 mL bottles. *Zactran®*; (Rx). FDA-approved (NADA 141-328) for use in cattle (see below).

There is a website (dailymed.nlm.nih.gov) with the FDA-approved veterinary product's label: *Zactran®*.

Withdrawal times/restrictions: USA labeling: Do not treat cattle within 35 days of slaughter. Because a discard time in milk has not been established, do not use in female dairy cattle 20 months of age or older. A withdrawal period has not been established for this product in pre-ruminating calves. Do not use in calves to be processed for veal. U.K. labeling: Meat and offal withdrawal period: 64 days. Not authorised for use in lactating animals producing milk for human consumption. Do not use in pregnant cows or heifers, which are intended to produce milk for human consumption, within 2 months of expected parturition.

HUMAN-LABELED PRODUCTS: NONE.

Revisions/References

Monograph written July 2013.

anon (2011). Zactran® [Product Label]. Secondary Zactran® [Product Label]. Secondary anon. Harlow Essex, Merial U.K. Volume
anon (2012a). Zactran® [Package Insert]. Secondary Zactran® [Package Insert]. Secondary anon. Duluth, GA, Merial. Volume
anon (2012b). Zactran® [Technical Manual]. Secondary Zactran® [Technical Manual]. Secondary anon. Duluth, GA, Merial. Volume
Berghaus, L. J., et al. (2012). Plasma pharmacokinetics, pulmonary distribution, and in vitro activity of gamithromycin in foals. J. Vet. Pharmacol. Ther. 35(1): 59-66.
Giguere, S., et al. (2011). Disposition of gamithromycin in plasma, pulmonary epithelial lining fluid, bronchoalveolar cells, and lung tissue in cattle. American Journal of Veterinary Research 72(3): 326-30.
Huang, R. A., et al. (2010). Pharmacokinetics of gamithromycin in cattle with comparison of plasma and lung tissue concentrations and plasma antibacterial activity. J. Vet. Pharmacol. Ther. 33(3): 227-37.
Michael, G. B., et al. (2012). Increased MICs of gamithromycin and tildipirosin in the presence of the genes erm(42) and msr(E)-mph(E) for bovine Pasteurella multocida and Mannheimia haemolytica. Journal of Antimicrobial Chemotherapy 67(6): 1555-7.

Gemcitabine HCl

(jem-site-ah-ben)   Gemzar®

Antineoplastic

Prescriber Highlights

▶ Antineoplastic agent that may potentially be useful for treating several cancers in dogs or cats.
▶ Very limited clinical use & research performed thus far.
▶ GI effects and myelosuppression (neutropenia) most likely adverse effects.
▶ Very expensive.

Uses/Indications

Very limited clinical use and research performed with this drug to date has demonstrated limited clinical efficacy. However, it potentially may be useful as a radiosensitizer for non-resectable tumors, as part of combination protocols, or as a single agent for tumors not amenable to more accepted therapies. Combining low-dosage (2 mg/kg) gemcitabine with carboplatin for post-amputation appendicular osteosarcoma in dogs did not appear to improve outcome from studies using carboplatin alone (McMahon et al. 2011). In dogs with transitional cell bladder carcinoma, gemcitabine combined with piroxicam did not significantly improve survival time when compared to carboplatin or cisplatin-based treatment protocols, but did have fewer adverse effects (Marconato et al. 2011). A retrospective study in cats with exocrine pancreatic carcinoma showed that 82% cats treated with gemcitabine (± carboplatin) had a decrease in clinical signs associated with their malignancies, but due to the retrospective nature of the study any determination of actual improvement of quality of life was questionable (Linderman et al. 2013).

In humans, gemcitabine has shown some efficacy in treating pancreatic carcinoma, small-cell lung carcinoma, lymphoma, bladder and other soft tissue carcinomas.

Pharmacology/Actions

Gemcitabine exhibits cell phase specificity and acts primarily on the S phase. It also inhibits cell progression through the G1/S-phase boundary.

Gemcitabine is metabolized intracellularly to diflurodeoxycytidine monophosphate (dFdCMP) that is then converted into diphosphate (dFdCDP) and triphosphate (dFdCTP) forms, the metabolites that give the drug its activity. The diphosphate inhibits ribonucleotide reductase. The triphosphate competes with deoxycytidine triphosphate (dTCP; the "normal" nucleotide) for incorporation into DNA strands.

Pharmacokinetics

In dogs, gemcitabine exhibits first order elimination and has a terminal half-life of about 1.5-3.2 hours. Volume of distribution (steady-state) is around 1 L/kg. Approximately 80% of the drug is excreted in the urine within 24 hours of dosing, primarily as the uracil metabolite.

In humans, gemcitabine levels achieve steady state in about 15 minutes during a 30-minute infusion. Protein binding is negligible. Volume of distribution is about 50 L/m². Less than 10% of the drug is excreted unchanged in the urine.

Contraindications/Precautions/Warnings

Gemcitabine is contraindicated in patients hypersensitive to it. It should be used with caution in patients with diminished renal or hepatic function.

Adverse Effects

Gemcitabine may cause myelosuppression and can affect red cell, white cell, and platelet cell lines, but neutrophils and platelets appear to be most affected. Neutrophil nadirs usually occur 3-7 days post treatment. GI effects have been reported in animals receiving the drug, but are usually mild. Retinal hemorrhage could occur in animals receiving gemcitabine.

In a pilot study (Kosarek et al. 2005) in 19 dogs receiving up to 675 mg/m^2 biweekly demonstrated "minimal and acceptable toxicity." Another study (Turner et al. 2006) where dogs with lymphoma were given gemcitabine as single agent therapy at 400 mg/m^2 weekly for 3 weeks and then off one week, showed significant decreases in neutrophils and platelets 7 days post treatment. 15 of the 21 dogs in the study required dosage reduction or delay in retreatment. Only 7 of the 21 dogs finished the initial 4-week cycle and a second cycle did not result in any objective therapeutic response. In a study where gemcitabine was combined with carboplatin treatment for carcinomas in dogs, adverse effects included mild to moderate GI and hematologic toxicity; 32% of dogs developed grade 3 or 4 neutropenia, 24% developed thrombocytopenia and 73% developed mild to moderate, self-limiting GI toxicity. (Dominguez et al. 2009)

In cats treated with double therapy (carboplatin/gemcitabine), 21% or 50% of treated cats, depending on the dosing protocol used, developed grade 3 or 4 neutropenia or thrombocytopenia and 7% developed grade 3 or 4 GI toxicity. (Martinez-Ruzafa et al. 2009)

Reproductive/Nursing Safety

In pregnant humans, gemcitabine is designated by the FDA as a category **D** drug (*There is evidence of human fetal risk, but the potential benefits from the use of the drug in pregnant women may be acceptable despite its potential risks.*)

It is unknown whether gemcitabine is excreted in maternal milk.

Overdosage/Acute Toxicity

There is no known antidote to gemcitabine in an overdose situation. Myelosuppression should be expected. Treatment is supportive.

Drug Interactions

No specific drug interactions were noted, but toxic effects (myelosuppression, GI) could be additive when used with other drugs that also cause those effects.

Laboratory Considerations

- No specific laboratory interactions or considerations noted.

Doses

- **DOGS/CATS:**

    NOTE: Because of the potential toxicity of this drug to patients, veterinary personnel and clients, and since chemotherapy indications, treatment protocols, monitoring and safety guidelines often change, the following dosages should be used only as a general guide. Consultation with a veterinary oncologist and referral to current veterinary oncology [e.g., (Withrow et al. 2012); (Dobson et al. 2011); (Henry et al. 2009); (North et al. 2009); (Argyle et al. 2008)] are strongly recommended. Relatively safe and effective dosages for gemcitabine in veterinary patients with potentially susceptible tumors is not truly known, and depending on the study, clinician and protocol dosages for dogs and cats have ranged widely from 45 mg/m^2 – 800 mg/m^2, usually given IV over 30-60 minutes every 7-14 days. Some studies combining it with carboplatin in dogs and cats have used 2 mg/kg IV over 20-30 minutes no more than once every 7 days.

Monitoring

- CBC before each treatment.
- Fundic exam weekly while on therapy.
- Prior to therapy, baseline renal and hepatic function and periodically thereafter.

Client Information

- Owners should understand that veterinary experience with this drug is limited.
- Gemcitabine residues can be detected in urine up to 7 days after a dose. If owners must clean up urine from treated dogs, take proper precautions such as wearing disposable gloves.

Chemistry/Synonyms

A synthetic pyrimidine nucleoside cytarabine analog antineoplastic agent, gemcitabine HCl occurs as white to off-white solid. It is soluble in water and practically insoluble in ethanol or polar organic solvents. Its chemical name is 2,2'-diflurodeoxycytidine.

Gemcitabine may also be known as: dFdC, LY-288022, *Abine®*, *Antoril®*, *Gemcite®*, or *Gemtrol®* and *Gemzar®*.

Storage/Stability

Store unreconstituted gemcitabine at controlled room temperature (20-25°C; 68-77°F). After reconstitution with 0.9% sodium chloride injection without preservatives, the resulting solution may be stored at room temperature for up to 24 hours. Reportedly, when frozen at -20°C, the reconstituted solution is stable for 7 days. Do not refrigerate or re-crystallization may occur. Reconstituted solution should not be greater than 40 mg/mL (at least 5 mL of diluent for 200 mg vial; 25 mL diluent for 1 gram vial). Additional diluent may be added to yield concentrations as low as 0.1 mg/mL.

Compatibility/Compounding Considerations

Gemcitabine injection is reportedly physically **incompatible** with the following medications when used via Y-site injection: acyclovir, amphotericin B, cefoperazone, cefotaxime sodium, furosemide, imipenem, methotrexate, methylprednisolone sodium succinate, mitomycin, piperacillin, and prochlorperazine.

Dosage Forms/Regulatory Status

VETERINARY-LABELED PRODUCTS: NONE.

HUMAN-LABELED PRODUCTS:

Gemcitabine HCl lyophilized Powder for Injection: 200 mg (in 10 mL single-use vials) and 1 g (in 50 mL single-use vials); *Gemzar®*, generic; (Rx)

Revisions/References

Monograph revised/updated January 2014.

Argyle, D., et al. (2008). *Decision Making in Small Animal Oncology*, Wiley-Blackwell.
Dobson, J. & D. Lascelles (2011). *BSAVA Manual of Canine and Feline Oncology*, BSAVA.
Dominguez, P. A., et al. (2009). Combined Gemcitabine and Carboplatin Therapy for Carcinomas in Dogs. Journal of Veterinary Internal Medicine 23(1): 130-7.
Henry, C. & M. Higginbotham (2009). *Cancer Management in Small Animal Practice*, Saunders.
Kosarek, C., et al. (2005). Clinical evaluation of gemcitabine in dogs with spontaneously occurring malignancies. J Vet Intern Med 19(1): 81-6.
Linderman, M. J., et al. (2013). Feline exocrine pancreatic carcinoma: a retrospective study of 34 cases. Veterinary and Comparative Oncology 11(3): 208-18.
Marconato, L., et al. (2011). Toxic effects and antitumor response of gemcitabine in combination with piroxicam treatment in dogs with transitional cell carcinoma of the urinary bladder. Journal of the American Veterinary Medical Association 238(8): 1004-10.
Martinez-Ruzafa, I., et al. (2009). Tolerability of Gemcitabine and Carboplatin Doublet Therapy in Cats with Carcinomas. Journal of Veterinary Internal Medicine 23(3): 570-7.
McMahon, M., et al. (2011). Adjuvant Carboplatin and Gemcitabine Combination Chemotherapy Postamputation in Canine Appendicular Osteosarcoma. Journal of Veterinary Internal Medicine 25(3): 511-7.
North, S. & T. Banks (2009). *Small Animal Oncology: An Introduction*, Saunders.
Turner, A., et al. (2006). Single agent gemcitabine chemotherapy in dogs with spontaneously occurring lymphoma. J Vet Intern Med 20(6): 1384-88.
Withrow, S., et al. (2012). Withrow and MacEwen's Small Animal Clinical Oncology, 5th Ed., Saunders.

Gemfibrozil

(jem-fih-broh-zil)   Lopid®

Oral Antihyperlipidemic

Prescriber Highlights

▶ May be useful as adjunctive therapy (with low fat diet) to treat hypertriglyceridemia in dogs or cats.

▶ Very limited experience & no published clinical studies in dogs or cats; efficacy or safety is not established.

Uses/Indications

Gemfibrozil may be useful to reduce serum triglycerides in those dogs or cats with hypertriglyceridemia and when diet modifications alone have been unsuccessful. One reference (Elliott 2005) suggests not adding drug therapy to treat hypertriglyceridemia unless the serum triglyceride concentration exceeds 500 mg/dL with associated clinical signs. Another states that because side effects are believed to occur rarely, gemfibrozil is commonly recommended in dogs in combination with dietary therapy when the latter fails to lower triglyceride levels below 5.65 mmol/L (500 mg/dL) (Xenoulis et al. 2010).

Gemfibrozil has been shown to reduce influenza-related mortality in mice and may become an adjunctive treatment for severe influenza.

Pharmacology/Actions

Gemfibrozil inhibits lipolysis in adipose issue and reduces hepatic uptake of plasma free fatty acids causing reduced production of triglycerides. Secondarily, gemfibrozil inhibits the synthesis of very low-density lipoprotein (VLDL) carrier apolipoprotein B, which reduces VLDL production and incorporation of long-chain fatty acids into triglycerides.

Pharmacokinetics

No pharmacokinetic data for dogs or cats was found. In humans, gemfibrozil is rapidly and completely absorbed from the GI tract. The rate and extent of absorption are greatest when administered 30 minutes before a meal. It is highly bound to plasma protein and highest concentrations of the drug are found in the liver and kidneys. In the liver, 4 major metabolites are formed in humans, which are primarily excreted in the urine. Elimination half-life is about 1.5 hours. Reductions in plasma VDL levels are noted within 5 days; peak reductions occur about 4 weeks after starting therapy.

Contraindications/Precautions/Warnings

Contraindications for using gemfibrozil in dogs or cats are not known. In humans, gemfibrozil is contraindicated in patients with severe hepatic or renal dysfunction or with known hypersensitivity to gemfibrozil.

Use with caution in dogs or cats as very limited safety data is available for this medication.

Adverse Effects

Because no clinical studies have been published regarding gemfibrozil use in dogs and cats and clinical use has been quite limited, an accurate adverse effect profile is not known. Anecdotal reports are that the drug has been well tolerated in the few patients that have received the medication, but abdominal pain, vomiting, diarrhea, and abnormal liver function tests have been reported.

In humans, the most common adverse effects reported are GI related (dyspepsia, nausea, vomiting, diarrhea, etc.) and CNS related (headache, paresthesias, somnolence, dizziness, fatigue). Other adverse effects reported include myositis, taste alterations, blurred vision, eczema and decreased libido/impotence. Rarely, hypersensitivity reactions, bone marrow depression, and increases in liver function test values (AST, ALT, Alk Phos, bilirubin) have been re-

ported. Long-term studies in rats have demonstrated an increased rate of benign and malignant liver tumors when doses were approximately 1.3X of the human dose.

Reproductive/Nursing Safety

Gemfibrozil administered to female rats prior to and during gestation at 0.6-2X the human dose, showed decreased fertility rates and their offspring had an increased incidence of skeletal abnormalities. When given to pregnant rabbits at 1-3X the human dose, litter sizes were decreased and at the highest dose (3X), parietal bone variations were noted. In humans, the FDA categorizes gemfibrozil as category C for use during pregnancy (*Animal studies have shown an adverse effect on the fetus, but there are no adequate studies in humans; or there are no animal reproduction studies and no adequate studies in humans.*)

It is not known if gemfibrozil enters milk and safe use during nursing cannot be assured.

Overdosage/Acute Toxicity

Limited information is available. One 7-year-old child ingested up to 9 grams and recovered with supportive treatment. The reported LD50 (oral) in rats is 1414 mg/kg. Consider gut-emptying protocols for recent large oral ingestions and support as required. Monitor for dehydration and electrolyte imbalance if vomiting and/or diarrhea is severe or persists. Monitor liver function tests.

Drug Interactions

The following drug interactions have either been reported or are theoretical in humans or animals receiving gemfibrozil and may be of in veterinary patients. Unless otherwise noted, use together is not necessarily contraindicated, but weigh the potential risks and perform additional monitoring when appropriate.

- **THIAZIDE DIURETICS, BETA-BLOCKERS,** and **ESTROGENS**: May possibly increase triglyceride concentrations.
- **URSODIOL**: May reduce effectiveness of gemfibrozil.
- **WARFARIN**: Gemfibrozil may potentiate anticoagulant effects.

Laboratory Considerations

- No specific concerns associated with gemfibrozil; see Monitoring section below.

Doses

- **DOGS/CATS:**

  For hypertriglyceridemia that has not been controlled with diet alone (extra-label): There is little information published on the safety and efficacy of this agent in dogs or cats. Anecdotal dosage recommendations for dogs are generally 150 – 300 mg per dog (**not** mg/kg) PO twice daily and for cats 7.5 – 10 mg/kg PO twice daily.

Monitoring

- Plasma triglycerides; realistic goal for therapy is 400 mg/dL or less.
- Baseline and periodic: CBC, liver function tests.
- Adverse effects.
- If treatment is less effective than hoped, assure that clients have adhered to prescribed diet and dosing schedule before altering dosage.

Client Information

- Clients must understand the use of this drug in animals is "investigational"; although FDA-approved for use in people, little information is known about it for use in dogs or cats.
- Gemfibrozil is used in conjunction with diet modification; lack of adherence to dietary recommendations will likely negate the benefits of using this medication.
- Report any significant adverse effects to the veterinarian, including changes in behavior, activity level, gastrointestinal effects

(vomiting, diarrhea, lack of appetite), yellowish eyes or mucous membranes, etc.

Chemistry/Synonyms

Gemfibrozil is a fibric acid derivative that occurs as a waxy, crystalline solid that is practically insoluble in water, but soluble in alcohol.

Gemfibrozil may also be known as: CI-719, gemfibrozilo, or gemfibrozilium; many international trade names are available.

Storage/Stability

Gemfibrozil tablets or capsules should be stored below 30°C in tight containers.

Dosage Forms/Regulatory Status

VETERINARY-LABELED PRODUCTS: NONE.

HUMAN-LABELED PRODUCTS:

Gemfibrozil Oral Tablets: 600 mg; *Lopid®*, generic; (Rx). **Note:** 300 mg capsules are available in Canada.

Revisions/References

Monograph revised/updated January 2014.

Elliott, D. (2005). Dietary and medical considerations in hyperlipidemia. *Textbook of Veterinary Internal Medicine.* S. Ettinger and E. Feldman, Elsevier: 592-5.
Xenoulis, P. G. & J. M. Steiner (2010). Lipid metabolism and hyperlipidemia in dogs. *Veterinary Journal* 183(1): 12-21.

Gentamicin Sulfate, Systemic

(jen-ta-mye-sin)   Gentocin®, Garamycin®

Aminoglycoside Antibiotic

Prescriber Highlights

▶ Parenteral-aminoglycoside antibiotic that is active against a variety of bacteria, predominantly gram-negative aerobic bacilli, but also many staphylococci strains.

▶ Because of potential adverse effects when given systemically, usually reserved for serious infections.

▶ Adverse effect profile: Nephrotoxicity, ototoxicity, neuromuscular blockade.

▶ Cats may be more sensitive to toxic effects, especially vestibular effects.

▶ Risk factors for nephrotoxicity: Preexisting renal disease, age (both neonatal & geriatric), fever, treatment duration, hypokalemia, sepsis, & dehydration.

▶ Usually dosed once daily in dogs, cats and horses with uncompromised renal function.

Uses/Indications

The potential for toxicity of the aminoglycosides limits their systemic (parenteral) use to the treatment of serious infections when there is either a documented lack of susceptibility to other less toxic antibiotics or when the clinical situation dictates immediate treatment of a presumed gram-negative infection before culture and susceptibility results can be reported.

Various gentamicin products are FDA-approved for parenteral use in dogs, cats, chickens, turkeys, and swine though the injectable small animal products no longer appear to be marketed. Although routinely used parenterally in horses, gentamicin is only FDA-approved for intrauterine infusion in this species. Oral products are FDA-approved for gastrointestinal infections in swine and turkeys. For more information, refer to the Dosage section below or the approved product label.

Pharmacology/Actions

Gentamicin has a mechanism of action and spectrum of activity (primarily gram-negative aerobes) similar to the other aminoglycosides. Like the other aminoglycoside antibiotics, it acts on susceptible bacteria presumably by irreversibly binding to the 30S ribo-

somal subunit thereby inhibiting protein synthesis. It is considered a bactericidal concentration-dependent antibiotic. A ratio of 10 or greater for peak plasma concentration to MIC is believed optimal for antibacterial efficacy. Once daily dosing is now the norm for patients with uncompromised renal function. Gentamicin's spectrum of activity includes coverage against many aerobic gram-negative and some aerobic gram-positive bacteria, including most species of *E. coli*, Klebsiella, Proteus, Pseudomonas, Salmonella, Enterobacter, Serratia, and Shigella, Mycoplasma, and Staphylococcus (methicillin-resistant strains may be resistant). Several strains of *Pseudomonas aeruginosa*, Proteus, and Serratia that are resistant to gentamicin may still be susceptible to amikacin. While gentamicin has *in vitro* activity against *Rhodococcus equi*, its water-soluble nature does not allow it to penetrate intracellularly but liposomal forms show promise.

Antimicrobial activity of the aminoglycosides is enhanced in an alkaline environment. The presence of pus, necrotic tissue or cellular debris reduce aminoglycoside efficacy.

The aminoglycoside antibiotics are inactive against fungi, viruses and most anaerobic bacteria.

Pharmacokinetics

Gentamicin, like other aminoglycosides, is not appreciably absorbed after oral or intrauterine administration, but is absorbed from topical administration (not skin or urinary bladder) when used in irrigations during surgical procedures. Patients receiving oral aminoglycosides with hemorrhagic or necrotic enteritises may absorb appreciable quantities of the drug. After IM administration to dogs and cats, peak levels occur from 1/2 to 1 hour later. Subcutaneous injection results in slightly delayed peak levels and more variability than after IM injection. Bioavailability from extravascular injection (IM or SC) is greater than 90%.

After absorption, aminoglycosides are distributed primarily in the extracellular fluid. They are found in ascitic, pleural, pericardial, peritoneal, synovial and abscess fluids and high levels are found in sputum, bronchial secretions and bile. Aminoglycosides are minimally protein bound (<20%, streptomycin 35%) to plasma proteins. Aminoglycosides do not readily cross the blood-brain barrier or penetrate ocular tissue. CSF levels are unpredictable and range from 0-50% of those found in the serum. Therapeutic levels are found in bone, heart, gallbladder and lung tissues after parenteral dosing. Aminoglycosides tend to accumulate in certain tissues, such as the inner ear and kidneys, which may help explain their toxicity. Volumes of distribution have been reported to be 0.15 – 0.3 L/kg in adult cats and dogs, and 0.26 – 0.58 L/kg in horses. Volumes of distribution may be significantly larger in neonates and juvenile animals due to their higher extracellular fluid fractions. Aminoglycosides cross the placenta, but one study showed no detectable levels in foals when gentamicin was administered to mares at term. In other species, fetal concentrations range from 15-50% of those found in maternal serum.

Elimination of aminoglycosides after parenteral administration occurs almost entirely by glomerular filtration. The elimination half-lives for gentamicin have been reported to be 1.82-3.25 hours in horses, 2.2-2.7 hours in calves, 2.4 hours in sheep, 1.8 hours in cows, 1.9 hours in swine, 1 hour in rabbits, and 0.5-1.5 hours in dogs and cats. Patients with decreased renal function can have significantly prolonged half-lives. In humans with normal renal function, elimination rates can be highly variable with the aminoglycoside antibiotics.

Contraindications/Precautions/Warnings

Aminoglycosides are contraindicated in patients who are hypersensitive to them. Because these drugs are often the only effective agents in severe gram-negative infections there are no other absolute contraindications to their use. However, they should be used with extreme caution in patients with preexisting renal disease with concomitant monitoring and dosage interval adjustments made. Other risk factors for the development of toxicity include age (both neonatal and geriatric patients), fever, hypokalemia, treatment duration, sepsis and dehydration.

In dogs and cats, urinalysis (specific gravity, glucose, protein, sediment, urine protein/serum creatinine ratio), serum creatinine, serum electrolytes (sodium, potassium), hematocrit/total protein, body weight, and blood pressure have all been recommended for evaluation prior to and during aminoglycoside treatment. If signs of acute kidney injury (AKI) are noted (*e.g.*, renal casts in urine sediment, glucosuria, low urine specific gravity, azotemia) therapy should be halted if possible and alternative antibiotic therapy instituted.

Because aminoglycosides can cause irreversible ototoxicity, they should be used with caution in "working" or service dogs (*e.g.*, "seeing-eye", herding, dogs for the hearing impaired, etc.).

Aminoglycosides should be used with caution in patients with neuromuscular disorders (*e.g.*, myasthenia gravis) due to their neuromuscular blocking activity. They should not be used in animals with botulism.

Sighthound dogs may require reduced dosages of aminoglycosides as they have significantly smaller volumes of distribution.

Because aminoglycosides are eliminated primarily through renal mechanisms, they should be used cautiously, preferably with serum monitoring and dosage adjustment in neonatal or geriatric animals.

IM injections in horses have caused muscle irritation and IV injections are preferred. The risk for antibiotic associated diarrhea/colitis in horses due to gentamicin is thought to be low. But gentamicin may promote Beta-2 toxin production by *C. perfringens* and may increase the severity of colitis (McGorum et al. 2010).

Aminoglycosides are often considered contraindicated in rabbits as they adversely affect the GI flora balance in these animals; use with extreme caution.

Adverse Effects

The aminoglycosides' nephrotoxic and ototoxic effects are well known. The nephrotoxic (tubular necrosis) mechanisms of these drugs are not completely understood, but are probably related to interference with phospholipid metabolism in the lysosomes of proximal renal tubular cells, resulting in leakage of proteolytic enzymes into the cytoplasm. Nephrotoxicity is usually manifested by increases in: BUN, creatinine, non-protein nitrogen in the serum, and decreases in urine specific gravity and creatinine clearance. Proteinuria and cells or casts may also be seen in the urine. Nephrotoxicity is usually reversible once the drug is discontinued, but development of oliguric acute kidney injury portends a poor prognosis. While gentamicin may be more nephrotoxic than some other aminoglycosides, the risk for nephrotoxicity with all systemic aminoglycosides requires equal caution and monitoring. Strategies to reduce the potential for nephrotoxicity in animals with uncompromised renal function include: Once daily administration, renal function monitoring, hydration and electrolyte balance, avoiding use of other nephrotoxic drugs, and employing therapeutic drug monitoring to adjust dosages and/or dosage intervals to maintain high peak serum levels (>20 mcg/mL) and low troughs (preferably <1 mcg/mL).

Aminoglycoside ototoxicity (8th cranial nerve toxicity) can manifest by either auditory and/or vestibular clinical signs and may be irreversible. Vestibular clinical signs are more frequent with streptomycin, gentamicin, or tobramycin. Auditory clinical signs are more frequent with amikacin, neomycin, or kanamycin, but other forms can occur with any of the drugs. Cats are apparently very sensitive to the vestibular effects of the aminoglycosides and can exhibit signs of vertigo, head tilt, ataxia, impaired righting reflex, and post-rotatory righting reflex.

High oral doses of gentamicin (in combination with paromomycin) in cats with cryptosporidiosis have caused systemic adverse effects.

Aminoglycosides can also cause neuromuscular blockade, facial edema, pain and inflammation at the injection site, peripheral neuropathy and hypersensitivity reactions. Rarely, GI clinical signs, hematologic, and hepatic effects have been reported.

Reproductive/Nursing Safety

Aminoglycosides can cross the placenta and, while rare, may cause 8th cranial nerve toxicity or nephrotoxicity in fetuses. Because the drug should only be used in serious infections, the benefits of therapy may exceed the potential risks. In humans, the FDA categorizes this drug as category *D* for use during pregnancy (*There is evidence of human fetal risk, but the potential benefits from the use of the drug in pregnant women may be acceptable despite its potential risks.*). In a separate system evaluating the safety of drugs in canine and feline pregnancy (Papich 1989), this drug is categorized as class: *C* (*These drugs may have potential risks. Studies in people or laboratory animals have uncovered risks, and these drugs should be used cautiously as a last resort when the benefit of therapy clearly outweighs the risks.*)

While small amounts of gentamicin may be excreted into milk, the risk to nursing offspring appears minimal.

Overdosage/Acute Toxicity

Should an inadvertent overdosage be administered, three treatments have been recommended. 1) Hemodialysis is very effective in reducing serum levels of the drug, but is not a viable option for most veterinary patients; 2) Peritoneal dialysis also will reduce serum levels, but is much less effective; 3) Complexation of drug with ticarcillin (12 – 20 g/day in humans) is reportedly nearly as effective as hemodialysis.

Drug Interactions

The following drug interactions have either been reported or are theoretical in humans or animals receiving gentamicin and may be of in veterinary patients. Unless otherwise noted, use together is not necessarily contraindicated, but weigh the potential risks and perform additional monitoring when appropriate.

- **BETA-LACTAM ANTIBIOTICS (penicillins, cephalosporins):** May have synergistic effects against some bacteria; some potential for inactivation of aminoglycosides *in vitro* (do not mix together) and *in vivo* (patients in renal failure).
- **CEPHALOSPORINS:** The concurrent use of aminoglycosides with cephalosporins is somewhat controversial. Potentially, cephalosporins could cause additive nephrotoxicity when used with aminoglycosides, but this interaction has only been well documented with cephaloridine and cephalothin (both no longer marketed).
- **DIURETICS, LOOP** (*e.g.,* **furosemide, torsemide**) or **OSMOTIC** (*e.g.,* **mannitol**): Concurrent use with loop or osmotic diuretics may increase the nephrotoxic or ototoxic potential of the aminoglycosides.
- **NEPHROTOXIC DRUGS, OTHER** (*e.g.,* **cisplatin, amphotericin B, polymyxin B, or vancomycin**): Potential for increased risk for nephrotoxicity.
- **NEUROMUSCULAR BLOCKING AGENTS & ANESTHETICS, GENERAL:** Concomitant use with general anesthetics or neuromuscular blocking agents could potentiate neuromuscular blockade.

Laboratory Considerations

- **Gentamicin serum concentrations** may be falsely decreased if the patient is also receiving beta-lactam antibiotics and the serum is stored prior analysis. It is recommended that if assay is delayed, samples be frozen and, if possible, drawn at times when the beta-lactam antibiotic is at a trough.

Doses

Note: Most infectious disease clinicians now agree that aminoglycosides should be dosed once a day in most patients (mammals) with uncompromised renal function. This dosing regimen yields higher peak levels with resultant greater bacterial kill, and as aminoglycosides exhibit a "post-antibiotic effect", surviving susceptible bacteria generally do not replicate as rapidly even when antibiotic concentrations are below MIC. Periods where levels are low may decrease the "adaptive resistance" (bacteria take up less drug in the presence of continuous exposure) that can occur. Once daily dosing may also decrease the toxicity of aminoglycosides as lower urinary concentrations may mean less-uptake into renal tubular cells. However, patients that are neutropenic (or otherwise immunosuppressed) may benefit from more frequent dosing (q8h). Therapeutic drug monitoring is highly recommended particularly for patients with sepsis or that have risk factors for nephrotoxicity.

- **DOGS:**

For susceptible infections (extra-label): Dosage recommendations vary, but initial dosages of 9 – 12 mg/kg IV, IM or SQ once a day (q24h) is reasonable for most breeds and infections. Consider higher dosages (up to 15 mg/kg for life-threatening infections; *e.g.*, sepsis) or dividing the daily dose and administering q8h) in immunocompromised or neutropenic patients. Dosage adjustments using therapeutic drug monitoring (see Monitoring section) should be considered to maximize efficacy and reduce the potential for nephrotoxicity. Lower initial dosages for Greyhounds and probably other Sighthound breeds has been recommended: 6 mg/kg IV q24h or 9 mg/kg SC/IM q24h. (KuKanich 2008)

- **CATS:**

For susceptible infections (extra-label): Similarly to dog dosages above, but recommended initial dosages are generally lower: 5 – 8 mg/kg IV, IM or SC q24h.

- **FERRETS:**

For susceptible infections (extra-label): Similarly to dog dosages above, but recommended initial dosages are generally lower: 5 – 8 mg/kg IV, IM or SC q24h.

- **RABBITS/RODENTS/SMALL MAMMALS:**

a) **Rabbits:** 5 – 8 mg/kg daily dose (may divide into q8h-q24h) SC, IM or IV. Increased efficacy and decreased toxicity if given once daily. If given IV, dilute into 4 mL/kg of saline and give over 20 minutes. (Ivey et al. 2000)

b) **Chinchillas, Gerbils, Guinea pigs, Hamsters, Mice, Rats:** 2 – 4 mg/kg SC or IM q8–24h. (Adamcak et al. 2000)

- **HORSES:**

For susceptible infections (parenteral administration; extra-label): Adults: Recent studies indicate that initial dosages in adult horses should generally be higher than previously thought and given once daily IV: 7.7 – 9.7 mg/kg IV q24h has been recommended (Read et al. 2011). Higher dosages (11 – 15 mg/kg IV q24h) have been suggested if treating septic arthritis. IM administration may cause muscle irritation. TDM is recommended to guide therapy.

Foals: Initial dosages in foals less than 2 weeks old: 12 mg/kg IV q36h. In foals greater than 2 weeks old: 6.6 mg/kg IV q24h should be adequate (Burton et al. 2013). Ideally, TDM should be used to reduce risk for nephrotoxicity and optimizing efficacy. (Corley et al. 2009)

For susceptible uterine infections (intrauterine infusion):

a) Labeled Dose (FDA-approved): 2 – 2.5 grams (20-25 mL) diluted in 200 – 500 mL sterile normal saline and infused aseptically into uterus once daily for 3-5 days during estrus. (Adapted from label)

b) Extra-label: Irrigate uterus for 2-3 days prior to antibiotic infusion to remove inflammatory debris. Gentamicin dosed at 1 – 2 grams IU. Buffer with bicarbonate (equal volume of 7.5% bicarbonate and diluted in saline) or large volume (200 mL) of saline. Mares with bacterial endometritis should be treated with IU antibiotics for 3-7 days. Treatment length is dependent on history, chronicity of infection, bacteria isolated, and mare's ability to clear uterine fluid. (LeBlanc 2009)

- **SWINE:**

For susceptible infections (labeled dose, FDA-approved):

a) For colibacillosis in neonates: 5 mg PO or IM once. (Label directions; *Garacin® Pig Pump* and *Piglet Injection*—Schering)

b) For weanlings and other swine: Colibacillosis: 1.1 mg/kg/day in drinking water (concentration of 25 mg/gallon) for 3 days. Swine dysentery (*Treponema hyodysenteriae*): 2.2 mg/kg/day in drinking water (concentration of 50 mg/gallon) for 3 days (Label directions; *Garacin® Soluble Powder* and *Oral Solution*—Schering)

- **BIRDS:**

For susceptible infections (extra-label): In companion birds: Amikacin is the preferred aminoglycoside, but gentamicin can be used to reduce expense: 2.5 – 5 mg/kg once per day (**Note:** *route not listed, IM assumed as author lists IM doses for amikacin—Plumb*). In severely immunocompromised birds, twice daily administration with a beta-lactam antibiotic may improve treatment success. Birds often show polyuria during treatment, but it usually resolves after short duration (<7 days) of therapy. Concurrent SC fluids may reduce nephrotoxicity. (Flammer 2006)

- **REPTILES:**

For susceptible infections (extra-label):

a) For bacterial gastritis in **snakes**: gentamicin 2.5 mg/kg IM every 72 hours with oral neomycin 15 mg/kg plus oral live lactobacillus. (Burke 1986)

b) For bacterial shell diseases in **turtles**: 5 – 10 mg/kg daily in water turtles, every other day in land turtles and tortoises for 7-10 days. Used commonly with a beta-lactam antibiotic. Recommend beginning therapy with 20 mL/kg fluid injection. Maintain hydration and monitor uric acid levels when possible. (Rosskopf 1986)

Monitoring

- Efficacy (cultures, clinical signs associated with infection).
- Renal toxicity; baseline urinalysis, serum creatinine/BUN. Casts in the urine are often the initial sign of impending nephrotoxicity. Casts or increased serum creatinine may not be good markers in neonates. Frequency of monitoring during therapy is somewhat controversial but daily urinalysis and serum creatinine may not be too frequent. Assess the hydration status of the patient (body weight, total plasma protein concentration and hematocrit) at least once weekly. After drug discontinuation, continue monitoring for nephrotoxic signs for one week.
- Gross monitoring for vestibular or auditory toxicity is recommended, especially in cats.
- Therapeutic drug monitoring (TDM) when possible in patients with uncompromised renal function; highly recommended for patients with risk factors for nephrotoxicity. Generally, peak lev-

els (approximately 30-60 minutes post IV dose) should be greater than 20 mcg/mL and trough levels less than 1 mcg/mL. As a general rule, a 4-hour post dose level should generally be less than 10 mcg/mL and an 8-hour level in the 4-5 mcg/mL range. Your clinical laboratory may be able to assist in sample-time determination and dosage amount/frequency adjustment.

Client Information

- To treat infections in the body, this drug must be injected; it is only given orally (by mouth) to reduce the amount of bacteria in animals' intestines before intestinal surgery.
- Given once daily either in the vein (by veterinarian) or under the skin (subcutaneously). If injecting at home, be sure you understand how to properly inject it.
- Can damage the nerves, hearing, and kidneys. Cats may be more likely to have damage to hearing.
- Can be used topically for ear, skin or eye infections.

Chemistry/Synonyms

An aminoglycoside obtained from cultures of *Micromonaspora purpurea*, gentamicin sulfate occurs as a white to buff powder that is soluble in water and insoluble in alcohol. The commercial product is actually a combination of gentamicin sulfate C_1, C_2, and C_3, but all these compounds apparently have similar antimicrobial activities. Commercially available injections have a pH from 3-5.5.

Gentamicin may also be known as: gentamicin sulphate, gentamicini sulfas, NSC-82261, and Sch-9724; many trade names are available.

Storage/Stability

Gentamicin sulfate for injection and the oral solution should be stored at room temperature (15-30°C); freezing or temperatures above 40°C should be avoided. The soluble powder should be stored from 2-30°C. Do not store or offer medicated-drinking water in rusty containers or the drug may be destroyed.

Compatibility/Compounding Considerations

While the manufacturer does not recommend that gentamicin be mixed with other drugs, it is reportedly physically **compatible** and stable in all commonly used intravenous solutions and with the following drugs: bleomycin sulfate, cefoxitin sodium, cimetidine HCl, clindamycin phosphate, metronidazole (with and without sodium bicarbonate), penicillin G sodium, and verapamil HCl.

The following drugs or solutions are reportedly physically **incompatible** or only compatible in specific situations with gentamicin: amphotericin B, ampicillin sodium, dopamine HCl, furosemide, and heparin sodium. Compatibility is dependent upon factors such as pH, concentration, temperature and diluent used; consult specialized references or a hospital pharmacist for more specific information.

In vitro inactivation of aminoglycoside antibiotics by beta-lactam antibiotics is well documented. Gentamicin is very susceptible to this effect and it is recommended to avoid mixing with these compounds.

Dosage Forms/Regulatory Status

VETERINARY-LABELED PRODUCTS:

Gentamicin Sulfate Solution (for intrauterine infusion): 100 mg/mL in 100 mL and 250 mL vials; multiple trade names, generic; (Rx). FDA-approved for horses.

Gentamicin Sulfate Injection: 100 mg/mL (poultry only) in 100 mL vials; *Garasol® Injection, Gentapoult®*; (OTC). For use only in day-old chickens (slaughter withdrawal = 5 weeks) and 1-3 day-old turkeys (slaughter withdrawal = 9 weeks).

Gentamicin Sulfate Injection: 5 mg/mL in 250 mL vials; *Garacin® Piglet Injection*; (OTC). FDA-approved for use in piglets up to 3 days

of age. Slaughter withdrawal (when used as labeled) = 40 days.

Gentamicin Sulfate Oral Solution: 5 mg/mL in 118 mL bottles with pump applicator; generic; (Rx). FDA-approved for use in neonatal swine only. Slaughter withdrawal = 14 days.

Gentamicin Soluble Powder: 333.33 mg/g in 360 g jars. FDA-approved for use in weanling swine. Slaughter withdrawal = 10 days. *Gen-Gard® Soluble Powder*; (OTC)

Gentamicin Sulfate Soluble Powder: 2 g gentamicin/30 g of powder in 360 g jar; *Garacin® Soluble Powder*; (OTC). FDA-approved for use in swine. Slaughter withdrawal (when used as labeled) = 10 days.

Veterinary FDA-approved injections for chickens and turkeys plus a water additive for egg dipping may also be available. Ophthalmic, otic, and topical preparations are available with veterinary labeling.

HUMAN-APPROVED PRODUCTS:

Partial listing:

Gentamicin Sulfate Injection: 10 mg/mL and 40 mg/mL (as sulfate) in vials and cartridge-needle units and in various concentrations (0.8-1.6 mg/mL) pre-mixed in saline in 50 mL and 100 mL single-dose containers; generic; (Rx)

Topical, otic and ophthalmic-labeled products are also available.

Revisions/References

Monograph revised/updated February 2014.

Adamcak, A. & B. Otten (2000). Rodent Therapeutics. Vet Clin NA: Exotic Anim Pract **3:1**(Jan): 221-40.
Burke, T. J. (1986). Regurgitation in snakes. *Current Veterinary Therapy (CVT) IX Small Animal Practice*. R. W. Kirk. Philadelphia, WB Saunders: 749-50.
Burton, A. J., et al. (2013). Effect of age on the pharmacokinetics of a single daily dose of gentamicin sulfate in healthy foals. Equine Veterinary Journal **45**(4): 507-11.
Corley, K. T. T. & A. R. Hollis (2009). Antimicrobial therapy in neonatal foals. Equine Veterinary Education **21**(8): 436-48.
Flammer, K. (2006). Antibiotic drug selection in companion birds. Journal of Exotic Pet Medicine **15**(3): 166-76.
Ivey, E. & J. Morrisey (2000). Therapeutics for Rabbits. Vet Clin NA: Exotic Anim Pract **3:1**(Jan): 183-216.
KuKanich, B. (2008). Canine breed specific differences in clinical pharmacology. Proceedings: WVC. accessed via Veterinary Information Network; vin.com
LeBlanc, M. M. (2009). The current status of antibiotic use in equine reproduction. Equine Veterinary Education **21**(3): 156-67.
McGorum, B. C. & R. S. Pirie (2010). Antimicrobial associated diarrhoea in the horse. Part 2: Which antimicrobials are associated with AAD in the horse? Equine Veterinary Education **22**(1): 43-50.
Read, J. R., et al. (2011). Plasma Peak and Trough Gentamicin Concentrations in Hospitalized Horses Receiving Once Daily Gentamicin. ACVIM. accessed via Veterinary Information Network; vin.com
Rosskopf, W. J. (1986). Shell diseases in turtles and tortoises. *Current Veterinary Therapy (CVT) IX Small Animal Practice*. R. W. Kirk. Philadelphia, WB Saunders: 751-9.

Glimepiride

(glye-meh-per-ide)   Amaryl®

Sulfonylurea Antidiabetic Agent

Prescriber Highlights

▶ Oral, once-daily, anti-hyperglycemic agent; could be useful in the adjunctive treatment of non-insulin dependent diabetes mellitus (NIDDM) in cats.
▶ Very limited experience in cats.
▶ Contraindicated: Patients hypersensitive to it or with diabetic ketoacidosis.
▶ Hypoglycemia may occur.
▶ Potentially, significant drug interactions.
▶ Do not confuse glipizide, glimepiride & glyburide.

Uses/Indications

Glimepiride may potentially be a useful adjunct in the treatment of non-insulin dependent diabetes mellitus (NIDDM) in cats. Its duration of action in humans allows it to be dosed once daily, which could be of benefit. Glimepiride may also have fewer side effects than glipizide.

Pharmacology/Actions

Glimepiride is a medium- to long-acting secretagogue sulfonylurea. It increases pancreatic release of insulin from functioning beta cells and, with continued use, may also increase peripheral tissue sensitivity to insulin. The exact mechanism for these effects is not well understood.

Pharmacokinetics

No pharmacokinetic data for cats was located. But when 0.5 mg glimepiride was administered orally to healthy cats followed by an intravenous glucose tolerance test 3-6 hours later, glucose levels were lowest at 3 hours post dose and insulin levels peaked twice, first at 60 minutes and a smaller peak at 4 hours (Mori et al. 2009).

In humans, glimepiride is completely absorbed from the GI tract. Peak levels occur in 2-3 hours; food delays the peak somewhat and lowers AUC by about 9%. Volume of distribution is 0.11 L/kg; the drug is greater than 99% bound to plasma proteins. Glimepiride is hepatically metabolized to at least two major metabolites. One of these, M1, has activity at about 1/3 that of the parent compound; clearance is 48 mL/min and elimination half-life about 9 hours. Approximately 60% of the drug (as metabolites) is excreted into the urine and the remainder in the feces. The drug has a 24-hour duration of activity in humans.

Contraindications/Precautions/Warnings

Glimepiride is contraindicated in patients hypersensitive to it or with diabetic ketoacidosis.

Do not confuse gliMEPIRIDE with glyBURIDE or glipiZIDE.

Adverse Effects

Hypoglycemia has been reported in about 1% of human patients taking the drug. Dizziness and asthenia have been reported; rarely, liver function impairment, allergic respiratory reactions, dermatologic reactions, or hematologic reactions have been reported in humans.

Reproductive/Nursing Safety

In humans, the FDA categorizes glimepiride as a category *C* drug for use during pregnancy (*Animal studies have shown an adverse effect on the fetus, but there are no adequate studies in humans; or there are no animal reproduction studies and no adequate studies in humans*). In rabbits and rats, glimepiride did not cause teratogenic effects when given at high dosages. There were some intrauterine deaths if drug-induced maternal hypoglycemia occurred.

Some glimepiride is excreted into maternal milk of rats. The manufacturer states to discontinue the drug in nursing, human mothers.

Overdosage/Acute Toxicity

Overdoses may result in hypoglycemia, ranging from mild to severe. Treatment consists of glucose administration and intensive monitoring. Because of the drug's long duration of activity, patients may need to be supported with glucose for at least 48 hours post-ingestion, even after apparent recovery.

Drug Interactions

The following drug interactions have either been reported or are theoretical in humans or animals receiving glimepiride and may be of in veterinary patients. Unless otherwise noted, use together is not necessarily contraindicated, but weigh the potential risks and perform additional monitoring when appropriate.

- **ANTIFUNGALS, AZOLE** (*e.g.*, ketoconazole, itraconazole, fluconazole): May increase plasma levels of glimepiride.
- **BETA-BLOCKERS:** May potentiate hypoglycemic effect.
- **CHLORAMPHENICOL:** May displace glimepiride from plasma proteins.

- **CORTICOSTEROIDS:** May reduce efficacy.
- **DIURETICS, THIAZIDE:** May reduce hypoglycemic efficacy.
- **ISONIAZID:** May reduce hypoglycemic efficacy.
- **NIACIN:** May reduce hypoglycemic efficacy.
- **PHENOTHIAZINES:** May reduce hypoglycemic efficacy.
- **PHENYTOIN:** May reduce hypoglycemic efficacy.
- **SULFONAMIDES:** May displace glimepiride from plasma proteins.
- **SYMPATHOMIMETIC AGENTS:** May reduce hypoglycemic efficacy.
- **WARFARIN:** May displace glimepiride from plasma proteins.

Laboratory Considerations

- No specific laboratory interactions or considerations were noted.

Doses

- **CATS:**

  For treatment of non-insulin dependent diabetes mellitus (extra-label): Very little evidence to support use, but for cats/owners that cannot tolerate insulin injections, 2 mg per cat PO once daily can be tried in conjunction with dietary modifications (low carbohydrate; high protein).

Monitoring

- Efficacy: Standard methods of monitoring efficacy for diabetes treatment should be followed (*e.g.*, fasting blood glucose, appetite, attitude, body condition, PU/PD resolution and, perhaps, serum fructosamine and/or glycosylated hemoglobin levels).
- Adverse effects.

Client Information

- May be useful for treating diabetes in cats; limited experience in veterinary medicine.
- Give about the same time each day. May be given with or without food. If your animal vomits or acts sick after getting it on an empty stomach, give with food or small treat to see if this helps. If vomiting continues, contact your veterinarian.
- Watch for signs of blood sugar that's too low (hypoglycemia; uncommon): Seizures (convulsions), collapsing/fainting, rear leg weakness or paralysis, muscle twitching, unsteadiness, lack of energy, or depression. If any of these are seen, contact your veterinarian right away.
- Has not been used in many cats so other side effects could occur. Report anything unusual to your veterinarian.

Chemistry/Synonyms

A sulfonylurea antidiabetic agent, glimepiride occurs as a white to yellowish-white, crystalline, odorless to practically odorless powder. It is practically insoluble in water.

Glimepiride may also be known as: HOE-490, *Amarel®*, *Amaryl®*, *Amarylle®*, *Euglim®*, *Glimepil®*, *Solosa®*, and *Roname®*.

Storage/Stability

Glimepiride tablets should be stored between 15-30°C (59-86°F) in well closed containers.

Dosage Forms/Regulatory Status

VETERINARY-LABELED PRODUCTS: NONE.

HUMAN-LABELED PRODUCTS:

Glimepiride Oral Tablets: 1 mg, 2 mg, & 4 mg; *Amaryl®*, generic; (Rx)

Revisions/References

Monograph revised/updated February 2014.

Mori, A., et al. (2009). Effect of glimepiride and nateglinide on serum insulin and glucose concentration in healthy cats. Veterinary Research Communications 33(8): 957-70.

Glipizide

(glip-i-zide)   Glucotrol®

Sulfonylurea Antidiabetic Agent

Prescriber Highlights

▶ Human oral antidiabetic agent (Type II) that may be useful in cats. May take 4-8 weeks before full effects are seen.

▶ Contraindications: Severe burns/trauma/infection, diabetic coma or other hypoglycemic conditions, major surgery, ketosis, ketoacidosis or other significant acidotic conditions. Caution: Untreated adrenal or pituitary insufficiency; thyroid, renal or hepatic function impairment; prolonged vomiting; high fever; malnourishment or debilitated condition.

▶ Adverse Effects: **Cats:** GI (*i.e.*, anorexia, vomiting), hypoglycemia, liver toxicity.

▶ Drug interactions.

▶ Do not confuse glipizide, glimepiride & glyburide.

Uses/Indications

Glipizide may be of benefit in treating cats with type II diabetes if they have a population of functioning beta cells. Perhaps 20%-30% of newly diagnosed cats may benefit (improvement in hyperglycemia) from glipizide, but there is no way to predict which cats will benefit in advance of a trial. It has been suggested that there are two situations when a glipizide trial can be recommended: 1) If an owner refuses to consider using insulin usually due to a fear of needles, and 2) the cat appears to be relatively well controlled on quite small doses of insulin and the owner would strongly prefer to no longer give insulin (Feldman 2005).

While glipizide potentially could be useful in treating canine patients with type II or III diabetes, by the time dogs present with hyperglycemia, they are absolutely or relatively insulinopenic and glipizide would unlikely be effective.

Pharmacology/Actions

Glipizide is a second-generation sulfonylurea. Sulfonylureas lower blood glucose concentrations in both diabetics and non-diabetics. The exact mechanism of action is not known, but these agents are thought to exert the effect primarily by stimulating the beta cells in the pancreas to secrete additional endogenous insulin. Extrapancreatic effects include enhanced tissue sensitivity of circulating insulin. Ongoing use of the sulfonylureas appears to enhance peripheral sensitivity to insulin and reduce the production of hepatic basal glucose. The mechanisms causing these effects are yet to be fully explained, however.

Prolonged hyperglycemia may cause beta cell "exhaustion" and permanent damage to beta cells contributing to their death. It has been suggested that by treating all cats initially with insulin to rapidly reduce hyperglycemia, increases in beta cell sensitivity and insulin release may occur with time and potentially increase success using glipizide (Sparkes 2009).

Pharmacokinetics

Glipizide is rapidly and practically completely absorbed after oral administration. Transdermal administration on cats does not appear to be adequately absorbed to be useful. The absolute bioavailability reported in humans ranges from 80-100%. Food will alter the rate, but not the extent, of absorption. Glipizide is very highly bound to plasma proteins. It is primarily biotransformed in the liver to inactive metabolites that are then excreted by the kidneys. In humans, half-life is about 2-4 hours. Effects on insulin levels in cats tend to be short-lived. Effects peak in about 15 minutes and return to baseline after about 60 minutes.

Contraindications/Precautions/Warnings

Oral antidiabetic agents are considered contraindicated with the following conditions: severe burns, trauma or infection, diabetic coma or other hypoglycemic conditions, major surgery, ketosis, ketoacidosis or other significant acidotic conditions. Glipizide should only be used when its potential benefits outweigh its risks when the following are present: untreated adrenal or pituitary insufficiency; thyroid, renal or hepatic function impairment; prolonged vomiting; high fever; malnourishment or debilitated condition.

While glipizide may initially be effective, it may become ineffective in weeks to months after starting therapy; insulin will then be required.

Some patients with type II or type III diabetes may have their disease complicated by the production of excessive amounts of cortisol or growth hormone which may antagonize insulin's effects. These causes should be ruled out before initiating oral antidiabetic therapy.

Do not confuse glipiZIDE with glyBURIDE or gliMEPIRIDE.

Adverse Effects

Approximately 15% of cats receiving glipizide develop gastrointestinal adverse effects (*i.e.*, anorexia, vomiting). Vomiting usually occurs shortly after dosing and will subside in 2-5 days. If it persists or is severe, decrease dose or frequency and, if necessary, discontinue.

Some cats receiving this drug have developed hypoglycemia, but severe hypoglycemia appears to be rare. Should hypoglycemia occur, discontinue glipizide and recheck glucose in one week; may restart at a lower dose or dosing frequency if hyperglycemia is noted.

Increased amyloid deposit formation can occur with glipizide, which can potentially cause further destruction of functional beta cells.

Effects on the liver have been reported. Approximately 8% of cats treated with glipizide may develop cholestatic jaundice and have increased liver enzymes. Serum hepatic enzymes should be checked every 1-2 weeks initially. Discontinue glipizide in cats with elevated enzymes if they develop lethargy, anorexia, vomiting, or if ALT exceeds 500 IU/L. Should icterus occur, discontinue glipizide and restart at a lower dose once icterus resolves; discontinue use should icterus reoccur.

Other adverse effects that are possible (noted in humans) include allergic skin reactions and bone marrow suppression.

Glipizide does not appear to be effective in cats demonstrating insulin resistance.

Reproductive/Nursing Safety

Safe use during pregnancy has not been established. Glipizide was found to be mildly fetotoxic in rats when given at doses at 5 – 50 mg/kg, however no other teratogenic effects were noted. Use in pregnancy only when benefits outweigh potential risks. In humans, the FDA categorizes this drug as category C for use during pregnancy (*Animal studies have shown an adverse effect on the fetus, but there are no adequate studies in humans; or there are no animal reproduction studies and no adequate studies in humans.*)

It is unknown if glipizide enters milk.

Overdosage/Acute Toxicity

Oral LD_{50}'s are greater than 4 g/kg in all animal species tested. Profound hypoglycemia is the greatest concern after an overdose. Gut emptying protocols should be employed when warranted. Because of its shorter half-life than chlorpropamide, prolonged hypoglycemia is less likely with glipizide, but blood glucose monitoring and treatment with parenteral glucose may be required for several days. Massive overdoses may also require additional monitoring (blood gases, serum electrolytes) and supportive therapy.

Drug Interactions

The following drug interactions have either been reported or are theoretical in humans or animals receiving glipizide and may be of in veterinary patients. Unless otherwise noted, use together is not necessarily contraindicated, but weigh the potential risks and perform additional monitoring when appropriate.

- **ALCOHOL:** A disulfiram-like reaction (anorexia, nausea, vomiting) has been reported in humans who have ingested alcohol within 48-72 hours of receiving glipizide.
- **ANTIFUNGALS, AZOLE (ketoconazole, itraconazole, fluconazole):** May increase plasma levels of glipizide.
- **BETA-BLOCKERS:** May potentiate hypoglycemic effect.
- **CHLORAMPHENICOL:** May displace glipizide from plasma proteins.
- **CIMETIDINE:** May potentiate hypoglycemic effect.
- **CORTICOSTEROIDS:** May reduce efficacy.
- **DIURETICS, THIAZIDE:** May reduce hypoglycemic efficacy.
- **ISONIAZID:** May reduce hypoglycemic efficacy.
- **MAO INHIBITORS:** May potentiate hypoglycemic effect.
- **NIACIN:** May reduce hypoglycemic efficacy.
- **PHENOTHIAZINES:** May reduce hypoglycemic efficacy.
- **PHENYTOIN:** May reduce hypoglycemic efficacy.
- **PROBENECID:** May potentiate hypoglycemic effect.
- **SULFONAMIDES:** May displace glipizide from plasma proteins.
- **SYMPATHOMIMETIC AGENTS:** May reduce hypoglycemic efficacy.
- **THYROID AGENTS:** May reduce hypoglycemic effect.
- **WARFARIN:** May displace glipizide from plasma proteins.

Doses

- **CATS:**

  For diabetes mellitus (extra-label): Rarely recommended (see Uses/Indications) and evidence to support any dosage regimen is low. When decision is made to try the drug, most recommendations are to start at 2.5 mg per cat PO twice daily with food. The following is an example dosage regimen: In non-ketotic cats that are relatively healthy: Initially monitor weight, urine/glucose/ketones, and several blood glucose measurements. Then give 2.5 mg PO per cat twice daily in conjunction with a meal. During first 24 hours of therapy perform spot blood glucose measurements (every 3-4 hours for the initial 12-18 hours) to check for hypoglycemia. After 2 weeks, monitor again and if hyperglycemia is still present and adverse reactions (vomiting, icterus) have not occurred, increase dose to 5 mg twice daily. Therapy is continued as long as cat is stable. If cat is euglycemic or hypoglycemia develops, the dosage may be tapered down or discontinued, and blood glucose concentrations re-evaluated 1 week later to assess the need for the drug. If hyperglycemia recurs, the dosage is increased or glipizide is reinitiated, with a reduction in dosage in those cats previously developing hypoglycemia. Discontinue and initiate insulin therapy if clinical signs continue to worsen, the cat becomes ill, develops ketoacidosis, blood glucose concentrations remain greater than 15 mmol/L (270 mg/dL) after one or two months of therapy, or the owners become dissatisfied with the treatment. (Herrtage 2009)

Monitoring

- Weekly exams during first month of therapy, including PE, body weight, urine glucose/ketones, and several blood glucose exams.
- Adverse effects (anorexia, vomiting, icterus), and occasional liver enzymes and CBC.

Client Information

- Give with meals; usually twice per day.
- About 15% of cats will vomit after starting this drug, but this usually gets better after a few days.
- May take 1-2 months to see if the drug is working properly.
- Rarely, it can cause jaundice or blood sugar to be too low (hypoglycemia). Watch for seizures (convulsions), collapsing/fainting, rear leg weakness or paralysis, muscle twitching, unsteadiness, lack of energy, or depression.

Chemistry/Synonyms

A sulfonylurea antidiabetic agent, glipizide (also known as glydiazinamide) occurs as a whitish powder. It is practically insoluble in water and has pK_a of 5.9.

Glipizide may also be known as: CP-28720, glipizidum, glydiazinamide, or K-4024; many international trade names are available.

Storage/Stability

Tablets should be stored in tight, light-resistant containers at room temperature.

Dosage Forms/Regulatory Status

VETERINARY-LABELED PRODUCTS: NONE.

HUMAN-LABELED PRODUCTS:

Glipizide Oral Tablets: 5 mg, & 10 mg; *Glucotrol®*, generic (Rx)

Glipizide Oral Extended Release Tablets: 2.5 mg, 5 mg, & 10 mg; *Glucotrol XL®*, generic; (Rx). **Note:** This product is generally not used in veterinary medicine.

Glipizide/Metformin Hydrochloride Tablets (film-coated): 2.5 mg glipizide/250 mg or 500 mg metformin; 5 mg glipizide/500 mg metformin; *Metaglip®*, generic; (Rx). **Note:** This product is generally not used in veterinary medicine.

Revisions/References

Monograph revised/updated February 2014.

Feldman, E. (2005). Management of Diabetes Mellitus in Dogs and Cats: I, II, & III. Proceedings: Western Vet Conf. accessed via Veterinary Information Network; vin.com
Herrtage, M. (2009). New Strategies in the Management of Feline Diabetes Mellitus. Proceedings: WSAVA. accessed via Veterinary Information Network; vin.com
Sparkes, A. (2009). Long-Term Care of Diabetic Cats: Home Monitoring and Hospital. Proceedings: BSAVA. accessed via Veterinary Information Network; vin.com

Glucagon

(gloo-ka-gon)   GlucoGen®

Hormonal Agent

Prescriber Highlights

▶ Hormone to increase blood glucose that may be useful for treating hypoglycemia in small animals & potentially, fatty liver syndrome in dairy cows.

▶ May be effective in treating beta-blocker or calcium channel overdoses, or when patients being treated for anaphylaxis have received beta-blockers.

▶ Must be parenterally administered.

▶ When used as CRI, must be in a setting where blood glucose can be monitored.

▶ Unlikely to cause adverse effects; sedation is possible.

Uses/Indications

In small animals, the primary use for glucagon is to increase blood glucose in patients with excessive insulin levels, either endogenously produced (insulinoma) or exogenously administered (insulin overdose). There is significant interest in its potential subcutaneous use in emergency home treatment of hypoglycemia in small animals (Niessen 2012).

In human medicine and potentially for veterinary patients, glucagon can be used in treating the cardiac manifestations of beta-blocker, calcium-channel blocker, and tricyclic antidepressant overdoses. One study (Kerns et al. 1997) in dogs however, demonstrated insulin to be superior to glucagon in treating experimental propranolol overdoses. Glucagon can also be used in conjunction with epinephrine for treating anaphylaxis in patients that have received beta-blockers and it has potential in the treatment of fatty liver syndrome in dairy cattle.

Glucagon is used to treat "steakhouse syndrome" (food bolus lodged in esophagus) in human patients.

Pharmacology/Actions

Glucagon's main pharmacologic activities are to increase blood glucose and relax smooth muscles of the GI tract. It primarily increases blood glucose by stimulating hepatic glycogenolysis, but can also increase glucose via hepatic gluconeogenesis from available amino acid substrates. In healthy dogs, glucagon can overcome the inhibitory activity of insulin on hepatic glucose production; intravenous (not SC) glucagon can also cause transient increases in ACTH and cortisol (Zeugswetter et al. 2012). Glucagon does not stimulate reactive release of insulin or cause rebound hypoglycemia.

The mechanisms of action for its GI effects are not well understood.

Pharmacokinetics

Glucagon must be administered parenterally; it is destroyed in the gut after oral dosing. In healthy beagles, 1 mg given SC caused plasma glucose to increase significantly within 10 minutes and peak at 20 minutes. Glucose levels were still approximately 60% above baseline at 30 minutes. After intravenous injection, maximum glucose levels were attained approximately 20 minutes later (Zeugswetter et al. 2012).

Glucagon is degraded in the plasma, liver and kidneys. In humans, hyperglycemic effects persist up to 90 minutes after dosing and plasma half-life is around 10 minutes.

Contraindications/Precautions/Warnings

Glucagon should usually not be used in patients with pheochromocytoma as catecholamines may be released leading to hypertension. When used for insulinoma, it must be in a setting where blood glucose can be closely monitored. While glucagon may be useful for blood glucose elevation in insulinoma patients, in humans its use for this is cautioned as it can increase insulin production, leading to greater hypoglycemia once the drug is discontinued.

Adverse Effects

Glucagon is usually well tolerated, but sedation may occur. Potentially, nausea and vomiting soon after administration are possible. Hypokalemia and hypersensitivity reactions (very rare) are unlikely, but possible.

Reproductive/Nursing Safety

In humans, glucagon is designated by the FDA as a category *B* drug (*Animal studies have not demonstrated risk to the fetus, but there are no adequate studies in pregnant women; or animal studies have shown an adverse effect, but adequate studies in pregnant women have not demonstrated a risk to the fetus during the first trimester of pregnancy, and there is no evidence of risk in later trimesters.*) As an endogenously produced hormone, it is unlikely to cause significant risk to offspring.

It is unknown if glucagon enters maternal milk, but it is unlikely to cause harm to nursing offspring.

Overdosage/Acute Toxicity

Adverse effects seen with overdose include nausea, vomiting, diarrhea, gastric hypotonicity and, possibly, hypokalemia. Because glucagon's elimination half-life is so short, treatment may not be necessary and would be symptomatic in nature. If the patient is also receiving beta-blockers, greater increases in blood pressure and heart rate may be seen.

Drug Interactions

The following drug interactions have either been reported or are theoretical in humans or animals receiving glucagon and may be of in veterinary patients. Unless otherwise noted, use together is not necessarily contraindicated, but weigh the potential risks and perform additional monitoring when appropriate.

- **ANTICOAGULANTS:** May have their effects increased when glucagon is concurrently administered; this effect may be delayed. It is suggested to monitor for bleeding and prothrombin activity if glucagon is necessary.

Laboratory Considerations

- No glucagon-related laboratory interactions noted.

Doses

- **DOGS/CATS:**

  Intravenous dosing for severe hypoglycemia (extra-label): There are two primary recommended dosing regimens; available evidence does not support one over the other:

  Regimen 1: 1 mg of glucagon is reconstituted per manufacturer directions and then added to 1000 mL of 0.9% Sodium Chloride; this results in a 1000 ng/mL (nanograms/mL) solution. [**Note:** Some references state not to mix or dilute with saline solutions, but use D5W only.] Initially, give a 50 nanogram/kg IV bolus and then administer at a constant rate infusion (CRI) using a suitable pump at a rate of 10 – 15 nanograms/kg/minute. May need to increase up to 40 nanograms/kg/minute to maintain euglycemia.

  Regimen 2: Prepare solution as above, but give as a CRI at an initial infusion rate of 5 nanograms/kg/minute and adjust according to the blood glucose values; can be increased to 13 nanograms/kg/minute.

  Subcutaneous emergency home dosing for severe hypoglycemia (extra-label): At the time of writing (01/2014), there is not enough published information to recommend clinical use for either dogs or cats. A study done in 5 normal beagles and a subsequent editorial suggest that the treatment does warrant additional research to determine if it is safe and effective for home use in dogs and/or cats. (Niessen 2012; Zeugswetter et al. 2012)

- **CATTLE:**

  For treatment of fatty liver in early lactation dairy cows older than 3.5 years: 5 mg glucagon in 60 mL of normal saline SC q8h (15 mg/day) for 14 days. (Bobe et al. 2003)

Monitoring

- Blood glucose.
- Serum potassium if used other than for acute treatment.

Client Information

- Glucagon could potentially be used for outpatient emergency initial treatment of hypoglycemia, but oral glucose is probably more appropriate (and cheaper) for use by clients.

Chemistry/Synonyms

A hormone secreted by the alpha$_2$ cells of the pancreas, glucagon is a straight chain polypeptide that contains 29 amino acids whose sequence is consistent throughout mammalian species. It has a molecular weight of 3483. When in crystalline form it is a white- to off-white powder that is relatively insoluble in water at physiologic pH, but is soluble at pH of less than 3 and greater than 9.5. Glucagon may be expressed in terms of International Units (IU; expressed as Units in this reference) or by weight. One International Unit (IU) is equivalent to one milligram of glucagon. Commercially available glucagon is now obtained via recombinant DNA sources.

Glucagon may also be known as glucagonum or HGF, and *GlucaGen®*.

Storage/Stability

The commercially available powder for reconstitution should be stored at room temperature between 20-25°C (68-77°F); avoid freezing and protect from light. Once reconstituted with the supplied diluent the solution should be clear with a water-like consistency and used immediately; any unused portion should be discarded. If the solution contains any gel formation or particles, it should be discarded.

Compatibility/Compounding Considerations

To prepare glucagon for a continuous rate infusion, dilute 1 mg with the supplied diluent or sterile water; roll gently until dissolved, this may then be further diluted in D5W. May be given through a Y-tube or 3-way stopcock if a dextrose solution is running.

Dosage Forms/Regulatory Status

VETERINARY-LABELED PRODUCTS: NONE.

HUMAN-LABELED PRODUCTS:

Glucagon (human rDNA-origin) Powder for Injection: 1 mg (1 unit) with 1 mL diluent in vials & syringes; *GlucaGen®*, *GlucaGen HypoKit®*, *Glucagon Emergency Kit*; (Rx)

Revisions/References

Monograph revised/updated February 2014.

Bobe, G., et al. (2003). Potential treatment of fatty liver with 14-day subcutaneous injections of glucagon. J Dairy Sci **86**: 3138-47.

Kerns, W., et al. (1997). Insulin improves survival in a canine model of acute beta-blocker toxicity. Ann Emerg Med. **29**(6): 748-57.

Niessen, S. J. M. (2012). Glucagon: Are we missing a (life-saving) trick? J. Vet. Emerg. Crit. Care **22**(5).

Zeugswetter, F. K., et al. (2012). Metabolic and hormonal responses to subcutaneous glucagon in healthy beagles. J. Vet. Emerg. Crit. Care **22**(5): 558-63.

Glucocorticoid Agents, General Information

Glucocorticoid Comparison Table

Drug	Equiv. Antiinflammatory Dose (mg)	Relative Anti-inflammatory potency	Relative mineral-corticoid activity	Plasma Half-Life Dogs (min) [Humans]	Duration of action after oral/IV	Ester Form: Solubility/Release Durations (IM)
Hydrocortisone (Cortisol)	20	1	1–2	52–57 [90]	<12 hrs (8-12)	Sodium Succinate: Very/Minutes
Betamethasone	0.6	25	0	[300+]	>36 (36-54) hrs	Sodium Succinate or phosphate: Very/Minutes
Dexamethasone	0.75	30	0	119–136 [200–300+]	>36 hours (36-54) hrs	Sodium Succ or Sod. Phos: Very/Minutes Phenylpropionate or Isonicotinate: Mod./Days to weeks
Flumethasone	1.5	15–30	?	?		Very/Minutes
Isoflupredone		17				Acetate: Duration of action up to 48 hours
Methylprednisolone	4	5	0	91 [200]	12–36 hrs	Sod. Succinate: Very/Minutes Acetate: Mod./Days to weeks
Prednisolone	5	4	1	69–197 [115–212]	12–36 hrs	Sodium Succinate: Very/Minutes Acetate: Mod./Days to weeks
Prednisone	5	4	1	[60]	12–36 hrs	
Triamcinolone	4	5	0	[200+]	24-48 hrs	Acetonide: Poorly/Weeks

Uses/Indications

Glucocorticoids have been used in an attempt to treat practically every malady that afflicts man or animal, but there are four broad uses and dosage ranges for use of these agents. 1) Replacement of glucocorticoid activity in patients with adrenal insufficiency; 2) as an antiinflammatory agent; 3) as a cytotoxic/antineoplastic agent; and 4) as an immunosuppressive. Some of the uses for glucocorticoids include treatment of: endocrine conditions (*e.g.*, adrenal insufficiency), rheumatic diseases (*e.g.*, rheumatoid arthritis), collagen diseases (*e.g.*, systemic lupus), allergic states, respiratory diseases (*e.g.*, asthma), dermatologic diseases (*e.g.*, pemphigus, allergic dermatoses), hematologic disorders (*e.g.*, thrombocytopenias, autoimmune hemolytic anemias), neoplasias, nervous system disorders, GI diseases (*e.g.*, ulcerative colitis exacerbations), and renal diseases (*e.g.*, nephrotic syndrome). Some glucocorticoids are used topically in the eye and skin for various conditions or are injected intra-articularly or intra-lesionally. The above listing is certainly not complete. For specific dosages and indications refer to the Doses section for each glucocorticoid drug monograph.

Glucocorticoids have been used for CNS trauma (especially spinal chord injury) or shock, but their use for these indications are controversial as there is little evidence supporting their use. Relative adrenal insufficiency may occur in critically ill animals, and low or physiologic doses of corticosteroids (having both glucocorticoid and mineralocorticoid activity, *e.g.*, hydrocortisone) may be indicated in patients that have not responded to pressor agents.

Pharmacology/Actions

Glucocorticoids have effects on virtually every cell type and system in mammals. An overview of the effects of these agents follows:

Cardiovascular System: Glucocorticoids can reduce capillary permeability and enhance vasoconstriction. A relatively clinically insignificant positive inotropic effect can occur after glucocorticoid administration. Increased blood pressure can result from both the drugs' vasoconstrictive properties and increased blood volume that may be produced.

Cells: Glucocorticoids inhibit fibroblast proliferation, macrophage response to migration inhibiting factor, sensitization of lymphocytes and the cellular response to mediators of inflammation. Glucocorticoids stabilize lysosomal membranes.

CNS/Autonomic Nervous System: Glucocorticoids can lower seizure threshold, alter mood and behavior, diminish the response to pyrogens, stimulate appetite and maintain alpha rhythm. Glucocorticoids are necessary for normal adrenergic receptor sensitivity.

Endocrine System: When animals are not stressed, glucocorticoids will suppress the release of ACTH from the anterior pituitary, thereby reducing or preventing the release of endogenous corticosteroids. Stress factors (*e.g.*, renal disease, liver disease, diabetes) may sometimes nullify the suppressing aspects of exogenously administered steroids. Release of thyroid-stimulating hormone (TSH), follicle-stimulating hormone (FSH), prolactin, and luteinizing hormone (LH) may all be reduced when glucocorticoids are administered at pharmacological doses. Conversion of thyroxine (T_4) to triiodothyronine (T_3) may be reduced by glucocorticoids; and plasma levels of parathyroid hormone increased. Glucocorticoids may inhibit osteoblast function. Vasopressin (ADH) activity is reduced at the renal tubules and diuresis may occur. Glucocorticoids inhibit insulin binding to insulin-receptors and the post-receptor effects of insulin.

Hematopoietic System: Glucocorticoids can increase the numbers of circulating platelets, neutrophils and red blood cells, but platelet aggregation is inhibited. Decreased amounts of lymphocytes (peripheral), monocytes and eosinophils are seen as glucocorticoids can sequester these cells into the lungs and spleen and prompt decreased release from the bone marrow. Removal of old red blood cells becomes diminished. Glucocorticoids can cause involution of lymphoid tissue.

GI Tract and Hepatic System: Glucocorticoids increase the secretion of gastric acid, pepsin, and trypsin. They alter the structure of mucin and decrease mucosal cell proliferation. Iron salts and calcium absorption are decreased while fat absorption is increased. Hepatic changes can include increased fat and glycogen deposits within hepatocytes, increased serum levels of alanine aminotransferase (ALT), and gamma-glutamyl transpeptidase (GGT). Significant increases can be seen in serum alkaline phosphatase levels. Glucocorticoids can cause minor increases in BSP (bromosulfophthalein) retention time.

Immune System (also see Cells and Hematopoietic System): Glucocorticoids can decrease circulating levels of T-lymphocytes; inhibit lymphokines; inhibit neutrophil, macrophage, and monocyte migration; reduce production of interferon; inhibit phagocytosis and chemotaxis; antigen processing; and diminish intracellular killing. Specific acquired immunity is affected less than nonspecific immune responses. Glucocorticoids can also antagonize the complement cascade and mask the clinical signs of infection. Mast cells are decreased in number and histamine synthesis is suppressed. Many of these effects only occur at high or very high doses and there are species differences in response.

Metabolic effects: Glucocorticoids stimulate gluconeogenesis. Lipogenesis is enhanced in certain areas of the body (*e.g.*, abdomen) and adipose tissue can be redistributed away from the extremities to the trunk. Fatty acids are mobilized from tissues and their oxidation is increased. Plasma levels of triglycerides, cholesterol, and glycerol are increased. Protein is mobilized from most areas of the body (not the liver).

Musculoskeletal: Glucocorticoids may cause muscular weakness (also caused if there is a lack of glucocorticoids), atrophy, and osteoporosis. Bone growth can be inhibited via growth hormone and somatomedin inhibition, increased calcium excretion and inhibition of vitamin D activation. Resorption of bone can be enhanced. Fibrocartilage growth is also inhibited.

Ophthalmic: Prolonged corticosteroid use (both systemic or topically to the eye) can cause increased intraocular pressure and glaucoma, cataracts, and exophthalmos.

Renal, Fluid, & Electrolytes: Glucocorticoids can increase potassium and calcium excretion, sodium and chloride reabsorption, and extracellular fluid volume. Hypokalemia and/or hypocalcemia rarely occur. Diuresis may develop following glucocorticoid administration.

Skin: Thinning of dermal tissue and skin atrophy can be seen with glucocorticoid therapy. Hair follicles can become distended and alopecia may occur.

Contraindications/Precautions/Warnings

Systemic use of glucocorticoids is generally considered contraindicated in systemic fungal infections (unless used for replacement therapy in Addison's), when administered IM in patients with idiopathic thrombocytopenia, and in patients hypersensitive to a particular drug. Use of sustained-release injectable glucocorticoids is considered contraindicated for chronic corticosteroid therapy of systemic diseases.

Animals that have received glucocorticoids systemically, other than with "burst" therapy, should be tapered off the drugs. Patients who have received the drugs chronically should be tapered off slowly as endogenous ACTH and corticosteroid function may return slowly. Should the animal undergo a "stressor" (*e.g.*, surgery, trauma, illness, etc.) during the tapering process or until normal adrenal and pituitary function resume, additional glucocorticoids should be administered.

Adverse Effects

Adverse effects are generally associated with long-term administration of these drugs, especially if given at high dosages or not on an alternate day regimen. Effects generally manifest as clinical signs of hyperadrenocorticism. When administered to young, growing animals, glucocorticoids can retard growth. Many of the potential effects, adverse and otherwise, are outlined above in the Pharmacology section.

In dogs, high parenteral dosages may be associated with significant GI toxicity. Polydipsia (PD), polyphagia (PP), and polyuria (PU) may all be seen with short-term "burst" therapy as well as with alternate-day maintenance therapy on days when the drug is given. Adverse effects in dogs can include: dull, dry haircoat, weight gain, panting, vomiting, diarrhea, elevated liver enzymes, pancreatitis, GI ulceration, lipidemias, activation or worsening of diabetes mellitus, muscle wasting and behavioral changes (depression, lethargy, viciousness). Discontinuation of the drug may be necessary; changing to an alternate steroid may also alleviate the problem. With the exception of PU/PD/PP, adverse effects associated with short-term antiinflammatory therapy occur relatively uncommonly. Adverse effects associated with immunosuppressive doses are more common and potentially more severe.

In dogs, glucocorticoids can increase liver enzymes (SAP>ALT) and cause vacuolar hepatopathy. Cats may show mild vacuolar changes, but enzymes are generally not affected.

Cats generally require higher dosages than dogs for clinical effect, but tend to develop fewer adverse effects. Occasionally, polydipsia, polyuria, polyphagia with weight gain, diarrhea, or depression can be seen. Long-term, high dose therapy can lead to "Cushingoid" effects, however.

Administration of dexamethasone or triamcinolone may play a role in the development of laminitis in horses.

Reproductive/Nursing Safety

Glucocorticoids are probably necessary for normal fetal development. They may be required for adequate surfactant production, myelin, retinal, pancreatic, and mammary development. Excessive dosages early in pregnancy may lead to teratogenic effects. In horses and ruminants, exogenous steroid administration may induce parturition when administered in the latter stages of pregnancy.

Glucocorticoids unbound to plasma proteins will enter milk. High dosages or prolonged administration to mothers may potentially inhibit the growth of nursing newborns. In humans, several studies suggest that amounts excreted in human breast milk are negligible with prednisone or prednisolone doses of 20 mg/day or less, or methylprednisolone doses less than or equal to 8 mg/day. Large doses for short periods may not harm the infant. Waiting 3-4 hours after the dose before nursing, and using prednisolone rather than prednisone may result in a lower corticosteroid dose to offspring.

Overdosage/Acute Toxicity

Glucocorticoids when given short-term are unlikely to cause harmful effects, even in massive dosages. One incidence of a dog developing acute CNS effects after accidental ingestion of glucocorticoids has been reported. Should clinical signs occur, use supportive treatment if required.

Chronic usage of glucocorticoids can lead to serious adverse effects. Refer to Adverse Effects above for more information.

Drug Interactions

The following drug interactions have either been reported or are theoretical in humans or animals receiving glucocorticoids and may be of in veterinary patients. Unless otherwise noted, use together is not necessarily contraindicated, but weigh the potential risks and perform additional monitoring when appropriate.

- **AMPHOTERICIN B:** When administered concomitantly with glucocorticoids may cause hypokalemia.
- **ANTICHOLINESTERASE AGENTS** (*e.g.*, **pyridostigmine, neostigmine**, etc.): In patients with myasthenia gravis, concomitant glucocorticoid with these agents may lead to profound muscle weakness. If possible, discontinue anticholinesterase medication at least 24 hours prior to corticosteroid administration.
- **ASPIRIN** (**salicylates**): Glucocorticoids may reduce salicylate blood levels.
- **CYCLOPHOSPHAMIDE:** Glucocorticoids may also inhibit the hepatic metabolism of cyclophosphamide; dosage adjustments may be required.
- **CYCLOSPORINE:** Concomitant administration of may increase the blood levels of each, by mutually inhibiting the hepatic metabolism of each other; clinical significance of this interaction is not clear.
- **DIGOXIN:** Secondary to hypokalemia, increased risk for arrhythmias.
- **DIURETICS, POTASSIUM-DEPLETING** (*e.g.*, **furosemide, thiazides**): When administered concomitantly with glucocorticoids may cause hypokalemia.
- **EPHEDRINE:** May increase metabolism.
- **ESTROGENS:** The effects of hydrocortisone, and possibly other glucocorticoids, may be potentiated by concomitant administration with estrogens.
- **INSULIN:** Requirements may increase in patients receiving glucocorticoids.
- **KETOCONAZOLE:** May decrease metabolism.
- **MITOTANE:** May alter the metabolism of steroids; higher than usual doses of steroids may be necessary to treat mitotane-induced adrenal insufficiency.
- **NSAIDS:** Administration of other ulcerogenic drugs with glucocorticoids may increase ulceration risk.
- **PHENOBARBITAL:** May increase the metabolism of glucocorticoids.
- **PHENYTOIN:** May increase the metabolism of glucocorticoids.
- **RIFAMPIN:** May increase the metabolism of glucocorticoids.
- **VACCINES:** Patients receiving corticosteroids at immuno-suppressive dosages should generally not receive live attenuated-virus vaccines as virus replication may be augmented; a diminished immune response may occur after vaccine, toxoid, or bacterin administration in patients receiving glucocorticoids.

Laboratory Considerations

- Glucocorticoids may increase serum **cholesterol** and **urine glucose** levels.
- Certain glucocorticoids (e.g., prednisone, prednisolone, hydrocortisone) will interfere with **cortisol assays** (**ACTH stimulation tests**, etc.). Dexamethasone does not interfere.
- Glucocorticoids may decrease serum **potassium**.
- Glucocorticoids can suppress the release of thyroid stimulating hormone (TSH) and reduce T_3 & T_4 values. Thyroid gland atrophy has been reported after chronic glucocorticoid administration. Uptake of I^{131} by the thyroid may be decreased by glucocorticoids.
- Reactions to **skin tests** may be suppressed by glucocorticoids.
- False-negative results of the **nitroblue tetrazolium test for systemic bacterial infection**s may be induced by glucocorticoids.

Monitoring

Monitoring of glucocorticoid therapy is dependent on its reason for use, dosage, agent used (amount of mineralocorticoid activity), dosage schedule (daily versus alternate day therapy), duration of therapy, and the animal's age and condition. The following list may not be appropriate or complete for all animals; use clinical assessment and judgment should adverse effects be noted:

- Weight, appetite, signs of edema.
- Serum and/or urine electrolytes.
- Total plasma proteins, albumin.
- Blood glucose.
- Growth and development in young animals.
- ACTH stimulation test, if necessary.

Client Information

- Clients should carefully follow the dosage instructions and should not discontinue the drug abruptly without consulting with veterinarian beforehand.
- Clients should be briefed on the potential adverse effects that can be seen with these drugs and instructed to contact the veterinarian should these effects progress or become severe.

Glucosamine/Chondroitin Sulfate

(gloo-kose-a-meen/kon-droy-tin sul-fayt)   Cosequin®

Nutritional Supplement

Prescriber Highlights

▶ Nutritional supplement that may be useful as an adjunctive treatment for osteoarthritis or other painful conditions in horses, cats, dogs, etc.; FLUTD in cats.
▶ Well tolerated, but efficacy is uncertain.
▶ Not a regulated drug; choose products carefully; large variation in commercially available products.

Uses/Indications

These compounds may be useful in treating osteoarthritis or other painful conditions in domestic animals, but large, well-designed controlled clinical studies proving efficacy were not located. Additionally, since there is no FDA-approval process or oversight for these products, product quality and bioavailability may be highly variable. One study in dogs (McCarthy et al. 2007) showed some positive effect, but this study was not placebo controlled and compared responses versus carprofen. Another placebo-controlled, blinded study in dogs (Moreau et al. 2003), did not demonstrate statistically significant improvement after 60 days of treatment. An article reviewing the quality of evidence supporting the use of glucosamine-based nutraceuticals in equine joint disease concluded that "...the quality of these studies is generally low. A poorly defined experimental paradigm makes balanced interpretation of individual studies difficult, and analysis of the body of literature as a whole virtually impossible" (Pearson et al. 2009).

These compounds potentially could be of benefit in cats with FLUTD (feline lower urinary tract disease) because of the presence of glycosaminoglycans as part of the protective layer of the urinary tract. Controlled studies have shown some positive effects in some cats, but overall it did not appear to make a significant difference.

Pharmacology/Actions

Cartilage cells use glucosamine to produce glycosaminoglycans and hyaluronan. Glucosamine also regulates synthesis of collagen and proteoglycans in cartilage and has mild antiinflammatory effects due to its ability to scavenge free radicals. Chondrocytes normally produce ample quantities of glucosamine from glucose and amino acids, but this ability may diminish with age, disease, or trauma. Exogenously administered glucosamine appears to be able to be utilized by chondrocytes.

Chondroitin sulfate possesses several pharmacologic effects. It appears to inhibit destructive enzymes in joint fluid and cartilage. Thrombi formation in microvasculature may be reduced. In joint cartilage, it stimulates the production of glycosaminoglycans and proteoglycans.

While in vitro evidence exists, there is not solid evidence that using these compounds together improves clinical effect over either alone, but in vivo studies are ongoing. Onset of any clinical efficacy may require 2-6 weeks of treatment.

Pharmacokinetics

The pharmacokinetics of these compounds are difficult to evaluate due to the different salts, lack of standards, etc. Both glucosamine HCl and glucosamine sulfate can be absorbed in the gut after the salt is cleaved in the stomach, but bioavailability may be very low. One study done in six mature horses fed diets with pure glucosamine and chondroitin top-dressed on their feed did not detect any absorption into plasma (Welch et al. 2012). There exists controversy as to whether either salt of glucosamine is superior to the other. Most clinical studies in veterinary species have been done with the HCl salt.

Contraindications/Precautions/Warnings

No absolute contraindications were located for these compounds. As hypersensitivity reactions are a theoretical possibility, animals demonstrating prior hypersensitivity reactions to these compounds should not receive them.

In humans, glucosamine may exacerbate symptoms associated with asthma. Although this has not yet been reported in veterinary patients, caution is advised in patients with bronchoconstrictive conditions.

Adverse Effects

These products appear to be very well tolerated in dogs, cats, and horses. Adverse effects could potentially include some minor gastrointestinal effects (flatulence, stool softening). Since these products are often derived from natural sources, hypersensitivity reactions could occur.

Reproductive/Nursing Safety

No studies on the safety of these compounds in pregnant or lactating animals have been performed.

Overdosage/Acute Toxicity

Oral overdosage is unlikely to cause significant problems. The LD_{50} for the combined compound in rats is greater than 5 g/kg. Gastrointestinal effects may result. Changes in coagulation parameters could occur, but have not been documented to date.

Products that contain manganese could lead to manganese toxicity if given in very high dosages (above label recommendations) chronically.

Drug Interactions

No clinically significant drug interactions have been reported to date in animals. By reducing **doxorubicin** or **etoposide** inhibition of topoisomerase II, glucosamine may induce resistance to these agents. High dose chondroitin sulfate and/or glucosamine potentially could enhance the effects of **warfarin**, **heparin**, or other drugs that affect coagulation.

Laboratory Considerations

- High dose chondroitin and glucosamine theoretically could increase International Normalized Ratio (**INR**) in patients taking warfarin.

Doses

Note: Because of the variability in products available, lack of controlled studies clearly documenting efficacy, or FDA-approval, use of these products for controlling chronic pain conditions is controversial. If a therapy trial is made it is recommended to choose a product that has been tested in the species for which it is marketed; consult the product's label for specific label information.

- **DOGS/CATS:**

    For adjunctive treatment of chronic pain conditions (extra-label; not FDA-approved products): Anecdotal recommendations are usually to treat initially at 15 – 30 mg/kg (of the chondroitin component). After 4-6 weeks, if a positive response is seen dosage may be halved or given every other day.

Monitoring

- Clinical efficacy.

Client Information

- May be given with or without food. If your animal vomits or acts sick after getting it on an empty stomach, give with food or small treat to see if this helps. If vomiting continues, contact your veterinarian.
- May take 2-6 weeks of treatment to see if drug is helping.
- Do not switch brands from that prescribed without first contacting your veterinarian. The amount of each drug might not be the same.
- Side effects are unlikely, but mild gastrointestinal upset has been reported in small animals.

Chemistry/Synonyms

Glucosamine is most often available as either glucosamine HCl or glucosamine sulfate. It is an amino sugar that is synthesized in vivo by animal cells from glucose and glutamine.

Glucosamine (HCl or Sulfate) may also be known as: chitosamine, NSC-758, 2-amino-2-deoxy-beta-D-glucopyranose, G6SD-glucosamine, glucose-6-phosphate, or amino monosaccharide.

Chondroitin sulfate is an acid mucopolysaccharide/glycosaminoglycan that is found in most cartilaginous tissues. It is a long chain compound that contains Units of galactosamine and glucuronic acid.

Chondroitin sulfate may also be known as chondroitin 4-sulfate, chondroitin sulfate A, chondroitin sulfate B, chondroitin sulfate C, chondroitin sulfate sodium, CSA, sodium chondroitin sulfate, chondroitin polysulfate, CDA, CSCSC, GAG, or galactosaminogluconoglycan sulfate.

Storage/Stability

Because of the multiple products and product formulations available, check label for storage and stability (expiration date) information. Chondroitin sulfate is an extremely hygroscopic compound and, generally, these products should be stored in tight containers at room temperature. Avoid storing in direct sunlight.

Compatibility/Compounding Considerations

No specific information was noted; refer to the product label for more information.

Dosage Forms/Regulatory Status

VETERINARY-LABELED PRODUCTS:

None as pharmaceuticals. Supplements are available from a wide variety of sources and dosage forms include tablets, capsules and powder in a variety of concentrations. There are specific products marketed for use in animals, including *Cosequin®*, *Restor-A-Flex®*, *OsteO-3®*, *Arthri-Nu®*, *ProMotion®*, *Seraquin®*, *Oste-O-Guard®*, *Caniflex®*, *Equi-Phar Flex®*, etc.

Glucosamine and chondroitin sulfate are considered nutritional supplements by the FDA. No standards have been accepted for potency, purity, safety or efficacy by regulatory bodies. Bioequivalence between products cannot be assumed and independent analysis has shown a wide variation in products.

HUMAN-LABELED PRODUCTS:

None as pharmaceuticals.

Revisions/References

Monograph revised/updated February 2014.

McCarthy, G., et al. (2007). Randomised double-blind, positive-controlled trial to assess the efficacy of glucosamine/chondroitin sulfate for the treatment of dogs with osteoarthritis. Vet J **174**(1): 54-61.
Moreau, M., et al. (2003). Clinical evaluation of a nutraceutical, carprofen and meloxicam for the treatment of dogs with osteoarthritis. Vet Rec **152**(11): 323-9.
Pearson, W. & M. Lindinger (2009). Low quality of evidence for glucosamine-based nutraceuticals in equine joint disease: Review of in vivo studies. Equine Veterinary Journal **41**(7): 706-12.
Welch, C. A., et al. (2012). Plasma Concentration of Glucosamine and Chondroitin Sulfate in Horses after an Oral Dose. Journal of Equine Veterinary Science **32**(1): 60-4.

Glutamine

(gloo-ta-meen)   L-Glutamine

Nutritional

Prescriber Highlights

► Amino acid that may be useful in preventing/treating GI epithelium damage or pancreatitis (exocrine function).
► Little documentation for efficacy, but adverse effects unlikely.

Uses/Indications

Glutamine has been used as a GI protectant and in an attempt to enhance GI healing in conditions where GI epithelium is damaged (Parvo enteritis, chemotherapy, etc.), pancreatitis, or when patients are under severe stress (critically ill). Animals that have an adequate dietary protein intake are unlikely to benefit from exogenously administered glutamine unless in catabolic or stressed states.

A study that evaluated the efficacy of glutamine supplementation in cats with methotrexate-induced enteritis found no difference between cats supplemented with glutamine and those that were not (Marks et al. 1999).

An oral human-labeled prescription product (*NutreStore®*) is indicated for treatment of Short Bowel Syndrome (SBS) in patients receiving specialized nutritional support when used in conjunction with a recombinant human growth hormone.

Pharmacology/Actions

Glutamine is a conditionally essential amino acid that is produced primarily in skeletal muscle and then released into the circulation.

Glutamine is required for proper function of the immune system, GI tract, kidneys, and liver. Glutamine also serves as a precursor for glutathione, glutamate, purines, pyrimidines, and other amino acids.

Glutamine's effects on the gastrointestinal tract are of interest for therapeutic use as an exogenously administered drug. When the body is under severe stress, it consumes more glutamine than it can produce and progressive muscle wasting occurs as it attempts to meet glutamine requirements. There is some evidence that glutamine may have a role in intestinal cell proliferation and determination. Glutamine is the preferred energy source for enterocytes and supplementation may improve function and repair of intestinal mucosa. When glutamine is depleted, intestinal epithelium can atrophy, ulcerate, or become necrotic. If in glutamine deficit secondary to liver dysfunction or catabolic states such as sepsis, translocation of gram-negative bacteria from the gut may occur and expose the liver to increased amounts of endotoxin. In patients undergoing cancer chemotherapy or radiotherapy, diminished glutamine levels in the gastrointestinal tract can cause increased GI toxicity. Supplementation of exogenous glutamine may help protect the GI from these effects.

Pharmacokinetics

Pharmacokinetic data for domestic animals was not located. In healthy humans, peak levels occur about 30 minutes after administration.

Contraindications/Precautions/Warnings

Because it is partially metabolized into ammonia and glutamate, use with caution in patients with severe hepatic insufficiency, severe behavior disorders or epilepsy.

Adverse Effects

Glutamine is well tolerated when used orally or intravenously. Potentially, it may have some CNS effects at high dosages.

Reproductive/Nursing Safety

There is insufficient data available documenting the safe use of glutamine during pregnancy or nursing.

Overdosage/Acute Toxicity

Overdosages are unlikely to be harmful. Doses of up to 40 grams per day IV have been tolerated in humans without ill effects. Because glutamine is partially metabolized to ammonia, patients with hepatic insufficiency may be adversely affected.

Drug Interactions

The following drug interactions have either been reported or are theoretical in humans or animals receiving glutamine and may be of in veterinary patients. Unless otherwise noted, use together is not necessarily contraindicated, but weigh the potential risks and perform additional monitoring when appropriate.

■ **ANTICONVULSANT MEDICATIONS:** Glutamine could potentially affect the efficacy of antiseizure medications (**phenobarbital**, **potassium bromide**, etc.). It is partially converted into glutamate, which can act as an excitatory neurotransmitter. This interaction is not well documented.

■ **LACTULOSE:** Theoretically, glutamine may antagonize the effects of lactulose in patients with hepatic encephalopathy.

Laboratory Considerations

■ Glutamine may increase **serum ammonia** or **glutamate** levels.

Doses

■ **DOGS & CATS:**

For adjunctive treatment of GI inflammatory conditions (extra-label): Dosages are not well established. Anecdotally, 0.5 grams/kg per day have been recommended. This is usually divided and given 2-3 times per day either in food or in drinking water.

Monitoring

- Efficacy.

Client Information

- Can be mixed with food if animal is able to eat; otherwise powder can be mixed into drinking water.
- Normally this drug does not cause side effects.

Chemistry/Synonyms

Glutamine is an aliphatic amino acid. It occurs as white crystals or crystalline powder and is soluble in water and practically insoluble in alcohol.

Glutamine may also be known as: glutamic acid, GLN, glutamate, glutaminate, levoglutamide, levoglutamine, L-glutamic acid, L-glutamic acid 5-amide, l-glutamine, L-glutamine, and Q.

Storage/Stability

Glutamine tablets and powder should be stored in tight containers at room temperature. When mixed into water at usual pH (6-8), glutamine has a degradation rate of less than 2% per day (Khan et al. 1991).

Compatibility/Compounding Considerations

When purchased as powder for mixing in water, a fresh mixture should be prepared daily.

Dosage Forms/Regulatory Status

VETERINARY-LABELED PRODUCTS: NONE.

HUMAN-LABELED PRODUCTS:

Glutamine is considered a nutrient. There is a 5 gram powder packet product *NutreStore®* that is labeled as a prescription drug and has FDA-approved labeling. Glutamine may be purchased without prescription as L-glutamine 500 mg tablets or capsules, glutamine powder in 5 or 10 gram packets. It may also be found as glutamic acid in 500 mg tablets or powder. Glutamic acid is rapidly degraded in the body to glutamine. Parenteral forms of glutamate may be available in other countries.

Revisions/References

Monograph revised/updated February 2014.

Khan, K. & M. Elia (1991). Factors Affecting the Stability of L-Glutamine in Solution Clinical Nutrition **10**(4): 186-92.

Marks, S., et al. (1999). Effects of glutamine supplementation of an an amino acid-based purified diet on intestinal mucosal integrity in cats with methotrexate-induced enteritis. Am J Vet Res **60**(6): 755-73.

Glyburide

(glye-byoor-ide)   DiaBeta®, Micronase®

Sulfonylurea Antidiabetic Agent

Prescriber Highlights

▶ Human oral antidiabetic agent (Type II) that may be useful in cats.

▶ Glipizide used more often when oral hypoglycemics are tried; glyburide may be useful if glipizide unavailable or if once a day dosing is important.

▶ Contraindications: Severe burns, severe trauma, severe infection, diabetic coma or other hypoglycemic conditions, major surgery, ketosis, ketoacidosis or other significant acidotic conditions.

▶ Caution: Untreated adrenal or pituitary insufficiency; thyroid, renal, or hepatic function impairment; prolonged vomiting; high fever; malnourishment or debilitated condition.

▶ Adverse Effects: <u>Cats</u>: GI (*i.e.*, vomiting), hypoglycemia, liver toxicity.

▶ Drug interactions.

▶ Do not confuse glipizide, glimepiride & glyburide.

Uses/Indications

Glyburide is an alternative oral treatment for non-insulin dependent diabetes mellitus (NIDDM) in cats, particularly if glipizide is unavailable or if twice daily administration of glipizide is not tolerated (by cat or owner). Insulin therapy for cats with diabetes is generally preferred over oral treatments.

Pharmacology/Actions

Like glipizide and other oral sulfonylureas, glyburide lowers blood glucose concentrations in both diabetic and normal patients. While it is unknown how glyburide precisely lowers glucose, it initially stimulates secretion of endogenous functional beta cells in the pancreas. It also may enhance insulin activity at post receptor sites and reduce basal hepatic glucose production that may explain its effectiveness with long-term administration.

Pharmacokinetics

Glyburide appears to be well absorbed but bioavailability data is lacking. Food apparently does not have an effect on the absorptive characteristics of the drug. Glyburide is distributed throughout the body, including into the brain and across the placenta. Glyburide is apparently completely metabolized, presumably in the liver. Metabolites are excreted in both the feces and urine. While its elimination half-life in cats is not known, once a day dosing appears to be effective in cats with NIDDM.

Contraindications/Precautions/Warnings

Oral antidiabetic agents are considered contraindicated with the following conditions: severe burns, severe trauma, severe infection, diabetic coma or other hypoglycemic conditions, major surgery, ketosis, ketoacidosis or other significant acidotic conditions. Glyburide should only be used when its potential benefits outweigh its risks in patients with untreated adrenal or pituitary insufficiency; thyroid, renal, or hepatic function impairment; prolonged vomiting; high fever; malnourishment or in debilitated condition.

Some patients with type II diabetes may have their disease complicated by the production of excessive amounts of cortisol or growth hormone that may antagonize insulin's effects. These causes should be ruled out before initiating oral antidiabetic therapy.

Do not confuse glyBURIDE with glipiZIDE or gliMEPIRIDE.

Adverse Effects

Experience with glyburide is limited in veterinary medicine. Hypoglycemia, vomiting, icterus, and increased ALT (SGPT) levels are all potentially possible. Should toxicity develop, reinstitution of drug therapy may be attempted at a lower dosage after clinical signs resolve.

Other adverse effects that are possible (noted in humans) include: allergic skin reactions, arthralgia, bone marrow suppression, or cholestatic jaundice.

Glyburide may not be effective in cats demonstrating insulin resistance.

Reproductive/Nursing Safety

In humans, the FDA categorizes this drug as category C for use during pregnancy (*Animal studies have shown an adverse effect on the fetus, but there are no adequate studies in humans; or there are no animal reproduction studies and no adequate studies in humans.*)

It is unknown if glyburide is excreted in milk.

Overdosage/Acute Toxicity

Profound hypoglycemia is the greatest concern after an overdose. In humans, severe hypoglycemia has occurred at relatively low dosages. Gut emptying protocols should be employed when warranted. Because its half-life is longer than glipizide, prolonged hypoglycemia may occur and blood glucose monitoring and treatment with parenteral glucose may be required for several days. Massive overdoses may also require additional monitoring (blood gases, serum electrolytes) and supportive therapy.

Drug Interactions

The following drug interactions have either been reported or are theoretical in humans or animals receiving glyburide and may be of in veterinary patients. Unless otherwise noted, use together is not necessarily contraindicated, but weigh the potential risks and perform additional monitoring when appropriate.

- **ALCOHOL**: A disulfiram-like reaction (anorexia, nausea, vomiting) is possible.
- **ANTIFUNGALS, AZOLE (ketoconazole, itraconazole, fluconazole)**: May increase plasma levels of glyburide.
- **BETA-BLOCKERS**: May potentiate hypoglycemic effect.
- **CHLORAMPHENICOL**: May displace glyburide from plasma proteins.
- **CIMETIDINE**: May potentiate hypoglycemic effect.
- **CIPROFLOXACIN (and potentially other quinolones)**: May potentiate hypoglycemic effect of glyburide.
- **CORTICOSTEROIDS**: May reduce efficacy.
- **DIURETICS, THIAZIDE**: May reduce hypoglycemic efficacy.
- **ISONIAZID**: May reduce hypoglycemic efficacy.
- **MAO INHIBITORS**: May potentiate hypoglycemic effect.
- **NIACIN**: May reduce hypoglycemic efficacy.
- **PHENOTHIAZINES**: May reduce hypoglycemic efficacy.
- **PHENYTOIN**: May reduce hypoglycemic efficacy.
- **PROBENECID**: May potentiate hypoglycemic effect.
- **SULFONAMIDES**: May displace glyburide from plasma proteins.
- **SYMPATHOMIMETIC AGENTS**: May reduce hypoglycemic efficacy.
- **THYROID AGENTS**: May reduce hypoglycemic effect.
- **WARFARIN**: May displace glyburide from plasma proteins.

Doses

- **CATS:**

  For non-insulin dependent diabetes mellitus (extra-label): There is little information published on using this medication in cats, and evidence to support clinical use is very weak. Two anecdotal dosage suggestions have been noted:
  a) Initial dose at 0.625 mg (1/2 of a 1.25 mg tablet) per cat PO once daily. (Nelson 2000)
  b) If cat is generally well, weight loss is mild, is not ketoacidotic, and does not have peripheral neuropathy, may try glyburide at: 2.5 mg per cat PO twice a day. (Daminet 2003)

Monitoring

- Weekly exams during first month of therapy including PE, body weight, urine glucose/ketones and several blood glucose exams.
- Adverse effects (vomiting, icterus), and occasional liver enzymes and CBC.

Client Information

- May be useful for treating diabetes in cats; limited experience in veterinary medicine.
- Give about the same time each day. May be given with or without food. If your animal vomits or acts sick after getting it on an empty stomach, give with food or small treat to see if this helps. If vomiting continues, contact your veterinarian.
- Watch for signs of blood sugar that's too low (hypoglycemia; uncommon): Seizures (convulsions), collapsing/fainting, rear leg weakness or paralysis, muscle twitching, unsteadiness, lack of energy, or depression. If any of these are seen, contact your veterinarian right away.

- Has not been used in many cats so other side effects could occur. Report anything unusual to your veterinarian.

Chemistry/Synonyms

An oral sulfonylurea antidiabetic agent, glyburide occurs as a white or nearly white, odorless or almost odorless, crystalline powder. As pH increases, solubility increases. At a pH of 4, solubility in water is about 4 micrograms/mL and at pH of 9, solubility is 600 micrograms/mL. Glyburide has a pKa of 6.8.

Glyburide may also be known as: glibenclamide, glibenclamidum, glybenclamide, glybenzcyclamide, HB-419, and U-26452; many trade names are available.

Storage/Stability

Glyburide oral tablets should be stored in well-closed containers at room temperature.

Compatibility/Compounding Considerations

No specific information noted.

Dosage Forms/Regulatory Status

VETERINARY-LABELED PRODUCTS: NONE.

HUMAN-LABELED PRODUCTS:

Glyburide Oral Tablets: 1.25 mg, 2.5 mg, & 5 mg; micronized tablets: 1.5 mg, 3 mg, 4.5 mg & 6 mg; *Glynase® PresTab, DiaBeta®*; generic; (Rx)

Fixed dose combinations of glyburide and metformin are also available.

Revisions/References

Monograph revised/updated February 2014.

Daminet, S. (2003). Canine and Feline Diabetes Mellitus. Proceedings: World Small Animal Veterinary Assoc. World Congress. accessed via Veterinary Information Network; vin.com

Nelson, R. (2000). Diabetes Mellitus. *Textbook of Veterinary Internal Medicine: Diseases of the Dog and Cat*. S. Ettinger and E. Feldman. Philadelphia, WB Saunders. 2: 1438-60.

Glycerin, Oral

(gli-ser-in)   Glycerol, Osmoglyn®

Osmotic Agent

Prescriber Highlights

▶ Oral osmotic that reduces intraocular & CSF pressure.
▶ Contraindications: Patients with known hypersensitivity, anuria (well established), severe dehydration, severe cardiac decompensation, acute pulmonary edema. Caution: Hypovolemia, cardiac disease, or diabetes.
▶ Adverse Effects: Vomiting (most common).

Uses/Indications

Oral glycerin is used primarily for the short-term reduction of IOP in small animals with acute glaucoma. It may also be considered for use to reduce increased CSF pressure.

The IOP-lowering effect of glycerin may be more variable than with mannitol, but since it may be given orally, it may be more advantageous to use in certain cases.

Pharmacology/Actions

Glycerin in therapeutic oral doses increases the osmotic pressure of plasma so that water from extracellular spaces is drawn into the blood. This can decrease intraocular pressure (IOP). The amount of decrease in IOP is dependent upon the dose of glycerin, and the cause and extent of increased IOP. Glycerin also decreases extracellular water content from other tissues and can cause dehydration and decreased CSF pressure.

Pharmacokinetics

Glycerin is rapidly absorbed from the GI tract and decreases in IOP can be seen within 30 minutes; peak serum levels generally occur within 90 minutes and maximum decreases in IOP usually occur within an hour of dosing and persist for 5-12 hours. Glycerin is distributed throughout the blood and is primarily metabolized by the liver. About 10% of the drug is excreted unchanged in the urine. Serum half-life in humans is about 30-45 minutes.

Contraindications/Precautions/Warnings

Glycerin is contraindicated in patients hypersensitive to it. It is also contraindicated in patients with well-established anuria, that are severely dehydrated, severely cardiac decompensated, or with frank or impending acute pulmonary edema.

Glycerin should be used with caution in animals when the blood:ocular barrier is not intact (hyphema, uveitis), and in those with hypovolemia, cardiac disease, or diabetes. One reference states that glycerine is contraindicated in dogs with diabetes mellitus, dehydration, and cardiac or renal disease (Reinstein et al. 2009). Another states that heart failure is a contraindication and use should be avoided in patients with chronic renal failure or compromised renal function (Pickett 2009). Acute urinary retention should be avoided during the preoperative period.

Adverse Effects

Vomiting after dosing is the most common adverse effect seen with glycerin use. In humans, headache, nausea, thirst, and diarrhea have also been reported.

Reproductive/Nursing Safety

The safety of this drug in pregnant animals is unknown; use only when potential benefits outweigh the risks of therapy. In humans, the FDA categorizes this drug as category *C* for use during pregnancy (*Animal studies have shown an adverse effect on the fetus, but there are no adequate studies in humans; or there are no animal reproduction studies and no adequate studies in humans.*)

No specific information on glycerin was located for lactation safety.

Overdosage/Acute Toxicity

No specific information was located, but cardiac arrhythmias, non-ketotic hyperosmolar coma, and severe dehydration have been reported with the drug.

Drug Interactions

The following drug interactions have either been reported or are theoretical in humans or animals receiving glycerin and may be of in veterinary patients. Unless otherwise noted, use together is not necessarily contraindicated, but weigh the potential risks and perform additional monitoring when appropriate.

- **CARBONIC ANHYDRASE INHIBITORS** (*e.g.*, **acetazolamide, dichlorphenamide**): Concomitant administration of carbonic anhydrase inhibitors or topical miotic agents may prolong the IOP-reducing effects of glycerin.
- **MIOTIC AGENTS, TOPICAL:** Concomitant administration topical miotic agents may prolong the IOP-reducing effects of glycerin.

Doses

- **DOGS & CATS:**

  For acute glaucoma as an "emergency drug" in place of aqueous centesis to rapidly reduce IOP (extra-label): Most recommend using 1 – 2 grams/kg PO. This would be approximately 1.1 – 2.2 mL/kg of the 90% solution. To reduce the risk for vomiting, diluting to a 45-50% concentration with water, milk or ice cream is often recommended. In patients where it would not be contraindicated, withholding water or fluids for 3-4 hours after administering can increase efficacy. Adapted from (Herring 2003), (Reinstein et al. 2009), (Collins 2006), (Pickett 2009)

Monitoring

- IOP.
- Urine output.
- Hydration status.

Chemistry/Synonyms

A trihydric alcohol, glycerin occurs as clear, sweet-tasting, syrupy, hygroscopic liquid that has a characteristic odor. It is miscible with water and alcohol, but not miscible in oils. Glycerin solutions are neutral to litmus.

Glycerin may also be known as: E422, glycerol, glicerol, glycerin, glycerine, and glycerolum; many trade names are available.

Storage/Stability

Glycerin oral solution should be stored in tight containers at room temperature; protect from freezing.

Compatibility/Compounding Considerations

90% glycerin USP can be mixed into water, milk or ice cream to reduce the potential for vomiting and improve palatability. To convert 90% glycerin to a 50% concentration, 1 mL of 90% glycerin can be diluted to a 50% concentration by the addition of 0.8 mL of diluent. Practically, many clinicians will dilute with equal parts of diluent to obtain a 45% concentration.

Dosage Forms/Regulatory Status

VETERINARY-LABELED PRODUCTS: NONE FOR SYSTEMIC USE.

HUMAN-LABELED PRODUCTS:

The 50% oral solution that was approved for oral use has been discontinued and there are no commercial approved products being marketed. USP glycerin 90% could be used for oral use in small animals (see doses above).

Glycerin is also available in a topical ophthalmic solution and as suppositories or liquid for rectal laxative use.

Revisions/References

Monograph revised/updated February 2014.

Collins, B. (2006). Update for glaucoma. Proceedings; Western Vet Conf. accessed via Veterinary Information Network; vin.com

Herring, I. (2003). Glaucoma. *Handbook of Small Animal Practice, 4th Ed.* R. Morgan, R. Bright and M. Swartout. Phila., Saunders: 988-94.

Pickett, J. (2009). The canine glaucomas. Proceedings: ABVP. accessed via Veterinary Information Network; vin.com

Reinstein, S. L., et al. (2009). Canine Glaucoma: Medical and Surgical Treatment Options. Compendium-Continuing Education for Veterinarians **31**(10): 454-8.

Glyceryl Guaiacolate; GG – see Guaifenesin

Glycopyrrolate

(glye-koe-pye-roe-late)   Robinul®

Anticholinergic (Antimuscarinic)

Prescriber Highlights

▶ Synthetic antimuscarinic agent similar to atropine available both orally & parenterally; used for a variety of indications (bradycardia, premed, antidote, etc.).

▶ Contraindicated in conditions where anticholinergic effects would be detrimental (*e.g.*, narrow angle glaucoma, tachycardias, ileus, urinary obstruction, etc.). Not recommended for treating bradycardia secondary to dexmedetomidine.

▶ Adverse effects are dose related & anticholinergic in nature, including: dry secretions; initial bradycardia, then tachycardia; slowing of gut & urinary tract motility; mydriasis/cycloplegia.

▶ Drug interactions.

Uses/Indications

Glycopyrrolate injection is FDA-approved for use in dogs and cats. The FDA-approved indication for these species is as a preanesthetic anticholinergic agent, but today it is generally not used routinely in dogs or cats. Glycopyrrolate may be of benefit in young animals when cardiac output is dependent on heart rate or when potent opioids are used. The drug is also used in an extra-label manner to treat sinus bradycardia, sinoatrial arrest, and incomplete AV block, where anticholinergic therapy may be beneficial. When cholinergic agents such as neostigmine or pyridostigmine are used to reverse neuromuscular blockade due to non-depolarizing muscle relaxants, glycopyrrolate may be administered simultaneously to prevent the peripheral muscarinic effects of the cholinergic agent. A study in horses, suggested that glycopyrrolate was superior to reducing the cholinergic adverse effects of imidocarb (Donnellan et al. 2013).

Pharmacology/Actions

An antimuscarinic with similar actions as atropine, glycopyrrolate is a quaternary ammonium compound and unlike atropine, does not cross appreciably into the CNS. Therefore CNS adverse effects should not be exhibited to the same extent. For further information, refer to the atropine monograph.

Pharmacokinetics

Quaternary anticholinergic agents are not completely absorbed after oral administration, but quantitative data reporting the rate and extent of absorption of glycopyrrolate is not available. In dogs, following IV administration, the onset of action is generally within one minute. After IM or SC administration, peak effects occur approximately 30-45 minutes post injection. The vagolytic effects persist for 2-3 hours and the antisialagogue (reduced salivation) effects persist for up to 7 hours. After oral administration, the anticholinergic effects of glycopyrrolate may persist for 8-12 hours.

Little information is available regarding glycopyrrolate's distribution characteristics. Being a quaternary ammonium compound it is completely ionized and therefore has poor lipid solubility and does not readily penetrate into the CNS or eye. Glycopyrrolate crosses the placenta only marginally; it is unknown if it is excreted into milk.

For horses, the pharmacokinetics of intravenous glycopyrrolate have been described. After 1 mg (1.72 – 1.93 microgram/kg) was given IV, the following median values were reported: Volume of distribution (SS): 1.43 L/kg; clearance: 14.2 mL/kg/min; terminal half-life: 7.4 hours. Plasma clearance of the drug in horses appears to be similar to hepatic blood flow (Rumpler et al. 2011).

In humans, glycopyrrolate is eliminated rapidly from the serum after IV administration and virtually no drug remains in the serum 30 minutes to 3 hours after dosing. Only a small amount is metabolized; the majority is eliminated unchanged in the feces and urine.

Contraindications/Precautions/Warnings

The veterinary product label states the drug is contraindicated in dogs and cats hypersensitive to glycopyrrolate and that it should not be used in pregnant animals.

Antimuscarinic agents should be used with extreme caution in patients with known or suspected GI infections. Atropine or other antimuscarinic agents can decrease GI motility and prolong retention of the causative agent(s) or toxin(s) resulting in prolonged clinical signs. Antimuscarinic agents must also be used with extreme caution in patients with autonomic neuropathy. Anticholinergic agents such as atropine or glycopyrrolate are not recommended to treat bradycardias secondary to dexmedetomidine; the reversal agent atipamezole is preferred.

Antimuscarinic agents should be used with caution in patients with hepatic or renal disease, geriatric or pediatric patients, hyperthyroidism, hypertension, hypertrophic cardiomyopathy/CHF, tachyarrhythmias, prostatic hypertrophy, or esophageal reflux. These drugs can produce sinus tachycardia and predispose hypotensive patients to cardiac arrhythmias (including ventricular fibrillation).

Antimuscarinics (e.g., atropine, glycopyrrolate) are not routinely administered to reptiles, as it can cause increased viscosity of respiratory tract secretions with resultant risks for airway obstruction or endotracheal tube occlusion.

Adverse Effects

With the exceptions of rare CNS adverse effects and being slightly less arrhythmogenic, glycopyrrolate can be expected to have a similar adverse effect profile as atropine; and are generally dose-related extensions of the drug's pharmacologic effects. At usual doses, effects tend to be mild in relatively healthy patients. The more severe effects listed tend to occur with high or toxic doses. GI effects can include dry mouth (xerostomia), increased viscosity of secretions, dysphagia, constipation, vomiting, and thirst. GU effects may include urinary retention or hesitancy. Ophthalmic effects including blurred vision, pupil dilation, cycloplegia, and photophobia are possible, but less likely than with atropine. Cardiovascular effects include sinus tachycardia (at higher doses), increased myocardial work and oxygen consumption, bradycardia (initially, or at very low doses), hypertension, hypotension, arrhythmias (ectopic complexes), and circulatory failure.

The veterinary drug label only lists mydriasis, tachycardia, and xerostomia as adverse effects in dogs and cats at labeled doses.

Reproductive/Nursing Safety

While the veterinary label states that the drug should not be used during pregnancy, it likely does not pose much risk as it only marginally crosses the placenta. For humans, the FDA categorizes this drug as category *B* for use during pregnancy (*Animal studies have not yet demonstrated risk to the fetus, but there are no adequate studies in pregnant women; or animal studies have shown an adverse effect, but adequate studies in pregnant women have not demonstrated a risk to the fetus in the first trimester of pregnancy, and there is no evidence of risk in later trimesters.*) In a separate system evaluating the safety of drugs in canine and feline pregnancy (Papich 1989), this drug is categorized as class: *B* (*Safe for use if used cautiously. Studies in laboratory animals may have uncovered some risk, but these drugs appear to be safe in dogs and cats or these drugs are safe if they are not administered when the animal is near term.*)

No specific lactation safety information was found; however, it is unlikely to be excreted into milk in substantial quantities because of its quaternary structure.

Overdosage/Acute Toxicity

In dogs, the LD_{50} for glycopyrrolate is reported to be 25 mg/kg IV. Doses of 2 mg/kg IV daily for 5 days per week for 4 weeks demonstrated no signs of toxicity. In the cat, the LD_{50} after IM injection is 283 mg/kg. Because of its quaternary structure, it would be expected that minimal CNS effects would occur after an overdose of glycopyrrolate when compared to atropine. See the information listed in the atropine monograph for more information.

Drug Interactions

Glycopyrrolate would be expected to have a similar drug interaction profile as atropine. The following drug interactions have either been reported or are theoretical in humans or animals receiving atropine or glycopyrrolate and may be of in veterinary patients. Unless otherwise noted, use together is not necessarily contraindicated, but weigh the potential risks and perform additional monitoring when appropriate.

- **AMITRAZ:** Glycopyrrolate may aggravate some signs seen with amitraz toxicity leading to hypertension and further inhibition of peristalsis.
- **ANTACIDS:** May decrease PO absorption; give oral glycopyrrolate at least 1 hour prior to oral antacids.

- **BETA-BLOCKERS:** Glycopyrrolate may increase oral bioavailability.
- **DIGOXIN (tablets):** Glycopyrrolate may increase serum digoxin levels; use oral liquid.
- **METOCLOPRAMIDE:** Atropine and its derivatives may antagonize the actions of metoclopramide.
- **POTASSIUM CHLORIDE, ORAL (solid dosage forms):** May significantly increase the amount of potassium absorbed.

The following drugs may enhance the activity or toxicity of glycopyrrolate:

- **AMANTADINE**
- **ANTICHOLINERGIC AGENTS (OTHER)**
- **ANTICHOLINERGIC MUSCLE RELAXANTS**
- **ANTIHISTAMINES** (*e.g.,* diphenhydramine)
- **MEPERIDINE**
- **PHENOTHIAZINES**
- **PROCAINAMIDE**
- **PRIMIDONE**
- **TRICYCLIC ANTIDEPRESSANTS** (*e.g.,* amitriptyline, clomipramine)

Doses

- **DOGS:**

As an adjunct to anesthesia:

Labeled-dose (FDA-approved): 0.011 mg/kg IV, IM, or SC. (Package Insert; *Robinul®-V*)

Extra-label: Not routinely used, but may be of benefit in pediatric patients or when using potent opioids. When used, it is usually as part of a premed with 0.01 mg/kg IV, IM, or SC most commonly recommended, but dosages as low as 0.003 mg/kg have been noted at the low range.

As a vagolytic for bradyarrhythmias (extra-label): To determine if increased vagal tone is contributing to a bradyarrhythmias: 0.01 mg/kg IV. To treat vagally-induced bradyarrhythmias it is usually dosed at 0.005 – 0.01 mg/kg IV. If given IM or SC, slightly higher dosages (up to 0.02 mg/kg) may be considered.

For adjunctive treatment of muscarinic signs associated with carbamate or organophosphate intoxication (extra-label): 0.01 – 0.02 mg/kg IV; repeat as necessary.

- **CATS:**

As an adjunct to anesthesia:

Labeled-dose (FDA-approved): 0.011 mg/kg IM, for maximum effect give 15 minutes prior to anesthetic administration 0.011 mg/kg IV, IM, or SC. (Package Insert; *Robinul®-V*)

Extra-label: Not routinely used, but may be of benefit in pediatric patients or when using potent opioids. When used, it is usually as part of a premed with 0.01 mg/kg IV, IM, or SC most commonly recommended, but dosages as low as 0.003 mg/kg have been noted at the low range.

As a vagolytic for bradyarrhythmias (extra-label): To determine if increased vagal tone is contributing to a bradyarrhythmias: 0.01 mg/kg IV; to treat vagally-induced bradyarrhythmias it is usually dosed at 0.005 – 0.01 mg/kg IV. If given IM or SC, slightly higher dosages (up to 0.02 mg/kg) may be considered.

For adjunctive treatment of muscarinic signs associated with carbamate or organophosphate intoxication (extra-label): 0.01 – 0.02 mg/kg IV; repeat as necessary.

- **FERRETS:**

As a premed (extra-label): 0.01 – 0.02 mg/kg IM, SC or IV.

- **RABBITS/RODENTS/SMALL MAMMALS:**

As a preanesthetic (extra-label): **Rodents:** 0.01 – 0.02 mg/kg SC or IM. **Rabbits:** 0.01 – 0.1 mg/kg IM or SC. As part of an injectable anesthesia protocol in rabbits: acepromazine (0.2 mg/kg), plus oxymorphone (0.1 mg/kg), plus glycopyrrolate (0.01 mg/kg) IM. (Bennett 2009)

As an adjunctive drug for CPR in rabbits: A retrospective study found the median dosage used was 0.01 mg/kg IV. (Buckley et al. 2011)

- **HORSES:** (NOTE: ARCI UCGFS CLASS 3 DRUG)

For treatment of bradyarrhythmias (extra-label): 0.005 – 0.01 mg/kg (5 – 10 micrograms/kg) IV is usually recommended, but a lower end of the dosing range (0.0025 mg/kg) has been noted in some references.

To control muscarinic adverse effects associated with imidocarb therapy (extra-label): 0.0025 mg/kg IV. (Donnellan et al. 2003), (Donnellan et al. 2013)

- **REPTILES:**

For bradycardia (prolonged or profound) associated with anesthesia (extra-label): 0.01 mg/kg IM, IV or IC (intracoelemic). (Mehler 2009)

Monitoring

- Dependent on route of administration, dose, and reason for use. See the atropine monograph for more information.

Client Information

- Injectable glycopyrrolate administration is best performed by professional staff where adequate cardiac monitoring is available.
- If animal is receiving glycopyrrolate tablets, allow animal free access to water and encourage drinking if dry mouth is a problem. Can be given with or without food. If your animal vomits or acts sick after getting it on an empty stomach, give with food or small treat to see if this helps. If vomiting continues, contact your veterinarian.

Chemistry/Synonyms

A synthetic quaternary ammonium antimuscarinic agent, glycopyrrolate occurs as a bitter-tasting, practically odorless, white, crystalline powder with a melting range of 193-198°C. One gram is soluble in 20 mL of water; 30 mL of alcohol. The commercially available injection is adjusted to a pH of 2-3 and contains 0.9% benzyl alcohol as a preservative.

Glycopyrrolate may also be known as: glycopyrronium bromide, AHR-504, *Acpan®*, *Gastrodyn®*, *Glycostigmin®*, and *Robinul®*.

Storage/Stability

Glycopyrrolate tablets should be stored in tight containers and both the injection and tablets should be stored at room temperature (15-30°C).

Glycopyrrolate is stable under ordinary conditions of light and temperature. It is most stable in solution at an acidic pH and undergoes ester hydrolysis at pH's above 6.

Compatibility/Compounding Considerations

Although stability information was not located: glycopyrrolate injection has been mixed in syringes with acepromazine, buprenorphine, morphine and ketamine.

Glycopyrrolate injection is physically **stable** in the following IV solutions: D5W, D5/half normal saline, Ringer's injection, and normal saline. Glycopyrrolate may be administered via the tubing of an IV running lactated Ringer's, but rapid hydrolysis will occur if it is added to an IV bag of LRS. The following drugs are reportedly physically **compatible** with glycopyrrolate: atropine sulfate, chlorpromazine HCl, codeine phosphate, diphenhydramine HCl, hydromorphone, hydroxyzine HCl, lidocaine HCl, meperidine HCl, morphine sulfate, neostigmine methylsulfate, oxymorphone HCl, procaine HCl, prochlorperazine HCl, promazine HCl, promethazine HCl, pyridostigmine Br, and scopolamine HBr.

The following drugs are reportedly physically **incompatible** with glycopyrrolate: chloramphenicol sodium succinate, dexamethasone sodium phosphate, diazepam, dimenhydrinate, methohexital sodium, methylprednisolone sodium succinate, pentazocine lactate, pentobarbital sodium, sodium bicarbonate, and thiopental sodium. Other alkaline drugs (*e.g.*, thiamylal) would also be **expected to be incompatible** with glycopyrrolate. Compatibility is dependent upon factors such as pH, concentration, temperature, and diluent used; consult specialized references for more specific information.

Dosage Forms/Regulatory Status

VETERINARY-LABELED PRODUCTS:

Glycopyrrolate for Injection: 0.2 mg/mL; (Rx). While approved products for dogs and cats are still listed in the FDA-Green Book, they may not be commercially marketed.

The ARCI (Racing Commissioners International) has designated this drug as a class 3 substance. See the appendix for more information.

HUMAN-LABELED PRODUCTS:

Glycopyrrolate Tablets: 1 mg & 2 mg; *Robinul*® & *Robinul Forte*®, generic; (Rx)

Glycopyrrolate Oral Solution: 1 mg/5 ml (0.2 mg/mL); *Cuvposa*®; (Rx)

Glycopyrrolate Injection: 0.2 mg/mL in 1 mL, 2 mL, 5 mL, & 20 mL vials; *Robinul*®, generic; (Rx)

Revisions/References

Monograph revised/updated February 2014.

Bennett, R. (2009). Small Mammal Anesthesia--Rabbits and Rodents. Proceedings: ACVC. accessed via Veterinary Information Network; vin.com

Buckley, G. J., et al. (2011). Cardiopulmonary Resuscitation in Hospitalized Rabbits: 15 cases. Journal of Exotic Pet Medicine **20**(1): 46-50.

Donnellan, C., et al. (2003). Effect of atropine and glycopyrrolate in ameliorating the side effects caused by imidocarb diproprionate administration in horses. Proceedings: ACVIM Forum. accessed via Veterinary Information Network; vin.com

Donnellan, C. M. B., et al. (2013). Comparison of glycopyrrolate and atropine in ameliorating the adverse effects of imidocarb dipropionate in horses. Equine Veterinary Journal **45**(5): 625-9.

Mehler, S. (2009). Anaesthesia and care of the reptile. Proceedings: BSAVA. accessed via Veterinary Information Network; vin.com

Rumpler, M. J., et al. (2011). Pharmacokinetics of glycopyrrolate following intravenous administration in the horse. J. Vet. Pharmacol. Ther. **34**(6): 605-8.

Gonadorelin

(goe-nad-oe-rell-in)   GnRH

Hormonal Agent

Prescriber Highlights

▶ Hypothalamic hormone used to treat ovarian cysts & other reproductive disorders in a variety of species. In cattle, FDA restricts use for fixed time artificial insemination (FTAI) in combination with prostaglandins to specific approved products.

▶ Duration of action is very short (minutes).

▶ Contraindications & adverse effects: None reported.

▶ No slaughter or milk withdrawal when used as labeled.

Uses/Indications

Gonadorelin is indicated (FDA-approved) for the treatment of ovarian follicular cysts in cattle. Two products, *GONABreed*® and *Factrel*®, are approved with cloprostenol or dinoprost respectively to synchronize estrous cycles to allow for fixed time artificial insemination (FTAI) in lactating dairy cows and beef cows.

Additionally, gonadorelin has been used in cattle to reduce the time interval from calving to first ovulation and increase the number of ovulations within the first 3 months after calving. This may be particularly important in increasing fertility in cows with retained placenta.

In dogs, gonadorelin has been used experimentally to help diagnose reproductive disorders or to identify intact animals versus castrated ones by maximally stimulating FSH and LH production. It has also been used experimentally in dogs to induce estrus through pulsatile dosing. While apparently effective, specialized administration equipment is required for this method.

Gonadorelin has been used in cats as an alternate therapy to FSH or hCG to induce estrus in cats with prolonged anestrus.

In Europe, a synthetic analogue buserelin has been used in horses to stimulate cyclic estrus. Its efficacy rates poorly when compared to an artificial light program, however.

In human medicine, gonadorelin has been used for the diagnosis of hypothalamic-pituitary dysfunction, cryptorchidism, and depression secondary to prolonged severe stress.

Pharmacology/Actions

Gonadorelin is a synthetic form of GnRH and stimulates the production and release of FSH and LH from the anterior pituitary. Secretion of endogenous GnRH from the hypothalamus is thought to be controlled by several factors, including circulating sex hormones.

Gonadorelin causes a surge-like release of FSH and LH after a single injection. In cows and ewes, this can induce ovulation, but not in estrus mares. A constant infusion of gonadorelin will initially stimulate LH and FSH release, but after a period of time, levels will return to baseline.

Pharmacokinetics

After intravenous injection in pigs, gonadorelin is rapidly distributed to extracellular fluid, with a distribution half-life of about 2 minutes. The elimination half-life of gonadorelin is approximately 13 minutes in the pig.

After intravenous injection in humans, gonadorelin reportedly has a plasma half-life of only a few minutes. Within one hour, approximately half the dose is excreted in the urine as metabolites.

Contraindications/Precautions/Warnings

None are noted on the label.

Adverse Effects

No reported adverse reactions were located for this agent. Synthetically prepared gonadorelin should not cause any hypersensitivity reactions. This may not be the case with pituitary-obtained LH preparations or hCG.

Reproductive/Nursing Safety

In humans, the FDA categorizes this drug as category *B* for use during pregnancy (*Animal studies have not yet demonstrated risk to the fetus, but there are no adequate studies in pregnant women; or animal studies have shown an adverse effect, but adequate studies in pregnant women have not demonstrated a risk to the fetus in the first trimester of pregnancy, and there is no evidence of risk in later trimesters.*)

No specific lactation safety information was listed for this drug.

Overdosage/Acute Toxicity

In doses of up to 120 micrograms/kg, no untoward effects were noted in several species of test animals. Gonadorelin is unlikely to cause significant adverse effects after inadvertent overdosage.

Drug Interactions

▪ None noted.

Doses

▪ **DOGS:**

GnRH stimulation test to differentiate castration from cryptorchidism (extra-label): Take pre-sample, give 50 micrograms gonadorelin (GnRH) per dog IM, 2-3 hours later take post-injection sample. Castrated dogs have testosterone concentrations <0.1 ng/mL; GnRH does not stimulate testosterone production. (Pinto 2007)

GnRH stimulation test to determine if dog has retained testicle (extra-label): Take pre-sample, give gonadorelin 2.5 micrograms/kg IM (if very small dog use 25 micrograms total dose instead) and take second sample in 60-90 minutes. (Freshman 2009)

To increase libido in male dogs (extra-label): Anecdotally, 50 – 100 micrograms IM weekly for 4-6 weeks may improve libido. (Freshman 2002)

For cystic ovarian disease in bitches (extra-label): 3.3 micrograms/kg IM once daily for 3 days. An elevated progesterone level (>2 ng/mL) measured 1-2 weeks post treatment verifies success. (Purswell 1999)

■ **CATS:**

For infertility, reduced libido, testis descent in male cats (extra-label): 1 microgram/kg every 2-3 days. (Verstegen 2000)

To detect ovarian remnants in queens after ovariohysterectomy (extra-label): 25 micrograms per cat. A progesterone level (>1 ng/mL) measured 1-2 weeks post treatment verifies presence of ovarian tissue in the abdomen. (Purswell 1999)

■ **CATTLE:**

For the treatment of ovarian cysts in cattle (labeled dose; FDA-approved): 100 micrograms per cow IM or IV. (**Note:** *Factrel®* is labeled for IM use only).

For use with dinoprost tromethamine to synchronize estrous cycles to allow fixed-time artificial insemination (FTAI) in lactating dairy cows (labeled dose for *Factrel®*; FDA-approved— see FDA "Dear Dr." information in Dosage Forms): Administer 100 – 200 micrograms (2 – 4 mL; *Factrel®*) per cow IM at Day 0. Administer 25 mg dinoprost, (as dinoprost tromethamine) IM 6-8 days after the first dose of *Factrel®*. Administer a second dose (2 – 4 mL) of *Factrel®* 30-72 hours after the dinoprost. Perform FTAI 0-24 hours after the second dose of *Factrel®* or inseminate cows on detected estrus using standard herd practices. (Adapted from label; *Factrel®*)

For use with cloprostenol sodium to synchronize estrous cycles to allow fixed-time artificial insemination (FTAI) in lactating dairy cows (labeled dose for *GONABreed®*; FDA-approved—see FDA "Dear Dr." information in Dosage Forms): Administer 100 micrograms (1 mL; *GONABreed®*) per cow IV or IM at Day 0. Administer 500 micrograms cloprostenol (as cloprostenol sodium) IM 6-8 days after the first dose of *GONABreed®*. Administer a second dose (1 mL) of *GONABreed®* 3-72 hours after the cloprostenol. Perform FTAI 0-24 hours after the second dose of *GONABreed®* or inseminate cows on detected estrus using standard herd practices. (Adapted from label; *GONABreed®*)

Monitoring
■ Dependent on reason for use; efficacy.

Client Information
■ In small animals, gonadorelin is best administered by a veterinarian.

Chemistry/Synonyms
A hormone produced by the hypothalamus, gonadorelin is obtained from natural sources or is synthetically produced. It is a decapeptide that occurs as white or faintly yellowish-white powder. One gram is soluble in 25 mL of water or in 50 mL of methyl alcohol. 50 micrograms of gonadorelin acetate is approximately equivalent to 31 Units. The commercially available products in the United States are the diacetate decahydrate (*Cystorelin®*, others) and HCl (*Factrel®*) salts.

Gonadorelin may also be known as: follicle stimulating hormone-releasing factor, GnRH, gonadoliberin, gonadorelinum, gonadotrophin-releasing hormone, Hoe-471, LH/FSH-RF, LH/FSH-RH, LH-RF, LH-RH, luliberin, luteinising hormone-releasing factor, *Cryptocur®*, *Cystorelin®*, *Factrel®*, *Fertagyl®*, *Fertiral®*, *HRF®*, *Kryptocur®*, *LRH®*, *Luforan®*, *Luteoliberina®*, *Lutrefact®*, *Ovacyst®*, *Parlib®*, *Pulsti®*, *Relefact LH-RH®*, and *Stimu-LH®*.

Storage/Stability
The manufacturers recommend storing gonadorelin in the refrigerator (2-8°C). There is very little information available on the stability and compatibility of gonadorelin. Because bacterial contamination can inactivate the product, it has been recommended that multi-dose vials be used completely and as rapidly as possible.

Dosage Forms/Regulatory Status
VETERINARY-LABELED PRODUCTS:
Note: The FDA sent out a "Dear Dr. letter" to bovine veterinarians in 2013 that stated in part: "Six gonadorelin (GnRH) products are FDA-approved to treat cystic ovaries in dairy cows. Of these six products, only *Factrel®* (with dinoprost tromethamine) and *GONABreed®* (with cloprostenol sodium) are also FDA-approved for use in combination with another drug for synchronizing estrous cycles in lactating dairy cows. Other than the two combinations (*Factrel®* with dinoprost tromethamine; *GONABreed®* with cloprostenol sodium), it is illegal to use GnRH products in combination with another drug for estrous synchrony".

Gonadorelin (diacetate tetrahydrate) for Injection: 50 mcg/mL (gonadorelin), 2 mL single-use or 10 mL multi-dose vials; *Cystorelin®*, *Fertagyl®*, *Fertalin®*, *Ovacyst®*; (Rx). FDA-approved for use in dairy cattle for cystic ovaries. There are no withdrawal times required for either milk or slaughter.

Gonadorelin HCl Solution for Injection: 50 micrograms/mL (gonadorelin) in 2 mL single-use, and 20 mL multi-dose vials; *Factrel®*; (Rx). FDA-approved for the treatment of ovarian follicular cysts in cattle and in combination with dinoprost tromethamine to synchronize estrous cycles to allow fixed-time artificial insemination in lactating dairy cows. No withdrawal period required.

Gonadorelin Acetate 100 micrograms/mL (gonadorelin) in 20 mL & 100 mL multidose vials; *GONABreed®*; (Rx). FDA-approved for the treatment of ovarian follicular cysts in dairy cattle and in combination with cloprostenol sodium to synchronize estrous cycles to allow for fixed time artificial insemination in lactating dairy and beef cows. No withdrawal period required.

HUMAN-LABELED PRODUCTS:
Gonadorelin HCl Powder for Injection (lyophilized): 100 micrograms/vial & 500 micrograms/vial (as hydrochloride) with 2 mL sterile diluent; *Factrel®*; (Rx)

Revisions/References
Monograph revised/updated February 2014.

Freshman, J. (2002). When Boys Won't Be Boys: Clinical Diagnosis Of Infertility In The Stud Dog. Proceedings: ACVIM. accessed via Veterinary Information Network; vin.com
Freshman, J. (2009). "Dosage for gonadotropin releasing hormone stimulation test to determine if dog is cryptorchid." *VIN Boards* http://goo.gl/IScA0.
Pinto, C. (2007). Cryptorchidism. *Blackwell's Five-Minute Veterinary Consult: Canine & Feline.* L. Tilley and F. Smith, Blackwell: 318.
Purswell, B. (1999). Pharmaceuticals used in canine theriogenology - Part 1 & 2. Proceedings: Central Veterinary Conference, Kansas City. accessed via Veterinary Information Network; vin.com
Verstegen, J. (2000). Feline Reproduction. *Textbook of Veterinary Internal Medicine: Diseases of the Dog and Cat.* S. Ettinger and E. Feldman. Philadelphia, WB Saunders. 2: 1585-98.

Gonadotropin, Chorionic — See Chorionic Gonadotropin

Granisetron HCl

(gran-iss-eh-tron)   Kytril®

5-HT3 Antagonist Antiemetic

Prescriber Highlights

▶ 5-HT3 receptor antagonist for the treatment of severe vomiting or emesis prophylaxis before chemotherapy.

▶ Appears safe, but not commonly used in veterinary medicine.

▶ Relatively expensive.

Uses/Indications

Granisetron is an alternative to other 5-HT3 receptor antagonists (*e.g.*, ondansetron or dolasetron) for the treatment of severe vomiting or prophylaxis before administering antineoplastic drugs such as cisplatin that can cause severe vomiting.

Pharmacology/Actions

Granisetron, like ondansetron or dolasetron, exerts its anti-nausea and antiemetic actions by selectively antagonizing 5-hydroxytryptamine3 (5-HT3; serotonin3) receptors. These receptors are found primarily in the CNS chemoreceptor trigger zone, on vagal nerve terminals and enteric neurons in the GI tract. Chemotherapy associated vomiting in cats is believed primarily due to activation of 5-HT3 receptors in the chemoreceptor trigger zone (CTZ), but in dogs, enteric and vagal receptors may be more important.

Pharmacokinetics

No pharmacokinetic data for dogs or cats was located. In humans, granisetron is rapidly absorbed after oral dosing and peak levels occur in about 2 hours. Oral bioavailability is only 60% due to first-pass metabolism in the liver. The presence of food can decrease AUC by 5%, but increase peak levels by 30%. Granisetron has a volume of distribution of about 3 L/kg and plasma protein binding is approximately 65%. The drug is metabolized in the liver, primarily via demethylation and oxidation and then conjugation. Less than 20% is excreted unchanged in the urine; the remainder is eliminated in the urine and feces as metabolites. Elimination half-life varies considerably, with reported values from about 1-30 hours. Cancer patients appear to have longer elimination half-lives than do healthy adults.

Contraindications/Precautions/Warnings

There are no known contraindications to using this medication in dogs or cats. In humans, granisetron is contraindicated in patients hypersensitive to it and it should not be used to treat vomiting associated with apomorphine (see Drug Interactions).

No dosage adjustments are required in elderly patients or those with impaired renal or hepatic function. Granisetron may mask the signs associated with progressive ileus and/or gastric distention; it should not replace required nasogastric suction.

Adverse Effects

Because of limited use in dogs and cats, a comprehensive adverse effect profile for granisetron is not known, however, it appears to be tolerated well.

In humans, the most common adverse effect reported is headache. Other adverse effects that may occur include abdominal pain, constipation or diarrhea, asthenia, or somnolence. Rarely, hypersensitivity reactions or cardiovascular effects (arrhythmias, chest pain, hypotension) have been reported.

Reproductive/Nursing Safety

Safety in pregnancy is not clearly established, but high dose studies in rodents and rabbits did not demonstrate overt fetal toxicity or teratogenicity. In humans, the FDA categorizes this drug as category *B* for use during pregnancy (*Animal studies have not yet demonstrated risk to the fetus, but there are no adequate studies in pregnant women; or animal studies have shown an adverse effect, but adequate studies in pregnant women have not demonstrated a risk to the fetus in the first trimester of pregnancy, and there is no evidence of risk in later trimesters.*)

It is not known if granisetron enters milk, but it is probably safe to use during nursing.

Overdosage/Acute Toxicity

Limited information is available. An overdose of 38.5 mg in a person caused only a slight headache. Observation and, if required, supportive treatment are suggested.

Drug Interactions

The following drug interactions have either been reported or are theoretical in humans or animals receiving granisetron and may be of in veterinary patients. Unless otherwise noted, use together is not necessarily contraindicated, but weigh the potential risks and perform additional monitoring when appropriate.

▪ **APOMORPHINE:** Profound hypotension can occur.

▪ **KETOCONAZOLE:** May inhibit the metabolism of granisetron.

▪ **PHENOBARBITAL:** Can induce the metabolism of granisetron.

Laboratory Considerations

▪ No specific laboratory concerns associated with granisetron.

Doses

▪ **DOGS/CATS:**

As an antiemetic (extra-label): Little is published on the clinical use of this drug in animals; dosages of 0.1 – 0.5 mg/kg PO or IV q12–24h have been suggested. IV administration may be more effective than PO.

Monitoring

▪ Clinical efficacy.

Client Information

▪ This drug is usually used on an inpatient basis or during outpatient visits for chemotherapy.

▪ If used orally on an outpatient basis, have client contact veterinarian for further instructions if vomiting is not controlled or if the dose is vomited up after administrating.

Chemistry/Synonyms

Granisetron HCl occurs as a white or almost white powder that is freely soluble in water. Dosages are expressed in terms of the base; 1.12 mg of granisetron HCl is equivalent to 1 mg of granisetron base.

Granisetron may also be known as: granistroni, granisetrono, or BRL-43694A, *Aludal®, Eumetic®, Granicip®, Granitron®, Kytril®, Kevatril®, Rigmoz®* or *Setron®*.

Storage/Stability

The commercially available tablets and oral solution should be stored at room temperature (15-30°C) in tight containers and protected from light. The oral solution should be stored in an upright position. The injectable solution should be stored between 15-30°C; preferably at 25°C. Protect from light and do not freeze solution. Once the multi-dose vial is penetrated, it must be used within 30 days.

Compatibility/Compounding Considerations

The injectable solution is **compatible** with sodium chloride 0.9%, dextrose 5% in sodium chloride 0.45% or 0.9%, and dextrose 5% in water. It is compatible with many drugs at intravenous Y-sites, but is **incompatible** with amphotericin B.

Dosage Forms/Regulatory Status

VETERINARY-LABELED PRODUCTS: NONE.

HUMAN-LABELED PRODUCTS:

Granisetron Oral Tablets: 1 mg (1.12 mg as HCl); generic; (Rx)

Granisetron Oral Solution: 1 mg/5 mL (1.12 mg/5 mL as HCl; orange flavor; contains sorbitol) in 30 mL bottles; *Granisol®*; (Rx)

Granisetron Injection Solution: 0.1 mg/mL (0.112 mg/mL as HCl) preservative-free, may contain sodium chloride 9 mg in 1 mL single-use vials; 1 mg/mL (1.12 mg/mL as HCl), regular & preservative-free, in 1 mL single-dose & 4 mL multi-dose vials; generic; (Rx)

Granisetron Transdermal Patch: 3.1 mg/24 hours (34.3 mg/52 cm²); *Sancuso®*; (Rx)

Revisions/References

Monograph revised/updated February 2014.

Griseofulvin

(gri-see-oh-ful-vin)   Fulvicin®

Antifungal Agent

Prescriber Highlights

▶ Fungistatic antibiotic used primarily for ringworm & other dermatophytic infections; no effect on other fungi. Terbinafine and azole antifungal agents have largely supplanted griseofulvin for treating small animals.

▶ Contraindications: Pregnancy, known hypersensitivity, or hepatocellular failure. Known teratogen in cats. Caution: Kittens may be overly sensitive to the drug; cats with FIV.

▶ Adverse Effects: Anorexia, vomiting, diarrhea, anemia, neutropenia, leukopenia, thrombocytopenia, depression, ataxia, hepatotoxicity, or dermatitis/photosensitivity.

▶ Only new hair & nail growth resistant to fungi after treating.

▶ Dosing is different for microsize & ultramicrosize forms.

▶ Availability becoming an issue.

Uses/Indications

In veterinary species, griseofulvin has been FDA-approved for use in dogs and cats to treat dermatophytic fungal (see below) infections of the skin, hair and claws, and to treat ringworm (caused by *T. equinum* and *M. gypseum*) in horses. It has also been used in laboratory animals and ruminants for the same indications. The oral tablets FDA-approved for dogs and cats are no longer marketed in the USA, but human dosage forms are available. Secondary to the availability of potentially more effective and less toxic drugs, griseofulvin is infrequently recommended today for use in small animals, especially cats.

Pharmacology/Actions

Griseofulvin acts on susceptible fungi by disrupting the structure of the cell's mitotic spindle, arresting the metaphase of cell division. Griseofulvin has activity against species of *Trichophyton*, *Microsporum* and *Epidermophyton*. Only new hair and nail growth is resistant to infection. It has no antibacterial activity and is not clinically useful against other pathogenic fungi, including Malassezia yeasts.

Pharmacokinetics

The microsized form of the drug is absorbed variably (25-70%); dietary fat will enhance absorption. The ultramicrosize form of the drug may be nearly 100% absorbed. Generally, the ultramicrosize form is absorbed 1.5 times as well as the microsized form for a given patient.

Griseofulvin is concentrated in skin, hair, nails, fat, skeletal muscle, and the liver, and can be found in the stratum corneum within 4 hours of dosing.

Griseofulvin is metabolized by the liver via oxidative demethylation and glucuronidation to 6-desmethylgriseofulvin, which is not active. In humans, the half-life is 9-24 hours. A serum half-life of 47 minutes has been reported for dogs. Less than 1% of the drug is excreted unchanged in the urine.

Contraindications/Precautions/Warnings

Griseofulvin is contraindicated in patients hypersensitive to it or with hepatocellular failure. It should not be used in pregnant animals. It must not be used in horses intended for food.

Because kittens may be overly sensitive to the adverse effects associated with griseofulvin, they should be monitored carefully if treatment is instituted. Cats should be tested for FIV before using griseofulvin because of the possible neutropenic or panleukopenic effects of the drug.

Adverse Effects

Griseofulvin can cause anorexia, vomiting, diarrhea, anemia, neutropenia, leukopenia, thrombocytopenia, depression, ataxia, hepatotoxicity, dermatitis, photosensitivity, and toxic epidermal necrolysis. The drug has a disagreeable taste so dosing may be difficult. With the exception of GI clinical signs, adverse effects are uncommon in dogs at usual doses. Cats, particularly kittens, may be more susceptible to adverse effects (*e.g.*, bone marrow depression) than other species. This could be due to this species' propensity to more slowly form glucuronide conjugates and thus metabolize the drug at a slower rate than either dogs or humans.

Reproductive/Nursing Safety

Griseofulvin is a known teratogen in cats and, probably, in dogs and horses as well. Dosages of 35 mg/kg given to cats during the first trimester caused cleft palate and other skeletal and brain malformations in kittens. Griseofulvin may also inhibit spermatogenesis. Because dermatophytic infections are not generally life-threatening and alternative therapies are available, use of the drug should be considered contraindicated during pregnancy. However, griseofulvin has been used in mares during the later stages of pregnancy without noted ill effect (Davis 2008).

In humans, the FDA categorizes this drug as category *C* for use during pregnancy (*Animal studies have shown an adverse effect on the fetus, but there are no adequate studies in humans; or there are no animal reproduction studies and no adequate studies in humans.*) In a separate system evaluating the safety of drugs in canine and feline pregnancy (Papich 1989), this drug is categorized as class: *D* (*Contraindicated. These drugs have been shown to cause congenital malformations or embryotoxicity.*)

No lactation safety information was found.

Overdosage/Acute Toxicity

No specifics regarding griseofulvin overdosage or acute toxicity were located. It is suggested that significant overdoses be handled with gut emptying, charcoal and cathartic administration unless contraindicated. Contact an animal poison control center for more information.

Horses have received 100 mg/kg PO for 20 days without apparent ill effect.

Drug Interactions

The following drug interactions have either been reported or are theoretical in humans or animals receiving griseofulvin and may be of in veterinary patients. Unless otherwise noted, use together is not necessarily contraindicated, but weigh the potential risks and perform additional monitoring when appropriate.

■ **ALCOHOL:** Griseofulvin may potentiate the effects of alcohol.

■ **ASPIRIN:** Griseofulvin may decrease salicylate levels.

■ **CYCLOSPORINE:** Griseofulvin may decrease cyclosporine levels.

- PHENOBARBITAL: Phenobarbital and other barbiturates have been implicated in causing decreased griseofulvin blood concentrations, presumably by inducing hepatic microsomal enzymes and/or reducing absorption. If phenobarbital and griseofulvin are given concurrently, griseofulvin dosage adjustment may be necessary.
- THEOPHYLLINE: In some patients, griseofulvin may decrease theophylline half-life and levels.
- WARFARIN: Coumarin anticoagulants may have their anticoagulant activity reduced by griseofulvin; anticoagulant adjustment may be required.

Doses

■ DOGS:

For dermatophytosis (extra-label): Griseofulvin is not frequently recommended today and dosage forms suitable for dogs may be difficult to obtain. Dosage recommendations have usually been: Microsize forms: 50 mg/kg PO once daily or divided and given twice daily. Ultramicrosize forms: 5 – 10 mg/kg PO once daily. Both forms should be given with or immediately following a fatty meal, or administered with corn oil. Treatment may be required for many months. Treat for at least two weeks following clinical cure and 2 negative skin cultures taken at least one week apart.

■ CATS:

For dermatophytosis (extra-label): Usually not recommended for use in cats secondary to potential for serious adverse effects. When used, it is usually dosed similarly as for dogs.

■ RABBITS/RODENTS/SMALL MAMMALS:

For dermatophytosis (extra-label): There are several anecdotal dosage recommendations published for a variety of species; these generally mimic the dog dosage above.

■ HORSES:

For susceptible dermatophytic infections (extra-label): Using the microsize (not ultra-microsize) products: 5 mg/kg PO once daily. Smaller doses (1.25 grams) should be used for foals or ponies. If using ultra-microsize (human) formulations the dose should be reduced by 50%. (Davis 2008)

Monitoring

- Clinical efficacy; fungal culture.
- Adverse effects.
- CBC; before therapy and q1-3 weeks during therapy.
- Liver enzymes (if indicated).

Client Information

- Clients should be instructed in procedures used to prevent reinfection (destruction of old bedding, disinfection, periodic reexaminations, hair clipping, etc.), and the importance of compliance with the dosage regimen.
- Should be given with fatty foods/oils (*e.g.,* cheese, cream, butter, corn oil, etc.).
- Lack of appetite (eating less or not at all), vomiting, & diarrhea are the most common side effects.
- Kittens are more sensitive to the drug and harmful effects on bone marrow are possible.
- Pregnant women should handle this drug with care; griseofulvin has caused birth defects in animals and may do so in humans.

Chemistry/Synonyms

A fungistatic antibiotic produced by species of penicillium (primarily *P. griseofulvum*), griseofulvin occurs as an odorless or nearly odorless, bitter tasting, white to creamy white powder. It is very slightly soluble in water and sparingly soluble in alcohol.

Two forms of the drug have been available commercially. Micro-

size griseofulvin contains particles with a predominant size of 4 micrometers in diameter, while the ultramicrosize form particle size averages less than 1 micron in diameter. For human medicine, only ultramicrosize oral tablets are still being marketed.

Griseofulvin may also be known as: curling factor, griseofulvina, and griseofulvinum; many trade names are available.

Storage/Stability

Although griseofulvin is relatively thermostable, products should be stored at less than 40°C, preferably at 15-30°C. Griseofulvin suspension should be stored in tight, light-resistant containers. Microsize tablets and capsules should be stored in tight containers; the ultramicrosize tablets should be stored in well-closed containers.

Compatibility/Compounding Considerations

As commercial pharmaceutical dosage forms are becoming less available, compounding may be required. If obtaining compounded dosage forms, understand which form (microsize or ultra-microsize) of griseofulvin is being supplied and adjust dosage accordingly.

Dosage Forms/Regulatory Status

VETERINARY-LABELED PRODUCTS:

Griseofulvin (Microsize) Powder: 2.5 g griseofulvin in 15 g sachets; generic; (Rx). FDA-approved for use in horses not intended for food. Marketing status is unknown.

The FDA's "Green Book" still lists several other veterinary FDA-approved griseofulvin products, but it does not appear they are presently being marketed. Compounding pharmacies may be able to provide.

HUMAN-LABELED PRODUCTS:

Griseofulvin Ultramicrosize Tablets: 125 mg & 250 mg; *Gris-PEG®*; (Rx)

Revisions/References

Monograph revised/updated February 2014.
Davis, J. (2008). The use of antifungals. Comp Equine(April): 128-33.

Guaifenesin, Intravenous

(gwye-fen-e-sin) GG, Guailaxin®

Parenteral Muscle Relaxant

Prescriber Highlights

▶ Muscle relaxant (parenteral) adjunctive for anesthesia.

▶ Contraindications: None noted except concurrent use with physostigmine. Must be used with caution in induction protocols.

▶ Adverse Effects: Mild hypotensive effect & increase in cardiac rate, thrombophlebitis possible.

▶ Availability is an issue for the injection.

Uses/Indications

In veterinary medicine, guaifenesin is used to induce muscle relaxation and restraint as an adjunct to anesthesia for short procedures (30-60 minutes) in large and small animal species. There are combination oral products containing guaifenesin for treating respiratory conditions in horses.

In human medicine, guaifenesin has long been touted as an oral expectorant, but definitive proof for its efficacy is lacking.

Pharmacology/Actions

While the exact mechanism of action for the muscle relaxant effect is not known, it is believed that guaifenesin acts centrally by depressing or blocking nerve impulse transmission at the internuncial neuron level of the subcortical areas of the brain, brainstem and spinal cord. It relaxes both the laryngeal and pharyngeal muscles, thus allowing easier intubation. Guaifenesin also has mild intrinsic analgesic and sedative qualities, but does not cause unconsciousness or provide analgesia significant enough to affect painful stimuli.

Guaifenesin causes an excitement-free induction and recovery from anesthesia in horses. It produces relaxation of skeletal muscles but does not affect diaphragmatic function and has little, if any, effect on respiratory function at usual doses. Possible effects on the cardiovascular system include transient mild decreases in blood pressure and increases in cardiac rate. Gastrointestinal motility may be increased, but generally no adversity is seen with this.

Guaifenesin can potentiate the activity of preanesthetic and anesthetic agents.

Pharmacokinetics

The pharmacokinetics of guaifenesin have not been thoroughly studied in most species. When administered alone to horses IV, recumbency usually occurs within 2 minutes and light (not surgical level) restraint persists for about 6 minutes. Muscle relaxation reportedly persists for 10-20 minutes after a single dose.

Guaifenesin is conjugated in the liver and excreted into the urine. A gender difference in the elimination half-life of guaifenesin in ponies has been demonstrated, with males having a half-life of approximately 85 minutes, and females a half-life of about 60 minutes. Guaifenesin reportedly crosses the placenta, but adverse effects in newborns of mothers who received guaifenesin have not been described.

Contraindications/Precautions/Warnings

- The veterinary label states that the use of physostigmine is contraindicated with guaifenesin (see Drug Interactions).
- While guaifenesin has some sedative and mild analgesic effects, it must be used intraoperatively with other suitable anesthetic and analgesic agents.
- Because it can cause significant tissue damage if given perivascularly, guaifenesin should always be administered through an intravenous catheter.
- When used as part of an induction protocol in horses, guaifenesin must be used with extreme caution; appropriate numbers of personnel and equipment (*e.g.*, induction swing-gate) should be available. Muscle relaxation/ataxia can occur dramatically and timing of the administration of a drug like ketamine is critical. Therefore it has been recommended to NOT use guaifenesin as part of induction for field anesthesia (Sinclair 2013).
- Avoid giving ruminants concentrations of guaifenesin greater than 5% as hemolysis can occur.

Adverse Effects

- At usual doses, side effects are transient and generally minor. A mild decrease in blood pressure and increase in cardiac rate can be seen.
- Thrombophlebitis has been reported after IV injection, and perivascular administration may cause some tissue reaction.
- Hemolysis may occur in solutions containing greater than a 5% concentration of guaifenesin, but some sources state this is insignificant at even a 15% concentration. Hemolysis may be more of an issue in ruminants than in horses.

Reproductive/Nursing Safety

In humans, the FDA categorizes this drug as category C for use during pregnancy (*Animal studies have shown an adverse effect on the fetus, but there are no adequate studies in humans; or there are no animal reproduction studies and no adequate studies in humans.*)

It is not known whether guaifenesin is excreted in milk.

Overdosage/Acute Toxicity

The margin of safety is reportedly 3X the usual dose. Clinical signs associated with toxic levels of parenteral guaifenesin include opisthotonus, apneustic breathing, nystagmus, hypotension, and contradictory muscle rigidity. Should any of these signs occur, it is recommended to stop the infusion and give supportive care as needed.

There were 64 oral exposures to guaifenesin reported to the ASPCA Animal Poison Control Center (APCC) during 2005-2009. In these cases 64 were dogs with only 5 showing clinical signs and 6 cases were cats with only 3 showing clinical signs. The dog received a dosage estimated between 415 and 830 mg/kg and exhibited hypothermia, mild tremors, ataxia and vomiting. The cat received a dosage of 132 mg/kg and exhibited lethargy and anorexia.

No specific antidote is available. It is suggested that treatment be supportive until the drug is cleared to sub-toxic levels.

Drug Interactions

Drug interactions with parenteral guaifenesin are not well studied. The following drug interactions have either been reported or are theoretical in animals receiving guaifenesin and may be of in veterinary patients. Unless otherwise noted, use together is not necessarily contraindicated, but weigh the potential risks and perform additional monitoring when appropriate.

- **PHYSOSTIGMINE:** The veterinary label states that physostigmine is contraindicated in horses receiving guaifenesin, but does not elucidate on the actual interaction. It may be logical to assume that other anticholinesterase agents (**neostigmine, pyridostigmine, edrophonium**) may also be contraindicated.

Doses

Note: Various protocols combining guaifenesin with other drugs are too numerous to list in this reference. The following listings are examples for horses, small ruminants, and new world camelids. Additional protocols for other drug combinations and species can be found in other anesthesia references. Referring to these references or consulting with a veterinary anesthesiologist is highly recommended when considering using this agent as an anesthetic adjunct.

- **HORSES:** (NOTE: ARCI UCGFS CLASS 4 DRUG)

  As a muscle relaxant as <u>part of induction protocols</u> (extra-label): **Note:** Must be used with caution; not recommended for field anesthesia. The following is one example using xylazine as the alpha-2 agonist in the protocols. There are numerous others that use other alpha-2 agonists (*e.g.*, detomidine, romifidine), butorphanol, acepromazine, etc. See equine anesthesia references for additional information.

  <u>For normal healthy patients:</u> Administer xylazine (0.44 – 0.66 mg/kg IV, or 200 – 300 mg/450 kg horse). <u>Wait</u> for sedation and muscle relaxation to occur (approximately 5 minutes). Guaifenesin (5% solution, or 50 mg/mL) is then rapidly infused using pressurization until marked sedation and muscle relaxation is achieved (generally a total dose of 30 – 50 mg/kg). Ketamine (2.2 mg/kg IV, 1000 mg/450 kg) should be administered at a point that allows for its slow onset to occur without the patient becoming excessively weak and collapsing from effects of guaifenesin. Recumbency generally occurs approximately 60 seconds following ketamine administration. The slow administration of guaifenesin described below can also be used in normal healthy patients in place of a supplemental dose of xylazine when the level of initial sedation is inadequate.

  <u>For compromised patients:</u> Try to use a very modest dose of xylazine (0.22 – 0.44 mg/kg IV, or 100 – 200 mg/450 kg horse) depending on status and demeanor to minimize its cardiovascular effects in compromised patients. Slow administration of

guaifenesin (5% solution) can be used to gradually create the desired level of sedation. It is still important to allow adequate time for centralization of cardiac output to progress sufficiently prior to initiating the rapid phase of guaifenesin administration that precedes the induction bolus. Guaifenesin has a slow onset of action, when used to augment the level of pre-induction sedation. SLOW administration is important to avoid creating an overly weak and ataxic patient while waiting for centralization to progress sufficiently. Guaifenesin is then rapidly infused using pressurization until marked sedation and muscle relaxation is achieved (generally a total dose of 30 – 50 mg/kg IV). Ketamine (dose decreases as degree of compromise increases, 1.34 – 1.55 mg/kg IV, or 600 – 700 mg/450 kg) for extremely compromised patients should be administered at a point that allows for its slow onset to occur without the patient becoming excessively weak and collapsing from the growing effects of guaifenesin. Experience may be required to get the timing right. Recumbency takes even longer (up to a couple minutes) when ketamine dose is reduced in compromised patients. (Abrahamsen 2007)

As a muscle relaxant as part of a general anesthesia <u>after induction</u> (extra-label): **Note:** When used as part of total intravenous anesthetic protocols, guaifenesin is used in triple drip mixtures that also contain an alpha-agonists (xylazine, detomidine, romifidine) and ketamine. These can be particularly useful for field use with short procedures (up to 60 minutes). Additional information can found in anesthesia references, including *Total Intravenous Anesthesia in Horses* (Lerche 2013). The following is an example of a dosage recommendation:

To augment muscle relaxation in horses that are too light or too tense after alpha-2 agonist + ketamine ± benzodiazepine induction, and do not respond sufficiently to additional increments of alpha-2 agonist or ketamine: Approximately 25 – 50 mg/kg (250 – 500 mL of a 5% solution) IV.

For long-term IV (>30 minutes) anesthesia using "GKX" or "triple-drip": Guaifenesin (50 mg/mL), ketamine (1 – 2 mg/mL; 2 mg/mL concentration used for more painful or noxious procedures), and xylazine (0.5 mg/mL). Most practitioners prefer to induce with xylazine/ketamine or xylazine/diazepam/ketamine and then use GKX for maintenance. Typically the CRI runs at 1.5 – 2.2 mL /kg/hr depending on the procedure, patient response and ketamine concentration.

An alternative to "GKX" is "GKD" where detomidine is substituted for the xylazine and the concentrations of guaifenesin and ketamine are increased: Guaifenesin (100 mg/mL), ketamine (4 mg/mL), and detomidine (0.04 mg/mL). The CRI runs at 0.8 mL/kg/hr for the first hour and 0.6 mL/kg/hour for the final 30 minutes. (Wagner 2009b)

■ **SHEEP, GOATS:**

For general anesthesia (extra-label):

a) Using "GKX" for induction/maintenance: Mix 1000 mL of 5% (50 mg/mL) guaifenesin with 1000 mg of ketamine ± 0 – 100 mg of xylazine. Induce with 2.2 mL/kg IV (calculate dose; do NOT overdose!). Maintain with approximately 2.2 mL/kg/hr IV (calculate drip rate, adjust as needed). (Wagner 2009a)

b) Using "GKX": To a 500 mL bag of 5% guaifenesin, add 50 mg of xylazine and 500 mg ketamine. Administer at a rate of 2 – 4 mL/kg IV. Given rapidly until animal is recumbent and then slowed to maintain desired anesthesia plane. Monitor drip to prevent overdosing. (Rings 2005)

■ **CAMELIDS:**

For general anesthesia using "GKX" for induction/maintenance (extra-label): Mix 1000 mL of 5% (50 mg/mL) guaifenesin with 1000 mg of ketamine ± 200 mg of xylazine. Induce with 2.2 mL/kg IV (calculate dose; do NOT overdose!). Maintain with approximately 2.2 mL/kg/hr IV (calculate drip rate, adjust as needed). (Wagner 2009a)

Monitoring

Monitoring patients during general anesthesia is vital and guaifenesin-based injectable anesthesia can affect multiple systems. Monitoring depth of anesthesia, muscle relaxation, respiratory rates/oxygenation, cardiac rates, and blood pressure are all warranted. Refer to specific anesthesia references for more information.

Client Information

Injectable guaifenesin must be given by a veterinarian.

Chemistry/Synonyms

Formerly known as glyceryl guaiacolate, guaifenesin occurs as a white to slightly gray, crystalline powder that may have a characteristic odor. It is nonhygroscopic and melts between 78°-82°C. One g is soluble in 15 mL of water and soluble in alcohol, propylene glycol and glycerin.

Guaifenesin may also be known as: GG, glyceryl guaiacolate, glycerylguayacolum, guaiacol glycerol ether, guaiacyl glyceryl ether, guaifenesina, guaifenesinum, guaiphenesin, and guajacolum glycerolatum; many trade names are available.

Storage/Stability

Guaifenesin is stable in light and heat (less than melting point). It should be stored in well-closed containers.

When dissolved into aqueous solutions, guaifenesin may slightly precipitate out of solution when the temperature is less than 22°C (72°F). Slight warming and agitation generally resolubilizes the drug. A microwave oven has been suggested for heating and dissolving the drug. It is recommended that the solution be prepared freshly before use, but a 10% solution (in sterile water) may apparently be stored safely at room temperature for up to one week with only slight precipitation occurring.

Parenteral 5% guaifenesin does not contain preservatives and should be for single-use only.

Compatibility/Compounding Considerations

Guaifenesin is physically **compatible** with sterile water or D5W. It is also reportedly **compatible** with ketamine, pentobarbital, thiamylal, thiopental, and xylazine.

As there apparently are no commercially available injections being marketed in the USA, compounding an injection product from a USP grade powder may be the only way to obtain a parenteral dosage form. Compounding pharmacies with appropriate facilities, equipment, and procedures may be able to prepare a sterile product. The commercially available products contained per mL: Guaifenesin 50 mg, dextrose (anhydrous) 50 mg, propylene glycol 20 mg, dimethyl acetamide 50 mg, edetate disodium 0.75 mg, water for injection q.s. For stability, it is highly recommended that the compounding pharmacy use this or another validated formula.

Dosage Forms/Regulatory Status

VETERINARY-LABELED PRODUCTS:

Guaifenesin Injection: 50 mg/mL in 500 mL & 1000 mL. There are several GG 5% injection products still listed as FDA-approved in the FDA's Green Book, but it is believed there are no products presently being marketed. Compounding pharmacies may be available to provide (see Compatibility/Compounding above).

The ARCI (Racing Commissioners International) has designated this drug as a class 4 substance. See the appendix for more information.

HUMAN-LABELED PRODUCTS:

No parenteral preparations are FDA-approved. There are many OTC oral expectorant/cough preparations on the market.

Revisions/References

Monograph revised/updated February 2014.

Abrahamsen, E. (2007). Analgesia in equine practice. Proceedings: Western Vet Conference. accessed via Veterinary Information Network; vin.com

Lerche, P. (2013). Total Intravenous Anesthesia in Horses. Veterinary Clinics of North America-Equine Practice **29**(1): 123-+.

Rings, D. (2005). Anesthesia and Surgical Procedures for Small Ruminants I & II. Proceedings: WVC.

Sinclair, M. (2013). Equine Field Anesthesia with Triple Drip Mixtures. 65th Convention of the Canadian Veterinary Medical Association. accessed via Veterinary Information Network; vin.com

Wagner, A. E. (2009a). Anaesthesia for Small Ruminants and Camelids. Proceedings: AVA. accessed via Veterinary Information Network; vin.com

Wagner, A. E. (2009b). Injectable Field Anaesthesia in the Horse. Proceedings: AVA. accessed via Veterinary Information Network; vin.com

HCG – see Chorionic Gonadotropin

Hemoglobin Glutamer-200 (Bovine)

(hee-moe-gloe-bin gloo-ta-mer)

HG-200, Hb-200, HBOC-301, Oxyglobin®

Semi-Synthetic Hemoglobin Replacer; Colloid

Prescriber Highlights

▶ Bovine-source polymerized hemoglobin product for the treatment of anemia.

▶ Contraindications: Advanced cardiac disease, renal impairment with oliguria or anuria.

▶ Many potential adverse effects; most are not serious (see below).

▶ Potential drug-lab interactions.

▶ Availability has been an issue. At time of writing (2/2014) not available in USA.

Uses/Indications

Hemoglobin glutamer-200 [bovine] (HB-200, HG-200, HBOC-301, *Oxyglobin*®) is indicated for the treatment of dogs with anemia, regardless of the cause of anemia (hemolysis, blood loss, or ineffective erythropoiesis). From a prognostic standpoint, the drug should be more valuable in dogs with regenerative anemias (versus nonregenerative anemias). It has also been used extra-label in other species as well, such as cats or foals for neonatal isoerythrolysis. Its primary benefit is for the patient that is anemic and difficult to transfuse due to unavailability of blood, or when no suitable donors are identified on crossmatch(Jandrey 2007). It has also been used in an extra-label manner in other species for treating anemia and as a colloid for treating hypotension in dogs and cats. Dogs with gastric dilatation-volvulus (GDV) resuscitated with HB-200 reached resuscitation end points more rapidly and required significantly smaller volumes of crystalloid and colloid than those resuscitated with hetastarch 6% (Haak et al. 2012).

Pharmacology/Actions

The bovine hemoglobin in the product is polymerized into larger molecules to increase safety, efficacy, and intravascular persistence; it is shipped in a deoxygenated state and becomes oxygenated once circulated through the lungs. HG-200 does not contain red blood cells and is stroma free. HG-200 releases oxygen to tissue in a mechanism similar to endogenous hemoglobin thereby increasing plasma and total hemoglobin concentrations and systemic oxygen content. Because of its small size (in comparison to normal RBC's), it may better deliver oxygen to cells supplied by severely constricted arteries. HG-200 shifts the oxygen dissociation curve to the right, so oxygen is transferred to tissues more easily. In experimental-

ly-induced hypovolemic shock in dogs, HG-200 caused severe vasoconstriction and decreased cardiac output (Driessen et al. 2001).

HG-200 also has colloidal properties similar to dextran 70 and hetastarch.

Pharmacokinetics

In dogs receiving 15 mL/kg, peak hemoglobin concentrations increased approximately 2.5 g/dL; at 30 mL/kg, approximately 4 mg/dL. Duration of effect continues for at least 24 hours. The half-life in dogs at labeled dosages is approximately 18-43 hours and HG-200 can be detected in plasma for 5-7 days after a single dose.

As with endogenous hemoglobin, HG-200 is metabolized and eliminated by the reticuloendothelial system. Small amounts of unstabilized hemoglobin (<5%) may be excreted through the kidneys, causing discoloration (reddening) of the urine.

Contraindications/Precautions/Warnings

As safe use of *Oxyglobin*® has not been tested for the following conditions and plasma expanders are generally contraindicated in them, the product is labeled as contraindicated in dogs with advanced cardiac disease (*i.e.*, congestive heart failure) or otherwise severely impaired cardiac function or renal impairment with oliguria or anuria. The safety and efficacy of *Oxyglobin*® has not been evaluated in dogs with DIC, thrombocytopenia with active bleeding, hemoglobinemia and hemoglobinuria, or autoagglutination.

HG-200 is a potent colloid and can cause vasoconstriction. Care must be taken not to volume overload patients when giving this drug as hydrostatic pressures may be increased and cause pulmonary overload (pleural effusion, pulmonary edema). This is particularly important in cats.

Because of its vasoconstrictive properties, the amount of HG-200 required for fluid resuscitation in trauma patients is approximately 1/3 that of hetastarch (Rudloff et al. 2009).

Administration of any foreign protein has the potential to cause immunologic reactions. While low levels of IgG antibodies have been detected after multiple dosages, no anaphylactic reactions have been reported thus far. If an immediate hypersensitivity reaction occurs, infusion should be immediately discontinued and appropriate treatment administered. If a delayed type of hypersensitivity reaction occurs, immunosuppressant therapy is recommended.

Adverse Effects

The package insert lists the following frequency of adverse reactions that occurred in greater than 4% of dogs treated with *Oxyglobin*® (**Note:** first figure is % of dogs treated; in parentheses: is the % treated with hemolytic anemia): Discolored mucous membranes 69% (47%); discolored sclera (yellow, red, brown) 56% (48%); discolored urine (orange, red, brown) 52% (41%); discolored skin (yellow) 12% (83%); increased central venous pressure (CVP) 33% (47%); ventricular arrhythmias (AV block, tachycardia, ventricular premature contractions) 15% (78%); ecchymosis/petechiae 8% (50%); bradycardia 6% (67%); vomiting 35% (72%); diarrhea 15% (50%); anorexia 8% (25%); tachypnea 15% (50%); dyspnea 14% (71%); pulmonary edema 12% (67%); harsh lung sounds/crackles 8% (50%); pleural effusion 6% (67%); fever 17% (40%); death/euthanasia 15% (63%); peripheral edema 8% (25%); hemoglobinuria 6% (67%); dehydration 6% (33%).

Adverse reactions occurring in 4% of the dogs treated with *Oxyglobin*® include coughing, disseminated intravascular coagulopathy, melena, nasal discharge/crusts (red), peritoneal effusion, respiratory arrest, and weight loss (5-7% body weight). Adverse reactions occurring in less than 2% of the dogs treated with *Oxyglobin*® included: abdominal discomfort on palpation, acidosis, cardiac arrest, cardiovascular volume overload (by echocardiography), collapse, cystitis, dark stool, discolored soft stool (red-brown) and tongue (purple), focal hyperemic areas on gums, forelimb cellulitis/lameness, hematemesis or hemoptysis (unable to differentiate), hypernatremia, hypotension, hypoxemia, lack of neurologic responses, left forebrain signs, nystagmus, pancreatitis, pendulous abdomen, polyuria, pulmonary thromboembolism, ptosis, reddened pinnae with papules/head shaking, reduction in heart rate, thrombocytopenia (worsening), and venous thrombosis.

Increases in IgG antibodies have been detected in dogs receiving multiple courses of HG-200, but no documented cases of anaphylaxis have been reported.

Small amounts of unstabilized hemoglobin (<5%) may be excreted through the kidneys, resulting in transient discoloration (reddening) of the urine following the infusion. This discoloration of the urine should not be interpreted as due to intravascular hemolysis and has no effect on renal function.

In clinical use, *Oxyglobin®* has not been demonstrated to affect platelet function or impair coagulation.

Cats may be susceptible to pulmonary edema or pleural effusion particularly with rapid infusions of large (dog) dosages. However, a retrospective study using in low dosages in 44 cats with hypotension, reported the following adverse effects: respiratory changes (8), vomiting (2), and pigmented serum (30), but most incidences that could be potentially associated with HB-200 were not considered to be clinically significant (Wehausen et al. 2011).

Increases in aspartate aminotransferase (AST) and alanine aminotransferase (ALT) not associated with histopathologic changes in the liver, increase in serum total protein, and hemoglobinuria may also be seen.

Reproductive/Nursing Safety
Safe use in breeding dogs and pregnant or lactating bitches has not been determined.

Overdosage/Acute Toxicity
The clinical signs associated with *Oxyglobin®* administered to dogs at 1, 2, and 3 times the recommended dose twice, 3 days apart included yellow-orange discoloration of skin, ear canals, pinnae, mucous membranes (gums), and sclera, red-dark-green-black discoloration of feces, brown-black discoloration of urine, red spotting of skin and/or lips (less common), decreased appetite and thirst, vomiting, diarrhea, and decreased skin elasticity. The frequency and/or intensity of these signs increased with repeated and increasing doses. Healthy dogs administered 3X overdoses twice, all survived.

Overdosage or an excessively rapid administration rate (*i.e.*, >10 mL/kg/hr) may result in circulatory overload.

Drug Interactions
Other than concerns with compatibility, no specific drug interactions have been noted.

Laboratory Considerations
- Hemoglobin-based oxygen carriers (HBOCs) can impact several laboratory tests. The manufacturer maintains a website: www.HBOCLab.com to help guide laboratories and clinicians.
- The presence of HG-200 in serum may cause artifactual increases or decreases in the results of **serum chemistry tests**, depending on the type of analyzer and reagents used. May cause false increases in AST, or creatinine. May cause false decreases in LDH. May cause unacceptable interference with GGT, albumin, or bilirubin.
- There is reportedly no interference with directly measured hemoglobin tests, but due to the dilutional effects of HG-200, PCV and RBC count are not accurate measures of the degree of anemia for 24 hours following administration. **Prothrombin time** (PT) and **activated partial thromboplastin time** (aPTT) determined using methods that are mechanical, magnetic and

light scattering are accurate, but optical methods are not reliable while HG-200 is present.
- **Urine dipstick** measurements (*i.e.*, pH, glucose, ketones, protein) are inaccurate while gross discoloration of the urine is present.

Doses
- **DOGS:**

For anemia, regardless of the cause of anemia (hemolysis, blood loss, or ineffective erythropoiesis) (labeled-dose; FDA approved): One-time dose of 10 – 30 mL/kg IV at a rate of up to 10 mL/kg/hr. May be warmed to 37°C prior to administration. Blood transfusions are not contraindicated in dogs which receive *Oxyglobin®* nor is *Oxyglobin®* contraindicated in dogs which have previously received a blood transfusion. There is no need for typing or crossmatching before use. Should be administered using aseptic technique via a standard intravenous infusion set and catheter through a central or peripheral vein at a rate of 10 mL/kg/hr. Do not administer with other fluids or drugs via the same infusion set. Do not add medications or other solutions to the bag. Do not combine the contents of more than one bag. (Package Insert; *Oxyglobin®*—Biopure)

To provide a "bridge" until immunosuppressive drugs take effect in dogs with IMHA with a transfusion reaction: (extra-label): 7 – 10 mL/kg q12h can maintain hemoglobin levels above 3.5 g/dL; higher doses 30 mL/kg may provide oxygen carrying support for 48-72 hours. (Macintire 2006)

For trauma/resuscitation (all are extra-label):
a) For resuscitation of trauma patients in shock with or without hemorrhage: Empirically, 3 – 5 mL/kg with concurrent crystalloid at 1/2 to 2 times maintenance. (Gfeller 2002)
b) As an option to provide oxygen carrying capacity in the trauma patient: 10 – 15 mL/kg IV given over several hours. Care must be taken not to cause fluid overload. (Waddell 2009)
c) As a vasopressor once there is adequate intravascular volume in trauma patients: 3 – 5 mL/kg IV. (Rudloff et al. 2009)

- **CATS:**

For treating hypotension (extra-label): From a retrospective study of 44 cases. The mean IV bolus dose and administration time was 3.1 mL/kg and 25 minutes. Mean increase of systemic arterial pressure (SAP) > 20 mm Hg after the bolus. Most also received CRIs after bolus with a mean volume administered of 0.8 ± 0.5 mL/kg/hour. Mean SAP during CRI was 92 ± 18 mm Hg. (Wehausen et al. 2011)

As an option to provide oxygen carrying capacity in the trauma patient (extra-label): 5 – 10 mL/kg IV given over several hours. Care must be taken not to cause fluid overload, especially in cats. (Waddell 2009)

Monitoring
- Hgb; clinical signs of adequate tissue oxygenation.
- Signs of circulatory overload (CVP).
- Other adverse effects (see above).

Client Information
- Clients should be informed of the cost/risk/benefit profile for this agent before use. It must be administered by a veterinarian.

Chemistry/Synonyms
Hemoglobin glutamer-200 (bovine)—*Oxyglobin®* is a sterile, clear, dark purple solution containing 13 g/dL purified, polymerized hemoglobin of bovine origin in a modified lactated Ringer's solution. It has an osmolality of 300 mOsm/kg and a pH of 7.8. Less than 5% of the hemoglobin are as unstabilized tetramers, and approximately 50% have a molecular weight between 65 and 130 kD, with no more

than 10% having a molecular weight >500 kD. The product contains less than the detectable level of 3.5 micrograms/mL free-glutaraldehyde and 0.05 EU/mL, endotoxin.

Hemoglobin glutamer-200 (bovine) may also be known as HBOC-301, Hb-200, or HG-200.

Storage/Stability

The product remains stable at room temperature or refrigerated (2°-30°C) for up to 3 years; expiration date is printed on the bag. Outdated product is not returnable. Do not freeze. It must remain in its over wrap during storage; once removed, it should be used within 24 hours. The foil over wrap serves as an oxygen barrier, protecting the hemoglobin from conversion to methemoglobin.

Compatibility/Compounding Considerations

The manufacturer states that *Oxyglobin®* is physically **compatible** with any other IV fluid, but should not be mixed with other solutions or medications in the bag. Other intravenous solutions and medications may be administered via a separate site and line.

Dosage Forms/Regulatory Status

VETERINARY-LABELED PRODUCTS:

Hemoglobin Glutamer-200 (bovine) in 60 mL and 125 mL ready to use infusion bags; *Oxyglobin®*; (Rx). FDA-approved for use in dogs. At time of writing (2/2014), not currently available in USA. It reportedly may be available in Europe.

The ARCI (Racing Commissioners International) has designated this drug as a class 2 substance. It is prohibited to be at racing premises. See the appendix for more information.

HUMAN-LABELED PRODUCTS: NONE.

Revisions/References

Monograph revised/updated February 2014.

Driessen, B., et al. (2001). Inadequacy of low-volume resuscitation with hemoglobin-based oxygen carrier hemoglobin glutamer-200 (bovine) in canine hypovolemia. J. Vet. Pharmacol. Ther. 24(1): 61-71.

Gfeller, R. (2002). Traumatic shock resuscitation-What now? Proceedings: ACVIM Forum. accessed via Veterinary Information Network; vin.com

Haak, C. E., et al. (2012). Comparison of Hb-200 and 6% hetastarch 450/0.7 during initial fluid resuscitation of 20 dogs with gastric dilatation-volvulus. J. Vet. Emerg. Crit. Care 22(2): 201-10.

Jandrey, K. (2007). Principles and practice of transfusion medicine. Proceedings: UCD Canine Medicine Symposium. accessed via Veterinary Information Network; vin.com

Macintire, D. (2006). Immune-mediated hemolytic anemia--a metabolic disaster. Proceedings: ACVC. accessed via Veterinary Information Network; vin.com

Rudloff, E. & J. Devey (2009). Assessment and Management of the Multi-trauma Patient. Proceedings: IVECCS. accessed via Veterinary Information Network; vin.com

Waddell, L. S. (2009). Fluid therapy in the trauma patient. Proceedings: WVC.

Wehausen, C. E., et al. (2011). Evaluation of the effects of bovine hemoglobin glutamer-200 on systolic arterial blood pressure in hypotensive cats: 44 cases (1997‚Äì2008). Journal of the American Veterinary Medical Association 238(7): 909-14.

Heparin Sodium

(hep-ah-rin)   *Unfractionated Heparin, UHF*

Anticoagulant

Prescriber Highlights

▶ Parenteral anticoagulant used primarily for thromboprophylaxis and adjunctive treatment of thromboembolic disease.

▶ Contraindications: Known hypersensitivity, severe thrombocytopenia, or uncontrollable bleeding (caused by something other than DIC).

▶ Adverse Effects: Most common are bleeding & thrombocytopenia.

▶ Protamine may reverse effects.

▶ Monitoring is necessary; but specific guidelines are not yet clear for veterinary patients.

Uses/Indications

Heparin's primary uses in small animal medicine have been treatment of disseminated intravascular coagulation (DIC) and prophylaxis of thromboembolic disease. The most recent evidence is strong that prophylactic heparin can reduce incidence in patients at high risk for developing macrovascular thromboembolism. Use for treating DIC has become increasingly controversial and current evidence suggests that heparin should not be used during DIC in patients with concurrent inflammatory processes.

In horses, it has been used in the treatment of DIC and as prophylactic therapy for laminitis. To date, there are no controlled prospective studies that demonstrate efficacy for these indications. Heparin has also been administered systemically (IV, SC) or as an intraperitoneally administered lavage solution to prevent intestinal adhesion formation after surgery. Its efficacy for this indication is questionable.

Pharmacology/Actions

Heparin acts on coagulation factors in both the intrinsic and extrinsic coagulation pathways. Low concentrations of heparin when combined with antithrombin III inactivate factor X_a and prevent the conversion of prothrombin to thrombin. In higher doses, heparin inactivates thrombin, blocks the conversion of fibrinogen to fibrin and when combined with antithrombin III, inactivates factors IX, X, XI, XII. By inhibiting the activation of factor XIII (fibrin stabilizing factor), heparin prevents the formation of stable fibrin clots. While heparin will inhibit the reactions that lead to clotting, it does not significantly change the concentrations of clotting factors. Heparin does not lyse clots but it can prevent the growth of existing clots.

Heparin causes increased release of lipoprotein lipase thereby increasing the clearance of circulating lipids and boosting plasma levels of free fatty acids.

Pharmacokinetics

Heparin is not absorbed by the gut when administered orally; it must be given parenterally to be effective. Anticoagulant activity begins immediately after direct IV bolus injection, but may take up to one hour after deep SC injection. When heparin is given by continuous IV infusion, an initial bolus must be administered for full anticoagulant activity to begin.

Heparin is extensively protein bound, primarily to fibrinogen, low-density lipoproteins and globulins. It does not appreciably cross the placenta or enter milk.

Heparin's metabolic fate is not completely understood. The drug is apparently partially metabolized by the liver and also inactivated by the reticuloendothelial system. Serum half-lives in humans averages 1-2 hours.

In healthy dogs, bioavailability after subcutaneous injection is about 50%. When 200 Units/kg were administered to healthy dogs SC, plasma heparin concentrations were in the therapeutic range between 1 and 6 hours after administration. (Diquelou et al. 2005)

Contraindications/Precautions/Warnings

Heparin is contraindicated in patients hypersensitive to it, having severe thrombocytopenia or uncontrollable bleeding (caused by something other than DIC). One author (Green 1989) states that with DIC "heparin should not be given to actively bleeding patients that have severe factor depletion and thrombocytopenia, as fatal hemorrhage may result."

Use for treating DIC has become increasingly controversial. The most recent evidence suggests that heparin should not be used during DIC in patients with concurrent inflammatory processes. Until further evidence suggests practices to the contrary, heparin should be used with extreme caution in both human and veterinary patients with dysfunctional interactions between inflammatory and hemostatic systems and the endothelium (Bateman 2005).

Do not administer IM as heparin may cause hematoma formation. Hematomas, pain, and irritation may occur after deep SC dosing.

Dogs with renal insufficiency may have lower plasma levels and faster elimination rates of heparin; dosage adjustment may be required.

Adverse Effects

Bleeding and thrombocytopenia are the most common adverse effects associated with heparin therapy. Because heparin is derived from bovine or porcine tissues, hypersensitivity reactions may be possible. Less commonly encountered adverse effects that have been reported in animals and/or humans include vasospastic reactions (after several days of therapy), osteoporosis and diminished renal function (after long-term, high-dose therapy), rebound hyperlipidemia, hyperkalemia, alopecia, suppressed aldosterone synthesis and priapism.

The most common adverse effect associated with heparin therapy in horses is anemia, which is probably due to erythrocyte agglutination. Erythrocyte counts return to normal within 96 hours after heparin is stopped. Other adverse effects reported in horses include hemorrhage, thrombocytopenia, and pain at injection sites.

Reproductive/Nursing Safety

While heparin does not cross the placenta and is generally felt to be the anticoagulant of choice during pregnancy, its safe use in pregnancy has not been firmly established and pregnancy outcomes may be unfavorable. It should be used cautiously and only when clearly necessary. In humans, the FDA categorizes this drug as category C for use during pregnancy (*Animal studies have shown an adverse effect on the fetus, but there are no adequate studies in humans; or there are no animal reproduction studies and no adequate studies in humans.*)

Heparin is not excreted into milk.

Overdosage/Acute Toxicity

Overdosage of heparin is associated with bleeding. Clinical signs that could be seen before frank bleeding occurs include hematuria, tarry stools, petechiae, bruising, etc. Protamine can reverse heparin's effects; see the Protamine monograph for more information.

Drug Interactions

The following drug interactions have either been reported or are theoretical in humans or animals receiving heparin and may be of in veterinary patients. Unless otherwise noted, use together is not necessarily contraindicated, but weigh the potential risks and perform additional monitoring when appropriate.

- **ASPIRIN:** May increase the risk for hemorrhage.
- **DEXTRAN:** May increase the risk for hemorrhage.
- **NSAIDS:** May increase the risk for hemorrhage.
- **WARFARIN:** May increase the risk for hemorrhage.
- The following drugs may partially counteract heparin's anticoagulant effects: ANTIHISTAMINES, NITROGLYCERIN (IV), PROPYLENE GLYCOL, DIGOXIN, and TETRACYCLINES.

Laboratory Considerations

- Unless heparin is administered by continuous infusion, it can alter prothrombin time, (PT), which can be misleading in patients also receiving a coumarin or an indanedione anticoagulant.
- Heparin can interfere with the results of the BSP (sulfobromophthalein, bromosulfophthalein) test by changing the color intensity of the dye and shifting the absorption peak from 580 nm to 595 nm.
- Heparin can cause falsely elevated values of serum **thyroxine** if using competitive protein binding methods of determination. Radioimmunoassay (RIA) and protein bound iodine methods

are apparently unaffected by heparin.

- When heparin is used as an anticoagulant *in vitro* (*e.g.*, in **blood collection containers**), white cell counts should be performed within 2 hours of collection. Do not use heparinized blood for platelet counts, erythrocyte sedimentation rates, erythrocyte fragmentation tests, or for any tests involving complement or isoagglutinins. Errors in blood gas determinations for CO_2 pressure, bicarbonate concentration, or base excess may occur if heparin encompasses 10% or more of the blood sample.

Doses

- **DOGS:**

For thromboprophylaxis in patients with immune-mediated hemolytic anemia (extra-label): A recently published 'State of the Art Review' concluded that while heparin, aspirin, and clopidogrel have been used for thromboprophylaxis in dogs with IMHA, a lack of validated therapeutic endpoints and controlled studies make it difficult to determine if survival is affected or if one drug is more effective than another (Kidd et al. 2013). A small (N=15), but controlled study comparing a constant dose regimen versus adjusting dosage based upon anti-Xa monitoring found highly variable dosages (150 – 566 Units/kg q6h SC) were required to reach target anti-factor Xa activity. At day 180 of the study, 1 dog (of 7) was alive in the constant dose group; in the dosage adjustment group, 7 of 8 were still alive (Helmond et al. 2010). Until further guidelines on monitoring and dosing heparin have been determined, the following dosage recommendation may be considered: 150 – 300 Units/kg SC q6-8h. Each individual animal may respond differently to this dose, and therapy must be monitored by serial physical examination and by PTT or other coagulation assay (*e.g.*, thromboelastography).

In critically ill animals, a constant rate IV infusion (CRI) of UFH is more likely to result in consistent anti-coagulation and prolongation of PTT. A loading dose of 100 Units/kg is followed by a CRI from 20 – 50 Units/kg/hr. Small changes in the dose can result in large changes in PTT, and it is recommended to start at a low dose and slowly titrate higher in increments of 5 Units/kg/hr. To help prevent rebound hypercoagulability it is recommended to taper the dose gradually, decreasing by 50 Units/kg per dose day over 3-4 days (Brainard 2008).

- **CATS:**

For thromboprophylaxis in cats at risk for arterial thrombosis or thromboembolism (ATE); (extra-label): No outcome-based studies have evaluated any heparin dose for cats with ATE, and dosage recommendations are highly variable. Most cats receive either 50 – 100 Units/kg ("low-dose") or 200 – 300 Units/kg ("high-dose") SC q6-8h. There is wide individual variation in heparin pharmacokinetics in cats with ATE, with some requiring very high doses (up to 475 Units/kg) to maintain plasma concentrations within the therapeutic range. (Smith 2012)

- **HORSES:**

For thromboprophylaxis (extra-label): Dosages are not well established and recommendations range widely. 20 – 125 Units/kg SC or IV q6-12h have been noted.

In an attempt to prevent abdominal adhesions (extra-label): 30,000 – 50,000 Units heparin in 10 L of lavage fluid (warm LRS) and administered intraperitoneally via a 32 french fenestrated trocar catheter placed in the right ventral abdomen at the time of surgery. Lavage performed at 12, 18, 36, and 48 hours post-surgery and allowed to drain through a Heimlich valve. Drain removed after final lavage or it becomes occluded. (Eggleston et al. 2003)

Monitoring

Note: What constitutes appropriate monitoring in veterinary patients receiving heparin is controversial and no outcome-based guidelines have been accepted.

- While anti-factor Xa activity, whole blood clotting time (WBCT), partial thromboplastin time (PTT), and activated partial thromboplastin times (aPTT) may all be used to monitor therapy, aPTT is most often recommended for dogs or cats, but adjusting heparin therapy based on aPTT (1.5-2.5X prolongation target) may not correlate with anti-Xa activity in dogs (especially those with inflammatory diseases). Newer tests (*e.g.*, thromboelastography) are being evaluated, but the presence of anemia can affect results.
- Platelet counts and hematocrit (PCV) should be done periodically.
- Occult blood in stool and urine; other observations for bleeding.
- Clinical efficacy.

Client Information

- This medication must be injected subcutaneously (SC, under the skin); be sure you understand how to correctly give the injection. Several shots a day may be required.
- Bleeding can occur. If you see any bleeding, contact veterinarian immediately.
- If your animal is very listless (lacking energy or interest in things), appears to be having trouble breathing, has trouble walking or loses the use of its rear legs, contact your veterinarian immediately as blood clots may have formed.

Chemistry/Synonyms

Heparin is an anionic, heterogeneous sulfated glycosaminoglycan molecule with an average molecular weight of 12,000 that is found naturally in mast cells. It is available commercially as the sodium salt and is obtained from either porcine intestinal mucosa or bovine lung tissue (sodium salt only). Heparin sodium occurs as white or pale-colored, amorphous, hygroscopic powder having a faint odor. It is soluble in water and practically insoluble in alcohol; the commercial injections have a pH of 5-7.5. Heparin potency is expressed in terms of USP Heparin Units and values are obtained by comparing against a standard reference from the USP. The USP requires that potencies be not less than 120 Units/mg on a dried basis for heparin derived from lung tissue, and 140 Units/mg when derived from all other tissue sources.

Heparin sodium may also be as: heparinum natricum, sodium heparin, and soluble heparin; many trade names are available.

Storage/Stability

Heparin solutions should be stored at room temperature (15-30°C) and not frozen. Avoid excessive exposure to heat.

Compatibility/Compounding Considerations

Heparin sodium is reportedly physically **compatible** with the following intravenous solutions and drugs: amino acids 4.25%-dextrose 25%, dextrose-Ringer's combinations, dextrose-lactated Ringer's solutions, fat emulsion 10%, Ringer's injection, Normosol R, aminophylline, amphotericin B with or without hydrocortisone sodium phosphate, ascorbic acid injection, bleomycin sulfate, calcium gluconate, cephapirin sodium, chloramphenicol sodium succinate, clindamycin phosphate, dimenhydrinate, dopamine HCl, erythromycin gluceptate, isoproterenol HCl, lidocaine HCl, methylprednisolone sodium succinate, metronidazole with sodium succinate, norepinephrine bitartrate, potassium chloride, prednisolone sodium succinate, promazine HCl, sodium bicarbonate, verapamil HCl, and vitamin B-complex with or without vitamin C.

Heparin **compatibility information conflicts** or is dependent on diluent or concentration factors with the following drugs or solutions: dextrose-saline combinations, dextrose in water, lactated Ringer's injection, saline solutions, ampicillin sodium, dobutamine HCl, hydrocortisone sodium succinate, oxytetracycline HCl, penicillin G sodium/potassium, and tetracycline HCl. Compatibility is dependent upon factors such as pH, concentration, temperature and diluent used; consult specialized references or a hospital pharmacist for more specific information.

Heparin sodium is reported physically **incompatible** when mixed with the following solutions or drugs: sodium lactate 1/6 M, amikacin sulfate, chlorpromazine HCl, codeine phosphate, cytarabine, daunorubicin HCl, diazepam, doxorubicin HCl, erythromycin lactobionate, gentamicin sulfate, hyaluronidase, levorphanol bitartrate, meperidine HCl, methadone HCl, morphine sulfate, pentazocine lactate, phenytoin sodium, polymyxin B sulfate, and vancomycin HCl.

Dosage Forms/Regulatory Status

VETERINARY-LABELED PRODUCTS: NONE.

HUMAN-LABELED PRODUCTS:

Heparin Sodium Injection: 1000 Units/mL, 2000 Units/mL, 2500 Units/mL, 5000 Units/mL, 10,000 Units/mL, 20,000 Units/mL, & 40,000 Units/mL in 0.5 mL, 1 mL, 2 mL, 4 mL, 5 mL, 10 mL, and 30 mL vials; generic; (Rx).

Heparin Unit-Dose Sodium Injection: 1000 Units/dose, 2500 Units/dose, 5000 Units/dose, 7500 Units/dose, 10,000 Units/dose and 20,000 Units/dose in 1 mL, 10 mL, & 30 mL *Dosette* vials, 0.5 mL & 1 mL *Tubex*, 0.5 mL, 1 mL, 4 mL & 10 mL vials, and 1 mL fill in 2 mL *Carpuject* (depending on concentration and manufacturer); generic; (Rx)

Heparin Sodium and 0.9% Sodium Chloride Injection: 1000 & 2000 Units in 500 mL and 1000 mL, respectively; generic; (Rx)

Heparin Sodium and 0.45% Sodium Chloride Injection: 12,500 in 250 mL & 25,000 Units in 250 mL & 500 mL; generic; (Rx)

Heparin Sodium Lock Flush (IV use) Injection: 1 Unit/mL in 1, 2, 2.5, 5 & 10 mL syringes; 10 Units/mL and 100 Units/mL in 1, 2, 5, 10 mL (regular and preservative free), 30 mL & 50 mL vials; 1 mL (regular and preservative free) & 2 mL *Dosette* vials; 1 mL & 2.5 mL *Dosette* cartridge needle units; 1 mL amps; 1 mL, 2 mL, 2.5 mL, 3 mL, and 5 mL disposable syringes; generic; (Rx)

Revisions/References

Monograph revised/updated February 2014.

Bateman, S. (2005). DIC and Heparin. Proceedings: IVECCS. accessed via Veterinary Information Network; vin.com

Brainard, B. (2008). Practical anticoagulation. Proceedings: IVECCS. accessed via Veterinary Information Network; vin.com

Diquelou, A., et al. (2005). Pharmacokinetics and pharmacodynamics of a therapeutic dose of unfractionated heparin (200 I/kg) administered subcutaneously or intravenously to healthy dogs. Vet Clin Path 34(3): 237-42.

Eggleston, R. B. & P. O. E. Mueller (2003). Prevention and treatment of gastrointestinal adhesions. Veterinary Clinics of North America-Equine Practice 19(3): 741-+.

Helmond, S. E., et al. (2010). Treatment of Immune-Mediated Hemolytic Anemia with Individually Adjusted Heparin Dosing in Dogs. Journal of Veterinary Internal Medicine 24(3): 597-605.

Kidd, L. & N. Mackman (2013). Prothrombotic mechanisms and anticoagulant therapy in dogs with immune-mediated hemolytic anemia. J. Vet. Emerg. Crit. Care 23(1): 3-13.

Smith, S. A. (2012). Antithrombotic Therapy. Topics in Companion Animal Medicine 27(2): 88-94.

Hetastarch—See Hydroxyethyl Starch

Hyaluronate Sodium
Sodium Hyaluronate
Hyaluronan

(hy-al-yoo-ron-nate) Hyalovet®, Hyvisc®, Legend®

Mucopolysaccharide

Prescriber Highlights

▶ Parenteral, high viscosity mucopolysaccharide used for synovitis.

▶ Contraindications: None on label.

▶ Adverse Effects: Local reactions possible.

▶ Different products have different dosages, etc.; check label before using.

Uses/Indications

Hyaluronate sodium (HS) is useful in the treatment of synovitis not associated with severe degenerative joint disease. It may be helpful to treat secondary synovitis in conditions where full thickness cartilage loss exists.

The choice of a high molecular weight product (MW >1×10^6) versus a low molecular weight one is quite controversial. One author (Nixon 1992) states "…low molecular weight products (which tend to be less expensive) can be equally efficacious in ameliorating signs of joint disease. When synovial adhesions and pannus are to be avoided (as in most surgeries for carpal and fetlock fracture fragment removal), higher molecular weight preparations are recommended because they inhibit proliferation of synovial fibroblasts." However, at the time of writing (2014), there are no controlled studies directly comparing the various products for treating joint disease and product choice is primarily a result of a clinician's personal preference.

There is considerable interest in oral hyaluronate administration for treating equine joint disease. One blinded, controlled study found the use of an oral gel "nutraceutical" significantly reduced synovial effusion in tarsocrural joints post-arthroscopic surgery for osteochondritis dissecans (OCD) (Bergin et al. 2006).

Pharmacology/Actions

Hyaluronate sodium (HS) is found naturally in the connective tissue of both man and animals and is identical chemically regardless of species. Highest concentrations found naturally are in the synovial fluid, vitreous of the eye and umbilical cord. Surfaces of articular cartilage are covered with a thin layer of a protein-hyaluronate complex; hyaluronate is also found in synovial fluid and the cartilage matrix. The net effects in joints include a cushioning effect, reduction of protein and cellular influx into the joint, and a lubricating effect. Hyaluronate has a direct antiinflammatory effect in joints by scavenging free radicals and suppressing prostaglandins.

Pharmacokinetics

In the equine joint the half-life of hyaluronate has been reported to be 96 hours.

Contraindications/Precautions/Warnings

No contraindications to HS's use are noted on the label. HS should not be used as a substitute for adequate diagnosis; radiographic examinations should be performed to rule out serious fractures. Do not perform intra-articular injections through skin that has been recently fired or blistered, or that has excessive scurf and counterirritants on it.

Adverse Effects

Some patients may develop local reactions manifested by heat, swelling, and/or effusion. Effects generally subside within 24-48 hours; some animals may require up to 96 hours for resolution. No treatment for this effect is recommended. When used in combination with other drugs, incidence of flares may actually be higher. No systemic adverse effects have been noted.

Reproductive/Nursing Safety

While HS is unlikely to cause problems, safe use in breeding animals has not been established and most manufacturers caution against its use in these animals.

Overdosage/Acute Toxicity

Acute toxicology studies performed in horses have demonstrated no systemic toxicity associated with overdoses.

Drug Interactions/Laboratory Considerations

▪ None were noted.

Doses

▪ **HORSES:**

Note: Because of the differences in the commercially available products, see each individual product's label for specific dosing information. The following are recommended doses from a review article (Goodrich et al. 2006) on the medical treatment of osteoarthritis in the horse:

Hylartin-V®: 20 mg IA (intra-articularly)

Hyvisc®: 20 mg IA

Equron®: 10 mg IA

Synacid®: 50 mg IA

Hyalovet®: 20 mg IA

Legend®: 40 mg IV (also labeled for IA injection: 20 mg)

To reduce joint effusion post-arthroscopic surgery for osteochondritis dissecans (OCD): 100 mg PO (as an oral gel; *Conquer®*) once daily for 30 days. (Bergin et al. 2006)

▪ **DOGS:**

For the adjunctive treatment of synovitis (rather than the presence of a damaged articular cartilage): Using a high molecular weight compound: 3 – 5 mg IA using sterile technique at weekly intervals. Long-term effects are not achieved. (Bloomberg 1992)

Client Information

▪ HS should be administered by a veterinarian only, using aseptic technique.

Chemistry/Synonyms

Hyaluronate sodium (HS) is the sodium salt of hyaluronic acid which is a naturally occurring high-viscosity mucopolysaccharide. Much of the commercially available hyaluronic acid products are derived from the combs of roosters.

Hyaluronate sodium may also be known as: HA, hyaluronan, "rooster juice", hyaluronic acid, and natrii hyaluronas; many trade names are available.

Storage/Stability

Store at room temperature or refrigerate depending on the product used—check label; do not freeze. Protect from light.

Compatibility/Compounding Considerations

Unless the product's label states otherwise, do not mix with other drugs.

Dosage Forms/Regulatory Status

VETERINARY-LABELED PRODUCTS:

Hyaluronate Sodium: There are many equine products for intraarticular administration available in various molecular weights, concentrations and package sizes including: *Hyalovet®*, *Legend®*, *NexHA®*; *Hyvisc®*, *Equron®*, *Hylartin®V*, and *Synacid®*; (Rx) FDA-approved for use in horses not intended for food.

Hyaluronate Sodium Oral Gel: 10 mg/mL (100 mg/10 mL) (apple-flavored) in 60 mL tubes; *Conquer®* Equine Gel. This product is labeled as a nutritional supplement and is not FDA-approved.

There may also be other hyaluronate products marketed as topical solutions, semen extenders, and oral supplements. These products are not necessarily approved by the FDA.

HUMAN-LABELED PRODUCTS: NONE.

Revisions/References

Monograph revised/updated February 2014.

Bergin, B. J., et al. (2006). Oral hyaluronan gel reduces post operative tarsocrural effusion in the yearling Thoroughbred. Equine Veterinary Journal 38(4): 375-8.

Bloomberg, M. (1992). Pharmacokinetics of musculoskeletal drugs (Polysulfated Glycosaminoglycans, DMSO, Orgotein, and Hyaluronic Acid). Minnesota Veterinary Medicine Association: Annual Conference, Bloomington. accessed via Veterinary Information Network; vin.com

Goodrich, L. R. & A. J. Nixon (2006). Medical treatment of osteoarthritis in the horse - A review. Veterinary Journal 171(1): 51-69.

Hydralazine HCl

(hye-dral-a-zeen)   Apresoline®

Vasodilator

Prescriber Highlights

► Vasodilator drug used primarily for hypertension or adjunctive treatment of heart failure.

► Contraindications: Known hypersensitivity, coronary artery disease, hypovolemia or preexisting hypotension.

► Caution: Severe renal disease, intracerebral bleeding, preexisting autoimmune diseases.

► Adverse Effects: Hypotension, reflex tachycardia, sodium/water retention (if not given concurrently with a diuretic), or GI distress (vomiting, diarrhea).

► Drug interactions.

Uses/Indications

The primary uses of hydralazine in veterinary medicine have been as an afterload reducer for the adjunctive treatment in CHF and as an antihypertensive agent in dogs and cats. Hydralazine is not particularly useful in treating heart failure when myocardial disease is present, but may be of benefit if mitral valve insufficiency is the primary cause of heart failure when an ACE inhibitor is not effective in improving clinical signs. Additionally, it may be useful in dogs and cats with large septal defects or severe aortic regurgitation. When used to treat systemic hypertension, hydralazine is generally used in combination with other drugs (*e.g.*, beta-blockers) to offset hydralazine's tendency to cause reflex tachycardia and fluid retention.

Pharmacology/Actions

Hydralazine acts upon vascular smooth muscle and reduces peripheral resistance and blood pressure. Hydralazine is a semicarbazide-sensitive amine oxidase (SSAO) inhibitor. It is believed that hydralazine alters cellular calcium metabolism in smooth muscle, thereby interfering with calcium movements and preventing the initiation and maintenance of the contractile state. Hydralazine has more effect on arterioles than on veins.

In patients with CHF, hydralazine significantly increases cardiac output, and decreases systemic vascular resistance. Cardiac rate may be slightly increased or unchanged while blood pressure, pulmonary venous pressure, and right atrial pressure may be decreased or unchanged.

When used to treat hypertensive patients (without CHF), increased heart rate, cardiac output and stroke volume can be noted. The renin-angiotensin system can be activated with a resultant increase in sodium and water retention if not given with diuretics or sympathetic blocking drugs.

Parenteral hydralazine administration can cause respiratory stimulation.

Pharmacokinetics

In dogs, hydralazine is rapidly absorbed after oral administration with an onset of action within one hour and peak effects at 3-5 hours. There is a high first-pass effect after oral administration. The presence of food may enhance the bioavailability of hydralazine tablets.

Hydralazine is widely distributed in body tissues. In humans, approximately 85% of the drug in the blood is bound to plasma proteins. Hydralazine crosses the placenta and very small amounts are excreted into the milk.

Hydralazine is extensively metabolized in the liver and approximately 15% is excreted unchanged in the urine. The half-life in humans is usually 2-4 hours, but may be as long as 8 hours.

Specific pharmacokinetic parameters for this drug in veterinary species are limited, but the duration of action of hydralazine in dogs after oral administration is reportedly 11-13 hours. Vasodilating effects occur within one hour and peak within 3 hours of dosing. Food decreases oral bioavailability in dogs by about 63%. At lower doses there is relatively high first pass effect but this is apparently a saturable process as bioavailability increases with dose. N-acetylation is a primary enzymatic pathway for hydralazine metabolism and this pathway is mostly absent in dogs leading to concerns for increased risks for toxicity.

Contraindications/Precautions/Warnings

Hydralazine is contraindicated in patients hypersensitive to it and those with coronary artery disease. The drug is listed as contraindicated in human patients with mitral valvular rheumatic disease, but it has been recommended for use in small animal patients with mitral valve insufficiency. It is not recommended to use the drug in patients with hypovolemia or preexisting hypotension.

Doses need to be titrated upwards carefully as severe hypotension can result.

Hydralazine should be used with caution in patients with renal disease. Secondary to reduced renal blood flow, hydralazine can activate the renin angiotensin aldosterone system (RAAS) and exacerbate renal injury; pretreatment with an ACE inhibitor and spironolactone is often advised to reduce this risk.

Hydralazine should be used with caution in patients with intracerebral bleeding. In humans, a syndrome resembling systemic lupus erythematosus (SLE) has been documented after hydralazine use. While this syndrome has not been documented in veterinary patients, the drug should be used with caution in patients with preexisting autoimmune diseases.

Do not confuse hydrALAzine with hydrOXYzine.

Adverse Effects

The most prevalent adverse effects seen in small animals are hypotension, weakness/lethargy and syncope particularly when doses are increased too fast. Reflex tachycardia, sodium/water retention (if not given concurrently with a diuretic), and GI distress (vomiting, diarrhea) can also occur. If necessary, tachycardias may be treated with digoxin or a beta-blocker (Caution: beta-blockers may reduce cardiac performance). Hydralazine can increase creatinine levels. Other adverse effects documented in humans that could occur include: an SLE-like syndrome, lacrimation, conjunctivitis, peripheral neuritis, blood dyscrasias, urinary retention, constipation, and hypersensitivity reactions.

Reproductive/Nursing Safety

In humans, the FDA categorizes this drug as category *C* for use during pregnancy (*Animal studies have shown an adverse effect on the fetus, but there are no adequate studies in humans; or there are no animal reproduction studies and no adequate studies in humans*).

In a separate system evaluating the safety of drugs in canine and feline pregnancy (Papich 1989), this drug is categorized as class: *B* (*Safe for use if used cautiously. Studies in laboratory animals may have uncovered some risk, but these drugs appear to be safe in dogs and cats or these drugs are safe if they are not administered when the animal is near term.*)

Hydralazine is excreted in milk. According to the American Academy of Pediatrics, hydralazine is compatible with breastfeeding, but exercise caution.

Overdosage /Acute Toxicity

Overdoses may be characterized by severe hypotension, tachycardia or other arrhythmias, skin flushing, and myocardial ischemia. Cardiovascular system support is the primary treatment modality. Evacuate gastric contents and administer activated charcoal using standard precautionary measures if the ingestion was recent and cardiovascular status has been stabilized. Treat shock using volume expanders without using pressor agents if possible. If a pressor agent is required to maintain blood pressure, the use of a minimally arrhythmogenic agent (*e.g.*, phenylephrine or methoxamine) is recommended. Digitalis agents may be required. Monitor blood pressure and renal function diligently.

Drug Interactions

The following drug interactions have either been reported or are theoretical in humans or animals receiving hydralazine and may be of in veterinary patients. Unless otherwise noted, use together is not necessarily contraindicated, but weigh the potential risks and perform additional monitoring when appropriate.

- **ACE-INHIBITORS:** May cause additive hypotensive effect; usually used for therapeutic advantage.
- **BETA-BLOCKERS:** May cause additive hypotensive effect; usually used for therapeutic advantage.
- **DIAZOXIDE:** Potentially could cause profound hypotension.
- **DIURETICS:** May cause additive hypotensive effect; usually used for therapeutic advantage.
- **FUROSEMIDE:** Hydralazine may increase furosemide's renal effects.
- **MAO INHIBITORS:** May cause additive hypotensive effect.
- **SYMPATHOMIMETICS** (*e.g.*, **epinephrine**): Hydralazine may cause decreased pressor effect and additive tachycardia.

Doses

Because of the sodium/water retention associated with this drug, it is often used concurrently with a diuretic when used for adjunctive treatment of heart failure. When used for hypertension, a diuretic may not be required.

DOGS:

For adjunctive therapy in treatment of heart failure secondary to valve disease (extra-label): Published high-level evidence is not available to support any dosage, but many cardiologists believe the drug may be useful in certain circumstances, particularly in dogs with refractory CHF. The following dosage regimen is one example:

Effective dose is 0.5 – 3 mg/kg PO q12h. Dose must be titrated, starting with a low dose and titrating upwards.

In dogs that are not receiving ACE inhibitors: Get initial baseline assessment (mucous membrane color, capillary refill time, murmur intensity, cardiac size on radiographs, and severity of pulmonary edema). Starting dose is 1 mg/kg PO q12h and repeat assessments made in 12-48 hours. If no response identified, increase dosage to 2 mg/kg q12h. Repeat assessments as above and increase to 3 mg/kg PO q12h if no response. Can be titrated with or without blood pressure monitoring. If BP cannot be

monitored, titration is performed more slowly and clinical and radiographic signs are monitored.

If blood pressure measurement available, dosage titration can be made more rapidly than above: Measure baseline blood pressure. Administer 1 mg/kg PO. Repeat BP in 1-2 hours and if it has decreased by at least 15 mmHg, administer q12h from then on. If response is inadequate, give another 1 mg/kg and repeat BP measurement in 1-2 hours. This may be repeated until a cumulative dose of 3 mg/kg has been given within a 12-hour period. The resulting cumulative dose becomes the dosage to be given q12h.

In dogs that are receiving ACE inhibitors: Give hydralazine with caution as severe hypotension may occur if dosage not titrated carefully. Begin dosing at 0.5 mg/kg with blood pressure monitoring and increase in 0.5 mg/kg increments until a response is identified to a maximum of 3 mg/kg. Consider referral.

For dogs with acute, fulminant heart failure due to severe mitral regurgitation and not receiving ACE inhibitors: 2 mg/kg along with IV furosemide. May cause hypotension, but the risks of not effectively treating fulminant pulmonary edema outweigh the risks of treating. (Kittleson 2000, 2007)

For treatment of systemic hypertension (extra-label): For severe, acute hypertension, hydralazine can be considered as an alternative to nitroprusside. Parenteral doses of 0.5 – 3 mg/kg IV q12h or a 0.1 mg/kg IV loading dose, followed by a CRI of 1.5 – 5 micrograms/kg/minute has been noted (Ross 2011). Oral dosages of 0.5 – 3 mg/kg PO q12h to effect have also been reported. For chronic use, refer to the heart failure (Kittleson) dose above.

- **CATS:**

For adjunctive therapy in treatment of heart failure (extra-label): See the dog dose above for heart failure, but start titration at 2.5 mg (total dose) and if necessary, increase up to 10 mg. (Kittleson 1985)

For treatment of systemic hypertension (extra-label): For severe, acute hypertension: Parenteral doses of: 2.5 mg per cat SC; may be repeated in 15-30 minutes if systolic BP has not decreased; or 0.1 mg/kg IV loading dose, followed by a CRI of 1.5 – 5 micrograms/kg/minute have been noted. Oral dosages of 2.5 mg per cat PO q12h to effect have also been recommended. For chronic treatment of hypertension in cats, hydralazine is usually considered as a "third or fourth step" drug after amlodipine, ACE inhibitors, and possibly spironolactone. It is usually dosed at 2.5 mg per cat (1/4 of a 10 mg tablet) PO twice daily.

- **HORSES:** (NOTE: ARCI UCGFS CLASS 3 DRUG)

For adjunctive therapy in treatment of heart failure (afterload reducer); (extra-label): Not commonly used in horses. One dosage recommendation is: 0.5 mg/kg IV; for long-term therapy use 0.5 – 1.5 mg/kg PO q12h. (Mogg 1999)

Monitoring

- Baseline thoracic radiographs.
- Mucous membrane color.
- Serum electrolytes.
- If possible, arterial blood pressure and venous PO_2. A mean arterial pressure (MAP) of between 60-80 mmHg has been recommended when used in dogs for the short-term treatment of CHF secondary to valve disease (Erling et al. 2008).
- Because blood dyscrasias are a possibility, an occasional CBC should be considered.

Client Information

- Give this medication with food.
- When starting your animal on this medication, your veterinari-

an may start with a low dose and gradually increase it over time. Be sure you are giving your animal the right dose.

- If given initially in too large a dose, hydralazine may cause low blood pressure and cause your animal's condition to get worse. Loss of appetite, depression, lack of energy or muscle weakness can indicate that blood pressure is too low.

Chemistry/Synonyms

A phthalazine-derivative antihypertensive and vasodilating agent, hydralazine HCl occurs as an odorless, white to off-white crystalline powder with a melting point between 270-280°C and a pK_a of 7.3. One gram is soluble in approximately 25 mL of water or 500 mL of alcohol. The commercially available injection has a pH of 3.4-4.

Hydralazine may also be known as: apressinum, hydralazini, hydrallazine, idralazina, *or Apresoline®*.

Storage/Stability

Hydralazine tablets should be stored in tight, light resistant containers at room temperature. The injectable product should be stored at room temperature; avoid refrigeration or freezing.

When mixed with most infusion solutions a color change can occur which does not necessarily indicate a loss in potency (if occurred over 8-12 hours).

Compatibility/Compounding Considerations

Hydralazine is reported to be physically **compatible** with the following infusion solutions/drugs: dextrose-Ringer's combinations, dextrose-saline combinations, Ringer's injection, lactated Ringer's injection, sodium chloride solutions, and dobutamine HCl.

Hydralazine is reported to be physically **incompatible** when mixed with 10% dextrose or fructose and is reported to be physically **incompatible** when mixed with the following drugs: aminophylline, ampicillin sodium, chlorothiazide sodium, edetate calcium disodium, hydrocortisone sodium succinate, phenobarbital sodium, and verapamil HCl. Compatibility is dependent upon factors such as pH, concentration, temperature, and diluent used; consult specialized references for more specific information.

Dosage Forms/Regulatory Status

VETERINARY-LABELED PRODUCTS: NONE.

The ARCI (Racing Commissioners International) has designated this drug as a class 3 substance. See the appendix for more information.

HUMAN-LABELED PRODUCTS:

Hydralazine HCl Oral Tablets: 10 mg, 25 mg, 50 mg & 100 mg; generic; (Rx)

Hydralazine Injection: 20 mg/mL in 1 mL vials; generic; (Rx)

Revisions/References

Monograph revised/updated February 2014.

Erling, P. & E. M. Mazzaferro (2008). Left-sided congestive heart failure in dogs: Treatment and monitoring of emergency patients. Compendium-Continuing Education for Veterinarians 30(2): 94-+.

Kittleson, M. (2000). Therapy of Heart Failure. *Textbook of Veterinary Internal Medicine: Diseases of the Dog and Cat.* S. Ettinger and E. Feldman. Philadelphia, WB Saunders. 1: 713-37.

Kittleson, M. (2007). Management of Heart Failure. *Small Animal Medicine Cardiology Textbook, 2nd Ed.,* Accessed Online via the Veterinary Drug Information Network.

Kittleson, M. D. (1985). Pathophysiology and treatment of heart failure. *Manual of Small Animal Cardiology.* L. P. Tilley and J. M. Owens. New York, Churchill Livingstone: 308-32.

Mogg, T. (1999). Equine Cardiac Disease: Clinical pharmacology and therapeutics. The Veterinary Clinics of North America: Equine Practice 15:3(December).

Ross, L. (2011). Acute Kidney Injury in Dogs and Cats. Veterinary Clinics of North America-Small Animal Practice 41(1): 1-+.

Hydrochlorothiazide

(hye-droe-klor-oh-thye-a-zide)   HydroDIURIL®

Thiazide Diuretic

Prescriber Highlights

▶ Thiazide diuretic used for nephrogenic diabetes insipidus, hypertension, calcium oxalate urolith prevention, hypoglycemia, & as a diuretic for heart failure.

▶ Contraindications: Hypersensitivity; pregnancy (relative contraindication).

▶ Extreme Caution/Avoid: Severe renal disease, preexisting electrolyte/water balance abnormalities, impaired hepatic function, hyperuricemia, SLE, diabetes mellitus.

▶ Adverse Effects: Hypokalemia, hypochloremic alkalosis, other electrolyte imbalances, hyperuricemia, GI effects.

▶ Many possible drug interactions; lab test interactions.

Uses/Indications

In veterinary medicine, furosemide has largely supplanted the use of thiazides as a general diuretic (edema treatment). But there are times when they can be very useful drugs. Thiazides are still used for the treatment of systemic hypertension, ascites, hypermagnesemia, nephrogenic diabetes insipidus, and to help prevent the recurrence of calcium oxalate uroliths in dogs, and potentially in cats. In horses, hydrochlorothiazide may be used as an alternative to acetazolamide for hyperkalemic periodic paralysis (HyPP) when dietary therapy alone does not control episodes.

Pharmacology/Actions

Thiazide diuretics act by interfering with the transport of sodium ions across renal tubular epithelium possibly by altering the metabolism of tubular cells. The principle site of action is at the cortical diluting segment of the nephron. Enhanced excretion of sodium, chloride, and water results. Thiazides increase the excretion of potassium, magnesium, phosphate, iodide, and bromide and decrease the glomerular filtration rate (GFR). Plasma renin and resulting aldosterone levels are increased which contribute to the hypokalemic effects of the thiazides. Bicarbonate excretion is increased, but effects on urine pH are usually minimal. Thiazides initially have a hypercalciuric effect, although with continued therapy calcium excretion is significantly decreased. Uric acid excretion is decreased by the thiazides. Thiazides can cause or exacerbate hyperglycemia in diabetic patients or induce diabetes mellitus in prediabetic patients.

The antihypertensive effects of thiazides are well known and these agents are used extensively in human medicine for treating essential hypertension. The exact mechanism for this effect has not been established.

Thiazides paradoxically reduce urine output in patients with diabetes insipidus (DI). They have been used as adjunctive therapy in patients with neurogenic DI and are the only drug therapy for nephrogenic DI.

Pharmacokinetics

The pharmacokinetics of the thiazides have apparently not been studied in domestic animals. In humans, hydrochlorothiazide is about 65-75% absorbed after oral administration. The onset of diuretic activity occurs in 2 hours; peaks at 4-6 hours. The serum half-life is approximately 5.6-14.8 hours and the duration of activity is 6-12 hours. The drug is apparently not metabolized and is excreted unchanged into the urine. Like all thiazides, the antihypertensive effects of hydrochlorothiazide may take several days to occur.

Contraindications/Precautions/Warnings

Hydrochlorothiazide is contraindicated in patients with anuria or hypersensitive to any thiazide. Although many sources state that thiazides are contraindicated in patients hypersensitive to sulfonamides, clear evidence for cross-reactivity has not been established in humans or animals. In humans, their use is inappropriate during pregnancy in women who are otherwise healthy and have only mild edema.

Do not use in dogs with absorptive (intestinal) hypercalcuria as hypercalcemia may result.

Thiazides should be used with extreme caution, if at all, in patients with severe renal disease or with preexisting electrolyte (including hypercalcemia) or water balance abnormalities, impaired hepatic function (may precipitate hepatic coma), hyperuricemia, lupus (SLE), or diabetes mellitus. Patients with conditions that may lead to electrolyte or water balance abnormalities (*e.g.*, vomiting, diarrhea, etc.) should be monitored carefully.

Adverse Effects

- Gastrointestinal effects (vomiting, diarrhea, etc.) are possible and may be more prevalent in animals with mild azotemia.
- Hypokalemia is possible, but rarely causes clinical signs or progresses. However, monitoring of potassium is recommended with chronic therapy. Hypochloremic alkalosis (with hypokalemia) may develop, especially if there are other causes of potassium and chloride loss (*e.g.*, vomiting, diarrhea, potassium-losing nephropathies, etc.) or the patient has cirrhotic liver disease.
- Dilutional hyponatremia and hypomagnesemia may occur.
- Hyperparathyroid-like effects of hypercalcemia and hypophosphatemia have been reported in humans, but have not led to effects such as nephrolithiasis, bone resorption, or peptic ulceration.
- Hyperuricemia can occur, but is usually asymptomatic.
- Other possible adverse effects include: hypersensitivity/dermatologic reactions, GU reactions (polyuria), hematologic toxicity, hyperglycemia, hyperlipidemias, and orthostatic hypotension.

Reproductive/Nursing Safety

In humans, the FDA categorizes this drug as category *B* for use during pregnancy (*Animal studies have not yet demonstrated risk to the fetus, but there are no adequate studies in pregnant women; or animal studies have shown an adverse effect, but adequate studies in pregnant women have not demonstrated a risk to the fetus in the first trimester of pregnancy, and there is no evidence of risk in later trimesters.*) In a separate system evaluating the safety of drugs in canine and feline pregnancy (Papich 1989), thiazides are categorized as class: *C* (*These drugs may have potential risks. Studies in people or laboratory animals have uncovered risks, and these drugs should be used cautiously as a last resort when the benefit of therapy clearly outweighs the risks.*)

Thiazides may appear in milk and there have been case reports of newborn human infants developing thrombocytopenia when their mothers received thiazides.

Overdosage/Acute Toxicity

Acute overdosage may cause electrolyte and water balance problems, CNS effects (lethargy to coma and seizures), and GI effects (hypermotility, GI distress). Transient increases in BUN have been reported.

Treatment consists of emptying the gut after recent oral ingestion using standard protocols. Avoid giving concomitant cathartics as they may exacerbate the fluid and electrolyte imbalances that may ensue. Monitor and treat electrolyte and water balance abnormalities supportively. Additionally, monitor respiratory, CNS, and cardiovascular status; treat supportively and symptomatically if required.

Drug Interactions

The following drug interactions have either been reported or are theoretical in humans or animals receiving hydrochlorothiazide and may be of in veterinary patients. Unless otherwise noted, use together is not necessarily contraindicated, but weigh the potential risks and perform additional monitoring when appropriate.

- **AMPHOTERICIN B:** Use with thiazides can lead to an increased risk for severe hypokalemia.
- **CORTICOSTEROIDS, CORTICOTROPIN:** Use with thiazides can lead to an increased risk for severe hypokalemia.
- **DIAZOXIDE:** Increased risk for hyperglycemia, hyperuricemia, and hypotension.
- **DIGOXIN:** Thiazide-induced hypokalemia, hypomagnesemia, and/or hypercalcemia may increase the likelihood of digitalis toxicity.
- **INSULIN:** Thiazides may increase insulin requirements.
- **LITHIUM:** Thiazides can increase serum lithium concentrations.
- **METHENAMINE:** Thiazides can alkalinize urine and reduce methenamine effectiveness.
- **NSAIDS:** Thiazides may increase risk for renal toxicity and NSAIDs may reduce diuretic actions of thiazides.
- **NEUROMUSCULAR BLOCKING AGENTS:** Tubocurarine or other nondepolarizing neuromuscular blocking agents response or duration of effect may be increased.
- **PROBENECID:** Blocks thiazide-induced uric acid retention (used to therapeutic advantage).
- **QUINIDINE:** Half-life may be prolonged by thiazides (thiazides can alkalinize the urine).
- **VITAMIN D or CALCIUM SALTS:** Hypercalcemia may be exacerbated if thiazides are concurrently administered.

Laboratory Considerations

- **AMYLASE:** Thiazides can increase serum amylase values in asymptomatic patients and those in the developmental stages of acute pancreatitis (humans).
- **CORTISOL:** Thiazides can decrease the renal excretion of cortisol.
- **ESTROGEN, URINARY:** Hydrochlorothiazide may falsely decrease total urinary estrogen when using a spectrophotometric assay.
- **HISTAMINE:** Thiazides may cause false-negative results when testing for pheochromocytoma.
- **PARATHYROID-FUNCTION TESTS:** Thiazides may elevate serum calcium; recommend discontinuing thiazides prior to testing.
- **PHENOLSULFONPHTHALEIN (PSP):** Thiazides can compete for secretion at proximal renal tubules.
- **PHENTOLAMINE TEST:** Thiazides may give false-negative results.
- **PROTEIN-BOUND IODINE:** Thiazides may decrease values.
- **TRIIODOTHYRONINE RESIN UPTAKE TEST:** Thiazides may slightly reduce uptake.
- **TYRAMINE:** Thiazides can cause false-negative results.

Doses

- **DOGS:**

  For prevention of recurrent calcium oxalate uroliths with renal hypercalcuria: (extra-label): Usually added when dietary therapy does not adequately control calcium oxalate crystalluria. Most recommend 2 – 2.2 mg/kg PO q12h. Although an upper dosage limit of 4 mg/kg PO q12h has been noted.

As a diuretic (extra-label):

For adjunctive treatment of heart failure when patients become refractory to furosemide alone: Several dosage regimens have been recommended, but evidence is weak supporting any specific one. Most recommendations are between 1 – 4 mg/kg PO q12h. Many recommend starting at the low end (1 – 2 mg/kg and giving PO q12h) and then titrating dosage upwards if required. Some patients may only require once a day dosing at 1 – 2 mg/kg. Some use with spironolactone, particularly if hypokalemia is an issue.

For ascites in patients with liver disease using the fixed-dose (1:1) combination with spironolactone (*aka Aldactazide®*): Dosed empirically based on the spironolactone content at 0.5 – 1 mg/kg PO twice daily. (Trepanier 2008)

For treatment of systemic hypertension (extra-label): As a second choice agent, 1 mg/kg PO q12-24h; may combine with spironolactone (1 – 2 mg/kg PO q12 hours) to reduce potassium loss. (Brown et al. 2000), (Brown 2008)

For treatment of nephrogenic diabetes insipidus (extra-label): Based on a case report: 2 mg/kg PO twice daily with a low sodium diet. (Takemura 1998)

- **CATS:**

  As a diuretic (extra-label): For heart failure in combination with furosemide in patients who have become refractory to furosemide alone: 1 – 2 mg/kg PO q12h. (Kittleson 2000), (Kittleson 2006)

  For ascites in patients with liver disease using the fixed-dose (1:1) combination with spironolactone (*aka Aldactazide®*): Dosed empirically based on the spironolactone content at 0.5 – 1 mg/kg PO twice daily. (Trepanier 2008)

  To reduce calcium oxalate saturation in urine (extra-label): Study done in normal cats, unknown what effect HCTZ will have in cats with spontaneously occurring calcium oxalate urolithiasis: 1 mg/kg PO q12h. (Hezel et al. 2007)

- **HORSES:** (NOTE: ARCI UCGFS CLASS 4 DRUG)

  For adjunctive therapy of hyperkalemic periodic paralysis (HyPP); (extra-label): 0.5 – 1 mg/kg PO q12h when diet adjustment does not control episodes. (Valberg 2008)

Monitoring

- Serum electrolytes, BUN, creatinine, glucose.
- Hydration status.
- Blood pressure, if indicated.
- Hemograms, if indicated.

Client Information

- When beginning this medicine your animal may urinate more often than normal.
- May be given with or without food. Allow access to water at all times; encourage normal food intake. If your animal vomits or acts sick after getting it on an empty stomach, give with food or small treat to see if this helps. If vomiting continues, contact your veterinarian.
- Because this drug can change electrolytes (salts) in the blood, your veterinarian will probably want to do more frequent testing.
- Contact veterinarian immediately if excessive thirst, muscle weakness or collapsing/fainting, head tilt, lack of urination, or a racing heartbeat is noticed.

Chemistry/Synonyms

Hydrochlorothiazide occurs as a practically odorless, slightly bitter-tasting, white, or practically white, crystalline powder with pK$_a$s of 7.9 and 9.2. It is slightly soluble in water and soluble in alcohol.

Hydrochlorothiazide may also be known as: HCTZ, hidroclorotiazida, or hydrochlorothiazidum; many trade names are available.

Storage/Stability

Hydrochlorothiazide capsules and tablets should be stored at room temperature in well-closed containers.

Compatibility/Compounding Considerations

Compounded preparation stability: A method for compounding a spironolactone and hydrochlorothiazide oral suspension compounded from commercially available tablets has been published (Allen et al. 1996). Triturating twenty-four (24) spironolactone and hydrochlorothiazide 25/25 mg tablets with 60 mL of *Ora-Plus®* and qs ad to 120 mL with *Ora-Sweet®* (or *Ora-Sweet® SF*) yields a 5 mg/mL suspension of both spironolactone and hydrochlorothiazide that retains >90% potency for 60 days stored at both 5°C and 25°C. Compounded preparations of hydrochlorothiazide should be protected from light.

Dosage Forms/Regulatory Status

VETERINARY-LABELED PRODUCTS: NONE.

The ARCI (Racing Commissioners International) has designated this drug as a class 4 substance. See the appendix for more information.

HUMAN-LABELED PRODUCTS:

Hydrochlorothiazide Oral Tablets: 12.5 mg, 25 mg, & 50 mg; generic; (Rx)

Hydrochlorothiazide Oral Capsules: 12.5 mg; *Microzide® Capsules*; generic; (Rx)

Spironolactone/Hydrochlorothiazide Oral Tablets: 25 mg/25 mg & 50 mg/50 mg; generic; (Rx)

There are other fixed dose combinations with hydrochlorothiazide, including (partial list) with: amlodipine, benazepril, candesartan, irbesartan, lisinopril, losartan, metoprolol, and triamterene.

Revisions/References

Monograph revised/updated February 2014.

Allen, L. V. & M. A. Erickson (1996). Stability of labetalol hydrochloride, metoprolol tartrate, verapamil hydrochloride, and spironolactone with hydrochlorothiazide in extemporaneously compounded oral liquids. Am J Health Syst Pharm 53(19): 2304-9.

Brown, S. (2008). Current Knowledge in the Field of Renoprotection: Blood Pressure Control. Proceedings: ECVIM. accessed via Veterinary Information Network; vin.com

Brown, S. & R. Henik (2000). Therapy for Systemic Hypertension in Dogs and Cats. *Kirk's Current Veterinary Therapy: XIII Small Animal Practice*. J. Bonagura. Philadelphia, WB Saunders: 838-41.

Hezel, A., et al. (2007). Influence of Hydrochlorothiazide on Urinary Calcium Oxalate Relative Supersaturation in Healthy Young Adult Female Domestic Shorthaired Cats.

Kittleson, M. (2000). Therapy of Heart Failure. *Textbook of Veterinary Internal Medicine: Diseases of the Dog and Cat*. S. Ettinger and E. Feldman. Philadelphia, WB Saunders. 1: 713-37.

Kittleson, M. (2006). "Chapt 10: Management of Heart Failure." *Small Animal Cardiology, 2nd Ed* Veterinary Information Network.

Takemura, N. (1998). Successful long-term treatment of congenital nephrogenic diabetes insipidus in a dog. Journal of Small Animal Practice 39(12): 592-4.

Trepanier, L. (2008). Choosing therapy for chronic liver disease. Proceedings: WSAVA. accessed via Veterinary Information Network; vin.com

Valberg, S. (2008). Muscle Tremors in Horses. Proceedings: Western Veterinary Conference. accessed via Veterinary Information Network; vin.com

Hydrocodone Bitartrate

(hye-droe-koe-done)   Tussigon®, Hycodan®

Opiate

Prescriber Highlights

▶ Opiate agonist available only in USA in combination with homatropine or acetaminophen. Used primarily as an antitussive in dogs, but potentially useful as an oral analgesic for moderate pain in dogs.

▶ Contraindications: Hypersensitivity to narcotic analgesic, patients receiving monoamine oxidase inhibitors (MAOIs; selegiline?), diarrhea caused by a toxic ingestion. **Any combination product containing acetaminophen must NOT be used in cats.**

▶ Caution: Patients with hypothyroidism, severe renal insufficiency, adrenocortical insufficiency (Addison's), head injuries or increased intracranial pressure, acute abdominal conditions, & geriatric or severely debilitated patients. Use extreme caution in patients suffering from respiratory diseases when respiratory secretions are increased or when liquids are nebulized into the respiratory tract.

▶ Adverse Effects: Sedation, constipation (with chronic therapy), vomiting, or other GI disturbances.

▶ May mask the clinical signs (cough) of respiratory disease.

▶ Combination products are C-II controlled substances.

Uses/Indications

Used principally in canine medicine as an antitussive for cough secondary to conditions such as collapsing trachea, bronchitis, or canine upper respiratory infection complex (C-URI, "kennel cough", canine infectious tracheobronchitis). Its use is generally reserved for harsh, dry, non-productive coughs.

The human combination products containing hydrocodone and acetaminophen potentially could be useful oral analgesics in dogs (**NOT** in cats).

Pharmacology/Actions

While hydrocodone exhibits the characteristics of other opiate agonists, it tends to have a slightly greater antitussive effect than codeine (on a weight basis). The mechanism of this effect is thought to be a result of direct suppression of the cough reflex on the cough center in the medulla. Hydrocodone tends to have a drying effect on respiratory mucosa and the viscosity of respiratory secretions may be increased; the addition of homatropine MBr (in *Hycodan®* and others) may enhance this effect. Hydrocodone may also be more sedating than codeine, but is not more constipating.

Pharmacokinetics

In dogs (greyhounds; N=6), oral doses of approximately 0.5 mg/kg hydrocodone bitartrate (in combination with acetaminophen) produced mean peak levels of hydrocodone in about 45 minutes and hydromorphone—the active metabolite in about 1.5 hours. Plasma concentrations of hydromorphone remained above 1.6 ng/mL through the 8 hours of the study. This is above the concentration thought to be therapeutic in humans. Mean elimination half-life of hydromorphone was about 3 hours (KuKanich et al. 2013). Hydrocodone has an oral bioavailability of approximately 40%-80% in dogs. The antitussive and analgesic actions of hydrocodone are thought to persist for 6-12 hours, but PK/PD studies correlating oral hydrocodone's antinociceptive effects in dogs are not currently available.

In humans, hydrocodone is well absorbed after oral administration and has a serum half-life of about 3.8 hours; antitussive effect usually lasts 4-6 hours in adults.

Contraindications/Precautions/Warnings

Hydrocodone is contraindicated in cases where the patient is hypersensitive to narcotic analgesics and those with diarrhea caused by a toxic ingestion (until the toxin is eliminated from the GI tract). All opiates should be used with caution in patients with hypothyroidism, severe renal insufficiency, adrenocortical insufficiency (Addison's), and in geriatric or severely debilitated patients.

Commercially marketed hydrocodone products are available only as combination products. Those containing acetaminophen (*e.g., Vicodin®, Lortab®,* etc.) must not be used in cats and those containing ibuprofen should not be used in dogs or cats. Because of dosage form concerns and a lack of evidence supporting its use in cats for any purpose, it cannot be recommended for feline patients.

Hydrocodone should be used with caution in patients with head injuries or increased intracranial pressure and acute abdominal conditions as it may obscure the diagnosis or clinical course of these conditions. It should be used with extreme caution in patients suffering from respiratory diseases when respiratory secretions are increased or when liquids are nebulized into the respiratory tract.

Hydrocodone products have a relatively high abuse potential in humans and veterinarians are advised to be on the lookout for drug seeking clients.

Adverse Effects

Side effects that may be encountered with hydrocodone therapy in dogs include sedation, constipation (with chronic therapy), vomiting or other GI disturbances.

Hydrocodone may mask the clinical signs (cough) of respiratory disease and should not take the place of appropriate specific treatments for the underlying cause of coughs.

Reproductive/Nursing Safety

In humans, the FDA categorizes this drug as category C for use during pregnancy (*Animal studies have shown an adverse effect on the fetus, but there are no adequate studies in humans; or there are no animal reproduction studies and no adequate studies in humans*).

It is unknown if hydrocodone enters milk; use with caution.

Overdosage/Acute Toxicity

The initial concern with a very large overdose of *Hycodan®* (or equivalent) would be CNS, cardiovascular and respiratory depression secondary to the opiate effects.

There were 72 single agent exposures to hydrocodone reported to the ASPCA Animal Poison Control Center (APCC) during 2009-2013. Of the 66 dogs, 27 were symptomatic with 70% lethargic/sedated, 33% vocalizing, 15% hyperactive, 15% vomiting, and 11% ataxic.

If the ingestion was recent, emptying the gut using standard protocols should be performed and treatment with naloxone instituted as necessary. The homatropine ingredient may give rise to anticholinergic effects that may complicate the clinical picture, but its relatively low toxicity may not require any treatment. For further information on handling opiate or anticholinergic overdoses, refer to the meperidine and atropine monographs, respectively.

Drug Interactions

The following drug interactions have either been reported or are theoretical in humans or animals receiving hydrocodone and may be of in veterinary patients. Unless otherwise noted, use together is not necessarily contraindicated, but weigh the potential risks and perform additional monitoring when appropriate.

■ **ACEPROMAZINE:** Acepromazine and hydrocodone may cause additive hypotension in dogs with collapsing trachea.

■ **ANTICHOLINERGIC DRUGS:** May cause additive anticholinergic effects.

- **ANTIDEPRESSANTS, TRICYCLIC & MOA INHIBITORS:** Use with hydrocodone may potentiate the adverse effects associated with the antidepressant.
- **CNS DEPRESSANTS, OTHER:** Other CNS depressants (*e.g.,* anesthetic agents, antihistamines, phenothiazines, barbiturates, tranquilizers, alcohol, etc.) may cause increased CNS or respiratory depression when used with hydrocodone.

Doses

- **DOGS:**

  As an antitussive (extra-label): 0.2 – 0.5 mg/kg PO q6-12h is usually recommended, but dosages up to 1 mg/kg PO q6h have been noted. The goal of therapy is to suppress cough without excessive sedation. (Johnson 2000)

  As an analgesic (extra-label): The strength of evidence supporting use is low, but limited pharmacokinetics studies and clinical experience suggest it may be an effective analgesic for mild to moderate pain in dogs. One dosage recommendation is: Using the fixed dose combination products with acetaminophen: 0.22 – 0.5 mg/kg (of the hydrocodone component) PO q8-12h. Do not exceed 15 mg/kg of the acetaminophen component q8h (KuKanich 2008). This dosage can be practically administered to dogs by using tablets that each contain 10 mg of hydrocodone bitartrate and 300 mg acetaminophen (*e.g., Vicodin® HP* 10/300) and administering ¼ tablet per 5 kg (11 lb.) bodyweight PO q8-12h.

- **CATS:**

  Note: Commercially marketed hydrocodone products are available only as combination products and any product containing acetaminophen (*e.g.; Vicodin®*) is contraindicated in cats. While hydrocodone (alone) may be an effective opioid agent in cats, at this time it cannot be recommended for use in cats.

Monitoring

- Clinical efficacy.
- Adverse effects.

Client Information

- Any product that also contains acetaminophen (*Tylenol®*, APAP, *Vicodin®*, etc.) must **NEVER** be used in **cats**. If you are unsure whether a product containing hydrocodone is safe to use in cats, ask your veterinarian.
- Can give with or without food. If your animal vomits or acts sick after getting it on an empty stomach, give with food or small treat to see if this helps. If vomiting continues, contact your veterinarian.
- Sedation (sleepiness/fatigue) and constipation are the most likely side effects. Watch for adverse effects and contact veterinarian immediately if your animal stops eating, if the whites of the eyes become yellowish, continues to vomit or has diarrhea, or blood is seen in vomit or stool.
- Do NOT give more than veterinarian prescribes. Unless veterinarian instructs, do NOT give other pain or fever medicines.
- Hydrocodone in combination with acetaminophen or homatropine are controlled substances (C-III) in the USA. It is a federal offense to give or sell this medication to anyone other than the patient for which it was prescribed.

Chemistry/Synonyms

A phenanthrene-derivative opiate agonist, hydrocodone bitartrate occurs as fine, white crystals or crystalline powder. One gram is soluble in about 16 mL of water; it is slightly soluble in alcohol.

Hydrocodone bitartrate may also be as: hydrocodone tartrate, dihydrocodeinone acid tartrate, hydrocodone acid tartrate, hydrocodoni bitartras, or hydrocone bitartrate.

Storage/Stability

Products should be protected from light.

Compatibility/Compounding Considerations

No specific information noted.

Dosage Forms/Regulatory Status

VETERINARY-LABELED PRODUCTS: NONE.

The ARCI (Racing Commissioners International) has designated this drug as a class 1 substance. See the appendix for more information.

HUMAN-LABELED PRODUCTS:

In the USA, there are no hydrocodone products available as a sole ingredient. All commercially available products containing hydrocodone are Class-II controlled substances.

Hydrocodone Bitartrate Oral Tablets: 5 mg with Homatropine MBr 1.5 mg; *Tussigon®*, generic; (Rx, C-II)

Hydrocodone Bitartrate Oral Syrup: 5 mg with Homatropine MBr 1.5 mg (per 5 mL) in 473 mL and 3.8 L; *Hydromet® Syrup*, generic (Rx, C-II)

The following are representative oral dosage forms containing hydrocodone and acetaminophen and include those most likely to be of benefit (higher ratios of hydrocodone to acetaminophen) in treating dogs and are usually stocked at human pharmacies. **WARNING:** These products must **NOT** be used in cats.

Hydrocodone/Acetaminophen Oral Tablets: 5 mg/300 mg, 5 mg/325 mg, 7.5 mg/300 mg, 7.5 mg/325 mg, 10 mg/300 mg, & 10 mg/325 mg. An oral solution containing hydrocodone 2.5 mg/5 mL in combination with acetaminophen 167 mg/5 mL (0.5 mg/mL hydrocodone and 33.3 mg/mL of acetaminophen) is also readily available. Commonly used trade names for these products include: *Vicodin®, Norco®,* and *Lortabs®*.

There are also oral tablets and liquids with hydrocodone available in combination with chlorpheniramine, or ibuprofen.

Revisions/References

Monograph revised/updated February 2014.

Johnson, L. (2000). Diseases of the Bronchus. *Textbook of Veterinary Internal Medicine: Diseases of the Dog and Cat.* S. Ettinger and E. Feldman. Philadelphia, WB Saunders. **2**: 1055-61.

KuKanich, B. (2008). Beyond NSAIDs and Opioids. Proceedings: WVC. accessed via Veterinary Information Network; vin.com

KuKanich, B. & J. Spade (2013). Pharmacokinetics of hydrocodone and hydromorphone after oral hydrocodone in healthy Greyhound dogs. Veterinary Journal **196**(2): 266-8.

Hydrocortisone
Hydrocortisone Sodium Succinate

(hye-droe-kor-ti-zone)   Cortef®, Solu-Cortef®

Glucocorticoid

Prescriber Highlights

- ▶ "Benchmark" injectable, oral, & topical glucocorticoid (depending on salt). IV form (sodium succinate) most commonly used when immediate mineralocorticoid & glucocorticoid activity is desired (e.g., Addisonian crisis, CIRCI).
- ▶ Primary adverse effects are "Cushingoid" in nature with sustained use.
- ▶ Many potential drug & lab interactions.
- ▶ Can be expensive.

Uses/Indications

Because of its rapid effect and relatively high mineralocorticoid effect, hydrocortisone sodium succinate (*Solu-Cortef®*) IV is the most commonly used form of this medication when an acute glucocorticoid/mineralocorticoid effect is desired (*e.g.*, acute adrenal insufficiency; critical illness-related corticosteroid insufficiency; CIRCI). While oral forms are available, they are not routinely used in veterinary patients.

Pharmacology/Actions
Glucocorticoids have effects on virtually every cell type and system in mammals. See the Glucocorticoid General Information monograph for more information.

Pharmacokinetics
In humans, hydrocortisone is readily absorbed after oral administration. Hydrocortisone sodium succinate is administered parenterally, and absorption is rapid after IM administration. Duration of activity is 8-12 hours.

Contraindications/Precautions/Warnings
Glucocorticoid agents used systemically are generally considered contraindicated in systemic fungal infections (unless used for replacement therapy in Addison's), when administered IM in patients with idiopathic thrombocytopenia, and those hypersensitive to a particular drug.

Patients that have received the drug chronically should be tapered off slowly as endogenous ACTH and corticosteroid function may return slowly. Should the animal undergo a "stressor" (*e.g.*, surgery, trauma, illness, etc.) during the tapering process or until normal adrenal and pituitary function resume, additional glucocorticoids should be administered.

Adverse Effects
Adverse effects are generally associated with long-term administration of glucocorticoids, especially if given at high dosages or not on an alternate day regimen. Effects generally manifest as clinical signs of hyperadrenocorticism.

When hydrocortisone is used intravenously at recommended dosages for acute hypoadrenocorticism or CIRCI, the adverse effect profile for dogs and cats is not well described. When used in humans in the ICU setting (CIRCI), potential important adverse effects include immune suppression with increased risk for infection, impaired wound healing, hyperglycemia, myopathy, hypokalemic metabolic acidosis, psychosis, and HPA axis and glucocorticoid receptor suppression (Marik 2012).

Reproductive/Nursing Safety
Glucocorticoids are probably necessary for normal fetal development. They may be required for adequate surfactant production, myelin, retinal, pancreatic, and mammary development. Excessive dosages early in pregnancy may lead to teratogenic effects. In horses and ruminants, exogenous steroid administration may induce parturition when administered in the latter stages of pregnancy. In humans, the FDA categorizes this drug as category *C* for use during pregnancy (*Animal studies have shown an adverse effect on the fetus, but there are no adequate studies in humans; or there are no animal reproduction studies and no adequate studies in humans.*)

Glucocorticoids unbound to plasma proteins will enter milk. High dosages or prolonged administration to mothers may potentially inhibit the growth of nursing newborns.

Overdosage/Acute Toxicity
Glucocorticoids when given short-term are unlikely to cause harmful effects, even in massive dosages. One incidence of a dog developing acute CNS effects after accidental ingestion of glucocorticoids has been reported. Should clinical signs occur, use supportive treatment if necessary.

Drug Interactions
The following drug interactions have either been reported or are theoretical in humans or animals receiving hydrocortisone and may be of in veterinary patients. Unless otherwise noted, use together is not necessarily contraindicated, but weigh the potential risks and perform additional monitoring when appropriate.

- **AMPHOTERICIN B**: Administered concomitantly with glucocorticoids may cause hypokalemia; in humans, there have been cases of CHF and cardiac enlargement reported after using hydrocortisone to treat Amphotericin B adverse effects.
- **ANTICHOLINESTERASE AGENTS** (*e.g.*, **pyridostigmine, neostigmine**, etc.): In patients with myasthenia gravis, concomitant glucocorticoid and anticholinesterase agent administration may lead to profound muscle weakness. If possible, discontinue anticholinesterase medication at least 24 hours prior to hydrocortisone administration.
- **ASPIRIN**: Glucocorticoids may reduce salicylate blood levels and increase risk for GI ulceration/bleeding.
- **BARBITURATES**: May increase the metabolism of glucocorticoids and decrease flumethasone blood levels.
- **CYCLOPHOSPHAMIDE**: Glucocorticoids may inhibit the hepatic metabolism of cyclophosphamide; dosage adjustments may be required.
- **CYCLOSPORINE**: Concomitant administration of glucocorticoids and cyclosporine may increase the blood levels of each by mutually inhibiting the hepatic metabolism of each other; the clinical significance of this interaction is not clear.
- **DIURETICS, POTASSIUM-DEPLETING** (*e.g.*, **spironolactone, triamterene**): Administered concomitantly with glucocorticoids may cause hypokalemia.
- **EPHEDRINE**: May reduce hydrocortisone blood levels.
- **ESTROGENS**: The effects of hydrocortisone and, possibly, other glucocorticoids, may be potentiated by concomitant administration with estrogens.
- **INSULIN**: Insulin requirements may increase in patients receiving glucocorticoids.
- **KETOCONAZOLE** and other **AZOLE ANTIFUNGALS**: May decrease the metabolism of glucocorticoids and increase hydrocortisone blood levels; ketoconazole may induce adrenal insufficiency when glucocorticoids are withdrawn by inhibiting adrenal corticosteroid synthesis.
- **MACROLIDE ANTIBIOTICS** (*e.g.*, **erythromycin, clarithromycin**): May decrease the metabolism of glucocorticoids and increase hydrocortisone blood levels.
- **MITOTANE**: May alter the metabolism of steroids; higher than usual doses of steroids may be necessary to treat mitotane-induced adrenal insufficiency.
- **NSAIDs**: Administration of ulcerogenic drugs with glucocorticoids may increase the risk of gastrointestinal ulceration.
- **PHENOBARBITAL**: May increase the metabolism of glucocorticoids and decrease hydrocortisone blood levels.
- **RIFAMPIN**: May increase the metabolism of glucocorticoids and decrease hydrocortisone blood levels.
- **VACCINES**: Patients receiving corticosteroids at immunosuppressive dosages should generally not receive live attenuated-virus vaccines as virus replication may be augmented; a diminished immune response may occur after vaccine, toxoid, or bacterin administration in patients receiving glucocorticoids.
- **WARFARIN**: Hydrocortisone may affect INR's; monitor.

Laboratory Considerations
- Hydrocortisone can cross react with cortisol in ACTH response test. This test must be performed before hydrocortisone is administered or 24 hours after the last dose of hydrocortisone. (**Note**: Dexamethasone does not cross react).
- Glucocorticoids may increase **serum cholesterol**.
- Glucocorticoids may increase **urine glucose** levels.

- Glucocorticoids may decrease **serum potassium.**
- Glucocorticoids can suppress the release of thyroid stimulating hormone (TSH) and reduce T_3 & T_4 values. Thyroid gland atrophy has been reported after chronic glucocorticoid administration. Uptake of I^{131} by the thyroid may be decreased by glucocorticoids.
- Reactions to **skin tests** may be suppressed by glucocorticoids.
- False-negative results of the **nitroblue tetrazolium** test for systemic bacterial infections may be induced by glucocorticoids.
- Glucocorticoids may cause **neutrophilia** within 4-8 hours after dosing and return to baseline within 24-48 hours after drug discontinuation.
- Glucocorticoids can cause **lymphopenia** that can persist for weeks after drug discontinuation in dogs.

Doses

- **DOGS/CATS:**

  For adjunctive therapy for acute adrenocortical insufficiency (extra-label): Most recommendations are: After ACTH stimulation test is completed, 0.3 – 0.5 mg/kg/hour IV as a CRI or 2 – 4 mg/kg IV q6-8h. Once GI function has returned and patient is eating and drinking normally, therapy can be changed to oral steroid supplementation.

  For relative adrenal insufficiency (RAI); critical illness-related corticosteroid insufficiency (CIRCI); (extra-label): At present, there is not strong evidence for use of any corticosteroid in veterinary patients for this indication and no consensus guidelines have been published, but based upon research done in critically ill humans, it is reasonable to consider treating. One recommended dosage is: Hydrocortisone sodium succinate at a total daily dose of 1 – 4.3 mg/kg. This total daily dose can be divided into 4 equal doses and given IV every 6 hours or as a constant-rate infusion. Because the HPA dysfunction in CIRCI is thought to be transient, lifelong therapy with corticosteroids is not required and dosage is tapered by 25% each day after resolution of critical illness. An ACTH stimulation test should be repeated to confirm the return of normal adrenocortical function following the resolution of critical illness and discontinuation of corticosteroid supplementation (Martin 2011). Human data suggests that CRI's may provide better glycemic control, but may cause greater HPA axis suppression than if given episodically.

  For patients that have been resuscitated after CPCR (extra-label): From the RECOVER consensus guidelines: Routine administration of corticosteroids is not recommended. Use may be considered in patients that remain hemodynamically unstable despite administration of fluids and inotropes/pressors. Hydrocortisone sodium succinate: Initially 1 mg/kg IV followed by either 1 mg/kg q6h IV or as a CRI at 0.15 mg/kg/hour and then tapered as the patient's condition allows. (Fletcher et al. 2012)

Monitoring

Monitoring of glucocorticoid therapy is dependent on its reason for use, dosage, agent used (amount of mineralocorticoid activity), dosage schedule (daily versus alternate day therapy), duration of therapy, and the animal's age and condition. The following list may not be appropriate or complete for all animals; use clinical assessment and judgment should adverse effects be noted.

- Weight, appetite, signs of edema.
- Serum and/or urine electrolytes.
- Total plasma proteins, albumin.
- Blood glucose.
- ACTH stimulation test if necessary, preferably 24 hours after last hydrocortisone dose.

Client Information

- If using oral tablets at home, clients should carefully follow the dosage instructions and should not discontinue the drug abruptly without consulting with the veterinarian beforehand.

Chemistry/Synonyms

Also known as compound F or cortisol, hydrocortisone is secreted by the adrenal gland. Hydrocortisone occurs as an odorless, white to practically white, crystalline powder. It is very slightly soluble in water and sparingly soluble in alcohol. Hydrocortisone is administered orally.

Hydrocortisone sodium succinate occurs as an odorless, white to nearly white, hygroscopic, amorphous solid. It is very soluble in both water and alcohol. Hydrocortisone sodium succinate injection is administered via IM or IV routes.

Hydrocortisone may also be known as: antiinflammatory hormone, compound F, cortisol, hydrocortisonum, 17-hydroxycorticosterone, and NSC-10483; many trade names are available.

Storage/Stability

Hydrocortisone sodium succinate (HSS) in intact containers should be stored at controlled room temperatures of 68-77°F (20-25°C). After reconstitution, solutions are stable if protected from light and kept at, or below controlled room temperature. The solution should only be used if clear; discard unused solutions after 3 days. Hydrocortisone sodium succinate is heat labile and cannot be autoclaved. Reconstituted HSS 500 mg/4 mL solution kept frozen for 4 weeks showed no loss of potency.

Hydrocortisone tablets should be stored in well-closed containers. The cypionate oral suspension should be stored in tight, light resistant containers. All products should be stored at room temperature (15-30°C); avoid freezing the suspensions or solutions. After reconstituting solutions, only use products that are clear. Discard unused solutions after 3 days.

Compatibility/Compounding Considerations

Hydrocortisone sodium succinate is reportedly physically **compatible** with the following solutions and drugs: dextrose-Ringer's injection combinations, dextrose-Ringer's lactate injection combinations, dextrose-saline combinations, dextrose injections, Ringer's injection, lactated Ringer's injection, sodium chloride injections, amikacin sulfate, aminophylline, amphotericin B (limited quantities), calcium chloride/gluconate, chloramphenicol sodium succinate, clindamycin phosphate, corticotropin, daunorubicin HCl, dopamine HCl, erythromycin gluceptate, erythromycin lactobionate, lidocaine HCl, mephentermine sulfate, metronidazole with sodium bicarbonate, penicillin G potassium/sodium, piperacillin sodium, polymyxin B sulfate, potassium chloride, prochlorperazine edisylate, sodium bicarbonate, vancomycin HCl, verapamil HCl, and vitamin B-complex with C.

Hydrocortisone sodium succinate is reportedly physically **incompatible** when mixed with the following solutions and drugs: ampicillin sodium, bleomycin sulfate, dimenhydrinate, diphenhydramine HCl, doxorubicin HCl, ephedrine sulfate, heparin sodium, hydralazine HCl, metaraminol bitartrate, oxytetracycline HCl, pentobarbital sodium, phenobarbital sodium, promethazine HCl, and tetracycline HCl.

Compatibility is dependent upon factors such as pH, concentration, temperature and diluent used; consult specialized references or a hospital pharmacist for more specific information.

Dosage Forms/Regulatory Status

VETERINARY-LABELED PRODUCTS:

There are no products containing hydrocortisone (or its salts) known for systemic use. There are a variety of hydrocortisone veterinary products for topical use. A 10 ppb tolerance has been established for hydrocortisone (as the succinate or acetate) in milk.

The ARCI (Racing Commissioners International) has designated this drug as a class 4 substance. See the appendix for more information.

HUMAN-LABELED PRODUCTS:

Hydrocortisone Oral Tablets: 5 mg, 10 mg, & 20 mg; *Cortef*®, generic; (Rx)

Hydrocortisone Sodium Succinate Injection: 100 mg/vial, 250 mg/vial, 500 mg/vial, 1000 mg/vial (as sodium succinate); *Solu-Cortef*®, *A-Hydrocort*® ; (Rx)

There are many OTC and Rx topical and anorectal products available in a variety of dosage forms.

Revisions/References

Monograph revised/updated February 2014.

Fletcher, D. J., et al. (2012). RECOVER evidence and knowledge gap analysis on veterinary CPR. Part 7: Clinical guidelines. J. Vet. Emerg. Crit. Care **22**.

Marik, P. (2012). Critical Illness-Related Corticosteroid Insufficiency. ACVIM. accessed via Veterinary Information Network; vin.com

Martin, L. G. (2011). Critical Illness–Related Corticosteroid Insufficiency in Small Animals. Vet Clin Small Anim **41**: 767-82.

Hydrogen Peroxide 3% (Oral)

(hye-droe-jen per-oks-ide)

Oral Emetic, Topical Antiseptic

Also see the Decontamination information in the appendix.

Prescriber Highlights

▶ Topical antiseptic that is used orally as a home-administered emetic in dogs when clients cannot transport the patient to a veterinary hospital in a timely manner. Not a reliable emetic in cats.

▶ Can cause esophageal irritation or other gastric effects; aspiration is possible.

▶ Many contraindications for use as an emetic.

Uses/Indications

Hydrogen peroxide 3% solution can be used as an orally administered emetic in dogs, cats, pigs and ferrets. It is best reserved for those cases when animals cannot be transported to a veterinary hospital in a timely way and immediate emesis is required. Apomorphine for dogs and xylazine/dexmedetomidine for cats are the generally preferred emetic agents administered in a veterinary practice. A prospective observational study found that 3% hydrogen peroxide successful induced emesis in 90% of treated dogs and was equally as effective as apomorphine (Khan et al. 2012).

Pharmacology/Actions

Orally administered hydrogen peroxide solution (3%) induces a vomiting reflex via direct irritant effects of the oropharynx and gastric lining. After administering PO to dogs, emesis usually ensues within 10-15 minutes. It is estimated that about 50% of ingested agents are recovered after inducing emesis with either apomorphine or hydrogen peroxide (Khan et al. 2012).

Pharmacokinetics

No pharmacokinetic information located. Emetic effects may persist up to 45 minutes after administering PO to dogs.

Contraindications/Precautions/Warnings

Do not induce emesis in those dogs or cats that are already vomiting, severely lethargic, comatose, debilitated (*e.g.*, respiratory distress, decreased swallowing reflex, bradycardia, etc.), seizuring or hyperactive, have had recent abdominal surgery or with megaesophagus. Emesis is generally contraindicated after ingestions of corrosives/caustics (*e.g.*, acids, alkalis), sharp objects, or bagged illicit drugs. Emesis is usually contraindicated after ingestion of a hydrocarbon or petroleum distillate.

Use caution when attempting to induce emesis in a dog that has ingested a compound that can cause seizures or CNS depression as CNS status may rapidly deteriorate.

Before inducing emesis, obtain a complete history of the ingestion and ensure that vital signs are stable.

Administration and emesis generally must occur within 4 hours (some say 2 hours or 6 hours maximum) of the toxic ingestion.

Do not use emetics in rodents or rabbits.

If home administration of hydrogen peroxide is necessary, be sure that clients use only the 3% medical grade solution and not another more concentrated hydrogen peroxide product.

Because aspiration and/or bradycardia are possible, animals should be closely observed after administration. Suctioning, respiratory and cardiovascular support (*e.g.*, atropine) should be available. Do not allow animal to re-ingest vomitus.

Successful induction of emesis does not ensure that stomach contents have been emptied and significant quantities of the ingested drug/toxin may remain or already been absorbed.

Adverse Effects

In dogs, diarrhea, lethargy and protracted nausea/vomiting are possible; antiemetic agents administered after desired emesis occurs may alleviate nausea/vomiting in severely affected dogs. Aspiration of hydrogen peroxide solution during administration or stomach contents after inducing emesis is possible, but thought to occur only rarely in dogs. Cats can be particularly susceptible to hemorrhagic gastritis or esophagitis. Inducing emesis in animals with cardiovascular compromise may cause a vasovagal (bradycardic) response. Gastric dilatation-volvulus in dogs has been reported.

Reproductive/Nursing Safety

No specific information was located. While orally administered 3% hydrogen peroxide is unlikely to cause reproductive harm, weigh the risks to the dam and offspring of the ingested toxin versus the risks associated with inducing emesis.

Overdosage/Acute Toxicity

Hydrogen peroxide 3% solution is relatively non-toxic (see Adverse Effects) after oral ingestion. Hydrogen peroxide in concentrations of 10% or greater can be very corrosive (severe burns to oral/gastric mucosa) and induce oxygen emboli after oral ingestion.

Drug Interactions

■ **ACETYLCYSTEINE (oral):** Hydrogen peroxide can oxidize acetylcysteine in the gut and although clinical significance is unclear, alternative emetics (*e.g.*, apomorphine, xylazine) are preferred for acetaminophen overdoses.

■ **ANTIEMETICS (*e.g.*, ondansetron, maropitant, etc.):** Preadministration or ingestion of these products may negate the emetic effects of hydrogen peroxide.

Laboratory Considerations

■ No specific concerns were noted.

Doses

■ **DOGS:**

As an emetic (extra-label): In an observational study in dogs, hydrogen peroxide 3% was dosed at 2.2 mL/kg PO, to a maximum of 45 mL/dog. If vomiting was not induced after 10-15 minutes, dosage was repeated once. 90% of treated dogs were successfully treated (vs. 94% with apomorphine) (Khan et al. 2012). **Note:** Not a reliable emetic in cats and generally is not recommended secondary to possible gastric/esophageal adverse effects; potentially could be effective in pot-bellied pigs and ferrets.

Monitoring

- Efficacy (emesis, signs associated with toxicity of the substance ingested, blood levels of toxicants if applicable).
- Heart rate/respiration rate & auscultation after emesis.

Client Information

- Use only under the direct instructions of a veterinarian or an animal poison control center.
- Only use hydrogen peroxide 3%; stronger concentrations can be very toxic.
- Carefully administer; do not allow patient to "inhale" the liquid.
- Observe animal after giving hydrogen peroxide, do not allow them to re-ingest the vomited material (vomitus).
- Save all vomitus for the veterinarian to examine.

Chemistry/Synonyms

Hydrogen peroxide 3% solution is a clear, colorless liquid containing 2.5-3.5% w/v hydrogen peroxide. Up to 0.05% of the liquid may contain preservatives.

Hydrogen peroxide 3% solution may also be known as dilute hydrogen peroxide solution, hydrogen peroxide solution 10-volume (**Note: NOT** 10%), or hydrogen peroxide topical solution.

Storage/Stability

Store 3% solutions in airtight containers at room temperature and protected from light.

Hydrogen peroxide 3% can deteriorate with time; outdated or improperly stored products may not be effective as an emetic.

Compatibility/Compounding Considerations

Any compounded emetic for home use should be made from 3% hydrogen peroxide and not stronger concentrations.

Dosage Forms/Regulatory Status

VETERINARY-LABELED PRODUCTS:

None as an oral emetic.

HUMAN-LABELED PRODUCTS:

None as an oral emetic. Hydrogen Peroxide 3% Solution is readily available over-the-counter from a variety of manufacturers. It is usually sold in pint bottles.

Revisions/References

Monograph revised/updated February 2014.

Khan, S. A., et al. (2012). Effectiveness and adverse effects of the use of apomorphine and 3% hydrogen peroxide solution to induce emesis in dogs. Javma-Journal of the American Veterinary Medical Association **241**(9): 1179-84.

Hydromorphone

(hye-droe-**mor**-fone)   Dilaudid®

Opiate Agonist

Prescriber Highlights

▶ Injectable opiate sedative/restraining agent, analgesic, & preanesthetic similar to oxymorphone. May be less expensive than oxymorphone.

▶ Adverse Effects **Dogs:** Nausea/vomiting, defecation, panting, vocalization, & sedation are common. CNS depression, respiratory depression, & bradycardia; decreased GI motility with resultant constipation (with chronic use) possible.

▶ Adverse Effects **Cats:** Nausea common. Ataxia, hyperesthesia, hyperthermia, & behavioral changes (without concomitant tranquilization) possible.

▶ Drug-drug; drug-lab interactions.

▶ C-II controlled substance.

Uses/Indications

Like oxymorphone, hydromorphone is used in dogs and cats as a sedative/restraining agent, analgesic and preanesthetic. It may also be useful as an analgesic in horses and other species. In dogs and cats, hydromorphone is generally less sedating that morphine, usually causes minimal histamine release after IV administration, and rarely causes vasodilation and hypotension. One randomized, blinded, clinical trial in dogs and cats found hydromorphone's analgesic efficacy and duration of action similar to oxymorphone, but the incidence of nausea and vomiting was higher with hydromorphone (Bateman et al. 2008).

Pharmacology/Actions

Receptors for opiate analgesics are found in high concentrations in the limbic system, spinal cord, thalamus, hypothalamus, striatum, and midbrain. They are also found in tissues such as the gastrointestinal tract, urinary tract, and other smooth muscle.

Hydromorphone is approximately 5 times more potent an analgesic on a per weight basis when compared to morphine and approximately equal in potency to oxymorphone. The morphine-like agonists (morphine, meperidine, oxymorphone, hydromorphone) have primary activity at the *mu* receptors, with some activity possible at the delta receptor. The primary pharmacologic effects of these agents include: analgesia, antitussive activity, respiratory depression, sedation, emesis, physical dependence, and intestinal effects (constipation/defecation). Analgesic effects in dogs and cats begin approximately 1-5 minutes after IV injection, and depending on dose and pain severity, usually persist for 2-4 hours.

Secondary pharmacologic effects include: CNS: euphoria, sedation, and confusion. Cardiovascular: bradycardia due to central vagal stimulation, alpha-adrenergic receptors may be depressed resulting in peripheral vasodilation, decreased peripheral resistance, and baroreceptor inhibition. Orthostatic hypotension and syncope may occur. Urinary: Increased bladder sphincter tone can induce urinary retention.

Various species may exhibit contradictory effects from these agents. For example, horses, cattle, swine, and cats may develop excitement and dogs may defecate after morphine injections. These effects are in contrast to the expected effects of sedation and constipation. Dogs and humans may develop miosis, while other species (especially cats) may develop mydriasis.

While sedation associated with hydromorphone use in dogs is often reported as an attribute/adverse effect (see Adverse Effects), a prospective, randomized, blinded, controlled trial found that clinically normal dogs receiving hydromorphone (alone) at 0.1 mg/kg IM did not have significantly higher sedation scores than placebo, while acepromazine (alone) and acepromazine/hydromorphone caused significant levels of sedation (Hofmeister et al. 2010).

Respiratory depression can occur especially in debilitated, neonatal, or geriatric patients. Bradycardia, as well as a slight decrease in cardiac contractility and blood pressure, may be seen. Like oxymorphone, hydromorphone does initially increase the respiratory rate (panting in dogs) while actual oxygenation may be decreased and blood CO_2 levels may increase by 10 mmHg or more. Gut motility is decreased with resultant increases in stomach emptying times. Unlike either morphine or meperidine, hydromorphone may only infrequently cause mild histamine release in dogs or cats after IV injection. Unlike morphine or fentanyl, hydromorphone does not appear to affect the immune system or stimulate HPA axis/cortisol-release (Odunayo et al. 2010).

In horses there is marked individual variation in responses. Opioids can induce eating behavior (at low doses) and dose-dependent locomotor activity with incoordination at high doses (Clutton 2010).

Pharmacokinetics

Hydromorphone is absorbed when given by IV, IM, SC, and rectal routes. After hydromorphone is administered subcutaneously to dogs, peak levels occur between 10-30 minutes after dosing. The volume of distribution in dogs is high > 4 L/kg both with IV and SC dosing. Terminal half-lives are rapid and appear to be route and dose dependent; half-lives are about 35 minutes to an hour long (KuKanich et al. 2008). In cats, the elimination half-life is approximately 1.5-2 hours. The drug is metabolized in the liver, primarily by glucuronidation. Because cats are deficient in this metabolic pathway, half-lives in cats are probably prolonged. The glucuronidated metabolite is excreted by the kidneys.

Contraindications/Precautions/Warnings

All opiates should be used with caution in patients with hypothyroidism, severe renal insufficiency, adrenocortical insufficiency (Addison's), and in geriatric or severely debilitated patients. Hydromorphone is contraindicated in patients hypersensitive to narcotic analgesics, and generally in patients with diarrhea caused by a toxic ingestion (until the toxin is eliminated from the GI tract).

Because it may cause vomiting, hydromorphone used as a preanesthetic medication in animals with suspected gastric dilation, volvulus, or intestinal obstruction is usually considered contraindicated, but pretreatment with maropitant has been shown to help prevent vomiting in dogs treated with hydromorphone (Kraus 2013).

Hydromorphone should be used with extreme caution in patients with head injuries, increased intracranial pressure, and acute abdominal conditions (*e.g.*, colic) as it may obscure the diagnosis or clinical course of these conditions. It should be used with extreme caution in patients suffering from respiratory disease or acute respiratory dysfunction (*e.g.*, pulmonary edema secondary to smoke inhalation).

Hydromorphone can cause bradycardia and therefore should be used cautiously in patients with preexisting bradyarrhythmias.

Neonatal, debilitated, or geriatric patients may be more susceptible to the effects of hydromorphone and may require lower dosages. Patients with severe hepatic disease may have prolonged duration of action of the drug.

Hyperthermia has been reported in cats with hydromorphone use and some recommend to avoid using this drug in cats (Hansen 2008), but others believe this is a misconception and that many cats have received hydromorphone without complications. If used in cats at high dosages, it has been recommended to give concurrently with a tranquilizing agent, as hydromorphone can produce bizarre behavioral changes in this species. Generally this is recommended when using other *mu*-agonist opiate agents in cats (*e.g.*, morphine) as well.

Opiate analgesics are contraindicated in patients who have been stung by the scorpion species *Centruroides sculpturatus Ewing* and *C. gertschi Stahnke* as it may potentiate these venoms.

Adverse Effects

Hydromorphone has a similar adverse effect profile to oxymorphone or morphine in dogs and cats. In dogs, vomiting, sedation, panting, whining/vocalization, and defecation can be noted. A randomized clinical study in dogs, concluded that maropitant given at 1 mg/kg SC 1-hour prior to, or 2 mg/kg PO at least two-hours prior to hydromorphone (0.1 mg/kg IM) prevented vomiting (Kraus 2013). Vomiting, nausea and defecation reportedly may occur more frequently after SC dosing versus IV dosing. CNS depression may be greater than desired, particularly when treating moderate to severe pain. In dogs, constant rate IV infusions of >0.05 mg/kg/hr administered for more than 12 hours may cause sedation and adverse effects severe enough to require reducing the rate (Hansen 2008).

Dose related respiratory depression is possible and more likely during general anesthesia. Panting (may occur more often than with oxymorphone) and cough suppression (may be of benefit) can occur.

Secondary to enhanced vagal tone, hydromorphone can cause bradycardia. This apparently occurs on par with morphine or oxymorphone.

Hydromorphone may cause histamine release that, while significantly less then with morphine and usually clinically insignificant, may be significant in critically ill animals.

Constipation is possible with chronic dosing.

In cats, opioids may cause excitement and increase body temperature. One study done in eight cats showed that hydromorphone, morphine, butorphanol, and buprenorphine all cause an increase in body temperature and that hydromorphone increased body temperature equivalently to those other drugs. The increased body temperature in all of the experimental treatments was self-limiting, and the majority returned to normal within 5 hours. No apparent morbidity or mortality was noted. Administration of ketamine or isoflurane in addition to hydromorphone did not produce a clinically relevant increase in body temperature compared with that of administration of hydromorphone alone (Posner et al. 2010). Should hyperthermia occur, naloxone has been used to rapidly reduce body temperature in cats.

Reproductive/Nursing Safety

In humans, the FDA categorizes this drug as category **C** for use during pregnancy (*Animal studies have shown an adverse effect on the fetus, but there are no adequate studies in humans; or there are no animal reproduction studies and no adequate studies in humans.*)

Most opiates are excreted into milk, but effects on nursing offspring may not be significant.

Overdosage/Acute Toxicity

Massive overdoses may produce profound respiratory and/or CNS depression in most species. Other effects may include cardiovascular collapse, hypothermia, and skeletal muscle hypotonia. Mania may be seen in cats. Naloxone is the agent of choice in treating respiratory depression. In massive overdoses, naloxone doses may need to be repeated and animals should be closely observed as naloxone's effects can diminish before sub-toxic levels of oxymorphone are attained. Mechanical respiratory support should be considered in cases of severe respiratory depression.

In susceptible patients, moderate overdoses may require naloxone and supportive treatment as well.

Drug Interactions

The following drug interactions have either been reported or are theoretical in humans or animals receiving hydromorphone and may be of in veterinary patients. Unless otherwise noted, use together is not necessarily contraindicated, but weigh the potential risks and perform additional monitoring when appropriate.

- **BUTORPHANOL, NALBUPHINE:** Potentially could antagonize opiate effects.
- **CNS DEPRESSANTS, OTHER:** Additive CNS effects possible.
- **DIURETICS:** Opiates may decrease efficacy in CHF patients.
- **MONOAMINE OXIDASE INHIBITORS** (*e.g.*, **amitraz** and potentially, **selegiline**): Severe and unpredictable opiate potentiation may be seen; not recommended (in humans) if MAO inhibitor has been used within 14 days.
- **MUSCLE RELAXANTS, SKELETAL:** Hydromorphone may enhance effects.
- **PHENOTHIAZINES:** Some phenothiazines may antagonize analgesic effects and increase risk for hypotension.

- TRICYCLIC ANTIDEPRESSANTS (clomipramine, amitriptyline, etc.): Hydromorphone may exacerbate the effects of tricyclic antidepressants.
- WARFARIN: Opiates may potentiate anticoagulant activity.

Laboratory Considerations
- As they may increase biliary tract pressure, opiates can increase plasma amylase and lipase values up to 24 hours following their administration.

Doses
- **DOGS:**

As an analgesic (extra-label): Recommendations vary somewhat, but generally are: 0.1 – 0.2 mg/kg IV, IM or SC q2-4h or given as a CRI with an initial dose of 0.05 – 0.1 mg kg IV and then as CRI at 0.01 – 0.05 mg/kg/hour.

When used as a sedative/premed prior to painful procedures (extra-label): Used in combination with another agent. The following is one dosage protocol:

In young, healthy patients: Hydromorphone at 0.1 mg/kg; may be combined with acepromazine (0.02 – 0.05 mg/kg). As a sedative/restraint agent for fractious or aggressive dogs: 0.1 – 0.2 mg/kg mixed with acepromazine (0.05 mg/kg) IM. Maximal effect usually reached in about 15 minutes, but waiting another 15 minutes may be necessary in some dogs.

As an alternate induction method (especially in critical patients): hydromorphone 0.05 – 0.2 mg/kg IV, slowly to effect followed by diazepam 0.02 mg/kg IV (do not mix two drugs together). Endotracheal intubation may be possible after administration, if not, delivery of an inhalant by facemask will give a greater depth of anesthesia. Positive pressure ventilation likely will be necessary. If bradycardia requires treatment, use either glycopyrrolate (0.01 – 0.02 mg/kg IV) or atropine (0.02 – 0.04 mg/kg IV). (Pettifer et al. 2000)

- **CATS:**

As an analgesic (extra-label): Recommendations vary somewhat, but generally are: 0.05 – 0.1 mg/kg IV, IM or SC q2-6h or given as a CRI with an initial dose of 0.025 mg kg IV and then as CRI at 0.01 – 0.05 mg/kg/hour (start at low end of range). Monitor body temperature.

As a premed prior to moderately painful procedures (extra-label): Not commonly used, but the following is one recommendation:

In young, healthy patients: 0.1 mg/kg; may be combined with acepromazine (0.05 – 0.2 mg/kg).

As an alternate induction method (especially in critical patients): hydromorphone 0.05 – 0.2 mg/kg IV, slowly to effect followed by diazepam 0.02 mg/kg IV (do not mix two drugs together). Endotracheal intubation may be possible after administration, if not, delivery of an inhalant by facemask will give a greater depth of anesthesia. Positive pressure ventilation likely will be necessary. If bradycardia requires treatment, use either glycopyrrolate (0.01 – 0.02 mg/kg IV) or atropine (0.02 – 0.04 mg/kg IV). (Pettifer et al. 2000)

- **FERRETS:**

As an analgesic (extra-label): 0.1 – 0.2 mg/kg IV, IM or SC q6-8h or as a CRI with a 0.05 mg/kg IV loading dose, then 0.05 – 0.1 mg/kg/hr.

- **SMALL MAMMALS:**

As an analgesic (extra-label): Most recommended dosages are 0.05 – 0.2 mg/kg SC, IM q6-8h.

- **REPTILES:**

As an analgesic (extra-label): Most recommended dosages are 0.5 – 1 mg/kg SC, IM q24h.

Monitoring
- Respiratory rate/depth (pulse oximetry highly recommended).
- CNS level of depression/excitation.
- Blood pressure (especially with IV use).
- Cardiac rate.
- Analgesic efficacy.

Client Information
- When given parenterally, this agent should be used in an inpatient setting or with direct professional supervision

Chemistry/Synonyms
A semi-synthetic phenanthrene-derivative opiate related to morphine, hydromorphone HCl occurs as white, fine, crystalline powder. It is freely soluble in water. The commercial injection has a pH of 4-5.5.

Hydromorphone may also be known as: dihydromorphinone hydrochloride, *Dolonovag®*, *Hydal®*, *HydroStat IR®*, *Hydromorph®*, *Opidol®*, *Palladon®*, *Palladone®*, and *Sophidone®*.

Storage/Stability
The injection should be stored at room temperature and protected from light. A slight yellowish tint to the solution may occur, but does not indicate loss of potency. The injection remains stable for at least 24 hours when mixed with commonly used IV fluids if protected from light.

Hydromorphone tablets should be stored at room temperature in tight, light resistant containers. The suppositories should be kept in the refrigerator.

Compatibility/Compounding Considerations
Hydromorphone injection is **compatible** in commonly used IV fluids (for 24 hours when protected from light at 25°C) and with midazolam, ondansetron, potassium chloride, and heparin sodium. Hydromorphone injection mixed in the same syringe with atropine and medetomidine (*Domitor®*) for use as a pre-op in dogs prior to sevoflurane or propofol anesthesia has been described (Ko 2005). Hydromorphone is **incompatible** with sodium bicarbonate, or thiopental.

Dosage Forms/Regulatory Status
VETERINARY-LABELED PRODUCTS: NONE.

HUMAN-LABELED PRODUCTS:

Hydromorphone HCl Injection: 1 mg/mL in 1 mL amps & syringes, 2 mg/mL in 1 mL vials, amps & syringes, 20 mL vials & multidose vials; 4 mg/mL in 1 mL amps & syringes; and 10 mg/mL (concentrate) in 1 mL, & 5 mL, single-dose vials & amps and 50 mL single-dose vials; *Dilaudid®* & *Dilandid-HP®*, generic; (Rx, C-II)

Hydromorphone HCl Powder for Injection, lyophilized: 250 mg (10 mg/mL after reconstitution) preservative-free in single-dose vials; *Dilaudid-HP®*; (Rx, C-II)

Hydromorphone HCl Oral Tablets: 2 mg, 4 mg, & 8 mg; generic; (Rx, C-II)

Hydromorphone HCl Oral Capsules (extended-release): 8 mg, 12 mg, & 16 mg; *Exalgo®*; (Rx, C-II)

Hydromorphone HCL Oral Liquid: 1 mg/1 mL in 4 mL & 8 mL UD patient cups; 250 mL & 473 mL (may contain sodium metabisulfite); *Dilaudid®*, generic; (Rx, C-II)

Hydromorphone Suppositories: 3 mg; generic; (Rx, C-II)

Revisions/References

Monograph revised/updated February 2014.

Bateman, S. W., et al. (2008). Comparison of the analgesic efficacy of hydromorphone and oxymorphone in dogs and cats: a randomized blinded study. Veterinary Anaesthesia and Analgesia 35(4): 341-7.

Clutton, R. E. (2010). Opioid Analgesia in Horses. Veterinary Clinics of North America-Equine Practice 26(3): 493-+.

Hansen, B. (2008). Analgesia for the Critically Ill Dog or Cat: An Update. Veterinary Clinics of North America-Small Animal Practice 38(6): 1353-+.

Hofmeister, E. H., et al. (2010). Effects of acepromazine, hydromorphone, or an acepromazine-hydromorphone combination on the degree of sedation in clinically normal dogs. Journal of the American Veterinary Medical Association 237(10): 1155-9.

Ko, J. (2005). New anesthesia-analgesia injectable combinations in dogs and cats. Proceedings: ACVC. accessed via Veterinary Information Network; vin.com

Kraus, B. L. H. (2013). Efficacy of maropitant in preventing vomiting in dogs premedicated with hydromorphone. Veterinary Anaesthesia and Analgesia 40(1): 28-34.

KuKanich, B., et al. (2008). Pharmacokinetics of hydromorphone hydrochloride in healthy dogs. Veterinary Anaesthesia and Analgesia 35(3): 256-64.

Odunayo, A., et al. (2010). State-of-the-Art-Review: Immunomodulatory effects of opioids. J. Vet. Emerg. Crit. Care 20(4): 376-85.

Pettifer, G. & D. Dyson (2000). Hydromorphone: A cost-effective alternative to the use of oxymorphone. Can Vet Jnl 41(2): 135-7.

Posner, L. P., et al. (2010). Effects of opioids and anesthetic drugs on body temperature in cats. Veterinary Anaesthesia and Analgesia 37(1): 35-43.

Hydroxychloroquine Sulfate

(hye-**drox**-ee-klor-oh-kwin)   Plaquenil®

Antimalarial; Immunomodulator

Prescriber Highlights

► Oral antimalarial/immunomodulating drug with potential to treat variants of canine cutaneous lupus erythematous.

► Very little clinical experience or published for veterinary use; use with caution.

Uses/Indications

There is very limited information available on the safety and efficacy of this agent in dogs, but hydroxychloroquine may potentially be useful for treating variants of canine cutaneous lupus erythematous. Only a few case reports have been published to date (Mauldin et al. 2010; Oberkirchner et al. 2012), and while the drug may prove beneficial, its use at present must be considered 'experimental'.

Pharmacology/Actions

Hydroxychloroquine is an orally administered aminoquinoline with antimalarial and immunomodulatory properties. The exact immunomodulatory mechanism is unknown, but it is thought to inhibit neutrophil phagocytosis and superoxide production, chemotaxis, and toll-like receptor (TLR)-9 stimulation. Other actions that may contribute to its effects for treating lupus erythromatosus include decreasing ultraviolet light sensitivity, and antiplatelet and antihyperlipidemic effects.

Pharmacokinetics

No information was located for dogs. In humans, hydroxychloroquine has an oral bioavailability of 74%. Elimination half-life is very long (40 days).

Contraindications/Precautions/Warnings

Hydroxychloroquine is contraindicated in patients hypersensitive to the drug or to other aminoquinoline compounds. Patients with pre-existing cardiac abnormalities (*e.g.,* rhythm disturbances) should receive the drug with caution.

In humans, it is contraindicated if retinal or visual field changes are attributable to any 4-aminoquinoline and for long-term therapy in children. It should be used with caution in human patients with hepatic function impairment, psoriasis or other dermatoses, porphyria, elderly patients, and children.

Adverse Effects

There is not enough clinical experience in dogs with this drug to characterize an adverse effect profile. In the limited numbers dogs treated it has been tolerated well.

In humans, common adverse effects include: ocular effects; skeletal muscle myopathy or neuromyopathy; GI effects (anorexia, diarrhea, nausea, abdominal cramps, vomiting); CNS effects (headache, dizziness); dermatologic effects. The risk for retinal changes in humans is low when dosages are 6.5 mg/kg/per day or less.

Reproductive/Nursing Safety

In humans, when used at antimalarial dosages the CDC considers the drug safe for use during pregnancy, but it is unknown if it is safe at higher dosages. Hydroxychloroquine is excreted into milk and nursing safety is not known when it is used at higher (non-malarial prophylaxis) dosages.

Overdosage/Acute Toxicity

Overdoses can be very serious and toxic quinidine-like effects can be noted within 30 minutes of ingestion. In patients where it is not contraindicated and potential overdose is large, consider GI decontamination; contact a veterinary poison control center. Signs of overdose/toxicity in humans include: headache, drowsiness, visual disturbances, cardiovascular collapse, seizures, hypokalemia, rhythm and conduction disorders including QT prolongation, torsades de pointes, ventricular tachycardia and ventricular fibrillation followed by sudden, potentially fatal, respiratory and cardiac arrest.

Drug Interactions

The following drug interactions have either been reported or are theoretical in humans or animals receiving hydroxychloroquine and may be of in veterinary patients. Unless otherwise noted, use together is not necessarily contraindicated, but weigh the potential risks and perform additional monitoring when appropriate.

- **AUROTHIOGLUCOSE:** In humans, use together is contraindicated as there may be an increased risk for blood dyscrasias.
- **CIMETIDINE:** Potentially increases pharmacological effects of hydroxychloroquine; dosage adjustment may be required.
- **CYCLOSPORINE:** Increased serum levels of cyclosporine possible.
- **DIGOXIN:** Increased digoxin levels and effects possible.
- **MAGNEISUM SALTS (ORAL):** May reduce hydroxychloroquine absorption; separate dosages by at least two hours.
- **METOPROLOL:** Hydroxychloroquine may increase effects.
- **RABIES VACCINE:** In human patients, hydroxychloroquine may decrease immune response. Veterinary significance is not known.

Laboratory Considerations

- No specific information noted.

Doses

- **DOGS:**

  For adjunctive treatment of canine cutaneous lupus erythromatosus (extra-label): There is little information available on doses, efficacy or adverse effects. The following is derived from two case reports of 4 dogs total [(German shorthaired pointers (3) & Chinese crested dog (1)]: 5 – 10 mg/kg PO q24h. (Mauldin et al. 2010; Oberkirchner et al. 2012)

Monitoring

- Efficacy.
- Because there is little information on the safety of this drug in dogs, consider regular monitoring with eye exams, CBC, serum chemistry profiles.

- Consider ECG/cardiac exams in dogs with pre-existing cardiac abnormalities.

Client Information

- Give with food.
- Not much experience when used in animals, report any side effects to veterinarian.
- Keep away from children and other animals; overdoses can be very serious.

Chemistry/Synonyms

Hydroxychloroquine is a 4-aminoquinoline antimalarial agent that occurs as a white or practically white, odorless, crystalline powder. It exists in two forms, one form (usually used as the pharmaceutical) melting at about 240° and another other form that melts at about 198°. It is freely soluble in water and practically insoluble in alcohol, chloroform, and ether. Solutions in water have a pH of about 4.5.

Hydroxychloroquine sulfate may also be known as WIN-1258-2. A common trade name is *Plaquenil®*.

Storage/Stability

Hydroxychloroquine tablets can be stored at temperatures up to 30°C (86°F) in light-resistant containers.

Compatibility/Compounding Considerations

Tablets may be split. Dogs weighing less than 5 kg (11 lb.) require the dosage form to be compounded for accurate dosing (¼ tablet is approximately 50 mg; upper end of suggested dosage is 10 mg/kg).

Dosage Forms/Regulatory Status

VETERINARY-LABELED PRODUCTS: NONE.

HUMAN-LABELED PRODUCTS:

Hydroxychloroquine Sulfate Oral Tablets: 200 mg; *Plaquenil®*, generic; (Rx). Dosages for animals may need to be compounded.

Revisions/References

Monograph written February 2014.

Mauldin, E. A., et al. (2010). Exfoliative cutaneous lupus erythematosus in German short-haired pointer dogs: disease development, progression and evaluation of three immuno-modulatory drugs (ciclosporin, hydroxychloroquine, and adalimumab) in a controlled environment. Veterinary Dermatology 21(4): 373-82.

Oberkirchner, U., et al. (2012). Successful treatment of a novel generalized variant of canine discoid lupus erythematosus with oral hydroxychloroquine. Veterinary Dermatology 23(1): 65-E16.

Hydroxyethyl Starch Colloids (HES)

Colloid Volume Expander   Hetastarch, Tetrastarch, Pentastarch

NOTE: Nomenclature for these products can be confusing. Be certain when using HES products that you are familiar with the specific product and its respective cautions and uses.

Prescriber Highlights

▶ Volume expanders used to treat hypovolemia when colloidal therapy is required.

▶ Different HES molecular weight/degree of substitution products available.

▶ Contraindications: Severe heart failure, severe bleeding disorders, & patients in oliguric or anuric renal failure. Caution: Thrombocytopenia, patients undergoing CNS surgery; liver disease.

▶ May cause volume overload: Use with caution in patients with renal dysfunction, congestive heart failure, or pulmonary edema.

▶ Adverse Effects: Coagulopathies possible; too rapid administration to small animals (especially cats) may cause nausea/vomiting; hypersensitivity reactions possible but very rare.

Uses/Indications

Hydroxyethyl starch colloids (HES) are intravenous fluids that can be used to increase blood pressure and support colloid osmotic pressure (COP). There are two primary reasons to choose HES therapy over crystalloid therapy. The first is their better intravascular persistence and more prolonged volume expanding effects, and secondly, for use in patients with "capillary leak syndromes" where HES can reduce vascular permeability and down-regulate expression of pro-inflammatory mediators (Boag 2007). Additionally, HES are likely less prone to cause hypersensitivity reactions in animals than (human) albumin products. In hypovolemic patients where total protein is less than 3.5 g/dL and crystalloid therapy is likely to reduce this level further, colloid therapy (plasma, dextran or HES) is often considered as part of intravascular volume restoration particularly when blood products are unavailable or time is of the essence and the wait for crossmatching is unacceptable. Specific indications for considering colloid therapy in small animals include: traumatic brain injury (with hypertonic saline), non-cardiogenic pulmonary edema (CRI of diuretics, oxygen therapy, and, potentially, colloids), and hypoalbuminemia (Powell 2013).

In experimental isoflurane-induced hypotension in dogs, hetastarch administration was found superior to LRS (Aarnes et al. 2009).

In horses, hetastarch may be useful in increasing plasma oncotic pressure and volume expansion in hypoproteinemic conditions (*e.g.,* acute colitis) and may reduce endotoxin-induced vascular permeability better then plasma. A study in anesthetized horses found that administration of hetastarch 6% 2.5 mL/kg IV over one hour in combination with LRS did not attenuate the decrease in COP typically seen during anesthesia with crystalloid administration alone (Wendt-Hornickle et al. 2011). Hetastarch (10 ml/kg) and plasma (10 ml/kg) increased plasma COP comparatively in healthy horses for up to 48 hours (Esser et al. 2012).

The most commonly used hydroxyethyl starch solution in North America has been the high molecular weight (MW) product, hetastarch (6% HES 450/0.7) in normal saline with the trade name, *Hespan®*. The low-MW product, tetrastarch (6% HES 130/0.4) in normal saline is available as both an FDA-approved (USA) human product (*Voluven®*) and a veterinary-labeled product (*Vetstarch®*). It potentially causes less coagulation altering effects then the high-MW product. There is also a very high-MW product, (HES 670/0.75) in LRS, *Hextend®*, but little information on its use in veterinary patients is available. In many European countries and Canada, an HES 200/0.5 product, often called pentastarch, is commonly used.

Pharmacology/Actions

HESs acts as a plasma volume expander by increasing the oncotic pressure within the intravascular space similarly to either dextran or albumin. Maximum volume expansion occurs within a few minutes of the completion of infusion. Duration of effect is variable, but may persist for 24 hours or more for hetastarch (450/0.7) and approximately 12 hours for tetrastarch (130/0.04). When added to whole blood in humans, hetastarch causes an increase in erythrocyte sedimentation rate.

Pharmacokinetics

Lower molecular weight molecules, (less than 50,000) are rapidly excreted by the kidneys; larger molecules are slowly degraded enzymatically to a size where they then can be excreted. About 40% of a dose is excreted in the first 24 hours after infusion. After about 2 weeks, practically all the drug is excreted. In hypoproteinemic horses, colloidal pressure may be increased up to 24 hours after dosing. A study in healthy llamas, found that that administration of 15 mL/kg of hetastarch (450/0.7) during a 60-minute IV infusion significantly increased plasma COP for 96 hours (Carney et al. 2011).

Contraindications/Precautions/Warnings

The veterinary labeled product (*Vetstarch®*) lists the following contraindications: Patients with known hypersensitivity to hydroxyethyl starch, fluid overload (hyperhydration) and especially in cases of pulmonary edema and congestive heart failure; renal failure with oliguria or anuria not related to hypovolemia; patients receiving dialysis treatment; severe hypernatremia or severe hyperchloremia; or intracranial bleeding.

It is believed that significant bleeding can occur if HES are used in animals with compromised coagulation systems. For example, use in patients with von Willebrand's disease could significantly increase the risk for bleeding. Because of their effect on platelets, HES should be used with caution in patients with thrombocytopenia and with extreme caution in patients undergoing CNS surgery.

As they haves no oxygen carrying capacity, HES are not a replacement for whole blood or red blood cells.

In humans, there is a potential of risk for acute kidney injury with HES, particularly in acute sepsis patients. It is unknown if this risk also occurs in veterinary patients. Use HES with caution in patients with liver disease due to their effects on indirect serum bilirubin levels.

Because of the danger of volume overload, use of HES for the treatment of shock not accompanied by hypovolemia may be hazardous; they should be used in caution in patients with renal dysfunction, congestive heart failure or pulmonary edema. Additionally, animals with sepsis, systemic inflammatory response syndrome (SIRS) or severe trauma may extravasate colloids such as HES into the lungs that could potentially, cause or worsen pulmonary edema. Monitoring for clinical signs of pulmonary edema and if possible, blood gases is mandatory in these circumstances.

In humans, HES are contraindicated in patients with severe heart failure, severe bleeding disorders and patients in oliguric or anuric renal failure.

Adverse Effects

HES can affect platelet function and coagulation times and alter Factor VIII (FVIII) and von Willebrand Factor. At recommended dosages, HES may cause changes in clotting times and platelet counts due to direct (precipitation of Factor VIII) and dilutional causes. A retrospective study in dogs, showed that hetastarch can significantly increase PTT's, but did not affect survival rates (Helmbold et al. 2009). Clinically, these effects may be insignificant, but patients with preexisting coagulopathies may be predisposed to further bleeding. Dosages of HES exceeding 20 mL/kg/day are more likely to cause coagulation abnormalities. Potentially, tetrastarch (HES 130/0.4) may have less effect on coagulation then hetastarch (HES 450/0.7 or HES 670/0.75). One *in vitro* study did find that HES 130/0.4 did affect canine platelet function, but the authors concluded that the clinical relevance of these *in vitro* findings is not obvious (Classen et al. 2012). Another found that HES 200/0.5 (not commercially available in USA), but NOT HES 130/0.4 significantly increased closure time (Ct) beyond the dilutional effect (McBride et al. 2013). An *in vivo* study in dogs, found that HES 670/0.75 at clinically relevant dosages, prolonged closure time for up to 24 hours (Chohan et al. 2011).

HES are less antigenic than dextran, but can cause sensitivity reactions and interfere with antigen-antibody testing. Anaphylactic reactions and severe coagulopathies are thought to occur rarely, however.

When given via rapid infusion to cats, hetastarch may cause signs of nausea and vomiting; if administered over 15-30 minutes, these signs are eliminated.

Circulatory overload leading to pulmonary edema is possible, particularly when large dosages are administered to patients with diminished renal function. Do not give intramuscularly as bleeding, bruising, or hematomas may occur.

When HES infusions are stopped a "rebound effect" can occur; colloid that has leaked into interstitial spaces can pull additional fluid from the intravascular space.

In humans, increases in serum indirect bilirubin have occurred occasionally. No effect on other liver function tests were noted and the increases subsided over several days. Serum amylase levels may be falsely elevated for several days after HES are administered. While clinically insignificant, the changes may preclude using serum amylase to diagnosis or monitor patients with acute pancreatitis.

Reproductive/Nursing Safety

HES safety during pregnancy has not been established, but no untoward effects have apparently been reported. In humans, the FDA categorizes this drug as category *C* for use during pregnancy (*Animal studies have shown an adverse effect on the fetus, but there are no adequate studies in humans; or there are no animal reproduction studies and no adequate studies in humans.*)

It is not known whether HESs are excreted in milk, but they are unlikely to pose much risk to offspring.

Overdosage/Acute Toxicity

Overdosage could result in volume overload in susceptible patients. Dose and monitor fluid status carefully.

Drug Interactions

The following drug interactions have either been reported or are theoretical in humans or animals receiving <u>hydroxyethyl starch colloids</u> and may be of in veterinary patients. Unless otherwise noted, use together is not necessarily contraindicated, but weigh the potential risks and perform additional monitoring when appropriate.

- **WARFARIN**: High dosages of HES may increase risk for bleeding.

The following drug interactions have either been reported or are theoretical in humans or animals receiving <u>hetastarch in lactated electrolytes</u> (*Hextend®*) and may be of in veterinary patients. Unless otherwise noted, use together is not necessarily contraindicated, but weigh the potential risks and perform additional monitoring when appropriate.

- **ANGIOTENSIN RECEPTOR BLOCKERS** (ARBs; *e.g.*, **losartan, irbesartan**); **POTASSIUM SPARING DIURETICS** (*e.g.*, **spironolactone**): Potential for increased serum potassium; increased monitoring warranted.
- **CEFTRIAXONE**: In human neonates, use with calcium-containing IV fluids is contraindicated.

Laboratory Considerations

- Hetastarch (670/0.75) can falsely elevate **urine** concentration (**specific gravity**) in dogs (Smart et al. 2009).
- **Serum amylase** concentrations may be temporarily increased and interfere with pancreatitis diagnosis.
- At high dosages, the dilutional effects may result in decreased levels of **coagulation factors**, other **plasma proteins** and a decrease in **hematocrit**.

Doses

NOTE: All doses are for hetastarch (6% HES 450/0.7; *Hespan®*) unless otherwise noted.

- **DOGS/CATS:**

  To increase blood pressure and support colloid osmotic pressure (COP) Note: Rate of administration is determined by individual patient requirements (*i.e.*, blood volume, indication, and patient response); adequate monitoring for successful treatment of shock is mandatory. The following dosages are **NOT** "Give and forget"; they should be used as general guidelines for treatment.

Using 6% HES 450/0.7 (*Hespan®*); (extra-label): Recommendations vary somewhat; generally: Shock bolus (resuscitation): 10 – 20 mL/kg in dogs and 5 – 10 mL/kg in cats IV usually over 15-30 minutes. A CRI can follow at 1 – 2 mL/kg/hour; not to exceed 20 mL/kg/day (some recommend not exceeding 10 mL/kg/day in cats).

Using 6% HES 130/0.4 (*Vetstarch®*); (labeled dose): Adult Dose: As a general recommendation, up to 20 mL/kg per day in small animal patients. The initial 10 – 20 mL should be infused slowly, keeping the patient under close observation due to possible anaphylactoid reactions. The daily dose and rate of infusion depend on the patient's blood loss, on the maintenance or restoration of hemodynamics and on the hemodilution (dilution effect); can be administered repetitively over several days. The use of 6% hydroxyethyl starch 130/0.4 has been dosed at 50 mL/kg/day in human studies. (Adapted from label; *Vetstarch®*).

- **HORSES:**

  When colloids are selected for volume replacement (extra-label): hetastarch at 3 – 10 mL/kg can be used. Total daily doses of 10 mL/kg should not be exceeded due to risk for coagulopathies. (Magdesian 2010)

  For colloidal support for fluid resuscitation and management of hypoproteinemia (extra-label): 8 – 10 mL/kg IV bolus or as a CRI at 0.5 – 1 mL/kg/hr (max. of 10 mL/kg/day). (Naylor et al. 2009)

- **BIRDS:**

  As a colloid (extra-label): 10 – 15 mL/kg over 20-40 minutes, up to four times daily, OR 10 – 15 mL/kg bolus over 20-40 minutes followed by 1 – 2 mL/kg/hr continuous rate infusion. Recommended maximum dose is 20 mL/kg/24 hours, but author notes that she has exceeded this dose with no side effects noted. For small volume replacement/CPCR resuscitation: For the shocky debilitated patient, hypertonic saline is administered (3 – 5 mL/kg) over 5 minutes, followed by hetastarch (3 – 5 mL/kg over 5 min). This combination prior to crystalloid administration enables fluids to stay within the vascular space. Blood pressure should be monitored closely. Follow with small boluses of crystalloid fluids (LRS, Plasma-Lyte at 15 – 20 mL/kg) along with hetastarch at 3 – 5 mL/kg over 15 minutes, and reassess the bird every 15 minutes. The crystalloids and hetastarch can be combined in the same syringe or bag. This process is repeated every 15-20 minutes until temperature normalizes and blood pressure is over 120 mmHg. (Antinoff 2009)

- **CAMELIDS:**

  As a colloid: A study done in healthy llamas showed that 15 mL/kg significantly increased COP for up to 96 hours. Transient, mild hemodilution and mild increases in PT and PTT were noted. (McKenzie et al. 2009)

Monitoring

- Other than the regular monitoring performed in patients that would require volume expansion therapy, there is no inordinate monitoring required specific to hetastarch therapy, but consider monitoring coagulation parameters particularly in high risk patients or when using high dosages of hetastarch.

Client Information

- As these fluids are used in an in-patient setting only, the two factors to consider when communicating with clients are the drug's cost and the reasons for using colloid therapy.

Chemistry/Synonyms

A synthetic polymer derived from a waxy starch, HES is composed primarily of amylopectin. Hetastarch occurs as a white powder. It is very soluble in water and insoluble in alcohol.

To avoid degradation by serum amylase, hydroxyethyl ether groups are added to the glucose Units. Commercially available HES solutions are classified by their mean molecular weight (MW) and degree of substitution (DS). The DS refers to the average number of hydroxyethyl groups per glucose unit within the branched-chain polymer.

The most commonly used HES solution is HES 450/0.7 (*Hespan®*) and therefore has an average MW of 450 kD and a DS of 0.75. While the average molecular weight is 450,000, commercial HES solutions contain a vide variation in molecule sizes, ranging from a few thousand to a few million Daltons distributed in a concentration/size ratio more or less as a bell-shaped curve. The commercially available colloidal solution appears as a clear, pale yellow to amber solution. In 500 mL of the commercial preparation containing HES (450/0.7) 6% and 0.9% sodium chloride, it contains 77 mEq of sodium and 77 mEq of chloride. It has an osmolality of 310 mOsm/L and a pH of about 5.5.

The HES (670/0.75) product in lactated electrolyte solution (*Hextend®*) contains 143 mEq/L of sodium, 124 mEq/L of chloride, 28 mEq/L of lactate, 5 mEq/L of calcium, 3 mEq/L of potassium, 0.9 mEq/L of magnesium, and 0.99 grams/L of dextrose. These values approximate what is found in human plasma.

The lower MW product HES 6% (130/0.4) in sterile saline (*Vetstarch®, Voluven®*) has an average molecular weight of 130 kD, a DS of 0.4 (range 0.38-0.45) and a pH of 4-5.5. It contains 154 mEq/L sodium, and 154 mEq/L chloride. Calculated osmolarity is 308.

Pentastarch 10% in 0.9% sodium chloride (*Pentaspan®*) molecular weight ranges from 200-300 kD, has a DS range of 0.4-0.5 and a pH of approximately 5. Calculated osmolarity is 326.

Hetastarch may also be known by the following synonyms: etherified starches, HES, and hydroxyethyl starch; many trade names are available.

Storage/Stability

Hetastarch 6% in 0.9% NaCl or lactated electrolyte should be stored at temperatures less than 40°C; freezing should be avoided. Exposure to temperature extremes may result in formation of a crystalline precipitate or a color change to a turbid deep brown. Do not use should this occur.

Compatibility/Compounding Considerations

The following drugs are reported **compatible** at Y-sites with hetastarch (450/0.7) 6% in normal saline: cimetidine, diltiazem, enalaprilat, and ertapenem. For *Hextend®*: Do not administer simultaneously with blood through the same administration set as there is a risk of coagulation.

Dosage Forms/Regulatory Status

VETERINARY-LABELED PRODUCTS:

Hydroxyethyl starch (tetrastarch) 6% (6 g/100 mL) 130/0.4 in isotonic sodium chloride injection in 250 mL and 500 mL polyolefin bags; *Vetstarch®*; (Rx). This product is not "officially" an FDA-approved product for use in animals, but the label information has been approved by FDA.

HUMAN-LABELED PRODUCTS:

Hetastarch Injection: 6% (6 g/100 mL) HES (450/0.7) in 0.9% sodium chloride in 500 mL IV infusion bottles, polyolefin bags & single-dose containers; *Hespan®*; 6% Hetastarch; (Rx)

Hetastarch Injection: 6% (6 g/100 mL) HES (670/0.75) in lactated electrolyte in 500 mL IV infusion single-dose containers; *Hextend®*, generic; (Rx)

Hydroxyethyl starch (tetrastarch) 6% (6 g/100 mL) 130/0.4: in 0.9% sodium chloride in 500 mL polyolefin bags; *Voluven®*; (Rx)

In some countries (not in USA): Pentastarch 10% in 0.9% sodium chloride in 250 ml & 500 mL plastic bags; *Pentaspan®*; (Rx)

Revisions/References

Monograph revised/updated February 2014.

Aarnes, T. K., et al. (2009). Effect of intravenous administration of lactated Ringer's solution or hetastarch for the treatment of isoflurane-induced hypotension in dogs. American Journal of Veterinary Research 70(11): 1345-53.

Antinoff, N. (2009). Avian Critical Care: What's Old, What's New. Proceedings: IVECCS. accessed via Veterinary Information Network; vin.com

Boag, A. (2007). Hetastarch: Not All Starches Are the Same. Proceedings: IVECCS. accessed via Veterinary Information Network; vin.com

Carney, K. R., et al. (2011). Evaluation of the effect of hetastarch and lactated Ringer's solution on plasma colloid osmotic pressure in healthy llamas. Javma-Journal of the American Veterinary Medical Association 238(6): 768-72.

Chohan, A. S., et al. (2011). Effects of 6% hetastarch (600/0.75) or lactated Ringer's solution on hemostatic variables and clinical bleeding in healthy dogs anesthetized for orthopedic surgery. Veterinary Anaesthesia and Analgesia 38(2): 94-105.

Classen, J., et al. (2012). In vitro effect of hydroxyethyl starch 130/0.42 on canine platelet function. American Journal of Veterinary Research 73(12): 1908-12.

Esser, M., et al. (2012). Effect of Hetastarch and Plasma on Colloid Osmotic Pressure of Healthy Horses. IVECCS. accessed via Veterinary Information Network; vin.com

Helmbold, K., et al. (2009). Effects of hetastarch on coagulation parameters and clinical outcome in dogs. Proceedings: IVECC. accessed via Veterinary Information Network; vin.com

Magdesian, K. G. (2010). Replacement Fluid Therapy for the Critical Equine Patient. Proceedings: ACVIM. accessed via Veterinary Information Network; vin.com

McBride, D., et al. (2013). Effect of hydroxyethyl starch 130/0.4 and 200/0.5 solutions on canine platelet function in vitro. American Journal of Veterinary Research 74(8): 1133-7.

McKenzie, E., et al. (2009). Hetastarch on the colloid osmotic pressure of healthy llamas. Proceedings: IVECC. accessed via Veterinary Information Network; vin.com

Naylor, R. J. & B. Dunkel (2009). The treatment of diarrhoea in the adult horse. Equine Veterinary Education 21(9): 494-504.

Powell, L. (2013). Colloid therapy and concentrated albumn transfusions. ACVIM. accessed via Veterinary Information Network; vin.com

Smart, L., et al. (2009). The Effect of Hetastarch (670/0.75) on Urine Specific Gravity and Osmolality in the Dog. Journal of Veterinary Internal Medicine 23(2): 388-91.

Wendt-Hornickle, E. L., et al. (2011). The effects of lactated Ringer's solution (LRS) or LRS and 6% hetastarch on the colloid osmotic pressure, total protein and osmolality in healthy horses under general anesthesia. Veterinary Anaesthesia and Analgesia 38(4): 336-43.

Hydroxyurea

(hye-drox-ee-yor-ee-a)   Hydrea®, Droxia®, Mylocel®

Antineoplastic

Prescriber Highlights

▶ Antineoplastic used for treatment of polycythemia vera, mastocytomas, & leukemias in dogs & cats.

▶ Caution: Anemia, bone marrow depression, history of urate stones, infection, impaired renal function, or in patients who have received previous chemotherapy or radiotherapy.

▶ Adverse Effects: GI effects, stomatitis, sloughing of nails, alopecia, & dysuria; most serious are bone marrow depression & pulmonary fibrosis.

▶ Proven teratogen.

Uses/Indications

Hydroxyurea may be useful in the treatment of polycythemia vera, mast cell tumors, and leukemias in dogs and cats. A prospective, open label study in dogs with mast cell tumors found an overall response rate of 28% (Rassnick et al. 2010). It has been used to treat dogs with chronic myelogenous leukemia no longer responsive to busulfan. Hydroxyurea, potentially, may be of benefit in the treatment of feline hypereosinophilic syndrome and in the adjunctive treatment of canine meningiomas. It can also be used in dogs for the adjunctive medical treatment (to reduce hematocrit) of right to left shunting patent ductus arteriosus or tetralogy of Fallot.

Pharmacology/Actions

While the exact mechanism of action for hydroxyurea has not been determined, it appears to interfere with DNA synthesis without interfering with RNA or protein synthesis. Hydroxyurea apparently inhibits thymidine incorporation into DNS and may directly damage DNA. It is an S-phase inhibitor but may also arrest cells at the G_1-S border.

Hydroxyurea inhibits urease but is less potent than acetohydroxamic acid. Hydroxyurea can stimulate production of fetal hemoglobin.

Pharmacokinetics

Hydroxyurea is well absorbed after oral administration and crosses the blood-brain barrier. Approximately 50% of an absorbed dose is excreted unchanged in the urine and about 50% is metabolized in the liver and then excreted in the urine.

Contraindications/Precautions/Warnings

Risk versus benefit should be considered before using hydroxyurea in patients with the following conditions: anemia, bone marrow depression, history of urate stones, current infection, impaired renal function, or in patients who have received previous chemotherapy or radiotherapy.

Adverse Effects

Potential adverse effects include GI effects (anorexia, vomiting, diarrhea), stomatitis, sloughing of nails, alopecia, and dysuria. While hydroxyurea can cause vomiting, it is usually not severe. The most serious adverse effects associated with hydroxyurea are bone marrow depression (anemia, thrombocytopenia, leukopenia) and pulmonary fibrosis. If myelotoxicity occurs, it is recommended to halt therapy until values return to normal. Methemoglobinemia has been reported in cats given high dosages (>500 mg) (Rassnick et al. 2010).

Reproductive/Nursing Safety

Hydroxyurea is a teratogen. Use only during pregnancy when the benefits to the mother outweigh the risks to the offspring. Hydroxyurea can suppress gonadal function; arrest of spermatogenesis has been noted in dogs. In humans, the FDA categorizes this drug as category *D* for use during pregnancy (*There is evidence of human fetal risk, but the potential benefits from the use of the drug in pregnant women may be acceptable despite its potential risks.*)

Although hydroxyurea distribution into milk has not been documented, nursing puppies or kittens should receive milk replacer when the dam is receiving hydroxyurea.

Overdosage/Acute Toxicity

Cats given hydroxyurea in doses greater than 500 mg (total) may develop methemoglobinemia.

There were 45 single agent exposures to hydroxyurea reported to the ASPCA Animal Poison Control Center (APCC) during 2009-2013. Of the 37 exposed dogs, 22 were symptomatic. The most common clinical signs included: vomiting (32%), ataxia (27%), methemoglobinemia (27%), tachycardia (27%), lethargy (23%), and hypothermia (18%).

Because of the potential toxicity of the drug, overdoses should be treated aggressively with gut emptying protocols employed when possible. Acetylcysteine or methylene blue (not for cats) has been suggested for treating methemoglobinemia (Khan 2012). For further information, contact an animal poison control center.

Drug Interactions

The following drug interactions have either been reported or are theoretical in humans or animals receiving hydroxyurea and may be of in veterinary patients. Unless otherwise noted, use together is not necessarily contraindicated, but weigh the potential risks and perform additional monitoring when appropriate.

■ **BONE MARROW DEPRESSANT DRUGS, OTHER** (*e.g.*, other **antineoplastics**, **chloramphenicol**, **flucytosine**, **amphotericin**

B, or **colchicine**): Other bone marrow depressant drugs may cause additive myelosuppression when used with hydroxyurea.

Laboratory Considerations

- Hydroxyurea may raise serum **uric acid** levels; drugs such as allopurinol may be required to control hyperuricemia

Doses

Note: Hydroxyurea is not commonly used in veterinary medicine and published dosage recommendations can vary widely. Because there is little evidence to support any particular dosage the following dosages should be used only as a general guide. Consultation with a veterinary oncologist is highly recommended.

- **DOGS:**

  For polycythemia vera (PV); chronic myelogenous leukemia, mast cell tumors (extra-label): Depending on the reference, dosage recommendations vary considerably. Generally, initial daily dosages (q24h) are 50 – 60 mg/kg once a day (or divided twice daily) PO for 1-2 weeks (for PV until hematocrit is below 60%) and then every other day (for PV tapered to lowest effective dosage frequency).

- **CATS:**

  For polycythemia vera (PV); chronic myelogenous leukemia (extra-label): Depending on the reference, dosage recommendations vary considerably. Generally, initial daily dosages (q24h) are 30 mg/kg once a day or 10 – 15 mg/kg twice daily PO for 1-2 weeks (for PV until hematocrit is below 60%) and then every other day (for PV tapered to lowest effective dosage frequency).

Monitoring

Note: Cats may require more frequent monitoring than dogs.
- CBC with platelets at least every 1-2 weeks until stable; then every 3 months.
- BUN/Serum Creatinine; initially before starting treatment and then every 3-4 months.

Client Information

- Hydroxyurea is a chemotherapy (cancer) drug. The drug and its byproducts can be hazardous to other animals and people that come in contact with it. On the day your animal gets the drug and then for a few days afterward, all bodily waste (urine, feces, litter), blood, or vomit should only be handled while wearing disposable gloves. Seal the waste in a plastic bag and then place both the bag and gloves in with the regular trash.
- Can be very toxic to the gastrointestinal tract (vomiting, diarrhea, ulcers and stomach upset) and cause lung damage.
- Can cause loss of toenails and fur.
- Give with food.

Chemistry/Synonyms

Structurally similar to urea and acetohydroxamic acid, hydroxyurea occurs as white, crystalline powder that is freely soluble in water. It is moisture labile.

Hydroxyurea may also be known as: hydroxycarbamide, hydroxycarbamidum, NSC-32065, SQ-1089, WR-83799, *Dacrodil®, Droxiurea®, Hydrea®, Droxia®, Hydrine®, Litalir®, Medroxyurea®, Neodrea®, Onco-Carbide®, Oxeron®,* and *Syrea®.*

Storage/Stability

Capsules should be stored in tight containers at room temperature. Avoid excessive heat.

Compatibility/Compounding Considerations

Because of limited available dosage forms, compounded preparations may be necessary to accurately dose small animals.

Compounded preparation stability: Hydroxyurea oral suspension compounded from commercially available capsules has been published (Heeney et al. 2004). Triturating ten (10) hydroxyurea 500 mg capsules with room temperature water, stirring, filtering and bringing to a final volume of 50 mL with *Syrpalta®* yields a 100 mg/mL suspension that retains >95% potency for 180 days when stored at 25°C. Suspensions of hydroxyurea heated to 41°C result in an immediate 40% loss of drug potency. Compounded preparations of hydroxyurea should be protected from light.

Dosage Forms/Regulatory Status

VETERINARY-LABELED PRODUCTS: NONE.

HUMAN-LABELED PRODUCTS:

Hydroxyurea Oral Capsules: 200 mg, 300 mg, 400 mg & 500 mg; *Hydrea®, Droxia®,* generic (500 mg only); (Rx)

Revisions/References

Monograph revised/updated February 2014.

Heeney, M. M., et al. (2004). Chemical and functional analysis of hydroxyurea oral solutions. J Pediatr Hematol Oncol 26(3): 179-84.
Khan, S. A. (2012). Common Reversal Agents/Antidotes in Small Animal Poisoning. Veterinary Clinics of North America-Small Animal Practice 42(2): 403-+.
Rassnick, K. M., et al. (2010). Phase II open-label study of single-agent hydroxyurea for treatment of mast cell tumours in dogs*. Veterinary and Comparative Oncology 8(2): 103-11.

Hydroxyzine HCl
Hydroxyzine Pamoate

(hye-drox-i-zeen)   Atarax®, Vistaril®

Antihistamine;

Prescriber Highlights

▶ Used principally for antihistaminic, antipruritic, & sedative/tranquilization qualities. Must be given on a regular basis as a preventative for atopic dermatitis.

▶ Contraindications: Hypersensitivity to the drug. Caution in patients with prostatic hypertrophy, bladder neck obstruction, severe cardiac failure, angle-closure glaucoma, or pyeloduodenal obstruction.

▶ Adverse Effects: Sedation most likely; **Dogs** (rarely): Tremors, seizures; **Cats:** Polydipsia, depression, or behavioral changes.

Uses/Indications

Hydroxyzine is used principally for its antihistaminic, antipruritic, and sedative/tranquilization qualities, often in atopic patients. Efficacy for treating acute flares of canine atopic dermatitis 'after the fact' is unlikely, and there is little evidence to support use for chronic atopic dermatitis. However, hydroxyzine (and cetirizine) have demonstrated an inhibitory effect after intradermal histamine injections in dogs. If a trial for treatment is desired, it should be given as a preventative on a regular basis (Olivry et al. 2010).

Pharmacology/Actions

Like other H_1-receptor antihistamines, hydroxyzine acts by competing with histamine for sites on H_1-receptor sites on effector cells. Antihistamines do not block histamine release, but can antagonize its effects. In addition to its antihistaminic effects, hydroxyzine possesses anticholinergic, sedative, tranquilizing, antispasmodic, local anesthetic, mild bronchodilative, and antiemetic activities.

Pharmacokinetics

In dogs, hydroxyzine (pamoate) has an oral bioavailability of about 70%, but there was high interpatient variability. Peak levels occur about 3 hours after dosing and elimination half-life is approximately 18 hours. Hydroxyzine is rapidly metabolized to cetirizine (active), which has an elimination half-life of about 11 hours. Area under the curve (AUC) for cetirizine was about 10X that for hydroxyzine (Bizikova et al. 2008).

Contraindications/Precautions/Warnings

Hydroxyzine is contraindicated in patients hypersensitive to it. It should be used with caution in patients with prostatic hypertrophy, bladder neck obstruction, severe cardiac failure, angle-closure glaucoma, or pyeloduodenal obstruction.

Adverse Effects

The most likely adverse effect associated with hydroxyzine is sedation. In dogs, this is usually mild and transient. Occasionally antihistamines can cause a hyperexcitability reaction. Dogs have reportedly developed fine rapid tremors, whole body tremors and, rarely, seizures while receiving this drug. Cats may develop polydipsia, depression, or behavioral changes while on this medication.

Reproductive/Nursing Safety

At doses substantially greater than those used therapeutically, hydroxyzine has been shown to be teratogenic in lab animals. Use during pregnancy (particularly during the first trimester) only when the benefits outweigh the risks. In humans, the FDA categorizes this drug as category C for use during pregnancy (*Animal studies have shown an adverse effect on the fetus, but there are no adequate studies in humans; or there are no animal reproduction studies and no adequate studies in humans.*)

It is unknown if hydroxyzine enters maternal milk; cetirizine a metabolite of hydroxyzine, has been detected in milk.

Overdosage/Acute Toxicity

Overdoses would be expected to cause increased sedation and perhaps, hypotension. At high doses, fine rapid tremors and rarely seizures have been reported. There were 280 single agent exposures to hydroxyzine reported to the ASPCA Animal Poison Control Center (APCC) during 2009-2013. Of the 256 dogs, 74 were symptomatic with 32% lethargic, 23% hyperthermic, 20% tremoring, 15% tachycardic, 12% ataxic, and 9% seizuring. There are no specific antidotes available. Gut emptying protocols should be considered with large or unknown quantity overdoses. Supportive and symptomatic treatment is recommended if necessary.

Drug Interactions

The following drug interactions have either been reported or are theoretical in humans or animals receiving hydroxyzine and may be of in veterinary patients. Unless otherwise noted, use together is not necessarily contraindicated, but weigh the potential risks and perform additional monitoring when appropriate.

- **ANTICHOLINERGIC AGENTS:** Additive anticholinergic effects may occur when hydroxyzine is used concomitantly with other anticholinergic agents.
- **CNS DEPRESSANT DRUGS, OTHER:** Additive CNS depression may be seen if combining hydroxyzine with other CNS depressant medications, such as barbiturates, tranquilizers, etc.
- **EPINEPHRINE:** Hydroxyzine may inhibit or reverse the vasopressor effects of epinephrine; use norepinephrine or metaraminol instead.

Laboratory Considerations

- False increases have been reported in **17-hydroxycorticosteroid** urine values after hydroxyzine use.
- Intradermal allergy testing. Discontinue hydroxyzine 10-14 days prior to test.

Doses

- **DOGS:**

  As an antipruritic/antihistamine (extra-label): Based upon a pharmacokinetic study and pharmacologic modeling: 2 mg/kg PO q12h. Data suggests that increasing dosage or frequency of administration would not result in greater histamine inhibition (Bizikova et al. 2008). Antihistamines should be given on a regular basis to help maintain histamine-1 receptors in an inactive state. (Olivry et al. 2010)

- **CATS:**

  As an antipruritic/antihistamine (extra-label): 5 – 10 mg per cat PO q12h.

- **FERRETS:**

  As an antipruritic/antihistamine (extra-label): 2 mg/kg PO 3 times daily. (Williams 2000)

- **HORSES:** (NOTE: ARCI UCGFS CLASS 2 DRUG)

  As an antipruritic/antihistamine (extra-label):

  a) 0.5 – 1 mg/kg IM or PO twice daily. (Robinson 1992)

  b) Using the pamoate salt: 0.67 mg/kg PO twice daily. (Duran 1992)

- **BIRDS:**

  For pruritus associated with allergies, feather picking, or self-mutilation (extra-label):

  a) 2 mg/kg q8h PO or 1.5 – 2 mg per 4 oz of drinking water daily; adjust dose to minimize drowsiness and maximize effect. (Hillyer 1994)

  b) 2 mg/kg PO q12h. (Siebert 2003)

Monitoring

- Efficacy.
- Adverse effects.

Client Information

- Antihistamines are normally used on a regular, ongoing basis in animals that respond to them. They work better if used before exposure to an allergen.
- Most common side effect is drowsiness/sleepiness, which may be useful in some animals.
- Dry mouth, decreased gastrointestinal activity, and trouble urinating are possible.
- May be given with or without food. If your animal drools, vomits or acts sick after getting it on an empty stomach, give with food or small treat to see if this helps. If vomiting continues, contact your veterinarian.

Chemistry/Synonyms

A piperazine-derivative antihistamine, hydroxyzine HCl occurs as a white, odorless powder. It is very soluble in water and freely soluble in alcohol. Hydroxyzine pamoate occurs as a light yellow, practically odorless powder. It is practically insoluble in water or alcohol.

Hydroxyzine may also be known as: hydroxyzine embonate, hydroxyzine pamoate, hydroxyzine HCl, hydroxyzini HCl, *Vistaril®*, *Atarax®* or *Masmoran®*.

Storage/Stability

Hydroxyzine oral products should be stored at room temperature in tight, light-resistant containers. Avoid freezing all liquid products.

Compatibility/Compounding Considerations

The HCl injection has been reported to be physically **compatible** with the following drugs when mixed in syringes: atropine sulfate, butorphanol tartrate, chlorpromazine HCl, cimetidine HCl, codeine phosphate, diphenhydramine HCl, doxapram HCl, droperidol, fentanyl citrate, glycopyrrolate, hydromorphone HCl, lidocaine HCl, meperidine HCl, metoclopramide HCl, midazolam HCl, morphine sulfate, oxymorphone HCl, pentazocine lactate, procaine HCl, prochlorperazine edisylate, promazine HCl, promethazine HCl, and scopolamine HBr. Compatibility is dependent upon factors such as pH, concentration, temperature and diluent used; consult specialized references or a hospital pharmacist for more specific information.

Dosage Forms/Regulatory Status

VETERINARY-LABELED PRODUCTS: NONE.

The ARCI (Racing Commissioners International) has designated this drug as a class 2 substance. See the appendix for more information.

HUMAN-LABELED PRODUCTS:

Hydroxyzine HCl Oral Tablets: 10 mg, 25 mg & 50 mg; generic; (Rx)

Hydroxyzine HCl Oral Syrup/Solution: 10 mg/5 mL (2 mg/mL) in 118 mL & 473 mL (may contain alcohol); generic; (Rx)

Hydroxyzine HCl Injection: 25 mg/mL (may contain benzyl alcohol) in 1 mL & 2 mL vials and 50 mg/mL (may contain benzyl alcohol) in 1 mL, 2 mL & 10 mL vials; generic; (Rx)

Hydroxyzine Pamoate Oral Capsules (equivalent to hydroxyzine HCl): 25 mg, 50 mg, & 100 mg (as pamoate); *Vistaril*®, generic; (Rx)

Revisions/References

Monograph revised/updated February 2014.

Bizikova, P., et al. (2008). Hydroxyzine and cetirizine pharmacokinetics and pharmacodynamics after oral and intravenous administration of hydroxyzine to healthy dogs. Veterinary Dermatology **19**(6): 348-57.

Duran, S. (1992). Personal Communication.

Hillyer, E. (1994). Avian dermatology. *Saunders Manual of Small Animal Practice*. S. Birchard and R. Sherding. Philadelphia, W.B. Saunders Company: 1271-81.

Olivry, T., et al. (2010). Treatment of canine atopic dermatitis: 2010 clinical practice guidelines from the International Task Force on Canine Atopic Dermatitis. Veterinary Dermatology **21**(3): 233-48.

Robinson, N. (1992). Table of Drugs: Approximate Doses. *Current Therapy in Equine Medicine 3*. N. Robinson. Philadelphia, W.B. Saunders Co.: 815-21.

Siebert, L. (2003). Psittacine feather picking. Proceedings: Western Veterinary Conference. accessed via Veterinary Information Network; vin.com

Williams, B. (2000). Therapeutics in Ferrets. Vet Clin NA: Exotic Anim Pract **3**:1(Jan): 131-53.

Hyoscyamine Sulfate

(hye-oh-**sye**-ah-meen *or* hye-**ah**-ska-meen)   Levsin®

Oral and Injectable Anticholinergic

Prescriber Highlights

▶ Anticholinergic that may be useful for treating hypermotile GI conditions such as irritable bowel syndrome or bradycardia in dogs.

▶ Limited use or experience in veterinary medicine.

▶ Adverse effects can include mydriasis, xerostomia, constipation, urinary retention, & xerophthalmia.

Uses/Indications

Although not commonly used in veterinary medicine, hyoscyamine may be useful as an alternative to other anticholinergic drugs such as glycopyrrolate for treating bradycardia or hypermotile GI conditions such as irritable bowel syndrome in dogs. It potentially could be useful for treating hypersalivation, urinary spasms, vomiting, or reducing secretions perioperatively, but little is known regarding safety and efficacy in animals when used for these conditions.

In humans, hyoscyamine is used primarily for its effects in reducing GI tract motility or to decrease pharyngeal, bronchial and tracheal secretions.

Pharmacology/Actions

Hyoscyamine is an anticholinergic agent similar to atropine, but more potent both in central and peripheral effects. It inhibits acetylcholine at tissues innervated by postganglionic nerves and smooth muscles that respond to acetylcholine but do not have cholinergic innervation. It does not have action on autonomic ganglia. Pharmacologic effects include dose-related reductions in secretions, gas-trointestinal and urinary tract motility, mydriasis, and increased heart rate.

Pharmacokinetics

No pharmacokinetic data was located for veterinary species. In humans, hyoscyamine is rapidly and nearly completely absorbed after oral or sublingual administration. Extended release oral dosage forms may have somewhat reduced oral bioavailability. It is distributed throughout the body, enters the CNS and crosses the placenta. Hyoscyamine is partially hydrolyzed in the liver to tropic acid and tropine. The majority of the drug is excreted unchanged in the urine. Elimination half-life is about 3.5 hours; about 7 hours for the sustained-release product, *Levsinex*®. Average duration of action in humans is approximately 4-6 hours.

Contraindications/Precautions/Warnings

Hyoscyamine is contraindicated in patients hypersensitive to it. Patients sensitive to one belladonna alkaloid or derivative may be sensitive to another.

Use with caution in patients with renal dysfunction as hyoscyamine elimination may be reduced. Use of anticholinergics should be carefully considered before using in patients with tachyarrhythmias, cardiac valve disease or congestive heart failure. Patients with myasthenia gravis may have their condition aggravated with concurrent use of hyoscyamine. Other contraindications for using hyoscyamine in humans include: glaucoma (narrow or wide angle), intestinal obstruction, toxic megacolon, intestinal atony, severe ulcerative colitis, obstructive uropathy, or acute hemorrhage.

Adverse Effects

Adverse effects can include mydriasis, xerostomia, constipation, urinary retention, and xerophthalmia. Higher dosages may cause CNS effects (somnolence or excitement) or tachycardia.

Reproductive/Nursing Safety

There is limited information available on the drug's use during pregnancy. While hyoscyamine crosses the placenta, reproductive studies in animals have not been performed. Two limited studies (322 & 281 pregnancies) in humans have been published evaluating hyoscyamine safety during pregnancy. One study showed no increase in congenital malformations, but the other showed a slight increase above normally expected malformations in infants. In humans, the FDA categorizes hyoscyamine as category C for use during pregnancy (*Animal studies have shown an adverse effect on the fetus, but there are no adequate studies in humans; or there are no animal reproduction studies and no adequate studies in humans.*)

Only traces of hyoscyamine are detected in milk. While no problems have been reported and risk to offspring cannot be ruled out, it is probably safe to use in nursing patients.

Overdosage/Acute Toxicity

The LD50 for hyoscyamine in rats is 375 mg/kg. Significant overdosage in animals may be serious and contacting an animal poison control center is advised. Toxicity is exhibited by intensified and prolonged anticholinergic effects; signs include: increased heart rate, CNS effects (behavior changes, depression, seizures), urinary retention, decreased gut sounds/motility, and mydriasis. Protocols to decrease oral absorption should be considered if overdose was recent. Severe anticholinergic effects can be treated with physostigmine or neostigmine, but it is suggested to do so only under the guidance of an animal poison control center. In humans, delirium or excitement has been treated with small doses of short-acting barbiturates or benzodiazepines. Hyoscyamine can be removed by hemodialysis.

Drug Interactions

The following drug interactions have either been reported or are theoretical in humans or animals receiving hyoscyamine and may be of in veterinary patients. Unless otherwise noted, use together is not necessarily contraindicated, but weigh the potential risks and perform additional monitoring when appropriate.

- **ANTACIDS containing magnesium, aluminum or calcium salts:** May interfere with hyoscyamine absorption.
- **ANTICHOLINERGICS, OTHER (atropine, glycopyrrolate, etc.):** Additive actions and adverse effects can occur.
- **ANTIHISTAMINES, FIRST GENERATION** (*e.g.,* **diphenhydramine**): Additive actions and adverse effects can occur.
- **PROKINETIC AGENTS** (*e.g.,* **cisapride, metoclopramide**): Hyoscyamine may counteract their effects.

Laboratory Considerations

- No specific concerns noted with hyoscyamine.

Doses

- **DOGS:**

  Note: The following dosage is assumed to be for the immediate release oral dosage forms. Potentially, the extended release tablets or capsules could be effective and reduce dosing frequency particularly in larger dogs, but no data was located for using them.

  As an antimuscarinic for irritable bowel syndrome, sinus node disease, etc. (extra-label): There is little published evidence or information to support use. Noted dosages are generally 0.003 – 0.006 mg/kg PO q8h.

Monitoring

- Clinical efficacy.
- Adverse effects (*e.g.,* heart rate, bowel or urinary elimination difficulties).

Client Information

- May be given with or without food. If your animal vomits or acts sick after getting it on an empty stomach, give with food or small treat to see if this helps. If vomiting continues, contact your veterinarian.
- Common side effects include dry mouth, dry eyes, constipation, trouble urinating, and faster heartbeat.
- Be sure animal has access to water at all times.
- Contact veterinarian immediately if seizures (convulsions), collapsing/fainting or large changes in behavior (*e.g.,* hyperexcitability (overly excited) or depression, etc.) occur.
- If using a sustained-release capsule or tablet, do not split, crush or allow the animal to chew it.

Chemistry/Synonyms

Hyoscyamine sulfate is a tertiary amine that occurs as white, odorless crystals or crystalline powder. One gram is soluble in 0.5 mL of water or in 1 mL of alcohol. It is practically insoluble in ether.

Hyoscyamine may also be known as: daturin, duboisine, tropine-L-tropate. International trade names include: *Egazil Duretter®* and *Neo-Allospasmin®*.

Storage/Stability

Unless otherwise advised by the manufacturer, hyoscyamine sulfate oral products should be stored at room temperature, in tight containers, and protected from light. The injectable product should be stored at room temperature and protected from freezing.

Compatibility/Compounding Considerations

No specific information noted.

Dosage Forms/Regulatory Status

VETERINARY-LABELED PRODUCTS:

None as single ingredient products.

HUMAN-LABELED PRODUCTS:

Hyoscyamine Oral Tablets: 0.125 mg (regular & chewable), & 0.15 mg; Many trade names are available including: *Anaspaz®, ED-SPAZ®, HyoMax®, Levsin®, Cystospaz®*, generic; (Rx)

Hyoscyamine Orally Disintegrating Tablets: 0.125 mg, & 0.25 mg; *Neosol®, NuLev®, Symax FasTab®, Mar-Spas®*; (Rx)

Hyoscyamine Sublingual Oral Tablets: 0.125 mg; *Levsin/SL®, Symax-SL®*, generic; (Rx)

Hyoscyamine Extended/Sustained-Release Oral Tablets: 0.25 mg (0.125 mg immediate-release) & 0.375 mg; *Levbid®, Symax-SR®* and *Symax Duotab®*, generic; (Rx)

Hyoscyamine Extended/Timed-Release Oral Capsules: 0.375 mg; *Levsinex®*, generic; (Rx)

Hyoscyamine Oral Solution: 0.125 mg/mL in 15 mL; generic; (Rx)

Hyoscyamine Oral Elixir: 0.025 mg/mL (0.125mg/5mL) in pint bottles; generic; (Rx)

Hyoscyamine Oral Spray: 0.125 mg/spray in 30 mL; *IB-Stat®*; (Rx)

Hyoscyamine Injection: 0.05 mg/mL in 1 mL amps & 10 mL vials; *Levsin®*; (Rx)

Revisions/References

Monograph revised/updated February 2014.

Hypertonic Saline (7% – 7.5%)

(hye-per-ton-ik say-leen)   HTS, Sodium Chloride 7%- 7.5%

Prescriber Highlights

► Hypertonic saline (HTS) can provide immediate intravascular expansion in hypovolemic shock and reduce intracerebral pressure in traumatic brain injury. Administer with colloids to increase persistence of intravascular expansion.

► Must be administered IV slowly; CRI's not recommended. Follow with isotonic crystalloids to replenish body water.

► Veterinary-labeled product is not an FDA-approved drug. If compounding from concentrated sodium chloride, use extreme caution.

Uses/Indications

Hypertonic saline solutions (HTS) with concentrations of 7-7.5% are most commonly used in veterinary medicine. HTS is used as an alternative to isotonic crystalloids for resuscitation in previously normovolemic healthy patients with intravascular hypovolemic shock, and in patients with burns or hypovolemic traumatic brain injury (TBI). HTS is particularly useful in conditions where large fluid volumes of crystalloids can cause interstitial edema (e.g., traumatic brain injury, spinal chord trauma, pancreatitis, burns). HTS is also used as a hyperosmolar agent for intracerebral pressure reduction after TBI or to reduce spinal edema after spinal chord trauma.

Use in combination with a synthetic colloid (e.g., dextran, hydroxyethyl starch) is somewhat controversial. Duration of extravascular expansion can be significantly prolonged, but in 2 studies of experimental controlled hemorrhagic shock in dogs, HTS-colloid solutions were shown inferior for improving systemic and regional tissue oxygenation to either lactated Ringer's or hydroxyethyl starch alone (both given in various ratios with shed blood) (Barros et al. 2011), (Braz et al. 2004).

In horses, a study comparing isotonic saline versus HTS (7.2%) for fluid resuscitation after an endurance ride, found that HTS-treated horses had greater decreases in PCV, total protein, albumin, and globulin concentrations, and had a shorter time to urination with lower urine specific gravity (Fielding et al. 2011).

Calves with noninfectious diarrhea and metabolic acidosis treated with HTS (7.5%) and an oral PO isotonic electrolyte solution had faster decreases in hematocrit, total protein/albumin concentration, urea nitrogen concentration, and plasma volume, and faster increases in blood pH, bicarbonate concentration, and central venous pressure than calves treated with oral PO isotonic electrolyte solution alone (Leal et al. 2012).

Pharmacology/Actions

Small bolus doses of HTS can cause immediate intravascular volume expansion. High sodium concentration increases plasma osmolarity causing movement of water from the interstitial space into the intravascular space. Intravascular volume expansion can be in excess of the amount of HTS infused. Equilibrium between the intravascular and interstitial spaces is restored by intracellular water moving into the interstitial space.

HTS may have additional benefits when used for trauma resuscitation including positive immunomodulatory effects due to alterations of neutrophil-endothelial interactions, reduced albumin leakage, reduced endothelial cell swelling, improved cardiac function, improved microcirculation, and reduced edema formation.

Pharmacokinetics

Volume expansion occurs immediately, and is highest at the end of the infusion. Volume expansion effects are relatively transient and may only persist for 30 minutes to 3 hours. Effects may last longer than 3 hours if combined with a colloid (e.g., dextran or hydroxyethyl starch).

Contraindications/Precautions/Warnings

Hypertonic saline is contraindicated in patients with significant hypernatremia, hyperosmolality, hyperchloremia, hypokalemia or intravascular overload. It must be used with extreme caution in dehydrated patients, and after HTS infusion isotonic crystalloid therapy is required to replenish interstitial and intracellular water.

Adequate patient monitoring is mandatory as HTS' effects are transient and critically ill patients can rapidly decompensate.

Hypertonic saline can improve perfusion but it is not a replacement for blood products.

Use with caution, especially at higher than recommended dosages in patients with coagulopathies, thrombocytopenia, or platelet dysfunction. Until it is evaluated further, HTS administered via a constant rate infusion (CRI) is not recommended (Kyes et al. 2011).

Hypertonic saline is a high-risk medication and mistakenly administering hypertonic saline instead of isotonic crystalloids can be extremely hazardous. Limiting the available concentrations available, standardizing dosing and monitoring, keeping the solution separate from other fluids in controlled-access cabinets, colored labeling, and oversight by pharmacists have all been recommended to ensure patient safety in human hospitals (Patanwala et al. 2010).

Adverse Effects

When used at dosages less than 5 mL/kg IV and at infusion rates not greater than 1 mL/kg/minute HTS is considered relatively safe in patients where it is not contraindicated. If infused at a higher rate, arteriolar vasodilation with transient (<1 minute) reductions in mean arterial pressure and vagally mediated bradycardia can occur.

Fluid and electrolyte disturbances (hypokalemia, hypernatremia, hyperchloremia) are possible especially when used repeatedly, at high doses, or if adequate fluid replenishment is not administered.

At concentrations less than 10% infused at recommended rates into peripheral veins, HTS is not likely to cause phlebitis. Consider administering via a central line if available.

In vitro studies have shown that hypertonic saline infusions exceeding 5 mL/kg may prolong clotting or cause clinical coagulopathies.

Reproductive/Nursing Safety

When used appropriately in critically ill patients, use of HTS in pregnant animals should not be a clinical concern.

Overdosage/Acute Toxicity

Inadvertent overdosage can cause electrolyte imbalance (hypernatremia, hyperchloremia, hypokalemia), edema, and aggravation of existing acidosis.

Drug Interactions

- No specific drug interactions noted.

Laboratory Considerations

- No specific concerns noted.

Doses

- **DOGS/CATS:**

  Note: All dosages are for hypertonic saline (sodium chloride) 7%- 7.5%. Many use the veterinary labeled 7.2% product, but there is no evidence to suggest that using concentrations from 7% – 7.5% would be unacceptable.

  For low volume resuscitation using HTS alone (extra-label): Dosage recommendations vary slightly. Using 7 – 7.5% HTS, 4 – 6 mL/kg IV at a rate not to exceed 1 mL/kg/minute is recommended. However, dosages ranging from 2 – 8 mL/kg have been noted. Some state that cats should receive dosages at the low end of the range. Follow with crystalloid therapy to maintain adequate tissue hydration.

  For low volume resuscitation using HTS with a colloid (extra-label): Mixing 23.4% concentrated sodium chloride solution with hetastarch in a 1:2 ratio (1 part sodium chloride 23.4% to 2 parts hetastarch 6%) and administering 4 – 5 mL/kg over 5 minutes has been recommended.

  For neurologic trauma using HTS alone: Dosage recommendations vary but 2- 4 mL/kg IV over 15-20 minutes has been noted. Follow with crystalloids.

- **HORSES:**

  For small volume resuscitation (extra-label): In the study (after an endurance ride) treated horses received an initial bolus of 2 liters of 7.2% HTS and 5 liters of lactated Ringer's solution (also contained 250 mL of 23% calcium gluconate) followed with additional LRS as deemed necessary by the treating veterinarian. (Fielding et al. 2011)

- **CATTLE:**

  For adjunctive treatment of neonatal diarrhea in calves (extra-label): In the study calves received 7.2% HTS 5 mL/kg IV over 3-10 minutes and 60 mL of an isotonic electrolyte solution PO (repeated twice at 8 and 16 hours). (Leal et al. 2012)

- **BIRDS:**

  For small volume replacement/CPCR resuscitation (extra-label): For the shocky debilitated patient, hypertonic saline is administered (3 – 5 mL/kg) over 5 minutes, followed by hetastarch (3 – 5 mL/kg over 5 min). This combination prior to crystalloid administration enables fluids to stay within the vascular space. Blood pressure should be monitored closely. Follow with small boluses of crystalloid fluids (LRS, Plasma-Lyte at 15 – 20 mL/kg) along with hetastarch at 3 – 5 mL/kg over 15 minutes, and reassess the bird every 15 minutes. The crystalloids and hetastarch can be combined in the same syringe or bag. This process is repeated every 15-20 minutes until temperature normalizes and blood pressure is over 120 mmHg. (Antinoff 2009)

Monitoring

- Efficacy: blood pressure, central venous pressure (if possible), and clinical parameters (e.g., heart rate, pulse quality, mucous membrane color, capillary refill time, mental acuity, body temperature).
- Serum electrolytes (sodium, potassium, chloride), serum osmolality, urine output, hematocrit.

Client Information

- Hypertonic saline should only be used in an inpatient setting with appropriate monitoring.

Chemistry/Synonyms

7.2% sodium chloride for injection solution contains 1232 mEq/liter (1.23 mEq/mL) of sodium and 1232 mEq/liter (1.23 mEq/mL) of chloride. Osmolarity is 2464 mOsm/L. Colloid osmotic pressure (COP) is 0.

Storage/Stability

Sodium chloride 7.2% injection should be stored at controlled room temperature between 15°-30°C (59°-86°F). It does not contain a preservative and is appropriate for single-use only. Discard any unused solution.

Sodium Chloride 14.6%, 23.4% (for additive use) should be stored at controlled room temperature and protected from excessive heat and freezing.

Compatibility/Compounding Considerations

The veterinary labeled 7.2% product does not contain a preservative and is appropriate for one-time use only.

Concentrated sodium chloride solutions for IV additive use (14.6 & 23.4%) are thought compatible with hydroxyethyl starch compounds.

Dosage Forms/Regulatory Status

VETERINARY-LABELED PRODUCTS:

Hypertonic Saline (sodium chloride 7.2%) Injection Solution: in 1000 mL bottles; generic; (Rx). Contains no preservative and is labeled for single-use. Labeled (not FDA-approved) for use in horses and cattle. The product (MWI/VetOne) information on the dailymed.nlm.nih.gov website has the following: "**Note:** This drug has not been found by FDA to be safe and effective, and this labeling has not been approved by FDA."

HUMAN-LABELED PRODUCTS:

Sodium Chloride Solution Concentrate 14.6%, 23.4%; generic; (Rx). For IV additive use only; must be diluted before use.

Revisions/References

Monograph written June 2014.

Antinoff, N. (2009). Avian Critical Care: What's Old, What's New. Proceedings: IVECCS. accessed via Veterinary Information Network; vin.com

Barros, J. M. P., et al. (2011). The Effects of 6% Hydroxyethyl Starch-Hypertonic Saline in Resuscitation of Dogs with Hemorrhagic Shock. Anesthesia and Analgesia **112**(2): 395-404.

Braz, J. R. C., et al. (2004). The early systemic and gastrointestinal oxygenation effects of hemorrhagic shock resuscitation with hypertonic saline and hypertonic saline 6% dextran-70: A comparative study in dogs. Anesthesia and Analgesia **99**(2): 536-46.

Fielding, C. L. & K. G. Magdesian (2011). A Comparison of Hypertonic (7.2%) and Isotonic (0.9%) Saline for Fluid Resuscitation in Horses: A Randomized, Double-blinded, Clinical Trial. Journal of Veterinary Internal Medicine **25**(5): 1138-43.

Kyes, J. & J. Johnson (2011). Hypertonic Saline Solutions in Shock Resuscitation. Comp CE; Accessed via vetlearn.com(March): E1-E9.

Leal, M. L. R., et al. (2012). Intravenous hypertonic saline solution (7.5%) and oral electrolytes to treat of calves with noninfectious diarrhea and metabolic acidosis (vol 26, pg 1042, 2012). Journal of Veterinary Internal Medicine **26**(5): 1236-.

Patanwala, A. E., et al. (2010). Use of hypertonic saline injection in trauma. American Journal of Health-System Pharmacy **67**(22): 1920-8.

Ifosfamide

(eye-foss-fa-mide)   Ifex®

Antineoplastic

Prescriber Highlights

- ▶ Alkylating agent that may be useful in treating lymphomas & sarcomas in dogs & cats.
- ▶ Limited veterinary clinical experience to date. Dosage for cats is much greater than for dogs.
- ▶ May be very toxic (myelosuppression, nephrotoxic, bladder toxicity, neurotoxicity, GI, etc.).
- ▶ Must be given with saline diuresis & bladder-protective agent (mesna).

Uses/Indications

In small animals, ifosfamide may be of benefit as part of treatment protocols for a variety of neoplasms. Treatment of lymphomas and soft tissue sarcomas with ifosfamide in dogs and cats has been investigated to some extent; some efficacy has been demonstrated although it does not appear to be efficacious as a single agent for treating lymphoma. A phase II study in cats with vaccine associated sarcoma, demonstrated a measurable response in 41% of treated cats (Rassnick, Rodriguez, et al. 2006).

In humans, ifosfamide is used in various treatment protocols for testicular neoplasms, bone and soft tissue sarcomas, bladder cancer, lung cancer, cervical cancer, ovarian cancer, and some types of lymphomas.

Pharmacology/Actions

Ifosfamide appears to act similarly to other alkylating agents. Its active metabolites interfere with DNA replication and transcription of RNA, thereby disrupting nucleic acid function. It is cycle-phase nonspecific.

Pharmacokinetics

As ifosfamide is a prodrug and does not have pharmacologic activity, it must be biotransformed into active metabolites. Ifosfamide's pharmacokinetics are very complex and not well understood. While normally given IV, it is well absorbed after SC injection or oral administration; bioavailabilities via these routes are 90% or greater. Ifosfamide and its metabolites are widely distributed and enter into both bone and CNS. Ifosfamide is converted into its metabolites primarily via oxidative pathways found in the liver and, to a smaller extent, in the lungs. It then is catalyzed (primarily in cells) into the primary active alkylating agent, ifosfamide mustard. Ifosfamide and its metabolites are primarily excreted via the kidney into urine.

Contraindications/Precautions/Warnings

Because of its toxicity, ifosfamide should only be used by clinicians experienced with the use of cytotoxic agents and able to adequately monitor the effects of therapy. Ifosfamide is contraindicated in patients hypersensitive to it or with severely depressed bone marrow function or active hemorrhagic cystitis. Ifosfamide should be used with extreme caution in patients with impaired renal function. Patients that cannot tolerate forced saline diuresis (*e.g.*, severe heart disease) should not receive the drug.

Ifosfamide must be used in conjunction with mesna to reduce the risk for hemorrhagic cystitis. Should secondary urinary tract infections occur, it has been recommended that even with clinical resolution it (or cyclophosphamide) must not be used again in that patient.

Adverse Effects

Dose related myelosuppression occurs with ifosfamide use; neutropenia generally occurs at 5-7 days post treatment, but may be delayed (14-21 days) particularly with repeated dosing. Nadirs in cats are seen typically at day 7 or 8. Platelets can also be significantly impacted.

Ifosfamide can damage bladder epithelium, and cause nephrotoxicity with resultant electrolyte abnormalities. Renal toxicity is primarily focused on proximal and distal tubular damage, but glomerular effects may occur. To reduce the incidence of nephrotoxicity and bladder toxicity, saline diuresis is performed (see dosages) and mesna given concomitantly to reduce bladder epithelial toxicity (see below). Volume overload with pulmonary edema may result, however, particularly in patients with preexisting cardiac disease. Gastrointestinal effects including nausea, drooling, vomiting have been reported, especially during drug administration. Treatment with antiemetics may be required. Other adverse effects that may occur include: hypersensitivity (anaphylactoid) reactions, anorexia, neurotoxicity (somnolence to confusion, coma, encephalopathy), alopecia, and abnormal liver function tests.

In studies in cats, when doses were at 900 mg/m^2 or less, neutrophil counts of <1,000 cells/microL were seen in about 33% of treated cats, but no secondary infections were noted. Some cats did show some mild, self-limiting GI effects (lack of appetite, vomiting, diarrhea). Signs of nausea during IV infusion were seen in about 1/3rd of those treated; pulmonary edema, and hypersensitivity were seen in single cats. Nephrotoxicity was seen in two cats (Rassnick, Moore, et al. 2006), (Rassnick, Rodriguez, et al. 2006).

Administering mesna with ifosfamide significantly reduces the incidence and severity of ifosfamide-induced hemorrhagic cystitis and hematuria. Mesna interacts with metabolites of ifosfamide that cause the toxicity. Because mesna is hydrophilic, it does not enter most cells and, therefore, does not appear to significantly reduce the anti-tumor efficacy of ifosfamide. Mesna does not prevent or reduce the incidence of other adverse effects associated with ifosfamide (*e.g.*, myelosuppression, GI effects, neurotoxicity, renal toxicity).

Like other cytotoxic drugs, ifosfamide should be handled and disposed of appropriately.

Reproductive/Nursing Safety

In pregnant humans, ifosfamide is designated by the FDA as a category D drug (*There is evidence of human fetal risk, but the potential benefits from the use of the drug in pregnant women may be acceptable despite its potential risks.*) Teratogenic and fetotoxic effects have been demonstrated at usual doses in humans and laboratory animals.

Ifosfamide is excreted in maternal milk. If this drug is being used in lactating mothers, consider using milk replacer.

Overdosage/Acute Toxicity

There is limited information available on acute overdoses. It would be expected that toxicity would be exacerbations of the adverse effects seen at usual doses. No specific antidote (including mesna) is known; treatment is supportive. Methylene blue (50 mg in a 1-2% aqueous solution IV over 5 minutes) has been suggested to treat ifosfamide-induced encephalopathy in humans.

Drug Interactions

The following drug interactions have either been reported or are theoretical in humans or animals receiving ifosfamide and may be of in veterinary patients. Unless otherwise noted, use together is not necessarily contraindicated, but weigh the potential risks and perform additional monitoring when appropriate.

- **BENZODIAZEPINES:** One study where mice received benzodiazepines (**diazepam**, **chlordiazepoxide**, **oxazepam**) prior to receiving ifosfamide showed increased concentrations of active ifosfamide and increased toxicity to the drug; clinical significance has not been determined for human (or dog or cat) patients.

- **CISPLATIN:** Ifosfamide may enhance cisplatin-induced ototoxicity and nephrotoxicity.

- **MYELOSUPPRESSIVE DRUGS, OTHER** (*e.g.*, other **antineoplastics, chloramphenicol, flucytosine, amphotericin B,** or **colchicine**): Other bone marrow depressant drugs may cause additive myelosuppression when used with ifosfamide.

Laboratory Considerations

- No specific laboratory interactions or considerations were noted.

Doses

Note: Because of the potential toxicity of this drug to patients, veterinary personnel and clients, and since chemotherapy indications, treatment protocols, monitoring and safety guidelines often change, the following dosages should be used only as a general guide. Consultation with a veterinary oncologist and referral to current veterinary oncology [e.g., (Withrow et al. 2012); (Dobson et al. 2011); (Henry et al. 2009); (North et al. 2009); (Argyle et al. 2008)] are strongly recommended.

- **DOGS:**

  For adjunctive treatment of lymphomas and sarcomas (extra-label):

  a) Normal (0.9%) saline IV diuresis at a fluid rate of 6X maintenance over 30 minutes. Ifosfamide 375 mg/m^2 diluted to 20 mg/mL or less, IV over 20 minutes. Normal saline IV diuresis at 6X maintenance over 5 hours. MESNA urothelial protectant dosed at 20% of the patient's calculated mg dose of ifosfamide and administered at time zero (immediately before ifosfamide administration), and then repeated 2 and 5 hours after ifosfamide. This therapy may be repeated on a 21-day basis (Kitchell 2008). **Note:** Some sources say treatment can be repeated every 2-3 weeks.

  b) Give IV saline at 18.3 mL/kg/hr for 6 hours. Give ifosfamide at 350 mg/m^2 (if patient weighs less than 10 kg), 375 mg/m^2 (if greater than 10 kg) IV during the second 30 minutes of the 6-hour infusion. Mesna at a dose of 20% of the ifosfamide dose is given as an IV bolus at the start of the IV infusion and again 2 and 5 hours after the ifosfamide infusion. Repeat every 3 weeks (Brewer 2003). **Note:** Some sources say treatment can be repeated every 2-3 weeks.

- **CATS:**

  For adjunctive treatment of lymphomas and sarcomas (extra-label):

  a) Based upon a phase I safety study and a phase II trial for vaccine-related sarcomas, the authors recommend a dose of 900 mg/m^2 every 3 weeks. Mesna bolus and saline diuresis (30 minutes at 18.3 mL/kg/hr) were first given, then ifosfamide and saline diuresis continued for 5 hours after ifosfamide administration completed. (Rassnick, Moore, et al. 2006; Rassnick, Rodriguez, et al. 2006)

  b) Normal (0.9%) saline IV diuresis at a fluid rate of 6X maintenance over 30 minutes. Ifosfamide 900 mg/m^2 diluted to 20 mg/mL or less, IV over 20 minutes. Normal saline IV diuresis at 6X maintenance over 5 hours. MESNA urothelial protectant dosed at 20% of the patient's calculated mg dose of ifosfamide and administered at time zero (immediately before ifosfamide administration), and then repeated 2 and 5 hours after ifosfamide. This therapy may be repeated on a 21-day basis. (Kitchell 2008)

Monitoring

- CBC with platelets (baseline and before re-dosing).
- Renal function with electrolytes (baseline and before re-dosing).
- Urinalysis (baseline and periodic).

- Liver function (baseline and periodic).
- Other adverse effects (volume overload/pulmonary edema, neurotoxicity, GI toxicity).
- Efficacy.

Client Information

- Ifosfamide is a chemotherapy (cancer) drug. The drug and its byproducts can be hazardous to other animals and people that come in contact with it. On the day your animal gets the drug and then for a few days afterward, all bodily waste (urine, feces, litter), blood, or vomit should only be handled while wearing disposable gloves. Seal the waste in a plastic bag and then place both the bag and gloves in with the regular trash.
- See the Adverse Effects section for important information.

Chemistry/Synonyms

An alkylating agent structurally related to cyclophosphamide, ifosfamide occurs as a white, crystalline powder with a melting point of 40°C. It is freely soluble in water and very soluble in alcohol. A 10% solution in water has a pH between 4-7.

Ifosfamide may also be known as: MJF-9325, NSC-109724, Z-4942, and *Ifex*®.

Storage/Stability

Ifosfamide powder for injection should be stored at 20-25°C (68-77°F). It should be protected from temperatures greater than 30°C (86°F) as the drug may liquefy at temperatures greater than 35°C (95°F). Once reconstituted with sterile water for injection or bacteriostatic water for injection the solution is stable for 24 hours when refrigerated. **Note**: One reference states that bacteriostatic water for injection containing benzyl alcohol caused the solution to become turbid at concentrations of ifosfamide greater than 60 mg/mL. No such incompatibility occurred when using bacteriostatic water for injection containing parabens.

Compatibility/Compounding Considerations

The reconstituted drug is **compatible** with D_5W, normal saline, or lactated Ringer's and is stable for up to 24 hours when refrigerated. Ifosfamide is compatible and stable when mixed with mesna in D_5W or lactated Ringer's.

Dosage Forms/Regulatory Status

VETERINARY-LABELED PRODUCTS: NONE.

HUMAN-LABELED PRODUCTS:

Ifosfamide Powder for IV infusion: 1 gram with 200 mg amps of Mesnex (mesna) in single dose vials; 3 grams with 400 mg amps of Mesnex (mesna) in single dose vials; *Ifex*®, generic; (Rx)

Revisions/References

Monograph revised/updated February 2014.

Argyle, D., et al. (2008). *Decision Making in Small Animal Oncology*, Wiley-Blackwell.
Brewer, W. (2003). New, Promising Chemotherapy Agents. Proceedings: Western Veterinary Conference. accessed via Veterinary Information Network; vin.com
Dobson, J. & D. Lascelles (2011). *BSAVA Manual of Canine and Feline Oncology*, BSAVA.
Henry, C. & M. Higginbotham (2009). *Cancer Management in Small Animal Practice*, Saunders.
Kitchell, B. (2008). Advances in feline oncology. Proceedings: WSAVA. accessed via Veterinary Information Network; vin.com
North, S. & T. Banks (2009). *Small Animal Oncology: An Introduction*, Saunders.
Rassnick, K. M., et al. (2006). Phase I trial and pharmacokinetic analysis of ifosfamide in cats with sarcomas. American Journal of Veterinary Research **67**(3): 510-6.
Rassnick, K. M., et al. (2006). Results of a phase II clinical trial on the use of ifosfamide for treatment of cats with vaccine-associated sarcomas. American Journal of Veterinary Research **67**(3): 517-23.
Withrow, S., et al. (2012). *Withrow and MacEwen's Small Animal Clinical Oncology*, 5th Ed., Saunders.

Imepitoin

(ih-meh-pi-toyn)   Pexion®

Anticonvulsant

Prescriber Highlights

▶ New, novel anticonvulsant for idiopathic epilepsy in dogs. Not currently (March 2014) available in USA.

▶ Appears to be efficacious in some dogs and well tolerated, but little currently is published on clinical efficacy or long-term safety. Tolerance development and drug interaction potential do not appear to be major concerns.

Uses/Indications

Imepitoin is available in the U.K. and E.U. and is indicated for the reduction of the frequency of generalized seizures due to idiopathic epilepsy in dogs after careful evaluation of alternative treatment options. The product label states: "The pharmacological response to imepitoin may vary and efficacy may not be complete. Nevertheless imepitoin is considered to be a suitable treatment option in some dogs because of its safety profile." Safety or efficacy as an "add-on" drug is not known.

Pharmacology/Actions

Imepitoin is a low-affinity partial agonist at benzodiazepine binding sites of the $GABA_A$-receptor. Affinity at the site is approximately 600X less than diazepam. When compared to full agonists, this has the potential advantage of causing less severe adverse effects and a lower risk for tolerance and dependence development (Loscher et al. 2013). $GABA_A$-receptor mediated inhibitory effects on neurons is potentiated, thereby preventing seizures. Additionally, a weak inhibition of neuronal calcium channels may contribute to its anticonvulsant activity. Imepitoin also possesses anxiolytic effects.

Pharmacokinetics

In dogs (beagles), imepitoin demonstrates linear kinetics over the therapeutic dosing range. It is slowly, but well absorbed after oral administration (fasted) with a bioavailability of approximately 92%. Peak levels occur about two hours after dosing. The presence of food may reduce the total AUC by 30%, but does not significantly affect peak levels or time to peak. Volume of distribution ranges from 0.6-1.6 L/kg; protein binding is relatively low (60-70%). It is extensively metabolized via oxidative mechanisms to four major inactive metabolites. Clearance ranges from 260-570 mL/hrs/kg. Elimination half-life is about 1.5-2 hours. The majority of a dose is eliminated via fecal routes (Rundfeldt et al. 2014).

Contraindications/Precautions/Warnings

Imepitoin is contraindicated in patients hypersensitive to it, with severely impaired hepatic function or severe renal or cardiovascular disorders.

Efficacy for status epilepticus and cluster seizures in dogs has not been investigated so it should not be used as primary treatment in dogs with cluster seizures and status epilepticus.

Safety has not been tested in dogs weighing less than 5 kg or in dogs with renal, liver, cardiac, gastrointestinal or other disease.

As mild behavioral or muscular signs may be observed in dogs upon abrupt termination of treatment, consider withdrawing the drug gradually if appropriate.

The product label states "Use of the veterinary medicinal product is not recommended in male breeding dogs or in female dogs during pregnancy and lactation."

Adverse Effects

Thus far, adverse effects are not commonly noted and are generally mild and transient. The following have been observed in pre-clinical and clinical studies (listed in decreasing frequency): polyphagia (especially at the beginning of treatment), hyperactivity, polyuria, polydipsia, somnolence, hypersalivation, vomiting, ataxia, apathy, diarrhea, prolapsed nictitating membrane, decreased sight and sensitivity to sound.

Mild elevations in plasma creatinine and cholesterol levels have been noted but did not exceed normal reference ranges and were not associated with clinically significant observations or events.

Reproductive/Nursing Safety

Reproductive safety or safety during nursing is not known. The product label states: ". . . is not recommended in male breeding dogs or in female dogs during pregnancy and lactation." Male dogs administered 10X dosages, diffuse atrophy of seminiferous tubules in the testes and associated decreased sperm counts were seen.

Overdosage/Acute Toxicity

The acute toxicity of PO imepitoin was assessed in rats and mice after oral administration; no mortality was noted in either species up to 2105 mg/kg. The TD_{50} for motor impairment in the rotarod test is about 1 g/kg PO in rats (Bialer et al. 2013).

In dogs where repeated overdoses of up to 5X the highest recommended dose, central nervous system effects (loss of righting reflex, decreased activity, eyelid closure, lacrimation, dry eye and nystagmus), GI effects, and reversible prolongation of the QT interval have been noted. These are not usually life-threatening and generally resolve within 24 hours with supportive and symptomatic treatment.

The benzodiazepine antagonist, flumazenil could potentially be used to reverse severe central nervous effects associated with an overdose, and also to eliminate the drug's anticonvulsant action.

Drug Interactions

The U.K. product label states: "The product has been used in combination with phenobarbital in a small number of cases and no harmful clinical interactions were observed." Imepitoin has a very low drug interaction potential and interactions with highly protein bound or enzyme-inducing drugs are not expected (Rundfeldt et al. 2014). The following drug interactions have either been reported or are theoretical in humans or animals receiving imepitoin and may be of in veterinary patients. Unless otherwise noted, use together is not necessarily contraindicated, but weigh the potential risks and perform additional monitoring when appropriate.

- **FLUMAZENIL:** Could antagonize the anxiolytic and anticonvulsant effects of imepitoin (Bialer et al. 2013).

Laboratory Considerations

- No specific laboratory interactions or considerations were noted.

Doses

- **DOGS:**

  For the reduction of the frequency of generalized seizures due to idiopathic epilepsy in dogs after careful evaluation of alternative treatment options (extra-label in USA): Initially, 10 mg/kg PO twice daily (approximately 12 hours apart). Bioavailability is greater when administered to fasted dogs; maintain consistent administration time in relation to feeding. Tablets can be halved. If seizures are not adequately reduced following a minimum of 1-week of treatment at the current dose, patient should be re-assessed by veterinarian. Dosages vary and range from 10 – 30 mg/kg PO twice daily depending on severity of the seizure disorder. If patient tolerates the drug, dosages may be increased in 50-100% increments to a maximum of 30 mg/kg twice daily. (Adapted from label information—*Pexion*®; B-I U.K.)

Monitoring

- Clinical efficacy.
- Adverse effects.

- Consider baseline renal function tests and occasional serum creatinine.

Client Information

- Best given on an empty stomach about 12 hours apart but if animal vomits after getting the drug, try giving it with food.
- To be effective, the drug must be given on a regular basis as instructed by your veterinarian.
- Possible side effects in dogs include: increased appetite and thirst, increased urination increased drooling, vomiting, and changes in behavior or activity level. Contact veterinarian if these are severe or continue.

Chemistry/Synonyms

An imidaolinone, imepitoin occurs as a white to almost white, solid, non-hygroscopic, odorless, non-bitter tasting substance. It is practically insoluble in water.

Imepitoin may also be known AWD 131—138, ELB 138, or 1-(4-chlorophenyl)- 4-morpholino-imidazolin-2-one). The canine product trade name is *Pexion*®.

Storage/Stability

This veterinary product does not require any special storage conditions. A 3-year shelf life has been assigned to the product.

Compatibility/Compounding Considerations

No specific information noted.

Dosage Forms/Regulatory Status

VETERINARY-LABELED PRODUCTS: NONE IN USA.

Imepitoin Oral Tablets (scored): 100 mg & 400 mg; *Pexion*®; (POM-V). Licensed and available in the U.K. and E.U.

HUMAN-LABELED PRODUCTS: NONE.

Revisions/References

Monograph written March 2014.

Bialer, M., et al. (2013). Progress report on new antiepileptic drugs: A summary of the Eleventh Eilat Conference (EILAT XI). Epilepsy Research 103(1): 2-30.

Loscher, W., et al. (2013). The novel antiepileptic drug imepitoin compares favourably to other GABA-mimetic drugs in a seizure threshold model in mice and dogs. Pharmacological Research 77: 39-46.

Rundfeldt, C., et al. (2014). Imepitoin as novel treatment option for canine idiopathic epilepsy: pharmacokinetics, distribution, and metabolism in dogs. J. Vet. Pharmacol. Ther.: n/a-n/a.

Imidacloprid — See the listing in the Topical Dermatologic section

Imidacloprid/Moxidectin — See Moxidectin and the Imidacloprid listing (in the Topical Dermatologic section)

Imidapril

(ih-mid-a-pril)   Prilium®

Angiotensin-Converting Enzyme (ACE) Inhibitor

Prescriber Highlights

▶ Veterinary ACE inhibitor (not presently available in the USA) labeled (in the U.K.) for dogs for the treatment of moderate to severe heart failure by mitral regurgitation or by dilated cardiomyopathy. Dosed once daily.

▶ Product label has several contraindications listed including: hypersensitivity to ACE inhibitors, low blood pressure, acute renal insufficiency, congenital heart disease, obstructive hypertrophic cardiomyopathy and patients with hemodynamically relevant stenoses (aortic stenosis, mitral valve stenosis, pulmonal stenosis).

▶ Caution: pregnancy, renal insufficiency (doses may need to be reduced), patients with hyponatremia, coronary or cerebrovascular insufficiency, preexisting hematologic abnormalities or a collagen vascular disease (*e.g.*, SLE).

▶ Adverse Effects: GI distress (anorexia, vomiting, diarrhea). Potentially: weakness, hypotension, renal dysfunction & hyperkalemia.

Uses/Indications

Imidapril is labeled (in the U.K.) for use in dogs for the treatment of moderate to severe heart failure by mitral regurgitation or by dilated cardiomyopathy (Anon. 2014). Like other ACE inhibitors, it could also be useful for treating dogs with protein-losing nephropathy.

Pharmacology/Actions

Like enalapril, imidapril is a prodrug and is converted in the liver to the active compound imidaprilat. Imidaprilat prevents the formation of angiotensin-II (a potent vasoconstrictor) by competing with angiotensin-I for the enzyme angiotensin-converting enzyme (ACE). ACE has a much higher affinity for enalaprilat than for angiotensin-I. Because angiotensin-II concentrations are decreased, aldosterone secretion is reduced and plasma renin activity is increased.

The cardiovascular effects of ACE inhibitors in patients with CHF include: decreased total peripheral resistance, pulmonary vascular resistance, mean arterial and right atrial pressures, and pulmonary capillary wedge pressure, no change or decrease in heart rate, and increased cardiac index and output, stroke volume, and exercise tolerance.

ACE inhibitors increase renal blood flow and decrease glomerular efferent arteriole resistance. In animals with glomerular disease, ACE inhibitors decrease proteinuria and may help to preserve renal function. Imidapril partially blocks amlodipine's activation of the renin-angiotensin-aldosterone system (RAAS) in dogs (Atkins et al. 2007).

Pharmacokinetics

Following oral administration in the dog, imidapril is rapidly absorbed but bioavailability is decreased by the presence of food. Maximum plasma concentration occurs less than one hour after dosing and elimination half-life is about 2 hours. Imidapril is mainly hydrolyzed in the liver and kidney to its active metabolite, imidaprilat. Peak imidaprilat plasma concentrations occur in about 5 hours; elimination half-life is more than 10 hours. Protein binding of imidapril and imidaprilat is moderate (85% and 53%, respectively). After oral administration of radio labeled imidapril, about 40% of total radioactivity is excreted in urine and about 60% in the feces. After multiple dosing, plasma imidaprilat concentrations are about

3X higher after the second dose than after the first, but no additional increase is observed with subsequent doses.

Contraindications/Precautions/Warnings

The product label has several contraindications for use in dogs including: hypersensitivity to ACE inhibitors, low blood pressure, acute renal insufficiency, congenital heart disease, obstructive hypertrophic cardiomyopathy and those with hemodynamically relevant stenoses (aortic stenosis, mitral valve stenosis, pulmonal stenosis).

Use ACE inhibitors with caution in patients with hyponatremia or sodium depletion, coronary or cerebrovascular insufficiency, preexisting hematologic abnormalities, or a collagen vascular disease (*e.g.*, SLE). Patients with severe CHF should be monitored very closely upon initiation of therapy.

Adverse Effects

Imidapril's adverse effect profile in dogs is not well described. The product label states that: "Diarrhea, hypotension and related symptoms such as fatigue, dizziness or anorexia can occur in rare cases. Vomiting can also occur in very rare cases. In such cases treatment should be discontinued until the patient's condition has returned to normal. The use of ACE inhibitors in dogs with hypovolemia/dehydration can lead to acute hypotension. In such cases the fluid and electrolyte balance should be restored immediately and treatment suspended until it has been stabilized. Parameters used for monitoring renal function should be checked at the beginning of the treatment and at regular time intervals thereafter." Other ACE inhibitors primary adverse effect in dogs is GI distress (anorexia, vomiting, diarrhea). Potentially, weakness, hypotension, renal dysfunction and hyperkalemia could occur. Because it lacks a sulfhydryl group (unlike captopril), there is less likelihood that immune-mediated reactions will occur, but rashes, neutropenia, and agranulocytosis have been reported in humans with other ACE inhibitors. In humans, ACE inhibitors commonly cause coughs, but this occurs rarely in dogs or cats.

Reproductive/Nursing Safety

The product label states: "Laboratory studies in rats and rabbits did not produce any evidence of teratogenic, embryotoxic or maternotoxic effects, or effects on reproductive performances, when imidapril was administered at the therapeutic dose. In the absence of data, do not use in pregnant or lactating bitches or in breeding dogs." For humans, a related drug enalapril has a "black box" warning to discontinue enalapril as soon as possible when pregnancy is detected. High doses in rodents have caused decreased fetal weights and increases in fetal and maternal death rates; teratogenic effects have not been reported. In humans, the FDA categorizes this drug as <u>category C for use during pregnancy in the first trimester</u> (*Animal studies have shown an adverse effect on the fetus, but there are no adequate studies in humans; or there are no animal reproduction studies and no adequate studies in humans.*) In humans, the FDA categorizes this drug as <u>category D for use during pregnancy in second and third trimesters</u> (*There is evidence of human fetal risk, but the potential benefits from the use of the drug in pregnant women may be acceptable despite its potential risks.*) as ACE inhibitors may cause abnormal fetal and postnatal kidney development.

It is not known if imidapril/imidaprilat enters maternal milk. Safe use during nursing cannot be assumed.

Overdosage/Acute Toxicity

In dogs, doses up to 5 mg/kg of imidapril (20X) have been well tolerated in healthy dogs. Hypotension may occur as a symptom of overdosage with signs of apathy and ataxia. The treatment is symptomatic.

Drug Interactions

The product labels states that: "… diuretics and a low sodium diet potentiate the effect of ACE inhibitors by activating the renin-angiotensin-aldosterone system (RAAS). Diuretics used at high doses and a low sodium diet are thus not recommended during treatment with ACE inhibitors in order to avoid hypotension with clinical signs such as apathy, ataxia, rare syncope and kidney failure. In case of joint administration with potassium retaining diuretics, potassium must be monitored because there is a risk of hyperkalemia."

The following drug interactions have either been reported or are theoretical in humans or animals receiving ACE inhibitors and may be of significance in veterinary patients receiving imidapril:

- **ANTIDIABETIC AGENTS (insulin, oral agents)**: Possible increased risk for hypoglycemia; enhanced monitoring recommended.
- **DIURETICS** (*e.g.,* **furosemide, hydrochlorothiazide**): Potential for increased hypotensive effects.
- **DIURETICS, POTASSIUM-SPARING** (*e.g.,* **spironolactone, triamterene**): Increased hyperkalemic effects, enhanced monitoring of serum potassium recommended.
- **HYPOTENSIVE AGENTS, OTHER**: Potential for increased hypotensive effect.
- **LITHIUM**: Increased serum lithium levels possible; increased monitoring required.
- **NSAIDS**: May reduce the anti-hypertensive or positive hemodynamic effects of imidapril; may increase risk for reduced renal function. Clinical significance has not been demonstrated in dogs receiving the related ACE-inhibitor enalapril and an NSAID.
- **POTASSIUM SUPPLEMENTS**: Increased risk for hyperkalemia.

Laboratory Considerations

- When using iodohippurate sodium I^{123}/I^{134} or Technetium Tc^{99} pentetate **renal imaging** in patients with renal artery stenosis, ACE inhibitors may cause a reversible decrease in localization and excretion of these agents in the affected kidney, which may lead to confusion in test interpretation.

Doses

- **DOGS:**

  For adjunctive treatment of moderate to severe heart failure by mitral regurgitation or by dilated cardiomyopathy (extra-label in USA): 0.25 mg/kg PO once daily. (Adapted from label; *Prilium*® U.K.)

Monitoring

- Clinical signs of CHF.
- Serum electrolytes, creatinine, BUN, urine protein.
- CBC with differential, periodic.
- Blood pressure (if treating hypertension or clinical signs associated with hypotension arise).

Client Information

- Imidapril is used to treat heart failure, high blood pressure and some forms of kidney disease in dogs and cats.
- Usually well tolerated, but vomiting and diarrhea can occur. May be given with or without food. If your animal vomits, stops eating, or acts sick after getting it on an empty stomach, give with food or small treat to see if this helps. If vomiting continues, contact your veterinarian.
- If a rash or signs of infection occur (*e.g.,* fever) contact your veterinarian immediately.
- Very important to give as prescribed. Do not stop or reduce dosage without veterinarian's guidance.
- Your animal will likely need to have blood pressure and lab tests performed.

Chemistry/Synonyms

Angiotensin-converting enzyme (ACE) inhibitors, imidapril and imidaprilat are structurally related to captopril. Imidapril is a pro-drug and is converted *in vivo* by the liver to imidaprilat. Imidapril occurs as a fine, white powder.

Imidapril may also be known as imidaprilum. *Tanatril*® and *Prilium*® are two trade names.

Storage/Stability

Before reconstitution, do not store above 25°C. After reconstitution, store at 2°-8°C (in the refrigerator) for up to 77 days.

Compatibility/Compounding Considerations

Preparation of the oral solution: Remove the nipple and the stopper of the vial containing the powder and fill with tap water up to the 30 mL mark which is indicated by a raised ring around the body of the bottle, place the child proof cap and screw on tightly.

Dosage Forms/Regulatory Status

VETERINARY-LABELED PRODUCTS:

None in the USA. In the U.K. and some other countries: Imidapril Powder for Oral Solution: 2.5 mg/mL (75 mg per bottle); 5 mg/mL (150 mg per bottle), & 10 mg/mL (300 mg per bottle) in 30 mL bottles; *Prilium*®; POM-V (U.K.).

HUMAN-LABELED PRODUCTS: NONE.

Revisions/References

Monograph written February 2014.

Anon. (2014). Prilium® Product Label. Vetoquinol U.K.
Atkins, C. E., et al. (2007). The effect of amlodipine and the combination of amlodipine and enalapril on the renin-angiotensin-aldosterone system in the dog. J. Vet. Pharmacol. Ther. 30(5): 394-400.

Imidocarb Dipropionate

(i-mid-oh-karb)   Imizol®

Antiprotozoal

Prescriber Highlights

▶ Antiprotozoal with activity for Babesia & related parasites.

▶ Contraindications: Patients exposed to cholinesterase-inhibiting drugs (*e.g.,* pyridostigmine), pesticides, or chemicals.

▶ Caution: Impaired lung, hepatic or renal function; safety in puppies, pregnant, lactating, or breeding animals has not been established.

▶ Adverse Effects: Most common are pain during injection & mild cholinergic signs (salivation, nasal drip, & brief episodes of vomiting); less common: panting, diarrhea, injection site inflammation (rarely ulceration), & restlessness. Cholinergic effects may be lessened with antimuscarinic drugs.

▶ Not for intravenous administration.

Uses/Indications

Imidocarb is FDA-approved for use to treat *Babesia canis* infections (babesiosis) in dogs, but the drug may also be efficacious against other Babesia species (*B. Conradae* and North Carolina Babesia species). Imidocarb appears to be more effective against *B. canis* than *B. gibsoni*. A prospective, unmasked study in dogs with *B. gibsoni* comparing atovaquone/azithromycin (AA) with a protocol using clindamycin, diminazene and imidocarb (CDI) found that CDI had higher recovery and lower relapse rates, albeit longer therapy duration and slower reduction in parasite numbers than AA. The authors concluded that CDI was effective for initial therapy and when the M121I gene in *B. Gibsoni* had mutated (Lin et al. 2012). Imidocarb has been used to treat ehrlichiosis (*E. canis*) but one study found that when used alone, it did not clear the organism (Eddlestone et al. 2006). Imidocarb appears to be effective for hepatozoonosis (*H. canis*) in dogs and it has also been suggested as a treatment for American canine hepatozoonosis (*H. americanum*), but it does not clear the encysted stage.

In cats, imidocarb therapy has been recommended for treating cytauxzoonosis (*C. felis*) but currently atovaquone with azithromycin is the treatment of choice.

In horses, imidocarb dipropionate is considered to be the most effective treatment for piroplasmosis, including the strains of the *B. equi/T. equi* currently causing infections in horses in the USA (Knowles et al. 2013; Wise et al. 2013).

Imidocarb may be of benefit in treating Babesia and related parasitic diseases in a variety of other domestic and exotic animals.

Pharmacology/Actions

Imidocarb is thought to act by combining with nucleic acids of DNA in susceptible organisms, causing the DNA to unwind and denature. This damage to DNA is believed to inhibit cellular repair and replication.

Pharmacokinetics

After IM injection of imidocarb dipropionate in horses, imidocarb rapidly distributes and is not detected in plasma 12 hours after dosing. However urine levels are similar to peak plasma levels up to 36 hours and the drug is detectable in feces up to 10 days, suggesting that it is rapidly sequestered into tissues.

Contraindications/Precautions/Warnings

Do not use imidocarb in patients exposed to cholinesterase-inhibiting drugs, pesticides, or chemicals. The manufacturer states to consider risks versus benefits before treating dogs with impaired lung, hepatic, or renal function. Donkeys and mules appear to be more sensitive to the toxic effects of the drug than are horses.

Do **NOT** administer intravenously. In cats, puppies and debilitated dogs, pretreatment with atropine or glycopyrrolate has been advised.

Adverse Effects

Most commonly reported adverse effects in dogs include pain during injection and mild cholinergic signs (salivation, nasal drip and brief episodes of vomiting). Less commonly reported effects include panting, diarrhea, injection site inflammation (rarely ulceration), and restlessness. Rarely, severe renal tubular or hepatic necrosis, and severe cholinergic signs have occurred. Adverse effects in cats include salivation, lacrimation, vomiting, diarrhea, muscle tremors, restlessness, tachycardia, and dyspnea. Cholinergic adverse effects can be treated with an antimuscarinic (*e.g.,* atropine, glycopyrrolate) if necessary.

Horses given therapeutic dosages (2.4 mg/kg) can show signs of abdominal pain/colic, diarrhea, lacrimation, sweating, and serous nasal discharge after treatment. Antimuscarinic agents (atropine, glycopyrrolate, or N-butylscopolammonium) have been used to mitigate these effects.

Imidocarb has reportedly caused an increase incidence of tumor formation in rats.

Reproductive/Nursing Safety

Safety in puppies, pregnant, lactating, or breeding animals has not been established.

Imidocarb is detectable in mare's milk 2 hours after a single dose of 2.4 mg/kg IM. Safety has not established for nursing foals.

Overdosage/Acute Toxicity

Dogs receiving a dosage of 9.9 mg/kg (1.5X labeled dose) showed signs of liver injury (slightly increased liver enzymes), pain and swelling at the injection site, and vomiting. Overdoses or chronic toxicity may present with cholinergic signs (vomiting, weakness, lethargy, salivation) or adverse changes in liver, kidney, lung, or intestinal function. Treatment with atropine may be useful to treat cholinergic signs associated with imidocarb.

The LD-50 in horses is reportedly 16 mg/kg.

Drug Interactions

The manufacturer warns not use imidocarb in patients exposed to **cholinesterase-inhibiting drugs, pesticides,** or **chemicals.**

Laboratory Considerations

- Imidocarb IM injections may cause significant increases in **creatine kinase (CK).**

Doses

- **DOGS:**

For treatment of babesiosis:

Labeled Dose (FDA-approved): 6.6 mg/kg IM or SC; repeat dose in 2 weeks. (Package Insert; *Imizol®*)

Extra-label Doses:

a) *For B. canis*: Dosage recommendations vary somewhat and range from 5 – 7.5 mg/kg IM or SC; repeat in 2 weeks. Some will re-treat in 7 days if dog is doing poorly clinically.

b) For *B. gibsoni* when the M121I gene had mutated (extra-label; based on a prospective, unmasked study): Clindamycin 30 mg/kg PO q12h; diminazene aceturate 3.5 mg/kg IM once on the day of presentation; imidocarb diproprionate 6 mg/kg SC once on the day after the diminazene was administered. (Lin et al. 2012)

For treatment of Ehrlichiosis (extra-label): Use is generally reserved unless doxycycline or minocycline is demonstrated to be ineffective. Two studies (Eddlestone et al. 2005; Eddlestone et al. 2006) demonstrated that imidocarb alone was not effective in clearing *Ehrlichia canis* from the blood of experimentally infected dogs. If it is tried, the following dosage could be considered: In particularly severe cases, imidocarb at 5 mg/kg SC (in a single injection or two injections 15 days apart) with doxycycline at 10 mg/kg/day for 28 days. (Sainz 2002)

For treatment of hepatozoonosis (*H. canis*); (extra-label): Most recommend 5 – 6 mg/kg IM or SC; every 14 days until gamonts clear from blood smears and remain absent for 2-3 consecutive months (Baneth 2011). However, PCR or buffy-coat smears are much more sensitive to detect the presence of parasitemia for *H. canis* than blood smears (Sasanelli et al. 2010). The prognosis for dogs with low levels of parasitemia is usually good with repeated injections, but prognosis is guarded in dogs with higher levels of parasitemia.

- **CATS:**

For treatment of *Cytauxzoon felis* (extra-label): At present, treatment with atovaquone with azithromycin is considered superior to treatment with imidocarb. If therapy attempted with imidocarb, dosage recommendations generally are: 2 – 4 mg/kg IM once and repeated in 7-14 days. Consider pre-treatment with atropine or another antimuscarinic. Aggressive supportive therapy (IV fluids, prophylactic heparin, nutritional/nursing care, analgesia, and potentially transfusion) is required.

For feline babesiosis (large babesia); (extra-label): Primaquine is usually the drug choice. Imidocarb at 2.5 mg/kg IM once alone, or with co-administration with doxycycline may be effective for treating *B. canis* subspecies *presentii* and *B. herpailuri*. Does not appear to have efficacy against *B. felis*. (Ayoob et al. 2010)

For treatment of feline hemoplasmosis (Nomenclature is in flux: *Haemobartonella felis, Mycoplasma haemofelis; Candidatus*

Mycoplasma, Candidatus M. turicensis); (extra-label): Doxycycline is preferred, but in cats intolerant to that, marbofloxacin, enrofloxacin, or orbifloxacin may be effective. Alternatively imidocarb at 5 mg/kg, IM, every 2 weeks for at least 2 injections was used successfully in the management of five naturally infected cats that had failed treatment with other drugs. Blood transfusion should be given if clinically indicated. Most drug protocols have failed to eliminate infection and so at this time there is no clinical utility to repeat PCR testing. The owners should be warned that recurrence might occur. (Lappin 2006; Lappin 2011)

■ **HORSES:**

For treatment of equine piroplasmosis (*Babesia caballi; Babesia equi/Theileria equi*) (extra-label): Reported dosages for alleviation of clinical signs vary; most sources indicate that 2.2 – 4.4 mg/kg given IM once effective. If necessary, lower dosages can be repeated at 24-72 hour intervals for 2-3 treatments. In non-endemic areas where chemotherapeutic clearance of the organism is desired, animals infected with *B. caballi* or *T. equi* can be cleared with a dose of 4.4 mg/kg IM every 72 hours for 4 treatments. (Wise et al. 2013)

Monitoring

■ Efficacy. Usually via blood smear, but PCR tests if available, appear much more sensitive for detecting parasite presence.

■ Adverse effect profile.

■ Renal and hepatic function tests; baseline and periodically after treatment until stable.

Client Information

Imidocarb is best administered by a veterinarian. Side effects that can be seen after a dose include:

■ Dogs: Common: Salivation/drooling, nasal drip and brief episodes of vomiting. Less common: Panting, diarrhea, injection site inflammation (rarely ulceration), and restlessness.

■ Cats: Salivation/drooling, lacrimation/tearing, vomiting, diarrhea, muscle tremors, restlessness, fast heart rate and difficulty breathing.

■ Horses: Abdominal pain/colic, diarrhea, lacrimation/tearing, sweating, and nasal discharge.

■ Your veterinarian may give another medicine to counteract some of these side effects if they are severe.

Chemistry/Synonyms

Imidocarb dipropionate is a diamidine of the carbanalide series of antiprotozoal compounds.

Imidocarb may also be known as 4A65 (imidocarb hydrochloride) and *Imizol®*.

Storage/Stability

The injection should be stored between 2°-25°C (36°-77°F) and protected from light.

Compatibility/Compounding Considerations

Do not mix imidocarb injection with other medications.

Dosage Forms/Regulatory Status

VETERINARY-LABELED PRODUCTS:

Imidocarb Dipropionate for IM or SC Injection: 120 mg/mL in 10 mL multi-dose vials; *Imizol®*; (Rx). FDA-approved for use in dogs.

HUMAN-LABELED PRODUCTS: NONE.

Revisions/References

Monograph revised/updated February 2014.

Ayoob, A. L., et al. (2010). Feline babesiosis. J. Vet. Emerg. Crit. Care 20(1): 90-7.
Baneth, G. (2011). Perspectives on canine and feline hepatozoonosis. Veterinary Parasitology 181(1): 3-11.
Eddlestone, S., et al. (2005). Failure of imidocarb dipropionate to clear experimentally induced Ehrlichia canis in dogs. Proceedings: ACVIM. accessed via Veterinary Information Network; vin.com
Eddlestone, S. M., et al. (2006). Failure of imidocarb dipropionate to clear experimentally induced Ehrlichia canis infection in dogs. Journal of Veterinary Internal Medicine 20(4): 840-4.
Knowles, D. P. & L. N. Wise (2013). Theileria equi: A Review of Clearance Therapeutics and Novel Diagnostic Techniques. ACVIM. accessed via Veterinary Information Network; vin.com
Lappin, M. (2006). Update on Flea-associated agents of cats: Bartonella Spp., Hemoplasma Spp., and Rickettsia felis. Proceedings: WSAVA World Congress. accessed via Veterinary Information Network; vin.com
Lappin, M. R. (2011). Flea-Associated Diseases in the Cat: Update on the Diagnosis and Treatment of Haemoplasmas and Rickettsia spp. World Small Animal Veterinary Association World Congress Proceedings. accessed via Veterinary Information Network; vin.com
Lin, E. C. Y., et al. (2012). The therapeutic efficacy of two antibabesial strategies against Babesia gibsoni. Veterinary Parasitology 186(3-4): 159-64.
Sainz, A. (2002). Clinical and therapeutic aspects of canine ehrlichiosis. Proceedings: World Small Animal Veterinary Association World Congress. accessed via Veterinary Information Network; vin.com
Sasanelli, M., et al. (2010). Failure of imidocarb dipropionate to eliminate Hepatozoon canis in naturally infected dogs based on parasitological and molecular evaluation methods. Veterinary Parasitology 171(3-4): 194-9.
Wise, L. N., et al. (2013). Review of Equine Piroplasmosis. Journal of Veterinary Internal Medicine 27(6): 1334-46.

Imipenem-Cilastatin Sodium

(ih-me-peh-nem sye-la-sta-tin)   Primaxin®

Carbapenem Antibiotic

Prescriber Highlights

▶ Parenteral broad spectrum antibiotic/deactivating enzyme inhibitor combination used for serious infections where a single agent is desired.

▶ Contraindications/Cautions: Patients hypersensitive to it or other beta-lactams, with renal impairment (dosages adjustment may be required), or CNS disorders (*e.g.*, seizures, head trauma).

▶ Adverse Effects: GI effects, CNS toxicity (seizures, tremors), hypersensitivity, & infusion reactions (thrombophlebitis).

▶ Too rapid IV infusions may cause GI or CNS toxicity, or other untoward effects; Rarely: increases in serum creatinine, BUN, hepatic enzymes; hypotension or tachycardia.

Uses/Indications

Imipenem may be useful in equine or small animal medicine to treat serious infections when other less expensive antibiotics are ineffective or have unacceptable adverse effect srofiles. The carbapenems, including imipenem, ertapenem, and meropenem can be valuable when treating serious gram-negative infections, particularly when multi-drug resistant bacteria are documented to be susceptible to imipenem. However, the BSAVA/PROTECT guidelines state "There are very strong arguments that antimicrobials with restricted use in human medicine (*e.g.*, imipenem, linezolid, teicoplanin, vancomycin) should not be used in animals under any circumstances."

Pharmacology/Actions

This fixed combination of a carbapenem antibiotic (imipenem) and an inhibitor (cilastatin) of dehydropeptidase I (DHP I) has a very broad spectrum of activity. Imipenem is generally considered to be a time-dependent bactericidal agent, but may be bacteriostatic against some bacteria. It has an affinity for and binds to most penicillin-binding protein sites, thereby inhibiting bacterial cell wall synthesis.

Imipenem has activity against a wide variety of bacteria, including gram-positive aerobic cocci (including some bacteriostatic activity against some enterococci), gram-positive aerobic bacilli (including static activity against Listeria), gram-negative aerobic bacteria (Haemophilus, Enterobacteriaceae, many strains of *Pseudomonas aeruginosa*), and anaerobes (including some strains of Bacteroides).

Imipenem is not efficacious for treating infections caused by methicillin-resistant staphylococci or resistant strains of *Enterococcus faecium*.

Cilastatin inhibits the metabolism of imipenem by DHP 1 on the brush borders of renal tubular cells. This serves two functions: it allows higher urine levels and may protect against proximal renal tubular necrosis that can occur when imipenem is used alone.

Pharmacokinetics

Neither drug is absorbed appreciably from the GI tract and, therefore, they are given parenterally. In dogs, bioavailability of imipenem after SC injection is complete and elimination half-life is about an hour (Barker et al. 2003).

In cats, 5 mg/kg (using the IV form) SC and IM bioavailability was high (>90%). Elimination half-life is between 1-2 hours after IV, SC, or IM administration (Albarellos et al. 2013).

Imipenem is distributed widely throughout the body, with the exception of the CSF. Imipenem crosses the placenta and is distributed into milk. When given with cilastatin, imipenem is eliminated by both renal and non-renal mechanisms. Approximately 75% of a dose is excreted in the urine and about 25% is excreted by unknown non-renal mechanisms. Half-lives in patients with normal renal function range from 1-3 hours on average. In horses elimination half-life is about 70 minutes.

Contraindications/Precautions/Warnings

The potential risks versus benefits should be carefully weighed before using imipenem/cilastatin in patients hypersensitive to it or other beta-lactam antibiotics (*e.g.*, penicillins or cephalosporins as partial cross-reactivity may occur), with renal function impairment (dosages may need to be reduced or time between doses lengthened), or with CNS disorders (*e.g.*, seizures, head trauma) as CNS adverse effects are more likely.

Do not give this drug via rapid IV infusion, as seizures are possible. In humans, it is recommended to give doses of 500 mg or less over 20-30 minutes, and doses over 500 mg over 40-60 minutes.

Adverse Effects

Potential adverse effects include: GI effects (vomiting, anorexia, diarrhea), CNS toxicity (seizures, tremors), hypersensitivity (pruritus, fever to anaphylaxis) and infusion reactions (thrombophlebitis; too rapid IV infusions may cause GI or CNS toxicity). Rapid IV infusion or multiple high doses to animals with reduced renal function (including neonates and geriatric animals) may increase the risk for seizures.

SC or IM administration may be painful. There was a separate IM form available, but that product has been discontinued; it could cause severe pain at the injection site and neurovascular damage. Rarely, hypotension, tachycardia, or transient increases in renal (BUN or serum creatinine values) or hepatic (AST/ALT/Alk Phosphatase) function tests may be noted.

Reproductive/Nursing Safety

While no teratogenic effects have been noted in animal studies, safe use during pregnancy has not been firmly established. In humans, the FDA categorizes this drug as category *C* for use during pregnancy (*Animal studies have shown an adverse effect on the fetus, but there are no adequate studies in humans; or there are no animal reproduction studies and no adequate studies in humans.*)

While imipenem enters milk, no adverse effects attributable to it have been noted in nursing offspring.

Overdosage/Acute Toxicity

Little information is available. The LD_{50} of imipenem:cilastatin in a 1:1 ratio in mice and rats is approximately 1 gram/kg/day. Acute overdoses should be handled by halting therapy then treating supportively and symptomatically.

Drug Interactions

The following drug interactions have either been reported or are theoretical in humans or animals receiving imipenem-cilastatin and may be of in veterinary patients. Unless otherwise noted, use together is not necessarily contraindicated, but weigh the potential risks and perform additional monitoring when appropriate.

- **AMINOGLYCOSIDES:** Additive effects or synergy may result when aminoglycosides are added to imipenem/cilastatin therapy, particularly against Enterococcus, *Staph. aureus*, and *Listeria monocytogenes*. There is apparently neither synergy nor antagonism when used in combination against Enterobacteriaceae, including *Pseudomonas aeruginosa*.
- **BETA-LACTAM ANTIBIOTICS:** Antagonism may occur when used in combination with other beta lactam antibiotics against several Enterobacteriaceae (including many strains of *Pseudomonas aeruginosa* and some strains of Klebsiella, Enterobacter, Serratia, Enterobacter, Citrobacter, and Morganella); clinical importance of this interaction is unclear, but at present it is **not** recommended to use imipenem in conjunction with other beta-lactam antibiotics.
- **CHLORAMPHENICOL:** May antagonize the antibacterial effects of imipenem (*in vitro* evidence).
- **CYCLOSPORINE:** Increased potential for CNS effects.
- **GANCICLOVIR:** Increased risk for seizures.
- **PROBENECID:** May increase concentrations and elimination half-life of cilastatin, but not imipenem; concurrent use not recommended.
- **TRIMETHOPRIM/SULFA:** Synergy may occur against *Nocardia asteroides* when imipenem is used in combination with trimethoprim/sulfa.

Laboratory Considerations

- Imipenem may cause a false-positive **urine glucose** determination when using the cupric sulfate solution test (*e.g.*, Clinitest®), Benedict' solution or Fehling's solution. Enzymatic glucose oxidase based tests are not affected (*e.g.*, Tes-Tape®, Clinistix®).

Doses

- **DOGS & CATS:**

  For susceptible infections (extra-label): 5 – 10 mg/kg IV q6-8h. Anecdotally, imipenem/cilastatin has been administered SC, but the solubility (11 mg/mL) of imipenem and relatively short time the reconstituted solution is stable are limitations to this practice. Meropenem may be more suitable for SC administration.

- **HORSES:**

  For susceptible infections (extra-label):

  Adult horses: 10 – 20 mg/kg via slow IV (over a 10 minute period) q6h; alternatively a CRI of 16 micrograms/kg/minute should maintain synovial concentrations greater than 1 microgram/mL. (Orsini et al. 2005)

  Foals: 10 – 15 mg/kg IV q6-12h; IM if diluted into 1% lidocaine. May give as a CRI at 0.4 – 0.8 mg/kg/hr. (Corley et al. 2009)

Monitoring

- Efficacy.
- Adverse effects (including renal and hepatic function tests if treatment is prolonged or patient's renal or hepatic functions are in question).

Client Information

- Imipenem/cilastatin should be administered in an inpatient setting by a veterinarian.

Chemistry/Synonyms

Imipenem monohydrate is a carbapenem antibiotic that occurs as white or off-white, non-hygroscopic, crystalline compound. At room temperature, 11 mg are soluble in 1 mL of water. Cilastatin sodium, an inhibitor of dehydropeptidase I (DHP I), occurs as an off-white to yellowish, hygroscopic, amorphous compound. More than 2 grams are soluble in 1 mL of water.

The commercially available injections are available in a 1:1 fixed dose ratio. The solutions are clear to yellowish in color; pH after reconstitution ranges from 6.5-7.5. These products have sodium bicarbonate added as a buffer.

Imipenem may also be known as: N-formimidoyl thienamycin, imipemide, MK-787, and MK-0787; multi-ingredient preparations: *Imipem®, Klonam®, Primaxin®, Tenacid®, Tienam®, Tracix®*, and *Zienam®*.

Storage/stability

Commercially available sterile powders for injection should be stored at room temperature (<25°C). After reconstitution, the solution is stable for 4 hours at room temperature; 10 hours when refrigerated. If other diluents are used, stability times may be reduced (see package insert). Do not freeze solutions. The manufacturer does not recommend admixing with other drugs.

Compatibility/Compounding Considerations

The following drugs are reportedly **compatible** with imipenem/cilastatin for IV infusion at a Y-site: aztreonam, cefepime, diltiazem, famotidine, insulin, ondansetron, and propofol.

Dosage Forms/Regulatory Status

VETERINARY-LABELED PRODUCTS: NONE.

HUMAN-LABELED PRODUCTS:

Imipenem/Cilastatin Powder for Injection: 250 mg imipenem equivalent and 250 mg cilastatin equivalent (0.8 mEq sodium); 500 mg imipenem equivalent and 500 mg cilastatin equivalent (1.6 mEq sodium); *Primaxin® I.V.*, generic; (Rx)

Revisions/References

Monograph revised/updated February 2014.

Albarellos, G. A., et al. (2013). Pharmacokinetics of imipenem after intravenous, intramuscular and subcutaneous administration to cats. Journal of Feline Medicine and Surgery **15**(6): 483-7.

Barker, C. W., et al. (2003). Pharmacokinetics of imipenem in dogs. American Journal of Veterinary Research **64**(6): 694-9.

Corley, K. T. T. & A. R. Hollis (2009). Antimicrobial therapy in neonatal foals. Equine Veterinary Education **21**(8): 436-48.

Orsini, J., et al. (2005). Pharmacokinetics of imipenem-cilastatin following intravenous administration in healthy horses. J Vet Phamacol Ther **28**: 355-61.

Imipramine

(im-ip-ra-meen)   Tofranil®

Tricyclic Antidepressant

Prescriber Highlights

▶ Human-labeled tricyclic "antidepressant" used primarily in dogs and cats for urinary incontinence, cataplexy and tricyclic-responsive behavior disorders. Like other tricyclics it may be useful for the adjunctive treatment of chronic pain. In horses, has been tried to treat narcolepsy & ejaculatory dysfunction.

▶ May reduce seizure thresholds in epileptic animals.

▶ Can be very toxic in overdoses to both animals & humans.

▶ May be teratogenic.

▶ Adverse Effects: Sedation & anticholinergic effects (tachycardia, hyperexcitability, tremors) most likely.

Uses/Indications

In dogs and cats, imipramine has been used for urinary incontinence, cataplexy and tricyclic-responsive behavior disorders. Like other tricyclics it may be useful for the adjunctive treatment of chronic pain. In horses, imipramine has been used to treat narcolepsy and ejaculatory dysfunction (no parenteral dosage forms available).

Pharmacology/Actions

Imipramine and its active metabolite, desipramine, have a complicated pharmacologic profile. From a slightly oversimplified viewpoint, they have 3 main characteristics: blockage of the amine pump, thereby increasing neurotransmitter levels (principally serotonin, but also norepinephrine), sedation, and central and peripheral anticholinergic activity. While not completely understood, it is thought that the antienuretic activity of imipramine is related to its anticholinergic effects, but imipramine may also have some alpha-adrenergic agonist activity. In animals, tricyclic antidepressants are similar to the actions of phenothiazines in altering avoidance behaviors.

Pharmacokinetics

Imipramine is rapidly absorbed from both the GI tract and parenteral injection sites. Peak levels occur within 1-2 hours after oral dosing. Imipramine and desipramine enter the CNS and maternal milk in levels equal to that found in maternal serum. The drug is metabolized in the liver to several metabolites, including desipramine, which is active. In humans the terminal half-life is approximately 8-16 hours.

Contraindications/Precautions/Warnings

These agents are contraindicated if prior sensitivity has been noted with any other tricyclic. Concomitant use with monoamine oxidase inhibitors is generally contraindicated.

Use with caution in patients with seizure disorders; imipramine may lower seizure threshold.

Adverse Effects

While there is little experience with this drug in domestic animals, the most predominant adverse effects seen with the tricyclics are related to their sedating and anticholinergic (dry mouth, constipation, tachycardia, hyperexcitability, tremors) properties. They can cause CNS stimulation (seizures) however, and adverse effects can run the entire gamut of systems including hematologic (bone marrow suppression), GI (diarrhea, vomiting), endocrine, etc.

Reproductive/Nursing Safety

Isolated reports of limb reduction abnormalities have been noted; restrict use to pregnant animals only when the benefits clearly outweigh the risks. In humans, the FDA categorizes this drug as category **D** for use during pregnancy (*There is evidence of human fetal risk, but the potential benefits from the use of the drug in pregnant women may be acceptable despite its potential risks.*)

Imipramine is excreted into milk in low concentrations (approximate milk:plasma ratio of 0.4-1.5).

Overdosage/Acute Toxicity

Overdosage with tricyclics can be life-threatening (arrhythmias, cardiorespiratory collapse). Because the toxicities and therapies for treatment are complicated and controversial, it is recommended to contact an animal poison control center for further information in any potential overdose situation.

Drug Interactions

The following drug interactions have either been reported or are theoretical in humans or animals receiving imipramine and may be of in veterinary patients. Unless otherwise noted, use together is not necessarily contraindicated, but weigh the potential risks and perform additional monitoring when appropriate.

- **ANTICHOLINERGIC AGENTS:** Because of additive effects, use with imipramine cautiously.
- **CIMETIDINE:** May inhibit tricyclic antidepressant metabolism and increase the risk of toxicity.
- **CISAPRIDE:** Increased risk for prolonged QT interval.
- **CLONIDINE:** Tricyclics may increase blood pressure.
- **CNS DEPRESSANTS:** Because of additive effects, use with imipramine cautiously.
- **LEVODOPA:** Imipramine may decrease levodopa oral absorption.
- **MEPERIDINE, PENTAZOCINE:** Increased risk for serotonin syndrome.
- **PHENOBARBITAL:** May decrease tricyclic levels.
- **QUINIDINE:** Increased risk for QTc interval prolongation and tricyclic adverse effects.
- **RIFAMPIN:** May decrease tricyclic blood levels.
- **SSRIs** (*e.g.,* **fluoxetine, paroxetine, sertraline,** etc.): Increased risk for serotonin syndrome; avoid use with imipramine.
- **SYMPATHOMIMETIC AGENTS:** Use in combination with sympathomimetic agents may increase the risk of cardiac effects (arrhythmias, hypertension, hyperpyrexia).
- **MONOAMINE OXIDASE INHIBITORS** (including **amitraz,** and possibly **selegiline**): Concomitant use (within 14 days) with monoamine oxidase inhibitors is generally contraindicated (serotonin syndrome).
- **THYROID AGENTS:** May increase risk for cardiac arrhythmias.

Laboratory Considerations
- **ECG:** Tricyclics can widen QRS complexes, prolong PR intervals and invert or flatten T-waves on ECG.
- **GLUCOSE, BLOOD:** Tricyclics may alter (increase or decrease) blood glucose levels.

Doses
- **DOGS:**

  For urethral incompetence (extra-label): No controlled studies were noted documenting efficacy; most recommend 5 – 15 mg per dog PO q12h (twice a day); some recommend dosages up to 20 mg per dog twice a day.

  For cataplexy (extra-label): Studies are not available to document efficacy. One suggested dose is 0.5 – 1 mg/kg PO q8h; titrate dose based on clinical effect. (Coleman 1999)

  For behavior-related conditions (extra-label): Not often recommended as clomipramine (approved) or amitriptyline are the most commonly used when a tricyclic is employed. One recommended dosage is: For adjunctive treatment of separation anxiety or other tricyclic antidepressant-responsive behavior disorders: 2.2 – 4.4 mg/kg PO once to twice daily. (Marder 1991)

  For adjunctive treatment of chronic pain (extra-label): No controlled studies located documenting efficacy. Recommended dosage is 0.5 – 1 mg/kg PO q8h.

- **CATS:**

  For urethral incompetence or adjunctive treatment of chronic pain (extra-label): No controlled studies were noted documenting efficacy; most recommend 2.5 – 5 mg per cat PO q12h (twice a day).

- **HORSES:** (NOTE: ARCI UCGFS CLASS 2 DRUG)

  Note: The injectable product is no longer marketed in the USA. Compounded preparations may be available.

  For pharmacologic induced ejaculation (extra-label): 2 mg/kg IV. If imipramine alone does not induce erection and ejacula-

tion in 10-15 minutes, give xylazine 0.2 – 0.3 mg/kg IV. (Samper 2004)

For narcolepsy/cataplexy (extra-label): 0.55 mg/kg IV or 250 – 750 mg (total dose) orally. PO administration produces inconsistent results. (Andrews et al. 2004)

Monitoring
- Efficacy.
- Adverse effects.

Client Information
- May be given with or without food. If your animal vomits or acts sick after getting it on an empty stomach, give with food or small treat to see if this helps. If vomiting continues, contact your veterinarian.
- May take several days or even weeks to determine if the drug is effective.
- Most common side effects are: drowsiness/sleepiness, dry mouth and constipation; be sure your animal has access to water at all times.
- Rare side effects that can be serious: abnormal bleeding or fever, seizures, very fast or irregular heartbeat. Contact your veterinarian immediately if you see any of these.
- Overdoses can be very serious; keep out of the reach of animals and children.
- If your animal wore a flea collar in the past two weeks, let your veterinarian know. Do not use one on your animal while it's getting this medicine without first talking to your veterinarian.

Chemistry/Synonyms
A tricyclic antidepressant agent, imipramine is available commercially in either the hydrochloride or pamoate salts. Imipramine HCl occurs as an odorless or practically odorless, white to off-white crystalline powder that is freely soluble in water or alcohol. Imipramine pamoate occurs as a fine yellow powder that is practically insoluble in water, but soluble in alcohol. The HCl injection has a pH of 4-5.

Imipramine HCl may also be known as: imipramini chloridum, imipramini hydrochloridum, imizine, and *Tofranil®*.

Storage/Stability
Imipramine HCl tablets and the pamoate capsules should be stored in tight, light resistant containers, preferably at room temperature. The HCl injection should be stored at temperatures less than 40°C and freezing should be avoided. Expiration dates for oral HCL products are from 3-5 years after manufacture; for the pamoate, 3 years.

Imipramine HCl will turn yellow to reddish on exposure. Slight discoloration will not affect potency, but marked changes in color are associated with a loss of potency.

Compatibility/Compounding Considerations
No specific information noted.

Dosage Forms/Regulatory Status
VETERINARY-LABELED PRODUCTS: NONE.

The ARCI (Racing Commissioners International) has designated this drug as a class 2 substance. See the appendix for more information.

HUMAN-LABELED PRODUCTS:

Imipramine HCl Tablets: 10 mg, 25 mg & 50 mg; *Tofranil®*, generic; (Rx)

Imipramine Pamoate Capsules: 75 mg, 100 mg, 125 mg & 150 mg; *Tofranil®-PM*, generic; (Rx)

Revisions/References

Monograph revised/updated February 2014.

Andrews, F. & H. Matthews (2004). Seizures, narcoplexy, and cataplexy. *Equine Internal Medicine, 2nd Ed.* S. Reed, W. Bayly and D. Sellon. Philadelphia, Saunders: 560-79.

Coleman, E. (1999). Canine narcolepsy and the role of the nervous system. Comp CE 21(7): 641-50.

Marder, A. (1991). Psychotropic drugs and behavioral therapy. Veterinary Clinics of North America: Small Animal Practice 21(2): 329-42.

Samper, J. (2004). The stallion. *Equine Internal Medicine, 2nd Ed.* S. Reed, W. Bayly and D. Sellon. Philadelphia, Saunders: 1135-68.

Imiquimod – see the Topical Dermatologic section in the appendix

Immune Globulin (Human), Intravenous

(im-myoon glob-yoo-lin)   IGIV, IVIG, hIVIG

Immune Serum

Prescriber Highlights

▶ Potentially useful for canine immune-mediated diseases (*e.g.,* IMHA, pIMT, immune-mediated dermatopathies).
▶ Limited experience in dogs.
▶ Hypersensitivity reactions possible. Potentially could increase risk for thrombosis in dogs with IMHA.
▶ Very expensive.

Uses/Indications

No consensus has been reached on indications, appropriate dosages, or safety of human intravenous immune globulin (IVIG) in veterinary medicine (Spurlock et al. 2011). Definitive studies evaluating the safety and efficacy of IVIG in veterinary patients are not available and because of the drug's significant expense are unlikely in the foreseeable future. Some question whether the drug should be used at all in veterinary patients since supply is limited and some countries ration its use in humans.

However IVIG may be useful for treating immune-mediated hemolytic (IMHA), immune-mediated dermatopathies, immune-mediated thrombocytopenia (pIMT), and Evans' syndrome, particularly in patients that have failed other treatments. Limited retrospective and prospective studies have demonstrated mixed results, but the data while very limited, suggests that IVIG may be most useful in treating primary immune-mediated thrombocytopenia in dogs. However, a prospective, randomized study in 20 dogs with ITP comparing vincristine versus IVIG found that there were no significant differences between both groups in median platelet recovery time (2.5 days) or median hospitalization time for dogs that survived (4 days). Seven of 10 dogs in the IVIG group and 10 of 10 in the vincristine group survived to discharge. There were no significant differences for survival at discharge, 6 months, and 1 year. No adverse effects were reported in either group. The authors concluded that vincristine should be the first-line adjunctive treatment for the acute management of canine ITP because of lower cost and ease of administration (Balog et al. 2013).

A prospective, randomized, double-blinded, controlled trial of IVIG (with glucocorticoids) in 28 dogs with recently diagnosed IMHA found no statistically significant differences between the treated and placebo groups in survival, length of hospitalization, time to hematocrit stabilization, and transfusion requirements. While the study population was relatively small, the authors concluded that the cost of the treatment does not lend support to its use as an early intervention treatment in dogs (Whelan et al. 2009).

In humans, IVIG has been used for a variety of immune system-related conditions including primary and secondary immunodeficiencies, graft versus host disease, Guillain-Barre syndrome, chronic inflammatory demyelinating polyneuropathy, autoimmune hemolytic anemia, juvenile idiopathic arthritis, myasthenia gravis, toxic epidermal necrolysis, systemic vasculitis, and sepsis.

Pharmacology/Actions

Immunoglobulins are produced by B lymphocytes as part of the humoral response to foreign antigens. IVIG antibodies act through a variety of mechanisms, including antimicrobial or antitoxin neutralization. Its efficacy for treating autoimmune disorders may be due to: providing anti-idiotypic antibodies that neutralize autoantibodies; negative feedback and down-regulation of antibody production; binding to CD5 receptors, interleukin (IL)-1a, IL-6, tumor necrosis factor-alpha, and T-cell receptors; and suppressing pathogenic cytokines and phagocytes.

Pharmacokinetics

Elimination half-life in dogs is reported to be 7-9 days. In humans, the onset of actions is rapid. Immunoglobulins are primarily eliminated by catabolism and the mean half-life is about 3 weeks. Fever or infection may decrease antibody half-life because of increased catabolism or consumption.

Contraindications/Precautions/Warnings

Dogs that have had prior hypersensitivity reactions after receiving human albumin, should not receive IVIG. Trace amounts of human albumin may be found in IVIG.

In humans, many adverse reactions are associated with administering IVIG at rates higher than recommended. Follow infusion rate guidelines carefully. At doses used in dogs (0.5 – 1.5 grams/kg), IVIG is generally infused over a 6-12 hour period. A study in healthy dogs that showed that IVIG promoted hypercoagulability and an inflammatory state which raises concerns about using it in dogs with IMHA (Tsuchiya et al. 2009).

The FDA has placed a "Black Box Warning" on the labeling of IVIG for use in humans as it has been associated with renal dysfunction, acute renal failure, osmotic nephrosis, and death.

Adverse Effects

In dogs, IVIG can cause increased blood pressure. Local reactions at or near the injection site are possible. Anecdotal reports of anaphylaxis have been reported in dogs receiving IVIG. IVIG can contain trace amounts of human albumin that has been associated with hypersensitivity reactions in dogs. As IVIG can have colloid-like properties, volume overload is possible. Thrombotic events have been reported in humans and are possible in dogs. One study done in healthy dogs, demonstrated that IVIG promoted hypercoagulability and an inflammatory state (Tsuchiya et al. 2009).

In humans, adverse effects of IVIG in people are relatively uncommon and most are transient, self-limiting and include fever, chills, facial flushing, headache, and nausea. Thrombotic events have been reported. Rarely, acute renal failure, acute tubular necrosis, osmotic nephrosis, and proximal tubular nephropathy have been reported in humans. Increases in creatinine and BUN have been seen as soon as 1-2 days following infusion. Hypersensitivity reactions, including anaphylaxis have been reported, but are very rare in human patients.

Reproductive/Nursing Safety

In humans, the FDA has placed IVIG in category C for use during pregnancy (*Animal studies have shown an adverse effect on the fetus, but there are no adequate studies in humans; or there are no animal reproduction studies and no adequate studies in humans.* However, there does not appear to be a significant risk to offspring.

The drug appears to be safe for use during lactation and nursing.

Overdosage/Acute Toxicity

Fluid volume overload is possible. Other reactions could include pain and tenderness at the injection site.

Drug Interactions

The following drug interactions have either been reported or are theoretical in humans or animals receiving IVIG and may be of in veterinary patients. Unless otherwise noted, use together is not necessarily contraindicated, but weigh the potential risks and perform additional monitoring when appropriate.

- **VACCINES, LIVE:** IVIG may interfere with immune response and efficacy.

Laboratory Considerations

- **BLOOD GLUCOSE:** Falsely elevated blood glucose measurements can occur when using the glucose dehydrogenase pyrroloquinoline quinone (GDH-PQQ) based test. Consider using tests that are not affected, including the glucose oxidase, glucose dehydrogenase nicotine adenine dinucleotide (GDH-NAD), or glucose dehydrogenase flavin adenine dinucleotide (GDH-FAD) methods.
- **COOMBS TEST:** In humans, the transitory rise of the various passively transferred antibodies may cause positive serological testing results, potentially altering the test's results and interpretation.

Doses

- **DOGS:**

Note: Various dosages have been used in dogs ranging from 0.3 – 1.5 grams/kg which translates into an estimated $400 to $1500 associated with the cost of the drug alone. Recommendations that IVIG should be considered when dogs with IMHA or ITP fail to respond to conventional therapy must be weighed against the additional cost clients have already spent. From a healthcare system point of view this would appear to be unjustifiable and probably would not be recommended, however, on an individual patient basis, clients and clinicians may find such therapy offers some degree of hope and cost-analyses may not dissuade its usage (Chan 2009).

For immune-mediated hemolytic anemia (IMHA) in dogs refractory to other immunosuppressive therapies (extra-label): Note: See Contraindications/Cautions regarding hypercoagulability. IVIG has shown some benefit in IMHA patients that are refractory to conventional treatment. It is given at a dose of 0.5 – 1.5 grams/kg IV over 4-12 hours. (Macintire 2006)

For primary immune-mediated thrombocytopenia (pIMT) (extra-label): The optimal dose of IVIG for ITP remains to be identified, and a wide variety of doses have been reported, ranging from 0.28 – 1.3 g/kg (Nakamura et al. 2012). A recent study recommended using vincristine as first-line adjunctive treatment for the acute management of canine ITP because of similar efficacy but lower cost and ease of administration (Balog et al. 2013). In one prospective study, dogs in the treatment group received IVIG at 0.5 g/kg as a 6% concentration over 6-12 hours IV once. The authors concluded that compared with corticosteroids alone, adjunctive emergency therapy of a single IVIG infusion was safe and associated with a significant reduction in platelet count recovery time and duration of hospitalization without increasing the expense of medical care (Bianco et al. 2009).

For refractory cases of erythema multiforme, Stevens-Johnson syndrome/toxic epidermal necrolysis, and other cutaneous adverse drug reactions (extra-label): No controlled studies were located and dosage recommendations are based upon case reports. One suggested dosage is: a 5-6% solution is given at 0.5 – 1 g/kg IV over a 4-6 hour period, 1-2 times, 24 hours apart. This treatment may need to be repeated for 3-4 days in a row. Further study is needed. (Jazic 2010)

Monitoring

- Vital signs: including blood pressure, temperature prior to infusion and frequently during administration.
- Lung auscultation to assess for volume overload.
- Renal function tests and urine output.
- Efficacy (depending on purpose for use).

Client Information

- Clients should understand that this drug is not commonly used in veterinary medicine, plus the costs and risks associated with its use.

Chemistry/Synonyms

IVIG consists of fractionated immunoglobulins, and is primarily intact IgG. It is obtained from pooled human plasma (1,000 – 60,000 human donors). It may also contain trace amounts of IgM, IgA, soluble CD4, CD8 and HLA molecules, and some cytokines. Further processing is performed to inactivate viruses and remove IgG aggregates and other contaminants. Stabilizing agents can include polyethylene glycol, glycine, sorbitol, polysorbate 80, and sugars (maltose, glucose, sucrose).

Immune globulin (human) may also be known as hIVIG, IVIG, IGIV, immunoglobulin, immunglobuline, or immunoglobulinas.

Storage/Stability

IVIG products are usually stored at room temperature, but specific storage requirements may vary with each product; refer to the label. These products should not be frozen.

Compatibility/Compounding Considerations

Each product may have differing instructions for mixing, dilution, etc. Refer to the product label for specific directions. Generally, IVIG should not be mixed with other medications. One product's label (*Privigen®*) states that it can be diluted with 5% dextrose in water (D5W) if necessary. Lyophilized products can usually be reconstituted with sterile water, dextrose 5% or sterile saline. Do not shake; excessive shaking will cause foaming. Any undissolved particles should respond to careful rotation of the bottle; avoid foaming.

Dosage Forms/Regulatory Status

VETERINARY-LABELED PRODUCTS: NONE.

HUMAN-LABELED PRODUCTS:

Immune Globulin (Human) Injection: 5% (50 mg/mL) preservative-free in 10 mL, 20 mL, 50 mL, 100 mL, & 200 mL (0.5 gram, 1 gram, 2.5 grams, 5 grams, & 10 grams—depending on product) single use bottles; *Flebogamma®*, *Gammaplex®*; (Rx)

Immune Globulin (Human) Injection: 10% (100 mg/mL) preservative-free in 10 mL, 20 mL, 50 mL, 100 mL, & 200 mL (1 gram, 2 grams, 10 grams, & 20 grams—depending on product) single use bottles; *Gamunex-C®*, *Gammagard®*, *Gammaked®*, *Bivigam®*, *Privigen®*; (Rx)

Immune Globulin (Human) Lyophilized Powder for Solution: 2.5 gram, 3 grams, 6 grams & 12 grams—depending on product; *Carimune NF®*, *Gammagard S/D®*; (Rx)

Revisions/References

Monograph revised/updated February 2014.

Balog, K., et al. (2013). A Prospective Randomized Clinical Trial of Vincristine versus Human Intravenous Immunoglobulin for Acute Adjunctive Management of Presumptive Primary Immune-Mediated Thrombocytopenia in Dogs. Journal of Veterinary Internal Medicine 27(3): 536-41.
Bianco, D., et al. (2009). A Prospective, Randomized, Double-Blinded, Placebo-Controlled Study of Human Intravenous Immunoglobulin for the Acute Management of Presumptive Primary Immune-Mediated Thrombocytopenia in Dogs. Journal of Veterinary Internal Medicine 23(5): 1071-8.
Chan, D. (2009). Immunoglobulin Therapy: Worth the Cost? Proceedings: IVECCS. accessed via Veterinary Information Network; vin.com

Jazic, E. (2010). The Great Chameleon: Diagnosis and Management of Cutaneous Adverse Drug Reactions in Dogs and Cats. Proceedings: WVC. accessed via Veterinary Information Network; vin.com

Macintire, D. (2006). New therapies for immune-mediated hemolytic anemia. Proceedings: ACVIM 2006. accessed via Veterinary Information Network; vin.com

Nakamura, R. K., et al. (2012). Therapeutic options for immune-mediated thrombocytopenia. J. Vet. Emerg. Crit. Care 22(1): 59-72.

Spurlock, N. K. & J. E. Prittie (2011). A review of current indications, adverse effects, and administration recommendations for intravenous immunoglobulin. J. Vet. Emerg. Crit. Care 21(5): 471-83.

Tsuchiya, R., et al. (2009). Prothrombotic and Inflammatory Effects of Intravenous Administration of Human Immunoglobulin G in Dogs. Journal of Veterinary Internal Medicine 23(6): 1164-9.

Whelan, M. F., et al. (2009). Use of human immunoglobulin in addition to glucocorticoids for the initial treatment of dogs with immune-mediated hemolytic anemia. J. Vet. Emerg. Crit. Care 19(2): 158-64.

INSULIN
–Regular (Crystalline Zinc)
–Lispro
–Isophane
–Protamine Zinc
–Porcine Zinc
–Glargine
–Detemir

Hormone

Note: Insulin preparations available to the practitioner are in a constant state of change. It is highly recommended to review current references or sources of information pertaining to insulin therapy for dogs and cats to maximize efficacy of therapy and reduce the chance for errors.

Prescriber Highlights

▶ Pancreatic hormone used to treat diabetic ketoacidosis, uncomplicated diabetes mellitus, & as adjunctive therapy in treating hyperkalemia.

▶ Contraindications: No absolute contraindications except during episodes of hypoglycemia.

▶ Adverse Effects: Hypoglycemia, insulin-induced hyperglycemia ("Somogyi effect"), insulin antagonism/resistance, rapid insulin metabolism, & local reactions to the "foreign" proteins.

▶ Do not confuse insulin types, strengths, syringes.

▶ Drug Interactions.

Monograph by Dinah Jordan, PharmD, DICVP

Uses/Indications

Insulin preparations are used for the adjunctive treatment of diabetic ketoacidosis (DKA), uncomplicated diabetes mellitus, and as adjunctive therapy in treating hyperkalemia. Veterinary use of insulin has been primarily in dogs and cats, although there are documented reports in a number of other species, including, but not limited to, birds, guinea pigs, ferrets, horses, camelids and cattle.

Regular insulin is commonly used for stabilization of the diabetic patient and is the only formulation labeled for intravenous administration (IV); it is also administered by intramuscular (IM) and subcutaneous (SC) injection. Intravenous administration of regular insulin is recommended in patients with poor tissue perfusion, shock, or cardiovascular collapse, or in patients requiring insulin for the treatment of severe, life-threatening hyperkalemia causing cardiotoxicity (*i.e.*, >8 mEq/L). While historically, regular insulin was the only insulin preparation recommended for treatment of DKA in veterinary patients, new information suggests that other preparations, including glargine, lispro, and aspart may be equally effective. Two separate studies demonstrated that lispro insulin (Sears et al. 2012) or insulin aspart (Walsh et al. 2012) administered as an intravenous continuous rate infusion were safe and effective alternatives to regular insulin treatment in dogs with DKA. Other studies demonstrated that intramuscular administration of glargine is effective for treatment of feline DKA (Marshall et al. 2010) and that a combination of glargine administered subcutaneously every 12 hours and regular insulin administered IM up to every 8 hours resolved DKA faster in cats than a protocol using regular insulin in a CRI (Buob et al. 2010). Once the patient is stabilized, longer acting insulin products are given subcutaneously for maintenance insulin therapy.

Pharmacology

Insulin is a hormone secreted by the beta cells of the pancreatic islets of Langerhans. Eliciting multiple biological responses, insulin initiates its actions by binding to cell-surface receptors, present in varying numbers in virtually all mammalian cells. This binding results in a cascade of intracellular events that can be studied in detail by consulting a physiology text. In avian species, patients with hyperglycemia can have insulin levels that are low, normal or high and relative glucagon excess may be the cause for diabetes in birds.

Insulin is the primary hormone responsible for controlling the uptake, utilization, and storage of cellular nutrients. Insulin affects primarily liver, muscle, and adipose tissues, but also exerts potent regulatory effects on other cell types as well. Insulin stimulates carbohydrate metabolism in cardiac, skeletal, and adipose tissue by facilitating the uptake of glucose by these cells. Other tissues, such as brain, nerve, intestinal, liver, and kidney tubules, do not require insulin for glucose transport. Liver cells do need insulin to convert glucose to glycogen (for storage), and the hypothalamus requires insulin for glucose entry into the satiety center. Insulin has a direct effect on fat and protein metabolism. The hormone stimulates lipogenesis, increases protein synthesis, and inhibits lipolysis and free fatty acid release from adipose tissues. Insulin promotes an intracellular shift of potassium and magnesium. Exogenous insulin elicits all the pharmacologic responses usually produced by endogenous insulin.

Pharmacokinetics

Insulin is metabolized mainly by the liver and kidneys (also muscle and fat to a lesser degree) by enzymatic reduction to form peptides and amino acids. About 50% of the insulin that reaches the liver via the portal vein is destroyed and never reaches the general circulation. Insulin is filtered by the renal glomeruli and is reabsorbed by the tubules, which also degrade it. Severe impairment of renal function appears to affect the rate of clearance of circulating insulin to a greater extent than hepatic disease. Hepatic degradation of insulin operates near its maximal capacity and cannot compensate for diminished renal breakdown of the hormone. The half-life of endogenous insulin is less than ten minutes in normal subjects and in patients with uncomplicated diabetes.

Note: The pharmacokinetics of various insulin formulations can vary widely from published values among species, among individuals within a species, and within the same individual patient from day to day. Therefore, the values should only be used as a general reference guide.

<u>Regular insulin injection:</u> When the recombinant human insulin product is given IV to dogs and cats, it has an immediate onset of action, with maximum effects occurring at 0.5-2 hours; duration of action is 1-4 hours. Following IM administration, onset is 10-30 minutes; peak 1-4 hours; and duration 3-8 hours. After subcutaneous administration, onset is generally 10-30 minutes; peak from 1-5 hours; duration 4-10 hours. In alpacas, regular insulin has an immediate onset of action, but the duration of action is less than one hour (Cebra 2001).

Although the kinetics of all insulin products vary markedly for the individual product among species, regular insulin appears to exhibit the most similar properties.

Insulin lispro injection: While published studies are lacking, the pharmacokinetics of lispro and regular insulin in dogs and cats when administered intravenously appear to be comparable to humans.

Isophane insulin suspension (NPH): NPH insulin is administered by the subcutaneous route only. Following SC administration of the recombinant human insulin product, onset is 0.5-2 hours in dogs and cats; peak is 2-10 hours in dogs and 2-8 hours in cats; and duration is 6-18 hours in dogs and 4-12 hours in cats. Following SC administration of the recombinant human insulin product to 10 diabetic dogs, onset was 30 minutes to 4 hours (median 1.5 hours); peak was 1 to >10 hours (median 4 h); duration was 3.1 to >10 (median 8.5 hours) (Palm et al. 2009).

Porcine insulin zinc suspension (Lente): Classified as intermediate-acting, it has two peaks of activity following subcutaneous administration in diabetic dogs (the first at 2-6 hours and the second at 8-14 hours). These peaks are helpful in controlling the postprandial hyperglycemia seen in many diabetic dogs. The duration of activity varies between 14 and 24 hours. The peak(s), duration of activity, and dose required to adequately control diabetic signs will vary among dogs. In diabetic cats, there is a single peak that occurs 1.5-8 hours following SC administration. Duration of activity varies from 8-12 hours (*Vetsulin*® package insert). **Protamine zinc suspension (PZI)**: Following SC administration, onset is 1-4 hours in dogs and cats; peak is 4-8 hours; duration is 6-28 hours in dogs; 6-24 hours in cats. No pharmacokinetic studies using the final formulation of *ProZinc*® have been conducted in dogs & cats; however, data on protamine zinc insulin (PZI) and other human and animal–origin insulins can be extrapolated to *ProZinc*® (anon 2013).

Insulin glargine injection: Following subcutaneous injection, the acidic solution is neutralized and microprecipitates are formed that slowly release small amounts of insulin glargine. This action results in a relatively constant concentration/time profile over 24 hours with no pronounced peak in humans. A small study compared equal doses of insulin glargine, PZI (mixed beef/pork), and purified pork lente insulin in 9 healthy cats. Results showed no significant difference in onset of action or nadir glucose concentrations among the insulins; time to reach nadir glucose concentration was longer for glargine (~16 hours) vs. PZI (~6 hours) and lente (~4.5 hours). Duration was significantly shorter for lente than for glargine or PZI, with glargine and PZI not significantly different. The study in healthy cats also showed there were definite peaks in insulin concentration and glucose lowering effects of glargine. (Marshall et al. 2004) If glargine is diluted or administered either IM or IV, microprecipitates are not formed producing a rapid release of insulin similar to regular insulin.

Insulin detemir injection: A comparison study of glargine and detemir in 10 young healthy cats showed that following administration of 0.5 Units/kg SC, the, onset of action was 1.8 ± 0.8 and 1.3 ± 0.5 hours for insulin detemir and insulin glargine respectively. End of action of insulin detemir was reached at 13.5 ± 3.5 hours and for insulin glargine at 11.3 ± 4.5 hours. Time-to-peak action of insulin detemir was reached at 6.9 ± 3.1 hours and for insulin glargine at 5.3 ± 3.8 hours. The time-action curves of both insulin analogs varied between relatively flat curves in some cats and peaked curves in others (Gilor et al. 2010).

Contraindications/Precautions/Warnings

Because there are no alternatives for insulin when it is used for diabetic indications, there are no absolute contraindications to its use except during episodes of hypoglycemia. If animals develop hyper-sensitivity (local or otherwise) or should insulin resistance develop, a change in type or species of insulin should be tried. Pork insulin is identical to canine insulin and is considered the insulin source of choice for diabetic dogs. Human insulin has a low potential for producing insulin antibodies in dogs (~5%), while beef/pork insulin produces antibody formation in a higher percentage of dogs (~45%) and is associated with insulin resistance and poor or erratic glycemic control. Dogs known to have a systemic allergy to pork or pork products should not be treated with *Vetsulin*®. The incidence of insulin antibody production related to insulin source is low in cats, and overt insulin resistance occurs in less than 5% of cats treated with recombinant human insulin; approximately the same rate as in cats treated with beef/pork insulin.

Do not inject insulin at the same site day after day or lipodystrophic reactions can occur.

Do not abbreviate Units as "U" as it has been shown to increase the rate of transcription and dosage errors. In human medicine, insulin is considered a "high alert" medication (medications that require special safeguards to reduce the risk of errors). Consider instituting practices such as redundant drug dosage and volume checking, special alert labels, etc.

Adverse Effects

Adverse effects of insulin therapy may include hypoglycemia (see overdosage below), insulin-induced hyperglycemia ("Somogyi effect"), insulin antagonism/resistance, rapid insulin metabolism, and local reactions to the "foreign" proteins.

Reproductive/Nursing Safety

In humans, the FDA categorizes purified pork, all human insulin, and human insulin analog lispro as category *B* for use during pregnancy (*Animal studies have not yet demonstrated risk to the fetus, but there are no adequate studies in pregnant women; or animal studies have shown an adverse effect, but adequate studies in pregnant women have not demonstrated a risk to the fetus in the first trimester of pregnancy, and there is no evidence of risk in later trimesters.*) In humans, the FDA categorizes insulin glargine and detemir as category *C* for use during pregnancy (*Animal studies have shown an adverse effect on the fetus, but there are no adequate studies in humans; or there are no animal reproduction studies and no adequate studies in humans.*)

Insulin is compatible with nursing.

Overdosage/Acute Toxicity

Overdosage of insulin can lead to various degrees of hypoglycemia. Signs may include weakness, shaking, head tilting, lethargy, ataxia, seizures, blindness, bizarre behavior, and coma. Other signs may include restlessness, hunger, and muscle fasciculations. Prolonged hypoglycemia can result in permanent brain damage or death.

Mild hypoglycemia can be treated by offering the animal its usual food. More serious signs (such as seizures) should be treated with oral dextrose solutions (*e.g.*, *Karo*® syrup) rubbed on the oral mucosa (not poured down the throat) or by intravenous injections of 50% dextrose solutions (small amounts, slowly administered—usually 2 – 15 mL). If the animal is seizuring, fingers should not be placed in the animal's mouth. Once the animal's hypoglycemia is alleviated (response usually occurs within 1-2 minutes), it should be closely monitored (both by physical observation and serial blood glucose levels) to prevent a recurrence of hypoglycemia (especially with the slower absorbed products) and to prevent hyperglycemia from developing. Future insulin dosages or feeding habits should be adjusted to prevent further occurrences of hypoglycemia.

Drug Interactions

The following drug interactions have either been reported or are theoretical in humans or animals receiving insulin and may be of in veterinary patients. Unless otherwise noted, use together is not necessarily contraindicated, but weigh the potential risks and perform additional monitoring when appropriate.

- **BETA-ADRENERGIC BLOCKERS** (*e.g.,* **propranolol**): Can have variable effects on glycemic control and can mask the signs associated with hypoglycemia.
- **CLONIDINE; RESERPINE**: Can mask the signs associated with hypoglycemia.
- **DIGOXIN**: Because insulin can alter serum potassium levels, patients receiving concomitant cardiac glycoside (e.g., digoxin) therapy should be closely monitored; especially true in patients receiving concurrent diuretic therapy.

The following drugs or drug classes may <u>potentiate</u> the hypoglycemic activity of insulin:

- **ALCOHOL.**
- **ANABOLIC STEROIDS** (*e.g.,* stanozolol, boldenone).
- **ANGIOTENSIN CONVERTING ENZYME INHIBITORS** (*e.g.,* captopril, enalapril).
- **ASPIRIN OR OTHER SALICYLATES.**
- **DISOPYRAMIDE.**
- **FLUOXETINE.**
- **MONOAMINE OXIDASE INHIBITORS.**
- **SOMATOSTATIN DERIVATIVES** (*e.g.,* octreotide).
- **SULFONAMIDES.**

The following drugs or drug classes may <u>decrease</u> the hypoglycemic activity of insulin:

- **CALCIUM CHANNEL BLOCKERS** (*e.g.,* diltiazem).
- **CORTICOSTEROIDS.**
- **DANAZOL.**
- **DIURETICS.**
- **ISONIAZID.**
- **NIACIN.**
- **PHENOTHIAZINES.**
- **THYROID HORMONES** (can elevate blood glucose levels in diabetic patients when thyroid hormone therapy is first initiated).

Doses

Note: Treatment of diabetes mellitus and in particular, diabetic ketoacidosis is complex. Insulin is only one component of therapy; fluid and electrolytes, acid/base, and if necessary, antimicrobial therapy must also be employed. Adequate patient monitoring is mandatory. The reader is strongly encouraged to refer to more thorough discussions of treatment in veterinary endocrinology or internal medicine references for additional information. All dosages are extra-label except for FDA-approved veterinary products in the approved species (e.g., *Vetsulin*®, *ProZinc*®).

- **DOGS:**

  For adjunctive therapy of diabetic ketoacidosis:

  a) Using regular insulin, choose either the intermittent IM technique or low-dose IV infusion technique.

  Intermittent IM technique: Initial Dose: 0.2 Units/kg IM into muscles of the rear legs; repeat IM doses of 0.1 Units/kg hourly. Initial doses (first 2 to 3 injections) may be reduced by 25-50% in animals with severe hypokalemia. Goal is to slowly lower blood glucose to 200 – 250 mg/dL over a 6-10 hour period. As blood glucose approaches 250 mg/dL, switch to IM regular insulin at 0.1 – 0.3 Units/kg q4-6h or subcutaneous (if hydration status is good) q6-8h. Goal is to keep blood glucose in the 150 – 300 mg/dL range. Giving 5% dextrose IV is necessary during this stage.

  Constant Low-Dose Infusion Technique: Administer insulin infusion in an IV line separate from that for fluid therapy. Initial doses may be reduced by 25-50% in animals with severe hypokalemia. Adjust infusion rate based upon hourly blood glucose determinations. An hourly reduction in blood glucose by 50 – 100 mg/dL is ideal. Once blood glucose approaches 250 mg/dL switch to IM regular insulin every 4-6 hours or to subcutaneous regular insulin at 0.1 – 0.4 Units/kg q6-8h if hydration status is good. Goal is to keep blood glucose in the 150 – 300 mg/dL range. Giving 5% dextrose IV is necessary during this stage. Alternatively, may continue IV infusion at a decreased rate until exchanged for a longer-acting product. (Nelson et al. 2003a; Nelson 2008)

  b) **For IV infusion:** Preparation of insulin infusion by adding 2.2 Units/kg <u>regular insulin or insulin lispro</u> to 250 mL of 0.9% sterile saline for injection. Run approximately 50 mL of the insulin-containing fluid through the drip set prior to administration (See adsorption). (Hess 2008)

Blood Glucose Concentration (mg/dL)	IV Fluid	Rate of Administration (mL/hr)
>250	0.9% NaCl	10
200-250	0.45% NaCl + 2.5% dextrose	7
150-200	0.45% NaCl + 2.5% dextrose	5
100-150	0.45% NaCl + 5% dextrose	5
<100	0.45% NaCl + 5% dextrose	Stop fluid administration

For adjunctive treatment of severe hyperkalemia (>8 mEq/L): Give <u>regular insulin</u> 0.25 – 0.5 Units/kg slow IV bolus followed by 50% dextrose (4 mL/U of administered insulin); or give regular 0.5 – 1 Units/kg in parenteral fluids plus 2 grams dextrose per unit insulin administered (Nelson et al. 2003b)

For initial insulin treatment of uncomplicated diabetes mellitus:

<u>Porcine zinc (lente)</u>: 0.25 Units/kg SC q12h with equal sized meals at time of insulin injection. (Rucinsky et al. 2010)

Vetsulin®: 0.5 Units/kg SC once daily concurrently with or right after a meal. Revaluate at appropriate intervals and adjust dose based on clinical signs, urinalysis results, and glucose curve values until adequate glycemic control has been attained. Twice daily therapy should be initiated if the duration of insulin action is determined to be inadequate. If twice-daily treatment is initiated, the two doses should be 25% less than the once daily dose required to attain an acceptable nadir. For example, if a dog receiving 20 Units of *Vetsulin*® once daily has an acceptable nadir but inadequate duration of activity, the *Vetsulin*® dose should be changed to 15 Units twice daily. (*Vetsulin*® product package insert)

<u>NPH</u>: 0.25 Units/kg SC q12h (AAHA 2010)

<u>PZI</u>: 0.5 Units/kg SC q12h. Decrease to once daily if blood glucose nadir is consistently 12 hours or longer after administration. (Della Maggiore et al. 2012)

<u>Glargine</u>: 0.25 – 0.5 Units/kg SC q12h. (Fracassi et al. 2010) Insulin <u>glargine</u> (*Lantus*®) is used in poorly-controlled diabetic dogs where NPH and Lente insulin are ineffective because of problems with too short a duration of insulin effect. (Nelson 2006)

<u>Detemir</u>: 0.1 – 0.2 Units/kg SC q12h. **Note** the lower starting dose for detemir. Canine insulin receptors appear to be 4X more sensitive than human receptors to detemir. (Ford et al. 2010)

- **CATS:**

For adjunctive therapy of diabetic ketoacidosis:

<u>Regular insulin</u>: Use the same protocols as described above for dogs. (Nelson et al. 2003a; Hess 2010)

<u>Glargine</u>: 2 Units per cat SC and 1 Unit per cat IM (regardless of body weight) initially; repeat the IM dose 4 or more hours later if the blood glucose concentration is greater than 14-16 mMol/L (250-290 mg/dL); repeat the SC dose q12h. (Rand 2010a)

For adjunctive treatment of severe hyperkalemia: Regular insulin: 0.5 to 1 Unit/kg IM plus 2 grams dextrose per unit of insulin IV. (Feldman et al. 2010)

For initial insulin treatment of uncomplicated diabetes mellitus: Note: Cats are very unpredictable in their response to insulin therapy, and no single type of insulin is routinely effective in maintaining glycemic control, even with twice daily dosing. Cats should be closely monitored during the first month of insulin therapy.

<u>ProZinc®</u>: 0.2 – 0.7 Units/kg SC every 12 hours given concurrently with or right after a meal. Monitor clinical signs & blood glucose nadirs. Goal: glucose nadir (9 hr glucose curve) between 80 & 150 mg/dL & improvement in clinical signs. (ProZinc® product package insert)

<u>Glargine, detemir, or PZI insulin:</u>

Blood glucose <360 mg/dL (<20 mmol/L): 0.25 Units/kg of ideal body weight SC q12h;

Blood glucose ≥360 mg/dL (>20 mmol/L): 0.5 Units/kg of ideal body weight SC q12h;

Monitor response to therapy for first 3 days then increase or decrease the insulin dose weekly as needed. If no monitoring is occurring in the first week, begin with 1 Unit per cat every 12 hours. (Rand 2010b)

<u>PZI or glargine</u>: starting dose is 1 to 2 Units per cat SC every 12 hours (initial dose should not exceed 2 Units per cat even in very large cats). Decrease dose by 0.5 Units if blood glucose is <150 mg/dL any time during the day. Do not increase dose for 7 days after initiation or change in insulin dose. (Rucinsky et al. 2010)

<u>Vetsulin®</u>: Starting dose: 1 – 2 Units per cat SC twice daily at approximately 12 hour intervals. For cats fed twice daily, the injections should be given concurrently with, or right after each meal. For cats fed *ad libitum*, no change in feeding schedule is needed. (Vetsulin® product package insert)

Note: <u>Porcine zinc (lente) insulin is not recommended</u> for initial treatment for cats due to its short duration of action and poor control of clinical signs. (Rucinsky et al. 2010)

- **BIRDS:**

Treatment of diabetes mellitus: Insulin therapy is sometimes hindered by the highly variable dose needed for individual birds, the development of insulin resistance, and development of pancreatic atrophy/insufficiency. If bird is hospitalized, <u>regular insulin</u> at 0.1 – 0.2 Units/kg can be administered. Serum glucose concentrations are monitored every 1-2 hours; dosage is adjusted until blood glucose concentration is maintained within normal range. When the bird is stable or when hospitalization is not required, therapy with longer-acting <u>NPH insulin</u> is begun; in birds that were not been previously hospitalized a serial blood glucose curve should be obtained, adjusting the insulin dosage until blood glucose concentration is maintained within the normal range. Dosages will vary significantly between birds and should be individually titrated. An extremely wide range of dosages have been reported: from 0.067 – 3.3 Units/kg IM q12-24h. In most cases, twice daily injections are necessary. The goals of long-term home management are to eliminate weight loss and reduce the clinical signs of polyphagia, polyuria, and polydipsia. If urine is used to monitor insulin therapy at home, it is usually necessary to maintain a slight hyperglycemia with subsequent polyuria to obtain a urine sample to test. The urine is monitored with test reagent strips 2-3 times daily (at the time of each insulin injection and once in the middle of the day). Urine glucose should be maintained at slight positive or "trace" and the insulin dosage adjusted accordingly. It is important to advise the owner of the signs of hypoglycemia, home treatment for these events, and under what circumstances hospitalization is necessary. As with diabetic mammals, a high fiber diet should be offered. Ideally, the bird should return to the hospital for serial blood glucose monitoring several days after the initiation of insulin therapy, since it is likely that several days are required for glucose homeostasis to equilibrate (as is the case in mammals). The serial blood glucose curve should also be re-evaluated whenever clinical signs of diabetes and glycosuria become persistent, or every 2-3 months in the well controlled bird. The lack of knowledge of the pathophysiologic mechanism behind diabetes mellitus in avian species that are commonly kept as pets requires strict monitoring and flexibility on the part of the veterinarian. (Oglesbee 2003)

- **FERRETS:**

Treatment of diabetes mellitus:

a) <u>NPH</u>: 0.5 – 1 Unit per ferret SC twice daily. Goal of therapy is negative ketones and a small amount of glucose in the urine. (Quesenberry et al. 2004; Quesenberry et al. 2012)

b) <u>NPH</u>: 0.1 – 0.5 Units/kg IM or SC twice daily to start; adjust to optimal dose. May require insulin to be diluted; monitor urine for glucose/ketones. (Williams 2000)

c) <u>Glargine</u>: 0.5 Units per ferret SC between the scapulae q12h if urine dipstick positive for glucose. (Hess 2012)

- **SMALL MAMMALS**

Treatment of diabetes mellitus in Guinea pigs: <u>NPH</u>: 1 Unit per guinea pig SC every 12 hours. Monitor urine for glucose & ketones and adjust dose if needed. (Vannevel 1998)

- **CAMELIDS:**

Treatment of severe hyperlipemia:

<u>Regular</u>: 0.2 Units/kg IV with glucose, most commonly q6h; maximum frequency q1h. (Waitt et al. 2008)

<u>PZI</u>: 0.2 – 0.4 Units/kg SC with glucose q12-24h. Generally, duration is 8 to 16 hours. (Cebra 2002)

- **CATTLE:**

For adjunctive treatment of ketosis: PZI insulin 200 Units (total dose per animal) SC q48h (every other day). (Smith 2002; Smith 2009)

- **HORSES:**

For diabetes mellitus: Stabilization: Regular insulin 0.1 Units/kg IM every 6-12 hours or CRI infused at 0.1 Units/kg/hour. Chronic management: Glargine (expensive!) or NPH at 0.2 – 0.4 Units/kg SC q24h. (Giri et al. 2011)

For treatment of hyperlipemia in ponies:

a) For a 200 kg pony: <u>PZI</u> 30 Units (total dose) IM q12h on odd days (given with 100 grams glucose orally once daily); PZI 15 Units (total dose) IM q12h on even days (given with 100 grams galactose orally once daily) until hyperlipemia resolves. (Smith 2002; Smith 2009)

b) <u>PZI</u>: 0.4 Units/kg SC or IM q24h. (Knottenbelt 2006)

c) <u>PZI</u>: 0.1 – 0.3 Units/kg SC or IM q12-24h. (Munroe et al. 2011)

For management of hyperglycemia in critically ill foals during parenteral nutrition support: Regular insulin CRI infused at 0.07 Units/kg/hour. If BG >150mg/dL after 2 hours, increase rate by 50% at 2 hour intervals until BG is below 150mg/dL (Reed et al. 2010)

Monitoring Parameters
- Blood glucose.
- Patient weight, appetite, fluid intake/output.
- Blood, urine ketones (if warranted).
- Glycosylated hemoglobin and fructosamine [goal = fructosamine <450 micromol/L] (if available and warranted).

Client Information
- Keep insulin products away from temperature extremes. If stored in the refrigerator, allow to come to room temperature in syringe before injecting.
- Proper injection techniques should be taught and practiced with the client before the animal's discharge. Emphasis should be placed on matching the appropriate syringe and insulin concentration (*e.g.*, Do not interchange U-40 insulin/syringes with U-100 insulin/syringes).
- Insulin prescriptions should be labeled with appropriate handling procedures according to individual product labels. For example, insulin suspensions should be rolled gently until thoroughly mixed, not shaken to avoid bubbles and the potential for inaccurate dosing. The exception is *Vetsulin®*, which should be shaken thoroughly until a uniform, milky suspension is formed.
- All insulin products should be visually inspected prior to use. Insulin solutions should be clear and colorless without visible particles. Insulin suspensions should appear as uniform milky suspensions. Do not use insulin suspensions if clumps or white particles persist after mixing.
- The clinical signs of hypoglycemia should be thoroughly reviewed with the owner.
- A written protocol outlining monitoring procedures and treatment steps for hypoglycemia should be sent home with the owner.
- When traveling, insulin should not be left in carry-on luggage that will pass through airport surveillance equipment. Generally, insulin stability is not affected by a single pass through surveillance equipment; however, longer than normal exposure or repeated passes through surveillance equipment may alter insulin potency.

Chemistry/Synonyms
The endocrine component of the pancreas is organized as discrete islets (islets of Langerhans) that contain four cell types, each of which produces a different hormone. Insulin is produced in the beta cells, which comprise 60-80% of the islet. Insulin is a protein consisting of two chains, designated A and B, with 21 and 30 amino acids respectively that are connected by two disulfide bonds. The amino acid composition of insulin has been determined in various species of animals. The insulin of dogs, pigs, and certain whales (sperm and fin) is identical in structure; sheep insulin is identical to goat. Cattle, sheep, horses, and dogs differ only in positions 8, 9, and 10 of the A chain. Porcine insulin differs from human insulin by one amino acid [alanine instead of threonine at the carboxy terminal of the B chain (*i.e.*, in position B 30)], and bovine insulin differs by two additional alterations in the A chain (threonine and isoleucine in positions A8 and A10 are replaced by alanine and valine, respectively). Of the domestic species, feline insulin is most similar to bovine insulin, differing by only 1 amino acid (at position 18 of the A chain). Human insulin differs from rabbit insulin by a single amino acid. There is a single insulin gene and a single protein product in most mammalian species (multiple insulins appear to occur frequently among fishes).

For therapeutic purposes, doses and concentrations of insulin are expressed in Units. This is sometimes abbreviated as "U", but this practice is discouraged to reduce the chance for transcription and dosage errors. One unit of insulin is equal to the amount required to reduce the concentration of blood glucose in a fasting rabbit to 45 mg/dL (2.5 mM). All commercial preparations of human insulin currently manufactured in the U.S. are supplied in solution or suspension at a concentration of 100 Units/mL, which is approximately 3.6 mg of insulin per milliliter; likewise, one unit of insulin equals about 36 micrograms of insulin.

Insulin is a small protein; human insulin has a molecular weight of 5808. Insulin secretion is a tightly regulated process designed to provide stable concentrations of glucose in blood during fasting and feeding. This regulation is achieved by the coordinated interplay of various nutrients, gastrointestinal and pancreatic hormones, and autonomic neurotransmitters. The primary stimulus for secretion of endogenous insulin is glucose.

Regular insulin human injection, USP (rDNA origin) is structurally identical to human insulin and is synthesized through rDNA technology in a special non-disease-producing laboratory strain of *Escherichia coli* bacteria (*Humulin®*-R) or *Saccharomyces cerevisiae* yeast (*Novolin®*-R). It is a rapid-acting sterile, clear and colorless or almost colorless solution. Discoloration, turbidity, or unusual viscosity indicates deterioration or contamination.

Insulin lispro injection, USP (rDNA origin) is a human insulin analog that is rapid-acting and is synthesized in a special non-pathogenic laboratory strain of *Escherichia coli* that has been genetically altered. It is created when the amino acids at positions 28 and 29 on the B chain are reversed. The sterile solution consists of zinc-insulin lispro crystals dissolved in a clear aqueous fluid.

Isophane insulin, more commonly known as NPH, is an intermediate-acting, sterile suspension of zinc insulin crystals and protamine sulfate in buffered water for injection.

Porcine Lente insulin is a sterile aqueous suspension of purified pork Lente insulin consisting of 35% amorphous zinc insulin and 65% crystalline zinc insulin. It is available only as a U-40 insulin concentration and is a cloudy or milky suspension of a mixture of characteristic crystals and particles with no uniform shape.

Protamine zinc insulin is a sterile aqueous protamine zinc suspension of recombinant human insulin produced with recombinant DNA technology in the yeast *Pichia pastoris*.

Insulin glargine is a long-acting human insulin analog produced by recombinant DNA technology utilizing a non-pathogenic laboratory strain of *E. coli*. It differs from human insulin in that the amino acid asparagine at position A21 is replaced by glycine, and two arginines are added to the C-terminus of the B chain. The injection consists of insulin glargine dissolved in a clear aqueous fluid. It is available only as a U-100 insulin concentration.

Insulin detemir is a long-acting human insulin analog produced by recombinant DNA technology using a genetically modified strain of *Saccharomyces cerevisiae*. Insulin detemir differs from human insulin in that the amino acid threonine in position B30 has been omitted, and a C14 fatty acid chain has been attached to the amino acid B29. It is a clear, colorless, aqueous solution.

All human and purified pork insulin products have a neutral pH of approximately 7-7.8 except for insulin glargine, which has an acidic pH of approximately 4.

Stability/Storage
Manufacturers of insulin recommend that all insulin products be stored in the refrigerator but protected from freezing temperatures (do not store at temperatures <36°F (<2°C). Freezing may al-

ter the protein structure, decreasing potency. Particle aggregation and crystal damage may be visible to the naked eye or may require microscopic examination. Higher temperature (>86°F; >30°C) extremes and direct exposure to sunlight should be avoided (such as might occur when insulin is stored in a car glove compartment or on a window sill), since insulin transformation products and fibril formation may occur. Manufacturers recommend a maximum of 30 days storage at room temperature (except for detemir, which is 42 days). The manufacturer's label for *ProZinc®* does not contain a discard date for punctured vials other than the expiration date on the vial. Pet owners should be advised to visually inspect and discard any unused insulin if there are visual signs of contamination before each use.

Unused *Vetsulin®* should be discarded 42 days after initial puncture of the vial, according to the manufacturer's label.

According to the manufacturer's label, insulin glargine has a discard date of 28 days after the initial puncture of the vial, although clinical reports indicate that opened vials stored in the refrigerator have been used for up to 6 months in veterinary patients if not contaminated; discard vial immediately if there is any discoloration. Bacterial contamination and precipitation associated with pH change can cause cloudiness (Rand 2010b). For animals requiring small doses of glargine, the 3 mL cartridge may be preferable to the 10 mL vial to prevent the need for extended use beyond the recommended discard date.

Flocculation of NPH human insulin may appear 3-6 weeks after opening the vial. Deterioration in glycemic control may appear before frosting of the vial. If unexplained hyperglycemia is observed, a new vial of insulin should be used.

Regular and NPH insulin may be stored in plastic or glass syringes under refrigeration or at room temperature for 28 days without loss of potency; however, the antibacterial preservatives present in the insulin formulations may be lost if stored at room temperature (Trissel 2013). It is generally accepted that syringes of insulin can be stored for 28 days under refrigeration without fear of potency loss.

Compatibility/Compounding Considerations

Regular insulin is reportedly physically **compatible** with following drugs/solutions: normal saline, TPN solutions (4% amino acids, 25% dextrose with electrolytes and vitamins; must occasionally shake bag to prevent separation), cimetidine HCl, lidocaine HCl, oxytetracycline HCl, and verapamil HCl. Regular insulin may be mixed with other insulin products (except for glargine) used in veterinary medicine (e.g., NPH, PZI, etc.).

Regular insulin is reportedly physically **incompatible** when mixed with the following drugs/solutions: aminophylline, chlorothiazide sodium, cytarabine, dobutamine HCl, pentobarbital sodium, phenobarbital sodium, phenytoin sodium, sodium bicarbonate, sulfisoxazole sodium, and thiopental sodium. Compatibility is dependent upon factors such as pH, concentration, temperature, and diluent used; consult specialized references for more specific information.

Diluting insulin: Other than for immediate use, insulin should only be diluted using product-specific sterile diluents supplied by the manufacturers. Diluents for Regular insulin (*Humulin®-R*) and NPH insulin (*Humulin®-N*) and sterile vials can be obtained by telephoning Eli Lilly. *Insulin Diluting Medium for NovoLog®* is used to dilute *Novolin®-N* or *Novolog®* and may be obtained from Novo Nordisk. Diluted insulin (10 Units/mL) is stable for 4 weeks and should be stored in the refrigerator, although refrigeration is not required (anon 2010). For immediate use, insulin products (except glargine) can be diluted with normal saline for injection, but the potency cannot be predicted after 24 hours. Insulin glargine must not be diluted or mixed with any other insulin or solution for sub-

cutaneous use because the prolonged action is dependent on its pH.

Adsorption: The adsorption of regular insulin to the surfaces of IV infusion solution containers, glass and plastic (including PVC, ethylene vinyl acetate, polyethylene, and other polyolefins), tubing, and filters has been demonstrated. Estimates of loss of potency range from 20-80%, although reports of 20-30% are more common. The percent adsorbed is inversely proportional to the concentration of the insulin, and may include other factors such as the amount of container surface area, the fill volume of the solution, the type of solution, type and length of administration set, temperature, previous exposure of tubing to insulin, and the presence of other drugs, blood, etc. The adsorption process is instantaneous, with the bulk of insulin adsorption occurring within the first 30-60 minutes. To saturate binding sites and deliver a more predictable dose to the patient through an IV infusion, it is recommended that the first 50 mL be run through the IV tubing and discarded.

Insulin Syringes: Syringes are designed for use with a specific strength of insulin, with the needle covers color-coded according to strength. U-40 syringes have a red top, while U-100 syringes have an orange top. U-40 syringes contain 1/2 cc (equivalent to 0.5 mL) and have 20 unit marks. Measuring U-40 insulin to the one unit mark in a U-40 syringe will contain 1U of insulin. U-100 syringes are available in 0.3 mL, 0.5 mL, and 1 mL size. Measuring U-100 insulin to one mark in a U-100 syringe will contain 1 Unit of insulin.

Tuberculin syringes can also be used, but are not generally recommended because the potential for confusion is substantial. If using 100 Units/mL or TB syringes to measure 40 Units/mL insulin doses:

- Determine the required dose in units.
- If using U-100 insulin syringes (orange top), multiply the required Units of U-40 insulin by 2.5 (*e.g.* If required dose is 10 units, 10 x 2.5=25 units).
- If using TB syringes, multiply the required Units of U-40 insulin x 0.025 (*e.g.*, If the required dose is 10 Units, 10 x 0.025 = 0.25 mL).

Reuse of Insulin Syringes: Reuse of disposable insulin syringes has been suggested to reduce client costs. However, disposable insulin syringes are usually siliconized, and reuse can result in contamination of vials of insulin with silicone oil, causing a white precipitate and impairment of biological effects. Also, needles become dull with more than one use and can cause pain at the injection site.

Dosage Forms/Regulatory Status

VETERINARY-LABELED PRODUCTS:

Porcine insulin zinc suspension 40 Units/mL, intermediate-acting; *Vetsulin®* & *VetPen®* cartridge system; (Rx). FDA-approved for use in dogs and cats. *Caninsulin®* is available in Canada & Europe.

Protamine zinc (rDNA) insulin (PZI) aqueous suspension 40 Units/mL in 10 mL vials; *ProZinc®*; (Rx). FDA-approved for use in cats.

HUMAN-LABELED PRODUCTS:

Note: Partial listing; includes only those products generally used in veterinary medicine.

Short-Acting:

Insulin, Regular Injection Human (rDNA): 100 Units/mL in 10 mL vials; *Humulin®-R*, *Novolin®-R*; (OTC in humans; requires prescription under extra-label provisions of AMDUCA when used in animals)

Insulin Lispro Injection Human (rDNA): 100 Units/mL in 3 mL & 10 mL vials, *Humalog®*; (Rx)

Intermediate-Acting:

Isophane (Neutral Protamine Hagedorn; NPH) Human (rDNA):

100 Units/mL in 10 mL vials, 5 x 1.5 mL prefilled syringes & 5 x 3 mL pen insulin delivery devices; *Humulin®-N, Novolin®-N*; (OTC in humans; requires prescription under extra-label provisions of AMDUCA when used in animals)

NPH/Regular Insulin Mixtures:

Human (rDNA) 100 Units/mL 70% isophane insulin (NPH) & 30 % insulin injection (regular) in 5 x 3 mL disposable pen insulin delivery devices, 10 mL vials & 5 x 1.5 mL prefilled syringes; *Humulin®* 70/30, *Novolin®* 70/30; (OTC in humans; requires prescription under extra-label provisions of AMDUCA when used in animals)

Human (rDNA) Injection (suspension): 100 Units/mL; 50% isophane insulin (NPH) & 50% insulin injection (regular) in 10 mL vials; *Humulin®* 50/50; (OTC in humans; requires prescription under extra-label provisions of AMDUCA when used in animals)

Long-Acting:

Insulin Glargine Injection Human (rDNA) 100 Units/mL in 10 mL vials & 3 mL cartridge system; *Lantus®*; (Rx)

Insulin Detemir Injection Human (rDNA) 100 Units/mL in 10 mL vials & 3 mL cartridge system; *Levemir®*; (Rx)

Revisions/References

Monograph revised/updated May 2014.
anon (2010). Novo Nordisk (3/30/2010) Technical Services Doc. ASP024. Secondary Novo Nordisk (3/30/2010) Technical Services Doc. ASP024. Secondary anon. Volume
anon (2013). European Medicines Agency: CVMP assessment report for ProZinc (EMEA/V/C/002634). Secondary European Medicines Agency: CVMP assessment report for Pro-Zinc (EMEA/V/C/002634). Secondary anon. Volume
Buob, S., et al. (2010). An Intermittent Insulin Protocol Improves Metabolic Acidosis Faster Than a Continuous Rate Infusion of Regular Insulin in Feline Diabetic Ketoacidosis. Proceedings: ACVIM. accessed via Veterinary Information Network; vin.com
Cebra, C. (2002). Abnormal Energy Metabolism in New World Camelids. Proceedings ACVIM. accessed via Veterinary Information Network; vin.com
Cebra, C. K. (2001). Effects of exogenous insulin on glucose tolerance in alpacas. American Journal of Veterinary Research **62**: 1544-47.
Della Maggiore, A., et al. (2012). Efficacy of Protamine Zinc Recombinant Human Insulin for Controlling Hyperglycemia in Dogs with Diabetes Mellitus. Journal of Veterinary Internal Medicine **26**(1): 109-15.
Feldman, E. & D. Church (2010). Electrolyte Disorders: Potassium (Hyper/Hypokalemia). *Textbook of Veterinary Internal Medicine, 7th Ed*. S. Ettinger and E. Feldman. St Louis, Saunders: 303-8.
Ford, S., et al. (2010). Evaluation of Detemir Insulin in Diabetic Dogs Managed with Home Blood Glucose Monitoring. Proceedings: ACVIM. accessed via Veterinary Information Network; vin.com
Fracassi, F., et al. (2010). Use of Insulin Glargine in Dogs with Diabetes Mellitus. Proceedings: ECVIM. accessed via Veterinary Information Network; vin.com
Gilor, C., et al. (2010). Pharmacodynamics of Insulin Detemir and Insulin Glargine Assessed by an Isoglycemic Clamp Method in Healthy Cats. Journal of Veterinary Internal Medicine **24**(4): 870-4.
Giri, J. K., et al. (2011). Insulin-dependent diabetes mellitus associated with presumed autoimmune polyendocrine syndrome in a mare. Canadian Veterinary Journal-Revue Veterinaire Canadienne **52**(5): 506-12.
Hess, L. (2012). Insulin glargine treatment of a ferret with diabetes mellitus. Javma-Journal of the American Veterinary Medical Association **241**(11): 1490-4.
Hess, R. (2010). Diabetic Emergencies. *Consultations in Feline Internal Medicine*. J. August. St Louis, Saunders: 297-303.
Hess, R. S. (2008). Canine Diabetic Ketoacidosis. Proceedings: ACVIM. accessed via Veterinary Information Network; vin.com
Knottenbelt, D. (2006). *Saunders Equine Formulary*, Elsevier. Liverpool.
Marshall, R. & J. Rand (2004). Comparison of the pharmacokinetics and pharmacodynamics of glargine, protamine zinc and porcine lente insulins in normal cats. Proceedings: ACVIM Forum. accessed via Veterinary Information Network; vin.com
Marshall, R., et al. (2010). Glargine Administered Intramuscularly is Effective for Treatment of Feline Diabetic Ketoacidosis. Proceedings: ACVIM. accessed via Veterinary Information Network; vin.com
Munroe, G. & S. Weese (2011). Equine Clinical Medicine, Surgery, & Reproduction, Manson. London.
Nelson, R. (2006). Canine Diabetes Mellitus. Proceedings: UCDCMC2006. accessed via Veterinary Information Network; vin.com
Nelson, R. (2008). Managing Diabetic Ketoacidosis. Proceedings: WVC. accessed via Veterinary Information Network; vin.com
Nelson, R. & D. Elliott (2003a). Endocrine disorders. *Small Animal Internal Medicine, 3rd Ed*. R. Nelson and C. Couto. St Louis, Mosby: 660-815.
Nelson, R. & D. Elliott (2003b). Metabolic and electrolyte disorders. *Small Animal Internal Medicine, 3rd Ed*. R. Nelson and C. Couto. St Louis, Mosby: 816-46.
Oglesbee, B. (2003). Approach to the Polydipsic/Polyuric Bird. Proceedings: Western Veterinary Conference. accessed via Veterinary Information Network; vin.com
Palm, C. A., et al. (2009). An Investigation of the Action of Neutral Protamine Hagedorn

Human Analogue Insulin in Dogs with Naturally Occurring Diabetes Mellitus. Journal of Veterinary Internal Medicine **23**(1): 50-5.
Quesenberry, K. & D. M. Carpenter (2012). Ferrets, Rabbits, and Rodents Clinical Medicine and Surgery 3rd ed, Saunders. St Louis.
Quesenberry, K. & J. Carpenter (2004). Ferrets, Rabbits, and Rodents Clinical Medicine and Surgery 2nd ed, Saunders. St Louis.
Rand, J. (2010a). Diabetes Mellitus: Ketoacidosis. *The Feline Patient, 4th Ed*. G. Norsworthy, S. Grace, M. Crystal and L. Tilley, Wiley-Blackwell.
Rand, J. (2010b). Use of Longa-Acting Insulin in the Treatment of Diabetes Mellitus. *Consultations in Feline Internal Medicine*. J. August. St Louis: 286-96.
Reed, S. M., et al. (2010). *Equine Internal Medicine, 3rd Ed.*, Saunders. St. Louis.
Rucinsky, R., et al. (2010). AAHA Diabetes Management Guidelines. J. Am. Anim. Hosp. Assoc. **46**(3): 215-24.
Sears, K. W., et al. (2012). Use of lispro insulin for treatment of diabetic ketoacidosis in dogs. J. Vet. Emerg. Crit. Care **22**(2): 211-8.
Smith, B. (2002). Large Animal Internal Medicine, 3rd edition, Mosby. St Louis.
Smith, B. H. E. (2009). *Large Animal Internal Medicine 4th Ed.*, Mosby. St. Louis.
Trissel, L. 2013. Handbook on Injectable Drugs - 17th Edition. Accessed via STAT!Ref; Teton Data Systems
Vannevel, J. (1998). Diabetes mellitus in a 3-year-old, intact, female guinea pig. Canadian Veterinary Journal-Revue Veterinaire Canadienne **39**(8): 503-.
Waitt, L. H. & C. K. Cebra (2008). Characterization of hypertriglyceridemia and response to treatment with insulin in llamas and alpacas: 31 cases (1995-2005). Javma-Journal of the American Veterinary Medical Association **232**(9): 1362-7.
Walsh, E. S., et al. (2012). Aspart insulin constant rate infusion for treatment of dogs with diabetic ketoacidosis. Journal of Veterinary Internal Medicine **26**(3): 755-.
Williams, B. (2000). Therapeutics in Ferrets. Vet Clin NA: Exotic Anim Pract **3:1**(Jan): 131-53.

Interferon Alfa, Human Recombinant

(in-ter-feer-on)   huIFN-alfa Intron-A®

Immunomodulator

Prescriber Highlights

▶ Cytokine used to alleviate clinical effects of certain viral diseases; little solid evidence available to document safety/efficacy in small animals.

▶ Adverse Effects: In cats, adverse effects are apparently uncommon with PO; higher dosages given parenterally may cause malaise; fever, allergic reactions, myelotoxicity & myalgia are possible.

Uses/Indications

In veterinary medicine interferon alfa has primarily been used in cats to treat a variety of virus-induced diseases using either SC or oral/buccal administration. Despite rapid antibody development when injected parenterally and little, if any, absorption after oral administration, the drug does appear to have some efficacy for certain diseases, either via direct antiviral action or more likely, an immunomodulatory effect. Interferon-alfa has been used in dogs for the adjunctive treatment of viral- or immunosuppression-related conditions, such as papillomas, pododermatitis, or digital keratomas. Some work has been done in dogs evaluating it as an adjunctive treatment for certain neoplastic diseases (*e.g.*, hemangiosarcoma).

At the time of writing (2014), there is little published documenting clear efficacy via prospective, placebo-controlled studies in clinically ill animals. A placebo-controlled, blinded study evaluating the efficacy of huIFN-2alfa and zidovudine (AZT) separately and together in cats infected naturally with FeLV found no statistic differences for clinical or immunological parameters in any of the treatment groups versus placebo (Stuetzer et al. 2013). In summarizing the *in vitro*, controlled study and clinical efficacy status *in vivo* for human interferon-alfa use in virus infected cats, one author (Hartmann 2008) reports: High dose SC administration to cats does not appear to be clinically effective for FIV or FeLV infections. Low dose oral treatment does appear to have some efficacy for FIV in cats. Low dose oral therapy does not appear to be effective for FeLV, FHV-1, or FCV (feline calicivirus), and is contraindicated in

FIP. Topical administration to FHV-1 infected cats may have some efficacy (see topical ophthalmology section). Feline interferon-omega has recently become available in several countries and it may be useful in treating viral diseases in both cats and dogs. A separate monograph for that agent follows this one.

Pharmacology/Actions

The pharmacologic effects of the interferons are widespread and complex. Suffice it to say, that interferon alfa has antiviral, antiproliferative, and immunomodulating effects. Its antiproliferative and antiviral activities are thought to be due to its effects on the synthesis of RNA, DNA, and cellular proteins (oncogenes included). The mechanisms for its antineoplastic activities are not well understood, but are probably related these effects as well.

Pharmacokinetics

Interferon alfa is poorly absorbed after oral administration due to its degradation by proteolytic enzymes and studies have not detected measurable levels in the systemic circulation, however, there may be some absorption via upper GI mucosa. It may have some immunomodulating effect via stimulation of local lymphoid tissues.

Interferon alfa is widely distributed throughout the body, although it does not penetrate into the CNS well. It is unknown if it crosses the placenta. Interferon alfa is freely filtered by the glomeruli, and is absorbed by the renal tubules where it is metabolized by brush border or lysosomes. Hepatic metabolism is of minor importance. The plasma half-life in cats has been reported as 2.9 hours.

Contraindications/Precautions/Warnings

When used parenterally, consider the risks versus benefits in patients with preexisting autoimmune disease, severe cardiac disease, pulmonary disease, "brittle" diabetes, Herpes infections, hypersensitivity to the drug, or CNS disorders.

One author states that low dose oral therapy is contraindicated in cats with FIP (Hartmann 2008).

Adverse Effects

When used orally in cats, adverse effects are apparently uncommon. Higher dosages given parenterally to cats may cause malaise; fever, allergic reactions, myelotoxicity, and myalgia are possible. Cats given human interferon-alfa parenterally may develop significant antibodies to it after 3-7 weeks of treatment with resultant loss of efficacy.

When used systemically in humans, adverse effects have included anemia, leukopenias, thrombocytopenia, hepatotoxicity, neurotoxicity, taste sensation changes, anorexia, nausea, vomiting, diarrhea, dizziness, "flu-like" syndrome, transient hypotension, skin rashes, and dry mouth. Except for the "flu-like "syndrome, most adverse effects are dose-related and may vary depending on the condition treated.

Reproductive/Nursing Safety

Safety during pregnancy has not been established; high parenteral doses in monkeys did not cause teratogenic effects but did increase abortifacient activity. In humans, the FDA categorizes this drug as category *C* for use during pregnancy (*Animal studies have shown an adverse effect on the fetus, but there are no adequate studies in humans; or there are no animal reproduction studies and no adequate studies in humans.*)

It is not known whether this drug is excreted in milk.

Overdosage/Acute Toxicity

No information was located. Determine dosages carefully.

Drug Interactions

The following drug interactions have either been reported or are theoretical in humans or animals receiving interferon alfa and may be of in veterinary patients. Unless otherwise noted, use together is not necessarily contraindicated, but weigh the potential risks and perform additional monitoring when appropriate.

- **ACYCLOVIR, ZIDOVUDINE, VIDARABINE:** Additive or synergistic antiviral effects may occur when interferon alfa is used in conjunction with zidovudine (AZT) or acyclovir. This effect does not appear to occur with vidarabine, although increased toxicities may occur. The veterinary significance of these potential interactions is unclear.

Doses

Note: All dosages are extra-label and evidence for safety and efficacy is relatively weak (EBM Grades 3 or 4). All dosages are for human interferon alfa-2b as interferon alfa-2a is no longer marketed.

- **DOGS:**

  For cutaneus T-cell lymphoma and severe cases of oral/cutaneus papillomas: $1.5 - 2$ million Units/m^2 SC 3 times weekly. (White 2000)

  As an immunostimulant for the adjunctive treatment of certain dermatologic conditions (*e.g.,* pododermatitis, papillomas, digital keratomas): 1000 Units PO once daily (given as 1000 Unit/mL solution). (Yu 2008)

- **CATS:**

  For treatment of virus infections (extra-label):

  a) FeLV, calcivirus, FHV-1 or FIV-infected cats: <u>Low-dose oral</u>: No controlled studies were located documenting efficacy, but anecdotally some clinicians feel it has helped some patients. Most recommendations are for using $30 - 50$ Units per cat, PO or buccally once daily. Some have treated 7 days on, 7 days off.

  b) For FCV or FHV-1: <u>High-dose SC Injection</u>: 10,000 Units/kg (diluted in saline) once daily for up to 14 days has led to clinical resolution of disease in some cats treated in the study. (Fenimore et al. 2012; Lappin 2012)

Client Information

- Owners should be made aware of the "investigational" nature of this compound and understand that efficacy and safety have not necessarily been established.

- For oral use: Compounded liquid given orally (by mouth) or inside the cheek (buccally). Best not to mix with food. If your animal vomits or acts sick after getting it on an empty stomach, give with food or small treat to see if this helps. If vomiting continues, contact your veterinarian.

- Usually very well tolerated

Chemistry/Synonyms

Prepared from genetically engineered cultures of *E. coli* with genes from human leukocytes, interferon alfa-2b is commercially available as a sterile solution or sterile powder. Human interferon alfa is a complex protein that contains 165 or 166 amino acids.

Interferon may also be known as: IFN-alpha, interferon-alpha, Sch-30500 (interferon alfa-2b); there are many internationally registered trade names available.

Storage/stability

Commercially available products should be stored in the refrigerator; do not freeze the accompanying diluent. Do not expose solutions to room temperature for longer than 24 hours. Do not vigorously shake solutions.

An article proposing using this product in cats for the treatment of FeLV states that after dilution of 3 million Units in one liter of sterile saline, the resultant solution remains active for years if frozen or for months if refrigerated. However, data corroborating this is apparently not available.

Compatibility/Compounding Considerations

<u>Preparation of solution for 30 Units/mL oral administration</u>: Using the 3 million Unit vial (see below), dilute the entire contents into a 1 L bag of sterile normal saline; mix well. Resulting solution contains approximately 3,000 Units/mL. Divide into aliquots of either 1 mL or 10 mL and freeze. By diluting further 100 fold (1 mL of 3000 Units/mL solution with 100 mL of sterile saline, or 10 mL with 1000 mL of sterile saline) a 30 Units/mL solution will result. Some have advised aliquoting the diluted solution into 1 mL volumes for freezing up to a year; defrost as necessary. Once defrosted, the drug can be refrigerated up to one week. Freezing the most dilute solutions is associated with loss in activity unless protein such as albumin (see above) is added during dilution. (Greene et al. 2006)

Dosage Forms/Regulatory Status

VETERINARY-LABELED PRODUCTS: NONE.

HUMAN-LABELED PRODUCTS:

Interferon Alfa-2b (human recombinant) (IFN-alpha2; rIFN-a2; a-2-interferon) Powder for Injection: 10 million Units/vial; 18 million Units/vial; & 50 million Units/vial in vials with diluent; *Intron A®*; (Rx)

Interferon Alfa-2b (human recombinant) (IFN-alpha2; rIFN-a2; a-2-interferon) Injection: 6 million Units/mL in 3.6 mL vials & 10 million Units/mL in 3.2 mL vials; *Intron A®*; (Rx)

Interferon Alfa-2a (*Roferen® A*), which was used in veterinary medicine has been discontinued.

Revisions/References

Monograph revised/updated February 2014.

Fenimore, A., et al. (2012). Treatment of Chronic Rhinitis in Shelter Cats with Parenteral Alpha-Interferon or an Intranasal Feline Herpesvirus 1 and Feline Calicivirus Vaccine. ACVIM. accessed via Veterinary Information Network; vin.com

Greene, C., et al. (2006). Appendix 8: Antimicrobial Drug Formulary. *Infectious Disease of the Dog and Cat.* C. Greene, Elsevier: 1186-333.

Hartmann, K. (2008). Antiviral chemotherapy in veterinary medicine. Proceedings: ACVIM. accessed via Veterinary Information Network; vin.com

Lappin, M. R. (2012). Treatment & Prevention of Infectious Causes of Feline Upper Respiratory Disease Complex. Western Veterinary Conference. accessed via Veterinary Information Network; vin.com

Stuetzer, B., et al. (2013). A trial with 3 '-azido-2 ',3 '-dideoxythymidine and human interferon-alpha in cats naturally infected with feline leukaemia virus. Journal of Feline Medicine and Surgery 15(8): 667-71.

White, S. (2000). Veterinary Dermatology: New Treatments, 'New' Diseases. Proceedings: The North American Veterinary Conference, Orlando. accessed via Veterinary Information Network; vin.com

Yu, A. (2008). Pododermatitis I: Infectious. Proceedings: WVC. accessed via Veterinary Information Network; vin.com

---

Interferon-ω (omega), Feline Origin

(in-ter-feer-on oh-may-ga)   Virbagen Omega®, Recombinant

Omega Interferon of Feline Origin, rFeIFN-ωω

Immunomodulator

Prescriber Highlights

▶ Immunomodulating cytokine labeled (in Europe) for treating FeLV & FIV in cats & Parvo in dogs; not commercially available in USA. May potentially be effective in treating canine atopic dermatitis.

▶ Appears to be well tolerated; adverse effects include: hyperthermia, vomiting, diarrhea (cats), fatigue (cats).

▶ Increases in ALT & decreases in RBC, WBC, & platelet counts have been seen.

▶ Treatment may be very expensive.

Uses/Indications

Omega interferon (feline; rFeIFN-ω) is labeled (in the EU) for dogs 1 month of age or older for the reduction in mortality and clinical signs of parvovirus (enteric form). In cats 9 weeks of age or older, it is labeled for treating FeLV and/or FIV in non-terminal clinical stages. It may be of benefit in treating canine distemper, canine atopic dermatitis, acute feline calicivirus infections, FIP, or topically for feline herpetic keratitis, but data is still being gathered to document efficacy. In an article evaluating the evidence for safety and efficacy for treatments for canine atopic dermatitis (AD), the authors concluded that based on one randomized clinical trial there is only low-quality evidence of the efficacy and safety of injectable recombinant feline interferon-omega to treat canine AD (Olivry et al. 2013).

In summarizing the *in vitro*, controlled study and clinical efficacy status *in vivo* for feline interferon-omega use in virus infected cats and dogs, one author (Hartmann 2008) reports that controlled studies have been done for FIV (ineffective), FeLV (some effect), and canine parvovirus (effective). Controlled studies have not been performed for FHV-1 (possibly effective), FCV (possibly effective), FIP (possibly effective) or feline panleukovirus (likely effective). In an open label study of 16 naturally infected cats with FIV/FeLV given labeled doses of rFeIFN-ω, improved clinical signs and decreased concurrent virus excretion was noted (Gil et al. 2013).

Pharmacology/Actions

Omega interferon is a type 1 interferon related to alpha interferon. Its principle action is not as a direct anti-viral, but by acting on virus-infected cells inhibiting mRNA and translation proteins thereby inhibiting viral replication. It may also nonspecifically enhance immune defense mechanisms.

Pharmacokinetics

It has been stated that omega interferon pharmacokinetics in dogs and cats is similar to that of human interferons. After intravenous injection, omega interferon is rapidly bound to specific receptor sites on a variety of cells. Highest tissue levels are found in the liver and kidneys. Interferon is filtered in the renal glomeruli and catabolized in the kidneys. In dogs, volume of distribution at steady state is about 0.1L/kg. Biphasic elimination occurs with an alpha half-life of 3.14 hours and a beta half-life of 0.24 hours. Total body clearance is 6.9 mL/min/kg.

Contraindications/Precautions/Warnings

The manufacturer cautions against vaccinating dogs currently being treated with omega interferon and not to vaccinate until the patient appears to have recovered. As both FeLV and FIV infections are known to be immunosuppressive, the manufacturer states that cat vaccinations are contraindicated during and after omega interferon treatment.

There are several different interferons available for use in humans (several sub-types of alpha, beta, or gamma interferon); one cannot be substituted for another.

Adverse Effects

In cats and dogs, hyperthermia (3–6 hours post-dose) and vomiting have been reported. Slight decreases in RBCs, platelets and WBCs, and increased ALT have been observed but, reportedly, these indices return to normal within a week of the last injection.

Additionally, soft feces/mild diarrhea and transient fatigue may be noted in cats. Intravenous administration to cats may cause increased incidence and severity of adverse effects, but in cats, adverse effects occur uncommonly.

Dogs may develop antibodies to interferon omega if treatment is prolonged (beyond labeled dosage period) or repeated.

Reproductive/Nursing Safety

Safety during pregnancy or lactation has not been established.

Overdosage/Acute Toxicity

10X overdoses in dogs and cats caused mild lethargy/somnolence, slight hyperthermia, slight increases in respiratory and heart rates.

In animals tested, signs resolved within 7 days and no treatment was required.

Drug Interactions

No reported drug interactions at the time of writing, but use caution when using other drugs that can be hepatotoxic or myelosuppressive.

Laboratory Considerations

- No specific concerns were noted.

Doses

- **DOGS:**

  For treatment of parvovirus as labeled (extra-label in USA): 2.5 million Units/kg IV once daily for 3 days. The earlier the dog is treated, the more likely of success. (Label information; *Virbagen Omega*®—Virbac UK)

  For treatment of atopic dermatitis (extra-label): Per injection: Dogs 8-15 kg = 1 million Units; 15-29 kg = 2 million Units; 29-40 kg = 3 million Units; 29-40 kg = 4 million Units. In the study, doses were administered. In the study, dogs were dosed SC on days: 0, 3, 7, 14, 21, 35, 56, 90, 120, & 150. Further larger-scale studies needed to confirm that low dose rFeIFN-omega is cost-effective and safe option for long-term treatment. (Carlotti et al. 2009)

- **CATS:**

  For treatment of FeLV or FV as labeled (extra-label in USA): 1 million Units/kg SC once daily for 5 days. Three separate 5-day treatments performed at day 0, day 14, and day 60. (Label information; *Virbagen Omega*®—Virbac UK)

  For FHV-1 facial dermatitis (extra-label): From a case report treating a cat with FHV-1 facial dermatitis: Day 0: Cat sedated with propofol and rFeIFN-ω 1.5 million Units/kg injected, half of which was injected peri-lesionally and intradermally and the other half subcutaneously on the lateral thorax. Day 2 and day 9: 1.5 million Units/kg injected SC on the lateral thorax. On days 19, 21, and 23: 0.75 million Units/kg injected peri-lesionally and intradermally as well as 0.75 million Units/kg SC on the lateral thorax. The cat was sedated as described above when peri-lesional and intradermal injections made. (Gutzwiller et al. 2007)

Monitoring

- Monitor for efficacy for infection treated.
- CBC and hepatic function tests suggested.

Client Information

- This drug is best administered on an inpatient basis where the patient may be observed and supported.

Chemistry/Synonyms

Interferon omega of feline origin is a type 1 recombinant interferon obtained from silkworms after inoculation with a recombinant baculovirus. It is provided commercially as a lyophilisate powder with a separate solvent.

Recombinant omega interferon of feline origin may also be known as: Interferon omega, omega interferon, interferon-ω, IFN-ω, IFN-ω (feline recombinant), rFeIFN-ω, and *Virbagen Omega*®.

Storage/stability

The commercial veterinary product should be stored in its original carton refrigerated (4°C ± 2°C) and protected from freezing. It has a designated shelf life of 2 years when properly stored. Once reconstituted with the supplied isotonic sodium chloride solution, it should be used immediately as it contains no preservative, however, the solution is reported to be stable for at least 3 weeks when refrigerated. No data was located on the stability of the reconstituted solution when frozen.

Compatibility/Compounding Considerations

The manufacturer states: Do not mix with any other vaccine/immunological product, except the solvent supplied for use with the product.

Dosage Forms/Regulatory Status

VETERINARY-LABELED PRODUCTS:

None in the USA. In the EU: Recombinant Omega Interferon of Feline Origin 10 million Units/vial; *Virbagen Omega*®; (Rx). Licensed for dogs and cats. A 5 million Unit vial may be available in some countries.

HUMAN-LABELED PRODUCTS: NONE.

Revisions/References

Monograph revised/updated February 2014.

Carlotti, D. N., et al. (2009). The use of recombinant omega interferon therapy in canine atopic dermatitis: a double-blind controlled study. Veterinary Dermatology **20**(5-6): 405-11.

Gil, S., et al. (2013). Relevance of feline interferon omega for clinical improvement and reduction of concurrent viral excretion in retrovirus infected cats from a rescue shelter. Research in Veterinary Science **94**(3): 753-63.

Gutzwiller, M. E. R., et al. (2007). Feline herpes dermatitis treated with interferon omega. Veterinary Dermatology **18**(1): 50-4.

Hartmann, K. (2008). Antiviral chemotherapy in veterinary medicine. Proceedings: ACVIM. accessed via Veterinary Information Network; vin.com

Olivry, T. & P. Bizikova (2013). A systematic review of randomized controlled trials for prevention or treatment of atopic dermatitis in dogs: 2008-2011 update. Veterinary Dermatology **24**(1): 97-+.

Intravenous Lipid Emulsion — See Fat Emulsion, Intravenous

Iodide, Sodium
Iodide, Potassium

(eye-oh-dide)   SSKI, Iodoject®

Antifungal, Nutritional

Prescriber Highlights

- ▶ Iodides have been used for actinobacillosis in ruminants and sporotrichosis in horses, dogs, & cats.
- ▶ Contraindications: Iodide hypersensitivity, lactating animals, hyperthyroidism, renal failure, or dehydration. May cause abortion in cattle.
- ▶ Very metallic taste, patient acceptance can be problematic.
- ▶ Do not inject IM; in horses give IV slowly & with caution as severe generalized reactions have been reported.
- ▶ Adverse Effects: Iodism: Excessive tearing, vomiting, anorexia nasal discharge, muscle twitching, cardiomyopathy, scaly haircoats/dandruff, hyperthermia, decreased milk production & weight gain, coughing, inappetence, & diarrhea.
- ▶ Cats may be more prone to developing toxicity.

Uses/Indications

The primary use for sodium iodide is in the treatment of actinobacillosis and actinomycosis in cattle. It has been used as an expectorant with little success in a variety of species and occasionally as a supplement for iodine deficiency disorders. In horses, dogs and cats, oral sodium or potassium iodide has been used in the treatment of sporotrichosis.

Use in cats is controversial as they may be prone to developing adverse effects; cats may require other antifungal (*e.g.*, itraconazole) therapy. A recent study using oral potassium iodide (alone) for sporotrichosis reported a cure rate of 48% and a treatment failure rate of 37% (Reis et al. 2012).

Pharmacology/Actions

While the exact mode of action for its efficacy in treating actinobacillosis is unknown, iodides probably have some effect on the granulomatous inflammatory process. Iodides have little, if any, *in vitro* antibiotic activity.

Pharmacokinetics

Little published information appears to be available. Therapeutic efficacy of intravenous sodium iodide for actinobacillosis is rapid, with beneficial effects usually seen within 48 hours of therapy.

Contraindications/Precautions/Warnings

Sodium iodide injection labels state that it should not be given to lactating animals or those with hyperthyroidism. Do not inject intramuscularly (IM).

Iodides given parenterally should be administered slowly intravenously and with caution to horses; severe generalized reactions have been reported.

Should not be used in animals in renal failure or that are severely dehydrated.

Adverse Effects

In ruminants, the adverse effect profile is related to excessive iodine (see Overdosage below). Young animals may be more susceptible to iodism than adults.

Foals have developed goiter when mares have been excessively supplemented.

Chronic use or overdoses may cause iodism. Cats are apparently more prone to developing this than other species. Signs can include vomiting, inappetence, depression/lethargy, twitching, hypothermia, and cardiovascular failure. In a recent study, 27% of treated cats had increased liver enzymes and about half of those cats exhibited signs of hepatotoxicity (Reis et al. 2012).

The taste of the liquid is very unpleasant and animals may avoid dosing. Giving with food or a fatty liquid (*e.g.,* whole milk, ice cream) may improve palatability and reduce nausea and vomiting. Cats reportedly tolerate the taste of sodium iodide better then potassium iodide. Potassium iodide oral tablets 130 mg (available OTC for reducing risk for thyroid cancer after radioactive isotope exposure) or compounded capsules may be useful in small dogs or cats that cannot tolerate oral solutions.

Reproductive/Nursing Safety

Anecdotal reports that iodides can cause abortion in cattle persist and label information of some veterinary products state not to use in pregnant animals. Clearly, potential risks versus benefits of therapy must be weighed. In humans, the FDA categorizes this drug as category *D* for use during pregnancy (*There is evidence of human fetal risk, but the potential benefits from the use of the drug in pregnant women may be acceptable despite its potential risks.*)

Iodides are excreted in milk. If iodides are required in the nursing dam, switch to milk replacer.

Overdosage/Acute Toxicity

Excessive iodine in animals can cause excessive tearing, vomiting, anorexia, nasal discharge, muscle twitching, cardiomyopathy, scaly haircoats/dandruff, hyperthermia, decreased milk production and weight gain, coughing, inappetence, and diarrhea.

Drug Interactions

The following drug interactions have either been reported or are theoretical in humans or animals receiving iodide and may be of in veterinary patients. Unless otherwise noted, use together is not necessarily contraindicated, but weigh the potential risks and perform additional monitoring when appropriate.

- **ANTITHYROID MEDICATIONS:** Iodides may decrease the efficacy of antithyroid medications.
- **THYROID SUPPLEMENTS:** Iodides may enhance the efficacy of thyroid medications.

Doses

- **DOGS:**

  For sporotrichosis (extra-label): Using potassium iodide (SSKI): 40 mg/kg PO q12h with food; itraconazole less likely to have adverse effects. (Grooters 2005)

- **CATS:**

  For sporotrichosis (extra-label): Generally, azole antifungal agents are recommended, but as a low cost alternative treatment (from an observational cohort study): Using potassium iodide compounded into capsules, initially at 2.5 mg/kg PO q24h. Then, doses were progressively increased at each 5-day period until a clinical response was achieved or signs of toxicity appeared as follows: 5 mg/kg, 10 mg/kg, 15 mg/kg and 20 mg/kg q24h. Cats with mild adverse clinical effects had therapy suspended for 7 days and resumed 2.5 mg/kg dose increments until the highest dose that did not induce toxicity was attained. (Reis et al. 2012)

- **CATTLE, SHEEP & GOATS:**

  For treatment of actinobacillosis (woody tongue); (extra-label): 70 mg/kg IV given as a 10% or 20% solution; repeat at least one more time at a 7-10 day interval. Refractory cases may require more frequent (2-3 day interval) treatment. Severe, generalized, or refractory cases may require adjunctive treatment with antibiotics (sulfas, aminoglycoside or tetracyclines). (Smith 1996)

- **HORSES:**

  For sporotrichosis (extra-label): Loading dose of sodium iodide at 20 – 40 mg/kg IV for 2-5 days, then 20 – 40 mg/kg PO once daily for at least 3 weeks after all clinical lesions disappear. May administer via oral syringe or mixed in sweet feed. Topical hot packs of 20% sodium iodide may be used on open wounds. (Rees 2004)

  For conidiobolomycosis (extra-label): From a case report: A mare with *C. coronatus* granulomatous tracheitis was successfully treated with 20% sodium iodide at 44 mg/kg IV for 7 days, then ethylenediamine dihydroiodide (iodide powder, granules) at 1.3 mg/kg PO q12h for 4 months, then q24h for 1 year, then once per week. Excessive lacrimation was occasionally noted, but resolved if the drug was held for one day. (Stewart et al. 2005)

Monitoring

- Clinical efficacy.
- Signs of iodism (excessive tearing, nasal discharge, scaly haircoats/dandruff, hyperthermia, decreased milk production and weight gain, coughing, inappetence, and diarrhea.
- Liver enzymes.

Client Information

- Nausea and vomiting (dogs, cats), unpleasant taste (which may make your animal difficult to dose) occurs commonly, especially if given on an empty stomach. Give with cream or high fat food. Compounded capsules may be easier to administer in some animals.
- Excessive tearing (lacrimation/tearing); may need to skip a dose if this is a problem.
- Long term use or high dosages can cause iodide toxicity (iodism); see adverse effects below.
- If liquid turns brownish-yellow do not use.

Chemistry/Synonyms

Sodium iodide occurs as colorless, odorless crystals or white crystalline powder. It develops a brown tint upon degradation. Approximately 1 gram is soluble in 0.6 mL of water and 2 mL of alcohol.

Potassium iodide occurs as a clear to white granular powder. Approximately 1 gram is soluble in 0.7 mL of water. One gram (one mL) of SSKI contains 6 mEq of potassium.

Potassium iodide oral solution may also be known as SSKI (super saturated potassium iodide), or *Pima®*.

Storage/stability

Commercially available veterinary injectable products should generally be stored at room temperature (15-30° C).

Supersaturated potassium iodide (SSKI) solution should be stored below 40°C (104°F) and preferably between 15-30°C (59-86°F) in a tight, light-resistant container; protect from freezing. Crystallization can occur, particularly if stored at low temperatures; re-warming the contents and shaking will usually redissolve the crystals. If oxidation occurs, the solution will turn brownish yellow in color; discard should this occur.

Compatibility/Compounding Considerations

Sodium iodide injection is reportedly physically **incompatible** with vitamins B and C injection.

Dosage Forms/Regulatory Status

VETERINARY-LABELED PRODUCTS:

Sodium Iodide Injection: 20 g/100 mL (20%; 200 mg/mL) in 250 mL vials—available as multi- or single use vials; generic; (Rx). Labeled for use in non-lactating cattle.

Oral iodide powders/granules for addition to feeds are available. Active ingredient is ethylenediamine dihydroiodide.

HUMAN-LABELED PRODUCTS:

Potassium Iodide Solution: 1 gram potassium iodide/mL (SSKI); generic; (Rx)

Potassium Iodide Oral Syrup: 62.5 mg potassium iodide/mL (325 mg/5 mL) in pints and gallons; *Pima®*; (Rx)

Potassium Iodide Oral Tablets 65 mg, & 130 mg; *Thyrosafe®*, *Iosat®*; (OTC)

There are also radioactive iodine compounds available for thyroid diagnostic and treatment.

Revisions/References

Monograph revised/updated February 2014.

Grooters, A. (2005). Deep fungal infections. Proceedings; ACVIM. accessed via Veterinary Information Network; vin.com

Rees, C. (2004). Disorders of the skin. *Equine Internal Medicine 2nd Ed.* S. Reed, W. Bayly and D. Sellon. Philadelphia, Saunders: 667-720.

Reis, E. G., et al. (2012). Potassium iodide capsule treatment of feline sporotrichosis. Journal of Feline Medicine and Surgery 14(6): 399-404.

Smith, B. (1996). Actinomycosis. *Large Animal Internal Medicine 2nd Ed.* B. Smith. St Louis, Mosby: 796-7.

Stewart, A. & T. Salazar (2005). Fungal infections of the respiratory tract. Proceedings: ACVIM. accessed via Veterinary Information Network; vin.com

Iodixanol

(eye-oh-**dix**-ah-nol)   Visipaque®

Contrast Agent

Prescriber Highlights

▶ Contrast agent used in medical imaging and potentially to estimate GFR.

▶ Fewer adverse effects than with older ionic iodine contrast agents; may have less nephrotoxic potential than iohexol, but presently more expensive.

Uses/Indications

Iodixanol can be used as a contrast agent for variety of radiographic imaging procedures in veterinary patients, and can be used as a marker agent for estimating glomerular filtration rates (GFR) in animals, including dogs, cats, rabbits, calves and horses (Imai et al. 2011; Satoh et al. 2011; Imai et al. 2012; Katayama et al. 2012; Michigoshi et al. 2012). Iodixanol may have even less nephrotoxic potential than iohexol.

Pharmacology/Actions

Like iohexol, iodixanol is a near ideal marker for estimating glomerular filtration rate and thereby, renal function. Its protein binding is negligible; nearly 100% is excreted unchanged in the urine within 24 hours and can be measured in plasma using a variety of assays.

When used as a radio contrast agent, organic iodine is relatively radiopaque and can help define adjacent structures.

Pharmacokinetics

No pharmacokinetic information was found for domestic animals. In humans, the volume of distribution is 0.26 L/kg (consistent with extracellular space) with little or no protein binding. Plasma and urine levels suggest that clearance is primarily due to renal mechanisms. In adult humans, approximately 97% of injected doses are excreted unchanged in urine within 24 hours. Less than 2% is excreted in feces. Elimination half-life in young, healthy adult males is about 2 hours. Renal clearance of iodixanol was equivalent to GFR.

Contraindications/Precautions/Warnings

In the pediatric (human) population, prolonged fasting and the administration of a laxative before iodixanol injection are contraindicated. Not for intrathecal use. Other labeled warnings or precautions include human patients with: pheochromocytoma, coagulation disorders, hyperthyroidism, multiple myeloma, dehydration, CHF, and severe renal or hepatic impairment.

Avoid extravasation.

Adverse Effects

When used intravascularly, iodixanol appears to be well tolerated, but usage in animals has been limited. Hypersensitivity reactions with iodixanol can occur, but in humans, only very rarely. Nephrotoxicity from iodixanol is potentially possible but the risk appears slight. Iodixanol is considered one of the agents used for contrast studies with the lowest toxicity for humans.

Reproductive/Nursing Safety

The human product label states that adequate and well-controlled studies in pregnant women have not been conducted. Use this drug during pregnancy only if clearly needed. The FDA has designated it as a category *B* drug (*Animal studies have not demonstrated risk to the fetus, but there are no adequate studies in pregnant women; or animal studies have shown an adverse effect, but adequate studies in pregnant women have not demonstrated a risk to the fetus during the first trimester of pregnancy, and there is no evidence of risk in later trimesters.*)

It is not known if iodixanol is distributed into milk but many similar contrast agents are in very low quantities. No adverse effects have been reported in breastfeeding infants whose mothers received the related drug iohexol and the American Academy of Pediatrics considers that iohexol is usually compatible with breastfeeding.

Overdosage/Acute Toxicity

The adverse effects of intravenous overdosage can be serious and life-threatening and primarily affect the pulmonary and cardiovascular systems. Clinical signs can include: cyanosis, bradycardia, acidosis, pulmonary hemorrhage, convulsions, coma, and cardiac arrest. Treatment is supportive.

Drug Interactions

The following drug interactions have either been reported or are theoretical in humans or animals receiving iodixanol and may be of in veterinary patients. Unless otherwise noted, use together is not necessarily contraindicated, but weigh the potential risks and perform additional monitoring when appropriate.

- **IODINE ISOTOPES:** Iodixanol may alter binding to thyroid tissue for at least 16 days.
- **METFORMIN:** Use together is contraindicated in humans; lactic acidosis may result.

Laboratory Considerations

- **Thyroid Function Tests:** If iodine-containing isotopes are to be used for diagnosing thyroid disease, prior use of iodixanol can reduce the iodine-binding capacity of thyroid tissue for at least 16 days (in humans). Thyroid function tests that do not depend on iodine estimation (*e.g.* T3 resin uptake and total or free thyroxine/T4 assays) are not affected.
- False positive **urine protein** when using *Multistix®* can occur. The Coomassie blue method has been shown to give accurate results.
- **Urine specific gravity** results may be falsely high; refractometry or urine osmolality may be substituted.

Doses

To estimate GFR: At the time of writing (2014), widespread clinical use or usefulness for limited- or single-sample iodixanol clearance or concentration determination to estimate GFR in domestic animals has yet to be realized, but research is ongoing and results look promising for future use in clinical settings. Follow the current literature and scientific proceedings for more information as it becomes available. **Note:** Dosages are expressed as organically bound iodine. For example if using *Visipaque®* 320, the concentration of organically bound iodine is 320 mg/mL. Most studies are using dosages of 20 – 40 mg/kg IV. (Imai et al. 2011; Satoh et al. 2011; Imai et al. 2012; Katayama et al. 2012; Michigoshi et al. 2012)

Monitoring

- No specific monitoring outside of adverse effects.

Client Information

This medication is administered only by veterinarians.

Chemistry/Synonyms

Iodixanol is a nonionic iodinated contrast agent that occurs as a white to off-white, amorphous, odorless, hygroscopic powder. It is freely soluble in water. Commercial products list the concentration of the product as organic iodine concentration per mL.

Visipaque® 270 contains iodixanol 550 mg/mL, equivalent to 270 mg/mL of organically bound iodine. Visipaque® 320 contains iodixanol 652 mg/mL, equivalent to 320 mg/mL of organically bound iodine.

Iodixanol may also be known as 2-5410-3A, iodixanolum, jodiksanoli or jodixanol. A common trade name is *Visipaque®*.

Storage/Stability

Iodixanol should be stored between 20°-25°C (68°-77°F); excursions permitted between 15°-30°C. Do not open foil overwrap, which serves as a moisture and light barrier, from flexible containers until immediately before injecting. Protect vials, glass and polymer bottles, and flexible containers from strong daylight and direct exposure to sunlight. Only vials and glass and polymer bottles may be stored at 37°C (98.6°F) for up to 1 month in a contrast agent warmer utilizing circulating warm air. Special handling and storage for polymer bottles only: Do not freeze or use if the product is inadvertently frozen. Freezing may compromise the closure integrity of these packages.

Compatibility/Compounding Considerations

The manufacturer does not recommend mixing or administering with any other drugs, solutions or total parenteral nutritional solutions.

Dosage Forms/Regulatory Status

VETERINARY-LABELED PRODUCTS: NONE.

HUMAN-LABELED PRODUCTS:
Iodixanol Injection (dosage expressed as organically bound iodine): 270 mg/mL & 320 mg/mL; *Visipaque®*; (Rx)

Revisions/References

Monograph written February 2014.

Imai, K., et al. (2011). Serum Clearance of Iodixanol for Estimating Glomerular Filtration Rate in Calves. Journal of Veterinary Medical Science 73(12): 1625-8.

Imai, K., et al. (2012). Estimation of glomerular filtration rate in calves using the contrast medium iodixanol. Veterinary Journal 193(1): 174-9.

Katayama, R., et al. (2012). Simplified procedure for the estimation of glomerular filtration rate following intravenous administration of iodixanol in cats. American Journal of Veterinary Research 73(9): 1344-9.

Michigoshi, Y., et al. (2012). Estimation of glomerular filtration rate in rabbits by a single-sample method using iodixanol. Laboratory Animals 46(4): 341-4.

Satoh, H., et al. (2011). Optimum conditions for serum clearance of iodixanol, applicable to the estimation of glomerular filtration rate in horses. Veterinary Research Communications 35(7): 463-8.

Iohexol

(eye-oh-hex-ol)   Omnipaque®

Contrast Agent

Prescriber Highlights

▶ Contrast agent used in medical imaging and to estimate GFR.
▶ Fewer adverse effects than with older ionic iodine contrast agents.

Uses/Indications

Iohexol can be used as a contrast agent for variety of radiographic imaging procedures in veterinary patients, and can be used as a marker agent for estimating glomerular filtration rates (GFR) in dogs or cats. The current usual laboratory measures of renal function (plasma/serum creatinine, plasma/blood urea nitrogen) are not very sensitive indicators for detecting early kidney disease or monitoring real-time renal function status, so other tests are needed. This is an area of intense research interest; it is hoped that, ultimately, results from a simple one or two sample test incorporated with patient characteristics that estimate extra-cellular fluid volume (*e.g.*, age, weight, breed, etc.) might be inserted into an equation that then can be used to reasonably estimate renal function status. Iohexol clearance closely mimics inulin clearance, but iohexol has the advantages of being readily available in dosage forms amenable for clinical use, less expensive than inulin, and being stable in plasma or urine.

Iohexol, when used as a contrast agent can be administered (depending on product and procedure) via intravascular (venous and arterial), intrathecal, intracavitary, or oral routes.

Pharmacology/Actions

Iohexol is a near ideal marker for measuring glomerular filtration rate and thereby, renal function. Its protein binding is negligible, it is nearly 100% excreted unchanged in the urine within 24 hours and can be measured in plasma using a variety of assays.

When used as a radio contrast agent, organic iodine is relatively radiopaque and can help define adjacent structures.

Iohexol has a lower osmolality when compared with conventional (ionic) radio contrast agents, and has been associated (in humans) with a lower incidence of side effects such as pain, heat sensations, adverse hemodynamic changes, EKG changes, endothelial and erythrocyte damage.

Pharmacokinetics

After intravascular administration, iohexol is rapidly distributed throughout the circulation. Protein binding is very low (<1%). Within 24 hours, nearly 100% of a dose is excreted in the urine in patients with normal renal function. In dogs, mean pharmacokinetic parameters reported include: volume of distribution (Vd_{SS}):

221 mL/kg; clearance in dogs is about 2.5 – 2.9 mL/kg/min; mean residence time: 82 minutes; elimination half-life: 75 minutes (Heiene et al. 2010), (Goy-Thollot et al. 2006). Mean clearance of iohexol in cats reported include: 2.3 mL/kg/min (Heiene et al. 2009), and 2.75 mL/kg/min (Goy-Thollot et al. 2006).

Iohexol has an elimination half-life of about 2 hours in human patients.

Contraindications/Precautions/Warnings

Iohexol is contraindicated in patients with a prior hypersensitivity reaction.

Adverse Effects

When used intravascularly, iohexol appears to be well tolerated, but usage in dogs or cats has been limited. Hypersensitivity reactions with iohexol can occur, but in humans, only very rarely. Nephrotoxicity from iohexol is potentially possible, but the risk appears slight. Iohexol is considered to be one of the agents used for contrast studies with the lowest toxicity for humans.

Reproductive/Nursing Safety

While iohexol use in the latter stages of pregnancy potentially carries some fetal risk (thyroid function in newborns), the FDA has designated it as a category *B* drug (*Animal studies have not demonstrated risk to the fetus, but there are no adequate studies in pregnant women; or animal studies have shown an adverse effect, but adequate studies in pregnant women have not demonstrated a risk to the fetus during the first trimester of pregnancy, and there is no evidence of risk in later trimesters.*)

Iohexol is distributed into milk in very low quantities, but no adverse effects have been seen in breastfeeding infants whose mothers received iohexol; the American Academy of Pediatrics considers that iohexol is usually compatible with breastfeeding.

Overdosage/Acute Toxicity

The adverse effects of intravenous overdosage can be serious and life-threatening and primarily affect the pulmonary and cardiovascular systems. Clinical signs can include: cyanosis, bradycardia, acidosis, pulmonary hemorrhage, convulsions, coma, and cardiac arrest; treatment is supportive.

Drug Interactions

The following drug interactions have either been reported or are theoretical in humans or animals receiving iohexol and may be of in veterinary patients. Unless otherwise noted, use together is not necessarily contraindicated, but weigh the potential risks and perform additional monitoring when appropriate.

- **DRUGS THAT MAY PROLONG QTc INTERVALS** (*e.g.,* **amiodarone, cisapride, procainamide, quinidine, sotalol, cisapride, dolasetron, moxifloxacin**): Iohexol may cause additive prolongation of QTc interval. Iohexol does not cause as much QTc prolongation (in humans) as diatrizoate.
- **IODINE ISOTOPES**: Iohexol may alter binding to thyroid tissue for up to two weeks.
- **PHENOTHIAZINES**: Iohexol (especially when used intrathecally) may increase risk for lowering seizure threshold.

Laboratory Considerations

- **Thyroid Function Tests**: If iodine-containing isotopes are to be used for diagnosing thyroid disease, prior use of iohexol can reduce the iodine-binding capacity of thyroid tissue for up to 2 weeks. Thyroid function tests that do not depend on iodine estimation are not affected.

Doses

- **DOGS/CATS:**

  To estimate GFR: At the time of writing (2014), the widespread clinical use or usefulness for limited-sample iohexol clearance

determination in dogs and cats has yet to be realized, but for use in clinical settings the following illustrate that results are promising. Follow the current literature and scientific proceedings for more information as it becomes available. For more information on protocols, etc. contact your clinical laboratory service. It is reported that the Diagnostic Center Laboratory at Michigan State University will perform assays for iohexol—see http://www.dcpah.msu.edu for more information.

a) Dogs: Comparing iohexol clearance using a limited sampling (2-4 sample) method versus a 9-sample method; study done in healthy dogs: Using iohexol 300 mg/mL given IV over a minute. Doses administered varied from 129 – 658 mg/kg of iohexol. The lower doses were initially given to dogs early in the study due to concerns for toxicity, but resulted in many samples with plasma concentrations too low for accurate analysis. No toxicity was seen at the higher dose. Using the 2-sample method, samples were obtained at 2 and 3 hours post dose; 3-sample method at 2, 3, and 4 hours post-dose. Clearance was predicted via a trapezoidal method using an empirical polynomial regression equation. Authors concluded that limited sample methods for iohexol clearance may be acceptable in most situations in which available resources do not allow determination of the complete plasma disappearance curve. (Heiene et al. 2010)

b) Dogs and Cats: Using a single sampling method to estimate iohexol clearance: In the study, dogs were administered iohexol 300 mg/mL at a dose of 90 mg iodine content/kg in non-azotemic animals and 45 mg iodine content/kg in azotemic animals IV. Three samples were drawn (at 120, 180, & 240 minutes in non-azotemic animals; 120, 240, & 360 minutes in azotemic animals). The 120 minute sample was used to assess the validity of a single-sample method. After receiver operating characteristics (ROC) analysis was performed to assess the sensitivity and specificity of the single sampling methods for detection of decreasing GFR in dogs and cats, results for sensitivity and specificity for dogs were 98% and 93%, respectively, and in cats, the sensitivity and specificity were 98% and 93%, respectively. No adverse effects were in the dogs or cats studied (N = 779 dogs; 339 cats). (Miyagawa et al. 2010)

As a contrast agent for patients with suspected GI perforation (extra-label): In cats, the recommended dose is a 1:3 dilution of iohexol 240 at 10 mL/kg of body weight. In dogs, a similar dosage is recommended (700 – 875 mg Iodine/kg, 10 mL/kg). Best administered via orogastric tube (dogs) or nasogastric/nasoesophogeal tube (cats). Radiographs should be obtained immediately following the administration of contrast material; additional sets of radiographs can be obtained at 15, 30, and 60 minutes. (Saunders 2008)

- **BIRDS:**

As a contrast agent (extra-label): Indications for contrast imaging may include differentiation of abdominal masses, organ placement or displacement, assessment of GI abnormalities (perforation, foreign body), or GI transit time (proventricular dilatation disease). Contrast agents safe for use in the avian patient include barium sulfate or iohexol administered directly into the crop by gavage. (Retrograde administration of contrast medium directly into the cloaca may help to evaluate cloacal abnormalities.) Survey radiographs (without contrast) should precede the use of contrast agents. The number of images and intervals are based on the agent used and the purpose of the study. If perforation is suspected, iohexol is preferred over barium sulfate.

Dosing is based on the estimated crop volume of 25-30 mL/kg. Iohexol may be diluted 1:1 with water. (Murray 2008)

Monitoring
- No specific monitoring outside of adverse effects.

Client Information
- This medication is administered by veterinarians only.

Chemistry/Synonyms

Iohexol is a nonionic iodinated contrast agent that occurs as a white to off-white, hygroscopic, odorless powder; it is very soluble in water and in methyl alcohol; practically insoluble or insoluble in chloroform and ether. Commercial products list the concentration of the product as organic iodine concentration per mL. For example, *Omnipaque® 180* contains iohexol 288 mg/mL, equivalent to 180 mg/mL of organic iodine content. Physical properties of iohexol injection include:

Concentration (mg/mL) organic iodine	Osmolality (mOsm/kg H$_2$O)	Viscosity @ 20°C	Viscosity @ 37°C	Specific Gravity (grams/mL) @37°C
180	408	3.1	2	1.209
210	460	4.2	2.5	1.244
240	520	5.8	3.4	1.280
300	672	11.8	6.3	1.349
350	844	20.4	10.4	1.406

Iohexol may also be known as WIN-39424, iohexolum, ioheksoli, or ioheksolis. A common trade name is *Omnipaque®*.

Storage/Stability

Iohexol should be stored at room temperature 25°C (68°F); excursions permitted between 15°-30°C. Protect from light.

Compatibility/Compounding Considerations

Depending on concentration, the following drugs are reported **compatible** with iohexol: ampicillin, chloramphenicol sodium succinate, cimetidine, diazepam, diphenhydramine, epinephrine, gentamicin, heparin, hydrocortisone sodium succinate, lidocaine, methylprednisolone sodium succinate, nitroglycerin, protamine, and vasopressin. Because compatibility depends on several factors and is time dependent, it is advisable to contact a hospital pharmacist before admixing drugs.

Dosage Forms/Regulatory Status

VETERINARY-LABELED PRODUCTS: NONE.

HUMAN-LABELED PRODUCTS:

Iohexol Injection (preservative-free; concentrations are listed as organic iodine content per mL): 180 mg/mL, 240 mg/mL, 300 mg/mL & 350 mg/mL in 10 mL, 20 mL, 30 mL, 50 mL, 100 mL, 150 mL, 200 mL, & 500 mL vials, bottles, syringes or cartridges (depending on concentration); *Omnipaque®*; (Rx)

Revisions/References

Monograph revised/updated February 2014.

Goy-Thollot, I., et al. (2006). Iohexol plasma clearance in healthy dogs and cats. Veterinary Radiology & Ultrasound 47(2): 168-73.

Heiene, R., et al. (2010). Glomerular filtration rate in dogs as estimated via plasma clearance of inulin and iohexol and use of limited-sample methods. American Journal of Veterinary Research 71(9): 1100-7.

Heiene, R., et al. (2009). Estimation of glomerular filtration rate via 2-and 4-sample plasma clearance of iohexol and creatinine in clinically normal cats. American Journal of Veterinary Research 70(2): 176-85.

Miyagawa, Y., et al. (2010). Assessments of Factors that Affect Glomerular Filtration Rate and Indirect Markers of Renal Function in Dogs and Cats. Journal of Veterinary Medical Science 72(9): 1129-36.

Murray, J. (2008). Avian Radiographic Imaging. Proceedings: AAV. accessed via Veterinary Information Network; vin.com

Saunders, A. B. (2008). Team Approach to Treating the Emergency Patient with GI Emergencies: Imaging. Proceedings: IVECCS. accessed via Veterinary Information Network; vin.com

Ipodate
(eye-poe-date)

Antithyroid Agent

Prescriber Highlights
▶ Organic iodine compound that may be useful in some cats for medical treatment of hyperthyroidism.
▶ Very limited experience.
▶ Less effective for cats with severe hyperthyroidism.
▶ Efficacy may be transient.
▶ Dosage forms must be compounded and may be difficult to locate.

Uses/Indications

Ipodate may be useful in some cats for the short-term medical treatment of mild hyperthyroidism when methimazole (or carbimazole) cannot be tolerated. Because it uses a different mechanism of action than methimazole, ipodate may potentially be useful in reducing methimazole dosages (and hence toxicity). Efficacy is limited and likely transient. An open label study using iopanoic acid, a related compound, for treating spontaneous hyperthyroidism in cats found that while mean serum T3 concentrations decreased compared to baseline and five (of eleven) cats had a partial response during the initial 4 weeks of therapy, effects were transient and no significant improvements in clinical signs or physical exam findings were noted (Gallagher et al. 2011).

Pharmacology/Actions

Ipodate's efficacy in treating hyperthyroidism is thought to be primarily due to inhibition of the conversion of T$_4$ to T$_3$. Ipodate may also block T$_3$ receptors and thereby protect the heart from the hypertrophic effects of hyperthyroidism. It may block the actions of TSH.

Pharmacokinetics

The drug is well absorbed after oral administration. Other pertinent pharmacokinetic data for cats is unavailable.

Contraindications/Precautions/Warnings

Ipodate is contraindicated in patients with known hypersensitivity to it. It should be used with caution in patients who have had previous reactions to iodine compounds. Humans with hepatic dysfunction should not receive multiple doses of the drug as renal toxicity has resulted in a few patients. It is recommended to use with caution in human patients with hyperuricemia (possible uric acid nephropathy).

Adverse Effects

Cats reportedly tolerate ipodate well, but may become refractory to treatment after a relatively short time. Oral iodine containing products can cause GI distress (nausea, vomiting, diarrhea, cramping, inappetence). Drug-induced pemphigus is a possibility. Skin rashes, itching, dizziness and headache have been reported by human patients.

Reproductive/Nursing Safety

If administered to pregnant cats, congenital hypothyroidism is a possibility.

Overdosage/Acute Toxicity

No specific information located. Cats have reportedly tolerated daily doses up to 400 mg.

Drug Interactions

The following drug interactions have either been reported or are theoretical in humans or animals receiving ipodate and may be of in veterinary patients. Unless otherwise noted, use together is not necessarily contraindicated, but weigh the potential risks and perform additional monitoring when appropriate.

- **IODINE, RADIOACTIVE:** Ipodate may interfere with radioactive iodine therapy. It is suggested to treat no sooner than 2 weeks after discontinuing ipodate (3-4 weeks or more if possible).

Laboratory Considerations

- Ipodate may increase BSP retention times and **serum bilirubin** levels.
- False positive **urine protein** determinations may occur.
- Ipodate can interfere with **thyroid scanning**.

Doses

- **CATS:**

  For short-term medical treatment of hyperthyroidism in patients who cannot tolerate methimazole and whose owners will not permit surgery or radioiodine therapy (extra-label): Very limited efficacy and may be difficult to obtain. Most dosage recommendations are initially 50 mg per cat PO q12h. Dosage may be increased in 50 mg increments up to 200 mg per day. The dosage is usually divided q12h, but some state 100 – 200 mg per cat can be given once daily.

Monitoring

- Clinical efficacy (heart rate, body weight, etc.).
- Serum T3 (**Note:** T4 did not change—remained high in study group).

Client Information

- It must be stressed to owners that this drug will decrease excessive thyroid hormones, but does not cure the condition and compliance with the treatment regimen is necessary for success.
- Long-term efficacy is questionable.

Chemistry/Synonyms

An orally administered radiopaque organic iodine compound, ipodate sodium occurs as a white to off-white, fine crystalline powder. It is freely soluble in alcohol and water. Each 500 mg capsule contains 61.4% (or 333.4 mg) of iodine.

Ipodate calcium may also be known as: calcium iopodate, calcium ipodate, ipodate calcium, *Solu-Biloptin®*, and *Solubiloptine®*.

Ipodate sodium may also be known as: sodium iopodate, sodium ipodate, NSC-106962, *Bilivist®*, *Biloptin®*, and *Oragrafin®*.

Storage/Stability

Store capsules in tight containers and protect from light.

Compatibility/Compounding Considerations

No specific information noted.

Dosage Forms/Regulatory Status

VETERINARY-LABELED PRODUCTS: NONE.

HUMAN-LABELED PRODUCTS:

None; must obtained via a compounding pharmacy.

Note: Most of the studies using ipodate in cats have been done with calcium ipodate. It is likely that sodium ipodate would be fairly equivalent. If the compounding pharmacy has access to calcium ipodate, it is suggested to use that form. Other options that have been used anecdotally in cats at similar dosages include iopanoic acid or diatrizoate meglumine (Trepanier 2006).

Revisions/References

Monograph revised/updated May 2014.

Gallagher, A. E. & D. L. Panciera (2011). Efficacy of iopanoic acid for treatment of spontaneous hyperthyroidism in cats. Journal of Feline Medicine and Surgery 13(6): 441-7.

Trepanier, L. A. (2006). Medical management of hyperthyroidism. Clinical Techniques in Small Animal Practice 21(1): 22-8.

Ipratropium Bromide

(eye-prah-troh-pee-um)   Atrovent®

Inhaled Antimuscarinic

Prescriber Highlights

▶ Inhaled antimuscarinic agent for adjunctive treatment of bronchoconstrictive conditions.

▶ Very little information available for use in small animals.

▶ Likely safe.

▶ May need to be administered quite often; duration of activity is relatively short.

Uses/Indications

Locally administered (inhaled) ipratropium bromide can be used for the adjunctive treatment of bronchospastic conditions (RAO; heaves). While ipratropium has been shown to have bronchodilatory effects in experimentally induced bronchoconstriction in cats (Leemans et al. 2006; Leemans et al. 2009; Leemans et al. 2012) and may prove beneficial for the short-term treatment of bronchospasm, additional research is required to determine its role for clinical use.

Pharmacology/Actions

Ipratropium inhibits vagally mediated reflexes by antagonizing acetylcholine. Increases in intracellular concentrations of cyclic guanosine monophosphate (cyclic GMP) secondary to acetylcholine are prevented, thereby reducing bronchial smooth muscle constriction. Unlike atropine, ipratropium does not reduce mucociliary clearance.

Pharmacokinetics

Because the medication is inhaled, minimal drug is absorbed in the systemic circulation. In humans, elimination half-life is about 2 hours. In healthy cats with experimentally induced bronchospasm, inhaled (neb) ipratropium gave maximal efficacy for about 4 hours. When combined with albuterol (salbutamol), increased efficacy resulted (Leemans et al. 2006). In horses, onset of action is approximately 30 minutes and duration of effect is approximately 4-6 hours.

Contraindications/Precautions/Warnings

Ipratropium is contraindicated in patients hypersensitive to it or other atropine derivatives.

It should be used with caution in other conditions where antimuscarinics may be harmful, including narrow-angle glaucoma, bladder-neck obstruction, or prostatic hypertrophy.

Adverse Effects

Adverse effects are unlikely to be significant. Tracheal or bronchial irritation (coughing) has been reported on occasion. Allergic responses are possible and some patients develop anticholinergic effects.

Reproductive/Nursing Safety

Large oral dosages in laboratory animals did not cause teratogenic effects. In humans, the FDA categorizes ipratropium as category *B* for use during the first two trimesters of pregnancy (*Animal studies have not yet demonstrated risk to the fetus, but there are no adequate studies in pregnant women; or animal studies have shown an adverse effect, but adequate studies in pregnant women have not demonstrated a risk to the fetus in the first trimester of pregnancy, and there is no evidence of risk in later trimesters.*)

Ipratropium is likely to be safe to use during nursing.

Overdosage/Acute Toxicity

Overdosage is unlikely to be a cause for concern. The drug is not well absorbed orally or after inhalation and oral LD50 values for laboratory animals were greater than 1 g/kg.

Drug Interactions

The following drug interactions have either been reported or are theoretical in humans or animals receiving ipratropium and may be of in veterinary patients. Unless otherwise noted, use together is not necessarily contraindicated, but weigh the potential risks and perform additional monitoring when appropriate.

- **ANTICHOLINERGIC DRUGS**: May cause additive antimuscarinic effects.
- **BETA-ADRENERGIC AGONISTS** (*e.g.*, **albuterol**): May have additive therapeutic effects.

Laboratory Considerations

- No specific concerns were noted.

Doses

- **HORSES:**

  For adjunctive treatment of RAO, heaves (mild to moderate disease); (extra-label): For adult horses, most recommend 180 micrograms aerosol per horse inhaled via an equine specific mask every 6 hours (range q4-8h). A study in 6 adult horses with heaves, found 0.3 mg (300 micrograms) per horse via inhalation that some indices of airway function were improved for between 6-24 hours after ipratropium administration, however clinical scores for breathing effort were not clinically significant (McGorum et al. 2013). A reported dosage for foals with severe bronchospasm is 2 – 3 micrograms/kg via aerosol q6-8h. (Rush 2007)

- **SMALL MAMMALS:**

  As a bronchodilator in rats (extra-label): One puff into nebulization chamber twice daily. (Monks et al. 2009)

Monitoring

- Clinical efficacy.

Client Information

- If using the aerosol metered dose inhalers, do not use after 200 inhalations (puffs) even if there appears to be medication remaining; active ingredient cannot be assured; do not shake the HFA canister before using.
- Normally given as an aerosol into the lungs, often with other drugs, to help your animal breathe better. Special masks for dogs, cats, and horses are usually used.
- Ipratropium is usually very safe but irritation of the throat and lungs can occur.
- No need to shake aerosol before each use. Prime (2 sprays) before first using or if not used in past 3 days.
- Do not store aerosol canister in hot places or dispose of it by burning it.

Chemistry/Synonyms

Ipratropium bromide occurs as a white or almost white crystalline powder. It is soluble in water and slightly soluble in alcohol. The pH of a 1% solution is between 5-7.5.

Ipratropium bromide may also be known as Sch-1000; many trade names are available including *Atrovent®*.

Storage/stability

The solution for inhalation should be stored at room temperature and protected from light. Keep in foil pouch until time of use. The metered dose inhalers should be stored at room temperature.

Compatibility/Compounding Considerations

The solution for nebulization may be mixed with albuterol or metaproterenol if used within one hour.

Dosage Forms/Regulatory Status

VETERINARY-LABELED PRODUCTS: NONE.

HUMAN-LABELED PRODUCTS:

Ipratropium Bromide Solution for Inhalation: 0.02% (500 micrograms/vial) preservative free in 25 & 60 unit-dose vials (2.5 mL UD "nebs"); generic; (Rx)

Ipratropium Bromide Aerosol for Inhalation: each actuation delivers 17 micrograms in 12.9 grams metered dose inhaler w/mouthpiece (approx. 200 inhalations); *Atrovent® HFA*; (Rx)

Nasal sprays are available, and in combination with albuterol as nebs: *DuoNeb®* and as a metered dose inhaler, *Combivent®*.

Revisions/References

Monograph revised/updated February 2014.

Leemans, J., et al. (2009). A pilot study comparing the antispasmodic effects of inhaled salmeterol, salbutamol and ipratropium bromide using different aerosol devices on muscarinic bronchoconstriction in healthy cats. Veterinary Journal 180(2): 236-45.

Leemans, J., et al. (2012). A comparison of in vitro relaxant responses to ipratropium bromide, beta-adrenoceptor agonists and theophylline in feline bronchial smooth muscle. Veterinary Journal 193(1): 228-33.

Leemans, J., et al. (2006). Bronchoprotective effect of inhaled salmeterol, salbutamol and ipratropium bromide using different devices on muscarinic bronchoconstriction in healthy cats. Proceedings: ECVIM. accessed via Veterinary Information Network; vin.com

McGorum, B. C., et al. (2013). Bronchodilator activity of the selective muscarinic antagonist revatropate in horses with heaves. Veterinary Journal 195(1): 80-5.

Monks, D. & M. Cowan (2009). Chronic respiratory disease in rats. Proceedings: AAVC-UEP. accessed via Veterinary Information Network; vin.com

Rush, B. (2007). Foal Pneumonia. Proceedings: ABVP. accessed via Veterinary Information Network; vin.com

Irbesartan

(ihr-beh-sar-tan)   Avapro®

Angiotensin-II Receptor Blocker (ARB)

Prescriber Highlights

▶ ARB that may be useful in treating dogs or cats with hypertension secondary to renal insufficiency.

▶ Very limited experience in veterinary medicine.

▶ Not safe during pregnancy.

Uses/Indications

Although experience in veterinary medicine is minimal, irbesartan may prove useful in treating canine or feline hypertension associated with renal insufficiency and along with an ACE inhibitor, for proteinuria associated with glomerular disease. It may be effective in the adjunctive treatment of heart failure when dogs are unable to tolerate ACE inhibitors, but documentation for this use is lacking. One study, using very high irbesartan dosages (60 mg/kg PO twice daily) in dogs with subacute mitral regurgitation, demonstrated no improvement in left ventricular function or prevention of left ventricular remodeling (Perry et al. 2002). An experimental study in cats, showed that irbesartan at 2, 6, or 10 mg/kg at 90 minutes significantly reduced blood pressure associated with exogenously administered angiotensin (Coleman et al. 2013).

Pharmacology/Actions

Irbesartan is an angiotensin-II receptor blocker (ARB). By selectively blocking the AT1 receptor, aldosterone synthesis and secretion is reduced causing vasodilation and decreased potassium and increased sodium excretion. While plasma concentrations of renin and angiotensin-II are increased, this does not counteract the blood pressure lowering effects of irbesartan. Irbesartan does not interfere with substance P or bradykinin responses.

Irbesartan does not need to be converted to an active metabolite as does the ARB, losartan (*Cozaar®*). Dogs, unlike humans, reportedly do not convert losartan to the active metabolite.

Pharmacokinetics

After single 30 mg/kg oral doses in dogs with experimentally induced renal hypertension, irbesartan peak levels occurred between 3-4 hours later and elimination half-life was approximately 9 hours. After 30 mg/kg doses PO once daily for 8 days, the elimination half-life was approximately 21 hours (Huang et al. 2005).

In humans, absorption is rapid and bioavailability ranges from 60-80%. Peak levels occur in about 1.5-2 hours. Bioavailability is not altered by the presence of food. The drug is 90% bound to plasma proteins and crosses the blood-brain barrier and placenta in small quantities. Irbesartan is metabolized in the liver via glucuronidation and oxidation; metabolites are not active. Both metabolites and unchanged drug are eliminated primarily in the feces and to a lesser extent, urine. Terminal elimination half-life ranges from 11-15 hours. Dosages do not need to be adjusted in patients with renal dysfunction.

Contraindications/Precautions/Warnings

Patients who are volume or sodium depleted should have these corrected before starting therapy. Do not use in hypotensive patients. In humans, the drug is contraindicated in patients hypersensitive to it. It should not be used during pregnancy (see Reproductive Safety).

Adverse Effects

An adverse effect profile for dogs is not known due to limited use of this medication. In humans, the most commonly reported adverse effects include diarrhea, dyspepsia, fatigue, and orthostatic dizziness/hypotension.

Reproductive/Nursing Safety

Irbesartan is not safe to use during pregnancy. Studies in pregnant rats given high doses demonstrated a variety of fetal abnormalities (renal pelvic cavitation, hydroureter, absence of renal papilla). Smaller doses in rabbits caused increased maternal death and spontaneous abortion. In humans, the drug is considered teratogenic, particularly during the 2nd and 3rd trimesters. During this time, the FDA categorizes irbesartan as category **D** for use during pregnancy (*There is evidence of human fetal risk, but the potential benefits from the use of the drug in pregnant women may be acceptable despite its potential risks.*) If pregnancy is detected in patients receiving irbesartan, the drug should be discontinued as soon as possible.

Because small amounts of irbesartan have been detected in rat milk and there is significant concern about the safety of the drug in neonates, the manufacturer recommends that it not be used in nursing women.

Overdosage/Acute Toxicity

Rats and mice survived acute oral overdoses in excess of 2000 mg/kg. Likely effects seen in an overdose situation include hypotension and either bradycardia or tachycardia; treatment is supportive. Contact an animal poison control center for further information.

Drug Interactions

The following drug interactions have either been reported or are theoretical in humans or animals receiving irbesartan and potentially could be of in veterinary patients. Unless otherwise noted, use together is not necessarily contraindicated, but weigh the potential risks and perform additional monitoring when appropriate.

- **ACE INHIBITORS (benazepril, enalapril**, etc.): Increased risk for adverse effects (e.g.; hypotension, hyperkalemia, renal function changes); increased monitoring may be warranted.
- **ASPIRIN**: Possible reduced antihypertensive effect of irbesartan and increased risk for renal impairment; increased monitoring may be warranted.
- **NSAIDs** (*e.g.,* **carprofen, meloxicam**, etc.): Possible reduced antihypertensive effect of irbesartan and increased risk for renal impairment; increased monitoring may be warranted.
- **POTASSIUM PREPARATIONS, POTASSIUM–SPARING DIURETICS** (*e.g.,* **spironolactone**): Increased risk for hyperkalemia; increased monitoring of serum potassium may be warranted.

Laboratory Considerations

- No specific concerns were noted.

Doses

- **DOGS/CATS:**

  Note: At the time of update (2/2014), dosage recommendations for clinical use of irbesartan for hypertension, proteinuria or heart failure in dogs and/or cats are very preliminary. 5 mg/kg PO q12-24h has been recommended anecdotally for dogs. This is not unreasonable based upon a PK/PD study in healthy beagles where the authors concluded that although further studies are necessary, 5 mg/kg seems to be the more appropriate dose (versus 2 mg/kg) to obtain a hypotensive effect in Beagles (Carlucci et al. 2013). Dosages for cats are still mostly unknown although the drug does seem to have efficacy for angiotensin-induced hypertension (Coleman et al. 2013).

Monitoring

- Blood pressure, heart rate.
- Serum electrolytes, BUN, creatinine.
- Adverse Effects: possibly GI (diarrhea), somnolence/activity changes.

Client Information

- This medication may be given with or without food. If your animal vomits or acts sick after getting it on an empty stomach, give with food or small treat to see if this helps. If vomiting continues, contact your veterinarian.
- Because this medication has not been used very often in dogs or cats, watch carefully for any side effects and report them to your veterinarian. Possible side effects include: diarrhea, vomiting, lack of appetite, fatigue (tiredness), and low blood pressure (*e.g.,* fainting, muscle weakness, can't exercise, etc.).
- This drug has caused birth defects and should not be used in pregnant animals. If a human in the household is pregnant, they should be very careful not to ingest these tablets and wear disposable gloves when administering doses and wash hands after touching these tablets.

Chemistry/Synonyms

Irbesartan is a nonpeptide angiotensin-II antagonist and occurs as white to off-white, crystalline powder. It is practically insoluble in water and slightly soluble in alcohol.

Irbesartan may also be known as: BMS 186295, SR 47436, Irbesartanum, *Aprovel®, Arbit®, Avalide®, Avapro®, Cavapro®, Coaproval®, Ecard®, Ibsan®, Irban®, Irbes®, Iretensa®, Irovel®, Irvell®, Isart®,* and *Karvea®.*

Storage/Stability

Irbesartan tablets should be stored at room temperature (15-30°C).

Compatibility/Compounding Considerations

No specific information noted.

Dosage Forms/Regulatory Status

VETERINARY-LABELED PRODUCTS: NONE.

The ARCI (Racing Commissioners International) has designated this drug as a class 3 substance.

HUMAN-LABELED PRODUCTS:
Irbesartan Tablets: 75 mg, 150 mg, & 300 mg; *Avapro*®, generic; (Rx)

Irbesartan 150 mg with Hydrochlorothiazide 12.5 mg Tablets, Irbesartan 300 mg with Hydrochlorothiazide 12.5 mg or 25 mg Tablets; *Avalide*®, generic; (Rx)

Revisions/References
Monograph revised/updated February 2014.

Carlucci, L., et al. (2013). Pharmacokinetics and pharmacodynamics (PK/PD) of irbesartan in Beagle dogs after oral administration at two dose rates (Abstract). Polish Journal of Veterinary Sciences **16**(3): 555-61.

Coleman, A. E., et al. (2013). Attenuation of the Pressor Response to Exogenous Angiotensin by Angiotensin Receptor Blockers in Normal Cats (Abstract). ACVIM. accessed via Veterinary Information Network; vin.com

Huang, X., et al. (2005). Pharmacokinetic and pharmacodynamic interaction between irbesartan and hydrochlorothiazide in renal hypertensive dogs. J Cardiovasc Pharmacol **46**(6): 863-9.

Perry, G., et al. (2002). Angiotensin II receptor blockade does not improve left ventricular function and remodeling in subacute mitral regurgitation in the dog. J AM Coll Cardiol **39**(8): 1374-9.

Iron Dextran
(eye-urn dex-tran)

Injectable Hematinic

Prescriber Highlights

▶ Injectable hematinic. Used with EPO in small animals.

▶ Contraindications: Do not give IV or SC. Known hypersensitivity to iron dextran, or with any anemia other than iron deficiency anemia; acute renal infections, in conjunction with oral iron supplements.

▶ Adverse Effects: Pain with IM injection. Prostration & muscular weakness, anaphylactoid reactions.

▶ High dosages may cause increased incidences of teratogenicity & embryotoxicity.

▶ Pigs born of vitamin E/selenium-deficient sows may demonstrate nausea, vomiting, & sudden death within 1 hour of injection.

▶ IM use in pigs after 4 weeks of age may cause muscle tissue staining.

Uses/Indications

Iron dextran is used in the treatment and prophylaxis of iron deficiency anemias, primarily in neonatal food-producing animals. It is also commonly employed when dogs or cats receive erythrocyte-stimulating agents such as epoetin (EPO) or darbepoetin (DPO).

Pharmacology/Actions

Iron is necessary for myoglobin and hemoglobin in the transport and utilization of oxygen. While neither stimulating erythropoiesis nor correcting hemoglobin abnormalities not caused by iron deficiency, iron administration does correct both physical signs and decreased hemoglobin levels secondary to iron deficiency.

Ionized iron is a component in the enzymes cytochrome oxidase, succinic dehydrogenase, and xanthine oxidase.

Pharmacokinetics

After IM injection, iron dextran is slowly absorbed primarily via the lymphatic system. About 60% of the drug is absorbed within 3 days of injection and up to 90% of the dose is absorbed after 1-3 weeks. The remaining drug may be absorbed slowly over several months.

After absorption, the reticuloendothelial cells of the liver, spleen, and bone marrow gradually clear the drug from plasma. The iron is cleaved from the dextran component and the dextran is then metabolized or excreted. The iron is immediately bound to protein elements to form hemosiderin, ferritin or transferrin. Iron crosses the placenta, but in what form is unknown. Only traces of iron are excreted in milk.

Iron is not readily eliminated from the body. Iron liberated by the destruction of hemoglobin is reused by the body and only small amounts are lost by the body via hair and nail growth, normal skin desquamation, and GI tract sloughing. Accumulation can result with repeated dosing as only trace amounts of iron are eliminated in the feces, bile, or urine.

Contraindications/Precautions/Warnings

Iron dextran is contraindicated in patients with known hypersensitivity to it or with any anemia other than iron deficiency anemia. It is not to be used in patients with acute renal infections, and should not be used in conjunction with oral iron supplements.

Observe patient after dosing as rarely, anaphylaxis can occur.

Adverse Effects

The manufacturers of iron dextran injection for use in pigs state that occasionally pigs may react after injection with iron dextran, characterized by prostration and muscular weakness. Rarely, death may result from an anaphylactoid reaction. Iron dextran used in pigs born of vitamin E/selenium-deficient sows may demonstrate nausea, vomiting, and sudden death within 1 hour of injection. Iron dextran injected IM in pigs after 4 weeks of age may cause muscle tissue staining.

In dogs or cats, pain on IM injection can occur. Anaphylaxis is rare, but can occur. Chronic overdoses can cause hepatic cirrhosis in dogs.

Large SC doses have been associated with the development of sarcomas in laboratory animals (rabbits, mice, rats, and hamsters).

Reproductive/Nursing Safety

High dosages may cause increased incidences of teratogenicity and embryotoxicity. Use only when clearly necessary at recommended doses in pregnant animals. In humans, the FDA categorizes this drug as category *C* for use during pregnancy (*Animal studies have shown an adverse effect on the fetus, but there are no adequate studies in humans; or there are no animal reproduction studies and no adequate studies in humans.*)

Traces of unmetabolized iron dextran are excreted in milk.

Overdosage/Acute Toxicity

Depending on the size of the dose, inadvertent overdose injections may require chelation therapy. For more information, refer to the Ferrous Sulfate monograph for information on using deferoxamine and other treatments for iron toxicity.

Drug Interactions

The following drug interactions have either been reported or are theoretical in humans or animals receiving iron and may be of in veterinary patients. Unless otherwise noted, use together is not necessarily contraindicated, but weigh the potential risks and perform additional monitoring when appropriate.

■ **CHLORAMPHENICOL:** Because chloramphenicol may delay the response to iron administration, avoid using it in patients with iron deficiency anemia.

Laboratory Considerations

■ Large doses of injectable iron may discolor the serum brown that can cause falsely elevated **serum bilirubin** values and falsely decreased **serum calcium** values.

■ After large doses of iron dextran, **serum iron** values may not be meaningful for up to 3 weeks.

Doses

■ **DOGS:**

For iron supplementation in association with erythrocyte stimulating agents (EPO, DPO); (extra-label): At the time EPO or DPO therapy is initiated, most recommend 50 – 300 mg per dog IM; approximately 10 – 20 mg/kg (max. of 300 mg per dog). A single injection may be all that is needed, but 50 – 300 mg per dog IM as needed—generally no more than once monthly—can be considered.

For iron deficiency anemia: Iron dextran 10 – 20 mg/kg once, followed by oral therapy with ferrous sulfate (see ferrous sulfate monograph). (Weiser 1989)

- **CATS:**

For iron supplementation in association with erythrocyte stimulating agents (EPO, DPO); (extra-label): At the time EPO or DPO therapy is initiated, most recommend 50 per cat IM; approximately 10 mg/kg. A single injection may be all that is needed, but 50 mg per cat IM as needed—generally no more than once monthly—can be considered.

For prevention of transient neonatal iron deficiency anemia (extra-label): 50 mg iron dextran injection at 18 days of age. (Weiser 1989)

- **FERRETS:**

For iron deficiency (extra-label): 10 mg/kg IM once weekly. (Williams 2000)

- **SWINE:**

For prevention of iron deficiency anemia in baby pigs (2-4 days of age); (labeled-dose): Administer an initial intramuscular injection of 100 mg of elemental iron to each animal at 2-4 days of age. Dosage may be repeated in 14-21 days. (Label directions; *Ferrextran-100®*)

- **BIRDS:**

For iron deficiency anemia or following hemorrhage (extra-label): 10 mg/kg IM; repeat in 7-10 days if PCV fails to return to normal. (McDonald 1989)

Monitoring
- If indicated: CBC, RBC indices.
- Adverse reactions.

Client Information
- In pigs, inject IM in the back of the ham.
- In small animals veterinarians administer iron dextran.

Chemistry/Synonyms
Iron dextran is a complex of ferric oxyhydroxide and low molecular weight partially hydrolyzed dextran derivative. The commercially available injection occurs as a dark brown, slightly viscous liquid that is completely miscible with water or normal saline and has a pH of 5.2-6.5.

Iron dextran may also be known as: iron-dextran complex, *Cosmofer®, DexFerrum®, Dexiron®, Driken®, Fercayl®, Ferrocel®, Ferroin®, Ferrum Hausmann®, Fexiron®, Imferdex®, Imferon®, InFeD®, Uniferon®* and *Infufer®*.

Storage/stability
Iron dextran injection should be stored at room temperature (15-30°C); avoid freezing.

Compatibility/Compounding Considerations
Iron dextran injection is reportedly physically **incompatible** when mixed with oxytetracycline HCl and sulfadiazine sodium.

Dosage Forms/Regulatory Status/Withdrawal Times
VETERINARY-LABELED PRODUCTS:
Iron Dextran Injection: 100 mg of elemental iron/mL and 200 mg of elemental iron/mL in 100 mL vials; various manufacturers and trade names; (OTC). FDA-approved for use in swine. No slaughter withdrawal time required.

HUMAN-LABELED PRODUCTS:
Iron Dextran Injection: 50 mg of elemental iron/mL (as dextran) in 1 mL & 2 mL single-dose vials; *InFeD®, DexFerrum®*; (Rx)

Revisions/References
Monograph revised/updated February 2014.

McDonald, S. E. (1989). Summary of medications for use in psittacine birds. JAAV 3(3): 120-7.

Weiser, M. G. (1989). Erythrocytes and Associated Disorders. *The Cat: Diseases and Clinical Management.* R. G. Sherding. New York, Churchill Livingstone. 1: 529-56.

Williams, B. (2000). Therapeutics in Ferrets. Vet Clin NA: Exotic Anim Pract 3:1(Jan): 131-53.

Isoflupredone Acetate

(eye-so-floo-preh-dohn)   Predef 2X®

Injectable Glucocorticoid

For topical or otic use of isoflupredone, see the Topical Dermatological Agents, and Otic Appendixes

Prescriber Highlights
▶ Injectable glucocorticoid labeled for use in cattle, horses & swine for antiinflammatory & immunosuppressive effects.
▶ Less likely to cause early parturition than dexamethasone or betamethasone, but avoid use in pregnancy.
▶ May have mineralocorticoid effects in horses & cattle; hypokalemia has been noted.

Uses/Indications
Isoflupredone acetate is a potent glucocorticoid and like other glucocorticoids can be used for its antiinflammatory or immunosuppressive effects. Labeled indications for isoflupredone include: adjunctive treatment of bovine ketosis, alleviating pain and lameness associated with musculoskeletal conditions, acute hypersensitivity reactions, adjunctive treatment of overwhelming infections with severe toxicity, shock, supportive therapy in the treatment of stress conditions (*e.g.,* surgery), dystocia, retained placenta, inflammatory ocular conditions, snakebite and parturient paresis.

A study evaluating the effects of isoflupredone (20 mg IM) with or without insulin (ultralente 100 Units) on energy metabolism, milk production and overall health in dairy cows during the early lactation phase showed that isoflupredone with or without insulin "offered no metabolic, production, or reproductive benefits in lactating dairy cattle" (Seifi et al. 2007). A study evaluating oxytetracycline with or without isoflupredone acetate for treating experimentally-induced bronchopneumonia in heifers found only animals receiving the combination prevented a reduction in dry-matter intake and average daily gain (ADG) (Hewson et al. 2011). However, the author of that study has subsequently stated that "based on the existing literature, it is currently still not possible to fully determine whether corticosteroids have a clinical application in managing BRD. Differences in treatment outcomes between the limited corticosteroids that have been studied thus far may reflect the method used for BRD diagnosis in the feedlot setting, timing of medical intervention with respect to onset of infection, involvement of multiple respiratory pathogens in naturally occurring respiratory disease, or simply effects specific to the corticosteroids used" (Hewson 2013).

In horses, isoflupredone has been used parenterally to reduce inflammation associated with recurrent airway obstruction (RAO, "heaves", COPD).

While the drug could be used in small animals, it is recommended to use other glucocorticoid agents instead, where there has been more experience and other FDA-approved products for dogs and cats are available.

Pharmacology/Actions

Isoflupredone's antiinflammatory potency is approximately 17X that of hydrocortisone (cortisol). The label states that the glucocorticoid activity of isoflupredone is 50X that of hydrocortisone and 10X that of prednisolone as measured by liver glycogen deposition in rats. Isoflupredone reportedly has some mineralocorticoid effects, and can cause hypokalemia.

For more information on the pharmacologic actions associated with glucocorticoids, see the *Glucocorticoid Agents, General Information* monograph.

Pharmacokinetics

No specific pharmacokinetic values were located. The manufacturer states that gluconeogenic activity persists for 48 hours after dosing in cattle.

Contraindications/Precautions/Warnings

Systemic use of glucocorticoids is generally considered contraindicated in systemic fungal infections (unless used for replacement therapy in Addison's), when administered IM in patients with idiopathic thrombocytopenia, and in patients hypersensitive to a particular compound. Because of their ulcerogenic potential, glucocorticoids should be used with extreme caution in patients with active GI ulcers or those susceptible to them. Use cautiously in patients with diabetes mellitus.

Because it can cause hypokalemia, it should not be used in downer cows or animals susceptible to the effects of hypokalemia.

Chronic use in young, growing animals must be undertaken cautiously, as decreased growth may occur.

Not to be used in calves to be processed into veal.

See Reproductive/Nursing Safety section for information on use during pregnancy.

Adverse Effects

Adverse effects are generally associated with long-term administration of glucocorticoids, particularly if given at higher dosages; these effects generally are manifested as signs of hyperadrenocorticism. Recent research has indicated, however, that even single doses administered to dairy cattle can cause hypokalemia. Potential adverse effects include: reduced milk production, hypokalemia, delayed wound healing, GI ulceration, increased infection rates, diabetes mellitus exacerbation/hyperglycemia, pancreatitis, hepatopathy, renal dysfunction, osteoporosis, laminitis (horses), hypothyroidism, and hyperlipidemia. When administered to young, growing animals, glucocorticoids can retard growth.

Reproductive/Nursing Safety

Avoid using isoflupredone during pregnancy. Glucocorticoids can induce abortion or early parturition in the later stages of pregnancy; most commonly seen in ruminants. While isoflupredone appears to have a much lower abortifacient potential (like hydrocortisone, prednisolone, & triamcinolone) than steroids such as dexamethasone, betamethasone or flumethasone, it may induce premature parturition with retained placenta and its use should generally be avoided during the later stages of pregnancy.

Glucocorticoids used during the first trimester have been linked to a variety of teratogenic effects in dogs and laboratory animals.

Glucocorticoid administration may reduce milk production. Glucocorticoids unbound to plasma proteins will enter milk. High dosages or prolonged administration to mothers may potentially inhibit the growth of nursing newborns.

Overdosage/Acute Toxicity

A single overdose of isoflupredone is unlikely to cause harmful effects. Should clinical signs require intervention, use supportive treatment.

Chronic usage of glucocorticoids can lead to serious adverse effects. Refer to the Adverse Effects section for more information.

Drug Interactions

The following drug interactions have either been reported or are theoretical in humans or animals receiving isoflupredone or other glucocorticoids and may be of in veterinary patients. Unless otherwise noted, use together is not necessarily contraindicated, but weigh the potential risks and perform additional monitoring when appropriate.

- **DIGITALIS GLYCOSIDES (digoxin):** Increased chance of digitalis toxicity may occur should hypokalemia develop; diligent monitoring of potassium and digitalis glycoside levels is recommended.
- **POTASSIUM-DEPLETING DIURETICS (furosemide, thiazides):** Administered concomitantly with glucocorticoids may cause hypokalemia.
- **SALICYLATES:** Glucocorticoids may reduce salicylate blood levels.
- **ULCEROGENIC DRUGS** (*e.g.*, **NSAIDs**): With glucocorticoids may increase the risk of gastrointestinal ulceration.
- **VACCINES, TOXOIDS, BACTERINS:** A diminished immune response may occur after vaccine, toxoid, or bacterin administration; patients receiving corticosteroids at immunosuppressive dosages should generally not receive live attenuated-virus vaccines as virus replication may be augmented.

Laboratory Considerations

- Glucocorticoids may increase **serum cholesterol** and **serum and urine glucose** levels.
- Isoflupredone may decrease **serum potassium.**
- Glucocorticoids can suppress the release of thyroid stimulating hormone (TSH) and reduce **T3 & T4** values; thyroid gland atrophy has been reported after chronic glucocorticoid administration.
- Reactions to **skin tests** may be suppressed by glucocorticoids.
- Glucocorticoids may cause false-negative results of the **nitroblue tetrazolium test** for systemic bacterial infections.

Doses

- **CATTLE:**

  For labeled systemic indications (FDA-approved): 10 – 20 mg (total dose) IM, according to the size of the animal and severity of the condition. The dose may be repeated in 12-24 hours if indicated. (Label information; *Predef 2X®*)

- **HORSES:** (NOTE: RCI CLASS 4)

  For labeled systemic indications (FDA-approved): 5 – 20 mg (total dose) IM repeated as necessary. For intrasynovial administration: 5 – 20 mg or more depending on the size of the joint cavity. (Label information; *Predef 2X®*)

  For intraarticular administration (extra-label): 4 – 20 mg; has a short to medium duration of action. (Goodrich 2006)

  For treatment of "heaves" (RAO) (extra-label): In the study 0.03 mg/kg IM once daily was used. Patients were treated for 14 days and developed significant decreases in serum potassium. (Picandet et al. 2003)

- **SWINE:**

  For labeled systemic indications (FDA-approved): 5 mg (total dose) IM for a 300 lb. animal. Adjust dose proportionally for a smaller or larger animal. (Label information; *Predef 2X®*)

Monitoring

- Single injections may not require monitoring beyond observation of the patient for efficacy and adverse effects, but consider evaluating serum potassium.
- Ongoing usage requires enhanced monitoring including: renal and liver function, CBC, blood glucose and serum electrolytes.

- ACTH stimulation tests may be indicated to determine extent of HPA axis suppression.
- Consider thyroid hormone monitoring if use is prolonged or patient exhibits signs associated with thyroid hormone deficiency.

Client Information

- If used in dairy cattle, warn producer that milk production may be affected.
- If owners are to administer the medication, caution them to only administer as the veterinarian directs.
- Adverse effects become more likely the longer it is used and when used at higher dosages.

Chemistry/Synonyms

Isoflupredone acetate is a fluorinated synthetic corticosteroid with a molecular weight of 420.5. The commercial injection is in an aqueous suspension that also contains sodium citrate, polyethylene glycol 3350, and povidone.

Isoflupredone acetate may also be known as: U-6013, 9alpha-fluoroprednisolone acetate, and *Predef 2x®*.

Storage/Stability

The injection should be stored at controlled room temperature 20°-25°C.

Compatibility/Compounding Considerations

No specific information noted.

Dosage Forms/Regulatory Status

VETERINARY-LABELED PRODUCTS:

Isoflupredone acetate 2 mg/mL aqueous suspension for injection in 10 mL and 100 mL vials; *Predef 2x®*; (Rx). In the USA, *Predef 2x®* is FDA-approved for use in cattle, horses and swine.

Meat withdrawal time is 7 days; it is not to be used in calves to be processed for veal. There is no milk withdrawal time for isoflupredone in the USA, but in Canada a 72-hour withdrawal time is specified.

Isoflupredone is also found in some topical and otic products. For more information see the *Dermatological Agents, Topical* and *Otic* Appendixes.

The ARCI (Racing Commissioners International) has designated this drug as a class 4 substance.

HUMAN-LABELED PRODUCTS: NONE.

Revisions/References

Monograph revised/updated February 2014.

Goodrich, L. (2006). Current therapies for osteoarthritis. Proceedings: Western Veterinary Conf 2006, Accessed via the Veterinary Information Network Jan 2007. accessed via Veterinary Information Network; vin.com

Hewson, J. (2013). Managing the Collateral Damage of Inflammation to Optimize Outcome in Cattle with Respiratory Disease. 65th Convention of the Canadian Veterinary Medical Association. accessed via Veterinary Information Network; vin.com

Hewson, J., et al. (2011). Impact of isoflupredone acetate treatment on clinical signs and weight gain in weanling heifers with experimentally induced Mannheimia haemolytica bronchopneumonia. American Journal of Veterinary Research 72(12): 1613-21.

Picandet, V., et al. (2003). Comparison of efficacy and tolerability of isoflupredone and dexamethasone in the treatment of horses affected with recurrent airway obstruction (RAO). Equine Vet J 35(4): 419-24.

Seifi, H. A., et al. (2007). Effect of isoflupredone acetate with or without insulin on energy metabolism, reproduction, milk production, and health in dairy cows in early lactation. Journal of Dairy Science 90(9): 4181-91.

Isoflurane

(eye-soe-flure-ane)   Isoflo®, Iso-Thesia®
General Anesthetic, Inhalant

Prescriber Highlights

- ▶ Inhalant general anesthetic.
- ▶ Contraindications: History or predilection towards malignant hyperthermia.
- ▶ Caution with increased CSF or head injury, or myasthenia gravis.
- ▶ Adverse Effects: Dose related hypotension, respiratory depression, & GI effects (nausea, vomiting, ileus); cardiodepression generally is minimal at doses causing surgical planes of anesthesia. Arrhythmias are rare.
- ▶ May be fetotoxic.
- ▶ Drug interactions.

Uses/Indications

As halothane is no longer available, isoflurane is now the primary inhalant anesthetic used in veterinary medicine. When compared with older anesthetics such as halothane or methoxyflurane, isoflurane has less myocardial depressant and catecholamine sensitizing effects and it can be used safely in patients with hepatic or renal disease. The newer inhalant anesthetics, sevoflurane (ability to change depth of anesthesia faster; not as respiratory irritating; mask inductions possible) and desflurane (very fast onset, faster recoveries) have some advantages over isoflurane, but are more expensive. Isoflurane with oxygen can be used for refractory status epilepticus in dogs that are refractory to benzodiazepine boluses, but can cause increased CSF pressure.

Pharmacology/Actions

The precise mechanism of how inhalant anesthetics produce their general anesthetic effects is not known. They may interfere with the functioning of nerve cells in the brain by acting at the lipid matrix of the membrane. Some key pharmacologic effects noted with isoflurane include: CNS depression, depression of body temperature regulating centers, increased cerebral blood flow, respiratory depression, hypotension, vasodilatation, myocardial depression (less so than with halothane), and muscular relaxation.

Minimal Alveolar Concentration (MAC; %) in oxygen reported for isoflurane in various species: Dog = 1.5; Cat = 1.2; Horse = 1.31; Human = 1.2. Several factors may alter MAC (acid/base status, temperature, other CNS depressants on board, age, ongoing acute disease, etc.).

Pharmacokinetics

Isoflurane is rapidly absorbed from the alveoli. It is rapidly distributed into the CNS and crosses the placenta. The vast majority of the drug is eliminated via the lungs; only about 0.17% is metabolized in the liver and only very small amounts of inorganic fluoride is formed.

Contraindications/Precautions/Warnings

Isoflurane is contraindicated in patients with a history or predilection towards malignant hyperthermia. It should be used with caution (benefits vs. risks) in patients with increased CSF or head injury, or myasthenia gravis.

Because of its respiratory depressant effects, intermittent positive pressure ventilation may be required to achieve anesthesia, particularly in horses; overdose risks are increased, however.

Both isoflurane and desflurane can be irritating to the respiratory system and are not recommended for mask induction (Clarke 2008).

Adverse Effects

At usual concentrations, hypotension secondary to vasodilation may occur and is considered to be dose related. Hypotension usually responds to fluids, but profound hypotension may require the use of vasopressors. A study in dogs, found that hetastarch was superior to LRS for treating isoflurane-induced hypotension (Aarnes et al. 2009). While cardiodepression is usually not clinically significant at doses causing surgical planes of anesthesia, it can occur. Arrhythmias have rarely been reported.

Dose-dependent respiratory depression, and GI effects (nausea, vomiting, ileus) have been reported.

Reproductive/Nursing Safety

Some animal studies have indicated that isoflurane may be fetotoxic. Use during pregnancy with caution. In a system evaluating the safety of drugs in canine and feline pregnancy (Papich 1989), this drug is categorized as class: *B* (*Safe for use if used cautiously. Studies in laboratory animals may have uncovered some risk, but these drugs appear to be safe in dogs and cats or these drugs are safe if they are not administered when the animal is near term.*)

Drug Interactions

The following drug interactions have either been reported or are theoretical in humans or animals receiving isoflurane and may be of in veterinary patients. Unless otherwise noted, use together is not necessarily contraindicated, but weigh the potential risks and perform additional monitoring when appropriate.

- **AMINOGLYCOSIDES:** Use with caution with halogenated anesthetic agents as additive neuromuscular blockade may occur.
- **ACE INHIBITORS OR OTHER HYPOTENSIVE AGENTS:** Concomitant use may increase risks for hypotension. Enalapril caused significant decreases in systolic blood pressure in cats and dogs undergoing isoflurane anesthesia (Ishikawa, Uechi and Ishikawa 2007), (Ishikawa, Uechi and Hori 2007).
- **OPIOIDS:** Intraoperative opioids can reduce MAC requirements.
- **LINCOSAMIDES:** Use with caution with halogenated anesthetic agents as additive neuromuscular blockade may occur.
- **NON-DEPOLARIZING NEUROMUSCULAR BLOCKING AGENTS:** Additive neuromuscular blockade may occur.
- **SUCCINYLCHOLINE:** With inhalation anesthetics, may induce increased incidences of cardiac effects (bradycardia, arrhythmias, sinus arrest and apnea) and, in susceptible patients, malignant hyperthermia.
- **SYMPATHOMIMETICS (dopamine, epinephrine, norepinephrine, ephedrine, metaraminol,** etc.**):** While isoflurane sensitizes the myocardium to the effects of sympathomimetics less so than halothane, arrhythmias may still result. If these drugs are needed, they should be used with caution and in significantly reduced dosages with intensive monitoring.

Doses

Note: General anesthesia using inhalants must be performed with adequate monitoring and support and cannot be dosed in "cookbook" fashion. MAC can be significantly reduced by administration of other agents that affect the CNS. Concentrations are dependent upon fresh gas flow rate; generally the lower the flow rate, the higher the concentration required. Isoflurane should be used in areas with adequate ventilation to prevent the accumulation of anesthetic vapors.

- **DOGS:**

  For general anesthesia (labeled dosage; FDA-approved): Induction: 2 – 2.5% isoflurane alone with oxygen following an injectable anesthetic induction agent is usually employed. Maintenance: Surgical levels of anesthesia may be sustained with a 1.5 – 1.8% concentration of isoflurane in oxygen. (Adapted from label; *IsoFlo®*) Note: The labeled doses are relatively old and may not reflect current thinking in veterinary anesthesia especially for use for induction; refer to current anesthesia references for more information.

- **CATS:**

  For general anesthesia (extra-label): In a systematic review of the literature, the MAC for isoflurane ranged from $1.20 \pm 0.13\%$ to $2.22 \pm 0.35\%$ and the average MAC was $1.71 \pm 0.07\%$. MAC is affected by many variables, including the type and location of stimulus, type of ventilation, type of breathing system, and age of the animal (younger cats had higher MAC values).

- **FERRETS/SMALL MAMMALS:**

  For general anesthesia (extra-label):

  a) **Mice, Rats, Gerbils, Hamsters, Guinea pigs, Chinchillas:** Using a non-rebreathing system: Induction: 2 – 3%, maintenance: 0.25 – 2%. (Anderson 1994); (Adamcak et al. 2000)

  b) **Ferrets:** After premed with medetomidine at 50 – 100 micrograms/kg. Atropine at 0.05 mg/kg SC is used to counteract hypersalivation and bradycardia. Starting isoflurane at 1 – 2% will be less irritating to the ferret and cause less of a struggle. Use a non-rebreathing system. Consider intubation in procedures lasting longer than 30 minutes. For post-op pain either butorphanol at 0.1 mg/kg SC or buprenorphine at 0.02 mg/kg SC. (Johnson 2006)

- **HORSES:**

  For general anesthesia (labeled dosage; FDA-approved): Induction: 3 – 5% isoflurane alone with oxygen following an injectable anesthetic induction agent are usually employed. Maintenance: Surgical levels of anesthesia may be sustained with a 1.5 – 1.8% concentration of isoflurane in oxygen. (Adapted from label; *Aerrane®*) Note: The labeled doses are relatively old and may not reflect current thinking in veterinary anesthesia; refer to current anesthesia references for more information.

- **SMALL RUMINANTS:**

  For general anesthesia (extra-label): Inhalational anesthesia is seldom feasible or economically justified in small ruminants, but it is by far the safest and most satisfactory in debilitated, pregnant, very young or aged animals, or for prolonged (i.e., >1 hour) and complicated surgical procedures. Vaporizer should be set to 4% – 6% when isoflurane is used for induction and adjusted to 1.5% – 3% during maintenance. Oxygen flow rate should be 2 – 4 L/min during induction and reduced to 0.5 – 1 L/min during maintenance. (Galatos 2011)

- **REPTILES:**

  For general anesthesia (extra-label):

  a) It is preferable to induce reptiles with injectable agents and then maintain anesthesia with inhalant gases. For maintenance of general anesthesia most reptiles require concentrations of 2% – 3% of isoflurane. In green iguanas MAC is reportedly 1.8 – 2.1%. (Sladky et al. 2012)

  b) Give 5% isoflurane and oxygen in a clear plastic bag or induction chamber. Fill chamber with gas and seal. Induction time may take 30-60 minutes, but can be shortened to 15-30 minutes with increased depth of anesthesia if animal is injected with 10 – 20 mg/kg of ketamine (SC or IM). Patient should be kept warm by placing on a water blanket. Surgical anesthesia can be determined by the loss of righting reflex. After induction, use either a mask, ET tube, or leave head in chamber. Maintenance levels are 3 – 5% (if isoflurane used alone). If apnea occurs during or after anesthesia, discontinue gas anesthetic and apply gentle manual ventilation 2-4 times per minute with small doses of doxapram IV. Normal respiration generally resumes in 3-5 minutes. Righting reflex generally recovers in an hour, but animal may be tranquilized for up to 24 hours. (Gillespie 1994)

c) Anesthetic gas of choice for reptiles. Induction can be with a face mask, or with a "cat box." Animal may be intubated, especially if has been preanesthetized with ketamine or *Telazol®*, and "bag" it down with positive pressure ventilation. Maintenance is usually 1.5 – 3%. (Funk 2002)

■ **BIRDS:**

For general anesthesia (extra-label): Induction occurs within 1-2 minutes at a concentration of 3 – 5%. Maintenance at 1.5 – 2% is adequate for most birds. Anesthetic of choice for birds; heart rate may decrease, but not to the same degree as halothane. Recovery very rapid; most patients are standing and cage safe within 5 min. after anesthesia discontinued, but there seems to be a direct relationship between anesthesia time and recovery time. (Bennett 2002)

Monitoring
■ Respiratory and ventilatory status.
■ Cardiac rate/rhythm; blood pressure (particularly with "at risk" patients).
■ Level of anesthesia.

Client Information
Isoflurane is used for general anesthesia only by veterinarians.

Chemistry/Synonyms
An inhalant general anesthetic agent, isoflurane occurs as a colorless, nonflammable, stable liquid. It has a characteristic mildly pungent musty, ethereal odor. At 20°C, isoflurane's specific gravity is 1.496 and vapor pressure is 238 mm Hg. Its boiling point is 48.5°C and solubility coefficients are blood-gas: 1.4 and oil-gas: 91.

Isoflurane may also be known as: compound 469, isofluranum, *AErrane®, Forene®, Forenium®, Forthane®, Isoflo®, Isofor®, Isoforine®, Isosol®, Isothane®, Iso-Thesia®, Lisorane®, Sofloran®, Tensocold®, Terrell®* and *Zuflax®*.

Storage/stability
Isoflurane should be stored at room temperature; it is relatively unaffected by exposure to light, but should be stored in a tight, light-resistant container. Isoflurane does not attack aluminum, brass, tin, iron, or copper.

Compatibility/Compounding Considerations
No specific information noted.

Dosage Forms/Regulatory Status
VETERINARY-LABELED PRODUCTS:
Isoflurane for Inhalation: 99.9%/mL in 100 mL & 250 mL; *Aerrane®, Isoflo®, Isosol®*, generic; (Rx). Products may be FDA-approved for use in horses (those not intended for food) and dogs.

HUMAN-LABELED PRODUCTS:
Isoflurane Liquid for Inhalation in 100 mL & 250 mL; *Forane®, Terrell®*, generic; (Rx)

Revisions/References
Monograph revised/updated February 2014.

Aarnes, T. K., et al. (2009). Effect of intravenous administration of lactated Ringer's solution or hetastarch for the treatment of isoflurane-induced hypotension in dogs. American Journal of Veterinary Research 70(11): 1345-53.
Adamcak, A. & B. Otten (2000). Rodent Therapeutics. Vet Clin NA: Exotic Anim Pract 3:1(Jan): 221-40.
Anderson, N. (1994). Basic husbandry and medicine of pocket pets. *Saunders Manual of Small Animal Practice*. S. Birchard and R. Sherding. Philadelphia, W.B. Saunders Company: 1363-89.
Bennett, R. (2002). Avian Anesthesia. Proceedings: Western Veterinary Conference. accessed via Veterinary Information Network; vin.com
Clarke, K. W. (2008). Options for inhalation anaesthesia. In Practice 30(9): 513-8.

Funk, R. (2002). Anesthesia in reptiles. Proceedings: Western Veterinary Conf. accessed via Veterinary Information Network; vin.com
Galatos, A. D. (2011). Anesthesia and Analgesia in Sheep and Goats. Veterinary Clinics of North America-Food Animal Practice 27(1): 47-+.
Gillespie, D. (1994). Reptiles. *Saunders Manual of Small Animal Practice*. S. Birchard and R. Sherding. Philadelphia, W.B. Saunders Company: 1390- 411.
Ishikawa, Y., et al. (2007). Effect of Isoflurane Anesthesia on Hemodynamics Following Administration of an Angiotensin-Converting Enzyme Inhibitor in Dogs. Proceedings: ACVIM. accessed via Veterinary Information Network; vin.com
Ishikawa, Y., et al. (2007). Effect of Isoflurane Anesthesia on Hemodynamics Following Administration of an Angiotensin-Converting Enzyme Inhibitor in Cats. Proceedings: ACVIM. accessed via Veterinary Information Network; vin.com
Johnson, D. (2006). Ferrets: the other companion animal. Proceedings: ACVC. accessed via Veterinary Information Network; vin.com
Papich, M. (1989). Effects of drugs on pregnancy. *Current Veterinary Therapy X: Small Animal Practice*. R. Kirk. Philadelphia, Saunders: 1291-9.
Sladky, K. K. & C. Mans (2012). Clinical anesthesia in reptiles. Journal of Exotic Pet Medicine 21(1): 17-31.

Isoniazid (INH)

(eye-so-nye-ah-zid)   Isonicotinic acid hydrazide

Antimycobacterial

Prescriber Highlights
▶ Antimycobacterial that may be used for chemoprophylaxis of *M. bovis* or *M. tuberculosis* in small animals.
▶ Has been used in cattle for paratuberculosis (MAP, Johne's).
▶ Treating active infections is controversial because of potential public health risks associated with the infections.
▶ Hepatotoxicity & neurotoxicity possible; narrow therapeutic index.

Uses/Indications
Isoniazid (INH) is sometimes used for chemoprophylaxis in small animals in households having a human with tuberculosis. It potentially can be used in combination with other antimycobacterial drugs to treat infections of *M. bovis* or *M. tuberculosis* in dogs or cats. But because of the public health risks, particularly in the face of increased populations of immunocompromised people, treatment of mycobacterial (*M. bovis, M. tuberculosis*) infections in domestic or captive animals is controversial. In addition, INH has a narrow therapeutic index and toxicity is a concern (see Adverse Effects).

Isoniazid, alone or in combination, has been used to treat (not cure) *Mycobacterium avium* subsp. *paratuberculosis* (MAP; Johne's Disease) in cattle that are of significant economic, genetic or sentimental value (Fecteau et al. 2011).

In humans, isoniazid (INH) is routinely used alone to treat latent tuberculosis infections (positive tuberculin skin test) and in combination with other antimycobacterial agents to treat active disease.

Pharmacology/Actions
Isoniazid inhibits the synthesis of mycoloic acids, a component of mycobacterial cell walls; its exact mechanism is not well understood. It is most active against mycobacteria that are actively dividing and affects both extracellular and intracellular mycobacteria.

Isoniazid is only active against *M. tuberculosis*, *M. bovis* and some strains of *M. kansasii*. In humans, resistance develops rapidly if used alone against active clinical disease, but not when used for prophylactic treatment.

Pharmacokinetics
No information was located on the pharmacokinetics of INH in dogs or cats. It is reported that the drug is absorbed after oral administration to ruminants.

In humans, isoniazid is rapidly absorbed after oral administration; food can decrease absorption somewhat and INH may undergo significant first pass metabolism. The drug is highly distributed in the body and crosses into the CSF and caseous material. It is distributed into milk and crosses the placenta. It is only slightly (10%) bound to plasma proteins. In humans, the drug is initially primarily acetylated in the liver. The N-acetylated form is then further biotransformed to isonicotinic acid and monoacetylhydrazine. Monoacetylhydrazine is thought to play a role in the drug's hepatic toxicity. As dogs, like some humans, lack N-acetyltransferase, increased potential for INH toxicity may occur in this species. Elimination half-life in fast acetylators (humans) is 0.5-1.6 hours and 2-5 hours in slow acetylators. Patients with acute or chronic liver disease may have substantially longer half-lives (2X). The drug is mostly eliminated in the urine as inactive metabolites.

Contraindications/Precautions/Warnings

Isoniazid is contraindicated in patients with acute liver disease or those that developed hepatopathy while taking the medication in the past.

It should be used with caution in patients with decreased hepatic function or severe renal disease.

Adverse Effects

The primary adverse effect associated with INH in dogs is hepatotoxicity with increased serum liver enzymes. Additional adverse effects reported in dogs include CNS stimulation, peripheral neuropathy and thrombocytopenia. Ataxia, seizures, salivation, diarrhea, vomiting and arrhythmias have been reported after overdoses in dogs. Adverse effects reported in cats include hepatotoxicity and peripheral neuritis. In humans, urticaria, hepatotoxicity and peripheral neuropathy are commonly reported; rarely, blood dyscrasias, SLE, and seizures have been reported.

In cattle, toxic signs (refusal to eat, decreased milk product, rear leg stiffness) can be noted at 30 mg/kg. At 60 mg/kg severe ataxia can be seen and death can occur at doses of 100 mg/kg.

Reproductive/Nursing Safety

Isoniazid crosses the placenta and has been found to be embryocidal in some laboratory species, but teratogenic effects have not been detected in mice, rabbits, or rats. In humans, the FDA categorizes isoniazid as category *C* for use during pregnancy (*Animal studies have shown an adverse effect on the fetus, but there are no adequate studies in humans; or there are no animal reproduction studies and no adequate studies in humans.*)

Isoniazid potentially can induce abortion in cattle.

Isoniazid is excreted in milk in low concentrations (approx. 1-2% of maternal serum concentrations in humans) and it is thought to be safe to use during nursing. Ingested levels via milk are not high enough to serve as prophylaxis for tuberculosis in nursing infants.

Overdosage/Acute Toxicity

Overdosage of INH can be very serious. In dogs, the reported LD50 is 50 mg/kg; serious toxicity can occur with as little as one 300 mg tablet ingested. Ataxia, seizures, myocardial necrosis, metabolic acidosis, rhabdomyolysis, salivation, diarrhea, vomiting, and arrhythmias have been reported after overdoses in dogs; it is strongly recommended to contact an animal poison control center in the event of any inadvertent ingestion. Treatment may include enterogastric lavage, activated charcoal and drugs such as diazepam or phenobarbital to control seizures. Fluids and acidemia may need correction.

Pyridoxine (Vitamin B-6) has been suggested to be administered intravenously (preferably over 30-60 minutes) on a mg per mg of INH-ingested basis. It is commercially available as a 100 mg/mL 1 mL vial, but it may be difficult to obtain in an emergency situation. A local human hospital may stock it.

Drug Interactions

Drug interactions have not been reported with isoniazid in animals. The following drug interactions have either been reported or are theoretical in humans receiving INH and may be of in veterinary patients. Unless otherwise noted, use together is not necessarily contraindicated, but weigh the potential risks and perform additional monitoring when appropriate.

- **ALFENTANIL:** Prolonged alfentanil duration of action.
- **ANTACIDS** (especially those containing **aluminum**): Decreased INH absorption.
- **BENZODIAZEPINES:** INH may reduce benzodiazepine metabolism.
- **CORTICOSTEROIDS:** May reduce INH efficacy.
- **KETOCONAZOLE:** INH may reduce ketoconazole serum concentrations.
- **OTHER HEPATOTOXIC DRUGS** (*e.g.,* **acetaminophen, itraconazole, fluconazole, methimazole, ketoconazole, phenothiazines, sulfonamides, estrogens,** etc.): Increased risk of hepatotoxicity.
- **OTHER NEUROTOXIC DRUGS:** Increased risk of neurotoxicity.
- **PYRIDOXINE:** INH may antagonize or increase the excretion of pyridoxine and increased pyridoxine may be required; increased peripheral neuritis may occur secondary to pyridoxine/INH interaction.
- **PHENYTOIN:** INH may inhibit metabolism and increase risks for phenytoin toxicity.
- **RIFAMPIN:** Increased risk for hepatotoxicity.
- **THEOPHYLLINE:** Increased risk of theophylline toxicity.
- **FOOD INTERACTIONS** in humans: **cheese** (Swiss, Cheshire, etc.) or **fish** (Tuna, Skipjack, Sardinella): INH may interfere with metabolism of tyramine and histamine found in fish and cheese.

Laboratory Considerations

- INH may cause false-positive **urine glucose determinations** when using cupric sulfate solution (Benedict's Solution, *Clinitest®*); tests utilizing glucose oxidase (*Tes-Tape®, Clinistix®*) are not affected.

Doses

Note: It is recommended to contact local veterinary or public health authorities before treating any animal with a confirmed mycobacterial infection.

- **DOGS:**

  For *M. tuberculosis* chemoprophylaxis (extra-label): 10 mg/kg PO once daily. Drug can be hepatotoxic and dose is extrapolated from human data. Treatment *of M. tuberculosis* or *M. bovis* infections in dogs and cats is not recommended. (Greene et al. 2006)

- **CATS:**

  As a second-line treatment (reserved for resistant infections) for feline TB (extra-label): 10 – 20 mg/kg PO once daily. (Gunn-Moore 2008)

- **CATTLE/RUMINANTS:**

  To attempt to induce clinical remission of paratuberculosis (Johne's; JD) in cattle or other ruminants that are of significant economic, genetic or sentimental value (extra-label): 11 – 25 mg/kg PO once daily. Treatment typically must be maintained for the life of the animal and treated animals usually continue to shed MAP. Owner must be fully informed about the implications of keeping an animal with clinical JD on the premises. Strongly advise having owner sign a document stating that the milk and meat from the animal will never be used for human consumption. (Fecteau et al. 2011)

Monitoring

- Baseline and periodic physical exam, including clinical efficacy and adverse effect queries.
- Baseline and periodic: CBC, liver function, renal function.

Client Information

- Best to administer on an empty stomach.
- If this medication is to be effective, it must be given regularly as directed.
- If a dose is missed, do not double the next dose.
- Store well out of reach of children or pets; overdoses can be very serious.
- Contact veterinarian if any of the following occur: vomiting, decreased appetite/weight loss, diarrhea or loose stools, changes in behavior or activity, yellowing of whites of eyes or mucous membranes, or difficulty running or going up/down stairs.

Chemistry/Synonyms

Isoniazid occurs as colorless, or white, odorless crystals. It is freely soluble in water and sparingly soluble in alcohol. It is recommended not to use sugars such as glucose, fructose or sucrose in compounded oral solutions, as a condensation product can be formed that can impair absorption.

Isoniazid may also be known as: INH, INAH, isonicotinic acid hydrazide, isonicotinylhydrazide, isonicotinylhydrazine, or tubazid. INH is available throughout the world in many trade names, some of the more commonly used names include *Isotamine®*, *Laniazid®*, or *Nydrazid®*. **Caution:** *Isopyrin®* is one isoniazid trade name that in some countries contains ramifenazone and not isoniazid.

Storage/Stability

Isoniazid tablets should be stored at temperatures below 40°C, preferably between 15-30°C, in well-closed, light-resistant containers. The oral syrup should be stored at temperatures below 40°C, preferably between 15-30°C, in well-closed, light-resistant containers protected from freezing. The injection should be stored at temperatures below 40°C, preferably between 15-30°C; protected from light and freezing. At low temperatures, crystals may form in the injectable solution; crystals should redissolve upon warming to room temperature.

Compatibility/Compounding Considerations

No specific information noted.

Dosage Forms/Regulatory Status

VETERINARY-LABELED PRODUCTS: NONE.

HUMAN-LABELED PRODUCTS:

Isoniazid Oral Tablets: 100 mg & 300 mg; generic; (Rx)

Isoniazid Oral Syrup: 10 mg/mL (50 mg/mL) in pints; generic; (Rx)

Isoniazid Injection Solution: 100 mg/mL in 10 mL multidose vials; generic; (Rx)

Combination Products:

Tablets: Rifampin 120 mg, Isoniazid 50 mg, & Pyrazinamide 300 mg; *Rifater®*; (Rx)

Capsules: Rifampin 300 mg & Isoniazid 150 mg; *IsonaRif®*, *Rifamate®*; (Rx)

Revisions/References

Monograph revised/updated February 2014.

Fecteau, M.-E. & R. H. Whitlock (2011). Treatment and Chemoprophylaxis for Paratuberculosis. Veterinary Clinics of North America-Food Animal Practice 27(3): 547-+.

Greene, C. & D. Gunn-Moore (2006). Mycobacterial Infections: Infections caused by slow-growing mycobacteria. *Infectious Diseases of the Dog and Cat, 3rd Ed.* C. Greene, Elsevier: 462-77.

Gunn-Moore, D. (2008). Feline Mycobacterial Infections. Proceedings: WSAVA. accessed via Veterinary Information Network; vin.com

Isoproterenol HCl

(eye-soe-proe-ter-e-nole)   Isoprenoline®, Isuprel®

Beta-Adrenergic Agonist

Prescriber Highlights

▶ Non-specific beta agonist used rarely for acute bronchial constriction, cardiac arrhythmias (complete AV block), & as adjunctive therapy in shock or heart failure.

▶ Contraindications: Tachycardias or AV block caused by cardiac glycoside intoxication, ventricular arrhythmias that do not require increased inotropic activity.

▶ Caution: Coronary insufficiency, hyperthyroidism, renal disease, hypertension, or diabetes; not a substitute for adequate fluid replacement in shock.

▶ Adverse Effects: Tachycardia, anxiety, tremors, excitability, headache, weakness, & vomiting; more arrhythmogenic than dopamine or dobutamine.

▶ Short duration of activity (including adverse effects).

Uses/Indications

Isoproterenol is infrequently used in veterinary medicine in the treatment of acute bronchial constriction, cardiac arrhythmias (complete AV block) and, occasionally, as adjunctive therapy in shock or heart failure (limited use because of increases in heart rate and ventricular arrhythmogenicity).

Pharmacology/Actions

Isoproterenol is a synthetic beta$_1$- and beta$_2$-adrenergic agonist that has no appreciable alpha activity at therapeutic doses. It is thought that isoproterenol's adrenergic activity is a result of stimulating cyclic-AMP production. Its primary actions are increased inotropism and chronotropism, relaxation of bronchial smooth muscle, and peripheral vasodilatation. Isoproterenol may increase perfusion to skeletal muscle (at the expense of vital organs in shock). Isoproterenol will inhibit the antigen-mediated release of histamine and slow releasing substance of anaphylaxis (SRS-A).

Hemodynamic effects noted include decreased total peripheral resistance, increased cardiac output, increased venous return to the heart, and increased rate of discharge by cardiac pacemakers.

Pharmacokinetics

Isoproterenol is rapidly inactivated by the GI tract and metabolized by the liver after oral administration. Sublingual administration is not reliably absorbed and effects may take up to 30 minutes to be seen. Intravenous administration results in immediate effects, but only persists for a few minutes after discontinuation.

It is unknown if isoproterenol is distributed into milk. The pharmacologic actions of isoproterenol are ended primarily through tissue uptake. Isoproterenol is metabolized in the liver and other tissues by catechol-O-methyltransferase (COMT) to a weakly active metabolite.

Contraindications/Precautions/Warnings

Isoproterenol is contraindicated in patients that have tachycardias or AV block caused by cardiac glycoside intoxication. It is also contraindicated in ventricular arrhythmias that do not require increased inotropic activity.

Use isoproterenol with caution in patients with coronary insufficiency, hyperthyroidism, renal disease, hypertension or diabetes. Isoproterenol is not a substitute for adequate fluid replacement in shock.

Adverse Effects

Isoproterenol can cause tachycardia, anxiety, tremors, excitability, headache, weakness, and vomiting. Because of isoproterenol's short duration of action, adverse effects are usually transient and do not require cessation of therapy, but may require lowering the dose or infusion rate. Isoproterenol is considered more arrhythmogenic than either dopamine or dobutamine, so it is rarely used in the treatment of heart failure.

Reproductive/Nursing Safety

In humans, the FDA categorizes this drug as category *C* for use during pregnancy (*Animal studies have shown an adverse effect on the fetus, but there are no adequate studies in humans; or there are no animal reproduction studies and no adequate studies in humans.*) In a separate system evaluating the safety of drugs in canine and feline pregnancy (Papich 1989), this drug is categorized as class: *C* (*These drugs may have potential risks. Studies in people or laboratory animals have uncovered risks, and these drugs should be used cautiously as a last resort when the benefit of therapy clearly outweighs the risks.*).

No specific lactation safety information was found, however, as isoproterenol is rapidly deactivated in the gut, it is unlikely to pose much risk to nursing offspring.

Overdosage/Acute Toxicity

In addition to the signs listed in the Adverse Effects section, high doses may cause an initial hypertension, followed by hypotension as well as tachycardias and other arrhythmias. Besides halting or reducing the drug, treatment is considered to be supportive. Should tachycardias persist, a beta-blocker could be considered for treatment (if patient does not have a bronchospastic disease).

Drug Interactions

The following drug interactions have either been reported or are theoretical in humans or animals receiving isoproterenol and may be of in veterinary patients. Unless otherwise noted, use together is not necessarily contraindicated, but weigh the potential risks and perform additional monitoring when appropriate.

- **ANESTHETICS, GENERAL:** An increased risk of arrhythmias developing can occur if isoproterenol is administered to patients who have received cyclopropane or a halogenated hydrocarbon anesthetic agent. Propranolol may be administered should these occur.
- **BETA-BLOCKERS:** May antagonize isoproterenol's cardiac, bronchodilating, and vasodilating effects by blocking the beta effects of isoproterenol. Beta-blockers may be administered to treat the tachycardia associated with isoproterenol use, but use with caution in patients with bronchospastic disease.
- **DIGOXIN:** An increased risk of arrhythmias may occur if isoproterenol is used concurrently with digitalis glycosides.
- **OXYTOCIC AGENTS:** Hypertension may result if isoproterenol is used with oxytocic agents.
- **SELEGILINE:** Increased hypertensive effects possible.
- **SYMPATHOMIMETIC AGENTS, OTHER:** Isoproterenol should not be administered with other sympathomimetic agents (*e.g.*, **phenylpropanolamine**) as increased toxicity may result.
- **THEOPHYLLINE:** Isoproterenol may reduce theophylline levels.

Doses

Note: Because of the cardiostimulatory properties of isoproterenol, its parenteral use in human medicine for the treatment of bronchospasm has been largely supplanted by other more beta$_2$ specific drugs (*e.g.*, terbutaline) and administration methods (nebulization). Use with care.

- **DOGS/CATS:**

  For sinoatrial arrest, sinus bradycardia, complete AV block, or as an alternative to atropine for calcium channel blocker overdose (extra-label): Dilute injection as described for IV infu-

sion below in Compatibility/Compounding Considerations (*e.g.*, 1 mg into 500 mL of D5W yields a 2 microgram/mL solution) and infuse as a CRI to effect. Most commonly dosages of 0.04 – 0.08 micrograms/kg/minute are recommended. For example: If diluted to a concentration of 2 micrograms/mL, a 10 kg dog at 0.04 micrograms/kg/min would correspond to a 12 mL/hr IV infusion pump setting. A dynamic drip rate table creation tool can be found at Global RPh: http://www.globalrph.com/drip.htm

Monitoring

- Cardiac rate/rhythm.
- Respiratory rate/auscultation during anaphylaxis.
- Urine flow, if possible.
- Blood pressure, and blood gases if indicated and possible.

Client Information

- Isoproterenol for injection should be used only by trained personnel in a setting where adequate monitoring can be performed.

Chemistry/Synonyms

Isoproterenol HCl is a synthetic beta-adrenergic agent that occurs as a white to practically white, crystalline powder that is freely soluble in water and sparingly soluble in alcohol. The pH of the commercially available injection is 3.5-4.5.

Isoproterenol HCl may also be known as: isoprenaline hydrochloride, isopropylarterenol hydrochloride, isopropylnoradrenaline hydrochloride, *Imuprel®*, *Isolin®*, *Isuprel®*, *Lenoprel®*, *Norisodrine Aerotrol®*, *Proterenal*, *Saventrine®*, and *Vapo-iso®*.

Storage/Stability

Store isoproterenol preparations in tight, light-resistant containers. It is stable indefinitely at room temperature. Isoproterenol salts will darken with time upon exposure to air, light, or heat. Sulfites or sulfur dioxide may be added to preparations as an antioxidant. Solutions may become pink or brownish-pink if exposed to air, alkalies, or metals. Do not use solutions that are discolored or contain a precipitate. If isoproterenol is mixed with other drugs or fluids that result in a solution with a pH greater than 6, it is recommended that it be used immediately.

Compatibility/Compounding Considerations

Isoproterenol for injection is reported to be physically **compatible** with all commonly used IV solutions (except 5% sodium bicarbonate), and the following drugs: calcium chloride/gluceptate, cimetidine HCl, dobutamine HCl, heparin sodium, magnesium sulfate, multivitamin infusion, oxytetracycline HCl, potassium chloride, succinylcholine chloride, tetracycline HCl, verapamil HCl, and vitamin B complex with C.

It is reported to be physically **incompatible** when mixed with: aminophylline or sodium bicarbonate. Compatibility is dependent upon factors such as pH, concentration, temperature, and diluent used; consult specialized references for more specific information.

The commercially available injection is available as 0.2 mg/mL. For direct IV injection, dilute 1 mL of the commercially available injection to a volume of 10 mL with 0.9% sodium chloride injection or 5% dextrose injection. For IV infusion, solutions may be prepared by diluting 1-10 mL of the 0.2 mg/mL injection with 500 mL of 5% dextrose, 0.9% sodium chloride, or LRS injection to provide infusion solutions containing 0.4 – 4 micrograms/mL. For example, 5 mL (1 mg) of the 0.2 mg/mL injection in 500 mL of D5W would yield a concentration of 2 micrograms/mL. As the injection concentrate contains no bacteriostatic or antimicrobial agent, each vial/ampule is intended for single use only; any unused solution should be discarded.

Dosage Forms/Regulatory Status

VETERINARY-LABELED PRODUCTS: NONE.

HUMAN-LABELED PRODUCTS:

Isoproterenol HCl for Injection: 1:5000 solution (0.2 mg/mL) in 1 mL & 5 mL ampules; *Isuprel®*; (Rx)

Revisions/References

Monograph revised/updated February 2014.

Papich, M. (1989). Effects of drugs on pregnancy. *Current Veterinary Therapy X: Small Animal Practice.* R. Kirk. Philadelphia, Saunders: 1291-9.

Isosorbide Dinitrate
Isosorbide Mononitrate

(eye-soe-sor-bide)   Isordil®, Ismo®, Imdur®

Vasodilator

Prescriber Highlights

▶ Limited clinical experience; but could have some utility in small animal medicine for adjunctive treatment of heart failure. Efficacy and adverse effect profile are unknown in dogs or cats.

Uses/Indications

Isosorbide mononitrate (ISMN) and dinitrate (ISDN) are organic nitrates potentially useful as preload reducing agents in treating heart failure in small animals, however, research and clinical experience demonstrating clinical efficacy are lacking in dogs or cats. Limited research available indicates that dogs may require much higher dosages of isosorbide to achieve therapeutic effects than do humans.

In humans, isosorbide nitrates are used for treating or preventing angina, treating esophageal spasm, and as an adjunctive treatment in CHF.

Pharmacology/Actions

Organic nitrates (*e.g.,* isosorbide nitrates, nitroglycerin) share a similar pharmacologic profile. They relax vascular smooth muscles causing vasodilation, predominantly on the venous side, but somewhat on arteries/arterioles as well. The mechanism of action is related to their conversion to free radical nitric oxide. Nitric acid is thought to activate guanylate cyclase, thus increasing cyclic GMP and eventually leading to dephosphorylating light chain myosin, causing vasodilation. In humans, nitrates reduce myocardial oxygen demand, but the exact mechanism for this effect is not well understood. Nitrates functionally antagonize the effects of acetylcholine, norepinephrine and histamine. Additionally, nitrates relax all smooth muscles including biliary (including biliary ducts, sphincter of Oddi), bronchial, GI (including the esophagus), ureteral and uterine.

Serum concentrations of isosorbide mononitrate above 100 ng/mL minimum concentration of the drug are believed required for hemodynamic effects in dogs and humans. However, a study (Adin et al. 2001) in both normal dogs and those with CHF, demonstrated no hemodynamic effects (blood pressure, heart rate, PCV, thoracic blood volume percentage, abdominal blood volume percentage) at doses that yielded peak levels as high as 2,352 ± 701 ng/mL.

In a study performed in dogs with experimentally induced mitral regurgitation, oral dosages of a sustained-release isosorbide dinitrate product at 8 mg/kg and above resulted in significant decreases in preload and afterload with increased cardiac output. Effects were sustained for at least 10 hours after dosing (Nagasawa et al. 2003). In a subsequent study in beagles with experimentally-induced mitral regurgitation, a sustained-release form of isosorbide dinitrate significantly reduced left arterial pressure (LAP) for at least 11 hours when dosed at 10 mg/kg PO. Significantly reduced LAP at 5 mg/kg

doses was only noted at 3 and 4 hours post dose (Yamamoto et al. 2013).

Pharmacokinetics

In dogs, isosorbide mononitrate oral bioavailability is approximately 70% after oral administration. Oral doses with standard tablets above 2 mg/kg yield peak plasma levels above 100 ng/mL, which is believed to be the minimum concentration of the drug required for hemodynamic effects in dogs and humans. Elimination half-life in dogs with standard tablets is about 1.5 hours. Dogs (24-31kg BW) given 60 mg sustained-release tablets (*Imdur®*) had peak plasma levels of approximately 550 ng/mL 3 hours after dosing. No pharmacokinetic information was located for cats.

Limited information on isosorbide dinitrate pharmacokinetics in small animals is available; it is reported that pharmacokinetics are similar in dogs and humans. In humans, both isosorbide dinitrate and mononitrate are well absorbed after oral administration. Food may delay the rate, but not the extent, of absorption. Isosorbide dinitrate undergoes extensive first-pass metabolism primarily to isosorbide mononitrate. Isosorbide mononitrate is metabolized primarily in the liver, but does not undergo first pass metabolism. Metabolites do not appear to have pharmacologic activity and are principally excreted in the urine.

Contraindications/Precautions/Warnings

Isosorbide nitrates should not be used in patients in shock or used alone in treating heart failure. Use with extreme caution in patients with low blood pressure or hypovolemia.

Adverse Effects

As there is limited experience in using these drugs in animals, an adverse effect profile is not well known.

In humans, the most common adverse effects are headache and postural hypotension. Tachycardia, restlessness or gastrointestinal effects are not uncommon. There have been rare cases of patients who are hypersensitive to organic nitrates.

Reproductive/Nursing Safety

Isosorbide nitrates are probably safe to use at therapeutic dosages during pregnancy. Dose-related increases in embryotoxicity occurred in rabbits given isosorbide dinitrate at 35-150X human dosages and there were some effects noted in rats (litter size, pup survival, prolonged gestation/parturition) given 125X doses of isosorbide mononitrate. Isosorbide mononitrate administered to rats and rabbits at 250 mg/kg/day (75X human dose) demonstrated no untoward effects. In humans, the FDA categorizes isosorbide nitrates as category C for use during pregnancy (*Animal studies have shown an adverse effect on the fetus, but there are no adequate studies in humans; or there are no animal reproduction studies and no adequate studies in humans.*)

It is unknown if isosorbide nitrates enter milk. Safe use during lactation cannot be guaranteed, but it is unlikely these drugs would pose significant risk to nursing offspring.

Overdosage/Acute Toxicity

Isosorbide mononitrate caused significant lethality in rats and mice at dosages of 2000 mg/kg and 3000 mg/kg, respectively. The primary concerns with an overdosage of isosorbide nitrates would be venous pooling, decreased cardiac output, and hypotension. Treatment is basically supportive; drug therapies with agents such as epinephrine are not recommended. Increasing central fluid volume may be useful but in patients with CHF, must be used with extreme caution.

Drug Interactions

The following drug interactions have either been reported or are theoretical in humans or animals receiving isosorbide and may be of in veterinary patients. Unless otherwise noted, use together is not necessarily contraindicated, but weigh the potential risks and perform additional monitoring when appropriate.

- **ANTIHYPERTENSIVE DRUGS:** Possible additive hypotensive effects.
- **PHENOTHIAZINES:** Possible additive hypotensive effects.
- **SELECTIVE PHOSPHODIESTERASE INHIBITORS** (*e.g.*, sildenafil): Profound hypotension (use is contraindicated).

Laboratory Considerations

- Serum cholesterol levels may be falsely decreased by nitrates when using the Zlatkis-Zak color reaction method

Doses

- **DOGS/CATS:**

  For adjunctive treatment of heart failure (extra-label): Efficacy is unknown and suspect. Some have suggested that dosages (of isosorbide dinitrate or mononitrate) at 0.5 – 2 mg PO q8-12h can be used, but limited experimental data and clinical use suggests that these dosages may not be effective. More recent experimental data (Nagasawa et al. 2003; Yamamoto et al. 2013) suggest that sustained release forms of isosorbide dinitrate at 8 – 10 mg/kg PO q12h in dogs may have efficacy, but it is unknown if therapeutic efficacy would be sustained or the adverse effects of these dosages.

Monitoring

- Clinical efficacy.

Client Information

- Inform clients of the limited experience in veterinary medicine with this medication.
- May be given with or without meals.

Chemistry/Synonyms

To minimize the risk for explosion, dry isosorbide dinitrate is mixed with lactose, mannitol or other inert excipients. To further stabilize the mixture, up to 1% ammonium phosphate or other suitable stabilizer can be used. The resultant dry mixture contains approximately 25% isosorbide dinitrate and is called diluted isosorbide dinitrate. It is an ivory-white, odorless powder that is very slightly soluble in water and sparingly soluble in alcohol.

Undiluted isosorbide mononitrate occurs as a white, crystalline powder that is freely soluble in water or alcohol. It is diluted with lactose or another suitable excipient to stabilize the powder and permit safe handling.

Isosorbide dinitrate may also be known as: ISD, ISDN, EV-151, sorbide nitrate, *Dilatrate-SR®*, *Isochron®*, *Isordil Titradose®*; many international trade name products are available.

Isosorbide mononitrate may also be known as: AHR-4698, BM-22145, IS-5-MN, or isosorbide-5-mononitrate, *Imdur®*, *Ismo®*, and *Monoket®*; many international trade name products are available.

Storage/Stability

Isosorbide dinitrate oral tablets, chewable tablets, extended-release tablets, and sublingual tablets should be stored in well-closed containers, below 40°C and preferably between 15-30°C. Heat and moisture accelerates loss of potency.

Isosorbide mononitrate tablets should be stored in tight containers, below 40°C and preferably between 15°-30°C. Isosorbide mononitrate extended-release tablets should be stored in tight containers, between 2°-30°C. Heat and moisture accelerates loss of potency.

Compatibility/Compounding Considerations

No specific information noted.

Dosage Forms/Regulatory Status

VETERINARY-LABELED PRODUCTS: NONE.
The ARCI (Racing Commissioners International) has designated this drug as a class 4 substance.

HUMAN-LABELED PRODUCTS:

Isosorbide Dinitrate Oral Tablets: 5 mg, 10 mg, 20 mg, 30 mg, & 40 mg; generic, *Isordil Titradose®*; (Rx)

Isosorbide Dinitrate Sublingual Oral Tablets: 2.5 mg, & 5 mg; generic; (Rx)

Isosorbide Dinitrate Extended-Release Oral Tablets: 40 mg; *Isochron®*, generic; (Rx)

Isosorbide Dinitrate Sustained-Release Oral Capsules: 40 mg; *Dilatrate-SR®*); (Rx)

Isosorbide Mononitrate Tablets: 10 mg, & 20 mg; generic, *Monoket®*; *Ismo®*; (Rx)

Isosorbide Mononitrate Extended-Release Tablets: 30 mg, 60 mg, & 120 mg; *Imdur®*, generic; (Rx)

Revisions/References

Monograph revised/updated February 2014.

Adin, D., et al. (2001). Efficacy of a single oral dose of isosorbide 5-mononitrate in normal dogs and in dogs with congestive heart failure. J Vet Intern Med 15: 105-11.
Nagasawa, Y., et al. (2003). Effect of sustained release isosorbide dinitrate (EV151) in dogs with experimentally-induced mitral insufficiency. J Vet Med Sci 65(5): 615-8.
Yamamoto, Y., et al. (2013). Effects of a Sustained-Release Form of Isosorbide Dinitrate on Left Atrial Pressure in Dogs with Experimentally Induced Mitral Valve Regurgitation. Journal of Veterinary Internal Medicine 27(6): 1421-6.

Isotretinoin

(eye-so-tret-i-noyn)   Accutane®

Retinoid

Prescriber Highlights

▶ Synthetic retinoid that may be useful in treatment a variety of dermatology diseases associated with epithelial cell proliferation & differentiation.

▶ Cautions (risk vs. benefit): Serum hypertriglyceridemia, hypersensitivity to drug; known teratogen.

▶ Adverse Effects: Most common adverse effect seen in dogs is keratoconjunctivitis sicca (KCS); apparently not a problem in cats. Other potential adverse effects in small animals include: GI effects (anorexia, vomiting, abdominal distention), CNS effects (lassitude, hyperactivity, collapse), pruritus, erythema of feet & mucocutaneous junctions, polydipsia, swollen tongue.

▶ Obtaining the medication for veterinary patients may be difficult and cost may be prohibitive.

▶ Pregnant women must avoid contact with medication; should not be dispensed to households where pregnant women present.

Uses/Indications

Isotretinoin may be useful in treating a variety of dermatologic-related conditions, including canine lamellar ichthyosis, cutaneus T-cell lymphoma, intracutaneous cornifying epitheliomas, multiple epidermal inclusion cysts, comedo syndrome in Schnauzers, and sebaceous adenitis seen in standard poodles. There is little scientific evidence available to support its use in veterinary patients, however.

Because of the concerns of teratogenic effects in humans, availability to veterinarians may be restricted by manufacturers and drug distributors; obtaining the medication for veterinary patients may be difficult.

Pharmacology/Actions

A retinoid, isotretinoin's major pharmacologic effects appear to be regulation of epithelial cell proliferation and differentiation. It affects monocyte and lymphocyte function, which can cause changes in cellular immune responses. The effects on skin include reduction of sebaceous gland size and activity, thereby reducing sebum production. It also has anti-keratinization and antiinflammatory activity and may indirectly reduce bacterial populations in sebaceous pores.

Pharmacokinetics

Isotretinoin is rapidly absorbed from the gut once the capsule disintegrates and the drug is dispersed in the GI contents. This may require up to 2 hours after dosing. Animal studies have shown that only about 25% of a dose reaches the systemic circulation, but food or milk in the gut may increase this amount. Isotretinoin is distributed into many tissues, but is not stored in the liver (unlike vitamin A). It crosses the placenta and is highly bound to plasma proteins. It is unknown if it enters milk. Isotretinoin is metabolized in the liver and is excreted in the urine and feces. In humans, terminal half-life is about 10-20 hours.

Contraindications/Precautions/Warnings

Isotretinoin should only be used when the potential benefits outweigh the risks when the following conditions exist: hypertriglyceridemia, severe renal or hepatic disease, or sensitivity to isotretinoin.

Isotretinoin is a known teratogen. Major anomalies have been reported in children of women taking the medication and it is not advised to use the medication in households where pregnant women are present.

Adverse Effects

There appears to be a low incidence of adverse effects, particularly in dogs. The most common adverse effect seen in dogs is keratoconjunctivitis sicca (KCS). This apparently is not a problem in cats. Other potential adverse effects include: GI effects (anorexia, vomiting, diarrhea, abdominal distention), CNS effects (lassitude, hyperactivity, behavioral changes, collapse), stiffness of limbs, pruritus, exfoliative dermatitis, erythema of feet and mucocutaneous junctions/cheilitis, polydipsia, and swollen tongue.

Incidence of adverse effects may be higher in cats. Effects reported include: blepharospasm, periocular crusting, erythema, diarrhea and, especially, weight loss secondary to anorexia. If cats develop adverse effects, the time between doses may be prolonged (*e.g.*, every other week give every other day) to reduce the total dose given.

Reproductive/Nursing Safety

Isotretinoin is a known teratogen. Major anomalies have been reported in children of women taking the medication. It is absolutely contraindicated in pregnant veterinary patients as well. Isotretinoin also appears to inhibit spermatogenesis. In humans, the FDA categorizes this drug as category *X* for use during pregnancy (*Studies in animals or humans demonstrate fetal abnormalities or adverse reaction; reports indicate evidence of fetal risk. The risk of use in pregnant women clearly outweighs any possible benefit.*)

It is not known whether this drug is excreted in breast milk. At this time, it is not recommended for use in nursing mothers.

Overdosage/Acute Toxicity

There were 147 exposures to isotretinoin reported to the ASPCA Animal Poison Control Center (APCC) during 2008-2009. In these cases 140 were dogs with 5 showing clinical signs and the remaining 7 reported cases were cats showing no clinical signs. Common findings in dogs included hypersalivation. Because of the drug's potential adverse effects, gut emptying should be considered with acute overdoses when warranted.

Drug Interactions

The following drug interactions have either been reported or are theoretical in humans or animals receiving isotretinoin and may be of in veterinary patients. Unless otherwise noted, use together is not necessarily contraindicated, but weigh the potential risks and perform additional monitoring when appropriate.
- **VITAMIN A** or **OTHER RETINOIDS**: Isotretinoin used with other retinoids (**etretinate**, **tretinoin**, or **vitamin A**) may cause additive toxic effects.
- **CYCLOSPORINE**: Isotretinoin may increase cyclosporine levels.
- **TETRACYCLINES**: Use with tetracyclines may increase the potential for the occurrence of pseudotumor cerebri (cerebral edema and increased CSF pressure).

Laboratory Considerations
- Increases in serum **triglyceride** and **cholesterol** levels may be noted that can be associated with corneal lipid deposits.
- **Platelets** may be increased.
- **ALT** (SGOT), **AST** (SGPT), and **LDH** levels may be increased.

Doses
- **DOGS:**

  For sebaceous adenitis, Schnauzer comedo syndrome, keratocanthoma, ichthyosis, sebaceous gland hyperplasia and adenoma (extra-label): Dosage can vary and no prospective, well-controlled, clinical studies were located to support any dosage regimen. Most recommend an initial dose of 1 mg/kg PO once or twice daily. Should be given with food. Any clinical efficacy may not be seen for 6-8 weeks. If efficacy is noted, may decrease dosage to 0.5 mg/kg or increase the time between dosages to every other day. Long-term treatment may be required.

  For epitheliotropic lymphoma (extra-label): Higher dosages have been suggested than those listed above. 3 – 4 mg/kg PO once daily or divided twice daily.

- **CATS:**

  For feline acne (extra-label): 5 – 10 mg per cat PO once daily have been suggested.

  For epitheliotropic lymphoma (extra-label): 10 mg per cat once daily has been suggested.

Monitoring
See Lab Considerations and Adverse Effects.
- Efficacy.
- Liver function tests (baseline and if signs appear).
- Dogs: Schirmer Tear tests (monthly—especially in older dogs).
- Cats: Weight.

Client Information
- Isotretinoin should not be handled by pregnant females and use in households where pregnant women are present is not advised. **Pregnant women must not be exposed to this drug;** severe birth defects can result. Veterinarians must take the personal responsibility to educate clients of the potential risk of ingestion by pregnant females.
- Best given with foods high in fat. Give the same way (with food or without) each time. If your animal vomits or acts sick after getting it on an empty stomach, give with food or small treat to see if this helps. If vomiting continues, contact your veterinarian.
- Dogs tolerate it better than cats. Most common side effect in dogs is dry eye syndrome (KCS); in cats, gastrointestinal effects (*e.g.*, loss of appetite, diarrhea, weight loss, etc.) may limit use.

Chemistry/Synonyms
A synthetic retinoid, isotretinoin occurs as a yellow-orange to orange, crystalline powder. It is insoluble in both water and alcohol. Commercially, it is available in soft gelatin capsules as a suspension in soybean oil.

Isotretinoin may also be known as: isotretinoinum, 13-cis-retinoic acid, Ro-4-3780, and *Accutane®*.

Storage/stability

Capsules should be stored at room temperature in tight, light resistant containers. The drug is photosensitive and will degrade with light exposure. Expiration dates of 2 years are assigned after manufacture.

Compatibility/Compounding Considerations

No specific information noted.

Dosage Forms/Regulatory Status

VETERINARY-LABELED PRODUCTS: NONE.

HUMAN-LABELED PRODUCTS:

Isotretinoin Oral Capsules: 10 mg, 20 mg, 30 mg & 40 mg (regular & soft gel); *Claravis*®; *Amnesteem*®); *Sotret*®; (Rx)

Note: Because of the concerns of teratogenic effects in humans availability to veterinarians may be restricted by manufacturers and drug distributors; obtaining the medication for veterinary patients may be difficult.

Revisions/References

Monograph revised/updated February 2014.

Isoxsuprine HCl

(eye-sox-suh-preen)   Vasodilan®

Prescriber Highlights

▶ Peripheral vasodilator that may have some efficacy in treatment of navicular disease in horses; efficacy in doubt when used orally. No commercially manufactured parenteral dosage forms are available in the USA.

▶ May be beneficial for Raynaud's-like syndrome in dogs.

▶ Contraindications: Immediately post-partum or in the presence of arterial bleeding.

▶ Adverse Effects: After injection, CNS stimulation (uneasiness, hyperexcitability, nose-rubbing) or sweating. Adverse effects are unlikely after oral administration.

Uses/Indications

Isoxsuprine is used in veterinary medicine principally for the treatment of navicular disease in horses, however, recent studies have shown disappointing efficacy when used orally. Dosages that cause vasodilation in horses are likely to induce neurologic adverse effects. Isoxsuprine has been used in humans for the treatment of cerebral vascular insufficiency, dysmenorrhea, and premature labor, but efficacies are unproven for these indications.

There have been anecdotal reports of isoxsuprine being helpful for treating dogs with a Raynaud's-like syndrome (periodic digital cyanosis, onychogryphosis) (Carlotti 2002) and to improve microcirculation in birds.

Pharmacology/Actions

Isoxsuprine causes direct vascular smooth muscle relaxation primarily in skeletal muscle. While it stimulates beta-adrenergic receptors it is believed that this action is not required for vasodilatation to occur. In horses with navicular disease, isoxsuprine will raise distal limb temperatures significantly. Isoxsuprine will relax uterine smooth muscle and may have positive inotropic and chronotropic effects on the heart. At high doses, isoxsuprine can decrease blood viscosity and reduce platelet aggregation. Isoxsuprine does not appear to possess significant analgesia properties in horses (Lizarraga et al. 2004).

Pharmacokinetics

In humans, isoxsuprine is almost completely absorbed from the GI tract, but in one study that looked at the cardiovascular and pharmacokinetic effects of isoxsuprine in horses (Matthews 1986),

bioavailability was low after oral administration, probably due to a high first-pass effect. After oral dosing of 0.6 mg/kg, the drug was non-detectable in plasma and no cardiac changes were detected. This study did not evaluate cardiovascular effects in horses with navicular disease nor did it attempt to measure changes in distal limb blood flow. After IV administration in horses, the elimination half-life is between 2.5-3 hours.

Contraindications/Precautions/Warnings

Isoxsuprine should not be administered to animals immediately post-partum or in the presence of arterial bleeding.

Adverse Effects

After parenteral administration, horses may show signs of CNS stimulation (uneasiness, hyperexcitability, nose-rubbing) or sweating. Adverse effects are unlikely after oral administration but hypotension, tachycardia, and GI effects are possible.

Reproductive/Nursing Safety

In humans, the FDA categorizes this drug as category *C* for use during pregnancy (*Animal studies have shown an adverse effect on the fetus, but there are no adequate studies in humans; or there are no animal reproduction studies and no adequate studies in humans.*)

No specific lactation safety information was found.

Overdosage/Acute Toxicity

Serious toxicity is unlikely in horses after an inadvertent oral overdose, but signs listed in the Adverse Effects section above could be seen. Treat signs if necessary. CNS hyperexcitability could be treated with diazepam, and hypotension with fluids.

Drug Interactions

No clinically significant drug interactions have been reported for this agent.

Laboratory Considerations

▪ None were noted.

Doses

▪ **HORSES:** (NOTE: ARCI UCGFS CLASS 4 DRUG)

For treatment of orthopedic conditions, such as navicular disease (extra-label): Unlikely to provide benefit. Dosage recommendations in the past have usually been 1.2 mg/kg PO q8-12h initially, and then time between dosages is increased to once a day and then every other day.

▪ **DOGS:**

For treatment of "Raynaud-like" disease (extra-label): 1 mg/kg per day PO. (Carlotti 2002)

Monitoring

▪ Clinical efficacy.
▪ Adverse effects (tachycardia, GI disturbances, CNS stimulation).

Client Information

▪ May be given with or without food. If your animal (dog) vomits or acts sick after getting it on an empty stomach, give with food or small treat to see if this helps. If vomiting continues, contact your veterinarian. Tablets may be crushed and made into a slurry, suspension, or paste by adding corn syrup, cherry syrup, etc., just before administration.

▪ May cause gastrointestinal effects (*e.g.,* lack of appetite, vomiting, diarrhea, etc.). Fast heart rates or low blood pressure are possible, but not common.

▪ Central nervous system stimulation (uneasiness, nose-rubbing, overly excited), rapid heart rate, low blood pressure are possible in overdoses or when given IV.

Chemistry/Synonyms

A peripheral vasodilating agent, isoxsuprine occurs as an odorless, bitter-tasting, white, crystalline powder with a melting point of about 200°C. It is slightly soluble in water and sparingly soluble in alcohol.

Isoxsuprine HCl may also be known as: Caa-40, isoxsuprini hydrochloridum, phenoxyisopropylnorsuprifen, *Dilum®, Duvadilan®, Fadaespasmol®, Fenam®, Inibina®, Isodilan®, Isotenk®, Uterine®, Vadosilan®, Vasodilan®, Vasolan®, Vasosuprina Ilfi®, Voxsuprine®,* and *Xuprin®.*

Storage/Stability

Tablets should be stored in tight containers at room temperature (15-30°C).

Compatibility/Compounding Considerations

No specific information noted.

Dosage Forms/Regulatory Status

VETERINARY-LABELED PRODUCTS: NONE.

The ARCI (Racing Commissioners International) has designated this drug as a class 4 substance. See the appendix for more information.

HUMAN-LABELED PRODUCTS:

Isoxsuprine HCl Tablets: 10 mg & 20 mg; generic; (Rx)

Revisions/References

Monograph revised/updated February 2014.

Carlotti, D.-N. (2002). Claw diseases in dogs and cats. Proceedings: World Small Animal Veterinary Association World Congress. accessed via Veterinary Information Network; vin.com

Lizarraga, I., et al. (2004). An analgesic evaluation of isoxsuprine in horses. Journal of Veterinary Medicine Series a-Physiology Pathology Clinical Medicine 51(7-8): 370-4.

Matthews, H. (1986). Cardiovascular and pharmacokinetic effects of isoxsuprine in the horse. Am J Vet Res 47(10): 2110-3.

Itraconazole

(ey-tra-kon-a-zole)   Sporanox®, Intrafungol®

Antifungal

Prescriber Highlights

▶ Synthetic oral triazole antifungal used for systemic and cutaneous mycoses.

▶ Not amenable to compounding; be wary of compounded itraconazole dosage forms as bulk powder itraconazole may not be absorbed.

▶ Contraindications (relative: risk vs. benefit): Hypersensitivity to it or other azole antifungal agents, hepatic impairment, or achlorhydria (or hypochlorhydria).

▶ Adverse Effects: **Dogs:** Anorexia is the most common, but hepatic toxicity and vasculitis are most significant adverse effects. At the higher dosage rate, some develop ulcerative skin lesions/vasculitis & limb edema. Rare, serious erythema multiforme or toxic epidermal necrolysis.

▶ Adverse Effects: **Cats:** Dose related; GI effects (anorexia, weight loss, vomiting), hepatotoxicity (increased ALT, jaundice), & depression.

▶ Maternotoxicity, fetotoxicity, & teratogenicity in lab animals at high dosages (5-20X labeled).

▶ Drug interactions.

Uses/Indications

Itraconazole is used in veterinary medicine in the treatment of systemic mycoses, including aspergillosis, cryptococcal meningitis, blastomycosis, coccidioidomycosis, sporotrichosis, and histoplasmosis. It can be useful as adjunctive treatment for pythiosis, lagendosis, zygomycosis, phaeohyphomycosis, and hyalohyphomycosis. Itraconazole is often considered first-line treatment for non–life threatening systemic mycoses that do not involve the central nervous system. Levels adequate to treat CNS or ocular infection can occur if there is associated inflammation and compromise of the barriers (Foy et al. 2010). It may also be useful for dermatophytosis, onychomycosis, and Malassezia dermatitis. Itraconazole does not have appreciable effects (unlike ketoconazole) on hormone synthesis and likely has fewer side effects than ketoconazole in small animals.

In horses, itraconazole may be useful in the treatment of sporotrichosis and *Coccidioides immitis* osteomyelitis.

Pharmacology/Actions

Itraconazole is a fungistatic triazole compound. Triazole-derivative agents, like the imidazoles (clotrimazole, ketoconazole, etc.), presumably act by altering the cellular membranes of susceptible fungi, thereby increasing membrane permeability and allowing leakage of cellular contents and impaired uptake of purine and pyrimidine precursors. Itraconazole has efficacy against a variety of pathogenic fungi, including yeasts and dermatophytes. *In vivo* studies using laboratory models have shown that itraconazole has fungistatic activity against many strains of Candida, Aspergillus, Cryptococcus, Histoplasma, Blastomyces, and *Trypanosoma cruzi.*

Itraconazole has immune-suppressing activity, probably via suppressing T-lymphocyte proliferation.

Pharmacokinetics

Itraconazole absorption is highly dependent on gastric pH and presence of food. When given on an empty stomach, bioavailability may only be 50% or less; with food, it may approach 100%. The commercially available capsules are specially formulated to increase oral bioavailability. Compounding capsules from bulk powders will likely not be absorbed. The commercially available liquid preparation possesses adequate oral bioavailability in dogs, cats and other species and may produce fewer GI adverse effects. The oral solution appears to be much better absorbed than capsules in horses. Use of human generic capsules of itraconazole (versus *Sporanox®*) in dogs and cats is somewhat controversial. However, a recent study comparing the pharmacokinetics of itraconazole in healthy dogs using generic versus brand name capsules concluded that generic itraconazole is bioequivalent to the innovator *Sporanox®* in dogs (Mawby et al. 2013).

Itraconazole has very high protein binding and is widely distributed throughout the body, particularly to tissues high in lipids (drug is highly lipophilic). Skin, sebum, the female reproductive tract, and pus all have concentrations greater than those found in the serum. Only minimal concentrations are found in CSF, urine, aqueous humor, and saliva. However, many fungal infections in the CNS, eye, or prostate can be effectively treated with itraconazole.

Itraconazole is metabolized by the liver to many different metabolites including to hydroxyitraconazole, which is active. In humans, itraconazole's serum half-life ranges from 21-64 hours. Elimination may be a saturable process. Because of its long half-life, itraconazole does not reach steady-state plasma levels for at least 6 days after starting therapy. If loading doses are given, levels will approach those of steady-state sooner.

Contraindications/Precautions/Warnings

Itraconazole should not be used in patients hypersensitive to it or other azole antifungal agents.

Use itraconazole in patients with hepatic impairment or achlorhydria (or hypochlorhydria) only when the potential benefits outweigh the risks.

Itraconazole may have a negative inotropic effect; use with caution in animals with reduced cardiac function.

African grey Parrots appear to be extremely sensitive to itraconazole and can develop anorexia and depression. Other antifungals or reduced dosages of itraconazole are recommended for use in this species.

Compounding capsules from bulk powders may not yield a dosage form that is absorbed.

Adverse Effects

In dogs, anorexia is the most common adverse effect seen, especially at higher dosages, but hepatic toxicity and vasculitis appear to be the most significant adverse effects. Approximately 10% of dogs receiving 10 mg/kg/day and 5% of dogs receiving 5 mg/kg/day developed hepatic toxicosis serious enough to discontinue treatment, at least temporarily. Hepatic injury is determined by an increased ALT activity. Anorexia is often the symptomatic marker for toxicity and usually occurs in the second month of treatment. Some dogs (7+%) given itraconazole at the higher dosage rate (10 mg/kg/day) may develop ulcerative skin lesions/vasculitis and limb edema that may require dosage reduction. These generally resolve following drug discontinuation. Rarely, serious erythema multiforme or toxic epidermal necrolysis reactions have been noted.

In cats, adverse effects appear to be dose related. GI effects (anorexia, weight loss, vomiting), hepatotoxicity (increased ALT, jaundice) and depression have been noted. As with dogs, doses above 10 mg/kg may be associated with a greater frequency of adverse effects, including hepatotoxicity.

Should adverse effects occur and ALT is elevated, the drug should be discontinued. Increased liver enzymes in the absence of other signs do not necessarily mandate dosage reduction or drug discontinuation. Once ALT levels return to normal and other adverse effects have diminished, if necessary, the drug may be restarted at a lower dosage or use longer dosing intervals with intense monitoring.

Reproductive/Nursing Safety

In laboratory animals, itraconazole has caused dose-related maternotoxicity, fetotoxicity and teratogenicity at high dosages (5-20X labeled). As safety has not been established, use only when the benefits outweigh the potential risks. In humans, the FDA categorizes this drug as category C for use during pregnancy (*Animal studies have shown an adverse effect on the fetus, but there are no adequate studies in humans; or there are no animal reproduction studies and no adequate studies in humans.*)

Itraconazole enters maternal milk; significance is unknown.

Overdosage/Acute Toxicity

There is very limited information on the acute toxicity of itraconazole. Giving oral antacids may help reduce absorption. If a large overdose occurs, consider gut emptying and give supportive therapy as required. Itraconazole is not removed by dialysis, but may be amenable to intravenous lipid emulsion therapy.

Drug Interactions

The following drug interactions have either been reported or are theoretical in humans or animals receiving itraconazole and may be of in veterinary patients. Unless otherwise noted, use together is not necessarily contraindicated, but weigh the potential risks and perform additional monitoring when appropriate.

- **AMPHOTERICIN B:** Lab animal studies have shown that itraconazole used concomitantly with amphotericin B may be antagonistic against Aspergillus or Candida; the clinical importance of these findings is not yet clear.
- **ANTACIDS:** May reduce oral absorption of itraconazole; administer itraconazole at least 1 hour before or 2 hours after antacids.
- **BENZODIAZEPINES** (*e.g.,* **alprazolam, diazepam, midazolam, triazolam**): Itraconazole may increase levels.
- **BUSPIRONE:** Plasma concentrations may be elevated.
- **BUSULFAN:** Itraconazole may increase levels.

- **CALCIUM-CHANNEL BLOCKING AGENTS** (*e.g.,* **amlodipine, verapamil**): Itraconazole may increase levels.
- **CISAPRIDE:** Itraconazole may increased cisapride levels and possibility for toxicity; use together contraindicated in humans.
- **CORTICOSTEROIDS:** Itraconazole may inhibit the metabolism of corticosteroids; potential for increased adverse effects.
- **CYCLOPHOSPHAMIDE:** Itraconazole may inhibit the metabolism of cyclophosphamide and its metabolites; potential for increased toxicity.
- **CYCLOSPORINE:** Increased cyclosporine levels.
- **DIGOXIN:** Itraconazole may increase digoxin levels; use together considered contraindicated in humans.
- **FENTANYL/ALFENTANIL:** Itraconazole may increase fentanyl or alfentanil levels.
- **H2-BLOCKERS** (**ranitidine, famotidine**, etc.): Increased gastric pH may reduce itraconazole absorption.
- **IVERMECTIN:** Itraconazole may increase risk for neurotoxicity.
- **MACROLIDE ANTIBIOTICS** (**erythromycin, clarithromycin,** etc.): May increase itraconazole concentrations.
- **PHENOBARBITAL/PHENYTOIN:** May decrease itraconazole levels.
- **PROTON-PUMP INHIBITORS** (**omeprazole**, etc.): Increased gastric pH may reduce itraconazole absorption.
- **QUINIDINE:** Increased risk for quinidine toxicity.
- **RIFAMPIN:** May decrease itraconazole levels; itraconazole may increase rifampin levels.
- **SULFONYLUREA ANTIDIABETIC AGENTS** (*e.g.,* **glipizide, glyburide**): Itraconazole may increase levels; hypoglycemia possible.
- **TRICYCLIC ANTIDEPRESSANTS** (**clomipramine, amitriptyline,** etc.): Itraconazole may decrease metabolism and increase tricyclic levels.
- **VINCRISTINE/VINBLASTINE:** Itraconazole may inhibit vinca alkaloid metabolism and increase levels.
- **WARFARIN:** Itraconazole may cause increased prothrombin times in patients receiving warfarin or other coumarin anticoagulants.

Laboratory Considerations

- Itraconazole may cause **hypokalemia** or increases in **liver function tests** in a small percentage of patients.

Doses

- **DOGS:**

  For systemic mycoses (extra-label): The "usual dose" in dogs is 5 – 10 mg/kg PO once daily (or divided q12h) with food; recommendations for treatment duration vary and are determined by the infective agent and site of infection. In general, treatment for systemic mycoses should be maintained for at least 30 days (some say 60 days) after clinical resolution. 10 mg/kg PO once daily with amphotericin B has been recommended for histoplasmosis. Infections such as pythiosis, lagendosis, zygomycosis, phaoehyphomycosis, hyalohyphomycosis may require dosages of 10 – 15 mg/kg PO once daily for many months along with surgical resection and additional antifungal agents (*e.g.,* terbinafine). Dosages of 10 mg/kg per day and above are associated with an increased risk for adverse effects.

  For dermatophytosis, onychomycosis (extra-label): 5 – 10 mg/kg PO q24h. Alternatively a pulse therapy protocol can be used: 5 – 10 mg/kg PO q24h on an every other week schedule. Duration of therapy should continue until at least 2 consecutive negative cultures 1-2 weeks apart.

For **Malassezia dermatitis** (extra-label): 5 mg/kg PO q24h and continued for 1 week after complete resolution of clinical signs.

- **CATS:**

For susceptible systemic mycoses (extra-label): The "usual dose" in cats is 5 – 10 mg/kg PO once daily (or divided q12h) with food. Treatment duration may be for many months (2-3 or more) and treatment is generally recommended to continue for at least 30-60 days after resolution of clinical signs. Certain infections may require additional surgical treatment or additional antifungals (amphotericin B, terbinafine, etc.).

For generalized dermatophytosis:

a) Caused by *Microsporum canis* (extra-label in USA): 5 mg/kg PO once daily for 7 days on, 7 days off; repeat 3 times. Cats must be treated during weeks 1, 3 and 5 and left untreated during weeks 2 and 4. In cases where a positive culture is obtained 4 weeks after the end of administration, the treatment should be repeated once at the same dosage regimen. In such cases where the cat is also immunosuppressed, treatment should be repeated and the underlying disease addressed. (Label Information—*Intrafungol*®; Janssen. U.K.)

b) In shelter cats (extra-label): 5 mg/kg PO once daily for 21 days with concurrent twice-weekly lime sulfur rinses. Treating otherwise healthy cats without biochemical monitoring is reasonable and cost effective. However, if cats become depressed or anorexic, biochemical monitoring is indicated. (Newbury et al. 2011; Moriello et al. 2013)

For Malassezia dermatitis (extra-label): 5 mg/kg PO q24h. Alternatively a pulse therapy protocol can be used: 5 mg/kg PO q24h for 2 consecutive days per week. Continue therapy until 1 week after complete resolution of clinical signs.

- **RABBITS, RODENTS, SMALL MAMMALS:**

Note: All are extra-label.

Mice: For blastomycosis: 50 – 150 mg/kg q24h.

Rats: For vaginal candidiasis (extra-label): 2.5 – 10 mg/kg q24h.

Guinea pigs: For systemic candidiasis: 5 mg/kg q24h. (Adamcak et al. 2000)

- **HORSES:**

For guttural pouch mycosis, mycotic rhinitis or osteomyelitis (extra-label): Using the oral solution at 5 mg/kg PO q24h should be sufficient for treatment. (Davis 2007)

- **BIRDS:**

Note: All are extra-label.

a) 5 – 10 mg/kg PO q12-24h. Use with caution in African grey parrots. (Tully 2008)

b) For aspergillosis: 5 – 10 mg/kg PO once daily in Amazon parrots; 2.5 – 5 mg/kg PO once daily in African grey Parrots. (Oglesbee 2009)

- **REPTILES:**

For susceptible fungal diseases (extra-label): 10 – 20 mg/kg PO q24h. (Schumacher 2011)

Monitoring

- Clinical Efficacy.
- With long-term therapy, routine liver function tests are recommended (monthly ALT).
- Appetite.
- Physical assessment for ulcerative skin lesions in dogs.

Client Information

- Compliance with treatment recommendations must be stressed.

- Give capsules or capsule contents with a fatty food (*e.g.*, butter, cream, ice cream, cheese, etc.). Preferably, give oral solution on an empty stomach in mammals.
- Interacts with many other drugs; do not give other medications without first talking to your veterinarian.
- Vomiting and loss of appetite are the most common side effects seen in dogs and cats. Liver toxicity and serious skin effects are possible (see adverse effects below).

Chemistry/Synonyms

A synthetic triazole antifungal, itraconazole is structurally related to fluconazole. It has a molecular weight of 706 and pKa of 3.7. It is practically insoluble in water and highly lipophilic.

Itraconazole may also be known as: itraconazolum, oriconazole, R-51211, or *Sporanox*®; many other trade names are available.

Storage/stability

Itraconazole capsules should be stored between 15-25°C and protected from light and moisture.

Itraconazole oral solution should be stored at temperatures less than 26°C, and protected from freezing.

Compatibility/Compounding Considerations

Compounding capsules or solutions from bulk chemicals or powders likely will not yield dosage forms that are absorbed. The oral bioavailability and solubility of itraconazole is dependent upon complexation with cyclodextrin molecules, a technology used in the brand (*Sporanox*®) and generic commercially produced human drug products for itraconazole, but not in compounded dosage forms. Two recent studies (Smith et al. 2010; Mawby et al. 2013) demonstrated that itraconazole compounded from the bulk chemical produces inferior blood levels in Black-footed penguins compared to FDA-approved itraconazole products. Inferior blood levels of itraconazole may contribute to treatment failure and fatality if compounded itraconazole is utilized in life-threatening infections such as blastomycosis or pythiosis. Unless itraconazole dosage forms are formulated from FDA-approved dosage forms, it is recommended not to use compounded itraconazole products unless prepared from commercial capsules or documented bioavailability and stability data are provided.

Compounded preparation stability: Two methods of preparing a stable (not necessarily bioavailable) itraconazole oral suspension prepared from commercially available capsules have been published. **1)** Triturating twenty-four (24) itraconazole 100 mg capsules with 5 mL ethanol 95%, allowing to stand 3-4 minutes, grinding to paste and then bringing to a final volume of 60 mL with simple syrup yields a 40 mg/mL oral suspension that retains >95% potency for 35 days stored at 4°C and protected from light (Jacobson et al. 1995). **2)** Triturating forty (40) itraconazole 100 mg capsules with 15 mL of ethanol 95%, allowing to stand 3-4 minutes, grinding to paste, adding 100 mL of *Ora-Plus*® and bringing to volume of 200 mL *Ora-Sweet*® yields a 20 mg/mL itraconazole suspension (Abdel-Rahmen et al. 1998). Solutions of itraconazole have a pH of 2.

Dosage Forms/Regulatory Status

VETERINARY-LABELED PRODUCTS: NONE IN THE USA.

In several countries, itraconazole oral liquid 10 mg/mL in 52 mL bottles with dosing syringe; *Intrafungol*®; (Rx). Labeled for use in cats (in the UK).

HUMAN-LABELED PRODUCTS:

Itraconazole Capsules: 100 mg; *Sporanox*®; generic; (Rx)

Itraconazole Tablets 100 mg; *Onmel*®; (Rx)

Itraconazole Oral Solution: 10 mg/mL in 150 mL; *Sporanox*®; (Rx)

Revisions/References

Monograph revised/updated February 2014.

Abdel-Rahmen, S. & M. C. Nahata (1998). Stability of itraconazole in an extemporaneous suspension. J Pediatr Pharm Pract 3: 115-8.

Adamcak, A. & B. Otten (2000). Rodent Therapeutics. Vet Clin NA: Exotic Anim Pract 3:1(Jan): 221-40.

Davis, J. L. (2007). Update on Antifungal Therapies in Horses. Proceedings: ACVIM. accessed via Veterinary Information Network; vin.com

Foy, D. S. & L. A. Trepanier (2010). Antifungal Treatment of Small Animal Veterinary Patients. Veterinary Clinics of North America-Small Animal Practice 40(6): 1171-+.

Jacobson, P. A., et al. (1995). Stability of Itraconazole in an Extemporaneously Compounded Oral Liquid. American Journal of Health-System Pharmacy 52(2): 189-91.

Mawby, D. I., et al. (2013). Bioequivalence of itraconazole formulations in healthy dogs (Abs.). Journal of Veterinary Internal Medicine 27(3): 748-9.

Moriello, K. A. & M. Verbrugge (2013). Changes in serum chemistry values in shelter cats treated with 21 consecutive days of oral itraconazole for dermatophytosis. Veterinary Dermatology 24(5): 557-8.

Newbury, S., et al. (2011). Use of itraconazole and either lime sulphur or Malaseb Concentrate Rinse (R) to treat shelter cats naturally infected with Microsporum canis: an open field trial. Veterinary Dermatology 22(1): 75-9.

Oglesbee, B. (2009). Working up the pet bird with upper respiratory tract disorders. Proceedings: WVC. accessed via Veterinary Information Network; vin.com

Schumacher, J. (2011). Respiratory Medicine of Reptiles. Vet Clin Exot Anim 14: 207-24.

Smith, J. A., et al. (2010). Effects Of Compounding On Pharmacokinetics Of Itraconazole In Black-Footed Penguins (Spheniscus Demersus). Journal of Zoo and Wildlife Medicine 41(3): 487-95.

Tully, T. (2008). Treating avian fungal diseases. Proceedings: Atlantic Coast Veterinary Conf. accessed via Veterinary Information Network; vin.com

---

Ivermectin

(eye-ver-mek-tin)   Heartgard®, Ivomec®

Antiparasitic

Prescriber Highlights

▶ Prototype avermectin drug used in a variety of species as an antiparasiticide.

▶ Contraindications: Label specific due to lack of safety data (foals, puppies, etc.) or public health safety (lactating dairy animals).

▶ Caution in breeds susceptible to *ABCB1-1Δ* (formerly MDR1-allele) mutation (Collies, Australian Shepherds, Shelties, Long-haired Whippet, "white feet"); at higher risk for CNS toxicity.

▶ Use very cautiously (or avoid) with other drugs affecting p-glycoprotein (P-gp)—see Drug Interactions.

▶ Adverse Effects: **Horses:** Swelling & pruritus at the ventral mid-line can be seen approximately 24 hours after ivermectin administration due to a hypersensitivity reaction to dead *Onchocerca* spp. microfilaria. **Dogs:** May exhibit a shock-like reaction when ivermectin is used as a microfilaricide, presumably due to a reaction associated with the dying microfilaria. **Cattle:** Ivermectin can induce serious adverse effects by killing the larva when they are in vital areas; may also cause discomfort or transient swelling at the injection site. **Mice & rats:** May cause neurologic toxicity at doses slightly more than usually prescribed. **Birds:** Death, lethargy, or anorexia may be seen. Orange-cheeked Waxbill Finches & budgerigars may be more sensitive to ivermectin than other species.

Uses/Indications

Ivermectin is FDA-approved in horses for the control of: large adult strongyles (*Strongylus vulgaris, S. edentatus, S. equinus, Triodontophorus* spp.), small strongyles, pinworms (adults and 4th stage larva), ascarids (adults), hairworms (adults), large-mouth stomach worms (adults), neck threadworms (microfilaria), bots (oral and gastric stages), lungworms (adults and 4th stage larva), intestinal threadworms (adults), and summer sores (cutaneous 3rd stage larva) secondary to *Hebronema* or *Draschia* spp.

In cattle, ivermectin is FDA-approved for use in the control of gastrointestinal roundworms (adults and 4th stage larva), lungworms (adults and 4th stage larva), cattle grubs (parasitic stages), sucking lice, and mites (scabies). For a listing of individual species covered, refer to the product information.

In swine, ivermectin is FDA-approved for use to treat GI roundworms, lungworms, lice, and mange mites. For a listing of individual species covered, refer to the product information.

In reindeer, ivermectin is FDA-approved for use in the control of warbles. In American Bison, ivermectin is FDA-approved for use in the control of grubs.

In dogs, ivermectin is FDA-approved only for use as a preventative for heartworm. In cats, it is FDA-approved for heartworm prevention and control of hookworms. It has also been used as a microfilaricide, ectoparasiticide, and endoparasiticide. Ivermectin and doxycycline individually suppress embryogenesis and weaken adult heartworms and when used together provide more rapid adulticidal activity than either drug alone. The American Heartworm Society does <u>not</u> recommend using macrocyclic lactones at prophylactic doses as a slow-kill adulticide method for *D. immitis* (Nelson et al. 2014).

Pharmacology/Actions

Ivermectin enhances the release of gamma amino butyric acid (GABA) at presynaptic neurons. GABA acts as an inhibitory neurotransmitter and blocks the post-synaptic stimulation of the adjacent neuron in nematodes or the muscle fiber in arthropods. By stimulating the release of GABA, ivermectin causes paralysis of the parasite and eventual death. As liver flukes and tapeworms do not use GABA as a peripheral nerve transmitter, ivermectin is ineffective against these parasites.

Ivermectin can kill *D. immitis* larval stages 3 & 4, kill microfilaria, and reduce the lifespan of adult heartworms. Resistance by *D. immitis* (MP3 strain) to macrocyclic lactones is a concern and research is ongoing to characterize the issue in more detail. The American Heartworm Society has stated that: "It is now generally accepted that pockets of resistant heartworms exist. The extent, the degree of spread, and the reasons for resistance are not understood and are controversial. All agree that owner compliance is the biggest factor in the "failure" of preventives" (Nelson et al. 2014).

Pharmacokinetics

In simple-stomached animals, ivermectin is up to 95% absorbed after oral administration. Ruminants only absorb 1/4-1/3 of a dose due to inactivation of the drug in the rumen. While there is greater bioavailability after SC administration, absorption after oral dosing is more rapid than SC. It has been reported that ivermectin's bioavailability is lower in cats than in dogs, necessitating a higher dosage for prophylaxis of heartworm in this species.

Ivermectin is well distributed to most tissues, but does not readily penetrate into the CSF, thereby minimizing its toxicity. Dogs with the ABCB-1 gene defect allow more ivermectin into the CNS than is seen in other tested mammalian species.

Ivermectin has a long terminal half-life in most species (see below). It is metabolized in the liver via oxidative pathways and is primarily excreted in the feces. Less than 5% of the drug (as parent compound or metabolites) is excreted in the urine.

Pharmacokinetic parameters of ivermectin have been reported for various species:

Cattle: Volume of distribution = 0.45 – 2.4 L/kg; elimination half-life = 2-3 days; total body clearance = 0.79 L/kg/day.

Dogs: Bioavailability = 0.95; volume of distribution = 2.4 L/kg; elimination half-life = 2 days.

Swine: Volume of distribution = 4 L/kg; elimination half-life = 0.5 days.

Sheep: Bioavailability = 1 (intra-abomasal), 0.25 (intra-ruminal); volume of distribution = 4.6 L/kg; elimination half-life = 2-7 days.

Contraindications/Precautions/Warnings

The manufacturer recommends that ivermectin not be used in foals less than 4 months old as safety of the drug in animals this young has not been firmly established. However, foals less than 30 days of age have tolerated doses as high as 1 mg/kg without signs of toxicity.

Ivermectin is not recommended for use in puppies less than 6 weeks old. After receiving heartworm prophylaxis doses, the manufacturer recommends observing Collie-type breeds for at least 8 hours after administration. Secondary to a defective blood-brain barrier, *ABCB1-1Δ* (MDR1-allele) mutant/mutant dogs can show adverse neurologic signs after a single doses >120 micrograms/kg and develop life-threatening neurologic toxicity at doses of 300 micrograms/kg (Mealey 2013). When used at extra-label dosages in dogs, most clinicians feel that ivermectin should not be used in breeds susceptible (Collies, Shelties, Australian shepherds, etc.) to the *ABCB1-1Δ* mutation unless the patient has been tested and found not to have the gene defect. A specific test for identifying dogs that have the gene defect is available; contact the veterinary clinical pharmacology lab at www.vetmed.wsu.edu. At higher dosages, neurotoxicity can occur rarely in dogs tested normal/normal so it is advised to continually monitor for adverse effects. When used at labeled heartworm preventative dosages, toxicity is rarely observed. It is recommended that should they occur, ivermectin be discontinued.

Ivermectin is reportedly contraindicated in chelonians, Indigo snakes and skinks. Milbemycin has reportedly been given safely to chelonians.

Because milk withdrawal times have not been established, the drug is not FDA-approved for use in lactating dairy animals or females of breeding age.

The injectable products for use in cattle and swine should be given subcutaneously only; do **not** give IM or IV.

If using a product in a species not labeled for that product (extra-label), be certain of the dosage and/or dilutions. There are many reports of overdoses in small animals when large animal injectable products have been used.

Adverse Effects

In horses, swelling and pruritus at the ventral mid-line can be seen approximately 24 hours after ivermectin administration due to a hypersensitivity reaction to dead *Onchocerca* spp. microfilaria. The reaction is preventable by administering a glucocorticoid just prior to, and for 1-2 days after, ivermectin. If untreated, swelling usually subsides within 7-10 days and pruritus will resolve within 3 weeks.

Neurotoxicity is possible in dogs, particularly in those with the gene defect (deletion mutation of the *ABCB1* (formerly MDR1) gene) that has been seen in certain genetic lines of Collie-type breeds. There are case reports of dogs without the *ABCB1* mutation developing neurotoxicity after receiving ivermectin at demodicosis doses. Dogs may exhibit a shock-like reaction when ivermectin is used as a microfilaricide, presumably due to a reaction associated with the dying microfilaria. Other adverse effects when used as a microfilaricide include depression, hypothermia, and vomiting. Pretreatment with diphenhydramine (2 mg/kg IM) and dexamethasone (0.25 mg/kg IV) can help prevent adverse reactions (Atkins 2005).

When used to treat *Hypoderma bovis* larva (Cattle grubs) in cattle, ivermectin can induce serious adverse effects by killing the larva when they are in vital areas. Larva killed in the vertebral canal can cause paralysis and staggering. Larva killed around the gullet can induce salivation and bloat. These effects can be avoided by treating for grubs immediately after the Heal fly (Warble fly) season or after the stages of grub development where these areas would be affected. Cattle may experience discomfort or transient swelling at

the injection site. Using a maximum of 10 mL at any one-injection site can help minimize these effects.

There are case reports of horses developing neurotoxicity after receiving recommended oral dosages (Swor et al. 2009).

In mice and rats, ivermectin may cause neurologic toxicity at doses slightly more than usually prescribed (less than 0.5 mg/kg).

In birds, death, lethargy or anorexia may be seen. Orange-cheeked Waxbill Finches and budgerigars may be more sensitive to ivermectin than other species.

For additional information refer to the Overdosage/Acute Toxicity section below.

Reproductive/Nursing Safety

Ivermectin is considered safe to use during pregnancy. Reproductive studies performed in dogs, horses, cattle and swine have not demonstrated adverse effects to fetuses. Reproductive performance in male animals is apparently unaltered. In humans, the FDA categorizes this drug as category C for use during pregnancy (*Animal studies have shown an adverse effect on the fetus, but there are no adequate studies in humans; or there are no animal reproduction studies and no adequate studies in humans.*) In a separate system evaluating the safety of drugs in canine and feline pregnancy (Papich 1989), this drug is categorized as class: *A (Probably safe. Although specific studies may not have proved the safety of all drugs in dogs and cats, there are no reports of adverse effects in laboratory animals or women.*)

Ivermectin is excreted in milk in low concentrations; it is unlikely to pose significant risk to nursing offspring.

Overdosage/Acute Toxicity

There were 733 single agent exposures to ivermectin reported to the ASPCA Animal Poison Control Center (APCC) during 2009-2013. Of the 658 dogs, 502 were symptomatic with ataxia (70%), mydriasis (49%), blindness (43%), tremors (38%), vomiting (20%), and seizures (9%) being the most common signs. Of the 53 cats, 37 were symptomatic with ataxia (76%), mydriasis (68%), blindness (32%), tremors (24%) and vomiting (19%) being the most common.

In dogs (non-sensitive breeds), signs of acute toxicity rarely occur at single dosages of 1 mg/kg (1000 micrograms/kg) or less. At 2.5 mg/kg, mydriasis occurs, and at 5 mg/kg, tremors occur. At doses of 10 mg/kg, severe tremors and ataxia are seen. Deaths occurred when dosages exceeded 40 mg/kg, but the LD50 is 80 mg/kg. Dogs (Beagles) receiving 0.5 mg/kg PO for 14 weeks developed no signs of toxicity, but at 1 – 2 mg/kg for the same time period, developed mydriasis and had some weight decreases. Half of the dogs receiving 2 mg/kg/day for 14 weeks developed signs of depression, tremors, ataxia, anorexia, and dehydration.

Ivermectin is actively transported by the p-glycoprotein pump and certain breeds susceptible to MDR1-allele mutation (Collies, Australian Shepherds, Shelties, Long-haired Whippets, etc.) are at higher risk for CNS toxicity. At the dosage recommended for heartworm prophylaxis, it is generally believed that the drug is safe to use in these animals. In cases of overdoses signs can develop within 4 hours in sensitive breeds.

Dogs that receive an overdosage of ivermectin or develop signs of acute toxicity (CNS effects, GI, cardiovascular, hypercapnea) should receive supportive and symptomatic therapy. Emptying the gut should be considered for recent massive oral ingestions in dogs or cats. For both oral and injected ivermectin overdoses, the use of repeated activated charcoal doses has been advised to interrupt enterohepatic recirculation.

Intravenous fat emulsion has been successfully used to treat dogs, cats or ponies with large ivermectin overdoses or neurotoxicity (Clarke et al. 2011; Fernandez et al. 2011; Bruenisholz et al. 2012; Gwaltney-Brant et al. 2012; Held et al. 2012; Bates et al. 2013; Epstein et al. 2013; Kidwell et al. 2014). This therapy is still in the developmental stage; contact an animal poison center for further guidance if considering this treatment.

Ivermectin has a large safety margin in cats. Kittens receiving doses of at least 110 mcg/kg and adult cats receiving at least 750 mcg/kg showed no untoward effects. The margin of safety is narrower in kittens as significant clinical signs have been seen at 300 micrograms/kg. Acute toxic signs associated with massive overdoses in cats will appear within 10 hours of ingestion. Signs may include agitation, vocalization, anorexia, mydriasis, rear limb paresis, tremors, and disorientation. Blindness, head pressing, wall climbing, absence of oculomotor menace reflex, and a slow and incomplete response to pupillary light may also be seen. Neurologic signs usually diminish over several days and most animals completely recover within 2-4 weeks. Symptomatic and supportive care is recommended.

In horses, doses of 1.8 mg/kg (9X recommended dose) PO did not produce signs of toxicity, but doses of 2 mg/kg caused signs of visual impairment, depression and ataxia. In cattle, toxic effects generally do not appear until dosages of 30X those recommended are injected. At 8 mg/kg, cattle showed signs of ataxia, listlessness, and occasionally, death occurred.

Sheep have shown signs of ataxia and depression at ivermectin doses of 4 mg/kg.

Swine have shown signs of toxicosis (lethargy, ataxia, tremors, lateral recumbency, and mydriasis) at doses of 30 mg/kg. Neonatal pigs may be more susceptible to ivermectin overdoses, presumably due to a more permeable blood-brain barrier. Accurate dosing practices are recommended.

Drug Interactions

The following drug interactions have either been reported or are theoretical in humans or animals receiving ivermectin and may be of in veterinary patients. Unless otherwise noted, use together is not necessarily contraindicated, but weigh the potential risks and perform additional monitoring when appropriate.

- **BENZODIAZEPINES:** Effects may be potentiated by ivermectin; use together not advised in humans.
- **KETAMINE:** It has been recommended not to use ivermectin in reptiles within 10 days of ketamine (Bays 2009).

Caution is advised if using other drugs that can inhibit **P-glycoprotein**. Dogs at risk for *ABCB*1-1Δ (formerly MDR1 allele) mutation (Collies, Australian Shepherds, Shelties, Long-haired Whippet, etc., "white feet") should probably not receive ivermectin with the following drugs, unless tested "normal". Drugs and drug classes involved include:

- **AMIODARONE**
- **BROMOCRIPTINE**
- **CARVEDILOL**
- **CETIRIZINE:** In horses, pre-treatment (12 hours before cetirizine, but not 1.5 hours) with ivermectin increased cetirizine plasma AUC, mean residence time and terminal half-life significantly (Olsen et al. 2007). Because of cetirizine's large therapeutic index, clinical significance is not likely.
- **CLARITHROMYCIN**
- **CYCLOSPORINE**
- **DILTIAZEM**
- **ERYTHROMYCIN**
- **FLUOXETINE, PAROXETINE**
- **GRAPEFRUIT JUICE**
- **ITRACONAZOLE**
- **KETOCONAZOLE:** At least one reference states that ivermectin should never be used with ketoconazole in dogs (Waisglass 2009).

- **METHODONE, PENTAZOCINE**
- **QUINIDINE**
- **SOLANUM spp.** (Nightshades): Horses ingesting Nightshade species and receiving oral ivermectin developed neurotoxicity. Authors suggest that *Solanum* spp. may alter P-gp in horses or other mammalian species (Norman et al. 2012).
- **SPIRONOLACTONE**
- **SPINOSAD:** It has been recommended not to use with the high extra-label doses of ivermectin (Kuhl 2009); in healthy beagles spinosad has been shown to alter ivermectin pharmacokinetics and may alter blood-brain barrier permeability and increase risk for neurotoxicity (Dunn et al. 2011).
- **ST. JOHNS WORT**
- **TACROLIMUS**
- **TAMOXIFEN**
- **VERAPAMIL**

Laboratory Considerations

- When used at microfilaricide dosages, ivermectin may yield false-negative results in animals with occult heartworm infection.

Doses

For dosages of combination products, refer to the product label for specific approved dosage suggestions.

- **DOGS:**

Note: When used for prophylaxis or treatment of dirofilariasis it is recommended to review the guidelines published by the American Heartworm Society at www.heartwormsociety.org

As a preventative for heartworm (labeled-dose; FDA-approved): Minimum dosage of 6 micrograms/kg (0.006 mg/kg) PO per month (Package insert; *Heartgard30®*). To be maximally effective, heartworm prophylaxis should be given year-round, but if seasonal treatment is chosen, administration should begin at least one month prior to the anticipated start of heartworm transmission and should continue for at least 3 months after transmission typically ceases. (Nelson et al. 2014)

As adjunctive treatment for heartworm disease (extra-label): On a regular basis, The American Heartworm Society publishes specific guidelines for the treatment of heartworms. In the 2014 update as one part of the guidelines, approved heartworm preventatives are given at labeled dosages on day 1 of the treatment protocol and repeated every 30 days. For more information refer to www.heartwormsociety.org

As an ectoparasiticide (miticide): **Warning:** Do not use in ABCB1-1Δ (formerly MDR1-allele) mutation susceptible breeds unless tested "normal/normal" for mutation (www.vetmed.wsu.edu). If normal/normal, drug reaction is very unlikely but still possible; continue to monitor for adverse effects.

a) **For generalized demodicosis** (extra-label): The usual target dose recommended is 0.6 mg/kg (600 micrograms/kg) PO once daily until 4 weeks past 2 negative skin scrapings taken 4-6 weeks apart. Start at a low dosage and increase: **Day 1:** 0.05 mg/kg (50 micrograms/kg) PO. **Day 2:** 0.1 mg/kg (100 micrograms/kg) PO. **Day 3:** 0.15 mg/kg (150 micrograms/kg) PO. **Day 4:** 0.2 mg/kg (200 micrograms/kg) PO. **Day 5:** 0.3 mg/kg (300 microgram/kg) PO. Then increase by 0.1 mg/kg (100 mcg/kg) every 3-7 days until the final target dose is reached. Treatment may be required for several months. Advise the owner to discontinue immediately if there is evidence of ivermectin toxicity (especially lethargy, ataxia, mydriasis and gastrointestinal signs). If there is no reaction at a lower but therapeutic dose (above

0.3 mg/kg), some will attempt treating at that lower dose but on an alternate day treatment schedule. Adapted from: (Waisglass 2009; Koch et al. 2011; Mueller et al. 2012)

b) **For sarcoptic mange, cheyletiellosis** (extra-label): <u>SC Dose</u>: If positive skin scrapings 0.2 – 0.4 mg/kg (200 – 400 micrograms/kg) SC every 2 weeks for 3 treatments. If skin scrapings not taken or are negative and performing a therapeutic trial: if after the 2nd injection there are positive results, give 3rd injection. If no response, reconsider diagnosis. Alternatively a <u>PO dose</u> for sarcoptic mange can be considered: 0.2 – 0.4 mg/kg (200 – 400 mcg/kg) PO once weekly for 4 treatments. Adapted from: (Koch et al. 2011)

c) **For otodectic acariosis** (extra-label): 0.3 mg/kg (300 micrograms/kg) SC every 2 weeks or topical application of 0.5 mL (Using 0.1 mg/mL concentration) per ear for 1-2 treatments. (Koch et al. 2011)

d) **For nasal mites**: 0.3 mg/kg (300 micrograms/kg) SC every 1-2 weeks for 2-3 treatments. (Koch et al. 2011)

■ **CATS:**

Note: When used for prophylaxis or treatment of dirofilariasis it is recommended to review the guidelines published by the American Heartworm Society at www.heartwormsociety.org

As a preventative for heartworm and control of hookworm (labeled dose; FDA-approved): The individual minimum monthly prophylactic dose of ivermectin is 24 micrograms/kg (adapted from: *Heartgard®* for Cats). Preventives should be started in kittens at 8 weeks of age and administered to all cats in heartworm endemic areas during the heartworm season. Use is not precluded by antibody or antigen seropositivity (Jones et al. 2014).

■ **FERRETS:**

For prevention of heartworm disease (extra-label): 0.02 mg/kg PO monthly. (Hoeffer 2000)

To treat heartworm disease using the very slow protocol (extra-label): 50 micrograms PO once a month. (Hernandez-Divers 2007)

■ **RABBITS/RODENTS/SMALL MAMMALS:**

Note: All are extra-label.

a) **Rabbits:** For *Sarcoptes scabiei, Notoedres cati*: 0.3 – 0.4 mg/kg SC, repeat in 14 days. For ear mites (Psoroptes) 0.2 – 0.44 mg/kg PO, SC repeat in 8-18 days. (Ivey et al. 2000)

b) **Rabbits:** For treatment of ear mites: 200 micrograms/kg SC and repeated in two weeks. All rabbits in colony should be treated and cages cleaned and disinfected. (Burke 1999)

c) **Rodents and lagomorphs:** For treatment of sarcoptoid and some fur mites: 200 – 250 micrograms/kg SC. Cages should be thoroughly cleaned and disinfected. (Burke 1999)

d) **Mice, Rats, Gerbils, Guinea pigs, Chinchillas:** 200 micrograms/kg SC or PO every 7 days for 3 weeks. **Hamsters:** 200 – 500 micrograms/kg SC or PO every 14 days for 3 weeks. (Adamcak et al. 2000)

e) **Guinea pigs** for *Trixacarus caviae* mites: 500 micrograms/kg SC, repeated at 14 and 28 days. (Johnson 2006)

■ **CATTLE:**

For susceptible parasites (labeled dose; FDA-approved): For gastrointestinal roundworms (including inhibited *Ostertagia ostertagi* in cattle), lungworms, grubs, sucking lice, and mange mites: 200 micrograms/kg (0.2 mg/kg) SC under the loose skin in front of or behind the shoulder. (Product Information; *Ivomec® Inj. for Cattle 1%*)

■ **HORSES:**

For susceptible parasites (labeled dose; FDA-approved): 200 micrograms/kg (0.2 mg/kg) PO using oral paste or oral liquid. (Product Information; *Eqvalan®*)

■ **SWINE:**

For susceptible parasites (gastrointestinal roundworms, lungworms, lice, and mange mites (labeled-dose, FDA-approved): 300 micrograms/kg (0.3 mg/kg) SC in the neck immediately behind the ear. (Product Information; *Ivomec® Inj. for Swine 1%*)

■ **SHEEP/GOATS:**

For susceptible parasites:

a) **For gastrointestinal roundworms** (*Haemonchus contortus, Ostertagia circumcincta, Trichostrongylus axei T. colubriformis, Cooperia curticei, Nematodirus spathiger, N. battus,* and *Oesophagostomum columbianum*); **Lungworms** (*Dictyocaulus filarial*); and all the larval stages of Nasal Bot (*Oestrus ovis*). Also treatment and control of adult forms only of *Haemonchus placei, Cooperia oncophora, Strongyloides papillosus, Oesophagostomum venulosum, Trichuris ovis,* and *Chabertia ovina* (labeled dose; FDA-approved for sheep): Using the approved oral drench for sheep is administered orally at a dose of 3 mL (2.4 mg ivermectin) per 26 lb. body weight or 200 mcg/kg PO. (Adapted from label: Ivomec® Oral Drench 0.08%)

b) **For adjunctive treatment of meningeal worm** (*Parelaphostrongylus tenuis*); (extra-label): To prevent further migration: Ivermectin at 0.3 mg/kg SC once daily for 5 days with fenbendazole (50 mg/kg PO once daily for 5 days). (Edmondson 2009)

■ **CAMELIDS:**

For GI helminths (extra-label): In new world camelids: 0.2 mg/kg PO once. (Wolff 2009)

For adjunctive treatment of meningeal worm (*Parelaphostrongylus tenuis*); (extra-label): To prevent further migration: Fenbendazole at 50 mg/kg PO once daily for 5 days and ivermectin at 0.3 mg/kg SC once daily for 5 days. Camelids very susceptible to GI ulcers; give prophylaxis or treat with omeprazole or ranitidine. (Edmondson 2009)

■ **BIRDS:**

For susceptible parasites (all are extra-label):

a) **For ascarids, Capillaria and other intestinal worms,** *Knemidocoptes pilae* (scaly face and leg mites): Dilute to a 2 mg/mL concentration. After diluting product, use immediately. <u>Most birds</u>: Inject 220 micrograms/kg IM; <u>Amazons</u>: 0.1 mg IM; <u>Macaws</u>: 0.2 mg IM; <u>Finches</u>: 0.02 mg. (Stunkard 1984)

b) **For ascarids, coccidia and other intestinal nematodes,** Oxysipura, gapeworms, *Knemidocoptes pilae* (scaly face and leg mites); (extra-label) Dilute bovine preparation (10 mg/mL) 1:4 with propylene glycol. <u>For most species</u>: 200 micrograms/kg IM or orally, repeat in 10-14 days; <u>Budgerigars</u>: 0.01 mL of diluted product (see above) IM or PO. (Clubb 1986)

■ **REPTILES:**

For most nematodes, ectoparasites (extra-label): For <u>lizards, snakes, and alligators</u>: 0.2 mg/kg (200 micrograms/kg) IM, SC, or PO once; repeat in 2 weeks. A third treatment can be given if still positive after the second treatment. **Note:** Ivermectin is toxic to chelonians, indigo snakes, skinks. (Gauvin 1993; de la Navarre 2003)

Monitoring

- Clinical efficacy.
- Adverse effects/toxicity (see Adverse Effects and Overdosage Sections).

Client Information

- When using large animal products the manufacturer recommends not eating or smoking and to wash hands after use. Avoid contact with eyes. Do not use large animal products in small animals.
- May be given with or without food. If your animal vomits or acts sick after getting it on an empty stomach, give with food or small treat to see if this helps. If vomiting continues, contact your veterinarian.
- Overdoses can be serious; measure dosages carefully and keep chewable/flavored tablets out of reach of children and animals.
- Usually tolerated very well; if CNS signs (see adverse effects) are seen, contact your veterinarian immediately.
- Dispose of unused product carefully; can be very toxic to fish and wildlife.

Chemistry/Synonyms

An avermectin anthelmintic, ivermectin occurs as an off-white to yellowish powder. It is very poorly soluble in water (4 micrograms/mL), but is soluble in propylene glycol, polyethylene glycol, and vegetable oils.

Ivermectin may also be known as MK 933, ivermectine, ivermectinum or ivermectina; many trade names are available.

Storage/stability

Ivermectin is photolabile in solution; protect from light. Unless otherwise specified by the manufacturer, store ivermectin products at room temperature (15-30°C).

Ivermectin 1% oral solution (equine tube wormer product) is stable at 1:20 and 1:40 dilutions with water for 72 hours when stored in a tight container, at room temperature, and protected from light.

Compatibility/Compounding Considerations

If compounding from the concentrated injectable forms, institute multiple check systems to reduce the chance for overdoses.

Dosage Forms/Regulatory Status

VETERINARY PRODUCTS:

Note: As ivermectin is no longer patent protected in the USA; there are a variety of "generic" products available with many trade names. The following may not be a complete listing.

Ivermectin for Injection: 10 mg/mL (1%) in 50 mL, 200 mL, 500 mL bottles; *Ivomec® 1% Injection for Cattle* and *Swine*, generic; (OTC). FDA-approved for use in cattle (not female dairy cattle of breeding age) and swine. Slaughter (when used as labeled): cattle = 35 days, swine = 18 days, reindeer = 56 days, bison = 56 days. No milk withdrawal time has been established.

Ivermectin for Injection: 2.7 mg/mL (0.27%) in 200 mL bottles; *Ivomec® 0.27% Injection for Feeder* and *Grower Pigs*; (OTC). FDA-approved for use in swine. Slaughter (when used as labeled) = 18 days.

Ivermectin Oral Paste: 1.87% (18.7 mg/gram) in 6.08 gram syringes; *Equimectrin® Paste 1.87%, Eqvalan® Paste 1.87% Zimectrin® Paste*, generic; (OTC). FDA-approved for use in horses (not intended for food purposes).

Oral Paste: containing 1.87% ivermectin and 14.03% of praziquantel in oral syringes (sufficient to treat one 1320 lb. horse); *Equimax®*; (OTC). FDA-approved for use in horse or ponies not intended for food purposes.

Oral Paste: containing 1.55% ivermectin and 7.75% of praziquantel in oral syringes; *Zimecterin Gold®*; (OTC). FDA-approved for use in horse or ponies not intended for food purposes.

Ivermectin Liquid: 1% (10 mg/mL) in 50 mL and 100 mL btls (for tube administration; **not** for injection); *Eqvalan® Liquid*, generic; (Rx). FDA-approved for use in horses (not intended for food purposes).

Ivermectin Oral Tablets: 68 mcg, 136 mcg, 272 mcg (Plain or Chewable) in 6 chewables/carton; *Heartgard® Tablets*, generic; (Rx). FDA-approved for use in dogs.

Ivermectin Oral Chewable Tablets: 55 mcg or 165 mcg in cartons of 6; *Heartgard® for Cats*; (Rx). FDA-approved for use in cats.

Ivermectin Oral Solution: 0.08% in 960 mL and 4,800 mL containers; *Ivomec® Sheep Drench*; (OTC). FDA-approved for use in sheep. Slaughter withdrawal time = 11 days.

Ivermectin Bolus: 1.72 gram; *Ivomec® SR Bolus*; (OTC). FDA-approved for use in cattle (not female dairy cattle of breeding age). Slaughter withdrawal time = 180 days. No milk withdrawal time has been established.

Ivermectin Topical Parasiticide Pour-on for Cattle: 5 mg/mL; *Ivomec® Pour-on for Cattle*, generic; (OTC). FDA-approved for use in cattle (not female dairy cattle of breeding age). Slaughter withdrawal time = 48 days; milk withdrawal has not been established.

Ivermectin Medicated feeds: *Ivomec® Premix for Swine Type A Medicated Article*) 0.6% in 50 lb.; *Ivomec® Premix for Swine Type C Medicated Feed 0.02%* in 20 lb. one-ton bag and 40 lb. two-ton bag; *Ivomec® Premix for Swine Type C medicated feed 0.1%* in 20 lb. one-ton bag. FDA-approved for use in swine. Slaughter withdrawal = 5 days.

Combination Products:

Ivermectin for Injection: 10 mg/mL (1%) and Clorsulon 100 mg/mL; *Ivomec® Plus Injection for Cattle*, generic; (OTC). FDA-approved for use in cattle (not female dairy cattle of breeding age). Slaughter withdrawal (at labeled doses) = 40 days. No milk withdrawal has been established.

Ivermectin/Pyrantel Oral Tablets: 68 mcg/57 mg, 136 mcg/114 mg, 272 mcg/228 mg; *Heartgard® Plus Chewables*, generic; (Rx). FDA-approved for use in dogs.

An otic product *Acarexx®* is also available.

HUMAN-LABELED PRODUCTS:

Ivermectin Tablets: 3 mg and 6 mg; *Stromectol®*; (Rx)

A topical 0.5% topical lotion (*Sklice®*) pediculocide is also available.

Revisions/References

Monograph revised/updated February 2014.

Adamcak, A. & B. Otten (2000). Rodent Therapeutics. Vet Clin NA: Exotic Anim Pract 3:1(Jan): 221-40.

Atkins, C. (2005). Recent Advances, Controversies and Complications with Canine Heartworm Disease. Proceedings: ACVIM. accessed via Veterinary Information Network; vin.com

Bates, N., et al. (2013). Lipid infusion in the management of poisoning: a report of 6 canine cases. Veterinary Record 172(13).

Bays, T. (2009). Practice tips for exotic animals. Proceedings: WVC. accessed via Veterinary Information Network; vin.com

Bruenisholz, H., et al. (2012). Treatment of Ivermectin Overdose in a Miniature Shetland Pony Using Intravenous Administration of a Lipid Emulsion. Journal of Veterinary Internal Medicine 26(2): 407-11.

Burke, T. (1999). Husbandry and Medicine of Rodents and Lagomorphs. Proceedings: Central Veterinary Conference, Kansas City. accessed via Veterinary Information Network; vin.com

Clarke, D. L., et al. (2011). Use of intravenous lipid emulsion to treat ivermectin toxicosis in a Border Collie. Javma-Journal of the American Veterinary Medical Association 239(10): 1328-33.

Clubb, S. L. (1986). Therapeutics: Individual and Flock Treatment Regimens. *Clinical Avian Medicine and Surgery*. G. J. Harrison and L. R. Harrison. Philadelphia, W.B. Saunders: 327-55.

de la Navarre, B. (2003). Common parasitic diseases of reptiles and amphibians. Proceedings: Western Veterinary Conf. accessed via Veterinary Information Network; vin.com

Dunn, S. T., et al. (2011). Pharmacokinetic Interaction of the Antiparasitic Agents Ivermectin and Spinosad in Dogs. Drug Metabolism and Disposition 39(5): 789-95.

Edmondson, M. (2009). Internal parasites of goats, sheep, and camelids. ABVP. accessed via Veterinary Information Network; vin.com

Epstein, S. E. & S. R. Hollingsworth (2013). Ivermectin-induced blindness treated with intravenous lipid therapy in a dog. J. Vet. Emerg. Crit. Care 23(1): 58-62.

Fernandez, A., et al. (2011). The Use of Intravenous Lipid Emulsion as an Antidote in Toxicology: A Review. J Vet Emerg Crit Care **Pending Publication.**

Gauvin, J. (1993). Drug therapy in reptiles. Seminars in Avian & Exotic Med 2(1): 48-59.

Gwaltney-Brant, S. & I. Meadows (2012). Use of Intravenous Lipid Emulsions for Treating Certain Poisoning Cases in Small Animals. Veterinary Clinics of North America-Small Animal Practice 42(2): 251-+.

Held, S., et al. (2012). Lipid-infusion therapy of avermectin-induced neurotoxicosis in two dogs with homozygous nt230(del4) MDR1 mutation. Kleintierpraxis 57(6): 313-+.

Hernandez-Divers, S. J. (2007). Conundrums in Ferret Medicine. Proceedings: ACVC. accessed via Veterinary Information Network; vin.com

Hoeffer, H. (2000). Heart Disease in Ferrets. Kirk's Current Veterinary Therapy: XIII Small Animal Practice. J. Bonagura. Philadelphia, WB Saunders: 1144-8.

Ivey, E. & J. Morrisey (2000). Therapeutics for Rabbits. Vet Clin NA: Exotic Anim Pract 3:1(Jan): 183-216.

Johnson, D. (2006). Guinea Pig Medicine Primer. Proceedings: ACVC. accessed via Veterinary Information Network; vin.com

Jones, S., et al. (2014). Current Feline Guidelines for the Prevention, Diagnosis, and Management of Heartworm (Dirofilaria immitis) Infection in Cats. American Heartworm Society.

Kidwell, J. H., et al. (2014). Use of IV Lipid Emulsion for Treatment of Ivermectin Toxicosis in a Cat. J. Am. Anim. Hosp. Assoc. 50(1): 59-61.

Koch, S., et al. (2011). Small Animal Dermatology Drug Handbook, Wiley-Blackwell. Ames.

Kuhl, K. (2009). Integrated Parasite Control in Dogs. Proceedings: WVC. accessed via Veterinary Information Network; vin.com

Mealey, K. L. (2013). Adverse Drug Reactions in Veterinary Patients Associated with Drug Transporters. Veterinary Clinics of North America-Small Animal Practice 43(5): 1067-+.

Mueller, R. S., et al. (2012). Treatment of demodicosis in dogs: 2011 clinical practice guidelines. Veterinary Dermatology 23(2): 86-+.

Nelson, C., et al. (2014). Current Canine Guidelines for the Prevention, Diagnosis, and Management of Heartworm (Dirofilaria immitis) Infection in Dogs. American Heartworm Society.

Norman, T. E., et al. (2012). Concurrent Ivermectin and Solanum spp. Toxicosis in a Herd of Horses. Journal of Veterinary Internal Medicine 26(6): 1439-42.

Olsen, L., et al. (2007). Cetirizine in horses: pharmacokinetics and effect of ivermectin pretreatment. J. Vet. Pharmacol. Ther. 30(3): 194-200.

Papich, M. (1989). Effects of drugs on pregnancy. Current Veterinary Therapy X: Small Animal Practice. R. Kirk. Philadelphia, Saunders: 1291-9.

Stunkard, J. M. (1984). Diagnosis, Treatment and Husbandry of Pet Birds, Stunkard Publishing. Edgewater, MD.

Swor, T. M., et al. (2009). Ivermectin toxicosis in three adult horses. Javma-Journal of the American Veterinary Medical Association 235(5): 558-62.

Waisglass, S. (2009). Demodicosis Update--Some Considerations to Increase Your Success Rate. Proceedings: WVC. accessed via Veterinary Information Network; vin.com

Wolff, P. (2009). Camelid Medicine. Proceedings: AAZV. accessed via Veterinary Information Network; vin.com

Kaolin/Pectin

(kay-oh-lin/pek-tin)   Kaopectolin

GI Adsorbent/Protectant

Prescriber Highlights

▶ Adsorbent for treatment of diarrhea & GI toxins; questionable efficacy.

▶ Contraindications: Should not be relied on to control severe diarrheas or replace adequate fluid/electrolyte monitoring or as replacement therapy in severe or chronic diarrheas.

▶ Adverse Effects: Transient constipation.

▶ Drug Interactions.

Uses/Indications

Although its efficacy is in question, kaolin/pectin is used primarily in veterinary medicine as an oral anti-diarrheal agent. It has also been used as an adsorbent agent following the ingestion of certain toxins. Administration may be difficult due to the large volumes that may be necessary to give orally. No studies documenting the clinical efficacy of this combination in either human or veterinary species were located.

Pharmacology/Actions

Kaolin/pectin is thought to possess adsorbent and protective qualities. Presumably, bacteria and toxins are adsorbed in the gut and the coating action of the suspension may protect inflamed GI mucosa. The pectin component, by forming galacturonic acid, has been demonstrated to decrease pH in the intestinal lumen. Kaolin can improve stool consistency within 24-48 hours, but it does not reduce the amount of fluid lost from the GI tract.

In one study in children with acute nonspecific diarrhea stool fluidity was decreased but stool frequency, water content, and weight remained unchanged.

Pharmacokinetics

Neither kaolin nor pectin are absorbed after oral administration. Up to 90% of the pectin administered may be decomposed in the gut.

Contraindications/Precautions/Warnings

There are no absolute contraindications to kaolin/pectin therapy, but it should not be relied on to control severe diarrheas. Kaolin/pectin should not replace adequate fluid/electrolyte monitoring or replacement therapy in severe or chronic diarrheas.

Adverse Effects

At usual doses, kaolin/pectin generally has no adverse effects. Constipation may occur, but is usually transient and associated with high dosages. High doses in debilitated or very old or young patients may rarely cause fecal impaction. In rats, kaolin/pectin has been demonstrated to increase fecal sodium loss in diarrhea.

In humans, kaolin/pectin is recommended for use only under the direct supervision of a physician in patients less than 3 years of age or if it must be used longer than 48 hours.

Reproductive/Nursing Safety

Adsorbent (only) anti-diarrheal products should be safe to use during pregnancy and lactation. The addition of other active ingredients (*e.g.,* opiates) may alter this recommendation.

Overdosage/Acute Toxicity

Overdosage is unlikely to cause any serious effects, but constipation requiring treatment may occur.

Drug Interactions

The following drug interactions have either been reported or are theoretical in humans or animals receiving kaolin/pectin and may be of significance in veterinary patients. Unless otherwise noted, use together is not necessarily contraindicated, but weigh the potential risks and perform additional monitoring when appropriate.

■ **DIGOXIN:** Some evidence exists that kaolin/pectin may impair the oral absorption of digoxin. Separate doses by at least two hours.

■ **CLINDAMYCIN, LINCOMYCIN:** Kaolin/pectin may inhibit oral absorption. If both drugs are to be used, administer kaolin/pectin at least 2 hours before or 3-4 hours after the antibiotic dose.

■ **PENICILLAMINE:** Kaolin/pectin may inhibit oral absorption. Separate dosages by at least two hours.

■ **TRIMETHOPRIM/SULFA:** Kaolin/pectin may inhibit oral absorption. Separate dosages by at least two hours.

Doses

Note: Evidence to support efficacy of kaolin/pectin is weak. All dosages are anecdotal and extra-label as no products have undergone the FDA-approval process for use in animals.

■ **DOGS/CATS:**

For diarrhea/loose stools: 1 – 2 mL/kg PO 4-6 times daily as needed.

- **FERRETS:**

  For diarrhea/loose stools: 1 – 2 mL/kg PO 3-4 times daily. (Williams 2000)

- **RABBITS/RODENTS/SMALL MAMMALS:**

  For diarrhea/loose stools in guinea pigs: 0.2 mL PO 3-4 times a day. (Adamcak *et al.* 2000)

- **CATTLE:**

  For diarrhea/loose stools: Adult: 4 – 10 fl. oz. PO; **Calves:** 2 – 3 fl. oz PO; repeat every 2-4 hours or as indicated until condition improves. If no improvement in 48 hours, additional treatment is indicated. (Label Directions; *Kao-Forte®*—Vet-A-Mix)

- **HORSES:**

  For diarrhea/loose stools:

  a) 2 – 4 quarts PO per 450 kg body weight twice daily. (Robinson 1987)

  b) 1 oz. per 8 kg body weight PO 3-4 times a day. (Clark *et al.* 1987)

  c) Foals: 3 – 4 oz PO q6-8h (authors believe that bismuth subsalicylate is superior). (Martens *et al.* 1982)

- **SWINE:**

  For diarrhea/loose stools: 1/2 – 2 fl. oz. PO; repeat every 2-4 hours or as indicated until condition improves. If no improvement in 48 hours, additional treatment is indicated. (Label Directions; *Kao-Forte®*—Vet-A-Mix)

- **BIRDS:**

  a) **Canary or parakeet:** 1 drop PO twice daily; or 1 and 1/2 dropperful placed in 2/3 oz. drinking water. **Medium-sized birds:** 0.5 mL PO. **Large birds:** 1 mL PO 1-4 times a day. (Stunkard 1984)

  b) 2 mL/kg PO 2-4 times a day. (Clubb 1986)

Monitoring

- Clinical efficacy.
- Fluid and electrolyte status in severe diarrhea.

Client Information

- Shake well before using.
- If diarrhea persists, or if animal appears listless or develops a high fever, contact veterinarian.

Chemistry/Synonyms

Kaolin is a naturally occurring hydrated aluminum silicate that is powdered and refined for pharmaceutical use. Kaolin is a white/light, odorless, almost tasteless powder that is practically insoluble in water. Light kaolin is preferred for use in pharmaceutical preparations.

Pectin is a carbohydrate polymer consisting primarily of partially methoxylated polygalacturonic acids. Pectin is a course or fine, yellowish-white, almost odorless with a mucilaginous flavor. It is obtained from the inner rind of citrus fruits or from apple pomace. One gram of pectin is soluble in 20 mL of water and forms a viscous, colloidal solution.

In the United States, the two compounds generally are used together in an oral suspension formulation in most proprietary products.

Kaolin may also be known as: bolus alba, E559, hydrated aluminum silicate, China clay, porcelain clay, white bole, argilla, weisser ton, Kao-Pec®, Kao-Pect®, Kao-Pront®, Kaogel®; many multi-ingredient trade names are available.

Storage/Stability

Kaolin/pectin should be stored in airtight containers; protect from freezing.

Compatibility/Compounding Considerations

It is physically **incompatible** when mixed with alkalis, heavy metals, salicylic acid, tannic acid, or strong alcohol. If using raw kaolin powder, wear an appropriate particulate mask as pneumonitis can occur if inhaled.

Dosage Forms/Regulatory Status

There are a variety of kaolin/pectin products available without prescription. Several products are labeled for veterinary use; their approval status is not known. Many products that formerly contained kaolin (*e.g.*, *Kaopectate®*) no longer contain any kaolin. In the USA, *Kaopectate®* now contains bismuth subsalicylate as its active ingredient.

VETERINARY-LABELED PRODUCTS:

Kaolin Pectin 90 grams kaolin/2 grams pectin per fluid oz. in 1 quart and 1 gallon containers; generic, (OTC). Products may be labeled for use in horses, cattle, dogs and cats.

Kaolin Pectin 90 grams kaolin/4 grams pectin per fl. oz. in 1 gallon containers; generic; (OTC)

HUMAN-LABELED PRODUCTS:

Kaolin, Pectin Antidiarrheal Suspension: 90 grams kaolin, 2 grams pectin/30 mL in 180 mL and 360 mL, pt. and UD 30 mL; *Kapectolin* (various), generic; (OTC)

Revisions/References

Monograph revised/updated March 2014.

Adamcak, A. & B. Otten (2000). Rodent Therapeutics. Vet Clin NA: Exotic Anim Pract 3:1(Jan): 221-40.

Clark, E. S. & J. L. Becht (1987). Clinical Pharmacology of the Gastrointestinal Tract. Vet Clin North Am (Equine Practice) 3(1): 101-22.

Clubb, S. L. (1986). Therapeutics: Individual and Flock Treatment Regimens. *Clinical Avian Medicine and Surgery*. G. J. Harrison and L. R. Harrison. Philadelphia, W.B. Saunders: 327-55.

Martens, R. J. & W. L. Scrutchfield (1982). Foal Diarrhea: Pathogenesis, Etiology, and Therapy. Comp Cont Ed 4(4): S175-S86.

Robinson, N. E. (1987). Table of Common Drugs: Approximate Doses. *Current Therapy in Equine Medicine, 2*. N. E. Robinson. Philadelphia, W.B. Saunders: 761.

Stunkard, J. M. (1984). *Diagnosis, Treatment and Husbandry of Pet Birds*, Stunkard Publishing. Edgewater, MD.

Williams, B. (2000). Therapeutics in Ferrets. Vet Clin NA: Exotic Anim Pract 3:1(Jan): 131-53.

Ketamine HCl

(kee-ta-meen)   Ketaset®, Ketaflo®, Vetalar®

Dissociative General Anesthetic; NMDA-Receptor Antagonist

Prescriber Highlights

▶ Dissociative general anesthetic; also inhibits NMDA-receptors so may be adjunctively useful to control pain.

▶ Contraindications: Prior hypersensitivity reactions, animals to be used for human consumption, alone for general anesthesia, increased CSF pressure/head trauma. Relative contraindications: Significant blood loss, malignant hyperthermia, increased intra-ocular pressure or open globe injuries, procedures involving the pharynx, larynx, or trachea. Caution: Significant hypertension, heart failure, & arterial aneurysms, hepatic or renal insufficiency, seizure disorders.

▶ Adverse Effects: Hypertension, hypersalivation, respiratory depression, hyperthermia, emesis, vocalization, erratic & prolonged recovery, dyspnea, spastic jerking movements, seizures, muscular tremors, hypertonicity, opisthotonos, & cardiac arrest; pain after IM injection may occur.

▶ Cats' eyes remain open after ketamine; protect.

▶ Minimize exposure to handling or loud noises during the recovery period, but monitor adequately.

▶ Drug interactions.

▶ Determine dosages carefully. Do not confuse CRI dosages: mg/kg/hour vs. micrograms/kg/minute.

Uses/Indications

Ketamine has been FDA-approved for use in humans, sub-human primates, and cats, although it has been used in many other species (see Dosage section). The FDA-approved indications for cats include, "for restraint, or as the sole anesthetic agent for diagnostic, or minor, brief, surgical procedures that do not require skeletal muscle relaxation... and in subhuman primates for restraint." (Package Insert; *Ketaset®*).

Ketamine can inhibit NMDA receptors in the CNS and can decrease "wind-up" effect. There is increasing interest in using it to prevent exaggerated pain associated with surgery or chronic pain states in animals.

Pharmacology/Actions

Ketamine is a rapid acting general anesthetic that has significant analgesic activity and a relative lack of cardiopulmonary depressant effects in healthy animals. It is thought to induce both anesthesia and amnesia by functionally disrupting the CNS through over-stimulating the CNS or inducing a cataleptic state. Ketamine inhibits GABA, and may block serotonin, norepinephrine, and dopamine in the CNS. The thalamoneocortical system is depressed while the limbic system is activated. It induces anesthetic stages I and II, but not stage III. In cats, it causes a slight hypothermic effect as body temperatures decrease on average by 1.6° C after therapeutic doses.

Ketamine possesses analgesic effects at sub-anesthetic doses. Analgesia is secondary to effects on NMDA excitatory glutamate receptors by decreasing the activity of areas in the CNS that respond to pain-invoking stimuli. At these lower dosages adverse effects are generally minimal in most species. Ketamine's analgesic effects can be synergistic with other analgesics.

In some species, ketamine has demonstrated antiinflammatory effects. In response to endotoxin stimulation in dogs, reductions in tumor necrosis factor-alpha were noted (DeClue *et al.* 2008).

Effects on muscle tone are described as being variable, but ketamine generally either causes no changes in muscle tone or increased tone. Ketamine does not abrogate the pinnal and pedal reflexes, nor the photic, corneal, laryngeal or pharyngeal reflexes.

Ketamine's effects on the cardiovascular system include increased cardiac output, heart rate, mean aortic pressure, pulmonary artery pressure, and central venous pressure. Its effects on total peripheral resistance are described as being variable. Cardiovascular effects are secondary to increased sympathetic tone; ketamine has negative inotropic effects if the sympathetic system is blocked.

Ketamine can cause apneustic breathing (rapid breaths followed by breath-holding). It does not cause significant respiratory depression at usual doses, but at higher doses it can cause respiratory rates to decrease. Ketamine can cause bronchodilation and in humans with asthma, ketamine causes decreased airway resistance.

Pharmacokinetics

After IM injection in the cat, peak levels occur in approximately 10 minutes. Administration of a ketamine spray sublingually to cats appears to be absorbed enough to have pharmacologic action (Issabeagloo 2008). Ketamine is distributed into all body tissues rapidly, with highest levels found in the brain, liver, lung, and fat. Plasma protein binding is approximately 50% in the horse, 53% in the dogs, and 37-53% in the cat.

In most species, ketamine is metabolized in the liver principally by demethylation and hydroxylation and these metabolites, along with unchanged ketamine, are eliminated in the urine. In dogs, CYP2B11 plays an active role in metabolizing ketamine. One active metabolite, nor-ketamine, has 10-30% of the activity of the parent compound. In cats, ketamine is almost exclusively excreted unchanged in the urine. Ketamine will induce hepatic microsomal enzymes, but there appears to be little clinical significance associated with this effect. The elimination half-life in cats, calves, and horses is approximately 1 hour; in humans, 2-3 hours. Like the thiobarbiturates, the redistribution of ketamine out of the CNS is more of a factor in determining duration of anesthesia than elimination half-life. In horses, S-ketamine is eliminated faster than the racemic mixture.

By increasing dosages of ketamine, duration of anesthesia can be prolonged, but not its intensity.

Contraindications/Precautions/Warnings

Ketamine is contraindicated in patients who have exhibited prior hypersensitivity reactions to it and animals to be used for human consumption. Use in patients with significant hypertension, heart failure, and arterial aneurysms could be hazardous. The manufacturer warns against its use in patients with hepatic or renal insufficiency but in humans with renal insufficiency, the duration of action is not prolonged. Because ketamine does not provide good muscle relaxation, it is contraindicated when used alone for major surgery.

Ketamine can cause increases in CSF pressure and should not be used in cases with elevated pressures or when head trauma has occurred. When used at lower dosages as an analgesic adjunct, there is less potential for increases in intracranial pressure.

Because of its epileptogenic potential, ketamine should generally not be used (unless very cautiously) in animals with preexisting seizure disorders. As myelography can induce seizures, ketamine should be used cautiously in animals undergoing this procedure. However, ketamine may be beneficial in treating so-called self-sustaining status epilepticus (SSSE) in humans and dogs.

Ketamine is considered to be relatively contraindicated when increased intra-ocular pressure or open globe injuries exist, and for procedures involving the pharynx, larynx, or trachea. Animals that have lost significant amounts of blood, may require significantly reduced ketamine dosages.

While ketamine has been used safely in humans with malignant hyperthermia, its use in animals susceptible to this condition is controversial.

Ketamine can increase heart rate, blood pressure and myocardial oxygen consumption; its use should be avoided in cats with hypertrophic cardiomyopathy (HCM) or other patients where an increase in heart rate, blood pressure and myocardial oxygen consumption can be detrimental (*e.g.*, unstable shock or congestive heart failure). Its effects on respiratory function may be enhanced in patients with unstable cardiopulmonary function. Because of ketamine's tendencies to increase sympathetic tone (increased norepinephrine release), it should be used with caution in animals where increased sympathetic tone concurrently exists (*e.g.*, pheochromocytoma, hyperthyroidism). Hyperthyroid human patients and those receiving exogenous thyroid replacement may be susceptible to developing severe hypertension and tachycardia when given ketamine. The veterinary significance of this potential problem is unknown.

Cats' eyes can remain open after receiving ketamine, and should be protected from injury plus an ophthalmic lubricant (*e.g.*, *Lacri-Lube®*) should be applied to prevent excessive drying of the cornea.

Because ketamine is excreted almost exclusively via renal mechanisms, it should be used with caution in cats with reduced renal function.

To minimize the incidences of emergence reactions, it is recommended to minimize exposure to handling or loud noises during the recovery period. The monitoring of vital signs should still be performed during the recovery phase, however.

In horses, it has been recommended to avoid excessive ketamine dosages close to recovery so to reduce the potential for muscle rigidity or CNS excitement (Valverde 2013).

Because ketamine can increase blood pressure, careful control of post-surgical (*e.g.*, declawing) hemorrhage should be managed. It is not essential to withhold food or water prior to surgery, but in elective procedures it is recommended to withhold food for 6 hours prior to surgery.

In human medicine, ketamine is considered a "high alert" medication (medications that require special safeguards to reduce the risk of errors). Consider instituting practices such as redundant drug dosage and volume checking, special alert labels, etc.

Adverse Effects

In species where the drug is FDA-approved, the following adverse reactions are listed by the manufacturer: "respiratory depression… following high doses, emesis, vocalization, erratic and prolonged recovery, dyspnea, spastic jerking movements, convulsions, muscular tremors, hypertonicity, opisthotonos and cardiac arrest. In the cat, myoclonic jerking and/or tonic/clonic convulsions can be controlled by ultrashort-acting barbiturates or acepromazine. These latter drugs must be given intravenously, cautiously, and slowly, to effect (approximately 1/6 to 1/4 the normal dose may be required)." (Package Insert; *Ketaset®*—Fort Dodge)

When used alone ketamine may induce seizures. Seizures have been reported to occur in up to 20% of cats that receive ketamine (alone) at therapeutic dosages. Diazepam is suggested if treatment is necessary. It has been reported to rarely cause a variety of other CNS effects (mild CNS effects to blindness and death). Ketamine has been documented to cause hyperthermia in cats; low doses of acepromazine (0.01 – 0.02 mg/kg IV) may alleviate this effect. Anecdotal reports of ketamine causing acute CHF in cats with mild to moderate heart disease have been reported.

Pain after IM injection may occur.

To reduce the incidence of hypersalivation and other autonomic signs, atropine or glycopyrrolate is sometimes administered.

Reproductive/Nursing Safety

In humans, the FDA categorizes this drug as category *C* for use during pregnancy (*Animal studies have shown an adverse effect on the fetus, but there are no adequate studies in humans; or there are no animal reproduction studies and no adequate studies in humans.*) In a separate system evaluating the safety of drugs in canine and feline pregnancy (Papich 1989), this drug is categorized as class: *B* (*Safe for use if used cautiously. Studies in laboratory animals may have uncovered some risk, but these drugs appear to be safe in dogs and cats or these drugs are safe if they are not administered when the animal is near term.*)

No specific lactation information was found.

Overdosage/Acute Toxicity

Ketamine is considered to have a wide therapeutic index (approximately 5X greater when compared to pentobarbital). When given too rapidly or in excessive doses, significant respiratory depression may occur. Treatment using mechanically assisted respiratory support is recommended versus the use of analeptic agents. In cats, yohimbine with 4-aminopyridine has been suggested for use as a partial antagonist.

Drug Interactions

The following drug interactions have either been reported or are theoretical in humans or animals receiving ketamine and may be of significance in veterinary patients. Unless otherwise noted, use together is not necessarily contraindicated, but weigh the potential risks and perform additional monitoring when appropriate.

- **CHLORAMPHENICOL** (**parenteral**): May prolong the anesthetic actions of ketamine. Chloramphenicol did not prolong anesthesia in dogs receiving xylazine/ketamine in one study.
- **CNS DEPRESSANTS**: Narcotics, barbiturates, or benzodiazepines may prolong the recovery time after ketamine anesthesia.
- **HALOTHANE**: When used with halothane, ketamine recovery rates may be prolonged and the cardiac stimulatory effects of ketamine may be inhibited; close monitoring of cardiac status is recommended when using ketamine with halothane.
- **IVERMECTIN**: It has been recommended not to use ivermectin in reptiles within 10 days of ketamine (Bays 2009).
- **MEDETOMIDINE**: In dogs, medetomidine potentially could reduce the metabolism of ketamine via inhibition of CYB2B11 (*in vitro*). Any clinical significance is not clear at this time. Dexmedetomidine (used in dogs) would be expected to reduce interaction risks considerably (Baratta *et al.* 2010).
- **NEUROMUSCULAR BLOCKERS** (*e.g.*, **succinylcholine** and **tubocurarine**): May cause enhanced or prolonged respiratory depression.
- **THEOPHYLLINE**: In humans, ketamine may lower theophylline seizure threshold; veterinary significance is unknown.
- **THYROID HORMONES**: When given concomitantly with ketamine, thyroid hormones have induced hypertension and tachycardia in humans; beta-blockers (*e.g.*, propranolol) may be of benefit in treating these effects.

Doses

Note: Ketamine is used in many different combinations with other agents. The following are representative, but not necessarily inclusive; it is suggested to refer to a recent veterinary anesthesia reference for more information. Do NOT confuse CRI dosages listed as <u>mg/kg/hour</u> with those listed as <u>micrograms/kg/minute.</u>

- **DOGS:**

  As an adjunct to anesthesia (extra-label):

  For use in combination with an opioid and ketamine (so-called "doggie magic") **to provide anesthesia and pain management** (**Note:** reference has dosing tables for conversion of patient weight to various micrograms/m² doses of dexmedetomidine; opioid concentrations used in the reference are: Butorphanol 10 mg/mL, Hydromorphone 2 mg/mL, Morphine 15 mg/mL, & Buprenorphine 0.3 mg/mL. Ketamine concentration is 100 mg/mL. As these drugs may be available in other concentrations, only use those products with the above concentrations if using this protocol.):

  For geriatric dogs, dogs with renal or liver dysfunction as a premed prior to propofol or face mask induction, followed by maintenance on isoflurane or sevoflurane: dexmedetomidine at 62.5 micrograms/m². Combine with equal volumes of one of the opioids noted above and ketamine. May administer IM or IV.

  For slightly heavier sedation in ASA class II or II dogs requiring sedation for radiographic procedures: Dexmedetomidine at 125 micrograms/m². Combine with equal volumes of one of the opioids noted above and ketamine. May administer IM or IV.

  For dogs undergoing minor surgery, Penn hip or OFA-types of radiographic procedures that require significant muscle relaxation: Dexmedetomidine at 250 micrograms/m². Combine with equal volumes of one of the opioids noted above and ketamine. May administer IM or IV.

  To induce a surgical plane of anesthesia for OHE, castration, or other abdominal surgery: Dexmedetomidine at 375 micrograms/m². Combine with equal volumes of one of the opioids noted above and ketamine. May administer IM or IV. Provides rapid immobilization; lateral recumbency in 5-8 minutes. Dogs can be intubated and maintained on oxygen. Supplemental low doses of isoflurane (0.5%) or sevoflurane (1%) can be used.

For immobilizing extremely fractious dogs and wolf-hybrid dogs: Dexmedetomidine at 500 micrograms/m². Combine with equal volumes of one of the opioids noted above and ketamine. Administer IM. This dose is rarely required.

To reverse above: atipamezole IM at the same volume as the dexmedetomidine. (Ko, J. 2009)

As a premed before surgery or an anesthetic adjunct (extra-label): Note: there are many potential combinations that have been suggested; the following are examples and not inclusive. For additional information refer to other anesthesia-specific references such as *Handbook of Veterinary Anesthesia*, 5th Ed., Muir & Hubbell, Elsevier 2012; *Essentials of Small Animal Anesthesia & Analgesia*, Grimm et al, Wiley-Blackwell 2011 or the website Veterinary Anesthesia & Analgesia Support Group (vasg.org). In the study, efficacy and cardiorespiratory effects of a combination of dexmedetomidine (15 micrograms/kg), ketamine (3 mg/kg) and either buprenorphine (40 micrograms/kg), butorphanol, or hydromorphone as a single IM injection (with or without reversal by atipamezole) in dogs undergoing castration. Supplemental isoflurane used when anesthesia was considered inadequate during surgery. Authors concluded that the most suitable combination was with buprenorphine and that atipamezole shortened recovery times. (Barletta *et al.* 2011)

As an NMDA antagonist for adjunctive pain control (extra-label): Note: When using as a CRI do NOT confuse dosages listed as mg/kg/hour with micrograms/kg/minute.

a) 0.5 mg/kg IV loading dose, followed by a CRI of 0.1 – 0.6 mg/kg/hr IV CRI. (Lamont 2008)

b) **For intraoperative use:** If anesthesia was induced with a drug other than ketamine, give a loading dose of 0.5 mg/kg IV, then an infusion of 10 – 20 micrograms/kg/minute. A CRI of 2 – 10 micrograms/kg/minute can be used post-op. (Hellyer 2006)

c) **In combination with opioids or lidocaine:** 0.5 mg/kg IV loading bolus followed by 10 micrograms/kg/min CRI during surgery and 2 micrograms/kg/min for 24 hours following surgery. (Shaffran 2009)

- **CATS:**

In combination as a preop or immobilizing agent (extra-label): Note: There are many potential combinations that have been suggested; the following are examples and not inclusive. For additional information refer to other anesthesia-specific references such as *Handbook of Veterinary Anesthesia*, 5th Ed., Muir & Hubbell, Elsevier 2012; *Essentials of Small Animal Anesthesia & Analgesia*, Grimm et al, Wiley-Blackwell 2011 or the website Veterinary Anesthesia & Analgesia Support Group (vasg.org).

a) **For use in combination with an opioid and ketamine (so-called "kitty magic", "DKT" or "Triple Combination") to provide sedation and analgesia** (Note: Opioid concentrations used in the reference are: Butorphanol 10 mg/mL, Hydromorphone 2 mg/mL, Morphine 15 mg/mL, & Buprenorphine 0.3 mg/mL. Ketamine concentration is 100 mg/mL. Dexmedetomidine concentration is 0.5 mg/mL. As these drugs may be available in other concentrations, only use those products with the above concentrations if using this protocol.):

For the chart below: MILD = For sedation or as a premed prior to propofol or facemask induction; MODERATE = For castration or minor surgical procedures; PROFOUND = In-

vasive surgical procedures including OHE and declaws. Cats can be reversed immediately with an equal volume (of the dexmedetomidine dose) of atipamezole. (Ko, J. 2009)

Cat Weight		Volume (of each) of: Dexmedetomidine-Opioid-Ketamine			IM Route
Lbs.	Kg	MILD	MODERATE	PROFOUND	
4-7	2-3	0.025 mL	0.05 mL	0.1 – 0.15 mL	
7-9	3-4	0.05 mL	0.1 mL	0.2 – 0.25 mL	
9-13	4-6	0.1 mL	0.2 mL	0.3 – 0.35 mL	
14-15	6-7	0.2 mL	0.3 mL	0.4 – 0.45 mL	
15-18	7-8	0.3 mL	0.4 mL	0.5 – 0.55 mL	

b) **Combining butorphanol, ketamine, midazolam and medetomidine** (extra-label): In the study (assessing analgesia after OHE), one of the protocols used was: Ten minutes prior to surgery, Ketamine 60 mg/m² (~3 mg/kg), midazolam 3 mg/m² (~0.2 mg/kg), medetomidine 600 micrograms/m² (~30 micrograms/kg), and butorphanol 6 mg/m² (~0.4 micrograms/kg) combined and given as a single IM injection in quadriceps muscles. Additionally, either carprofen (4 mg/kg) or meloxicam (0.3 mg/kg) were given subcutaneously. All protocols in the study provided adequate analgesia. (Polson *et al.* 2012)

c) **Combining butorphanol and midazolam with ketamine or dexmedetomidine** (extra-label): In a small (n=6) healthy cat crossover study, the combination of butorphanol (0.4 mg/kg), midazolam (0.4 mg/kg) and ketamine (3 mg/kg) combined and given IM, the authors concluded that it provided acceptable sedation and minimal cardiovascular changes. Substituting dexmedetomidine (5 micrograms/kg) for the ketamine produced excellent sedation/recovery, but caused more cardiovascular depression and hematologic changes. (Biermann *et al.* 2012)

d) **Combining butorphanol, dexmedetomidine, and ketamine** (extra-label): The study evaluated efficacy and cardiorespiratory effects of a combination of dexmedetomidine (25 micrograms/kg), ketamine (3 mg/kg) and either butorphanol (0.2 mg/kg), hydromorphone (0.05 mg/kg) or buprenorphine (30 micrograms/kg) as a single IM injection, (with or without reversal by atipamezole) in cats undergoing castration. Cats also received meloxicam (0.2 mg/kg SC) immediately prior to the conclusion of surgery. Supplemental isoflurane used when anesthesia was considered inadequate during surgery. Authors concluded that combinations including butorphanol or hydromorphone were suitable injectable anesthetic protocols for castration in cats commencing at 10 minutes after injection. Atipamezole shortened recovery times. (Ko, J.C. *et al.* 2011)

e) **Labeled-dose:** 11 mg/kg IM for restraint; 22 – 33 mg/kg for diagnostic or minor surgical procedures not requiring skeletal muscle relaxation. (Package Insert; *Ketaset®*)

In combination as an immobilizing agent: For cats requiring more sedation when insufficient sedation from opioid, higher doses of medetomidine, and midazolam: butorphanol 0.2 mg/kg; medetomidine 0.015 – 0.02 mg/kg; midazolam 0.05 – 0.2 mg/kg; ketamine 1 – 5 mg/kg; all are given IM. For painful procedures consider adding buprenorphine at 0.02 – 0.04 mg/kg or substituting butorphanol or buprenorphine with either morphine 0.5 mg/kg or hydromorphone 0.1 mg/kg. More information available from: www.vsag.org

For highly aggressive cats, 1 mL of ketamine can be sprayed into the open mouth or directed into the cat's mouth using a feline urethral catheter through the cage bars. The drug should be sprayed quickly so the cat does not chew and swallow the catheter. (Moffat 2008)

As a premed before surgery (extra-label): In the study (assessing analgesia after OHE), one of the protocols used was: Ten minutes prior to surgery, ketamine 60 mg/m² (~3 mg/kg), midazolam 3 mg/m² (~0.2 mg/kg), medetomidine 600 micrograms/m² (~30 micrograms/kg), and buprenorphine 180 micrograms/m² (~9 micrograms/kg) combined and given as a single IM injection in quadriceps muscles. Additionally, either carprofen (4 mg/kg) or meloxicam (0.3 mg/kg) were given subcutaneously. All protocols in the study provided adequate analgesia. (Polson *et al.* 2012)

As an NMDA antagonist for adjunctive pain control (extra-label):

a) 0.5 mg/kg IV loading dose, followed by a CRI of 0.1 – 0.6 mg/kg/hr IV CRI. (Lamont 2008)

b) **For intraoperative use**: If anesthesia was induced with a drug other than ketamine, give a loading dose of 0.5 mg/kg IV, then an infusion of 10 – 20 micrograms/kg/minute. A CRI of 2 – 10 micrograms/kg/minute can be used post-op. (Hellyer 2006)

c) **In combination with opioids or lidocaine**: **Note**: Cats are reportedly very sensitive to the CNS effects of lidocaine and can develop cardio-depression. There are several sources that state that lidocaine should not be used in cats as an injectable analgesic, but others use it routinely. If using in cats, monitor carefully. 0.5 mg/kg IV loading bolus followed by 10 micrograms/kg/min CRI during surgery and 2 micrograms/kg/min for 24 hrs. following surgery.

d) **Using the MLK (morphine/lidocaine/ketamine) mixture**: To a 500 mL bag of LRS add 10 mg morphine sulfate, 120 mg lidocaine, and 100 mg ketamine. Infuse at a rate of 10 mL/kg/hr (will provide morphine at 0.2 mg/kg/hr, lidocaine 40 micrograms/kg/minute, and ketamine 2 mg/kg/hr). Can add dexmedetomidine if needed. (Shaffran 2009)

■ **RABBITS/RODENTS/SMALL MAMMALS:**

For chemical restraint (extra-label):

a) **Mice**: Alone: 50 –100 mg/kg IM or IP, 50 mg/kg IV; In combination with diazepam: Ketamine 200 mg/kg with Diazepam 5 mg/kg IM or IP; In combination with xylazine: Ketamine 100 mg/kg with Xylazine 5 – 15 mg/kg IM or IP. (Burke 1999)

b) **Rats**: Alone: 50 –100 mg/kg IM or IP, 40 – 50 mg/kg IV; In combination with diazepam: Ketamine 40 – 60 mg/kg with Diazepam 5 – 10 mg/kg IP; In combination with xylazine: Ketamine 40 – 75 mg/kg with Xylazine 5 – 12 mg/kg IM or IP. (Burke 1999)

c) **Hamsters/Gerbils**: 100 mg/kg IM; In combination with diazepam: Ketamine 50 mg/kg with Diazepam 5 mg/kg IM; In combination with xylazine: Not recommended. (Burke 1999)

d) **Guinea pig**: Alone: 10 – 30 mg/kg IM; In combination with diazepam: Ketamine 60 – 100 mg/kg with Diazepam 5 – 8 mg/kg IM; In combination with xylazine: Ketamine 85 mg/kg with Xylazine 12 – 13 mg/kg IM. (Burke 1999)

e) **Rabbits**: Alone: 20 – 60 mg/kg IM or IV; In combination with diazepam: Ketamine 60 – 80 mg/kg with Diazepam 5 – 10 mg/kg IM; In combination with xylazine: Ketamine 10 mg/kg with Xylazine 3 mg/kg IV. (Burke 1999)

f) **Rabbits**: Alone: 20 – 50 mg/kg IM or 15 – 20 mg/kg IV; In combination with diazepam for induction: Diazepam 5 – 10 mg/kg IM give ketamine 30 minutes after diazepam at 20 – 40 mg/kg IM or Diazepam 0.2 – 0.5 mg/kg and Ketamine 10 – 15 mg/kg (to effect) IV; In combination with diazepam for anesthesia without inhalants: Diazepam 5 – 10 mg/kg IM plus ketamine 60 – 80 mg/kg IM 30 minutes later; In combination with xylazine: NOT recommended for pet rabbits. (Ivey *et al.* 2000)

g) **For Injectable anesthesia**: **Rodents**: midazolam (5 mg/kg) + ketamine (100 mg/kg) + buprenorphine (0.05 mg/kg) IP. **Rabbits**: Midazolam (0.05 mg/kg) + buprenorphine (0.03 mg/kg) + ketamine (10 mg/kg) IM. (Bennett 2009)

■ **FERRETS:**

For injectable anesthesia (extra-label): Butorphanol 0.1 mg/kg, ketamine 5 mg/kg, medetomidine 80 micrograms/kg. Combine in one syringe and give IM. May need to supplement with isoflurane (0.5 – 1.5%) for abdominal surgery. (Finkler 1999)

As a post-operative analgesic adjunct: In a CRI combination with fentanyl. Ketamine at 0.3 – 0.4 mg/kg/hour combined with fentanyl (2.5 – 5 micrograms/kg/hour) CRI. (Lichtenberger 2006)

■ **CATTLE/RUMINANTS:**

Note: FARAD recommends a 3-day meat withdrawal and 3-day milk withdrawal for ketamine (Smith 2013).

For chemical restraint (mild sedation of standing patients to semi-anesthetized recumbency as "ketamine stun"); (extra-label): **Note**: The following are abbreviated suggested initial dosages. See the reference in Vet Clin Food Anim 29 (2013) 209-227 (Abrahamsen, E.J. 2013) for a thorough discussion including dosages for other combinations using ketamine and re-dosing recommendations.

Ketamine stun IV recumbent (for short procedures requiring a high level of systemic analgesia and/or patient cooperation such as castrations, biopsies, flushing joints, casting, etc.): A combination of xylazine (0.025 – 0.05 mg/kg), butorphanol (0.05 – 0.1 mg/kg), and ketamine (0.3 – 0.5 mg/kg) IV. Author generally uses the upper end of the dosage range unless contraindicated.

Ketamine stun IM, SC recumbent: A combination of butorphanol (0.025 mg/kg), xylazine (0.05 mg/kg), and ketamine (0.1 mg/kg) is administered IM or SC. Provides a longer, less intense chemical restraint than IV.

Ketamine stun IV standing: First sedate with xylazine at 0.02 – 0.0275 mg/kg IV depending on initial demeanor of patient. Then slowly administer ketamine (0.05 – 0.1 mg/kg IV). Can add an opioid to augment the level of systemic analgesia and patient control (butorphanol at 0.05 – 0.1 mg/kg IV or IM in smaller ruminants, or 0.02 – 0.05 mg/kg IV or IM in larger ruminants), or (morphine 0.05 – 0.1 mg/kg IV or IM).

Ketamine stun IM, SC standing: A combination of butorphanol (0.01 mg/kg), xylazine (0.02 mg/kg), and ketamine (0.04 mg/kg) IM or SC. In a 500 kg cow this is 5 mg of butorphanol, 10 mg of xylazine and 20 mg of ketamine ("5-10-20").

For injectable anesthesia (extra-label): In the above cited reference (Abrahamsen, E.J. 2013), the author discusses several protocols using ketamine in combination with other anesthetic and analgesic compounds including IM, IV, and CRI protocols. The reader is referred to the full article for details on ketamine use for this purpose.

For adjunctive analgesia (extra-label): 0.4 – 1.2 mg/kg/hr as a CRI. (Miesner 2009)

■ **HORSES:** (NOTE: ARCI UCGFS CLASS 2 DRUG)

Note: There are a plethora of protocols published for use of ketamine in combination with other agents for equine anesthesia. A survey published in 2010 of American Association of Equine Practitioners (AAEP) found that the preferred agents for an induction protocol for short-term anesthesia (20 minutes or less) was xylazine administered as a sedative first and then followed by ketamine and diazepam. However, other alpha-2 agonists (detomidine, romifidine, etc.) or benzodiazepines (*e.g.,* midazolam) have been substituted. For longer procedures requiring anesthesia (>30 minute duration) protocols using guaifenesin, ketamine and xylazine (GKX), or isoflurane were used most commonly. The following are some examples of published protocols. A thorough discussion of balanced anesthesia, partial and total intravenous anesthesia for horses can be found in Vet Clin Equine 29 (2013) 89-122 (Valverde 2013), Vet Clin Equine 29 (2013) 123-129 (Lerche 2013)7 or other equine anesthesia references. The following are some examples of published protocols:

For field anesthesia: (extra-label): Sedate with xylazine (1 mg/kg IV; 2 mg/kg IM) given 5-10 minutes (longer for IM route) before induction of anesthesia with ketamine (2 mg/kg IV). Horse must be adequately sedated (head to the knees) before giving the ketamine (ketamine can cause muscle rigidity and seizures). If adequate sedation does not occur, either: **1)** Re-dose xylazine: up to half the original dose; or **2)** Add butorphanol (0.02 – 0.04 mg/kg IV). Butorphanol can be given with the original xylazine if you suspect that the horse will be difficult to tranquilize (*e.g.,* high-strung Thoroughbreds) or added before the ketamine. This combination will improve induction, increase analgesia and increase recumbency time by ≈5-10 minutes; or **3)** give diazepam (0.03 mg/kg IV). Mix the diazepam with the ketamine. This combination will improve induction when sedation is marginal, improve muscle relaxation during anesthesia and prolong anesthesia by ≈5-10 minutes; or **4)** Guaifenesin (5% solution administered IV to effect) can also be used to increase sedation and muscle relaxation. (Mathews 1999)

As part of induction protocols (extra-label): **Note:** Must be used with caution; not recommended for field anesthesia.

For normal healthy patients: Administer xylazine (0.44 – 0.66 mg/kg IV, or 200 – 300 mg/450 kg horse). Wait for sedation and muscle relaxation to occur (approximately 5 minutes). Guaifenesin (5% solution, or 50 mg/mL) is then rapidly infused using pressurization until marked sedation and muscle relaxation is achieved (generally a total dose of 30 – 50 mg/kg). Ketamine (2.2 mg/kg IV, 1000 mg/450 kg) should be administered at a point that allows for its slow onset to occur without the patient becoming excessively weak and collapsing from effects of guaifenesin. Recumbency generally occurs approximately 60 seconds following ketamine administration. The slow administration of guaifenesin described below can also be used in normal healthy patients in place of a supplemental dose of xylazine when the level of initial sedation is inadequate.

For compromised patients: Try to use a very modest dose of xylazine (0.22 – 0.44 mg/kg IV, or 100 – 200 mg/450 kg horse) depending on status and demeanor to minimize its cardiovascular effects in compromised patients. Slow administration of guaifenesin (5% solution) can be used to gradually create the desired level of sedation. It is still important to allow adequate time for centralization of cardiac output to progress sufficiently prior to initiating the rapid phase of guaifenesin administration that precedes the induction bolus. Guaifenesin has a slow onset of action, when used to augment the level of pre-induction sedation. SLOW administration is important to avoid creating an overly weak and ataxic patient while waiting for centralization to progress sufficiently. Guaifenesin is then rapidly infused using pressurization until marked sedation and muscle relaxation is achieved (generally a total dose of 30 – 50 mg/kg IV). Ketamine (dose decreases as degree of compromise increases, 1.34 – 1.55 mg/kg IV, or 600 – 700 mg/450 kg) for extremely compromised patients should be administered at a point that allows for its slow onset to occur without the patient becoming excessively weak and collapsing from the growing effects of guaifenesin. Experience may be required to get the timing right. Recumbency takes even longer (up to a couple minutes) when ketamine dose is reduced in compromised patients. (Abrahamsen, E. 2007)

Using ketamine and propofol after xylazine sedation: From a retrospective study (n=100). All horses were sedated with xylazine at 0.99 ± 0.2 mg/kg IV. Some also received IV butorphanol. After visually apparent sedation, a combination of propofol 0.40 ± (0.1) mg/kg and ketamine 2.8 ± (0.3) mg/kg were given via IV bolus. The order of administration was not standardized and in some cases, the two drugs were mixed together before administration. Following induction, six horses required a onetime administration of additional ketamine (0.7±0.4 mg/kg). Anesthesia was maintained with GKX (see below) in 34 horses and with isoflurane in oxygen in 66 horses. (Posner *et al.* 2013)

For long-term IV (>30 minutes) anesthesia using "GKX" or "triple-drip" (extra-label): Guaifenesin (50 mg/mL), ketamine (1 – 2 mg/mL; 2 mg/mL concentration used for more painful or noxious procedures), and xylazine (0.5 mg/mL). Most practitioners prefer to induce with xylazine/ketamine or xylazine/diazepam/ketamine and then use GKX for maintenance. Typically the CRI runs at 1.5 – 2.2 mL/kg/hr depending on the procedure, patient response and ketamine concentration.

An alternative to "GKX" is "GKD" where detomidine is substituted for the xylazine and the concentrations of guaifenesin and ketamine are increased: Guaifenesin (100 mg/mL), ketamine (4 mg/mL), and detomidine (0.04 mg/mL). The CRI runs at 0.8 mL/kg/hr for the first hour and 0.6 mL/kg/hour for the final 30 minutes. (Wagner 2009)

■ **SWINE:**

a) Give atropine, then ketamine at 11 mg/kg IM. To prolong anesthesia and increase analgesia give additional ketamine 2 – 4 mg/kg IV. Local anesthetics injected at the surgical site (*e.g.,* 2% lidocaine) may enhance analgesia. (Thurmon *et al.* 1986)

b) Ketamine (22 mg/kg) combined with acepromazine (1.1 mg/kg) IM. (Swindle 1985)

c) 4.4 mg/kg IM or IV after sedation. (Mandsager 1988)

■ **CAMELIDS (LLAMAS AND ALPACAS):**

As an anesthetic (extra-label): butorphanol 0.07 – 0.1 mg/kg; ketamine 0.2 – 0.3 mg/kg; xylazine 0.2 – 0.3 mg/kg **IV** or butorphanol 0.05 – 0.1 mg/kg; ketamine 0.2 – 0.5 mg/kg; xylazine 0.2 – 0.5 mg/kg **IM.** (Wolff 2009)

For procedural pain (*e.g.,* castrations) when recumbency (up to 30 minutes) is desired (extra-label): **Alpacas:** butorphanol 0.046 mg/kg; xylazine 0.46 mg/kg; ketamine 4.6 mg/kg. **Llamas:** butorphanol 0.037 mg/kg; xylazine 0.37 mg/kg; ketamine 3.7 mg/kg. All drugs are combined in one syringe and given IM. May administer 50% of original dose of ketamine and xylazine during anesthesia to prolong effect up to 15 minutes.

If doing mass castrations on 3 or more animals, can make up bottle of the "cocktail". Add 10 mg (1 mL) of butorphanol and 100 mg (1 mL) xylazine to a 1 gram (10 ml) vial of ketamine. This mixture is dosed at 1 mL/40 lbs. (18 kg) for alpacas, and 1 mL per 50 lbs. (22 kg) for llamas. Handle quietly and allow plenty of time before starting procedure. Expect 20 minutes of surgical time; patient should stand 45 minutes to 1 hour after injection. (Miesner 2009)

- **REPTILES:**

Medium to small land Tortoises: Medetomidine 100 – 150 micrograms/kg with ketamine 5 – 10 mg/kg IV or IM;

Freshwater Turtles: Medetomidine 150 – 300 micrograms/kg with ketamine 10 – 20 mg/kg IV or IM;

Giant Land Tortoises: 200 kg Aldabra tortoise: Medetomidine 40 micrograms/kg with ketamine 4 mg/kg IV or IM;

Smaller Aldabra tortoises: Medetomidine 40 – 80 micrograms/kg with ketamine 4 – 8 mg/kg IV or IM. Wait 30-40 minutes for peak effect;

Iguanas: Medetomidine 100 – 150 micrograms/kg with ketamine 5 – 10 mg/kg IV or IM;

Reversal of all dosages with atipamezole is 4-5 times the medetomidine dose. (Heard 1999)

- **BIRDS:**

a) Birds weighing:

<100 grams (canaries, finches, budgies): 0.1 – 0.2 mg/gm IM;

250 – 500 grams (parrots, pigeons): 0.05 – 0.1 mg/gm IM;

500 grams – 3 kg (chickens, owls, hawks): 0.02 – 0.1 mg/gm IM;

>3 kg (ducks, geese, swans): 0.02 – 0.05 mg/gm IM. (Booth 1988)

b) **In combination with xylazine:** Ketamine 10 – 30 mg/kg IM; Xylazine 2 – 6 mg/kg IM; birds less than 250 grams require a higher dosage (per kg) than birds weighing >250 g. Xylazine is not recommended to be used in debilitated birds because of its cardiodepressant effects.

In combination with diazepam: Ketamine 10 – 50 mg/kg IM; Diazepam 0.5 – 2 mg/kg IM or IV; doses can be halved for IV use.

In combination with acepromazine: Ketamine 25 – 50 mg/kg IM; Acepromazine 0.5 – 1 mg/kg IM. (Wheler 1993)

- **ZOO, EXOTIC, WILDLIFE SPECIES:**

For use of ketamine in zoo, exotic and wildlife medicine refer to specific references, including:

a) *Zoo Animal and Wildlife Immobilization and Anesthesia.* West, G, Heard, D, Caulkett, N. (eds.). Blackwell Publishing, 2007.

b) *Handbook of Wildlife Chemical Immobilization, 3rd Ed.* Kreeger, T.J. and J.M. Arnemo. 2007.

c) *Restraint and Handling of Wild and Domestic Animals.* Fowler, M (ed.), Iowa State University Press, 1995

d) *Exotic Animal Formulary, 3rd Ed.* Carpenter, J.W., Saunders. 2005

e) The 2009 American Association of Zoo Veterinarian Proceedings by D. K. Fontenot also has several dosages listed for restraint, anesthesia, and analgesia for a variety of drugs for carnivores and primates. VIN members can access them at: http://goo.gl/BHRih or http://goo.gl/9UJse

Monitoring

- Level of anesthesia/analgesia.
- Respiratory function; cardiovascular status (rate, rhythm, BP if possible).
- Monitor eyes to prevent drying or injury.
- Body temperature.

Client Information

- Should only be administered by individuals familiar with its use.

Chemistry/Synonyms

A congener of phencyclidine, ketamine HCl occurs as white, crystalline powder. It has a melting point of 258-261°C, a characteristic odor, and will precipitate as the free base at high pH. One gram is soluble in 5 mL of water, and 14 mL of alcohol. The pH of the commercially available injections are between 3.5-5.5.

Ketamine HCl may also be known as: CI-581, CL-369, CN-52372-2, ketamini hydrochloridum, *Amtech®*, *Brevinaze®*, *Calypsol®*, *Cost®*, *Inducmina®*, *Keta®*, *Keta-Hameln®*, *Ketaject®*, *Ketalin®*, *Ketanest®*, *Ketaset®*, *Ketasthesia®*, *Keta-sthetic®*, *Ketava®*, *Ketina®*, *Ketmin®*, *Ketolar®*, *Velonarcon®*, *VetaKet®*, and *Vetalar®*.

Storage/Stability

Ketamine injection should be stored between 15-30°C (59-86°F) and protected from light.

Solution may darken upon prolonged exposure to light, which does not affect the drug's potency. Do not use if precipitates appear.

Ketamine may be mixed with sterile water for injection, D5W, and normal saline for diluent purposes. Do not mix ketamine with barbiturates or diazepam in the same syringe or IV bag as precipitation may occur.

Compatibility/Compounding Considerations

Ketamine may be mixed with sterile water for injection, D5W, and normal saline for diluent purposes. Ketamine is physically **compatible in the same syringe** with xylazine, morphine, fentanyl, dexamethasone sodium phosphate, lidocaine, bupivacaine and doxapram (if used within 9 hours).

Mixing ketamine with barbiturates or diazepam in the same syringe or IV bag is NOT recommended as precipitation may occur. Although there are many anecdotal reports of mixing ketamine with diazepam, or ketamine with midazolam in the same syringe just prior to injection there does not appear to be any published information documenting the stability of the drugs after mixing. Do not use if a visible precipitate forms.

A study (Taylor *et al.* 2009) evaluating the stability, sterility, pH, particulate formation and efficacy in laboratory rodents of compounded ketamine, acepromazine and xylazine ("KAX") supported the finding that the drugs are stable and efficacious for at least 180 days after mixing if stored in the dark at room temperature.

Information "on file" with the manufacturer states that dexmedetomidine 0.5 mg/mL solution for injection can be mixed with butorphanol 2 mg/mL or with ketamine 50 mg/mL solution, or with butorphanol 2 mg/mL solution and ketamine 50 mg/mL solution, in the same syringe and possesses no pharmacological risk.

Dosage Forms/Regulatory Status

VETERINARY-LABELED PRODUCTS:

Ketamine HCl for Injection: 100 mg/mL in 10 mL vials; *Ketaject®*, *Ketaset®*, *Keta-sthetic®*, *Vetalar®*; *VetaKet®*, generic; (Rx, C-III). FDA-approved for use in cats and sub-human primates.

The ARCI (Racing Commissioners International) has designated this drug as a class 2 substance. See the appendix for more information.

The recommended milk and meat withdrawal time for ketamine in cattle is 72-hours (3 days) (Smith 2013).

HUMAN-LABELED PRODUCTS:

Ketamine HCl Injection: 10 mg/mL in 20 mL vials; 50 mg/mL in 10 mL vials & 100 mg/mL in 5 mL vials; *Ketalar®*, generic; (Rx, C-III).

Revisions/References

Monograph revised/updated March 2014.

Abrahamsen, E. (2007). Analgesia in equine practice. Proceedings: Western Vet Conference. accessed via Veterinary Information Network; vin.com

Abrahamsen, E. J. (2013). Chemical Restraint and Injectable Anesthesia of Ruminants. Veterinary Clinics of North America-Food Animal Practice 29(1): 209-+.

Baratta, M. T., et al. (2010). Canine CYP2B11 metabolizes and is inhibited by anesthetic agents often co-administered in dogs. J. Vet. Pharmacol. Ther. 33(1): 50-5.

Barletta, M., et al. (2011). Evaluation of dexmedetomidine and ketamine in combination with opioids as injectable anesthesia for castration in dogs. Journal of the American Veterinary Medical Association 238(9): 1159-67.

Bays, T. (2009). Practice tips for exotic animals. Proceedings: WVC. accessed via Veterinary Information Network; vin.com

Bennett, R. (2009). Small Mammal Anesthesia--Rabbits and Rodents. Proceedings: ACVC. accessed via Veterinary Information Network; vin.com

Biermann, K., et al. (2012). Sedative, cardiovascular, haematologic and biochemical effects of four different drug combinations administered intramuscularly in cats. Veterinary Anaesthesia and Analgesia 39(2): 137-50.

Booth, N. H. (1988). Drugs Acting on the Central Nervous System. *Veterinary Pharmacology and Therapeutics - 6th Ed.* N. H. Booth and L. E. McDonald. Ames, Iowa State University Press: 153-408.

Burke, T. (1999). Husbandry and Medicine of Rodents and Lagomorphs. Proceedings: Central Veterinary Conference, Kansas City. accessed via Veterinary Information Network; vin.com

DeClue, A. E., et al. (2008). Effects of subanesthetic doses of ketamine on hemodynamic and immunologic variables in dogs with experimentally induced endotoxemia. American Journal of Veterinary Research 69(2): 228-32.

Finkler, M. (1999). Anesthesia in Ferrets. Proceedings: Central Veterinary Conference, Kansas City. accessed via Veterinary Information Network; vin.com

Heard, D. (1999). Advances in Reptile Anesthesia. The North American Veterinary Conference, Orlando. accessed via Veterinary Information Network; vin.com

Hellyer, P. (2006). Pain assessment and multimodal analgesic therapy in dogs and cats. Proceedings: ABVP. accessed via Veterinary Information Network; vin.com

Issabeagloo, E. (2008). Comparison of sedative effects of oral ketamine and alprazolam in cat (Poster Session). Intl Jnl Psychophysiology 69: 276-316.

Ivey, E. & J. Morrisey (2000). Therapeutics for Rabbits. Vet Clin NA: Exotic Anim Pract 3:1(Jan): 183-216.

Ko, J. (2009). Dexmedetomidine and its injectable anesthetic-pain management combinations. Proceedings: ACVC. accessed via Veterinary Information Network; vin.com

Ko, J. C., et al. (2011). Evaluation of dexmedetomidine and ketamine in combination with various opioids as injectable anesthetic combinations for castration in cats. Javma-Journal of the American Veterinary Medical Association 239(11): 1453-62.

Lamont, L. A. (2008). Adjunctive Analgesic Therapy in Veterinary Medicine. Veterinary Clinics of North America-Small Animal Practice 38(6): 1187-+.

Lerche, P. (2013). Total Intravenous Anesthesia in Horses. Veterinary Clinics of North America-Equine Practice 29(1): 123-+.

Lichtenberger, M. (2006). Anesthesia Protocols and Pain Management for Exotic Animal Patients. Proceedings: Western Vet Conf. accessed via Veterinary Information Network; vin.com

Mandsager, R. E. (1988). Personal Communication.

Mathews, N. (1999). Anesthesia in large animals— Injectable (field) anesthesia: How to make it better. Proceedings: Central Veterinary Conference, Kansas City. accessed via Veterinary Information Network; vin.com

Miesner, M. (2009). Field anesthesia techniques in camelids. Proceedings: WVC. accessed via Veterinary Information Network; vin.com

Moffat, K. (2008). Addressing canine and feline aggression in the veterinary clinic. Vet Clin NA: Sm Anim Pract 38: 983-1003.

Papich, M. (1989). Effects of drugs on pregnancy. *Current Veterinary Therapy X: Small Animal Practice.* R. Kirk. Philadelphia, Saunders: 1291-9.

Polson, S., et al. (2012). Analgesia after feline ovariohysterectomy under midazolam-medetomidine-ketamine anaesthesia with buprenorphine or butorphanol, and carprofen or meloxicam: a prospective, randomised clinical trial. Journal of Feline Medicine and Surgery 14(8): 553-9.

Posner, L. P., et al. (2013). Propofol with ketamine following sedation with xylazine for routine induction of general anaesthesia in horses. Veterinary Record 173(22): 550-+.

Shaffran, N. (2009). Leaps and Bounds in Pain Management with CRIS. Proceedings: IVECCS. accessed via Veterinary Information Network; vin.com

Smith, G. (2013). Extralabel Use of Anesthetic and Analgesic Compounds in Cattle. Veterinary Clinics of North America-Food Animal Practice 29(1): 29-+.

Swindle, M. M. (1985). Anesthesia in Swine. Charles River Tech Bul 3(3).

Taylor, B. J., et al. (2009). Beyond-Use Dating of Extemporaneously Compounded Ketamine, Acepromazine, and Xylazine: Safety, Stability, and Efficacy over Time. Journal of the American Association for Laboratory Animal Science 48(6): 718-26.

Thurmon, J. C. & G. J. Benson (1986). Anesthesia in ruminants and swine. *Current Veterinary Therapy 2: Food Animal Practice.* J. L. Howard. Philadelphia, WB Saunders: 51-71.

Valverde, A. (2013). Balanced Anesthesia and Constant-Rate Infusions in Horses. Veterinary Clinics of North America-Equine Practice 29(1): 89-+.

Wagner, A. E. (2009). Injectable Field Anaesthesia in the Horse. Proceedings: AVA. accessed via Veterinary Information Network; vin.com

Wheler, C. (1993). Avian anesthetics, analgesics, and tranquilizers. Seminars in Avian & Exotic Med 2(1): 7-12.

Wolff, P. (2009). Camelid Medicine. Proceedings: AAZV. accessed via Veterinary Information Network; vin.com

Ketoconazole, Systemic

(kee-toe-kah-na-zole)   Nizoral®

Azole Antifungal

Prescriber Highlights

▶ Original imidazole oral antifungal historically used for systemic mycoses, but now newer agents are generally preferred. Still a low-cost/effective treatment for Malassezia dermatitis in dogs including aspergillosis, cryptococcal meningitis, blastomycosis, & histoplasmosis; also used to reduce dose/costs of cyclosporine therapy and as an alternative treatment of hyperadrenocorticism in dogs.

▶ Contraindications: Known hypersensitivity; some believe ketoconazole is contraindicated in cats.

▶ Caution: Hepatic disease or thrombocytopenia.

▶ Potentially teratogenic & embryotoxic; weigh risks vs. benefits.

▶ May cause infertility in male dogs by decreasing testosterone synthesis.

▶ Adverse Effects: GI (anorexia, vomiting, &/or diarrhea) most common & more prevalent in cats; hepatic toxicity, thrombocytopenia, reversible lightening of haircoat, transient dose-related suppressant effect on gonadal & adrenal steroid synthesis.

▶ Long-term treatment may be required.

▶ Many drug interactions.

Uses/Indications

Because of ketoconazole's comparative lack of toxicity when compared to amphotericin B, oral administration, and relatively good efficacy, it has been used to treat several types of fungal infections in dogs, cats, and other small species. Today, newer antifungal agents (*e.g.,* fluconazole, itraconazole) are usually preferred as they have advantages over ketoconazole, including less toxicity and/or enhanced efficacy. However, ketoconazole can be significantly less expensive than the newer agents. Ketoconazole is considered by some to still be the drug of choice for treating histoplasmosis in dogs.

Use of ketoconazole in cats is controversial due to its potential for causing hepatotoxicity; some say it should not be used in cats.

Ketoconazole has also been used clinically for the medical treatment of hyperadrenocorticism in dogs, but other treatments are more commonly recommended (mitotane or trilostane). However, it may be particularly useful for palliative therapy in dogs with large, malignant, or invasive tumors where surgery is not an option. As it is a reversible inhibitor of steroidogenesis, it is usually not a viable option for long-term treatment.

Ketoconazole interferes with the metabolism of cyclosporine and some another drugs that are metabolized via CYP-450 isoenzymes. This drug interaction has been used in dogs to reduce cyclosporine dosage/cost.

Pharmacology/Actions

At usual doses and serum concentrations, ketoconazole is fungistatic against susceptible fungi. At higher concentrations for prolonged periods of time or against very susceptible organisms, ketoconazole may be fungicidal. It is believed that ketoconazole increases cellular membrane permeability and causes secondary metabolic effects and growth inhibition. The exact mechanism for these effects has not been determined, but may be due to ketoconazole interfering with ergosterol synthesis. The fungicidal action of ketoconazole may be due to a direct effect on cell membranes.

Ketoconazole has activity against most pathogenic fungi, including Blastomyces, Coccidioides, Cryptococcus, Histoplasma,

Microsporum, and Trichophyton. Higher levels are necessary to treat most strains of Aspergillus and Sporothrix. Resistance to ketoconazole has been documented for some strains of *Candida albicans*.

Ketoconazole has *in vitro* activity against *Staphylococcus aureas* and *epidermidis*, Nocardia, enterococci, and herpes simplex virus types 1 and 2. The clinical implications of this activity are unknown.

Via inhibition of 5-lipooxygenase, ketoconazole possesses some antiinflammatory activity. The drug can suppress the immune system, probably by suppressing T-lymphocytes proliferation.

Ketoconazole also has endocrine effects; steroid synthesis is directly inhibited by blocking several P-450 enzyme systems. Measurable reductions in testosterone or cortisol synthesis can occur at dosages used for antifungal therapy, but higher dosages are generally required to reduce levels of testosterone or cortisol to be clinically useful in the treatment of prostatic carcinoma or hyperadrenocorticism. Effects on mineralocorticoids are negligible.

Pharmacokinetics

Although it is reported that ketoconazole is well absorbed after oral administration, oral bioavailability of ketoconazole tablets in dogs is highly variable. One study (Baxter *et al.* 1986) in six normal dogs, found bioavailabilities ranging from 0.04-0.89 (4-89%) after 400 mg (19.5 – 25.2 mg/kg) was administered to fasted dogs. Peak serum concentrations occur between 1-4.25 hours after dosing and peak serum levels ranged from 1.1-45.6 micrograms/mL. This wide interpatient variation may have significant clinical implications from both a toxicity and efficacy standpoint, particularly since ketoconazole is often used in life-threatening infections, and assays for measuring serum levels are not readily available. Administration with food may increase absorption.

Oral absorption of tablets in horses is poor. Single doses of 30 mg/kg yielded nondetectable blood levels. But if given via NG tube in a 0.2 Normal hydrochloric acid solution, bioavailability increased to 23%. The commercially available oral solution is reportedly 60% bioavailable.

Ketoconazole absorption is enhanced in an acidic environment and should not be administered (at the same time) with H_2 blockers or antacids (see Drug Interactions below). Whether to administer ketoconazole with meals or during a fasted state to maximize absorption is controversial. The manufacturer recommends giving with food in human patients. Dogs or cats that develop anorexia/vomiting during therapy may benefit from administration with meals.

After absorption, ketoconazole is distributed into the bile, cerumen, saliva, urine, synovial fluid, and CSF. CSF levels are generally less than 10% of those found in the serum, but may be increased if the meninges are inflamed. High levels of the drug are found in the liver, adrenals, and pituitary gland, while more moderate levels are found in the kidneys, lungs, bladder, bone marrow, and myocardium. At usual doses (10 mg/kg), attained levels are probably inadequate in the brain, testis, and eyes to treat most infections; higher dosages are required. Ketoconazole is 84-99% bound to plasma proteins and crosses the placenta (at least in rats). The drug is found in bitch's milk.

Ketoconazole is extensively metabolized into several inactive metabolites by the liver. These metabolites are excreted primarily into the feces via the bile. About 13% of a given dose is excreted into the urine and only 2-4% of the drug is excreted unchanged in the urine. Half-life in dogs is ≈1-6 hours (avg. 2.7 hours).

Contraindications/Precautions/Warnings

Ketoconazole is contraindicated in patients with known hypersensitivity to it. It should be used with caution in patients with hepatic disease or thrombocytopenia. Because of its effects on cortisol synthesis, it should be used with caution in dogs undergoing stressful events (*e.g.*, surgery, trauma, critical illness).

Use in cats is controversial as hepatotoxic effects are possible.

There are many potential drug interactions possible with ketoconazole. It is a potent inhibitor of CYP3A12 (and possibly other isoenzymes) and can inhibit p-glycoprotein.

Adverse Effects

Gastrointestinal signs of anorexia, vomiting, and/or diarrhea are the most common adverse effects seen with ketoconazole therapy and are more prevalent in cats. Dividing the dose and/or giving it with meals may minimize anorexia. Appetite stimulants such as oxazepam or cyproheptadine may also be of benefit in cats.

Hepatic toxicity consisting of cholangiohepatitis and increased liver enzymes has been reported with ketoconazole, and may be either idiosyncratic in nature or a dose-related phenomenon. Cats may be more prone to developing hepatotoxicity than dogs. While liver enzymes should be monitored during therapy, an increase does not necessarily mandate dosage reduction or discontinuation unless concomitant anorexia, vomiting, diarrhea, or abdominal pain is present. Thrombocytopenia has also been reported with ketoconazole therapy, but is rarely encountered. A reversible lightening of haircoat may also occur in patients treated with ketoconazole.

Ketoconazole has a transient dose-related suppressant effect on gonadal and adrenal steroid synthesis. Doses as low as 10 mg/kg depressed serum testosterone levels in dogs within 3-4 hours after dosing, but levels returned to normal within 10 hours. Doses of 30 mg/kg/day have been demonstrated to suppress serum cortisol levels in dogs with hyperadrenocorticism (see Dosages section). Dogs undergoing high dose antifungal therapy may need additional glucocorticoid support during periods of acute stress.

Reproductive/Nursing Safety

Ketoconazole is a known teratogen and embryotoxin in rats. There have been reports of mummified fetuses and stillbirths in dogs who have been treated. Ketoconazole should not be considered absolutely contraindicated in pregnant animals, however, as it is often used in potentially life-threatening infections. The benefits of therapy should be weighed against the potential risks. Ketoconazole may cause infertility in male dogs by decreasing testosterone synthesis. Testosterone production rebounds once the drug is discontinued.

In humans, the FDA categorizes this drug as category *C* for use during pregnancy (*Animal studies have shown an adverse effect on the fetus, but there are no adequate studies in humans; or there are no animal reproduction studies and no adequate studies in humans.*) In a separate system evaluating the safety of drugs in canine and feline pregnancy (Papich 1989), this drug is categorized as class: *B* (*Safe for use if used cautiously. Studies in laboratory animals may have uncovered some risk, but these drugs appear to be safe in dogs and cats or these drugs are safe if they are not administered when the animal is near term.*)

Ketoconazole is excreted in milk; use with caution in nursing dams.

Overdosage/Acute Toxicity

No reports of acute toxicity associated with overdosage were located. The oral LD_{50} in dogs after oral administration is >500 mg/kg. Should an acute overdose occur, the manufacturer recommends employing supportive measures, including gastric lavage with sodium bicarbonate.

Drug Interactions

The following drug interactions have either been reported or are theoretical in humans or animals receiving ketoconazole and may be of significance in veterinary patients. Unless otherwise noted, use together is not necessarily contraindicated, but weigh the potential risks and perform additional monitoring when appropriate.

- **ALCOHOL:** Ethanol may interact with ketoconazole and produce a disulfiram-like reaction (vomiting).
- **ANTACIDS:** May reduce oral absorption of ketoconazole; administer ketoconazole at least 1 hour before or 2 hours after.
- **ANTIDEPRESSANTS, TRICYCLIC** (*e.g.,* **amitriptyline, clomipramine**): Ketoconazole may reduce metabolism and increase adverse effects.
- **BENZODIAZEPINES** (*e.g.,* **midazolam, triazolam**): Ketoconazole may increase levels. A study in greyhounds showed that ketoconazole significantly decreased the elimination of midazolam (KuKanich *et al.* 2010).
- **BUSPIRONE:** Plasma concentrations may be elevated.
- **BUSULFAN:** Ketoconazole may increase levels.
- **CALCIUM-CHANNEL BLOCKING AGENTS** (*e.g.,* **amlodipine, verapamil**): Ketoconazole may increase levels.
- **CISAPRIDE:** Ketoconazole may increase cisapride levels and possibility for toxicity; use together contraindicated in humans.
- **CORTICOSTEROIDS:** Ketoconazole may inhibit the metabolism of corticosteroids; potential for increased adverse effects.
- **CYCLOPHOSPHAMIDE:** Ketoconazole may inhibit the metabolism of cyclophosphamide and its metabolites; potential for increased toxicity.
- **CYCLOSPORINE:** Increased cyclosporine levels.
- **DIGOXIN:** Ketoconazole may increase digoxin levels.
- **FENTANYL/ALFENTANIL:** Ketoconazole may increase fentanyl or alfentanil levels.
- **H2-BLOCKERS** (**ranitidine, famotidine**, etc.): Increased gastric pH may reduce ketoconazole absorption.
- **HEPATOTOXIC DRUGS, OTHER:** Because ketoconazole can cause hepatotoxicity, it should be used cautiously with other hepatotoxic agents.
- **ISONIAZID:** May affect ketoconazole levels and concomitant use not recommended in humans.
- **IVERMECTIN:** Ketoconazole may increase risk for neurotoxicity. At least one reference states that ivermectin should never be used with ketoconazole in dogs (Waisglass 2009).
- **MACROLIDE ANTIBIOTICS** (**erythromycin, clarithromycin**, etc.): May increase ketoconazole concentrations.
- **MITOTANE:** Mitotane and ketoconazole are not recommended for use together to treat hyperadrenocorticism as the adrenolytic effects of mitotane may be inhibited by ketoconazole's inhibition of cytochrome P450 enzymes.
- **PHENYTOIN:** May decrease ketoconazole levels.
- **PROTON-PUMP INHIBITORS** (**omeprazole**, etc.): Increased gastric pH may reduce ketoconazole absorption.
- **QUINIDINE:** Ketoconazole may increase quinidine levels.
- **RIFAMPIN:** May decrease ketoconazole levels; ketoconazole may increase rifampin levels.
- **SUCRALFATE:** May reduce absorption of ketoconazole.
- **SULFONYLUREA ANTIDIABETIC AGENTS** (*e.g.,* **glipizide, glyburide**): Ketoconazole may increase levels; hypoglycemia possible.
- **THEOPHYLLINE:** Ketoconazole may decrease serum theophylline concentrations in some patients; theophylline levels should be monitored.
- **VINCRISTINE/VINBLASTINE:** Ketoconazole may inhibit vinca alkaloid metabolism and increase levels.
- **WARFARIN:** Ketoconazole may cause increased prothrombin times in patients receiving warfarin or other coumarin anticoagulants.

Laboratory Considerations

- Ketoconazole can reduce serum cortisol levels and affect adrenal function tests. After stopping ketoconazole, cortisol levels usually return to baseline within 24 hours.

Doses

Note: All dosages are extra-label.

- **DOGS:**

  Note: Oral ketoconazole has been used historically to treat various systemic mycoses, including blastomycosis and histoplasmosis. However, to obtain efficacy comparable to itraconazole alone, it must be combined with amphotericin B. Triazole antifungals (*e.g.,* itraconazole, fluconazole) are now generally recommended. Ketoconazole may be considered for these infections when drug cost determines whether treatment occurs. It does continue to be a low-cost and effective treatment for Malassezia dermatitis. (Foy *et al.* 2010)

  For Malassezia dermatitis: Based on a review of published evidence, the authors concluded that fair evidence exists to recommend ketoconazole at 5 – 10 mg/kg once daily PO (Negre *et al.* 2009). Most recommend treatment for 2-4 weeks.

  To reduce the dosage requirements of cyclosporine; (consider monitoring cyclosporine levels): 5 – 10 mg/kg PO once daily has been often suggested and may be appropriate when cyclosporine is used as an Immunomodulator for conditions such as IMHA. However when used for canine atopic dermatitis, a recent study measuring cyclosporine levels in whole blood and skin of normal dogs after receiving cyclosporine and ketoconazole at either 2.5 mg/kg or 5 mg/kg of each drug concluded, "it is anticipated that administration of cyclosporine and ketoconazole concurrently at 2.5 mg/kg per day may be as effective as cyclosporine alone at 5 mg/kg/day for treating canine atopic dermatitis." The authors then went on to caution that whether ketoconazole at 5 mg/kg/day translates into increased efficacy deserves further investigation and may result in higher cyclosporine levels than needed. The resulting significantly higher whole blood CSA concentrations may cause an increased risk of adverse effects. (Gray *et al.* 2013)

  For treatment of hyperadrenocorticism: Not commonly recommended. The following dosage regimen has been reported: Author (Merchant) usually uses mitotane therapy, but if animal fails to respond can try ketoconazole: Initiate therapy at 5 – 10 mg/kg PO twice daily. The patient is monitored as for mitotane—water consumption or first sign of side effects (vomiting, diarrhea or anorexia), which can be seen as a result of the drug or secondary to hypocortisolemia. An idiosyncratic hepatopathy can also be seen (rare?). If no side effects are seen or the patient was not PU/PD initially, then the medication is given for 7-14 days and the patient is reevaluated with an ACTH stimulation test. The goal of therapy is to have an ACTH stimulation test in the low normal to slightly below normal range. If there is a continued exaggerated response, then ketoconazole dose is increased to 15 mg/kg PO twice daily and the patient reevaluated as above. The patient is maintained on the same dose that brought the ACTH stimulation test into the normal or subnormal range (*e.g.,* 5 – 15 mg/kg PO twice daily). The ACTH stimulation test is then performed every 3-4 months. (Merchant 2009)

  For treatment of systemic mycoses when drug cost for other

antifungal treatments is prohibitive: 5 – 10 mg/kg PO q12-24h. Treatment duration can vary, but generally should continue for least 1 month after complete resolution of clinical signs.

- **CATS:**

Note: Use is controversial and some clinicians recommend that ketoconazole not be used in cats because of its toxic potential. Consider using other antifungals (*e.g.*, fluconazole, itraconazole, etc.) in its place. However, ketoconazole may be considered when drug cost is the overriding factor for treatment.

For susceptible systemic mycoses when drug costs are the primary concern: Usually dosed at 10 mg/kg (or 50 mg per cat) q12-24h. Treatment may be required for many months. Administer with food. Hepatotoxicity possible; monitor liver enzymes.

- **HORSES:**

For susceptible yeasts and *Aspergillus* spp.: Using the commercial oral solution (**Note:** Not marketed in the USA): 5 mg/kg PO once daily.

For *Scopulariopsis* pneumonia: Oral tablets may be administered via NG tube by mixing them with 0.2 Normal hydrochloric acid and dosed at 30 mg/kg q12h. (Stewart *et al.* 2008a, b)

- **RABBITS/RODENTS/SMALL MAMMALS:**

Rabbits: 10 – 40 mg/kg per day PO for 14 days. (Ivey *et al.* 2000)

Hamsters, Gerbils, Mice, Rats, Guinea pigs, Chinchillas: For systemic mycoses/candidiasis: 10 – 40 mg/kg per day PO for 14 days. (Adamcak *et al.* 2000)

- **BIRDS:**

For susceptible fungal infections:

a) **For severe refractory candidiasis in Psittacines:** 5 – 10 mg/kg as a gavage twice daily for 14 days. For local effect in crop dissolve 1/4 tablet (50 mg) in 0.2 mL of 1 Normal hydrochloric acid and add 0.8 mL of water. Solution turns pale pink when dissolved. Add mixture to food for gavage.

To add to water for most species: 200 mg/L for 7-14 days. As drug is not water soluble at neutral pH, dissolve in acid prior to adding to water (see above).

To add to feed for most species: 10 – 20 mg/kg for 7-14 days. Add to favorite food or add to mash. (Clubb 1986)

b) 20 – 30 mg/kg PO twice daily (based on the kinetics determined in a single trial of Moluccan Cockatoos). (Flammer 2003)

- **REPTILES:**

For susceptible fungal infections in most species: 15 – 30 mg/kg PO once daily for 2-4 weeks. (Gauvin 1993)

Monitoring

- Liver enzymes with chronic therapy (at least every 2 months; some clinicians say monthly).
- CBC with platelets.
- Efficacy and other adverse effects.

Client Information

- Give with food especially foods high in fat (*e.g.,* cream, cheese, butter, cheese, etc.).
- Gastrointestinal effects (*e.g.,* lack of appetite, vomiting, etc.) are the most likely side effect seen (especially in cats).
- Liver toxicity is possible; watch for severe vomiting, no appetite, yellowing of gums or whites of the eyes. If seen, stop giving the drug and contact your veterinarian immediately.
- May cause birth defects in animals and reduce fertility in males; use only when absolutely necessary in pregnant or breeding animals. Pregnant women should use caution when handling.

Chemistry/Synonyms

An imidazole antifungal agent, ketoconazole occurs as a white to slightly beige powder with pK_as of 2.9 and 6.5. It is practically insoluble in water.

Ketoconazole may also be known as ketoconazolum, and R-41400; many trade names are available.

Storage/Stability

Ketoconazole tablets should be stored at room temperature in well-closed containers.

Compatibility/Compounding Considerations

Compounded preparation stability: Ketoconazole oral suspension compounded from the commercially available tablets has been published (Allen *et al.* 1996). Triturating twelve (12) ketoconazole 200 mg tablets with 60 mL of *Ora Plus*® and *qs ad* to 120 mL with *Ora Sweet*® or *Ora-Sweet-SF*® yields a 20 mg/mL ketoconazole oral suspension that retains >95% potency for 60 days when stored at both 5°C and 25°C and protected from light.

Dosage Forms/Regulatory Status

VETERINARY-LABELED PRODUCTS: NONE FOR SYSTEMIC USE.

HUMAN-LABELED PRODUCTS:

Ketoconazole Tablets: 200 mg (scored); generic; (Rx)

Topical forms are also available.

Revisions/References

Monograph revised/updated March 2014.

Adamcak, A. & B. Otten (2000). Rodent Therapeutics. Vet Clin NA: Exotic Anim Pract 3:1(Jan): 221-40.

Allen, L. V. & M. A. Erickson (1996). Stability of ketoconazole, metolazone, metronidazole, procainamide hydrochloride, and spironolactone in extemporaneously compounded oral liquids. Am J Health Syst Pharm 53(17): 2073-8.

Baxter, J. G., et al. (1986). Pharmacokinetics of ketoconazole administered intravenously to dogs and orally as tablet and solution to humans and dogs. J Pharm Sci 75(5): 443-7.

Clubb, S. L. (1986). Therapeutics: Individual and Flock Treatment Regimens. *Clinical Avian Medicine and Surgery*. G. J. Harrison and L. R. Harrison. Philadelphia, W.B. Saunders: 327-55.

Flammer, K. (2003). Antifungal therapy in avian medicine. Proceedings: Western Veterinary Conference. accessed via Veterinary Information Network; vin.com

Foy, D. S. & L. A. Trepanier (2010). Antifungal Treatment of Small Animal Veterinary Patients. Veterinary Clinics of North America-Small Animal Practice 40(6): 1171-+.

Gauvin, J. (1993). Drug therapy in reptiles. Seminars in Avian & Exotic Med 2(1): 48-59.

Gray, L. L., et al. (2013). The effect of ketoconazole on whole blood and skin ciclosporin concentrations in dogs. Veterinary Dermatology 24(1): 118-+.

Ivey, E. & J. Morrisey (2000). Therapeutics for Rabbits. Vet Clin NA: Exotic Anim Pract 3:1(Jan): 183-216.

KuKanich, B. & M. Hubin (2010). The pharmacokinetics of ketoconazole and its effects on the pharmacokinetics of midazolam and fentanyl in dogs. J. Vet. Pharmacol. Ther. 33(1): 42-9.

Merchant, S. (2009). Diagnosis and Long Term Management of Canine Cushing's Disease. Proceedings: ACVC. accessed via Veterinary Information Network; vin.com

Negre, A., et al. (2009). Evidence-based veterinary dermatology: a systematic review of interventions for Malassezia dermatitis in dogs. Veterinary Dermatology 20(1): 1-12.

Papich, M. (1989). Effects of drugs on pregnancy. *Current Veterinary Therapy X: Small Animal Practice*. R. Kirk. Philadelphia, Saunders: 1291-9.

Stewart, A., et al. (2008a). Fungal infections of the upper respiratory tract. Compendium Equine(May): 208-.

Stewart, A., et al. (2008b). Pulmonary and systemic fungal infections. Compendium Equine(June): 260-72.

Waisglass, S. (2009). Demodicosis Update--Some Considerations to Increase Your Success Rate. Proceedings: WVC. accessed via Veterinary Information Network; vin.com

Ketoprofen

(kee-toe-proe-fen)   Ketofen®, Anafen®

Non-Steroidal Antiinflammatory Agent

Prescriber Highlights

▶ Nonsteroidal antiinflammatory agent used in horses, cats (short-term) & dogs.

▶ Cautions: GI ulceration or bleeding, hypoproteinemia, breeding animals (especially late in pregnancy), significant renal or hepatic impairment; may mask the signs of infection (inflammation, hyperpyrexia).

▶ Adverse Effects: **Horses:** Potentially, gastric mucosal damage & GI ulceration, renal crest necrosis, & mild hepatitis may occur. **Dogs:** Vomiting, anorexia, & GI ulcers.

▶ Do not administer intra-arterially & avoid SC injections.

▶ Drug-drug; drug-lab interactions.

Uses/Indications

In the USA, ketoprofen is approved for IV use in horses for the alleviation of inflammation and pain associated with musculoskeletal disorders. Like flunixin (and other NSAIDs) ketoprofen potentially has many other uses in a variety of species and conditions.

There are approved dosage forms of ketoprofen for dogs, cats, cattle, and swine in the U.K. and elsewhere, but not in the USA. Ketoprofen was considered by some to be the NSAID of choice for use short-term for analgesia in cats, but the availability of robenacoxib for cats in the USA has now altered its status. In Canada, ketoprofen has labeled indications for use in dogs and cats for the alleviation of inflammation, lameness and pain due to osteoarthritis, hip dysplasia, disc disease, spondylosis, panosteitis, trauma, and related musculoskeletal diseases; for the management of post-surgical pain; and for the symptomatic treatment of fever. It is labeled to be used with appropriate anti-infective therapy when inflammation and/or fever are associated with a primary infectious process.

Pharmacology/Actions

Ketoprofen exhibits actions similar to that of other nonsteroidal antiinflammatory agents in that it possesses antipyretic, analgesic and antiinflammatory activity. Its purported mechanism of action is the inhibition of cyclooxygenase catalysis of arachadonic acid to prostaglandin precursors (endoperoxides), thereby inhibiting the synthesis of prostaglandins in tissues. Ketoprofen purportedly has inhibitory activity on lipoxygenase, whereas flunixin reportedly does not at therapeutic doses, but the evidence for this action is weak as *in vitro* studies have not confirmed lipoxygenase activity in studied species.

The S (+) enantiomer is associated with anti-prostaglandin activity and toxicity and the R (-) form analgesia without the GI effects.

Pharmacokinetics

In species studied (rats, dog, man), ketoprofen is rapidly and nearly completely absorbed after oral administration. The presence of food or milk decreases oral absorption. Oral absorption is poor in horses. It has been reported that when comparing IV vs. IM injections in horses, the areas under the curve are relatively equivalent. Volume of distribution is low in adult horses. Volume of distribution is reportedly higher in foals and doses may need to be higher (1.5X) with longer durations between doses in neonates (Wilcke *et al.* 1998). The drug enters synovial fluid and is highly bound to plasma proteins (99% in humans, and approximately 93% in horses). In horses, the manufacturer reports that the onset of activity is within 2 hours and peak effects 12 hours post dose.

Ketoprofen is eliminated via the kidneys both as a conjugated metabolite (primarily glucuronidation in dogs and horses) and

unchanged drug. In cats, thioesterification is proposed as a major elimination mechanism. The elimination half-life in horses is ≈1.5 hours and in adult cats it is approximately 1-1.5 hours. The S- form half-life in dogs is ≈1.6 hours.

Contraindications/Precautions/Warnings

For horses the manufacturer states that there are no contraindications to the drug's use (other than previous hypersensitivity to ketoprofen). However it should be used only when the potential benefits outweigh the risks in cases where GI ulceration or bleeding is evident or in patients with significant renal or hepatic impairment. It is not labeled for use in breeding animals. Do not use in horses intended for human consumption.

Ketoprofen may mask the clinical signs of infection (inflammation, hyperpyrexia). Because ketoprofen is highly protein bound, patients with hypoproteinemia may have increased levels of free drug, thereby increasing the risks for toxicity.

Because there are approved NSAIDs for use in dogs and cats in the USA, extra-label use of ketoprofen is not recommended.

Adverse Effects

Ketoprofen appears to have low toxicity in horses and reports indicate that ketoprofen appears relatively safe to use in horses and may have a lower incidence of adverse effects than either phenylbutazone or flunixin. Potentially, gastric mucosal damage and GI ulceration, renal crest necrosis, and mild hepatitis may occur.

Do not administer intra-arterially and avoid SC injections. While not labeled for IM use in horses, it reportedly is effective and may only cause occasional inflammation at the injection site.

In dogs or cats, ketoprofen may cause vomiting, anorexia, and GI ulcers. When used perioperatively in dogs, ketoprofen can decrease platelet aggregation but this may not have clinical significance.

Reproductive/Nursing Safety

The manufacturer cautions against ketoprofen's use in breeding horses because effects on fertility, pregnancy, or fetal health have not been established. However, rat and mice studies have not demonstrated increased teratogenicity or embryotoxicity. Rabbits receiving twice the human dose exhibited increased embryotoxicity, but not teratogenicity. Because non-steroidal antiinflammatory agents inhibit prostaglandin synthesis, adversely affecting neonatal cardiovascular systems (premature closure of patent ductus), ketoprofen should not be used late in pregnancy. Studies in male rats demonstrated no changes in fertility. In humans, the FDA categorizes this drug as category *B* for use during the first two trimesters of pregnancy (*Animal studies have not yet demonstrated risk to the fetus, but there are no adequate studies in pregnant women; or animal studies have shown an adverse effect, but adequate studies in pregnant women have not demonstrated a risk to the fetus in the first trimester of pregnancy, and there is no evidence of risk in later trimesters.*)

It is presently unknown whether ketoprofen enters equine milk. Ketoprofen does enter canine milk; use with caution.

Overdosage/Acute Toxicity

Humans have survived oral ingestions of up to 5 grams. The LD$_{50}$ in dogs after oral ingestion has been reported to be 2000 mg/kg, but exposures as low as 0.44 mg/kg in dogs have caused GI ulcers. Cats have developed renal toxicity at doses as low as 0.7 mg/kg. Horses given ketoprofen at doses up to 11 mg/kg administered IV once daily for 15 days exhibited no signs of toxicity. Severe laminitis was observed in a horse given 33 mg/kg/day (15X over labeled dosage) for 5 days. Anorexia, depression, icterus, and abdominal swelling were noted in horses given 55 mg/kg/day (25X labeled dose) for 5 days. Upon necropsy, gastritis, nephritis, and hepatitis were diagnosed in this group.

There were 16 exposures to ketoprofen reported to the ASPCA

Animal Poison Control Center (APCC) during 2008-2009. In these cases 9 were dogs with 2 showing clinical signs and the remaining 7 cases with 2 showing clinical signs. Common findings in dogs recorded included vomiting.

This medication is a NSAID. As with any NSAID, overdosage can lead to gastrointestinal and renal effects. Decontamination with emetics and/or activated charcoal is appropriate. For doses where GI effects are expected, the use of gastrointestinal protectants is warranted. If renal effects are also expected, fluid diuresis is warranted.

Drug Interactions

The following drug interactions have either been reported or are theoretical in humans or animals receiving ketoprofen and may be of significance in veterinary patients. Unless otherwise noted, use together is not necessarily contraindicated, but weigh the potential risks and perform additional monitoring when appropriate.

- **AMINOGLYCOSIDES (gentamicin, amikacin,** etc.): Increased risk for nephrotoxicity.
- **ANTICOAGULANTS (heparin, LMWH, warfarin):** Increased risk for bleeding possible.
- **ASPIRIN:** When aspirin is used concurrently with ketoprofen, plasma levels of ketoprofen could decrease and an increased likelihood of GI adverse effects (blood loss) could occur. Concomitant administration of aspirin with ketoprofen cannot be recommended.
- **BISPHOSPHONATES (alendronate,** etc.): May increase risk for GI ulceration.
- **CORTICOSTEROIDS:** Concomitant administration with NSAIDs may significantly increase the risks for GI, platelet or renal adverse effects especially in dogs.
- **CYCLOSPORINE:** May increase risk for nephrotoxicity.
- **FLUCONAZOLE:** May increase NSAID levels.
- **FUROSEMIDE:** Ketoprofen may reduce the saluretic and diuretic effects of furosemide.
- **HIGHLY PROTEIN BOUND DRUGS** (*e.g.,* **phenytoin, valproic acid, oral anticoagulants,** other **antiinflammatory agents, salicylates, sulfonamides,** and the **sulfonylurea antidiabetic agents):** Because ketoprofen is highly bound to plasma proteins (99%), it potentially could displace other highly bound drugs; increased serum levels and duration of actions may occur. Although these interactions are usually of little concern clinically, use together with caution.
- **METHOTREXATE:** Serious toxicity has occurred in humans when NSAIDs have been used concomitantly with methotrexate; use together with extreme caution.
- **PROBENECID:** May cause a significant increase in serum levels and half-life of ketoprofen.

Laboratory Considerations

Ketoprofen may cause:
- Falsely elevated **blood glucose** values when using the glucose oxidase and peroxidase method using ABTS as a chromogen.
- Falsely elevated **serum bilirubin** values when using DMSO as a reagent.
- Falsely elevated **serum iron** concentrations using the Ramsey method, or falsely decreased serum iron concentrations when using bathophenanthroline disulfonate as a reagent.

Doses

- **DOGS:**

    As an antiinflammatory/analgesic (all are extra-label in USA):

    Canada label: Injection at a dose of 2 mg/kg IM, IV or SC injection for one day, and continue with ketoprofen tablets PO at a lower maintenance dose of 1 mg/kg once a day for four more

days. (Adapted from label information—*Anafen®*; Merial-Canada)

U.K. label: For acute indications: 2 mg/kg SC, IM, IV once daily for up to 3 consecutive days. If preferred after one injection treatment may be followed on the next day with tablets at 1 mg/kg PO per day and continued on successive days for up to 4 days (*i.e.,* up to 5 days in total). For chronic pain: 0.25 mg/kg PO once daily for up to 30 days. (Label Information *Ketofen 1%*; *Ketofen® Tablets*—Merial U.K.)

- **CATS:**

    As an antiinflammatory/analgesic (all are extra-label in USA):

    Canada label: Injection at a dose of 2 mg/kg SC for one day, and continue with ketoprofen tablets PO at a lower maintenance dose of 1 mg/kg once a day for 4 more days. In severe cases, the parenteral loading dose of 2 mg/kg can be given for up to 3 consecutive days. (Label information; *Anafen®*—Merial-Canada)

    U.K. label: 2 mg/kg SC once daily for up to 3 consecutive days. If preferred after one injection treatment may be followed on the next day with tablets at 1 mg/kg and continued on successive days for up to 4 days (i.e., up to 5 days in total). (Label Information *Ketofen® 1%*; *Ketofen® Tablets*—Merial U.K.)

- **FERRETS:**

    As a post-operative analgesic (extra-label): 1 – 2 mg/kg *(route not indicted; suggest SC or IM as per cats—Plumb)* q24h. (Lichtenberger 2008)

- **RABBITS/RODENTS/SMALL MAMMALS:**

    a) **Rabbits:** For chronic pain/antiinflammatory: 1 mg/kg IM q12-24h. (Ivey *et al.* 2000)

    b) **Rats:** 5 mg/kg SC. (Adamcak *et al.* 2000)

    c) **Rabbits:** 3 mg/kg IM, estimated duration of action 12-24 hours. (Flecknell 2008)

- **HORSES:** (NOTE: ARCI UCGFS CLASS 4 DRUG)

    For the alleviation of inflammation and pain associated with musculoskeletal disorders (FDA-approved): 2.2 mg/kg (1 mL/100 lbs.) IV once daily for up to 5 days. (Package insert; *Ketofen®*)

- **CATTLE:**

    For antiinflammatory and analgesic treatment of mammary gland disorders; reduction of pyrexia associated with respiratory disease in conjunction with antimicrobial treatment (extra-label in USA): 3 mg/kg IV or deep IM once daily for up to 3 days; withdrawal times (U.K.) are meat: 4 days; milk: 0 days. (Label information *Comforion Vet®*—Merial U.K.) **Note:** The Food Animal Residue Avoidance Databank (FARAD) has recommended a meat withdrawal interval of 7 days and a milk withdrawal interval of 24 hours following dosages of up to 3.3 mg/kg every 24 hours for 3 days. However, because flunixin is approved, ketoprofen's use in cattle in the USA would not be allowed under the current guidelines for extra-label drug use; therefore it is not considered appropriate for use in supportive treatment of a cow with toxemia (Smith 2013).

- **SWINE:**

    For the reduction of pyrexia in respiratory tract disorders and supportive treatment of post-partum dysgalactiae syndrome (MMA-syndrome—mastitis, metritis, agalactia) in conjunction with antibiotic therapy (extra-label USA): 3 mg/kg deep IM once daily for up to 3 days; withdrawal times (U.K.) for meat: 4 days. (Label information *Comforion Vet®*—Merial U.K.)

- **BIRDS:**

    As an antiinflammatory/analgesic (extra-label): 2 mg/kg IM or SC q8-24h. (Echols 2008)

- **ZOO, EXOTIC, WILDLIFE SPECIES:**

  For use of ketoprofen in zoo, exotic and wildlife medicine refer to specific references, including:

  a) *Exotic Animal Formulary, 3rd Ed.* Carpenter JW. Saunders. 2005

  b) The 2009 American Association of Zoo Veterinarian Proceedings by D. K. Fontenot also has several dosages listed for restraint, anesthesia, and analgesia for a variety of drugs for carnivores and primates. VIN members can access them at: http://goo.gl/BHRih or http://goo.gl/9UJse

Monitoring

- Efficacy.
- Adverse Effects (occasional liver or renal function tests are recommended with long-term therapy).

Client information

- Give with food to small animals. Do not inject this drug into an artery or subcutaneously (SC, under the skin) in horses.
- Must only be used for a few days in cats or serious side effects can occur.
- Most common side effects are gastrointestinal-related (*e.g.*, reduced appetite, vomiting, diarrhea in small animals). Ulcers, bleeding, liver and kidney problems can also occur (see side effects section).

Chemistry/Synonyms

A propionic acid derivative nonsteroidal antiinflammatory agent (NSAID), ketoprofen occurs as an off-white to white, fine to granular powder. It is practically insoluble in water, but freely soluble in alcohol at 20°C. Ketoprofen has a pK_a of 5.9 in a 3:1 methanol:water solution. Ketoprofen has both an S enantiomer and R enantiomer. The commercial product contains a racemic mixture of both. The S (+) enantiomer has greater antiinflammatory potency than the R (-) form.

Ketoprofen may also be known as ketoprofenum and RP-19583; many trade names are available.

Storage/Stability

Ketoprofen oral capsules should be stored at room temperature in tight, light resistant containers. The veterinary injection should be stored at room temperature. Compatibility studies with injectable ketoprofen and other compounds have apparently not been published.

Compatibility/Compounding Considerations

No specific information noted.

Dosage Forms/Regulatory Status

VETERINARY-LABELED PRODUCTS:

Ketoprofen Injection: 100 mg/mL in 50 mL and 100 mL multi-dose vials; *Ketofen®*, generic, (Rx). FDA-approved for use in horses not intended for food.

In Canada and the U.K., there are approved oral dosage forms and injectable forms for use in dogs and cats. Trade names include *Anafen®* and *Ketofen®*.

The ARCI (Racing Commissioners International) has designated this drug as a class 4 substance. See the appendix for more information.

HUMAN-LABELED PRODUCTS:

Ketoprofen Capsules: 50 mg & 75 mg; generic; (Rx)

Ketoprofen Extended-Release Capsules: 200 mg; generic; (Rx)

Revisions/References

Monograph revised/updated March 2014.

Adamcak, A. & B. Otten (2000). Rodent Therapeutics. Vet Clin NA: Exotic Anim Pract **3:**1(Jan): 221-40.

Echols, M. (2008). Avian Anesthesia and Analgesia. Proceedings: IVECCS. accessed via Veterinary Information Network; vin.com

Flecknell, P. (2008). Analgesia and perioperative care. Proceedings: World Veterinary Congress. accessed via Veterinary Information Network; vin.com

Ivey, E. & J. Morrisey (2000). Therapeutics for Rabbits. Vet Clin NA: Exotic Anim Pract **3:**1(Jan): 183-216.

Lichtenberger, M. (2008). Anesthesia and Analgesia for the Exotic Pets. Proceedings: WVC. accessed via Veterinary Information Network; vin.com

Smith, G. (2013). Extralabel Use of Anesthetic and Analgesic Compounds in Cattle. Veterinary Clinics of North America-Food Animal Practice 29(1): 29-+.

Wilcke, J. R., et al. (1998). Pharmacokinetics of ketoprofen in healthy foals less than twenty-four hours old. American Journal of Veterinary Research 59(3): 290-2.

Ketorolac Tromethamine

(kee-toe-role-ak)   Toradol®

Non-Steroidal Antiinflammatory Agent

Prescriber Highlights

► NSAID used primarily for short-term analgesia. It is also used topically as an ophthalmic (see Ophthalmology section).

► Contraindications: Active GI ulcers or history of hypersensitivity to the drug.

► Relatively contraindicated: Hematologic, renal, or hepatic disease.

► Caution: History of gastric ulcers, heart failure.

► Adverse Effects: GI ulcers & perforation, renal effects possible with chronic use; consider co-dosing with misoprostol/sucralfate in dogs to reduce chances of ulcers.

Uses/Indications

Ketorolac is used primarily for its analgesic effects for short-term treatment of mild to moderate pain in dogs and rodents. The duration of analgesic effect in dogs is ≈8-12 hours, but because of the availability of approved, safer NSAIDs for dogs, its use is questionable.

Pharmacology/Actions

Like other NSAIDs, ketorolac exhibits analgesic, antiinflammatory, and antipyretic activity probably through its inhibition of cyclooxygenase with resultant impediment of prostaglandin synthesis. Ketorolac may exhibit a more potent analgesic effect than some other NSAIDs. It inhibits both COX-1 and COX-2 receptors.

Pharmacokinetics

After 0.5 mg/kg IV injection in dogs, ketorolac's volume of distribution is ≈1 L/kg and elimination half-life averaged about 11 hours (Cagnardi *et al.* 2013). After oral administration, ketorolac is rapidly absorbed; in dogs peak levels occur in ≈50 minutes and oral bioavailability is ≈50-75%.

Ketorolac is distributed marginally through the body. It does not appear to cross the blood-brain barrier and is highly bound to plasma proteins (99%). The volume of distribution in dogs is reported to be ≈0.33-0.42 L/kg (similar in humans). The drug does cross the placenta.

Ketorolac is primarily metabolized via glucuronidation and hydroxylation. Both unchanged drug and metabolites are excreted mainly in the urine. Patients with diminished renal function will have longer elimination times than normal. In normal dogs, the elimination half-life is between 4-8 hours.

Contraindications/Precautions/Warnings

Ketorolac is relatively contraindicated in patients with a history of, or preexisting, hematologic, renal or hepatic disease. It is contraindicated in patients with active GI ulcers or a history of hypersensitivity to the drug. It should be used cautiously in patients with a history of GI ulcers, or heart failure (may cause fluid retention), and in geriatric patients. Animals suffering from inflammation secondary to concomitant infection, should receive appropriate antimicrobial therapy.

Because ketorolac has a tendency to cause gastric erosion and ulcers in dogs, long-term use (>3 days) is not recommended in this species.

Do not confuse ketorolac with *Ketalar*® (ketamine).

Adverse Effects

Ketorolac use is limited in domestic animals because of its adverse effect profile and a lack of veterinary-labeled products. The primary issue in dogs is its GI toxicity. GI ulceration can be common if the drug is used chronically. Most clinicians who have used this medication in dogs limit treatment to less than 3 days and give misoprostol with or without sucralfate concurrently. Like other NSAIDS, platelet inhibition, renal, and hepatic toxicity are also possible with this drug.

Reproductive/Nursing Safety

Ketorolac does cross the placenta. In humans, the FDA categorizes this drug as category *C* for use during the first two trimesters of pregnancy (*Animal studies have shown an adverse effect on the fetus, but there are no adequate studies in humans; or there are no animal reproduction studies and no adequate studies in humans.*) In humans, all NSAIDs are assigned to category *D* for use during pregnancy during the third trimester or near delivery (*There is evidence of human fetal risk, but the potential benefits from the use of the drug in pregnant women may be acceptable despite its potential risks.*)

Most NSAIDs are excreted in milk. Ketorolac was detected in human breast milk at a maximum milk:plasma ratio of 0.037. It is unlikely to pose great risk to nursing offspring.

Overdosage/Acute Toxicity

Limited information is available. Cats have developed renal toxicity at doses as low as 0.7 mg/kg. The oral LD_{50} is 200 mg/kg in mice. GI effects, including GI ulceration are likely in overdoses in small animals. Metabolic acidosis was reported in one human patient. Consider GI emptying in large overdoses; patients should be monitored for GI bleeding. Treat ulcers with sucralfate; consider giving misoprostol early.

Drug Interactions

The following drug interactions have either been reported or are theoretical in humans or animals receiving ketorolac and may be of significance in veterinary patients. Unless otherwise noted, use together is not necessarily contraindicated, but weigh the potential risks and perform additional monitoring when appropriate.

- **ACE INHIBITORS:** Increased risk for nephrotoxicity.
- **ALPRAZOLAM:** Hallucinations reported in some human patients taking with ketorolac.
- **AMINOGLYCOSIDES (gentamicin, amikacin, etc.):** Increased risk for nephrotoxicity.
- **ANTICOAGULANTS (heparin, LMWH, warfarin):** Increased risk for bleeding possible.
- **ASPIRIN:** Increased likelihood of GI adverse effects (blood loss).
- **BISPHOSPHONATES (alendronate, etc.):** May increase risk for GI ulceration.
- **CORTICOSTEROIDS:** Concomitant administration with NSAIDs may significantly increase the risks for GI adverse effects.
- **CYCLOSPORINE:** May increase risk for nephrotoxicity.
- **FLUCONAZOLE:** May increase NSAID levels.
- **FLUOXETINE:** Hallucinations reported in some human patients taking with ketorolac.

- **FUROSEMIDE:** Ketorolac may reduce the saluretic and diuretic effects of furosemide.
- **METHOTREXATE:** Serious toxicity has occurred when NSAIDs have been used concomitantly with methotrexate; use together with extreme caution.
- **MUSCLE RELAXANTS, NONDEPOLARIZING:** Ketorolac may potentiate effects.
- **PROBENECID:** May cause a significant increase in serum levels and half-life of ketorolac.

Doses

- **DOGS:**

  As a post-operative analgesic (extra-label): In the study, ketorolac at 0.5 mg/kg IV bolus after intubation and 20 minutes prior surgery. Based upon the drug's apparent pharmacokinetic profile and pain scores following surgery, analgesic activity was maintained until 6-7 hours after administration (≈4-5 hours after surgery completion). Readministration 6 hours after the first dose may maintain a higher analgesic efficacy. Because ketorolac had limited efficacy during the intraoperative period, consider use only post-operatively. A repeated dosage study would better clarify efficacy, kinetics, and dosage regimens. (Cagnardi *et al.* 2013)

- **RABBITS/RODENTS/SMALL MAMMALS:**

  As an analgesic (extra-label): Mice: 0.7 – 10 mg/kg PO once daily. **Rats:** 3 – 5 mg/kg PO 1-2 times a day; 1 mg/kg IM 1-2 times a day. (Huerkamp 2000)

Monitoring

- Analgesic/antiinflammatory efficacy.
- GI: appetite, feces (occult blood, diarrhea).

Client Information

- Human NSAID that can be used for the short-term treatment of pain in dogs or small mammals.
- Give oral doses with food.
- Gastrointestinal (*e.g.,* vomiting, ulcers, bleeding, etc.) are highly possible if used for more than a few days. Liver, kidney and blood problems can also occur.
- Notify veterinarian if signs of GI distress (lack of appetite, vomiting, diarrhea, black feces, or blood in stool) occur, or if the animal becomes depressed.

Chemistry/Synonyms

A carboxylic acid derivative nonsteroidal antiinflammatory (NSAID), ketorolac tromethamine occurs as an off-white crystalline powder with a pKa of 3.54 (in water). More than 500 mg are soluble in one mL of water at room temperature. The commercially available injection is a clear, slightly yellow solution with a pH of 6.9-7.9. Sodium chloride is added to make the solution isotonic.

Ketorolac tromethamine may also be known as RS-37619-00-31-3; many trade names are available.

Storage/Stability

Both the tablets and injection should be stored at room temperature and protected from light. Protect the tablets from excessive humidity. The injection is stable for at least 48 hours in commonly used IV solutions.

Compatibility/Compounding Considerations

Do not mix with other drugs in the same syringe.

Dosage Forms/Regulatory Status

VETERINARY-LABELED PRODUCTS: NONE.

The ARCI (Racing Commissioners International) has designated this drug as a class 3 substance. See the appendix for more information.

Ketorolac Tromethamine Tablets: 10 mg; generic; (Rx)

Ketorolac Tromethamine Injection: 15 mg/mL & 30 mg/mL in 1 mL, 2 mL single-dose vials, & 10 mL multiple-dose vials; generic; (Rx)

A topical ophthalmic preparation is also available; see the ophthalmology section in the appendix for further information.

Revisions/References

Monograph revised/updated March 2014.

Cagnardi, P., et al. (2013). Pharmacokinetics and perioperative efficacy of intravenous ketorolac in dogs. J. Vet. Pharmacol. Ther. **36**(6): 603-8.

Huerkamp, M. (2000). The use of analgesics in rodents and rabbits. Emory University, Division of Animal Resources.

L-Theanine

(el thee-ah-neen)   Suntheanine®, Anxitane®, Composure®

Nutritional Anxiolytic Agent

Prescriber Highlights

▶ Used as a calming (anxiolytic) agent in dogs and cats. Very limited evidence documenting efficacy. Nutraceutical; not an approved drug.

▶ Appears to be tolerated well.

Uses/Indications

L-theanine is a nutritional supplement that is used as an anxiolytic for dogs and cats. There is very limited published data that documents efficacy in animals. A study in 5 beagles with anxiety towards humans showed greater human interaction and approach than the placebo control group (Araujo *et al.* 2010). Another open-label pilot study concluded that L-theanine improved anxiety-related emotional disorders in cats (Dramard *et al.* 2007).

For human use, *Natural Standard* (Anon 2013) has assigned the following grades (A-F scale) of scientific evidence for common/studied uses for L-theanine: Anxiety=C, Blood pressure control=C, Mood=C, Cognition=D.

Pharmacology/Actions

L-theanine is thought to increase serotonin, dopamine, and gamma-aminobutyric acid (GABA) levels in the CNS. Rat studies have found that theanine significantly lowered levels of 5-hydroxyindole in the brain and that it may inhibit glutamic acid excitotoxicity (Anon 2013).

Pharmacokinetics

Only pharmacokinetic data for lab animals was located. The L-form of theanine is preferentially absorbed from the intestine with peak levels occurring approximately 1-2 hours post-dose. In rats, it is hydrolyzed by phosphate-independent glutaminase in kidneys to glutamic acid and ethylamine. No drug is detectable after 24 hours.

Contraindications/Precautions/Warnings

L-theanine is contraindicated in patients hypersensitive to it. A veterinary-labeled product (*Anxitane*®) warns: "Not intended for use in animals with severe phobias, separation anxiety or in animals with a known history of aggression."

Do not confuse L-THEAnine with L-THREOnine.

Adverse Effects

L-theanine is relatively safe and adverse effects are not frequently reported in animals or humans. Some human patients taking L-theanine have reported headaches, reduced blood pressure, or alterations in cognition.

Reproductive/Nursing Safety

No specific information was noted, while likely safe, use with caution during pregnancy or nursing.

Overdosage/Acute Toxicity

Limited information is available, but it is likely relatively non-toxic. A 13-week study in rats determined no-observed-adverse-effect-level (NOAEL) of 4000 mg/kg/day, the highest dose tested (Borzelleca *et al.* 2006). Products containing L-theanine may contain other ingredients that may have toxic potential.

Drug Interactions

The following drug interactions have either been reported or are theoretical in humans or animals receiving L-theanine and may be of significance in veterinary patients. Unless otherwise noted, use together is not necessarily contraindicated, but weigh the potential risks and perform additional monitoring when appropriate.

▪ **ANTIHYPERTENSIVE AGENTS:** L-theanine potentially can reduce blood pressure and cause additive effects.

▪ **D-THEANINE; D,L-THEANINE:** Can reduce the absorption of L-theanine.

Doses

▪ **DOGS/CATS:**

As an anxiolytic agent (Not FDA-approved):

a) For cats and dogs weighing less than 10 kg = 25 mg; dogs 10-25 kg = 50 mg; dogs>25 kg = 100 mg. Give PO q12h and 2 hours before anxiety-producing event and every 6 hours during the event. Use in conjunction with concurrent behavior therapy. (Adapted from label—*Anxitane*®)

b) For dogs or cats weighing up to 25 lbs. (11.4 kg) – one mini chew (10.5 mg of L-theanine); 25-50 lbs. – one chew (21 mg of L-theanine); 50-100 lbs. – two chews (42 mg of L-theanine); over 100 lbs. – three chews (63 mg of L-theanine). Give PO once daily. During times of increased stress, it is safe to double or triple the above amount, as needed. (Adapted from label –*Composure*®)

Monitoring

▪ Efficacy.

Client Information

▪ Follow label directions or give as your veterinarian has recommended.

▪ Shake liquid well before use.

Chemistry/Synonyms

Theanine is a nonprotein amino acid found primarily in tea leaves. Younger and fresher tea leaves tend to be richer in caffeine, while older, drier leaves may have higher theanine levels. The L-form is used in nutritional supplements, as it appears to be better absorbed from the gut. Standardized methods of determining L-theanine have not been established.

L-theanine may also be known as glutamylethylamide, or L-N-ethylglutamine. *Suntheanine*® is common trade name.

Storage/Stability

Store bulk powder, tablets or capsules at room temperature away from moisture. Keep chewable tablets away from children or animals. The *Anxitane*® label states to keep tablets in original blister pack until used.

Compatibility/Compounding Considerations

No information noted.

Dosage Forms/Regulatory Status

VETERINARY-LABELED PRODUCTS:

The following are considered nutritionals by the FDA and are not approved drugs. Other products containing l-theanine may be marketed for use in dogs and cats.

L-theanine Tablets (chewable): 50 mg & 100 mg; *Anxitane*® S (50 mg) and *M&L* (100 mg); (OTC)

L-theanine Tablets (chewable): 10.5 mg (with thiamine 67 mg & colostrum calming complex 11 mg) & 21 mg (with thiamine 134 mg & colostrum calming complex 22 mg); *Composure®* (*Mini*; 10.5 mg) & (regular; 21 mg) *Bite-sized Chews*; (OTC)

Liquid: L-theanine 21 mg/2.5 mL (with thiamine 134 mg/2.5 mL & colostrum calming complex 22 mg/2.5 mL); *Composure® Max Liquid*; (OTC)

HUMAN-LABELED PRODUCTS:

No FDA-approved products noted. Nutritional supplements as bulk powder or capsules containing 100 mg, 150 mg or 200 mg of L-theanine are available. *Suntheanine®* is a common trade name.

Revisions/References

Monograph written March 2014.

Anon (2013). *Theanine (L-theanine) [Monograph]*, Natural Standard Professional Database; Foods, Herbs & Supplements. Somerville, MA.

Araujo, J. A., et al. (2010). ANXITANE (R) tablets reduce fear of human beings in a Laboratory model of anxiety-related behavior. Journal of Veterinary Behavior-Clinical Applications and Research 5(5): 268-75.

Borzelleca, J. F., et al. (2006). A 13-week dietary toxicity and toxicokinetic study with L-theanine in rats. Food and Chemical Toxicology 44(7): 1158-66.

Dramard, V., et al. (2007). Clinical efficacy of L-theanine tablets to reduce anxiety-related emotional disorders in cats: A pilot open-label clinical trial. J Vet Behav 2(3): 85-6.

L-Asparaginase – see Asparaginase

L-Thyroxine – see Levothyroxine Sodium

Lactated Ringer's – see the appendix section on intravenous fluids

---

Lactulose

(lak-tyoo-lose)   Cephulac®

Disaccharide Laxative/Ammonia Reducer

Prescriber Highlights

▶ Disaccharide laxative & reducer of blood ammonia levels.

▶ Adverse Effects: Flatulence, gastric distention, cramping, etc.; diarrhea & dehydration are signs of overdosage.

▶ Cats dislike the taste of lactulose liquid & administration may be difficult; lactulose crystals (*Kristalose®*) mixed into cat food may be more accepted.

▶ May alter insulin requirements in diabetics.

Uses/Indications

The primary use of lactulose in veterinary medicine is to reduce ammonia blood levels in the prevention and treatment of hepatic encephalopathy (portal-systemic encephalopathy; PSE) in small animals, pet birds and potentially, horses. It is also used as a laxative in small animals.

Pharmacology/Actions

Lactulose is a disaccharide (galactose/fructose) that is not hydrolyzable by mammalian and, probably, avian gut enzymes. Upon reaching the colon, lactulose is metabolized by the resident bacteria resulting in the formation of low molecular weight acids (lactic, formic, acetic) and CO_2. These acids have a dual effect; they increase osmotic pressure drawing water into the bowel causing a laxative effect and also acidify colonic contents. The acidification causes ammonia NH_3 (ammonia) to migrate from the blood into the colon where it is trapped as $[NH_4]^+$ (ammonium ion) and expelled with the feces.

Pharmacokinetics

In humans, less than 3% of an oral dose of lactulose in absorbed (in the small intestine). The absorbed drug is not metabolized and excreted unchanged in the urine within 24 hours.

Contraindications/Precautions/Warnings

Lactulose syrup contains some free lactose and galactose, and may alter the insulin requirements in diabetic patients. In patients with preexisting fluid and electrolyte imbalances, lactulose may exacerbate these conditions if it causes diarrhea; use cautiously.

Adverse Effects

Signs of flatulence, gastric distention, cramping, etc. are not uncommon early in therapy, but generally abate with time. Diarrhea and dehydration are signs of overdosage; dosage should be reduced.

Cats dislike the taste of lactulose syrup and administration may be difficult. Lactulose granules (crystals) have been more successfully administered after mixing into food.

Reproductive/Nursing Safety

In humans, the FDA categorizes this drug as category *B* for use during pregnancy (*Animal studies have not yet demonstrated risk to the fetus, but there are no adequate studies in pregnant women; or animal studies have shown an adverse effect, but adequate studies in pregnant women have not demonstrated a risk to the fetus in the first trimester of pregnancy, and there is no evidence of risk in later trimesters.*)

It is not known whether lactulose is excreted in milk, but it would be unexpected.

Overdosage/Acute Toxicity

Excessive doses may cause flatulence, diarrhea, cramping, and dehydration. Replace fluids and electrolytes if necessary.

Drug Interactions

The following drug interactions have either been reported or are theoretical in humans or animals receiving lactulose and may be of significance in veterinary patients. Unless otherwise noted, use together is not necessarily contraindicated, but weigh the potential risks and perform additional monitoring when appropriate.

■ **ANTACIDS, ORAL**: Antacids (non-absorbable) may reduce the colonic acidification effects (efficacy) of lactulose.

■ **LAXATIVES, OTHER**: Do not use lactulose with other laxatives as the loose stools that are formed can be falsely attributed to the lactulose with resultant inadequate therapy for hepatic encephalopathy.

■ **NEOMYCIN, GENTAMICIN (ORAL)**: Theoretically, orally administered antibiotics could eliminate the bacteria responsible for metabolizing lactulose, thereby reducing its efficacy. However, some data suggests that synergy may occur when lactulose is used with an oral antibiotic for the treatment of hepatic encephalopathy; enhanced monitoring of lactulose efficacy is probably warranted in cases if an oral antibiotic is added to the therapy.

Doses

■ **DOGS:**

Note: If using the crystals for oral solution: one gram of the crystals is equivalent to 1.5 mL of the liquid.

For hepatic encephalopathy (extra-label): <u>Orally</u>: 0.25 – 0.5 mL/kg PO q6-8h until stools are loose. <u>Enema</u>: Make a solution of 3 parts lactulose and 7 parts warm water and give 1 – 10 mL/kg as a retention enema for 20-30 minutes. Measure post-enema fluid and repeat if pH > 6. (McCord *et al.* 2011) **Note:** The PO dose could also be employed as a laxative.

■ **CATS:**

Note: If using the crystals for oral solution: one gram of the crystals is equivalent to 1.5 mL of the liquid.

For hepatic encephalopathy (extra-label): <u>Orally</u>: 0.25 – 0.5 mL/kg PO q6-8h until stools are loose. <u>Enema</u>: Make a solution of 3 parts lactulose and 7 parts warm water and give 1 – 10 mL/kg as a retention enema for 20-30 minutes. Measure post-enema fluid and repeat if pH > 6. (McCord *et al.* 2011)

For constipation (extra-label): Liquid: 0.5 mL/kg (usually 2-3 mLs per cat) PO 2-3 times daily. Crystals: ½ – ¾ teaspoonful (2.5 – 3.75 mL) twice daily mixed with food is commonly recommended. Dosages are adjusted to obtain the stool quality desired. For acute, severe constipation can also be administered as an enema as for hepatic encephalopathy.

- **BIRDS:**

  For hepatic encephalopathy; to stimulate appetite, improve intestinal flora (extra-label): **Cockatiel:** 0.03 mL PO 2-3 times a day; **Amazon:** 0.1 mL PO 2-3 times a day. Reduce dosage if diarrhea develops. May be used for weeks. (Clubb 1986)

- **REPTILES:**

  As a laxative (extra-label): **Green Iguana:** 0.3 mL/kg PO q12h. (Wilson 2002)

Monitoring

- Clinical efficacy (2-3 soft stools per day) when used for PSE.
- In long-term use (months) or in patients with preexisting fluid/electrolyte problems, serum electrolytes should be monitored.

Client Information

- Most commonly used to reduce ammonia levels in small animals and birds. Also used to treat constipation.
- Lactulose is generally well tolerated, especially after using a while. Contact your veterinarian if your animal develops diarrhea.
- When lactulose is used for hepatic encephalopathy, contact veterinarian if signs worsen or less than 2-3 soft stools are produced per day.

Chemistry/Synonyms

A synthetic derivative of lactose, lactulose is a disaccharide containing one molecule of galactose and one molecule of fructose. It occurs as a white powder that is very slightly soluble in alcohol and very soluble in water. The commercially available solutions are viscous, sweet liquids with an adjusted pH of 3-7.

One gram of the lactulose crystals for oral solution (*Kristalose®*) is equivalent to 1.5 mL of the liquid.

Lactulose may also be known as lactulosum; many trade names are available including *Cephulac®*.

Storage/Stability

Lactulose syrup should be stored in tight containers, preferably at room temperature; avoid freezing. If exposed to heat or light, darkening or cloudiness of the solution may occur, but apparently this does not affect drug potency.

Compatibility/Compounding Considerations

For use as an enema, the human approved products recommended mixing 300 mL lactulose solution with 700 mL water or physiologic saline.

Dosage Forms/Regulatory Status

VETERINARY-LABELED PRODUCTS: NONE.

HUMAN-LABELED PRODUCTS:

Lactulose Solution: 1 gram/1.5 mL (labeled as 10 grams/15 mL or 20 grams/30 mL); (<1.6 grams galactose, <1.2 grams lactose and ≤1.2 grams of other sugars); *Generlac®*, *Constulose®* and *Enulose®*, generic; (Rx)

Lactulose Crystals for Oral Solution: Lactulose (<0.3 grams galactose and lactose/10 g) in 10 grams and 20 gram packets; *Kristalose®*; (Rx)

Revisions/References

Monograph revised/updated March 2014.

Clubb, S. L. (1986). Therapeutics: Individual and Flock Treatment Regimens. *Clinical Avian Medicine and Surgery*. G. J. Harrison and L. R. Harrison. Philadelphia, W.B. Saunders: 327-55.

McCord, K. W. & C. B. Webb (2011). Hepatic Dysfunction. Veterinary Clinics of North America-Small Animal Practice 41(4): 745-+.

Wilson, H. (2002). Disease management of the Green Iguana. Proceedings: Atlantic Coast Veterinary Conference. accessed via Veterinary Information Network; vin.com

Lanthanum Carbonate

(lan-tha-num)   Fosrenol®, Lantharenol®

Oral Phosphate Binding Agent

Prescriber Highlights

- ▶ Orally administered phosphate binder; products labeled for use in cats in some countries.
- ▶ Limited experience and relatively little published in veterinary literature.
- ▶ Appears safe; vomiting nausea/inappetence possible.

Uses/Indications

Lanthanum carbonate is potentially useful as an orally administered phosphate binding agent for patients with chronic renal disease. While phosphorous dietary restrictions are the mainstay of controlling hyperphosphatemia in small animals, binding agents such as aluminum, sevelamer, or lanthanum can be considered for use in patients whose phosphate levels are not controlled with diet alone or that will not consume very-low phosphorous diets. Lanthanum has a potential advantage over calcium or aluminum containing phosphate binders in that it does not appear to be absorbed, even at high dosages or with continued use, though palatability can be an issue.

Pharmacology/Actions

Lanthanum carbonate's mechanism of action to reduce hyperphosphatemia is by dissociating in the acid environment of the upper GI tract to release lanthanum ions. These ions bind to dietary phosphate and form highly insoluble lanthanum phosphate complexes that are then eliminated in the feces.

Pharmacokinetics

Following oral doses, lanthanum bioavailability is very low (less than 0.002%). In humans, systemically available lanthanum is very highly bound to plasma proteins (>99%). Studies in dogs, mice, and rats have shown that lanthanum levels in tissues increase over time and can be several orders of magnitude higher than that found in the plasma. Highest tissue levels are found in the GI tract, bone, and liver. In rats, absorbed lanthanum is cleared primarily via biliary excretion into the feces. In dogs, mean recovery of an oral dose of lanthanum averages 94%.

Contraindications/Precautions/Warnings

There are no listed contraindications for lanthanum carbonate, but it should be used with caution in patients where the GI tract is not intact (*e.g.*, GI ulcers, colitis, etc.) as there is an increased chance for oral absorption.

Adverse Effects

Limited information is available for dogs and cats but it appears that lanthanum is well tolerated. Vomiting has been reported in some cats and food avoidance can occur when lanthanum carbonate is mixed into food.

Healthy cats given 1 g/kg PO over 3 months did not show any bone histological changes (Nunamaker *et al.* 2012).

In humans, adverse effects most commonly reported include nausea and vomiting. These are generally self-limiting and usually abate with continued use.

Reproductive/Nursing Safety

It is likely that lanthanum is safe to use during pregnancy. For humans, the FDA has placed it in category *C* for use during pregnancy (*Animal studies have shown an adverse effect on the fetus, but there are no adequate studies in humans; or there are no animal reproduction studies and no adequate studies in humans. However, there does not appear to be a significant risk to offspring.*)

Lanthanum should be safe to use in nursing dams.

Overdosage/Acute Toxicity

No specific information was located. It is likely that an acute overdose would be tolerated, with the chance that it might cause GI effects. Only supportive treatment should be required. In a poster presentation of a dose escalation study in cats, cats tolerated oral dosages up to 1 gram/kg, but vomited repeatedly after receiving 2 grams/kg (Schmidt *et al.* 2009).

Drug Interactions

Drug interactions with lanthanum carbonate have not been reported, but as it is a binding agent similar to aluminum, it seems prudent to separate by at least 2 hours dosing lanthanum and the following:

- **ALLOPURINOL**
- **CHLOROQUINE**
- **CORTICOSTEROIDS**
- **DIGOXIN**
- **ETHAMBUTOL**
- **FLUOROQUINOLONES**
- **H-2 ANTAGONISTS** (Ranitidine, Famotidine, etc.)
- **IRON SALTS**
- **ISONIAZID**
- **PENICILLAMINE**
- **PHENOTHIAZINES**
- **TETRACYCLINES**
- **THYROID HORMONES**

Laboratory Considerations

- No specific concerns.

Doses

- **CATS:**

    As a phosphate binder (extra-label in USA): **Note:** dosages are "to effect".

    a) Initially, 30 mg/kg/day PO divided 2-3 times a day and on or in food. A common dose is 200 mg PO twice daily.

    b) Using the proprietary product *Renalzin*®: The standard recommended dosage is 2 mLs (400 mg) applied in the cat's food, once or twice daily depending on the cat's feeding regimen. (*Renalzin*®—Bayer-UK)

Monitoring

- Serum phosphorous (and other electrolytes such as potassium, calcium, bicarbonate, chloride).

Client Information

- Used to bind up phosphorous found in food and prevent it from being absorbed.
- Mix into or sprinkle on top of food. If using tablets, crush them before mixing into food.
- Sometimes can cause vomiting.

Chemistry/Synonyms

Lanthanum is a chemical element with the symbol La and atomic number 57. When used pharmacologically, it is administered as lanthanum carbonate. Lanthanum carbonate may also be known as: Bay-78-1887, and by the trade names *Lantharenol*®, *Renalzin*®, and *Fosrenol*®.

Storage/Stability

Store tablets at room temperature (25°C, 77°F); excursions are permitted to 15°-30°C (59°-86°F). Protect from moisture.

Compatibility/Compounding Considerations

No specific information noted.

Dosage Forms/Regulatory Status

VETERINARY-LABELED PRODUCTS: NONE IN USA.

A lanthanum carbonate (octa-hydrate), kaolin, and vitamin E labeled product (*Renalzin*®) for use in cats is available in several countries (not USA). It does not appear to be a licensed product, but is a food additive/supplement in those countries. Confirmed concentrations of the ingredients were not found, but it has been reported that 1 mL contains 200 mg of lanthanum carbonate. Available as a pump gel/paste in 50 mL and 150 mL pump containers; *Renalzin*®.

HUMAN-LABELED PRODUCTS:

Lanthanum Carbonate Oral Chewable Tablet: 500 mg, 750 mg, & 1,000 mg; *Fosrenol*®; (Rx)

Revisions/References

Monograph revised/updated March 2014.

Nunamaker, E. A. & J. G. Sherman (2012). Oral administration of lanthanum dioxycarbonate does not alter bone morphology of normal cats. J. Vet. Pharmacol. Ther. 35(2): 193-7.

Schmidt, B. H. & U. Spiecker-Hauser (2009). Overdose acceptance and tolerance of Lantharenol (R) in adult healthy cats. J. Vet. Pharmacol. Ther. 32: 129-.

Laxatives, Hyperosmotic — See Lactulose; Saline Cathartics; PEG 3350; & Sorbitol

Laxatives, Stimulant — See Bisacodyl

Leflunomide

(le-floo-noh-myde)   Arava®

Immunomodulating Agent

Prescriber Highlights

▶ Immunomodulating drug that in small animal medicine can be useful as immune suppressant particularly in patients that are refractory to treatment with conventional medications or when glucocorticoids are contraindicated.

▶ Appears well-tolerated by dogs and cats, but numbers treated are low.

▶ Teratogenic (Category X).

▶ Active metabolite can persist in body for years.

▶ Treatment expense may be an issue.

Uses/Indications

Leflunomide is an immunomodulating drug that in small animal medicine can be useful as immune suppressant for treating a variety of immune-related conditions, particularly in patients that are refractory to treatment with conventional medications or when glucocorticoids are contraindicated. Conditions where it may be useful include IMHA, systemic and cutaneous reactive histiocytosis, immune-mediated polyarthritis (Colopy *et al.* 2010), Evans syndrome (Bianco *et al.* 2009), granulomatous meningoencephalitis, etc. and as part of transplant rejection protocols in dogs. Leflunomide has been used with methotrexate to treat rheumatoid arthritis in cats.

Pharmacology/Actions

Leflunomide inhibits autoimmune T-cell proliferation and autoantibody production by B cells. Leflunomide acts almost exclusively via its active metabolite teriflunomide (A77 1726; M1). This metabolite reversibly inhibits the mitochondrial enzyme dihydroorotate dehydrogenase thereby preventing the formation of ribonucleotide uridine monophosphate (rUMP). This causes decreased DNA and

RNA synthesis, inhibition of cell proliferation, and G1 cell cycle arrest.

Pharmacokinetics

In healthy dogs (n=4) after a single oral dosage of 4 mg/kg, the following mean values for teriflunomide (A77 1726) were reported: time to peak level (Tmax)=5 hrs.; peak level (Cmax)= 5 mcg/mL; elimination half-life (t1/2)=21.3 hours; mean residence time (MRT)=27 hours. It is not understood why the apparent half-life for dogs is so much shorter (approx. 1 day) than it is for humans (15 days) (Singer *et al.* 2011).

In healthy cats (n=6) after single IV dosages of 4 mg/kg of teriflunomide (A77 1726) the following mean values for teriflunomide were reported: volume of distribution (Vd$_{ss}$)= 97 mL/kg); clearance=1.1 mL/kg/hr; elimination half-life (t1/2)= 58 hrs. Oral dosages of leflunomide at 4 mg/kg had 100% bioavailability, peak levels of teriflunomide occurred ≈8 hours after dosing, and elimination half-life was similar (59 hrs.) to IV values (Mehl *et al.* 2012).

In humans, leflunomide is rapidly converted to the active metabolite teriflunomide (A77 1726; M1) in the GI mucosa and liver. Peak levels of A77 1726 occur between 6-12 hours after an oral dose. The presence of food in the gut does not appear to affect oral bioavailability. Teriflunomide is highly bound to albumin (>99%). It is further degraded in the liver as glucuronides and an oxalinic acid compound that are excreted in the urine and bile. Half-life is ≈15 days, but teriflunomide (A77 1726) can be detectable in patients up to 2 years after it is discontinued.

Contraindications/Precautions/Warnings

Leflunomide is contraindicated during pregnancy and in patients hypersensitive to it. It should be used with extreme caution in patients with immunodeficiency and in patients with significant renal impairment.

Adverse Effects

Leflunomide appears to be well tolerated by dogs, particularly when administered at dosages of ≤ 4 mg/kg PO per day. Adverse effects reported include decreased appetite, lethargy, vomiting, lymphopenia, thrombocytopenia, hypercholesterolemia, and anemia.

In humans, gastrointestinal effects (diarrhea, nausea), alopecia and rash are most commonly reported. Serious adverse effects that have been reported include hematologic toxicity, dermatologic effects (TEN, Stevens-Johnson, etc.), and hepatotoxicity.

Reproductive/Nursing Safety

Leflunomide should not be used during pregnancy. A variety of teratogenic effects in laboratory animals have been detailed at doses used clinically. In humans, the FDA categorizes this drug as category *X* for use during pregnancy (*Studies in animals or humans demonstrate fetal abnormalities or adverse reaction; reports indicate evidence of fetal risk. The risk of use in pregnant women clearly outweighs any possible benefit.*)

It is not known whether leflunomide is excreted in milk; it is suggested to use milk replacer if the dam is receiving the drug.

Overdosage/Acute Toxicity

Acute toxicologic studies in mice and rats have demonstrated that the minimally toxic dose is 200 mg/kg and 100 mg/kg, respectively. Cholestyramine or activated charcoal are recommended to accelerate elimination. Contact an animal poison control center for more information.

Drug Interactions

The following drug interactions have either been reported or are theoretical in humans or animals receiving leflunomide and may be of significance in veterinary patients. Unless otherwise noted, use together is not necessarily contraindicated, but weigh the potential risks and perform additional monitoring when appropriate.

- **CHARCOAL, ACTIVATED:** Can increase elimination and decrease teriflunomide (A77 1726) drug concentrations; may be used when more rapid elimination is desirable.
- **CHOLESTYRAMINE:** Can increase elimination and decrease teriflunomide (A77 1726) drug concentrations; may be used when more rapid elimination is desirable.
- **HEPATOTOXIC AGENTS, OTHER:** Increased risk for toxicity.
- **METHOTREXATE:** Increased adverse effects and ALT possible.
- **PHENYTOIN:** Leflunomide can increase phenytoin levels.
- **RIFAMPIN:** Can increase teriflunomide (A77 1726) peak levels.
- **VACCINES, LIVE VIRUS:** Live virus vaccines should be used with caution, if at all, during leflunomide therapy.
- **WARFARIN:** Leflunomide may increase INR.

Doses

- **DOGS:**

  As an immunosuppressive (extra-label): Most recommendations for initial dosages range from 3 – 4 mg/kg PO once daily (q24h). Some recommend monitoring blood levels in 4-6 weeks (see Monitoring) and adjust dosage based upon trough level, clinical signs and adverse effects. Depending on the reason for use (condition) and response to treatment, dosage reduction (or increased time between dosages) can be considered in time. A dosage (from a case report) for treatment of Evans' Syndrome in a diabetic dog is: In combination with human intravenous immunoglobulin (hIVIG), leflunomide was initiated at a dosage of 2 mg/kg PO q12h (based on the nontoxic dosage of 4 mg/kg per day used in studies of the canine renal transplantation model). Leflunomide dosage was decreased by 25% every 4 weeks for the first 4 months in order to achieve a trough level of approximately 20 micrograms/mL (leflunomide trough levels were based on studies of the canine renal transplantation model); then the dosage was decreased every 8 weeks until discontinuation after 10 months of therapy. (Bianco *et al.* 2009)

- **CATS:**

  As an immunosuppressive (extra-label): Based upon limited PK/PD information (Mehl *et al.* 2012) an initial dosage of 2 – 3 mg/kg (practical dosage 10 mg per cat) PO once daily is reasonable. Some recommend monitoring blood levels in 4-6 weeks (see Monitoring) and adjusting dosage based upon trough level, clinical signs and adverse effects. Depending on the reason for use (condition) and response to treatment, dosage reduction (or increased time between dosages) can be considered in time. An anecdotal dosage for treating rheumatoid arthritis with methotrexate is: Initially, leflunomide at 10 mg (total dose) PO once daily and methotrexate at 2.5 mg (total dose) PO three times on one day per week. When significant improvement occurs, reduce doses of leflunomide to 10 mg PO twice weekly and methotrexate to 2.5 mg PO once weekly. (Bennett 2005)

Monitoring

- Clinical efficacy.
- Adverse effects (CBC, liver enzymes).
- Trough levels of teriflunomide (A771 1726) may be considered; 20 micrograms/mL is the target for human patients; it is not known if this applies to veterinary patients.

Client Information

- May be given either with food or on an empty stomach. Give with food if animal vomits or acts "sick" after getting a dose.
- Side effects can include decreased appetite, lethargy (tiredness), vomiting, and problems with blood cells.

- Contact your veterinarian right away if you see bleeding or signs of infection (e.g., fever, extreme tiredness, etc.). Pregnant women must use caution when handling; can cause birth defects.

Chemistry/Synonyms

Leflunomide is an isoxasole immunomodulator with a melting point of 165-166°C. It is poorly soluble in water (21 mg/L).

Leflunomide may also be known as HWA 486, RS 34821, or SU 101; a common trade name is *Arava*®.

Storage/Stability

Leflunomide tablets should be stored at room temperature (15-30°C) and protected from light.

Compatibility/Compounding Considerations

No specific information noted.

Dosage Forms/Regulatory Status

VETERINARY-LABELED PRODUCTS: NONE.

HUMAN-LABELED PRODUCTS:

Leflunomide Tablets: 10 mg & 20 mg; *Arava*®, generic; (Rx)

Revisions/References

Monograph revised/updated March 2014.

Bennett, D. (2005). Immune-mediated and infective arthritis. *Textbook of Veterinary Internal Medicine, 6th Ed.* S. Ettinger and E. Feldman, Elsevier: 1958-65.

Bianco, D. & R. M. Hardy (2009). Treatment of Evans' Syndrome With Human Intravenous Immunoglobulin and Leflunomide in a Diabetic Dog. J. Am. Anim. Hosp. Assoc. 45(3): 147-50.

Colopy, S. A., et al. (2010). Efficacy of leflunomide for treatment of immune-mediated polyarthritis in dogs: 14 cases (2006-2008). Javma-Journal of the American Veterinary Medical Association 236(3): 312-8.

Mehl, M. L., et al. (2012). Pharmacokinetics and pharmacodynamics of A77 1726 and leflunomide in domestic cats. J. Vet. Pharmacol. Ther. 35(2): 139-46.

Singer, L. M., et al. (2011). Leflunomide pharmacokinetics after single oral administration to dogs. J. Vet. Pharmacol. Ther. 34(6): 609-11.

Leucovorin Calcium

(loo-koe-vor-in)   Folinic Acid, Citrovorum Factor, Calcium Folinate

Oral or Injectable Folic Acid Derivative

Prescriber Highlights

▶ Primarily used in veterinary medicine to help reverse neurotoxicity or hematologic toxicity associated with dihydrofolate reductase inhibitors (*e.g.*, pyrimethamine, trimethoprim, or ormetoprim).

▶ Leucovorin does not require conversion by dihydrofolate reductase for it to be active.

Uses/Indications

Leucovorin calcium is the calcium salt of folinic acid and is used as an antidote for toxicity from folic acid antagonists (*e.g.*, methotrexate, pyrimethamine, trimethoprim, ormetoprim). It is used routinely in human medicine as a rescue agent for high-dose methotrexate chemotherapy, but the drug is rarely used for this in veterinary medicine. More commonly, it is used in dogs, cats or horses to help reverse or prevent hematologic toxicity associated with pyrimethamine, trimethoprim, or ormetoprim.

Pharmacology/Actions

Reduced folates act as coenzymes in the synthesis of purine and pyrimidine nucleotides that are necessary for DNA synthesis. Folates are also required for maintenance of normal erythropoiesis.

Leucovorin is a reduced form of folic acid that does not require dihydrofolate reductase conversion, as does folic acid, for it to become biologically active. It is further converted to active reduced forms, of which 5-methyltetrahdyrofolate (5-methyl THF) is predominantly responsible for its activity. Although, leucovorin is a mixture of diastereoisomers, only the (-)-L-isomer (citrovorum factor) becomes biologically active.

Leucovorin inhibits thymidylate synthase by stabilizing the binding of fluorodeoxyuredylic acid to the enzyme. This can potentiate the activity, but also the toxicity of fluorouracil (5-FU).

Pharmacokinetics

There is limited information available on the pharmacokinetics of leucovorin in animals. In dogs, the elimination half-life of the L-isomer (active) of leucovorin is ≈50 minutes. It is extensively metabolized and then excreted into the urine. The D-form (not biologically active) elimination half-life is ≈2.5 hours. Apparent volume of distribution for both forms is ≈0.6 L/kg.

In humans, oral bioavailability of leucovorin is reduced as dosage is increased above 25 mg. A 25 mg dose in an adult has a bioavailability of 97%, while 50 mg and 100 mg doses have bioavailabilities of 75% and 37%, respectively. IM bioavailability is similar to IV. Oral doses of 25 mg yield peak levels of leucovorin in ≈60 minutes and peaks of the active reduced folates occur between 1.7-2.4 hours after dosing. After intravenous administration, peak total reduced folate levels occur in ≈10 minutes. About 50% of oral body stores of reduced folates are found in the liver. Elimination occurs in the urine, primarily as 10-formyl-THF or 5,10-methyl-THF. Elimination half-life is approximately 5-6 hours for total reduced folates.

Contraindications/Precautions/Warnings

Leucovorin is contraindicated only when known intolerance to the drug is documented. In humans, cobalamin (B-12) levels may be reduced with megaloblastic anemias and folinic acid therapy may mask the signs associated with it.

Use with extreme caution in patients receiving systemic fluorouracil (see Drug Interactions).

Because of its calcium content, large intravenous doses should be given slowly and not bolused.

Do not confuse leucovorin with *Leukeran*®, foLINIC acid with foLIC acid, or foLINATE with foLATE.

Reproductive/Nursing Safety

Leucovorin reproductive studies have not been performed nor is it known if it enters milk, however, it is likely safe to administer during pregnancy or nursing.

Adverse Effects

Adverse effects have not been noted when leucovorin has been used in animals. In humans, gastrointestinal effects can be seen when the drug is given orally and, very rarely, seizures or hypersensitivity reactions may occur.

Overdosage/Acute Toxicity

Except in situations where drug interactions are possible, an inadvertent overdose is unlikely to be of concern.

Drug Interactions

The following drug interactions have either been reported or are theoretical in humans or animals receiving leucovorin and may be of significance in veterinary patients. Unless otherwise noted, use together is not necessarily contraindicated, but weigh the potential risks and perform additional monitoring when appropriate.

- **BARBITURATES, PRIMIDONE, PHENYTOIN:** Large doses of leucovorin may reduce the antiseizure efficacy of these agents.
- **FLUOROURACIL:** Leucovorin may increase both the antineoplastic efficacy and toxicity of 5-FU.
- **TRIMETHOPRIM, ORMETOPRIM, PYRIMETHAMINE** (drugs that inhibit dihydrofolate reductase): Leucovorin may reduce efficacy somewhat, however, protozoa cannot utilize leucovorin.

Laboratory Considerations

- No specific concerns were noted.

Doses

- **DOGS/CATS:**

   For folate deficiency/bone marrow depression associated with pyrimethamine, trimethoprim, ormetoprim, etc. (extra-label): Little is published to define dosages for animals. Extrapolating from human dosages, a dosage of 0.1 – 0.3 mg/kg PO once daily could be considered. A practical dosage would be to round up to the nearest ½ tablet of a commercial dosage form (5 mg, 10 mg, 15 mg, 25 mg tablets).

   For methotrexate overdoses (extra-label):

   a) Most effective if given within 48 hours of overdose. The dose of leucovorin is dependent on the serum methotrexate concentration. Dogs with serum methotrexate levels $>10^{-7}$ M at 48 hours have toxic reactions. Leucovorin dosage ranges from 25 – 200 mg/m² parenterally every 6 hours until methotrexate levels are less than 1×10^{-8} M. In one study, dogs tolerated methotrexate dosages up to 3 grams/m² when leucovorin was given at 15 mg/m² IV q 3 hours for 8 doses, then IM q6h hours for 8 doses. Higher doses of methotrexate may be tolerated if higher doses of leucovorin are given. (O'Keefe *et al.* 1990)

   b) From a report of two cases (dogs); MTX assay was not available. Following GI decontamination (apomorphine; charcoal/sorbitol times 3 over 6 hours), leucovorin calcium was given at 200 mg/m² IV q6h for 8 doses. Forced alkaline diuresis, and N-acetylcysteine (IV) were also administered. (Lewis *et al.* 2010)

- **HORSES:**

   For macrocytic anemia and neutropenia associated with pyrimethamine and/or trimethoprim (especially in pregnant mares); (extra-label): 0.1 – 0.3 mg/kg PO once daily. A more practical approach would be to ensure that the horse receives green hay or pasture (high tetrahydrofolate levels in green roughage). (Divers 2002)

Monitoring

- CBC.
- Methotrexate serum levels (contact a local human hospital) if used for methotrexate overdoses.

Client Information

- If being used for methotrexate toxicity, this medication should only be administered in an inpatient setting.
- Oral leucovorin may be administered with or without meals.
- When used to treat or prevent hematologic (bone marrow) toxicity, it is very important to not skip or miss doses.

Chemistry/Synonyms

Leucovorin calcium occurs as a yellowish-white or yellow, odorless powder. It is very soluble in water and practically insoluble in alcohol. It is a mixture of diastereoisomers of 5-formyl tetrahydrofolic acid.

Leucovorin calcium may also be known as: folinic acid, citrovorum factor, 5-formyl tetrahydrofolate, citrovorin, folidan, folinic, FTHF, NSC-3590, calcium folinate, calcifolin, calfonat, or folinic acid calcium salt; many international trade names are available.

Storage/Stability

Leucovorin calcium tablets should be stored below 40°C, preferably between 15-30°C in a well-closed container; protect from light.

Leucovorin solution for injection should be stored refrigerated between 2°-8°C; protect from light.

Leucovorin Powder for reconstitution and injection should be stored below 40°C, preferably between 15-30°C; protect from light.

Compatibility/Compounding Considerations

The powder for injection is reconstituted by adding 5 or 10 mL of bacteriostatic water for injection or sterile water for injection. As bacteriostatic water for injection contains benzyl alcohol, it is not recommended in neonates or very small animals. If reconstituting with sterile water for injection, the resulting solution should be administered immediately; solutions made with bacteriostatic water for injection are stable up to 7 days.

Intravenous solutions containing leucovorin calcium are stable up to 24 hours at room temperature in Ringer's lactate, Ringer's, or 0.9% sodium chloride. Leucovorin calcium is **not compatible** with solutions containing fluorouracil.

Dosage Forms/Regulatory Status

VETERINARY-LABELED PRODUCTS: NONE.

HUMAN-LABELED PRODUCTS:

Note: Strengths listed are in terms of leucovorin base.

Leucovorin Calcium Oral Tablets: 5 mg, 10 mg, 15 mg, & 25 mg; generic; (Rx)

Leucovorin Calcium Injection Solution: 10 mg/mL in vials; generic; (Rx)

Leucovorin Calcium Powder for Injection: 50 mg, 100 mg, 200 mg & 350 mg in vials; generic; (Rx)

Revisions/References

Monograph revised/updated March 2014.

Divers, T. (2002). Management and treatment of equine protozoal myeloencephalitis (EPM). Proceedings: ACVIM 2002. accessed via Veterinary Information Network; vin.com

Lewis, D. H., et al. (2010). Use of calcium folinate in the management of accidental methotrexate ingestion in two dogs. Javma-Journal of the American Veterinary Medical Association 237(12): 1450-4.

O'Keefe, D. A. & C. L. Harris (1990). Toxicology of Oncologic Drugs. Vet Clinics of North America: Small Animal Pract 20(2): 483-504.

Leuprolide

(loo-proe-lide)   Lupron®

GnRH-analog Agonist

Prescriber Highlights

▶ For medical treatment of adrenal associated endocrinopathy in ferrets, & to suppress gonadal activity in birds.

▶ Depot form must not be confused with once a day injectable; doses below are for depot. Effects generally are shorter in ferrets and birds than human-label states for 3-6 month products.

▶ Teratogenic, contraindicated in pregnancy.

▶ Extremely costly (especially for ferrets); may be obtained in smaller aliquots from compounding pharmacies.

▶ Lab interactions/considerations.

Uses/Indications

The primary uses for leuprolide at present are for the medical treatment of adrenal associated endocrinopathy in ferrets. Vulvular swelling, pruritus, dysuria, and aggression can be reduced/diminished within days to weeks, while regrowth of hair can take 1-2 months (Chen *et al.* 2014). Leuprolide may be more effective earlier in the disease-process than later, and treating ferrets with adrenal hyperplasia or adenomas rather than adenocarcinoma.

In captive birds leuprolide the 30-day depot injection can suppress gonadal activity for 2-3 weeks (Mans *et al.* 2014). It has also been used to treat malignant ovarian neoplasias in birds.

In dogs and cats, leuprolide has been used experimentally to induce estrus and treat hormone-responsive incontinence.

Pharmacology/Actions

Leuprolide is a luteinizing hormone-releasing hormone agonist. Via negative feedback, leuprolide inhibits the release of luteinizing hormone and follicle stimulating hormone from the pituitary. Both estrogen and androgen levels are decreased in the serum.

Pharmacokinetics

No veterinary data was located. The depot forms appear to have sustained effects in birds and ferrets. Duration of effect in ferrets varies but when using the 30-day formulation, clinical effects can persist from 1.5-8 months (Chen *et al.* 2014). In birds when using the 30-day formulation, the duration of effect may last up to 3 weeks.

Contraindications/Precautions/Warnings

Contraindicated in pregnancy.

Adverse Effects

In ferrets, adverse effects reported include pain/irritation at injection site, dyspnea, and lethargy. Tachyphylaxis (higher dosages required over time to obtain same effect) has been reported.

Little information is available on the adverse effect profile of leuprolide birds. At this point, it appears safe at the recommended doses. There is a case report of a suspected anaphylactic reaction/ death in 2 elf owls (*Micrathene whitneyi*).

Reproductive/Nursing Safety

Leuprolide is considered contraindicated in pregnancy. Major fetal abnormalities may result. In humans, the FDA categorizes this drug as category *X* for use during pregnancy (*Studies in animals or humans demonstrate fetal abnormalities or adverse reaction; reports indicate evidence of fetal risk. The risk of use in pregnant women clearly outweighs any possible benefit.*)

It is not known whether leuprolide is excreted in milk; use with caution.

Overdosage/Acute Toxicity

Because of its expense and method of dosing, it is unlikely an acute overdose would occur. Studies in lab animals at dosages of up to 5 grams/kg IM produced no untoward effects.

Drug Interactions

No documented adverse drug interactions with leuprolide were located.

Laboratory Considerations

- Diagnostic tests measuring **pituitary gonadotrophic** and **gonadal functions** may be misleading during, and for several months after discontinuing therapy.

Doses

- **FERRETS:**

  For treatment of adrenal associated endocrinopathy (extra-label): Dosages are for the 30-day depot formulation and vary by the source. No published evidence currently supports one dosage over another. Initially, 100 – 200 micrograms per ferret (some say 100 micrograms in females or those under 1 kg and 200 micrograms in males or those >1kg) IM q4-6 weeks. All patients may require 200 micrograms in time and some become refractory to treatment at any dosage. Adapted from: (Chen *et al.* 2014), (Johnson-Delaney 2009)

- **BIRDS:**

  As a GnRH-agonist (extra-label): The 1-month product is used most frequently in avian medicine; duration of effect in birds is generally less than 4 weeks. A wide-range of dosages have been reported for birds, ranging from 100 micrograms/kg to 1.2 mg/kg. For palliative treatment of ovarian neoplasias in cockatiels or macro-orchidism, very high dosages (1.5 – 3.5 mg/kg) have been recommended by some. However, most prefer dosages between 400 and 1000 micrograms/kg IM

repeated every 2-3 weeks. Adapted from: (Hernandez-Divers 2009; Nernetz 2009; Mans *et al.* 2014)

Monitoring

- Clinical effects (Birds: decreased egg-laying; Ferrets: decreases in vulvar swelling, pruritus, undesirable sexual behaviors, aggression, and increased hair regrowth).

Client Information

- Leuprolide is a treatment and will not cure adrenal diseases in ferrets. Life-long treatment is necessary.
- Can be very expensive.

Chemistry/Synonyms

A synthetic nonapeptide analog of GnRH (gonadotropin releasing hormone, gonadorelin, luteinizing hormone-releasing hormone), leuprolide acetate occurs as a white to off-white powder. In water more than 250 mg are soluble in 1 mL.

Leuprolide may also be known as: leuprorelin, leuprorelinum, abbott-43818, leuprolide acetate, TAP-144, *Carcinil®, Daronda®, Eligard®, Elityran®, Enanton®, Enantone®, Enantone-Gyn®, Ginecrin®, Lectrum®, Leuplin®, Lucrin®, Lupride®, Lupron®, Procren®, Procrin®, Prostap®, Reliser®, Trenantone®, Uno-Enantone®,* and *Viadur®.*

Storage/Stability

The injection should be stored below room temperature (<78°F); do not freeze and protect from light (store in carton until use). The depot form may be stored at room temperature. After reconstituting the suspension is stable for 24 hours, but as it contains no preservative it is recommended for immediate use.

Compatibility/Compounding Considerations

The issue whether the solution containing microspheres (depot forms) can be frozen for later use is somewhat controversial as some have frozen the solution and state that it is still effective. However, the manufacturer states that the depot form is not to be frozen as the microspheres are destroyed and no studies are known that support the stability of the depot activity when frozen and thawed. Some compounding pharmacies may divide the lyophilized powder into individual dosages in vials. If it is decided to freeze the solution, most recommend putting individual aliquots into tuberculin syringes before freezing; do not re-freeze once thawed.

Dosage Forms/Regulatory Status

VETERINARY-LABELED PRODUCTS: NONE.

HUMAN-LABELED PRODUCTS:

Leuprolide Acetate Injection: 1 mg/0.2 mL; generic; (Rx)

Leuprolide Acetate Injection Kits for SC Use: 7.5 mg (regular—30 day), 22.5 mg (3 month), 30 mg (4 month), & 60 mg (6 month); *Eligard®*; (Rx)

Leuprolide Acetate Microspheres for Injection (kits): 3.75 mg, 7.5 mg, 11.25 mg (regular—30 day & 3 month), 15 mg, 22.5 mg (3 month), 30 mg (4 month), & 60 mg (6 month); *Lupron® Depot* and *Lupron® Depot-Ped* and *Lupron® Depot-3, -4,* or *-6 Month*; (Rx)

Revisions/References

Monograph revised/updated March 2014.

Chen, S., et al. (2014). Nonsurgical Management of Hyperadrenocorticism in Ferrets. Vet Clin Exot Anim 17: 35-49.

Hernandez-Divers, S. (2009). Avian reproductive medicine and surgery. Proceedings: AAZV. accessed via Veterinary Information Network; vin.com

Johnson-Delaney, C. (2009). Endocrine System and Diseases of Exotic Companion Mammals. Proceedings: ABVP. accessed via Veterinary Information Network; vin.com

Mans, C. & A. Pilny (2014). Use of GnRH-agonists for Medical Management of Reproductive Disorders in Birds. Vet Clin Exot Anim 17: 23-33.

Nernetz, L. (2009). Management of Macroorchidism Using Leuprolide Acetate. Proceedings: AAV. accessed via Veterinary Information Network; vin.com

Levamisole

(leh-vam-i-sole)   Levasole®, Tramisol®

Antiparasitic, Immune Stimulant

Prescriber Highlights

▶ Antinematodal parasiticide that also may be useful as an immune stimulant; infrequently used today.

▶ Contraindications: Milk-producing animals (not approved).

▶ Very cautiously, if at all: Severely debilitated, or significant renal or hepatic impairment; in cattle that are stressed due to vaccination, dehorning, or castration.

▶ Numerous adverse effects.

Uses/Indications

Levamisole use today as an antiparasitic agent veterinary medicine is limited. While there are still several products approved for use in various species, many of them are not commercially marketed ostensibly due to increased resistance and the potential for adverse effects. Depending on the product licensed, levamisole is indicated for the treatment of many nematodes in cattle, sheep and goats, swine, poultry. In sheep and cattle, levamisole has relatively good activity against abomasal nematodes, small intestinal nematodes (not particularly good against *Strongyloides* spp.), large intestinal nematodes (not *Trichuris* spp.), and lungworms. Adult forms of species that are usually covered by levamisole, include: *Haemonchus* spp., *Trichostrongylus* spp., *Osteragia* spp., *Cooperia* spp., *Nematodirus* spp., *Bunostomum* spp., *Oesophagostomum* spp., *Chabertia* spp., and *Dictyocaulus vivapurus*. Levamisole is less effective against the immature forms of these parasites, and generally ineffective in cattle (but not sheep) against arrested larval forms.

In swine, levamisole is indicated for the treatment of *Ascaris suum*, *Oesophagostomum* spp., Strongyloides, Stephanurus, and Metastrongylus.

In horses with equine protozoal myeloencephalitis, levamisole may be useful for the control of clinical signs secondary to inflammation after treatment with antiprotozoal therapy.

Levamisole has been used in dogs as a microfilaricide to treat *Dirofilaria immitis* infection in the past, but is rarely used today. It has also garnered some interest as an immunostimulant in the adjunctive therapy of various neoplasms or in combination with steroids for treating systemic lupus erythematosus (SLE).

Because of its narrow margin for safety and limited efficacy against many equine parasites, levamisole is not generally used in horses as an antiparasitic agent. It has been tried as an immune stimulant, however.

Pharmacology/Actions

Levamisole stimulates the parasympathetic and sympathetic ganglia in susceptible worms. At higher levels, levamisole interferes with nematode carbohydrate metabolism by blocking fumarate reduction and succinate oxidation. The net effect is a paralyzing effect on the worm that is then expelled alive. Levamisole's effects are considered to be nicotine-like in action.

Levamisole's mechanism of action for its immunostimulating effects are not well understood. It is believed it restores cell-mediated immune function in peripheral T-lymphocytes and stimulates phagocytosis by monocytes. Its immune stimulating effects appear to be more pronounced in animals that are immune-compromised.

Pharmacokinetics

Levamisole is absorbed from the gut after oral dosing and through the skin after dermal application, although bioavailabilities are variable. It is reportedly distributed throughout the body. Levamisole is primarily metabolized with less than 6% excreted unchanged in the urine. Plasma elimination half-lives have been determined for several veterinary species: Cattle, 4-6 hours; Dogs, 1.8-4 hours; and Swine, 3.5-6.8 hours. Metabolites are excreted in both the urine (primarily) and feces.

Contraindications/Precautions/Warnings

Levamisole is contraindicated in lactating animals (not approved). It should be used cautiously, if at all, in animals that are severely debilitated, or significant renal or hepatic impairment.

Use cautiously or, preferably, delay use in cattle that are stressed due to vaccination, dehorning, or castration.

Levamisole use in goats is somewhat controversial as there is evidence it is toxic in fiber-producing goats. Oral routes are preferred; IM administration is contraindicated, but some have administered it SC.

Levamisole is not indicated for use as a dirofilarial adulticide.

Avoid if possible, administering levamisole intramuscularly to birds.

One reference states that levamisole is contraindicated in cats with FIV or FIP and likely ineffective in cats with FeLV (Hartmann 2009).

Adverse Effects

Adverse effects that may be seen in cattle can include muzzle foaming or hypersalivation, excitement or trembling, lip-licking and head shaking. These effects are generally noted with higher than recommended doses or if levamisole is used concomitantly with organophosphates. Signs generally subside within 2 hours. When injecting into cattle, swelling may occur at the injection site. This will usually abate in 7-14 days, but may be objectionable in animals that are close to slaughter.

In sheep, levamisole may cause a transient excitability in some animals after dosing. In goats, levamisole may cause depression, hyperesthesia, and salivation. Injecting levamisole SC in goats apparently causes a stinging sensation.

In swine, levamisole may cause salivation or muzzle foaming. Swine infected with lungworms may develop coughing or vomiting.

Adverse effects that may be seen in dogs include GI disturbances (usually vomiting, diarrhea), neurotoxicity (panting, shaking, agitation or other behavioral changes), immune-mediated anemia, agranulocytosis, dyspnea, pulmonary edema, immune-mediated skin eruptions (erythroedema, erythema multiforme, toxic epidermal necrolysis), and lethargy.

Adverse effects seen in cats include hypersalivation, excitement, mydriasis, and vomiting.

Reproductive/Nursing Safety

There is little information available regarding the safety of this drug in pregnant animals. Levamisole has been implicated in causing abortion in goats. Although levamisole is considered relatively safe to use in large animals that are pregnant, use only if the potential benefits outweigh the risks. In humans, the FDA categorizes this drug as category **C** for use during pregnancy (*Animal studies have shown an adverse effect on the fetus, but there are no adequate studies in humans; or there are no animal reproduction studies and no adequate studies in humans.*) In a separate system evaluating the safety of drugs in canine and feline pregnancy (Papich 1989), this drug is categorized class: **C** (*These drugs may have potential risks. Studies in people or laboratory animals have uncovered risks, and these drugs should be used cautiously as a last resort when the benefit of therapy clearly outweighs the risks.*)

Levamisole is excreted in cows' milk; use with caution in nursing dams.

Overdosage/Toxicity

Signs of levamisole toxicity often mimic those of organophosphate toxicity. Signs may include hypersalivation, hyperesthesias and irritability, clonic seizures, CNS depression, dyspnea, defecation, urination, and collapse. These effects are best treated by supportive means as animals generally recover within hours of dosing. Acute levamisole overdosage can result in death due to respiratory failure. Should respiratory failure occur, artificial ventilation with oxygen should be instituted until recovery occurs. Cardiac arrhythmias may also be seen. If the ingestion was oral, emptying the gut and/or administering charcoal with cathartics may be indicated.

Levamisole is considered to be more dangerous when administered parenterally than when given orally or topically. Intravenous administration is particularly hazardous, and is never recommended.

In pet birds (cockatoos, budgerigars, Mynah birds, parrots, etc.), 40 mg/kg has been reported as a toxic dose when administered SC. IM injections may cause more severe toxicity. Depression, ataxia, leg and wing paralysis, mydriasis, regurgitation, and death may be seen after a toxic dose in birds.

Drug Interactions

The following drug interactions have either been reported or are theoretical in humans or animals receiving levamisole and may be of significance in veterinary patients. Unless otherwise noted, use together is not necessarily contraindicated, but weigh the potential risks and perform additional monitoring when appropriate.

- **ASPIRIN:** Levamisole may increase salicylate levels.
- **CHLORAMPHENICOL:** Fatalities have been reported after concomitant levamisole and chloramphenicol administration; avoid using these agents together.
- **CHOLINESTERASE-INHIBITING DRUGS** (*e.g.,* **organophosphates, neostigmine**): Could theoretically enhance the toxic effects of levamisole; use together with caution.
- **NICOTINE-LIKE COMPOUNDS** (*e.g.,* **pyrantel, morantel, diethylcarbamazine**): Could theoretically enhance the toxic effects of levamisole; use together with caution.
- **WARFARIN:** Increased risk for bleeding.

Doses

- **DOGS:**

  As adjunctive therapy for SLE (extra-label): Give 0.5 – 1 mg/kg prednisone PO q12h with levamisole at 2 – 5 mg/kg (maximum of 150 mg per dog) PO q48h (every other day). Taper prednisone dosage over 1-2 months. Continue levamisole for 4 months or longer if a relapse occurs. (Johnson *et al.* 2012)

- **HORSES:**

  As adjunctive treatment for EPM (extra-label):

  a) Dosages have ranged from 2.5 mg/kg injected at 7 day intervals, and 2.2 mg/kg PO every 24 hours for 3 days, then off for 4 days for a period of 4-6 weeks. Anecdotal reports of beneficial effects in the treatment of nasal viral papillomas, COPD, and EPM have been suggested. (Bentz 2006)

  b) 1 – 2 mg/kg per day PO. (MacKay 2008)

- **CATTLE:**

  Note: Note for dairy animals of breeding age.

  For treatment of susceptible nematodes (refer to specific label directions for FDA-approved products); (FDA-approved): Slaughter withdrawal = 48 hours.

  a) **Using the 46.8 g/packet powder**: As a standard oral drench: Place the contents of each packet in a 1-quart (960 mL; 32 fl. oz.) container, fill with water; swirl until dissolved. Administer as a single drench dose of 15 mL (1/2 fl. oz.) per 200 lbs. body weight. As a concentrated drench solution using a 20 mL automatic syringe: Place the contents of each packet in a standard household measuring container and add water to the 8 & ¾ fl. oz. (260 mL) level. Swirl until dissolved. Give 2 mL (milliliter) per 100 lbs. body weight.

  b) **Using the 544.5 g bottle:** When ready to use, add water to the powder in the bottle up to the 3-liter mark. Swirl to mix thoroughly before using. If any solution is left over, it may be stored for up to 3 months in this tightly capped bottle, shake well before using. Administer as single drench dose of 2 mL per 100 lbs. body weight.

- **SHEEP:**

  For treatment of susceptible nematodes (refer to specific label directions for FDA-approved products); (FDA-approved): Slaughter withdrawal = 72 hours.

  a) **Using the 46.8 g/packet powder:** As a standard oral drench. Place the contents of each packet in a 1-gallon (12 fl. oz.) container, fill with water; swirl until dissolved. Administer as a single drench dose of 15 mL (1/2 fl. oz.) per 50 lbs. body weight. As a concentrated drench solution using a 20 mL automatic syringe. Place the contents of each packet in a standard household measuring container and add water to the 17 & ½ fl. oz. (520 mL) level. Swirl until dissolved. Give 2 mL (milliliter) per 50 lbs. body weight.

  b) **Using the 544.5 g bottle:** When ready to use, add water to the powder in the bottle up to the 3-liter mark. Swirl to mix thoroughly before using. If any solution is left over, it may be stored for up to 3 months in this tightly capped bottle, shake well before using. Administer as single drench dose of 1 mL per 50 lbs. body weight.

- **GOATS:**

  As an anthelmintic (extra-label): Use is somewhat controversial. One source recommends using 1.5X the sheep dosage. Avoid injectable products, but if the injection is the only dosage form available, give SC (not IM). (Hoste *et al.* 2011)

- **REPTILES:**

  As an anthelmintic (extra-label): Nematodes: 5 – 10 mg/kg PO; repeat in 2 weeks followed by a fecal exam 14 days after the 2nd dose. If positive, a 3rd dose is given. Acanthocephalans, or Pentastomes: as above, but may also be given SC or ICe. (de la Navarre 2003)

Monitoring

- Clinical efficacy.
- Adverse effects/toxicity observation.

Client Information

- Follow directions on the product label unless otherwise directed by veterinarian.
- When given orally (by mouth), giving with food may help prevent vomiting in dogs. Do not administer injectable products IV.
- Most common side effects seen in small animals: vomiting, dilated/big pupils, diarrhea, drooling, & lethargy (lack of energy).
- Serious side effects can occur, including bone marrow toxicity, skin rashes, central nervous system effects, etc. See adverse effects for more information. Report serious adverse effects to veterinarian.
- Can be very toxic when overdosed; follow dosages carefully.
- Avoid skin contact with liquid forms as the drug can be absorbed through skin.
- Levamisole is not FDA-approved for use in dairy animals of breeding age.

Chemistry/Synonyms

The levo-isomer of dl-tetramisole, levamisole has a greater safety margin than does the racemic mixture. It is available commercially in two salts, a phosphate and a hydrochloride. Levamisole hydrochloride occurs as a white to pale cream colored, odorless or nearly odorless, crystalline powder. One gram is soluble in 2 mL of water.

Levamisole HCl may also be known as: cloridrato de levamizol, ICI-59623, levamisoli hydrochloridum, NSC-177023, R-12564, RP-20605, l-tetramisole hydrochloride, *Amtech®*, *Ascaridil®*, *Decaris®*, *Ergamisol®*, *Immunol®*, *Ketrax®*, *Levasole®;*, *Meglum®*, *Prohibit®*, *Solaskil®*, *Vermisol®*, and *Vizole®*.

Storage/Stability

Levamisole hydrochloride products should be stored at room temperature (15-30°C), unless otherwise instructed by the manufacturer; avoid temperatures >40°C. Levamisole phosphate injection should be stored at temperatures at or below 21°C (70°F); refrigeration is recommended and freezing should be avoided.

Compatibility/Compounding Considerations

Compounded preparation stability: Levamisole oral solution compounded from the commercially available tablets and active pharmaceutical ingredient powder has been published (Chiadmi *et al.* 2005). Triturating 2500 mg (2.5 grams) of levamisole hydrochloride powder with 100 mL sterile water yields a 25 mg/mL levamisole hydrochloride oral solution that retains >97% potency for 90 days when stored at both 4°C and 25°C and protected from light.

Dosage Forms/Regulatory Status

In cattle, sheep, and swine a level of 0.1 ppm has been established for negligible residues in edible tissues.

VETERINARY-LABELED PRODUCTS:

Note: FDA's "Green book" still lists many approved levamisole products, but most are no longer marketed. At the time of writing (March 2014), the following product was apparently still available.

Levamisole Hydrochloride Soluble Drench Powder 46.8 grams/packet; 544.5 grams/21.34 oz bottle. *Prohibit®* (OTC). FDA-approved for use in cattle and sheep. Slaughter withdrawal (at labeled dosages) cattle = 48 hours, sheep = 72 hours. To prevent residues in milk, do not administer to dairy animals of breeding age.

HUMAN-LABELED PRODUCTS: NONE.

Revisions/References

Monograph revised/updated March 2014.

Bentz, B. (2006). Antiviral therapies in the horse. Proceedings: ABVP. accessed via Veterinary Information Network; vin.com
Chiadmi, F., et al. (2005). Stability of levamisole oral solutions prepared from tablets and powder. J Pharm Pharm Sci 8(2): 322-5.
de la Navarre, B. (2003). Common parasitic diseases of reptiles and amphibians. Proceedings: Western Veterinary Conf. accessed via Veterinary Information Network; vin.com
Hartmann, K. (2009). Immunomodulators in Veterinary Medicine--Is There Evidence of Efficacy? Proceedings: ACVIM. accessed via Veterinary Information Network; vin.com
Hoste, H., et al. (2011). Control of Endoparasitic Nematode Infections in Goats. Veterinary Clinics of North America-Food Animal Practice 27(1): 163-+.
Johnson, K. C. & A. Mackin (2012). Canine Immune-Mediated Polyarthritis PART 2: DIAGNOSIS AND TREATMENT. J. Am. Anim. Hosp. Assoc. 48(2): 71-82.
MacKay, R. (2008). Equine Protozoal Myeloencephalitis: Managing Relapses. Comp Equine(Jan/Feb): 24-7.
Papich, M. (1989). Effects of drugs on pregnancy. *Current Veterinary Therapy X: Small Animal Practice*. R. Kirk. Philadelphia, Saunders: 1291-9.

Levarterenol — See Norepinephrine

Levetiracetam

(lee-ve-tye-ra-se-tam)   Keppra®

Anticonvulsant

Prescriber Highlights

► A "broad spectrum" anticonvulsant, levetiracetem may be useful as a 3rd drug adjunct for refractory canine epilepsy or when either phenobarbital or bromides are not tolerated. Dogs may become refractory to therapy with time.

► In cats, probably a 2nd-line drug when phenobarbital alone does not control seizures, but can be tried as sole therapy when phenobarbital is not tolerated.

► Appears to be well tolerated; adverse effects (may be transient) include sedation in dogs, and lethargy and decreased appetite in cats.

► Phenobarbital may cause significant drug interaction with levetiracetam in dogs.

► Dosage frequency (three times daily) problematic.

► Cost has been an issue, but costs decreasing with availability of generics.

Uses/Indications

Levetiracetam has been shown to be useful for treating status epilepticus (SE) and acute repetitive seizures (ARS; cluster seizures) in dogs in a small, double-masked, placebo controlled study (Hardy *et al.* 2012). Additionally, IV levetiracetem was used successfully to treat refractory seizures in a dog that ingested a lethal dose of fluorouracil (5-FU) (Friedenberg *et al.* 2013). SC dosing at home may be useful for those dogs that develop SE or ARS that do not always respond sufficiently to diazepam (per rectum and/or intranasal). For refractory epilepsy it can be useful as an add-on drug for dogs that are not well controlled with, or cannot tolerate phenobarbital and bromide. Some evidence suggests that in dogs suffering from phenobarbital liver toxicity, the addition of levetiracetam will allow reduction of their phenobarbital dosage without increasing seizure frequency (Munana *et al.* 2012). Recent reports in dogs of reduced efficacy with time ("honeymoon effect") and that phenobarbital can significantly affect levetiracetam pharmacokinetics in dogs are concerning.

Levetiracetam may also be useful as add-on therapy in cats when phenobarbital does not control seizures or alone in cats that are unable to tolerate phenobarbital.

Preliminary data in horses has demonstrated that it may be efficacious when given orally (Cesar *et al.* 2013).

Pharmacology/Actions

The exact mechanism for levetiracetam's antiseizure activity is not well understood. It appears to affect the release of neurotransmitters by selective binding to the presynaptic protein SVA2 and may selectively prevent hypersynchronization of epileptiform burst-firing and propagation of seizure activity. It does not affect normal neuronal excitability.

Pharmacokinetics

In dogs, levetiracetam (regular tablet) is well absorbed after oral dosing and peak levels occur in ≈2 hours. Levetiracetam elimination half-life is ≈2-6 hours and volume of distribution is ≈0.9 L/kg. Repeated dosages (over 7 days) do not appreciably alter pharmacokinetic values (Moore, S.A. *et al.* 2010), but concurrent administration of phenobarbital significantly increased levetiracetam clearance, reduced half-life and peak levels (Moore, S.A. *et al.* 2011). The pharmacokinetics of the extended-release tablets (*Keppra XR®*) have been evaluated in dogs, but at the time of writing (2013) only abstracts/proceedings were available. In fed dogs, bioavailability was higher than when receiving regular tablets, but elimination half-life with the extended-release tablets was similar to regular tablets. Data suggest that a q12h dosing schedule should maintain therapeutic levels and in some dogs q24h may be acceptable (Platt *et al.* 2011; Beasely *et al.* 2012).

In cats, oral bioavailability of levetiracetem is high and elimination half-life is around 3 hours. The authors concluded that 20 mg/kg administered IV or orally every 8 hours should be adequate for most cats (Carnes *et al.* 2011).

In horses, oral bioavailability is high for both regular and extended-release tablets. However, the extended-release tablets were crushed which may have affected its pharmacokinetic profile. Elimination half-life was approximately 17 hours (regular tablets). The authors concluded that oral administration of 30 mg/kg of either the regular or extended-release tablets in healthy adult horses is likely to achieve therapeutic concentrations for at least 18 hours (Cesar *et al.* 2013).

In humans, levetiracetam is rapidly, and nearly completely, absorbed after oral administration. Peak levels occur ≈60 minutes after dosing. Presence of food in the gut delays the rate but not the extent of drug absorbed and it can be administered without regard to feeding status. Less than 10% of the drug is bound to plasma proteins. While not extensively metabolized, the drug's acetamide group is enzymatically hydrolyzed to the carboxylic acid metabolite that is apparently not active. Hepatic CYP P450 isoenzymes are not involved. Half-life in humans is ≈7 hours; ≈66% of a given dose is excreted unchanged via renal mechanisms, primarily glomerular filtration and active tubular secretion. Clearance can be significantly reduced in patients with impaired renal function.

Contraindications/Precautions/Warnings

Levetiracetam is contraindicated in patients who have previously exhibited hypersensitivity to it or any of its components. It should be used with caution in patients with renal impairment; dosage amounts or dosing frequency changes should be considered. In humans, renal elimination of levetiracetam correlates with creatinine clearance.

In dogs, it is unknown if all extended-release tablets are bioequivalent. Anecdotally it has been reported that generic extended-release tablets may not fully disintegrate in the canine GI tract.

Do not confuse levETIRAcetam with levOCARNitine or levO-FLOXacin.

Adverse Effects

Levetiracetam appears to be very well tolerated in dogs and cats. Most common adverse effects reported include sedation and ataxia in dogs and reduced appetite, hypersalivation, and lethargy in cats. These effects may be transient. Changes in behavior, and gastrointestinal effects could occur.

In humans, it is recommended to withdraw the drug slowly to prevent "withdrawal" seizures.

Reproductive/Nursing Safety

In pregnant dogs or cats, levetiracetam should be used with caution. In humans, the FDA categorizes levetiracetam as a category *C* drug for use during pregnancy (*Animal studies have shown an adverse effect on the fetus, but there are no adequate studies in humans; or there are no animal reproduction studies and no adequate studies in humans*). At high dosages, levetiracetam has caused increased embryofetal mortality in rabbits and rats. At dosages equivalent to the maximum human therapeutic dose, levetiracetam caused minor skeletal abnormalities and retarded offspring growth in rats.

Levetiracetam is excreted into maternal milk and its safety in nursing offspring is unknown. Use with caution in nursing patients.

Overdosage/Acute Toxicity

Levetiracetam is a relatively safe agent. Dogs given 1200 mg/kg/day (approximately 20X therapeutic dosage) developed only salivation and vomiting. Human patients given 6000 mg/kg during drug testing developed only drowsiness. Other effects noted in human overdoses (doses not specified) after the drug was released include depressed levels of consciousness, agitation, aggression and respiratory depression.

There were 114 single agent exposures to levetiracetam reported to the ASPCA Animal Poison Control Center (APCC) during 2009-2013. Of the 108 dogs, 13 were symptomatic with lethargy (69%), hyperthermia (15%), recumbency (15%) and vomiting (15%) being the most common clinical signs.

Treatment is basically supportive; the drug can be removed with hemodialysis. In the circumstance of a significant overdose in animals, contact an animal poison control center for further recommendations.

Drug Interactions

The following drug interactions have either been reported or are theoretical in humans or animals receiving levetiracetam and may be of significance in veterinary patients. Unless otherwise noted, use together is not necessarily contraindicated, but weigh the potential risks and perform additional monitoring when appropriate.

- **NSAIDS:** In humans, naproxen and ketorolac have been implicated with increasing the risk for seizures in patients with epilepsy. Veterinary significance is not clear.
- **PHENOBARBITAL:** In dogs, ongoing (21 days in the study) phenobarbital use significantly increased levetiracetam clearance and reduced half-life (from 3.43 hrs. without phenobarbital to 1.73 hrs. after 21 days of phenobarbital); dosage adjustments may be required. (Moore, S. *et al.* 2009)

Laboratory Considerations

- No specific laboratory interactions or considerations noted.

Doses

- **DOGS:**

  For treatment of refractory epilepsy (extra-label):
  a) <u>Using regular tablets</u>: Based on pharmacokinetic studies and presumed therapeutic levels most recommend 20 mg/kg PO q8h although recommendations up to 30 mg/kg PO q8h have been noted. Some have suggested that because of the drug's safety, dosages may be increased further until efficacy is achieved, side effects become apparent, or drug cost becomes prohibitive. If using as an add-on to phenobarbital therapy levetiracetem half-life may be shortened and dosage adjustment may be necessary.
  b) <u>Using extended-release tablets</u>: Based upon pharmacokinetic studies in dogs using *Keppra XR®*: 30 mg/kg PO q12h. Once daily dosing may be acceptable in some dogs, although monitoring is recommended to confirm. Do not split or crush. The smallest extended-release tablet is 500 mg so it cannot be practically dosed in small dogs. (Platt *et al.* 2011; Beasely *et al.* 2012)

  For status epilepticus or acute repetitive (cluster) seizures (extra-label): Doses of 30 mg/kg or 60 mg/kg IV were effective in 56% of treated dogs. While levetiracetem was safe in these patients and potentially is effective for the treatment of SE and ARS, larger, controlled clinical trials are needed (Hardy *et al.* 2012). From a single-dose pharmacokinetic study: In normal dogs, a 60 mg/kg IV bolus dose of levetiracetam is well tolerated and achieves plasma drug concentrations within or above the therapeutic range reported for humans for at least 8 hours after administration (Dewey *et al.* 2008).

For home SC administration in dogs that do not always respond sufficiently to diazepam (per rectum and/or intranasally); (extra-label): 60 mg/kg SC; based on a pilot study in healthy dogs. (Hardy *et al.* 2011)

- **CATS:**

For epilepsy (extra-label): Based on the drug's pharmacokinetics in cats and the presumed therapeutic levels for the drug, an initial dose of 20 mg/kg IV, PO q8h should be adequate for most cats. However, for some cats the trough level may be too low and doubling the dose to approximately 40 mg/kg PO q8h be necessary (Carnes *et al.* 2011). As an add-on to phenobarbital treatment: Initially, 20 mg/kg PO three times daily. Monitor as below. If ineffective, increase dose in 20 mg/kg increments (Bailey *et al.* 2008), (Bailey *et al.* 2009).

Monitoring

- The therapeutic range for animals has not been specifically determined, but it is thought that it is similar to humans, 5 – 45 micrograms/mL. Because the drug appears to be very safe, therapeutic drug monitoring is used primarily to adjust dosage (Bailey *et al.* 2009).
- Veterinarians should have the owner keep a record of seizure activity to document efficacy and report any potential levetiracetam-associated adverse effects.
- Routine CBC, basic metabolic panel every 6 months.

Client Information

- May be given with or without food. If your animal vomits or acts sick after getting it on an empty stomach, give with food or small treat to see if this helps. If vomiting continues, contact your veterinarian.
- May need to be given three times a day. It may not work if it is given less often.
- Lethargy (tiredness; lack of energy) and reduced appetite are the most likely side effects.
- Do not crush or allow your pet to chew extended-release tablets.

Chemistry/Synonyms

A pyrrolidone-derivative antiepileptic agent, levetiracetam occurs as an odorless, bitter-tasting, white to off-white crystalline powder. It is very soluble in water and soluble in ethanol. It is a chiral molecule with one asymmetric carbon atom. Levetiracetam is not related chemically to other antiseizure medications.

Levetiracetam may also be known as: S-Etriacetam, UCB-22059, UCB-L059, and *Keppra*®.

Storage/Stability

Levetiracetam tablets or oral solution should be stored at 25°C (77°F); excursions permitted to 15-30°C (59-86°F).

Compatibility/Compounding Considerations

Extended-release tablets are labeled: "Should be taken whole and not chewed, broken, or crushed."

Dosage Forms/Regulatory Status

VETERINARY-LABELED PRODUCTS: NONE.

HUMAN-LABELED PRODUCTS:

Levetiracetam Oral Tablets (film-coated, scored): 250 mg, 500 mg, 750 mg & 1000 mg; *Keppra*®, generic; (Rx)

Levetiracetam Extended-Release Oral Tablets: 500 mg & 750 mg; *Keppra XR*®, generic; (Rx). Do not crush or split.

Levetiracetam Oral Solution: 100 mg/mL in 473 mL, 480 mL & 500 mL; *Keppra*®, generic; (Rx). Also contains acesulfame K, ammonium glycyrrhizinate and maltitol.

Levetiracetam Concentrate for Injection: 100 mg/mL in 5 mL single-use vials, 5 mg/mL in 100 mL, and 10 mg/mL in 100 mL; *Keppra*®, generic; (Rx)

Revisions/References

Monograph revised/updated March 2014.

Bailey, K. S. & C. W. Dewey (2009). The Seizuring Cat: Diagnostic work-up and therapy. Journal of Feline Medicine and Surgery 11(5): 385-94.

Bailey, K. S., et al. (2008). Levetiracetam as an adjunct to phenobarbital treatment in cats with suspected idiopathic epilepsy. Javma-Journal of the American Veterinary Medical Association 232(6): 867-72.

Beasely, M. J. & D. M. Boothe (2012). The Pharmacokinetics of Single Dose Extended Release Keppra® With and Without Food in Healthy Adult Dogs. ACVIM Proceedings. accessed via Veterinary Information Network; vin.com

Carnes, M. B., et al. (2011). Pharmacokinetics of levetiracetam after oral and intravenous administration of a single dose to clinically normal cats. American Journal of Veterinary Research 72(9): 1247-52.

Cesar, F. B., et al. (2013). Disposition of levetiracetam in healthy adult horses. Journal of Veterinary Internal Medicine 27(3): 667-8.

Dewey, C. W., et al. (2008). Pharmacokinetics of single-dose intravenous levetiracetam administration in normal dogs. J. Vet. Emerg. Crit. Care 18(2): 153-7.

Friedenberg, S. G., et al. (2013). Successful treatment of a dog with massive 5-fluorouracil toxicosis. J. Vet. Emerg. Crit. Care 23(6): 643-7.

Hardy, B. T., et al. (2011). Subcutaneous administration of levetiracetam in healthy dogs. Journal of Veterinary Internal Medicine 25(3): 741-.

Hardy, B. T., et al. (2012). Double-Masked, Placebo-Controlled Study of Intravenous Levetiracetam for the Treatment of Status Epilepticus and Acute Repetitive Seizures in Dogs. Journal of Veterinary Internal Medicine 26(2): 334-40.

Moore, S., et al. (2009). The Pharmacokinetics of Levetiracetam in Dogs Concurrently Receiving Phenobarbital. Proceedings: ACVIM. accessed via Veterinary Information Network; vin.com

Moore, S. A., et al. (2010). Levetiracetam pharmacokinetics in healthy dogs following oral administration of single and multiple doses. American Journal of Veterinary Research 71(3): 337-41.

Moore, S. A., et al. (2011). The pharmacokinetics of levetiracetam in healthy dogs concurrently receiving phenobarbital. J. Vet. Pharmacol. Ther. 34(1): 31-4.

Munana, K. R., et al. (2012). Evaluation of Levetiracetam as Adjunctive Treatment for Refractory Canine Epilepsy: A Randomized, Placebo-Controlled, Crossover Trial. Journal of Veterinary Internal Medicine 26(2): 341-8.

Platt, S. R., et al. (2011). Pharmacokinetic evaluation of extended release levetiracetam in dogs. Journal of Veterinary Internal Medicine 25(3): 729-.

Levothyroxine Sodium

(lee-voe-thye-rox-een)   Soloxine®, Synthroid®

Thyroid Hormone

Prescriber Highlights

▶ Thyroid hormone for hypothyroidism in all species.

▶ Contraindications: Acute myocardial infarction, thyrotoxicosis, or untreated adrenal insufficiency.

▶ Caution: Concurrent hypoadrenocorticism (treated), cardiac disease, diabetes, or elderly patients.

▶ Adverse Effects: Only associated with OD's (tachycardia, polyphagia, PU/PD, excitability, nervousness, & excessive panting); some cats may appear apathetic.

▶ Drug-drug; drug-lab interactions.

Uses/Indications

Levothyroxine sodium is indicated for the treatment of hypothyroidism in all species. In horses, it has been used to treat equine metabolic syndrome.

Pharmacology/Actions

Thyroid hormones affect the rate of many physiologic processes including: fat, protein, and carbohydrate metabolism, increasing protein synthesis, increasing gluconeogenesis, and promoting mobilization and utilization of glycogen stores. Thyroid hormones also increase oxygen consumption, body temperature, heart rate and cardiac output, blood volume, enzyme system activity, and growth and maturity. Thyroid hormone is particularly important for adequate development of the central nervous system. While the exact mechanisms how thyroid hormones exert their effects are not fully understood, it is known that thyroid hormones (primarily triiodothyronine) act at the cellular level.

In humans, triiodothyronine (T3) is the primary hormone responsible for activity. Approximately 80% of T3 found in the peripheral tissues is derived from thyroxine (T4) which is the principle hormone released by the thyroid.

Pharmacokinetics

In dogs orally administered levothyroxine has relatively low bioavailability and short elimination half-life when compared to humans. Peak serum concentrations after oral dosing reportedly occur 4-12 hours after administration and the serum half-life is approximately 12-16 hours. However, there can be wide interpatient variability in pharmacokinetic parameters. Concerns that various tablet formulations can have substantially different bioavailability in dogs with possible resultant treatment failure have led to recommendations by some to use "brand name" products for dogs and to not change brands once the patient is stabilized. However, no recent studies were located documenting different bioavailabilities for tablets in dogs. An oral liquid formulated for dogs, (*Leventa®*) does appear to be absorbed differently than tablet formulations. It has an oral bioavailability of approximately 22% in fasted, healthy dogs. Giving with food reduced this significantly, time to peak level was increased and peak level was decreased (Le Traon *et al.* 2008). When oral levothyroxine liquid (*Leventa®*) was mixed in four various dry canine diets, no significant differences in thyroxine pharmacokinetics occurred between the groups (Iemura *et al.* 2013). When comparing oral tablets dosed at 200 mcg twice daily with the oral liquid at 200 mcg once daily, the relative bioavailability of the liquid was 206% (median) that of the tablets (Le Traon *et al.* 2008).

Contraindications/Precautions/Warnings

Levothyroxine (and other replacement thyroid hormones) are contraindicated in patients with acute myocardial infarction, thyrotoxicosis, or untreated adrenal insufficiency. It should be used with caution, and at a lower initial dosage, in patients with concurrent hypoadrenocorticism (treated), cardiac disease, diabetes mellitus, or in very elderly patients. For these patients, the recommendation for reduction in initial dosage of levothyroxine varies and ranges from 25-75% of usual. Dogs with hypoadrenocorticism should receive replacement of mineralocorticoid and glucocorticoid therapy before receiving levothyroxine as an increased basal metabolic rate may exacerbate electrolyte disturbances.

Adverse Effects

When administered at an appropriate dose to patients requiring thyroid hormone replacement, there should not be any adverse effects associated with therapy. For adverse effects associated with overdosage, see below. Case reports of rare incidences of fixed drug eruptions and erythema multiforme have been reported in dogs that were treated with levothyroxine.

Reproductive/Nursing Safety

In humans, the FDA categorizes this drug as category *A* for use during pregnancy (*Adequate studies in pregnant women have not demonstrated a risk to the fetus in the first trimester of pregnancy, and there is no evidence of risk in later trimesters.*)

Minimal amounts of thyroid hormones are excreted in milk and should not affect nursing offspring.

Overdosage/Acute Toxicity

Chronic overdosage will produce signs of hyperthyroidism, including tachycardia, polyphagia, PU/PD, excitability, nervousness and excessive panting. Dosage should be reduced and/or temporarily withheld until signs subside. Some (10%?) cats may exhibit signs of "apathetic" (listlessness, anorexia, etc.) hyperthyroidism.

A single acute overdose in small animals is less likely to cause severe thyrotoxicosis than with chronic overdosage. Vomiting, diarrhea, hyperactivity to lethargy, hypertension, tachycardia, tachypnea, dyspnea, and abnormal pupillary light reflexes may be noted in dogs and cats. In dogs, clinical signs may appear within 1-9 hours after ingestion. If ingestion occurred within 2 hours, treatment to reduce absorption of drug should be accomplished using standard protocols (emetics, cathartics, charcoal) unless contraindicated by the patient's condition. Treatment is supportive and symptomatic. Oxygen, artificial ventilation, cardiac glycosides, beta-blockers (*e.g.*, propranolol), fluids, dextrose, and antipyretic agents have all been suggested for use if necessary; contact an animal poison control center for further guidance.

Drug Interactions

The following drug interactions have either been reported or are theoretical in humans or animals receiving levothyroxine and may be of significance in veterinary patients. Unless otherwise noted, use together is not necessarily contraindicated, but weigh the potential risks and perform additional monitoring when appropriate.

- **AMIODARONE:** May decrease the metabolism of T4 to T3.
- **ANTACIDS, ORAL:** May reduce levothyroxine absorption; separate doses by 4 hours.
- **ANTIDEPRESSANTS, TRICYCLIC/TETRACYCLIC:** Increased risk for CNS stimulation and cardiac arrhythmias.
- **ANTIDIABETIC AGENTS (insulin, oral agents):** Levothyroxine may increase requirements for insulin or oral agents.
- **CHOLESTYRAMINE:** May reduce levothyroxine absorption; separate doses by 4 hours.
- **CORTICOSTEROIDS** (high dose): Decreased conversion of T4 to T3.
- **DIGOXIN:** Potential for reduced digoxin levels.
- **FERROUS SULFATE:** May reduce levothyroxine absorption; separate doses by 4 hours.
- **HIGH FIBER DIET:** May reduce levothyroxine absorption.
- **KETAMINE:** May cause tachycardia and hypertension.
- **PHENOBARBITAL:** Possible increased metabolism of thyroxine; dosage adjustments may be needed.
- **PROPYLTHIOURACIL:** Decreased conversion of T4 to T3.
- **RIFAMPIN:** Possible increased metabolism of thyroxine; dosage adjustments may be needed.
- **SERTRALINE:** May increase levothyroxine requirements.
- **SUCRALFATE:** May reduce levothyroxine absorption; separate doses by 4 hours.
- **SYMPATHOMIMETIC AGENTS (epinephrine, norepinephrine, etc.):** Levothyroxine can potentiate effects.
- **WARFARIN:** Thyroid hormones increase the catabolism of vitamin K-dependent clotting factors that may increase the anticoagulation effects in patients on warfarin.

Laboratory Considerations

- **Renal Function Tests:** Hypothyroid dogs can have decreased GFR (creatinine clearance); restoration to a euthyroid state can increase GFR and reduce serum creatinine levels.

The following drugs may have effects on thyroid function tests; evaluate results accordingly:

- <u>Effects on serum T4:</u> aminoglutethimide↓, anabolic steroids/androgens↓, antithyroid drugs (PTU, methimazole)↓, asparaginase↓, barbiturates↓, corticosteroids↓, danazol↓, diazepam↓, estrogens↑ (**Note:** estrogens may have no effect on canine T3 or T4 concentrations), fluorouracil↑, heparin↓, insulin↑, lithium carbonate↓, mitotane (o,p-DDD)↓, nitroprusside↓, phenylbutazone↓, phenytoin↓, propranolol↑, salicylates (large doses)↓, sulfonamides↓, and sulfonylureas↓.
- <u>Effects on serum T3:</u> antithyroid drugs (PTU, methimazole)↓, barbiturates↓, corticosteroids↓, estrogens↑, fluorouracil↑, hep-

arin↓, lithium carbonate↓, phenytoin↓, propranolol↓, salicylates (large doses)↓, sulfonamides↓, and thiazides↑.

- **Effects on T₃ uptake resin**: anabolic steroids/androgens↑, antithyroid drugs (PTU, methimazole)↓, asparaginase↑, corticosteroids↑, danazol↑, estrogens↓, fluorouracil↓, heparin↑, lithium carbonate↓, phenylbutazone↑, and salicylates (large doses)↑.

- **Effects on serum TSH**: aminoglutethimide↑, antithyroid drugs (PTU, methimazole)↑, corticosteroids↓, danazol↓, lithium carbonate↑, and sulfonamides↑.

- **Effects on Free Thyroxine Index (FTI)**: antithyroid drugs (PTU, methimazole)↓, barbiturates↓, corticosteroids↓, heparin↑, lithium carbonate↓, and phenylbutazone↓.

Doses

- **DOGS:**

For hypothyroidism (extra-label):

For myxedema crisis (extra-label): 5 micrograms/kg (0.005 mg/kg) IV q12h during crises. Consider a lower dosage in dogs with underlying heart disease or heart failure. If parenteral levothyroxine is unavailable, can attempt to give via nasoesophogeal or orogastric tube. Once patient is stabilized and can swallow, begin PO therapy. Adapted from: (Koenig 2013), (Scott-Moncrieff, J.C. 2012)

Oral therapy: Note: Initial dosages vary by the author and the formulation that is used. There does not seem to be good published evidence or general consensus that supports one recommendation over the other. Commonly, initial dosages of 0.02 mg/kg (20 micrograms/kg) PO on an empty stomach q12h have been noted. A maximum initial dosage of 0.8 mg per dog q12h is often recommended. There is some evidence that 0.02 mg/kg of the oral liquid (*Leventa®*) may be administered once daily. Lower dosages are recommended for dogs with certain concurrent conditions (see Contraindications). If it is not possible to give on an empty stomach, give with consistent timing with regard to food intake. Monitoring recommendations for adjusting dosages and dosage frequency vary considerably; see Monitoring (below) for examples.

To confirm diagnosis of hypothyroidism using a trial of levothyroxine (extra-label): It is not recommended to initiate treatment without performing thyroid function testing and ruling out non-thyroidal illness but if this is to be done, the following protocol should provide the most accurate assessment of response to treatment. Obtain history and perform physical examination. Give levothyroxine at 0.02 mg/kg PO q12h. If a positive response is obtained within 2 months of treatment, treatment should be temporarily withdrawn and the dog re-examined in 4-6 weeks. A diagnosis of hypothyroidism is made when clinical signs improve or resolve during treatment and reoccur after cessation of treatment. Other treatments should be avoided during this trial period. If there is no response to treatment after 2-3 months levothyroxine, and 4- to 6-hour post-dose serum T4 (total) concentration is within the appropriate therapeutic range, therapy should be withdrawn and other diagnoses pursued. Adapted from: (Panciera 2009), (Scott-Moncrieff, J.C. 2012)

- **CATS:**

For hypothyroidism (extra-label): 0.05 – 0.1 mg (per cat) PO once daily. Monitoring and dosage adjustments as for dogs. (Scott-Moncrieff, J. *et al.* 2000)

Post antithyroid medication, thyroidectomy, or radioiodine treatment (extra-label): Cats with hyperthyroidism and CKD (IRIS stage 2 & 3) treated with radioiodine that received levothyroxine at 0.1 mg/kg PO q24h had significantly lower increases in serum Cr and BUN over the next 12 months than non-treated cats. (Broome *et al.* 2013)

- **HORSES:**

For hypothyroidism or post thyroidectomy (extra-label): 0.02 mg/kg (20 micrograms/kg) PO once daily has traditionally been used, but recent studies suggest that doses as high as 0.05 – 0.1 mg/kg (50 – 100 micrograms/kg) PO per day may be well tolerated, at least for a short period. Horses in those studies were administered levothyroxine in a small meal of grain, which may have affected absorption. Dosages may vary, depending on whether it is given to fasted horses or if it is fed with a meal. Serum thyroid hormone concentrations should be monitored during supplementation so that dosages can be adjusted to maintain thyroid hormone levels in the normal range. If a sensitive TSH assay becomes commercially available, dosages should be adjusted to normalize TSH. (Breuhaus 2011)

For adjunctive treatment of equine metabolic syndrome (extra-label): When administered at high dosages levothyroxine induces weight loss in horses, and this is accompanied by an increase in insulin sensitivity. Levothyroxine is administered at an approximate dose of 0.1 mg/kg, which is rounded to 48 mg per day for horses weighing 450-525 kg. Weight loss can be enhanced during treatment by restricting caloric intake and increasing exercise. Horses should not be permitted to graze on pasture because levothyroxine is likely to induce hyperphagia, which offsets its effects on body weight. Levothyroxine is primarily administered for the purpose of accelerating weight loss in obese horses, and can be prescribed for 3-6 months while other management practices are instituted. (Frank 2011)

- **BIRDS:**

For hypothyroidism (extra-label): One 0.1 mg tablet in 30 mL – 120 mL of water daily; stir water and offer for 15 minutes and remove. Use high dose for budgerigars and low dose for water drinkers. Used for respiratory clicking, vomiting in budgerigars and thyroid responsive problems. (Clubb 1986)

- **REPTILES:**

For hypothyroidism in tortoises (extra-label): 0.02 mg/kg PO every other day. (Gauvin 1993)

Monitoring

Levothyroxine monitoring in <u>dogs</u> to determine efficacy and for dosage adjustment varies by the author. The following are examples:

- Patient is revaluated 1-2 months after initiating therapy and dosage is adjusted based on clinical response and results of the TT4. When interpreting the result of TT4, time of sampling compared to the administration of the medication should be taken into consideration. Most commonly, blood is taken 3-6 hours after the last medication is administered (post-tablet test) and peak concentrations are measured. In this case, TT4 is expected to be within the reference range (upper half limit), and a TT4 value just above the reference range is acceptable. In most patients, follow-up of TSH does not offer a significant advantage over a measurement of T4 solely. (Daminet 2010).

- Monitoring includes evaluation of clinical response, serum T4 concentrations, and serum TSH concentration. Concentrations are typically evaluated 4-6 hours after levothyroxine administration. Trough levels are recommended if levothyroxine is being given once a day. Serum T4 and TSH concentrations should be measured 4 weeks after initiating therapy, whenever signs of thyrotoxicosis develop, or if there has been minimal or no response to therapy. After a dosage adjustment is made in dogs showing a poor response to treatment, measure concentrations 2-4 weeks later. Ideally, serum T4 and TSH concentrations should be in the reference range when measured 4-6 hours after a levothyroxine dose, but post-dosing serum T4 concentrations are frequently above the reference range. This is not an absolute indication to reduce the dose of levothyroxine, especially if there are no clinical signs of thyrotoxicosis. However, a reduction in the dose is recommended whenever serum T4 concentrations exceed 55 nmol/L. Post-dosing serum T4 concentrations may also be less than 20 nmol/L. In this situation, an increase in the dose or frequency of administration of levothyroxine is indicated if clinical manifestations of hypothyroidism persist, the serum TSH concentration remains increased, or both, but is not necessarily indicated if the clinical response is good and the serum TSH concentration is in the reference range. Resolution of clinical signs and a satisfied owner are the most important parameters when considering adjusting the levothyroxine dose. (Nelson 2013)

- Monitoring of T4 or TSH is not routinely needed unless there is a poor response to therapy or signs of thyrotoxicosis are present. Wait one month after starting therapy or changing dosage. Inquire about owner compliance and expiration date of medication. Measure serum T4 immediately prior to next dose (trough). Normalization of serum TSH levels may be the best way to monitor therapy, but this requires that an elevated TSH existed prior to therapy. Samples for TSH may be obtained 2-3 weeks after starting supplementation, and concentrations are not dependent on the time the sample is obtained relative to the dosing of thyroxine. (Bruyette 2012)

- Therapy is titrated using routine measurement of T4, initially monthly until clinical signs resolve and the T4 is within or just above reference range 4-6 hours after dosing, then 1-2 times yearly in an otherwise asymptomatic and clinically well patient. Because of individual variability in T4 absorption and serum half-life, the dose should be adjusted based on the measured serum T4 concentration 4-6 hours after dosing. Therapy should be individualized based on clinical response, presence of concurrent illness, age, and concurrent drug administration. If clinical signs resolve and T4 concentrations are within the therapeutic range after 4-8 weeks of therapy, the frequency of T4 administration can be decreased to once daily. Therapeutic monitoring also minimizes the effect of any differences in potency and bioavailability between different brands of L-thyroxine. Improvement in activity should be evident within the first 1-2 weeks of treatment; weight loss should be evident within 8 weeks. Achievement of a normal hair coat may take several months and the coat may initially appear worse as telogen hairs are shed. Neurologic deficits improve rapidly after treatment but complete resolution may take 8-12 weeks. (Scott-Moncrieff, J.C. 2012)

Client Information

- Dogs require much higher doses than humans. Cat doses may be similar to what an adult human would take.

- Side effects are only associated with giving too much drug and include fast or racing heart rate, greater appetite, thirst and urination, excitability/nervousness, and panting (in dogs). Cats may appear withdrawn or apathetic (uncaring).

- May be given with or without food, but give the same way every day. Clients should be instructed in the importance of compliance with therapy as prescribed.

Chemistry/Synonyms

Prepared synthetically for commercial use, levothyroxine sodium is the levo isomer of thyroxine that is the primary secretion of the thyroid gland. It occurs as an odorless, light yellow to buff-colored, tasteless, hygroscopic powder that is very slightly soluble in water and slightly soluble in alcohol. The commercially available powders for injection also contain mannitol.

100 micrograms of levothyroxine is approximately equivalent to 65 mg (1 grain) of desiccated thyroid.

Levothyroxine sodium may also be known as: T4, T4 thyroxine sodium, levothyroxin natrium, levothyroxinum natricum, 3,5,3',5'-tetra-iodo-L-thyronine sodium, thyroxine sodium, L-thyroxine sodium, thyroxinum natricum, tirossina, and tiroxina sodica; many trade names are available.

Storage/Stability

Levothyroxine sodium preparations should be stored at room temperature in tight, light-resistant containers. The injectable product should be reconstituted immediately before use; unused injection should be discarded after reconstituting.

Before first use, the oral solution should be stored refrigerated at 2°-8°C (37°-46°F) and protected from light. After first opening, store at room temperature 20°-25°C (68°-77°F) and use within 2 months.

Levothyroxine sodium is reportedly **unstable** in aqueous solutions. If using a commercial liquid preparation, it is suggested to obtain validated stability data for the product.

Compatibility/Compounding Considerations

Do **NOT** mix levothyroxine sodium injection with other drugs or IV fluids.

Dosage Forms/Regulatory Status

All levothyroxine products require a prescription, but are not necessarily FDA-approved; no veterinary product found during a search on the FDA's Green Book. There have been bioavailability differences between products reported. It is recommended to use a reputable product and not to change brands indiscriminately.

VETERINARY-LABELED PRODUCTS:

Levothyroxine Sodium Tablets: 0.1 mg, 0.2 mg, 0.3 mg, 0.4 mg, 0.5 mg, 0.6 mg, 0.7 mg, 0.8 mg, & 1 mg; many trade name products may be available and include: *Soloxine®, Levosyn®, Thyro-Tabs®, Thyrosyn®, Thyroxine-L Tablets®, Thyrozine®, Thyrokare®*, generic; (Rx). Labeled for use in dogs.

Levothyroxine Sodium Tablets Chewable (Veterinary): 0.1 mg, 0.2 mg, 0.3 mg, 0.4 mg, 0.5 mg, 0.6 mg, 0.7 mg, 0.8 mg; Products that may be available include: *Canine Thyroid Chewable Tablets®, Nutrived® T-4 Chewable Tablets, Thyromed® Chewable Tablets*; (Rx). Labeled for use in dogs.

Levothyroxine Oral Solution: 1 mg/mL in 30 mL bottles: *Leventa® Oral Solution*; (Rx). Labeled for use in dogs.

Levothyroxine Sodium Powder (Veterinary): 0.22% (1 gram of T4 in 454 grams of powder): One level teaspoonful contains 12 mg of T4. Available in 1 lb. and 10 lbs. containers; many trade name products may be available and include: *Equine Thyroid Supplement®, Thyrozine Powder®, Levoxine® Powder); Thyro-L®, Throxine-L® Powder, Thyrosyn Powder®, Thyrokare® Powder*; (Rx). Labeled for use in horses.

HUMAN-LABELED PRODUCTS:

Levothyroxine Sodium Tablets: 0.025 mg (25 micrograms), 0.05 mg (50 micrograms), 0.075 mg (75 micrograms), 0.088 mg (88 micrograms), 0.1 mg (100 micrograms), 0.112 mg (112 micrograms), 0.125 mg (125 micrograms), 0.137 mg (137 micrograms), 0.15 mg (150 micrograms), 0.175 mg (175 micrograms), 0.2 mg (200 micrograms) & 0.3 mg (300 micrograms); *Synthroid®, Levoxyl®, Unithroid®*, generic; (Rx)

Levothyroxine Sodium Liquid-filled Oral Capsules: 13 micrograms (0.013 mg), 25 micrograms (0.025 mg), 50 micrograms (0.05 mg), 75 micrograms (0.075 mg), 88 micrograms (0.088 mg), 100 micrograms (0.1 mg),

112 micrograms (0.112 mg), 125 micrograms (0.125 mg), 137 micrograms (0.137 mg) & 150 micrograms (0.15 mg); *Tirosint®*; (Rx)

Levothyroxine Powder for Injection lyophilized: 200 micrograms (0.2 mg) & 500 micrograms (0.5 mg) in 10 mL vials; generic; (Rx)

Revisions/References

Monograph revised/updated March 2014.

Breuhaus, B. A. (2011). Disorders of the Equine Thyroid Gland. Veterinary Clinics of North America-Equine Practice 27(1): 115-+.

Broome, M. R. & M. E. Peterson (2013). Use of L-thyroxine supplementation after radioiodine therapy helps blunt the worsening of azotemia in hyperthyroid cats with pre-existing kidney disease (ACVIM Forum Abstract). J Vet Intern Med 27: 604-756.

Bruyette, D. S. (2012). Canine Hypothyroidism. Atlantic Coast Veterinary Conference. accessed via Veterinary Information Network; vin.com

Clubb, S. L. (1986). Therapeutics: Individual and Flock Treatment Regimens. *Clinical Avian Medicine and Surgery.* G. J. Harrison and L. R. Harrison. Philadelphia, W.B. Saunders: 327-55.

Daminet, S. (2010). Canine Hypothyroidism: Update on Diagnosis and Treatment. Proceedings: WSAVA. accessed via Veterinary Information Network; vin.com

Frank, N. (2011). Equine Metabolic Syndrome. Veterinary Clinics of North America-Equine Practice 27(1): 73-+.

Gauvin, J. (1993). Drug therapy in reptiles. Seminars in Avian & Exotic Med 2(1): 48-59.

Iemura, R., et al. (2013). Effects of type of diet on pharmacokinetics of levothyroxine sodium oral solution. Research in Veterinary Science 94(3): 695-7.

Koenig, A. (2013). Endocrine Emergencies in Dogs and Cats. Veterinary Clinics of North America: Small Animal Practice 43(4): 869-97.

Le Traon, G., et al. (2008). Pharmacokinetics of total thyroxine in dogs after administration of an oral solution of levothyroxine sodium. J. Vet. Pharmacol. Ther. 31(2): 95-101.

Nelson, R. W. (2013). How I Treat: Canine Hypothyroidism. WSAVA World Congress Proceedings. accessed via Veterinary Information Network; vin.com

Panciera, D. (2009). Diagnostic Testing and Treatment Options for Canine Hypothyroidism. Proceedings: ACVC. accessed via Veterinary Information Network; vin.com

Scott-Moncrieff, J. & L. Guptill-Yoran (2000). Hypothyroidism. *Textbook of Veterinary Internal Medicine: Diseases of the Dog and Cat.* S. Ettinger and E. Feldman. Philadelphia, WB Saunders. 2: 1419-29.

Scott-Moncrieff, J. C. (2012). Thyroid Disorders in the Geriatric Veterinary Patient. Veterinary Clinics of North America-Small Animal Practice 42(4): 707-+.

Lidocaine HCl (I.V.; Systemic)

(lye-doe-kane)   Xylocaine®, Lignocaine

Antiarrhythmic/Local Anesthetic

Prescriber Highlights

▶ Local anesthetic & antiarrhythmic (ventricular tachycardia) agent; may be useful as an IV anesthetic/analgesic adjunct.

▶ Contraindications: Known hypersensitivity to the amide-class local anesthetics, severe degree of SA, AV, or intraventricular heart block (if not being artificially paced), or Adams-Stokes syndrome.

▶ Caution: Cats appear more sensitive to cardiodepressant and CNS effects of lidocaine; many clinicians avoid lidocaine use in cats. Use with caution in patients with liver disease, congestive heart failure, shock, hypovolemia, severe respiratory depression, marked hypoxia, bradycardia, or incomplete heart block having VPC's, unless the heart rate is first accelerated.

▶ Patients susceptible to malignant hyperthermia should receive intensified monitoring.

▶ Adverse Effects: Most common adverse effects reported are dose related (serum level) & mild. CNS signs include drowsiness, depression, ataxia, muscle tremors, etc.; nausea & vomiting (usually transient). Adverse cardiac effects usually only at high plasma concentrations in most species, but cats are susceptible.

▶ When an IV bolus is given too rapidly, hypotension may occur. Seizures are possible.

▶ Do **NOT** use the product containing epinephrine intravenously.

▶ Drug interactions.

Uses/Indications

Besides its use as a local and topical anesthetic agent, lidocaine is sometimes used to treat ventricular arrhythmias, principally ventricular tachycardia and ventricular premature complexes in all species. It may also have benefit in dogs to terminate supraventricular tachycardia in the presence or absence of an accessory pathway and paroxysmal atrial fibrillation initiated by elevated vagal tone in large breed dogs with normal cardiac function. Cats may be more sensitive to the drug and some clinicians feel that it should not be used in this species as an antiarrhythmic, but this remains controversial. In critically ill dogs, lidocaine may be beneficial secondary to its free radical scavenging abilities, analgesic effects, and antiarrhythmic properties. It potentially could be useful in dogs with gastric dilatation volvulus (GDV) to reduce cardiac arrhythmias, acute kidney injury and hospitalization times (Bruchim *et al.* 2012)

In horses, lidocaine has been used as part of partial intravenous anesthesia (PIVA) protocols for its analgesic, antiinflammatory and prokinetic effects. It may be useful to prevent post-operative ileus and reperfusion injury and for the adjunctive treatment of endotoxemia.

Low dose intravenous lidocaine infusions for hyperalgesia and neuropathic pain states induced by trauma or surgical procedures have been documented to be useful. Intravenous lidocaine (at usual dosages; 1 – 4 mg/kg) is relatively safe in rabbits and guinea pigs (Schnellbacher *et al.* 2012).

Pharmacology/Actions

Lidocaine is considered to be a class IB antidysrhythmic agent (membrane-stabilizing). It is thought that lidocaine acts by combining with fast sodium channels when inactive which inhibits recovery after repolarization. Class IB agents demonstrate rapid rates of attachment and dissociation to sodium channels. At therapeutic levels, lidocaine causes phase 4 diastolic depolarization attenuation, decreased automaticity, and either a decrease or no change in membrane responsiveness and excitability. These effects will occur at serum levels that will not inhibit the automaticity of the SA node, and will have little effect on AV node conduction or His-Purkinje conduction.

Lidocaine's analgesic effects are not well understood but are likely via several mechanisms, including reducing ectopic activity of damaged afferent neurons.

Lidocaine apparently has some enhancing effects on intestinal motility in patients with postoperative ileus. The mechanism for this effect is not well understood, but probably involves more than just blocking increased sympathetic tone.

Lidocaine has been shown to be a scavenger of reactive oxygen species (ROS) and lipid peroxidation.

Pharmacokinetics

Lidocaine is not effective orally as it has a high first-pass effect. If very high oral doses are given, toxic signs occur (due to active metabolites?) before therapeutic levels can be reached. Following a therapeutic IV bolus dose, the onset of action is generally within 2 minutes and has duration of action of 10-20 minutes. If a constant infusion is begun without an initial IV bolus, it may take up to an hour for therapeutic levels to be reached. IM injections may be given every 1.5 hours in the dog, but because monitoring and adjusting dosages are difficult, it should be reserved for cases where IV infusions are not possible.

After injection, the drug is rapidly redistributed from the plasma into highly perfused organs (kidney, liver, lungs, heart) and distributed widely throughout body tissues. It has a high affinity for fat and adipose tissue and is bound to plasma proteins, primarily alpha$_1$-acid glycoprotein. It has been reported that lidocaine binding to this protein is highly variable and concentration dependent in the dog and may be higher in dogs with inflammatory disease. Lidocaine is distributed into milk. The apparent volume of distribution (V_d) has been reported to be 4.5 L/kg in the dog.

Lidocaine is rapidly metabolized in the liver to active metabolites (MEGX and GX). The terminal half-life of lidocaine in humans is 1.5-2 hours and has been reported to be 0.9 hours in dogs and approximately 1 hour in horses.

The half-lives of lidocaine and MEGX may be prolonged in patients with cardiac failure or hepatic disease. Less than 10% of a parenteral dose is excreted unchanged in the urine.

Contraindications/Precautions/Warnings

Cats tend to be more sensitive to the CNS and cardiodepressant effects of lidocaine; use with caution. Cats with concurrent illnesses or under general anesthesia may be particularly sensitive to lidocaine's effects. Some clinicians avoid the use of lidocaine entirely in cats, while others suggest that at the lower CRI dosage rates for analgesia, it can be safely used.

Lidocaine is contraindicated in patients with known hypersensitivity to the amide-class local anesthetics, a severe degree of SA, AV or intraventricular heart block (if not being artificially paced), or Adams-Stokes syndrome. The use of lidocaine in patients with Wolff-Parkinson-White (WPW) syndrome is controversial. Some manufacturers state its use is contraindicated, but several physicians have used the drug in people.

Lidocaine should be used with caution in patients with liver disease, congestive heart failure, shock, hypovolemia, severe respiratory depression, or marked hypoxia. Consider reducing dosages by 50% in animals with liver dysfunction. It should also be used with caution in patients with bradycardia or incomplete heart block having VPC's unless the heart rate is first accelerated. Patients susceptible to developing malignant hyperthermia should receive lidocaine with intensified monitoring.

When preparing lidocaine for intravenous injection, be certain of the concentration and do NOT use products containing epinephrine.

Adverse Effects

At usual doses and if the serum level remains within the proposed therapeutic range (1-5 micrograms/mL), serious adverse reactions are quite rare. The most common adverse effects reported are dose related (serum level) and mild. CNS signs include drowsiness, depression, ataxia, muscle tremors, etc. Nausea and vomiting may occur, but are usually transient. Adverse cardiac effects generally only occur at high plasma concentrations and are usually associated with PR and QRS interval prolongation and QT interval shortening. Lidocaine may increase ventricular rates if used in patients with atrial fibrillation. If an IV bolus is given too rapidly, hypotension may occur. Horses are less sensitive than other species to lidocaine's adverse cardiovascular effects.

Do NOT to use the product that contains epinephrine intravenously.

Reproductive/Nursing Safety

In humans, the FDA categorizes systemic lidocaine as category *B* for use during pregnancy (*Animal studies have not yet demonstrated risk to the fetus, but there are no adequate studies in pregnant women; or animal studies have shown an adverse effect, but adequate studies in pregnant women have not demonstrated a risk to the fetus in the first trimester of pregnancy, and there is no evidence of risk in later trimesters.*) In a separate system evaluating the safety of drugs in canine and feline pregnancy (Papich 1989), systemic lidocaine is categorized class: *B* (*Safe for use if used cautiously. Studies in laboratory animals may have uncovered some risk, but these drugs appear to be safe in dogs and cats or these drugs are safe if they are not administered when the animal is near term.*)

Lidocaine is excreted in concentrations of approximately 40% of that found in the serum and would unlikely to pose significant risk to nursing offspring.

Overdosage/Acute Toxicity

In dogs, if serum levels of >8 micrograms/mL are attained, toxicity may result. Signs may include ataxia, nystagmus, depression, seizures, bradycardia, hypotension and, at very high levels, circulatory collapse. Because lidocaine is rapidly metabolized, cessation of therapy or reduction in infusion rates with monitoring may be all that is required for minor signs. Seizures or excitement may be treated with diazepam, or a short or ultrashort acting barbiturate. Longer acting barbiturates should be avoided (*e.g.*, pentobarbital). Should circulatory depression occur, treat with fluids, pressor agents and, if necessary, begin CPR. A lidocaine overdose in a cat was successfully treated with intravenous lipid emulsion (ILE) (O'Brien *et al.* 2010).

Drug Interactions

The following drug interactions have either been reported or are theoretical in humans or animals receiving lidocaine and may be of significance in veterinary patients. Unless otherwise noted, use together is not necessarily contraindicated, but weigh the potential risks and perform additional monitoring when appropriate.

- **ANESTHETICS, GAS:** Lidocaine infusions perioperatively have been shown to reduce MAC requirements in dogs, horses and cats. In dogs and horses, this may be of benefit but in cats, additive cardiodepression has been shown. However in horses, lidocaine with inhalant anesthetics can cause tremors/ataxia and affect the quality of anesthetic recovery, it has been recommended to discontinue lidocaine CRI's at least 30 minutes before the start of the recovery period.
- **ANTIARRHYTHMICS, OTHER** (*e.g.*, **procainamide, quinidine, propranolol, phenytoin**): When administered with lidocaine may cause additive or antagonistic cardiac effects and toxicity may be enhanced.
- **BETA-BLOCKERS:** Lidocaine levels or effects may be increased.
- **CIMETIDINE:** Lidocaine levels or effects may be increased.
- **FUROSEMIDE (or other drugs that can cause hypokalemia):** Hypokalemia may reduce the antiarrhythmic effects of lidocaine.
- **KETAMINE:** Lidocaine may increase ataxic effects in horses.
- **PHENOBARBITAL, PHENYTOIN:** May increase lidocaine metabolism; decrease levels.
- **SUCCINYLCHOLINE:** Large doses of lidocaine may prolong succinylcholine-induced apnea.
- **XYLAZINE (and other ALPHA-2 AGONISTS):** Lidocaine may increase the ataxic effects of alpha-2 agonists in horses.

Laboratory Considerations

- Lidocaine may cause increased **creatine kinase** levels (CK).

Doses

Note: Do not confuse CRI dosages listed as **micrograms/kg/minute** with those listed as **mg/kg/hour**.

- **DOGS:**

  As an antiarrhythmic agent:

  For refractory ventricular fibrillation (VF)/pulseless ventricular tachycardia (VT); (extra-label): The treatment of choice is electrical defibrillation, but patients with VF refractory to defibrillation may benefit from treatment with amiodarone. If amiodarone is not available, lidocaine at 2 mg/kg slow IV/IO push may be of benefit. (Fletcher *et al.* 2012)

  For ventricular tachycardia (extra-label): For rapid conversion of life-threatening, sustained, and/or unstable ventricular tachycardia. Dosage recommendations vary and consensus does not exist for a dosing protocol, but consider an initial dosage of 2 – 4 mg/kg IV over 1-2 minutes while monitoring ECG. If sinus rhythm is achieved or ectopy satisfactorily reduced during the IV bolus, stop administering and begin a CRI of 25 – 100 micrograms/kg/minute (1.5 – 6 mg/kg/hour) adjusting rate to maintain efficacy while minimizing adverse effects. Prepare to re-bolus at half the initial effective dosage if arrhythmia recurs within 5-10 minutes. This can be repeated every 5-10 minutes up to a maximum total dose of 8 mg/kg while waiting for the CRI to be effective. (Kittleson 2014)

For adjunctive treatment of GDV or other critical illnesses: Loading dose of 1 – 2 mg/kg IV, then a CRI at 17 – 50 micrograms/kg/minute (1 – 3 mg/kg/hour).

As an analgesic agent (extra-label):

a) When used alone, lidocaine is often given as a slow (over 2-3 minutes) IV bolus of 1 – 2 mg/kg IV, followed by a CRI ranging from 25 – 100 micrograms/kg/minute (1.5 – 6 mg/kg/hour).

b) "MLK": Low-dose CRI's of a combination (MLK) of morphine (3.3 micrograms/kg/min), lidocaine (50 micrograms/kg/min), and ketamine (10 micrograms/kg/min), decreases isoflurane MAC in dogs and were not associated with adverse hemodynamic effects (Muir *et al.* 2003). Additional information on MLK CRI's can be found on the Veterinary Anesthesia & Analgesia Support Group website at http://www.vasg.org/constant_rate_infusions. htm for using the MLK (combination of morphine (or other opiates), lidocaine, & ketamine) CRI use in dogs and cats. Another "recipe" can be found in the Compatibility/Compounding Considerations section below.

As an epidural (extra-label): 4 – 5 mg/kg epidurally. Onset of action <10 minutes; duration 1.5 hours. Can be combined with alpha2 agonists or opioids. Adding epinephrine prolongs duration of action. (Valverde, A 2008)

- **CATS:**

Caution: Cats are reportedly very sensitive to the CNS effects of lidocaine and can develop cardiodepression. There are several sources that state that lidocaine should not be used in cats as an injectable analgesic, but others use it routinely. If using in cats, monitor carefully.

As an analgesic agent (extra-label): "MLK": See the information on the Veterinary Anesthesia & Analgesia Support Group website at http://www.vasg.org/constant_rate_infusions.htm for using the MLK (combination of morphine (or other opiates), lidocaine, & ketamine) CRI use in dogs and cats.

As an antiarrhythmic (extra-label): Initially, IV bolus of 0.25 – 0.5 mg/kg given slowly; can repeat at 0.15 – 0.25 mg/kg in 5-20 minutes; if effective, 10 – 20 micrograms/kg/minute (0.6 – 1.2 mg/kg/hour) as a constant rate IV infusion. (Ware 2000)

- **HORSES:** (NOTE: ARCI UCGFS CLASS 2 DRUG)

For ventricular tachyarrhythmias (extra-label): During anesthesia, if VPCs are frequent or polymorphic (*i.e.*, 2 or more different abnormal QRS-T configurations can be identified), if the HR is fast enough that diastolic filling time and cardiac output seem to be suffering (*e.g.*, pale mucous membranes, prolonged CRT, hypotension), or if the R-on-T phenomenon (the VPC overlaps the T wave of the previous P-QRS-T complex) occurs: lidocaine at 0.25 – 0.5 mg/kg IV slowly; can repeat in 5-10 minutes. Avoid giving more than 2 mg/kg (totaled doses) as boluses. If multiple boluses are required, a CRI at 50 micrograms/kg/minute (3 mg/kg/hour) can be started. Adapted from: (Boesch 2013)

For postoperative ileus/colic (extra-label): Initially, IV bolus of 1.3 – 1.4 mg/kg followed by a CRI at 30 – 50 micrograms/kg/minute (1.8 – 3 mg/kg/hr) for 24 hours (for post-operative ileus). Adapted from: (Malone *et al.* 1999), (Valverde, A 2008), (Hallowell 2008)

For PIVA (extra-label): Based upon the drug's pharmacokinetics an IV loading dose of 1.5 – 5 mg/kg followed by a CRI of 75 micrograms/kg/min (4.5 mg/kg/hour) should yield a plasma concentration of 3000 ng/mL (3 mcg/mL) and provide an approximate 30% reduction in MAC. The rate of administration of the loading dose has varied in studies ranging from 1-20 minutes. Administration rate is more relevant in conscious horses but is less so in anesthetized horses because lidocaine's neurologic effects (ataxia, vision disturbances) are blunted and not observed. Discontinue the CRI at least 30 minutes prior to the start of recovery. Has been used in PIVA protocols with ketamine or medetomidine or morphine. (Valverde, A. 2013)

Monitoring

- ECG.
- Signs of toxicity (see Adverse Effects and Overdosage).
- If available and indicated, serum levels may be monitored. Therapeutic levels are considered to range from 1-6 micrograms/mL.

Client Information

- This drug should only be used systemically by professionals familiar with its use and in a setting where adequate patient monitoring can be performed.

Chemistry/Synonyms

A potent local anesthetic and antiarrhythmic agent, lidocaine HCl occurs as a white, odorless, slightly bitter tasting, crystalline powder with a melting point between 74°-79°C and a pK_a of 7.86. It is very soluble in water and alcohol. The pH of the commercial injection is adjusted to 5-7, and the pH of the commercially available infusion in dextrose 5% is adjusted to 3.5-6.

Lidocaine may also be known as: lidocaini hydrochloridum, and lignocaine hydrochloride; many trade names are available; a common trade name is *Xylocaine®* (Astra).

Storage/Stability

Lidocaine for injection should be stored at temperatures less than 40°C and preferably between 15-30°C; avoid freezing.

Compatibility/Compounding Considerations

Lidocaine is physically **compatible** with most commonly used IV infusion solutions, including D5W, lactated Ringer's, saline, and combinations of these. It is also reportedly physically **compatible** with: aminophylline, calcium chloride/gluceptate/gluconate, chloramphenicol sodium succinate, chlorothiazide sodium, cimetidine HCl, dexamethasone sodium phosphate, dexmedetomidine, digoxin, diphenhydramine HCl, dobutamine HCl, ephedrine sulfate, erythromycin lactobionate, fentanyl, glycopyrrolate, heparin sodium, hydrocortisone sodium succinate, hydroxyzine HCl, ketamine, insulin (regular), metoclopramide HCl, morphine sulfate, oxytetracycline HCl, penicillin G potassium, pentobarbital sodium, phenylephrine HCl, potassium chloride, procainamide HCl, prochlorperazine edisylate, promazine HCl, sodium bicarbonate, sodium lactate, verapamil HCl, and Vitamin B-Complex with C.

Lidocaine **may not be compatible** with dopamine, epinephrine, isoproterenol, or norepinephrine as these require low pH for stability. Lidocaine is reportedly physically **incompatible** when mixed with ampicillin sodium, cefazolin sodium, methohexital sodium, or phenytoin sodium. Compatibility is dependent upon factors such as pH, concentration, temperature, and diluent used; consult specialized references or a hospital pharmacist for more specific information.

- **"MLK" Recipe:** Also see http://www.vasg.org/constant_rate _infusions.htm

To prepare IV infusion solution using the veterinary 2% solution add 1 gram (50 mL of 2% solution to 1 liter of D5W or other compatible solution, this will give an approximate concentration of 1 mg/mL (1000 micrograms/mL). When using a mini-drip (60 drops/mL) IV set, each drop will contain approximately 17 micrograms. In small dogs and cats, a less concentrated solution may be used for greater dosage accuracy. When preparing solutions be certain that you are not using the lidocaine product that contains epinephrine.

A combination intravenous infusion for analgesia and sedation in vigorous postoperative patients (dogs, <u>NOT</u> cats) that require sedation to sleep the night after surgery is described (Hansen 2008): For this technique, plan on adding the drugs to a bag of fluids for which the administration rate will not change, which usually means picking a fluid and administration rate calculated to provide maintenance needs for water. For example, to calculate a drug plan for a 20-kg dog that is to receive morphine, lidocaine, ketamine, and medetomidine for the first 8-24 hours postoperatively, drug doses to consider might include:

Morphine: 0.1 mg/kg/hr x 20 kg = 2 mg/hr.

Lidocaine: 2.5 mg/kg/hr x 20 kg = 50 mg/hr.

Ketamine: 0.1 mg/kg/hr x 20 kg = 2 mg/hr.

Medetomidine: 2 micrograms/kg/hr x 20 kg = 40 micrograms/hr (**Note:** This is <u>not</u> the dose for <u>dexmedetomidine; see the dexmedetomidine monograph or vasg.org for use as a CRI</u>).

The maintenance fluid administration rate for a dog this size lying quietly in a cage is roughly 800 mL/day or 33 mL/hr. Therefore, a 1-L bag contains approximately 30 hour's worth of treatment, and to a 1-L bag one must add:

Morphine: 2 mg/hr x 30 hours = 60 mg = 4 mL (if using 15 mg/mL morphine).

Lidocaine: 50 mg/hr x 30 hours = 1500 mg = 75 mL [if using 2% (20 mg/mL) lidocaine].

Ketamine: 2 mg/hr x 30 hours = 60 mg = 0.6 mL (if using 100 mg/mL ketamine).

Medetomidine: 40 micrograms/hr x 30 hours = 1200 micrograms = 1.2 mL (if using 1000 micrograms/mL medetomidine).

If the drugs are added to a 1-L bag of fluid, the final volume is >1 liter—in this case 1081 mL. Therefore, 81 mL should be removed from the bag before addition of the medications. (Hansen 2008)

Dosage Forms/Regulatory Status

VETERINARY-LABELED PRODUCTS:

There are injectable lidocaine products labeled for use in veterinary medicine (dogs, cats, horses, and cattle) as an injectable anesthetic, but it is not FDA-approved for use as an antiarrhythmic agent. Information regarding its use in food-producing species is conflicting; when using a food animal it is suggested to contact FARAD (see appendix).

Lidocaine HCl for Injection: 2% (20 mg/mL) in 100 mL & 250 mL multi-use vials; (contains preservatives); generic; (Rx)

The ARCI (Racing Commissioners International) has designated this drug as a class 2 substance. See the appendix for more information.

HUMAN-LABELED PRODUCTS:

Lidocaine Hydrochloride Injection: 0.5%, 1%, 1.5%, 2% & 4% in 5 mL, 10 mL, 20 mL, 30 mL & 50 mL single- & multi-dose vials, 2 mL & 5 mL amps, 5 mL syringes & cartridges; *Xylocaine®* & *Xylocaine MPF®*, generic; (Rx)

Lidocaine Hydrochloride with Dextrose Injection: 1.5% with 7.5% dextrose & 5% with 7.5 % dextrose in 2 mL amps & single-dose amps; *Xylocaine MPF®*, generic; (Rx)

Premixed with D5W for IV infusion in concentrations of 2 mg/mL, 4 mg/mL, and 5 mg/mL, injections with epinephrine, topical liquids, patches, ointment, cream, lotion, gel, spray, & jelly available.

Revisions/References

Monograph revised/updated March 2014.

Boesch, J. M. (2013). Anesthesia for the Horse with Colic. Veterinary Clinics of North America-Equine Practice **29**(1): 193-+.

Bruchim, Y., et al. (2012). Evaluation of lidocaine treatment on frequency of cardiac arrhythmias, acute kidney injury, and hospitalization time in dogs with gastric dilatation volvulus. J. Vet. Emerg. Crit. Care **22**(4).

Fletcher, D. J., et al. (2012). RECOVER evidence and knowledge gap analysis on veterinary CPR. Part 7: Clinical guidelines. J. Vet. Emerg. Crit. Care **22**.

Hallowell, G. (2008). Update on Current and New Treatments for Colic Patients. Proceedings: ACVIM. accessed via Veterinary Information Network; vin.com

Hansen, B. (2008). Analgesia for the Critically Ill Dog or Cat: An Update. Veterinary Clinics of North America-Small Animal Practice **38**(6): 1353-+.

Kittleson, M. D. (2014). Personal Communication.

Malone, E., et al. (1999). Intravenous lidocaine for the treatment of equine ileus (abstract). Proceedings: American College of Veterinary Internal Medicine: 17th Annual Veterinary Medical Forum, Chicago. accessed via Veterinary Information Network; vin.com

Muir, W. W., et al. (2003). Effects of morphine, lidocaine, ketamine, and morphine-lidocaine-ketamine drug combination on minimum alveolar concentration in dogs anesthetized with isoflurane. American Journal of Veterinary Research **64**(9): 1155-60.

O'Brien, T. Q., et al. (2010). Infusion of a lipid emulsion to treat lidocaine intoxication in a cat. Javma-Journal of the American Veterinary Medical Association **237**(12): 1455-8.

Papich, M. (1989). Effects of drugs on pregnancy. *Current Veterinary Therapy X: Small Animal Practice*. R. Kirk. Philadelphia, Saunders: 1291-9.

Schnellbacher, R., et al. (2012). Emergency presentations associated with cardiovascular disease in exotic herbivores. Journal of Exotic Pet Medicine **21**(4): 316-27.

Valverde, A. (2008). Epidural analgesia and anesthesia in dogs and cats. Vet Clin NA: Sm Anim Pract **38**: 1205-30.

Valverde, A. (2013). Balanced Anesthesia and Constant-Rate Infusions in Horses. Veterinary Clinics of North America-Equine Practice **29**(1): 89-+.

Ware, W. (2000). Therapy for Critical Arrhythmias: New Advances. Proceedings: The North American Veterinary Conference, Orlando. accessed via Veterinary Information Network; vin.com

Lincomycin HCl

(lin-koe-**mye**-sin)   Lincocin®, Lincomix®

Lincosamide Antibiotic

Prescriber Highlights

▶ Lincosamide antibiotic similar to clindamycin; broad spectrum against many anaerobes, gram-positive aerobic cocci, Toxoplasma, etc.

▶ Contraindications: Horses, rodents, ruminants, lagomorphs; hypersensitivity to lincosamides.

▶ Caution: Liver or renal dysfunction; consider reducing dosage if severe.

▶ Adverse Effects: Gastroenteritis, pain at injection site if given IM; rapid IV administration can cause hypotension & cardiopulmonary arrest.

▶ Distributed into milk; may cause diarrhea in nursing animals.

▶ Drug interactions.

Uses/Indications

Lincomycin has dosage forms FDA-approved for use in dogs, cats, swine, and in combination with other agents for chickens. Because clindamycin is generally better absorbed, more active, and probably less toxic, it has largely supplanted the use of lincomycin for oral and injectable therapy in small animals, but some clinicians believe that clindamycin does not offer enough clinically significant improvements over lincomycin to justify its higher cost. For further information, refer to the Pharmacology or Doses sections.

Pharmacology/Actions

The lincosamide antibiotics lincomycin and clindamycin, share mechanisms of action and have similar spectrums of activity although lincomycin is usually less active against susceptible organisms. Complete cross-resistance occurs between the two drugs; at least partial cross-resistance occurs between the lincosamides and erythromycin. They may act as bacteriostatic or bactericidal agents, depending on the concentration of the drug at the infection site and the susceptibility of the organism. Lincosamides can accumulate in cells (*e.g.*, leukocytes, macrophages, etc.). They are believed to act by binding to the 50S ribosomal subunit of susceptible bacteria, thereby inhibiting peptide bond formation.

Most aerobic gram-positive cocci are susceptible to the lincosamides (*Strep. faecalis* is not), including staphylococcus and streptococci. Many strains of *S. pseudintermedius* are resistant. Other organisms that are generally susceptible include: *Corynebacterium diphtheriae, Nocardia asteroides*, Erysepelothrix, and *Mycoplasma* spp. Anaerobic bacteria that may be susceptible to lincomycin include: *Clostridium perfringens. C. tetani* (not *C. difficile*), Bacteroides (including many strains of *B. fragilis*), Fusobacterium, Peptostreptococcus, Actinomyces, and Peptococcus. Most enterococci are resistant.

Pharmacokinetics

The pharmacokinetics of lincomycin have not apparently been extensively studied in veterinary species.

In cats, after IV or oral doses of 15 mg/kg the following pharmacokinetic parameters (means) were reported: Bioavailability (oral): 82%; volume of distribution (steady-state): 0.98 L/kg; clearance: 0.17 L/kg/hr; elimination half-life: 4.2 hours. The skin to plasma ratio 2-hours post dose was about 2:1 (Albarellos *et al.* 2013). Protein binding in cats is low (<20%). IM dosage of 10 mg/kg had a mean bioavailability of 83%. Bone to serum ratio measured 30-45 minutes after IM dosing was ≈0.7:1 (Albarellos *et al.* 2012).

Unless otherwise noted, the following information applies to humans. The drug is rapidly absorbed from the gut, but only ≈30-40% of the total dose is absorbed. Food both decreases the extent and the rate of absorption. Peak serum levels are attained ≈2-4 hour after oral dosing. IM administration gives peak levels about double those reached after oral dosing, and peak at ≈30 minutes post injection.

Lincomycin is distributed into most tissues. Therapeutic levels are achieved in bone, synovial fluid, bile, pleural fluid, peritoneal fluid, skin, and heart muscle. CNS levels may reach 40% of those in the serum if meninges are inflamed. Lincomycin is bound from 57-72% to plasma proteins, depending on the drug's concentration. The drug crosses the placenta and can be distributed into milk at concentrations equal to those found in plasma.

Lincomycin is partially metabolized in the liver. Unchanged drug and metabolites are excreted in the urine, feces and bile. Half-lives can be prolonged in patients with renal or hepatic dysfunction. The elimination half-life of lincomycin is reportedly 3-4 hours in small animals.

Contraindications/Precautions/Warnings

Although there have been case reports of parenteral administration of lincosamides to horses, cattle and sheep, the lincosamides are considered **contraindicated** for use in **rabbits**, **hamsters**, **guinea pigs**, **horses**, and **ruminants** because of serious gastrointestinal effects that may occur, including death.

Lincomycin is contraindicated in patients with known hypersensitivity to it or having a preexisting monilial infection.

Lincomycin is generally not recommended for use in neonatal animals because of its effects on gut flora.

In patients with hepatic insufficiency, consider dosage reduction or using alternative drugs.

Adverse Effects

Adverse effects reported in dogs and cats include gastroenteritis (emesis, loose stools, and infrequently bloody diarrhea in dogs). IM injections reportedly cause pain at the injection site. Rapid intravenous administration can cause hypotension and cardiopulmonary arrest.

Swine may develop gastrointestinal disturbances while receiving the medication.

Reproductive/Nursing Safety

Lincomycin crosses the placenta and cord blood concentrations are approximately 25% of those found in maternal serum. Safe use during pregnancy has not been established, but neither has the drug been implicated in causing teratogenic effects.

In humans, the FDA categorizes this drug as category *B* for use during pregnancy (*Animal studies have not yet demonstrated risk to the fetus, but there are no adequate studies in pregnant women; or animal studies have shown an adverse effect, but adequate studies in pregnant women have not demonstrated a risk to the fetus in the first trimester of pregnancy, and there is no evidence of risk in later trimesters.*) In a separate system evaluating the safety of drugs in canine and feline pregnancy (Papich 1989), this drug is categorized class: *A* (*Probably safe. Although specific studies may not have proved the safety of all drugs in dogs and cats, there are no reports of adverse effects in laboratory animals or women.*)

Because lincomycin is distributed into milk, nursing animals of mothers given lincomycin may develop diarrhea.

Overdosage/Acute Toxicity

There is little information available regarding overdoses of this drug. In dogs, oral doses of up to 300 mg/kg/day for up to one year or parenterally at 60 mg/kg/day apparently did not result in toxicity.

Drug Interactions

The following drug interactions have either been reported or are theoretical in humans or animals receiving lincomycin and may be of significance in veterinary patients. Unless otherwise noted, use together is not necessarily contraindicated, but weigh the potential risks and perform additional monitoring when appropriate.

- **CYCLOSPORINE**: Lincomycin may reduce levels.
- **ERYTHROMYCIN**: *In vitro* antagonism when used with lincomycin; concomitant use should probably be avoided.
- **KAOLIN**: Kaolin (found in several over-the-counter antidiarrheal preparations) has been shown to reduce the absorption of lincomycin by up to 90% if both are given concurrently; if both drugs are necessary, separate doses by at least 2 hours.
- **NEUROMUSCULAR BLOCKING AGENTS** (*e.g.*, **pancuronium**): Lincomycin possesses intrinsic neuromuscular blocking activity and should be used cautiously with other neuromuscular blocking agents.

Laboratory Considerations

- Slight increases in **liver function tests** (AST, ALT, Alk. Phosph.) may occur. There is apparently not any clinical significance associated with these increases.

Doses

- **DOGS:**

  For susceptible infections:

  Labeled dose (FDA-approved): <u>For the treatment of skin infections</u> (pustular dermatitis, abscesses, infected wounds [including bite and fight wounds]), <u>upper respiratory tract infections</u> (tonsillitis, laryngitis), <u>metritis, and secondary bacterial infections</u> associated with the canine distemper-hepatitis complex: 15.4 mg/kg PO q8h or 22 mg/kg PO q12h; 11 mg/kg q12h or 22 mg/kg q24h IV (diluted and administered as a slow infusion) or IM. (Adapted from label; *Lincocin®*) **Note:** Some have given it SC in an extra-label manner.

  Extra-label dose: <u>For pyoderma</u> (susceptible staphylococci):

20 – 25 mg/kg PO q12h. Some recommend up to 30 mg/kg PO q12h.

- **CATS:**

For susceptible infections

Labeled dose: (FDA-approved): For the treatment of localized infections, such as abscesses, pneumonitis, and feline rhinotracheitis: 15.4 mg/kg PO q8h or 22 mg/kg PO q12h; 11 mg/kg q12h or 22 mg/kg q24h IV (diluted and administered as a slow infusion) or IM. (Adapted from label; *Lincocin®*) **Note**: Some have given it SC in an extra-label manner.

Extra-label dose: For skin infections: Based on pharmacokinetic values and reported MIC's a dosage of 15 mg/kg PO q12h is supported for treating skin infections. (Albarellos *et al.* 2013)

- **FERRETS:**

For susceptible infections (extra-label): 10 – 15 mg/kg PO three times daily; 10 mg/kg IM twice daily. (Williams 2000)

- **SWINE:**

For susceptible infections:

a) **For mycoplasmal (*M. hyopneumoniae*) pneumonia**: Fed at 200 grams per ton of feed for 21 days or 11 mg/kg IM once daily (Amass 1999)

b) 11 mg/kg IM once daily for 3-7 days; or added to drinking water at a rate of 250 mg/gallon (average of 8.36 mg/kg/day). (Label directions; *Lincocin®*)

Monitoring

- Clinical efficacy.
- Adverse effects; particularly severe diarrheas.

Client Information

- Used for infections of skin, wounds, and bone.
- Report severe, continued, or bloody diarrhea to the veterinarian immediately.
- Do **NOT** give to horses, rabbits, mice, rats, hamsters, guinea pigs, cattle, sheep, goats or deer as it may cause fatal diarrhea.
- May give with or without food, but do not "dry pill" or it may cause throat burns. Give a small amount of food or a very small amount of water (little over a teaspoonful) after pilling.
- Very bitter taste; may require disguising in food to get animal to take it.

Chemistry/Synonyms

An antibiotic obtained from cultures of *Streptomyces lincolnensis*, lincomycin is available commercially as the monohydrate hydrochloride. It occurs as a white to off-white, crystalline powder that is freely soluble in water. The powder may have a faint odor and has a pK_a of 7.6. The commercially available injection has a pH of 3-5.5 and occurs as a clear to slightly yellow solution.

Lincomycin may also be as: U-10149, NSC-70731, *Lincomix®* or *Lincocin®*.

Storage/Stability

Lincomycin capsules, tablets and soluble powder should be stored at room temperature (15-30°C) in tight containers. Lincomycin injectable products should be stored at room temperature; avoid freezing.

Compatibility/Compounding Considerations

Lincomycin HCl for injection is reportedly physically **compatible** for at least 24 hours in the following IV infusion solutions and drugs: D_5W, D_5W in sodium chloride 0.9%, $D_{10}W$, sodium chloride 0.9%, Ringer's injection, amikacin sulfate, chloramphenicol sodium succinate, cimetidine HCl, cytarabine, heparin sodium, penicillin G potassium/sodium (4 hours only), polymyxin B sulfate, tetracycline HCl, and vitamin B-complex with C.

Drugs that are reportedly physically **incompatible** when mixed with lincomycin, data conflicts, or compatibility is concentration and/or time dependent include: ampicillin sodium, carbenicillin disodium, and phenytoin sodium. Compatibility is dependent upon factors such as pH, concentration, temperature and diluent used; consult specialized references or a hospital pharmacist for more specific information.

Dosage Forms/Regulatory Status

VETERINARY-LABELED PRODUCTS:

Lincomycin Oral Tablets: 100 mg, 200 mg, 500 mg; *Lincocin®*; (Rx). FDA-approved for use in dogs and cats.

Lincomycin Oral Solution: 50 mg/mL in 20 mL dropper bottles; *Lincocin® Aquadrops*; (Rx). FDA-approved for use in dogs and cats.

Lincomycin Sterile Injection: 100 mg/mL in 20 mL vials; *Lincocin®*; (Rx). FDA-approved for use in dogs and cats.

Lincomycin Sterile Injection: 25 mg/mL, 100 mg/mL & 300 mg/mL in 100 mL vials; FDA-approved for use in swine. Slaughter withdrawal (when used as labeled) = 48 hours. *Lincocin® Sterile Solution*, *Lincomix® Injectable*, generic; (OTC)

There are also several lincomycin combination feed/water additive products for use in swine and/or poultry.

HUMAN-LABELED PRODUCTS:

Lincomycin Injection: 300 mg (as hydrochloride)/mL in 2 mL & 10 mL vials; *Lincocin®*; (Rx)

Revisions/References

Monograph revised/updated March 2014.

Albarellos, G. A., et al. (2013). Pharmacokinetics and skin concentrations of lincomycin after intravenous and oral administration to cats. Journal of the South African Veterinary Association-Tydskrif Van Die Suid-Afrikaanse Veterinere Vereniging **84**(1).

Albarellos, G. A., et al. (2012). Pharmacokinetics and bone tissue concentrations of lincomycin following intravenous and intramuscular administrations to cats. J. Vet. Pharmacol. Ther. **35**(6): 534-40.

Amass, S. (1999). A review of mycoplasmal pneumonia. Proceedings: The North American Veterinary Conference, Orlando. accessed via Veterinary Information Network; vin.com

Papich, M. (1989). Effects of drugs on pregnancy. *Current Veterinary Therapy X: Small Animal Practice*. R. Kirk. Philadelphia, Saunders: 1291-9.

Williams, B. (2000). Therapeutics in Ferrets. Vet Clin NA: Exotic Anim Pract **3**:1(Jan): 131-53.

Liothyronine Sodium

(lye-oh-**thye**-roe-neen)

Triiodothyronine, Cytomel®, Triostat®

Thyroid Hormone

Prescriber Highlights

▶ Form of T3 (active thyroid hormone) used for hypothyroidism, but usually only when patients are unresponsive to levothyroxine; shorter duration of effect than levothyroxine.

▶ Also used in cats as part of the T3 suppression test for diagnosing hyperthyroidism.

Uses/Indications

Because of its shorter duration of effect (requires 3 times daily administration) and is more likely to cause iatrogenic hyperthyroidism, liothyronine is generally not recommended for treating hypothyroidism in dogs. On occasion, animals not responding to levothyroxine secondary to inadequate GI absorption, may respond to liothyronine. Liothyronine is not recommended for initial therapy because only serum T3 concentrations are normalized while T4 levels remain low.

In cats, liothyronine is used in the T3 suppression test for diagnosing hyperthyroidism.

Pharmacology/Actions

Thyroid hormones affect the rate of many physiologic processes including: fat, protein, and carbohydrate metabolism, increasing protein synthesis, increasing gluconeogenesis, and promoting mobilization and utilization of glycogen stores. Thyroid hormones also increase oxygen consumption, body temperature, heart rate and cardiac output, blood volume, enzyme system activity, and growth and maturity. Thyroid hormone is particularly important for adequate development of the central nervous system. While the exact mechanisms how thyroid hormones exert their effects are not well understood, it is known that thyroid hormones (primarily triiodothyronine) act at the cellular level.

In humans, triiodothyronine (T3) is the primary hormone responsible for activity. Approximately 80% of T3 found in the peripheral tissues is derived from thyroxine (T4) which is the principle hormone released by the thyroid.

Pharmacokinetics

In dogs, peak plasma levels of liothyronine occur 2-5 hours after oral dosing. The plasma half-life is approximately 5-6 hours. In contrast to levothyroxine, it is believed that liothyronine is nearly completely absorbed by dogs and absorption is not as affected by stomach contents, intestinal flora changes, etc.

Contraindications/Precautions/Warnings

Liothyronine (and other replacement thyroid hormones) are contraindicated in patients with acute myocardial infarction, thyrotoxicosis, or untreated adrenal insufficiency. It should be used with caution and at a lower initial dosage in patients with concurrent hypoadrenocorticism (treated), cardiac disease, diabetes, or in elderly patients.

Adverse Effects

When administered at an appropriate dose to patients requiring thyroid hormone replacement, there should not be any adverse effects associated with therapy. For adverse effects associated with overdosage, see below.

Reproductive/Nursing Safety

In humans, the FDA categorizes this drug as category *A* for use during pregnancy (*Adequate studies in pregnant women have not demonstrated a risk to the fetus in the first trimester of pregnancy, and there is no evidence of risk in later trimesters.*)

Minimal amounts of thyroid hormones are excreted in milk and should not adversely affect nursing offspring.

Overdosage/Acute Toxicity

Chronic overdosage will produce signs of hyperthyroidism, including tachycardia, polyphagia, PU/PD, excitability, nervousness, and excessive panting. Dosage should be reduced and/or temporarily withheld until signs subside. Some (10%?) cats may exhibit signs of "apathetic" (listlessness, anorexia, etc.) hyperthyroidism.

Acute massive overdosage can produce signs resembling thyroid storm. After oral ingestion, treatment to reduce absorption of drug should be accomplished using standard protocols (emetics or gastric lavage, cathartics, charcoal) unless contraindicated by the patient's condition. Treatment is supportive and symptomatic. Oxygen, artificial ventilation, cardiac glycosides, beta-blockers (*e.g.*, propranolol), fluids, dextrose, and antipyretic agents have all been suggested for use if necessary.

Drug Interactions

The following drug interactions have either been reported or are theoretical in humans or animals receiving liothyronine and may be of significance in veterinary patients. Unless otherwise noted, use together is not necessarily contraindicated, but weigh the potential risks and perform additional monitoring when appropriate.

- **ANTIDEPRESSANTS, TRICYCLIC/TETRACYCLIC:** Increased risk for CNS stimulation and cardiac arrhythmias.
- **ANTIDIABETIC AGENTS (insulin, oral agents):** Levothyroxine may increase requirements for insulin or oral agents.
- **CHOLESTYRAMINE:** May reduce liothyronine absorption; separate doses by 4 hours.
- **DIGOXIN:** Potential for reduced digoxin levels.
- **KETAMINE:** May cause tachycardia and hypertension.
- **SYMPATHOMIMETIC AGENTS (epinephrine, norepinephrine, etc.):** Levothyroxine can potentiate effects.
- **WARFARIN:** Thyroid hormones increase the catabolism of vitamin K-dependent clotting factors that may increase the anticoagulation effects in patients on warfarin.

Laboratory Considerations

Refer to the levothyroxine monograph for information and the T3 suppression test in the dosage section for cats.

Doses

- **DOGS:**

  For hypothyroidism (extra-label): Initial starting dose is 4 – 6 micrograms/kg PO q8h. Liothyronine is only indicated in those few situations when T4 supplementation has failed to achieve a response in a dog with confirmed hypothyroidism, perhaps due to impaired GI T4 absorption. Dogs receiving T3 supplementation may be more susceptible to iatrogenic thyrotoxicosis since serum T4 concentrations are important in the feedback regulation of the hypothalamic-pituitary-thyroid axis. Combination products that contain both T3 and T4 should be avoided for similar reasons. (Scott-Moncrieff, J. *et al.* 2000) (Scott-Moncrieff, J.C. 2009)

- **CATS:**

  T3 suppression test to diagnose hyperthyroidism (extra-label): Baseline T3 and T4 concentrations are measured. Liothyronine is then given at 25 micrograms per cat PO q8h for 7 doses. T3 and T4 concentrations are then measured again 2-6 hours after the last dose. In euthyroid cats, the 2nd T4 concentration should be less than 1.5 micrograms/dL or more than 50% lower than the baseline T4 concentration. Cats with hyperthyroidism fail to suppress. T3 concentrations are measured before and after T3 administration to confirm good client compliance and adequate absorption of the drug. (Scott-Moncrieff, J.C. 2012)

  For hypothyroidism (extra-label): Initially, 4.4 micrograms/kg PO 2-3 times a day. (Feldman *et al.* 1987)

Monitoring

- Similar to levothyroxine, but T4 levels will remain low. When monitoring T3 levels, draw serum just prior to dosing and again 2-4 hours after administering the drug.

Client Information

- Clients should be instructed in the importance of compliance with therapy as prescribed.
- Also, review the signs that can be seen with too much thyroid supplementation.

Chemistry/Synonyms

A synthetically prepared sodium salt of the naturally occurring hormone T3, liothyronine sodium occurs as an odorless, light tan crystalline powder. It is very slightly soluble in water and slightly soluble in alcohol. Each 25 micrograms of liothyronine is approximately equivalent to 60-65 mg (1 grain) of thyroglobulin or desiccated thyroid and 100 micrograms or less of levothyroxine.

Liothyronine sodium may also be known as: T3, T3 thyronine sodium, L-triiodothyronine, sodium L-triiodothyronine, liothyroninum natricum, sodium liothyronine, l-tri-iodothyronine sodium, 3,5,3'-Tri-iodo-L-thyronine sodium or *Cytomel®*.

Storage/Stability

Liothyronine tablets should be stored at room temperature (15-30°C) in tight containers.

The injection should be stored refrigerated (2-8°C).

Compatibility/Compounding Considerations

No specific information noted.

Dosage Forms/Regulatory Status

VETERINARY-LABELED PRODUCTS: NONE.

HUMAN-LABELED PRODUCTS:

Liothyronine Sodium Tablets: 5 mcg, 25 mcg & 50 mcg; *Cytomel®*, generic; (Rx)

Liothyronine Sodium Injection Solution: 10 micrograms/mL in 1 mL vials; *Triostat®*, generic; (Rx)

Revisions/References

Monograph revised/updated March 2014.

Feldman, E. C. & R. W. Nelson (1987). Hypothyroidism. *Canine and Feline Endocrinology and Reproduction.* Philadelphia, WB Saunders: 55-90.

Scott-Moncrieff, J. & L. Guptill-Yoran (2000). Hypothyroidism. *Textbook of Veterinary Internal Medicine: Diseases of the Dog and Cat.* S. Ettinger and E. Feldman. Philadelphia, WB Saunders. 2: 1419-29.

Scott-Moncrieff, J. C. (2009). Canine Hypothyroidism. Proceedings: WVC. accessed via Veterinary Information Network; vin.com

Scott-Moncrieff, J. C. (2012). Thyroid Disorders in the Geriatric Veterinary Patient. Veterinary Clinics of North America-Small Animal Practice 42(4): 707-+.

Lipid Emulsion, Intravenous — See Fat Emulsion, Intravenous

Lisinopril

(lye-**sin**-oh-pril)   Prinivil®, Zestril®

Angiotensin-Converting Enzyme (ACE) Inhibitor

Prescriber Highlights

▶ ACE inhibitor similar to enalapril or benazepril used primarily as a vasodilator in the treatment of heart failure or hypertension; may also be of benefit in the treatment of chronic renal failure or protein losing nephropathies.

▶ May be less expensive than other ACE inhibitors & possibly can be dosed once daily. When compared to enalapril and benazepril, not as much information available or clinical experience for dogs or cats.

▶ Caution: Renal insufficiency (doses may need to be reduced), patients with hyponatremia, coronary or cerebrovascular insufficiency, preexisting hematologic abnormalities, or a collagen vascular disease (*e.g.*, SLE).

▶ Adverse Effects: GI distress (anorexia, vomiting, diarrhea); Potentially: weakness, hypotension, renal dysfunction, & hyperkalemia.

Uses/Indications

The principle uses of lisinopril in veterinary medicine at present are as a vasodilator in the treatment of heart failure or hypertension. Recent studies have demonstrated that ACE inhibitors, particularly when used in conjunction with furosemide, do improve the quality of life in dogs with heart failure. It is not clear, however, whether it has any significant effect on survival times. Lisinopril may also be of benefit in treating the effects associated with valvular heart disease (mitral regurgitation) and left to right shunts. It is being explored as adjunctive treatment in chronic renal failure and protein losing nephropathies.

Lisinopril may have advantages over other ACE inhibitors in that it may be dosed once daily and is less expensive. Disadvantages are that it is only available in human labeled dosage forms and there is

much less published information on its use (efficacy, safety, dosing) in veterinary species.

Pharmacology/Actions

Unlike enalapril, lisinopril does not need to be converted in the liver to an active metabolite. Lisinopril prevents the formation of angiotensin-II (a potent vasoconstrictor) by competing with angiotensin-I for the enzyme angiotensin-converting enzyme (ACE). ACE has a much higher affinity for lisinopril than for angiotensin-I. Because angiotensin-II concentrations are decreased, aldosterone secretion is reduced and plasma renin activity is increased. Lisinopril has a higher affinity for ACE than either enalaprilat or captopril.

The cardiovascular effects of lisinopril in patients with CHF include decreased total peripheral resistance, pulmonary vascular resistance, mean arterial and right atrial pressures, and pulmonary capillary wedge pressure, no change or decrease in heart rate, and increased cardiac index and output, stroke volume, and exercise tolerance. Renal blood flow can be increased with little change in hepatic blood flow. In animals with glomerular disease, ACE inhibitors probably decrease proteinuria and help to preserve renal function.

Pharmacokinetics

In dogs, lisinopril's bioavailability ranges from 25-50% with peak levels occurring ≈4 hours after dosing. Lisinopril is distributed poorly into the CNS. It is unknown if it is distributed into maternal milk, but it does cross the placenta. Half-lives are increased in patients with renal failure or severe CHF. Duration of action in dogs has been described as being 24 hours, but effects tend to drop off with time.

No information was located for cats.

Contraindications/Precautions/Warnings

Lisinopril is contraindicated in patients who have demonstrated hypersensitivity to the ACE inhibitors. It should be used with caution and close supervision in patients with renal insufficiency and doses may need to be reduced.

Lisinopril should be used with caution in patients with hyponatremia or sodium depletion, coronary or cerebrovascular insufficiency, preexisting hematologic abnormalities, or a collagen vascular disease (*e.g.*, SLE). Patients with severe CHF should be monitored very closely upon initiation of therapy.

Adverse Effects

Lisinopril's adverse effect profile in dogs is reportedly similar to other ACE inhibitors, principally GI distress (anorexia, vomiting, diarrhea). Potentially, cough, weakness, hypotension, renal dysfunction, and hyperkalemia could occur. Because it lacks a sulfhydryl group (unlike captopril), there is less likelihood that immune-mediated reactions will occur, but rashes, neutropenia, and agranulocytosis have been reported in humans.

Reproductive/Nursing Safety

Lisinopril crosses the placenta. High doses in rodents have caused decreased fetal weights and increases in fetal and maternal death rates; teratogenic effects have not been reported.

Current recommendations for humans are to discontinue ACE inhibitors as soon as pregnancy is detected. In humans, the FDA categorizes this drug as category *C* for use during the 1st trimester of pregnancy (*Animal studies have shown an adverse effect on the fetus, but there are no adequate studies in humans; or there are no animal reproduction studies and no adequate studies in humans.*) In humans, the FDA categorizes this drug as category *D* for use during the 2nd and 3rd trimesters of pregnancy (*There is evidence of human fetal risk, but the potential benefits from the use of the drug in pregnant women may be acceptable despite its potential risks.*)

It is not known whether lisinopril is excreted in milk; use with caution.

Overdosage/Acute Toxicity

The ASPCA Animal Poison Control Center (APCC) has over 3500 lisinopril exposure cases in its files, mostly involving dogs, but some birds and cats. The lowest dosage documented to cause hypotension in dogs is 27 mg/kg. Generally dosages below 20 mg/kg cause mild signs only, most commonly vomiting and lethargy. Higher dosages warrant decontamination. Only a single cat out of 218 cats developed hypotension at a dosage of 4.9 mg/kg. In birds, only mild somnolence occurred at 41 mg/kg.

There were 1882 single agent exposures to lisinopril reported to the ASPCA Animal Poison Control Center (APCC) during 2009-2013. There were 1781 dogs exposed and 156 that became symptomatic. The most common clinical signs included: lethargy (24%), tachycardia (18%), vomiting (14%) and hypotension (13%). Of the 98 cats, 7 were symptomatic with 29% hypertensive, 29% tachycardic and 29% vomiting.

In overdose situations, the primary concern is hypotension; supportive treatment with volume expansion with normal saline is recommended to correct blood pressure. Because of the drug's long duration of action, prolonged monitoring and treatment may be required. Recent overdoses should be managed using gut-emptying protocols when warranted.

Drug Interactions

The following drug interactions have either been reported or are theoretical in humans or animals receiving lisinopril and may be of significance in veterinary patients. Unless otherwise noted, use together is not necessarily contraindicated, but weigh the potential risks and perform additional monitoring when appropriate.

- **ANTIDIABETIC AGENTS (insulin, oral agents):** Possible increased risk for hypoglycemia; enhanced monitoring recommended.
- **DIURETICS** (*e.g.,* **furosemide, hydrochlorothiazide):** Potential for increased hypotensive effects.
- **DIURETICS, POTASSIUM-SPARING** (*e.g.,* **spironolactone, triamterene):** Increased hyperkalemic effects, enhanced monitoring of serum potassium recommended.
- **HYPOTENSIVE AGENTS, OTHER:** Potential for increased hypotensive effect.
- **LITHIUM:** Increased serum lithium levels possible; increased monitoring required.
- **NSAIDS:** May reduce the anti-hypertensive or positive hemodynamic effects of lisinopril; may increase risk for reduced renal function.
- **POTASSIUM SUPPLEMENTS:** Increased risk for hyperkalemia.

Laboratory Considerations

- ACE inhibitors may cause a reversible decrease in localization and excretion of **iodohippurate sodium** I^{123}/I^{134}, or **Technetium Tc^{99}** pententate renal imaging in the affected kidney in patients with renal artery stenosis, that may lead to confusion in test interpretation.

Doses

- **DOGS:**

   For adjunctive treatment of heart failure or for other uses when an ACE inhibitor is indicated: Because PK/PD studies have not confirmed that lisinopril can be given once daily in dogs, it may need to be dosed twice daily similarly to enalapril. Suggested dosages usually are 0.5 mg/kg PO 1-2 times daily.

- **CATS:**

   For adjunctive treatment of heart failure or for other uses when an ACE inhibitor is indicated: Dosage is not well established or supported by published evidence: 0.25 – 0.5 mg/kg PO once daily has been suggested.

Monitoring

- Clinical signs of CHF.
- Serum electrolytes, creatinine, BUN, urine protein.
- CBC with differential, periodic.
- Blood pressure (if treating hypertension or signs associated with hypotension arise).

Client Information

- Lisinopril is used to treat heart failure, high blood pressure and some forms of kidney disease in dogs and cats.
- Usually well tolerated, but vomiting and diarrhea can occur. Give with food if vomiting or lack of appetite becomes a problem. If a rash or signs of infection occur (*e.g.,* fever) contact your veterinarian immediately.
- Very important to give lisinopril as prescribed. Do not stop or reduce dosage without veterinarian's guidance.
- Your animal will likely need to have blood pressure and lab tests performed while receiving lisinopril.

Chemistry/Synonyms

An oral angiotensin-converting enzyme inhibitor (ACE inhibitor) lisinopril is directly active and not a prodrug like enalapril. It occurs as a white crystalline powder. One mg is soluble in 10 mL of water; 70 mL of methanol. It is practically insoluble in alcohol, chloroform, or ether.

Lisinopril may also be known as: L-154826, lisinoprilum, and MK-521; many trade names are available.

Storage/Stability

Store lisinopril tablets at room temperature in tight containers, unless otherwise directed by manufacturer.

Compatibility/Compounding Considerations

Compounded preparation stability: Lisinopril oral suspension compounded from the commercially available tablets has been published (Nahata *et al.* 2004). Triturating ten (10) lisinopril 10 mg tablets with 50 mL of *Ora Plus®* and qs ad to 100 mL with *Ora Sweet®* yields a 1 mg/mL lisinopril oral suspension that retains >95% potency for 91 days when stored at 4°C and protected from light.

Dosage Forms/Regulatory Status

VETERINARY-LABELED PRODUCTS: NONE.

The ARCI (Racing Commissioners International) has designated this drug as a class 3 substance. See the appendix for more information.

HUMAN-LABELED PRODUCTS:

Lisinopril Oral Tablets: 2.5 mg, 5 mg, 10 mg, 20 mg, 30 mg & 40 mg; *Prinivil®, Zestril®*; (Rx)

Also available are fixed dose combinations of lisinopril with hydrochlorothiazide.

Revisions/References

Monograph revised/updated March 2014.

Nahata, M. C. & R. S. Morosco (2004). Stability of lisinopril in two liquid dosage forms. Ann Pharmacother 38(3): 396-9.

Lithium Carbonate
Lithium Citrate

(lith-ee-um)   Eskalith®, Lithobid®

Hematopoietic; Antimanic

Prescriber Highlights

▶ Lithium could potentially help treat anemia and/or neutropenia in dogs. Little information is known about usage in veterinary medicine and the potential risk for toxicity is quite high.

▶ NOT recommended for use in cats.

▶ Dosed orally in dogs, usually twice per day.

▶ Monitoring lithium levels is mandatory. Adverse effects are usually GI, renal or CNS-related and associated with higher serum levels.

Uses/Indications

In dogs, lithium may be useful in treating neutropenia or anemia secondary to bone marrow depressant drugs (estrogens, chemotherapy drugs, etc.). Very limited information is published for use of lithium in dogs and its efficacy and safety are not well understood in canine patients.

Cases of possible successful lithium treatment of dogs with estrogen-induced anemia have been reported. A small (5 dogs) uncontrolled study of dogs with pure red cell aplasia demonstrated that lithium could have assisted remission in 2 dogs (Trehy *et al.* 2011).

In a small, preliminary study in dogs with lomustine-induced myelosuppression, the 2 dogs treated with lithium did not show efficacy but did have lithium-associated adverse effects (Abrams-Ogg 2011). In a similar study in clinically normal dogs, lithium did stimulate thrombocyte formation, but did not significantly affect carboplatin-induced thrombocytopenia (Leclerc *et al.* 2010).

Use of lithium carbonate for the adjunctive treatment of dogs with immune-mediated thrombocytopenia or immune-mediated hemolytic anemia has been described as "not recommended...while lithium carbonate is inexpensive, significant effect is unlikely, lithium levels must be monitored, and there is significant potential for serious side effects."(Abrams-Ogg 2012)

In humans, lithium's primary uses have been for treating bipolar disorder (maintenance and manic episodes) and for augmenting antidepressants. It has also been used to treat anemia or neutropenia secondary to antineoplastic drugs but this is still controversial, and some claim that although it increases white blood cells, effect on outcome is variable. Lithium has also been used, primarily in the past, for the treatment of inappropriate secretion of antidiuretic hormone (SIADH).

Pharmacology/Actions

Lithium competes at a variety of cellular sites with sodium, potassium, calcium, and magnesium ions. At cell membranes, lithium passes through sodium channels and can block potassium channels at high concentrations. It has a variety of effects in the CNS, but the mechanisms for its anti-manic and antidepressant actions in humans are not well understood.

Lithium can stimulate production of red cells, neutrophils and platelets. The exact mechanisms for these effects are not fully understood, but are probably secondary to direct stimulation of hematopoietic cells and enhanced activity of hematopoietic colony-stimulating factors. In humans, lithium-induced leukocytosis peaks within 7-10 days of initiating therapy and the WBC count will return to baseline 7-10 days after discontinuing lithium.

Pharmacokinetics

After oral administration of lithium carbonate (powder in gelatin capsules) to mixed breed-dogs mean bioavailability was ≈80%, but there was wide inter-subject variability (2 of the 8 dogs had bioavailability values of 26% and 39%). Half-life was around 21 hours. The authors concluded that based upon the kinetics data from the study that a dosage schedule of 12.24 mg/kg q12h should maintain serum lithium concentrations in the desired range of serum lithium concentrations of 0.8 – 1.5 mEq/L (Rosenthal *et al.* 1986). The same authors also did a pharmacokinetic study in purpose-bred beagles and found similar steady-state volumes of distribution (approx. 0.6 L/kg), but significantly different elimination rate constants and half-lives (11.2 hours) in beagles (Rosenthal *et al.* 1989).

No information on the pharmacokinetics of extended-release tablets in dogs was located.

In humans, oral bioavailability of lithium carbonate capsules, conventional tablets and lithium citrate solutions is nearly complete. Extended-release tablets are 60-90% absorbed. Food does affect oral bioavailability. Lithium is not bound to plasma proteins and is widely distributed in the body, including into bone, eye, CNS, erythrocytes and thyroid tissue. It freely crosses the placenta and milk concentrations are approximately 50% of what is found in the plasma. Lithium is not metabolized and elimination of absorbed drug is primarily via renal mechanisms. Elimination half-life in healthy adults is around 24 hours. Half-life in patients with impaired renal function and the elderly can be significantly prolonged (40-50 hours). It can be removed by hemodialysis, but not peritoneal dialysis.

Contraindications/Precautions/Warnings

For canine patients, contraindications to lithium have not been well delineated. For humans, the FDA-approved label has the following Black Box Warning: "Lithium toxicity is closely related to serum lithium levels, and can occur at doses close to therapeutic levels. Facilities for prompt and accurate serum lithium determinations should be available before initiating therapy." As there is a very high risk for lithium toxicity, lithium is contraindicated or relatively contraindicated in humans with significant renal or cardiovascular disease, severe debilitation, dehydration, sodium depletion, or concomitant therapy with diuretics. Because lithium can decrease thyroid hormone synthesis it should be used with caution in dogs with low thyroid levels.

Anything that affects water balance can quickly cause lithium problems. Dehydration from any cause must be avoided.

Adverse Effects

In dogs, lithium's adverse effect profile and its relationship to serum lithium concentrations is not well known. In limited published information the following have been reported when dogs were receiving lithium (causation not proved): diarrhea, hypersalivation/ptyalism, seizures, increased liver enzymes, and polyuria/polydipsia with changes in urine specific gravity.

In humans, lithium has the potential for a litany of adverse effects but most are dose-related and usually involve CNS/Neuromuscular, GI tract, and kidneys. More rarely, cardiovascular effects can occur (*e.g.,* bradycardia). Steady-state 12-hour post-dose serum concentrations of 1 mEq/L or greater are most commonly associated with adverse effects. Gastrointestinal effects (nausea, vomiting, anorexia, abdominal pain, etc.) are the most commonly reported adverse effects and are usually mild and may be reduced by giving with food, changing dosage forms or altering dosage administration strategy (*e.g.,* dividing dose). The most common renal effect is a nephrogenic diabetes insipidus manifesting as polyuria/polydipsia (night time urination may be an early sign). The most commonly reported central nervous system and neuromuscular effects include lethargy/fatigue, confusion, muscle weakness and tremor.

Reproductive/Nursing Safety

In humans, the FDA categorizes lithium as category *D* for use during pregnancy (*There is evidence of human fetal risk, but the potential benefits from the use of the drug in pregnant women may be acceptable despite its potential risks.*) and its use in pregnant animals cannot be recommended.

Lithium is distributed into milk and either nursing or the drug should be discontinued.

Overdosage/Acute Toxicity

Acute toxicity of lithium is usually less severe than chronic toxicity but depending on the amount ingested, lithium overdoses can still be extremely serious and mortality has been reported in humans. Often the initial signs on presentation are not attributed to lithium ingestion. It is recommended that any overdose situation be evaluated and managed in conjunction with an animal poison control center.

There were 189 single agent exposures to lithium reported to the ASPCA Animal Poison Control Center (APCC) during 2009-2013. Of the 155 dogs, 36 were symptomatic with 61% vomiting and 33% lethargic. Of the 35 cats, 9 were symptomatic with 67% vomiting.

Serum levels above 3 (some say 2.5) mEq/L are considered a medical emergency in humans. Activated charcoal is not effective in binding lithium in the gut, but sodium polystyrene sulfonate (SPS; *Kayexalate®*) can reduce the absorption of lithium. Hemodialysis and/or forced alkaline diuresis may be considered to increase renal excretion.

Lithium-containing button-type battery ingestion can be very serious. After 30 minutes of contact, one 3-volt battery can cause severe necrosis in the gastrointestinal tract. It is highly recommended that a veterinary poison center be immediately consulted when lithium-containing batteries are ingested.

Drug Interactions

The following drug interactions have either been reported or are theoretical in humans or animals receiving lithium and may be of significance in veterinary patients. Unless otherwise noted, use together is not necessarily contraindicated, but weigh the potential risks and perform additional monitoring when appropriate.

- **ACE INHIBITORS** (*e.g.*, **enalapril, benazepril**): Increased lithium levels possible, avoid using together or increase lithium level monitoring.
- **BETA-BLOCKERS:** May mask lithium-induced tremor (an early sign of toxicity in some patients) and have additional bradycardic effects in patents with lithium toxicity induced bradycardia.
- **CALCIUM-CHANNEL BLOCKERS** (*e.g.*, **diltiazem, verapamil**): May decrease lithium levels and/or increase lithium's toxic effects; increased monitoring recommended.
- **DIURETICS:** Not all diuretics affect lithium renal clearance equally. Lithium serum concentrations are likely to decrease with osmotic diuretics and carbonic anhydrase inhibitors, increase with thiazides, and unlikely to change with loop diuretics (*e.g.*, furosemide), but any effect on water balance can cause lithium toxicity.
- **IODIDE:** Could potentiate hypothyroid effect.
- **METRONIDAZOLE:** Could increase lithium levels.
- **NON-STEROIDAL ANTIINFLAMMATORY DRUGS (NSAIDs):** Increased lithium levels possible.
- **OPIATES:** Could reduce opiate analgesic effects.
- **SELECTIVE SEROTONIN-REUPTAKE INHIBITORS (SSRIs):** Possibility for increased risk of serotonin syndrome or increased lithium levels; avoid use together or increase monitoring. In human medicine, lithium and SSRI's are often used together to augment antidepressant action and serotonin syndrome does

not commonly occur, but early clinical signs (*e.g.*, myoclonus/muscle contractions) for it are still monitored.
- **SODIUM:** Sodium intake can significantly alter lithium renal clearance. Increased sodium intake can increase lithium renal clearance (and reduce serum levels) and decreased sodium intake can decrease clearance (and increase serum levels).
- **THEOPHYLLINE:** May increase urinary excretion and decrease lithium serum levels.
- **URINARY ALKALINIZERS** (*e.g.*, **sodium bicarbonate, potassium/sodium citrate**): Can increase renal clearance of lithium.

Laboratory Considerations

- **Serum or urinary sodium.** Lithium can falsely elevate serum and/or urinary sodium values when using some analyzers (Microlyte—Kone OY; Electrolyte 2-Beckman). A 1 mEq/L lithium serum level can increase serum sodium by 2.8 mEq/L. Inform the laboratory doing the testing that the patient is receiving lithium when submitting samples for sodium determination.

Dosages

- **DOGS:**

To stimulate hematopoiesis: 10 – 11 mg/kg PO q12h using conventional tablets or capsules. There can be significant interpatient variability in dosage requirements to achieve 'therapeutic' yet non-toxic serum levels; serum concentration monitoring is required to adjust dosage and reduce chances for toxicity (see Monitoring). While potentially the extended-release tablets could be used, no information was located on their use in dogs. **Note:** Switching between oral tablets (lithium carbonate) and liquid forms (lithium citrate) requires dosage conversion as different drug concentration systems are used. Lithium carbonate uses mg/tablet and lithium citrate is expressed in mEq/mL. They are **NOT** interchangeable. If using lithium citrate solution, convert lithium carbonate dosage to mEq of lithium (1 mg lithium carbonate = 0.027 mEq lithium) and convert to an equivalent amount of solution. Commercially available lithium citrate solution contains 1.6 mEq lithium/mL (*e.g.*, Dosing a 13.6 kg/dog at 11 mg/kg would give an approximate lithium carbonate dosage of 150 mg which is 4.06 mEq of lithium and approximately equivalent to 2.5 mLs of oral lithium citrate solution.)

Monitoring

- **Lithium serum levels.** The optimal lithium serum/plasma concentration to stimulate hematopoiesis in dogs (or other species) is unknown, but one review article on estrogen-induced myelotoxicity in dogs suggested that therapeutic levels were 0.5-1.8 mmol/L (0.5-1.8 mEq/L) and that serum/plasma levels be monitored weekly (Sontas *et al.* 2009). However, it should be noted that in humans, serum concentrations above 1.5 mEq/L are regularly associated with signs of toxicity and patients that are more sensitive to lithium (*e.g.*, elderly humans) may exhibit signs of toxicity at serum levels of 1 mEq/L. Lithium levels are usually measured at the 'trough' approximately 12 hours (± 2 hours) after the previous dose, but blood draws should be the same approximate time after a dose to reduce variability. Clients must be forewarned not to give the AM dose if an AM lithium level is scheduled.
- Complete blood counts/platelets to determine efficacy.
- Renal function (serum creatinine; BUN), initially and ongoing, particularly if treatment is prolonged.
- Consider monitoring baseline and ongoing urine specific gravity.
- Serum sodium. Alterations in serum sodium can affect lithium clearance.
- Adverse effects/toxicity.

Client Information

- Lithium must be given 2 times a day (and sometimes more often); to prevent the chance for stomach upset it is best to give with food.
- Lithium blood levels and side effects can be affected by 'water balance' in your dog. Be sure your dog has access to clean water at all times. Anything that affects your dog's ability to drink adequate water or causes increased need for larger amounts of water (like fever, diarrhea, high temperatures) should be reported to your veterinarian right away.
- Lithium can be very toxic if dosages are too high; lithium blood levels must be measured to determine the best dose. So that your veterinarian can best use the information from these blood tests, all prescribed doses must be given. Tell your veterinarian if you have missed giving some doses (and when the last dose was given before this visit for blood test) so that they can decide whether to do the blood test.
- If your veterinarian has prescribed an extended-release tablet it should be given whole; do not crush, or split the tablet and do not allow your dog to chew it.
- Lithium is not used very often in dogs so let your veterinarian know about any side effects you notice.

Chemistry/Synonyms

Lithium carbonate (CAS registry: 554-13-2; ATC:N05AN01) occurs as a white or almost white, odorless, granular powder. It is sparingly soluble in water and very slightly soluble in alcohol. Lithium carbonate dissolves, with effervescence, in dilute mineral acids. One gram of lithium carbonate contains 27 mEq of lithium (1 mg = 0.027 mEq).

Lithium Citrate (CAS Registry: 6080-58-6) occurs as a crystalline powder that has a slight saline taste. It is very soluble in water and practically insoluble in alcohol. One gram of anhydrous lithium citrate contains approximately 14.3 mEq of lithium (1 mg ≈ 0.0143 mEq). Lithium citrate oral solution has a pH of 4-5.

Lithium carbonate may also be known as carbonic acid dilithium salt, dilithium carbonate, CP-15467-61, or NSC-169895. It has been marketed under a variety of trade names including *Eskalith*®, *Lithobid*®, and *Lithonate*®.

Storage/Stability

Lithium carbonate capsules, tablets and extended-release tablets should be stored at room temperature of 25°C (77° F); excursions are permitted between 15-30°C (59-86°F). Protect from moisture.

Compatibility/Compounding Considerations

No specific information noted.

Dosage Forms/Regulatory Status

VETERINARY-LABELED PRODUCTS: NONE.

HUMAN-LABELED PRODUCTS:

Lithium Carbonate Oral Tablets: 300 mg (8.12 mEq of lithium); generic (Rx)

Lithium Carbonate Oral Capsules: 150 mg (4.06 mEq of lithium), 300 mg (8.12 mEq of lithium), 600 mg (14.24 mEq of lithium); generic; (Rx)

Lithium Carbonate Extended-Release (ER) Tablets: 300 mg (8.12 mEq of lithium), 450 mg (12.8 mEq of lithium); *Lithobid*®, generic; (Rx)

Lithium Citrate Oral Solution 8 mEq/5mL (1.6 mEq/mL); generic; (Rx)

Revisions/References

Monograph written August 2013.

Abrams-Ogg, A. C. G. (2011). The use of lithium carbonate to prevent lomustine-induced myelosuppression in dogs: A pilot study. Canadian Journal of Veterinary Research-Revue Canadienne De Recherche Veterinaire 75(1): 73-6.

Abrams-Ogg, A. C. G. (2012). Standard-of-Care for Treatment of Immune-Mediated Hemolytic Anemia and Immune-Mediated Thrombocytopenia in Dogs. 64th Convention of the Canadian Veterinary Medical Association. accessed via Veterinary Information Network; vin.com

Leclerc, A., et al. (2010). Effects of lithium carbonate on carboplatin-induced thrombocytopenia in dogs. American Journal of Veterinary Research 71(5): 555-63.

Rosenthal, R. C. & G. D. Koritz (1989). Pharmacokinetics of Lithium in Beagles. J. Vet. Pharmacol. Ther. 12(3): 330-3.

Rosenthal, R. C., et al. (1986). Pharmacokinetics of Lithium in the Dog. J. Vet. Pharmacol. Ther. 9(1): 81-7.

Sontas, H. B., et al. (2009). Estrogen-induced myelotoxicity in dogs: A review. Canadian Veterinary Journal-Revue Veterinaire Canadienne 50(10): 1054-8.

Trehy, M., et al. (2011). The Use of Lithium Carbonate in the Treatment of Pure Red Cell Aplasia in Dogs: 5 Cases (2006-2010). British Small Animal Veterinary Congress. accessed via Veterinary Information Network; vin.com

Lomustine (CCNU)

(loe-**mus**-teen)   CeeNu®

Oral Antineoplastic

Prescriber Highlights

▶ Oral antineoplastic usually used for CNS neoplasms, mast cell tumors, histiocytic sarcomas or as a rescue agent for lymphoma protocol (LOPP, LOPP-UF).

▶ Cautions (risk vs. benefit): Anemia, bone marrow depression, pulmonary function impairment, current infection, impaired renal function, sensitivity to lomustine, or patients that have received previous chemotherapy or radiotherapy.

▶ Adverse Effects: GI effects (anorexia, vomiting, diarrhea)—more so in dogs, stomatitis, alopecia, corneal de-epithelization, &, rarely, renal toxicity, hepatotoxicity—more so in dogs, & pulmonary infiltrates or fibrosis. Most serious: bone marrow depression (anemia, thrombocytopenia, leukopenia); nadirs in dogs generally occur ≈1-3 weeks after treatment.

▶ Teratogenic.

Uses/Indications

Lomustine may be useful in the adjunctive treatment of CNS neoplasms, lymphomas, and mast cell tumors in dogs and cats. Lomustine is usually dosed in a pulse fashion (higher dose every 2-6 weeks depending on the protocol), but metronomic (low dose, daily) dosing potentially could be useful in dogs that do not have other standard-care treatment options (Tripp *et al.* 2011).

Pharmacology/Actions

While lomustine's mechanism of action is not totally understood, it is believed it acts as an alkylating agent; however, other mechanisms such as carbamoylation and cellular protein modification may be involved; net effects are DNA and RNA synthesis inhibition. Lomustine is cell cycle-phase nonspecific.

Cross-resistance may occur between lomustine and carmustine.

Pharmacokinetics

Lomustine is absorbed rapidly and extensively from the GI tract and some absorption occurs after topical administration. Lomustine or its active metabolites are widely distributed in the body. While lomustine is not detected in the CSF, its active metabolites are detected in substantial concentrations. Lomustine is metabolized extensively in the liver to both active and inactive metabolites that are then eliminated primarily in the urine. Lomustine half-life in humans is very short (≈15 minutes), but its biologic activity is significantly longer due to the longer elimination times of active metabolites.

Contraindications/Precautions/Warnings
Lomustine should be used only when its potential benefits outweigh its risks with the following conditions: anemia, bone marrow depression, pulmonary function impairment, current infection, impaired renal function, sensitivity to lomustine, or patients who have received previous chemotherapy or radiotherapy.

Adverse Effects
Lomustine treatment can cause fatal adverse effects, particularly when used at higher dosages and for prolonged treatment periods. The most serious adverse effects are bone marrow depression (anemia, thrombocytopenia, leukopenia) and hepatotoxicity. CBC nadirs in dogs generally occur ≈1-2 weeks, but can range from 1-6 weeks after treatment has begun. In dogs, lomustine may cause delayed, cumulative dose-related, chronic, irreversible hepatotoxicity (Kristal *et al.* 2004). Neutropenia in cats (nadir is variable, usually 1-4 weeks but can range from 1-6 weeks) is usually the dose-limiting factor for lomustine, however, there is apparently significant interpatient variation in cats for dosage toleration. While neutropenia is relatively common, secondary infections or sepsis is relatively uncommon.

Because some rat studies have shown that alpha-lipoic acid may reduce the incidence/severity of hepatotoxicity associated with some chemotherapeutic agents, alpha-lipoic acid (5 mg/kg PO q12h) has been used in some treatment protocols using lomustine (Fahey *et al.* 2011). There is also a report using SAMe and silymarin (*Denamarin*®) for the same purpose (Skorupski *et al.* 2011; Vandeweerd *et al.* 2013) but that study was criticized as having significant limitations (Vandeweerd *et al.* 2013). Hepatotoxicity reportedly is less common in cats than in dogs (Musser *et al.* 2012).

Other potential adverse effects include GI effects (anorexia, vomiting, diarrhea), stomatitis, alopecia, corneal de-epithelization and, rarely, renal toxicity and pulmonary infiltrates or fibrosis. GI effects are more commonly seen in dogs than in cats.

A retrospective study of 185 dogs receiving lomustine reported following adverse effect incidences: neutropenia (57%), increased ALT (49%), GI toxicosis (38%; approximately two-thirds of that percentage was due to vomiting), anemia (34%), thrombocytopenia (14%), azotemia (12%), and hepatic failure (1.2%). The authors concluded that lomustine-induced toxicity is common in dogs, but usually is not life-threatening (Heading *et al.* 2011).

Reproductive/Nursing Safety
Lomustine is a teratogen in lab animals. Use only during pregnancy when the benefits to the mother outweigh the risks to the offspring. Lomustine can suppress gonadal function. In humans, the FDA categorizes this drug as category *D* for use during pregnancy (*There is evidence of human fetal risk, but the potential benefits from the use of the drug in pregnant women may be acceptable despite its potential risks.*)

Lomustine and its metabolites have been detected in maternal milk. Nursing puppies should receive milk replacer when the bitch is receiving lomustine.

Overdosage/Acute Toxicity
No specific information was located. Because of the potential toxicity of the drug, overdoses should be treated aggressively with gut emptying protocols employed when possible. For further information, refer to an animal poison control center.

Drug Interactions
The following drug interactions have either been reported or are theoretical in humans or animals receiving lomustine and may be of significance in veterinary patients. Unless otherwise noted, use together is not necessarily contraindicated, but weigh the potential risks and perform additional monitoring when appropriate.

- **IMMUNOSUPPRESSIVE DRUGS, OTHER** (*e.g.*, **azathioprine, cyclophosphamide, corticosteroids**): Use with other immunosuppressant drugs may increase the risk of infection.
- **MYELOSUPPRESSIVE DRUGS, OTHER** (*e.g.*, **chloramphenicol, flucytosine, amphotericin B**, or **colchicine**): The principal concern with lomustine is with its concurrent use with other drugs that are also myelosuppressive, including many of the other antineoplastics and bone marrow depressant drugs. Bone marrow depression may be additive.
- **VACCINES, LIVE VIRUS:** Live virus vaccines should be used with caution, if at all, during lomustine therapy.

Doses
Note: Because of the potential toxicity of this drug to patients, veterinary personnel and clients, and since chemotherapy indications, treatment protocols, monitoring and safety guidelines often change, the following dosages should be used only as a general guide. Consultation with a veterinary oncologist and referral to current veterinary oncology references [*e.g.*, (Withrow *et al.* 2012); (Dobson *et al.* 2011); (Henry *et al.* 2009); (North *et al.* 2009); (Argyle *et al.* 2008)] are strongly recommended.

- **DOGS/CATS**

    The following is a usual dose or dose range for this drug and should be used only as a general guide: Depending on the indication and protocol, lomustine is usually dosed in dogs from 50 – 90 mg/m² (**NOT** mg/kg) every 2-6 weeks and in cats at 40 – 60 mg/m² every 3-6 weeks or as a single 10 mg dose every 3 weeks. All dosages are extra-label use.

Monitoring
- CBC with platelets one week after dosing and prior to next dose; if platelets less than 200,000/mcL; stop therapy until thrombocytopenia is resolved.
- Biochem (including liver function indicators), baseline and before each treatment (especially in dogs).

Client Information
- Lomustine is a chemotherapy (cancer) drug. The drug and its byproducts can be hazardous to other animals and people that come in contact with it. On the day your animal gets the drug and then for a few days afterward, all bodily waste (urine, feces, litter), blood, or vomit should only be handled while wearing disposable gloves. Seal the waste in a plastic bag and then place both the bag and gloves in with the regular trash.
- Liver and bone marrow toxicity are possible; contact veterinarian immediately if patient develops an infection, runs a fever, bleeds, has yellowing of the whites of the eyes, has persistent vomiting or becomes ill.
- Lomustine may cause severe lung damage.

Chemistry/Synonyms
A nitrosourea derivative alkylating agent, lomustine occurs as a yellow powder that is practically insoluble in water and soluble in alcohol.

Lomustine may also be known as: CCNU, lomustinum, NSC-79037, RB-1509, WR-139017, and *CeeNu*®.

Storage/Stability
Store capsules in well-closed containers at room temperature. Expiration dates of 2 years are assigned after manufacture.

Compatibility/Compounding Considerations
Precautions (*e.g.*, biological safety cabinet) must be taken to avoid exposure from capsule contents when compounding dosage forms from commercially available capsules.

Dosage Forms/Regulatory Status
VETERINARY-LABELED PRODUCTS: NONE.

Lomustine Capsules: 10 mg, 40 mg & 100 mg with mannitol; generic; (Rx)

Revisions/References

Monograph revised/updated March 2014.

Argyle, D., et al. (2008). *Decision Making in Small Animal Oncology*, Wiley-Blackwell.

Dobson, J. & D. Lascelles (2011). *BSAVA Manual of Canine and Feline Oncology*, BSAVA.

Fahey, C. E., et al. (2011). Evaluation of the University of Florida lomustine, vincristine, procarbazine, and prednisone chemotherapy protocol for the treatment of relapsed lymphoma in dogs: 33 cases (2003-2009). Javma-Journal of the American Veterinary Medical Association **239**(2): 209-15.

Heading, K. L., et al. (2011). CCNU (lomustine) toxicity in dogs: a retrospective study (2002-07). Australian Veterinary Journal **89**(4): 109-16.

Henry, C. & M. Higginbotham (2009). *Cancer Management in Small Animal Practice*, Saunders.

Kristal, O., et al. (2004). Hepatotoxicity associated with CCNU (lomustine) Chemotherapy in Dogs. J Vet Intern Med **18**: 75-80.

Musser, M. L., et al. (2012). Low apparent risk of CCNU (lomustine)-associated clinical hepatotoxicity in cats. Journal of Feline Medicine and Surgery **14**(12): 871-5.

North, S. & T. Banks (2009). *Small Animal Oncology: An Introduction*, Saunders.

Skorupski, K. A., et al. (2011). Prospective Randomized Clinical Trial Assessing the Efficacy of Denamarin for Prevention of CCNU-Induced Hepatopathy in Tumor-Bearing Dogs. Journal of Veterinary Internal Medicine **25**(4): 838-45.

Tripp, C. D., et al. (2011). Tolerability of Metronomic Administration of Lomustine in Dogs with Cancer. Journal of Veterinary Internal Medicine **25**(2): 278-84.

Vandeweerd, J. M., et al. (2013). Nutraceuticals for Canine Liver Disease: Assessing the Evidence. Vet Clin Small Anim **43**: 1171-9.

Withrow, S., et al. (2012). Withrow and MacEwen's Small Animal Clinical Oncology, 5th Ed., Saunders.

Loperamide HCl

(loe-**per**-a-mide)   Imodium®

Opiate Antidiarrheal

Prescriber Highlights

▶ Synthetic opiate GI motility modifier used for symptomatic treatment of diarrhea, primarily in dogs.

▶ Contraindications: Dogs with *ABCB1*-1Δ (MDR1) mutation (mutant/mutant). Known hypersensitivity to narcotic analgesics, diarrhea caused by a toxic ingestion until the toxin is eliminated from the GI tract. Avoid use if cause is due to invasive microorganisms.

▶ Caution: Respiratory disease, hepatic encephalopathy, hypothyroidism, severe renal insufficiency, adrenocortical insufficiency (Addison's), head injuries, or increased intracranial pressure, & acute abdominal conditions (*e.g.*, colic), & in geriatric or severely debilitated patients; avoid use in untested dogs of breeds ("white-feet") susceptible to MDR1 mutation and at reduced dosages for dogs that are heterozygous for the mutation.

▶ Adverse Effects: **Dogs:** Constipation, bloat, & sedation. Potential for: paralytic ileus, toxic megacolon, pancreatitis, & CNS effects. **Cats:** Use is controversial, may exhibit excitatory behavior.

▶ Dose very carefully in small dogs and cats.

Uses/Indications

Loperamide is used as a GI motility modifier in small animals. Some have found that loperamide is useful for treating or helping to reduce chemotherapy-induced (*e.g.,* toceranib) diarrhea in dogs (London 2010), (Vail 2009). Use in cats is controversial and many clinicians do not recommend using in cats.

Pharmacology/Actions

Among their other actions, opiates inhibit GI motility and excessive GI propulsion. They also decrease intestinal secretion induced by cholera toxin, prostaglandin E_2 and diarrheas caused by factors in which calcium is the second messenger (non-cyclic AMP/GMP mediated). Opiates may also enhance mucosal absorption.

Pharmacokinetics

In dogs, loperamide reportedly has a faster onset of action and longer duration of action than diphenoxylate, but clinical studies confirming this appear to be lacking. In humans, loperamide's half-life is ≈11 hours. It is unknown if the drug enters milk or crosses the placenta.

Contraindications/Precautions/Warnings

Because loperamide is potentially a neurotoxic substrate of P-glycoprotein, it is contraindicated in dogs tested positive (mutant/mutant) for the *ABCB1*-1Δ (MDR1) mutation. Alternative antidiarrheals should be considered in untested dogs of herding breeds (*e.g.*, Collies, Shelties, Australian shepherds, etc.) that may have the gene mutation. Dogs that are heterozygous for the mutation should receive loperamide at reduced dosages if it is absolutely required.

Opiate GI motility modifiers should be avoided if diarrhea etiology is due to invasive microorganisms or by an ingested toxin. All opiates should be used with caution in patients with hypothyroidism, severe renal insufficiency, adrenocortical insufficiency, (Addison's), and in geriatric or severely debilitated patients.

Opiate antidiarrheals should be used with caution in patients with head injuries or increased intracranial pressure and acute abdominal conditions (*e.g.*, colic), as it may obscure the diagnosis or clinical course of these conditions. It should be used with extreme caution in patients suffering from respiratory disease or from acute respiratory dysfunction (*e.g.*, pulmonary edema secondary to smoke inhalation). Opiate antidiarrheals should be used with extreme caution in patients with hepatic disease with CNS clinical signs of hepatic encephalopathy. Hepatic coma may result.

Many clinicians recommend that diphenoxylate or loperamide not be used in dogs weighing less than 10 kg, but this is probably a result of the potency of the tablet or capsule forms of the drugs. Dosage titration using the liquid forms of these agents should allow their safe use in dogs when indicated.

Adverse Effects

In dogs, constipation, bloat, and sedation are the most likely adverse reactions encountered when usual doses are used. Potentially, paralytic ileus, toxic megacolon, pancreatitis, and CNS effects could be seen. Dogs the *ABCB1*-1Δ mutation (mutant/mutant) can develop severe CNS depression after receiving loperamide. Naloxone may reverse these effects.(Mealey 2013)

Use of antidiarrheal opiates in cats is controversial; this species may react with excitatory behavior.

Reproductive/Nursing Safety

In humans, the FDA categorizes loperamide as category *B* for use during pregnancy (*Animal studies have not yet demonstrated risk to the fetus, but there are no adequate studies in pregnant women; or animal studies have shown an adverse effect, but adequate studies in pregnant women have not demonstrated a risk to the fetus in the first trimester of pregnancy, and there is no evidence of risk in later trimesters.*)

It is not known whether loperamide is excreted in maternal milk. Safety during nursing has not been established.

Overdosage/Acute Toxicity

In dog toxicity studies, doses of 1.25 – 5 mg/kg/day produced vomiting, depression, severe salivation, and weight loss. Breeds with a defective MDR-1 gene are more sensitive to CNS depression with loperamide than other breeds and have shown signs at 0.06 mg/kg per the APCC database.

There were 766 single agent exposures to loperamide reported to the ASPCA Animal Poison Control Center (APCC) during 2009-2013. Of the 732 dogs, 519 were symptomatic with 81% vomiting, 46% lethargic, 26% with diarrhea, 17% hypersalivation, 13% hypothermic, and 9% bradycardic. Of the 23 cats, 7 were symptomatic with vomiting (43%), lethargy (29%) and mydriasis (29%) being the most common.

Treatment should follow standard decontamination protocols, although the use of apomorphine for emesis should be avoided since it can have additive CNSA or respiratory depressant effects. Naloxone may be used to treat severe depression; higher than usual doses may be required. Intravenous lipid (ILE) rescue may be useful.

Drug Interactions

The following drug interactions have either been reported or are theoretical in humans or animals receiving loperamide and may be of significance in veterinary patients. Unless otherwise noted, use together is not necessarily contraindicated, but weigh the potential risks and perform additional monitoring when appropriate.

- **AMIODARONE:** By inhibiting P-gp may increase loperamide plasma concentrations.
- **CARVEDILOL:** By inhibiting P-gp may increase loperamide plasma concentrations.
- **CYP2B11 SUBSTRATES** (*e.g.,* **propofol, progesterone, midazolam, ketamine**): Loperamide can inhibit metabolism of this isoenzyme in dogs and potentially increase blood levels of substrates.
- **CYP2D15 SUSBTRATES** (*e.g.,* **imipramine, propranolol, metoprolol**): Loperamide can inhibit metabolism of this isoenzyme in dogs and potentially increase blood levels of substrates.
- **CYP3A12 SUBSTRATES** (*e.g.,* **erythromycin, cyclosporine, tacrolimus, medetomidine**): Loperamide can inhibit metabolism of this isoenzyme in dogs and potentially increase blood levels of substrates.
- **ERYTHROMYCIN:** By inhibiting P-gp may increase loperamide plasma concentrations.
- **KETOCONAZOLE, ITRACONAZOLE:** By inhibiting P-gp may increase loperamide plasma concentrations.
- **QUINIDINE:** By inhibiting P-gp may increase loperamide plasma concentrations.
- **TAMOXIFEN:** By inhibiting P-gp may increase loperamide plasma concentrations.
- **VERAPAMIL:** By inhibiting P-gp may increase loperamide plasma concentrations.

Laboratory Considerations

- Plasma **amylase** and **lipase** values may be increased for up to 24 hours following administration of opiates.

Doses

- **DOGS:**

  Note: Collies, related breeds, or other dogs susceptible to the ABCB1 (MDR1) mutation may be overly sensitive to loperamide; avoid use. See Contraindications.

  As an antidiarrheal (extra-label): Anecdotal dosage recommendations vary and no published evidence supporting one over the other was found. Most recommend 0.08 – 0.1 mg/kg PO three times daily as needed, but dosages as high as 0.2 mg/kg PO 3-4 times daily have been noted.

- **CATS:**

  As an antidiarrheal (extra-label): Not commonly used in cats and its use is controversial; cats may react with excitatory behavior. Anecdotal dosages ranging from 0.04 – 0.16 mg/kg PO q12h have been noted. The oral liquid dosage form is necessary to dose accurately.

- **RABBITS, RODENTS, SMALL MAMMALS:**

  To reduce gut motility (extra-label):

  Rabbits: 0.1 mg/kg in 1 mL of water PO q8h for 3 days, then once daily for 2 days. (Ivey *et al.* 2000)

  Mice, Rats, Gerbils, Hamsters, Guinea pigs, Chinchillas: 0.1 mg/kg PO q8h for 3 days, then once daily for 2 days; give in 1 mL of water. (Adamcak *et al.* 2000)

Monitoring

- Clinical efficacy.
- Fluid and electrolyte status in severe diarrhea.
- CNS effects.

Client Information

- Used to treat diarrhea.
- Loperamide is generally well tolerated with few side effects. But it can be toxic in some dogs with a certain genetic mutation (ABCB1-1Δ or MDR1) most commonly found in "white feet" breeds.
- If diarrhea continues or if animal appears listless or develops a high fever, contact veterinarian right away.
- Loperamide is available OTC (over-the-counter; without a prescription). Do not give loperamide (or any other OTC medications) to your animal without first consulting a veterinarian.

Chemistry/Synonyms

A synthetic piperidine-derivative antidiarrheal, loperamide occurs as a white to faintly yellow powder with a pK_a of 8.6 that is soluble in alcohol and slightly soluble in water.

Loperamide may also be known as PJ 185, or R 18553; a common trade name is *Imodium*®.

Storage/Stability

Loperamide capsules or oral solution should be stored at room temperature in well-closed containers. It is recommended that the oral solution not be diluted with other solvents.

Compatibility/Compounding Considerations

No specific information noted.

Dosage Forms/Regulatory Status

VETERINARY-LABELED PRODUCTS: NONE.

HUMAN-LABELED PRODUCTS:

Loperamide HCl Oral Liquid: 1 mg/5 mL (0.2 mg/mL), & 1 mg/7.5 mL in 60 mL, 90 mL, 118 mL and 120 mL; *Imodium*® A-D, generic; (OTC)

Loperamide HCl Capsules and Tablets: 2 mg; *Imodium*® A-D Caplets; other proprietary named products are available as well as generics; (OTC & Rx)

Revisions/References

Monograph revised/updated March 2014.

Adamcak, A. & B. Otten (2000). Rodent Therapeutics. Vet Clin NA: Exotic Anim Pract 3:1(Jan): 221-40.
Ivey, E. & J. Morrisey (2000). Therapeutics for Rabbits. Vet Clin NA: Exotic Anim Pract 3:1(Jan): 183-216.
London, C. A. (2010). Tyrosine Kinase Inhibitor (TKI) Therapy in Companion Animals: Year One. Proceedings: ACVIM. accessed via Veterinary Information Network; vin.com
Mealey, K. L. (2013). Adverse Drug Reactions in Veterinary Patients Associated with Drug Transporters. Veterinary Clinics of North America-Small Animal Practice 43(5): 1067-+.
Vail, D. M. (2009). Supporting the Veterinary Cancer Patient on Chemotherapy: Neutropenia and Gastrointestinal Toxicity. Topics in Companion Animal Medicine 24(3): 122-9.

Loratadine

(lor-at-eh-deen)   Claritin®, Alavert®

Antihistamine

Prescriber Highlights

▶ Oral non-sedating antihistamine.

▶ Very limited experience in dogs or cats; efficacy (if any) not determined.

Uses/Indications

Loratadine is a 2nd-generation antihistamine and at usual dosages it is non-sedating in humans. While it potentially could be useful in treating histamine-mediated conditions in dogs or cats, no evidence was located documenting efficacy.

Pharmacology/Actions

Loratadine is a long-acting oral antihistamine that can block peripheral histamine(H1)-receptors. At therapeutically used dosages it does not have significant antimuscarinic activity.

Pharmacokinetics

No information was located for dogs or cats.

In humans, loratadine is rapidly absorbed from the GI tract; peak plasma concentrations occur in ≈1 hour. Food decreases time to peak, but overall bioavailability is increased. It is extensively metabolized in the liver and its primary metabolite (desloratadine) is active. Loratadine is highly bound to plasma proteins (98%); plasma protein binding for desloratadine is lower. Minimal levels enter the CNS at therapeutic dosages. Severe renal impairment does not appreciably alter blood levels of the drug or its active metabolite. Elimination half-life is approximately 9 hours (loratadine) and 28 hours (desloratadine). Elimination is mostly as metabolites via urine and feces.

Contraindications/Precautions/Warnings

Loratadine is contraindicated in patients that are hypersensitive to it or desloratadine. Use with caution in dogs with dry-eye syndrome as loratadine has been shown to decrease tear production in humans. It is labeled to be used with caution in humans with hepatic or kidney impairment.

Adverse Effects

Adverse effects are not well documented for loratadine in small animals. Potentially, at higher dosages it could have CNS effects (sedation, lethargy, contradictory excitement), GI effects (vomiting) and cause tachycardia. Dry mouth and decreased tear production are possible.

Reproductive/Nursing Safety

Animal safety during pregnancy or nursing has not been established, but for humans, loratadine is listed in FDA category *B* (*Animal studies have revealed no evidence of harm to the fetus, however, there are no adequate and well-controlled studies in pregnant women. (OR) Animal studies have shown an adverse effect, but adequate and well-controlled studies in pregnant women have failed to demonstrate a risk to the fetus.*); the American Academy of Pediatrics has listed loratadine as compatible with breast-feeding.

Overdosage/Acute Toxicity

Mild overdoses of loratadine are generally not serious, but moderate to severe overdoses can cause cardiac and CNS effects. Clinical signs usually occur within 30 minutes to 7-hours post ingestion and can persist 12-24 hours or more. Clinical signs in dogs have been noted as low as 0.25 mg/kg, but doses as high as 72 mg/kg have been tolerated without serious effects or death (Murphy 2001). There were 525 single agent exposures to loratadine reported to the ASPCA Animal Poison Control Center (APCC) during 2009-2013.

Of the 485 dogs, 115 were symptomatic with tachycardia (40%), lethargy (22%) and vomiting (20%) being the most common clinical signs. Consider decontamination for very large ingestions. Treatment is supportive; hemodialysis does not appear to be an effective in removing loratadine or desloratadine from the body. Contact a veterinary poison control center for further guidance.

Drug Interactions

The following drug interactions have either been reported or are theoretical in humans or animals receiving loratadine and may be of significance in veterinary patients. Unless otherwise noted, use together is not necessarily contraindicated, but weigh the potential risks and perform additional monitoring when appropriate.

■ **AMIDOARONE**: In humans, QT-interval prolongation and torsades de pointes have been reported; clinical monitoring has been recommended.

■ **CIMETIDINE**: May increase loratadine (and desloratadine) levels; no clinical effects noted in humans.

■ **KETOCONAZOLE**: May increase loratadine (and desloratadine) levels; no clinical effects noted in humans.

Laboratory Considerations

■ Loratadine may interfere with intradermal allergy testing. Antihistamine withdrawal is usually recommended for at least 1 week prior to allergy testing.

Doses

■ **DOGS:**

As an antihistamine (extra-label): No published evidence was located supporting efficacy and safety for pruritus or atopic dermatitis. Anecdotal dosages ranging from: 0.25 – 1.1 mg/kg PO once daily or divided twice daily have been noted. Practically it could be dosed: <u>Small dogs</u>: 5 mg per dog PO once daily; <u>Medium-sized dogs</u>: 10 mg per dog PO once daily; <u>Large dogs</u>: 10 mg per dog PO twice daily.

■ **CATS:**

As an antihistamine (extra-label): No published evidence was located supporting use for upper respiratory signs associated with allergies. An anecdotal dosage 0.5 mg/kg PO once daily has been noted.

Monitoring

■ No specific monitoring is required beyond clinical efficacy and adverse effects.

Client Information

■ Antihistamines should be used on a regular, ongoing basis in animals that respond to them. They work better if used before exposure to an allergen.

■ Causes less drowsiness/sleepiness than some other antihistamines.

■ Not used commonly in veterinary medicine so possible side effects are not well known.

Chemistry/Synonyms

Loratadine is a piperidine-derivative related structurally to azatadine. The USP 36 description for it is: loratadine is a white to off-white powder. Insoluble in water; freely soluble in acetone, chloroform, methyl alcohol, and toluene.

Loratadine may also be known as SCh-29851, loratadiini, loratadin, loratadinum or loratadyna.

Storage/Stability

Loratadine syrup or tablets should be stored in tight, light-resistant containers. The orally dispersing tablets should be protected from humidity. Tablets should be stored between 2-30°C; syrup and orally disintegrating tablets should be stored at 225°C.

Compatibility/Compounding Considerations
▪ No specific information noted.

Dosage Forms/Regulatory Status
VETERINARY-LABELED PRODUCTS: NONE.

HUMAN-LABELED PRODUCTS:

Loratadine Tablets, Oral Dispersible Tablets, Chewable Tablets: 5 mg & 10 mg; generic; (OTC). Many proprietary brands are available, two common ones are *Claritin*® and *Alavert*®. **Note:** Oral dispersible tablets may contain xylitol (unknown quantity).

Loratadine Oral Solution/Syrup: 1 mg/mL (labeled as 5 mg/5 mL); generic; (OTC). Many proprietary brands are available, two common ones are *Claritin*® and *Alavert*®.

Revisions/References
Monograph written March 2014.
Murphy, L. (2001). Antihistamine Toxicosis. Veterinary Medicine(October 2001).

Lorazepam
(lor-**ayz**-eh-pam)   Ativan®

Benzodiazepine

Prescriber Highlights
▶ Benzodiazepine that can be useful as an anxiolytic in dogs & cats or as an alternative to diazepam for treating status epilepticus.

▶ Can be administered intranasally or IV for status epilepticus.

▶ Adverse Effects (most likely): Increased appetite, activity or behavior changes (lethargy/somnolence to hyperexcitability/aggression).

Uses/Indications
Lorazepam may be useful in treating status epilepticus in dogs and the adjunctive treatment of behavior disorders (fears, phobias, anxiety) in dogs and cats. When compared with diazepam, there is much less experience with lorazepam in small animal medicine but it has some advantages. Since lorazepam is not metabolized into active metabolites by the liver it can be used more safely in patients with liver dysfunction, and obese, or geriatric patients. It appears as effective as diazepam, may have longer anticonvulsant duration of action (not proven in dogs), and may be easier to administer (intranasal, sublingual/buccal). It is not recommended for rectal administration for status epilepticus.

In human medicine, lorazepam is now often used in place of diazepam for treating status epilepticus and anxiolytic indications. It is also used for treating cancer chemotherapy-induced nausea and emesis, alcohol withdrawal, and akathisia secondary to antipsychotic medications.

Pharmacology/Actions
Lorazepam is considered a long-acting benzodiazepine in humans, but it has a much shorter half-life in dogs. It and other benzodiazepines depress the subcortical levels of the CNS (primarily limbic, thalamic, and hypothalamic) thus producing anxiolytic, sedative, skeletal muscle relaxant, and anticonvulsant effects. The exact mechanism of action is unknown, but postulated mechanisms include: antagonism of serotonin, increased release of and/or facilitation of gamma-aminobutyric acid (GABA) activity, and diminished release or turnover of acetylcholine in the CNS. Benzodiazepine specific receptors have been located in the mammalian brain, kidney, liver, lung, and heart. Receptors are lacking in the white matter in all species studied.

Pharmacokinetics
In dogs, intravenous administration of 0.2 mg/kg gave peak levels of ≈165 ng/mL and remained above 30 ng/mL (considered necessary for anticonvulsant activity in humans) for 60 minutes. After intranasal administration of 0.2 mg/kg to dogs (Mariani *et al.* 2003), peak levels of ≈106 ng/mL were achieved; in 3/6 dogs studied, levels stayed above 30 ng/mL for 60 minutes. Levels reached 30 ng/mL between 3-9 minutes after intranasal administration. While elimination half-life has been reported as approximately 1 hour in dogs, concentrations in the brain may persist longer than in the serum as lorazepam has a high affinity for benzodiazepine receptors in the CNS. Rectal administration of lorazepam in dogs does not appear to yield serum concentrations high enough for efficacious treatment of status epilepticus due to a high first-pass effect. Lorazepam is converted into glucuronide forms in the liver in most species. These metabolites are not active. Primary elimination route is via the urine in dogs.

In cats, lorazepam is efficiently glucuronidated; elimination is approximately 50% in the urine (primarily as the glucuronide) and 50% in the feces.

In humans, absolute bioavailability is ≈90% after oral administration and, unlike diazepam, it is relatively rapidly and completely absorbed after IM dosing. Sublingual administration has similar bioavailability as oral dosing, but serum levels peak sooner. Elimination half-life appears to be much longer in humans (12 hours) than in dogs (≈1 hour).

Contraindications/Precautions/Warnings
Lorazepam is contraindicated in patients known to be hypersensitive to benzodiazepines, or with severe respiratory insufficiency unless they are being mechanically ventilated.

When using for negative behaviors, withdraw the drug gradually or a rebound effect may occur. Physical dependency has been induced in dogs. If long-term regular usage has occurred, withdraw the drug gradually.

Injectable lorazepam must not be given intra-arterially; arteriospasm may occur resulting in necrosis. Use repeated high doses or CRI's with caution as the injection contains propylene glycol and benzyl alcohol.

Do not confuse LORazepam with other sound-alike/look-alike drugs (*e.g.*, CLONazepam, ALPRAZolam).

Adverse Effects
In small animals, benzodiazepines can cause increased appetite, aggression, increased activity/excitement, and vocalization. With initiation of therapy, dosage increases, or at higher dosages, ataxia, somnolence and lethargy can occur.

Lorazepam injection contains both propylene glycol 400 (0.18 mL per mL of injection) and 2% benzyl alcohol. Repeated high dosages or CRI's may have toxic effects in dogs and cats.

Reproductive/Nursing Safety
For humans, lorazepam is designated by the FDA as category *D* for use during pregnancy (*There is evidence of human fetal risk, but the potential benefits from the use of the drug in pregnant women may be acceptable despite its potential risks.*) However, studies in animals generally suggest that the drug is relatively safe for use during pregnancy at usual dosages. Except in one study in mice that were given approximately 400X the human dose producing offspring with an increased rate of cleft palate formation, animal studies have not shown significant increased rates of teratogenicity. If high doses are used just prior to delivery, "floppy infant" syndrome has been seen in humans.

Small amounts of lorazepam are distributed into milk, but it should be safe to use during nursing.

Overdosage/Acute Toxicity
Overdoses of lorazepam are generally limited to CNS depression (confusion, lethargy, somnolence, decreased reflexes, etc.). Very large overdoses can cause ataxia, hypotension, coma, and death

(very rare). Repeated high dosages or CRI's of the injection may cause propylene glycol or benzyl alcohol toxicity.

There were 644 single agent exposures to lorazepam reported to the ASPCA Animal Poison Control Center (APCC) during 2009-2013. Of the 538 dogs, 109 were symptomatic. The most common clinical signs were 29% sedated/lethargic, 17% hyperactive, 15% ataxic and 13% vomiting. Of the 102 cats, 71 were symptomatic with 79% ataxic, 24% lethargic, 18% vocalizing and 11% agitated.

Treatment of acute orally ingested toxicity consists of standard protocols for removing and/or binding the drug in the gut and supportive systemic measures. In patients with normal renal function, forced diuresis with intravenous fluids/electrolytes and mannitol may enhance excretion of lorazepam. The use of analeptic agents (CNS stimulants such as caffeine) is generally not recommended. Flumazenil may be considered for adjunctive treatment of serious overdoses of benzodiazepines, but its use does not replace proper supportive therapy. Flumazenil is not recommended in patients with seizure-disorders as it may induce seizures.

Drug Interactions

The following drug interactions have either been reported or are theoretical in humans or animals receiving lorazepam and may be of significance in veterinary patients. Unless otherwise noted, use together is not necessarily contraindicated, but weigh the potential risks and perform additional monitoring when appropriate.

- **CNS DEPRESSANTS** (*e.g.*, **opiates, barbiturates, sedatives, anticonvulsants**): Additive CNS effects.
- **PROBENECID:** Decreased renal clearance of lorazepam.
- **SCOPOLAMINE:** Increased CNS depression, irrational behavior.
- **THEOPHYLLINE:** Decreased sedation from lorazepam.
- **VALPROATE:** Increased lorazepam serum concentration.

Laboratory Considerations

- No specific concerns noted.

Doses

- **DOGS:**

  For status epilepticus (extra-label): Lorazepam can be used as an alternative to diazepam. Dosage recommendation is 0.2 mg/kg IV. The same dosage (0.2 mg/kg) can also be administered intranasally. This route can be an alternative to at-home rectal administration of diazepam. Onset of effect after intranasal administration is usually within 3 minutes and effects can persist for 60+ minutes.

  For behavior indications (*e.g.*, **fears, anxieties, phobias, night waking**); (extra-label): Anecdotal dosage recommendations vary somewhat but usually range from 0.02 – 0.2 mg/kg 1-3 times a day or on an as needed basis. However, dosages ranging from 0.02 – 0.5 mg/kg q8-24h have been noted. No published evidence was located supporting any one dosage over the other. It is suggested to start therapy at the lower end of the dosing range and choosing a practical dose for the patient that is closest to ½ or one 0.5 mg or 1 mg tablet (per dog); titrate upwards if necessary.

- **CATS:**

  For behavior indications (*e.g.*, **fears, anxieties, phobias, night waking**); (extra-label): Anecdotal dosage recommendations vary somewhat but usually range from 0.025 – 0.08 mg/kg 1-2 times a day or on an as needed basis. However, dosages ranging from 0.025 – 0.25 mg/kg q8-24h have been noted. No published evidence was located supporting any one dosage over the other. It is suggested to start therapy at the lower end of the dosing range choosing a practical dose for the patient that is closest to ¼ or ½ 0.5 mg tablet (0.125 – 0.25 mg per cat); titrate upwards if necessary.

Monitoring

- No specific monitoring is required beyond clinical efficacy and adverse effects.

Client Information

- When using for thunderstorm phobias or other triggers (*e.g.*, owners separation anxiety, etc.) that upset your animal try to give about an hour before the event or trigger.
- Tablets are relatively tasteless and readily disintegrate in saliva. If pilling is difficult, place inside the patient's cheek and follow in a minute or so with a small treat to facilitate swallowing of saliva/medication.
- If you see yellowing of the whites of the eyes or the gums have a yellowish tint; contact veterinarian immediately.
- Sleepiness is most common side effect, but sometimes the drug can change behavior or work in the opposite way from what is expected.
- This drug may increase appetite, especially in cats.
- Contact your veterinarian immediately if your cat stops eating or seems depressed.

Chemistry/Synonyms

Lorazepam occurs as a white or practically white, practically odorless powder. It is insoluble in water and sparingly soluble in alcohol. Each mL of lorazepam for injection contains 0.18 mL of polyethylene glycol 400 and 2% benzyl alcohol in propylene glycol.

Lorazepam may also be known as BRN-07599084, CB-8133, Ro-7-8408, Wy-4036, lorazapamum, anxiedin, azurogen, bonatranquan, delormetazepam, lorazin, lorazon, lorenin, norlormetazepam, novhepar, novolorazem, o-Chloroxazepam, sinestron, *Ativan*®, and *Lorazepam Intensol*®; many international trade names are available.

Storage/Stability

Lorazepam tablets should be stored in well-closed containers at room temperature (20-25°C). The oral solution and injection should be stored refrigerated (2-8°C) and protected from light.

The injection must be further diluted just prior before to intravenous injection with an equal volume of D5W, normal saline, or sterile water for injection. Do not shake the syringe vigorously, but gently invert repeatedly until the injection is diluted and completely mixed in solution. Do not use if solution is discolored or a precipitate forms. IV injections should be administered slowly, 2 mg over 2-5 minutes.

Although not part of the label information, lorazepam can be further diluted in D5W or NS for IV infusion. When used in this manner, lorazepam injection is most soluble in final concentrations from 0.1 – 0.2 mg/mL. For example, if using the 2 mg/mL injection, further dilution with 9 mL or 19 mL of D5W or NS would yield a final concentration of 0.2 or 0.1 mg/mL. The injection is very viscous; mix well before use. As precipitation/crystallization can occur, observe the solution before and during the infusion. D5W may be less prone to crystallization formation than is NS. Solutions for infusion mixed in this manner should be used within 12 hours of preparation.

Compatibility/Compounding Considerations

Medications reported to be **compatible** with lorazepam injection (partial listing):

- **Syringe:** hydromorphone, dimenhydrinate.
- **Y-Site:** albumin, amikacin, amphotericin B cholesteryl, atracurium, cefotaxime, ciprofloxacin, cisplatin, dexamethasone, diltiazem, diphenhydramine, dobutamine, doxorubicin, famotidine, fentanyl, fosphenytoin, furosemide, gentamicin, heparin, hetastarch, hydromorphone, levetiracetem, methadone, metroni-

dazole, morphine, piperacillin-tazobactam, propofol, ranitidine, vancomycin, and vecuronium.

It is **incompatible** with (partial listing):

- **Syringe:** buprenorphine and pantoprazole.
- **Y-Site:** aztreonam, gallium nitrate, imipenem-cilastatin, omeprazole, and ondansetron.

Dosage Forms/Regulatory Status

VETERINARY-LABELED PRODUCTS: NONE.

The ARCI (Racing Commissioners International) has designated this drug as a class 2 substance. See appendix for more information.

HUMAN-LABELED PRODUCTS:

Lorazepam Tablets: 0.5 mg, 1 mg, & 2 mg; *Ativan®*, generic; (Rx; C-IV)

Lorazepam Concentrated Oral Solution: 2 mg/mL in 10 mL and 30 mL with dropper; *Lorazepam Intensol®*; (Rx; C-IV)

Lorazepam Injection: 2 mg/mL & 4 mg/mL in 1 mL prefilled syringes, 1 mL single use vials & 10 mL multidose vials; *Ativan®*, generic; (Rx; C-IV)

Revisions/References

Monograph revised/updated March 2014.

Mariani, C., et al. (2003). A comparison of intranasal and intravenous lorazepam in normal dogs. Proceedings: ACVIM 2003. accessed via Veterinary Information Network; vin.com

Losartan Potassium

(loe-**sar**-tan)   Cozaar®

Angiotensin-II Receptor Blocker (ARB)

Prescriber Highlights

▶ ARB that potentially could be useful in dogs and cats for the adjunctive treatment of proteinuria, hypertension secondary to renal insufficiency, or congestive heart failure.

▶ Very limited experience in veterinary medicine; little data on efficacy, safety, adverse effects, etc. At this point, little data to support clinical use in dogs or cats.

▶ Not safe during pregnancy.

Uses/Indications

Losartan is a human-approved angiotensin-II AT1-receptor blocker that potentially could be useful for the adjunctive treatment of hypertension, proteinuria and cardiomyopathies in dogs and cats, but very little information on its safety and efficacy are known for veterinary species.

Any potential clinical usefulness in cats is in question as one study done in 6 cats with experimentally-induced (angiotensin-I given IV) hypertension did not show that losartan had any significant or consistent effect on blood pressure or pressor response (Reynolds *et al.* 2002).

In dogs, potential clinical usefulness is tempered with the concern that dogs do not metabolize much losartan into an active metabolite (E-3174; EXP-3174) (Christ *et al.* 1994), which in humans is thought to produce much of the drug's therapeutic effect and allow once per day dosing. A study measuring hemodynamic functions in dogs with experimentally-induced tachycardia-induced canine heart failure, demonstrated that losartan was ≈3X less potent than E-1374 in improving some measured functions (reduced pulmonary artery pressure, mean arterial pressure, pulmonary capillary wedge pressure and peripheral resistance, and increased stroke volume) (Suzuki *et al.* 2001). Additional studies are clearly necessary to determine where losartan fits into the veterinary drug armamentarium.

Pharmacology/Actions

Losartan is an angiotensin-II receptor blocker (ARB). By selectively blocking the AT1-receptor, aldosterone synthesis and secretion is reduced causing vasodilation and decreased potassium and increased sodium excretion. While plasma concentrations of renin and angiotensin-II are increased, this does not counteract the blood pressure lowering effects of losartan. Losartan does not interfere with substance P or bradykinin responses.

In humans, losartan is converted in the liver probably via P-450 2C9 into an active metabolite (E-3174), which appears to be a reversible, noncompetitive inhibitor of the AT_1 receptor and is approximately 40X more potent (by weight) than losartan. Dogs do not appear to produce much of the active metabolite (Christ *et al.* 1994) which may, when compared to human patients, considerably alter the dosing strategy, adverse effects and efficacy for the drug.

Pharmacokinetics

In dogs, losartan given as single oral doses was rapidly absorbed with peak levels occurring within one hour and had a bioavailability of 23-33%. Volume of distribution was 0.3 L/kg and plasma protein binding was ≈97% with free drug between 2-3%. Elimination half-life was between 2-3 hours. It is thought the majority of drug is eliminated in the bile/feces, but significant enterohepatic recirculation occurs (Christ *et al.* 1994).

No losartan pharmacokinetic data was located for cats.

In humans, the pharmacokinetics of losartan differs markedly from what is seen in dogs. After oral dosing, absorption is rapid with a bioavailability of the parent compound around 33%. Presence of food can slow absorption, but does not affect the extent. Significant first-pass metabolism converts much of the absorbed drug into a carboxylic metabolite (E-3174), which is responsible for much of the drug's therapeutic efficacy. Bioavailability of E-3174 is ≈14% of the administered dose. Peak levels of the losartan and E-3174 occur at ≈1 and 4 hours, respectively. Free fractions of losartan/E-3174 are 1.3%/0.2%. Terminal half-lives are approximately 2 hours for losartan and 8 hours for E-3174. Area under the curve for E-3174 is ≈4X that of the parent compound. Approximately 10% of the drug and active metabolite are excreted unchanged in the urine with the remainder excreted primarily via bile/feces and as other metabolites in urine.

Contraindications/Precautions/Warnings

Losartan is contraindicated in patients that are allergic (hypersensitive) to it. It is not known if cross-reactivity occurs between other ARBs and losartan. Hypotensive patients should not receive the drug. Patients that are volume or electrolyte depleted should not receive the drug until volume/electrolytes have been replenished/corrected.

Losartan should be used with caution in patients with moderate hepatic impairment; dosage reduction may be warranted.

The human label has the following Black Box Warning: "Fetal toxicity: When pregnancy is detected, discontinue losartan as soon as possible. Drugs that act directly on the renin-angiotensin system can cause injury and even death to the developing fetus." See the Reproductive Safety section for more information.

Adverse Effects

The adverse effect profile for this drug when used clinically in veterinary species is not known. In humans, adverse effects are not common. Adverse effects reported include dry cough (much less likely to occur than with lisinopril) and orthostatic dizziness/hypotension. Changes in renal function and hyperkalemia are possible. Very rarely in humans, hypersensitivity and hepatopathy/increased liver enzymes have been reported.

Reproductive/Nursing Safety

Losartan is not considered safe to use during pregnancy. Studies in pregnant rats given high doses of ARBs demonstrated a variety of fetal abnormalities (renal pelvic cavitation, hydroureter, absence of renal papilla). Smaller doses in rabbits caused increased maternal death and spontaneous abortion. In humans, the drug is considered teratogenic, particularly during the 2nd and 3rd trimesters. During this time, the FDA categorizes losartan as category *D* for use during pregnancy (*There is evidence of human fetal risk, but the potential benefits from the use of the drug in pregnant women may be acceptable despite its potential risks.*) If pregnancy is detected in patients receiving losartan, the drug should be discontinued as soon as possible.

Because losartan and its active metabolite have been detected in substantial quantities in rat milk, there is significant concern about the safety of the drug during nursing.

Overdosage/Acute Toxicity

Significant lethality was observed in mice and rats after oral administration of 1 gram/kg. Hemodialysis is not effective in removing losartan or its active metabolites.

Drug Interactions

The following drug interactions have either been reported or are theoretical in humans or animals receiving losartan and may be of significance in veterinary patients. Unless otherwise noted, use together is not necessarily contraindicated, but weigh the potential risks and perform additional monitoring when appropriate.

- **ACE INHIBITORS: (benazepril, enalapril**, etc.): Increased risk for adverse effects (*e.g.*, hypotension, hyperkalemia, renal function changes); increased monitoring may be warranted. However, using ACE inhibitors with ARBs may be useful in treating proteinuria and allow dosage reductions of the drugs being used.
- **ASPIRIN:** Possible reduced antihypertensive effect of losartan and increased risk for renal impairment; increased monitoring may be warranted.
- **NSAIDs** (*e.g.*, **carprofen, meloxicam,** etc.): Possible reduced antihypertensive effect of losartan and increased risk for renal impairment; increased monitoring may be warranted.
- **RIFAMPIN:** May decrease plasma concentrations of losartan (and its active metabolite).
- **POTASSIUM PREPARATIONS, POTASSIUM–SPARING DIURETICS** (*e.g.*, **spironolactone**): Increased risk for hyperkalemia; increased monitoring of serum potassium may be warranted.

Laboratory Considerations

None noted.

Dosages

- **DOGS:**

  Note: There is very little clinical experience using this drug in animal patients and almost nothing published on its clinical usage; consider use at this time as 'experimental'—use with caution. The active metabolite thought to produce much of the drug's effect and duration of action is found in much lower quantities in dogs than in humans, so dosages may need to be higher and given more frequently in dogs (unconfirmed).

  For adjunctive treatment of proteinuria and/or hypertension in dogs with glomerular disease (extra-label): The International Renal Interest Society (IRIS) has published their consensus recommended dosages: <u>Azotemic dogs</u>: Initial dose of 0.125 mg/kg PO per day and an escalating dose of 0.5 mg/kg per day. <u>Non-azotemic dogs</u>: 0.5 mg/kg per day and an escalating dose of 1 mg/kg per day. Concurrent administration of an ACE inhibitor is generally recommended (Brown *et al.* 2013).

Monitoring

- Depending on reason for use and patient's clinical condition: renal function, urine protein, blood pressure, serum potassium levels, volume status, and liver function tests. IRIS recommends: Urine protein-to-creatinine ratio (UPC), urinalysis, systemic arterial blood pressure (BP), and serum albumin, creatinine, and potassium concentrations (in fasting samples) should be monitored at least quarterly in all dogs being treated for glomerular disease (Brown *et al.* 2013).

Client Information

- This medication may be given with or without food.
- Because this medication has not been often used in dogs or cats, side effects are not well known; watch carefully for any side effects and report them to your veterinarian. Possible side effects could include: diarrhea, vomiting, lack of appetite, fatigue (tiredness), and low blood pressure (fainting, weakness, can't exercise, etc.).
- This drug has caused birth defects and should not be used in pregnant animals. If a human in the household is pregnant, they should be very careful not to ingest these tablets and should wear disposable gloves when administering doses and wash their hands after touching these tablets.

Chemistry/Synonyms

Losartan potassium [CAS Registry: 114798-26-4 (losartan); 124750-99-8 (losartan potassium); ATC: C09CA01] occurs as a white to off-white, hygroscopic crystalline powder. It is freely soluble in water and methyl alcohol; soluble in isopropyl alcohol and slightly soluble in acetonitrile.

Losartan potassium may also be known as: DuP-753, E-3340, or MK-0954. A common trade name is *Cozaar®*.

Storage/Stability

Store losartan tablets at room temperature (up to 30°C; 86F) and protect from light.

Compatibility/Compounding Considerations

The manufacturer of the human label tablets (Merck & Co.) describes a method to prepare an extemporaneous suspension containing losartan potassium 2.5 mg/mL: Add 10 mL of purified water to a 240 mL polyethylene terephthalate (PET) bottle containing ten 50 mg tablets of losartan potassium; shake contents for ≥2 minutes. Allow concentrated suspension to stand for 60 minutes following reconstitution, then shake for an additional minute. Prepare a mixture containing equal parts (by volume) of syrup (*Ora-Sweet®*) and suspending vehicle (*Ora-Plus®*) separately. Dilute the concentrated suspension of losartan potassium with 190 mL of the *Ora-Sweet®* and *Ora-Plus®* mixture; shake the container an additional minute to disperse ingredients. Shake suspension before dispensing each dose. Store in the refrigerator (2-8°C) for up to 30 days.

Dosage Forms/Regulatory Status

VETERINARY-LABELED PRODUCTS: NONE.

HUMAN-LABELED PRODUCTS:

Oral Tablets: 25 mg, 50 mg, 100 mg; *Cozaar®*, generic; (Rx)

Combination products containing losartan potassium and hydrochlorothiazide are also available. There is a website (dailymed.nlm.nih.gov) listing FDA-approved (human drug) labels for losartan potassium products.

References

Monograph written August 2013; updated March 2014.

Brown, S., et al. (2013). Consensus Recommendations for Standard Therapy of Glomerular Disease in Dogs. Journal of Veterinary Internal Medicine 27: S27-S43.

Christ, D. D., et al. (1994). The Pharmacokinetics and Pharmacodynamics of the Angiotensin-II Receptor Antagonist Losartan Potassium (Dup 753/Mk 954) in the Dog. Journal of Pharmacology and Experimental Therapeutics 268(3): 1199-205.

Reynolds, V., et al. (2002). Losartan fails to block angiotensin pressor response in cats with induced renal insufficiency. ACVIM Forumn. accessed via Veterinary Information Network; vin.com

Suzuki, J., et al. (2001). Acute effects of E-3174, a human active metabolite of losartan, on the cardiovascular system in tachycardia-induced canine heart failure. Hypertension Research 24(1): 65-74.

Lufenuron

(loo-fen-yur-on)   Program®, Sentinel®

Chitin Synthesis Inhibitor

Prescriber Highlights

▶ Used for flea control in dogs & cats; potentially an antifungal agent. Found in several antiparasitic products combined w/milbemycin± praziquantel or packaged in combination with nitenpyram.

▶ Adverse Effects are rarely seen at recommended oral doses. Injectable can cause a local tissue reaction in cats.

Uses/Indications

Lufenuron is FDA-approved for use in dogs and cats 6 weeks of age and older for the control of flea populations. The 6-month injectable for cats is indicated for flea control in cats 6 weeks old or older. The combination product of lufenuron and milbemycin (*Sentinel®*) is indicated for use in puppies and dogs 4 weeks and older for prevention and control flea populations, prevention of heartworm disease, control of adult hookworms, and the removal and control of adult roundworms and whipworms. The oral chewable tablet product (*Sentinel Spectrum®*) for dogs combining milbemycin, lufenuron and praziquantel adds the additional indication for tapeworms.

In evaluating lufenuron used solely as an ectoparasiticide, advantages include: convenient, can be administered orally, safe environmentally and to patient. Disadvantages: Treated animals must not come into contact with any untreated animal, must be given with food, no repellant activity, does not kill adult fleas of pupae, adult flea must feed on animal to ingest the drug, no activity on ticks, lag period of several weeks to months (often 60-90 days), can be expensive in multi-pet households. One source (Ihrke 2009) recommends lufenuron to be used with spot-ons or with newer oral products for long-term control, not for use as sole therapy unless very closed environment.

Lufenuron has been proposed as a potential treatment or preventative for *E. cuniculi* infections in rabbits, but no studies are available evaluating its use for this indication.

Lufenuron showed initial promise as a treatment for fungal infections but the early enthusiasm has dampened considerably as efficacy appears limited.

Pharmacology/Actions

Lufenuron acts by inhibiting chitin synthesis, polymerization, and deposition in fleas, thereby preventing eggs from developing into adults. Lufenuron does not kill adult fleas. It is believed that lufenuron's nonspecific effect on chitin synthesis is related to serine protease inhibition. Lufenuron's mechanism of action, theoretically, would also have effect on fungi.

Pharmacokinetics

Approximately 40% of an oral dose is absorbed with the remainder eliminated in the feces. To maximize oral absorption, the manufacturer recommends administering in conjunction with or immediately after (within 30 minutes) a full meal. The drug is absorbed in the small intestine and stored in lipose tissue that acts as a depot reservoir to slowly redistribute the drug back into the circulation. While the drug concentrates in the milk of lactating animals, it apparently does not cause ill effects in nursing animals.

After cats receive the injectable product, 2-3 weeks are required before blood levels attain effective concentrations. Cats require a substantially higher oral dosage per kg than do dogs for equivalent efficacy. The drug is apparently not metabolized, but excreted unchanged into the bile and eliminated in the feces.

Contraindications/Precautions/Warnings

The cat labeled injectable product should not be used in dogs; severe local reactions are possible.

Adverse Effects

Adverse effects reported in dogs and cats after oral lufenuron include: vomiting, lethargy/depression, pruritus/urticaria, diarrhea, dyspnea, anorexia, and reddened skin. The manufacturer reports that the adverse reaction rate is less than 5 animals in one million doses.

After receiving the injectable product, a small lump or tissue reaction at the injection site has been noted in some cats. A few weeks may be required for this to dissipate. Studies in rats demonstrated that injectable lufenuron primarily induced infiltrates of macrophages, and not lymphocytes, plasma cells or neutrophils. Some have cautioned that sarcomas can occur at the injection site, however only a single-case report was located. The FDA's adverse drug experience (ADE) database noted that "injection site neoplasm" had been reported 13 times between 1987 and April 30, 2013.

Reproductive/Nursing Safety

The oral lufenuron products are considered safe to use in pregnant, breeding, or lactating animals; safety of the injectable product in reproducing cats has not been formally established at this time.

Overdosage/Acute Toxicity

Growing puppies were dosed at levels up to 30X for 10 months without overt effect on growth or viability noted. Cats receiving oral dosages of up to 17X apparently were unaffected.

Drug Interactions

Limited data available; the manufacturer states that when used with a variety of adulticides, vaccines, antibiotics, anthelmintics, and steroids no adverse effects or interactions were noted in either dogs or cats.

Doses

■ **DOGS:**

Labeled Indications:

For control of flea populations: See the label directions for Program with Capstar for using lufenuron with nitenpyram.

For control of fleas, heartworm prevention, hookworms, ascarids and whipworms: see the label directions for Lufenuron/Milbemycin with Nitenpyram (*Sentinel®* and *Capstar®*—Novartis)

For control of fleas, heartworm prevention, hookworm, ascarids, whipworms and tapeworms: See the label directions for Lufenuron/Milbemycin/Praziquantel (*Sentinel® Spectrum®*—Novartis)

Extra-label Doses: For adjunctive therapy for dermatophytosis: While efficacy is questionable, the following has been suggested: 65 – 100 mg/kg PO once every 2 weeks for 2 treatments. If significant improvement is not seen, a different antifungal agent should be selected. If improvement is seen, re-treat monthly thereafter until at least 2 negative fungal cultures are obtained.

■ **CATS:**

Labeled Indications: For control of flea populations: See the label directions *Program Injectable®*, *Program®* and *Program with Capstar®* for using lufenuron with or without nitenpyram.

Extra-label Doses: For adjunctive treatment of dermatophytosis: While efficacy is questionable, the following have been suggested: 80 mg/kg PO for house cats; 100 mg/kg PO for cats housed in catteries. Re-treat after 14 days and monthly thereafter until at least 2 negative fungal cultures are obtained.

- **RABBITS/RODENTS/SMALL MAMMALS:**
  Rabbits: 30 mg/kg PO every month. (Ivey *et al.* 2000)

Monitoring

- Efficacy.

Client Information

- Helps to control fleas by preventing development of flea eggs; does not kill adult fleas unless used with another drug that kills adult fleas.
- Oral products must be used every 30 days to maximize efficacy. Give with, or mix in with food.
- All animals in a household should be treated.
- Usually no side effects when given orally (by mouth), but side effects have been reported. Vomiting after a dose is the most common side effect. If animal vomits within 2 hours after dosing, the drug should be re-dosed.
- If a dose is missed, re-dose and then resume a monthly dosage regimen.
- Do not split tablets unless instructed to do so.

Chemistry/Synonyms

A benzoylphenylurea derivative, lufenuron is classified as an insect development inhibitor. The drug is lipophilic.

Lufenuron may also be known as CGA-184699, *Capstar®*, *Program®* and *Sentinel®*.

Storage/Stability

The commercially available tablets and suspension should be stored at room temperature (15-30°C). The manufacturer states that intermittent exposure or exposure less than 48 hours to temperatures outside of storage recommendations for the tablets or suspension should not affect potency. Lufenuron tablets are assigned a 4 year expiration date after manufacture; the suspension, 3 years after manufacture; and *Sentinel®* tablets, 3 years after manufacture. Opened pouches of the suspension are not recommended for storage or use for the following dosing cycle.

Compatibility/Compounding Considerations

- No specific information noted.

Dosage Forms/Regulatory Status

VETERINARY-LABELED PRODUCTS:

Lufenuron Oral Suspension: in six tube packs; 135 mg (for cats up to 10 lbs.,—orange), 270 mg (for cats 11-20 lbs.,—green), cats over 20 lbs. are provided the appropriate combination of packs.; *Program® Suspension*; (Rx). FDA-approved for use in cats and kittens (6 weeks of age or older).

Lufenuron 6 Month Injectable for Cats: 100 mg/mL in 10 syringe packages: 0.4 mL (40 mg) prefilled syringe (for cats up to 8.8 lbs.), 0.8 mL (80 mg) prefilled syringe (for cats 8.9-17.6 lbs.); *Program® 6 Month Injectable*; (Rx). FDA-approved for use in cats and kittens 6 weeks of age or older.

Lufenuron Oral Flavor Tabs for Dogs and Cats: For dogs up to 10 lbs: 45 mg; For dogs 11-20 lbs: 90 mg; For dogs 21-45 lbs: 204.9 mg; For dogs 46-90 lbs: 409.8 mg; Dogs over 90 lbs. receive the appropriate combination of tablets; For cats up to 6 lbs. 90 mg; 7-15 lbs: 204.9 mg; cats over 15 lbs. receive the appropriate combination of tablets. *Program® Flavor Tabs*; (OTC). FDA-approved for use in dogs, puppies, cats, & kittens (4 weeks of age or older).

Lufenuron and Nitenpyram Oral Tablets for Dogs: For dogs up to 10 lbs: 45 mg lufenuron, 11.4 mg nitenpyram; For dogs 11-20 lbs.: 90 mg lufenuron, 11.4 mg nitenpyram; For dogs 21-25 lbs: 204.9 mg lufenuron, 11.4 mg nitenpyram; For dogs 26-45 lbs: 204.9 mg lufenuron, 57 mg nitenpyram; For dogs 46-90 lbs: 409.8 mg lufenuron, 57 mg nitenpyram; Dogs over 90 lbs. receive the appropriate combination of lufenuron tablets and 57 mg nitenpyram tablets; *Program® Flavor Tabs* and *Capstar® Flea Management System for Dogs*. (OTC). FDA-approved for use in dogs and puppies (6 weeks of age or older).

Lufenuron and Nitenpyram Oral Tablets for Cats: For cats 2–6 lbs.: 90 mg lufenuron, 11.4 mg nitenpyram; For cats 7-15 lbs.: 204.9 mg lufenuron, 11.4 mg nitenpyram; For cats 16-25 lbs: appropriate combination of tabs provided lufenuron, 11.4 mg nitenpyram; *Program® Flavor Tabs* (OTC); and *Capstar® Flea Management System for Cats*; (OTC)

Milbemycin/Lufenuron Oral Tablets: For dogs: 2-10 lbs.: 2.3 mg/46 mg; 11-25 lbs.: 5.75 mg/115 mg; 26-50 lbs.: 11.5 mg/230 mg; 51-100 lbs.: 23 mg/460 mg; *Sentinel®* Flavor Tabs; (Rx). FDA-approved for use in dogs and puppies 4 weeks of age or older. Also available in combination with nitenpyram (*Capstar®*).

Milbemycin/Lufenuron/Praziquantel Chewable Oral Tablets: For dogs 2-8 lbs.: 2.3 mg/46 mg/22.8 mg; For dogs 8.1-25 lbs: 5.75 mg/115 mg/57 mg; For dogs 25.1-50 lbs.: 11.5 mg/230 mg/114 mg; For dogs 50.1-100 lbs.: 23 mg/460 mg/228 mg; *Sentinel® Spectrum®* (Rx). FDA-approved for use in dogs and puppies 6 weeks of age or older.

HUMAN-APPROVED PRODUCTS: NONE.

Revisions/References

Monograph revised/updated March 2014.

Ihrke, P. (2009). Managing flea allergy- Where are we in 2009? Proceedings: WVC. accessed via Veterinary Information Network; vin.com

Ivey, E. & J. Morrisey (2000). Therapeutics for Rabbits. Vet Clin NA: Exotic Anim Pract **3:1**(Jan): 183-216.

Lysine
L-Lysine

(lye-seen)

Nutritional Amino Acid; Anti-Feline Herpes Virus

Prescriber Highlights

▶ Amino acid that may be effective in suppressing FHV-1 infections in cats.

▶ Long-term treatment required.

Uses/Indications

Lysine may be effective in suppressing FHV-1 infections in cats. Three published studies (Drazenovich *et al.* 2009), (Maggs *et al.* 2007), (Rees *et al.* 2008) however, have not shown lysine to be effective to prevent or reduce the recurrence of upper respiratory tract infections in shelter cats and in two of these studies, cats receiving lysine supplementation had increases in disease severity and detection of FHV-1 DNA. Although no clinical benefit has been proven in shelter cats, client-owned cats are likely subjected to less stress and it may of be of use in this population, provided the stress of administering the drug does not outweigh any benefit (Reed 2014).

Pharmacology/Actions

Lysine is an amino acid that is thought to compete with arginine for incorporation into many herpes viruses. As it is believed that arginine is required for producing infective viral particles, when lysine is incorporated, the virus becomes less infective.

Pharmacokinetics

No specific information was located.

Contraindications/Precautions/Warnings

No specific contraindications.

Adverse Effects

Adverse effects are unlikely when mixed with food, although several recommended that lysine be given as an oral "bolus" to cats. Human patients taking lysine have occasionally complained of abdominal pain and diarrhea; one patient developing tubulointerstitial nephritis has been reported.

Reproductive/Nursing Safety

Lysine showed no teratogenic effects when given to pregnant rats, although safety has not been established in other species.

Overdosage/Acute Toxicity

Significant toxicity is unlikely. Gastrointestinal effects (nausea, vomiting, diarrhea) may occur.

Drug Interactions

The following drug interactions have either been reported or are theoretical in humans or animals receiving lysine and may be of significance in veterinary patients. Unless otherwise noted, use together is not necessarily contraindicated, but weigh the potential risks and perform additional monitoring when appropriate.

- **ARGININE:** Arginine may negate the anti-herpesvirus effects of lysine. It is unlikely that the concentration of arginine found in feline diets would be significant.
- **CALCIUM, ORAL:** Concomitant use of lysine with calcium supplements may increase calcium absorption from the gut and decrease calcium loss in the urine.

Laboratory Considerations

- No specific concerns noted.

Doses

- **CATS:**

  To prevent or reduce recurrent feline herpesvirus infections (extra-label): While efficacy is not proven, many recommend its use for household cats. Most commonly 250 – 500 mg per cat PO twice daily is recommended although many say 500 mg (only) PO twice daily. Some state not to mix with food, while others say mixing with a small amount of soft, moist food is acceptable.

Monitoring

- No specific monitoring is required for lysine except those that would be required to monitor the herpes infection in the patient.

Client Information

- Nutritional agent that can be tried to suppress feline herpesvirus-1 infections in cats. Not a cure.
- Mix with a small amount of soft, moist food unless veterinarian tells you not to do so.
- Side effects are not likely. Diarrhea is possible.
- Treatment may be long-term.

Chemistry/Synonyms

An aliphatic amino acid, lysine has the chemical name L-2,6-di-aminohexanoic acid and has a molecular weight of 146.2. It may be commercially available as the acetate or hydrochloride salts, or as the base.

Lysine may also be known as: L-lysine, L-*Lysine Powder-Pure*®, *Enisyl*®, *Incremin*®, and *Viralys*®.

Storage/Stability

Unless otherwise specified on the label, lysine should be stored at room temperature in tight containers.

Compatibility/Compounding Considerations

- No specific information noted.

Dosage Forms/Regulatory Status

VETERINARY-LABELED PRODUCTS:

Note: There are many products containing lysine as one of many ingredients. No lysine products were located in FDA's Green Book of approved animal drugs. The following products were located with veterinary labeling where lysine is the sole active ingredient:

L-lysine Gel: 250 mg per 1.25 mL: *Viralys*® *Gel*; (OTC). Labeled for use in cats and kittens.

L-lysine Powder: (in a palatable base) approximately 250 mg per rounded scoop: *Viralys*® *Powder*; (OTC). Labeled for use in cats and kittens.

L-Lysine Powder Feed Additive: in 16 oz. jars and 5 lb. pails; L-*Lysine Powder-Pure*®; (OTC) Labeled for use in horses.

HUMAN-LABELED PRODUCTS:

L-Lysine Tablets & Capsules: 312 mg, 334 mg, 500 mg & 1000 mg; *Enisyl*®, generic; (OTC)

Lysine is considered a nutrient in the USA, therefore, it is exempt from FDA drug approval requirements. There are many products available including tablets and capsules that usually range in strengths from 250 mg to 1000 mg. Combination products are also available.

Revisions/References

Monograph revised/updated March 2014.

Drazenovich, T. L., et al. (2009). Effects of dietary lysine supplementation on upper respiratory and ocular disease and detection of infectious organisms in cats within an animal shelter. American Journal of Veterinary Research 70(11): 1391-400.

Maggs, D. J., et al. (2007). Effects of dietary lysine supplementation in cats with enzootic upper respiratory disease. Journal of Feline Medicine and Surgery 9(2): 97-108.

Reed, N. (2014). Chronic Rhinitis in the Cat. Veterinary Clinics of North America-Small Animal Practice 44(1): 33-+.

Rees, T. M. & J. L. Lubinski (2008). Oral supplementation with L-lysine did not prevent upper respiratory infection in a shelter population of cats. Journal of Feline Medicine and Surgery 10(5): 510-3.

Magnesium Citrate; Magnesium Sulfate (oral); Magnesium Oxide — see Saline Cathartics

Magnesium Hydroxide Magnesium/Aluminum Antacids

(mag-**nee**-zee-um hye-**droks**-ide)

Oral Antacid/Laxative

Prescriber Highlights

▶ Used as a gastric antacid for ulcers, etc.; use largely supplanted by newer agents.

▶ In ruminants, can be useful to increase rumen pH; powder much more effective than boluses.

▶ Magnesium salts contraindicated in patients with renal disease. In cattle, rumen pH should be determined before use.

▶ Magnesium salts may cause diarrhea.

▶ Chronic use may lead to electrolyte abnormalities.

▶ Many potential drug interactions with orally administered drugs.

Uses/Indications

Magnesium hydroxide (oxide) alone, or in combination with aluminum salts, has been used in veterinary medicine for the adjunctive treatment of esophagitis, gastric hyperacidity, peptic ulcer and gastritis. In foals and small animals, because of difficulty in administration, the frequent dosing that is often required, and availability of the histamine-2 blocking agents (ranitidine, etc.), proton-pump inhibitors (*e.g.*, omeprazole) and sucralfate, antacids have largely been relegated to adjunctive roles for these indications.

Magnesium hydroxide alone (milk of magnesia) is sometimes used as an oral laxative in small animals.

In ruminants, magnesium hydroxide is used to increase rumen pH and as a laxative in the treatment of rumen overload syndrome (*aka* acute rumen engorgement, rumen acidosis, grain overload, engorgement toxemia, rumen impaction).

Pharmacology/Actions

Oral antacids used in veterinary medicine are generally relatively non-absorbable salts of aluminum, calcium or magnesium. Up to 20% of an oral dose of magnesium can be absorbed. Antacids decrease HCl concentrations in the GI. One gram of these compounds generally neutralizes 20-35 mEq of acid (*in vitro*). Although the pH of the gastric fluid can rarely be brought to near-neutral conditions, at a pH of 3.3, 99% of all gastric acid is neutralized, thereby reducing gastric acid back-diffusion through the gastric mucosa and reducing the amount of acid presented to the duodenum. Pepsin proteolytic activity is reduced by raising the pH and can be minimized if the pH of the gastric contents can be increased to >4.

In cattle, orally administered magnesium hydroxide can act as a rumen alkalinizing agent and decrease rumen antimicrobial activity.

Contraindications/Precautions/Warnings

Magnesium-containing antacids are contraindicated in patients with renal disease. Some products have significant quantities of sodium or potassium and should be used cautiously in patients who should have these electrolytes restricted in their diet. Aluminum-containing antacids may inhibit gastric emptying; use cautiously in patients with gastric outlet obstruction.

Oral magnesium hydroxide should only be used clinically in ruminants with documented rumen acidosis and should not be used for treatment of other suspected rumen disorders or hypomagnesemia. (Smith *et al.* 2004).

Adverse Effects

In monogastric animals, the most common side effects of antacid therapy are constipation with aluminum- and calcium-containing antacids, and diarrhea or frequent loose stools with magnesium containing antacids. Many products contain both aluminum and magnesium salts in the attempt to balance the constipating and laxative actions of the other.

If the patient is receiving a low phosphate diet, hypophosphatemia can develop if the patient chronically receives aluminum-containing antacids. Magnesium-containing antacids can cause hypermagnesemia in patients with severe renal insufficiency.

In ruminants, alkalinization of the rumen may enhance the absorption of ammonia, histamine or other basic compounds.

Reproductive/Nursing Safety

In a system evaluating the safety of drugs in canine and feline pregnancy (Papich 1989), these drugs are categorized as class: *A* (*Probably safe. Although specific studies may not have proved the safety of all drugs in dogs and cats, there are no reports of adverse effects in laboratory animals or women.*)

Overdosage/Acute Toxicity

See the Adverse Effects section above. If necessary, GI and electrolyte imbalances that can occur with chronic or acute overdose should be treated symptomatically.

Drug Interactions

The following drug interactions have either been reported or are theoretical in humans or animals receiving oral magnesium hydroxide and may be of significance in veterinary patients. Unless otherwise noted, use together is not necessarily contraindicated, but weigh the potential risks and perform additional monitoring when appropriate.

- **QUINIDINE:** Increased absorption or pharmacologic effect may occur.
- **SODIUM POLYSTYRENE SULFONATE** (*Kayexalate®*): Antacids may decrease the potassium lowering effectiveness of the drug and in patients in renal failure, may cause metabolic alkalosis.
- **SUSTAINED-** or **EXTENDED-RELEASE MEDICATIONS:** When magnesium hydroxide is used at laxative dosages, it may alter the absorption of these drugs by altering GI transit times.
- **SYMPATHOMIMETIC AGENTS:** Increased absorption or pharmacologic effect may occur.

Oral magnesium salts can **decrease** the amount absorbed or the pharmacologic effect the drugs listed below; separate oral doses of oral magnesium salts and these drugs by 2 hours to help reduce this interaction.

- **ALLOPURINOL**
- **AZOLE ANTIFUNGALS** (**ketoconazole, itraconazole,** etc.)
- **CHLOROQUINE**
- **CORTICOSTEROIDS**
- **DIGOXIN**
- **ETHAMBUTOL**
- **FLUOROQUINOLONES**
- **H-2 ANTAGONISTS** (**ranitidine, famotidine,** etc.)
- **IRON SALTS**
- **ISONIAZID**
- **PENICILLAMINE**
- **PHENOTHIAZINES**
- **TETRACYCLINES**
- **THYROID HORMONES**

Doses

- **DOGS:**

  For adjunctive treatment of hypomagnesemia in dogs with GI disease and severe hypocalcemia (extra-label): Oral magnesium hydroxide (milk of magnesia) at 5 – 15 mL/per dog per 24 hours. (Marks 2009)

- **CATS:**

  As an antacid: Magnesium hydroxide (Milk of Magnesia) (extra-label): 5 – 15 mL PO 1-2 times daily. (Morgan 1988)

- **CATTLE:**

  For rumen overload syndrome (extra-label): For <u>adult animals</u>: Up to 1 gram/kg (MgOH) mixed in 2-3 gallons of warm water and given PO per tube. May repeat (use smaller doses) at 6-12 hour intervals. If the rumen has been evacuated, do not exceed 225 grams initially. Dehydration and systemic acidosis must be concomitantly corrected. <u>Calves:</u> As above but use 1/8th – 1/4th the amount. (Wass *et al.* 1986)

- **HORSES:**

  For adjunctive gastroduodenal ulcer therapy in foals (extra-label): Aluminum/magnesium hydroxide suspension: 15 mL 4 times a day. (Clark *et al.* 1987)

- **SHEEP & GOATS:**

  For rumen overload syndrome (extra-label): As above for cattle, but use 1/8th – 1/4th the amount. (Wass *et al.* 1986)

Monitoring

- Monitoring parameters are dependent upon the indication for the product. Patients receiving high dose or chronic therapy should be monitored for electrolyte imbalances outlined above.

Client Information

- Oral magnesium hydroxide products are available without prescription (OTC); do not give on a regular basis without veterinary supervision.
- Generally well tolerated; constipation or diarrhea can occur.

Compatibility/Compounding Considerations

- No specific information noted.

Dosage Forms/Regulatory Status

VETERINARY-LABELED PRODUCTS:

Note: No oral magnesium hydroxide/oxide products were located in FDA's "Green book" as approved animal drugs.

Oral Boluses 17.9 – 27 grams of magnesium hydroxide (**Note:** products may also contain ginger, capsicum and methyl salicylate). The following may be available: *Magnalax®, Carmilax®, Polymag®, Rumen Bolus®, Instamag®, Magnalax®, Polyox®II, Laxade®*; (OTC)

Oral Powder, each pound of powder contains: 350 – 361 grams of magnesium hydroxide (**Note:** products may also contain ginger, capsicum and methyl salicylate). The following may be available: *Carmilax Powder®, Magnalax®, Polyox®, Laxade®*; (OTC)

Milk of Magnesia (Magnesium Hydroxide) 80 mg/mL in gallons; generic; (OTC). Additional information can be found in the monograph: Saline Cathartics.

HUMAN-LABELED PRODUCTS:

The following is a list of some magnesium hydroxide products available, it is not meant to be all-inclusive.

Magnesium Hydroxide

Tablets chewable: 311 mg & 400 mg; *Phillips' Chewable®, Pedia-Lax®*; (OTC)

Liquid, Oral (also called Milk of Magnesia): 400 mg/5 mL in 129 mL, 355 mL, 360 mL, 780 mL, pt, gal and UD 15 mL & 30 mL; liquid concentrate: 800 mg/5 mL in 240 mL & 1,200 mg/5 mL in 400 mL; generic; (OTC). Additional information can be found in the monograph: Saline Cathartics.

Aluminum Hydroxide and Magnesium Hydroxide

Suspension (**Note:** There are too many products and concentrations to list in this reference; a representative product is *Maalox®* Suspension contains 225 mg aluminum hydroxide and 200 mg magnesium hydroxide per 5 mL.

All aluminum and magnesium hydroxide preparations are OTC. Other dosage forms that are available commercially include: tablets, chewable tablets, and aerosol foam suspension.

Revisions/References

Monograph revised/updated March 2014.

Clark, E. S. & J. L. Becht (1987). Clinical Pharmacology of the Gastrointestinal Tract. Vet Clin North Am (Equine Practice) 3(1): 101-22.

Marks, S. L. (2009). Diagnosis and management of protein-losing enteropathies. Proceedings: WVC. accessed via Veterinary Information Network; vin.com

Morgan, R. V., Ed. (1988). *Handbook of Small Animal Practice.* New York, Churchill Livingstone.

Papich, M. (1989). Effects of drugs on pregnancy. *Current Veterinary Therapy X: Small Animal Practice.* R. Kirk. Philadelphia, Saunders: 1291-9.

Smith, G. W. & M. T. Correa (2004). The effects of oral magnesium hydroxide administration on rumen fluid in cattle. Journal of Veterinary Internal Medicine 18(1): 109-12.

Wass, W. M., et al. (1986). Diseases of the ruminant forestomach. *Current Veterinary Therapy 2: Food Animal Practice.* J. L. Howard. Philadelphia, WB Suanders: 715-23.

Magnesium, Intravenous

(mag-**nee**-zee-um)

Parenteral Electrolyte

For information on the use of oral magnesium hydroxide, refer to the previous monograph. Oral magnesium sulfate and magnesium citrate are detailed in the monograph for Saline Cathartics.

Prescriber Highlights

▶ Parenteral electrolyte for hypomagnesemia, for adjunctive therapy of malignant hyperthermia in swine, as an anticonvulsant, & for refractory ventricular arrhythmias.

▶ Contraindications: Significant myocardial damage or heart block. Caution: Impaired renal function.

▶ Adverse Effects: Usually as a result of OD (drowsiness or other CNS depressant effects, muscular weakness, bradycardia, hypotension, respiratory depression, & increased Q-T intervals on ECG). Very high levels: Neuromuscular blocking activity &, eventually, cardiac arrest.

▶ Must monitor to avoid hypermagnesemia.

▶ Do not confuse mEq/mL & mg/mL concentrations & dosages.

Uses/Indications

Magnesium sulfate is the salt usually used as a source of magnesium and is given via the IV route in magnesium deficient states (hypomagnesemia), for adjunctive therapy of malignant hyperthermia in swine, and also as an anticonvulsant. In humans, intravenous magnesium has been used as a treatment of hypertensive crisis in patients with pheochromocytoma. A case report of using intravenous magnesium in a dog with generalized tetanus has been published (Simmonds *et al.* 2011). In dogs and cats, routine use of magnesium during CPR is not recommended for cardiac arrhythmias, but may be considered for treatment of torsades de pointes (Fletcher *et al.* 2012).

Pharmacology/Actions

Magnesium is used as a cofactor in a variety of enzyme systems and plays a role in muscular excitement and neurochemical transmission.

Pharmacokinetics

IV magnesium results in immediate effects; IM administration may require ≈1 hour for effect. Magnesium is ≈30-35% bound to proteins and the remainder exists as free ions. It is excreted by the kidneys at a rate proportional to the serum concentration and glomerular filtration.

Contraindications/Precautions/Warnings

Parenteral magnesium is contraindicated in patients with myocardial damage or heart block. Magnesium should be given with caution to patients with impaired renal function as hypermagnesemia can result. Dosage reductions of 50-75% have been suggested.

When using IV for hypomagnesemia, consider reducing potassium supplementation or hyperkalemia may result.

Patients receiving parenteral magnesium, especially with reduced renal function, should be observed (loss of deep tendon reflexes, hypotension, respiratory paralysis) and monitored carefully to avoid hypermagnesemia.

Magnesium sulfate for injection is considered a "high-risk medication"; additional dosage determination and dosage preparation safety checks should be employed.

Adverse Effects

Magnesium sulfate (parenteral) adverse effects are generally the result of magnesium overdosage and may include drowsiness or other CNS depressant effects, muscular weakness, bradycardia, hypotension, hypocalcemia, respiratory depression and increased Q-T intervals on ECG. Very high magnesium levels may cause neuromuscular blocking activity and, eventually, cardiac arrest.

Reproductive/Nursing Safety

In humans, the FDA categorizes this drug as category *C* for use during pregnancy (*Animal studies have shown an adverse effect on the fetus, but there are no adequate studies in humans; or there are no animal reproduction studies and no adequate studies in humans.*) The possibility of fetal harm appears remote; however, use only if clearly needed.

Magnesium is excreted in milk, but is unlikely to pose significant risk to nursing offspring.

Overdosage/Acute Toxicity

See Adverse Effects above. Treatment of hypermagnesemia is dependent on the serum magnesium level and any associated clinical effects. Ventilatory support and administration of intravenous calcium [10 – 50 mg/kg IV; (Macintire 2003)] may be required for severe hypermagnesemia.

Drug Interactions

The following drug interactions have either been reported or are theoretical in humans or animals receiving parenteral magnesium sulfate or HCl and may be of significance in veterinary patients. Unless otherwise noted, use together is not necessarily contraindicated, but weigh the potential risks and perform additional monitoring when appropriate.

- **CALCIUM**: Concurrent use of calcium salts may negate the effects of parenteral magnesium.
- **CNS DEPRESSANT DRUGS** (*e.g.*, **barbiturates**, **general anesthetics**): Additive CNS depression may occur.
- **DIGOXIN**: Because serious conduction disturbances can occur, parenteral magnesium should be used with extreme caution with digitalis cardioglycosides.
- **NEUROMUSCULAR BLOCKING AGENTS**: Excessive neuromuscular blockade possible.

Doses

Note: Do not confuse mEq/mL, mEq/kg, mmol/mL, mmol/kg, mg/mL, and mg/kg concentrations and dosages. One gram of magnesium sulfate hexahydrate contains 8.1 mEq of magnesium; 1 mg magnesium sulfate injection contains 0.0081 mEq of magnesium. Magnesium chloride contains 9.25 mEq of magnesium per gram. In adult humans, it is recommended to administer magnesium sulfate IV slowly and cautiously and except for certain conditions (*e.g.*, seizures during eclampsia) not to exceed 150 mg/minute (approximately 2 mg/kg/minute for an average adult human). Extrapolating these recommendations to animals would be approximately 0.016 mEq/kg/minute or 0.027 mg/kg/minute of magnesium sulfate.

- **DOGS/CATS:**

    For hypomagnesemia (extra-label):

    Supplemental magnesium for animals with refractory hypokalemia or endocrine diseases (*e.g.*, **diabetic crises, DKA**), **or critically ill animals** (extra-label): Hypomagnesemia can be difficult to diagnose (see monitoring) so parenteral magnesium is used routinely in these patients at 0.75 mEq/kg/day IV (or 0.375 mmol/kg/day) IV. Used in addition to potassium. (Mazzaferro *et al.* 2013)

    For suspected (or confirmed), severe hypomagnesemia (hypocalcemia, etc.); (extra-label): Dosage recommendations vary; most recommend giving a loading dose of 0.15 – 0.3 mEq/kg (equivalent to 18.5 – 37 mg/kg of magnesium sulfate) IV slowly over 10-20 minutes. Then a CRI is started to give 0.75 – 1 mEq/kg/day (equivalent to 92 –123 mg/kg/day of magnesium sulfate). Daily dose can be given over 12-24 hours. Dos-

ages should be reduced in animals with renal insufficiency. Some suggest reducing daily dosages after the first day. Monitor for signs of hypermagnesemia (see Monitoring).

For refractory ventricular arrhythmias (extra-label): Not recommended for routine use during CPR (Fletcher *et al.* 2012); 0.15 – 0.3 mEq/kg may be administered over 5-15 minutes. (Holland *et al.* 1995)

- **HORSES:**

    For hypomagnesemia (extra-label): <u>Intravenous:</u> Magnesium sulfate and magnesium chloride are the solutions of choice for intravenous administration. For oral treatment, magnesium oxide, magnesium carbonate and magnesium sulfate can be used. For magnesium sulfate, a dose of 100 mg/kg will provide 9.7 mg/kg of Mg^{++} while for magnesium chloride a dose of 100 mg/kg will provide 25.5 mg/kg of Mg^{++}. This is critical as overdosing can be fatal. Excessive oral (nasogastric) supplementation with magnesium sulfate can act as a laxative and induce CNS depression. Recommended IV dose rates for magnesium sulfate in adult horses are 25 – 150 mg/kg/IV/day diluted in 0.9% NaCl, dextrose or polyionic isotonic solutions. Constant rate infusions (CRI) of magnesium sulfate at 100 – 150 mg/kg/day should meet the daily requirements of foals and adult horses. Magnesium sulfate is also used to treat ventricular arrhythmias, in particular quinidine intoxication (torsades de pointes), and should be considered in horses with refractory ileus and synchronous diaphragmatic flutter. Doses of 50 – 100 mg/kg over 30 minutes are considered safe. This is equivalent to 25 – 50 grams of magnesium sulfate for an adult horse. In foals with ischemic encephalopathy, an initial magnesium sulfate dose of 50 mg/kg in the first hour, followed by a CRI of 25 mg/kg/hr has been proposed. This regime can be continued for several days, adjusting the dose based on serum magnesium concentrations. <u>Oral supplementation</u> with magnesium oxide, magnesium carbonate or magnesium sulfate should be considered in animals with chronic hypomagnesemia, malabsorption, renal disease, and exercise-associated hypomagnesemia. Recommended doses are 30 – 50 mg/kg/day for magnesium oxide, 60 – 80 mg/kg/day for magnesium carbonate, or 80 – 100 mg/kg/day for magnesium sulfate. These doses are safe for horses, particularly when compared to the cathartic doses of magnesium sulfate (0.5 – 1 gram/kg). (Toribio 2009)

    For adjunctive treatment of perinatal asphyxia syndrome in foals (extra-label): Magnesium sulfate 50 mg/kg diluted to 1% and given IV over one hour, then decrease to 25 mg/kg/hour as a constant rate infusion for 24 hours (Vaala 2003) or for 1-3 days. (Bentz 2006)

- **RUMINANTS:**

    For hypomagnesemia (grass and other magnesium-related tetanies); (extra-label):

    a) <u>Cattle</u> (presentation was specifically on beef cattle): A typical treatment to an adult cow has been slow intravenous administration (over at least 5 minutes) of 100 mL of the 25% Epsom salt solution, this provides 2.5 grams of magnesium (0.025 grams of magnesium/mL of solution). This solution is highly hypertonic (2028 mOsm/L). Hypomagnesemia is most commonly treated using commercially available combined calcium, magnesium, and phosphorous solutions, 500 mL of these solutions typically contain 1.6 to 2.7 grams of magnesium in the form of a borogluconate, chloride, or hypophosphite salt (the phosphorous in hypophosphite salt form is unavailable to ruminants and therefore worthless). Combined calcium and magnesium solutions are preferred for intravenous administration to 25% Epsom salt solution because ruminants with hypomagnesemia frequently have hypocalcemia, and hypercalcemia provides some protection against the toxic effects of hypermagnesemia. The maximum safe rate of administration of magnesium in cattle is 0.04 mL of 25% Epsom salt solution/kg body weight/minute. For a 500 kg beef cow with hypomagnesemia, this corresponds to a maximum safe rate of administration of 20 mL/minute.

Subcutaneous administration can cause necrosis of the skin. Only combined solutions containing calcium and magnesium solutions should be given subcutaneously.

In a seizuring, hypomagnesemic beef cow, rectal administration may be the only safe and practical way to administer magnesium. After evacuating the rectal contents, an enema containing 60 grams of Epsom Salts (magnesium sulfate heptahydrate) or magnesium chloride in 200 mL of water can be placed in the descending colon (NOT the rectum) and the tail held down for 5 minutes; this increases plasma magnesium concentrations within 10 minutes. Enema solutions can be prematurely evacuated, eliminating the chance for therapeutic success, and some degree of colonic mucosal injury is expected because of the high osmolarity of 30% solutions (approximately 2400 mOsm/L). (Constable 2008)

b) Cattle: 350 mL (250 mL of 25% calcium borogluconate and 100 mL of 10% of magnesium sulfate) by slow IV. If not a proprietary mixture, give calcium first. Relapses occur frequently after IV therapy, and 350 mL SC of magnesium sulfate 20% may give more sustained magnesium levels. Alternating calcium and magnesium may prevent adverse effects. Continue control measures for 4-7 days to prevent relapse. Sheep and Goats: 50 – 100 mL of above solution (calcium/magnesium). (Merrall *et al.* 1986)

- **SWINE:**

  For adjunctive therapy of malignant hyperthermia syndrome (extra-label): Magnesium sulfate 50%: Incremental doses of 1 gram injected slowly IV until heart rate and muscle tone are reduced. Use calcium if magnesium-related cardiac arrest occurs. (Booth *et al.* 1988)

Monitoring

- Serum magnesium. Total serum magnesium (tMg) measures magnesium in the serum in its 3 forms (ionized, bound, and complexed). Unfortunately it does not correlate well with total body magnesium, but may be useful especially when suspecting hypermagnesemia. Ionized magnesium (iMg) is preferred by some, but alone may not be clinically useful due to methodology concerns and the low percentages of total body magnesium it represents. The iMg/tMg ratio may be more useful. In patients with normal renal function, pre-magnesium levels (iMg/tMg) are compared with levels after an IV loading dose. If the ratio is elevated, it suggests that a larger portion of stored body magnesium is being mobilized in response to a decrease in whole body magnesium content. Alternatively, after an IV load a 24-hour urine magnesium collection can be obtained. Retention of >20% of the magnesium loading dose is considered suggestive of cellular magnesium depletion and >50% retention is considered diagnostic (Hoareau 2013).Physical signs associated with hypomagnesemia or hypermagnesemia (loss of deep tendon reflexes, hypotension, respiratory paralysis).
- Serum calcium, potassium if indicated.

Client Information

Injectable magnesium is given by veterinarians only.

Chemistry/Synonyms

Magnesium sulfate occurs as small, usually needle-like, colorless crystals with a cool, saline, bitter taste. It is freely soluble in water and sparingly soluble in alcohol. Magnesium sulfate injection has a pH of 5.5-7. One gram of magnesium sulfate hexahydrate contains 8.1 mEq of magnesium. Magnesium chloride contains 9.25 mEq of magnesium per gram.

When using commercially available magnesium sulfate injections:

- Magnesium sulfate 4% (40 mg/mL) Injection contains 0.325 mEq/mL of elemental magnesium
- Magnesium sulfate 8% (80 mg/mL) Injection contains 0.65 mEq/mL of elemental magnesium
- Magnesium sulfate 50% (500 mg/mL) Injection contains 4 mEq/mL of elemental magnesium
- Magnesium sulfate 1% in Dextrose 5% Injection contains 0.081 mEq/mL elemental magnesium
- Magnesium sulfate 2% in Dextrose 5% Injection contains 0.162 mEq/mL elemental magnesium
- Magnesium chloride 200 mg/mL Injection contains 1.97 mEq/mL of elemental magnesium.

Magnesium Sulfate may also be known as: 518, epsom salts, magnesii sulfas, magnesium sulfuricum heptahydricum, magnesium sulphate, sal amarum, sel anglais, and sel de sedlitz; many trade names are available.

Storage/Stability

Magnesium sulfate and magnesium chloride for injection should be stored at room temperature (15-30°C); avoid freezing. Refrigeration may result in precipitation or crystallization.

Compatibility/Compounding Considerations

Magnesium sulfate 50% must be diluted to 20% or less before administration. Dextrose 5% injection and sodium chloride 0.9% injection are commonly used as diluents.

Magnesium sulfate is reportedly physically **compatible** with the following intravenous solutions: dextrose 5%, LRS, and Normal saline. It is also **compatible** with calcium gluconate (low concentrations of both—if contemplating mixing with calcium contact a hospital pharmacist), chloramphenicol sodium succinate, cisplatin, hydrocortisone sodium succinate, isoproterenol HCl, metoclopramide HCl (in syringes), norepinephrine bitartrate, penicillin G potassium, potassium phosphate, and verapamil HCl. Additionally, at Y-sites: acyclovir sodium, amikacin sulfate, ampicillin sodium, cefazolin sodium, cefotaxime sodium, cefoxitin sodium, clindamycin phosphate, doxycycline phosphate, erythromycin lactobionate, esmolol HCl, gentamicin sulfate, heparin sodium, labetalol HCl, metronidazole (RTU), oxacillin sodium, piperacillin sodium, potassium chloride, tetracycline HCl, tobramycin sulfate, trimethoprim/sulfamethoxazole, vancomycin HCl, and vitamin B-complex with C.

Magnesium sulfate is reportedly physically **incompatible** when mixed with alkali hydroxides, alkali carbonates, salicylates and many metals, including the following solutions or drugs: fat emulsion 10 %, calcium gluceptate, dobutamine HCl, polymyxin B sulfate, procaine HCl, and sodium bicarbonate. Compatibility is dependent upon factors such as pH, concentration, temperature and diluent used; consult specialized references or a hospital pharmacist for more specific information.

Dosage Forms/Regulatory Status

VETERINARY-LABELED PRODUCTS:

There are no parenteral magnesium-only products FDA-approved for veterinary medicine. There are, however, several proprietary magnesium-containing products available that may also include calcium, phosphorus, potassium, and/or dextrose; refer to the individual product's labeling for specific dosage information. Trade names for these products include: *Norcalciphos®*, *Cal-Dextro® Special*, and *#2* and *CMPK®*, and *Cal-Phos® #2*; (Rx)

HUMAN-LABELED PRODUCTS:

Magnesium Sulfate Injection, Solution in 5% Dextrose: 1% (10 mg/mL; 0.081 mEq/mL) in single-dose containers; 2% (20 mg/mL; 0.162 mEq/mL) in 500 mL & 1,000 mL single-dose containers; generic; (Rx)

Magnesium Sulfate Injection, solution: 4% (40 mg/mL; 0.325 mEq/mL) in 50 mL, 100 mL, 500 mL & 1,000 mL; 8% (80 mg/mL; 0.65 mEq/mL) in 50 mL; 50% (500 mg/mL; 4 mEq/mL) in 2 mL, 10 mL, 20 mL & 50 mL vials; generic; (Rx)

Magnesium Chloride Injection: 20% (200 mg/mL; 1.97 mEq/mL) in 50 mL multi-dose vials; generic; (Rx)

There are many oral magnesium products in various dosage forms available.

Revisions/References

Monograph revised/updated March 2014.

Bentz, B. (2006). Current management practices for critically ill foals. Proceedings: ABVP. accessed via Veterinary Information Network; vin.com

Booth, N. H. & L. E. McDonald, Eds. (1988). *Veterinary Pharmacology and Therapeutics.* Ames, Iowa State University Press.

Constable, P. D. (2008). Metabolic Disease of Beef Cattle: Diagnosis, Treatment, & Prevention. Western Veterinary Conference. accessed via Veterinary Information Network; vin.com

Fletcher, D. J., et al. (2012). RECOVER evidence and knowledge gap analysis on veterinary CPR. Part 7: Clinical guidelines. J. Vet. Emerg. Crit. Care **22**.

Hoareau, G. L. (2013). Are you missing low magnesium? Proceedings: International Veterinary Emergency and Critical Care Symposium. accessed via Veterinary Information Network; vin.com

Holland, M. & C. Chastain (1995). Uses & misuses of aspirin. *Kirk's Current Veterinary Therapy:XII.* J. Bonagura. Philadelphia, W.B. Saunders: 70-3.

Macintire, D. (2003). Metabolic derangements in critical patients. Proceedings: ACVIM Forum. accessed via Veterinary Information Network; vin.com

Mazzaferro, E. & L. L. Powell (2013). Fluid Therapy for the Emergent Small Animal Patient: Crystalloids, Colloids, and Albumin Products. Veterinary Clinics of North America: Small Animal Practice **43**(4): 721-34.

Merrall, M. & D. M. West (1986). Rumiant hypomagnesemic tetanies. *Current Veterinary Therapy: Food Animal Practice 2.* J. L. Howard. Philadelphia, W.B. Saunders: 328-32.

Simmonds, E. E., et al. (2011). Magnesium sulfate as an adjunct therapy in the management of severe generalized tetanus in a dog. J. Vet. Emerg. Crit. Care **21**(5): 542-6.

Toribio, R. (2009). Disorders of the Equine Calcium & Magnesium Metabolism. Proceedings: ACVIM. accessed via Veterinary Information Network; vin.com

Vaala, W. (2003). Perinatal asphyxia syndrome in foals. *Current Therapy in Equine Medicine 5.* N. Robinson and E. Carr. Phila., Saunders: 644-9.

Mannitol

(**man**-i-tole)

Osmotic Diuretic

Prescriber Highlights

▶ Osmotic diuretic used for acute oliguric renal failure, to reduce intraocular & intracerebral pressures, to enhance urinary excretion of some toxins &, with other diuretics, to rapidly reduce edema or ascites (caution).

▶ Contraindications: Anuria secondary to renal disease, severe dehydration, severe pulmonary congestion, or pulmonary edema.

▶ Halt treatment if progressive heart failure, pulmonary congestion, or progressive renal failure/damage develop.

▶ Adverse Effects: Fluid & electrolyte imbalances, GI (nausea, vomiting), cardiovascular (pulmonary edema, CHF, tachycardia), & CNS effects (dizziness, headache, etc.).

▶ Adequate urine output, fluid, & electrolyte monitoring & treatment mandatory.

▶ Be certain crystals are dissolved in solution before administering; in-line IV filter (5 micron) is recommended.

Uses/Indications

Mannitol is used to promote diuresis in acute oliguric renal failure, reduce intraocular and intracerebral pressures, enhance urinary excretion of some toxins, (*e.g.*, aspirin, some barbiturates, bromides, ethylene glycol) and, in conjunction with other diuretics, to rapidly reduce edema or ascites when appropriate (see Contraindications-Precautions below). In stable cats with calcium oxalate stones and minimal renal compromise, mannitol has been used for intravenous fluid diuresis expulsion therapy (Palm *et al.* 2011). In humans, it is also used as an irrigating solution during transurethral prostatic resections.

Pharmacology/Actions

After intravenous administration, mannitol is freely filtered at the glomerulus and poorly reabsorbed in the tubule. The increased osmotic pressure prevents water from being reabsorbed at the tubule. To be effective, there must be sufficient renal blood flow and filtration for mannitol to reach the tubules. Although water is proportionately excreted at a higher rate, sodium, other electrolytes, uric acid, and urea excretions are also enhanced.

Mannitol may have a nephro-protective effect by preventing the concentration of nephrotoxins from accumulating in the tubular fluid. Additionally, it may minimize renal tubular swelling via its osmotic properties, increase renal blood flow and glomerular filtration by causing renal arteriole dilatation, decreased vascular resistance, and decreased blood viscosity.

Mannitol does not appreciably enter the eye or the CNS, but can decrease intraocular and CSF pressure through its osmotic effects. Mannitol has immediate plasma-expanding effects, thereby decreasing blood viscosity and improving erythrocyte oxygen delivery to the CNS. Mannitol also has some free radical scavenging effects. Mannitol can reduce intracranial pressure for 2-5 hours; intraocular pressure is usually reduced for 4-12 hours. Rebound increases in CSF pressures may occur after the drug is discontinued.

Pharmacokinetics

Although long believed to be unabsorbed from the GI, up to 17% of an oral dose is excreted unchanged in the urine after oral dosing in humans. After intravenous dosing, mannitol is distributed to the extracellular compartment and does not penetrate the eye. Unless the patient has received very high doses, is acidotic, or there is loss of integrity of the blood-brain barrier, it does not cross into the CNS.

Only 7-10% of mannitol is metabolized, the remainder is excreted unchanged in the urine. The elimination half-life of mannitol is approximately 100 minutes in adult humans. Half-lives in cattle and sheep are reported to be between 40-60 minutes.

Contraindications/Precautions/Warnings

Mannitol is contraindicated in patients with anuria secondary to renal disease, severe dehydration, severe pulmonary congestion or pulmonary edema. In humans, mannitol is labeled as contraindicated in patients with intracranial bleeding (unless during craniotomy), but there does not appear to be any clinical evidence to support this contraindication and it is often used in human patients with intracranial bleeding.

Use with extreme caution in hypovolemic patients as mannitol can enhance hypotension. Hypertonic saline may be a better choice to treat increased CSF pressure and increase intravascular volume in these patients. Adequate fluid replacement must be administered to dehydrated animals before mannitol therapy is started. Do not administer more than a test dose of mannitol until determining whether the patient has some renal function and urine output.

Use mannitol with caution when treating ethylene glycol toxicity or other hyperosmolar states as it can add to intravascular hyperosmolarity. Mannitol can cause false positive test results for ethylene glycol, so EG testing should occur before mannitol is administered.

Mannitol therapy should be stopped if progressive heart failure, pulmonary congestion, progressive renal failure or damage (including increasing oliguria and azotemia) develops after mannitol therapy is instituted.

Use mannitol with caution for treating secondary glaucomas, as it may cross the damaged "blood-aqueous barrier" and increase intraocular pressure (IOP).

Do not give mannitol with whole blood products, unless at least 20 mEq/L of sodium chloride is added to the solution or pseudo-agglutination may result.

Be certain any crystals in solution are re-dissolved before administering; an in-line IV filter (5 micron) is also recommended.

Adverse Effects

Fluid (volume depletion, volume overload in oliguric patients), electrolyte (hypernatremia, hypokalemia, pseudo-hyponatremia), and acid-base (metabolic acidosis) imbalances are the most severe adverse effects generally encountered during mannitol therapy. When used for oliguric renal failure, the potential exists for volume overload if oliguria persists.

Adequate monitoring and support are imperative.

Other adverse effects that may be encountered include GI (nausea, vomiting), cardiovascular (pulmonary edema, CHF, tachycardia), acute kidney injury (if osmolality >320 mOsm/L), and CNS effects (dizziness, headache, etc.).

Reproductive/Nursing Safety

In humans, the FDA categorizes this drug as category *C* for use during pregnancy (*Animal studies have shown an adverse effect on the fetus, but there are no adequate studies in humans; or there are no animal reproduction studies and no adequate studies in humans.*)

It is not known whether this drug is excreted in milk, but it is unlikely that it would pose significant risk to nursing offspring.

Overdosage/Acute Toxicity

Inadvertent overdosage can cause excessive excretion of sodium, potassium, and chloride. If urine output is inadequate, water intoxication or pulmonary edema may occur. Treat by halting mannitol administration and monitoring and correcting electrolyte and fluid imbalances. Hemodialysis is effective in clearing mannitol.

Drug Interactions

The following drug interactions have either been reported or are theoretical in humans or animals receiving mannitol and may be of significance in veterinary patients. Unless otherwise noted, use together is not necessarily contraindicated, but weigh the potential risks and perform additional monitoring when appropriate.

- **FUROSEMIDE:** Use with mannitol can increase risk for hypovolemia; evidence conflicts whether any benefit occurs in treating increased CSF pressure.
- **LITHIUM:** Mannitol can increase the renal elimination of lithium.
- **SOTALOL:** Mannitol's effects on potassium and magnesium may increase the risk for QT prolongation.

Laboratory Considerations

- Mannitol can interfere with **blood inorganic phosphorus** concentrations and **blood ethylene glycol** determinations.
- Mannitol can give a false positive **ethylene glycol test**.

Doses

- **DOGS/CATS:**

  For treatment of oliguric renal failure (extra-label): Only use after correcting fluid, electrolyte, acid/base balance and determining that the patient is not anuric. Most recommend 0.25 – 0.5 grams/kg as a slow IV bolus over 10-20 minutes.

  (Recommendations vary and range from 0.25 – 1 gram/kg IV over 10-40 minutes, but no evidence was located that supports one recommendation over the other.) If substantial diuresis occurs, can either start a CRI at 60 – 120 mg/kg/hour IV or give as intermittent repeated boluses (0.25 – 0.5 grams/kg) every 4-6 hours. Some recommend that total daily dose should not exceed 2 grams/kg per day. Intensive monitoring of fluid and electrolyte status required.

  For adjunctive treatment of acute glaucoma (extra-label): Topical therapy using prostaglandin analogs, carbonic anhydrase inhibitors, beta-blockers and/or miotics have usually replaced the need for intravenous mannitol therapy, but emergency osmotic therapy with mannitol is often still necessary in animals refractory to topical medication. Most recommend 0.5 – 1 gram/kg as a slow IV bolus over 10-20 minutes. (Recommendations vary and range from 0.5 – 2 grams/kg IV over 20-30 minutes, but no evidence was located that supports one recommendation over the other.) Withholding water for 1-4 hours post-dose is often recommended. Effects begin ≈20-30 minutes post-dose, peak around 90 minutes and can persist for several hours.

  For adjunctive treatment of increased CSF pressure/cerebral edema (extra-label): Only use after correcting fluid, electrolyte, acid/base balance and determining that the patient is not anuric. Most recommend 0.5 grams/kg IV/IO over 15-20 minutes. Effects for lowering CSF pressure begin within 30 minutes and can last up to 6 hours. If required, repeat boluses may be administered (usually q6-8h); CRI's are not recommended. Intensive monitoring of fluid and electrolyte status required; avoid hypovolemia. On source states: "Mannitol administration should always be followed by isotonic crystalloid and/or colloid therapy to avoid hypovolemia..." (DiFazio *et al.* 2013).

- **CATTLE, SWINE, SHEEP, GOATS:**

  For adjunctive treatment of cerebral edema (extra-label): 1 – 3 gram/kg IV (usually with steroids and/or DMSO). (Dill 1986)

  As a diuretic for oliguric renal failure (extra-label): 1 – 2 gram/kg (5 – 10 mL of 20% solution) IV after rehydration; monitor urine flow and fluid balance. (Osweiler 1986)

- **HORSES:**

  Adjunctive treatment of hypoxicischemic encephalopathy (HIE) in foals; (extra-label): 0.25 – 1 g/kg IV q6-12h. (Valla 2013)

  For increased intracranial pressure from traumatic brain injury (TBI); (extra-label): Intermittent IV bolus doses of 0.25 – 1 gram/kg. Mannitol produces immediate reduction of ICP by decreasing hematocrit and viscosity, improving CBF, and decreasing blood vessel diameter. Cerebral oxygenation improves because of improved red cell oxygen transport. These effects are best accomplished with rapid bolus administration rather than continuous administration. The patient must be monitored to avoid hypovolemia and hypotension. Risks of mannitol therapy are the development of acute renal failure, rebound cerebral edema, and blood brain barrier disruption with repeated or high dosages. The efficacy of mannitol wanes with repeated administration. In humans, mannitol is avoided if serum osmolality is >320 mOsm/L to prevent the risk of acute renal failure. (Aleman 2007)

Monitoring

- Serum electrolytes (especially sodium), osmolality (especially if multiple doses or CRI's are administered).
- BUN, serum creatinine.
- Urine output.

- Central venous pressure, if possible.
- Lung auscultation.

Client Information

- Mannitol should only be administered by professional staff in a setting where adequate monitoring can occur.

Chemistry/Synonyms

An osmotic diuretic, mannitol occurs as an odorless, sweet-tasting, white, crystalline powder with a melting range of 165°-168° and a pK$_a$ of 3.4. One gram is soluble in ≈5.5 mL of water (at 25°C); it is very slightly soluble in alcohol. The commercially available injectable products have approximate pH of 4.5-7.

Mannitol may also be known as: cordycepic acid, E421, manita, manitol, manna sugar, mannite, mannitolum, or Eufusol M.

Storage/Stability

Mannitol solutions are recommended to be stored at room temperature; avoid freezing.

Crystallization may occur at low temperatures in concentrations >15%. Resolubolization of the crystals can be accomplished by heating the bottle in hot (up to 80°C) water. Cool to body temperature before administering. An in-line IV filter is recommended when administering concentrated mannitol solutions. Alternatively, heated storage chambers (35°-50°C) have been suggested to assure that soluble product is available at all times. Microwaving glass ampules/vials has been suggested, but explosions have been documented and this procedure cannot be recommended. Supersaturated solutions of mannitol in PVC bags may show a white flocculent precipitate that will tend to reoccur even after heating.

Compatibility/Compounding Considerations

Drugs reported to be physically **compatible** with mannitol include: amikacin sulfate, cefoxitin sodium, cimetidine HCl, dopamine HCl, gentamicin sulfate, metoclopramide HCl, tobramycin sulfate, and verapamil HCl.

Mannitol should NOT be added to whole blood products to be used for transfusion. Sodium or potassium chloride can cause mannitol to precipitate out of solution when mannitol concentrations are 20% or greater. Mannitol may be physically **incompatible** when mixed with strongly acidic or alkaline solutions.

Mannitol is reportedly stable when mixed with cisplatin for a short period of time, but advanced premixing of the drugs should be avoided because a complex may form.

Dosage Forms/Regulatory Status

VETERINARY-LABELED PRODUCTS:

There are no FDA-approved products listed in the "Green Book" (on date of review: 04/2014). Unapproved, veterinary-labeled products may be available.

HUMAN-LABELED PRODUCTS:

Mannitol for Injection

Mannitol Injection: 5% (50 mg/mL; 275 mOsm/L) in 1000 mL;

10% (100 mg/mL; 550 mOsm/L) in 500 mL and 1000 mL;

15% (150 mg/mL; 825 mOsm/L) in 500 mL;

20% (200 mg/mL; 1100 mOsm/L) in 250 mL and 500 mL;

25% (250 mg/mL; 1375 mOsm/L) in 50 mL vials and syringes (12.5 grams/vial); generic; (Rx)

Mannitol Solution (irrigant): 5 grams/100 mL in distilled water (275 mOsm/L) in 2000 mL; generic; (Rx)

Revisions/References

Monograph revised/updated March 2014.

Aleman, M. (2007). Pharmacotherapy for neurologic disorders. Proceedings: IVECCS. accessed via Veterinary Information Network; vin.com

DiFazio, J. & D. J. Fletcher (2013). Updates in the Management of the Small Animal Patient with Neurologic Trauma. Veterinary Clinics of North America: Small Animal Practice 43(4): 915-40.

Dill, S. G. (1986). Polioencephalomalacia in Ruminants. *Current Veterinary Therapy: Food Animal Practice 2*. J. L. Howard. Philadelphia, W.B. Saunders: 868-9.

Osweiler, G. D. (1986). Nephrotoxic Plants. *Current Veterinary Therapy: Food Animal Practice 2*. J. L. Howard. Philadelphia, W.B. Saunders: 401-4.

Palm, C. & J. Westropp (2011). Cats and calcium oxalate: Strategies for managing lower and upper tract stone disease. Journal of Feline Medicine and Surgery 13(9): 651-60.

Valla, W. (2013). The Problem Pregnancy: Recognition and Therapy. Proceedings: ABVP. accessed via Veterinary Information Network; vin.com

Marbofloxacin

(mar-boe-**flox**-a-sin)   Zeniquin®

Fluoroquinolone Antibiotic

Prescriber Highlights

▶ Veterinary oral fluoroquinolone antibiotic effective against a variety of pathogens.

▶ Not effective against anaerobes.

▶ Contraindications: Hypersensitivity to fluoroquinolones; Relatively contraindicated for young, growing animals due to cartilage abnormalities.

▶ Caution: Hepatic or renal insufficiency, seizure patients, or dehydration.

▶ Adverse Effects: GI distress; does not appear to cause ocular toxicity in cats.

▶ Drug interactions.

Uses/Indications

Marbofloxacin is labeled for the treatment of susceptible bacterial infections in dogs and cats. In the published guidelines for treatment of urinary tract disease in dogs and cats, the Antimicrobial Guidelines Working Group of the International Society for Companion Animal Infectious Diseases recommends that marbofloxacin be reserved for documented resistant UTIs, but it is a good first-line choice for pyelonephritis (Weese *et al.* 2011). In dogs, marbofloxacin appears to have some efficacy for treating the clinical signs associated with canine leishmaniasis (Rougier *et al.* 2012).

Pharmacology/Actions

Marbofloxacin is a bactericidal agent. The bactericidal activity of marbofloxacin is concentration dependent, with susceptible bacteria cell death occurring within 20-30 minutes of exposure. Like other fluoroquinolones, marbofloxacin has demonstrated a significant post-antibiotic effect for both gram-negative and gram-positive bacteria and is active in both stationary and growth phases of bacterial replication.

Its mechanism of action is not thoroughly understood, but it is believed to act by inhibiting bacterial DNA-gyrase (a type-II topoisomerase), preventing DNA supercoiling and DNA synthesis.

Marbofloxacin has a similar spectrum of activity as the other veterinary commercially available agents although marbofloxacin is considered the most active veterinary fluoroquinolone against *Pseudomonas aeruginosa*. Fluoroquinolones agents have good activity against many gram-negative bacilli and cocci, including most species and strains of *Pseudomonas aeruginosa*, *Klebsiella* spp., *E. coli*, Enterobacter, Campylobacter, Shigella, Salmonella, Aeromonas, Haemophilus, Proteus, Yersinia, Serratia, and Vibrio species. Other organisms that are generally susceptible include *Brucella* spp., *Chlamydia trachomatis*, Staphylococci (including penicillinase-producing and methicillin-resistant strains), Mycoplasma, and *Mycobacterium* spp. (not the etiologic agent for Johne's Disease).

The fluoroquinolones have variable activity against most streptococci and are not usually recommended to use for these infections. These drugs have weak activity against most anaerobes and are ineffective in treating anaerobic infections.

Resistance does occur by mutation, particularly with *Pseudomonas aeruginosa*, *Klebsiella pneumonia*, Acinetobacter, and Enterococci, but plasmid-mediated resistance is thought to occur only rarely.

Marbofloxacin's leishmanicidal activity is via the TNF-alpha and nitric oxide synthase pathways (Rougier *et al.* 2012).

Pharmacokinetics

In dogs, marbofloxacin is characterized as being rapidly absorbed after oral administration with a bioavailability of 94%. Peak plasma levels occur in ≈1.5 hours. Protein binding is low and the apparent volume of distribution is 1.2-1.9 L/kg. Relatively high levels can be found in prostatic fluid. Elimination half-life averages 9-12 hours. The drug is eliminated unchanged in the urine (40%) and bile/feces. Only ≈15% of a dose is metabolized in the liver.

In cats, absorption after oral dosing is nearly complete and peak serum levels occur ≈1-2 hours post-dose. Terminal elimination half-life is ≈13 hours.

Renal impairment does not significantly alter dosing requirements.

Contraindications/Precautions/Warnings

Like other quinolones, marbofloxacin is labeled as contraindicated in small and medium breed dogs up to 8 months of age, large breeds to 12 months old, and giant breeds to 18 months old. It is also labeled as contraindicated in cats less than 12 months of age. Quinolones are also contraindicated in patients hypersensitive to them.

Marbofloxacin can (rarely) cause CNS stimulation and should be used with caution in patients with seizure disorders.

The FDA has prohibited the use of this drug in food-producing animals.

Adverse Effects

With the exception of potential cartilage abnormalities in young animals (see Contraindications above), the adverse effect profile of marbofloxacin is usually limited to GI distress (vomiting, anorexia, soft stools, diarrhea) and decreased activity.

Other fluoroquinolones have, in rare incidences, caused elevated hepatic enzymes, ataxia, seizures, depression, lethargy, and nervousness in dogs. Hypersensitivity reactions or crystalluria could potentially occur.

It is not known if marbofloxacin can also cause the ocular toxicity that has been reported with high dose enrofloxacin in cats. While unlikely, FDA's Adverse Drug Reaction database has received 14 reports (as of July 3, 2007) of blindness associated with marbofloxacin. Causal effect cannot be proven, but use higher dosages carefully.

Reproductive/Nursing Safety

Safety of marbofloxacin during pregnancy has not been established.

Overdosage/Acute Toxicity

It is unlikely an acute overdose of marbofloxacin would result in signs more serious than either anorexia or vomiting, but the adverse effects noted above could occur. Dogs receiving 55 mg/kg per day for 12 days developed anorexia, vomiting, dehydration, tremors, red skin, facial swelling, lethargy, and weight loss.

Drug Interactions

The following drug interactions have either been reported or are theoretical in humans or animals receiving marbofloxacin or related fluoroquinolones and may be of significance in veterinary patients. Unless otherwise noted, use together is not necessarily contraindicated, but weigh the potential risks and perform additional monitoring when appropriate.

- **ANTACIDS/DAIRY PRODUCTS**: Containing cations (Mg++, Al+++, Ca++) may bind to marbofloxacin and prevent its absorption; separate doses of these products by at least 2 hours.

- **ANTIBIOTICS, OTHER (aminoglycosides, 3rd-generation cephalosporins, penicillins—extended-spectrum)**: Synergism may occur, but is not predictable, against some bacteria (particularly *Pseudomonas aeruginosa*) with these compounds. Although marbofloxacin has minimal activity against anaerobes, *in vitro* synergy has been reported when used with **clindamycin** against strains of Peptostreptococcus, Lactobacillus and *Bacteroides fragilis*.

- **CYCLOSPORINE**: Fluoroquinolones may exacerbate the nephrotoxicity and reduce the metabolism of cyclosporine (used systemically).

- **FLUNIXIN**: Has been shown in dogs to increase the AUC and elimination half-life of enrofloxacin and enrofloxacin increases the AUC and elimination half-life of flunixin; it is unknown if marbofloxacin also causes this effect or if other NSAIDs interact with marbofloxacin in dogs.

- **GLYBURIDE**: Severe hypoglycemia possible.

- **IRON, ZINC (oral)**: Decreased marbofloxacin absorption; separate doses by at least 2 hours.

- **METHOTREXATE**: Increased MTX levels possible with resultant toxicity.

- **NITROFURANTOIN**: May antagonize the antimicrobial activity of the fluoroquinolones and their concomitant use is not recommended.

- **PHENYTOIN**: Marbofloxacin may alter phenytoin levels.

- **PROBENECID**: Blocks tubular secretion of ciprofloxacin and may also increase the blood level and half-life of marbofloxacin.

- **QUINIDINE**: Increased risk for cardiotoxicity.

- **SUCRALFATE**: May inhibit absorption of marbofloxacin; separate doses of these drugs by at least 2 hours.

- **THEOPHYLLINE**: Marbofloxacin may increase theophylline blood levels; this interaction is more likely with enrofloxacin than with marbofloxacin (Martin-Jimenez 2009).

- **WARFARIN**: Potential for increased warfarin effects.

Laboratory Considerations

- In some human patients, the fluoroquinolones have caused increases in liver enzymes, BUN, and creatinine and decreases in hematocrit. The clinical relevance of these mild changes is not known at this time.

Doses

- **DOGS:**

For susceptible infections (urinary tract, skin and soft tissue); (labeled dose; FDA-approved): 2.75 – 5.5 mg/kg PO once daily. Give for 2-3 days beyond cessation of clinical signs (skin/soft tissue infections) and for at least 10 days (urinary tract). If no improvement noted after 5 days, reevaluate diagnosis. Maximum duration of treatment is 30 days. (Package insert; *Zeniquin®*) **Note:** When treating Pseudomonas infections, most recommend using at the higher end of the dosing range.

For susceptible *Pseudomonas* otitis in patients with otitis media, severe proliferative chronic otitis externa, ulcerative otitis externa, where inflammatory cells are seen cytologically (indicating deeper skin involvement), whose owners cannot administer topical therapy or that have previously had an adverse reaction to topically administered antimicrobial agents (extra-label): Dose at the high end of the flexible dosing label (**Note:** high end = 5.5 mg/kg PO once daily). (Cole 2008)

For leishmaniasis (extra-label): 2 mg/kg PO once daily for 28 days. At one-year follow-up, marbofloxacin showed some efficacy in 70% of treated dogs. At 3 months, there was a 61% decrease in the sum of clinical scores. Though clinically improved, dogs remained parasitologically positive. (Rougier *et al.* 2012)

■ **CATS:**

For susceptible infections (urinary tract, skin and soft tissue); (labeled dose; FDA-approved): 2.75 – 5.5 mg/kg PO once daily. Give for 2-3 days beyond cessation of clinical signs (skin/soft tissue infections); and for at least 10 days (urinary tract). If no improvement noted after 5 days, reevaluate diagnosis. Maximum duration of treatment is 30 days. (Package insert; *Zeniquin®*)

First-line treatment (pending definitive diagnosis) for feline tuberculosis (extra-label): If decision is made to treat cases of localized cutaneous infections or non-tuberculous mycobacteria (NTM); 2 mg/kg PO once daily. Not effective against MAC infection. (Gunn-Moore 2008)

For hemoplasmosis (extra-label): 2.75 mg/kg PO once daily (q24h) for 14-28 days. (Treatment up to 8 weeks with a goal to achieve a negative PCR has been suggested.) (Dowers 2009), (Abrams-Ogg 2012)

■ **REPTILES:**

From a pharmacokinetic study done in Ball pythons (*Python regius*): 10 mg/kg PO at least every 48 hours. Further studies required to determine effective doses and toxicity. (Coke *et al.* 2006)

Monitoring
- Clinical efficacy.
- Adverse effects.

Client Information
- This drug is best given without food on an empty stomach, but if your animal vomits or acts sick after getting it, give with food or small treat (no dairy products, antacids or iron supplements) to see if this helps. If vomiting continues, contact your veterinarian.
- Do not give at the same time with other drugs or vitamins that contain calcium, iron, or aluminum (including sucralfate) as these can reduce the amount of drug absorbed.
- May stunt bone growth or cause joint abnormalities if used in young animals, during pregnancy or while nursing.
- Most common side effects are vomiting, nausea, or diarrhea.
- Give as the veterinarian prescribes; do not stop treating just because the animal appears well.

Chemistry/Synonyms
A synthetic fluoroquinolone antibiotic, marbofloxacin is soluble in water, but solubility decreases as pH increases.

Marbofloxacin may also be known as Ro 9-1168, *Marbocyl®*, or *Zeniquin®*.

Storage/Stability
Marbofloxacin tablets should be stored below 30°C.

Compatibility/Compounding Considerations
- No specific information noted.

Dosage Forms/Regulatory Status
VETERINARY-LABELED PRODUCTS:
Marbofloxacin Oral Tablets: 25 mg, 50 mg, 100 mg, 200 mg; *Zeniquin®*; (Rx). FDA-approved for use in dogs and cats. Must not be used in food animals (USA).

There are several injectable marbofloxacin products licensed in Europe for use in cattle and pigs. Extra-label use of fluoroquinolones is illegal in food animals in the USA.

HUMAN-LABELED PRODUCTS: NONE.

Revisions/References
Monograph revised/updated March 2014.

Abrams-Ogg, A. C. G. (2012). Regenerative anemia in cats. 64th Convention of the Canadian Veterinary Medical Association. accessed via Veterinary Information Network; vin.com
Coke, R. L., et al. (2006). Preliminary single-dose pharmacokinetics of marbofloxacin in ball pythons (Python regius). Journal of Zoo and Wildlife Medicine **37**(1): 6-10.
Cole, L. (2008). Pseudomonas Otitis: Diagnosis, Treatment, and Prognosis. Peroceedings: AVA. accessed via Veterinary Information Network; vin.com
Dowers, K. (2009). Causes of feline anemia: old and new? Proceedings: ACVIM. accessed via Veterinary Information Network; vin.com
Gunn-Moore, D. (2008). Feline Mycobacterial Infections. Proceedings: WSAVA. accessed via Veterinary Information Network; vin.com
Martin-Jimenez, T. (2009). Antimicrobial Drug-Drug Interactions--Synergy & Antagonism. Proceedings: ACVIM. accessed via Veterinary Information Network; vin.com
Rougier, S., et al. (2012). One-year clinical and parasitological follow-up of dogs treated with marbofloxacin for canine leishmaniosis. Veterinary Parasitology **186**(3-4): 245-53.
Weese, J. S., et al. (2011). Antimicrobial Use Guidelines for Treatment of Urinary Tract Disease in Dogs and Cats: Antimicrobial Guidelines Working Group of the International Society for Companion Animal Infectious Diseases. Veterinary Medicine International.

Maropitant Citrate

(ma-**rahp**-it-ent)   Cerenia®

Neurokinin (NK₁) Receptor Antagonist Antiemetic

Prescriber Highlights
▶ Veterinary FDA-approved antiemetic for use in dogs (8 weeks old or older) and cats (16 weeks old or older).
▶ Acts at the emetic center; therefore effective for emesis mediated via either peripheral or central mechanisms.
▶ Subcutaneous injection is FDA-approved for the prevention & treatment of acute vomiting (dogs) and treatment of vomiting (cats). SC injections may cause pain and swelling at injection site. Refrigerating the injection may reduce pain.
▶ Oral dose is higher than subcutaneous dose due to decreased bioavailability of the oral tablet.

Uses/Indications
Maropitant citrate injectable solution is indicated for the prevention and treatment of acute vomiting in dogs (8 weeks old or older); maropitant citrate tablets are indicated for the prevention of acute vomiting and vomiting due to motion sickness in dogs.

In cats, the injection is approved for treatment of vomiting in cats 16 weeks or older.

Maropitant has been effective to control vomiting secondary to a variety of stimuli, including xylazine (cats), hydromorphone (dogs), morphine (dogs), cisplatin (chemotherapy; dogs), copper sulfate and apomorphine (dogs).

Pharmacology/Actions
Maropitant is a neurokinin-1 (NK₁) receptor antagonist that acts in the central nervous system by inhibiting Substance P, the key neurotransmitter involved in vomiting. Maropitant suppresses both peripheral & centrally mediated emesis. Maropitant has been shown to reduce the MAC requirements of sevoflurane and reduce visceral pain in dogs as NK-1 receptors are stimulated by substance P (Boscan *et al.* 2009). Maropitant does not affect gastric emptying times or intestinal transit times, but it can decrease small intestine contraction pressure patterns (McCord *et al.* 2009).

Pharmacokinetics
In dogs, maropitant is rapidly absorbed after oral (PO) & subcutaneous (SC) administration. Peak plasma concentrations (Tmax) occur in less than 1 hour following 1 mg/kg subcutaneous administration and less than 2 hours after oral administration of 2 or 8 mg/kg. After oral administration bioavailability is 24% (2 mg/kg) and 37% (8 mg/kg), suggesting first pass metabolism that becomes saturated at the higher dose. Feeding status does not affect bioavailability.

Maropitant follows non-linear pharmacokinetics (PK) at oral

therapeutic doses but approximately linear PK at higher doses (20 – 50 mg/kg). Bioavailability is 91% following subcutaneous administration of 1 mg/kg. An accumulation ratio of 1.5 occurs after once daily use of maropitant for 5 consecutive days at 1 mg/kg SC or 2 mg/kg PO. Accumulation ratio is 2.18 after 2 consecutive days at 8 mg/kg PO daily.

Hepatic metabolism of maropitant involves two cytochrome P450 enzymes: CYP2D15 (low capacity, high affinity) and CYP 3A12 (high capacity, low affinity). The non-linear kinetics at oral doses of 2 – 16 mg/kg may be due to saturation of the low capacity enzyme and increased involvement of CYP3A12 at higher doses. Twenty-one metabolites have been identified with the major (pharmacologically active) metabolite being CJ-18,518, a product of hydroxylation. Plasma protein binding of maropitant is high (99.5%). Half-life is 8.84 hours (range: 6.07-17.7 hrs.) for 1 mg/kg SC; 4.03 hours (range: 2.58-7.09 hrs.) for 2 mg/kg. Maropitant is eliminated primarily by the liver. Urinary recovery of maropitant and its major metabolite is minimal (<1%). Large inter-patient pharmacokinetic variations have been observed.

In cats, bioavailability is ≈50% (PO) and 91% (SC). Protein plasma binding is high (99%). Maropitant displays linear kinetics when administered subcutaneously within the 0.25 – 3 mg/kg dose range. There appears to be an age-related effect on pharmacokinetics, as kittens (16 weeks) appear to have a faster clearance of maropitant than adults. Terminal elimination half-life is approximately 15 hours. Feline-related isoforms of CYP1A and CYP3A enzymes are involved in the hepatic biotransformation of maropitant in cats. Less than 1% of a dose is excreted unchanged in urine or feces (Hickman *et al.* 2008); (Cerenia® label information).

Contraindications/Precautions/Warnings

Safe use has not been evaluated in dogs or cats with gastrointestinal obstruction or that have ingested toxins.

If vomiting persists despite treatment, re-evaluate the case in the attempt to determine the cause.

Maropitant can cause prolongation of the QT interval due to blockade of cardiac potassium channels. The safety of maropitant has not been reported in patients with underlying cardiac disease, when administered with cardiac antiarrhythmic drugs, or when administered with doxorubicin (KuKanich 2012).

Maropitant is most effective in preventing vomiting associated with chemotherapy if administered prior to the chemotherapeutic agent.

Use with caution in patients with hepatic dysfunction as maropitant is hepatically metabolized. One suggestion is to reduce the dosage by 50% if using in patients with hepatic dysfunction.

Use with caution with other medications that are highly protein bound, although clinical significance has not been determined.

Use with caution in puppies less than 11 weeks old; a higher frequency and greater severity of histological evidence of bone marrow hypoplasia was seen in puppies treated with maropitant than in control puppies.

Adverse Effects

Maropitant appears to be well tolerated in dogs and cats. Allergic reactions are possible, but very rare and typically resolve with treatment within 48 hours after discontinuing the drug.

In dogs, pre-travel vomiting and hypersalivation are the two most common side effects seen after administration of the tablets at the higher dosage required for prevention of motion sickness. Swelling or pain at the injection site has been reported following SC administration of the drug. One study found that when the injection was stored in the refrigerator and immediately injected, dogs had less pain at the injection site (Narishetty *et al.* 2007). Other adverse effects reported to the FDA include depression/lethargy, anorexia,

diarrhea, anaphylaxis/anaphylactoid reactions (including swelling of the head/face), ataxia, and convulsions.

In cats, adverse effects reported to the FDA include depression/lethargy, anorexia, injection site pain, and hypersalivation.

Reproductive/Nursing Safety

The safe use of maropitant has not been evaluated in dogs or cats used for breeding, pregnant or lactating bitches or queens. Maropitant should only be used in pregnant or lactating bitches or queens following a benefit/risk assessment by the veterinarian.

Overdosage/Acute Toxicity

Single dose toxicity was studied in mice and rats after oral and intravenous administration. No adverse events were reported after oral administration of up to 30 mg/kg (mice) and 100 mg/kg (rats) and after IV administration of 6.5 mg/kg (mice) and 2.5 mg/kg (rats). The clinical signs of overdosage in mice and rats were similar and independent from the route of administration and included decreased activity, irregular or labored respiration, ataxia and tremors. Salivation, nasal discharge and "raspy" breathing were also noted in rats after oral dosing, while the excretion of reddish urine was observed in some mice and rats following intravenous administration.

In dogs, tolerance has been confirmed in doses of up to 3X the recommended oral dose of 8 mg/kg, for 3 times longer than the proposed maximum duration of treatment. A GLP compliant study revealed no adverse events in dogs after repeated oral doses delivered by oral gavage (5 mg/kg PO q24h x 93 days). In the same study at 20 mg/kg/day, effects included emesis in 2 females on day 1, body weights losses of 8-15% when compared to those at start of study, ECG changes (slight increases in P-R interval, P wave duration and QRS amplitude were noted over the course of treatment), slightly lower serum albumin and slightly higher adrenal weights (females) at 20 mg/kg/day in both sexes.

Oral toxicokinetic studies with the primary metabolite were conducted in mice, rats, rabbits and dogs, indicating that the metabolite was well tolerated.

Drug Interactions

Drug interactions with maropitant have not been thoroughly investigated. During field safety and efficacy studies, a number of medications were used concomitantly with maropitant. Many dogs received multiple medications. The most common concomitant medication was metronidazole. Other commonly used concomitant medications included: dextrose/Ringers solution IV, sodium chloride IV, amoxicillin, ampicillin, cefazolin, cephalexin, enrofloxacin, sulfamethoxazole/trimethoprim, famotidine, sucralfate, cimetidine, dexamethasone, ivermectin, ivermectin/pyrantel, pyrantel, lufenuron/milbemycin, milbemycin, moxidectin, vitamin B, and vaccines. There were no problems observed with any of these drugs in conjunction with maropitant.

Because maropitant is biotransformed in the liver by CYP-450 enzymes and is highly bound to plasma proteins, it may be susceptible to interactions with drugs such **chloramphenicol, phenobarbital, erythromycin, ketoconazole, itraconazole, NSAIDs, etc.**

Laboratory Considerations

- No specific concerns noted.

Doses

Note: When injecting subcutaneously, the label states: Use of refrigerated product may reduce the pain response associated with the injection.

- **DOGS:**

    Labeled Doses (FDA-approved):

    Prevention of acute vomiting: 1 mg/kg SC given at least one hour prior to anticipated emetogenic event and q24h thereafter for up to 5 consecutive days. At a minimum of 2 mg/kg PO given at least 2 hours prior to anticipated emetogenic event and q24h thereafter for up to 5 consecutive days.

Treatment of acute vomiting: 1 mg/kg SC q24h for up to 5 consecutive days. If a longer duration of therapy is needed, a 48-hour washout period is recommended due to accumulation of the drug.

Prevention of vomiting due to motion sickness: At a minimum of 8 mg/kg PO given at least 2 hours prior to travel and q24h for up to 2 consecutive days. Dogs should be fasted 1 hour prior to dosing. (Label Information; *Cerenia*®)

- **CATS:**

Labeled Dose (FDA-approved) **for treatment of vomiting**: 1 mg/kg SC q24h for up to 5 consecutive days. (Label Information; *Cerenia*®)

Extra-label Dose: The labeled dose (1 mg/kg SC) or 1 mg/kg PO are also used in an extra-label manner for prevention of vomiting and motion sickness in cats.

Monitoring
- Clinical efficacy measured by decreased episodes of vomiting.
- Adverse effects.

Client Information
- When using to prevent motion sickness: 3 hours before traveling feed your animal a small meal or snack, then 1 hour later (2 hours before travelling) give maropitant.
- A few dogs may vomit after taking this medication, but giving with a small amount of food will help prevent this.
- Do not wrap the pills tightly in food snacks as this can prevent the drug from being released into the stomach.
- If giving fractions (½, ¼) of a tablet, wrap the remaining portion of the split tablet tightly in foil and store away from children and other animals until you are ready to give it.
- Don't use in puppies less than 8 weeks old as bone marrow problems can occur.
- Side effects are unusual; contact veterinarian if drooling, lethargy (lack of energy), drowsiness/sleepiness, lack of appetite or diarrhea occur.

Chemistry/Synonyms
Classified as a substituted quinuclidine, maropitant's molecular weight is 678.81. The chemical name is (2S,3S)-2-benzhydryl-N-(5-tert-butyl-2-methoxybenzyl) quinuclidin-3-amine citrate.

Maropitant may also be known as CJ-11,972.

Storage/Stability
Maropitant injectable solution contains a preservative and is designed for multi-dose use. The product label states the injectable solution should be stored at controlled room temperature 20-25°C (68-77°F) with excursions between 15-30°C (59-86°F) permitted. After first vial puncture, it should be stored at refrigerated temperature 2-8°C (36-46°F). Use within 90 days of first vial puncture. Stopper may be punctured a maximum of 25 times.

Maropitant tablets are packaged in foil to protect them from moisture uptake, which was observed in less-protective packaging. A European stability study indicated that tablets removed from the blister pack and halved showed no loss of potency during the 48-hour testing period.

Compatibility/Compounding Considerations
No drug-drug compatibility information was located for maropitant.

Dosage Forms/Regulatory Status
VETERINARY-LABELED PRODUCTS:

Maropitant Citrate Injectable Solution: 10 mg/mL in 20 mL multi-dose vials; *Cerenia*®; (Rx). FDA-approved for use in dogs and cats.

Maropitant Citrate Oral Tablets: 16 mg, 24 mg, 60 mg, and 160 mg in blister packs (4 tablets per pack; carton of 10); *Cerenia*®; (Rx). Labeled for use in dogs.

HUMAN-LABELED PRODUCTS: NONE.

Revisions/References
Monograph revised/updated March 2014.

Boscan, P., et al. (2009). Maropitant, a NK-1 Antagonist Decreases the Sevoflurane MAC During Visceral Stimulation in Dogs. Proceedings: IVECCS. accessed via Veterinary Information Network; vin.com
Hickman, M. A., et al. (2008). Safety, pharmacokinetics and use of the novel NK-1 receptor antagonist maropitant (Cerenia(TM)) for the prevention of emesis and motion sickness in cats. J. Vet. Pharmacol. Ther. 31(3): 220-9.
KuKanich, B. (2012). Geriatric Veterinary Pharmacology. Veterinary Clinics of North America-Small Animal Practice 42(4): 631-+.
McCord, K., et al. (2009). Comparison of Gastrointestinal Motility in Dogs Treated with Metoclopramide, Cisapride, Erythromycin or Maropitant Using theSmartpillTM. Proceedings: ACVIM. accessed via Veterinary Information Network; vin.com
Narishetty, S., et al. (2007). "Effect of Refrigeration of the Antiemetic Cerenia (Maropitant) on Pain on Injection." vetlearn.com.

Masitinib Mesylate

(mass-a-**tin**-ib)   Kinavet CA-1®, Masivet®

Tyrosine-Kinase Inhibitor Antineoplastic

Prescriber Highlights

▶ Tyrosine kinase inhibitor antineoplastic agent approved for use in dogs for some forms of mast cell tumors.

▶ Indications and contraindications for masitinib use narrow potential patient pool considerably.

▶ Many potential side effects with GI effects very common. Ongoing monitoring of renal function (including urine protein), CBCs, serum albumin, and liver enzymes are required.

▶ Potentially many drug interactions possible, but little specific information is available to determine potential for clinical significance; use cautiously with other drugs.

▶ Clients must handle drug carefully and avoid contact with dog's excretions, etc.

Uses/Indications

Masitinib oral tablets are labeled as indicated for the treatment of recurrent (post-surgery) or non-resectable Grade II or III cutaneous mast cell tumors in dogs that have not previously received radiotherapy and/or chemotherapy except corticosteroids. At present, the FDA has conditionally approved masitinib for this use.

Masitinib may also prove to be effective alone or in combination with other agents in dogs for treating other tumors or conditions including: osteosarcoma (Fahey *et al.* 2013), hemangiosarcoma (Lyles *et al.* 2012), inflammatory bowel disease (Procoli 2010), and atopic dermatitis (Cadot *et al.* 2011). Before considering clinical (non-research) use of masitinib for these indications, additional research and safety data are needed.

In cats, preliminary findings indicates that masitinib may potentially be effective for treating neoplastic disease such as injection site sarcomas (Lawrence *et al.* 2012), or inflammatory conditions such as feline asthma (Lee-Fowler *et al.* 2012) or inflammatory bowel disease, but more safety/efficacy information must be available before clinical use can be recommended.

A phase-I preclinical study in 20 healthy cats, found that 65% (90% in the once per day group; 40% in the every other day group) developed gastrointestinal effects, but 10% of treated cats developed proteinuria and 15% developed neutropenia (Daly *et al.* 2011).

Pharmacology/Actions

Masitinib is an inhibitor of receptor tyrosine kinase, a protein kinase. Because protein kinases help control several key cellular processes, including cell survival, growth, differentiation and migration, they are an important part of normal cell biology. By binding with growth factors, receptor tyrosine kinases are stimulated. In certain cancer cells, protein kinases may be abnormally activated and enhance cancer cell and blood vessel growth (angiogenesis). Masitinib competitively binds the receptor's ATP-binding site of the intracellular kinase domain, which inhibits phosphorylation and activation of the receptor. Specifically, masitinib's targets include c-KIT, platelet-derived growth factor receptors, and the cytoplasmic kinase Lyn, fibroblast growth factor receptor 3 (FGFR3), and the focal adhesion kinase (FAK) pathway. Mutations in the c-KIT gene have been observed in approximately 25-50% of intermediate and high-grade canine mast cell tumors.

Resistance by cancer cells to tyrosine kinase inhibitors often develops after initial efficacy and relapses are not infrequent.

Mast cells play a key role in allergic reactions, anaphylaxis and inflammation via their release of cytokines and other inflammatory mediators. Masitinib targets c-Kit on mast cells and potentially could treat mast cell mediated allergic or inflammatory conditions.

An *in vitro* study showed that masitinib can reverse doxorubicin-resistance in lymphoid cells via P-glycoprotein inhibition (Zandvliet *et al.* 2013).

Pharmacokinetics

In normal healthy Beagles, masitinib has an oral bioavailability of approximately 80%. It is rapidly absorbed after oral administration with peak levels occurring ≈2-3 hours after a dose. The presence of food increases absorption by ≈15-35%. Volume of distribution is 17 L/kg; the drug is ≈90% bound to plasma proteins. Masitinib is metabolized in the liver predominantly by N-dealkylation, and elimination is principally via the bile and gastrointestinal tract. Total body clearance is 14 mL/min/kg and terminal elimination half-life ranges from 3-11 hours (Anon 2010).

In cats, masitinib (10 mg/kg PO) has a bioavailability of approximately 60%; peak plasma concentrations occur between 1-2 hours post-dose. Volume of distribution ranges from 14-21 L/kg. Terminal half-life is between 3-5 hours; and the clearance is approximately 3 L/hr/kg (Bellamy *et al.* 2009).

Contraindications/Precautions/Warnings

Labeled contraindications for dogs include:

- Dogs weighing less than 4 kg as they cannot be accurately and safely dosed (European label). The USA label states that the drug cannot be safely dosed in dogs weighing less than 7 kg.
- Dogs less than 6 months old (European label). The USA label states that safe use has not been evaluated in dogs less than 2 years old.
- Hypoalbuminemia (serum albumin <1X lower limit of normal).
- Proteinuria (urine protein to creatinine [UPC] ratio >1).
- Azotemia (elevated blood urea nitrogen or creatinine >1X upper limit of normal).
- Anemia (hematocrit < 30% or hemoglobin <10 g/dL).
- Neutropenia (<2,000/mcL)
- AST or ALT elevations (>3X upper limit of normal).
- Hyperbilirubinemia (>1.5X upper limit of normal).
- Hypersensitivity to masitinib.
- Dogs that are pregnant or nursing (See Reproductive Safety).

Additionally, masitinib should be used with caution in dogs with mild to moderate hepatic or renal impairment, and with other potentially nephrotoxic or gastrointestinal toxic drugs (including NSAIDs).

Adverse Effects

In dogs, masitinib can cause a litany of adverse effects, some of them serious that can require dosage reduction or drug discontinuation. Most commonly, gastrointestinal effects (vomiting, anorexia and diarrhea) and increases in ALT are seen. Some clinicians prescribe drugs such as H2-blockers, proton pump inhibitors and opiate antidiarrheals (*e.g.*, loperamide—caution in MDR1-sensitive breeds) to help control GI signs. Mild to moderate lethargy, cough, lymphadenopathy and alopecia are also fairly common. Renal toxicity (increased serum creatinine, proteinuria), neutropenia, anemia (non-regenerative and hemolytic), decreased serum albumin, increased liver enzymes can occur and ongoing monitoring for these effects is required. Many other adverse effects have been described (see package insert). A case report of a dog with masitinib-associated minimal change disease with acute tubular necrosis has been published (Brown *et al.* 2013).

A phase-I preclinical study in 20 healthy cats, found that 65% (90% in the once per day group; 40% in the every other day group) developed gastrointestinal effects, but 10% of treated cats developed proteinuria and 15% developed neutropenia (Daly *et al.* 2011).

Reproductive/Nursing Safety

The drug label states: "Do not use in dogs that are pregnant, lactating, or intended for breeding." Studies in rats have shown evidence of impaired female fertility at doses of 100 mg/kg/day, and embryotoxicity and developmental toxicity (delayed ossification) at doses above 30 mg/kg/day. Studies in rabbits did not show embryotoxicity or developmental toxicity.

Overdosage/Acute Toxicity

Masitinib has a narrow margin of safety, but acute toxicity data is not readily available. In the event of an acute overdose, guidance from an animal poison control center is advised.

Drug Interactions

Specific drug interactions with masitinib are not well defined, but there is a potential for masitinib to interact with other drugs metabolized by cytochrome P450 isoenzymes and/or drugs that are also highly protein bound to plasma proteins. These interactions could result in higher or lower plasma levels of masitinib or the other affected drug; use with caution. Drugs/drug classes potentially affected include: azole antifungals, benzodiazepines, beta blockers, calcium channel blockers, cisapride, cyclosporine, doxorubicin, macrolide antibiotics, NSAIDs, SSRI's, tricyclic antidepressants, and warfarin.

The efficacy of masitinib might be reduced in dogs previously treated with chemotherapy and/or radiotherapy. No information relating to potential cross-resistance with other cytostatic products is available.

Laboratory Considerations

- No laboratory interactions noted.

Dosages

- **DOGS:**

    For the treatment of recurrent (post-surgery) or non-resectable Grade II or III cutaneous mast cell tumors that have not previously received radiotherapy and/or chemotherapy except corticosteroids (labeled dose; conditionally approved by FDA): Initial Dose for dogs weighing 7 kg or more and that are at least 2 years old: 12.5 mg/kg/day PO with food. Dose reductions to 9 mg/kg/day (for dogs weighing at least 10.5 kg) and dose interruptions may be utilized, if needed, to manage adverse reactions (see table below). Do not split or crush tablets. The package insert has tables for determining the appropriate tablets to use for a given weight.

Adverse Reaction Class	Toxicity	Dose Adjustment
Gastrointestinal Toxicity	Vomiting: >5 vomiting episodes in 24 hours or vomiting for >4 days; Diarrhea: >6 stools per day over baseline	If the current dose is 12.5 mg/kg, discontinue treatment until resolution, then resume treatment at 9 mg/kg.
Hepatic Toxicity	ALT or AST: >3X upper limit of normal; Bilirubin: >1.5X upper limit of normal	
Neutropenia	Neutrophils: <1500/mcL	If the current dose is 9 mg/kg, permanently discontinue treatment.
Renal Toxicities and Protein Loss Syndrome	Hypoalbuminemia: serum albumin <0.75X lower limit of normal; Proteinuria: UPC >1; Azotemia: BUN or Creatinine >1.5X upper limit of normal)	
Non-Regenerative Anemia and Hemolytic Anemia	Hematocrit: <30% Hemoglobin: <10 g/dL	Permanently discontinue treatment
Other Adverse Reactions	Severe weight loss	

Monitoring

Note: See the dosage adjustment/drug discontinuation guidelines in the table above.

- Every 2 weeks: Hypoalbuminemia and proteinuria.
- Every 4 weeks: Azotemia, anemia, neutropenia, elevated AST or ALT, and hyperbilirubinemia.
- In the case of a positive semi-quantitative test for proteinuria (dipstick protein ≥30 mg/dL) or clinical signs of anemia or hemolysis, urine protein should be confirmed with a quantitative test (UPC ratio) and the dog should be tested for hypoalbuminemia, anemia, and azotemia.
- Patient Weight.
- Gastrointestinal effects (vomiting, diarrhea).

Client Information

- A client information sheet for this product should be provided when dispensed.
- This drug should be given with food.
- Do not crush or split tablets.
- Masitinib can cause severe vomiting and diarrhea. If your dog vomits more than 5 times in one day or vomits for more than 4 days, or has more than 6 stools (diarrhea) in a day; contact your veterinarian right away.
- Your veterinarian will need to do regular blood and urine tests to be sure this drug is not causing toxic effects to your animal.
- Not for use in humans. People with known hypersensitivity to masitinib should not handle the product. Keep this and all medications out of the reach of children; children should not come into contact with the drug and should be kept away from feces, urine, litter or vomit of treated dogs. Do not allow treated animals to lick humans for a few days after the last dose. To avoid exposure to drug, wash hands with soap and water after administering and wear protective gloves to prevent contact with feces, urine, vomit, and broken or crushed tablets. Place all waste material in a plastic bag and seal before disposal in the regular trash. If eyes are accidentally exposed to the drug, immediately rinse eyes with water. In case of accidental ingestion by a person, immediately seek medical advice and show the package insert or label to the physician. Pregnant women, women who may become pregnant, or nursing mothers should pay special attention to these handling precautions as masitinib may harm an unborn baby (cause birth defects) or a nursing baby.

Chemistry/Synonyms

Masitinib (CAS Registry: 0790299-79-5; ATCvet code: QL01XE90) occurs as a crystalline solid. It is soluble in DMSO at 200 mg/mL.

Masitinib may also be known as AB-1010 or masitinibum. Trade names include *Masivet®* and *Kinavet CA-1®*.

Storage/Stability

Masitinib tablets should be stored at controlled room temperature (15-25°C; 59-77°F); protect from heat sources or humidity.

Compatibility/Compounding Considerations

Tablets should not be split or crushed.

Dosage Forms/Regulatory Status

VETERINARY-LABELED PRODUCTS:

Oral Tablets: 50 mg & 150 mg; *Kinavet-CA1®*; (Rx). Conditionally approved by FDA (NADA-141-308) for use in dogs for the treatment of recurrent (post-surgery) or non-resectable Grade II or III cutaneous mast cell tumors in dogs that have not previously received radiotherapy and/or chemotherapy except corticosteroids (Anon 2010). The product's trade name in Europe is *Masivet®*.

HUMAN-LABELED PRODUCTS: NONE.

Revisions/References

Monograph written August 2013; updated March 2014.

Anon (2010). Kinavet-CA1® (Masitinib) [Package Insert]. Secondary Kinavet-CA1® (Masitinib) [Package Insert]. Secondary Anon. Short Hills, NJ, AB Science USA. Volume

Bellamy, F., et al. (2009). Pharmacokinetics of masitinib in cats. Veterinary Research Communications 33(8): 831-7.

Brown, M. R., et al. (2013). Masitinib-Associated Minimal Change Disease with Acute Tubular Necrosis Resulting in Acute Kidney Injury in a Dog. Journal of Veterinary Internal Medicine 27(6): 1622-6.

Cadot, P., et al. (2011). Masitinib decreases signs of canine atopic dermatitis: a multicentre, randomized, double-blind, placebo-controlled phase3trial. Veterinary Dermatology 22(6): 554-64.

Daly, M., et al. (2011). Safety of Masitinib Mesylate in Healthy Cats. Journal of Veterinary Internal Medicine 25(2): 297-302.

Fahey, C. E., et al. (2013). Apoptotic effects of the tyrosine kinase inhibitor, masitinib mesylate, on canine osteosarcoma cells. Anti-Cancer Drugs 24(5): 519-26.

Lawrence, J., et al. (2012). Masitinib demonstrates anti-proliferative and pro-apoptotic activity in primary and metastatic feline injection-site sarcoma cells. Veterinary and Comparative Oncology 10(2): 143-54.

Lee-Fowler, T. M., et al. (2012). The Tyrosine Kinase Inhibitor Masitinib Blunts Airway Inflammation and Improves Associated Lung Mechanics in a Feline Model of Chronic Allergic Asthma. Int. Arch. Allergy Immunol. 158(4): 369-74.

Lyles, S. E., et al. (2012). In vitro effects of the tyrosine kinase inhibitor, masitinib mesylate, on canine hemangiosarcoma cell lines. Veterinary and Comparative Oncology 10(3): 223-35.

Procoli, F. (2010). Clinical trial on the efficacy of masitinib in canine IBD. Veterinary Record 167(19): 760-.

Zandvliet, M., et al. (2013). Masitinib reverses doxorubicin resistance in canine lymphoid cells by inhibiting the function of P-glycoprotein. J. Vet. Pharmacol. Ther. 36(6): 583-7.

Mavacoxib

(mav-ah-**cox**-ib)   Trocoxil®

Long-Acting NSAID

Prescriber Highlights

- ▶ Very long acting NSAID for dogs; half life averages 16-17 days. At time of writing (2014) not available in the USA.
- ▶ Limited clinical experience, but appears to be relatively safe and effective.
- ▶ Adverse effect profile expected to be similar to other canine-approved NSAIDs.
- ▶ Primary benefit appears to be for patients whose owners have difficulty adhering to a daily oral dosing regimen; but adverse effects may persist as well.

Uses/Indications

Mavacoxib is a very long acting oral NSAID that is licensed for use in dogs in the UK, Europe and elsewhere. In the UK it is labeled "for the treatment of pain and inflammation associated with degenerative joint disease in dogs aged 12 months or more in cases where continuous treatment exceeding one month is indicated." At present, its place in the NSAID armamentarium for canine use is yet to be determined. It could be of benefit in those cases where owners have difficulty adhering to a daily oral dosing regimen, but because of its long half-life and duration of action, adverse effects could persist for many weeks after the drug was last given.

In a study comparing the safety and efficacy of mavacoxib with carprofen in 124 dogs, efficacy comparing the two were statistically equivalent and each had a similar rate and profile of adverse effects (Johnson *et al.* 2009).

Pharmacology/Actions

In dogs, mavacoxib appears to be a relative selective inhibiting cyclooxygenase (COX)-1 versus COX-2. It is believed to predominantly inhibit cyclooxygenase-2 (COX-2) and spare COX-1 at therapeutic dosages. This, theoretically, would inhibit production of the prostaglandins that contribute to pain and inflammation (COX-2) and spare those that maintain normal gastrointestinal and renal function (COX-1). However, COX-1 and COX-2 inhibition studies are done *in vitro* and do not necessarily correlate perfectly with clinical effects seen in actual patients.

Pharmacokinetics

Pharmacokinetic values for mavacoxib in dogs are widely patient variable. Average bioavailability after oral dosing is ≈46% when fasted, but nearly doubles (87%) when given with food. Peak levels occur in ≈11 hours, but range widely. In most dogs, blood levels of those thought to be therapeutic occur in approximately one hour after dosing when given with food. Apparent volume of distribution (steady-state) averaged 1.6 L/kg and the drug is highly bound to canine plasma proteins (98%). Total body clearance was a very low 2.7 mL/hour/kg and it is primarily cleared by biliary excretion. The average terminal half-life was 16.6 days (range: 8-39 days) (Cox, S. *et al.* 2010a). A population pharmacokinetic study by the same research group, reported a typical elimination half-life of 44 days, but ≈5% of patients had Bayesian estimates of >80 days (Cox, S.R. *et al.* 2011).

Contraindications/Precautions/Warnings

The UK labels lists the following contraindications: Dogs less than 12 months of age and/or less than 5 kg body weight, dogs with GI disorders including ulceration and bleeding, evidence of a hemorrhagic disorder, impaired renal or hepatic function, cardiac insufficiency, (history of) hypersensitivity to the active substance, sulfonamides or to any of the excipients. Do not use in pregnant, breeding or lactating animals or use concomitantly with glucocorticoids or other NSAIDs. Do not administer other NSAIDs within 1 month of the last administration of mavacoxib. It also states to avoid use in any dehydrated, hypovolemic or hypotensive animal, as there is a potential risk of increased renal toxicity. Concurrent administration of potentially nephrotoxic medicinal products should be avoided.

Animals should not become dehydrated when receiving this or other NSAIDs.

Adverse Effects

As mavacoxib is a new agent, its adverse effect profile has not been fully determined in dogs; field studies have indicated that it causes similar adverse effects seen with other NSAIDs, but it is not known if this drug will have fewer or greater incidences of adverse effects when compared with other FDA-approved NSAIDs. NSAID adverse effects in dogs can include inappetence, diarrhea, vomiting, depression and renal toxicity.

Reproductive/Nursing Safety

The safety of mavacoxib has not been established during pregnancy and lactation. The UK label states: Do not use in pregnant, breeding or lactating animals. Studies in pregnant rabbits with another coxib-class NSAID (firocoxib) at dosages approximating those given to dogs, demonstrated maternotoxic and fetotoxic effects.

Overdosage/Acute Toxicity

In overdose safety studies performed in dogs, repeated doses (at labeled dosage frequency) of 5 and 10 mg/kg did not demonstrate adverse events, abnormal clinical chemistry or significant histological abnormalities. At 15 mg/kg, vomiting, softened/mucoid feces and increases in clinical chemistry parameters reflecting decreased renal function were noted. Doses of 25 mg/kg cause GI ulceration. One study dog died from GI perforation and peritonitis at the 25 mg/kg dose (Krautmann *et al.* 2009).

Oral acute overdoses of mavacoxib, should be managed as with other NSAID toxicity, but because of the drug's very long duration of effect, prolonged monitoring and treatment may be required; consulting a veterinary poison center or the drug sponsor's hotline seems prudent until more experience has been gained with this agent.

As with any NSAID, overdosage can lead to gastrointestinal and renal effects. The ASPCA Animal Poison Control Center (APCC) has not yet set a dosage level of concern for renal damage for dogs or cats. Decontamination with emetics and/or activated charcoal is appropriate. For doses where GI effects are expected, the use of gastrointestinal protectants is warranted. If renal effects are also expected, fluid diuresis is warranted.

Drug Interactions

At the time of writing, no drug interactions have been reported with mavacoxib, but the manufacturer warns that use in conjunction with other **NSAIDs** or **corticosteroids** be avoided. It is also possible mavacoxib could cause increased renal dysfunction if used with other drugs that can cause or contribute to **renal dysfunction** (*e.g.*, **diuretics, aminoglycosides**), but the clinical significance of this potential interaction is unclear. The following drug interactions are either expected or are for dogs receiving mavacoxib and may be of clinical significance:

- **ACE INHIBITORS** (*e.g.*, **enalapril, benazepril**): Some NSAIDs can reduce effects on blood pressure. Because ACE inhibitors potentially can reduce renal blood flow, use with NSAIDs could increase the risk for renal injury. However, one study in dogs receiving tepoxalin did not show any adverse effect. It is unknown what effects, if any, occur if other NSAIDs and ACE inhibitors are used together in dogs.
- **ASPIRIN**: May increase the risk of gastrointestinal toxicity (*e.g.*, ulceration, bleeding, vomiting, diarrhea). Washout periods several weeks long are probably warranted when switching from mavacoxib to aspirin therapy in dogs.
- **CORTICOSTEROIDS** (*e.g.*, **prednisone**): May increase the risk of gastrointestinal toxicity (*e.g.*, ulceration, bleeding, vomiting, diarrhea).
- **DIGOXIN**: NSAIDS may increase serum levels.
- **FLUCONAZOLE**: Administration has increased plasma levels of celecoxib in humans and potentially could also affect mavacoxib levels in dogs.
- **FUROSEMIDE**: NSAIDs may reduce saluretic and diuretic effects.
- **METHOTREXATE**: Serious toxicity has occurred when NSAIDs have been used concomitantly with methotrexate; use together with extreme caution.
- **NEPHROTOXIC DRUGS** (*e.g.*, **furosemide, aminoglycosides, amphotericin B**, etc.): May enhance the risk of nephrotoxicity development.
- **NSAIDS, OTHER**: May increase the risk of gastrointestinal tox-

icity (*e.g.*, ulceration, bleeding, vomiting, diarrhea). The UK label states: "Should another NSAID be administered after *Trocoxil®* treatment, a treatment-free period of at least ONE MONTH should be ensured to avoid adverse effects." However, because of its very long half-life (up to 39 hours in one study dog) (Cox, S.R. *et al.* 2010b), mavacoxib may have a conservative washout time of 195 days (KuKanich *et al.* 2012).

Laboratory Considerations
- None identified.

Doses
- **DOGS:**

  U.K. Label: **For the treatment of pain and inflammation associated with degenerative joint disease in dogs aged 12 months or more in cases where continuous treatment exceeding one month is indicated** (extra-label in USA): 2 mg/kg PO given immediately before or with the dog's main meal. Care should be taken to ensure that the tablet is ingested. The treatment should be repeated 14 days later; thereafter the dosing interval is ONE MONTH. A treatment cycle should not exceed 7 consecutive doses (6.5 months). THIS IS NOT A DAILY NSAID. (Label Information—*Trocoxil®*; Pfizer U.K.)

Monitoring
- Baseline and periodic CBC and serum chemistry (including BUN/serum creatinine, and liver function assessment).
- Baseline history and physical.
- Efficacy of therapy.
- Adverse effect monitoring via client.

Client Information
- Give doses exactly as directed by veterinarian, do not give extra doses or increase the dose without veterinarian's guidance. This drug is NOT given every day. After the first 2 doses given 2 weeks apart, it is given once a month for up to 5 doses, then an extra month off the drug is needed if it is to be started again.
- Do not administer other NSAIDs within 1 month of the last dose of mavacoxib (*e.g.*, carprofen, deracoxib, meloxicam, etc.).
- Give the medication with the dog's largest meal of the day. The drug is much better absorbed from the stomach if given with food.
- Contact the veterinarian if any of the following adverse effects persist or are severe: loss of appetite, vomiting, change in bowel movements (*e.g.*, stool color), change in behavior, decrease in water consumption, or urination; these could potentially occur after many weeks after the last dose was given. Immediately report to the veterinarian if any of the following adverse effects occur: bloody stool/diarrhea, bloody vomiting, or allergic reaction (facial swelling face, hives, red, itchy skin).
- Do not allow dog to become dehydrated while receiving this drug.
- Since dogs may find the chewable tablets' taste desirable, the drug should be stored out of reach of animals and children.

Chemistry/Synonyms
Mavacoxib is structurally related to the human NSAID celecoxib and categorized as a diaryl substituted pyrazole. Mavacoxib's solubility in water is relatively low (0.006 mg/mL).

Mavacoxib may also be known as mavacoxibum; PHA 739,521; or UNII-YFT7X7SR77. A common trade name is *Trocoxil®*.

Storage/Stability
Store in the original packaging at room temperature out of reach of pets and children.

Compatibility/Compounding Considerations
No specific information noted.

Dosage Forms/Regulatory Status
VETERINARY-LABELED PRODUCTS:
None in USA at time of writing. In the UK and Europe: Mavacoxib Oral Chewable Tablets: 6 mg, 20 mg, 30 mg, 75 mg, & 95 mg; *Trocoxil®*; (Rx)

HUMAN-LABELED PRODUCTS: NONE.

Revisions/References
Monograph revised/updated March 2014.

Cox, S., et al. (2010a). The pharmacokinetics of mavacoxib, a long-acting COX-2 inhibitor, in young adult laboratory dogs. J Vet Pharmacol Ther **33**: 461-70.
Cox, S. R., et al. (2010b). The pharmacokinetics of mavacoxib, a long-acting COX-2 inhibitor, in young adult laboratory dogs. J. Vet. Pharmacol. Ther. **33**(5): 461-70.
Cox, S. R., et al. (2011). Population pharmacokinetics of mavacoxib in osteoarthritic dogs. J. Vet. Pharmacol. Ther. **34**(1): 1-11.
Johnson, M., et al. (2009). Determination of the Efficacy and Safety of Mavacoxib Tablets Administered Monthly at 2 mg/Kg BW in the Treatment of Pain and Inflammation Associated with Osteoarthritis in Dogs. Proceedings: BSAVA. accessed via Veterinary Information Network; vin.com
Krautmann, M., et al. (2009). Target animal safety studies of mavacoxib in dogs. J Vet Pharmacol Ther **32**(Suppl.1): 46-7.
KuKanich, B., et al. (2012). Clinical pharmacology of nonsteroidal anti-inflammatory drugs in dogs. Veterinary Anaesthesia and Analgesia **39**(1): 69-90.

Mechlorethamine HCl
(me-klor-**eth**-a-meen)   Mustargen®
Antineoplastic

Prescriber Highlights
▶ Antineoplastic for lymphoreticular neoplasms or pleural & peritoneal effusions (intracavitary).
▶ Contraindications (relative; risk vs. benefit): Anemia, bone marrow depression, tumor cell infiltration into bone marrow, current infection, sensitivity to mechlorethamine, or patients who have received previous chemotherapy or radiotherapy.
▶ Adverse Effects: Bone marrow depression, GI effects (vomiting, nausea), ototoxicity (high dosages or regional perfusions). Potentially: alopecia, hyperuricemia, hepatotoxicity, peripheral neuropathy, & GI ulcers.
▶ Teratogen.
▶ Avoid extravasation.

Uses/Indications
In small animals, mechlorethamine may be useful for the adjunctive treatment of lymphoreticular neoplasms or, with intracavitary administration, for treating pleural and peritoneal effusions. A change in owners of the pharmaceutical product has reportedly resulted in very large price increases for this medication and some veterinary oncologists are substituting dactinomycin for the mechlorethamine in MOPP rescue protocols.

Pharmacology/Actions
Mechlorethamine is an alkylating agent, thereby interfering with DNA replication, RNA transcription, and protein synthesis. It is cell cycle-phase nonspecific.

With intracavitary administration, mechlorethamine causes sclerosing and an inflammatory response on serous membranes, thereby causing adherence of serosal surfaces.

Pharmacokinetics
Because mechlorethamine is so irritating to tissues it must be given IV for systemic use. It is incompletely absorbed after intracavitary administration. After injection, mechlorethamine is rapidly (within minutes) inactivated.

Contraindications/Precautions/Warnings

Mechlorethamine is contraindicated in patients with a known infection or that have had a prior anaphylactic reaction to the drug.

Mechlorethamine should be used only when its potential benefits outweigh its risks with the following conditions: anemia, bone marrow depression, tumor cell infiltration into bone marrow, sensitivity to mechlorethamine, or patients who have received previous chemotherapy or radiotherapy.

Adverse Effects

Bone marrow depression (leukopenia, thrombocytopenia) and GI effects (vomiting, nausea) are quite common and can be serious enough to halt therapy. Ototoxicity may occur with either high dosages or regional perfusions. Other potential effects include alopecia, hyperuricemia, hepatotoxicity, peripheral neuropathy, and GI ulcers.

Because severe tissue sloughing may occur, avoid extravasation.

Reproductive/Nursing Safety

Mechlorethamine is a teratogen in lab animals. Use only during pregnancy when the benefits to the mother outweigh the risks to the offspring. Mechlorethamine can suppress gonadal function. In humans, the FDA categorizes this drug as category *D* for use during pregnancy (*There is evidence of human fetal risk, but the potential benefits from the use of the drug in pregnant women may be acceptable despite its potential risks.*)

While it is not known whether mechlorethamine enters maternal milk, nursing puppies or kittens should receive milk replacer when the dam is receiving mechlorethamine.

Overdosage/Acute Toxicity

Because of the toxic potential of this agent, overdoses must be avoided. Determine dosages carefully.

Drug Interactions

The following drug interactions have either been reported or are theoretical in humans or animals receiving mechlorethamine and may be of significance in veterinary patients. Unless otherwise noted, use together is not necessarily contraindicated, but weigh the potential risks and perform additional monitoring when appropriate.

- **IMMUNOSUPPRESSANT DRUGS** (*e.g.,* **azathioprine, cyclophosphamide, corticosteroids**): Use with other immunosuppressant drugs may increase the risk of infection.
- **MYELOSUPPRESSIVE DRUGS** (*e.g.,* **chloramphenicol, flucytosine, amphotericin B,** or **colchicine**): Use extreme caution when used concurrently with other drugs that are also myelosuppressive, including many of the other antineoplastics and other bone marrow depressant drugs. Bone marrow depression may be additive.
- **VACCINES, LIVE:** Live virus vaccines should be used with caution, if at all, during therapy.

Laboratory Considerations

- Mechlorethamine may raise **serum uric acid** levels. Drugs such as allopurinol may be required to control hyperuricemia.

Doses

Note: Because of the potential toxicity of this drug to patients, veterinary personnel and clients, and since chemotherapy indications, treatment protocols, monitoring and safety guidelines often change, the following dosages should be used only as a general guide. Consultation with a veterinary oncologist and referral to current veterinary oncology references [*e.g.,* (Withrow *et al.* 2012); (Dobson *et al.* 2011); (Henry *et al.* 2009); (North *et al.* 2009); (Argyle *et al.* 2008)] are strongly recommended.

- **DOGS/CATS:**
Mechlorethamine is usually dosed as part of a lymphoma rescue protocol that includes vincristine (or vinblastine), procarbazine and prednisone (or prednisolone), the so-called MOPP protocol. Doses of mechlorethamine are usually 3 mg/m² (**NOT** mg/kg) IV given on days 1 and 7 of a 28-day protocol, but some are giving it on days 1 and 14 to better allow bone marrow to recover.

Monitoring

- CBC with platelets at least every 1-2 weeks until stable; then every 3 months.
- Liver function tests; initially before starting treatment and then every 3-4 months.
- Injection site for signs of extravasation.

Client Information

- Mechlorethamine is a chemotherapy (cancer) drug. The drug and its byproducts can be hazardous to other animals and people that come in contact with it. On the day your animal gets the drug and then for a few days afterward, all bodily waste (urine, feces, litter), blood, or vomit should only be handled while wearing disposable gloves. Seal the waste in a plastic bag and then place both the bag and gloves in with the regular trash.

Chemistry/Synonyms

A bifunctional alkylating agent, mechlorethamine occurs as a hygroscopic, white, crystalline powder that is very soluble in water. After reconstitution with sterile water or sterile saline, the resultant solution is clear and has a pH of 3-5.

Mechlorethamine may also be known as: nitrogen mustard, mustine, HN_2, chlormethine hydrochloride, chlorethazine hydrochloride, HN2 (mustine [chlormethine]), mechlorethamine hydrochloride, mustine hydrochloride, nitrogen mustard (mustine [chlormethine]), NSC-762, WR-147650, *Caryolysine®*, *Mustargen®* and *Onco-Cloramin®*.

Storage/Stability

Store the powder for injection at room temperature. Mechlorethamine is highly unstable in neutral or alkaline aqueous solutions and rapidly degrades. While more stable in an acidic environment, the drug should be administered immediately after preparation.

Compatibility/Compounding Considerations

It is **NOT** recommended to mix mechlorethamine with any other medication or to dilute further beyond what is described in the package insert.

Drugs that have been reported to be **compatible** with mechlorethamine when given via an IV Y-site include aztreonam, filgrastim, granisetron, melphalan, and ondansetron.

Unused portions of reconstituted drug can be neutralized by adding equal volumes of 5% sodium thiosulfate and 5% sodium bicarbonate. This solution is allowed to stand for 45 minutes and then can be discarded appropriately.

Dosage Forms/Regulatory Status

VETERINARY-LABELED PRODUCTS: NONE.

HUMAN-LABELED PRODUCTS:

Mechlorethamine Powder for Injection: 10 mg; *Mustargen®*; (Rx)

Revisions/References

Monograph revised/updated March 2014.

Argyle, D., et al. (2008). *Decision Making in Small Animal Oncology*, Wiley-Blackwell.
Dobson, J. & D. Lascelles (2011). *BSAVA Manual of Canine and Feline Oncology*, BSAVA.
Henry, C. & M. Higginbotham (2009). *Cancer Management in Small Animal Practice*, Saunders.
North, S. & T. Banks (2009). *Small Animal Oncology: An Introduction*, Saunders.
Withrow, S., et al. (2012). Withrow and MacEwen's *Small Animal Clinical Oncology*, 5th Ed., Saunders.

Meclizine HCl

(mek-li-zeen)   Antivert®

Antihistamine, Antiemetic

Prescriber Highlights

▶ Antihistamine with sedative & antiemetic effects, used primarily for motion sickness.

▶ Caution: Prostatic hypertrophy, bladder neck obstruction, severe cardiac failure, angle-closure glaucoma, or pyeloduodenal obstruction.

▶ Adverse Effects: Sedation; less frequently anticholinergic effects may be noted (dry mucous membranes, eyes, tachycardia, etc.); contradictory CNS stimulation possible.

Uses/Indications

Meclizine is principally used in small animals as an antiemetic and for the treatment and prevention of motion sickness.

Pharmacology/Actions

Meclizine is a piperazine antihistamine. In addition to its antihistamine activity, it has antiemetic, CNS depressant, antispasmodic, and local anesthetic effects. The exact mechanisms of action for its antiemetic and anti-motion-sickness effects are not completely understood, but it is thought they are a result of the drug's central anticholinergic and CNS depressant activity. The antiemetic effect is probably mediated through the chemoreceptor trigger zone (CTZ).

Pharmacokinetics

Very little information is available. Meclizine is metabolized in the liver and has a serum half-life of ≈6 hours.

Contraindications/Precautions/Warnings

Meclizine is contraindicated in patients hypersensitive to it. It should be used with caution in patients with prostatic hypertrophy, bladder neck obstruction, severe cardiac failure, angle-closure glaucoma, or pyeloduodenal obstruction.

Adverse Effects

The usual adverse effect noted with meclizine is sedation; less frequently anticholinergic effects may be noted (dry mucous membranes, eyes, tachycardia, etc.). Contradictory CNS stimulation has also been reported. Cats may develop inappetence while receiving this medication.

Reproductive/Nursing Safety

Meclizine is considered teratogenic at high dosages in laboratory animals and cleft palates have been noted in rats at 25-50 times higher than labeled dosages. However, in humans, it has been suggested that meclizine possesses the lowest risk for teratogenicity for antiemetic drugs and that it is the drug of first choice to treat nausea/vomiting associated with pregnancy. In humans, the FDA categorizes this drug as category *B* for use during pregnancy (*Animal studies have not yet demonstrated risk to the fetus, but there are no adequate studies in pregnant women; or animal studies have shown an adverse effect, but adequate studies in pregnant women have not demonstrated a risk to the fetus in the first trimester of pregnancy, and there is no evidence of risk in later trimesters.*)

It is unknown if meclizine enters milk; its anticholinergic activity may, potentially, inhibit lactation.

Overdosage/Acute Toxicity

Moderate overdosage may result in drowsiness alternating with hyperexcitability. Massive overdosages may result in profound CNS depression, hallucinations, seizures and other anticholinergic effects (tachycardia, urinary retention, etc.).

There were 182 single agent exposures to meclizine reported to the ASPCA Animal Poison Control Center (APCC) during 2009-2013. Of the 176 dogs, 29 were symptomatic with 28% demonstrating tachycardia, 24% vomiting and 21% lethargic.

Treatment is considered symptomatic and supportive. Consider gut emptying when patients present soon after ingestion. Avoid respiratory depressant medications.

Drug Interactions

The following drug interactions have either been reported or are theoretical in humans or animals receiving meclizine and may be of significance in veterinary patients. Unless otherwise noted, use together is not necessarily contraindicated, but weigh the potential risks and perform additional monitoring when appropriate.

■ **CNS DEPRESSANTS:** Use with other CNS depressants may cause additive sedation.

■ **ANTICHOLINERGIC DRUGS:** Other anticholinergic drugs may cause additive anticholinergic effects.

Laboratory Considerations

■ Because these drugs are antihistamines, they may affect the results of **skin tests** using allergen extracts. Do not use within 3-7 days before testing.

Doses

■ **DOGS:**

For vertigo (vestibular disease), prevention of motion sickness/vomiting (extra-label): No controlled studies supporting any dosage regimen were located, anecdotally: 4 mg/kg PO once daily. Practically, 12.5 mg – 50 mg per dog PO once daily.

■ **CATS:**

For vertigo (vestibular disease), prevention of motion sickness/vomiting (extra-label): No controlled studies supporting any dosage regimen were located, anecdotally: 6.25 – 12.5 mg per cat (1/2 – one 12.5 mg tablet) PO once daily.

■ **RABBITS, RODENTS, SMALL MAMMALS:**

Rabbits: For Rolling, torticollis, motion sickness head tilt ("wry neck"); (extra-label): 2 – 12 mg/kg PO once daily (Ivey *et al.* 2000); 12.5 mg per rabbit PO q12-24h. (Johnson 2006)

Monitoring

■ Efficacy.

■ Adverse effects.

Client Information

■ May give with or without food. Giving with a small amount of food or treat may help prevent vomiting.

■ When using for motion sickness prevention, give medication 30-60 minutes before travel.

■ Most common side effect is sedation (drowsiness/sleepiness).

Chemistry/Synonyms

Meclizine HCl is a piperazine derivative antiemetic antihistamine.

Meclizine may also be known as: meclozine, meclizinium, meclozine, or parachloramine. *Antivert*® & *Bonine*® are common trade names.

Storage/Stability

Meclizine products should be stored at room temperature in well-closed containers.

Compatibility/Compounding Considerations

No specific information noted.

Dosage Forms/Regulatory Status

VETERINARY-LABELED PRODUCTS: NONE.

The ARCI (Racing Commissioners International) has designated this drug as a class 4 substance. See the appendix for more information.

Meclizine HCl Oral Tablets: 12.5 mg, 25 mg (plain and chewable) & 32 mg; *Vertin-32®*, *Dramamine® Less Drowsy Formula*, *Bonine®*, *UniVert®*, generic; (Rx and OTC).

Revisions/References
Monograph revised/updated March 2014.

Ivey, E. & J. Morrisey (2000). Therapeutics for Rabbits. Vet Clin NA: Exotic Anim Pract 3:1(Jan): 183-216.
Johnson, D. (2006). Rabbit Medicine and Surgery. Proceedings: ACVC. accessed via Veterinary Information Network; vin.com

Medetomidine HCl

(mee-de-**toe**-mi-deen)   Domitor®

Alpha-2 Adrenergic Agonist

Prescriber Highlights

▶ Alpha₂-adrenergic sedative analgesic used primarily in dogs & cats, but also may be useful in small mammals, exotics, etc.

▶ Contraindications: Cardiac disease, respiratory disorders, liver or kidney diseases, shock, severe debilitation, or animals stressed due to heat, cold or fatigue. Caution in very old or young animals.

▶ **NOT** recommended for use during pregnancy.

▶ Adverse Effects: Bradycardia, occasional AV blocks, decreased respiration, hypothermia, urination, vomiting, hyperglycemia, & pain on injection (IM). Rarely: prolonged sedation, paradoxical excitation, hypersensitivity, apnea & death from circulatory failure.

▶ Drug interactions.

▶ Do **NOT** confuse with detomidine or dexmedetomidine.

Uses/Indications
Medetomidine is an alpha-2 agonist used as a sedative, premedicant/anesthesia adjunct and analgesic in dogs, cats and other small animals. Commercial dosage forms may not be available in the USA, but multiple products are licensed in Europe.

Pharmacology/Actions
An alpha adrenergic receptor, medetomidine has an alpha₂:alpha₁ selectivity factor of 1620, and when compared to xylazine is reportedly 10X more specific for alpha₂ receptors versus alpha₁ receptors. The pharmacologic effects of medetomidine include: depression of CNS (sedation, anxiolysis), GI (decreased secretions, varying affects on intestinal muscle tone) and endocrine functions, peripheral and cardiac vasoconstriction, bradycardia, respiratory depression, diuresis, hypothermia, analgesia (somatic and visceral), muscle relaxation (but not enough for intubation), and blanched or cyanotic mucous membranes. Effects on blood pressure are variable, but medetomidine can cause hypertension longer than does xylazine. Medetomidine also induces sedation for a longer period than does xylazine. Sedative effects persist longer than analgesic effects.

Pharmacokinetics
After IV or IM injection, onset of effect is rapid (5 min. for IV; 10-15 min. for IM). After SC injection, responses are unreliable and this method of administration cannot be recommended. The drug is absorbed via the oral mucosa when administered sublingually in dogs, but efficacy at a given dose may be less than IM dosing.

Contraindications/Precautions/Warnings
The label states that medetomidine is contraindicated in dogs having the following conditions: cardiac disease, respiratory disorders, liver or kidney diseases, shock, severe debilitation, or dogs stressed due to heat, cold, or fatigue.

Dogs that are extremely agitated or excited may have a decreased response to medetomidine; the manufacturer suggests allowing these dogs to rest quietly before administration of the drug. Dogs not responding to medetomidine should not be re-dosed. Use in very young or older dogs should be done with caution.

Do not confuse medetomidine with detomidine or dexmedetomidine

Adverse Effects
The adverse effects reported with medetomidine are essentially extensions of its pharmacologic effects including bradycardia, occasional AV blocks, decreased respiration, hypothermia, urination, vomiting, hyperglycemia, and pain on injection (IM). Rare effects have also been reported, including prolonged sedation, paradoxical excitation, hypersensitivity, apnea, and death from circulatory failure.

Reproductive/Nursing Safety
The drug is not recommended to use in pregnant dogs or those used for breeding purposes because safety data for use during pregnancy is insufficient; therefore, use only when the benefits clearly outweigh the drug's risks.

Overdosage/Acute Toxicity
Single doses of up to 5X (IV) and 10X (IM) were tolerated in dogs, but adverse effects can occur (see above). Death has occurred rarely in dogs (1 in 40,000) receiving 2X doses.

Because of the potential of additional adverse effects occurring (heart block, PVC's, or tachycardia), treatment of medetomidine-induced bradycardia with anticholinergic agents (atropine or glycopyrrolate) is usually not recommended. Atipamezole is probably a safer choice to treat any medetomidine-induced effect.

Drug Interactions
The following drug interactions have either been reported or are theoretical in humans or animals receiving medetomidine and may be of significance in veterinary patients. Unless otherwise noted, use together is not necessarily contraindicated, but weigh the potential risks and perform additional monitoring when appropriate.

Note: Before attempting combination therapy with medetomidine, it is strongly advised to access references from veterinary anesthesiologists familiar with the use of this product.

▪ **ATROPINE, GLYCOPYRROLATE:** The use of atropine or glycopyrrolate to prevent or treat medetomidine-caused bradycardia is controversial as tachycardia and hypertension may result. This is more important when using higher doses of medetomidine (>20 micrograms/kg) and concomitant use is discouraged.

▪ **OPIATES:** Enhancement of sedation and analgesia may occur when medetomidine is used concurrently with fentanyl, butorphanol, or meperidine, but adverse effects may be pronounced as well. Reduced dosages and monitoring are advised if contemplating combination therapy.

▪ **PROPOFOL:** When propofol is used after medetomidine, hypoxemia may occur. Dosage adjustments may be required along with adequate monitoring.

▪ **YOHIMBINE:** May reverse the effects of medetomidine; but atipamezole is preferred for clinical use to reverse the drug's effects.

Laboratory Considerations
▪ Medetomidine can inhibit ADP-induced **platelet aggregation** in cats.

Doses
Note: Dosages are expressed as medetomidine HCl. There are several products licensed for use in the UK and other countries. Access to the full label datasheets for these products can be accessed via: http://www.noahcompendium.co.uk

- **DOGS:**

For sedation/premedication: Labeled Dose (U.K.); (extra-label in USA): For sedation: 750 micrograms/m^2 IV or 1000 micrograms/m^2 (1 mg/m^2) IM. This corresponds to 20 – 100 micrograms/kg (**Note**: Dosage per kg goes down as animal weight increases).

For premedication, use 50% of the sedation dosage. The exact dose depends on the combination of drugs used and the dosage(s) of the other drug(s). The dose should furthermore be adjusted to the type of surgery, length of procedure and patient temperament/weight. Premedication with medetomidine will significantly reduce the dosage of the induction agent required and will reduce volatile anesthetic requirements for maintenance anesthesia. All anesthetic agents used for induction or maintenance of anesthesia should be administered to effect. Before using any combinations, product literature for the other products should be consulted (Adapted from label; *Dorbene®*—Zoetis U.K.). The *Domitor®*—Elanco label has dosages combining medetomidine with butorphanol and for subsequent use of propofol as a general anesthetic.

- **CATS:**

For sedation to facilitate handling; premedication, and in combination with ketamine for general anesthesia for minor surgical procedures of short duration: Labeled Dose (U.K.); (extra-label in USA): For moderate-deep sedation and restraint 50 – 150 micrograms/kg IM or SC. Using the 1 mg/mL medetomidine HCl injection this would correspond to an amount of 0.05 – 0.15 mL/kg. The speed of induction is slower when SC administration is used. For anesthesia: medetomidine HCl at 80 micrograms/kg and ketamine at 2.5 – 7.5 mg/kg. Using this dosage anesthesia occurs within 3-4 minutes and is apparent for 20-50 minutes. For longer lasting procedures administration has to be repeated by using ½ of the initial dose (*i.e.,* 40 micrograms/kg of medetomidine HCl and ketamine at 2.5 – 3.75 mg/kg or ketamine at 3 mg/kg can be used alone). Alternatively, for longer lasting procedures anesthesia may be extended by use of the inhalation agent isoflurane, with oxygen or oxygen/nitrous oxide. (Adapted from label; *Dorbene®*—Zoetis U.K.). Other products (*e.g., Dormilan®*—Dechra; *Sedanorm®*—Bimeda) have IV administration for cats on the label. The *Domitor®*—Elanco label has dosages combining medetomidine with butorphanol and butorphanol/ketamine and for subsequent use of alfaxalone as a general anesthetic.

- **FERRETS:**

As a sedative/premedicant/anesthetic adjunct (extra-label): 15 minutes prior to medetomidine, give atropine (0.05 mg/kg) or glycopyrrolate (0.01 mg/kg) then give medetomidine at 60 – 80 micrograms/kg IM or SC. Sedation lasts up to 3 hours. May be reversed with atipamezole (400 micrograms/kg IM); For injectable anesthesia: Butorphanol 0.1 mg/kg, Ketamine 5 mg/kg, Medetomidine 80 micrograms/kg. Combine in one syringe and give IM. May need to supplement with isoflurane (0.5-1.5%) for abdominal surgery. (Finkler 1999)

- **BIRDS:**

For sedation/analgesia (extra-label): 0.1 mg/kg IM; limited data available on duration of effect, adverse effects, etc. (Clyde *et al.* 2000)

- **REPTILES:**

For sedation/analgesia (extra-label):

Medium to small land Tortoises: Medetomidine 100 – 150 micrograms/kg with ketamine 5 – 10 mg/kg IV or IM;

Freshwater Turtles: Medetomidine 150 – 300 micrograms/kg with ketamine 10 – 20 mg/kg IV or IM;

Giant Land Tortoises: 200 kg Aldabra tortoise: Medetomidine 40 micrograms/kg with ketamine 4 mg/kg IV or IM;

Smaller Aldabra tortoises: Medetomidine 40 – 80 micrograms/kg with ketamine 4 – 8 mg/kg IV or IM. Wait 30-40 minutes for peak effect;

Iguanas: Medetomidine 100 – 150 micrograms/kg with ketamine 5 – 10 mg/kg IV or IM;

Reversal of all dosages with atipamezole is 4-5 times the medetomidine dose. (Heard 1999)

- **ZOO, EXOTIC, WILDLIFE SPECIES:**

For use of medetomidine in zoo, exotic and wildlife medicine refer to specific references, including:

a) *Zoo Animal and Wildlife Immobilization and Anesthesia.* West, G., Heard, D., Caulkett, N. (eds.). Blackwell Publishing, 2007.

b) Handbook of Wildlife Chemical Immobilization, 3rd Ed. Kreeger, T.J. and J.M. Arnemo. 2007.

c) Fowler's Zoo and Wild Animal Medicine Current Therapy, Volume 7, Miller, R.E., Fowler, M.E., Saunders. 2011.

d) *Exotic Animal Formulary, 4th Ed.* Carpenter, J.W., Saunders. 2012.

e) The 2009 American Association of Zoo Veterinarian Proceedings by D. K. Fontenot also has several dosages listed for restraint, anesthesia, and analgesia for a variety of drugs for carnivores and primates. VIN members can access them at: http://goo.gl/NNIWQ or http://goo.gl/9UJse

Monitoring

- Level of sedation and analgesia; heart rate; body temperature.
- Heart rhythm, blood pressure, respiration rate, and pulse oximetry should be considered, particularly in higher risk patients if the drug is to be used.

Client Information

- This drug should be administered and monitored by veterinary professionals only.
- Clients should be made aware of the potential adverse effects associated with its use, particularly in dogs at risk (older, preexisting conditions).

Chemistry/Synonyms

An alpha$_2$-adrenergic agonist, medetomidine occurs as a white or almost white crystalline substance. It is soluble in water. While the compound exists as two stereoisomers, only the D-isomer is active. 1 mg of medetomidine HCL is equivalent to 0.85 mg of medetomidine base. Dosages are expressed as medetomidine HCl.

Medetomidine HCl may also be known as MPV-785 and *Domitor®*.

Storage/Stability

The commercially available injection should be stored at room temperature (15-30°C) and protected from freezing.

Compatibility/Compounding Considerations

See the dosage section for acceptable combinations; more information may also be found in the dexmedetomidine monograph.

Dosage Forms/Regulatory Status

VETERINARY-LABELED PRODUCTS:

Medetomidine HCl for Injection: 1 mg/mL in 10 mL multidose vials; *Domitor®*; (Rx). FDA-approved for use in dogs over 12 weeks of age. Although still listed in the FDA's Green Book, it may not be currently marketed in the USA. There are several products that may be licensed and marketed for dogs and cats in the U.K., Europe and AUS/NZ.

The ARCI (Racing Commissioners International) has designated this drug as a class 3 substance. See the appendix for more information.

HUMAN-LABELED PRODUCTS: NONE.

Revisions/References
Monograph revised/updated March 2014.
Clyde, V. & J. Paul-Murphy (2000). Avian Analgesia. *Kirk's Current Veterinary Therapy: XIII Small Animal Practice.* J. Bonagura. Philadelphia, WB Saunders: 1126-8.
Finkler, M. (1999). Anesthesia in Ferrets. Proceedings: Central Veterinary Conference, Kansas City. accessed via Veterinary Information Network; vin.com
Heard, D. (1999). Advances in Reptile Anesthesia. The North American Veterinary Conference, Orlando. accessed via Veterinary Information Network; vin.com

Medium Chain Triglycerides (MCT Oil)
Nutritional

Prescriber Highlights
► Lipid sometimes used to provide calories & fatty acids to dogs with restricted fat intake due to chronic infiltrative disease of small intestine or fat malabsorption syndromes present.
► Most clinicians use dietary therapy instead of MCT oil today.
► Cautions: Significant hepatic disease (*e.g.*, portacaval shunts, cirrhosis, etc.).
► Adverse Effects: Unpalatability (dogs), bloating, flatulence, & diarrhea. May be associated with hepatic lipidosis in cats.

Uses/Indications
MCT oil as a separate compound (not as an ingredient in commercial foods) is sometimes used to offset the caloric reduction when long-chain triglycerides found in dietary fat are restricted, usually in chronic infiltrative diseases of the small intestine or when there is fat malabsorption of any cause. Because of expense and unpalatability to dogs, many clinicians are bypassing MCT oil and having their clients prepare homemade, highly digestible, ultra-low fat diets (*e.g.*, white turkey meat plus rice/potato) or using very low fat prescription diets.

MCT oil may be useful as a base-vehicle to administer drugs to cats. A study evaluating the acceptance of low-dose (0.1 mL/kg) MCT oil, gelatin capsules, or thin-film dissolving strips, found that owner-perceived acceptability by cats of MCT oil and thin-film strips cats was significantly higher than gelatin capsules (Traas *et al.* 2010).

MCT's in diets may play a supporting role in prevention or treating cognitive dysfunction syndromes in dogs and cats (Pan 2011).

Pharmacology/Actions
Medium chain triglycerides (MCT) are more readily hydrolyzed than conventional food fat. They also require less bile acids for digestion, are not dependent for chylomicron formation or lymphatic transport, and are transported by the portal vein. Medium chain triglycerides are not a source for essential fatty acids.

MCT oil supplementation (as coconut oil) to the diet of cats did not cause food aversion or significant effects on lipid metabolism (Trevizan *et al.* 2010).

Pharmacokinetics
No specific information located; see Pharmacology above.

Contraindications/Precautions/Warnings
MCT oil should be used with caution in patients with significant hepatic disease (*e.g.*, portacaval shunts, cirrhosis, etc.). Medium chain triglycerides are rapidly absorbed via the portal vein and if their hepatic clearance is impaired, significantly high systemic blood and CSF levels of medium chain fatty acids can occur. This may precipitate or exacerbate hepatic coma.

Adverse Effects
Adverse effects seen with MCT oil in small animals include unpalatability, bloating, flatulence, and diarrhea. In cats, higher dosages of MCT oil may induce hepatic lipidosis. These may be transient and minimized by starting doses at the low end of the spectrum and then gradually increasing the dose. Fat-soluble vitamin supplementation (Vitamins A, D, E, and K) by using a commercial feline or canine vitamin-mineral supplement has been recommended.

Reproductive/Nursing Safety
Although, no reproductive safety data was located, MCT oil would likely not cause problems.

Overdosage/Acute Toxicity
Overdosage would likely exacerbate the GI adverse effects noted above. Treat severe diarrhea supportively if necessary.

Drug Interactions
■ None listed, but MCT oil could, theoretically, affect absorption of drugs that are dependent on fat for oral absorption (*e.g.*, griseofulvin, fat soluble vitamins, etc.).

Doses
■ **DOGS:**
To offset the caloric reduction when long-chain triglycerides found in dietary fat are restricted (extra-label): Most prefer to use dietary (foods with additional MCT's in their formulation) therapy, but 0.5 – 2 mL/kg/day added to food has been noted. Palatability and diarrhea may be issues.

Monitoring
■ Adverse Effects.
■ Efficacy (weight, stool consistency).

Client Information
■ Because of the unpalatability of the oil, it should be mixed with small quantities of food before offering to the patient.

Chemistry/Synonyms
MCT Oil is a lipid fraction of coconut oil consisting principally of the triglycerides C_8 (approx. 67%) and C_{10} (approx. 23%) saturated fatty acids. Each 15 mL contains 115 kCal (7.67 kCal/mL).

Medium chain triglycerides may also be known as triglycerida saturata media.

Storage/Stability
Unless otherwise noted by the manufacturer, store at room temperature in glass bottles.

Compatibility/Compounding Considerations
No specific information noted.

Dosage Forms/Regulatory Status
VETERINARY-LABELED PRODUCTS: NONE.

HUMAN-LABELED PRODUCTS:
Medium Chain Triglycerides Oil: in quart bottles; *MCT*®; (OTC)

Revisions/References
Monograph revised/updated March 2014.
Pan, Y. L. (2011). Enhancing Brain Functions in Senior Dogs: A New Nutritional Approach. Topics in Companion Animal Medicine **26**(1): 10-6.
Traas, A. M., et al. (2010). Ease of oral administration and owner-perceived acceptability of triglyceride oil, dissolving thin film strip, and gelatin capsule formulations to healthy cats. American Journal of Veterinary Research **71**(6): 610-4.
Trevizan, L., et al. (2010). Effects of dietary medium-chain triglycerides on plasma lipids and lipoprotein distribution and food aversion in cats. American Journal of Veterinary Research **71**(4): 435-40.

Medroxyprogesterone Acetate

(me-**drox**-ee-proe-**jess**-te-rone)   Provera®

Progestin

Prescriber Highlights

▶ Synthetic progestin used primarily to treat sexually dimorphic behavior problems such as roaming, inter-male aggressive behaviors, spraying, mounting, etc.; sometimes used to treat feline psychogenic dermatitis & alopecia X in dogs.

▶ Because of its serious adverse effect profile, particularly in small animals, consider safer alternatives first.

▶ Contraindications: Do not use in pre-pubescent cats or dogs, diabetics, pseudopregnant bitches, females in diestrus or with prolonged heat, uterine hemorrhage or discharge.

▶ Adverse Effects: Increased thirst, appetite, weight gain, depression, lethargy, personality changes, adrenocortical depression, mammary changes (including enlargement, milk production, & neoplasms), diabetes mellitus, pyometra, & temporary inhibition of spermatogenesis.

▶ SC injection may cause permanent local alopecia, atrophy & depigmentation may occur.

▶ Drug-lab (including pathology) interactions.

Uses/Indications

In cats, medroxyprogesterone acetate (MPA) has been used when either castration is ineffective or undesirable to treat sexually dimorphic behavior problems such as roaming, inter-male aggressive behaviors, spraying, mounting, etc. MPA has also been used as a tranquilizing agent to treat syndromes such as feline psychogenic dermatitis and alopecia, but treatment with "true" tranquilizing agents may be preferable.

In dogs, MPA may be useful for treating progestin-responsive dermatitis, aggressive behaviors, long-term reproductive control, treatment of young German shepherd dwarfs, short-term treatment of benign prostatic hypertrophy, and luteal insufficiency. An open study in 8 Pomeranian dogs with alopecia X, found that MPA administration resulted in partial hair regrowth in 3 of 8 and complete hair regrowth in 1 of 8 dogs treated (Frank *et al.* 2013).

Progesterones have been used in horses for many purposes, including management of the spring transition period, prevention of estrus behavior, induction of estrous cycle synchrony, pregnancy maintenance, and modification of stallion behavior (Dascanio 2009). However, MPA does not appear to effectively suppress estrous behavior or follicular activity in normal cycling mares (Gee *et al.* 2008).

In humans, parenteral MPA has been used as a long-acting contraceptive in females, to decrease sexually deviant behavior in males, and as an antineoplastic agent for some carcinomas (see Pharmacology section above). Oral MPA is used in human females to treat secondary amenorrhea or abnormal uterine bleeding secondary to hormone imbalances.

Pharmacology/Actions

Progestins are primarily produced endogenously by the corpus luteum. They transform proliferative endometrium to secretory endometrium, enhance myometrium hypertrophy and inhibit spontaneous uterine contraction. Progestins have a dose-dependent inhibitory effect on the secretion of pituitary gonadotropins and can have an anti-insulin effect. Medroxyprogesterone has exhibited a pronounced adrenocorticoid effect in animals (species not listed) and can suppress ACTH and cortisol release. MPA is anti-estrogenic and will also decrease plasma testosterone levels in male humans and dogs.

MPA has antineoplastic activity against endometrial carcinoma and renal carcinoma (efficacy in doubt) in human patients. The mechanism for this activity is not known.

Pharmacokinetics

No specific pharmacokinetic parameters in veterinary species were located for this drug. It has been reported (Beaver 1989) that injectable MPA has an approximate duration of action of 30 days when used to treat behavior disorders in cats. When administered IM to women, MPA has contraceptive activity for at least 3 months.

Contraindications/Precautions/Warnings

Progestagen therapy can cause serious adverse effects (see below). Safer alternative treatments should be considered when possible, otherwise, weigh the potential risks versus benefits before instituting therapy. Many clinicians believe that progestogens are grossly overused.

Do not use MPA prior to puberty in cats as chronic, severe, mammary hypertrophy may result. Use in dogs before puberty may precipitate subclinical uterine or endocrine conditions (*e.g.*, cystic endometrial hyperplasia-pyometra; diabetes).

This agent should not be used during pregnancy or to treat bitches with pseudo-pregnancy. Females should not be treated during diestrus, or with uterine hemorrhage. Do not use in females with prolonged heat unless cystic ovarian disease is confirmed and surgery or GNRH or hCG are not viable options. Animals with diabetes should not receive medroxyprogesterone.

Because this drug can suppress adrenal function, exogenous steroids may need to be administered if the patient is stressed (*e.g.*, surgery, trauma).

When used for reproductive control, patients should 1) undergo a thorough reproductive history to rule out occurrence of estrus within the last 1-2 months (female in diestrus); 2) a complete physical exam; 3) palpation of mammary glands to rule out mammary nodules; 4) a vaginal smear to rule out presence of estrus (Romagnoli 2002).

Adverse Effects

If MPA is administered subcutaneously, permanent local alopecia, atrophy, and depigmentation may occur. If injecting SC, it is recommended to use the inguinal area to avoid these manifestations. Adverse reactions that are possible in dogs and cats include: increased appetite with increases in body weight and/or thirst, depression, lethargy, personality changes, adrenocortical depression, mammary changes (including enlargement, milk production, and neoplasms), diabetes mellitus, hypothyroidism, pyometra, and temporary inhibition of spermatogenesis. In dogs, acromegaly and increased growth hormone levels have been seen when used in patients with diabetes mellitus.

Reproductive/Nursing Safety

See the dog dose "a", and the horse dose below, for more information on use of MPA during canine or equine pregnancy.

In humans, the FDA categorizes this drug as category *X* for use during pregnancy—especially the first 4 months: (*Studies in animals or humans demonstrate fetal abnormalities or adverse reaction; reports indicate evidence of fetal risk. The risk of use in pregnant women clearly outweighs any possible benefit.*)

Medroxyprogesterone can be detected in maternal milk, but in humans, no adverse effects in nursing infants have been noted.

Overdosage/Acute Toxicity

No reports or information was located on inadvertent overdosage with this agent. Refer to the Adverse Effects section above.

Drug Interactions

The following drug interactions have either been reported or are theoretical in humans or animals receiving medroxyprogesterone and may be of significance in veterinary patients. Unless otherwise noted, use together is not necessarily contraindicated, but weigh the potential risks and perform additional monitoring when appropriate.

- **FELBAMATE:** May increase medroxyprogesterone metabolism.
- **RIFAMPIN:** A potential interaction exists with rifampin, which may decrease progestin activity if administered concomitantly. This is presumably due to microsomal enzyme induction with resultant increase in progestin metabolism. The clinical significance of this potential interaction is unknown.

Laboratory Considerations

- In humans, progestins in combination with estrogens (*e.g.*, oral contraceptives) have been demonstrated to increase thyroxine-binding globulin (TBG) with resultant increases in total circulating thyroid hormone. Decreased T_3 resin uptake also occurs, but free T_4 levels are unaltered. Liver function tests may also be altered.
- The manufacturer recommends notifying the pathologist of patient medroxyprogesterone exposure when submitting relevant specimens.

Doses

- **DOGS:**

  For apparent luteal insufficiency in bitches (extra-label): 0.1 mg/kg PO once daily. Treatment is discontinued several days prior to the expected due date to avoid prolonged gestation. In humans, progestins have caused congenital heart defects, limb-reduction deformities, hypospadias in male fetuses, and mild virilization of the external genitalia of female fetuses, especially when administered to women during the first 4 months of pregnancy. Facial deformities were reported in one of the four pups in a litter from a bitch treated with MPA for hypoluteoidism. In most instances, the potential benefits of progesterone treatment for hypoluteoidism during the second half of pregnancy outweigh the maternal and fetal risks. (Gorlinger *et al.* 2005), (Johnson 2008)

  For long-term reproductive control (extra-label): 2.5 – 3 mg/kg IM q5 months. (Romagnoli 2002, 2006, 2009)

  For alopecia X (extra-label): Study done in Pomeranians. MPA at 5 or 10 mg/kg SC every 4 weeks for 4 treatments resulted in partial hair regrowth in 3 of 8, and complete hair regrowth in 1 of 8 dogs treated; no adverse effects reported. Authors concluded that prolonged treatment could result in improved success with careful monitoring for adverse effects. (Frank *et al.* 2013)

- **CATS:**

  To treat behavioral disorders (extra-label): To reduce marking in neutered male cats when all other drugs have been unsuccessful: Medroxyprogesterone acetate at 5 – 20 mg/kg SC or IM three to four times yearly. (Landsberg 2007)

  For long-term reproductive control (extra-label): 2 mg/kg IM q5 months. (Romagnoli 2002, 2006, 2009)

- **HORSES:**

  Extra-label: Progesterones have been used in horses for many purposes, including management of the spring transition period, prevention of estrus behavior, induction of estrous cycle synchrony, pregnancy maintenance, and modification of stallion behavior. MPA (*Depo-Provera®*) is dosed at ≈500 – 800 mg IM. The interval between shots varies between horses. Most injections last 2-3 months. This drug will not prevent pregnancy loss and does not stop cyclicity. (Dascanio 2009). However, MPA does not appear to effectively suppress estrous behavior or follicular activity in normal cycling mares (Gee *et al.* 2008).

Monitoring

- Weight.
- Blood glucose (draw baseline before therapy).
- Mammary gland physical examination.
- Adrenocortical function.
- Efficacy.

Client Information

- Side effects in dogs and cats can include: Loss of hair/fur at site of injection, increased appetite with increases in body weight and/or thirst, depression and lethargy, changes in behavior, mammary changes (including enlargement, milk production, and tumors), diabetes mellitus, hypothyroidism, uterine infection (females), and temporary inhibition of sperm production (males).

Chemistry/Synonyms

A synthetic progestin, medroxyprogesterone acetate (MPA) occurs as an odorless, white to off-white, crystalline powder. It is insoluble in water and sparingly soluble in alcohol. It has a melting range of 200-210°C.

Medroxyprogesterone acetate may also be known as: MPA, MAP, acetoxymethylprogesterone, medroxyprogesteroni acetas, methylacetoxyprogesterone, metipregnone, and NSC-26386; many trade names are available.

Storage/Stability

Medroxyprogesterone acetate suspensions for injection should be stored at room temperature (15-30°C); avoid freezing and temperatures above 40°C. MPA tablets should be stored in well-closed containers at room temperature.

Compatibility/Compounding Considerations

No specific information noted.

Dosage Forms/Regulatory Status

VETERINARY-LABELED PRODUCTS: NONE.

HUMAN-LABELED PRODUCTS:

Medroxyprogesterone Acetate Tablets (scored): 2.5 mg, 5 mg & 10 mg; *Provera®*, generic; (Rx)

Medroxyprogesterone Acetate Injection: 104 mg (160 mg/mL) in 0.65 mL prefilled syringes; 150 mg/mL in 1 mL vials; 400 mg/mL in 2.5 mL& 10 mL vials and 1 mL *U-ject*; *Depo-SubQ provera 104®*, *Depo-Provera®*, generic; (Rx)

Revisions/References

Monograph revised/updated March 2014.

Dascanio, J. (2009). Hormonal Control of Reproduction. Proceedings: ABVP. accessed via Veterinary Information Network; vin.com

Frank, L. A. & J. B. Watson (2013). Treatment of alopecia X with medroxyprogesterone acetate. Veterinary Dermatology 24(6): 624-+.

Gee, E. K., et al. (2008). Efficacy of medroxyprogesterone acetate in suppression of estrous behavior and follicular activity. Theriogenology 70(3): 588-.

Gorlinger, S., et al. (2005). Hypoluteoidism in a bitch. Theriogenology 64(1): 213-9.

Johnson, C. A. (2008). High-risk pregnancy and hypoluteoidism in the bitch. Theriogenology 70(9): 1424-30.

Landsberg, G. (2007). Drug and natural alternatives for marking cats. Proceedings: Western Vet Conference. accessed via Veterinary Information Network; vin.com

Romagnoli, S. (2002). Clinical use of hormones in the control of reproduction in the bitches and queens. Proceedings: World Small Animal Veterinary Association World Congress. accessed via Veterinary Information Network; vin.com

Romagnoli, S. (2006). Control of reproduction in dogs and cats: Use and misuse of hormones. Proceedings: WSAVA World Congress. accessed via Veterinary Information Network; vin.com

Romagnoli, S. (2009). Non-Surgical Contraception in Dogs and Cats. Proceedings: WSAVA World Congress. accessed via Veterinary Information Network; vin.com

Megestrol Acetate

(me-**jess**-trole)   Ovaban®, Megace®

Progestin

Prescriber Highlights

▶ Synthetic progestin used in **dogs (female):** for postponement of estrus & the alleviation of false pregnancy; **Dogs (male):** benign prostatic hypertrophy. **Cats:** Many dermatologic & behavior-related conditions.

▶ Contraindications: Pregnant animals or with uterine disease, diabetes mellitus, or mammary neoplasias; should not be used to treat bitches with pseudo-pregnancy; females should not be treated during diestrus, or with uterine hemorrhage.

▶ Caution: Thrombophlebitis.

▶ Adverse Effects: **Cats:** Profound adrenocortical suppression, adrenal atrophy, transient diabetes mellitus, polydipsia/polyuria, personality changes, increased weight, endometritis, cystic endometrial hyperplasia, mammary hypertrophy, neoplasias, & hepatotoxicity possible. **Dogs:** Increased appetite & weight gain, lethargy, change in behavior or hair color, mucometra, endometritis, cystic endometrial hyperplasia, mammary enlargement & neoplasia, acromegaly, adrenocortical suppression, or lactation (rare).

Uses/Indications

Megestrol acetate (MA; *Ovaban®*) is FDA-approved for use in dogs only for the postponement of estrus and the alleviation of false pregnancy. In male dogs, it has been used for benign prostatic hypertrophy. MA has been used clinically for many dermatologic and behavior-related conditions, primarily in cats. Low-dose MA may be an alternative to surgery for contraception in free roaming cats, but questions of safety, efficacy, regulatory pathways and ethics remain to be answered (Greenberg *et al.* 2013).

Megestrol acetate is indicated in humans for the palliative treatment of advanced carcinoma of the breast or endometrium.

Pharmacology/Actions

Megestrol acetate possesses the pharmacologic actions expected of other progestationals (*e.g.*, medroxyprogesterone acetate). It has significant anti-estrogen and glucocorticoid activity (with resultant adrenal suppression). It does not have anabolic or masculinizing effects on the developing fetus.

Pharmacokinetics

Megestrol acetate is well absorbed from the GI tract and appears to be metabolized completely in the liver to conjugates and free steroids.

The half-life of megestrol acetate is reported to be 8 days in the dog.

Contraindications/Precautions/Warnings

Megestrol acetate is contraindicated in pregnant animals or in animals with uterine disease, diabetes mellitus, or mammary neoplasias. It has been recommended that MA not be used in dogs prior to their first estrous cycle or for anestrus therapy in dogs with abnormal cycles. The manufacturer (Schering) recommends that mating be prevented should estrus occur within 30 days of cessation of MA therapy.

This agent should not be used during pregnancy or to treat bitches with pseudo-pregnancy. Females should not be treated during diestrus, or with uterine hemorrhage. Do not use in females with prolonged heat unless cystic ovarian disease is confirmed and surgery or GNRH or hCG are not viable options. Animals with diabetes should not receive megestrol.

Because this drug can suppress adrenal function, exogenous steroids may need to be administered if the patient is stressed (*e.g.*, surgery, trauma).

For estrus control, the manufacturer recommends that drug must be given for the full treatment regimen to be effective. The package insert states that "*Ovaban®* should not be given for more than 2 consecutive treatments," but the reasons for this are unclear; some theriogenologists question the need for this precaution.

When used for reproductive control, it has been recommended that patients undergo: **1)** a thorough reproductive history to rule out occurrence of estrus within the last 1-2 months (female in diestrus); **2)** a complete physical exam; **3)** palpation of mammary glands to rule out mammary nodules; **4)** a vaginal smear to rule out presence of estrus (Romagnoli 2002, 2009).

In humans, megestrol acetate is to be used with caution in patients with thrombophlebitis and is contraindicated as a test for pregnancy.

Adverse Effects

In dogs, increased appetite and weight gain, lethargy, change in behavior or hair color, mucometra, endometritis, pyometra, cystic endometrial hyperplasia, mammary enlargement and neoplasia, acromegaly, adrenocortical suppression or lactation (rare) may occur. One dog reportedly developed diabetes mellitus after use. The reported incidence is 0.8% for pyometra in dogs that are treated per the label of the veterinary-labeled product (*Ovaban®*) (Kustritz 2012).

In cats, megestrol acetate can induce a profound adrenocortical suppression, adrenal atrophy, and an iatrogenic "Addison's" syndrome can develop at "standard" dosages (2.5 – 5 mg every other day) within 1-2 weeks. Once the drug has been discontinued, serum cortisol levels (both resting and ACTH-stimulated) will return to normal levels within a few weeks. Clinical signs of adrenocortical insufficiency (*e.g.*, vomiting, lethargy) are uncommon, but exogenous steroid support should be considered if the animal is stressed (surgery, trauma, etc.). Cats may develop a transient diabetes mellitus while receiving MA. Polydipsia/polyuria, personality changes, increased weight, endometritis, cystic endometrial hyperplasia, mammary hypertrophy and neoplasias may also occur. Increased appetite and weight gain are not consistently seen, but MA is occasionally used as an appetite stimulant. Rarely, megestrol acetate can cause hepatotoxicity (increased alkaline phosphatase) in cats. Megestrol potentially can exacerbate latent viral infections (*e.g.*, FHV-1).

Limited clinical studies have suggested that megestrol acetate may cause less cystic endometrial hyperplasia than other progestational agents, but cautious use and vigilant monitoring is still warranted.

Reproductive/Nursing Safety

No effects were noted in either the bitch or litter when pregnant dogs received 0.25 mg/kg/day for 32 days during the first half of pregnancy; reduced litter sizes and puppy survival were detected when the dose was given during the last half of pregnancy. Fetal hypospadias are possible if progestational agents are administered during pregnancy.

During the first 4 months of pregnancy in humans, the FDA categorizes this drug as category *X* for use during pregnancy (*Studies in animals or humans demonstrate fetal abnormalities or adverse reaction; reports indicate evidence of fetal risk. The risk of use in pregnant women clearly outweighs any possible benefit.*) During the last 5 months of pregnancy in humans, the FDA categorizes this drug as category *D* for use during pregnancy (*There is evidence of human fetal risk, but the potential benefits from the use of the drug in pregnant women may be acceptable despite its potential risks.*)

Detectable amounts of progestins enter the milk of mothers receiving these agents. Effects on nursing infants have not been established.

Overdosage/Acute Toxicity

No information was located regarding acute overdosage of megestrol acetate. In humans, dosages of up to 800 mg/day caused no observable adverse reactions.

Toxicity studies performed in dogs at dosages of 0.1 – 0.25 mg/kg/day PO for 36 months yielded no gross abnormalities in the study population. Histologically, cystic endometrial hyperplasia was noted at 36 months, but resolved when therapy was discontinued. At dosages of 0.5 mg/kg/day PO for 5 months, a reversible uterine hyperplasia was seen in treated dogs. Dosages of 2 mg/kg/day demonstrated early cystic endometritis in biopsies done on dogs at 64 days.

Drug Interactions

- **CORTICOSTEROIDS**: Megestrol used with corticosteroids (long-term) may exacerbate adrenocortical suppression and diabetes mellitus.
- **RIFAMPIN**: May decrease progestin activity if administered concomitantly. This is presumably due to microsomal enzyme induction with resultant increase in progestin metabolism. The clinical significance of this potential interaction is unknown.

Doses

- **DOGS:**

  For estrus control (extra-label): Either low dose at 0.55 mg/kg PO once daily for 32 days during anestrus or at a high dose 2.2 mg/kg PO once daily for 8 days during the first 3 days of proestrus. If used properly during anestrus, return to subsequent proestrus will be postponed for ≈3 months. If used properly during proestrus, physical manifestations of proestrus and estrus, and breeding behavior will subside within days and the bitch will not ovulate on that cycle. (Kustritz 2012)

  For benign prostatic hypertrophy (extra-label): 0.1 – 0.5 mg/kg per day for 3-8 weeks; best used to maintain breeding potential for short time prior to castration; use with caution. (Lane 2006)

  For treatment for subinvolution of placental sites (SIPS); (extra-label): From a small non-blinded study in 9 dogs (7 treated; 2 control): 0.1 mg/kg PO once daily for the first week and then 0.05 mg/kg PO once daily for the 2nd week. All treated dogs' vaginal discharge ceased within treatment period and 5 of 6 that were subsequently mated became pregnant. No adverse effects were noted. (Voorhorst et al. 2013)

- **CATS:**

  For suppression of estrus (extra-label): In anestrus: 5 mg/cat PO every 2 weeks or 2.5 mg/cat per week (better if divided into 2 doses given every 3.5 days); In proestrus: 5 mg/cat per day for 4 days, then 5 mg PO every 2 weeks. (Romagnoli 2006, 2009)

  As a "last ditch" (because of potential side effects) **alternative for treating feline atopy** (extra-label): Remission of clinical signs can often be achieved with an oral dose of 2.5 – 5 mg per cat PO every 48 hours for 1-3 weeks. This dose is then used once weekly. (Rosychuk 2007)

  To reduce marking in neutered male cats when all other drugs have been unsuccessful (extra-label): 2.5 – 10 mg per cat PO once daily for one week, then reduce to once or twice weekly. (Landsberg 2007)

Monitoring

- Weight.
- Blood glucose (draw baseline before therapy).
- Mammary gland development and appearance.
- Adrenocortical function.
- Liver enzymes if long-term treatment.
- Efficacy.

Client Information

- May give with food or on an empty stomach, but giving with food may help prevent vomiting.
- Megestrol can have many side effects, some of them serious. In particular watch for changes in mammary glands/nipples or any vaginal discharge.
- Pregnant women should use caution when handling this medication.

Chemistry/Synonyms

A synthetic progestin, megestrol acetate (MA) occurs as an essentially odorless, tasteless, white to creamy white, crystalline powder that is insoluble in water, sparingly soluble in alcohol, and slightly soluble in fixed oils. It has a melting range of 213-219°C over a 3° range and a specific rotation of +8° to +12°.

Megestrol acetate may also be known as: BDH-1298, compound 5071, megestroli acetas, NSC-71423, SC-10363, *Megace®*, and *Ovaban®* are common trade names.

Storage/Stability

Megestrol acetate tablets should be stored in well-closed containers at a temperature of less than 40°C. The tablets may be crushed and administered with food. The veterinary manufacturer recommends storing the tablets from 2°-30°C (36°-86°F).

Compatibility/Compounding Considerations

No specific information noted.

Dosage Forms/Regulatory Status

VETERINARY-LABELED PRODUCTS:

Megestrol Acetate Oral Tablets: 5 mg, 20 mg; available in bottles of 250 and 500 tablets, and in 30 foil strips of 8 and packaged in cartons of 240 tablets; *Ovaban®*; (Rx). FDA-approved for use in dogs only. **Note:** This product is still listed in FDA's "Green Book" of approved animal drugs, but may no longer be marketed in the USA.

HUMAN-LABELED PRODUCTS:

Megestrol Acetate Tablets: 20 mg & 40 mg; *Megace®*, generic; (Rx)

Megestrol Acetate Suspension: 40 mg/mL & 125 mg/mL; *Megace®*, *Megace ES®*, generic (40 mg/mL); (Rx)

Revisions/References

Monograph revised/updated March 2014.

Greenberg, M., et al. (2013). Low-dose megestrol acetate revisited: A viable adjunct to surgical sterilization in free roaming cats? Veterinary Journal 196(3): 304-8.

Kustritz, M. V. R. (2012). Managing the Reproductive Cycle in the Bitch. Veterinary Clinics of North America-Small Animal Practice 42(3): 423-37.

Landsberg, G. (2007). Drug and natural alternatives for marking cats. Proceedings: Western Vet Conference. accessed via Veterinary Information Network; vin.com

Lane, I. (2006). Update on prostatic disorders. Proceedings: Western Vet Conf. accessed via Veterinary Information Network; vin.com

Romagnoli, S. (2002). Clinical use of hormones in the control of reproduction in the bitches and queens. Proceedings: World Small Animal Veterinary Association World Congress. accessed via Veterinary Information Network; vin.com

Romagnoli, S. (2006). Control of reproduction in dogs and cats: Use and misuse of hormones. Proceedings: WSAVA World Congress. accessed via Veterinary Information Network; vin.com

Romagnoli, S. (2009). Non-Surgical Contraception in Dogs and Cats. Proceedings: WSAVA World Congress. accessed via Veterinary Information Network; vin.com

Rosychuk, R. (2007). Dermatologic Diseases of the Head - Part I. Proceedings: AAFP. accessed via Veterinary Information Network; vin.com

Voorhorst, M. J., et al. (2013). Successful Treatment for Subinvolution of Placental Sites in the Bitch with Low Oral Doses of Progestagen. Reproduction in Domestic Animals 48(5): 840-3.

Meglumine Antimoniate

(**meg**-loo-meen an-tih-**mohne**-ee-ate)

Glucantime®, N-methyl-glucamine antimoniate

Pentavalent Antimony Antileishmanial

Prescriber Highlights

▶ Pentavalent antimony compound used for treating leishmaniasis (with or without allopurinol) in dogs.

▶ Not available in USA.

▶ Extreme caution (relatively contraindicated) in patients with cardiac, hepatic or renal insufficiency.

▶ Primary adverse effects noted in dogs with meglumine antimoniate are injection site reactions, lethargy & gastrointestinal effects (inappetence, vomiting).

▶ Resistance to treatment has been reported.

▶ Treatment is prolonged & cost may be substantial.

Uses/Indications

Meglumine antimoniate is used alone or in combination with allopurinol to treat leishmaniasis in dogs. At present, this combination appears to be the treatment of choice for treating dogs with confirmed infection. It is available commercially in some Mediterranean and South American countries but not in the USA.

Meglumine antimoniate may be useful for treating feline leishmaniasis, but more evidence for safety and efficacy are needed before suggesting its use.

Pharmacology/Actions

Pentavalent antimony compounds such as meglumine antimoniate and sodium stibogluconate selectively inhibit the leishmanial enzymes required for glycolytic and fatty acid oxidation. Pentavalent antimony compounds rarely are successful in completely eradicating *Leishmania* organisms in infected dogs. When used with allopurinol, synergy for treating leishmaniasis and reduced risk for antimonial drug-resistance development can occur.

Pharmacokinetics

After subcutaneous or intramuscular injections in dogs systemic bioavailability is ≈92%; highest tissue concentrations are found in the liver, spleen, and skin. Elimination half-life is relatively short (approx. 2 hours when given SC). Within 9 hours of dosing, 80% of the antimony is excreted in the urine. Reduced renal function can cause increased antimoniate half-lives.

Contraindications/Precautions/Warnings

Patients with renal, hepatic or cardiac failure are more likely to develop serious adverse effects with this agent; weigh the potential risks versus benefits carefully before treating. Decreased renal function in particular, may lead to drug accumulation and an increased risk for toxicity. In dogs with severe renal failure (IRIS stages III-IV) the correction of fluid and acid-base imbalances prior to treatment with allopurinol alone has been recommended (Koutinas *et al.* 2007).

Hypersensitivity reactions have been reported in people, and any patient with previous hypersensitivity to meglumine antimoniate should not receive the drug.

Adverse Effects

Primary adverse effects noted in dogs are injection site reactions (cutaneous abscesses/cellulitis), lethargy, and gastrointestinal effects (inappetence, vomiting). Transient increases in liver enzymes have been reported.

Potentially, the drug may be nephrotoxic in dogs, but this is difficult to evaluate in clinically-infected dogs as renal dysfunction is one of the likely consequences of the infection. A study done in healthy dogs showed diffuse proximal tubule cell vacuolization and multifocal areas with coagulative necrosis under light microscopy. Electron microscopy showed reduced organellar content, loss or attenuation of brush border, cellular detachment from the basement membrane, apical blebbing and individual cell necrosis. The authors concluded that meglumine antimoniate caused severe tubular damage (Brovida *et al.* 2009).

Drug resistance may occur. After several courses of treatment, decreased sensitivity of *L. infantum* to meglumine antimoniate or antimonials has been reported.

In humans, increased serum lipase, amylase, creatinine, urea nitrogen, and increased QT interval on ECG, have been reported. Occasionally, decreases in white blood cell counts and hemoglobin have been reported in humans. In a study in 28 dogs with clinical disease treated with meglumine antimoniate (75 mg/kg q12h for 60 days) when compared pre-treatment and post-treatment (day 60), significant changes in serum cardiac troponin I concentrations or corrected QT intervals were not found (Luciani *et al.* 2013).

Reproductive/Nursing Safety

There is limited information available. Pregnant rats given up to 300 mg/kg on days 6-15 caused increased fetal resorptions and increased rates of abnormalities of the atlas bone. A case report of a bitch that received meglumine antimoniate during pregnancy has been published (Spada *et al.* 2011). Pregnancy and delivery were deemed normal. Three puppies died within 2 days of delivery, but the two surviving puppies were followed clinically, serologically and with real-time PCR until one year old. Neither puppy had clinical or serological evidence of *L. infantum* despite *L. infantum* DNA-evidence being found in the uterine tissue of the bitch. The authors concluded that meglumine antimoniate may have prevented vertical transmission of leishmaniasis.

Weigh the risks versus benefits when deciding to treat during pregnancy. It is unknown if the drug enters maternal milk.

Overdosage/Acute Toxicity

No specific overdose information was located. Depending on the dosage, a single overdose could potentially cause renal, hepatic, pancreatic, and hematologic effects, but gastrointestinal effects (vomiting) and lethargy would be the most likely outcomes. It is recommended to observe the patient and contact an animal poison control center for further guidance with an overdose situation.

Drug Interactions

The following drug interactions have either been reported or are theoretical in humans or animals receiving meglumine antimoniate and may be of significance in veterinary patients (dogs):

■ **AGENTS THAT CAN PROLONG QT INTERVAL** (*e.g.*, **tricyclic antidepressants, disopyramide, quinidine, procainamide**, etc.): Meglumine antimoniate may prolong QT interval further with increased risk for arrhythmias.

■ **OTHER POTENTIALLY NEPHROTOXIC DRUGS** (e.g., **amphotericin B, aminoglycosides**): Avoid or use with caution in dogs with clinical leishmaniasis and kidney disease being treated with meglumine antimoniate (Torres *et al.* 2011).

Laboratory Considerations

■ No specific laboratory interactions or considerations noted.

Doses

■ **DOGS:**

For leishmaniasis (extra-label): 100 mg/kg SC once daily for 4 weeks is the most commonly reported treatment regimen. However, because of the short half-life, giving 50 mg/kg SC twice daily for 4-8 weeks could be more effective. Combining with allopurinol (10 mg/kg PO twice daily for at least 6 months) may yield a longer period of clinical remission than if treated with either drug alone. (Oliva *et al.* 2010), (Goldstein *et al.* 2013)

Monitoring

- Clinical and serological (PCR preferred) efficacy.
- CBC (baseline and periodic).
- Liver enzymes; renal function tests (serum creatinine, BUN); serum lipase and amylase (baseline and periodic).
- Urinalysis (baseline and periodic).

Client Information

- Clients should understand that treatment with this drug can be prolonged and expensive, and that a "cure" (complete eradication) is unlikely.

Chemistry/Synonyms

Meglumine antimoniate is 1-Deoxy-1-methylamino-D-glucitol antimoniate. It has a molecular weight of 366. One gram contains approximately 272 mg of antimony.

Meglumine antimoniate may also be known as: meglumine antimonate, N-methylglucamine antimoniate, RP-2168, antimony meglumine, Protostib, 1-Deoxy-1-methylamino-D-glucitol antimoniate, *Glucantime®* and *Glucantim®*.

Storage/Stability

Unless otherwise specified by the manufacturer, commercially available ampules should be stored below 40°C, preferably between 15°-30°C; protect from freezing.

Compatibility/Compounding Considerations

No specific information noted.

Dosage Forms/Regulatory Status

VETERINARY-LABELED PRODUCTS:

None in the USA. May be available via the CDC, see: http://www.cdc.gov/ncidod/srp/drugs/drug-service.html

HUMAN-LABELED PRODUCTS: NONE IN THE USA.

Meglumine antimoniate may be available in several countries, including Brazil, Venezuela, and in Europe; trade names include: *Glucantime®* and *Glucantim®*. Commercially it is available as a solution containing 1.5 grams of meglumine antimoniate (425 mg pentavalent antimony) per 5 mL.

Revisions/References

Monograph revised/updated April 2014.

Brovida, C., et al. (2009). Evaluation of Nephrotoxic Effects of Miltefosine and Meglumine Antimonate in 8 Healthy Beagles. Proceedings: ECVIM. accessed via Veterinary Information Network; vin.com

Goldstein, R. E., et al. (2013). Consensus Recommendations for Treatment for Dogs with Serology Positive Glomerular Disease. Journal of Veterinary Internal Medicine 27: S60-S6.

Koutinas, A. & C. Koutinas (2007). Renal function in canine leishmaniasis. Proceedings: ECVIM. accessed via Veterinary Information Network; vin.com

Luciani, A., et al. (2013). Evaluation of the cardiac toxicity of N-methyl-glucamine antimoniate in dogs with naturally occurring leishmaniasis. Veterinary Journal 196(1): 119-21.

Oliva, G., et al. (2010). Guidelines for treatment of leishmaniasis in dogs. Journal of the American Veterinary Medical Association 236(11): 1192-8.

Spada, E., et al. (2011). First Report of the Use of Meglumine Antimoniate for Treatment of Canine Leishmaniasis in a Pregnant Dog. J. Am. Anim. Hosp. Assoc. 47(1): 67-71.

Torres, M., et al. (2011). Long term follow-up of dogs diagnosed with leishmaniosis (clinical stage II) and treated with meglumine antimoniate and allopurinol. Veterinary Journal 188(3): 346-51.

Melarsomine

(mee-**lar**-soe-meen)   Immiticide®

Arsenical Antiparasitic

Prescriber Highlights

▶ Organic arsenical adulticide for heartworm disease in dogs. American Heartworm Society recommends 3-dose protocol (except for dogs with caval syndrome) with prior treatment with doxycycline and a macrocyclic lactone.

▶ Contraindications: Class IV (very severe) heartworm disease; weigh risk vs. potential benefits in pregnant, lactating, or breeding dogs. Reportedly very toxic to cats; not currently recommended.

▶ Adverse Effects: Many possible, most common are: injection site reactions coughing/gagging, depression/lethargy, anorexia/inappetence, excessive salivation, fever, lung congestion, vomiting, pulmonary thromboembolism.

▶ Calculate dosages very carefully. Proper IM injection technique required; do not give IV or SC. Avoid human exposure.

▶ Strict cage rest after treatment essential.

Uses/Indications

Melarsomine is indicated for the treatment of stabilized class I, II, and III heartworm disease caused by immature (4 month old, stage L5) to mature adult infections of *D. immitis* in dogs. When compared with thiacetarsamide, melarsomine appears to be more efficacious, less irritating to tissues, and does not cause hepatic necrosis.

The American Heartworm Society recommends that regardless of the severity of the disease (with the exception of caval syndrome), due to increased safety and efficacy only the three-dose protocol be used. Additionally they recommend administering doxycycline (10 mg/kg PO twice daily for 4 weeks prior to melarsomine) and a macrocyclic lactone (at heartworm preventative dosages for 2-3 months prior to melarsomine treatment). Doxycycline helps to reduce subsequent microfilaremia by eliminating *Wolbachia*, a bacterium associated with embryogenesis in *D. immitis*. The macrocyclic lactone will reduce new infections, eliminate existing susceptible larvae, and allow older worms (between 2 and 4 months of age) to mature to an age where they would be more susceptible to melarsomine (Nelson *et al.* 2014).

Melarsomine may also be useful for treating ferrets; it has been suggested to contact the manufacturer before using the drug in this species.

Pharmacology/Actions

While melarsomine is an arsenical compound, its exact mechanism of action is not known. Both laboratory and field studies have demonstrated that melarsomine is 90-99% effective in killing adult and L5 larvae of *D. immitis* in dogs at recommended dosages. The 2 injection method kills only about 90% of adult worms while the 3 injection method will kill 98% (Nelson *et al.* 2014).

Pharmacokinetics

Melarsomine is reportedly rapidly absorbed after IM injection in dogs; time to peak plasma concentration is ≈11 minutes. The apparent volume of distribution is ≈0.7 L/kg; terminal half-life is approximately 3 hours.

Contraindications/Precautions/Warnings

Melarsomine is contraindicated in dogs with class IV (very severe) heartworm disease. Class IV is having caval syndrome (heartworms present in venae cavae and right atrium). Melarsomine is reportedly very toxic to cats and at this time its use cannot be recommended for feline patients.

Older dogs (>8 years) may be more susceptible to adverse effects than younger dogs.

Do **NOT** give IV or SC; significant toxicity or tissue damage may occur. Administer only deep IM as directed (lumbar epaxial muscles (L3-L5). Do not administer at any other site. Some giant breed dogs (*e.g.,* Great Danes) that require large dosages may be more susceptible to tissue damage. Consider contacting Merial's product support (888-637-4251) for treatment advice.

While all dogs with heartworm disease are at risk for post-treatment pulmonary thromboembolism, those with severe pulmonary artery disease are at increased risk for post treatment morbidity and mortality.

Strictly adhering to the manufacturer's instructions for administration is imperative and exercise restriction during the recovery period is <u>essential</u> for minimizing cardiopulmonary complications (Nelson *et al.* 2014). Cage rest (2-4 weeks) in the veterinary clinic is recommended if feasible. If clinic cage rest and observation are not possible, owners should be advised that unless the patient's exercise is restricted, thrombolic events are more likely and can be fatal. Wash hands after use or wear gloves. Avoid drug contact with animal's eyes; if exposed wash with copious amounts of water. Avoid human exposure. If human exposure occurs, contact a physician.

Adverse Effects

Approximately 1/3 of dogs show signs of injection site reactions (pain, swelling, tenderness, reluctance to move) after receiving melarsomine. This can be minimized by ensuring the injection is deposited deep into the belly of the epaxial musculature with a needle newly changed after the drug is drawn into the syringe and that is an appropriate length and gauge for the size of dog and body condition (Nelson *et al.* 2014). Most injection site signs resolve within weeks, but, rarely, severe injection reactions can occur. Firm nodules at the injection site can persist indefinitely. SC or IV injections must be avoided. The most severe local reactions are usually seen if the drug leaks back from the injection site into subcutaneous tissues. Applying firm pressure to the injection site after administration may reduce the risk for this problem.

Other reactions reported in 5% or more dogs treated include: coughing/gagging (22% incidence; average day of onset after treatment = 10); depression/lethargy (15% incidence; average day of onset after treatment = 5); anorexia/inappetence (13% incidence; average day of onset after treatment = 5); fever (7%); lung congestion (6%); vomiting (5%). There is significant interpatient variance in both the date of onset and duration for the above effects. Dogs may also exhibit excessive salivation after dosing.

There are a plethora of other adverse effects in dogs with reported incidences less than 3%, including paresis and paralysis. Refer to the package insert for specifics.

Animals not exhibiting adverse effects after the first dose or course of therapy may demonstrate them after the 2nd dose or course of therapy.

Reproductive/Nursing Safety

Safety has not been established for use in pregnant, lactating, or breeding dogs. Risks versus potential benefits of therapy should be weighed before use.

Overdosage/Acute Toxicity

There is low margin of safety with melarsomine dosages. A 3X dose (7.5 mg/kg) in healthy dogs has demonstrated respiratory inflammation and distress, excessive salivation, restlessness, panting, vomiting, edema, tremors, lethargy, ataxia, cyanosis, stupor, and death. Signs of diarrhea, excessive salivation, restlessness, panting, vomiting, and fever have been noted in infected dogs that have received inadvertent overdoses (2X).

Treatment with dimercaprol (BAL in Oil) may be considered to treat melarsomine overdoses. Clinical efficacy of melarsomine may be reduced, however.

Drug Interactions

The manufacturer reports that during clinical field trials, melarsomine was given to dogs receiving antiinflammatory agents, antibiotics, insecticides, heartworm prophylactic medications, and various other drugs commonly used to stabilize and support dogs with heartworm disease and that no adverse drug interactions were noted.

- **ASPIRIN:** Has been shown not to reduce adverse effects and may complicate therapy; use is not recommended.
- **CNS DEPRESSANT DRUGS:** Drugs that have similar adverse effects (*e.g.,* depression caused by CNS depressants, etc.) may cause additive adverse effects or increase their incidence when used with melarsomine.

Doses

CAUTION: Because of the low margin of safety; calculate dosages very carefully. Do not confuse mg/lb with mg/kg!

- **DOGS:**

It is suggested to review the guidelines published by the American Heartworm Society at www.heartwormsociety.org for more information. The *Immiticide*® (Merial) product support phone number: 888-637-4251.

For treatment of heartworm disease:

<u>Labeled Dose</u> (FDA-approved): After diagnosis, determine the class (stage) of the disease. **Note:** The manufacturer provides worksheets that assist in the classification and treatment regime determination. It is highly recommended to use these treatment records to avoid confusion and document therapy.

Class I, & II: 2.5 mg/kg deep IM as directed (lumbar epaxial muscles; L3-L5) twice 24 hours apart and rest. Use alternating sides with each administration. In 4 months, the regimen may be repeated.

Class III: 2.5 mg/kg deep IM as directed (lumbar epaxial muscles; L3-L5). Strict rest and give all necessary systemic treatment. One month later, give 2.5 mg/kg deep IM as directed (lumbar epaxial muscles; L3-L5) twice 24 hours apart.

Note: Recommended needle size for dogs 10 kg or less = 23 gauge 1 inch; 10 kg or more body weight = 22 gauge 1.5 inch. (Package Insert; *Immiticide*®—Merial)

<u>Extra-label Protocol (American Heartworm Society) for treatment of heartworm disease in both symptomatic (not caval syndrome) and asymptomatic dogs</u>: The American Heartworm Society has a detailed management program table (including diagnostic, nursing, and monitoring guidelines) that can be accessed at www.heartwormsociety.org. The following is a summary: Prior to use administer a macrocyclic lactone (at heartworm preventative dosages for 2-3 months prior to melarsomine treatment; Days 1, 30, 60) and doxycycline (10 mg/kg PO twice daily for 4 weeks prior to melarsomine; Days 1-28). Use the three-dose regimen of melarsomine described above (Class III; one injection of 2.5 mg/kg body weight followed one month later by 2 injections of the same dose 24 hours apart; days 60, 90, & 91). To reduce the risk for thromboembolism after melarsomine treatment is started, glucocorticoids are often used in dogs located in highly endemic areas where they are more likely to have significant worm burdens. Prednisone is routinely dosed at 0.5 mg/kg twice a day for the first week, then 0.5 mg/kg once daily for the 2nd week, followed by 0.5 mg/kg every other day for 1-2 weeks. Symptomatic dogs also get prednisone (same dosage regiment) at time of diagnosis (Day 0). (Nelson *et al.* 2014)

Monitoring

- Adverse effects. Signs of thromboembolism include: low grade fever, cough, hemoptysis, and exacerbation of right heart failure.
- Cardiac biomarkers (cardiac troponin I, MB isoenzyme of creatine kinase, myoglobin) may be useful to monitor the effects of worms and adulticide treatment on the heart, but additional research is necessary to confirm utility (Carreton *et al.* 2013).
- Clinical efficacy.
- Microfilaria. Test 30 days after last melarsomine dose.
- Antigen test. Test 6 months after last melarsomine dose.

Client Information

- Strict exercise restriction after dosing is essential.
- Because of the seriousness of the disease and the potential for morbidity and mortality associated with the treatment, clients should give informed consent before electing to treat.

Chemistry/Synonyms

An organic arsenical compound, melarsomine dihydrochloride has a molecular weight of 501 and is freely soluble in water.

Melarsomine may also be known as *Immiticide®*. Its CAS registry is 128470-15-5.

Storage/Stability

The unreconstituted powder should be stored upright at room temperature. Once reconstituted, the solution should be kept in the original container and kept refrigerated for up to 24 hours. Do not freeze. Do not mix with any other drug.

Compatibility/Compounding Considerations

Reconstitute with 2 mL of the diluent provided (sterile water for injection) with a resultant concentration of 25 mg/mL. Once reconstituted, the solution should be kept in the original container and kept refrigerated for up to 24 hours. Do not freeze.

Dosage Forms/Regulatory Status

VETERINARY-LABELED PRODUCTS:

Melarsomine Dihydrochloride Powder for Injection: 50 mg/vial; *Immiticide®*; (Rx). FDA-approved for use in dogs.

HUMAN-LABELED PRODUCTS: NONE.

Revisions/References

Monograph revised/updated April 2014.

Carreton, E., et al. (2013). Utility of cardiac biomarkers during adulticide treatment of heartworm disease (Dirofilaria immitis) in dogs. Veterinary Parasitology 197(1-2): 244-50.

Nelson, C., et al. (2014). Current Canine Guidelines for the Prevention, Diagnosis, and Management of Heartworm (Dirofilaria immitis) Infection in Dogs. American Heartworm Society.

Melatonin

(mel-a-**tone**-in)   Regulin®

Hormone

Prescriber Highlights

▶ Oral & implantable pineal gland hormone.

▶ Potential uses include: As a reversible estrus suppression agent in cats, treatment of alopecia in dogs, sleep & behavior disorders in cats & dogs, adjusting seasonally controlled fertility in sheep, goats, & horses, & adjunctive treatment for adrenal disease in ferrets.

▶ Adverse effects appear to be minimal, but little experience.

▶ Potential contraindications include: Pregnancy, sexually immature animals, & liver dysfunction.

Uses/Indications

The only FDA-approved indication for melatonin is for SC implants in healthy male and female kits and adult female mink (*Mustela vison*) to accelerate the fur priming cycle. While published evidence is weak to support clinical use of melatonin for clinical conditions in animals, it has been proposed for many purposes. Many clinicians will use it on a trial basis since the potential for adverse effects is very low.

In dogs, melatonin may be useful to treat Alopecia-X in Nordic breeds, canine pattern baldness, or canine recurrent flank alopecia. It has been used for the treatment of sleep cycle disorders, cognitive dysfunction syndrome, phobias and separation anxiety, and idiopathic vacuolar hepatopathy. Melatonin potentially could stimulate platelet production.

In sheep and goats (and potentially in horses) implants are used to improve early breeding and ovulation rates (Abecia *et al.* 2011), (Faya *et al.* 2011).

In cats, melatonin has been used for the treatment of sleep cycle disorders. Preliminary evidence suggests that melatonin implants (18 mg) can provide short-term estrus control.

In ferrets, melatonin is widely used and appears to be effective in alleviating clinical signs associated with adrenal neoplasia, including alopecia, aggressive behavior, vulvar swelling, and prostatomegaly. It does not appear to alter tumor growth.

In pigs, one study (Bubenik, Ayles et al. 1998) demonstrated that 5 mg/kg in feed reduced the incidence of gastric ulcers in young pigs.

For horses, melatonin has been suggested for treating seasonal head shaking syndrome.

Pharmacology/Actions

Melatonin is involved with the neuroendocrine control of photoperiod dependent molting, hair growth and pelage color. Melatonin stimulates winter coat growth and spring shedding occurs when melatonin decreases. The mechanism of how melatonin induces these effects is not well understood. It may have direct effects on the hair follicle or alter the secretion of prolactin and/or melanocyte stimulating hormone.

Melatonin also increases serum prolactin levels, growth hormone, and increases response to growth hormone releasing hormone. Long-term use may decrease luteinizing hormone. Melatonin is also ostensibly a free radical scavenger.

Pharmacokinetics

No specific information was located for animals. In humans, melatonin has a short half-life (20-50 minutes); plasma levels return to baseline within 24 hours of a dose even after long-term dosing of <10 mg/day.

Contraindications/Precautions/Warnings

Melatonin implants are considered contraindicated in pregnant or sexually immature animals. There are very specific times for administration depending on latitude, hemisphere, and breed. Animals that are nursing young may not benefit from implant therapy.

In humans, melatonin is considered contraindicated in patients with hepatic insufficiency as it is cleared hepatically. Use with caution in patients with renal impairment. Because of its CNS depressant qualities, melatonin is sometimes stated that it should be used with caution in patients with a history of cerebrovascular disease, depression or neurological disorders.

Adverse Effects

Melatonin appears to be quite safe in dogs. Side effects in dogs when given orally are rare but the hormone may cause sedation, and affect sex hormone secretion and fertility. Subcutaneous implants in dogs have been associated with sterile abscesses.

Adverse effects in ferrets are not commonly reported. Potentially, weight gain and lethargy could occur.

Adverse effects reported in humans include altered sleep patterns, hypothermia, sedation, tachycardia, confusion, headache, and pruritus.

Reproductive/Nursing Safety

No information was located; use with caution. The mink implant label states: Do not implant in breeding stock.

Overdosage/Acute Toxicity

Little information is available; unlikely to cause significant morbidity after a single overdose.

Drug Interactions

The following drug interactions have either been reported or are theoretical in humans or animals receiving melatonin and may be of significance in veterinary patients. Unless otherwise noted, use together is not necessarily contraindicated, but weigh the potential risks and perform additional monitoring when appropriate.

- **BENZODIAZEPINES:** Melatonin may potentiate effects.
- **SUCCINYLCHOLINE:** Melatonin may potentiate effects.

Laboratory Considerations

- Melatonin can reduce cortisol and estradiol levels.

Doses

- **DOGS:**

  For dermatologic conditions such as Alopecia-X in Nordic breeds, canine pattern baldness, color dilution alopecia, recurrent or seasonal flank alopecia; (extra-label): No published studies were located to document efficacy, but the potential for serious adverse effects is very low. Anecdotal dosage recommendations vary, but oral dosages usually range from 3 mg – 12 mg (depending on the dog's size) PO 2-3 times a day. Perform a trial for at least 4 months before evaluating response. If using the implants, the following has been suggested: 8 mg (dogs less than 9 kg), 12 mg (dogs 9-18 kg) and 18 mg (dogs more than 18 kg) implanted SC. Re-treatment may be necessary 1-2 times a year.

  For sleep disorders (nocturnal activity), phobias (extra-label): Dosage recommendations vary somewhat; no evidence was located supporting one over the other. Consider 0.1 mg/kg PO 1-3 times a day initially. Practically, round dosage up to the nearest 1 mg. A single dose (from 1 – 9 mg per dog depending on dog's size) approximately 30 minutes before bedtime may be sufficient to help with night waking.

  For adjunctive treatment of thrombocytopenia (ITP); (extra-label): In some human cases with ITP, platelet production is impaired (low thrombopoietin levels) and there is some evidence that melatonin can stimulate platelet production and theoretically, could be of benefit. A dosage of 3 mg PO q12h for dogs <20 kg, and 6 mg PO q12h for dogs >20 kg has been suggested. (Abrams-Ogg 2012)

- **CATS:**

  For sleep disorders (nocturnal activity); (extra-label): Practically, 1.5 – 6 mg PO per cat before bedtime.

  For suppression of estrus; (extra-label): 18 mg implant SC suppressed estrus for 2-4 months. (Gimenez *et al.* 2009) Another study found that the interestrus period averaged only 64 days and the authors concluded that from a practical perspective, this short cycle suppression in mature animals was deemed insufficient; further work using higher melatonin doses, a longer release formulation, or repeated administrations, are needed (Faya *et al.* 2011).

- **FERRETS:**

  For adjunctive treatment of adrenal disease to help control clinical signs (extra-label): PO doses: Anecdotally, 0.5 – 1 mg per ferret PO once daily 7-9 hours after sunrise. Implants: 2.7 mg (under 600 gram body weight) or 5.4 mg (over 600 grams body weight) SC q3-4 months.

- **HORSES**

  Head Shaking syndrome for seasonal headshakers that begin in spring and stop in late fall or winter (extra-label): Starting November 1 (Northern hemisphere) give 12 – 15 mg melatonin PO once daily at 5PM (1700). Give this dose all year round; horse may not shed and need body clipping. (Madigan 2011)

Monitoring

- Clinical efficacy.

Client Information

- For use in small animals, must be administered as directed to be effective.
- For oral melatonin: May give with or without food.
- Usually very well tolerated; sedation/sleepiness may occur.

Chemistry/Synonyms

A naturally occurring hormone produced in the pineal gland, melatonin occurs as a pale yellow, crystalline solid and has a molecular weight of 232. It can be derived from natural sources or by synthetic means.

Melatonin may also be known as: n-acetyl-5-methoxytryptamine, MEL, MLT, or pineal hormone.

Storage/Stability

Unless otherwise labeled, store at room temperature in tight containers.

Dosage Forms/Regulatory Status

VETERINARY-LABELED PRODUCTS:

Melatonin implant 2.7 mg; *PrimeX*®; (OTC). FDA-approved (NADA 140-846) for use in mink.

The following products are marketed for ferret and dog use. Their approval status is not known and they are not listed in FDA's Green Book of approved animal drugs. More information can be found at: www.melatek.net

Melatonin 2.7 mg & 5.4 mg implant product marketed for ferrets; *Ferretonin*®.

Melatonin 8 mg, 12 mg, 18 mg implant product marketed for dogs; *Dermatonin*®.

An 18 mg implant for sustained subcutaneous release is available in a variety of countries. One trade name is *Regulin*®. It is labeled for use in sheep (UK and AUS/NZ) and goats (AUS/NZ) to improve early breeding and ovulation rates.

HUMAN-LABELED PRODUCTS:

Melatonin tablets are available in a variety of strengths from a variety of sources. Common strengths available range from 0.5 to 3 mg tablets. Sustained release capsules (3 mg) and oral liquid (500 micrograms/mL) may also be available. Because melatonin is considered a "nutrient" there is no official labeling or central quality control systems for it in the USA. Purchase from reputable sources.

Revisions/References

Monograph revised/updated April 2014.

Abecia, J. A., et al. (2011). Pharmaceutical Control of Reproduction in Sheep and Goats. Veterinary Clinics of North America-Food Animal Practice 27(1): 67-+.

Abrams-Ogg, A. C. G. (2012). Standard-of-Care for Treatment of Immune-Mediated Hemolytic Anemia and Immune-Mediated Thrombocytopenia in Dogs. 64th Convention of the Canadian Veterinary Medical Association. accessed via Veterinary Information Network; vin.com

Faya, M., et al. (2011). Long-term melatonin treatment prolongs interestrus, but does not delay puberty, in domestic cats. Theriogenology 75(9): 1750-4.

Gimenez, F., et al. (2009). Suppression of estrus in cats with melatonin implants. Theriogenology 72(4): 493-9.

Madigan, J. E. (2011). Headshaking Syndrome in Horses - Trigeminal Nerve Electrophysiological Findings and New Therapeutics. Australian Veterinary Association Proceedings accessed via Veterinary Information Network; vin.com

Meloxicam

(mel-**ox**-i-kam)   Metacam®
Nonsteroidal Antiinflammatory Agent (NSAID)

Prescriber Highlights

▶ NSAID used in many species; COX-2 preferential. Chronic (ongoing) use in cats is controversial (at least in the USA).

▶ Available as both injectable & oral (including transmucosal spray) products.

▶ Primary adverse effects are GI and renal-related, but idiosyncratic hepatotoxicity has rarely occurred in dogs.

Uses/Indications

Meloxicam is used for treating pain, inflammation and osteoarthritis in dogs. Short-term (single dose injectable; administered prior to surgery) use is also FDA-approved (in the USA) for cats for the control of postoperative pain and inflammation associated with orthopedic surgery, ovariohysterectomy and castration. Meloxicam is licensed for longer-term use (at lower dosages) in cats in several countries.

Recent work in calves suggests that oral meloxicam may be a cost-effective agent to treat painful procedures such as castration or dehorning (Coetzee *et al.* 2009).

Pharmacology/Actions

Meloxicam has antiinflammatory, analgesic, and antipyretic activity similar to other NSAIDs. Like other NSAIDs, meloxicam exhibits analgesic, antiinflammatory, and antipyretic activity probably through its inhibition of cyclooxygenase, phospholipase A_2, and inhibition of prostaglandin synthesis. It is considered COX-2 preferential (not COX-2 specific) as at higher dosages its COX-2 specificity is diminished.

Acute dosing studies in dogs have not demonstrated any untoward renal or hepatic toxicity.

Pharmacokinetics

In dogs, meloxicam is well absorbed after oral administration. Food does not alter absorption. The oral transmucosal spray product is bioequivalent to the canine-approved oral suspension (Lees *et al.* 2013). Peak blood levels occur in ≈7-8 hours after administration. The volume of distribution in dogs is 0.3 L/kg and ≈97% is bound to plasma proteins. Meloxicam is extensively biotransformed to several different metabolites in the liver; none of these appear to have pharmacologic activity. The majority of these (and unchanged drug) are eliminated in the feces. A significant amount of enterohepatic recirculation occurs. Elimination half-life is species specific. The elimination half-life in dogs averages 24 hours (range: 12-36 hours); other species: pigs: 4 hours; horses: 3 hours; cattle: 13 hours.

In cats, subcutaneous injection is nearly completely absorbed. Peak levels occur ≈1.5 hours after injection. Meloxicam is relatively highly bound to feline plasma proteins (97%) and volume of distribution is ≈0.27 L/kg. After a single dose, total systemic clearance is ≈130 mL/hr/kg and elimination half life is ≈15 hours. Major pathway for biotransformation is oxidation and the major elimination route is fecal.

Oral meloxicam tablets in horses appear to be well absorbed regardless of feeding status. Reported serum half-life in horses: 3-5 hours.

In ruminant calves (approx. 3 months old) oral meloxicam at 1 mg/kg was well absorbed and had an elimination half-life of about one day (Coetzee *et al.* 2009).

Contraindications/Precautions/Warnings

Meloxicam is contraindicated in animals hypersensitive to it. Safe use has not been evaluated in dogs less than 6 months old. The European label states that safe use has not been evaluated in dogs less than 6 weeks old. Although not part of the label, it should probably not be used or used with extreme caution in dogs with active GI ulceration, bleeding, or receiving glucocorticoids. Meloxicam, like all NSAIDs, should be used with caution in patients with impaired hepatic, cardiac or renal function and hemorrhagic disorders. Hypotension, high dosages, hypovolemia, sodium depletion, hypotension, and inhalant anesthesia all appear to increase the risk for renal toxicity of NSAIDs (KuKanich, B. *et al.* 2012).

Due to its long half-life in dogs, a 5-7 day washout period after stopping meloxicam has been recommended before starting a new NSAID (KuKanich, B 2008).

Meloxicam is contraindicated in cats with known hypersensitivity to meloxicam or other NSAIDs. The manufacturer warns that additional doses of meloxicam or other NSAIDs are contraindicated as no safe dosage for repeated NSAID administration has been established. Safe use in cats less than 4 months of age has not been established. Use preoperatively for cats undergoing major surgery where hypotensive episodes are possible; may be at higher risk for renal damage.

The human label states that no dosage adjustment is necessary in patients with mild to moderate hepatic or renal impairment.

Adverse Effects

Experience in Europe and Canada has demonstrated a relatively safe adverse effect profile for meloxicam at labeled dosages in healthy dogs. GI distress is the most commonly reported adverse effect, and in US field trials vomiting, soft stools, diarrhea, and inappetence were the most common adverse effects reported. Renal toxicity appears to be quite low in animals with normal renal blood flow. Post-approval reported adverse effects have included: GI effects (vomiting, anorexia, diarrhea, melena, ulceration), elevated liver enzymes/hepatotoxicity, pruritus, azotemia, elevated creatinine, and renal failure. When NSAIDs are used chronically in dogs, gastroprotectant drugs (PPIs, H2 blockers, or misoprostol) have been used in an attempt to prevent or limit GI adverse effects but it is still not clear what effect they actually have in this regard. Like other COX-2 NSAIDs, meloxicam may have effects on platelet function. A case report of a dog developing vasculitis with ulcers, vesicles, and erosions has been published (Niza *et al.* 2007). In cats, single doses of meloxicam appear relatively safe. In field trials some cats developed elevated BUN, post-treatment anemia and, rarely, residual pain at the injection site. In other studies, meloxicam has caused GI effects (vomiting, diarrhea, inappetence), behavior changes, and lethargy. Repeated use of meloxicam in cats is controversial, as repeated doses have been associated with renal failure and death. Recently, the FDA has changed the label in the USA to warn against repeated doses in cats. However, low dose chronic use is licensed in some countries and the ISFM & AAFP guidelines for long-term NSAID use in cats suggests that benefits of treatment often outweigh the risks (Sparkes *et al.* 2010).

When used at recommended dosages, it is relatively safe in other species (horses, cattle, swine, rabbits, small ruminants, camelids, etc.).

Reproductive/Nursing Safety

Safe use has not been established in dogs or cats used for breeding, or in pregnant or lactating animals. In humans, the FDA categorizes this drug as category C for use during pregnancy (*Animal studies have shown an adverse effect on the fetus, but there are no adequate studies in humans; or there are no animal reproduction studies and no adequate studies in humans.)*

Most NSAIDs are excreted in milk; use cautiously.

Overdosage/Acute Toxicity

The manufacturer warns to prevent accidental overdosing in small dogs. When dosing by the drop, put drops on food and not directly into the mouth. Overdoses should be treated symptomatically and supportively.

Drug Interactions

The following drug interactions have either been reported or are theoretical in humans or animals receiving meloxicam and may be of significance in veterinary patients. Unless otherwise noted, use together is not necessarily contraindicated, but weigh the potential risks and perform additional monitoring when appropriate.

- **ACE INHIBITORS** (*e.g.,* **enalapril, benazepril**): Some NSAIDs can reduce effects on blood pressure.
- **ANESTHETICS, INHALANT**: May increase the risk for renal hypotension and NSAID renal toxicity.
- **ANTICOAGULANTS** (*e.g.,* **heparin, warfarin**, etc.): Increased chance for bleeding.
- **ASPIRIN**: May increase the risk of gastrointestinal toxicity (*e.g.,* ulceration, bleeding, vomiting, diarrhea).
- **CORTICOSTEROIDS** (*e.g.,* **prednisone**): May increase the risk of gastrointestinal toxicity (*e.g.,* ulceration, bleeding, vomiting, diarrhea); avoid use with NSAIDs.
- **DIGOXIN**: NSAIDS may increase serum levels.
- **FLUCONAZOLE**: Administration has increased plasma levels of celecoxib in humans and potentially could also affect meloxicam levels in dogs.
- **FUROSEMIDE**: NSAIDs may reduce saluretic and diuretic effects of furosemide. Furosemide may increase the risks for NSAID renal toxicity.
- **METHOTREXATE**: Serious toxicity has occurred when NSAIDs have been used concomitantly with methotrexate; use together with extreme caution.
- **NEPHROTOXIC DRUGS** (*e.g.,* **furosemide, aminoglycosides, amphotericin B**, etc.): May enhance the risk of nephrotoxicity.
- **NSAIDS, OTHER**: May increase the risk of gastrointestinal toxicity (*e.g.,* ulceration, bleeding, vomiting, diarrhea).

Doses

When doses are listed in "drops" use with caution; drug concentration per drop may be different in products marketed in various countries.

- **DOGS:**

  For osteoarthritis, analgesia, inflammatory conditions (labeled-dose; FDA-approved):

  PO, IV, SC: Initially 0.2 mg/kg PO, IV or SC on the first day of treatment, subsequent doses of 0.1 mg/kg PO once daily in food or placed directly into mouth—do not place directly in the mouth when dosing by the drop. (Adapted from label; *Metacam® Injection/Oral Suspension*)

  Transmucosal Oral: Administer 0.1 mg/kg transmucosally once daily using the metered dose pump. (Adapted from label; *Oro-CAM®*)

- **CATS:**

  For pain (labeled-dose; FDA-approved): For labeled indications: 0.3 mg/kg as a single one-time administration subcutaneous dose that should not be followed by additional doses of meloxicam or other NSAIDs. (Label information; *Metacam® Injection for Cats*)

Note: The following dosages for cats are extra-label in the USA and in 2010 the drug sponsor (BIVI-USA) and the FDA issued the following: "*WARNING: Repeated use of meloxicam in cats has been associated with acute renal failure and death. Do not administer additional doses of injectable or oral meloxicam to cats. See Contraindications, Warnings and Precautions for detailed information.*" However, in another document published in 2010, the *ISFM and AAFP Consensus Guidelines: Long-Term Use of NSAIDs in Cats* (available at: http://www.icatcare.org/vets/guidelines) in their summary points they state: "It is only recently that NSAIDs have become licensed for long-term use in cats in some countries. The panel believe that these drugs have a major role to play in the management of chronic pain in cats, but at present only limited feline-specific data are available. To date published studies of the medium- to long-term use of the COX-1 sparing drug meloxicam in older cats and cats with chronic kidney disease provide encouraging data that these drugs can be used safely and should be used to relieve pain when needed. While further data are needed, and would undoubtedly lead to refinement of the guidelines presented here, the panel hope that these recommendations will encourage rational and safe long-term use of NSAIDs in cats, thereby improving patients' quality of life in the face of painful disease conditions." (Sparkes *et al.* 2010)

Acute musculoskeletal disorders (extra-label in USA): Initial treatment is a single oral dose of 0.2 mg/kg on the first day. Treatment is to be continued once daily by oral administration (at 24-hour intervals) at a dose of 0.05 mg meloxicam/kg body weight for as long as acute pain and inflammation persist. (Adapted from datasheet: *Metacam® Oral Suspension for Cats—BI-U.K.*)

For mild to moderate post-operative pain and inflammation following surgical procedures (extra-label in USA): 0.2 mg/kg SC once before surgery. To continue treatment for up to five days, this initial dose may be followed 24 hours later by administration of oral suspension at 0.05 mg/kg PO q24h (once daily) for up to a total of four PO doses. For cats that will not be receiving additional PO doses, a single SC injection of 0.3 mg/kg has also been shown to be safe and efficacious. (Adapted from datasheet: *Metacam® Injection for Cats—BI-U.K.*)

Chronic musculoskeletal disorders (extra-label in USA): Initial treatment is a single oral dose of 0.1 mg meloxicam/kg body weight on the first day. Treatment is to be continued once daily by oral administration (at 24-hour intervals) at a maintenance dose of 0.05 mg meloxicam/kg body weight. A clinical response is normally seen within 7 days. Treatment should be discontinued after 14 days at the latest if no clinical improvement is apparent. (Adapted from datasheet: *Metacam® Oral Suspension for Cats—BI-U.K.*). Many cats may experience pain relief at even lower doses given every 2-3 days. Titrating to the lowest effective dose may help avoid adverse effects (Little 2013), (Bennett *et al.* 2012).

- **HORSES:**

  For inflammation and pain associated with musculoskeletal disorders or colic pain (IV); (extra-label in USA): IV: Single intravenous injection at a dosage of 0.6 mg/kg; may follow with oral dosing after 24 hours. Oral: Either mixed with food or directly into the mouth at a dosage of 0.6 mg/kg PO once daily, up to 14 days. Where the product is mixed with food, it should be added to a small quantity of food, prior to feeding. Withdrawal periods: Meat/Offal: 5 days. (Adapted from label; *Metacam® Injection & Oral Suspension for Horses—BIVI-UK*)

  For pain/inflammation (foals); (extra-label): Based on a pharmacokinetic study done in healthy foals, the authors concluded that 0.6 mg/kg PO q12h would likely be therapeutic in foals less than 7 weeks of age. (Raidal *et al.* 2013)

- **CATTLE:**

Injectable: For use in acute respiratory infection with appropriate antibiotic therapy to reduce clinical signs in cattle. For use in diarrhea, in combination with oral rehydration therapy, to reduce clinical signs in calves of over one week of age and young non-lactating cattle. For adjunctive therapy in the treatment of acute mastitis, in combination with antibiotic therapy (extra-label in USA): Single SC or IV injection at a dose rate of 0.5 mg/kg (in combination with antibiotic therapy or with oral rehydration therapy as appropriate. U.K. Withdrawal periods: Meat/Offal: 15 days; Milk: 120 hours. (*Metacam®* Injection—BIVI-UK)

Oral: For surgical pain; analgesia (extra-label): 0.5 – 1 mg/kg PO q24-48h. (Anderson *et al.* 2013) **Note:** Conservative 21-day meat withdrawal and 5-day milk withdrawal times have been recommended (Smith 2013).

- **SMALL RUMINANTS:**

For pain/inflammation (extra-label): Sheep: 0.5 mg/kg IV q12h. 2 mg/kg PO on first day, and then 1 mg/kg PO once daily. Goats: 0.5 mg/kg IV q8h; 0.5 mg/kg IM or PO once daily. (Plummer *et al.* 2013), (Stock *et al.* 2013)

- **CAMELIDS:**

For pain/inflammation (extra-label): 0.5 mg/kg IV; 1 mg/kg PO every 3rd day. (Plummer *et al.* 2013)

- **SWINE:**

For use in non-infectious locomotor disorders to reduce the symptoms of lameness and inflammation. For adjunctive therapy in the treatment of puerperal septicemia and toxemia (mastitis-metritis-agalactia syndrome) with appropriate antibiotic therapy (extra-label in USA): Single IM injection at a dosage of 0.4 mg/kg in combination with antibiotic therapy, as appropriate. If required, a second administration of meloxicam can be given after 24 hours. Withdrawal periods: Meat/Offal: 5 days. (*Metacam®* Injection—BIVI-UK)

- **FERRETS:**

As an antiinflammatory/analgesic (extra-label) For post-surgical pain: 0.2 mg/kg PO or SC once. (Schoemaker 2008)

- **SMALL MAMMALS:**

For Pain and inflammation (extra-label): **Rabbits:** A study in 6 healthy rabbits receiving 1 mg/kg PO once daily for 29 days, concluded that meloxicam at this dosage and treatment duration may be safe and effective. (Delk *et al.* 2013), (Fredholm *et al.* 2013)

- **BIRDS:**

As an analgesic (extra-label): 0.5 mg/kg IM is also commonly used in birds and may be the safest of the NSAID analgesics for avian species. As the side effects of all analgesics have not been studied in birds, these drugs should be used carefully in avian patients (Echols 2008). Another source states: "Injectable forms of meloxicam and carprofen will cause myositis/muscle necrosis and therefore oral formulations are recommended... however oral bioavailability of NSAIDs varies greatly between avian species. Therefore it is critical to monitor response to dosage and frequency of NSAID treatment for each avian patient (Paul-Murphy 2013)."

- **REPTILES**

For pain/inflammation (extra-label): 0.2 mg/kg PO daily for 5 days may achieve therapeutic levels over a few days. Subsequent dosing should be 0.2 mg/kg every other day. If used chronical-ly, evaluate patient for renal disease on a regular basis. A study in Ball pythons failed to demonstrate analgesic effects when meloxicam was used at 0.3 mg/kg. (Eatwell 2013)

- **ZOO, EXOTIC, WILDLIFE SPECIES:**

For additional dosages of meloxicam in zoo, exotic and wildlife medicine refer to specific references, including:

a) Fowler's Zoo and Wild Animal Medicine Current Therapy, Volume 7, Miller, R.E., Fowler, M.E., Saunders. 2011.

b) *Exotic Animal Formulary, 4th Ed.* Carpenter, J.W., Saunders. 2012.

c) The 2009 American Association of Zoo Veterinarian Proceedings by D. K. Fontenot also has several dosages listed for restraint, anesthesia, and analgesia for a variety of drugs for carnivores and primates. VIN members can access them at: http://goo.gl/BHRih or http://goo.gl/9UJse

Monitoring

- Clinical efficacy.
- Adverse effects, especially GI effects in dogs.
- Renal function and hepatic function if used chronically. One recommendation is to do baseline renal and hepatic panels; repeat within the first 2 weeks and periodically thereafter (KuKanich, B. *et al.* 2012). When liver enzymes are elevated and concern for liver function is present, liver function tests (serum bile acids, plasma ammonia concentration) should be performed (Fox 2013).

Client Information

- Oral Liquid: Shake well before using. Carefully measure dose (oral liquid); do not confuse the markings on the syringe (provided by the manufacturer). Give with food; depending on size of the animal it can be given either on top of food or directly into the mouth (see the instructions in the manufacturer provided information sheet for clients).
- Oral spray is sprayed inside the cheek space (see the instructions in the manufacturer provided information sheet for clients).
- Most animals tolerate it very well, but rarely some will develop ulcers or serious kidney (especially cats) and liver problems. Watch for these: Eating more or less than normal, vomiting, changes in bowel movements, changes in behavior or activity (more or less active than normal), weakness (*e.g.,* stumbling, clumsiness, etc.), seizures (convulsions) or aggression (threatening behavior/actions), yellowing of gums, skin, or whites of the eyes (jaundice), changes in drinking habits (frequency, amount consumed) or urination habits (frequency, color, or smell). If animal develops adverse effects, contact the veterinarian.
- Store honey-flavored oral liquid well out of reach of animals and children.
- Periodic lab tests to check for liver and kidney side effects are required.

Chemistry/Synonyms

A COX-2 receptor preferential NSAID, meloxicam occurs as a pale yellow powder. It is in the oxicam class, related to piroxicam.

Meloxicam may also be known as: UH-AC-62, and UH-AC-62XX; many trade names are available.

Storage/Stability

Unless otherwise labeled, store the injection and oral liquid at room temperature.

Dosage Forms/Regulatory Status

VETERINARY-LABELED PRODUCTS:

Meloxicam Oral Suspension: 1.5 mg/mL (0.05 mg per drop in the USA product) in a honey-flavored base: 10 mL, 32 mL, 100 mL dropper bottles with measuring syringe (marked in 5 lb. body weight increments); *Metacam®*; (Rx). FDA-approved for use in dogs.

Meloxicam 5 mg/mL Transmucosal Oral Spray: *OroCAM®*; (Rx). FDA-approved for use in dogs.

Meloxicam 5 mg/mL for Injection: 10 mL vial; *Metacam® Injection for Dogs*, *Loxicom®*; (Rx). FDA-approved for use in dogs.

Meloxicam 5 mg/mL for Injection: 10 mL vial; *Metacam® Injection for Cats*, *Loxicom®*; (Rx). FDA-approved for use in cats.

In the UK and Europe, there are dosage forms licensed for use in horses, cattle, pigs, The ARCI (Racing Commissioners International) has designated this drug as a class 3 substance. See the appendix for more information.

HUMAN-LABELED PRODUCTS:

Meloxicam Tablets: 7.5 mg & 15 mg; *Mobic®*, generic; (Rx)

Meloxicam Oral Suspension: 7.5 mg/5 mL in 100 mL; *Mobic®*, generic; (Rx)

In Canada, *Mobicox®*; (Rx)

Revisions/References

Monograph revised/updated April 2014.

Anderson, D. E. & M. A. Edmondson (2013). Prevention and Management of Surgical Pain in Cattle. Veterinary Clinics of North America-Food Animal Practice **29**(1): 157-+.

Bennett, D., et al. (2012). Osteoarthritis in the cat 2. How should it be managed and treated? Journal of Feline Medicine and Surgery **14**(1): 76-84.

Coetzee, J., et al. (2009). Pharmacokinetics of intravenous and oral meloxicam in ruminant calves. Vet Therapeutics **10**(4).

Delk, K., et al. (2013). Pharmacokinetics of Meloxicam Administered Orally Long-Term in the PETRabbit (Oryctolagus cuniculus). Association of Exotic Mammal Veterinarians Conference. accessed via Veterinary Information Network; vin.com

Eatwell, K. (2013). Recognising and Controlling Pain in Reptiles. British Small Animal Veterinary Congress. accessed via Veterinary Information Network; vin.com

Echols, M. (2008). Avian Anesthesia and Analgesia. Proceedings: IVECCS. accessed via Veterinary Information Network; vin.com

Fox, S. (2013). NSAIDs - The Most Frequently Scripted Drugs in Veterinary Medicine. Western Veterinary Conference. accessed via Veterinary Information Network; vin.com

Fredholm, D. V., et al. (2013). Pharmacokinetics of meloxicam in rabbits after oral administration of single and multiple doses. American Journal of Veterinary Research **74**(4): 636-41.

KuKanich, B. (2008). NSAIDs in Dogs. Proceedings: WVC. accessed via Veterinary Information Network; vin.com

KuKanich, B., et al. (2012). Clinical pharmacology of nonsteroidal anti-inflammatory drugs in dogs. Veterinary Anaesthesia and Analgesia **39**(1): 69-90.

Lees, P., et al. (2013). Bioequivalence in dogs of a meloxicam formulation administered as a transmucosal oral mist with an orally administered pioneer suspension product. J. Vet. Pharmacol. Ther. **36**(1): 78-84.

Little, S. (2013). Managing Arthritis in Senior Cats. International Society of Feline Medicine. accessed via Veterinary Information Network; vin.com

Niza, M., et al. (2007). Cutaneous and ocular adverse reactions in a dog following meloxicam administration. Vet Derm **18**: 45-9.

Paul-Murphy, J. (2013). Which NSAIDs Are For the Birds. American Association of Zoo Veterinarians Conference. accessed via Veterinary Information Network; vin.com

Plummer, P. J. & J. A. Schleining (2013). Assessment and Management of Pain in Small Ruminants and Camelids. Veterinary Clinics of North America-Food Animal Practice **29**(1): 185-+.

Raidal, S. L., et al. (2013). Pharmacokinetics and Safety of Oral Administration of Meloxicam to Foals. Journal of Veterinary Internal Medicine **27**(2): 300-7.

Schoemaker, N. (2008). What every veterinarian should know about ferret medicine. Proceedings: BSAVA. accessed via Veterinary Information Network; vin.com

Smith, G. (2013). Extralabel Use of Anesthetic and Analgesic Compounds in Cattle. Veterinary Clinics of North America-Food Animal Practice **29**(1): 29-+.

Sparkes, A. H., et al. (2010). ISFM AND AAFP CONSENSUS GUIDELINES Long-term use of NSAIDs in cats. Journal of Feline Medicine and Surgery **12**(7): 521-38.

Stock, M. L., et al. (2013). Pharmacokinetics of intravenously and orally administered meloxicam in sheep. American Journal of Veterinary Research **74**(5): 779-83.

Melphalan

(mel-fa-lan)   Alkeran®

Antineoplastic

Prescriber Highlights

▶ Alkylating agent antineoplastic used for ovarian carcinoma, lymphoreticular neoplasms, osteosarcoma, mammary or pulmonary neoplasms, & multiple myeloma.

▶ Contraindications (relative; risk vs. benefit): Anemia, bone marrow depression, current infection, impaired renal function, tumor cell infiltration of bone marrow, sensitivity to drug, or patients who have received previous chemotherapy or radiotherapy.

▶ Adverse Effects: GI effects (anorexia, vomiting, diarrhea), pulmonary infiltrates or fibrosis, bone marrow depression (anemia, thrombocytopenia, leukopenia).

▶ Potential teratogen.

▶ Determine dosages carefully.

Uses/Indications

Melphalan may be useful in the treatment of a variety of neoplastic diseases, including ovarian carcinoma, lymphoreticular neoplasms, osteosarcoma, and mammary or pulmonary neoplasms. When combined with prednisone, it is considered the drug of choice for treating multiple myeloma. Melphalan can be used for treating primary (essential) thrombocythemia in dogs or cats. It has been used successfully in a rescue protocol combining dexamethasone, melphalan, dactinomycin and cytarabine to treat relapsed multicentric lymphoma in dogs.

Pharmacology/Actions

Melphalan is a bifunctional alkylating agent and interferes with RNA transcription and DNA replication, thereby disrupting nucleic acid function. Because it is bifunctional, it has affect on both dividing and resting cells. Melphalan does not require activation by the liver (unlike cyclophosphamide).

Pharmacokinetics

Melphalan absorption is variable and often incomplete. It is distributed throughout the body water, but it is unknown whether it crosses the placenta, blood brain barrier or enters maternal milk. Melphalan is eliminated principally by hydrolysis in plasma. In humans, terminal half-lives average ≈90 minutes.

Contraindications/Precautions/Warnings

Melphalan should be used with the following conditions only when its potential benefits outweigh its risks: anemia, bone marrow depression, current infection, impaired renal function, tumor cell infiltration of bone marrow, sensitivity to melphalan or patients who have received previous chemotherapy or radiotherapy.

Adverse Effects

The most serious adverse effect likely with melphalan is bone marrow depression (anemia, thrombocytopenia, leukopenia). Potential adverse effects include GI effects (anorexia, vomiting, diarrhea), pulmonary infiltrates or fibrosis, or neurotoxic effects.

Reproductive/Nursing Safety

Safe use of melphalan during pregnancy has not been established; other alkylating agents are known teratogens. Use only during pregnancy when the benefits to the mother outweigh the risks to the offspring. Melphalan can suppress gonadal function.

While it is unknown whether melphalan enters maternal milk, nursing puppies or kittens should receive milk replacer when the bitch or queen is receiving melphalan.

Overdosage/Acute Toxicity

Because of the toxic potential of this agent, overdoses must be avoided. Determine dosages carefully.

Drug Interactions

The following drug interactions have either been reported or are theoretical in humans or animals receiving melphalan and may be of significance in veterinary patients. Unless otherwise noted, use together is not necessarily contraindicated, but weigh the potential risks and perform additional monitoring when appropriate.

- **CYCLOSPORINE:** There are anecdotal reports of melphalan causing increased nephrotoxicity associated with systemic cyclosporine use in humans.

- **IMMUNOSUPPRESSANT DRUGS** (*e.g.*, **azathioprine, cyclophosphamide, corticosteroids**): Use with other immunosuppressant drugs may increase the risk of infection.

- **MYELOSUPPRESSIVE DRUGS** (*e.g.*, **chloramphenicol, flucytosine, amphotericin B,** or **colchicine**): Use extreme caution when used concurrently with other drugs that are also myelosuppressive, including many of the other antineoplastics and other bone marrow depressant drugs. Bone marrow depression may be additive.

- **VACCINES, LIVE:** Live virus vaccines should be used with caution, if at all, during therapy.

Laboratory Considerations

- Melphalan may raise serum **uric acid** levels. Drugs such as allopurinol may be required to control hyperuricemia.

Doses

Note: Because of the potential toxicity of this drug to patients, veterinary personnel and clients, and since chemotherapy indications, treatment protocols, monitoring and safety guidelines often change, the following dosages should be used only as a general guide. <u>Consultation with a veterinary oncologist and referral to current veterinary oncology</u> references [*e.g.*, (Withrow *et al.* 2012); (Dobson *et al.* 2011); (Henry *et al.* 2009); (North *et al.* 2009); (Argyle *et al.* 2008)] are strongly recommended.

- **DOGS:**

  Melphalan dosages for dogs vary depending on the source, the disease treated, and the protocol being used. As a general guide, it is usually dosed from 1.5 – 2 mg/m² or 0.1 – 0.2 mg/kg in dogs, but higher dosages have been used. Dosage frequencies range from daily to every other day, to pulse dosing (daily for 7-10 days, then 3 weeks off, etc.). The following are examples:

  a) **For multiple myeloma:** Several dosing schedules have been developed to treat canine multiple myeloma with melphalan. One recommended dosing regimen is 0.1 mg/kg PO q24h for 10 days, followed by 0.05 mg/kg PO q48h thereafter. Another source recommends 0.25 mg/kg/day PO for 4 days and 2 – 4 mg/day PO maintenance. Pulse therapy is another reported option (7 mg/m² PO q24h for 5 days every 21 days). The recommended intravenous dose is 16 mg/m² every 2 weeks for 4 doses and then every 4 weeks. A 50% dose reduction is recommended for animals with preexisting renal insufficiency. Clinical response can be assessed by improved clinical signs and reduced serum immunoglobulin. Melphalan should be administered indefinitely until clinical relapse, which may involve worsened bone pain, recurrence of bleeding diathesis, funduscopic changes, or elevated serum immunoglobulins. (Kitchell *et al.* 2004)

  b) **As part of a rescue protocol (DMAC) to treat relapsed multicentric lymphoma:** Dactinomycin (0.75 mg/m² IV), Cytarabine (300 mg/m² IV over 4 hours or SC) and dexamethasone (1 mg/kg PO) on day 0 and melphalan (20 mg/m² PO) and dexamethasone (1 mg/kg PO) on day 7. The cycle is repeated continuously every 2 weeks as long as a complete or partial remission is achieved. After four cycles, chlorambucil was substituted for melphalan at the same dose. If complete remission achieved, protocol was discontinued after 5-8 cycles and maintenance therapy with the LMP (chlorambucil, methotrexate, prednisone) or lomustine/prednisone protocols were instituted. If dogs developed grades 3 or 4 toxicosis, DMAC was discontinued and maintenance protocol was started. (Alvarez *et al.* 2006; Rassnick 2006)

- **CATS:**

  Melphalan dosages for cats vary depending on the source, the disease treated, and the protocol being used. As a general guide, it is usually dosed from 1.5 – 2 mg/m² or 0.5 mg per cat. Dosage frequencies range from daily to every other day, to pulse dosing (daily for 7-10 days, then 3 weeks off, etc.). The following listed indication and dosage is an example:

  For chronic lymphocytic leukemia (extra-label): 2 mg/m² PO every other day with or without prednisone at 20 mg/m² PO every other day. (Peterson *et al.* 1994)

Monitoring

- CBC with platelets at least every week for 2 weeks and then monthly thereafter. Significant myelosuppression requires an alteration in dose or frequency of administration.

Client Information

- Wear gloves when handling the medication and give it with food.
- Melphalan is a chemotherapy (cancer) drug. The drug and its byproducts can be hazardous to other animals and people that come in contact with it. On the day your animal gets the drug and then for a few days afterward, all bodily waste (urine, feces, litter), blood, or vomit should only be handled while wearing disposable gloves. Seal the waste in a plastic bag and then place both the bag and gloves in with the regular trash.
- Melphalan must be given as the veterinarian has directed; immediately report any signs associated with toxicity (*e.g.*, abnormal bleeding, bruising, urination, depression, infection, shortness of breath, etc.).

Chemistry/Synonyms

A nitrogen mustard derivative, melphalan occurs as an off-white to buff-colored powder that is practically insoluble in water.

Melphalan may also be known as: CB-3025, NSC-8806, PAM, L-PAM, L-phenylalanine mustard, phenylalanine mustard, phenylalanine nitrogen mustard, L-sarcolysine, WR-19813, *Alkeran®* or *Alkerana®*.

Storage/Stability

Store melphalan tablets in well-closed, light-resistant, glass containers in the refrigerator (2-8°C). It is recommended to dispense the tablets in glass containers.

Once reconstituted, the injectable product should not be refrigerated or a precipitate may form. It is stable at room temperature for 90 minutes after reconstitution. For administration, the reconstituted solution should be further diluted with sterile 0.9% sodium chloride to a concentration of not more than 0.45 mg/mL. This diluted solution is stable for 60 minutes at room temperature.

Dosage Forms/Regulatory Status

VETERINARY-LABELED PRODUCTS: NONE.

HUMAN-LABELED PRODUCTS:

Melphalan Oral Tablets: 2 mg; *Alkeran®*; (Rx)

Melphalan Powder for Injection (lyophilized): 50 mg in single use vials with 10 mL vial of sterile diluent; *Alkeran®*, generic; (Rx)

Revisions/References

Monograph revised/updated April 2014.

Alvarez, F., et al. (2006). Dexamethasone, melphalan, actinomycin D, cytosine arabinoside (DMAC) protocol for dogs with relapsed lymphoma. J Vet Intern Med **20**: 1178-83.

Argyle, D., et al. (2008). *Decision Making in Small Animal Oncology*, Wiley-Blackwell.

Dobson, J. & D. Lascelles (2011). *BSAVA Manual of Canine and Feline Oncology*, BSAVA.

Henry, C. & M. Higginbotham (2009). *Cancer Management in Small Animal Practice*, Saunders.

Kitchell, B. & A. Wiedemann (2004). "Pharm Profile: Melphalan." vetlearn.com.

North, S. & T. Banks (2009). *Small Animal Oncology: An Introduction*, Saunders.

Peterson, J. & C. Couto (1994). Lymphoid leukemias. *Consultations in Feline Internal Medicine: 2*. J. August. Philadelphia, W.B. Saunders Company: 509-13.

Rassnick, K. (2006). Rescue chemotherapy protocols for dogs with lymphoma. Proceedings: ACVIM. accessed via Veterinary Information Network; vin.com

Withrow, S., et al. (2012). Withrow and MacEwen's Small Animal Clinical Oncology, 5th Ed., Saunders.

Meperidine HCl

(me-**per**-i-deen)   Demerol®, Pethidine

Opiate Agonist

Prescriber Highlights

▶ Opiate analgesic; infrequently used as it has a short duration of analgesia & may cause more adverse effects than other commonly used injectable opiates.

▶ Contraindications: Hypersensitivity to it, diarrhea caused by a toxic ingestion. Extreme Caution: Respiratory disease or acute respiratory dysfunction.

▶ Caution: Hypothyroidism, severe renal insufficiency, adrenocortical insufficiency, geriatric or severely debilitated patients, head injuries or increased intracranial pressure, & acute abdominal conditions (*e.g.*, colic).

▶ Adverse Effects: Respiratory depression, histamine release, bronchoconstriction, CNS depression, GI (nausea, vomiting, & decreased intestinal peristalsis), mydriasis (dogs), salivation (esp. cats); physical dependence (chronic use). Horses (in addition): Tachycardia with PVC's, profuse sweating, hyperpnea; may potentiate intestinal obstruction secondary to reduced intestinal motility.

▶ Give very slowly if using IV (many state not to use IV); may be irritating if given SC.

▶ Overdoses can cause CNS excitatory effects (agitation to seizures); naloxone may enhance these effects.

▶ C-II controlled substance.

Uses/Indications

Although no product is licensed in the United States for veterinary use, this agent has been used as an analgesic in several different species. While meperidine has been used as sedative/analgesic in small animals for both post-operative pain and medical conditions such as acute pancreatitis and thermal burns, usually other opiates are preferred since meperidine has a short analgesic duration of activity and can cause significant histamine release. It is occasionally used in equine medicine in the treatment of colic and in other large animal species for pain control.

Pharmacology/Actions

Meperidine is a *mu* (OP$_3$)-receptor (MOR) agonist opioid with approximately 20-25% the potency of morphine. Receptors for opiate analgesics are found in high concentrations in the limbic system, spinal cord, thalamus, hypothalamus, striatum, and midbrain. They are also found in tissues such as the gastrointestinal tract, urinary tract, and in other smooth muscle.

The morphine-like agonists (morphine, meperidine, oxymorphone) have primary activity at the *mu* receptors, with some activity possible at the delta receptor. The primary pharmacologic effects of these agents include: analgesia, antitussive activity, respiratory depression, sedation, emesis, physical dependence, and intestinal effects (constipation/defecation). Secondary pharmacologic effects include: CNS: euphoria, sedation, and confusion. Cardiovascular: bradycardia due to central vagal stimulation, alpha-adrenergic receptors may be depressed resulting in peripheral vasodilation, decreased peripheral resistance, and baroreceptor inhibition. Orthostatic hypotension and syncope may occur. Urinary: Increased bladder sphincter tone can induce urinary retention.

Meperidine produces equivalent respiratory depression at equi-analgesic doses as morphine. Like morphine, it can cause histamine release. It does not have antitussive activity at doses lower than those causing analgesia. Meperidine is the only used opioid that has vagolytic and negative inotropic properties at clinically used doses. One study in ponies demonstrated changes in jejunal activity after meperidine administration, but no effects on transit time or colonic electrical activity were noted.

Refer to the monograph: Narcotic (opiate) Analgesic Agonists, Pharmacology of, for more information.

Pharmacokinetics

Although generally well absorbed orally, a marked first-pass effect limits the oral effectiveness of meperidine and it is rarely used PO clinically. Oral bioavailability in dogs (beagles; n=3) ranged from 3-25%. After injection by IM or SC routes the peak analgesic effects occur between 30-60 minutes, with the IM route having a slightly faster onset. Duration of action is variable with effects generally lasting from 1-6 hours in most species. In dogs and cats, analgesic duration of only <2 hours and often <1 hour at clinically used doses. The drug is metabolized primarily in the liver (mostly hydrolysis with some conjugation) and approximately 5% is excreted unchanged in the urine. One metabolite is normeperidine, which is active with approximately 50% of the analgesic effects of the parent compound. More importantly is its CNS excitatory effects that appear to be mediated by other than opiate *mu*-receptors and is not amenable to reversal by naloxone or other *mu*-antagonists.

Contraindications/Precautions/Warnings

Meperidine is contraindicated in cases where the patient is hypersensitive to narcotic analgesics, or in patients receiving monoamine oxidase inhibitors (MAOIs). It is also contraindicated in patients with diarrhea caused by a toxic ingestion until the toxin is eliminated from the GI tract. All opiates should be used with caution in patients with hypothyroidism, severe renal insufficiency, adrenocortical insufficiency (Addison's disease), and in geriatric or severely debilitated patients.

Use with caution in cats. Some recommend that meperidine not be used in feline patients.

Many recommend that meperidine not be administered intravenously. If given IV, it must be given very slowly or severe hypotension can result.

Consider using an alternate analgesic in patients with seizure disorders. A metabolite of meperidine (normeperidine) can cause CNS excitement.

Meperidine should be used with caution in patients with head injuries or increased intracranial pressure and acute abdominal conditions (*e.g.*, colic) as it may obscure the diagnosis or clinical course of these conditions. It should be used with extreme caution in patients suffering from respiratory disease or from acute respiratory dysfunction (*e.g.*, pulmonary edema secondary to smoke inhalation).

Opiate analgesics are also contraindicated in patients who have been stung by the scorpion species *Centruroides sculpturatus Ewing* and *C. gertschi Stahnke* as they may potentiate these venoms. Meperidine should not be used for pain secondary to envenomations from Gila monsters or Mexican beaded lizards (Hackett 2007).

Adverse Effects

Meperidine may be irritating when administered subcutaneously and must be given very slowly IV or it may cause severe hypotension. It can cause pronounced histamine release, particularly with IV administration. At usual doses, the primary concern is the effect the opioids have on respiratory function. Decreased tidal volume, depressed cough reflex, and the drying of respiratory secretions may all have a detrimental effect on a susceptible patient. Bronchoconstriction following IV doses has been noted in dogs. Gastrointestinal effects may include: nausea, vomiting, and decreased intestinal peristalsis. In dogs, meperidine causes mydriasis (unlike morphine). If given orally, the drug may be irritating to the buccal mucosa and cause salivation; this is of particular concern in cats. Chronic administration can lead to physical dependence.

In horses undergoing general anesthesia, meperidine has been associated with a reaction that manifests as tachycardia with PVC's, profuse sweating, and hyperpnea. IV meperidine may induce urticaria presumably due to histamine release. Meperidine can reduce colonic activity and increase the risk for post anesthetic colic. Higher dosages >2mg/kg may induce locomotor activity; 5 mg/kg can initially cause incoordination, shaking, immobility, followed by a substantial locomotor response (Clutton 2010).

Reproductive/Nursing Safety

Meperidine is more lipophilic and can cross the placenta more readily than several other opiates (*e.g.* morphine or hydromorphone). It generally is not recommended for use in pregnant animals. In humans, the FDA categorizes this drug as category *C* for use during pregnancy (*Animal studies have shown an adverse effect on the fetus, but there are no adequate studies in humans; or there are no animal reproduction studies and no adequate studies in humans.*) In a separate system evaluating the safety of drugs in canine and feline pregnancy (Papich 1989), this drug is categorized as class: *B* (*Safe for use if used cautiously. Studies in laboratory animals may have uncovered some risk, but these drugs appear to be safe in dogs and cats or these drugs are safe if they are not administered when the animal is near term.*)

Most opiates are excreted into milk. Meperidine enters human breast milk at concentrations slightly higher than those found in serum, but effects on nursing offspring may not be significant.

Overdosage/Acute Toxicity

In most species, overdosage may produce profound respiratory and/or CNS depression. Other effects can include cardiovascular collapse, hypothermia, and skeletal muscle hypotonia. A metabolite of meperidine, normeperidine can have CNS excitatory effects (agitation, hyperreflexia, seizures), and these effects can predominate in meperidine overdoses. While naloxone (at low dosages) can be used for treating profound respiratory depression when ventilator support is unavailable, it is not recommended when treating suspected normeperidine-induced CNS excitotoxicity (Golder *et al.* 2010). Benzodiazepines or barbiturates may be considered if treatment of CNS excitement signs is needed. Use caution as additive effects on respiratory depression can occur.

Drug Interactions

The following drug interactions have either been reported or are theoretical in humans or animals receiving meperidine and may be of significance in veterinary patients. Unless otherwise noted, use together is not necessarily contraindicated, but weigh the potential risks and perform additional monitoring when appropriate.

- **BUTORPHANOL; NALOXONE:** May contribute to CNS excitatory effects of normeperidine (see overdoses). In cases where normeperidine excitotoxicity is suspected, avoid use of naloxone or butorphanol, unless severe respiratory depression is present without a method of ventilatory support (Golder *et al.* 2010).
- **CNS DEPRESSANTS, OTHER** (*e.g.*, anesthetic agents, antihistamines, phenothiazines, barbiturates, tranquilizers, alcohol, etc.): May cause increased CNS or respiratory depression when used with meperidine.
- **DIURETICS:** Opiates may decrease efficacy in CHF patients.
- **ISONIAZID:** Meperidine may enhance INH adverse effects.
- **MONAMINE OXIDASE (MAO) INHIBITORS** (*e.g.*, **amitraz**, possibly **selegiline**): Meperidine is contraindicated in patients receiving monamino oxidase (MAO) inhibitors for at least 14 days after receiving MAO inhibitors in humans. Some human patients have exhibited signs of opiate overdose after receiving therapeutic doses of meperidine while taking MAOIs.
- **MUSCLE RELAXANTS, SKELETAL:** Meperidine may enhance neuromuscular blockade.
- **TRICYCLIC ANTIDEPRESSANTS** (**clomipramine, amitriptyline,** etc.): Meperidine may exacerbate the effects of tricyclic antidepressants.
- **WARFARIN:** Opiates may potentiate anticoagulant activity.

Laboratory Considerations

- As they may increase biliary tract pressure, opiates can increase plasma amylase and lipase values up to 24 hours following their administration.

Doses

- **DOGS:**

As an analgesic (extra-label): Dosage recommendations vary, but usually are 3 – 5 mg/kg (up to 11 mg/kg has been noted) IM or SC. Analgesic duration in dogs usually lasts 30 minutes to 2 hours.

- **CATS:**

As an analgesic for perioperative pain (extra-label): Dosage recommendations vary, but usually are 2 – 5 mg/kg IM, SC. Duration of effect from 30-60+ minutes. **Note:** Usually not recommended for cats.

- **FERRETS:**

As an analgesic (extra-label): 5 – 10 mg/kg SC or IM every 2-3 hours. (Williams 2000)

- **RABBITS, RODENTS, SMALL MAMMALS:**

As an analgesic (extra-label):

a) **Rabbits for moderate pain:** 5 – 10 mg/kg SC, IM q2-3h. Using Banana flavored oral syrup: 0.2 mg/mL in drinking water. (Ivey *et al.* 2000)

b) **Small mammals:** 5 – 10 mg/kg q2-4h IM, IV, SC. (Bays 2013)

- **CATTLE:**

As a perioperative analgesic (extra-label): 3.3 – 4.4 mg/kg SC or IM. (Anderson *et al.* 2013)

- **HORSES:**

As an analgesic (extra-label): Most commonly meperidine is suggested to be dosed at 1 – 2 mg/kg IM, although an IV dose of 0.3 – 0.6 mg/kg IV (slowly) has been noted. A study comparing meperidine (1 mg/kg IM) vs. placebo for treating pain associated with experimental laminitis found meperidine was more effective, but analgesic effects only lasted for 2-3.7 hours. The authors concluded that it could be used as an alternative analgesic for acute foot pain with efficacy lasting from 2-3 hours. (Foreman *et al.* 2013) **Note:** Meperidine may cause CNS excitement or ataxia in horses. Some recommend pretreatment with acepromazine (0.02 – 0.04 mg/kg IV), or xylazine (0.3 – 0.5 mg/kg IV) to reduce the behavioral changes caused by these drugs. **Warning:** Narcotic analgesics can mask the behavioral and cardiovascular signs associated with mild colic.

- **SWINE:**

As a restraining agent/premed (extra-label): Given alone meperidine does not give much restraint in large animals. Has been used in combination with promazine (2 mg/kg IM) and atropine (0.07 – 0.09 mg/kg IM) at a dose of 1 – 2 mg/kg IM as a preanesthetic 45-60 minutes before barbiturate/inhalant anesthesia. All the above should be given in separate sites. (Booth 1988)

Monitoring

- Respiratory rate/depth.
- CNS level of depression/excitation.
- Blood pressure (especially with IV use).
- Analgesic activity.

Client Information

- Oral dosage forms may cause mouth irritation.
- When given by injection, this agent should be given by a veterinarian or with direct professional supervision.

Chemistry/Synonyms

A synthetic opiate analgesic, meperidine HCl is a fine, white, crystalline, odorless powder that is very soluble in water, sparingly soluble in ether and soluble in alcohol. It has a pK_a of 7.7-8.15 and a melting range of 186-189°C. The pH of the commercially available injectable preparation is between 3.5-6.

Meperidine HCl may also be known as: pethidine HCl, isonipecaine, meperidine hydrochloride, pethidini hydrochloridum; or *Demerol*®.

Storage/Stability

Meperidine is stable at room temperature. Avoid freezing the injectable solution and protect from light during storage. Meperidine has not exhibited significant adsorption to PVC IV bags or tubing in studies to date.

Compatibility/Compounding Considerations

Meperidine is reported to be physically **compatible** with the following fluids and drugs: sodium chloride 0.45 and 0.9%, Ringer's injection, lactated Ringer's injection, dextrose 2.5, 5 and 10% for injection, dextrose/saline combinations, dextrose/Ringers lactated solutions, atropine, butorphanol, chlorpromazine, dimenhydrinate, diphenhydramine HCl, dobutamine, fentanyl citrate, glycopyrrolate, metoclopramide, pentazocine lactate, promazine HCl, succinylcholine, and verapamil HCl.

Meperidine is reported to be physically **incompatible** when mixed with the following agents: aminophylline, heparin sodium, hydrocortisone sodium succinate, methylprednisolone sodium succinate, morphine sulfate, nitrofurantoin sodium, oxytetracycline HCl, pentobarbital sodium, phenobarbital sodium, phenytoin sodium, sodium iodide, tetracycline HCl, and thiopental.

Dosage Forms/Regulatory Status

VETERINARY-LABELED PRODUCTS: NONE.

HUMAN-LABELED PRODUCTS:

Meperidine HCl Injection: 25 mg/mL, 50 mg/mL, 75 mg/mL & 100 mg/mL; *Demerol*®, generic; (Rx, C-II)

Meperidine HCl Tablets: 50 mg & 100 mg; *Demerol*®, generic; (Rx, C-II)

Meperidine HCl Syrup/Oral Solution: 50 mg/5 mL (10 mg/mL); *Demerol*®, generic; (Rx, C-II)

Note: Meperidine is listed as a Class-II controlled substance and all products require a prescription. Very accurate record keeping is required as to use and disposition of stock.

Revisions/References

Monograph revised/updated April 2014.

Anderson, D. E. & M. A. Edmondson (2013). Prevention and Management of Surgical Pain in Cattle. Veterinary Clinics of North America-Food Animal Practice **29**(1): 157-+.

Bays, T. (2013). Recognizing Signs of Pain and Pain Management in Exotics. 65th Convention of the Canadian Veterinary Medical Association. accessed via Veterinary Information Network; vin.com

Booth, N. H. (1988). Drugs Acting on the Central Nervous System. *Veterinary Pharmacology and Therapeutics - 6th Ed.* N. H. Booth and L. E. McDonald. Ames, Iowa State University Press: 153-408.

Clutton, R. E. (2010). Opioid Analgesia in Horses. Veterinary Clinics of North America-Equine Practice **26**(3): 493-+.

Foreman, J. H. & R. Ruemmler (2013). Efficacy of intramuscular meperidine hydrochloride versus placebo in experimental foot lameness in horses. Equine Veterinary Journal **45**: 48-53.

Golder, F. J., et al. (2010). Suspected acute meperidine toxicity in a dog. Veterinary Anaesthesia and Analgesia **37**(5): 471-7.

Hackett, T. (2007). Spiders and Snakes: Recognizing and Treating Envenomations.

Ivey, E. & J. Morrisey (2000). Therapeutics for Rabbits. Vet Clin NA: Exotic Anim Pract **3**:1(Jan): 183-216.

Papich, M. (1989). Effects of drugs on pregnancy. *Current Veterinary Therapy X: Small Animal Practice.* R. Kirk. Philadelphia, Saunders: 1291-9.

Williams, B. (2000). Therapeutics in Ferrets. Vet Clin NA: Exotic Anim Pract **3**:1(Jan): 131-53.

Mercaptopurine

(mer-kap-toe-**pyoor**-een)   6-Mercaptopurine, Purinethol®

Antineoplastic; Immunosuppressant

Prescriber Highlights

▶ Oral antineoplastic/immunosuppressant rarely used in dogs for adjunctive treatment of lymphosarcoma, acute leukemias, & severe rheumatoid arthritis or other autoimmune conditions (*e.g.,* unresponsive ulcerative colitis).

▶ Caution (risk versus benefit): In patients with hepatic dysfunction, bone marrow depression, infection, renal function impairment (adjust dosage), or with a history of urate urinary stones.

▶ Adverse Effects: GI effects (nausea, anorexia, vomiting, diarrhea) most likely; bone marrow suppression, hepatotoxicity, pancreatitis, GI (including oral) ulceration &, potentially, dermatologic reactions.

▶ Teratogenic; use milk replacer in nursing animals.

▶ Drug interactions.

Uses/Indications

Rarely used in veterinary medicine. Veterinary uses of mercaptopurine have included adjunctive therapy of lymphosarcoma, acute leukemias, and severe rheumatoid arthritis. It may have potential benefit in treating other autoimmune conditions (*e.g.,* unresponsive ulcerative colitis) as well.

Pharmacology/Actions

Intracellularly, mercaptopurine is converted into a ribonucleotide that acts as a purine antagonist, thereby inhibiting RNA and DNA synthesis. Mercaptopurine acts as an immunosuppressant, primarily inhibiting humoral immunity.

Pharmacokinetics

Absorption after oral dosing is variable and incomplete. Mercaptopurine is distributed throughout the total body water and is rapidly taken up by lymphocytes and erythrocytes. The drug crosses the blood-brain barrier, but not in levels significant enough to treat CNS neoplasms. It is unknown whether mercaptopurine enters milk. Mercaptopurine remaining in the plasma is then further metabolized to several other compounds that are excreted by the kidneys. Only minimal amounts of mercaptopurine are excreted unchanged. Two primary methods are used to inactivate mercaptopurine; one is oxidation to 6-thiouric acid via xanthine oxidase and the other is via thiol methylation, which is catalyzed by the polymorphic enzyme TPMT, to form the inactive metabolite methyl-

6mercaptopurine. Cats have low activity of thiopurine methyl-transferase (TPMT) and dogs have variable TMPT activity levels similar to that seen in humans. This may explain why some canine breeds/patients respond better and/or develop more myelotoxicity with azathioprine or mercaptopurine than others. TPMT activity is lower in giant schnauzers and much higher in Alaskan mala-mutes than in other breeds. One study in dogs however, did not show significant correlation between TMPT activity in red blood cells and drug toxicity (Rodriguez *et al.* 2004). Approximately 11% of humans have low thiopurine methyltransferase activity. These individuals have a greater incidence of bone marrow suppression, but also greater efficacy with treatment.

Contraindications/Precautions/Warnings

Mercaptopurine is contraindicated in patients hypersensitive to it. The drug should be used cautiously (risk versus benefit) in patients with hepatic dysfunction, bone marrow depression, infection, renal function impairment (adjust dosage), or a history of urate urinary stones.

Like azathioprine, mercaptopurine is best avoided in cats. Additionally, use with caution in dog breeds that potentially have low TPMT activity (*e.g.*, giant Schnauzers).

Adverse Effects

At usual doses, GI effects (nausea, anorexia, vomiting, diarrhea) are most likely seen in small animals. However, bone marrow suppression, hepatotoxicity, pancreatitis, GI (including oral) ulceration, and dermatologic reactions are, potentially, possible.

Reproductive/Nursing Safety

Mercaptopurine is mutagenic and teratogenic and is not recommended for use during pregnancy. In humans, the FDA categorizes this drug as category *D* for use during pregnancy (*There is evidence of human fetal risk, but the potential benefits from the use of the drug in pregnant women may be acceptable despite its potential risks.*)

It is not known whether mercaptopurine is excreted in milk, but use of milk replacer is recommended for nursing bitches or queens.

Overdosage/Acute Toxicity

Toxicity may present acutely (GI effects) or be delayed (bone marrow depression, hepatotoxicity, gastroenteritis). It is suggested to use standard protocols to empty the GI tract if ingestion was recent and to treat supportively.

Drug Interactions

The following drug interactions have either been reported or are theoretical in humans or animals receiving mercaptopurine and may be of significance in veterinary patients. Unless otherwise noted, use together is not necessarily contraindicated, but weigh the potential risks and perform additional monitoring when appropriate.

- **ALLOPURINOL:** The hepatic metabolism of mercaptopurine may be decreased by concomitant administration of allopurinol. In humans, it is recommended to reduce the mercaptopurine dose to 1/4-1/3 usual if both drugs are to be used together.
- **AMINOSALICYLATES** (*e.g.*, **mesalamine, sulfasalazine**): May increase risk for mercaptopurine toxicity.
- **HEPATOTOXIC DRUGS** (*e.g.*, **ketoconazole, valproic acid, phenobarbital, primidone**, etc.): Mercaptopurine should be used cautiously with other drugs that can cause hepatotoxicity. In humans, one study demonstrated increased hepatotoxicity when mercaptopurine was used in conjunction with doxorubicin.
- **IMMUNOSUPPRESSIVE DRUGS** (*e.g.*, **azathioprine, cyclophosphamide, corticosteroids**): Use with other immunosuppressing drugs may increase the risk of infection.
- **MYELOSUPPRESSIVE DRUGS** (*e.g.*, **antineoplastics, chloramphenicol, flucytosine, amphotericin B, colchicine, trimetho-**prim/sulfa, etc.): Use extreme caution when used concurrently with other drugs that are also myelosuppressive, including many of the other antineoplastics and other bone marrow depressant drugs; bone marrow depression may be additive. In humans, enhanced bone marrow depression has occurred when used concomitantly with trimethoprim/sulfa.
- **VACCINES, LIVE:** Live virus vaccines should be used with caution, if at all, during therapy.
- **WARFARIN:** Mercaptopurine may reduce anticoagulant effect.

Laboratory Considerations

- Mercaptopurine may give falsely elevated **serum glucose** and **uric acid** values when using a SMA (sequential multiple analyzer) 12/60.

Doses

- **DOGS:**

  As an **immunosuppressant/antineoplastic agent (leukemias)**; (extra-label): Rarely recommended for use as azathioprine is generally preferred. Dosages are usually 2 – 2.2 mg/kg once daily initially, if efficacious and adverse effects are tolerated (see Monitoring), dosage frequency is titrated down to every other day or less often. Usually used in combination with glucocorticoids (prednisone).

Monitoring

- Hemograms (including platelets) should be monitored closely; initially every 1-2 weeks and every 1-2 months once on maintenance therapy. It is recommended by some clinicians that if the WBC count drops to between 5,000-7,000 cells/mm³ the dose be reduced by 25%. If WBC count drops below 5,000 cells/mm³ treatment should be discontinued until leukopenia resolves.
- Liver function tests; serum amylase, if indicated.
- Efficacy.

Client Information

- Wear gloves when handling this medication and give it with food.
- Mercaptopurine is a chemotherapy (cancer) drug. The drug and its byproducts can be hazardous to other animals and people that come in contact with it. On the day your animal gets the drug and then for a few days afterward, all bodily waste (urine, feces, litter), blood, or vomit should only be handled while wearing disposable gloves. Seal the waste in a plastic bag and then place both the bag and gloves in with the regular trash.
- Mercaptopurine can be very toxic to the gastrointestinal tract and cause vomiting, loss of appetite, diarrhea and gastrointestinal upset. Contact veterinarian if abnormal bleeding, bruising, anorexia, vomiting, or infection occurs.

Chemistry/Synonyms

A purine analog, mercaptopurine occurs as a slightly yellow, crystalline powder. It is insoluble in water and has a pKa of 7.6.

Mercaptopurine may also be known as: 6-mercaptopurine, 6-MP, 6MP, mercaptopurinum, NSC-755, purinethiol, WR-2785, and *Purinethol*®.

Storage/Stability

Mercaptopurine tablets should be stored at room temperature in well-closed containers.

Compatibility/Compounding Considerations

Note: Compound cautiously since mercaptopurine is an antineoplastic agent. For mercaptopurine 50 mg/mL oral suspension, crush thirty 50 mg oral tablets completely. Combine with 1:1 mixture of methylcellulose 1% and syrup to form a paste. Dilute with a sufficient amount of methylcellulose/syrup mixture for a final total volume of 30 mL. Simple syrup or cherry syrup may be used. Shake suspension well before using. (Nahata *et al.* 2003)

Dosage Forms/Regulatory Status

VETERINARY-LABELED PRODUCTS: NONE.

HUMAN-LABELED PRODUCTS:

Mercaptopurine Tablets: 50 mg; *Purinethol*®, generic; (Rx)

Revisions/References

Monograph revised/updated April 2014.

Nahata, M. C., et al. (2003). *Pediatric Drug Formulations. 5th ed.*, Harvey Whitney Books. Cincinnati.

Rodriguez, D., et al. (2004). Relationship between red blood cell thiopurine methyltransferase activity and myelotoxicity in dogs receiving azathioprine. J Vet Intern Med 18(3): 339-45.

Meropenem

(mare-oh-**pen**-ehm)   Merrem IV®

Carbapenem Antibiotic

Prescriber Highlights

▶ Parenteral carbapenem antibiotic similar to imipenem, but it does not cause seizures & may be more effective against some resistant gram-negative infections.

▶ Can be administered more rapidly and with less volume (could be given SC) than imipenem.

▶ Use should be reserved for empiric therapy for severe sepsis/septic shock or when documented resistant infections &/or when aminoglycosides not indicated (renal dysfunction, CNS infections).

▶ Seems well tolerated in animals.

▶ Prices may now be decreasing as generics are available.

Uses/Indications

Meropenem may be useful in treating resistant gram-negative bacterial infections, particularly when aminoglycoside use would be risky (*i.e.*, renal failure) or not effective (*i.e.*, resistance or CNS infections). Meropenem could potentially be used as an outpatient drug, as reconstituted volumes are amenable for SC administration. In the published guidelines for treatment of urinary tract disease in dogs and cats, the Antimicrobial Guidelines Working Group of the International Society for Companion Animal Infectious Diseases recommends that meropenem be reserved for treatment of multi-drug-resistant infections, particularly those caused by Enterobacteriaceae or *Pseudomonas aeruginosa*. They also recommend consultation with a urinary or infectious disease veterinary specialist or veterinary pharmacologist prior to use (Weese *et al.* 2011).

Pharmacology/Actions

Meropenem has a broad antibacterial spectrum similar to that of imipenem, but meropenem is more active against Enterobacteriaceae and less so against gram-positive bacteria. Synergy against *Pseudomonas aeruginosa* could occur when used with aminoglycosides. In dogs and cats in North America, *E. coli* strains resistant to meropenem are still relatively uncommon. Oxacillin-resistant Staphylococci are usually resistant to meropenem. Because meropenem is more stable to renal dehydropeptidase-I than is imipenem, it does not require the addition of cilastatin to inhibit that enzyme. Meropenem may also have less potential to induce seizures than imipenem or ertapenem.

Pharmacokinetics

Meropenem must be administered via parenteral means. After SC injection in dogs, bioavailability is 84%. After IV injection in dogs, meropenem's volume of distribution is approximately 0.37 L/kg and protein binding ≈12%; half-life ≈is 40 minutes, and clearance is≈ 6.5 mL/min/kg. Concentrations of unbound drug in tissue fluid and

plasma are similar (Bidgood *et al.* 2002). In ewes, after IM injection meropenem was rapidly absorbed and had a bioavailability equal to that of intravenous dosing. Volume of distribution at steady state was 0.06 L/kg and protein binding ≈43%; elimination half-life was ≈43 minutes. 91% of the drug was recovered in the urine over 24 hours after IM injection.

Pharmacokinetic data for humans include: wide distribution in body tissues and fluids, including into the CSF and bile; very low protein binding; in patients with normal renal function, elimination half-life is ≈1 hour. One inactive metabolite has been identified, but the majority of the drug is eliminated via renal mechanisms (tubular secretions and glomerular filtration) and 70% of a dose is recovered unchanged in the urine over 12 hours.

Contraindications/Precautions/Warnings

Meropenem is contraindicated in patients hypersensitive to it or other carbapenems, and those that have developed anaphylaxis after receiving any beta-lactam antibiotic.

Adverse Effects

Meropenem is usually very well tolerated. Animals given the drug SC may show slight hair loss over injection sites. In human patients receiving meropenem, only GI effects (nausea, vomiting, diarrhea) have been reported to occur in >1% of patients treated.

Reproductive/Nursing Safety

In humans, meropenem is designated by the FDA as a category *B* drug (*Animal studies have not demonstrated risk to the fetus, but there are no adequate studies in pregnant women; or animal studies have shown an adverse effect, but adequate studies in pregnant women have not demonstrated a risk to the fetus during the first trimester of pregnancy, and there is no evidence of risk in later trimesters.*)

Meropenem is likely safe to use during lactation.

Overdosage/Acute Toxicity

Overdoses of meropenem are unlikely to occur in patients with normal renal function. In human trials, doses of 2 grams every 8 hours failed to demonstrate any significant adversity. Should an overdose occur, the drug can be discontinued if necessary or the next dose could be delayed by a few hours. Meropenem can be removed via hemodialysis when necessary.

Drug Interactions

The following drug interactions have either been reported or are theoretical in humans or animals receiving meropenem and may be of significance in veterinary patients. Unless otherwise noted, use together is not necessarily contraindicated, but weigh the potential risks and perform additional monitoring when appropriate.

▪ **PROBENECID:** May increase serum concentrations and elimination half-life of meropenem.

Laboratory Considerations

▪ No specific laboratory interactions were noted for meropenem.

Doses

▪ **DOGS/CATS:**

For treatment of documented multidrug-resistant urinary tract infections, particularly those caused by Enterobacteriaceae *or Pseudomonas aeruginosa* (extra-label): 8.5 mg/kg q12h SC or q8h IV. Recommend consultation with a urinary or infectious disease veterinary specialist or veterinary pharmacologist prior to use. (Weese *et al.* 2011)

For treatment of documented multidrug-resistant systemic or soft tissue infections, particularly those caused by Enterobacteriaceae *or Pseudomonas aeruginosa* (extra-label): Same dosages and caveats as above.

For severe sepsis/septic shock: After cultures are taken, meropenem at 12 mg/kg IV q8h can be considered for empiric therapy. Usually administered IV over 15-30 minutes, although low volumes can be given over 3-5 minutes. Once patient is hemodynamically stable, 8-12 mg/kg SC q8-12h could be considered. If culture and susceptibility results indicate an acceptable, less broad-spectrum antibiotic would be effective, consider "de-escalating" the antibiotic therapy.

Monitoring

- There are no specific monitoring requirements for meropenem except to monitor for clinical efficacy.

Client Information

- Meropenem must be injected in the vein (IV) or under the skin (SC, subcutaneous); it does not work if given by mouth.
- Fur may become thinner or change color over the injection site.

Chemistry/Synonyms

A synthetic carbapenem antibiotic, meropenem occurs as a clear to white to pale yellow powder or crystals. It is very slightly soluble in water or hydrated alcohol and practically insoluble in acetone or ether. When the commercially available injection is reconstituted the resulting pH is between 7.3 and 8.3.

Meropenem may also be known as: ICI-194660, SM-7338, *Meronem®*, *Meropen®*, *Merrem®*, *Optinem®*, or *Zeropenem®*.

Storage/Stability

The powder for injection should be stored at controlled room temperature (20-25°C; 69-77°F). When the commercially available powder for injection is reconstituted with sterile water for injection (up to a concentration of 50 mg/mL), it is labeled as stable (per the manufacturer) for up to 2 hours at room temperature; up to 12 hours when refrigerated. The package insert lists several options for dilution with several different solutions in plastic IV bags, syringes, minibags, etc. The longest time the drug the manufacturer states the drug is stable, is 48 hours when diluted in normal saline or sterile water for injection at concentrations from 1 – 20 mg/mL in plastic syringes and kept refrigerated.

The manufacturer recommends that solutions of meropenem not be frozen, but meropenem concentrations of 1 and 22 mg/mL in dextrose 5% and sodium chloride 0.9% have been stored frozen at -20°C for up to 14 days with a calculated loss of potency of 10%.

For subcutaneous administration in veterinary patients, meropenem has been diluted to a concentration of 20 mg/mL in sterile sodium chloride 0.9%. The solution should be protected from light and is reportedly stable (90% or greater of the original drug concentration) if kept refrigerated (5°C) for up to 5 days (Smith *et al.* 2004). Once the refrigerated solution is brought back to room temperature it should be used within 6 hours (Jordan 2004).

Compatibility/Compounding Considerations

Meropenem has been reported **compatible** with vancomycin, ranitidine, morphine sulfate, metoclopramide, heparin, gentamicin, furosemide, dopamine, dobutamine, dexamethasone sodium phosphate, atropine, and aminophylline. Compatibility is dependent upon factors such as pH, concentration, temperature and diluent used; consult specialized references or a hospital pharmacist for more specific information.

Dosage Forms/Regulatory Status

VETERINARY-LABELED PRODUCTS: NONE.

HUMAN-LABELED PRODUCTS:

Meropenem Powder for solution for Injection: 500 mg & 1 gram in 20 mL, & 30 mL vials; *Merrem® IV*, generic; (Rx)

Revisions/References

Monograph revised/updated April 2014.

Bidgood, T. & M. G. Papich (2002). Plasma pharmacokinetics and tissue fluid concentrations of meropenem after intravenous and subcutaneous administration in dogs. American Journal of Veterinary Research 63(12): 1622-8.

Jordan, D. (2004). Personal Communication.

Smith, D. L., et al. (2004). Stability of meropenem in polyvinyl chloride bags and an elastomeric infusion device. American Journal of Health-System Pharmacy 61(16): 1682-5.

Weese, J. S., et al. (2011). Antimicrobial Use Guidelines for Treatment of Urinary Tract Disease in Dogs and Cats: Antimicrobial Guidelines Working Group of the International Society for Companion Animal Infectious Diseases. Veterinary Medicine International.

Metergoline

(meh-**tir**-goe-leen)   Contralac®, Liserdol®

Serotonin Antagonist; Prolactin Inhibitor

Prescriber Highlights

▶ Serotonin antagonist prolactin inhibitor used primarily for pseudopregnancy in dogs.

▶ Not available commercially in USA.

▶ Primary adverse effects are GI (esp. vomiting) and behavior-related.

Uses/Indications

Metergoline is an ergot-derivative drug that is used for pseudopregnancy in dogs. It is available as a veterinary product in several European and South American countries. Metergoline has been investigated as an abortifacient in dogs at high doses (0.4 – 0.6 mg/kg), similarly to other ergot prolactin inhibitors it can only used reliably for this effect during the last 3 weeks of gestation (Nothling *et al.* 2003).

In humans, metergoline has been used for hyperprolactemia, prolactinomas, and the prophylactic treatment of migraine headaches.

Pharmacology/Actions

Metergoline reduces prolactin primarily via its serotonin antagonism effects. It differs from cabergoline and bromocriptine in that it has both strong central and peripheral anti-serotonin effects, and only weak direct dopamine-2 agonist effects. Like those drugs, it also is an antagonist at dopamine-1 receptors. Potentially, metergoline could be used to induce estrus or treat pyometra in bitches.

Pharmacokinetics

Little information was located for dogs. Metergoline half-life is reportedly quite short (approx. 4 hours) and twice daily dosing is required.

In humans, metergoline oral bioavailability is ≈25% and volume of distribution is 0.8 L/kg. It is metabolized in the liver to at least one active metabolite (1-desmethylmetergoline), which attains plasma levels higher than that of the parent drug. Elimination half-life of the parent drug is ≈50 minutes; 1-desmethylmetergoline, 80-100 minutes.

Contraindications/Precautions/Warnings

Metergoline is contraindicated in dogs and cats that are pregnant unless abortion is desired (see indications). It should not be used in patients who are hypersensitive to ergot derivatives. Patients that do not tolerate cabergoline or bromocriptine may or may not tolerate metergoline. Patients with significantly impaired liver function should receive the drug with caution and, if required, possibly at a lower dosage.

Adverse Effects

Reported adverse effects for metergoline in dogs include behavior-related effects (anxiety, aggressiveness, depression, hyperexcitation, whining and escaping) and GI effects (anorexia, vomiting, nausea). One source states "...even very high doses of metergoline do not induce vomiting in bitches" (Kutzler 2007).

Reproductive/Nursing Safety

Metergoline is contraindicated in dogs and cats that are pregnant unless abortion is desired (see indications). Because it suppresses prolactin, it should not be used in nursing mothers.

Overdosage/Acute Toxicity

Little information is available. Vomiting is the most likely effect that would be seen in overdose situations.

Drug Interactions

The following drug interactions have either been reported or are theoretical in humans or animals receiving metergoline and may be of significance in veterinary patients. Unless otherwise noted, use together is not necessarily contraindicated, but weigh the potential risks and perform additional monitoring when appropriate.

- **BROMOCRIPTINE, CABERGOLINE:** May cause additive effects if used with metergoline.
- **CYPROHEPTADINE:** May cause additive effects if used with metergoline.
- **METOCLOPRAMIDE:** Use with metergoline may reduce the efficacy of both drugs and should be avoided.
- **SSRIs** (*e.g.*, **fluoxetine, paroxetine, sertraline**, etc.): Potentially could reduce the efficacy of each drug.

Laboratory Considerations

- No particular laboratory interactions or considerations were located for this drug.

Doses

- **DOGS:**

  For treatment of pseudopregnancy: 0.5 mg/kg (500 micrograms/kg) PO twice a day. Administration for 4-5 days is effective in treating pseudopregnancy signs and reducing milk production in most bitches. Occasional failures can be dealt with by repeating the treatment protocol and extending it to 8-10 days, or by using joint protocols of cabergoline plus metergoline or cabergoline plus bromocriptine. (Romagnoli 2009)

  For pregnancy termination (extra-label): 400–500 micrograms/kg PO once daily for 5 days. (Lamm *et al.* 2012)

  To induce estrus (extra-label): Cabergoline and bromocriptine have consistently given positive results, while metergoline's results have been more variable depending on dosage. Using low dose (0.1 mg/kg PO twice a day) the commercial oral preparation of metergoline administered from 100 days after ovulation until the following proestrus, the interestrus interval can be significantly shortened. (Romagnoli 2006)

- **CATS:**

  For treatment of pseudopregnancy or to halt post-partum lactation (extra-label in USA): 0.125 mg/kg PO twice a day for 4-8 days. (Label Information—*Contralac*®; Virbac-Switzerland)

Monitoring

- Efficacy and adverse effects.
- If used long term, liver function tests.

Client Information

- Give this medication with food; contact veterinarian if vomiting persists.
- Keep this an all medications away from pets and animals.

Chemistry/Synonyms

Metergoline is an ergot derivative and has the chemical name: Benzyl (8S,10S)-(1,6-dimethylergolin-8-ylmethyl)carbamate.

Metergoline may also be known as: FI-6337, MCE, Metergoliini, Metergolin, Metergolina, Métergoline, Metergolinum, or Methergoline. Common trade names are *Contralac*® (veterinary) and *Liserdol*® (human).

Storage/Stability

Metergoline tablets should be stored at room temperature; protected from light.

Compatibility/Compounding Considerations

No specific information noted.

Dosage Forms/Regulatory Status

VETERINARY-LABELED PRODUCTS:

None in the USA, in several countries in Europe and South America: Metergoline 0.5 mg & 2 mg oral tablets are available; *Contralac*® (Virbac)

HUMAN-LABELED PRODUCTS:

None in USA. In some countries: Metergoline 4 mg tablets are available.

Revisions/References

Monograph revised/updated April 2014.

Kutzler, M. A. (2007). Estrus induction and synchronization in canids and felids. Theriogenology 68(3): 354-74.

Lamm, C. G. & C. L. Makloski (2012). Current Advances in Gestation and Parturition in Cats and Dogs. Vet Clin Small Anim 42: 445-56.

Nothling, J. O., et al. (2003). Abortifacient and endocrine effects of metergoline in beagle bitches during the second half of gestation. Theriogenology 59(9): 1929-40.

Romagnoli, S. (2006). Control of reproduction in dogs and cats: Use and misuse of hormones. Proceedings: WSAVA World Congress. accessed via Veterinary Information Network; vin.com

Romagnoli, S. (2009). An update on pseudopregnancy. Proceedings: WSAVA. accessed via Veterinary Information Network; vin.com

Metformin HCl

(met-**fore**-min)   Glucophage®

Antihyperglycemic

Prescriber Highlights

► Oral anti-hyperglycemic agent that potentially could be useful in the adjunctive treatment of insulin resistance associated with equine metabolic syndrome. Use is controversial in cats for treating non-insulin dependent diabetes mellitus (NIDDM).

► Contraindicated in patients hypersensitive to it; with renal dysfunction, metabolic acidosis, or temporarily when iodinated contrast agents are to be used (see Drug Interactions).

► Adverse effects may include lethargy, inappetence, vomiting, & weight loss.

► Potentially significant drug interactions.

► Human dosage forms may be difficult to accurately dose in cats.

Uses/Indications

Metformin may be useful in the adjunctive treatment of non-insulin dependent diabetes mellitus in cats. Only limited trials of the drug have been performed in cats, with only very limited success when the drug is used alone. Currently, metformin should only be used in cats with functional beta cells known to have type-2 diabetes mellitus (Palm *et al.* 2013). Studies comparing its safety and efficacy with other oral antihyperglycemics (*e.g.*, glipizide or insulin) were not located.

There has been some research evaluating metformin for treating insulin resistance associated with equine metabolic syndrome in horses, but data conflicts regarding its efficacy (Durham 2012), (Rendle *et al.* 2013). Because of the drug's low cost and low adverse effect profile, further investigation of its clinical usefulness is warranted.

Pharmacology/Actions

Metformin's actions are multifaceted. At usual dosages, it increases insulin's ability to transport glucose across cell membranes in skeletal muscle without increasing lactate production and inhibits formation of advanced glycosylation end-products. Metformin decreases hepatic glucose production, and may decrease intestinal absorption of glucose. It does not stimulate insulin production or release from the pancreas and, therefore, does not cause hypoglycemia.

In horses, metformin has poor oral bioavailability (around 5%) and is not likely to act systemically, however there is some indication that metformin may act locally and limit gut glucose uptake. A recently published study in 7 normal horses found that metformin at 30 mg/kg via NG tube 1 hour prior to an oral glucose challenge test (dextrose powder 0.5 g/kg PO in feed) reduced glycemic and insulinemic responses. Further work is required to determine whether these effects may translate into clinical benefits in horses with EMS and hyperinsulinemia (Rendle *et al.* 2013).

Pharmacokinetics

A pharmacokinetic study done in cats (Chastain *et al.* 1999) showed that metformin is variably absorbed after oral administration 35-67%. In cats, steady-state volume of distribution was 0.55 L/kg; elimination half-life ≈12 hours and total clearance was 0.15 L/hr/kg. Metformin is primarily eliminated via the kidneys. The authors concluded that the drug's pharmacokinetics are similar to that seen in humans, and that a dosage of 2 mg/kg twice daily would give plasma concentrations known to be effective in humans.

In a small (4 subjects) pharmacokinetic study in horses, metformin demonstrated very low oral bioavailability (4% fed, 7% fasted). Maximum blood levels were around 0.4 micrograms/mL. Elimination half-life after IV dosing was ≈25 minutes. (Hustace *et al.* 2009)

Contraindications/Precautions/Warnings

In humans (and presumably cats), metformin is contraindicated in patients hypersensitive to it, with renal dysfunction or metabolic acidosis. It is also temporarily contraindicated when iodinated contrast agents are to be used (see Drug Interactions).

Adverse Effects

In cats, metformin may cause lethargy, inappetence, vomiting, and weight loss. In a study evaluating metformin in diabetic cats (Nelson *et al.* 2004), 1 of 5 diabetic cats studied died 11 days after receiving metformin. As the cause of death was undetermined, metformin could not be ruled out as a causative factor. Hypoglycemia would not be an expected adverse effect when metformin is used as a single agent.

Reproductive/Nursing Safety

In pregnant humans, metformin is designated by the FDA as a category **B** drug (*Animal studies have not demonstrated risk to the fetus, but there are no adequate studies in pregnant women; or animal studies have shown an adverse effect, but adequate studies in pregnant women have not demonstrated a risk to the fetus during the first trimester of pregnancy, and there is no evidence of risk in later trimesters.*)

Metformin is excreted in maternal milk in levels equivalent to those found in plasma. While adverse effects in nursing kittens would be unlikely, use with caution in lactating queens.

Overdosage/Acute Toxicity

In small animals hypoglycemia is not commonly seen in overdoses with metformin alone, but it has a narrow margin of safety regarding GI upset. Vomiting commonly occurs with ingestions of metformin in small animals. There were 627 single agent exposures to metformin reported to the ASPCA Animal Poison Control Center (APCC) during 2009-2013. Of the 591 dogs, 77 were symptomatic with vomiting (61%) and lethargy (18%) most commonly seen.

Massive overdoses in humans (100 grams) caused hypoglycemia only 10% of the time, but lactic acidosis occurred. Lactic acidosis has been seen in human overdoses of 7 and 20 grams (total dose). It is unknown at what dose acidosis may occur in domestic animals. Ingestion of up to 1700 mg by children is not usually associated with significant toxicity. Enhancement of metformin elimination may be amenable to dialysis.

Drug Interactions

The following drug interactions have either been reported or are theoretical in humans or animals receiving metformin and may be of significance in veterinary patients. Unless otherwise noted, use together is not necessarily contraindicated, but weigh the potential risks and perform additional monitoring when appropriate.

- **ACE INHIBITORS:** May increase risk for hypoglycemia.
- **CIMETIDINE:** In humans, cimetidine can cause a 60% increase in peak metformin plasma levels and a 40% increase in AUC.
- **CORTICOSTEROIDS:** May reduce efficacy.
- **DIURETICS, THIAZIDE:** May reduce hypoglycemic efficacy.
- **FUROSEMIDE:** Can increase the AUC and plasma levels of metformin by 22% in humans; metformin can decrease the peak plasma concentrations and AUC of furosemide.
- **IODINATED CONTRAST AGENTS, PARENTERAL:** May cause acute renal failure and lactic acidosis if used within 48 hours of a metformin dose.
- **ISONIAZID:** May reduce hypoglycemic efficacy.
- **SYMPATHOMIMETIC AGENTS:** May reduce hypoglycemic efficacy.

Laboratory Considerations

- No specific laboratory interactions or considerations noted.

Doses

- **CATS:**

  For non-insulin dependent diabetes mellitus (patients with detectable concentrations of insulin); (extra-label): 25 or 50 mg per cat PO twice daily (Palm *et al.* 2013). If using tablets, must be compounded. No information on the use of the oral liquid (100 mg/mL) or extended-release tablets for use in cats was noted.

- **HORSES:**

  For adjunctive treatment of equine metabolic syndrome (extra-label): **Note:** Use is controversial and evidence for efficacy conflicts. Reserve metformin treatment for horses and ponies with markedly increased OST (oral sugar test; corn syrup-based) insulin concentrations, even after loss of body fat mass and dietary management. Current recommendations are metformin 30 mg/kg PO every 8-12h, preferably 30-60 minutes before the horse is fed. (Rendle *et al.* 2013), (Frank *et al.* 2014)

Monitoring

- Efficacy: Standard methods of monitoring efficacy for diabetes treatment should be followed (*e.g.*, fasting blood glucose, appetite, attitude, body condition, PU/PD resolution, and perhaps serum fructosamine and/or glycosylated hemoglobin levels).
- Renal function (baseline and annually).
- Adverse effects.

Client Information

- Clients should understand the relative "investigational" nature of using this compound in cats and report any untoward effects to the veterinarian.

Chemistry/Synonyms

A biguanide oral anti-hyperglycemic agent, metformin HCl occurs as white to off-white crystals that are slightly soluble in alcohol and freely soluble in water. It is a weak base; a 1% aqueous solution of metformin HCl has a pKa of 6.68 and metformin base has a pKa of 12.4.

Metformin HCl may also be known as dimethylbiguanide HCl or metforimini hydrochloridium. There are many proprietary names outside of the USA for this drug.

Storage/Stability

Metformin HCl oral products (oral tablets, sustained-release tablets, and fixed dose combination products with glipizide or rosiglitazone) should be stored protected from light at a controlled room temperature of 20-25°C (68-77°F), excursions permitted to 15-30°C (59-86°F). The combination product containing metformin HCL and glyburide should be stored at temperatures up to 25°C (77°F) and protected from light.

Compatibility/Compounding Considerations

No specific information noted.

Dosage Forms/Regulatory Status

VETERINARY-LABELED PRODUCTS: NONE.

HUMAN-LABELED PRODUCTS:

Metformin HCl Oral Tablets: 500 mg, 850 mg & 1000 mg; *Glucophage®*, generic; (Rx)

Metformin HCl Extended-Release Oral Tablets: 500 mg, 750 mg & 1000 mg; *Glucophage XR®*, *Glumetza®*, *Fortamet®*, generic; (Rx)

Metformin HCl Oral Solution: 500 mg/5 mL (100 mg/mL) in 118 mL & 473 mL; *Riomet®*; (Rx)

The are also fixed-dose oral tablet combination products available containing metformin and glyburide or glipizide.

Revisions/References

Monograph revised/updated April 2014.

Chastain, C., et al. (1999). Pharmacokinetics of the antihyperglycemic agent metformin in cats. Am Jnl Vet Res **60**: 738-42.
Durham, A. E. (2012). Metformin in equine metabolic syndrome: An enigma or a dead duck? Veterinary Journal **191**(1): 17-8.
Frank, N. & R. Geor (2014). Current best practice in clinical management of equine endocrine patients. Equine Veterinary Education **26**(1): 6-9.
Hustace, J. L., et al. (2009). Pharmacokinetics and bioavailability of metformin in horses. American Journal of Veterinary Research **70**(5): 665-8.
Nelson, R., et al. (2004). Evaluation of the oral antihyperglycemic drug metformin in normal and diabetic cats. J Vet Intern Med **18**(1): 18-24.
Palm, C. A. & E. C. Feldman (2013). Oral Hypoglycemics in Cats with Diabetes Mellitus. Veterinary Clinics of North America-Small Animal Practice **43**(2): 407-+.
Rendle, D. I., et al. (2013). Effects of metformin hydrochloride on blood glucose and insulin responses to oral dextrose in horses. Equine Veterinary Journal **45**(6): 751-4.

Methadone HCl

(meth-a-done)   Dolophine®

Opiate Agonist

Prescriber Highlights

▶ Narcotic agonist that may be used as an alternative to morphine in dogs, cats, horses, etc.
▶ Causes less histamine-release (with IV), sedation & vomiting than morphine.
▶ Depending on the country, it may be significantly more expensive than morphine.
▶ C-II controlled substance in USA.

Uses/Indications

Methadone may be used as an alternative opioid preanesthetic or analgesic in dogs or cats. It is also being investigated for epidural use for horses. Poor oral bioavailability precludes oral dosing in dogs. (KuKanich *et al.* 2011)

Pharmacology/Actions

In small animals methadone acts similarly to morphine with regard to its degree of analgesia and duration of action. Methadone is a *mu*-receptor (OP3; MOR) agonist that also is a non-competitive inhibitor of NMDA (n-methyl-d-aspartate) receptors. Methadone can also reduce re-uptake of norepinephrine and serotonin, which may contribute to its analgesic effects. Due to these other actions, methadone potentially may be more efficacious than other *mu* agonists (*e.g.*, morphine) particularly for neuropathic or chronic pain. Methadone is more lipid-soluble than is morphine and approximately 1-1.5X as potent. It does not cause significant histamine release when administered intravenously.

Refer to the monograph: Narcotic (opiate) Analgesic Agonists, Pharmacology of, for more information.

Pharmacokinetics

Limited information is available on the pharmacokinetics of methadone in domestic animals. In dogs, methadone has poor oral bioavailability and ketoconazole or omeprazole alone do not significantly affect oral bioavailability. Unlike in humans, CYP3A does not appear to be a major metabolic pathway for methadone biotransformation in dogs (KuKanich *et al.* 2005). However the co-administration of multiple CYP450 inhibitors (ketoconazole, fluoxetine, trimethoprim, chloramphenicol presumably affecting different isoenzymes in dogs) has been shown to significantly increase AUC and plasma concentrations of methadone in dogs (KuKanich *et al.* 2011). Subcutaneous administration has a bioavailability of ≈80% and peak levels occur around an hour after dosing. Terminal elimination half-life after intravenous dosing is ≈1.75-4 hours in dogs; clearance is ≈25-30 mL/kg/min. After SC administration, half-life is closer to 11 hours, but there was wide inter-patient variation (Ingvast-Larsson *et al.* 2010).

In cats, after administration of methadone IV (0.3 mg/kg) or via oral transmucosal (OTM) administration (0.6 mg/kg), peak levels occurred at 10 minutes (IV) and 2 hours (OTM). This study was more focused on the physiological and antinociceptive/behavioral effects, rather than the pharmacokinetics of methadone in cats. Antinociceptive effects were detected at 10 minutes (IV & OTM) and persisted ≥ 2 hours (IV) and ≥ 4 hours (OTM) (Ferreira *et al.* 2011).

In horses, orally administered methadone appears to be well absorbed after oral administration, but bioavailability is approximately 3X lower when administered intragastrically. P-glycoprotein may play a role in the poor intestinal absorption of methadone *in vivo*. Methadone is rapidly eliminated (half-life around 1 hour) in horses (Linardi, R. *et al.* 2008), (Linardi, R.L. *et al.* 2012), (Linardi, R.L. *et al.* 2013).

In goats, methadone has a high bioavailability after SC administration; half-life is ≈1.5 hours (Olsen *et al.* 2013).

In humans, methadone is well absorbed from the GI tract (PO), and after subcutaneous or intramuscular injection. It is widely distributed and extensively bound to plasma proteins (60-90%). Methadone is metabolized in the liver primarily by the cytochrome P450 CYP3A isoenzyme, but other isoenzymes also play a role. Metabolites do not have activity. Methadone's half-life is widely variable in humans (15-60 hours); elimination half-lives may be extended if giving multiple doses.

Contraindications/Precautions/Warnings

All opiates should be used with caution in patients with heart failure, hypertension, head injuries, elevated CSF pressures, and in geriatric or severely debilitated patients.

Adverse Effects

Adverse effects from methadone can include panting, whining, sedation, defecation, constipation, bradycardia, and respiratory depression. Methadone tends to cause less sedation or vomiting than morphine.

Methadone in cats appears to cause less excitation or vomiting than some other *mu* agonists.

In horses, methadone at IV doses of 0.1 mg/kg or greater has caused pronounced CNS excitement.

Reproductive/Nursing Safety

Methadone is relatively safe to use at low dosages for short periods during the first two trimesters of pregnancy, but it should be avoided late in term as significant respiratory depression and increased rates of stillbirths have been noted in humans. Infants of humans who have been taking methadone for opiate addiction, have shown high rates of moderate to severe opiate withdrawal signs during the neonatal period, and long-term developmental problems.

Although methadone enters maternal milk, the American Academy of Pediatrics considers methadone compatible with breast-feeding in women.

Overdosage/Acute Toxicity

Overdosage may produce profound respiratory and/or CNS depression in most species. Newborns may be more susceptible to these effects than adult animals. Other toxic effects can include cardiovascular collapse, hypothermia, and skeletal muscle hypotonia. Naloxone is the agent of choice in treating respiratory depression. In massive overdoses, naloxone doses may need to be repeated. Animals should be closely observed since naloxone's effects might diminish before sub-toxic levels of methadone are attained. Mechanical respiratory support should be considered in cases of severe respiratory depression. Dialysis, charcoal hemoperfusion, or forced diuresis do not appear to be beneficial in treating methadone overdoses.

Drug Interactions

The following drug interactions have either been reported or are theoretical in humans or animals receiving methadone and may be of significance in veterinary patients. Unless otherwise noted, use together is not necessarily contraindicated, but weigh the potential risks and perform additional monitoring when appropriate.

- **ANTIARRHYTHMICS, CLASS I & III** (*e.g.*, **lidocaine, procainamide, quinidine, amiodarone**): Use with methadone may increase risks for arrhythmias.
- **ALPHA2-AGONISTS** (*e.g.*, **medetomidine, xylazine**): In a small study done in dogs, methadone potentiated the sedative and analgesic effects of medetomidine in dogs, but severe hypoxemia was seen in dogs breathing room air (Raekallio *et al.* 2009). Results from another study combining xylazine and methadone, suggested that methadone is a good alternative for sedation in dogs when combined with acepromazine or xylazine. A satisfactory degree of sedation was achieved with both combinations. The combination of methadone and xylazine appeared to result in better analgesia compared to xylazine alone (Monteiro *et al.* 2008).
- **AZOLE ANTIFUNGALS** (*e.g.*, **fluconazole, itraconazole, ketoconazole**): May increase methadone levels.
- **CALCIUM CHANNEL BLOCKERS**: Use with methadone may increase risks for arrhythmias.
- **CHLORAMPHENICOL**: May increase methadone levels.
- **CNS DEPRESSANTS, OTHER** (*e.g.*, **anesthetic agents, antihistamines, phenothiazines, barbiturates, tranquilizers, alcohol,** etc.): May cause increased CNS or respiratory depression when used with methadone.
- **CORTICOSTEROIDS (MINERALOCORTICOIDS)**: Use with methadone may increase potential for electrolyte abnormalities.
- **DIURETICS**: Opiates may decrease efficacy in CHF patients.
- **MACROLIDE ANTIBIOTICS** (*e.g.*, **erythromycin, clarithromycin**): May inhibit metabolism of methadone and increase levels.
- **MONAMINE OXIDASE (MAO) INHIBITORS** (*e.g.*, **amitraz,** possibly **selegiline**): Meperidine with MAOIs in humans has caused severe CNS/behavior reactions and potentially could do the same with methadone; avoid concomitant use.

- **MUSCLE RELAXANTS, SKELETAL**: Methadone may enhance neuromuscular blockade.
- **PHENOBARBITAL, PHENYTOIN**: May decrease methadone levels.
- **RIFAMPIN**: May decrease methadone levels (Probably does not affect dogs).
- **SSRI ANTIDEPRESSANTS** (**fluoxetine, sertraline,** etc.): May increase methadone levels.
- **St JOHN'S WORT**: May decrease methadone levels.
- **TRICYCLIC ANTIDEPRESSANTS** (**clomipramine, amitriptyline,** etc.): Methadone may exacerbate the effects of tricyclic antidepressants.
- **TRIMETHOPRIM**: May increase methadone levels.
- **WARFARIN**: Opiates may potentiate anticoagulant activity.
- **ZIDOVUDINE**: Methadone may increase zidovudine levels.

Laboratory Considerations

- As they may increase biliary tract pressure, opiates can increase plasma **amylase** and **lipase** values up to 24 hours following their administration.
- The following drugs can reportedly cause false-positive results on **urine screening tests for methadone**: Chlorpromazine, clomipramine, diphenhydramine, doxylamine, quetiapine, thioridazine, and verapamil.

Doses

- **DOGS:**

  For perioperative pain control (extra-label): From a study where 38 dogs received meloxicam (0.2 mg/kg at induction), and acepromazine (0.03 mg/kg) combined either with methadone (0.5 mg/kg) or buprenorphine (20 micrograms/kg) as a premedication prior to orthopedic surgery. Authors concluded that at the doses investigated, methadone produced superior analgesia to buprenorphine for 8 hours postoperatively (Hunt *et al.* 2013).

  For analgesia (extra-label): As a CRI: Loading dose of 0.1 – 0.2 mg/kg IV; followed by a CRI at 0.12 mg/kg/hour. Practically, add 60 mg methadone HCl (6 mL of the 10 mg/mL injection) to 500 mL IV fluid and run at 1 mL/kg/hour. Can be combined with ketamine and/or lidocaine (Grubb 2013). As an intermittent dose: Dosage recommendations vary, but usually range from 0.1 – 1 mg/kg q4-8h IV, SC or IM.

- **CATS:**

  For perioperative pain control (extra-label): In a prospective, randomized study in 22 cats (10 butorphanol, 12 methadone) undergoing OHE; methadone at 0.6 mg/kg with acepromazine at 0.02 mg/kg SC as pre-operative combination resulted in pain scores that were significantly lower than in the butorphanol group; 3 of 12 methadone-treated cats, compared with 6 of 10 butorphanol-treated cats required rescue analgesia within 6 hours of the dose. Authors concluded that methadone appeared to be a better postoperative analgesic than butorphanol and provided effective analgesia for 6 hours following ovariohysterectomy in most cats (Warne *et al.* 2013).

  For analgesia (extra-label): As a CRI: Loading dose of 0.1 – 0.2 mg/kg IV; followed by a CRI at 0.12 mg/kg/hour. Practically, add 60 mg methadone HCl (6 mL of the 10 mg/mL injection) to 500 mLs IV fluid and run at 1 mL/kg/hour. Can be combined with ketamine and/or lidocaine (Grubb 2013). As an intermittent dose: Dosage recommendations vary, but usually range from 0.05 – 0.5 mg/kg q4-6h IV, SC or IM.

Monitoring

- Analgesic or preanesthetic efficacy.
- At higher dosages, monitor for respiratory depression.

Client Information

- When given parenterally, this agent should be used in an inpatient setting or with direct professional supervision.
- If being used orally for pain control, be sure to keep out of reach of children and pets.

Chemistry/Synonyms

A synthetic diphenylheptane-derivative narcotic agonist, methadone HCl occurs as an odorless, colorless or white crystalline powder. It is freely soluble in water, chloroform, or alcohol and practically insoluble in ether or glycerol. The pH of a 1% solution in water is between 4.5-6.5. The commercially available injection has a pH from 3-6.5. The dispersible tablet formulation (*Diskets®*) contains insoluble ingredients that deter their use for injection.

Methadone may also be known as: Amidine HCl, amidone HCl, methadoni hydrochloridum, Phenadone, *Adolan®*, *Biodone®*, *Cloro Nona®*, *Dolmed®*, *Eptadone®*, *Gobbidona®*, *Heptadon®*, *Ketalgine®*, *Metadol®*, *Metasedin®*, *Methaddict®*, *Methadose®*, *Methatabs®*, *Methex®*, *Pallidone®*, *Phymet®*, *Physeptone®*, *Pinadone®*, *Sedo®*, *Symoron®*, or *Synastone®*.

Storage/Stability

Unless otherwise labeled, methadone products should be stored at room temperature and protected from light.

Compatibility/Compounding Considerations

Methadone injection is reportedly stable when mixed in a syringe with acepromazine. The injection is reportedly **not compatible** with pentobarbital, phenobarbital, or thiopental.

Dosage Forms/Regulatory Status

VETERINARY-LABELED PRODUCTS: NONE.

The ARCI (Racing Commissioners International) has designated this drug as a class 1 substance. See the appendix for more information.

HUMAN-LABELED PRODUCTS:

Methadone HCl Injection: 10 mg/mL in 20 mL multidose vials; generic; (Rx, C-II)

Methadone HCl Oral Tablets: 5 mg & 10 mg; Dispersible Tablets 40 mg; *Dolophine®*, *Methadose®*, generic; (Rx, C-II)

Methadone HCl Oral Solution/Liquid Concentrate: 1 mg/mL, 2 mg/mL & 10 mg/mL in 30 mL (w/calibrated dropper), 500 mL, 946 mL, 1 L & 15 L; *Methadose®*, generic; (Rx, C-II)

All methadone-containing products are C-II controlled substances in the USA. When used as an analgesic, methadone may be dispensed by any pharmacy or practitioner registered with the DEA for Class-II narcotics. When methadone is used to treat narcotic addiction, specialized approval must be obtained from the FDA and, usually, state regulators.

Revisions/References

Monograph revised/updated April 2014.

Ferreira, T. H., et al. (2011). Plasma concentrations and behavioral, antinociceptive, and physiologic effects of methadone after intravenous and oral transmucosal administration in cats. American Journal of Veterinary Research 72(6): 764-71.

Grubb, T. (2013). Analgesia Drop by Drop: Constant-Rate Infusions Made Easy & Fun! Proceedings: Atlantic Coast Veterinary Conference 2013. accessed via Veterinary Information Network; vin.com

Hunt, J. R., et al. (2013). Comparison of premedication with buprenorphine or methadone with meloxicam for postoperative analgesia in dogs undergoing orthopaedic surgery. Journal of Small Animal Practice 54(8): 418-24.

Ingvast-Larsson, C., et al. (2010). Clinical pharmacology of methadone in dogs. Veterinary Anaesthesia and Analgesia 37(1): 48-56.

KuKanich, B., et al. (2011). The effects of concurrent administration of cytochrome P-450 inhibitors on the pharmacokinetics of oral methadone in healthy dogs. Veterinary Anaesthesia and Analgesia 38(3): 224-30.

KuKanich, B., et al. (2005). The effects of inhibiting cytochrome P450 3A, p-glycoprotein, and gastric acid secretion on the oral bioavailability of methadone in dogs. J. Vet. Pharmacol. Ther. 28(5): 461-6.

Linardi, R., et al. (2008). Oral Absorption and Pharmacokinetics of Methadone HCl in Horses. Proceedings: IVECCS. accessed via Veterinary Information Network; vin.com

Linardi, R. L., et al. (2013). The effect of P-Glycoprotein on methadone hydrochloride flux in equine intestinal mucosa. J. Vet. Pharmacol. Ther. 36(1): 43-50.

Linardi, R. L., et al. (2012). Bioavailability and pharmacokinetics of oral and injectable formulations of methadone after intravenous, oral, and intragastric administration in horses. American Journal of Veterinary Research 73(2): 290-5.

Monteiro, E. R., et al. (2008). Effects of methadone, alone or in combination with acepromazine or xylazine, on sedation and physiologic values in dogs. Veterinary Anaesthesia and Analgesia 35(6): 519-27.

Olsen, L., et al. (2013). Methadone in healthy goats - Pharmacokinetics, behaviour and blood pressure. Research in Veterinary Science 95(1): 231-7.

Raekallio, M. R., et al. (2009). Effects of medetomidine, l-methadone, and their combination on arterial blood gases in dogs. Veterinary Anaesthesia and Analgesia 36(2): 158-61.

Warne, L. N., et al. (2013). Comparison of perioperative analgesic efficacy between methadone and butorphanol in cats. Javma-Journal of the American Veterinary Medical Association 243(6): 844-50.

Methazolamide

(meth-a-**zoe**-la-mide)   Neptazane®

Carbonic Anhydrase Inhibitor

Prescriber Highlights

- ► Oral carbonic anhydrase inhibitor used primarily for open angle glaucoma. Reportedly is becoming difficult to obtain at an affordable cost.
- ► Contraindicated in patients with significant hepatic, renal, pulmonary or adrenocortical insufficiency, hyponatremia, hypokalemia, hyperchloremic acidosis, or electrolyte imbalance.
- ► Primary adverse effects are GI-related, hypokalemia, metabolic acidosis. Cats may be more susceptible to developing adverse effects.
- ► Give oral doses with food if GI upset occurs.
- ► Monitor with tonometry for glaucoma; check electrolytes.

Uses/Indications

Orally administered methazolamide is used for the medical treatment of glaucoma. Topical carbonic anhydrase inhibitors (*e.g.*, dorzolamide) are more commonly used today as they can lower IOP as effectively as systemic drugs and have fewer adverse effects.

Pharmacology/Actions

The carbonic anhydrase inhibitors act by a noncompetitive, reversible inhibition of the enzyme carbonic anhydrase. This reduces the formation of hydrogen and bicarbonate ions from carbon dioxide and reduces the availability of these ions for active transport into body secretions.

Pharmacologic effects of the carbonic anhydrase inhibitors include decreased formation of aqueous humor, thereby reducing intraocular pressure; increased renal tubular secretion of sodium and potassium and, to a greater extent, bicarbonate, leading to increased urine alkalinity and volume; anticonvulsant activity, which is independent of its diuretic effects (mechanism not fully understood, but may be due to carbonic anhydrase or a metabolic acidosis effect).

Pharmacokinetics

Little information is available. Methazolamide is absorbed from the GI tract albeit more slowly than acetazolamide. It is distributed throughout the body, including the CSF and aqueous humor. Methazolamide is at least partially metabolized in the liver.

Contraindications/Precautions/Warnings

Carbonic anhydrase inhibitors are contraindicated in patients with significant hepatic disease (may precipitate hepatic coma), renal or adrenocortical insufficiency, hyponatremia, hypokalemia, hyperchloremic acidosis, or electrolyte imbalance. They should not be used in patients with severe pulmonary obstruction unable to increase alveolar ventilation or those that are hypersensitive to them. Long-term use of carbonic anhydrase inhibitors is contraindicated in patients with chronic, noncongestive, angle-closure glaucoma as angle closure may occur and the drug may mask the condition by lowering intra-ocular pressures.

Do not confuse methazolamide with methimazole, or methenamine.

Adverse Effects

Potential adverse effects that may be encountered include GI disturbances (vomiting, diarrhea, inappetence), metabolic acidosis (with heavy panting), CNS effects (sedation, depression, disorientation, excitement, etc.), hypokalemia, hematologic effects (bone marrow depression, thrombocytopenia), renal effects (crystalluria, dysuria, renal colic, polyuria, polydipsia), hyperglycemia, hyponatremia, hyperuricemia, hepatic insufficiency, dermatologic effects (rash, etc.), and hypersensitivity reactions. Electrolyte imbalances may manifest as weakness or cardiac arrhythmias.

Cats may be more prone to developing adverse effects than are dogs.

Combining methazolamide (oral dosing) with topical (ophthalmic) dorzolamide does not apparently yield additive reductions in intraocular pressure and may cause increased adverse effects.

Reproductive/Nursing Safety

In humans, the FDA categorizes this drug as category C for use during pregnancy (*Animal studies have shown an adverse effect on the fetus, but there are no adequate studies in humans; or there are no animal reproduction studies and no adequate studies in humans.*)

Safety for use during nursing has not been established. But a related compound, acetazolamide, is excreted in the milk in concentrations unlikely to have pharmacologic effect.

Overdosage/Acute Toxicity

Information regarding overdosage of this drug is not readily available. It is suggested to monitor serum electrolytes, blood gases, volume status, and CNS status during an acute overdose. Treat symptomatically and supportively.

Drug Interactions

The following drug interactions have either been reported or are theoretical in humans or animals receiving methazolamide and may be of significance in veterinary patients. Unless otherwise noted, use together is not necessarily contraindicated, but weigh the potential risks and perform additional monitoring when appropriate.

- **ANTIDEPRESSANTS, TRICYCLIC:** Alkaline urine caused by methazolamide may decrease excretion.
- **ASPIRIN** (or other **salicylates**): Increased risk of methazolamide accumulation and toxicity and metabolic acidosis; methazolamide increases salicylate excretion.
- **DIGOXIN:** As methazolamide may cause hypokalemia, increased risk for toxicity.
- **INSULIN:** Rarely, carbonic anhydrase inhibitors interfere with the hypoglycemic effects of insulin.
- **METHENAMINE COMPOUNDS:** Methazolamide may negate effects in the urine.
- **POTASSIUM, DRUGS AFFECTING (corticosteroids, amphotericin B, corticotropin, or other diuretics):** Concomitant use may exacerbate potassium depletion.
- **PHENOBARBITAL:** May increase urinary excretion and reduce phenobarbital levels.
- **PRIMIDONE:** Decreased primidone concentrations as per phenobarbital.
- **QUINIDINE:** Alkaline urine caused by methazolamide may decrease excretion.

Laboratory Considerations

- By alkalinizing the urine, carbonic anhydrase inhibitors may cause false positive results in determining **urine protein** using bromphenol blue reagent (*Albustix®, Albutest®, Labstix®*), sulfosalicylic acid (*Bumintest®, Exton's® Test Reagent*), nitric acid ring test, or heat and acetic acid test methods.
- Carbonic anhydrase inhibitors may **decrease iodine uptake** by the thyroid gland in hyperthyroid or euthyroid patients.

Doses

- **DOGS:**

  For medical treatment of glaucoma (extra-label): Dosages usually range from 2 – 5 mg/kg PO 2-3 times a day.

- **CATS:**

  For medical treatment of glaucoma (extra-label): Dosages usually range from 1 – 4 mg/kg PO 2-3 times a day.

Monitoring

- Intraocular pressure/tonometry.
- Serum electrolytes, pH. May need to supplement potassium.
- Baseline CBC with differential and periodic retests if using chronically.
- Other adverse effects.

Client Information

- Must be given 2-3 times a day.
- If GI upset (vomiting, lack of appetite, etc.) occurs, give with food.
- Notify veterinarian if abnormal bleeding or bruising occurs or if animal develops tremors or a rash.

Chemistry/Synonyms

A carbonic anhydrase inhibitor similar to dichlorphenamide, methazolamide occurs as a white to slightly yellow crystalline powder. It is very slightly soluble in water.

Methazolamide may also be known as: *GlaucTabs®, Glaumetax®, MZM®*, and *Neptazane®*.

Storage/Stability

Methazolamide tablets should be stored at room temperature in well-closed containers. Methazolamide tablets have an expiration date of 5 years after manufacture.

Compatibility/Compounding Considerations

No specific information noted.

Dosage Forms/Regulatory Status

VETERINARY-LABELED PRODUCTS: NONE.

The ARCI (Racing Commissioners International) has designated this drug as a class 4 substance. See the appendix for more information.

HUMAN-LABELED PRODUCTS:

Methazolamide Tablets: 25 mg & 50 mg; generic; (Rx)

Revisions/References

Monograph revised/updated April 2014.

Methenamine

(meth-**en**-a-meen)   Hiprex®, Urex®

Urinary Antiseptic

Prescriber Highlights

▶ Theoretically, converted into an urinary antiseptic; efficacy somewhat questionable in small animals.

▶ Contraindications: Metabolic acidosis, hypersensitivity to it, renal insufficiency, severe hepatic impairment (due to ammonia production), or severe dehydration.

▶ Adverse Effects: GI irritation; dysuria possible if used long-term.

▶ Urine pH must be below 6.5 and ideally <6, to be effective.

Uses/Indications

Methenamine is used as an antimicrobial agent for prophylaxis of recurrent urinary tract infection. It is not commonly used in veterinary medicine and little good evidence is available to confirm its efficacy in dogs or cats.

Pharmacology/Actions

In an acidic urinary environment (pH <6.5), methenamine is converted to formaldehyde. Formaldehyde is a non-specific antibacterial agent that exerts a bactericidal effect. It can have activity against a variety of bacteria, including both gram-positive (*Staphylococcus aureus, S. epidermidis,* Enterococcus) and gram-negative organisms (*E. Coli,* Enterobacter, Klebsiella, Proteus, and *Pseudomonas aeruginosa*), but may be less effective against those that produce urease (increased pH). Reportedly, methenamine has activity against fungal urinary tract infections.

Hippuric acid is added primarily to help acidify the urine, but it also has some non-specific antibacterial activity. Bacterial resistance to formaldehyde or hippuric acid does not usually occur.

Pharmacokinetics

Human data: While methenamine and its salts are well absorbed from the GI tract, up to 30% of a dose may be hydrolyzed by gastric acid to ammonia and formaldehyde. With enteric-coated tablets, the amount hydrolyzed in the gut is reduced. While absorbed, plasma concentrations of both formaldehyde and methenamine are very low and have negligible systemic antibacterial activity. Methenamine does cross the placenta and is distributed into milk.

Within 24 hours, 70-90% of a dose is excreted unchanged into the urine. In acidic urine, conversion to ammonia and formaldehyde takes place. Peak formaldehyde concentrations occur in the urine at ≈2 hours post-dose (3-8 hours with enteric-coated tablets).

Contraindications/Precautions/Warnings

Methenamine and its salts are contraindicated in patients known to be hypersensitive to it, with renal insufficiency, metabolic acidosis, severe hepatic impairment (due to ammonia production), or severe dehydration.

Do not confuse methenamine with methionine.

Adverse Effects

The most likely adverse effect noted is gastrointestinal upset, with nausea, vomiting, and anorexia predominant. Some patients may develop dysuria, probably secondary to irritation due to high formaldehyde concentrations. Cats reportedly do not tolerate methenamine as well as dogs. Lipoid pneumonitis has been reported in some humans receiving prolonged therapy with the suspension. Potentially, systemic acidosis could occur.

Because methenamine requires acid urine to be beneficial, urine pH should ideally be kept at or below 5.5. Some urea-splitting bacteria (*e.g.,* Proteus and some strains of staphylococci, Enterobacter

and Pseudomonas) may increase urine pH. Addition of a urinary acidification program may be required using dietary modification and acidifying drugs (*e.g.,* ascorbic acid, methionine, sodium biphosphate, ammonium chloride).

Reproductive/Nursing Safety

While methenamine crosses the placenta and lab animal studies have not demonstrated any teratogenic effects, it should be used with caution during pregnancy. In humans, the FDA categorizes this drug as category *C* for use during pregnancy (*Animal studies have shown an adverse effect on the fetus, but there are no adequate studies in humans; or there are no animal reproduction studies and no adequate studies in humans.*)

Methenamine enters milk, but adverse effects have not been reported in nursing children of mothers taking methenamine.

Overdosage/Acute Toxicity

Dogs have received single IV dosages of up to 600 mg/kg of methenamine hippurate without overt toxic effects. Large oral overdoses should be handled using established gut emptying protocols, maintaining hydration status and supporting as required.

Drug Interactions

The following drug interactions have either been reported or are theoretical in humans or animals receiving methenamine and may be of significance in veterinary patients. Unless otherwise noted, use together is not necessarily contraindicated, but weigh the potential risks and perform additional monitoring when appropriate.

▪ **SULFONAMIDES:** Use of methenamine with sulfonamides is not recommended. An insoluble precipitate may form in urine.

▪ **URINE ALKALINIZING DRUGS** (*e.g.,* **calcium or magnesium containing antacids, carbonic anhydrase inhibitors, citrates, sodium bicarbonate, thiazide diuretics**): Use of urinary alkalinizing drugs may reduce the efficacy of the methenamine.

Laboratory Considerations

▪ Urinary values of the following compounds may be falsely elevated: **catecholamines, vanillylmandelic acid (VMA), 17-hydrocorticosteroid.**

▪ Falsely decreased urinary values of **estriol** or **5-HIAA** may occur.

▪ Methenamine may cause may cause false-positive **urine glucose determinations** when using cupric sulfate solution (Benedict's Solution, *Clinitest*®) and false-negative tests utilizing the glucose oxidase (*Tes-Tape*®, *Clinistix*®) method.

Doses

▪ **DOGS/CATS:**

For recurrent UTI (extra-label): There is little evidence to support clinical use in dogs, but it theoretically could be effective. Recommended anecdotal doses usually range from 10 – 20 mg/kg PO q8-12h. Practically, this is rounded off to the nearest 250 mg (as usually only available in 1 gram tablets). Requires acidic urine (pH ≤6; optimally <5.5) for efficacy and an acidifying diet and/or urinary acidifiers may be required. It reportedly is not tolerated very well in cats but some have recommended 250 mg per cat PO twice daily.

Monitoring

▪ Urine pH.

▪ Efficacy.

Client Information

▪ Give with food to prevent stomach upset. Tablets are very large, but can be split.

▪ Vomiting, nausea (acting 'sick'), and reduced appetite are common. Cats may not tolerate the drug as well as dogs.

- Requires urine to be acidic to work properly. Your veterinarian may recommend other drugs (*e.g.*, vitamin C, methionine, etc.) or dietary changes to increase urine acidity.

Chemistry/Synonyms

Methenamine is chemically unrelated to other anti-infective agents. It is commercially available as methenamine hippurate or methenamine mandelate. Methenamine mandelate occurs as a white, crystalline powder and contains approximately 48% methenamine and 52% mandelic acid. It is very soluble in water. Methenamine hippurate occurs as a white, crystalline powder with a sour taste and contains approximately 44% methenamine and 56% hippuric acid. It is freely soluble in water.

Methenamine may also be known as: hexamine amygdalate, hexamine mandelate, mandelato de metenamina, *Aci-steril®*, *Mandelamine®*, *Hiprex®*, *Reflux®*, *Urocedulamin®*, and *Urex®*.

Storage/Stability

Commercially available methenamine products should be stored at room temperature. Because acids hydrolyze methenamine to formaldehyde and ammonia, do not mix with acidic vehicles before administering.

Compatibility/Compounding Considerations

Methenamine is physically **incompatible** when mixed with most alkaloids and metallic salts (*e.g.*, ferric, mercuric or silver salts). Ammonium salts or alkalis will darken methenamine.

Dosage Forms/Regulatory Status

VETERINARY-LABELED PRODUCTS: NONE.

HUMAN-LABELED PRODUCTS:

Methenamine Hippurate Oral Tablets: 1 gram; *Hiprex®*, *Urex®*; (Rx)

Methenamine Mandelate Tablets: 0.5 gram & 1 gram; generic; (Rx). There may be methenamine mandelate products being marketed, but they are not listed as an FDA-approved drug.

Revisions/References

Monograph revised/updated April 2014.

Methimazole

(meth-**im**-a-zole)   Tapazole®

Antithyroid

Prescriber Highlights

► Used for medical treatment of feline hyperthyroidism.

► Potentially, transdermal gels with methimazole may have efficacy in cats (or owners) that cannot tolerate oral dosing.

► Contraindications: Hypersensitivity to it.

► Caution: History of, or concurrent: hematologic abnormalities, liver disease, or autoimmune disease.

► Adverse Effects: Most occur within first 3 mos. of treatment: vomiting, anorexia, & depression most frequent. Eosinophilia, leukopenia, & lymphocytosis are usually transient. Rare, but serious: self-induced excoriations, bleeding, hepatopathy, thrombocytopenia, agranulocytosis, positive direct antiglobulin test, & acquired myasthenia gravis.

► Place kittens on milk replacer if mother receiving drug.

► Very bitter taste.

Uses/Indications

Methimazole is considered by most clinicians in North America as the drug of choice when using medications to treat feline hyperthyroidism. Sustained-release carbimazole is not presently available commercially and propylthiouracil has significantly higher inci-

dences of adverse reactions when compared to methimazole and is rarely used today.

Transdermal methimazole (in PLO gel; 2.5 mg twice daily) has been used with some therapeutic success in cats that do not tolerate oral dosing. Efficacy may require four or more weeks to detect. Studies are ongoing.

Methimazole may be useful for the prophylactic prevention of cisplatin-induced nephrotoxicity in dogs.

Pharmacology/Actions

Methimazole interferes with iodine incorporation into tyrosyl residues of thyroglobulin, thereby inhibiting the synthesis of thyroid hormones. It also inhibits iodinated tyrosyl residues from coupling to form iodothyronine. Methimazole has no effect on the release or activity of thyroid hormones already formed or in the general circulation.

Pharmacokinetics

Information on the pharmacokinetics of methimazole in cats is available (Trepanier, L.A. *et al.* 1989). These researchers reported that in normal cats, the bioavailability of the drug is highly variable (45-98%), as is the volume of distribution (0.12 – 0.84 L/kg). After oral dosing, plasma elimination half-life ranges from 2.3-10.2 hours. There is usually a 1-3 week lag time between starting the drug and significant reductions in serum T4.

A study in cats using compounded (PLO-base) transdermal methimazole (either 2.5 mg/kg twice daily or 5 mg/kg once daily), found at 1 and 3 weeks after starting treatment all cats showed sustained suppression of T4 concentration during the 10-hours after administration. In both groups T4 concentrations measured immediately before the next methimazole treatment were not significantly different when compared with any time point after application (Boretti *et al.* 2013).

In dogs, methimazole has a serum half-life of 8-9 hours. Methimazole apparently concentrates in canine thyroid tissue.

Contraindications/Precautions/Warnings

Methimazole is contraindicated in patients who are hypersensitive to it, carbimazole, or the excipient, polyethylene glycol. The veterinary label also states that it is contraindicated in cats with autoimmune disease, primary liver disease, renal failure, hematologic disorders or coagulopathies, or pregnant or lactating queens. Cats with liver disease could potentially receive the drug at low dosages with dose titration with liver function tests intensely monitored. Treatment of hyperthyroid cats with methimazole can unmask underlying renal disease.

Do not confuse methimazole with methazolamide or metolazone.

Adverse Effects

Most adverse effects associated with methimazole use in cats occur within the first 3 months of therapy with vomiting, anorexia, and depression/lethargy occurring most frequently. GI effects occur in about 10% of treated cats may be related to the drug's bitter taste or direct gastric irritation and are usually transient. Cats that cannot tolerate GI adverse effects may tolerate transdermal methimazole.

Eosinophilia, leukopenia, thrombocytopenia, and lymphocytosis may be noted in approximately 15% of cats treated within the first 8 weeks of therapy. These hematologic effects usually are also transient and generally do not require drug withdrawal. But blood dyscrasias (severe thrombocytopenia/bleeding, neutropenia, agranulocytosis) can occur in approximately 4% of cats and typically occur within the first 1-2 months of treatment. Methimazole re-challenge can cause recurrence (Trepanier, L. A. 2013).

Methimazole treated cats can develop pruritus and facial excoriations. Incidence is reported as 2-3% with the majority of cases afflicted within the first 3 weeks of treatment (Trepanier, L. A. 2013). However, an incidence rate of up to 15% has been reported (Voie *et al.* 2012).

Other serious but rare adverse effects include: hepatopathy (1.5%), and positive direct antiglobulin test (1.9%). These effects generally require withdrawal of the drug and adjunctive therapy.

Up to 50% of cats receiving methimazole chronically (>6 months) will develop a positive ANA, requiring dosage reduction.

Rarely, cats will develop an acquired myasthenia gravis that requires either withdrawal or concomitant glucocorticoid therapy.

A guide for <u>Prevention and Management for Methimazole Toxicity</u> has been published (Trepanier, L. A. 2013). It includes:

- Counsel owners to monitor for lethargy, vomiting, inappetence, jaundice, or pruritus.
- Stop drug at first potential sign of adverse reaction.
- Evaluate cat as soon as possible: 1) Physical examination for skin excoriations; 2) Rule out blood dyscrasia (complete blood count); 3) Rule out hepatotoxicity (ALT, bilirubin, SAP)—compare with pretreatment liver enzymes (often reversibly increased in hyperthyroid cats); 4) Evaluate for renal decompensation (blood urea nitrogen–BUN, creatinine, serum T4).
- If simple gastrointestinal (GI) upset (blood work is normal): Plan dose reduction or switch to transdermal methimazole, which has a lower incidence of GI upset than oral methimazole.
- If blood dyscrasia, hepatopathy, or facial excoriation: Plan radioiodine, or if not available, thyroidectomy with atenolol pretreatment. **Note:** The efficacy of glutathione precursors or glucocorticoids has not been evaluated for methimazole in this setting.

Reproductive/Nursing Safety

High levels of methimazole cross the placenta and may induce hypothyroidism in kittens born of queens receiving the drug. The veterinary label states that the drug should not be used in pregnant or lactating queens as laboratory studies in mice and rats have shown evidence of teratogenic and embryotoxic effects.

In humans, the FDA categorizes this drug as category *D* for use during pregnancy (*There is evidence of human fetal risk, but the potential benefits from the use of the drug in pregnant women may be acceptable despite its potential risks.*)

Levels higher than those found in plasma are detected in human breast milk. It is suggested that kittens be placed on a milk replacer after receiving colostrum from mothers on methimazole.

Overdosage/Acute Toxicity

Acute toxicity that may be seen with overdosage include those that are listed above under Adverse Effects. Agranulocytosis, hepatopathy, and thrombocytopenias are perhaps the most serious effects that may be seen. Treatment consists of following standard protocols in handling an oral ingestion (empty stomach, if not contraindicated, administer charcoal, etc.) and to treat symptomatically and supportively.

Drug Interactions

The following drug interactions have either been reported or are theoretical in humans or animals receiving methimazole and may be of significance in veterinary patients. Unless otherwise noted, use together is not necessarily contraindicated, but weigh the potential risks and perform additional monitoring when appropriate.

- **BENZIMIDAZOLE ANTIPARASITICS:** Methimazole can reduce hepatic oxidation of benzimidazoles and increase blood levels.
- **BETA-BLOCKERS:** Veterinary label states: A reduction in dose may be needed when the patient becomes euthyroid.
- **BUPROPION:** Potential for increased risk for hepatotoxicity; increased monitoring (LFT's) necessary.

- **DIGOXIN:** Methimazole may decrease digoxin efficacy, but the veterinary label states: A reduction in dose may be needed when the patient becomes euthyroid.
- **PHENOBARBITAL:** Veterinary label states: Concurrent use of phenobarbital may reduce the clinical effectiveness.
- **THEOPHYLLINE:** Veterinary label states: A reduction in dose may be needed when the patient becomes euthyroid.
- **WARFARIN:** In human hyperthyroid patients, the metabolism of vitamin K clotting factors is increased, resulting in increased sensitivity to oral anticoagulants. By reducing the effects of hyperthyroidism, methimazole may decrease clotting factor metabolism reduce the effects of warfarin. However, patients that are euthyroid on methimazole and receiving warfarin may develop hypoprothrombinemia if methimazole is stopped and they once again become thyrotoxic. The veterinary label states: Anticoagulants may be potentiated by methimazole. Recommendation: If methimazole and warfarin are used together, increased monitoring anticoagulant effect is warranted.

Doses

- **CATS:**

For hyperthyroidism:

Labeled Dose (FDA-approved): The starting dose is 2.5 mg per cat administered every 12 hours. Following 3 weeks of treatment, the dose should be titrated to effect based on individual serum total T4 (TT4) levels and clinical response. Dose adjustments should be made in 2.5 mg increments. The maximum total dosage is 20 mg per day divided, not to exceed 10 mg as a single administration. (Adapted from label Information; *Felimazole®*—Dechra)

Extra-Label Doses:

<u>Oral</u>: The panel of the publication *"Best practice for the pharmacological management of hyperthyroid cats with antithyroid drugs"* (Daminet *et al.* 2014) recommends an initial dosage of using 2.5 mg per cat PO twice a day; an initial dose of 5 mg/kg PO twice a day can be used in cases of extremely elevated total T4 (TT4). TT4 is evaluated 2-3 weeks after starting therapy. Most cats will become euthyroid after this time. Dosages are titrated in 2.5 mg/day increments to obtain and maintain circulating total thyroxine (TT4) concentrations in the lower half of the reference interval. Once euthyroidism is achieved, once a day dosing can be considered. (Daminet *et al.* 2014)

<u>Transdermal</u>: Methimazole (50 mg/mL; 5 mg/0.1 mL) in PLO for <u>transdermal administration</u>: 2.5 mg to inner pinna q12h. Person applying should wear gloves or finger cots. Somewhat lower efficacy than PO (67% vs. 82% euthyroid at 4 weeks). Lower incidence of GI effects with transdermal (4% vs. 24%). No difference in facial excoriation, neutropenia, hepatotoxicity, or thrombocytopenia. Drawbacks for transdermal administration include: erythema at application site, increased cost, and stability of compounded medication (2 weeks guaranteed stable) (Trepanier, L. 2006). The aforementioned *"Best practices…"* panel states: Topical preparations, when available, could be useful for uncooperative cats, and the same or a slightly higher starting dose as for the oral route should be used (Daminet *et al.* 2014).

- **SMALL MAMMALS**

For hyperthyroidism in Guinea pigs: From a case report of 3 animals treated medically. Initial dose was 2 mg/kg PO once daily. Based on these cases, the authors concluded that all animals showed improvement of clinical signs during therapy, but not until the dosage or frequency of administration was increased. Therefore, regular monitoring of circulating total T4 concentrations might be required to determine appropriate dosage and dosage frequency. (Kunzel *et al.* 2013)

Monitoring

Also see the guide for <u>Prevention and Management for Methimazole Toxicity</u> (Trepanier, L. A. 2013) in the Adverse Effects section.

During first 3 months of therapy (baseline values and every 2-3 weeks):

- CBC, platelet count.
- Serum T4.
- If indicated by symptomatology: liver function tests, ANA.

After stabilized (at least 3 months of therapy):

- Total T4 (TT4) at 3-6 month intervals.
- Other diagnostic tests as dictated by adverse effects.
- The label for the feline-approved product states: Hematology, biochemistry, and TT4 should be evaluated prior to initiating treatment and monitored after 3 and 6 weeks of treatment. Thereafter, bloodwork should be monitored every 3 months and the dose adjusted as necessary. Cats receiving doses >10 mg per day should be monitored more frequently.

Client Information

- This drug will decrease excessive thyroid hormones, but does not cure the condition; following the treatment regimen is necessary for success.
- The manufacturer warns that: Pregnant women or women who may become pregnant, and nursing mothers should wear gloves when handling tablets, litter or bodily fluids of treated cats.
- Available in different dosage forms, including a topical gel.
- Most side effects, including vomiting, decreased appetite, or lethargy (tiredness; lack of energy) occur in the first 3 months of therapy.

Chemistry/Synonyms

A thioimidazole-derivative antithyroid drug, methimazole occurs as a white to pale buff crystalline powder, having a faint characteristic odor and a melting point of 144-147°C. It is freely soluble (1 gram in 5 mL) in water or alcohol.

Methimazole may also be known as: thiamazole, mercazolylum, methylmercaptoimidazole, thiamazolum; tiamazol, *Felimazole®* and *Tapazole®*.

Storage/Stability

Methimazole tablets should be stored in well-closed, light-resistant containers at room temperature; protect from moisture.

Compatibility/Compounding Considerations

No specific information noted.

Dosage Forms/Regulatory Status

VETERINARY-LABELED PRODUCTS:

Methimazole Tablets (sugar-coated): 2.5 mg & 5 mg; *Felimazole®*; (Rx). FDA-approved (NADA 141-292) for use in cats.

HUMAN-LABELED PRODUCTS:

Methimazole Tablets (plain & scored): 5 mg & 10 mg; *Tapazole®*, generic; (Rx)

Revisions/References

Monograph revised/updated April 2014.

Boretti, F. S., et al. (2013). Duration of T4 Suppression in Hyperthyroid Cats Treated Once and Twice Daily with Transdermal Methimazole. Journal of Veterinary Internal Medicine 27(2): 377-81.
Daminet, S., et al. (2014). Best practice for the pharmacological management of hyperthyroid cats with antithyroid drugs. Journal of Small Animal Practice 55(1): 4-13.
Kunzel, F., et al. (2013). Hyperthyroidism in four guinea pigs: clinical manifestations, diagnosis, and treatment. Journal of Small Animal Practice 54(12): 667-71.
Trepanier, L. (2006). Transdermal medication in cats: Can it be done? Proceedings: ECVIM-CA Congress. accessed via Veterinary Information Network; vin.com
Trepanier, L. A. (2013). Idiosyncratic Drug Toxicity Affecting the Liver, Skin, and Bone Marrow in Dogs and Cats. Veterinary Clinics of North America-Small Animal Practice 43(5): 1055-+.
Trepanier, L. A., et al. (1989). Methimazole Pharmacokinetics in the Normal Cat. Proceedings: American College of Veterinary Internal Medicine. accessed via Veterinary Information Network; vin.com
Voie, K. L., et al. (2012). Drug Hypersensitivity Reactions Targeting the Skin in Dogs and Cats. Journal of Veterinary Internal Medicine 26(4): 863-74.

Methionine
dl-Methionine

(me-thye-oh-neen)   Racemethionine

Urinary Acidifier; Nutritional

Prescriber Highlights

▶ Used primarily as a urinary acidifier; questionable efficacy in reducing stone formation.
▶ Contraindications: Renal failure, pancreatic disease, hepatic insufficiency, preexisting acidosis, oxalate or urate calculi; not recommended for kittens.
▶ Adverse Effects: Gastrointestinal distress (food may alleviate), Heinz-body hemolytic anemia (cats).
▶ Drug interactions.

Uses/Indications

In small animals, methionine has been used primarily for its urine acidification effects in the treatment and prevention of certain types (*e.g.*, struvite) of stone formation and to reduce ammoniacal urine odor. Use is generally not recommended unless urine pH is >6.5. In food animals, it has been used as a nutritional supplement in swine and poultry feed and in the treatment of ketosis in cattle. It has been touted as a treatment for laminitis in horses and cattle (purportedly provides a disulfide bond substrate to maintain the hoof-pedal bone bond), but definitive studies demonstrating its effectiveness for this indication are lacking. It potentially may be useful as a urinary acidifier to reduce uroliths in male (wethers) goats.

Methionine is used in humans to reduce urine ammonia (pH) and odor.

Pharmacology/Actions

Methionine has several pharmacologic effects. It is an essential amino acid (l-form) and nutrient, a lipotrope (prevents or corrects fatty liver in choline deficiency), and a urine acidifier. Two molecules of methionine can be converted to one molecule of cysteine. Methionine supplies both sulfhydryl and methyl groups to the liver for metabolic processes. Choline is formed when methionine supplies a methyl group to ethanolamine. After methionine is metabolized, sulfate is excreted in the urine as sulfuric acid, thereby acidifying it.

Pharmacokinetics

No information is available on the pharmacokinetics of this agent in veterinary species or humans.

Contraindications/Precautions/Warnings

Methionine (in therapeutic doses) is contraindicated in patients with renal failure or pancreatic disease. If used in patients with frank hepatic insufficiency, methionine can cause increased production of mercaptan-like compounds and intensify the signs of hepatic dementia or coma. Methionine should not be given to animals with preexisting acidosis, oxalate or urate calculi. It is not recommended for use in kittens.

Do not confuse methionine with methenamine or S-adenosyl-L-methionine (SAMe).

Adverse Effects

At usual doses, gastrointestinal distress can occur; give with food to alleviate this effect and to enhance efficacy. Methionine may cause Heinz-body hemolytic anemia in cats. See Overdosage (below) for other potential adverse effects.

Unmonitored use with an acidifying diet (*e.g.*, s/d, c/d), may lead to signs associated with overdose.

Reproductive/Nursing Safety

No specific information was located; methionine could, potentially, cause fetal acidosis.

Overdosage/Acute Toxicity

Methionine may be toxic to kittens who consume other cats' food in which methionine has been added. When methionine was administered at a dose of 2 grams orally per day to mature cats, anorexia, methemoglobinemia, Heinz body formation (with resultant hemolytic anemia), ataxia and cyanosis were noted. Metabolic acidosis, particularly in combination with an acidifying diet may occur with overdoses in any species. No specific information was located on the treatment of methionine overdosage.

Drug Interactions

The following drug interactions have either been reported or are theoretical in humans or animals receiving methionine and may be of significance in veterinary patients. Unless otherwise noted, use together is not necessarily contraindicated, but weigh the potential risks and perform additional monitoring when appropriate.

- **AMINOGLYCOSIDES (gentamicin, amikacin**, etc.): The aminoglycosides are more effective in an alkaline medium; urine acidification may diminish these drugs effectiveness in treating bacterial urinary tract infections.

- **ERYTHROMYCIN**: Is more effective in an alkaline medium; urine acidification may diminish erythromycin effectiveness in treating bacterial urinary tract infections.

- **QUINIDINE**: Urine acidification may increase the renal excretion of quinidine.

Doses

- **DOGS:**

    For urine acidification/struvite dissolution (extra-label): At approximately 100 mg/kg PO q12h methionine is safe and effective in dissolving presumed infection-induced struvite uroliths in dogs in combination with an appropriate anti-microbial agent without using a struvite dissolution diet. Successful dissolution occurs when uroliths decrease in size by at least 50% at the 1-month re-evaluation. If uroliths do not decrease in size by at least 50% at the 1 month re-evaluation, then consideration should be given to (1) lack of compliance, (2) inappropriate dosage, (3) difficulty in controlling the bacterial urinary tract infection, or (4) uroliths being composed of other minerals, most likely calcium oxalate, in addition to or instead of struvite. (Bartges *et al.* 2010)

- **CATS:**

    For urine acidification (urine pH >6.5); (extra-label): If diet and antimicrobials do not reduce pH, 1000 – 1500 mg per cat per day given in the food once daily. (Lewis *et al.* 1987). **Note:** Use with caution in kittens and do not overdose.

- **SMALL RUMINANTS**

    For urine acidification (extra-label): From a small study (n=5) done in male goats (wethers): 200 mg/kg/day PO in feed. Authors concluded that methionine has potential promise as a more palatable alternative for urine acidification in small ruminants that is worthy of further investigation. (Grissett *et al.* 2012)

Monitoring

- Urine pH (Urine pH's of ≤6.5 have been recommended as goal of therapy).
- Blood pH if signs of toxicity are present.

- CBC in cats exhibiting signs of toxicity.

Client Information

- Give with meals or mixed in food, unless otherwise instructed by veterinarian.

Chemistry/Synonyms

A sulfur-containing amino acid, methionine occurs as a white, crystalline powder with a characteristic odor. One gram is soluble in ≈30 mL of water and it is very slightly soluble in alcohol. 74.6 mg is equivalent to 1 mEq of methionine.

Methionine may also be known as: dl-methionine, racemethionine, M, s-methionine, l-methionine, methioninum, *Ammonil*®, *Methigel*®, *Methio-Form*®, *Pedameth*® and *Uracid*®.

Storage/Stability

Methionine should be stored at room temperature.

Compatibility/Compounding Considerations

No specific information noted.

Dosage Forms/Regulatory Status

VETERINARY-LABELED PRODUCTS:

Methionine is labeled for use in dogs, cats, and horses in pharmaceutical dosage forms, but at the time of review (04/14), there were no methionine products listed in the FDA's "Green Book" of approved products. Products labeled as nutritionals may be approved for use in other species. Depending on the product, methionine may be available without prescription. Methionine is an ingredient in many other nutritional products.

Methionine Tablets: 200 mg and 500 mg; *Ammonil*® *Tablets*, generic; (Rx). Labeled for use in cats and dogs.

Methionine Tablets Chewable: 500 mg; *Methio-Form*®; (Rx). Labeled for use in cats and dogs.

Methionine Powder (concentration varies with product); May also be called: d-l-Methionine Powder. Labeled for use in dogs and cats.

Methionine Gel: 400 mg (8%) in 120.5 gram tubes; *Methigel*®; (OTC). Labeled for use in cats and dogs.

HUMAN-LABELED PRODUCTS:

Methionine Capsules & Tablets: 500 mg; generic; (OTC)

Methionine Oral Powder 100 mg/packet; generic; (OTC)

Topical Ointments, cream, lotion, pads and powder available.

Revisions/References

Monograph revised/updated April 2014.

Bartges, J. & T. Moyers (2010). Evaluation of D, L-Methionine and Antimicrobial Agents for Medical Dissolution of Spontaneously Occurring Infection-Induced Struvite Urocystoliths in Dogs. Proceedings: ACVIM. accessed via Veterinary Information Network; vin.com

Grissett, G., et al. (2012). Evaluation of Orally Supplemented D, L-Methionine as a Urine Acidifier for Small Ruminants. Proceedings: ACVIM. accessed via Veterinary Information Network; vin.com

Lewis, L. D., et al. (1987). Feline Urological Syndrome. *Small Animal Clinician Nutrition III.* Topeka, Mark Morris Assoc.

Methocarbamol

(meth-oh-**kar**-ba-mole)   Robaxin®

Muscle Relaxant

Prescriber Highlights

▶ Oral & injectable centrally acting muscle relaxant; appears useful in treating muscle tremors associated with toxic agents.

▶ Contraindications: Food animals, renal disease (injectable only), hypersensitivity to it.

▶ Adverse Effects: Sedation, salivation, emesis, lethargy, weakness, & ataxia.

▶ Give IV slowly (don't exceed 2 mL/min); avoid extravasation; do not give SC.

▶ Injectable is becoming expensive and availability is an issue.

Uses/Indications

In dogs and cats, methocarbamol is indicated (FDA approved) "as adjunctive therapy of acute inflammatory and traumatic conditions of the skeletal muscle and to reduce muscular spasms." In horses, intravenous use is indicated (FDA approved) "as adjunctive therapy of acute inflammatory and traumatic conditions of the skeletal muscle to reduce muscular spasms, and effect striated muscle relaxation" (Package insert; *Robaxin®V*). Intravenous methocarbamol has been found useful in treating tremors and muscle fasciculations associated with various toxicities in dogs and cats.

Pharmacology/Actions

Methocarbamol's exact mechanism of causing skeletal muscle relaxation is unknown. It is thought to work centrally, perhaps by general depressant effects. It has no direct relaxant effects on striated muscle, nerve fibers, or the motor endplate. It will not directly relax contracted skeletal muscles. The drug has a secondary sedative effect.

Pharmacokinetics

Limited pharmacokinetic data is available in veterinary species. In humans, methocarbamol has an onset of action of ≈30 minutes after oral administration. Peak levels occur approximately 2 hours after dosing. Serum half-life is ≈1-2 hours. The drug is metabolized and the inactive metabolites are excreted into the urine and the feces (small amounts).

In horses, an older study showed that methocarbamol plasma clearance appeared to be dose dependent after IV administration as lower clearances were measured after higher doses were given. The serum half-life of methocarbamol in that study was approximately 60-70 minutes (Muir, Sams, and Ashcraft 1984). A more recent study where both IV (15 mg/kg) and oral pharmacokinetics were evaluated found an elimination half-life of ≈3 hours and an oral bioavailability of around 50% (Rumpler *et al.* 2014).

Guaifenesin is a minor metabolite of methocarbamol and was quantifiable after oral dosing, which may have racing regulatory ramifications. However, it probably has little clinical effect.

Contraindications/Precautions/Warnings

Because the injectable product contains polyethylene glycol 300, the manufacturer lists known or suspected renal pathology as a contraindication to injectable methocarbamol therapy. Polyethylene glycol 300 has been noted to increase preexisting acidosis and urea retention in humans with renal impairment.

Methocarbamol should not be used in patients hypersensitive to it or in animals to be used for food purpose.

Do not administer subcutaneously and avoid extravasation. Do not exceed 2 mL per minute when injecting IV in dogs and cats.

Adverse Effects

Side effects can include sedation, salivation, emesis, lethargy, weakness, and ataxia in dogs and cats. Sedation and ataxia are possible in horses. Because of its CNS depressant effects, methocarbamol may impair the abilities of working animals.

Reproductive/Nursing Safety

Methocarbamol should be used with caution during pregnancy as studies demonstrating its safety during pregnancy are lacking. In humans, the FDA categorizes this drug as category *C* for use during pregnancy (*Animal studies have shown an adverse effect on the fetus, but there are no adequate studies in humans; or there are no animal reproduction studies and no adequate studies in humans.*). In a separate system evaluating the safety of drugs in canine and feline pregnancy (Papich 1989), this drug is categorized as class: *C* (*These drugs may have potential risks. Studies in people or laboratory animals have uncovered risks, and these drugs should be used cautiously as a last resort when the benefit of therapy clearly outweighs the risks.*)

It is not known whether methocarbamol is excreted in milk. Exercise caution, but the American Academy of Pediatrics classifies methocarbamol as compatible with women breastfeeding.

Overdosage/Acute Toxicity

Overdosage is generally characterized by CNS depressant effects (loss of righting reflex, prostration). Excessive doses in dogs and cats may be represented by emesis, salivation, weakness, and ataxia.

There were 70 single agent exposures to methocarbamol reported to the ASPCA Animal Poison Control Center (APCC) during 2009-2013. There were 64 dogs, 15 of which were symptomatic. The most common signs were lethargy (27%), vomiting (27%) and ataxia (20%).

If the overdose is after oral administration, emptying the gut may be indicated if the overdose was recent. Do not induce emesis if the patient's continued consciousness is not assured. Other clinical signs should be treated if severe and in a supportive manner.

Drug Interactions

The following drug interactions have either been reported or are theoretical in humans or animals receiving methocarbamol and may be of significance in veterinary patients. Unless otherwise noted, use together is not necessarily contraindicated, but weigh the potential risks and perform additional monitoring when appropriate.

- **CNS DEPRESSANTS, OTHER**: Additive depression may occur when given with other CNS depressant agents.
- **PYRIDOSTIGMINE**: One human patient, with myasthenia gravis and taking pyridostigmine, developed severe weakness after receiving methocarbamol.

Laboratory Considerations

- Urinary values of the following compounds may be falsely elevated: **vanillylmandelic acid (VMA)**, or **5-HIAA**.

Doses

- **DOGS/CATS:**

  Labeled dose (FDA-approved): **Injectable:** <u>For relief of moderate conditions</u>: 44 mg/kg IV; <u>For controlling severe effects of strychnine and tetanus</u>: 55 – 220 mg/kg IV, do not exceed 330 mg/kg/day. Administer half the estimated dose rapidly, then wait until animal starts to relax and continue administration to effect. **Oral (tablets):** Initially, 132 mg/kg/day PO divided q8h-q12h, then 61 – 132 mg/kg divided q8-12h. If no response in 5 days, discontinue. (Package insert; *Robaxin®-V*)

  Extra-label doses for adjunctive treatment of poisonings (or intoxications) associated with muscle tremors (pyrethroids, metaldehyde, strychnine, CNS stimulants [caffeine, amphetamines,

Guarna, etc.], SSRIs, compost ingestions, etc.): Although there are no controlled studies documenting efficacy in animals, consider using an initial IV bolus followed by a CRI or multiple (if required) IV boluses. Initially give 40 – 50 mg/kg IV slowly over 3-5 minutes to clinical effect (resolution or near-resolution of clinical signs). Then repeat as necessary or follow with a CRI at an initial rate of 10 mg/kg/hr. Titrate the bolus dose/frequency or CRI administration rate, to clinical effect. The labeled maximum of 330 mg/kg/day can be exceeded if necessary, but patient must be monitored for profound CNS depression, seizures and hypotension.

■ **HORSES:** (NOTE: ARCI UCGFS CLASS 4 DRUG)
Labeled-dose (FDA-approved): For moderate conditions: 4.4 – 22 mg/kg IV to effect; for severe conditions: 22 – 55 mg/kg IV. (Package insert, *Robaxin*®-*V*)

Monitoring
■ Level of muscle relaxation/sedation.

Client Information
■ May be given with or without food.
■ Drowsiness/sedation is the most common side effect.
■ May cause dark urine, but this is not a problem.

Chemistry/Synonyms
A centrally acting muscle relaxant related structurally to guaifenesin, methocarbamol occurs as a fine, white powder with a characteristic odor. In water, it has a solubility of 25 mg/mL. The pH of commercial injection is approximately 4-5.

Methocarbamol may also be known as: guaiphenesin carbamate, *Robinax*® and *Robaxin*®.

Storage/Stability
Methocarbamol tablets should be stored at room temperature in tight containers; the injection should be stored at room temperature and not frozen. Solutions prepared for IV infusion should not be refrigerated as a precipitate may form. Because a haze or precipitate may form, all diluted intravenous solutions should be physically inspected before administration.

Compatibility/Compounding Considerations
No specific information noted.

Dosage Forms/Regulatory Status
VETERINARY-LABELED PRODUCTS:
Note: As of April 2014, the two veterinary products below are still listed in the FDA's Green Book, but their marketing status is uncertain. The injectable is listed in the "Fort Dodge to Pfizer" acquired product listing, but is not listed on the Zoetis Animal Health website.

Methocarbamol Tablets: 500 mg; *Robaxin*®*V*; (Rx). FDA-approved for use in dogs and cats.

Methocarbamol Injection: 100 mg/mL in vials of 20 mL & 100 mL; *Robaxin*®-*V*; (Rx). FDA-approved for use in dogs, cats, and horses not intended for food.

The ARCI (Racing Commissioners International) has designated this drug as a class 4 substance. See the appendix for more information.

HUMAN-LABELED PRODUCTS:
Methocarbamol Tablets: 500 mg & 750 mg; *Robaxin*® & *Robaxin-750*®, generic; (Rx)

Methocarbamol Injection: 100 mg/mL in 10 mL vials; *Robaxin*®; (Rx)

Revisions/References
Monograph revised/updated April 2014.
Papich, M. (1989). Effects of drugs on pregnancy. *Current Veterinary Therapy X: Small Animal Practice.* R. Kirk. Philadelphia, Saunders: 1291-9.
Rumpler, M. J., et al. (2014). The pharmacokinetics of methocarbamol and guaifenesin after single intravenous and multiple-dose oral administration of methocarbamol in the horse. J. Vet. Pharmacol. Ther. 37(1): 25-34.

Methohexital Sodium
(meth-oh-**hex**-i-tal)   Brevital®
Ultra-Short Acting Barbiturate

Prescriber Highlights
▶ Infrequently used ultra-short acting barbiturate for anesthesia induction, or for anesthesia for very short procedures, especially in sight hounds. No analgesic or muscle relaxant properties. Can cause very rough recoveries in dogs if used alone; premed or continuation of gas anesthesia during methohexital recovery may help reduce/prevent rough recoveries.
▶ Contraindications: Absolute contraindications: absence of suitable veins for IV administration, history of hypersensitivity reactions to barbiturates, status asthmaticus. Relative contraindications: severe cardiovascular disease or preexisting ventricular arrhythmias, shock, increased intracranial pressure, myasthenia gravis, asthma, & conditions where hypnotic effects may be prolonged (*e.g.*, severe hepatic disease, myxedema, severe anemia, excessive premedication, etc.)
▶ Avoid extravasation.
▶ Adverse Effects: Apnea, hypotension, tremors, or seizures during recovery.
▶ C-IV Controlled Substance; relatively expensive.

Uses/Indications
Methohexital is sometimes used in small animals as an ultrashort acting anesthetic agent, but propofol has largely supplanted methohexital's use in small animals. However, because it is not dependent on redistribution to fat to reverse its effect, it may be useful in sight hound breeds. Because methohexital can induce anesthesia very rapidly, it may also be useful when general anesthesia must be administered to a patient with a full stomach, as an ET tube may be placed rapidly before aspiration of vomitus can occur.

Pharmacology/Actions
Methohexital is an ultra-short acting methylated oxybarbiturate anesthetic agent. It is about twice as potent as thiopental and its duration of action about half as long. Like all the barbiturates, methohexital acts by depressing the reticular activating center of the brain.

Pharmacokinetics
After IV injection, methohexital rapidly causes anesthesia (15-60 seconds). Its distribution half-life is 5-6 minutes. When used alone, a single dose will cause surgical anesthesia for 5-15 minutes. Unlike the thiobarbiturates, methohexital is rapidly metabolized by the liver and not dependent on redistribution to fat to reverse its effects. No drug is detectable in the body 24 hours after administration. Its elimination half-life is reported to be 3-5 hours. Recovery times in small animals average 30 minutes.

Contraindications/Precautions/Warnings
Contraindicated in patients hypersensitive to barbiturates or that do not have adequate veins for safe IV administration. Relative contraindications include: seizure-prone animals, severe cardiovascular disease or preexisting ventricular arrhythmias, shock, increased intracranial pressure, myasthenia gravis, asthma, and conditions where hypnotic effects may be prolonged (*e.g.*, severe hepatic disease, myxedema, severe anemia, excessive premedication, etc.).

These relative contraindications do not preclude the use of methohexital, but dosage adjustments must be considered and the drug must be given slowly and cautiously.

Repeated dosing or using an IV infusion are not recommended as recovery times can be significantly prolonged and increase the risk for complications.

Because of its unpredictability in cattle, it is not recommended for use in this species.

Adverse Effects

Methohexital can cause profound respiratory depression. The lethal dose may only be 2-3 times2-3X that of the anesthetic dose. Because excitation (including muscle tremors and seizures) can occur upon recovery, methohexital is generally recommended for use with a premed. Postoperative seizures have been reported and can be treated with IV diazepam.

In small animals (especially dogs), methohexital may induce rougher recoveries when compared to thiopental or other anesthetics. Premedication or using gas anesthetics during methohexital recovery phase may be helpful to reduce or prevent this occurrence.

Because of its rapid elimination and very short action, there is a possibility that methohexital's effects may diminish before inhalant anesthesia takes full effect.

Too rapid an injection may lead to apnea and hypotension. Barbiturates do not provide analgesia or any muscle relaxation.

Because it can be very irritating to tissues and localized necrosis can occur in soft tissue, methohexital solutions must be only given IV, and perivascular injection must be avoided. Extravasation injuries can be treated with multiple infiltrates of sterile normal saline. Lidocaine can be injected to reduce pain.

Reproductive/Nursing Safety

While safety of methohexital has not been established in pregnancy, doses of up to 7X those of humans given to pregnant rabbits and rats resulted in no overt teratogenicity or fetal harm. In humans, the FDA categorizes this drug as category *B* for use during pregnancy (*Animal studies have not yet demonstrated risk to the fetus, but there are no adequate studies in pregnant women; or animal studies have shown an adverse effect, but adequate studies in pregnant women have not demonstrated a risk to the fetus in the first trimester of pregnancy, and there is no evidence of risk in later trimesters.*)

Small amounts of thiopental have been detected in milk following administration of large doses to humans. It is unlikely that methohexital poses much risk to nursing offspring.

Overdosage/Acute Toxicity

See Adverse Effects above; figure dosages carefully.

Drug Interactions

The following drug interactions have either been reported or are theoretical in humans or animals receiving methohexital and may be of significance in veterinary patients. Unless otherwise noted, use together is not necessarily contraindicated, but weigh the potential risks and perform additional monitoring when appropriate.

- **CNS DEPRESSANT DRUGS** (*e.g.*, **ALPHA2-AGONISTS, OPIOIDS, etc.**): When used with other CNS depressant drugs, methohexital may have additive effects. Use with a pre-med is usually preferred to reduce methohexital dosage required for inductions and to decrease rough recoveries.

Doses

- **DOGS/CATS:**

  For anesthetic induction or light anesthesia for very short procedures (extra-label): <u>Dogs: For induction with premedication:</u> 5 mg/kg; give 1/2 to 3/4 of dose over 10 seconds. In 30 seconds if adequate plane is not reached to allow intubation, give additional drug. Delay will result in poor induction due to rapid redistribu-

tion. (McKelvey *et al.* 2000); <u>For induction or sole anesthetic in non-premedicated dogs or cats:</u> 11 mg/kg IV, give approximately 1/2 the dose rapidly and then titrate to effect. If premedicated, give 5.5 – 6.6 mg/kg IV, 10-30% is given rapidly IV and then the remainder titrated to effect. (Paddleford 1999)

Monitoring

- Plane of anesthesia.
- Respiratory rate/depth.
- Cardiac rate, rhythm and blood pressure.
- Upon recovery, monitor for CNS stimulation (seizures).

Client Information

- Methohexital should be used in a setting only where adequate monitoring and support are available.

Chemistry/Synonyms

An ultra-short acing barbiturate agent, methohexital occurs as a white, crystalline powder. It is freely soluble in water.

Methohexital sodium may also be known as: compound 25398, enallynymalnatrium, methohexitone sodium, *Brevimytal®*, *Brevital®*, and *Brietal®*.

Storage/Stability

Methohexital sodium powder for injection should be stored at room temperature (<25°C). Preferably, reconstitute the powder for injection with sterile water for injection. D5W or 0.9% sodium chloride may also be used, particularly when making concentrations of 0.2% (to avoid extreme hypotonicity). While the manufacturer states not to make concentrations >1%, some veterinary anesthesiologists will make concentrations of up 6% (especially when using in large animals). Do not use solutions with bacteriostatic agents to prepare the solution.

The labeling for this product was changed to reduce the permitted time after reconstitution to 24 hours primarily since the product did not contain preservatives. Formerly, the labeling stated that after reconstituting with sterile water for injection, solutions are stable for at least 6 weeks at room temperature and as long as the solution remains clear and colorless, it is permissible to use. Solutions of D5W or normal saline are not stable for much more than 24 hours after reconstituting. A study demonstrated that solutions reconstituted with sterile water to a concentration of 10 mg/mL were stable up to 6 weeks when refrigerated and did not show any antimicrobial growth (Beeman *et al.* 1994).

Compatibility/Compounding Considerations

Methohexital solutions are alkaline. Do **NOT** mix with acidic drugs (*e.g.*, atropine or succinylcholine). Refer to specialized references before attempting to mix methohexital with another drug. Methohexital is **incompatible** with silicone. Do not allow contact with silicone-treated rubber stoppers or silicone treated parts of disposable syringes.

Dosage Forms/Regulatory Status

VETERINARY-LABELED PRODUCTS: NONE.

The ARCI (Racing Commissioners International) has designated this drug as a class 2 substance. See the appendix for more information.

HUMAN-LABELED PRODUCTS:

Methohexital Sodium Powder for Injection: 500 mg & 2.5 grams in 50 mL multiple dose vials; *Brevital® Sodium*; (Rx, C-IV)

Revisions/References

Monograph revised/updated April 2014.

Beeman, C. S., et al. (1994). Stability of reconstituted methohexital sodium. Journal of Oral and Maxillofacial Surgery 52(4): 393-6.

McKelvey, D. & K. Hollingshead (2000). *Small Animal Anesthesia and Analgesia*, Mosby. St Louis.

Paddleford, R. (1999). *Manual of Small Animal Anesthesia*, WB Saunders. Philadelphia.

Methotrexate
Methotrexate Sodium

(meth-oh-**trex**-ate)   MTX, Amethopterin

Antineoplastic, Immunosuppressive

Prescriber Highlights

▶ Antineoplastic/immunosuppressant used primarily for lymphomas & some solid tumors in dogs & cats.

▶ Contraindications: Preexisting bone marrow depression, severe hepatic or renal insufficiency, or hypersensitivity to MTX.

▶ Caution: If patient susceptible or has preexisting clinical signs associated with the adverse reactions associated with this drug.

▶ Adverse Effects: GI (diarrhea, nausea, & vomiting); Higher dosage: listlessness, GI toxicity (ulcers, mucosal sloughing, stomatitis), hematopoietic toxicity (nadir at 4-6 days), hepatopathy, renal tubular necrosis, alopecia, depigmentation, pulmonary infiltrates & fibrosis; anaphylaxis (rare).

▶ Teratogenic; may affect spermatogenesis. Avoid human exposure.

▶ Determine dosages accurately.

▶ Drug interactions.

Uses/Indications

Methotrexate is used (as part of multi-drug protocols) for treating lymphomas and some solid tumors in dogs, cats, and ferrets.

Although there is little clinical experience using methotrexate as an immunomodulating drug in animals, low-dose methotrexate has been used as an alternate immunosuppressive when other immunosuppressive drugs (*e.g.* prednisone, azathioprine, etc.) have not been effective, or as an add-on to enhance efficacy or allow dosage reductions of other drugs.

Pharmacology/Actions

An S-phase specific antimetabolite antineoplastic agent, methotrexate competitively inhibits folic acid reductase, preventing the reduction of dihydrofolate to tetrahydrofolate and affecting production of purines and pyrimidines. Rapidly proliferating cells (*e.g.,* neoplasms, bone marrow, GI tract epithelium, fetal cells, etc.) are most sensitive to the drug's effects.

Dihydrofolate reductase has a much greater affinity for methotrexate than either folic acid or dihydrofolic acid and coadministration of folic acid will not reduce methotrexate's effects. Leucovorin calcium, a derivative of tetrahydrofolic acid, can block the effects of methotrexate.

Methotrexate also has immunosuppressive activity, possibly due to its effects on lymphocyte replication. Tumor cells have been noted to develop resistance to methotrexate that may be due to decreased cellular uptake of the drug.

Pharmacokinetics

Methotrexate is well absorbed from the GI tract after oral administration of dosages <30 mg/m^2 with a bioavailability of ≈60%. In humans, peak levels occur within 4 hours after oral dosing, and between 30 minutes and 2 hours after IM injection.

Methotrexate is widely distributed in the body and is actively transported across cell membranes. Highest concentrations are found in the kidneys, spleen, gallbladder, liver, and skin. When given orally or parenterally, methotrexate does not reach therapeutic levels in the CSF. When given intrathecally, methotrexate attains therapeutic levels in the CSF and also passes into the systemic circulation. Methotrexate is ≈50% bound to plasma proteins and crosses the placenta.

Methotrexate is excreted almost entirely by the kidneys via both glomerular filtration and active transport. Serum half-life is <10 hours and generally between 2-4 hours.

Contraindications/Precautions/Warnings

Methotrexate is contraindicated in patients with preexisting bone marrow depression, severe hepatic or renal insufficiency, or hypersensitivity to the drug. It should be used with caution in patients that are susceptible to, or have preexisting clinical signs associated with, the adverse reactions associated with this drug.

When administering MTX, either wear gloves or immediately wash hands after handling. Gloves are particularly important if handling split, broken, or crushed tablets. Preparation of intravenous solutions should ideally be performed in a vertical laminar flow hood.

In human medicine, methotrexate is considered a "high alert" medication (medications that require special safeguards to reduce the risk of errors). Consider instituting practices such as redundant drug dosage and volume checking, special alert labels, etc.

Adverse Effects

In dogs and cats, gastrointestinal side effects are most prevalent with diarrhea, nausea, inappetence (especially cats) and vomiting (especially dogs) seen. Higher dosages may lead to listlessness, GI toxicity (ulcers, mucosal sloughing, stomatitis), hematopoietic toxicity (nadir at 4-6 days), hepatopathy, renal tubular necrosis, alopecia, depigmentation, pulmonary infiltrates, and fibrosis. CNS toxicity (encephalopathy) may be noted if methotrexate is given intrathecally. Rarely, anaphylaxis may be seen.

Reproductive/Nursing Safety

Methotrexate is teratogenic, embryotoxic, and may affect spermatogenesis in male animals. In humans, the FDA categorizes this drug as category *X* for use during pregnancy (*Studies in animals or humans demonstrate fetal abnormalities or adverse reaction; reports indicate evidence of fetal risk. The risk of use in pregnant women clearly outweighs any possible benefit.*) In a separate system evaluating the safety of drugs in canine and feline pregnancy (Papich 1989), this drug is categorized as class: *C* (*These drugs may have potential risks. Studies in people or laboratory animals have uncovered risks, and these drugs should be used cautiously as a last resort when the benefit of therapy clearly outweighs the risks.*)

Methotrexate is contraindicated in nursing mothers. It is excreted in breast milk in low concentrations with a milk:plasma ratio of 0.08:1. Nursing offspring should be switched to milk replacer if the dam requires methotrexate.

Overdosage/Acute Toxicity

Acute overdosage in dogs is associated with exacerbations of the adverse effects outlined above, particularly myelosuppression and acute renal failure. Acute tubular necrosis is secondary to drug precipitation in the tubules. In dogs, the maximally tolerated dose is reported to be 0.12 mg/kg q24h for 5 days. 10 mg/kg is considered a lethal dose if leucovorin rescue is not performed. Because of the serious sequelae associated with MTX overdoses, refer to an animal poison center for guidance on assessment and management.

There were 117 single agent exposures to methotrexate reported to the ASPCA Animal Poison Control Center (APCC) during 2009-2013. Of the 110 dogs, 26 were symptomatic with 58% vomiting, 31% lethargic, and 27% anorexic.

Treatment of acute oral overdoses include emptying the gut and preventing absorption using standard protocols if the ingestion is recent. Additionally, oral neomycin has been suggested to help prevent absorption of MTX from the intestine. In order to minimize renal damage, forced alkaline diuresis should be considered. Urine pH should be maintained between 7.5-8 by the addition of 0.5 – 1 mEq/kg of sodium bicarbonate per 500 mL of IV fluid.

Leucovorin calcium is specific therapy for methotrexate overdoses. It should be given as soon as possible, preferably within the first hour and, definitely, within 48 hours. Doses of leucovorin required are dependent on the MTX serum concentration. Refer to the leucovorin monograph or an animal poison center for more information.

Drug Interactions

Methotrexate has been shown to be a substrate of the drug transporter ABCG2 and there are potentially many interactions with other drugs that may be clinically significant. The following drug interactions have either been reported or are theoretical in humans or animals receiving methotrexate (MTX) and may be of significance in veterinary patients. Unless otherwise noted, use together is not necessarily contraindicated, but weigh the potential risks and perform additional monitoring when appropriate.

- **AMIODARONE:** Prolonged PO administration of amiodarone (>2 weeks) may inhibit MTX metabolism.
- **ASPARAGINASE:** Asparaginase given concomitantly with MTX may decrease MTX efficacy.
- **AZATHIOPRINE:** Potential for increased risk for hepatic toxicity.
- **CHLORAMPHENICOL:** May displace MTX from plasma proteins increasing risk for toxicity, but also may reduce MTX absorption and enterohepatic recirculation.
- **CISPLATIN:** May have synergistic action with MTX, but alter the renal elimination of MTX.
- **CYCLOSPORINE:** May increase MTX levels.
- **FOLIC ACID:** May reduce MTX efficacy, but folate deficiency increases MTX toxicity.
- **NEOMYCIN (oral):** Oral neomycin may decrease the absorption of oral methotrexate if given concomitantly.
- **NSAIDS, SALICYLATES:** In humans, severe hematologic and GI toxicity has resulted in patients receiving both MTX and non-steroidal antiinflammatory agents; avoid or use very cautiously in dogs on MTX.
- **PENICILLINS:** May decrease MTX renal elimination.
- **PROBENECID:** May inhibit the tubular secretion of MTX and increase its half-life.
- **PYRIMETHAMINE:** Pyrimethamine, a similar folic acid antagonist, may increase MTX toxicity and should not be given to patients receiving MTX.
- **RETINOIDS:** Potential for increased risk for hepatic toxicity.
- **SULFASALAZINE:** Potential for increased risk for hepatic toxicity.
- **SULFONAMIDES:** May displace MTX from plasma proteins increasing risk for toxicity.
- **TETRACYCLINES:** May displace MTX from plasma proteins increasing risk for toxicity, but also may reduce MTX absorption and enterohepatic recirculation.
- **THEOPHYLLINES:** MTX may reduce theophylline elimination.
- **TRIMETHOPRIM/SULFA:** Rarely, may increase myelosuppression of MTX.
- **VACCINES, LIVE:** Live virus vaccines should be used with caution, if at all during therapy.

Laboratory Considerations

- Methotrexate may interfere with the microbiologic assay for **folic acid**.

Doses

Note: Dosages and dosage forms of methotrexate sodium are expressed in terms of methotrexate. Because of the potential toxicity of methotrexate when used at antineoplastic dosages, to patients, veterinary personnel and clients, and since chemotherapy indications, treatment protocols, monitoring and safety guidelines often change, the following dosages should be used only as a general guide. Consultation with a veterinary oncologist and referral to current veterinary oncology references [e.g., (Withrow *et al.* 2012); (Dobson *et al.* 2011); (Henry *et al.* 2009); (North *et al.* 2009); (Argyle *et al.* 2008)] are strongly recommended.

- **DOGS:**

  For susceptible neoplastic diseases (usually as part of a multidrug protocol) (extra-label):

  a) As part of the LMP protocol for maintenance of canine lymphoma: Chlorambucil 20 mg/m^2 PO every 15 days; Methotrexate 2.5 – 5 mg/m^2 PO twice a week; Prednisone 20 mg/m^2 PO every other day. When Vincristine is added it is at a dose of 0.5 – 0.7 mg/m^2 and is given every 15 days alternating weeks with the chlorambucil. (Berger 2005)

  b) In combination with other antineoplastics (per protocol): 5 mg/m^2 PO twice weekly or 0.8 mg/kg IV every 21 days; alternatively 2.5 mg/m^2 PO daily. (USPC 1990)

  As an immunosuppressive agent (extra-label): There is not much experience using MTX as an immunosuppressant agent in animals. Anecdotal dosages noted include 2.5 mg/m^2 PO q24h.

- **CATS:**

  For susceptible neoplastic diseases (usually as part of a multidrug protocol); (extra-label): 2.5 mg/m^2 PO 2-3 times weekly; 0.3 – 0.8 mg/m^2 IV every 7 days. (O'Keefe *et al.* 1990)

  As an immunosuppressive agent (extra-label): There is not much experience using MTX as an immunosuppressant agent in animals, anecdotal dosages noted include: 2.5 mg/m^2 PO 2-3 times per week; 7.5 mg per cat PO once weekly with leflunomide.

Monitoring

- Efficacy.
- Toxicity:

  a) Monitor for clinical signs of GI irritation and ulceration.

  b) Complete blood counts (with platelets) should be performed weekly early in therapy and eventually every 4-6 weeks when stabilized. If WBC is <4000/mm^3 or platelet count is <100,000/mm^3 therapy should be discontinued.

  c) Baseline renal function tests. Continue to monitor if abnormal.

  d) Baseline hepatic function tests. Monitor liver enzymes on a regular basis during therapy.

Client Information

- Give with food.
- Wear disposable gloves when administering tablets (particularly if crushed or split); if gloves are not used, wash hands thoroughly after handling tablets.
- Methotrexate is a chemotherapy (cancer) drug. The drug and its byproducts can be hazardous to other animals and people that come in contact with it. On the day your animal gets the drug and then for a few days afterward, all bodily waste (urine, feces, litter), blood, or vomit should only be handled while wearing disposable gloves. Seal the waste in a plastic bag and then place both the bag and gloves in with the regular trash.
- Contact the veterinarian if the patient exhibits clinical signs of profound depression, abnormal bleeding (including bloody diarrhea) and/or bruising.

Chemistry/Synonyms

A folic acid antagonist, methotrexate is available commercially as the sodium salt. It occurs as a yellow powder that is soluble in water. Methotrexate sodium injection has a pH of 7.5-9.

Methotrexate and methotrexate sodium may also be known as: MTX, amethopterin, 4-Amino-4-deoxy-10-methylpteroyl-L-glutamic acid, 4-Amino-10-methylfolic acid, CL-14377, alpha-methopterin, methotrexatum, metotrexato, NSC-740, WR-19039; there are many trade names available.

Storage/Stability

Methotrexate sodium tablets should be stored at room temperature (15-30°C) in well-closed containers and protected from light. The injection and powder for injection should be stored at room temperature (15-30°C) and protected from light.

Compatibility/Compounding Considerations

Methotrexate sodium is reportedly physically **compatible** with the following intravenous solutions and drugs: Amino acids 4.25%/dextrose 25%, D5W, sodium bicarbonate 0.05 M, cytarabine, mercaptopurine sodium, sodium bicarbonate, and vincristine sulfate. In syringes, methotrexate is physically **compatible** with: bleomycin sulfate, cyclophosphamide, doxorubicin HCl, fluorouracil, furosemide, leucovorin calcium, mitomycin, vinblastine sulfate, and vincristine sulfate.

Methotrexate sodium **compatibility information conflicts** or is dependent on diluent or concentration factors with the following drugs or solutions: heparin sodium and metoclopramide HCl. Compatibility is dependent upon factors such as pH, concentration, temperature and diluent used; consult specialized references or a hospital pharmacist for more specific information.

Methotrexate sodium is reportedly physically **incompatible** when mixed with the following solutions or drugs: bleomycin sulfate (as an IV additive only; compatible in syringes and Y-lines), fluorouracil (as an IV additive only; compatible in syringes and Y-lines), prednisolone sodium phosphate, and ranitidine HCl.

Dosage Forms/Regulatory Status

VETERINARY-LABELED PRODUCTS: NONE.

The ARCI (Racing Commissioners International) has designated this drug as a class 2 substance. See the appendix for more information.

HUMAN-LABELED PRODUCTS:

Methotrexate Sodium Tablets (plain & scored): 2.5 mg; generic; (Rx)

Methotrexate Injection (preservative-free) for SC Use (Auto-injector): 10 mg/0.4 mL, 15 mg/0.4 mL, 20 mg/0.4 mL, 25 mg/0.4 mL; *Otrexup®*; (Rx)

Methotrexate Sodium Injection: 25 mg/mL (as base) in 2 mL & 10 mL vials; preservative-free in 2 mL, 4 mL, 8 mL, 10 mL, 20 mL, & 40 mL single-use vials; *Methotrexate LPF® Sodium*, generic; (Rx)

Methotrexate Powder for Injection, lyophilized: 1 gram preservative-free in single-use vials; generic; (Rx)

Revisions/References

Monograph revised/updated April 2014.

Argyle, D., et al. (2008). *Decision Making in Small Animal Oncology*, Wiley-Blackwell.
Berger, F. (2005). Rescue treatment of canine lymphoma. Proceedings: WSAVA World Congress. accessed via Veterinary Information Network; vin.com
Dobson, J. & D. Lascelles (2011). *BSAVA Manual of Canine and Feline Oncology*, BSAVA.
Henry, C. & M. Higginbotham (2009). *Cancer Management in Small Animal Practice*, Saunders.
North, S. & T. Banks (2009). *Small Animal Oncology: An Introduction*, Saunders.
O'Keefe, D. A. & C. L. Harris (1990). Toxicology of Oncologic Drugs. Vet Clinics of North America: Small Animal Pract **20**(2): 483-504.
Papich, M. (1989). Effects of drugs on pregnancy. *Current Veterinary Therapy X: Small Animal Practice*. R. Kirk. Philadelphia, Saunders: 1291-9.
USPC (1990). Veterinary Information- Appendix III. *Drug Information for the Health Professional*. Rockville, United States Pharmacopeial Convention. **2**: 2811-60.
Withrow, S., et al. (2012). Withrow and MacEwen's Small Animal Clinical Oncology, 5th Ed., Saunders.

Methylene Blue

(meth-i-leen)

Antidote

Prescriber Highlights

▶ Thiazine dye used to primarily treat methemoglobinemia in ruminants, but can be used in dogs.
▶ Contraindications: Cats (most agree), lactating dairy animals, renal insufficiency; hypersensitive to methylene blue; or given as an intraspinal (intrathecal) injection.
▶ Not very effective in horses.
▶ Adverse Effects: Heinz body anemia or other red cell morphological changes, methemoglobinemia, & decreased red cell life spans. Cats most sensitive, but to a lesser degree, dogs & horses also.
▶ A 180-day slaughter withdrawal time has been suggested, but 14 days may be sufficient (see doses).

Uses/Indications

Methylene blue is used primarily for treating methemoglobinemia secondary to oxidative agents (nitrates, chlorates) in ruminants. It is also employed occasionally as adjunctive or alternative therapy for cyanide toxicity.

In dogs, methylene blue may be considered for treating methemoglobinemia secondary to drugs or toxins (*e.g.*, phenol, mothballs, hydroxyurea, phenazopyridine).

Intra-operative methylene blue can be used to preferentially stain islet-cell tumors of the pancreas in dogs in order to aid in their surgical removal or in determining the animal's prognosis. However, IV methylene blue is rarely used for this purpose due to its adverse effects and delayed effect colorizing pancreatic cells.

Pharmacology/Actions

Methylene blue is rapidly converted to leucomethylene blue in tissues. This compound serves as a reducing agent that helps to convert methemoglobin (Fe^{+++}) to hemoglobin (Fe^{++}). Methylene blue is an oxidating agent, and, if high doses (species dependent) are administered, may actually cause methemoglobinemia.

Pharmacokinetics

Methylene blue is absorbed from the GI tract, but is usually administered parenterally in veterinary medicine. It is excreted in the urine and bile, primarily in the colorless form, but some unchanged drug may be also excreted.

Contraindications/Precautions/Warnings

Methylene blue is contraindicated in patients with renal insufficiency, or are hypersensitive to methylene blue. It cannot be given as an intraspinal (intrathecal) injection. Because cats may develop Heinz body anemia and methemoglobinemia secondary to methylene blue it is considered contraindicated by most clinicians. Methylene blue is considered relatively ineffective in reducing methemoglobin in horses.

Adverse Effects

The greatest concerns with methylene blue therapy are the development of Heinz body anemia or other red cell morphological changes, methemoglobinemia, and decreased red cell life spans. Cats tend to be very sensitive to these effects and some consider it contraindicated in feline patients, but dogs and horses can also develop hematologic adverse effects at relatively low dosages.

Methylene blue has the potential to cause serotonin syndrome.

Necrotic abscesses may develop if injected SC or extravasation occurs during IV administration.

Reproductive/Nursing Safety

Safe use of this agent during pregnancy has not been demonstrated. In humans, the FDA categorizes this drug as category *C* for use during pregnancy (*Animal studies have shown an adverse effect on the fetus, but there are no adequate studies in humans; or there are no animal reproduction studies and no adequate studies in humans.*) No information on lactation safety was found.

Overdosage/Acute Toxicity

In sheep, the IV LD_{50} for 3% methylene blue is approximately 43 mg/kg.

Drug Interactions

- None reported.

Laboratory Considerations

- Methylene blue can cause a green-blue color in urine and may affect the accuracy of **urinalysis**.
- **Pulse oximetry.** Methemoglobinemia interferes with the accuracy of pulse oximeters.

Doses

- **DOGS:**

To preferentially stain islet-cell tumors of the pancreas (extra-label): 3 mg/kg in 250 mL sterile normal saline and administered IV over 30-40 minutes intraoperatively. Initial tumor staining requires approximately 20 minutes after infusion has begun and is maximal at $\approx$25-35 minutes after infusion is started. Tumors generally appear to be a reddish-violet in color versus a dusky blue (background staining). (Fingeroth *et al.* 1988)

To treat severe methemoglobinemia (extra-label): 1 – 1.5 mg/kg as a 1% solution given slowly IV over several minutes. A dramatic response should occur during the first 30 minutes after treatment. It may be repeated if necessary, but it should be used cautiously as it can cause Heinz body anemia. Measure hematocrit for 3 days after treatment (Harvey 2006). A case report of a dog receiving 4 mg/kg for phenazopyridine intoxication has been reported (Gerken *et al.* 1997).

- **CATS:**

To treat severe methemoglobinemia (extra-label): **Note:** Use with extreme caution in cats; many say that methylene blue is contraindicated. 1 – 1.5 mg/kg IV infusion slowly (over several minutes) one time only.

- **RUMINANTS:**

Note: When used in food animals, FARAD recommends a minimum milk withdrawal time of 4 days after the last treatment. Because of concerns of carcinogenicity, an extremely conservative withdrawal time for meat of 180 days has been recommended; however, available data suggest that a much shorter withdrawal time of 14 days would be sufficient (Haskell *et al.* 2005).

For methemoglobin-producing toxins (nitrites, nitrates, chlorates); (extra-label): Using a 1% solution, methylene blue is given at 4 – 15 mg/kg IV q6h. (Osweiler 2007)

- **HORSES:**

For methemoglobinemia secondary to chlorate toxicity; (extra-label): 4.4 mg/kg as 1% solution by intravenous drip; may repeat in 15-30 minutes if clinical response is not obtained. (Schmitz 2004)

Monitoring

- Methemoglobinemia using co-oximetry; pulse oximetry is not reliable.
- Red cell morphology, red cell indices, hematocrit, hemoglobin.

Client Information

- Because of the potential toxicity of this agent and the seriousness of methemoglobin-related intoxications, this drug should be used with close professional supervision only.
- Methylene blue may be very staining to clothing or skin. Removal may be accomplished using hypochlorite solutions (bleach).

Chemistry/Synonyms

A thiazine dye, methylene blue occurs as dark green crystals or crystalline powder that has a bronze-like luster. It may have a slight odor and is soluble in water and sparingly soluble in alcohol. When dissolved, a dark blue solution results. Commercially available methylene blue injection (human-labeled) has a pH from 3-4.5.

Methylene blue may also be known as: methylthioninium chloride, azul de metileno, blu di metilene, CI basic blue 9, colour index no. 52015, methylenii caeruleum, methylthioninii chloridum, schultz no. 1038, tetramethylthionine chloride trihydrate, *Azul Metile®, Collubleu®, Desmoidpillen®, Vitableu®, Urolene Blue®* and *Zumetil®.*

Storage/Stability

Unless otherwise instructed by the manufacturer, store methylene blue at room temperature.

Compatibility/Compounding Considerations

Methylene blue is reportedly physically **incompatible** when mixed with caustic alkalies, dichromates, iodides, and oxidizing or reducing agents.

Dosage Forms/Regulatory Status

VETERINARY-LABELED PRODUCTS:

No FDA-approved products as pharmaceuticals for internal use. A non-sterile 1% (10 mg/mL) methylene blue solution is labeled for animal use as a dye, laboratory indicator and reagent. It is available in pint and gallon bottles. Methylene Blue, USP powder may be available from chemical supply houses.

HUMAN-LABELED PRODUCTS:

Methylene Blue Injection: 1% (10 mg/mL) in 1 mL & 10 mL amps; generic; (Rx)

Revisions/References

Monograph revised/updated April 2014.

Fingeroth, J. M. & D. D. Smeak (1988). Intravenous methylene blue infusion for intraoperative identification of pancreatic islet-cell tumors in dogs. Part II: Clinical trials and results in four dogs. J Am Anim Hosp Assoc **24**(2): 175-82.

Gerken, D., et al. (1997). Phenazopyridine toxicosis in a dog. Proceedings of the 40th Annual Meeting American Association of Veterinary Laboratory Diagnosticians. accessed via Veterinary Information Network; vin.com

Harvey, J. (2006). Toxic hemolytic anemias. Proceedings: ACVIM. accessed via Veterinary Information Network; vin.com

Haskell, S., et al. (2005). Farad Digest: Antidotes in Food Animal Practice. JAVMA **226**(6): 884-7.

Osweiler, G. (2007). Detoxification and Antidotes for Ruminant Poisoning. Proceedings: ACVIM. accessed via Veterinary Information Network; vin.com

Schmitz, D. (2004). Toxicologic problems. *Equine Internal Medicine 2nd Ed.* S. Reed, W. Bayly and D. Sellon. Philadelphia, Saunders: 1441-512.

Methylphenidate

(meth-ill-**fen**-i-date)   Ritalin®

CNS Stimulant

Prescriber Highlights

▶ Amphetamine-like drug that may be useful for treating cataplexy/narcolepsy or hyperkinesis/hyperactivity in dogs.

▶ Use with caution in dogs with seizure disorders, cardiac disease/hypertension, or in aggressive animals.

▶ Adverse effects are primarily CNS stimulation-related.

▶ Class-II controlled drug in USA.

Uses/Indications

Methylphenidate may be useful for diagnosing and treating cataplexy/narcolepsy or hyperactivity in dogs.

Pharmacology/Actions

Methylphenidate has stimulating effects on the central nervous and respiratory systems similar to that of amphetamines. It also has weak sympathomimetic activity, and at normal dosages has little effect on peripheral circulation.

Pharmacokinetics

In dogs, there is limited information available. Single PO doses of immediate-release 20 mg tablets to 7-19 kg beagles gave peak levels of ≈60 micrograms/mL in ≈15 minutes after dosing. Clearance was ≈0.27 L/hr and elimination half-life around an hour. With 20 mg sustained-release tablets there was much more inter-patient variation, serum concentrations peaked around 30 minutes after dosing, peak levels of 19 micrograms/mL were much lower then the immediate-release tablets. Clearance was ≈0.97 L/hr and elimination half-life was approximately 40 minutes. For reference, the therapeutic plasma concentration of methylphenidate is thought to be between 1-10 micrograms/mL (Giorgi *et al.* 2010).

In humans, methylphenidate (regular tablets) is rapidly and well absorbed from the GI tract. Food in the GI tract may increase the rate, but not the extent, of drug absorbed. Peak levels occur ≈2 hours post-dose. The drug is extensively metabolized during the first-pass; protein binding is low. Terminal elimination half-life is approximately 3 hours; <1% is excreted unchanged in the urine.

Contraindications/Precautions/Warnings

The risks associated with methylphenidate should be carefully considered before using this drug in dogs with seizure disorders, cardiac disease/hypertension, or in aggressive animals.

Be alert for drug-seeking individuals as methylphenidate is a controlled drug (C-II in the USA). A written prescription (30 day supply maximum) is required each time the drug is dispensed by a pharmacy.

Adverse Effects

Most likely adverse effects to be encountered include increased heart and respiratory rates, anorexia, tremors and hyperthermia (particularly exercised-induced). CNS stimulation can occur (see Overdosage).

Reproductive/Nursing Safety

In humans, the FDA categorizes methylphenidate as a category C drug for use during pregnancy (*Animal studies have shown an adverse effect on the fetus, but there are no adequate studies in humans; or there are no animal reproduction studies and no adequate studies in humans*). Methylphenidate was associated with teratogenic effects in rabbits, but at massive dosages (200 mg/kg/day).

It is unknown if methylphenidate enters maternal milk.

Overdosage/Acute Toxicity

In dogs, even relatively low dosages can cause serious toxicosis. Dosages of 1 mg/kg (or below) have caused toxic reactions and there is one report of a fatality after a dog ingested 3.1 mg/kg. However, research dogs have survived doses of 20 mg/kg/day for 90 days. A detailed retrospective review of methylphenidate toxicosis in dogs has been published (Genovese *et al.* 2010).

A cat given a 5 mg tablet of methylphenidate, showed signs of tremors, agitation, mydriasis, tachycardia, tachypnea and hypertension; signs resolved 25 hours post-ingestion with supportive care (dark cage, diazepam, fluids) (Genovese *et al.* 2010).

Expected signs associated with an overdose in dogs are generally CNS over-stimulation and excessive sympathomimetic effects and can include: hyperactivity, salivation, diarrhea, head bobbing, agitation, tachycardia, hypertension, tremors, seizures, and hyperthermia. Consider the dosage form (extended-release vs. regular tablets) when considering treatment options and expected onset and duration of effects.

There were 1215 single agent exposures to methylphenidate reported to the ASPCA Animal Poison Control Center (APCC) during 2009-2013. Of the 1060 dogs, 198 were symptomatic with 38% agitated, 28% tachycardic, and 16% hyperthermic. Of the 153 cats, 86 were symptomatic with 47% tachycardic, 40% mydriatic and 30% agitated.

Usual gut decontamination protocols can be considered, but as CNS signs can rapidly occur, emetics should be used with caution. Treatment is basically supportive by controlling signs associated with toxicity. Phenothiazines (*e.g.*, acepromazine, chlorpromazine) may be useful in controlling agitation. Benzodiazepines (e.g., diazepam) potentially could increase the severity of agitation and are typically avoided. Seizures may be controlled with propofol followed by barbiturates if necessary. Additional treatments that may be considered include: injectable methocarbamol for tremors; beta-blockers for tachycardia; prazosin, amlodipine, nitroprusside, or hydralazine for hypertension; external cooling for hyperthermia; and cyproheptadine to help prevent serotonin syndrome.

Drug Interactions

The following drug interactions have either been reported or are theoretical in humans or animals receiving methylphenidate and may be of significance in veterinary patients. Unless otherwise noted, use together is not necessarily contraindicated, but weigh the potential risks and perform additional monitoring when appropriate.

- **ANTICONVULSANTS** (*e.g.,* **phenobarbital, primidone, phenytoin**): Methylphenidate may increase serum levels.
- **CLONIDINE**: Rare cases (in humans) of cardiovascular effects (including death); mechanism not understood and causality not established.
- **HYPOTENSIVE DRUGS**: Methylphenidate may reduce effects.
- **MAO INHIBITORS** (including **amitraz** and potentially, **selegiline**): Could lead to hypertensive crisis.
- **SSRI ANTIDEPRESSANTS** (*e.g.,* **fluoxetine, sertraline**, etc.): Methylphenidate may inhibit metabolism and increase levels.
- **TRICYCLIC ANTIDEPRESSANTS** (*e.g.,* **amitriptyline, clomipramine**, etc.): Methylphenidate may inhibit metabolism and increase levels.
- **WARFARIN**: Methylphenidate may inhibit warfarin metabolism and increase INR.

Laboratory Considerations

- No specific laboratory interactions were noted for this drug.

Doses

- **DOGS:**

  For adjunctive treatment of narcolepsy/cataplexy (extra-label): Dosage recommendations of 0.25 – 0.5 mg/kg PO or 5 – 10 mg (per dog) PO q12-24h have been noted.

  For diagnosis and treatment of hyperkinesis (extra-label): For diagnosis (behavior returns to normal), dosages 5 – 20 mg (per dog; depending on dog's size) PO q8-12h is given for 3 days and patient is assessed for improvement of target behaviors (anxiety, overactivity, learning ability). If effective, can begin at a lower dosage 1-2 times a day (and increased if necessary) while training and behavior modification therapy is performed. Drug holidays (no dose given) can occur on days when dog's behavior does not matter. Adapted from: (Siebert 2003), (Virga 2002), (Beaver 2010)

Monitoring

- Clinical efficacy.
- Occasional physical exam to monitor vital signs, body weight.
- In humans, it is recommended to do periodic CBC with differential and platelet counts during prolonged therapy.

Client Information

- A common side effect is decreased appetite.
- If your animal wore a flea collar in the past 2 weeks, let your veterinarian know. Do not use one on your animal while it's getting this medicine without first talking to your veterinarian.
- Contact your veterinarian immediately if your animal has a seizure while taking this medication.
- Methylphenidate has significant potential for abuse by humans and should be kept safely secure.
- If using an extended-release product, do not crush tablet or capsule.

Chemistry/Synonyms

A CNS stimulant related to amphetamines, methylphenidate HCl occurs as fine, white odorless, crystalline powder. It is freely soluble in water and soluble in alcohol.

Methylphenidate may also be known as: *Attenta®, Daytrana®, Equasym®, Focalin®, Metadate ER®, Methylin®, Rilatine®, Riphenidate®, Ritalina®, Ritalin®, Ritaline®, Ritaphen®, Rubifen®,* or *Tranquilyn®.*

Storage/Stability

Unless otherwise noted on the label, methylphenidate tablets and extended-release tablets and capsules should be stored in tight, light-resistant containers at room temperature.

Compatibility/Compounding Considerations

No specific information noted.

Dosage Forms/Regulatory Status

VETERINARY-LABELED PRODUCTS: NONE.

The ARCI (Racing Commissioners International) has designated this drug as a class 1 substance. See the appendix for more information.

HUMAN-LABELED PRODUCTS:

Methylphenidate Oral Tablets: 5 mg, 10 mg & 20 mg; Chewable Tablets: 2.5 mg, 5 mg & 10 mg; Extended-Release Tablets: 10 mg, 18 mg, 20 mg, 27 mg, 36 mg & 54 mg; Extended-Release Capsules: 20 mg, 30 mg, 40 mg, 50 mg & 60 mg; Trade names include: *Methylin®, Ritalin®, Ritalin® LA,* & *Ritalin-SR®; Metadate ER®* & *Metadate CD®, Concerta®,* generic; (Rx; C-II)

Methylphenidate Oral Solution: 5 mg/5 mL (1 mg/mL) & 10 mg/5 mL (2 mg/mL); *Methylin®,* generic; (Rx; C-II)

There is also a Methylphenidate Transdermal Patch.

Revisions/References

Monograph revised/updated April 2014.

Beaver, B. (2010). ADHD in Small Animals. Proceedings; Wild West Veterinary Conference 2010. accessed via Veterinary Information Network; vin.com

Genovese, D. W., et al. (2010). Methylphenidate toxicosis in dogs: 128 cases (2001-2008). Javma-Journal of the American Veterinary Medical Association 237(12): 1438-43.

Giorgi, M., et al. (2010). Pharmacokinetics of methylphenidate following two oral formulations (immediate and sustained release) in the dog. Veterinary Research Communications 34: S73-S7.

Siebert, L. (2003). Psychoactive drugs in behavioral medicine. Western Veterinary Conference. accessed via Veterinary Information Network; vin.com

Virga, V. (2002). Which drug and why: An update on psychopharmacology. Proceedings: Atlantic Coast Veterinary Conference. accessed via Veterinary Information Network; vin.com

Methylprednisolone
Methylprednisolone Acetate
Methylprednisolone Sodium Succinate

(meth-ill-pred-**niss**-oh-lone)   Medrol®, Depo-Medrol®

Glucocorticoid

Prescriber Highlights

▶ Oral & parenteral glucocorticoid that is 4-5X more potent than hydrocortisone; no appreciable mineralocorticoid activity.

▶ Contraindicated (relatively): Systemic fungal infections, manufacturer lists: "in viral infections, ...animals with arrested tuberculosis, peptic ulcer, acute psychoses, corneal ulcer, & Cushingoid syndrome. The presence of diabetes, osteoporosis, chronic psychotic reactions, predisposition to thrombophlebitis, hypertension, CHF, renal insufficiency, & active tuberculosis necessitates carefully controlled use."

▶ Acetate can cause significant HPA axis suppression. In cats, extracellular hyperglycemia can cause volume expansion and may predispose cats to congestive heart failure. IM administration generally reserved when owners cannot adhere to oral treatment regimens.

▶ Usual therapy goal is to use as much as is required & as little as possible for as short an amount of time as possible.

▶ Primary adverse effects are "Cushingoid" in nature with sustained use.

▶ Many potential drug & lab interactions.

Uses/Indications

Methylprednisolone is similar to prednisone or prednisolone, but slightly more potent.

Glucocorticoids have been used in an attempt to treat practically every malady that afflicts man or animal, but there are three broad uses and dosage ranges for use of these agents: 1) Replacement of glucocorticoid activity in patients with adrenal insufficiency, 2) as an antiinflammatory agent, and 3) as an immunosuppressive. Glucocorticoids are used in the treatment of endocrine conditions (*e.g.,* adrenal insufficiency), rheumatic diseases (*e.g.,* rheumatoid arthritis), collagen diseases (*e.g.,* systemic lupus), allergic states/anaphylaxis, envenomation, inducing fetal maturation, respiratory diseases (*e.g.,* asthma), dermatologic diseases (*e.g.,* pemphigus, allergic dermatoses), hematologic disorders (*e.g.,* thrombocytopenias, autoimmune hemolytic anemia), neoplasias, nervous system disorders (increased CSF pressure), GI diseases (*e.g.,* ulcerative colitis exacerbations), and renal diseases (*e.g.,* nephrotic syndrome). Some glucocorticoids are used topically in the eye and skin for various conditions or are injected intra-articularly or intra-lesionally. This listing is certainly not complete. High dose (*e.g.,* 30 mg/kg IV), fast-acting corticosteroids are no longer recommended for use in shock or CNS trauma (still controversial); recent studies have not demonstrated significant benefit and it actually may cause increased deleterious effects.

Pharmacology/Actions

Methylprednisolone may be administered either orally or parenterally (IV sodium succinate; acetate IM only). Its relative anti-inflammatory potency is approximately 5X that of cortisol. It has negligible to very slight mineralocorticoid activity. Once in the systemic circulation it has an approximate duration of activity of 12-36 hours. Duration of activity is not dependent on elimination half-life.

Glucocorticoids have effects on virtually every cell type and system in mammals. For more information, refer to the Glucocorticoid Agents, General Information monograph.

Pharmacokinetics

Methylprednisolone administered orally is relatively well absorbed and extensively distributed. The liver is the primary site for metabolism (oxidation); most of the drug is excreted renally as metabolites. Elimination half-life is multiphasic and does not appreciably effect duration of action.

The sodium succinate IV injection is water soluble and considered very fast acting.

The acetate IM injection is slowly absorbed and can have duration of effect of weeks to months. After IA administration of 100 mg or 200 mg in horses, a study found the last quantifiable plasma concentrations for methylprednisolone at 7 days (100 mg) and 18 days (200 mg) (Menendez *et al.* 2012).

Contraindications/Precautions/Warnings

The original manufacturer's (Upjohn Veterinary) label states that the drug (tablets) should not be used in dogs or cats "in viral infections, …animals with arrested tuberculosis, peptic ulcer, acute psychoses, corneal ulcer, and Cushingoid syndrome. The presence of diabetes, osteoporosis, chronic psychotic reactions, predisposition to thrombophlebitis, hypertension, CHF, renal insufficiency, and active tuberculosis necessitates carefully controlled use." A study in cats (n=8) with feline herpesvirus 1 (FHV-1) administered 5 mg/kg methylprednisolone acetate IM on day 0 and day 21, reported that clinical signs of activated FHV-1 occurred in some cats, but in most it was mild and self-limited (Lappin *et al.* 2011).

The injectable acetate product is contraindicated as outlined above when used systemically. When injected intrasynovially, intratendinously, or by other local means, it is contraindicated in the "presence of acute local infections." Because of its long duration of action and increased risks for adverse effects, most do not recommend use of methylprednisolone acetate IM when alternate day oral glucocorticoid therapy could be used. In difficult-to-pill cats however, it may be a viable alternative to oral glucocorticoids.

Systemic use of glucocorticoids is generally considered contraindicated in systemic fungal infections (unless used for replacement therapy in Addison's), when administered IM in patients with idiopathic thrombocytopenia and those hypersensitive to a particular drug. Use of sustained-release injectable glucocorticoids is considered contraindicated for chronic corticosteroid therapy of systemic diseases.

Unless very short-term burst therapy is used, patients that have received systemic glucocorticoids systemically should be tapered off the drug. Tapers should be slow if the patient has been receiving a glucocorticoid chronically as endogenous ACTH and corticosteroid function may return slowly. Should the animal undergo a "stressor" (*e.g.*, surgery, trauma, illness, etc.) during the tapering process and/or until normal adrenal and pituitary function resume, additional glucocorticoids should be administered.

Animals, particularly cats, at risk for diabetes mellitus or with concurrent cardiovascular disease should receive glucocorticoids with caution due to these agents' potent hyperglycemic effect.

To reduce risk for confusing with other sound-alike/look-alike drugs, FDA recommends using tall-man lettering for this drug: methylPREDNISolone.

Adverse Effects

Serious adverse effects are generally associated with long-term administration, especially if given at high dosages or not on an alternate day regimen. Adverse effects associated with chronic therapy commonly manifest as clinical signs of hyperadrenocorticism. Acute use of high dosages, particularly in dogs, can produce serious effects including GI ulceration/perforation, bleeding and potentially, infections.

Glucocorticoids can retard growth in young animals.

In dogs, polydipsia (PD), polyphagia (PP), and polyuria (PU) may all be seen with short-term "burst" therapy as well as with alternate-day maintenance therapy on days when receiving the drug. Adverse effects in dogs can include dull, dry haircoat, weight gain, panting, vomiting, diarrhea, elevated liver enzymes, pancreatitis, GI ulceration, lipidemias, activation or worsening of diabetes mellitus, muscle wasting, and behavioral changes (depression, lethargy, viciousness). Discontinuation of the drug may be necessary; changing to an alternate steroid may also alleviate the problem. With the exception of PU/PD/PP, adverse effects associated with antiinflammatory therapy are relatively uncommon. Adverse effects associated with immunosuppressive doses are more common and, potentially, more severe.

Cats generally require higher dosages than dogs for clinical effect, but tend to develop fewer adverse effects. Occasionally, polydipsia, polyuria, polyphagia with weight gain, diarrhea, or depression can be seen. Long-term high dose therapy can lead to "Cushingoid" effects, however. In cats, the long-acting acetate salt has been implicated in causing extracellular hyperglycemia leading to volume expansion and may predispose patients to congestive heart failure; however, current evidence for this effect is not strong.

Corticosteroid-related diabetes mellitus may be related to increased urinary excretion of chromium and potentially could respond to chromium supplementation.

Many other potential effects, adverse and otherwise, are outlined above in the Glucocorticoid Agents, General Information monograph.

Reproductive/Nursing Safety

Glucocorticoids are probably necessary for normal fetal development. They may be required for adequate surfactant production, myelin, retinal, pancreas and mammary development. Excessive dosages early in pregnancy may lead to teratogenic effects. In horses and ruminants, exogenous steroid administration may induce parturition when administered in the latter stages of pregnancy. In humans, the FDA categorizes this drug as category **C** for use during pregnancy (*Animal studies have shown an adverse effect on the fetus, but there are no adequate studies in humans; or there are no animal reproduction studies and no adequate studies in humans.*)

Use with caution in nursing dams. Glucocorticoids unbound to plasma proteins will enter milk. High dosages or prolonged administration to mothers may, potentially, inhibit growth, interfere with endogenous corticosteroid production or cause other unwanted effects in nursing offspring. However, in humans, several studies suggest that amounts excreted in breast milk are negligible when methylprednisolone doses are ≤8 mg/day. Larger doses for short periods may not harm the infant.

Overdosage/Acute Toxicity

Glucocorticoids when given short-term are unlikely to cause harmful effects, even in massive dosages. One incidence of a dog developing acute CNS effects after accidental ingestion of glucocorticoids has been reported. Should clinical signs occur, use supportive treatment if required.

Chronic usage of glucocorticoids can lead to serious adverse effects. Refer to Adverse Effects above for more information.

Drug Interactions

The following drug interactions have either been reported or are theoretical in humans or animals receiving methylprednisolone and may be of significance in veterinary patients. Unless otherwise noted, use together is not necessarily contraindicated, but weigh the potential risks and perform additional monitoring when appropriate.

- **AMPHOTERICIN B:** Administered concomitantly with glucocorticoids may cause hypokalemia; in humans, there have been cases of CHF and cardiac enlargement reported after using methylprednisolone to treat Amphotericin B adverse effects.
- **ANALGESICS, OPIATE** and/or **ANESTHETICS, LOCAL** (**epidural injections**): Combination with glucocorticoids in epidurals has caused serious CNS injuries and death; do not use more volume than very small intrathecal test doses of these agents with glucocorticoids.
- **ANTICHOLINESTERASE AGENTS** (*e.g.,* **pyridostigmine, neostigmine**, etc.): In patients with myasthenia gravis, concomitant glucocorticoid and anticholinesterase agent administration may lead to profound muscle weakness. If possible, discontinue anticholinesterase medication at least 24 hours prior to corticosteroid administration.
- **ASPIRIN:** Glucocorticoids may reduce salicylate blood levels.
- **BARBITURATES:** May increase the metabolism of glucocorticoids and decrease blood levels.
- **CYCLOPHOSPHAMIDE:** Glucocorticoids may inhibit the hepatic metabolism of cyclophosphamide; dosage adjustments may be required.
- **CYCLOSPORINE:** Concomitant administration of glucocorticoids and cyclosporine may increase the blood levels of each, by mutually inhibiting the hepatic metabolism of each other; the clinical significance of this interaction is not clear.
- **DIURETICS, POTASSIUM-DEPLETING** (*e.g.,* **spironolactone, triamterene**): Administered concomitantly with glucocorticoids may cause hypokalemia.
- **EPHEDRINE:** May reduce methylprednisolone blood levels.
- **ESTROGENS:** The effects of methylprednisolone, and possibly other glucocorticoids, may be potentiated by concomitant administration with estrogens.
- **INSULIN:** Insulin requirements may increase in patients receiving glucocorticoids.
- **KETOCONAZOLE** and other **AZOLE ANTIFUNGALS:** May decrease the metabolism of glucocorticoids and increase methylprednisolone blood levels; ketoconazole may induce adrenal insufficiency when glucocorticoids are withdrawn by inhibiting adrenal corticosteroid synthesis.
- **MACROLIDE ANTIBIOTICS** (*e.g.,* **erythromycin, clarithromycin**): May decrease the metabolism of glucocorticoids and increase methylprednisolone blood levels.
- **MITOTANE:** May alter the metabolism of steroids; higher than usual doses of steroids may be necessary to treat mitotane-induced adrenal insufficiency.
- **NSAIDs:** Administration of ulcerogenic drugs with glucocorticoids may increase the risk of gastrointestinal ulceration.
- **PHENOBARBITAL:** May increase the metabolism of glucocorticoids and decrease methylprednisolone blood levels.
- **RIFAMPIN:** May increase the metabolism of glucocorticoids and decrease methylprednisolone blood levels.
- **VACCINES:** Patients receiving corticosteroids at immunosuppressive dosages should generally not receive live attenuated-virus vaccines as virus replication may be augmented; a diminished immune response may occur after vaccine, toxoid, or bacterin administration in patients receiving glucocorticoids.
- **WARFARIN:** Methylprednisolone may affect INR's; monitor.

Laboratory Considerations

- **ACTH stimulation test:** Methylprednisolone can cross-react with the **cortisol assay** and spurious results can occur. Dexamethasone does not interfere with the assay for cortisol.
- Reactions to **intradermal allergy skin tests** may be suppressed by glucocorticoids. Suggested methylprednisolone withdrawal times prior to testing are: tablets = 3-4 weeks; IM methylprednisolone acetate = 8 weeks.
- False-negative results of the **nitroblue tetrazolium** test for systemic bacterial infections may be induced by glucocorticoids.
- Glucocorticoids may increase **serum cholesterol.**
- Glucocorticoids may increase **serum and urine glucose** levels.
- Glucocorticoids may decrease **serum potassium.**
- Glucocorticoids can suppress the release of thyroid stimulating hormone (TSH) and reduce T_3 & T_4 values. Thyroid gland atrophy has been reported after chronic glucocorticoid administration. Uptake of I^{131} by the thyroid may be decreased by glucocorticoids.
- Glucocorticoids may cause **neutrophilia** within 4–8 hours after dosing and return to baseline within 24-48 hours after drug discontinuation.
- Glucocorticoids can cause **lymphopenia** that can persist for weeks after drug discontinuation in dogs.

Doses

There are a plethora of doses and protocols associated with many specific indications for systemic administration of glucocorticoids, but there are four primary uses and dose ranges: 1) replacement or supplementation (*e.g.,* relative adrenal insufficiency associated with septic shock) of glucocorticoid effects secondary to hypoadrenocorticism, 2) as an antiinflammatory, 3) as an immunosuppressive, and 4) as an antineoplastic agent. Current evidence does not support high dose use for hemorrhagic or hypovolemic shock, head trauma, spinal cord trauma, or sepsis.

Note: If using methylprednisolone tablets orally or methylprednisolone sodium succinate for IV injection, refer to the prednis(ol)one dose section to determine an appropriate dose for the condition treated. A near equivalent dose for methylprednisolone can be determined by dividing it by 1.25 (*e.g.,* if the dose is 5 mg of prednisone or prednisolone, the methylprednisolone dose would be 4 mg).

- **DOGS:**

  For labeled uses (FDA-approved): Oral: Dogs weighing 5-15 lbs: 2 mg; Dogs weighing 15-40 lbs: 2 – 4 mg; Dogs weighing 40-80 lbs: 4 – 8 mg; these total daily doses should be divided and given 6-10 hours apart. Intramuscularly (methylprednisolone acetate): 2 – 120 mg IM (average 20 mg); depending on breed (size), severity of condition, and response. May repeat at weekly intervals or in accordance with the severity of the condition and the response. (Label information; *Medrol®, Depo-Medrol®*) The manufacturer has specific directions for use of the drug intrasynovially. It is recommended to refer directly to the package insert for more information.

  For adjunctive treatment of canine atopic dermatitis (extra-label): Initial dosage of approximately 0.4 – 0.5 mg/kg PO once to twice daily to be tapered as needed. Multiple high-quality random, controlled trials have shown consistent efficacy, with minor and predictable adverse effects (Olivry *et al.* 2013).

For adjunctive treatment of anaphylaxis (extra-label): Methylprednisolone sodium succinate 2 – 6 mg/kg IV. Not a substitute for epinephrine. Pre-treatment does NOT prevent anaphylaxis. (Shmuel *et al.* 2013)

For intralesional (sub-lesional) use (extra-label): A sufficient volume of 20 mg/mL methylprednisolone acetate is used to undermine the lesion (10 – 40 mg total dose). (Scott 1982)

- **CATS:**

For labeled uses (FDA-approved): Oral: Cats weighing 5-15 lbs: 2 mg; Cats weighing >15 lbs: 2 – 4 mg. These total daily doses should be divided and given 6-10 hours apart. Intramuscularly using methylprednisolone acetate (*Depo-Medrol*®): up to 20 mg (average 10 mg) IM; depending on breed (size), severity of condition, and response. May repeat at weekly intervals or in accordance with the severity of the condition and the response. (Label information; *Medrol*®, *Depo-Medrol*®)

For adjunctive treatment of pruritus in allergic cats (extra-label): From a double-blinded, randomized, prospective study. Initial induction dosage was 4 mg per cat PO once daily for cats weighing ≤5 kg, and 6 mg per cat PO once daily for cats >5 kg. Cats that did not achieve remission by day 7 had their once daily induction dose doubled for the next 7 days. Mean dosage required for induction of remission was 1.41 mg/kg (range 0.8 – 2.2 mg/kg) PO once daily; 88% of treated cats achieved remission by the end of the second week. Dosages used to achieve remission were then given every other day and tapered (from 100% to 25% of induction dose in 25% increments) to the lowest every other day dosage that maintained remission. 67% of cats that achieved remission were maintained at 25% of the induction dose given every other day. (Ganz *et al.* 2012)

For adjunctive treatment of anaphylaxis (extra-label): Methylprednisolone sodium succinate 2 – 6 mg/kg IV. Not a substitute for epinephrine. Pre-treatment does NOT prevent anaphylaxis. (Shmuel *et al.* 2013)

For intralesional (sub-lesional) use (extra-label): A sufficient volume of 20 mg/mL methylprednisolone acetate is used to undermine the lesion (10 – 40 mg total dose). (Scott 1982)

- **HORSES:**

As an antiinflammatory (glucocorticoid effects); (labeled dose; FDA-approved): Methylprednisolone acetate 200 mg IM repeated as necessary (Package insert; *Depo-Medrol*®). The manufacturer has specific directions for use of the drug intrasynovially. It is recommended to refer directly to the package insert for more information.

For intra-articular use (extra-label): Methylprednisolone acetate 100 mg IA. (McClure 2002)

Monitoring

Monitoring of glucocorticoid therapy is dependent on its reason for use, dosage, agent used (amount of mineralocorticoid activity), dosage schedule (daily versus alternate day therapy), duration of therapy, and the animal's age and condition. The following list may not be appropriate or complete for all animals; use clinical assessment and judgment should adverse effects be noted:

- Weight, appetite, signs of edema.
- Serum and/or urine electrolytes.
- Total plasma proteins, albumin.
- Blood glucose.
- Growth and development in young animals.
- ACTH stimulation test if necessary. **Note:** Methylprednisolone can interfere with cortisol assay.

Client Information

- Give oral products with food.
- Goal is to find the lowest dose possible and use for the shortest period of time.
- Many side effects are possible (see below), especially when the medication is used long term. Most common ones are greater appetite, thirst, and need to urinate.
- In dogs, stomach or intestinal ulcers, perforation or bleeding can occur. If your animal stops eating, or you notice a high fever, black tarry stools or bloody vomit, contact your veterinarian right away.
- Do not stop therapy abruptly (cold turkey) without a veterinarian's guidance as serious side effects could occur.

Chemistry/Synonyms

Methylprednisolone is a synthetically produced glucocorticoid. Both the free alcohol and the acetate ester occur as odorless, white or practically white, crystalline powder. They are practically insoluble in water and sparingly soluble in alcohol.

Methylprednisolone sodium succinate occurs as an odorless, white or nearly white, hygroscopic, amorphous solid. It is very soluble in both water and alcohol.

Methylprednisolone may also be known as: 6alpha-methylprednisolone, methylprednisolonum, NSC-19987, *A-Methapred*®, *Depo-Medrol*®, *Medrol*® or *Solu-Medrol*®.

Storage/Stability

Commercially available products of methylprednisolone should be stored at room temperature (15-30°C); avoid freezing the acetate injection. After reconstituting the sodium succinate injection, store at room temperature and use within 48 hours; only use solutions that are clear.

Compatibility/Compounding Considerations

Methylprednisolone sodium succinate injection is reportedly physically **compatible** with the following fluids and drugs: amino acids 4.25%/dextrose 25%, amphotericin B (limited amounts), chloramphenicol sodium succinate, cimetidine HCl, clindamycin phosphate, dopamine HCl, heparin sodium, metoclopramide, norepinephrine bitartrate, penicillin G potassium, and verapamil.

The following drugs and fluids have either been reported to be physically **incompatible** when mixed with methylprednisolone sodium succinate, compatible dependent upon concentration, or **data conflicts**: D5/half normal saline, D5 normal saline (80 mg/L reported compatible), D5W (up to 5 grams/L reported compatible), Lactated Ringer's (up to 80 mg/L reported compatible), normal saline (data conflicts; some reports of up to 60 grams/Liter compatible), calcium gluconate, glycopyrrolate, insulin, penicillin G sodium, and tetracycline HCl. Compatibility is dependent upon factors such as pH, concentration, temperature, and diluent used; consult specialized references or a hospital pharmacist for more specific information.

Dosage Forms/Regulatory Status

VETERINARY-LABELED PRODUCTS:

Methylprednisolone Tablets: 4 mg tablets, *Medrol*®; (Rx). FDA-approved for use in dogs and cats.

Methylprednisolone Acetate Injection: 20 mg/mL in 10 mL and 20 mL vials, and 40 mg/mL in 5 mL vials; *Depo-Medrol*®, generic; (Rx). FDA-approved for IM and intrasynovial injection in dogs and horses; for IM injection in cats.

The ARCI (Racing Commissioners International) has designated this drug as a class 4 substance. See the appendix for more information.

A 10 ppb tolerance has been established for methylprednisolone in milk.

HUMAN-LABELED PRODUCTS:

Methylprednisolone Oral Tablets: 2 mg, 4 mg, 8 mg, 16 mg, & 32 mg; *Medrol*®, generic; (Rx)

Methylprednisolone Acetate Injection: 20 mg/mL, 40 mg/mL, 80 mg/mL suspension in 1 mL (40 & 80 mg only), 5 mL & 10 mL vials; *Depo-Medrol*®, generic; (Rx)

Methylprednisolone Sodium Succinate Powder for Injection: 40 mg, 125 mg, 500 mg, 1 gram, & 2 gram vials for reconstitution; *Solu-Medrol*®, *A-Methapred*®, generic; (Rx)

Revisions/References

Monograph revised/updated April 2014.

Ganz, E. C., et al. (2012). Evaluation of methylprednisolone and triamcinolone for the induction and maintenance treatment of pruritus in allergic cats: a double-blinded, randomized, prospective study. Veterinary Dermatology 23(5).

Lappin, M. R. & L. M. Roycroft (2011). Effect of Cyclosporine and Methylprednisolone Acetate on Cats with Chronic Feline Herpesvirus 1 Infection. Proceedings: ACVIM. accessed via Veterinary Information Network; vin.com

McClure, S. (2002). An opinion on joint therapy. Proceedings: Western Veterinary Conf. accessed via Veterinary Information Network; vin.com

Menendez, M. I., et al. (2012). Pharmacokinetics of methylprednisolone acetate after intra-articular administration and subsequent suppression of endogenous hydrocortisone secretion in exercising horses. American Journal of Veterinary Research 73(9): 1453-61.

Olivry, T. & P. Bizikova (2013). A systematic review of randomized controlled trials for prevention or treatment of atopic dermatitis in dogs: 2008-2011 update. Veterinary Dermatology 24(1): 97-+.

Scott, D. W. (1982). Dermatologic Use of Glucocorticoids: Systemic and Topical. Vet Clin of North America: Small Anim Prac 12(1): 19-32.

Shmuel, D. L. & Y. Cortes (2013). Anaphylaxis in dogs and cats. J. Vet. Emerg. Crit. Care 23(4): 377-94.

4-Methylpyrazole—see Fomepizole

Methyltestosterone

(meth-ill-tess-**toss**-ter-ohn)   Android®, Methitest®

Androgenic/Anabolic

Prescriber Highlights

▶ Rarely used androgenic & anabolic agent that may be useful in dogs to treat testosterone-responsive alopecia, incontinence, and pseudopregnancy.

▶ Most serious adverse effect is hepatotoxicity. Use in cats is controversial as hepatotoxicity may be more prevalent.

▶ Contraindicated in pregnancy or hepatic dysfunction.

▶ Controlled drug in USA.

Uses/Indications

Methyltestosterone is only rarely recommended for animal patients due to potential toxicity (especially hepatotoxicity) and abuse-potential by humans.

In female dogs, methyltestosterone has been used for treating estrogen-dependent mammary tumors, pseudopregnancy, or certain hormonal-dependent alopecias. In male dogs, it has been used for treating deficient libido, testosterone-responsive incontinence, and certain hormonal alopecias in older, neutered dogs. Using methyltestosterone to suppress estrus in racing greyhounds is controversial and not recommended.

In cats, methyltestosterone has been tried for certain hormonal-dependent alopecias and increasing libido in toms.

Pharmacology/Actions

Methyltestosterone is an androgen with anabolic effects. It has a methyl-group at the 17 position of the steroid nucleus of testosterone, resulting in better oral absorption and slower hepatic metabolism than testosterone. Androgens are required for both the development and maintenance of male sexual characteristics and function. The anabolic effects of methyltestosterone include stimulating erythropoiesis, enhancing nitrogen balance and protein anabolism (in the presence of sufficient protein and calories) and retention of potassium, sodium, and phosphorus.

Pharmacokinetics

Methyltestosterone is absorbed from the GI tract and oral mucosa. It undergoes less first pass metabolism than orally administered testosterone. In dogs, methyltestosterone is metabolized in the liver. Principle metabolites found in urine are glucuronidated forms (both conjugated and free) of methyltestosterone. Unlike in humans, sulfated forms are not a major metabolic component.

In humans, peak levels occur ≈2 hours after oral dosing; elimination half-life is approximately 3 hours.

Contraindications/Precautions/Warnings

Methyltestosterone is contraindicated in patients with hepatic dysfunction and during pregnancy (see Reproductive Safety). It should be used with extreme caution in animals with heart failure. Prolonged use in young animals can cause premature epiphyseal closure. It is not recommended for use in cats.

Methyltestosterone is a controlled drug in the USA; be alert for drug-seeking clients.

Adverse Effects

Adverse effects in dogs include: hepatotoxicity, seborrhea oleosa, virilization of females (clitoral hypertrophy), vaginal discharge, prostatic hyperplasia, and increased aggression in males. Chronic dosing in dogs of 2 – 6 mg/kg/day for 27 weeks caused hepatotoxicity characterized by enlarged periportal hepatocytes, and hemosiderin in macrophages. Cats may be more susceptible to hepatic injury than are dogs.

Reproductive/Nursing Safety

Spermatogenesis suppression in males may occur with high dosage methyltestosterone secondary to a negative feedback mechanism. Methyltestosterone may suppress estrus in females (see Uses). After the drug is discontinued, normal reproductive function usually returns in both males and females.

Methyltestosterone is contraindicated during pregnancy. Dose-related genital masculinization of female fetuses is well described. In humans, the FDA categorizes this drug as category *X* for use during pregnancy (*Studies in animals or humans demonstrate fetal abnormalities or adverse reaction; reports indicate evidence of fetal risk. The risk of use in pregnant women clearly outweighs any possible benefit.*)

Overdosage/Acute Toxicity

Information on the acute toxicity of methyltestosterone is limited. Nausea and edema are the most likely effects of a single overdose. Consider liver function monitoring with large overdoses.

Drug Interactions

The following drug interactions have either been reported or are theoretical in humans or animals receiving methyltestosterone and may be of significance in veterinary patients. Unless otherwise noted, use together is not necessarily contraindicated, but weigh the potential risks and perform additional monitoring when appropriate.

▪ **CYCLOSPORINE:** Methyltestosterone may increase serum cyclosporine levels.

▪ **INSULIN; ORAL ANTIDIABETIC AGENTS:** Methyltestosterone may decrease serum glucose levels.

▪ **WARFARIN:** Methyltestosterone may increase anticoagulant effects.

Laboratory Considerations

▪ Methyltestosterone or other androgens can decrease **thyroxine-binding globulin** concentrations. This can cause decreased serum levels of **total T4** and increased resin uptake of T4 and T3. Clinically, this is unimportant, as free thyroid hormone concentrations are not affected.

Doses

- **DOGS:**

  For testosterone-responsive alopecia in neutered male dogs (extra-label): Rarely recommended; no studies were located documenting safety and efficacy. Anecdotal dosages generally range from 1 – 1.1 mg/kg (maximum of 30 mg per dog) PO once daily or every other day until hair-regrowth is noted (usually 1-3 months). Dosage frequency is then reduced over weeks to months to maintenance dosage (1-2 times per week). Liver profile must be monitored.

  For testosterone-responsive urinary incontinence in neutered male dogs (extra-label): Rarely recommended; no studies were located documenting safety and efficacy. An anecdotal dosage of 0.5 mg/kg PO once daily has been noted.

Monitoring

- Hepatic function (liver enzymes, icterus, anorexia/weight loss/vomiting).

Client Information

- Liver toxicity is biggest concern; cats may be more susceptible. Other possible side effects include: masculinization or vaginal discharge in females, prostate problems and aggression in males.
- Pregnant women should handle this medication with caution.
- Controlled substance (C-III) in USA. It is a federal offense to give or sell this medication to others than for whom it was prescribed.

Chemistry/Synonyms

Methyltestosterone occurs as white or creamy-white, odorless, crystals or crystalline powder. It is slightly hygroscopic, practically insoluble in water, freely soluble in alcohol, and sparingly soluble in vegetable oils.

Methyltestosterone may also be known as NSC-9701 or by its chemical name, 17beta-Hydroxy-17alpha-methyladrost-4-ene-3one, *Android*®, *Methitest*®, *Testred*® and *Virilon*®. A trade name for a veterinary product formerly available in the U.K. is *Orandrone*®.

Storage/Stability

Unless otherwise specified by the manufacturer, methyltestosterone tablets or capsules should be stored below 40°C, preferably between 15-30°C in well-closed containers.

Compatibility/Compounding Considerations

No specific information noted.

Dosage Forms/Regulatory Status

VETERINARY-LABELED PRODUCTS: NONE.

The ARCI (Racing Commissioners International) has designated this drug as a class 4 substance. See appendix for more information.

Methyltestosterone Tablets: 10 mg & 25 mg; *Methitest*®; (Rx, C-III)

Methyltestosterone Capsules: 10 mg; *Testred*® & *Android*®; (Rx, C-III)

Revisions/References

Monograph revised/updated April 2014.

Metoclopramide HCl

(met-oh-kloe-**pra**-mide)   Reglan®

GI Prokinetic Agent

Prescriber Highlights

▶ Stimulates upper GI motility & has antiemetic properties; more potent as an antiemetic (in dogs) than a prokinetic agent. May be a poor antiemetic in cats.

▶ Contraindications: GI hemorrhage, obstruction or perforation, hypersensitivity. Relatively contraindicated: Seizure disorders, pheochromocytoma.

▶ Adverse Effects: **Dogs:** Changes in mentation & behavior, constipation; **Cats:** Signs of frenzied behavior or disorientation, constipation; **Horses:** IV use, severe CNS effects, behavioral changes & abdominal pain; **Foals:** Adverse effects less common.

▶ Several potentially serious drug interactions.

Uses/Indications

Metoclopramide has been used in veterinary species for both its GI stimulatory and antiemetic properties. It has been used clinically for gastric stasis disorders, gastroesophageal reflux, to allow intubation of the small intestine, as a general antiemetic (for parvovirus, bilious vomiting syndrome, uremic gastritis, etc.), and an antiemetic to prevent or treat chemotherapy-induced vomiting. While widely accepted as an antiemetic in dogs, controlled studies documenting safety and efficacy for this purpose in dogs (or cats) was not located. Distinct differences of antiemetic and prokinetic effects can be seen depending on the species. Antiemetic effects appear more pronounced in dogs than cats, while distal esophageal motility effects are greater in cats. Metoclopramide has gastric prokinetic effects in both species.

Pharmacology/Actions

The primary pharmacologic effects of metoclopramide are associated with the GI tract and the CNS. In the GI tract, metoclopramide stimulates motility of the upper GI without stimulating gastric, pancreatic or biliary secretions. While the exact mechanisms for these actions are unknown, it appears that metoclopramide sensitizes upper GI smooth muscle to the effects of acetylcholine. Intact vagal innervation is not necessary for enhanced motility, but anticholinergic drugs will negate metoclopramide's effects. Gastrointestinal effects seen include increased tone and amplitude of gastric contractions, relaxed pyloric sphincter, and increased duodenal and jejunal peristalsis. Gastric emptying and intestinal transit times can be significantly reduced. There is little or no effect on colon motility. Additionally, metoclopramide will increase lower esophageal sphincter pressure and prevent or reduce gastroesophageal reflux, but a study did not show any reduction in gastroesophageal reflux in dogs undergoing anesthesia (acepromazine, propofol, isoflurane) (Favarato *et al.* 2012). Metoclopramide's stimulatory effects on distal esophageal peristalsis are species specific with more effect in humans, cats, and guinea pigs; less in dogs.

In the CNS, metoclopramide apparently antagonizes dopamine (D_2) at receptor sites. It is also a weak inhibitor of 5-HT_3 and an agonist for 5-HT_4 receptors. These actions help explain its sedative, central anti-emetic, extrapyramidal, and prolactin secretion stimulation effects.

Antiemetic effects of metoclopramide are secondary to both central and peripheral (local) effects. Cats reportedly have few CNS dopamine receptors and therefore metoclopramide may be a poor antiemetic choice in this species (Twedt 2008).

Metoclopramide can induce transient increases in aldosterone levels thereby increasing sodium and fluid retention.

In a study in horses comparing the effects of certain drugs (metoclopramide, cisapride, mosapride) on gastric emptying, and small intestinal and cecal motility, metoclopramide promoted jejunal motility but did not significantly affect gastric emptying or cecal motility (Okamura *et al.* 2009).

Pharmacokinetics

Metoclopramide is absorbed well after oral administration, but a significant first-pass effect in some human patients may reduce systemic bioavailability to 30%. There apparently is a great deal of interpatient variation with this effect. Bioavailability after intramuscular administration has been measured to be 74-96%. After oral dosing, peak plasma levels generally occur within 2 hours.

The drug is well distributed in the body and enters the CNS. Metoclopramide is only weakly bound to 13-22% of plasma proteins. The drug also crosses the placenta and enters the milk in concentrations approximately twice those of plasma.

Metoclopramide is primarily excreted in the urine in humans. Approximately 20-25% of the drug is excreted unchanged in the urine. The majority of the rest of the drug is metabolized to glucuronidated or sulfated conjugate forms and then excreted in the urine. Approximately 5% is excreted in the feces. The half-life of metoclopramide in the dog has been reported to be approximately 90 minutes.

Contraindications/Precautions/Warnings

Metoclopramide is contraindicated in patients with GI hemorrhage, obstruction (should be ruled out before use) or perforation, and in those hypersensitive to it. It is relatively (some say absolutely) contraindicated in patients with seizure disorders or head trauma. In patients with pheochromocytoma, metoclopramide may induce a hypertensive crisis.

Several veterinary references state that metoclopramide is contraindicated with concurrent phenothiazine therapy (see Drug Interactions). Depending on the reference (human), metoclopramide use together with the following drugs and drug classes may be contraindicated: tricyclic antidepressants (amitriptyline, clomipramine, etc.), SSRI-type antidepressants (paroxetine, fluoxetine, sertraline, etc.), or mirtazapine. Major drug interactions with tramadol and selegiline are possible.

Metoclopramide should be avoided in dogs with pseudopregnancy as it can cause prolactin release (Romagnoli 2009).

Due to its effects on aldosterone, it should be used with caution in patients with congestive heart failure.

Dosage adjustment may be required when used as a CRI in patients with renal failure. One reference suggests based upon anecdotal experience, reducing the CRI 25-50% of standard dosage (Trepanier 2008).

Adverse Effects

In dogs, the most common (although infrequent) adverse reactions seen are changes in mentation and behavior (motor restlessness, involuntary spasms, aggression, and hyperactivity to drowsiness/depression). Metoclopramide can increase detrusor muscle contractility and reduce bladder capacity.

Cats may exhibit signs of frenzied behavior or disorientation. Both species can develop constipation while receiving this medication.

In adult horses, IV metoclopramide administration has been associated with the development of severe CNS effects. Alternating periods of sedation and excitement, behavioral changes and abdominal pain have been noted. These effects appear to be less common in foals.

Other adverse effects that have been reported in humans and are potentially plausible in animals include extrapyramidal effects, nausea, diarrhea, transient hypertension, and elevated prolactin levels.

Reproductive/Nursing Safety

In humans, the FDA categorizes this drug as category *B* for use during pregnancy (*Animal studies have not yet demonstrated risk to the fetus, but there are no adequate studies in pregnant women; or animal studies have shown an adverse effect, but adequate studies in pregnant women have not demonstrated a risk to the fetus in the first trimester of pregnancy, and there is no evidence of risk in later trimesters.*) In a separate system evaluating the safety of drugs in canine and feline pregnancy (Papich 1989), this drug is categorized as class: *B* (*Safe for use if used cautiously. Studies in laboratory animals may have uncovered some risk, but these drugs appear to be safe in dogs and cats or these drugs are safe if they are not administered when the animal is near term.*)

Metoclopramide is excreted into milk and may concentrate at about twice the plasma level, but there does not appear to be significant risk to nursing offspring.

Overdosage/Acute Toxicity

The oral LD_{50} doses of metoclopramide in mice, rats, and rabbits are 465 mg/kg, 760 mg/kg and 870 mg/kg, respectively. Because of the high dosages required for lethality, it is unlikely an oral overdose will cause death in a veterinary patient. Likely clinical signs of overdosage include sedation, ataxia, agitation, extrapyramidal effects, nausea, vomiting, and constipation. Serotonin syndrome is possible.

There were 84 single agent exposures to metoclopramide reported to the ASPCA Animal Poison Control Center (APCC) during 2009-2013. Of the 59 dogs, 25 were symptomatic with 20% having diarrhea, 24% agitation and 16% vomiting. Of the 24 cats, 16 were symptomatic with 31% vocalizing and 25% agitated.

There is no specific antidotal therapy for metoclopramide intoxication. If an oral ingestion was recent, the stomach should be emptied using standard protocols. Metoclopramide may affect efficacy of apomorphine as an emetic. Anticholinergic agents (diphenhydramine 2.2 mg/kg IV, benztropine, etc.) that enter the CNS may be helpful in controlling extrapyramidal effects. Peritoneal dialysis or hemodialysis is not thought to be effective in enhancing the removal of the drug.

Drug Interactions

The following drug interactions have either been reported or are theoretical in humans or animals receiving oral metoclopramide and may be of significance in veterinary patients. Unless otherwise noted, use together is not necessarily contraindicated, but weigh the potential risks and perform additional monitoring when appropriate.

- **ASPIRIN, ACETAMINOPHEN, ALCOHOL:** In overdose situations in humans, metoclopramide has enhanced absorption of these agents.
- **ANESTHETICS:** If metoclopramide is used concurrently IV, acute hypotension has been reported.
- **APOMORPHINE:** Metoclopramide may negate the emetic effects of apomorphine. Hydrogen peroxide (PO; dogs) may be an effective alternative.
- **ATROPINE (and related anticholinergic compounds):** May antagonize the GI motility effects of metoclopramide.
- **CEPHALEXIN:** In dogs, oral metoclopramide was shown to increase cephalexin peak plasma concentrations and area under the curve. No dosage adjustments are required. (Prados *et al.* 2007)
- **CHOLINERGIC DRUGS** (*e.g.*, **bethanechol**): May enhance metoclopramide's GI effects.

- **CNS DEPRESSANTS** (*e.g.*, **anesthetic agents, antihistamines, phenothiazines, barbiturates, tranquilizers, alcohol**, etc.): Metoclopramide may enhance CNS depressant effects.
- **CYCLOSPORINE:** Metoclopramide potentially could increase the rate and extent of GI absorption of cyclosporine, however this does not appear to be an issue in dogs (Radwanski *et al.* 2011).
- **DOPAMINE:** Metoclopramide could theoretically interact with IV dopamine, but clinical significance has not been established.
- **OPIATE ANALGESICS:** May antagonize the GI motility effects of metoclopramide and enhance metoclopramide's CNS effects.
- **MAO INHIBITORS** (including **amitraz**): Could cause hypertension.
- **MIRTAZAPINE:** Increased risk for extrapyramidal adverse effects; use together is contraindicated in humans.
- **PHENOTHIAZINES** (*e.g.*, **acepromazine, chlorpromazine**, etc.) and **BUTYROPHENONES** (*e.g.*, **droperidol, azaperone**): May potentiate the extrapyramidal effects of metoclopramide.
- **PROPOFOL:** In humans, metoclopramide reduces induction requirements of propofol by 20-25%.
- **SELEGILINE:** Use together may increase risk for hypertensive crisis.
- **SSRI & TRICYCLIC ANTIDEPRESSANTS** (*e.g.*, **amitriptyline, clomipramine, fluoxetine, sertraline, paroxetine**, etc.): Potential for enhanced extrapyramidal effects or neuroleptic malignant syndrome. Use together is contraindicated in humans.
- **TETRACYCLINES:** Metoclopramide can increase the rate and extent of GI absorption.
- **TRAMADOL:** Use together may increase risk for seizures.
- **XYLAZINE:** In cats, metoclopramide may reduce the emetic effects of xylazine (Kolahian *et al.* 2010).

Laboratory Considerations
- **Vasopressin.** Metoclopramide may induce secretion of vasopressin and alter fluid and electrolyte values.

Doses
- **DOGS:**

  As an antiemetic and gastric prokinetic (extra-label): 0.2 – 0.5 mg/kg q6-8h PO, SC or IM; or 0.01 – 0.09 mg/kg hour as a continuous IV infusion (CRI). When used as an antiemetic for chemotherapy induced emesis, higher dosages (1 mg/kg SC, IM) may be required.

  To induce milk let-down for secondary agalactia (extra-label): oxytocin 0.25 – 1 Unit (total dose) SC q2h. Neonates are removed for 30 minutes post-injection, and then encouraged to suckle, or gentle stripping of the glands performed. Metoclopramide at 0.1 – 0.2 mg/kg SC q12h (dopamine antagonist) can be used to promote milk production. Therapy is usually rewarding within 24 hours. (Davidson 2009)

- **CATS:**

  As an antiemetic and gastric prokinetic (extra-label): Usually other antiemetics (ondansetron, dolasetron, maropitant, etc.) and prokinetic agents (*e.g.*, cisapride) are used, but the dosages for dogs could be tried.

- **RABBITS, RODENTS, SMALL MAMMALS:**

  Anecdotal dosages of 0.2 – 1 mg/kg PO, IM or SC q8-24h have been noted.

Monitoring
- Clinical efficacy.
- Adverse effects, including monitoring for tremors.

Client Information
- May give by mouth with or without food. Sometimes given under the skin (SC, subcutaneously) especially when vomiting in small animals is being treated/prevented.
- Usually tolerated well by dogs and cats. Contact veterinarian if animal develops severe restlessness/hyperactivity, rigid posture, spasms, aggression, or severe drowsiness/depression. Bladder capacity can be reduced and more frequent urination necessary. Cats may show signs of frenzied behavior or disorientation. Both dogs and cats can become constipated.

Chemistry/Synonyms
A derivative of para-aminobenzoic acid, metoclopramide HCl occurs as an odorless, white, crystalline powder with pK_as of 0.6 and 9.3. One gram is approximately soluble in 0.7 mL of water or 3 mL of alcohol. The injectable product has a pH of 3-6.5.

Metoclopramide HCl may also be known as: AHR-3070-C, DEL-1267, metoclopramidi hydrochloridum, and MK-745; many trade names are available.

Storage/Stability
Metoclopramide is photosensitive and must be stored in light resistant containers at room temperature. Metoclopramide tablets should be kept in tight containers.

The injection is reportedly stable in solutions of a pH range of 2-9 and with the following IV solutions: D_5W, 0.9% sodium chloride, D_5-1/2 normal saline, Ringer's, and lactated Ringer's injection.

Compatibility/Compounding Considerations
The following drugs have been stated to be physically **compatible** with metoclopramide for at least 24 hours: aminophylline, ascorbic acid, atropine sulfate, chlorpromazine HCl, cimetidine HCl, clindamycin phosphate, cyclophosphamide, cytarabine, dexamethasone sodium phosphate, dimenhydrinate, diphenhydramine HCl, doxorubicin HCl, fentanyl citrate, heparin sodium, hydrocortisone sodium phosphate, hydroxyzine HCl, insulin (regular), lidocaine HCl, magnesium sulfate, mannitol, meperidine HCl, methylprednisolone sodium succinate, morphine sulfate, multivitamin infusion (MVI), pentazocine lactate, potassium acetate/chloride/phosphate, prochlorperazine edisylate, ranitidine, TPN solution (25% dextrose with 4.25% *Travasol*® with or without electrolytes), verapamil, and vitamin B-complex with vitamin C.

Metoclopramide is reported to be physically **incompatible** when mixed with the following drugs: ampicillin sodium, calcium gluconate, chloramphenicol sodium succinate, cisplatin, erythromycin lactobionate, methotrexate sodium, penicillin G potassium, sodium bicarbonate, and tetracycline. Compatibility is dependent upon factors such as pH, concentration, temperature, and diluent used; consult specialized references or a hospital pharmacist for more specific information.

Dosage Forms/Regulatory Status
VETERINARY-LABELED PRODUCTS: NONE.

The ARCI (Racing Commissioners International) has designated this drug as a class 4 substance. See the appendix for more information.

HUMAN-LABELED PRODUCTS:

All are expressed in terms of metoclopramide monohydrate.

Metoclopramide HCl Oral Tablets: 5 mg & 10 mg; *Reglan*®, generic; (Rx)

Metoclopramide Oral Dispersible Tablets (ODT): 5 mg; *Metozolv*®, generic; (Rx)

Metoclopramide HCl Oral Syrup: 1 mg/mL; generic; (Rx)

Metoclopramide HCl Injection Solution: 5 mg/mL; generic; (Rx)

Revisions/References

Monograph revised/updated April 2014.

Davidson, A. (2009). Postpartum disorders in the bitch and queen. Proceedings: WVC. accessed via Veterinary Information Network; vin.com

Favarato, E. S., et al. (2012). Evaluation of metoclopramide and ranitidine on the prevention of gastroesophageal reflux episodes in anesthetized dogs. *Research in Veterinary Science* 93(1): 466-7.

Kolahian, S. & S. Jarolmasjed (2010). Effects of metoclopramide on emesis in cats sedated with xylazine hydrochloride. *Journal of Feline Medicine and Surgery* 12(12): 899-903.

Okamura, K., et al. (2009). Effects of mosapride citrate, metoclopramide hydrochloride, lidocaine hydrochloride, and cisapride citrate on equine gastric emptying, small intestinal and caecal motility. *Research in Veterinary Science* 86(2): 302-8.

Papich, M. (1989). Effects of drugs on pregnancy. *Current Veterinary Therapy X: Small Animal Practice.* R. Kirk. Philadelphia, Saunders: 1291-9.

Prados, A. P., et al. (2007). Metoclopramide modifies oral cephalexin pharmacokinetics in dogs. *J. Vet. Pharmacol. Ther.* 30(2): 127-31.

Radwanski, N. E., et al. (2011). Effects of powdered whole grapefruit and metoclopramide on the pharmacokinetics of cyclosporine in dogs. *American Journal of Veterinary Research* 72(5): 687-93.

Romagnoli, S. (2009). An update on pseudopregnancy. Proceedings: WSAVA. accessed via Veterinary Information Network; vin.com

Trepanier, L. (2008). Case presentations: Drug dose adjustments. Proceedings: ACVIM. accessed via Veterinary Information Network; vin.com

Twedt, D. (2008). Antiemetics, prokinetics & antacids. Proceedings: ACVIM. accessed via Veterinary Information Network; vin.com

Metoprolol Tartrate
Metoprolol Succinate

(me-**toe**-pro-lole)   Lopressor®, Toprol XL®

Beta-Adrenergic Blocker

Prescriber Highlights

▶ Beta$_1$-blocker used for supraventricular tachyarrhythmias, premature ventricular contractions (PVC's, VPC's), systemic hypertension, & treatment in cats with hypertrophic cardiomyopathy.

▶ Probably safer to use than propranolol in animals with bronchoconstrictive disease.

▶ Contraindications: Overt or unstable heart failure, hypersensitivity beta-blockers, greater than 1st-degree heart block, or sinus bradycardia.

▶ Caution: Significant hepatic insufficiency, bronchospastic lung disease, CHF, hyperthyroidism (masks clinical signs, but may be useful for treatment), labile diabetics, & sinus node dysfunction.

▶ Adverse Effects: Most common in geriatric animals or those that have acute decompensating heart disease, include: bradycardia, lethargy & depression, impaired AV conduction, CHF or worsening of heart failure, hypotension, hypoglycemia, bronchoconstriction, syncope, & diarrhea.

▶ Try to wean off drug gradually.

Uses/Indications

Because metoprolol is relatively safe to use in animals with bronchospastic disease, it is often chosen over propranolol. It may be effective in supraventricular tachyarrhythmias, premature ventricular contractions (PVC's, VPC's), systemic hypertension, and treating cats with hypertrophic cardiomyopathy.

There is no consensus for use of beta-blockers in dogs with non-congestive heart failure. One retrospective study showed increased survival times when dogs were given metoprolol, but definitive prospective, double-blinded studies have not been reported documenting the benefit (increased survival) of beta-blockers in dogs with heart failure. In the American College of Veterinary Internal Medicine (ACVIM) Consensus Panel *Guidelines for the Diagnosis and Treatment of Canine Chronic Valvular Heart Disease*, the panel recommends that if beta-blocker therapy is to be instituted in Class C2 (dogs with either clinical signs mild enough to allow home therapy or dogs previously stabilized during hospitalization for acute CHF) myxomatous mitral valve disease (MMVD), their use should be limited to dogs that have been stabilized and the dosage gradually increased with careful monitoring. Dogs in this class with atrial fibrillation are another reason to consider beta-blockers to help control heart rate (Atkins, C. *et al.* 2009; Atkins, C.E. *et al.* 2012).

Pharmacology/Actions

Metoprolol is a relatively specific beta$_1$-blocker and is sometimes characterized as a 2nd-generation beta-blocker. At higher dosages, this specificity may be lost and beta$_2$-blockade can occur. Metoprolol does not possess any intrinsic sympathomimetic activity like pindolol nor does it possess membrane-stabilizing activity like pindolol or propranolol. Cardiovascular effects secondary to metoprolol's negative inotropic and chronotropic actions include: decreased sinus heart rate, slowed AV conduction, diminished cardiac output at rest and during exercise, decreased myocardial oxygen demand, reduced blood pressure, and inhibition of isoproterenol-induced tachycardia.

Pharmacokinetics

Metoprolol tartrate is rapidly and nearly completely absorbed from the GI tract, but it has a relatively high first pass effect (50%) so systemic bioavailability is reduced. The drug has very low protein binding characteristics (5-15%) and is distributed well into most tissues. Metoprolol crosses the blood-brain barrier and CSF levels are ≈78% of those found in the serum. It crosses the placenta and levels in milk are 3-4X higher than those found in plasma. Metoprolol is primarily biotransformed in the liver; unchanged drug and metabolites are then principally excreted in the urine. Reported half-lives in various species: Dogs: 1.6 hours; Cats: 1.3 hours; Humans 3-4 hours.

No information on the pharmacokinetics of human metoprolol succinate extended-release dosage forms was located for dogs or cats.

Contraindications/Precautions/Warnings

Metoprolol is contraindicated in patients with overt or unstable heart failure, hypersensitivity to this class of agents, greater than 1st-degree heart block, or sinus bradycardia. The ACVIM Consensus Panel unanimously advised against the using beta-adrenergic blockers in dogs with active CHF (Atkins, C. *et al.* 2009). Non-specific beta-blockers are also relatively contraindicated in patients with bronchospastic lung disease.

Metoprolol should be used cautiously in patients with significant hepatic insufficiency or sinus node dysfunction.

Metoprolol (at high dosages) can mask the clinical signs associated with hypoglycemia. It can also cause hypoglycemia or hyperglycemia and, therefore, should be used cautiously in labile diabetic patients.

Metoprolol can mask the clinical signs associated with thyrotoxicosis, but it may be used clinically to treat the clinical signs associated with this condition.

Do not confuse metoprolol succinate with metoprolol tartrate.

Adverse Effects

It is reported that adverse effects most commonly occur in geriatric animals or those that have acute decompensating heart disease. Adverse effects considered clinically relevant include: bradycardia, lethargy, weakness and depression, impaired AV conduction, CHF or worsening of heart failure, hypotension, hypoglycemia, and bronchoconstriction (less so with beta$_1$-specific drugs like metoprolol). Syncope and diarrhea have also been reported in canine patients with beta-blockers. Cats with hypertrophic cardiomyopathy may be at an increased risk for pulmonary edema.

Exacerbation of clinical signs has been reported following abrupt cessation of beta-blockers in humans. When possible, it is recommended to withdraw therapy gradually in patients that have been receiving the drug on a chronic basis.

Reproductive/Nursing Safety

Safe use during pregnancy has not been established, but adverse effects to fetuses have apparently not been documented. In humans, the FDA categorizes this drug as category *C* for use during pregnancy (*Animal studies have shown an adverse effect on the fetus, but there are no adequate studies in humans; or there are no animal reproduction studies and no adequate studies in humans.*)

Metoprolol is excreted in milk in very small quantities and is unlikely to pose significant risk to nursing offspring.

Overdosage/Acute Toxicity

There is limited information available on metoprolol overdosage. Humans have apparently survived dosages of up to 5 grams. The most predominant clinical signs expected would be extensions of the drug's pharmacologic effects: hypotension, bradycardia, bronchospasm, cardiac failure, and, potentially, hypoglycemia.

There were 1079 single agent exposures to metoprolol reported to the ASPCA Animal Poison Control Center (APCC) during 2009-2013. Of the 995 exposed dogs, 97 were symptomatic. The most common clinical signs included: lethargy (23%), tachycardia (20%), vomiting (18%) and bradycardia (16%). Of the 80 cats, 12 were symptomatic with 17% being bradycardic, mydriatic or tachycardic.

If overdose is secondary to a recent oral ingestion, emptying the gut and charcoal administration may be considered. Use caution inducing emesis as coma and seizures may develop rapidly. Monitor: ECG, blood glucose, potassium, and, blood pressure. Treatment of the cardiovascular effects is symptomatic. Use fluids and pressor agents to treat hypotension. Bradycardia may be treated with atropine. If atropine fails, isoproterenol, given cautiously, has been recommended. Use of a transvenous pacemaker may be necessary. Cardiac failure can be treated with a digitalis glycosides, diuretics, and oxygen. Glucagon (5 – 10 mg IV—Human dose) may increase heart rate and blood pressure and reduce the cardiodepressant effects of metoprolol. Intravenous lipid (ILE) infusions are not likely to affect metoprolol intoxication.

Drug Interactions

The following drug interactions have either been reported or are theoretical in humans or animals receiving metoprolol and may be of significance in veterinary patients. Unless otherwise noted, use together is not necessarily contraindicated, but weigh the potential risks and perform additional monitoring when appropriate.

- **ANESTHETICS, GENERAL (with myocardial depressant effects)**: Increased risk for heart failure and hypotension.
- **CALCIUM-CHANNEL BLOCKERS** (*e.g.*, **diltiazem, verapamil, amlodipine**): Concurrent use of beta-blockers with calcium channel blockers (or other negative inotropics) should be done with caution, particularly in patients with preexisting cardiomyopathy or CHF.
- **DIGOXIN**: Use with metoprolol may increase negative effects on SA or AV node conduction.
- **DIURETICS (thiazides, furosemide)**: May increase hypotensive effect of metoprolol.
- **HYDRALAZINE**: May increase the risks for pulmonary hypertension in uremic patients.
- **QUINIDINE**: May increase metoprolol plasma concentrations.
- **RESERPINE**: Potential for additive effects (hypotension, bradycardia).
- **SSRI ANTIDEPRESSANTS** (*e.g.,* **fluoxetine, sertraline, paroxetine**): May increase metoprolol plasma concentrations.
- **SYMPATHOMIMETICS (metaproterenol, terbutaline, beta-effects of epinephrine, phenylpropanolamine, etc.)**: May

have their actions blocked by metoprolol and they may, in turn, reduce the efficacy of atenolol.

Doses

- **DOGS:**

    As an oral beta blocker for adjunctive treatment of non-congestive heart failure or heart rate control in dogs with atrial fibrillation (extra-label): Using metoprolol tartrate (regular tablets): Usually dosages are started low at approximately 0.2 mg/kg PO q12h and slowly titrated upwards (as tolerated) every 2-3 weeks. Practically, the dosage per dog will be a minimum of 6.25 mg (1/4 of a 25 mg tablet) unless dosage forms are compounded. Commonly, dosages of 0.4 – 1 mg/kg PO q8-12h are used, but dosages as high as 6.6 mg/kg PO 3 times daily have been noted. However, many dogs will not tolerate upward dosage titration. Sustained-release metoprolol succinate tablets could be considered, but pharmacokinetic data supporting their use in dogs is not available.

- **CATS:**

    As an oral beta-blocker (extra-label): Anecdotal dosages of 2 – 15 mg per cat PO q8h have been noted. As the smallest commercial dosage form available is a 25 mg tablet, dosages may need to be compounded for cats.

Monitoring

- Cardiac function, pulse rate, ECG if necessary, BP if indicated.
- Toxicity (see Adverse Effects/Overdosage).

Client Information

- To be effective, the animal must receive all doses as prescribed. Can be given with or without food.
- Most common side effects include lethargy (tiredness/lack of energy) and weakness. Low blood pressure is possible. Too slow a heart rate with and heart symptoms that get worse can occur if dose is too high. Notify veterinarian if animal becomes exercise intolerant, has shortness of breath or cough, or develops a change in behavior or attitude.
- When starting this drug, your veterinarian may start with a low dose and gradually increase it over time to see how your animal reacts to it. Do not administer more at one time than your veterinarian prescribes.
- Very important not to stop the drug abruptly without veterinarian's guidance.

Chemistry/Synonyms

A beta$_1$-specific adrenergic blocker, metoprolol tartrate occurs as a white, crystalline powder having a bitter taste. It is very soluble in water. Metoprolol succinate occurs as a white, crystalline powder and is freely soluble in water.

Metoprolol may also be known as: CGP-2175E, H-93/26, and metoprolol; many trade names are available.

Storage/Stability

Store all products protected from light. Store tablets in tight, light-resistant containers at room temperature. Avoid freezing the injection.

Compatibility/Compounding Considerations

The injection is **compatible** with D5W and normal saline, and at Y-sites with morphine sulfate.

Compounded preparation stability: Metoprolol oral suspension compounded from the commercially available tablets has been published (Allen *et al.* 1996). Triturating twelve (12) metoprolol tartrate 100 mg tablets with 60 mL of *Ora-Plus®* and *qs ad* to 120 mL with *Ora-Sweet®* or *Ora-Sweet SF®* yields a 10 mg/mL metoprolol tartrate oral suspension that retains >95% potency for 60 days when stored at both 4°C and 25°C and protected from light.

Dosage Forms/Regulatory Status

VETERINARY-LABELED PRODUCTS: NONE.

The ARCI (Racing Commissioners International) has designated this drug as a class 3 substance. See the appendix for more information.

HUMAN-LABELED PRODUCTS:

Metoprolol Tartrate Oral Tablets: 25 mg, 50 mg & 100 mg; *Lopressor®*, generic; (Rx)

Metoprolol Succinate Extended-Release Tablets: 25 mg, 50 mg, 100 mg & 200 mg; *Toprol XL®*, generic; (Rx)

Metoprolol Tartrate Injection: 1 mg/mL; *Lopressor®*, generic; (Rx)

Revisions/References

Monograph revised/updated April 2014.

Allen, L. V. & M. A. Erickson (1996). Stability of labetalol hydrochloride, metoprolol tartrate, verapamil hydrochloride, and spironolactone with hydrochlorothiazide in extemporaneous compounded oral liquids. Am J Health Syst Pharm 53(19): 2304-9.
Atkins, C., et al. (2009). Guidelines for the Diagnosis and Treatment of Canine Chronic Valvular Heart Disease. Journal of Veterinary Internal Medicine 23(6): 1142-50.
Atkins, C. E. & J. Haggstrom (2012). Pharmacologic management of myxomatous mitral valve disease in dogs. Journal of veterinary cardiology : the official journal of the European Society of Veterinary Cardiology 14(1).

Metronidazole

(me-troe-ni-da-zole)   Flagyl®

Antibiotic, Antiparasitic

Prescriber Highlights

▶ Injectable & oral antibacterial (anaerobes) & antiprotozoal agent.

▶ Prohibited by the FDA for use in food animals.

▶ Contraindications: Hypersensitivity to it or other nitroimidazole derivatives. Extreme caution: in severely debilitated, pregnant or nursing animals; hepatic dysfunction. May be a teratogen, especially in early pregnancy.

▶ Adverse Effects: Neurologic disorders, lethargy, weakness, neutropenia, hepatotoxicity, hematuria, anorexia, nausea, vomiting, & diarrhea.

▶ Very bitter, metronidazole benzoate may be more palatable when compounded.

Uses/Indications

Although there are no veterinary-approved metronidazole products, the drug has been used extensively in the treatment of Giardia in both dogs and cats. It is also used clinically in small animals for the treatment of other parasites (Trichomonas and *Balantidium coli*) as well as treating both enteric and systemic anaerobic infections. It is commonly employed as a perioperative surgical prophylaxis antibiotic where anaerobes are likely (*e.g.*, colon; periodontal).

In horses, metronidazole has been used clinically for the treatment of anaerobic infections.

Pharmacology/Actions

Metronidazole is a concentration-dependent bactericidal agent against susceptible bacteria. Its exact mechanism of action is not completely understood, but it is taken-up by anaerobic organisms where it is reduced to an unidentified polar compound. It is believed that this compound is responsible for the drug's antimicrobial activity by disrupting DNA and nucleic acid synthesis in the bacteria. Metronidazole has activity against most obligate anaerobes including *Bacteroides* spp. (including *B. fragilis*), Fusobacterium, Veillonella, *Clostridium* spp., Peptococcus, and Peptostreptococcus. Actinomyces is frequently resistant to metronidazole. Some isolates of *C. difficile* may be resistant.

Metronidazole is also trichomonacidal and amebicidal in action

and acts as a direct amebicide. Its mechanism of action for its antiprotozoal activity is not understood. It has therapeutic activity against *Entamoeba histolytica*, Trichomonas, Giardia, and *Balantidium coli*. It acts primarily against the trophozoite forms of Entamoeba rather than encysted forms.

Metronidazole has some inhibitive actions on cell-mediated immunity that may play a role in its use for treating inflammatory bowel disease.

Pharmacokinetics

Metronidazole is relatively well absorbed after oral administration. Metronidazole is rather lipophilic and is rapidly and widely distributed after absorption. It is distributed to most body tissues and fluids, including bone, abscesses, the CNS, and seminal fluid. Metronidazole is <20% bound to plasma proteins in humans. Metronidazole is primarily metabolized in the liver via several pathways. Both the metabolites and unchanged drug are eliminated in the urine and feces.

The oral bioavailability in dogs is high, but interpatient variable, with ranges from 50-100% reported. If given with food, absorption is enhanced in dogs, but delayed in humans. Peak levels occur ≈1 hour after oral dosing.

In a single-dose study in cats (Sekis *et al.* 2009), the oral bioavailability of metronidazole benzoate is variable, but averages around 65%. Peak levels after oral dosing appear to be highly variable in cats (ranging from 1-8 hours) and peak serum concentrations are somewhat lower in cats than in dogs or humans. Mean systemic clearance is slower in cats than dogs (2.49 mL/kg/min vs. 1.53 mL/kg/min). Despite the concern that glucuronidation is a metabolic pathway for metronidazole, terminal elimination half-life is only slightly (not significantly) longer (5-6 hours) in cats.

The oral bioavailability of the drug in horses averages ≈80% (range 57-100%). In adult horses, food does not appreciably alter oral absorption (Britzi *et al.* 2010). If administered rectally to horses, bioavailability is decreased by ≈50%. Elimination half-life in the horse is ≈2.9-4.3 hours.

Contraindications/Precautions/Warnings

Metronidazole is prohibited for use in food animals by the FDA.

Metronidazole is contraindicated in animals hypersensitive to the drug or nitroimidazole derivatives. It has been recommended not to use the drug in severely debilitated, pregnant or nursing animals. Metronidazole should be used with caution in animals with hepatic dysfunction. If the drug must be used in animals with significant liver impairment, consider reducing the total daily dose to 1/3 of standard anti-anaerobe dosage and dose once daily (Trepanier 2013).

Because of the risk for neurotoxicity in dogs, total daily doses of metronidazole should not exceed 65 mg/kg per day (Tams 2007).

Adverse Effects

Adverse effects reported in dogs include neurologic disorders, lethargy, weakness, neutropenia, hepatotoxicity, hematuria, anorexia, nausea, vomiting, and diarrhea. Rare cases of cutaneous vasculitis associated with metronidazole have been reported. Neurologic toxicity in dogs may occur after acute high dosages or more likely, with chronic moderate to high-dose therapy. Clinical signs reported are described below in the Overdosage section.

In cats, vomiting, inappetence, hepatotoxicity and rarely, central nervous toxicity can occur with metronidazole therapy (Scorza *et al.* 2004). Genotoxicity was detected in peripheral blood mononuclear cells collected from cats after 7 days of oral metronidazole, but resolved within 6 days of discontinuing the drug. Clinical significance, particularly with chronic therapy, is yet to be determined (Sekis *et al.* 2009).

In horses, metronidazole may occasionally cause anorexia, ataxia and depression, particularly when used at higher dosages. There have been reported cases of *C. difficile* and *C. perfringens* diarrhea and death after use of metronidazole.

Metronidazole tablets have a sharp, metallic taste that animals find unpleasant. Placing in capsules or using compounded oral suspensions may alleviate the problem of dosing avoidance.

Reproductive/Nursing Safety

Metronidazole's potential for teratogenicity is somewhat controversial; some references state that it has been teratogenic in some laboratory animal studies, but others state that it has not. However, unless the benefits to the mother outweigh the risks to the fetus(es), it should not be used during pregnancy, particularly during the first 3 weeks of gestation. In humans, the FDA categorizes this drug as category *B* for use during pregnancy (*Animal studies have not yet demonstrated risk to the fetus, but there are no adequate studies in pregnant women; or animal studies have shown an adverse effect, but adequate studies in pregnant women have not demonstrated a risk to the fetus in the first trimester of pregnancy, and there is no evidence of risk in later trimesters.*) In a separate system evaluating the safety of drugs in canine and feline pregnancy (Papich 1989), this drug is categorized as class: *C* (*These drugs may have potential risks. Studies in people or laboratory animals have uncovered risks, and these drugs should be used cautiously as a last resort when the benefit of therapy clearly outweighs the risks.*)

Because of the potential for tumorigenicity, consider using alternative therapy or switching to milk replacer for nursing patients.

Overdosage/Acute Toxicity

Signs of intoxication associated with metronidazole in dogs and cats, include anorexia and/or vomiting, depression, mydriasis, nystagmus, ataxia, head-tilt, deficits of proprioception, joint knuckling, disorientation, tremors, seizures, bradycardia, rigidity and stiffness. These effects may be seen with acute overdoses, doses in dogs above 60 mg/kg per day, or in some animals on chronic therapy when using older "recommended" doses (*e.g.*, 30 mg/kg/day).

In dogs, common signs of metronidazole toxicity include generalized ataxia with a very rapid positional nystagmus. Most often, dogs have neurological deficits localized to the central vestibular system and/or cerebellum. Dogs with mild to moderate clinical signs usually improve rapidly within 1-2 days, once metronidazole has been discontinued (Vernau 2009).

Diazepam has been used successfully to decrease the CNS effects associated with metronidazole toxicity, but has not been evaluated in a controlled manner. See the Diazepam monograph or the reference by Evans, Levesque, et al for more information (Evans *et al.* 2002).

Acute overdoses should be handled by attempting to limit the absorption of the drug using standard protocols. Extreme caution should be used before attempting to induce vomiting in patients demonstrating CNS effects or aspiration may result. If acute toxicity is seen after chronic therapy, the drug should be discontinued and the patient treated supportively and symptomatically. Neurologic clinical signs may require several days before showing signs of resolving.

Drug Interactions

The following drug interactions have either been reported or are theoretical in humans or animals receiving metronidazole and may be of significance in veterinary patients. Unless otherwise noted, use together is not necessarily contraindicated, but weigh the potential risks and perform additional monitoring when appropriate.

- **ALCOHOL:** May induce a disulfiram-like (nausea, vomiting, cramps, etc.) reaction when given with metronidazole.
- **BUSULFAN:** May result in increased busulfan levels and toxicity.

- **CIMETIDINE:** May decrease the metabolism of metronidazole and increase the likelihood of dose-related side effects.
- **CYCLOSPORINE:** Use with metronidazole may increase cyclosporine levels.
- **FLUOROURACIL (5-FU):** May result in increased fluorouracil levels and toxicity.
- **PHENOBARBITAL** or **PHENYTOIN:** May increase the metabolism of metronidazole, thereby decreasing blood levels.
- **WARFARIN:** Metronidazole may prolong the PT in patients receiving warfarin or other coumarin anticoagulants. Avoid concurrent use if possible; otherwise, intensify monitoring.

Laboratory Considerations

- Metronidazole can cause falsely decreased readings of **AST** (SGOT) and **ALT** (SGPT) when determined using methods measuring decreases in ultraviolet absorbance when NADH is reduced to NAD.

Doses

Note: Doses are for <u>metronidazole base</u> unless otherwise noted. If using <u>metronidazole benzoate</u> adjust dosages unless provided by pharmacy as "mg/mL of the base". 1 mg of metronidazole base = 1.6 mg of metronidazole benzoate.

- **DOGS:**

  For treatment of giardiasis (extra-label): The Companion Animal Parasite Council (CAPC) recommends fenbendazole (50 mg/kg PO once daily for 5 days) as its first choice drug, but fenbendazole can be used in combination with metronidazole at 25 mg/kg PO twice daily for 5 days. This combination therapy may result in better resolution of clinical disease and cyst shedding. If treatment combined with bathing (see Control and Prevention) does not eliminate infection (as evidenced by testing feces for persistence of cysts), treatment with either fenbendazole alone or in combination with metronidazole may be extended for another 10 days. If other pets live with an infected dog or cat, all those of the same species may also be treated with a single course of anti-giardial therapy. Repeated courses of treatment are not indicated in dogs or cats without clinical signs. (CAPC 2014)

  For other protozoal infections (extra-label): *Entamoeba histolytica* or *Pentatrichomas hominis*: 25 mg/kg PO q12h for 8 days. (Lappin 2000)

  For perioperative surgical prophylaxis (colorectal surgery); (extra-label): There is no consensus for dosages in veterinary medicine, but consider metronidazole 15 mg/kg IV over 30-60 minutes and completed approximately 1 hour before surgery. Usually used in conjunction with cefazolin.

  For anaerobic infections (extra-label): **For sepsis:** 15 mg/kg IV q12h; for less severe anaerobic infections 10 – 15 mg/kg q8-12h can be considered.

  For clostridial enteritis: 10–15 mg/kg orally every 8-12 hours for 5 days. 15 mg/kg IV q12h for 5 days can be used if PO is not an option.

  For adjunctive therapy of inflammatory GI conditions (IBD); (extra-label): 10 – 15 mg/kg PO twice daily. Long-term therapy has potential risks for neurotoxicosis and hepatotoxicosis.

  For treating Helicobacter gastritis infections (extra-label): Using triple therapy: Metronidazole 15.4 mg/kg q8h, amoxicillin 11 mg/kg q8h and bismuth subsalicylate (original *Pepto-Bismol®*) 0.22 mL/kg PO q4-6h. Give each for 3 weeks. (Hall 2000)

- **CATS:**

  For treatment of giardiasis (extra-label): The Companion Animal Parasite Council (CAPC) states: Data on treatment of cats with *Giardia* are lacking. However, cats may be treated with either fenbendazole at 50 mg/kg PO once daily for 5 days or metronidazole at 25 mg/kg PO twice daily for 5 days, or a combination of the two as described for dogs. There is anecdotal evidence that metronidazole benzoate is tolerated better in cats than metronidazole (USP). If other pets live with an infected dog or cat, all those of the same species may also be treated with a single course of anti-giardial therapy. Repeated courses of treatment are not indicated in dogs or cats without clinical signs. (CAPC 2014)

For feline trichomoniasis (*Tritrichomonas foetus*—most prevalent; *Pentatrichomonas hominis*); (extra-label): Metronidazole at 30 – 50 mg/kg PO twice daily for 3-14 days has been used in the past for *T. foetus*, but clearance of infections appears less common than when ronidazole is used. (CAPC 2014)

For perioperative surgical prophylaxis (colorectal surgery); (extra-label): There is no consensus for dosages in veterinary medicine, but consider metronidazole 15 mg/kg IV over 30-60 minutes and completed approximately 1 hour before surgery. Usually used in conjunction with cefazolin.

For treating *H. pylori* (extra-label): Metronidazole 10 – 15 mg/kg PO twice daily; clarithromycin 7.5 mg/kg PO twice daily; amoxicillin 20 mg/kg PO twice daily for 14 days. (Simpson 2003)

For anaerobic infections (extra-label): For sepsis: 15 mg/kg IV q12h; for less severe anaerobic infections 10 – 15 mg/kg PO q12h or 15 – 25 mg/kg PO once daily can be considered. Practically, ¼ of a 250 mg (62.5 mg) per cat is often chosen for a PO dose; but because of the drug's extreme bitterness consider using compounded metronidazole benzoate or putting the quartered tablet in an empty gelatin capsule.

For clostridial enteritis: 62.5 mg per cat PO q12h for 5 days.

For adjunctive therapy of inflammatory GI conditions (IBD); extra-label): 10 – 15 mg/kg PO twice daily. Long-term therapy has potential risks for neurotoxicity and hepatotoxicity.

■ **FERRETS:**

For treating *Helicobacter mustelae* gastritis infections (extra-label): Amoxicillin 30 mg/kg PO q8h, metronidazole 20 mg/kg PO q8h, & bismuth subsalicylate 7.5 mg/kg PO q8h. All are given for 21-28 days. (Johnson-Delaney 2008)

For anaerobic infections (extra-label): 10 – 30 mg/kg PO 1-2 times daily. Very bitter; mask flavor. (Williams 2000)

For inflammatory bowel disease (extra-label): 50 mg/kg PO once daily. (Johnson-Delaney 2008)

■ **RABBITS, RODENTS, SMALL MAMMALS:**

a) **Rabbits: For anaerobic infections:** 20 mg/kg PO q12h for 3–5 days or 40 mg/kg PO once daily; 5 mg/kg slow IV q12h. (Ivey *et al.* 2000)

b) **Mice:** 3.5 mg/mL in water for 5 days. **Rats:** 10 – 40 mg per rat PO once daily. **Chinchillas, Guinea pigs:** 10 – 40 mg/kg PO once daily. **Gerbils, Hamsters:** 7.5 mg/70-90 grams of body weight PO q8h. Add sucrose to improve palatability. (Adamcak *et al.* 2000)

c) **Mice:** For *S. muris:* 10 – 40 mg/kg PO twice, 5 days apart. (Huynh *et al.* 2013)

■ **HORSES:**

For clostridial enterocolitis in foals (extra-label): Dosage recommendations vary, but 15 mg/kg PO q8-12h appears reasonable. Intravenous route can be used if PO not possible. Consider lower dosages (*i.e.* 10 mg/kg q12h) in newborn foals (<5-days old).

For metritis secondary to *B. fragilis* (extra-label): 15 – 25 mg/kg PO q12h. (LeBlanc 2009)

For *L. intracellularis* infections (extra-label): metronidazole 10 – 15 mg/kg PO q8-12h with either oxytetracycline (10 – 18 mg/kg via slow IV q24h) or chloramphenicol (44 mg/kg PO q6-8h). (Frazer 2007)

■ **BIRDS:**

For susceptible infections (anaerobes; giardia): 10 – 50 mg/kg PO q12h. (Oglesbee 2009)

■ **REPTILES/AMPHIBIANS:**

In reptiles and amphibians for treatment of amoebae, flagellates and ciliates (extra-label): Typically with metronidazole at 100 mg/kg PO repeated in 2 weeks; or 50 mg/kg PO once daily for 3-5 days; repeat prn. As is the case with all medications used in reptiles and amphibians, each animal has to be treated on a case-by-case basis for all medications; in the literature there are several different doses as well as treatment schedules listed. (de la Navarre 2003)

For anaerobic respiratory infections in reptiles (extra-label): 20 mg/kg PO q48h (every other day). (Schumacher 2011)

Monitoring
■ Clinical efficacy.
■ Adverse effects (clients should report any neurologic signs).

Client Information
■ Report any neurologic clinical signs to veterinarian (see Overdose section).

Chemistry/Synonyms
A synthetic, nitroimidazole antibacterial and antiprotozoal agent, metronidazole occurs as white to pale yellow crystalline powder or crystals with a pK_a of 2.6. It is sparingly soluble in water or alcohol. Metronidazole base is commercially available as tablets or solution for IV injection and metronidazole HCl is available as injectable powder for reconstitution. The hydrochloride is very soluble in water.

Metronidazole benzoate is the benzoic ester of metronidazole. It occurs as a white to slightly yellow, crystalline powder that is practically insoluble in water, slightly soluble in alcohol, and soluble in acetone. As it is less soluble in aqueous solutions than is the base, it does not taste as bad.

Metronidazole may also be known as: Bayer-5360, metronidazolum, SC-32642, NSC-50364, RP-8823, and SC-10295; many trade names are available.

Storage/Stability
Metronidazole tablets and HCl powder for injection should be stored at temperatures <30°C and protected from light. The injection should be protected from light and freezing and stored at room temperature.

Specific recommendations on the reconstitution, dilution, and neutralization of metronidazole HCl powder for injection are detailed in the package insert of the drug and should be referred to if this product is used. Do not use aluminum hub needles to reconstitute or transfer this drug as a reddish-brown discoloration may result in the solution.

Compatibility/Compounding Considerations
The following drugs and solutions are reportedly physically **compatible** with metronidazole ready-to-use solutions for injection: amikacin sulfate, aminophylline, cefazolin sodium, cefotaxime sodium, cefoxitin sodium, cefuroxime sodium, chloramphenicol sodium succinate, clindamycin phosphate, disopyramide phosphate, gentamicin sulfate, heparin sodium, hydrocortisone sodium succinate, hydromorphone HCl, magnesium sulfate, meperidine HCl, morphine sulfate, multielectrolyte concentrate, multivitamins, penicillin G sodium, and tobramycin sulfate. Compatibility is de-

pendent upon factors such as pH, concentration, temperature, and diluent used; consult specialized references or a hospital pharmacist for more specific information.

The following drugs and solutions are reportedly physically **incompatible** (or compatibility data conflicts) with metronidazole ready-to-use solutions for injection: aztreonam, cefamandole naftate, and dopamine HCl.

Metronidazole hydrochloride is very bitter tasting and even with taste masking or flavoring agents is universally unpalatable to veterinary patients. Although not commercially available in the United States, the metronidazole ester of benzoic acid, metronidazole benzoate, is relatively palatable to animal patients and is often used in extemporaneously compounded suspensions, particularly for cats to reduce the drug's bitterness. If using metronidazole benzoate adjust dosages from those for the base unless provided by pharmacy as "mg/mL of the base". One mg of metronidazole base ≈ 1.6 mg of metronidazole benzoate. Crystallization and sedimentation can occur in aqueous metronidazole benzoate suspensions when conversion from the anhydrous to the monohydrate form occurs.

Compounded preparation stability: One method for compounding a metronidazole benzoate suspension (80 mg/mL) that is stable (when protected from light, ambient temperature) for at least a year, has been published (Vu *et al.* 2008). To make 750 mL of an 80 mg/mL suspension: Place metronidazole benzoate powder 60 grams in a suitable mortar. The powder is then triturated with 1.25 grams of Propylene Glycol, NF to a smooth paste, then add increasing amounts of *SyrSpend SF* (Gallipot) until the suspension is pour-able. The liquid suspension should then be transferred to a suitable graduated container and the mortar rinsed with three small aliquots of *SyrSpend SF*, which are then added to the suspension. Add additional *SyrSpend SF* to bring the suspension to the final volume of 750 mL. Store in light-resistant containers refrigerated or at room temperature.

Another published method is to triturate 9.6 grams (9,600 mg) of metronidazole benzoate powder with 60 mL of *Ora-Plus®* and *qs ad* to 120 mL with *Ora-Sweet®* or *Ora-Sweet SF®* to yield a 80 mg/mL metronidazole benzoate oral suspension (equivalent to 50 mg/mL metronidazole hydrochloride) that retains >90% potency for 90 days when stored at both 4°C and 25°C and protected from light (Mathew *et al.* 1994).

Dosage Forms/Regulatory Status

VETERINARY-LABELED PRODUCTS: NONE.
Metronidazole is prohibited for use in food animals by the FDA.

HUMAN-LABELED PRODUCTS:

Metronidazole Oral Tablets: 250 mg & 500 mg; *Flagyl®*, generic; (Rx)

Metronidazole Oral Capsules: 375 mg; *Flagyl 375®*, generic; (Rx)

Metronidazole Extended-Release Oral Tablets: 750 mg; *Flagyl ER®*; (Rx)

Metronidazole Injection: 5 mg/mL in 100 mL vials and single-dose containers and 500 mg pre-mixed in sodium chloride for injection; (Rx)

Lotions, gels, vaginal products and creams also available.

Revisions/References

Monograph revised/updated April 2014.
Adamcak, A. & B. Otten (2000). Rodent Therapeutics. Vet Clin NA: Exotic Anim Pract 3:1(Jan): 221-40.
Britzi, M., et al. (2010). Bioavailability and pharmacokinetics of metronidazole in fed and fasted horses. J. Vet. Pharmacol. Ther. 33(5): 511-4.
CAPC (2014). Companion Animal Parasite Council (CAPC) Recommendations, CAPCvet. org.
de la Navarre, B. (2003). Common parasitic diseases of reptiles and amphibians. Proceedings: Western Veterinary Conf. accessed via Veterinary Information Network; vin.com
Evans, J., et al. (2002). The use of diazepam in the treatment of metronidazole toxicosis in the dog. Proceedings: ACVIM Forum. accessed via Veterinary Information Network; vin. com
Frazer, M. (2007). A review of Lawsonia intracellularis: A significant equine pathogen. Proceedings: ACVIM. accessed via Veterinary Information Network; vin.com
Hall, J. (2000). Diseases of the Stomach. *Textbook of Veterinary Internal Medicine: Diseases of the Dog and Cat.* S. Ettinger and E. Feldman. Philadelphia, WB Saunders. 2: 1154-82.
Huynh, M. & C. Pignon (2013). Gastrointestinal disease in exotic small mammals. Journal of Exotic Pet Medicine 22(2): 118-31.
Ivey, E. & J. Morrisey (2000). Therapeutics for Rabbits. Vet Clin NA: Exotic Anim Pract 3:1(Jan): 183-216.
Johnson-Delaney, C. (2008). Gastrointestinal Diseases in Ferrets. Proceedings: WVC. accessed via Veterinary Information Network; vin.com
Lappin, M. (2000). Protozoal and Miscellaneous Infections. *Textbook of Veterinary Internal Medicine: Diseases of the Dog and Cat.* S. Ettinger and E. Feldman. Philadelphia, WB Saunders. 1: 408-17.
LeBlanc, M. M. (2009). The current status of antibiotic use in equine reproduction. Equine Veterinary Education 21(3): 156-67.
Mathew, M., et al. (1994). Stability of metronidazole benzoate in suspensions. J Clin Pharm Ther 19(1): 31-4.
Oglesbee, B. (2009). Vomiting & Diarrhea in Pet Birds: Where do I Start? Proceedings: WVC. accessed via Veterinary Information Network; vin.com
Papich, M. (1989). Effects of drugs on pregnancy. *Current Veterinary Therapy X: Small Animal Practice.* R. Kirk. Philadelphia, Saunders: 1291-9.
Schumacher, J. (2011). Respiratory Medicine of Reptiles. Vet Clin Exot Anim 14: 207-24.
Scorza, A. V. & M. R. Lappin (2004). Metronidazole for the treatment of feline giardiasis. Journal of Feline Medicine and Surgery 6(3): 157-60.
Sekis, I., et al. (2009). Single-dose pharmacokinetics and genotoxicity of metronidazole in cats. Journal of Feline Medicine and Surgery 11(2): 60-8.
Simpson, K. (2003). Intragastric warfare in Helicobacter infected cats. Proceedings: ACVIM Forum. accessed via Veterinary Information Network; vin.com
Tams, T. (2007). Giardiasis, Clostridium perfringens Enterotoxicosis, Tritrichomonas foetus, and Cryptosporidiosis. Prpoceedings: ABVP. accessed via Veterinary Information Network; vin.com
Trepanier, L. A. (2013). Applying Pharmacokinetics to Veterinary Clinical Practice. Veterinary Clinics of North America-Small Animal Practice 43(5): 1013-+.
Vernau, K. (2009). Cerebellar Disease. Veterinary Neurology Symposium; Univ. of Calif.-Davis. accessed via Veterinary Information Network; vin.com
Vu, N., et al. (2008). Stability of Metronidazole Benzoate in SyrSpend SF One-Step Suspension System. Intl Jnl Pharmaceutical Cmpd 12(6): 558-64.
Williams, B. (2000). Therapeutics in Ferrets. Vet Clin NA: Exotic Anim Pract 3:1(Jan): 131-53.

Metyrapone

(me-**teer**-a-pone)   Metopirone®
Adrenal Steroid Inhibitor

Prescriber Highlights

▶ Adrenal steroid synthesis inhibitor primarily used in cats with hyperadrenocorticism; may be most useful for short-term treatment to stabilize patient before adrenalectomy.
▶ Seems well tolerated in cats at recommended doses.
▶ May alter insulin requirements; monitor blood glucose closely.
▶ Has had availability issues.

Uses/Indications

Metyrapone may be useful to treat cats with hyperadrenocorticism, especially short-term in an attempt to stabilize the patient prior to adrenalectomy. Clinical experience is quite limited, but it appears to give consistent results and not be overly toxic to cats. Resolving hypercortisolism should reduce insulin antagonism and reduce or eliminate the need for exogenous insulin in some cats (Feldman 2009). Metyrapone may potentially be useful in treating hyperadrenocorticism in ferrets and small mammals (*e.g.*, hamsters), but there is little, if any, information available on its use in these species.

In humans, metyrapone is used with other biochemical and laboratory evaluations in the diagnostic evaluation of hypothalamic-pituitary adrenal corticotropin hormone-function. It is also used for treatment of Cushing's Syndrome (not an FDA-approved indication).

Pharmacology/Actions

Metyrapone reduces cortisol and corticosterone production by inhibiting hydroxylation of 11-deoxycortisol to cortisol in the adrenal cortex. ACTH production can increase as the negative feedback mechanism is inhibited. With time, this may override the effects of metyrapone on the adrenal gland. Metyrapone can also suppress synthesis of aldosterone, and cause a mild natriuresis. Continued inhibition stimulates increased ACTH production that can ultimately override the inhibitory effects. Mineralocorticoid deficiency does not usually occur with long-term metyrapone therapy because inhibition of the 11-beta-hydroxylation reaction increases production of 11-desoxycorticosterone, a mineralocorticoid that can cause hypertension in patients receiving long-term metyrapone therapy.

Pharmacokinetics

No information on the pharmacokinetics of metyrapone was located for cats. In humans, metyrapone is well absorbed after oral administration. Peak levels occur in about an hour; however, pharmacological response to metyrapone does not occur immediately. It is rapidly cleared from the plasma and has an average elimination half-life of around 2 hours. Metyrapone's major metabolite, metyrapol, is active and formed via reduction; it has a half-life about twice as long as metyrapone. Both metyrapol and metyrapone are conjugated with glucuronide in humans. As cats are unable to effectively glucuronidate, it is unclear what metabolic path(s) metyrapone takes in this species.

Contraindications/Precautions/Warnings

Metyrapone should not be used in animals that are hypersensitive to it or have adrenal cortical insufficiency.

Use cautiously (enhanced monitoring) in cats with concurrent diabetes; monitor blood glucose closely as hypoglycemia can develop rapidly.

Adverse Effects

Metyrapone appears be relatively well tolerated in cats. Dosages ranging from 195 – 250 mg/cat/day (divided) have been used in cats with hyperadrenocorticism without observed toxicity (Bruyette 2010). The following adverse effects have been reported in human patients taking metyrapone: headache, dizziness, sedation, allergic rash, nausea, vomiting, and abdominal pain. Rarely, metyrapone can cause bone marrow depression.

Reproductive/Nursing Safety

Metyrapone should be given to pregnant queens only if clearly needed. Animal reproduction studies have not been conducted with metyrapone. In women given the drug in the 2nd and 3rd trimester, evidence of fetal pituitary response to the enzymatic block was detected. The FDA has assigned metyrapone to category C for use during pregnancy (*Animal studies have shown an adverse effect on the fetus, but there are no adequate studies in humans; or there are no animal reproduction studies and no adequate studies in humans.*)

Metyrapone's safety in lactating animals and their offspring is not known.

Overdosage/Acute Toxicity

The oral LD_{50} in rats (mg/kg) was 521 mg/kg. Metyrapone overdoses likely would cause GI effects and, possibly, acute adrenocortical insufficiency. Other effects that may be seen include: hypoglycemia, hyponatremia, hypochloremia, hyperkalemia, cardiac arrhythmias, hypotension, dehydration, and impairment of consciousness. There is no specific antidote. Standard decontamination protocols should be considered with intravenous hydrocortisone, saline and glucose. Monitoring and support for several days may be required. Contact an animal poison control center for more information and guidance.

Drug Interactions

The following drug interactions have either been reported or are theoretical in humans or animals receiving metyrapone and may be of significance in veterinary patients. Unless otherwise noted, use together is not necessarily contraindicated, but weigh the potential risks and perform additional monitoring when appropriate.

- **ACETAMINOPHEN (Do NOT use in cats)**: In humans, there is an increased risk for acetaminophen toxicity.
- **CORTICOSTEROIDS**: Decreases the efficacy of metyrapone.

Laboratory Considerations

- In humans, the following drugs have been reported to interfere with the results of the metyrapone test: antidepressants such as amitriptyline, antithyroid drugs, phenothiazines, barbiturates, corticosteroids, cyproheptadine, and hormones such as estrogens and progesterone.
- The metyrapone test may not be reliable in humans with hyper- or hypothyroidism.

Doses

- **CATS:**

  For hyperadrenocorticism (extra-label): Metyrapone has been used to successfully treat hyperadrenocorticism in the cat, but results are variable; recommended dose is 65 mg/kg PO q12h. Practically, one 250 mg capsule would be used for each dose. If effective, results are generally noted within 5 days.

Monitoring

- Blood glucose should be closely monitored in cats, particularly those that are diabetic.
- Clinical signs associated with hyperadrenocorticism or hypoadrenocorticism.

Client Information

- May be given with or without food, but with food is preferred as it may help prevent vomiting.
- May also be useful in ferrets, hamsters, etc. but little is known about the drug in these species.
- Experience in cats is limited, but it seems to be tolerated well. Cats with diabetes will need their blood glucose monitored carefully while receiving this drug. Report any unusual symptoms you see to your veterinarian.
- Will need to be made (compounded) into a dosage form appropriate for cats, etc. Follow storage recommendations for the compounded product.

Chemistry/Synonyms

Metyrapone occurs as a white to light amber, fine, crystalline powder, with a characteristic odor. It is sparingly soluble in water; soluble in chloroform and methyl alcohol.

Metyrapone may also be known as SU-4885, metirapon, metirapona, or metyraponum. A common trade name is *Metopirone®*.

Storage/Stability

Store metyrapone at room temperature in a well-closed, light-resistant container.

Compatibility/Compounding Considerations

No specific information noted.

Dosage Forms/Regulatory Status

VETERINARY-LABELED PRODUCTS: NONE.

HUMAN-LABELED PRODUCTS:

Metyrapone Oral Capsules: 250 mg; *Metopirone®*; (Rx)

Revisions/References

Monograph revised/updated April 2014.

Bruyette, D. (2010). Feline Adrenal Disease: Exploring the Unexplored. Proceedings: WVC. accessed via Veterinary Information Network; vin.com

Feldman, E. C. (2009). Diagnosis & Treatment of Hyperadrenocorticism in Cats. Proceedings: Western Veterinary Conference. accessed via Veterinary Information Network; vin.com

Mexiletine HCl

(mex-**ill**-i-teen)   Mexitil®

Oral Antiarrhythmic

Prescriber Highlights

▶ Oral antiarrhythmic with similar effects as lidocaine; used for V tach, PVC's; often used with sotalol in dogs. Low therapeutic index, availability, expense, and dosing frequency are all problematic for clinical use in animals.

▶ Extreme caution: Pre-existing 2nd or 3rd degree AV block (without pacemaker), or in patients with cardiogenic shock. Caution: Dog breeds susceptible to *ABCB*-1 gene defect. Patients with severe congestive heart failure or acute myocardial infarction, hepatic function impairment, hypotension, intraventricular conduction abnormalities, sinus node function impairment, seizure disorder, or sensitivity to the drug.

▶ Adverse Effects: GI distress, including vomiting (give with meals to alleviate). Potentially: CNS effects (trembling, unsteadiness, dizziness, depression), shortness of breath, PVC's & chest pain could occur; rarely (reported in humans): seizures, agranulocytosis, & thrombocytopenia.

▶ Drug-drug; drug-lab interactions.

Uses/Indications

Mexiletine may be useful to treat some ventricular arrhythmias, including PVC's and ventricular tachycardia in dogs. Ventricular tachycardias that have responded to lidocaine may respond to mexiletine. Limited, controlled or retrospective studies have shown some evidence for efficacy for certain dogs (Boxers, German shepherds) (Prosek *et al.* 2006; Gelzer *et al.* 2010; Caro-Vadillo *et al.* 2013), but the drug's low therapeutic index, availability, expense, and dosing frequency are all problematic.

Mexiletine may be useful treating certain myopathies in dogs such as myotonia congenita (most studied in miniature schnauzers and Chow Chows) and myokymia in Jack Russell Terriers.

Pharmacology/Actions

Mexiletine is considered a class IB antiarrhythmic agent and is similar to lidocaine in its mechanism of antiarrhythmic activity. It inhibits the inward sodium current (fast sodium channel), thereby reducing the rate of rise of the action potential, Phase O. In the Purkinje fibers, automaticity is decreased, action potential is shortened and, to a lesser extent, effective refractory period is decreased. Usually conduction is unaffected, but may be slowed in patients with preexisting conduction abnormalities.

Pharmacokinetics

There is limited information available for dogs. Mexiletine is relatively well absorbed from the gut and has a low first-pass effect. A preliminary report of a study done in 6 healthy dogs (4 Beagles, 2 hounds) reported that sotalol (2.5 mg/kg PO twice daily) combined with mexiletine (8 – 10 mg/kg PO twice daily) for 10 days, resulted in mexiletine serum levels within the described therapeutic range (humans) for the 12-hour post-dose period in the 3 dogs weighing >10kg (Scollan *et al.* 2013).

In humans, it is moderately bound to plasma proteins (60-75%), and metabolized in the liver to inactive metabolites with an elimination half-life of ≈10-12 hours. Half-lives may be significantly increased in patients with moderate to severe hepatic disease, or in those having severely reduced cardiac outputs. Half-lives may be slightly prolonged in patients with severe renal disease or after acute myocardial infarction.

Contraindications/Precautions/Warnings

Mexiletine should be used with extreme caution, if at all, in patients with pre-existing 2nd or 3rd degree AV block (without pacemaker), or with cardiogenic shock. It should be used only when the benefits of therapy outweigh the risks when the following medical conditions exist: severe congestive heart failure or acute myocardial infarction, hepatic function impairment, hypotension, intraventricular conduction abnormalities, sinus node function impairment, seizure disorder, or sensitivity to the drug.

Dogs that are homozygous for the *ABCB*-1 gene defect may be susceptible to mexiletine toxicity. It is recommended to test before using in susceptible breeds.

It is anecdotally reported that cats are more sensitive than dogs to mexiletine's adverse effects.

Adverse Effects

The most likely adverse effect noted in animals is GI distress, including vomiting. Giving with meals may alleviate GI effects. Potentially (reported in humans): CNS effects (trembling, unsteadiness, dizziness, depression), shortness of breath, PVC's and chest pain could occur. Rarely, seizures, agranulocytosis, and thrombocytopenia have been reported in humans.

Reproductive/Nursing Safety

Lab animal studies have not demonstrated teratogenicity. In humans, the FDA categorizes this drug as category *C* for use during pregnancy (*Animal studies have shown an adverse effect on the fetus, but there are no adequate studies in humans; or there are no animal reproduction studies and no adequate studies in humans.*)

Because mexiletine is secreted into maternal milk, it has been recommended to use milk replacer if the mother is receiving the drug.

Overdosage/Acute Toxicity

Toxicity associated with overdosage may be significant. Case reports in humans have noted that CNS signs always preceded cardiovascular signs. Treatment should consist of GI tract emptying protocols when indicated, acidification of the urine to enhance urinary excretion, and supportive therapy. Atropine may be useful if hypotension or bradycardia occur.

Drug Interactions

The following drug interactions have either been reported or are theoretical in humans or animals receiving mexiletine and may be of significance in veterinary patients. Unless otherwise noted, use together is not necessarily contraindicated, but weigh the potential risks and perform additional monitoring when appropriate.

- **ANTACIDS, ALUMINUM-MAGNESIUM:** May slow the absorption of mexiletine.
- **ATROPINE:** May reduce the rate of oral absorption.
- **CIMETIDINE:** May increase or decrease mexiletine blood levels.
- **GRISEOFULVIN:** May accelerate the metabolism of mexiletine.
- **LIDOCAINE:** May cause additive adverse effects
- **METOCLOPRAMIDE:** May accelerate the absorption of mexiletine.
- **OPIATES:** May slow the absorption of mexiletine.
- **PHENOBARBITAL, PRIMIDONE, PHENYTOIN:** May accelerate the metabolism of mexiletine.
- **RIFAMPIN:** May accelerate the metabolism of mexiletine.
- **SOTALOL:** May increase mexiletine plasma concentrations (Gelzer *et al.* 2010). This may be used for therapeutic effect, but also could increase potential for adverse effects.
- **THEOPHYLLINE (aminophylline):** Metabolism may be reduced by mexiletine, thereby leading to theophylline toxicity.
- **URINARY ACIDIFYING DRUGS** (*e.g.*, **methionine, ammoni-**

um chloride, potassium phosphate, sodium phosphate): May accelerate the renal excretion of mexiletine.

- **URINARY ALKALINIZING DRUGS** (*e.g.,* citrates, bicarb, carbonic anhydrase inhibitors): May reduce the urinary excretion of mexiletine.

Laboratory Considerations

- Some human patients (1-3%) have had **AST** values increase by as much as 3X or more above the upper limit of normal. This is reportedly a transient effect and asymptomatic.

Doses

- **DOGS:**

  For treating or attempt to prevent ventricular arrhythmias (extra-label): Dosages range from 5 – 10 mg/kg PO q8h. When used with sotalol or atenolol some recommend 8 mg/kg as the upper end of the dosing range.

  For treating myotonia congenital in Chow Chows and miniature schnauzers or myokymia in Jack Russell terriers (extra-label): 8.3 mg/kg PO q8h. (Lorenz 2007)

Monitoring

- In humans, therapeutic plasma concentrations are: 0.5 – 2 micrograms/mL; toxicity may be noted at therapeutic levels.
- ECG.
- Adverse effects.

Client Information

- Needs to be given 3 times a day.
- Give with food to reduce the risk of vomiting or nausea (acting 'sick').
- Vomiting is the most likely side effect; contact veterinarian if it is serious, or continues.

Chemistry/Synonyms

A class IB antiarrhythmic, mexiletine HCl occurs as a white or almost white, odorless, crystalline powder. It is freely soluble in water.

Mexiletine may also be known as: Ko-1173, mexiletini hydrochloridum, *Mexilen®*, *Mexitil®*, *Mexitilen®*, *Myovek®*, and *Ritalmex®*.

Storage/Stability

Mexiletine capsules should be stored in tight containers at room temperature.

Compatibility/Compounding Considerations

No specific information noted.

Dosage Forms/Regulatory Status

VETERINARY-LABELED PRODUCTS: NONE.
The ARCI (Racing Commissioners International) has designated this drug as a class 4 substance. See the appendix for more information.

HUMAN-LABELED PRODUCTS:

Mexiletine Oral Capsules: 150 mg, 200 mg & 250 mg; generic; (Rx)

Revisions/References

Monograph revised/updated April 2014.

Caro-Vadillo, A., et al. (2013). Arrhythmogenic right ventricular cardiomyopathy in boxer dogs: a retrospective study of survival. Veterinary Record 172(10).

Gelzer, A. R. M., et al. (2010). Combination therapy with mexiletine and sotalol suppresses inherited ventricular arrhythmias in German shepherd dogs better than mexiletine or sotalol monotherapy: A randomized cross-over study. Journal of Veterinary Cardiology 12(2): 93-106.

Lorenz, M. (2007). Section 1: Motor unit disorders/Peripheral neuropathies/Myopathies. Proceedings: Western Vet Conference. accessed via Veterinary Information Network; vin.com

Prosek, R., et al. (2006). Comparison of sotalol and mexiletine versus stand alone sotalol in treatment of Boxer dogs with ventricular arrhythmias. Proceedings: ACVIM. accessed via Veterinary Information Network; vin.com

Scollan, K. & D. Sisson (2013). Mexiletine Serum Levels with Twice-Daily Dosing in Combination with Sotalol in Healthy Dogs. Proceedings: 23rd ECVIM-CA Congress. accessed via Veterinary Information Network; vin.com

Mibolerone

(mye-**boe**-le-rone) Cheque® Drops

Androgen; Anabolic

Prescriber Highlights

- ▶ Availability an issue; now a controlled substance in the USA.
- ▶ Androgenic, anabolic, antigonadotropic used to suppress estrus, treat pseudocyesis (false pregnancy) or severe galactorrhea in dogs.
- ▶ Contraindications: Perianal adenoma, perianal adenocarcinoma or other androgen-dependent neoplasias, pregnant or lactating bitches, ongoing or history of liver or kidney disease. The manufacturer also recommends not using the drug in Bedlington terriers.
- ▶ **NOT** for use in cats.
- ▶ Adverse Effects: Prepuberal females: premature epiphyseal closure, clitoral enlargement, & vaginitis. Adult bitch: mild clitoral hypertrophy, vulvovaginitis, increased body odor, abnormal behavior, urinary incontinence, voice deepening, riding behavior, enhanced clinical signs of seborrhea oleosa, epiphora (tearing), hepatic changes (intranuclear hyaline bodies), & increased kidney weight (without pathology), hepatic dysfunction (rare).

Uses/Indications

Cheque® Drops was labeled as indicated "for estrous (heat) prevention in adult female dogs not intended primarily for breeding purposes." In clinical trials it was 90% effective in suppressing estrus.

Although not approved, mibolerone at dosages of 50 micrograms/day will prevent estrus in the cat, but its use is generally not recommended because of the very narrow therapeutic index of the drug in this species (see the Adverse Effects and Overdosage sections for more information).

Pharmacology/Actions

Mibolerone acts by blocking the release of luteinizing hormone (LH) from the anterior pituitary via a negative feedback mechanism. Because of the lack of LH, follicles will develop to a certain point, but will not mature and hence no ovulation or corpus luteum development occurs. The net result is a suppression of the estrous cycle if the drug is given prior to (as much as 30 days) the onset of proestrus. After discontinuation of the drug, the next estrus may occur within 7-200 days (avg. 70 days).

Pharmacokinetics

Mibolerone is reported to be well absorbed from the intestine after oral administration and rapidly metabolized in the liver to over 10 separate metabolites. Excretion is apparently equally divided between the urine and feces.

Contraindications/Precautions/Warnings

Mibolerone is contraindicated in female dogs with perianal adenoma, perianal adenocarcinoma or other androgen-dependent neoplasias. It is also contraindicated in patients with ongoing, or a history of, liver or kidney disease. The manufacturer recommends not using the drug in Bedlington Terriers.

If use begins 30 days or closer to the first day of proestrus, "silent heat" may occur and increase risk of unwanted breeding.

Adverse Effects

Immature females (dogs) may be more prone to develop adverse reactions than more mature females. In prepuberal females, mibolerone can induce premature epiphyseal closure, clitoral enlargement, and vaginitis. Adverse effects that may be seen in the adult bitch include mild clitoral hypertrophy (may be partially reversible), vulvovaginitis, increased body odor, abnormal behavior, urinary incontinence, voice deepening, riding behavior, enhanced clinical signs of seborrhea oleosa, epiphora (tearing), hepatic changes (intranuclear hyaline bodies), and increased kidney weight (without pathology). Although reported, overt hepatic dysfunction would be considered to occur rarely in dogs. With the exception of residual mild clitoral hypertrophy, adverse effects will generally resolve after discontinuation of therapy. Uterine wall thinning has been reported after long-term (years) use in bitches.

In the cat, dosages of 60 micrograms/day have caused hepatic dysfunction and 120 micrograms/day have caused death. Other adverse effects that have been noted in cats include clitoral hypertrophy, thyroid dysfunction, os clitorides formation, cervical dermis thickening, and pancreatic dysfunction.

Reproductive/Nursing Safety

Mibolerone should not be used in pregnant bitches; masculinization of the female fetuses will occur. Alterations seen may include: changes in vagina patency, multiple urethral openings in the vagina, a phallus-like structure instead of a clitoris, formation of testes-like structures, and fluid accumulation in the vagina and uterus. Because it may inhibit lactation, it should not be used in nursing bitches.

The manufacturer recommends discontinuing the product after 24 months of use. It should not be used to try to attempt to abbreviate an estrous period or in bitches prior to their first estrous period.

Overdosage/Acute Toxicity

Many toxicology studies have been performed in dogs. The drug did not cause death in doses up to 30,000 micrograms/kg/day when administered to beagles for 28 days. For a more detailed discussion of the toxicology of the drug, the reader is referred to the package insert for Cheque® Drops.

In the cat, dosages as low as 120 micrograms/day have resulted in fatalities.

Drug Interactions

Increased seizure activity has been reported in a dog after receiving mibolerone who was previously controlled on **phenytoin**. Mibolerone should generally not be used concurrently with **progestins** or **estrogens**.

Laboratory Considerations

- Mibolerone has been reported to cause **thyroid** dysfunction in cats.

Doses

- **DOGS:**

  For suppression of estrus (treatment must begin at least 30 days prior to proestrus); (labeled dose; FDA-approved): Bitches weighing: 0.5-11 kg: 30 micrograms PO per day; 12-22 kg: 60 micrograms PO per day; 23-45 kg: 120 micrograms PO per day; >45 kg: 180 micrograms PO per day; German shepherds or German shepherd crosses: 180 micrograms PO per day; regardless of weight (Information from label; Cheque® Drops—Upjohn)

  For cystic endometrial hyperplasia (CEH) (extra-label): 30 micrograms/25 lb. body weight PO daily during 6 months. (Fontbonne 2006)

- **CATS:**

  WARNING: Because of the very low margin of safety with this drug in cats, it cannot be recommended for use.

Monitoring

- Clinical signs of estrus.
- Liver function tests (baseline, annual, or as needed).
- Physical examination of genitalia.

Client Information

- It must be stressed to owners that compliance with dosage and administration direction is crucial for this agent to be effective.

Chemistry/Synonyms

A non-progestational, androgenic, anabolic, antigonadotropic, 19-nor-steroid, mibolerone occurs as a white, crystalline solid.

Mibolerone may also be known as: dimethyl-nortestosterone, NSC-72260, and U-10997.

Storage/Stability

The original manufacturer (Upjohn) states that the compound in Cheque® Drops is stable under ordinary conditions and temperatures. If using a compounded preparation, follow specific instructions from the pharmacy.

Compatibility/Compounding Considerations

No specific information noted.

Dosage Forms/Regulatory Status

VETERINARY-LABELED PRODUCTS:

Commercially prepared mibolerone preparations are apparently no longer being marketed although it is still listed in FDA's Green Book (April 2014). Mibolerone may be available from compounding pharmacies. Mibolerone is now categorized as a Class-III controlled substance in the USA.

HUMAN-LABELED PRODUCTS: NONE.

Revisions/References

Monograph revised/updated April 2014.
Fontbonne, A. (2006). Infertility in the bitch. Proceedings: WSAVA. accessed via Veterinary Information Network; vin.com

---

Midazolam HCl

(mid-**ay**-zoe-lam)   Versed®

Parenteral Benzodiazepine

Prescriber Highlights

▶ Injectable benzodiazepine used primarily as a pre-op med; unlike diazepam may be given IM for seizures.

▶ Contraindications: Hypersensitivity to benzodiazepines; acute narrow-angle glaucoma. Caution: Hepatic or renal disease, debilitated or geriatric patients, & those in coma, shock, or with significant respiratory depression.

▶ Adverse Effects: Potential for respiratory depression is of most concern. Cats may develop"excited" behaviors; use with sedatives/tranquilizers.

▶ Avoid intra-carotid injection.

▶ Drug interactions.

Uses/Indications

In veterinary patients, midazolam is used principally for its sedative, anxiolytic and muscle relaxant properties as a premedicant in combination with other drugs prior to induction of general anesthesia. Alone, it does not appear to provide predictable sedation in dogs, cats or horses, but sedation may be adequate in rabbits, ferrets and some birds. Animals may become sedated or dysphoric and excited. Cats may be more prone to develop the "excited" effect/disinhibition more so than dogs. When used in combination with other drugs (*e.g.,* opioids, ketamine, acepromazine, dexmedetomidine), midazolam does provide more predictable sedation. It has been suggested that if midazolam is used in place of diazepam in pre-ops, to dose it on mg/mg basis for the diazepam in the protocol.

Midazolam may also be of benefit to treat status epilepticus when given either IV, IM, or intranasally (but not rectally). In dogs, bioavailability after IM injection can be substantially lower than IV.

In humans, midazolam has been suggested for use as a premedicant before surgery, and as a conscious sedative when combined with potent analgesic/anesthetic drugs (*e.g.*, ketamine or fentanyl). In humans, midazolam reduces the incidences of "dreamlike" emergence reactions and increases in blood pressure and cardiac rate caused by ketamine.

Pharmacology/Actions

Midazolam exhibits similar pharmacologic actions as other benzodiazepines. The subcortical levels (primarily limbic, thalamic, and hypothalamic) of the CNS are depressed thus producing the anxiolytic, sedative, skeletal muscle relaxant, and anticonvulsant effects seen. The exact mechanism of action is unknown, but postulated mechanisms include: antagonism of serotonin, increased release of and/or facilitation of gamma-aminobutyric acid (GABA) activity, and diminished release or turnover of acetylcholine in the CNS. Benzodiazepine specific receptors have been located in the mammalian brain, kidney, liver, lung, and heart. In all species studied, receptors are lacking in the white matter.

Midazolam's unique solubility characteristics (water soluble injection but lipid soluble at body pH) give it a very rapid onset of action after injection. When compared to diazepam, midazolam has approximately twice the affinity for benzodiazepine receptors, is nearly 3 times as potent, and has a faster onset of action and a shorter duration of effect.

Pharmacokinetics

In healthy dogs after IM administration bioavailability was approximately 47% and peak levels occurred around 7-8 minutes post. The authors concluded that IM midazolam could be useful in treating seizures in dogs when venous access is unavailable, but that higher dosages may be necessary (Schwartz *et al.* 2012). In dogs, midazolam is absorbed when the commercially available injection is administered intranasally and peak levels are higher than when it is administered rectally. A 50 mg/mL compounded gel (0.2% hydroxypropylmethylcellulose) demonstrated significantly higher peak levels after intranasal administration than when the injection was administered rectally or intranasally to dogs (Eagleson *et al.* 2010). Midazolam elimination half-lives in dogs average 77 minutes. Midazolam is metabolized in the liver via the cytochrome P450 enzyme system. The isoenzyme that appears to be responsible in dogs is CYP2B11. This in contrast to humans, where CYP3A4 and CYP3A5 are largely responsible for midazolam's metabolism.

In horses, after doses of 0.05 or 0.1 mg/kg IV total clearance was 10.6 mL/min/kg (median); volume of distribution (SS) was 2-3 L/kg; terminal half-life varied widely ranging from 120-924 minutes (medians were 216 minutes after 0.05 mg/kg and 408 minutes after 0.1 mg/kg). Cardiorespiratory parameters and sedation scores did not change, but agitation, postural sway, and weakness were noted and one horse became recumbent after a 0.1 mg/kg dose (Hubbell *et al.* 2013).

In alpacas, after midazolam was given 0.05 mg/kg IM or IV, IM bioavailability was 92% and peak levels were ≈3X lower than after IV. Elimination half-life (mean) was 98 minutes (IV) and 234 minutes (IM). The authors concluded that at present, it appears that midazolam provides a short duration of action with moderate levels of sedation and minimal cardiovascular or behavioral adverse effects in alpacas (Aarnes *et al.* 2013).

In humans, the onset of action following IV administration is very rapid due to the high lipophilicity of the agent and the loss of the lash reflex or counting occurs within 30-97 seconds of administration. Following IM injection, midazolam is rapidly and nearly completely (91%) absorbed. It is well absorbed after oral administration (no oral products are marketed), but because of a rapid first-pass effect, bioavailabilities suffer (31-72%).

The drug is highly protein bound (94-97%) and rapidly crosses the blood-brain barrier. Because only unbound drug will cross into the CNS, changes in plasma protein concentrations and resultant protein binding may significantly alter the response to a given dose. Midazolam is metabolized in the liver, principally by microsomal oxidation. An active metabolite (alpha-hydroxymidazolam) is formed, but because of its very short half-life and lower pharmacologic activity, it probably has negligible clinical effects. The serum half-life and duration of activity of midazolam in humans is considerably shorter than that of diazepam. Elimination half-life in humans is ≈2 hours (vs. approx. 30 hours for diazepam).

Contraindications/Precautions/Warnings

The manufacturer lists the following contraindications for use in humans: hypersensitivity to benzodiazepines, or acute narrow-angle glaucoma. Additionally, intra-carotid artery injections must be avoided.

Use cautiously in patients with hepatic or renal disease, and debilitated or geriatric patients. Patients with congestive heart failure or hepatic dysfunction may eliminate the drug more slowly and prolonged effects can occur. The drug should be administered to patients in coma, shock, or with significant respiratory depression very cautiously.

When used alone, midazolam does not possess significant effects on cardiorespiratory function, but in combination with other agents, cardiorespiratory effects may be noted. Increased heart rate and blood pressure may be noted when used with ketamine. If this combination is used after an opioid has been administered, these effects may be diminished. If isoflurane will be used as the general anesthetic, use ketamine/midazolam with caution as bradycardia, hypotension and reduced cardiac output are possible.

Midazolam/opioid combinations can cause less cardiovascular depression, but greater respiratory depression, than acepromazine/opioid.

Midazolam and butorphanol used during isoflurane anesthesia can cause decreased blood pressure, heart rate and enhanced respiratory depression.

Midazolam with etomidate should be used with caution in dogs undergoing ocular surgery. A study found this combination caused clinically relevant miosis, significantly increased intraocular pressure, and commonly induced ptyalism, gagging, and abdominal heaving. Midazolam and propofol caused only a minor decrease in pupil diameter (Gunderson *et al.* 2013).

Adverse Effects

The primary concern using midazolam in veterinary patients is the possibility of respiratory depression.

In dogs, after morphine/acepromazine pre-op, midazolam given at 0.2 mg/kg IV prior to propofol anesthesia caused excitement in some patients (Covey-Crump *et al.* 2008), (Hopkins *et al.* 2014).

Few adverse effects have been reported in human patients receiving midazolam. Most frequently, effects on respiratory rate, cardiac rate and blood pressure have been reported. Respiratory depression has been reported in patients who have received narcotics or have COPD. The following adverse effects have been reported in >1%, but <5% of patients receiving midazolam: pain on injection, local irritation, headache, nausea, vomiting, and hiccups.

Reproductive/Nursing Safety

Although midazolam has not been demonstrated to cause fetal abnormalities, in humans, other benzodiazepines have been implicated in causing congenital abnormalities if administered during the 1st trimester of pregnancy. Infants born of mothers receiving large doses of benzodiazepines shortly before delivery have been reported to suffer from apnea, impaired metabolic response to cold stress, difficulty in feeding, hyperbilirubinemia, hypotonia, etc. Withdrawal symptoms have occurred in infants whose mothers chronically took benzodiazepines during pregnancy. The veterinary significance of these effects is unclear, but the use of these agents during the 1st trimester of pregnancy should only occur when the benefits clearly outweigh the risks associated with their use. In humans, the FDA categorizes this drug as category **D** for use during pregnancy (*There is evidence of human fetal risk, but the potential benefits from the use of the drug in pregnant women may be acceptable despite its potential risks.*)

Midazolam is excreted in milk and may cause CNS effects in nursing neonates. Exercise caution when administering to a nursing mother.

Overdosage/Acute Toxicity

Very limited information is currently available. The IV LD$_{50}$ in mice has been reported to be 86 mg/kg. It is suggested that accidental overdoses be managed in a supportive manner, similar to diazepam. Flumazenil could be used to antagonize midazolam effects, but because of midazolam's short duration of effect and flumazenil's high cost, supportive therapy may be more suitable in all but the largest overdoses.

Drug Interactions

See the precautions noted above (Contraindications/Precautions) when using midazolam with other agents for preoperative use in small animals. The following drug interactions have either been reported or are theoretical in humans or animals receiving midazolam and may be of significance in veterinary patients. Unless otherwise noted, use together is not necessarily contraindicated, but weigh the potential risks and perform additional monitoring when appropriate.

- **ANESTHETICS, INHALATIONAL:** Midazolam may decrease the dosages required.
- **AZOLE ANTIFUNGALS** (*e.g.*, **ketoconazole, itraconazole, fluconazole**): May increase midazolam levels by decreasing hepatic clearance; prolonged effects may occur. A study in greyhounds showed that ketoconazole significantly decreased the elimination of midazolam (KuKanich *et al.* 2010).
- **CALCIUM CHANNEL BLOCKERS** (*e.g.*, **diltiazem, verapamil**): May increase midazolam levels.
- **CIMETIDINE:** May increase midazolam levels.
- **CNS DEPRESSANTS, OTHER:** May increase the risk of respiratory depression.
- **MACROLIDES** (*e.g.*, **erythromycin, clarithromycin**): May increase midazolam levels.
- **LOPERAMIDE:** May increase midazolam levels by decreasing hepatic clearance.
- **OPIATES:** May increase the hypnotic effects of midazolam; hypotension has been reported when midazolam is used with meperidine.
- **PHENOBARBITAL:** May decrease peak levels and AUC of midazolam.
- **RIFAMPIN:** May decrease peak levels and AUC of midazolam.
- **THIOPENTAL:** Midazolam may decrease the dosages required.

Doses

- **DOGS:**

  As a preoperative agent (extra-label): Used in combination with other premeds (*e.g.*, ketamine, acepromazine, opioids, alpha2 agonists). Typical dosage range: 0.1 – 0.3 mg/kg SC, IM, IV.

  For status epilepticus (extra-label): Dosage recommendations vary and no evidence was located that supports one over the other.

  IV, or IM: Most recommend 0.1 – 0.3 mg/kg, but dosages range from 0.07 – 0.5 mg IM or IV; IM dosages may need to be higher than IV dosages. Dosages up to 0.5 mg/kg may be repeated twice if no response. If seizures recur, re-bolus and consider a CRI.

  Intranasal: 0.2 – 0.5 mg/kg intranasal. Re-dose as above.

  As a CRI: Dosage recommendations vary; most recommend a range of approximately 0.05 – 0.5 mg/kg/hour, but up to 2 mg/kg/hour has been noted. Generally, start at low end and increase rate until seizures are controlled. Midazolam IV CRI's may cause thrombophlebitis less often than diazepam CRI's.

- **CATS:**

  As a preoperative agent (extra-label): Used in combination with other premeds (*e.g.*, ketamine, acepromazine, opioids, alpha2 agonists). Typical dosage range: 0.1 – 0.3 mg/kg SC, IM, IV. Midazolam with butorphanol combination may cause anxiousness, aggressiveness and difficulty in restraint in some cats and is best reserved for geriatric or very ill cats (Biermann *et al.* 2012).

- **RABBITS, RODENTS, SMALL MAMMALS:**

  Note: All are extra-label.

  a) **Hamsters, Gerbils, Mice, Rats, Guinea pigs, Chinchillas:** 1 – 2 mg/kg IM. (Adamcak *et al.* 2000)

  b) **As a preanesthetic: Rabbits:** 0.5 – 5 mg/kg IM or IV; **Rodents:** 3 – 5 mg/kg IM or IV; often beneficial to minimize stress, anxiety and patient struggling. May be reversed with flumazenil if necessary (0.1 mg/kg IV, but may precipitate seizures). (Bennett 2009)

  c) **Injectable anesthesia: Rodents:** midazolam (5 mg/kg) + ketamine (100 mg/kg) + buprenorphine (0.05 mg/kg) IP. **Rabbits:** Midazolam (0.05 mg/kg) + buprenorphine (0.03 mg/kg) + ketamine (10 mg/kg) IM. (Bennett 2009)

  d) **As an induction agent in rabbits:** 0.05 – 0.5 mg/kg IV (typically via a marginal ear vein). The low end of the dosage range is usually given and topped up as necessary. In non-sedated animals, prior preparation of the area with topical local anesthetics may be useful. Intravenous midazolam leads to further sedation of the patient, sufficient to allow intubation, but may also induce apneic side effects. This, together with fentanyl's respiratory depression, can potentially compound the possibility of hypoxia. It is important therefore, that midazolam is given to effect and that pre-oxygenation is performed. Intubation is considered essential when using this protocol. **Note:** Not all patients require midazolam induction for purposes of intubation. An assessment of the patient can be made in the first 10 minutes post premedicant delivery. Some rabbits may be sufficiently sedated to allow intubation at this point. (Vella 2009)

- **HORSES:**

  As a preoperative agent/TIVA (extra-label): Midazolam may be used or substituted for diazepam in protocols with ketamine ± xylazine. See Ketamine and Diazepam monographs for more information.

  For seizure control in foals (extra-label): 2 – 5 mg (not mg/kg) for a 50 kg foal IV, IM. Rapid IV administration may result in apnea and hypotension. Repeat as necessary. A CRI may be used at a dose of 1 – 3 mg/hour (not mg/kg/hour) for a 50 kg foal. Adapted from: (Bentz 2006), (Toppin 2007)

- **BIRDS:**

  As a sedative/restraining agent (intranasal); (extra-label): A study in Hispaniolan Amazon Parrots given 2 mg/kg intranasally 15 minutes prior to manual restraint found that sedation occurred within 3 minutes of administration, and vocalization, flight, and defense responses were significantly reduced when compared to control (saline) birds during capture. Additionally, treated birds had significantly lower cloacal temperature, and mean respiratory rates were significantly lower for up to 12 minutes. Flumazenil antagonized the effects of midazolam within 10 minutes. No overt clinical adverse effects to intranasal midazolam and flumazenil administration were observed. Authors suggest further studies on safety of intranasal midazolam and flumazenil reversal in this species. (Mans *et al.* 2012)

As a pre-med for anxious or easily stressed birds (*e.g.*, macaws, African greys, raptors and many wild birds); (extra-label): 1 mg/kg IM. This will cause mild sedation and relaxation. Doses as high as 6 mg/kg have been reported resulting in considerable sedation. (Morrisey 2010)

As part of an injectable anesthetic regimen (extra-label): Injectable anesthetics are only occasionally used in birds for short procedures or in situations where inhalant anesthetics are not available. Ketamine at 10 – 30 mg/kg and midazolam at 2 – 6 mg/kg can be used. The midazolam can be reversed with flumazenil (0.1 mg/kg) if necessary. Butorphanol can be added for analgesia at a dose of 1 – 2 mg/kg. (Morrisey 2010)

- **ZOO, EXOTIC, WILDLIFE SPECIES:**

For use of midazolam in zoo, exotic and wildlife medicine refer to specific references, including:

a) *Zoo Animal and Wildlife Immobilization and Anesthesia.* West, G., Heard, D., Caulkett, N. (eds.). Blackwell Publishing, 2007.

b) *Handbook of Wildlife Chemical Immobilization, 3rd Ed.* Kreeger, T.J. and J.M. Arnemo. 2007.

c) *Fowler's Zoo and Wild Animal Medicine Current Therapy, Volume 7*, Miller, R.E., Fowler, M.E., Saunders. 2011.

d) *Exotic Animal Formulary, 4th Ed.* Carpenter, J.W., Saunders. 2012.

e) The 2009 American Association of Zoo Veterinarian Proceedings by D. K. Fontenot also has several dosages listed for restraint, anesthesia, and analgesia for a variety of drugs for carnivores and primates. VIN members can access them at: http://goo.gl/NNIWQ or http://goo.gl/9UJse

Monitoring
- Level of sedation.
- Respiratory and cardiac signs.

Client Information
- When injected, midazolam should be used in an inpatient setting only or with direct professional supervision where cardiorespiratory support services are available.
- If giving intranasally to stop a seizure in dogs, follow your veterinarian's instructions exactly and contact your veterinarian immediately for further advice.

Chemistry/Synonyms
Midazolam HCL is a benzodiazepine that occurs as a white or yellowish crystalline powder. Solubility in water is dependent upon pH. At a pH of 3.4 (approximately the pH of commercial injection), 10.3 mg are soluble in one mL of water.

Midazolam HCl may also be known as Ro-21-3981/003, or *Versed®*.

Storage/Stability
It is recommended to store midazolam injection at room temperature (15-30°C) and protected from light. After being frozen for 3 days and allowed to thaw at room temperature, the injectable product was physically stable. Midazolam is stable at a pH from 3-3.6.

Compatibility/Compounding Considerations
Midazolam is reportedly physically **compatible** when mixed with the following products: D5W, normal saline, lactated Ringer's, atracurium, atropine sulfate, buprenorphine, butorphanol, cefuroxime, chlorpromazine, ciprofloxacin, fentanyl citrate, gentamicin, glycopyrrolate, hydromorphone, hydroxyzine, ketamine, meperidine, metoclopramide, morphine sulfate, nalbuphine, ondansetron, promethazine HCl, sufentanil citrate, and scopolamine HBr.

Midazolam is physically **incompatible** with dexamethasone sodium phosphate, dimenhydrinate, heparin, pantoprazole, pentobarbital, prochlorperazine, and ranitidine. Compatibility is dependent upon factors such as pH, concentration, temperature, and diluent used; consult specialized references or a hospital pharmacist for more specific information.

Midazolam hydrochloride oral suspension compounded from the commercially available injectable solution has been published (Steedman *et al.* 1992). Diluting midazolam 5 mg/mL injection in a 1:1 ratio with *Syrpalta®* yields a 2.5 mg/mL midazolam hydrochloride oral solution that retains >90% potency for 56 days when stored at 7°C, 20°C, and 40°C and protected from light.

Dosage Forms/Regulatory Status
VETERINARY-LABELED PRODUCTS: NONE.

The ARCI (Racing Commissioners International) has designated this drug as a class 2 substance. See the appendix for more information.

HUMAN-LABELED PRODUCTS:

Midazolam HCl Injection: 1 mg (as HCl)/mL; 5 mg (as HCl)/mL; generic; (Rx, C-IV)

Midazolam HCl Syrup: 2 mg/mL; generic; (Rx, C-IV)

Revisions/References
Monograph revised/updated April 2014.

Aarnes, T. K., et al. (2013). Pharmacokinetics and pharmacodynamics of midazolam after intravenous and intramuscular administration in alpacas. American Journal of Veterinary Research 74(2): 294-9.

Adamcak, A. & B. Otten (2000). Rodent Therapeutics. Vet Clin NA: Exotic Anim Pract 3:1(Jan): 221-40.

Bennett, R. (2009). Small Mammal Anesthesia--Rabbits and Rodents. Proceedings: ACVC. accessed via Veterinary Information Network; vin.com

Bentz, B. (2006). Current management practices for critically ill foals. Proceedings: ABVP. accessed via Veterinary Information Network; vin.com

Biermann, K., et al. (2012). Sedative, cardiovascular, haematologic and biochemical effects of four different drug combinations administered intramuscularly in cats. Veterinary Anaesthesia and Analgesia 39(2): 137-50.

Covey-Crump, G. L. & P. J. Murison (2008). Fentanyl or midazolam for co-induction of anaesthesia with propofol in dogs. Veterinary Anaesthesia and Analgesia 35(6): 463-72.

Eagleson, J., et al. (2010). Pharmacokinetics of a Novel Intranasal Midazolam Gel in Dogs. Proceedings: ACVIM. accessed via Veterinary Information Network; vin.com

Gunderson, E. G., et al. (2013). Effects of anesthetic induction with midazolam-propofol and midazolam-etomidate on selected ocular and cardiorespiratory variables in clinically normal dogs. American Journal of Veterinary Research 74(4): 629-35.

Hopkins, A., et al. (2014). Midazolam, as a co-induction agent, has propofol sparing effects but also decreases systolic blood pressure in healthy dogs. Veterinary Anaesthesia and Analgesia 41(1): 64-72.

Hubbell, J. A. E., et al. (2013). Pharmacokinetics of midazolam after intravenous administration to horses. Equine Veterinary Journal 45(6): 721-5.

KuKanich, B. & M. Hubin (2010). The pharmacokinetics of ketoconazole and its effects on the pharmacokinetics of midazolam and fentanyl in dogs. J. Vet. Pharmacol. Ther. 33(1): 42-9.

Mans, C., et al. (2012). Sedation and Physiologic Response to Manual Restraint After Intranasal Administration of Midazolam in Hispaniolan Amazon Parrots (Amazona ventralis). Journal of Avian Medicine and Surgery 26(3): 130-9.

Morrisey, J. K. (2010). Avian Analgesia and Anesthesia. Proceedings: WVC. accessed via Veterinary Information Network; vin.com

Schwartz, M., et al. (2012). Pharmacokinetics of Midazolam After Intravenous, Rectal, and Intramuscular Administration in Dogs. Proceedings: ACVIM. accessed via Veterinary Information Network; vin.com

Steedman, S. L., et al. (1992). Stability of midazolam hydrochloride in a flavored, dye-free oral solution. Am J Hosp Pharm 49(3): 615-8.

Toppin, S. (2007). ICU activities and procedures for the newborn foal: I-III. Proceedings: Western Vet Conf. accessed via Veterinary Information Network; vin.com

Vella, D. (2009). Rabbit General Anesthesia. Proceedings: AAVAC-UEP. accessed via Veterinary Information Network; vin.com

Milbemycin Oxime

(mil-beh-**my**-sin)

Macrolide Antiparasitic

For information on the combination products with lufenuron (*Sentinel®*, *Sentinel Spectrum®*) see the Lufenuron monograph. For information on the combination product with spinosad (*Trifexis®*), see the Spinosad monograph.

Prescriber Highlights

▶ At time of writing (April 2014) only available in combination products (*e.g.*, *Sentinel®*, *Sentinel Spectrum®*, *Trifexis®*).

▶ GABA inhibitor in invertebrates used for heartworm prophylaxis, microfilaricide, & treat demodicosis, etc.

▶ Contraindications: No absolute contraindications.

▶ Adverse Effects: Animals with circulating microfilaria may develop a transient shock-like syndrome; at higher doses, neuro signs become more likely.

Uses/Indications

Milbemycin tablets are labeled as a once-a-month heartworm preventative (*Dirofilaria immitis*) and for hookworm control (*Ancylostoma caninum*). It has activity against a variety of other parasites, including adult hookworms (*A. caninum*), adult roundworms (*T. canis, T. leonina*) and whipworms (*Trichuris vulpis*).

Pharmacology/Actions

Milbemycin is thought to act by disrupting the transmission of the neurotransmitter gamma amino butyric acid (GABA) in invertebrates.

Pharmacokinetics

No specific information was located. At labeled doses, milbemycin is considered effective for at least 45 days after infection by *D. immitis* larva.

Contraindications/Precautions/Warnings

Because some dogs with a high number of circulating microfilaria will develop a transient, shock-like syndrome after receiving milbemycin, the manufacturer recommends testing for preexisting heartworm infections.

If using milbemycin at doses greater than labeled in breeds susceptible to the *ABCB1* genetic mutation, genetic testing is recommended before initiating therapy.

The manufacturer states to only use the product (*Interceptor®*) in dogs 4 weeks of age or older, and at least 2 lbs. body weight.

Adverse Effects

At labeled doses, adverse effects appear to be infrequent in microfilaria-free dogs, including breeds susceptible to neurologic toxicity (see Overdosage below). In a recent study where dogs of breeds susceptible to the *ABCB1* mutation were given milbemycin at doses from 1 – 2.2 mg/kg PO daily, all *ABCB1* mutant/mutant dogs experienced CNS toxicity, while no *ABCB1* wild-type/wild-type or *ABCB1* mutant/wild-type dogs experienced toxicity (Barbet *et al.* 2009).

Eight week old puppies receiving 2.5 mg/kg (5X label) for 3 consecutive days showed no clinical signs after the first day, but after the second or third consecutive dose, showed some ataxia and trembling.

Reproductive/Nursing Safety

The manufacturer states that safety in breeding, pregnant, and lactating queens and breeding toms has not been established.

Studies in pregnant dogs at daily doses 3X those labeled showed no adverse effects to offspring or bitch.

Milbemycin does enter maternal milk; at standard doses, no adverse effects have been noted in nursing puppies.

Overdosage/Acute Toxicity

Beagles have tolerated a single oral dose of 200 mg/kg (200X monthly rate). Rough-coated collies have tolerated doses of 10 mg/kg (20X labeled) without adversity. Toxic doses can cause mydriasis, hypersalivation, lethargy, ataxia, pyrexia, seizures, coma and death. There is no specific antidotal treatment and supportive therapy is recommended.

Drug Interactions

The manufacturer states that the drug was used safely during testing in dogs receiving other frequently used veterinary products, including vaccines, anthelmintics, antibiotics, steroids, flea collars, shampoos and dips.

The following drug interactions have either been reported or are theoretical in humans or animals receiving GABA agonists and may be of significance in veterinary patients. Unless otherwise noted, use together is not necessarily contraindicated, but weigh the potential risks and perform additional monitoring when appropriate.

- **BENZODIAZEPINES**: Effects may be potentiated by milbemycin; use together not advised in humans

Caution is advised if using other drugs that can inhibit **p-glycoprotein** particularly in those dogs at risk for *ABCB1*-1Δ (formerly MDR1-allele) mutation (Collies, Australian Shepherds, Shelties, Long-haired Whippet, etc. "white feet"), unless tested "normal": Drugs and drug classes involved include:

- **AMIODARONE**
- **AZOLE ANTIFUNGALS** (*e.g.*, **ketoconazole**)
- **CARVEDILOL**
- **CYCLOSPORINE**
- **DILTIAZEM**
- **ERYTHROMYCIN; CLARITHROMYCIN**
- **QUINIDINE**
- **SPIRONOLACTONE**
- **TAMOXIFEN**
- **VERAPAMIL**

Doses

- **DOGS:**

For prophylaxis and treatment of dirofilariasis, it is suggested to review the guidelines published by the American Heartworm Society at www.heartwormsociety.org.

As a parasiticide (labeled dosages; FDA-approved):

For Milbemycin alone: For heartworm prophylaxis, control of adult hookworms (*A. caninum*), adult roundworms (*T. canis, T. leonina*) and whipworms (*Trichuris vulpis*) in dogs 4 weeks of age or older and at least 2 lbs. body weight: Minimum dosage is 0.5 mg/kg PO once a month. (Label information; *Interceptor®*—Novartis)

For Milbemycin/Lufenuron (*Sentinel®*); Milbemycin/Lufenuron/Praziquantel (*Sentinel Spectrum®*) or Milbemycin/Spinosad (*Trifexis®*): Products come in a variety of tablet sizes for given weights of dogs. They are dosed PO on a monthly basis.

- **CATS:**

For prevention of heartworm; treat adult hookworm and adult roundworms (labeled dose; FDA-approved): 2 mg/kg PO once monthly. (Label directions; *Interceptor® Flavor Tabs for Cats*—Novartis)

Client Information

- Used monthly in dogs and cats for heartworm control, roundworms, hookworms, and in dogs for whipworms.
- Appears very safe when used as a heartworm preventative.

- Store flavored tablets out of reach of children and animals; may be toxic to wildlife so dispose of unused tablets properly.
- Review importance of compliance with therapy and to be certain that the dose was consumed.

Chemistry/Synonyms

Milbemycin oxime consists of ≈80% of the A4 derivatives and 20% of the A3 derivatives of 5-didehydromilbemycin. Milbemycin is considered to be a macrolide antibiotic structurally.

Milbemycin may also be known as CGA-179246, *Interceptor®*.

Storage/Stability

Store milbemycin oxime tablets at room temperature.

Compatibility/Compounding Considerations

No specific information noted.

Dosage Forms/Regulatory Status

VETERINARY-LABELED PRODUCTS:

Milbemycin Oxime Oral Tablets: 2.3 mg (brown, 2-10 lbs.), 5.75 mg (green, 11-25 lbs.), 11.5 mg (yellow, 26-50 lbs.), 23 mg (white, 51-100 lbs.), dogs >100 lbs. are provided the appropriate combination of tablets; *Interceptor® Flavor Tabs*; (Rx). FDA-approved for use in dogs and puppies >4 weeks of age and 2 lbs. or greater. **Note:** At time of writing (April 2014) this product is still listed on FDA's Green Book, but may not be commercially available.

Milbemycin Oxime Oral Tablets: 5.75 mg (cats weighing 1.5-6 lbs.), 11.5 mg (6.1-12 lbs.), 23 mg (white, 12.1-25 lbs.); *Interceptor® Flavor Tabs*; (Rx). FDA-approved for cats and kittens >6 wks. old and >1.5 lbs. **Note:** At time of writing (April 2014) this product is still listed on FDA's Green Book, but may not be commercially available.

Milbemycin/Lufenuron Oral Tablets: For dogs: 2-10 lbs.: 2.3 mg/46 mg; 11-25 lbs.: 5.75 mg/115 mg; 26-50 lbs.: 11.5 mg/230 mg; 51-100 lbs.: 23 mg/460 mg milbemycin/lufenuron; *Sentinel® Flavor Tabs*; (Rx). FDA-approved for use in dogs and puppies 4 weeks of age or older. Also available in combination with nitenpyram (*Capstar®*).

Milbemycin/Lufenuron/Praziquantel Chewable Oral Tablets: For dogs: 2-8 lbs.: 2.3 mg/46 mg/22.8 mg; 8.1-25 lbs: 5.75 mg/115 mg/57 mg; 25.1-50 lbs.: 11.5 mg/230 mg/114 mg; 50.1-100 lbs.: 23 mg/460 mg/228 mg; *Sentinel® Spectrum®* (Rx). FDA-approved for use in dogs and puppies 6 weeks of age or older.

Milbemycin/Spinosad Chewable Oral Tablets: For dogs: 5-10 lbs. (140 mg spinosad and 2.3 mg milbemycin oxime); 10.1-20 lbs. (270 mg spinosad and 4.5 mg milbemycin oxime); 20.1-40 lbs. (560 mg spinosad and 9.3 mg milbemycin oxime); 40.1-60 lbs. (810 mg spinosad and 13.5 mg milbemycin oxime); 60.1-120 lbs. (1620 mg spinosad and 27 mg milbemycin oxime); *Trifexis®*; (Rx). FDA-approved for use in dogs and puppies 8 weeks of age or older and at least 5 lbs. of weight.

There is also a milbemycin 0.1% otic solution (*Milbemite®*) available.

HUMAN-LABELED PRODUCTS: NONE.

Revisions/References

Monograph revised/updated April 2014.

Barbet, J. L., et al. (2009). ABCB1-1 Delta (MDR-1 Delta) genotype is associated with adverse reactions in dogs treated with milbemycin oxime for generalized demodicosis. Veterinary Dermatology 20(2): 111-4.

Milk Thistle – see Silymarin

Miltefosine

(mil-**tef**-oh-seen)   Milteforan®, Impavido®

Antileishmanial

Prescriber Highlights

▶ Oral treatment for canine leishmaniasis.
▶ Not available commercially in USA (human orphan drug).
▶ Vomiting very common.
▶ Like other drugs, unlikely to fully clear the organism, but can reduce clinical implications.
▶ Appears to be more effective when used with allopurinol.

Uses/Indications

Originally developed as an antineoplastic agent, miltefosine can be used alone or with allopurinol to treat canine leishmaniasis (CanL). Like other drugs, it does not completely clear the organism in dogs, but can substantially reduce the parasitic load. Clinical efficacy is improved when used with allopurinol.

Pharmacology/Actions

While the exact mechanism of action for miltefosine against *Leishmania infantum* is not understood, it is thought that it inhibits the penetration of the organism into macrophages by interacting with glycosomes and glycosylphosphatidyl-inositol anchors that are essential for the survival of Leishmania intracellularly. Also by inhibiting phospholipase, miltefosine disrupts Leishmania membrane signal transduction. Miltefosine has antineoplastic, immunomodulatory, and antiviral activity.

Pharmacokinetics

After oral administration in dogs, miltefosine has a bioavailability of 94% with peak plasma levels occurring around 5 hours post-dose. The drug is distributed throughout the major organs, including the brain. Intravascularly, it is nearly evenly distributed between plasma and erythrocytes. Miltefosine is mainly eliminated via the feces, with ≈10% of a dose eliminated unchanged. Renal elimination appears negligible. Miltefosine has a very long half-life of around 6.5 days.

Contraindications/Precautions/Warnings

Miltefosine is labeled as contraindicated in patients hypersensitive to it and in pregnant, lactating or breeding animals.

Use with caution in patients with severe hepatic dysfunction. Do not under dose as it may increase the risk for drug resistance to occur.

Adverse Effects

Vomiting is the most common adverse effect seen in dogs. Other GI signs (inappetence, diarrhea) may also be seen. Miltefosine potentially may cause nephrotoxicity and/or hepatotoxicity, but as leishmaniasis can cause kidney and liver damage, it is difficult to ascribe any specific risk for these potential adverse effects in dogs. One study in healthy Beagles, found that 2 mg/kg/day PO of miltefosine in 8 dogs did not cause renal tubular damage, but 100 mg/kg/day SC of meglumine antimoniate caused severe tubular damage (cell necrosis and apoptosis) (Bianciardi *et al.* 2009).

In humans, the most common (>10%) adverse effects are vomiting, diarrhea and an increase in liver enzymes. Nephrotoxicity has also been reported in humans treated with miltefosine for leishmaniasis.

Reproductive/Nursing Safety

Miltefosine is labeled as contraindicated in pregnant, lactating and breeding animals and during pregnancy and breastfeeding in humans. When pregnant rats were dosed at 1.2 mg/kg/day and higher during the early embryonic development (up to day 7 of pregnancy), an increased risk for embryotoxic, fetotoxic and teratogenic effects was determined. In pregnant rabbits given 2.4 mg/kg/day and higher during the organogenesis phase, embryotoxic and fetotoxic effects were also seen.

Male rats given miltefosine daily at 8.25 mg/kg showed testicular atrophy and impaired fertility; this was reversible within 10 weeks.

It is not known if miltefosine is excreted into milk. The canine and human labels state that it should not be used in nursing mothers.

Overdosage/Acute Toxicity

Overdoses likely would cause GI signs (vomiting, etc.). Potentially, hepatic, renal, and retinal toxicity are possible in large overdoses. A specific antidote for miltefosine overdose is not known.

Drug Interactions

No drug interactions have been reported for miltefosine at present.

Laboratory Considerations

- No specific concerns noted.

Doses

- **DOGS:**

  For canine leishmaniasis (extra-label in USA):

  a) The product should be administered at 2 mg/kg PO, poured onto food, with a full or partial meal once a day for 28 days. (From the translated label Information—*Milteforan®*; Virbac-France)

  b) As an alternative treatment to meglumine antimoniate and allopurinol: Miltefosine 2 mg/kg PO once daily for 28 days with allopurinol (10 mg/kg PO q12h, orally for at least 6 months). (Miro *et al.* 2009), (Zini 2010)

Monitoring

- Baseline and periodic renal function and hepatic enzymes.
- Adverse effects (especially vomiting); patient weight.

Client Information

- Give with food, to help reduce the chance for vomiting.
- If vomiting or severe diarrhea occur, contact veterinarian.
- Wear disposable gloves when administering this product as it has caused skin reactions.
- Because this drug has caused birth defects, it should not be handled by pregnant women.
- Do not allow treated dogs to lick persons immediately after intake of the medication.
- To avoid foaming, do not shake the vial.

Chemistry/Synonyms

Miltefosine is a phospholipid derivative (alkylphosphocholine) that is structurally related to the phospholipid components of cell membranes. The commercially available canine product (*Milteforan®*) is a clear, colorless, viscous solution containing 20 mg/mL of miltefosine. Excipients in the solution include hydroxypropylcellulose, propylene glycol, and water.

Miltefosine may also be known as D-18506, HDPC, hexadecilfosfocolina, hexadecylphosphocholine, miltefosiini, miltefosina, miltéfosine, or miltefosinum. Trade names include: *Milteforan®*, *Miltex®* and *Impavido®*.

Storage/Stability

This veterinary medicinal product does not require any special storage conditions. Avoid freezing the solution.

Compatibility/Compounding Considerations

No specific information noted.

Dosage Forms/Regulatory Status

VETERINARY-LABELED PRODUCTS:

None in the USA. Elsewhere, a canine licensed product may be available. Miltefosine Oral Solution: 20 mg/mL in 30 mL, 50 mL & 90 mL vials; *Milteforan®*; (Rx)

HUMAN-LABELED PRODUCTS:

Impavido® is approved as an orphan drug by FDA. In countries where leishmaniasis in humans is endemic, 10 mg and 50 mg capsules (*Impavido®*) may be marketed.

Revisions/References

Monograph revised/updated April 2014.

Bianciardi, P., et al. (2009). Administration of Miltefosine and Meglumine Antimoniate in Healthy Dogs: Clinicopathological Evaluation of the Impact on the Kidneys. Toxicologic Pathology 37(6): 770-5.

Miro, G., et al. (2009). Multicentric, controlled clinical study to evaluate effectiveness and safety of miltefosine and allopurinol for canine leishmaniosis. Veterinary Dermatology 20(5-6): 397-404.

Zini, E. (2010). Canine Leishmaniasis - Challenging Treatment of a Multifaceted Disease. Proceedings: ECVIM. accessed via Veterinary Information Network; vin.com

Mineral Oil

White Petrolatum, Liquid Paraffin

Lubricant Laxative

Prescriber Highlights

- ▶ Cautions: Debilitated or pregnant patients, & patients with hiatal hernia, dysphagia, esophageal or gastric retention.
- ▶ Use caution when administering by tube to avoid aspiration.
- ▶ Adverse Effects: Lipid pneumonitis if aspirated; granulomatous reactions in liver etc. if significant amounts are absorbed from gut; oil leakage from the anus; long-term use may lead to decreased absorption of fat-soluble vitamins (A, D, E, & K).
- ▶ Drug interactions.

Uses/Indications

Mineral oil is commonly used in horses to treat constipation and fecal impactions. It is also employed as a laxative in other species as well, but used less frequently. Mineral oil has been administered after ingesting lipid-soluble toxins (*e.g.*, kerosene, metaldehyde) to retard the absorption of these toxins through its laxative and solubility properties.

Petrolatum containing products (*e.g.*, *Felaxin®*, *Laxatone®*, *Kat-A-Lax®*, etc.) may be used in dogs and cats as a laxative or to prevent/reduce "hair-balls" in cats.

Pharmacology/Actions

Mineral oil and petrolatum act as laxatives by lubricating fecal material and the intestinal mucosa. They also reduce reabsorption of water from the GI tract, thereby increasing fecal bulk and decreasing intestinal transit time.

Pharmacokinetics

It has been reported that after oral administration, emulsions of mineral oil may be up to 60% absorbed, but most reports state that mineral oil preparations are only minimally absorbed from the gut.

Contraindications/Precautions/Warnings

No specific contraindications were noted with regard to veterinary patients. In humans, mineral oil (orally administered) is considered contraindicated in patients <6 yrs. old, debilitated or pregnant patients, and patients with hiatal hernia, dysphagia, esophageal or gastric retention. Use caution when administering by tube to avoid aspiration, especially in debilitated or recalcitrant animals. To avoid aspiration in small animals, orally administered mineral oil should not be attempted when there is an increased risk of vomiting, regurgitation, or other preexisting swallowing difficulty. Many clinicians believe that mineral oil should not be administered orally to small animals due to the risk for aspiration and, if used as a laxative, should be administered rectally.

In horses, mineral oil and docusate are contraindicated for use to remove an esophageal blockage as aspiration can occur.

Adverse Effects

When used on a short-term basis and at recommended doses, mineral oil or petrolatum should cause minimal adverse effects. The most serious effect that could be encountered is aspiration of the oil with resultant lipid pneumonitis; prevent this by using the drug only in appropriate cases, when "tubing", ascertain that the tube is in the stomach, and administrate the oil at a reasonable rate.

Granulomatous reactions have occurred in the liver, spleen and mesenteric lymph nodes when significant quantities of mineral oil are absorbed from the gut. Oil leakage from the anus may occur and be of concern in animals with rectal lesions or house pets. Long-term administration of mineral oil/petrolatum may lead to decreased absorption of fat-soluble vitamins (A, D, E, and K). No reports were found documenting clinically significant hypovitaminosis in cats receiving long-term petrolatum therapy, however.

Reproductive/Nursing Safety

In humans, the FDA categorizes this drug as category C for use during pregnancy (*Animal studies have shown an adverse effect on the fetus, but there are no adequate studies in humans; or there are no animal reproduction studies and no adequate studies in humans.*)

Oral mineral oil should be safe to use during nursing.

Overdosage/Acute Toxicity

No specific information was located regarding overdoses of mineral oil; but it would be expected that with the exception of aspiration, the effects would be self-limiting. See adverse effects section for more information.

Drug Interactions

The following drug interactions have either been reported or are theoretical in humans or animals receiving mineral oil and may be of significance in veterinary patients. Unless otherwise noted, use together is not necessarily contraindicated, but weigh the potential risks and perform additional monitoring when appropriate.

- **DOCUSATE:** Theoretically, mineral oil should not be given with docusate (DSS) as enhanced absorption of the mineral oil could occur. However, this does not appear to be of significant clinical concern with large animals.
- **VITAMINS A, D, E, & K:** Chronic administration of mineral oil may affect Vitamin K and other fat-soluble vitamin absorption. It has been recommended to administer mineral oil products between meals to minimize this problem.

Doses

- **DOGS/CATS:**

 As a lubricant laxative (extra-label): Because of the risk for aspiration, liquid mineral oil is rarely recommended for PO administration today. Occasionally, some administer liquid mineral oil rectally (5 – 30 mL dogs; 5 – 10 mL cats). Cat laxative (petrolatum-based) products are sometimes recommended at 1 – 5 mL per cat per day.

- **RABBITS, RODENTS, SMALL MAMMALS:**

 As a laxative/remove hairballs (extra-label): **Rabbits:** Using feline laxative product: 1 – 2 mL/day for 3-5 days. (Ivey *et al.* 2000)

- **CATTLE:**

 As a laxative (extra-label): <u>Adults</u>: 0.5 – 4 liters, <u>Calves</u>: 60 – 120 mLs via stomach tube.

- **HORSES:**

 As a laxative (extra-label):

 For large colon impactions: Via nasogastric tube: <u>Adults</u>: 2 – 4 liters, may be repeated q12h; <u>Foals</u>: 60 – 240 mL. Not recommended for foals <24 hours old.

 For sand colic: In this experimental study, 0.5 kg psyllium was mixed with 1 liter of mash and given twice daily and 2 liters of mineral oil via NG tube were administered once daily. This combination was more effective (measured ash content of feces) than giving mineral oil alone. (Hotwagner *et al.* 2008).

- **SWINE:**

 As a laxative (extra-label): 50 – 100 mL; administer via stomach tube. (Howard 1986)

- **SHEEP & GOATS:**

 As a laxative (extra-label): 100 – 500 mL; administer via stomach tube. (Howard 1986)

- **BIRDS:**

 Use as a laxative and to aid in the removal of lead from the gizzard (extra-label): 1 – 3 drops per 30 grams of body weight or 5 mL/kg PO once. Repeat as necessary. Give via tube or slowly to avoid aspiration. (Clubb 1986)

Monitoring

- Clinical efficacy.
- If possibility of aspiration: auscultate, radiograph if necessary.

Client Information

- Follow veterinarian's instructions or label directions for "cat laxative" products.
- Do not increase dosage or prolong treatment beyond veterinarian's recommendations.

Chemistry/Synonyms

Mineral oil, also known as liquid petrolatum, liquid paraffin or white mineral oil occurs as a tasteless, odorless (when cold), transparent, colorless, oily liquid that is insoluble in both water and alcohol. It is a mixture of complex hydrocarbons and is derived from crude petroleum. For pharmaceutical purposes, heavy mineral oil is recommended over light mineral oil, as it is believed to have a lesser tendency to be absorbed in the gut or aspirated after oral administration.

White petrolatum, also known as white petroleum jelly or white soft paraffin, occurs as a white or faintly yellow unctuous mass. It is insoluble in water and almost insoluble in alcohol. White petrolatum differs from petrolatum only in that it is further refined to remove more of the yellow color.

Mineral Oil may also be known as: liquid paraffin, 905 (mineral hydrocarbons), dickflussiges paraffin, heavy liquid petrolatum, huile de vaseline epaisse, liquid petrolatum, oleum petrolei, oleum vaselini, paraffinum liquidum, paraffinum subliquidum, vaselinol, vaselinum liquidum, and white mineral oil; many trade names are available.

Storage/Stability

Petrolatum products should be stored at temperatures <30°C.

Compatibility/Compounding Considerations

No specific information noted.

Dosage Forms/Regulatory Status

VETERINARY-LABELED PRODUCTS:

Mineral oil products have not been formally FDA-approved for use in food animals. These products and preparations are available without a prescription (OTC).

<u>Petrolatum Oral Preparations:</u>

Liquid Mineral Oil: available in gallons or 55 gallon drums.

Cat "Laxative" Products: Products may vary in actual composition; some contain liquid petrolatum in place of white petrolatum and may have various flavors (tuna, caviar, malt, etc.). There are many proprietary products marketed.

HUMAN-LABELED PRODUCTS:

Mineral Oil Liquid: in 180 mL and 473 mL; generic; (OTC)

Mineral Oil Emulsions: There are several products available that are emulsions of mineral oil and may be more palatable for oral administration. Trade names include: *Kondremul® Plain*; (OTC). Various generic products are available.

Revisions/References

Monograph revised/updated April 2014.

Clubb, S. L. (1986). Therapeutics: Individual and Flock Treatment Regimens. *Clinical Avian Medicine and Surgery*. G. J. Harrison and L. R. Harrison. Philadelphia, W.B. Saunders: 327-55.

Hotwagner, K. & C. Iben (2008). Evacuation of sand from the equine intestine with mineral oil, with and without psyllium. Journal of Animal Physiology and Animal Nutrition 92(1): 86-91.

Howard, J. L., Ed. (1986). *Current Veterinary Therapy 2, Food Animal Practice*. Philadelphia, W.B. Saunders.

Ivey, E. & J. Morrisey (2000). Therapeutics for Rabbits. Vet Clin NA: Exotic Anim Pract 3:1(Jan): 183-216.

Minocycline HCl

(mi-noe-**sye**-kleen)   Minocin®

Tetracycline Antibiotic

Prescriber Highlights

► Oral & parenteral tetracycline antibiotic; potential alternative to doxycycline.

► Less likely to cause bone & teeth abnormalities than other tetracyclines, but avoid use in pregnancy & young animals.

► May be used in patients with renal insufficiency.

► Adverse Effects are most commonly GI-related.

► Drug-drug; drug-lab interactions.

Uses/Indications

Minocycline may be useful for treating Brucellosis (in combination with aminoglycosides), Lyme disease, and certain nosocomial infections where other more commonly used drugs are ineffective. It is potentially an alternative for doxycycline and may be effective for treating some methicillin-resistant strains of *Staphylococcus pseudintermedius* (MRSP).

Minocycline has been investigated as adjunctive therapy for treating hemangiosarcomas, but early results have been disappointing.

Pharmacology/Actions

Tetracyclines are time-dependent, bacteriostatic antibiotics. They act by inhibiting protein synthesis by reversibly binding to 30S ribosomal subunits of susceptible organisms, thereby preventing binding to those ribosomes of aminoacyl transfer-RNA. Tetracyclines can alter cytoplasmic membrane permeability in susceptible organisms. In high concentrations, tetracyclines can inhibit protein synthesis by mammalian cells.

For dogs and cats, there are not established breakpoints for minocycline and using human breakpoints may not apply because of the drug's apparent high protein binding in dogs and cats. While doxycycline and minocycline are sometimes considered interchangeable there are differences in pharmacokinetics and antibacterial activity. A retrospective review of methicillin-resistant *Staphylococcus pseudintermedius* (MRSP) found that of the 107 isolates tested, 36% were susceptible to tetracycline, 38% to doxycycline and 65% to minocycline (Weese *et al*. 2013). If treating MRSP, minocycline susceptibility should be performed. Resistance to minocycline indicates presence of the tet(M) gene, while susceptibility to minocycline but resistance to tetracycline indicates presence of the tet(K) gene (Frank *et al*. 2012).

As a class, the tetracyclines have activity against most mycoplasma, spirochetes (including the Lyme disease organism), Chlamydia, and Rickettsia. Against gram-positive bacteria, the tetracyclines have activity against some strains of staphylococci and streptococci, but resistance of these organisms is increasing (Weese *et al*. 2013). Gram-positive bacteria that are usually covered by tetracyclines, include *Actinomyces* spp., *Bacillus anthracis*, *Clostridium perfringens* and tetani, *Listeria monocytogenes*, and Nocardia. Among gram-negative bacteria that tetracyclines usually have *in vitro* and *in vivo* activity include *Bordetella* spp., Brucella, Bartonella, *Haemophilus* spp., *Pasteurella multocida*, Shigella, and *Yersinia pestis*. Many or most strains of *E. coli*, Klebsiella, Bacteroides, Enterobacter, Proteus, and *Pseudomonas aeruginosa* are resistant to the tetracyclines.

Minocycline and doxycycline have significant inhibitory properties against the activity of matrix metalloproteinases (collagenase, gelatinase) and can act as a disease-modifying agent for osteoarthritis.

Pharmacokinetics

There is limited information available on the pharmacokinetics of minocycline in dogs and cats. Minocycline appears to be well absorbed after oral absorption regardless of the presence of food. A study done in 6 Beagles reported a mean oral bioavailability of ≈50%, but bioavailability ranged from 28-74% (Maaland *et al*. 2014). It is highly lipid soluble and distributed widely throughout the body. It appears that in dogs, minocycline is cleared more rapidly than doxycycline. Therapeutic levels can be found in the CSF (whether meninges are inflamed or not), prostate, saliva, and eye. Minocycline is extensively metabolized in the liver and primarily excreted as inactive metabolites in the feces and urine. Less than 20% is excreted unchanged in the urine. The half-life in dogs is ≈4 hours after an oral dose (Maaland *et al*. 2014).

In horses, when compared to doxycycline, minocycline appears to have higher oral bioavailability, and as it is less bound to plasma proteins attains higher concentrations in CSF and aqueous fluids. In a single-dose (2.2 mg/kg) IV study in adult horses, mean volume of distribution (SS) was 1.53 L/kg; plasma protein binding was 68%, volume of distribution (SS) was 1.53 L/kg, total body clearance was 0.16 L/h/kg, and the elimination half-life was ≈8 hours. Plasma concentration of free minocycline was 0.12 mcg/mL at 12 hours. A 5-dose (0.4 mg/kg PO q12h) oral study found a steady-state elimination half-life of ≈12 hours. (Schnabel *et al*. 2012), (Divers 2013), (Nagata *et al*. 2010)

Contraindications/Precautions/Warnings

Minocycline should be considered contraindicated in patients hypersensitive to tetracyclines, those that are pregnant or nursing, or in animals <6 months old. Minocycline is considered to be less likely to cause these abnormalities than other more water-soluble tetracyclines (*e.g.*, tetracycline, oxytetracycline). Unlike either oxytetracycline or tetracycline, minocycline can be used in patients with moderate renal insufficiency without dosage adjustment. Oliguric renal failure may require dosage adjustment.

Because urine levels are low, minocycline is not recommended for treating urinary tract infections.

If using orally in cats, follow the doxycycline recommendations to reduce the risk for oro-esophageal erosions. If using oral tablets or capsules "pilling" should be followed by at least 6 mL of water or food. Do not dry pill.

Adverse Effects

The most commonly reported side effects of oral minocycline therapy in dogs and cats are nausea and vomiting. To alleviate these effects, the drug could be given with food without clinically significant reductions in drug absorption. Dental or bone staining can occur when minocycline exposure occurs in utero or in early life. More rarely, increases in hepatic enzymes and ototoxicity are possible.

Like doxycycline, oral minocycline could cause esophagitis and esophageal strictures in cats. See Warnings for more information.

IV injections of minocycline in dogs have caused urticaria, shivering, hypotension, dyspnea, cardiac arrhythmias, and shock when given rapidly. Give IV slowly.

Tetracycline therapy (especially long-term) may result in overgrowth (superinfections) of non-susceptible bacteria or fungi.

In humans, minocycline (or other tetracyclines) has also been associated with photosensitivity reactions and, rarely, hepatotoxicity or blood dyscrasias. CNS effects (dizziness, lightheadedness) have been reported in people taking minocycline. A blue-gray pigmentation of skin and mucous membranes may occur.

Reproductive/Nursing Safety
Because tetracyclines can retard fetal skeletal development and discolor deciduous teeth, they should only be used in the last half of pregnancy when the benefits outweigh the fetal risks. Minocycline has been shown to impair fertility in male rats. In humans, the FDA categorizes this drug as category *D* for use during pregnancy (*There is evidence of human fetal risk, but the potential benefits from the use of the drug in pregnant women may be acceptable despite its potential risks.*)

Tetracyclines are excreted in milk. Milk:plasma ratios vary between 0.25 and 1.5. While minocycline probably has less effect on teeth and bones than other tetracyclines, its use should be avoided during nursing.

Overdosage/Acute Toxicity
Minocycline oral overdoses would most likely be associated with GI disturbances (vomiting, anorexia, and/or diarrhea). Although it is less vulnerable to chelation with cations than other tetracyclines, oral administration of divalent or trivalent cation antacids may bind some of the drug and reduce GI distress. Should the patient develop severe emesis or diarrhea, fluids and electrolytes should be monitored and replaced if necessary.

Drug Interactions
The following drug interactions have either been reported or are theoretical in humans or animals receiving minocycline and may be of significance in veterinary patients. Unless otherwise noted, use together is not necessarily contraindicated, but weigh the potential risks and perform additional monitoring when appropriate.

- **ANTACIDS, ORAL:** When orally administered, tetracyclines can chelate divalent or trivalent cations that can decrease the absorption of the tetracycline or the other drug if it contains these cations. Oral antacids, saline cathartics, or other GI products containing aluminum, calcium, magnesium, zinc, or bismuth cations are most commonly associated with this interaction. Minocycline has a relatively low affinity for divalent or trivalent cations, but it is recommended that all oral tetracyclines be given at least 1-2 hours before or after the cation-containing product.
- **BISMUTH SUBSALICYLATE, KAOLIN, PECTIN:** May reduce absorption.
- **IRON, ORAL:** Oral iron products are associated with decreased tetracycline absorption, and administration of iron salts should preferably be given 3 hours before or 2 hours after the tetracycline dose.
- **ISOTRETINOIN:** When used with minocycline may increase the risk for nervous system effects.
- **PENICILLINS:** Bacteriostatic drugs, like the tetracyclines, may interfere with bactericidal activity of the penicillins, cephalospo-

rins, and aminoglycosides. There is a fair amount of controversy regarding the actual clinical significance of this interaction, however.
- **RIFAMPIN:** Synergistic activity against *R. equi* in foals may occur.
- **SUCRALFATE:** Significantly decreased the oral bioavailability of minocycline in healthy dogs. Administering 2 hours after minocycline did not have a significant impact on absorption of minocycline. (KuKanich *et al.* 2014)
- **WARFARIN:** Tetracyclines may depress plasma prothrombin activity and patients on anticoagulant therapy may need dosage adjustment.

Laboratory Considerations
- Tetracyclines reportedly can cause false-positive **urine glucose** results if using the cupric sulfate method of determination (Benedict's reagent, *Clinitest®*), but this may be the result of ascorbic acid that is found in some parenteral formulations of tetracyclines.
- Tetracyclines reportedly have caused false-negative results in determining **urine glucose** when using the glucose oxidase method (*Clinistix®, Tes-Tape®*).
- Minocycline may interfere with the fluorescence test for **urinary catecholamines** causing falsely elevated values.

Doses
- **DOGS:**

For minocycline susceptible infections (extra-label): At time of writing (April-July 2014) there are not clear guidelines for dosing minocycline in dogs, but recently published research suggests that it may be effective at dosages slightly lower than those for doxycycline. A 10 mg/kg PO twice daily dose had been suggested in the interim (Boothe 2013). A small pharmacokinetic/drug interaction study in 5 healthy greyhounds found that a dose of 7.5 mg/kg PO q12h achieved the pharmacodynamic index for a bacterial (MIC) of 0.25 mcg/mL (AUC:MIC ≥33.9), but the authors cautioned that this was not an efficacy study and that further studies were required (KuKanich *et al.* 2014). Another study in 6 Beagles, concluded that minocycline at a dosage of 5 mg/kg PO twice daily is sufficient to inhibit *S. pseudintermedius* isolates with MICs ≤ 0.25 mcg/mL making minocycline a useful second-tier drug for treatment of canine infections caused by MRSP ST71 and other multidrug-resistant strains harboring tetracycline resistance gene tet(K) (Maaland *et al.* 2014). Practically, doses would be rounded to the nearest 25 mg if using commercially available solid, non-extended release dosage forms.

- **CATS:**

For minocycline susceptible infections (extra-label): At time of writing (April 2014) there is very little information on the pharmacokinetics of minocycline in cats and no clear guidelines for dosing. Anecdotal dosing recommendations range from 5 – 25 mg/kg PO twice daily, while 5 – 12.5 mg/kg PO twice daily is most commonly noted. Practically, doses would be rounded to the nearest 25 mg if using commercially available solid, non-extended release dosage forms.

- **HORSES:**

For susceptible (MIC ≤0.25 mcg/mL) non-ocular infections (extra-label): 4 mg/kg PO q12h. From a PK study in adult, normal horses. (Schnabel *et al.* 2012)

Monitoring
- Clinical efficacy.
- Adverse effects.

Client Information

- Oral minocycline products can be given without regard to feeding. Milk or other dairy products do not significantly alter the amount of minocycline absorbed.

- Do not give as a "dry pill". Give with a moist treat or small amount of liquid to be sure that it reaches the stomach; this is especially important for cats. Minocycline may cause ulcers in the throat and esophagus if it gets stuck there before it reaches the stomach. If your animal has trouble swallowing or eating, contact your veterinarian immediately.

- May upset stomach. To help prevent this, give with a small amount of food.

- Do not give antacids including sucralfate, oral iron or antidiarrheal medicines within 2 hours before or after giving minocycline. These products will reduce its effectiveness.

- This drug may make your animal's skin more sensitive to sunlight and increase the risk of sunburn on hairless areas such as the nose and around the eyelids and ears. Tell your veterinarian if you notice any reddening/sunburn on the skin while your animal is on this medication.

Chemistry/Synonyms

A semisynthetic tetracycline, minocycline HCl occurs as a yellow, crystalline powder. It is soluble in water and slightly soluble in alcohol.

Minocycline may also be known as: minocyclini hydrochloridum, *Arestin®*, *Minocin®*, or *Solodyn®*; many other trade names are available.

Storage/Stability

Store the oral preparations at room temperature in tight containers. Do not freeze the oral suspension. The injectable should be stored at room temperature and protected from light. After reconstituting with sterile water for injection, solutions with a concentration of 20 mg/mL are stable for 24 hours at room temperature.

Compatibility/Compounding Considerations

While minocycline is **compatible** with the usual intravenous fluids (including Ringer's and lactated Ringer's) do not add any other calcium containing fluid as precipitation could result.

Dosage Forms/Regulatory Status

VETERINARY-LABELED PRODUCTS: NONE.

HUMAN-LABELED PRODUCTS:

Minocycline HCl Oral Tablets: 50 mg, 75 mg & 100 mg; generic; (Rx)

Minocycline Extended-Release Tablets: 55 mg, 65 mg, 80 mg, 90 mg, 105 mg, 115 mg & 135 mg; *Solodyn®*, generic; (Rx)

Minocycline HCl Oral Capsules: 50 mg, 75 mg & 100 mg; generic; (Rx)

Minocycline HCl Pellet-filled Oral Capsules: 50 mg & 100 mg; *Minocin®*; (Rx)

Minocycline HCl Powder for Injection: 100 mg in vials; *Minocin®*; (Rx)

Minocycline HCl Powdered Microspheres, Extended-Release, dental: 1 mg; *Arestin®*; (Rx)

Revisions/References

Monograph revised/updated April 2014.

Boothe, D. M. (2013). Doxycycline for veterinary use during shortage. Javma-Journal of the American Veterinary Medical Association 242(10): 1340-.

Divers, T. J. (2013). Equine Lyme Disease. Journal of Equine Veterinary Science 33(7): 488-92.

Frank, L. A. & A. Loeffler (2012). Meticillin-resistant Staphylococcus pseudintermedius: clinical challenge and treatment options. Veterinary Dermatology 23(4): 283-E56.

KuKanich, K. S., et al. (2014). Effect of sucralfate on oral minocycline absorption in healthy dogs. J Vet Phamacol Ther **doi: 10.1111/jvp.12116.**

Maaland, M. G., et al. (2014). Minocycline pharmacokinetics and pharmacodynamics in dogs: dosage recommendations for treatment of meticillin-resistant Staphylococcus pseudintermedius infections. Veterinary Dermatology 25(3): 182-+.

Nagata, S.-i., et al. (2010). Pharmacokinetics and tissue distribution of minocycline hydrochloride in horses. American Journal of Veterinary Research 71(9): 1062-6.

Schnabel, L. V., et al. (2012). Pharmacokinetics and distribution of minocycline in mature horses after oral administration of multiple doses and comparison with minimum inhibitory concentrations. Equine Veterinary Journal 44(4): 453-8.

Weese, J. S., et al. (2013). Evaluation of minocycline susceptibility of methicillin-resistant Staphylococcus pseudintermedius. Veterinary Microbiology 162(2-4): 968-71.

Mirtazapine

(mir-**taz**-ah-peen)   Remeron®

Tetracyclic Antidepressant; 5-HT₃ Antagonist

Prescriber Highlights

▶ Used in veterinary medicine primarily as an appetite stimulant & antiemetic in dogs & cats with chronic kidney disease.

▶ Can be used in conjunction with other antiemetics.

▶ Primary side effect is sedation. In cats vocalization and increased affection can be noted.

▶ Use lowest effective dose to reduce sedative properties.

▶ Do not exceed 30 mg per day when used for appetite stimulation.

Uses/Indications

In cats and dogs, mirtazapine's main use to date has been as an appetite stimulant and antiemetic in animals with chronic kidney disease. When compared with placebo, cats ingested significantly more food when on mirtazapine. No difference in food ingestion was noted between the dosage groups, but high doses (3.75 mg) were associated with significantly more noticeable behavior changes (Quimby, J. *et al.* 2009), (Quimby, J.M. *et al.* 2011b). Other potential veterinary uses of mirtazapine could include treatment of chemotherapy-induced nausea and vomiting (CINV), behavior-related conditions, congestive heart failure, gastro-intestinal disorders, liver disease, or neoplasia.

Pharmacology/Actions

The antidepressant activity of mirtazapine appears to be mediated by antagonism at central pre-synaptic alpha₂-receptors, which normally acts as a negative feedback mechanism that inhibits further norepinephrine (NE) release. By blocking these receptors, mirtazapine overcomes the negative feedback loop and results in a net increase in NE. This mechanism may also contribute to the appetite stimulating effects of the medication since NE acts at other alpha-receptors to increase appetite. Additionally, mirtazapine antagonizes several serotonin (5HT) receptor subtypes. The drug is a potent inhibitor of the 5HT₂ and 5HT₃ receptors and of histamine (H₁) receptors. Antagonism at the 5HT₃ receptors accounts for the anti-nausea and antiemetic effects of the drug, and its action at H₁-receptors produces prominent sedative effects. It is a moderate peripheral alpha₁ adrenergic antagonist, a property that may explain the occasional orthostatic hypotension associated with its use; it is a moderate antagonist of muscarinic receptors, which may explain the relatively low incidence of anticholinergic effects.

Pharmacokinetics

In healthy cats, after oral dosing of either 1.88 mg (low dose; LD) or 3.75 mg (high dose, HD), median elimination half-lives were 15.9 hours (HD) and 9.2 hours (LD). Mean clearance was 10.5 mL/kg/min (LD) and 18 mL/kg/min (HD). A single low dose of mirtazapine was well tolerated and resulted in a half-life that is compatible with 24 hour dosing intervals in healthy cats. Mirtazapine does not appear to have linear kinetics in cats. A study in cats with chronic kidney disease (n=6) found that mean half-life was 15.2 hours and mean clearance/F was 0.6 L/hr/kg. The authors concluded the results were compatible with q48h (every other day dosing) in cats with chronic kidney disease (Quimby, J.M. *et al.* 2011a).

In dogs, a pilot study reported that after 20 mg PO per dog (Beagles; n=6), mean clearance of mirtazapine was 1193 mL/h/kg and mean half-life was 6.17 hours (Giorgi *et al.* 2012).

In horses after a single PO dose of 2 mg/kg (fed or fasted), peak levels occurred at 1.3 hours (fasted) and 2.2 hours (fed). Mirtazapine mean residence time was 4-6 hours and elimination half-life was ≈4-5 hours. The authors concluded that mirtazapine may be amenable for long-term oral administration, but additional information concerning safety and efficacy is critical before it is used clinically (Rouini *et al.* 2013).

Following oral administration in humans, mirtazapine is rapidly and completely absorbed. Studies in rats showed a linear relationship between the effects of mirtazapine and measured plasma and brain concentrations. Peak plasma concentrations are reached within ≈2 hours after an oral dose in humans. Food has minimal effects on both the rate and extent of absorption and does not require adjustments in the dose. Oral bioavailability of mirtazapine is ≈20% for rats and dogs, and ≈50% for humans.

Mirtazapine is metabolized via multiple pathways and varies by species. In all species tested (humans and laboratory animals), the drug was metabolized via the following mechanisms: 8-hydroxlaton followed by conjugation, N-oxidation, and demethylation followed by conjugation. Humans and guinea pigs also produce metabolites via N+-glucuronidation, whereas mice were the only species found to utilize demethylation followed by CO_2 addition and conjugation, and 13-hydroxylation followed by conjugation as methods of mirtazapine breakdown. These processes are conducted primarily by CYP2D6, CYP1A2, and CYP3A4, yet mirtazapine exerts minimal inhibition on any of these cytochromes. Several metabolic pathways of mirtazapine involve conjugation with glucuronide (glucuronidation). Since cats have a limited capacity for glucuronidation, mirtazapine is cleared less rapidly from the system and, therefore, an extended dosing may be required.

It is estimated that the active metabolite of mirtazapine contributes only 3-6% of the total pharmacodynamic profile of the drug since it is ≈10-fold less active than mirtazapine and affects the AUC minimally. Therefore, only the levels of the parent compound are considered clinically relevant.

The extent of binding of drugs to plasma proteins sometimes differs considerably among animal species. Plasma protein binding (PPB) for mirtazapine appears to be ≈70-72% for mice, rats, and dogs, whereas for humans and rabbits it is ≈85%. Despite the interspecies differences in PPB, no displacement interactions or dosage adjustments for mirtazapine are expected due to its large therapeutic window and nonspecific and relative low affinity for plasma proteins.

Human literature documents that elimination occurs via the urine (75%) and the feces (15%), renal impairment may reduce elimination by 30-50% compared to normal subjects, and hepatic impairment may reduce clearance by up to 30%. Human studies show the elimination half-life of mirtazapine to be long and range from 20-40 hours across age and gender subgroups, so dosage increases should take place no sooner than every 7-14 days. Females (both human and animal) of all ages exhibit significantly longer elimination half-lives than males (mean half-life of 37 hours for females vs. 26 hours for males in humans).

Contraindications/Precautions/Warnings

Mirtazapine is contraindicated in patients with hypersensitivity to mirtazapine or that have received monoamine oxidase inhibitors (*e.g.,* selegiline) in the past 14 days.

Mirtazapine has been associated with orthostatic hypotension

in humans and should, therefore, be used with caution in patients with known cardiac disease or cerebrovascular disease that could be exacerbated by hypotension. Patients with renal impairment, renal failure, or hepatic disease should be monitored while on mirtazapine therapy.

Abrupt discontinuation of mirtazapine after long-term administration has resulted in withdrawal symptoms such as nausea, headache and malaise in humans. In general, antidepressants may affect blood glucose concentrations because of their indirect effects on the endocrine system; use with caution in patients with diabetes mellitus.

Mirtazapine exhibits very weak anticholinergic activity, consequently, vigilance should be used in patients who might be more susceptible to these effects, such as those with urinary retention, prostatic hypertrophy, acute, untreated closed-angle glaucoma or increased intraocular pressure, or GI obstruction or ileus. Also, effects of mirtazapine may be additive to anticholinergic medications.

Extra care should be taken with active animals as mirtazapine may impair concentration and alertness. Although extremely rare, mirtazapine has been associated with blood dyscrasias in humans and should be used cautiously in patients with pre-existing hematological disease, especially leukopenia, neutropenia, or thrombocytopenia.

Adverse Effects

Mirtazapine appears to be well tolerated in both dogs and cats, but use has been limited. Besides the desirable side effect of appetite stimulation, other currently reported side effects in animals include: drowsiness/sedation, vocalization, increased affection in cats, hypotension, and tachycardia (all dose-dependent). Increases in liver enzymes have been reported in some cats receiving mirtazapine.

Reproductive/Nursing Safety

In humans, mirtazapine is FDA pregnancy category *C (animal studies have shown an adverse effect on the fetus, but there are no adequate studies in humans; or there are no animal reproduction studies and no adequate studies in humans)*. However, reproductive studies in rats, rabbits, and dogs have shown no evidence of teratogenicity. Additional studies in hamsters, rabbits, and rats showed no evidence of fetal genetic mutation or reduction in parental fertility, although there were increases in post-implantation losses and pup deaths, as well as decreased pup birth weight. No fetal harm was reported in any of several case reports of mirtazapine use during pregnancy or in animal studies.

In animals, mirtazapine is excreted in very small amounts in milk, the implications of which are currently unknown; consequently, it may be prudent to use caution in nursing mothers. Mirtazapine is distributed into human breast milk and safe use in humans during nursing cannot be assured. In one case report mirtazapine concentrations were detected in breast milk, but the examining neuropediatrician detected no adverse effects (including weight gain or sedation) in the infant.

Overdosage/Acute Toxicity

There were 235 single agent exposures to mirtazapine reported to the ASPCA Animal Poison Control Center (APCC) during 2009-2013. Of the 58 dogs, 21 were symptomatic with 52% agitated, 29% lethargic, 19% vocalizing, 19% panting and 14% tremoring. Of the 178 cats, 131 were symptomatic with 57% vocalizing, 38% agitated, 23% vomiting, 21% tachycardic, 15% ataxic and 11% lethargic.

Mirtazapine ingestion of upwards of 10-fold therapeutic dose in humans exhibits minimal toxicity requiring no acute intervention and only 6 hours of observation. Similar effects were seen in patients receiving up to 30X the recommended dose. However, serotonin syndrome is possible and the package insert for mirtazapine recommends that activated charcoal be administered in addition to other standard monitoring activities in an overdose situation.

Drug Interactions

The following drug interactions have either been reported or are theoretical in humans or animals receiving mirtazapine and may be of significance in veterinary patients. Unless otherwise noted, use together is not necessarily contraindicated, but weigh the potential risks and perform additional monitoring when appropriate.

- **CLONIDINE:** Mirtazapine may cause increases in blood pressure.
- **CYPROHEPTADINE:** May negate the effects mirtazapine.
- **DIAZEPAM** (and other **benzodiazepines**): Minimal effects on mirtazapine blood levels, but may cause additive impairment of motor skills.
- **FLUVOXAMINE:** May cause increased serum concentrations of mirtazapine.
- **LINEZOLID:** Increased risk for serotonin syndrome.
- **SELEGILINE, AMITRAZ:** Increased risk for serotonin syndrome; MAO inhibitors considered contraindicated with mirtazapine.
- **TRAMADOL:** Increased risk for serotonin syndrome.

In vitro studies identify mirtazapine as a substrate for several hepatic cytochrome CYP450 isoenzymes including 2D6, 1A2, and 3A4. Mirtazapine is not a potent inhibitor of any of these enzymes; clinically significant pharmacokinetic interactions are not likely with drugs metabolized by CYP enzymes.

Laboratory Considerations

- No specific concerns noted.

Doses

- **DOGS:**

  As an appetite stimulant and/or antiemetic (extra-label): There is little data on mirtazapine pharmacokinetics or efficacy in dogs. Anecdotal dosages ranging from 3.75 – 30 mg (depending on dog size) PO once daily have been suggested.

- **CATS:**

  As an appetite stimulant and/or antiemetic (extra-label): 1.88 mg (practically 1/4 of a 7.5 mg tablet; 1/8th of a 15 mg tablet) per cat PO every other day. A masked placebo-controlled crossover clinical trial in cats with chronic kidney disease demonstrated that mirtazapine significantly increased appetite and activity and significantly decreased vomiting (Quimby, J.M. *et al.* 2013). Some will advise giving this dose once daily in cats with normal renal function.

Monitoring

- Clinical efficacy measured by the following parameters: increased appetite, decreased episodes of vomiting, and weight gain.
- Liver enzymes in cats.
- Adverse Effects (behavior).

Client Information

- May be given with or without food. If your animal vomits after receiving it on an empty stomach, give with food or treat to see if this helps. If vomiting continues, contact your veterinarian.
- Tolerated very in well dogs. More side effects in cats and dosage may need to be adjusted if they occur. Common side effects include: vocalization, behavior changes, and tremors/shaking. Report excessive drowsiness or vocalization to your veterinarian.
- If your animal is receiving the orally disintegrating tablets, make sure hands are dry before handling the tablet. Place the tablet under the animal's tongue and hold mouth closed for several

seconds to allow it to dissolve (should occur quickly). After the tablet has melted, offer the patient water.

Chemistry/Synonyms

A member of the piperazino-azepine group of compounds, mirtazapine is classified as an atypical tetracyclic antidepressant and is not chemically related to other antidepressants. Mirtazapine, with a molecular weight of 265.36, occurs as a white to creamy white crystalline powder that is slightly soluble in water.

Mirtazapine may also be known as 6-azamianserin, Org-3770, mepirzapine and *Remeron®*; many trade names for international products are available.

Storage/Stability

The coated tablets and the orally disintegrating tablets should be stored at 25°C (77°F) with excursions permitted to 15-30°C (59-86°F). Protect from light and moisture. The stability of the orally disintegrating tablets once removed from the tablet blister is unknown and immediate use is recommended.

Compatibility/Compounding Considerations

No specific information noted.

Dosage Forms/Regulatory Status

VETERINARY-LABELED PRODUCTS: NONE.

HUMAN-LABELED PRODUCTS:

Mirtazapine Oral Tablets: 7.5 mg, 15 mg, 30 mg & 45 mg; *Remeron®*, generic; (Rx)

Mirtazapine Orally Disintegrating Tablets: 15 mg, 30 mg & 45 mg; *Remeron SolTab®*, generic; (Rx). **Note:** Some generic ODT's may contain xylitol (unknown quantity).

Revisions/References

Monograph revised/updated April 2014.

Giorgi, M. & H. Yun (2012). Pharmacokinetics of mirtazapine and its main metabolites in Beagle dogs: A pilot study. Veterinary Journal 192(2): 239-41.

Quimby, J., et al. (2009). The Pharmacokinetics of Mirtazapine in Healthy Cats. Proceedings: ACVIM. accessed via Veterinary Information Network; vin.com

Quimby, J. M., et al. (2011a). The Pharmacokinetics of Mirtazapine in Cats with Chronic Kidney Disease and In Age-Matched Control Cats. Journal of Veterinary Internal Medicine 25(5): 985-9.

Quimby, J. M., et al. (2011b). Studies on the pharmacokinetics and pharmacodynamics of mirtazapine in healthy young cats. J. Vet. Pharmacol. Ther. 34(4): 388-96.

Quimby, J. M. & K. F. Lunn (2013). Mirtazapine as an appetite stimulant and anti-emetic in cats with chronic kidney disease: A masked placebo-controlled crossover clinical trial. Veterinary Journal 197(3): 651-5.

Rouini, M. R., et al. (2013). Pharmacokinetics of Mirtazapine and Its Main Metabolites after Single Oral Administration in Fasting/Fed Horses. Journal of Equine Veterinary Science 33(6): 410-4.

Misoprostol

(mye-soe-**prost**-ole)   Cytotec®

Prostaglandin E₁ Analog

Prescriber Highlights

▶ Prostaglandin E₁ analog for treating or preventing gastric ulcers, especially associated with NSAIDs; may also be useful as an abortifacient adjunct.

▶ Contraindications: Pregnancy (but has been used in horses mid-gestation and intravaginally in humans during labor/delivery); nursing mothers (diarrhea in the nursing offspring).

▶ Caution: Sensitivity to prostaglandins or prostaglandin analogs; patients with cerebral or coronary vascular disease.

▶ Adverse Effects: GI distress (diarrhea, abdominal pain, vomiting, & flatulence); Potentially, uterine contractions & vaginal bleeding in female dogs.

▶ Pregnant women should handle with caution.

Uses/Indications

Misoprostol may be useful as primary or adjunctive therapy in treating or preventing GI adverse effects (anorexia, vomiting) or gastro-duodenal ulceration, especially when caused or aggravated by non-steroidal antiinflammatory drugs (NSAIDs). While it can be used for treating gastric ulcers, other drugs are probably just as effective and less expensive. It does not appear to be very effective in reducing gastric ulceration secondary to high-dose corticosteroid therapy.

There is some evidence for efficacy for misoprostol as antiallergic medications in dogs, but due to the modest benefits, relatively high costs and adverse effects associated with these medications, they probably should not be used as first line medications to treat dogs with atopic dermatitis (Olivry, T. et al. 2010).

Misoprostol's effects on uterine contractibility and cervical softening/opening make it effective as an adjunctive treatment in pregnancy termination.

Pharmacology/Actions

Misoprostol has two main pharmacologic effects that make it a potentially useful agent. By a direct action on parietal cells, it inhibits basal and nocturnal gastric acid secretion as well as gastric acid secretions that are stimulated by food, pentagastrin or histamine. Pepsin secretion is decreased under basal conditions, but not when stimulated by histamine.

Misoprostol also has a cytoprotective effect on gastric mucosa. Probably by increasing production of gastric mucosa and bicarbonate, increasing turnover and blood supply of gastric mucosal cells, misoprostol enhances mucosal defense mechanisms and healing in response to acid-related injuries.

Other pharmacologic effects of misoprostol include increased amplitude and frequency of uterine contractions, cervical thinning and relaxation, stimulating uterine bleeding, and causing total or partial expulsion of uterine contents in pregnant animals.

Pharmacokinetics

Approximately 88% of an oral dose of misoprostol is rapidly absorbed from the GI tract, but a significant amount is metabolized via the first-pass effect. The presence of food and antacids will delay the absorption of the drug. Misoprostol is rapidly de-esterified to misoprostol acid, which is the primary active metabolite. Misoprostol and misoprostol acid are thought equal in their effects on gastric mucosa. Both misoprostol and the acid metabolite are fairly well bound to plasma proteins (≈90% bound). It is not believed that misoprostol enters maternal milk, but it is unknown whether the acid enters milk.

Misoprostol acid is further biotransformed via oxidative mechanisms to pharmacologically inactive metabolites. These metabolites, the free acid and small amounts of unchanged drug are principally excreted into the urine. In humans, the serum half-life of misoprostol is ≈30 minutes and its duration of pharmacological effect is ≈3-6 hours.

Contraindications/Precautions/Warnings

It should be used in patients with the following conditions only when its potential benefits outweigh the risks: Sensitivity to prostaglandins or prostaglandin analogs; patients with cerebral or coronary vascular disease. Although not reported with misoprostol, some prostaglandins and prostaglandin analogs have precipitated seizures in epileptic human patients, and have caused hypotension, which may adversely affect patients with seizure disorders, or cerebral or coronary vascular disease.

Do not confuse misoprostol with mifepristone.

Adverse Effects

The most prevalent adverse effect seen with misoprostol is GI distress, usually manifested by diarrhea, abdominal pain, vomiting, and flatulence. Adverse effects are often transient and resolve over several days or may be minimized by dosage adjustment or giving doses with food. Potentially, uterine contractions and vaginal bleeding could occur in female dogs.

Reproductive/Nursing Safety

Misoprostol is generally considered contraindicated during pregnancy due to its potential abortifacient activity, although in humans it is used intravaginally during labor and delivery. In humans, the FDA categorizes this drug as category X for use during pregnancy (*Studies in animals or humans demonstrate fetal abnormalities or adverse reaction; reports indicate evidence of fetal risk. The risk of use in pregnant women clearly outweighs any possible benefit.*) In a separate system evaluating the safety of drugs in canine and feline pregnancy (Papich 1989), this drug is categorized as class: D (*Contraindicated. These drugs have been shown to cause congenital malformations or embryotoxicity.*)

In horses, a study in mid-gestational pregnant mares that received a 5-day course of oral misoprostol (5 micrograms/kg PO twice daily) as a GI mucosal cytoprotectant during colic found that pregnancy was not disrupted nor were any adverse effects noted. Cervical tone, ultrasonographic characteristics of the uterus, cervix and conceptus, and progesterone and estrone sulfate concentrations were similar prior to that measured before misoprostol. Authors concluded that additional investigation of treatment at earlier and later stages of gestation, for longer-term treatment, and evaluating neonates for developmental disturbances, would add further information on safety of misoprostol during gestation (Jacobson et al. 2013).

It is unlikely that misoprostol is excreted in milk because it is rapidly metabolized, however, it is not known if the active metabolite (misoprostol acid) is excreted in milk. Misoprostol is not recommended for nursing mothers as it potentially could cause significant diarrhea in the nursing offspring.

Overdosage/Acute Toxicity

There is limited information available. Overdoses in laboratory animals have produced diarrhea, GI lesions, emesis, tremors, focal cardiac, hepatic or renal tubular necrosis, seizures, and hypotension.

There were 86 single agent exposures to misoprostol reported to the ASPCA Animal Poison Control Center (APCC) during 2009-2013. Of these animals, 85 were dogs, with 21 being symptomatic. The most common sign was vomiting (62%).

Overdoses should be treated seriously and standard gut emptying techniques employed when applicable. Resultant toxicity should be treated symptomatically and supportively.

Drug Interactions

The following drug interactions have either been reported or are theoretical in humans or animals receiving misoprostol and may be of significance in veterinary patients. Unless otherwise noted, use together is not necessarily contraindicated, but weigh the potential risks and perform additional monitoring when appropriate.

- **ANTACIDS, MAGNESIUM-CONTAINING:** Magnesium-containing antacids may aggravate misoprostol-induced diarrhea. If an antacid is required, an aluminum-only antacid may be a better choice. Antacids and food do reduce the rate of misoprostol absorption and may reduce the systemic availability, but probably do not affect therapeutic efficacy.
- **OXYTOCIN:** Misoprostol may enhance effects.

Doses

- ### DOGS:

  For the prevention and treatment of GI ulcers/NSAID GI adverse effects (extra-label):

  For prevention of aspirin-induced gastric injury: Study suggests that misoprostol 3 micrograms/kg PO q12h is as effective as misoprostol 3 micrograms/kg PO q8h. (Ward *et al.* 2003)

  For other NSAIDs: No controlled studies documenting safety and efficacy were located and no clear evidence currently is available that supports any dosage in dogs. Anecdotal dosage recommendations usually range from 2 – 5 micrograms/kg PO q8-12h although some have suggested that longer times between doses may be effective and that dosages above 3 mcg/kg may be associated with more GI adverse effects.

  For reproductive system indications (all are extra-label):

  As part of an abortifacient protocol: Aglepristone 10 mg/kg SC on 2 consecutive days and misoprostol 200 micrograms (for bitches weighing ≤20 kg) or 400 micrograms for bitches weighing >20 kg) intravaginally once daily until completion of abortion. In the study all bitches in this treatment group aborted within 6 days. (Agaoglu *et al.* 2011)

  As part of an abortifacient protocol: Misoprostol 1 – 3 micrograms/kg once daily administered as a vaginal suppository to promote cervical dilation. This allows for a reduced dinoprost (PGF2 alpha) dose (0.1 mg/kg SC q8h for 2 days, then 0.2 mg/kg q8h SC to effect). Abortion usually occurs after 5 days. (Shaw 2007)

  For treating pyometra/metritis: Give aglepristone 10 mg/kg SC on days 1, 2, 8, 15, 29. Give misoprostol 10 micrograms/kg PO twice daily on days 3 through 12. Approximately 75% of cases show significant clinical improvement without developing the adverse effects associated with the prostaglandins (PGF2alpha, cloprostenol). (Fontbonne 2007)

  As an adjunctive therapy for atopic dermatitis (extra-label): Target dosage of 5 micrograms/kg PO 3 times daily. Modest improvement in clinical signs. (Olivry, T *et al.* 2003)

- ### CATS

  For GI adverse effects associated with NSAID use (extra-label): No controlled studies documenting safety or efficacy in cats were located. The ISFM and AAFP consensus guidelines: *Long-term use of NSAIDs in cats* recommends that when adverse GI events are observed in cats, NSAID therapy be withheld, and appropriate supportive therapy introduced, until any mucosal lesions have healed. If therapy is re-instituted, it should be done so at the lowest effective dose with consideration given to the concomitant use of omeprazole (0.7 – 1 mg/kg PO q24h) or misoprostol (5 micrograms/kg PO q8h), and/or a different NSAID where licensing permits. (Sparkes *et al.* 2010)

- ### HORSES:

  As a GI mucosal cytoprotectant (extra-label): 5 micrograms/kg PO q8-12h.

  To induce cervical relaxation (extra-label): From a case report of post-breeding endometritis in a maiden mare in which the cervix remained closed during estrus and acted as a barrier to uterine clearance: After uterus was lavaged and catheter removed, 1000 micrograms (total dose) of misoprostol as a compounded cream was applied to the caudal os and lumen of the cervix. Oxytocin (20 Units IM) was administered immediately following lavage and again every 6 hours until the following morning. (Nie *et al.* 2003)

Monitoring

- Efficacy.
- Adverse effects.

Client Information

- Give with food.
- Common side effects include diarrhea, abdominal/stomach pain, vomiting, and flatulence (gas). These may only last a few days and giving with food may help, but if any of these are severe, get worse or continue to be a problem, contact your veterinarian.
- Pregnant women should avoid handling medication; can cause miscarriage.

Chemistry/Synonyms

A synthetic prostaglandin E_1 analog, misoprostol occurs as a yellow, viscous liquid having a musty odor.

Misoprostol may also be known as: SC-29333, *Arthrotec®*, or *Cytotec®*.

Storage/Stability

Misoprostol tablets should be stored in well-closed containers at room temperature. After manufacture, misoprostol has an expiration date of 18 months.

Compatibility/Compounding Considerations

No specific information noted.

Dosage Forms/Regulatory Status

VETERINARY-LABELED PRODUCTS: NONE.

The ARCI (Racing Commissioners International) has designated this drug as a class 5 substance. See the appendix for more information.

HUMAN-LABELED PRODUCTS:

Misoprostol Tablets: 100 micrograms & 200 micrograms; *Cytotec®*, generic; (Rx)

Revisions/References

Monograph revised/updated April 2014.

Agaoglu, A. R., et al. (2011). The intravaginal application of misoprostol improves induction of abortion with aglepnstone. Theriogenology 76(1): 74-82.

Fontbonne, A. (2007). Anti-Progestins Compounds in Reproduction. Proceedings: World Small Animal Veterinary Association Congress. accessed via Veterinary Information Network; vin.com

Jacobson, C. C., et al. (2013). Mid-gestation pregnancy is not disrupted by a 5-day gastrointestinal mucosal cytoprotectant oral regimen of misoprostol. Equine Veterinary Journal 45(1): 91-3.

Nie, G. J. & A. J. Barnes (2003). Use of prostaglandin E-1 to induce cervical relaxation in a maiden mare with post breeding endometritis. Equine Veterinary Education 15(4): 172-4.

Olivry, T., et al. (2010). Treatment of canine atopic dermatitis: 2010 clinical practice guidelines from the International Task Force on Canine Atopic Dermatitis. Veterinary Dermatology 21(3): 233-48.

Olivry, T., et al. (2003). A randomized controlled trial of misoprostol monotherapy for canine atopic dermatitis: effects on dermal cellularity and cutaneous tumor necrosis factor-alpha. Vet Derm 14: 37-46.

Papich, M. (1989). Effects of drugs on pregnancy. *Current Veterinary Therapy X: Small Animal Practice*. R. Kirk. Philadelphia, Saunders; 1291-9.

Shaw, S. (2007). Dealing with Reproductive Emergencies. Proceedings: IVECCS. accessed via Veterinary Information Network; vin.com

Sparkes, A. H., et al. (2010). ISFM AND AAFP CONSENSUS GUIDELINES Long-term use of NSAIDs in cats. Journal of Feline Medicine and Surgery 12(7): 521-38.

Ward, D. M., et al. (2003). The effect of dosing interval on the efficacy of misoprostol in the prevention of aspirin-induced gastric injury. Journal of Veterinary Internal Medicine 17(3): 282-90.

Mitotane

(mye-toe-tane)   Lysodren®, o,p'-DDD

Adrenal Cytotoxic; Antineoplastic

Prescriber Highlights

▶ Adrenal cytotoxic agent used for medical treatment of pituitary-dependent hyperadrenocorticism.

▶ Caution: Pregnancy, diabetes, & preexisting renal or hepatic disease.

▶ Adverse Effects: Lethargy, ataxia, weakness, anorexia, vomiting, &/or diarrhea; liver changes possible.

▶ Relapses are not uncommon.

▶ All dogs receiving mitotane therapy should receive additional glucocorticoid supplementation if undergoing a stress (*e.g.*, surgery, trauma, acute illness).

▶ Monitoring is mandatory.

▶ Avoid human exposure.

Uses/Indications

In veterinary medicine, mitotane is used primarily for the medical treatment of pituitary-dependent hyperadrenocorticism (PDH), principally in dogs. An in-depth review of mitotane versus trilostane for the medical management of pituitary-dependent hyperadrenocorticism (PDH) in dogs, has been published (Reine 2012). A retrospective study of 37 dogs, found no statistical difference in survival times in dogs treated with mitotane or trilostane (Helm *et al.* 2011). Mitotane has also been used for the palliative treatment of adrenal carcinoma in humans and dogs. (Reine 2012)

Pharmacology/Actions

While mitotane is considered an adrenal cytotoxic agent, it apparently can also inhibit adrenocortical function without causing cell destruction. The exact mechanisms of action for these effects are not clearly understood.

In dogs with pituitary-dependent hyperadrenocorticism (PDH), mitotane has been demonstrated to cause severe, progressive necrosis of the zona fasciculata and zona reticularis. These effects occur quite rapidly (usually within 5-10 days of starting therapy). It has been stated that mitotane spares the zona glomerulosa and therefore aldosterone synthesis is unaffected. This is only partially true, as the zona glomerulosa may also be affected by mitotane therapy, but it is uncommon for clinically significant effects on aldosterone production to be noted with therapy.

Pharmacokinetics

In dogs, the systemic bioavailability of mitotane is poor. Oral absorption can be enhanced by giving the drug with food (especially food high in oil/fat content). In humans, ≈40% of an oral dose of mitotane is absorbed after dosing, with peak serum levels occurring ≈3-5 hours after a single dose. Distribution of the drug occurs to virtually all tissues in the body. The drug is stored in the fat and does not accumulate in the adrenal glands. A small amount may enter the CSF. It is unknown if the drug crosses the placenta or is distributed into milk.

Mitotane has a very long plasma half-life in humans, with values ranging from 18-159 days being reported. Serum half-lives may increase in a given patient with continued dosing, perhaps due to a depot effect from adipose tissue releasing the drug. The drug is metabolized in the liver and is excreted as metabolites in the urine and bile. Approximately 15% of an oral dose is excreted in the bile, and 10% in the urine within 24 hours of dosing.

Contraindications/Precautions/Warnings

Mitotane is contraindicated in patients known to be hypersensitive to it. Patients with concurrent diabetes mellitus may have rapidly changing insulin requirements during the initial treatment period. These animals should be closely monitored until they are clinically stable.

Dogs with preexisting renal or hepatic disease should receive the drug with caution and with more intense monitoring. It has been stated (Scott-Moncrieff 2010) that "Mitotane should never be administered in animals that are not eating well."

It has been stated: "…hyperadrenocorticism is a clinical condition. No dog should be treated for this condition unless there are obvious clinical signs, consistent with the diagnosis, that are worrisome to the owner" (Feldman 2007).

Some clinicians recommend giving prednisolone at 0.2 mg/kg/day during the initial treatment period (0.4 mg/kg/day to diabetic dogs) to reduce the potential for side effects from acute endogenous steroid withdrawal. Other clinicians have argued that routinely administering steroids masks the clinical markers that signify when the endpoint of therapy has been reached and must be withdrawn 2-3 days before ACTH stimulation tests can be done. Since in adequately observed patients adverse effects requiring glucocorticoid therapy may only be necessary in 5% of patients, the benefits of routine glucocorticoid administration may not be warranted.

Adverse Effects

Most common adverse effects seen with initial therapy in dogs include lethargy, ataxia, weakness, anorexia, vomiting, and/or diarrhea. Neurologic signs can be seen, but are not common. Adverse effects are commonly associated with plasma cortisol levels of <1 micrograms/dL or a too rapid decrease of plasma cortisol levels into the normal range. Adverse effects may also be more commonly seen in dogs weighing <5 kg, which may be due to the inability to accurately dose. The incidence of one or more of these effects is ≈25% and they are usually mild. If adverse effects are noted, it is recommended to temporarily halt mitotane therapy and supplement with glucocorticoids. Owners should be provided with a small supply of predniso(lo)ne tablets to initiate treatment. Should the clinical signs persist 3 hours after steroids are supplemented, consider other medical problems.

Liver changes (congestion, centrolobular atrophy, and moderate to severe fatty degeneration) have been noted in dogs given mitotane. Although not commonly associated with clinical symptomatology, these effects may be more pronounced with long-term therapy or in dogs with preexisting liver disease.

In perhaps 5% of dogs treated, long-term glucocorticoid and sometimes mineralocorticoid replacement therapy may be required. All dogs receiving mitotane therapy should receive additional glucocorticoid supplementation if undergoing a stress (*e.g.*, surgery, trauma, acute illness).

Relapses are not uncommon in canine patients treated for Cushing's with mitotane.

Reasons for treatment failure include misdiagnosis (*e.g.*, iatrogenic hyperadrenocorticism), adrenal tumors unresponsive to mitotane, loss of drug potency, or inadequate dose for that particular patient.

Reproductive/Nursing Safety

In humans, the FDA categorizes this drug as category *C* for use during pregnancy (*Animal studies have shown an adverse effect on the fetus, but there are no adequate studies in humans; or there are no animal reproduction studies and no adequate studies in humans.*) In a separate system evaluating the safety of drugs in canine and feline pregnancy (Papich 1989), this drug is categorized as class: *D* (*Contraindicated. These drugs have been shown to cause congenital malformations or embryotoxicity.*)

It is not known whether this drug is excreted in maternal milk.

Because of the potential for adverse reactions in nursing offspring, decide whether to discontinue nursing or discontinue the drug.

Overdosage/Acute Toxicity

No specific recommendations were located regarding overdoses of this medication. Because of the drug's toxicity and long half-life, emptying the stomach and administering charcoal and a cathartic should be considered after a recent ingestion. It is recommended that the patient be closely monitored and given glucocorticoids if necessary.

Drug Interactions

The following drug interactions have either been reported or are theoretical in humans or animals receiving mitotane and may be of significance in veterinary patients. Unless otherwise noted, use together is not necessarily contraindicated, but weigh the potential risks and perform additional monitoring when appropriate.

- **CNS DEPRESSANT DRUGS**: If mitotane is used concomitantly with drugs that cause CNS depression, additive depressant effects may be seen.
- **INSULIN**: Diabetic dogs receiving insulin may have their insulin requirements decreased when mitotane therapy is instituted.
- **PHENOBARBITAL**: Can induce enzymes and reduce the efficacy of mitotane, conversely mitotane can induce hepatic microsomal enzymes and increase the metabolism of phenobarbital.
- **SPIRONOLACTONE**: In dogs, spironolactone has been demonstrated to block the action of mitotane; it is recommended to use an alternate diuretic if possible.

Laboratory Considerations

- Mitotane will bind competitively to thyroxine-binding globulin and decreases the amount of serum protein-bound iodine. Serum **thyroxine** concentrations may be unchanged or slightly decreased, but free thyroxine values remain in the normal range. Mitotane does not affect the results of the resin triiodothyronine uptake test.
- Mitotane can reduce the amounts measurable **17-OHCS** in the urine, which may or may not reflect a decrease in serum cortisol levels or adrenal secretion.

Doses

- **DOGS:**

    For medical treatment of pituitary-dependent hyperadrenocorticism (bilateral adrenal hyperplasia); (extra-label): Note: Treatment with mitotane can be very complex and potentially serious adverse effects can occur. Use requires vigilance by the veterinarian and owner for monitoring therapy. The following are synopses of published dosing protocols. The reader is well-advised to refer to the original references for more detail, to the review by Reine (Reine 2012), or to the *Lysodren®* FAQ on VIN (Wilson 2010).

    a) <u>Induction phase</u> 30 – 50 mg/kg/day PO with a meal once daily or divided q12h for 7-10 days. If adverse effects (lethargy, vomiting, weakness, diarrhea) occur, discontinue mitotane and give glucocorticoids (prednis(ol)one at 0.15 – 0.25 mg/kg/day) until dog can be evaluated. If decreased appetite occurs discontinue mitotane and evaluate with an ACTH stimulation test. Perform ACTH stimulation test at end of 10 day period or sooner if adverse effects occur. Goal is to have basal and post-ACTH cortisol between 1-5 micrograms/dL (normal for most labs). If basal and post ACTH cortisol falls below 1 microgram/dL, temporarily suspend mitotane and supplement with glucocorticoids until circulating cortisol normalizes (usually 2-4 weeks, but may take several weeks to months). If basal or post ACTH cortisol is above normal, continue daily mitotane and recheck ACTH

stimulation tests at 5-10 day intervals until serum cortisol falls within normal resting range. <u>Begin maintenance</u> when desired cortisol concentrations are documented by ACTH stimulation testing. Mitotane given initially at 35 – 50 mg/kg per week in 2-3 divided doses. Should adverse effects, discontinue mitotane and supplement with glucocorticoids until dog can be evaluated by serum electrolytes and ACTH stimulation test. (Kintzer, P. 2007)

b) <u>Initial dose</u> of 50 mg/kg divided q12h. Glucocorticoids are not usually administered concurrently, but a small supply of prednisone should be made available to the owner for emergencies. Continue until water consumption decreases to <100 mL/kg/day, or until a decreased appetite, depression, diarrhea, or vomiting are observed. The time for clinical response is quite variable but most dogs respond within 3-7 days. At this point the dog should be reevaluated and an ACTH stimulation test performed. Prednisone treatment (0.2 mg/kg) should be initiated in patients that are showing clinical signs of hypocortisolemia, until the results of the ACTH stimulation test are known. In patients that are not polydipsic prior to therapy, where water consumption cannot be monitored, and whose polydipsia is due to another cause (*e.g.,* diabetes mellitus), mitotane should be administered for a maximum of 5-7 days prior to ACTH stimulation testing. The goal of treatment is to have both the pre- and post-cortisol measurement in the normal resting range (2-6 micrograms/dL). <u>Maintenance therapy</u> (50 mg/kg every 7-10 days) is started once the ACTH stimulation test shows adequate suppression and prednisone therapy (if necessary) has been discontinued. Failure to use maintenance therapy will result in re-growth of the adrenal cortex and recurrence of clinical signs. Efficacy of maintenance therapy is monitored by an ACTH stimulation test after one month of maintenance treatment and then every 3 months. The dose of mitotane required for long-term maintenance is very variable (26 – 330 mg/kg/week). (Scott-Moncrieff 2010)

c) <u>Intentionally causing complete destruction of the adrenal cortex as an alternative to the traditional mitotane treatment:</u> Mitotane at 75 – 100 mg/kg per day for 25 consecutive days, given in 3-4 doses per day with food. Lifelong prednisone at 0.1 – 0.5 mg/kg PO twice daily initially and mineralocorticoid therapy is begun at the start of mitotane therapy. Prednisone dose is tapered after completion of the 25-day protocol. Relapse is common and periodic ACTH stimulation testing is necessary. May be considerably more expensive than traditional therapy because of the expense associated with treating Addisonian dogs. (Nelson 2003)

d) <u>For total adrenal ablation for management of Cushing's</u>: Mitotane 100 mg/kg/day divided twice daily for 30 days. Supplemental cortisone acetate 2 mg/kg/day divided twice daily and fludrocortisone acetate 0.1 mg/10 lb of body weight PO once daily are begun on day 1 of mitotane therapy. Diet is supplemented with 1 – 5 grams of sodium chloride per day. One week after induction phase with mitotane, cortisone acetate is reduced to 1 mg/kg/day. Electrolytes and ACTH stimulation test are performed at end of induction, every 6 months, and at any time animal demonstrates signs compatible with either hypo- or hyperadrenocorticism. This form of management requires close patient monitoring and life-long daily therapy. Close attention during stress and non-adrenal illnesses required. (Bruyette 2002)

For palliative medical treatment of adrenal carcinomas or medical treatment of adrenal adenomas (extra-label): Initially,

50 – 75 mg/kg PO in daily divided doses for 10-14 days. May supplement with predniso(lo)ne at 0.2 mg/kg/day. Stop therapy and evaluate dog if adverse effects occur. After initial therapy run ACTH-stimulation test (do not give predniso(lo)ne the morning of the test). If basal or post-ACTH serum cortisol values are decreased, but still above the therapeutic end-point (<1 micrograms/dL), repeat therapy for an additional 7-14 days and repeat testing. If post-ACTH serum cortisol values remain greatly elevated or unchanged, increase mitotane to 100 mg/kg/day and repeat ACTH-stimulation test at 7-14 day intervals. If ACTH continues to remain greatly elevated, increase dosage by 50 mg/kg/day every 7-14 days until response occurs or drug intolerance ensues. Adjust dosage as necessary as patient tolerates or ACTH-responsive dictates. Once undetectable or low-normal post-ACTH cortisol levels are attained, continue mitotane at 100 – 200 mg/kg/week in divided doses with glucocorticoid supplementation (predniso(lo)ne 0.2 mg/kg/day). Repeat ACTH-stimulation test in 1-2 months. Continue at present dose if cortisol remains below 1 micrograms/dL. Should cortisol increase to 1-4 micrograms/dL, increase maintenance dose by 50%. If basal or post-ACTH cortisol goes above 4 micrograms/dL, restart daily treatment (50 – 100 mg/kg/day) as outlined above. Once patient is stabilized, repeat ACTH-stimulation tests at 3-6 month intervals. (Kintzer, P.P. *et al.* 1989)

- **FERRETS:**

  For medical treatment of hyperadrenocorticism where surgery has not been performed or tumor has not been fully resected (extra-label): 50 mg per ferret PO once daily for 1 week, then 50 mg PO 2-3 times per week. Have a compounding pharmacy make 50 mg capsules. Capsules can be easily administered if coated with a substance such as *Nutrical*. (Rosenthal *et al.* 2000)

Monitoring

Initially and as needed (see doses above):
- Physical exam and history (including water and food consumption, weight).
- BUN, CBC, Liver enzymes, Blood glucose, ACTH response test, serum electrolytes (Na$^+$/K$^+$).

Client Information

- <u>Mitotane treatment requires intensive monitoring and close supervision by your veterinarian.</u> Be sure you understand what signs acute hypoadrenocorticism can cause.
- The drug should be given with food, especially foods high in fat.
- Usually see positive effects (eats, drinks and urinates less) in 5-14 days after starting drug.
- The most common side effects are stomach upset (acting 'sick'), diarrhea and vomiting. Your veterinarian will tell you what to do when you see side effects (*e.g.,* hold the next dose, give prednisone, or contact veterinarian immediately).
- Pregnant women should not handle drug; others should wear disposable gloves whenever handling the drug.
- Dispose of unused drug appropriately.

Chemistry/Synonyms

Mitotane, also commonly known in veterinary medicine as o,p'-DDD, is structurally related to the infamous insecticide, chlorophenothane (DDT). It occurs as a white, crystalline powder with a slightly aromatic odor. It is practically insoluble in water and soluble in alcohol.

Mitotane may also be known as: CB-313, o,p'DDD, NSC-38721, WR-13045, *Lysodren®*, or *Lisodren®*.

Storage/Stability

Mitotane tablets should be stored at room temperature (15-30°C), in tight, light resistant containers.

Compatibility/Compounding Considerations

No specific information noted.

Dosage Forms/Regulatory Status

VETERINARY-LABELED PRODUCTS: NONE.

HUMAN-LABELED PRODUCTS:

Mitotane Tablets (scored): 500 mg; *Lysodren®*; (Rx)

Revisions/References

Monograph revised/updated April 2014.

Bruyette, D. (2002). Diagnosis and Treatment of Canine Cushing's Syndrome. Western Veterinary Conference. accessed via Veterinary Information Network; vin.com

Feldman, E. (2007). Medical management of canine hyperadrenocorticism: A comparison of trilostane to mitotane. Proceedings: UCD Canine Medicine Symposium. accessed via Veterinary Information Network; vin.com

Helm, J. R., et al. (2011). A Comparison of Factors that Influence Survival in Dogs with Adrenal-Dependent Hyperadrenocorticism Treated with Mitotane or Trilostane. Journal of Veterinary Internal Medicine 25(2): 251-60.

Kintzer, P. (2007). Treatment challenges in canine hyperadrenocorticism. Proceedings: Western Vet Conference. accessed via Veterinary Information Network; vin.com

Kintzer, P. P. & M. E. Peterson (1989). Mitotane (o,p'-DDD) treatment of cortisol-secreting adrenocortical neoplasia. *Current Veterinary Therapy X: Small Animal Practice.* R. W. Kirk. Philadelphia, WB Saunders: 1034-7.

Nelson, R. (2003). Treatment Options for Canine Cushing's Disease. Proceedings: World Small Animal Veterinary Association. accessed via Veterinary Information Network; vin.com

Papich, M. (1989). Effects of drugs on pregnancy. *Current Veterinary Therapy X: Small Animal Practice.* R. Kirk. Philadelphia, Saunders: 1291-9.

Reine, N. J. (2012). Medical Management of Pituitary-Dependent Hyperadrenocorticism: Mitotane versus Trilostane. Topics in Companion Animal Medicine 27(1): 25-30.

Rosenthal, K. & M. Peterson (2000). Hyperadrenocorticism in the ferret. *Kirk's Current Veterinary Therapy: XIII Small Animal Practice.* J. Bonagura. Philadelphia, WB Saunders: 372-4.

Scott-Moncrieff, J. C. (2010). Update on treatment of hyperadrenocorticism: What is the current recommendation? Proceedings: ACVIM Forum. accessed via Veterinary Information Network; vin.com

Wilson, S. Lysodren Protocols FAQ.

Mitoxantrone HCl

(mye-toe-**zan**-trone)   Novantrone®

Antineoplastic

Prescriber Highlights

▶ Antineoplastic that may be useful for a variety of neoplastic diseases. Renal clearance of drug is minimal. More myelosuppressive than doxorubicin but has less risk of causing nephrotoxicity.

▶ Contraindications (relative): Myelosuppression, concurrent infection, impaired cardiac function, and those that have received prior cytotoxic drug or radiation exposure. Caution: Sensitivity to drug, hyperuricemia or hyperuricuria, impaired hepatic function.

▶ Adverse Effects: Dose-dependent GI distress (vomiting, diarrhea, anorexia), bone marrow depression, lethargy, & seizures (cats). Extravasation injuries possible.

▶ Relatively expensive.

Uses/Indications

Mitoxantrone may be useful in the treatment of several neoplastic diseases in dogs and cats, including lymphosarcoma mammary adenocarcinoma, squamous cell carcinoma, renal adenocarcinoma, fibroid sarcoma, thyroid or prostate carcinoma, and hemangiopericytoma. When used with piroxicam, mitoxantrone has shown efficacy for treating transitional cell bladder carcinoma in dogs.

Because renal clearance of the drug is minimal (10%), it may be administered to cats with renal insufficiency much more safely than doxorubicin.

Pharmacology/Actions

By intercalation between base pairs and a nonintercalative electrostatic interaction, mitoxantrone binds to DNA and inhibits both DNA and RNA synthesis. Mitoxantrone is not cell-cycle phase specific, but appears to be most active during the S phase.

Pharmacokinetics

Mitoxantrone is rapidly and extensively distributed after intravenous infusion. Highest concentrations of the drug are found in the liver, heart, thyroid, and red blood cells. In humans, it is ≈78% bound to plasma proteins. Mitoxantrone is metabolized in the liver, but the majority of the drug is excreted unchanged in the urine. In humans, half-life averages ≈5 days as a result of the drug being taken up, bound, and then slowly released, by tissues.

Contraindications/Precautions/Warnings

Mitoxantrone is relatively contraindicated (weigh risk vs. benefit) in patients with myelosuppression, concurrent infection, impaired cardiac function, or those that have received prior cytotoxic drug or radiation exposure. It should be used with caution in patients with sensitivity to mitoxantrone, hyperuricemia or hyperuricuria, or impaired hepatic function.

Adverse Effects

In dogs and cats, effects include dose-dependent GI distress (vomiting, anorexia, diarrhea) and bone marrow depression (sepsis). Non-regenerative anemias may be detected and white cell nadirs generally occur on day 10. Some evidence exists that by giving recombinant granulocyte-colony stimulating factor bone marrow depression severity and duration may be reduced. Lethargy may also be noticed. Some cats receiving this drug have developed seizures.

Unlike doxorubicin, cardiotoxicity has not yet been reported in dogs and only rarely occurs in humans. Other adverse effects less frequently or rarely noted in humans and, potentially possible in dogs, include conjunctivitis, jaundice, renal failure, seizures, allergic reactions, thrombocytopenia, irritation or phlebitis at injection site. Tissue necrosis associated with extravasation has only been reported in a few human cases.

Reproductive/Nursing Safety

In humans, the FDA categorizes this drug as category *D* for use during pregnancy (*There is evidence of human fetal risk, but the potential benefits from the use of the drug in pregnant women may be acceptable despite its potential risks.*)

Mitoxantrone is excreted in maternal milk and significant concentrations (18 ng/mL) have been reported for 28 days after the last administration to humans. Because of the potential for serious adverse reactions in offspring, it is recommended to use milk replacer if mitoxantrone is administered.

Overdosage/Acute Toxicity

Because of the potential serious toxicity associated with this agent, dosage determinations must be made carefully.

Drug Interactions

Mitoxantrone is a substrate for ABCB1 (P-glycoprotein) and ABCG2 and it is likely that there are other interacting drugs yet to be identified. The following drug interactions have either been reported or are theoretical in humans or animals receiving mitoxantrone and may be of significance in veterinary patients. Unless otherwise noted, use together is not necessarily contraindicated, but weigh the potential risks and perform additional monitoring when appropriate.

- **CYCLOSPORINE:** May increase mitoxantrone's toxic effects.
- **DOXORUBICIN, DAUNORUBICIN, or RADIATION THERAPY:** Cardiotoxicity risks may be enhanced in patients that have previously received doxorubicin, daunorubicin, or radiation therapy to the mediastinum.
- **IMMUNOSUPPRESSANT DRUGS** (*e.g.,* **azathioprine, cyclophosphamide, corticosteroids**): Use with other immunosuppressant drugs may increase the risk of infection.
- **MYELOSUPPRESSIVE DRUGS** (*e.g.,* **chloramphenicol, flucytosine, amphotericin B,** or **colchicine**): Use extreme caution when used concurrently with other drugs that are also myelosuppressive, including many of the other antineoplastics and other bone marrow depressant drugs; bone marrow depression may be additive.
- **VACCINES, LIVE:** Live virus vaccines should be used with caution, if at all, during therapy.

Laboratory Considerations

- Mitoxantrone may raise serum **uric acid** levels. Drugs such as allopurinol may be required to control hyperuricemia.
- **Liver function tests** may become abnormal, indicating hepatotoxicity.
- Mitoxantrone may discolor **urine** to a green-blue color.

Doses

Note: Because of the potential toxicity of mitoxantrone when used at antineoplastic dosages, to patients, veterinary personnel and clients, and since chemotherapy indications, treatment protocols, monitoring and safety guidelines often change, the following dosages should be used only as a general guide. Consultation with a veterinary oncologist and referral to current veterinary oncology references [e.g., (Withrow *et al.* 2012); (Dobson *et al.* 2011); (Henry *et al.* 2009); (North *et al.* 2009); (Argyle *et al.* 2008)] are strongly recommended.

- **DOGS:**

  As an alternative agent for the treatment of a variety of neoplastic diseases (see Indications above): Usually used in chemotherapy protocols with other agents; commonly dosed at 5 – 6 mg/m² (not mg/kg) IV once every 3 weeks (q21 days). Should be administered IV into a running saline infusion or D5W infusion over a minimum of 5 minutes.

- **CATS:**

  As an alternative agent for the treatment of a variety of neoplastic diseases (extra-label): Usually dosed at 5.5 – 6.5 mg/m² (not mg/kg) IV once every 3 weeks (q21 days). Should be administered IV into a running saline or D5W infusion over a minimum of 5 minutes.

Monitoring

- CBC with differential and platelets (see Adverse Effects section).
- Efficacy.
- Chest radiographs, ECG or other cardiac function tests if cardiac symptomatology present.
- Liver function tests if jaundice or other clinical signs of hepatotoxicity present.
- Serum uric acid levels for susceptible patients.

Client Information

- Mitoxantrone or its metabolites may be detected in urine up to 6 days, and in feces up to 7 days after administration. Mitoxantrone is a chemotherapy (cancer) drug. The drug and its byproducts can be hazardous to other animals and people that come in contact with it. On the day your animal gets the drug and then for a few days afterward, all bodily waste (urine, feces, litter), blood, or vomit should only be handled while wearing disposable gloves. Seal the waste in a plastic bag and then place both the bag and gloves in with the regular trash.
- A blue-green color to urine or a bluish color to the whites of the eyes can be seen but is not a problem.
- If you see severe vomiting, bloody diarrhea, or redness or swelling where the drug was injected call your veterinarian immediately.
- Bone marrow suppression can occur and affect blood cells; watch your pet for: muscle weakness, fever, bruising and bleeding. If you see any of these, contact your veterinarian immediately.

Chemistry/Synonyms

Mitoxantrone HCl is a synthetic anthracenedione antineoplastic. It occurs as a dark-blue powder that is sparingly soluble in water, practically insoluble in acetone, acetonitrile, and chloroform, and slightly soluble in methyl alcohol.

Mitoxantrone may also be known as: L-232315, DHAD, dihydroxyanthracenedione dihydrochloride, mitoxantroni hydrochloridum, NSC-301739, or *Novantrone®*.

Storage/Stability

Mitoxantrone HCl should be stored at room temperature. While the manufacturer recommends not to freeze, one study (Mauldin 2002) demonstrated that the drug maintained its cytotoxic effects when frozen and thawed at various intervals over a 12 month period. Do not mix or use the same IV line with heparin infusions (precipitate may form). At present, it is not recommended to mix with other IV drugs.

Compatibility/Compounding Considerations

Do not mix or use the same IV line with heparin infusions (precipitate may form). At present, it is recommended to not mix with other IV drugs.

Dosage Forms/Regulatory Status

VETERINARY-LABELED PRODUCTS: NONE.

HUMAN-LABELED PRODUCTS:

Mitoxantrone HCl for Injection Solution Concentrate: 2 mg/mL, preservative free in 10 mL, 12.5 mL, & 15 mL multi-dose vials; generic; (Rx)

Revisions/References

Monograph revised/updated April 2014.

Argyle, D., et al. (2008). *Decision Making in Small Animal Oncology*, Wiley-Blackwell.
Dobson, J. & D. Lascelles (2011). *BSAVA Manual of Canine and Feline Oncology*, BSAVA.
Henry, C. & M. Higginbotham (2009). *Cancer Management in Small Animal Practice*, Saunders.
Mauldin, G. (2002). Evaluation of the in vitro cytotoxicity of mitoxantrone following repeated freeze-thaw cycles. Vet Therapeutics 3(3): 290-6.
North, S. & T. Banks (2009). *Small Animal Oncology: An Introduction*, Saunders.
Withrow, S., et al. (2012). Withrow and MacEwen's Small Animal Clinical Oncology, 5th Ed., Saunders.

Montelukast Sodium

(mon-teh-**loo**-kast)   Singulair®

Leukotriene Antagonist

Prescriber Highlights

▶ Leukotriene inhibitor; potentially may be useful in cats for feline asthma, IBD, upper respiratory disease, and heartworm-associated respiratory disease syndrome.

▶ Good evidence not yet available to support use in cats.

▶ No significant adverse effects reported in cats to date.

Uses/Indications

In veterinary medicine, montelukast has been used primarily in cats. Potential indications include: feline asthma, upper respiratory disease, inflammatory bowel disease and heartworm disease. Its use in treating feline asthma has been disappointing, and few recommend it for this purpose. At the time of writing, only anecdotal evidence exists for efficacy for this class of drugs in cats. A small trial in horses with RAO did not show efficacy (Robinson 2010).

In humans, montelukast is FDA-approved for allergic rhinitis and asthma. It is used off-label for atopic dermatitis, urticaria (chronic and NSAID-induced), and eosinophilic esophagitis.

Pharmacology/Actions

Montelukast is a leukotriene antagonist that inhibits at the cysteinyl leukotriene (CysLT1) receptor. The cysteinyl leukotrienes (LTC4, LTD4, LTE4) are pro-inflammatory products of arachadonic acid metabolism released from certain cells, including mast cells and eosinophils.

Pharmacokinetics

No pharmacokinetic information for cats was located.

In humans, oral bioavailability is 64% and peak levels occur 3-4 hours after dosing. The presence of food does not affect bioavailability. Montelukast is highly bound (99+%) to human plasma proteins. It is extensively metabolized in the liver via cytochrome P450 isoenzymes CYP3A4, CYP2A6, and CYP2C9. Based on *in vitro* studies in human liver microsomes, therapeutic plasma concentrations of montelukast do not inhibit CYP-450 isoenzymes 3A4, 2C9, 1A2, 2A6, 2C19, or 2D6. Metabolites are excreted primarily in the bile and eliminated in the feces. In healthy young adults, plasma half-life averages around 4 hours.

Contraindications/Precautions/Warnings

Montelukast is contraindicated in patients hypersensitive to it or to any component of the product. Humans are warned not use it to attempt to reverse acute bronchospasm.

Adverse Effects

No adverse effects were noted for cats but the drug has not been extensively studied or used in cats.

In humans, the drug is usually well tolerated with minimal adverse effects reported. Rarely, behavioral effects (aggression, suicidal thoughts), palpitations, cholestatic hepatitis and allergic granulomatous angiitis have been reported.

Reproductive/Nursing Safety

Montelukast appears safe to use during pregnancy. No teratogenicity was observed in rats at oral dosages of up to 100X, or rabbits at 110X the human dose. The FDA has designated it as a category *B* drug (*Animal studies have not demonstrated risk to the fetus, but there are no adequate studies in pregnant women; or animal studies have shown an adverse effect, but adequate studies in pregnant women have not demonstrated a risk to the fetus during the first trimester of pregnancy, and there is no evidence of risk in later trimesters.*)

While studies in rats have shown that montelukast is excreted in milk, it is likely safe to use during nursing.

Overdosage/Acute Toxicity

Montelukast is relatively safe in overdose situations. Rats and mice survived oral doses of approximately 230X and 335X of the usual human adult dose. Reports of human adults and children receiving doses as high as 1,000 mg have been reported and the majority of overdoses had no adverse effects. The most frequent adverse experiences observed in humans are: headache, vomiting, psychomotor hyperactivity, thirst, somnolence, mydriasis, hyperkinesia, and abdominal pain. Treatment is basically supportive.

Drug Interactions

The following drug interactions have either been reported or are theoretical in humans receiving montelukast and may be of significance in veterinary patients. Unless otherwise noted, use together is not necessarily contraindicated, but weigh the potential risks and perform additional monitoring when appropriate.

■ **CYP-450 ENZYME INDUCERS** (*e.g.,* **phenobarbital, rifampin**): May reduce the montelukast plasma concentrations and efficacy.

■ **PREDNISONE, PREDNISOLONE:** Severe peripheral edema has been reported in a human receiving both drugs, presumably due to increased renal tubular sodium and fluid retention. After prednisone was discontinued, edema resolved; clinical significance is not clear.

Laboratory Considerations

- None noted.

Doses

- **CATS:**

  For adjunctive treatment of feline asthma, allergic rhinitis, mild cases of IBD, atopy, or feline heartworm (extra-label): There is no clear evidence that montelukast is effective for any of these indications. Anecdotal suggested dosages usually range from 0.25 – 1 mg/kg PO once daily. Practically this would be 1/8th – ¼ of a 10 mg tablet per cat PO once daily.

Monitoring

- Clinical efficacy.

Client Information

- May be given with or without food. Food may help if animal vomits or acts 'sick' after getting the drug. If vomiting continues, contact your veterinarian.
- Does not reverse an active asthma attack; it is not useful for immediate treatment of asthma.
- No significant side effects reported when used in cats, but the drug has not been used in many. Contact veterinarian if side effects occur.

Chemistry/Synonyms

Montelukast is a cyclopropaneacetic acid derivative leukotriene inhibitor. It is freely soluble in ethanol, methanol, and water.

Montelukast may also be known as MK-476, L-706631, or montelukastum.

Storage/Stability

Store tablets or granules at room temperature; excursions are permitted to 15°-30°C (59°-86°F). Protect from moisture and light.

Compatibility/Compounding Considerations

No specific information noted.

Dosage Forms/Regulatory Status

VETERINARY-LABELED PRODUCTS: NONE.

HUMAN-LABELED PRODUCTS:

Montelukast Sodium Oral Tablets: 4 mg (chewable), 5 mg (chewable), 10 mg; oral granules 4 mg/packet; *Singulair®*, generic; (Rx)

Revisions/References

Monograph revised/updated April 2014.

Robinson, N. E. (2010). Airway Obstructive Disorders: Are Humans Good Models for Horses? Proceeedings: ACVIM. accessed via Veterinary Information Network; vin.com

---

Morantel Tartrate

(mor-an-tel)   Rumatel®

Antiparasitic Agent

Prescriber Highlights

▶ Infrequently used anthelmintic for ruminants.

▶ Contraindications: None.

▶ Adverse Effects: Large safety margin; clinical signs of OD include increased respiratory rates, profuse sweating, ataxia or other cholinergic effects.

Uses/Indications

Morantel is labeled for the removal of the following parasites in cattle: Mature forms of: *Haemonchus* spp., *Ostertagia* spp., *Trichostrongylus* spp., *Nematodirus* spp., *Cooperia* spp. and *Oesophagostomum radiatum*. In goats it is indicated for the removal and control of mature gastrointestinal nematode infections including *Haemonchus contortus, Ostertagia (Teladorsagia) circumcincta*, and *Trichostrongylus axei*.

Pharmacology/Actions

Like pyrantel, morantel acts as a depolarizing neuromuscular blocking agent in susceptible parasites, thereby paralyzing the organism. The drug possesses nicotine-like properties and acts similarly to acetylcholine. Morantel also inhibits fumarate reductase in *Haemonchus* spp.

Morantel is slower than pyrantel in its onset of action, but is ≈100X as potent.

Pharmacokinetics

After oral administration, morantel is absorbed rapidly from the upper abomasum and small intestine. Peak levels occur ≈4-6 hours after dosing. The drug is promptly metabolized in the liver. Within 96 hours of administration, 17% of the drug is excreted in the urine with the remainder in the feces.

Contraindications/Precautions/Warnings

There are no absolute contraindications to using this drug.

Adverse Effects

At recommended doses, adverse effects are not commonly seen. For more information, see Overdosage section below.

Reproductive/Nursing Safety

Morantel is considered generally safe to use during pregnancy.

Overdosage/Acute Toxicity

Morantel tartrate has a large safety margin. In cattle, dosages of up to 200 mg/kg (20X recommended dose) resulted in no toxic reactions. The LD_{50} in mice is 5 grams/kg. Clinical signs of toxicity that might possibly be seen include increased respiratory rates, profuse sweating (in species with sweat glands), ataxia or other cholinergic effects.

Chronic toxicity studies have been conducted in cattle and sheep. Doses of 4X recommended were given to sheep with no detectable deleterious effects. Cattle receiving 2.5X recommended dose for 2 weeks showed no toxic signs.

Drug Interactions

- **BENTONITE:** Do not add to feeds containing bentonite.
- **LEVAMISOLE, PYRANTEL:** Because of similar mechanisms of action (and toxicity), morantel is not recommended for use concurrently with pyrantel or levamisole.
- **ORGANOPHOSPHATES, DIETHYLCARBAMAZINE:** Observation for adverse effects should be intensified if used concomitantly with an organophosphate or diethylcarbamazine.
- **PIPERAZINE:** Has antagonistic mechanism of action; do not use with morantel.

Doses

- **CATTLE:**

  For susceptible parasites (labeled-dose; FDA-approved): Use a single therapeutic treatment. Medicated feed is to be fed at the rate of 0.44 grams of morantel tartrate per 100 lbs. of body weight. The medicated feed mix should be consumed within 6 hours. May be fed as the sole ration or mixed with 1-2 parts of complete feed or as a top dress. When used as a top dress the medication as well as the underlying feed should be evenly distributed. Animals should be grouped by size for optimum efficacy. Fresh water should be available at all times. When all medicated feed is consumed resume normal feeding. Conditions of constant worm exposure may require retreatment within 2-4 weeks. (Label Directions; *Rumatel®-88*)

- **SHEEP & GOATS:**

  For susceptible parasites (Labeled-dose; FDA-approved): Goats: As a single therapeutic treatment at 0.44 grams morantel tartrate per 100 lbs. body weight. Fresh water should be available at all times. Conditions of constant worm exposure may require retreatment in 2-4 weeks. (Label directions; *Goat Care-2X®*—Durvet)

Client Information

- Follow all label directions and withdrawal times.

Chemistry/Synonyms

A tetrahydropyrimidine anthelmintic, morantel tartrate occurs as a practically odorless, off-white to pale yellow, crystalline solid that is soluble in water. It has a melting range of 167-171°C. The tartrate salt is equivalent to 59.5% of base activity.

Morantel tartrate may also be known as: CP-12009-18, moranteli hydrogenotartras, or UK-2964-18, *Goat Care-2X®* and *Rumatel®*.

Storage/Stability

Morantel tartrate products should be stored at room temperature (15-30°C, 59-86°F) and protected from light unless otherwise instructed by the manufacturer.

Compatibility/Compounding Considerations

No specific information noted.

Dosage Forms/Regulatory Status

VETERINARY-LABELED PRODUCTS:

Morantel Tartrate Medicated Pellets: 0.194% (880 mg/lbs.) in 3 lbs. (treats 12-50 lb. goats) and 10 lbs. (treats 40-50 lb. goats). *Goat Care-2X®*; (OTC); 30-day slaughter withdrawal. Do not mix in feeds containing bentonite.

Morantel Tartrate Medicated Premix: 19.4%; 88 grams morantel tartrate per lb. in 25 lb. bags: *Rumatel®-88 Medicated Premix*; (OTC). FDA-approved for use in beef or dairy cattle. Milk withdrawal (at labeled doses) = none; Slaughter withdrawal (at labeled doses) = 14 days (cattle); 30 days (goats).

HUMAN-LABELED PRODUCTS: NONE.

Revisions/References

Monograph revised/updated April 2014.

Morphine Sulfate

(mor-feen)

Opiate Agonist

Prescriber Highlights

▶ Classic opiate analgesic. Response varies by species.

▶ Contraindications: Hypersensitivity to morphine, diarrhea caused by a toxic ingestion. Extreme Caution: Respiratory disease or from acute respiratory dysfunction.

▶ Caution: Hypothyroidism, severe renal insufficiency (acute uremia), adrenocortical insufficiency, geriatric or severely debilitated patients, head injuries or increased intracranial pressure, & acute abdominal conditions (*e.g.*, colic).

▶ Adverse Effects: Histamine release/vasodilatation (especially with rapid IV injection), respiratory depression, bronchoconstriction, CNS depression, physical dependence (chronic use), hyperthermia (cattle, goats, horses & cats), hypothermia (dogs, rabbits); GI Gastrointestinal effects may include: (nausea, vomiting, & decreased intestinal peristalsis), defecation (dogs).

▶ C-II controlled substance.

Uses/Indications

Morphine is used for the treatment of acute pain in dogs, cats, horses, swine, sheep, and goats. It is used as a preanesthetic agent in several species. For sedation and analgesia in critically ill small animals, in combination with a sedative agent (e.g., midazolam),

mu-opioids (*e.g.*, morphine, hydromorphone or oxymorphone) are often preferred as premedicants because of their minimal effect on cardiac output, systemic blood pressure, and oxygen delivery. Additionally, sedative effects can be reversed with naloxone if necessary (Quandt 2013). Additionally, morphine has been used as an antitussive, antidiarrheal, and adjunctive therapy for some cardiac abnormalities (see doses) in dogs. Due to its poor oral bioavailability in dogs, oral morphine is not recommended in canine patients.

Intra-articular administration of morphine as part of a balanced analgesic protocol may be beneficial in horses (and other species) for synovitis or after joint surgery.

Pharmacology/Actions

The morphine-like agonists (*e.g.*, morphine, meperidine, oxymorphone) have primary activity at the *mu* receptors, with some activity possible at the delta receptor. The primary pharmacologic effects of these agents are species specific but can include: analgesia, antitussive activity, respiratory depression, sedation, emesis, physical dependence, and intestinal effects (constipation/defecation). Secondary pharmacologic effects include: *CNS*: euphoria, sedation, and confusion. *Cardiovascular*: bradycardia due to central vagal stimulation, alpha-adrenergic receptors may be depressed resulting in peripheral vasodilation, decreased peripheral resistance, and baroreceptor inhibition. Orthostatic hypotension and syncope may occur. *Urinary*: Increased bladder sphincter tone can induce urinary retention.

When administered intra-articularly (0.05 mg/kg IA) in horses with experimentally-induced synovitis, morphine demonstrated antiinflammatory effects (reduced swelling, reduced synovial total protein, serum amyloid and white blood cell counts) (Lindegaard *et al.* 2010). Another study injecting 120 mg into the talocrural joint 1-hour after inducing synovitis found significant decreases in synovial white blood cell count, prostaglandin E2 and bradykinin levels, and improvement in clinical lameness, kinematic and behavioral parameters when compared to placebo (Van Loon *et al.* 2010).

Morphine's CNS effects are irregular and are species specific. Cats, horses, sheep, goats, cattle, and swine may exhibit stimulatory effects after morphine injection, while dogs, humans, and other primates exhibit CNS depression. Both dogs and cats are sensitive to the emetic effects of morphine, but significantly higher doses are required in cats before vomiting occurs as a result of a direct stimulation of the chemoreceptor trigger zone (CTZ). Other species (horses, ruminants, and swine) do not respond to the emetic effects of morphine. Like meperidine, morphine can affect the release of histamine from mast cells.

Morphine is an effective centrally acting antitussive in dogs. Following morphine administration, hypothermia may be seen in dogs and rabbits, while hyperthermia may be seen in cattle, goats, horses, and cats. Morphine can cause miosis (pinpoint pupils) in humans and rabbits. While miosis is listed as a pharmacologic effect of morphine in dogs, in a recent study in normal dogs, intravenous doses of morphine (dose not specified), did not significantly affect pupil size or intraocular pressure (Pirie *et al.* 2008).

While morphine is considered a respiratory depressant, respirations are stimulated initially in dogs. Panting may ensue that may be a result of increased body temperature. Often however, body temperature may be reduced due to a resetting of the "body's thermostat." As CNS depression increases and the hyperthermia resolves, respirations can become depressed. Morphine at moderate to high doses can also cause bronchoconstriction in dogs.

The cardiovascular effects of morphine in dogs are in direct contrast to its effects on humans. In dogs, morphine causes coronary vasoconstriction with resultant increase in coronary vascular resistance, and a transient decrease in arterial pressure. Both bradycardias and tachycardias have been reported in dogs. While morphine has been used for years as a sedative/analgesic in the treatment of myocardial infarction and congestive heart failure in humans, its effects on dogs make it a less than optimal choice in canine patients with clinical signs of cardiopulmonary failure.

The effects of morphine on the gastrointestinal (GI) tract consist primarily of a decrease in motility and secretions. Horses administered doses as low as 0.05 mg/kg had decreased gastrointestinal motility 1-2 hours after IM administration (Figueiredo *et al.* 2012). Dogs however, can defecate following an injection of morphine, then exhibit the signs of decreased intestinal motility and, ultimately, constipation can result. Both biliary and gastric secretions are reduced following administration of morphine, but gastric secretion of HCl will later be compensated by increased (above normal) acid secretion.

Initially, morphine can induce micturition, but with higher doses (>2.4 mg/kg IV) urine secretion can be substantially reduced by an increase in anti-diuretic hormone (ADH) release. Morphine may cause bladder hypertonia, which can lead to increased difficulty in urination (Lindegaard *et al.* 2010).

Pharmacokinetics

Morphine is absorbed when given by IV, IM, SC, and rectal routes. Although absorbed when given orally, bioavailability is reduced, probably because of a high first-pass effect. Very low oral bioavailability (<20%) in dogs, limits the clinical usefulness of orally administered morphine in canines. Morphine concentrates in the kidney, liver, and lungs; lower levels are found in the CNS. Although at lower levels then in the parenchymatous tissues, the majority of free morphine is found in skeletal muscle. Morphine crosses the placenta and narcotized newborns can result if mothers are given the drug before giving birth. These effects can be rapidly reversed with naloxone. Small amounts of morphine will also be distributed into the milk of nursing mothers.

The major route of elimination of morphine is by metabolism in the liver, primarily by glucuronidation. Because cats are deficient in this metabolic pathway, half-lives in cats are probably prolonged (reported to be ≈3 hours). The glucuronidated metabolite M6G (active), is excreted by the kidney.

After IV administration in dogs, morphine has a volume of distribution of ≈7.5 L/kg and a clearance of ≈83 mL/min/kg. Its elimination half-life is slightly longer than 1 hour. The oral bioavailability of the extended release tablets is widely variable and this dosage form of the drug is erratically absorbed in dogs (KuKanich *et al.* 2005).

In horses, the serum half-life of morphine has been reported to be 1.5 hours after a dose of 0.1 mg/kg IV or IM (Devine *et al.* 2013). At this dose the drug was detectable in serum for 48 hours and urine for up to 6 days. When morphine was administered epidurally to horses, rapid, short-lasting serum concentrations and delayed, long-lasting CSF concentrations (elimination half-life of approx. 8 hours) resulted. Isoflurane anesthesia did not significantly alter values (Bellei *et al.* 2008).

Contraindications/Precautions/Warnings

All opiates should be used with caution in patients with hypothyroidism, severe renal insufficiency, adrenocortical insufficiency (Addison's), and in geriatric or severely debilitated patients. Morphine is contraindicated in cases where the patient is hypersensitive to narcotic analgesics, receiving monamino oxidase inhibitors (MAOIs), or with diarrhea caused by a toxic ingestion until the toxin is eliminated from the GI tract. Morphine should be avoided in envenomation situations, as clinical signs associated with histamine-release can be confused with anaphylaxis. It has been advised that morphine or other respiratory depressants should not be used

in coral snake envenomation in dogs or cats (Perez *et al.* 2012). Opiate analgesics are contraindicated in patients who have been stung by the scorpion species *Centuroides sculpturatus Ewing* and *C. gertschi Stahnke* as they can potentiate these venoms.

Morphine should be used with extreme caution in patients with head injuries, increased intracranial pressure, and acute abdominal conditions (*e.g.*, colic) as it may obscure the diagnosis or clinical course of these conditions. Morphine may also increase intracranial pressure secondary to cerebral vasodilatation as a result of increased p_aCO_2 stemming from respiratory depression. It should be used with extreme caution in patients suffering from respiratory disease or from acute respiratory dysfunction (*e.g.*, pulmonary edema secondary to smoke inhalation).

Because of its effects on vasopressin (ADH), morphine must be used cautiously in patients suffering from acute uremia. Urine flow has been reported to decrease by as much as 90% in dogs given large doses of morphine. If administering IV, morphine must be given slowly or significant hypotension can result.

Neonatal, debilitated, or geriatric patients may be more susceptible to the effects of morphine and require lower dosages. Patients with severe hepatic disease may have prolonged duration of action of the drug. Anecdotally, some have suggested that brachycephalic dog breeds may be potentially sensitive to morphine's adverse effects, but no scientific documentation for this was located.

Adverse Effects

At usual doses, the primary concern is the effect the opioids have on respiratory function. Decreased tidal volume, depressed cough reflex, and the drying of respiratory secretions may all have a detrimental effect on a susceptible patient. Bronchoconstriction (secondary to histamine release?) following IV doses has been noted in dogs. Significant hypotension can occur if administered rapidly IV. Panting is often seen in dogs after morphine administration.

Gastrointestinal effects may include: nausea, vomiting, and decreased intestinal peristalsis. Dogs may defecate after an initial dose of morphine, but this is not usually seen when used post-operatively. Horses exhibiting signs of mild colic may have their clinical signs masked by the administration of narcotic analgesics. In ferrets, morphine can induce nausea and vomiting and it is often avoided in this species.

The CNS effects of morphine are dose and species specific. Animals that are stimulated by morphine may elucidate changes in behavior (*e.g.*, 'morphine mania" in cats, increased locomotor activity in horses, etc.), appear restless and, at very high doses, have convulsions. The CNS depressant effects seen in dogs may encumber the abilities of working animals.

Body temperature changes may be seen. Cattle, goats, horses, and cats may exhibit signs of hyperthermia, while rabbits and dogs may develop hypothermia.

Chronic administration may lead to physical dependence.

Reproductive/Nursing Safety

Placental transfer of opiates is rapid. In humans, the FDA categorizes this drug as category *C* for use during pregnancy (*Animal studies have shown an adverse effect on the fetus, but there are no adequate studies in humans; or there are no animal reproduction studies and no adequate studies in humans.*) In a separate system evaluating the safety of drugs in canine and feline pregnancy (Papich 1989), this drug is categorized as class: *B* (*Safe for use if used cautiously. Studies in laboratory animals may have uncovered some risk, but these drugs appear to be safe in dogs and cats or these drugs are safe if they are not administered when the animal is near term.*)

Morphine appears in maternal milk, but effects on offspring may not be significant when used for short periods. Withdrawal symptoms have occurred however in breastfeeding infants when maternal administration of an opioid-analgesic stopped. Decide whether to accept the risks, discontinue nursing or to discontinue the drug, taking into account the importance of the drug to the mother.

Overdosage/Acute Toxicity

Overdosage may produce profound respiratory and/or CNS depression in most species. Newborns may be more susceptible to these effects than adult animals. Parenteral doses >100 mg/kg are thought to be fatal in dogs. Other toxic effects can include cardiovascular collapse, hypothermia, and skeletal muscle hypotonia. Some species such as horses, cats, swine, and cattle may demonstrate CNS excitability (hyperreflexia, tremors) and seizures at high doses or if given rapidly intravenously. Naloxone is the agent of choice in treating respiratory depression. In massive overdoses, naloxone doses may need to be repeated. Animals should be closely observed as naloxone's effects might diminish before sub-toxic levels of morphine are attained. Mechanical respiratory support should be considered in cases of severe respiratory depression.

Pentobarbital has been suggested as a treatment for CNS excitement and seizures in cats. Extreme caution should be used as barbiturates and narcotics can have additive effects on respiratory depression.

Drug Interactions

The following drug interactions have either been reported or are theoretical in humans or animals receiving morphine and may be of significance in veterinary patients. Unless otherwise noted, use together is not necessarily contraindicated, but weigh the potential risks and perform additional monitoring when appropriate.

- **CNS DEPRESSANTS, OTHER** (*e.g.*, **anesthetic agents, antihistamines, phenothiazines, barbiturates, tranquilizers, alcohol,** etc.): May cause increased CNS or respiratory depression when used with morphine.
- **DIURETICS:** Opiates may decrease efficacy in CHF patients.
- **MONAMINE OXIDASE (MAO) INHIBITORS** (*e.g.*, **amitraz,** possibly **selegiline**): Use MAOI's with morphine with extreme caution as meperidine (a related opiate) is contraindicated in human patients receiving monamino oxidase (MAO) inhibitors for at least 14 days after receiving MAO inhibitors. Some human patients have exhibited signs of opiate overdose after receiving therapeutic doses of meperidine while taking MAOIs.
- **MUSCLE RELAXANTS, SKELETAL:** Morphine may enhance neuromuscular blockade.
- **TRICYCLIC ANTIDEPRESSANTS (clomipramine, amitriptyline,** etc.): Morphine may exacerbate the effects of tricyclic antidepressants.
- **WARFARIN:** Opiates may potentiate anticoagulant activity.

Laboratory Considerations

- As they may increase biliary tract pressure, opiates can increase plasma amylase and lipase values up to 24 hours following their administration.

Doses

Note: For additional doses/protocols for using morphine in combination with other drugs (*e.g.*, ketamine, lidocaine, dexmedetomidine) for pain/sedation in dogs or cats, see the doses and their accompanying references in the dexmedetomidine, ketamine, and lidocaine monographs. An additional online resource is: vasg.org

- **DOGS:**

For analgesia (acute pain, parenteral); (extra-label):

Pulsed Dosing: Morphine is usually dosed ranging from 0.5 – 2 mg/kg IM, SC, or IV (slowly). Lower dosages may be necessary in geriatric or severely debilitated animals and higher dosages required for excruciating pain. Duration of effect can vary, and often re-dosing is needed after 2 hours.

CRI Dosing: After an initial loading dose of 0.3 mg IV (slowly) followed by a CRI of 0.1 – 0.2 mg/kg/hour. Higher infusion rates may be required for excruciating pain. Adverse effects may be pronounced at higher infusion rates or if duration of use is prolonged.

For analgesia (palliative care; oral); (extra-label): Although in dogs oral absorption can be very low and sustained-release oral products have been shown to have highly variable absorption rates, oral products can be tried for palliative care. One recommendation is: In dogs, the starting oral dose of regular morphine is 1 mg/kg PO q4-6h. Sustained-release morphine is used in dogs at 2 – 5 mg/kg PO twice a day. When using sustained-release morphine, be sure to educate pet owners not to break or crush the tablets under any circumstances. Breaking or crushing turns sustained-release morphine into immediate-release and can result in overdose and death. (Downing 2011)

For analgesia (epidural administration); (extra-label): Morphine (use preservative-free if possible): 0.1 mg/kg in 0.3 mL/kg (max of 6 mL). Opioids provide analgesia without loss of hind limb function or muscle tone. Analgesia has a fairly long duration and can be maintained with an epidural catheter (although placement and maintenance of the catheter may be difficult). One advantage of epidural morphine is that the analgesia will migrate cranially and be effective up to ≈18 hrs. (Matthews 2008)

In combination as a preanesthetic or perioperative sedative analgesic (extra-label): **Note:** Morphine is generally used in combination with other sedative/anesthetics.

As a premedicant: There are many combinations used. Morphine is usually dosed between 0.1 – 0.5 mg/kg IM in combination with drugs such as acepromazine, midazolam, dexmedetomidine, ketamine, etc. Lower dosages (0.05 mg/kg) may be necessary in old, debilitated, or critically ill animals. Giving acepromazine 20 minutes prior to morphine can significantly reduce vomiting.

'MLK' Low-dose CRI's: A combination (MLK) of morphine (3.3 micrograms/kg/min), lidocaine (50 micrograms/kg/min), and ketamine (10 micrograms/kg/min), decreases isoflurane MAC in dogs and were not associated with adverse hemodynamic effects (Muir *et al.* 2003). Additional information on MLK CRI's can be found on the Veterinary Anesthesia & Analgesia Support Group website at http://www.vasg.org/constant_rate_infusions.htm for using the MLK (combination of morphine (or other opiates), lidocaine, ketamine) CRI use in dogs and cats.

- **CATS:**

For analgesia (acute pain, parenteral); (extra-label):

Pulsed Dosing: Morphine is sometimes used in cats, but it does not appear to be as effective as in dogs and alone it does not produce good sedation. Usually dosed ranging from 0.05 – 0.4 mg/kg IM, SC every 3-6 hours as needed. Duration of effect can vary, and often re-dosing is needed after 3 hours.

CRI Dosing: Not usually used in cats.

For analgesia (epidural administration); (extra-label): In the study, 0.1 mg/kg morphine diluted with saline to a volume of 0.22 mL/kg was administered over 60 seconds. Both epidural tramadol and morphine provided adequate analgesia to the level of noxious stimulation produced in this study, but morphine provided superior analgesia for hours 6-12 post-administration (Castro *et al.* 2009). **Note:** Use preservative-free morphine if possible.

- **RABBITS, RODENTS, SMALL MAMMALS:**

As an analgesic/sedative (extra-label):

Rats: 2.5 mg/kg SC q4h. **Mice:** 2.5 mg/kg SC q2-4h. **Guinea pigs:** 2 – 5 mg/kg SC, IM q4h. (Miller *et al.* 2011)

Rabbits: 2 – 5 mg/kg IM, SC q2-4h; epidurally it has been used at 0.1 mg/kg. (Barter 2011)

- **HORSES:** (NOTE: ARCI UCGFS CLASS 1 DRUG)

Note: Narcotics may cause CNS excitement in the horse. Some clinicians recommend pretreatment with acepromazine, detomidine, or xylazine to reduce the behavioral changes these drugs can cause. **Warning:** Narcotic analgesics can mask the behavioral and cardiovascular clinical signs associated with mild colic.

For analgesia (extra-label):

a) 0.1 mg/kg IM q4h; this dose reduces morphine's impact on GI motility, but patients must be observed for problems following morphine use. To cover the excitatory effects of morphine, small doses of acepromazine (0.011 – 0.022 mg/kg IM, or 5 – 10 mg/450 kg) are generally included with the morphine injection. (Abrahamsen 2007)

b) Morphine may be used IV (0.012 – 0.66 mg/kg) as an analgesic agent in combination with alpha2 agonists. When used IV as a sole analgesic agent, it may result in profound excitation. Anecdotally, IM morphine use is not associated with CNS excitation and this may represent an under-appreciated analgesic option. (Sellon 2007)

Epidural Injection (extra-label):

a) In the study 6 hours after inducing carpal synovitis in ponies, 0.1 mg/kg morphine (diluted in a 0.9% NaCl solution to a final volume of 0.15 mL/kg of body weight) administered by epidural at a rate of one ml per 10 seconds. Authors concluded that epidural morphine produced analgesia that lasted for more than 12 hours without side effects and would be a valuable analgesic option to alleviate joint pain in the thoracic limbs in ponies (Freitas *et al.* 2011).

b) Morphine may be administered epidurally on its own or in combination with detomidine (0.03 – 0.06 mg/kg) to provide effective analgesia of the caudal half of the body. Morphine is typically used at doses of 0.1 – 0.2 mg/kg diluted to 10 – 20 mL with 0.9% saline (total volume of 0.04 mL/kg body weight). Analgesic effects are seen within 20-30 minutes and may last 8-24 hours without adverse effects on motor function. (Sellon 2007)

c) <u>Adult horses:</u> 0.1 – 0.2 mg/kg using conventional morphine injection (15 mg/mL). Use a freshly opened vial. Suggest diluting with saline to a total volume of 0.04 mL/kg or 20 mL/450kg. <u>Foals:</u> Using preservative free morphine at 0.1 mg/kg. If no preservative free morphine available, dilute to a volume of 0.2 mL/kg. (Abrahamsen 2007)

For intra-articular injection for acute inflammatory joint pain (extra-label): Two single dose experimental studies (Lindegaard *et al.* 2010; Van Loon *et al.* 2010) suggest that IA morphine has antiinflammatory effects for acute synovitis. One study used 0.05 mg/kg (radiocarpal joint) and the other 120 mg diluted in 20 mL saline (talocrural joint).

- **CAMELIDS:**

Epidural (extra-label): 0.1 – 0.3 mg/kg of preservative-free morphine diluted to 12 mL. (Cebra 2009)

- **ZOO, EXOTIC, WILDLIFE SPECIES:**

For use of morphine in zoo, exotic and wildlife medicine refer to specific references, including:

- *Zoo Animal and Wildlife Immobilization and Anesthesia.*

West, G., Heard, D., Caulkett, N. (eds.). Blackwell Publishing, 2007.

- *Handbook of Wildlife Chemical Immobilization, 3rd Ed.* Kreeger, T.J. and J.M. Arnemo. 2007.

- *Fowler's Zoo and Wild Animal Medicine Current Therapy, Volume 7,* Miller, R.E., Fowler, M.E., Saunders. 2011.

- *Exotic Animal Formulary, 4th Ed.* Carpenter, J.W., Saunders. 2012.

- The 2009 American Association of Zoo Veterinarian Proceedings by D. K. Fontenot also has several dosages listed for restraint, anesthesia, and analgesia for a variety of drugs for carnivores and primates. VIN members can access them at: http://goo.gl/NNIWQ or http://goo.gl/9UJse

Monitoring

- Respiratory rate/depth.
- CNS level of depression/excitation.
- Blood pressure (especially with IV use).
- Analgesic activity.

Client Information

- When given parenterally, this agent should be used in an inpatient setting or with direct professional supervision.

Chemistry/Synonyms

The sulfate salt of a natural (derived from opium) occurring opiate analgesic, morphine sulfate occurs as white, odorless, crystals. Solubility: 1 gram in 16 mL of water (62.5 mg/mL), 570 mL (1.75 mg/mL) of alcohol. It is insoluble in chloroform or ether. The pH of morphine sulfate injection ranges from 2.5-6.

Morphine sulfate may also be known as morphini sulfas, *Astramorph PF®, Avinza®, DepoDur®, Infumorph®, Kadian®, MSIR®, MS Contin®, Oramorph SR, RMS®,* and *Roxanol®.*

Storage/Stability

Oral morphine products should be stored at in tight, light-resistant containers at room temperature unless otherwise labeled. Morphine injection should be stored at room temperature, protected from light; do not freeze. Morphine gradually darkens in color when exposed to light; protect from prolonged exposure to bright light. Morphine does not appear to adsorb to plastic or PVC syringes, tubing or bags.

Compatibility/Compounding Considerations

Morphine sulfate has been shown to be physically **compatible** at a concentration of 16.2 mg/L with the following intravenous fluids: Dextrose 2.5%, 5%, 10% in water; Ringer's injection and Lactated Ringer's injection; Sodium Chloride 0.45% and 0.9% for injection. Compatibility is dependent upon factors such as pH, concentration, temperature, and diluent used; consult specialized references or a hospital pharmacist for more specific information.

The following drugs have been shown to be physically **incompatible** when mixed with morphine sulfate: aminophylline, heparin sodium, meperidine, pentobarbital sodium, phenobarbital sodium, phenytoin sodium, sodium bicarbonate, and thiopental sodium. Morphine sulfate has been demonstrated to be generally physically **compatible** when mixed with the following agents: Atropine sulfate, benzquinamide HCl, butorphanol tartrate, chlorpromazine HCl, diphenhydramine HCl, dobutamine HCl, droperidol, fentanyl citrate, glycopyrrolate, hydroxyzine HCl, metoclopramide, pentazocine lactate, promazine HCl, scopolamine HBr, and succinylcholine chloride.

Dosage Forms/Regulatory Status

VETERINARY-LABELED PRODUCTS: NONE.

The ARCI (Racing Commissioners International) has designated this drug as a class 1 substance. See the appendix for more information.

HUMAN-LABELED PRODUCTS:

Morphine Sulfate for Injection: 1 mg/mL, 5 mg/mL, 8 mg/mL, 10 mg/mL, 15 mg/mL, 25 mg/mL, 50 mg/mL in amps, vials, syringes, and pre-filled IV bags in sizes that range from 1 mL to 250 mL depending on manufacturer and concentration. (Rx; C-II)

Morphine Sulfate Liposomal Extended-release Injection: 10 mg/mL in 1 mL, 1.5 mL, & 2 mL single-use vials; *DepoDur®*; (Rx, C-II)

Morphine Sulfate for Injection (preservative-free): 0.5 mg/mL: 2 mL amps, & 10 mL amps and vials; 1 mg/mL: 10 mL amps and vials; 10 mg/mL (200 mg) in 20 mL amps; 25 mg/mL (500 mg) in 20 mL amps; *Infumorph®, Astramorph PF®*; (Rx, C-II)

Morphine Sulfate Soluble Tablets for Injection: 10 mg, 15 mg & 30 mg; generic; (Rx, C-II)

Morphine Sulfate Oral Tablets: 15 mg & 30 mg; generic; (Rx, C-II)

Morphine Sulfate Extended/Controlled Release Tablets: 15 mg, 30 mg, 60 mg, 100 mg & 200 mg; *MS Contin®, Oramorph SR®*, generic; (Rx, C-II)

Morphine Sulfate Extended/Sustained Release Capsules: 20 mg, 30 mg, 45 mg, 50 mg, 60 mg, 75 mg, 80 mg, 90 mg, 100 mg, 120 mg & 200 mg; *Avinza®, Kadian®*; (Rx, C-II)

Morphine Sulfate Oral Solution: 2 mg/mL in 100 mL, 500 mL and UD 5mL & 10 mL; 4 mg/mL in 100 mL, 120 mL & 500 mL; 20 mg/mL (concentrate) in 15 mL, 30 mL, 120 mL & 240 mL/calibrated dropper or spoon; *MSIR®, Roxanol®, -T, & -100*, generic; (Rx; C-II)

Morphine Sulfate Rectal Suppositories: 5 mg, 10 mg, 20 mg, & 30 mg; *RMS®*, generic; (various); (Rx, C-II)

Note: All morphine products are Rx and a Class-II controlled substance. Very accurate record keeping is required as to use and disposition of stock.

Revisions/References

Monograph revised/updated April 2014.

Abrahamsen, E. (2007). Analgesia in equine practice. Proceedings: Western Vet Conference. accessed via Veterinary Information Network; vin.com

Barter, L. S. (2011). Rabbit Analgesia. Vet Clin Exot Anim 14: 93-104.

Bellei, M., et al. (2008). Pharmacokinetics of Epidural Morphine in Awake and Isoflurane-Anesthetized Horses. Proceedings: IVECCS. accessed via Veterinary Information Network; vin.com

Castro, D. S., et al. (2009). Comparison between the analgesic effects of morphine and tramadol delivered epidurally in cats receiving a standardized noxious stimulation. Journal of Feline Medicine and Surgery 11(12): 948-53.

Cebra, C. K. (2009). Abdominal Discomfort in Llamas & Alpacas: Diagnosis & Treatment. Proceedings: ACVIM. accessed via Veterinary Information Network; vin.com

Devine, E. P., et al. (2013). Pharmacokinetics of intramuscularly administered morphine in horses. Javma-Journal of the American Veterinary Medical Association 243(1): 105-12.

Downing, R. (2011). Pain Management for Veterinary Palliative Care and Hospice Patients. Veterinary Clinics of North America-Small Animal Practice 41(3): 531-+.

Figueiredo, J. P., et al. (2012). Cardiorespiratory, gastrointestinal, and analgesic effects of morphine sulfate in conscious healthy horses. American Journal of Veterinary Research 73(6): 799-808.

Freitas, G., et al. (2011). Epidural analgesia with morphine or buprenorphine in ponies with lipopolysaccharide (LPS)-induced carpal synovitis. Canadian Journal of Veterinary Research 75: 141-6.

KuKanich, B., et al. (2005). Pharmacokinetics of morphine and plasma concentrations of morphine-6-glucuronide following morphine administration to dogs. J Vet Phamacol Ther 28: 371-6.

Lindegaard, C., et al. (2010). Anti-inflammatory effects of intra-articular administration of morphine in horses with experimentally induced synovitis. American Journal of Veterinary Research 71(1): 69-75.

Matthews, N. (2008). Perioperative Analgesia: Part 1. Concepts and Drugs. Proceedings: ACVC. accessed via Veterinary Information Network; vin.com

Miller, A. L. & C. Richardson (2011). Rodent Analgesia. Vet Clin Exot Anim 14: 81-92.

Muir, W. W., et al. (2003). Effects of morphine, lidocaine, ketamine, and morphine-lidocaine-ketamine drug combination on minimum alveolar concentration in dogs anesthetized with isoflurane. American Journal of Veterinary Research 64(9): 1155-60.

Papich, M. (1989). Effects of drugs on pregnancy. Current Veterinary Therapy X: Small Animal Practice. R. Kirk. Philadelphia, Saunders: 1291-9.

Perez, M. L., et al. (2012). A retrospective evaluation of coral snake envenomation in dogs and cats: 20 cases (1996-2011). J. Vet. Emerg. Crit. Care 22(6): 682-9.

Pirie, C., et al. (2008). The Effect of Intravenous Hydromorphone, Butorphanol, Morphine, and Buprenorphine on Pupil Size and Intraocular Pressure in Normal Dogs. Proceedings: ACVO. accessed via Veterinary Information Network; vin.com

Quandt, J. (2013). Analgesia, Anesthesia, and Chemical Restraint in the Emergent Small Animal Patient. Veterinary Clinics of North America-Small Animal Practice 43(4): 941-+.

Sellon, D. (2007). New Alternatives for Pain Management in Horses. Proceedings: New Alternatives for Pain Management in Horses. accessed via Veterinary Information Network; vin.com

Van Loon, J. P. A. M., et al. (2010). Intra-articular opioid analgesia is effective in reducing pain and inflammation in an equine LPS induced synovitis model. Equine Veterinary Journal 42(5): 412-9.

Moxidectin

(mox-i-**dek**-tin)   Cydectin®, ProHeart®, Advantage® Multi

Avermectin Antiparasitic

Prescriber Highlights

▶ Avermectin antiparasitic with products FDA-approved for cattle, dogs, cats, ferrets, sheep, & horses.

▶ Contraindications (oral; topical): **Dogs:** Hypersensitive to drug; **Cattle:** Female dairy cattle of breeding age; **Horses:** Intended for food purposes or in foals younger than 4 months of age.

▶ Adverse Effects (topical; oral): **Dogs** (potentially): Lethargy, vomiting, ataxia, anorexia, diarrhea, nervousness, weakness, increased thirst, & itching. **Cattle:** Adverse effects minimal. **Horses:** At labeled doses, appear minimal.

▶ Apparently safe to use in *ABCB1-1Δ* (formerly MDR1-allele) gene mutation dog breeds at labeled doses; higher doses may cause neurotoxicity in these dogs.

Uses/Indications

In dogs, a 6-month injectable product (*ProHeart® 6*) is FDA-approved for use (in the USA) for use in dogs six months of age and older for the prevention of heartworm disease caused by *Dirofilaria immitis* and for the treatment of existing larval and adult hookworm (*Ancylostoma caninum* and *Uncinaria stenocephala*) infections.

The topically applied combination with imidacloprid (*Advantage Multi®*) is labeled in dogs and cats as a once a month topical preventative for the prevention of heartworm, flea adulticide, and treatment for hookworms and roundworms. In cats it is approved for treating ear mites. In dogs, it is approved for treating whipworms, sarcoptic mange, and to treat circulating heartworm microfilaria. In ferrets it is labeled for adult fleas and flea infestations and to prevent heartworm disease. Orally administered moxidectin and increased frequency of administration of the canine topical product have also been used in an extra-label manner as a treatment for generalized demodicosis in dogs; results have been mixed and it appears to be most effective in dogs with mild disease; high dose oral treatment can be highly neurotoxic in dogs, particularly in those with the *ABCB-1* mutation.

In cattle, moxidectin is indicated for the treatment and control of the following internal [adult and fourth stage larvae (L4)] and external parasites: <u>Gastrointestinal roundworms</u>: *Ostertagia ostertagi* (adult and L4, including inhibited larvae), *Haemonchus placei* (adult), *Trichostrongylus axei* (adult and L4), *Trichostrongylus colubriformis* (adult), *Cooperia oncophora* (adult), *Cooperia punctata* (adult), *Bunostomum phlebotomum* (adult), *Oesophagostomum radiatum* (adult), *Nematodirus helvetianus* (adult); <u>Lungworm</u>: *Dictyocaulus viviparus* (adult and L4); <u>Cattle Grubs</u>: *Hypoderma bovis*, *Hypoderma lineatum* <u>Mites</u>: *Chorioptes bovis*, *Psoroptes ovis* (*Psoroptes communis var. bovis*); <u>Lice</u>: *Linognathus vituli*, *Haematopinus eurysternus*, *Solenopotes capillatus*, *Damalinia bovis*; <u>Horn flies</u>: *Haematobia irritans*. It is also used to control infections and protect from reinfection from *Ostertagia ostertagi* for 28 days after treatment and from *Dictyocaulus viviparus* for 42 days after treatment.

In sheep, oral moxidectin is indicated for the control of *Haemonchus contortus* (adult and L4), *Teladosrsagia circumcincta & trifurcata* (adult and L4), *Trichostrongylus colubriformis, axei, & vitrinius* (adult & L4), *Cooperia curticei & oncophora* (adult and L4), *Oesophagostomum columbianum & venolosum* (adult & L4), and *Nematodirus battus, filicollis, & spathiger* (adult & L4).

In horses and ponies 6 months of age or older, moxidectin is indicated for the treatment and control of the following stages of gastrointestinal parasites: Large strongyles: *Strongylus vulgaris* (adults and L4L5 arterial stages); *Strongylus edentatus* (adults and tissue stages); *Triodontophorus brevicauda* (adults); *Triodontophorus serratus* (adults); Small strongyles (adults and larvae): *Cyathostomum* spp. *(adults); Cylicocyclus* spp. (adults); *Cylicostephanus* spp. (adults); *Gyalocephalus capitatus* (adults); undifferentiated lumenal larvae; Encysted cyathostomes: late L3 and L4 mucosal cyathostome larvae; Ascarids: *Parascaris equorum* (adults and L4 larval stages); Pin worms: *Oxyuris equi* (adults and L4 larval stages); Hair worms: *Trichostrongylus axei* (adults); Large-mouth stomach worms: *Habronema muscae* (adults); Horse stomach bots: *Gasterophilus intestinalis* (2nd and 3rd instars). When combined with praziquantel, additional coverage against *Anoplocephala* spp. occurs. Resistance to antiparasitic agents is an ongoing problem. It is recommended to perform fecal egg count reduction testing (FECRT) for strongyle nematodes. A value of <95% in 5-10 horses is the suggested cut-off for determining resistance on a given farm (Nielsen *et al.* 2009).

Pharmacology/Actions

The primary mode of action of avermectins like moxidectin is to affect chloride ion channel activity in the nervous system of nematodes and arthropods. The drug binds to receptors that increase membrane permeability to chloride ions. This inhibits the electrical activity of nerve cells in nematodes and muscle cells in arthropods and causes paralysis and death of the parasites. Avermectins also enhance the release of gamma amino butyric acid (GABA) at presynaptic neurons. GABA acts as an inhibitory neurotransmitter and blocks the post-synaptic stimulation of the adjacent neuron in nematodes or the muscle fiber in arthropods. Avermectins are generally not toxic to mammals, since they do not have glutamate-gated chloride channels and these compounds do not readily cross the blood-brain barrier where mammalian GABA receptors occur.

Pharmacokinetics

Minimal information was located. In cattle, the drug apparently has a long duration of plasma residence (14-15 days). After SC injection, ≈5% of the dose given to the cow can be passed to the suckling calf.

In horses, moxidectin may have a period of action of up to 12 weeks.

Moxidectin is very lipophilic (100X that of ivermectin), so volumes of distribution would likely be very high. Animals with very low body fat (neonates, cachexia) could potentially have serum levels much higher than normal patients.

Contraindications/Precautions/Warnings

Dogs: Contraindicated in dogs hypersensitive to it. The manufacturer warns to only use the oral product in dogs tested negative for heartworm infection. Adult heartworms and microfilaria should be removed prior to therapy. If more than 2 months pass between dosages of this or other once a month heartworm preventative medications, the dog should be tested for heartworm infection before receiving the next dose. Oral formulation doses (3 mg/kg/month) and topical formulation heartworm prevention doses (2500 micrograms/kg/month) are safe for all *ABCB*1 genotypes (Mealey 2008).

For the 6-month injectable product (*ProHeart*® 6): Contraindicated in patients previously found hypersensitive to the drug, or are sick, debilitated, underweight or who have a history of weight loss. Use with caution in dogs with pre-existing allergic disease, including food allergy, atopy, and flea allergy dermatitis. Caution should be used when administering concurrently with vaccinations. Adverse reactions, including anaphylaxis, have been reported following the concomitant use of *ProHeart*® 6 and vaccinations. Caution should be used when administering to heartworm positive dogs; prior to administration, dogs should be tested for existing heartworm infections. Safety and effectiveness has not been evaluated in dogs less than 6 months of age.

For *Advantage Multi*®: For the first 30 minutes after application: ensure that dogs cannot lick the product from application sites on themselves or other treated dogs, and separate treated dogs from one another and other pets to reduce the risk of accidental ingestion. Ingestion of this product by dogs may cause serious adverse reactions including depression, salivation, dilated pupils, incoordination, panting, and generalized muscle tremors. In avermectin sensitive dogs, the signs may be more severe and may include coma and death.

Cats/Ferrets: Do not use on sick, debilitated or underweight animals.

Do not allow children to come in contact with the application area for at least 2 hours (30 minutes for the cat product).

Cattle: Not for use in female dairy cattle of breeding age.

Horses: Not for horses intended for food purposes and is not labeled for use in foals younger than 4 months of age.

Animals with very low body fat (neonates, cachexia) could be more prone to develop adverse reactions.

Adverse Effects

Dogs: The topically applied product (w/imidacloprid) appears to be very well tolerated in dogs, regardless of their *ABCB*1 genotype.

The injectable product (*ProHeart*® 6) has been implicated in serious adverse effects in the past. In 2004, at the request FDA, the manufacturer instituted a voluntary recall of *ProHeart*® 6, after reports of serious adverse events in dogs that included anaphylaxis, liver disease, autoimmune hemolytic disease, convulsions and death. After data analysis and label revision, the product re-entered the market. For further information contact the manufacturer (Zoetis) or refer to the label (package insert). It may be found at the Zoetis website.

Cats: In field studies, behavioral changes (*e.g.*, agitated, excessive grooming, hiding, pacing, spinning), discomfort (*e.g.*, scratching, rubbing, head-shaking, lethargy, hypersalivation, polydipsia, and coughing or gagging were noted in some animals.

Ferrets: pruritus/scratching, scabbing, redness, wounds and inflammation at the treatment site; lethargy; and chemical odor.

Cattle: Thus far at labeled doses, adverse effects appear to nonexistent or minimal.

Horses: Thus far at labeled doses, adverse effects appear to be nonexistent or minimal. A case report where three foals developed CNS depression and coma after receiving high dosages has been reported. Two of these three animals were less than 2 weeks of age and all received much higher than labeled dosages.

Reproductive/Nursing Safety

Dogs, Cats: Reproductive studies have demonstrated no evidence of adverse effects on fertility, reproductive performance, or offspring. Safety has not been established in breeding, pregnant, and lactating ferrets.

Cattle & Horses: Reproductive studies performed thus far have demonstrated no evidence of adverse effects on fertility, reproductive performance, or offspring in cattle or horses treated.

Overdosage/Acute Toxicity

Dogs: The drug apparently has a very wide margin of safety in dogs when administered topically at the labeled dosage. In dogs with the *ABCB*1 (mutant/mutant) genotype, dosages of 90 micrograms/kg can cause neurologic toxicity. Dogs administered inadvertent over-doses during a clinical study treating demodicosis showed signs of dysorexia, hypersalivation, mydriasis, and fasciculations and ataxia of the pelvic limbs.

<u>Cats</u>: Topical overdoses as low as 3X caused lethargy, ataxia and disorientation in one healthy 9 week-old kitten tested. Oral ingestion of the topical solution (at maximum labeled dose) caused vomiting and hypersalivation.

There were 172 exposures to moxidectin reported to the ASPCA Animal Poison Control Center (APCC) during 2005-2006. In these cases, 171 were dogs with 42 showing clinical signs and the remaining case was 1 cat that showed clinical signs. Common findings in dogs recorded in decreasing frequency included tremors, ataxia, seizures, vomiting and hyperesthesia. Common findings in cats recorded included recumbency.

<u>Cattle</u>: In studies done on cattle, application of the pour-on solution at 5X the recommended dose for 5 consecutive days, 10X for 2 consecutive days and 25X for 1 day did not produce any significant adverse clinical or pathological effects.

<u>Horses</u>: In one study, 3 of 8 foals given the 3X dose became depressed or ataxic after one treatment. The author has received an anecdotal report of a miniature horse developing seizures after receiving a full tube of *Quest®*.

Intravenous fat emulsion (IFE) has been used in dogs to treat toxicity associated with moxidectin and other highly lipid soluble drugs (Bates *et al.* 2013), (Crandell *et al.* 2009).

Drug Interactions

While no specific drug interactions for moxidectin have been reported, the following drug interactions have either been reported or are theoretical in humans or animals receiving ivermectin (a related compound) and may be of significance in veterinary patients. Unless otherwise noted, use together is not necessarily contraindicated, but weigh the potential risks and perform additional monitoring when appropriate.

- **BENZODIAZEPINES**: Effects may be potentiated by moxidectin; use together not advised in humans

Caution is advised if using other drugs that can inhibit **p-glycoprotein**. Those dogs at risk for *ABCB1-1Δ* (formerly MDR1-allele) mutation (Collies, Australian Shepherds, Shelties, Long-haired Whippet, etc. "white feet") should probably not receive moxidectin with the following drugs, unless tested "normal". Drugs and drug classes involved include:

- **AMIODARONE**
- **CARVEDILOL**
- **CLARITHROMYCIN**
- **CYCLOSPORINE**
- **DILTIAZEM**
- **ERYTHROMYCIN**
- **ITRACONAZOLE**
- **KETOCONAZOLE**
- **QUINIDINE**
- **SPINOSAD**
- **SPIRONOLACTONE**
- **TAMOXIFEN**
- **VERAPAMIL**

Laboratory Considerations

- In horses, when performing a **fecal egg count reduction test** (**FECRT**) it is preferable to wait at least 12 weeks before collecting a pretreatment sample. (Vaala 2013)

Doses

- **DOGS:**

For *Advantage Multi®* labeled indications: Recommended minimum dose is 10 mg/kg imidacloprid with 2.5 mg/kg moxidectin once a month by topical administration (**Note:** See package insert for specific instructions on application and safety). For dogs 3-9 lbs. = 0.4 mL; 9.1-20 lbs. = 1 mL; 20.1-55 lbs. = 2.5 mL, 55.1-88 lbs. = 4 mL; dogs over 88 lbs. should be treated with appropriate combination for their weight. (Label directions; *Advantage Multi®* for Dogs—Bayer)

For *ProHeart®* 6 labeled indications: **Note:** Owners should be given the Client Information Sheet for *ProHeart®* 6 to read before the drug is administered and should be advised to observe their dogs for potential drug toxicity described in the sheet. The recommended subcutaneous dose is 0.05 mL of the constituted suspension/kg body weight. This provides 0.17 mg moxidectin/kg bodyweight. To ensure accurate dosing, calculate each dose based on the dog's weight at the time of treatment. Do not overdose growing puppies in anticipation of their expected adult weight. A dosage chart is found in the package insert that may be used as a guide. <u>Injection Technique</u>: The two-part sustained release product must be mixed at least 30 minutes prior to the intended time of use. Once constituted, swirl the bottle gently before every use to uniformly re-suspend the microspheres. Withdraw 0.05 mL of suspension/kg body weight into an appropriately sized syringe fitted with an 18G or 20G hypodermic needle. Dose promptly after drawing into dosing syringe. If administration is delayed, gently roll the dosing syringe prior to injection to maintain a uniform suspension and accurate dosing. Using aseptic technique, inject the product subcutaneously in the left or right side of the dorsum of the neck cranial to the scapula. No more than 3 mL should be administered in a single site. The location(s) of each injection (left or right side) should be noted so that prior injection sites can be identified and the next injection can be administered on the opposite side. <u>Frequency of Treatment</u>: *ProHeart®* 6 prevents infection by *D. immitis* for six months. It should be administered within one month of the dog's first exposure to mosquitoes. Follow-up treatments may be given every six months if the dog has continued exposure to mosquitoes and continues to be healthy without weight loss. When replacing another heartworm preventive product, *ProHeart®* 6 should be given within one month of the last dose of the former medication. (Label Information; *ProHeart®* 6—Pfizer)

For canine demodicosis (extra-label): **Warning:** Because serious neurotoxicity can occur at these dosages in dogs with the *ABCB-1* mutation, it is highly recommended to test for this before using avermectins for treating demodicosis in dogs; a negative test (normal/normal) however does not ensure that toxicity will not occur. The 2011 clinical practice guidelines for treatment of demodicosis in dogs (Mueller *et al.* 2012) states: "Based on the published evidence, moxidectin at 0.2 – 0.5 mg/kg PO daily can be recommended as an effective therapy for canine demodicosis an initial gradual dose increase and careful monitoring are recommended, similar to oral ivermectin. The spot-on containing 2.5% moxidectin and 10% imidacloprid can be recommended as weekly treatment for dogs with juvenile-onset and mild forms of the disease. If significant improvement is not seen within the first few weeks, other therapy may be indicated." **Note:** The weekly topical treatment for this indication is approved in some countries (not USA).

- **CATS:**

For labeled indications (*Advantage Multi®* for Cats): Recommended minimum dose is 10 mg/kg imidacloprid/1 mg/kg moxidectin once a month by topical administration (**Note:** See package insert for specific instructions on application and safety). For cats 2-5 lbs. = 0.23 mL; 5.1-9 lbs. = 0.4 mL; 9.1-18 lbs. = 0.8 mL; cats over 18 lbs. should be treated with appropriate combination for their weight. (Label directions; *Advantage Multi® for Cats*)

For feline aelurostrongylosis (*Aelurostrongylus abstrusus*); (extra-label): 1-3 topical applications of 1 mg/kg moxidectin (in combination with imidacloprid) appeared to be effective in the treatment of 8 cats infected with *A. abstrusus*. (Conboy 2009)

For notoedric mange (feline scabies); (extra-label): In the study, when applied topically at the minimal therapeutic dose of 10 mg imidacloprid/1 mg moxidectin/kg efficacy was 100% at 28 days post-treatment. (Capari *et al.* 2013)

- **FERRETS:**

For labeled indications (*Advantage Multi® for Cats*): Indicated for ferrets that weigh at least 2 lbs. body weight. Recommended minimum dose for a ferret is 9 mg/lb (20 mg/kg) imidacloprid and 0.9 mg/lb (2 mg/kg) moxidectin, once a month, by topical administration. Only the 0.4 mL applicator tube volume should be used on ferrets. Do not apply to irritated skin. (Label directions; *Advantage Multi® for Cats*)

- **CATTLE:**

For labeled indications (pour-on topical): 1 mL (5 mg)/10 kg (22 lbs.) bodyweight applied directly to the hair and skin along the top of the back from the withers to the base of the tail. Application should be made to healthy skin avoiding mange scabs, skin lesions or extraneous foreign matter. (Label Directions; *Cydectin® Pour-On*)

For labeled indications (subcutaneously): 0.2 mg/kg [1 mL for each 110 lbs. (50 kg) of bodyweight] subcutaneously under the loose skin in front of or behind the shoulder. Needles 1/2-3/4 inch in length and 16-18 gauge are recommended. (Label Directions; *Cydectin® Injection*)

- **SHEEP/GOATS:**

For labeled indications in sheep: 0.2 mg/kg [1 mL per 11 lbs. (1 mL per 5 kg) bodyweight] PO (drench). (*Cydectin® Oral Drench for Sheep*)

Goats (extra-label): Moxidectin should be used at 2 times the sheep dose if it is deemed necessary for use (Snyder 2009); 1.5 times the injectable sheep dose in countries where the injection is licensed for use in sheep (Hoste *et al.* 2011).

- **HORSES:**

For labeled indications using the combination oral gel with or without praziquantel: Dial in the weight of the animal on the syringe. Administer gel by inserting the syringe applicator into the animal's mouth through the interdental space and depositing the gel in the back of the mouth near the base of the tongue. Once the syringe is removed, the animal's head should be raised to insure proper swallowing of the gel. Horses weighing more than 1150 lbs. (1250 lbs. for *Quest Plus®*) require additional gel from a second syringe. (Label Directions; *Quest®*; *Quest® Plus*)

- **CAMELIDS (NWC):**

As an antiparasitic agent (extra-label): Oral treatment with ivermectin or moxidectin at 0.2 mg/kg is generally felt to be the regimen of choice for gastrointestinal helminthes. (Wolff 2009)

Monitoring

- Efficacy & adverse effects.

Client Information

- Give the client information sheet for the appropriate product to the client.
- Children should not come into contact with the topical small an-

imal products for at least 2 hours (30 minutes for the cat product) after application. For the first 30 minutes after application: Ensure that dogs cannot lick the product from application sites on themselves or other treated dogs, and separate treated dogs from one another and other pets to reduce the risk of accidental ingestion. Ingestion of this product by dogs may cause serious adverse reactions including depression, salivation, dilated pupils, incoordination, panting, and generalized muscle tremors. In avermectin sensitive dogs, the signs may be more severe and may include coma and death.

- For horses: Oral pastes are very safe to use when used as directed.

Chemistry/Synonyms

An avermectin-class antiparasitic agent, moxidectin is a semi-synthetic methoxime derivative of nemadectin.

Moxidectin may also be known as CL-301423, *Advantage Multi®*, *Advocate®*, *ComboCare®*, *Cydectin®*, and *Quest®*.

Storage/Stability

For the sustained-release injection (*ProHeart® 6*), store the unconstituted product at or below 25°C (77°F). Do not expose to light for extended periods of time. After constitution, the product is stable for 4 weeks stored under refrigeration at 2°-8°C (36°-46°F).

The commercially available injection and the oral drench for sheep should be stored at, or below 77°F (25°C) and protected from light.

The topical solution for cattle should be stored at or below room temperature. Do not allow prolonged exposure to temperatures above 77°F. If product becomes frozen, thaw completely and shake well before using.

The oral gel for horses should be stored at or near room temperature (59°F-86°F); avoid freezing. If product becomes frozen, thaw completely before using. Partially used syringes should have the cap tightly secured.

Compatibility/Compounding Considerations

When constituting the sustained-release injectable product (*ProHeart® 6*) the provided diluent must be used and there are very specific direction for proper preparation. Refer to the package insert for more information.

Dosage Forms/Regulatory Status

VETERINARY-LABELED PRODUCTS:

Moxidectin 10% Sustained-Release (microspheres) Injectable: 598 mg/vial with 17 mL diluent vial; *ProHeart® 6*; (Rx). FDA-approved for use in dogs 6 weeks or older.

Moxidectin 0.5% (5 mg/mL) Pour-On for Cattle in 500 mL, 1 L, 2.5 L, 5 L, and 10 L containers; *Cydectin®*; (OTC). FDA-approved for use in cattle; not to be used in veal calves. No meat or milk withdrawal times required, but FDA has established tolerances of 50 ppb and 200 ppb for parent moxidectin in muscle and liver, respectively, for cattle.

Moxidectin 10 mg/mL Injectable Solution in 200 mL and 500 mL; *Cydectin® Injectable Solution*; (OTC). FDA-approved for cattle. Not to be used in female dairy cattle of breeding age, veal calves, and calves <8 weeks of age. Meat withdrawal = 21 days.

Moxidectin 1 mg/mL Oral Drench Solution in 1 L and 4 L; *Cydectin® Oral Drench for Sheep*; (OTC). FDA-approved for sheep. Not to be used in female sheep providing milk for human consumption. Meat withdrawal = 7 days.

Moxidectin Oral Gel containing 20 mg/mL in 11.3 gram syringes (sufficient to treat one 1150 lb. horse); *Quest®*; (OTC). FDA-approved for use in horse or ponies not intended for food purposes.

Combination products:

Moxidectin 20 mg/mL and Praziquantel 125 mg/mL Oral Gel in 11.6 gram syringes (sufficient to treat one 1250 lb. horse); *Quest Plus*®; (OTC). FDA-approved for use in horse or ponies not intended for food purposes.

Moxidectin 1% (10 mg/mL) and Imidacloprid 10% (100 mg/mL) Topical Solution in 3—0.23 mL tubes, 6—0.4 mL tubes & 6—0.8 mL tubes; *Advantage Multi*® *for Cats*; (Rx). FDA-approved for use on cats 9 weeks of age or older, and >2 lbs. body weight. Approved (0.4 mL only) for ferrets weighing 2 lbs. or more.

Moxidectin 2.5% (25 mg/mL) and Imidacloprid 10% (100 mg/mL) Topical Solution in 6—0.4 mL tubes, 6—1 mL tubes, 6—2.5 mL tubes, & 6—4 mL tubes; *Advantage Multi*® *for Dogs*; (Rx). FDA-approved for use on dogs 7 weeks of age or older, and >3 lbs. body weight. This products may be known as *Advocate*® in some countries.

HUMAN-LABELED PRODUCTS: NONE.

Revisions/References

Monograph revised/updated April 2014.

Bates, N., et al. (2013). Lipid infusion in the management of poisoning: a report of 6 canine cases. Veterinary Record 172(13).

Capari, B., et al. (2013). Treatment of Naturally Notoedres cati-Infested Cats with a Combination of Imidacloprid 10%/Moxidectin 1% Spot-On (Advocate/Advantage Multi Bayer). Proceedings; International Society of Feline Medicine. accessed via Veterinary Information Network; vin.com

Conboy, G. (2009). Helminth Parasites of the Canine and Feline Respiratory Tract. Veterinary Clinics of North America-Small Animal Practice 39(6): 1109-+.

Crandell, D. E. & G. L. Weinberg (2009). Moxidectin toxicosis in a puppy successfully treated with intravenous lipids. J. Vet. Emerg. Crit. Care 19(2): 181-6.

Hoste, H., et al. (2011). Control of Endoparasitic Nematode Infections in Goats. Veterinary Clinics of North America-Food Animal Practice 27(1): 163-+.

Mealey, K. L. (2008). Canine ABCB1 and macrocyclic lactones: Heartworm prevention and pharmacogenetics. Veterinary Parasitology 158(3): 215-22.

Mueller, R. S., et al. (2012). Treatment of demodicosis in dogs: 2011 clinical practice guidelines. Veterinary Dermatology 23(2): 86-+.

Nielsen, M. & R. M. Kaplan (2009). Diagnosis & Management of Anthelmintic Resistance in Equid Parasites. Proceedings: ACVIM. accessed via Veterinary Information Network; vin.com

Snyder, J. (2009). Management of Internal Parasites in Sheep I & II. Proceedings: WVC. accessed via Veterinary Information Network; vin.com

Vaala, W. (2013). Strategic Equine Parasite Control for Foals and Adults. Proceedings; ABVP. accessed via Veterinary Information Network; vin.com

Wolff, P. (2009). Camelid Medicine. Proceedings: AAZV. accessed via Veterinary Information Network; vin.com

Mycobacterial Cell Wall Fraction Immunomodulator

(my-koe-bak-**tear**-ee-al)   Regressin®-V, Equimune® I.V.

Immunostimulant

Prescriber Highlights

▶ Biologic used in dogs as a locally infiltrated injection for immunotherapy treatment of mixed mammary tumor & mammary adenocarcinomas.

▶ In horses, used for immunotherapy treatment of sarcoids (local infiltration), ERCD (IV) or as an aid in the treatment of equine metritis caused by *Streptococcus zooepidemicus* (IV, IU).

▶ Adverse effects include: Transient fever, depression, decreased appetite, localized pain. Hypersensitivity & systemic inflammatory reactions possible.

▶ Efficacy for systemic use is not well established.

Uses/Indications

Mycobacterial cell wall fraction immunomodulator is commercially available as three products with veterinary labeling, *Immunocidin*®, *Equimune*®*-IV* and *Settle*®. *Immunocidin*® is labeled as a locally infiltrated injection for immunotherapy treatment of mixed mammary tumor and mammary adenocarcinomas in dogs, and for

immunotherapy treatment of sarcoids in horses. *Equimune*®*-IV* is labeled for use in horses only as an immunotherapeutic agent for the treatment of Equine Respiratory Disease Complex (ERDC). *Settle*® is labeled as an aid in the treatment of equine metritis caused by *Streptococcus zooepidemicus* (IV, IU) in horses.

Although not labeled indications, *Equimune*®*-IV* has reportedly been used in horses as an adjuvant for EPM treatment and as an adjuvant for herpesvirus vaccines when injected IM at a separate site from the vaccine. Documentation of efficacy for these uses was not located.

Pharmacology/Actions

Mycobacterial fractionated compounds require a functional immune system for efficacy. They have a non-specific immune stimulatory primarily on cell-mediated immune mechanisms and macrophage activation. Interleukin-1 release from macrophages is thought to be the primary mediator for their actions.

Pharmacokinetics

No information was located.

Contraindications/Precautions/Warnings

These drugs should not be used in patients with prior hypersensitivity to mycobacterial cell wall compounds or those with mycobacterial infections.

The manufacturer warns that patients receiving cortisone or ACTH may not respond to treatment; in case of an anaphylactic reaction, administer epinephrine.

Adverse Effects

Horses: Adverse effects include fever, drowsiness and diminished appetite for 1-2 days after injection. Local infiltrations can cause pain and tenderness at injection site. Anaphylaxis and severe respiratory inflammatory reactions have also been reported.

Dogs: Adverse effects include fever, drowsiness and diminished appetite for 1-2 days after injection. Local infiltrations can cause pain and tenderness at injection site. Later necrosis and draining may occur. Anaphylaxis or hypersensitivity reactions are possible.

Reproductive/Nursing Safety

The manufacturer states that *Regressin*®*-V (Immunocidin*®) and *Equimune*®*-I.V.* are safe to use in pregnant mares. No other information was located.

Overdosage/Acute Toxicity

No information was located.

Drug Interactions

▪ **CORTICOSTEROIDS, ACTH, IMMUNOSUPPRESSIVE DRUGS** (*e.g.,* **cyclosporine**): May reduce the effectiveness of mycobacterial cell wall immunostimulants.

Laboratory Considerations

▪ None identified.

Doses

▪ **DOGS:**

For immunotherapy of mixed mammary tumor and mammary adenocarcinoma: Using *Immunocidin*® (administered only by intratumoral injection): The entire tumor and a small region of adjacent and underlying tissue must be thoroughly infiltrated using no larger than a 20 gauge needle. Injection without careful infiltration of the tumor may not be effective. It is important to mix the emulsion thoroughly and inject the tumor as quickly as possible because the emulsion separates soon after mixing. The tumor tissue may be very firm and excessive pressure on the syringe plunger may be required to infiltrate it. The injection may produce pain in some animals; anesthetics or additional analgesics may be used. Dosage varies with tumor size but 1 mL should be considered a minimum dose. Tumors may be treated once, 2-4 weeks before surgery. If surgery is not to be used, repeat treatment every 1-3 weeks. If no response after 4 treatments, discontinue. (Adapted from label information; *Immunocidin*®—Bioniche)

- **HORSES:**

Using *Regressin*®-V for immunotherapy of sarcoids: Large pedunculated sarcoids should be de-bulked by partial excision prior to treatment. Using no larger than a 20-gauge needle, infiltrate entire tumor and a small region of adjacent and underlying tissue. Dosage varies with tumor size, but 1 mL should be considered a minimum dose. Be certain the emulsion is mixed thoroughly and inject quickly as emulsion can separate rapidly (see Stability information for more information on mixing.) As pain may occur, additional anesthetics or analgesics may be used. Repeat treatment every 1-3 weeks. If no response after 4 treatments, discontinue. (Label information; *Regressin*®-V—Bioniche)

Using *Equimune*®I.V. as an immunotherapeutic agent for the treatment of Equine Respiratory Disease Complex (ERDC): 1.5 mL (one syringe) IV into the jugular vein. May be repeated in 1-3 weeks. (Label information; *Equimune*®I.V.—Bioniche)

Using *Settle*® as an aid in the treatment of equine metritis caused by *Streptococcus zooepidemicus:* Intravenous use: 1.5 mL (one syringe) IV into the jugular vein during the early estrus period. Or administer via intrauterine instillation: Dilute 1.5 mL of *Settle*® in sterile LRS, normal saline, water for injection or semen extender to provide a final volume of 25 – 50 mL. Aseptically administer the diluted solution into the uterus using a sterile catheter. (Label information; *Settle*®—Bioniche)

Monitoring

- Clinical Efficacy (tumor size, metritis improvement, or respiratory infection improvement).
- Adverse Effects (fever, local reactions, appetite).

Client Information

- Intratumoral injection may cause pain or tenderness at the injection site. Tumors may drain or become necrotic indicating effectiveness; if this occurs and is bothersome, contact veterinarian for further instructions on management.
- Treated animals may be depressed, develop fever, or have reduced appetite for a few days after treatment; if these persist or are severe, contact veterinarian.

Chemistry/Synonyms

Regressin®-V, *Equimune*®-I.V. and *Settle*® are oil-in-water emulsions containing purified cell wall fractions obtained from Mycobacteria (species not described) that are non-pathogenic. Concentration is not listed for either product. *Regressin*®-V also contains procaine HCl 0.2% w/v as a local anesthetic and a green tracking dye solution (not identified) 0.1% w/v used to indicate area infiltrated.

Mycobacterial cell wall fraction may also be known as mycobacterial cell wall extract, bacillus Calmette-Guerin, or BCG, *Equimune*®, *Regressin*®, and *Settle*®.

Storage/Stability

These products should be stored refrigerated (2-7°C), but not frozen. Unused product from vials not labeled for multi-dose use should be discarded after use.

The emulsion "breaks" upon standing and the product must be re-emulsified before administration. To re-emulsify to a milky appearance, shake vial, roll syringe between hands, or heat in hot water (150°F, 65°C).

Compatibility/Compounding Considerations

No specific information noted.

Dosage Forms/Regulatory Status

VETERINARY-LABELED PRODUCTS:

Note: These products are USDA-licensed biologics and are not FDA-approved products. *Equimune*®I.V. and *Regressin*®-V are not to be used in food producing animals. The label for *Settle*® states that it should not be administered to horses within 21 days of slaughter.

Mycobacterial Cell Wall Fraction Immunomodulator for IV Injection in 1.5 mL single use vials and 4.5 mL multi-dose vials; *Equimune*®IV. Labeled for use in horses.

Mycobacterial Cell Wall Fraction Immunomodulator for Intrauterine instillation in 1.5 mL single use vials; *Settle*®. Contains gentamicin as a preservative. Labeled for use in horses.

Mycobacterial Cell Wall Fraction Immunomodulator for Tumor Infiltration in 10 mL vials; *Immunocidin*®. Also contains procaine and a green dye. Labeled for use in horses and dogs.

HUMAN-LABELED PRODUCTS: NONE.

Revisions/References

Monograph revised/updated April 2014.

Mycophenolate Mofetil

(my-koh-**fen**-oh-layt)   Cellcept®, MMF

Immunosuppressant

Prescriber Highlights

▶ Immunosuppressive drug that may be useful for treating dogs with IMHA, glomerulonephritis, myasthenia gravis, pemphigus foliaceus or inflammatory bowel disease in dogs; potentially useful in cats, but little information available on safety or efficacy.

▶ Very limited experience in veterinary medicine, especially in cats or for long-term use.

▶ Gastrointestinal effects (diarrhea, vomiting, anorexia) most likely adverse effects & can be severe.

▶ Treatment may be expensive and it may need to be compounded into appropriate dosage forms.

Uses/Indications

While there has been limited clinical experience using mycophenolate (MMF) in veterinary medicine and no large well-controlled studies were located, it potentially could be useful in the treatment of a variety of autoimmune diseases, including immune-mediated hemolytic anemia (IMHA), myasthenia gravis, glomerulonephritis, and pemphigus foliaceus. While mycophenolate has been suggested for use in treating inflammatory bowel disease in dogs, the drug's primary adverse effects in dogs are gastritis, diarrhea, and intestinal inflammation, which may be problematic. Mycophenolate is also used in anti-rejection protocols for organ transplants in animals.

In humans, although it is used "off label" for a variety of autoimmune disease indications, the drug is only labeled for use to prevent transplant rejection.

Pharmacology/Actions

Mycophenolate mofetil (MMF) is a prodrug that must be converted (hydrolyzed) *in vivo* to mycophenolic acid (MPA) for it to be pharmacologically active. MPA non-competitively, but reversibly, inhibits inosine monophosphate dehydrogenase (IMPDHA). This is the rate-limiting enzyme in *de novo* synthesis of guanosine nucleotides. As T- and B-cells are dependent on *de novo* synthesis of purines (*e.g.*, guanosine) and unlike other cells cannot use salvage pathways, proliferative responses of T- and B-cells are inhibited and suppression of B-cell formation of antibodies occur. Via its effects,

MPA can inhibit leukocyte recruitment to inflammatory sites and allotransplant tissues.

Pharmacokinetics

After oral administration mycophenolate mofetil is absorbed, but limited bioavailability studies in dogs have shown both a wide inter-patient and inter-dose variation. One study done in a single dog showed bioavailabilities of 54%, 65%, and 87% after doses of 10, 15, and 20 mg/kg of MMF were administered (Lupu *et al.* 2006). In humans, oral bioavailability averages 94%; food reduces peak levels of MPA by up to 40%. After absorption, MMF is rapidly hydrolyzed to mycophenolic acid.

In a study in dogs comparing mycophenolic acid's (MPA) pharmacokinetic parameters with its pharmacodynamic effects on inosine monophosphate dehydrogenase activity in lymphocytes (Langman *et al.* 1996), volume of distribution at steady-state was ≈5 L/kg, but there was wide inter-patient variability (±4.5). Elimination half-life for MPA was ≈8 hours (±4 hours). Mycophenolic acid is primarily excreted in the urine, both unchanged (≈5%) and as the glucuronide metabolite (≈90%). In this study, the authors concluded that the pharmacokinetic/pharmacodynamic profile of MMF in dogs suggests that an every 8-hour dosing schedule would be required for optimization of immunosuppressive efficacy.

Contraindications/Precautions/Warnings

Do not use in patients with documented hypersensitivity reactions to mycophenolate. Patients with severe renal dysfunction may require dosage adjustment. Because MMF can cause diarrhea, use with caution in patients with inflammatory bowel disease.

Intravenous mycophenolate must be administered over at least 2 hours; it is not to be given as an IV bolus or via rapid IV infusion.

In humans, the active metabolite, MPA is primarily excreted as the MPA-glucuronide metabolite. As cats are deficient in this metabolic process, it should be used with caution in this species.

For humans, mycophenolate has a "black box" warning regarding potential increased risk for lymphoma associated with its use.

Adverse Effects

Because of the limited experience with mycophenolate in veterinary patients, the adverse effect profile is not well established. At "usual doses" (10 mg/kg PO twice daily) it is usually tolerated well in dogs. Dose-dependent diarrhea appears to be the most common adverse effect, but vomiting, anorexia, lethargy/reduced activity, lymphopenia, and increased rates of dermal infections can be seen. Mild hypersensitivity reactions after intravenous administration are possible. Because of the drug's immunosuppressive actions, increased systemic infection and malignancy rates are possible, especially with long-term use. A study (Chanda *et al.* 2002) comparing adverse effects in dogs with mycophenolate mofetil capsules and mycophenolate sodium enteric-coated tablets demonstrated significantly greater occurrences and severity of diarrhea, weight loss and hypo-activity in the dogs that received the sodium salt enteric-coated tablets.

Very little information is available on mycophenolate adverse effects in cats.

In humans, the most common adverse effects include GI effects (constipation, diarrhea, nausea, vomiting) and headache. Hypertension and peripheral edema occur in about 30% of patients. Leukopenia has been reported in 25-45% of patients taking the medication. Other effects that occur more rarely include: GI bleeding, severe neutropenia, cough, confusion, tremor, infection and malignant lymphoma (0.4-1%).

Reproductive/Nursing Safety

At doses significantly lower than those used in humans, increased resorptions and malformations were noted in rabbits and rats; it is recommended that the drug be avoided, if at all possible, during pregnancy.

Mycophenolic acid is distributed in rat milk. It is unknown if it is safe to use during nursing.

Overdosage/Acute Toxicity

In oral acute studies performed in mice and monkeys, no deaths occurred in dosages up to 4,000 mg/kg and 1,000 mg/kg, respectively. In small animals, acute GI disturbances could be expected. Treat supportively, if required.

Drug Interactions

The following drug interactions have either been reported or are theoretical in humans or animals receiving mycophenolate mofetil and may be of significance in veterinary patients. Unless otherwise noted, use together is not necessarily contraindicated, but weigh the potential risks and perform additional monitoring when appropriate.

- **ACYCLOVIR**: Increased serum concentrations of acyclovir and the phenolic glucuronide of mycophenolic acid.
- **AMINOGLYCOSIDES** (*e.g.*, **gentamicin, amikacin**): In rats, use together induced greater nephrotoxicity.
- **ANTACIDS** (**aluminum** or **magnesium containing**): Decreased absorption of mycophenolate; separate dosing by at least 2 hours.
- **ASPIRIN** (or **other salicylates**): Potentially increased concentrations of free mycophenolic acid.
- **AZATHIOPRINE**: Increased risk for bone marrow suppression; use together not recommended in humans.
- **IRON** (**oral**): Decreased absorption of mycophenolate; separate dosing by at least 2 hours.
- **PROBENECID**: Potentially increased serum levels of mycophenolic acid and the phenolic glucuronide of mycophenolic acid.
- **VACCINES** (**live virus**): May be less effective; avoid use.

Laboratory Considerations

- No issues noted.

Doses

- **DOGS:**

  For immune-mediated hemolytic anemia (extra-label): From a retrospective study of 30 dogs. Authors concluded that immunosuppression with mycophenolate at 10 mg/kg IV or PO q12h, appears safe in dogs with idiopathic IMHA. The combination of glucocorticoids and MMF provides similar short-term outcomes and potentially fewer adverse side effects compared with other immunosuppressive protocols used to treat this disease. (Wang *et al.* 2013)

  For adjunctive immunosuppressive treatment of glomerular disease based on established pathology (extra-label): The International Renal Interest Society (IRIS) consensus statement recommends mycophenolate alone or in combination with prednisolone for peracute and/or rapidly progressive glomerular disease: mycophenolate 10 mg/kg PO q12h. For stable or slowly progressive glomerular diseases they recommend mycophenolate alone. In the absence of overt adverse effects, therapy should continue for at least 8 weeks before altering or discontinuing the drug. Therapy should be continued in dogs demonstrating a complete or partial response to initial treatment for a minimum of 12-16 weeks. Thereafter, consideration should be given to tapering the treatment to a dose/schedule that maintains the response without worsening of the proteinuria, azotemia, or clinical signs. (Segev *et al.* 2013)

  For myasthenia gravis (extra-label): 10 – 20 mg/kg PO q12h has been suggested, but one retrospective study found that when compared to using pyridostigmine alone, MMF with pyridostigmine did not significantly affect remission rate, time to remission, or survival time (Dewey *et al.* 2010). A case report in 3 dogs used MMF as a rescue agent for generalized myasthenia gravis: Initially, dogs received 500 mg (15 – 20 mg/kg) diluted and given IV over 2-4 hours. Dogs were given daily IV treatments for 1-3 days until they could adequately swallow oral meds. They were then switched to oral mycophenolate at doses between 10 – 11 mg/kg PO q12h. Subsequently, doses were adjusted based upon clinical response and AChR titers. (Abelson *et al.* 2009)

For pemphigus foliaceus (extra-label): Anecdotally, 20 – 40 mg/kg divided into 3 daily doses PO can have a steroid saving effect.

For aplastic anemia (extra-label): From a case report in one dog: 10 mg/kg PO q12h. The first effects (improvements in hematocrit) were observed 2 weeks later, and complete remission of all blood cell counts were obtained in ≈3 weeks. (Yuki *et al.* 2007)

- **CATS:**

  For adjunctive treatment of IMHA (extra-label): From a case report of 2 cats: 10 mg/kg PO q12h. (Bacek *et al.* 2011)

Monitoring

- Efficacy.
- CBC, renal and hepatic function, serum electrolytes; baseline and periodically (frequency depending on reason for treatment).
- Gastrointestinal effects (weight, client's report).

Client Information

- Preferably give on an empty stomach; if vomiting or lack of appetite occurs, give with food to see if it improves.
- Very limited experience in veterinary medicine, especially in cats or for long-term use.
- Gastrointestinal effects (diarrhea, vomiting, anorexia) most likely adverse effects & can be severe. If diarrhea persists or is severe, contact veterinarian.
- Because of concerns that this drug can cause birth defects, the manufacturer recommends that tablets or capsules not be crushed, split, or opened.

Chemistry/Synonyms

Mycophenolate mofetil occurs as a white or almost white, crystalline powder. It is practically insoluble in water and sparingly soluble in alcohol.

Mycophenolate mofetil may also be known as: RS-61443 or MMF. International trade names include: *CellCept®*, *Cellmune®*, *Imuxgen®*, *Munotras®*, *Mycept®*, *Myfortic®*, and *Refrat®*.

Storage/Compatibility

Mycophenolate mofetil tablets and capsules should be stored between 15-30°C and protected from light.

Mycophenolate mofetil powder for oral suspension should be stored between 15-30°C; preferably at 25°C. Once reconstituted with 94 mL of water it may be stored at room temperature or in the refrigerator; do not freeze. Unused drug should be discarded after 60 days.

The injectable product should be stored between 15-30°C; preferably at 25°C. Each vial should be reconstituted with 14 mL of 5% dextrose injection; final volume is approximately 15 mL. Gently agitate to dissolve the powder. For human use, the manufacturer recommends further diluting with dextrose 5% to a concentration of 6 mg/mL for IV administration. This would be an additional 70 mL of dextrose 5% per vial. Mycophenolate injection should not be mixed or given with any other medication or diluent. It is recommended to administer within 6 hours of dilution. The drug must be administered over at least 2 hours and is not to be given as an IV bolus or via rapid IV infusion.

Compatibility/Compounding Considerations

Mycophenolate injection should not be mixed or given with any other medication or diluent.

Dosage Forms/Regulatory Status

VETERINARY-LABELED PRODUCTS: NONE.

HUMAN-LABELED PRODUCTS:

Mycophenolate Mofetil Oral Capsules: 250 mg; *CellCept®*, generic; (Rx)

Mycophenolate Mofetil Oral Tablets: 500 mg; *CellCept®*, generic; (Rx)

Mycophenolate Mofetil Powder for Oral Suspension: 200 mg/mL (reconstituted) in 225 mL bottles; *CellCept®*; (Rx)

Mycophenolate Mofetil Lyophilized Powder for Injection: 500 mg in 20 mL vials; *CellCept®*; (Rx)

Mycophenolate is also available as the sodium salt of mycophenolic acid in oral, delayed-release tablets in 180 mg and 360 mg strengths; *Myfortic®*, generic; (Rx). It does not appear that this dosage form will be useful for veterinary patients.

Revisions/References

Monograph revised/updated April 2014.

Abelson, A. L., et al. (2009). Use of mycophenolate mofetil as a rescue agent in the treatment of severe generalized myasthenia gravis in three dogs. J. Vet. Emerg. Crit. Care **19**(4): 369-74.

Bacek, L. M. & D. K. Macintire (2011). Treatment of primary immune-mediated hemolytic anemia with mycophenolate mofetil in two cats. J. Vet. Emerg. Crit. Care **21**(3): 285-.

Chanda, S., et al. (2002). Comparative gastrointestinal effects of mycophenolate mofetil capsules and enteric-coated tablets of sodium mycophenolic acid in beagle dogs. Transplantation Proceedings **34**(8): 3387-92.

Dewey, C. W., et al. (2010). Mycophenolate mofetil treatment in dogs with serologically diagnosed acquired myasthenia gravis: 27 cases (1999-2008). Javma-Journal of the American Veterinary Medical Association **236**(6): 664-8.

Langman, L., et al. (1996). Pharmacodynamic assessment of mycophenolic acid-induced immunosuppression by measurement of inosine monophosphate dehydrogenase activity in a canine model. Transplantation **61**(1): 87-92.

Lupu, M., et al. (2006). Pharmacokinetics of oral mycophenolate mofetil in dog: Bioavailability studies and the impact of antibiotic therapy. Biology of Blood and Marrow Transplantation **12**(12): 1352-4.

Segev, G., et al. (2013). Consensus Recommendations for Immunosuppressive Treatment of Dogs with Glomerular Disease Based on Established Pathology. Journal of Veterinary Internal Medicine **27**: S44-S54.

Wang, A., et al. (2013). Treatment of canine idiopathic immune-mediated haemolytic anaemia with mycophenolate mofetil and glucocorticoids: 30 cases (2007 to 2011). Journal of Small Animal Practice **54**(8): 399-404.

Yuki, M., et al. (2007). Recovery of a dog from aplastic anaemia after treatment with mycophenolate mofetil. Australian Veterinary Journal **85**(12): 495-7.

N-Butylscopolammonium Bromide (Hyoscine Butylbromide)

(en-**byoo**-tel-skoe-**pahl**-ah-**moe**-nee-um **broe**-mide)   Buscopan®

Quaternary Ammonium Antispasmodic & Anticholinergic

Prescriber Highlights

► Injectable anticholinergic used in horses labeled for treating colic associated with spasmodic colic, flatulent colic, & simple impactions. May be an alternative to atropine or glycopyrrolate for treating bradycardia or acute RAO.

► Shorter acting than atropine; only labeled for a single (one-time) dose IV. Extra-label IM dosing has a longer duration of action.

► Not for use in patients with ileus or when decreased GI motility may be harmful.

► Adverse effects include transient tachycardia, pupil dilation, decreased secretions, & dry mucous membranes.

Uses/Indications

N-butylscopolammonium bromide (NBB) injection is indicated (per the label) for control of abdominal pain (colic) associated with spasmodic colic, flatulent colic, and simple impactions in horses. It may also be of benefit in horses in combination with oxytocin to treat esophageal obstruction (choke), and as an aid to performing rectal exams, including colonoscopy. In horses with detomidine-induced bradycardia, NBB (0.2 mg/kg IV) positive chronotropic duration of action was shorter than atropine, but it did not cause prolong reductions in intestinal motility. The authors concluded that NBB could be considered an alternative to atropine as a positive chronotropic agent in horses (Pimenta *et al.* 2011). In horses with recurrent airway obstruction (RAO), NBB (0.3 mg/kg IV) demonstrated potent bronchodilatory effects that peaked at 10 minutes and dissipated within one hour (Couetil *et al.* 2012).

Pharmacology/Actions

N-butylscopolammonium reduces gastrointestinal peristalsis and rectal pressure via its anti-cholinergic actions by competitively inhibiting muscarinic receptors on smooth muscle. It has some bronchodilatory and chronotropic effects in horses. N-butylscopolammonium has shorter duration of action than atropine. It appears to have brief (15-20 minutes) visceral colorectal distention antinociceptive effects in horses (Sanchez *et al.* 2008).

Pharmacokinetics

Limited information is available for horses. After an intravenous dose, the drug is eliminated within 48 hours in urine and feces equally. Estimated elimination half-life is ≈6 hours.

Contraindications/Precautions/Warnings

N-butylscopolammonium is labeled as contraindicated in horses with impaction colics associated with ileus or those with glaucoma.

This medication is not to be used in horses intended for food purposes.

The manufacturer has not studied the safety of IM administration, but one source has stated: "Although there was a difference between the IV and IM routes in terms of induction to affect and recovery of gastrointestinal sounds the findings were clinically comparable. An increased duration may be expected with use of the IM route. In terms of heart rate, the initial affect was greatly diminished in the IM vs. the IV route. The IM route appears to be a safe and effective means of administration" (Bertone 2012).

Because NBB can increase heart rate, use with caution in horses with systemic cardiovascular compromise (Morton *et al.* 2011).

Adverse Effects

Adverse effects include transient tachycardia and decreased borborygmal sounds that last for ≈20-30 minutes after IV dosing. Transient pupil dilation can be noted. Other effects include decreased secretions and dry mucous membranes.

Because this drug can cause increases in heart rate, heart rate cannot be used as a valid pain indicator for 30 minutes after injection.

When used for labeled indications, a lack of response may indicate a more serious problem that may require surgery or more aggressive care (White 2005).

Reproductive/Nursing Safety

As no data is available to document safety, the manufacturer does not recommend use in nursing foals or pregnant or lactating mares.

Overdosage/Acute Toxicity

Dosages up to 10X (3 mg/kg) were administered to horses as part of pre-approval studies. Clinical effects noted included dilated pupils (returned to normal in 4-24 hours), tachycardia (returned to normal within 4 hours) and dry mucous membranes (returned to normal in 1-2 hours). Gut motility was inhibited, but returned to baseline within 4 hours and normal feces were seen within 6 hours. Two of the four horses treated at 10X dosage developed mild signs of colic that resolved without further treatment.

Drug Interactions

The following drug interactions have either been reported or are theoretical in animals receiving N-butylscopolammonium bromide and may be of significance in veterinary patients. Unless otherwise noted, use together is not necessarily contraindicated, but weigh the potential risks and perform additional monitoring when appropriate.

- **ATROPINE or other anticholinergic agents**: May cause additive effects if used with N-butylscopolammonium.
- **METOCLOPRAMIDE and other drugs that have cholinergic-like actions on the GI tract**: These drugs and N-butylscopolammonium may counteract one another's actions on GI smooth muscle.
- **XYLAZINE**: In healthy horses, NBB with xylazine can cause significant hypertension and cardiac tachyarrhythmias; may falsely influence surgical decision-making and prognostication in horses with colic. (Morton *et al.* 2011)

Laboratory Considerations
- No specific concerns noted.

Doses
- **HORSES:**

  For labeled indications (FDA-approved): 0.3 mg/kg (30 mg or 1.5 mL per 100 kg of body weight) via slow IV, one time (Label information; *Buscopan*®). May also use IM (extra-label). (Bertone 2012).

  To treat esophageal obstruction (extra-label): 0.3 mg/kg IV once with oxytocin (0.11 – 0.22 Units/kg IV once). Oxytocin use should be avoided in mares, or dose significantly reduced. Do not use in pregnant mares. (Beard 2008)

Monitoring
- Heart rate (**Note**: Heart rate cannot be used as indicator for pain for the first 30 minutes after administration).
- GI motility via gut sounds and feces output.

Client Information
- Because an accurate patient assessment must be performed prior to the use of this medication and it requires intravenous administration and subsequent monitoring, this drug should only be administered by veterinarians.

Chemistry/Synonyms

N-butylscopolammonium bromide, a derivative of scopolamine, is a synthetic, quaternary ammonium antispasmodic-anticholinergic agent. It occurs as a white crystalline substance that is soluble in water.

N-butylscopolammonium bromide may also be known as: butylscopolamine bromide, hyosine butylbromide, hysocine N-butylbromide, scopolamini butylbromidum, hyoscini butylbromidum, *Buscopan*® or *Buscapina*®.

Storage/Stability

The commercially available injection should be stored at room temperature (15-30°C).

Compatibility/Compounding Considerations

No specific information noted.

Dosage Forms/Regulatory Status
VETERINARY-LABELED PRODUCTS:

N-butylscopolammonium bromide Injection: 20 mg/mL in 50 mL multi-dose vials; *Buscopan*®; (Rx). FDA-approved for use in horses.

In the UK, *Buscopan Compositum*® (BI) is commercially available. This product contains metamizole (a form of dipyrone) 500 mg/mL and hyoscine butylbromide (synonym for N-butylscopolammonium Br) 4 mg/mL. It is labeled for use in horses, cattle and dogs.

None in the USA. There are several products with the trade name *Buscopan®* or *Buscapina®* available in many countries. Refer to actual product labels as ingredients and concentrations may vary.

Revisions/References
Monograph revised/updated April 2014.

Nalbuphine HCl

(**nal**-byoo-feen)   Nubain®

Opiate Partial Agonist

Prescriber Highlights

▶ Injectable opiate agonist/antagonist used in combination as a 'pre-med' in small animals. Relatively short duration of action in dogs and cats, but could also be used for mild to moderate pain relief or to reverse effects of other opiate drugs without complete elimination of analgesia.

▶ Not very much information known about its use in veterinary medicine but appears to be relatively safe and effective in small animals.

▶ Not a DEA-controlled drug (in USA) and may be less expensive than butorphanol or buprenorphine.

Uses/Indications

Nalbuphine is an injectable opiate *kappa*-receptor agonist and *mu*-receptor antagonist that can be used as a 'pre-med' prior to surgical procedures. It could be used for analgesia but it is only effective for mild to moderate pain and its relatively short duration of effect make it a relatively poor choice. It could be used to reverse the adverse effects of *mu*-agonists (*e.g.*, morphine) and still offer some analgesia. When compared with other agonist/antagonists (*e.g.*, butorphanol or buprenorphine) nalbuphine's potential benefits are that it is not a DEA-controlled drug (in the USA) and may be less expensive, however, there is considerably less clinical experience and published information on its use in animals.

Pharmacology/Actions

Nalbuphine is a synthetic opioid agonist-antagonist analgesic of the phenanthrene series. Nalbuphine binds to *kappa*, *mu*, and *delta* opiate receptors, but not to *sigma* receptors. Its primary analgesic pharmacologic activity is due its agonist activity at *kappa* receptors and partial antagonism at *mu* receptors. Nalbuphine can cause respiratory depression, but above a certain dose (30 mg in adult humans), further respiratory depression does not occur.

Nalbuphine does not increase plasma histamine in dogs (Muldoon *et al.* 1983).

Pharmacokinetics

Nalbuphine has a similar pharmacokinetic profile as morphine (Riviere *et al.* 2009). However, it must be administered parenterally as it has very low oral bioavailability secondary to GI mucosal metabolism and a high-first pass effect. In humans, onset of action is usually within 3 minutes after IV administration and 15 minutes after subcutaneous or intramuscular doses. In humans, plasma half-life is ≈5 hours. Analgesic effects usually last from 3-6 hours after a dose. Analgesic duration of action in dogs and cats has been reported anecdotally as significantly shorter than in humans.

In birds (Hispaniolan parrots), IM dosages of nalbuphine HCl had complete bioavailability. After IV administration, measured volume of distribution was 2 L/kg, and clearance ≈70 mL/min/kg. Terminal half-life (≈20 minutes) was very fast for both IV and IM doses (Keller *et al.* 2011). A follow-up study using a sustained-release intramuscular form (nalbuphine decanoate 37.5 mg/kg IM) showed a mean terminal half-life of 20.4 hours. Plasma concentrations that could be associated with antinociception (20 ng/mL) were maintained for 24 hours after injection (Guzman *et al.* 2013).

Contraindications/Precautions/Warnings

Nalbuphine is contraindicated in patients hypersensitive to it. Severe pain should be treated with other analgesics (*e.g.*, *mu*-agonist opioids). Use cautiously in patients with hepatic or renal impairment, bradyarrhythmias or head trauma.

When use alone, nalbuphine rarely causes clinically significant respiratory depression, but it should be used with caution in patients with impaired respiratory function or when used concomitantly with other CNS- or respiratory-depressant agents; respiratory depression can be severe in these patients—adequate monitoring is required. Naloxone can reverse nalbuphine-induced respiratory depression.

Nalbuphine can precipitate withdrawal signs in patients that are physically dependent on opioid drugs. While the potential for abuse of nalbuphine by humans is less than with other opiates (especially *mu*-receptor agents), there have been reports of diversion, abuse, and dependence. Although there are no special recordkeeping or storage requirements, veterinarians should be alert to this potential.

Adverse Effects

Respiratory depression is unlikely but can occur (see Warnings above). Other adverse effects that can be seen with nalbuphine include excitement (high dosages), dysphoria, vomiting, and bradycardia.

Reproductive/Nursing Safety

Safe use of nalbuphine during pregnancy has not been established. In humans, the FDA categorizes this drug as category *B* for use during pregnancy (*Animal studies have not yet demonstrated risk to the fetus, but there are no adequate studies in pregnant women; or animal studies have shown an adverse effect, but adequate studies in pregnant women have not demonstrated a risk to the fetus in the first trimester of pregnancy, and there is no evidence of risk in later trimesters.*)

Very little drug is excreted into milk and nalbuphine is considered safe to use while nursing.

Overdosage/Acute Toxicity

Overdoses of nalbuphine are rarely serious, particularly when used on an inpatient basis and with adequate monitoring when used with other CNS/respiratory depressant drugs. Respiratory depression can be reversed with naloxone. In humans, subcutaneous single doses of 72 mg nalbuphine administered to healthy subjects caused sedation/sleepiness and mild dysphoria. Oral ingestions are not serious as the drug has very low oral bioavailability.

Drug Interactions

The following drug interactions have either been reported or are theoretical in humans or animals receiving nalbuphine and may be of significance in veterinary patients. Unless otherwise noted, use together is not necessarily contraindicated, but weigh the potential risks and perform additional monitoring when appropriate.

- **CIMETIDINE:** Increased nalbuphine effects possible.
- **CNS or RESPIRATORY DEPRESSANTS:** Additive CNS and/or respiratory depression can occur.

Laboratory Considerations

- Opioid **screening tests.** Nalbuphine may interfere with enzymatic tests.

Dosages

- **DOGS/CATS:**

  As a component of a pre-operative sedative/analgesic combination with other drugs (*e.g.*, midazolam, acepromazine, alpha-2 agonists, etc.); (extra-label): Nalbuphine could replace butorphanol at similar dosages in 'pre-med cocktails' at 0.2 - 0.4 mg/kg.

As a solo agent for mild-to moderate pain (extra-label): Of limited efficacy and relatively short duration (1+ hours) of action, similar to butorphanol. Dosages of 0.2 – 0.5 mg/kg IV, IM, SC (up to 2 mg/kg IV, IM has been suggested for use in dogs).

- **SMALL MAMMALS:**

    As an analgesic (extra-label):

    Rabbits, Ferrets: 0.5 – 1.5 mg/kg IV, IM q4h.

    Guinea Pigs: 1 – 4 mg/kg IM, SC q3h.

    Gerbils, Mice, Rats, Hamsters: 1 – 2 mg/kg IM, SC q2-4h (dosages have been recommended up to 8 mg/kg IM).

Monitoring

- Sedation/analgesia.
- Respiratory status when used in combination with other respiratory depressant drugs.

Client Information

- Nalbuphine is only used in an inpatient setting.

Chemistry/Synonyms

Nalbuphine HCl is a synthetic opiate agonist/antagonist in the phenanthrene series and structurally related to both naloxone (opiate antagonist) and oxymorphone (opiate agonist). Nalbuphine HCl is soluble in water and ethanol; insoluble in chloroform and ether.

The commercially available injection in 10 mL vials also contains in vials also contains sodium citrate hydrous 0.94%, citric acid anhydrous 1.26%, methyl- and propylparabens 0.2%, and hydrochloric acid to adjust pH to 3.5-3.7.

Nalbuphine HCl may also be known as EN-2234A. A 'street name' is "Nubian" and a common trade name is *Nubain*®.

Storage/Stability

Intact vials and ampules should be stored at 15-30°C (59-86°F) and protected from light.

Compatibility/Compounding Considerations

Nalbuphine HCl injection has been found **compatible** with the following intravenous solutions: dextrose 5% in sodium chloride 0.9% (D5NS); dextrose 10% (D10), lactated Ringer's solution (LRS), and sodium chloride 0.9% (NS) (Trissel 2013).

At usual concentrations, nalbuphine has been found **compatible** with the following drugs (partial listing) when mixed in syringes: atropine sulfate, diphenhydramine, glycopyrrolate, hydroxyzine, lidocaine, midazolam and ranitidine. Diazepam, ketorolac, and pentobarbital are incompatible. Propofol is compatible at a 1:1 ratio at Y-site (Trissel 2013). There are anecdotal reports of syringe mixtures successfully combining nalbuphine with acepromazine, dexmedetomidine or medetomidine, although published stability data was not located.

Dosage Forms/Regulatory Status

VETERINARY-LABELED PRODUCTS: NONE.

HUMAN-LABELED PRODUCTS:

Nalbuphine HCl Injectable Solution: 10 mg/mL & 20 mg/mL in 1 mL ampules and 10 mL multi-dose vials; generic; (Rx)

Revisions/References

Monograph written August 2013; revised April 2014.
Note: An online resource with additional information on nalbuphine use, including videos of its use in veterinary patients can be found at Veterinary Anesthesia & Analgesia Support Group (vasg.org).

Beard, L. (2008). Respiratory disease in the geriatric patient. Proceedings: WVC. accessed via Veterinary Information Network; vin.com

Bertone, J. (2012). Buscopan: Colic, Choke, Rectal Palpation, IM & Other Uses. Proceedings: Western Veterinary Conference. accessed via Veterinary Information Network; vin.com

Couetil, L., et al. (2012). Effects of N-Butylscopolammonium Bromide on Lung Function in Horses with Recurrent Airway Obstruction. Journal of Veterinary Internal Medicine 26(6): 1433-8.

Guzman, D. S. M., et al. (2013). Pharmacokinetics of long-acting nalbuphine decanoate after intramuscular administration to Hispaniolan Amazon parrots (Amazona ventralis). American Journal of Veterinary Research 74(2): 191-5.

Keller, D. L., et al. (2011). Pharmacokinetics of nalbuphine hydrochloride after intravenous and intramuscular administration to Hispaniolan Amazon parrots (Amazona ventrails). American Journal of Veterinary Research 72(6): 741-5.

Morton, A. J., et al. (2011). Cardiovascular effects of N-butylscopolammonium bromide and xylazine in horses. Equine Veterinary Journal 43: 117-22.

Muldoon, S. M., et al. (1983). Plasma Histamine Levels In Nalbuphine And Morphine Treated Dogs. Federation Proceedings 42(4): 904-.

Pimenta, E. L. M., et al. (2011). Comparative study between atropine and hyoscine-N-butylbromide for reversal of detomidine induced bradycardia in horses. Equine Veterinary Journal 43(3): 332-40.

Riviere, J. E. & M. G. Papich, Eds. (2009). *Veterinary Pharmacology and Therapeutics, Ninth Edition*. Ames, IA, Wiley-Blackwell.

Sanchez, L. C., et al. (2008). Effect of acepromazine, butorphanol, or N-butylscopolammonium bromide on visceral and somatic nociception and duodenal motility in conscious horses. American Journal of Veterinary Research 69(5): 579-85.

Trissel, L. 2013. Handbook on Injectable Drugs - 17th Edition. Accessed via STAT!Ref; Teton Data Systems

White, N. (2005). Medical Treatment of Colic. Western Veterinary Conference: Proceedings. accessed via Veterinary Information Network; vin.com

Naloxone HCl

(nal-**ox**-one)   Narcan®

Antidote; Opiate Antagonist

Prescriber Highlights

► Injectable opiate antagonist.
► Caution: Preexisting cardiac abnormalities or opioid dependent. At 'reversal' dosages, can negate opioid analgesic effects.
► Reversal effect may last for a shorter time than opioid effect; monitor & re-dose as needed.

Uses/Indications

Naloxone is used in veterinary medicine almost exclusively for its opiate reversal effects, but the drug is being investigated for treating other conditions (*e.g.*, septic, hypovolemic or cardiogenic shock). Some have found ultra low-dosage naloxone useful in treating post-anesthetic dysphoria associated with perioperative opioids but this practice is somewhat controversial due to the difficulty in distinguishing hyperalgesia from dysphoria in animal patients. Naloxone may also be employed as a test drug to see if endogenous opiate blockade will result in diminished tail chasing or other self-mutilating behaviors.

Pharmacology/Actions

Naloxone is considered a pure opiate antagonist and it has no analgesic activity at usual dosages. The exact mechanism for its activity is not understood, but it is believed that the drug acts as a competitive antagonist by binding to the *mu*, *kappa*, and *sigma* opioid receptor sites. The drug apparently has its highest affinity for the *mu* receptor. There is some evidence that at sub-reversal dosages naloxone may enhance the analgesic effects of opioids. One study in cats however, did not find any increased nociceptive effects when buprenorphine and naloxone were given at a 15:1 ratio (Slingsby *et al.* 2012).

Naloxone reverses the majority of effects associated with high-dose opiate administration (respiratory and CNS depression). In dogs, naloxone apparently does not reverse the emetic actions of apomorphine.

Naloxone may be useful in treating adverse effects associated with overdoses of propoxyphene, pentazocine, buprenorphine and loperamide, but larger naloxone doses may be required.

Naloxone has other pharmacologic activity at high doses, including effects on dopaminergic mechanisms (increases dopamine levels) and GABA antagonism.

Pharmacokinetics

Naloxone is only minimally absorbed when given orally as it is rapidly destroyed in the GI tract. Much higher doses are required if using this route of administration for any pharmacologic effect. When given IV, naloxone has a very rapid onset of action (usually 1-2 minutes). If given IM, the drug generally has an onset of action within 5 minutes of administration. The duration of action usually persists from 45-90 minutes, but may act for up to 3 hours.

Naloxone is distributed rapidly throughout the body with high levels found in the brain, kidneys, spleen, skeletal muscle, lung, and heart. The drug also readily crosses the placenta.

Naloxone is metabolized in the liver, principally via glucuronidative conjugation, with metabolites excreted into the urine. In humans, the serum half-life is ≈60-100 minutes.

Contraindications/Precautions/Warnings

Naloxone is contraindicated in patients hypersensitive to it. It should be used cautiously in animals that have preexisting cardiac abnormalities or that may be opioid dependent. The veterinary manufacturer of the product once marketed for veterinary use states to use the drug "…cautiously in animals who have received exceedingly large doses of narcotics…it may produce an acute withdrawal syndrome and smaller doses should be employed." (Package Insert; *P/M® Naloxone HCl Injection*)

Naloxone is reportedly not effective for reversing meperidine-induced seizures. Benzodiazepines and/or barbiturates may be necessary. In a case of a dog that received an overdose (10X) of meperidine, naloxone administration elicited CNS excitement. The authors recommend that naloxone (and butorphanol) should be avoided when normeperidine (active metabolite of meperidine) excitotoxicity is suspected, unless severe respiratory depression is present without a method of ventilatory support available (Golder *et al.* 2010).

Naloxone has not been shown to be an effective therapy to reverse apnea of newborns and its routine use is not recommended. However, if the dam received opiates during parturition, it may reverse opiate-induced respiratory depression. Naloxone is not a good reversal agent for buprenorphine. Doses of 100X-usual have been required to reverse effects in a normal dog.

When used to reduce post-operative dysphoria associated with perioperative opioids, naloxone dosage and administration rate must be carefully titrated or hyperalgesia can occur.

Adverse Effects

At usual doses, naloxone is relatively free of adverse effects in non-opioid dependent patients; however, when using to reverse opiates' effects, it can also reverse any analgesic activity of the opiate (see Warnings above).

Because the duration of action of naloxone may be shorter than that of the narcotic being reversed, animals that are being treated for opioid intoxication or with clinical signs of respiratory depression should be closely monitored as additional doses of naloxone and/or ventilatory support may be required.

Reproductive/Nursing Safety

In humans, the FDA categorizes this drug as category *B* for use during pregnancy (*Animal studies have not yet demonstrated risk to the fetus, but there are no adequate studies in pregnant women; or animal studies have shown an adverse effect, but adequate studies in pregnant women have not demonstrated a risk to the fetus in the first trimester of pregnancy, and there is no evidence of risk in later trimesters.*) In a separate system evaluating the safety of drugs in canine and feline pregnancy (Papich 1989), this drug is categorized as class: *A* (*Probably safe. Although specific studies may not have proved he safety of all drugs in dogs and cats, there are no reports of adverse effects in laboratory animals or women.*)

It is not known whether the drug is excreted in maternal milk. Use caution when administering to nursing patients.

Overdosage/Acute Toxicity

Naloxone is considered a very safe agent with a very wide margin of safety, but very high doses have initiated seizures (secondary to GABA antagonism?) in a few patients.

Drug Interactions

The following drug interactions have either been reported or are theoretical in humans or animals receiving naloxone and may be of significance in veterinary patients. Unless otherwise noted, use together is not necessarily contraindicated, but weigh the potential risks and perform additional monitoring when appropriate.

- **MEPERIDINE (OVERDOSE):** Naloxone may contribute to CNS excitatory effects of normeperidine (meperidine metabolite). In cases where normeperidine excitotoxicity is suspected, avoid use of naloxone (or butorphanol), unless severe respiratory depression is present without a method of ventilatory support (Golder *et al.* 2010).
- **OPIOID PARTIAL-AGONISTS** (*e.g.*, **buprenorphine, butorphanol**, **pentazocine**, or **nalbuphine**): Naloxone may also antagonize the effects of these agents (respiratory depression, analgesia). It should not be relied upon to treat respiratory depression caused by buprenorphine.
- **CLONIDINE**: Naloxone may reduce the hypotensive and bradycardic effects of clonidine; potentially useful for clonidine overdoses.
- **YOHIMBINE**: Naloxone may increase the CNS effects of yohimbine (anxiety, tremors, nausea, palpitations) and increase plasma cortisol levels.

Doses

- **DOGS & CATS:**

For opioid reversal (extra-label):

a) 0.01 – 0.04 mg/kg IV, IM, SC or IO; repeat as necessary. If given IM or SC effects may be delayed up to 5 minutes. If necessary, intranasal or intratracheal (endotracheal) administration can be considered, dosages of 0.04 – 0.1 mg/kg have been suggested for animal patients.

b) For newborns when opioids given to dam: 1 drop (of the 0.4 mg/mL injection) can be given under tongue; repeat as necessary. Alternatively can be dosed parenterally as above.

c) During CPR in cases of opioid toxicity or if recent opioids were administered: 0.04 mg/kg IV, IO may be considered. (Fletcher *et al.* 2012)

d) For post-operative dysphoria: If the patient is clearly dysphoric or returns to a whining state shortly after additional opioid administration, or if suspicion exists related to the use of high doses of opioid during surgery, a slow titration of IV naloxone can be given to effect. Depending on the size of the patient either dilute 0.1 mL of the 0.4 mg/mL injection (0.04 mg; 40 micrograms) into 5 mL sterile saline (8 micrograms/mL) or 0.25 mL of the 0.4 mg/mL injection (0.1 mg; 100 micrograms) into 10 mL sterile saline (10 micrograms/mL). Give 1 mL of the dilution IV over 30-60 seconds at the Y-site injection port nearest to the patient. Observe patient carefully during infusion. Once patient calms or sleeps, stop infusion. Most patients do not require the full 1 mL. Overdosing can induce hyperalgesia. If dysphoria recurs, may need to repeat. Adapted from (Dyson 2008), (Mathews 2013)

For adjunctive treatment of hyperthermia in cats (extra-label): Post-anesthesia hyperthermia (exceeding 41.1°C; 106°F) has been treated with naloxone at 0.01 mg/kg IM or SC. Temperatures have returned to normal <30 minutes. (Posner *et al.* 2010)

- **RABBITS, RODENTS, SMALL MAMMALS:**
  For opioid reversal (extra-label): Wide range of anecdotal dosages noted (0.005 – 0.1 mg/kg); consider an initial dose of 0.01 – 0.02 mg/kg IV, IM, SC, or IP; repeat as necessary.

- **HORSES:** (NOTE: ARCI UCGFS CLASS 3 DRUG)
  For opioid reversal (extra-label): 0.01 – 0.05 mg/kg IV; low end of dosing range can limit opioid-induced locomotor activity; upper end may stimulate colonic propulsion. Duration of effect can be very short (under 30 minutes).

Monitoring

- Respiratory rate/depth.
- CNS function.
- Pain associated with opiate reversal.

Client Information

- Should be used with direct professional supervision only.

Chemistry/Synonyms

An opiate antagonist, naloxone HCl is structurally related to oxymorphone. It occurs as a white to slightly off-white powder with a pK_a of 7.94. Naloxone is soluble in water and slightly soluble in alcohol. The pH ranges of commercially available injectable solutions are from 3-4.5.

Naloxone HCl may also be known as: N-allylnoroxymorphone, naloxona, EN-15304, naloxoni and by the trade name, *Narcan®*.

Storage/Stability

Naloxone HCl for injection should be stored at room temperature (15-30°C) and protected from light.

Sterile water for injection is the recommended diluent for naloxone injection. When given as an IV infusion, either D_5W or normal saline should be used.

Compatibility/Compounding Considerations

Naloxone HCl injection **should not** be mixed with solutions containing sulfites, bisulfites, long-chain or high molecular weight anions or any solutions at alkaline pH.

Dosage Forms/Regulatory Status

VETERINARY-LABELED PRODUCTS: NONE.

There were approved products in the past but these have been discontinued. The ARCI (Racing Commissioners International) has designated this drug as a class 3 substance—see the appendix for more information.

HUMAN-LABELED PRODUCTS:

Naloxone HCl Injection: 0.4 mg/mL (400 micrograms/mL) & 1 mg/mL; generic; (Rx)

Revisions/References

Monograph revised/updated April 2014.

Dyson, D. H. (2008). Perioperative Pain Management in Veterinary Patients. Veterinary Clinics of North America-Small Animal Practice 38(6): 1309-+.

Fletcher, D. J., et al. (2012). RECOVER evidence and knowledge gap analysis on veterinary CPR. Part 7: Clinical guidelines. J. Vet. Emerg. Crit. Care 22.

Golder, F. J., et al. (2010). Suspected acute meperidine toxicity in a dog. Veterinary Anaesthesia and Analgesia 37(5): 471-7.

Mathews, K. A. (2013). Is It Pain or Dysphoria? How to Tell. Proceedings: IVECCS. accessed via Veterinary Information Network; vin.com

Papich, M. (1989). Effects of drugs on pregnancy. *Current Veterinary Therapy X: Small Animal Practice.* R. Kirk. Philadelphia, Saunders: 1291-9.

Posner, L. P., et al. (2010). Effects of opioids and anesthetic drugs on body temperature in cats. Veterinary Anaesthesia and Analgesia 37(1): 35-43.

Slingsby, L. S., et al. (2012). Buprenorphine in combination with naloxone at a ratio of 15:1 does not enhance antinociception from buprenorphine in healthy cats. Veterinary Journal 192(3): 523-4.

Naltrexone HCl

(nal-**trex**-ohne)   Trexan®, ReVia®
Opiate Antagonist

Prescriber Highlights

▶ Oral opiate antagonist that might be useful in determining if adverse behaviors have a significant endorphin component & for the short-term treatment of same. Compounded injection may be an alternative to naloxone for reversing opioid effects.

▶ Contraindications: Patients physically dependent on opiate drugs, in hepatic failure, or with acute hepatitis. Caution: hepatic dysfunction or who have had a history of allergic reaction to naltrexone or naloxone.

▶ Adverse Effects: Relatively free of adverse effects. Potentially: Abdominal cramping, nausea & vomiting, nervousness, insomnia, joint or muscle pain, skin rashes, & pruritus. Dose-dependent hepatotoxicity is possible.

▶ May cause clinical signs of withdrawal in physically dependent patients.

▶ Oral treatment can be expensive.

Uses/Indications

Naltrexone might be useful in determining if adverse behaviors (*e.g.*, self-mutilating or tail-chasing) in dogs or cats have a significant endorphin component. Its relative expense and other more accepted treatments have largely supplanted the use of this drug in animals for treatment of behavioral disorders. Compounded injectable naltrexone may be an acceptable replacement for reversing opioids when commercial naloxone injection is not available. A study in cats, found that hourly IV injections of 600 micrograms/kg antagonized the dysphoric and antinociceptive effects of hourly, high doses of remifentanil (Pypendop *et al.* 2011).

Pharmacology/Actions

Naltrexone is an orally available narcotic antagonist. It competitively binds to opiate receptors in the CNS, thereby preventing both endogenous opiates (*e.g.*, endorphins) and exogenously administered opiate agonists or agonist/antagonists from occupying the site. Naltrexone may be more effective in blocking the euphoric aspects of the opiates and less effective at blocking the respiratory depressive or miotic effects.

Naltrexone may also increase plasma concentrations of luteinizing hormone (LH), cortisol, and ACTH. In dogs with experimentally-induced hypovolemic shock, naltrexone (like naloxone) given IV in high dosages increased mean arterial pressure, cardiac output, stroke volume, and left ventricular contractility.

Pharmacokinetics

In humans, naltrexone is rapidly and nearly completely absorbed, but undergoes a significant first-pass effect as only 5-12% of a dose reaches the systemic circulation. Naltrexone circulates throughout the body and CSF levels are ≈30% of those found in plasma. Only ≈20-30% is bound to plasma proteins. It is unknown whether naltrexone crosses the placenta or enters milk. Naltrexone is metabolized in the liver primarily to 6-beta-naltrexol, which has some opiate blocking activity. Naltrexone's metabolites are eliminated primarily via the kidney. In humans, serum half-life of naltrexone is ≈4 hours and ≈13 hours for 6-beta-naltrexol.

Contraindications/Precautions/Warnings

Naltrexone is contraindicated in patients physically dependent on opiate drugs, in hepatic failure, or with acute hepatitis. The benefits of the drug versus its risks should be weighed in patients with hepatic dysfunction or with a history of allergic reaction to naltrexone or naloxone.

Adverse Effects

At usual doses, naltrexone is relatively free of adverse effects in non-opioid dependent patients. Some human patients have developed abdominal cramping, nausea and vomiting, nervousness, insomnia, joint or muscle pain, skin rashes, and pruritus. Dose-dependent hepatotoxicity has been described in humans on occasion.

Naltrexone will block the analgesic, antidiarrheal, and antitussive effects of opiate agonist or agonist/antagonist agents. Withdrawal clinical signs may be precipitated in physically dependent patients.

Reproductive/Nursing Safety

In humans, the FDA categorizes this drug as category *D* for use during pregnancy (*There is evidence of human fetal risk, but the potential benefits from the use of the drug in pregnant women may be acceptable despite its potential risks.*) Very high doses have caused increased embryotoxicity in some laboratory animals. It should be used during pregnancy only when the benefits outweigh any potential risks.

Naltrexone enters into milk of humans and sheep. Use caution when administering to nursing patients.

Overdosage/Acute Toxicity

Naltrexone appears to be relatively safe even after very large doses. The LD_{50} in dogs after subcutaneous injection has been reported to be 200 mg/kg. Oral LD_{50}'s in species tested range from 1.1 grams/kg in mice to 3 grams/kg in monkeys (dogs or cats not tested). Deaths at these doses were a result of respiratory depression and/or tonic-clonic seizures. Massive overdoses should be treated using gut-emptying protocols when warranted and giving supportive treatment.

Drug Interactions

The following drug interactions have either been reported or are theoretical in humans or animals receiving naltrexone and may be of significance in veterinary patients. Unless otherwise noted, use together is not necessarily contraindicated, but weigh the potential risks and perform additional monitoring when appropriate.

- **YOHIMBINE:** Naltrexone may increase the CNS effects of yohimbine (anxiety, tremors, nausea, palpitations) and increase plasma cortisol levels.

Laboratory Considerations

- Naltrexone reportedly does not interfere with TLC, GLC, or HPLC methods of determining **urinary opiates**, or quinine, but can interfere with some enzymatic assays
- Naltrexone may cause increases in **hepatic function tests** (*e.g.*, AST, ALT) (see Adverse Effects above).

Doses

- **DOGS/CATS:**

  As adjunctive therapy in behavior disorders (*e.g.*, stereotypy); (extra-label): Limited evidence to support use. Dosage recommendations vary but 2 – 5 mg/kg PO once or divided twice daily have been noted. If using commercially available tablets (50 mg) dosage is typically rounded to nearest 25 mg. Tablets can be bitter tasting.

- **ZOO, EXOTIC, WILDLIFE SPECIES:**

  For use of compounded injectable naltrexone as an opioid reversal agent in zoo, exotic and wildlife medicine refer to specific references, including:

  a) Zoo Animal and Wildlife Immobilization and Anesthesia. West, G., Heard, D., Caulkett, N. (eds.). Blackwell Publishing, 2007.

  b) Handbook of Wildlife Chemical Immobilization, 3rd Ed. Kreeger, T.J. and J.M. Arnemo. 2007.

  c) Fowler's Zoo and Wild Animal Medicine Current Therapy, Volume 7, Miller, R.E., Fowler, M.E., Saunders. 2011.

  d) Exotic Animal Formulary, 4th Ed. Carpenter, J.W., Saunders. 2012.

  e) The 2009 American Association of Zoo Veterinarian Proceedings by D. K. Fontenot also has several dosages listed for restraint, anesthesia, and analgesia for a variety of drugs for carnivores and primates. VIN members can access them at: http://goo.gl/NNIWQ or http://goo.gl/9UJse

Monitoring

- Efficacy.
- Liver enzymes if using very high dose with prolonged therapy.

Client Information

- Stress the importance of compliance with prescribed dosing regimen.
- Additional behavior modification techniques may be required to alleviate clinical signs.

Chemistry/Synonyms

A synthetic opiate antagonist, naltrexone HCl occurs as white crystals having a bitter taste. 100 mg are soluble in 1 mL of water.

Naltrexone may also be known as EN-1639A, *ReVia*® and *Vivitrol*®.

Storage/Stability

Naltrexone tablets should be stored at room temperature in well-closed containers.

Compatibility/Compounding Considerations

No specific information noted.

Dosage Forms/Regulatory Status

VETERINARY-LABELED PRODUCTS: NONE.

The ARCI (Racing Commissioners International) has designated this drug as a class 3 substance. See the appendix for more information.

Compounded naltrexone for injection may be available.

HUMAN-LABELED PRODUCTS:

Naltrexone HCl Oral Tablets: 50 mg; *ReVia*®, generic; (Rx)

Naltrexone HCl Powder for Suspension Extended-Release Injection: 380 mg/vial in single-use vials w/4 mL diluent; *Vivitrol*®; (Rx). **Note:** No information on using this product in veterinary medicine was located.

Revisions/References

Monograph revised/updated April 2014.

Pypendop, B. H., et al. (2011). Use of naltrexone to antagonize high doses of remifentanil in cats: a dose-finding study. Veterinary Anaesthesia and Analgesia 38(6): 594-7.

Nandrolone

(**nan**-droe-lone)   Laurabolin®

Parenteral Anabolic Steroid

Prescriber Highlights

▶ Injectable anabolic steroid; may be useful to stimulate erythropoiesis or to stimulate appetite. Rarely recommended or used today.

▶ Contraindications: Hepatic dysfunction, hypercalcemia, history of myocardial infarction, pituitary insufficiency, prostate carcinoma, mammary carcinoma, benign prostatic hypertrophy, & during the nephrotic stage of nephritis.

▶ Adverse Effects: Sodium, calcium, potassium, water, chloride, & phosphate retention; hepatotoxicity, behavioral (androgenic) changes, & reproductive abnormalities (oligospermia, estrus suppression).

▶ Known teratogen. Drug Interactions.

▶ C-III Controlled Substance. No FDA-approved products marketed in USA; may be available from compounding pharmacies. Nandrolone laurate or nandrolone phenylpropianate may be available in some markets.

Uses/Indications

The principle use of nandrolone in veterinary medicine has been to stimulate erythropoiesis in patients with certain anemias (*e.g.*, secondary to renal failure, aplastic anemias). It has also been suggested for use as an appetite stimulant. Anabolic steroids are rarely recommended or used today in veterinary medicine.

Pharmacology/Actions

Nandrolone exhibits similar actions as other anabolic agents. In the presence of adequate protein and calories, anabolic steroids promote body tissue building processes and can reverse catabolism. As these agents are either derived from or closely related to testosterone, the anabolics have varying degrees of androgenic effects. Endogenous testosterone release may be suppressed by inhibiting luteinizing hormone (LH). Large doses can impede spermatogenesis by negative feedback inhibition of FSH.

Anabolic steroids can stimulate erythropoiesis. The mechanism for this effect may occur by stimulating erythropoietic stimulating factor. Anabolics can cause nitrogen, sodium, potassium, and phosphorus retention and decrease the urinary excretion of calcium. Many veterinary and human clinicians feel that nandrolone is clinically superior to other anabolics in its ability to stimulate erythropoiesis. It is believed that nandrolone may enhance red cell counts by directly stimulating red cell precursors in the bone marrow, increasing red cell 2,3-diphosphoglycerate and erythropoietin production in the kidney.

Pharmacokinetics

No specific information was located for this agent. The decanoate salt is generally recommended for both small animals and humans to be dosed on a weekly basis; the laurate salt is dosed every 3 weeks.

Contraindications/Precautions/Warnings

Nandrolone should not be used in pregnant animals. It should be used with caution in animals with hepatic dysfunction.

In humans, anabolic agents are contraindicated in patients with hepatic dysfunction, hypercalcemia, patients with a history of myocardial infarction (can cause hypercholesterolemia), pituitary insufficiency, prostate carcinoma, in selected patients with breast carcinoma, benign prostatic hypertrophy, and during the nephrotic stage of nephritis.

Adverse Effects

Potential (from human data) adverse reactions of the anabolic agents in dogs and cats include: sodium, calcium, potassium, water, chloride, and phosphate retention; hepatotoxicity, behavioral (androgenic) changes, and reproductive abnormalities (oligospermia, estrus suppression). May cause cat urine to have a strong odor.

Reproductive/Nursing Safety

In humans, the FDA categorizes this drug as category *X* for use during pregnancy (*Studies in animals or humans demonstrate fetal abnormalities or adverse reaction; reports indicate evidence of fetal risk. The risk of use in pregnant women clearly outweighs any possible benefit.*) Anabolic steroids can cause masculinization of the fetus.

It is not known whether anabolic steroids are excreted in maternal milk. Because of the potential for serious adverse reactions in nursing offspring, decide whether to discontinue nursing or the drug.

Overdosage/Acute Toxicity

No information was located for this specific agent. In humans, sodium and water retention can occur after overdosage of anabolic steroids. It is suggested to treat supportively and monitor liver function should an inadvertent overdose be administered.

Drug Interactions

The following drug interactions have either been reported or are theoretical in humans or animals receiving nandrolone and may be of significance in veterinary patients. Unless otherwise noted, use together is not necessarily contraindicated, but weigh the potential risks and perform additional monitoring when appropriate.

- **ANTICOAGULANTS (warfarin):** Anabolic agents as a class may potentiate the effects of anticoagulants; monitoring of INR and dosage adjustment of the anticoagulant (if necessary) are recommended.

- **CORTICOSTEROIDS, ACTH:** Anabolics may enhance the edema that can be associated with ACTH or adrenal steroid therapy.

- **INSULIN:** Diabetic patients receiving insulin may need dosage adjustments if anabolic therapy is added or discontinued; anabolics may decrease blood glucose and decrease insulin requirements.

Laboratory Considerations

- Concentrations of **protein bound iodine** (PBI) can be decreased in patients receiving androgen/anabolic therapy, but the clinical significance of this is probably not important.

- Androgen/anabolic agents can decrease amounts of **thyroxine-binding globulin** and decrease **total T_4** concentrations and increase **resin uptake of T_3 and T_4**; free thyroid hormones are unaltered and, clinically, there is no evidence of dysfunction.

- Both **creatinine** and **creatine excretion** can be decreased by anabolic steroids.

- Anabolic steroids can increase the urinary excretion of **17-ketosteroids**.

- Androgenic/anabolic steroids may alter **blood glucose** levels.

- Androgenic/anabolic steroids may suppress **clotting factors II, V, VII, and X.**

- Anabolic agents can affect **liver function tests** (BSP retention, SGOT, SGPT, bilirubin, and alkaline phosphatase).

Doses

- **DOGS/CATS:**

  For the supportive management of chronic renal failure (extra-label in USA): Nandrolone laurate at 2 – 5 mg/kg IM or SC; may repeat every 21 days. (Label information; *Laurabolin®*—

MSD Animal Health U.K.)

For anabolic effects (extra-label): Nandrolone decanoate: Recommended doses are usually 1 – 3 mg/kg IM once weekly; some have recommended 5 mg/kg (maximum of 200 mg) once weekly for aplastic anemia.

- **REPTILES:**

To reduce protein catabolism in renal disease of lizard species (extra-label): Nandrolone decanoate: 1 mg/kg IM every 7-28 days. (de la Navarre 2003)

Monitoring

- Androgenic side effects.
- Fluid and electrolyte status, if indicated.
- Liver function tests if indicated.
- Red blood cell count, indices, if indicated.
- Weight, appetite.

Client Information

- Because of the potential for abuse of anabolic steroids by humans, this agent is a controlled (C-III) drug. It should be kept in a secure area and out of the reach of children.

Chemistry/Synonyms

An injectable anabolic steroid, nandrolone decanoate occurs as a white, to creamy white, crystalline powder. It is odorless or may have a slight odor and melts between 33-37°C. Nandrolone decanoate is soluble in alcohol and vegetable oils and is practically insoluble in water. The commercial injectable products were generally solutions of nandrolone decanoate dissolved in sesame oil.

Nandrolone may also be known as nortestosterone.

Storage/Stability

Nandrolone decanoate for injection should be stored at temperatures <40°C preferably between 15-30°C (59-86°F) and protected from freezing and light.

Nandrolone laurate for injection should stored protected from light. Do not store above 25°C. At low temperatures the product may become viscous. Warming the product in the hand will return the contents to the normal state.

Compatibility/Compounding Considerations

No specific information noted. Do not mix injection with other drugs.

Dosage Forms/Regulatory Status

VETERINARY-LABELED PRODUCTS:

There are no commercial products available in the USA. Potentially, it may be available from compounding pharmacies. The ARCI (Racing Commissioners International) has designated this drug as a class 4 substance. See the appendix for more information.

Nandrolone Laurate injection 25 mg/mL may be available in Europe. Trade name is *Laurabolin®*.

HUMAN-LABELED PRODUCTS: NONE.

Revisions/References

Monograph revised/updated April 2014.

de la Navarre, B. (2003). Acute and chronic renal disease (specifically in lizard species). Proceedings: Western Veterinary Conference. accessed via Veterinary Information Network; vin.com

Naproxen

(na-**prox**-en)   *Naprosyn®, Aleve®*

Nonsteroidal Antiinflammatory Agent

Prescriber Highlights

▶ NSAID; rarely used in animal patients as there are approved less toxic NSAIDs available.

▶ Contraindications: Patients with active GI ulcers or history of hypersensitivity to the drug. Relatively Contraindicated: Hematologic, renal or hepatic disease. Caution: History of gastric ulcers, heart failure.

▶ Adverse Effects: Relatively uncommon in **Horses:** Possible GI (distress, diarrhea, ulcers), hematologic (hypoproteinemia, decreased hematocrit), renal (fluid retention), & CNS (neuropathies). **Dogs:** GI ulcers & perforation, renal effects (nephritis/nephrotic syndrome), & hepatic (increased liver enzymes) effects.

▶ Drug Interactions.

Uses/Indications

A NSAID that is commonly used in humans, naproxen is rarely recommended for veterinary patients. There are effective, safer, and approved alternatives.

Pharmacology/Actions

Like other NSAIDs, naproxen exhibits analgesic, antiinflammatory, and antipyretic activity probably through its inhibition of cyclooxygenase with resultant impediment of prostaglandin synthesis.

Pharmacokinetics

In horses, the drug is reported to have a 50% bioavailability after oral dosing and a half-life of ≈4 hours. Absorption does not appear to be altered by the presence of food. It may take 5-7 days to see a beneficial response after starting treatment. Following a dose, the drug is metabolized in the liver. It is detectable in the urine for at least 48 hours in the horse after an oral dose.

In dogs, absorption after oral dosing is rapid and bioavailability is between 68-100%. The drug is highly bound to plasma proteins. The average half-life in dogs is very long at 74 hours.

In humans, naproxen is highly bound to plasma proteins (99%). It crosses the placenta and enters milk in levels of ≈1% of those found in serum.

Contraindications/Precautions/Warnings

Naproxen is relatively contraindicated in patients with a history of or preexisting hematologic, renal, or hepatic disease. It is contraindicated in patients with active GI ulcers, or with a history of hypersensitivity to the drug. It should be used cautiously in patients with a history of GI ulcers, or heart failure (may cause fluid retention). Animals suffering from inflammation secondary to concomitant infection, should receive appropriate antimicrobial therapy.

Adverse Effects

Adverse effects are apparently uncommon in horses. The possibility exists for GI (distress, diarrhea, ulcers), hematologic (hypoproteinemia, decreased hematocrit), renal (fluid retention), and CNS (neuropathies) effects.

Reports of GI ulcers and perforation associated with naproxen have occurred in dogs. Dogs may also be overly sensitive to the adverse renal (nephritis/nephrotic syndrome) and hepatic effects (increased liver enzymes) of naproxen. Because of the apparently very narrow therapeutic index and the seriousness of the potential adverse reactions that can be seen in dogs, many clinicians feel that the drug should not be used in this species.

Reproductive/Nursing Safety

In humans, the FDA categorizes this drug as category *B* for use during pregnancy (*Animal studies have not yet demonstrated risk to the fetus, but there are no adequate studies in pregnant women; or animal studies have shown an adverse effect, but adequate studies in pregnant women have not demonstrated a risk to the fetus in the first trimester of pregnancy, and there is no evidence of risk in later trimesters.*) In studies in rodents and in limited studies in horses, no evidence of teratogenicity or adverse effects in breeding performance have been detected following the use of naproxen. Weigh the potential benefits of therapy against the potential risks of its use in pregnant animals.

Most NSAIDs are excreted in maternal milk. Naproxen appears at ≈1% of maternal serum concentration.

Overdosage/Acute Toxicity

There is limited information regarding acute overdoses of this drug in humans and domestic animals. The reported oral LD50 in dogs is >1000 mg/kg. In dogs, PO ingestions of >5 mg/kg can cause gastrointestinal signs and GI ulceration; >25 mg/kg (some dogs as low as 10 mg/kg) can cause significant renal damage, and >50 mg/kg can result in neuro signs.

One report of a dog that received 5.6 mg/kg for 7 days has been published (Gilmour *et al.* 1987). The dog presented with clinical signs of melena, vomiting, depression, regenerative anemia, and pale mucous membranes. Laboratory indices of note included neutrophilia with a left shift, BUN of 66 mg/dL, serum creatinine of 2.1 mg/dL, serum protein to albumin ratio of 4.0:2.1 grams/dL. The dog recovered following treatment with fluids/blood, antibiotics, vitamin/iron supplementation, oral antacids, and cimetidine.

There were 817 exposures to naproxen reported to the ASPCA Animal Poison Control Center (APCC) during 2008-2009. In these cases 764 were dogs with 335 dogs showing clinical signs, 49 cats with 13 showing clinical signs, 2 rodents with 1 showing clinical signs and the remaining 2 cases were 1 bird and 1 bovine showing no clinical signs. Common findings in dogs recorded in decreasing frequency included vomiting, lethargy, anorexia, bloody vomitus, diarrhea, melena, and anemia. Common findings in cats recorded in decreasing frequency included vomiting, lethargy, and anorexia.

As with any NSAID, overdosage can lead to gastrointestinal and renal effects. Decontamination with emetics and/or activated charcoal is appropriate. For doses where GI effects are expected, the use of gastrointestinal protectants, including misoprostol and sucralfate should be considered GI protectant treatment is generally recommended for 10-14 days post-exposure. If renal effects are also expected, fluid diuresis should be considered. Supportive treatment should be instituted as necessary. Monitor electrolyte and fluid balance carefully and manage renal failure using established guidelines.

Drug Interactions

The following drug interactions have either been reported or are theoretical in humans or animals receiving naproxen and may be of significance in veterinary patients. Unless otherwise noted, use together is not necessarily contraindicated, but weigh the potential risks and perform additional monitoring when appropriate.

- **AMINOGLYCOSIDES (gentamicin, amikacin**, etc.): Increased risk for nephrotoxicity.
- **ANTICOAGULANTS (heparin, LMWH, warfarin**): Increased risk for bleeding possible.
- **ASPIRIN**: When aspirin is used concurrently with naproxen, plasma levels of naproxen could decrease and an increased likelihood of GI adverse effects (blood loss) could occur. Concomitant administration of aspirin with naproxen cannot be recommended.
- **BISPHOSPHONATES (alendronate**, etc.): May increase risk for GI ulceration.
- **CORTICOSTEROIDS**: Concomitant administration with NSAIDs may significantly increase the risks for GI adverse effects.
- **FUROSEMIDE**: Naproxen may reduce the saluretic and diuretic effects of furosemide.
- **HIGHLY PROTEIN BOUND DRUGS** (*e.g.,* **phenytoin, valproic acid, oral anticoagulants, other antiinflammatory agents, salicylates, sulfonamides**, and the **sulfonylurea antidiabetic agents**): Because naproxen is highly bound to plasma proteins (99%), it potentially could displace other highly bound drugs; increased serum levels and duration of actions may occur. Although these interactions are usually of little concern clinically, use together with caution.
- **METHOTREXATE**: Serious toxicity has occurred when NSAIDs have been used concomitantly with methotrexate; use together with extreme caution.
- **PROBENECID**: May cause a significant increase in serum levels and half-life of naproxen.

Doses

- **DOGS:**

  For pain and inflammation (extra-label): **Note:** Because of the difficulty in accurately dosing naproxen and its potential for adverse effects, the use of this drug in dogs should only be considered when FDA-approved and safer NSAIDs have been ineffective and the client is aware that serious adverse effects can occur. An anecdotal dosage of 2 mg/kg PO every other day (q48h) has been noted.

- **RABBITS, RODENTS, SMALL MAMMALS:**

  For septic arthritis pain; inflammation in rabbits (extra-label): 2.4 mg/mL in drinking water for 21 days. (Ivey *et al.* 2000)

- **HORSES:** (NOTE: ARCI UCGFS CLASS 4 DRUG)

  For pain and inflammation: 5 mg/kg by slow IV, then 10 mg/kg, PO (top dressed in feed) twice daily for up to 14 days or 10 mg/kg, PO (top dressed in feed) twice daily for up to 14 consecutive days. (Package Insert; *Equiproxen*®; **Note:** No longer commercially available)

Monitoring

- Analgesic/antiinflammatory efficacy.
- GI: appetite, feces (occult blood, diarrhea).
- PCV (packed cell volume), hematocrit if indicated or on chronic therapy.
- WBC's if indicated or on chronic therapy.

Client Information

- Notify veterinarian if clinical signs of GI distress (anorexia, vomiting, diarrhea, black feces, or blood in stool) occur, or if animal becomes depressed.

Chemistry/Synonyms

Naproxen is a propionic acid derivative, having similar structure and pharmacologic profiles as ibuprofen and ketoprofen. It is a white to off-white crystalline powder with an apparent pKa of 4.15. It is practically insoluble in water and freely soluble in alcohol. The sodium salt is also available commercially for human use.

Naproxen may also be known as: naproxeneum, RS-3540, RS-3650, *Aleve*®, *Anaprox*®, *EC-Naprosyn*®, *Midol*®, *Naprelan*® and *Naprosyn*®.

Storage/Stability

Naproxen should be stored in well-closed, light resistant containers at room temperature. Temperatures above 40° C (104°F) should be avoided.

Compatibility/Compounding Considerations

No specific information noted.

Dosage Forms/Regulatory Status

VETERINARY-LABELED PRODUCTS:

None; the equine product is no longer marketed in the USA. The ARCI (Racing Commissioners International) has designated this drug as a class 4 substance. See the appendix for more information.

HUMAN-LABELED PRODUCTS:

Naproxen Oral Tablets or Capsules: 200 mg (220 mg naproxen sodium), 250 mg (275 mg naproxen sodium), 375 mg, 500 mg (550 mg naproxen sodium); there are many proprietary named products including: *Naprosyn®*, *Anaprox®*, *Aleve®*, generic; (Rx and OTC–220 mg naproxen sodium only)

Naproxen Delayed/Controlled-release Tablets: 375 mg, 500 mg & 750 mg; *EC-Naprosyn®*, *Naprelan®*, Naproxen DR®, generic; (Rx)

Naproxen Oral Suspension: 125 mg/5 mL in 15 mL, 20 mL, 473 mL & 500 mL; *Naprosyn®*; (Rx)

Revisions/References

Monograph revised/updated April 2014.

Gilmour, M. A. & R. Walshaw (1987). Naproxen-induced toxicosis in a dog. JAVMA **191**(11): 1431-2.

Ivey, E. & J. Morrisey (2000). Therapeutics for Rabbits. Vet Clin NA: Exotic Anim Pract **3:1**(Jan): 183-216.

Narcotic (Opiate) Agonist Analgesics, Pharmacology of

Receptors for opiate analgesics are found in high concentrations in the limbic system, spinal cord, thalamus, hypothalamus, striatum, and midbrain. They are also found in tissues such as the gastrointestinal tract, urinary tract, and in other smooth muscle.

Opiate receptors are further broken down into five main subgroups. *Mu* receptors are found primarily in the pain regulating areas of the brain. They are thought to contribute to the analgesia, euphoria, respiratory depression, physical dependence, miosis, and hypothermic actions of opiates. *Kappa* receptors are located primarily in the deep layers of the cerebral cortex and spinal cord. They are responsible for analgesia, sedation, and miosis. *Sigma* receptors are thought to be responsible for the dysphoric effects (struggling, whining), hallucinations, respiratory and cardiac stimulation, and mydriatic effects of opiates. *Delta* receptors, located in the limbic areas of the CNS, and epsilon receptors have also been described, but their actions have not been well explained at this time.

The morphine-like agonists (morphine, meperidine, oxymorphone) have primary activity at the *mu* receptors, with some activity possible at the *delta* receptor. The primary pharmacologic effects of these agents include: analgesia, antitussive activity, respiratory depression, sedation, emesis, physical dependence, and intestinal effects (constipation/defecation). Secondary pharmacologic effects include, <u>CNS</u>: euphoria, sedation, and confusion. <u>Cardiovascular</u>: bradycardia due to central vagal stimulation, alpha-adrenergic receptors may be depressed resulting in peripheral vasodilation, decreased peripheral resistance, and baroreceptor inhibition. Orthostatic hypotension and syncope may occur. <u>Urinary</u>: Increased bladder sphincter tone can induce urinary retention.

Various species may exhibit contradictory effects from these agents. For example, horses, cattle, swine, and cats may develop excitement after morphine injections and dogs may defecate after morphine. These effects are in contrast to the expected effects of sedation and constipation. Dogs and humans may develop miosis, while other species (especially cats) may develop mydriasis. For more information see the individual monographs for each agent.

N-Butylscopolammonium Bromide — Monograph is found at the beginning of the N's

Neomycin Sulfate

(nee-o-mye-sin)   Biosol®, Neomix®

Oral Aminoglycoside Antibiotic

Prescriber Highlights

▶ Aminoglycoside antibiotic usually used orally (gut "sterilization"). Also found in topical formulations.

▶ Contraindications: Hypersensitivity to aminoglycosides, intestinal blockage, rabbits.

▶ Adverse Effects: Chronic use can lead to GI superinfections. Rarely, oral neomycin may cause ototoxicity, nephrotoxicity, severe diarrhea, & intestinal malabsorption. Horses may be susceptible to enterocolitis from neomycin.

▶ Minimal amounts absorbed via GI (if intact).

Uses/Indications

Because neomycin is more nephrotoxic and less effective against several bacterial species than either gentamicin or amikacin, its use is generally limited to topical formulations for skin, eyes, and ears, oral treatment of enteric infections, to reduce microbe numbers in the colon prior to colon surgery, and oral or enema administration to reduce ammonia-producing bacteria in the treatment of hepatic encephalopathy.

Pharmacology/Actions

Neomycin has a mechanism of action and spectrum of activity (primarily gram-negative aerobes) similar to the other aminoglycosides, but in comparison to either gentamicin or amikacin, it is significantly less effective against several species of gram-negative organisms, including strains of Klebsiella, *E. coli*, and Pseudomonas. However, most strains of neomycin-resistant bacteria of these species remain susceptible to amikacin. More detailed information on the aminoglycosides mechanism of action and spectrum of activity is outlined in the amikacin monograph.

Pharmacokinetics

Approximately 3% of a dose of neomycin is absorbed after oral or rectal (retention enema) administration, but this can be increased if gut motility is slowed or if the bowel wall is damaged. Therapeutic levels are not attained in the systemic circulation after oral administration.

After IM administration, therapeutic levels can be attained with peak levels occurring within 1 hour of dosing. The drug apparently distributes to tissues and is eliminated like the other aminoglycosides (refer to Amikacin monograph for more details). Orally administered neomycin is nearly all excreted unchanged in the feces.

Contraindications/Precautions/Warnings

Oral neomycin is contraindicated in the presence of intestinal obstruction or if the patient is hypersensitive to aminoglycosides.

In neonates, orally administered neomycin can yield high systemic levels; avoid use in neonatal patients.

Aminoglycosides are generally considered contraindicated in rabbits/hares, as they adversely affect the GI flora balance in these animals. Oral neomycin has been associated with antibiotic-associated diarrhea (enterocolitis) in horses and is not commonly used in this species.

Chronic usage of oral aminoglycosides may result in bacterial or fungal superinfections.

Adverse Effects

Antibiotic-associated diarrhea can occur and some species may be more susceptible (*e.g.*, horses). Rarely, oral neomycin may cause ototoxicity, nephrotoxicity, severe diarrhea, and intestinal malabsorption.

Reproductive/Nursing Safety

In humans, the FDA categorizes this drug as category *C* for use during pregnancy (*Animal studies have shown an adverse effect on the fetus, but there are no adequate studies in humans; or there are no animal reproduction studies and no adequate studies in humans.*) In a separate system evaluating the safety of drugs in canine and feline pregnancy (Papich 1989), this drug is categorized as class: *A* (*Probably safe. Although specific studies may not have proved he safety of all drugs in dogs and cats, there are no reports of adverse effects in laboratory animals or women.*)

Neomycin is excreted in cow's milk following a single IM injection. If used orally, it is unlikely neomycin poses significant systemic risk to nursing offspring, but may negatively alter gut flora and cause diarrhea.

Drug Interactions

The following drug interactions have either been reported or are theoretical in humans or animals receiving oral neomycin and may be of significance in veterinary patients. Unless otherwise noted, use together is not necessarily contraindicated, but weigh the potential risks and perform additional monitoring when appropriate.

- **DIGOXIN:** Oral neomycin with orally administered digoxin may result in decreased absorption. Separating the doses of the two medications may not alleviate this effect. Some human patients (<10%) metabolize digoxin in the GI tract and neomycin may increase serum digoxin levels in these patients. It is recommended that enhanced monitoring be performed if oral neomycin is added or withdrawn from the drug regimen of a patient stabilized on a digitalis glycoside.
- **METHOTREXATE:** Absorption may be reduced by oral neomycin but is increased by oral kanamycin (found in *Amforal®*).
- **OTOTOXIC, NEPHROTOXIC DRUGS:** Although only minimal amounts of neomycin are absorbed after oral or rectal administration, the concurrent use of other ototoxic or nephrotoxic drugs with neomycin should be done with caution.
- **PENICILLIN VK (oral):** Oral neomycin should not be given concurrently with oral penicillin VK as malabsorption of the penicillin may occur.
- **WARFARIN:** Oral neomycin may decrease the amount of vitamin K absorbed from the gut; this may have ramifications for patients receiving oral anticoagulants.

Laboratory Considerations

- No specific concerns noted.

Doses

- **DOGS/CATS:**

For adjunctive treatment of hepatic encephalopathy (extra-label):

a) A check list for acute management of hepatic encephalopathy includes: **1)** Lactulose (orally, or by enema if stupor or seizures; see lactulose monograph for dosages); **2)** NPO for 12-24 hours. **3)** If no response, add metronidazole orally at 15 mg/kg/day. **4)** If no response, add neomycin orally at 20 mg/kg PO 3 times daily. **5)** Provide IV fluids with potassium (and dextrose for patients with portosystemic shunts or severe cirrhosis). **6)** Add anti-ulcer therapy (GI bleeding is a protein load in hepatic encephalopathy), and add vitamin K1 if jaundiced. **7)** Withhold any glucocorticoids until encephalopathy is resolved. **8)** Give as much dietary protein as tolerated; increase the lactulose dosage if needed. (Trepanier 2008)

b) Animals that are neurologically and systemically stable should be treated with orally-administered nonabsorbable antibiotics in order to decrease the numbers of urease-producing bacteria within the gastrointestinal tract. If using neomycin: 20 mg/kg PO q12h. Avoid neomycin if any evidence of intestinal bleeding, ulcerations, or renal failure. The use of oral lactulose therapy, in conjunction with or as an alternative to antibiotics, is also beneficial in neurologically stable animals. The combination of neomycin and lactulose may be synergistic. (Silverstein 2009)

For GI tract infections (extra-label): For campylobacteriosis: 20 mg/kg PO q12h. (Willard 2003)

- **FERRETS:**

For susceptible enteric infections (extra-label): 10 – 20 mg/kg, PO 2-4 times daily. (Williams 2000)

- **RODENTS, SMALL MAMMALS:**

Note: Contraindicated in rabbits/hares, hamsters. Best to avoid use in any hindgut fermenter.

- **HORSES:**

For hyperammonemia (extra-label): 20 – 30 mg/kg PO q6h.

- **CATTLE:**

For oral administration to treat susceptible enteral infections (labeled-dose): **Note:** One reference states: "Published studies do not support the oral administration of potentiated sulfonamides, tetracyclines or neomycin in the treatment of calf scours" (Coetzee 2013). Labeled dose: Feed at levels of 70 – 140 grams/ton of feed or mix the appropriate dose in the drinking water that will be consumed by animals in 12 hours to provide 11 mg/kg or mix with reconstituted milk replacers to provide 200 – 400 mg/gallon. (Label directions; *Neomix Ag® 325*—Upjohn)

- **SHEEP & GOATS:**

For oral administration to treat susceptible enteral infections (labeled-dose): Feed at levels of 70 – 140 grams/ton of feed or mix the appropriate dose in the drinking water that will be consumed by animals in 12 hours to provide 11 mg/kg or mix with reconstituted milk replacers to provide 200 – 400 mg/gallon. (Label directions; *Neomix Ag® 325*—Upjohn)

- **BIRDS:**

For bacterial enteritis (labeled-dose): Chickens, turkeys, ducks: Feed at levels of 70 – 140 grams/ton of feed or mix the appropriate dose in the drinking water that will be consumed by animals in 12 hours to provide 11 mg/kg. (Label directions; *Neomix Ag® 325*—Upjohn)

- **REPTILES:**

For bacterial gastritis in snakes (extra-label): Gentamicin 2.5 mg/kg IM every 72 hours with oral neomycin 15 mg/kg plus oral live lactobacillus. (Burke 1986)

Monitoring

For oral use:

- Clinical efficacy.
- Systemic and GI adverse effects with prolonged use.

Client Information

- Oral antibiotic used to reduce bacteria in GI tract before surgery or to reduce ammonia-producing bacteria. Should **not** be given to hamsters, rabbits or hares.
- May be given by mouth with or without food. If your animal vomits or acts sick after getting it on an empty stomach, give with food or small treat to see if this helps. If vomiting continues, contact your veterinarian.
- When used by mouth for short periods, neomycin usually is tolerated well. Not much is absorbed orally, but still can damage the

nerves, hearing, and kidneys especially if used for a long time or in animals that have ulcers in their intestines. Cats may be more likely to have damage to hearing.

■ Can cause diarrhea.

Chemistry/Synonyms

An aminoglycoside antibiotic obtained from *Streptomyces fradiae*, neomycin is actually a complex of three separate compounds, neomycin A (neamine; inactive), neomycin C, and neomycin B (framycetin). The commercially available product almost entirely consists of the sulfate salt of neomycin B. It occurs as an odorless or almost odorless, white to slightly yellow, hygroscopic powder or cryodessicated solid. It is freely soluble in water and very slightly soluble in alcohol. One mg of pure neomycin sulfate is equivalent to not less than 650 Units.

Neomycin sulfate may also be known as: fradiomycin sulfate, neomycin sulphate, or neomycini sulfas, *Neo-325®*, *Neo-fradin®*, *Neo-Sol 50®*, and *Neovet®*.

Storage/Stability

Neomycin sulfate oral solution should be stored at room temperature (15-30°C) in tight, light-resistant containers. Unless otherwise instructed by the manufacturer, oral tablets/boluses should be stored in tight containers at room temperature.

In the dry state, neomycin is stable for at least 2 years at room temperature.

Compatibility/Compounding Considerations

No specific information noted.

Dosage Forms/Regulatory Status

VETERINARY-LABELED PRODUCTS:

Neomycin Sulfate; Oral Liquid: 200 mg/mL (140 mg neomycin base/mL); generic; (OTC). Depending on labeling FDA-approved for use in cattle, swine, sheep, goats, turkeys, laying hens, and broilers. Check labels for slaughter withdrawals; may vary with product. General withdrawal times (when used as labeled): Cattle = 1 day; Sheep = 2 days and swine and goats = 3 days. Withdrawal period has not been established in pre-ruminating calves. Do not use in calves to be processed for veal. A milk discard period has not been established in lactating dairy cattle. Do not use in female dairy cattle 20 months of age or older.

Neomycin Sulfate Soluble Powder: 325 grams/lb: *Neo-325® Soluble Powder, Neovet® 325/100 & NeoVet® 325 AG Grade* (includes turkey label), *Neo-Sol 50®*; (OTC). FDA-approved for use in cattle and goats (not veal calves), swine, sheep, goats and turkeys (some products). Check labels for slaughter withdrawals; may vary with product. General slaughter withdrawal times (when used as labeled): Cattle = 1 day; Turkeys = 0 days; Sheep = 2 days; Swine and Goats = 3 days.

HUMAN-LABELED PRODUCTS:

Neomycin Sulfate Tablets: 500 mg; generic; (Rx)

Revisions/References

Monograph revised/updated April 2014.

Burke, T. J. (1986). Regurgitation in snakes. *Current Veterinary Therapy (CVT) IX Small Animal Practice*. R. W. Kirk. Philadelphia, WB Saunders: 749-50.

Coetzee, H. (2013). Treatment and Prevention of Calf Scours. Proceedings: 65th Convention of the Canadian Veterinary Medical Association. accessed via Veterinary Information Network; vin.com

Papich, M. (1989). Effects of drugs on pregnancy. *Current Veterinary Therapy X: Small Animal Practice*. R. Kirk. Philadelphia, Saunders: 1291-9.

Silverstein, D. (2009). Management of hepatic encephalopathy. Proceedings: Western Veterinary Conf. accessed via Veterinary Information Network; vin.com

Trepanier, L. (2008). Choosing therapy for chronic liver disease. Proceedings: WSAVA. accessed via Veterinary Information Network; vin.com

Willard, M. (2003). Disorders of the intestinal tract. *Small Animal Internal Medicine, 3rd Ed.* R. Nelson and C. Couto. St Louis, Mosby: 431-65.

Williams, B. (2000). Therapeutics in Ferrets. *Vet Clin NA: Exotic Anim Pract* **3:1**(Jan): 131-53.

Neostigmine

(nee-oh-**stig**-meen)   Prostigmin®

Parasympathomimetic (Cholinergic)

Prescriber Highlights

▶ Parasympathomimetic used to initiate peristalsis, empty the bladder, & stimulate skeletal muscle contractions. Also for diagnosis & treatment of myasthenia gravis & treatment/reversal of non-depolarizing neuromuscular blocking agents (curare-type) overdose.

▶ Contraindications: Peritonitis, mechanical intestinal or urinary tract obstructions, late stages of pregnancy, hypersensitivity to this class of compounds, or if treated with other cholinesterase inhibitors.

▶ Adverse Effects: Cholinergic in nature & dose related (nausea, vomiting, diarrhea, excessive salivation & drooling, sweating, miosis, lacrimation, increased bronchial secretions, bradycardia or tachycardia, cardiospasm, bronchospasm, hypotension, muscle cramps & weakness, agitation, restlessness, or paralysis).

▶ Cholinergic crisis & myasthenic crisis must not be confused.

Uses/Indications

Neostigmine as a veterinary product is labeled as indicated for rumen atony, initiating peristalsis, emptying the bladder, and stimulating skeletal muscle contractions in cattle, horses, sheep, and swine (Package insert; *Stiglyn® 1:500-P/M*—Mallinckrodt). It has been used in the diagnosis and treatment of myasthenia gravis and in treating non-depolarizing neuromuscular blocking agents (curare-type) overdoses in dogs.

Pharmacology/Actions

Neostigmine competes with acetylcholine for acetylcholinesterase. As the neostigmine-acetylcholinesterase complex is hydrolyzed at a slower rate than that of the acetylcholine-enzyme complex, acetylcholine will accumulate with a resultant exaggeration and prolongation of its effects. These effects can include increased tone of intestinal and skeletal musculature, stimulation of salivary and sweat glands, bronchoconstriction, ureter constriction, miosis and bradycardia. Neostigmine also has a direct cholinomimetic effect on skeletal muscle.

In horses, it has been reported that neostigmine decreases jejunal activity and delays gastric emptying, but a study where horses were administered neostigmine at 0.008 mg/kg/hr as a CRI reported increased fecal production and urination frequency and that it did not decrease gastric emptying. They also found that neostigmine stimulated contractile activity of jejunum and pelvic flexure smooth muscle strips *in vitro* (Nieto et al. 2013). Neostigmine's use for treating colon impactions and post-operative ileus is controversial and more studies are necessary to determine its clinical usefulness for these indications in horses.

Pharmacokinetics

Information on the pharmacokinetics of neostigmine in veterinary species was not located. In humans, neostigmine bromide is poorly absorbed after oral administration with only 1-2% of the dose absorbed. Neostigmine effects on peristaltic activity in humans begin within 10-30 minutes after parenteral administration and can persist for up to 4 hours.

Neostigmine is 15-25% bound to plasma proteins. It has not been detected in human milk nor would it be expected to cross the placenta when given at usual doses.

In humans, the half-life of the drug is ≈1 hour. It is metabolized in the liver and hydrolyzed by cholinesterases to 3-OH PTM, which is weakly active. When administered parenterally, ≈80% of the drug is excreted in the urine within 24 hours, with 50% excreted unchanged.

Contraindications/Precautions/Warnings

Neostigmine is contraindicated in patients with peritonitis, mechanical intestinal or urinary tract obstructions, in animals hypersensitive to this class of compounds or treated with other cholinesterase inhibitors.

Use neostigmine with caution in patients with epilepsy, peptic ulcer disease, bronchial asthma, cardiac arrhythmias, hyperthyroidism, vagotonia, or megacolon.

Adverse Effects

Adverse effects of neostigmine are dose-related and cholinergic in nature. A case report of a dog developing a cholinergic crisis after receiving a dose of 0.05 mg/kg SC has been published (Foy *et al.* 2011). For more information on cholinergic signs, see the overdosage section below.

Reproductive/Nursing Safety

In humans, the FDA categorizes this drug as category *C* for use during pregnancy (*Animal studies have shown an adverse effect on the fetus, but there are no adequate studies in humans; or there are no animal reproduction studies and no adequate studies in humans.*)

Because it is ionized at physiologic pH, neostigmine would not be expected to be excreted in maternal milk.

Overdosage/Acute Toxicity

Overdosage of neostigmine can induce a cholinergic crisis. Clinical signs can include: nausea, vomiting, diarrhea, excessive salivation and drooling, sweating (in animals with sweat glands), miosis, lacrimation, increased bronchial secretions, bradycardia or tachycardia, cardiospasm, bronchospasm, hypotension, muscle cramps and weakness, agitation, restlessness, or paralysis. In patients with myasthenia gravis, it may be difficult to distinguish between a cholinergic crisis and myasthenic crisis. A test dose of edrophonium should differentiate between the two.

Treat cholinergic crisis by temporarily ceasing neostigmine therapy and instituting treatment with atropine. Maintain adequate respirations using mechanical assistance if necessary.

Drug Interactions

The following drug interactions have either been reported or are theoretical in humans or animals receiving neostigmine and may be of significance in veterinary patients. Unless otherwise noted, use together is not necessarily contraindicated, but weigh the potential risks and perform additional monitoring when appropriate.

- **ATROPINE:** Atropine will antagonize the muscarinic effects of neostigmine and some clinicians routinely use the two together, but concurrent use should be used cautiously as atropine can mask the early clinical signs of cholinergic crisis.
- **CORTICOSTEROIDS:** May decrease the anticholinesterase activity of neostigmine; after stopping corticosteroid therapy, neostigmine may cause increased anticholinesterase activity.
- **DEXPANTHENOL:** Theoretically, dexpanthenol may have additive effects when used with neostigmine.
- **MAGNESIUM:** Anticholinesterase therapy may be antagonized by administration of parenteral magnesium therapy, as it can have a direct depressant effect on skeletal muscle.
- **MUSCLE RELAXANTS:** Neostigmine may prolong the Phase I block of depolarizing muscle relaxants (*e.g.,* **succinylcholine, decamethonium**) and edrophonium antagonizes the actions of non-depolarizing neuromuscular blocking agents (*e.g.,* **pancuronium, tubocurarine, gallamine, vecuronium, atracurium,** etc.).

Laboratory Considerations

- No specific concerns noted.

Doses

- **DOGS/CATS:**

    For treatment of myasthenia gravis (extra-label): If pyridostigmine is not available or oral medication cannot be given in actively regurgitating animals: 0.04 mg/kg IM, SC q6h.

    For diagnosis of myasthenia gravis (extra-label): When edrophonium (*Tensilon®*) is not available: 0.04 mg/kg SC, IM or 0.02 mg/kg IV. Some pre-treat with atropine, but this must be done with caution as it can mask the early signs associated with a cholinergic crisis. If clinical improvement occurs in 15-30 minutes it is suggestive of a diagnosis.

- **CATTLE:**

    For rumen atony; initiating peristalsis to cause evacuation of the bowel; emptying the urinary bladder; and stimulating skeletal muscle contractions (labeled-dose): 1 mg/100 lbs. of body weight SC; repeat as indicated. (Package Insert; *Stiglyn® 1:500-P/M*)

- **HORSES:** (NOTE: ARCI UCGFS CLASS 3 DRUG)

    For initiating peristalsis to cause evacuation of the bowel; emptying the urinary bladder; and stimulating skeletal muscle contractions (labeled-dose): 1 mg/100 lbs. of body weight SC; repeat as indicated. (Package Insert; *Stiglyn® 1:500-P/M*)

    As a reversal agent for neuromuscular blockers (extra-label): Reversal is not attempted until some degree of spontaneous recovery has been established. A dose of 0.007 mg/kg has been used in some studies with mild rocuronium-induced blockade. (Auer *et al.* 2011), (Auer *et al.* 2007), (Martin-Flores 2013)

- **SWINE:**

    For initiating peristalsis to cause evacuation of the bowel; emptying the urinary bladder; and stimulating skeletal muscle contractions (labeled-dose): 2 – 3 mg/100 lbs. of body weight IM; repeat as indicated. (Package Insert; *Stiglyn® 1:500-P/M*)

- **SHEEP:**

    For rumen atony; initiating peristalsis that causes evacuation of the bowel; emptying the urinary bladder; and stimulating skeletal muscle contractions (labeled-dose): 1 – 1.5 mg/100 lbs. of body weight SC; repeat as indicated. (Package Insert; *Stiglyn® 1:500-P/M*)

Monitoring

Dependent on reason for use.

- Adverse reactions (see Adverse Effects and Overdosage above).
- Clinical efficacy.

Client Information

- This drug should only be used in a setting where professionals can monitor the drug's effects.

Chemistry/Synonyms

Synthetic quaternary ammonium parasympathomimetic agents, neostigmine bromide and neostigmine methylsulfate both occur as odorless, bitter-tasting, white, crystalline powders that are very soluble in water and soluble in alcohol. The melting point of neostigmine methylsulfate is from 144-149°. The pH of the commercially available neostigmine methylsulfate injection is from 5-6.5.

Neostigmine methylsulfate may also be known as: neostigmine metilsulfate, neostigmine methylsulphate, neostigmini metilsulfas, proserinum, or *Prostigmin®, Prostigmina®, or Stiglyn®.*

Storage/Stability

Neostigmine bromide tablets should be stored at room temperature in tight containers. Neostigmine methylsulfate injection should be stored at room temperature and protected from light; avoid freezing.

Compatibility/Compounding Considerations

Neostigmine methylsulfate injection is reportedly physically **compatible** with the commonly used IV replacement solutions and the following drugs: glycopyrrolate, pentobarbital sodium, and thiopental sodium.

Dosage Forms/Regulatory Status

VETERINARY-LABELED PRODUCTS: NONE.

Historically, there was an approved injectable product (*Stiglyn*® 1:500), and although still listed in FDA's Green book, it does not appear to be marketed. The ARCI (Racing Commissioners International) has designated this drug as a class 3 substance. See the appendix for more information.

HUMAN-LABELED PRODUCTS:

Neostigmine Methylsulfate Injection: 1:1000 (1 mg/mL) in 10 mL vials, 1:2000 (0.5 mg/mL) in 1 mL amps & 10 mL vials; *Prostigmin*®, generic; (Rx)

Neostigmine Bromide Oral Tablets: 15 mg; *Prostigmin*®; (Rx)

Revisions/References

Monograph revised/updated April 2014.

Auer, U. & Y. Moens (2011). Neuromuscular blockade with rocuronium bromide for ophthalmic surgery in horses. Vet. Ophthalmol. **14**(4): 244-7.

Auer, U., et al. (2007). Observations on the muscle relaxant rocuronium bromide in the horse - a dose-response study. Veterinary Anaesthesia and Analgesia **34**(2): 75-81.

Foy, D. S., et al. (2011). Cholinergic crisis after neostigmine administration in a dog with acquired focal myasthenia gravis. J. Vet. Emerg. Crit. Care **21**(5): 547-51.

Martin-Flores, M. (2013). Neuromuscular Blocking Agents and Monitoring in the Equine Patient. Veterinary Clinics of North America-Equine Practice **29**(1): 131-+.

Nieto, J. E., et al. (2013). In vivo and in vitro effects of neostigmine on gastrointestinal tract motility of horses. American Journal of Veterinary Research **74**(4): 579-88.

Niacinamide

(nye-a-**sin**-a-mide)   Nicotinamide

Immunomodulator; Nutritional

Prescriber Highlights

▶ Used in canine medicine in combination with a tetracycline for treatment of a variety of sterile inflammatory skin conditions.

▶ Possible Contraindications: Liver disease, active peptic ulcers, or hypersensitivity to it.

▶ Adverse Effects: Anorexia, vomiting, & lethargy; occasionally increases in liver enzymes seen. Giving with food may help limit GI effects.

▶ Improvement may be gradual & take 6-8+ weeks.

▶ Inexpensive, but 3 times a day dosing may be problematic.

Uses/Indications

When used in conjunction with tetracycline or doxycycline (or minocycline), niacinamide may be useful in controlling a variety of sterile inflammatory skin conditions in dogs including: discoid lupus erythematosus (DLE), sterile granulomatous/pyogranulomatous syndrome, sterile nodular panniculitis, cutaneous reactive histiocytosis, cutaneous vesicular lupus erythematosus, pemphigus erythematosus, pemphigus foliaceus, lupoid onychodystrophy/onychitis, German shepherd dog metatarsal fistulae, vasculitis, arteritis of the nasal philtrum, sebaceous adenitis and dermatomyositiss (Koch *et al.* 2011). Controlled studies demonstrating clear efficacy are lacking, but anecdotally it appears effective in some patients including up to 2/3 of dogs that are treated for DLE. Often used in conjunction with other immunomodulating drugs, especially in the initial treatment phase. Nicainamide (with a tetracycline) may make take 1-2 months before efficacy is noted.

Pharmacology/Actions

While niacinamide is an essential nutrient in humans (necessary for lipid metabolism, tissue respiration, and glycogenolysis) its primary pharmacologic use (in combination with a tetracycline) for sterile inflammatory skin disorders in dogs is secondary to its action of blocking IgE-induced histamine release and degranulation of mast cells. When used with tetracycline, niacinamide may suppress leukocyte chemotaxis secondary to complement activation by antibody-antigen complexes. It also inhibits phosphodiesterases and decreases the release of proteases. While niacinamide and niacin act identically as vitamins, niacinamide does not affect blood lipid levels or the cardiovascular system.

Pharmacokinetics

Niacinamide is absorbed well after oral administration and widely distributed to body tissues. Niacinamide is metabolized in the liver to several metabolites that are excreted into the urine. At physiologic doses, only a small amount of niacinamide is excreted into the urine unchanged, but as dosages increase, larger quantities are excreted unchanged.

Contraindications/Precautions/Warnings

In humans, niacinamide therapy is contraindicated in patients with liver disease, active peptic ulcers, or hypersensitivity to the drug. Use niacinamide/tetracycline with caution in dogs with a seizure history.

Adverse Effects

Adverse effects of niacinamide in dogs are uncommon, but may include anorexia, vomiting, and lethargy. Occasionally, increases in liver enzymes may be noted. There have been some anecdotal reports of increased seizure frequencies in dogs. Because niacinamide is used clinically in combination with a tetracycline, adverse effects noted may be due to niacinamide and/or the tetracycline.

Reproductive/Nursing Safety

While niacinamide alone should be safe to use in pregnant and lactating animals, its use in combination with tetracycline may not be safe.

Overdosage/Acute Toxicity

There is unlikely to be a problem with niacinamide overdoses other than acute GI distress.

Niacinamide may interfere with intradermal and serum allergy testing. If possible, consider withdrawing the drug at least 2 weeks prior to allergy testing.

Drug Interactions

Niacinamide and tetracycline treatment does not interfere with antibody production associated with routine vaccinations in dogs. Also see the tetracycline, doxycycline or minocycline monographs for additional drug interactions if using combination therapy.

The following drug interactions have either been reported or are theoretical in humans or animals receiving niacinamide and may be of significance in veterinary patients. Unless otherwise noted, use together is not necessarily contraindicated, but weigh the potential risks and perform additional monitoring when appropriate.

■ **INSULIN/ORAL ANTIDIABETIC AGENTS:** In diabetic humans, dosage adjustments for insulin or oral antidiabetic agents have sometimes been necessary after initiating niacinamide therapy.

Laboratory Considerations

■ Potentially could interfere with intradermal or serum **allergy testing**. If possible, consider withdrawing the drug 1-2 weeks before testing.

Doses

■ **DOGS:**

For adjunctive treatment of sterile inflammatory dermatoses (extra-label): Used with a tetracycline. Recommended dosages are empirical and vary somewhat. Practically, for dogs weighing

5 kg or less: 100 mg niacinamide per dog PO 3 times a day; for dogs weighing 5-10 kg: 250 mg (1/2 of a 500 mg tablet) niacinamide per dog PO 3 times a day; for dogs weighing more than 10 kg: 500 mg niacinamide per dog PO 3 times a day. If efficacy/remission occurs, may reduce to twice daily administration and then tapered further over time when possible.

If using tetracycline HCl, dose at the same amount of niacinamide PO 3 times daily. If using doxycycline consider 5 – 10 mg/kg PO twice daily. If using minocycline consider 7.5 mg/kg PO twice daily.

Monitoring

- Efficacy.
- Adverse effects (baseline and occasional monitoring of liver enzymes is suggested).

Client Information

- Used in dogs in combination with tetracycline for treatment of a variety of serious skin and other autoimmune diseases.
- Give as directed; usually 3 times a day at first. Improvement may be gradual & take 6-8 weeks.
- Side effects from niacinamide alone are rare. Vomiting and reduced appetite (eating less than normal) are the most likely side effects. When used in combination with a tetracycline, risk for side effects is greater and include lethargy (tiredness or lack of energy) and rarely liver problems.

Chemistry/Synonyms

Niacinamide, also commonly known as nicotinamide, occurs as a white crystalline powder. It is odorless or nearly odorless and has a bitter taste. It is freely soluble in water or alcohol.

Niacinamide may also be known as: nicotinamide, nicotinamidum, nicotinic acid amide, nicotylamide, Vitamin B(3), or Vitamin PP.

Storage/Stability

Store niacinamide tablets in tight containers at room temperature unless otherwise labeled. Niacinamide is **incompatible** with alkalis or strong acids.

Compatibility/Compounding Considerations

No specific information noted.

Dosage Forms/Regulatory Status

VETERINARY-LABELED PRODUCTS: NONE.

HUMAN-LABELED PRODUCTS:

Niacinamide (Nicotinamide) Tablets: 100 mg & 500 mg; generic; (OTC)

Revisions/References

Monograph revised/updated April 2014.
Koch, S., et al. (2011). *Small Animal Dermatology Drug Handbook*, Wiley-Blackwell. Ames.

Nitazoxanide

(nye-tah-**zox**-ah-nide)

Antiparasitic Agent

Prescriber Highlights

▶ Drug that has activity against a variety of protozoa, nematodes, bacteria, & trematodes, including *Sarcocystis neurona*, giardia, cryptosporidia, & *Helicobacter pylori*.

▶ Was approved for use in horses (EPM), but veterinary paste no longer marketed.

▶ Interest in using in other companion animals (*e.g.*, dogs, cats), but data is lacking to support use.

▶ Adverse effects in dogs (GI, hypersalivation) may be therapy limiting; but very well tolerated in humans.

Uses/Indications

Nitazoxanide may be useful as an alternative treatment for cryptosporidia in cats. In humans, nitazoxanide is FDA-approved for use in treating diarrhea caused by *Cryptosporidium parvum* and *Giardia lamblia* in pediatric patients from ages 1-11 years old. Because of the drug's spectrum of activity and apparent safety, there is considerable interest in using it in a variety of companion animal species, but data is lacking for specific indications and dosages.

Nitazoxanide oral paste was approved for the treatment of horses with equine protozoal myeloencephalitis (EPM) caused by *Sarcocystis neurona*, but is no longer marketed in the USA.

Pharmacology

While the precise mechanism of action of nitazoxanide is unknown, its active metabolites tizoxanide and tizoxanide glucuronide, are thought to inhibit the pyruvate ferredoxin oxidoreductase (PFOR) enzyme-dependent electron transfer reactions essential to anaerobic energy metabolism. Nitazoxanide has activity against a variety of protozoa, nematodes, bacteria, and trematodes, including *Sarcocystis neurona*, giardia, cryptosporidia, and *Helicobacter pylori*.

Pharmacokinetics

Following oral administration in horses, nitazoxanide is absorbed and rapidly converted to tizoxanide (desacetyl-nitazoxanide). Peak levels of tizoxanide are attained between 2-3 hours and are not detectable by 24 hours post dosing. In humans, nitazoxanide is not detectable in plasma, but peak levels of tizoxanide and tizoxanide glucuronide occur ≈3-4 hours post dose. More than 99% of tizoxanide is bound to plasma proteins. Tizoxanide is excreted in the urine, bile, and feces; the glucuronide metabolite is secreted in the urine and bile.

Contraindications/Precautions/Warnings

Safety for use in animals with compromised renal or hepatic function has not been established; use with caution.

Adverse Effects

In cats, GI irritation can occur.

In a study using nitazoxanide in dogs with naturally occurring *Giardia* spp. infections, 5 of 9 in the study developed excessive salivation, vomiting, or diarrhea that resulted in removal from the study (Lappin *et al.* 2008).

In humans, nitazoxanide appears to be well tolerated and adverse effect rates are similar to placebo. Rarely, sclera may turn yellow secondary to drug disposition, but return to normal after drug discontinuation.

Reproductive/Nursing Safety

In pregnant humans, nitazoxanide is designated by the FDA as a category **B** drug (*Animal studies have not demonstrated risk to the fetus, but there are no adequate studies in pregnant women; or animal studies have shown an adverse effect, but adequate studies in pregnant women have not demonstrated a risk to the fetus during the first trimester of pregnancy, and there is no evidence of risk in later trimesters.*) Nitazoxanide did not affect male or female fertility in rats given ≈66X the human dose. It did not cause fetal harm in pregnant rats or rabbits given 48X and 3X the human dose, respectively. It is unknown if tizoxanide is excreted into milk.

Overdosage/Acute Toxicity

There is limited information available on the acute toxicity of nitazoxanide. It has been reported that overdoses of 2.5X in horses has been associated with fatalities. The oral LD_{50} for cats and dogs is >10 grams/kg. Repeated doses of 450 mg/kg in rats caused intense salivation and increased liver and spleen weights. In horses given ≈5X the labeled dose, all developed anorexia, diarrhea, and lethargy, and testing was halted after 4 days of study. Human volunteers have taken doses of up to 4 grams without significant adverse effects occurring. In the event of an overdose, it is suggested to observe the patient closely and treat adverse effects in a supportive manner.

Drug Interactions

No specific drug interactions have been noted to date, but the veterinary and human manufacturers warn to use with caution if the patient is receiving other drugs that are highly protein bound and with a narrow therapeutic index.

Laboratory Considerations

- No specific laboratory interactions or considerations noted.

Doses

- **CATS:**

  For cryptosporidia-associated diarrhea (extra-label): 10 – 25 mg/kg PO q12-24h. No drug is consistently effective. In cats, *Cryptosporidium* spp. associated diarrhea sometimes resolves after administration of tylosin, paromomycin, or nitazoxanide. (Lappin 2011)

- **HORSES:**

  For equine protozoal myeloencephalitis (EPM) caused by *Sarcocystis neurona*: For a 28 day course of therapy: Days 1-5: 25 mg/kg (11.36 mg/lb) PO once daily; Days 6-28: 50 mg/kg (22.72 mg/lb) PO once daily. See directions for use in client information section that follows. (Package insert; *Navigator®*—Idexx). **Note:** Product has been withdrawn from the US market.

Monitoring

- Clinical efficacy.
- Weekly body weight.
- Adverse reactions.

Client Information

- This drug has not been commonly used in dogs or cats and adverse effects may occur, including excessive salivation, vomiting, or diarrhea.

Chemistry/Synonyms

A nitrothiazolyl-salicylamide derivative antiparasitic agent, nitazoxanide occurs as a light yellow powder. It is slightly soluble in ethanol and practically insoluble in water.

Nitazoxanide may also be known as: PH-5776, *Alinia®*, *Daxon®*, *Heliton®*, and *Navigator®*.

Storage/Stability

The human-approved powder for oral suspension should be stored at 25°C (77°F); excursions permitted to 15-30°C (59-86°F). Once suspended with tap water, the oral suspension should be kept in tightly closed containers at room temperature and discarded after 7 days.

Compatibility/Compounding Considerations

No specific information noted.

Dosage Forms/Regulatory Status

VETERINARY-LABELED PRODUCTS:

None. Nitazoxanide oral paste (32%) *Navigator®* was FDA-approved in the USA for horses, but the drug is no longer manufactured or marketed and approval has been withdrawn.

HUMAN-LABELED PRODUCTS:

Nitazoxanide Oral Tablets: 500 mg; *Alinia®*; (Rx)

Nitazoxanide Powder for Oral Suspension: 20 mg/mL (100 mg/5 mL after reconstitution) in 60 mL; *Alinia®*; (Rx)

Revisions/References

Monograph revised/updated April 2014.

Lappin, M. R. (2011). Diagnosis and Treatment of Cryptosporidium and Isospora in Cats. Proceedings: World Small Animal; Veterinary Association World Congress. accessed via Veterinary Information Network; vin.com

Lappin, M. R., et al. (2008). Treatment of Healthy Giardia Spp. Positive Dogs with Fenbendazole or Nitazoxanide. accessed via Veterinary Information Network; vin.com

Nitenpyram

(nye-ten-**pye**-rum)   Capstar®

Oral Insecticide

Prescriber Highlights

▶ Oral insecticide used primarily as a flea adulticide in dogs & cats; may also have efficacy for other conditions (*e.g.*, maggots). Not effective alone for flea eggs or other immature forms.

▶ Relatively safe. Over-the-counter.

Uses/Indications

Nitenpyram is indicated as a flea adulticide in dogs and cats that are, at a minimum, 2 pounds in weight and 4 weeks old. It does not repel fleas or ticks and does not reliably kill ticks, flea eggs, larvae or immature fleas. Nitenpyram may be effective for treating fly larvae (maggots) of various species. Fleas begin to fall from treated animals about 30 minutes after dosing and a single dose can protect animals for 1-2 days.

Pharmacology/Actions

Nitenpyram is in the class of neonicotinoid insecticides. It enters the systemic circulation of the adult flea after consuming blood from a treated animal. It binds to nicotinic acetylcholine receptors in the postsynaptic membranes and blocks acetylcholine-mediated neuronal transmission causing paralysis and death of the flea. Nitenpyram is 3500X more selective for insect alpha-4beta-2 nicotinic receptors than in vertebrate receptors. It does not inhibit acetylcholinesterase. Efficacy appears to be >99% (kill rate) in dogs or cats within 3-6 hours of treatment. When combined with an insect growth regulator (*e.g.*, lufenuron), immature stages of fleas may also be controlled.

Pharmacokinetics

Nitenpyram is rapidly and practically completely absorbed after oral administration. Peak levels occur ≈80 minutes after dosing in dogs; ≈40 minutes in cats. Elimination half-lives are: ≈3 hours for dogs; 8 hours for cats. Nitenpyram is excreted primarily as conjugated metabolites in the urine and excretion is complete within 48 hours of dosing. In dogs, ≈3% of a dose is excreted in the feces; in cats ≈5% is excreted in the feces.

Contraindications/Precautions/Warnings

Nitenpyram is not to be used in animals under 2 pounds of body weight or under 4 weeks of age. Use with caution in animals under 8 weeks old.

Adverse Effects

Nitenpyram is usually tolerated well, but serious adverse effects have been reported. Based on post-approval adverse drug experience reporting, the following adverse events (listed in decreasing order of frequency) have been reported:

Cats: Hyperactivity, panting, lethargy, itching, vocalization, vomiting, fever, decreased appetite, nervousness, diarrhea, difficulty breathing, salivation, incoordination, seizures, pupil dilation, increased heart rate, and trembling.

Dogs: Lethargy/depression, vomiting, itching, decreased appetite, diarrhea, hyperactivity, incoordination, trembling, seizures, panting, allergic reactions including hives, vocalization, salivation, fever, and nervousness.

The frequency of serious signs, including neurologic signs and death, was greater in animals under 2 pounds of body weight, less than 8 weeks of age, and/or reported to be in poor body condition.

Reproductive/Nursing Safety

Nitenpyram is probably safe to use in most breeding, pregnant, or lactating animals, but in some instances, birth defects and fetal/neonatal loss were reported after treatment of pregnant and/or lactating animals.

Overdosage/Acute Toxicity

Nitenpyram is relatively safe in high dosages to mammals. The oral LD_{50} in rats is $\approx$1.6 grams/kg. Cats or dogs given 10X the usual dose for 14 days showed no untoward effects. In the circumstance of a massive overdose, contact an animal poison control center for additional guidance.

Drug Interactions

No specific drug interactions were located. Nitenpyram has reportedly been used safely with a variety of other medications and other flea products.

Laboratory Considerations

- No specific laboratory interactions or considerations noted.

Doses

- **DOGS:**

    As a flea adulticide: For dogs weighing 2-25 lbs. (0.9-11.36 kg): Give one 11.4 mg tablet PO. May be given as often as once per day. For dogs weighing 25-125 lbs. (11.36-56.8kg): Give one 57 mg tablet PO. May be given as often as once per day. May be given with or without food. (Label directions; *Capstar*®—Novartis)

- **CATS:**

    As a flea adulticide: For cats weighing 2-25 lbs. (0.9-11.36 kg): Give one 11.4 mg tablet PO. May be given as often as once per day. May be given with or without food. (Label directions; *Capstar*®—Novartis)

- **REPTILES:**

    For maggots (extra-label): crush one 11.4 mg tablet into powder and give PO, as an enema, or on wound one time. (Klaphake 2005)

Monitoring

- Efficacy.

Client Information

- Oral insecticide used primarily as a flea adulticide in dogs & cats; may also have efficacy for other conditions (*e.g.,* maggots). Not effective alone for flea eggs or other immature forms so usually used in combination with other products that will control those forms of fleas.
- Usually dosed once a day to once per week. Best given after a meal.
- Usually tolerated well in dogs and cats. Serious side effects are rare and occur most often in animals that weigh less than 2 lbs., are less than 8 weeks old or in poor health.
- Treat all animals in the household.
- Keep tablets out of reach of children. Dispose of unused tablets appropriately.

Chemistry/Synonyms

A neonicotinoid insecticide, nitenpyram occurs as a pale yellow crystalline powder and is very soluble in water (840 mg/mL).

Nitenpyram may also be known as: TI-304, (E)-Nitenpyram, *Bestguard*®, and *Capstar*®.

Storage/Stability

Commercially available nitenpyram tablets should be stored at room temperature (15-30°C; 59-86°F). Shelf life is reported to be 3 years if stored below 25°C (76°F).

Compatibility/Compounding Considerations

No specific information noted.

Dosage Forms/Regulatory Status

VETERINARY-LABELED PRODUCTS:

Nitenpyram Oral Tablets: 11.4 mg and 57 mg in boxes containing blister packs of 6 tablets; *Capstar*®; (OTC); FDA-approved for use in dogs and cats.

Also available in combination packs with Lufenuron [*Program*® *Flavor Tabs* and *Capstar*® *Flea Management System for Dogs* and *Program*® *Flavor Tabs* (OTC); and *Capstar*® *Flea Management System for Cats* (OTC)] and in combination with milbemycin and lufenuron [*Sentinel*® *Flavor Tabs* and *Capstar*® *Flea Management System for Dogs* (Rx)].

HUMAN-LABELED PRODUCTS: NONE.

Revisions/References

Monograph revised/updated April 2014.

Klaphake, E. (2005). Reptilian Parasites. Proceedings: Western Vet Conf. accessed via Veterinary Information Network; vin.com

Nitrofurantoin

(nye-troe-fyoor-**an**-toyn)   Macrodantin®, Macrobid®

Urinary Antimicrobial

Prescriber Highlights

▶ Antibacterial infrequently used for susceptible UTI's.

▶ Contraindications: Renal impairment; hypersensitivity to nitrofurantoin.

▶ Adverse Effects: Gastrointestinal disturbances, peripheral neuropathy & hepatopathy of most concern.

▶ Potentially teratogenic, may cause infertility in males and be toxic to neonates.

Uses/Indications

Considered a urinary tract antiseptic, nitrofurantoin is used primarily in small animals, but also occasionally in horses in the treatment of lower urinary tract infections caused by susceptible bacteria. In the published guidelines for treatment of urinary tract disease in dogs and cats, the Antimicrobial Guidelines Working Group of the International Society for Companion Animal Infectious Diseases recommends that nitrofurantoin is a "good second-line option for simple uncomplicated UTI, particularly when multidrug-resistant pathogens are involved" (Weese *et al.* 2011). Nitrofurantoin is not effective in treating renal cortical or perinephric abscesses or other systemic infections.

Pharmacology/Actions

Nitrofurantoin usually acts as a bacteriostatic antimicrobial, but it may be bactericidal depending on the concentration of the drug and the susceptibility of the organism. The exact mechanism of action of nitrofurantoin has not been fully elucidated, but the drug apparently inhibits various bacterial enzyme systems, including acetyl coenzyme A. Nitrofurantoin has greater antibacterial activity in acidic environments.

Nitrofurantoin has activity against several gram-negative and some gram-positive organisms, including many strains of *E. coli*, Klebsiella, Enterobacter, Enterococci, *Staphylococcus aureus* and *epidermidis*, Enterobacter, Citrobacter, Salmonella, Shigella, and Corynebacterium. It has little or no activity against most strains of Proteus, Serratia, or Acinetobacter and has no activity against *Pseudomonas* spp.

Pharmacokinetics

There are three commercial (human label) oral forms of the drug. Regular nitrofurantoin in an oral suspension, macrocrystalline capsules and monohydrate/macrocrystals capsules. No pharmacokinetic studies comparing these forms in dogs or cats were located. In humans, nitrofurantoin is rapidly absorbed from the GI tract; the presence of food may enhance the absorption of the drug. Macrocrystalline (*e.g., Macrodantin®*) capsules are more slowly absorbed but it is still dosed 3-4 times daily for treating urinary tract infections in humans. Monohydrate macrocrystalline forms of the drug (*e.g., Macrobid®*) are absorbed even more slowly with less GI upset. Because of its slower absorption, urine levels of the drug may be prolonged with the monohydrate macrocrystalline form and so it is dosed twice daily in humans.

Therapeutic levels in the systemic circulation are not maintained due to the rapid elimination of the drug after absorption. Approximately 20-60% of the drug is bound to serum proteins. Peak urine levels occur within 30 minutes of dosing. The drug crosses the placenta and only minimal quantities of the drug are found in milk.

Approximately 40-50% of the drug is eliminated into urine unchanged via both glomerular filtration and tubular secretion. Some of the drug is metabolized, primarily in the liver. Elimination half-lives in humans with normal renal function average 20 minutes.

Contraindications/Precautions/Warnings

Nitrofurantoin is contraindicated in patients with renal impairment as the drug is much less efficacious and the development of toxicity is much more likely. The drug is also contraindicated in patients hypersensitive to it.

Rats can develop neurotoxicity when given nitrofurantoin; avoid using in this species.

Adverse Effects

In dogs and cats, gastrointestinal disturbances (primarily vomiting), peripheral neuropathies (reversible) and hepatopathy can occur. Chronic active hepatitis, hemolytic anemia, and pneumonitis have been described in humans, but are believed to occur very rarely in animals.

Reproductive/Nursing Safety

In humans, the drug is contraindicated in pregnant patients at term and neonates as hemolytic anemia can occur secondary to immature enzyme systems. Safe use of the drug during earlier stages of pregnancy has not been determined. Nitrofurantoin has been implicated in causing infertility in male dogs. Use only when the benefits of therapy outweigh the potential risks.

Nitrofurantoin is excreted into maternal milk in very low concentrations. Safety for use in the nursing mother or offspring has not been established.

Overdosage/Acute Toxicity

No specific information was located. Because the drug is rapidly absorbed and excreted, patients with normal renal function should require little therapy when mild overdoses occur. If the ingestion was relatively recent, massive overdoses should be handled by emptying the gut using standard protocols; patient should then be monitored for adverse effects (see above).

Drug Interactions

The following drug interactions have either been reported or are theoretical in humans or animals receiving nitrofurantoin and may be of significance in veterinary patients. Unless otherwise noted, use together is not necessarily contraindicated, but weigh the potential risks and perform additional monitoring when appropriate.

- **FLUOROQUINOLONES** (*e.g.,* **enrofloxacin, ciprofloxacin**):

Nitrofurantoin may antagonize the antimicrobial activity of the fluoroquinolones and concomitant use is best avoided.

- **FOOD** or **ANTICHOLINERGIC DRUGS:** May increase the oral bioavailability of nitrofurantoin.
- **MAGNESIUM TRISILICATE CONTAINING ANTACIDS:** May inhibit the oral absorption of nitrofurantoin.
- **PROBENECID:** May inhibit the renal excretion of nitrofurantoin potentially increasing its toxicity and reducing its effectiveness in urinary tract infections.
- **SPIRONOLACTONE:** Nitrofurantoin may increase hyperkalemic effects.

Laboratory Considerations

- Nitrofurantoin may cause false-positive **urine glucose** determinations if using cupric-sulfate solutions (Benedict's reagent, *Clinitest®*). Tests using glucose oxidase methods (*Tes-Tape®, Clinistix®*) are not affected by nitrofurantoin.
- Nitrofurantoin may cause decreases in **blood glucose**, and increases in **serum creatinine**, **bilirubin** and **alkaline phosphatase**.

Doses

- **DOGS/CATS:**

  Note: Neither reference below states which form is being used: macrocrystalline (*e.g., Macrodantin®*) or monohydrate (*e.g., Macrobid®*). Unless otherwise noted assume it is the macrocrystalline form.

  For simple uncomplicated UTI, particularly when multidrug-resistant pathogens are involved (extra-label): 4.4 – 5 mg/kg PO q8h. Typically, uncomplicated UTIs are treated for 7-14 days. However, a shorter treatment time (≤ 7 days) may be effective. Accordingly, in the absence of objective data, 7 days of appropriate antimicrobial treatment is reasonable. (Weese *et al.* 2011)

  For prevention of re-infections with gram-negative organisms (extra-label): Dogs: 4 mg/kg PO once a day immediately before bedtime after dog has urinated. May rarely cause drug-induced hepatopathy and liver enzymes should be evaluated if any adverse effects are suspected. Preventative therapy for repeated reinfection (> 2 per 6 months) should only be utilized after an extensive search for any underlying cause. This approach will not resolve existing UTI and should only be used after effective treatment using full therapeutic doses. (Adams 2009)

Monitoring

- Clinical efficacy.
- Adverse effects.
- Periodic liver function tests should be considered with chronic therapy.

Client Information

- Give with food.
- Can discolor urine to a brownish color. This is normal.
- Stomach upset (acting 'sick') and vomiting are the most common side effects, but muscle weakness may indicate nerve toxicity (serious).

Chemistry/Synonyms

A synthetic, nitrofuran antibacterial, nitrofurantoin occurs as a bitter tasting, lemon-yellow, crystalline powder with a pK_a of 7.2. It is very slightly soluble in water or alcohol.

Nitrofurantoin may also be known as: furadoninum or nitrofurantoinum, *Furadantin®, Macrobid®,* and *Macrodantin®*.

Storage/Stability

Nitrofurantoin preparations should be stored in tight containers at room temperature and protected from light. The oral suspension should not be frozen. Nitrofurantoin will decompose if it comes into contact with metals other than aluminum or stainless steel.

Compatibility/Compounding Considerations

No specific information noted.

Dosage Forms/Regulatory Status

VETERINARY-LABELED PRODUCTS: NONE.

HUMAN-LABELED PRODUCTS:

Nitrofurantoin Macrocrystalline Oral Capsules: 25 mg, 50 mg & 100 mg (as macrocrystals); *Macrodantin®*; (Rx)

Nitrofurantoin Monohydrate Macrocrystals Oral Capsules: 100 mg; *Macrobid®*, generic; (Rx)

Nitrofurantoin Oral Suspension: 5 mg/mL (25 mg/5 mL) in 470 mL; *Furadantin®*, generic; (Rx)

Revisions/References

Monograph revised/updated April 2014.

Adams, L. (2009). Recurrent Urinary Tract Infections: Bad Bugs That Won't Go Away. Proceedings: WVC. accessed via Veterinary Information Network; vin.com

Weese, J. S., et al. (2011). Antimicrobial Use Guidelines for Treatment of Urinary Tract Disease in Dogs and Cats: Antimicrobial Guidelines Working Group of the International Society for Companion Animal Infectious Diseases. Veterinary Medicine International.

Nitroglycerin, Transdermal

(nye-troe-gli-ser-in)   NTG, Nitro-bid®, Minitran®

Venodilator; Afterload Reducer

Prescriber Highlights

▶ Transdermal, oral, & injectable venodilator; occasionally used topically in veterinary medicine for CHF or hypertension.

▶ Continuous use results in tolerance after 48-72 hours.

▶ Adverse Effects: rashes at the application sites; hypotension is possible. Transient headaches (common in humans); may be a problem for some animals.

▶ Rotate application sites.

▶ Wear gloves when applying; avoid human skin contact.

Uses/Indications

Transdermal nitroglycerin (NTG) in small animal medicine is used primarily as an adjunctive vasodilator in heart failure and cardiogenic edema. Because of questionable efficacy and rapid development of tolerance, topical nitroglycerine is not commonly used in veterinary medicine today. When parenteral treatment is required for critical animals, most will use nitroprusside. In humans, NTG is also used as an anti-anginal agent, antihypertensive (acute), and topically to treat Raynaud's disease.

For horses, topical nitroglycerin is ineffective in increasing digital blood flow in laminitis.

Pharmacology/Actions

Nitroglycerin relaxes vascular smooth muscle primarily on the venous side, but a dose related effect on arterioles is possible. Preload (left end-diastolic pressure) is reduced from the peripheral pooling of blood and decreased venous return to the heart. Because of its arteriolar effects, depending on the dose, afterload may also be reduced. Myocardial oxygen demand and workload are reduced and coronary circulation can be improved.

Pharmacokinetics

Nitroglycerin transdermal ointment is absorbed through the skin, with an onset of action usually within 1 hour and duration of action of 2-12 hours. It is generally dosed in dogs and cats q6-8 hours (3-4 times a day). The transdermal patches have a wide inter-patient

bioavailability. Reportedly, the topical paste can be absorbed when rubbed on the gums of dogs and cats. Nitroglycerin has a very short half-life (1-4 minutes in humans) and is metabolized in the liver. At least two metabolites have some vasodilator activity and have longer half-lives than NTG.

Contraindications/Precautions/Warnings

Nitrates are contraindicated in patients with severe anemia or those hypersensitive to them. They should be used with caution (if at all) in patients with cerebral hemorrhage or head trauma, diuretic-induced hypovolemia or other hypotensive conditions.

Adverse Effects

Most common side effect seen is a rash at the application site. If hypotension is a problem, reduce dosage. Transient headaches are a common side effect seen in humans and may be a problem for some animals.

Continuous use (48-72 hours) of nitroglycerin results in the rapid development of tolerance to the effects of the drug.

Reproductive/Nursing Safety

In humans, the FDA categorizes this drug as category *C* for use during pregnancy (*Animal studies have shown an adverse effect on the fetus, but there are no adequate studies in humans; or there are no animal reproduction studies and no adequate studies in humans.*) In a separate system evaluating the safety of drugs in canine and feline pregnancy (Papich 1989), this drug is categorized as class: *C* (*These drugs may have potential risks. Studies in people or laboratory animals have uncovered risks, and these drugs should be used cautiously as a last resort when the benefit of therapy clearly outweighs the risks.*)

It is not known whether nitrates are excreted in maternal milk; use with caution in nursing animals.

Overdosage/Acute Toxicity

If severe hypotension results after topical administration, wash the site of application to prevent any more absorption of ointment. Fluids may be administered if necessary. Epinephrine is contraindicated as it is ineffective and may complicate the animal's condition.

Drug Interactions

The following drug interactions have either been reported or are theoretical in humans or animals receiving nitroglycerin and may be of significance in veterinary patients. Unless otherwise noted, use together is not necessarily contraindicated, but weigh the potential risks and perform additional monitoring when appropriate.

■ **ANTIHYPERTENSIVE DRUGS, OTHER:** Use of nitroglycerin with other antihypertensive drugs may cause additive hypotensive effects.

■ **PHENOTHIAZINES:** May increase hypotensive effects.

■ **SILDENAFIL (and other PDE INHIBITORS):** May profoundly increase risk for hypotension.

Doses

Note: Transdermal nitroglycerin is not used alone for the treatment of acute heart failure; must be used with a loop diuretic (*e.g.*, furosemide). There is very limited evidence of the efficacy of topical nitroglycerin in dogs and cats, but it is unlikely to cause harm.

■ **DOGS/CATS:**

For adjunctive treatment of acute heart failure using the transdermal ointment (*Nitro-bid®*); (extra-label): Dosed semi-quantitatively based on animal size. Cats: 1/8th – 1/4 inch; small dogs: ¼ – ½ inch; medium dogs: ½ – 1 inch; large dogs: 1 – 2 inches q6-12h for first 24-48 hours. Applied with a gloved finger to the inner ear pinnae, groin or axilla. Some have suggested that it can be applied oral mucous membranes and is absorbed and tolerated well.

- **FERRETS:**

  For adjunctive therapy for heart failure (extra-label): 1/8th inch strip applied to inside of pinna q12h for the first 24 hours of therapy. (Hoeffer 2000)

Monitoring
- Clinical efficacy.
- Sites of application for signs of rash.
- Blood pressure, particularly if hypotensive effects are seen.

Client Information
- Dosage is measured in inches of ointment; use papers supplied with product to measure appropriate dose. Wear gloves (non-permeable) when applying.
- Do not pet animal where ointment has been applied.
- Rotate application sites. Recommended application sites include: groin, inside the ears, and thorax. Rub ointment into skin well. If rash develops, do not use on that site again until it's cleared. Sometimes, veterinarians will have you rub it onto the gums of your animal.
- Contact veterinarian if rash persists or animal's condition deteriorates.
- There is no danger of explosion or fire with the use of this product.

Chemistry/Synonyms
Famous as an explosive, nitroglycerin (NTG) occurs undiluted as a thick, volatile, white-pale yellow flammable, explosive liquid with a sweet, burning taste. The undiluted drug is soluble in alcohol and slightly soluble in water. Because of obvious safety reasons, nitroglycerin is diluted with lactose, dextrose, propylene glycol, alcohol, etc. when used for pharmaceutical purposes.

Nitroglycerin may also be known as: glyceryl trinitrate, glonoine, GTN; nitroglycerol, NTG, trinitrin, or trinitroglycerin, *Minitran®*, *Nitro-bid®*, and *Nitro-Dur®*.

Storage/Stability
The topical ointment should be stored at room temperature and the cap firmly attached. For storage/stability and compatibility for dosage forms other than the topical ointment, see specialized references or the package inserts for each product.

Compatibility/Compounding Considerations
No specific information noted.

Dosage Forms/Regulatory Status
VETERINARY-LABELED PRODUCTS: NONE.

The ARCI (Racing Commissioners International) has designated this drug as a class 3 substance. See the appendix for more information.

HUMAN-LABELED PRODUCTS:

Note: Many dosage forms of nitroglycerin are available for human use, including sublingual tablets, buccal tablets, lingual spray, extended-release oral capsules and tablets, and parenteral solutions for IV infusion. Because the use of nitroglycerin in small animal medicine is practically limited to the use of topical ointment or transdermal patches, those other dosage forms are not listed here.

Nitroglycerin Topical Ointment: 2% in a lanolin-white petrolatum base in 30 gram & 60 gram tubes and UD 1 gram; *Nitro-bid®*; (Rx)

Nitroglycerin Transdermal Systems (patches): 0.1 mg/hr, 0.2 mg/hr, 0.3 mg/hr, 0.4 mg/hr, 0.6 mg/hr & 0.8 mg/hr; *Minitran®*, *Nitro-Dur®*, generic; (Rx) **Note:** Various products contain differing quantities of nitroglycerin and patch surface area size, but release rates of drug are identical for a given mg/hr.

Revisions/References
Monograph revised/updated April 2014.

Hoeffer, H. (2000). Heart Disease in Ferrets. *Kirk's Current Veterinary Therapy: XIII Small Animal Practice.* J. Bonagura. Philadelphia, WB Saunders: 1144-8.

Papich, M. (1989). Effects of drugs on pregnancy. *Current Veterinary Therapy X: Small Animal Practice.* R. Kirk. Philadelphia, Saunders: 1291-9.

Nitroprusside Sodium

(nye-troe-**pruss**-ide)   Nitropress®, Sodium Nitroprusside

Vasodilator

Prescriber Highlights
▶ Vascular, smooth muscle relaxant used for acute/severe hypertension; acute heart failure secondary to mitral regurgitation & in combination with dobutamine for refractory CHF. Use only in an ICU setting; monitoring essential, including continuous measurement of direct or, less ideally, indirect arterial blood pressure.

▶ Contraindications: Compensatory hypertension, inadequate cerebral circulation, or during emergency surgery in patients near death. Caution: Geriatric patients, hepatic insufficiency, severe renal impairment, hyponatremia, or hypothyroidism.

▶ Adverse effects: Hypotensive effects; potentially: nausea, retching, restlessness, apprehension, muscle twitching, dizziness.

▶ May be irritating at the infusion site; avoid extravasation.

▶ Continued use at high dosages may lead to potential thiocyanate & cyanide toxicity.

Uses/Indications
Nitroprusside is used for adjunctive treatment of severe, acute heart failure, and hypertensive crisis when blood pressure must be reduced relatively rapidly. Its use in veterinary medicine is generally reserved for the treatment of critically ill patients only when constant blood pressure monitoring can be performed. In patients with dilated cardiomyopathy, administering dobutamine first to improve contractility and increase cardiac output can offset the hypotensive effects of sodium nitroprusside (Erling *et al.* 2008).

Pharmacology/Actions
Nitroprusside is an immediate acting intravenous hypotensive agent that directly causes peripheral vasodilation (arterial and venous) independent of autonomic innervation. It produces a lowering of blood pressure, an increase in heart rate, a mild decrease in cardiac output, and a significant reduction in total peripheral resistance. Preload, afterload and left ventricular end-diastolic pressures are reduced. Unlike the organic nitrates, tolerance does not develop to nitroprusside.

Pharmacokinetics
After starting an IV infusion of nitroprusside, reduction in blood pressure and other pharmacologic effects begin almost immediately. Blood pressure will return to pretreatment levels within 1-10 minutes following cessation of therapy.

Nitroprusside is metabolized non-enzymatically in the blood and tissues to cyanogen (cyanide radical). Cyanogen is converted in the liver to thiocyanate where it is eliminated in the urine, feces, and exhaled air. The half-life of cyanogen is 2.7-7 days if renal function is normal, but prolonged in patients with impaired renal function or with hyponatremia.

Contraindications/Precautions/Warnings
Nitroprusside is contraindicated in patients with compensatory hypertension (*e.g.*, AV shunts or coarctation of the aorta; Cushing's reflex), inadequate cerebral circulation, or during emergency surgery in patients near death.

Nitroprusside must be used with caution in patients with hepatic insufficiency, severe renal impairment, hyponatremia, or hypothyroidism. When nitroprusside is used for controlled hypotension during surgery, patients may have less tolerance to hypovolemia, anemia, or blood loss. Geriatric patients may be more sensitive to the hypotensive effects of nitroprusside.

Do **NOT** flush IV line or severe hypotension can result.

The FDA label (human use) includes a "black box" warning that includes: "After reconstitution, nitroprusside is not suitable for direct injection. The reconstituted solution must be further diluted in dextrose 5% injection before infusion. Nitroprusside can cause precipitous decreases in blood pressure. In patients not properly monitored, these decreases can lead to irreversible ischemic injuries or death. Use only when available equipment and personnel allow blood pressure to be continuously monitored. Except when used briefly or at low (<2 mcg/kg/min) infusion rates, nitroprusside injection gives rise to important quantities of cyanide ion, which can reach toxic, potentially lethal levels. The usual dose rate is 0.5 to 10 mcg/kg/min, but infusion at the maximum dose rates should never last more than 10 minutes. If blood pressure has not been adequately controlled after 10 minutes of infusion at the maximum rate, terminate administration immediately. Although acid-base balance and venous oxygen concentration should be monitored and may indicate cyanide toxicity, these laboratory tests provide imperfect guidance."

Nitroprusside is considered a "high alert" medication (medications that require special safeguards to reduce the risk of errors). Consider instituting practices such as redundant drug dosage and volume checking, special alert labels, etc.

Adverse Effects

Most adverse reactions from nitroprusside are associated with its hypotensive effects, particularly if blood pressure is reduced too rapidly. Clinical signs such as nausea, retching, restlessness, apprehension, muscle twitching, and dizziness have been reported in humans. These effects disappear when the infusion rate is reduced or stopped. Nitroprusside may be irritating at the infusion site; avoid extravasation.

Continued use may lead to potential thiocyanate and cyanide toxicity (see Overdosage section). Cats may be more susceptible to nitroprusside-induced oxidative damage; use minimum dosage required for efficacy.

Reproductive/Nursing Safety

In humans, the FDA categorizes this drug as category C for use during pregnancy (*Animal studies have shown an adverse effect on the fetus, but there are no adequate studies in humans; or there are no animal reproduction studies and no adequate studies in humans.*) In a separate system evaluating the safety of drugs in canine and feline pregnancy (Papich 1989), this drug is categorized as class: C (*These drugs may have potential risks. Studies in people or laboratory animals have uncovered risks, and these drugs should be used cautiously as a last resort when the benefit of therapy clearly outweighs the risks.*)

It is not known whether nitroprusside and its metabolites are excreted in maternal milk.

Overdosage/Acute Toxicity

Acute overdosage is manifested by a profound hypotension. Treat by reducing or stopping the infusion and giving fluids. Monitor blood pressure constantly.

Excessive doses, prolonged therapy, a depleted hepatic thiosulfate (sulfur) supply, or severe hepatic or renal insufficiency may lead to profound hypotension, cyanogen, or thiocyanate toxicity. Acid/base status should be monitored to evaluate therapy and to detect metabolic acidosis (early sign of cyanogen toxicity). Toler-

ance to therapy is also an early sign of nitroprusside toxicity. Hydroxocobalamin (Vitamin B_{12a}) may prevent cyanogen toxicity. Thiocyanate toxicity may be exhibited as delirium in dogs. Serum thiocyanate levels may need to be monitored in patients on prolonged therapy, especially in those patients with concurrent renal dysfunction. Serum levels >100 micrograms/mL are considered toxic. It is suggested to refer to other references or contact an animal poison control center for further information should cyanogen or thiocyanate toxicity be suspected.

Drug Interactions

The following drug interactions have either been reported or are theoretical in humans or animals receiving nitroprusside and may be of significance in veterinary patients. Unless otherwise noted, use together is not necessarily contraindicated, but weigh the potential risks and perform additional monitoring when appropriate.

- **ANESTHETICS, GENERAL:** The hypotensive effects of nitroprusside may be enhanced by concomitant administration of general anesthetics (*e.g.*, **halothane, enflurane**), or other circulatory depressants.
- **DOBUTAMINE:** Synergistic effects (increased cardiac output and reduced wedge pressure) may result if dobutamine is used with nitroprusside.
- **HYPOTENSIVE AGENTS, OTHER:** Patients receiving other hypotensive agents (*e.g.*, **beta-blockers, ACE inhibitors**, etc.) may be more sensitive to the hypotensive effects of nitroprusside.

Doses

Note: Must be diluted before use. See Compounding Considerations for information on preparing the infusion. An online drip rate table generator is available at: http://www.globalrph.com/drip.htm

- **DOGS/CATS:**

  For hypertensive crisis (systolic arterial BP >200 mm Hg); (extra-label): As a CRI, begin infusion at 0.5 micrograms/kg/minute, titrate upwards every 5 minutes until a predetermined target BP is attained. Reduce blood pressure 25% over 4-hour period.

  For adjunctive treatment of acute heart failure (cardiogenic shock; fulminant pulmonary edema) (extra-label): infusion at: Dogs: 1 microgram/kg/minute; Cats: 0.5 microgram/kg/minute. Continuously monitor blood pressure. Targeting a mean blood pressure of 70 mm Hg or systolic blood pressure of 90-100 mm Hg, titrate dosage upwards to effect in 0.5 – 1 microgram/kg increments every 10-15 minutes as long as blood pressure remains stable and until perfusion and pulmonary function improves. Maximum CRI rate is 10 micrograms/kg/minute, but most recommend a much lower maximum (*e.g.*, 5 micrograms/kg/min). Dobutamine can be used to treat or prevent hypotension if severe heart failure is confirmed by echocardiogram. If hypotension occurs, stop nitroprusside infusion and restart at a lower rate if therapy is continued. Maintain effective dosage for 12+ hours while continuously monitoring. Prolonged therapy increases risk for cyanide/thiocyanate toxicity and nitroprusside is rarely used longer than 24 hours. When patient is clinically improved (respiratory effort, lung auscultation, normal heart rate and capillary refill time, pink mucous membranes, and normal blood pressure) Nitroprusside is tapered off over 4-6 hours, ACE inhibitors started, followed by dobutamine weaning. Adapted from (Lichtenberger 2006), (Macintire 2006), (Proulx 2003), (Sumner *et al.* 2013)

Monitoring

- Blood pressure must be constantly monitored. Direct arterial blood pressure monitoring is recommended; however, if an arterial catheter cannot be placed (*e.g.*, smaller dogs and cats), continuous indirect blood pressures (*e.g.*, Doppler) can be used.

- Acid/base balance.
- Electrolytes (especially Na⁺).

Client Information

- Must only be used by professionals in a setting where precise IV infusion and constant blood pressure monitoring can be performed.

Chemistry/Synonyms

A vascular smooth muscle relaxant, nitroprusside sodium occurs as practically odorless, reddish-brown crystals or powder. It is freely soluble in water and slightly soluble in alcohol. After reconstitution in D_5W, solution may have a brownish, straw, or light orange color and have a pH of 3.5-6.

Nitroprusside sodium may also be known as: natrii nitroprussias, sodium nitroferricyanide dihydrate, sodium nitroprusside, or sodium nitroprussiate, and *Nitropress®*.

Storage/Stability

Nitroprusside sodium powder for injection should be stored protected from light and moisture and kept at room temperature (15-30°C). Nitroprusside solutions exposed to light will cause a reduction of the ferric ion to the ferrous ion with a resultant loss in potency and a change from a brownish-color to a blue color. Degradation is enhanced with nitroprusside solutions in *Viaflex®* (Baxter) plastic bags exposed to fluorescent light. After reconstitution, protect immediately by covering vial or infusion bag with aluminum foil or other opaque material. Discard solutions that turn to a blue, dark red, or green color. Solutions protected from light will remain stable for 24 hours after reconstitution. IV infusion tubing does not need to be protected from light while the infusion is running. It is not recommended to use IV infusion solutions other than D_5W or to add any other medications to the infusion solution.

Compatibility/Compounding Considerations

It is not recommended to use IV infusion solutions other than D_5W or to add any other medications to the prepared infusion solution. However, nitroprusside is considered **compatible at Y-sites** with the following drugs: atracurium, dexmedetomidine, diltiazem, dopamine, enalaprilat, esmolol, furosemide, heparin, lidocaine, midazolam, morphine, norepinephrine, potassium chloride, propofol, and vecuronium. Dobutamine Y-site compatibility with nitroprusside is variable depending on drug concentration. Nitroprusside solutions with concentrations up to 1.2 mg/mL were compatible with dobutamine 12.5 mg/mL solutions for 48 hours in one study (Seto *et al.* 2001).

<u>Directions for preparation of infusion</u>: Add 2 – 3 mL D5W to 50 mg vial to dissolve powder. Add dissolved solution to 1000 mL of D5W and promptly protect solution from light (using aluminum foil or other opaque covering). Resultant solution contains 50 micrograms/mL of nitroprusside. Different concentrations may be necessary for precise administration and/or restricting IV fluids. The administration set (IV line) does not need to be protected from light. Solution may have a slight brownish tint, but discard solutions that turn to a blue, dark red or green color. Solution is stable for 24 hours after reconstitution. Do not add any other medications to IV running nitroprusside. Avoid extravasation at IV site. Use an accurate flow control device (pump, controller, etc.) for administration. If a mini-drip IV set must be used: 60 drops ≈ 1 mL; 1 drop contains ≈0.83 micrograms of nitroprusside.

Dosage Forms/Regulatory Status

VETERINARY-LABELED PRODUCTS: NONE.

HUMAN-LABELED PRODUCTS:

Nitroprusside Sodium Powder for Injection: 50 mg/vial in 2 mL and 5 mL vials; *Nitropress®*; (Rx)

Revisions/References

Monograph revised/updated April 2014.

Erling, P. & E. M. Mazzaferro (2008). Left-sided congestive heart failure in dogs: Treatment and monitoring of emergency patients. Compendium-Continuing Education for Veterinarians 30(2): 94-+.

Lichtenberger, M. (2006). CHF in the ER: Keeping them alive. Proceedings: IVECCS. accessed via Veterinary Information Network; vin.com

Macintire, D. (2006). Cardiac Emergencies. Proceedings: ACVC 2006. accessed via Veterinary Information Network; vin.com

Papich, M. (1989). Effects of drugs on pregnancy. *Current Veterinary Therapy X: Small Animal Practice*. R. Kirk. Philadelphia, Saunders: 1291-9.

Proulx, J. (2003). Intensive management of heart failure. Proceedings: Western Veterinary Conference. accessed via Veterinary Information Network; vin.com

Seto, W., et al. (2001). Visual compatibility of sodium nitroprusside with other injectable medications given to pediatric patients. Am J Health-Syst Pharm 58: 1422-6.

Sumner, C. & E. Rozanski (2013). Management of Respiratory Emergencies in Small Animals. Veterinary Clinics of North America: Small Animal Practice 43(4): 799-815.

Nizatidine

(ni-**za**-ti-dine)   Axid®

H2-Receptor Antagonist; Prokinetic

Prescriber Highlights

▶ H_2 receptor antagonist similar to ranitidine; used primarily for its prokinetic activity; may be useful in preventing hemorrhagic necrosis in cats with pancreatitis. Not frequently used in veterinary medicine.

▶ Caution: Geriatric patients or those with hepatic or renal insufficiency.

▶ Adverse Effects are rare.

Uses/Indications

While nizatidine acts similarly to cimetidine and ranitidine as an H_2 blocker to reduce gastric acid secretion in the stomach, in small animal medicine its use has been primarily for its prokinetic effects. It may be useful to treat delayed gastric emptying, pseudo-obstruction of the intestine and constipation.

H_2 blockers may be useful in preventing hemorrhagic necrosis in feline pancreatitis.

Pharmacology/Actions

At the H_2 receptors of the parietal cells, nizatidine competitively inhibits histamine, thereby reducing gastric acid output both during basal conditions and when stimulated by food, amino acids, pentagastrin, histamine, or insulin.

While nizatidine can cause gastric emptying times to be delayed, it more likely will stimulate GI motility and gastric emptying by inhibiting acetylcholinesterase (thereby increasing acetylcholine at muscarinic receptors). It may also have direct agonist effects on M_3 muscarinic receptors. Lower esophageal sphincter pressures may be increased by nizatidine. By decreasing the amount of gastric juice produced, nizatidine decreases the amount of pepsin secreted.

Pharmacokinetics

In dogs, oral absorption is rapid and nearly complete with minimal first pass effect. Food can enhance the absorption of nizatidine, but this is not considered clinically important. The drug is only marginally bound to plasma proteins. It is unknown if it enters the CNS. Nizatidine is metabolized in the liver to several metabolites, including at least one that has some activity. In animals with normal renal function over half the drug is excreted in the urine unchanged.

Contraindications/Precautions/Warnings

Nizatidine is contraindicated in patients who are hypersensitive to it. It should be used cautiously and, possibly, at reduced dosage in patients with diminished renal function. Nizatidine has caused increased serum ALT levels in humans receiving high IV doses for longer than 5 days. The manufacturer recommends that in high dose, chronic therapy, serum ALT values be monitored.

Adverse Effects

Nizatidine appears to be very well tolerated. Very rarely, anemia has been reported in humans taking the drug. CNS effects have been noted (headache, dizziness) but incidence is similar to those taking placebo. Rash and pruritus have also been reported in a few humans taking nizatidine.

Reproductive/Nursing Safety

Doses of up to 275 mg/kg per day in pregnant rabbits did not reveal any teratogenic or fetotoxic effects. Safety during pregnancy not firmly established, so use only when clearly warranted. In humans, the FDA categorizes this drug as category *B* for use during pregnancy (*Animal studies have not yet demonstrated risk to the fetus, but there are no adequate studies in pregnant women; or animal studies have shown an adverse effect, but adequate studies in pregnant women have not demonstrated a risk to the fetus in the first trimester of pregnancy, and there is no evidence of risk in later trimesters.*)

Nizatidine is excreted in maternal milk in a concentration of 0.1% of the oral dose in proportion to plasma concentrations and unlikely to cause significant effects in nursing offspring.

Overdosage/Acute Toxicity

Single oral doses of up to 800 mg/kg were not lethal in dogs. Adverse effects could include cholinergic effects (lacrimation, salivation, emesis, miosis and diarrhea); suggest treating supportively and symptomatically.

Drug Interactions

The following drug interactions have either been reported or are theoretical in humans or animals receiving nizatidine and may be of significance in veterinary patients. Unless otherwise noted, use together is not necessarily contraindicated, but weigh the potential risks and perform additional monitoring when appropriate.

- **ANTICHOLINERGIC AGENTS (atropine, propantheline** etc.): May negate the prokinetic effects of nizatidine.
- **ASPIRIN:** Nizatidine may increase salicylate levels in patients receiving high doses of aspirin (or **other salicylates**).

Laboratory Considerations

- False positive tests for **urobilinogen** may occur with patients receiving nizatidine.

Doses

- **DOGS/CATS:**

  As a prokinetic agent (primarily gastric emptying) or an H$_2$ blocker (extra-label): Dosages not well established. Anecdotal dosages of 2.5 – 5 mg/kg PO once or twice daily are commonly noted, but up to 3 times daily is reported. For colonic prokinetic effects in cats use with cisapride may be considered.

Monitoring

- Clinical efficacy (dependent on reason for use); monitored by decrease in symptomatology, endoscopic examination, blood in feces, etc.

Client Information

- Used to treat or prevent stomach ulcers or to help the stomach to empty.
- When given once a day, works best if given before the first meal of the day.
- Nizatidine is available OTC (over the counter; without a prescription), but only give it to your animal if your veterinarian recommends.

Chemistry/Synonyms

Nizatidine occurs as an off-white to buff-colored crystalline powder. It has a bitter taste and a slight sulfur-like odor. Nizatidine is sparingly soluble in water.

Nizatidine may also be known as: LY-139037, nizatidinum, and *Axid®*.

Storage/Stability

Nizatidine oral tablets and capsules should be stored in tight, light-resistant containers at room temperature.

Compatibility/Compounding Considerations

No specific information noted.

Dosage Forms/Regulatory Status

VETERINARY-LABELED PRODUCTS: NONE.

The ARCI (Racing Commissioners International) has designated this drug as a class 5 substance. See the appendix for more information.

HUMAN-LABELED PRODUCTS:

Nizatidine Tablets: 75 mg; *Axid® AR;* (OTC)

Nizatidine Capsules: 150 mg & 300 mg; *Axid®*, generic; (Rx)

Nizatidine Oral Solution: 15 mg/mL in 480 mL; *Axid®*, generic; (Rx)

Revisions/References

Monograph revised/updated April 2014.

Norepinephrine Bitartrate

(nor-epeh-**nef**-rin)   Noradrenaline, Levarterenol, Levophed®

Alpha & Beta Adrenergic Pressor Agent

Prescriber Highlights

▶ Pressor agent for persistent, profound shock (after fluids replaced); potentially useful for isoflurane-induced hypotension.

▶ ICU drug, requires CRI and continuous monitoring.

▶ Extravasation injuries possible.

Uses/Indications

Norepinephrine is a direct-acting sympathomimetic vasopressor and cardiac inotrope that may be indicated for treating profound hypotension—especially septic shock, or post-cardiac arrest hypotension due to vasodilation. In patients with persistent shock after adequate fluid volume replacement, it can be used as a cardiac stimulant and to raise blood pressure. Norepinephrine has been shown to decrease hypotension in dogs and foals secondary to isoflurane anesthesia (Craig *et al.* 2007), (Valverde *et al.* 2006), (Henao-Guerrero *et al.* 2013). Norepinephrine may also be of useful when administered intragastrically or intraperitoneally for treating upper GI bleeding.

Pharmacology/Actions

Norepinephrine has strong affinity for beta$_1$-, alpha$_1$-, & alpha$_2$-adrenergic receptors. Norepinephrine acts as a peripheral vasoconstrictor (alpha-adrenergic) and inotropic cardiostimulant and coronary artery dilator (betaadrenergic). Total peripheral resistance is increased, resulting in increased systolic and diastolic blood pressure. Perfusion to vital organs, skin, and skeletal muscle can be reduced especially at higher dosages.

Pharmacokinetics

When administered intravenously, norepinephrine's onset of action occurs within 1-2 minutes and persists for an additional 1-2 minutes. It can cause tissue damage and is poorly absorbed subcutaneously. After oral administration, norepinephrine is destroyed in the GI tract and not absorbed. After uptake by sympathetic nerve endings, it is rapidly metabolized via catechol-*O*-methyltransferase (COMT) and monoamine oxidase (MAO) to inactive metabolites.

Contraindications/Precautions/Warnings

Pressors are not a substitute for adequate blood, fluid or electrolyte replacement. Norepinephrine should not be given to patients that are hypotensive from blood volume deficits except as an emergency measure to maintain coronary and cerebral artery perfusion until blood volume replacement therapy can be completed. If used in the absence of blood volume replacement severe peripheral and visceral vasoconstriction, decreased renal perfusion and urine output, and poor systemic blood flow despite "normal" blood pressure can occur. Norepinephrine should not be used if severe peripheral vasoconstriction exists since it may be ineffective and cause further reductions in blood flow to vital organs. Because it increases myocardial oxygen demand, use during cardiac events may outweigh the drug's benefits.

Norepinephrine is a critical care (ICU) drug. Patients must be observed and dosage rates titrated. Avoid abrupt withdrawal of the infusion.

Do NOT confuse NOREPInephrine with EPInephrine. Norepinephrine is considered a "high alert" medication (medications that require special safeguards to reduce the risk of errors). Consider instituting practices such as redundant drug dosage and volume checking, special alert labels, etc.

Adverse Effects

If used in the absence of blood volume replacement, the following may occur: Severe peripheral and visceral vasoconstriction, decreased renal perfusion and urine output, and poor systemic blood flow despite "normal" blood pressure. Higher dosages can cause arrhythmias and seizures. Cats may be more susceptible to these adverse effects. In humans, reported adverse effects for norepinephrine include: headache, weakness, dizziness, tremor, pallor, respiratory difficulty or apnea, and precordial pain.

The human label has a "black box warning" regarding extravasation injuries from norepinephrine. To prevent sloughing and necrosis in areas in which extravasation has taken place, the area should be infiltrated as soon as possible with 10 – 15 mL of saline solution containing from 5 – 10 mg of phentolamine, an adrenergic blocking agent (**Note:** This may need to be obtained from a human hospital pharmacy). A syringe with a fine hypodermic needle should be used, with the solution being infiltrated liberally throughout the area, which is easily identified by its cold, hard, and pallid appearance. Sympathetic blockade with phentolamine causes immediate and conspicuous local hyperemic changes if the area is infiltrated within 12 hours. Therefore, phentolamine should be given as soon as possible after the extravasation is noted.

Reproductive/Nursing Safety

In humans, the FDA categorizes this drug as category *C* for use during pregnancy (*Animal studies have shown an adverse effect on the fetus, but there are no adequate studies in humans; or there are no animal reproduction studies and no adequate studies in humans.*) In a separate system evaluating the safety of drugs in canine and feline pregnancy (Papich 1989), this drug is categorized as class: *C* (*These drugs may have potential risks. Studies in people or laboratory animals have uncovered risks, and these drugs should be used cautiously as a last resort when the benefit of therapy clearly outweighs the risks.*)

It is not known if norepinephrine enters maternal milk.

Overdosage/Acute Toxicity

Overdosage with norepinephrine bitartrate can result in severe hypertension, reflex bradycardia, cardiac ischemia, increase in peripheral resistance with resulting decreased perfusion to vital organs, and decreased cardiac output.

Drug Interactions

The following drug interactions have either been reported or are theoretical in humans or animals receiving norepinephrine and may be of significance in veterinary patients. Unless otherwise noted, use together is not necessarily contraindicated, but weigh the potential risks and perform additional monitoring when appropriate.

- **ATROPINE:** May block the reflex bradycardia caused by norepinephrine and enhances the pressor response.
- **BETA-BLOCKERS:** May result in higher blood pressures secondary to blocking beta-2 arteriole dilation. Can antagonize cardiac stimulating effects; propranolol may be used to treat norepinephrine-induced cardiac arrhythmias.
- **DIGOXIN:** Increased risk for arrhythmias.
- **DIPHENHYDRAMINE:** May potentiate pressor effects.
- **FUROSEMIDE:** May decrease arterial responsiveness to norepinephrine.
- **LINEZOLID:** Norepinephrine effects may be increased.
- **MAO INHIBITORS:** Hypertension can result.
- **TRICYCLIC ANTIDEPRESSANTS** (*e.g.,* **amitriptyline, clomipramine,** etc.): Hypertension, cardiac arrhythmias, tachycardia can result.

Doses

Note: Dosages and drug concentrations are listed as norepinephrine base. Injectable product concentration is labeled as norepinephrine base. An online drip rate table generator is available at: http://www.globalrph.com/drip.htm

- **DOGS/CATS:**

  For persistent, profound hypotension after adequate fluid volume replacement (extra-label): An initial dosage of 0.05 – 0.1 micrograms/kg/minute as a CRI then titrated to desired effect; most recommend a maximum rate of 1 – 2 micrograms/kg/minute. If using a 4 microgram/mL dilution (4 mg in a 1 liter bag of a dextrose 5% containing fluid), the initial rate would be 0.75 – 1.5 mLs/kg/hour. Often used in combination with dopamine, dobutamine or vasopressin.

- **HORSES:**

  For hypotension in critically ill foals (extra-label): Initially 0.1 microgram/kg/minute as a CRI then titrated to desired effect. If using a 4 microgram/mL dilution (4 mg in a 1 liter bag of a dextrose 5% containing fluid) the initial rate would be 1.5 mLs/kg/hour. Upper end of dosage range is approximately 1.5 microgram/kg/minute. (Corley 2004). Use with dobutamine could be considered (Dickey *et al.* 2010).

  For isoflurane–induced hypotension in neonatal foals (extra-label): In the study, hypotension was induced by isoflurane and norepinephrine, dobutamine and vasopressin were evaluated. Norepinephrine was dosed at 0.3 and 1 micrograms/kg/min. Norepinephrine improved cardiac index and O2 delivery; high dosage significantly increased blood pressure. Authors concluded that norepinephrine and dobutamine are better alternatives than vasopressin for restoring cardiovascular function and maintaining splanchnic circulation during isoflurane-induced hypotension in neonatal foals. Effects of combining dobutamine and norepinephrine were not evaluated. (Valverde *et al.* 2006)

Monitoring

Norepinephrine is a critical care (ICU) drug. Patients must be observed and dosage rates titrated. Avoid abrupt withdrawal of the infusion.

- Blood pressure. Preferably including central venous pressure or pulmonary arterial diastolic pressure. Maintain mean arterial pressure >65 mm Hg.
- Heart rate/rhythm
- Blood gases, if available.

- Urine output.

Client Information

- Must only be used by professionals in a setting where precise IV infusion and constant blood pressure monitoring can be performed.

Chemistry/Synonyms

Norepinephrine bitartrate (noradrenaline acid tartrate) occurs as a white or faintly grey, odorless, crystalline powder that slowly darkens on exposure to air and light. One part is soluble in 2.5 parts water. Solutions in water have a pH of ≈3.5. The bitartrate injection contains sulfites.

Norepinephrine may also be known as levarterenol, noradrenaline, or L-arterenol. A commonly known trade name is *Levophed®*.

Storage/Stability

Store at room temperature (25°C; 77°F); excursions are permitted to 15-30°C (59-86°F). Protect from light.

Compatibility/Compounding Considerations

Avoid contact with iron salts, alkalis, or oxidizing agents. Norepinephrine is **not compatible** with aminophylline or sodium bicarbonate. Administer whole blood or plasma separately (via a Ytube and individual containers if given simultaneously).

The following drugs are listed as **compatible** with norepinephrine infusions: amikacin sulfate, calcium chloride/gluconate, ciprofloxacin, dimenhydrinate, dobutamine HCl, heparin sodium, hydrocortisone sodium succinate, magnesium sulfate, meropenem, methylprednisolone sodium succinate, multivitamins, potassium chloride, succinylcholine chloride, and verapamil HCl. Compatibility is dependent upon factors such as pH, concentration, temperature, and diluent used; consult specialized references or a hospital pharmacist for more specific information.

Dilute norepinephrine in dextrose 5% or D5/NS. Administration in saline solution alone is not recommended as significant loss of potency can occur due to oxidation. Dextrose containing fluids can help prevent oxidation. A 4 mL vial (4 mg) is added to a 250 mL, 500 mL, or 1000 mL bag of a dextrose 5%-containing IV solution. Each mL of this dilution then contains either 16 mcg/mL (250 mL bag), 8 mcg/mL (500 mL bag), or 4 mcg/mL (1 L bag) of norepinephrine bitartrate base. Do not use if solution color is pinkish, darker than slightly yellow, or if it contains a precipitate.

Dosage Forms/Regulatory Status

VETERINARY-LABELED PRODUCTS: NONE.

HUMAN-LABELED PRODUCTS:

Norepinephrine Bitartrate for injection (must be diluted before use): 1 mg/mL in 4 mL vials; *Levophed®*, generic; (Rx). Concentrations are listed as norepinephrine base.

Revisions/References

Monograph written April 2014.

Corley, K. T. T. (2004). Inotropes and vasopressors in adults and foals. Veterinary Clinics of North America-Equine Practice 20(1): 77-+.
Craig, C. A., et al. (2007). The cardiopulmonary effects of dobutamine and norepinephrine in isoflurane-anesthetized foals. Veterinary Anaesthesia and Analgesia 34(6): 377-87.
Dickey, E. J., et al. (2010). Use of pressor therapy in 34 hypotensive critically ill neonatal foals. Australian Veterinary Journal 88(12): 472-7.
Henao-Guerrero, N., et al. (2013). Comparison of Dobutamine, Norepinephrine, Vasopressin and Hetastarch for Treatment of Isoflurane-Induced Hypotension in Normovolemic Dogs. Proceedings: International Veterinary Emergency and Critical Care Symposium. accessed via Veterinary Information Network; vin.com
Papich, M. (1989). Effects of drugs on pregnancy. Current Veterinary Therapy X: Small Animal Practice. R. Kirk. Philadelphia, Saunders: 1291-9.
Valverde, A., et al. (2006). Effects of dobutamine, norepinephrine, and vasopressin on cardiovascular function in anesthetized neonatal foals with induced hypotension. American Journal of Veterinary Research 67(10): 1730-7.

Novobiocin Sodium

(noe-ve-**bye**-oh-sin)   Albaplex®

Antibiotic

Prescriber Highlights

▶ Antibiotic primarily effective against some gram-positive cocci. Potentially could be useful for treating staphylococci (including some methicillin-resistant strains) associated with pyoderma in dogs, but commercial oral dosage forms apparently are no longer marketed (in USA).

▶ Contraindications: hypersensitivity to it; Extreme caution: hepatic or hematopoietic dysfunction.

▶ Adverse Effects: Systemic use: Fever, GI (nausea, vomiting, diarrhea), rashes, & blood dyscrasias.

Uses/Indications

Novobiocin is FDA-approved in combination with penicillin G for use in dry dairy cattle as a mastitis tube. Novobiocin was formerly available in combination with tetracycline (± prednisolone) for oral use in dogs.

Pharmacology/Actions

Novobiocin is believed to act in several ways in a bactericidal manner. It inhibits bacterial DNA gyrase, interfering with protein and nucleic acid synthesis and also interferes with bacterial cell wall synthesis. Activity of the drug is enhanced in an alkaline medium.

The spectrum of activity of novobiocin includes some gram-positive cocci (Staphylococci, *Streptococcus pneumonia*, and some group A streptococci). Activity is variable against other streptococci and weak against the Enterococci. Most gram-negative organisms are resistant to the drug, but some *Haemophilus* spp., *Neisseria* spp., and *Proteus* spp. may be susceptible. A small study evaluating *in vitro* susceptibility of methicillin-resistant (MRS) and methicillin-susceptible (MSS) staphylococci found on dogs with superficial pyoderma, found that 93% of MSS strains were susceptible and 80% of MRS strains were susceptible. Resistance to novobiocin was 18X more likely if isolate was also resistant to clindamycin and 10X more likely if also resistant to cefpodoxime (Fulham *et al.* 2011).

Pharmacokinetics

After oral administration, novobiocin is well absorbed from the GI tract. Peak levels occur within 1-4 hours. The presence of food can decrease peak concentrations of the drug.

Novobiocin is only poorly distributed to body fluids with concentrations in synovial, pleural, and ascitic fluids less than those found in plasma. Only minimal quantities of the drug cross the blood-brain barrier, even when meninges are inflamed. Highest concentrations of novobiocin are found in the small intestine and liver. The drug is ≈90% protein bound and is distributed into milk.

Novobiocin is primarily eliminated in the bile and feces. Approximately 3% is excreted into the urine; urine levels are usually less than those found in serum.

Contraindications/Precautions/Warnings

Novobiocin is contraindicated in patients hypersensitive to it. Additionally, the drug should be used with extreme caution in patients with preexisting hepatic or hematopoietic dysfunction.

Adverse Effects

Adverse effects reported with the systemic use of this drug include fever, GI disturbances (nausea, vomiting, diarrhea), rashes, and blood dyscrasias. In humans, occurrences of hypersensitivity reactions, hepatotoxicity, and blood dyscrasias have significantly limited the use of this drug.

Reproductive/Nursing Safety

Safety during pregnancy has not been established; use only when clearly indicated.

Overdosage/Acute Toxicity

Little information is available regarding overdoses of this drug. It is suggested that large oral overdoses be handled by emptying the gut following standard protocols; monitor and treat adverse effects symptomatically if necessary.

Drug Interactions

The following drug interactions have either been reported or are theoretical in humans or animals receiving novobiocin and may be of significance in veterinary patients. Unless otherwise noted, use together is not necessarily contraindicated, but weigh the potential risks and perform additional monitoring when appropriate.

- **BETA-LACTAM ANTIBIOTICS:** Novobiocin reportedly acts similarly to probenecid by blocking the tubular transport of drugs. Although the clinical significance of this is unclear, the elimination rates of drugs excreted in this manner (*e.g.*, **penicillins, cephalosporins**) could be decreased and half-lives prolonged.

Laboratory Considerations

- Novobiocin can be metabolized into a yellow-colored product that can interfere with **serum bilirubin** determinations.
- Novobiocin may interfere with the determination **BSP** (bromosulfophthalein, sulfobromophthalein) uptake tests by altering BSP uptake or biliary excretion.

Doses

- **DOGS:**

  For susceptible infections using the combination product (with tetracycline): 22 mg/kg of each antibiotic PO q12h. (Package insert; *Albaplex*®—Upjohn)

- **CATTLE:**

  For treatment of subclinical mastitis in dry cows (labeled-dose; FDA-approved): Infuse contents of one syringe into each quarter at the time of drying off; not later than 30 days prior to calving. Shake well before using. (Package directions; *Albadry Plus*®—Pharmacia & Upjohn)

Monitoring

- Clinical efficacy.
- Adverse effects.
- Periodic liver function tests and CBC's are recommended if using long-term systemically.

Client Information

- Shake mastitis tubes well before using.
- Do not exceed dosage recommendations or length of treatment.

Chemistry/Synonyms

An antibiotic obtained from *Streptomyces niveus* or *spheroides*, novobiocin sodium occurs as white to light yellow, crystalline powder and is very soluble in water.

Novobiocin or novobiocin sodium may also be known as: crystallinic acid, PA-93, streptonivicin, U-6591, novobiocinum natricum, sodium novobiocin, *Albadry Plus*®, *Albamycin*®, *Biodry*® and *Delta Albaplex*®.

Storage/Stability

Novobiocin should be stored at room temperature in tight containers unless otherwise directed.

Compatibility/Compounding Considerations

No specific information noted.

Dosage Forms/Regulatory Status

VETERINARY-LABELED PRODUCTS:

Novobiocin Combination Products:

Novobiocin (as the sodium salt): 400 mg and Penicillin G Procaine 200,000 Units per 10 mL *Plastet*® Syringe; *Albadry Plus*®; (OTC). FDA-approved for use in dry cows only. Do not use 30 days prior to calving. Milk must not be used for 72 hours after calving. Slaughter withdrawal (at labeled doses) = 30 days.

Novobiocin Sodium 60 mg, Tetracycline HCl 60 mg; Novobiocin Sodium 180 mg, Tetracycline HCl 180 mg; *Albaplex*® and *Albaplex*® *3X*; (Rx). FDA-approved for use in dogs. These products are still listed in FDA's "Green Book", but apparently are no longer marketed. Another product that also contained prednisolone (*Delta Albaplex*®) was also historically available.

HUMAN-LABELED PRODUCTS: NONE.

Revisions/References

Monograph revised/updated April 2014.

Fulham, K. S., et al. (2011). In vitro susceptibility testing of meticillin-resistant and meticillin-susceptible staphylococci to mupirocin and novobiocin. Veterinary Dermatology 22(1): 88-94.

Nystatin (Oral)

(nye-**stat**-in)

Antifungal (Candida/Yeasts)

Prescriber Highlights

- Oral & topical antifungal (Candida); not absorbed systemically after PO.
- Adverse Effects: GI effects possible at high dosages; hypersensitivity possible.

Uses/Indications

Orally administered nystatin is used primarily for the treatment of oral or gastrointestinal tract Candida infections/overgrowth in dogs, cats, and birds; it has been used less commonly in other species for the same indications.

Pharmacology/Actions

Nystatin has a mechanism of action similar to that of amphotericin B. It binds to sterols in the membrane of the fungal cell altering the permeability of the membrane allowing intracellular potassium and other cellular constituents to "leak out." When given orally, the drug must come into contact with the organism to be effective.

Nystatin has activity against a variety of fungal organisms, but is clinically used against topical, oropharyngeal, and gastrointestinal Candida infections.

Pharmacokinetics

Nystatin is not measurably absorbed after oral administration and almost entirely excreted unchanged in the feces. The drug is not used parenterally because it is reportedly extremely toxic to internal tissues.

Contraindications/Precautions/Warnings

Nystatin is contraindicated in patients with known hypersensitivity to it.

Do not confuse nystatin with HMG-CoA reductase inhibitors ("statin drugs" *e.g.*, simvastatin, etc.).

Adverse Effects

Occasionally, high dosages of nystatin may cause GI upset (anorexia, vomiting, diarrhea). Rarely, hypersensitivity reactions have been reported in humans.

Reproductive/Nursing Safety

Although the safety of the drug during pregnancy has not been firmly established, the lack of appreciable absorption or case reports associating the drug with teratogenic effects appear to make it safe to use. In humans, the FDA categorizes this drug as category *B* for use during pregnancy (*Animal studies have not yet demonstrated risk to the fetus, but there are no adequate studies in pregnant women; or animal studies have shown an adverse effect, but adequate studies in pregnant women have not demonstrated a risk to the fetus in the first trimester of pregnancy, and there is no evidence of risk in later trimesters.*)

It is not known whether nystatin is excreted in maternal milk, but because the drug is not absorbed after oral administration it is unlikely to be of concern.

Overdosage/Acute Toxicity

Because the drug is not absorbed after oral administration, acute toxicity after an oral overdose is extremely unlikely, but transient GI distress may result.

Drug Interactions

- No significant interactions reported for oral nystatin.

Doses

- **DOGS/CATS:**

  For oral treatment of candidiasis (extra-label): Dosages are not well established. Anecdotal dosages from 0.1 – 0.15 million units per dog or cat PO 3-4 times a day have been noted.

- **HORSES:**

  For intrauterine infusion for Candidal overgrowth (extra-label): 250,000 – 1,000,000 IU; Mix with sterile water; precipitates in saline. Little science is available for recommending doses, volume infused, frequency, diluents, etc. Most intrauterine treatments are commonly performed every day or every other day for 3-7 days. (Perkins 1999)

- **BIRDS:**

  For crop mycosis and mycotic diarrhea (*Candida albicans*) **for growing turkeys** (FDA-approved): Feed at 50 grams per ton (*Pharmastatin*®-20) or at 100 grams/ton for 7–10 days. (Label directions; *Pharmastatin*®-20 Type A Medicated Article —Zoetis)

  For enteric yeast (Candidal) infections (extra-label):

  a) 200,000 – 300,000 Units/kg PO q8-12h. Relatively large volume must be administered (2 – 3 mL). May also be used prophylactically to prevent yeast infection in nestling birds treated with broad-spectrum antibiotics. Oral lesions may be missed if bird is tubed. (Flammer 2003)

  b) **For neonates on antibiotic therapy:** Crush one fluconazole 100 mg tablet and mix with 20 mL of nystatin 100,000 Units/mL oral suspension. Dose at 0.5 mL/1000g of body weight PO twice daily for duration of antibiotic therapy. (Wissman 2003)

  c) **For treatment of candidiasis after antibiotic or in conjunction with antibiotics:** One mL of the 100,000 Units/mL suspension per 300 grams body weight PO 1-3 times daily for 7-14 days. If treating mouth lesions do not give by gavage. Hand-fed babies should receive antifungal therapy if being treated with antibiotics. (Clubb 1986)

- **REPTILES:**

  For candidiasis (extra-label):

  a) **For turtles with enteric yeast infections:** 100,000 Units/kg PO once daily for 10 days. (Gauvin 1993)

  b) **All species:** 100,000 Units/kg PO once daily. (Jacobson 1999)

Monitoring

- Clinical efficacy.

Client Information

- Shake suspension well before administering.

Chemistry/Synonyms

A polyene antifungal antibiotic produced by *Streptomyces noursei*, nystatin occurs as a yellow to light tan, hygroscopic powder having a cereal-like odor. It is very slightly soluble in water and slightly to sparingly soluble in alcohol. One mg of nystatin contains not less than 4400 Units of activity. According to the USP, nystatin used in the preparation of oral suspensions should not contain less than 5000 Units per mg.

Nystatin may also be known as: fungicidin, nistatina, or nystatinum, *Mycostatin*®, and *Nilstat*®.

Storage/Stability

Nystatin tablets and oral suspension should be stored at room temperature (15-30°C) in tight, light-resistant containers. Avoid freezing the oral suspension or exposing to temperatures >40°C.

Nystatin deteriorates when exposed to heat, light, air or moisture.

Compatibility/Compounding Considerations

No specific information noted.

Dosage Forms/Regulatory Status

VETERINARY-LABELED PRODUCTS:

A Type A medicated feed (*Pharmastatin*®-20 Type A Medicated Article) for use in turkeys is approved.

For topical use, see the topical dermatologic section in the appendix.

HUMAN-LABELED PRODUCTS:

Nystatin Oral Suspension: 0.1 Million Units/mL in 5 mL, 60 mL, 473 mL and 480 mL; generic; (Rx)

Nystatin Bulk powder: 50 million Units, 150 million Units, 500 million Units, 1 billion Units, 2 billion Units & 5 billion Units; *Bio-statin*®, generic, (Rx)

Nystatin Oral Tablets: 0.5 million Units; generic; (Rx)

Nystatin Oral Capsules 0.5 & 1 million Units; *Bio-Statin*®; (Rx)

Also available in oral troches, vaginal tablets, topical creams, powders and ointments.

Revisions/References

Monograph revised/updated April 2014.

Clubb, S. L. (1986). Therapeutics: Individual and Flock Treatment Regimens. *Clinical Avian Medicine and Surgery*. G. J. Harrison and L. R. Harrison. Philadelphia, W.B. Saunders: 327-55.

Flammer, K. (2003). Antifungal therapy in avian medicine. Proceedings: Western Veterinary Conference. accessed via Veterinary Information Network; vin.com

Gauvin, J. (1993). Drug therapy in reptiles. Seminars in Avian & Exotic Med 2(1): 48-59.

Jacobson, E. (1999). Bacterial infections and antimicrobial treatment in reptiles. The North American Veterinary Conference, Orlando. accessed via Veterinary Information Network; vin.com

Perkins, N. (1999). Equine reproductive pharmacology. The Veterinary Clinics of North America: Equine Practice **15**:3(December): 687-704.

Wissman, M. (2003). Avian pediatrics. Western Veterinary Conference. accessed via Veterinary Information Network; vin.com

Oclacitinib

(ok- la-**sit**-ti-nib)   Apoquel®

Janus Kinase (JAK) Inhibitor, Antipruritic

Prescriber Highlights

▶ JAK1 & JAK3 inhibitor for treating pruritus in dogs.

▶ New drug so full adverse effect profile is unknown. Most commonly reported adverse effects are gastrointestinal related (vomiting, diarrhea, inappetence), polydipsia, and lethargy. Serious adverse effects including susceptibility to infections (*e.g.*, pneumonia, demodicosis), neoplasia, and skin disorders are possible.

▶ Dosed twice a day for up to 2 weeks and then backed down to once daily.

Uses/Indications

Oclacitinib is FDA-approved in dogs (at least 1-year old) for the control of pruritus associated with allergic dermatitis and control of atopic dermatitis (Anon 2013a).

In a large (436 dogs), randomized, double-blinded, placebo-controlled, pre-authorization study evaluating the safety and efficacy of oclacitinib for the control of pruritus associated with allergic dermatitis, both owner- and veterinarian-scored visual analog scale scores for pruritus were significantly better for oclacitinib treated dogs versus those treated with placebo (Cosgrove *et al.* 2013a). Another similar study in 299 dogs with chronic atopic dermatitis found that when compared to the placebo group, treated dogs had significantly higher reductions in VAS scores (owner-scored) and Canine AD Extent and Severity Index (CADESI-02; dermatologist-scored) (Cosgrove *et al.* 2013b).

Pharmacology/Actions

Oclacitinib inhibits Janus kinase (JAK) 1-dependent and JAK3-dependent cytokines, including interleukin (IL)-2, IL-4, IL-6 IL-13, and IL-31. These cytokines are thought to play a significant role in inflammatory, pruritic, and allergic processes. Oclacitinib does not significantly inhibit JAK2-dependent cytokines that are important for hematopoiesis.

Onset of antipruritic efficacy can be noted within 12 hours of the first dose.

Pharmacokinetics

After oral administration to dogs, oclacitinib maleate has a bioavailability of 89% and peak plasma concentrations occur in less than 1-hour. Feeding state did not affect pharmacokinetics. Oclacitinib is not significantly bound to plasma proteins in dogs (66-69%). Apparent volume of distribution (steady-state) was 942 mL/kg and total body plasma clearance was 5.3 mL/min/kg. Terminal half-life is 3.5 hours (IV) and 4.1 hours (PO). Oclacitinib is metabolized to several metabolites with an oxidative form being the major metabolite. Less than 4% of the drug is excreted unchanged in the urine within 24 hours of dosing (Collard *et al.* 2012a; Collard *et al.* 2012b).

Contraindications/Precautions/Warnings

The product label states that it is not for use in dogs <12 months of age, those with serious infections, breeding dogs, or pregnant or lactating bitches. Additionally, oclacitinib is labeled that it may increase susceptibility to infection, including demodicosis, and exacerbate neoplastic conditions (Anon 2013a).

While not stated on the label, marketing information from the drug sponsor states that oclacitinib has been safely used in conjunction with vaccines (Anon 2013b). A pre-authorization vaccine response study concluded that at 3X (1.8 mg/kg) doses, there were adequate serological immune responses to a multivalent modified live vaccine (MLV) containing canine distemper virus (CDV), canine parvovirus (CPV), canine adenovirus (CAV), and canine parainfluenza virus (CPI), and to a killed-virus rabies vaccine. However at this dosage rate, 5 of 8 treated dogs developed enlarged lymph nodes, interdigital furunculosis, cysts and mild to severe pododermatitis. One dog was euthanized and was found to have had acute pneumonia and chronic lymphadenitis of mesenteric lymph nodes (Anon 2013c).

Adverse Effects

Due to its recent approval and limited clinical use, oclacitinib's adverse effect profile is not fully known. Most commonly gastrointestinal effects (vomiting, diarrhea, anorexia), polydipsia or lethargy have been noted but other potentially serious adverse effects, including susceptibility to infections (*e.g.,* pneumonia, demodicosis), neoplasia, and skin disorders are possible.

Reproductive/Nursing Safety

Safe use during pregnancy, breeding or nursing has not been established. The drug's label states that it should not be used in breeding dogs, or pregnant or lactating bitches.

Overdosage/Acute Toxicity

Limited information is available on acute toxicity. In pre-approval margin of safety studies, dogs receiving 5X dosages (3 mg/kg PO twice daily for 6 weeks, then once daily for 20 weeks) clinically observed adverse effects attributable to the drug included vomiting, diarrhea, interdigital furunculosis/dermatitis, papillomas and peripheral node lymphadenopathy. No deaths or serious effects were reported (Anon 2013c).

Drug Interactions

No specific drug interactions have been reported. The package insert states that use has not been evaluated in combination with glucocorticoids, cyclosporine, or other systemic immunosuppressive agents. Oclacitinib is not highly bound to plasma proteins and does not inhibit canine cytochrome P450 enzymes. Marketing information from the drug sponsor states that oclacitinib has been safely used in conjunction with other common medications including vaccines, NSAIDs, antibiotics, parasiticides, anticonvulsants, and allergen immunotherapy (Anon 2013b), but this information could not be found on the drug label.

Laboratory Considerations

- Marketing information from the drug sponsor states that oclacitinib can be used in combination with allergy testing (Anon 2013b), but this information could not be found on the current drug label.

Dosages

- **DOGS:**

  For the control of pruritus associated with allergic dermatitis and control of atopic dermatitis (labeled-dose; FDA-approved): 0.4 – 0.6 mg/kg PO twice daily for up to 14 days, and then once daily for maintenance therapy. May be administered with or without food. A dosing chart showing the appropriate number and size of tablets to be administered for the dog's bodyweight can be found in the package insert. (Adapted from Label Information: *Apoquel*®)

Monitoring

- Clinical efficacy.
- Monitor for the development of infections, including demodicosis, and neoplasia.

Client Information

- For use in dogs only; not for human use. Wash hands immediately after handling the tablets. In case of accidental eye contact, flush immediately with water or saline for at least 15 minutes and then seek medical attention. In case of accidental ingestion, seek medical attention immediately (Anon 2013a).

- May give with or without food. If dog vomits or acts 'sick' after a dose, try giving with some food.
- If your dog shows signs of infection, pneumonia (*e.g.*, difficulty breathing or is listless) or has a fever, contact your veterinarian immediately.
- If you see abnormal skin changes or growths, contact your veterinarian.

Chemistry/Synonyms

Oclacitinib maleate (CAS Registry 1208319-26-9; ATC:QD11AH90) is a synthetic sulfonamide-derivative inhibitor of Janus Kinase (JAK).

Oclacitinib may also be known as PF-03394197-11. The trade name is *Apoquel®*.

Storage/Stability

Tablets should be stored at room temperature (20-25°C; 68-77°F). Excursions are allowed between 15-40°C (59-104°F).

Compatibility/Compounding Considerations

No specific information noted.

Dosage Forms/Regulatory Status

VETERINARY-LABELED PRODUCTS:

Oclacitinib Oral Tablets (scored): 3.6 mg, 5.4 mg, & 16 mg; *Apoquel®*; (Rx). Approved for use in dogs (NADA 141-345).

HUMAN-LABELED PRODUCTS: NONE.

Revisions/References

Monograph written August 2013; revised May 2014.

Anon (2013a). Apoquel Tablets (Oclacitinib Maleate) [Package Insert]. Secondary Apoquel Tablets (Oclacitinib Maleate) [Package Insert]. Secondary Anon, Zoetis Inc. Volume

Anon (2013b). Apoquel® (Oclacitinib Tablet): A Rapid and Safe New Treatment for the Control of Pruritus. Secondary Apoquel® (Oclacitinib Tablet): A Rapid and Safe New Treatment for the Control of Pruritus. Secondary Anon, Zoetis Inc. Volume

Anon (2013c). Food and Drug Administration - Freedom of Information Summary: Apoquel (Oclacitinib Tablet; NADA 141-345).

Collard, T., et al. (2012a). The absorption, distribution, metabolism, and elimination of oclacitinib maleate, a novel Janus kinase inhibitor, in the dog. J. Vet. Pharmacol. Ther. 35: 139-40.

Collard, T., et al. (2012b). The pharmacokinetics of oclacitinib maleate, a novel Janus kinase inhibitor, in the dog. J. Vet. Pharmacol. Ther. 35: 58-9.

Cosgrove, S. B., et al. (2013a). Efficacy and safety of oclacitinib for the control of pruritus and associated skin lesions in dogs with canine allergic dermatitis. Veterinary Dermatology: n/a-n/a.

Cosgrove, S. B., et al. (2013b). A blinded, randomized, placebo-controlled trial of the efficacy and safety of the Janus kinase inhibitor oclacitinib (Apoquel (R)) in client-owned dogs with atopic dermatitis. Veterinary Dermatology 24(6): 587-+.

Octreotide Acetate

(ok-**trye**-oh-tide) Sandostatin®

Somatostatin Analog

Prescriber Highlights

▶ Injectable long acting somatostatin analog that may be useful for adjunctive treatment of insulinomas & gastrinomas.

▶ Limited experience, but appears safe. Reduced appetite/anorexia may occur in dogs. May affect GI fat absorption.

▶ Multiple daily SC injections are required. No information for veterinary use of depot IM form.

▶ Can be expensive (especially in large dogs).

Uses/Indications

Octreotide may be useful in the diagnosis and symptomatic treatment of gastrinomas in dogs or cats and in the adjunctive treatment of hyperinsulinemia in patients with insulinomas (especially dogs and ferrets). For insulinomas, duration of effect can be short and response is variable, presumably dependent on whether the tumor

cells have receptors for somatostatin. A case report of successful treatment using octreotide in a dog with necrolytic migratory erythema (NME; superficial necrolytic dermatitis) due to metastatic glucagonoma has been published (Oberkirchner *et al.* 2010).

More research is needed before octreotide can be recommended for this use in veterinary patients with acute pancreatitis. Octreotide has not been effective in reducing growth hormone levels or enhancing insulin sensitivity in cats with acromegaly.

Pharmacology/Actions

Octreotide is a synthetic long acting analog of somatostatin. It inhibits the secretion of insulin (in both normal and neoplastic beta cells), glucagon, secretin, growth hormone, gastrin and motilin. In humans, octreotide may bind to any one of 5 subtypes of somatostatin receptors found on neoplastic beta cells, but dogs only have one subtype. However, canine insulinoma cells receptors can have a high affinity for octreotide. In dogs with insulinomas, increased glycemic effects may be transient and persist for only 3-4 hours.

Pharmacokinetics

Octreotide is absorbed and distributed rapidly from the injection site after SC administration. Half lives in humans average ≈ 2 hours with duration of effect up to 12 hours. Treated dogs or ferrets generally require 2-3 injections per day to maintain blood glucose. About 32% of a dose is excreted unchanged in the urine and patients with severe renal dysfunction may need dosage adjustment.

Contraindications/Precautions/Warnings

Octreotide is contraindicated in patients hypersensitive to it. It should be used with caution in patients with biliary tract disorders.

Adverse Effects

Very limited experience in domestic animals, although it appears to be well tolerated thus far. Anorexia has been reported in some dogs. GI effects (including biliary tract effects) are most commonly noted in human patients, particularly those with acromegaly.

Reproductive/Nursing Safety

In humans, the FDA categorizes this drug as category *B* for use during pregnancy (*Animal studies have not yet demonstrated risk to the fetus, but there are no adequate studies in pregnant women; or animal studies have shown an adverse effect, but adequate studies in pregnant women have not demonstrated a risk to the fetus in the first trimester of pregnancy, and there is no evidence of risk in later trimesters.*)

It is not known whether this drug is excreted in maternal milk.

Overdosage/Acute Toxicity

Serious adverse effects are unlikely. Human subjects have received up to 120 mg IV over 8 hours with no untoward effects.

Drug Interactions

The following drug interactions have either been reported or are theoretical in humans or animals receiving octreotide and may be of significance in veterinary patients. Unless otherwise noted, use together is not necessarily contraindicated, but weigh the potential risks and perform additional monitoring when appropriate.

- **BETA-BLOCKERS:** Octreotide may cause additive bradycardic effects.
- **BROMOCRIPTINE:** Octreotide may increase oral bioavailability.
- **CALCIUM-CHANNEL BLOCKERS:** Octreotide may cause additive bradycardic effects.
- **CYCLOSPORINE:** Octreotide may reduce cyclosporine levels.
- **DIURETICS (and other agents that affect fluid/electrolyte balance):** Octreotide may enhance fluid/electrolyte imbalances.
- **FOOD:** Octreotide may reduce fat absorption.

- INSULIN, ORAL HYPOGLYCEMICS: Octreotide may inhibit insulin.
- QUINIDINE: Octreotide may reduce the quinidine clearance.

Doses

Note: All doses are for "regular" octreotide injection (not the human depot form) unless otherwise noted.

- **DOGS:**

  For adjunctive medical treatment of insulinoma (beta cell tumor) particularly in patients refractory to or unable to tolerate other medical or surgical therapy (extra-label): Based on very limited numbers of dogs. For acute treatment: 20 – 40 micrograms/kg SC q8-12h. For chronic treatment: 2 – 4 micrograms/kg SC q8-12h. (Goutal *et al.* 2012)

  For adjunctive medical treatment of gastrinoma, or necrolytic migratory erythema (NME; 2° to glucagonoma) (extra-label): Based on very limited numbers of dogs. 1 – 20 micrograms/kg SC 3-4 times day.

- **FERRETS:**

  For medical treatment of insulinoma (particularly in patients refractory to or unable to tolerate other medical or surgical therapy); (extra-label): 1 – 2 micrograms/kg SC 2-3 times a day. (Meleo *et al.* 2000)

Monitoring

- Blood glucose (for insulinoma treatment).
- Clinical efficacy.

Client Information

- There is very limited experience with this medication in dogs and ferrets and therapy must be considered experimental.
- Injections must be given 2-3 times a day per veterinarian instructions.
- The expense associated with this medication can be considerable.

Chemistry/Synonyms

Octreotide acetate is a synthetic polypeptide related to somatostatin. It is commercially available in injectable forms for subcutaneous or IV injection, and as an extended release suspension for IM administration.

Octreotide acetate may also be known as: SMS-201-995, *Longastatina®, Samilstin®, Sandostatin®, Sandostatina®,* or *Sandostatine®*.

Storage/Stability

When stored at room temperature and protected from light, octreotide acetate injection remains stable for 14 days. For long-term storage, keep refrigerated. If injecting solution that has been in the refrigerator, allow it to come to room temperature in the syringe before injecting. Do not use artificial warming techniques. It is recommended to use multidose vials within 14 days of initial use.

Dosage Forms/Regulatory Status

VETERINARY-LABELED PRODUCTS: NONE.

HUMAN-LABELED PRODUCTS:

Octreotide Acetate for Injection: 0.05 mg/mL (50 mcg/mL), 0.1 mg/mL (100 micrograms/mL), 0.2 mg/mL (200 micrograms/mL), 0.5 mg/mL (500 micrograms/mL) & 1 mg/mL (1,000 micrograms/mL) in 1 mg amps, single-dose vials and 5 mL multidose vials; *Sandostatin®*, generic; (Rx)

Octreotide Acetate Powder for Injectable Suspension: 10 mg/5 mL, 20 mg/5 mL & 30 mg/5mL in single-use kits; *Sandostatin® LAR Depot*; (Rx)

Revisions/References

Monograph revised/updated May 2014.

Goutal, C. M., et al. (2012). Insulinoma in Dogs: A Review. J. Am. Anim. Hosp. Assoc. 48(3): 151-63.

Meleo, K. & E. Caplan (2000). Treatment of insulinoma in the dogs, cat, and ferret. *Kirk's Current Veterinary Therapy: XIII Small Animal Practice.* J. Bonagura. Philadelphia, WB Saunders: 357-61.

Oberkirchner, U., et al. (2010). Successful treatment of canine necrolytic migratory erythema (superficial necrolytic dermatitis) due to metastatic glucagonoma with octreotide. Veterinary Dermatology 21(5): 510-6.

Olsalazine Sodium

(ole-**sal**-a-zeen)   Dipentum®

Antiinflammatory (Local GI Tract)

Prescriber Highlights

▶ Used for treatment of chronic colitis in dogs that either are unresponsive to or cannot tolerate sulfasalazine; limited experience.

▶ Keratoconjunctivitis sicca (KCS) has been reported in some dogs.

▶ Converted to 2 molecules of 5-ASA (mesalamine) in colon.

▶ Expensive compared to sulfasalazine.

Uses/Indications

Olsalazine is used for treatment of dogs with chronic colitis that either cannot tolerate the adverse effects associated with sulfasalazine or the response to sulfasalazine has been ineffective.

Pharmacology/Actions

Olsalazine is cleaved in the intestine into 5-aminosalicylic acid (5-ASA, mesalamine) by bacteria in the gut. While its exact mechanism is unknown, mesalamine is thought to have efficacy for chronic colitis secondary to its antiinflammatory activity.

Pharmacokinetics

Olsalazine is poorly absorbed; ≈ 98% of a dose reaches the colon intact and what drug is absorbed is rapidly eliminated. Serum half-life is ≈ 1 hour.

Contraindications/Precautions/Warnings

Olsalazine is contraindicated in patients hypersensitive to it or to salicylates. Use with caution in animals with renal disease as renal toxicity has developed, though rarely, in human patients.

Adverse Effects

While keratoconjunctivitis sicca (KCS) is occasionally reported in dogs receiving olsalazine, it probably occurs less frequently than with sulfasalazine therapy. In humans, ≈ 17% of patients developed more serious diarrhea (than they had prior to treatment) after receiving olsalazine.

Reproductive/Nursing Safety

In high dose rat studies, some fetal abnormalities were seen. Use during pregnancy only when benefits outweigh the risks. In humans, the FDA categorizes this drug as category *C* for use during pregnancy (*Animal studies have shown an adverse effect on the fetus, but there are no adequate studies in humans; or there are no animal reproduction studies and no adequate studies in humans.*)

Oral olsalazine given to lactating rats in doses 5-20X the human dose produced growth retardation in their pups. Use with caution in nursing patients.

Overdosage/Acute Toxicity

Overdosage in dogs may cause vomiting, diarrhea and decreased motor activity; treat symptomatically and supportively. Dosages up to 2 grams/kg were not lethal in dogs.

Drug Interactions

The following drug interaction has either been reported or is theoretical in humans or animals receiving olsalazine and may be of significance in veterinary patients. Unless otherwise noted, use together is not necessarily contraindicated, but weigh the potential risks and perform additional monitoring when appropriate.

- **WARFARIN:** Olsalazine may increase prothrombin times in patients receiving warfarin.

Laboratory Considerations

- Olsalazine may cause increases in **ALT** or **AST**.

Doses

- **DOGS:**

  For treatment of inflammatory bowel disease (extra-label): Not commonly recommended unless dogs cannot tolerate sulfasalazine; (extra-label): 5 – 20 mg/kg PO 3 times a day. If a tolerated dose is effective; attempt to slowly titrate down to the lowest effective dose.

Monitoring

- Clinical efficacy.
- Adverse effects.

Client Information

- Should be given with food in evenly spaced doses (if possible).
- Side effects include vomiting, worsening diarrhea, and dry eye syndrome.

Chemistry/Synonyms

Olsalazine sodium occurs as a yellow crystalline powder that is soluble in water and stable under physiologic acidic and alkaline conditions. It is basically 2 molecules of mesalamine (5-ASA) connected at the azo bonding site.

Olsalazine sodium may also be known as: azodisal sodium, dimesalamine, CI mordant yellow 5, CI No. 14130, CJ-91B, olsalazinum natricum, sodium azodisalicylate, *Dipentum®* or *Rasal®*.

Storage/Stability

Store capsules at room temperature.

Dosage Forms/Regulatory Status

VETERINARY-LABELED PRODUCTS: NONE.

The ARCI (Racing Commissioners International) has designated this drug as a class 4 substance. See the appendix for more information.

HUMAN-LABELED PRODUCTS:

Olsalazine Sodium Oral Capsules: 250 mg; *Dipentum®*; (Rx)

Revisions/References

Monograph revised/updated May 2014.

Omeprazole

(oh-**meh**-prah-zahl)   Gastrogard®, Prilosec®

Proton Pump Inhibitor

Prescriber Highlights

▶ Proton pump inhibitor used for GI ulcers & erosions.

▶ May need to adjust dosage in animals with hepatic or renal disease.

▶ Adverse Effects: **Horses:** Unlikely; potential hypersensitivity. **Small Animals:** Appears to be well tolerated. Potentially: GI distress (anorexia, colic, nausea, vomiting, flatulence, diarrhea), hematologic abnormalities, urinary tract infections, proteinuria, or CNS disturbances.

Uses/Indications

Omeprazole is potentially useful in treating both gastroduodenal ulcer disease and preventing or treating gastric erosions caused by ulcerogenic drugs (*e.g.*, aspirin, NSAIDs). Omeprazole was superior to famotidine when used to prevent exercise-induced gastritis in racing Alaskan sled dogs (Williamson *et al.* 2010). When given at 1.5 – 2.6 mg/kg PO q24h it significantly suppressed gastric acid better in dogs than famotidine given at 1 – 1.3 mg/kg PO q12h (Tolbert *et al.* 2011). It has been used as part of triple therapy (with clarithromycin and amoxicillin) for successfully treating Helicobacter infections in dogs (Mirzaeian *et al.* 2013). Omeprazole may reduce cerebrospinal fluid (CSF) production in dogs and be useful in conditions causing intracranial hypertension (hydrocephalus, syringomyelia).

An oral paste product is labeled for the treatment and prevention of recurrence of gastric ulcers in horses. A study in 62 young thoroughbreds during the training phase found that 1 of 31 treated horses (omeprazole 1 mg/kg PO oral paste once daily for 28 days) developed gastric ulcers, while 12 of 31 horses in the control group did. Authors concluded that omeprazole was efficacious in preventing gastric ulcers in young Thoroughbreds during the training period (Endo *et al.* 2012). Another study in thoroughbreds demonstrated that healing and improvement was much better when omeprazole is used for squamous gastric ulcers (ESGUS) than glandular gastric ulcers (EGGUS) (Sykes *et al.* 2013).

Pharmacology/Actions

Omeprazole is a substituted benzimidazole gastric acid (proton) pump inhibitor. In an acidic environment, omeprazole is activated to a sulphenamide derivative that binds irreversibly at the secretory surface of parietal cells to the enzyme, H^+/K^+ ATPase. There it inhibits the transport of hydrogen ions into the stomach. Omeprazole reduces acid secretion during both basal and stimulated conditions. There is a lag time between administration and efficacy. In dogs, ≈ 3-5 days is required for maximum gastric acid reduction. Omeprazole also inhibits the hepatic cytochrome P-450 mixed function oxidase system (see Drug Interactions below).

Pharmacokinetics

Omeprazole is rapidly absorbed from the gut; the human commercial product is in an enteric-coated granule form as the drug is rapidly degraded by acid. The equine paste is not enteric coated. In humans, peak serum levels occur within 0.5-3.5 hours and onset of action within 1 hour. Omeprazole is distributed widely, but primarily in gastric parietal cells. In humans, ≈ 95% is bound to albumin and alpha$_1$-acid glycoprotein.

Omeprazole is extensively metabolized in the liver to at least six different metabolites. These are excreted principally in the urine, but also via the bile into feces. Significant hepatic dysfunction will reduce the first pass effect of the drug. In humans and dogs with normal hepatic function, serum half-life averages ≈ 1 hour, but the duration of therapeutic effect may persist for 24-72 hours or more. Effects on acid production in horses can last up to 27 hours, depending upon dose.

Contraindications/Precautions/Warnings

Omeprazole is contraindicated in patients hypersensitive to it. In patients with hepatic or renal disease, the drug's half-life may be prolonged and dosage adjustment may be necessary if the disease is severe.

Do not confuse omeprazole with fomepizole.

Adverse Effects

The manufacturer does not note any adverse effects for use in horses at labeled dosages. Potentially in foals, calcium absorption may be reduced; clinical significance is not clear. There is an anecdotal case report of one horse developing urticaria after receiving omeprazole.

Omeprazole appears to be well tolerated in both dogs and cats at effective dosages. Potentially, GI distress (anorexia, colic, nausea, vomiting, flatulence, diarrhea) could occur, as well as hematologic abnormalities (rare in humans), proteinuria, or CNS disturbances. Chronic very high doses in rats caused enterochromaffin-like cell hyperplasia and gastric carcinoid tumors; effects occurred in dose related manner. The clinical significance of these findings for long-term low-dose clinical usage is not known, however, at the current time in humans, dosing for longer than 8 weeks is rarely recommended unless the benefits of therapy outweigh the potential risks. In dogs, omeprazole use is believed safe for at least 4 weeks of therapy. Treatment of horses for up to 90 days is believed safe.

Reproductive/Nursing Safety
Omeprazole's safety during pregnancy has not been established, but a study done in rats at doses of up to 345X those recommended did not demonstrate any teratogenic effects; however, increased embryo–lethality has been noted in lab animals at very high dosages. In humans, the FDA categorizes this drug as category *C* for use during pregnancy (*Animal studies have shown an adverse effect on the fetus, but there are no adequate studies in humans; or there are no animal reproduction studies and no adequate studies in humans.*)

It is not known whether these agents are excreted in maternal milk. In rats, omeprazole administration during late gestation and lactation at doses of 35–345X the human dose resulted in decreased weight gain in pups. In humans, because of the potential for serious adverse reactions in nursing infants, and the potential for tumorigenicity shown in rat carcinogenicity studies, nursing is discouraged if the drug is required.

Overdosage/Acute Toxicity
The LD_{50} in rats after oral administration is reportedly >4 grams/kg. Humans have tolerated oral dosages of 360 mg/day without significant toxicity. Should a massive overdose occur, treat symptomatically and supportively.

Drug Interactions
The following drug interactions have either been reported or are theoretical in humans or animals receiving omeprazole and may be of significance in veterinary patients. Unless otherwise noted, use together is not necessarily contraindicated, but weigh the potential risks and perform additional monitoring when appropriate.

- BENZODIAZEPINES (*e.g.*, diazepam): Omeprazole may potentially alter benzodiazepine metabolism and prolong CNS effects.
- CLARITHROMYCIN: Increased levels of omeprazole, clarithromycin and 14-hydroxyclarithromycin are possible.
- CLOPIDOGREL: Omeprazole may reduce the transformation of clopidogrel to its active metabolite. Consider using pantoprazole in place of omeprazole.
- CYANOCOBALAMIN (oral): Omeprazole may decrease oral absorption.
- CYCLOSPORINE: Omeprazole may reduce cyclosporine metabolism.
- DIGOXIN: Omeprazole may increase digoxin bioavailability.
- DRUGS REQUIRING DECREASED GASTRIC PH FOR OPTIMAL ABSORPTION (*e.g.,* ketoconazole, itraconazole, iron, ampicillin esters): Omeprazole may decrease drug absorption.
- RIFAMPIN: Omeprazole serum levels may be decreased.
- WARFARIN: Omeprazole may increase anticoagulant effect.

Laboratory Considerations
- Omeprazole may cause increased **liver enzymes.**
- Omeprazole will increase **serum gastrin** levels early in therapy.

Doses
Dose dependent on formulation, equine paste and human oral forms may not be interchangeable. Be wary of compounded formulations; bioequivalence is not assured.

- **DOGS:**

  For GI ulcer management/prevention (extra-label): Usually dosed at 0.5 – 1 mg/kg PO once daily. Practically rounding to the nearest 10 mg within this range. For severe esophagitis some have recommended giving twice a day (up to 2 mg/kg).

  To prevent exercise-induced gastritis in racing Alaskan sled dogs (extra-label): In the study, dogs were dosed at approx. 0.85 mg/kg (one 20 mg tablet) once daily ≈ 30 minutes before being fed. Dosing began ≈ 48 hours before exercise. (Williamson *et al.* 2010)

  For Helicobacter infection/gastritis (extra-label): Omeprazole 0.5 – 1 mg/kg PO once daily, amoxicillin 20 mg/kg PO twice daily, and clarithromycin 7.5 mg/kg PO twice daily for 21 days. (Mirzaeian *et al.* 2013)

- **CATS:**

  For GI ulcer management/prevention (extra-label): Usually dosed at 0.5 – 1 mg/kg PO once daily. Practically rounding to the nearest 10 mg within this range. For severe esophagitis some have recommended giving twice a day (up to 1.5 mg/kg).

- **FERRETS:**

  For short-term treatment of gastroenteritis (extra-label): 0.7 mg/kg PO q24h. (Johnson-Delaney 2009)

- **HORSES:** (NOTE: ARCI UCGFS CLASS 5 DRUG)

  For gastric ulcers (labeled-dose; FDA-approved): <u>For treatment</u> of gastric ulcers: 4 mg/kg PO once daily for 4 weeks; <u>to prevent recurrence</u> treat for at least another 4 weeks at 2 mg/kg PO once daily. (Label Directions; *Gastrogard®*)

  For prevention of gastric ulcers in Thoroughbreds in training (extra-label): 1 mg/kg PO q24h (study was for 28 days) (Endo *et al.* 2012). Another study found that dosages as low as 0.5 mg/kg PO once daily were as effective as the higher dose (Sykes *et al.* 2012).

  Foals: For treatment or prophylaxis of gastric ulcers (extra-label): 4 mg/kg PO once daily for treatment, 1 – 2 mg/kg PO once daily for prophylaxis. (Wilkins 2004)

- **SWINE:**

  For ulcer management (extra-label): 40 mg of PO daily for two days; fasted for 48 hours. (DeMint 1999)

Monitoring
- Efficacy.
- Adverse effects.

Client Information
- Used to treat or prevent stomach ulcers and usually only short-term.
- Works best if given before the first meal of the day.
- Do not open capsules, break or cut tablets unless instructed to. Talk with your veterinarian or pharmacist if you need a different dosage form.

Chemistry/Synonyms
A substituted benzimidazole proton pump inhibitor, omeprazole has a molecular weight of 345.4 and pK_a's of 4 and 8.8.

Omeprazole may also be known as: H-168/68, or omeprazolum, *Gastrogard®*, *Prilosec®*, *Ulcergard®* and *Zegerid®*.

Storage/Stability
Omeprazole oral paste should be stored below 86°F. Transient exposure to temperatures up to 104°F is permitted. Omeprazole tab-

lets should be stored at room temperature in light-resistant, tight containers. Omeprazole pellets found in the capsules are fragile and should not be crushed. If needed to administer as a slurry, it has been suggested to mix the pellets carefully with fruit juices, not water, milk or saline.

Compatibility/Compounding Considerations

Use caution when using compounded omeprazole products; bioequivalence has been an issue with some compounded preparations. Omeprazole capsules or tablets should not be crushed or chewed. If reducing the dose of the commercially available capsules, the capsule contents should be re-inserted into a gelatin capsule so they cannot be chewed.

Compounded preparation stability: Omeprazole oral suspension compounded from the commercially available powder packets has been published (Johnson *et al.* 2007). Dissolving one (1) omeprazole 20 mg powder packet *qs ad* to 10 mL in sterile water yields 2 mg/mL omeprazole oral suspension that retains >98% potency for 45 days when stored at 4°C; however, the resulting low concentration and strawberry flavoring may not be suitable for administration to veterinary patients. The efficacy of omeprazole 40 mg/mL oral suspension compounded by diluting commercially available equine paste 1:9 with sesame oil for use in dogs has been published (Tolbert *et al.* 2011). While the long-term stability of this preparation has not yet been assayed, it meets the default beyond-use-date criteria of 180 days for non-aqueous oral suspensions.

Dosage Forms/Regulatory Status

VETERINARY-LABELED PRODUCTS:

Omeprazole Oral Paste, 2.28 g per syringe; *Gastrogard®*, (Rx); *Ulcergard®*; (OTC)

The ARCI (Racing Commissioners International) has designated this drug as a class 5 substance. See the appendix for more information.

HUMAN-LABELED PRODUCTS:

Omeprazole Oral Delayed-Release Capsules: 10 mg, 20 mg (tablets & capsules) & 40 mg; *Prilosec®*, *Prilosec® OTC* (*Losec®* in Canada), generic; (Rx & OTC)

Omeprazole Oral Suspension: 2 mg/mL; *First-Omeprazole®*, *Omeprazole+Syrspend SF Alka®*; (Rx).

Omeprazole/Sodium Bicarbonate Oral Capsules (Immediate Release): 20 mg omeprazole/1,100 mg sodium bicarbonate; 40 mg omeprazole/1,100 mg sodium bicarbonate; *Zegerid®*; (Rx)

Omeprazole/Sodium Bicarbonate Powder for Oral Suspension: 20 mg omeprazole/1,680 sodium bicarbonate; 40 mg omeprazole/1,680 sodium bicarbonate in 30 unit-dose packets; *Zegerid®*; (Rx)

Revisions/References

Monograph revised/updated May 2014.

DeMint, J. (1999). Gastric Ulcers. Proceedings: Central Veterinary Conference, Kansas City. accessed via Veterinary Information Network; vin.com

Endo, Y., et al. (2012). Efficacy of Omeprazole Paste in the Prevention of Gastric Ulcers in 2 Years Old Thoroughbreds. Journal of Veterinary Medical Science 74(8): 1079-81.

Johnson, C. E., et al. (2007). Stability of partial doses of omeprazole-sodium bicarbonate oral suspension. Ann Pharmacother 41(12): 1954-61.

Johnson-Delaney, C. (2009). Gastrointestinal physiology and disease of carnivorous exotic companion animals. Proceedings: ABVP. accessed via Veterinary Information Network; vin.com

Mirzaeian, S., et al. (2013). Eradication of gastric Helicobacter spp. by triple therapy in dogs. Veterinarni Medicina 58(11): 582-6.

Sykes, B. W. & G. D. Hallowell (2012). A comparison of two doses of omeprazole in the treatment of gastric ulceration in thoroughbred racehorses. Journal of Veterinary Internal Medicine 26(3): 737-.

Sykes, B. W., et al. (2013). A comparison of three doses of omeprazole in the treatment of gastric ulceration in throughbred racehorses. Journal of Veterinary Internal Medicine 27(3): 652-.

Tolbert, K., et al. (2011). Efficacy of Oral Famotidine and 2 Omeprazole Formulations for the Control of Intragastric pH in Dogs. J Vet Intern Med 25(1): 47-54.

Wilkins, P. (2004). Disorders of foals. Equine Internal Medicine, 2nd Ed. S. Reed, W. Bayly and D. Sellon. Philadelphia, Saunders: 1381-431.

Williamson, K. K., et al. (2010). Efficacy of Omeprazole versus High-Dose Famotidine for Prevention of Exercise-Induced Gastritis in Racing Alaskan Sled Dogs. Journal of Veterinary Internal Medicine 24(2): 285-8.

Ondansetron HCl

(on-**dan**-sah-tron)   Zofran®

5-HT₃ Receptor Antagonist

Prescriber Highlights

▶ 5-HT₃ receptor antagonist for severe vomiting.

▶ Appears to be well tolerated.

Uses/Indications

Ondansetron is an antiemetic used for severe vomiting in dogs and cats. It can be particularly effective for treating chemotherapy associated-vomiting. A study in cats found that ondansetron (0.22 mg/kg IM) administered with dexmedetomidine and buprenorphine (in the same syringe) reduced the incidence ($\approx$ 33%) and severity of nausea and vomiting when compared to ondansetron given 30 minutes prior to dexmedetomidine and buprenorphine (67%) or when ondansetron was not given (76%) (Santos *et al.* 2011).

Pharmacology/Actions

Ondansetron is a 5-HT₃ (serotonin type 3) receptor antagonist. 5-HT₃ receptors are found peripherally on vagal nerve terminals and centrally in the chemoreceptor trigger zone (CTZ). It is not clear if ondansetron's effects are mediated centrally, peripherally or both.

Pharmacokinetics

In cats, ondansetron's oral bioavailability is $\approx$ 32%, but 75% when injected SC. Elimination half-life is $\approx$ 2 hours (IV), 1.2 hours (PO), and 3.2 hours (SC) (Quimby *et al.* 2013).

No canine data was located for ondansetron pharmacokinetics, but it has been reported that oral bioavailability is low. In humans, ondansetron is well absorbed from the GI tract, but exhibits some first pass hepatic metabolism. Bioavailability is $\approx$ 50-60%. Peak plasma levels occur $\approx$ 2 hours after an oral dose. Ondansetron is extensively metabolized in the liver. Elimination half-lives are $\approx$ 3-4 hours, but are prolonged in elderly patients.

Contraindications/Precautions/Warnings

Ondansetron is contraindicated in patients hypersensitive to it or other agents in this class. Ondansetron may mask ileus or gastric distention; it should not be used in place of nasogastric suction. Use with caution in patients with hepatic dysfunction as half-life may be prolonged.

In humans, ondansetron is pumped by P-glycoprotein (the protein encoded by the MDR1/*ABCB*1 gene), but there is currently no data stating whether it is pumped by canine P-glycoprotein. It is suggested to use caution when administering ondansetron to dogs with the MDR1 mutation (Anon 2009).

Adverse Effects

Ondansetron appears to be well tolerated. Constipation, sedation, extrapyramidal clinical signs (head shaking), arrhythmias and hypotension are possible (incidence in humans <10%).

Reproductive/Nursing Safety

Safety in pregnancy not clearly established, but high dose studies in rodents did not demonstrate overt fetal toxicity or teratogenicity. In humans, the FDA categorizes this drug as category *B* for use during pregnancy (*Animal studies have not yet demonstrated risk to the fetus, but there are no adequate studies in pregnant women; or animal studies have shown an adverse effect, but adequate studies in pregnant women have not demonstrated a risk to the fetus in the first trimester of pregnancy, and there is no evidence of risk in later trimesters.*)

Ondansetron is excreted in the maternal milk of rats. Exercise caution when 5-HT$_3$ antagonists are administered to nursing patients.

Overdosage/Acute Toxicity

Overdoses of up to 10X did not cause significant morbidity in human subjects. If an overdose occurs, treat supportively.

Drug Interactions/Laboratory Considerations

- **APOMORPHINE:** A human patient that received ondansetron and apomorphine developed severe hypotension. In humans, use together is contraindicated.
- **CISPLATIN:** Plasma cisplatin concentrations may be decreased.
- **CYCLOPHOSPHAMIDE:** Plasma cyclophosphamide concentrations may be decreased.
- **DRUGS AFFECTING QTc INTERVAL** (*e.g.,* **amiodarone, cisapride, halothane, isoflurane, sotalol**): Theoretically, ondansetron may have additive effects on QTc interval; possible serious arrhythmias may result.
- **TRAMADOL:** In humans, use together may reduce the efficacy of both drugs. Veterinary significance is not known.

Doses

- **DOGS:**

    As an antiemetic (*extra-label*): Most recommend dosages of 0.5 – 1 mg/kg PO or IV (slowly over 2-15 minutes) q12h. However, IV dosages of 0.1 – 0.2 mg/kg have been noted and are closer to human pediatric recommendations. If being used before chemotherapy, give IV (slowly) 30 minutes prior; may repeat q8-12h.

- **CATS:**

    For acute vomiting (*extra-label*): Dosage recommendations vary somewhat; 0.1 – 1 mg/kg IV (slowly), SC, IM or PO q6-12h. Based upon a recent pharmacokinetic study (Quimby *et al.* 2013), oral dosages may need to be towards the high end and given more frequently than IV or SC. If being used before chemotherapy, give IV (slowly) 30 minutes prior to chemo; may repeat q6-12h.

    To reduce the incidence and severity of vomiting associated with dexmedetomidine/buprenorphine premed (*extra-label*): 0.22 mg/kg (IM) administered with dexmedetomidine and buprenorphine (in the same syringe). (Santos *et al.* 2011)

Monitoring

- Clinical efficacy.

Client Information

- Used to treat or prevent severe vomiting. May give oral products with or without food.
- Usually tolerated very well.
- If using compounded topical gel, wear gloves when applying.
- If using orally disintegrating tablets, protect the tablets from moisture and be sure hands are dry whenever handling them.

Chemistry/Synonyms

A selective inhibitor of serotonin type 3 (5-HT$_3$), ondansetron HCl dihydrate occurs as a white to off-white powder that is soluble in water.

Ondansetron HCl may also be known as: GR-38032F or ondansetroni hydrochloridum, and *Zofran®*.

Storage/Stability

Unless otherwise labeled, store oral products in tight, light-resistant containers between 2-30°C. The injection should be stored between 2-30°C and protected from light.

Compatibility/Compounding Considerations

Drugs reported to be **compatible** with ondansetron when combined in a syringe and administered via a Y-site, include: alfentanil, atropine, fentanyl, glycopyrrolate, metoclopramide, midazolam, morphine, naloxone, neostigmine, and propofol.

Ondansetron is reported **compatible** with the following drugs when administered via a Y-site: amikacin, azithromycin, bleomycin, carboplatin, carmustine, cefotaxime, ceftazidime, cefuroxime, cisplatin, clindamycin, cyclophosphamide, cytarabine, dacarbazine, dactinomycin, daunorubicin, dexamethasone sodium phosphate, dexmedetomidine, diphenhydramine, dopamine, doxorubicin HCL (also liposome form), doxycycline, famotidine, filgrastim, fluconazole, gemcitabine, gentamicin, heparin, hydromorphone, hydroxyzine, ifosfamide, imipenem-cilastatin, mannitol, mesna, methotrexate, methylprednisolone sodium succinate, metoclopramide, mitoxantrone, morphine, piperacillin-tazobactam, potassium chloride, prochlorperazine, promethazine, ranitidine, vancomycin, vinblastine, vincristine, and zidovudine.

Compatibility is dependent upon factors such as pH, concentration, temperature, and diluent used; consult specialized references or a hospital pharmacist for more specific information.

Dosage Forms/Regulatory Status

VETERINARY-LABELED PRODUCTS: NONE.

HUMAN-LABELED PRODUCTS:

Ondansetron HCl Tablets: 4 mg, 8 mg, 16 mg & 24 mg; *Zofran®*, generic; (Rx)

Ondansetron Orally Disintegrating Tablets or Oral Film: 4 mg & 8 mg (as base); *Zofran® ODT, Zuplenz®*, generic; (Rx)

Ondansetron HCl Oral Solution: 0.8 mg/ml (4 mg/5 mL) in 50 mL; *Zofran®*, generic; (Rx)

Ondansetron HCl Injection: 2 mg/mL in 2 mL single-dose & 20 mL multi-dose vials; *Zofran®*, generic; (Rx)

Revisions/References

Monograph revised/updated May 2014.

Anon (2009). Problem Drugs, Veterinary Clinical Pharmacology Lab, College of Vet Med, Washington State University.

Quimby, J. M., et al. (2013). Oral, subcutaneous and intravenous pharmacokinetics of ondansetron in healthy cats. Journal of Veterinary Internal Medicine 27(3): 749-50.

Santos, L. C. P., et al. (2011). A randomized, blinded, controlled trial of the antiemetic effect of ondansetron on dexmedetomidine-induced emesis in cats. Veterinary Anaesthesia and Analgesia 38(4): 320-7.

o,p-DDD – see Mitotane

Opiate Antidiarrheals – See Separate Monographs for Diphenoxylate/Atropine, Loperamide, or Paregoric

Orbifloxacin

(or-bi-**flox**-a-sin)   Orbax®

Fluoroquinolone Antibiotic

Prescriber Highlights

▶ Fluoroquinolone antibiotic labeled for dogs & cats.
▶ Contraindications: Immature dogs during the rapid growth phase; known hypersensitivity to this class of drugs. Caution: Known or suspected CNS disorders.
▶ Adverse Effects: GI effects most likely.
▶ Drug Interactions.

Uses/Indications

Orbifloxacin is indicated for treatment in dogs and cats for susceptible bacterial infections. Orbifloxacin may also be of benefit in treating susceptible gram-negative infections in horses.

Pharmacology/Actions

Orbifloxacin is a concentration-dependent bactericidal agent. It acts by inhibiting bacterial DNA-gyrase (a type-II topoisomerase), thereby preventing DNA supercoiling and DNA synthesis. The net result is disruption of bacterial cell replication.

Orbifloxacin has good activity against many gram-negative and gram-positive bacilli and cocci, including most species and strains of *Klebsiella* spp., *Staphylococcus* pseudintermedius or *aureus*, *E. coli*, Enterobacter, Campylobacter, Shigella, Proteus, Pasteurella species. Some strains of *Pseudomonas aeruginosa* and *Pseudomonas* spp. are resistant to orbifloxacin and most *Enterococcus* spp. are resistant. Like other fluoroquinolones, orbifloxacin has weak activity against most anaerobes and is not a good choice when treating known or suspected anaerobic infections.

Pharmacokinetics

After oral administration in dogs or cats, orbifloxacin is apparently nearly completely absorbed. The drug is distributed well (V_d=1.5 L/kg in dogs and 1.4 L/kg in cats) and only slightly bound to plasma proteins (8% dogs; 15% cats). Orbifloxacin is eliminated primarily via the kidneys. Approximately 50% of the drug is excreted unchanged. Serum half-life is ≈ 4-6 hours in both dogs and cats. Urine levels remain well above MIC's for susceptible organisms for at least 24 hours after dosing.

In horses, orbifloxacin is well absorbed after oral administration (bioavailability is ≈ 70%) and distributes in many body fluids and endometrial tissue. Protein binding is relatively low (approx. 20%). Elimination half-life is ≈ 6 hours.

Contraindications/Precautions/Warnings

Orbifloxacin, like other fluoroquinolones, can cause arthropathies in immature, growing animals. Because dogs appear to be more sensitive to this effect, the manufacturer states that the drug is contraindicated in immature dogs during the rapid growth phase (between 2-8 months in small and medium-sized breeds and up to 18 months in large and giant breeds). The drug is also contraindicated in dogs and cats known to be hypersensitive to orbifloxacin or other drugs in its class (quinolones).

The manufacturer states that orbifloxacin should be used with caution in animals with known or suspected CNS disorders (*e.g.*, seizure disorders) as, rarely, drugs in this class have been associated with CNS stimulation.

Adverse Effects

While the manufacturer reports that no adverse effects were reported during clinical studies (at 2.5 mg/kg dosing) in adult animals, higher doses or additional experience with use of the drug may demonstrate additional adverse effects. Gastrointestinal effects (anorexia, vomiting, diarrhea) would most likely be the first adverse effects noted.

Ophthalmic adverse effects are not likely in cats, but the FDA's Adverse Drug Reaction database has received 28 reports (cumulative; as of April 30, 2013) of blindness associated with orbifloxacin. Causal effect cannot be proven, but use higher dosages carefully.

Reproductive/Nursing Safety

Safety in breeding or pregnant dogs or cats has not been established. It is not known whether orbifloxacin enters maternal milk.

Overdosage/Acute Toxicity

Dogs and cats receiving up to 5X (37.5 mg/kg) for 30 days did not result in any significant adverse effects. Cats receiving the higher dosages exhibited soft feces and decreased body weight gains. Retinal toxicity/blindness in cats is possible.

Drug Interactions

The following drug interactions have either been reported or are theoretical in humans or animals receiving orbifloxacin or related fluoroquinolones and may be of significance in veterinary patients. Orbifloxacin has been shown to inhibit CYP1A activity in dogs (Regmi *et al.* 2005). Unless otherwise noted, use together is not necessarily contraindicated, but weigh the potential risks and perform additional monitoring when appropriate.

- **ANTACIDS/DAIRY PRODUCTS:** Containing cations (Mg^{++}, Al^{+++}, Ca^{++}) may bind to orbifloxacin and prevent its absorption; separate doses of these products by at least 2 hours.
- **ANTIBIOTICS, OTHER (aminoglycosides, 3rd-generation cephalosporins, penicillins—extended-spectrum):** Synergism may occur, but is not predictable, against some bacteria (particularly *Pseudomonas aeruginosa*) with these compounds. Although orbifloxacin has minimal activity against anaerobes, *in vitro* synergy has been reported when used with **clindamycin** against strains of Peptostreptococcus, Lactobacillus and *Bacteroides fragilis*.
- **CYCLOSPORINE:** Fluoroquinolones may exacerbate the nephrotoxicity, and reduce the metabolism of systemically administered cyclosporine.
- **FLUNIXIN:** Has been shown in dogs to increase the AUC and elimination half-life of enrofloxacin and enrofloxacin increases the AUC and elimination half-life of flunixin; it is unknown if orbifloxacin also causes this effect or if other NSAIDs interact with orbifloxacin in dogs.
- **GLYBURIDE:** Severe hypoglycemia possible.
- **IRON, ZINC (oral):** Decreased orbifloxacin absorption; separate doses by at least two hours.
- **METHOTREXATE:** Increased MTX levels possible with resultant toxicity.
- **NITROFURANTOIN:** May antagonize the antimicrobial activity of the fluoroquinolones and their concomitant use is not recommended.
- **PHENYTOIN:** Orbifloxacin may alter phenytoin levels.
- **PROBENECID:** Blocks tubular secretion of ciprofloxacin and may also increase the blood level and half-life of orbifloxacin.
- **SUCRALFATE:** May inhibit absorption of orbifloxacin; separate doses of these drugs by at least 2 hours.
- **THEOPHYLLINE:** Orbifloxacin may increase theophylline blood levels.
- **WARFARIN:** Potential for increased warfarin effects.

Doses

- **DOGS/CATS:**

  For susceptible infections (labeled dose; FDA-approved):

  Tablets: Dogs and cats: 2.5 mg/kg – 7.5 mg/kg, once daily PO. Higher end of the dosing range may be necessary in hospitalized patients, those with underlying disease (*e.g.*, malignancy) or structural alterations (*e.g.*, burns, complicated urinary tract infections, foreign body infections), infections associated with vascular compromise and infections caused by "problem" pathogens. (Package Insert; *Orbax®*)

  Suspension: Dogs: For the treatment of urinary tract infections (cystitis) and skin and soft tissue infections (wounds and abscesses) caused by susceptible bacteria (see package insert for actual species): 2.5 – 7.5 mg/kg PO once daily.

  Cats: For the treatment of skin infections (wounds and abscesses) caused by susceptible strains of *S. aureus, E. coli,* and *P. multocida*: 7.5 mg/kg PO once daily. (Package insert; *Orbax® Suspension*)

- **HORSES:**

  For susceptible infections (extra-label): Little documentation exists for clinical use in horses. Two PK studies suggested

5 mg/kg PO once daily (Davis *et al.* 2006), and 7.5 mg/kg PO once daily (Haines *et al.* 2001).

- **BIRDS:**

For Japanese Quail (extra-label): From a PK/PD study: Authors concluded that 20 mg/kg PO once daily would be a rational dose to treat susceptible infections in Japanese quail not intended for food; for more sensitive organisms, 15 mg/kg PO may also be effective. (Hawkins *et al.* 2011)

Monitoring

- Efficacy.
- Adverse effects.

Client Information

- This drug is best given without food on an empty stomach, but if your animal vomits or acts sick after getting it, give with small amount of food or small treat (**no** dairy products, antacids or anything containing iron) to see if this helps. If vomiting continues, contact your veterinarian.
- Do not give at the same time with other drugs or vitamins that contain calcium, iron, or aluminum as these can reduce the amount of drug absorbed.
- Most common side effects are vomiting, nausea (acts 'sick'), or diarrhea.
- Give as long as your veterinarian tells you to even if your animal appears well.

Chemistry/Synonyms

A 4-fluoroquinolone antibiotic, orbifloxacin is slightly soluble in water at neutral pH. Solubility increases in either an acidic or basic medium.

Orbifloxacin may also be known as marufloxacin or *Orbax®*.

Storage/Stability

The commercially available tablets should be stored between 2-30°C (36-86°F) and protected from excessive moisture.

The oral suspension should be stored between 2-25°C (36-77°F). It does not require refrigeration. Store upright. Shake well before use.

Compatibility/Compounding Considerations

An orbifloxacin 22.7 mg tablet crushed and mixed with molasses, dark corn syrup, water from canned tuna, Kame fish sauce, *Ora-Plus®*, *Syrplata®*, or simple syrup was relatively stable (>85% expected value) for up to 7 days when stored unrefrigerated, but protected from light. Mixing with oral supplements that contain calcium or magnesium (*e.g., Lixotinic®*) showed significant inactivation of orbifloxacin by 4 days (Kukanich *et al.* 2003).

Dosage Forms/Regulatory Status

VETERINARY-LABELED PRODUCTS:
Orbifloxacin Oral Tablets: 5.7 mg (yellow) in btls of 250; 22.7 mg (green; E-Z Break) in btls of 250; 68 mg (blue; E-Z Break) in btls of 100; *Orbax®*; (Rx). FDA-approved for use in dogs and cats. Federal law prohibits the use of the drug in food-producing animals.

Orbifloxacin Oral Suspension: 30mg/mL in 20 mL btls; *Orbax® Suspension*; (Rx). FDA-approved for use in dogs and cats. Federal law prohibits the use of the drug in food-producing animals.

HUMAN-LABELED PRODUCTS: NONE.

Revisions/References
Monograph revised/updated May 2014.

Davis, J., et al. (2006). The pharmacokinetics of orbifloxacin in the horse following oral and intravenous administration. J Vet Phamacol Ther **29**(3): 191-7.

Haines, G., et al. (2001). Pharmacokinetics of orbifloxacin and its concentration in body fluids and in endometrial tissues of mares. Can J Vet Res **65**(3): 181-7.

Hawkins, M. G., et al. (2011). Pharmacokinetic–pharmacodynamic integration of orbifloxacin in Japanese quail (Coturnix japonica) following oral and intravenous administration. J. Vet. Pharmacol. Ther. **34**(4): 350-8.

Kukanich, B. & M. Papich (2003). Fluoroquinolone stability in vehicles for oral administration. Proceedings: ACVIM Forum. accessed via Veterinary Information Network; vin.com

Regmi, N. L., et al. (2005). Inhibitory effect of several fluoroquinolones on hepatic microsomal cytochrome P-450 1A activities in dogs. J. Vet. Pharmacol. Ther. **28**(6): 553-7.

Ormetoprim – see Sulfadimethoxine/Ormetoprim

Osaterone Acetate

(oh-**sat**-eh-rone)   *Ypozane®*

Antiandrogenic; Progestational

Prescriber Highlights

▶ For benign prostatic hypertrophy in intact male dogs; not commercially available in USA.

▶ Treatment is labeled for 7 days; efficacy can persist for several months.

▶ Most common side effects include transient appetite stimulation and behavioral changes. Can decrease cortisol levels and affect ACTH stimulation tests.

Uses/Indications

Osaterone acetate is used to treat benign prostatic hypertrophy (BPH) in dogs. It may be of particular usefulness in young, breeding dogs with BPH. Available in the UK and Europe, but at time of writing it is not available it the USA.

Osaterone is also being investigated as a treatment for Alopecia X in dogs.

Pharmacology/Actions

Osaterone acetate is structurally related to progesterone and has anti-androgenic effects. It is thought to act primarily by decreasing testosterone transport into the prostate and competitively binding to prostate androgen receptors. The 15-beta hydroxylated metabolite (PB-4) also has anti-androgenic activity. Although osaterone has weak affinity for glucocorticoid receptors, PB-4 can cause some adrenosuppression. Osaterone has some progestational activity, but does not have mineralocorticoid activity.

Pharmacokinetics

In dogs, osaterone is rapidly absorbed after oral administration; peak levels occur ≈ 2 hours after dosing. Plasma protein binding is around 90% for osaterone and 80% for its active metabolite (PB-4). Osaterone is primarily metabolized via hydroxylation to PB-4 (Minato *et al.* 2005). Elimination half-life is around 80 hours and elimination is primarily in feces via biliary excretion and to a lesser extent, in urine. After a single dose, osaterone/metabolites can be detected in urine and feces for up to 14 days.

Contraindications/Precautions/Warnings

No labeled contraindications. The drug should not be used in female animals or animals hypersensitive (allergic) to it. Osaterone should be used with caution in animals with hepatic dysfunction.

Adverse Effects

The most common adverse effect reported in dogs is a temporary increase in appetite. Transient behavioral changes, including changes in activity level and sociability are common. Polyuria/polydipsia, mammary glad hyperplasia (rare), hair coat changes (very rare) and gastrointestinal effects (vomiting, diarrhea) have been reported. Decreased cortisol plasma levels occur commonly early in treatment and can persist for several weeks. In dogs with hypoadrenocorticism or that are under physiological stress (post-surgery, post-trauma, etc.) consider additional monitoring and glucocorticoid support, if required.

Reproductive/Nursing Safety

Osaterone should not be used in female animals; in laboratory animals it has caused adverse effects on reproductive function.

While the label states that effects on semen quality have not been reported (Anon 2007; Fontaine *et al.* 2010), an early study in Beagles reported transient abnormalities in semen quality probably secondary to decreased testosterone effects on the epididymis (Tsutsui *et al.* 2001).

Overdosage/Acute Toxicity

Little information is available for clinical overdoses. Dosages >10 mg/kg may cause ataxia/tremors. Dogs given 1.25 mg/kg (2.5X labeled dose) for 10 days only showed decrease plasma cortisol levels. One human male ingesting 40 mg had decreased levels of LH, FSH, and testosterone, but no associated clinical signs.

Drug Interactions

The product label states that there are no known interactions and the product can be administered concurrently with antimicrobials. (Anon 2007)

Laboratory Considerations

- Plasma cortisol levels may decrease after starting treatment and continue for several weeks. ACTH stimulation tests may be suppressed.

Dosages

- **DOGS:**

  For treatment of benign prostatic hypertrophy (BPH) in male dogs (extra-label in USA): 0.25 - 0.5 mg/kg PO once a day for 7 days. *Ypozane®* label; (Anon 2007)

Monitoring

- Clinical efficacy (reduced prostate size, improvement in constipation, difficulty urinating).
- Liver enzymes (ALT, ALP) in dogs with a history or signs of hepatic dysfunction.
- Plasma cortisol in dogs with a history or signs of hypoadrenocorticism.

Client Information

- Can be given with or without food.
- Osaterone is usually given for 7 days and then stopped. Improvement is usually seen within 2 weeks and can last for 5 months or more. Your veterinarian will usually want to evaluate your dog 5 months after treatment or sooner if the effects of the drug wear off.
- Often increases appetite or changes in activity level/sociability in treated dogs, these usually stop after a while.
- Wash hands after administration. In the case of accidental ingestion by a person, seek medical advice immediately and show the package leaflet or the label to the physician. Women of childbearing age should avoid contact with, or wear disposable gloves, when administering the product.

Chemistry/Synonyms

Osaterone acetate (CAS Registry: 0010549-04-0; ATCvet: QG-04CX) is structurally related to progesterone and is a derivative of chlormadinone. The commercially available tablets also contain (as excipients): pre-gelatinized starch, carmellose calcium, corn (maize) starch, talc, and magnesium stearate.

Osaterone acetate may also be known as TZP-4238 or 17alpha-acetoxy-6-chloro-2-oxa-4,6-pregnadiene-3, 20-dione. A trade name is *Ypozane®*.

Storage/Stability

Osaterone tablets should be stored at room temperature (15-30°C; 59-86°F). Expiration dates of 3 years post-manufacture are assigned.

Compatibility/Compounding Considerations

No specific information noted.

Dosage Forms/Regulatory Status

VETERINARY-LABELED PRODUCTS: NONE IN THE USA.

In the U.K and some other countries: Oral Tablets: 1.875 mg, 3.75 mg, 7.5 mg, & 15 mg; *Ypozane®*; (Rx, POM-V). Approved for use in dogs.

HUMAN-LABELED PRODUCTS: NONE.

Revisions/References

Monograph written August 2013; revised May 2014.

Anon (2007). Ypozane® [Label Information]. Secondary Ypozane® [Label Information]. Secondary Anon. Suffolk, UK, Virbac Limited. Volume

Fontaine, E., et al. (2010). Fertility after osaterone acetate treatment in breeding dogs suffering from prostatic diseases. Reproduction in Domestic Animals 45: 60-.

Minato, K., et al. (2005). Metabolism of osaterone acetate in dogs and humans. Steroids **70**(9): 563-72.

Tsutsui, T., et al. (2001). Effect of osaterone acetate administration on prostatic regression rate, peripheral blood hormone levels and semen quality in dogs with benign prostatic hypertrophy. Journal of Veterinary Medical Science **63**(4): 453-6.

Oseltamivir Phosphate

(oh-sell-**tam**-ih-vir)   Tamiflu®

Neuraminidase Inhibitor Antiviral

Prescriber Highlights

▶ Neuraminidase inhibitor antiviral for influenza A & B viruses. Potentially could be useful for parvovirus infections in dogs or other mixed bacterial/viral infections, but evidence supporting use is very scant; two studies have not demonstrated efficacy in reducing morbidity or mortality.

▶ Very limited information on efficacy & safety in animals.

▶ Public health concerns; use in veterinary medicine is controversial.

▶ Expense an issue, especially for treating horses.

Uses/Indications

Oseltamivir has been suggested as a treatment for canine parvovirus infections. A published small (n=35; 19 in treatment group), prospective, randomized, blinded, placebo-controlled clinical trial study, treated dogs showed statistically significant differences versus untreated dogs in weight gain and maintenance of white blood cell count (untreated dogs WBC's decreased), but no significant decreases in hospitalization time, treatments needed, clinical scores, morbidity, or mortality. No major adverse effects were noted in the treated group. The authors concluded that while a clear advantage to oseltamivir treated dogs was not established, and the true role of oseltamivir for the treatment of parvovirus enteritis remains speculative, further investigation is warranted (Savigny *et al.* 2010). Another study in 50 dogs, also did not show any significant reduction in mortality or morbidity (Papaioannou *et al.* 2013). Oseltamivir may be of benefit for adjunctive treatment of other viral infections, particularly those with associated secondary bacterial components, but research or experience is lacking. A recent study performed in horses experimentally infected with equine influenza A (H3N8) documented some efficacy in the attenuation of clinical signs (pyrexia), viral shedding, and secondary bacterial pneumonias (Yamanaka *et al.* 2006).

Because oseltamivir is the primary antiviral agent proposed for treatment or prophylaxis for an H5N1 influenza ("bird flu") pandemic in humans, its use in veterinary patients is controversial, particularly due to concerns of adequate drug supply for the human population and the potential for influenza virus resistance development. In 2006, the FDA banned the extra-label use of oseltamivir and other influenza antivirals in chickens, turkeys and ducks.

Pharmacology/Actions

Oseltamivir phosphate is a prodrug that is converted after absorption into oseltamivir carboxylate, the active form of the drug. Oseltamivir carboxylate competitively inhibits influenza virus neuraminidase, an enzyme that is required for viral replication, release of virus from infected cells and the prevention of formation of viral aggregates after release from cells. Resistance to oseltamivir has been induced in the laboratory and from post-treatment isolates from infected humans. Oseltamivir or oseltamivir carboxylate do not act as substrates or inhibitors for any CYP-450 isoenzymes.

It has been postulated that oseltamivir may limit the ability of canine parvovirus to pass through intestinal mucosa and infect intestinal crypt cells. There is some evidence that oseltamivir has this effect (increased mucous inactivation) on influenza viruses in the respiratory tract of humans. Additionally, it may reduce GI bacteria colonization, translocation and toxin production.

Pharmacokinetics

No information was located for the pharmacokinetic profiles of oseltamivir in dogs or cats.

In horses, oseltamivir and oseltamivir carboxylate (active metabolite) pharmacokinetics were evaluated after NG administration of 2 mg/kg. The drug was rapidly absorbed and peak levels were attained between 1-2 hours post-dose. Elimination half-lives were ≈ 2 hours for oseltamivir and 2.5 hours of the carboxylate. When dosed at 2 mg/kg, the authors concluded that to maintain levels above the inhibitory concentrations against equine influenza A viruses administration intervals should be <10 hrs (Yamanaka *et al.* 2007).

In humans, oseltamivir phosphate is readily absorbed and converted into the carboxylate (active) form predominantly via liver esterases. The bioavailability of oseltamivir carboxylate is ≈ 75%; it is minimally bound to plasma proteins. Elimination of oseltamivir carboxylate is primarily via renal mechanisms, both glomerular filtration and tubular secretion. Elimination half-life is ≈ 6-10 hours in patients with normal renal function. Up to 20% of a dose may be eliminated in the feces.

Contraindications/Precautions/Warnings

Oseltamivir should not be used in patients with documented hypersensitivity to it. For efficacy, treatment must begin as early as possible. Delay in treatment beyond 40 hours after the onset of clinical signs in humans with influenza is associated with minimal efficacy. Dosages may need adjustment in patients with severe renal insufficiency.

Studies where neonatal rats were administered 1 gram/kg levels of the prodrug in the brain were 1500X greater and the active metabolite was 3X higher than those found in adult rats. Potentially, newborn puppies could exhibit similar findings; neurotoxicity is a possibility.

In 2006, the FDA banned the extra-label use of oseltamivir and other influenza antivirals in chickens, turkeys and ducks.

The UC-Davis Koret Shelter Medicine Program website (accessed October 2010) states: Oseltamivir is a drug developed for treatment of influenza in humans. This drug should not be used for treatment of canine influenza at this time. There are several reasons for this. We do not currently know the appropriate dose and duration for treatment of dogs. For best effect in humans, the drug needs to be started within 48 hours of infection. We rarely recognize canine flu this early. Most importantly, *Tamiflu*® represents a primary line of defense against a human influenza pandemic. Use of this drug may soon be restricted in order to best reserve its use for protection of human health.

Adverse Effects

Adverse effect profile in animals is not known. In the study mentioned above performed in horses, no adverse effects were noted.

In humans, oseltamivir can cause gastrointestinal effects (nausea, vomiting), insomnia and vertigo. Bronchitis has been reported, but may be an artifact associated with influenza infection. Gastrointestinal effects are usually transient and may be alleviated by giving the medication with food.

Reproductive/Nursing Safety

Oseltamivir appears to be relatively safe during pregnancy. In rabbits, doses of 150 and 500 mg/kg (13X, 100X) caused dose-dependent increases of minor skeletal abnormalities. In humans, the FDA categorizes oseltamivir as category C for use during pregnancy (*Animal studies have shown an adverse effect on the fetus, but there are no adequate studies in humans; or there are no animal reproduction studies and no adequate studies in humans.*)

Oseltamivir and oseltamivir carboxylate have been detected in the milk of lactating rats. Safety during nursing cannot be guaranteed, but it is unlikely to pose significant risk in nursing veterinary patients.

Overdosage/Acute Toxicity

Oseltamivir has relatively low toxic potential. In humans, overdoses of up to 1000 mg have caused only nausea and vomiting.

Drug Interactions

The following drug interactions have either been reported or are theoretical in humans or animals receiving oseltamivir and may be of significance in veterinary patients. Unless otherwise noted, use together is not necessarily contraindicated, but weigh the potential risks and perform additional monitoring when appropriate.

- **PROBENECID:** May increase 2-fold the exposure to oseltamivir carboxylate (active metabolite) by reducing tubular secretion. This could potentially be useful in reducing drug dosages or dosing frequency, or increasing serum concentrations at the usual dosage, however supporting data is not readily available. Because of the implications associated with treating H5N1 influenza in humans, expect more information to be published on this interaction in the future. See the Probenecid monograph for more information.

- **VACCINES, INFLUENZA (live):** Oseltamivir may potentially reduce the immune response to live influenza virus vaccines. There does not appear to be any effect on inactivated (killed) vaccines.

Laboratory Considerations

- No specific concerns noted.

Doses

- **DOGS:**

  For adjunctive treatment of canine parvovirus enteritis (extra-label): From a small (n=35), prospective, randomized, blinded, placebo-controlled clinical trial: Dogs in treatment group received 2 mg/kg PO q12h for 5 days. No significant reduction in morbidity or mortality was noted. (Savigny *et al.* 2010)

- **HORSES:**

  For treatment of equine Influenza A (extra-label): 2 mg/kg PO twice daily for 5 days. Must be given early in the course of the disease to obtain satisfactory outcome. Dose used in this experimental study was based upon human pediatric dosage not equine pharmacokinetic or pharmacodynamic data. This study also showed efficacy in reducing the clinical effects of influenza when used prophylactically. Dosage used was 2 mg/kg PO once daily for 5 days, but the authors concluded that this dosage may need to be given longer or changed for better prophylaxis. (Yamanaka *et al.* 2006).

Monitoring

- Efficacy.

Client Information

- If used in veterinary patients, clients should understand the experimental nature of using this treatment.

Chemistry/Synonyms

Oseltamivir phosphate occurs as a white crystalline solid. Molecular weights are 312.4 for the free base and 410.4 for the phosphate salt.

Oseltamivir phosphate may also be known as GS-4104/002, or Ro-64-0796/002 and *Tamiflu®*.

Storage/Stability

Oseltamivir capsules should be stored at 25°C, excursions are permitted to 15-30°C. The oral powder for reconstitution should be stored between 15-30°C. Once reconstituted with 23 mL of water, it should be stored at room temperature (15-30°C) or in the refrigerator (2-8°C) and protected from freezing. After reconstitution, it is stable for 10 days.

Compatibility/Compounding Considerations

A method of preparing an extemporaneously compounded oral suspension (15 mg/mL) has been published by the manufacturer of *Tamiflu®* at: http://goo.gl/pHCVk

Dosage Forms/Regulatory Status

VETERINARY-LABELED PRODUCTS: NONE.

In 2006, the FDA banned the extra-label use of oseltamivir and other influenza antivirals in chickens, turkeys and ducks.

HUMAN-LABELED PRODUCTS:

Oseltamivir Phosphate Oral Capsules: 30 mg, 45 mg, & 75 mg (as base); *Tamiflu®*; (Rx)

Oseltamivir Phosphate Powder for Oral Suspension: 12 mg/mL (as base) after reconstitution in 25 mL bottles; *Tamiflu®*; (Rx)

Revisions/References

Monograph revised/updated May 2014.
Papaioannou, E., et al. (2013). The Potential Role of Oseltamivir in the Management of Canine Parvoviral Enteritis in
50 Natural Cases. British Small Animal Veterinary Congress 2013. accessed via Veterinary Information Network; vin.com
Savigny, M. R. & D. K. Macintire (2010). Use of oseltamivir in the treatment of canine parvoviral enteritis. J. Vet. Emerg. Crit. Care 20(1): 132-42.
Yamanaka, T., et al. (2006). Efficacy of oseltamivir phosphate to horses inoculated with equine influenza A virus. J Vet Med Sci 68(9): 923-8.
Yamanaka, T., et al. (2007). Clinical pharmacokinetics of oseltamivir and its active metabolite oseltamivir carboxylate after oral administration in horses. Journal of Veterinary Medical Science 69(3): 293-6.

Oxacillin Sodium

(ox-a-**sill**-in)

Anti-Staphylococcal Penicillin

Prescriber Highlights

▶ Anti-staphylococcal penicillin; only parenteral dosage forms being marketed in USA.
▶ Predominant adverse effects are GI in nature.

Uses/Indications

The veterinary use of these agents has been primarily in the treatment of bone, skin, and other soft tissue infections in small animals when penicillinase-producing Staphylococcus species have been isolated. Because of its rapid elimination with required frequent dosing and the present unavailability of oral dosage forms, it is rarely used in animals.

Pharmacology/Actions

Cloxacillin, dicloxacillin and oxacillin have nearly identical spectrums of activity and can be considered therapeutically equivalent when comparing *in vitro* activity. These penicillinase-resistant penicillins have a narrower spectrum of activity than the natural penicillins. Their antimicrobial efficacy is aimed directly against penicillinase-producing strains of gram-positive cocci, particularly staphylococcal species. They are sometimes called anti-staphylococcal penicillins. There are documented strains of Staphylococcus that are resistant to these drugs (so-called methicillin-resistant or oxacillin-resistant Staph), but these strains have only begun to be a significant problem in veterinary species. While this class of penicillins does have activity against some other gram-positive and gram-negative aerobes and anaerobes, other antibiotics are usually better choices. The penicillinase-resistant penicillins are inactive against Rickettsia, mycobacteria, fungi, Mycoplasma, and viruses.

Pharmacokinetics

Oxacillin sodium is resistant to acid inactivation in the gut, but is only partially absorbed after oral administration. The bioavailability after oral administration in humans has been reported to range from 30-35%, and, if given with food, both the rate and extent of absorption is decreased. After IM administration, oxacillin is rapidly absorbed and peak levels generally occur within 30 minutes.

The drug is distributed to the lungs, kidneys, bone, bile, pleural fluid, synovial fluid, and ascitic fluid. The volume of distribution is reportedly 0.4 L/kg in human adults and 0.3 L/kg in dogs. As with the other penicillins, only minimal amounts are distributed into the CSF, but levels are increased with meningeal inflammation. In humans, ≈ 89-94% of the drug is bound to plasma proteins.

Oxacillin is partially metabolized to both active and inactive metabolites. These metabolites and the parent compound are rapidly excreted in the urine via both glomerular filtration and tubular secretion mechanisms. A small amount of the drug is also excreted in the feces via biliary elimination. The serum half-life in humans with normal renal function ranges from ≈ 18-48 minutes. In dogs, the elimination half-life has been reported as 20-30 minutes.

Contraindications/Precautions/Warnings

Penicillins are contraindicated in patients with a history of hypersensitivity to them. Because there may be cross-reactivity, use penicillins cautiously in patients who are documented hypersensitive to other beta-lactam antibiotics (*e.g.*, cephalosporins, cefamycins, carbapenems).

Do not administer systemic antibiotics orally in patients with septicemia, shock, or other grave illnesses as absorption of the medication from the GI tract may be significantly delayed or diminished. Parenteral (preferably IV) routes should be used for these cases.

Adverse Effects

Adverse effects with the penicillins are usually not serious and have a relatively low frequency of occurrence.

Hypersensitivity reactions unrelated to dose can occur with these agents and can manifest as rashes, fever, eosinophilia, neutropenia, agranulocytosis, thrombocytopenia, leukopenia, anemias, lymphadenopathy, or full-blown anaphylaxis. In humans, it is estimated that 1-15% of patients hypersensitive to cephalosporins will also be hypersensitive to penicillins. The incidence of cross-reactivity in veterinary patients is unknown.

When given orally, penicillins may cause GI effects (anorexia, vomiting, diarrhea). Because the penicillins may also alter gut flora, antibiotic-associated diarrhea can occur and allow the proliferation of resistant bacteria in the colon (superinfections).

Neurotoxicity (*e.g.*, ataxia in dogs) has been associated with very high doses or very prolonged use. Although the penicillins are not considered hepatotoxic, elevated liver enzymes have been reported. Other effects reported in dogs include tachypnea, dyspnea, edema, and tachycardia.

Reproductive/Nursing Safety

Penicillins have been shown to cross the placenta and safe use of them during pregnancy has not been firmly established, but neither have there been any documented teratogenic problems associated with these drugs; however, use only when the potential benefits outweigh the risks. In humans, the FDA categorizes this drug as category *B* for use during pregnancy (*Animal studies have not yet demonstrated risk to the fetus, but there are no adequate studies in pregnant women; or animal studies have shown an adverse effect, but adequate studies in pregnant women have not demonstrated a risk to the fetus in the first trimester of pregnancy, and there is no evidence of risk in later trimesters.*) In a separate system evaluating the safety of drugs in canine and feline pregnancy (Papich 1989), this drug is categorized as class: *A* (*Probably safe. Although specific studies may not have proved the safety of all drugs in dogs and cats, there are no reports of adverse effects in laboratory animals or women.*)

Penicillins are excreted in maternal milk in low concentrations; use may cause diarrhea, candidiasis, or allergic response in nursing offspring.

Overdosage/Acute Toxicity

Acute oral penicillin overdoses are unlikely to cause significant problems other than GI distress, but other effects are possible (see Adverse effects). In humans, very high dosages of parenteral penicillins, especially in patients with renal disease, have induced CNS effects.

Drug Interactions

The following drug interactions have either been reported or are theoretical in humans or animals receiving oxacillin and may be of significance in veterinary patients. Unless otherwise noted, use together is not necessarily contraindicated, but weigh the potential risks and perform additional monitoring when appropriate.

- **AMINOGLYCOSIDES:** *In vitro* evidence of synergism with oxacillin against *S. aureus* strains.
- **CYCLOSPORINE:** Oxacillin may reduce levels.
- **PROBENECID:** Competitively blocks the tubular secretion of oxacillin, thereby increasing serum levels and serum half-lives.
- **TETRACYCLINES:** Theoretical antagonism; use together usually not recommended.
- **WARFARIN:** Oxacillin may cause decreased warfarin efficacy.

Laboratory Considerations

- As penicillins and other beta-lactams can inactivate aminoglycosides *in vitro* (and *in vivo* in patients in renal failure), serum concentrations of **aminoglycosides** may be falsely decreased if the patient is also receiving beta-lactam antibiotics and the serum is stored prior to analysis. It is recommended that if the assay is delayed, samples be frozen and, if possible, drawn at times when the beta-lactam antibiotic is at a trough.

Doses

Note: Oxacillin is only available commercially in the USA for use as a parenteral injection. For oral therapy, dicloxacillin capsules may be substituted for oxacillin.

- **DOGS/CATS:**
  For susceptible infections (extra-label): 22 – 40 mg/kg PO, SC, IM, or IV q8h. (Lappin 2003)

- **HORSES:**
  For susceptible infections (extra-label): Foals: 20 – 30 mg/kg IV q6-8h (Dose extrapolated from adult horse data; use lower dose or longer interval in premature foals or those <7 days old). (Caprile *et al.* 1987; Brumbaugh 1999)

Monitoring

- Because penicillins usually have minimal toxicity associated with their use, monitoring for efficacy is usually all that is required unless toxic signs develop. Serum levels and therapeutic drug monitoring are not routinely done with these agents.

Client Information

- Unless otherwise instructed by the veterinarian, this drug should be given to an animal with an empty stomach, at least 1 hour before feeding or 2 hours after.

Chemistry/Synonyms

An isoxazolyl-penicillin, oxacillin sodium is a semi-synthetic penicillinase-resistant penicillin. It is available commercially as the monohydrate sodium salt, which occurs as a fine, white, crystalline powder that is odorless or has a slight odor. It is freely soluble in water and has a pK_a of ≈ 2.8. One mg of oxacillin sodium contains not less than 815-950 micrograms of oxacillin. Each gram of the commercially available powder for injection contains 2.8-3.1 mEq of sodium.

Oxacillin sodium may also be known as: sodium oxacillin, methylphenyl isoxazolyl penicillin, (5-methyl-3-phenyl-4-isoxazolyl) penicillin sodium, oxacillinum natricum, oxacillinum natrium, P-12, or SQ-16423.

Storage/Stability

Oxacillin sodium powder for oral solution, and powder for injection should be stored at room temperature (15-30°C) in tight containers. After reconstituting with water, refrigerate and discard any remaining oral solution after 14 days. If kept at room temperature, the oral solution is stable for 3 days.

After reconstituting the sterile powder for injection with sterile water for injection or sterile sodium chloride 0.9%, the resultant solution with a concentration of 167 mg/mL is stable for 3 days at room temperature or 7 days if refrigerated. The manufacturer recommends using different quantities of diluent depending on whether the drug is to be administered IM, IV directly, or IV (piggyback). Refer to the package insert for specific instructions.

Compatibility/Compounding Considerations

Oxacillin sodium injection is reportedly physically **compatible** with the following fluids/drugs: dextrose 5% and 10% in water, dextrose 5% and 10% in sodium chloride 0.9%, lactated Ringer's injection, sodium chloride 0.9% amikacin sulfate, cephapirin sodium, chloramphenicol sodium succinate, dopamine HCl, potassium chloride, sodium bicarbonate, and verapamil.

Oxacillin sodium injection is reportedly physically **incompatible** with the following fluids/drugs: oxytetracycline HCl and tetracycline HCl. Compatibility is dependent upon factors such as pH, concentration, temperature, and diluent used; consult specialized references or a hospital pharmacist for more specific information.

Dosage Forms/Regulatory Status

VETERINARY-LABELED PRODUCTS: NONE.

HUMAN-LABELED PRODUCTS:

Oxacillin Sodium Powder for Injection: 1 gram, 2 gram, & 10 gram, *Bactocill*®, generic; (Rx)

Revisions/References

Monograph revised/updated May 2014.

Brumbaugh, G. (1999). Clinical Pharmacology and the Pediatric Patient. 45th Annual AAEP Convention, Albuquerque. accessed via Veterinary Information Network; vin.com

Caprile, K. A. & C. R. Short (1987). Pharmacologic considerations in drug therapy in foals. Vet Clin North Am (Equine Practice) 3(1): 123-44.

Lappin, M. (2003). Infectious disease. *Small Animal Internal Medicine, 3rd Ed.* R. Nelson and C. Couto. St Louis, Mosby: 12229-1321.

Papich, M. (1989). Effects of drugs on pregnancy. *Current Veterinary Therapy X: Small Animal Practice.* R. Kirk. Philadelphia, Saunders: 1291-9.

Oxazepam

(ox-a-ze-pam)   Serax®

Benzodiazepine

Prescriber Highlights

▶ Benzodiazepine used primarily as an appetite stimulant in cats, but may also be useful to treat behavior problems in dogs or cats.

▶ Contraindications: Known benzodiazepine hypersensitivity, acute narrow angle glaucoma. Caution: Myasthenia gravis, hepatic dysfunction, seizure disorders.

▶ Adverse Effects: Primarily sedation & occasionally, ataxia.

▶ Possibly teratogenic.

▶ C-IV Controlled substance.

Uses/Indications

Oxazepam is used most frequently in small animal medicine as an appetite stimulant in cats and dogs. It may also be useful as an oral anxiolytic agent for adjunctive therapy of behavior-related disorders for both dogs and cats. Like lorazepam, it does not have any active metabolites so it may be a good choice for treating geriatric patients and those with liver dysfunction. Use in feline patients with liver dysfunction is somewhat controversial as it has been anecdotally reported that oxazepam has been associated with fulminant hepatic failure.

Pharmacology/Actions

Oxazepam is classified as an intermediate acting benzodiazepine. The subcortical levels (primarily limbic, thalamic, and hypothalamic) of the CNS are depressed by oxazepam and other benzodiazepines thus producing the anxiolytic, sedative, skeletal muscle relaxant and anticonvulsant effects seen. The exact mechanism of action is unknown, but postulated mechanisms include: antagonism of serotonin, increased release of gamma-aminobutyric acid (GABA) and/or facilitation of GABA activity, and diminished release or turnover of acetylcholine in the CNS. Benzodiazepine specific receptors have been located in the mammalian brain, kidney, liver, lung, and heart. In all species studied, receptors are lacking in the white matter.

Pharmacokinetics

Oxazepam is absorbed from the GI tract, but it is one of the more slowly absorbed oral benzodiazepines. Oxazepam, like other benzodiazepines is widely distributed; it is highly bound to plasma proteins (97% in humans). While not confirmed, oxazepam may cross the placenta and enter maternal milk. Oxazepam is principally conjugated in the liver via glucuronidation to an inactive metabolite. Serum half-life in humans ranges from 3-21 hours.

Contraindications/Precautions/Warnings

Oxazepam is contraindicated in patients who are hypersensitive to it or other benzodiazepines or have acute narrow angle glaucoma. Benzodiazepines have been reported to exacerbate myasthenia gravis. While oxazepam is less susceptible to accumulation than many other benzodiazepines in patients with hepatic dysfunction, it should be used with caution nonetheless.

Use in feline patients with liver dysfunction is somewhat controversial, as it has been anecdotally reported that rarely, oxazepam has been associated with fulminant hepatic failure in cats.

Adverse Effects

The most prevalent adverse effects seen with oxazepam in small animals are sedation, and occasionally, ataxia. These may be transient and dosage adjustment may be required to alleviate them. Paradoxical effects such as excitability, vocalization or aggression are possible. When used to treat negative behaviors a rebound effect can occur, particularly if the drug is not withdrawn slowly.

Rarely, oxazepam has reportedly precipitated tonic-clonic seizures; use with caution in susceptible patients. Potentially, oxazepam could cause hepatic toxicity in cats, but this occurs very rarely.

Reproductive/Nursing Safety

Safe use during pregnancy has not been established; teratogenic effects of similar benzodiazepines have been noted in rabbits and rats. In humans, the FDA categorizes this drug as category *D* for use during pregnancy (*There is evidence of human fetal risk, but the potential benefits from the use of the drug in pregnant women may be acceptable despite its potential risks.*)

Benzodiazepines are excreted in maternal milk. Since neonates metabolize benzodiazepines more slowly than adults do, accumulation of the drug and its metabolites to toxic levels is possible. Chronic diazepam use in nursing mothers reportedly caused human infants to be lethargic and lose weight; avoid the use of benzodiazepines in nursing patients.

Overdosage/Acute Toxicity

When used alone, oxazepam overdoses are generally limited to significant CNS depression (confusion, coma, decreased reflexes, etc.). Treatment of significant overdoses consists of standard protocols for removing and/or binding the drug (if taken orally) in the gut, and supportive systemic measures. The use of analeptic agents, (CNS stimulants such as caffeine, amphetamines, etc.) are generally not recommended. Flumazenil could potentially be used in life-threatening overdoses.

Drug Interactions

The following drug interactions have either been reported or are theoretical in humans or animals receiving oxazepam and may be of significance in veterinary patients. Unless otherwise noted, use together is not necessarily contraindicated, but weigh the potential risks and perform additional monitoring when appropriate.

- **CNS DEPRESSANT DRUGS:** If oxazepam administered with other CNS depressant agents (**barbiturates, narcotics, anesthetics,** etc.) additive effects may occur.
- **PHENYTOIN:** May decrease oxazepam concentrations.
- **PROBENECID:** May impair glucuronide conjugation (in dogs) and prolong effects.
- **RIFAMPIN:** May induce hepatic microsomal enzymes and decrease the pharmacologic effects of benzodiazepines.
- **ST. JOHN'S WORT:** May decrease oxazepam effectiveness.
- **THEOPHYLLINES:** May decrease oxazepam effectiveness.

Laboratory Considerations

- Benzodiazepines may decrease the thyroidal uptake of I^{123} or I^{131}.

Doses

Note: Because 10 mg capsules are the smallest dosage form available, dosages may need to be compounded, especially for cats and smaller dogs.

- **DOGS:**

  For treating fears and phobias (extra-label): Dosage recommendations vary somewhat and no published evidence supporting one over the other was located. Most recommend a range from 0.2 – 1 mg/kg PO q12-24h.

- **CATS:**

  For behavior-related conditions or as an appetite stimulant (extra-label): Dosage recommendations vary somewhat and no published evidence supporting one over the other was located. Most recommend a range from 0.2 – 0.5 mg/kg PO q12-24h.

Monitoring

- Efficacy.
- Adverse effects.

Client Information

- When using for thunderstorm phobias or other triggers (*e.g.,* separation anxiety, etc.) that upset your animal, try to give it about an hour before the event or trigger.
- If you see yellowing of the whites of the eyes or the gums have a yellowish tint; contact veterinarian immediately.
- Sleepiness is most common side effect, but sometimes the drug can change the animal's behavior or work in the opposite way from what is expected.
- This drug may increase appetite, especially in cats.
- Contact your veterinarian immediately if your animal stops eating or seems depressed.

Chemistry/Synonyms

A benzodiazepine, oxazepam occurs as a creamy white to pale yellow powder. It is practically insoluble in water.

Oxazepam may also be known as: oxazepamum, Wy-3498, and *Serax®*.

Storage/Stability

Store oxazepam capsules and tablets at room temperature in well-closed containers.

Dosage Forms/Regulatory Status

VETERINARY-LABELED PRODUCTS: NONE.

The ARCI (Racing Commissioners International) has designated this drug as a class 2 substance. See the appendix for more information.

HUMAN-LABELED PRODUCTS:

Oxazepam Capsules: 10 mg, 15 mg & 30 mg; generic; (Rx; C-IV)

Revisions/References

Monograph revised/updated May 2014.

Oxfendazole

(ox-**fen**-da-zole)   Synanthic®

Antiparasitic Agent (Anthelmintic)

Prescriber Highlights

▶ Benzimidazole anthelmintic used primarily in cattle.
▶ Contraindications: Not for use in female dairy cattle of breeding age.
▶ Caution: Debilitated or sick horses; 7 day slaughter withdrawal in cattle.
▶ Adverse Effects: Unlikely; hypersensitivity possible.

Uses/Indications

Oxfendazole (*Synanthic®*) is indicated in cattle for the removal and control of lungworms, roundworms (including inhibited forms of *Ostertagia ostertagi*) and tapeworms. See the label for actual species covered for the indication.

Oxfendazole marketed as *Benzelmin®* was indicated (no longer marketed in the USA) for the removal of the following parasites in horses: large roundworms (*Parascaris equorum*), large strongyles (*S. edentatus, S. equinus, S. vulgaris*), small strongyles, and pinworms (*Oxyuris equi*).

Pharmacology/Actions

Benzimidazole antiparasitic agents have a broad spectrum of activity against a variety of pathogenic internal parasites. In susceptible parasites, their mechanism of action is believed due to disrupting intracellular microtubular transport systems by binding selectively and damaging tubulin, preventing tubulin polymerization, and inhibiting microtubule formation. Benzimidazoles also act at higher concentrations to disrupt metabolic pathways within the helminth and inhibit metabolic enzymes including malate dehydrogenase

and fumarate reductase.

Pharmacokinetics

Limited information is available regarding this compound's pharmacokinetics. Unlike most of the other benzimidazole compounds, oxfendazole is absorbed more readily from the GI tract. The elimination half-life has been reported to be ≈ 7.5 hours in sheep and 5.25 hours in goats. Absorbed oxfendazole is metabolized to the sulfone and to the active compound fenbendazole (sulfoxide).

After a single oral dose of 50 mg/kg to dogs, oxfendazole levels peaked at 8 hours. Elimination half-lives for the parent compound and the sulfoxide metabolite (active) were both ≈ 5.5 hours. In dogs, oxfendazole plasma concentrations were significantly higher and resident times longer than that of either fenbendazole or albendazole following single oral administration at the same dose (50 mg/kg) (Gokbulut *et al.* 2007).

Contraindications/Precautions/Warnings

Not for use in female dairy cattle of breeding age. A 7-day slaughter withdrawal is required when using at labeled doses.

There are no contraindications to using this drug in horses, but it is recommended to use oxfendazole cautiously in debilitated or sick horses.

Adverse Effects

When used as labeled, it is unlikely any adverse effects will be noted. Hypersensitivity reactions secondary to antigen release by dying parasites are theoretically possible, particularly at high dosages.

Reproductive/Nursing Safety

Oxfendazole may be safely used in pregnant mares and foals. It is not labeled for use in for use in female dairy cattle of breeding age.

Overdosage/Acute Toxicity

Doses of 10X those recommended elicited no adverse reactions in horses tested. It is unlikely that this compound would cause serious toxicity when given alone.

Drug Interactions

The following drug interactions have either been reported or are theoretical in humans or animals receiving oxfendazole and may be of significance in veterinary patients. Unless otherwise noted, use together is not necessarily contraindicated, but weigh the potential risks and perform additional monitoring when appropriate.

- **BROMSALAN FLUKICIDES (dibromsalan, tribromsalan):** Oxfendazole should not be given concurrently with these agents; abortions in cattle and death in sheep have been reported after using these compounds together

Doses

- **HORSES:**

   For susceptible parasites: 10 mg/kg PO. (Roberson 1988), (Package insert; *Benzelmin®*) **Note:** No longer marketed.

- **CATTLE:**

   For the removal and control of lungworms, roundworms (including inhibited forms of *Ostertagia ostertagi*) and tapeworms. See the label for actual species covered for the indication. (labeled dose; FDA-approved): 4.5 mg/kg either PO or via intraruminal injection (22.5% only). May repeat in 4-6 weeks. Dose of the 9.06% suspension is 2.5 mL per 100 lb (50 kg) of body weight PO. Dose of the 22.5% suspension is 1 mL per 100 lb (50 kg) of body weight either PO or intraruminal injection. See package label for specific directions if giving by intraruminal injection. (Adapted from label; *Synanthic®* 9.06% and 22.5%)

- **SWINE:**

   For adult stages of *A. suum, Oesophagostomum* spp., *T. suis* and *Metastrongylus* spp. (extra-label): 30 mg/kg PO once. (Alvarez *et al.* 2013)

Monitoring

- Efficacy.

Client Information

- Not to be used in horses intended for food purposes.
- Shake suspension well.
- Slaughter withdrawal in cattle is 7 days; not FDA-approved for lactating dairy cattle.

Chemistry/Synonyms

A benzimidazole anthelmintic, oxfendazole occurs as white or almost white powder possessing a characteristic odor. It is practically insoluble in water. Oxfendazole is the sulfoxide metabolite of fenbendazole.

Oxfendazole may also be known as RS 8858; there are many international trade names.

Storage/Stability

Unless otherwise directed by the manufacturer, oxfendazole products should be stored at room temperature and protected from light. The manufacturer recommends discarding any unused suspension 24 hours after it has been reconstituted.

Dosage Forms/Preparations/Regulatory Status

VETERINARY-LABELED PRODUCTS:

Oxfendazole Oral Suspension: 9.06% in 1 liter and 4 liter; *Synanthic®*; (OTC). FDA-approved for use in beef cattle and female dairy cattle not of breeding age. Because a withdrawal time in milk has not been established, do not use in female dairy cattle of breeding age. At recommended dosages, slaughter withdrawal is 7 days.

Oxfendazole Oral Suspension: 22.5% in 500 mL and 1 liter; *Synanthic®*; (OTC). FDA-approved for use in beef cattle and female dairy cattle not of breeding age. Because a withdrawal time in milk has not been established, do not use in female dairy cattle of breeding age. At recommended dosages, slaughter withdrawal is 7 days.

HUMAN-LABELED PRODUCTS: NONE.

Revisions/References

Monograph revised/updated May 2014.

Alvarez, L., et al. (2013). Efficacy of a single high oxfendazole dose against gastrointestinal nematodes in naturally infected pigs. Veterinary Parasitology **194**(1): 70-4.
Gokbulut, C., et al. (2007). Comparative plasma disposition of fenbendazole, oxfendazole and albendazole in dogs. Veterinary Parasitology **148**(3-4): 279-87.
Roberson, E. L. (1988). Antinematodal Agents. *Veterinary Pharmacology and Therapeutics.* N. H. Booth and L. E. McDonald. Ames, Iowa State University Press: 882-927.

Oxibendazole

(ox-i-**ben**-da-zole)   Anthelcide EQ®

Antiparasitic Agent (Anthelmintic)

Prescriber Highlights

▶ Benzimidazole anthelmintic used primarily in horses.
▶ Resistance development an ongoing issue.
▶ Contraindications: Severely debilitated horses or horses suffering from colic, toxemia or infectious disease.
▶ Adverse Effects: Unlikely; hypersensitivity possible.

Uses/Indications

Oxibendazole is indicated (labeled) for the removal of the following parasites in horses: large roundworms (*Parascaris equorum*), large strongyles (*S. edentatus, S. equinus, S. vulgaris*), small strongyles, threadworms, and pinworms (*Oxyuris equi*). Resistance to antiparasitic agents is an ongoing problem. It is recommended to perform fecal egg count reduction testing (FECRT) for strongyle nematodes. A value of <90% in 5-10 horses is the suggested cut-off for determining resistance on a given farm (Kaplan *et al.* 2010).

Oxibendazole has also been used in rabbits for adjunctive treatment of *E. cuniculi*.

Pharmacology/Actions

Benzimidazole antiparasitic agents have a broad spectrum of activity against a variety of pathogenic internal parasites. In susceptible parasites, their mechanism of action is believed due to disrupting intracellular microtubular transport systems by binding selectively and damaging tubulin, preventing tubulin polymerization, and inhibiting microtubule formation. Benzimidazoles also act at higher concentrations to disrupt metabolic pathways within the helminth, and inhibit metabolic enzymes, including malate dehydrogenase and fumarate reductase.

Pharmacokinetics

No information was located.

Contraindications/Precautions/Warnings

The label states: Contraindicated in severely debilitated horses or horses suffering from colic, toxemia, or infectious disease.

Adverse Effects

When used in horses at recommended doses, it is unlikely any adverse effects would be seen. Hypersensitivity reactions secondary to antigen release by dying parasites are theoretically possible, particularly at high dosages.

Oxibendazole in combination with diethylcarbamazine (*Filaribits Plus®*) was implicated in causing periportal hepatitis in dogs when it was marketed (1980's).

Bone marrow suppression can occur in rabbits.

Reproductive/Nursing Safety

Oxibendazole is considered safe to use in pregnant mares.

Overdosage/Acute Toxicity

Doses of 60X those recommended elicited no adverse reactions in horses tested. It is unlikely that this compound would cause serious toxicity when given alone to horses.

Drug Interactions

- No significant interactions have been reported.

Doses

- **HORSES:**

   For susceptible parasites (labeled dose; FDA-approved): 10 mg/kg PO; 15 mg/kg PO for strongyloides; horses maintained on premises where reinfection is likely to occur should be retreated in 6-8 weeks. (Package insert; *Anthelcide EQ®*)

- **RABBITS:**

   For adjunctive treatment of *E. cuniculi* (extra-label): Published evidence is scant; bone marrow suppression has been reported. Suggested dosage is 30 mg/kg PO q24h for 7-14 days, then 15 mg/kg once daily for 30-60 days. For palliative treatment of larval migrans 60 mg/kg PO once daily indefinitely has been suggested.

Monitoring

- Efficacy.
- For rabbits, consider CBC after 14 days of treatment.

Client Information

- Protect suspension from freezing. Shake suspension well before using.
- Not for use in horses intended for food.
- Side effects are unlikely.

Chemistry/Synonyms

A benzimidazole anthelmintic, oxibendazole occurs as a white powder that is practically insoluble in water.

Oxibendazole may also be known as SKF-30310 and *Anthelcide EQ®* and in the U.K. by the proprietary names: *Dio®, Equidin®, Equitac®* or *Loditac®*.

Storage/Stability

Unless otherwise directed by the manufacturer, oxibendazole products should be stored at room temperature; protect from freezing.

Dosage Forms/Regulatory Status

VETERINARY-LABELED PRODUCTS:

Oxibendazole Suspension: 100 mg/mL (10%) in gallons. *Anthelcide EQ® Suspension*; (Rx). FDA-approved for use in horses not used for food.

Oxibendazole Oral Paste: 227 mg/gram (22.7%) in 24-gram syringes. *Anthelcide EQ® Paste*; (OTC). FDA-approved for use in horses not used for food.

HUMAN-LABELED PRODUCTS: NONE.

Revisions/References

Monograph revised/updated May 2014.

Kaplan, R. M. & M. K. Nielsen (2010). An evidence-based approach to equine parasite control: It ain't the 60s anymore. Equine Veterinary Education 22(6): 306-16.

Oxybutynin Chloride

(ox-i-**byoo**-tin-in)   Ditropan®, Oxytrol®

Genitourinary Smooth Muscle Relaxant

Prescriber Highlights

▶ Urinary antispasmodic potentially useful in dogs or cats.

▶ Cautions (risk vs. benefit): Obstructive GI tract disease or intestinal atony/paralytic ileus, angle closure glaucoma, hiatal hernia, cardiac disease (particularly associated with mitral stenosis, associated arrhythmias, tachycardia, CHF, etc.), myasthenia gravis, hyperthyroidism, prostatic hypertrophy, severe ulcerative colitis, urinary retention, or other obstructive uropathies.

▶ Adverse Effects: Diarrhea, constipation, urinary retention, hypersalivation, & sedation.

Uses/Indications

Oxybutynin may be useful for the adjunctive therapy of detrusor hyperreflexia in dogs and in cats with FeLV-associated detrusor instability.

Pharmacology/Actions

Considered a urinary antispasmodic, oxybutynin has direct antimuscarinic (atropine-like) and spasmolytic (papaverine-like) effects on smooth muscle. Spasmolytic effects appear to be most predominant on the detrusor muscle of the bladder and small and large intestine. It does not have appreciable effects on vascular smooth muscle. Studies done in patients with neurogenic bladders showed that oxybutynin increased bladder capacity, reduced the frequency of uninhibited contractions of the detrusor muscle and delayed initial desire to void. Effects were more pronounced in patients with uninhibited neurogenic bladders than in patients with reflex neurogenic bladders. Other effects noted in lab animal studies include moderate antihistaminic, local anesthetic, mild analgesic, very low mydriatic, and antisialagogue effects.

Pharmacokinetics

Oxybutynin is apparently rapidly and well absorbed from the GI tract. Studies done in rats show the drug distributed into the brain, lungs, kidneys, and liver. While elimination characteristics have not been well documented, oxybutynin apparently is metabolized in the liver and excreted in the urine. In humans, the duration of action is from 6-10 hours after a dose.

Contraindications/Precautions/Warnings

Because of the drug's pharmacologic actions, oxybutynin should be used when its benefits outweigh its risks if the following conditions are present: obstructive GI tract disease or intestinal atony/para-lytic ileus, angle closure glaucoma, hiatal hernia, cardiac disease (particularly associated with mitral stenosis, associated arrhythmias, tachycardia, CHF, etc.), myasthenia gravis, hyperthyroidism, prostatic hypertrophy, severe ulcerative colitis, urinary retention or other obstructive uropathies.

Adverse Effects

While use in small animals is limited, diarrhea, constipation, urinary retention, hypersalivation, and sedation have been reported. Other adverse effects reported in humans, and potentially seen in animals, primarily result from the drug's pharmacologic effects, including: dry mouth or eyes, tachycardia, anorexia, vomiting, weakness, or mydriasis.

Reproductive/Nursing Safety

While safety during pregnancy has not been firmly established, studies in a variety of lab animals have demonstrated no teratogenic effect associated with the drug. In humans, the FDA categorizes this drug as category *B* for use during pregnancy (*Animal studies have not yet demonstrated risk to the fetus, but there are no adequate studies in pregnant women; or animal studies have shown an adverse effect, but adequate studies in pregnant women have not demonstrated a risk to the fetus in the first trimester of pregnancy, and there is no evidence of risk in later trimesters.*)

It is not known whether this drug is excreted in maternal milk. While oxybutynin may inhibit lactation, no documented problems associated with its use in nursing offspring have been noted.

Overdosage/Acute Toxicity

Overdosage may cause CNS effects (*e.g.*, restlessness, excitement, seizures), cardiovascular effects (*e.g.*, hyper- or hypotension, tachycardia, circulatory failure), fever, nausea or vomiting. Massive overdoses may lead to paralysis, coma, respiratory failure and death. Treatment of overdoses should consist of general techniques to limit absorption of the drug from the GI tract and supportive care as required; intravenous physostigmine may be useful. See the atropine monograph for more information on the use of physostigmine.

There were 82 single agent exposures to oxybutynin reported to the ASPCA Animal Poison Control Center (APCC) during 2009-2013. Of these animals 74 were dogs, with 20 being symptomatic (25% vomiting).

Drug Interactions

The following drug interactions have either been reported or are theoretical in humans or animals receiving oxybutynin and may be of significance in veterinary patients. Unless otherwise noted, use together is not necessarily contraindicated, but weigh the potential risks and perform additional monitoring when appropriate.

- **ANTICHOLINERGIC AGENTS** (*e.g.*, **atropine, propantheline, scopolamine, isopropamide, glycopyrrolate, hyoscyamine, tricyclic antidepressants, disopyramide, procainamide, antihistamines,** etc.): May intensify oxybutynin's anticholinergic effects.

- **AZOLE ANTIFUNGALS** (**ketoconazole,** etc.): May increase oxybutynin levels.

- **CNS DEPRESSANTS:** Other sedating drugs may exacerbate the sedating effects of oxybutynin.

- **MACROLIDE ANTIBIOTICS** (**erythromycin, clarithromycin,** etc.): May increase oxybutynin levels.

Doses

Note: All dosages are for using 'regular' 5 mg oxybutynin tablets or oral syrup unless otherwise noted. There are also sustained-release tablets (q24h for humans), and transdermal gels/patches commercially available. No dosages for these products for dogs or cats were found.

- **DOGS:**

  For **refractory incontinence (detrusor hyperreflexia)** (extra-label): 0.2 mg/kg PO q8-12h; practically most dogs are dosed at (1.25 mg – 3.75 mg; ¼ - one 5 mg tablet) per dog PO q8-12h.

- **CATS:**

  For **refractory incontinence (detrusor hyperreflexia)** (extra-label): 0.5 – 1.25 mg (approximately 1/8ᵗʰ to ¼ of a 5 mg tablet) per cat PO q8-12h.

Monitoring

- Efficacy.
- Adverse effects.

Client Information

- In dogs and cats, oxybutynin is used to help stop bladder spasms that cause leaking of urine.
- Side effects include: diarrhea or constipation, urinary retention (trouble urinating), hypersalivation/drooling, sedation/drowsiness.

Chemistry/Synonyms

A synthetic tertiary amine, oxybutynin chloride occurs as white to off-white crystals. It is freely soluble in water.

Oxybutynin chloride may also be known as: oxybutinyn HCl, 5058, MJ-4309-1, oxybutynini hydrochloridum, *Ditropan®* and *Oxytrol®*.

Storage/Stability

Tablets and oral solution should be stored at room temperature in tight containers. Protect oral solution from light. Tablets have an expiration date of 4 years after manufacture.

Dosage Forms/Regulatory Status

VETERINARY-LABELED PRODUCTS: NONE.

HUMAN-LABELED PRODUCTS:

Oxybutynin Chloride Oral Tablets: 5 mg; generic; (Rx)

Oxybutynin Chloride Oral Extended-release tablets: 5 mg, 10 mg & 15 mg; *Ditropan®* XL, generic; (Rx)

Oxybutynin Chloride Oral Syrup: 1 mg/mL in 473 mL; generic; (Rx)

Oxybutynin Chloride Transdermal System, Topical: 36 mg of oxybutynin delivering 3.9 mg/day in 39 cm² system; *Oxytrol®*; (Rx)

Oxybutynin Topical Gel: 10% in 1 gram sachets; *Gelnique®*; (Rx)

Revisions/References

Monograph revised/updated May 2014.

Oxymorphone HCl

(ox-ee-**mor**-fone)   Numorphan®

Opiate Agonist

Prescriber Highlights

▶ Injectable opiate sedative/restraining agent, analgesic, & preanesthetic.

▶ Availability & expense are issues and most use hydromorphone in its place.

▶ C-II controlled substance.

Uses/Indications

Oxymorphone is used in dogs and cats as a sedative/restraining agent, analgesic, and preanesthetic; occasionally in horses as an analgesic and anesthesia induction agent. It may also be used in swine as an adjunctive analgesic with ketamine/xylazine anesthesia and small rodents as an analgesic/anesthetic for minor surgical procedures.

Oxymorphone is effective for moderate to severe pain and its effects on the cardiovascular system are usually not clinically significant. It causes less histamine release than morphine.

In a study done in dogs, oxymorphone was comparable to hydromorphone in potency and efficacy for pain control. Patients receiving hydromorphone vomited more than when oxymorphone was used, but hydromorphone was significantly less expensive (Bateman *et al.* 2008).

Pharmacology/Actions

Oxymorphone is *mu*-receptor opioid agonist and is ≈ 10X more potent an analgesic on a per weight basis when compared to morphine. Receptors for opiate analgesics are found in high concentrations in the limbic system, spinal cord, thalamus, hypothalamus, striatum, and midbrain. They are also found in tissues such as the gastrointestinal tract, urinary tract, and other smooth muscle.

The morphine-like agonists (morphine, meperidine, oxymorphone) have primary activity at the *mu* receptors, with some activity possible at the *delta* receptor. The primary pharmacologic effects of these agents include: analgesia, antitussive activity, respiratory depression, sedation, emesis, physical dependence, and intestinal effects (constipation/defecation). Secondary pharmacologic effects include: CNS: euphoria, sedation, and confusion. Cardiovascular: bradycardia due to central vagal stimulation, alpha-adrenergic receptors may be depressed resulting in peripheral vasodilation, decreased peripheral resistance, and baroreceptor inhibition. Orthostatic hypotension and syncope may occur. Urinary: Increased bladder sphincter tone can induce urinary retention.

Various species may exhibit contradictory effects from these agents. For example, horses, cattle, swine, and cats may develop excitement after morphine injections and dogs may defecate after morphine. These effects are in contrast to the expected effects of sedation and constipation. Dogs and humans may develop miosis, while other species (especially cats) may develop mydriasis. For more information, see the individual monographs for each agent.

Oxymorphone has less antitussive activity than morphine. In humans, it has more of a tendency to cause increased nausea and vomiting than does morphine, while in dogs the opposite appears to be true. At the usual doses employed, oxymorphone alone has good sedative qualities in the dog. Respiratory depression can occur especially in debilitated, neonatal or geriatric patients. Bradycardia, as well as a slight decrease in cardiac contractility and blood pressure, may also be seen. Like morphine, oxymorphone does initially increase the respiratory rate (panting in dogs) while actual oxygenation may be decreased and blood CO_2 levels may increase by 10 mmHg or more. Oxymorphone may cause more panting in dogs than morphine. Gut motility is decreased with resultant increases in stomach emptying times. Unlike either morphine or meperidine, oxymorphone does not appear to cause histamine release when administered IV and may cause less excitement than morphine.

Pharmacokinetics

Oxymorphone is absorbed when given by IV, IM, SC, and rectal routes. Although absorbed when given orally, bioavailability is reduced, probably from a high first-pass effect. After IV administration, analgesic efficacy usually occurs within 3-5 minutes. After 0.1 mg/kg IM administration to dogs, onset of action is ≈ 15 minutes and duration of effect ≈ 2-4 hours.

In cats, has moderate volume of distribution at steady state (≈ 2.5 L/kg); clearance ≈ 26 mL/min/kg); and a short elimination half-life of ≈ 1.5 hours (Siao *et al.* 2011). After buccal administration to cats, bioavailability is only about 17% (Pypendop *et al.* 2013).

Like morphine, oxymorphone concentrates in the kidney, liver, and lungs; lower levels are found in the CNS. Oxymorphone crosses the placenta and narcotized newborns can result if mothers are given the drug before giving birth, but these effects can be rapidly reversed with naloxone.

The drug is metabolized in the liver; primarily by glucuronidation. Because cats are deficient in this metabolic pathway, half-lives in cats are probably prolonged. The kidneys excrete the glucuronidated metabolite.

Contraindications/Precautions/Warnings

All opiates should be used with caution in patients with hypothyroidism, severe renal insufficiency, adrenocortical insufficiency (Addison's), and in geriatric or severely debilitated patients. Oxymorphone is contraindicated in patients hypersensitive to narcotic analgesics, and generally in patients with diarrhea caused by a toxic ingestion (until the toxin is eliminated from the GI tract).

Because it may cause vomiting, oxymorphone used as a preanesthetic medication in animals with suspected gastric dilation, volvulus, or intestinal obstruction is usually considered contraindicated, but pretreatment with maropitant has been shown to help prevent vomiting in dogs treated with hydromorphone (and presumably oxymorphone) (Kraus 2013).

Oxymorphone should be used with extreme caution in patients with head injuries, increased intracranial pressure, and acute abdominal conditions (*e.g.*, colic) as it may obscure the diagnosis or clinical course of these conditions. It should be used with extreme caution in patients suffering from respiratory disease or acute respiratory dysfunction (*e.g.*, pulmonary edema secondary to smoke inhalation).

Oxymorphone can cause bradycardia and therefore should be used cautiously in patients with preexisting bradyarrhythmias.

Neonatal, debilitated, or geriatric patients may be more susceptible to the effects of oxymorphone and may require lower dosages. Patients with severe hepatic disease may have prolonged duration of action of the drug.

In horses, opiates can mask the behavioral and cardiovascular clinical signs associated with mild colic.

If used in cats at high dosages, it has been recommended to give concurrently with a tranquilizing agent, as oxymorphone can produce bizarre behavioral changes in this species. Generally this is recommended when using other *mu*-agonist opiate agents in cats (*e.g.*, morphine) as well.

Opiate analgesics are also contraindicated in patients who have been stung by the scorpion species *Centruroides sculpturatus Ewing* and *C. gertschi Stahnke* as it may potentiate these venoms.

Adverse Effects

Oxymorphone has a similar adverse effect profile to hydromorphone or morphine in dogs and cats. In dogs, vomiting, sedation, panting, whining/vocalization, and defecation can be noted. Vomiting, nausea and defecation reportedly may occur more frequently after SC dosing versus IV dosing. CNS depression may be greater than desired, particularly when treating moderate to severe pain. In dogs, constant rate IV infusions of >0.05 mg/kg/hr administered for more than 12 hours may cause sedation and adverse effects severe enough to require reducing the rate (Hansen 2008).

Dose related respiratory depression is possible and more likely during general anesthesia. Panting (may occur less often than with hydromorphone) and cough suppression (may be of benefit) may occur.

Secondary to enhanced vagal tone, hydromorphone can cause bradycardia. This apparently occurs on par with morphine or oxymorphone.

Oxymorphone may cause histamine release that, while significantly less then with morphine and usually clinically insignificant, may be significant in critically ill animals.

Constipation is possible with chronic dosing.

When used in cats at high dosages, oxymorphone may cause ataxia, hyperesthesia, and behavioral changes such as hyperexcitability or aggression (without concomitant tranquilization).

In horses, opiates may cause CNS excitement and pretreatment with drugs such as xylazine are usually administered to reduce the behavioral changes these drugs can cause.

Reproductive/Nursing Safety

In humans, the FDA categorizes this drug as category *C* for use during pregnancy (*Animal studies have shown an adverse effect on the fetus, but there are no adequate studies in humans; or there are no animal reproduction studies and no adequate studies in humans.*) In a separate system evaluating the safety of drugs in canine and feline pregnancy (Papich 1989), this drug is categorized as class: *B* (*Safe for use if used cautiously. Studies in laboratory animals may have uncovered some risk, but these drugs appear to be safe in dogs and cats or these drugs are safe if they are not administered when the animal is near term.*)

Most opioids appear in maternal milk, but effects on offspring may not be significant. Withdrawal symptoms have occurred in breastfeeding human infants when maternal administration of an opioid-analgesic is stopped.

Overdosage/Acute Toxicity

Massive overdoses may produce profound respiratory and/or CNS depression in most species. Other effects may include cardiovascular collapse, hypothermia, and skeletal muscle hypotonia. Naloxone is the agent of choice in treating respiratory depression. In massive overdoses, naloxone doses may need to be repeated, and animals should be closely observed as naloxone's effects sometimes diminish before sub-toxic levels of oxymorphone are attained. Mechanical respiratory support should be considered in cases of severe respiratory depression.

Drug Interactions

The following drug interactions have either been reported or are theoretical in humans or animals receiving oxymorphone and may be of significance in veterinary patients. Unless otherwise noted, use together is not necessarily contraindicated, but weigh the potential risks and perform additional monitoring when appropriate.

- **BUTORPHANOL, BUPRENORPHINE, & NALBUPHINE:** Potentially could antagonize opiate effects.
- **CNS DEPRESSANTS, OTHER:** Additive CNS effects possible.
- **DIURETICS:** Opiates may decrease efficacy in CHF patients.
- **MONOAMINE OXIDASE INHIBITORS** (*e.g.*, **amitraz**, possibly **selegiline**): Use MAOI's with oxymorphone with extreme caution as meperidine (a related opiate) is contraindicated in human patients receiving monoamine oxidase (MAO) inhibitors for at least 14 days after receiving MAO inhibitors. Some human patients have exhibited signs of opiate overdose after receiving therapeutic doses of meperidine while taking MAOIs.
- **MUSCLE RELAXANTS, SKELETAL:** Oxymorphone may enhance effects.
- **PHENOTHIAZINES:** Some phenothiazines may antagonize analgesic effects and increase risk for hypotension
- **TRICYCLIC ANTIDEPRESSANTS** (**clomipramine**, **amitriptyline**, etc.): Oxymorphone may exacerbate the effects of tricyclic antidepressants.
- **WARFARIN:** Opiates may potentiate anticoagulant activity.

Laboratory Considerations

- As they may increase biliary tract pressure, opiates can increase plasma **amylase** and **lipase** values up to 24 hours following their administration.

Doses

- **DOGS/CATS:**

  For analgesic sedation/premedication (extra-label): 0.05 – 0.2 mg/kg IV, IM, or SC. Used in combination with a sedative.

  For analgesia (acute pain); (extra-label):

  a) 0.05 – 0.2 mg/kg IV, IM, or SC q1-6h as necessary.

  b) For epidural administration in dogs: 0.05 mg/kg. Recommend to dilute with sterile saline to a volume not to exceed 0.3 mL/kg to a maximum of 6 mL. Use of preservative-free opioids is best. (Matthews 2008)

- **FERRETS:**

  As an analgesic (extra-label): 0.05 – 0.2 mg/kg IV, IM, SC q6-12h.

- **SMALL MAMMALS:**

  As an analgesic (extra-label):

  Rabbits: 0.1 – 0.3 mg/kg IM, SC, IV q2-4h.

  Hamsters, Gerbils, Mice, Rats, Guinea pigs, Chinchillas: 0.2 – 0.5 mg/kg SC q6-12h.

- **HORSES:** (NOTE: ARCI UCGFS CLASS 1 DRUG)

  As an analgesic (extra-label): 0.01 – 0.03 mg/kg IV or IM. **Note:** Opiates (oxymorphone included) may cause CNS excitement in the horse. Pretreatment with acepromazine or xylazine often recommended to reduce the severity of CNS excitement .

- **BIRDS:**

  As a premed (in most species) (extra-label): 0.05 – 0.2 mg/kg IV, IM, SC.

- **ZOO, EXOTIC, WILDLIFE SPECIES:**

  For use in zoo, exotic and wildlife medicine refer to specific references, including:

  a) *Zoo Animal and Wildlife Immobilization and Anesthesia.* West, G., Heard, D., Caulkett, N. (eds.). Blackwell Publishing, 2007.

  b) Handbook of Wildlife Chemical Immobilization, 3rd Ed. Kreeger, T.J. and J.M. Arnemo. 2007.

  c) Fowler's Zoo and Wild Animal Medicine Current Therapy, Volume 7, Miller, R.E., Fowler, M.E., Saunders. 2011.

  d) *Exotic Animal Formulary, 4th Ed.* Carpenter, J.W., Saunders. 2012.

  e) The 2009 American Association of Zoo Veterinarian Proceedings by D. K. Fontenot also has several dosages listed for restraint, anesthesia, and analgesia for a variety of drugs for carnivores and primates. VIN members can access them at: http://goo.gl/NNIWQ or http://goo.gl/9UJse

Monitoring

- Respiratory rate/depth.
- CNS level of depression/excitation.
- Blood pressure (especially with IV use).
- Analgesic activity.
- Cardiac rate.

Client Information

- When given parenterally, this agent should be used in an inpatient setting or with direct professional supervision.

Chemistry/Synonyms

A semi-synthetic phenanthrene narcotic agonist, oxymorphone HCl occurs as odorless white crystals or white to off-white powder. It will darken in color with prolonged exposure to light. One gram of oxymorphone HCl is soluble in 4 mL of water; it is sparingly soluble in alcohol or ether. The commercially available injection has a pH of 2.7-4.5.

Oxymorphone HCl may also be known as: 7,8-Dihydro-14-hydroxymorphinone hydrochloride, or oximorphone hydrochloride, *Numorphan®* and *Opana®*.

Storage/Stability

The injection should be stored protected from light and at room temperature (15-30°C); avoid freezing. The commercially available suppositories should be stored at temperatures between 2-15°C.

Compatibility/Compounding Considerations

Oxymorphone has been reported to be physically **compatible** when mixed with acepromazine, atropine, glycopyrrolate, and ranitidine. It is physically **incompatible** when mixed with barbiturates or diazepam.

Dosage Forms/Regulatory Status

VETERINARY-LABELED PRODUCTS: NONE.

The ARCI (Racing Commissioners International) has designated this drug as a class 1 substance. See the appendix for more information.

HUMAN-LABELED PRODUCTS:

Oxymorphone HCl Oral Tablets: 5 mg & 10 mg; *Opana®*, generic; (Rx, C-II)

Oxymorphone HCl Extended-Release Oral Tablets: 5 mg, 7.5 mg, 10 mg, 15 mg, 20 mg, 30 mg & 40 mg; *Opana® ER*, generic; (Rx, C-II)

Oxymorphone HCl for Injection: 1 mg/mL in 1 mL amps; *Opana®*; (Rx, C-II)

Note: Oxymorphone is a Class-II controlled substance. Very accurate record keeping is required as to use and disposition of stock.

Revisions/References

Monograph revised/updated May 2014.

Bateman, S. W., et al. (2008). Comparison of the analgesic efficacy of hydromorphone and oxymorphone in dogs and cats: a randomized blinded study. Veterinary Anaesthesia and Analgesia 35(4): 341-7.

Hansen, B. (2008). Analgesia for the Critically Ill Dog or Cat: An Update. Veterinary Clinics of North America-Small Animal Practice 38(6): 1353-+.

Kraus, B. L. H. (2013). Efficacy of maropitant in preventing vomiting in dogs premedicated with hydromorphone. Veterinary Anaesthesia and Analgesia 40(1): 28-34.

Matthews, N. (2008). Perioperative Analgesia: Part 1. Concepts and Drugs. Proceedings: ACVC. accessed via Veterinary Information Network; vin.com

Papich, M. (1989). Effects of drugs on pregnancy. *Current Veterinary Therapy X: Small Animal Practice.* R. Kirk. Philadelphia, Saunders: 1291-9.

Pypendop, B. H., et al. (2013). Bioavailability of Oxymorphone, Hydromorphone, Morphine, and Methadone Following Buccal Administration in Cats (Abstract). International Veterinary Emergency and Critical Care Symposium 2013. accessed via Veterinary Information Network; vin.com

Siao, K. T., et al. (2011). Pharmacokinetics of oxymorphone in cats. J. Vet. Pharmacol. Ther. 34(6): 594-8.

Oxytetracycline
Oxytetracycline HCl

(ox-it-tet-ra-**sye**-kleen)   Terramycin®

Tetracycline Antibiotic

Prescriber Highlights

▶ Tetracycline antibiotic; while many bacteria are now resistant, it still may be very useful to treat mycoplasma, rickettsia, spirochetes, & Chlamydia.

▶ Many products and formulations available; when used in food animals refer to actual product labels for indications, restrictions, dosages and withdrawal times.

▶ Contraindications: Hypersensitivity to the tetracyclines. Extreme Caution: Pregnancy. Caution: Liver, renal insufficiency.

▶ Adverse Effects: GI distress, staining of developing teeth & bones, superinfections, photosensitivity; long-term use may cause uroliths. **Cats** do not tolerate very well. **Horses:** if stressed may break with diarrheas (oral use). **Ruminants:** high oral doses can cause ruminal microflora depression & ruminoreticular stasis. Rapid IV of undiluted propylene glycol-based products can cause intravascular hemolysis & cardiodepressant effects. IM: local reactions, yellow staining & necrosis may be seen at the injection site.

Uses/Indications

Certain oxytetracycline products are FDA-approved for use in dogs and cats (no known products are being marketed), calves, non-lactating dairy cattle, sheep, beef cattle, swine, fish, honeybees, and poultry. For cattle, there are several injectable oxytetracycline products, concentrations and formulations. Depending on the product they may be indicated for infectious diseases such as Bovine Respiratory Disease (BRD), diphtheria, foot rot, and infectious bovine keratoconjunctivitis (pinkeye), bacterial enteritis (scours), wooden tongue, leptospirosis, wound infections, and acute metritis. Concentrated formulations (200 mg/mL and 300 mg/mL) have been used for metaphylactic therapy in cattle at high risk for BRD. For more information, refer to the Doses section or the actual product label.

Pharmacology/Actions

Tetracyclines generally act as bacteriostatic antibiotics and inhibit protein synthesis by reversibly binding to 30S ribosomal subunits of susceptible organisms, preventing binding to those ribosomes of aminoacyl transfer-RNA. Tetracyclines also are believed to reversibly bind to 50S ribosomes and additionally alter cytoplasmic membrane permeability in susceptible organisms. In high concentrations, tetracyclines can also inhibit protein synthesis by mammalian cells.

As a class, the tetracyclines have activity against most mycoplasma, spirochetes (including the Lyme disease organism), Chlamydia, and Rickettsia. Against gram-positive bacteria, the tetracyclines have activity against some strains of staphylococci and streptococci, but resistance of these organisms is increasing. Gram-positive bacteria that are usually covered by tetracyclines, include *Actinomyces* spp., *Bacillus anthracis*, *Clostridium perfringens* and *tetani*, *Listeria monocytogenes*, and Nocardia. Among gram-negative bacteria that tetracyclines usually have *in vitro* and *in vivo* activity include *Bordetella* spp., Brucella, Bartonella, *Haemophilus* spp., *Pasteurella multocida*, Shigella, and *Yersinia pestis*. Many or most strains of *E. coli*, Klebsiella, Bacteroides, Enterobacter, Proteus and *Pseudomonas aeruginosa* are resistant to the tetracyclines. While most strains of *Pseudomonas aeruginosa* show *in vitro* resistance to tetracyclines, those compounds attaining high urine levels (*e.g.*, tet-racycline, oxytetracycline) have been associated with clinical cures in dogs with UTI secondary to this organism.

Oxytetracycline and tetracycline share nearly identical spectrums of activity and patterns of cross-resistance. A tetracycline susceptibility disk is usually used for *in vitro* testing for oxytetracycline susceptibility.

Oxytetracycline appears to have immunomodulatory effects that may contribute to its clinical efficacy. In horses, oxytetracycline appears to be a potent inhibitor of matrix metalloproteinase-9 and a modest inhibitor of matrix metalloproteinase-2 (Fugler *et al.* 2009).

Pharmacokinetics

Both oxytetracycline and tetracycline are readily absorbed after oral administration to fasting animals. Bioavailabilities are ≈ 60-80%. The presence of food or dairy products can significantly reduce the amount of tetracycline absorbed, with reductions of 50% or more possible. After IM administration of oxytetracycline (not long-acting) peak levels may occur in 30 minutes to several hours, depending on the volume and site of injection. The long-acting product (*LA-200®*) has significantly slower absorption after IM injection.

Tetracyclines as a class are widely distributed in the body, including to the heart, kidney, lungs, muscle, pleural fluid, bronchial secretions, sputum, bile, saliva, urine, synovial fluid, ascitic fluid, and aqueous and vitreous humor. Only small quantities of tetracycline and oxytetracycline are distributed to the CSF and therapeutic levels may not be attainable. While all tetracyclines distribute to the prostate and eye, doxycycline or minocycline penetrate better into these and most other tissues. Tetracyclines cross the placenta, enter fetal circulation and are distributed into milk. The volume of distribution of oxytetracycline is ≈ 2.1 L/kg in small animals, 1.4 L/kg in horses, and 0.8 L/kg in cattle. The amount of plasma protein binding is ≈ 10-40% for oxytetracycline. Oxytetracycline tissue concentrations are higher in diseased lung than in healthy lung and concentrations in milk are higher than serum when mammary glands are inflamed.

Both oxytetracycline and tetracycline are eliminated unchanged primarily via glomerular filtration. Patients with impaired renal function can have prolonged elimination half-lives and may accumulate the drug with repeated dosing. These drugs apparently are not metabolized, but are excreted into the GI tract via both biliary and nonbiliary routes and may become inactive after chelation with fecal materials. The elimination half-life of oxytetracycline is ≈ 4-6 hours in dogs and cats, 4.3-9.7 hours in cattle, 10.5 hours in horses, 6.7 hours in swine, and 3.6 hours in sheep.

Contraindications/Precautions/Warnings

Oxytetracycline is contraindicated in patients hypersensitive to it or other tetracyclines. Because tetracyclines can retard fetal skeletal development and discolor deciduous teeth, they should only be used in the last half of pregnancy when the benefits outweigh the fetal risks. Oxytetracycline and tetracycline are considered more likely to cause these abnormalities than either doxycycline or minocycline.

In patients with renal insufficiency or hepatic impairment, oxytetracycline and tetracycline must be used cautiously. Lower than usual dosages are recommended with enhanced monitoring of renal and hepatic function. Avoid concurrent administration of other nephrotoxic or hepatotoxic drugs with tetracyclines. Monitoring of serum levels should be considered if long-term therapy is required.

Oral administration of tetracycline, chlortetracycline, or oxytetracycline appears safe in mice and rats, but little appears to be absorbed. These drugs administered orally to hamsters, gerbils, guinea pigs, and rabbits may either be toxic or not absorbed (Donnelly 2012).

Adverse Effects

Oxytetracycline and tetracycline given to young animals can cause a yellow, brown, or gray discoloration of bones and teeth. High dosages or chronic administration may delay bone growth and healing. Tetracyclines in high levels can exert an antianabolic effect, which can cause an increase in BUN and/or hepatotoxicity, particularly in patients with preexisting renal dysfunction. As renal function deteriorates secondary to drug accumulation, this effect may be exacerbated.

In ruminants, high oral doses can cause ruminal microflora depression and ruminoreticular stasis. Rapid intravenous injection of undiluted propylene glycol-based products can cause intravascular hemolysis with resultant hemoglobinuria. Propylene glycol based products have also caused cardiodepressant effects when administered to calves. When administered IM, local reactions, yellow staining, and necrosis may be seen at the injection site.

In small animals, tetracyclines can cause nausea, vomiting, anorexia, and diarrhea. Cats do not tolerate oral tetracycline or oxytetracycline very well, and may present with clinical signs of colic, fever, hair loss, and depression. There are reports that long-term tetracycline use may cause urolith formation in dogs, but this is thought to occur very rarely.

Diarrhea in horses is possible.

Tetracycline therapy (especially long-term) may result in overgrowth (superinfections) of non-susceptible bacteria or fungi.

Tetracyclines have also been associated with photosensitivity reactions and, rarely, hepatotoxicity or blood dyscrasias.

Reproductive/Nursing Safety

In humans, the FDA categorizes this drug as category *D* for use during pregnancy (*There is evidence of human fetal risk, but the potential benefits from the use of the drug in pregnant women may be acceptable despite its potential risks.*) In a separate system evaluating the safety of drugs in canine and feline pregnancy (Papich 1989), this drug is categorized as class: *D* (*Contraindicated. These drugs have been shown to cause congenital malformations or embryotoxicity.*)

Tetracyclines are excreted in maternal milk. Milk to plasma ratios varies between 0.25 to 1.5. Because of the potential for serious adverse reactions, decide whether to discontinue nursing or discontinue the drug.

Overdosage/Acute Toxicity

Tetracyclines are generally well tolerated after acute overdoses. Dogs given more than 400 mg/kg/day orally or 100 mg/kg/day IM of oxytetracycline did not demonstrate any toxicity. Oral overdoses would most likely be associated with GI disturbances (vomiting, anorexia, and/or diarrhea). Should the patient develop severe emesis or diarrhea, fluids and electrolytes should be monitored and replaced if necessary. Chronic overdoses may lead to drug accumulation and nephrotoxicity.

High oral doses given to ruminants, can cause ruminal microflora depression and ruminoreticular stasis. Rapid intravenous injection of undiluted propylene glycol-based products can cause intravascular hemolysis with resultant hemoglobinuria.

Rapid intravenous injection of tetracyclines has induced transient collapse and cardiac arrhythmias in several species, presumably due to chelation with intravascular calcium ions. Overdose quantities of drug could exacerbate this effect if given too rapidly IV. If the drug must be given rapidly IV (<5 minutes), some clinicians recommend pre-treating the animal with intravenous calcium gluconate.

Drug Interactions

The following drug interactions have either been reported or are theoretical in humans or animals receiving oxytetracycline and may be of significance in veterinary patients. Unless otherwise noted, use together is not necessarily contraindicated, but weigh the potential risks and perform additional monitoring when appropriate.

- **ATOVAQUONE:** Tetracyclines have caused decreased atovaquone levels.
- **BETA-LACTAM or AMINOGLYCOSIDE ANTIBIOTICS:** Bacteriostatic drugs, like the tetracyclines, may interfere with bactericidal activity of the penicillins, cephalosporins, and aminoglycosides; actual clinical significance of this interaction is in doubt.
- **DIGOXIN:** Tetracyclines may increase the bioavailability of digoxin in a small percentage of human patients and lead to digoxin toxicity. These effects may persist for months after discontinuation of the tetracycline.
- **DIVALENT or TRIVALENT CATIONS (oral antacids, saline cathartics** or other **GI products containing aluminum, calcium, iron, magnesium, zinc,** or **bismuth cations):** When orally administered, tetracyclines can chelate divalent or trivalent cations that can decrease the absorption of the tetracycline or the other drug if it contains these cations; it is recommended that all oral tetracyclines be given at least 1-2 hours before or after the cation-containing products.
- **WARFARIN:** Tetracyclines may depress plasma prothrombin activity and patients on anticoagulant therapy may need dosage adjustment.

Laboratory Considerations

- Tetracyclines (not minocycline) may cause falsely elevated values of **urine catecholamines** when using fluorometric methods of determination.
- Tetracyclines reportedly can cause false-positive **urine glucose** results if using the cupric sulfate method of determination (Benedict's reagent, *Clinitest®*), but this may be the result of ascorbic acid, which is found in some parenteral formulations of tetracyclines. Tetracyclines have also reportedly caused false-negative results in determining urine glucose when using the glucose oxidase method (*Clinistix®*, *Tes-Tape®*).

Doses

- **DOGS/CATS:**

  For susceptible systemic infections (extra-label): 10 mg/kg IV q12h; 20 mg/kg PO q8-12h.

  For adjunctive treatment of Salmon poisoning (*Neorickettsia helmintheca*) (extra-label): 7 mg/kg IV every 8 h for 3-5 days. (Headley *et al.*)

  As a chelating antibiotic for medial canthus syndrome (tear staining) (extra-label): 25 – 50 mg (total dose) PO once per day 2 weeks on and off and on. (Krohne 2008)

  For diagnosis and treatment of idiopathic antibiotic-responsive diarrhea (extra-label): 10 – 20 mg/kg PO q8h; can be given with food. If helpful, usually continued for 4 weeks and then discontinuing antibiotics may result in dietary management alone being sufficient. (Allenspach 2009), (Hall 2011), (Donnelly 2012)

  For hemotropic mycoplasmosis/feline hemoplasmosis in cats (extra-label): 10 – 25 mg/kg PO, IV q8h for 5-7 days (Greene *et al.* 2006). Oxytetracycline does not seem to clear the infection, as parasites may still be present three months after therapy. (Lobetti 2007)

- **CATTLE:**

  For susceptible infections (labeled doses):

  a) Using *Liquamycin LA-200®:* For bacterial pneumonia caused by *Pasteurella* spp. (shipping fever) in calves and yearlings, where retreatment is impractical due to husbandry conditions, such as cattle on range, or where their repeated restraint is inadvisable, or infectious bovine keratoconjunctivitis (pinkeye) caused by (M. bovis): 9 mg/lb (20 mg/kg) SC or IM once. Can also be given at 3 – 5 mg/lb (6.6 – 11 mg/kg) IM, SC, or IV once daily. In the treatment of severe foot rot and advanced cases of other indicated diseases, a dosage level of 5 mg/lb (11 mg/kg) per day is recommended. Treatment should be continued 24-48 hours following remission of disease signs; however, treatment should not exceed a total of 4 consecutive days. (Label information; *Liquamycin LA-200®*)

b) Using *Tetradure-300®*: For the control of respiratory disease in cattle at high risk of developing BRD associated with *Mannheimia (Pasteurella) haemolytica*: 13.6 mg/lb (30 mg/kg) IM or SC once. For bacterial pneumonia caused by *Pasteurella* spp (shipping fever) in calves and yearlings where retreatment is impractical due to husbandry conditions, such as cattle on range, or where their repeated restraint is inadvisable, or infectious bovine keratoconjunctivitis (pink eye) caused by *Moraxella bovis*: 9 – 13.6 mg/lb (20 – 30 mg/kg) IM or SC once.

For other indications (see label): 3 – 5 mg/lb (6.6 – 11 mg/kg) IM, SC or IV (IV slowly over a period of at least 5 minutes) once daily. In treatment of footrot and advanced cases of other indicated diseases, a dosage level of 5 mg/lb (11 mg/kg) per day is recommended. Treatment should be continued 24-48 hours following remission of disease signs, however, not to exceed a total of 4 consecutive days. If improvement is not noted within 24-48 hours of the beginning of treatment, diagnosis and therapy should be re-evaluated.

Do not administer intramuscularly in the neck of small calves due to lack of sufficient muscle mass. Use extreme care when administering this product by intravenous injection. Perivascular injection or leakage from an intravenous injection may cause severe swelling at the injection site. (Label information; *Tetradure-300®*)

c) Using the combination product with flunixin (*Hexasol®*): 1 mL per 22 lb. body weight (13.6 mg oxytetracycline and 0.9 mg flunixin per lb.) IM or SC once. Do not administer more than 10 mL per injection site (1-2 mL per site in small calves). Recommended where retreatment of calves and yearlings is impractical due to husbandry conditions, such as cattle on range, or where their repeated restraint is inadvisable. (adapted from label; *Hexasol®*)

For listeriosis (*L. monocytogenes*); (extra-label): Requires administration of very high doses to be effective; recommended oxytetracycline treatment scheme requires doses as high as 10 mg/kg per day for at least five days. (Wiedmann 2007)

■ **HORSES:**

For susceptible infections (all are extra-label): Dosage recommendations can vary considerably. For "regular" oxytetracycline injection, 6.6 – 10 mg/kg IV once daily is commonly seen. Some use 5 – 6.6 mg/kg IV q12h. The following are representative indications and dosages:

Foals: 5 – 10 mg/kg IV q12h diluted and given slowly, or 10 – 20 mg/kg IV q24h diluted and given slowly. Monitor creatinine and UA. (Bentz 2007)

For equine monocytic or granulocytic ehrlichiosis: 6.6 – 7 mg/kg IV q24h for 5-7 days; to safeguard against adverse effects (muscle tremors, agitation or acute collapse) dilute at least in a 1:1 ratio and give IV slowly, or deliver it as an infusion in 500 mL or 1 liter of fluids. (Bentz 2007), (Madigan *et al.* 2000)

For Lyme disease: A common intensive treatment scenario has been to give IV oxytetracycline, 6.6 mg/kg q12h for 7-10 days, followed by PO doxycycline at 10 mg/kg q12h for 1-2 months.

For Potomac Horse Fever (*Neorickettsia risticii*) early in the clinical course of the disease: 6.6 mg/kg IV twice a day. Usually no more than 5 days treatment is necessary. (Madigan *et al.* 2000)

For proliferative enteropathy (*Lawsonia intracellularis*) in foals (extra-label): 6.6 mg/kg IV (slowly) q24h; typically administered for 2-4 weeks (Giguere 2013). Alternatively, 5 – 6.6. mg/kg IV q12h for 3-7 days followed by doxycycline (10 mg/kg PO q12h for 7-17 days). (Sampieri *et al.* 2006)

For intrauterine infusion: 1 – 5 grams; use povidone based products only. Little science is available for recommending doses, volume infused, frequency, diluents, etc. Most intrauterine treatments are commonly performed every day or every other day for 3-7 days. (Perkins 1999)

For adjunctive treatment of flexural limb deformities in foals (extra-label): 44 – 70 mg/kg (3 grams for a 50 kg foal) diluted in 250 – 500 mL of normal saline and given IV. May repeat q24h for 2-3 doses.

■ **SWINE:**

For susceptible infections:

a) Using *Tetradure-300®*: For bacterial pneumonia caused by *Pasteurella multocida* where retreatment is impractical due to husbandry conditions or where repeated restraint is inadvisable: 9 mg/lb (20 mg/kg) IM once. May also be used at 3 – 5 mg/lb (6.6 – 11 mg/kg) IM once per day. Treatment should be continued 24-48 hours following remission of disease signs; however, not to exceed a total of four (4) consecutive days. If improvement is not noted within 24-48 hours of the beginning of treatment, diagnosis and therapy should be re-evaluated. For sows as an aid in the control of infectious enteritis in baby pigs: 3 mg/lb (6.6.mg/kg) IM once approximately 8 hours before farrowing or immediately after completion of farrowing. For swine weighing 25 lbs (11.4 kg) or less, administer undiluted for treatment at 9 mg/lb (20 mg/kg), but should be administered diluted (see label for guidelines) for treatment at 3 or 5 mg/lb (6.6 – 11 mg/kg). (Label information; *Tetradure-300®*)

b) If using 50 mg/mL or 100 mg/mL product: 10 mg/kg IM initially, then 7.5 mg/kg IM once daily. (Baggot 1983)

■ **SHEEP & GOATS:**

For enteritis (*E. coli*) and pneumonia (*P. multocida*): 22 mg/kg in water daily for 7-14 days. (Fajt 2008)

For *C. abortus* in pregnant ewes: In the face of an outbreak, all pregnant ewes should be treated. Long acting oxytetracycline at 20 mg/kg can be used successfully. (Stuen *et al.* 2011)

For *C. burnetii* (Q fever): Aborting animals and other animals in late pregnancy receive 2 injections of oxytetracycline (20 mg/kg) during the last month of gestation. Treatment does not totally suppress abortions and shedding of *C. burnetii* at lambing. (Stuen *et al.* 2011)

■ **BIRDS:**

For chlamydiosis (Psittacosis); (extra-label): Using 200 mg/mL product (*LA-200®*): 50 mg/kg IM once every 3-5 days in birds suspected or confirmed of having disease. Used in conjunction with other forms of tetracyclines. IM injections may cause severe local tissue reactions. (McDonald 1989)

■ **REPTILES:**

For susceptible infections (extra-label): For turtles and tortoises: 10 mg/kg PO once daily for 7 days (useful in ulcerative stomatitis caused by Vibrio). (Gauvin 1993)

Monitoring

- Adverse effects.
- Clinical efficacy.
- Long-term use or in susceptible patients: periodic renal, hepatic, hematologic evaluations.

Client Information

- When given orally it should be given on an empty stomach spaced 1-2 hours apart from food, milk, other dairy products, and minerals such as calcium or iron. If animal vomits or acts sick after getting it on an empty stomach, give with food or a small treat to see if this helps. If vomiting continues, contact your veterinarian.
- May permanently stain teeth and developing bones in young animals.
- This drug may make your animal's skin more sensitive to sunlight and increase the risk of sunburn on hairless areas such as the nose and around the eyelids and ears. Tell your veterinarian if you notice any reddening/sunburn on the skin while your animal is on this medication.
- Injectable forms may be painful and stain skin and muscle.

Chemistry/Synonyms

A tetracycline derivative obtained from *Streptomyces rimosus*, oxytetracycline base occurs as a pale yellow to tan, crystalline powder that is very slightly soluble in water and sparingly soluble in alcohol. Oxytetracycline HCl occurs as a bitter-tasting, hygroscopic, yellow, crystalline powder that is freely soluble in water and sparingly soluble in alcohol. Commercially available 50 mg/mL and 100 mg/mL oxytetracycline HCl injections are usually available in either propylene glycol or povidone-based products.

Oxytetracycline may also be known as: glomycin, hydroxytetracycline, oxytetracyclinum, riomitsin, terrafungine, *Biomycin®*, *Liquamycin®*, *Medamycin®*, *Oxyject®*, *Oxytet®*, and *Terramycin®*.

Storage/Stability

Unless otherwise directed by the manufacturer, oxytetracycline HCl and oxytetracycline products should be stored in tight, light-resistant containers at temperatures of <40°C (104°F) and preferably at room temperature (15-30°C); avoid freezing.

Compatibility/Compounding Considerations

The following information pertains to regular (not sustained-release) forms of oxytetracycline HCl. It is generally considered to be physically **compatible** with most commonly used IV infusion solutions, including D_5W, sodium chloride 0.9%, and lactated Ringer's, but can become relatively unstable in solutions with a pH >6, particularly in those containing calcium. This is apparently more of a problem with the veterinary injections that are propylene glycol based rather than those that are povidone based. Other drugs that are reported to be physically **compatible** with oxytetracycline for injection include: corticotropin, dimenhydrinate, insulin (regular), isoproterenol HCl, norepinephrine bitartrate, potassium chloride, tetracycline HCl, and vitamin B-complex with C.

Drugs that are reportedly physically **incompatible** with oxytetracycline, data conflicts, or compatibility is concentration/time dependent, include: amikacin sulfate, aminophylline, amphotericin B, calcium chloride/gluconate, chloramphenicol sodium succinate, erythromycin gluceptate, heparin sodium, hydrocortisone sodium succinate, iron dextran, methohexital sodium, oxacillin sodium, penicillin G potassium/sodium, pentobarbital sodium, phenobarbital sodium, and sodium bicarbonate. Compatibility is dependent

upon factors such as pH, concentration, temperature, and diluent used; consult specialized references or a hospital pharmacist for more specific information.

Dosage Forms/Regulatory Status

VETERINARY-LABELED PRODUCTS:

Oxytetracycline HCl 50 mg/mL, 100 mg/mL Injection: There are many FDA-approved oxytetracycline products marketed in these concentrations. Some trade names for these products include: *Terramycin®*, *Liquamycin®*, *Biomycin®*, *Medamycin®*, *Biocyl®*, *Oxyject®*, and *Oxytet®*. Some are labeled for Rx (prescription) use only, while some are over-the-counter (OTC). Depending on the actual product, this drug may be FDA-approved for use in swine, cattle, beef cattle, chickens or turkeys. Products may also be labeled for IV, IM, or SC use. Withdrawal times vary with regard to individual products; when used as labeled, slaughter withdrawal times vary in cattle from 15-22 days, swine 20-26 days, and 5 days for chickens and turkeys. Refer to the actual labeled information for the product used for more information.

Oxytetracycline base 200 mg/mL Injection in 100, 250, and 500 mL bottles; *Liquamycin® LA-200, Biomycin®-200* generic; (OTC or Rx). FDA-approved for use in swine and cattle. When used as labeled, slaughter withdrawal = 28 days for swine and cattle; Milk withdrawal = 96 hours

Oxytetracycline base 300 mg/mL Injection in 100 mL, 250 mL and 500 mL vials; *Noromycin® 300-LA, 300 Pro® LA, Tetradure®-300*; (OTC or Rx). FDA-approved for use in beef cattle, non-lactating dairy cattle, calves, including pre-ruminating (veal) calves, and swine. When used as labeled, slaughter withdrawal = 28 days

Oxytetracycline Oral Tablets (Boluses) 250 mg & 500 mg tablets; *Terramycin® Scours Tablets*; (OTC). FDA-approved for use in non-lactating dairy and beef cattle. Withdrawal periods may vary; refer to the product label.

Combination Products:

Oxytetracycline 300 mg/mL and Flunixin (as flunixin meglumine) 20 mg/mL in 100 mL, 250 mL and 500 mLs; *Hexasol®*; (Rx)

Oxytetracycline is also available in feed additive, premix, ophthalmic, and intramammary products.

Established residue tolerances: Uncooked edible tissues of swine, cattle, salmonids, catfish and lobsters: 0.10 ppm. Uncooked kidneys of chickens or turkeys: 3 ppm. Uncooked muscle, liver, fat or skin of chickens or turkeys: 1 ppm.

HUMAN-LABELED PRODUCTS: NONE.

Revisions/References

Monograph revised/updated May 2014.

Allenspach, K. (2009). Treatment of IBD. Proceediings: BSAVA. accessed via Veterinary Information Network; vin.com

Baggot, J. D. (1983). Systemic antimicrobial therapy in large animals. *Pharmacological Basis of Large Animal Medicine*. J. A. Bogan, P. Lees and A. T. Yoxall. Oxford, Blackwell Scientific Publications: 45-69.

Bentz, B. (2007). Antimicrobial selections for foals. Proceedings: Western Vet Conf. accessed via Veterinary Information Network; vin.com

Donnelly, T. (2012). Rational Antimicrobial Therapeutics for Exotic Companion Mammals. ABVP Proceedings. accessed via Veterinary Information Network; vin.com

Fajt, V. R. (2008). Small Ruminant Antimicrobial Decision-Making: Regimen Design. Proceedings: ACVIM. accessed via Veterinary Information Network; vin.com

Fugler, L., et al. (2009). Evaluation of Various Matrix Metalloproteinase Inhibitors (MMPIS) in the Horse. Proceedings: ACVIM. accessed via Veterinary Information Network; vin.com

Gauvin, J. (1993). Drug therapy in reptiles. Seminars in Avian & Exotic Med 2(1): 48-59.

Giguere, S. (2013). Update on Infections Caused by *Lawsonia intracellularis* in Foals. 65th Convention of the Canadian Veterinary Medical Association. accessed via Veterinary Information Network; vin.com

Greene, C., et al. (2006). Appendix 8: Antimicrobial Drug Formulary. *Infectious Disease of the Dog and Cat*. C. Greene, Elsevier: 1186-333.

Hall, E. J. (2011). Antibiotic-Responsive Diarrhea in Small Animals. Veterinary Clinics of North America-Small Animal Practice **41**(2): 273-+.

Headley, S. A., et al. Neorickettsia helminthoeca and salmon poisoning disease: A review. The Veterinary Journal **In Press, Corrected Proof.**

Krohne, S. (2008). Tear Staining & Pigment & Hairs--Oh My: Treating Medial Canthus Syndrome in Dogs. Proceedings: World Veterinary Conference. accessed via Veterinary Information Network; vin.com

Lobetti, R. (2007). Feline Haemoplasmosis. Provceedings: Feline Haemoplasmosis. accessed via Veterinary Information Network; vin.com

Madigan, J. & N. Pusterla (2000). Ehrlichial Diseases. The Veterinary Clinics of North America: Equine Practice **16**:3(December).

McDonald, S. E. (1989). Summary of medications for use in psittacine birds. JAAV **3**(3): 120-7.

Papich, M. (1989). Effects of drugs on pregnancy. *Current Veterinary Therapy X: Small Animal Practice.* R. Kirk. Philadelphia, Saunders: 1291-9.

Perkins, N. (1999). Equine reproductive pharmacology. The Veterinary Clinics of North America: Equine Practice **15**:3(December): 687-704.

Sampieri, F., et al. (2006). Tetracycline therapy of Lawsonia intracellularis enteropathy in foals. Equine Veterinary Journal **38**(1): 89-92.

Stuen, S. & D. Longbottom (2011). Treatment and Control of Chlamydial and Rickettsial Infections in Sheep and Goats. Veterinary Clinics of North America-Food Animal Practice **27**(1): 213-+.

Wiedmann, M. (2007). Listeria Monocytogenes: Transmission and Disease in Ruminants. Proceedings: ACVIM. accessed via Veterinary Information Network; vin.com

Oxytocin

(ox-i-**toe**-sin)   Pitocin®

Hormonal Agent

Prescriber Highlights

▶ Hypothalamic hormone used for induction or enhancement of uterine contractions at parturition, postpartum retained placenta & metritis, uterine involution after manual correction of prolapsed uterus in dogs, & agalactia.

▶ Contraindications: Known hypersensitivity, dystocia due to abnormal presentation of fetus(es) unless correction is made. When used prepartum, oxytocin should be used only when the cervix is relaxed naturally or by the prior administration of estrogens.

▶ Treat hypoglycemia or hypocalcemia before using.

▶ Adverse Effects: Usually occur only when used in inappropriate patients or at too high a dosage.

▶ Drug Interactions.

Uses/Indications

In veterinary medicine, oxytocin has been used for induction or enhancement of uterine contractions at parturition, treatment of postpartum retained placenta and metritis, uterine involution after manual correction of prolapsed uterus in dogs, and in treating agalactia.

Pharmacology/Actions

By increasing the sodium permeability of uterine myofibrils, oxytocin stimulates uterine contraction. The threshold for oxytocin-induced uterine contraction is reduced with pregnancy duration, in the presence of high estrogen levels and in patients already in labor.

Oxytocin can facilitate milk ejection, but does not have any galactopoietic properties. While oxytocin only has minimal antidiuretic properties, water intoxication can occur if it is administered at too rapid a rate and/or if excessively large volumes of electrolyte-free intravenous fluids are administered.

Pharmacokinetics

Oxytocin is destroyed in the GI tract and, therefore, must be administered parenterally. After IV administration, uterine response occurs almost immediately. Following IM administration, the uterus responds generally within 3-5 minutes. The duration of effect in dogs after IV or IM/SC administration has been reported to be 13 minutes and 20 minutes, respectively. While oxytocin can be administered intranasally, absorption can be erratic. Oxytocin is distributed throughout the extracellular fluid. It is believed that small quantities of the drug cross the placenta and enter the fetal circulation.

In humans, plasma half-life of oxytocin is ≈ 3-5 minutes. In goats, this value has been reported to be ≈ 22 minutes. Oxytocin is metabolized rapidly in the liver and kidneys and a circulating enzyme, oxytocinase, can also destroy the hormone. Very small amounts of oxytocin are excreted in the urine unchanged.

Contraindications/Precautions/Warnings

Oxytocin is considered contraindicated in animals with dystocia due to abnormal presentation of fetus(es), unless correction is made. When used prepartum, oxytocin should be used only when the cervix is relaxed naturally or by the prior administration of estrogens (**Note:** Most clinicians avoid the use of estrogens, as natural relaxation is a better indicator for the proper time to induce contractions.) Oxytocin is also contraindicated in patients who are hypersensitive to it.

Before using oxytocin, treat hypoglycemia or hypocalcemia if present.

Oxytocin is ineffective for treatment of primary uterine inertia (uterine muscles do not contract normally at parturition).

In humans, oxytocin is contraindicated in patients with significant cephalopelvic disproportion, unfavorable fetal positions, in obstetrical emergencies when surgical intervention is warranted, severe toxemia, or when vaginal delivery is contraindicated. Nasally administered oxytocin is contraindicated in pregnancy.

In human medicine, IV oxytocin is considered a "high alert" medication (medications that require special safeguards to reduce the risk of errors). Consider instituting practices such as redundant drug dosage and volume checking, special alert labels, etc.

Adverse Effects

When used appropriately at reasonable dosages, oxytocin rarely causes significant adverse reactions. Most adverse effects are a result of using the drug in inappropriate individuals (adequate physical exam and monitoring of patient are essential) or at too high doses (see Overdosage below). Most of the older dosage recommendations for dogs or cats are obsolete, as mini-doses have been found to improve the frequency of uterine contractility, and are less hazardous to the bitch (uterine rupture) and the fetuses (placental compromise). Hypersensitivity reactions are a possibility in non-synthetically produced products. Repeated bolus injections of oxytocin may cause uterine cramping and discomfort.

Overdosage/Acute Toxicity

Effects of overdosage on the uterus depend on the stage of the uterus and position of the fetus(es). Hypertonic or tetanic contractions can occur leading to tumultuous labor, uterine rupture, fetal injury, or death.

Water intoxication can occur if large doses are infused for a long period, especially if large volumes of electrolyte-free intravenous fluids are concomitantly being administered. Early clinical signs can include listlessness or depression. More severe intoxication clinical signs can include coma, seizures and eventually death. Treatment for mild water intoxication is stopping oxytocin therapy and restricting water access until resolved. Severe intoxication may require the use of osmotic diuretics (mannitol, urea, dextrose) with or without furosemide.

Reproductive/Nursing Safety

In humans, oxytocin is contraindicated in patients with significant cephalopelvic disproportion, unfavorable fetal positions, in obstetrical emergencies when surgical intervention is warranted, severe toxemia, or when vaginal delivery is contraindicated. Nasally administered oxytocin is contraindicated in pregnancy.

No known indications for use in the first trimester exist other than in relation to spontaneous or induced abortion. Oxytocin is not expected to present a risk of fetal abnormalities when use as indicated.

Oxytocin may be found in small quantities in maternal milk but is unlikely to have significant effects.

Drug Interactions

The following drug interactions have either been reported or are theoretical in humans or animals receiving oxytocin and may be of significance in veterinary patients. Unless otherwise noted, use together is not necessarily contraindicated, but weigh the potential risks and perform additional monitoring when appropriate.

- **THIOPENTAL:** One case in humans has been reported where thiopental anesthesia was delayed when oxytocin was being administered. The clinical significance of this interaction has not been firmly established.

- **VASOCONSTRICTORS:** If sympathomimetic agents or other vasoconstrictors are used concurrently with oxytocin post-partum hypertension may result. Monitor and treat if necessary.

Doses

Note: Unless otherwise indicated all dosages are extra-label.

- **DOGS/CATS:**

For uterine inertia: Use uterine and fetal monitors to guide oxytocin and calcium gluconate therapy. Generally, the administration of oxytocin increases the frequency of uterine contractions, while the administration of calcium increases their strength. Calcium is given before oxytocin in most cases, improving contraction strength before increasing frequency. Additionally, the action of oxytocin appears to be improved when given 15 minutes after calcium. Calcium gluconate 10% solution (0.465 mEq of calcium/mL) is given SC at 1 mL/5.5 kg of body weight (BW) as indicated by the strength of uterine contractions, generally no more frequently than every 4-6 hours. Oxytocin is effective at mini-doses, starting with 0.25 Units (per bitch or queen) SC or IM to a maximum dose of 4 Units per bitch or queen. Higher doses of oxytocin or intravenous boluses can cause tetanic, ineffective uterine contractions that can further compromise fetal oxygen supply by placental compression. The frequency of oxytocin administration is dictated by the labor pattern, and generally not given more frequently than hourly. (Davidson 2009a)

For secondary agalactia: 0.25 – 1 Unit (per bitch or queen) SC q2h. Neonates are removed for 30 minutes post-injection, and then encouraged to suckle, or gentle stripping of the glands performed. Metoclopramide is given at 0.1 – 0.2 mg/kg SC q12h (dopamine antagonist) to promote milk production. Therapy is usually rewarding within 24 hours. (Davidson 2009b)

For adjunctive treatment of acute metritis: Dam started on a broad-spectrum antibiotic with good tissue penetration into the reproductive tract, while waiting for the culture and sensitivity results. Institute fluid therapy if patient is dehydrated or in shock. Oxytocin at 0.5 – 5 Units (per bitch or queen) IM may be used if birth has occurred <hours prior or dinoprost (0.25 mg/kg SQ) may be used at any time to promote evacuation of the uterus. (Traas *et al.* 2009)

To promote uterine involution after uterine prolapse manual reduction:

a) Digital manipulation can be attempted to replace the uterus using general and/or epidural anesthesia. If the tissue is very swollen, hyperosmotic fluids such as 50% dextrose or mannitol may assist in replacement. In some cases an episiotomy is required to successfully reduce the prolapse. Following reduction, oxytocin 0.5 – 5 Units IM will promote uterine involution. If the uterus cannot be reduced manually, laparotomy may be necessary. If tissue damage is significant, the potential for uterine vessel rupture and hemo-abdomen is increased and ovariohysterectomy is indicated. (Traas *et al.* 2009)

b) Anesthetize patient and apply sterile lubricant liberally to the exposed tissue. The uterine horn is flushed with sterile saline under pressure. Mannitol or hypertonic saline can be used to reduce edema if necessary before attempting reduction. Once the uterus is replaced, give 5 – 10 Units (total dose) of oxytocin IM to cause uterine involution. If the uterus stays in for 24 hours, further risk of prolapse is unlikely because the cervix should be closed. (Shaw 2007)

- **RABBITS, RODENTS, SMALL MAMMALS:**

Mice, Rats, Gerbils, Hamsters, Guinea pigs, Chinchillas: 0.2 – 3 Units/kg IV, IM or SC. (Adamcak *et al.* 2000)

- **CATTLE:**

For retained placenta:

a) 40 – 60 Units oxytocin q2h (often in conjunction with intravenous calcium therapy) as necessary. Of limited value after 48 hours postpartum as uterine sensitivity is reduced. (McClary 1986)

b) To reduce incidence of retained placenta: 20 Units IM immediately following calving and repeated 2-4 hours later. (Hameida *et al.* 1986)

For mild to moderate cases of acute post-partum metritis: 20 Units IM 3-4 times a day for 2-3 days. (Hameida *et al.* 1986)

To augment uterine contractions during parturition:

a) 30 Units IM; repeat no sooner than 30 minutes if necessary. (Wheaton 1989)

b) For obstetrical use in cows: 100 Units IV, IM or SC. (Package Insert; Oxytocin Injection—Anthony Products)

For milk let-down: 10 – 20 Units IV. (Package Insert; Oxytocin Injection—Anthony Products)

- **HORSES:**

To augment or initiate uterine contractions during parturition in properly evaluated mares (extra-label): Ideally, prior to induction, colostrum should be present in the udder, the cervix should be soft and dilating and the mare should be as close to her own normal "due" date as possible. The optimal dose of and route of administration for induction remains controversial. Three protocols have been suggested: 1) Low doses 2.5 – 5 Units IV q15-30 minutes; 2) Continuous IV infusion at a rate of 1 Unit/minute; 3) Multiple smaller doses: 15 Units IM q15-20 minutes. (Vaala 2013)

To prevent luteolysis (extra-label): To prolong corpus luteum lifespan, oxytocin is given from day 7 to day 14 post-ovulation at a dose of 60 Units (3 mL) IM once daily. Mares have stayed out of heat for up to 45-60 days with this protocol. The negative aspect to using oxytocin in this manner is that ovulation must be documented (or estimated really closely). (Dascanio 2009)

For evacuation of uterine fluid (extra-label): 20 Units IV or IM 1-3 times a day. (McCue 2003)

To aid in removal of retained fetal membranes (extra-label): 20 Units IV or IM given every hour beginning 2-3 hours after foaling. Repeat as needed. (McCue 2003)

To treat esophageal obstruction ("choke"); (extra-label): N-butylscopolammonium bromide (*Buscopan*®) at 0.3 mg/kg IV once and oxytocin 0.11 – 0.22 Units/kg IV once. Oxytocin use should be avoided in mares, or dose significantly reduced. Do not use in pregnant mares. (Beard 2008)

- **SWINE:**

  For adjunctive treatment of agalactia syndrome (MMA): 20 – 50 Units IM or 5 – 10 Units IV. (Einarsson 1986)

  For retained placenta in patients with uterine atony: 20 – 30 Units oxytocin q2-3h as necessary (with broad-spectrum antibiotics). (McClary 1986)

  To augment uterine contractions during parturition: 10 Units IM; repeat no sooner than 30 minutes if necessary. (Wheaton 1989)

  For mild to moderate cases of acute post-partum metritis: 5 Units IM; may need to be repeated as effect may be as short as 30 minutes. (Meredith 1986)

  For milk let-down in sows: 5 – 20 Units IV. (Package Insert; Oxytocin Injection—Anthony Products)

- **SHEEP & GOATS:**

  For retained placenta in patients with uterine atony: 10 – 20 Units oxytocin. Of limited value after 48 hours postpartum as uterine sensitivity is reduced. If signs of metritis develop, treat with antibiotics. (McClary 1986)

  For mild to moderate cases of acute post-partum metritis: 5 – 10 Units IM 3-4 times a day for 2-3 days. (Hameida *et al.* 1986)

  To control post-extraction cervical and uterine bleeding after internal manipulations (*e.g.*, fetotomy, etc.): Goats: 10 – 20 Units IV, may repeat SC in 2 hours. (Franklin 1986)

- **CAMELIDS (NW):**

  For retained placenta: 5 – 10 Units oxytocin may be given IM at 10-minute intervals with or without gentle traction. Strenuous traction may induce uterine prolapse. (Adams 2008)

- **BIRDS:**

  As a uterotonic agent (extra-label): 0.5 Units/kg IM; may repeat in 60 minutes. (Pollock 2007)

- **REPTILES:**

  For egg binding in combination with calcium: Calcium glubionate (10 – 50 mg/kg IM as needed until calcium levels back to normal or egg binding is resolved); oxytocin: 1 – 10 Units/kg IM. Use care when giving multiple injections. Not as effective in lizards as in other species. (Gauvin 1993)

  To induce oviposition: Doses range from 1 – 30 Units/kg. A dose of 10 Units/kg appears to be effective in many chelonians. May have to repeat in several hours, but there is a risk of oviduct rupture if cloaca is obstructed or eggs cannot pass for other reasons. (Lewbart 2001)

Monitoring

- Uterine contractions, status of cervix.
- Fetal monitoring if available and indicated.

Client Information

- Oxytocin should only be used by individuals able to adequately monitor its effects.

Chemistry/Synonyms

A nonapeptide hypothalamic hormone stored in the posterior pituitary (in mammals), oxytocin occurs as a white powder that is soluble in water. The commercially available preparations are highly purified and have virtually no antidiuretic or vasopressor activity when administered at usual doses. Oxytocin potency is standardized according to its vasopressor activity in chickens and is expressed in USP Posterior Pituitary Units. One unit is equivalent of ≈ 2-2.2 micrograms of pure hormone.

Commercial preparations of oxytocin injection have their pH adjusted with acetic acid to 2.5-4.5 and multi-dose vials generally contain chlorobutanol 0.5% as a preservative.

Oxytocin may also be known as: alpha-hypophamine, or oxytocinum and *Pitocin®*.

Storage/Stability

Oxytocin injection should be stored at temperatures of <25°C, but not frozen. Some manufacturers recommend storing the product under refrigeration (2-8°C), but some products have been demonstrated to be stable for up to 5 years when stored at <26°C.

Compatibility/Compounding Considerations

Oxytocin is reportedly physically **compatible** with most commonly used intravenous fluids and the following drugs: chloramphenicol sodium succinate, sodium bicarbonate, tetracycline HCl, thiopental sodium, and verapamil HCl.

Oxytocin is reportedly physically **incompatible** with the following drugs: fibrinolysin, norepinephrine bitartrate, prochlorperazine edisylate, and warfarin sodium. Compatibility is dependent upon factors such as pH, concentration, temperature, and diluent used; consult specialized references or a hospital pharmacist for more specific information.

Dosage Forms/Regulatory Status

VETERINARY-LABELED PRODUCTS:

Oxytocin for Injection: 20 USP Units/mL in 10 mL, 30 mL, and 100 mL vials; available labeled generically from several manufacturers; (Rx). Oxytocin products are labeled for several species, including horses, dairy cattle, beef cattle, sheep, swine, cats, and dogs. There are no milk or meat withdrawal times specified for oxytocin.

HUMAN-LABELED PRODUCTS:

Oxytocin Solution for Injection: 10 Units/mL in 1 mL amps, 3 mL & 10 mL vials and 10 mL multiple-dose vials; *Pitocin®*, generic; (Rx)

Revisions/References

Monograph revised/updated May 2014.

Adamcak, A. & B. Otten (2000). Rodent Therapeutics. Vet Clin NA: Exotic Anim Pract 3:1(Jan): 221-40.

Adams, G. (2008). Eutocia, Dystocia and Post-Partum Care of the Dam and Neonatal Llama & Alpaca. Proceedings: WVC. accessed via Veterinary Information Network; vin.com

Beard, L. (2008). Respiratory disease in the geriatric patient. Proceedings: WVC. accessed via Veterinary Information Network; vin.com

Dascanio, J. (2009). Hormonal Control of Reproduction. Proceedings: ABVP. accessed via Veterinary Information Network; vin.com

Davidson, A. (2009a). Medical and Surgical Management of Dystocia. Proceedings: WVC. accessed via Veterinary Information Network; vin.com

Davidson, A. (2009b). Postpartum disorders in the bitch and queen. Proceedings: WVC. accessed via Veterinary Information Network; vin.com

Einarsson, S. (1986). Agalactia in Sows. Current Therapy in Theriogenology 2: Diagnosis, Treatment and Prevention of Reproductive Diseases in Small and Large Animals. D. A. Morrow. Philadelphia, WB Saunders: 935-7.

Franklin, J. S. (1986). Dystocia and obstetrics in goats. Current Therapy in Theriogenology 2: Diagnosis, Treatment and Prevention of Reproductive Diseases in Small and Large Animals. D. A. Morrow. Philadelphia, WB Saunders: 590-2.

Gauvin, J. (1993). Drug therapy in reptiles. Seminars in Avian & Exotic Med 2(1): 48-59.

Hameida, N. A., et al. (1986). Therapy of uterine infections: Alternatives to antibiotics. *Current Therapy in Theriogenology 2: Diagnosis, Treatment and Prevention of Reproductive Diseases in Small and Large Animals*. D. A. Morrow. Philadelphia, WB Saunders: 45-7.

Lewbart (2001). Reptile Formulary. Proceedings: Atlantic Coast Veterinary Conference. accessed via Veterinary Information Network; vin.com

McClary, D. (1986). Retained Placenta. *Current Veterinary Therapy: Food Animal Practice 2*. J. L. Howard. Philadelphia, W.B. Saunders: 773-5.

McCue, P. (2003). Hormone therapy: new aspects. Proceedings: Western Veterinary Conference. accessed via Veterinary Information Network; vin.com

Meredith, M. J. (1986). Bacterial endometritis. Current Therapy in Theriogenology 2: Diagnosis, Treatment and Prevention of Reproductive Diseases in Small and Large Animals. D. A. Morrow. Philadelphia, WB Saunders: 953-6.

Pollock, C. (2007). Avian Reproductive Diseases. Proceedings: Western Vet Conf. accessed via Veterinary Information Network; vin.com

Shaw, S. (2007). Dealing with Reproductive Emergencies. Proceedings: IVECCS. accessed via Veterinary Information Network; vin.com

Traas, A. & C. O'Conner (2009). Postpartum Emergencies. Peroceedings: IVECCS. accessed via Veterinary Information Network; vin.com

Vaala, W. (2013). The Problem Pregnancy: Recognition and Therapy. Proceedings: ABVP. accessed via Veterinary Information Network; vin.com

Wheaton, L. G. (1989). Drugs that affect uterine motility. *Current Veterinary Therapy X: Small Animal Practice*. R. W. Kirk. Philadelphia, WB Saunders: 1299-302.

Paclitaxel

(pa-cli-**tax**-el)   Paccal Vet®-CA1

Antineoplastic

Prescriber Highlights

▶ Conditionally approved taxane-class antineoplastic for dogs with certain mammary and squamous cell carcinomas. Extra-label use prohibited.

▶ Not interchangeable with human dosage forms; do not use human dosage forms in dogs.

▶ Serious adverse effects commonly occur; neutropenia and severe GI effects are most frequently observed. Appropriate monitoring and management are mandatory.

Uses/Indications

Paclitaxel for injection (*Paccal Vet®-CA1*) is conditionally approved (pending a full demonstration of effectiveness) for the treatment of non-resectable stage III, IV or V mammary carcinoma in dogs that have not received previous chemotherapy or radiotherapy, and for resectable and non-resectable squamous cell carcinoma in dogs that have not received previous chemotherapy or radiotherapy (Anon 2014). As a conditionally approved drug it is a violation of federal law (USA) to use this product other than as directed in the labeling.

For grade II or III non-resectable mast cell tumors, soluble micellar paclitaxel (*Paccal Vet®*) was shown to have better anti-tumor activity and safety when compared to lomustine (Vail *et al.* 2012).

Pharmacology/Actions

Paclitaxel is a taxane-class antimicrotubule antineoplastic agent that suppresses spindle microtubule dynamics. The precise mechanism of action of paclitaxel is not fully understood, but it disrupts the dynamic equilibrium within the microtubule system, blocks cells in the late G_2 phase and M phase of the cell cycle, inhibits cell replication from tubulin dimers, and stabilizes microtubules by preventing depolymerization. Additionally, paclitaxel enhances the cytotoxic effects of ionizing radiation and may induce cell death by triggering apoptosis.

Pharmacokinetics

In dogs, paclitaxel exhibits similar pharmacokinetics to other species studied. After intravenous injection it undergoes extensive tissue distribution with a rapid (3-5 hours) initial redistribution to the peripheral compartment. 3-7% of the administered dose remains in tissues and slowly (up to 12 hours) depletes. Drug accumulation does not occur when administered once every three weeks at labeled dosages. Systemic drug exposure is directly proportional to dose within the dosing range of 130 – 150 mg/m².

In humans, between 89%-98% is bound to plasma proteins. Paclitaxel is extensively metabolized in the liver. Its major metabolite in humans is 6α-hydroxypaclitaxel, which is catalyzed via CYP2C8; two of its minor metabolites are catalyzed via CYP3A4.

Contraindications/Precautions/Warnings

- Do not use in dogs that have a neutropenia (< 2000 cells/microL) or a concurrent serious infection.

- Not for use in dogs that are pregnant, lactating, or intended for breeding.

- Monitor patients carefully for vomiting, diarrhea and dehydration. Provide supportive care as clinically indicated.

- Do not use human dosage forms in dogs (see Dosage Forms/Regulatory Status).

- Do not confuse PACLitaxel with *Paxil®* or DOCEtaxel.

- Should be administered under the supervision of a veterinarian experienced in the use of cancer chemotherapeutic agents.

- Avoid extravasation.

- Pregnant or nursing women should not prepare or administer the product. Humans that are sensitive to retinoids should avoid contact.

- Wear protective gloves to prevent contact with feces, urine, vomit and saliva for three days after the dog has received treatment. Place all waste material in a plastic bag and seal before disposal.

- See the product label for additional information to prevent human exposure and management should exposure occur.

Adverse Effects

Paclitaxel has a narrow margin of safety. All treated dogs are likely to exhibit adverse effects and serious adverse effects commonly occur. Appropriate monitoring and management are mandatory.

- Neutropenia can occur in 80-90% of treated dogs with nadirs usually seen at days 4-7.

- Gastrointestinal mucosal toxicity occurs in the majority of patients treated. Associated clinical signs include vomiting, anorexia, diarrhea and dehydration.

- In pre-approval field trials the following additional adverse effects were noted in >10% of treated patients: lethargy (69%), alopecia (39%), dehydration (26%), dermatitis (24%), hepatopathy (19%), edema (14%), pyrexia (13%), and lameness (12%). See the product label for additional adverse effects.

- Extravasation injuries are possible. The following recommendations are for human patients but may be considered/adapted to canine patients: If signs of extravasation occur, stop the infusion immediately. If possible, withdraw 3-5 mL of blood to remove some of the drug. Remove the infusion needle. Apply ice compresses may be applied to the site for 15 minutes every 6 hours for 48 hours. Delineate the infiltrated area on the patient's skin with a felt-tip marker. Elevate for 48 hours above heart level using a sling or stockinette dressing with an observation window cut in the dressing. Avoid pressure or friction. Do not rub the area. Observe for signs of increased erythema, pain, or skin necrosis. If increased symptoms occur, consult a plastic surgeon. After 48 hours, encourage the patient to use the extremity normally to promote full range of motion.

Reproductive/Nursing Safety

The veterinary product label states: "Do not use in dogs that are pregnant, lactating, or intended for breeding. Paclitaxel is a teratogen and can affect female and male fertility. Laboratory studies in the rat have shown reduced fertility, embryotoxicity, teratogenicity, and maternal toxicity."

In pregnant humans, the FDA lists paclitaxel as a category *D* drug (*There is evidence of human fetal risk, but the potential benefits from the use of the drug in pregnant women may be acceptable despite its potential risks.*)

Overdosage/Acute Toxicity

No specific information noted for canine overdoses. In humans overdosage is associated with bone marrow suppression, peripheral neurotoxicity, and mucositis.

Conventional hemodialysis and peritoneal dialysis are not effective (0%-24%) in removing paclitaxel.

Drug Interactions

The canine product label states: "Drug interaction studies have not been performed. Paclitaxel is metabolized by cytochrome P450 isoenzymes and is a P-glycoprotein (P-gp) substrate. Exercise caution when administering paclitaxel with medications that inhibit or induce cytochrome P450 isoenzymes or with medications that are P-gp substrates." The following drug interactions have either been reported or are theoretical in humans or animals receiving paclitaxel and may be of significance in veterinary patients. Unless otherwise noted, use together is not necessarily contraindicated, but weigh the potential risks and perform additional monitoring when appropriate.

- CISPLATIN: If paclitaxel is given after cisplatin, myelosuppression may be greater than if paclitaxel given before cisplatin.
- CLARITHROMYCIN, ERYTHROMYCIN: Metabolism of paclitaxel may be decreased increasing paclitaxel plasma levels.
- DOXORUBICIN: Doxorubicin and its active metabolite doxorubicinol levels may be increased.
- KETOCONAZOLE, ITRACONAZOLE: Metabolism of paclitaxel may be decreased increasing paclitaxel plasma levels.
- RIFAMPIN: Paclitaxel levels may be decreased.

Laboratory Considerations
- No specific concerns noted.

Doses
- **DOGS:**

  For non-resectable stage III, IV or V mammary carcinoma or non-resectable squamous cell carcinoma, in dogs that have not received previous chemotherapy or radiotherapy (labeled dose; FDA-approved): 150 mg/m^2 body surface area (BSA) IV over 15-30 minutes, once every 3 weeks for up to 4 doses. Dose reductions of 10 mg/m^2 or dose delays may be used to manage adverse reaction. **Note:** The FDA does not permit extra-label use for this conditionally approved drug. (Adapted from label; *Paccal Vet*®-CA1)

Monitoring
- CBC; myelosuppression. Neutropenic effects generally occur at 4-7 days. Neutrophil nadirs for canine patients were at day 4 in one study (Vail *et al.* 2012). In humans, median neutrophil nadir is 11 days.
- GI toxicity; hydration status.
- Other adverse effects.

Client Information
- The product label states: "Always provide the Client Information Sheet to the dog owner with each dose administration."
- Advise dog owners about possible adverse reactions and when to contact a veterinarian.
- Wear protective gloves to prevent contact with feces, urine, vomit and saliva for 3 days after the dog has received treatment. Place all waste material in a plastic bag and seal before disposal.

Chemistry/Synonyms
Taxanes are a natural product extracted from various species of yews (*Taxus spp.*) or produced using a semisynthetic process Paclitaxel occurs as white to off-white powder. It is insoluble in water and soluble in alcohol.

The veterinary product for injection is made water soluble via a mixed micellar preparation with a surfactant based retinoic acid derivatives. It is supplied as a greenish-yellow to yellow sterile lyophilized powder in the form of a cake. Each single use vial contains 60 mg of paclitaxel, 40 mg of N-(all-trans-retinoyl)-L-cysteic acid methyl ester sodium salt and 40 mg of N-(13-cis-retinoyl)-L-cysteic acid methyl ester sodium salt (XR-17). After reconstitution paclitaxel concentration is 1 mg/mL. In the aqueous solution for infusion these constituents are soluble and form micellar nanoparticles with a size of ≈ 20-40 nm.

Paclitaxel may also be known as BMS-181339-01, NSC-125973, Taxol®, Taxol A, Abraxane®, or Paccal-Vet®.

Storage/Stability
Store unopened *Paccal-Vet*® vials refrigerated at 2-8°C (36-46°F). Retain in the original package to protect from light. As the product contains no preservatives, use immediately after reconstitution.

Human products have different storage requirements and stability characteristics.

Compatibility/Compounding Considerations
The manufacturer recommends using lactated Ringer's injection for reconstitution. Do not mix with other fluids or drugs.

Paccal Vet®-CA1 is supplied as a sterile powder for reconstitution before use. After reconstitution the solution contains 1 mg of paclitaxel/mL. Protect from light throughout the preparation process. Preparation for use should be done with aseptic technique and the reconstituted product should be used immediately. Reconstitution instructions:

1. Obtain the desired number of vials from the refrigerator. The powder should be greenish-yellow to yellow. In case of discoloration, discard the vial. Let the vials stand protected from light at room temperature for ≈ 20-30 minutes. The room temperature should not exceed 25°C (77°F).

2. Using a sterile syringe, inject 60 mL of Lactated Ringer's solution, USP, into a vial of *Paccal Vet*®-CA1. Pressure must be equilibrated by a needle or vial spike before injection. The Lactated Ringer's solution should be injected slowly, directed onto the inside wall of the vial and not directly onto the powder as this will result in foaming.

3. Gently swirl the vial by hand for 20-30 seconds. Protect from light and allow the vial to stand for 3-5 minutes. Gently and slowly swirl and/or invert the vial until the powder is completely dissolved. Do not shake, this will result in foaming. If foam develops, allow the solution to stand for several minutes. Reconstitution can continue even if all of the foam has not dissipated. If undissolved product is present, the vial should be placed on a shaker and rotated for up to 15 minutes, while protecting from light.

5. The solution should be clear and greenish-yellow without visible precipitates. If precipitates or discoloration (orange-reddish) are observed, the solution should be discarded.

6. Inject the appropriate amount of reconstituted *Paccal Vet*®-CA1 into an empty, sterile, EVA (ethyl vinyl acetate) infusion bag. Protect the reconstituted product in the EVA infusion bag from light. The reconstituted product should be used immediately. Compatibility of administration sets containing DEHP (di(2-ethylhexyl) phthalate) has not been demonstrated.

Dispose of any unused product or waste materials in accordance with proper procedures for cytotoxic drugs

Dosage Forms/Regulatory Status
VETERINARY-LABELED PRODUCTS:

Paclitaxel (water-soluble micellar nanoparticles) 60 mg per vial (1 mg/mL after reconstitution); *Paccal Vet*®-CA1; (Rx). FDA conditionally approved for use in dogs only. It is a violation of federal law (USA) to use this product other than as directed in the labeling.

HUMAN-LABELED PRODUCTS:

There are two forms of parenteral human paclitaxel products but these are not recommended for use in animals. One is a human albumin-bound form and the other contains polyoxyethylated castor oil (Cremaphor EL), a compound that causes allergic or anaphylactic hypersensitivity reactions in the majority of treated dogs.

Revisions/References
Monograph written May 2014.

Anon (2014). Paccal Vet-CA1 (Paclitaxel for Injection) [Package Insert]. Secondary Paccal Vet-CA1 (Paclitaxel for Injection) [Package Insert]. Secondary Anon, Abbott Animal Health. Volume

Vail, D. M., et al. (2012). A Randomized Trial Investigating the Efficacy and Safety of Water Soluble Micellar Paclitaxel (Paccal Vet) for Treatment of Nonresectable Grade 2 or 3 Mast Cell Tumors in Dogs. Journal of Veterinary Internal Medicine **26**(3): 598-607.

Pamidronate Disodium

(pah-**mih**-dro-nate)   Aredia®

Bisphosphonate

Prescriber Highlights

▶ Bisphosphonate used IV for treating hypercalcemia and for adjuvant analgesia treatment of osteosarcoma.

▶ Must be given IV in saline over several hours.

▶ Potentially can cause electrolyte abnormalities, anemias, or renal toxicity.

Uses/Indications

Pamidronate may be useful in treating refractory idiopathic hypercalcemia, and hypercalcemia associated with malignancy or vitamin D-related toxicoses. Several studies suggest that pamidronate may be useful as an adjunctive analgesic for treating bone pain associated with osteosarcoma in dogs (Fan 2009), but one retrospective study found that mean survival time was reduced if pamidronate was combined with radiation therapy ± chemotherapy .

Pharmacology/Actions

Bisphosphonates at therapeutic levels inhibit bone resorption and do not inhibit bone mineralization via binding to hydroxyapatite crystals. They impede osteoclast activity, and induce osteoclast apoptosis. Pamidronate has ≈ 100X greater relative antiresorptive potency when compared to etidronate.

Bisphosphonates *in vitro* have direct cytotoxic or cytostatic effects on human osteosarcoma cell lines. They may also have antiangiogenic effects and inhibit cell migration in certain cancers.

Pharmacokinetics

After intravenous infusion in rats, 50-60% of the dose is rapidly absorbed by bone. Bone uptake is highest in areas of rapid bone turnover. The kidneys very slowly eliminate the drug. Terminal half-life is on the order of 300 days in rats. When used for hypercalcemia, pamidronate's onset of action is in 24-48 hours and its duration of effect ranges from 2-4 weeks.

Contraindications/Precautions/Warnings

Pamidronate is contraindicated in patients hypersensitive to it or any of the bisphosphonate drugs. It should be used with caution in patients with impaired renal function; the drug has been associated with renal toxicity. In humans, it has not been tested in patients with serum creatinine levels >5 mg/dL.

Adverse Effects

Electrolyte abnormalities may occur with pamidronate therapy. One case of a dog developing hypomagnesemia and arrhythmias after pamidronate has been reported (Kadar *et al.* 2004). Pamidronate potentially can cause renal toxicity in dogs, but it is thought this can be minimized or avoided by infusing the drug over at least 2 hours. In humans, ophthalmic syndromes (*e.g.,* scleritis), transient bone pain, hypocalcemia, anemia, thrombocytopenia and agranulocytosis have been reported.

Reproductive/Nursing Safety

In pregnant humans, the FDA lists pamidronate as a category *D* drug (*There is evidence of human fetal risk, but the potential benefits from the use of the drug in pregnant women may be acceptable despite its potential risks.*) Pamidronate has produced both maternal and embryo/fetal toxicity in laboratory animals when given at dosages therapeutically used in human patients. If it is used in pregnant veterinary patients, informed consent by the owner accepting the risks to both mother and offspring is recommended.

It is unknown if pamidronate is excreted into milk. Use with caution in nursing mothers.

Overdosage/Acute Toxicity

Overdosage of pamidronate may cause hypocalcemia, including tetany. Should this occur, treat with short-term, intravenous calcium.

Drug Interactions

The following drug interactions have either been reported or are theoretical in humans or animals receiving pamidronate and may be of significance in veterinary patients. Unless otherwise noted, use together is not necessarily contraindicated, but weigh the potential risks and perform additional monitoring when appropriate.

■ **AMINOGLYCOSIDES:** May enhance hypocalcemic effects of pamidronate; monitor.

■ **CALCIUM-AFFECTING DRUGS** (*e.g.,* **furosemide, corticosteroids**): Pamidronate must be used carefully (with monitoring) when used in conjunction with other drugs that can affect calcium.

■ **NEPHROTOXIC DRUGS** (*e.g.,* **cisplatin, aminoglycosides**): Use with caution, potential for increased risk for nephrotoxicity.

■ **NSAIDS:** Use with caution, potential for increased risk for nephrotoxicity and GI toxicity.

Laboratory Considerations

■ No specific laboratory interactions or considerations noted.

Doses

■ **DOGS/CATS:**

For refractory hypercalcemia (extra-label): If possible remove the underlying cause. For acute treatment, hydration (IV saline), furosemide, glucocorticoids, and calcitonin are often recommended first, if these do not resolve hypercalcemia, pamidronate may be considered. Dosages range from 1.3 – 2.3 mg/kg (diluted in 150-250 mL of 0.9% sodium chloride) and administered IV over 2-4 hours. May be repeated every 21-28 days.

For treatment of vitamin D (cholecalciferol, calcipotriene and related compounds) induced hypercalcemia: 1.3 – 2 mg/kg slow IV infusion. In most cases, a single dose will lower calcium levels back to normal levels. Recommended to monitor calcium levels daily for at least 10 days after they have returned to normal and some patients may need to be retreated in 5-7 days. (Gwaltney-Brant 2003), (DeClementi *et al.* 2012)

For palliative adjunctive analgesia for osteosarcoma bone pain (extra-label): 1 – 2 mg/kg; diluted into 250 mL of 0.9% sodium chloride and administered as a CRI over 2 hours every 28 days (Fan *et al.* 2003), (Fan *et al.* 2007). **Note:** Some sources anecdotally recommend giving as frequently as once per week.

Monitoring

■ Renal function (serum creatinine, etc.) and hydration status should be monitored before treating and prior to each dose.

■ Serum calcium, phosphate, magnesium, potassium.

■ CBC; baseline and continued if ongoing treatment.

■ Urinalysis.

Client Information

■ The medication must be given in an inpatient setting.

■ Clients should understand the costs for the medication, care, and monitoring associated with its use.

Chemistry/Synonyms

Pamidronate disodium a bisphosphonate inhibitor of bone resorption occurs as a white, crystalline powder that is soluble in water and practically insoluble in organic solvents.

Pamidronate may also be known as: ADP sodium, AHPrBP sodium, GCP-23339A, *Aminomux*®, *Aredia*®, *Aredronet*®, *Ostepam*®, or *Pamidran*®.

Storage/Stability

Do not store at temperatures >30°C (86°F).

Once the lyophilized powder for injection is reconstituted (10 mL) with sterile water for injection, it may be stored in the refrigerator for 24 hours. Be sure drug is completely dissolved before withdrawing into syringe.

Compatibility/Compounding Considerations

Do not mix pamidronate with any intravenous fluid containing calcium (*e.g.*, Ringer's). It is recommended to use a dedicated IV solution (0.45% or 0.9% NaCl, or D_5W) and intravenous line.

Dosage Forms/Regulatory Status

VETERINARY-LABELED PRODUCTS: NONE.

HUMAN-LABELED PRODUCTS:

Pamidronate Disodium Lyophilized Powder for Injection (IV infusion): 30 mg & 90 mg with 375 mg or 470 mg mannitol in vials; generic; (Rx)

Pamidronate Disodium Injection: 3 mg/mL, 6 mg/mL & 9 mg/mL (may contain mannitol) in 10 mL vials; generic; (Rx)

Revisions/References

Monograph revised/updated May 2014.

DeClementi, C. & B. R. Sobczak (2012). Common Rodenticide Toxicoses in Small Animals. Veterinary Clinics of North America-Small Animal Practice 42(2): 349-+.

Fan, T. & L.-P. de Lorimier (2003). Bisphosphonates: molecular mechanisms and therapeutic uses in veterinary oncology. Proceedings: ACVIM Forum. accessed via Veterinary Information Network; vin.com

Fan, T., et al. (2007). Single-agent pamidronate for palliative therapy of canine appendicular osteosarcoma bone pain. J Vet Intern Med 21(431-439).

Fan, T. M. (2009). Intravenous Aminobisphosphonates for Managing Complications of Malignant Osteolysis in Companion Animals. Topics in Companion Animal Medicine 24(3): 151-6.

Gwaltney-Brant, S. (2003). Terrible Toxicants. Proceedings: IVECC2003. accessed via Veterinary Information Network; vin.com

Kadar, E., et al. (2004). Electrolyte disturbances and cardiac arrhythmias in a dog following pamidronate, calcitonin, and furosemide administration for hypercalcemia of malignancy. J Am Anim Hosp Assoc 40(1): 75-81.

Pancrelipase

(pan-kree-**lih**-pase) Viokase®, Lipase/Protease/Amylase

Pancreatic Enzymes

Prescriber Highlights

▶ Pancreatic enzymes used to treat exocrine pancreatic enzyme deficiency or to test for pancreatic insufficiency secondary to chronic pancreatitis.

▶ Contraindications: Hypersensitivity to pork products.

▶ Adverse Effects: High doses may cause GI distress.

▶ Avoid inhalation of powder; may cause skin irritation; wash off if gets on hands.

Uses/Indications

Pancrelipase is used to treat patients with exocrine pancreatic enzyme insufficiency (EPI).

The serum trypsin-like immunoreactivity (TLI) assay is used to establish the diagnosis in dogs. Dogs may have EPI and not respond to pancreatic enzyme replacement because: a) the enzyme product is poorly effective, b) the diet is too high in fat, and/or c) the dog has concurrent antibiotic responsive enteropathy. About 15% of dogs with EPI simply will not respond to therapy and have a bad prognosis (Willard 2009).

It may also be used in the attempt to test for pancreatic insufficiency secondary to chronic pancreatitis.

Pharmacology/Actions

The enzymes found in pancrelipase help to digest and absorb fats, proteins, and carbohydrates.

Contraindications/Precautions/Warnings

Pancrelipase products are contraindicated in animals that are hypersensitive to pork proteins.

Do not inhale the powder or bronchial/lung irritation can occur. Avoid contact with mucous membranes or skin.

Adverse Effects

High doses may cause GI distress (diarrhea, cramping, nausea). Concentrated pancreatic enzymes can cause oral or esophageal ulcers; follow dosing with food or water. Oral bleeding has been reported in dogs after receiving pancrelipase (Rutz *et al.* 2002). Dose reduction and moistening the food pancreatic/powder mix may also decrease the incidence of this adverse effect.

Reproductive/Nursing Safety

In humans, the FDA categorizes this drug as category *C* for use during pregnancy (*Animal studies have shown an adverse effect on the fetus, but there are no adequate studies in humans; or there are no animal reproduction studies and no adequate studies in humans.*)

These enzymes are unlikely to be excreted in maternal milk or pose risk to offspring.

Overdosage/Acute Toxicity

Overdosage may cause diarrhea or other intestinal upset. The effects should be temporary; treat by reducing dosage and supportively if diarrhea is severe.

Drug Interactions

The following drug interactions have either been reported or are theoretical in humans or animals receiving pancrelipase and may be of significance in veterinary patients. Unless otherwise noted, use together is not necessarily contraindicated, but weigh the potential risks and perform additional monitoring when appropriate.

- **ANTACIDS (magnesium hydroxide, calcium carbonate)**: May diminish the effectiveness of pancrelipase.
- **CIMETIDINE (or other H_2 antagonists)**: May increase the amount of pancrelipase that reaches the duodenum.

Doses

- **DOGS:**

  For pancreatic exocrine insufficiency (extra-label):

  a) Initially, one teaspoon per 10 kg body weight per meal. Oral bleeding has recently been reported in 3 of 25 dogs with EPI treated with pancreatic enzyme supplements. The oral bleeding stopped in all 3 dogs after the dose of pancreatic enzymes was decreased. Moistening the food pancreatic/powder mix also appears to decrease the frequency of this side effect. When clinical signs have resolved, the amount of pancreatic enzymes given can be gradually decreased to the lowest effective dose, which may vary from patient to patient and from batch to batch of the pancreatic supplement. (Steiner 2008)

  b) 1 – 2 teaspoonsful of powder or finely crushed nonenteric-coated tablets to each of two meals of balanced canine ration. It is not necessary to incubate the enzyme preparation before feeding. Tailor regimen to maintain optimal body weight. (Bunch 2003)

- **CATS:**

  For pancreatic exocrine insufficiency (extra-label): **Note:** Cats reportedly "hate" the taste of the powder but may accept the powder if mixed with fish/tuna oil and then thoroughly mixed with a canned food. If using solid dosage forms (enteric-coated tablets or compounded capsules made from powder or crushed tablets) be certain that immediately after dosing, water or food is consumed to reduce the risk for esophageal damage.

  a) 1 teaspoonful of powder or finely crushed nonenteric-coated tablets to each of two meals of balanced feline ration. Cats that refuse to eat food treated with powder may be dosed with capsules filled with powder or crushed non-enteric coated tablets. It is not necessary to incubate the enzyme preparation before feeding. Tailor regimen to maintain optimal body weight. (Bunch 2003)

b) Initially, one teaspoon per cat per meal. When clinical signs have resolved, the amount of pancreatic enzymes given can be gradually decreased to the lowest effective dose, which may vary from patient to patient and from batch to batch of the pancreatic supplement. (Steiner 2008)

- **RABBITS, RODENTS, SMALL MAMMALS:**

Rabbits, for gastric trichobezoars (extra-label): 1 teaspoonful (5 mL) pancrelipase powder plus 3 teaspoonsful (15 mL) of yogurt; let stand for 15 minutes, then give 2 – 3 mL PO q12h. Questionable efficacy for removing "hairballs", but might help dissolve the protein matrix surrounding hair. (Ivey *et al.* 2000)

- **BIRDS:**

For pancreatic exocrine insufficiency (used in birds that are polyphagic "going light", passing whole seeds, and slow in emptying crops); (extra-label): 1/8 teaspoon per kg. Mix with moistened feed or administer by gavage. Incubate with food for 15 minutes prior to gavage. (Clubb 1986)

Monitoring

- Animal's weight.
- Stool consistency, frequency.

Client Information

- Pancrelipase powder or crushed tablets are usually mixed in the food and left to stand for 15-20 minutes before feeding. Your veterinarian may instruct you to mix it into food and offer it to your animal without waiting.
- Cats often "hate" the taste of the powder and may be more easily dosed using solid dosage forms (enteric-coated tablets or capsules made (compounded) from powder or crushed tablets). Some cats will eat food mixed with one brand of veterinary powder and refuse another.
- If using solid dosage forms (capsules, tablets), be certain that your animal gets water or food right after dosing to reduce the risk for esophageal damage.
- Use caution to avoid inhaling powder; can cause lung irritation and asthma. If you skin comes into contact with the powder, wash it off immediately.

Chemistry/Synonyms

Pancrelipase contains pancreatic enzymes, primarily lipase but also amylase and protease, and is obtained from the pancreas of hogs. Each mg of pancrelipase contains not less than 24 USP Units of lipase activity, not less than 100 USP Units of protease activity, and not less than 100 USP Units of amylase activity. When compared on a per weight basis, pancrelipase has at least 4X the trypsin and amylase content of pancreatin, and at least 12X the lipolytic activity of pancreatin.

Pancrelipase may also be known as pancrelipasa, *Epizyme®, Panakare®, Pancrepowder Plus®, Pancreved®, Pancrezyme®,* and *Viokase®.*

Storage/Stability

Unless otherwise recommended by the manufacturer, store at room temperature in a dry place in tight containers. When present in quantities greater than trace amounts, acids will inactivate pancrelipase.

Dosage Forms/Regulatory Status

Note: There are several dosage forms (both human and veterinary-label) available containing pancrelipase, including oral capsules, oral delayed-release capsules, tablets, and delayed-released tablets. Most small animal practitioners believe the oral powder is most effective in dogs.

VETERINARY-LABELED PRODUCTS:

Pancrelipase Powder containing ≈ 2.8 grams per teaspoonful: 71,400 Units lipase; 388,000 Units protease; 460,000 Units amylase; in 8 oz bottle; *Viokase®-V Powder, Pancrezyme® Powder, Pancrepowder Plus®, Pancreved® Powder, Epizyme® Powder, Panakare® Plus Powder;* (Rx). Labeled for use in dogs and cats.

HUMAN-LABELED PRODUCTS:

There are capsules, tablets, and powders available containing lipase, protease, and amylase in varying units available for human consumption from many distributors.

Revisions/References

Monograph revised/updated May 2014.

Bunch, S. (2003). Hepatobiliary and exocrine pancreatic disorders. *Small Animal Internal Medicine, 3rd Ed.* R. Nelson and C. Couto. St Louis, Mosby: 472-567.
Clubb, S. L. (1986). Therapeutics: Individual and Flock Treatment Regimens. *Clinical Avian Medicine and Surgery.* G. J. Harrison and L. R. Harrison. Philadelphia, W.B. Saunders: 327-55.
Ivey, E. & J. Morrisey (2000). Therapeutics for Rabbits. Vet Clin NA: Exotic Anim Pract **3:1**(Jan): 183-216.
Rutz, G. M., et al. (2002). Oral bleeding associated with pancreatic enzyme supplementation in three dogs with exocrine pancreatic insufficiency. Journal of the American Veterinary Medical Association **221**(12): 1716-8.
Steiner, J. M. (2008). How I Treat--Exocrine Pancreatic Insufficiency. Proceedings: WSAVA. accessed via Veterinary Information Network; vin.com
Willard, M. (2009). Canine Chronic Diarrheas: Diagnosis/Management of Non-Infiltrative Disorders. Proceedings: ACVIM. accessed via Veterinary Information Network; vin.com

Pancuronium Bromide

(pan-kue-**roe**-nee-um)   Pavulon®

Non-Depolarizing Neuromuscular Blocker

Prescriber Highlights

- ▶ Non-depolarizing neuromuscular blocker used as an adjunct to general anesthesia. Rarely used today.
- ▶ Extreme Caution: Myasthenia gravis. Caution: Renal dysfunction, hepatic or biliary disease; patients where tachycardias may be deleterious.
- ▶ No analgesic or sedative/anesthetic actions.
- ▶ Adverse Effects: Slight elevations in cardiac rate & blood pressure, hypersalivation (if not pretreated with an anticholinergic agent), prolonged or profound muscular weakness, & respiratory depression. Very Rarely: Histamine release with resultant hypersensitivity reaction.
- ▶ Drug Interactions.

Uses/Indications

Pancuronium is sometimes used as an adjunct to general anesthesia to produce muscle relaxation during surgical procedures or mechanical ventilation and to facilitate endotracheal intubation. Use today is rare; vecuronium, atracurium or rocuronium are generally preferred.

Pharmacology/Actions

Pancuronium is a nondepolarizing neuromuscular blocking agent and acts by competitively binding at cholinergic receptor sites at the motor endplate, inhibiting the effects of acetylcholine. It is considered 5X as potent as d-tubocurarine and 1/3 as potent as vecuronium (some sources say that pancuronium is equipotent with vecuronium in animals). It has little effect on the cardiovascular system other than increasing heart rate slightly, and only rarely does it cause histamine release.

Pharmacokinetics

After intravenous administration, muscle relaxation sufficient for endotracheal intubation occurs generally within 2-3 minutes, but is dependent on the actual dose administered. Duration of action may persist 30-45 minutes, but this again is dependent on the dose. Additional doses may slightly increase the magnitude of the blockade and will significantly increase the duration of action.

In humans, pancuronium is ≈ 87% bound to plasma proteins, but it may be used in hypoalbuminemic patients. Activity is non-affected substantially by either plasma pH or carbon dioxide levels.

The half-life in humans ranges from 90-161 minutes. Approximately 40% of the drug is excreted unchanged by the kidneys. The remainder is excreted in the bile (11%) or metabolized by the liver. In patients with renal failure, plasma half-lives are doubled; atracurium may be a better choice for these patients.

Contraindications/Precautions/Warnings

Pancuronium is contraindicated in patients hypersensitive to it. It should be used with caution in patients with renal dysfunction, or where tachycardias may be deleterious. Lower doses may be necessary in patients with hepatic or biliary disease. Pancuronium has no analgesic or sedative/anesthetic actions. In patients with myasthenia gravis, neuromuscular blocking agents should be used with extreme caution, if at all.

Do not confuse pancuronium with *Panacur®*.

Adverse Effects

Adverse reactions seen with pancuronium include: slight elevations in cardiac rate and blood pressure, hypersalivation (if not pretreated with an anticholinergic agent), occasional rash (humans), and prolonged or profound muscular weakness and respiratory depression. Very rarely, pancuronium will cause substantial histamine release with resultant hypersensitivity reactions.

Reproductive/Nursing Safety

In humans, the FDA categorizes this drug as category *C* for use during pregnancy (*Animal studies have shown an adverse effect on the fetus, but there are no adequate studies in humans; or there are no animal reproduction studies and no adequate studies in humans.*) In a separate system evaluating the safety of drugs in canine and feline pregnancy (Papich 1989), this drug is categorized as class: *B* (*Safe for use if used cautiously. Studies in laboratory animals may have uncovered some risk, but these drugs appear to be safe in dogs and cats or these drugs are safe if they are not administered when the animal is near term.*)

It is not known whether these drugs are excreted in maternal milk.

Overdosage/Acute Toxicity

Monitoring muscle twitch response to peripheral nerve stimulation can minimize overdosage possibilities. Increased risks of hypotension and histamine release occur with overdoses, as well as prolonged duration of muscle blockade.

Besides treating conservatively (mechanical ventilation, O_2, fluids, etc.), reversal of blockade may be accomplished by administering an anticholinesterase agent (edrophonium, physostigmine, or neostigmine) with an anticholinergic (atropine or glycopyrrolate). A suggested dose for neostigmine is 0.06 mg/kg IV after atropine 0.02 mg/kg IV.

Drug Interactions

The following drug interactions have either been reported or are theoretical in humans or animals receiving pancuronium and may be of significance in veterinary patients. Unless otherwise noted, use together is not necessarily contraindicated, but weigh the potential risks and perform additional monitoring when appropriate.

- **AZATHIOPRINE:** May reverse pancuronium's neuromuscular blocking effects.

- **AMINOGLYCOSIDES (gentamicin, etc.):** May enhance the neuromuscular blocking activity of pancuronium.
- **ANESTHETICS, INHALATIONAL:** May enhance the neuromuscular blocking activity of pancuronium.
- **CALCIUM (IV):** May reverse the effects of nondepolarizing neuromuscular blocking agents.
- **CYCLOSPORINE:** May enhance the neuromuscular blocking activity of pancuronium.
- **KETAMINE:** Heart rate may increase and myocardial perfusion decreased.
- **LINCOSAMIDES: (clindamycin, etc.):** May enhance the neuromuscular blocking activity of pancuronium.
- **MAGNESIUM SULFATE or HCl:** May enhance the neuromuscular blocking activity of pancuronium
- **QUINIDINE:** May enhance the neuromuscular blocking activity of pancuronium.
- **SUCCINYLCHOLINE:** Other muscle relaxant drugs may cause a synergistic or antagonistic effect. Succinylcholine may speed the onset of action and enhance the neuromuscular blocking actions of pancuronium. Do not give pancuronium until succinylcholine effects have subsided.
- **THEOPHYLLINE:** May inhibit or reverse the neuromuscular blocking action of pancuronium and possibly induce arrhythmias.
- **VERAPAMIL:** May enhance the neuromuscular blocking activity of pancuronium.

Doses

- **DOGS/CATS:**

   As a neuromuscular blocker (extra-label)

   a) **As a paralytic during mechanical ventilation:** 0.05 – 0.1 mg/kg IV; lasts ≈ 1 hour, must give sedation as well. (Carr 2003)

   b) **On occasions when anesthesia maintenance with IV or regional techniques are not adequate to prevent spontaneous movement and the addition of inhalational agents results in severe hypotension (not corrected with fluid therapy):** 0.02 – 0.04 mg/kg IV provides 30-45 minutes of muscle relaxation. (Day 2005)

Monitoring

- Level of neuromuscular blockade.
- Cardiac rate.

Client Information

- This drug should only be used by professionals familiar with using neuromuscular blocking agents in a supervised setting with adequate ventilatory support.

Chemistry/Synonyms

A synthetic, non-depolarizing neuromuscular blocker, pancuronium bromide occurs as a white, odorless, bitter-tasting, hygroscopic, fine powder. It has a melting point of 215°C and one gram is soluble in 100 mL of water; it is very soluble in alcohol. Acetic acid is used to adjust the commercially available injection to a pH of ≈ 4.

Pancuronium bromide may also be known as: NA-97, Org-NA-97, or pancuronii bromidum.

Storage/Stability

Pancuronium injection should be stored under refrigeration (2-8°C), but, according to the manufacturer, it is stable for 6 months at room temperature.

Do not store pancuronium in plastic syringes or containers as it may be adsorbed to plastic surfaces. It may be administered in plastic syringes, however.

Compatibility/Compounding Considerations

It is recommended that pancuronium NOT be mixed with barbiturates, as a precipitate may form, although data conflicts on this point. No precipitate was seen when pancuronium was mixed with succinylcholine, meperidine, neostigmine, gallamine, tubocurarine, or promethazine.

Dosage Forms/Regulatory Status

VETERINARY-LABELED PRODUCTS: NONE.

The ARCI (Racing Commissioners International) has designated this drug as a class 2 substance. See the appendix for more information.

HUMAN-LABELED PRODUCTS:

Pancuronium Bromide for Injection: 1 mg/mL in 10 mL vials; 2 mg/mL in 2 mL & 5 mL vials & amps; generic; (Rx)

Revisions/References

Monograph revised/updated May 2014.

Carr, A. (2003). Short-term ventilator management: A practical discussion. Proceedings: IVECCS. accessed via Veterinary Information Network; vin.com

Day, T. (2005). Anesthesia for the septic patient. Proceedings: IVECCS. accessed via Veterinary Information Network; vin.com

Papich, M. (1989). Effects of drugs on pregnancy. *Current Veterinary Therapy X: Small Animal Practice.* R. Kirk. Philadelphia, Saunders: 1291-9.

Pantoprazole

(pan-**toe**-prah-zohl)   Protonix®, Pantoloc®

Proton Pump Inhibitor

Prescriber Highlights

▶ Proton pump inhibitor similar to omeprazole; also available in IV dosage form.

▶ May be useful in treating or preventing gastric acid-related pathologies in dogs, cats, foals & camelids.

▶ Relatively limited research & experience in veterinary medicine, particularly when compared with PO omeprazole.

▶ Appears well tolerated.

Uses/Indications

Pantoprazole may be useful in treating or preventing gastric acid-related pathologies in dogs, cats, foals and camelids, particularly when the intravenous route is preferred. Pantoprazole is available in both intravenous and oral tablet (delayed-release) formulations. One study (Bersenas *et al.* 2005) performed in dogs, comparing the gastric pH effects of intravenous pantoprazole with oral omeprazole, intravenous ranitidine, and intravenous famotidine, found at the dosages used that pantoprazole was more effective than ranitidine but similar to famotidine, and that oral omeprazole was more effective in maintaining intragastric pH >3 for a longer period than pantoprazole.

Pantoprazole has been shown to directly reduce *in vitro* counts of *H. pylori* and is used in some *H. pylori* treatment protocols for humans.

Pharmacology/Actions

Pantoprazole is a substituted benzimidazole, similar to omeprazole and the other proton pump inhibitors (PPIs). At the secretory surface of gastric parietal cells, pantoprazole forms a covalent bond at two sites of the H$^+$/K$^+$ ATPase (proton pump) enzyme system. There it inhibits the transport of hydrogen ions into the stomach. Pantoprazole reduces acid secretion during both basal and stimulated conditions.

Pharmacokinetics

No specific information was located for pantoprazole pharmacokinetics in dogs or cats.

In neonatal foals, intragastric (IG) administered pantoprazole

bioavailability was 41% and drug was detected in plasma within 5 minutes of administration. Mean hourly gastric pH was increased for 2-24 hours versus untreated foals after either IV or IG administration, but IV administration increased pH significantly greater than IG administration, presumably due to low GI bioavailability (Ryan *et al.* 2005).

In alpacas, pantoprazole has a high SC bioavailability (>100% in some animals). A dosage of 2 mg/kg (SC) produced significantly higher AUC's and longer half-life than IV, but half-life is still short (mean of 0.58 hours) (Smith *et al.* 2010).

In humans, it is rapidly absorbed after oral administration with an oral bioavailability of 77%. Food can reduce the rate of absorption, but does not appear to affect the extent of absorption. On average, 51% of gastric acid secretion is inhibited at 2.5 hours after a single dose and 85% is inhibited after the seventh day of daily administration. Protein binding is 98%, primarily to albumin. The drug is metabolized in the liver, primarily by CYP2C19 isoenzymes. CYP3A4, 2D6, 2C9, or 1A2 are minor components of pantoprazole biotransformation; pantoprazole does not appear to clinically affect (either induce or inhibit) the metabolism of other drugs using these isoenzymes for biotransformation. Metabolites of pantoprazole do not appear to have pharmacologic activity. Elimination half-life for both oral and IV administration is only ≈ 1 hour, but the drug's pharmacologic action can persist for 24 hours or more, presumably due to irreversible binding at the receptor site. About 71% of a dose is excreted as metabolites in the urine, with the remainder in the feces as metabolites and unabsorbed drug.

Contraindications/Precautions/Warnings

Pantoprazole is contraindicated in patients known to be hypersensitive to it or other substituted benzimidazole PPIs.

Parenteral pantoprazole must be administered IV; do not give IM or SQ. Reconstituted injection (4 mg/mL) must be administered intravenously over not less than 2 minutes.

Adverse Effects

Use has been limited in small animals and an adverse effect profile is not well established; however, the drug appears to be tolerated well.

In humans, the most commonly reported adverse effects are diarrhea and headache. Hyperglycemia has been reported in ≈ 1% of patients. Proton pump inhibitors have been associated with an increased risk of developing community-acquired pneumonia in humans. Injection site reactions (thrombophlebitis, abscess) have occurred with IV administration.

Reproductive/Nursing Safety

When pantoprazole was dosed in rats (98X human dose) and rabbits (16X), no affects on fertility or teratogenic effects were noted. In humans, the FDA categorizes pantoprazole as category *B* for use during pregnancy (*Animal studies have not yet demonstrated risk to the fetus, but there are no adequate studies in pregnant women; or animal studies have shown an adverse effect, but adequate studies in pregnant women have not demonstrated a risk to the fetus in the first trimester of pregnancy, and there is no evidence of risk in later trimesters.*)

Pantoprazole and its metabolites have been detected in milk, but it should be relatively safe to use in nursing veterinary patients.

Overdosage/Acute Toxicity

There is limited information available. A single oral dose of 887 mg/kg was lethal in dogs. Acute toxic signs included ataxia, hypo-activity, and tremor. In humans, single oral overdoses of up to 600 mg have been reported without adversity. In the event of a large overdose, it is recommended to contact an animal poison control center for guidance.

Drug Interactions

The following drug interactions have either been reported or are theoretical in humans or animals receiving pantoprazole and may be of significance in veterinary patients. Unless otherwise noted, use together is not necessarily contraindicated, but weigh the potential risks and perform additional monitoring when appropriate.

- **DRUGS REQUIRING DECREASED GASTRIC PH FOR OPTIMAL ABSORPTION** (*e.g.,* ketoconazole, itraconazole, iron, ampicillin esters): Pantoprazole may decrease drug absorption.
- **SUCRALFATE:** May decrease bioavailability of orally administered pantoprazole.
- **WARFARIN:** Pantoprazole may increase anticoagulant effect.

Laboratory Considerations

- Although not likely to be important for veterinary patients, pantoprazole may cause false-positive results for **urine screening tests for THC** (tetrahydrocannabinol).

Doses

- **DOGS/CATS:**

  As a parenteral proton-pump inhibitor (extra-label): 0.7 – 1 mg/kg IV over 15 minutes q24h (once daily). (Marks 2008)

- **HORSES:**

  For gastric acid suppression in neonatal foals: 1.5 mg/kg IV once daily. **Note:** From an experimental study evaluating the pharmacokinetics and pharmacodynamics in normal neonatal foals. Further studies are required to investigate the use of this drug in critically ill patients. (Ryan *et al.* 2005)

- **CAMELIDS (NW)**

  For gastric ulcers (extra-label): From a pharmacokinetic and efficacy study in alpacas. Authors concluded, "Although not evaluated in this study, based on the high bioavailability, lower dosages (1 – 1.5 mg/kg) SC may be efficacious in decreasing gastric acid production and could lower the daily treatment cost. The use of lower doses of pantoprazole should be evaluated in future studies." (Smith *et al.* 2010)

Monitoring

- Efficacy.
- Adverse effects (vomiting, diarrhea, injection site reactions if used IV).

Client Information

- Used to treat or prevent stomach ulcers. Usually treatment is only short-term.
- Works best if given before the first meal of the day.
- Do not break or cut tablets.

Chemistry/Synonyms

Pantoprazole sodium sesquihydrate occurs as a white to off-white crystalline powder and is racemic. It is freely soluble in water and very slightly soluble in phosphate buffer at a pH of 7.4. Stability of aqueous solutions is pH dependent. At room temperature, solutions of pH 5 are stable for ≈ 3 hours; at a pH of 7.8, 220 hours.

Pantoprazole may also be known as BY-1023, or SKF-96022. International trade names include: *Controloc®, Pantoloc®, Zurcal®, Pantozol®, Pantop®, Protonix®, Protium®, Somac-MA®*, and many others.

Storage/Stability

Delayed-release tablets should be stored between 15-30°C.

The powder for injection should be stored protected from light at 20-25°C; excursions are permitted to 15-30°C.

The product is labeled: "Reconstituted solutions (10 mL) are stable for up to 2 hours at room temperature. If further diluted (per 15 minute infusion), it is stable for up to 22 hours at room tem-

perature. Reconstituted solutions do not need to be protected from light. Do not freeze. Do not use the IV solution if discoloration or precipitates are seen; should these be observed during the infusion, stop immediately." However a study (Donnelly 2011) demonstrated that pantoprazole 4 mg/mL was stable (least 90% of initial concentration) for 3 days when stored in glass vials at 20-25°C or for 28 days when stored in polypropylene syringes at 2-8°C. Pantoprazole 0.4 mg/mL diluted in D5W and stored in PVC minibags was stable for 2 days at 20-25°C or for 14 days at 2-8°C. At 0.8 mg/mL, pantoprazole in D5W was stable for 3 days at 20-25°C or 28 days at 2-8°C. Pantoprazole diluted to either 0.4 or 0.8 mg/mL in normal saline and stored in PVC minibags was stable for 3 days at 20-25°C or 28 days at 2-8°C.

Compatibility/Compounding Considerations

At Y-sites, pantoprazole injection is **not compatible** with dobutamine, esmolol, mannitol, midazolam, and multivitamins and may not be compatible with solutions containing zinc. It is reportedly **compatible** (at Y-sites) with ampicillin, cefazolin, ceftriaxone, dimenhydrinate, dopamine, epinephrine, furosemide, morphine, nitroglycerin, potassium chloride and vasopressin.

For a 2-minute IV infusion; reconstitute with 10 mL of 0.9% sodium chloride injection. To prepare the injection for a 15-minute IV infusion, reconstitute with 10 mL of 0.9% sodium chloride injection, then dilute further with 100 mL of D5W, 0.9% sodium chloride or lactated Ringer's injection to a final concentration of ≈ 0.4 mg/mL.

Dosage Forms/Regulatory Status

VETERINARY-LABELED PRODUCTS: NONE.

The ARCI (Racing Commissioners International) has designated this drug as a class 5 substance. See the appendix for more information.

HUMAN-LABELED PRODUCTS:

Pantoprazole Sodium Delayed-Release Tablets: 20 mg (as base) & 40 mg (as base); *Protonix®*, generic; (Rx)

Pantoprazole Lyophilized Powder for Injection Solution: 40 mg (as base) in vials; *Protonix I.V.®*, generic; (Rx)

Pantoprazole Sodium Delayed-Release Granules for Suspension: 40 mg; *Protonix®*; (Rx)

Revisions/References

Monograph revised/updated May 2014.

Bersenas, A., et al. (2005). Effects of ranitidine, famotidine, pantoprazole, and omeprazole on intragastric pH in dogs. AJVR **66**(3): 425-31.

Donnelly, R. (2011). Stability of pantoprazole sodium in glass vials, polyvinyl chloride minibags, and polypropylene syringes. Can J Hosp Pharm **64**(3): 192-8.

Marks, S. (2008). GI Therapeutics: Which Ones and When? Proceedings; IVECCS. accessed via Veterinary Information Network; vin.com

Ryan, C., et al. (2005). Pharmacokinetics and pharmacodynamics of pantoprazole in clinically normal neonatal foals. Proceedings: ACVIM 2005. accessed via Veterinary Information Network; vin.com

Smith, G. W., et al. (2010). Efficacy and Pharmacokinetics of Pantoprazole in Alpacas. Journal of Veterinary Internal Medicine **24**(4): 949-55.

Parapox Ovis Virus Immunomodulator

(pair-ah-**poks** oh-vis)   Inactivated *Parapoxvirus ovis*, Zylexis®

Immunostimulant

Prescriber Highlights

▶ Biologic immunostimulant labeled for use in healthy horses 4 months of age & older as an aid in reducing upper respiratory disease caused by equine herpesvirus types 1 & 4.

▶ Limited published information available on safety & clinical efficacy.

Uses/Indications

Parapox ovis virus immunomodulator (inactivated *parapoxvirus ovis*, iPPVO) is commercially available in the USA labeled for "use in healthy horses 4 months of age and older as an aid in reducing upper respiratory disease caused by equine herpesvirus types 1 and 4."

A placebo-controlled study in foals (N=59; age range: 24-48 hours) on a farm with endemic *R. equi* infections, found no significant difference in the pneumonia incidence between treated foals (2 mL *Zylexis*®; repeated in 1 & 9 days later) and the placebo group (Sturgill *et al.* 2011). Published evidence that supports iPPVO's clinical efficacy for reducing the incidence of equine respiratory disease complex (ERDC) conflicts, but a recent review (Paillot 2013) concluded that "an increasing amount of studies and reports that support the efficient use of non-specific immune-modulators such as iPPVO or *P. acnes* as adjuncts to conventional management of ERDC. Their activity is mostly based on non-specific stimulation of innate immune response. They may not provide protection against direct infection or transmission of respiratory pathogens but they seem to contribute to the reduction of the disease severity, subsequently reducing the frequency of complications and improving the rate of recovery. In the case of iPPVO, its anti-herpetic function may provide a valuable contribution in prevention of equine herpesviruses infection."

A parapoxvirus product (*Baypamun*®) is reportedly available in some European countries for use in small animals.

Pharmacology/Actions

Parapox ovis (parapoxvirus ovis) is the virus responsible for "orf" in sheep, a contagious pustular dermatitis. The virus is inactivated in the commercial product. Parapoxvirus products are so-called "paramunity inducers" and are believed to prevent viral infection by pathogenic viruses via viral interference. By "infecting" host cells with a defective (non-replicating) virus, interference with infection by the pathogenic virus can occur. Postulated mechanisms of action include induction of interferons, cytokines and colony-stimulating factors, and activation of natural killer cells.

Pharmacokinetics

Effects on the immune system are reported to occur 4-6 hours after treating; effects persist for 1-2 weeks.

Contraindications/Precautions/Warnings

Do not be use in patients with prior hypersensitivity to the agent. The manufacturer warns that in the case of an anaphylactic reaction, administer epinephrine or equivalent.

Reproductive/Nursing Safety

No information was located.

Adverse Effects

No adverse effects are listed in the package insert, but hypersensitivity or anaphylaxis is possible.

Overdosage/Acute Toxicity

No information was located.

Drug Interactions

- None noted.

Laboratory Considerations

- None identified.

Doses

- **HORSES:**

  For an aid in reducing upper airway disease caused by herpesvirus types 1 and 4 (labeled dose): After reconstituting with the sterile diluent provided, administer 2 mL IM. Repeat doses on days 2 and 9 following the initial dose. Retreatment is recom-

mended during subsequent disease episodes or prior to stress inducing situations. (Label information; *Zylexis*®)

Monitoring

- Clinical Efficacy (respiratory infection improvement).

Chemistry/Synonyms

Zylexis® is provided commercially as a freeze-dried inactivated (killed) virus component with separate 2 mL vial of sterile diluent.

Parapox ovis virus immunomodulator may also be known as: iPPVO, PPOV, PIND-ORF, or *Baypamune*® and *Zylexis*®.

Storage/Stability

Zylexis® should be stored refrigerated (2-8°C), but not be frozen. After reconstituting, entire contents should be used.

Dosage Forms/Regulatory Status

VETERINARY-LABELED PRODUCTS:

Parapox Ovis Virus Immunomodulator Injection in boxes of 5-single dose vials for reconstitution with 5- 2mL vials of sterile diluent; *Zylexis*®. Labeled for use in horses.

Note: This product is a USDA-licensed biologic and is not FDA-approved. The label for *Zylexis*® states that it should not be administered to horses within 21 days of slaughter.

HUMAN-LABELED PRODUCTS: NONE.

Revisions/References

Monograph revised/updated May 2014.

Paillot, R. (2013). A systematic review of the immune-modulators Parapoxvirus ovis and Propionibacterium acnes for the prevention of respiratory disease and other infections in the horse. Veterinary Immunology and Immunopathology 153(1-2): 1-9.
Sturgill, T. L., et al. (2011). Effects of inactivated parapoxvirus ovis on the cumulative incidence of pneumonia and cytokine secretion in foals on a farm with endemic infections caused by Rhodococcus equi. Veterinary Immunology and Immunopathology 140(3-4): 237-43.

Paregoric

(par-eh-**gore**-ik); Camphorated Tincture of Opium

Opiate Antidiarrheal

Prescriber Highlights

▶ Opiate GI motility modifier for diarrhea.

▶ Contraindications: Known hypersensitivity to narcotic analgesics, patients receiving monoamine oxidase inhibitors (MAOIs), diarrhea caused by a toxic ingestion until the toxin is eliminated from the GI tract. Caution: Respiratory disease, hepatic encephalopathy, hypothyroidism, severe renal insufficiency, adrenocortical insufficiency (Addison's), head injuries, or increased intracranial pressure, acute abdominal conditions (*e.g.*, colic), & in geriatric or severely debilitated patients.

▶ Adverse Effects: **Dogs:** Constipation, bloat, & sedation. Potential for: paralytic ileus, toxic megacolon, pancreatitis, & CNS effects. **Cats:** Use is controversial, may exhibit excitatory behavior. **Horses:** With GI bacterial infection, may delay the disappearance of the microbe from the feces & prolong the febrile state.

▶ Dose carefully in small animals; do not confuse with opium tincture.

▶ Paregoric is a C-III controlled substance.

Uses/Indications

Paregoric is occasionally used as a motility modifier for animals with diarrhea. Opiates as an antidiarrheal treatment in cats is controversial and many clinicians do not recommend their use in this species.

Pharmacology/Actions

Among their other actions, opiates inhibit GI motility and excessive GI propulsion. They also decrease intestinal secretion induced by cholera toxin, prostaglandin E_2 and diarrheas caused by factors in which calcium is the second messenger (non-cyclic AMP/GMP mediated). Opiates may also enhance mucosal absorption.

Pharmacokinetics

The morphine in paregoric is absorbed in a variable fashion from the GI tract. It is rapidly metabolized in the liver and serum morphine levels are considerably less than when morphine is administered parenterally.

Contraindications/Precautions/Warnings

All opiates should be used with caution in patients with hypothyroidism, severe renal insufficiency, adrenocortical insufficiency, (Addison's), in geriatric patients or those that are severely debilitated. Opiate antidiarrheals are contraindicated in cases where the patient is hypersensitive to narcotic analgesics, those receiving monoamine oxidase inhibitors (MAOIs), and with diarrhea caused by a toxic ingestion until the toxin is eliminated from the GI tract.

Opiate antidiarrheals should be used with caution in patients with head injuries or increased intracranial pressure and acute abdominal conditions (*e.g.*, colic), as it may obscure the diagnosis or clinical course of these conditions. It should be used with extreme caution in patients suffering from respiratory disease or acute respiratory dysfunction (*e.g.*, pulmonary edema secondary to smoke inhalation). Opiate antidiarrheals should be used with extreme caution in patients with hepatic disease with CNS clinical signs of hepatic encephalopathy; hepatic coma may result.

Paregoric (camphorated tincture of opium) should not be confused with opium tincture (tincture of opium), which contains 50 mg/5 mL of anhydrous morphine equivalent (25X more potent than paregoric).

Adverse Effects

In dogs, constipation, bloat, and sedation are the most likely adverse reactions encountered when usual doses are used. Potentially, paralytic ileus, toxic megacolon, pancreatitis, and CNS effects could be seen.

Use of antidiarrheal opiates in cats is controversial; this species may react with excitatory behavior.

Opiates used in horses with acute diarrhea (or in any animal with a potentially bacterial-induced diarrhea) may have a detrimental effect. Opiates may enhance bacterial proliferation, delay the disappearance of the microbe from the feces, and prolong the febrile state.

Reproductive/Nursing Safety

Opium tincture is classified as category *C* for use during pregnancy (*Animal studies have shown an adverse effect on the fetus, but there are no adequate studies in humans; or there are no animal reproduction studies and no adequate studies in humans.*)

Safe use of paregoric during breastfeeding in women has not been established; use with caution in nursing animals.

Overdosage/Acute Toxicity

Acute overdosage of the opiate antidiarrheals could result in CNS, cardiovascular, GI, or respiratory toxicity. Because the opiates may significantly reduce GI motility, absorption from the GI may be delayed and prolonged. For more information, refer to the meperidine and morphine monographs found in the CNS section. Naloxone may be necessary to reverse the opiate effects.

Drug Interactions

The following drug interactions have either been reported or are theoretical in humans or animals receiving opiate antidiarrheals and may be of significance in veterinary patients. Unless otherwise noted, use together is not necessarily contraindicated, but weigh the potential risks and perform additional monitoring when appropriate.

- **CNS DEPRESSANT DRUGS** (*e.g.*, **anesthetic agents, antihistamines, phenothiazines, barbiturates, tranquilizers, alcohol,** etc.): May cause increased CNS or respiratory depression when used with opiate antidiarrheal agents.
- **MONOAMINE OXIDASE INHIBITORS** (including **amitraz,** and possibly **selegiline**): Opiate antidiarrheal agents are contraindicated in human patients receiving monoamine oxidase (MAO) inhibitors for at least 14 days after receiving MAO inhibitors.

Laboratory Considerations

- Plasma **amylase** and **lipase** values may be increased for up to 24 hours following administration of opiates.

Doses

- **DOGS/CATS:**

  As an antidiarrheal (extra-label): 0.05 – 0.06 mg/kg PO 2-3 times daily. **Note:** Use of antidiarrheal opiates in cats is controversial; this species may react with excitatory behavior.

Monitoring

- Clinical efficacy.
- Fluid and electrolyte status in severe diarrhea.
- CNS effects if using high dosages.

Client Information

- Used to treat diarrhea; **NOT** for diarrhea caused by a toxin or poison.
- Possible side effects are sedation and constipation.
- If diarrhea continues or animal appears listless or develops a high fever, contact veterinarian.
- Paregoric is a C-III controlled substance. It is a federal offense to give or sell this medication to others than for whom it was prescribed.

Chemistry/Synonyms

Paregoric contains 2 mg/5 mL of the equivalent of anhydrous morphine (usually as powdered opium or opium tincture). Also included (per 5 mL) are 0.02 mL anise oil, 0.2 mL glycerin, 20 mg benzoic acid, 20 mg camphor, and a sufficient quantity of diluted alcohol to make a total of 5 mL. Paregoric should not be confused with opium tincture (tincture of opium), which contains 50 mg of anhydrous morphine equivalent per 5 mL (25X more potent than paregoric).

Paregoric is also known as camphorated tincture of opium or tinctura opii camphorata.

Storage/Stability

Paregoric should be stored in tight, light-resistant containers. Avoid exposure to excessive heat or direct exposure to sunlight.

Dosage Forms/Regulatory Status

VETERINARY-LABELED PRODUCTS: NONE.

HUMAN-LABELED PRODUCTS:

Paregoric (camphorated tincture of opium): 2 mg of morphine equiv. per 5 mL (45% alcohol) in 473 mL; generic; (Rx; C-III)

Note: Do not confuse with opium tincture, which contains 25X more morphine per mL than paregoric.

Revisions/References

Monograph revised/updated May 2014.

Paromomycin Sulfate

(pair-oh-moe-**my**-sin)   Aminosidine, Humatin®

Oral Aminoglycoside Antiparasitic

Prescriber Highlights

▶ Oral aminoglycoside used primarily as treatment of cryptosporidiosis in small animals.

▶ Not appreciably absorbed in dogs when dosed orally if gut is intact. Some state the drug is contraindicated in cats secondary to toxicity.

▶ Adverse effects are usually limited to GI effects (nausea, vomiting, diarrhea); cats may be susceptible to renal & ophthalmic toxicity.

▶ Use with caution in patients with intestinal ulceration.

Uses/Indications

Paromomycin (aminosidine) may be useful as a treatment for cryptosporidiosis in dogs and cats. While some consider it to a be second-line treatment for dogs and should be avoided in cats, a recent review states: "Considering the results from different drugs tested, paromomycin appears to be the drug of choice for the treatment of cryptosporidiosis in dogs and cats"(Shahiduzzamana *et al.* 2012).

In dogs, paromomycin is also used topically to treat cutaneous Leishmaniasis. Subcutaneously administered paromomycin (no dosage forms available in USA) in combination with meglumine antimoniate is used in some protocols for treating systemic Leishmaniasis, but serious adverse effects limit usefulness.

In humans, paromomycin has been used as an alternative oral treatment for giardiasis, *Dientamoeba fragilis*, and hepatic coma.

Pharmacology/Actions

Paromomycin has an antimicrobial spectrum of activity similar to neomycin, but its primary therapeutic uses are for the treatment of protozoa, including *Leishmania* spp., *Entamoeba histolytica*, and *Cryptosporidium* spp. It also has activity against a variety of tapeworms, but there are better choices available for clinical use.

Pharmacokinetics

Like neomycin, paromomycin is very poorly absorbed when given orally. Potentially systemic toxicity (nephrotoxicity, ototoxicity, pancreatitis) could occur if used in patients with significant ulcerative intestinal lesions or for a prolonged period at high dosages.

Contraindications/Precautions/Warnings

Paromomycin is contraindicated in patients with:

■ Known hypersensitivity to the drug.

■ Ileus or intestinal obstruction, GI ulceration, or blood in stool; increased likelihood of systemic absorption with resultant toxic effects.

Use with caution in cats; because of potential toxicity, some clinicians avoid using in cats.

Do not confuse *Humatin®* with *Humalin®*.

Adverse Effects

■ Gastrointestinal effects (nausea, inappetence, vomiting, diarrhea) are the most likely adverse effects to be noted with therapy.

■ Because paromomycin can affect gut flora, nonsusceptible bacterial or fungal overgrowths are a possibility.

■ In patients with significant gut ulceration or degradation of GI mucosal barriers, paromomycin may be absorbed systemically with resultant nephrotoxicity, ototoxicity, or pancreatitis.

■ Use in cats has been associated with renal dysfunction, ototoxicity and blindness.

■ Similarly to neomycin (parenteral), SC administration of paromomycin can cause renal and vestibular toxicity.

Reproductive/Nursing Safety

Because minimal amounts are absorbed when administered orally, paromomycin should be safe to use during pregnancy. It should not be used parenterally during pregnancy.

When used orally, paromomycin should be safe to use during lactation.

Overdosage/Acute Toxicity

Because paromomycin is not appreciably absorbed after oral administration, acute overdose adverse effects should be limited to gastrointestinal distress in patients with an intact GI system. Chronic overdoses may lead to systemic toxicity.

Drug Interactions

The following drug interactions have either been reported or are theoretical in humans or animals receiving paromomycin and may be of significance in veterinary patients. Unless otherwise noted, use together is not necessarily contraindicated, but weigh the potential risks and perform additional monitoring when appropriate.

■ **DIGOXIN:** Paromomycin may reduce digoxin absorption.

■ **METHOTREXATE:** Paromomycin may reduce methotrexate absorption.

Laboratory Considerations

■ None were noted.

Doses

■ **DOGS:**

For treatment of cryptosporidiosis (extra-label): A dosing range of 125 – 165 mg/kg PO twice daily for 5 days has been suggested (Blagburn 2003); commonly 150 mg/kg PO once daily for 5 days is recommended.

■ **CATS:**

For treatment of cryptosporidiosis (extra-label): **Note:** Higher dosages of paromomycin have caused renal or otic toxicity and/or blindness in some treated cats. Consider using an alternate treatment first (*e.g.*, azithromycin) or paromomycin at an initially reduced dosage level. Some recommend the canine dose. Another recommendation is 150 mg/kg PO q12-24hr. Paromomycin can be nephrotoxic if absorbed. If the cat is responding to the first 7 days of therapy and toxicity has not been noted, continue treatment for 1 week past clinical resolution of diarrhea. (Lappin 2008)

■ **CAMELIDS (NEW WORLD):**

For treatment of cryptosporidiosis in crias (extra-label): 50 mg/kg PO (*dosing interval not specified, assume once per day—Plumb*) for 5-10 days. (Walker 2009)

■ **REPTILES:**

For treatment of cryptosporidiosis (extra-label): 300 – 800 mg/kg PO q24-48h for 7-14 days or as needed. (de la Navarre 2003)

Monitoring

■ Efficacy.

■ GI adverse effects.

■ If used in cats, monitor renal function.

Client Information

■ Unless otherwise instructed, give with food.

Chemistry/Synonyms

An aminoglycoside antibiotic, paromomycin sulfate occurs as an odorless, creamy white to light yellow, hygroscopic, amorphous powder having a saline taste. Paromomycin is very soluble in water (>1 gram/mL).

Paromomycin may also be known as: aminosidin sulphate, aminosidine sulphate, catenulin sulphate, crestomycin sulphate; estomycin sulphate, hydroxymycin sulphate, monomycin A sulphate, neomycin E sulphate, paucimycin sulphate, and *Humatin*®.

Storage/Stability

Paromomycin capsules should be stored at room temperature (15-30°C; 59-86°F) in tight containers.

Dosage Forms/Regulatory Status

VETERINARY-LABELED PRODUCTS: NONE.

HUMAN-LABELED PRODUCTS:

Paromomycin Sulfate Oral Capsules: 250 mg; generic; (Rx)

Revisions/References

Monograph revised/updated May 2014.

Blagburn, B. (2003). Current recognition, control and prevention of protozoan parasites affecting dogs and cats. Proceedings: Western Veterinary Conference. accessed via Veterinary Information Network; vin.com
de la Navarre, B. (2003). Common parasitic diseases of reptiles and amphibians. Proceedings: Western Veterinary Conf. accessed via Veterinary Information Network; vin.com
Lappin, M. R. (2008). Giardia and Cryptosporidium Spp. Infections of Cats: Clinical and Zoonotic Aspects. Proceedings: ECVIM. accessed via Veterinary Information Network; vin.com
Shahiduzzamana, M. & A. Daugschiesb (2012). Therapy and prevention of cryptosporidiosis in animals. Veterinary Parasitology 188: 203-14.
Walker, P. (2009). Differential Diagnosis of Diarrhea in Camelid Crias. Proceedings: ACVIM. accessed via Veterinary Information Network; vin.com

Paroxetine HCl

(pah-**rox**-a-teen)   Paxil®

Selective Serotonin Reuptake Inhibitor (SSRI) Antidepressant

Prescriber Highlights

▶ Selective serotonin reuptake inhibitor antidepressant related to fluoxetine used in dogs & cats for variety of behavior disorders.

▶ Contraindications: Patients with known hypersensitivity or receiving monoamine oxidase inhibitors. Caution: Patients with severe cardiac, renal or hepatic disease. Dosages may need to be reduced in patients with severe renal or hepatic impairment. If patient is on the drug for an extended period, gradual withdrawal recommended.

▶ Adverse effect profile is not well established; potentially in **Dogs:** Anorexia, lethargy, GI effects, anxiety, irritability, insomnia/hyperactivity, or panting. Aggressive behavior in previously unaggressive dogs possible. **Cats:** May exhibit behavior changes (anxiety, irritability, sleep disturbances), anorexia, constipation & changes in elimination patterns.

Uses/Indications

Paroxetine may be beneficial for the treatment of canine aggression, and stereotypic or other obsessive-compulsive behaviors. It has been used occasionally in cats as well.

Pharmacology/Actions

Paroxetine is a highly selective inhibitor of the reuptake of serotonin (SSRI) in the CNS, thus potentiating the pharmacologic activity of serotonin. Paroxetine apparently has little effect on other neurotransmitters (*e.g.*, dopamine or norepinephrine).

Pharmacokinetics

No data for cats or dogs was located.

In grey parrots, paroxetine HCl dissolved in water given PO was slowly absorbed and had a bioavailability (mean) of 31%, but there was significant interpatient variation. Repeated administration increased bioavailability. Terminal elimination half-life was ≈ 5 hours (van Zeeland *et al.* 2013).

In humans, paroxetine is slowly, but nearly completely, absorbed from the GI tract. Because of a relatively high first pass-effect, relatively small amounts reach the systemic circulation unchanged. Food does not impair absorption.

The drug is ≈ 95% bound to plasma proteins. Paroxetine is extensively metabolized, probably in the liver. Half-life in humans ranges from 7-65 hours and averages ≈ 24 hours.

Contraindications/Precautions/Warnings

Paroxetine is contraindicated in patients with known hypersensitivity to it or those receiving monoamine oxidase inhibitors (see Drug Interactions below). Use with caution in patients with seizure disorders, severe cardiac, hepatic, or renal disease. Dosages may need to be reduced in patients with severe hepatic or renal impairment.

If paroxetine is rapidly discontinued, withdrawal reactions can occur. If the patient has been receiving the drug for an extended period, a gradual withdrawal is recommended.

Do not confuse paroxetine with fluoxetine or piroxicam. Do not confuse *Paxil*® with paclitaxel.

Adverse Effects

In dogs, paroxetine can cause lethargy, salivation, GI effects, anxiety, irritability, insomnia/hyperactivity, or panting. Anorexia is a common side effect in dogs (usually transient and may be negated by temporarily increasing the palatability of food and/or hand feeding). Some dogs have persistent anorexia that precludes further treatment. Aggressive behavior in previously unaggressive dogs has been reported. SSRIs may also cause changes in blood glucose levels and potentially, reduce seizure threshold.

Paroxetine in cats can cause behavior changes (anxiety, irritability, sleep disturbances), anorexia, constipation and changes in elimination patterns.

Reproductive/Nursing Safety

Paroxetine's safety during pregnancy has not been established. Preliminary studies done in rats demonstrated no overt teratogenic effects. In humans, the FDA categorizes this drug as category C for use during pregnancy (*Animal studies have shown an adverse effect on the fetus, but there are no adequate studies in humans; or there are no animal reproduction studies and no adequate studies in humans.*)

The drug is excreted into milk but at low levels; caution is advised in nursing patients.

Overdosage/Acute Toxicity

While not as toxic as the tricyclic antidepressants, fatalities and significant morbidity have occurred after paroxetine overdoses. In one retrospective study in dogs, a median dose of 7.7 mg/kg (range: 0.3 – 25.9 mg/kg; n = 5) was associated with clinical signs in overdoses, but no clinical significance could be differentiated from dosages that did not cause clinical signs (Thomas *et al.* 2012). Another retrospective review in dogs found the following overdoses and associated clinical signs: 1 – 3 mg/kg: vomiting, drooling, and lethargy; >3 mg/kg: agitation and seizures; <4 mg/kg (sustained-release product): sedation, drooling, and vomiting; >4.5 mg/kg (sustained-release product): agitation—no seizures reported from the sustained-release product (Mohammad-Zadeh *et al.* 2008).There were 222 single agent exposures to paroxetine reported to the ASPCA Animal Poison Control Center (APCC) during 2009-2013. Of the 194 dogs, 33 were symptomatic with lethargy (36%) and vomiting (18%) being the most common. Of the 30 cats, 9 were symptomatic with 56% having behavior changes and 44% being mydriatic.

In overdoses in small animals, contact an animal poison control center for additional guidance. When ingestion amounts are associated with significant morbidity or when the ingested amount is unknown, consider GI decontamination (if not contraindicated). Activated charcoal can be very effective in binding paroxetine. Treat supportively. Phenothiazines and cyproheptadine can be effective in controlling serotonin syndrome.

Drug Interactions

The following drug interactions have either been reported or are theoretical in humans or animals receiving paroxetine and may be of significance in veterinary patients. Unless otherwise noted, use together is not necessarily contraindicated, but weigh the potential risks and perform additional monitoring when appropriate.

- **BUSPIRONE:** Increased risk for serotonin syndrome.
- **CYPROHEPTADINE:** May decrease or reverse the effects of SSRIs.
- **DIAZEPAM, ALPRAZOLAM:** Paroxetine may increase diazepam levels.
- **DIURETICS:** Increased risk for hyponatremia.
- **INSULIN:** May alter insulin requirements.
- **ISONIAZID:** Increased risk for serotonin syndrome.
- **MAO INHIBITORS** (including **amitraz** and potentially, **selegiline**): High risk for serotonin syndrome; use contraindicated; in humans, a 5 week washout period is required after discontinuing paroxetine and a 2 week washout period if first discontinuing the MAO inhibitor.
- **NONSTEROIDAL ANTIINFLAMMATORY DRUGS (NSAIDS, ASPIRIN):** SSRI's may increase the risk for GI ulceration.
- **PENTAZOCINE:** Serotonin syndrome-like adverse effects possible.
- **PHENYTOIN:** Increased plasma levels of phenytoin possible.
- **PROPRANOLOL, METOPROLOL:** Paroxetine may increase these beta-blocker's plasma levels; atenolol may be safer to use if paroxetine is required.
- **ST JOHNS WORT:** Increased risk for serotonin syndrome.
- **TRAMADOL:** SSRI's can inhibit the metabolism of tramadol to the active metabolites decreasing its efficacy and increasing the risk of toxicity (serotonin syndrome, seizures).
- **TRICYCLIC ANTIDEPRESSANTS** (*e.g.*, **clomipramine**, **amitriptyline**): Paroxetine may increase TCA blood levels and the risk for serotonin syndrome.
- **TRAZODONE:** Increased plasma levels of trazodone possible.
- **WARFARIN:** Paroxetine may increase the risk for bleeding.

Doses

- **DOGS:**

For SSRI-responsive behavior problems (extra-label): Using regular tablets: 0.5 – 2 mg/kg PO once daily (q24h). Used in conjunction with behavior modification. Usually start at the low-end of the dosing range and treat for ≈ 2 months; evaluate and adjust dosage if necessary.

- **CATS:**

For SSRI-responsive behavior problems (extra-label): 0.5 – 1 mg/kg q24h; practically 1.25 – 5 mg (1/8th – ½ of a regular 10 mg tablet) per cat once daily (q24h). Usually start at the low-end of the dosing range and treat for ≈ 2 months; evaluate and adjust dosage if necessary.

- **BIRDS:**

For stress- or anxiety-related behavioral disorders (*e.g.*, feather picking); (extra-label): From a pharmacokinetic study in Grey parrots: Paroxetine HCl dissolved in water (human oral suspension was not consistently absorbed), given at 4 mg/kg PO twice daily seems sufficient to reach plasma concentrations that are reported to be effective in humans. Large inter-individual differences occur (may be gender-related) and can be associated with efficacy or adverse effects. Clinical trials should first be performed to demonstrate whether parrots with stress- or anxiety-related behavioral disorders actually benefit from SSRI's;

more investigations are needed to correlate kinetic parameters with efficacy for distinct clinical indications (van Zeeland *et al.* 2013).

Monitoring

- Efficacy.
- Adverse effects; including appetite (weight).

Client Information

- May take several days to weeks to determine if the drug is effective.
- Most common side effects are: drowsiness/sleepiness, and reduced appetite.
- Rare side effects that can be serious (contact veterinarian immediately): seizures, aggression (threatening behavior/actions).
- Overdoses can be very serious; keep out of the reach of animals and children.
- If your animal wore a flea collar in the past two weeks, let your veterinarian know. Do not use one on your animal while it's getting this medicine without first talking to your veterinarian.

Chemistry/Synonyms

A selective serotonin reuptake inhibitor (SSRI) antidepressant, paroxetine HCl occurs as an off-white, odorless powder. Its solubility in water is 5.4 mg/mL and pKa is 9.9.

Paroxetine may also be known as: BRL-29060, FG-7051 and *Paxil®*.

Storage/Stability

Paroxetine oral tablets should be stored at 15-30°C. The oral suspension should be stored below 25°C.

Dosage Forms/Regulatory Status

VETERINARY-LABELED PRODUCTS: NONE.

The ARCI (Racing Commissioners International) has designated this drug as a class 2 substance. See the appendix for more information.

HUMAN-LABELED PRODUCTS:

Paroxetine Oral Tablets: 10 mg, 20 mg, 30 mg & 40 mg; *Paxil®*, *Pexeva®*, generic; (Rx)

Paroxetine Oral Tablets Controlled-release: 12.5 mg, 25 mg & 37.5 mg; *Paxil® CR*, generic; (Rx)

Paroxetine Oral Suspension: 2 mg/mL in 250 mL; *Paxil®*, generic; (Rx)

Revisions/References

Monograph revised/updated May 2014.

Mohammad-Zadeh, L. F., et al. (2008). Serotonin: a review. J. Vet. Pharmacol. Ther. **31**(3): 187-99.

Thomas, D. E., et al. (2012). Retrospective evaluation of toxicosis from selective serotonin reuptake inhibitor antidepressants: 313 dogs (2005-2010). J. Vet. Emerg. Crit. Care **22**(6): 674-81.

van Zeeland, Y. R. A., et al. (2013). Pharmacokinetics of paroxetine, a selective serotonin reuptake inhibitor, in Grey parrots (Psittacus erithacus erithacus): influence of pharmaceutical formulation and length of dosing. J. Vet. Pharmacol. Ther. **36**(1): 51-8.

PEG 3350 Products – see Polyethylene Glycol 3350

Penicillamine

(pen-i-**sill**-a-meen)   Depen®, Cuprimine®

Antidote; Chelating Agent

Prescriber Highlights

▶ Chelating agent used primarily for copper-storage hepatopathies (dogs). Can be considered for lead poisoning or cystine urolithiasis, but other therapies are preferred.

▶ Contraindications: History of penicillamine-related blood dyscrasias; lead present in GI tract. Potentially teratogenic.

▶ Adverse Effects: Nausea, vomiting, & depression. Can reduce GI dietary mineral (zinc, iron, copper, and calcium) absorption and cause deficiencies; Rarely: Fever, lymphadenopathy, skin hypersensitivity reactions, or immune-complex glomerulonephropathy.

▶ Pyridoxine deficiency may occur; consider supplementation.

▶ Food significantly reduces oral bioavailability. Give on an empty stomach (if it can be tolerated).

Uses/Indications

Penicillamine is used primarily for its chelating ability in veterinary medicine. It is the drug of choice for Copper storage-associated hepatopathies in dogs, but clinical improvement may require weeks to months of therapy. It can also be used for the long-term oral treatment of lead, or mercury poisoning or in cystine urolithiasis.

Because it has anti-fibrotic effects, penicillamine may be of benefit in chronic hepatitis, but doses necessary for effective treatment are likely too high to be tolerated.

Pharmacology/Actions

Penicillamine chelates a variety of metals, including copper, lead, iron, and mercury, forming stable water soluble complexes that are excreted by the kidneys and combines chemically with cystine to form a stable, soluble complex that can be readily excreted.

Penicillamine has antirheumatic activity. The exact mechanisms for this action are not understood, but the drug apparently improves lymphocyte function, decreases IgM rheumatoid factor and immune complexes in serum and synovial fluid.

Penicillamine possesses antifibrotic activity via inhibition of collagen crosslinking thereby causing collagen to be more susceptible to degradation.

Although penicillamine is a degradation product of penicillins, it has no antimicrobial activity.

Pharmacokinetics

In dogs, giving with food reduces bioavailability by ≈ 70% compared to the fasted state with resultant significant reductions in peak levels and area-under-the-curve (24h hr) (Langlois *et al.* 2013).

In humans, penicillamine is well absorbed after oral administration and peak serum levels occur ≈ 1 hour after dosing. The drug apparently crosses the placenta but, otherwise, little information is known about its distribution. Penicillamine that is not complexed with either a metal or cystine is thought metabolized by the liver and excreted in the urine and feces.

Contraindications/Precautions/Warnings

Penicillamine is contraindicated in patients with a history of penicillamine-related blood dyscrasias. Penicillamine potentially can cause enhanced absorption of lead from the gastrointestinal tract. If lead is still present in the gut, it should not be administered.

Adverse Effects

In dogs, the most prevalent adverse effects associated with penicillamine are:

■ Nausea, vomiting, and depression. While penicillamine should be given on an empty stomach (at least 30 minutes before feeding), if the animal develops problems with vomiting or anorexia, four remedies have been suggested:

1) Give the same total daily dose, but divide into smaller individual doses and give more frequently.

2) Temporarily reduce the daily dose and gradually increase to recommended dosage.

3) Give a long-acting antiemetic one-hour before dosing.

4) Give with a small amount of food (*e.g.,* cheese or bread) if one of the first three do not alleviate vomiting.

■ Although thought infrequent or rare, fever, lymphadenopathy, skin hypersensitivity reactions, or immune-complex glomerulonephropathy may occur. A case of hemolytic anemia in a cat has been reported.

■ Penicillamine can reduce GI dietary mineral (zinc, iron, copper, and calcium) absorption and cause deficiencies with long-term use. Pyridoxine deficient states may occur; supplementation advised.

Reproductive/Nursing Safety

Penicillamine has been associated with the development of birth defects in offspring of rats given 10X the recommended dose. There are also some reports of human teratogenicity. In humans, the FDA categorizes this drug as category *D* for use during pregnancy (*There is evidence of human fetal risk, but the potential benefits from the use of the drug in pregnant women may be acceptable despite its potential risks.*)

Lactation safety has not been established.

Overdosage/Acute Toxicity

No specific acute toxic dose has been established for penicillamine and toxic effects generally occur in patients taking the drug chronically. Any relationship of toxicity to dose is unclear; patients on small doses may develop toxicity.

Drug Interactions

The following drug interactions have either been reported or are theoretical in humans or animals receiving penicillamine and may be of significance in veterinary patients. Unless otherwise noted, use together is not necessarily contraindicated, but weigh the potential risks and perform additional monitoring when appropriate.

■ **4-AMINOQUINOLINE DRUGS** (*e.g.,* **chloroquine**, **quinacrine**): Concomitant administration with these agents may increase the risks for severe dermatologic adverse effects.

■ **CATIONS, ORAL including ZINC, IRON, CALCIUM, & MAGNESIUM**: May decrease the effectiveness of penicillamine if given orally together. Long-term use of penicillamine may induce deficient states.

■ **FOOD, ANTACIDS**: The amount of penicillamine absorbed from the GI tract may be significantly reduced by the concurrent administration of food or antacids.

■ **GOLD COMPOUNDS**: May increase the risk of hematologic and/or renal adverse reactions.

■ **IMMUNOSUPPRESSANT DRUGS** (*e.g.,* **cyclophosphamide**, **azathioprine**, but **not corticosteroids**): May increase the risk of hematologic and/or renal adverse reactions.

■ **PHENYLBUTAZONE**: May increase the risk of hematologic and/or renal adverse reactions.

■ **PYRIDOXINE**: Penicillamine may induce deficient states. Supplementation is advised in human patients.

Laboratory Considerations

■ When using **technetium Tc 99m gluceptate** to visualize the kidneys, penicillamine may chelate this agent and form a compound that is excreted via the hepatobiliary system resulting in gallbladder visualization that could confuse the results.

Doses

- **DOGS:**

  For copper-associated hepatopathy (extra-label): The "standard" recommended dosage is 10 – 15 mg/kg PO twice daily on an empty stomach (at least 20-30 minutes before feeding). However, in a recent pharmacokinetic study the authors suggest that a lower dosage (7 mg/kg PO twice daily on an empty stomach) might be efficacious while reducing drug cost and the incidence of vomiting. Alternatively, a long acting antiemetic could be administered 1 hour before dosing in dogs that have a proclivity to vomit. (Langlois *et al.* 2013)

  For cystine urolithiasis (extra-label): 15 mg/kg: PO twice daily with food. (Lage *et al.* 1988)

  For lead poisoning (extra-label): As an alternate or adjunct to CaEDTA: 110 mg/kg/day divided q6-8h PO 30 minutes before feeding for 1-2 weeks. If vomiting is a problem, may pre-medicate with dimenhydrinate (2 – 4 mg/kg PO). Alternatively, may give 33 – 55 mg/kg/day divided as above. Dissolving medication in juice may facilitate administration. (Nicholson 2000)

- **CATS:**

  For primary copper hepatopathy (extra-label): From a retrospective study where 5 cats received penicillamine: 10 – 15 mg/kg PO q12h. One cat developed hemolytic anemia. (Hurwitz *et al.* 2014)

- **RUMINANTS:**

  Note: When used in food animals, FARAD recommends a minimum milk withdrawal time of 3 days after the last treatment and a 21-day preslaughter withdrawal. (Haskell *et al.* 2005)

  For copper toxicity in small ruminants (extra-label): 26 – 52 mg/kg PO once daily for 6 days. (Boileau 2009)

  For lead or mercury toxicity (extra-label): 110 mg/kg PO for 1-3 weeks. To prevent continued metal absorption, must clear GI tract of toxic metal before therapy. (Osweiler 2007)

- **BIRDS:**

  For adjunctive treatment of lead poisoning (extra-label): 55 mg/kg PO q12h for 1-2 weeks. It has been suggested that combining CaEDTA and penicillamine for several days until symptoms dissipate, followed by a 3-6 week treatment with penicillamine is the best regimen for lead toxicity. (Jones 2007)

Monitoring

- Monitoring for efficacy with penicillamine therapy is dependent upon the reason for its use (*e.g.*, liver copper levels, blood lead concentrations, etc.)
- Adverse effects.

Client Information

- Used to remove excess metals (*e.g.*, copper, lead, mercury) from the body.
- Can cause nausea (acting 'sick') and vomiting.
- Should be given on an empty stomach, at least 30 minutes before feeding.
- Does not have any antibiotic activity.

Chemistry/Synonyms

A monothiol chelating agent that is a degradation product of penicillins, penicillamine occurs as a white or practically white, crystalline powder with a characteristic odor. Penicillamine is freely soluble in water and slightly soluble in alcohol with pK_a values of 1.83, 8.03, and 10.83.

Penicillamine may also be known as: D-Penicillamine, beta,be-

ta-Dimethylcysteine, D-3-Mercaptovaline, penicillaminum, *Depen*® and *Cuprimine*®.

Storage/Stability

Penicillamine should be stored at room temperature (15-30°C). The capsules should be stored in tight containers; tablets in well-closed containers.

Dosage Forms/Regulatory Status

VETERINARY-LABELED PRODUCTS: NONE.

HUMAN-LABELED PRODUCTS:

Penicillamine Titratable Oral Tablets: 250 mg (scored); *Depen*®; (Rx)

Penicillamine Oral Capsules: 250 mg; *Cuprimine*®; (Rx)

Revisions/References

Monograph revised/updated May 2014.

Boileau, M. (2009). Challenging cases in small ruminant medicine. Proceedings: ACVIM. accessed via Veterinary Information Network; vin.com

Haskell, S., et al. (2005). Farad Digest: Antidotes in Food Animal Practice. JAVMA 226(6): 884-7.

Hurwitz, B. M., et al. (2014). Presumed primary and secondary hepatic copper accumulation in cats. Javma-Journal of the American Veterinary Medical Association 244(1): 68-77.

Jones, M. (2007). Avian Toxicology. Proceedings: Western Vet Conf. accessed via Veterinary Information Network; vin.com

Lage, A. L., et al. (1988). Diseases of the Bladder. *Handbook of Small Animal Practice.* R. V. Morgan. New York, Churchill Livingstone: 605-20.

Langlois, D. K., et al. (2013). Pharmacokinetics and Relative Bioavailability of d-Penicillamine in Fasted and Nonfasted Dogs. Journal of Veterinary Internal Medicine 27(5): 1071-6.

Nicholson, S. (2000). Toxicology. *Textbook of Veterinary Internal Medicine: Diseases of the Dog and Cat.* S. Ettinger and E. Feldman. Philadelphia, WB Saunders. 1: 357-63.

Osweiler, G. (2007). Detoxification and Antidotes for Ruminant Poisoning. Proceedings: ACVIM. accessed via Veterinary Information Network; vin.com

Penicillins, General Information

(pen-i-sill-in)

Uses/Indications

Penicillins have been used for a wide range of infections in various species. FDA-approved indications/species, as well as non-FDA-approved uses, are listed in the Uses/Indications and Dosage section for each drug.

Pharmacology/Actions

Penicillins are usually bactericidal against susceptible bacteria and act by inhibiting mucopeptide synthesis in the cell wall resulting in a defective barrier and an osmotically unstable spheroplast. The exact mechanism for this effect has not been definitively determined, but beta-lactam antibiotics have been shown to bind to several enzymes (carboxypeptidases, transpeptidases, endopeptidases) within the bacterial cytoplasmic membrane that are involved with cell wall synthesis. The different affinities that various beta-lactam antibiotics have for these enzymes (also known as penicillin-binding proteins; PBPs) help explain the differences in spectrums of activity the drugs have that are not explained by the influence of beta-lactamases. Like other beta-lactam antibiotics, penicillins are generally considered more effective against actively growing bacteria.

The clinically available penicillins encompass several distinct classes of compounds with varying spectrums of activity: The so-called natural penicillins including penicillin G and V; the penicillinase-resistant penicillins including cloxacillin, dicloxacillin, oxacillin; the aminopenicillins including ampicillin, amoxicillin & hetacillin; extended-spectrum penicillins including carbenicillin, ticarcillin, piperacillin, and azlocillin; and the potentiated penicillins including amoxicillin-potassium clavulanate, ampicillin-sulbactam, piperacillin-tazobactam, and ticarcillin-potassium clavulanate.

The natural penicillins (G and K) have similar spectrums of activity, but penicillin G is slightly more active *in vitro* on a weight basis against many organisms. This class of penicillin has *in vitro* activity against most spirochetes and gram-positive and gram-negative aerobic cocci, but not penicillinase-producing strains. They have activity against some aerobic and anaerobic gram-positive bacilli such as *Bacillus anthracis*, *Clostridium* spp. (not *C. difficile*), Fusobacterium, and Actinomyces. The natural penicillins are customarily inactive against most gram-negative aerobic and anaerobic bacilli, and all Rickettsia, mycobacteria, fungi, Mycoplasma, and viruses.

The penicillinase-resistant penicillins have a narrower spectrum of activity than the natural penicillins. Their antimicrobial efficacy is aimed directly against penicillinase-producing strains of gram-positive cocci, particularly staphylococcal species; these drugs are sometimes called anti-staphylococcal penicillins. There are documented strains of Staphylococcus that are resistant to these drugs (so-called methicillin-resistant or oxacillin-resistant Staph), but these strains have only begun to be a significant problem in veterinary species. While this class of penicillins does have activity against some other gram-positive and gram-negative aerobes and anaerobes, other antibiotics are usually better choices. The penicillinase-resistant penicillins are inactive against Rickettsia, mycobacteria, fungi, Mycoplasma, and viruses.

The aminopenicillins, also called the "broad-spectrum" or ampicillin penicillins, have increased activity against many strains of gram-negative aerobes not covered by either the natural penicillins or penicillinase-resistant penicillins including some strains of *E. coli*, Klebsiella, and Haemophilus. Like the natural penicillins, they are susceptible to inactivation by beta-lactamase-producing bacteria (*e.g.*, Staph aureus). Although not as active as the natural penicillins, they do have activity against many anaerobic bacteria, including Clostridial organisms. Organisms that are generally not susceptible include *Pseudomonas aeruginosa*, Serratia, Indole-positive Proteus (*Proteus mirabilis* is susceptible), Enterobacter, Citrobacter, and Acinetobacter. The aminopenicillins also are inactive against Rickettsia, mycobacteria, fungi, Mycoplasma, and viruses.

The extended-spectrum penicillins, sometimes called anti-pseudomonal penicillins, include both alpha-carboxypenicillins (carbenicillin and ticarcillin) and acylaminopenicillins (piperacillin, azlocillin, and mezlocillin). These agents have similar spectrums of activity as the aminopenicillins but with additional activity against several gram-negative organisms of the family Enterobacteriaceae, including many strains of *Pseudomonas aeruginosa*. Like the aminopenicillins, these agents are susceptible to inactivation by beta-lactamases.

In order to reduce the inactivation of penicillins by beta-lactamases, potassium clavulanate and sulbactam have been developed to inactivate these enzymes and extend the spectrum of those penicillins. When used with penicillin, these combinations are often effective against many beta-lactamase-producing strains of otherwise resistant *E. coli*, *Pasteurella* spp., *Staphylococcus* spp., Klebsiella, and Proteus. Type I beta-lactamases are often associated with *E. coli*, Enterobacter, and Pseudomonas, and not generally inhibited by clavulanic acid.

Pharmacokinetics (General)

The oral absorption characteristics of the penicillins are dependent upon its class. Penicillin G is the only available oral penicillin that is substantially affected by gastric pH and can be completely inactivated at a pH <2. The other orally available penicillins are resistant to acid degradation but bioavailability can be decreased (not amoxicillin) by the presence of food. Of the orally administered penicillins, penicillin V and amoxicillin tend to have the greatest bioavailability in their respective classes.

Penicillins are generally distributed widely throughout the body. Most drugs attain therapeutic levels in the kidneys, liver, heart, skin, lungs, intestines, bile, bone, prostate, and peritoneal, pleural, and synovial fluids. Penetration into the CSF and eye only occur with inflammation and may not reach therapeutic levels. Penicillins are bound in varying degrees to plasma proteins and cross the placenta.

Most penicillin's are rapidly excreted largely unchanged by the kidneys into the urine via glomerular filtration and tubular secretion. Probenecid can prolong half-lives and increase serum levels by blocking the tubular secretion of penicillins. Except for nafcillin and oxacillin, hepatic inactivation and biliary secretion is a minor route of excretion.

Contraindications/Precautions/Warnings

Penicillins are contraindicated in patients with a history of hypersensitivity to them. Because there may be cross-reactivity, use penicillins cautiously in patients who are documented hypersensitive to other beta-lactam antibiotics (*e.g.*, cephalosporins, cefamycins, carbapenems).

Do not administer systemic antibiotics orally in patients with septicemia, shock, or other grave illnesses, as absorption of the medication from the GI tract may be significantly delayed or diminished. Parenteral (preferably IV) routes should be used for these cases. Certain species (snakes, birds, turtles, Guinea pigs, and chinchillas) are reportedly sensitive to procaine penicillin G.

High doses of penicillin G sodium or potassium, particularly in small animals with a preexisting electrolyte abnormality, renal disease, or congestive heart failure may cause electrolyte imbalances. Other injectable penicillins, such as ticarcillin, carbenicillin, and ampicillin, have significant quantities of sodium per gram and may cause electrolyte imbalances when used in large dosages in susceptible patients.

Adverse Effects

Adverse effects with the penicillins are usually not serious and have a relatively low frequency of occurrence.

Hypersensitivity reactions unrelated to dose can occur with these agents and manifest as rashes, fever, eosinophilia, neutropenia, agranulocytosis, thrombocytopenia, leukopenia, anemias, lymphadenopathy, or full-blown anaphylaxis. In humans, it is estimated that up to 15% of patients hypersensitive to cephalosporins will also be hypersensitive to penicillins. The incidence of cross-reactivity in veterinary patients is unknown.

When given orally, penicillins may cause GI effects (anorexia, vomiting, diarrhea). Because the penicillins may also alter gut flora, antibiotic-associated diarrhea can occur and allow the proliferation of resistant bacteria in the colon (superinfections).

Neurotoxicity (*e.g.*, ataxia in dogs) has been associated with very high doses or very prolonged use. Although the penicillins are not considered hepatotoxic, elevated liver enzymes have been reported. Other effects reported in dogs include tachypnea, dyspnea, edema, and tachycardia.

Some penicillins (ticarcillin, carbenicillin, azlocillin, mezlocillin, piperacillin and nafcillin) have been implicated in causing bleeding problems in humans. These drugs are infrequently used systemically in veterinary species so the ramifications of this effect are unclear.

Reproductive/Nursing Safety

Penicillins have been shown to cross the placenta and safe use of them during pregnancy has not been firmly established, but neither have there been any documented teratogenic problems associated with these drugs. In humans, the FDA categorizes this drug as category *B* for use during pregnancy (*Animal studies have not yet demonstrated risk to the fetus, but there are no adequate studies in pregnant women; or animal studies have shown an adverse effect, but adequate studies in pregnant women have not demonstrated a risk to the fetus in the first trimester of pregnancy, and there is no evidence of risk in later trimesters.)* However, use only when the potential benefits outweigh the risks.

Penicillins are excreted in maternal milk in low concentrations; use potentially could cause diarrhea, candidiasis, or allergic response in the nursing offspring.

Overdosage/Acute Toxicity

Acute oral penicillin overdoses are unlikely to cause significant problems other than GI distress, but other effects are possible (see Adverse effects). In humans, very high dosages of parenteral penicillins, especially in patients with renal disease, have induced CNS effects.

Drug Interactions

The following drug interactions have either been reported or are theoretical in humans or animals receiving penicillins and may be of significance in veterinary patients. Unless otherwise noted, use together is not necessarily contraindicated, but weigh the potential risks and perform additional monitoring when appropriate.

- **AMINOGLYCOSIDES:** *In vitro* studies have demonstrated that penicillins can have synergistic or additive activity against certain bacteria when used with aminoglycosides or cephalosporins.
- **BACTERIOSTATIC ANTIBIOTICS** (*e.g.*, **chloramphenicol, erythromycin, tetracyclines**): Use with penicillins is generally not recommended, particularly in acute infections where the organism is proliferating rapidly as penicillins tend to perform better on actively growing bacteria.
- **PROBENECID:** Competitively blocks the tubular secretion of most penicillins, thereby increasing serum levels and serum half-lives.

Laboratory Considerations

- Penicillins may cause false-positive **urine glucose** determinations when using cupric-sulfate solution (Benedict's Solution, *Clinitest®*). Tests utilizing glucose oxidase (*Tes-Tape®*, *Clinistix®*) are not affected by penicillin.
- In humans, clavulanic acid and high dosages of piperacillin have caused a false-positive direct **Combs' test**.
- As penicillins and other beta-lactams can inactivate aminoglycosides *in vitro* (and *in vivo* in patients in renal failure), serum concentrations of **aminoglycosides** may be falsely decreased if the patient is also receiving beta-lactam antibiotics and the serum is stored prior to analysis. It is recommended that if the assay is delayed, samples be frozen and, if possible, drawn at times when the beta-lactam antibiotic is at a trough.

Monitoring

- Because penicillins usually have minimal toxicity associated with their use, monitoring for efficacy is usually all that is required unless toxic signs develop.
- Serum levels and therapeutic drug monitoring are not routinely done with these agents.

Client Information

- Owners should be instructed to give oral penicillins on an empty stomach, unless using amoxicillin or GI effects (anorexia, vomiting) can occur.
- Compliance with the therapeutic regimen should be stressed.
- Reconstituted oral suspensions should be kept refrigerated and discarded after 14 days, unless labeled otherwise.

Penicillin G

(pen-i-sill-in jee)

Penicillin Antibiotic

Prescriber Highlights

- ► Prototypical penicillin agent used for susceptible gram-positive aerobes & anaerobes; best used parenterally.
- ► Contraindications: Known hypersensitivity (unless no other options).
- ► Adverse Effects: Hypersensitivity possible. Very high doses may cause CNS effects.
- ► Benzathine penicillin only effective against extremely sensitive agents.
- ► Certain species may be sensitive to procaine penicillin G.

Uses/Indications

Natural penicillins remain the drugs of choice for a variety of bacteria, including group A beta-hemolytic streptococci, many gram-positive anaerobes, spirochetes, gram-negative aerobic cocci and some gram-negative aerobic bacilli. Generally, if bacteria remain susceptible to a natural penicillin, either penicillin G or V is preferred for treating that infection as long as adequate penetration of the drug to the site of the infection occurs and the patient is not hypersensitive to penicillins.

Pharmacology/Actions

Penicillins are usually bactericidal against susceptible bacteria and act by inhibiting mucopeptide synthesis in the cell wall resulting in a defective barrier and an osmotically unstable spheroplast. The exact mechanism for this effect has not been definitively determined, but beta-lactam antibiotics have been shown to bind to several enzymes (carboxypeptidases, transpeptidases, endopeptidases) within the bacterial cytoplasmic membrane that are involved with cell wall synthesis. The different affinities that various beta-lactam antibiotics have for these enzymes (also known as penicillin-binding proteins; PBPs) help explain the differences in spectrums of activity the drugs have that are not explained by the influence of beta-lactamases. Like other beta-lactam antibiotics, penicillins are generally considered more effective against actively growing bacteria. Penicillins are considered time dependent antibiotics as efficacy depends on the length of time that plasma (or tissue) concentrations exceed the MIC of pathogens.

The natural penicillins (G and K) have similar spectrums of activity, but penicillin G is slightly more active *in vitro* on a weight basis against many organisms. This class of penicillin has *in vitro* activity against most spirochetes and gram-positive and gram-negative aerobic cocci, but not penicillinase producing strains. They have activity against some aerobic and anaerobic gram-positive bacilli such as *Bacillus anthracis*, *Clostridium* spp. (not *C. difficile*), Fusobacterium, and Actinomyces. The natural penicillins are customarily inactive against most gram-negative aerobic and anaerobic bacilli, and all Rickettsia, mycobacteria, fungi, Mycoplasma, and viruses.

Pharmacokinetics

Penicillin G potassium is poorly absorbed orally because of rapid acid-catalyzed hydrolysis. When administered on an empty (fasted) stomach, oral bioavailability is only ≈ 15-30%. If given with food, absorption rate and extent will be decreased.

Penicillin G potassium and sodium salts are rapidly absorbed after IM injections and yield high peak levels usually within 20 minutes of administration. In horses, equivalent doses given either IV or IM demonstrated that IM dosing will provide serum levels above

0.5 micrograms/mL for ≈ 2X as long as IV administration [approx. 3-4 hours (IV) vs. 6-7 hours (IM)].

Procaine penicillin G is slowly hydrolyzed to penicillin G after IM injection. Peak levels are much lower than with parenterally administered aqueous penicillin G sodium or potassium, but serum levels are more prolonged.

Benzathine penicillin G is also very slowly absorbed after IM injections after being hydrolyzed to the parent compound. Serum levels can be very prolonged, but levels attained generally only exceed MIC's for the most susceptible streptococci, and the use of benzathine penicillin G should be limited to these infections when other penicillin therapy is impractical.

After absorption, penicillin G is widely distributed throughout the body with the exception of the CSF, joints and milk. In lactating dairy cattle, the milk to plasma ratio is ≈ 0.2. CSF levels are generally only 10% or less of those found in the serum when meninges are not inflamed. Levels in the CSF may be greater in patients with inflamed meninges or if probenecid is given concurrently. Binding to plasma proteins is ≈ 50% in most species.

Penicillin G is principally excreted unchanged into the urine through renal mechanisms via both glomerular filtration and tubular secretion. Elimination half-lives are very rapid and are usually one hour or less in most species (if normal renal function exists).

Contraindications/Precautions/Warnings

Penicillins are contraindicated in patients with a history of hypersensitivity to them. Because there may be cross-reactivity, use penicillins cautiously in patients who are documented hypersensitive to other beta-lactam antibiotics (*e.g.*, cephalosporins, cefamycins, carbapenems).

Do not administer systemic antibiotics orally in patients with septicemia, shock, or other grave illnesses as absorption of the medication from the GI tract may be significantly delayed or diminished; parenteral (preferably IV) routes should be used for these cases.

High doses of penicillin G sodium or potassium, particularly in small animals with a preexisting electrolyte abnormality, renal disease, or congestive heart failure may cause electrolyte imbalances. Other injectable penicillins, such as ticarcillin, carbenicillin, and ampicillin, have significant quantities of sodium per gram and may cause electrolyte imbalances when used in large dosages in susceptible patients.

Certain species (snakes, birds, turtles, Guinea pigs, and chinchillas) are reportedly sensitive to procaine penicillin G.

Adverse Effects

Adverse effects with the penicillins are usually not serious and have a relatively low frequency of occurrence.

Hypersensitivity reactions unrelated to dose can occur with these agents and manifest as rashes, fever, eosinophilia, neutropenia, agranulocytosis, thrombocytopenia, leukopenia, anemias, lymphadenopathy, or full-blown anaphylaxis. In humans, it is estimated that up to 15% of patients hypersensitive to cephalosporins will also be hypersensitive to penicillins. The incidence of cross-reactivity in veterinary patients is unknown.

When given orally, penicillins may cause GI effects (anorexia, vomiting, diarrhea). Because the penicillins may also alter gut flora, antibiotic-associated diarrhea can occur and allow the proliferation of resistant bacteria in the colon (superinfections).

Neurotoxicity (*e.g.*, ataxia in dogs) has been associated with very high doses or very prolonged use. Although the penicillins are not considered hepatotoxic, elevated liver enzymes have been reported. Other effects reported in dogs include tachypnea, dyspnea, edema and tachycardia.

Reproductive/Nursing Safety

Penicillins have been shown to cross the placenta and safe use of them during pregnancy has not been firmly established, but neither has there been any documented teratogenic problems associated with these drugs; however, use only when the potential benefits outweigh the risks.

In humans, the FDA categorizes this drug as category *B* for use during pregnancy (*Animal studies have not yet demonstrated risk to the fetus, but there are no adequate studies in pregnant women; or animal studies have shown an adverse effect, but adequate studies in pregnant women have not demonstrated a risk to the fetus in the first trimester of pregnancy, and there is no evidence of risk in later trimesters.*) In a separate system evaluating the safety of drugs in canine and feline pregnancy (Papich 1989), this drug is categorized as class: *A (Probably safe. Although specific studies may not have proved the safety of all drugs in dogs and cats, there are no reports of adverse effects in laboratory animals or women.*)

Penicillins are excreted in maternal milk in low concentrations; use could potentially cause diarrhea, candidiasis, or allergic responses in nursing offspring.

Overdosage/Acute Toxicity

Acute oral penicillin overdoses are unlikely to cause significant problems other than GI distress, but other effects are possible (see Adverse Effects). In humans, very high dosages of parenteral penicillins, especially those with renal disease, have induced CNS effects.

Drug Interactions

The following drug interactions have either been reported or are theoretical in humans or animals receiving penicillin G and may be of significance in veterinary patients. Unless otherwise noted, use together is not necessarily contraindicated, but weigh the potential risks and perform additional monitoring when appropriate.

- **AMINOGLYCOSIDES:** *In vitro* studies have demonstrated that penicillins can have synergistic or additive activity against certain bacteria when used with aminoglycosides or cephalosporins.
- **BACTERIOSTATIC ANTIBIOTICS** (*e.g.*, **chloramphenicol, erythromycin, tetracyclines**): Use with penicillins is generally not recommended, particularly in acute infections where the organism is proliferating rapidly as penicillins tend to perform better on actively growing bacteria. However, actual clinical significance is in question.
- **METHOTREXATE:** Penicillins may decrease renal elimination of MTX.
- **PROBENECID:** Competitively blocks the tubular secretion of most penicillins, thereby increasing serum levels and serum half-lives.

Laboratory Considerations

- As penicillins and other beta-lactams can inactivate **aminoglycosides** *in vitro* (and *in vivo* in patients in renal failure), serum concentrations of aminoglycosides may be falsely decreased if the patient is also receiving beta-lactam antibiotics and the serum is stored prior to analysis. It is recommended that if the assay is delayed, samples be frozen and, if possible, drawn at times when the beta-lactam antibiotic is at a trough.
- Penicillin G can cause falsely elevated **serum uric acid** values if the copper-chelate method is used; phosphotungstate and uricase methods are not affected.
- Penicillins may cause false-positive **urine glucose** determinations when using cupric-sulfate solution (Benedict's Solution, *Clinitest*®). Tests utilizing glucose oxidase (*Tes-Tape*®, *Clinistix*®) are not affected by penicillin.

Doses

- **DOGS/CATS:**

  For susceptible infections (extra-label):

  <u>Penicillin G sodium or potassium</u>: 20,000 – 40,000 Units/kg IV or IM q4-8h

  <u>Penicillin G procaine</u>: 20,000 – 40,000 Units/kg IM, SC q12-24h.

  <u>Penicillin G benzathine</u>: 40,000 Units/kg IM q5 days.

- **FERRETS:**

  For susceptible infections (extra-label): <u>Procaine Penicillin G</u>: 20,000 – 40,000 Units/kg IM 1-2 times/day; <u>Sodium or potassium Penicillin G</u>: 20,000 Units/kg SC, IM or IV q4h or 40,000 Units/kg PO 3 times daily. (Williams 2000)

- **RABBITS, RODENTS, SMALL MAMMALS:**

  Rabbits (extra-label): <u>Penicillin G Procaine</u>: 20,000 – 84,000 Units/kg SC, IM q24h for 5-7 days for venereal spirochetosis. (Ivey *et al.* 2000)

  Hedgehogs: (extra-label): <u>Penicillin G Procaine</u>: 40,000 Units/kg IM once daily. (Smith 2000)

- **CATTLE (AND OTHER RUMINANTS UNLESS SPECIFIED):**

  Note: When procaine penicillin G is administered in an extra-label manner, dosage, dosage frequency, treatment duration, injection site, and injection route (IM vs. SC) all can affect drug residues (DeDonder *et al.* 2013). Veterinarians seeking information for determination of a withdrawal interval following extra-label drug use should contact the Food Animal Residue Avoidance Databank (FARAD) for assistance.

  For susceptible infections (extra-label): <u>Penicillin G procaine</u>: 24,000 – 66,000 Units/kg IM once per day. (USPC 1990)

  For clostridial abomasitis and enteritis in calves: Procaine Penicillin G: 10,000 – 20,000 Units/kg PO q12-24 for 1-4 days. Oral penicillin is preferred over systemic as it is poorly absorbed from the GI tract and will provide activity in the intestinal lumen where the bacteria reside. (Callan *et al.* 2003)

- **HORSES:**

  For susceptible infections (extra-label):

  For gram-positive aerobes: <u>Penicillin G potassium or sodium</u>: 10,000 – 20,000 Units/kg IV or IM q6h. <u>Penicillin G procaine</u>: 22,000 – 44,000 Units/kg IM q12h.

  For serious gram-positive infections (*e.g.*, tetanus, botulism, *C. difficile* enterocolitis in foals): <u>Penicillin G sodium or potassium</u>: 22,000 – 44,000 Units/kg IV q6h. (Whittem 1999)

  Treatment of carriers with *S. equi* infections of the gutteral pouches (extra-label): Administration of both systemic and topical penicillin G appears to improve treatment success rate. Before topical therapy, remove all visible inflammatory material removed from gutteral pouch. To make a gelatin/penicillin G mix of 50 mL for gutteral pouch instillation:

  1) Weigh out 2 grams gelatin (Sigma G-6650 or household) and add 40 mL of sterile water.

  2) Heat or microwave to dissolve. Cool to 45-50°C.

  3) Add 10 mL sterile water to a 10 million Units <u>sodium penicillin G</u> for injection vial and mix with the cooled gelatin to total volume of 50 mL.

  4) Dispense into syringes and leave overnight in the refrigerator.

     Instillation is easiest through a catheter inserted up the nose and endoscopically guided into the pouch opening with the last inch bent at an angle to aid entry under the pouch flap. Elevate horse's head for 20 minutes after infusion. (Verheyen *et al.* 2000).

  Foals (extra-label): <u>Potassium penicillin G</u>: 22,000 Units/kg q6h IV, IM (Excellent gram-positive coverage, expensive, high blood levels); <u>Procaine penicillin G</u>: 22,000 Units/kg q12h IM (painful, lower blood levels). (Stewart 2008)

- **SWINE:**

  Note: When used in an extra-label manner veterinarians seeking information for determination of a withdrawal interval following extra-label drug use should contact the Food Animal Residue Avoidance Databank (FARAD) for assistance.

  For susceptible infections (extra-label): <u>Procaine penicillin G</u>: 40,000 Units/kg IM once daily. <u>Procaine penicillin G/benzathine penicillin G</u> combination: 40,000 Units/kg IM once. (Howard 1986)

- **BIRDS:**

  For susceptible infections (extra-label): In turkeys: Procaine penicillin G/benzathine penicillin G combination: 100 mg/kg IM of each drug once a day or every 2 days. Use cautiously in small birds as it may cause procaine toxicity. (Clubb 1986)

Monitoring

- Because penicillins usually have minimal toxicity associated with their use, monitoring for efficacy is usually all that is required unless toxic signs develop. Serum levels and therapeutic drug monitoring are not routinely done with these agents.

Client Information

- Penicillin G is not usually given by mouth.
- Procaine Penicillin G should not be given in the vein.
- Injectable liquid solutions may cause stinging when injected under the skin (SC, subcutaneously).

Chemistry/Synonyms

Penicillin G is considered natural penicillin and is obtained from cultures *Penicillium chrysogenum* and available in several different salt forms. Penicillin G potassium (also known as benzylpenicillin potassium, aqueous or crystalline penicillin) occurs as colorless or white crystals, or white crystalline powder. It is very soluble in water and sparingly soluble in alcohol. Potency of penicillin G potassium is usually expressed in terms of Units. One mg of penicillin G potassium is equivalent to 1440-1680 USP Units (1355-1595 USP Units for the powder for injection). After reconstitution, penicillin G potassium powder for injection has a pH of 6-8.5, and contains 1.7 mEq of potassium per 1 million Units.

Penicillin G sodium (also known as benzylpenicillin sodium, aqueous or crystalline penicillin) occurs as colorless or white crystals, or white to slightly yellow, crystalline powder. Approximately 25 mg are soluble in 1 mL of water. Potency of penicillin G sodium is usually expressed in terms of Units. One mg of penicillin G sodium is equivalent to 1500-1750 USP Units (1420-1667 USP Units for the powder for injection). After reconstitution, penicillin G sodium powder for injection has a pH of 6-7.5, and contains 2 mEq of sodium per 1 million Units.

Penicillin G procaine (also known as APPG, Aqueous Procaine Penicillin G, Benzylpenicillin Procaine, Procaine Penicillin G, Procaine Benzylpenicillin) is the procaine monohydrate salt of penicillin G. *In vivo* it is hydrolyzed to penicillin G and acts as a depot, or repository form, of penicillin G. It occurs as white crystals or very fine, white crystalline powder. Approximately 4-4.5 mg are soluble in 1 mL of water and 3.3 mg are soluble in 1 mL of alcohol. Potency of penicillin G procaine is usually expressed in terms of Units. One mg of penicillin G procaine is equivalent to 900-1050 USP Units. The commercially available suspension for injection is buffered with sodium citrate and has a pH of 5-7.5. It is preserved with methylparaben and propylparaben.

Penicillin G Benzathine (also known as Benzathine Benzylpenicillin, Benzathine Penicillin G, Benzylpenicillin Benzathine, Dibenzylethylenediamine Benzylpenicillin) is the benzathine tetrahydrate salt of penicillin G. It is hydrolyzed *in vivo* to penicillin G and acts as a long-acting form of penicillin G. It occurs as an odorless, white, crystalline powder. Solubility's are 0.2-0.3 mg/mL of water and 15 mg/mL of alcohol. One mg of penicillin G benzathine is equivalent to 1090-1272 USP Units. The commercially available suspension for injection is buffered with sodium citrate and has a pH of 5-7.5. It is preserved with methylparaben and propylparaben.

Penicillin G may also be known as: benzylpenicillin, crystalline penicillin G, penicillin, *Bicillin C-R®*, and *Pfizerpen®*.

Storage/Stability

Penicillin G sodium and potassium should be protected from moisture to prevent hydrolysis of the compounds. Penicillin G potassium tablets and powder for oral solution should be stored at room temperature in tight containers; avoid exposure to excessive heat. After reconstituting, the oral powder for solution should be stored from 2-8°C (refrigerated) and discarded after 14 days.

Penicillin G sodium and potassium powder for injection can be stored at room temperature (15-30°C). After reconstituting, the injectable solution is stable for 7 days when kept refrigerated (2-8°C) and for 24 hours at room temperature.

Penicillin G procaine should be stored at 2-8°C; avoid freezing. Benzathine penicillin G should be stored at 2-8°C.

Compatibility/Compounding Considerations

All commonly used IV fluids (some Dextran products are physically **incompatible**) and the following drugs are reportedly physically **compatible** with penicillin G potassium: ascorbic acid injection, calcium chloride/gluconate, chloramphenicol sodium succinate, cimetidine HCl, clindamycin phosphate, corticotropin, dimenhydrinate, diphenhydramine HCl, ephedrine sulfate, erythromycin gluceptate/lactobionate, hydrocortisone sodium succinate, lidocaine HCl, methicillin sodium, methylprednisolone sodium succinate, metronidazole with sodium bicarbonate, nitrofurantoin sodium, polymyxin B sulfate, potassium chloride, prednisolone sodium phosphate, procaine HCl, prochlorperazine edisylate, sodium iodide, and verapamil HCl.

The following drugs/solutions are either physically **incompatible** or **data conflicts** regarding compatibility with penicillin G potassium injection: amikacin sulfate, aminophylline, chlorpromazine HCl, dopamine HCl, heparin sodium, hydroxyzine HCl, lincomycin HCl, metoclopramide HCl, oxytetracycline HCl, pentobarbital sodium, prochlorperazine mesylate, promazine HCl, promethazine HCl, sodium bicarbonate, tetracycline HCl, and vitamin B-complex with C.

The following drugs/solutions are reportedly physically **compatible** with penicillin G sodium injection: Dextran 40 10%, dextrose 5% (some degradation may occur if stored for 24 hours), sodium chloride 0.9% (some degradation may occur if stored for 24 hours), calcium chloride/gluconate, chloramphenicol sodium succinate, cimetidine HCl, clindamycin phosphate, diphenhydramine HCl, erythromycin lactobionate, gentamicin sulfate, hydrocortisone sodium succinate, polymyxin B sulfate, prednisolone sodium phosphate, procaine HCl, verapamil HCl, and vitamin B-complex with C.

The following drugs/solutions are either physically **incompatible** or **data conflicts** regarding compatibility with penicillin G sodium injection: amphotericin B, bleomycin sulfate, chlorpromazine HCl, heparin sodium, hydroxyzine HCl, lincomycin HCl, methylprednisolone sodium succinate, oxytetracycline HCl, potassium chloride, prochlorperazine mesylate, promethazine HCl and tetracycline HCl. Compatibility is dependent upon factors such as pH,

concentration, temperature and diluent used; consult specialized references or a hospital pharmacist for more specific information.

Dosage Forms/Regulatory Status

VETERINARY-LABELED PRODUCTS:

Note: Withdrawal times are for labeled dosages only. Contact FARAD when used in an extra-label manner for assistance in determining a withdrawal interval.

Penicillin G Procaine Injection 300,000 Units/mL in 100 mL and 250 mL vials: Variety of trade names available. Depending on product, FDA-approved for use in: cattle, sheep, horses, and swine. Not intended for use in horses used for food. Do not exceed 7 days of treatment in non-lactating dairy cattle, beef cattle, swine or sheep; 5 days in lactating dairy cattle. Treatment should not exceed 4 consecutive days.

Withdrawal times vary depending on the product are for the labeled dosage of 6,600 Units/kg once daily (rarely used clinically today). Actual withdrawal times may be longer. Milk withdrawal times (at labeled doses) = 48 hours. Slaughter withdrawal: Calves (non-ruminating) = 7 days; cattle = 4-10 days; sheep = 8-9 days; swine = 6-7 days; refer to label for more information.

There are also mastitis syringes in combination with novobiocin (*Albadry Plus®*).

Penicillin G Benzathine 150,000 Units/mL with Penicillin G Procaine Injection 150,000 Units/mL for Injection in 100 mL and 250 mL vials: Variety of trade names available. FDA-approved (most products) in horses and beef cattle. Not FDA-approved for horses intended for food use. Slaughter withdrawal: cattle = 30 days (at labeled doses). Actual species approvals and withdrawal times may vary with the product; refer to the label of the product you are using.

HUMAN-LABELED PRODUCTS:

Penicillin G (Aqueous) Sodium Powder for Injection: 5 million & 20 million Units; generic; (Rx)

Penicillin G (Aqueous) Potassium Injection: 5 million 20 million Units; *Pfizerpen-G®*, generic; (Rx)

Penicillin G Procaine Injection: 600,000 Units/vial in 1 mL *Tubex* & 1.2 million Units/vial in 2 mL *Tubex*; generic; (Rx)

Penicillin G Benzathine Injection: 600,000 Units/dose in 1 mL *Tubex*; 1.2 million Units/dose in 2 mL; 2.4 million Units/dose in 4 mL pre-filled syringes; *Bicillin L-A®*; (Rx)

Revisions/References

Monograph revised/updated May 2014.

Callan, M. B. & V. T. Rentko (2003). Clinical application of a hemoglobin-based oxygen-carrying solution. Veterinary Clinics of North America-Small Animal Practice 33(6): 1277-+.

Clubb, S. L. (1986). Therapeutics: Individual and Flock Treatment Regimens. *Clinical Avian Medicine and Surgery*. G. J. Harrison and L. R. Harrison. Philadelphia, W.B. Saunders: 327-55.

DeDonder, K. D., et al. (2013). Effects of new sampling protocols on procaine penicillin G withdrawal intervals for cattle. Javma-Journal of the American Veterinary Medical Association 243(10): 1408-12.

Howard, J. L., Ed. (1986). *Current Veterinary Therapy 2, Food Animal Practice*. Philadelphia, W.B. Saunders.

Ivey, E. & J. Morrisey (2000). Therapeutics for Rabbits. Vet Clin NA: Exotic Anim Pract 3:1(Jan): 183-216.

Papich, M. (1989). Effects of drugs on pregnancy. *Current Veterinary Therapy X: Small Animal Practice*. R. Kirk. Philadelphia, Saunders: 1291-9.

Smith, A. (2000). General husbandry and medical care of hedgehogs. *Kirk's Current Veterinary Therapy: XIII Small Animal Practice*. J. Bonagura. Philadelphia, WB Saunders: 1128-33.

Stewart, A. (2008). Equine Neonatal Sepsis. Proceedings: WVC. accessed via Veterinary Information Network; vin.com

USPC (1990). Veterinary Information- Appendix III. *Drug Information for the Health Professional*. Rockville, United States Pharmacopeial Convention. 2: 2811- 60.

Verheyen, K., et al. (2000). Elimination of guttural pouch infection and inflammation in asymptomatic carriers of Streptococcus equi. Equine Vet J 32(6): 527-32.

Whittem, T. (1999). Appendix: Formulary of Common Equine Drugs. The Veterinary Clinics of North America: Equine Practice **15**:3(December): 747-68.

Williams, B. (2000). Therapeutics in Ferrets. Vet Clin NA: Exotic Anim Pract **3**:1(Jan): 131-53.

Penicillin V Potassium

(pen-i-**sill**-in **vee**) *Phenoxymethylpenicillin*

Oral Penicillin Antibiotic

Prescriber Highlights

▶ Oral natural penicillin. Not commonly used in veterinary medicine.

▶ Contraindications: Known hypersensitivity (unless no other options).

▶ Adverse Effects: GI effects or hypersensitivity possible.

▶ Best to give on an empty stomach.

Uses/Indications

Penicillin V is a "natural" penicillin that is still active against many streptococci, but is rarely used today in veterinary medicine.

Pharmacology/Actions

The natural penicillins (G and K) have similar spectrums of activity, but penicillin G is slightly more active *in vitro* on a per weight basis against many organisms. This class of penicillin has *in vitro* activity against most spirochetes and gram-positive and gram-negative aerobic cocci, but not penicillinase producing strains. They have activity against some aerobic and anaerobic gram-positive bacilli such as *Bacillus anthracis*, *Clostridium* spp. (not *C. difficile*), Fusobacterium, and Actinomyces. The natural penicillins are customarily inactive against most gram-negative aerobic and anaerobic bacilli, and all Rickettsia, mycobacteria, fungi, Mycoplasma, and viruses. Although penicillin V may be slightly less active than penicillin G against organisms susceptible to the natural penicillins, its superior absorptive characteristics after oral administration make it a better choice against mild to moderately severe infections when oral administration is desired in monogastric animals.

Penicillins are usually bactericidal against susceptible bacteria and act by inhibiting mucopeptide synthesis in the cell wall resulting in a defective barrier and an osmotically unstable spheroplast. The exact mechanism for this effect has not been definitively determined, but beta-lactam antibiotics have been shown to bind to several enzymes (carboxypeptidases, transpeptidases, endopeptidases) within the bacterial cytoplasmic membrane that are involved with cell wall synthesis. The different affinities that various beta-lactam antibiotics have for these enzymes (also known as penicillin-binding proteins; PBPs) help explain the differences in spectrums of activity the drugs have that are not explained by the influence of beta-lactamases. Like other beta-lactam antibiotics, penicillins are generally considered more effective against actively growing bacteria.

Pharmacokinetics

The pharmacokinetics of penicillin V are very similar to penicillin G with the exception of oral bioavailability and the percent of the drug that is bound to plasma proteins. Penicillin V is significantly more resistant to acid-catalyzed inactivation in the gut and bioavailability after oral administration in humans is ≈ 60-73%. In veterinary species, bioavailability in calves is only 30%, but studies performed in horses and dogs demonstrated that therapeutic serum levels can be achieved after oral administration. In dogs, food will decrease the rate and extent of absorption.

Distribution of penicillin V follows that of penicillin G but, at least in humans, the drug is bound to a larger extent to plasma proteins (≈ 80% with penicillin V vs. 50% with penicillin G).

Like penicillin G, penicillin V is excreted rapidly in the urine via the kidney. Elimination half-lives are generally <1 hour in animals with normal renal function; an elimination half-life of 3.65 hours has been reported after oral dosing in horses (Schwark *et al.* 1983).

Contraindications/Precautions/Warnings

Penicillins are contraindicated in patients with a history of hypersensitivity to them. Because there may be cross-reactivity, use penicillins cautiously in patients who are documented hypersensitive to other beta-lactam antibiotics (*e.g.*, cephalosporins, cefamycins, carbapenems).

Do not administer systemic antibiotics orally in patients with septicemia, shock, or other grave illnesses as absorption of the medication from the GI tract may be significantly delayed or diminished. Parenteral (preferably IV) routes should be used for these cases.

Adverse Effects

Adverse effects with the penicillins are usually not serious and have a relatively low frequency of occurrence.

Hypersensitivity reactions unrelated to dose can occur with these agents and manifest as rashes, fever, eosinophilia, neutropenia, agranulocytosis, thrombocytopenia, leukopenia, anemias, lymphadenopathy, or full-blown anaphylaxis. In humans, it is estimated that up to 15% of patients hypersensitive to cephalosporins will also be hypersensitive to penicillins. The incidence of cross-reactivity in veterinary patients is unknown.

When given orally, penicillins may cause GI effects (anorexia, vomiting, diarrhea). Because the penicillins may also alter gut flora, antibiotic-associated diarrhea can occur and allow the proliferation of resistant bacteria in the colon (superinfections).

Neurotoxicity (*e.g.*, ataxia in dogs) has been associated with very high doses or very prolonged use. Although the penicillins are not considered hepatotoxic, elevated liver enzymes have been reported. Other effects reported in dogs include tachypnea, dyspnea, edema and tachycardia.

Reproductive/Nursing Safety

Penicillins have been shown to cross the placenta and safe use of them during pregnancy has not been firmly established, but neither has there been any documented teratogenic problems associated with these drugs; however, use only when the potential benefits outweigh the risks. Certain species (snakes, birds, turtles, Guinea pigs, and chinchillas) are reported to be sensitive to penicillins. High doses of penicillin G sodium or potassium, particularly in small animals with a preexisting electrolyte abnormality, renal disease, or congestive heart failure may cause electrolyte imbalances. Other injectable penicillins, such as ticarcillin, carbenicillin, and ampicillin, have significant quantities of sodium per gram and may cause electrolyte imbalances when used in large dosages in susceptible patients.

In humans, the FDA categorizes this drug as category *B* for use during pregnancy (*Animal studies have not yet demonstrated risk to the fetus, but there are no adequate studies in pregnant women; or animal studies have shown an adverse effect, but adequate studies in pregnant women have not demonstrated a risk to the fetus in the first trimester of pregnancy, and there is no evidence of risk in later trimesters*).

Penicillins are excreted in maternal milk in low concentrations; use could potentially cause diarrhea, candidiasis, or allergic response in nursing offspring.

Overdosage/Acute Toxicity

Acute oral penicillin overdoses are unlikely to cause significant problems other than GI distress, but other effects are possible (see Adverse effects). In humans, very high dosages of parenteral penicillins, especially in patients with renal disease, have induced CNS effects.

Drug Interactions

The following drug interactions have either been reported or are theoretical in humans or animals receiving penicillin V potassium and may be of significance in veterinary patients. Unless otherwise noted, use together is not necessarily contraindicated, but weigh the potential risks and perform additional monitoring when appropriate.

- **AMINOGLYCOSIDES:** *In vitro* studies have demonstrated that penicillins can have synergistic or additive activity against certain bacteria when used with aminoglycosides or cephalosporins.
- **BACTERIOSTATIC ANTIBIOTICS** (*e.g.,* **chloramphenicol, erythromycin, tetracyclines**): Use with penicillins is generally not recommended, particularly in acute infections where the organism is proliferating rapidly as penicillins tend to perform better on actively growing bacteria. The actual clinical significance of this interaction is in question.
- **METHOTREXATE:** Penicillins may decrease renal elimination of MTX
- **PROBENECID:** Competitively blocks the tubular secretion of most penicillins, thereby increasing serum levels and serum half-lives.

Laboratory Considerations

- As penicillins and other beta-lactams can inactivate **aminoglycosides** *in vitro* (and *in vivo* in patients in renal failure), serum concentrations of aminoglycosides may be falsely decreased if the patient is also receiving beta-lactam antibiotics and the serum is stored prior to analysis. It is recommended that if the assay is delayed, samples be frozen and, if possible, drawn at times when the beta-lactam antibiotic is at a trough.
- Penicillin V can cause falsely elevated **serum uric acid** values if the copper-chelate method is used; phosphotungstate and uricase methods are not affected.
- Penicillins may cause false-positive **urine glucose** determinations when using cupric-sulfate solution (Benedict's Solution, *Clinitest*®). Tests utilizing glucose oxidase (*Tes-Tape*®, *Clinistix*®) are not affected by penicillin.

Doses

- **DOGS/CATS:**

  For susceptible infections (extra-label): 10 mg/kg PO q8h for 7 days. (Greene *et al.* 2006)

- **HORSES:**

  For susceptible infections (extra-label): 110,000 Units/kg (68.75 mg/kg) PO q8h (may yield supra-optimal levels against uncomplicated infections by sensitive organisms). (Schwark *et al.* 1983)

Monitoring

- Because penicillins usually have minimal toxicity associated with their use, monitoring for efficacy is usually all that is required unless toxic signs develop. Serum levels and therapeutic drug monitoring are not routinely done with these agents.

Client Information

- Penicillin V is given by mouth in most animals and it works best when given on any empty stomach.
- Penicillin V should not be given by mouth to rabbits, guinea pigs, gerbils, hamsters, rodents, chinchillas, etc. as life-threatening diarrhea may occur.

Chemistry/Synonyms

A natural-penicillin, penicillin V is produced from *Penicillium chrysogenum* and usually commercially available as the potassium salt. Penicillin V potassium occurs as an odorless, white, crystalline powder that is very soluble in water and slightly soluble in alcohol. Potency of penicillin V potassium is usually expressed in terms of weight (in mg) of penicillin V, but penicillin V units may also be used. One mg of penicillin V potassium is equivalent to 1380-1610 USP Units of penicillin V. Manufacturers however generally state that 125 mg of penicillin V potassium is ≈ 200,000 USP units of penicillin V.

Penicillin V may also be known as: phenoxymethylpenicillin, fenoximetilpenicilina, penicillin, phenoxymethyl phenomycilline, phenoxymethyl penicillin, phenoxymethylpenicillinum, and *Veetids*®.

Storage/Stability

Penicillin V potassium tablets and powder for oral solution should be stored in tight containers at room temperature (15-30°C). After reconstitution, the oral solution should be stored at 2-8°C (refrigerated) and any unused portion discarded after 14 days.

Dosage Forms/Regulatory Status

VETERINARY-LABELED PRODUCTS: NONE.

HUMAN-LABELED PRODUCTS:

Penicillin V Potassium Tablets: 250 mg & 500 mg; generic; (Rx)

Penicillin V Potassium Powder for Oral Solution: 25 mg/mL (labeled as 125 mg/5 mL) & 50 mg/mL (labeled as 250 mg/5 mL) in 100 mL & 200 mL; generic; (Rx)

Revisions/References

Monograph revised/updated May 2014.

Greene, C., et al. (2006). Appendix 8: Antimicrobial Drug Formulary. *Infectious Disease of the Dog and Cat*. C. Greene, Elsevier: 1186-333.

Schwark, W. S., et al. (1983). Absorption and distribution patterns of oral phenoxymethyl penicillin (penicillin V) in the horse. Cornell Vet 73: 314-22.

Pentazocine Lactate
Pentazocine HCl

(pen-**taz**-oh-seen)   Talwin®

Partial Opiate Agonist

Prescriber Highlights

▶ Partial opiate agonist analgesic used in a variety of species; rarely recommended today.

▶ Contraindications: Known hypersensitivity. Caution: Head trauma, increased CSF pressure or other CNS dysfunction, hypothyroidism, severe renal insufficiency, adrenocortical insufficiency (Addison's), & geriatric or severely debilitated patients.

▶ Not a replacement for surgery or medical treatment for horses with colic.

▶ Adverse Effects: **Horses:** Transient ataxia, CNS excitement, increased pulse, & respiratory rate. **Dogs:** Salivation most prevalent; ataxia, fine tremors, seizures, emesis, & swelling at injection site possible. **Cats:** Use is controversial; may cause dysphoric reactions.

▶ C-IV controlled substance.

Uses/Indications

The formerly marketed veterinary product was labeled for the symptomatic relief of pain of colic in horses and the amelioration of pain accompanying postoperative recovery from fractures, trauma, and spinal disorders in dogs. It has also been used as an analgesic in other species. Currently, pentazocine is not commonly recommended for use in veterinary medicine.

Pharmacology/Actions

While considered a partial opiate agonist, pentazocine exhibits many of the same characteristics as the true opiate agonists. It is reported to have an analgesic potency of ≈ 1/2 that of morphine and 5X that of meperidine. It is a very weak antagonist at the *mu* opioid receptor when compared to naloxone. It will not antagonize the respiratory depression caused by drugs like morphine, but may induce symptoms of withdrawal in human patients physically dependent on narcotic agents. Pentazocine's mixed agonist/antagonist properties limit its maximal analgesic efficacy (ceiling effect).

Besides its analgesic properties, pentazocine can cause respiratory depression, decreased GI motility, sedation, and it possesses antitussive effects. Pentazocine tends to have less sedative qualities in animals than other opiates and is usually not used as a pre-operative medication.

In dogs, pentazocine can cause a transient decrease in blood pressure; in humans, increases in cardiac output, heart rate, and blood pressure can be seen.

Pharmacokinetics

Pentazocine is well-absorbed following oral, IM, or SC administration. Because of a high first-pass effect, only ≈ 20% of an oral dose will enter the systemic circulation in patients with normal hepatic function.

After absorption, the drug is distributed widely into tissues. In the equine, it has been shown to be 80% bound to plasma proteins. Pentazocine will cross the placenta and neonatal serum levels have been measured at 60-65% of maternal levels at delivery. It is not clearly known if or how much pentazocine crosses into milk.

The drug is primarily metabolized in the liver with resultant excretion by the kidneys of the metabolites. In the horse, ≈ 30% of a given dose is excreted as the glucuronide. Pentazocine and its metabolites have been detected in equine urine for up to 5 days following an injection. Apparently, < 15% of the drug is excreted by the kidneys in an unchanged form.

Plasma half-lives have been reported for various species: Humans = 2-3 hrs; Ponies = 97 min.; Dogs = 22 min.; Cats = 84 min.; Swine = 49 min. Volumes of distribution range from a high of 5.09 L/kg in ponies to 2.78 L/kg in cats. In horses, the onset of action has been reported to be 2-3 minutes following IV dosing with a peak effect at 5-10 minutes.

Contraindications/Precautions/Warnings

The drug is contraindicated in patients having known hypersensitivity to it. All opiates should be used with caution in patients with hypothyroidism, severe renal insufficiency, adrenocortical insufficiency (Addison's), and geriatric or severely debilitated patients.

Like other opiates, pentazocine must be used with extreme caution in patients with head trauma, increased CSF pressure or other CNS dysfunction (*e.g.*, coma). Pentazocine should not be used in place of appropriate therapy (medical &/or surgical) for equine colic, but only as adjunctive treatment for pain.

Adverse Effects

In dogs, the most predominant adverse reaction following parenteral administration is salivation. Other potential side effects at usual doses include fine tremors, emesis, and swelling at the injection site. At very high doses (6 mg/kg) dogs have been noted to develop ataxia, fine tremors, convulsions, and swelling at the injection site.

Horses may develop transient ataxia and clinical signs of CNS excitement. Pulse and respiratory rates may be mildly elevated.

Dysphoria has been reported in cats.

Reproductive/Nursing Safety

Because reproductive studies have not been done in dogs, the manufacturer does not recommend its use in pregnant bitches or bitches intended for breeding. Studies performed in laboratory animals have not demonstrated any indications of teratogenicity. In humans, the FDA categorizes this drug as category *C* for use during pregnancy (*Animal studies have shown an adverse effect on the fetus,*

but there are no adequate studies in humans; or there are no animal reproduction studies and no adequate studies in humans.)

Safety for use during lactation has not been established.

Overdosage/Acute Toxicity

There is little information regarding acute overdose situations with pentazocine. For oral ingestions, the gut should be emptied if indicated and safe to do so. Clinical signs should be managed by supportive treatment (O_2, pressor agents, IV fluids, mechanical ventilation) and respiratory depression can be treated with naloxone. Repeated doses of naloxone may be necessary.

Drug Interactions

The following drug interactions have either been reported or are theoretical in humans or animals receiving pentazocine and may be of significance in veterinary patients. Unless otherwise noted, use together is not necessarily contraindicated, but weigh the potential risks and perform additional monitoring when appropriate.

- **CNS DEPRESSANTS, OTHER** (*e.g.*, **anesthetic agents, antihistamines, phenothiazines, barbiturates, tranquilizers, alcohol,** etc.): May cause increased CNS or respiratory depression; dosage may need to be decreased.
- **FLUOXETINE** (and other SSRI'S): May be at increased risk for serotonin syndrome.

Laboratory Considerations

- Pentazocine may cause decreases for urinary **17-hydroxycorticosteroid** determinations.

Doses

- **DOGS:**

  For analgesia: Initially 1.65 mg/kg; up to 3.3 mg/kg IM. Duration of effect generally lasts 3 hours. If dose is repeated, use different injection site. (Package Insert; *Talwin®-V*; no longer marketed)

- **CATS:**

  Note: Pentazocine can cause dysphoria in cats; alternative analgesics are recommended.

- **FERRETS:**

  For analgesia (extra-label): 5 – 10 mg/kg SC or IM q4h. (Williams 2000)

- **RABBITS, RODENTS, SMALL MAMMALS:**

  Rabbits; post-operative analgesia (extra-label): 5 – 20 mg/kg SC, IV, or IM q4h. (Ivey *et al.* 2000)

- **HORSES:** NOTE: ARCI UCGFS CLASS 3 DRUG

  For analgesia: 0.33 mg/kg slowly in jugular vein. In cases of severe pain, a second dose (0.33 mg/kg) be given IM 15 minutes later (Package Insert; *Talwin®-V*; no longer marketed). **Note:** Studies have demonstrated that pentazocine is not as an effective analgesic as either butorphanol or flunixin in horses. Many clinicians no longer recommend its use.

Monitoring

- Analgesic efficacy.
- Respiratory rate/depth.
- Appetite/bowel function.
- CNS effects.

Client Information

- Clients should report any significant changes in behavior, appetite, bowel, or urinary function in their animals.

Chemistry/Synonyms

A synthetic partial opiate agonist, pentazocine is commercially available as two separate salts. The hydrochloride salt, which is found in oral dosage forms, occurs as a white, crystalline powder. It is soluble in water and freely soluble in alcohol. The commercial injection is prepared from pentazocine base with the assistance of lactic acid. This allows the drug to be soluble in water. The pH of this product is adjusted to a range of 4-5. Pentazocine is a weak base with an approximate pK$_a$ of 9.0.

Pentazocine may also be known as: NIH-7958, NSC-107430, pentazocinum, Win-20228, *Talacen®*, and *Talwin®*.

Storage/Stability

The tablet preparations should be stored at room temperature and in tight, light-resistant containers. The injectable product should be kept at room temperature; avoid freezing.

Compatibility/Compounding Considerations

The following agents have been reported to be physically **compatible** when mixed with pentazocine lactate: atropine sulfate, butorphanol tartrate, chlorpromazine HCl, dimenhydrinate, diphenhydramine HCl, fentanyl citrate, hydromorphone, hydroxyzine HCl, meperidine HCl, metoclopramide, morphine sulfate, perphenazine, prochlorperazine edisylate, promazine HCl, promethazine HCl, and scopolamine HBr.

The following agents have been reported to be physically **incompatible** when mixed with pentazocine lactate: aminophylline, flunixin meglumine, glycopyrrolate, pentobarbital sodium, phenobarbital sodium, and sodium bicarbonate.

Dosage Forms/Regulatory Status

VETERINARY-LABELED PRODUCTS: NONE.

The ARCI (Racing Commissioners International) has designated this drug as a class 3 substance. See the appendix for more information.

HUMAN-LABELED PRODUCTS:

Pentazocine Lactate Injection: 30 mg (as lactate)/mL; *Talwin®*; (Rx, C-IV)

Revisions/References

Monograph revised/updated May 2014.

Ivey, E. & J. Morrisey (2000). Therapeutics for Rabbits. Vet Clin NA: Exotic Anim Pract 3:1(Jan): 183-216.
Williams, D. (2000). Exocrine Pancreatic Disease. *Textbook of Veterinary Internal Medicine: Diseases of the Dog and Cat.* S. Ettinger and E. Feldman. Philadelphia, WB Saunders. 2: 1345-67.

Pentobarbital Sodium

(pen-toe-**bar**-bi-tal)   Nembutal®

Barbiturate

Note: *Pentobarbital and combinations with pentobarbital (e.g., phenytoin) for euthanasia have a separate monograph listed under Euthanasia Agents.*

Prescriber Highlights

▶ Barbiturate used therapeutically as a sedative/anesthetic, & treating intractable seizures; also used for euthanasia.

▶ Contraindications: Known hypersensitivity, severe liver disease, nephritis, or severe respiratory depression (large doses). Caution: Hypovolemia, anemia, borderline hypoadrenal function, or cardiac or respiratory disease. Use with caution in cats (sensitive to respiratory depression).

▶ Adverse Effects: respiratory depression (if using for anesthesia have ventilatory support available), hypothermia, or excitement post-anesthesia (dogs).

▶ When giving IV, administer SLOWLY (unless for euthanasia); very irritating if given SC or perivascularly; do not give IA.

▶ Numerous drug interactions.

Uses/Indications

Pentobarbital was once the principal agent used for general anesthesia in small animals, but has been largely supplanted by the use of inhalant and other injectable anesthetic agents. It continues to be useful as a sedative/restraining agent in animals being mechanically ventilated. Pentobarbital is commonly used as an anesthetic for rodents in laboratory situations.

Pentobarbital can be used for treating intractable seizures secondary to convulsant agents (*e.g.*, strychnine) or secondary to CNS toxins (*e.g.*, tetanus). It should not be used to treat seizures caused by lidocaine intoxication. For refractory status epilepticus not controlled with diazepam and phenobarbital, pentobarbital can be used. However, propofol or inhalant anesthetics are usually preferred today.

Pentobarbital has been used as a sedative and anesthetic agent in horses, cattle, swine, sheep, and goats.

Pentobarbital is a major active ingredient in several euthanasia solutions. This indication is discussed in the monograph for Euthanasia Agents.

Pharmacology/Actions

While barbiturates are generally considered CNS depressants, they can invoke all levels of CNS mood alteration from paradoxical excitement to deep coma and death. While the exact mechanisms for the CNS effects caused by barbiturates are unknown, they have been shown to inhibit the release of acetylcholine, norepinephrine, and glutamate. The barbiturates also have effects on GABA and pentobarbital has been shown to be GABA-mimetic. Pentobarbital may have neuroprotective effects via decreasing cerebral metabolic rate and oxygen consumption, scavenging of free radicals, and stabilization of endothelial and glial membranes. At high anesthetic doses, barbiturates have been demonstrated to inhibit the uptake of calcium at nerve endings.

The degree of depression produced is dependent on the dosage, route of administration, pharmacokinetics of the drug, and species treated. Additionally, effects may be altered by patient age, physical condition, or concurrent use of other drugs. The barbiturates depress the sensory cortex, lessen motor activity, and produce sedation at low dosages. In humans, it has been shown that barbiturates reduce the rapid-eye movement (REM) stage of sleep. Barbiturates have no true intrinsic analgesic activity.

In most species, barbiturates cause a dose-dependent respiratory depression, but, in some species, they can cause slight respiratory stimulation. At sedative/hypnotic doses, respiratory depression is similar to that during normal physiologic sleep. As doses increase, the medullary respiratory center is progressively depressed with resultant decreases in rate, depth, and volume. Respiratory arrest may occur at doses 4X lower than those that cause cardiac arrest. These drugs must be used very cautiously in cats; they are particularly sensitive to the respiratory depressant effects of barbiturates.

Besides the cardiac arresting effects of the barbiturates at euthanatizing dosages, the barbiturates have other cardiovascular effects. In the dog, pentobarbital has been demonstrated to cause tachycardia, decreased myocardial contractility and stroke volume, and decreased mean arterial pressure and total peripheral resistance.

The barbiturates cause reduced tone and motility of the intestinal musculature, probably secondary to its central depressant action. The thiobarbiturates (thiamylal, thiopental) may, after initial depression, cause an increase in both tone and motility of the intestinal musculature; however, these effects do not appear to have much clinical significance. Administration of barbiturates reduces the sensitivity of the motor end-plate to acetylcholine, thereby slightly relaxing skeletal muscle. Because the musculature is not completely relaxed, other skeletal muscle relaxants may be necessary for surgical procedures.

There is no direct effect on the kidney by the barbiturates, but severe renal impairment may occur secondary to hypotensive effects in overdose situations. Liver function is not directly affected when used acutely, but hepatic microsomal enzyme induction is well documented with extended barbiturate (especially phenobarbital) administration. Although barbiturates reduce oxygen consumption of all tissues, no change in metabolic rate is measurable when given at sedative dosages. Basal metabolic rates may be reduced with resultant decreases in body temperature when barbiturates are given at anesthetic doses.

Pharmacokinetics

Pentobarbital is absorbed quite rapidly from the gut after oral or rectal administration with peak plasma concentrations occurring between 30-60 minutes after oral dosing in humans. The onset of action usually occurs within 15-60 minutes after oral dosing and within 1 minute after IV administration.

Pentobarbital, like all barbiturates, distributes rapidly to all body tissues with highest concentrations found in the liver and brain. It is 35-45% bound to plasma proteins in humans. Although less lipophilic than the ultra-short acting barbiturates (*e.g.*, thiopental), pentobarbital is highly lipid soluble and patient fat content may alter the distributive qualities of the drug. All barbiturates cross the placenta and enter milk (at concentrations far below those of plasma). In neonates, pentobarbital may cross into the CNS at levels up to 6X those in adult animals.

Pentobarbital is metabolized in the liver principally by oxidation. Excretion of the drug is not appreciably enhanced by increased urine flow or alkalinizing the urine. Ruminants (especially sheep and goats) metabolize pentobarbital at a very rapid rate. The elimination half-life in the goat has been reported to be ≈ 0.9 hrs. Conversely, the half-life in dogs is ≈ 8 hours; in man, it ranges from 15-50 hours.

Contraindications/Precautions/Warnings

Barbiturates are contraindicated in patients with severe liver disease or who have demonstrated previous hypersensitivity reactions to them. Large doses are contraindicated in patients with nephritis or severe respiratory dysfunction. Use for cesarean section is not recommended because of fetal respiratory depression.

Use cautiously in patients that are hypovolemic, anemic, have borderline hypoadrenal function, or cardiac or respiratory disease. Use with caution in neonates, as pentobarbital levels in the CNS may be substantially higher than in adults. Cats tend to be particularly sensitive to the respiratory depressant effects of barbiturates; use with caution in this species. Female cats appear to be more susceptible to the effects of pentobarbital than males.

When administering IV, give SLOWLY. Barbiturates can be very irritating when administered SC or perivascularly; avoid these types of injections. Do not administer intra-arterially.

Do not confuse pentobarbital with phenobarbital.

Adverse Effects

Because of the respiratory depressant effects of pentobarbital, respiratory activity must be closely monitored and respiratory assistance must be readily available when using anesthetic dosages. Hypotension can occur at high dosages. Pentobarbital may cause excitement in dogs during recovery from anesthetic doses; this can be confused with seizure activity. Hypothermia may develop in animals receiving pentobarbital if exposed to temperatures below 27°C (80.6°F).

Reproductive/Nursing Safety

In humans, the FDA categorizes this drug as category *D* for use during pregnancy (*There is evidence of human fetal risk, but the potential benefits from the use of the drug in pregnant women may be acceptable despite its potential risks.*) In a separate system evaluating the safety of drugs in canine and feline pregnancy (Papich 1989), this drug is categorized as class: *D* (*Contraindicated. These drugs have been shown to cause congenital malformations or embryotoxicity.*)

Exercise caution when administering to the nursing mother, since small amounts are excreted in maternal milk. Drowsiness in nursing offspring has been reported.

Overdosage/Acute Toxicity

In dogs, the reported oral LD_{50} is 85 mg/kg and IV LD_{50} is 40 – 60 mg/kg. Fatalities from ingestion of meat from animals euthanized by pentobarbital have been reported in dogs. Treatment of pentobarbital overdose consists of removal of ingested product from the gut if appropriate and offering respiratory and cardiovascular support. Forced alkaline diuresis is of little benefit for this drug. Peritoneal or hemodialysis may be of benefit in severe intoxications.

Drug Interactions

Most clinically significant interactions have been documented in humans with phenobarbital; however, these interactions may also be of significance in animals receiving pentobarbital, especially if receiving it as chronic therapy.

- **ACETAMINOPHEN:** Increased risk for hepatotoxicity, particularly when large or chronic doses of barbiturates are given.
- **LIDOCAINE:** Fatalities have been reported when dogs suffering from lidocaine-induced seizures were treated with pentobarbital. Until this interaction is further clarified, it is suggested that lidocaine-induced seizures in dogs be treated initially with diazepam.
- **PHENYTOIN:** Barbiturates may affect the metabolism of phenytoin, and phenytoin may alter barbiturate levels; monitoring of blood levels may be indicated.
- **RIFAMPIN:** May induce enzymes that increase the metabolism of barbiturates.

The following drugs may <u>increase the effect</u> of pentobarbital:

- **ANTIHISTAMINES**
- **CHLORAMPHENICOL**
- **OPIATES**
- **PHENOTHIAZINES**
- **VALPROIC ACID**

Pentobarbital (particularly after chronic therapy) may <u>decrease the effect</u> of the following drugs/drug classes by lowering their serum concentrations:

- **ANTICOAGULANTS, ORAL (WARFARIN)**
- **BETA-BLOCKERS**
- **CHLORAMPHENICOL**
- **CLONAZEPAM**
- **CORTICOSTEROIDS**
- **CYCLOSPORINE**
- **DOXORUBICIN**
- **DOXYCYCLINE** (may persist for weeks after barbiturate discontinued)
- **ESTROGENS**
- **GRISEOFULVIN**
- **METHADONE**
- **METRONIDAZOLE**
- **QUINIDINE**
- **PAROXETINE**
- **PHENOTHIAZINES**
- **PROGESTINS**
- **THEOPHYLLINE**

- TRICYCLIC ANTIDEPRESSANTS
- VERAPAMIL

Laboratory Considerations

- Barbiturates may cause increased retention of **bromosulfoph-thalein** (BSP; sulfobromophthalein) and give falsely elevated results. It is recommended that barbiturates not be administered within the 24 hours before BSP retention tests.

Doses

Note: In order to avoid possible confusion, doses used for euthanasia are listed separately under the monograph for euthanasia solutions.

- **DOGS/CATS:**

  For chemical restraint in patients being mechanically ventilated (extra-label): For ventilator maintenance, pentobarbital is preferred and may be administered as a CRI from 1 – 3 mg/kg/hour IV; it is associated with relative cardiovascular stability, but may cause seizure-like movements during recovery from anesthesia. The author prefers to switch over to a shorter acting drug like propofol ≈ 12 hours prior to weaning from the ventilator; this will allow the pentobarbital levels to decrease and will help attenuate any seizure-like activity. (Brainard 2008)

  For intractable seizures refractory to benzodiazepine boluses (extra-label): Give 3 – 15 mg/kg IV slowly to effect. May require several minutes for full therapeutic effect. Once seizures controlled, consider a CRI of 0.5 – 5 mg/kg/hour. After seizures have been controlled for at least 6 hours patient may be slowly weaned from the CRI as standard anticonvulsant therapy is initiated.

- **SMALL MAMMALS/RODENTS:**

  For chemical restraint (extra-label):

  Mice: 30 – 80 mg/kg IP;

  Rats: 40 – 60 mg/kg IP;

  Hamsters/Gerbils: 70 – 80 mg/kg IP;

  Guinea pigs: 15 – 40 mg/kg IP; 30 mg/kg IV;

  Rabbits: 20 – 60 mg/kg IV. (Burke 1999)

- **HORSES:** NOTE: ARCI UCGFS CLASS 2 DRUG

  Note: Pentobarbital is generally not considered an ideal agent for use in the adult horse due to possible development of excitement and injury when the animal is "knocked down." Dosages of 3 – 18 mg/kg IV have been noted.

Monitoring

- Levels of consciousness and/or seizure control. EEG monitoring can be helpful in patients with intractable seizures.
- Respiratory and cardiac signs. Protect airway.
- Body temperature.

Client Information

- This drug is best used in an inpatient setting or with close professional supervision.
- If dosage forms are dispensed to clients, they must be in instructed to keep them away from children; dispense in child-resistant packaging.

Chemistry/Synonyms

Pentobarbital sodium occurs as odorless, slightly bitter tasting, white, crystalline powder or granules. It is very soluble in water and freely soluble in alcohol. The pK_a of the drug has been reported to range from 7.85-8.03 and the pH of the injection is from 9-10.5. Alcohol or propylene glycol may be added to enhance the stability of the injectable product.

Pentobarbital may also be known as: aethaminalum, mebubarbital, mebumal, pentobarbitalum, or pentobarbitone.

Storage/Stability

The injectable product should be stored at room temperature; the suppositories should be kept refrigerated. The aqueous solution is not very stable and should not be used if it contains a precipitate. Because precipitates may occur, pentobarbital sodium should not be added to acidic solutions.

Compatibility/Compounding Considerations

The following solutions and drugs have been reported to be physically **compatible** with pentobarbital sodium: dextrose IV solutions, Ringer's injection, lactated Ringer's injection, Saline IV solutions, dextrose-saline combinations, dextrose-Ringer's combinations, dextrose-Ringer's lactate combinations, amikacin sulfate, aminophylline, atropine sulfate (for at least 15 minutes, not 24 hours), calcium chloride, cephapirin sodium, chloramphenicol sodium succinate, hyaluronidase, hydromorphone HCl, lidocaine HCl, neostigmine methylsulfate, scopolamine HBr, sodium bicarbonate, sodium iodide, thiopental sodium, and verapamil HCl.

The following drugs have been reported to be physically **incompatible** with pentobarbital sodium: butorphanol tartrate, chlorpromazine HCl, cimetidine HCl, chlorpheniramine maleate, codeine phosphate, diphenhydramine HCl, droperidol, fentanyl citrate, glycopyrrolate, hydrocortisone sodium succinate, hydroxyzine HCl, insulin (regular), meperidine HCl, nalbuphine HCl, norepinephrine bitartrate, oxytetracycline HCl, penicillin G potassium, pentazocine lactate, phenytoin sodium, prochlorperazine edisylate, promazine HCl, and promethazine HCl. Compatibility is dependent upon factors such as pH, concentration, temperature, and diluent used; consult specialized references or a hospital pharmacist for more specific information.

Dosage Forms/Regulatory Status

VETERINARY-LABELED PRODUCTS: NONE.

The ARCI (Racing Commissioners International) has designated this drug as a class 2 substance. See the appendix for more information.

HUMAN-LABELED PRODUCTS:

Pentobarbital Sodium Injection: 50 mg/mL in 2 mL *Tubex*; generic; (Rx, C-II)

Pentobarbital is a Class-II controlled substance and detailed records must be maintained with regard to its use and disbursement.

Revisions/References

Monograph revised/updated May 2014.

Brainard, B. (2008). Long-term sedation for the ventilated patient. Proceedings: IVECCS. accessed via Veterinary Information Network; vin.com

Burke, T. (1999). Husbandry and Medicine of Rodents and Lagomorphs. Proceedings: Central Veterinary Conference, Kansas City. accessed via Veterinary Information Network; vin.com

Papich, M. (1989). Effects of drugs on pregnancy. *Current Veterinary Therapy X: Small Animal Practice*. R. Kirk. Philadelphia, Saunders: 1291-9.

Pentosan Polysulfate Sodium

(**pen**-toe-san) *PPS, Cartrophen-Vet®, Elmiron®*

Antiinflammatory, Osteoarthritis Disease-Modifier

Prescriber Highlights

▶ Injectable pentosan may be useful in treating osteoarthritis in dogs, cats, & horses.

▶ Oral product (human) possibly useful as adjunctive treatment of feline interstitial cystitis (feline idiopathic lower urinary tract disease—FLUTD) though efficacy for FLUTD is not well-documented and is in doubt. Adverse effects uncommon, but can cause bleeding, GI effects.

▶ Use with caution prior to surgery or with other drugs affecting coagulation.

Uses/Indications

Pentosan polysulfated sodium (sodium pentosan polysulfated; NaPPS) may be useful when injected IM or SC for treating osteoarthritis in dogs, cats, and horses. No products are approved for use in animals in the USA at present, but an injectable product (*Cartrophen-Vet®*) is licensed elsewhere, including in the UK and Canada (dogs), and Australia (dogs, horses).

A review of the clinical trial evidence for treating osteoarthritis in dogs (published in 2007), concluded that "Presently, a moderate level of comfort exists for pentosan polysulphate that the claimed relationship is scientifically valid. With the contradiction of results and the low number of controlled clinical trials, additional studies are necessary to construct a scientifically sound recommendation" (Aragon *et al.* 2007). However another review of evidence (published 2009) stated "There was weak or no evidence that the use of doxycycline, ESA, extra-corporeal shockwave therapy, gold wire acupuncture, hyaluronan, pentosan polysulphate, P54FP, tiaprofenic acid and tibial plateau-leveling osteotomy had significant or physiologically meaningful effects in the management of canine osteoarthritis. The studies involving these agents were generally of poor quality with too few animals" (Sanderson *et al.* 2009).

Horses with experimentally induced osteoarthritis (n=18; 9 in treatment group) were administered pentosan (NaPPS, *AU-PEN5000®*) 3 mg/kg IM once weekly for 4 weeks. Authors concluded, "Because NaPPS resulted in significant improvement in reducing articular cartilage fibrillation, near significant improvement in other variables was found, and no adverse effects were detected, the continued study of this therapeutic agent is justified" (McIlwraith *et al.* 2012).

Oral pentosan (human) been used anecdotally for the adjunctive treatment of feline interstitial cystitis (feline idiopathic lower urinary tract disease—FLUTD), but studies have demonstrated that it is not effective for short-term, acute lower urinary tract disease. A small study using injected pentosan (3 mg/kg SC on days 1, 2, 5 and 10) found no statistically significant differences between the treated or placebo-group cats in either short-term or long-term follow-up (Wallius *et al.* 2009).

Pharmacology/Actions

Pentosan has disease-modifying effects on osteoarthritic joints similar to polysulfated glycosoaminoglycans. It apparently modulates cytokine action, preserves preoteoglycan content and stimulates hyaluronic acid synthesis. Pentosan has antiinflammatory, hypolipidemic, anticoagulant (considerably weaker than heparin—1/15th), and fibrinolytic properties. These effects potentially could increase synovial blood flow and reduce joint inflammation. Proposed modes of action for pentosan's effects include increasing proteoglycan synthesis, reducing matrix metalloproteinase activity, inducing synoviocyte biosynthesis of high molecular weight hyaluronan, and increasing subchondral blood flow via thrombolytic activity (Ghosh 1999).

Pentosan has a mild analgesic effect when used for interstitial cystitis. The mechanism for its action in treating interstitial cystitis is not known, but it is postulated that it may adhere to bladder wall mucosal membranes and act as a "buffer" to prevent irritating compounds in urine from reaching bladder cells.

Pharmacokinetics

In rats, 10-20% of the calcium derivative (pentosan polysulfate calcium) is absorbed after oral dosing. In humans, only ≈ 3% of an oral dose of pentosan polysulfate sodium is absorbed. It distributes primarily to the uroepithelium of the genitourinary tract with smaller concentrations found in the liver, spleen, lung skin, bone marrow, and periosteum. About two-thirds of absorbed drug is desulfated in the liver and spleen within one hour; ≈ 3.5% of the absorbed drug is excreted into the urine.

Contraindications/Precautions/Warnings

Pentosan is contraindicated in patients hypersensitive to it.

The U.K. injectable product (*Cartrophen-Vet®*) licensed for use in dogs lists the following: Contraindicated for treatment of septic arthritis. Do not use in dogs with advanced liver or kidney impairment, evidence of infection, blood disorders, coagulation disorders, bleeding or malignancy (especially hemangiosarcoma). Do not use in the perioperative period as pentosan polysulfate has an anticoagulant effect. Do not use in the skeletally immature dog (*i.e.*, dogs whose long bone growth plates have not closed). Use with caution in dogs with history of pulmonary lacerations. Caution is also recommended in cases of hepatic impairment. No more than 3 courses of 4 injections should be administered in a 12-month period. Not recommended in pregnant dogs as safety has not been studied. Pentosan should not be used at the time of parturition due to its anticoagulant effects.

An Australian injectable equine product (*Arthropen® Vet 250*) lists the following contraindications: Contraindicated for use in horses with clotting defects, traumatic hemorrhage, infection, liver/kidney failure, or within 2 days of surgery.

Use this drug with caution in animals also receiving other medications that can affect coagulation, or having surgery in the near future.

Adverse Effects

Parenterally administered pentosan is usually well tolerated and adverse effects in veterinary species appear to be mild and transitory in nature. In dogs, vomiting, anorexia, lethargy, or mild depression are possible. Because pentosan has some anticoagulant effects, bleeding is possible in any species and may be more likely in animals receiving other drugs that affect coagulation (*e.g.*, aspirin) or undergoing stressful exercise. In horses, pentosan can cause dose-dependent increases in partial thromboplastin time (PTT) up to 24 hours post-dose.

When used orally in cats, pentosan seems to be tolerated well, but oral dosing twice daily can be problematic. In a small percentage (<2%) of humans taking the medication, transient increases in liver enzymes have been reported.

Reproductive/Nursing Safety

The U.K. label information for the injectable product (*Cartrophen-Vet®*) for use in dogs says the product is not recommended in pregnant dogs as safety has not been studied and that it should not be used at the time of parturition due to its anticoagulant effects.

In humans, pentosan is designated by the FDA as a category *B* drug (*Animal studies have not demonstrated risk to the fetus, but there are no adequate studies in pregnant women; or animal studies have shown an adverse effect, but adequate studies in pregnant wom-*

en have not demonstrated a risk to the fetus during the first trimester of pregnancy, and there is no evidence of risk in later trimesters.)

Pentosan is likely safe to use during nursing.

Overdosage/Acute Toxicity

Information regarding overdoses is not readily available. Potentially, overdoses could cause bleeding, thrombocytopenia, GI distress, and liver function abnormalities. At the present time, treatment recommendations are basically supportive in nature. If an oral overdose occurs, consider protocols for drug removal from the gut.

Drug Interactions

- No specific drug interactions were located; use this drug cautiously with other **drugs that can affect coagulation** (*e.g.*, **NSAIDs, aspirin, heparin**, etc.). The U.K. injectable product (*Cartrophen-Vet®*) licensed for use in dogs states: "NSAIDs and in particular aspirin should not be used in combination with pentosan polysulfate sodium as they may affect thrombocyte adhesion and potentiate the anticoagulant activity of the product. Corticosteroids have been shown to be antagonistic to a number of actions of pentosan polysulfate sodium. Furthermore, use of anti-inflammatory drugs may result in a premature increase in the dog's activity, which may interfere with the therapeutic activity of the product." The label also states: "Do not use concurrently with heparin, warfarin or other anti-coagulants."

Laboratory Considerations

- No laboratory interactions or considerations were noted.

Doses

- **DOGS:**

  As a chondroprotective for osteoarthritis (OA); (extra-label in USA): For the treatment of lameness and pain of degenerative joint disease/osteoarthrosis (non-infectious arthrosis) in the skeletally mature dog: 3 mg/kg SC on 4 occasions with an interval of 5-7 days between injections. (adapted from label information; *Cartrophen-Vet®*—Arthropharm U.K.) **Note:** Other products may be labeled in some markets for IM or SC use with an interval between injections of 5-7 days.

- **CATS:**

  As a chondroprotective for osteoarthritis (OA); (extra-label): 3 mg/kg SC or IM once weekly for 4 weeks has also been used anecdotally in cats. (Beale 2004)

- **HORSES:**

  As an aid in the treatment of non-infectious, inflammatory joint disease (extra-label in USA): Intramuscular administration: 3 mg/kg IM on 4 occasions with an interval of 5-7 days between injections. Intra-articular injection: 1 mL (250 mg). May be repeated at weekly intervals for 3-4 treatments. More than one joint may be treated at the one time. The horse should be rested for 2 weeks after the final injection, followed by a further 2 weeks of graded walking exercise before returning to work. (**Note:** See the label for specific directions on injection technique, etc.). (Label information; *Arthropen® Vet 250*; Australia)

Monitoring

- When used for veterinary indications clinical efficacy is the primary monitoring parameter.
- When administered into joints, animals should be assessed for intra-articular bleeding.

Client Information

- If administered at home, provide the client information leaflet accompanying the product.

Chemistry/Synonyms

A heparin-like compound, pentosan polysulfate sodium is a mixture of linear polymers of beta-1->4-linked xylose that are usual-ly sulfated at the 2- and 3- positions. Average molecular weight is between 4000 and 6000. It is not derived from animal sources, but from Beechwood hemicellulose.

Pentosan may also be known as: pentosan polysulphate sodium; PZ-68; sodium pentosan polysulphate; sodium xylanpolysulphate; SP-54, *Cartrophen-Vet®*, *AUPEN5000®*, *Zydax®* and *Elmiron®*.

Storage/Stability

Unless otherwise labeled, store oral pentosan products at controlled room temperature (15-30°C; 59-86°F) and injectable pentosan products under refrigeration (2-8°C) and protected from light.

Compatibility/Compounding Considerations

No specific information noted.

Dosage Forms/Regulatory Status

VETERINARY-LABELED PRODUCTS:

No products currently FDA-approved in USA.

In several other countries, injectable pentosan polysulfate sodium 100 mg/mL (*Cartrophen-Vet®* Injection) labeled for use in dogs and pentosan polysulfate sodium 250 mg/mL products (*e.g.*, *Arthropen Vet® 250*, *Cartrophen-Vet Forte®* Injection) labeled for horses are available in several countries.

HUMAN-LABELED PRODUCTS:

Pentosan Polysulfate Sodium Oral Capsules: 100 mg; *Elmiron®*; (Rx)

Revisions/References

Monograph revised/updated May 2014.

Aragon, C. L., et al. (2007). Systematic review of clinical trials of treatments for osteoarthritis in dogs. Javma-Journal of the American Veterinary Medical Association **230**(4): 514-21.

Beale, B. S. (2004). Use of nutraceuticals and chondroprotectants in osteoarthritic dogs and cats. Veterinary Clinics of North America-Small Animal Practice **34**(1): 271-+.

Ghosh, P. (1999). The pathobiology of osteoarthritis and the rationale for the use of pentosan polysulfate for its treatment. Seminars in Arthritis and Rheumatism **28**(4): 211-67.

McIlwraith, C. W., et al. (2012). Evaluation of intramuscularly administered sodium pentosan polysulfate for treatment of experimentally induced osteoarthritis in horses. American Journal of Veterinary Research **73**(5): 628-33.

Sanderson, R. O., et al. (2009). Systematic review of the management of canine osteoarthritis. Veterinary Record **164**(14): 418-24.

Wallius, B. M. & A. E. Tidholm (2009). Use of pentosan polysulphate in cats with idiopathic, non-obstructive lower urinary tract disease: a double-blind, randomised, placebo-controlled trial. Journal of Feline Medicine and Surgery **11**(6): 409-12.

Pentoxifylline

(pen-tox-**ih**-fi-leen)   *PTX*, Trental®

Hemorrheologic, Immunomodulatory Agent

Prescriber Highlights

- ▶ Compound that increases erythrocyte flexibility and reduces inflammation.
- ▶ Contraindications: Retinal or cerebral hemorrhage, intolerance or hypersensitivity to it or other xanthines (*i.e.*, theophylline).
- ▶ Caution: Severe hepatic or renal impairment, or at risk for hemorrhage.
- ▶ Adverse Effects: GI tract (vomiting/inappetence) most common. Potentially: Dizziness, other GI, CNS, or cardiovascular effects.

Uses/Indications

In horses, pentoxifylline has been used as adjunctive therapy for cutaneous vasculitis, placentitis, atopic dermatitis, endotoxemia and the treatment of navicular disease.

Pentoxifylline has been used in dogs to treat immune-mediated dermatologic conditions, enhance healing, and reduce inflammation caused by ulcerative dermatosis in Shelties and Collies and for other conditions where improved microcirculation may be of benefit. There is some evidence for efficacy for pentoxifylline and misoprostol as antiallergic medications in dogs but with their modest benefit, relatively high costs and adverse effects, these medications should probably not be used as first line medications to treat dogs with atopic dermatitis (Olivry *et al.* 2010). Pentoxifylline is being investigated for adjunctive therapy for dilated cardiomyopathy in Doberman pinschers and it has been tried in conjunction with prednisolone to decrease vasculitis associated with FIP in cats.

Pentoxifylline's major indications for humans include symptomatic treatment of peripheral vascular disease (*e.g.*, intermittent claudication, sickle cell disease, Raynaud's, etc.) and cerebrovascular diseases where blood flow may be impaired in the microvasculature.

Pharmacology/Actions

The mechanisms for pentoxifylline's actions are not fully understood. The drug increases erythrocyte flexibility probably by inhibiting erythrocyte phosphodiesterase and decreases blood viscosity by reducing plasma fibrinogen and increasing fibrinolytic activity. In horses, pentoxifylline appears to be a potent inhibitor of matrix metalloproteinase-9 and a modest inhibitor of matrix metalloproteinase-2 (Fugler *et al.* 2009).

Pentoxifylline is postulated to reduce negative endotoxic effects of cytokine mediators via its phosphodiesterase inhibition.

Pharmacokinetics

In horses, after PO administration of crushed, sustained-release tablets, pentoxifylline is rapidly absorbed with a wide interpatient variation of bioavailability that averages around 68%. Bioavailability may decrease with continued administration over several days. The authors concluded that 10 mg/kg q12h PO yields serum levels equivalent to those observed after administration of therapeutic doses to humans and horses.

In dogs, pentoxifylline reportedly has a bioavailability of ≈ 50% with peak levels occurring ≈ 1-3 hours after dosing. Serum half-life is ≈ 6-7 hours for the parent compound, 36 hours for active metabolite 1, and 8 hours for active metabolite 5.

In humans, pentoxifylline absorption from the gastrointestinal tract is rapid and almost complete but a significant first-pass effect occurs. Food affects the rate, but not the extent, of absorption. While the distributive characteristics have not been fully described, it is known that the drug enters maternal milk. Pentoxifylline is metabolized both in the liver and erythrocytes; all identified metabolites appear to be active.

Contraindications/Precautions/Warnings

Pentoxifylline should be considered contraindicated in patients that have been intolerant to the drug or xanthines (*e.g.*, theophylline, caffeine, theobromine) in the past and those with cerebral hemorrhage or retinal hemorrhage. It should be used cautiously in patients with severe hepatic or renal impairment and those at risk for hemorrhage.

Adverse Effects

In dogs and cats, most commonly reported adverse effects involve the GI tract (vomiting, inappetence, loose stools) or CNS (excitement, nervousness). In dogs, erythema multiforme may occur rarely.

In horses, IV administration may be associated with transient leukocytosis, muscle fasciculations, sweating on shoulders and flanks, and mild increases in heart rate. Oral dosing at 10 mg/kg or less appears to be well tolerated.

There are reports of dizziness and headache occurring in a small percentage of humans receiving the drug. Other adverse effects, primarily GI, CNS, and cardiovascular related, have been reported in people but are considered to occur rarely. Veterinary experience is limited with pentoxifylline and animal adverse effects may differ.

Reproductive/Nursing Safety

In humans, the FDA categorizes this drug as category *C* for use during pregnancy (*Animal studies have shown an adverse effect on the fetus, but there are no adequate studies in humans; or there are no animal reproduction studies and no adequate studies in humans.*) Pentoxifylline may be teratogenic at high dosages.

Pentoxifylline and its metabolites are excreted in maternal milk. Because of the potential for tumorigenicity (seen in rats), use cautiously in nursing patients.

Overdosage/Acute Toxicity

Humans overdosed with pentoxifylline have demonstrated signs of flushing, seizures, hypotension, unconsciousness, agitation, fever, somnolence, GI distress and ECG changes. One patient who ingested 80 mg/kg recovered completely. Overdoses should be treated using the usual methods of appropriate gut emptying and supportive therapies.

Drug Interactions

The following drug interactions have either been reported or are theoretical in humans or animals receiving pentoxifylline and may be of significance in veterinary patients. Unless otherwise noted, use together is not necessarily contraindicated, but weigh the potential risks and perform additional monitoring when appropriate.

- **ANTIHYPERTENSIVE DRUGS**: With pentoxifylline may increase hypotensive effect.
- **NSAIDS**: Use of non-steroidal antiinflammatory agents with pentoxifylline in horses is controversial. Some sources state that when used for endotoxemia in horses, pentoxifylline's beneficial effects are negated by NSAIDs, but one study showed superior efficacy when flunixin and pentoxifylline were used together, compared with either used alone.
- **PLATELET-AGGREGATION INHIBITORS** (*e.g.*, **aspirin, clopidogrel**): Increased risk for bleeding.
- **THEOPHYLLINE**: Serum levels may be increased when used concurrently with pentoxifylline.
- **WARFARIN**: When pentoxifylline is used with warfarin or other anticoagulants, increased risk of bleeding may result; use together with enhanced monitoring and caution.

Laboratory Considerations

- Pentoxifylline could potentially alter **intradermal allergen testing** results. It is advised to discontinue treatment at least one week prior to testing.

Doses

Note: The commercially available product is a 400 mg extended-release tablet. Cutting or crushing the tablets may negate the sustained-release characteristics and alter pharmacokinetics, but splitting tablets may be necessary to administer or accurately dose. Avoid crushing tablets for small animal use.

- **DOGS:**

  For inflammatory dermatologic conditions (*e.g.*, dermatomyositis, ear margin seborrhea/necrosis, ulcerative dermatitis of collies/shelties, contact dermatitis, atopy and any disease with underlying vasculitis): 10 – 30 mg/kg PO q8-12h. Typically 15 – 20 mg/kg PO q8-12h. A 2-month trial is warranted before evaluating response. (Koch *et al.* 2011)

  For ischemic dermatopathies (extra-label): 15 mg/kg PO q8h to 30 mg/kg PO q12h. One open label study used 25 mg/kg PO q12h (Rees *et al.* 2003). Usually used in combination with vitamin E (200 Units—small breeds, 400 units—medium breeds, 600 Units—large breeds PO every 12 hours) (Morris 2013).

- **CATS:**

  For inflammatory dermatologic conditions (extra-label): 100 mg per cat (1/4 of a 400 mg tablet) PO q12h. (Koch *et al.* 2011)

- **HORSES:** (NOTE: ARCI UCGFS CLASS 4 DRUG)

  For cutaneous vasculitis (extra-label): From a pharmacokinetic study. 10 mg/kg q12h PO yields serum levels equivalent to those observed after administration of therapeutic doses to humans and horses. OK to crush the sustained-release tablets and mix with molasses. If efficacy wanes with time, consider increasing the dose to 15 mg/kg PO twice daily or 10 mg/kg PO 3 times a day. In the experience of the authors, 10 mg/kg PO twice daily for 30 days results in clinical response in horses with cutaneous vasculitis. (Liska *et al.* 2006)

  For adjunctive treatment of atopic dermatitis (extra-label): 8 – 10 mg/kg PO q8-12h.

  For adjunctive treatment (experimental) of sepsis in foals (extra-label): 7.5 mg/kg IV bolus, followed by a CRI of 1.5 mg/kg/hour has been shown to increase regional blood flow and suppress coagulation. (McKenzie 2009)

  For placentitis (extra-label): From a study in pony mares with experimentally induced equine placentitis. Treated group was given trimethoprim/sulfamethoxazole (30 mg/kg PO q12h), pentoxifylline (8.5 mg/kg, PO q12h) and altrenogest (0.088 mg/kg PO q24h) from the onset of clinical signs to delivery of a live foal or abortion. 83% of treated mares delivered viable foals. (Bailey *et al.* 2010).

Monitoring

- Efficacy.
- Adverse effects.

Client Information

- Give with food.
- Usually well tolerated in horses when given by mouth; the most common side effects in dogs are vomiting and restlessness (won't settle down).

Chemistry/Synonyms

A synthetic xanthine derivative structurally related to caffeine and theophylline, pentoxifylline occurs as a white, odorless, bitter-tasting, crystalline powder. At room temperature, ≈ 77 mg are soluble in one mL of water and 63 mg in one mL of alcohol.

Pentoxifylline may also be known as: BL-191, oxpentifylline, or pentoxifyllinum and *Trental®*.

Storage/Stability

The commercially available tablets should be stored in well-closed containers, protected from light at 15-30°C.

Compatibility/Compounding Considerations

The commercially available product in the USA is a 400 mg extended-release tablet (labeled for human use). Cutting or crushing tablets may negate the sustained-release characteristics and alter pharmacokinetics. Splitting tablets may be necessary to administer or accurately dose. For horses crushing tablets may be required; avoid use of crushed tablets in dogs or cats as adverse effects (hyperexcitability, diarrhea) may occur.

Dosage Forms/Regulatory Status

VETERINARY-LABELED PRODUCTS: NONE.

The ARCI (Racing Commissioners International) has designated this drug as a class 4 substance. See the appendix for more information.

HUMAN-LABELED PRODUCTS:

Pentoxifylline Controlled/Extended Release Tablets: 400 mg; generic; (Rx)

Revisions/References

Monograph revised/updated May 2014.

Bailey, C. S., et al. (2010). Treatment efficacy of trimethoprim sulfamethoxazole, pentoxifylline and altrenogest in experimentally induced equine placentitis. Theriogenology 74(3): 402-12.

Fugler, L., et al. (2009). Evaluation of Various Matrix Metalloproteinase Inhibitors (MMPIS) in the Horse. Proceedings: ACVIM. accessed via Veterinary Information Network; vin.com

Koch, S., et al. (2011). *Small Animal Dermatology Drug Handbook*, Wiley-Blackwell. Ames.

Liska, D., et al. (2006). Pharmacokinetics of pentoxifylline and its 5-hydroxyethyl metabolite after oral and intravenous administration to healthy adult horses. AJVR 67(9): 1621-7.

McKenzie, E. (2009). Management of the Septic Foal. Proceedings: WVC. accessed via Veterinary Information Network; vin.com

Morris, D. O. (2013). Ischemic Dermatopathies. Veterinary Clinics of North America-Small Animal Practice 43(1): 99-+.

Olivry, T., et al. (2010). Treatment of canine atopic dermatitis: 2010 clinical practice guidelines from the International Task Force on Canine Atopic Dermatitis. Veterinary Dermatology 21(3): 233-48.

Rees, C. & D. M. Boothe (2003). Therapeutic response to pentoxifylline and its active metabolites in dogs with familial canine dermatomyositis. Vet Therapeutics 4(3): 234-41.

Pergolide Mesylate

(per-go-lide)   Prascend®

Dopamine Agonist

Prescriber Highlights

▶ Dopamine agonist that can help control signs associated with pituitary pars intermedia dysfunction (PPID, equine Cushing's disease).

▶ Apparently, very well tolerated in horses; anorexia occurs in up to 10% of patients.

▶ May be significant expense involved, since treatment is life-long.

Uses/Indications

The primary use for pergolide in veterinary medicine is in treatment of horses for pituitary pars intermedia dysfunction (PPID), commonly called equine Cushing's disease.

Pharmacology/Actions

Pergolide is a potent agonist at dopamine receptors D_1 and D_2 and is 10-1000X more potent than bromocriptine. It is thought that pituitary pars intermedia dysfunction (PPID) in horses is a dopaminergic degenerative disease and pergolide (or dopamine) can reduce expression of proopiomelanocortin (POMC) peptides from the pars intermedia. These peptides are implicated in causing the signs associated with PPID.

Pharmacokinetics

In horses (6 in the study), pergolide was rapidly absorbed following oral administration (0.01 mg/kg) with plasma concentrations reaching maximum levels within 1 hour of dosing. Maximum plasma levels ranged from 1.07-3.38 nanograms/mL. Pergolide appears to be rapidly and widely distributed. Elimination half-life averaged 27 hours, but there was high interpatient variation (Gehring *et al.* 2010).

In humans, the drug is orally absorbed (estimated 60% bioavailable) and 90% bound to plasma proteins. At least 10 different metabolites have been identified, some of which are active. The principle route of elimination is via the kidneys.

Contraindications/Precautions

Pergolide is contraindicated in patients hypersensitive to it or other ergot derivatives.

It has been reported that pergolide (*Prascend®*) tablets may cause eye irritation, an irritating smell, or headache when tablets are split or crushed; do not crush due to the potential for increased human exposure. Care should be taken to minimize exposure when splitting tablets.

Adverse Effects

Pergolide appears to be very well tolerated in horses. Decreased appetite is seen during the first week of therapy in ≈ 10% of horses treated; temporary dose reduction is often beneficial in alleviating this effect. Colic and diarrhea have been reported to occur more rarely.

Adverse effects reported in humans include: nervous system complaints (dyskinesia, hallucinations, somnolence and insomnia), gastrointestinal complaints (nausea, vomiting, diarrhea, constipation), transient hypotension, and rhinitis.

Reproductive/Nursing Safety

Safety of pergolide in pregnant horses has not been established. In humans, pergolide is designated by the FDA as a category *B* drug (*Animal studies have not demonstrated risk to the fetus, but there are no adequate studies in pregnant women; or animal studies have shown an adverse effect, but adequate studies in pregnant women have not demonstrated a risk to the fetus during the first trimester of pregnancy, and there is no evidence of risk in later trimesters.*)

It is not known if pergolide enters maternal milk; however, like other ergot-derivative dopamine agonists, it may interfere with lactation.

Overdosage/Acute Toxicity

There is limited information available on pergolide overdoses. Potential effects include GI disturbances, CNS effects, seizures, and hypotension.

There were 93 single agent exposures to pergolide mesylate reported to the ASPCA Animal Poison Control Center (APCC) during 2009-2013. Of the 81 dogs, 54 were symptomatic with vomiting (94%), lethargy (26%) and trembling (17%) being the most common. Of the 9 cats, 6 were symptomatic with 67% being hyperthermic, and 50% with mydriatic pupils or elevated third eyelids.

Treatment is supportive. Phenothiazines may decrease CNS stimulation effects.

Drug Interactions

The following drug interactions have either been reported or are theoretical in humans or animals receiving pergolide and may be of significance in veterinary patients. Unless otherwise noted, use together is not necessarily contraindicated, but weigh the potential risks and perform additional monitoring when appropriate.

- **DOPAMINE ANTAGONISTS** (*i.e.*, **phenothiazines**): May decrease the effects of pergolide.
- **METOCLOPRAMIDE**: May decrease the effects of pergolide.

Laboratory Considerations

- No specific laboratory interactions or considerations were noted for this drug.

Doses

- **HORSES:**

  For the control of clinical signs associated with Pituitary Pars Intermedia Dysfunction (PPID, Equine Cushing's Disease); (labeled-dose; FDA-approved): Administer orally at a starting dose of 2 micrograms/kg once daily. Dosage may be adjusted to effect, not to exceed 4 micrograms/kg daily. The tablets are scored and the calculated dosage should be provided to the nearest one-half tablet increment. For example, a 1000 lb. (454 kg) horse would receive one 1 mg tablet at 2 micrograms/kg and two 1 mg tablets at 4 micrograms/kg. The label has a dosing table for further reference. Titrate dose according to individual response to therapy to achieve the lowest effective dose. Dose titration is based on improvement in clinical signs associated with PPID and/or improvement or normalization of endocrine tests (*e.g.*, dexamethasone suppression test or endogenous ACTH test). If signs of dose intolerance develop, decrease dose by 50% for 3-5 days and then titrate back up in 2 microgram/kg increments every 2 weeks until the desired effect is achieved. (Adapted from label; *Prascend*®)

Monitoring

- Dexamethasone suppression test (baseline and at 4-8 weeks post pergolide therapy initiation, repeat in 4-8 weeks if dosage is adjusted).
- Blood glucose (baseline, and if abnormal and repeat as per dexamethasone suppression test).
- Clinical signs (hair coat, weight, PU/PD, etc.).
- Periodic CBC and clinical chemistry panel.

Client Information

- Pergolide does not cure the disease and it may take several weeks to months to see positive effects.
- Do not crush tablets.
- *Prascend*® (pergolide) should not be administered by persons who have had adverse reactions to ergotamine or other ergot derivatives. Pregnant or lactating women should wear gloves when administering this product.
- Reduced or lack of appetite is the most common side effect.
- Watch for unpredictable behavior, colic and signs of laminitis.

Chemistry/Synonyms

An ergot derivative, dopamine receptor agonist, pergolide occurs as white to off-white powder that is slightly soluble in water, dehydrated alcohol, or chloroform. It is very slightly soluble in acetone; practically insoluble in ether and sparingly soluble in methyl alcohol.

Pergolide mesylate may also be known as: LY-127809, pergolide mesilate, pergolidi mesilas, *Prascend*®, *Celance*®, *Nopar*®, *Parkotil*®, *Parlide*®, or *Pharken*®.

Storage/Stability

Store pergolide tablets in tight containers at room temperature (25°C; 77°F); excursions permitted to 15-30°C (59-86°F).

Compatibility/Compounding Considerations

An FDA-approved product (*Prascend*®) for horses is now commercially available and should be the first choice when prescribing pergolide for PPID. In certain circumstances (not based on drug cost) a compounded product may be preferable. When compounding, account for the molecular weight of the mesylate salt by using a conversion factor of 1.3 when calculating the amount of pergolide mesylate to obtain an equivalent amount of pergolide base. Pergolide aqueous suspensions are unstable after compounding. Compounded pergolide formulations in aqueous vehicles should be stored in dark containers, protected from light, and refrigerated. Do not use for more than 30 days after compounding. Formulations that have undergone a color change should be considered unstable and discarded (Davis *et al.* 2009).

Dosage Forms/Regulatory Status

VETERINARY-LABELED PRODUCTS:

Pergolide Mesylate Tablets: 1 mg; *Prascend*®; (Rx). FDA-approved (NADA 141-331) for use in horses.

HUMAN-LABELED PRODUCTS: NONE.

Due to an increased potential for heart valve damage associated with pergolide use in humans, all dosage forms were withdrawn from the US market in the spring of 2007.

Revisions/References

Monograph revised/updated June 2014.

Davis, J. L., et al. (2009). Effects of compounding and storage conditions on stability of pergolide mesylate. Javma-Journal of the American Veterinary Medical Association 234(3): 385-9.

Gehring, R., et al. (2010). Single-Dose Oral Pharmacokinetics of Pergolide Mesylate in Healthy Adult Mares. Vet Therapeutics 11(1): E1-E8.

Phenobarbital

(fee-noe-**bar**-bi-tal)   Phenobarbitone

Barbiturate

Prescriber Highlights

▶ Barbiturate used primarily as an antiseizure medication; also used as a sedative agent.

▶ Contraindications: Known hypersensitivity, severe liver disease, nephritis, or severe respiratory depression (large doses). Caution: Hypovolemia, anemia, borderline hypoadrenal function, or cardiac or respiratory disease; use with caution in cats (sensitive to respiratory depression).

▶ Adverse Effects: **Dogs:** Anxiety/agitation or lethargy (when initiating treatment); profound depression, (even at low doses) is possible. Sedation, ataxia, polydipsia, polyuria, polyphagia can be seen at moderate to high serum levels. Increase in liver enzymes possible, but overt hepatotoxicity relatively uncommon. Rare: Anemia, thrombocytopenia or neutropenia.

▶ Adverse Effects: **Cats:** Ataxia, lethargy, facial pruritus, polyphagia/weight gain & polydipsia/polyuria. Rare: Immune-mediated reactions & bone marrow hypoplasia.

▶ When administering IV, give SLOWLY; do not give SC or perivascularly (very irritating).

▶ Drug Interactions; drug-lab interactions.

▶ C-IV controlled substance.

Uses/Indications

Based on its efficacy, relative safety, reasonable dosing frequency (q12h) and low cost, phenobarbital is still considered first-line treatment for treating epilepsy in dogs and cats. As it has a slightly longer onset of action, phenobarbital is generally used for status epilepticus in dogs, cats, and horses, to prevent the recurrence of seizures after they have been halted with a benzodiazepine.

Phenobarbital may also useful in controlling excessive drooling in dogs and reducing feline vocalization while riding in automobiles. It is occasionally used as an oral sedative agent in both species but other agents are generally preferred for this indication.

In cattle, the microsomal enzyme stimulating properties of phenobarbital has been suggested for its use in speeding the detoxification of organochlorine (chlorinated hydrocarbon) insecticide poisoning. Additionally, phenobarbital has been used in the treatment and prevention of neonatal hyperbilirubinemia in human infants. It is unknown if hyperbilirubinemia is effectively treated in veterinary patients with phenobarbital.

Pharmacology/Actions

While barbiturates are generally considered CNS depressants, they can invoke all levels of CNS mood alteration from paradoxical excitement to deep coma and death. While the exact mechanisms for the CNS effects caused by barbiturates are unknown, they have been shown to inhibit the release of acetylcholine, norepinephrine, and glutamate. The barbiturates also have effects on GABA and pentobarbital has been shown to be GABA-mimetic. At high anesthetic doses, barbiturates have been demonstrated to inhibit the uptake of calcium at nerve endings.

The degree of depression produced is dependent on the dosage, route of administration, pharmacokinetics of the drug, and species treated. Additionally, effects may be altered by patient age, physical condition, or concurrent use of other drugs. The barbiturates depress the sensory cortex, lessen motor activity, and produce sedation at low dosages. In humans, it has been shown that barbiturates reduce the rapid-eye movement (REM) stage of sleep. Barbiturates have no true intrinsic analgesic activity.

In most species barbiturates cause a dose-dependent respiratory depression but in some species, they can cause slight respiratory stimulation. At sedative/hypnotic doses, respiratory depression is similar to that during normal physiologic sleep. As doses increase, the medullary respiratory center is progressively depressed with resultant decreases in rate, depth, and volume. Respiratory arrest may occur at doses 4X lower than those that cause cardiac arrest. These drugs must be used very cautiously in cats; they are particularly sensitive to the respiratory depressant effects of barbiturates.

The barbiturates cause reduced tone and motility of the intestinal musculature, probably secondary to its central depressant action. Administration of barbiturates reduces the sensitivity of the motor endplate to acetylcholine thereby slightly relaxing skeletal muscle. Because the musculature is not completely relaxed, other skeletal muscle relaxants may be necessary for surgical procedures.

There is no direct effect on the kidney by the barbiturates, but severe renal impairment may occur secondary to hypotensive effects in overdose situations. Liver function is not directly affected when used acutely but hepatic microsomal enzyme induction is well documented with extended barbiturate (especially phenobarbital) administration. Although barbiturates reduce oxygen consumption of all tissues, no change in metabolic rate is measurable when given at sedative dosages. Basal metabolic rates may be reduced with resultant decreases in body temperature when barbiturates are given at anesthetic doses.

Pharmacokinetics

The pharmacokinetics of phenobarbital have been thoroughly studied in humans and, in a more limited fashion, dogs, cats, and horses. Phenobarbital is slowly absorbed from the GI tract. Bioavailabilities range from 70-90% in humans, ≈ 90% in dogs, and absorption is practically complete in adult horses. Peak levels occur in 4-8 hours after oral dosing in dogs, and in 8-12 hours in humans.

Phenobarbital is widely distributed throughout the body, but because of its lower lipid solubility, it does not distribute as rapidly as most other barbiturates into the CNS. The amount of phenobarbital bound to plasma proteins has been reported to be 40-60%. The reported apparent volumes of distribution are: Horse ≈ 0.8 L/kg; Foals ≈ 0.86 L/kg; Dogs ≈ 0.75 L/kg.

The drug is metabolized in the liver primarily by hydroxylated oxidation to p-hydroxyphenobarbital; sulfate and glucuronide conjugates are also formed. The elimination half-lives reported in humans range from 2-6 days; in dogs from 12-125 hours with an average of ≈ 2 days. Because of its ability to induce the hepatic enzymes used to metabolize itself (and other drugs), elimination half-lives may decrease with time along with concomitant reductions in serum levels. Some dogs may have half lives <24 hours and may require 3X daily dosing for maximal control. An elimination half-life of 34-43 hours has been reported in cats. Elimination half-lives in horses are considerably shorter with values reported of ≈ 13 hours in foals and 18 hours in adult horses. Phenobarbital will induce hepatic microsomal enzymes and it can be expected that elimination half-lives will decrease with time. Approximately 25% of a dose is excreted unchanged by the kidney. Alkalinizing the urine and/or substantially increasing urine flow will increase excretion rates. Anuric or oliguric patients may accumulate unmetabolized drug; dosage adjustments may need to be made.

Changes in diet, body weight, and body composition may alter the pharmacokinetics of phenobarbital in dogs and necessitate dosage adjustment.

Contraindications/Precautions/Warnings

Use cautiously in patients that are hypovolemic, anemic, have borderline hypoadrenal function, or cardiac or respiratory disease. Large doses are contraindicated in patients with nephritis or severe respiratory dysfunction. Barbiturates are contraindicated in patients with severe liver disease or have demonstrated previous hypersensitivity reactions to them.

When administering IV, give slowly (not more than 60 mg/minute); too rapid IV administration may cause respiratory depression. Commercially available injectable preparations (excluding the sterile powder) must not be administered subcutaneously or perivascularly as significant tissue irritation and possible necrosis may result. Applications of moist heat and local infiltration of 0.5% procaine HCl solution have been recommended to treat these reactions.

Do not confuse phenobarbital with pentobarbital.

Adverse Effects

Dogs may exhibit increased clinical signs of anxiety/agitation or lethargy when initiating therapy. These effects are generally transitory in nature. Occasionally dogs will exhibit profound depression at lower dosage ranges (and plasma levels).

Polydipsia, polyuria, and polyphagia are also quite commonly displayed at moderate to high serum levels and may falsely infer a diagnosis of Cushing's disease; limiting intake of both food and water usually controls these signs. Sedation and/or ataxia often become significant concerns as serum levels reach the higher ends of the therapeutic range. Rarely, anemia, thrombocytopenia or neutropenia may occur which are reversible if detected early. Increases in liver enzymes are well described for phenobarbital in dogs and are not necessarily indicative of liver dysfunction, but if serum ALT or ALP is >4-5X the upper limit of normal, or if any elevation of AST and GGT are noted, it should raise concern. Phenobarbital should generally be discontinued if any increases in serum bilirubin, total serum bile acids or hypoalbuminemia are seen. Frank hepatic failure is uncommon and is usually associated with higher serum levels (>30-40 micrograms/mL).

Phenobarbital may rarely cause superficial necrolytic dermatitis (SND) in dogs associated with changes in hepatocytes (severe parenchymal collapse with glycogen-laden hepatocytes and moderate fibrosis sharply demarcated by nodules of normal hepatic parenchyma) distinct from that seen with phenobarbital hepatotoxicity.

Cats may develop ataxia, persistent sedation and lethargy, facial pruritus, polyphagia/weight gain, and polydipsia/polyuria. Rarely, immune-mediated reactions and bone marrow hypoplasia (thrombocytopenia, neutropenia) may be seen. Cats, unlike dogs, apparently do not have the issues of increased liver enzymes. Very high dosages (10 – 40 mg/kg/day) have caused coagulopathies in cats. Phenobarbital can potentially increase the metabolism of cortisol; it has been implicated in contributing to relative adrenal insufficiency.

Although there is much less information regarding its use in horses (and foals in particular), it would generally be expected that adverse effects would mirror those seen in other species.

Reproductive/Nursing Safety

Phenobarbital has been associated with rare congenital defects and bleeding problems in newborns, but may be safer than other anticonvulsants. In humans, the FDA categorizes this drug as category **D** for use during pregnancy (*There is evidence of human fetal risk, but the potential benefits from the use of the drug in pregnant women may be acceptable despite its potential risks.*) In a separate system evaluating the safety of drugs in canine and feline pregnancy (Papich 1989), this drug is categorized as class: **B** (*Safe for use if used cautiously. Studies in laboratory animals may have uncovered some risk, but these drugs appear to be safe in dogs and cats or these drugs are safe if they are not administered when the animal is near term.*)

Exercise caution when administering to a nursing mother since small amounts are excreted in maternal milk. Drowsiness in nursing offspring has been reported.

Overdosage/Acute Toxicity

There were 693 single agent exposures to phenobarbital reported to the ASPCA Animal Poison Control Center (APCC) during 2009-2013. Of the 613 dogs, 269 were symptomatic with 58% being ataxic, 55% lethargic/sedated, 13% hypothermic and 11% recumbent. Of the 80 cats, 41 were symptomatic with 68% ataxic, 32% lethargic/sedated and 10% hypothermic or mydriatic.

Treatment of a phenobarbital overdose consists of removal of ingested product from the gut, if appropriate, and giving respiratory and cardiovascular support. Activated charcoal has been demonstrated to be of considerable benefit in enhancing the clearance of phenobarbital, even when the drug was administered parenterally. Charcoal acts as a "sink" for the drug to diffuse from the vasculature back into the gut. Forced alkaline diuresis can also be of substantial benefit in augmenting the elimination of phenobarbital in patients with normal renal function. Peritoneal dialysis or hemodialysis may be helpful in severe intoxications or in anuric patients.

Drug Interactions

The following drug interactions have either been reported or are theoretical in humans or animals receiving phenobarbital and may be of significance in veterinary patients. Unless otherwise noted, use together is not necessarily contraindicated, but weigh the potential risks and perform additional monitoring when appropriate.

- **ACETAMINOPHEN:** Increased risk for hepatotoxicity, particularly when large or chronic doses of barbiturates are given.
- **CARPROFEN:** There may be an increased risk for hepatotoxicity secondary to carprofen metabolites. One source states: Patients should not receive phenobarbital or other hepatic drug metabolizing enzyme inducers when receiving this drug (Boothe 2005).
- **MONAMINE OXIDASE (MAO) INHIBITORS** (*e.g.*, **amitraz**, possibly **selegiline**): May prolong phenobarbital effects.
- **PHENYTOIN:** Barbiturates may affect the metabolism of phenytoin, and phenytoin may alter barbiturate levels; monitoring of blood levels may be indicated.
- **RIFAMPIN:** May induce enzymes that increase the metabolism of barbiturates.

The following drugs may <u>increase the effects</u> of phenobarbital:
- **ANTIHISTAMINES**
- **CHLORAMPHENICOL**
- **FELBAMATE**
- **OPIATES**
- **PHENOTHIAZINES**
- **URINARY ACIDIFIERS** (*e.g.*, ammonium chloride): Unchanged phenobarbital elimination in urine may be decreased with a resultant increase in serum half-life. (Fukunaga *et al.* 2008)
- **VALPROIC ACID**

Phenobarbital (particularly after chronic therapy) may <u>decrease the effects</u> of the following drugs/drug classes by lowering their serum concentrations:
- **ANTICOAGULANTS, ORAL (WARFARIN)**
- **BETA-BLOCKERS**
- **CHLORAMPHENICOL**
- **CLONAZEPAM**
- **CORTICOSTEROIDS**
- **CYCLOSPORINE**
- **DOXORUBICIN**
- **DOXYCYCLINE** (may persist for weeks after barbiturate discontinued).
- **ESTROGENS**

- **FELBAMATE:** Phenobarbital levels may increase and felbamate levels decrease.
- **GRISEOFULVIN**
- **ITRACONAZOLE**
- **LAMOTRIGINE**
- **LEVETIRACETAM:** In dogs, 21 days of phenobarbital reduced levetiracetam elimination half-life by ≈ 50%; 3.43 hrs to 1.73 hours. (Moore *et al.* 2009)
- **LEVOTHYROXINE**
- **MEDROXYPROGESTERONE**
- **METHADONE**
- **METRONIDAZOLE**
- **QUINIDINE**
- **PAROXETINE**
- **PHENOTHIAZINES**
- **PRAZIQUANTEL**
- **PROGESTINS**
- **THEOPHYLLINE**
- **TOPIRAMATE**
- **TRICYCLIC ANTIDEPRESSANTS**
- **URINARY ALKALINZERS** (*e.g.*, **potassium citrate**): Unchanged phenobarbital elimination in urine may be increased with a resultant decrease in serum half-life. (Fukunaga *et al.* 2008)
- **VALPROIC ACID** (may also increase risk for phenobarbital toxicity)
- **VERAPAMIL**
- **WARFARIN**
- **ZONISAMIDE** (Orito *et al.* 2008)

Laboratory Considerations

- Barbiturates may cause increased retention of **bromosulfophthalein** (BSP; sulfobromophthalein) and give falsely elevated results. It is recommended that barbiturates not be administered within the 24 hours before BSP retention tests or, if they must, (*e.g.*, for seizure control) the results be interpreted accordingly.
- Phenobarbital can alter **thyroid** testing. Decreased total and free T4, normal T3, and either normal or increased TSH have been reported. It has been suggested to wait at least 4 weeks after discontinuing phenobarbital to perform thyroid testing.
- In some dogs, phenobarbital may cause a false positive low dose **dexamethasone suppression test**, by increasing the clearance of dexamethasone. Phenobarbital apparently has no effect either on ACTH stimulation tests or on the hormonal equilibrium of the adrenal axis. As phenobarbital can potentially increase the metabolism of cortisol, it has been implicated in contributing to relative adrenal insufficiency.

Doses

- **DOGS:**

  For treatment of idiopathic epilepsy (extra-label): For initial therapy, dosage recommendations vary somewhat but usually are 2.5 – 3 mg/kg PO q12h. To achieve therapeutic levels sooner in dogs that are not receiving phenobarbital, some suggest an initial IV loading dose of 12 – 24 mg/kg (once). One source (Munana 2013) administers an initial dose of 12 mg/kg IV, followed by 2 – 4 mg/kg increments every 20-30 minutes to effect, with a maximum dose of 24 mg/kg . Adjust dosage based on drug levels, efficacy and adverse effects.

  For adjunctive treatment of status epilepticus (extra-label): After using benzodiazepines (diazepam, midazolam), phenobarbital at 5 – 8 mg/kg IV; continue to administer every 4-6 hours

until seizures are under control regardless of additional therapy. (Knipe 2009)

  For sialadenosis (extra-label): From a case report of sialadenosis after removal of an esophageal body: 1 mg/kg PO q12h. After 3 months, dog was slowly weaned off phenobarbital. (Gilor *et al.* 2010)

- **CATS:**

  Treatment of idiopathic epilepsy (extra-label): For initial therapy, dosage recommendations vary somewhat and range from 1 – 3 mg/kg PO q12h. No clear evidence supports any given dosage recommendation. Practically ½ – one 15 mg tablet per cat q12h is used. To achieve therapeutic levels sooner in cats that are not receiving phenobarbital (phenobarbital-naïve), some suggest an initial IV loading dose of 12 – 24 mg/kg (3– 4 mg/kg IV q20 minutes). Adjust dosage based on drug levels, efficacy and adverse effects.

  For adjunctive treatment of status epilepticus (extra-label): Emergency seizure control involves intravenous diazepam (0.5 mg/kg up to 3 doses), along with phenobarbital 3 mg/kg IV. Phenobarbital may be repeated every 20 minutes up to 24 mg/kg in a 24-hour period, or it can be given as a "loading" of 10 mg/kg IV bolus. (Abramson 2009)

  For sedation & controlling excessive feline vocalization for situational distress (*e.g.*, riding in automobiles); (extra-label): 2 – 3 mg/kg PO as needed. (Overall 2000)

- **FERRETS:**

  For seizures (extra-label): Loading dose of 16 – 20 mg/kg once IV; maintenance dose of 1 – 2 mg/kg PO q8-12h. (Knipe 2006), (Knipe 2009)

- **CATTLE:**

  For enzyme induction in organochlorine toxicity (extra-label): 5 grams PO for 3-4 weeks, off 3-4 weeks, then repeat for 3-4 more weeks. (Smith 1986)

- **HORSES: (NOTE: ARCI UCGFS CLASS 2 DRUG)**

  For seizures (extra-label): <u>Adult horses</u>: Loading dose of 16 – 20 mg/kg once IV; maintenance dose of 1 – 5 mg/kg PO twice daily. <u>Foals</u>: Loading dose of 16 – 20 mg/kg once IV; maintenance dose of 100 – 500 mg (total dose) PO twice daily. (Knipe 2006), (Knipe 2009)

Monitoring

- Anticonvulsant (or sedative) efficacy.
- Adverse effects (CNS related, PU/PD, weight gain).
- Serum phenobarbital levels. If phenobarbital was not "loaded", wait at least 5-6 half-lives (≈ 12-14 days in dogs and 9-10 days in cats) before measuring serum concentrations to confirm that therapeutic levels have been reached; time of sampling does not appear to be significant. Some recommend that all dogs have phenobarbital levels monitored once or twice a year and cats monitored every 6 months; consider re-checking levels more often if adverse reactions or reduced efficacy occurs. Although there is some disagreement, therapeutic serum levels in dogs and cats are thought to be similar to those in humans (15-45 mcg/mL; 65-194 mMol/L). A retrospective study of 30 cats found that 93% of cats had seizures controlled with a serum phenobarbital level between 15-45 mcg/mL (Finnerty *et al.* 2014). Optimum therapeutic levels of 23-30 mcg/mL (100-130 mMol/L) have been recommended in cats in an attempt to maximize seizure control with the lowest potential for side effects. Similarly, serum levels of 20-35 mcg/mL (86-150 mMol/L) have been recommended in dogs, with the decrease in the high end of the range reflecting suggested changes to minimize the potential for hepatotoxicity

(Munana 2010). Animals receiving both bromides and phenobarbital may require lower serum levels for seizure control.

- If used chronically, routine CBC's, liver enzymes (especially ALT and AST), and bilirubin at least every 6 months.

Client Information

- May give with or without food. If your animal vomits or acts sick after getting it on an empty stomach, give with food or small treat to see if this helps. If vomiting continues, contact your veterinarian.
- Do not skip doses; try to give doses at the same time each day.
- Sedation (sleepiness, lack of energy), greater thirst, appetite and need to urinate occur commonly when starting therapy.
- Liver problems in dogs can occur.
- Controlled drug in USA. It is against federal law to use, give away or sell this medication to others than for whom it was prescribed.

Chemistry/Synonyms

Phenobarbital, a barbiturate, occurs as white, glistening, odorless, small crystals or a white, crystalline powder with a melting point of 174°-178°C and a pK_a of 7.41. One gram is soluble in ≈ 1000 mL of water; 10 mL of alcohol. Compared to other barbiturates it has a low-lipid solubility.

Phenobarbital sodium occurs as bitter-tasting, white, odorless, flaky crystals or crystalline granules or powder. It is very soluble in water, soluble in alcohol, and freely soluble in propylene glycol. The injectable product has a pH of 8.5-10.5.

SI units (mMol/L) are multiplied by 0.232 to convert phenobarbital levels to conventional units (micrograms/mL); conversely, multiply conventional units by 4.31 to obtain SI units .

Phenobarbital may also be known as fenobarbital, phenemalum, phenobarbitalum, phenobarbitone, phenylethylbarbituric acid, phenylethylmalonylurea, *Luminal Sodium®* or *Solfoton®*.

Storage/Stability

Phenobarbital tablets should be stored in tight, light-resistant containers at room temperature (15-30°C); protect from moisture.

Phenobarbital elixir should be stored in tight containers at 20-20°C.

Phenobarbital sodium injection should be stored at room temperature (15-30°C).

Aqueous solutions of phenobarbital are not very stable. Propylene glycol is often used in injectable products to help stabilize the solution. Solutions of phenobarbital sodium should not be added to acidic solutions nor used if they contain a precipitate or are grossly discolored.

Compatibility/Compounding Considerations

The following solutions and drugs have been reported to be physically **compatible** with phenobarbital sodium: Dextrose IV solutions, Ringer's injection, lactated Ringer's injection, Saline IV solutions, dextrose-saline combinations, dextrose-Ringer's combinations, dextrose-Ringer's lactate combinations, amikacin sulfate, aminophylline, atropine sulfate (stable for at least 15 minutes, but not 24 hours), calcium chloride and gluconate, dimenhydrinate, polymyxin B sulfate, sodium bicarbonate, thiopental sodium, and verapamil HCl.

The following drugs have been reported to be physically **incompatible** with phenobarbital sodium: chlorpromazine HCl, codeine phosphate, ephedrine sulfate, fentanyl citrate, glycopyrrolate, hydralazine HCl, hydrocortisone sodium succinate, hydroxyzine HCl, insulin (regular), meperidine HCl, morphine sulfate, nalbuphine HCl, norepinephrine bitartrate, oxytetracycline HCl, pentazocine lactate, procaine HCl, prochlorperazine edisylate, promazine HCl, and promethazine HCl. Compatibility is dependent upon factors such as pH, concentration, temperature, and diluent used; consult

specialized references or a hospital pharmacist for more specific information.

Dosage Forms/Regulatory Status

VETERINARY-LABELED PRODUCTS: NONE.

The ARCI (Racing Commissioners International) has designated this drug as a class 2 substance. See the appendix for more information.

HUMAN-LABELED PRODUCTS:

Phenobarbital Tablets: 15 mg, 16.2 mg, 30 mg, 60 mg, 90 mg, & 100 mg; *Solfoton®*, generic; (Rx, C-IV)

Phenobarbital Elixir/Oral solution: 20 mg/5mL (4 mg/mL); generic; (Rx, C-IV)

Phenobarbital Sodium Injection: 65 mg/mL & 130 mg/mL; *Luminal Sodium®*, generic; (Rx; C-IV)

Revisions/References

Monograph revised/updated May 2014.

Abramson, C. J. (2009). Feline Neurology I. Proceedings: WVC. accessed via Veterinary Information Network; vin.com

Boothe, D. M. (2005). New information on nonsteroidal antiinflammatories: What every criticalist must know. Proceedings: IVECC. accessed via Veterinary Information Network; vin.com

Finnerty, K. E., et al. (2014). Evaluation of therapeutic phenobarbital concentrations and application of a classification system for seizures in cats: 30 cases (2004-2013). Javma-Journal of the American Veterinary Medical Association 244(2): 195-9.

Fukunaga, K., et al. (2008). Effects of urine pH modification on pharmacokinetics of phenobarbital in healthy dogs. J. Vet. Pharmacol. Ther. 31(5): 431-6.

Gilor, C., et al. (2010). Phenobarbital-Responsive Sialadenosis Associated With an Esophageal Foreign Body in a Dog. J. Am. Anim. Hosp. Assoc. 46(2): 115-20.

Knipe, M. (2006). The essential guide to seizures. Proceedings; Vet Neuro Symposium. accessed via Veterinary Information Network; vin.com

Knipe, M. (2009). The short and long of seizure management. Proceedings: UCD Veterinary Neurology Symposium. accessed via Veterinary Information Network; vin.com

Moore, S., et al. (2009). The Pharmacokinetics of Levetiracetam in Dogs Concurrently Receiving Phenobarbital. Proceedings: ACVIM. accessed via Veterinary Information Network; vin.com

Munana, K. (2010). Current Approaches to Seizure Management. Proceedings: ACVIM Forum. accessed via Veterinary Information Network; vin.com

Munana, K. R. (2013). Update Seizure Management in Small Animal Practice. Veterinary Clinics of North America-Small Animal Practice 43(5): 1127-+.

Orito, K., et al. (2008). Pharmacokinetics of zonisamide and drug interaction with phenobarbital in dogs. J. Vet. Pharmacol. Ther. 31(3): 259-64.

Overall, K. (2000). Behavioral Pharmacology. Proceedings: American Animal Hospital Association 67th Annual Meeting, Toronto. accessed via Veterinary Information Network; vin.com

Papich, M. (1989). Effects of drugs on pregnancy. *Current Veterinary Therapy X: Small Animal Practice*. R. Kirk. Philadelphia, Saunders: 1291-9.

Smith, J. A. (1986). Toxic encephalopathies in cattle. *Current Veterinary Therapy 2: Food Animal Practice*. J. L. Howard. Philadelphia, WB Saunders: 855-63.

Phenoxybenzamine HCl

(fen-ox-ee-**ben**-za-meen)   Dibenzyline®

Alpha-Adrenergic Blocker

Prescriber Highlights

▶ Alpha-adrenergic blocker used primarily in small animals for detrusor areflexia, and pheochromocytoma (hypertension).

▶ Contraindications: When hypotension would be deleterious; possibly glaucoma or diabetes mellitus, horses with clinical signs of colic. Caution: CHF or other heart disease, renal damage, or cerebral/coronary arteriosclerosis.

▶ Adverse Effects: Hypotension, hypertension (rebound), miosis, increased intraocular pressure, tachycardia, inhibition of ejaculation, nasal congestion, weakness/dizziness, and GI effects (*e.g.*, nausea, vomiting). Constipation may occur in horses.

▶ Availability and cost can be issues; may need to be obtained from compounding pharmacy.

▶ Drug Interactions.

Uses/Indications

Phenoxybenzamine is used primarily for its effect in reducing internal urethral sphincter tone when urethral sphincter hypertonus is present. It can also be used to treat the hypertension associated with pheochromocytoma prior to surgery or as adjunctive therapy in endotoxicosis.

Phenoxybenzamine has been anecdotally reported to increase acupuncture effectiveness.

In horses, phenoxybenzamine has been used to decrease urethral sphincter tone with bladder paresis. It has also been tried for preventing or treating laminitis in its early stages, and treating secretory diarrheas.

Pharmacology/Actions

Alpha-adrenergic response to circulating epinephrine or norepinephrine is noncompetitively blocked by phenoxybenzamine. The effect of phenoxybenzamine has been described as a "chemical sympathectomy." No effects on beta-adrenergic receptors or on the parasympathetic nervous system occur.

Phenoxybenzamine causes cutaneous blood flow to increase, but little effect is noted on skeletal or cerebral blood flow. Phenoxybenzamine can also block pupillary dilation, lid retraction, and nictitating membrane contraction. Both standing and supine blood pressures are decreased in humans.

Pharmacokinetics

No information was located on the pharmacokinetics of this agent in veterinary species. In humans, phenoxybenzamine is variably absorbed from the GI, with a bioavailability of 20-30%. Onset of action of the drug is slow (several hours) and increases over several days after regular dosing. Effects persist for 3-4 days after discontinuation of the drug.

Phenoxybenzamine is highly lipid soluble and may accumulate in body fat. It is unknown if it crosses the placenta or is excreted into milk. The serum half-life is ≈ 24 hours in humans. It is metabolized (dealkylated) and excreted in both the urine and bile.

Contraindications/Precautions/Warnings

Phenoxybenzamine is contraindicated in horses with clinical signs of colic and in patients when hypotension would be undesirable (e.g., shock, unless fluid replacement is adequate). One source (Labato 1989) listed glaucoma and diabetes mellitus as contraindications for the use of phenoxybenzamine in dogs.

Phenoxybenzamine should be used with caution in patients with CHF or other heart disease as drug-induced tachycardia can occur. It should be used cautiously in patients with renal damage or cerebral/coronary arteriosclerosis.

Adverse Effects

Adverse effects associated with alpha-adrenergic blockade include: hypotension, weakness/dizziness, GI effects (e.g., nausea, vomiting), miosis, increased intraocular pressure, tachycardia, sodium retention, inhibition of ejaculation, and nasal congestion.

When used in dogs for controlling hypertension prior to surgery for pheochromocytoma, phenoxybenzamine can cause prolonged postoperative hypotension; volume expansion may be required. Increased preoperative sodium intake has been suggested in human medicine.

Additionally, phenoxybenzamine can cause constipation in horses.

Reproductive/Nursing Safety

Phenoxybenzamine has been shown to cause abnormalities in the closure of the patent ductus in guinea pigs. In humans, the FDA categorizes this drug as category C for use during pregnancy (*Animal studies have shown an adverse effect on the fetus, but there are no adequate studies in humans; or there are no animal reproduction studies and no adequate studies in humans.*)

It is unknown if phenoxybenzamine is excreted into milk.

Overdosage/Acute Toxicity

Overdosage of phenoxybenzamine may yield signs of postural hypotension (dizziness, syncope), tachycardia, vomiting, lethargy, or shock.

Treatment should consist of emptying the gut if the ingestion was recent and there are no contraindications to those procedures. Hypotension can be treated with fluid support. Epinephrine is contraindicated (see Drug Interactions) and most vasopressor drugs are ineffective in reversing the effects of alpha-blockade. Intravenous norepinephrine (levarterenol) may be beneficial, however, if clinical signs are severe.

Drug Interactions

The following drug interactions have either been reported or are theoretical in humans or animals receiving phenoxybenzamine and may be of significance in veterinary patients. Unless otherwise noted, use together is not necessarily contraindicated, but weigh the potential risks and perform additional monitoring when appropriate.

- **EPINEPHRINE**: If used with drugs that have both alpha- and beta-adrenergic effects increased hypotension, vasodilatation or tachycardia may result.
- **PHENYLEPHRINE**: Phenoxybenzamine will antagonize the effects of alpha-adrenergic sympathomimetic agents.
- **RESERPINE**: Phenoxybenzamine can antagonize the hypothermic effects of reserpine.

Doses

- **DOGS:**

  To treat functional urethral obstruction by decreasing sympathetic-mediated urethral tone (extra-label): A common dosage recommendation is 0.25 mg/kg PO q12h, or practically 5 – 20 mg per dog PO q12h.

  Treatment of hypertension associated with pheochromocytoma (extra-label): Initially 0.25 – 0.5 mg/kg PO q12h. Dosage is gradually increased to a maximum of 2.5 mg/kg PO q12h or until clinical signs of hypotension (e.g., lethargy, weakness, syncope), adverse effects (e.g., vomiting) occur. Continue until surgery; close monitoring during the perioperative period is critical for a successful outcome.

- **CATS:**

  To treat functional urethral obstruction by decreasing sympathetic-mediated urethral tone (extra-label): A common dosage recommendation is 2.5 – 7.5 mg per cat PO once to twice a day.

- **HORSES:** (NOTE: ARCI UCGFS CLASS 3 DRUG)

  To decrease urethral sphincter tone in horses with bladder paresis (extra-label): 0.7 mg/kg PO 4 times a day (in combination with bethanechol at 0.25 – 0.75 mg/kg PO 2-4 times a day). (Schott II et al. 2003)

Monitoring

- Clinical efficacy (adequate urination, etc.).
- Efficacy for urinary problems may take a week or longer and the drug should be given for several weeks before determining it is not effective.
- Blood pressure.

Client Information

- May be given with or without food.
- Can cause GI effects (e.g., vomiting, diarrhea in small animals; constipation in horses), rapid heartbeat, pinpoint/tiny pupils, and runny nose.
- If your animal faints or collapses while receiving this medication, contact your veterinarian immediately.

Chemistry/Synonyms

An alpha-adrenergic blocking agent, phenoxybenzamine HCl occurs as an odorless, white crystalline powder with a melting range of 136°-141°C and a pK$_a$ of 4.4. Approximately 40 mg are soluble in 1 mL of water and 167 mg are soluble in 1 mL of alcohol.

Phenoxybenzamine may also be known as: SKF-688A, *Dibenyline®*, *Dibenzyran®*, or *Fenoxene®*.

Storage/Stability

Phenoxybenzamine capsules should be stored at room temperature in well-closed containers.

Dosage Forms/Regulatory Status

VETERINARY-LABELED PRODUCTS: NONE.

The ARCI (Racing Commissioners International) has designated this drug as a class 3 substance. See the appendix for more information.

HUMAN-LABELED PRODUCTS:

Phenoxybenzamine HCl Capsules: 10 mg; *Dibenzyline®*; (Rx)

Revisions/References

Monograph revised/updated May 2014.

Labato, M. A. (1989). Disorders of Micturation. *Handbook of Small Animal Practice*. R. V. Morgan. New York, Churchill Livingstone: 621-8.

Schott II, H. & E. Carr (2003). Urinary incontinence in horses. Proceedings: ACVIM Forum. accessed via Veterinary Information Network; vin.com

Phenylbutazone

(fen-ill-**byoo**-ta-zone)   Butazolidin®, *"Bute"*

Non-Steroidal Antiinflammatory Agent

Prescriber Highlights

▶ NSAID used primarily in horses; little reason to use in dogs today. Banned in dairy cattle.

▶ Contraindications: Known hypersensitivity, history of or preexisting hematologic or bone marrow abnormalities, preexisting GI ulcers, in food producing animals.

▶ Caution: Foals or ponies, preexisting renal disease, CHF, other drug allergies.

▶ Adverse Effects: **Horses:** Oral & GI erosions & ulcers, hypoalbuminemia, diarrhea, anorexia, & renal effects. **Dogs:** GI ulceration, sodium & water retention, diminished renal blood flow, blood dyscrasias.

▶ Do not give IM or SC; IA injections may cause seizures.

▶ Drug Interactions; lab interactions.

Uses/Indications

Phenylbutazone is a nonsteroidal antiinflammatory agent (NSAID) that is used primarily for treating pain and inflammation in horses. It has been used in other species (dogs, cattle, swine, etc.) but generally other NSAIDs are preferred.

Pharmacology/Actions

Phenylbutazone has analgesic, antiinflammatory, antipyretic, and mild uricosuric properties. The proposed mechanism of action is by the inhibition of cyclooxygenase, thereby reducing prostaglandin synthesis. Other pharmacologic actions phenylbutazone may induce include reduced renal blood flow and decreased glomerular filtration rate, decreased platelet aggregation, and gastric mucosal damage.

Pharmacokinetics

Following oral administration, phenylbutazone is absorbed from both the stomach and small intestine. The drug is distributed throughout the body with highest levels attained in the liver, heart, lungs, kidneys, and blood. Plasma protein binding in horses ex-

ceeds 99%. Both phenylbutazone and oxyphenbutazone cross the placenta and are excreted into milk.

The serum half-life in the horse ranges from 3.5-6 hours and, like aspirin is dose-dependent. Therapeutic efficacy, however, may last for more than 24 hours, probably due to the irreversible binding of phenylbutazone to cyclooxygenase. In horses and other species, phenylbutazone is nearly completely metabolized, primarily to oxyphenbutazone (active) and gamma-hydroxyphenylbutazone. Oxyphenbutazone has been detected in horse urine up to 48 hours after a single dose. Phenylbutazone is more rapidly excreted into alkaline than acidic urine.

Other serum half-lives reported for animals are: Cattle ≈ 40-55 hrs; Dogs ≈ 2.5-6 hrs; Swine ≈ 2-6 hrs.; Rabbits ≈ 3 hrs.

Contraindications/Precautions/Warnings

Phenylbutazone is contraindicated in patients with a history of or preexisting hematologic or bone marrow abnormalities, preexisting GI ulcers, and in food producing animals or lactating dairy cattle. Cautious use in both foals and ponies is recommended because of increased incidences of hypoproteinemia and GI ulceration. Foals with a heavy parasite burden or that are undernourished may be more susceptible to developing adverse effects.

Avoid use in horses with known or suspected EGUS; single doses of phenylbutazone will probably not result in catastrophic consequences, but repeated doses can exacerbate gastric ulcers (Videla *et al.* 2009).

Phenylbutazone may cause decreased renal blood flow and sodium and water retention; use cautiously in animals with preexisting renal disease or CHF.

Because phenylbutazone may mask clinical signs of lameness in horses for several days following therapy, unethical individuals may use it to disguise lameness for "soundness" exams. States may have different standards regarding the use of phenylbutazone in track animals. Complete elimination of phenylbutazone in horses may take 2 months and it can be detected in the urine for at least 7 days following administration. Phenylbutazone is contraindicated in patients demonstrating previous hypersensitivity reactions to it, and should be used very cautiously in patients with a history of allergies to other drugs.

Do not administer injectable preparation IM or SC; very irritating (swelling, to necrosis and sloughing). Intracarotid injections may cause CNS stimulation and seizures.

Phenylbutazone is labeled for use in horses that are not to be used for food. A recent, thorough evaluation of phenylbutazone residues and toxicology in humans and horses concluded that the illegal and erratic presence of trace amount residues of phenylbutazone in horse meat is not a public health issue (Lees *et al.* 2013).

Adverse Effects

While phenylbutazone is apparently a safer drug to use in horses and dogs than in people, serious adverse reactions can still occur. Toxic effects that have been reported in horses include oral and GI erosions and ulcers, hypoalbuminemia, diarrhea—right dorsal colitis, anorexia, and renal effects (azotemia, renal papillary necrosis). Unlike humans, it does not appear that phenylbutazone causes much sodium and water retention in horses at usual doses, but edema has been reported. In dogs, however, phenylbutazone may cause sodium and water retention and diminished renal blood flow. Phenylbutazone-induced blood dyscrasias and hepatotoxicity have also been reported in dogs.

Although gastric ulceration is frequently observed in adult horses and foals, evidence of an association between this disease and administration of NSAIDs such as phenylbutazone or flunixin at recommended dosages is lacking. On the basis of current evidence, prophylactic anti-ulcer medications for horses receiving therapeutic doses of NSAIDs is probably unnecessary in patients that are otherwise at low risk for gastric ulceration (Fennell *et al.* 2009).

IM or SC injection can cause swelling, necrosis and sloughing. Intracarotid injections may cause CNS stimulation and seizures.

Therapy should be halted at first signs of any toxic reactions (*e.g.*, anorexia, oral lesions, depression, reduced plasma proteins, increased serum creatinine or BUN, leukopenia, or anemias). The use of sucralfate or the H$_2$ blockers (*e.g.*, ranitidine, etc.) have been suggested for use in treating the GI effects. Misoprostol, a prostaglandin E analog, may also be useful in reducing the gastrointestinal effects of phenylbutazone.

The primary concerns with phenylbutazone therapy in humans include its bone marrow effects (agranulocytosis, aplastic anemia), renal and cardiovascular effects (fluid retention to acute renal failure), and GI effects (dyspepsia to perforated ulcers). Other serious concerns with phenylbutazone include hypersensitivity reactions, neurologic, dermatologic, and hepatic toxicities.

Reproductive/Nursing Safety

Although phenylbutazone has shown no direct teratogenic effects, rodent studies have demonstrated reduced litter sizes, increased neonatal mortality, and increased stillbirth rates. Phenylbutazone should, therefore, be used in pregnancy only when the potential benefits of therapy outweigh the risks associated with it.

In a system evaluating the safety of drugs in canine and feline pregnancy (Papich 1989), this drug is categorized as class: *C (These drugs may have potential risks. Studies in people or laboratory animals have uncovered risks, and these drugs should be used cautiously as a last resort when the benefit of therapy clearly outweighs the risks.)*

The safety of phenylbutazone during nursing has not been determined; use with caution.

Overdosage/Acute Toxicity

Manifestations (human) of acute overdosage with phenylbutazone include a prompt respiratory or metabolic acidosis with compensatory hyperventilation, seizures, coma, and acute hypotensive crisis. In an acute overdose, clinical signs of renal failure (oliguric, with proteinuria and hematuria), liver injury (hepatomegaly and jaundice), bone marrow depression, and ulceration (and perforation) of the GI tract may develop. Other symptoms reported in humans include: nausea, vomiting, abdominal pain, diaphoresis, neurologic and psychiatric symptoms, edema, hypertension, respiratory depression, and cyanosis.

There were 27 exposures to phenylbutazone reported to the ASPCA Animal Poison Control Center (APCC) during 2008-2009. In these cases 24 were dogs with 10 showing clinical signs, and 2 were equines with 1 showing clinical signs. The remaining reported case consisted of 1 cat that did not show any clinical signs. Common findings in dogs recorded in decreasing frequency included ataxia, seizures, tachycardia, trembling, and tremors.

Most common clinical signs in dogs (per unpublished APCC data) are tremors, seizures, ataxia, vomiting, and tachypnea. Oral LD50 in dogs is 332mg/kg (per RTECS 1988). Most common clinical signs in horses (per unpublished APCC data) are colic, anorexia, and ataxia.

Standard overdose procedures should be followed (empty gut following oral ingestion, etc.). Supportive treatment should be instituted as necessary and intravenous diazepam used to help control seizures. Monitor fluid therapy carefully, as phenylbutazone may cause fluid retention.

Drug Interactions

The following drug interactions have either been reported or are theoretical in humans or animals receiving phenylbutazone and may be of significance in veterinary patients. Unless otherwise not-

ed, use together is not necessarily contraindicated, but weigh the potential risks and perform additional monitoring when appropriate.

- **FUROSEMIDE**: Phenylbutazone may antagonize the increased renal blood flow effects caused by furosemide.
- **HEPATOTOXIC DRUGS**: Phenylbutazone administered concurrently with hepatotoxic drugs may increase the chances of hepatotoxicity developing.
- **NSAIDS**: Concurrent use with other NSAIDs may increase the potential for adverse reactions, however, some clinicians routinely use phenylbutazone concomitantly with flunixin in horses. One study did not show synergistic actions with flunixin, but did however, when phenylbutazone and ketoprofen were "stacked".
- **PENICILLAMINE**: May increase the risk of hematologic and/or renal adverse reactions.
- **PENICILLIN G**: Phenylbutazone may increase plasma half-life of penicillin G.
- **SULFONAMIDES**: Phenylbutazone could potentially displace sulfonamides from plasma proteins; increasing the risk for adverse effects.
- **WARFARIN**: Phenylbutazone could potentially displace warfarin from plasma proteins; increasing the risk for bleeding.

Laboratory Considerations

- Phenylbutazone and oxyphenbutazone may interfere with **thyroid function tests** by competing with thyroxine at protein binding sites or by inhibiting thyroid iodine uptake. Interpretation of thyroid function tests may be complicated.

Doses

- **DOGS:**

Note: With the release of safer FDA-approved NSAIDs, it is the author's (Plumb) opinion that there is little reason to use this drug in dogs today. Phenylbutazone tablets have had a labeled dosage at 14 mg/kg PO 3 times daily initially (maximum of 800 mg/day regardless of weight), titrate dose to lowest effective dose.

- **HORSES:**

Labeled dose (FDA-approved): 1 – 2 grams IV per 454 kg (1000 lb.) horse. Injection should be made slowly and with care. Limit IV administration to no more than 5 successive days of therapy. Follow with oral forms if necessary; or 2 – 4 grams PO per 454 kg (1000 lb.) horse. Do not exceed 4 grams/day. Use high end of dosage range initially, then titrate to lowest effective dose. (Package Insert; *Butazolidin®*)

Extra-label dose: Oral: 4.4 mg/kg q12h initially, followed by 2.2 mg/kg PO q12h. For maintenance, use the lowest dose required to produce the desired clinical response. IV: 2.2 – 4.4 mg/kg q12h. The dose is reduced after the first 48-96 hours. Administration should be limited to a maximum of 5 successive days. Oral administration may follow. (USPC 1990)

- **RUMINANTS:**

Note: The Food and Drug Administration (FDA) has issued an order prohibiting the extra-label use of phenylbutazone in female dairy cattle 20 months of age or older. In the USA there is zero tolerance for phenylbutazone residues in any edible tissue from any animal and many believe that phenylbutazone use in any food animal should be banned. FARAD has recommended a 55-60 day withdrawal interval following chronic oral administration (>10 days), and a minimum withdrawal interval of 55 days following IM in beef cattle (Smith 2013).

For surgical pain (extra-label; see above): 5 mg/kg PO q24-48h; 10 mg/kg PO q48-72h. (Anderson *et al.* 2013)

Monitoring

- Analgesic/antiinflammatory/antipyretic effect.
- Regular complete blood counts with chronic therapy (especially in dogs). The manufacturer recommends weekly CBC's early in therapy, and biweekly with chronic therapy.
- Urinalysis &/or renal function parameters (serum creatinine/BUN) with chronic therapy.
- Plasma protein determinations, especially in ponies, foals, and debilitated animals.

Client Information

For Horses:

- Give with food when given by mouth.
- Injections must only be in the vein (IV).
- Side effects can include: Mouth/stomach ulcers, kidney damage, loss of appetite, swelling/edema.

Chemistry/Synonyms

A synthetic pyrazolone derivative related chemically to aminopyrine, phenylbutazone occurs as a white to off-white, odorless crystalline powder that has a pK_a of 4.5. It is very slightly soluble in water and 1 gram will dissolve in 28 mL of alcohol. It is tasteless at first, but has a slightly bitter after-taste.

Phenylbutazone may also be known as: butadiene, fenilbutazona, bute, phenylbutazonum, or phenylbute.

Storage/Stability

Oral products should be stored in tight, child-resistant containers if possible. The injectable product should be stored in a cool place (46-56° F) or kept refrigerated.

Dosage Forms/Regulatory Status

VETERINARY-LABELED PRODUCTS:

Note: The Food and Drug Administration (FDA) has issued an order prohibiting the extra-label use of phenylbutazone animal and human drugs in female dairy cattle 20 months of age or older.

Phenylbutazone Tablets: 100 mg & 200 mg; many trade name and generic products available. FDA-approved for use in dogs. (Rx)

Phenylbutazone Tablets: 1 gram; many trade name and generic products available. (Rx). FDA-approved for use in horses. Not to be used in animals used for food.

Phenylbutazone Oral Powder: 1 gram in 10 grams of powder to be mixed into feed. *Phenylbute® Powder*; (Rx). Labeled for use in horses.

Phenylbutazone Paste Oral Syringes: containing 6 grams or 12 grams/syringe: Many trade name and generic products available. FDA-approved for use in horses not intended for food purposes. (Rx)

Phenylbutazone Injection: 200 mg/mL in 100 mL vials: Many trade name and generic products available. FDA-approved for use in horses. Not to be used in horses intended for food. (Rx)

HUMAN APPROVED PRODUCTS: NONE.

Revisions/References

Monograph revised/updated May 2014.

Anderson, D. E. & M. A. Edmondson (2013). Prevention and Management of Surgical Pain in Cattle. Veterinary Clinics of North America-Food Animal Practice 29(1): 157-+.

Fennell, L. C. & R. P. Franklin (2009). Do nonsteroidal anti-inflammatory drugs administered at therapeutic dosages induce gastric ulcers in horses? Equine Veterinary Education 21(12): 660-2.

Lees, P. & P. L. Toutain (2013). Pharmacokinetics, pharmacodynamics, metabolism, toxicology and residues of phenylbutazone in humans and horses. Veterinary Journal 196(3): 294-303.

Papich, M. (1989). Effects of drugs on pregnancy. *Current Veterinary Therapy X: Small Animal Practice*. R. Kirk. Philadelphia, Saunders: 1291-9.

Smith, G. (2013). Extralabel Use of Anesthetic and Analgesic Compounds in Cattle. Veterinary Clinics of North America-Food Animal Practice 29(1): 29-+.

USPC (1990). Veterinary Information- Appendix III. *Drug Information for the Health Professional*. Rockville, United States Pharmacopeial Convention. 2: 2811- 60.

Videla, R. & F. M. Andrews (2009). New Perspectives in Equine Gastric Ulcer Syndrome. Veterinary Clinics of North America-Equine Practice 25(2): 283-+.

Phenylephrine HCl, Parenteral

(fen-ill-**ef**-rin)   Neo-Synephrine®

Alpha-adrenergic Agonist

Prescriber Highlights

▶ Alpha-adrenergic used parenterally to treat hypotension without overt cardiostimulation.

▶ Contraindications: Severe hypertension, ventricular tachycardia, or hypersensitivity to it. Extreme Caution: Geriatric patients, patients with hyperthyroidism, bradycardia, partial heart block, or other heart disease.

▶ Not a replacement for adequate volume therapy in patients with shock.

▶ Adverse Effects: Reflex bradycardia, CNS effects (excitement, restlessness, headache), & rarely, arrhythmias. Hemorrhage possible in horses.

▶ Blood pressure must be monitored.

▶ Extravasation injuries with phenylephrine can be very serious.

Uses/Indications

Phenylephrine has been used to treat hypotension and shock (after adequate volume replacement), but many clinicians prefer to use an agent that also has cardiostimulatory properties. Phenylephrine is sometimes recommended for use to treat hypotension secondary to drug overdoses or idiosyncratic hypotensive reactions to drugs such as phenothiazines, adrenergic blocking agents, and ganglionic blockers. Its use to treat hypotension resulting from barbiturate or other CNS depressant agents is controversial. Phenylephrine has been used to increase blood pressure to terminate attacks of paroxysmal supraventricular tachycardia, particularly when the patient is also hypotensive. Phenylephrine has been used to treat hypotension and prolong the effects of spinal anesthesia.

In horses, phenylephrine has been used as adjunctive treatment of ascending colon displacement (McGovern *et al.* 2012). But a case series found that pretreatment with phenylephrine did not affect efficacy of rolling technique or surgery for nephrosplenic entrapment of the colon (Baker *et al.* 2011) and another retrospective study found that rolling was more effective than phenylephrine/exercise (Fultz *et al.* 2013).

Ophthalmic uses of phenylephrine include use for some diagnostic eye examinations, reducing posterior synechiae formation, and relieving pain associated with complicated uveitis. It has been applied intranasally in an attempt to reduce nasal congestion.

Pharmacology/Actions

Phenylephrine has predominantly post-synaptic alpha-adrenergic effects at therapeutic doses. At usual doses, it has negligible beta effects, but these can occur at high doses.

Phenylephrine's primary effects, when given intravenously, include peripheral vasoconstriction with resultant increases in diastolic and systolic blood pressures, small decreases in cardiac output, and an increase in circulation time. A reflex bradycardia (blocked by atropine) can occur. Most vascular beds are constricted (renal splanchnic, pulmonary, cutaneous), but coronary blood flow is increased. Its alpha effects can cause contraction of the pregnant uterus and constriction of uterine blood vessels.

Pharmacokinetics

After oral administration, phenylephrine is rapidly metabolized in the GI tract and cardiovascular effects are generally unattainable via this route of administration. Following IV administration, pressor effects begin almost immediately and will persist for up to 20 minutes. The onset of pressor action after IM administration is usually within 10-15 minutes, and will last for ≈ 60 minutes.

It is unknown if phenylephrine is excreted into milk. It is metabolized by the liver, and the effects of the drug are also terminated by uptake into tissues.

Contraindications/Precautions/Warnings

Phenylephrine is contraindicated in patients with severe hypertension, ventricular tachycardia or those who are hypersensitive to it. It should be used with extreme caution in geriatric patients, patients with hyperthyroidism, bradycardia, partial heart block or other heart disease. Phenylephrine is not a replacement for adequate volume therapy in patients with shock.

Adverse Effects

At usual doses, a reflex bradycardia, CNS effects (excitement, restlessness, headache) and, rarely, arrhythmias are seen. Blood pressure must be monitored to prevent hypertension. Hemorrhage is possible in horses (Frederick *et al.* 2010).

Extravasation injuries with phenylephrine can be very serious (necrosis and sloughing of surrounding tissue). Patient's IV sites should be routinely monitored. Should extravasation occur, infiltrate the site (ischemic areas) with a solution of 5 – 10 mg phentolamine (*Regitine*®) in 10-15 mL of normal saline. A syringe with a fine needle should be used to infiltrate the site with many injections.

Reproductive/Nursing Safety

In humans, the FDA categorizes this drug as category C for use during pregnancy (*Animal studies have shown an adverse effect on the fetus, but there are no adequate studies in humans; or there are no animal reproduction studies and no adequate studies in humans.*)

It is not known if these agents are excreted in maternal milk; exercise caution when administering to a nursing patient.

Overdosage/Acute Toxicity

There were 195 exposures to phenylephrine reported to the ASPCA Animal Poison Control Center (APCC) during 2008-2009. In these cases 189 were dogs with 51 showing clinical signs, 5 were cats with 1 showing clinic signs and 1 was a bird that did not show any clinical signs. Common findings in dogs recorded in decreasing frequency included vomiting, lethargy, depression, hyperactivity, and tachycardia.

Overdosage of phenylephrine can cause hypertension, seizures, vomiting, paresthesias, ventricular extrasystoles, and cerebral hemorrhage, but the margin of safety with phenylephrine overdose is fairly wide, especially after oral administration. Vomiting is commonly seen with overdoses. CNS stimulation (agitation, hyperactivity, and muscle tremors) or cardiovascular changes, most commonly tachycardia and hypertension are also seen. Cardiovascular changes often respond well to fluids. Beta-blockers or nitroprusside may be indicated when signs are refractory to fluids.

Drug Interactions

The following drug interactions have either been reported or are theoretical in humans or animals receiving phenylephrine (systemically) and may be of significance in veterinary patients. Unless otherwise noted, use together is not necessarily contraindicated, but weigh the potential risks and perform additional monitoring when appropriate.

- **ALPHA-ADRENERGIC BLOCKERS (phentolamine, phenothiazines, phenoxybenzamine)**: Higher dosages of phenylephrine may be required to attain a pressor effect if these agents have been used prior to therapy.
- **ANESTHETICS, GENERAL (halogenated)**: Phenylephrine potentially may induce cardiac arrhythmias when used with halothane anesthesia.

- **ATROPINE (and other anticholinergics)**: Block the reflex bradycardia caused by phenylephrine.
- **BETA-ADRENERGIC BLOCKERS**: The cardiostimulatory effects of phenylephrine can be blocked.
- **DIGOXIN**: Use with phenylephrine may cause increased myocardium sensitization.
- **MONAMINE OXIDASE (MAO) INHIBITORS** (*e.g.*, **amitraz**, possibly **selegiline**): Monoamine oxidase (MAO) inhibitors should not be used with phenylephrine because of a pronounced pressor effect.
- **OXYTOCIN**: When used concurrently with oxytocic agents, pressor effects may be enhanced.
- **SYMPATHOMIMETIC AGENTS (epinephrine)**: Tachycardia and serious arrhythmias are possible.

Doses

- **DOGS:**

  For hypotension (extra-label): Not commonly used; may be useful when profound vasodilation occurs (*e.g.*, septic shock). As a CRI: Low dose is 1 microgram/kg/min; high dose is 3 micrograms/kg/min. Increases peripheral vascular resistance and mean arterial blood pressure. May see reflex bradycardia, and vasoconstriction can lead to excessive decreases in blood flow to liver, GI tract, and kidneys, although coronary blood flow is increased. (Quandt 2009)

- **CATS:**

  For hypotension (extra-label): When it is advantageous to increase blood pressure by vasoconstriction, phenylephrine may be useful in patients with pronounced systemic vasodilation (*e.g.*, visceral inflammation) or to increase blood pressure when increasing myocardial contractility may be disadvantageous (*e.g.*, hypertrophic cardiomyopathy): 1 – 2 micrograms/kg/minute as a CRI. In this study, infusions of 1 microgram/kg/min significantly increased mean arterial pressure without a change in cardiac output. At 2 micrograms/kg/min, cardiac index also was increased with an increase in stroke volume index. (Pascoe *et al.* 2006)

- **HORSES:** (NOTE: ARCI UCGFS CLASS 3 DRUG)

  For adjunctive medical treatment of ascending (large) colon displacement (extra-label): 3 micrograms/kg/min for 15 minutes; repeated every 12 hours if the horse did not respond. (McGovern *et al.* 2012)

Monitoring

- Cardiac rate/rhythm.
- Blood pressure, and blood gases if possible.

Client Information

- Parenteral phenylephrine should only be used by professionals in a setting where adequate monitoring is possible.

Chemistry/Synonyms

An alpha-adrenergic sympathomimetic amine, phenylephrine HCl occurs as bitter-tasting, odorless, white to nearly white crystals with a melting point of 145-146°C. It is freely soluble in water and alcohol. The pH of the commercially available injection is 3-6.5.

Phenylephrine may also be known as: fenilefrina, phenylephrinum, m-synephrine, or *Neo-Synephrine*®.

Storage/Stability

The injectable product should be stored protected from light. Do not use solutions if they are brown or contain a precipitate. Oxidation of the drug can occur without a color change. To protect against oxidation, the air in commercially available ampules for injection is replaced with nitrogen and a sulfite added.

Compatibility/Compounding Considerations

Phenylephrine is reported to be physically **compatible** with all commonly used IV solutions and the following drugs: chloramphenicol sodium succinate, dobutamine HCl, lidocaine HCl, potassium chloride, and sodium bicarbonate. While stated to be physically **incompatible** with alkalis, it is stable with sodium bicarbonate solutions. Phenylephrine is reported to be **incompatible** with ferric salts, oxidizing agents, and metals.

Dosage Forms/Regulatory Status

VETERINARY-LABELED PRODUCTS:

There are oral combination products marketed as "cough" syrups for veterinary use that contain phenylephrine, pyrilamine (antihistamine), guaifenesin, sodium citrate, and sometimes ammonium chloride.

The ARCI (Racing Commissioners International) has designated this drug as a class 3 substance. See the appendix for more information.

HUMAN-LABELED PRODUCTS:

Phenylephrine HCl Injection: 1% (10 mg/mL); generic; (Rx)

Phenylephrine is also available in oral tablets (*e.g., Sudafed PE®*), oral solutions, ophthalmic and intranasal dosage forms and in combination with antihistamines, analgesics, decongestants, etc., for oral administration.

Revisions/References

Monograph revised/updated May 2014.

Baker, W. T., et al. (2011). Reevaluation of the Effect of Phenylephrine on Resolution of Nephrosplenic Entrapment by the Rolling Procedure in 87 Horses. Veterinary Surgery **40**(7): 825-9.

Frederick, J., et al. (2010). Severe phenylephrine-associated hemorrhage in five aged horses. Journal of the American Veterinary Medical Association **237**(7): 830-4.

Fultz, L. E., et al. (2013). Comparison of phenylephrine administration and exercise versus phenylephrine administration and a rolling procedure for the correction of nephrosplenic entrapment of the large colon in horses: 88 cases (2004-2010). Javma-Journal of the American Veterinary Medical Association **242**(8): 1146-51.

McGovern, K. F., et al. (2012). Attempted Medical Management of Suspected Ascending Colon Displacement in Horses. Veterinary Surgery **41**(3): 399-403.

Pascoe, P. J., et al. (2006). Effects of increasing infusion rates of dopamine, dobutamine, epinephrine, and phenylephrine in healthy anesthetized cats. American Journal of Veterinary Research **67**(9): 1491-9.

Quandt, J. (2009). The Use of Vasopressin & Positive Inotropes for the Treatment of Hypotension. Proceedings: ACVIM. accessed via Veterinary Information Network; vin.com

Phenylpropanolamine HCl

(fen-ill-proe-pa-**nole**-a-meen)   PPA, Proin®

Sympathomimetic

Prescriber Highlights

▶ Sympathomimetic used primarily for urethral sphincter hypotonus.

▶ Caution: Glaucoma, prostatic hypertrophy, hyperthyroidism, diabetes mellitus, cardiovascular disorders, or hypertension.

▶ Adverse Effects: Restlessness, irritability, hypertension, & anorexia.

Uses/Indications

In dogs, phenylpropanolamine (PPA) is approved for the control of urinary incontinence due to urethral sphincter hypotonus. It is also used in cats for the same indication. It has also been used in an attempt to treat nasal congestion in small animals.

Pharmacology/Actions

While the exact mechanisms of phenylpropanolamine's actions are undetermined, it is believed that it indirectly stimulates both alpha- and beta-adrenergic receptors by causing the release of norepinephrine. Prolonged use or excessive dosing frequency can deplete norepinephrine from its storage sites, and tachyphylaxis (decreased response) may ensue. Tachyphylaxis has not been documented in dogs or cats when used for urethral sphincter hypotonus, however.

Pharmacologic effects of phenylpropanolamine include increased vasoconstriction, heart rate, coronary blood flow, blood pressure, mild CNS stimulation, and decreased nasal congestion and appetite. Phenylpropanolamine can also increase urethral sphincter tone and produce closure of the bladder neck; its principle veterinary indications are because of these effects.

Pharmacokinetics

No information was located on the pharmacokinetics of this agent in veterinary species. In humans, phenylpropanolamine is readily absorbed after oral administration and has an onset of action (nasal decongestion) of ≈ 15-30 minutes with duration of effect lasting ≈ 3 hours (regular capsules or tablets).

Phenylpropanolamine is reportedly distributed into various tissues and fluids, including the CNS. It is unknown if it crosses the placenta or enters milk. The drug is partially metabolized to an active metabolite, but 80-90% is excreted unchanged in the urine within 24 hours of dosing. The serum half-life is ≈ 3-4 hours.

Contraindications/Precautions/Warnings

Phenylpropanolamine should be used with caution in patients with glaucoma, prostatic hypertrophy, hyperthyroidism, diabetes mellitus, cardiovascular disorders, kidney insufficiency or hypertension.

Adverse Effects

Most likely side effects include vomiting, anorexia, restlessness, anxiety, irritability, urine retention, tachycardia, and hypertension. Rare reports of "stroke" have occurred in dogs given therapeutic dosages of phenylpropanolamine.

Reproductive/Nursing Safety

Phenylpropanolamine may cause decreased ovum implantation; uncontrolled clinical experience, however, has not demonstrated any untoward effects during pregnancy.

Overdosage/Acute Toxicity

Clinical signs of overdosage may consist of an exacerbation of the adverse effects listed above or, if a very large over-dose, severe cardiovascular (hypertension to rebound hypotension, bradycardias to tachycardias, and cardiovascular collapse) or CNS effects (stimulation to coma) can be seen.

A dog ingesting 48 mg/kg of PPA has been reported (Crandell *et al.* 2005). Ventricular tachycardia and regions of myocardial necrosis were noted. All abnormalities resolved within 6 months. Another case report (Ginn *et al.* 2013) of a dog ingesting 56 – 69 mg/kg had clinical signs of anxiety, piloerection, mucosal ulceration, cardiac arrhythmia, mydriasis, hyphema, retinal detachment, elevated creatine kinase, AST, proteinuria, pigmenturia, ventricular tachycardia and severe systemic hypertension. Ventricular tachycardia and hypertension were successfully treated with phenoxybenzamine, sotalol, esmolol, and nitroprusside.

There were 1311 single agent exposures to phenylpropanolamine reported to the ASPCA Animal Poison Control Center (APCC) during 2009-2013. Of the 1286 dogs, 995 were symptomatic the hypertension (39%), vomiting (38%), bradycardia (31%), mydriasis (28%), piloerection (28%), agitation (15%), erythema (13%) and lethargy (11%) being the most common. Of the 26 cats, 10 were symptomatic with 30% vomiting, 20% hypertensive and 20% tachypneic.

If the overdose was recent, empty the stomach using the usual precautions and administer charcoal and a cathartic. Treat clinical signs supportively as they occur. Do not use propranolol to treat hypertension in bradycardic patients and do <u>not</u> use atropine to treat bradycardia. Hypertension may be managed with a phenothiazine (*e.g.,* acepromazine—very low dose such as 0.02 mg/kg IV or IM). If phenothiazines do not normalize blood pressure, consider using a

CRI of nitroprusside. Contact an animal poison control center for further guidance.

Drug Interactions

The following drug interactions have either been reported or are theoretical in humans or animals receiving phenylpropanolamine (PPA) and may be of significance in veterinary patients. Unless otherwise noted, use together is not necessarily contraindicated, but weigh the potential risks and perform additional monitoring when appropriate.

- **ASPIRIN:** PPA may potentiate decreased platelet aggregation.
- **ISOFLURANE, DESFULARANE & SEVOFLURANE:** PPA may increase potential for cardiac arrhythmias; use with caution.
- **MONAMINE OXIDASE (MAO) INHIBITORS** (*e.g.,* **amitraz,** possibly **selegiline**): Phenylpropanolamine should not be given within two weeks of a patient receiving monoamine oxidase inhibitors.
- **NSAIDS:** An increased chance of hypertension if given concomitantly with NSAIDs, including aspirin.
- **RESERPINE:** An increased chance of hypertension if given concomitantly.
- **SYMPATHOMIMETIC AGENTS, OTHER:** Phenylpropanolamine should not be administered with other sympathomimetic agents (*e.g.,* ephedrine) as increased toxicity may result.
- **TRICYCLIC ANTIDEPRESSANTS (clomipramine, amitriptyline,** etc.): An increased chance of hypertension if given concomitantly.

Doses

- **DOGS:**

  For control of urinary incontinence due to urethral sphincter hypotonus (labeled dose; FDA-approved): 2 mg/kg PO twice daily. The dosage should be calculated in half-tablet increments. (adapted from label—*Proin*®). **Note** (extra-label): Some dogs may require q8h dosing and some may respond adequately with once a day dosing.

  For retrograde ejaculation (extra-label): 3 – 4 mg/kg PO twice daily may be tried. (Fontbonne 2007)

- **CATS:**

  For urethral sphincter hypotonus (extra-label): 1 – 2.2 mg/kg PO 2-3 times daily; practically 12.5 mg per cat PO 2-3 times a day.

Monitoring

- Clinical effectiveness.
- Adverse effects (see above).
- Blood pressure.

Client Information

- May cause increased thirst; therefore, provide ample fresh water. Keep stored out of reach of dogs and children.
- May be given with or without food. Giving it with food may help if animal vomits or acts sick after getting the drug on an empty stomach.
- Tablets are liver flavored so be sure to keep out of reach of animals.

Chemistry/Synonyms

A sympathomimetic amine, phenylpropanolamine HCl occurs as a white crystalline powder with a slightly aromatic odor, a melting range between 191°-194°C, and a pK$_a$ of 9.4. One gram is soluble in ≈ 1.1 mL of water or 7 mL of alcohol.

Phenylpropanolamine may also be known as: (+/-)-norephedrine, dl-norephedrine or PPA, *Cystolamine*®, *Proin*®, *Propalin*®, *Uricon*®, and *Uriflex-PT*®.

Storage/Stability

Store phenylpropanolamine products at room temperature in light-resistant, tight containers.

Dosage Forms/Regulatory Status

VETERINARY-LABELED PRODUCTS:

Phenylpropanolamine Chewable Tablets: 25 mg, 50 mg, & 75 mg; *Proin*®; (Rx). FDA-approved for use in dogs (NADA 141-324).

The ARCI (Racing Commissioners International) has designated this drug as a class 3 substance. See the appendix for more information.

In the USA, phenylpropanolamine is classified as a list 1 chemical (drugs that can be used as precursors to manufacture methamphetamine) and in some states it may be a controlled substance or have other restrictions placed upon its sale. Be alert to persons desiring to purchase this medication.

HUMAN-LABELED PRODUCTS:

Note: Because of potential adverse effects in humans, phenylpropanolamine has been removed from the US market for human use.

Revisions/References

Monograph revised/updated May 2014.

Crandell, J. & W. Ware (2005). Cardiac toxicity from phenylpropanolamine overdose in a dog. J Am Anim Hosp Assoc 41(6): 413-20.

Fontbonne, A. (2007). Approach to infertility in the bitch and the dog. Proceedings: WSAVA World Congress. accessed via Veterinary Information Network; vin.com

Ginn, J. A., et al. (2013). Systemic Hypertension and Hypertensive Retinopathy Following PPA Overdose in a Dog. J. Am. Anim. Hosp. Assoc. 49(1): 46-53.

Phenytoin Sodium

(**fen-i-toe-in**) Dilantin®

Anticonvulsant, Antidysrhythmic

Prescriber Highlights

► Rarely used (in USA) as an anticonvulsant for treating seizures. Potentially useful as a treatment for ventricular dysrhythmias in horses or digoxin-induced arrhythmias in dogs or horses; may be useful in cats with myokemia and neuromyotonia.

► Contraindications: Hypersensitivity; IV use contraindicated for 2nd or 3rd degree heart block, sinoatrial block, Adams-Stokes syndrome, or sinus bradycardia.

► Adverse Effects: **Dogs:** Anorexia & vomiting, ataxia, sedation, gingival hyperplasia, hepatotoxicity. **Cats:** Ataxia, sedation, anorexia, dermal atrophy syndrome, thrombocytopenia.

► Potentially teratogenic; many drug interactions possible.

Uses/Indications

Because of its undesirable pharmacokinetic profiles in dogs and possibility for toxicity in cats, phenytoin as an anticonvulsant is rarely considered for long-term treatment of epilepsy. Potentially it could be useful (IV) in the treatment of canine seizure emergencies.

Although not commonly used, phenytoin has been employed as an oral or IV antiarrhythmic agent in both dogs and cats. It has been described as a drug of choice for digoxin-induced ventricular arrhythmias in dogs. A cat with myokemia and neuromyotonia was treated with phenytoin in a case report (Galano *et al.* 2005).

Phenytoin has been studied as a treatment for ventricular dysrhythmias in horses and preliminary reports demonstrate efficacy (Wijnberg *et al.* 2004). Oral phenytoin was used in two horses after quinidine atrial fibrillation conversion (Dicken *et al.* 2012).

Pharmacology/Actions

The anticonvulsant actions of phenytoin are thought to be caused by the promotion of sodium efflux from neurons, thereby inhibiting the spread of seizure activity in the motor cortex. It is believed that excessive stimulation or environmental changes can alter the sodium gradient, which may lower the threshold for seizure spread. Hydantoins tend to stabilize this threshold and limit seizure propagation from epileptogenic foci.

The cardiac electrophysiologic effects of phenytoin are similar (not identical) to that of lidocaine (Group 1B). It depresses phase O slightly and can shorten the action potential. Its principle cardiac use is in the treatment of digitalis-induced ventricular arrhythmias.

Phenytoin can inhibit insulin and vasopressin (ADH) secretion.

Pharmacokinetics

After oral administration, phenytoin is nearly completely absorbed in humans, but in dogs, bioavailabilities may only be ≈ 40%. Phenytoin is well distributed throughout the body and ≈ 78% bound to plasma proteins in dogs (vs. 95% in humans). Protein binding may be reduced in uremic patients. Small amounts of phenytoin may be excreted into the milk and it readily crosses the placenta.

The drug is metabolized in the liver with much of the drug conjugated to a glucuronide form and then excreted by the kidneys. Phenytoin will induce hepatic microsomal enzymes, which may enhance the metabolism of itself and other drugs. The serum half-life (elimination) differences between various species are striking. Phenytoin has reported half-lives of 2-8 hours in dogs, 8 hours in horses, 15-24 hours in humans, and 42-108 hours in cats. Because of the pronounced induction of hepatic enzymes in dogs, phenytoin metabolism is increased with shorter half-lives within 7-9 days after starting treatment. Puppies possess smaller volumes of distribution and shorter elimination half-lives (1.6 hours) than adult dogs.

The phenytoin prodrug fosphenytoin causes fewer IV administration related adverse events than phenytoin sodium injection in humans. After determining the pharmacokinetics in 4 dogs after 15 mg/kg (phenytoin equivalent) IV fosphenytoin, the authors concluded that this dosage appeared to be adequate to produce phenytoin levels predicted to be effective for the treatment of canine seizure emergencies; further studies are warranted (Craft *et al.* 2011).

Contraindications/Precautions/Warnings

Phenytoin is contraindicated in patients known to be hypersensitive to it or other hydantoins. Intravenous use of the drug is contraindicated in patients with 2nd or 3rd degree heart block, sinoatrial block, Adams-Stokes syndrome, or sinus bradycardia.

Most recommend not using phenytoin in cats.

Some data suggest that additive hepatotoxicity may result if phenytoin is used with either primidone or phenobarbital. Weigh the potential risks versus the benefits before adding phenytoin to either of these drugs in dogs.

Adverse Effects

Adverse effects in dogs associated with high serum levels include anorexia and vomiting, ataxia, and sedation. Liver function tests should be monitored in patients on chronic therapy as hepatotoxicity (elevated serum ALT, decreased serum albumin, hepatocellular hypertrophy and necrosis, hepatic lipidosis, and extramedullary hematopoiesis) have been reported. Gingival hyperplasia has been reported in dogs receiving chronic therapy. Oral absorption may be enhanced and GI upset decreased if given with food.

Cats exhibit ataxia, sedation, and anorexia secondary to accumulation of phenytoin and high serum levels. Cats have also been reported to develop thrombocytopenia and a dermal atrophy syndrome secondary to phenytoin.

High plasma concentrations of phenytoin in horses can cause excitement and recumbency.

Reproductive/Nursing Safety

In humans, the FDA categorizes this drug as category *D* for use during pregnancy (*There is evidence of human fetal risk, but the potential benefits from the use of the drug in pregnant women may be acceptable despite its potential risks.*) In a separate system evaluating the safety of drugs in canine and feline pregnancy (Papich 1989), this drug is categorized as class: *C* (*These drugs may have potential risks. Studies in people or laboratory animals have uncovered risks, and these drugs should be used cautiously as a last resort when the benefit of therapy clearly outweighs the risks.*)

Phenytoin is excreted in maternal milk. Because of the potential for serious adverse reactions in nursing offspring, consider whether to accept the risks, discontinue nursing or to discontinue the drug.

Overdosage/Acute Toxicity

Clinical signs of overdosage may include sedation, anorexia and ataxia at lower levels, and coma, hypotension and respiratory depression at higher levels. Treatment of overdoses in dogs is dependent on the severity of the clinical signs demonstrated since dogs rapidly clear the drug. Severe intoxications should be handled supportively.

Drug Interactions

The following drug interactions have either been reported or are theoretical in humans or animals receiving phenytoin and may be of significance in veterinary patients. Unless otherwise noted, use together is not necessarily contraindicated, but weigh the potential risks and perform additional monitoring when appropriate.

- **CHLORAMPHENICOL:** A case report of chloramphenicol increasing the serum half-life of phenytoin from 3-15 hours in a dog has been reported.
- **LITHIUM:** The toxicity of lithium may be enhanced.
- **MEPERIDINE:** Phenytoin may decrease the analgesic properties meperidine, but enhance its toxic effects.
- **PHENOBARBITAL/PRIMIDONE:** The pharmacologic effects of primidone may be altered. Some data suggest that additive hepatotoxicity may result if phenytoin is used with either primidone or phenobarbital. Weigh the potential risks versus the benefits before adding phenytoin to either of these drugs in dogs.

Note: The following interactions are from the human literature. Because of the significant differences in pharmacokinetics in dogs and cats, their significance, if any, will be variable veterinary medicine. This list includes only agents used in small animal medicine, in the human literature many more agents have been implicated.

The following agents <u>may increase the effects of phenytoin</u>: allopurinol, chloramphenicol, chlorpheniramine, cimetidine, diazepam, ethanol, isoniazid, phenylbutazone, salicylates, sulfonamides, trimethoprim and valproic acid.

The following agents <u>may decrease the pharmacologic activity of phenytoin</u>: antacids, antineoplastics, barbiturates, calcium (dietary and gluconate), diazoxide, enteral feedings, folic acid, nitrofurantoin, pyridoxine and theophylline.

<u>Phenytoin may decrease the pharmacologic activity</u> of the following agents: corticosteroids, disopyramide, dopamine, doxycycline, estrogens, furosemide and quinidine.

Doses

- **DOGS:**

  For treatment of ventricular arrhythmias (extra-label): 10 mg/kg slowly IV; 30 – 50 mg/kg PO q8h. (Ware 2003)

  For treatment (or prophylaxis) of digitalis intoxication (extra-label): 50 mg/kg PO q8h; long-term use may cause increases in serum alkaline phosphatase and increased hepatic cell size. (Kittleson 2006)

- **CATS:**

  Note: Because cats can easily accumulate this drug and develop clinical signs of toxicity, the use of phenytoin is very controversial in this species. and most recommend avoiding use in cats.

- **HORSES:** (NOTE: ARCI UCGFS CLASS 4 DRUG)

For persistent ventricular extra systoles or ventricular tachycardia where conventional treatment has failed (extra-label): 20 mg/kg PO q12h initially for the first 3-4 doses, followed by a maintenance dose of 10 – 15 mg/kg PO q12h. Suggest monitoring plasma concentrations. (Wijnberg *et al.* 2004)

To attempt to maintain normal sinus rhythm after quinidine cardioversion of atrial fibrillation (extra-label): From a case report (n=2). Initial phenytoin dose was 15 mg/kg PO q12h. Consider therapeutic drug monitoring to adjust dosage. (Dicken *et al.* 2012)

Monitoring

- Level of seizure control; sedation/ataxia.
- Body weight (anorexia).
- Liver enzymes (if chronic therapy) and serum albumin.
- Serum drug levels if signs of toxicity or lack of seizure control.

Client Information

- Must be dosed several times a day with food to dogs. Cats are dosed much less often and can easily develop toxic effects if dosages are too high.
- Side effects in dogs include: Lack of appetite, sedation (sleepiness), lethargy (lack of energy), incoordination/weakness (*e.g.*, stumbling, clumsiness, etc.) and vomiting can be seen, especially when blood levels of the drug are high; gum overgrowth and liver problems are possible.
- Side effects in cats include: Incoordination/weakness (*e.g.*, stumbling, clumsiness, etc.), sedation (sleepiness), lack of appetite, dermal atrophy (skin thinning) syndrome, and low blood platelet count.
- Pregnant women should handle this drug carefully.

Chemistry/Synonyms

A hydantoin-derivative, phenytoin sodium occurs as a white, hygroscopic powder which is freely soluble in water and warm propylene glycol, and soluble in alcohol.

Because phenytoin sodium slowly undergoes partial hydrolysis in aqueous solutions to phenytoin (base) with the resultant solution becoming turbid, the commercial injection contains 40% propylene glycol and 10% alcohol. The pH of the injectable solution is ≈ 12.

Phenytoin sodium is used in the commercially available capsules (both extended and prompt) and the injectable preparations. Phenytoin (base) is used in the oral tablets and suspensions. Each 100 mg of phenytoin sodium contains 92 mg of the base.

Phenytoin may also be known as: diphenylhydantoin, DPH, fenitoina, phenantoinum, or phenytoinum, *Dilantin*®, and *Phenytek*®.

Storage/Stability

Store capsules at room temperature (below 86°F) and protect from light and moisture. Store phenytoin sodium injection at room temperature and protect from freezing. If injection is frozen or refrigerated, a precipitate may form which should resolubolize when warmed. A slight yellowish color will not affect either potency or efficacy, but do not use precipitated solutions. Injectable solutions at less than a pH of 11.5 will precipitate. No problems with adsorption to plastic have been detected thus far.

Compatibility/Compounding Considerations

Phenytoin sodium injection is generally physically **incompatible** with most IV solutions (upon standing) and drugs. It has been successfully mixed with sodium bicarbonate and verapamil HCl. In human medicine, the phenytoin prodrug fosphenytoin is generally preferred when IV phenytoin treatment is desired. If phenytoin sodium is used for IV infusion recommendations are: **1)** use either normal saline or lactated Ringer's; **2)** a concentration of 1 mg/mL phenytoin be used; **3)** start infusion immediately and complete in a relatively short time; **4)** use a 0.22 μm in-line IV filter; **5)** watch the admixture carefully.

Dosage Forms/Regulatory Status

VETERINARY-LABELED PRODUCTS: NONE.

The ARCI (Racing Commissioners International) has designated this drug as a class 4 substance. See the appendix for more information.

HUMAN-LABELED PRODUCTS:

Phenytoin Sodium Extended-Release Capsules: 30 mg, 100 mg, 200 mg & 300 mg; *Dilantin*®, *Phenytek*®, generic; (Rx)

Phenytoin Oral Suspension: 25 mg/mL in 240 mL; *Dilantin-125*®, generic; (Rx)

Phenytoin Tablets: 50 mg (chewable); *Dilantin*® *Infa-Tabs*®; (Rx)

Phenytoin Sodium Injection: 50 mg/mL (46 mg/mL phenytoin) in 2 mL & 10 mL; generic; (Rx)

Fosphenytoin Sodium Injection: 50 mg (phenytoin equivalents)/mL; *Cerebyx*®, generic; (Rx)

Revisions/References

Monograph revised/updated May 2014.

Craft, E. M., et al. (2011). Pharmacokinetics and Tolerability of Intravenous Fosphenytoin in Four Healthy Dogs. Proceedings: ACVIM. accessed via Veterinary Information Network; vin.com

Dicken, M., et al. (2012). The use of phenytoin in two horses following conversion from atrial fibrillation. New Zealand Veterinary Journal **60**(3): 210-2.

Galano, H., et al. (2005). Myokymia and neuromyotonia in a cat. JAVMA **227**(10): 1608-12.

Kittleson, M. (2006). "Chapt 29: Drugs used in the treatment of cardiac arrhythmias." *Small Animal Cardiology, 2nd Ed* Veterinary Information Network.

Papich, M. (1989). Effects of drugs on pregnancy. *Current Veterinary Therapy X: Small Animal Practice.* R. Kirk. Philadelphia, Saunders: 1291-9.

Ware, W. (2003). Cardiovascular system disorders. *Small Animal Internal Medicine, 3rd Ed.* R. Nelson and C. Couto. St Louis, Mosby: 1-209.

Wijnberg, I. & F. Ververs (2004). Phenytoin sodium as a treatment for ventricular dysrhythmia in horses. J Vet Intern Med **18**(May/Jun): 350-3.

Pheromones

(fer-i-mones)   Feliway®, D.A.P.®

Pheromone Behavior Modifier

Prescriber Highlights

▶ Commercially available pheromones may be useful in **Cats** for urine marking or spraying, vertical scratching, avoidance of social contact, loss of appetite, stressful situations, or inter-cat aggression; **Dogs:** Behaviors associated with fear or stress or for calming in new environments or situations; **Horses:** Alleviating stressful situations.

▶ May need adjunctive therapy (behavior modification, drug therapy) for negative behaviors.

▶ Dog/Cat products are administered via the environment; Equine product administered intranasally.

▶ Appears to be safe.

Uses/Indications

Pheromones may be useful adjuncts to reduce anxiety and stress. In cats, FFP may be useful in treating urine marking or spraying, vertical scratching, avoidance of social contact, loss of appetite, stressful situations, or inter-cat aggression. Behavioral modification and/or concomitant drug therapy may be required.

In dogs, DAP may be useful in treating behaviors associated with fear or stress (*e.g.*, separation anxiety, destruction, excessive barking, house soiling, licking, phobias) or calming animals in new environments or situations.

In horses, EAP may be useful in alleviating stressful situations (*e.g.*, transport, shoeing, clipping, new environments, training).

Pharmacology/Actions

Appeasing pheromones produced during nursing are thought to exist with all mammals. They are detected by the Jacobson's organ or vomero-nasal organ (VNO). The VNO is more sensitive in young animals, but is believed to continue to function in older animals as well. It is not well understood what neurotransmitters or neurochemical processes are involved for pheromones to exhibit their effects. In most animals, pheromones have a general calming effect. In cats, the F3 facial pheromone is thought to inhibit urine marking, encourage feeding, and enhance exploratory behaviors in unfamiliar situations. The F4 pheromone is a so-called allomarking pheromone that calms and familiarizes the cat with its surroundings.

Pharmacokinetics

No information located.

Contraindications/Precautions/Reproductive Safety

No information located.

Adverse Effects

No significant adverse effects were located for these products and are unlikely to occur.

Overdosage/Acute Toxicity

No specific animal toxicity data was located. Although the ingredients in these products are not thought toxic, the manufacturer recommends that humans accidentally exposed resulting in an adverse reaction should report to a physician or poison control center.

Drug Interactions

- None were located. Effects may be reduced or negated by concurrent use of drugs that cause CNS stimulation.

Laboratory Considerations

- No information was located.

Doses

- **CATS:**

  Diffusers: Diffuser vial lasts ≈ 4 weeks and covers 500-650 sq. ft. Plug diffuser into electric outlet in the room most often used by the animal. Do not cover diffuser or place behind or under furniture. When plugged in, do not touch diffuser with wet hands or metal objects. Do not touch diffuser with uncovered hands during, or immediately after use. May require up to 72 hours to saturate area, so effects may not be immediate. (Label Information; *Feliway® Diffuser*)

  Spray: Do not spray directly on cats. Pump spray ≈ 4 inches from site, 8 inches from the floor. One spray per application site. Clean urine marks with clear water only. Urine marks and prominent objects (furniture, window or doorframes) should be sprayed 1-2 times daily for 30 days. If cat is observed rubbing its own facial pheromones onto a spot, treatment is no longer necessary at that location. Maintenance sprays every 2-3 days may be required. Inter-cat aggression problems may require behavior modification and concomitant drug therapy. (Label Information; *Feliway® Spray*)

- **DOGS:**

  Diffusers: Diffuser vial lasts ≈ 4 weeks and covers 500-650 sq. ft. Plug diffuser into electric outlet in the room most often used by the animal. Do not cover diffuser or place behind or under furniture. When plugged in, do not touch diffuser with wet hands or metal objects. Do not touch diffuser with uncovered hands during, or immediately after use. May require up to 72 hours to saturate area, so effects may not be immediate. (Label Information; *D.A.P.® Diffuser*)

  Spray: Do not spray directly on dogs. May spray in car, kennels, crates, carriers, or on neck bandanas. Spray ≈ 20 minutes prior to

travel, etc. When entering unfamiliar places/rooms, spray twice day in the area. (Label Information; *D.A.P.® Spray*)

- **HORSES:**

  Nasal spray: Administer 2 sprays into each nostril 1/2 hour before anticipated stress or event. After administration, keep horse in a non-stressful environment for 1/2 hour to achieve best results. (Label Information; *Modipher EQ® Spray*)

Monitoring

- Clinical efficacy.

Client Information

- Useful in treating behaviors associated with stress and anxiety. Administered to dogs and cats by sprays, diffusers, and collars.
- Appears to be safe with no known side effects.

Chemistry

Mammalian pheromones are fatty acids. Dog appeasing pheromone (DAP) is a synthetic derivative of bitch intermammary pheromone. Feline pheromone is a synthetic analog of feline cheek gland secretions (feline facial pheromone; FFP). The commercially available product available in the USA is an analog of the F3 fraction of the pheromone. Equine appeasing pheromone (EAP) is derived from maternal pheromones found in the "wax area" close to the mammae of nursing mares.

Storage/Stability

Unless otherwise labeled, store at room temperature and do not mix with other ingredients or substances. Keep products out of reach of children.

Compatibility/Compounding Considerations

No specific information noted.

Dosage Forms/Regulatory Status

VETERINARY-LABELED PRODUCTS:

Note: These products apparently have not been evaluated for safety or efficacy by the FDA. There may be additional products available.

Feline products include:

Feline Facial Pheromone (FFP-F3 fraction) Diffuser (electric diffuser plus a 2% FFP vial): 48 mL vial; *Feliway® Diffuser, Comfort Zone® Feline*; (OTC)

Feline Facial Pheromone (FFP-F3 fraction) Spray: 10% 75 mL bottle; *Feliway® Spray, Comfort Zone® Spray for Cats*; (OTC)

Canine products include:

Dog Appeasing Pheromone (DAP) Diffuser (electric diffuser plus a 2% DAP vial): 48 mL vial; *Adaptil® Diffuser, Comfort Zone®*; (OTC)

Dog Appeasing Pheromone 2% (DAP) Spray: 60 mL bottle; *Adpatil® Spray; Comfort Zone® Spray for Dogs*; (OTC)

Dog Appeasing Pheromone (DAP): 48 mL with or without plug in adapter; *Comfort Zone® Canine*; (OTC)

Dog Appeasing Pheromone Collar: *Adaptil® Collar*; (OTC)

Equine products include:

Equine Appeasing Pheromone (EAP): 0.1% Spray 7.5 mL bottle, *Modipher EQ® Mist with E.A.P*; (OTC)

A product (not currently available in the USA) called *FeliFriend®* contains a synthetic F4 fraction of FFP.

HUMAN-LABELED PRODUCTS: NONE.

Revisions/References

Monograph revised/updated May 2014.

Phosphate, Parenteral

(**fos**-fayt)

Electrolyte

Prescriber Highlights

▶ For treatment or prevention of hypophosphatemia. Available as either sodium or potassium salts.

▶ Contraindications: Hyperphosphatemia, hypocalcemia, oliguric renal failure, or if tissue necrosis is present; Potassium phosphate contraindicated if hyperkalemia present; sodium phosphate if hypernatremia present.

▶ Caution: Cardiac (esp. if receiving digoxin) or renal disease.

▶ Adverse Effects: Hyperphosphatemia, resulting in hypocalcemia, hypotension, renal failure or soft tissue mineralization; hyperkalemia or hypernatremia are possible.

▶ Dilute before giving IV.

Uses/Indications

Phosphate (IV) is useful in large volume parenteral fluids to correct or prevent hypophosphatemia when adequate oral phosphorous intake is not possible. Acute, severe hypophosphatemia can cause hemolytic anemia, thrombocytopenia, neuromuscular and CNS disorders, bone and joint pain, and decompensation in patients with cirrhotic liver disease.

Pharmacology/Actions

Phosphate is involved in several functions in the body, including calcium metabolism, acid-base buffering, B-vitamin utilization, bone deposition, and several enzyme systems.

Pharmacokinetics

Intravenously administered phosphate is eliminated via the kidneys. It is glomerularly filtered, but up to 80% is reabsorbed by the tubules.

Contraindications/Precautions/Warnings

Both potassium and sodium phosphate are contraindicated in patients with hyperphosphatemia, hypocalcemia, oliguric renal failure, or if tissue necrosis is present. Potassium phosphate is contraindicated in patients with hyperkalemia. Sodium or potassium phosphate should be used with caution in patients with cardiac or renal disease. Particular caution should be used in using potassium phosphate in patients receiving digitalis therapy. Sodium phosphate is contraindicated in patients with hypernatremia.

Adverse Effects

Overuse of parenteral phosphate can cause hyperphosphatemia, resulting in hypocalcemia (refer to the Overdose section for more information). Phosphate therapy can also result in hypotension, renal failure or soft tissue mineralization. Either hyperkalemia or hypernatremia may result in susceptible patients.

Reproductive/Nursing Safety

In humans, the FDA categorizes this drug as category *C* for use during pregnancy (*Animal studies have shown an adverse effect on the fetus, but there are no adequate studies in humans; or there are no animal reproduction studies and no adequate studies in humans.*)

It is not known whether this drug is excreted in maternal milk. It is unlikely to be of concern.

Overdosage/Acute Toxicity

Patients developing hyperphosphatemia secondary to intravenous therapy with potassium phosphate should have the infusion stopped and given appropriate parenteral calcium therapy to restore serum calcium levels. Serum potassium should be monitored and treated if required.

Drug Interactions

The following drug interactions have either been reported or are theoretical in humans or animals receiving phosphates and may be of significance in veterinary patients. Unless otherwise noted, use together is not necessarily contraindicated, but weigh the potential risks and perform additional monitoring when appropriate.

- **ALUMINUM** and **CALCIUM SALTS (oral)** and **SEVELAMER**: May reduce phosphorus levels.
- **ANGIOTENSIN CONVERTING ENZYME INHIBITORS (ACE Inhibitors)**: May cause potassium retention. When used with potassium products such as potassium phosphate, hyperkalemia can result.
- **BISPHOSPHONATES** (*e.g.*, **alendronate, etidronate, pamidronate, tiludronate**, etc.): Potentially could increase hypocalcemic effects of phosphates; monitor.
- **DIGOXIN**: Potassium salts (potassium phosphate) must be used very cautiously in patients on digitalis therapy and should not be used in digitalized patients with heart block.
- **POTASSIUM SPARING DIURETICS** (*e.g.*, **spironolactone**): May cause potassium retention. When used with potassium products such as potassium phosphate, hyperkalemia can result.

Doses

Both sodium and potassium phosphate injections must be diluted before intravenous administration.

- **DOGS/CATS:**

    For hypophosphatemia (extra-label): Most recommend administering parenteral phosphate in patients when serum phosphate <1.5 mg/L or when <2 mg/dL and clinical signs (*e.g.*, hemolysis, ileus, rhabdomyolysis, decreased contractility, or platelet dysfunction) are detected. Commonly 0.01 – 0.03 mMol/kg/hr IV is suggested, but for diabetic ketoacidosis (DKA) dosages ranging up to 0.12 mMol/kg/hr have been noted in some references. Dilute in a calcium-free intravenous solution (*i.e.*, **NOT** Lactated Ringer's, etc.). To provide parenteral phosphate, either potassium phosphate or sodium phosphate can be used (when not contraindicated); some recommend that when treating DKA that 1/3 to 1/2 of the supplemented phosphate be provided as potassium phosphate. Monitor serum phosphate levels initially every 4-6 hours and adjust infusion rate to maintain serum phosphate above 2 mg/dL. Do not induce hyperphosphatemia. Correct the underlying cause for hypophosphatemia if possible. Once patient is stabilized and levels are maintained above 2-2.5 mg/dL consider transitioning to oral phosphorus if continued phosphorous supplementation is needed.

Monitoring

- Serum inorganic phosphate (phosphorous).
- Other electrolytes, including calcium.

Chemistry

Potassium phosphate injection is a combination of 224 mg monobasic potassium phosphate and 236 mg dibasic potassium phosphate. The pH of the injection is 6.5 and has an osmolarity of 7357 mOsm/L.

Sodium phosphate injection is a combination of 276 mg monobasic sodium phosphate and 142 mg dibasic sodium phosphate. The pH of the injection is 5.7 and has an osmolarity of ≈ 7000 mOsm/L.

Because commercial preparations are a combination of monobasic and dibasic forms, prescribe and dispense in terms of mMoles of phosphate.

Storage/Stability

Unless otherwise instructed by the manufacturer, store potassium or sodium phosphate injection at room temperature; protect from freezing.

Compatibility/Compounding Considerations

Phosphates may be physically **incompatible** with metals such as calcium and magnesium.

Potassium phosphate injection is reportedly physically **compatible** with the following intravenous solutions and drugs: amino acids 4%/dextrose 25%, $D_{10}LRS$, $D_{10}Ringer's$, Dextrose 2.5%-10% injection, sodium chloride 0.45%-0.9%, magnesium sulfate, metoclopramide HCl, and verapamil HCl.

Potassium phosphate injection is reportedly physically **incompatible** with the following solutions or drugs: $D_{2.5}$ in half normal Ringer's or LRS, D_5 in Ringer's, D_{10}/sodium chloride 0.9%, Ringer's injection, LRS, and dobutamine HCl. Compatibility is dependent upon factors such as pH, concentration, temperature and diluent used; consult specialized references or a hospital pharmacist for more specific information.

Dosage Forms/Regulatory Status

VETERINARY-LABELED PRODUCTS: NONE.

There are no parenteral phosphate-only products FDA-approved for veterinary medicine. There are several proprietary phosphate-containing products labeled for large animals available that may also include calcium, magnesium, potassium, and/or dextrose; refer to the individual product's labeling for specific dosage information. Trade names for these products include: *Magnadex®*, *Norcalciphos®*, *Cal-Dextro® Special* and *#2*, *CMPK®*, and *Cal-Phos® #2*. They are Rx drugs.

HUMAN-LABELED PRODUCTS:

Potassium Phosphate (Dibasic) Injection; each mL provides 3 mM of phosphate (99.1 mg/dL of phosphorous) and 4.4 mEq of potassium per mL in 5, 10, 15, 30, and 50 mL vials; generic; (Rx)

Sodium Phosphate Injection; each mL provides 3 mM of phosphate (93 mg/dL of phosphorous) and 4 mEq of sodium per mL in 10, 15, 30, and 50 mL vials; generic; (Rx)

Revisions/References

Monograph revised/updated May 2014.

Physostigmine Salicylate

(fye-zoh-**stig**-meen sah-**lis**-ah-layt)   Antilirium®

Cholinesterase Inhibitor

Prescriber Highlights

▶ Cholinesterase inhibitor that may be used as a diagnostic aid for ivermectin toxicity in dogs, as a provocative agent for the diagnosis of narcolepsy in dogs & horses, and as a treatment for anticholinergic toxicity. Recent research suggests it may be useful in horses to improve recoveries after isoflurane anesthesia.

▶ Crosses into the CNS; effective for treating central anticholinergic toxicity, but also increases the risks for central physostigmine toxic effects (*e.g.*, seizures).

▶ Must be administered with direct patient supervision; adverse effects can be serious.

Uses/Indications

Physostigmine has been used as a diagnostic aid for detecting ivermectin toxicity in dogs, as a provocative agent for the diagnosis of narcolepsy in dogs and horses, and as a treatment for anticholinergic toxicity. Because of the potential for serious adverse effects, use of physostigmine as an antidote is generally reserved for very serious toxicity affecting the CNS. Otherwise, safer alternatives such as neostigmine or pyridostigmine are preferred.

A study in horses, demonstrated that physostigmine, but not neostigmine, may be useful for improving recovery and reducing emergence delirium after isoflurane general anesthesia (Wiese *et al.* 2014).

While physostigmine has been used to antagonize the CNS depressant effects of benzodiazepines in humans, it should not be used for this purpose because of the potential toxicity and non-specific action of physostigmine.

Pharmacology/Actions

Physostigmine reversibly inhibits the destruction of acetylcholine by acetylcholinesterase, thereby increasing acetylcholine at receptor sites. Because physostigmine is a tertiary amine, unlike the quaternary amine cholinesterase inhibitors neostigmine and pyridostigmine, it crosses the blood-brain barrier and inhibits acetylcholinesterase both centrally and peripherally. Pharmacologic effects include miosis, bronchial constriction, hypersalivation, muscle weakness, and sweating (in species with sweat glands). At higher dosages, cholinergic crisis can occur; seizures, bradycardia, tachycardia, asystole, nausea, vomiting, diarrhea, depolarizing neuromuscular block, pulmonary edema, and respiratory paralysis are possible.

Pharmacokinetics

Physostigmine is rapidly absorbed from the GI tract (no oral dosage form available), subcutaneous tissue or mucous membranes. After parenteral administration, physostigmine readily crosses the blood-brain barrier into the CNS. Peak effects occur within 5 minutes after IV administration; ≈ 25 minutes after IM dosing. The majority of administered drug is rapidly destroyed via hydrolysis by cholinesterases. Very small amounts can be eliminated unchanged into the urine. Duration of pharmacologic effects can be from 30 minutes to 5 hours; average duration is 30-60 minutes.

Contraindications/Precautions/Warnings

Contraindications for humans and, presumably, animal patients include: prior hypersensitivity reactions to physostigmine or sulfites, bronchoconstrictive disease (asthma), gangrene, diabetes mellitus, cardiovascular disease, mechanical obstruction of the GI or urinary tract, any vagotonic state, or the concurrent use of choline esters (*e.g.*, bethanechol, methacholine) or neuromuscular blocking agents (*e.g.*, succinylcholine)—see Drug Interactions.

When physostigmine is used in the absence of anticholinergic toxicity or to treat tricyclic or tetracyclic antidepressant overdoses, there is an increased risk for cholinergic crisis.

Rapid IV administration increases the potential for bradycardia, hypersalivation, or seizures. In humans, it should be given intravenously at a slow, controlled rate not exceeding 1 mg/minute (adults) and 0.5 mg/minute (children).

Because of the risks for toxicity, atropine should be readily available (see Overdosage).

Physostigmine injection contains benzyl alcohol that may be toxic in neonatal animals.

Adverse Effects

Adverse effects are a result of the drug's pharmacologic actions and, except for hypersensitivity reactions, are dose related depending upon concurrent anticholinergic effects secondary to anticholinergics on board. Pharmacologic effects include miosis, bronchial constriction, hypersalivation, muscle weakness, and sweating (in species with sweat glands). At higher dosages, cholinergic crisis can occur; seizures, bradycardia, tachycardia, hypotension, asystole, nausea, vomiting, diarrhea, depolarizing neuromuscular block, pulmonary edema, and respiratory paralysis are possible.

Reproductive/Nursing Safety

Little information is available, but it would be expected that physostigmine would cross the placenta. Teratogenic effects (behavioral, biochemical and metabolic) have reportedly been observed in mice studies. Weigh the potential risks of using physostigmine during pregnancy versus its potential benefits. In humans, the FDA categorizes alendronate as category *C* for use during pregnancy (*Animal studies have shown an adverse effect on the fetus, but there are no adequate studies in humans; or there are no animal reproduction studies and no adequate studies in humans.*)

It is not known if physostigmine enters milk, but it would unlikely pose much risk to nursing offspring.

Overdosage/Acute Toxicity

Overdoses or acute toxicity can be life-threatening (see Adverse Reactions), however, because of the short duration of effect, supportive care may be all that is required. Treatment of serious acute toxicity includes mechanical ventilation, repeated bronchial aspiration, and administration of IV atropine. Refer to the Atropine monograph for dosages for cholinergic toxicity. Readministration of atropine may be required. Pralidoxime (2-PAM) may be useful in reversing the ganglionic and skeletal muscle effects of physostigmine. Refer to the Pralidoxime monograph for more information. An animal poison control center may be helpful in assisting with case management.

Drug Interactions

The following drug interactions have either been reported or are theoretical in humans or animals receiving physostigmine and may be of significance in veterinary patients. Unless otherwise noted, use together is not necessarily contraindicated, but weigh the potential risks and perform additional monitoring when appropriate.

- **CHOLINE ESTERS (bethanechol, carbachol, methacholine):** Physostigmine may cause additive adverse effects.
- **ORGANOPHOSPHATES:** Physostigmine may cause additive adverse effects.
- **SUCCINYLCHOLINE:** Physostigmine can cause muscle fasciculations (at high doses) or depolarization block (at very high doses), which may be additive to the effects of succinylcholine-like neuromuscular blockers.

Laboratory Considerations
- None noted.

Doses

- **DOGS:**

   To temporarily reverse the CNS effects of ivermectin toxicosis in support of the diagnosis (extra-label): 1 mg (total dose per dog) IV. (Mealey 2006)

   Provocative test for narcolepsy/cataplexy if feeding test (*10 pieces of highly tasty food that the dog loves to eat in a row 12-24 inches apart; affected dogs will usually take 2 minutes or longer to eat the food and have several attacks*) is not successful (extra-label): Physostigmine at 0.025 mg/kg IV, wait 9-15 minutes and observe response to stimulus (food test or similar). If clinical signs do not appear, may try a higher dose of 0.05 mg/kg as above. Subsequent testing can be done at doses of 0.075 mg/kg and 1 mg/kg as above. Increased severity of signs that may persist for 15-45 minutes in response to stimulus is indicative of cataplexy/narcolepsy. (Shell 2003)

- **HORSES:** (NOTE: RCI CLASS 3 DRUG)

   Provocative test in diagnosing cataplexy or narcolepsy (extra-label): 0.05 – 0.08 mg/kg slow IV will precipitate a cataplectic attack within 3-10 minutes after administration in affected horses. Lack of positive response does not rule out diagnosis of narcolepsy. Diarrhea, colic or cholinergic stimulation are possible. Adapted from: (Andrews *et al.* 2004), (Mayhew 2005)

   To improve recovery after isoflurane anesthesia (extra-label): From a study in 14 horses: Physostigmine 0.04 mg/kg IV over

8-10 minutes during the anesthetic weaning process prior to moving a horse to the recovery stall. Authors concluded that while additional studies are necessary to define potential mechanisms, benefits and risks, "physostigmine may offer a means to improve anesthetic recovery quality in equine patients and thus decrease the exceptionally high perianesthetic morbidity and fatality rates in this species." (Wiese *et al.* 2014)

- **CATTLE:**

   For reversal of tall larkspur (*Delphinium barbeya*) poisoning (extra-label): 0.04 – 0.08 mg/kg IV rapidly; serial injections may be necessary. (Pfister *et al.* 1994)

Monitoring
- Direct patient supervision required for monitoring adverse effects.
- Heart rate, blood pressure; monitor heart rhythm if heart rate is abnormal.

Client Information
- This medication must be administered in a setting where direct veterinary supervision is available.

Chemistry/Synonyms

Physostigmine salicylate is made from an extract of *Physostigma venenosum* (Calabar Bean) seeds. It occurs as white, shining, odorless, crystals or crystalline powder. Upon exposure to heat, light, air, or exposure to traces of metals for a long period, it develops a red tint. One gram is soluble in 75 mL of water or 16 mL of alcohol. The injection has a pH of 3.5-5.

Physostigmine salicylate may also be known as eserine salicylate, physostigmine monosalicylate and *Anticholium®*.

Storage/Stability

The injection (ampules) should be stored below 40°C; preferably between 15-30°C. Protect from light and freezing.

Compatibility/Compounding Considerations

Physostigmine is labeled for human use to be administered IV undiluted. It may be given via a Y-site or stopcock port on IV set, but it should **not** be added to IV solutions.

Dosage Forms/Regulatory Status

VETERINARY-LABELED PRODUCTS: NONE.

The ARCI (Racing Commissioners International) has designated this drug as a class 3 substance. See the appendix for more information.

HUMAN-LABELED PRODUCTS:

Physostigmine Salicylate Injection: 1 mg/mL (contains benzyl alcohol 2% and 0.1% sodium metabisulfite) in 2 mL ampules; generic; (Rx)

Revisions/References
Monograph revised/updated May 2014.
Andrews, F. & H. Matthews (2004). Seizures, narcoplexy, and cataplexy. *Equine Internal Medicine, 2nd Ed.* S. Reed, W. Bayly and D. Sellon. Philadelphia, Saunders: 560-79.
Mayhew, J. (2005). Sleep disorders, seizures and epilepsy in horses. Proceedings: ACVIM2005. accessed via Veterinary Information Network; vin.com
Mealey, K. (2006). Ivermectin: Macrolide Antiparasitic Agents. *Small Animal Toxicology, 2nd Ed.* M. Peterson and P. Talcott, Elsevier: 785-94.
Pfister, J., et al. (1994). Reversal of tall larkspur (Delphinium barbeyi) poisoning in cattle with physostigmine. Vet Hum Toxicol 36(6): 511-14.
Shell, L. (2003). "Narcolepsy/Cataplexy." Veterinary Information Network.
Wiese, A. J., et al. (2014). Effects of acetylcholinesterase inhibition on quality of recovery from isoflurane-induced anesthesia in horses. American Journal of Veterinary Research 75(3): 223-30.

Phytonadione
Vitamin K₁

(fye-toe-na-**dye**-ohne)   Mephyton®

Antidote, Fat Soluble Vitamin

Prescriber Highlights

▶ Used for the treatment of anticoagulant rodenticide toxicity, dicumarol toxicity associated with sweet clover ingestion in ruminants, sulfaquinoxaline toxicity, & bleeding disorders associated with faulty formation of vitamin K-dependent coagulation factors.

▶ Contraindications: Hypersensitivity; does not correct hypoprothrombinemia due to hepatocellular damage.

▶ Adverse Effects: Anaphylactoid reactions after IV administration, IM use may result in acute bleeding from the site of injection during the early stages of treatment. SC injections or oral dosages may be slowly or poorly absorbed in hypovolemic animals.

▶ May require 6-12 hours for effect.

▶ Small gauge needles are recommended for use when injecting SC or IM.

Uses/Indications

The principal use of exogenously administered phytonadione (vitamin K1) is in the treatment of anticoagulant rodenticide toxicity. It is also used for treating dicumarol toxicity associated with sweet clover ingestion in ruminants, sulfaquinoxaline toxicity, and bleeding disorders associated with faulty formation of vitamin K-dependent coagulation factors.

Pharmacology/Actions

Vitamin K₁ is necessary for the synthesis of blood coagulation factors II, VII, IX, and X in the liver. It is believed that Vitamin K1 is involved in the carboxylation of the inactive precursors of these factors to form active compounds.

Pharmacokinetics

Phytonadione is absorbed from the GI tract in monogastric animals via the intestinal lymphatics, but only in the presence of bile salts. Oral absorption of phytonadione may be significantly enhanced by administration with fatty foods. The relative bioavailability of the drug is increased 4-5X in dogs given canned dog food with the dose. After oral administration, increases in clotting factors may not occur until 6-12 hours later.

In humans, oral administration may be more rapidly absorbed than with SC administration.

Phytonadione may concentrate in the liver for a short period of time, but is not appreciably stored in the liver or other tissues. Only small amounts are distributed across the placenta in pregnant animals. Exogenously administered phytonadione enters milk. The elimination of Vitamin K1 is not well understood.

Contraindications/Precautions/Warnings

Phytonadione is labeled as contraindicated in patients hypersensitive to it or any component of its formulation, but weigh the benefits for treating versus the risks.

Many sources state that the intravenous use of phytonadione is contraindicated in animals because of increased risk of anaphylaxis development and FDA-CVM has warned to avoid administering the drug IV. In human medicine, intravenous phytonadione is recommended (with caution) for severe bleeding associated with very high INR. In small animal patients, oral treatment is preferred unless the oral route is contraindicated (vomiting, just received activated charcoal, etc.).

Vitamin K does not correct hypoprothrombinemia due to hepatocellular damage.

Adverse Effects

Anaphylactoid reactions have been reported following IV administration of Vitamin K1; use with extreme caution (See Contraindications above). Anaphylactoid reactions also possible when injecting SC. IM or SC administration may result in acute bleeding from the site of injection during the early stages of treatment. Small gauge needles are recommended for use when injecting SC or IM. Subcutaneous injections or oral dosages may be slowly or poorly absorbed in animals that are hypovolemic.

Because 6-12 hours may be required for new clotting factors to be synthesized after phytonadione administration, emergency needs for clotting factors must be provided by giving blood products.

Reproductive/Nursing Safety

Phytonadione crosses the placenta only in small amounts, but its safety has not been documented in pregnant animals. In humans, the FDA categorizes this drug as category *C* for use during pregnancy (*Animal studies have shown an adverse effect on the fetus, but there are no adequate studies in humans; or there are no animal reproduction studies and no adequate studies in humans.*)

Vitamin K is excreted in maternal milk, but unlikely to have negative effects in nursing offspring.

Overdosage/Acute Toxicity

Phytonadione is relatively non-toxic, and it would be unlikely that toxic clinical signs would result after a single overdosage. However, refer to the Adverse Effects section for more information.

Drug Interactions

There are many drugs that may prolong or enhance the effects of coumarin anticoagulants and antagonize some of the therapeutic effects of phytonadione. Refer to the warfarin monograph for more details.

The following drug interactions have either been reported or are theoretical in humans or animals receiving phytonadione and may be of significance in veterinary patients. Unless otherwise noted, use together is not necessarily contraindicated, but weigh the potential risks and perform additional monitoring when appropriate.

- **ANTIBIOTICS, ORAL**: Although chronic antibiotic therapy should have no significant effect on the absorption of phytonadione, these drugs may decrease the numbers of vitamin K producing bacteria in the gut.

- **MINERAL OIL**: Concomitant administration of oral mineral oil may reduce the absorption of oral vitamin K.

- **WARFARIN**: Phytonadione antagonizes the anticoagulant effects of coumarin and indanedione agents.

Doses

- **SMALL ANIMALS:**

  For adjunctive treatment of anticoagulant rodenticide toxicity (extra-label): Asymptomatic patients: After decontamination (if appropriate) either, 1) begin prophylactic vitamin K1 at 1.5 – 2.5 mg/kg PO (with a fatty meal) twice daily without monitoring PT, or 2) monitor PT and give vitamin K1 only if PT becomes elevated. If PT is monitored, perform baseline (to determine if any prior exposure occurred) and repeat at 48 and 72 hours after exposure. If PT remains normal after 72 hours vitamin K1 is not needed. If any elevation occurs, full treatment with vitamin K1 is needed. For short-acting anticoagulant rodenticides (warfarin and pindone), minimum duration of treatment with vitamin K1 is 14 days; for bromadiolone: 21 days; for the other second-generation anticoagulant rodenticides (*e.g.*, brodifacoum, difethialone, & difenacoum): 28 days. If the ingested dose of anticoagulant is very high, more than 4 weeks of treatment with vitamin K1 may be necessary.

For bleeding patients, oxygen may be needed for dyspnea and transfusions with whole blood or fresh or fresh frozen plasma may be necessary to replace blood and clotting factors. Decontamination procedures are generally not worthwhile due to time delay between ingestion and onset of bleeding. Phytonadione at 2.5 mg/kg PO twice daily with a fatty meal should be administered for a minimum of 4 weeks. Other supportive measures may include broad-spectrum antibiotics, oxygen therapy and exercise restriction. Removing free blood from the thoracic cavity should only be performed when respiratory function is severely compromised.

In all patients, check the PT 48-72 hours after stopping phytonadione therapy and if the test result is prolonged, continue treatment for another week. Again, a patient must be tested for adequate clotting 48 hours after phytonadione has been discontinued. Adapted from: (Merola 2002), (Richardson *et al.* 2002), (Talcott 2008), (DeClementi *et al.* 2012)

- **CATTLE, SHEEP, GOATS, SWINE:**

  For anticoagulant rodenticide toxicity (extra-label): 0.5 – 2.5 mg/kg IM or SC once daily. Treatment duration may require several weeks. See Small Animal doses for estimated times.

  For sweet clover (*Melilotus* spp.) or lespedeza (*Lespedeza* spp.) toxicity (extra-label): 1 – 1.5 mg/kg SC once daily for several days, remove from source, avoid stress/injury. (Oehme 2009)

- **HORSES:**

  For anticoagulant rodenticide toxicity (extra-label): 2.5 mg/kg twice daily (SC or IM for 3 days and then switch to PO). Treatment duration depends on anticoagulant, see Small Animal dosages for estimated treatment times.

  For moldy sweet clover (dicumarol) toxicosis (extra-label): 1.5 mg/kg SC or IM twice daily for up to 3 days.

- **BIRDS:**

  For vitamin K-related hemorrhagic disorders (extra-label): 0.2 – 2.5 mg/kg IM as needed; usually only 1-2 injections are required. May also be used prophylactically when amprolium and sulfas are administered. (Clubb 1986)

Monitoring

- Clinical efficacy (lack of hemorrhage).
- One-stage prothrombin time (OSPT; PT); or PIVKA. For anticoagulant poisoning treatment regimens a PT should be checked 48-72 hours after the last phytonadione dose. If still elevated, continue treatment for an additional week and repeat as before.

Client Information

- Oral phytonadione is best given with food, preferably foods high in fat content.
- When given by mouth for anticoagulant rodenticide poisoning (mouse and rat poison), phytonadione is considered very safe.
- Do not skip doses or your animal may start to bleed. If you miss a dose, give it as soon as you remember. If it is time for the next dose, give both doses at that time.

Chemistry/Synonyms

A naphthoquinone derivative identical to naturally occurring vitamin K1, phytonadione occurs as a clear, yellow to amber, viscous liquid. It is insoluble in water, slightly soluble in alcohol and soluble in lipids.

Phytonadione may also be known as: methylphytylnaphthochinonum, phylloquinone, phytomenadionum, phytomenadione, vitamin K1, *Aqua-Mephyton®*, *K1®*, *K-Caps®*, *Konakion®*, or *Mephyton®*.

Storage/Stability

Phytonadione should be protected from light at all times, as it is quite sensitive to light. If used as an intravenous infusion, the container should be wrapped with an opaque material. Tablets and capsules should be stored in well-closed, light-resistant containers.

Compatibility/Compounding Considerations

Most veterinary clinicians state that phytonadione is contraindicated for intravenous use; consult specialized references or a hospital pharmacist for more specific information on compatibility of phytonadione with other agents.

Injectable phytonadione may be used orally. Draw up into a syringe; remove needle and squirt into mouth.

Dosage Forms/Regulatory Status

VETERINARY-LABELED PRODUCTS:

Note: The following products may not be FDA-approved as no phytonadione products were located in the FDA's "green book".

Phytonadione Oral Capsules: 25 mg & 50 mg; several trade names may be available; (Rx). Labeled for use in dogs and cats.

Phytonadione Oral Tablets, Chewable: 25 mg, 50 mg; *Vitamin K1 Chewable®*, *Vitamin K1 Chewablet®*, *K-Chews®*; (Rx). Labeled for use in dogs and cats.

Phytonadione Aqueous Colloidal Solution for Injection: 10 mg/mL in 30 mL and 100 mL vials; *K-Ject®*, *Veda-K1® Injection*, *Vita-Jec®*, *Vitamin K1*; (Rx). May be labeled for use dogs, cats, cattle, calves, horses, swine, sheep, and goats. No withdrawal times listed.

HUMAN-LABELED PRODUCTS:

Phytonadione Oral Tablets: 5 mg; *Mephyton®*; (Rx)

Phytonadione Injection, Emulsion: 2 mg/mL & 10 mg/mL in 0.5 mL & 1 mL amps; generic; (Rx)

Revisions/References

Monograph revised/updated June 2014.

Clubb, S. L. (1986). Therapeutics: Individual and Flock Treatment Regimens. *Clinical Avian Medicine and Surgery*. G. J. Harrison and L. R. Harrison. Philadelphia, W.B. Saunders: 327-55.

DeClementi, C. & B. R. Sobczak (2012). Common Rodenticide Toxicoses in Small Animals. Veterinary Clinics of North America-Small Animal Practice 42(2): 349-+.

Merola, V. (2002). Anticoagulant rodenticides: Deadly for pests, dangerous for pets. Vet Med(October): 716-22.

Oehme, F. (2009). The 10 Most Common Poisonings in Production Animals I. Proceedings: WVC. accessed via Veterinary Information Network; vin.com

Richardson, J. A. & S. Gwaltney-Brant (2002). Tips for treating anticoagulant rodenticide toxicity in small mammals. Exotic DVM 4(1): 5.

Talcott, P. (2008). Common and Uncommon Toxins for "Roaming Around" Pets. Proceedings: WVC. accessed via Veterinary Information Network; vin.com

Pimobendan

(pi-moe-**ben**-den)   Vetmedin®

Inodilator

Prescriber Highlights

▶ Oral drug that may be useful in treatment of congestive heart failure in dogs.

▶ Give on an empty stomach.

▶ May increase risks for arrhythmias.

Uses/Indications

Pimobendan is used to treat dogs with congestive heart failure (CHF) secondary to dilated cardiomyopathy (DCM) or chronic mitral valve insufficiency (CMVI), myxomatous/degenerative mitral valve disease (MMVD, DMVD). Two studies (Lombard *et al.* 2006; Häggström *et al.* 2008) reported that in dogs with MMVD and heart failure, pimobendan can improve survival times and quality of life when compared with standard treatment consisting of an ACE inhibitor and furosemide. The QUEST study concluded that while pimobendan and benazepril resulted in similar quality of life during the study, pimobendan treated patients had increased time before CHF treatment was intensified and resulted in smaller heart size, higher body temperature, and less retention of free water (Haggstrom *et al.* 2014).

A study done in Doberman Pinschers concluded that pimobendan should be used as first-line therapy in Doberman Pinschers for the treatment of CHF caused by DCM (O'Grady *et al.* 2008). The PROTECT study concluded that the administration of pimobendan to Dobermans with preclinical DCM prolongs the time to the onset of clinical signs and extends survival (Summerfield *et al.* 2012). Pimobendan has been shown that it may be viable as a first line or adjunctive treatment option for dogs with PHT secondary to mitral valve disease (Atkinson *et al.* 2009). In the 2009 ACVIM Consensus Statement: Guidelines for the Diagnosis and Treatment of Canine Chronic Valvular Heart Disease (Atkins *et al.* 2009) the panel recommended to incorporate pimobendan (0.25 – 0.3 mg/kg PO q12h) in the acute and chronic treatment of stage C heart failure (patients that have a structural abnormality and current or previous clinical signs of heart failure caused by CVHD). Extra-label high dose pimobendan (0.3 mg/kg PO q8h) used as 'rescue' therapy for refractory heart failure may be tolerated and potentially improve survival (Ames *et al.* 2013a).

Ongoing studies may help determine if pimobendan should be used in the occult or preclinical stage of heart failure, or if additional significant benefit occurs when used concurrently with an ACE inhibitor.

Pimobendan is not FDA-approved for use in cats and at the time writing (2014) there are no published, prospective, randomized clinical trials in cats with heart failure. However, there is some limited evidence for its use in restrictive and dilated cardiomyopathy. One retrospective study on pimobendan's effects on clinical outcome and survival of cats (n=32; cats received multiple therapies) with non-taurine responsive dilated cardiomyopathy concluded that pimobendan appeared to improve survival (Hambrook *et al.* 2012). Another retrospective study of 27 cats with heart failure concluded that while pimobendan appeared to be well tolerated in cats with heart failure characterized by ventricular systolic dysfunction of various etiologies, additional studies are needed to establish dosages for pimobendan and its effects before it can be recommended (Gordon *et al.* 2012). One source suggests that pimobendan can be considered in a cat with heart failure when left ventricular systolic dysfunction has been identified echocardiographically, there is significant pleural effusion, renal insufficiency, or severe refractory pulmonary edema (DeFrancesco 2013b) and that the "current impression is that most of our feline heart failure cases are being managed with pimobendan in combination with an ACE-inhibitor and furosemide" (DeFrancesco 2013a).

Pharmacology/Actions

Pimobendan is a so-called inodilator; it has both inotropic and vasodilator effects. Pimobendan usually decreases heart rate (negative chronotrope) in animals with CHF. Its inotropic effects occur via inhibition of phosphodiesterase III (PDE-III) and by increasing intracellular calcium sensitivity in the cardiac contractility apparatus. Cardiac contractility is enhanced without an increase in myocardial oxygen consumption, as pimobendan does not increase intracellular calcium levels. Commercially available pimobendan is a 50:50 mixture of *l*- and *d*-isomers. In dogs, the *l*-isomer of pimobendan has ≈ 1.5X greater inotropic activity than the *d*-isomer. Pimobendan's vasodilator effects are via vascular PDE-III inhibition and both arterial and venous dilation occur. In dogs, pimobendan at high dosages (0.6 mg/kg, PO q12h for 10 days) with furosemide (2 mg/kg PO q12h) did not substantially suppress or potentiate the renin-angiotensin-aldosterone system (Ames *et al.* 2013b). Pimobendan also possesses some antithrombotic activity, but at clinically used dosages it does not have effects on platelet function (Shipley *et al.* 2013).

Pharmacokinetics

In dogs, following a single oral administration of 0.25 mg/kg pimobendan peak levels of the parent compound and the active metabolite were observed 1-4 hours post-dose (mean: 2 and 3 hours, respectively). Food decreased the bioavailability of an aqueous solution of pimobendan, but the effect of food on the absorption of pimobendan from chewable tablets is unknown. The steady-state volume of distribution of pimobendan is 2.6 L/kg. Protein binding of pimobendan and the active metabolite in dog plasma is >90%. Pimobendan is oxidatively demethylated to a pharmacologically active metabolite that is then conjugated with sulfate or glucuronic acid and excreted mainly via feces. Clearance of pimobendan is ≈ 90 mL/min/kg, and the terminal elimination half-lives of pimobendan and the active metabolite are ≈ 0.5 hours and 2 hours, respectively. Plasma levels of pimobendan and the active metabolite were below quantifiable levels by 4 and 8 hours respectively after oral administration.

In healthy cats, the pharmacokinetics of pimobendan after single oral doses (≈0.28 mg/kg) have been determined. Peak levels occurred at 0.9 hours, apparent volume of distribution was high and mean elimination half-life was 1.3 hours (Hanzlicek *et al.* 2012).

In humans with heart failure, pimobendan is rapidly absorbed with peak levels occurring in <1 hour after dosing. The volume of distribution was ≈ 3.2 L/kg; clearance ≈ 25 mL/min/kg. Terminal half-life is slightly less than 3 hours.

Contraindications/Precautions/Warnings

Pimobendan is contraindicated in animals hypersensitive to it, with hypertrophic cardiomyopathy, aortic stenosis, or any other condition where an augmentation of cardiac output is inappropriate for functional or anatomic reasons. It should be used with caution in patients with uncontrolled cardiac arrhythmias.

The label states the drug has not been evaluated in dogs younger than 6 months of age, with congenital heart defects, diabetes mellitus or other serious metabolic diseases, dogs used for breeding, or pregnant or lactating bitches.

Adverse Effects

The primary adverse effects that have been noted in dogs are gastrointestinal effects. There is some evidence that pimobendan may increase the development of arrhythmias. Atrial fibrillation or increased ventricular ectopic beats have been reported in dogs on pimobendan, but because cardiomyopathy can cause arrhythmias, a causative effect has not been fully established. A small (n=6) study in small breed dogs with CHF, did not find evidence of increased incidence of cardiac arrhythmias (Ames *et al.* 2013a). A trial of pimobendan in humans with heart failure demonstrated an increased mortality rate while on the drug, but this result has not been duplicated in canine studies. In a US field trial (56 day) done in dogs, the adverse effect incidence (at least one occurrence reported per dog) was: poor appetite (38%), lethargy (33%), diarrhea (30%), dyspnea (29%), azotemia (14%), weakness and ataxia (13%), pleural effusion (10%), syncope (9%), cough (7%), sudden death (6%), ascites (6%), and heart murmur (3%). As experience with the drug continues, a more detailed adverse effect profile will be developed.

In a study comparing cardiac adverse effects of pimobendan with benazepril (Chetboul *et al.* 2007), dogs with mitral valve regurgitation had increases in systolic function but also developed worsening mitral valve disease and specific mitral valve lesions (acute hemorrhages, endocardial papilloform hyperplasia on the dorsal surfaces of the leaflets, and infiltration of *chordae tendinae* by glycosaminoglycans) not seen in the benazepril group. The authors recommend that patients with mitral valve disease that are treated chronically with pimobendan be regularly and cautiously examined for any worsening mitral valvular lesions and regurgitation.

A retrospective study concluded that cats with systolic anterior motion of the mitral valve may develop systemic hypotension when treated with pimobendan (Gordon *et al.* 2012).

Reproductive/Nursing Safety

The label states the drug has not been evaluated in dogs used for breeding, or pregnant or lactating bitches. When pimobendan was given in high dosages (300 mg/kg) to pregnant laboratory animals, increased resorptions occurred. Rabbits given 100 mg/kg showed no adverse fetal effects.

No information on the safety of pimobendan during nursing was located.

Overdosage/Acute Toxicity

A review of the Pet Poison Helpline database from 11/2004 to 04/2010 identified 98 cases of pimobendan toxicosis. Of those, 7 dogs that ingested between 2.6 – 21.3 mg/kg were selected for further evaluation. Clinical signs of cardiovascular abnormalities, including severe tachycardia (4/7), hypotension (2/7), and hypertension (2/7) were noted. In two dogs, no clinical signs were seen. In asymptomatic patients, prompt decontamination, including emesis induction and administration of activated charcoal is advised. Symptomatic and supportive care includes IV fluid therapy for hypotension and hydration requirements. Monitoring blood pressure and electrocardiogram is advised with high-dose toxicosis (Reinker *et al.* 2012).

There were 467 single agent exposures to pimobendan reported to the ASPCA Animal Poison Control Center (APCC) during 2009-2013. Of the 427 dogs, 111 were symptomatic with tachycardia (48%), vomiting (24%), hypertension (12%), lethargy (12%) and hypotension (9%) being the most common clinical signs. Of the 41 cats, only 6 were symptomatic with 33% vomiting.

Dose dependent increases in heart rate were seen at 2 and 8 mg/kg IV in a 4-week study in dogs. In a six-month toxicity study in dogs, mild heart murmurs developed in 1 dog at 3X (1.5 mg/kg) and in 2 dogs at 5X (2.5 mg/kg). The murmurs were non-clinical. Treatment: Decontamination (induce emesis and give activated charcoal early), monitor heart rate, blood pressure, and EKG if needed. Control hypotension with IV fluids and dopamine.

Drug Interactions

The drug is labeled as being used safely with furosemide, digoxin, enalapril, atenolol, nitroglycerin, hydralazine, diltiazem, antiparasitic products (including heartworm preventative), antibiotics, famotidine, theophylline, levothyroxin, diphenhydramine, hydrocodone, metoclopramide and butorphanol.

The U.K. label states "pimobendan-induced increases in contractility of the heart are attenuated in the presence of the calcium antagonist **verapamil** and the beta-antagonist **propranolol**." It is assumed that other drugs in these categories (*e.g.*, diltiazem, atenolol) may also have effect.

Milrinone, a human drug that also inhibits phosphodiesterase, has been used with a variety of other drugs (*e.g.*, cardiac glycosides, lidocaine, hydralazine, prazosin, quinidine, nitroglycerin, furosemide, warfarin, spironolactone, heparin, potassium) without apparent problems, but extrapolating this to pimobendan may not apply since pimobendan also increases calcium sensitivity.

Laboratory Considerations

- No laboratory interactions or special considerations were located.

Doses

- **DOGS:**

For management of the signs of mild, moderate or severe congestive heart failure due to AV valve insufficiency or dilated cardiomyopathy (labeled dose; FDA-approved): 0.5 mg/kg total daily dose. Divide daily dose into two portions that are not necessarily equal (using whole and half tablets) and administer approximately 12 hours apart. (Label directions; *Vetmedin®*)

For adjunctive treatment of acute or chronic stage D heart failure [patients have clinical signs of failure refractory to standard treatment for Stage C heart failure from CVHD (chronic valvular heart disease)] (extra-label): No consensus was reached by the panel regarding the following, but some panelists increase the pimobendan dose to 0.3 mg/kg PO 3 times (q8h) daily. Because this dosage recommendation is outside of the FDA-approved labeling for pimobendan, this use of the drug should be explained to, and approved by the client. (Atkins *et al.* 2009)

- **CATS:**

For the treatment of heart failure in cats with left ventricular systolic dysfunction, significant pleural effusion, renal insufficiency, or severe refractory pulmonary edema (extra-label): No prospective studies have evaluated pimobendan's safety and efficacy in cats, but it appears to be safe at dosages similar to those used in dogs: 0.25 mg/kg PO twice daily; practically, one 1.25 mg tablet per cat twice daily. Generally used in combination with an ACE-inhibitor and furosemide. (DeFrancesco 2013a)

Monitoring

- Cardiovascular parameters used to monitor heart function, including ECG (rate/rhythm), blood pressure, echo studies, clinical signs, etc.

Client Information

- This medication is best given on an empty stomach.
- GI effects (*e.g.*, poor appetite, diarrhea, etc.) are the most likely adverse effects, but if you see anything out of the ordinary, contact your veterinarian.
- Because this drug is used for a serious disease (heart failure), be sure to give exactly as prescribed.

Chemistry/Synonyms

A benzimidazole-derivative phosphodiesterase inhibitor, pimobendan occurs as a white or slightly yellowish, hygroscopic powder. It is practically insoluble in water and slightly soluble in acetone or methyl alcohol. Pimobendans's chemical name is: 4,5-Dihydro-6-[2-(p-methoxyphenyl)-5-benzimidazolyl]-5-methyl-3(2H) pyridazinone. It has a molecular weight of 334.4.

Pimobendan may also be known as: UDCG-115, *Acardi®*, and *Vetmedin®*.

Storage/Stability

Unless otherwise labeled, pimobendan chewable tablets or capsules should be stored at room temperature below 25°C (77°F) in a dry place.

Compatibility/Compounding Considerations

Compounded suspensions may not be stable; avoid use unless stability data is available.

Dosage Forms/Regulatory Status

VETERINARY-LABELED PRODUCTS:

Pimobendan Chewable Tablets: 1.25 mg, 2.5 mg and 5 mg; *Vetmedin®*; (Rx). FDA-approved for use in dogs.

HUMAN-LABELED PRODUCTS: NONE.

Revisions/References

Monograph revised/updated May 2014.

Ames, M. K., et al. (2013a). High-dose pimobendan in the treatment of refractory heart failure in dogs. Journal of Veterinary Internal Medicine 27(3): 640-.

Ames, M. K., et al. (2013b). Effect of furosemide and high-dosage pimobendan administration on the renin-angiotensin-aldosterone system in dogs. American Journal of Veterinary Research 74(8): 1084-90.

Atkins, C., et al. (2009). Guidelines for the Diagnosis and Treatment of Canine Chronic Valvular Heart Disease. Journal of Veterinary Internal Medicine 23(6): 1142-50.

Atkinson, K., et al. (2009). Evaluation of Pimobendan and N-Terminal Probrain Natriuretic Peptide in the Treatment of Pulmonary Hypertension Secondary to Degenerative Mitral Valve Disease in Dogs. Journal of Veterinary Internal Medicine 23(6): 1190-6.

Chetboul, V., et al. (2007). Comparative adverse cardiac effects of pimobendan and benazepril monotherapy in dogs with mild degenerative mitral valve disease: a prospective, controlled, blinded, and randomized study. J Vet Intern Med 21(4): 742-53.

DeFrancesco, T. (2013a). Basic Review of Cardiac Drugs for the ER and ICU. Proceedings: IVECCS. accessed via Veterinary Information Network; vin.com

DeFrancesco, T. C. (2013b). Management of Cardiac Emergencies in Small Animals. Veterinary Clinics of North America-Small Animal Practice 43(4): 817-+.

Gordon, S. G., et al. (2012). Effect of oral administration of pimobendan in cats with heart failure. Javma-Journal of the American Veterinary Medical Association 241(1): 89-94.

Haggstrom, J., et al. (2014). Longitudinal Analysis of Quality of Life, Clinical, Radiographic, Echocardiographic, and Laboratory Variables in Dogs with Myxomatous Mitral Valve Disease Receiving Pimobendan or Benazepril The QUEST Study. Kleintierpraxis 59(3): 117-+.

Häggström, J., et al. (2008). Effect of Pimobendan or Benazepril Hydrochloride on Survival Times in Dogs with Congestive Heart Failure Caused by Naturally Occurring Myxomatous Mitral Valve Disease: The QUEST Study. Journal of Veterinary Internal Medicine 22(5): 1124-35.

Hambrook, L. E. & P. F. Bennett (2012). Effect of pimobendan on the clinical outcome and survival of cats with non-taurine responsive dilated cardiomyopathy. Journal of Feline Medicine and Surgery 14(4): 233-9.

Hanzlicek, A., et al. (2012). Pharmacokinetics of oral pimobendan in healthy cats. Journal of Veterinary Cardiology 14: 489-96.

Lombard, C. W., et al. (2006). Clinical efficacy of pimobendan versus benazepril for the treatment of acquired atrioventricular valvular disease in dogs. J. Am. Anim. Hosp. Assoc. 42(4): 249-61.

O'Grady, M., et al. (2008). Effect of Pimobendan on Case Fatality Rate in Doberman Pinschers with Congestive Heart Failure Caused by Dilated Cardiomyopathy. Journal of Veterinary Internal Medicine 22(4): 897-904.

Reinker, L. N., et al. (2012). Clinical Signs of Cardiovascular Effects Secondary to Suspected Pimobendan Toxicosis in Five Dogs. J. Am. Anim. Hosp. Assoc. 48(4): 250-5.

Shipley, E. A., et al. (2013). In vitro effect of pimobendan on platelet aggregation in dogs. American Journal of Veterinary Research 74(3): 403-7.

Summerfield, N. J., et al. (2012). Efficacy of Pimobendan in the Prevention of Congestive Heart Failure or Sudden Death in Doberman Pinschers with Preclinical Dilated Cardiomyopathy (The PROTECT Study). Journal of Veterinary Internal Medicine 26(6): 1337-49.

Piperacillin Sodium + Tazobactam

(**pype**-er-ah-**sill**-in; tay-zoh-**bak**-tam)   Zosyn®

Extended Spectrum Penicillin + Beta-Lactamase Inhibitor

Prescriber Highlights

▶ Extended action parenteral penicillin with a beta lactamase inhibitor; piperacillin (alone) has been discontinued.

▶ Limited experience or research in veterinary medicine, but appears quite safe.

Uses/Indications

Although veterinary experience is limited with piperacillin/tazobactam, it has expanded coverage against many bacteria and may be suitable for empiric use until culture and susceptibility data are available or for surgical prophylaxis when gram-negative or mixed aerobic/anaerobic infections are concerns.

Pharmacology/Actions

Piperacillin is a bactericidal, extended action acylaminopenicillin that inhibits septum formation and cell wall synthesis in susceptible bacteria. It has a wide spectrum of activity against many aerobic and anaerobic gram-positive (including some enterococci—*E. faecalis*) and gram-negative bacteria. It has a similar spectrum of activity as the aminopenicillins, but with additional activity against several gram-negative organisms of the family Enterobacteriaceae, including *Enterobacter* spp. and many strains of *Pseudomonas aeruginosa. Klebsiella* spp. are often resistant. Like the aminope-

nicillins, it is susceptible to inactivation by beta-lactamases. The addition of a beta-lactamase inhibitor (tazobactam) in the product *Zosyn®* increases piperacillin's spectrum of activity against many beta lactamase producing strains of bacteria.

Tazobactam irreversibly binds to beta-lactamases thereby "protecting" the beta-lactam ring of piperacillin from hydrolysis. When tazobactam is combined with piperacillin, it extends piperacillin's spectrum of activity to those bacteria that produce beta-lactamases of Richmond-Sykes types II-V that would otherwise render it ineffective. It has slightly more activity than either clavulanate or sulbactam against some Type I beta-lactamases.

Tazobactam has minimal antibacterial activity when used alone, but in combination with piperacillin, synergistic effects may result. It is more potent than sulbactam and, unlike clavulanic acid, does not induce chromosomal beta-lactamases at serum concentrations achieved.

Pharmacokinetics

Limited information is available for veterinary species. In mares, piperacillin has an elimination half-life of ≈ 7 hours. IM bioavailability is 86% and protein binding $\approx 19\%$.

In humans, piperacillin is not appreciably absorbed from the gut so it must be administered parenterally. After IM administration peak levels occur in ≈ 30 minutes. The drug exhibits low protein binding and has a volume of distribution of 0.1 L/kg. It is widely distributed into many tissues and fluids including lung, gallbladder, intestinal mucosa, uterus, bile, and interstitial fluid. With inflamed meninges, piperacillin levels in the CSF are $\approx 30\%$ those in serum. If meninges are normal, CSF concentrations are only $\approx 6\%$ of serum levels. Piperacillin crosses the placenta and is distributed into milk in low concentrations. Piperacillin is metabolized somewhat in the liver to a desethyl metabolite that has only minimal antibacterial activity. Piperacillin is primarily (68%) eliminated unchanged in the urine via active tubular secretion and glomerular filtration; it is also excreted in the bile. Elimination half-life in humans is ≈ 1 hour.

Tazobactam's pharmacokinetics generally mirrors that of piperacillin. In dogs, piperacillin reduced the renal clearance of tazobactam, presumably due to competition for tubular secretion.

Contraindications/Precautions/Warnings

Piperacillin/tazobactam should not be used in patients with documented hypersensitive reactions to a beta-lactam or beta-lactamase inhibitor.

Because of sodium content, high dosages of piperacillin/tazobactam may adversely affect patients with cardiac failure or hypernatremic conditions.

Dosage adjustment may be required in patients with significantly decreased renal function (CrCl <40 mL/min).

Adverse Effects

Piperacillin/tazobactam is generally well tolerated. Hypersensitivity reactions are possible. Local effects (thrombophlebitis, etc.) associated with intravenous injection may occur. Alterations in gut flora may lead to antibiotic-associated diarrhea.

In humans, piperacillin has caused coagulation abnormalities on occasion, particularly in patients with renal failure. Very high doses may cause neurotoxicity (seizures); again, this is more likely in patients with diminished renal function. Superinfections with *Clostridium difficile* have been rarely reported.

Reproductive/Nursing Safety

Piperacillin/tazobactam is thought relatively safe to use during pregnancy. No teratogenic effects have been attributed to either drug in either humans or laboratory animals. In humans, the FDA categorizes piperacillin/tazobactam as category *B* for use during pregnancy (*Animal studies have not yet demonstrated risk to the fetus, but there are no adequate studies in pregnant women; or animal studies have shown an adverse effect, but adequate studies in pregnant women have not demonstrated a risk to the fetus in the first trimester of pregnancy, and there is no evidence of risk in later trimesters.)*

Piperacillin is distributed in milk in low concentrations. It is not known if tazobactam enters milk. This drug combination is likely safe to use during nursing.

Overdosage/Acute Toxicity

One-time overdoses are unlikely to pose much risk although very large overdoses may cause vomiting, diarrhea, or neurotoxicity. Dogs receiving up to 800 mg/kg/day of piperacillin/tazobactam for 6 months demonstrated no serious toxic effects. Doses ≥400 mg/kg/day caused some transient effects to the liver (glycogen granules in the cytoplasm and increases in smooth endoplasmic reticulum in hepatocytes) that were mostly reversed after one month.

Treatment for overdoses, if required, is supportive.

Drug Interactions

The following drug interactions have either been reported or are theoretical in humans or animals receiving piperacillin/tazobactam and may be of significance in veterinary patients. Unless otherwise noted, use together is not necessarily contraindicated, but weigh the potential risks and perform additional monitoring when appropriate.

- **AMINOGLYCOSIDES** (*e.g.*, **amikacin, gentamicin, tobramycin**): *In vitro* studies have demonstrated that penicillins can have synergistic or additive activity against certain bacteria when used with aminoglycosides. Beta-lactam antibiotics however, can inactivate aminoglycosides *in vitro* and *in vivo* in patients in renal failure or when penicillins are used in massive dosages. Amikacin is considered the most resistant aminoglycoside to this inactivation.
- **ANTICOAGULANTS**: Because piperacillin may rarely affect platelets, increased monitoring of coagulation parameters is suggested for patients on heparin or warfarin.
- **METHOTREXATE**: Piperacillin may increase MTX serum levels.
- **PROBENECID**: Can reduce the renal tubular secretion of both piperacillin and tazobactam, thereby maintaining higher systemic levels for a longer period of time; this potential "beneficial" interaction requires further investigation before dosing recommendations can be made for veterinary patients.
- **VECURONIUM**: Piperacillin may prolong neuromuscular blockade.

Laboratory Considerations

- **Urine glucose determinations** when using cupric sulfate solution (Benedict's Solution, *Clinitest®*): Piperacillin may cause false-positive results. Tests utilizing glucose oxidase (*Tes-Tape®, Clinistix®*) are not affected by piperacillin.
- **Aminoglycoside serum quantitative analysis**: As penicillins and other beta-lactams can inactivate aminoglycosides *in vitro* (and *in vivo* in patients in renal failure or when penicillins are used in massive dosages), serum concentrations of aminoglycosides may be falsely decreased if the patient is also receiving beta-lactam antibiotics and the serum is stored prior to analysis. It is recommended that if the aminoglycoside assay is delayed, samples be frozen and, if possible, drawn at times when the beta-lactam antibiotic is at a trough.
- **Direct antiglobulin (Coombs') tests**: False-positive results may occur.
- **Urine protein**: Piperacillin may produce false-positive urine protein results with the sulfosalicylic acid and boiling test, nitric

acid test, or the acetic acid test. Strips using bromophenol blue reagent (*e.g.*, *Multi-Stix®*) do not appear to be affected by high levels of penicillins in the urine.

Doses

- **DOGS/CATS:**

  For bacterial sepsis (extra-label): Very little information is available for use in veterinary medicine. Empirically, human pediatric dosages could be tried: 80 – 100 mg/kg (of the piperacillin component) IV (over 30 minutes) q8h. Potentially, CRI's would be effective.

- **REPTILES:**

  For susceptible respiratory tract infections (extra-label): 100 – 200 mg/kg IM q24h. 10 mg/mL in saline and nebulized (Schumacher 2011). **Note:** This reference was for using piperacillin alone; if using piperacillin/tazobactam figure dose per the piperacillin component.

- **BIRDS:**

  For susceptible infections (extra-label): Reconstitute to 200 mg/mL and administer at 100 mg/kg IM q8-12h; for severe polymicrobic bacteremia give 100 mg/kg IV q6h; for preoperative orthopedic or coelomic surgery: 100 mg/kg IM q12h. (Nemetz *et al.* 2006)

Monitoring

- Efficacy for the infection treated (CBC, clinical signs, etc.).

Client Information

- Limited experience in veterinary medicine.
- This medication cannot be given by mouth.
- Injectable solutions may cause stinging if given under the skin (SC, subcutaneous).

Chemistry/Synonyms

Piperacillin sodium/tazobactam sodium occurs as a white or almost white, cryodessicated powder. Tazobactam is structurally related to sulbactam and a penicillanic acid sulfone derivative. The commercially available piperacillin/tazobactam injection contains 2.79 mEq of sodium and 0.25 mg of EDTA per gram of piperacillin.

Tazobactam may also be known as: CL 298741, or YTR 830H. Piperacillin may also be known as piperacillinum, BL-P 1908, Cl 867, CL 227193, T 12220, and TA 058. International trade names for piperacillin/tazobactam include: *Tazobac®, Tazocin®, Zosyn®* and others.

Storage/Stability

Piperacillin/tazobactam injection vials and *ADD-Vantage* vials should be stored at controlled room temperature (20-25°C).

Conventional vials should be reconstituted with 5 mL of diluent per gram of piperacillin. Suitable diluents include 0.9% sodium chloride, sterile water for injection, and bacteriostatic saline or water for injection. Once reconstituted, further dilute for intravenous infusion with 50-150 mL of 0.9% sodium chloride, LRS (reformulated product only—see below) or D5W. IV infusion should be over at least 30 minutes.

Once reconstituted, vials should be used immediately. It is recommended to discard after 24 hours if kept at room temperature or 48 hours if stored in the refrigerator. The manufacturer recommends not freezing reconstituted vials. IV bags (50-150 mL) containing further diluted product are stable for up to 24 hours at room temperature and one week if refrigerated. As no preservatives are used, sterility is not assured in stored reconstituted products.

Compatibility/Compounding Considerations

Zosyn® (piperacillin/tazobactam) injection underwent a formulation change in 2006. Sodium citrate (buffer) and EDTA (metal chelator) were added that made it **compatible** with lactated Ringer's injection and via simultaneous Y-site administration at specific concentrations of gentamicin and amikacin (but not tobramycin). This reformulated product has a yellow background behind the *Zosyn®* name on the label. Refer to the package insert for specific information on diluent and concentration compatibility.

Dosage Forms/Regulatory Status

VETERINARY-LABELED PRODUCTS: NONE.

HUMAN-LABELED PRODUCTS:

Piperacillin Sodium & Tazobactam Injection (powder for solution); 2.25 grams (piperacillin 2 grams; tazobactam 0.25 g), 3.375 grams (piperacillin 3 grams; tazobactam 0.375 grams), 4.5 grams (piperacillin 4 grams; tazobactam 0.5 grams), 40.5 grams (piperacillin 36 grams; tazobactam 4.5 grams); *Zosyn®*, generic; (Rx).

Revisions/References

Monograph revised/updated June 2014.

Nemetz, L. & A. Lennox (2006). Zosyn: A replacement for Pipracil in the avian patient. Proceedings: AAV 2004. accessed via Veterinary Information Network; vin.com
Schumacher, J. (2011). Respiratory Medicine of Reptiles. Vet Clin Exot Anim 14: 207-24.

Piperazine

(pi-per-a-**zeen**)

Antiparasitic (Ascarids)

Prescriber Highlights

▶ Anthelmintic for ascarids in a variety of species. Limited efficacy. Rarely recommended today.

▶ Adverse Effects: Unlikely, but diarrhea, emesis, or ataxia possible.

Uses/Indications

Piperazine is sometimes used for the treatment of ascarids but more effective treatments are generally preferred. Piperazine is considered safe to use in animals with concurrent gastroenteritis and during pregnancy.

Pharmacology/Actions

Piperazine is thought to exert "curare-like" effects on susceptible nematodes thereby paralyzing or narcotizing the worm and allowing it to be passed out with the feces. The neuromuscular blocking effect is believed caused by blocking acetylcholine at the myoneural junction. In ascarids, succinic acid production is also inhibited.

Pharmacokinetics

Piperazine and its salts are reportedly readily absorbed from the proximal sections of the GI tract and the drug is metabolized and excreted by the kidneys. Absorptive, distribution, and elimination kinetics on individual species were not located.

Contraindications/Precautions/Warnings

Some recommend that piperazine not be used in puppies or kittens less than 6 weeks old. Piperazine is contraindicated in patients with chronic liver or kidney disease, and those with gastrointestinal hypomotility. There is some evidence in humans that high-dose piperazine may provoke seizures in patients with a seizure history or renal disease.

If used in horses with heavy infestations of *P. equorum*, rupture or blockage of intestines is possible due to the rapid death and detachment of the worm.

Adverse Effects

Adverse effects are uncommon at recommended doses, but diarrhea, emesis, and ataxia may be noted in dogs or cats. Horses and foals generally tolerate the drug quite well, even at high dosage rates, but a transient softening of the feces may be seen. Other adverse effects have been seen at toxic dosages; refer to the Overdosage section below for more information.

Reproductive/Nursing Safety

In a system evaluating the safety of drugs in canine and feline pregnancy (Papich 1989), this drug is categorized as class: *A (Probably safe. Although specific studies may not have proved the safety of all drugs in dogs and cats, there are no reports of adverse effects in laboratory animals or women.)*

No information was located on use during nursing, but it probably is safe to use.

Overdosage/Acute Toxicity

Acute massive overdosage can lead to paralysis and death, but the drug is generally considered to have a wide margin of safety. The oral LD_{50} of piperazine adipate in mice is 11.4 grams/kg.

In cats, adverse effects occur within 24 hours after a toxic dose is ingested. Emesis, weakness, dyspnea, muscular fasciculations of ears, whiskers, tail and eyes, rear limb ataxia, hypersalivation, depression, dehydration, head-pressing, positional nystagmus and slowed pupillary responses have all been described after toxic ingestions. Many of these effects may also be seen in dogs after toxic piperazine ingestions.

Treatment is symptomatic and supportive. If ingestion was recent, use of activated charcoal and a cathartic has been suggested. Intravenous fluid therapy and keeping the animal in a quiet, dark place is recommended. Recovery generally takes place within 3-4 days.

Drug Interactions

The following drug interactions have either been reported or are theoretical in humans or animals receiving piperazine and may be of significance in veterinary patients. Unless otherwise noted, use together is not necessarily contraindicated, but weigh the potential risks and perform additional monitoring when appropriate.

▪ **CHLORPROMAZINE:** Although data conflicts, piperazine and chlorpromazine may precipitate seizures if used concomitantly.

▪ **LAXATIVES:** The use of purgatives (laxatives) with piperazine is not recommended as the drug may be eliminated before its full efficacy is established.

▪ **PYRANTEL/MORANTEL:** Piperazine and pyrantel/morantel have antagonistic modes of action and should generally not be used together.

Laboratory Considerations

▪ Piperazine can have an effect on **uric acid** blood levels, but references conflict with regard to the effect. Both falsely high and low values have been reported; interpret results cautiously.

Doses

Caution: Piperazine is available in several salts that contain varying amounts of piperazine base (see Chemistry below). Refer to the label information for the product being used.

▪ **DOGS/CATS:**

For treatment of ascarids (extra-label): Rarely recommended today. 100 – 110 mg/kg PO once; repeat in 21 days.

▪ **RABBITS, RODENTS, SMALL MAMMALS:**

a) **Mice, Rats, Hamsters, Gerbils, and Rabbits for pinworms** (extra-label): Piperazine citrate in drinking water at 3 grams/liter for 2 weeks. (Burke 1999)

b) **Rabbits for pinworms** (extra-label): Piperazine citrate 100 mg/kg PO q24h for 2 days. Piperazine adipate: Adults: 200 – 500 mg/kg PO q24h for 2 days. **Young rabbits:** 750 mg/kg, PO once daily for 2 days. Wash the perianal area. (Ivey *et al.* 2000)

c) **Mice, Rats, Gerbils, Hamsters, Guinea pigs, Chinchillas for pinworms/tapeworms** (extra-label): Using piperazine citrate: 2 – 5 mg/mL drinking water for 7 days, off 7 days and repeat. (Adamcak *et al.* 2000)

- **BIRDS:**

  For *Ascaridia galli* in poultry (extra-label): 32 mg/kg (as base) (approximately 0.3 grams for each adult) given in each of 2 successive feedings or for 2 days in drinking water. Citrate or adipate salts are usually used in feed and the hexahydrate in drinking water. (Roberson 1988)

- **REPTILES:**

  For nematodes (extra-label): 40 – 60 mg/kg PO. Repeat in 2 weeks, followed by a fecal examination 14 days after the second dose. If positive for parasites, a third dose is given and the cycle continued until the parasites are cleared from the animal. (de la Navarre 2008)

Monitoring

- Clinical and/or laboratory efficacy.
- Adverse effects.

Client Information

- Wormer used for ascarids (roundworms); not effective against many other intestinal parasites.
- Adverse effects are unlikely, but diarrhea, vomiting and incoordination/weakness (*e.g.*, stumbling, clumsiness, etc.) are possible in dogs and cats.

Chemistry/Synonyms

Piperazine occurs as a white, crystalline powder that may have a slight odor. It is soluble in water and alcohol. Piperazine is available commercially in a variety of salts, including citrate, adipate, phosphate, hexahydrate, and dihydrochloride. Each salt contains a variable amount of piperazine (base): adipate (37%), chloride (48%), citrate (35%), dihydrochloride (50-53%), hexahydrate (44%), phosphate (42%), and sulfate (46%).

Piperazine may also be known as diethylendiamin, dispermin, hexahydropropyrazin, piperazinum, and *Pipa-Tabs®*.

Storage/Stability

Unless otherwise specified by the manufacturer, piperazine products should be stored at room temperature (15-30°C).

Dosage Forms/Regulatory Status

VETERINARY-LABELED PRODUCTS:

Piperazine Dihydrochloride tablets equivalent to 50 mg or 250 mg base; *Pipa-Tabs®*; (Rx). FDA-approved for use in dogs and cats.

Additional OTC products and combination products may be available for a variety of species. There are many trade names.

HUMAN-LABELED PRODUCTS: NONE.

Revisions/References

Monograph revised/updated June 2014.

Adamcak, A. & B. Otten (2000). Rodent Therapeutics. Vet Clin NA: Exotic Anim Pract 3:1(Jan): 221-40.

Burke, T. (1999). Husbandry and Medicine of Rodents and Lagomorphs. Proceedings: Central Veterinary Conference, Kansas City. accessed via Veterinary Information Network; vin.com

de la Navarre, B. (2008). Identification & treatment of common parasitic diseases of reptiles and amphibians. Proceedings: Western Veterinary Conf. accessed via Veterinary Information Network; vin.com

Ivey, E. & J. Morrisey (2000). Therapeutics for Rabbits. Vet Clin NA: Exotic Anim Pract 3:1(Jan): 183-216.

Papich, M. (1989). Effects of drugs on pregnancy. *Current Veterinary Therapy X: Small Animal Practice*. R. Kirk. Philadelphia, Saunders: 1291-9.

Roberson, E. L. (1988). Antinematodal Agents. *Veterinary Pharmacology and Therapeutics*. N. H. Booth and L. E. McDonald. Ames, Iowa State University Press: 882-927.

Pirlimycin HCl

(per-li-**mye**-sin)   Pirsue®

Intramammary Lincosamide Antibiotic

Prescriber Highlights

▶ Lincosamide antibiotic for intramammary use in dairy cattle.

▶ Milk withdrawal (at labeled doses) = 36 hours after last treatment; Meat withdrawal (at labeled doses) = 9 days.

Uses/Indications

Pirlimycin mastitis tubes are indicated for the treatment of clinical and subclinical mastitis caused by susceptible organisms in lactating dairy cattle.

Pharmacology/Actions

Like other lincosamides, pirlimycin acts by binding to the 50S ribosomal subunit of susceptible bacterial RNA, thus interfering with bacterial protein synthesis. It is primarily active against gram-positive bacteria, including a variety of species of staphylococcus (*S. aureus, S. epidermidis, S. chromogenes, S. hyicus, S. xylosus*), streptococcus (*S. agalactiae, S. dysgalactiae, S. uberis, S. bovis*) and *Enterococcus faecalis*.

Organisms with a MIC of ≤2 micrograms/mL are considered susceptible, and organisms with a MIC value of 4 micrograms/mL are considered resistant. If using a 2 microgram disk for Kirby-Bauer plate testing, a zone diameter of ≤12mm indicates resistance and a diameter of ≥13mm indicates susceptibility.

Pharmacokinetics

Little information is available; the manufacturer states that the drug penetrates the udder well and is absorbed systemically from the udder and then secreted into the milk of all four quarters. Tissue levels in treated quarters of pirlimycin are ≈ 2-3X those found in the extracellular fluid.

Contraindications/Precautions/Warnings

No information was noted.

Adverse Effects

No adverse affects, including udder irritation have been reported thus far.

Milk from untreated quarters must be disposed of during withdrawal time as residues may be detected from untreated quarters.

Reproductive/Nursing Safety

No information noted.

Overdosage/Acute Toxicity

No data was located.

Drug Interactions

- Because **erythromycin** and clindamycin have shown antagonism *in vitro*, this could also occur with pirlimycin.

Laboratory Considerations

- The established tolerance of pirlimycin in milk is 0.4 ppm.

Doses

- **CATTLE:**

  For the treatment of clinical and subclinical mastitis caused by susceptible organisms in lactating dairy cattle (labeled-dose; FDFA-approved): Infuse contents of one syringe into each affected quarter. Use proper teat end preparation, sanitation and intramammary infusion technique. Repeat treatment after 24 hours. Daily treatment may be repeated at 24-hour intervals for up to 8 consecutive days. (Package Insert; *Pirsue®*)

Monitoring
- Efficacy.
- Withdrawal periods.

Client Information
- Be sure clients understand dosage recommendations and withdrawal periods.
- Milk from untreated quarters must be disposed of during withdrawal time as residues may be detected from untreated quarters.

Chemistry/Synonyms
Pirlimycin HCl is a lincosamide antibiotic. It has a molecular weight of 465.4.

Pirlimycin HCl may also be known as U-57930E and *Pirsue®*.

Storage/Stability
Store syringes at or below 25°C (77°F); protect from freezing.

Dosage Forms/Regulatory Status
VETERINARY-LABELED PRODUCTS:

Pirlimycin HCl Sterile Solution: 50 mg (equiv. to free base) in a 10 mL disposable teat syringe; *Pirsue® Aqueous Gel*; (Rx). FDA-approved for use in lactating dairy cattle. Milk withdrawal (at labeled doses) = 36 hours after last treatment; Meat withdrawal if two infusions 24 hours apart are used = 9 days; following any extended duration of therapy (more than two infusions at a 24-hour interval, up to 8 consecutive days), animals must not be slaughtered for 21 days.

HUMAN-LABELED PRODUCTS: NONE.

Revisions/References
Monograph revised/updated June 2014.

Piroxicam
(peer-**ox**-i-kam)   Feldene®

Non-Steroidal Antiinflammatory (NSAID), Anti-Tumor

Prescriber Highlights
▶ NSAID primarily used for its antitumor (indirect) activity. There are safer and/or approved NSAIDs available for pain/inflammation for dogs & cats.

▶ Low dose metronomic (continuous) therapy with cyclophosphamide shows promise for preventing sarcoma recurrence in dogs with fewer adverse effects then high dose treatment.

▶ Contraindications: Hypersensitivity or severely allergic to aspirin or other NSAIDs. Extreme Caution: Active, or a history of GI ulcer disease or bleeding disorders. Caution: Severely compromised cardiac function.

▶ Use in cats is controversial; use with caution.

▶ Adverse Effects: GI ulceration & bleeding, renal papillary necrosis, & peritonitis.

Uses/Indications
In dogs and cats, piroxicam's primary use is as adjunctive treatment of bladder transitional cell carcinoma. It may also be of benefit in squamous cell carcinomas, mammary adenocarcinoma, and transmissible venereal tumor (TVT). Piroxicam may be beneficial in reducing the pain and inflammation associated with degenerative joint disease, but there are safer alternatives available.).

Pharmacology/Actions
Like other non-steroidal antiinflammatory agents, piroxicam has antiinflammatory, analgesic, and antipyretic activity. The drug's antiinflammatory activity is thought to be primarily due to its inhibition of prostaglandin synthesis, but additional mechanisms (*e.g.*, superoxide formation inhibition) may be important. As with other NSAIDs, piroxicam can affect renal function, cause GI mucosal damage, and inhibit platelet aggregation.

Piroxicam's antitumor effects are believed to be due to its action on the immune system and not because of direct effects on tumor cells.

Pharmacokinetics
After oral administration, piroxicam is well absorbed from the gut. While the presence of food will decrease the rate of absorption, it will not decrease the amount absorbed. It is not believed that antacids significantly affect absorption.

In dogs, piroxicam has high oral bioavailability (100%) with peak plasma levels reached ≈ 3 hours after dosing. Volume of distribution is ≈ 0.3 L/kg; total body clearance is 0.066 L/hour and elimination half-life is ≈ 40 hours (Galbraith *et al.* 1991).

After single oral doses in cats, piroxicam is well absorbed with an oral bioavailability of ≈ 80%. Peak levels occur in ≈ 3 hours. Elimination half-life after intravenous or oral dosing is ≈ 12-13 hours.

Piroxicam is highly bound to plasma proteins. In humans, synovial levels are ≈ 40% of those found in plasma. Maternal milk concentrations are only ≈ 1% of plasma levels.

In humans, piroxicam has a very long plasma half-life (≈ 50 hours). The drug is principally excreted as metabolites in the urine after hepatic biotransformation.

Contraindications/Precautions/Warnings
Piroxicam is contraindicated in patients hypersensitive to it or that are severely allergic to aspirin or other NSAIDs. It should be used only when its potential benefits outweigh the risks in patients with active or history of GI ulcer disease or bleeding disorders. Because peripheral edema has been noted in some human patients, it should be used with caution in patients with severely compromised cardiac function.

Piroxicam has not been evaluated for use in cats. It must be used with extreme caution, if at all, in this species.

Do not confuse piroxicam with PARoxetine.

Adverse Effects
Like other NSAIDs used in dogs, piroxicam has the potential for causing significant GI ulceration and bleeding. The therapeutic window for the drug is very narrow, as doses as low as 1 mg/kg given daily have caused significant GI ulceration, renal papillary necrosis, and peritonitis. Other adverse effects reported in humans and potentially possible in dogs include: CNS effects (headache, dizziness, etc.), otic effects (tinnitus), elevations in hepatic function tests, pruritus and rash, and peripheral edema. Renal papillary necrosis has been seen in dogs at post-mortem but, apparently, clinical effects have not been noted with these occurrences.

In cats, GI effects (vomiting, anorexia, diarrhea) may be seen, particularly early in therapy. There are anecdotal reports of piroxicam decreasing hematocrits in cats when dosed daily for 7-14 days. Renal toxicity is possible if used for prolonged periods.

Reproductive/Nursing Safety
Animal studies have not demonstrated any teratogenic effects associated with piroxicam. The drug is excreted into milk in very low concentrations (≈ 1% found in maternal plasma). In humans, the FDA categorizes this drug as category *C* for use during pregnancy (*Animal studies have shown an adverse effect on the fetus, but there are no adequate studies in humans; or there are no animal reproduction studies and no adequate studies in humans.*) If using in the third trimester or near delivery in humans, the FDA categorizes all NSAIDs as category *D* for use during pregnancy (*There is evidence of human fetal risk, but the potential benefits from the use of the drug in pregnant women may be acceptable despite its potential risks.*)

Most NSAIDs are excreted in maternal milk; use with caution in nursing patients.

Overdosage/Acute Toxicity

There is limited information available, but dogs may be more sensitive to the drugs ulcerative effects than are humans.

There were 63 exposures to piroxicam reported to the ASPCA Animal Poison Control Center (APCC) during 2008-2009. In these cases 58 were dogs with 12 showing clinical signs and 5 were cats with 1 showing clinical signs. Common findings in dogs recorded in decreasing frequency included vomiting, and bloody vomitus.

As with any NSAID, overdosage can lead to gastrointestinal and renal effects. Decontamination with emetics and/or activated charcoal is appropriate. For doses where GI effects are expected, the use of gastrointestinal protectants is warranted. If renal effects are also expected, fluid diuresis is should be considered. Patients ingesting significant overdoses should be monitored carefully and treated supportively.

Drug Interactions

The following drug interactions have either been reported or are theoretical in humans or animals receiving piroxicam and may be of significance in veterinary patients. Unless otherwise noted, use together is not necessarily contraindicated, but weigh the potential risks and perform additional monitoring when appropriate.

- **AMINOGLYCOSIDES (gentamicin, amikacin, etc.):** Increased risk for nephrotoxicity.
- **ANTICOAGULANTS (heparin, LMWH, warfarin, etc.):** Increased risk for bleeding possible.
- **ASPIRIN:** When aspirin is used concurrently with piroxicam, plasma levels of piroxicam could decrease and an increased likelihood of GI adverse effects (blood loss) could occur. Concomitant administration of aspirin with piroxicam cannot be recommended.
- **BISPHOSPHONATES (alendronate, etc.):** May increase risk for GI ulceration.
- **CISPLATIN:** Piroxicam may potentiate the renal toxicity of cisplatin when used in combination.
- **CORTICOSTEROIDS:** Concomitant administration with NSAIDs may significantly increase the risks for GI adverse effects.
- **FUROSEMIDE:** Piroxicam may reduce the saluretic and diuretic effects of furosemide.
- **HIGHLY PROTEIN BOUND DRUGS (e.g., phenytoin, oral anticoagulants, other antiinflammatory agents, salicylates, sulfonamides, and the sulfonylurea antidiabetic agents):** Because piroxicam is highly bound to plasma proteins (99%), it potentially could displace other highly bound drugs; increased serum levels and duration of actions may occur. Although these interactions are usually of little clinical concern, use together with caution.
- **METHOTREXATE:** Serious toxicity has occurred when NSAIDs have been used concomitantly with methotrexate; use together with extreme caution.

Laboratory Considerations

- Piroxicam may cause falsely elevated **blood glucose** values when using the glucose oxidase and peroxidase method using ABTS as a chromogen.

Doses

- **DOGS:**

  As an adjunctive therapy of neoplastic diseases (extra-label): 0.3 mg/kg PO with food once a day (preferred, if tolerated) or once every other day (q48h). Adding misoprostol may be considered in dogs that do not tolerate NSAID's GI effects.

  For adjunctive treatment of idiopathic lymphoplasmacytic rhinitis (LPR): Long-term administration of antibiotics having immunomodulatory effects (doxycycline 3 – 5 mg/kg PO q12h; or azithromycin 5 mg/kg PO q24h) combined with NSAIDs can be helpful in some dogs. Piroxicam 0.3 mg/kg PO q24h is recommended. If clinical improvement is observed within 2 weeks, daily piroxicam therapy is continued but the frequency of administration of doxycycline is reduced to once daily or azithromycin reduced to twice weekly. Therapy will likely be required for a minimum of 6 months, if not indefinitely. (Kuehn 2007b)

- **CATS:**

  As adjunctive therapy for neoplasia (extra-label): For adjunctive therapy of transitional cell carcinomas: 0.3 mg/kg PO q24-72h. Most will use q48h (every other day) dosing interval.

  As an antiinflammatory/analgesic (extra-label): 1 mg per cat PO q24h for a maximum of 7 days. (**Note:** After compounding, drug is stable for 10 days). (Gaynor 2008), (Rochette 2007)

  Idiopathic chronic rhinosinusitis (extra-label): Some cats' clinical signs can be reduced with piroxicam at 0.3 mg/kg PO once daily or every other day. (Kuehn 2007a)

- **HORSES:**

  For neoplastic diseases (extra-label):

  a) From a case report treating mucocutaneous squamous cell carcinoma: 80 mg (per horse) PO once daily; lip lesion resolved completely over 3 months, but patient developed colic signs twice. Dose was eventually reduced to every other day or every third day. (Moore *et al.* 2003)

  b) From a case report treating a squamous cell carcinoma of the third eyelid after surgical excision: 80 mg (per horse) PO once daily. (Iwabe *et al.* 2009)

- **RABBITS, RODENTS, SMALL MAMMALS:**

  Rabbits for fracture associated limb swelling (extra-label): 0.1 – 0.2 mg/kg PO q8h for 3 weeks. (Ivey *et al.* 2000)

Monitoring

- Adverse Effects (particularly GI bleeding).
- Liver function and renal function tests should be monitored occasionally with chronic use.

Client Information

- Best given with food to reduce the chance for stomach upset.
- Gastrointestinal (stomach) ulcers and bleeding and kidney problems (especially in cats) are possible.

Chemistry/Synonyms

An oxicam derivative non-steroidal antiinflammatory agent, piroxicam occurs as a white, crystalline solid. It is sparingly soluble in water. Piroxicam is structurally not related to other non-steroidal antiinflammatory agents.

Piroxicam may also be known as: CP-16171, piroxicamum or PIRO; many trade names are available.

Storage/Stability

Capsules should be stored at temperatures <30°C in tight, light-resistant containers. When stored as recommended, capsules have an expiration date of 36 months after manufacture.

Dosage Forms/Regulatory Status

VETERINARY-LABELED PRODUCTS: NONE.

The ARCI (Racing Commissioners International) has designated this drug as a class 4 substance. See the appendix for more information.

HUMAN-LABELED PRODUCTS:

Piroxicam Oral Capsules: 10 mg & 20 mg; *Feldene®*, generic; (Rx)

Revisions/References

Monograph revised/updated May 2014.

Galbraith, E. A. & Q. A. McKellar (1991). Pharmacokinetics and pharmacodynamics of piroxicam in dogs. Veterinary Record **128**(24): 561-5.

Gaynor, J. S. (2008). Control of Cancer Pain in Veterinary Patients. Veterinary Clinics of North America-Small Animal Practice **38**(6): 1429-+.

Ivey, E. & J. Morrisey (2000). Therapeutics for Rabbits. Vet Clin NA: Exotic Anim Pract **3**:1(Jan): 183-216.

Iwabe, S., et al. (2009). The use of piroxicam as an adjunctive treatment for squamous cell carcinoma in the third eyelid of a horse. Veterinaria Mexico **40**(4): 389-95.

Kuehn, N. (2007a). Chronic rhinitis in cats. Proceedings: ACVIM. accessed via Veterinary Information Network; vin.com

Kuehn, N. (2007b). Chronic rhinitis in dogs. Proceedings; ACVIM. accessed via Veterinary Information Network; vin.com

Moore, A. S., et al. (2003). Long-term control of mucocutaneous squamous cell carcinoma and metastases in a horse using piroxicam. Equine Veterinary Journal **35**(7): 715-8.

Rochette, J. (2007). Nerve Blocks and Management of Oral Pain. Proceedings: AAFP. accessed via Veterinary Information Network; vin.com

Plasma-Lyte – see the section on intravenous fluids in the Appendix

Polyethylene Glycol 3350 (PEG 3350)

Miralax®

Laxative, Hyperosmotic

Prescriber Highlights

▶ For constipation, bowel "cleansing" or to increase elimination of GI toxins.

▶ Contraindications: PEG 3350 solutions are contraindicated in patients with GI obstruction, gastric retention, bowel perforation, toxic colitis, or megacolon (humans).

▶ Adverse Effects: Cramping, nausea possible. Electrolyte disturbances possible, particularly with repeated use.

Uses/Indications

Polyethylene glycol 3350 (PEG 3350) used alone (*MiraLax®*, etc.) acts as an osmotic laxative agent. When balance electrolytes are added (*CoLyte®*, *GoLytely®*, etc.), it is used as a bowel cleansing solution. It could also be used to reduce intestinal transit time to reduce the absorption of orally ingested toxicants and poisons, but usually sorbitol is chosen for this indication.

Pharmacology/Actions

Polyethylene glycol 3350 is a non-absorbable compound, that when used alone (*MiraLax®*, etc.) acts as an osmotic laxative agent. When used as a bowel cleansing solution (*CoLyte®*, *GoLytely®*, etc.), additional electrolytes are added to help prevent electrolyte imbalance. Sodium sulfate is the primary sodium source so sodium absorption is minimized. Other electrolytes (bicarbonate potassium and chloride) are also added so that no net change occurs with either absorption or secretion of electrolytes or water in the gut.

Pharmacokinetics

Depending on dose and additional fluid consumed, PEG 3350 can have a laxative effect within one hour of dosing.

Contraindications/Precautions/Warnings

In humans, PEG 3350 solutions are contraindicated in patients that are hypersensitive to it or with GI obstruction, gastric retention, bowel perforation, toxic colitis, or megacolon.

Adverse Effects

Vomiting, nausea and cramping are possible. Long-term use could potentially cause hyponatremia, dehydration, or hyperkalemia. If PEG 3350 is absorbed, oxidative injury to red blood cells could occur in cats, but this has not been documented to date.

In humans, PEG 3350 has rarely caused hyponatremia secondary to syndrome of inappropriate vasopressin release (SIADH).

In one small study (n=6) in cats where PEG 3350 with electrolytes was given long-term (powder in food and dose titrated to produce soft, but formed stools), 1 cat sporadically vomited after dosing, mild erythrocytosis was noted in 1 cat, and 3 cats developed mild hyperkalemia. The authors concluded that PEG 3350 was a safe and palatable oral laxative in cats for long-term use; potential side effects include hyperkalemia and subclinical dehydration (Tam *et al.* 2010).

Reproductive/Nursing Safety

Minimal amounts are absorbed and it is likely that these products are safe to use in pregnant or lactating animals. Avoid inducing fluid or electrolyte imbalances.

Overdosage/Acute Toxicity

One time overdosage could cause diarrhea and fluid or electrolyte abnormalities.

Drug Interactions

No specific drug interactions were noted, but reduced absorption could occur of other oral drugs (especially extended-release) if given concomitantly.

Doses

- **DOGS:**

  <u>Polyethylene Glycol 3350-Electrolyte Solution (*e.g.,* CoLyte®, GoLytely®):</u>

  For colonic cleansing prior to colonoscopy (extra-label): Several slightly different protocols have been suggested. The following is an example: Keep animal from food for 24-36 hours. On the evening prior to a morning colonoscopy (or the morning for an afternoon colonoscopy), give 60 mL/kg *Go-Lytely®* via orogastric tube. Repeat in 2 hours. A warm water enema should follow each dose and a third enema given prior to anesthesia. (Leib 2003), (Leib 2006)

- **CATS:**

  <u>Polyethylene 3350 Powder (*e.g.,* Miralax®):</u>

  As a laxative (extra-label): 1/8th to ¼ teaspoonful twice daily in food.

  <u>Polyethylene Glycol 3350-Electrolyte Solution (*e.g.,* CoLyte®, GoLytely®):</u>

  For adjunctive treatment of obstipation/constipation (extra-label): From an observational study in 9 cats. *CoLyte®* was administered via naso-esophageal tube at rates between 6 – 10 mL/kg/hr. The median total dose given was 80 mL/kg (range 40 – 156 mL/kg). Median time to significant defecation was 8 hours (range 5-24). Side effects were limited to vomiting in 1 cat (was vomiting prior to admission). (Carr *et al.* 2010)

  For colonic cleansing prior to colonoscopy (extra-label): Keep animal from food for 24-36 hours. On the evening prior to a morning colonoscopy (or the morning for an afternoon colonoscopy), give 60 mL/kg *Go-Lytely®* via nasogastric tube. Repeat in 2 hours. A warm water enema should follow each dose and a third enema given prior to anesthesia. Metoclopramide (0.2 mg/kg SC 15-20 minutes before the first Go-Lytely® dose is given to reduce vomiting. (Leib 2003), (Leib 2006)

Monitoring

- Fluid and electrolyte status in susceptible patients, high doses, or chronic use.
- Clinical efficacy.

Client Information

- Used to treat constipation, bowel cleanse before procedures, or help remove toxins or poisons from GI tract.
- Polyethylene glycol 3350 (PEG 3350) powders need to be dis-

solved in liquid before using. Follow your veterinarians or pharmacists measuring instructions carefully.

- PEG 3350 is available OTC (over-the-counter; without a prescription). Do not give PEG 3350 (or any other OTC medications) to your animal without first consulting a veterinarian.
- Contact veterinarian if animal begins vomiting.

Chemistry/Synonyms

Polyethylene glycol 3350 is a non-absorbable compound that acts as an osmotic agent.

Storage/Stability

Store powder at 25°C (77°F); excursions are permitted from 15°-30°C (59°-86°F). Reconstituted PEG 3350 solutions (from powder by the pharmacy, client, clinic, etc.) should be kept refrigerated and used within 24 hours.

Dosage Forms/Regulatory Status

VETERINARY-LABELED PRODUCTS: NONE.

HUMAN-LABELED PRODUCTS:

Polyethylene Glycol 3350 Powder for solution: *MiraLax®*, *GlycoLax®*, *ClearLax®*, *Gavilax®*, *Dulcolax Balance®*, generic; (OTC). Available in either pre-measured 17 gram packets or bulk powder.

Polyethylene Glycol 3350 and Electrolyte Solutions (Rx):

There are a variety of "prep" products available. The following are representative:

OCL® Solution; (Rx) Oral Solution in 1500 mL: 146 mg sodium chloride, 168 mg sodium bicarbonate, 1.29 grams sodium sulfate decahydrate, 75 mg potassium chloride, 6 grams PEG-3350.

CoLyte®; (Rx); 1 gallon of Powder for Oral Solution in bottles: 227.1 grams PEG 3350, 5.53 grams sodium chloride, 6.36 grams sodium bicarbonate, 21.5 grams sodium sulfate, 2.82 grams potassium chloride; 4 L of solution: 240 grams PEG 3350, 22.72 grams sodium sulfate, 6.72 grams sodium bicarbonate, 5.84 grams NaCl, 2.98 grams KCL.

GoLYTELY®; (Rx); Powder for Oral Solution in jugs: 5.86 grams sodium chloride, 6.74 grams sodium bicarbonate, 22.74 grams sodium sulfate, 2.97 grams potassium chloride, 236 grams PEG 3350; Packets: 227.1 grams PEG 3350, 21.5 grams sodium sulfate, 6.36 grams sodium bicarbonate, 5.53 grams NaCl, 2.82 grams KCl.

NuLytely®, *TriLyte®*, (Rx); Powder for Reconstitution in 4 L jugs: 420 grams PEG 3350, 5.72 grams sodium bicarbonate, 11.2 grams NaCl, 1.48 grams KCl.

MoviPrep®; (Rx); Powder for Reconstitution in pouches: 100 grams PEG 3350, 7.5 grams sodium sulfate, 2.691 grams NaCl, 1.015 grams KCl.

Revisions/References

Monograph revised/updated June 2014.

Carr, A. & M. Gaunt (2010). Constipation Resolution with Administration of Polyethylene-Glycol Solution in Cats (Abstract). Proceedings: ACVIM. accessed via Veterinary Information Network; vin.com

Leib, M. (2003). Chronic diarrhea in dogs and cats: Parts 1 & 2. Proceedings: Atlantic Coast Veterinary Conference. accessed via Veterinary Information Network; vin.com

Leib, M. (2006). Colonoscopy. Proceedings: WVC. accessed via Veterinary Information Network; vin.com

Tam, F., et al. (2010). Safety and palatability of polyethylene glycol 3350 as an oral laxative in cats. Proceedings: ACVIM. accessed via Veterinary Information Network; vin.com

Polysulfated Glycosaminoglycan; (PSGAG)

(pol-ee-**sulf**-ayte-ed glye-**kose**-a-meen-ohe-**glye**-kan)

Adequan®, Chondroprotec®

Proteolytic Enzyme Inhibitor; Chondroprotectant

Prescriber Highlights

▶ Proteolytic enzyme inhibitor (*Adequan®* is FDA-approved) for IM or intra-articular treatment for non-infectious &/or traumatic joint dysfunction & associated lameness of the carpal joints in horses & non-infectious degenerative &/or traumatic arthritis in dogs.

▶ Contraindications: Intra-articular injection if patient hypersensitive to PSGAG. Should not be used in place of other treatments when infection suspected or present, or when surgery or joint immobilization required.

▶ Adverse Effects: **Horses:** IM use: Unlikely. Intra-articular: Post-injection inflammation possible. **Dogs:** Dose-related inhibition of coagulation/hemostasis possible.

Uses/Indications

Polysulfated glycosaminoglycan (PSGAG; *Adequan®*) administered to horses either IM or IA is indicated for the treatment of non-infectious and/or traumatic joint dysfunction and associated lameness of the carpal joints. Some studies have indicated that PSGAG is much less effective in joints where there has been acute trauma but no degradative enzymes are present.

PSGAG (*Adequan®*) is also FDA-approved for the control of signs associated with non-infectious degenerative and/or traumatic arthritis in dogs.

Pharmacology/Actions

In joint tissue, PSGAG inhibits proteolytic enzymes that can degrade proteoglycans (including naturally occurring glycosaminoglycans), thereby preventing or reducing decreased connective tissue flexibility, resistance to compression, and resiliency. By acting as a precursor, PSGAG increases the synthesis of proteoglycans, reduces inflammation by reducing concentrations of prostaglandin E_2 (released in response to joint injury) and increases hyaluronate concentrations in the joint, thereby restoring synovial fluid viscosity.

Pharmacokinetics

PSGAG is deposited in all layers of articular cartilage and preferentially taken up by osteoarthritic cartilage. When administered IM, articular levels will with time exceed those found in the serum. After IM injection, peak joint levels are reached in 48 hours and persist up to 96 hours. In small animals, some state that "SC dosing works as well as IM", however no published evidence supporting this was noted. No pharmacokinetic information was located for non-approved PSGAG products.

Contraindications/Precautions/Warnings

PSGAG is contraindicated for intra-articular administration in patients hypersensitive to it. While the manufacturer states there are no contraindications for IM use of the drug, the drug should not be used in place of other therapies in cases where infection is present or suspected, or in place of surgery or joint immobilization where indicated.

Some clinicians feel that PSGAG should not be used within one week of arthrotomy in dogs because it may cause increased bleeding. This effect apparently has not been confirmed in the literature.

Adverse Effects

Adverse effects are unlikely when using the IM route. Intra-articular administration may cause a post-injection inflammation (joint pain, effusion, swelling, and associated lameness) secondary to sensitivity reactions, traumatic injection technique, overdosage, or the number or frequency of the injections. Treatment consisting of antiinflammatory drugs, cold hydrotherapy, and rest is recommended. Although uncommon, joint sepsis secondary to intraarticular injection is possible; strict aseptic technique should be employed to minimize this occurrence. Several sources recommend adding 125 mg of amikacin if PSGAG is to be injected into joints of horses.

In dogs, a dose-related inhibition of coagulation/hemostasis has been described.

Reproductive/Nursing Safety

Reproductive studies have apparently not been performed; use with caution during pregnancy or in breeding animals (the manufacturer does not recommend use in breeding animals).

In humans, the FDA categorizes glycosaminoglycans as category B for use during pregnancy (*Animal studies have not yet demonstrated risk to the fetus, but there are no adequate studies in pregnant women; or animal studies have shown an adverse effect, but adequate studies in pregnant women have not demonstrated a risk to the fetus in the first trimester of pregnancy, and there is no evidence of risk in later trimesters.*)

It is not known whether glycosaminoglycans are excreted in maternal milk, but is unlikely to be of significant concern.

Overdosage/Acute Toxicity

Doses 5X those recommended (2.5 grams) given IM to horses twice weekly for 6 weeks revealed no untoward effects. Approximately 2% of horses receiving overdoses (up to 1250 mg) IA showed transient clinical signs associated with joint inflammation.

Drug Interactions

While specific drug interactions have not been detailed to date, using this product in conjunction with either steroids or non-steroidal antiinflammatory agents could mask the signs and clinical signs associated with septic joints.

There is some concern that since PSGAG is a heparin analog that it should not be used in conjunction with other NSAIDs or other anticoagulants. Clinical significance remains unclear, but use together with caution.

Doses

- **HORSES:**

    For the treatment of non-infectious and/or traumatic joint dysfunction and associated lameness of the carpal joints in horses (labeled-dose; FDA-approved): For IM administration: 500 mg IM (of IM product) every 4 days for 28 days. Thoroughly cleanse injection site before injecting. Do not mix with other drugs or chemicals. For intra-articular administration: 250 mg (of IA product) IA once a week for 5 weeks. Joint area should be shaved, and cleansed as if a surgical procedure, prior to injecting. Do not mix with other drugs or chemicals. (Package Inserts; *Adequan® I.M., Adequan® I.A.*)

- **DOGS:**

    For the treatment of non-infectious degenerative and/or traumatic arthritis (labeled-dose; FDA-approved): 4.4 mg/kg IM twice weekly for up to 4 weeks. (Label information; *Adequan® Canine*)

- **CATS:**

    As a chondroprotective drug (extra-label): 2 mg/kg IM every 3-5 days for 4 treatments; only anecdotal experience in cats (Kerwin 2007). Many protocols exist for administering *Adequan®* to cats, such as 5 mg/kg SC twice weekly for 4 weeks, then once weekly for 4 weeks, then once monthly. Results of clinical studies in other species are conflicting and no long-term data exist for cats (Little 2013).

- **RABBITS, RODENTS, SMALL MAMMALS:**

    Rabbits for arthritis (extra-label): 2.2 mg/kg SC or IM every 3 days for 21-28 days, then once every 2 weeks. (Ivey *et al.* 2000)

Monitoring

- Efficacy.
- Joint inflammation/infection if administered IA.

Client Information

- The IA product must be administered by veterinary professionals; the IM product could, with proper instruction, be administered by the owner.

Chemistry/Synonyms

Polysulfated glycosaminoglycan (PSGAG) is chemically similar to natural mucopolysaccharides found in cartilaginous tissues. PSGAG is reportedly an analog of heparin.

Polysulfated glycosaminoglycan is also known as PSGAG, *Adequan®* and *Chondroprotec®*.

Storage/Stability

Commercial products should be stored in a cool place 8-15°C (46-59°F). The manufacturer recommends discarding any unused portion from the vial or ampule and does not recommend mixing with any other drug or chemical.

Dosage Forms/Regulatory Status

VETERINARY-LABELED PRODUCTS:

Polysulfated Glycosaminoglycan for Intra-Articular Injection: 250 mg/mL in 1 mL single use vials, boxes of 6; *Adequan® I.A.*; (Rx). FDA-approved for use in horses (not in those intended for food).

Polysulfated Glycosaminoglycan for Intra-Muscular Injection: 100 mg/mL in 5 mL glass ampules or vials and 20 mL, 30 mL, and 50 mL multi-dose vials; *Adequan® I.M.*; (Rx). FDA-approved for use in horses (not in those intended for food).

Polysulfated Glycosaminoglycan for IM Injection: 100 mg/mL; *Adequan® Canine*; (Rx). FDA-approved for use in dogs.

There are also compounded products available. These are not FDA-approved drug products.

HUMAN-LABELED PRODUCTS: NONE.

Revisions/References

Monograph revised/updated June 2014.

Ivey, E. & J. Morrisey (2000). Therapeutics for Rabbits. Vet Clin NA: Exotic Anim Pract 3:1(Jan): 183-216.
Kerwin, S. (2007). Feline Osteoarthritis. Proceedings: Western Vet Conf. accessed via Veterinary Information Network; vin.com
Little, S. (2013). Managing Arthritis in Senior Cats. International Society of Feline Medicine. accessed via Veterinary Information Network; vin.com

Ponazuril

(poe-**naz**-yoor-ill)   Toltrazuril sulfone, Marquis®

Antiprotozoal

Prescriber Highlights

- Equine FDA-approved triazine for treating EPM.
- Adverse Effect profile not well established; in field trials: rashes, hives, blisters, or GI signs noted.
- Treatment is relatively expensive.

Uses/Indications

Ponazuril is indicated for the treatment of equine protozoal myeloencephalitis (EPM) caused by *Sarcocystis neurona*.

Ponazuril could potentially be useful in treating *Neospora caninum* and Toxoplasma or other protozoal infections in other species (*e.g.*, dogs, cats, birds, reptiles, ruminants).

Pharmacology/Actions

The triazine class of antiprotozoals is believed to target the "plastid" body, an organelle found in the members of the Apicomplexa phylum, including *Sarcocystis neurona*. *In vitro* levels required to kill *Sarcocystis neurona* range from 0.1-1 micrograms/mL. Ponazuril is coccidiocidal.

Pharmacokinetics

When administered orally to horses in water, ponazuril has a bioavailability of ≈ 30% and elimination half-life of 80 hours. After daily (5 mg/kg) oral administration to horses, ponazuril reaches its peak serum levels in ≈ 18 days and peak CSF levels in ≈ 15 days. Peak CSF levels are 1/20th (0.21 micrograms/mL) those found in the serum. Elimination half-life from serum averages ≈ 4.5 days. If ponazuril is given orally (2.2 mg/kg) dissolved in DMSO, bioavailability is significantly enhanced (Dirikolu *et al.* 2009a).

In cattle, 5 mg/kg oral doses of ponazuril are relatively well absorbed and have an approximate elimination half-life of 58 hours (Dirikolu *et al.* 2009b).

Contraindications/Precautions/Warnings

None were noted. Before treating, other conditions that can cause ataxia should be ruled out.

Adverse Effects

Field trials showed some animals developing blisters on nose and mouth or a rash/hives. Single animals developed diarrhea, mild colic or seizures.

Successful treatment may not negate all the clinical signs associated with EPM.

Keratoconjunctivitis sicca (KCS) has been reported in some dogs, especially those breeds with a predilection towards developing KCS or when the drug was given in overdose quantities.

Reproductive/Nursing Safety

Safety during pregnancy or in lactating mares has not been evaluated.

Overdosage/Acute Toxicity

Daily doses of up to 30 mg/kg (6X) primarily caused loose feces. Moderate edema of the uterine epithelium was noted on histopathology for female horses receiving the 6X dose.

Drug Interactions/Laboratory Considerations

- None noted.

Doses

- **DOGS/CATS:**

  For Neosporosis or Toxoplasmosis (extra-label): 7.5 – 15 mg/kg PO once daily for 28 days. Dose extrapolated between doses for horses and mice. (Greene *et al.* 2006)

  For coccidiosis (extra-label): Based upon a study in shelter dogs and cats. The authors concluded that extended courses (two 3-day courses) of ponazuril at 50 mg/kg PO q24h are sometimes necessary for fecal flotation results to become negative in dogs and cats with coccidiosis. (Litster *et al.* 2013)

- **SMALL MAMMALS:**

  Rabbits for adjunctive treatment of *Eimeria* species (extra-label): 20 mg/kg PO q24h for 7 days. (Kelleher 2008)

- **HORSES:**

  For EPM (labeled dose; FDA-approved): 5 mg/kg, PO once daily for 28 days. See the package insert for specific dosing instructions. (Package insert; *Marquis®*)

- **CAMELIDS (NEW WORLD):**

  For *Eimeria macusaniensis* in Crias (extra-label): 20 mg/kg, PO once daily for 3 days. Because E. mac can cause clinical disease or even death before oocysts are present in feces, prophylactic treatment should be considered in camelids that have unexplained weight loss with concurrent hypoproteinemia and without severe anemia. The commercially available paste (*Marquis®*) is too concentrated to be given to camelids and should be diluted before being administered. Recommend diluting the paste to 100 mg/mL by taking 40 grams of paste, *q.s.* with distilled water to 60 grams total and mixing well. It is very water-soluble and can be easily syringed into the animal. (Walker 2009)

- **BIRDS:**

  For Cryptosporidium respiratory disease in falcons (extra-label): Case report of two patients: 20 mg/kg PO (as a compounded suspension) once daily for 7 days. (Van Sant *et al.* 2009)

- **REPTILES:**

  For coccidiosis in Bearded dragons (extra-label): Anecdotal dosage recommendations vary considerably and include: For coccidians: 30 mg/kg PO twice 48 hours apart. (Mitchell 2008). Another recommendation is 30 – 45 mg/kg PO q24h for 28 days. Daily spot cleaning of the environment with weekly deep cleaning and disinfection is essential to prevent reinfection (Wright 2013).

Monitoring

- Clinical efficacy.

Client Information

- Very important not to miss any doses with this drug or it may not be effective.
- Can be given with or without food.
- Contact veterinarian if rashes, hives, blisters, or GI signs develop.

Chemistry/Synonyms

Related to other antiprotozoals such as toltrazuril, ponazuril is a triazine antiprotozoal (anticoccidial) agent. The commercially available oral paste is white to off-white in color and odorless; pH is 5.7-6. Solubility of ponazuril in DMSO is 250 mg/mL.

Ponazuril may also be known as: toltrazolone sulfone, toltrazuril sulfone, ICI-128436, *Marquis®*, and *Ponalrestat®*.

Storage/Stability

Store the paste at room temperature (15-30°C).

Compatibility/Compounding Considerations

For use in small animals, particularly in shelter situations various dilutions of the equine paste can be made. For practical purposes, 1 gram of paste is equivalent to 1 mL of paste and contains 150 mg of ponazuril. No specific stability data was located for these dilutions.

Dosage Forms/Regulatory Status

VETERINARY-LABELED PRODUCTS:

Ponazuril Oral Paste (15% w/w): 127-gram tubes; each gram of paste contains 150 mg of ponazuril; each syringe is enough to treat a 1200 lb. horse for 7 days. *Marquis®*; (Rx). Not for use in horses intended for food.

HUMAN-LABELED PRODUCTS: NONE.

Revisions/References

Monograph revised/updated May 2014.

Dirikolu, L., et al. (2009a). Synthesis and detection of toltrazuril sulfone and its pharmacokinetics in horses following administration in dimethylsulfoxide. J. Vet. Pharmacol. Ther. 32(4): 368-78.

Dirikolu, L., et al. (2009b). Detection, quantifications and pharmacokinetics of toltrazuril sulfone (Ponazuril) in cattle. J. Vet. Pharmacol. Ther. 32(3): 280-8.

Greene, C., et al. (2006). Appendix 8: Antimicrobial Drug Formulary. *Infectious Disease of the Dog and Cat.* C. Greene, Elsevier: 1186-333.

Kelleher, S. (2008). Rabbit GI Disease. Proceedings: WVC. accessed via Veterinary Information Network; vin.com

Litster, A., et al. (2013). Clinical trial to assess the efficacy of ponazuril for the treatment of coccidiosis in dogs and cats (Abstract). Journal of Veterinary Internal Medicine 27(3): 725-6.

Mitchell, M. A. (2008). Gastroenterology of Reptiles. Proceedings: ACVC. accessed via Veterinary Information Network; vin.com

Van Sant, F. & G. Stewart (2009). Ponazuril Used as a Treatment for Suspected Cryptosporidium Infection in 2 Hybrid Falcons. Proceedings: AAV. accessed via Veterinary Information Network; vin.com

Walker, P. (2009). Differential Diagnosis of Diarrhea in Camelid Crias. Proceedings: ACVIM. accessed via Veterinary Information Network; vin.com

Wright, K. (2013). Bearded Dragon Medicine & Surgery. Proceedings: ABVP. accessed via Veterinary Information Network; vin.com

Posaconazole

(poe-sa-**kon**-a-zole)   Noxafil®

Azole Antifungal

Prescriber Highlights

▶ Second generation triazole oral (suspension) antifungal with a wide spectrum of activity, but little information on clinical efficacy and safety published in veterinary medicine.

▶ Currently cost-prohibitive for most clients. May be cost-effective in cats and small dogs for itraconazole- or fluconazole-resistant infections.

▶ Adverse effect profile for animals is not known. Gastrointestinal effects most likely, but increases in liver enzymes have been reported.

▶ Treatment may be required for months and infection may not be fully cleared.

Uses/Indications

Posaconazole, a second generation triazole antifungal, could potentially be useful for treating systemic or severe fungal infections in dogs and cats, including aspergillosis, sporotrichosis, coccidioidomycosis, blastomycosis, histoplasmosis, zygomycosis and mucormycosis.

In humans, posaconazole is labeled for prophylaxis (in at-risk patients) or treatment of candidiasis or aspergillosis. It is also used in an extra-label manner for treatment of other fungal infections.

The currently available dosage form is very expensive and may prohibit its clinical use for many animals. The availability of a generic oral dosage form of posaconazole in the USA is not expected until at least 2019.

A topical veterinary otic preparation (*Posatex®*) containing orbifloxacin, posaconazole, and mometasone may also be available.

Pharmacology/Actions

Posaconazole is structurally related to itraconazole, but has a wider spectrum of activity and, at present, significantly less fungal resistance. Like other triazoles, posaconazole inhibits lanosterol 14-alfa demethylase (CYP51), which is responsible for ergosterol synthesis. Ergosterol is a component of fungal cell walls.

Posaconazole's spectrum of activity includes a variety of organisms, including many species/strains of Blastomyces, Coccidioides, Histoplasma, Aspergillus, Fusarium, Candida, Mucor and zygomycetes. Fungi that are resistant to posaconazole may also be resistant to other azole antifungals (*e.g.*, fluconazole, itraconazole).

Pharmacokinetics

In dogs, depending on which suspension was used, the oral bioavailability of posaconazole was 43-59%; food increased bioavailability (peak levels and area under the curve) ≈ 4X. Terminal half-life was 15 hours (after IV dosing). Multiple day dosing caused some accumulation of drug. Based upon the kinetics results and minimum fungicidal concentrations for most organisms, the authors

concluded that a dosage of 10 mg/kg per day should be effective (Nomeir *et al.* 2000).

No pharmacokinetic data for cats was located.

In humans, peak levels after oral administration occur in 3-6 hours. Bioavailability is significantly increased if given with food. Protein binding is high (98%). Posaconazole is metabolized, primarily via glucuronidation. Approximately 71% of a dose is eliminated in feces primarily as unchanged drug. About 13% of a dose is eliminated in the urine as metabolites. Elimination half-life averages 35 hours.

Contraindications/Precautions/Warnings

Contraindications for posaconazole use in small animals are not known. For human use, labeled contraindications for posaconazole include hypersensitivity to the drug or any component in the suspension, concomitant use with HMG-CoA reductase inhibitors (*e.g.*, atorvastatin, simvastatin), sirolimus, ergot alkaloids, or CYP3A4 substrates that can prolong QT interval (pimozide, quinidine). Dosage adjustment for patients with decreased renal function is not required but additional monitoring should be done to watch for breakthrough fungal infections. Hepatic impairment requires no alterations to therapy.

Adverse Effects

The adverse effect profile for posaconazole in dogs or cats is not established. The only side effect possibly associated with 16-week posaconazole treatment in a cat with orbital aspergillosis was facial and ear pruritus/erythema. In a retrospective study of cats with sino-nasal and sino-orbital aspergillosis that had received posaconazole, 2/10 cats developed transient 1.1-2X elevations in alanine aminotransferase activity, but it was otherwise well tolerated (Barrs *et al.* 2012).

The most commonly reported side effects in humans are GI-related and include nausea, vomiting, abdominal pain and diarrhea. Rare, but serious adverse effects include liver failure/cholestasis (associated with high dosages), prolonged QT interval/Torsade des pointes. Other side effects reported include skin rash, headache, tremors, hypertension, anorexia and weakness.

Mild to moderate increases in liver enzymes and bilirubin can be seen but are usually reversible with therapy discontinuation; monitor for development of more severe hepatic injury. Consider discontinuing the drug if clinical signs of liver disease occur.

Reproductive/Nursing Safety

Safe use of posaconazole during pregnancy or nursing has not been established. For humans, the FDA has classified this drug as Category C (*Animal studies have shown an adverse effect and there are no adequate studies in pregnant women; or no animal studies have been conducted and there are no adequate studies in pregnant women*). In rats, skeletal malformations were seen in some offspring of mothers given posaconazole while pregnant.

Posaconazole is excreted into rat milk, and safe use during nursing is not known.

Overdosage/Acute Toxicity

Acute toxicity in an overdose is unlikely. Humans have tolerated up to 1600 mg/day in clinical studies and one patient that ingested 1200 mg twice daily for 3 days did not develop adverse events.

Hemodialysis does not remove posaconazole.

Drug Interactions

Posaconazole can inhibit CYP3A4 and potentially could interact with drugs metabolized by CYP3A4 (increased plasma concentrations of CYP3A4 substrates). Posaconazole is also a substrate of the P-glycoprotein transport system and could potentially interact with other drugs that inhibit or induce this system.

The following drug interactions (partial list) have either been reported or are theoretical in humans or animals receiving posaconazole and may be of significance in veterinary patients. Unless otherwise noted, use together is not necessarily contraindicated, but weigh the potential risks and perform additional monitoring when appropriate.

- **BENZODIAZEPINES:** Increased benzodiazepine levels possible.
- **CIMETIDINE:** Decreased levels of posaconazole possible; avoid use together. No interactions reported with other H2 blockers (*e.g.,* famotidine).
- **CISAPRIDE:** Possible prolonged QT interval. In humans, use of cisapride and posaconazole together is contraindicated, but any clinical relevance for animal patients is unknown.
- **CYCLOSPORINE:** Increased cyclosporine levels possible.
- **DIGOXIN:** Possibility for increased digoxin levels.
- **METOCLOPRAMIDE:** Decreased levels of posaconazole possible.
- **PROTON-PUMP INHIBITORS** (*e.g.,* omeprazole): Decreased levels of posaconazole possible.
- **VINCA ALKALOIDS** (vincristine, vinblastine): Increased risk for vinca alkaloid toxicity possible.

Laboratory Considerations
No laboratory test interactions noted.

Dosages
- **DOGS:**

  For treatment of susceptible fungal infections: Anecdotal dosages range from 5 – 10 mg/kg PO q12-24h with food (preferably right after a high-fat meal); several months of treatment may be required. A preclinical study suggested that a dosage of 10 mg/kg per day should be effective (Nomeir *et al.* 2000).

- **CATS:**

  For treatment of susceptible fungal infections: Anecdotal dosages are usually reported as 5 – 7.5 mg/kg PO q24h or divided into two doses per day, with food (preferably right after a high-fat meal); several months of treatment may be required.

Monitoring
- Efficacy and adverse effects.
- Liver function tests; baseline and periodically during treatment.

Client Information
- Shake bottle well before measuring dosage.
- Give after food; a full meal if possible.
- May be dosed once per day, but if your animal vomits or acts 'sick' after a dose your veterinarian may have you give ½ of the daily dose twice per day.
- There is not much experience with this medication in animal patients so if you see any side effects, contact your veterinarian.

Chemistry/Synonyms
Posaconazole (CAS Registry: 171228-49-2; ATC:J02AC04) is a triazole antifungal that occurs as a white powder that is insoluble in water. The commercially available oral product is a white, cherry-flavored immediate-release oral suspension that contains polysorbate 80, simethicone, sodium benzoate, sodium citrate dihydrate, citric acid monohydrate, glycerin, xanthan gum, glucose, titanium dioxide, artificial cherry flavor and purified water.

Posaconazole may also be known as Sch-56592. Trade names include *Noxafil®* and *Spriafil®*.

Storage/Stability
The commercially available oral suspension should be stored at room temperature 25°C (77°F). It may be exposed to 15-30°C (59-86°F), but should not be allowed to freeze.

Compatibility/Compounding Considerations
No information noted.

Dosage Forms/Regulatory Status
VETERINARY-LABELED PRODUCTS: NONE IN USA.
An otic suspension may be available (*Posatex®*).

HUMAN-LABELED PRODUCTS:
Posaconazole Oral Suspension: 40 mg/mL in 105 ml bottles; *Noxafil®*; (Rx)

Revisions/References
Monograph written August 2013; revised June 2014.
Barrs, V. R., et al. (2012). Sinonasal and sino-orbital aspergillosis in 23 cats: Aetiology, clinicopathological features and treatment outcomes. Veterinary Journal **191**(1): 58-64.
Nomeir, A. A., et al. (2000). Pharmacokinetics of SCH 56592, a new azole broad-spectrum antifungal agent, in mice, rats, rabbits, dogs, and cynomolgus monkeys. Antimicrobial Agents and Chemotherapy **44**(3): 727-31.

Potassium Bromide – see Bromides

Potassium Iodide – see Iodide, Potassium

Potassium Chloride
Potassium Acetate
Potassium Gluconate
(po-**tass**-ee-um)

Electrolyte

Prescriber Highlights
▶ Parenteral and oral electrolyte used for treatment or prevention of hypokalemia.
▶ Contraindications: Hyperkalemia, renal failure or severe renal impairment, severe hemolytic reactions, untreated Addison's disease, acute dehydration, GI motility impairment (solid oral dosage forms). Caution: Patients on digoxin.
▶ Adverse Effects: Hyperkalemia. Oral therapy: GI distress; IV therapy may be irritating to veins.
▶ Intravenous potassium salts must be diluted before administering & drug must be given slowly.
▶ Acid/base, hydration status important.
▶ Drug Interactions.

Uses/Indications
Potassium supplementation is used to prevent or treat potassium deficits. Because it is safer, oral or nutritional therapy is generally preferred over parenteral potassium administration when feasible and appropriate.

Pharmacology/Actions
Potassium is the principal intracellular cation in the body. It is essential in maintaining cellular tonicity; nerve impulse transmission; smooth, skeletal and cardiac muscle contraction; and maintenance of normal renal function. Potassium is also used in carbohydrate utilization and protein synthesis.

Potassium requirements in mature dogs are approximately 3.7 mEq/kg/day, and in mature cats approximately 1.5 mEq/kg/day. Puppies and kittens require higher dietary potassium than do mature animals.

Pharmacokinetics
Approximately 98% of total body potassium is found in the intracellular fluid space while only 2% is in the extracellular fluid space. Plasma pH can alter distribution. Acidosis can shift potassium out of the intracellular space and conversely, alkalosis shifts potassium into the intracellular space. Potassium is primarily (80-90%) excreted via the kidneys with the majority of the remainder excreted in

the feces. Very small amounts may be excreted in perspiration (animals with sweat glands).

Contraindications/Precautions/Warnings

Potassium salts are contraindicated in patients with hyperkalemia, renal failure or severe renal impairment, severe hemolytic reactions, untreated Addison's disease, and acute dehydration. Cats with chronic kidney disease IRIS stages 2 and 3 often are hypokalemic and will require oral potassium supplementation. Solid oral dosage forms should not be used in patients where GI motility is impaired. Use cautiously in patients receiving digoxin (see Drug Interactions).

Because potassium is primarily an intracellular electrolyte, serum levels may not adequately reflect the total body stores of potassium. Acid-base balance may also mask the actual potassium picture. Patients with systemic acidosis conditions may appear to have hyperkalemia when, in fact, they may be significantly low in total body potassium. Conversely, alkalosis may cause a falsely low serum potassium value. Assess renal and cardiac function prior to therapy and closely monitor serum potassium levels. Supplementation should generally occur over 3-5 days to allow equilibration to occur between extracellular and intracellular fluids. Some clinicians feel that if acidosis is present or a concern, use potassium acetate, citrate or bicarbonate; if alkalosis is present, use potassium chloride.

Adverse Effects

The major problem associated with potassium supplementation is the development of hyperkalemia which is usually much more serious than hypokalemia. Clinical signs associated with hyperkalemia can range from muscular weakness and/or GI disturbances to cardiac conduction disturbances. Clinical signs can be exacerbated by concomitant hypocalcemia, hyponatremia, or acidosis. Intravenous potassium salts must be diluted before administering and given slowly (see Doses).

Oral therapy can cause GI distress and IV therapy may be irritating to veins.

Reproductive/Nursing Safety

Monitored potassium supplementation is unlikely to have negative effects during pregnancy or lactation.

Overdosage/Acute Toxicity

Fatal hyperkalemia may develop if potassium salts are administered too rapidly IV or if potassium renal excretory mechanisms are impaired. Clinical signs associated with hyperkalemia are noted in the Adverse Effects section above. Treatment of hyperkalemia is dependent upon the cause and/or severity of the condition and can consist of: discontinuation of the drug with ECG, acid/base and electrolyte monitoring, glucose/insulin infusions, sodium bicarbonate, calcium therapy, and polystyrene sulfonate resin. It is suggested to refer to other references appropriate for the species being treated for specific protocols for the treatment of hyperkalemia.

Drug Interactions

The following drug interactions have either been reported or are theoretical in humans or animals receiving potassium and may be of significance in veterinary patients. Unless otherwise noted, use together is not necessarily contraindicated, but weigh the potential risks and perform additional monitoring when appropriate.

- **ACE INHIBITORS** (*e.g.*, **enalapril**, etc.): Potassium retention may occur; increased risk for hyperkalemia.
- **DIGOXIN**: In patients with severe or complete heart block who are receiving digitalis therapy, it is often recommended not to use potassium salts.
- **NSAIDS**: Oral potassium given with non-steroidal antiinflammatory agents may increase the risk of gastrointestinal adverse effects.
- **POTASSIUM-SPARING DIURETICS** (*e.g.*, **spironolactone**): Potassium retention may occur; increased risk for hyperkalemia.

Doses

- **DOGS/CATS:**

    For hypokalemia (extra-label): **Note:** There are no exact formulas for calculating the total body potassium depletion, nor the requirement for supplementation. Guidelines should always be modified based on patient response. Patients with hypokalemia and an osmotic diuresis will have a much higher requirement for potassium than ones with normal urine output. Hypokalemia associated with diabetic ketoacidosis requires additional monitoring and treatment; refer to a specific reference for additional information.

    Treatment of chronic mild hypokalemia (3.0-3.5 mEq/L) can be accomplished with dietary measures or commercially available oral potassium supplement tablets and elixirs (diluted in water) at 0.5 – 1 mEq/kg mixed in food once or twice daily. If using the commercially available *Tumil-K®* powder, it is dosed at ¼ teaspoonful (2 mEq) per 4.5 kg body weight PO in food twice daily; adjust as necessary.

    For moderate to severe (<3.0 mEq/L) or acute hypokalemia with or without metabolic alkalosis requiring the administration of IV potassium; no accurate formulas available for calculating the exact amount of KCL needed to restore normokalemia. The rate of administration of intravenous KCL is more critical than the total amount administered. Under most circumstances the rate should not exceed 0.5 mEq/kg/hour. But under the most dire circumstances (serum potassium < 2.0 mEq/L), rate can be increased to 1.5 mEq/kg/hour along with close ECG (rate & rhythm) monitoring. While potassium administration should be determined on how much potassium to administer to the patient, not how much to add to a bag of fluid, suggested guidelines include: Serum K+ <2 mEq/L = 60 – 80 mEq/1000 mL IV fluid; Serum K+ 2-2.5 mEq/L = 40 – 60 mEq/1000 mL IV fluid; Serum K+ 2.5-3 mEq/L = 30 – 40 mEq/1000 mL IV fluid; Serum K+ 3-3.5 mEq/L = 20 – 30 mEq/1000 mL IV fluid.

    Amounts exceeding more than 10 mEq/hour to a small animal (<10 kg body weight) can be potentially life-threatening because of the effects of a more concentrated solution on the wall of the right ventricle if the solution is given through a central intravenous line. KCL supplemented fluids can also be safely given in patients weighing <10 kg. Isotonic fluids such as lactated Ringers or 0.9% saline containing 30 – 35 mEq/L KCl per Liter and administered at a dose of 150 mL SC every 12 hours. Adapted from: (Schaer 2009), (Devey 2009)

- **HORSES:**

    For hypokalemia (extra-label): To counteract potassium depletion in a completely anorectic horse, IV fluids should be supplemented with KCL (at least 50 mEq/hour in an adult horse). Hypertonic oral KCL pastes can be administered to horses with diarrhea. (Schott II 2009)

- **RUMINANTS:**

    For hypokalemia (extra-label): For severe hypokalemia (<2.3 mEq/L) with severe muscle weakness or recumbency: Isotonic potassium chloride (11.5 grams of potassium chloride per 1 liter of sterile water) at a rate of 4 mL/kg/hour. Combined with large doses of oral potassium salts (*i.e.*, 200 grams of KCl per day. (Smith 2006)

Monitoring

Level and frequency of monitoring associated with potassium therapy is dependent upon the cause and/or severity of hypokalemia, acid/base abnormalities, renal function, concomitant drugs administered, or disease states and can include:

- Serum potassium; other electrolytes.
- Acid/base status.
- Glucose.
- ECG.
- CBC.
- Urinalyses.

Client Information

For oral potassium:

- Oral potassium is best administered with food to help prevent stomach upset.
- Overdoses (both one-time and over a period of time) of potassium can be very serious; too much potassium in the body can cause serious problems.

Chemistry/Synonyms

Potassium chloride occurs as either white, granular powder or as colorless, elongated, prismatic, or cubical crystals. It is odorless and has a saline taste. One gram is soluble in $\approx$ 3 mL of water and is insoluble in alcohol. The pH of the injection ranges from 4-8. One gram of potassium chloride contains 13.4 mEq of potassium. A 2 mEq/mL solution has an osmolarity of 4000 mOsm/L. Potassium chloride may also be known as KCl.

Potassium gluconate occurs as white to yellowish white, crystalline powder or granules. It is odorless, has a slightly bitter taste, and is freely soluble in water. One gram of potassium gluconate contains 4.3 mEq of potassium.

Potassium Chloride may also be known as: KCl, cloreto de potassio, E508, kalii chloridum, or kalium chloratum.

Potassium Gluconate may also be known as: E577, *K-G Elixir®*, *Kaon®*, *Kaylixir®*, *Potasoral®*, *Potassiject®*, *Potassium-Rougier®*, *Renakare®*, *Sopa-K®*, *Tumil-K®*, and *Ultra-K®*.

Storage/Stability

Potassium gluconate oral products should be stored in tight, light resistant containers at room temperature (15-30°C), unless otherwise instructed by the manufacturer.

Unless otherwise directed by the manufacturer, potassium chloride products should be stored in tight, containers at room temperature (15-30°C); protect from freezing.

Compatibility/Compounding Considerations

Potassium chloride for injection is reportedly physically **compatible** with the following intravenous solutions and drugs (as an additive): all commonly used intravenous replacement fluids (not 10% fat emulsion), aminophylline, amiodarone HCl, calcium gluconate, chloramphenicol sodium succinate, cimetidine HCl, clindamycin phosphate, corticotropin (ACTH), cytarabine, dimenhydrinate, dopamine HCl, erythromycin gluceptate/lactobionate, heparin sodium, hydrocortisone sodium succinate, isoproterenol HCl, lidocaine HCl, metoclopramide HCl, norepinephrine bitartrate, oxacillin sodium, oxytetracycline HCl, penicillin G potassium, phenylephrine HCl, sodium bicarbonate, tetracycline HCl, thiopental sodium, vancomycin HCl, verapamil HCl, and vitamin B-complex with C.

Potassium chloride for injection **compatibility information conflicts** or is dependent on diluent or concentration factors with the following drugs or solutions: fat emulsion 10%, amikacin sulfate, dobutamine HCl, methylprednisolone sodium succinate (at Y-site), penicillin G sodium, and promethazine HCl (at Y-site). Compatibility is dependent upon factors such as pH, concentration, temperature, and diluent used; consult specialized references or a hospital pharmacist for more specific information.

Potassium chloride for injection is reportedly physically **incompatible** with the following solutions or drugs: amphotericin B, diazepam (at Y-site), and phenytoin sodium (at Y-site).

Dosage Forms/Regulatory Status

VETERINARY-LABELED PRODUCTS:

Parenteral Products: There are several products for parenteral use that contain potassium; refer to the tables in the appendix or individual proprietary veterinary products for additional information.

Potassium Chloride IV Solution: 2 mEq (149 mg) in 10 mL vials; *Potassiject®*, generic; (Rx)

Oral Products:

Potassium Gluconate Tablets: 2 mEq (468 mg); *Tumil-K®*, *Renakare®*; (Rx). Labeled for use in cats and dogs.

Potassium Gluconate Oral Powder: Each 0.65 gram 4 oz (1/4 teaspoonful) contains 2 mEq of potassium in 4 oz. Containers; *Renakare®*, *Tumil-K®*; (Rx). Labeled for use in dogs and cats.

Potassium Gluconate Gel: Each 2.34 grams (1/2 teaspoonful) contains 2 mEq of potassium in 5 oz tubes; *Tumil-K® Gel*, *Renakare®*; (Rx). Labeled for use in dogs and cats.

HUMAN-LABELED PRODUCTS: NOT A COMPLETE LIST.

Parenteral Products:

Potassium Chloride for Injection Concentrate (**Must be diluted before administering**): 0.4 mEq/mL, 1 mEq/mL, 2 mEq/mL, & 4 mEq/mL in multi-dose vials; generic; (Rx).

There are also pre-mixed IV bags of saline and dextrose (both separately and in various combinations) that contain (potassium) 10 mEq/liter, 20 mEq/liter, 30 mEq/liter, or 40 mEq/liter.

Potassium acetate for injection 2 mEq/mL and 4 mEq/mL (**Must be diluted before administering**); (Rx)

Potassium phosphate for injection (see Phosphate monograph) is also available.

Oral Products: There are a multitude of human-labeled potassium salts for oral use available in several dosage forms; refer to human drug references for more information on these products. Tablets, controlled/sustained release tablets and capsules, effervescent tablets, liquids, and powder in varying strengths available; (OTC and Rx)

Revisions/References

Monograph revised/updated May 2014.

Devey, J. (2009). What's All the Salt About? Understanding Sodium, Chloride and Potassium. Proceedings: ABVP. accessed via Veterinary Information Network; vin.com

Schaer, M. (2009). Hypokalemia--A Problem to Be Reckoned With. Proceedings: IVECCS. accessed via Veterinary Information Network; vin.com

Schott II, H. (2009). Disorders of Sodium & Potassium Balance in the Foal & Adult Horse. Proceedings: ACVIM. accessed via Veterinary Information Network; vin.com

Smith, G. (2006). Fluid therapy in adult ruminants. Proceedings: Western Vet Conference. accessed via Veterinary Information Network; vin.com

Potassium Citrate – see Citrate Salts

Pradofloxacin

(pra-doe-**flox**-a-sin)   *Veraflox®*

Fluoroquinolone Antibiotic

Prescriber Highlights

▶ Fluoroquinolone antibiotic approved for use in cats and dogs (not for dogs in USA).

▶ Unlike many fluoroquinolones, also has activity against anaerobes and enhanced activity against gram-positive (*e.g.*, *Staph. pseudintermedius*).

▶ Occasionally can cause gastrointestinal effects. Potentially could cause decreased white blood cell counts with prolonged use.

Uses/Indications

In cats, pradofloxacin oral suspension is labeled as indicated for the treatment of skin infections (wounds and abscesses) caused by susceptible strains of *Pasteurella multocida*, *Streptococcus canis*, *Staphylococcus aureus*, *Staphylococcus felis*, and *Staphylococcus pseudintermedius*. Pradofloxacin has also been used clinically in cats for the treatment of bacterial urinary tract infections, *Mycoplasma haemofelis* upper respiratory infections, and in combination with other antimycobacterial drugs for feline leprosy syndromes.

In dogs, pradofloxacin is labeled (in the UK) for the treatment of wound infections, superficial and deep pyoderma caused by susceptible strains of the *Staphylococcus pseudintermedius* group (including *S. pseudintermedius*); acute urinary tract infections caused by susceptible strains of *E. coli* and the *Staphylococcus pseudintermedius* group (including *S. pseudintermedius*) and as adjunctive treatment to mechanical or surgical periodontal therapy in the treatment of severe infections of the gingiva and periodontal tissues caused by susceptible strains of anaerobic organisms (*e.g.*, *Porphyromonas* spp. and *Prevotella* spp.). **Note**: At the time of writing (August 2013), the drug is not approved for use in dogs in the USA (see Contraindications below).

Pharmacology/Actions

Pradofloxacin is a broad spectrum third-generation fluoroquinolone bactericidal antibiotic. The bactericidal activity of pradofloxacin is concentration dependent. Its antibacterial action is via inhibition of DNA gyrase and topoisomerase IV affecting bacterial DNA.

Pradofloxacin is unique among veterinary fluoroquinolones in its gram-negative activity is similar to other fluoroquinolones, but additionally it has enhanced aerobic gram-positive activity and activity against anaerobes. This is similar to the human fluoroquinolone, moxifloxacin. Pradofloxacin, compared with other veterinary fluoroquinolones, also has enhanced activity against *Mycoplasma* species. It is the only antibiotic shown to date that can eliminate *Mycoplasma haemofelis* from the blood of experimentally inoculated cats (Dowers *et al.* 2009).

At present, development of bacterial resistance to pradofloxacin is relatively low, but cross-resistance with other fluoroquinolones can occur and multi-drug resistant strains are an ever-growing concern. At the time of writing (2013) no established (ALCS) breakpoints have been determined; proposed breakpoints during the approval process were: susceptible ≤1 mcg/mL & resistant ≥2 mcg/mL (Anon 2011). In an effort to slow the development of bacterial resistance to this drug the following formation can be found on the drug labels: "Prescribing antibacterial drugs in the absence of a proven or strongly suspected bacterial infection is unlikely to provide benefit to treated animals and may increase the risk of the development of drug-resistant animal pathogens (Anon 2012a)." "Whenever possible, the veterinary medicinal product should only be used based on susceptibility testing. Official and local antimicrobial policies should be taken into account when the veterinary medicinal product is used. Fluoroquinolones should be reserved for the treatment of clinical conditions which have responded poorly, or are expected to respond poorly, to other classes of antimicrobials (Anon 2012c)."

Unlike enrofloxacin, pradofloxacin does not cause retinal toxicity in cats (Messias *et al.* 2008).

Pharmacokinetics

In dogs, after oral administration pradofloxacin is rapidly absorbed with peak plasma levels occurring ≈ 2 hours after a dose. Bioavailability is reported to be high and not affected by tablet size or dose administered. Repeated dosages do not impact pharmacokinetics. Volume of distribution is >2 L/kg and only ≈ 35% of the drug is bound to plasma proteins. Peak drug concentrations are slightly higher in serum than in interstitial fluid (ISF), but persist at levels higher than in plasma for most of the 24-hour dosing period. Highest tissue levels are found in cartilage, liver and kidneys and measured 1-1.5 hours after a dose. Clearance is 0.24 l/hr/kg and plasma elimination half-life is ≈ 8 hours. Pradofloxacin is primarily metabolized via glucuronidation and sulfation; ≈ 40% of a dose is excreted in the urine. Approximately 85% of a dose is excreted into the urine within 24 hours—40% unchanged and the rest primarily as glucuronide metabolites. (Anon 2011; Korber-Irrgang *et al.* 2012; Hauschild *et al.* 2013; Lees 2013)

In cats, pradofloxacin is rapidly absorbed with peak plasma concentrations occurring within 1-2 hours. Oral bioavailability is ≈ 60% with the oral suspension and ≈ 70% with oral tablets. Repeat dosages do not significantly alter the pharmacokinetics. Volume of distribution is relatively high and only ≈ 30% of the drug is bound to plasma proteins. Like dogs, glucuronidation is the major metabolic pathway for cats. 70% of a dose is excreted into the urine within 24 hours, but only ≈ 10% of it as unchanged drug. Clearance is 0.27 L/hr/kg and terminal plasma elimination half-life has been variably reported from 3-8 hours (Hartmann *et al.* 2008; Anon 2011; Lees 2013).

Contraindications/Precautions/Warnings

Pradofloxacin is contraindicated in animals that are hypersensitive to it or other quinolones. Due to the lack of data, pradofloxacin should not be used in kittens <6 weeks old (UK label); the US label states "safety of pradofloxacin in cats younger than 12 weeks of age has not been evaluated." Pradofloxacin does not have effects on the developing cartilage of kittens 6 weeks of age and older, but it should not be used in cats with persisting articular cartilage lesions, as these lesions may worsen during treatment with fluoroquinolones (Anon 2012c).

The safety of pradofloxacin in immune-compromised cats (*i.e.*, cats infected with feline leukemia virus and/or feline immunodeficiency virus) has not been evaluated (Anon 2012a).

The UK label lists the following contraindications for dogs: "Because of effects on articular cartilage, pradofloxacin should not be use in dogs less than 12 months of age (most breeds), and in giant breeds less than 18 months old. It is also contraindicated in dogs with persisting articular cartilage lesions, central nervous system (CNS) disorders, such as epilepsy, and in dogs that are pregnant or lactating."

While Pradofloxacin is approved for use in dogs in the UK and Europe, the FDA-approved (USA) label states: "DO NOT USE IN DOGS. Pradofloxacin has been shown to cause bone marrow suppression in dogs. Dogs may be particularly sensitive to this effect, potentially resulting in severe thrombocytopenia and neutropenia." This topic is addressed in the European Medicines Agency: Veterinary Medicines and Product Data Management scientific discussion for *Veraflox®* document (Anon 2011). In evaluating target animal (dog) safety studies where the study design followed the relevant U.S. guidance documents they found that thrombocytopenia and leukopenia were induced at daily oral doses of 27 mg/kg (6X the maximum recommended dose) and above, but not at lower dosages (Anon 2011). However, because of the stern wording of the label, veterinarians in the USA should carefully consider the potential medico-legal consequences before using this drug in an extra-label manner in dogs.

Use with caution in animals with impaired renal function or severely impaired hepatic function.

Fluoroquinolones may cause photosensitization and prolonged exposure of bare skin (*e.g.*, nose) to direct sunlight should be avoided.

The artificial beef flavor used in the tablets originates from irradiated (to inactivate any viruses or microorganisms) pig livers. Dogs that are hypersensitive to pork products could potentially react to these proteins.

Adverse Effects

In dogs and cats, pradofloxacin at recommended dosages appears to be well tolerated with diarrhea/loose stools occasionally reported.

White blood cell decreases are possible in dogs and in cats (when used for longer than 7 days); (see Contraindications/Warnings above) (Anon 2012a).

In dogs, QT interval can be increased and pradofloxacin potentially could have proarrhythmic effects, especially in patients with coexisting risk factors (*e.g.*, hypothyroidism, bradycardia, ion disturbances, heart failure, liver or kidney disease) (Cepiel *et al.* 2013).

Reproductive/Nursing Safety

Based upon reproductive studies in rats and rabbits where some maternotoxic and fetotoxic effects were noted, pradofloxacin is labeled as contraindicated for use during pregnancy or lactation. The drug does not pose additional risk when used breeding animals (Anon 2011).

Overdosage/Acute Toxicity

Pradofloxacin appears to be quite safe in acute overdose situations with vomiting and diarrhea possible. The approximate LD_{50} after a single intraperitoneal application in rats was >50 mg/kg and single oral doses of 100 mg/kg were tolerated well in young cats, and in dogs. However in one dog there was temporary overloading of renal excretory capacity (Anon 2011).

Acute overdoses should be managed supportively. Consider performing baseline white blood cell counts in overdoses in dogs.

Drug Interactions

The following drug interactions have either been reported or are theoretical in humans or animals receiving pradofloxacin or other fluoroquinolones and may be of significance in veterinary patients. Unless otherwise noted, use together is not necessarily contraindicated, but weigh the potential risks and perform additional monitoring when appropriate.

- **ANTACIDS/DAIRY PRODUCTS** (containing cations (Mg^{++}, Al^{+++}, Ca^{++}): May bind to pradofloxacin and prevent its absorption; separate doses of these products by at least 2 hours.
- **CIMETIDINE:** "Cimetidine has been shown to interfere with the metabolism of quinolones and should be used with care when used concurrently."(Anon 2012a)
- **CYCLOSPORINE:** Fluoroquinolones may exacerbate the nephrotoxicity and reduce the metabolism of cyclosporine (used systemically). "Concurrent use of quinolones with oral cyclosporine should be avoided."(Anon 2012a)
- **DIGOXIN:** "The combined use of fluoroquinolones with digoxin should also be avoided because of potentially increased oral bioavailability of digoxin." (Anon 2012c)

- **NONSTEROIDAL ANTIINFLAMMATORY DRUGS (NSAIDS); FLUNIXIN:** Flunixin has been shown in dogs to increase the AUC and elimination half-life of enrofloxacin and enrofloxacin increases the AUC and elimination half-life of flunixin; it is unknown if pradofloxacin also causes this effect or if other NSAIDs interact with pradofloxacin in dogs. The UK labels states "…fluoroquinolones should not be used in combination with non-steroidal anti-inflammatory drugs (NSAIDs) in animals with a history of seizures because of potential pharmacodynamic interactions in the CNS."(Anon 2012c)
- **GLYBURIDE:** Severe hypoglycemia possible.
- **IRON, ZINC (oral):** Decreased pradofloxacin absorption; separate doses by at least 2 hours.
- **METHOTREXATE:** Increased MTX levels possible with resultant toxicity.
- **NITROFURANTOIN:** May antagonize the antimicrobial activity of the fluoroquinolones and their concomitant use is not recommended.
- **PHENYTOIN:** Pradofloxacin may alter phenytoin levels.
- **PROBENECID:** Blocks tubular secretion of ciprofloxacin and may also increase the blood level and half-life of pradofloxacin.
- **QUINIDINE:** Increased risk for cardiotoxicity.
- **SUCRALFATE:** May inhibit absorption of pradofloxacin; separate doses of these drugs by at least 2 hours.
- **THEOPHYLLINE:** Pradofloxacin may increase theophylline blood levels. The US label states: "The dosage of theophylline should be reduced when used concurrently with quinolones."(Anon 2012a) The UK labels states; "The combination of fluoroquinolones with theophylline could increase the plasma levels of theophylline by altering its metabolism and thus should be avoided."(Anon 2012a)
- **WARFARIN:** Potential for increased warfarin effects.

Laboratory Considerations

No specific concerns noted.

Dosages

- **DOGS:**

  Labeled doses:

  a) None in USA; see Contraindications above.

  b) **U.K. Label: For the treatment of wound infections, superficial and deep pyoderma caused by susceptible strains of the *Staphylococcus pseudintermedius* group (including *S. pseudintermedius*); acute urinary tract infections caused by susceptible strains of *E. coli* and the *Staphylococcus pseudintermedius* group (including *S. pseudintermedius*) and as adjunctive treatment to mechanical or surgical periodontal therapy in the treatment of severe infections of the gingiva and periodontal tissues caused by susceptible strains of anaerobic organisms (*e.g.*, *Porphyromonas* spp. and *Prevotella* spp.) (extra-label in USA): Oral tablets: 3 – 4.5 mg/kg PO once daily. The duration of the treatment depends on the nature and severity of the infection and on the response to treatment. For most infections the following treatment courses will be sufficient: Superficial pyoderma 14-21 days; Deep pyoderma 14-35 days; Wound infections 7 days; Acute infections of the urinary tract 7-21 days; Severe infections of the gingiva and periodontal tissues 7 days. The treatment should be re-considered if no improvement of the clinical conditions is observed within 3 days, or in cases of superficial pyoderma 7 days, and in cases of deep pyoderma 14 days, after starting the treatment. Adapted from: (Anon 2012c)**

■ **CATS:**

For the treatment of skin infections (wounds and abscesses) caused by susceptible strains of *Pasteurella multocida*, *Streptococcus canis*, *Staphylococcus aureus*, *Staphylococcus felis*, and *Staphylococcus pseudintermedius* (labeled dose; FDA-Approved): 7.5 mg/kg PO once daily for 7 consecutive days. Shake well before use. To ensure a correct dosage, body weight should be determined as accurately as possible. Use the syringe provided to ensure accuracy of dosing to the nearest 0.1 mL. Rinse syringe between doses. A sample of the lesion should be obtained for culture and susceptibility testing prior to beginning antibacterial therapy. Once results become available, continue with appropriate therapy. If acceptable response to treatment is not observed, or if no improvement is seen within 3 to 4 days, then the diagnosis should be re-evaluated and appropriate alternative therapy considered. Adapted from: (Anon 2012a)

UK label (extra-label in USA): Oral Suspension: 5 – 7.5 mg/kg PO once daily. Oral tablets: 3 – 4.5 mg/kg PO once daily. The duration of the treatment depends on the nature and severity of the infection and on the response to treatment. For most infections the following treatment courses will be sufficient: Wound infections and abscesses, 7 days; acute infections of the upper respiratory tract, 5 days. Adapted from: (Anon 2012b, c)

Monitoring

■ Clinical Efficacy.

■ If using at higher than labeled dosages, or if therapy continues past 7 days, consider performing periodic white blood cell counts. The label for the USA cat product states: "The administration of pradofloxacin for longer than 7 days induced reversible leukocyte, neutrophil, and lymphocyte decreases in healthy, 12-week-old kittens. If an unexplained drop in leukocyte, neutrophil, and/or lymphocyte counts is noted during pradofloxacin therapy, discontinuation of treatment is recommended." (Anon 2012a)

Client Information

■ Antibiotic approved only for use in cats in the USA; approved for use in dogs in some other countries.

■ Shake oral suspension container well before measuring each dose.

■ This drug is best given without food on an empty stomach, but if your animal vomits or acts sick after getting it, give with food or small treat (no dairy products, antacids or anything containing iron) to see if this helps. If vomiting continues, contact your veterinarian.

■ Do not give with other drugs that contain calcium, iron, or aluminum (including sucralfate) as these can reduce the amount of drug that gets absorbed.

■ May stunt bone growth or cause joint abnormalities if used in young animals, or during pregnancy or while nursing.

■ Most common side effects are vomiting, nausea (acting 'sick'), or diarrhea.

Chemistry/Synonyms

Pradofloxacin (CAS Registry 0195532-12-8; ATCvet: QJ01MA97, QJ01MA) is an 8-cyano fluoroquinolone antibiotic structurally similar to moxifloxacin. It occurs as a brownish, light yellow to yellow, fine crystalline powder. Pradofloxacin has four enantiomeric forms, but secondary to its high antimicrobial potency, the S,S-isomer is used in the pharmaceutical products.

The oral suspension contains 2 mg/mL sorbic acid (E200) as a preservative.

Pradofloxacin may also be known as UNII-6O0T5E048I. Its trade name is *Veraflox®*.

Storage/Stability

The oral suspension should be stored below 30°C (86°F) in the original container and kept tightly closed; after opening is stabile for at least 60 days (3 months on UK label). Oral tablets require no special storage conditions, but once the container is opened they should be protected from light and moisture.

Compatibility/Compounding Considerations

No information located.

Dosage Forms/Regulatory Status

VETERINARY-LABELED PRODUCTS:

Oral Suspension: 25 mg/mL in 15 mL & 30 mL bottles; *Veraflox®*; (Rx). Approved for use in cats (NADA 141-344).

There is a website (dailymed.nim.hih.gov) with the FDA-approved veterinary product's label: *Veraflox®*

Oral Tablets: 15 mg, 60 mg, 120 mg. Approved in UK and Europe for cats (15 mg only) and dogs (15 mg, 60 mg, 120 mg); POM-V; *Veraflox®*; (Rx)

HUMAN-LABELED PRODUCTS: NONE.

Revisions/References

Monograph written August 2013; revised June 2014.

Anon (2011). Veraflox® (Pradofloxacin) Scientific Discssion. Secondary Veraflox® (Pradofloxacin) Scientific Discssion. Secondary Anon, European Medicines Agency: Veterinary Medicines and Product Data Management. Volume

Anon (2012a). Veraflox® (pradofloxacin suspension) [Package Insert]. Secondary Veraflox® (pradofloxacin suspension) [Package Insert]. Secondary Anon. Shawnee Mission, KS, Bayer Healthcare. Volume

Anon (2012b). Veraflox® (pradofloxacin) 25 mg/mL Oral Suspension for Cats [Product Leaflet]. Secondary Veraflox® (pradofloxacin) 25 mg/mL Oral Suspension for Cats [Product Leaflet]. Secondary Anon. Newbury, Berkshire UK, Bayer Animal Health. Volume

Anon (2012c). Veraflox® (pradofloxacin) Tablets [Product Leaflet]. Secondary Veraflox® (pradofloxacin) Tablets [Product Leaflet]. Secondary Anon. Newbury, Berkshire UK, Bayer Animal Health. Volume

Cepiel, A., et al. (2013). Effect of oral administration of quinolones on ECG in dogs. Proceedings: 23rd ECVIM-CA Congress. accessed via Veterinary Information Network; vin.com

Dowers, K. L., et al. (2009). Use of pradofloxacin to treat experimentally induced Mycoplasma hemofelis infection in cats. American Journal of Veterinary Research 70(1): 105-11.

Hartmann, A., et al. (2008). Pharmacokinetics of pradofloxacin and doxycycline in serum, saliva, and tear fluid of cats after oral administration. J. Vet. Pharmacol. Ther. 31(2): 87-94.

Hauschild, G., et al. (2013). Pharmacokinetic study on pradofloxacin in the dog - Comparison of serum analysis, ultrafiltration and tissue sampling after oral administration. BMC Veterinary Research 9.

Korber-Irrgang, B., et al. (2012). Comparative activity of pradofloxacin and marbofloxacin against coagulase-positive staphylococci in a pharmacokinetic-pharmacodynamic model based on canine pharmacokinetics. J. Vet. Pharmacol. Ther. 35(6): 571-9.

Lees, P. (2013). Pharmacokinetics, pharmacodynamics and therapeutics of pradofloxacin in the dog and cat. J. Vet. Pharmacol. Ther. 36(3): 209-21.

Messias, A., et al. (2008). Retinal safety of a new fluoroquinolone, pradofloxacin, in cats: assessment with electroretinography. Documenta Ophthalmologica 116(3): 177-91.

Pralidoxime Chloride (2-PAM)

(pra-li-**dox**-eem)   Protopam Chloride®

Antidote; Cholinesterase Reactivator

Prescriber Highlights

▶ Cholinesterase reactivator used for adjunctive treatment of organophosphate poisoning.

▶ Contraindications: Hypersensitivity; generally not recommended for carbamate poisoning.

▶ Caution: Renal impairment, patients receiving anticholinesterase agents for the treatment of myasthenia gravis.

▶ Adverse Effects: Rapid IV injection may cause tachycardia, muscle rigidity, transient neuromuscular blockade, or laryngospasm.

▶ Most effective if given within 24 hours of exposure.

Uses/Indications

Pralidoxime is used in the treatment of organophosphate poisoning, often in conjunction with atropine and supportive therapy.

Pharmacology/Actions

Pralidoxime reactivates cholinesterase that has been inactivated by phosphorylation secondary to certain organophosphates. Via nucleophilic attack, the drug removes and binds the offending phosphoryl group attached to the enzyme, which is then excreted.

Pharmacokinetics

Pralidoxime is only marginally absorbed after oral dosing and oral dosage forms are no longer available in the United States. It is distributed primarily throughout the extracellular water. Because of its quaternary ammonium structure, it is not believed to enter the CNS in significant quantities, but recent studies and clinical responses have led some to question this.

Pralidoxime is thought to be metabolized by the liver and excreted as both metabolite(s) and unchanged drug in the urine.

Contraindications/Precautions/Warnings

Pralidoxime is contraindicated in patients hypersensitive to it. Pralidoxime is generally not recommended for use in instances of carbamate poisoning because inhibition is rapidly reversible, but there is some controversy regarding this issue.

Pralidoxime should be used with caution in patients receiving anticholinesterase agents for the treatment of myasthenia gravis as it may precipitate a myasthenic crisis. It should also be used cautiously and at a reduced dosage rate in patients with renal impairment.

Adverse Effects

At usual doses, pralidoxime generally is safe and free of significant adverse effects. Rapid IV injection may cause tachycardia, muscle rigidity, transient neuromuscular blockade, and laryngospasm.

Pralidoxime must generally be given within 24 hours of exposure to be effective, but some benefits may occur, particularly in large exposures, if given within 36-48 hours.

Reproductive/Nursing Safety

In humans, the FDA categorizes this drug as category C for use during pregnancy (*Animal studies have shown an adverse effect on the fetus, but there are no adequate studies in humans; or there are no animal reproduction studies and no adequate studies in humans.*)

It is not known whether this drug is excreted in maternal milk; exercise caution.

Overdosage/Acute Toxicity

The acute LD$_{50}$ of pralidoxime in dogs is 190 mg/kg and, at high dosages, causes signs associated with its own anticholinesterase activity. Clinical signs of toxicity in dogs may be exhibited as muscle weakness, ataxia, vomiting, hyperventilation, seizures, respiratory arrest, and death.

Drug Interactions

The following drug interactions have either been reported or are theoretical in humans or animals receiving pralidoxime and may be of significance in veterinary patients. Unless otherwise noted, use together is not necessarily contraindicated, but weigh the potential risks and perform additional monitoring when appropriate.

- **BARBITURATES:** Anticholinesterases can potentiate the action of barbiturates; use with caution.
- **CIMETIDINE, SUCCINYLCHOLINE, THEOPHYLLINE, RESERPINE,** and **RESPIRATORY DEPRESSANT DRUGS** (*e.g.,* **narcotics, phenothiazines**): Use should be avoided in patients with organophosphate toxicity.

Doses

Note: Often used in conjunction with atropine; refer to that monograph and/or the references below for more information.

- **DOGS & CATS:**

For organophosphate poisoning (extra-label): Usually used with atropine. After atropine is administered, pralidoxime initially at 20 mg/kg preferably IV (diluted in IV fluids and administered over not less than 5 minutes). IM can be used if IV is not available. Subsequent doses of 20 mg/kg IM, SC or IV (slowly) q6-12h until nicotinic signs are present. Discontinue after 3-4 treatments if no response or if nicotinic signs are aggravated.

- **RUMINANTS:**

Note: When used in food animals, FARAD recommends a 28-day meat and a 6-day milk withdrawal time. (Haskell *et al.* 2005)

For organophosphate poisoning (extra-label): Cattle: 30 mg/kg IM q8h. (Osweiler 2007)

- **HORSES:**

For organophosphate poisoning extra-label): 20 mg/kg (may require up to 35 mg/kg) IV and repeat q4-6h. (Oehme 1987)

- **BIRDS:**

For organophosphate poisoning (extra-label):
a) 10 – 20 mg/kg q8-12h (route not specified) with atropine (0.2 – 0.5 mg/kg IM q3-4h). (Jones 2007)
b) 10 – 100 mg/kg IM q24-48h or repeat once in 6 hours. (Johnson-Delaney *et al.* 2009)

Monitoring

- Pralidoxime therapy is monitored via the clinical signs associated with organophosphate poisoning. For more information, refer to one of the references outlined in the dosage section.

Client Information

- This agent should only be used with close professional supervision.

Chemistry/Synonyms

A quaternary ammonium oxime cholinesterase reactivator, pralidoxime chloride occurs as a white to pale yellow, crystalline powder with a pK$_a$ of 7.8-8. It is freely soluble in water. The commercially available injection has a pH of 3.5-4.5 after reconstitution.

Pralidoxime chloride may also be known as: 2-Formyl-1-methylpyridinium chloride oxime, 2-PAM, 2-PAM chloride, 2-PAMCl, 2-pyridine aldoxime methochloride and *Protopam*®.

Storage/Stability

Unless otherwise instructed by the manufacturer, pralidoxime chloride powder for injection should be stored at room temperature. After reconstituting with sterile water for injection, the solution should be used within a few hours. Do not use sterile water with preservatives added to reconstitute the powder for injection.

Compatibility/Compounding Considerations

Reconstitute with 20 mL of sterile water for injection to yield 50 mg/mL. For intravenous infusion, a concentration of 10 – 20 mg/mL in sodium chloride 0.9% is recommended. For intramuscular injection when intravenous administration is not feasible, reconstitute each vial with 3.3 mL of sterile water for injection (with no preservatives added) to yield 300 mg/mL.

Dosage Forms/Regulatory Status

VETERINARY-LABELED PRODUCTS: NONE.

HUMAN-LABELED PRODUCTS:

Pralidoxime Chloride Powder for Injection: 1 gram in 20 mL single-use vials; *Protopam® Chloride*; (Rx)

Also available in 600 mg/2 mL IM auto-injectors.

Revisions/References

Monograph revised/updated May 2014.

Haskell, S., et al. (2005). Farad Digest: Antidotes in Food Animal Practice. JAVMA **226**(6): 884-7.

Johnson-Delaney, C. & D. Reavill (2009). Toxicoses in Birds: Ante- and Postmortem Findings for Practitioners. Proceedings: AAV. accessed via Veterinary Information Network; vin.com

Jones, M. (2007). Avian Toxicology. Proceedings: Western Vet Conf. accessed via Veterinary Information Network; vin.com

Oehme, F. W. (1987). Insecticides. *Current Therapy in Equine Medicine.* N. E. Robinson. Philadelphia, WB Saunders: 658-60.

Osweiler, G. (2007). Detoxification and Antidotes for Ruminant Poisoning. Proceedings: ACVIM. accessed via Veterinary Information Network; vin.com

Praziquantel

(pra-zi-**kwon**-tel)   Droncit®

Anticestodal Antiparasitic

Prescriber Highlights

► Anticestodal anthelmintic also may be useful for some other parasites.

► Contraindications: Puppies <4 weeks old or kittens <6 weeks old; hypersensitivity to the drug.

► Adverse Effects: Uncommon after oral use; pain at injection site, anorexia, salivation, vomiting, lethargy, weakness, or diarrhea possible after using injectable.

For information on combination products containing praziquantel, see the Emodepside, Ivermectin, Milbemycin, Moxidectin, and Pyrantel monographs.

Uses/Indications

Praziquantel is indicated for (FDA-approved labeling) for the treatment of *Dipylidium caninum, Taenia pisiformis,* and *Echinococcus granulosis* in dogs, and *Dipylidium caninum* and *Taenia taeniaeformis* in cats. Fasting is not required nor recommended before dosing. A single dose is usually effective, but measures should be taken to prevent reinfection, particularly against *D. caninum.* Praziquantel can also be used for treating *Alaria* spp. in dogs and cats and *Spirometra mansonoides* infections in cats.

Praziquantel has been used in birds and other animals, but it is usually not economically feasible to use in large animals. In humans, praziquantel is used for schistosomiasis, other trematodes (lung, liver, intestinal flukes) and tapeworms. It is not routinely effective in treating *F. hepatica* infections in humans.

Combination products with praziquantel can control a wide spectrum of internal parasites in a variety of species.

Pharmacology/Actions

Praziquantel's exact mechanism of action against cestodes has not been determined, but it may be the result of interacting with phospholipids in the integument causing ion fluxes of sodium, potassium and calcium. At low concentrations *in vitro*, the drug appears to impair the function of their suckers and stimulates the worm's motility. At higher concentrations *in vitro*, praziquantel increases the contraction (irreversibly at very high concentrations) of the worm's strobilla (chain of proglottids). In addition, praziquantel causes irreversible focal vacuolization with subsequent cestodal disintegration at specific sites of the cestodal integument.

In schistosomes and trematodes, praziquantel directly kills the parasite, possibly by increasing calcium ion flux into the worm. Focal vacuolization of the integument follows and the parasite is phagocytized.

Pharmacokinetics

Praziquantel is rapidly and nearly completely absorbed after oral administration, but there is a significant first-pass effect. Peak serum levels are achieved between 30-120 minutes in dogs.

Praziquantel is distributed throughout the body. It crosses the intestinal wall and blood-brain barrier into the CNS.

Praziquantel is metabolized in the liver via CYP3A enzymes to metabolites of unknown activity. It is excreted primarily in the urine; elimination half-life is ≈ 3 hours in the dog. In dogs, orally administered grapefruit juice can increase the area under the curve by 150-200%.

Contraindications/Precautions/Warnings

The manufacturer recommends not using praziquantel in puppies <4 weeks old or kittens <6 weeks old. However, a combination product containing praziquantel and febantel from the same manufacturer is FDA-approved for use in puppies and kittens of all ages. No other contraindications are listed for this compound from the manufacturer. In humans, praziquantel is contraindicated in patients hypersensitive to the drug.

Adverse Effects

When used orally, praziquantel can cause anorexia, vomiting, lethargy, or diarrhea in dogs, but the incidence of these effects is <5%. In cats, adverse effects were quite rare (<2%) in field trials using oral praziquantel, with salivation and diarrhea being reported.

A greater incidence of adverse effects has been reported after using the injectable product. In dogs, pain at the injection site, vomiting, drowsiness, and/or a staggering gait were reported from field trials with the drug. Some cats (9.4%) showed clinical signs of diarrhea, weakness, vomiting, salivation, sleepiness, transient anorexia, and/or pain at the injection site.

Reproductive/Nursing Safety

Praziquantel is considered safe to use in pregnant dogs or cats. In humans, the FDA categorizes this drug as category *B* for use during pregnancy (*Animal studies have not yet demonstrated risk to the fetus, but there are no adequate studies in pregnant women; or animal studies have shown an adverse effect, but adequate studies in pregnant women have not demonstrated a risk to the fetus in the first trimester of pregnancy, and there is no evidence of risk in later trimesters.*) In a separate system evaluating the safety of drugs in canine and feline pregnancy (Papich 1989), this drug is categorized as class: *A* (*Probably safe. Although specific studies may not have proved the safety of all drugs in dogs and cats, there are no reports of adverse effects in laboratory animals or women.*)

Praziquantel appears in maternal milk at a concentration of ≈ 25% of that in maternal serum, but is unlikely to pose harm to nursing offspring.

Overdosage/Acute Toxicity

Praziquantel has a wide margin of safety. In rats and mice, the oral LD50 is at least 2 g/kg. An oral LD50 could not be determined in dogs, as at doses >200 mg/kg, the drug induced vomiting. Parenteral doses of 50 – 100 mg/kg in cats caused transient ataxia and depression; injected doses at 200 mg/kg were lethal in cats.

There were 22 exposures to praziquantel reported to the ASPCA Animal Poison Control Center (APCC) during 2001-2009. In these cases 12 were cats with 4 showing clinical signs. The remaining 10 were dogs that showed no clinical signs.

Drug Interactions

The following drug interactions have either been reported or are theoretical in humans or animals receiving praziquantel and may be of significance in veterinary patients. Unless otherwise noted, use together is not necessarily contraindicated, but weigh the potential risks and perform additional monitoring when appropriate.

■ **CIMETIDINE:** May increase the serum concentration of praziquantel.

■ **CYP3A4 INDUCERS** (*e.g.,* Rifampin): May decrease praziquantel levels. In humans it is recommended to discontinue rifampin 4 weeks prior to praziquantel.

■ **GRAPEFRUIT JUICE:** Can significantly increase praziquantel serum levels in Beagles. (Giorgi *et al.* 2003)

- **KETOCONAZOLE, ITRACONAZOLE:** May increase praziquantel levels.
- **OXAMINIQUINE:** Reportedly in humans, synergistic activity occurs with praziquantel and oxamniquine in the treatment of schistosomiasis. The clinical implications of this synergism in veterinary patients are not clear.

Doses

Note: For dosages of combination products containing praziquantel, see the Emodepside, Ivermectin, Lufenuron, Milbemycin, Moxidectin, and Pyrantel monographs.

- **DOGS:**

For susceptible cestodes (labeled-dose; FDA-approved):

Injectable: IM or SC using the 56.8 mg/mL injectable product: Body weight: Dose: ≤5 lbs: 17 mg (0.3 mL); 6-10 lbs: 28.4 mg (0.5 mL); 11-25 lbs: 56.8 mg (1 mL); ≥25 lbs: 0.2 mL/5 lb body weight; maximum 3 mL.

Oral: Using the 34 mg canine tablet: Body weight: Dose: ≤5 lbs: 17 mg (1/2 tab); 6-10 lbs: 34 mg (1 tab); 11-15 lbs: 51 mg (1.5 tabs); 16-30 lbs: 68 mg (2 tabs); 31-45 lbs: 102 mg (3 tabs); 46-60 lbs: 136 mg (4 tabs); ≥60 lbs: 170 mg (5 tabs maximum). (Package insert; *Droncit® Injectable* and *Tablets*—Bayer)

For removal of tapeworms (*Dipylidium caninum, Taenia pisiformis, Echinococcus granulosus*, and removal and control of *Echinococcus multilocularis*), **hookworms** (*Ancylostoma caninum, Uncinaria stenocephala*), **ascarids** (*Toxocara canis, Toxascaris leonina*), and **whipworms** (*Trichuris vulpis*) using *Drontal Plus®* (praziquantel, pyrantel, febantel); (labeled dose; FDA-approved): There are 3 tablet sizes available: Puppies and Small Dogs (2-25 lbs.), Medium Sized Dogs (26-60 lbs.); Large Dogs (≥45 lbs.). The package insert has a dosing table to determine the correct size tablet and dosage for a dog's weight. Not for use in puppies <3 weeks of age or dogs weighing <2 lbs. *Drontal Plus®* label information can be accessed via dailymed.nlm.nih.gov

Extra-label Doses:

a) For *Taenia, Echinococcus, Dipylidium caninum, Mesocestoides* (adult): 5 mg/kg PO or SC. (Conboy 2009)

b) For *Diphyllobothrium*: 7.5 mg/kg PO either once or for 2 days. (Conboy 2009)

c) For *Sparganum proliferum (adult)*: 7.5 mg/kg or 25 mg/kg PO or SC daily for 2 days. (Conboy 2009)

d) For *Spirometra mansonoides* or *Diphyllobothrium erinacei*: 7.5 mg/kg, PO once daily for 2 days. (Roberson 1988)

e) For treatment of Paragonimiasis (*Paragonimus kellicotti*): 23 – 25 mg/kg PO q8h for 3 days. (Reinemeyer 1995), (Hawkins 2000)

f) For treatment of liver flukes (Platynosum or Opisthorchiidae families): 20 – 40 mg/kg PO once daily for 3-10 days. (Taboada 1999)

g) For *Alaria* spp.: 20 mg/kg PO. (Ballweber 2004)

h) For adjunctive treatment of the flukes (*Nanophyetus salmincola*) associated with Salmon poisoning: Single dose of 10 – 30 mg/kg PO or SC. (Headley *et al.*)

i) For treatment of Giardia infections using *Drontal Plus®*: Use label dose once daily PO for 3 days (Lappin 2006). Give 2 small dog tablets of *Drontal Plus®* (febantel 113.4 mg; pyrantel 22.7 mg; praziquantel 22.7 mg) once daily PO for 5 days. (Scorza *et al.* 2004)

- **CATS:**

For susceptible cestodes (labeled-dose; FDA-approved): IM or SC using the 56.8 mg/mL **injectable product:**

Body weight: Dose; <5 lbs: 11.4 mg (0.2 mL); 5-10 lbs: 22.7 mg (0.4 mL); ≥10 lbs: 34.1 mg (0.6 mL maximum); **Oral:** Using the 23 mg feline tab Body weight: Dose <4 lbs: 11.5 mg (1/2 tab); 5-11 lbs: 23 mg (1 tab); >11 lbs: 34.5 mg (1.5 tabs). (Package insert; *Droncit® Injectable* and *Tablets*)

Extra-label Doses:

a) For treatment of Paragonimiasis (*Paragonimus kellicotti*): 23 – 25 mg/kg PO q8h for 3 days. (Reinemeyer 1995)(Hawkins 2000)

b) For *Diphyllobothrium* (adult): 35 mg/kg PO once has been recommended. (Conboy 2009)

c) For *Sparganum proliferum* (adult): 7.5 mg/kg or 25 mg/kg PO or SC daily for 2 days. (Conboy 2009)

d) For *Alaria* spp.: 20 mg/kg PO. (Ballweber 2004)

e) For *Taenia, Echinococcus, Dipylidium caninum, Mesocestoides* (adult): 5 mg/kg PO or SC. (Conboy 2009)

f) For *Spirometra mansonoides*: 30 – 35 mg/kg PO. (Bowman 2006)

g) For treatment of Giardia infections using *Drontal Plus®*: Give 2 small dog tablets of *Drontal Plus®* (febantel 113.4 mg; pyrantel 22.7 mg; praziquantel 22.7 mg) once daily PO for 5 days. (Scorza *et al.* 2004)

- **RABBITS, RODENTS, SMALL MAMMALS:**

Note: All are extra-label.

a) Chinchillas: 6 – 10 mg/kg PO. (Hayes 2000)

b) For tapeworms in mice, rats, hamsters and gerbils: 30 mg/kg, PO once (note the high dosage required). (Burke 1999)

c) For cestodes and trematodes on rabbits: 5 – 10 mg/kg PO once. (Bryan 2009)

- **SHEEP & GOATS:**

For all species of Moniezia, Stilesia, or Avitellina (extra-label): 10 – 15 mg/kg. (Roberson 1988)

- **HORSES:**

For *Anoplocephala perfoliata* (extra-label): At 1.5 – 2 mg/kg PO efficacy was 100% in treated horses. At 1 mg/kg PO efficacy was 99.7%. (Slocombe 2006)

- **CAMELIDS (NEW WORLD):**

For *D. Dendriticum* (extra-label): 50 mg/kg PO once. (**Note:** Product used was a concentrated [250 mg/mL] galenic paste formulation). (Dadak *et al.* 2013)

- **BIRDS:**

For susceptible parasites (tapeworms); (extra-label):

a) 1/4 of one 23 mg tablet/kg PO; repeat in 10-14 days. Add to feed or give by gavage. Injectable form is toxic to finches. (Clubb 1986)

b) For common tapeworms in chickens: 10 mg/kg. (Roberson 1988)

c) For cestodes and some trematodes: Direct dose: 5 – 10 mg/kg PO or IM as a single dose or 12 mg of crushed tablets baked into a 9"x 9"x 2" cake. **Finches** should have their regular food withheld and be pre-exposed to a non-medicated cake. (Marshall 1993)

- **REPTILES/AMPHIBIANS:**

Note: All are extra-label.

a) Reptiles: For cestodes and some trematodes in most species: 7.5 mg/kg PO once; repeat in 2 weeks PO. (Gauvin 1993)

b) For removal of common tapeworms in snakes: 3.5 – 7 mg/kg. (Roberson 1988)

c) **For cestodes and trematodes in reptiles and amphibians:** 7 – 8 mg/kg PO, IM, SC. (de la Navarre 2003)

Monitoring
- Clinical efficacy.

Client Information
- Can be given with or without food; tablets may be crushed or mixed with food.
- When given by mouth side effects are rare, but it can cause loss of appetite, salivation or drooling (in cats), vomiting, lethargy/tiredness/lack of energy, and diarrhea.
- Usually do not see dead tapeworms in feces after treating.

Chemistry/Synonyms
A prazinoisoquinoline derivative anthelmintic, praziquantel occurs as a white to practically white, hygroscopic, bitter tasting, crystalline powder, either odorless or having a faint odor. It is very slightly soluble in water and freely soluble in alcohol.

Praziquantel may also be known as: EMBAY-8440, praziquantelum, *Biltricide®*, *Bio-Cest®*, *Cercon®*, *Cesol®*, *Cestox®*, *Cisticid®*, *ComboCare®*, *Cysticide®*, *Droncit®*, *Drontal®*, *Ehliten®*, *Equimax®*, *Extiser Q®*, *Mycotricide®*, *Opticide®*, *Quest® Plus*, *Praquantel®*, *Prasikon®*, *Prazite®*, *Prozitel®*, *Sincerck®*, *Teniken®*, *Virbantel®*, *Waycital®*, or *Zifartel®* and *Zimecterin Gold Paste®*.

Storage/Stability
Unless otherwise instructed by the manufacturer, praziquantel tablets should be stored in tight containers at room temperature. Protect from light.

Dosage Forms/Regulatory Status
VETERINARY-LABELED PRODUCTS:
Praziquantel Tablets: 23 mg (feline); 34 mg (canine); *Droncit® Tablets*, generic; (Rx; OTC). FDA-approved for use in cats and dogs.

Praziquantel Injection: 56.8 mg/mL in 10 mL and 50 mL vials; *Droncit® Injection*, generic; (Rx). FDA-approved for use in cats and dogs.

Combination Products:

With Emodepside: Emodepside (1.98% w/w; 21.4 mg/mL) and Praziquantel (7.94% w/w; 85.8 mg/mL) Topical Solution in 0.35 mL (cats 2.2-5.5 lb.), 0.7 mL (cats >5.5-11 lb.) & 1.12 mL (cats >11-17.6 lb.) tubes; *Profender®*; (Rx). FDA-approved for use on cats.

With Febantel & Pyrantel: *Drontal Plus® Taste Tabs*: For Puppies and Small Dogs (2-25 lbs.): praziquantel 22.7 mg/pyrantel 22.7 mg/febantel, 113.4 mg; For Medium Sized Dogs (26-60 lbs.): praziquantel 68 mg/pyrantel 68 mg/febantel, 340.2 mg; For Large Dogs (≥45 lbs.): praziquantel 136 mg/pyrantel 136 mg/febantel, 680.4 mg; (Rx). Approved for use in dogs (NADA 141-007).

With Ivermectin: Oral Paste: containing 1.87% ivermectin and 14.03% of praziquantel in oral syringes (sufficient to treat one 1320 lb horse); *Equimax®*;; (OTC). FDA-approved for use in horse or ponies not intended for food purposes.

With Ivermectin: Oral Paste: containing 1.55% ivermectin and 7.75% of praziquantel in oral syringes; *Zimecterin Gold®*; (OTC). FDA-approved for use in horse or ponies not intended for food purposes.

With Milbemycin & Lufenuron: Milbemycin/Lufenuron/Praziquantel Chewable Oral Tablets: For dogs 2-8 lbs.: 2.3 mg/46 mg/22.8 mg; For dogs 8.1-25 lbs: 5.75 mg/115 mg/57 mg; For dogs 25.1-50 lbs.: 11.5 mg/230 mg/114 mg; For dogs 50.1-100 lbs.: 23 mg/460 mg/228 mg; *Sentinel® Spectrum®* (Rx). FDA-approved for use in dogs and puppies ≥6 weeks of age.

With Moxidectin: Moxidectin 20 mg/mL and Praziquantel 125 mg/mL Oral Gel in 11.6 gram syringes (sufficient to treat one 1250 lb. horse); *Quest Plus®*; (OTC). FDA-approved for use in horse or ponies not intended for food purposes.

With Pyrantel: Tablets: Praziquantel 13.6 mg/pyrantel pamoate 54.3 mg (as base) for 2-5.9 lb cats and kittens; Praziquantel 18.2 mg/pyrantel pamoate 72.6 mg (as base); Praziquantel 27.2 mg/pyrantel pamoate 108.6 mg (as base) for 6-24 lb. cats; *Drontal® Tablets*; some sizes may be available as generics or under various trade names (OTC). FDA-approved for use in cats and kittens that are ≥2 months of age and weigh ≥2 lb.

With Pyrantel: Chewable Tablets: Praziquantel 30 mg/pyrantel pamoate 30 mg; & Praziquantel 114 mg/pyrantel pamoate chewable tablets; *Virbantel Flavored Chewables®*; (OTC). FDA-approved for use in dogs.

With Ivermectin & Pyrantel: Ivermectin/Pyrantel Pamoate/Praziquantel Oral Chewable Tablets: 34mcg/28mg/28mg, 68mcg/57mg/57mg; 136mcg/114mg/114mg, 272mcg/228mg/228mg; *Iverhart® Max*; (Rx). FDA-approved for use in dogs.

HUMAN-LABELED PRODUCTS:
Praziquantel Oral Tablets (Film-coated): 600 mg; *Biltricide®*; (Rx)

Revisions/References
Monograph revised/updated May 2014.

Ballweber, L. (2004). Internal parasites in dogs and cats. Proceedings; Western Vet Conf. accessed via Veterinary Information Network; vin.com

Bowman, D. (2006). Feline gastrointestinal parasites. Proceedings: ACVC. accessed via Veterinary Information Network; vin.com

Bryan, J. (2009). Rabbit GI Physiology: What do I do now? Proceedings: WVC. accessed via Veterinary Information Network; vin.com

Burke, T. (1999). Husbandry and Medicine of Rodents and Lagomorphs. Proceedings: Central Veterinary Conference, Kansas City. accessed via Veterinary Information Network; vin.com

Clubb, S. L. (1986). Therapeutics: Individual and Flock Treatment Regimens. *Clinical Avian Medicine and Surgery*. G. J. Harrison and L. R. Harrison. Philadelphia, W.B. Saunders: 327-55.

Conboy, G. (2009). Cestodes of Dogs and Cats in North America. Veterinary Clinics of North America-Small Animal Practice 39(6): 1075-+.

Dadak, A. M., et al. (2013). Efficacy and safety of oral praziquantel against Dicrocoelium dendriticum in llamas. Veterinary Parasitology 197(1-2): 122-5.

de la Navarre, B. (2003). Common parasitic diseases of reptiles and amphibians. Proceedings: Western Veterinary Conf. accessed via Veterinary Information Network; vin.com

Gauvin, J. (1993). Drug therapy in reptiles. Seminars in Avian & Exotic Med 2(1): 48-59.

Giorgi, M., et al. (2003). Effects of liquid and freeze-dried grapefruit juice on the pharmacokinetics of praziquantel and its metabolite 4'-hydroxy-praziquantel in beagle dogs. Pharmacological Research 47: 82-92.

Hawkins, E. (2000). Pulmonary Parenchymal Diseases. *Textbook of Veterinary Internal Medicine: Diseases of the Dog and Cat*. S. Ettinger and E. Feldman. Philadelphia, WB Saunders. 2: 1061-91.

Hayes, P. (2000). Diseases of Chinchillas. *Kirk's Current Veterinary Therapy: XIII Small Animal Practice*. J. Bonagura. Philadelphia, WB Saunders: 1152-7.

Headley, S. A., et al. Neorickettsia helminthoeca and salmon poisoning disease: A review. The Veterinary Journal In Press, Corrected Proof.

Lappin, M. (2006). Giardia infections. Proceedings: WSAVA World Congress. accessed via Veterinary Information Network; vin.com

Marshall, R. (1993). Avian anthelmintics and antiprotozoals. Seminars in Avian & Exotic Med 2(1): 33-41.

Papich, M. (1989). Effects of drugs on pregnancy. *Current Veterinary Therapy X: Small Animal Practice*. R. Kirk. Philadelphia, Saunders: 1291-9.

Reinemeyer, C. (1995). Parasites of the respiratory system. *Kirk's Current Veterinary Therapy:XII*. J. Bonagura. Philadelphia, W.B. Saunders: 895-8.

Roberson, E. L. (1988). Anticestodal and antitrematodal drugs. *Veterinary Pharmacology and Therapeutics*. N. H. Booth and L. E. McDonald. Ames, Iowa State University Press: 928-49.

Scorza, A., et al. (2004). Efficacy of febantel/pyrantel/praziquantel for the treatment of giardia infection in cats. Proceedings: ACVIM Forum. accessed via Veterinary Information Network; vin.com

Slocombe, J. (2006). A modified critical test and its use in two dose titration trials to assess efficacy of praziquantel for Anoplocephala perfoliata in equids. Veterinary Parasitology 136(2): 127-35.

Taboada, J. (1999). How I treat gastrointestinal pythiosis. Proceedings: The North American Veterinary Conference, Orlando. accessed via Veterinary Information Network; vin.com

Prazosin HCl

(pra-zoe-**sin**) Minipress®

Alpha-1 Adrenergic Blocker

Prescriber Highlights

▶ Alpha₁-blocker that may be useful for adjunctive treatment of CHF, systemic hypertension, or pulmonary hypertension in dogs.

▶ Also used to reduce sympathetic tone to treat functional urethral obstruction in dogs & cats.

▶ Caution: Chronic renal failure or preexisting hypotensive conditions.

▶ Adverse Effects: Potentially hypotension, CNS (lethargy, dizziness, etc.) & GI effects.

Uses/Indications

Prazosin may be useful for treating functional urethral obstruction (VURD) in dogs. Its usefulness for this purpose in male cats is somewhat controversial (Lulich *et al.* 2013) and its efficacy is unknown.

For cardiac indications, prazosin is less well studied in dogs than hydralazine, and its capsule dosage form makes it less convenient for dosing. However, prazosin appears to cause less tachycardia, and its venous dilation effects may be an advantage over hydralazine when preload reduction is desired. Prazosin could be considered for therapy for the adjunctive treatment of CHF, particularly when secondary to mitral or aortic valve insufficiency, when hydralazine is ineffective or not tolerated. Prazosin may also be used for the treatment of systemic hypertension or pulmonary hypertension in dogs.

Pharmacology/Actions

Prazosin's effects are a result of its selective, competitive inhibition of alpha₁-adrenergic receptors. It reduces blood pressure and peripheral vascular resistance and, unlike hydralazine, has dilatory effects on both the arterial and venous side.

Prazosin significantly reduces systemic arterial and venous blood pressures, and right atrial pressure; cardiac output is increased in patients with CHF. Moderate reductions in blood pressure, pulmonary vascular resistance, and systemic vascular resistance are seen in these patients. Heart rates can be moderately decreased or unchanged. Unlike hydralazine, prazosin does not seem to increase renin release so diuretic therapy is not mandatory with this agent (but is usually beneficial in CHF). Prazosin did not antagonize medetomidine-induced diuresis in cats. (Murahata *et al.* 2014)

Pharmacokinetics

The pharmacokinetic parameters for this agent were not located for veterinary species. In humans, prazosin is variably absorbed after oral administration. Peak levels occur in 2-3 hours.

Prazosin is widely distributed throughout the body and is ≈97% bound to plasma proteins. Prazosin is minimally distributed into milk. It is unknown if it crosses the placenta.

Prazosin is metabolized in the liver and some metabolites have activity. Metabolites and some unchanged drug (5-10%) are primarily eliminated in feces via the bile.

Contraindications/Precautions/Warnings

Prazosin should be used with caution in patients with chronic renal failure or preexisting hypotensive conditions.

There are some anecdotal reports that dogs with the *ABCB1* mutation (MDR1) may be overly sensitive to the effects of prazosin; use with caution in breeds known to be susceptible to this mutation. Alternate drugs should be considered for dogs tested positive for this mutation until more information becomes available; if this is not possible, consider reducing the dosage and increase monitoring (particularly blood pressure).

Adverse Effects

An experimental study done in dogs using IV prazosin at 0.025 mg/kg caused significant decreases in systolic, diastolic and mean arterial blood pressures (Fischer *et al.* 2003). Whether this is a clinical concern when using prazosin orally to decrease urethral resistance is unclear. Other reported adverse effects include CNS effects (lethargy, dizziness, etc.) but they are usually transient in nature, GI effects (nausea, vomiting, diarrhea, constipation, etc.) and nictitans elevation. Tachyphylaxis (drug tolerance) has been reported in humans, but dosage adjustment, temporarily withdrawing the drug, &/or adding an aldosterone antagonist (*e.g.*, spironolactone) usually corrects this.

Syncope secondary to orthostatic hypotension has been reported in people after the first dose of the drug. This effect may persist if the dosage is too high for the patient.

Reproductive/Nursing Safety

In humans, the FDA categorizes this drug as category *C* for use during pregnancy (*Animal studies have shown an adverse effect on the fetus, but there are no adequate studies in humans; or there are no animal reproduction studies and no adequate studies in humans.*)

Prazosin is excreted in small amounts in maternal milk and unlikely to pose much risk to nursing offspring.

Overdosage/Acute Toxicity

There were 56 single agent exposures to prazosin reported to the ASPCA Animal Poison Control Center (APCC) during 2009-2013. Of the 30 dogs, 12 were symptomatic with 50% being ataxic, and 25% being lethargic or trembling. Of the 26 cats, 8 were symptomatic with hypotension (38%) being the most common.

Consider performing gut decontamination with activated charcoal using standard precautionary measures if the ingestion was recent and if cardiovascular status has been stabilized. Monitor heart rate and blood pressure. Treat shock using volume expanders and pressor agents if necessary. Monitor and support renal function.

Drug Interactions

The following drug interactions have either been reported or are theoretical in humans or animals receiving prazosin and may be of significance in veterinary patients. Unless otherwise noted, use together is not necessarily contraindicated, but weigh the potential risks and perform additional monitoring when appropriate.

- **BETA-BLOCKING AGENTS** (*e.g.*, **propranolol**): May enhance the postural hypotensive effects seen after the first dose of prazosin.
- **CLONIDINE**: May decrease prazosin antihypertensive effects.
- **SILDENAFIL** (and other **PDE INHIBITORS**): May increase risk for hypotension.
- **VERAPAMIL** or **NIFEDIPINE**: May cause synergistic hypotensive effects when used concomitantly with prazosin.

Doses

- **DOGS:**

  For adjunctive treatment of heart failure (extra-label): 1 mg per dog PO 3 times daily for dogs weighing <15 kg; 2 mg 3 times daily PO for dogs weighing >15 kg. (Kittleson 1985; Atkins 2007)

  For hypertension including hypertension associated with methylphenidate toxicosis (extra-label): 0.5 – 2 mg per dog PO q8-12h. Adapted from: (Ware 2003), (Genovese *et al.* 2010)

  To decrease urethral resistance in idiopathic vesico-urethral reflex dyssynergia (VURD); (extra-label): In the study (n=5), for the first 4 weeks in the study, 0.5 mg/kg PO twice daily. During the last 2 weeks, the dosage was reduced to 0.25 mg/kg twice daily. However, when side effects developed, the dosage was decreased by one-half. Moderate to good effect in 60% of the dogs treated. (Haagsman *et al.* 2013). Other (anecdotal) recommended dosages for dogs are 1 mg/15 kg of body weight PO 2-3 times a day.

- **CATS:**

  To decrease urethral resistance with functional urethral obstruction/urethral spasm (extra-label): Use is controversial and efficacy has been questioned (Lulich *et al.* 2013). Several dosages have been suggested, ranging from 0.25 – 0.5 mg per cat PO q12-24h (Coates 2004; Lulich 2004), (Vernau 2006); and 0.25 – 1 mg per cat PO q8-12h for urethral spasms; initially give for 5-7 days then wean off if possible (Gunn-Moore *et al.* 2009).

  For hypertension (extra-label): 0.25 – 0.5 mg per cat (not mg/kg) PO q 24h. (Clarke 2013)

Monitoring

- Baseline thoracic radiographs.
- Mucous membrane color; CRT.
- If possible, arterial blood pressure and venous PO_2.

Client Information

- Give with food.
- Most common side effect is lethargy (tiredness/lack of energy).
- May cause rapid heartbeat, hyperactivity or higher body temperature. Contact your veterinarian immediately if any of these occur.

Chemistry/Synonyms

A quinazoline-derivative postsynaptic $alpha_1$-adrenergic blocker, prazosin HCl occurs as a white to tan powder. It is slightly soluble in water and very slightly soluble in alcohol.

Prazosin may also be known as: CP-12299-1, furazosin hydrochloride, prazosini hydrochloridum; many trade names are available.

Storage/Stability

Prazosin capsules should be stored in well-closed containers at room temperature.

Dosage Forms/Regulatory Status

VETERINARY-LABELED PRODUCTS: NONE.

The ARCI (Racing Commissioners International) has designated this drug as a class 3 substance. See the appendix for more information.

HUMAN-LABELED PRODUCTS:

Prazosin Capsules: 1 mg, 2 mg & 5 mg (as base); *Minipress*®, generic; (Rx)

Revisions/References

Monograph revised/updated May 2014.

Atkins, C. (2007). Canine Heart Failure--Current concepts. Proceedings: WSAVA World Congress. accessed via Veterinary Information Network; vin.com

Clarke, D. (2013). Antihypertensives: When Pain Meds and ACE Don't Cut It. Proceedings; International Veterinary Emergency and Critical Care Symposium. accessed via Veterinary Information Network; vin.com

Coates, J. (2004). Neurogenic micturition disorders. Proceedings: ACVIM Forum. accessed via Veterinary Information Network; vin.com

Fischer, J. R., et al. (2003). Urethral pressure profile and hemodynamic effects of phenoxybenzamine and prazosin in non-sedated male beagle dogs. Canadian Journal of Veterinary Research-Revue Canadienne De Recherche Veterinaire 67(1): 30-8.

Genovese, D. W., et al. (2010). Methylphenidate toxicosis in dogs: 128 cases (2001-2008). Javma-Journal of the American Veterinary Medical Association 237(12): 1438-43.

Gunn-Moore, D. & R. Casey (2009). Feline Lower Urinary Tract Disease. Proceedings: BSAVA. accessed via Veterinary Information Network; vin.com

Haagsman, A. N., et al. (2013). Comparison of terazosin and prazosin for treatment of vesico-urethral reflex dyssynergia in dogs. Veterinary Record 173(2): 41-+.

Kittleson, M. D. (1985). Pathophysiology and treatment of heart failure. *Manual of Small Animal Cardiology.* L. P. Tilley and J. M. Owens. New York, Churchill Livingstone: 308-32.

Lulich, J. (2004). Managing functional urethral obstruction. Proceedings: ACVIM Forum. accessed via Veterinary Information Network; vin.com

Lulich, J. & C. Osborne (2013). Prazosin in cats with urethral obstruction. Javma-Journal of the American Veterinary Medical Association 243(9): 1240-.

Murahata, Y., et al. (2014). Antagonistic Effects of Atipamezole, Yohimbine and Prazosin on Medetomidine-Induced Diuresis in Healthy Cats. Journal of Veterinary Medical Science 76(2): 173-82.

Vernau, K. (2006). Dysuria: To pee or not to pee... Proceedings: UCD Veterinary Neurology Symposium. accessed via Veterinary Information Network; vin.com

Ware, W. (2003). Cardiovascular system disorders. *Small Animal Internal Medicine, 3rd Ed.* R. Nelson and C. Couto. St Louis, Mosby: 1-209.

Prednisolone
Prednisone
Prednisolone Sodium Succinate

(pred-**niss**-oh-lone); (pred-ni-zone)

For more information refer to the monograph: Glucocorticoids, General Information or to the manufacturer's product information for veterinary labeled products. See also the Trimeprazine Tartrate with Prednisolone monograph.

Note: Although separate entities, prednisone and prednisolone are often considered bioequivalent; most species rapidly convert prednisone to prednisolone in the liver. Horses, cats and patients in frank hepatic failure may not absorb or convert prednisone to prednisolone efficiently. Use either prednisolone or an alternative glucocorticoid in these patients when possible.

Prescriber Highlights

▶ Classic glucocorticoids used for many conditions in many species. Antiinflammatory activity is 4X more potent than hydrocortisone; has some mineralocorticoid activity.

▶ Contraindications (relative): Systemic fungal infections.

▶ Caution: Active bacterial infections, corneal ulcer, Cushingoid syndrome, diabetes, osteoporosis, chronic psychotic reactions, predisposition to thrombophlebitis, hypertension, CHF, renal insufficiency.

▶ Goal of therapy is to use as much as is required & as little as possible for as short an amount of time as possible.

▶ Prednisone poorly absorbed after oral use in horses; prednisone may not be readily converted to prednisolone in cats. Prednisolone is preferred in these two species.

▶ Primary adverse effects are "Cushingoid" in nature with sustained use.

▶ Many potential drug & lab interactions.

Uses/Indications

Glucocorticoids have been used in an attempt to treat practically every malady that afflicts man or animal, but for prednisolone/prednisone, there are there are four primary uses and dose ranges: **1)** replacement or supplementation (*e.g.*, relative adrenal insufficiency associated with septic shock) of glucocorticoid effects secondary to hypoadrenocorticism, **2)** as an antiinflammatory, **3)** as an immunosuppressive, and, **4)** as an antineoplastic agent. Current evidence does not support high dose use for hemorrhagic or hypovolemic shock, head trauma, spinal cord trauma, or sepsis. In general, when using glucocorticoids, the following principles should be followed:

- Glucocorticoids can mask disease! Try not to use them until you have a diagnosis.
- Make a specific diagnosis!
- Determine course from outset.
- Determine endpoint before you starting treating.
- Use the least potent form for the minimal time.
- Know when glucocorticoid use is inappropriate. (Behrend 2007)

Pharmacology/Actions

Prednisolone and prednisone are intermediate acting corticosteroids with a biologic "half-life" of 12-36 hours. Glucocorticoids have effects on virtually every cell type and system in mammals. For more information, refer to the Glucocorticoid Agents, General Information monograph.

Pharmacokinetics

In cats, prednisolone is much better absorbed when administered orally than prednisone. Reported bioavailabilities (of active prednisolone) are 100% and 21%, respectively. Over-conditioned cats had significantly higher plasma drug concentrations (2X) of prednisolone compared to normal-conditioned cats in one study.

Plasma half-life is not meaningful from a therapy standpoint when evaluating systemic corticosteroids. Prednisolone and prednisone are intermediate acting corticosteroids with a biologic "half-life" of 12-36 hours.

Contraindications/Precautions/Warnings

Systemic use of glucocorticoids is generally considered contraindicated in systemic fungal infections (unless used for replacement therapy in Addison's), when administered IM in patients with idiopathic thrombocytopenia, and those hypersensitive to a particular compound. Sustained-released injectable glucocorticoids are considered contraindicated for chronic corticosteroid therapy of systemic diseases.

The veterinary injectable product (*Solu-Delta-Cortef®*) label states: "contraindicated in animals with tuberculosis, Cushingoid syndrome, and peptic ulcer. Existence of congestive heart failure, diabetes, chronic nephritis, and osteoporosis are relative contraindications. In the presence of infection, appropriate antibacterial agents should also be administered and should be continued for at least 3 days after discontinuance of the hormone and disappearance of all signs of infection. Do not use in viral infections."

Use with caution in animals with concomitant renal disease as they may be at increased risk for GI adverse effects.

Animals that have received glucocorticoids systemically, other than with "burst" therapy, should be tapered off the drugs. Patients who have received the drugs chronically should be tapered off slowly as endogenous ACTH and corticosteroid function may return slowly. Should the animal undergo a "stressor" (*e.g.*, surgery, trauma, illness, etc.) during the tapering process or until normal adrenal and pituitary function resume, additional glucocorticoids should be administered.

Animals, particularly cats, at risk for diabetes mellitus or with concurrent cardiovascular disease should receive glucocorticoids with caution due to these agents' potent hyperglycemic effect.

Adverse Effects

Adverse effects are generally associated with long-term administration of these drugs, especially if given at high dosages or not on an alternate day regimen. Effects generally are manifested as clinical signs of hyperadrenocorticism. When administered to young, growing animals, glucocorticoids can retard growth. Many of the potential effects, adverse and otherwise, are outlined above in the Pharmacology section.

In dogs, polydipsia (PD), polyphagia (PP), and polyuria (PU) may all be seen with short-term "burst" therapy as well as with alternate-day maintenance therapy on days when giving the drug. Adverse effects in dogs can include: dull, dry haircoat, weight gain, panting, vomiting, diarrhea, elevated liver enzymes, GI ulceration (especially with high parenteral or oral dosages), hypercoagulability, lipidemias, activation or worsening of diabetes mellitus, muscle wasting, and behavioral changes (depression, lethargy, viciousness). Discontinuation of the drug may be necessary; changing to an alternate steroid may also alleviate the problem. With the exception of PU/PD/PP, adverse effects associated with antiinflammatory therapy are relatively uncommon. Adverse effects associated with immunosuppressive doses are more common and potentially more severe.

Cats generally require higher dosages than dogs for clinical effect, but tend to develop fewer adverse effects. Glucocorticoids appear to have a greater hyperglycemic effect in cats than other species. Occasionally, PU/PD/PP, with weight gain, diarrhea, or depression can be seen. Long-term, high dose therapy can lead to "Cushingoid" effects, however.

Reproductive/Nursing Safety

Corticosteroid therapy may induce parturition in large animal species during the latter stages of pregnancy. In humans, the FDA categorizes this drug as category C for use during pregnancy (*Animal studies have shown an adverse effect on the fetus, but there are no adequate studies in humans; or there are no animal reproduction studies and no adequate studies in humans.*) In a separate system evaluating the safety of drugs in canine and feline pregnancy (Papich 1989), this drug is categorized as class: C (*These drugs may have potential risks. Studies in people or laboratory animals have uncovered risks, and these drugs should be used cautiously as a last resort when the benefit of therapy clearly outweighs the risks.*)

Use with caution in nursing dams. Glucocorticoids unbound to plasma proteins will enter milk. High dosages or prolonged administration to mothers may potentially inhibit growth, interfere with endogenous corticosteroid production or cause other unwanted effects in nursing offspring. In humans, however, several studies suggest that amounts excreted in breast milk are negligible when prednisone or prednisolone doses in the mother are ≤20 mg/day or methylprednisolone doses are ≤8 mg/day. Larger doses for short periods may not harm the infant.

Overdosage/Acute Toxicity

Overdoses of glucocorticoids used alone are unlikely to cause harmful effects, but gastrointestinal signs that are sometimes severe, can be seen in dogs. Should clinical signs occur, use supportive treatment if required. Chronic usage of glucocorticoids can lead to serious adverse effects. Refer to Adverse Effects above for more information.

There were 175 exposures to prednisone reported to the ASPCA Animal Poison Control Center (APCC) during 2008-2009. In these cases, 164 were dogs with 16 showing clinical signs, and 10 were cats with 2 showing clinical signs. The remaining case was a bird that showed no clinical signs. Common findings in dogs included polydipsia and polyuria.

Drug Interactions

The following drug interactions have either been reported or are theoretical in humans or animals receiving oral prednisolone/prednisone and may be of significance in veterinary patients. Unless otherwise noted, use together is not necessarily contraindicated, but weigh the potential risks and perform additional monitoring when appropriate.

- **AMPHOTERICIN B:** When administered concomitantly with glucocorticoids may cause hypokalemia.
- **ANTICHOLINESTERASE AGENTS** (*e.g.*, **pyridostigmine, neostigmine**, etc.): In patients with myasthenia gravis, concomitant glucocorticoid with these agents may lead to profound muscle weakness. If possible, discontinue anticholinesterase medication at least 24 hours prior to corticosteroid administration.
- **ASPIRIN (salicylates):** Glucocorticoids may reduce salicylate blood levels. In dogs, prednisone with ultra low-dose (0.5 mg/kg) aspirin does not increase the severity of GI lesions when compared with prednisone alone, but may increase incidence of diarrhea (Graham *et al.* 2009).

- **CYCLOPHOSPHAMIDE:** Glucocorticoids may also inhibit the hepatic metabolism of cyclophosphamide; dosage adjustments may be required.
- **CYCLOSPORINE:** Concomitant administration of may increase the blood levels of each, by mutually inhibiting the hepatic metabolism of each other; clinical significance of this interaction is not clear.
- **DIGOXIN:** Secondary to hypokalemia, increased risk for arrhythmias.
- **DIURETICS, POTASSIUM-DEPLETING (furosemide, thiazides,** etc.): When administered concomitantly with glucocorticoids may cause hypokalemia.
- **EPHEDRINE:** May increase metabolism of glucocorticoids.
- **ESTROGENS:** The effects of hydrocortisone, and possibly other glucocorticoids, may be potentiated by concomitant administration with estrogens.
- **INSULIN:** Requirements may increase in patients receiving glucocorticoids.
- **KETOCONAZOLE:** May decrease metabolism of glucocorticoids.
- **MITOTANE:** May alter the metabolism of steroids; higher than usual doses of steroids may be necessary to treat mitotane-induced adrenal insufficiency.
- **NSAIDS:** Administration of other ulcerogenic drugs with glucocorticoids may increase risk.
- **PHENOBARBITAL:** May increase the metabolism of glucocorticoids.
- **PHENYTOIN:** May increase the metabolism of glucocorticoids.
- **RIFAMPIN:** May increase the metabolism of glucocorticoids.
- **VACCINES:** Patients receiving corticosteroids at immunosuppressive dosages should generally not receive live attenuated-virus vaccines as virus replication may be augmented; a diminished immune response may occur after vaccine, toxoid, or bacterin administration in patients receiving glucocorticoids.

Laboratory Considerations

- Glucocorticoids may increase serum **cholesterol** and **urine glucose** levels.
- Glucocorticoids may decrease serum **potassium**.
- Glucocorticoids can suppress the release of thyroid stimulating hormone (TSH) and reduce T_3 & T_4 values. Thyroid gland atrophy has been reported after chronic glucocorticoid administration. Uptake of I^{131} by the thyroid may be decreased by glucocorticoids.
- Reactions to allergen **intradermal skin tests** may be suppressed by glucocorticoids. A two-week (14 day) withdrawal time prior to intradermal skin testing is recommended for dogs and cats (Olivry *et al.* 2013), (Chang *et al.* 2011); no withdrawal time is required prior to serum IgE testing to identify sensitizing allergens in cats (Chang *et al.* 2011).
- False-negative results of the **nitroblue tetrazolium test for systemic bacterial infections** may be induced by glucocorticoids.

Doses

There are a plethora of doses and protocols associated with many specific indications for systemic administration of glucocorticoids, but there are four primary uses and dose ranges: **1)** replacement or supplementation (*e.g.*, relative adrenal insufficiency associated with septic shock) of glucocorticoid effects secondary to hypoadrenocorticism, **2)** as an antiinflammatory, **3)** as an immunosuppressive, and **4)** as an antineoplastic agent. Current evidence does not support high dose use for hemorrhagic or hypovolemic shock, head trauma, spinal cord trauma, or sepsis.

Unless cited to a veterinary-approved product, consider all dosages extra-label.

- **DOGS/CATS:**

Use PO prednisolone in place of prednisone in cats whenever possible as they do not absorb or convert prednisone to prednisolone as well as dogs. If PO prednisone must be used in cats, consider increasing the dose.

Note: If given daily, therapy for longer than one-two weeks will suppress the HPA axis and recovery will take longer than one week. Therefore, if corticosteroids are used for longer than a few days, dosage must be tapered off using alternate day therapy. Many glucocorticoid responsive diseases can be managed with chronic alternate day therapy; avoid if possible, doses >1 mg/kg (prednisolone equivalent) every other day. Larger doses saturate the dog's ability to fully metabolize the last dose before the next dose is given and can negate the benefits of alternate day therapy. However, to induce remission of clinical signs or manage their recurrence requires institution of daily therapy at an appropriate dose to control clinical signs, then tapering to reach a minimum daily dose that will control signs followed by alternate day therapy to manage the disease. Individuals vary greatly in their response to the therapeutic and adverse effects of glucocorticoids and there may be qualitative differences between the effects of different glucocorticoids in the same patient. (Maddison 2009)

As an antiinflammatory agent: 0.5 – 1 mg/kg PO per day. See above note for additional information.

As an immunosuppressive:

Dogs: Doses up to 2.2 mg/kg PO per day. Doses above 2.2 mg/kg/day do not give more immunosuppression but do cause more adverse effects. If further immunosuppression is required, an additional immunosuppressive drug is needed. Many internists believe that prednisone doses should not exceed 80 mg per day, regardless of dog's weight. A sample prednisone immunosuppressive protocol for dogs follows but doses and dosage schedule must be tailored to the ongoing requirements of the individual patient: 2.2 mg/kg/day (not to exceed 80 mg total dose per day) for 3 weeks, then 1 mg/kg/day for 3 weeks, then 0.5 mg/kg/day for 3 weeks, then 0.5 mg/kg every other day.

Cats: Often require up to 4.4 mg/kg/day PO for immunosuppression. If further immunosuppression is required, an additional immunosuppressive drug is needed. A sample prednisolone immunosuppressive protocol for cats follows but doses and dosage schedule must be tailored to the ongoing requirements of the individual patient: 4.4 mg/kg/day for 3 weeks, then 2.2 mg/kg/day for 3 weeks, then 1 mg/kg/day for 3 weeks, then 1 mg/kg every other day. (Wilson 2010, 2011)

As an antineoplastic/cytotoxic: When prednis(ol)one is used as an antineoplastic agent, whether alone or in a multi-drug chemotherapy protocol, the following dosages should be used only as a general guide. Consultation with a veterinary oncologist and referral to current veterinary oncology references [*e.g.*, (Withrow *et al.* 2012); (Dobson *et al.* 2011); (Henry *et al.* 2009); (North *et al.* 2009); (Argyle *et al.* 2008)] are strongly recommended.

Dogs: 2 mg/kg per day. Cats are relatively steroid resistant and require higher doses than dogs. Doses can usually be safely doubled compared to dogs. See above note for additional information (Maddison 2009). **Note:** When used with other cytotoxic agents in chemo protocols, prednis(ol)one doses may be reduced.

As adjunctive treatment for hypoadrenocorticism:

a) **Acute treatment:** After second blood draw for cortisol measurement (ACTH stimulation test), prednisolone sodium succinate 2 – 20 mg/kg IV. If animal is in shock, give steroids at shock doses instead of trying to get an immediate diagnosis, then give dexamethasone (0.05 – 0.1 mg/kg IV q12h) in IV fluids until able to switch to PO steroids.

For oral glucocorticoid replacement (ongoing, with a mineralocorticoid): Prednisone initially at 0.1 – 0.22 mg/kg, then taper to lowest dose to control clinical signs. (Scott-Moncrieff 2010)

b) **For physiologic replacement:** It is common for dogs to require no more than 0.1 mg/kg once per day of prednis(ol)one, and often less will be sufficient to prevent recurrence of signs of glucocorticoid insufficiency. When on fludrocortisone (*Florinef®*), approximately half of the cases do not require any additional prednisone as there is enough glucocorticoid activity in fludrocortisone for those dogs. However, if on desoxycorticosterone pivalate (*Percorten®*), all cases require additional prednisone as it only has mineralocorticoid activity. (Wilson 2010, 2011)

■ **CATTLE:**

For glucocorticoid activity: Prednisolone sodium succinate: 0.2 – 1 mg/kg IV or IM. (Howard 1986)

■ **RABBITS, RODENTS, SMALL MAMMALS:**

a) **Rabbits:** Rarely indicated. As an antiinflammatory: 0.5 – 2 mg/kg PO. (Ivey *et al.* 2000)

b) **Mice, Rats, Gerbils, Hamsters, Guinea pigs, Chinchillas:** 0.5 – 2.2 mg/kg IM or SC. (Adamcak *et al.* 2000)

■ **HORSES:** (NOTE: ARCI UCGFS CLASS 4 DRUG)

Note: Prednisone does not appear to be absorbed very well after oral dosing; use prednisolone or another oral steroid.

For adjunctive therapy of Recurrent Airway Obstruction (RAO; Heaves):

a) **For short term treatment with environmental control:** In the study, dexamethasone sodium phosphate was given (0.1 mg/kg IM once daily for 4 days, 0.075 mg/kg IM once daily for 4 days, and 0.05 mg/kg IM for 4 days) or oral prednisolone (1 mg/kg PO for 4 days, 0.75 mg/kg for 4 days, 0.5 mg/kg PO for 4 days). Except for bronchoalveolar lavage cytology, prednisolone was as effective as IM dexamethasone. (Courouce-Malblanc *et al.* 2008)

b) In this study, horses were under continuous antigen exposure: Dexamethasone was given (0.05 mg/kg PO once daily for 7 days) or prednisolone (2 mg/kg PO once daily for 7 days). Both were effective, but dexamethasone more so. (Leclere *et al.* 2010)

For pruritus: Topical therapy preferred, but for more severe cases oral prednisolone can be considered. Induction dose of 2 mg/kg PO once daily for 3-10 days. Once the pruritus is controlled, this dose can be tapered to 0.5 mg/kg every 48 hours. (Marsella 2013)

For adjunctive therapy of neoplasias: Prednisolone: Typical dose is 1 mg/kg PO every other day. (Mair *et al.* 2006).

For glucocorticoid effects (labeled-dose; FDA-approved): 50 – 100 mg per horse as an initial dose. This may either be given IV over a period of 1/2 to 1 minute, or IM, and may be repeated in inflammatory, allergic, or other stress conditions at intervals of 12, 24, or 48 hours, depending upon the size of the animal, the severity of the condition, and the response to treatment. (adapted from label: *Solu-Delta-Cortef®*)

■ **LLAMAS:**

For steroid-responsive pruritic dermatoses secondary to allergic origins: Prednisone: 0.5 – 1 mg/kg PO initially; gradually reduce dosage to lowest effective dose given every other day. (Rosychuk 1989)

■ **BIRDS:**

As an antiinflammatory (extra-label): Prednisolone: 0.2 mg/30 gram body weight, or dissolve one 5 mg tablet in 2.5 mL of water and administer 2 drops orally. Give twice daily. Decrease dosage schedule if using long-term. (Clubb 1986)

For treatment of shock (extra-label): Prednisolone sodium succinate (10 mg/mL): 0.1 – 0.2 mL/100 grams body weight. Repeat every 15 minutes to effect. In large birds, dosage may be decreased by 1/2. (Clubb 1986)

■ **REPTILES:**

For shock in most species using prednisolone sodium succinate (extra-label): 5 – 10 mg/kg IV as needed. (Gauvin 1993)

Monitoring

Monitoring of glucocorticoid therapy is dependent on its reason for use, dosage, agent used (amount of mineralocorticoid activity), dosage schedule (daily versus alternate day therapy), duration of therapy, and the animal's age and condition. The following list may not be appropriate or complete for all animals; use clinical assessment and judgment should adverse effects be noted:

■ Weight, appetite, signs of edema.
■ Serum and/or urine electrolytes.
■ Total plasma proteins, albumin.
■ Blood glucose.
■ Growth and development in young animals.
■ ACTH stimulation test if necessary.

Client Information

■ Give oral products with food.
■ Goal is to find the lowest dose possible and use it for the shortest period of time.
■ Many side effects are possible, especially when it is used long term. Most common ones are: greater appetite, thirst, and need to urinate.
■ In dogs, stomach or intestinal ulcers, perforation or bleeding can occur. If your animal stops eating or you notice a high fever, black tarry stools or bloody vomit, contact your veterinarian right away.
■ Do not stop therapy abruptly (cold turkey) without veterinarian's guidance as serious side effects could occur.

Chemistry/Synonyms

Prednisolone and prednisone are synthetic glucocorticoids. Prednisolone and prednisolone acetate occur as odorless, white to practically white, crystalline powders. Prednisolone is very slightly soluble in water and slightly soluble in alcohol. The acetate ester is practically insoluble in water and slightly soluble in alcohol. The sodium succinate ester is highly water-soluble.

Prednisone occurs as an odorless, white to practically white, crystalline powder. Prednisone is very slightly soluble in water and slightly soluble in alcohol.

Prednisolone is also known as deltahydrocortisone or metacortandralone.

Prednisone may also be known as: delta(1)-cortisone, 1,2-dehydrocortisone, deltacortisone, deltadehydrocortisone, metacortandracin, NSC-10023, prednisonum; many trade names are available.

Storage/Stability

Prednisolone and prednisone tablets should be stored in well-closed containers. All prednisone and prednisolone products should be stored at temperatures <40°; preferably between 15-30°C; avoid freezing liquid products. Do not autoclave. Oral liquid preparations of prednisone should be stored in tight containers. Do not refrigerate prednisolone syrup.

Prednisolone sodium succinate should be stored at room temperature and protected from light (store in carton). After reconstitution, the product is recommended for immediate use and not stored for later use. If the solution becomes cloudy after reconstituting, it should not be used intravenously.

Compatibility/Compounding Considerations

Little data appears to be available regarding the compatibility of prednisolone sodium succinate injection (*Solu-Delta Cortef®*) with other products. A related compound, prednisolone sodium phosphate is reportedly physically **compatible** with the following drugs/solutions: ascorbic acid injection, cytarabine, erythromycin lactobionate, fluorouracil, heparin sodium, penicillin G potassium/sodium, tetracycline HCl, and vitamin B-Complex with C. It is reportedly physically **incompatible** with: calcium gluconate/gluceptate, dimenhydrinate, metaraminol bitartrate, methotrexate sodium, prochlorperazine edisylate, polymyxin B sulfate, promazine HCl, and promethazine. Compatibility is dependent upon factors such as pH, concentration, temperature, and diluent used; consult specialized references or a hospital pharmacist for more specific information.

Dosage Forms/Regulatory Status

VETERINARY-LABELED PRODUCTS:

A zero tolerance of residues in milk for these compounds have been established for dairy cattle. All these agents require a prescription (Rx). Known FDA-approved-veterinary products for systemic use are indicated below.

The ARCI (Racing Commissioners International) has designated this drug as a class 4 substance. See the appendix for more information.

Prednisolone Tablets: 5 mg, 20 mg: *Prednis-Tab®* (various), generic; (Rx). FDA-approved for use in dogs.

Prednisolone Sodium Succinate for Injection *act-o-vial®* System 100 mg (equivalent to 10 mg prednisolone) & 500 mg (equivalent to 50 mg prednisolone) per 10 mL vial; *Solu-Delta-Cortef®*; (Rx). FDA-approved for use in dogs, cats, and horses.

Prednisolone & Trimeprazine Tartrate Tablets: each tablet contains trimeprazine 5 mg and prednisolone 2 mg; *Temaril-P®*; (Rx). FDA-approved for use in dogs.

HUMAN-LABELED PRODUCTS:

Prednisolone Oral Tablets: 5 mg; *Millipred®*, generic; (Rx)

Prednisolone Sodium Phosphate Orally Disintegrating Tablets: 10 mg, 15 mg & 30 mg (as base); *Orapred ODT®*; (Rx)

Prednisolone Syrup/Oral Liquid or Solution: 5 mg/5 mL (1 mg/mL), 6.7 mg/5 mL (1.34 mg/mL), 10 mg/5 mL (2 mg/mL), 15 mg/5 mL (3 mg/mL), 20 mg/5 mL (4 mg/mL), 25 mg/5 mL (5 mg/mL); *Pediapred®, Millipred®, Orapred®, Veripred® 20, Flo-Pred®*, generic; (Rx)

Prednisone Tablets: 1 mg, 2.5 mg, 5 mg, 10 mg, 20 mg & 50 mg; generic; (Rx)

Prednisone Oral Solution/Syrup: 5 mg/5 mL (1 mg/mL); *Prednisone* and *Prednisone Intensol® Concentrate*; (Rx)

Ophthalmic solutions/suspensions are available.

Revisions/References

Monograph revised/updated May 2014.

Adamcak, A. & B. Otten (2000). Rodent Therapeutics. Vet Clin NA: Exotic Anim Pract 3:1(Jan): 221-40.
Argyle, D., et al. (2008). *Decision Making in Small Animal Oncology*, Wiley-Blackwell.
Behrend, E. (2007). Approach to glucocorticoid therapy. Proceedings: Western Vet Conference. accessed via Veterinary Information Network; vin.com
Chang, C. H., et al. (2011). The impact of oral versus inhaled glucocorticoids on allergen specific IgE testing in experimentally asthmatic cats. Veterinary Immunology and Immunopathology 144(3-4): 437-41.
Clubb, S. L. (1986). Therapeutics: Individual and Flock Treatment Regimens. *Clinical Avian Medicine and Surgery*. G. J. Harrison and L. R. Harrison. Philadelphia, W.B. Saunders: 327-55.
Courouce-Malblanc, A., et al. (2008). Comparison of prednisolone and dexamethasone effects in the presence of environmental control in heaves-affected horses. Veterinary Journal 175(2): 227-33.
Dobson, J. & D. Lascelles (2011). *BSAVA Manual of Canine and Feline Oncology*, BSAVA.
Gauvin, J. (1993). Drug therapy in reptiles. Seminars in Avian & Exotic Med 2(1): 48-59.
Graham, A. H. & M. S. Leib (2009). Effects of Prednisone Alone or Prednisone with Ultralow-Dose Aspirin on the Gastroduodenal Mucosa of Healthy Dogs. Journal of Veterinary Internal Medicine 23(3): 482-7.
Henry, C. & M. Higginbotham (2009). *Cancer Management in Small Animal Practice*, Saunders.
Howard, J. L., Ed. (1986). *Current Veterinary Therapy 2, Food Animal Practice*. Philadelphia, W.B. Saunders.
Ivey, E. & J. Morrisey (2000). Therapeutics for Rabbits. Vet Clin NA: Exotic Anim Pract 3:1(Jan): 183-216.
Leclere, M., et al. (2010). Efficacy of oral prednisolone and dexamethasone in horses with recurrent airway obstruction in the presence of continuous antigen exposure. Equine Veterinary Journal 42(4): 316-21.
Maddison, J. (2009). Cortocosteroids--Friend or Foe? Proceedings: WSAVA. accessed via Veterinary Information Network; vin.com
Mair, T. S. & C. G. Couto (2006). The use of cytotoxic drugs in equine practice. Equine Veterinary Education 18(3): 149-56.
Marsella, R. (2013). Equine Allergy Therapy Update on the Treatment of Environmental, Insect Bite Hypersensitivity, and Food Allergies. Veterinary Clinics of North America-Equine Practice 29(3): 551-+.
North, S. & T. Banks (2009). *Small Animal Oncology: An Introduction*, Saunders.
Olivry, T., et al. (2013). Evidence-based guidelines for anti-allergic drug withdrawal times before allergen-specific intradermal and IgE serological tests in dogs. Veterinary Dermatology 24(2).
Papich, M. (1989). Effects of drugs on pregnancy. *Current Veterinary Therapy X: Small Animal Practice*. R. Kirk. Philadelphia, Saunders: 1291-9.
Rosychuk, R. A. W. (1989). Llama Dermatology. Vet Clin of North Amer: Food Anim Prac 5(1): 203-15.
Scott-Moncrieff, J. C. (2010). Hypoadrenocorticism in dogs and cats: Update on diagnosis & treatment. Proceedings: ACVIM Forum. accessed via Veterinary Information Network; vin.com
Wilson, S. (2010). VIN BOARDS: Diabetic with post lysodren treatment for Cushings.
Wilson, S. (2011). Personal Communication.
Withrow, S., et al. (2012). Withrow and MacEwen's Small Animal Clinical Oncology, 5th Ed., Saunders.

Pregabalin

(pre-**gab**-ah-lin)   *Lyrica®*

Anticonvulsant; Neuropathic Pain Agent

Prescriber Highlights

▶ Similar to gabapentin; may be useful as an anticonvulsant or to treat neuropathic pain.

▶ Little information available on safety and efficacy in dogs or cats.

▶ Most common adverse effects are sedation and ataxia.

▶ Currently very expensive.

Uses/Indications

Like gabapentin, pregabalin may be useful as adjunctive therapy for refractory or complex partial seizures and treating chronic pain, particularly neuropathic pain in small animals. In an open label, non-comparative study in dogs that were not controlled with phenobarbital and/or bromides, in 7/9 dogs pregabalin reduced seizures by ≈ 60%. Two dogs were considered non-responders to pregabalin (Dewey *et al.* 2009).

In humans, pregabalin is indicated for pain associated with diabetic peripheral neuropathy, partial-onset seizures, post-herpetic neuralgia, and fibromyalgia. Off-label uses include generalized anxiety, and it may reduce opiate demand for post-surgical analgesia and decrease postoperative nausea and vomiting.

Pharmacology/Actions

Pregabalin has antiepileptic, analgesic, and anxiolytic activity. Like gabapentin, pregabalin is a structural analog of the inhibitory neurotransmitter gamma-aminobutyric acid (GABA). The mechanism of action of pregabalin, for either its anticonvulsant or analgesic actions is not fully understood, but it appears to bind to CaVa2-d (alpha2-delta subunit of the voltage-gated calcium channels). By decreasing calcium influx, release of excitatory neurotransmitters (*e.g.*, substance P, glutamate, norepinephrine) is inhibited. It is 3-10X as potent as gabapentin.

Pharmacokinetics

After single oral doses in 6 dogs, pregabalin median parameters were: T max = 1.5 hours; Cmax = 7.15 micrograms/mL; elimination half-life = 6.9 hours (Salazar *et al.* 2009).

After single oral doses in 6 cats, pregabalin median parameters were: T max = 2.9 hours; Cmax = 8.3 micrograms/mL; elimination half-life = 10.4 hours (Cautela *et al.* 2009).

In humans, oral bioavailability is ≈ 90%. Presence of food can delay the rate, but not the amount absorbed and it can be administered regardless of feeding status. Pregabalin is not bound to plasma proteins and it has an apparent volume of distribution of ≈ 500 mL/kg. Hepatic metabolism is negligible and it does not appear to affect hepatic enzymes. The drug is almost exclusively cleared unchanged by renal routes with a renal clearance of 67-81 mL/minute in young, healthy subjects. Elimination half-life is ≈ 6 hours. Dosage adjustment may be required in patients with diminished renal function.

Contraindications/Precautions/Warnings

Pregabalin is contraindicated in patients hypersensitive to it. Use with caution in patients with renal insufficiency; if required, dosage adjustment should be considered. In humans, pregabalin doses are adjusted based on creatinine clearance. Pregabalin is used with caution in human patients with heart failure.

In humans, abrupt discontinuation may lead to increased seizure frequency, diarrhea, headache, insomnia, or nausea.

Adverse Effects

Most common adverse effects reported include sedation and ataxia. Because use to date is limited in animals, adverse effect profile may evolve with additional clinical experience.

In humans, the most common adverse effects reported are: somnolence, dizziness, ataxia, difficulty with concentration/attention/memory, blurred vision, dry mouth, peripheral edema, constipation and weight gain. Syncope and congestive heart failure have been reported less frequently. Rarely, renal failure (reversible) and rhabdomyolysis have been reported. Hypersensitivity reactions have included angioedema, rash, blisters, and wheezing. Pregabalin therapy has been associated with decreased platelet production or increased creatine kinase levels in some human patients.

Reproductive/Nursing Safety

In humans, the FDA categorizes this drug as category C for use during pregnancy (*Animal studies have shown an adverse effect on the fetus, but there are no adequate studies in humans; or there are no animal reproduction studies and no adequate studies in humans.*) Very high dosages of pregabalin have caused skeletal malformations in offspring when given to pregnant rats and rabbits. Pregabalin is excreted into milk, and safety has not been established. Weigh the potential risks of treating versus the benefits when using this drug in pregnant or nursing animals.

Overdosage/Acute Toxicity

There were 701 single agent exposures to pregabalin reported to the ASPCA Animal Poison Control Center (APCC) during 2009-2013. Of the 475 dogs, 130 were symptomatic with ataxia (43%) and lethargy (41%) being the most common. Of the 227 cats, 158 were symptomatic with ataxia (70%) and lethargy (43%) also being the most common.

One human ingested 8 grams without significant effect. There is no specific antidote for overdose with pregabalin. Standard decontamination protocols can be employed if indicated. Contact an animal poison center for more information.

Drug Interactions

The following drug interactions have either been reported or are theoretical in humans or animals receiving pregabalin and may be of significance in veterinary patients. Unless otherwise noted, use together is not necessarily contraindicated, but weigh the potential risks and perform additional monitoring when appropriate.

- **ACE INHIBITORS** (*e.g.*, **benazepril, enalapril**): In humans, co-administration with pregabalin may increase risks edema and hives.
- **CNS DEPRESSANTS:** Pregabalin may cause additive CNS depression.
- **NSAIDS:** In humans, ketorolac and naproxen have been cited as possibly reducing anticonvulsant effectiveness. Substantive evidence is weak, however.

Laboratory Considerations
- None noted.

Doses
- **DOGS:**

  For seizure disorders and potentially, neuropathic pain (extra-label): Generally used when seizure control cannot be obtained with a combination of phenobarbital and bromides. In a small single-dose pharmacokinetic study, the authors concluded that 4 mg/kg PO twice daily would produce plasma levels within the extrapolated (from humans) therapeutic range; further studies evaluating its safety and efficacy for the treatment of neuropathic pain and seizures in dogs is warranted. (Salazar *et al.* 2009) Several sources state to start at 2 mg/kg PO q12h to minimize sedation and titrate dosage upwards in 1 mg/kg increments per week to 3 – 4 mg/kg PO q8-12h.

- **CATS:**

  For seizure disorders and potentially, neuropathic pain (extra-label): There are anecdotal reports of pregabalin use in cats; 1 – 2 mg/kg PO q12h is most commonly mentioned (Munana 2010). Based on their single-dose pharmacokinetic study in 6 cats, the authors theorize that a dose of 1 – 2 mg/kg PO twice daily would be a reasonable starting dose. Further clinical trials are warranted based on a favorable pharmacokinetic profile. (Cautela *et al.* 2009)

Monitoring
- Efficacy/Adverse effects.
- At present, pregabalin plasma levels are not routinely monitored in human medicine. Levels >2.8 mcg/mL have been suggested as being "therapeutic".

Client Information
- May be given with or without food. If your animal vomits or acts sick after getting it on an empty stomach, try giving it with food or a small treat to see if this helps. If vomiting continues, contact your veterinarian.
- Drowsiness and loss of coordination (*e.g.*, stumbling/weakness, etc.) are the most likely side effects.
- Pregabalin is a controlled drug in the USA. It is against federal law to use, give away or sell this medication to others than for whom it was prescribed.

Chemistry/Synonyms

Pregabalin is (S)-3-(Aminomethyl)-5-methylhexanoic acid). It is freely soluble in water and in both basic and acidic aqueous solutions.

Pregabalin may also be known as CI-1008, PD-144723, pregabalina, prégabaline or pregabalinum. A common trade name is *Lyrica*®.

Storage/Stability
Store capsules and oral solution at room temperature, 25°C (77°F); excursions permitted between 15-30°C (59-86°F).

Use the oral solution within the first 45 days after opening the bottle.

Dosage Forms/Regulatory Status
VETERINARY-LABELED PRODUCTS: NONE.

HUMAN-LABELED PRODUCTS:

Pregabalin Oral Capsules: 25 mg, 50 mg, 75 mg, 100 mg, 150 mg, 200 mg, 225 mg, & 300 mg; *Lyrica®*; (Rx; C-V controlled substance)

Pregabalin Oral Solution: 20 mg/mL; *Lyrica®*; (Rx; C-V controlled substance)

Revisions/References
Monograph revised/updated May 2014.

Cautela, M., et al. (2009). Pharmacokinetics of oral pregabalin in catsa after single dose administration. Proceedings: ACVIM. accessed via Veterinary Information Network; vin.com

Dewey, C. W., et al. (2009). Pregabalin as an adjunct to phenobarbital, potassium bromide, or a combination of phenobarbital and potassium bromide for treatment of dogs with suspected idiopathic epilepsy. Javma-Journal of the American Veterinary Medical Association 235(12): 1442-9.

Munana, K. (2010). Current Approaches to Seizure Management. Proceedings: ACVIM Forum. accessed via Veterinary Information Network; vin.com

Salazar, V., et al. (2009). Pharmacokinetics of single-dose oral pregabalin administration in normal dogs. Veterinary Anaesthesia and Analgesia 36(6): 574-80.

Primaquine Phosphate
(prim-ah-kwin)

Antiprotozoal

Prescriber Highlights
▶ Antiprotozoal agent considered the drug of choice for treating *Babesia felis* in cats; does not apparently "cure" the infection; repeated courses of therapy may be necessary. May also be useful in treating *Hepatazoon canis* in dogs or *Plasmodium* spp. in birds.

▶ Most common adverse effect in cats is nausea; giving with food may help.

▶ Very narrow therapeutic index (safety margin); must be careful in determining dosages. Compounded preparations may be necessary for accurate dosing. Doses above 1 mg/kg in cats can be lethal.

▶ Monitoring CBC mandatory.

Uses/Indications
Primaquine is considered the drug of choice for treating *Babesia felis* in cats. Primaquine usually resolves the anemia and clinical signs of disease, but it often does not eliminate the infection; repeated courses of therapy may be necessary. Relapse rates of 20-80% have been reported but these are lower than other therapy protocols (Ayoob *et al.* 2010). Primaquine may be useful in treating *Hepatazoon canis* in dogs or *Plasmodium* spp. in birds. In humans, primaquine is used for treatment and prophylaxis for malaria and treating *Pneumocystis* pneumonia.

Pharmacology/Actions
Primaquine's antiprotozoal mechanism of action is not well understood, but it may be related to it binding and altering protozoal DNA. When used for *Babesia felis* in cats, decreased parasitemia and improvement in clinical signs is usually seen within 1-3 days.

Pharmacokinetics
No pharmacokinetic information was located for small animals. In humans, primaquine is rapidly absorbed with high (96%) systemic bioavailability. It is extensively distributed and rapidly metabolized in the liver to carboxyprimaquine. It is not known if this metabolite has any antiprotozoal activity. Elimination half-life is around 6 hours for primaquine; 24 hours for carboxyprimaquine.

Contraindications/Precautions/Warnings
Primaquine is contraindicated in patients with known hypersensitivity to it. In humans, it is contraindicated in patients receiving other bone marrow suppressant medications or patients susceptible to granulocytopenia (*e.g.*, lupus, rheumatoid arthritis). The CDC states the drug is contraindicated in individuals with G-6-PD deficiency, and during pregnancy or lactation (unless nursing infant determined not to be G-6-PD deficient).

Adverse Effects
Vomiting is the most common adverse effect in cats associated with primaquine; dosing with food may help alleviate this problem. Other concerns include myelosuppression, methemoglobinemia and hemolysis. Safety margin is particularly narrow with this drug in cats (see Overdoses).

Reproductive/Nursing Safety
The CDC recommends using chloroquine or mefloquine for humans during pregnancy and to defer using primaquine until after delivery primarily because primaquine can cause hemolytic anemia in G-6-PD deficient fetuses. It is also contraindicated during lactation in nursing infants unless they are determined not to be G-6-PD deficient. While significance for veterinary patients is not clear, primaquine should be avoided during pregnancy and lactation.

Overdosage/Acute Toxicity
In cats, it has been reported that dosages >1 mg/kg can be lethal. Overdoses should initially be handled aggressively using standardized protocols for removal of drug from the gut and to prevent absorption. Because of the potential seriousness of overdoses, it is recommended to contact an animal poison control center for guidance.

Drug Interactions
The following drug interactions have either been reported or are theoretical in humans or animals receiving primaquine and may be of significance in veterinary patients. Unless otherwise noted, use together is not necessarily contraindicated, but weigh the potential risks and perform additional monitoring when appropriate.

- **BONE MARROW DEPRESSANT DRUGS** (*e.g.*, **amphotericin B, azathioprine, chloramphenicol,** many **antineoplastic drugs**) or **HEMOLYSIS-INDUCING DRUGS** (*e.g.*, **acetohydroxamic acid, sulfonylureas, quinidine, sulfonamides**): Use with primaquine may cause increased risk for toxicity.
- **GRAPEFRUIT JUICE:** Can increase primaquine levels.
- **QUINACRINE:** May potentiate the toxicity of one another; use of primaquine within 3 months of quinacrine is not recommended.
- **RABIES VACCINE:** In humans, primaquine can decrease the immune response to rabies vaccine; recommend finishing rabies vaccine protocol in advance of primaquine, if not possible give via IM injection (vs. ID).

Laboratory Considerations
- No specific concerns noted.

Doses
- **CATS:**
  Note: Dosing for humans for primaquine is usually described in terms of primaquine base, but dosages for cats may not directly specify whether primaquine is being dosed as the phosphate or as the base. Because primaquine has an extremely narrow therapeutic index in cats, this is problematic as a 26.3 mg primaquine phosphate tablet contains 15 mg of primaquine base. Additionally, commercially available tablets are usually too concentrated to

be accurately dosed in domestic cats; a specialized compounding pharmacy should be employed to prepare a suitable dosage form. Be clear as to the amount of primaquine base or phosphate wanted per dose.

For *Babesia felis* (extra-label): Published dosages range from 0.5 – 1 mg/kg (as base) PO, IV, or IM once, or administered daily on 3 consecutive days. Long-term therapy has been reported to be safe although it should be emphasized that the duration of therapy should be based on hematologic variables and clinical signs rather than parasitemia. Do not exceed dosages of 1 mg/kg. (Ayoob *et al.* 2010)

Monitoring
- CBC; weekly while treating.
- Improved clinical signs (increased appetite and body weight, improvement in anemia).

Client Information
- This drug has a very low safety margin when used in cats; exact adherence with the prescribed dosage is very important; do not double-up the next dose if a dose was previously missed.
- Give dose with food to reduce chance for GI problems (vomiting).

Chemistry/Synonyms
Primaquine phosphate is an 8-amino-quinoline compound that occurs as an orange-red, odorless, bitter-tasting, crystalline powder. It is soluble (1 gram in 15 mL) in water and practically insoluble in alcohol. 1 mg of primaquine phosphate contains 0.57 mg of primaquine base.

Primaquine may also be known as primachina, primachinum, primaquina or SN 13272.

Storage/Stability
Primaquine phosphate tablets should be stored in a tight, light resistant container below 40°C, preferably between 15-30°C.

Dosage Forms/Regulatory Status
VETERINARY-LABELED PRODUCTS: NONE.

HUMAN-LABELED PRODUCTS:

Primaquine Phosphate Oral Tablets: 26.3 mg (equiv. to 15 mg primaquine base); generic; (Rx)

Revisions/References
Monograph revised/updated May 2014.
Ayoob, A. L., et al. (2010). Feline babesiosis. J. Vet. Emerg. Crit. Care **20**(1): 90-7.

Primidone

(pri-mi-done)   Mysoline®, Neurosyn®

Anticonvulsant

Prescriber Highlights
▶ Phenobarbital precursor that is used rarely for treating seizures in dogs; most recommend using phenobarbital instead. Most of the anticonvulsant activity comes from the phenobarbital metabolite of primidone. Primidone is likely more hepatotoxic than phenobarbital in dogs.

▶ Contraindications: Severe liver disease or patients with demonstrated previous hypersensitivity. **Large Doses Contraindicated:** Nephritis or severe respiratory dysfunction. **Extreme Caution: Cats. Caution:** Hypovolemic, anemic, have borderline hypoadrenal function, or cardiac or respiratory disease.

▶ Adverse Effects: **Dogs:** anxiety & agitation when initiating therapy, increases in liver enzymes, hepatic lipidosis, hepatocellular hypertrophy/necrosis, extramedullary hematopoiesis, depression, polydipsia, polyuria, & polyphagia, anorexia, tachycardia, dermatitis, episodic hyperventilation, urolith formation; rarely, megaloblastic anemia.

▶ Drug Interactions, lab interactions.

Uses/Indications
Primidone can be used for seizure control (idiopathic epilepsy, epileptiform convulsions) in dogs. Because it is rapidly converted into phenobarbital in this species (see Pharmacokinetics below), and has a greater incidence of hepatotoxicity and behavioral effects, most neurologists do not recommend its use. However, some believe that a percentage of animals not responding to phenobarbital do benefit from primidone therapy, perhaps as a result of the phenylethamalonamide (PEMA) metabolite. PEMA has been demonstrated to potentiate the anticonvulsant activity of phenobarbital in animals. When compared with phenobarbital, increased incidence of hepatotoxicity associated with primidone is considered the major limitation to long-term therapy with this agent.

Primidone is considered more toxic in rabbits and cats than in humans or dogs.

Pharmacology/Actions
Primidone and its active metabolites, phenylethamalonamide (PEMA) and phenobarbital have similar anticonvulsant actions. While the exact mechanism for this activity is unknown, these agents raise seizure thresholds or alter seizure patterns.

Pharmacokinetics
Primidone is slowly absorbed after oral administration in the dog, with peak levels occurring 2-4 hours after dosing. The bioavailability of primidone in humans has been reported as 60-80%.

Primidone is rapidly converted to PEMA and phenobarbital in the dog. Serum half-lives of primidone, PEMA, and phenobarbital have been reported to be 1.85 hrs, 7.1 hrs, and 41 hours, respectively (Yeary 1980). In dogs, the conversion rate of primidone to phenobarbital is ≈ 4:1; a 250 mg dose of primidone is ≈ 60 mg of phenobarbital (Platt 2005).

Primidone, like phenobarbital (possibly due to the phenobarbital?), can induce hepatic microsomal enzymes that can increase the rate of metabolism of itself and other drugs.

For more information on the pharmacokinetics of phenobarbital, refer to its monograph.

Contraindications/Precautions/Warnings
Many clinicians feel that primidone is contraindicated in cats; other clinicians dispute this, but it is recommended that primidone be

used in cats only with extreme caution. Use cautiously in patients that are hypovolemic, anemic, have borderline hypoadrenal function, or cardiac or respiratory disease. Large doses are contraindicated in patients with nephritis or severe respiratory dysfunction. Primidone is contraindicated in patients with severe liver disease or that have had hypersensitivity reactions.

When converting dogs from primidone to phenobarbital, it has been suggested do this slowly (1/4 of the dose each month) (Platt 2005).

Adverse Effects

Adverse effects in dogs are similar for both primidone and phenobarbital. Dogs may exhibit increased clinical signs of anxiety and agitation when initiating therapy. These effects may be transitory in nature and often will resolve with small dosage increases. Occasionally, dogs will exhibit profound depression at lower dosage ranges (and plasma levels). Polydipsia, polyuria, and polyphagia are quite commonly displayed at moderate to high serum levels; these are best controlled by limiting intake of both food and water. Sedation and/or ataxia often become significant concerns as serum levels reach the higher ends of the therapeutic range.

Increases in liver enzymes (ALT, ALP, glutamate dehydrogenase) and decreased serum albumin with chronic therapy are common (up to 70% of dogs treated), and more prevalent than with phenobarbital. Hepatic lipidosis, hepatocellular hypertrophy and necrosis, and extramedullary hematopoiesis can be seen after 6 months of therapy. Serious hepatic injury probably occurs in ≈ 6-14% of dogs treated.

In dogs, anorexia, tachycardia, dermatitis, episodic hyperventilation, urolith formation and, rarely, megaloblastic anemia have also been reported with primidone therapy.

A urolith consisting of primidone has been reported in one cat (Osborne *et al.* 1999).

Reproductive/Nursing Safety

The effects of primidone in pregnancy are unknown. In pregnant humans, primidone is designated by the FDA as a category *D* drug (*There is evidence of human fetal risk, but the potential benefits from the use of the drug in pregnant women may be acceptable despite its potential risks.*) In a separate system evaluating the safety of drugs in canine and feline pregnancy (Papich 1989), this drug is categorized as class: *C* (*These drugs may have potential risks. Studies in people or laboratory animals have uncovered risks, and these drugs should be used cautiously as a last resort when the benefit of therapy clearly outweighs the risks.*)

Primidone appears in maternal milk in substantial quantities. It is suggested that if somnolence occurs in nursing newborns to consider discontinue nursing.

Overdosage/Acute Toxicity

Because primidone is rapidly metabolized to phenobarbital in dogs, similar clinical signs (sedation to coma, anorexia, vomiting, nystagmus) are seen and corresponding procedures should be used for the treatment of acute primidone overdose. This includes the removal of ingested product from the gut if appropriate, and offering respiratory and cardiovascular support. Activated charcoal has been demonstrated to be of considerable benefit in enhancing the clearance of phenobarbital, even when the drug was administered parenterally. Charcoal acts as a "sink" for the drug to diffuse from the vasculature back into the gut. Forced alkaline diuresis can be of considerable benefit in augmenting the elimination of phenobarbital in patients with normal renal function. Peritoneal or hemodialysis may also be helpful in severe intoxications or anuric patients.

Drug Interactions

The following drug interactions have either been reported or are theoretical in humans or animals receiving primidone or pheno-barbital (primidone's active metabolite) and may be of significance in veterinary patients. Unless otherwise noted, use together is not necessarily contraindicated, but weigh the potential risks and perform additional monitoring when appropriate.

- **ACETAMINOPHEN**: Increased risk for hepatotoxicity, particularly when large or chronic doses of barbiturates are given.
- **CARBONIC ANHYDRASE INHIBITORS** (*e.g.*, **acetazolamide**): Oral administration may decrease the GI absorption of primidone.
- **MONAMINE OXIDASE (MAO) INHIBITORS** (*e.g.*, **amitraz**, possibly **selegiline**): May prolong phenobarbital effects.
- **PHENYTOIN**: Barbiturates may affect the metabolism of phenytoin, and phenytoin may alter barbiturate levels; monitoring of blood levels may be indicated.
- **RIFAMPIN**: May induce enzymes that increase the metabolism of barbiturates.

The following drugs may increase the effects of primidone (phenobarbital):

- **ANTIHISTAMINES**
- **CHLORAMPHENICOL**
- **OPIATES**
- **PHENOTHIAZINES**
- **VALPROIC ACID**

Primidone (phenobarbital), particularly after chronic therapy, may decrease the effect of the following drugs/drug classes by lowering their serum concentrations:

- **ANTICOAGULANTS, ORAL (WARFARIN)**
- **BETA-BLOCKERS**
- **CHLORAMPHENICOL**
- **CLONAZEPAM**
- **CORTICOSTEROIDS**
- **CYCLOSPORINE**
- **DOXORUBICIN**
- **DOXYCYCLINE** (may persist for weeks after barbiturate discontinued)
- **ESTROGENS**
- **GRISEOFULVIN**
- **METHADONE**
- **METRONIDAZOLE**
- **QUINIDINE**
- **PAROXETINE**
- **PHENOTHIAZINES**
- **PROGESTINS**
- **THEOPHYLLINE**
- **TRICYCLIC ANTIDEPRESSANTS**
- **VERAPAMIL**

Laboratory Considerations

- Barbiturates may cause increased retention of **bromosulfophthalein** (BSP; sulfobromophthalein) and give falsely elevated results. It is recommended that barbiturates not be administered within the 24 hours before BSP retention tests; or if they must, (*e.g.*, for seizure control) the results be interpreted accordingly.
- Primidone/phenobarbital can alter **thyroid** testing. Decreased total and free T4, normal T3, and either normal or increased TSH have been reported. It has been suggested to wait at least 4 weeks after discontinuing phenobarbital to perform thyroid testing.
- In some dogs, primidone/phenobarbital may cause a false positive low dose **dexamethasone suppression test**, by increasing the clearance of dexamethasone. Phenobarbital apparently has

no effect either on ACTH stimulation tests or on the hormonal equilibrium of the adrenal axis.

Doses

- **DOGS:**

For the control of convulsions associated with idiopathic epilepsy, epileptiform convulsions, viral encephalitis, distemper, and hardpad disease that occurs as a clinically recognizable lesion in certain entities in dogs (labeled-dose; FDA-approved): 55 mg/kg PO once daily or divided and administered at intervals. May be administered whole or crushed and mixed with the food. Reduction in dosage should be made gradually and never be abruptly discontinued. (adapted from label: *Mylepsin®*)

Monitoring

- Anticonvulsant efficacy.
- Adverse effects (CNS related, PU/PD, weight gain).
- Serum phenobarbital levels if lack of efficacy or adverse reactions noted. Although there is some disagreement, therapeutic serum levels in dogs are thought to mirror those in people at 15-40 micrograms/mL. See the phenobarbital monograph for more information.
- If used chronically, routine CBCs and liver enzymes at least every 6 months.

Client Information

- Compliance with therapy must be stressed to clients for successful epilepsy treatment. Encourage giving daily doses at same time each day.
- Veterinarian should be contacted if animal develops significant adverse reactions (including clinical signs of anemia and/or liver disease) or if seizure control is unacceptable.

Chemistry/Synonyms

An analog of phenobarbital, primidone occurs as a white, odorless, slightly bitter-tasting, crystalline powder with a melting point of 279°-284°C. One gram is soluble in ≈ 2000 mL of water or 200 mL of alcohol.

Primidone may also be known as: hexamidinum, primaclone, primidonum, *Mysoline®*, *Neurosyn®*, or *Mylepsin®*.

Storage/Stability

Tablets should be stored in well-closed containers preferably at room temperature. The oral suspension should be stored in tight, light-resistant containers preferably at room temperature; avoid freezing. Commercially available suspension and tablets generally have expiration dates of 5 years after manufacture.

Dosage Forms/Regulatory Status

VETERINARY-LABELED PRODUCTS:

Primidone Tablets: 50 mg and 250 mg; *Mylepsin®*, *Neurosyn®*, generic; (Rx). FDA-approved for use in dogs.

The ARCI (Racing Commissioners International) has designated this drug as a class 3 substance. See the appendix for more information.

HUMAN-LABELED PRODUCTS:

Primidone Tablets: 50 mg & 250 mg; *Mysoline®*, generic; (Rx)

Revisions/References

Monograph revised/updated May 2014.

Osborne, C. A., et al. (1999). Drug induced urolithiasis. Vet Clin NA: Sm Anim Pract 28(1): 251-66.

Papich, M. (1989). Effects of drugs on pregnancy. *Current Veterinary Therapy X: Small Animal Practice*. R. Kirk. Philadelphia, Saunders: 1291-9.

Platt, S. (2005). Anticonvulsant use for epileptics. Proceedings: WSAVA World Congress. accessed via Veterinary Information Network: vin.com

Yeary, R. A. (1980). Serum concentrations of primidone and its metabolites, phenylethyl-malonamide and phenobarbital in the dog. Am J Vet Res 41(10): 1643-5.

Probenecid

(proh-**ben**-eh-sid) Benemid®, Benuryl®

Uricosuric; Renal Tubular Secretion Inhibitor

Prescriber Highlights

▶ Uricosuric & renal tubular secretion inhibitor that may be useful for treating gout (particularly in reptiles).

▶ Probenecid is associated with many drug interactions as it inhibits the renal tubular secretion of numerous drugs, including several beta-lactam antibiotics; some interactions may be beneficial, others may increase potential for toxicity.

▶ Little experience using this drug in mammals other than humans.

Uses/Indications

Although there has been very limited clinical use or research on probenecid in veterinary medicine, it may be useful in treating gout (hyperuricemia), particularly in reptiles.

Probenecid's effect in inhibiting renal tubular secretion of certain beta-lactam antibiotics and other weak organic acids is of interest for increasing serum concentrations, or reducing doses and dosing frequency of these drugs. This may allow greater efficacy (but also toxic effects) and reduce the cost or dosing frequency of expensive human drugs. Probenecid has a significantly long elimination half-life in dogs (≈ 18 hours), which may make it particularly useful in this species, however, at present there is little research supporting this in veterinary patients.

Pharmacology/Actions

Probenecid reduces serum uric acid concentrations by enhancing uric acid excretion into the urine by competitively inhibiting urate reabsorption at the proximal renal tubules.

Probenecid competitively inhibits tubular secretion of weak organic acids including the penicillins, some cephalosporins (not ceftriaxone, ceftazidime, or cefoperazone), sulbactam and tazobactam (not clavulanic acid), oseltamivir, etc.

Pharmacokinetics

There is limited information available for veterinary species. In dogs, information on oral bioavailability was not located, but after intravenous administration the distribution half-life was 2.3 hours and apparent volume of distribution at steady state was 0.46 L/kg. In dogs, probenecid exhibits biphasic concentration-dependent plasma protein binding characteristics; probenecid plasma protein binding appears to be less than that occurring in humans. Plasma clearance was 0.343 mL/min/kg and elimination half-life was 17.7 hours, which is considerably longer than in humans (6.5 hrs) or sheep (1.55 hrs) (Kakizaki *et al.* 2005).

After administration to mares, probenecid had an oral bioavailability of ≈ 90%. The drug is highly bound (99.9%) to equine plasma proteins. Elimination half-life is ≈ 90-120 minutes.

In humans, absorption after oral administration is rapid and complete. The drug is converted in the liver to glucuronidated, carboxylated, and hydroxylated compounds that have uricosuric and renal tubular secretion inhibition activity. Elimination half-life is dosage dependent and large dosages (>500 mg) have longer half-lives.

Contraindications/Precautions/Warnings

Probenecid should not be used in patients with, or that are susceptible to, uric acid renal or bladder calculus formation or urate nephropathy (*e.g.*, cancer chemotherapy with rapidly cytolytic agents). Probenecid requires sufficient renal function to be effective; efficacy decreases with increasing renal function impairment. The drug has no efficacy in human patients with a creatine clearance of <30 mL per min.

Probenecid is not usually recommended for treating gout in birds as it can exacerbate the condition.

Adverse Effects

An accurate adverse effect profile for probenecid has not been determined for animal patients. In humans, probenecid occasionally causes headache, gastrointestinal effects (inappetence, nausea, mild vomiting), or rashes. When used for gout, it can initially cause an increased rate of gouty attacks unless prophylaxis with colchicine is used concurrently. Rarely, hypersensitivity, bone marrow suppression, hepatotoxicity, or nephrotic syndrome have been reported in humans.

Reproductive/Nursing Safety

Probenecid apparently crosses the placenta, but adverse effects to fetuses have not been reported. In humans, the FDA categorizes probenecid as category *B* for use during pregnancy (*Animal studies have not yet demonstrated risk to the fetus, but there are no adequate studies in pregnant women; or animal studies have shown an adverse effect, but adequate studies in pregnant women have not demonstrated a risk to the fetus in the first trimester of pregnancy, and there is no evidence of risk in later trimesters.*)

It is unknown if probenecid enters milk, but it is unlikely to pose much risk to nursing offspring.

Overdosage/Acute Toxicity

Limited information is available. One massive (>45 g) overdose in a human patient caused CNS stimulation, seizures, protracted vomiting and respiratory failure.

Consider contacting an animal poison control center for guidance with large overdoses. Generally, probenecid overdoses should initially be handled using standardized protocols for removal of drug from the gut and preventing absorption. Treat supportively, but use caution co-administrating drugs that may compete with probenecid for tubular secretion.

Drug Interactions

The following drug interactions have either been reported or are theoretical in humans or animals receiving probenecid and may be of significance in veterinary patients. Unless otherwise noted, use together is not necessarily contraindicated, but weigh the potential risks and perform additional monitoring when appropriate.

- **ACYCLOVIR:** Increased acyclovir serum concentrations; probenecid can decrease renal excretion.
- **ANTINEOPLASTICS (rapidly cytolytic):** Increased chance of uric acid nephropathy.
- **ASPIRIN (and other salicylates):** Salicylates antagonize the uricosuric effects of probenecid.
- **BENZODIAZEPINES (lorazepam, oxazepam, etc.):** Probenecid may prolong action or reduce time for onset of action.
- **BETA-LACTAM ANTIBIOTICS (including penicillins and some cephalosporins):** Probenecid may increase serum concentrations by reducing renal excretion.
- **BETA-LACTAMASE INHIBITORS (including sulbactam and tazobactam, but not clavulanic acid):** Probenecid may increase serum concentrations by reducing renal excretion.
- **CIPROFLOXACIN/ENROFLOXACIN:** Probenecid reduces renal tubular secretion of ciprofloxacin by ≈ 50%. In goats, probenecid significantly reduced renal excretion of enrofloxacin (Narayan *et al.* 2009).
- **DAPSONE:** Possible accumulation of dapsone or its active metabolites.
- **FUROSEMIDE:** Increased serum furosemide levels possible.
- **HEPARIN:** Probenecid may increase and prolong heparin's effects.

- **METHOTREXATE:** Probenecid may increase levels; increased risks for toxicity.
- **NSAIDS (including carprofen, ketoprofen & potentially others):** Probenecid may increase plasma levels and increase risks for toxicity.
- **NITROFURANTOIN:** Reduced urine levels; increased chance for systemic toxicity.
- **PENICILLAMINE:** May reduce penicillamine efficacy.
- **OSELTAMIVIR:** Probenecid may increase serum concentrations by reducing renal excretion.
- **RANITIDINE:** Probenecid may increase serum concentrations by reducing renal excretion.
- **RIFAMPIN:** Probenecid may reduce hepatic uptake of rifampin and serum levels can be increased; use together is not recommended as effect is inconsistent and can lead to toxicity.
- **SULFONAMIDES:** Probenecid decreases renal elimination of sulfonamides, but as free serum concentrations of sulfonamides are not increased this interaction is not therapeutically beneficial and may increase risks for sulfonamide toxicity.
- **THIOPENTAL:** Anesthesia may be extended or dose required for anesthesia decreased.
- **ZIDOVUDINE:** Probenecid may increase serum levels.

Laboratory Considerations

The following laboratory alterations have been reported in humans with probenecid and may be of significance in veterinary patients. Unless otherwise noted, use together is not necessarily contraindicated, but weigh the potential risks and perform additional monitoring when appropriate.

- **Urine glucose determinations:** When using cupric sulfate solution (Benedict's Solution, *Clinitest*®): Probenecid may cause false-positive results. Tests utilizing glucose oxidase (*Tes-Tape*®, *Clinistix*®) are not affected.
- **Theophylline levels:** Serum theophylline levels may be falsely elevated (Schack and Waxtler technique).
- **17-ketosteroid concentrations in urine:** May be decreased.
- **Phosphorus:** Probenecid may increase phosphorus reabsorption in hypoparathyroid patients.
- **Aminohippuric acid (PAH) or Phenolsulphonphthalein (PSP) clearance studies:** Probenecid decreases renal clearance.
- **Renal function studies using iodohippurate sodium I 123 or I 131, or technetium TC 99:** Decreased kidney uptake.
- **Homovanillic acid (HVA) or 5-Hydroxyindoleacetic acid (5-HIAA):** Probenecid inhibits transport from CSF into blood.

Doses

- **REPTILES:**

  For gout (extra-label): Dosages are not well defined for reptiles. 250 mg PO q12h; can be increased as needed. Suggested dosage based upon human data as dose is not established for reptiles (Johnson-Delaney 2005) or 40 mg/kg PO q12h (Coke 2004). (de la Navarre 2003)

Monitoring

- Depending on purpose for use: serum and urine uric acid, if concomitant urine alkalinization is used, consider monitoring acid-base balance.

Client Information

- In small animals, there is little scientific data supporting using probenecid for increasing blood levels of drugs that compete with probenecid for renal excretion; probenecid's adverse effects are not well known in these patients.

Chemistry/Synonyms

Probenecid is a sulfonamide derivative that occurs as a white, to practically white, practically odorless, fine, crystalline powder. It is practically insoluble in water and soluble in alcohol.

Probenecid may also be known as: probenecidas, probenecidum, *Benemid®* and *Benuryl®*.

Storage/Stability

Probenecid tablets should be stored at room temperature in well-closed containers. Expiration dates are generally 3-5 years after manufacture.

Dosage Forms/Regulatory Status

VETERINARY-LABELED PRODUCTS: NONE.

HUMAN-LABELED PRODUCTS:

Probenecid Tablets: 500 mg; generic; (Rx)

Revisions/References

Monograph revised/updated May 2014.

Coke, R. (2004). Practical reptile nutrition. Proceedings: Western Veterinary Conference. accessed via Veterinary Information Network; vin.com

de la Navarre, B. (2003). Acute and chronic renal disease (specifically in lizard species). Proceedings: Western Veterinary Conference. accessed via Veterinary Information Network; vin.com

Johnson-Delaney, C. (2005). Osteodystrophy and renal disease in reptiles. Proceedings: Atlantic Coast Veterinary Conference. accessed via Veterinary Information Network; vin.com

Kakizaki, T., et al. (2005). Probenecid: Its chromatographic determination, plasma protein binding, and in vivo pharmacokinetics in dogs. J Vet Med Sci **68**(4): 361-5.

Narayan, J., et al. (2009). Effect of probenecid on kinetics of enrofloxacin in lactating goats after subcutaneous administration. Indian J Exp Biol **47**(1): 53-6.

Procainamide HCl

(proe-kane-a-mide)   Pronestyl®

Antiarrhythmic

Prescriber Highlights

▶ Antiarrhythmic used primarily for treatment of atrial fibrillation, ventricular premature complexes (VPC's), ventricular tachycardia.

▶ **Contraindications:** Myasthenia gravis; hypersensitive to drug, procaine or other chemically related drugs; torsade de pointes; or 2nd or 3rd degree heart block (unless artificially paced). **Extreme Caution:** Cardiac glycoside intoxication, systemic lupus; **Caution:** Significant hepatic, renal disease or CHF.

▶ Adverse Effects: **Dogs:** Blood level related: GI effects, weakness, hypotension, negative inotropism, widened QRS complex & QT intervals, AV block, multiform ventricular tachycardias. Possible: fevers & leukopenias.

▶ Profound hypotension can occur if injected too rapidly IV. Consider dosage reduction in patients with renal failure, CHF, or critically ill.

▶ Availability becoming an issue. Oral products no longer commercially marketed; compounded preps may be available.

▶ Drug Interactions.

Uses/Indications

Procainamide potentially may be useful for the treatment of ventricular premature complexes (VPC's), ventricular tachycardia, or supraventricular tachycardias associated with wide QRS complexes. When a tachycardia with a wide QRS is seen that cannot be definitively identified as supraventricular or ventricular in origin, procainamide is an ideal first-line IV therapeutic agent because of its broad spectrum of activity for atrial and ventricular arrhythmias (Saunders *et al.* 2009).

Pharmacology/Actions

A class 1A antiarrhythmic agent, procainamide exhibits cardiac action similar to that of quinidine. It is considered both a supra-ventricular and ventricular antidysrhythmic. Procainamide prolongs the refractory times in both the atria and ventricles, decreases myocardial excitability, and depresses automaticity and conduction velocity. It has anticholinergic properties that may contribute to its effects. Procainamide's effects on heart rate are unpredictable, but it usually causes only slight increases or no change. It may exhibit negative inotropic actions on the heart, although cardiac outputs are generally not affected.

On ECG, QRS widening, and prolonged PR and QT intervals can be seen. The QRS complex and T wave may occasionally show some slight decreases in voltage.

Pharmacokinetics

After IM or IV administration, the onset of action is practically immediate. After oral administration in humans, ≈ 75-95% of a dose is absorbed in the intestine, but some patients absorb <50% of a dose. Food, delayed gastric emptying, or decreased stomach pH may delay oral absorption. In dogs, it has been reported that the oral bioavailability is ≈ 85% and the absorption half-life is 0.5 hours; however, there is an apparent large degree of variability in both bioavailability and half-life of absorption.

FDA-approved oral procainamide products are no longer available, but a small (n=6) pharmacokinetic study was performed in healthy dogs using a compounded delayed release formulation (Thomason *et al.* 2013). After dosing at 30 mg/kg PO the average time that procainamide serum levels were above 4 mcg/mL was 9.65 hours. The authors concluded: "Although specific dosing recommendations cannot be made from this data due to individual animal variability, it appears that twice daily administration of delayed-release procainamide could be efficacious in dogs. Due to individual patient variability, evaluation of serum trough concentrations should be considered to confirm concentrations within the reported therapeutic range."

Distribution of procainamide is highest into the CSF, liver, spleen, kidneys, lungs, heart and muscles. The volume of distribution in dogs is ≈ 1.4-3 L/kg. It is only ≈ 20% protein bound in humans and 15% in dogs. Procainamide can cross the placenta and is excreted into milk.

The elimination half-life in dogs has been reported to be variable; most studies report values between 2-3 hours. In humans, procainamide is metabolized to N-acetyl-procainamide (NAPA), an active metabolite. It appears, however, that dogs do not form appreciable amounts of NAPA from procainamide as they are unable to appreciably acetylate aromatic and hydrazine amino groups. In dogs, ≈ 90% (50-70% unchanged) of an intravenous dose is excreted in the urine as procainamide and metabolites within 24 hours after dosing.

Contraindications/Precautions/Warnings

Procainamide may be contraindicated in patients with myasthenia gravis (see Drug Interactions). Procainamide is contraindicated in patients hypersensitive to it, procaine or other chemically related drugs. In humans, procainamide is contraindicated in patients with systemic lupus erythematosus (SLE), but it is unknown if it adversely affects dogs with this condition. Procainamide should not be used in patients with torsade de pointes, or with 2nd or 3rd degree heart block (unless artificially paced).

Procainamide should be used with extreme caution, if at all, in patients with cardiac glycoside intoxication. It should be used with caution in patients with significant hepatic or renal disease or with congestive heart failure. Dosages should usually be reduced in patients with renal failure, congestive heart failure, or those that are critically ill.

It has been recommended to not use procainamide in Doberman pinschers and boxers with dilated cardiomyopathy or dogs with subaortic stenosis; the drug may be proarrhythmic in certain patients susceptible to tachyarrhythmic-induced sudden death (Kittleson 2006).

Adverse Effects

Adverse effects are generally dosage (blood level) related in the dog. Gastrointestinal effects may include anorexia, vomiting, or diarrhea. Effects related to the cardiovascular system can include weakness, hypotension, negative inotropism, widened QRS complex and QT intervals, AV block, multiform ventricular tachycardias. Fevers and leukopenias are a possibility. Profound hypotension can occur if injected too rapidly IV. In humans an SLE syndrome can occur, but its incidence has not been established in dogs.

Reproductive/Nursing Safety

In humans, the FDA categorizes this drug as category *C* for use during pregnancy (*Animal studies have shown an adverse effect on the fetus, but there are no adequate studies in humans; or there are no animal reproduction studies and no adequate studies in humans.*) In a separate system evaluating the safety of drugs in canine and feline pregnancy (Papich 1989), this drug is categorized as class: *B* (*Safe for use if used cautiously. Studies in laboratory animals may have uncovered some risk, but these drugs appear to be safe in dogs and cats or these drugs are safe if they are not administered when the animal is near term.*)

Both procainamide and NAPA are excreted in maternal milk and absorbed in nursing offspring. It should be used with caution in nursing patients; consider using milk replacer if the drug is to be continued.

Overdosage/Acute Toxicity

Clinical signs of overdosage can include hypotension, lethargy, confusion, nausea, vomiting, and oliguria. Cardiac signs may include widening of the QRS complex, junctional tachycardia, ventricular fibrillation, or intraventricular conduction delays.

If an oral ingestion, emptying of the gut and charcoal administration may be beneficial to remove any unabsorbed drug. IV fluids, plus dopamine, phenylephrine, or norepinephrine could be considered to treat hypotensive effects. A 1/6 molar intravenous infusion of sodium lactate may be used in an attempt to reduce the cardiotoxic effects of procainamide. Forced diuresis using fluids and diuretics along with reduction of urinary pH can enhance the renal excretion of the drug. Temporary cardiac pacing may be necessary should severe AV block occur.

Drug Interactions

The following drug interactions have either been reported or are theoretical in humans or animals receiving procainamide and may be of significance in veterinary patients. Unless otherwise noted, use together is not necessarily contraindicated, but weigh the potential risks and perform additional monitoring when appropriate.

Use with caution with other antidysrhythmic agents, as additive cardiotoxic or other toxic effects may result.

- **AMIODARONE:** May increase procainamide levels, procainamide dose may need to be reduced.
- **ANTICHOLINESTERASE AGENTS** (*e.g.,* **pyridostigmine, neostigmine**): Procainamide may antagonize effects in patients with myasthenia gravis.
- **CIMETIDINE, RANITIDINE:** May increase procainamide levels.
- **HYPOTENSIVE DRUGS:** Procainamide may enhance effect.
- **LIDOCAINE:** Toxic effects may be additive, and cardiac effects unpredictable.
- **NEUROMUSCULAR BLOCKING AGENTS:** Procainamide may potentiate or prolong the neuromuscular blocking activity.
- **QUINIDINE:** Toxic effects may be additive, and cardiac effects

unpredictable.
- **PHENYTOIN:** Toxic effects may be additive, and cardiac effects unpredictable.
- **PROPRANOLOL:** Toxic effects may be additive, and cardiac effects unpredictable.
- **TRIMETHOPRIM:** May increase procainamide levels.

Laboratory Considerations

- **Propranolol** can affect fluorescent tests for procainamide or NAPA.

Doses

- **DOGS:**

  For severe or symptomatic ventricular tachycardia (extra-label): Lidocaine is usually drug of first choice, but procainamide can be considered when lidocaine is ineffective and serum potassium and magnesium levels are adequate. Dosage recommendations vary somewhat. Consider procainamide slow IV boluses (over 2-5 minutes) of 2 – 4 mg/kg to a maximum of 20 mg/kg. If successful, followed with a CRI of 20 – 50 micrograms/kg/minute. If a CRI is not feasible, 7 – 10 mg/kg IM every 6-8 hours. Compounded oral delayed-release procainamide may be useful, but documentation of efficacy is lacking. One pharmacokinetic study (Thomason *et al.* 2013) using a compounded product at 30 mg/kg PO q12h concluded that q12h dosing could be efficacious, but evaluation of serum levels should be considered.

  For acute management of SVT's (extra-label): After drugs have been used to slow AV nodal conduction (*i.e.*, diltiazem), procainamide at 6 – 8 mg/kg IV over 3 minutes or 6 – 20 mg/kg IM may terminate atrial tachyarrhythmias. (Wright 2000)

- **HORSES:** (NOTE: ARCI UCGFS CLASS 4 DRUG)

  For atrial fibrillation (extra-label): Not as effective as quinidine; also has been used for ventricular tachycardia: IV at 1 mg/kg/min, not to exceed 20 mg/kg (20 minutes) total dose. Alternatively administer 25 – 35 mg/kg PO q8h. (Kimberly *et al.* 2006)

  For ventricular tachycardia (extra-label): A CRI at 1 mg/kg/minute IV up to a total dose of 20 mg/kg (20 minutes) has been suggested.

Monitoring

- ECG; continuously with IV dosing.
- Blood pressure, during IV administration.
- Clinical signs of toxicity (see Adverse Effects/Overdosage).
- Serum levels.

Because of the variability in pharmacokinetics reported in the dog, it is recommended to monitor therapy using serum drug levels. Because dogs apparently do not form the active metabolite NAPA in appreciable quantities, the therapeutic range for procainamide is controversial. Therapeutic ranges from 3-8 micrograms/mL to 8-20 micrograms/mL have been suggested. This author (Plumb) would suggest using the lower range as a guideline to initiate therapy, but not to hesitate increasing doses to attain the higher values if efficacy is not achieved and toxicity is not a problem. Digitalis-induced ventricular arrhythmias may require substantially higher blood levels for control. Trough levels are usually specified when monitoring oral therapy. Because NAPA is routinely monitored with procainamide in human medicine, it may be necessary to tell the laboratory that NAPA values need not be automatically run for canine patients.

In horses, therapeutic levels have been suggested as 4-10 micrograms/mL for procainamide and 10-30 micrograms/dL as procainamide and NAPA together (Kimberly *et al.* 2006).

Client Information

- Oral products should be administered at evenly spaced intervals throughout the day/night. Unless otherwise directed, give the medication at least 1 hour before feeding to animal with an empty stomach.
- Notify veterinarian if animal's condition deteriorates or clinical signs of toxicity (*e.g.*, vomiting, diarrhea, weakness, etc.) occur.

Chemistry/Synonyms

Structurally related to procaine, procainamide is used as an antiarrhythmic agent. Procainamide HCl differs from procaine by the substitution of an amide group for the ester group found on procaine. It occurs as an odorless, white to tan, hygroscopic, crystalline powder with a pK_a of 9.23 and a melting range from 165°-169°C. It is very soluble in water and soluble in alcohol. The pH of the injectable product ranges from 4-6.

Procainamide may also be known as: novocainamidum, procainamidi chloridum, procainamidi hydrochloridum, *Biocoryl®*, *Procan®*, *Procanbid®*, or *Pronestyl®*.

Storage/Stability

The solution may be used if the color is no darker than light amber. Refrigeration may retard the development of oxidation, but the solution may be stored at room temperature.

Compatibility/Compounding Considerations

The injectable product is reportedly physically **compatible** with sodium chloride 0.9% injection, and water for injection. Procainamide is also physically **compatible** with dobutamine HCl, lidocaine HCl, and verapamil HCl. Compatibility is dependent upon factors such as pH, concentration, temperature, and diluent used; consult specialized references or a hospital pharmacist for more specific information.

Dosage Forms/Regulatory Status

VETERINARY-LABELED PRODUCTS: NONE.

The ARCI (Racing Commissioners International) has designated this drug as a class 4 substance. See the appendix for more information.

HUMAN-LABELED PRODUCTS:

Procainamide HCl Injection Solution: 100 mg/mL & 500 mg/mL vials; generic; (Rx)

Revisions/References

Monograph revised/updated May 2014.

Kimberly, M. & K. McGurrin (2006). Update on antiarrhythmic therapy in horses. Proceedings; ACVIM. accessed via Veterinary Information Network; vin.com

Kittleson, M. (2006). "Chapt 29: Drugs used in the treatment of cardiac arrhythmias." *Small Animal Cardiology, 2nd Ed* Veterinary Information Network.

Papich, M. (1989). Effects of drugs on pregnancy. *Current Veterinary Therapy X: Small Animal Practice*. R. Kirk. Philadelphia, Saunders: 1291-9.

Saunders, A., et al. (2009). Canine Atrial Fibrillation. Comp CE(November): E1-E!).

Thomason, J. D., et al. (2013). Pharmacokinetic evaluation of a delayed-release procainamide preparation in dogs (Abstract). Journal of Veterinary Internal Medicine 27(3): 640-.

Wright, K. (2000). Assessment and treatment of supraventricular tachyarrhythmias. *Kirk's Current Veterinary Therapy: XIII Small Animal Practice*. J. Bonagura. Philadelphia, WB Saunders: 726-30.

Procarbazine HCl

(proe-**kar**-ba-zeen)   Matulane®

Antineoplastic

Prescriber Highlights

- ▶ Atypical alkylating agent that is used in MOPP lymphoma protocols for dogs/cats & for GME in dogs; enters CNS.
- ▶ Contraindications: Hypersensitivity to drug, inadequate bone marrow reserve. Teratogen.
- ▶ Caution: Hepatic/renal impairment, use with other CNS depressant drugs.
- ▶ Adverse Effects: GI (including hemorrhagic gastroenteritis), myelosuppression, central & peripheral nervous system, hepatic.
- ▶ Drug interactions.
- ▶ May need to be reformulated in an oil-based solution to dose appropriately; commercial preparation may be very expensive.

Uses/Indications

In veterinary medicine, procarbazine is used as part of MOPP protocols (mechlorethamine, vincristine, procarbazine, prednisone) to treat lymphomas in dogs and cats. It may be of benefit in treating granulomatous meningoencephalitis (GME) in dogs.

Pharmacology/Actions

Procarbazine's precise mode of action is not well understood, but it is considered by most to be an alkylating agent, as it appears to inhibit protein, RNA, and DNA synthesis. Procarbazine is auto-oxidized into hydrogen peroxide, which may also directly damage DNA.

Pharmacokinetics

No data specific for dogs or cats was located. In humans, procarbazine is well absorbed after oral administration and rapidly equilibrates between the CSF and plasma. Peak levels in plasma occur in ≈ 1 hour; in the CSF, ≈ 30-90 minutes after dosing. Procarbazine is almost entirely metabolized in the liver and kidney. Metabolic products are cytotoxic and excreted in the urine.

Contraindications/Precautions/Warnings

Procarbazine is contraindicated in patients known to be hypersensitive to it or with inadequate bone marrow reserve as determined by bone marrow aspirate.

Because procarbazine can cause CNS depression, use with extreme caution with other CNS depressant drugs.

Use with caution in patients with impaired renal or hepatic function.

Adverse Effects

When dosed as recommended for dogs and cats, procarbazine is relatively well tolerated. In dogs, procarbazine toxicity appears to mirror that seen in humans. Gastrointestinal effects (nausea, vomiting, hepatotoxicity) and myelosuppression (thrombocytopenia, leukopenia) can be seen. Thrombocytopenia nadirs usually occur at ≈ 4 weeks. Because it is often used in combination with other chemotherapy agents (MOPP), myelosuppression and GI effects (hemorrhagic gastritis) may be enhanced. Alternate day dosing or giving with metoclopramide have been suggested to alleviate severe anorexia in cats (Moore 2011). CNS effects may be noted and include sedation or agitation. Peripheral neuropathy can occur and include loss of tendon reflexes, paresthesias and myalgia.

In humans, it is recommended to discontinue therapy if any of the following occur: CNS signs, leukopenia (WBC <4000 mm³), thrombocytopenia (platelets <100,000 mm³), hypersensitivity, stomatitis (at sign of first ulceration), diarrhea, and hemorrhage or bleeding. Resume therapy at a lower dosage only when effects clear.

Reproductive/Nursing Safety

Procarbazine is potential teratogen. In pregnant humans, procarbazine is designated by the FDA as a category *D* drug (*There is evidence of human fetal risk, but the potential benefits from the use of the drug in pregnant women may be acceptable despite its potential risks.*)

It is unknown if procarbazine enters milk. It is recommended to use milk replacer if the dam requires procarbazine.

Overdosage/Acute Toxicity

The LD_{50} for laboratory animals range from 150 mg/kg (rabbits) to 1.3 grams/kg (mice). Treat overdoses aggressively to remove drug from the gut if overdose was within an hour or two. Anticipated adverse effects would be extensions of the drug's adverse effect profile (GI, bone marrow suppression, CNS effects). Monitor and support as necessary. Contact an animal poison control center for further guidance.

Drug Interactions

The following drug interactions have either been reported or are theoretical in humans or animals receiving procarbazine and may be of significance in veterinary patients. Unless otherwise noted, use together is not necessarily contraindicated, but weigh the potential risks and perform additional monitoring when appropriate.

- **ALCOHOL/ETHANOL:** May cause severe nausea and vomiting.
- **CNS DEPRESSANT DRUGS** (*e.g.,* **barbiturates, opiates, antihistamines, phenothiazines,** etc.): Because procarbazine can cause CNS depression, use with extreme caution with other CNS depressant drugs. Coma and death have been reported when procarbazine has been used with opiates.
- **FOODS WITH HIGH TYRAMINE CONTENT (aged cheese, yogurt):** Procarbazine exhibits some monoamine oxidase inhibitory (MAOI) activity; serious hypertension may result.
- **SYMPATHOMIMETICS (phenylpropanolamine,** etc.): Procarbazine exhibits some monoamine oxidase inhibitory (MAOI) activity; serious hypertension may result.
- **TRICYCLIC ANTIDEPRESSANTS** (*e.g.,* **clomipramine, amitriptyline,** etc.): Procarbazine exhibits some monoamine oxidase inhibitory (MAOI) activity. Do not use concurrently with tricyclic antidepressant drugs.

Laboratory Considerations

- None noted.

Doses

Note: Because of the potential toxicity of this drug to patients, veterinary personnel and clients, and since chemotherapy indications, treatment protocols, monitoring and safety guidelines often change, the following dosages should be used only as a general guide. Consultation with a veterinary oncologist and referral to current veterinary oncology references [*e.g.,* (Withrow *et al.* 2012); (Dobson *et al.* 2011); (Henry *et al.* 2009); (North *et al.* 2009); (Argyle *et al.* 2008)] are strongly recommended.

- **DOGS:**

  For lymphoma rescue (extra-label): When procarbazine is used, it is as part of a protocol in combination with other antineoplastic agents and usually given for the first 14 days of the treatment cycle. Usual dose for dogs is: 50 mg/m² PO.

  For treatment of granulomatous meningoencephalitis (GME); (extra-label): 25 – 50 mg/m² PO once daily, initially with prednisone treatment. After the first month of therapy, attempt to reduce procarbazine dose to every other day. Monitor CBC weekly for first month, and then monthly thereafter. Wear gloves when handling. To prepare a 10 mg/mL oil-based solution: Five 50 mg capsules, oil-based flavor (chicken, liver, fish) drops, 0.25 teaspoonful of silica gel (to keep in suspension), and gradually add sesame oil to a total of 25 mL. Assigned expiration date of 30 days. (Cuddon *et al.* 2002)

- **CATS:**

  For MOPP lymphoma rescue (extra-label): When procarbazine is used, it is as part of a protocol in combination with other antineoplastic agents and usually given for the first 14 days of the treatment cycle. Usual doses for cats are: 50 mg/m² PO or 10 mg per cat.

Monitoring

- Baseline: CBC, hepatic and renal function, urinalysis.
- Repeat CBC at least once weekly for the first month of treatment and then monthly.
- In humans, it is recommended to repeat urinalysis, transaminases/alkaline phosphatase, and BUN at least weekly.

Client Information

- Procarbazine is a chemotherapy (cancer) drug. The drug and its byproducts can be hazardous to other animals and people that come in contact with it. On the day your animal gets the drug and then for a few days afterward, all bodily waste (urine, feces, litter), blood, or vomit should only be handled while wearing disposable gloves. Seal the waste in a plastic bag and then place both the bag and gloves in with the regular trash.
- Relatively well tolerated by most dogs and cats, but can cause vomiting, gastrointestinal upset (*e.g.,* diarrhea, etc.), bone marrow depression, and liver toxicity.
- Procarbazine can also be toxic to the nerves and cause numbness, tingling or lameness.

Chemistry/Synonyms

A derivative of hydrazine, procarbazine HCl occurs as a white to pale yellow crystalline powder having a slight odor. It is soluble, but unstable in water or aqueous solutions.

Procarbazine may also be known as: Ibenzemethyzin, NSC-77213, Ro-4-6467/1, MIH, N-Methylhydrazine, *Matulane®, Natulan®,* and *Natulanar®.*

Storage/Stability

Procarbazine capsules should be stored in airtight containers, protected from light at temperatures <40°C (preferably between 15-30°C, (59-86°F). An expiration date of 4 years is assigned after the date of manufacture.

Dosage Forms/Regulatory Status

VETERINARY-LABELED PRODUCTS: NONE.

HUMAN-LABELED PRODUCTS:

Procarbazine HCl Capsules: 50 mg; *Matulane®*; (Rx)

Revisions/References

Monograph revised/updated May 2014.

Argyle, D., et al. (2008). *Decision Making in Small Animal Oncology,* Wiley-Blackwell.
Cuddon, P. & J. Coates (2002). New treatments for granulomatous meningoencephalitis. Proceedings: ACVIM Forum. accessed via Veterinary Information Network; vin.com
Dobson, J. & D. Lascelles (2011). *BSAVA Manual of Canine and Feline Oncology,* BSAVA.
Henry, C. & M. Higginbotham (2009). *Cancer Management in Small Animal Practice,* Saunders.
Moore, A. S. (2011). Feline Lymphoma: Time for a New Paradigm? Proceedings; ACVIM. accessed via Veterinary Information Network; vin.com
North, S. & T. Banks (2009). *Small Animal Oncology: An Introduction,* Saunders.
Withrow, S., et al. (2012). Withrow and MacEwen's Small Animal Clinical Oncology, 5th Ed., Saunders.

Prochlorperazine

(proe-klor-**per**-a-zeen)   Compazine®, Compro®
Phenothiazine Antiemetic

Prescriber Highlights

▶ Phenothiazine used alone as an antiemetic.
▶ Relative Contraindications: Hypovolemia/dehydration or shock & in patients with tetanus or strychnine intoxication. Caution: Hepatic dysfunction, cardiac disease, general debilitation, or very young animals.
▶ Adverse Effects: Sedation or hypotension.

Uses/Indications

Prochlorperazine as a single agent is used in dogs and cats as an antiemetic. Its mild sedative effect may be advantageous in an inpatient setting.

The only FDA-approved products for animals were combination products containing prochlorperazine, isopropamide, with or without neomycin (*Darbazine®, Neo-Darbazine®*). These products are no longer marketed in the USA. The FDA-approved indications for these products were: vomiting, non-specific gastroenteritis, drug induced diarrhea, infectious diarrhea, spastic colitis, and motion sickness in dogs and cats (injectable product only).

Pharmacology/Actions

The basic pharmacology of prochlorperazine is similar to that of the other phenothiazines with multiple mechanisms of action, including antagonism of dopamine, histamine type-1, alpha2-adrenergic, and muscarinic receptors. Antiemetic activity of prochlorperazine is due to its effects primarily in the brain's emetic center and chemoreceptor trigger zone, but it also has some peripheral activity. Prochlorperazine has weak anticholinergic effects, strong extrapyramidal effects, and moderate sedative effects.

Pharmacokinetics

Little information is available regarding the pharmacokinetics of prochlorperazine in animals, although it probably follows the general patterns of other phenothiazine agents in absorption, distribution, and elimination.

Contraindications/Precautions/Warnings

Animals may require lower dosages of general anesthetics following phenothiazines. Cautious use and smaller doses of phenothiazines should be given to animals with hepatic dysfunction, cardiac disease, or general debilitation. Because of their hypotensive effects, phenothiazines are relatively contraindicated in patients with hypovolemia/dehydration or shock. Phenothiazines may exacerbate depression in patients with CNS depression. It should not be used for tetanus or strychnine intoxication due to effects on the extrapyramidal system. Use cautiously in very young or debilitated animals.

Adverse Effects

Alone, prochlorperazine is most likely to cause sedation or hypotension. Muscle fasciculations/tremors, and prolactin release have been reported in small animals

Reproductive/Nursing Safety

In humans, the FDA categorizes this drug as category *C* for use during pregnancy (*Animal studies have shown an adverse effect on the fetus, but there are no adequate studies in humans; or there are no animal reproduction studies and no adequate studies in humans.*) In a separate system evaluating the safety of drugs in canine and feline pregnancy (Papich 1989), this drug is categorized as class: *B* (*Safe for use if used cautiously. Studies in laboratory animals may have uncovered some risk, but these drugs appear to be safe in dogs*

and cats or these drugs are safe if they are not administered when the animal is near term.*)

A related compound, chlorpromazine has been detected in maternal milk. Although few cases are documented, a milk:plasma ratio of 0.5-0.7 or less is reported. Prochlorperazine is unlikely to pose significant risk to nursing animals.

Overdosage/Acute Toxicity

Refer to the information listed in the acepromazine monograph. Acute extrapyramidal clinical signs (torticollis, tremor, salivation) have been successfully treated with injectable diphenhydramine in humans.

Drug Interactions

The following drug interactions have either been reported or are theoretical in humans or animals receiving prochlorperazine or other phenothiazines and may be of significance in veterinary patients. Unless otherwise noted, use together is not necessarily contraindicated, but weigh the potential risks and perform additional monitoring when appropriate.

▪ **ANTACIDS:** May cause reduced GI absorption of oral phenothiazines.
▪ **ANTIDIARRHEAL MIXTURES** (*e.g.,* **Kaolin/pectin, bismuth subsalicylate mixtures**): May cause reduced GI absorption of oral phenothiazines.
▪ **CNS DEPRESSANT AGENTS** (**barbiturates, narcotics, anesthetics**, etc.): May cause additive CNS depression if used with phenothiazines.
▪ **DOPAMINE:** Phenothiazines may decrease pressor effects.
▪ **EPINEPHRINE:** Phenothiazines block alpha-adrenergic receptors and concomitant epinephrine can lead to unopposed beta-activity causing vasodilation and increased cardiac rate.
▪ **METOCLOPRAMIDE:** Phenothiazines may potentiate the extrapyramidal effects of metoclopramide
▪ **OPIATES:** May enhance the hypotensive effects of the phenothiazines; dosages of prochlorperazine may need to be reduced when used with an opiate.
▪ **ORGANOPHOSPHATE AGENTS:** Phenothiazines should not be given within one month of worming with these agents as their effects may be potentiated.
▪ **PARAQUAT:** Toxicity of the herbicide paraquat may be increased by prochlorperazine.
▪ **PHENYTOIN:** Metabolism may be decreased if given concurrently with phenothiazines.
▪ **PHYSOSTIGMINE:** Toxicity may be enhanced by prochlorperazine.
▪ **PROCAINE:** Activity may be enhanced by phenothiazines.
▪ **PROPRANOLOL:** Increased blood levels of both drugs may result if administered with phenothiazines.
▪ **WARFARIN:** Prochlorperazine may decrease anticoagulant effect.

Doses

▪ **DOGS/CATS:**

As an antiemetic (extra-label): 0.1 – 0.5 mg/kg SC 6-8h; ensure adequate hydration. There is little published information to support clinical use (or this dosage) in dogs or cats.

Monitoring

▪ Cardiac rate/rhythm/blood pressure if indicated and possible to measure.
▪ Anti-emetic/anti-spasmodic efficacy; hydration and electrolyte status.
▪ Body temperature (especially if ambient temperature is very hot or cold).

Client Information

- Observe animal for at least one hour following dosing. Dry mouth may be relieved by applying small amounts of water to animal's tongue for 10-15 minutes.
- May discolor the urine to a pink or red-brown color; this is not abnormal.
- Protracted vomiting and diarrhea can be serious; contact veterinarian if clinical signs are not alleviated. Contact veterinarian if animal exhibits abnormal behavior, becomes rigid or displays other abnormal body movements.

Chemistry/Synonyms

Prochlorperazine, a piperazine phenothiazine derivative, is available commercially as the base in rectal formulations, the edisylate salt in injectable and oral solutions, and as the maleate salt in oral tablets and capsules. Each 8 mg of the maleate salt and 7.5 mg of the edisylate salt are ≈ 5 mg of prochlorperazine base.

The base occurs as a clear, to pale yellow, viscous liquid that is very slightly soluble in water and freely soluble in alcohol. The edisylate salt occurs as white to very light yellow, odorless, crystalline powder. 500 mg are soluble in 1 mL of water or 750 mL of alcohol. The maleate salt occurs as a white or pale yellow, practically odorless, crystalline powder. It is practically insoluble in water or alcohol.

The commercial injection is a solution of the edisylate salt in sterile water. It has a pH of 4.2-6.2.

Prochlorperazine may also be known as: chlormeprazine, prochlorpemazine, *Compazine®*, *Compro®*, *Prochlor®*, *Prorazin®*, *Stemetil®*, or *Tementil®*.

Storage/Stability

Store in tight, light resistant containers at room temperature. Avoid temperatures above 40°C and below freezing. A slight yellowing of the oral or injectable solution has no effects on potency or efficacy, but do not use if a precipitate forms or the solution is substantially discolored.

Compatibility/Compounding Considerations

The following products have been reported to be physically **compatible** when mixed with prochlorperazine edisylate injection: all usual IV fluids, ascorbic acid injection, atropine sulfate, butorphanol tartrate, chlorpromazine HCl, dexamethasone sodium phosphate, fentanyl citrate, glycopyrrolate, hydroxyzine HCl, lidocaine HCl, meperidine HCl, metoclopramide, morphine sulfate, nalbuphine HCl, pentazocine lactate, perphenazine, promazine HCl, promethazine, scopolamine HBr, sodium bicarbonate, and vitamin B complex with C.

The following drugs have been reported to be physically **incompatible** when mixed with prochlorperazine edisylate: aminophylline, amphotericin B, ampicillin sodium, calcium gluceptate, chloramphenicol sodium succinate, dimenhydrinate, hydrocortisone sodium succinate, methohexital sodium, penicillin G sodium, phenobarbital sodium, pentobarbital sodium, and thiopental sodium. Do not mix with other drugs/diluents having parabens as preservatives. Compatibility is dependent upon factors such as pH, concentration, temperature, and diluent used; consult specialized references or a hospital pharmacist for more specific information.

Dosage Forms/Regulatory Status

VETERINARY-LABELED PRODUCTS:

None; *Darbazine®* is no longer available.

The ARCI (Racing Commissioners International) has designated this drug as a class 2 substance. See the appendix for more information.

HUMAN-LABELED PRODUCTS:

Prochlorperazine for Injection: 5 mg/mL in 2 mL vials; generic; (Rx)

Prochlorperazine Tablets: 5 mg & 10 mg (as maleate); *Compazine®*, generic; (Rx)

Prochlorperazine (base) Suppositories: 25 mg; *Compro®*, generic; (Rx)

Revisions/References

Monograph revised/updated May 2014.

Papich, M. (1989). Effects of drugs on pregnancy. *Current Veterinary Therapy X: Small Animal Practice.* R. Kirk. Philadelphia, Saunders: 1291-9.

Promethazine HCl

(proe-**meth**-a-zeen)   Phenergan®

Phenothiazine

Prescriber Highlights

▶ Phenothiazine used as an antihistamine & antiemetic in small animals. Potential alternative to acepromazine in horses.
▶ Relatively little experience with this drug in veterinary medicine; not frequently recommended for use.
▶ Adverse Effects: sedation or anticholinergic effects.

Uses/Indications

Promethazine may be useful in dogs and cats as an antiemetic. A small study in cats, found that IM dosages of 2 mg/kg and 4 mg/kg given one-hour prior to xylazine, significantly reduced the frequency of emesis (Kolahian *et al.* 2012). Because of its antihistamine actions promethazine has been tried for treating pruritus in atopic dogs, but efficacy has been poor.

A study in standing horses that compared the sedative and hemodynamic effects of acepromazine (0.1 mg/kg IV) and promethazine (0.1, 0.2, & 0.3 mg/kg IV) found at the doses used, promethazine appeared to have less sedative and peripheral vasodilator effects than acepromazine. The authors concluded that it could be safer than acepromazine in horses with hypotension and postulated that if anti-inflammatory and anti-oxidative properties are confirmed *in vivo*, it could be of benefit in horses suffering from shock or cardiovascular depression (Pequito *et al.* 2012).

Pharmacology/Actions

The basic pharmacology of promethazine is similar to that of the other phenothiazines with multiple mechanisms of action including antagonism of dopamine (less than chlorpromazine), histamine type-1, alpha2-adrenergic, and muscarinic receptors. Antiemetic activity of promethazine is due to its effects primarily in the brain's emetic center and chemoreceptor trigger zone, but it also has some peripheral activity. It also has local anesthetic actions.

Pharmacokinetics

Little information is available regarding the pharmacokinetics of promethazine in animals, although oral bioavailability in dogs is very low (≈10%).

In humans, the drug is well absorbed following oral or rectal administration, and via IM injection. Sedative effects occur within minutes of IV administration and persist for several hours. The drug is metabolized in the liver and these metabolites are eliminated primarily in the urine. Elimination half-life in humans is ≈ 10 hours.

Contraindications/Precautions/Warnings

Animals may require lower dosages of general anesthetics following phenothiazines. Cautious use and smaller doses of phenothiazines should be given to animals with hepatic dysfunction, cardiac disease, or general debilitation. Because of their hypotensive effects, phenothiazines are relatively contraindicated in patients with hypovolemia or shock. Do not use in patients with tetanus or strychnine intoxication due to effects on the extrapyramidal system. Use cautiously in very young or debilitated animals.

In humans, promethazine has a "black box warning" to not use the medication in children <2 years old; fatal respiratory depression has occurred in that patient group.

Adverse Effects

Little experience has been reported with this drug in animals, but prochlorperazine would most likely cause sedation or anticholinergic effects (dry mouth, etc.).

Reproductive/Nursing Safety

In humans, the FDA categorizes this drug as category *C* for use during pregnancy (*Animal studies have shown an adverse effect on the fetus, but there are no adequate studies in humans; or there are no animal reproduction studies and no adequate studies in humans.*)

It is not known whether promethazine is distributed into milk; a related compound, chlorpromazine has been detected in maternal milk. Although few cases are documented, a milk to plasma ratio of 0.5-0.7 or less is reported. Promethazine is unlikely to pose significant risk to nursing animals.

Overdosage/Acute Toxicity

Refer to the information listed in the acepromazine monograph. Acute extrapyramidal clinical signs (torticollis, tremor, salivation) have been successfully treated with injectable diphenhydramine in humans.

Drug Interactions

The following drug interactions have either been reported or are theoretical in humans or animals receiving promethazine or other phenothiazines and may be of significance in veterinary patients. Unless otherwise noted, use together is not necessarily contraindicated, but weigh the potential risks and perform additional monitoring when appropriate.

- **ANTACIDS:** May cause reduced GI absorption of oral phenothiazines.
- **ANTIDIARRHEAL MIXTURES** (*e.g.*, **Kaolin/pectin, bismuth subsalicylate mixtures**): May cause reduced GI absorption of oral phenothiazines.
- **ATROPINE & OTHER ANTICHOLINERGICS:** May have additive effects when used with promethazine.
- **CNS DEPRESSANT AGENTS** (**barbiturates, narcotics, anesthetics**, etc.): May cause additive CNS depression if used with phenothiazines.
- **EPINEPHRINE:** Phenothiazines block alpha-adrenergic receptors and concomitant epinephrine can lead to unopposed beta-activity causing vasodilation and increased cardiac rate.
- **METOCLOPRAMIDE:** Phenothiazines may potentiate the extrapyramidal effects of metoclopramide.
- **MONOAMINE OXIDASE INHIBITORS:** May potentiate extrapyramidal effects.
- **OPIATES:** May enhance the hypotensive effects of the phenothiazines; dosages of prochlorperazine may need to be reduced when used with an opiate.
- **ORGANOPHOSPHATE AGENTS:** Phenothiazines should not be given within one month of worming with these agents as their effects may be potentiated.

Laboratory Considerations

- Promethazine can cause false positive results for **salicylates** in urine.
- Promethazine can cause false positive or false negative results for **chorionic gonadotropin** in urine.

Doses

- **DOGS:**

    As an antiemetic (extra-label): 0.2 – 0.5 mg/kg PO q6-8h. Generally used for prevention of motion sickness, but oral bioavailability is low so efficacy may be low. (KuKanich 2011)

- **CATS:**

    As an antiemetic (extra-label): In the study, 2 mg/kg IM given one-hour prior to xylazine significantly reduced the frequency of emesis. (Kolahian *et al.* 2012)

- **HORSES:**

    For possible anti-inflammatory and anti-oxidative effects in hypotensive horses (extra-label): From a study in 9 healthy horses. Authors concluded that if anti-inflammatory and antioxidant properties of acepromazine and promethazine are further confirmed, promethazine at 0.1 – 0.2 mg/kg IV could be an alternative to acepromazine in hypotensive horses. (Pequito *et al.* 2012).

Monitoring

- Efficacy.

Client Information

- Dry mouth may be relieved by applying small amounts of water to animal's tongue for 10-15 minutes.
- May cause sedation or behavior changes; contact veterinarian if these are a concern.
- Protracted vomiting or diarrhea can be serious; contact veterinarian if clinical signs are not alleviated.
- Contact veterinarian if animal exhibits abnormal movements or becomes rigid.

Chemistry/Synonyms

Promethazine HCl occurs as a white to faint yellow, practically odorless, crystalline powder. It slowly oxidizes and acquires a blue color on prolonged exposure to air. Promethazine HCl is freely soluble in water, hot dehydrated alcohol, or chloroform, but practically insoluble in acetone, ether, or ethyl acetate. The pH of a 5% solution in water is between 4-5.

Promethazine may also be known as: Lilly 01516, PM 284, RP 3277, prometazina or *Phenergan*®. There are many other trade names available.

Storage/Stability

Store tablets at room temperature (20-25°C) in tight, light resistant containers. The syrup should be stored from 15-25°C and protected from light.

The injection should be stored at room temperature 20-25°C and protected from light. Keep in covered carton until time of use. Do not use if a precipitate forms or the solution is discolored. Promethazine can be adsorbed to plastic IV bags and tubing.

Promethazine suppositories should be stored in the refrigerator (2-8°C).

Compatibility/Compounding Considerations

The following products have been reported to be physically **compatible** when promethazine injection is mixed with them: all usual IV fluids, amikacin, ascorbic acid, buprenorphine, butorphanol, cimetidine, diphenhydramine, fentanyl, fluconazole, glycopyrrolate, hydromorphone, hydroxyzine, meperidine, metoclopramide, midazolam, ondansetron, pancuronium, pentazocine, procainamide, and ranitidine.

Solutions of promethazine hydrochloride are **incompatible** with alkaline substances, which can precipitate promethazine base.

The following drugs have been reported to be physically **incompatible** when mixed with promethazine HCl: aminophylline, barbiturates, benzylpenicillin salts, chloramphenicol sodium succinate, dimenhydrinate, doxorubicin (in a liposomal formulation), furosemide, heparin sodium, hydrocortisone sodium succinate, morphine sulfate, and nalbuphine HCl. Compatibility is dependent upon factors such as pH, concentration, temperature, and diluent used; consult specialized references or a hospital pharmacist for more specific information.

Dosage Forms/Regulatory Status

VETERINARY-LABELED PRODUCTS: NONE.

The ARCI (Racing Commissioners International) has designated this drug as a class 3 substance. See the appendix for more information.

HUMAN-LABELED PRODUCTS:

Promethazine HCl for Injection: 25 mg/mL & 50 mg/mL in 1 mL amps; *Phenergan®*, generic; (Rx)

Promethazine HCl Oral syrup: 1.25 mg/mL in 473 mL; generic; (Rx)

Promethazine HCl Oral Tablets: 12.5 mg, 25 mg & 50 mg; *Phenergan®*, generic; (Rx)

Promethazine HCl Rectal Suppositories: 12.5 mg, 25 mg, & 50 mg; *Phenergan®*, *Phenadoz®*, *Promethegan®*, generic; (Rx)

Revisions/References

Monograph revised/updated May 2014.

Kolahian, S. & S. H. Jarolmasjed (2012). Antiemetic efficacy of promethazine on xylazine-induced emesis in cats. Canadian Veterinary Journal-Revue Veterinaire Canadienne 53(2): 193-5.

KuKanich, B. (2011). Antiemetics, What's New? Proceedings; Western Veterinary Conference. accessed via Veterinary Information Network; vin.com

Pequito, M., et al. (2012). Comparison of the Sedative and Hemodynamic Effects of Acepromazine and Promethazine in the Standing Horse. Journal of Equine Veterinary Science 32(12): 799-804.

Propantheline Bromide

(proe-**pan**-the-leen)   Pro-Banthine®

Quaternary Antimuscarinic

Prescriber Highlights

▶ Quaternary antimuscarinic agent used for its antispasmodic/antisecretory effects for the treatment of diarrhea, hyperreflexic detrusor or urge incontinence & anticholinergic responsive bradycardias. In horses, IV to reduce colonic peristalsis & relax rectum to allow easier examination & surgery.

▶ Contraindications: Hypersensitivity to anticholinergics, tachycardias secondary to thyrotoxicosis or cardiac insufficiency, myocardial ischemia, unstable cardiac status during acute hemorrhage, GI obstructive disease, paralytic ileus, severe ulcerative colitis, obstructive uropathy, or myasthenia gravis (unless used to reverse adverse muscarinic effects secondary to therapy).

▶ Extreme Caution: Known or suspected GI infections, autonomic neuropathy. Caution: hepatic or renal disease, hyperthyroidism, hypertension, CHF, tachyarrhythmias, prostatic hypertrophy, esophageal reflux, & geriatric or pediatric patients.

▶ Adverse Effects: Similar to atropine (dry mouth, dry eyes, urinary hesitancy, tachycardia, constipation, etc.), but less effects on eye or CNS. Cats may exhibit vomiting & hypersalivation. High doses may cause ileus.

Uses/Indications

In small animal medicine propantheline bromide has been used for its antispasmodic/antisecretory effects in the treatment of diarrhea. It is also employed in the treatment of hyperreflexic detrusor or urge incontinence and as an oral treatment in anticholinergic responsive bradycardias. In horses, propantheline has been used

intravenously to reduce colonic peristalsis and for relaxing the rectum to allow easier rectal examination and surgery.

Pharmacology/Actions

An antimuscarinic with similar actions as atropine, propantheline is a quaternary ammonium compound and does not cross appreciably into the CNS. It should not exhibit the same extent of CNS adverse effects that atropine possesses. After a 100 mg IV injection to horses, propantheline reduced gastrointestinal tract sounds for 2+ hours and elevated heart rate relative to the control. Maximum heart rates were noted between 60-90 minutes post-injection (Sundra *et al.* 2012).

Pharmacokinetics

Quaternary anticholinergic agents are not completely absorbed after oral administration because they are completely ionized. In humans, peak levels occur ≈ 2 hours after oral administration. Food apparently decreases the amount of drug absorbed. Propantheline is reportedly variably absorbed in dogs; dosages should be adjusted for each patient.

The distribution of propantheline has not been extensively studied, but like other quaternary antimuscarinics, propantheline is poorly lipid soluble and does not extensively penetrate into the CNS or eye.

Propantheline is believed to be prevalently metabolized in the GI and/or liver; <5% of an oral dose is excreted unchanged in the urine.

Contraindications/Precautions/Warnings

The equine product (Australia) is labeled as contraindicated in cases of tympanic colic. Do not use in cases of dry choke where saliva is deficient, as the anticholinergic properties will further inhibit secretion of saliva. Propantheline should be considered contraindicated if the patient has a history of hypersensitivity to anticholinergic drugs, tachycardias secondary to thyrotoxicosis or cardiac insufficiency, myocardial ischemia, unstable cardiac status during acute hemorrhage, GI obstructive disease, paralytic ileus, severe ulcerative colitis, obstructive uropathy, or myasthenia gravis (unless used to reverse adverse muscarinic effects secondary to therapy).

Antimuscarinic agents should be used with extreme caution in patients with known or suspected GI infections. Propantheline or other antimuscarinic agents can decrease GI motility and prolong retention of the causative agent(s) or toxin(s) resulting in prolonged clinical signs. Antimuscarinic agents must also be used with extreme caution in patients with autonomic neuropathy.

Antimuscarinic agents should be used with caution in patients with hepatic disease, renal disease, hyperthyroidism, hypertension, CHF, tachyarrhythmias, prostatic hypertrophy, esophageal reflux, and in geriatric or pediatric patients.

Adverse Effects

With the exception of fewer effects on the eye and the CNS, propantheline can be expected to have a similar adverse reaction profile as atropine (dry mouth, dry eyes, urinary hesitancy, tachycardia, constipation, etc.). Vomiting and hypersalivation have also been reported in cats. High doses may lead to the development of ileus with resultant bacterial overgrowth in susceptible animals. For more information, refer to the atropine monograph.

Reproductive/Nursing Safety

In humans, the FDA categorizes this drug as category *B* for use during pregnancy (*Animal studies have not yet demonstrated risk to the fetus, but there are no adequate studies in pregnant women; or animal studies have shown an adverse effect, but adequate studies in pregnant women have not demonstrated a risk to the fetus in the first trimester of pregnancy, and there is no evidence of risk in later trimesters.*)

Although anticholinergics (especially atropine) may be excreted in milk and cause toxicity and reduce milk production, it is unknown if propantheline enters maternal milk. Use with caution in nursing patients.

Overdosage/Acute Toxicity

Because of its quaternary structure, it would be expected that minimal CNS effects would occur after an overdose of propantheline when compared to atropine. See the information listed in the atropine monograph for more information on the clinical signs that may be seen following an overdose.

If a recent oral ingestion, emptying gut contents and administration of activated charcoal and saline cathartics may be warranted. Treat clinical signs supportively and symptomatically. Do not use phenothiazines as they may contribute to anticholinergic effects. Fluid therapy and standard treatments for shock may be instituted.

The use of physostigmine is controversial and should probably be reserved for cases where the patient exhibits either extreme agitation and is at risk for injuring themselves or others, or where supraventricular tachycardias and sinus tachycardias are severe or life threatening. The usual dose for physostigmine (human) is 2 mg IV slowly (for average sized adult); if no response may repeat every 20 minutes until reversal of toxic antimuscarinic effects or cholinergic effects takes place. The human pediatric dose is 0.02 mg/kg slow IV (repeat q10 minutes as above) and may be a reasonable choice for treatment of small animals. Physostigmine adverse effects (bronchoconstriction, bradycardia, seizures) may be treated with small doses of IV atropine.

Drug Interactions

The following drug interactions have either been reported or are theoretical in humans or animals receiving propantheline and may be of significance in veterinary patients. Unless otherwise noted, use together is not necessarily contraindicated, but weigh the potential risks and perform additional monitoring when appropriate.

- **ANTIHISTAMINES:** May enhance the activity of propantheline.
- **BENZODIAZEPINES:** May enhance the activity of propantheline.
- **CIMETIDINE:** Propantheline may decrease the absorption of cimetidine.
- **CORTICOSTEROIDS** (long-term use): May increase intraocular pressure.
- **MEPERIDINE:** May enhance the activity of propantheline.
- **NITRATES:** May potentiate the adverse effects of propantheline.
- **NITROFURANTOIN:** Propantheline may enhance actions.
- **PHENOTHIAZINES:** May enhance the activity of propantheline.
- **SYMPATHOMIMETICS:** Propantheline may enhance actions.
- **RANITIDINE:** Propantheline delays the absorption, but increases the peak serum level of ranitidine; the relative bioavailability of ranitidine may be increased by 23% when propantheline is administered concomitantly with ranitidine.
- **THIAZIDE DIURETICS:** Propantheline may enhance actions.

Doses

- **DOGS/CATS:**

  For detrusor hyperreflexia, urge incontinence (extra-label): Dogs: 7.5 – 30 mg per dog PO q8-24h. Cats: Suggested doses vary significantly ranging from 5 – 7.5 mg PO q8h to 7.5 mg per cat PO every 3 days. Use the lowest dose that will control clinical signs.

  For short-term treatment of sinus bradycardia, incomplete AV block, etc. (extra-label): Dogs: 7.5 – 30 mg per dog PO q8-12h. Cats: 7.5 mg per cat PO q8-12h. Usually well tolerated, but improvement is usually partial and often temporary. (Rishniw *et al.* 2000)

- **HORSES:**

  As a parasympatholytic (extra-label in USA): **For rectal palpation:** 50 - 100 mg (2 – 4 mL) IV. **Acute spasmodic colic:** 100 – 300 mg IV. **Rectal tears:** If rectal tears are suspected use immediately at a dose of 50 – 100 mg IV. Rectal relaxation will follow usually within one minute. (Adapted from label, *Propan B®*—Nature Vet; Australia)

Monitoring

Dependent on reason for use:
- Clinical efficacy.
- Heart rate and rhythm if indicated.
- Adverse effects.

Client Information

- Best to give on an empty stomach, but if animal vomits after getting a dose give with a small amount of food or treat to see if this helps. If vomiting continues, contact your veterinarian.
- Side effects can include: Dry mouth, dry eyes, trouble urinating or defecating, fast heartbeat, vomiting (in cats), drooling/hypersalivation (in cats).
- Dry mouth may be relieved by applying small amounts of water to animal's tongue for 10-15 minutes.
- Severe constipation can be serious. If your animal has not passed any stool for several days, contact your veterinarian right away.

Chemistry/Synonyms

A quaternary ammonium antimuscarinic agent, propantheline bromide occurs as bitter-tasting, odorless, white or practically white crystals, with a melting range of 156-162° (with decomposition). It is very soluble in both water and alcohol.

Propantheline bromide may also be known as: bromuro de propantelina, propanthelini bromidum, *Propan B®* or *Probanthine®*.

Storage/Stability

Propantheline bromide tablets should be stored at room temperature in tight containers.

The dry powder for reconstitution (*Propan B®*) should be stored below 25°C. Protect from light. Use prepared solution within 10 days.

Compatibility/Compounding Considerations

Reconstitute the powder for injection with 10 mL sterile water for injection. As there is no commercially available injectable product available in the USA, if a preparation is made from oral tablets it should be freshly prepared and filtered through a 0.22 micron-filter before administering. Use with caution. If using a compounded product, reconstitute as directed.

Dosage Forms/Regulatory Status

VETERINARY-LABELED PRODUCTS:

None in the USA. In Australia: Propantheline Bromide 300 mg sterile powder for reconstitution (for IV use) in 10 mL vials; *Propan B®*; S4-By Veterinary Prescription (APVMA 51275). Meat withholding period for horses is 28 days.

HUMAN-LABELED PRODUCTS:

Propantheline Bromide Tablets: 15 mg; generic; (Rx)

Revisions/References

Monograph revised/updated May 2014.

Rishniw, M. & W. Thomas (2000). Bradyarrhythmias. *Kirk's Current Veterinary Therapy: XIII Small Animal Practice*. J. Bonagura. Philadelphia, WB Saunders: 719-25.

Sundra, T. M., et al. (2012). The influence of spasmolytic agents on heart rate variability and gastrointestinal motility in normal horses. *Research in Veterinary Science* **93**(3): 1426-33.

Propionibacterium acnes Injection

(**proe**-pee-ohe-bak-**ter**-ee-um **ak**-nees)

Immunoregulin®, Eqstim®

Immunostimulant

Prescriber Highlights

▶ Immunostimulant for Staph pyoderma, FeLV, feline herpes, equine respiratory infections.

▶ Contraindications: Hypersensitivity to compound, canine lymphoma, or leukemias with CNS involvement. Caution: Cardiac dysfunction.

▶ Adverse Effects: Lethargy, hyperthermia, chills, & anorexia. Anaphylactic reactions are possible.

▶ Extravasation may cause local tissue inflammation.

Uses/Indications

The manufacturer's label notes the product (*Immunoregulin®*) is "… indicated in the dog as adjunct to antibiotic therapy in the treatment of chronic recurring canine pyoderma to decrease the severity and extent of lesions and increase the percentage of dogs free of lesions after the appropriate therapeutic period."

The equine product (*EqStim®*) is labeled as an immunostimulant for adjunctive therapy of primary or secondary viral or bacterial respiratory tract infections. A recent review (Paillot 2013) concluded that: "an increasing amount of studies and reports that support the efficient use of non-specific immune-modulators such as inactivated *parapoxvirus ovis* (iPPVO) or *P. acnes* injection as adjuncts to conventional management of equine respiratory disease complex (ERDC). Their activity is mostly based on non-specific stimulation of innate immune response. They may not provide protection against direct infection or transmission of respiratory pathogens but they seem to contribute to the reduction of the disease severity, subsequently reducing the frequency of complications and improving the rate of recovery. In the case of iPPVO, its anti-herpetic function may provide a valuable contribution in prevention of equine herpesviruses infection."

A study in neonatal foals (<30 days old) did not demonstrate any effect from *P. acnes* injection on interferon-gamma production (Sturgill *et al.* 2011). Another study in neonatal foals exposed *ex vivo* to *R. equi* had similar negative effects on interferon-gamma, but treated foals did have significantly less intracellular proliferation of *R. equi* within monocyte derived macrophages on day 12 compared to control foals (Ryan *et al.* 2010).

Additionally, *P. acnes* injection has been used as an immunostimulant for the adjunctive treatment of feline rhinotracheitis and feline leukemia virus-induced disease. In dogs, it may be of use in the adjunctive treatment of oral melanoma and mastocytoma. Unfortunately, controlled studies documenting efficacy were not located for these potential indications.

Pharmacology/Actions

A non-specific immunostimulant, non-viable *Propionibacterium acnes* injection may induce macrophage activation, lymphokine production, increase natural killer cell activity, and enhance cell-mediated immunity.

Pharmacokinetics

No information was noted.

Contraindications/Precautions/Warnings

Propionibacterium acnes injection is contraindicated in patients hypersensitive to it. It should also be considered contraindicated in canine lymphoma or leukemias with CNS involvement. Use with caution in patients with cardiac dysfunction. One source states that its use is contraindicated in cats with FIV or FIP (Hartmann 2009).

Adverse Effects

Occasionally within hours after injection, lethargy, increased body temperature, chills, and anorexia may be noted. Anaphylactic reactions have also been reported. Extravasation may cause local tissue inflammation. Long-term toxicity studies have demonstrated vomiting, anorexia, malaise, fever, acidosis, increased water consumption, and hepatitis.

Reproductive/Nursing Safety

Safe use during pregnancy has not been established.

Overdosage/Acute Toxicity

No overdosage information was noted; the manufacturer states that the antidote is epinephrine, presumably for the treatment of anaphylactic reactions.

Drug Interactions

The manufacturer states that the immunostimulant effects may be compromised if given concomitantly with **glucocorticoids** or **other immune suppressing drugs**; manufacturer recommends discontinuing steroids at least 7 days prior to initiating therapy.

Doses

■ **DOGS:**

For labeled indications (as adjunct to antibiotic therapy in the treatment of chronic recurring canine pyoderma): Shake well. Give via intravenous route at the following dosages: For animals weighing up to 15 lbs = 0.25 – 0.5 mL; 15-45 lbs = 0.25 – 1 mL; 45-75 lbs = 1 – 1.5 mL; >75 lbs = 1.5 – 2 mL. During the first two weeks, give 4 times at 3-4 day intervals, then once weekly until symptoms abate or stabilize. Maintenance doses once per month are recommended. (Package Insert; *Immunoregulin®*)

■ **CATS:**

For adjunctive therapy of feline retrovirus infections (extra-label): As an antiviral immunostimulant in cats to increase hematopoiesis in FeLV-positive cats: 5 lb cats: 0.25 mL IV, IP twice weekly for 2 weeks, then once weekly until remission and once monthly after that to maintain clinical improvement. For 10 lb cats: 0.5 mL IV, IP twice weekly for 2 weeks, then once weekly for 3 weeks and once monthly for 2 months for a total of nine injections after that to maintain clinical improvement. Some protocols suggest follow-up with injections once weekly for 20 weeks or longer as needed. Others suggest follow-up with once weekly until clinical remission, and then once per month. (Greene *et al.* 2006)

■ **HORSES:**

As an immunostimulant for adjunctive therapy of primary or secondary viral or bacterial respiratory tract infections: Using *EqStim®*: 1 mL per 114kg (250 lb) body weight IV. Repeat dosage on day 3 (or day 4), at day 7, and weekly as needed. (Label information; *Eqstim®*)

As an adjunctive treatment to improve fertility in mares with endometritis: Using *EqStim®*: 1 mL per 114 kg (250 lb) body weight IV. Given on days 0, 2, and 6. Best results in mares bred 2 days before to 8 days after initial administration. (Rohrbach *et al.* 2007; Dascanio 2009)

Monitoring

■ Efficacy.

■ Adverse effects (see above).

Chemistry/Synonyms

Propionibacterium acnes injection is an immunostimulant agent, containing nonviable *Propionibacterium acnes* suspended in 12.5% ethanol in saline.

Propionibacterium acnes may also be known as: *Corynebacterium parvum*; NSC-220537, *Arthrokehlan A®*, *Coparvax®*, *Cory-*

munun®, *Eqstim®*, *Imunoparvum®*, and *Immunoregulin®*.

Storage/Stability
Store refrigerated; do not freeze. Shake well before using.

Dosage Forms/Regulatory Status
VETERINARY-LABELED PRODUCTS:
Propionibacterium acnes (non-viable) IV: 0.4 mg/mL in 5 mL and 50 mL vials; *Immunoregulin®*; (OTC-biologic; manufacturer states that use is restricted to use by, or under the supervision of a veterinarian). Labeled for use in dogs. *Eqstim®* is labeled for use in horses and restricted to use by or under the supervision of a veterinarian.

HUMAN-LABELED PRODUCTS: NONE.

Revisions/References
Monograph revised/updated May 2014.
Dascanio, J. (2009). Hormonal Control of Reproduction. Proceedings: ABVP. accessed via Veterinary Information Network; vin.com
Greene, C., et al. (2006). Appendix 8: Antimicrobial Drug Formulary. *Infectious Disease of the Dog and Cat.* C. Greene, Elsevier: 1186-333.
Hartmann, K. (2009). Immunomodulators in Veterinary Medicine--Is There Evidence of Efficacy? Proceedings: ACVIM. accessed via Veterinary Information Network; vin.com
Paillot, R. (2013). A systematic review of the immune-modulators Parapoxvirus ovis and Propionibacterium acnes for the prevention of respiratory disease and other infections in the horse. Veterinary Immunology and Immunopathology 153(1-2): 1-9.
Rohrbach, B. W., et al. (2007). Effect of adjunctive treatment with intravenously administered Propionibacterium acnes on reproductive performance in mares with persistent endometritis. Javma-Journal of the American Veterinary Medical Association 231(1): 107-13.
Ryan, C., et al. (2010). Effects of two commercially available immunostimulants on leukocyte function of foals following ex vivo exposure to Rhodococcus equi. Veterinary Immunology and Immunopathology 138(3): 198-205.
Sturgill, T. L., et al. (2011). Effect of Propionibacterium acnes-containing immunostimulant on interferon-gamma (IFN gamma) production in the neonatal foal. Veterinary Immunology and Immunopathology 141(1-2): 124-7.

Propofol
(**proe**-po-fole)   Rapinovet®, PropoFlo®, Diprivan®
Injectable Anesthetic

Prescriber Highlights
▶ Short-acting injectable hypnotic agent.
▶ Contraindications: Hypersensitivity to it or any component of the product. Caution: Severe stress or having undergone trauma, hypoproteinemia, hyperlipidemia, seizures, or anaphylaxis history.
▶ Adverse Effects: Transient respiratory depression is common but usually clinically tolerable. Apnea possible, especially if given too rapidly. Can cause histamine release; anaphylactoid reactions possible. Hypotension, seizure-like clinical signs (paddling, opisthotonus, myoclonic twitching) during induction. Repeated doses in **Cats**: Increased Heinz body production (rare), slowed recoveries, anorexia, lethargy, malaise, & diarrhea.
▶ Little, if any, analgesia is provided.
▶ Consider dose reduction if using other CNS depressants.
▶ Sufficient monitoring & patient-support capabilities are mandatory.

Uses/Indications
In appropriate patients, propofol may be useful as an induction agent (especially before endotracheal intubation or an inhalant anesthetic), and as an anesthetic for outpatient diagnostic or minor procedures (*e.g.*, laceration repair, radiologic procedures, minor dentistry, minor biopsies, endoscopy, etc.). For relatively short procedures it can be used as a CRI for total intravenous anesthesia, but does not provide analgesia.

Propofol is used as a treatment for refractory status epilepticus, as it tends to cause less cardiovascular depression and recoveries can be smoother than with pentobarbital, but apnea is possible. Propofol may be of particular usefulness in patients with preexist-

ing cardiac dysrhythmias.

Propofol may be safely used in animals with liver or renal disease and mild to moderate cardiac disease.

In dogs, propofol's labeled indications are: 1) for induction of anesthesia; 2) for maintenance of anesthesia for up to 20 minutes; 3) for induction of general anesthesia where maintenance is provided by inhalant anesthetics.

Pharmacology/Actions
Propofol is a short acting hypnotic unrelated to other general anesthetic agents. Its mechanism of action is not well understood.

In dogs, propofol produces rapid yet smooth and excitement-free anesthesia induction (in 30-60 seconds) when given slowly IV. Sub-anesthetic dosages will produce sedation, restraint and an unawareness of surroundings. Anesthetic dosages produce unconsciousness and good muscle relaxation.

Propofol's cardiovascular effects include arterial hypotension, bradycardia, (especially in combination with opiate premedicants) and negative inotropism. It causes significant respiratory depression, particularly with rapid administration or very high dosages. Propofol can also increase intraocular pressure in dogs. Other possible effects include increased appetite and antiemetic action. It does not appear to precipitate malignant hyperthermia and has little or no analgesic properties.

Pharmacokinetics
After IV administration, propofol rapidly crosses the blood brain barrier and has an onset of action usually within one minute. Duration of action after a single bolus lasts ≈ 2-5 minutes. It is highly bound to plasma proteins (95-99%), crosses the placenta, is highly lipophilic, and reportedly enters maternal milk.

Propofol's short duration of action is principally due to its rapid redistribution from the CNS to other tissues. It is rapidly biotransformed in the liver via glucuronide conjugation to inactive metabolites, which are then excreted primarily by the kidneys.

In dogs, the steady state volume of distribution is >3 L/kg, elimination half-life ≈ 1.4 hours, and clearance ≈ 50 mL/kg/min. Canine CYP2B11 may be the isoenzyme responsible for propofol metabolism in dogs. Greyhounds (and other sighthound breeds?) clear propofol more slowly than mixed-breed or Beagle dogs (Zoran *et al.* 1993).

The addition of 2% benzyl alcohol does not appear to significantly alter propofol pharmacokinetics or alter pharmacodynamics (single dose induction) in cats (Griffenhagen *et al.* 2013b), (Griffenhagen *et al.* 2013a).

Contraindications/Precautions/Warnings
Propofol is contraindicated in patients hypersensitive to it or any component of the product. It should not be used in patients where general anesthesia or sedation is contraindicated.

In cats, propofol may be tolerated less well than in dogs as it is metabolized (and eliminated) more slowly. A new formulation of propofol (*PropoFlo 28®*) is labeled for dogs only and contains the preservative benzyl alcohol, which can potentially be toxic to cats at high doses. Anecdotally, it has been used safely in healthy cats with no indications of toxicity and normal recoveries. A small study concluded that addition of benzyl alcohol had no additional effect when propofol is used at normal-to-high clinical doses in healthy cats (Taylor *et al.* 2012). Propofol should only be used in facilities where sufficient monitoring and patient-support (intubation/ventilation) capabilities are available. Because patients that are in shock, under severe stress, or have undergone trauma may be overly sensitive to the cardiovascular and respiratory depressant effects of propofol, it should be used with caution in these patients. Using in combination with non-cardiodepressant premeds may allow lower dosages of propofol and thereby be safer to use in critically ill animals or those with cardiac disease. Adequate perfusion should be maintained before and during propofol anesthesia; dosage adjustments may be necessary.

When used in combination with other CNS depressant premedicants (*e.g.*, acepromazine, opioids, diazepam, etc.), a decrease in dosage of ≈ 25% (from the single agent dose) should be considered. In very thin animals, consider dosage reduction as well. A study in dogs found that administering propofol before midazolam resulted in less benzodiazepine-induced excitation and a greater reduction of total propofol requirements than when midazolam was given before propofol (Sanchez *et al.* 2013).

Induction of general anesthesia with propofol in overweight dogs may occur at lower doses than in normal weight dogs (Boveri *et al.* 2013).

Greyhounds (and other sighthound breeds?) clear propofol more slowly than mixed-breed or Beagle dogs.

As propofol is so highly bound to plasma proteins, patients with hypoproteinemia may be susceptible to untoward effects; general anesthetic agents may be a safer choice in these patients.

Propofol does not provide adequate analgesia and perioperative analgesics should be considered.

The benefits of propofol should be weighed against its risks in patients with a history of hyperlipidemia, seizures or anaphylactic reactions.

Adverse Effects

Transient respiratory depression is common but usually clinically tolerable. However, there is a relatively high incidence of apnea with resultant cyanosis if propofol is given too rapidly; it should be given slowly (25% of the calculated dose every 30 seconds until desired effect). Treat with assisted ventilation until spontaneous ventilation resumes.

Propofol has been documented to cause histamine release in some patients and anaphylactoid reactions (rare) have been noted in humans. Propofol has direct myocardial depressant properties and resultant arterial hypotension has been reported.

Occasionally, dogs may exhibit seizure-like clinical signs (paddling, opisthotonus, myoclonic twitching) during induction that if persistent, may be treated with intravenous diazepam. Propofol may have both anticonvulsant and seizure-causing properties. It should be used with caution in patients with a history of, or active seizure disorders, but some clinicians believe, however, that propofol is actually more appropriate to use in seizure patients or in high seizure-risk procedures (*e.g.*, myelography) than is thiopental.

When used repeatedly or as a prolonged CRI in cats, increased Heinz body production, slowed recoveries, anorexia, lethargy, malaise, and diarrhea have been noted, but do not occur commonly. Consecutive use in dogs appears to be safe.

Pain upon injection has been reported in humans, but does not appear to be a clinically significant problem for dogs or cats when using the macroemulsion products. Microemulsions of propofol (*e.g.*, *PropoClear®*) may be associated with pain on injection (Michou *et al.* 2012), especially with repeated administration (Minghella *et al.* 2010). Extravasation of propofol injection is not irritating nor does it cause tissue sloughing.

Reproductive/Nursing Safety

Propofol crosses the placenta and its safe use during pregnancy has not been established. High dosages (6X) in laboratory animals caused increased maternal death and decreased offspring survival rates after birth. In humans, the FDA categorizes this drug as category *B* for use during pregnancy (*Animal studies have not yet demonstrated risk to the fetus, but there are no adequate studies in pregnant women; or animal studies have shown an adverse effect, but adequate studies in pregnant women have not demonstrated a risk to the fetus in the first trimester of pregnancy, and there is no evidence of risk in later trimesters.*)

In humans, propofol is not recommended for use in nursing mothers because propofol is excreted in maternal milk and the effects of oral absorption of small amounts of propofol are not known. Use with caution in nursing veterinary patients.

Overdosage/Acute Toxicity

Overdosages are likely to cause significant respiratory depression and, potentially, cardiovascular depression. Treatment should consist of propofol discontinuation, artificial ventilation with oxygen and, if necessary, symptomatic and supportive treatment for cardiovascular depression (*e.g.*, intravenous fluids, pressors, anticholinergics, etc.).

Drug Interactions

The following drug interactions have either been reported or are theoretical in humans or animals receiving propofol and may be of significance in veterinary patients. Unless otherwise noted, use together is not necessarily contraindicated, but weigh the potential risks and perform additional monitoring when appropriate.

- **ANESTHETICS, INHALATION** (*e.g.*, **isoflurane**): Propofol serum concentrations may be increased.
- **ANESTHETICS, LOCAL**: Propofol dosage requirements for sedation or hypnosis reduced.
- **ANTICHOLINERGICS**: Propofol-induced bradycardia may be exacerbated in animals, particularly when opiate premedicants are used.
- **CHLORAMPHENICOL**: May decrease clearance of propofol and increase recovery times.
- **CLONIDINE**: When used as a premed, may reduce propofol dosage requirements.
- **CNS DEPRESSANTS**: Increased sedative, anesthetic, and cardiorespiratory depression possible.
- **DRUGS THAT INHIBIT THE HEPATIC P-450 ENZYME SYSTEM** (*e.g.*, **chloramphenicol, cimetidine, ketoconazole**, etc.): May potentially increase the recovery times associated with propofol; clinical significance is unclear, but it may be of significance in cats.
- **FENTANYL**: In pediatric (human) patients increased risk for bradycardia.
- **MEDETOMIDINE; DEXMEDETOMIDINE**: When propofol is used after medetomidine, hypoxemia may occur; dosage adjustments may be required along with adequate monitoring.
- **METOCLOPRAMIDE**: In humans, metoclopramide reduced the propofol dose required for induction by 20-25%.
- **MIDAZOLAM**: May have synergistic effects with propofol, midazolam plasma concentrations may be increased up to 20%.
- **OPIATES**: May increase the serum concentrations of both the opiate and propofol if used together.

Doses

- **DOGS:**

  ### Labeled Doses (FDA-Approved):

  For induction of general anesthesia using *PropoFlo® 28*: Dose should be titrated against the response of the patient over 30-60 seconds or until clinical signs show the onset of anesthesia. Rapid injection of propofol (<5 seconds) may be associated with an increased incidence of apnea. The average propofol induction dose rates for healthy dogs given propofol alone, or when propofol is preceded by a premedicant, are indicated in the table below. This table is for guidance only. The dose and rate should be based upon patient response.

<u>Induction Dosage Guidelines:</u>

Preanesthetic	Propofol Induction Dose: (mg/kg)	Propofol Rate of Administration		
		Seconds	mg/kg/min	mL/kg/min
None	5.5	40-60	5.5 – 8.3	0.55 – 0.83
Acepromazine	3.7	30-50	4.4 – 7.4	0.44 – 0.74
Acepromazine / Oxymorphone	2.6	30-50	3.1 – 5.2	0.31 – 0.52

Propofol doses and rates for the above premedicants were based upon the following average dosages which may be lower than the label directions for their use as a single medication: Acepromazine 0.06 mg/kg IM, SC, IV; Oxymorphone 0.09 mg/kg IM, SC, IV; Xylazine 0.33 IM, SC. The use of these drugs as preanesthetics markedly reduces propofol requirements. As with other sedative hypnotic agents, the amount of opioid and/or alpha2 agonist premedication will influence the response of the patient to an induction dose of propofol. In the presence of premedication, the dose of propofol may be reduced with increasing age of the animal. The dose of propofol should always be titrated against the response of the patient. During induction, additional low doses of propofol, similar to those used for maintenance with propofol, may be administered to facilitate intubation or the transition to inhalant maintenance anesthesia.

Maintenance of general anesthesia using *PropoFlo® 28*: <u>Intermittent Propofol Injections</u>: Anesthesia can be maintained by administering propofol in intermittent IV injections. Clinical response will be determined by the amount and the frequency of maintenance injections. The following table is provided for guidance:

Preanesthetic	Propofol Maintenance Dose: mg/kg	Propofol Rate of Administration		
		Seconds	mg/kg/min	mL/kg/min
None	2.2	10-30	4.4 – 13.2	0.44 – 1.32
Acepromazine	1.6	10-30	3.2 – 9.6	0.32 – 0.96
Acepromazine / Oxymorphone	1.8	10-30	3.6 – 10.8	0.36 – 1.08

Repeated maintenance doses of propofol do not result in increased recovery times or dosing intervals, indicating that the anesthetic effects of propofol are not cumulative.

B. <u>Maintenance by Inhalant Anesthetics</u>: Due to the rapid metabolism of propofol, additional low doses of propofol, similar to those used for maintenance with propofol, may be required to complete the transition to inhalant maintenance anesthesia. Clinical trials using propofol have shown that it may be necessary to use a higher initial concentration of the inhalant anesthetic halothane than is usually required following induction using barbiturate anesthetics, due to rapid recovery from propofol. (Label Information; *PropoFlo®*—Abbott)

<u>Extra-label Doses</u>: **Note:** The following dosages are for propofol macroemulsion unless otherwise noted.

For anesthetic induction and total intravenous anesthesia maintenance:

a) Propofol for induction is dosed to effect. Most recommend a dose between 6 – 8 mg/kg IV slowly (over approximately 60 seconds) to effect. Preanesthetic medications can reduce propofol requirements for induction by 25% (or more). General anesthesia can be maintained with a CRI of 0.1 – 0.5 mg/kg/minute. Must be monitored with 0$_2$/ventilation support. **Note:** Propofol alone does **NOT** have analgesic effects.

b) Study was done in healthy dogs undergoing OHE comparing propofol with alfaxalone. Dogs received acepromazine

(0.01 mg/kg) and morphine (0.4 mg/kg) SC approximately 30 minutes prior to general anesthesia. Induction was performed with propofol at approximately 6 mg/kg IV over about 40 seconds to effect. Patient intubated and O$_2$ given. General anesthesia was maintained with a CRI at 0.3 – 0.5 mg/kg/minute. Authors concluded that both alfaxalone and propofol in this protocol produced good quality anesthesia adequate for OHE. Ventilatory support during prolonged infusion periods with either agent is needed. (Suarez *et al.* 2012)

For refractory status epilepticus (extra-label): If seizures persist after diazepam and phenobarbital therapy propofol may be used as a substitute for pentobarbital if general anesthesia is required to control seizure activity. Because of its short duration of action, it must be given as a CRI: 6 mg/kg IV initial bolus followed by 0.1 – 0.6 mg/kg/minute CRI. Substantial respiratory depression and apnea can occur and anesthesia must be closely monitored with oxygen and ventilatory assistance when required. Propofol can also have pro-convulsant effects in some patients. Propofol dose should be kept as low, and duration of treatment as short, as possible. Maintain infusion for 6-12 hours and then gradually decrease. Maximum duration of propofol CRI is approximately 48 hours. Adapted from: (Knipe 2006), (Mariani 2010)

■ **CATS:**

<u>Extra-label doses</u>: **Note:** The following dosages are for propofol macroemulsion unless otherwise noted.

For anesthetic induction and total intravenous anesthesia maintenance: Propofol for induction is dosed to effect. Most recommend a dose between 6 – 8 mg/kg IV slowly (over approximately 60 seconds) to effect. Preanesthetic medications can reduce propofol requirements for induction by 25% (or more). General anesthesia can be maintained with a CRI of 0.1 – 0.5 mg/kg/minute, but cats may be susceptible to long recoveries when propofol is used alone as a CRI. Must be monitored with 0$_2$/ventilation support. **Note:** Propofol alone does **NOT** have analgesic effects.

For total intravenous anesthesia with ketamine (extra-label): Study was done in cats undergoing OHE. Anesthesia was induced with a ketamine (2 mg/kg) and propofol (2 mg/kg) combination IV (some cats also received dexmedetomidine 0.003 mg/kg). Anesthesia was maintained with an IV infusion of the 1:1 ketamine-propofol combination at a rate of 10 mg/kg/hour (for each drug) Authors concluded that total IV anesthesia with a ketamine-propofol combination, with or without dexmedetomidine, appeared to be effective in healthy cats. Short-term infusions produced smooth recovery and adequate analgesia during the postoperative period. (Ravasio *et al.* 2012)

For refractory status epilepticus (extra-label): Propofol may be used as a substitute for pentobarbital if general anesthesia is required to control seizure activity. Because of its short duration of action, it must be given as a CRI: 6 mg/kg IV initial bolus followed by 0.1 – 0.6 mg/kg/min (6 – 36 mg/kg/hour) CRI. Substantial respiratory depression can occur and anesthesia must be closely monitored. Also, propofol can have pro-convulsant effects in some patients. Carefully monitor PVC and CBC (Heinz body anemia, hemolytic anemia). Propofol dose should be kept as low, and duration of treatment as short as possible. Maintain infusion for 6-12 hours and then gradually decrease. Maximum duration of propofol CRI is approximately 48 hours. Adapted from: (Knipe 2006), (Mariani 2010)

■ **HORSES:**

For induction of general anesthesia using ketamine and propofol after xylazine sedation (extra-label): From a retrospective study (n=100). All horses were sedated with xylazine at 0.99 ± 0.2 mg/kg IV. Some also received IV butorphanol. After visually apparent sedation, a combination of propofol 0.40 ± (0.1) mg/kg and ketamine 2.8 ± (0.3) mg/kg were given via IV bolus. The order of administration was not standardized and in some cases, the two drugs were mixed together before administration. Following induction, 6 horses required a onetime administration of additional ketamine (0.7±0.4 mg/kg). Anesthesia was maintained with GKX in 34 horses and with isoflurane in oxygen in 66 horses. (Posner *et al.* 2013)

- **SHEEP, GOATS:**

For general anesthesia (goats) (extra-label): Induction: 3 – 7 mg/kg IV. Induction is smooth and rapid, although myoclonic activity of the face or limbs may occur; anesthesia lasts for 5-10 minutes and is suitable for endotracheal intubation. Anesthesia can be maintained with a CRI of 0.3 – 0.6 mg/kg/min. Propofol has no analgesic effect and apnea is common; supplemental oxygen and ventilation should be provided. (Galatos 2011)

- **RABBITS, RODENTS, SMALL MAMMALS:**

Rabbits: 5 – 14 mg/kg slow IV (20 mg/kg/minute) to effect; not recommended as the sole agent for maintenance. (Ivey *et al.* 2000)

Mice: 26 mg/kg IV. **Rats:** 10 mg/kg IV. (Adamcak *et al.* 2000)

- **REPTILES:**

For sedation (extra-label): Chelonians: 2- 5 mg IV (also provides light anesthesia); **Lizards:** 3 – 5 mg/kg IV or IO. **Snakes:** 3 – 5 mg/kg IV (can also provide light sedation). (Sladky *et al.* 2012)

For anesthesia induction (extra-label): 5 – 15 mg/kg IV or IO; in snakes intracardiac route is usually used. (Innis 2003)

- **ZOO, EXOTIC, WILDLIFE SPECIES:**

For use of propofol in zoo, exotic and wildlife medicine refer to specific references, including:

a) *Zoo Animal and Wildlife Immobilization and Anesthesia.* West, G., Heard, D., Caulkett, N. (eds.). Blackwell Publishing, 2007.

b) Handbook of Wildlife Chemical Immobilization, 3rd Ed. Kreeger, T.J. and J.M. Arnemo. 2007.

c) Fowler's Zoo and Wild Animal Medicine Current Therapy, Volume 7, Miller, R.E., Fowler, M.E., Saunders. 2011.

d) *Exotic Animal Formulary, 4th Ed.* Carpenter, J.W., Saunders. 2012.

e) The 2009 American Association of Zoo Veterinarian Proceedings by D. K. Fontenot also has several dosages listed for restraint, anesthesia, and analgesia for a variety of drugs for carnivores and primates. VIN members can access them at: http://goo.gl/NNIWQ or http://goo.gl/9UJse

Monitoring
- Level of anesthesia/CNS effects.
- Respiratory depression (respiratory rate, 02 saturation, etc.).
- Cardiovascular status (cardiac rate/rhythm; blood pressure).

Chemistry/Synonyms
Propofol is an alkylphenol derivative (2,6-diisopropylphenol). The commercially available injections are either a milky-white macroemulsion containing 100 mg/mL of soybean oil, 22.5 mg/mL of glycerol, and 12 mg/mL of egg lecithin with a pH of 7-8.5 or a clear (at room temperature) lipid-free microemulsion may contain disodium edetate, benzyl alcohol, or sodium metabisulfite as preservatives. 1% propofol macroemulsion is isotonic.

The human products *Diprivan®* and some generically labeled products are not identical. Disodium edetate is the antimicrobial agent in *Diprivan®* and generic products use either sodium metabisulfite or benzyl alcohol. *Diprivan®* and the generic propofol with benzyl alcohol have a pH range of 7-8.5. Products that use sodium metabisulfite, the pH is adjusted to 4.5-6.4.

Propofol may also be known as: disoprofol, ICI-35868, propofolum, *Ansiven®, Bioprofol®, Cryotol®, Diprofol®, Diprivan®, Disoprivan®, Fresofol®, Ivofol®, Klimofol®, Oleo-Lax®, Pofol®, Profolen®, Pronest®, Propoabbott®, Propocam®, PropoClear®, PropoFlo®, Propovan®, Provive®, Rapinovet®, Recofol®,* or *Recofol®.*

Storage/Stability
Macroemulsion (*PropoFlo® 28*): Store at room temperature. Once a vial is opened, the contents begin a 28-day shelf life. The opened vial should be labeled with "Date Opened" and "Use By" in the space provided. To avoid microbial overgrowth, the contents must be used within 28 days (4 weeks) of the date opened. The opened vial should be placed in a covered container, held at room temperature and used within the allotted 28-day timeframe. Refrigeration is not recommended. Any unused propofol remaining at the end of 28 days should be discarded. Shake the vial thoroughly before opening. Do not use if there is evidence of excessive creaming or aggregation, if large droplets are visible, or if there are other forms of phase separation indicating that the stability of the product has been compromised. Slight creaming, which should disappear after shaking, may be visible upon prolonged standing. Do not use if particulate matter and discoloration are present. Do not use if contamination is suspected.

Macroemulsion (human-labeled products): Store below 22°C (72°F), but not below 4°C (40°F.); do not refrigerate or freeze. Protect from light. Shake well before using. Do not use if the emulsion has separated. The manufacturer recommends discarding any unused portion at the end of the anesthetic procedure or after 6 hours, whichever occurs sooner. If using in-line filters, do not use sizes < 5 microns.

Microemulsion: Store propofol (microemulsion) injection protected from light at controlled room temperature. Do not store above 30°C and do not refrigerate. Exposure for an extended period to temperatures below 20°C may result in a cloudy appearance. A clear appearance will return upon allowing the product to warm to 20-30°C. Gentle agitation will speed the process. Do not administer if opaque or precipitates are noted. Discard unused portions 28 days after first use.

Compatibility/Compounding Considerations
Propofol (macroemulsion; *PropoFlo® 28*): Label states: "The emulsion should not be mixed with other therapeutic agents prior to administration."

Propofol (macroemulsion; *Diprivan®* human-label product): If dilution is necessary, only dilute with dextrose 5% injection and do not dilute to a concentration of <2 mg/mL. In diluted form, it is more stable when in contact with glass than with plastic (95% potency after 2 hours of running infusion in plastics).

Propofol macroemulsion (human-label) is physically **compatible** with the commonly used IV solutions (*e.g.*, LRS, D5W) when injected into a running IV line.

Drugs that are reported to be **compatible** with propofol (macroemulsion) at Y-site administration include (partial listing): alfentanil, ampicillin, butorphanol, calcium gluconate, cefazolin, cefoxitin, clindamycin, dexamethasone sodium phosphate, dexmedetomidine, diphenhydramine, dobutamine, dopamine, esmolol, epinephrine, fentanyl, furosemide, glycopyrrolate, heparin sodium, insulin, ketamine, lidocaine, lorazepam, magnesium sulfate, midazolam, morphine sulfate, mannitol, naloxone, nitroprusside sodium, norepinephrine, pentobarbital, phenobarbital, potassium chloride, propranolol, sodium bicarbonate, succinylcholine and vecuronium.

It is <u>incompatible</u> at Y-sites with amphotericin B, atracurium, calcium chloride, ceftazidime, diazepam, gentamicin, methylprednisolone sodium succinate, phenytoin, tobramycin and verapamil. Refer to specialized references or a hospital pharmacist for more information.

Dosage Forms/Regulatory Status

VETERINARY-LABELED PRODUCTS:

Propofol Injectable (macroemulsion): 10 mg/mL in 5 mL and 20 mL (single use) vials; *PropoFlo* 28®; (Rx). FDA-approved for use in dogs.

Propofol Injectable (microemulsion): 10 mg/mL in 20 mL, 50 mL and 100 mL multi-dose vials; *PropoClear*®; (Rx). FDA-approved for use in dogs and cats. At time of update, does not appear to be marketed in USA.

The ARCI (Racing Commissioners International) has designated this drug as a class 2 substance. See the appendix for more information.

HUMAN-LABELED PRODUCTS:

Propofol Injectable Emulsion: 10 mg/mL in 20 mL amps & vials, 50 mL & 100 mL vials; 50 mL & 100 mL infusion vials and 50 mL pre-filled single-use syringes; *Diprivan*®, *Fresenius Propoven*®, generic; (Rx)

Revisions/References

Monograph revised/updated June 2014.

Adamcak, A. & B. Otten (2000). Rodent Therapeutics. Vet Clin NA: Exotic Anim Pract **3**:1(Jan): 221-40.

Boveri, S., et al. (2013). The effect of body condition on propofol requirement in dogs. Veterinary Anaesthesia and Analgesia **40**(5): 449-54.

Galatos, A. D. (2011). Anesthesia and Analgesia in Sheep and Goats. Veterinary Clinics of North America-Food Animal Practice **27**(1): 47-+.

Griffenhagen, G., et al. (2013a). Pharmacodynamics of Intravenous Administration of a Single Induction Dose of Propofol With or Without 2% Benzyl Alcohol in Cats. Proceedings; IVECCS. accessed via Veterinary Information Network; vin.com

Griffenhagen, G., et al. (2013b). Pharmacokinetics of a Single Induction Dose of Propofol With or Without 2% Benzyl Alcohol Administered Intravenously in Cats. Proceedings: IVECCS. accessed via Veterinary Information Network; vin.com

Innis, C. (2003). Advances in anesthesia and analgesia in reptiles. Proceedings: Western Veterinary Conference. accessed via Veterinary Information Network; vin.com

Ivey, E. & J. Morrisey (2000). Therapeutics for Rabbits. Vet Clin NA: Exotic Anim Pract **3**:1(Jan): 183-216.

Knipe, M. (2006). Make it stop! Managing status epilepticus. Proceedings; Vet Neuro Symposium. accessed via Veterinary Information Network; vin.com

Mariani, C. (2010). Treatment of cluster seizures and stauts epilepticus. Proceedings: ACVIM Forum. accessed via Veterinary Information Network; vin.com

Michou, J. N., et al. (2012). Comparison of pain on injection during induction of anaesthesia with alfaxalone and two formulations of propofol in dogs. Veterinary Anaesthesia and Analgesia **39**(3): 275-81.

Minghella, E., et al. (2010). Pain after injection of a new formulation of propofol in six dogs. Veterinary Record **167**(22): 866-7.

Posner, L. P., et al. (2013). Propofol with ketamine following sedation with xylazine for routine induction of general anaesthesia in horses. Veterinary Record **173**(22): 550-+.

Ravasio, G., et al. (2012). Evaluation of a ketamine-propofol drug combination with or without dexmedetomidine for intravenous anesthesia in cats undergoing ovariectomy. Javma-Journal of the American Veterinary Medical Association **241**(10): 1307-13.

Sanchez, A., et al. (2013). Effects of altering the sequence of midazolam and propofol during co-induction of anaesthesia. Veterinary Anaesthesia and Analgesia **40**(4): 359-66.

Sladky, K. K. & C. Mans (2012). Clinical anesthesia in reptiles. Journal of Exotic Pet Medicine **21**(1): 17-31.

Suarez, M. A., et al. (2012). Comparison of alfaxalone and propofol administered as total intravenous anaesthesia for ovariohysterectomy in dogs. Veterinary Anaesthesia and Analgesia **39**(3): 236-44.

Taylor, P. M., et al. (2012). Evaluation of propofol containing 2% benzyl alcohol preservative in cats. Journal of Feline Medicine and Surgery **14**(8): 516-26.

Zoran, D. L., et al. (1993). Pharmacokinetics of propofol in mixed-breed dogs and greyhounds. American Journal of Veterinary Research **54**(5): 755-60.

Propranolol HCl

(proe-**pran**-oh-lole)   Inderal®

Beta-Adrenergic Blocker

Prescriber Highlights

▶ Non specific beta blocker primarily used in veterinary medicine as an antiarrhythmic agent. Sometimes used for short-term treatment of clinical signs associated with thyrotoxicosis or pheochromocytoma.

▶ Contraindications: Heart failure, hypersensitivity to this class of agents, greater than 1st degree heart block, or sinus bradycardia; generally contraindicated in patients with CHF unless secondary to a tachyarrhythmia responsive to beta-blockers or with bronchospastic lung disease. Caution: Significant renal or hepatic insufficiency, sinus node dysfunction, labile diabetic patients, digitalized or digitalis intoxicated patients.

▶ Adverse Effects: Bradycardia, lethargy, & depression, impaired AV conduction, CHF or worsening of heart failure, hypotension, syncope, diarrhea, hypoglycemia, & bronchoconstriction.

▶ If discontinuing drug, consider gradual withdrawal if it has been used chronically.

▶ Drug Interactions.

Uses/Indications

While propranolol is used for hypertension, migraine headache prophylaxis, and angina in human patients, it is used primarily in veterinary medicine for acute treatment of atrial premature complexes, ventricular premature complexes, supraventricular premature complexes and tachyarrhythmias, ventricular or atrial tachyarrhythmias secondary to digitalis, atrial tachycardia secondary to Wolff-Parkinson-White (WPW) with normal QRS complexes, and atrial fibrillation (generally in combination with digoxin). Other beta-blockers have largely supplanted its use due to propranolol's poor oral bioavailability, short half-life, and non-specificity.

Propranolol has also been used for the short-term treatment of hypertension and clinical signs associated with thyrotoxicosis in cats and pheochromocytoma in dogs.

Pharmacology/Actions

Propranolol blocks both $beta_1$- and $beta_2$-adrenergic receptors in the myocardium, bronchi, and vascular smooth muscle. Propranolol does not have any intrinsic sympathomimetic activity (ISA). Additionally, propranolol possesses membrane-stabilizing effects (quinidine-like) affecting the cardiac action potential and direct myocardial depressant effects. Cardiovascular effects secondary to propranolol include: decreased sinus heart rate, depressed AV conduction, diminished cardiac output at rest and during exercise, decreased myocardial oxygen demand, decreased hepatic and renal blood flow, reduced blood pressure, and inhibition of isoproterenol-induced tachycardia. Electrophysiologic effects on the heart include decreased automaticity, increased or no effect on effective refractory period, and no effect on conduction velocity.

Additional pharmacologic effects of propranolol, include increased airway resistance (especially in patients with bronchoconstrictive disease), prevention of migraine headaches, increased uterine activity (more so in the non-pregnant uterus), decreased platelet aggregability, inhibited glycogenolysis in cardiac and skeletal muscle, and increased numbers of circulating eosinophils.

Pharmacokinetics

Propranolol is well absorbed after oral administration, but a rapid first-pass effect through the liver reduces systemic bioavailability to ≈ 2-27% in dogs, thereby explaining the significant difference between oral and intravenous dosages. These values reportedly increase with chronic dosing. Hyperthyroid cats may have increased bioavailability of propranolol when compared with normal cats.

Propranolol is highly lipid soluble and readily crosses the blood-brain barrier. The apparent volume of distribution has been reported to 3.3-11 L/kg in the dog. Propranolol crosses the placenta and enters milk (at very low levels). In humans, propranolol is ≈ 90% bound to plasma proteins.

Propranolol metabolization occurs principally by the liver. The CYP2D15 isoenzyme is responsible for a significant percentage of propranolol's metabolism in dogs. An active metabolite, 4-hydroxypropranolol, has been identified after oral administration in humans. Less than 1% of a dose is excreted unchanged into the urine. The half-life in dogs has been reported to range from 0.77-2 hours, and in horses, <2 hours. It has been reported that hyperthyroid cats have a decreased clearance of propranolol when compared with normal cats.

Contraindications/Precautions/Warnings

Propranolol is contraindicated in patients with overt heart failure, hypersensitivity to this class of agents, greater than 1st degree heart block, or sinus bradycardia. Non-specific beta-blockers are generally contraindicated in patients with CHF unless secondary to a tachyarrhythmia responsive to beta-blocker therapy. They are also relatively contraindicated in patients with bronchospastic lung disease.

Propranolol should be used cautiously in patients with significant renal or hepatic insufficiency, or with sinus node dysfunction. In humans, it has been suggested to reduce dosage by 50% (or more) in patients with hepatic failure.

Propranolol can mask the clinical signs associated with hypoglycemia. It can also cause hypoglycemia or hyperglycemia and, therefore, should be used cautiously in labile diabetic patients.

Propranolol can mask the clinical signs associated with thyrotoxicosis, but it has been used clinically to treat the clinical signs associated with this condition.

Use propranolol cautiously with digoxin or in digoxin-intoxicated patients; severe bradycardias may result.

Adverse Effects

It is reported that adverse effects most commonly occur in geriatric animals or those that have acute decompensating heart disease. Clinically relevant adverse effects include: bradycardia, lethargy and depression, impaired AV conduction, CHF or worsening of heart failure, hypotension, hypoglycemia, and bronchoconstriction. Syncope and diarrhea have also been reported in canine patients.

Exacerbations of clinical signs have been reported following abrupt cessation of beta-blockers in humans. It is recommended to withdraw therapy gradually in patients who have been receiving the drug chronically.

Reproductive/Nursing Safety

In humans, the FDA categorizes this drug as category C for use during pregnancy (*Animal studies have shown an adverse effect on the fetus, but there are no adequate studies in humans; or there are no animal reproduction studies and no adequate studies in humans.*) In a separate system evaluating the safety of drugs in canine and feline pregnancy (Papich 1989), this drug is categorized as class: C (*These drugs may have potential risks. Studies in people or laboratory animals have uncovered risks, and these drugs should be used cautiously as a last resort when the benefit of therapy clearly outweighs the risks.*)

Propranolol is excreted in maternal milk. Use with caution in nursing patients.

Overdosage/Acute Toxicity

The most predominant clinical signs expected would be hypotension and bradycardia. Other possible effects could include: CNS (depressed consciousness to seizures), bronchospasm, hypoglycemia, hyperkalemia, respiratory depression, pulmonary edema, other arrhythmias (especially AV block), or asystole.

There were 243 single agent exposures to propranolol reported to the ASPCA Animal Poison Control Center (APCC) during 2009-2013. Of the 204 dogs, 26 were symptomatic with 27% having bradycardia. Of the 46 cats, 8 were symptomatic.

If overdose is secondary to a recent oral ingestion, emptying the gut and charcoal administration may be considered. Seizures are reported in people, but in a review of the APCC database, seizures were not reported in animals. Monitor patient's ECG, blood glucose, potassium and, if possible, blood pressure; treatment of the cardiovascular and CNS effects are symptomatic. Use fluids and pressor agents to treat hypotension. Bradycardia may be treated with atropine. If atropine fails, isoproterenol given cautiously has been recommended. Use of a transvenous pacemaker may be necessary. Cardiac failure can be treated with digoxin, diuretics, oxygen and, if necessary, IV aminophylline. Glucagon (5 – 10 mg IV; human dose) may increase heart rate and blood pressure and reduce the cardiodepressant effects of propranolol. Seizures generally will respond to IV diazepam.

Drug Interactions

The following drug interactions have either been reported or are theoretical in humans or animals receiving propranolol and may be of significance in veterinary patients. Unless otherwise noted, use together is not necessarily contraindicated, but weigh the potential risks and perform additional monitoring when appropriate.

- **ANTACIDS:** May reduce oral propranolol absorption; separate doses by at least one hour.
- **ANESTHETICS, GENERAL:** Additive myocardial depression may occur with the concurrent use of propranolol and myocardial depressant anesthetic agents.
- **ANTICHOLINERGICS:** May negate cardiac effects of beta-blockers.
- **CALCIUM CHANNEL BLOCKERS:** Concurrent use of beta-blockers with calcium channel blockers (or other negative inotropes) should be done with caution, particularly in patients with preexisting cardiomyopathy or CHF.
- **CIMETIDINE:** May decrease the metabolism of propranolol and increase blood levels.
- **DIURETICS:** May increase risk for hypotension.
- **EPINEPHRINE:** Unopposed alpha effects of epinephrine may lead to rapid increases in blood pressure and decrease in heart rate.
- **FLUOXETINE:** May decrease propranolol metabolism; complete heart block reported in one human.
- **INSULIN** and other **ANTIDIABETIC DRUGS:** Propranolol may prolong the hypoglycemic effects of insulin therapy.
- **LIDOCAINE:** Clearance may be impaired by propranolol.
- **METHIMAZOLE, PROPYLTHIOURACIL:** Propranolol doses may need to be decreased when initiating therapy.
- **PHENOBARBITAL:** May increase the metabolism of propranolol.
- **PHENOTHIAZINES:** May increase risk for hypotension.
- **RESERPINE:** May have additive effects with propranolol.
- **SUCCINYLCHOLINE, TUBOCURARINE:** Effects may be enhanced with propranolol therapy.
- **SYMPATHOMIMETICS** (*e.g.,* terbutaline, **beta effects of epinephrine, phenylpropanolamine,** etc.): May have their actions blocked by propranolol.
- **THEOPHYLLINE:** Effects of theophylline (bronchodilation) may be blocked by propranolol.

- THYROID HORMONES: May decrease the effects of beta blocking agents.

Doses

- **DOGS/CATS:**

Note: Because of a high-first pass effect after oral dosing, intravenous doses are approximately 10% of oral doses. Do not confuse the two.

For susceptible cardiac arrhythmias (extra-label): <u>IV Dose:</u> Initially at 0.02 mg/kg IV slowly over 2-3 minutes, titrate dose up to effect (to a maximum of 1 mg/kg). Can be repeated in 8 hours. <u>Oral dose dogs:</u> 0.1 – 0.2 mg/kg initially PO q8h (practically 2.5 – 10 mg per dog PO q8h), titrated to effect up to a maximum of 1.5 mg/kg q8h (practically 10 – 80 mg per dog PO q8h). <u>Oral dose cats:</u> 2.5 mg (up to 10 mg) per cat PO q8-12h.

For adjunctive treatment of severe thyrotoxicosis (thyroid storm); (extra-label): Cats: 5 mg per cat PO q8h or 0.02 mg/kg IV (over one minute). (Ward 2013)

- **FERRETS:**

For hypertrophic cardiomyopathy (extra-label): 0.5 – 2 mg/kg PO or SC once a day to twice a day. (Williams 2000)

- **HORSES:** (NOTE: ARCI UCGFS CLASS 3 DRUG)

For ventricular tachycardia (extra-label) 0.03 – 0.15 mg/kg IV or 0.3 – 0.7 mg/kg PO q8h. Considered not as effective as lidocaine; decreases ventricular rate even if it does not restore sinus rhythm. Toxic effects include bradycardia, AV block, proarrhythmic, negative inotrope and hypotension. Use with caution in animals with airway disease (bronchoconstriction). (Kimberly *et al.* 2006)

Monitoring

- ECG.
- Toxicity (see Adverse Effects/Overdosage).
- Blood pressure if administering IV.

Client Information

- Most common side effects include lethargy (tiredness/lack of energy/weakness) & diarrhea. A heartbeat that is too slow can occur if dose is too high and heart symptoms can get worse.
- When starting this drug, your veterinarian may start with a low dose and gradually increase the dose over time to see how your animal reacts.
- Very important not to stop the drug abruptly without veterinarian's guidance.

Chemistry/Synonyms

A non-specific beta-adrenergic blocking agent, propranolol HCl occurs as a bitter tasting, odorless, white to almost white powder with a pK_a of 9.45 and a melting point of ≈ 161°C. One gram of propranolol is soluble in ≈ 20 mL of water or alcohol. At a pH from 4-5, solutions of propranolol will fluoresce. The commercially available injectable solutions are adjusted with citric acid to a pH 2.8-3.5.

Propranolol may also be known as: AY-64043, ICI-45520, NSC-91523, propranololi hydrochloridum; many trade names are available.

Storage/Stability

All propranolol preparations should be stored at room temperature (15-30°C) and protected from light. Propranolol solutions will decompose rapidly at alkaline pH.

Compatibility/Compounding Considerations

Propranolol injection is reported to be physically **compatible** with D_5W, 0.9% sodium chloride, or lactated Ringer's injection. It is also physically **compatible** with dobutamine HCl and verapamil HCl.

Dosage Forms/Regulatory Status

VETERINARY-LABELED PRODUCTS: NONE.

HUMAN-LABELED PRODUCTS:

Propranolol HCl Oral Tablets: 10 mg, 20 mg, 40 mg, 60 mg & 80 mg; generic; (Rx)

Propranolol HCl Extended/Sustained-Release Capsules: 60 mg, 80 mg, 120 mg & 160 mg; *Inderal® LA* , *Inderal XL®*, *InnoPran® XL*, generic; (Rx)

Propranolol for Injection: 1 mg/mL in 1 mL amps or vials; *Inderal®*, generic; (Rx)

Propranolol Oral Solution: 4 mg/mL & 8 mg/mL in 500 mL; generic; (Rx)

Revisions/References

Monograph revised/updated June 2014.

Kimberly, M. & K. McGurrin (2006). Update on antiarrhythmic therapy in horses. Proceedings; ACVIM. accessed via Veterinary Information Network; vin.com

Papich, M. (1989). Effects of drugs on pregnancy. *Current Veterinary Therapy X: Small Animal Practice.* R. Kirk. Philadelphia, Saunders: 1291-9.

Ward, C. (2013). Feline Hyperthyroidism: The Usual and Unusual. Proceedings; ACVC. accessed via Veterinary Information Network; vin.com

Williams, B. (2000). Therapeutics in Ferrets. Vet Clin NA: Exotic Anim Pract 3:1(Jan): 131-53.

Prostaglandin F$_2$ alpha – see Dinoprost Tromethamine

Protamine Sulfate

(proe-ta-meen)

Antidote (Heparin)

Prescriber Highlights

▶ Protein that complexes with heparin (treatment of overdoses); may also be useful for Bracken Fern poisoning.

▶ Contraindications: Hypersensitivity to protamine.

▶ Adverse Effects: If injected IV too rapidly: Acute hypotension, bradycardia, pulmonary hypertension, & dyspnea; hypersensitivity possible.

▶ Monitor for heparin "rebound effect".

Uses/Indications

Protamine is used in all species for the treatment of heparin overdosage when significant bleeding occurs. While protamine will neutralize the anti-thrombin effects of low molecular weight heparins (*e.g.*, dalteparin or enoxaparin), it does not completely inhibit their anti-Xa activity. Laboratory animal studies however, show it does improve microvascular bleeding associated with LMWH overdoses. Protamine has been suggested for use for Bracken Fern toxicity in ruminants (see Doses).

Pharmacology/Actions

Protamine is strongly basic and heparin, strongly acidic; protamine complexes with heparin to form an inactive stable salt. Protamine has intrinsic anticoagulant activity, but its effects are weak and rarely cause problems.

Pharmacokinetics

After IV injection, protamine binds to heparin within 5 minutes. The exact metabolic fate of the heparin-protamine complex is not known, but there is evidence that the complex is partially metabolized and/or degraded by fibrinolysin thus freeing heparin.

Contraindications/Precautions/Warnings

Protamine is contraindicated in patients who have demonstrated hypersensitivity or intolerance to the drug in the past.

Adverse Effects

If protamine sulfate is injected IV too rapidly, acute hypotension, bradycardia, pulmonary hypertension, and dyspnea can occur.

These effects are usually absent or minimized when the drug is administered slowly (over 1-3 minutes). Hypersensitivity reactions have also been reported.

A heparin "rebound" effect has been reported where anticoagulation and bleeding occur several hours after heparin has apparently been neutralized. This may be due to either a release of heparin from extravascular compartments or the release of heparin from the protamine-heparin complex.

Reproductive/Nursing Safety

In humans, the FDA categorizes this drug as category C for use during pregnancy (*Animal studies have shown an adverse effect on the fetus, but there are no adequate studies in humans; or there are no animal reproduction studies and no adequate studies in humans.*)

It is not known whether this drug is excreted in milk.

Overdosage/Acute Toxicity

Because protamine has inherent anticoagulant activity, overdoses of protamine may, theoretically, result in hemorrhage; however, in one human study, overdoses of 600 – 800 mg resulted only in mild, transient effects on coagulation. The LD_{50} of protamine in mice is 100 mg/kg.

Drug Interactions; Laboratory Considerations

- None were located.

Doses

- **DOGS & CATS:**

  For heparin overdosage (life-threatening bleeding); (extra-label): Administer 1 mg protamine for each 100 Units of heparin to be inactivated. Decrease the protamine dose by 50% for every 30-60 minutes that has lapsed since heparin was administered. Give dose slowly IV, do not give at a rate faster than 50 mg over a 10-minute period.

- **CATTLE:**

  For Bracken Fern (*Pteridium* spp.) poisoning (extra-label): In combination with whole blood (2.25 – 4.5L), 1 injection of 10 mL of 1% protamine sulfate IV. (Osweiler *et al.* 1986)

Monitoring

- See the Heparin monograph.

Client Information

- Should only be used in a setting where adequate monitoring facilities are available.

Chemistry/Synonyms

Simple, low molecular weight, cationic proteins, protamines occur naturally in the sperm of fish. Commercially available protamine sulfate is produced from protamine obtained from the sperm or mature testes of salmon (or related species). It occurs as a fine, white to off-white crystalline or amorphous powder that is sparingly soluble in water and very slightly soluble in alcohol. The injection is available as either a prepared solution with a pH of 6-7 or a lyophilized powder that has a pH of 6.5-7.5 after reconstituting.

Protamine Sulfate may also be known as: protamine sulphate, protamini sulfas, sulfato de protamina, *Prosulf®*, or *Prota®*.

Storage/Stability

The powder for injection should be stored at room temperature (15-30°C), and the injection (liquid) in the refrigerator (2-8°C); avoid freezing. The injection is stable at room temperature for at least 2 weeks, however. The powder for injection should be used immediately if reconstituted with Sterile Water for Injection and within 72 hours if reconstituted with Bacteriostatic Water for Injection.

Compatibility/Compounding Considerations

It is recommended to use either D5W or normal saline for protamine sulfate infusions. Cimetidine and verapamil are reported to be physically **compatible** with protamine sulfate for injection.

Dosage Forms/Regulatory Status

VETERINARY-LABELED PRODUCTS: NONE.

HUMAN-LABELED PRODUCTS:

Protamine Sulfate Injection: 10 mg/mL preservative-free in 5 mL and 25 mL vials; generic; (Rx)

Revisions/References

Monograph revised/updated June 2014.

Osweiler, G. D. & L. P. Ruhr (1986). Plants affecting blood coagulation. *Current Veterinary Therapy: Food Animal Practice 2.* J. L. Howard. Philadelphia, W.B. Saunders: 404-6.

Pseudoephedrine HCl

(soo-doe-e-fed-rin)   Equiphed®, Sudafed®

Sympathomimetic

Prescriber Highlights

▶ Oral sympathomimetic that has been used primarily for urethral sphincter hypotonus. Toxic to dogs at dosages close to those used therapeutically; some state that it should NOT be used in dogs.

▶ Caution: Glaucoma, prostatic hypertrophy, hyperthyroidism, diabetes mellitus, cardiovascular disorders, or hypertension.

▶ Adverse Effects: Restlessness, irritability, hypertension, & anorexia. Overdoses can be serious.

▶ Restricted drug in USA; can be used as a precursor to manufacture methamphetamine.

Uses/Indications

Pseudoephedrine is used primarily as a substitute for phenylpropanolamine for the treatment of urinary incontinence (dribbling) in dogs. However, it is toxic to dogs at dosages that are close to those used therapeutically (see Overdosage). One study showed that it was not as effective and had more adverse effects then phenylpropanolamine in dogs with urinary incontinence (Byron *et al.* 2007). Since a FDA-approved phenylpropanolamine (PPA) product for dogs is available, there is little reason to consider use of pseudoephedrine unless PPA is unavailable.

Pseudoephedrine potentially could be useful as an oral decongestant or for treating retrograde ejaculation.

Pharmacology/Actions

While the exact mechanisms of pseudoephedrine's actions are undetermined, it is believed that it indirectly stimulates both alpha- and beta- (to a lesser degree) adrenergic receptors by causing the release of norepinephrine.

Pharmacologic effects of pseudoephedrine include increased vasoconstriction, heart rate, coronary blood flow, blood pressure, mild CNS stimulation, and decreased nasal congestion and appetite. Pseudoephedrine can also increase urethral sphincter tone and produce closure of the bladder neck.

Pharmacokinetics

Pseudoephedrine is rapidly and nearly completely absorbed from the GI tract. Food may delay the absorption somewhat, but not the extent. In children, the apparent volume of distribution is ≈ 2.5 L/kg. Pseudoephedrine is only partially metabolized and the bulk is excreted unchanged in the urine. Urine pH can affect excretion rates. Alkaline urine (pH 8) can prolong half-life while acidic urine (pH 5) can decrease it.

Contraindications/Precautions/Warnings

Pseudoephedrine should be used with caution in patients with glaucoma, prostatic hypertrophy, hyperthyroidism, diabetes mellitus, cardiovascular disorders or hypertension.

Adverse Effects

Adverse effects are dose related and adrenergic in nature with panting, decreased appetite, lethargy, and rapid heart rate the most likely to be seen at usual doses; CNS excitement/restlessness/insomnia are possible. Increases in blood pressure and arrhythmias can occur in susceptible individuals, particularly at high doses.

Because pseudoephedrine may be used to manufacture methamphetamine, be alert for clients wanting to purchase very large amounts of the drug.

Reproductive/Nursing Safety

Safe use has not been established during pregnancy; use with care. In humans, the FDA categorizes this drug as category C for use during pregnancy (*Animal studies have shown an adverse effect on the fetus, but there are no adequate studies in humans; or there are no animal reproduction studies and no adequate studies in humans.*)

In humans, it is not recommended to use systemic pseudoephedrine during breastfeeding as the drug enters maternal milk and infants may be very susceptible to the drug's effects. Use with caution in veterinary patients.

Overdosage/Acute Toxicity

Overdoses of pseudoephedrine can cause hyperthermia, mydriasis, tachycardia, hypertension, vomiting, disorientation, and seizures. In small animals, adverse reactions may develop at doses of 5 – 6 mg/kg. Deaths have occurred at doses >10 – 12 mg/kg.

There were 474 single agent exposures to pseudoephedrine reported to the ASPCA Animal Poison Control Center (APCC) during 2009-2013. Of the 453 dogs, 145 were symptomatic with 46% hyperactive/agitated, 21% tachycardic, 17% mydriatic and 15% hyperthermic.

Large overdoses should be treated with gastric evacuation (if not contraindicated); otherwise, treat supportively and symptomatically (*e.g.*, propranolol for tachycardia). Phenothiazines are preferred to treat hyperactivity, agitation, and tremors as diazepam may worsen dysphoria. It is recommended to contact an animal poison control center for further guidance in the case of a large pseudoephedrine overdose.

Drug Interactions

The following drug interactions have either been reported or are theoretical in humans or animals receiving pseudoephedrine and may be of significance in veterinary patients. Unless otherwise noted, use together is not necessarily contraindicated, but weigh the potential risks and perform additional monitoring when appropriate.

- **MONAMINE OXIDASE (MAO) INHIBITORS** (*e.g.*, **amitraz**, possibly **selegiline**): Pseudoephedrine should not be given within 2 weeks of a patient receiving monoamine oxidase inhibitors.
- **RESERPINE:** An increased chance of hypertension if given concomitantly.
- **SYMPATHOMIMETIC AGENTS, OTHER:** Phenylpropanolamine should not be administered with other sympathomimetic agents (*e.g.*, **ephedrine**) as increased toxicity may result.
- **TRICYCLIC ANTIDEPRESSANTS** (**clomipramine, amitriptyline**, etc.): An increased chance of hypertension if given concomitantly.

Doses

- **DOGS:**

    To increase urethral tone (extra-label): 1.5 mg/kg PO 2-3 times a day. (Dickinson 2010)

    For retrograde ejaculation (extra-label): 4 – 5 mg/kg PO 3 times daily or 1-3 hours before semen collection or attempted breeding may be tried. (Fontbonne 2007) **Note:** Dose carefully. Dosages

above 5 mg/kg have been associated with significant toxic effects (see Overdosage).

- **CATS:**

    As a decongestant (extra-label): 1 mg/kg PO q8h. (Scherk 2010)

Monitoring

- Efficacy.
- Adverse effects (heart rate, CNS stimulation, appetite).

Client Information

- Side effects include lack of appetite, restlessness (can't settle down), reduced energy, and rapid heartbeat.
- Overdoses can be serious; keep out of reach and give only as instructed.

Chemistry/Synonyms

A sympathomimetic, pseudoephedrine HCl is the stereoisomer of ephedrine. It occurs as a fine, white to off-white powder or crystals. Approximately 2 grams are soluble in 1 mL of water.

Pseudoephedrine may also be known as: pseudoephedrini, pseudoephedrina, and *Sudafed®*.

Storage/Stability

Oral pseudoephedrine products should be stored at room temperature in tight containers. Oral liquid preparations should be protected from light and freezing.

Dosage Forms/Regulatory Status

In the USA, pseudoephedrine is classified as a list 1 chemical (drugs that can be used as precursors to manufacture methamphetamine) and in some states it may be a controlled substance or have other restrictions placed upon its sale. Be alert to persons desiring to purchase this medication.

VETERINARY-LABELED PRODUCTS: NONE.

The ARCI (Racing Commissioners International) has designated this drug as a class 3 substance. See the appendix for more information.

HUMAN-LABELED PRODUCTS:

Pseudoephedrine HCl Tablets and Capsules: 30 mg & 60 mg; Extended/Controlled Release: 120 mg and 240 mg (immediate-release 60 mg, controlled-release 180 mg). A common trade name is *Sudafed®*, but there are many others and generically labeled pseudoephedrine is available. All are OTC, but sales are now restricted to "behind-the-counter" status.

Pseudoephedrine Liquid: 3 mg/mL and 6 mg/mL in 118 mL, 120 mL, 237 mL, 480 mL and 3.8 L. A common trade name is *Sudafed®*, but there are many others, including generically labeled pseudoephedrine available. All are OTC, restricted.

Pseudoephedrine Oral Drops: 7.5 mg/0.8 mL in 15 mL & 30 mL; *Kid Kare®*, Nasal Decongestant Oral (various); (OTC, restricted)

Revisions/References

Monograph revised/updated June 2014.

Byron, J. K., et al. (2007). Effect of phenylpropanolamine and pseudoephedrine on the urethral pressure profile and continence scores of incontinent female dogs. Journal of Veterinary Internal Medicine 21(1): 47-53.

Dickinson, P. (2010). Disorders of micturition and continence. Proceedings: UCD Veterinary Neurology Symposium. accessed via Veterinary Information Network; vin.com

Fontbonne, A. (2007). Approach to infertility in the bitch and the dog. Proceedings: WSAVA World Congress. accessed via Veterinary Information Network; vin.com

Scherk, M. (2010). Snots and Snuffles: Rational approach to chronic feline upper respiratory syndromes. Journal of Feline Medicine and Surgery 12(7): 548-57.

Psyllium Hydrophilic Mucilloid

(sill-i-yum hye-droe-fill-ik **myoo**-sill-oid)   Metamucil®

Bulk Forming GI Laxative/Antidiarrheal

Prescriber Highlights

▶ Bulk-forming agent used for treatment & prevention of sand colic in horses, as a laxative, & to increase stool consistency in patients with chronic, watery diarrhea.

▶ Contraindications: Rabbits. Where prompt intestinal evacuation is required, or when fecal impaction or intestinal obstruction is present.

▶ Adverse Effects: Flatulence; if insufficient liquid is given, increased possibility of esophageal or bowel obstruction.

Uses/Indications

Bulk forming laxatives are used in patients where constipation is a result a too little fiber in their diets or when straining to defecate may be deleterious. Psyllium is considered the laxative of choice in the treatment and prevention of sand colic in horses.

Psyllium has also been used to increase stool consistency in patients with chronic, watery diarrhea. The total amount of water in the stool remains unchanged.

Psyllium added to the diet could potentially be useful in helping to control metabolic syndrome in horses.

Pharmacology/Actions

By swelling after absorbing water, psyllium increases bulk in the intestine and is believed to induce peristalsis and decrease intestinal transit time. In the treatment of sand colic in horses, psyllium is thought to help collect sand and lubricate its passage through the GI tract.

In normal, non-obese, and unexercised horses, psyllium fed for 60 days was shown to reduce postprandial blood glucose (at 90, 180, & 270 g/day) and insulin levels (at 270 g/day) (Moreaux *et al.* 2011).

Pharmacokinetics

Psyllium is not absorbed when administered orally. Laxative action may take up to 72 hours to occur.

Contraindications/Precautions/Warnings

Bulk-forming laxatives should not be used in cases where prompt intestinal evacuation is required, or when fecal impaction (no feces being passed) or intestinal obstruction is present. Psyllium products are not recommended for use in rabbits as they may damage intestinal mucosa and cause blockage.

Adverse Effects

With the exception of increased flatulence, psyllium very rarely produces any adverse reactions if adequate water is given or is available to the patient. If insufficient liquid is given, there is an increased possibility of esophageal or bowel obstruction occurring.

Reproductive/Nursing Safety

Because there is no appreciable absorption of psyllium from the gut, it should be safe to use in pregnant animals. In humans, the FDA categorizes this drug as category *B* for use during pregnancy (*Animal studies have not yet demonstrated risk to the fetus, but there are no adequate studies in pregnant women; or animal studies have shown an adverse effect, but adequate studies in pregnant women have not demonstrated a risk to the fetus in the first trimester of pregnancy, and there is no evidence of risk in later trimesters.*)

Psyllium should be safe to administer to lactating animals.

Overdosage/Acute Toxicity

If administered with sufficient liquid, psyllium overdose should cause only an increased amount of soft or loose stools.

Drug Interactions

The following drug interactions have either been reported or are theoretical in humans or animals receiving psyllium and may be of significance in veterinary patients. Unless otherwise noted, use together is not necessarily contraindicated, but weigh the potential risks and perform additional monitoring when appropriate.

▪ **ASPIRIN** (and other **SALICYLATES**): Potential exists for psyllium to bind and reduce absorption if given at the same time; if possible, separate doses by 3 or more hours.

▪ **DIGOXIN**: Potential exists for psyllium to bind and reduce absorption if given at the same time; if possible, separate doses by 3 or more hours.

▪ **NITROFURANTOIN**: Potential exists for psyllium to bind and reduce absorption if given at the same time; if possible, separate doses by 3 or more hours

Doses

▪ **DOGS:**

For adjunctive treatment of idiopathic large bowel diarrhea (extra-label): For a trial using *Metamucil*®: Median dose is 2 tablespoonsful (30 mL) per day (1.33 grams/kg/day; range: 0.32 – 4.9 grams/kg/day) added to a highly digestible diet such as Hill's *i/d*®. (Leib 2004, 2005)

For constipation (extra-label): In dogs prone to constipation, 2% psyllium was added as part of diet. 80% of studied dogs had easier defecation process. (Tortola *et al.* 2009)

As an adjunct for treatment of hepatic encephalopathy (extra-label): 1 – 3 teaspoons per day as a source of soluble fiber. (Twedt 2009)

▪ **CATS:**

For chronic constipation (extra-label): 1 – 4 teaspoonsful per meal added to canned cat food. Be sure cat is properly hydrated. (Washabau 2001)

▪ **HORSES:**

For adjunctive treatment of sand colic (extra-label):

a) 1 gram/kg twice daily. Administration of psyllium, ≈ 1 lb, in powdered form can be given via nasogastric tube once the powder has been mixed with water; mix and administer immediately via NG tube or mixture will thicken. If giving orally to foals, esophageal obstruction can occur. Give small amounts of the mixture at a time and confirm that the foal swallows after each bolus. A liquid-like mixture versus paste-like mixtures can help also. Pelleted psyllium is also available and most horses find this form more palatable than if the powdered form is mixed with dry or moistened feed. If horse refuses the pelleted form, experimentation with different flavors and smells produced by different suppliers of psyllium pellets may be helpful. Another option is to try mixing the psyllium pellets with the horse's favorite treat or grain source to improve intake. (Tillotson *et al.* 2003)

b) In this experimental study, 0.5 kg psyllium was mixed with 1 liter of mash and given twice daily and 2 liters of mineral oil via NG tube were administered once daily. This combination was more effective (measured ash content of feces) than giving mineral oil alone. (Hotwagner *et al.* 2008).

Monitoring

▪ Stool consistency, frequency.

Client Information

▪ Be sure your animal always has plenty of clean water to drink while taking psyllium.

- Psyllium is available OTC (over-the-counter; without a prescription). Do not give psyllium (or any other OTC medications) to your animal without first consulting a veterinarian.
- Psyllium products are not recommended for use in rabbits.

Chemistry/Synonyms

Psyllium is obtained from the ripe seeds of varieties of Plantago species. The seed coating is high in content of hemicellulose mucilage that absorbs and swells in the presence of water.

Psyllium may also be known as *Metamucil®*; many other trade names are available.

Storage/Stability

Store psyllium products in tightly closed containers; protect from excess moisture or humidity.

Dosage Forms/Regulatory Status

VETERINARY-LABELED PRODUCTS:

Equine Enteric Colloid®, Equi-Phar® Sweet Psyllium; (not for horses intended for food); *Sandclear®, Anipsyll® Powder* (AHC), *Purepsyll® Powder, Vita-Flex Sand Relief®, Equa Aid Psyllium®*; (OTC). Products may be available in 28 oz, 56 oz, 1 lb, 10 lb and 30 lb pails and are labeled for use in horses.

Vetasyl Fiber Tablets for Cats® 500 mg, & 1000 mg tablets in bottles of 60 or 180; (OTC); Labeled for use in cats. Also contains barley malt extract powder, acacia and thiamine.

HUMAN-LABELED PRODUCTS:

There are many human-approved products containing psyllium, most products contain ≈ 3.4 grams of psyllium per rounded teaspoonful. Dosages of sugar-free products may be different from those containing sugar.

Revisions/References

Monograph revised/updated June 2014.

Hotwagner, K. & C. Iben (2008). Evacuation of sand from the equine intestine with mineral oil, with and without psyllium. Journal of Animal Physiology and Animal Nutrition **92**(1): 86-91.

Leib, M. (2004). Chronic idiopathic large bowel diarrhea in dogs. Proceedings: ACVIM Forum. accessed via Veterinary Information Network; vin.com

Leib, M. (2005). Idiopathic large intestinal diarrhea in dogs. Proceedings: Western Veterinary Conference 2005, Accessed via the Veterinary Information Network Jan 2007. accessed via Veterinary Information Network; vin.com

Moreaux, S. J. J., et al. (2011). Psyllium Lowers Blood Glucose and Insulin Concentrations in Horses. Journal of Equine Veterinary Science **31**(4): 160-5.

Tillotson, K. & J. Traub-Dargatz (2003). Gastrointestinal protectants and cathartics. Vet Clin Equine **19**: 599-615.

Tortola, L., et al. (2009). Psyllium (Plantago psyllium) Uses In The Management Of Constipation In Dogs. Proceedings: WSAVA. accessed via Veterinary Information Network; vin.com

Twedt, D. (2009). Treatment of liver disease. Proceedings: ACVC. accessed via Veterinary Information Network; vin.com

Washabau, R. (2001). Feline constipation, obstipation and megacolon: Prevention, diagnosis and treatment. Proceedings: World Small Animal Assoc. World Congress. accessed via Veterinary Information Network; vin.com

Pyrantel Pamoate

(pi-**ran**-tel **pam**-oh-ate)   Strongid T®, Nemex®

Antiparasitic

Prescriber Highlights

▶ Pyrimidine anthelmintic used primarily for ascarids in a variety of species.

▶ Contraindications: Severely debilitated animals.

▶ Adverse Effects: Unlikely, emesis possible in small animals.

Uses/Indications

Pyrantel has been used for the removal of the following parasites in dogs: ascarids (*Toxocara canis, T. leonina*), hookworms (*Ancylostoma caninum, Uncinaria stenocephala*), and stomach worm (*Physaloptera*). *A. caninum* resistance has been reported. Although not

FDA-approved for use in cats, it is useful for similar parasites and is considered safe to use.

Pyrantel is indicated (labeled) for the removal of the following parasites in horses: *Strongylus vulgaris* and *equinus, Parasacaris equorum*, and *Probstymayria vivapara*. It has variable activity against *Oxyuris equi, S. edentatus*, and small strongyles. Pyrantel is active against ileocecal tapeworm (*A. perfoliata*) when used at twice the recommended dose, although resistance has been reported. Resistance to antiparasitic agents is an ongoing problem. It is recommended to perform fecal egg count reduction testing (FECRT) for strongyle nematodes. A value of <90% in 5-10 horses is the suggested cut-off for determining resistance on a given farm (Nielsen *et al.* 2009).

Although there are apparently no pyrantel products FDA-approved for use in cattle, sheep, or goats, the drug is effective (as the tartrate) for the removal of the following parasites: *Haemonchus* spp., *Ostertagia* spp., *Trichostrongylus* spp., *Nematodirus* spp., *Chabertia* spp., *Cooperia* spp. and *Oesophagostomum* spp.

Pyrantel tartrate is indicated (labeled) for the removal or prevention of the following parasites in swine: large roundworms (*Ascaris suum*) and *Oesophagostomum* spp. The drug has activity against the swine stomach worm (*Hyostrongylus rubidus*).

Although not FDA-approved, pyrantel has been used in pet birds and llamas. See the Dosage section for more information.

Pharmacology/Actions

Pyrantel acts as a depolarizing, neuromuscular-blocking agent in susceptible parasites, which paralyzes the organism. The drug possesses nicotine-like properties and acts similarly to acetylcholine. It also inhibits cholinesterase.

In horses, resistance of cyathostomes to pyrantel is fairly common in North America.

Pharmacokinetics

Pyrantel pamoate is poorly absorbed from the GI tract, thus allowing it to reach the lower GI in dogs, cats and equines. Pyrantel tartrate is absorbed more readily than the pamoate salt. Pigs and dogs absorb pyrantel tartrate more so than do ruminants, with peak plasma levels occurring 2-3 hours after administration. Peak plasma levels occur at highly variable times in ruminants.

Absorbed drug is rapidly metabolized and excreted into the urine and feces.

Contraindications/Precautions/Warnings

Use with caution in severely debilitated animals. The manufacturers usually recommend not administering the drug to severely debilitated animals.

Adverse Effects

When administered at recommended doses, adverse effects are unlikely. Emesis may possibly occur in small animals receiving pyrantel pamoate.

Reproductive/Nursing Safety

In humans, the FDA categorizes this drug as category *C* for use during pregnancy (*Animal studies have shown an adverse effect on the fetus, but there are no adequate studies in humans; or there are no animal reproduction studies and no adequate studies in humans.*) In a separate system evaluating the safety of drugs in canine and feline pregnancy (Papich 1989), this drug is categorized as class: *A* (*Probably safe. Although specific studies may not have proved the safety of all drugs in dogs and cats, there are no reports of adverse effects in laboratory animals or women.*)

Pyrantel is considered safe to use in nursing veterinary patients.

Overdosage/Acute Toxicity

Pyrantel has a moderate margin of safety. Dosages up to ≈ 7X recommended generally result in no toxic reactions. In horses, doses of

20X yielded no adverse effects. The LD_{50} in mice and rats for pyrantel tartrate is 170 mg/kg; >690 mg/kg for pyrantel pamoate in dogs.

Chronic dosing of pyrantel pamoate in dogs resulted in clinical signs when given at 50 mg/kg/day, but not at 20 mg/kg/day over 3 months. Clinical signs of toxicity that may be seen include increased respiratory rates, profuse sweating (in species with sweat glands), ataxia or other cholinergic effects.

Drug Interactions

- **LEVAMISOLE:** Because of similar mechanisms of action (and toxicity), do not use concurrently with pyrantel.
- **MORANTEL:** Because of similar mechanisms of action (and toxicity), do not use concurrently with pyrantel.
- **ORGANOPHOSPHATES:** Increased risk for adverse effects.
- **PIPERAZINE:** Pyrantel and piperazine have antagonistic mechanisms of action; do not use together.

Doses

Note: All doses are for pyrantel pamoate unless otherwise noted. **Caution:** Listed dosages are often not specified as to whether using the salt or base.

For additional information using this drug in dogs in cats, see Companion Animal Parasite Council recommendations: http://goo.gl/wJBq1

- **DOGS:**

  For susceptible parasites:

  Labeled dose; FDA-Approved: For dogs weighing <5 lb: 10 mg/kg (as base) PO; for dogs weighing >5 lbs: 5 mg/kg (as base) PO. Treat puppies at 2, 3, 4, 6, 8, and 10 weeks of age. Treat lactating bitches 2-3 weeks after whelping. Do follow-up fecal 2-4 weeks after treating to determine need for retreatment. (Label directions; *Nemex® Tabs*)

  Extra-label doses:

  a) **For hookworms or roundworms:** 5 mg/kg PO after meals; repeat in 7-10 days. (Willard 2003)

  b) **Puppies:** To prevent environmental contamination, all pups should be routinely treated with pyrantel pamoate at 2, 4, 6, and 8 weeks of age and then placed on a monthly heartworm preventative with efficacy against *Toxocara* spp. (CAPC 2014)

  c) 20 mg/kg PO; be sure that liquid is well mixed before using; tablets may be broken for accurate dosing. (Blagburn 2005a)

- **CATS:**

  For susceptible parasites:

  Labeled dose; FDA-Approved for susceptible parasites using combination product with praziquantel (*Drontal®*): Administer a minimum dose of 2.27 mg praziquantel and 9.2 mg pyrantel pamoate per pound of body weight according to the dosing tables on labeling. May be given directly by mouth or in a small amount of food. Do not withhold food prior to or after treatment. If reinfection occurs, treatment may be repeated. (Package insert; *Drontal®*)

  Extra-label doses:

  a) 20 mg/kg PO; repeat when necessary. Not approved as single entity in cats, but data indicate that it is safe and effective. Assure that liquid is mixed prior to use. Tablets may be broken for accurate dosing. (Blagburn 2005b)

  b) **Kittens:** Can be treated as early as 2-3 weeks of age at 5 – 10 mg/kg PO; can be repeated every 2-3 weeks until at least 12 weeks of age. (Hoskins 2005)

- **RABBITS, RODENTS, SMALL MAMMALS:**

  Rabbits (extra-label): 15 – 10 mg/kg PO, repeat in 2-3 weeks. (Ivey *et al.* 2000)

- **HORSES:**

  For the removal and control of mature infections of large strongyles (*Strongylus vulgaris, S. edentatus, S. equinus*); small strongyles; pinworms (*Oxyuris equi*); and large roundworms (*Parascaris equorum*) in horses and ponies (labeled; dose; FDA-approved): 6.6 mg/kg PO. It is recommended that foals (2-8 months of age) be dosed every 4 weeks. To minimize the potential source of infection that the mare may pose to the foal, the mare should be treated 1 month prior to anticipated foaling date followed by retreatment 10 days to 2 weeks after birth of foal. Horses and ponies over 8 months of age should be routinely dosed every 6 weeks. (Adapted from label; *Strongid-T®*, *Strongid Paste®*)

  For control of cestodes (extra-label): Use 13.2 mg/kg PO (twice the labeled dose).

- **LLAMAS:**

  For susceptible parasites (extra-label): 18 mg/kg, PO for one day. (Cheney *et al.* 1989; Fowler 1989)

- **BIRDS:**

  For intestinal nematodes extra-label):

  a) **Psittacines:** In endemic areas, outdoor breeding birds and their offspring should be routinely dewormed for ascarids: 25 mg/kg PO q2 weeks. (Lightfoot 2008)

  b) 100 mg/kg, PO as a single dose in psittacines and passerines. (Marshall 1993)

Client Information

- May be given with or without food; can be mixed into food.
- Usually no side effects. Rarely, some small animals may vomit after getting it; give with food if this happens.
- In small animals, dose is usually repeated at various weekly intervals; follow your veterinarian's recommendation for best control of parasites.
- If using suspension, shake container well before each use; protect from sunlight.

Chemistry/Synonyms

A pyrimidine-derivative anthelmintic, pyrantel pamoate occurs as yellow to tan solid and is practically insoluble in water and alcohol. Each gram of pyrantel pamoate is ≈ 347 mg (34.7%) of the base.

Pyrantel may also be known as: CP-10423-16, pyrantel embonate, pirantel pamoate, *Anthel®, Antiminth®, Ascarical®, Aut®, Bantel®, Cobantril®, Combantrin®, Combantrin®, Early Bird®, Helmex®, Helmintox®, Jaa Pyral®, Lombriareu®, Nemex®, Nemocid®, Pin-X®, Pirantrim®, Pyrantin®, Pyrantrin®, Pyrapam®, Reese's® Pinworm, Strongid®, Trilombrin®,* or *Vertel®.*

Storage/Stability

Pyrantel pamoate products should be stored in tight, light-resistant containers at room temperature (15-30°C) unless otherwise directed by the manufacturer.

Dosage Forms/Regulatory Status

VETERINARY-LABELED PRODUCTS:

Note: Many products available; a partial listing of products follows:

Pyrantel Pamoate Tablets: 22.7 mg (of base), 113.5 mg (of base); (OTC). FDA-approved for use in dogs. A commonly known product is *Nemex® Tabs*.

Pyrantel Pamoate Oral Suspension: 4.54 mg/mL (as base) (for dogs only); in 60 mL, 120 mL 280 mL and 473 mL bottles. Many products are available; a commonly known trade name is *Nemex-2®*; (OTC)

Pyrantel Pamoate Oral Suspension: 50 mg/mL (of base); Many products are available; a commonly known trade name is *Strongid® T*; (OTC). FDA-approved for use in horses not intended for food.

Pyrantel Pamoate Oral Paste: 43.9% w/w pyrantel base in 23.6 grams (20 mL) paste (180 mg pyrantel base/mL); several products are available. A commonly known trade name is *Strongid® Paste*; (OTC). FDA-approved for use in horses not intended for food.

Pyrantel Tartrate 1.06% (4.8 grams/lb) Top Dress: in 25 lb pails: *Strongid C®*; (OTC). Labeled for use in horses (not intended for food).

Combination Products:

With Febantel & Praziquantel: *Drontal Plus® Taste Tabs*: For Puppies and Small Dogs (2-25 lbs.): praziquantel 22.7 mg/pyrantel 22.7 mg/febantel, 113.4 mg; For Medium Sized Dogs (26-60 lbs.): praziquantel 68 mg/pyrantel 68 mg/febantel, 340.2 mg; For Large Dogs (≥45 lbs.): praziquantel 136 mg/pyrantel 136 mg/febantel, 680.4 mg; (Rx). Approved for use in dogs (NADA 141-007)

With Praziquantel: Tablets: Praziquantel 13.6 mg/pyrantel pamoate 54.3 mg (as base) for 2-5.9 lb cats and kittens; Praziquantel 18.2 mg/pyrantel pamoate 72.6 mg (as base); Praziquantel 27.2 mg/pyrantel pamoate 108.6 mg (as base) for 6-24 lb. cats; *Drontal® Tablets*; some sizes may be available as generics or under various trade names (OTC). FDA-approved for use in cats and kittens that are ≥2 months of age and weigh ≥2 lb.

With Praziquantel: Chewable Tablets: Praziquantel 30 mg/pyrantel pamoate 30 mg; & Praziquantel 114 mg/pyrantel pamoate 114 mg chewable tablets; *Virbantel Flavored Chewables®*; (OTC). FDA-approved for use in dogs.

With Ivermectin: Ivermectin/Pyrantel Oral Tablets: 68 mcg/57 mg, 136 mcg/114 mg, 272 mcg/228 mg; *Heartgard® Plus Chewables*, generic; (Rx). FDA-approved for use in dogs.

With Ivermectin & Praziquantel: Ivermectin/Pyrantel Pamoate/Praziquantel Oral Chewable Tablets: 34mcg/28mg/28mg, 68mcg/57mg/57mg; 136mcg/114mg/114mg, 272mcg/228mg/228mg; *Iverhart® Max*; (Rx). FDA-approved for use in dogs.

HUMAN-LABELED PRODUCTS:

Pyrantel Pamoate Oral Suspension: 50 mg/mL & 144 mg/mL (equiv. to 50 mg/mL pyrantel base); *Reese's® Pinworm, Pin-X®*; (OTC)

Pyrantel Pamoate Oral Tablets: 180 mg & 720.5 mg (chewable); *Reese's Pinworm®, Pin-X®*; (OTC)

Revisions/References

Monograph revised/updated June 2014.

Blagburn, B. (2005a). Update on treatment and control of parasites and parasitic diseases of companion animals. Proceedings: ACVC2005. accessed via Veterinary Information Network; vin.com

Blagburn, B. L. (2005b). Expert Recommendations on Feline Parasite Control. Proceedings; Atlantic Veterinary Conference. accessed via Veterinary Information Network; vin.com

CAPC (2014). Companion Animal Parasite Council (CAPC) Recommendations, CAPCvet. org.

Cheney, J. M. & G. T. Allen (1989). Parasitism in Llamas. Vet Clin North America: Food Animal Practice 5(1): 217-32.

Fowler, M. E. (1989). *Medicine and Surgery of South American Camelids*, Iowa State University Press. Ames.

Hoskins, J. (2005). Veterinary pediatrics of the puppy and kitten. Proceedings: ACVC 2006. accessed via Veterinary Information Network; vin.com

Ivey, E. & J. Morrisey (2000). Therapeutics for Rabbits. Vet Clin NA: Exotic Anim Pract 3:1(Jan): 183-216.

Lightfoot, T. (2008). Pediatric Psittacine Diseases. Proceedings: WVC. accessed via Veterinary Information Network; vin.com

Marshall, R. (1993). Avian anthelmintics and antiprotozoals. Seminars in Avian & Exotic Med 2(1): 33-41.

Nielsen, M. & R. M. Kaplan (2009). Diagnosis & Management of Anthelmintic Resistance in Equid Parasites. Proceedings: ACVIM. accessed via Veterinary Information Network; vin.com

Papich, M. (1989). Effects of drugs on pregnancy. *Current Veterinary Therapy X: Small Animal Practice*. R. Kirk. Philadelphia, Saunders: 1291-9.

Willard, M. (2003). Digestive system disorders. *Small Animal Internal Medicine, 3rd Ed.* R. Nelson and C. Couto. St Louis, Mosby: 343-471.

Pyridostigmine Bromide

(peer-id-oh-**stig**-meen)   Mestinon®

Anticholinesterase Agent

Prescriber Highlights

▶ Anticholinesterase used for treatment of myasthenia gravis.

▶ Contraindications: hypersensitivity to this class of compounds or bromides, patients with mechanical or physical obstructions of the urinary or GI tract.

▶ Caution: bronchospastic disease, epilepsy, hyperthyroidism, bradycardia or other arrhythmias, vagotonia, or GI ulcer diseases.

▶ Adverse Effects: Usually dose related cholinergic effects GI (nausea, vomiting, diarrhea), salivation, sweating, respiratory (increased bronchial secretions, bronchospasm, pulmonary edema, respiratory paralysis), ophthalmic (miosis, blurred vision, lacrimation), cardiovascular (bradycardia or tachycardia, cardiospasm, hypotension, cardiac arrest), muscle cramps, & weakness.

Uses/Indications

Pyridostigmine is used in the treatment of myasthenia gravis (MG) in dogs (and rarely in cats). It is considered to be much more effective in acquired MG, than in congenital MG.

Pharmacology/Actions

Pyridostigmine inhibits the hydrolysis of acetylcholine by directly competing with acetylcholine for attachment to acetylcholinesterase. Because the pyridostigmine-acetylcholinesterase complex is hydrolyzed at a much slower rate than the acetylcholine-acetylcholinesterase complex, acetylcholine tends to accumulate at cholinergic synapses with resultant cholinergic activity.

At usual doses, pyridostigmine does not cross into the CNS (quaternary ammonium structure), but overdoses can cause CNS effects.

Pharmacokinetics

Pyridostigmine is only marginally absorbed from the GI tract and absorption may be more erratic with the sustained-release tablets than the regular tablets. The onset of action after oral dosing is generally within one hour.

At usual doses, pyridostigmine is apparently distributed to most tissues, but not to the brain, intestinal wall, fat or thymus. The drug crosses the placenta.

Pyridostigmine is metabolized by both the liver and hydrolyzed by cholinesterases.

Contraindications/Precautions/Warnings

Pyridostigmine is contraindicated in patients hypersensitive to this class of compounds or bromides, or in those who have mechanical or physical obstructions of the urinary or GI tract.

The drug should be used with caution in patients with bronchospastic disease, epilepsy, hyperthyroidism, bradycardia or other arrhythmias, vagotonia, or GI ulcer diseases.

Adverse Effects

Adverse effects associated with pyridostigmine are generally dose-related and cholinergic in nature such as increased GI motility, salivation, lacrimation, abdominal pain, diarrhea, bradycardia and increased lacrimation. These are usually mild and easily treatable with dosage reduction, but severe adverse effects are possible (see Overdosage below).

Reproductive/Nursing Safety

In humans, the FDA categorizes this drug as category *C* for use during pregnancy (*Animal studies have shown an adverse effect on the fetus, but there are no adequate studies in humans; or there are no animal reproduction studies and no adequate studies in humans.*)

Pyridostigmine is excreted in maternal milk; use with caution in nursing patients.

Overdosage/Acute Toxicity

Overdosage of pyridostigmine may induce a cholinergic crisis. Clinical signs of cholinergic toxicity can include: GI effects (nausea, vomiting, diarrhea), salivation, sweating (species with sweat glands), respiratory effects (increased bronchial secretions, bronchospasm, pulmonary edema, respiratory paralysis), ophthalmic effects (miosis, blurred vision, lacrimation), cardiovascular effects (bradycardia or tachycardia, cardiospasm, hypotension, cardiac arrest), muscle cramps, and weakness.

Overdoses in myasthenic patients can be very difficult to distinguish from the effects associated with a myasthenic crisis. The time of onset of clinical signs or an edrophonium challenge may help to distinguish between the two.

Treatment of pyridostigmine overdosage consists of both respiratory and cardiac supportive therapy and atropine if necessary. Refer to the atropine monograph for more information on its use for cholinergic toxicity.

Drug Interactions

The following drug interactions have either been reported or are theoretical in humans or animals receiving pyridostigmine and may be of significance in veterinary patients. Unless otherwise noted, use together is not necessarily contraindicated, but weigh the potential risks and perform additional monitoring when appropriate.

- **ATROPINE**: Atropine will antagonize the muscarinic effects of pyridostigmine but concurrent use should be used cautiously as atropine can mask the early clinical signs of cholinergic crisis.
- **CORTICOSTEROIDS**: May decrease the anticholinesterase activity of pyridostigmine. After stopping corticosteroid therapy, drugs like pyridostigmine may cause increased anticholinesterase activity.
- **DEXPANTHENOL**: Theoretically, dexpanthenol may have additive effects when used with pyridostigmine.
- **DRUGS WITH NEUROMUSCULAR BLOCKING ABILITY** (*e.g.*, **aminoglycoside antibiotics**): May necessitate increased dosages of pyridostigmine in treating or diagnosing myasthenic patients.
- **MAGNESIUM**: Anticholinesterase therapy may be antagonized by administration of parenteral magnesium therapy, as it can have a direct depressant effect on skeletal muscle.
- **MUSCLE RELAXANTS, SURGICAL**: Pyridostigmine may prolong the Phase I block of depolarizing muscle relaxants (*e.g.*, **succinylcholine, decamethonium**) and edrophonium antagonizes the actions of non-depolarizing neuromuscular blocking agents (*e.g.*, **pancuronium, tubocurarine, gallamine, vecuronium, atracurium**, etc.).

Doses

- **DOGS:**

  For adjunctive treatment of myasthenia gravis (MG): Once able to swallow, 0.5 – 3 mg/kg PO q8-12h with food. Practically, either round dose to nearest quarter of a regular 60 mg tablet or use the oral liquid for more precise dosing. Dosage is titrated to effect to minimize adverse effects and maximize muscle strength. For patients unable to swallow, especially in critically ill animals a CRI dosage of 0.01 – 0.03 mg/kg/hour has been noted.

- **CATS:**

  For myasthenia gravis (MG) (extra-label): Rarely used, but can be dosed similarly as dogs.

Monitoring

- Animals should be routinely monitored for clinical signs of cholinergic toxicity (see Overdosage section above) and efficacy of the therapy.

Client Information

- Can be given with or without food, but give the same way each time.
- Adjusting dosage is very important to avoid/reduce side effects. Report side effects such as excessive salivation, GI disturbances, weakness, or difficulty breathing (see side effects section) to veterinarian.
- Overdoses can be very serious, measure liquid doses very carefully and keep out of reach of children or animals.

Chemistry/Synonyms

An anticholinesterase agent, pyridostigmine bromide is a synthetic quaternary ammonium compound that occurs as an agreeable smelling, bitter tasting, hydroscopic, white or practically white, crystalline powder. It is freely soluble in water and alcohol. The pH of the commercially available injection is ≈ 5.

Pyridostigmine Bromide may also be known as: pyridostigmini bromidum, *Distinon*®, *Kalymin*®, *Mestinon*®, or *Regonol*®.

Storage/Stability

Unless otherwise instructed by the manufacturer, store pyridostigmine products at room temperature. The oral solution and injection should be protected from light and freezing. Pyridostigmine tablets should be kept in tight containers.

The extended-release tablets may become mottled with time, but this does not affect their potency.

Pyridostigmine injection is unstable in alkaline solutions. It contains 1% benzyl alcohol.

Compatibility/Compounding Considerations

Pyridostigmine injection is reportedly physically **compatible** with glycopyrrolate, heparin sodium, hydrocortisone sodium succinate, potassium chloride, and vitamin B-complex with C. Compatibility is dependent upon factors such as pH, concentration, temperature and diluent used; consult specialized references or a hospital pharmacist for more specific information.

Dosage Forms/Regulatory Status

VETERINARY-LABELED PRODUCTS: NONE.

The ARCI (Racing Commissioners International) has designated this drug as a class 3 substance. See the appendix for more information.

HUMAN-LABELED PRODUCTS:

Pyridostigmine Bromide Tablets: 60 mg; *Mestinon*®, generic, (Rx)

Pyridostigmine Bromide Extended-Release Tablets: 180 mg; *Mestinon*®; (Rx)

Pyridostigmine Bromide Syrup: 12 mg/mL (labeled as 60 mg/5 mL) in 480 mL; *Mestinon*®; (Rx)

Pyridostigmine Bromide Injection: 5 mg/mL in 2 mL amps; *Regonol*®; (Rx)

Revisions/References

Monograph revised/updated June 2014.

Pyridoxine HCl (Vitamin B-6)

(peer-ih-**dox**-een)

Nutritional B Vitamin, Antidote

Prescriber Highlights

▶ Pyridoxine may be beneficial in the treatment of isoniazid, crimidine, or hydrazine mushroom toxicity, delaying cutaneous toxicity of *Doxil*® (liposomal doxorubicin), or to supplement while patients are receiving penicillamine.

▶ Overdoses may cause peripheral neuropathy.

Uses/Indications

Pyridoxine use in veterinary medicine is relatively infrequent. It may be of benefit in the treatment of isoniazid (INH) or crimidine (an older rodenticide) toxicity. Pyridoxine deficiency is apparently extremely rare in dogs or cats able to ingest food. Cats with severe intestinal disease may have a greater requirement for pyridoxine in their diet. Experimentally, pyridoxine has been successfully used in dogs to reduce the cutaneous toxicity associated with doxorubicin containing pegylated liposomes (*Doxil*®). Pyridoxine has been demonstrated to suppress the growth of feline mammary tumors (cell line FRM) *in vitro*.

In humans, labeled uses for pyridoxine include pyridoxine deficiency and intractable neonatal seizures secondary to pyridoxine dependency syndrome. Unlabeled uses include premenstrual syndrome (PMS), carpal tunnel syndrome, tardive dyskinesia secondary to antipsychotic drugs, nausea and vomiting in pregnancy, hyperoxaluria type 1 and oxalate kidney stones, and for the treatment of isoniazid (INH), cycloserine, hydrazine or Gyromitra mushroom poisonings.

Pharmacology/Actions

In erythrocytes, pyridoxine is converted to pyridoxal phosphate and, to a lesser extent, pyridoxamine, which serve as coenzymes for metabolic functions affecting protein, lipid and carbohydrate utilization. Pyridoxine is necessary for tryptophan conversion to serotonin or niacin, glycogen breakdown, heme synthesis, synthesis of GABA in the CNS, and oxalate conversion to glycine. Pyridoxine can act as an antidote by enhancing the excretion of cycloserine or isoniazid.

Pyridoxine requirements increase as protein ingestion increases.

Pharmacokinetics

Pyridoxine is absorbed from the GI tract primarily in the jejunum. Malabsorption syndromes can significantly impair pyridoxine absorption. Pyridoxine is not bound to plasma proteins, but pyridoxal phosphate is completely bound to plasma proteins. Pyridoxine is stored primarily in the liver with smaller amounts stored in the brain and muscle. It is biotransformed in the liver and various tissues, and excreted almost entirely as metabolites into the urine. Elimination half-life in humans is ≈ 15-20 days.

Contraindications/Precautions/Warnings

Weigh potential risks versus benefits in patients with documented sensitivity to pyridoxine.

Adverse Effects

Pyridoxine is generally well tolerated unless doses are large (see Overdosage). In humans, paresthesias and somnolence have been reported. Reduced serum folic acid levels have occurred.

Reproductive/Nursing Safety

While pyridoxine is a nutritional agent and very safe at recommended doses during pregnancy, very large doses during pregnancy can cause a pyridoxine dependency syndrome in neonates.

Pyridoxine administration at low dosages should be safe during nursing. Pyridoxine requirements of the dam may be increased during nursing.

Overdosage/Acute Toxicity

Single overdoses are not considered overly problematic, unless they are massive. Laboratory animals given 3 – 4 grams/kg developed seizures and died. Beagles repeatedly given 3-gram oral daily doses developed uncoordinated gait and neurologic signs. Neuronal lesions were noted in sensory, dorsal root ganglia, and trigeminal ganglia. Signs generally resolved over a 2-month drug free period.

Drug Interactions

The following drug interactions have either been reported or are theoretical in humans or animals receiving pyridoxine and may be of significance in veterinary patients. Unless otherwise noted, use together is not necessarily contraindicated, but weigh the potential risks and perform additional monitoring when appropriate.

- **CHLORAMPHENICOL**: May cause increased pyridoxine requirements.
- **ESTROGENS**: May cause increased pyridoxine requirements.
- **HYDRALAZINE**: May cause increased pyridoxine requirements.
- **IMMUNOSUPPRESSANTS** (*e.g.,* **azathioprine, chlorambucil, cyclophosphamide, corticosteroids**): May cause increased pyridoxine requirements.
- **ISONIAZID**: May cause increased pyridoxine requirements.
- **PENICILLAMINE**: May cause increased pyridoxine requirements.
- **LEVODOPA**: Pyridoxine may reduce levodopa efficacy (no interaction when levodopa is used with carbidopa).
- **PHENOBARBITAL**: High dose pyridoxine may decrease phenobarbital serum levels.
- **PHENYTOIN**: High dose pyridoxine may decrease phenytoin serum concentration.

Laboratory Considerations

The following laboratory alterations have been reported in humans with pyridoxine and may be of significance in veterinary patients. Unless otherwise noted, use together is not necessarily contraindicated, but weigh the potential risks and perform additional monitoring when appropriate.

- **Urobilinogen in the spot test using Ehrlich's reagent**: Pyridoxine may cause false-positive results.
- **AST**: Excessive dosages of pyridoxine may elevate AST.

Doses

- **DOGS/CATS:**

  For isoniazid (INH) toxicity in dogs (extra-label): If quantity of INH ingested is known, give pyridoxine on a mg for mg (1:1) basis. If it is not known, give pyridoxine initially at 71 mg/kg as a 5-10% IV infusion over 30-60 minutes (some sources say it can be given as an IV bolus). Pyridoxine injection can usually be obtained from human hospital pharmacies. Do not use injectable B-complex vitamins. (Gwaltney-Brant 2003)

  To replace pyridoxine antagonized by crimidine ingestion (extra-label): 20 mg/kg IV. (Dalefield *et al.* 2006)

  For adjunctive treatment (acute seizures) of hydrazine mushroom (*Gyromitra* spp.) poisoning (extra-label): 75 – 150 mg/kg IV. (Puschner *et al.* 2012)

  For supplementation while on penicillamine (extra-label): 25 mg PO per dog once daily. (Center 2013)

  To delay the development of cutaneous toxicity (PPES; palmer-plantar-dyerythrodysesthesia) associated with doxorubicin containing pegylated liposomes (*Doxil*®) in dogs (extra-label):

50 mg PO 3 times daily during chemotherapy protocol period. (Vail *et al.* 1998)

Monitoring

- Other than evaluating efficacy for its intended use, no significant monitoring is required

Client Information

- Very safe; usually no side effects.
- Do not give more than the veterinarian has ordered.

Chemistry/Synonyms

Pyridoxine (vitamin B6) is a water-soluble vitamin present in many foods (liver, meat, eggs, cereals, legumes, and vegetables). The commercially available form (pyridoxine HCl) found in medications is obtained synthetically. Pyridoxine HCl occurs as white or practically white, crystals or crystalline powder with a slightly bitter, salty taste. It is freely soluble in water and slightly soluble in alcohol.

Pyridoxine or Vitamin B6 may also be known by the following synonyms or analogs: adermine, pyridoxal, pyridoxal-5-phosphate, pyridoxamine, pirodoxamina, piridossima, piridoxolum, piridossina, *Aminoxin®*, and *Vitelle Nestrex®*.

Storage/Stability

Unless otherwise specified by the manufacturer, pyridoxine tablets should be stored below 40°C (104°F), preferably between 15-30°C (59-86°F), in well-closed containers protected from light.

Pyridoxine HCl injection should be stored below 40°C (104°F), preferably between 15-30°C (59-86°F), protected from light and freezing.

Pyridoxine HCl injection can be administered undiluted or added to commonly used IV solutions. It is reportedly **compatible** with doxapram when mixed in a syringe and with fat emulsion 10%. It is reportedly **incompatible** with alkaline or oxidizing solutions, and iron salts.

Dosage Forms/Regulatory Status

VETERINARY-LABELED PRODUCTS:

No single ingredient pyridoxine products were located. There are a multitude of various veterinary-labeled products that contain pyridoxine as one of several ingredients.

HUMAN-LABELED PRODUCTS:

Pyridoxine Tablets 50 mg, 100 mg, 250 mg, & 500 mg; Vitamin B6; generic (various); (OTC)

Pyridoxine (as pyridoxal-5'-phosphate) Tablets (enteric-coated): 20 mg; *Aminoxin®*; (OTC)

Pyridoxine HCl Injection: 100 mg/mL in 1 mL vials; generic; (Rx)

Pyridoxine is also an ingredient in many combination products (*e.g.*, B-Complex, multivitamins).

Revisions/References

Monograph revised/updated May 2014.

Center, S. (2013). Canine Copper-Associated Hepatopathy. Proceedings; 23rd ECVIM-CA Congress. accessed via Veterinary Information Network; vin.com

Dalefield, R. & F. Oehme (2006). Antidotes for specific poisons. *Small Animal Toxicology*. M. Peterson and P. Talcott, Elsevier: 459-74.

Gwaltney-Brant, S. (2003). Terrible Toxicants. Proceedings: IVECC2003. accessed via Veterinary Information Network; vin.com

Puschner, B. & C. Wegenast (2012). Mushroom Poisoning Cases in Dogs and Cats: Diagnosis and Treatment of Hepatotoxic, Neurotoxic, Gastroenterotoxic, Nephrotoxic, and Muscarinic Mushrooms. *Vet Clin Small Anim* 42: 375-87.

Vail, D., et al. (1998). Efficacy of pyridoxine to ameliorate the cutaneous toxicity associated with doxorubicin containing pegylated (stealth) liposomes: A randomized, double-blind clinical trial using a canine model. *Clinical Cancer Res* 4(June): 1567-71.

Pyrilamine Maleate

(pye-ril-a-meen)   Histall®, Equiphed®

Antihistamine

Prescriber Highlights

- ▶ Injectable antihistamine.
- ▶ Contraindications: None noted.
- ▶ Adverse Effects: **Horses:** CNS stimulation (nervousness, insomnia, convulsions, tremors, ataxia), palpitation, GI disturbances, CNS depression (sedation), muscular weakness, anorexia, lassitude & incoordination.
- ▶ Drug Interactions.

Uses/Indications

Antihistamines are used in veterinary medicine to reduce or help prevent histamine mediated adverse effects; predominantly used in horses.

Pharmacology/Actions

Antihistamines (H_1-receptor antagonists) competitively inhibit histamine at H_1 receptor sites. They do not inactivate, nor prevent the release of histamine, but can prevent histamine's action on the cell. Besides their antihistaminic activity, these agents also have varying degrees of anticholinergic and CNS activity (sedation). Pyrilamine is considered to be less sedating and have fewer anticholinergic effects when compared to most other antihistamines.

Pharmacokinetics

The pharmacokinetics of this agent have apparently not been extensively studied in cattle, dogs or cats. In horses, pyrilamine is poorly bioavailable (18%) after oral administration. After IV administration, elimination half-life was ≈ 1.7 hours. After a single dose, pyrilamines principle metabolite, O-desmethylpyrilamine (O-DMP), can be detected in urine for at least two days, and possibly up to one week after dosing (Dirikolu *et al.* 2009).

Contraindications/Precautions/Warnings

The manufacturer indicates that the use of this product "…should not supersede the use of other emergency drugs and procedures."

Adverse Effects

Adverse effects in horses can include CNS stimulation (nervousness, insomnia, convulsions, tremors, ataxia), palpitation, GI disturbances, CNS depression (sedation), muscular weakness, anorexia, lassitude and incoordination.

Reproductive/Nursing Safety

At usual doses, pyrilamine is probably safe to use during pregnancy. Rats and mice treated with 10-20X the human dose had an increased frequency of embryonic, fetal or perinatal death, but a study in pregnant women, showed no increase in teratogenic or fetocidal rates.

It is unknown if pyrilamine enters milk.

Overdosage/Acute Toxicity

Treatment of overdosage is supportive and symptomatic. One manufacturer (*Histavet-P®*—Schering) suggests using "careful titration" of barbiturates to treat convulsions, and analeptics (caffeine, ephedrine, or amphetamines) to treat CNS depression. Most toxicologists however, recommend avoiding the use of CNS stimulants in the treatment of CNS depressant overdoses. Phenytoin (IV) is recommended in the treatment of seizures caused by antihistamine overdose in humans; barbiturates and diazepam are to be avoided.

Drug Interactions

The following drug interactions have either been reported or are theoretical in humans or animals receiving pyrilamine and may be of significance in veterinary patients. Unless otherwise noted, use

together is not necessarily contraindicated, but weigh the potential risks and perform additional monitoring when appropriate.

- **ANTICOAGULANTS (heparin, warfarin):** Antihistamines may partially counteract the anticoagulation effects of heparin or warfarin.
- **CNS DEPRESSANT DRUGS:** Increased sedation can occur if pyrilamine is combined with other CNS depressant drugs.
- **EPINEPHRINE:** Pyrilamine may enhance the effects of epinephrine.

Laboratory Considerations

- Antihistamines can decrease the wheal and flare response to antigen **skin testing.** In humans, it is suggested that antihistamines be discontinued at least 4 days before testing.

Doses

- **HORSES:** (NOTE: ARCI UCGFS CLASS 3 DRUG)

  As an antihistamine (labeled-dose; FDA-approved):

  Injectable: 0.88 – 1.32 mg/kg (2 – 3 mL of 20 mg/mL solution per 100 lbs body weight) IV (slowly), IM or SC; may repeat in 6-12 hours if necessary. **Foals:** 0.44 mg/kg (1 mL of 20 mg/mL solution per 100 lbs. body weight) IV (slowly), IM or SC; may repeat in 6-12 hours if necessary. (Package Insert; *Histavet-P*®)

  Oral (with Pseudoephedrine): 1/2 ounce (1 level tablespoon) per 1,000 lbs. body weight. Can be mixed with feed and repeated at 12-hour intervals if needed. (Label information; *Tri-Hist*® *Granules*). **Note:** Class 1 DEA chemical.

Monitoring

- Clinical efficacy.
- Adverse effects.

Chemistry/Synonyms

An ethylenediamine antihistamine, pyrilamine maleate occurs as a white, crystalline powder with a melting range of 99-103°. One gram is soluble in ≈ 0.5 mL of water or 3 mL alcohol.

Pyrilamine Maleate may also be known as: pyranisamine hydrochloride, pyrilamine hydrochloride, mepyramine hydrochloride, mepyramini maleas, myranisamine maleate, myrilamine maleate, mepyramine maleate, *Anihist*®, *Alergitanil*®, *Antemesyl*®, *Anthisan*®, *Anthisan*®, *Equi-Phar*® *Equi-Hist*®, *Equiphed*®, *Fluidasa*®, *Histall*®, *Histagranules*®, *Histamed*®, *Mepyraderm*®, *Mepyrimal*, *Pyramine*®, *Pyriped*®, *Relaxa-Tabs*®, and *Tri-Hist*®.

Storage/Stability

Avoid freezing the injectable product.

Dosage Forms/Regulatory Status

VETERINARY-LABELED PRODUCTS:

Note: The marketing status of these products is in flux and subject to change.

Pyrilamine Granules: 600 mg/oz in 20 oz containers; *Histall*®; (OTC). Labeled for use in horses. Do not use at least 72 hours before sporting events.

The following products contain pseudoephedrine. In the USA, pseudoephedrine is classified as a list 1 chemical (drugs that can be used as precursors to manufacture methamphetamine) and in some states it may be a controlled substance or have other restrictions placed upon its sale. Be alert to persons desiring to purchase this medication: Pseudoephedrine HCl 600 mg/oz and Pyrilamine maleate 600 mg/oz Granules: in 20 oz, 5 lb and 10 lb containers; *Equiphed*® (AHC), *Equi-Phar Equi-Hist 1200 Granules*®, *Tri-Hist Granules*®, *Histagranules*®; (Rx). Labeled for use in horses. Do not use at least 72 hours before sporting events.

Pyrilamine 600 mg/oz and Guaifenesin 2400 mg/oz Granules: in 20 oz, 5 lb and 25 lb containers; *Anihist*®, *Hist-EQ*®; (OTC). Labeled for use in horses. Do not use at least 72 hours before sporting events.

There are also combination cough syrups containing pyrilamine labeled for use in small animals.

The ARCI (Racing Commissioners International) has designated this drug as a class 3 substance. See the appendix for more information.

HUMAN-LABELED PRODUCTS: NONE.

Revisions/References

Monograph revised/updated May 2014.

Dirikolu, L., et al. (2009). Pyrilamine in the horse: detection and pharmacokinetics of pyrilamine and its major urinary metabolite O-desmethylpyrilamine. J. Vet. Pharmacol. Ther. 32(1): 66-78.

Pyrimethamine

(pye-ri-meth-a-meen)   Daraprim®

Antiprotozoal

Note: *Also see the Pyrimethamine/Sulfadiazine, and Sulfadiazine/Trimethoprim monographs*

Prescriber Highlights

▶ Folic acid inhibitor used primarily (in combination) for toxoplasmosis, *H. americanum*, neosporosis, & equine protozoal encephalomyelitis.

▶ Caution: Hematologic disorders; cats.

▶ Adverse Effects: **Small animals:** Anorexia, malaise, vomiting, depression, & bone marrow depression (anemia, thrombocytopenia, leukopenia). Cats may be more likely to develop adverse reactions. **Horses:** Leukopenias, thrombocytopenia, & anemias; Baker's yeast or folinic acid may treat/prevent.

▶ Potentially teratogenic; avoid use in pregnancy.

▶ Dosage form (25 mg tab only) may be inconvenient for accurate dosing; unpalatable to cats.

Uses/Indications

In veterinary medicine, pyrimethamine is used to treat *Hepatozoon americanum* infections, and toxoplasmosis in small animals (often in combination with sulfonamides). In horses, it is used to treat equine protozoal myeloencephalitis, sometimes called equine toxoplasmosis.

In humans, pyrimethamine is used for the treatment of toxoplasmosis and as a prophylactic agent for malaria.

Pharmacology/Actions

Pyrimethamine is a folic acid antagonist similar to trimethoprim. It acts by inhibiting the enzyme, dihydrofolate reductase that catalyzes the conversion of dihydrofolic acid to tetrahydrofolic acid. Pyrimethamine has *in vitro* activity against *T gondii*; adding sulfadiazine can enhance activity.

Pharmacokinetics

No pharmacokinetic data was located for veterinary species. In humans, pyrimethamine is well absorbed from the gut after oral administration. It is distributed primarily to the kidneys, liver, spleen, and lungs, but does cross the blood-brain barrier. It has a volume of distribution of ≈ 3 L/kg and is 80% bound to plasma proteins. Pyrimethamine enters milk in levels greater than those found in serum and can be detected in milk up to 48 hours after dosing.

In humans, plasma half-life is ≈ 3-5 days. It is unknown how or where the drug is metabolized, but metabolites are found in the urine.

Contraindications/Precautions/Warnings

Pyrimethamine is contraindicated in patients hypersensitive to it and should be used cautiously in patients with preexisting hematologic disorders. Some clinicians recommend avoiding its use in cats because of its adverse effect profile.

Adverse Effects

In small animals, anorexia, malaise, vomiting, depression, and bone marrow depression (anemia, thrombocytopenia, leukopenia) have been seen. Adverse effects may be more prominent in cats and noted 4-6 days after starting combination therapy. Some clinicians recommend avoiding its use in this species. Hematologic effects can develop rapidly and frequent monitoring is recommended, particularly if therapy persists longer than 2 weeks. Oral administration of folinic acid at 1 mg/kg PO, folic acid 5 mg/day, or Brewer's yeast 100 mg/kg/day has been suggested to alleviate adverse effects.

The drug is unpalatable to cats when mixed with food and the 25 mg tablet dosage size makes successful dosing a challenge.

In horses, pyrimethamine has caused leukopenias, thrombocytopenia and anemias when used in combination with sulfonamides. Baker's yeast and folinic acid have been suggested to antagonize these adverse effects. Alternatively, folic acid supplement may be used (an example is Folic Acid and Vitamin E Pak from Buckeye Feed Mills in Dalton, Ohio).

Reproductive/Nursing Safety

Pyrimethamine has been demonstrated to be teratogenic in rats. Fetal abnormalities have been seen in foals after mares have been treated, however, it has been used in treating women with toxoplasmosis during pregnancy. Clearly, the risks associated with therapy must be weighed against the potential for toxicity, the severity of the disease, and any alternative therapies available (*e.g.*, clindamycin in small animals). Concomitant administration of folinic acid has been recommended if the drug is to be used during pregnancy by some, but others state that pregnant mares should not receive folic acid during therapy as it may exacerbate fetal abnormalities or mortality. In humans, the FDA categorizes this drug as category C for use during pregnancy (*Animal studies have shown an adverse effect on the fetus, but there are no adequate studies in humans; or there are no animal reproduction studies and no adequate studies in humans.*)

Pyrimethamine is excreted in maternal milk; consider using milk replacer.

Overdosage/Acute Toxicity

Reports of acute overdosage of pyrimethamine in animals were not located. In humans, vomiting, nausea, anorexia, CNS stimulation (including seizures), and hematologic effects can be seen. Recommendations for treatment include: standard procedures in emptying the gut or preventing absorption, parenteral barbiturates for seizures, folinic acid for hematologic effects, and long-term monitoring (at least 1 month) of renal and hematopoietic systems.

Drug Interactions

The following drug interactions have either been reported or are theoretical in humans or animals receiving pyrimethamine and may be of significance in veterinary patients. Unless otherwise noted, use together is not necessarily contraindicated, but weigh the potential risks and perform additional monitoring when appropriate.

- **para-AMINOBENZOIC ACID (PABA):** PABA is reportedly antagonistic towards the activity of pyrimethamine; clinical significance is unclear.
- **SULFONAMIDES:** Pyrimethamine is synergistic with sulfonamides in activity against toxoplasmosis (and malaria).
- **TRIMETHOPRIM:** Use with pyrimethamine/sulfa is not recommended in humans as adverse effects may be additive. While this combination has been used clinically in horses it is currently not recommended as trimethoprim competitively inhibits pyrimethamine, thus decreasing the efficacy of the more effective dihydrofolate reductase inhibitor (Dirikolu *et al.* 2013).

Doses

- **DOGS:**

  For Toxoplasmosis (extra-label): Pyrimethamine (0.25 – 0.5 mg/kg) plus a sulfonamide (30 mg/kg twice daily for 2-4 weeks) also can be used to treat disseminated toxoplasmosis and to reduce oocyst shedding.

  For *Hepatazoon americanum* (extra-label): Trimethoprim/sulfa (15 mg/kg PO q12h), pyrimethamine (0.25 mg/kg PO q24h), and clindamycin (10 mg/kg q8h). Once remission attained, decoquinate (15 mg/kg mixed in food q12h for two years) can maintain. (Baneth 2007), (Baneth 2011)

  For canine neosporosis (extra-label): Trimethoprim/sulfadiazine (15-20 mg/kg PO every 12 hours for 4 weeks) in combination with pyrimethamine (1 mg/kg PO every 24 hours for 4 weeks). If observable clinical improvement is slow, treatment should be extended beyond the recommended 4 weeks until 2 weeks after clinical signs have plateaued. All littermates of affected puppies should be treated regardless of clinical signs. (CAPC 2014)

- **CATS:**

  Note: See warnings above (bone marrow depression).

  For toxoplasmosis (extra-label):

  a) For disseminated toxoplasmosis, pyrimethamine (0.25 – 0.5 mg/kg) plus a sulfonamide (30 mg/kg twice daily for 2-4 weeks) also can be used to treat disseminated toxoplasmosis and to reduce oocyst shedding. (CAPC 2014)

  b) In critical cases of pulmonary toxoplasmosis, clindamycin 12.5 mg/kg PO once daily (follow with food or water) and pyrimethamine 0.25 – 0.5 mg/kg PO q12h may be a better option than using clindamycin alone, especially in cats immunosuppressed with cyclosporine. (Foster *et al.* 2011)

- **HORSES:**

  See the next monograph (Pyrimethamine + Sulfadiazine)

- **BIRDS:**

  For coccidian organisms in raptors (extra-label): 0.5 mg/kg PO twice daily for 14-28 days (especially effective against Toxoplasmosis, Atoxoplasmosis and Sarcocystis). (Jones 2007)

Monitoring

- See adverse effects; CBC with platelet count.
- Clinical efficacy.

Client Information

- For dogs, cats, & birds: Can give with or without food. Very unpleasant tasting if mixed into food.
- Cats may be more likely to develop side effects while on this drug; use with caution.
- Side effects include: vomiting, lack of appetite, depression/malaise (tiredness/lack of energy), and bone marrow depression. If bleeding, extreme tiredness/lack of energy, infection, or fever are seen, contact veterinarian right away.
- Pregnant women should handle this drug very carefully.

Chemistry/Synonyms

An aminopyrimidine agent structurally related to trimethoprim, pyrimethamine occurs as an odorless, white, or almost white, crystalline powder or crystals. It is practically insoluble in water and slightly soluble in alcohol.

Pyrimethamine may also be known as: BW-50-63, pirimetamina, pyrimethaminum, RP-4753, *Daraprim®*, *Malocide®*, or *Pirimecidan®*.

Storage/Stability

Pyrimethamine tablets should be stored in tight, light-resistant containers.

Compatibility/Compounding Considerations

Pyrimethamine tablets may be crushed to make oral suspensions of the drug. Although stable in an aqueous solution, sugars tend to adversely affect the stability of pyrimethamine. If cherry syrup, corn syrup, or sucrose-containing liquids are used in the preparation of the suspension, it is recommended to store the suspension at room temperature and discard after 7 days.

Dosage Forms/Regulatory Status

VETERINARY-LABELED PRODUCTS: NONE.

HUMAN-LABELED PRODUCTS:

Pyrimethamine Tablets: 25 mg; *Daraprim®*; (Rx)

Revisions/References

Monograph revised/updated May 2014.

Baneth, G. (2007). Canine and Feline Hepatozoonosis--More than one disease. Proceedings: WSAVA World Congress. accessed via Veterinary Information Network; vin.com

Baneth, G. (2011). Perspectives on canine and feline hepatozoonosis. Veterinary Parasitology 181(1): 3-11.

CAPC (2014). Companion Animal Parasite Council (CAPC) Recommendations, CAPCvet. org.

Dirikolu, L., et al. (2013). Current therapeutic approaches to equine protozoal myeloencephalitis. Javma-Journal of the American Veterinary Medical Association 242(4): 482-91.

Foster, S. F. & P. Martin (2011). Lower respiratory tract infections in cats: Reaching beyond empirical therapy. Journal of Feline Medicine & Surgery 13(5): 313-32.

Jones, M. (2007). Falconry and raptor medicine. Proceedings: Western Vet Conf. accessed via Veterinary Information Network; vin.com

Pyrimethamine + Sulfadiazine

(pye-ri-**meth**-a-meen + sul-fa-**dye**-a-zeen)   ReBalance®

Antiprotozoal

Prescriber Highlights

▶ Tetrahydrofolic acid inhibitor suspension labeled for the treatment of horses with equine protozoal myeloencephalitis (EPM) caused by *Sarcocystis neurona*.

▶ May cause bone marrow suppression, GI effects, & "treatment crisis" (patient's signs worsen after beginning therapy).

▶ Daily treatment may be required for 3-9 months.

Uses/Indications

ReBalance® (pyrimethamine/sulfadiazine suspension in a 1:20 concentration) is labeled for the treatment of horses with equine protozoal myeloencephalitis (EPM) caused by *Sarcocystis neurona*. Some combine pyrimethamine and sulfadiazine with ponazuril or diclazuril in treating relapsing EPM.

Although not labeled for use in small animals it potentially could be useful for treating protozoal infections such as Toxoplasmosis in cats or Neosporosis in dogs.

Pharmacology/Actions

Sulfonamides inhibit the conversion of para-aminobenzoic acid (PABA) to dihydrofolic acid (DFA) by competing with PABA for dihydropteroate synthase. Pyrimethamine blocks the conversion of DFA to tetrahydrofolic acid by inhibiting dihydrofolate reductase. When sulfas and dihydrofolate reductase inhibitors (*e.g.*, trimethoprim, pyrimethamine) are used together, synergistic effects can occur. When comparing pyrimethamine and trimethoprim, pyrimethamine is more active against protozoal dihydrofolate reductase and trimethoprim is more active against bacterial dihydrofolate reductase.

When used (as labeled) for EPM in horses, estimated success rate is 60-70% with a 10% estimated relapse rate (Dirikolu *et al.* 2013).

Pharmacokinetics

No specific information was located for the pharmacokinetics of this drug combination and dosage form (oral suspension) in horses. Previous reports in horses using other dosage forms reported pyrimethamine oral bioavailability of ≈ 56% and elimination half-life of ≈ 12 hours. CNS levels are ≈ 25-50% of those found in plasma. Sulfadiazine is apparently well absorbed after oral administration to horses and enters the CSF. Volume of distribution is ≈ 0.58 L/kg; elimination half-life is ≈ 3-4 hours.

Contraindications/Precautions/Warnings

This drug combination is contraindicated in horses hypersensitive to either pyrimethamine or sulfadiazine. It should not be used in horses intended for human consumption. Because it may cause bone marrow suppression, use with caution in horses with preexisting hematologic abnormalities or those receiving other drugs that may cause bone marrow suppression.

Adverse Effects

Adverse effects in horses reported during field trials for pyrimethamine/sulfadiazine suspension include bone marrow suppression (anemia, leukopenia, neutropenia, thrombocytopenia), reduced appetite/anorexia, loose stools/diarrhea, and urticaria. CNS effects may be noted (seizures, depression), but are probably a result of the disease (EPM).

Baker's yeast or folinic acid have been suggested to antagonize the drug combination's bone marrow depressive effects, but efficacy has not been proven.

During the initial period (first few days) of treatment, neurologic signs may worsen—so-called treatment crisis—and may persist up to 5 weeks. It is thought this may be the result of an inflammatory reaction secondary to dying parasites in the central nervous system.

Reproductive/Nursing Safety

The label for *ReBalance®* (pyrimethamine/sulfadiazine suspension) states that the safe use of this product in horses for breeding purposes, during pregnancy, or in lactating mares has not been evaluated. Pyrimethamine has been demonstrated to be teratogenic in rats. Fetal abnormalities have been seen in foals after mares have been treated; however, it has been used in treating women with toxoplasmosis during pregnancy. Risks associated with therapy must be weighed against the potential for toxicity, the severity of the disease, and any alternative therapies available. Some have recommended concomitant administration of folinic acid if the drug is to be used during pregnancy, but others state that pregnant mares should not receive folic acid during therapy as it may exacerbate fetal abnormalities or mortality. In humans, the FDA categorizes pyrimethamine as category **C** for use during pregnancy (*Animal studies have shown an adverse effect on the fetus, but there are no adequate studies in humans; or there are no animal reproduction studies and no adequate studies in humans.*)

Sulfas cross the placenta and fetal serum levels may be up to 50% of that found in maternal serum. Teratogenicity has been reported in some laboratory animals when given at very high doses. Sulfas should be used in pregnant animals only when the benefits clearly outweigh the risks of therapy.

Sulfonamides are distributed into milk. Pyrimethamine is excreted in maternal milk and safety for nursing offspring has not been established; consider using milk replacer.

Overdosage/Acute Toxicity

Acute overdosage information for pyrimethamine/sulfadiazine in horses (>2X) was not located. *ReBalance®* (pyrimethamine/sulfadiazine suspension) was administered at 2X the labeled dose for 92 days to 49 horses. Signs noted included loose stools, slight increases in ALP in some horses, declines in RBC, HCT, Hgb, and PCV, and depressed appetite.

Drug Interactions

The label for *ReBalance®* (pyrimethamine/sulfadiazine suspension) states that the safety of this product with concomitant therapies in horses has not been evaluated.

In humans, the following drug interactions with sulfas and/or pyrimethamine have been reported or are theoretical and may be of significance in veterinary patients. Unless otherwise noted, use together is not necessarily contraindicated, but weigh the potential risks and perform additional monitoring when appropriate.

- **ANTACIDS:** May decrease the bioavailability of sulfonamides if administered concurrently.
- **HIGHLY PROTEIN-BOUND DRUGS** (*e.g.,* **methotrexate, phenylbutazone, thiazide diuretics, salicylates, probenecid, phenytoin, warfarin**): Sulfonamides may displace other highly bound drugs.
- **para-AMINOBENZOIC ACID (PABA):** PABA is reportedly antagonistic towards the activity of pyrimethamine; clinical significance is unclear.
- **TRIMETHOPRIM:** Use with pyrimethamine/sulfa is not recommended in humans as adverse effects may be additive. While this combination has been used clinically in horses it is currently not recommended as trimethoprim competitively inhibits pyrimethamine, thus decreasing the efficacy of the more effective dihydrofolate reductase inhibitor (Dirikolu *et al.* 2013).

Laboratory Considerations

The following laboratory alterations have been reported in humans taking sulfonamides and may be of significance in veterinary patients. Unless otherwise noted, use together is not necessarily contraindicated, but weigh the potential risks and perform additional monitoring when appropriate.

- **Urine glucose:** Sulfonamides may give false-positive results when using the Benedict's method.

Doses

- **HORSES:**

  For treatment of EPM:

  Labeled-dose (FDA-approved): 20 mg/kg sulfadiazine with 1 mg/kg pyrimethamine; equivalent to 4 mL of *ReBalance®* suspension per 50 kg (110 lb) body weight PO once daily at least 1 hour before feeding with hay or grain. Administer using a suitable oral dosing syringe; insert nozzle through the interdental space and deposit the dose on the back of the tongue by depressing the plunger. Treatment duration is based upon clinical response, but usually ranges from 90-270 days. (Label information; *ReBalance®*)

  Extra-label for horses that have had two relapses: Intermittent sulfa-pyrimethamine may be effective in maintaining clinical remission. After completing regular therapy for EPM, give pyrimethamine/sulfadiazine twice weekly (first and fourth day of each week). (MacKay 2008)

Monitoring

- CBC (including platelets): baseline and at least monthly during therapy.
- GI adverse effects.
- Clinical Efficacy: Improvement in neuro signs, CSF Western Blot test negative.

Client Information

- Shake well before each use.
- Give at least 1 hour before feeding with hay or grain.
- Using oral dosing syringe, place tip in the interdental space (entering side of the mouth behind front teeth) and apply the dose on the back of the tongue.

- During the first few days of treatment, neurologic signs (*e.g.,* weakness, trouble walking, etc.) may get worse and may last up to 5 weeks; this may be due to inflammation caused by dying parasites in the central nervous system.
- Adverse effects include: loose stools/diarrhea, reduced appetite, itching.
- If signs of bone marrow depression are seen (*e.g.,* bleeding, extreme tiredness/lack of energy, infection, fever, etc.), contact veterinarian right away.
- Pregnant women should handle this drug with caution.

Chemistry/Synonyms

Pyrimethamine is an aminopyrimidine agent structurally related to trimethoprim. It occurs as an odorless, white, or almost white, crystalline powder or crystals. It is practically insoluble in water and slightly soluble in alcohol.

Sulfadiazine occurs as an odorless or nearly odorless, white to slightly yellow powder. It is practically insoluble in water and sparingly soluble in alcohol.

Sulfadoxine and Pyrimethamine may also be known as *Fansidar®* and *ReBalance®*.

Storage/Stability

ReBalance® suspension should be stored at controlled room temperature (15-30°C) and protected from freezing.

Dosage Forms/Regulatory Status

VETERINARY-LABELED PRODUCTS:

Sulfadiazine (as the sodium salt) 250 mg/mL and Pyrimethamine 12.5 mg/mL Oral Suspension in quart (946.4 mL) bottles; *ReBalance® Antiprotozoal Oral Suspension*; (Rx) FDA-approved for use in horses; not for use in horses intended for human consumption.

HUMAN-LABELED PRODUCTS:

A related compound for humans that contained Sulfadoxine & Pyrimethamine *Fansidar®* has been discontinued in the US market.

Revisions/References

Monograph revised/updated May 2014.

Dirikolu, L., et al. (2013). Current therapeutic approaches to equine protozoal myeloencephalitis. Javma-Journal of the American Veterinary Medical Association 242(4): 482-91.
MacKay, R. (2008). Equine Protozoal Myeloencephalitis: Managing Relapses. Comp Equine(Jan/Feb): 24-7.

Quinacrine HCl

(**qwin**-a-krin)

Antiprotozoal

Prescriber Highlights

▶ Antiprotozoal that may be useful for treatment of Giardia, Leishmania, & coccidia. May improve clinical signs associated with giardial infection, but not eliminate infection.

▶ Contraindications (relative): Hepatic dysfunction; pregnancy.

▶ Adverse Effects: Yellowing of skin & urine color, (not of clinical importance); GI (anorexia, nausea, vomiting, diarrhea), abnormal behaviors ("fly biting", agitation), pruritus, & fever. Potentially: Hypersensitivity, hepatopathy, aplastic anemia, corneal edema, & retinopathy.

▶ Availability is an issue (USA); must be obtained from a compounding pharmacy.

▶ Give with meals; have liquid available.

Uses/Indications

Quinacrine has activity against a variety of protozoans and helminths. However in small animals, newer, safer or more effective agents have largely replaced quinacrine for all but its use as an alternative treatment for Giardia or Trichomonas. In humans, quinacrine may be used for treatment of mild to moderate discoid lupus erythromatosus, transcervically as a sterilizing agent, or in powder form as an intrapleural sclerosing agent.

Pharmacology/Actions

Quinacrine's mechanism of action for its antiprotozoal activity against Giardia is not understood, however it does bind to DNA by intercalation to adjacent base pairs thereby inhibiting RNA transcription and translocation. Additionally, quinacrine interferes with electron transport and inhibits succinate oxidation and cholinesterase. Quinacrine binds to nucleoproteins that (in humans at least) can suppress lupus erythromatosus (LE) cell factor.

Pharmacokinetics

Quinacrine is absorbed well from the GI tract or after intrapleural administration. It is distributed throughout the body, but CSF levels are only 1-5% of those found in plasma. Drug is concentrated in the liver, spleen, lungs, and adrenals. It is relatively highly bound to plasma proteins in humans (80-90%). Quinacrine crosses the placenta, but only small amounts enter maternal milk.

Quinacrine is eliminated very slowly (half life in humans: 5-14 days). Quinacrine is slowly metabolized, but primarily eliminated by the kidneys; acidifying the urine will increase renal excretion somewhat. Significant amounts may be detected in urine up to 2 months after drug discontinuation.

Contraindications/Precautions/Warnings

In humans, quinacrine is relatively contraindicated in patients with psychotic disorders, psoriasis, or porphyria as it may exacerbate these conditions. Veterinary relevance is unknown. The drug should be used with extreme caution in patients with hepatic dysfunction.

Adverse Effects

In small animals, a yellowing of skin and urine color can occur but is not of clinical importance (does not indicate jaundice). Additionally, gastrointestinal disturbances (anorexia, nausea, vomiting, diarrhea), abnormal behaviors ("fly biting", agitation), lethargy, pruritus, and fever have been noted.

Potentially hypersensitivity reactions, hepatopathy, aplastic anemia, corneal edema, and retinopathy could occur (all reported rarely in humans, primarily with high dose long-term use).

Reproductive/Nursing Safety

Quinacrine crosses the placenta and has been implicated in causing a case of renal agenesis and hydrocephalus in a human infant. In high doses, it has caused increased fetal death rates in rats. Weigh the potential benefits with the risks when considering use in pregnant animals.

In humans, the FDA categorizes this drug as category C for use during pregnancy (*Animal studies have shown an adverse effect on the fetus, but there are no adequate studies in humans; or there are no animal reproduction studies and no adequate studies in humans.*)

Overdosage/Acute Toxicity

Overdosage may be serious depending on the dose. In humans, a dose as low as 6.8 grams (administered intraduodenally) caused death. Clinical signs associated with acute toxicity include CNS excitation (including seizures), GI disturbances, vascular collapse, and cardiac arrhythmias. Treatment consists of gut emptying protocols, and supportive and symptomatic therapies. Urinary acidification with ammonium chloride and forced diuresis (with adequate fluid therapy) may be beneficial in enhancing urinary excretion of the drug.

Drug Interactions

The following drug interactions have either been reported or are theoretical in humans or animals receiving quinacrine HCl and may be of significance in veterinary patients. Unless otherwise not-

ed, use together is not necessarily contraindicated, but weigh the potential risks and perform additional monitoring when appropriate.
- **ALCOHOL**: Quinacrine may cause a "disulfiram-reaction" if used with alcohol.
- **HEPATOTOXIC DRUGS**: Quinacrine concentrates in the liver and should be used with caution with hepatotoxic drugs (clinical significance unknown).
- **PRIMAQUINE**: Quinacrine increases the toxicity of primaquine (generally not used in veterinary medicine), and the two should not be used simultaneously.

Laboratory Considerations
- When urine is acidic, quinacrine can cause it to turn a deep yellow color.
- By causing an interfering fluorescence, quinacrine can cause falsely elevated values of **plasma and urine cortisol** values.

Doses
- **DOGS:**
  As a second to third-line drug for treatment of Giardia or other susceptible protozoa (extra-label): 6.6 mg/kg PO q12h for 5 days. (Blagburn 2003, 2005)
- **CATS:**
  As a second to third-line drug for treatment of Giardia or other susceptible protozoa (extra-label): <u>Giardia</u>: 9 mg/kg PO once daily for 6 days; <u>Coccidiosis</u>: 10 mg/kg PO once daily for 5 days. (Blagburn 2003), (Blagburn 2005)
- **REPTILES:**
  For hemoprotozoal infections (extra-label): 19 – 100 mg/kg PO q48h (every other day) for 2-3 weeks. (de la Navarre 2003)

Monitoring
- Efficacy (fecal exams, reduction in diarrhea).
- Adverse effects.

Client Information
- Quinacrine should preferably be given after meals with plenty of liquids available.
- Make sure clients understand the importance of compliance with directions and to watch for signs of adverse effects.

Chemistry/Synonyms

A synthetic acridine derivative anthelmintic, quinacrine HCl occurs as a bright yellow, odorless, crystalline powder having a bitter taste. It is sparingly soluble in water.

Quinacrine HCl may also be known as mepacrine HCl.

Storage/Stability

Tablets should be stored in tight, light-resistant containers at room temperature. Quinacrine is not stable in solution for any length of time; however, it may be crushed and mixed with foods to mask its very bitter taste.

Compatibility/Compounding Considerations

No specific information noted.

Dosage Forms/Regulatory Status

VETERINARY-LABELED PRODUCTS: NONE.

HUMAN-LABELED PRODUCTS: NONE.

There currently are no quinacrine products being marketed in the USA. It may be available from compounding pharmacies.

Revisions/References

Monograph revised/updated August 2014.

Blagburn, B. (2003). Giardiasis and coccidiosis updates. Proceedings: Western Veterinary Conference. accessed via Veterinary Information Network; vin.com

Blagburn, B. (2005). Treatment and control of tick borne diseases and other important parasites of companion animals. Proceedings: ACVC2005. accessed via Veterinary Information Network; vin.com

de la Navarre, B. (2003). Common parasitic diseases of reptiles and amphibians. Proceedings: Western Veterinary Conf. accessed via Veterinary Information Network; vin.com

Quinidine

(qwin-i-deen)

Antiarrhythmic

Prescriber Highlights

▶ Antiarrhythmic agent used in small animals & horses.

▶ Contraindications: Hypersensitivity, myasthenia gravis; complete AV block with an AV junctional or idioventricular pacemaker; intraventricular conduction defects; digitalis intoxication with associated arrhythmias or AV conduction disorders; aberrant ectopic impulses; or abnormal rhythms secondary to escape mechanisms. Extreme Caution: Any form of AV block or if any clinical signs of digoxin toxicity are exhibited. Caution: Uncorrected hypokalemia, hypoxia, & disorders or acid-base balance; hepatic or renal insufficiency.

▶ Adverse Effects: **Dogs:** GI effects, weakness, hypotension (especially with too rapid IV administration), negative inotropism, widened QRS complex & QT intervals, AV block, & multiform ventricular tachycardias hypotension. **Horses:** inappetence, depression, swelling of the nasal mucosa, ataxia, diarrhea, colic, hypotension & rarely, laminitis, paraphimosis & the development of urticarial wheals; cardiac arrhythmias including AV block, circulatory collapse & sudden death.

▶ Consider monitoring blood levels.

▶ Administer at evenly spaced intervals throughout the day/night.

▶ GI upset may be decreased if administered with food. Do not allow animal to chew or crush sustained-release oral dosage forms.

▶ Many drug interactions.

Uses/Indications

Quinidine is used in small animal or equine medicine for the treatment of ventricular arrhythmias (VPCs, ventricular tachycardia), refractory supraventricular tachycardias, and supraventricular arrhythmias associated with anomalous conduction in Wolff-Parkinson-White (WPW) syndrome. Chronic use of quinidine for controlling ventricular arrhythmias and supraventricular tachycardia in dogs has diminished over the years as other drugs appear to be more effective. It is still used in dogs and horses to convert atrial fibrillation to sinus rhythm. Oral therapy is generally not used in cats.

Pharmacology/Actions

A class IA antiarrhythmic, quinidine has effects similar to that of procainamide. It depresses myocardial excitability, conduction velocity, and contractility. Quinidine will prolong the effective refractory period, which prevents the reentry phenomenon and increases conduction times. Quinidine also possesses anticholinergic activity, which decreases vagal tone and may facilitate AV conduction.

Pharmacokinetics

After oral administration, quinidine salts are nearly completely absorbed from the GI, however, the actual amount that reaches the systemic circulation will be reduced due to the hepatic first-pass effect. The extended-release formulations of quinidine sulfate and gluconate, as well as the polygalacturonate tablets, are more slowly absorbed than the conventional tablets or capsules.

Quinidine is distributed rapidly to all body tissues except the brain. Protein binding varies from 82-92%. The reported volumes of distribution in various species are: horses: ≈ 15.1 L/kg; cattle: ≈ 3.8 L/kg; dogs: ≈ 2.9 L/kg; cats: ≈ 2.2 L/kg. Quinidine is distributed into milk and crosses the placenta.

Quinidine is metabolized in the liver, primarily by hydroxylation. Approximately 20% of a dose may be excreted unchanged in the urine within 24 hours after dosing. Serum half-lives reported in various species are: horses ≈ 8.1 hours; cattle ≈ 2.3 hours; dogs ≈ 5.6 hours; cats ≈ 1.9 hours; swine ≈ 5.5 hours; goats ≈ 0.9 hours. Acidic urine (pH <6) can increase renal excretion of quinidine and decrease its serum half-life.

Contraindications/Precautions/Warnings

Quinidine is generally contraindicated in patients who have demonstrated previous hypersensitivity reactions to it; myasthenia gravis; complete AV block with an AV junctional or idioventricular pacemaker; intraventricular conduction defects (especially with pronounced QRS widening); digitalis intoxication with associated arrhythmias or AV conduction disorders; aberrant ectopic impulses; or abnormal rhythms secondary to escape mechanisms. It should be used with extreme caution, if at all, in any form of AV block or if any clinical signs of digitalis toxicity are exhibited.

Quinidine should be used with caution in patients with uncorrected hypokalemia, hypoxia, and disorders of acid-base balance. Use cautiously in patients with hepatic or renal insufficiency as accumulation of the drug may result.

When using to cardiovert horses with atrial fibrillation, monitor the ECG throughout treatment. Heart rates above 80 bpm, a widening of QRS beyond 125% of baseline, and abnormal complexes are all indicators to discontinue medication (McGurrin 2010).

Do not confuse quinidine with quinine.

Adverse Effects

In dogs, gastrointestinal effects may include anorexia, vomiting, or diarrhea. Effects related to the cardiovascular system can include weakness, hypotension (especially with too rapid IV administration), negative inotropism, widened QRS complex and QT intervals, AV block, and multiform ventricular tachycardias.

Horses may exhibit inappetence and depression commonly after quinidine therapy but this does not necessarily indicate toxicity. Signs of toxicity can include swelling of the nasal mucosa, ataxia, diarrhea, colic, ventricular rate exceeding 120 BPM, QRS broadening by 25% or more, hypotension and, rarely, laminitis, paraphimosis and the development of urticarial wheals. Urticaria or upper respiratory tract obstruction can be treated, if required, by discontinuing the drug and administering corticosteroids. If obstruction persists, nasotracheal tube placement or tracheostomy may be required. Horses may develop cardiac arrhythmias including AV block, circulatory collapse, and sudden death.

Patients exhibiting signs of toxicity or lack of response may be candidates for therapeutic serum monitoring. The therapeutic range is thought to be 2.5-5 micrograms/mL in dogs. Toxic effects usually are not seen unless levels are >10 micrograms/mL.

Reproductive/Nursing Safety

In humans, the FDA categorizes this drug as category *C* for use during pregnancy (*Animal studies have shown an adverse effect on the fetus, but there are no adequate studies in humans; or there are no animal reproduction studies and no adequate studies in humans.*) In a separate system evaluating the safety of drugs in canine and feline pregnancy (Papich 1989), this drug is categorized as class: *B (Safe for use if used cautiously. Studies in laboratory animals may have uncovered some risk, but these drugs appear to be safe in dogs and cats or these drugs are safe if they are not administered when the animal is near term.)*

Quinidine is excreted into maternal milk with a milk to serum ratio of ≈ 0.71. Use caution when quinidine is administered to nursing patients. The American Academy of Pediatrics considers quinidine compatible with breastfeeding.

Overdosage/Acute Toxicity

Clinical signs of overdosage can include depression, hypotension, lethargy, confusion, seizures, vomiting, diarrhea, and oliguria.

Cardiac signs may include depressed automaticity and conduction, or tachyarrhythmias. The CNS effects are often delayed after the onset of cardiovascular effects but may persist after the cardiovascular effects have begun to resolve.

If a recent oral ingestion, emptying of the gut and charcoal administration may be beneficial to remove any unabsorbed drug. IV fluids, plus metaraminol or norepinephrine, can be considered to treat hypotensive effects. A 1/6 molar intravenous infusion of sodium lactate may be used in an attempt to reduce the cardiotoxic effects of quinidine. Forced diuresis using fluids and diuretics along with reduction of urinary pH may enhance the renal excretion of the drug. Temporary cardiac pacing may be necessary should severe AV block occur. Hemodialysis will effectively remove quinidine, but peritoneal dialysis will not.

Drug Interactions

The following drug interactions have either been reported or are theoretical in humans or animals receiving quinidine and may be of significance in veterinary patients. Unless otherwise noted, use together is not necessarily contraindicated, but weigh the potential risks and perform additional monitoring when appropriate.

- **ACETAZOLAMIDE:** May reduce quinidine clearance.
- **AMIODARONE:** May increase quinidine levels (significantly).
- **ANTACIDS:** May delay oral absorption; separate dosages.
- **ANTIARRHYTHMIC AGENTS:** Use with caution with other antidysrhythmic agents, as additive cardiotoxic or other toxic effects may result.
- **ANTICHOLINESTERASES** (*e.g.,* **pyridostigmine, neostigmine**): Quinidine may antagonize the effects of anticholinesterases in patients with myasthenia gravis.
- **AUROTHIOGLUCOSE:** Increased risk for blood dyscrasias.
- **CIMETIDINE:** Cimetidine may increase the levels of quinidine by inhibiting hepatic microsomal enzymes.
- **CISAPRIDE:** Increased risk for QTc interval prolongation.
- **COLCHICINE:** Quinidine may increase colchicine levels.
- **CLARITHROMYCIN:** Increased risk for torsade de pointes.
- **DEXAMETHASONE:** In dogs, dexamethasone increased quinidine volume of distribution (49-78%) and elimination half-life (1.5-2.3X). (Zhang *et al.* 2006)
- **DIGOXIN:** Digoxin levels may increase considerably in patients stabilized on digoxin who receive quinidine. Some cardiologists recommend decreasing the digoxin dosage by 1/2 when adding quinidine. Therapeutic drug monitoring of both quinidine and digoxin may be warranted in these cases. Digoxin has been recommended for treating quinidine-induced profound hypotension or supraventricular tachycardia (>200 BPM) in horses (Divers 2013).
- **DILTIAZEM:** Possible decreased clearance; increased elimination half-life of quinidine. Diltiazem has been recommended for treating quinidine-induced profound hypotension or supraventricular tachycardia (>200 BPM) in horses (Divers 2013).
- **HYPOTENSIVE AGENTS:** Quinidine may potentiate the effects of other drugs having hypotensive effects.
- **FLUCONAZOLE, ITRACONAZOLE, & KETOCONAZOLE:** Increased risk for cardiotoxicity.
- **FLUOROQUINOLONE ANTIBIOTICS** (*e.g.,* **ciprofloxacin, enrofloxacin**, etc.): Increased risk for cardiotoxicity.
- **NEUROMUSCULAR BLOCKING AGENTS** (*e.g.,* **succinylcholine, tubocurarine, atracurium**, etc.): Quinidine may increase the neuromuscular blocking effects of drugs.
- **PHENOBARBITAL, PHENYTOIN:** May induce hepatic enzymes that metabolize quinidine thus reducing quinidine serum half-life by 50%.

- **PHENOTHIAZINES:** Additive cardiac depressant effects may be seen.
- **RIFAMPIN:** May induce hepatic enzymes that metabolize quinidine thus reducing quinidine serum half-life by 50%.
- **TRICYCLIC ANTIDEPRESSANTS** (*e.g.,* **amitriptyline, clomipramine, doxepin, imipramine**): Increased risk for QTc interval prolongation and tricyclic adverse effects.
- **URINARY ACIDIFIERS** (*e.g.,* **methionine, ammonium chloride**): Drugs that acidify the urine may increase the excretion of quinidine and decrease serum level.
- **URINARY ALKALINIZERS** (*e.g.,* **carbonic anhydrase inhibitors, thiazide diuretics, sodium bicarbonate, antacids**, etc.): Drugs that alkalinize the urine may decrease the excretion of quinidine, prolonging its half-life.
- **VERAPAMIL:** Possible decreased clearance; increased elimination half-life of quinidine; increased risk for hypotension.
- **WARFARIN:** Coumarin anticoagulants with quinidine may increase the likelihood of bleeding problems.

Doses

- **DOGS:**

  For VPC's or ventricular tachycardia (extra-label): 6 – 16 mg/kg PO or IM q6h (q8h with sustained release products). (Fox 2003)

  For conversion of atrial fib to sinus rhythm in dogs without underlying heart disease (extra-label): Initially attempted with quinidine gluconate at 6 – 11 mg/kg IM q6h. Some dogs will convert in the first 24 hours of therapy. If rapid ventricular response occurs, may give either digoxin or a beta-blocker to slow rate of conduction across AV node. (Russell *et al.* 1995), (Smith 2009)

- **HORSES:** (NOTE: ARCI UCGFS CLASS 4 DRUG)

  For atrial fibrillation in a horse without heart failure (extra-label): <u>Oral (via NG tube) Dosing:</u> give quinidine sulfate 22 mg/kg PO via nasogastric tube every 2 hours until cardioversion, toxic effects, or 6 doses have been given. If AF remains, continue administration every 6 hours until cardioversion or adverse effects. Alternate <u>IV dosing</u> method: 0.5 – 2.2 mg/kg IV bolus every 5-10 minutes to effect or until adverse effects seen. Maximum IV dose is 12 mg/kg. Conversion of ventricular tachycardia has occurred with a single 0.5 mg/kg dose. Monitor ECG throughout treatment. Heart rate in excess of 80 bpm, widening QRS complex >125% of baseline, or abnormal complexes are indicators to discontinue treatment.

  Toxic effects are variable. Mild signs include nasal edema, and mild depression. More severe signs include marked ataxia, hypotension, colic, diarrhea, seizures, sustained tachycardia, syncope and sudden death. Adverse effects not necessarily dose dependent. Hypokalemia increases risk for torsades de pointes. Therapeutic levels 3-5 micrograms/mL. (Kimberly *et al.* 2006)

  For sustained narrow-QRS tachycardia (extra-label): From a case report. Horse received 22 mg/kg via NG tube q2h for 3 doses. The rate of the tachycardia slowed gradually from 150 bpm to approximately 100 bpm. Approximately 1 hour after the third dose, the patient's cardiac rhythm abruptly converted to sinus tachycardia at a rate of 80 bpm. (Stern *et al.* 2012)

Monitoring

- ECG, continuous if possible.
- Blood pressure, during IV administration.
- Clinical signs of toxicity (see Adverse Reactions/Overdosage).
- Serum levels. Therapeutic serum levels are believed to range from 2-7 micrograms/mL (2-5 micrograms/mL in horses). Levels >10 micrograms/mL are considered toxic.

Client Information

- Oral products should be administered at evenly spaced intervals throughout the day/night. GI upset may be decreased if administered with food.
- Do not allow animal to chew or crush sustained-release oral dosage forms.
- Notify veterinarian if animal's condition deteriorates or signs of toxicity (e.g., vomiting, diarrhea, weakness, etc.) occur.

Chemistry/Synonyms

Used as an antiarrhythmic agent, quinidine is an alkaloid obtained from cinchona or related plants, or prepared from quinine. It is available commercially in two salts: gluconate or sulfate. Quinidine polygalacturonate is no longer commercially available.

Quinidine gluconate occurs as a very bitter tasting, odorless, white powder. It is freely soluble in water and slightly soluble in alcohol. The injectable form has a pH of 5.5-7. Quinidine gluconate contains 62% anhydrous quinidine alkaloid. Quinidine sulfate occurs as very bitter tasting, odorless, fine, needle-like, white crystals that may cohere in masses. One gram is soluble in ≈100 mL of water or 10 mL of alcohol. Quinidine sulfate contains 83% anhydrous quinidine alkaloid.

Quinidine gluconate may also be known as: quinidinium gluconate, *Duraquin*, *Quinaglute*, *Quinalan*, and *Quinate*.

Quinidine sulfate may also be known as: chinidini sulfas, chinidinsulfate, chinidinum sulfuricum, or quinidini sulfas; many trade names are available.

Storage/Stability

All quinidine salts darken upon exposure to light (acquire a brownish tint) and should be stored in light-resistant, well-closed containers. Use only colorless, clear solutions of quinidine gluconate for injection.

Quinidine gluconate injection is usually administered intramuscularly, but may be given very slowly (1 mL/minute) intravenously. It may be diluted by adding 10-40 mL of D5W.

Compatibility/Compounding Considerations

Quinidine gluconate is reported to be physically **compatible** with bretylium tosylate, cimetidine HCl, and verapamil HCl. It is reportedly physically **incompatible** with alkalies and iodides.

Dosage Forms/Regulatory Status

VETERINARY-LABELED PRODUCTS: NONE.
The ARCI (Racing Commissioners International) has designated this drug as a class 4 substance. See the appendix for more information.

HUMAN-LABELED PRODUCTS:

Quinidine Sulfate (83% anhydrous quinidine alkaloid) Tablets: 200 mg & 300 mg; generic; (Rx)

Quinidine Sulfate (83% anhydrous quinidine alkaloid) Sustained-Release Tablets: 300 mg; generic; (Rx)

Quinidine Gluconate (62% anhydrous quinidine alkaloid) Sustained-Release Tablets: 324 mg; generic; (Rx)

Quinidine Gluconate (62% anhydrous quinidine alkaloid) Injection: 80 mg/mL (50 mg/mL of quinidine base) in 10 mL multi-dose vials; generic; (Rx)

Revisions/References

Monograph revised/updated August 2014.

Divers, T. (2013). Treatment of Cardiopulmonary Disorders in Horses. Proceedings; International Veterinary Emergency and Critical Care Symposium. accessed via Veterinary Information Network; vin.com

Fox, P. (2003). Congestive heart failure: Clinical approach and management. Proceedings: World Small Animal Veterinary Assoc World Congress. accessed via Veterinary Information Network; vin.com

Kimberly, M. & K. McGurrin (2006). Update on antiarrhythmic therapy in horses. Proceedings; ACVIM. accessed via Veterinary Information Network; vin.com

McGurrin, M. (2010). Therapeutic Options in Atrial Fibrillation. Proceedings: ACVIM. accessed via Veterinary Information Network; vin.com

Papich, M. (1989). Effects of drugs on pregnancy. *Current Veterinary Therapy X: Small Animal Practice*. R. Kirk. Philadelphia, Saunders: 1291-9.

Russell, L. & J. Rush (1995). Cardiac Arrhythmias in Systemic Disease. *Kirk's Current Veterinary Therapy:XII*. J. Bonagura. Philadelphia, W.B. Saunders: 161-6.

Smith, F. (2009). Update on Antiarrhythmic Therapy. Proceedings: Western Veterinary Conference. accessed via Veterinary Information Network; vin.com

Stern, J. A., et al. (2012). Resolution of sustained narrow complex ventricular tachycardia and tachycardia-induced cardiomyopathy in a Quarter Horse following quinidine therapy. Journal of Veterinary Cardiology 14(3): 445-51.

Zhang, K. W., et al. (2006). Clinical oral doses of dexamethasone decreases intrinsic clearance of quinidine, a cytochrome P450 3A substrate in dogs. Journal of Veterinary Medical Science 68(9): 903-7.

Ramipril

(ram-ih-prill)   Altace®, Vasotop®

Angiotensin Converting Enzyme (ACE) Inhibitor

Prescriber Highlights

▶ ACE inhibitor used primarily as a vasodilator in the treatment of heart failure or hypertension; may be of benefit in the treatment of chronic renal failure or protein losing nephropathies.

▶ Not as much information or experience available as some other ACE inhibitors (e.g., enalapril, benazepril) in dogs or cats.

▶ Contraindications: Hypersensitivity to ACE inhibitors. Caution: Pregnancy, patients with hyponatremia, coronary or cerebrovascular insufficiency, preexisting hematologic abnormalities, or a collagen vascular disease (e.g., SLE).

▶ Adverse Effects: Appears well tolerated in both dogs & cats. GI effects (anorexia, vomiting, diarrhea) possible; potentially: weakness, hypotension, & hyperkalemia.

Uses/Indications

Ramipril is a long-acting angiotensin converting enzyme (ACE) inhibitor that may be useful in treating heart failure or hypertension in dogs or cats. It is an approved product in the UK for treating heart failure in dogs. In cats, ramipril has been used for treating arterial hypertension. A study (MacDonald *et al.* 2006) did not show any significant benefit using ramipril in treating Maine Coon cats with hypertrophic cardiomyopathy without heart failure.

Like other ACE inhibitors, it may potentially be useful as adjunctive treatment in chronic renal failure and protein losing nephropathies. In dogs with moderate renal impairment (such as might be found with CHF), there is apparently no need to adjust ramipril dosage.

In healthy horses, oral benazepril was found to be more effective than ramipril (0.3 or 0.1 mg/kg) at inhibiting serum ACE activity (Afonso *et al.* 2013).

Pharmacology/Actions

Ramipril is a pro-drug that has little pharmacologic activity until converted into ramiprilat. Ramiprilat prevents the formation of angiotensin-II (a potent vasoconstrictor) by competing with angiotensin-I for the enzyme angiotensin-converting enzyme (ACE). ACE has a much higher affinity for ramiprilat than for angiotensin-I. Because angiotensin-II concentrations are decreased, aldosterone secretion is reduced and plasma renin activity is increased.

The cardiovascular effects of ramiprilat in patients with CHF include decreased total peripheral resistance, pulmonary vascular resistance, mean arterial and right atrial pressures, and pulmonary capillary wedge pressure with no change or decrease in heart rate. Increased cardiac index and output, stroke volume, and exercise tolerance also occur. Renal blood flow can be increased with little change in hepatic blood flow. In animals with glomerular disease,

ACE inhibitors probably decrease proteinuria and help to preserve renal function.

Pharmacokinetics

After oral administration to dogs, ramipril is rapidly converted via de-esterification into ramiprilat. Bioavailability of ramiprilat after a dose of 0.25 mg/kg per day of ramipril is ≈ 6.7%. At this dose, ACE activity never exceeded 60% in either healthy dogs or those with experimentally induced renal dysfunction (GFR reduced 58%) (Lefebvre *et al.* 2006).

After oral administration to cats with ramipril doses ranging from 0.125 mg/kg to 1 mg/kg once daily for 9 days, ramipril peak concentrations occurred in ≈ 0.5 hours. Ramipril is rapidly converted into its active metabolite ramiprilat, which peaks at 1 hour post-administration. Repeated doses of 0.125 mg/kg inhibited serum ACE activity by 94% at maximum to 55% 24 hours post-dose. At a dose of 1 mg/kg, ACE activity was 97% inhibited at maximum, and 83% inhibited 24 hours post-dose (Coulet *et al.* 2002).

When cats were administered radiolabeled ramipril orally, 85-89% of the radioactivity was recovered in the feces. It is unclear how much of this represents unabsorbed drug or absorbed parent compound/metabolites eliminated in the feces. Approximately 10% of administered drug was recovered in the urine. Excretion of radiolabeled compounds was complete by 168 hours after dosing.

Contraindications/Precautions/Warnings

The labeling for the UK product approved for dogs (*Vasotop*®) states that it should not be used in clinical cases of vascular stenosis (*e.g.,* aortic stenosis), obstructive hypertrophic cardiomyopathy, or with potassium-sparing diuretics (see Drug Interactions).

Adverse Effects

While information is limited, ramipril appears to be well tolerated in dogs and cats. Gastrointestinal effects are probably the most likely adverse effects to be noted. Weakness, hypotension, or hyperkalemia are possible.

Reproductive/Nursing Safety

The labeling for the product approved in the UK (*Vasotop*®) suggests not using in bitches during pregnancy or lactation. Weigh the potential risks associated with using this medication (see human data below) in veterinary patients with the potential benefits of therapy. Dosages of up to 500 mg/kg/day did not impair fertility in rats. While no teratogenic effects have been detected with ramipril in studies performed in mice, rats, rabbits, and cynomolgus monkeys, fetal risk is increased in humans.

If used in humans during the 2nd and 3rd trimesters increased rates of fetal death, neonatal hypotension, skull hypoplasia, anuria, renal failure, oligohydramnios leading to fetal limb contractures, craniofacial deformation, and hypoplastic lung development were noted. In humans, ramipril has a "black box" warning regarding its use in pregnancy that states "When used in pregnancy during the second and third trimesters, angiotensin-converting enzyme (ACE) inhibitors can cause injury and even death to the developing fetus. When pregnancy is detected, ramipril should be discontinued as soon as possible." For humans, the FDA categorizes ramipril as category *D* for use during the 2nd and 3rd trimesters of pregnancy (*There is evidence of human fetal risk, but the potential benefits from the use of the drug in pregnant women may be acceptable despite its potential risks*) and as category *C* for use during the first trimester of pregnancy (*Animal studies have shown an adverse effect on the fetus, but there are no adequate studies in humans; or there are no animal reproduction studies and no adequate studies in humans.*)

It is unknown whether ramipril (or ramiprilat) enters milk. Both the veterinary label (UK) and human label recommended not using the drug during nursing.

Overdosage/Acute Toxicity

In dogs, ramipril appears quite safe; dosages as high as 1 gram/kg induced only mild GI distress. Lethal doses in rats and mice were noted at 10 – 11 grams/kg. No information was located on overdoses in cats. In overdose situations, the primary concern is hypotension; supportive treatment with volume expansion with normal saline is recommended to correct blood pressure. Because of the drug's long duration of action, prolonged monitoring and treatment may be required.

Drug Interactions

The following drug interactions have either been reported or are theoretical in humans or animals receiving ramipril and may be of significance in veterinary patients. Unless otherwise noted, use together is not necessarily contraindicated, but weigh the potential risks and perform additional monitoring when appropriate.

- **ASPIRIN**: Aspirin may potentially negate the decrease in systemic vascular resistance induced by ACE inhibitors. However, in one study in dogs using low-dose aspirin, hemodynamic effects of enalaprilat (active metabolite of enalapril—a related drug) were not affected.
- **ANTIDIABETIC AGENTS (insulin, oral agents)**: Possible increased risk for hypoglycemia; enhanced monitoring recommended.
- **DIURETICS** (*e.g.,* **furosemide, hydrochlorothiazide**): Potential for increased hypotensive effects.
- **DIURETICS, POTASSIUM SPARING** (*e.g.,* **spironolactone, triamterene**): Increased hyperkalemic effects, enhanced monitoring of serum potassium.
- **NSAIDS**: Potential for increased risk of renal dysfunction or hyperkalemia.
- **POTASSIUM SUPPLEMENTS**: Increased risk for hyperkalemia.

Laboratory Considerations

- ACE inhibitors may cause a reversible decrease in localization and excretion of **iodohippurate sodium I^{123}/I^{134}**, or **Technetium Tc^{99} pententate** renal imaging in the affected kidney in patients with renal artery stenosis, which could lead to confusion in test interpretation.

Doses

- **DOGS:**
  For treatment of heart failure (extra-label in USA): Initially, 0.125 mg/kg PO once daily; depending on the severity of pulmonary congestion, dose may be increased to 0.25 mg/kg PO once daily. (Label information; *Vasotop*®—Intervet UK)
- **CATS:**
  For treatment of arterial hypertension (extra-label): In the study cats were started at 0.125 mg/kg PO once daily. In cats where SBP was still above 160 mmHg on day 14 the dose was increased to 0.25 mg/kg PO once daily up to the end of the trial (day 63). 62% had a decrease in SBP of 20 mmHg or more; of these cats, 69% had a final SBP below 160 mmHg. (Van Israel *et al.* 2009)

Monitoring

- Clinical signs.
- Serum electrolytes, creatinine, BUN, urine protein.
- CBC with differential, periodic.
- Blood pressure (if treating hypertension or clinical signs associated with hypotension arise).

Client Information

- Ramipril is used to treat heart failure, high blood pressure and some forms of kidney disease in dogs and cats.
- Usually well tolerated, but vomiting and diarrhea can occur.

Give with food if vomiting or lack of appetite becomes a problem. If a rash or signs of infection occur (*e.g.*, fever) contact your veterinarian immediately.

- Very important to give exactly as prescribed. Do not stop or reduce dosage without first talking with your veterinarian.
- Your animal will likely need to have blood pressure and lab tests performed while on this medication.

Chemistry/Synonyms

Ramipril occurs as a white to almost white, crystalline powder that is sparingly soluble in water and freely soluble in methyl alcohol.

Ramipril may also be known as Hoe-498, ramiprilis, or ramiprilium. There are many international trade names including: *Altace*®, *Cardase*®, *Delix*®, *Ramase*®, *Triatec*®, and *Vasotop*®.

Storage/Stability

Capsules should be stored at room temperature (15-30°C) protected from light in tight containers.

Compatibility/Compounding Considerations

No specific information noted.

Dosage Forms/Regulatory Status

VETERINARY-LABELED PRODUCTS:

None in the USA; in the UK and in other European countries: Ramipril Tablets: 0.625 mg, 1.25 mg, 2.5 mg, & 5 mg; *Vasotop*®; (POM-V). Approved for use in dogs.

HUMAN-LABELED PRODUCTS:

Ramipril Oral Capsules: 1.25 mg, 2.5 mg, 5 mg, & 10 mg; *Altace*®, generic; (Rx)

Revisions/References

Monograph revised/updated August 2014.

Afonso, T., et al. (2013). Pharmacodynamic Evaluation of 4 Angiotensin-Converting Enzyme Inhibitors in Healthy Adult Horses. Journal of Veterinary Internal Medicine 27(5): 1185-92.

Coulet, M. & S. Burgaud (2002). Pharmacokinetics of ramipril and ramiprilat and angiotensin converting enzyme (ACE) activity after single and repeated oral administration of ramipril to cats. Proceedings: 12th ECVIM-CA Congress. accessed via Veterinary Information Network; vin.com

Lefebvre, H., et al. (2006). Pharmacokinetic and pharmacodynamic parameters of ramipril and ramiprilat in healthy dogs and dogs with reduced glomerular filtration rate. J Vet Intern Med 20: 499-507.

MacDonald, K., et al. (2006). The effect of ramipril on left ventricular mass, myocardial fibrosis, diastolic function, and plasma neurohormones in Maine Coon cats with familial hypertrophic cardiomyopathy without heart failure. J Vet Intern Med 20(5): 1093-105.

Van Israel, N., et al. (2009). Ramipril as a First Line Monotherapy for the Control of Feline Hypertension and Associated Clinical Signs. Proceedings: 19th ECVIM-CA Congress. accessed via Veterinary Information Network; vin.com

Ranitidine HCl

(rah-nit-a-deen)   Zantac®

H₂ Receptor Antagonist; Prokinetic

Prescriber Highlights

▶ H2 receptor antagonist similar to cimetidine, but fewer drug interactions; used to reduce acid output in stomach; also has prokinetic activity.

▶ Contraindications: Hypersensitivity. Caution: Geriatric patients, hepatic or renal insufficiency.

▶ Adverse Effects: Rare. IV boluses may cause vomiting. Potentially: Mental confusion, agranulocytosis, & transient cardiac arrhythmias (too rapid IV injection). Pain at the injection site after IM administration.

Uses/Indications

In veterinary medicine, ranitidine has been used for the treatment and/or prophylaxis of gastric, abomasal and duodenal ulcers, uremic gastritis, stress-related or drug-induced erosive gastritis, esophagitis, duodenal gastric reflux and esophageal reflux. One study did not demonstrate any reduction in the incidence of gastroesophageal reflux in anesthetized dogs from either ranitidine or metoclopramide (Favarato *et al.* 2012). Ranitidine has also been employed to treat hypersecretory conditions associated with gastrinomas and systemic mastocytosis. Because of its effects on gastric motility, ranitidine may be useful in increasing gastric emptying, particularly when delayed gastric emptying is associated with gastric ulcer disease. Ranitidine may also be useful to stimulate colonic activity in cats via its prokinetic effects.

Pharmacology/Actions

At the H2 receptors of the parietal cells, ranitidine competitively inhibits histamine, thereby reducing gastric acid output both during basal conditions and when stimulated by food, amino acids, pentagastrin, histamine, or insulin. Ranitidine is between 3-13X more potent (on a molar basis) as cimetidine.

Ranitidine may stimulate GI motility, especially in the stomach by inhibiting acetylcholinesterase (thereby increasing acetylcholine at muscarinic receptors). Lower esophageal sphincter pressures may be increased by ranitidine. By decreasing the amount of gastric juice produced, ranitidine decreases the amount of pepsin secreted.

Ranitidine, unlike cimetidine, does not appear to have any appreciable effect on serum prolactin levels, although it may inhibit the release of vasopressin.

Pharmacokinetics

In dogs, the oral bioavailability is approximately 81%, serum half-life is 2.2 hours and volume of distribution is 2.6 L/kg.

In horses, oral ranitidine has a bioavailability of ≈ 27% in adults and 38% in foals. Peak levels after oral dosing occur in ≈ 100 minutes in adults and 60 minutes in foals. Apparent volume of distribution is ≈ 1.1 L/kg and 1.5 L/kg in adults and foals, respectively. Clearance in adults is ≈ 10 mL/min/kg and 13.3 mL/min/kg in foals.

In humans, ranitidine is absorbed rapidly after oral administration, but undergoes extensive first-pass metabolism with a net systemic bioavailability of approximately 50%. Peak levels occur at ≈ 2-3 hours after oral dosing. Food does not appreciably alter the extent of absorption or the peak serum levels attained.

Ranitidine is distributed widely throughout the body and is only 10-19% bound to plasma proteins. Ranitidine is distributed into human milk at levels 25-100% of those found in plasma.

Ranitidine is both excreted in the urine by the kidneys (via glomerular filtration and tubular secretion) and metabolized in the liver to inactive metabolites; accumulation of the drug can occur in patients with renal insufficiency. The serum half-life of ranitidine in humans averages 2-3 hours. The duration of action at usual doses is from 8-12 hours.

Contraindications/Precautions/Warnings

Ranitidine is contraindicated in patients who are hypersensitive to it. It should be used cautiously and possibly at reduced dosage in patients with diminished renal function. Ranitidine has caused increased serum ALT levels in humans receiving high IV doses for longer than 5 days. The manufacturer recommends that with high-dose chronic therapy, serum ALT values be considered for monitoring.

Adverse Effects

Adverse effects appear to be very rare in animals at the dosages generally used. Potential adverse effects (documented in humans) that might be seen include mental confusion and headache. Rarely, agranulocytosis may develop and, if given rapidly IV, transient cardiac arrhythmias may be seen. Pain at the injection site may be noted after IM administration. IV boluses have been associated with vomiting in small animals and transient hypotension in cats.

Reproductive/Nursing Safety

In humans, the FDA categorizes this drug as category *B* for use during pregnancy (*Animal studies have not yet demonstrated risk to the fetus, but there are no adequate studies in pregnant women; or animal studies have shown an adverse effect, but adequate studies in pregnant women have not demonstrated a risk to the fetus in the first trimester of pregnancy, and there is no evidence of risk in later trimesters.*) In a separate system evaluating the safety of drugs in canine and feline pregnancy (Papich 1989), this drug is categorized as class: *B* (*Safe for use if used cautiously. Studies in laboratory animals may have uncovered some risk, but these drugs appear to be safe in dogs and cats or these drugs are safe if they are not administered when the animal is near term.*)

Ranitidine is excreted in human breast milk with milk:plasma ratios of approximately 5:1 to 12:1. The drug is not recommended to be used in nursing humans; use with caution in nursing veterinary patients.

Overdosage/Acute Toxicity

Clinical experience with ranitidine overdosage is limited. In laboratory animals, very high dosages (225 mg/kg/day) have been associated with muscular tremors, vomiting and rapid respirations. Single doses of 1 gram/kg in rodents did not cause death.

Treatment of overdoses in animals should be handled using standard protocols for oral ingestions of drugs; clinical signs may be treated symptomatically and supportively if necessary. Hemodialysis and peritoneal dialysis have been noted to remove ranitidine from the body.

Drug Interactions

Unlike cimetidine, ranitidine appears to have much less effect on the hepatic metabolism of drugs and is unlikely to cause clinically relevant drug interactions via this mechanism. The following drug interactions have either been reported or are theoretical in humans or animals receiving ranitidine and may be of significance in veterinary patients. Unless otherwise noted, use together is not necessarily contraindicated, but weigh the potential risks and perform additional monitoring when appropriate.

- **ACETAMINOPHEN:** Ranitidine (dose-dependent) may inhibit acetaminophen metabolism.
- **ANTACIDS** (high doses): May decrease the absorption of ranitidine; give at separate times (2 hours apart) if used concurrently.
- **KETOCONAZOLE, ITRACONAZOLE:** Absorption may be reduced secondary to increased gastric pH.
- **METOPROLOL:** Ranitidine may increase metoprolol half-life, and peak levels.
- **NIFEDIPINE:** Ranitidine may increase nifedipine AUC by 30%.
- **PROBENECID:** May reduce the excretion of ranitidine.
- **PROPANTHELINE:** Delays the absorption but increases the peak serum level of ranitidine; relative bioavailability of ranitidine may be increased by 23% when propantheline is administered concomitantly with ranitidine.
- **VITAMIN B-12:** Long-term ranitidine use may reduce oral absorption of B-12.

Laboratory Considerations

- Ranitidine may cause a false-positive **urine protein** reading when using *Multistix*. The sulfosalicylic acid reagent is recommended for determining urine protein when the patient is concomitantly receiving ranitidine.

Doses

- **DOGS:**
  For esophagitis, ulcer disease, gastritis, or gastric prokinetic (extra-label): Common anecdotal dosages generally range from 1 – 2 mg/kg PO, SC, IM or slow IV q8-12h, but one study (Berse-

nas *et al.* 2005) found that ranitidine at 2 mg/kg IV q12h did not significantly increase gastric pH when compared to saline. One source (Spillman 2012) states: "Therefore, current dose recommendations (0.5 – 2 mg/kg q8–12h) seem to be too low to be of any effect. Currently, clinical studies on the effect of ranitidine on gastric disorders in dogs and cats are lacking."

- **CATS:**
  For ulcer disease, esophagitis, or as a prokinetic agent to stimulate colonic motility (extra-label): Based on pharmacokinetic data: 2.5 mg/kg slow IV twice daily or 3.5 mg/kg PO twice daily. (Trepanier 2010)

- **FERRETS:**
  For *Helicobacter mustelae* (extra-label): Ranitidine bismuth citrate (**Note:** Not available commercially in USA; must be compounded) at 24 mg/kg PO q8-12h and clarithromycin (12.5 mg/kg PO q8-12h). Treat with both for 14 days. (Johnson-Delaney 2008)

- **HORSES:** (NOTE: ARCI UCGFS CLASS 5 DRUG)
  As a gastroprotectant/reduce stomach acid (extra-label): 1.5 – 2 mg/kg IV q8h or 6.6 – 10 mg/kg PO q8h.

- **SMALL MAMMALS:**
  Rabbits: As a prokinetic: 0.5 mg/kg IV q24 with cisapride (0.5 mg/kg PO q8h) (Lichtenberger 2008). **For suspected gastric ulceration:** 2 – 5 mg/kg PO twice daily. (Bryan 2009)

Monitoring

- Clinical efficacy (dependent on reason for use); monitored by decrease in clinical signs, endoscopic examination, blood in feces, etc.

Client Information

- Used to treat or prevent stomach ulcers.
- Works best if given before the first meal of the day.
- Ranitidine is available OTC (over the counter; without a prescription), but only give it to your animal if your veterinarian recommends.

Chemistry/Synonyms

An H_2 receptor antagonist, ranitidine HCl occurs as a white to pale-yellow granular substance with a bitter taste and a sulfur-like odor. The drug has pK_as of 8.2 and 2.7. One gram is soluble in approximately 1.5 mL of water or 6 mL of alcohol. The commercially available injection has a pH of 6.7-7.3.

Ranitidine HCl may also be known as: AH-19065, ranitidini hydrochloridum. Many trade names are available; a common trade name is *Zantac*.

Storage/Stability

Ranitidine tablets should be stored in tight, light-resistant containers at room temperature. The injectable product should be stored protected from light and at a temperature less than 30°C. A slight darkening of the injectable solution does not affect the potency of the drug.

Compatibility/Compounding Considerations

Ranitidine injection is reportedly stable up to 48 hours when mixed with the commonly used IV solutions (including 5% sodium bicarbonate).

Dosage Forms/Regulatory Status

VETERINARY-LABELED PRODUCTS: NONE.

The ARCI (Racing Commissioners International) has designated this drug as a class 5 substance. See the appendix for more information.

Revisions/References

Monograph revised/updated August 2014.

Bersenas, A., et al. (2005). Effects of ranitidine, famotidine, pantoprazole, and omeprazole on intragastric pH in dogs. AJVR 66(3): 425-31.

Bryan, J. (2009). Rabbit GI Physiology: What do I do now? Proceedings: WVC. accessed via Veterinary Information Network; vin.com

Favarato, E. S., et al. (2012). Evaluation of metoclopramide and ranitidine on the prevention of gastroesophageal reflux episodes in anesthetized dogs. Research in Veterinary Science 93(1): 466-7.

Johnson-Delaney, C. (2008). Gastrointestinal Diseases in Ferrets. Proceedings: WVC. accessed via Veterinary Information Network; vin.com

Lichtenberger, M. (2008). What's new in small mammal critical care. Proceedings: AAV. accessed via Veterinary Information Network; vin.com

Papich, M. (1989). Effects of drugs on pregnancy. *Current Veterinary Therapy X: Small Animal Practice*. R. Kirk. Philadelphia, Saunders: 1291-9.

Spillman, T. (2012). Antiemetics and Gastroprotective Drugs in Dogs: Fact and Fiction. Proceedings: WSAVA/FECAVA/BSAVA World Congress 2012. accessed via Veterinary Information Network; vin.com

Trepanier, L. (2010). Acute Vomiting in Cats: Rational treatment selection. Journal of Feline Medicine and Surgery 12(3): 225-30.

Remifentanil HCl

(rem-i-fen-ta-nil)   Ultiva®

Ultra-Short Acting Opioid Analgesic

Prescriber Highlights

▶ Opioid similar to fentanyl; used primarily as an anesthesia adjunct. Marginal veterinary clinical experience at present.

▶ Degraded by esterases in plasma, red cells, and tissues; can be used for prolonged procedures in patients with renal or hepatic dysfunction.

▶ Because of its short duration of action, may reduce recovery times.

▶ Currently much more expensive than fentanyl.

Uses/Indications

Remifentanil is a *mu*-opioid structurally related to fentanyl. Because remifentanil is primarily metabolized by tissue and red cell esterases, it can safely be used in patients with either hepatic or renal impairment. Its very short duration of action is also beneficial, because if adverse effects occur (*e.g.,* respiratory depression, bradycardia), reversal with naloxone should rarely be required. A possible advantage of using remifentanil versus fentanyl as an anesthesia adjunct is that recovery times may be faster with remifentanil.

Pharmacology/Actions

Remifentanil hydrochloride is a *mu*-opioid agonist with rapid onset of analgesic action and peak effect, and short duration of action. *Mu*-receptors are found primarily in the pain regulating areas of the brain. They are thought to contribute to the analgesia, euphoria, respiratory depression, physical dependence, miosis, and hypothermic actions of opiates. Receptors for opiate analgesics are found in high concentrations in the limbic system, spinal cord, thalamus, hypothalamus, striatum, and midbrain. They are also found in tissues such as the gastrointestinal tract, urinary tract, and other smooth muscles. The pharmacology of the opiate agonists is discussed in more detail in the monograph, Narcotic (opiate) Agonist Analgesics.

Unlike other opioids, remifentanil is rapidly metabolized by hydrolysis of the propanoic acid-methyl ester linkage by nonspecific blood and tissue esterases. Remifentanil is not appreciably metabolized by the liver or plasma cholinesterase (pseudocholinesterase). Adverse effects (bradycardia, respiratory depression, hypotension) are dose dependent and similar to other *mu*-opioids. When used as an anesthesia adjunct, remifentanil, like other opioids, has a ceiling effect (increased doses do not enhance analgesia).

Antagonists such as naloxone antagonize the opioid activity of remifentanil. Hourly dosages of naltrexone (600 mcg/kg IV) antagonized the behavioral and antinociceptive effects of a high dose of remifentanil in cats (Pypendop *et al.* 2011).

In dogs, remifentanil is equally efficacious but about half as potent as fentanyl; recovery from remifentanil anesthesia is much more rapid, especially after continuous infusions maintained for 6+ hours (Michelsen *et al.* 1996). Remifentanil reduced sevoflurane MAC similarly to fentanyl in dogs, but allowed shorter recovery times (Martinez *et al.* 2008). In another dog study, remifentanil given as a CRI reduced the dosage requirements of propofol for maintaining target-controlled infusion system–based anesthesia (Beier *et al.* 2009). A dose of 0.3 micrograms/kg/min resulted in nearly maximal isoflurane-sparing effect; a ceiling effect was observed at higher infusion rates (Monteiro *et al.* 2010). Remifentanil infusions of 0.25 – 0.5 micrograms/kg/minute combined with 0.2 mg/kg/minute of propofol produced minimal effects on arterial blood pressure, led to a good recovery, and analgesia was sufficient to control the nociceptive response applied by electrical stimulation (Gimenes *et al.* 2011). The principle carboxylic acid metabolite of remifentanil (GR90291) has been shown to be at least 4000X less potent in dogs as the parent drug (Hoke *et al.* 1997).

In cats, remifentanil reduced isoflurane MAC similarly (≈ 25% reduction) at the three doses studied (Ferreira *et al.* 2009). However in another cat study, remifentanil did not alter the MAC thresholds for isoflurane but did produce analgesia, reflected by increased thermal thresholds. The authors state that the extent or existence of an analgesic-MAC relationship cannot be assumed for all analgesics in all species. They concluded that measures of anesthetic immobility need not bear any relation to measures of analgesic efficacy. Consequently, MAC-sparing effects should not be used to infer analgesic effects without prior validation of the nature of such a relationship for a specific agent and species (Brosnan *et al.* 2009), (Pypendop *et al.* 2011).

Pharmacokinetics

In dogs, remifentanil is rapidly distributed into the CNS with a blood-brain equilibration half-life of 2.3-5.2 minutes. It has an terminal elimination half-life of 6 minutes (Hoke *et al.* 1997). Upon termination of an IV infusion, dogs recover in 5-20 minutes regardless of the infusion duration.

In cats, remifentanil has a moderately high volume of distribution (7.6 L/kg), a high clearance (766 mL/min/kg) and a short terminal elimination half-life (17.4 minutes). In anesthetized (isoflurane) cats, volume of distribution of remifentanil is decreased (1.65 L/kg), but elimination half-life is not significantly altered (Pypendop *et al.* 2008).

In humans after IV doses, remifentanil is rapidly distributed into the CNS and has a peak effect 1-3 minutes after administration. Remifentanil is approximately 70% bound to plasma proteins with the majority bound to alpha-1-acid-glycoprotein. Remifentanil has an effective biological half-life of 3-10 minutes in human patients. The pharmacokinetics of remifentanil are not appreciably altered in patients with renal or hepatic failure.

Contraindications/Precautions/Warnings

Remifentanil is contraindicated in patients hypersensitive to it or other fentanyl analogs. As the injection contains glycine, it is contraindicated for epidural or intrathecal administration.

Because of the possibility of significant respiratory depression or bradycardia, it should be administered only in a monitored anesthesia care setting. Continuous infusions should only be administered with an infusion device.

In morbidly obese patients, the drug dose should be based upon ideal body weight.

Adverse Effects

Remifentanil has an adverse effect profile similar to other *mu*-opioids. Respiratory depression, including apnea, bradyarrhythmias and hypotension are possible. Increased body temperatures in cats may be noted. Anaphylaxis is very rare, but possible.

In cats, dosages >1 microgram/kg/minute may be associated with dysphoria and frenetic locomotor activity.

Reproductive/Nursing Safety

Remifentanil appears to be relatively safe to use during pregnancy. No teratogenic effects were observed after administration of remifentanil at doses up to 5 mg/kg in rats and 0.8 mg/kg in rabbits. For humans, the FDA categorizes this drug as category C for use during pregnancy (*Animal studies have shown an adverse effect on the fetus, but there are no adequate studies in humans; or there are no animal reproduction studies and no adequate studies in humans.*)

It is unknown if remifentanil is excreted into milk, but clinical effect in offspring seems unlikely. However, weigh the potential risks of using this medication versus the benefits in pregnant or nursing animals.

Overdosage/Acute Toxicity

As with all potent opioid analgesics, overdosage should manifest as enhancement of the drug's non-analgesic pharmacological effects. Clinical signs may include: apnea, chest-wall rigidity, seizures, hypoxemia, hypotension, and bradycardia.

Discontinue drug administration and give supportive therapy including mechanical ventilation and oxygen administration. Oftentimes, this is all that is required since the drug is cleared so rapidly. Additional supportive therapy can include IV fluids, glycopyrrolate or atropine for bradycardia or hypotension. Naloxone may also be used to reverse the drug's *mu*-activity, but can lead to acute pain and sympathetic hyperactivity.

Drug Interactions

Remifentanil clearance is not altered by concomitant administration of thiopental, isoflurane, or propofol.

The following drug interactions have either been reported or are theoretical in humans or animals receiving the related drug, fentanyl and may apply to remifentanil and be of significance in veterinary patients. Unless otherwise noted, use together is not necessarily contraindicated, but weigh the potential risks and perform additional monitoring when appropriate.

- **CNS DEPRESSANTS, OTHER**: Additive CNS effects possible.
- **DIURETICS**: Opiates may decrease efficacy in CHF patients.
- **MONOAMINE OXIDASE INHIBITORS** (*e.g.*, **amitraz**, and possibly **selegiline**): Severe and unpredictable opiate potentiation may be seen; fentanyl not recommended (in humans) if MAO inhibitor has been used within 14 days.
- **MUSCLE RELAXANTS, SKELETAL**: Remifentanil may enhance neuromuscular blockade.
- **NITROUS OXIDE**: High remifentanil doses may cause cardiovascular depression.
- **TRICYCLIC ANTIDEPRESSANTS** (*e.g.*, **clomipramine, amitriptyline**, etc.): May exacerbate the effects of tricyclic antidepressants.
- **WARFARIN**: Opiates may potentiate anticoagulant activity.

Laboratory Considerations

- As they may increase biliary tract pressure, opiates can increase **plasma amylase** and **lipase values** up to 24 hours following their administration.

Doses

Note: Do not confuse microgram/kg/HOUR and microgram/kg/MINUTE CRI rates.

- **DOGS:**

  As an analgesic adjunct to general anesthesia (extra-label): 3 – 4 micrograms/kg bolus IV, followed by a CRI of 0.1 – 0.3 micrograms/kg/minute. Because of the drug's short duration of activity, consider additional analgesia upon termination of remifentanil if painful condition persists.

- **CATS:**

  As an analgesic adjunct to general anesthesia (extra-label): In one study, in propofol-anesthetized (0.3 micrograms/kg/minute) cats an infusion rate of remifentanil at 0.2 micrograms/kg/minute allowed ovariohysterectomies (OHE) to be performed; an infusion rate of 0.3 micrograms/kg/minute was required to reduce the incidence of stimulus-induced movement after electrical noxious stimulation (Correa *et al.* 2007). Another study for anesthesia during OHE used propofol (5 mg/kg induction, followed by 0.3 mg/kg/min) and remifentanil (0.24 ± 0.05 micrograms/kg/minute) (Padilha *et al.* 2011).

- **HORSES**

  As an adjunct for prolonged general anesthesia (extra-label): From a case report: After premed of xylazine, ketamine, and diazepam, mare was prepped with triple drip (ketamine, xylazine, guaifenesin). General anesthesia was maintained (for 13 hours) before and during surgery with sevoflurane, dexmedetomidine (1.5 micrograms/kg/hour), and remifentanil (3 micrograms/kg/hour). Dobutamine and fluids were used to maintain arterial pressure (MAP) above 70 mmHg. (Benmansour *et al.* 2013)

Monitoring

- Cardiac and respiratory rate.
- Pulse oximetry or other methods to measure blood oxygenation when used for anesthesia.
- Blood pressure.

Chemistry/Synonyms

Remifentanil hydrochloride has a pKa of 7.07 and partition coefficient n-octanol:water of 17.9 at pH 7.3. The commercially available injection has a pH of 2.5-3.5.

Remifentanil may also be known as: GI-87084B, remifentanilo, rémifentanil, or remifentanili. Trade names include: *Ultiva*® and *Remicit*®.

Storage/Stability

Prior to reconstitution, store lyophilized powder for solution between 2°-25°C (36°-77° F). It is stable for 24 hours at room temperature after reconstitution and further dilution to concentrations of 20 – 250 micrograms/mL with the following IV fluids: sterile water for injection; D₅W; D₅NS, 0.9% sodium chloride, 0.45% sodium chloride; D₅LR; it is stable for 4 hours at room temperature after reconstitution and further dilution to concentrations of 20 – 250 micrograms/mL with lactated Ringer's injection. The UK licensed product information states that it should **NOT** be mixed with lactated Ringer's injection with or without 5% glucose.

Compatibility/Compounding Considerations

To reconstitute solution, add 1 mL of diluent per mg of remifentanil. Shake well to dissolve. When reconstituted as directed, the solution contains approximately 1 mg of remifentanil activity per mL. It should then be further diluted to a final concentration of 20, 25, 50, or 250 micrograms/mL prior to administration. Do not administer remifentanil without dilution.

Dosage Forms/Regulatory Status

VETERINARY-LABELED PRODUCTS: NONE.

HUMAN-LABELED PRODUCTS:

Remifentanil HCl Powder for reconstitution (IV use only): 1 mg (3 mL vial), 2 mg (5 mL vial), 5 mg (10 mL vial); *Ultiva*®; (Rx, C-II controlled substance)

Revisions/References

Monograph revised/updated August 2014.

Beier, S. L., et al. (2009). Effect of remifentanil on requirements for propofol administered by use of a target-controlled infusion system for maintaining anesthesia in dogs. American Journal of Veterinary Research 70(6): 703-9.

Benmansour, P. & T. Duke-Novakovski (2013). Prolonged anesthesia using sevoflurane, remifentanil and dexmedetomidine in a horse. Veterinary Anaesthesia and Analgesia 40(5): 521-6.

Brosnan, R. J., et al. (2009). Effects of remifentanil on measures of anesthetic immobility and analgesia in cats. American Journal of Veterinary Research 70(9): 1065-71.

Correa, M. D., et al. (2007). Effects of remifentanil infusion regimens on cardiovascular function and responses to noxious stimulation in propofol-anesthetized cats. American Journal of Veterinary Research 68(9): 932-40.

Ferreira, T. H., et al. (2009). Effect of remifentanil hydrochloride administered via constant rate infusion on the minimum alveolar concentration of isoflurane in cats. American Journal of Veterinary Research 70(5): 581-8.

Gimenes, A. M., et al. (2011). Effect of intravenous propofol and remifentanil on heart rate, blood pressure and nociceptive response in acepromazine premedicated dogs. Veterinary Anaesthesia and Analgesia 38(1): 54-62.

Hoke, J. F., et al. (1997). Comparative pharmacokinetics and pharmacodynamics of remifentanil, its principle metabolite (GR90291) and alfentanil in dogs. Journal of Pharmacology and Experimental Therapeutics 281(1): 226-32.

Martinez, E. & M. Lepiz (2008). Effect of Remifentanil and Fentanyl on Minimum Alveolar Concentration and Recovery in Sevoflurane-Anesthetized Dogs. Proceedings: IVECCS. accessed via Veterinary Information Network; vin.com

Michelsen, L. G., et al. (1996). Anesthetic potency of remifentanil in dogs. Anesthesiology 84(4): 865-72.

Monteiro, E. R., et al. (2010). Hemodynamic effects in dogs anesthetized with isoflurane and remifentanil-isoflurane. American Journal of Veterinary Research 71(10): 1133-41.

Padilha, S. T., et al. (2011). A clinical comparison of remifentanil or alfentanil in propofol-anesthetized cats undergoing ovariohysterectomy. Journal of Feline Medicine and Surgery 13(10): 738-43.

Pypendop, B. H., et al. (2011). Use of naltrexone to antagonize high doses of remifentanil in cats: a dose-finding study. Veterinary Anaesthesia and Analgesia 38(6): 594-7.

Pypendop, B. H., et al. (2008). Pharmacokinetics of remifentanil in conscious cats and cats anesthetized with isoflurane. American Journal of Veterinary Research 69(4): 531-6.

Rifampin

(rif-am-pin)   Rifampicin

Antimicrobial

Prescriber Highlights

▶ Antimicrobial with activity against a variety of microbes (Rhodococcus, mycobacteria, staphylococci); has some antifungal & antiviral activity as well.

▶ Contraindications: Hypersensitivity to it or other rifamycins. Caution: Preexisting hepatic dysfunction (may need to reduce dosage). Dogs may be more susceptible to hepatotoxic effects.

▶ Adverse Effects: Increases in liver enzymes (especially dogs). Uncommon: potentially rashes, GI distress, and hepatitis.

▶ Preferably, give on an empty stomach.

▶ May cause red/orange urine, tears, & sweat (harmless, but can stain fabrics, etc.).

▶ Drug Interactions, lab interactions.

Uses/Indications

The principle use of rifampin (rifampicin) in veterinary medicine is in the treatment of *Rhodococcus equi* (*Corynebacterium equi*) infections in young horses. A consensus statement from the American College of Veterinary Internal Medicine recommended the combination of a macrolide (erythromycin, azithromycin, or clarithromycin) with rifampin as the preferred treatment for infection caused by *R. equi* (Giguere *et al.* 2011). However, a controlled, randomized, double-blinded clinical trial found no difference in efficacy between foals with mild pneumonia associated with *R. equi* that received azithromycin plus rifampin and those that received azithromycin alone (Venner *et al.* 2013). Rifampin may also be useful to treat proliferative enteropathy caused by *Lawsonia intracellularis* in foals.

In dogs, rifampin may be a useful drug for treating methicillin-resistant *S. pseudintermedius* pyoderma or as an alternative treatment of *E. canis*. When canine brucellosis treatment is attempted (not recommended), it may be used in combination with doxycycline and gentamicin. In small animals, rifampin is sometimes used combined with other antimycobacterial drugs to treat non-tubercular mycobacterial infections or with other antifungal agents (amphotericin B and 5-FC) in the treatment of histoplasmosis or aspergillosis with CNS involvement.

Pharmacology/Actions

Rifampin may act as either a bactericidal or bacteriostatic antimicrobial dependent upon the susceptibility of the organism and the concentration of the drug. For *R. equi* it is considered a time-dependent antibiotic. Rifampin acts by inhibiting DNA-dependent RNA polymerase in susceptible organisms thereby suppressing the initiation of chain formation for RNA synthesis. It does not inhibit the mammalian enzyme. Rifampin is active against a variety of mycobacterium species and staphylococci, Neisseria, Haemophilus, and *Rhodococcus equi* (*C. equi*).

Although the prevalence of equine *R. equi* isolates resistant to rifampin is currently relatively low, increased tolerance by *R. equi* with increasing MICs appears to be increasing. Commonly, rifampin is used in combination with another active antibiotic in the attempt to reduce the potential for resistance development, however this may not be beneficial with staphylococcal infections (Kadlec *et al.* 2011). Resistance is thought to occur via mutation with resistant strains spreading clonally.

At very high levels, rifampin has activity against poxviruses, adenoviruses, and *Chlamydia trachomatis*.

Rifampin has some antifungal activity when combined with other antifungal agents.

Pharmacokinetics

After oral administration, rifampin is relatively well absorbed from the GI tract. Oral bioavailability is reportedly ≈ 40-70% in horses and 37% in adult sheep. If food is given concurrently, peak plasma levels may be delayed and slightly reduced.

Rifampin is very lipophilic and readily penetrates most body tissues (including bone and prostate), cells and fluids (including CSF). It also penetrates abscesses and caseous material. Rifampin is 70-90% bound to serum proteins, is distributed into milk and crosses the placenta. Mean volume of distribution is ≈ 0.9 L/kg in horses, and 1.3 L/kg in sheep.

Rifampin is metabolized in the liver to a deacetylated form that also has antibacterial activity. Both this metabolite and unchanged drug are excreted primarily in the bile, but up to 30% may be excreted in the urine. The parent drug is substantially reabsorbed in the gut but the metabolite is not. Reported elimination half-lives for various species are: 6-8 hours (horses); 8 hours (dogs); 3-5 hours (sheep). Because rifampin can induce hepatic microsomal enzymes, elimination rates may increase with time.

Contraindications/Precautions/Warnings

Rifampin is contraindicated in patients hypersensitive to it or to other rifamycins. It should be used with caution in patients with preexisting hepatic dysfunction. Dogs may be more susceptible to hepatotoxicity than some other species. Small animals should be closely monitored for signs of hepatopathy (Kadlec *et al.* 2011).

Adverse Effects

Rifampin can cause red-orange colored urine, tears, sweat, and saliva. There are no harmful consequences from this effect. A retrospective study in dogs found that at dosages ranging from 2.9 – 16 mg/kg/day, 16% of treated dogs showed adverse effects including vomiting (7%), anorexia (6%) and lethargy (4%) (Bajwa *et al.* 2013). Commonly used dosages can cause increased liver enzymes (ALT) in ≈ 25% of treated dogs (Bajwa *et al.* 2013). Hepatitis has been reported in some treated dogs. Some have suggested that daily oral dosages not exceed 10 mg/kg in dogs to reduce chances for hepatopathy.

If using in cats for mycobacterial infections, signs of liver dysfunction including inappetence, vomiting or jaundice may occur. Hepatopathy can be fatal.

In some species (*e.g.*, humans) rashes, GI distress, and increases in liver enzymes may occur, particularly with long-term use.

Oral dosage forms may be unpalatable.

Adverse effects in horses are apparently rare, but when combined with erythromycin, mild diarrhea (self-limiting) to severe enterocolitis in foals and mares, hyperthermia, and acute respiratory distress can occur. Although not commercially available, intravenous rifampin has caused CNS depression, sweating, hemolysis, and anorexia in horses.

Reproductive/Nursing Safety

Rodents given high doses of rifampin 150 – 250 mg/kg/day resulted in some congenital malformations in offspring, but the drug has been used in pregnant women with no reported increases in teratogenicity. In humans, the FDA categorizes this drug as category *C* for use during pregnancy (*Animal studies have shown an adverse effect on the fetus, but there are no adequate studies in humans; or there are no animal reproduction studies and no adequate studies in humans.*)

Rifampin is excreted in maternal milk; use with caution in nursing veterinary patients.

Overdosage/Acute Toxicity

Clinical signs associated with overdosage of oral rifampin generally are extensions of the adverse effects outlined above (GI, orange-red coloring of fluids, and skin), but massive overdoses may cause hepatotoxicity.

There were 8 exposures to rifampin reported to the ASPCA Animal Poison Control Center (APCC) during 2008-2009. In these cases 4 were dogs with 2 showing clinical signs and 3 were cats with all 3 showing clinical signs. Common findings in dogs included central nervous system depression. Common findings in cats included erythema.

Should a massive oral overdosage occur, the gut should be emptied following standard protocols. Liver enzymes should be monitored and supportive treatment initiated if necessary.

Drug Interactions

There are a multitude of potential drug interactions with rifampin. The following drug interactions (partial listing) have either been reported or are theoretical in humans or animals receiving rifampin and may be of significance in veterinary patients. Unless otherwise noted, use together is not necessarily contraindicated, but weigh the potential risks and perform additional monitoring when appropriate.

- **Acetaminophen:** Rifampin may increase acetaminophen toxicity.
- **Isoniazid:** Increased risk for hepatotoxicity.
- **Fluoroquinolones:** *In vitro* antagonism has been reported when rifampin is used concurrently with fluoroquinolone antibiotics and concurrent use should be avoided.
- **IFOSFAMIDE:** Increased risk for nephrotoxicity/neurotoxicity.

Because rifampin has been documented to induce hepatic microsomal enzymes, drugs that are metabolized by these enzymes may have their elimination half-lives shortened and serum levels decreased. This effect may persist up to one month after rifampin is discontinued. Examples of drugs/classes that may be affected by this process include:

- **BARBITURATES**
- **BENZODIAZEPINES** (*e.g.*, **diazepam**)
- **BUSPIRONE**
- **CARVEDILOL**
- **CHLORAMPHENICOL**
- **CLARITHROMYCIN**
- **CORTICOSTEROIDS**
- **ENALAPRIL**
- **FLUCONAZOLE**
- **DAPSONE**
- **DILTIAZEM**
- **DOXORUBICIN**
- **KETOCONAZOLE**
- **MYCOPHENOLATE**
- **OPIOIDS** (*e.g.*, **fentanyl, hydrocodone, morphine, tramadol,** etc.)
- **PRAZIQUANTEL**
- **PROPRANOLOL**
- **QUINIDINE**
- **SERTRALINE**
- **THEOPHYLLINE**
- **VINCRISTINE**
- **VORICONAZOLE**
- **WARFARIN**

Laboratory Considerations

- Microbiologic methods of assaying serum **folate** and **vitamin B_{12}** are interfered with by rifampin.
- Rifampin can cause false-positive **BSP** (bromosulfophthalein, sulfobromophthalein) test results by inhibiting the hepatic uptake of the drug.

Doses

- **DOGS:**

  For superficial bacterial folliculitis (extra-label): When empirical selection of a first tier systemic antimicrobial agent (*e.g.*, cephalexin, amoxicillin/clavulanate, clindamycin, etc.) and topical therapy are not appropriate and when cultures indicate susceptibility: Rifampin 5 – 10 mg/kg PO twice daily. (Hillier *et al.* 2014)

  For canine leproid granuloma (extra-label): 10 – 15 mg/kg (maximum of 600 mg total) PO once daily. Combination antimicrobial therapy with agents known to be effective against slow-growing nontuberculous mycobacteria, such as rifampin, clofazimine, clarithromycin and either moxifloxacin or pradofloxacin, may facilitate disease resolution. A combination of rifampin (10 – 15 mg/kg PO once daily) and clarithromycin (7.5 – 12.5 mg/kg PO 2-3 times a day) is recommended for treating severe or refractory canine leproid granuloma in concert with topical silver sulfasalazine. (Malik *et al.* 2013)

  For treatment of canine brucellosis (extra-label): There are no known cures. Bacteria are sequestered inside cells and it is difficult for antibiotics to penetrate and eradicate this organism. Because the disease may recrudesce at times of stress and the animal can be a source of infection for other dogs and humans (especially children, elderly or immunosuppressed individuals), antibiotic therapy is not encouraged and euthanasia is the treatment of choice. If therapy is attempted: Infected dogs must be isolated form other dogs and breeding animals. Use combination therapy of doxycycline (10 mg/kg PO q12h), gentamicin (5 mg/kg SC q24h) and rifampin (5 mg/kg PO q24h) for 3 months. After this antibiotic trial, retest and repeat treatment until the patient has a negative test. After reaching a negative serology test, continue to test every 4-6 months and repeat treatment as necessary. (Makloski 2011)

- **CATS:**

For feline leprosy syndromes (extra-label): 10 – 15 mg/kg PO once daily. Combination antimicrobial therapy with agents known to be effective against slow-growing nontuberculous mycobacteria, such as rifampin, clofazimine, clarithromycin and either moxifloxacin or pradofloxacin, may facilitate disease resolution. (Malik *et al.* 2013)

- **HORSES:**

For treatment of *Rhodococcus equi* (*C. equi*) infections in foals (extra-label): There does not appear to be clear consensus on the treatment of choice for *R. equi* in foals. Commonly rifampin at 5 mg/kg PO twice daily will be used in combination with either: erythromycin (25 mg/kg PO q8h), clarithromycin (7.5 mg/kg PO q12h), or azithromycin (10 mg/kg PO q24h for 5 days, then q48h). GI effects may be higher with erythromycin. Duration of treatment may be required for 4-9 weeks, but can be reduced with early diagnosis and treatment.

For treatment of proliferative enteropathy caused by *Lawsonia intracellularis* in foals (extra-label): Erythromycin estolate (25 mg/kg PO q6-8h) alone or in combination with rifampin: 10 mg/kg PO once daily for a minimum of 21 days. (Lavoie *et al.* 2003)

Monitoring
- Clinical efficacy.
- For monitoring *C. equi* infections in foals and response to rifampin/macrolide: Chest radiographs and plasma fibrinogen levels have been suggested as prognostic indicators when done after 1 week of therapy.
- Adverse effects: especially clinical signs for hepatopathy in small animals. Liver function monitoring (especially in dogs or cats): Baseline LFT's and rechecks at 10-14 days, then at least monthly with long term therapy is suggested.

Client Information
- Best given on an empty stomach, but if it causes stomach upset/vomiting, give with food to see if this helps.
- Rifampin causes red/orange urine, tears, and saliva (and sweat in horses). This is not a problem but can stain fabrics.
- Can cause many serious drug interactions; be sure to tell your veterinarian and pharmacist about all the drugs your animal is getting.
- May cause liver damage. Effects on the liver may be worse in older animals. Your veterinarian may wish to do periodic blood tests to watch for this.

Chemistry/Synonyms
A semi-synthetic zwitterion derivative of rifamycin B, rifampin occurs as a red-brown, crystalline powder with a pK_a of 7.9. It is very slightly soluble in water and slightly soluble in alcohol.

Rifampin may also be known as: Rifampicin, Ba-41166/E, L-5103, NSC-113926, rifaldazine, rifampicinum, rifamycin AMP; many trade names are available.

Storage/Stability
Rifampin capsules should be stored in tight, light-resistant containers, preferably at room temperature (15-30°C).

Compatibility/Compounding Considerations
No specific information noted.

Dosage Forms/Regulatory Status
VETERINARY-LABELED PRODUCTS: NONE.
HUMAN-LABELED PRODUCTS:
Rifampin Oral Capsules: 150 mg & 300 mg; *Rifadin*®, generic; (Rx)

Rifampin Lyophilized Powder for Injection Solution: 600 mg; *Rifadin*®, generic; (Rx)

Revisions/References
Monograph revised/updated August 2014.

Bajwa, J., et al. (2013). Adverse effects of rifampicin in dogs and serum alanine aminotransferase monitoring recommendations based on a retrospective study of 344 dogs. Veterinary Dermatology 24(6): 570-+.
Giguere, S., et al. (2011). Diagnosis, Treatment, Control, and Prevention of Infections Caused by Rhodococcus equi in Foals. Journal of Veterinary Internal Medicine 25(6): 1209-20.
Hillier, A., et al. (2014). Guidelines for the diagnosis and antimicrobial therapy of canine superficial bacterial folliculitis (Antimicrobial Guidelines Working Group of the International Society for Companion Animal Infectious Diseases). Vet Derm.
Kadlec, K., et al. (2011). Molecular basis of rifampicin resistance in methicillin-resistant Staphylococcus pseudintermedius isolates from dogs. Journal of Antimicrobial Chemotherapy 66(6): 1236-42.
Lavoie, J.-P. & R. Drolet (2003). Proliferative enteropathy in foals. Proceedings: ACVIM Forum. accessed via Veterinary Information Network; vin.com
Makloski, C. L. (2011). Canine Brucellosis Management. Veterinary Clinics of North America-Small Animal Practice 41(6): 1209-+.
Malik, R., et al. (2013). Ulcerated and nonulcerated nontuberculous cutaneous mycobacterial granulomas in cats and dogs. Veterinary Dermatology 24(1): 146-+.
Venner, M., et al. (2013). Comparison of tulathromycin, azithromycin and azithromycin-rifampin for the treatment of mild pneumonia associated with Rhodococcus equi. Veterinary Record 173(16): 397-+.

Robenacoxib

(roe-ben-ah-cox-ib)   Onsior®

NSAID

Prescriber Highlights
- Coxib-class NSAID for cats (approved for up to 3 days in USA; 6 days in UK) and dogs (not approved in USA).
- Appears to be relatively COX-2 specific in both species.
- Limited clinical experience, but GI effects are the most likely adverse effect seen.

Uses/Indications
Robenacoxib is a coxib class non-steroidal anti-inflammatory drug (NSAID) that is available for use in cats and dogs some countries. In the USA, it is indicated for the control of postoperative pain and inflammation associated with orthopedic surgery, ovariohysterectomy, and castration, in cats ≥5.5 lbs. (2.5 kg) and ≥4 months of age; for up to a maximum of 3 days (*Onsior*®; USA label information). In the UK, the oral tablets are labeled as recommended for the treatment of pain and inflammation associated with chronic osteoarthritis in dogs and for the treatment of acute pain and inflammation associated with musculoskeletal disorders in cats. The injection is labeled for the treatment of pain and inflammation associated with orthopedic or soft tissue surgery in dogs and for the treatment of pain and inflammation associated with soft tissue surgery in cats (*Onsior*®; UK label information).

Robenacoxib appears to be a selective inhibitor for COX-2 in cats (Giraudel *et al.* 2009; Schmid *et al.* 2010a) and dogs (King *et al.* 2010). In a non-inferiority field trial in cats that compared robenacoxib flavored tablets with ketoprofen, robenacoxib had equivalent (non-inferior) efficacy and tolerability, and better palatability. The primary adverse effects in both groups were GI-related and included diarrhea and vomiting (Giraudel *et al.* 2010). In an acute synovitis model in dogs, robenacoxib had equivalent analgesic and antiinflammatory efficacy as meloxicam (Schmid *et al.* 2010b). In a multicenter, prospective, randomized, blinded field trial, the authors concluded that robenacoxib provided efficacy and tolerability similar to that of meloxicam for the management of perioperative pain and inflammation in dogs undergoing orthopedic surgery (Gruet *et al.* 2013).

Robenacoxib may potentially be of benefit in horses, but more research is necessary before it can be recommended.

Pharmacology/Actions

Like other NSAIDs in its class, robenacoxib is a selective inhibitor of the cyclooxygenase-2 enzyme (COX-2). COX-2 is the inducible form of the enzyme and primarily responsible for the production of mediators such as prostaglandin E that can induce pain, inflammation or fever.

In dogs and cats, robenacoxib is approximately 140X (dogs) and 500X (cats) selective for COX-2 as compared to COX-1 when using an *in vitro* whole blood assays for each species.

In dogs, robenacoxib (2 mg/kg SC 1 hour prior) decreased the sevoflurane minimum alveolar concentration for blunting adrenergic response (MAC-BAR) by ≈ 16% (Tamura *et al.* 2014).

Creatinine clearance in cats was not altered when determined immediately after a single dose (2 mg/kg SC) of robenacoxib or ketoprofen (Pelligand *et al.* 2010).

Pharmacokinetics

In dogs, peak blood concentrations occur ≈ 30 minutes after dosing; food decreases peak levels somewhat. It is highly bound to plasma proteins (>99%). In dogs, robenacoxib is metabolized by the liver; terminal half-life in blood is ≈ 1.2-1.7 hours. Robenacoxib persists longer and at higher concentrations at sites of inflammation than in blood. In dogs, robenacoxib resides longer at inflamed joints compared to blood in both healthy and dogs with osteoarthritis (Silber *et al.* 2010). Excretion is primarily via the biliary route (≈ 65%); remainder is excreted renally. Robenacoxib does not appear to induce hepatic enzymes in dogs.

In cats, bioavailability is ≈ 69% after SC administration. After oral administration peak blood concentrations of robenacoxib occur at ≈ 30 minutes and while the presence of a small amount of food does not significantly affect bioavailability, full rations may significantly reduce oral bioavailability (49%–fasted vs. 10%–full ration). As in dogs, robenacoxib is highly bound to plasma proteins (>99%) and extensively metabolized by the liver. Terminal elimination half-life is ≈ 1.7 hours. Elimination is 70% biliary and 30% renal.

Contraindications/Precautions/Warnings

Robenacoxib is contraindicated in patients with hypersensitivity to robenacoxib or known intolerance to NSAIDs, or with GI ulcers. It is also contraindicated in dogs with hepatic disease.

Use with caution in dogs or cats with impaired cardiac or renal function or that are dehydrated, hypovolemic or hypotensive and in cats with hepatic dysfunction. If use cannot be avoided in these cases, careful monitoring is required.

Robenacoxib should not be used concurrently with corticosteroids or other NSAIDs.

The US label states: Stop administration if appetite decreases or if the cat becomes lethargic. Use has not been evaluated in cats 4 months of age, cats weighing 5.5 lbs., cats used for breeding, or in pregnant or lactating cats, or in cats with cardiac disease (drug has been shown to prolong QT interval).

The U.K. label states: Pre-treatment with other anti-inflammatory medicines may result in additional or increased adverse effects and accordingly a treatment-free period with such substances should be observed for at least 24 hours before the commencement of treatment with robenacoxib. The treatment-free period, however, should take into account the pharmacokinetic properties of the products used previously. Use this product under strict veterinary monitoring in dogs or cats with a risk of gastrointestinal ulcers, or if

the animal previously displayed intolerance to other NSAIDs.

The manufacturer recommends that robenacoxib be used cautiously with other drugs that may affect renal blood flow (*e.g.*, diuretics, ACE inhibitors); additional clinical monitoring is recommended. They also recommend avoiding use with other potentially nephrotoxic drugs as there is a possibility for an increased risk for renal toxicity.

Adverse Effects

In pre-marketing field studies in cats, transient, mild diarrhea, soft feces or vomiting were commonly reported. US label states: Patients (cats) at greatest risk for adverse events are those that are dehydrated, on concomitant diuretic therapy, or those with existing renal, cardiovascular, and/or hepatic dysfunction. Safety trials in young, healthy cats receiving up to 10 mg/kg (≈ 5X; 10 mg/kg) PO once daily for 28 days or PO twice daily for 42 day showed that robenacoxib, relative to placebo, did not cause toxicologically significant effects on general observations of health, hematological and clinical chemistry variables, urinalyses, or on post- mortem organ weight, gross pathology or histopathology assessment (King *et al.* 2012).

In pre-marketing field studies in dogs, GI effects (decreased appetite, vomiting, soft feces, diarrhea) were commonly reported, but were usually mild and self-limiting. Blood in the feces was seen in some patients. In pre-clinical safety studies, dosages in beagles of up to 20X (40 mg/kg) PO for 1 month and 5X (10 mg/kg) for 6 months did not cause significant clinical adverse effects, hematological and clinical chemistry variables, or macroscopic or microscopic lesions at necropsy (King *et al.* 2011).

As there is limited clinical experience with this drug, the adverse effect profile will likely change with time. In a systematic review of NSAID adverse effects in dogs published in 2013, the authors state: "The safety of robenacoxib and, therefore, its adverse effects have only been reported in 4 studies. These manuscripts received high ratings and were performed in a large population of dogs that were consistent with a moderate ranking of classification. The current results were considered to be promising, and further studies and clinical trials will potentially strength its current evidence." (Monteiro-Steagall *et al.* 2013)

Reproductive/Nursing Safety

Because the safety of robenacoxib has not been established during pregnancy and lactation in dogs or cats used for breeding, the manufacturer does not recommended its use in pregnant or lactating dogs or cats.

Overdosage/Acute Toxicity

No acute toxicity data was located. Acute overdoses may potentially cause GI, kidney, or liver toxicity. In chronic toxicity studies in healthy young dogs (doses of up to 10 mg/kg/day for 6 months) of robenacoxib did not produce any signs of toxicity (King *et al.* 2011). In healthy young cats aged 10 months, once daily doses of 4 mg/kg (2X) SC for 2 days and 10 mg/kg (5X) SC for 3 consecutive days did not produce any signs of toxicity.

Symptomatic, supportive therapy including administration of gastrointestinal protective agents and forced diuresis may be appropriate. Contact an animal poison center for more information.

Drug Interactions

See the Contraindications section above for the manufacturer's warnings on use of robenacoxib with other medications. In addition, the following drug interactions have either been reported or are theoretical in humans or animals receiving NSAIDs and may be of significance in veterinary patients receiving robenacoxib. Unless otherwise noted, use together is not necessarily contraindicated, but weigh the potential risks and perform additional monitoring when appropriate.

- **ACE INHIBITORS** (*e.g.,* **enalapril, benazepril**): Some NSAIDs can reduce effects on blood pressure.

- **ASPIRIN:** May increase the risk of gastrointestinal toxicity (*e.g.,* ulceration, bleeding, vomiting, diarrhea).
- **CORTICOSTEROIDS** (*e.g.,* **prednisone**): May increase the risk of gastrointestinal toxicity (*e.g.,* ulceration, bleeding, vomiting, diarrhea).
- **DIGOXIN:** NSAIDS may increase serum levels.
- **FLUCONAZOLE:** Administration has increased plasma levels of celecoxib in humans and potentially could also affect robenacoxib levels in dogs.
- **FUROSEMIDE:** NSAIDs may reduce the saluretic and diuretic effects.
- **HIGHLY PROTEIN BOUND DRUGS (phenytoin, valproic acid, oral anticoagulants, other antiinflammatory agents, salicylates, sulfonamides, sulfonylurea antidiabetic agents):** As robenacoxib is highly bound to plasma proteins (>99%) in dogs and cats, it may displace other highly bound drugs or those agents could displace robenacoxib. Increased serum levels, duration of actions and toxicity could occur.
- **METHOTREXATE:** Serious toxicity has occurred when NSAIDs have been used concomitantly with **methotrexate**; use together with extreme caution.
- **NEPHROTOXIC DRUGS** (*e.g.,* **furosemide, aminoglycosides, amphotericin B**, etc.): May enhance the risk of nephrotoxicity development.

Laboratory Considerations
- None noted.

Doses
- **DOGS:**

  For pain and inflammation associated with chronic osteoarthritis (extra-label in USA): 1 mg/kg with a range of 1 – 2 mg/kg PO once daily (at the same time every day). A clinical response is normally seen within a week; discontinue after 10 days if no clinical improvement seen. For long-term treatment, can adjust to lowest effective dose for the patient. (Adapted from label information; *Onsior*®—Novartis. U.K.)

  For treatment of pain and inflammation associated with orthopedic or soft tissue surgery (extra-label in USA): 2 mg/kg SC <u>once</u> approximately 30 minutes before the start of surgery. (Adapted from label information; *Onsior Injection*®—Novartis. U.K.)

- **CATS:**

  For the control of postoperative pain and inflammation associated with orthopedic surgery, ovariohysterectomy, and castration in cats ≥5.5 lbs. and ≥4 months of age for up to a maximum of 3 days (labeled dose; FDA-approved): Cats weighing between: 5.5-13.2 lbs. (2.5-6 kg) 1 whole tablet PO once daily; between 13.3-26.4 lbs (6.1-12 kg) 2 whole tablets PO once daily. The first dose should be administered approximately 30 minutes prior to surgery, at the same time as the pre-anesthetic agents are given. May be given with or without food. Tablets are not scored and should not be broken. If a second and third dose is dispensed to the client to administer at home, doses should be dispensed in the dispensing envelope with the attached Information for Cat Owners sheet intact. Cats weighing ≥ 13.3 lbs. may require two blister cards, each dispensed in an individual dispensing envelope. (Adapted from label information; *Onsior*®—Novartis USA)

  For the treatment of acute pain and inflammation associated with musculoskeletal disorders for up to 6 days (extra-label in USA): 1 mg/kg; with a range of 1 – 2.4 mg/kg PO once daily (at the same time each day) for up to 6 days. Equates to 1 tablet for cats weighing 2.5 – <6 kg and 2 tablets for cats weighing 6 kg – <12 kg. Give either without food or with a small amount of food; tablets should not be divided or broken. (Adapted from label information; *Onsior*®—Novartis; U.K.)

  For treatment of pain and inflammation associated with soft tissue surgery (extra-label in USA): 2 mg/kg SC <u>once</u> approximately 30 minutes before the start of surgery. (Adapted from label information; *Onsior Injection*®—Novartis. U.K.)

Monitoring
- Baseline and periodic physical exam including clinical efficacy and adverse effect queries.
- Appetite in cats.
- Baseline and periodic: CBC, liver function, renal function, electrolytes, and urinalysis. For long term therapy in dogs, the manufacturer recommends that liver enzymes be monitored at the start of therapy, and after 2, 4 and 8 weeks; thereafter it is recommended to continue regular monitoring (every 3-6 months). Therapy should be discontinued if liver enzyme activities increase markedly or the dog shows clinical signs such as anorexia, apathy or vomiting in combination with elevated liver enzymes.

Client Information
- NSAID approved for cats short-term treatment (up to 3 days in USA) of pain and inflammation. Can be used long term in dogs.
- May be given to cats with or without food, but giving with food may help prevent stomach upset. Do not split tablets. When used as directed on the label, most cats tolerate the drug well and side effects are usually mild, but serious side effects can occur. If any of the following are seen, stop the drug and contact veterinarian right away: Decrease in appetite, vomiting, changes in bowel movements such as diarrhea, constipation or changes in stool color, changes in drinking or urination habits (*e.g.,* frequency, amounts, smell), changes in behavior (*e.g.,* depression or restlessness), seizures, or yellowing of gums, skin or white of the eyes (jaundice).
- For dogs, give at the same time each day. Best to give it about 30 minutes before letting the dog eat, but if dog vomits shortly after getting drug, try giving with food to see if this helps. If vomiting continues, contact your veterinarian. Most dogs tolerate it very well, but rarely some will develop ulcers or serious kidney and liver problems. Watch for these signs: Decreased or increased appetite, vomiting, change in bowel movements, change in behavior or activity (more or less active than normal), incoordination/weakness (*e.g.,* stumbling, clumsiness, etc.), seizures (convulsions) or aggression (threatening behavior/actions), yellowing of gums, skin, or whites of the eyes (jaundice), changes in drinking habits (frequency, amount consumed) or urination habits (frequency, color, or smell). Periodic lab tests to check for liver and kidney side effects are required.
- Store chewable tablets well out of reach of animals and children.
- The manufacturer recommends washing hands after contact with tablets; pregnant women who are near term should wear gloves when handling the drug.

Chemistry/Synonyms
A coxib-class NSAID, robenacoxib's chemical name is 5-ethyl-2-[(2,3,5,6-tetrafluorophenyl)amino]phenyl acetic acid. The commercially available injection is a clear, colorless to slightly pink solution.

Robenacoxib may also be known as robenacoxibum or robénacoxib. Its trade name is *Onsior*®.

Storage/Stability

Store the flavored canine tablets at 25°C (77°F) or less and the feline flavored tablets at no more than 30°C (86°F). The injection should be stored in the refrigerator (2°-8°C) in its original outer carton.

Compatibility/Compounding Considerations

The manufacturer states: In the absence of compatibility studies, this veterinary medicinal product must not be mixed with other veterinary medicinal products.

Dosage Forms/Regulatory Status

VETERINARY-LABELED PRODUCTS:

Robenacoxib Flavored (yeast) Tablets (not scored): 6 mg; *Onsior*; (Rx; POM-V). FDA-approved/licensed for use in cats.

Robenacoxib Flavored (yeast, artificial beef) Oral Tablets (not scored): 5 mg, 10 mg, 20 mg, 40 mg; *Onsior*; (POM-V). At time of writing (2014) not FDA-approved for dogs. Licensed in UK for use in dogs.

Robenacoxib Solution for Injection: 20 mg/mL in 20 mL multi-dose vials; *Onsior*; (POM-V). At time of writing (2014) not FDA-approved for dogs. Licensed in UK for use in dogs.

HUMAN-LABELED PRODUCTS: NONE.

Revisions/References

Monograph revised/updated August 2014.

Giraudel, J. M., et al. (2010). Evaluation of orally administered robenacoxib versus ketoprofen for treatment of acute pain and inflammation associated with musculoskeletal disorders in cats. American Journal of Veterinary Research 71(7): 710-9.

Giraudel, J. M., et al. (2009). Differential inhibition of cyclooxygenase isoenzymes in the cat by the NSAID robenacoxib. J. Vet. Pharmacol. Ther. 32(1): 31-40.

Gruet, P., et al. (2013). Robenacoxib versus meloxicam for the management of pain and inflammation associated with soft tissue surgery in dogs: a randomized, non-inferiority clinical trial. Bmc Veterinary Research 9.

King, J. N., et al. (2011). Robenacoxib in the dog: target species safety in relation to extent and duration of inhibition of COX-1 and COX-2. J. Vet. Pharmacol. Ther. 34(3): 298-311.

King, J. N., et al. (2012). Safety of oral robenacoxib in the cat. J. Vet. Pharmacol. Ther. 35(3): 290-300.

King, J. N., et al. (2010). In vitro and ex vivo inhibition of canine cyclooxygenase isoforms by robenacoxib: A comparative study. Research in Veterinary Science 88(3): 497-506.

Monteiro-Steagall, B. P., et al. (2013). Systematic Review of Nonsteroidal Anti-Inflammatory Drug-Induced Adverse Effects in Dogs. Journal of Veterinary Internal Medicine 27(5): 1011-9.

Pelligand, L., et al. (2010). Effect of Robenacoxib and Ketoprofen on Exogenous Serum Creatinine Clearance in Conscious Healthy Cats. Proceedings: ECVIM. accessed via Veterinary Information Network; vin.com

Schmid, V. B., et al. (2010a). In vitro and ex vivo inhibition of COX isoforms by robenacoxib in the cat: a comparative study. J. Vet. Pharmacol. Ther. 33(5): 444-52.

Schmid, V. B., et al. (2010b). Analgesic and anti-inflammatory actions of robenacoxib in acute joint inflammation in dog. J. Vet. Pharmacol. Ther. 33(2): 118-31.

Silber, H. E., et al. (2010). Population Pharmacokinetic Analysis of Blood and Joint Synovial Fluid Concentrations of Robenacoxib from Healthy Dogs and Dogs with Osteoarthritis. Pharmaceutical Research 27(12): 2633-45.

Tamura, J., et al. (2014). Sparing Effect of Robenacoxib on the Minimum Alveolar Concentration for Blunting Adrenergic Response (MAC-BAR) of Sevoflurane in Dogs. Journal of Veterinary Medical Science 76(1): 113-7.

Rocuronium Bromide

(roe-kyoo-roe-nee-um)   Zemuron®, Esmeron®

Non-depolarizing Neuromuscular Blocker

Prescriber Highlights

▶ Nondepolarizing neuromuscular blocking agent with a rapid to intermediate onset depending on dose and an intermediate duration of action.

▶ Faster onset of action than vecuronium or atracurium and fewer adverse effects than succinylcholine.

▶ Limited information and clinical experience in dogs, cats, or horses.

Uses/Indications

Rocuronium bromide is an aminosteroidal competitive, nondepolarizing neuromuscular blocking agent with a rapid to intermediate onset depending on dose and an intermediate duration of action. Rocuronium has minimal cardiovascular and histamine-releasing effects. It has a similar duration of action as vecuronium and atracurium but a faster onset of action (2-3X faster than vecuronium). Unlike both vecuronium and atracurium, it is stable in aqueous solutions. Rocuronium's onset of action is nearly as rapid as succinylcholine but it has fewer adverse effects. Clinical experience with rocuronium in veterinary patients is limited but it potentially can be used for rapid endotracheal intubation and muscle relaxation during surgery.

A study found in cats that could not be intubated after xylazine and tiletamine/zolazepam, that rocuronium (0.6 mg/kg IV) was an effective alternative to topical lidocaine spray to overcome the airway protective reflexes, but it required ventilatory support until paralysis wears off (Moreno-Sala *et al.* 2013).

Pharmacology/Actions

Rocuronium is a nondepolarizing neuromuscular blocking agent structurally similar to vecuronium, with a dose-dependent rapid to intermediate onset of action and an intermediate duration. Its mechanism of action is to compete for cholinergic receptors at the motor end plate. Effects are antagonized by acetylcholinesterase inhibitors (*e.g.*, edrophonium or neostigmine). Rocuronium does not appear to induce malignant hyperthermia (MH) as it did not cause hyperthermia in (MH)-susceptible swine. Rocuronium is mildly vagolytic and a slight, transient tachycardia is occasionally seen in human patients.

In dogs, a dose of 0.4 mg/kg IV produces complete neuromuscular blockade in $\approx$ 2-3 minutes (Dugdale *et al.* 2002). Cats administered 0.6 mg/kg IV caused complete neuromuscular blockade in 90% of cats in the study within 30-60 seconds and did not significantly affect HR in any of the animals. At doses of 0.6 mg/kg, rocuronium appears to have a longer duration of action in dogs (20 minutes) and horses (55 minutes) than in cats (13 minutes) (Auer *et al.* 2006; Auer *et al.* 2007).

Pharmacokinetics

Specific pharmacokinetic parameters for dogs, cats, or horses were not located. Onset of effect and duration of action are noted above. It has been reported that rocuronium is eliminated primarily by the liver in dogs and cats. The principle metabolite, 17-desacetyl-rocuronium has approximately 1/20th the neuromuscular-blocking potency of rocuronium in cats.

Contraindications/Precautions/Warnings

Rocuronium is contraindicated in patients hypersensitive to it or other neuromuscular blocking agents. It should only be used in settings where patients can be fully monitored and intubation, mechanical ventilation, oxygen therapy, and antagonist drugs are immediately available.

Rocuronium should only be used in patients that are adequately anesthetized or sedated.

There are conflicting reports whether rocuronium should be used in patients with hepatic or renal impairment and some have stated that atracurium is preferred in these patients.

Rocuronium is considered a "high alert" medication (medications that require special safeguards to reduce the risk of errors). Consider instituting practices such as redundant drug dosage/drug volume checking, special alert labels, etc.

Adverse Effects

Other than the effects associated with pharmacologic neuromuscular blockade, rocuronium appears to be well tolerated in the limited number of animals studied. Changes in heart rate and blood pressure may be noted. A more accurate picture of the drug's true adverse effect profile in veterinary patients may be forthcoming if it is more widely used.

In humans, the most common adverse reactions noted are effects on blood pressure (hypo- or hypertension). These are transient and usually mild and have been reported in only ≈ 2% of patients. Severe anaphylaxis has been reported in humans. While rocuronium is thought to possess little histamine releasing effects, histaminoid reactions have been reported. Because the drug reportedly can cause a severe burning pain at the injection site, it is recommended that rocuronium be given only when a deep stage of anesthesia has been achieved.

Reproductive/Nursing Safety

When administered to pregnant laboratory animals, rocuronium did not demonstrate teratogenic effects and it is likely safe to use as long as the patient does not become hypoxic during use. For humans, the FDA categorizes this drug as category *C* for use during pregnancy (*Animal studies have shown an adverse effect on the fetus, but there are no adequate studies in humans; or there are no animal reproduction studies and no adequate studies in humans.*)

The molecular weight of rocuronium is low enough for excretion into milk, but because the drug is ionized at physiologic pH, any clinical effect in offspring seems unlikely. However, weigh the potential risks of using this medication versus the benefits in pregnant or nursing animals.

Overdosage/Acute Toxicity

Overdosage with neuromuscular blocking agents may result in prolonged neuromuscular blockade. The primary treatment is maintenance of the patient's airway, mechanical ventilation and oxygenation, and adequate sedation until recovery function is assured. Only after evidence of recovery is seen should administration of an anticholinesterase drug with an anticholinergic agent be considered. Blood pressure and heart rate should be monitored during an overdose with any necessary supportive treatment performed.

Rocuronium's effects can be reversed by the drug sugammadex, a binding agent that is specific for rocuronium (and to a lesser extent vecuronium and pancuronium). However in 2008, the FDA (USA) rejected the new drug application for human use based upon concerns that it could cause anaphylaxis.

Drug Interactions

The following drug interactions have either been reported or are theoretical in humans or animals receiving rocuronium and may be of significance in veterinary patients. Unless otherwise noted, use together is not necessarily contraindicated, but weigh the potential risks and perform additional monitoring when appropriate.

- **NON-DEPOLARIZING MUSCLE RELAXANT DRUGS, OTHER**: May have a synergistic effect if used with rocuronium
- **SUCCINYLCHOLINE**: May speed the onset of action and enhance the neuromuscular blocking actions of rocuronium; do not give rocuronium until succinylcholine effects have subsided

The following agents may enhance or prolong the neuromuscular blocking activity of rocuronium:

- **AMINOGLYCOSIDES** (*e.g.,* **gentamicin, amikacin**)
- **ANESTHETICS** (**halothane, isoflurane, sevoflurane**, etc.)
- **CLINDAMYCIN, LINCOMYCIN**
- **DANTROLENE**
- **MAGNESIUM SALTS**
- **PIPERACILLIN, MEZLOCILLIN**
- **QUINIDINE**
- **TETRACYCLINES**
- **VERAPAMIL**

Laboratory Considerations

- No special considerations noted.

Doses

- **DOGS:**

  As a neuromuscular blocker (extra-label): In the study, rocuronium was given as a bolus dose of 0.5 mg/kg and then a CRI was started immediately at 0.2 mg/kg/hour. The authors concluded that rocuronium administered in this way was effective in dogs and easily applicable to clinical practice, but that further work is required on infusion titration. (Alderson *et al.* 2007)

- **CATS:**

  As a neuromuscular blocker (extra-label): In the study, the dose used was 0.6 mg/kg IV. The authors concluded that rocuronium appears to be an effective nondepolarizing muscle relaxant in cats; has a rapid onset and a short duration of action and does not cause significant changes in heart rate. (Auer *et al.* 2006)

- **HORSES:**

  As a neuromuscular blocker (extra-label): Although a formal dose-finding study for rocuronium has not yet been reported, doses ranging between 0.2 – 0.6 mg/kg have been used extensively in horses under inhalational anesthesia; doses of 0.2 mg/kg provides ≈ 90% twitch depression, and 0.4 – 0.6 mg/kg produces full blockade. Block lasts < 20 minutes at 0.2 mg/kg, and as long as 1-hour at 0.6 mg/kg. (Martin-Flores 2013)

Monitoring

- Degree of neuromuscular blockade; the manufacturer recommends use of a peripheral nerve stimulator to determine drug response, need for additional doses, and to evaluate recovery.

Chemistry/Synonyms

Rocuronium bromide is an aminosteroidal competitive, nondepolarizing neuromuscular blocking agent. It occurs as an almost white or pale yellow, slightly hygroscopic powder. It is freely soluble in water or dehydrated alcohol. A 1% solution (in water) has a pH 8.9-9.5. The commercially available injection is a sterile, non-pyrogenic, isotonic solution that is clear, colorless to yellow/orange. Each mL contains 10 mg rocuronium bromide and 2 mg sodium acetate and is adjusted to isotonicity with sodium chloride. The pH is adjusted to 4 with acetic acid and/or sodium hydroxide.

Rocuronium may also be known as: ORG-9426, rocuronii, rocuronio, rokuroniowy, or rokuronyum. Rocuronium may also be known by the trade names: *Zemuron*® or *Esmeron*®.

Storage/Stability

Store at 2°-8°C (36°-46°F). Do not freeze. When removed from refrigeration to room temperature storage conditions (25°C; 77°F), use within 60 days. Use opened vials of rocuronium within 30 days. Infusion solutions should be used within 24 hours of mixing. Unused portions of infusion solutions should be discarded.

Compatibility/Compounding Considerations

Rocuronium for injection is **compatible** in solution with: 0.9% NaCl, sterile water for injection, D_5W, D_5NS, and LRS. Rocuronium concentrations up to 5 mg/mL in these solutions are stable for 24 hours at room temperature in plastic bags, glass bottles, and plastic syringe pumps.

Rocuronium is physically **incompatible** when mixed with the following drugs: Amphotericin B, hydrocortisone sodium succinate, amoxicillin, insulin, azathioprine, lipid emulsion (Intralipid), cefazolin, ketorolac, cloxacillin, lorazepam, dexamethasone, methohexital, diazepam, methylprednisolone, erythromycin, thiopental, famotidine, trimethoprim, furosemide, and vancomycin.

Dosage Forms/Regulatory Status

VETERINARY-LABELED PRODUCTS: NONE.

HUMAN-LABELED PRODUCTS:
Rocuronium Bromide for Injection: 10 mg/mL in 5 mL & 10 mL
multi-dose vials; *Zemuron*®, generic; (Rx)

Revisions/References
Monograph revised/updated August 2014.
Alderson, B., et al. (2007). Use of rocuronium administered by continuous infusion in dogs.
  Veterinary Anaesthesia and Analgesia **34**(4): 251-6.
Auer, U. & M. Mosing (2006). A clinical study of the effects of rocuronium in isoflurane-an-
  aesthetized cats. Veterinary Anaesthesia and Analgesia **33**(4): 224-8.
Auer, U., et al. (2007). Observations on the muscle relaxant rocuronium bromide in the
  horse - a dose-response study. Veterinary Anaesthesia and Analgesia **34**(2): 75-81.
Dugdale, A. H. A., et al. (2002). The clinical use of the neuromuscular blocking agent rocu-
  ronium in dogs. Veterinary Anaesthesia and Analgesia **29**(1): 49-53.
Martin-Flores, M. (2013). Neuromuscular Blocking Agents and Monitoring in the Equine
  Patient. Veterinary Clinics of North America-Equine Practice **29**(1): 131-+.
Moreno-Sala, A., et al. (2013). Use of neuromuscular blockade with rocuronium bromide for
  intubation in cats. Veterinary Anaesthesia and Analgesia **40**(4): 351-8.

Romifidine HCl

(roe-mif-ih-deen)   Sedivet®

Alpha-2 Agonist Sedative Analgesic

Prescriber Highlights

▶ Alpha-2 agonist with sedative, muscle relaxant & analgesic effects.

▶ Indicated (in USA) for use in adult horses as a sedative & analgesic to facilitate handling, clinical examinations & procedures, minor surgical procedures, & as preanesthetic prior to the induction of general anesthesia.

▶ Labeled in some European countries for use in dogs & cats; has been used extra-label in foals & cattle.

▶ Adverse effects in **horses** include bradycardia (possibly profound), first- & second-degree atrioventricular heart block, sinus arrhythmias (dose dependent), initial hypertension followed by hypotension, ataxia, sweating, piloerection, salivation, muscle tremors, penile-relaxation, urination, swelling of face, lips & upper airways, stridor, decreased GI motility, flatulence & mild colic; anaphylaxis possible.

▶ In **dogs & cats**, romifidine may cause bradycardia, cardiac arrhythmias, hypotension, transient hyperglycemia, & alterations in thermoregulation. Dogs may pant, salivate, vomit (less likely than in cats), & develop muscle twitching. Vomiting in cats may be a problem.

▶ Adjust dosage if used with other CNS depressant drugs.

Uses/Indications

Romifidine is an alpha-2 agonist with sedative, muscle relaxant and analgesic effects. It is indicated (in the USA) for use in adult horses as a sedative and analgesic to facilitate handling, clinical examinations and procedures, minor surgical procedures, and as a preanesthetic prior to the induction of general anesthesia.

In certain European countries, it is approved for use in dogs and cats as a sedative/preanesthetic.

Although not approved, romifidine has been used in cattle and foals.

Pharmacology/Actions

A potent $alpha_2$-adrenergic agonist, romifidine is classified as a sedative/analgesic with muscle relaxant properties. Alpha-2 receptors are found in the CNS and several tissues peripherally; both presynaptically and postsynaptically. In the CNS, the primary action is a feedback inhibition of norepinephrine release. Opioids and alpha-2 agonists may have synergistic analgesic effects.

Pharmacologic effects of romifidine include sedation, analgesia, and reduced catecholamine release from the CNS. Thermoregulatory mechanisms may be altered. Peripherally, an initial vasoconstrictive response occurs with increases in blood pressure. Within minutes a hypotensive phase occurs. Heart rate can significantly decrease secondary to a vagal response to hypertension. A second-degree atrioventricular block may also occur. Antimuscarinic agents can prevent bradycardia, but their use is controversial as they can potentially cause hypertension, increased myocardial oxygen demand, and reduced GI motility. Alpha-2 agonists can transiently slow duodenal motility and increase micturition in horses and can inhibit insulin release from pancreatic islet cells resulting in hyperglycemia. Other effects seen in horses include sweating, mydriasis, decreases in hematocrit, and increased uterine pressure in non-pregnant mares.

In horses, when compared with other alpha-2 agonists (xylazine, detomidine, medetomidine), romifidine may not cause as much ataxia at sedative dosages and it has the longest duration of sedation. Duration of analgesia is shorter than the duration of sedation. Increasing dosage beyond a certain amount can increase the duration of sedation, but not its intensity (ceiling effect).

Pharmacokinetics

In horses, romifidine has a volume of distribution of approximately 2-3 L/kg, a clearance of ≈ 100 mL/min/kg and an elimination half-life ≈ 135 minutes (Wojtsiak-Wypart *et al.* 2008).

In dogs and cats, bioavailability after IM administration is 86% and 95%, respectively. Bioavailability after subcutaneous injection in dogs is 92%. Peak levels after IM injection occur in ≈ 50 minutes in dogs and 25 minutes in cats. After IV injection, volumes of distribution are ≈ 3 L/kg in dogs, and 6 L/kg in cats. Romifidine is biotransformed in the liver. In dogs, ≈ 80% of an administered dose is eliminated in the urine; 20% in the feces. Elimination half-lives are ≈ 2 hours for dogs, 6 hours for cats.

Contraindications/Precautions/Warnings

Romifidine should not be used in animals hypersensitive to it or in combination with intravenous potentiated sulfonamides. The label states that this medication should not be used in horses with respiratory disease, hepatic or renal disease, or other systemic conditions of compromised health. It also states that the effects of this medication have not been evaluated in horses with colic, or foals. Because of its effects on heart rhythm and blood pressure, use very cautiously in horses with preexisting cardiac conditions.

The manufacturer cautions that using with other sedatives, tranquilizers, or opioids may potentiate the adverse effects of romifidine and to avoid using epinephrine as it may potentiate the effects of alpha-2 agonists.

Although animals may appear to be deeply sedated, some may respond (kick, etc.) to external stimuli; use appropriate caution. Raising the horse's head can help prevent sudden kicking.

When used in dogs and cats, the label for *Romydis*® (*Virbac*®—Ireland) states: "Animals should be restrained to prevent injury, ensure that animals have sufficient fluid intake, and if undergoing prolonged sedation, animals should be prevented from becoming hypothermic. Additionally, care should be taken when used in animals in poor health, suffering from respiratory distress, or in cases of cardiovascular, renal, hepatic or pancreatic disease." Cats with pancreatitis should be closely monitored. Because dogs and, particularly, cats may vomit after receiving romifidine, the manufacturer recommends not feeding for at least 12 hours prior to use.

When used epidurally in dogs, romifidine causes cardiovascular effects similar to when it is administered IV and equivalent monitoring must be performed (Martin-Bouyer *et al.* 2010).

This medication can be absorbed through the skin and via oral routes. Persons administering the medication should handle it carefully and avoid self-exposure.

Adverse Effects

In horses, romifidine may cause bradycardia (possibly profound), first- and second-degree atrioventricular heart block, and sinus arrhythmias (dose dependent). Initially, hypertension may occur followed by hypotension. Other adverse effects can include: ataxia, sweating, piloerection, salivation, muscle tremors, penile-relaxation, urination (occurs ≈ 1 hour after dose), swelling of face, lips and upper airways, stridor, decreased GI motility, flatulence and mild colic. When used alone as a premedicant, romifidine can cause twitching. There is a possibility that horses may react paradoxically (excitation) to romifidine. Rarely, anaphylactic reactions to alpha-2 agonists have been reported in horses.

In dogs and cats romifidine may cause bradycardia, cardiac arrhythmias, hypotension, transient hyperglycemia, and alterations in thermoregulation (body temperature may increase or decrease depending on ambient temperature). Dogs may pant, salivate, vomit (less likely than in cats), and develop muscle twitching.

In cats, vomiting associated with romifidine use can be seen and persist up to 24 hours after dosing. Pancreatitis has been noted in some cats receiving the drug repeatedly every 2 days for 6 days; dose related increases in BUN have been observed. Localized injection site reactions have occurred in cats receiving the medication intramuscularly.

Reproductive/Nursing Safety

The label for the US product states that the effects of this medication have not been evaluated in pregnant mares, horses intended for breeding, or foals.

The labeling for the equine and small animal products approved in Europe states that the drug is contraindicated in pregnant horses during the last month of pregnancy and during pregnancy in dogs and cats.

Overdosage/Acute Toxicity

Horses have received up to 600 micrograms/kg (5X) in experimental studies. Signs exhibited included sinus bradycardia, 2nd degree heart block, occasional apnea and mild respiratory stridor, deep sedation, frequent urination, and sweating. No clinically significant alterations in blood gases, acid-base, hematological or chemical parameters were noted. If necessary, a reversal agent such as atipamezole (at a dose of 30 – 80 micrograms/kg) or yohimbine may be used to reduce the duration and extent of adverse effects associated with acute toxicity.

Dogs have been administered doses of up to 1 mg/kg (≈ 8-10X) IV daily for up to 4 weeks with no serious adverse effects reported.

Drug Interactions

The following drug interactions have either been reported or are theoretical in humans or animals receiving romifidine and may be of significance in veterinary patients. Unless otherwise noted, use together is not necessarily contraindicated, but weigh the potential risks and perform additional monitoring when appropriate.

- **INTRAVENOUS POTENTIATED SULFONAMIDES** (*e.g.*, **trimethoprim/sulfa**): The manufacturer warns against using this agent with intravenous potentiated sulfonamides as fatal dysrhythmias may occur.
- **OTHER ALPHA-2 AGONISTS** (*e.g.*, **xylazine, medetomidine, detomidine, clonidine** and including **epinephrine**): Not recommended to be used together with romifidine as effects may be additive.
- **PHENOTHIAZINES** (*e.g.*, **acepromazine**): Severe hypotension can result.
- **ANESTHETICS, OPIATES, SEDATIVE/HYPNOTICS**: Effects may be additive; dosage reduction of one or both agents may be required; potential for increased risk for arrhythmias when used in combination with thiopental, ketamine or halothane.

Laboratory Considerations

- **ADP-induced platelet aggregation**: Can be inhibited in cats by medetomidine (a related alpha-2 agonist); not known if romifidine can have this effect.

Doses

- **HORSES:**

For sedation and analgesia (in adults); (labeled dose; FDA-approved): 40 – 120 micrograms/kg IV slowly one time. This dose is equivalent to 0.4 – 1.2 mL per 100 kg (220 lb) body weight using the 1% (10 mg/mL) injection. Degree of sedation and analgesia is dose and time dependent. Onset of action occurs between 30 seconds to 5 minutes and gradually subsides during the next 2-4 hours. Duration of analgesia is shorter than the duration of sedation. See the package insert for expected onset and duration times for sedation and analgesia based upon dose. (Label information; *Sedavet*®—B-I)

As a preanesthetic (in adults); (labeled dose; FDA-approved): 100 micrograms/kg as slow, single IV injection. Induce anesthesia after maximal sedation is achieved. Mild to moderate sedation occurs in 2-4 minutes. Anesthetic doses may need to be decreased to prevent an overdose as romifidine has anesthesia-sparing effects. (Label information; *Sedavet*®—B-I)

As part of a 'GKR triple drip' total intravenous anesthesia (TIVA) protocol (extra-label): Add 40 mg romifidine and 3.3 g ketamine to 500 mL of 5% guaifenesin. Resultant solution contains: guaifenesin 50 mg/mL, ketamine 6.6 mg/mL, and romifidine 80 micrograms/mL. Infuse at a rate of 1 mL/kg/hour. (Lerche 2013)

As part of a ketamine/romifidine partial intravenous anesthesia (PIVA) protocol; (extra-label): In the study, horses received a pre-med of romifidine (50 micrograms/kg) and methadone (0.05 mg/kg) IV (over 1 minute). General anesthesia was induced after IV infusion of guaifenesin (administered by gravity drip to effect; maximal dose, 50 mg/kg) until muscle weakness was detected then followed by a rapid IV injection of ketamine (2.2 mg/kg). In the isoflurane, romifidine, ketamine (IRK) group, the anesthetic mixture included ketamine (6 mg/mL) and romifidine (0.06 mg/mL). The initial infusion rate was set at 6.6 **micro**L/kg/minute (≈ 0.4 mL/kg/hour) and adjusted. Mean infusion rate was approximately 5 **micro**L/kg/minute. Dobutamine was used for cardiovascular support, and thiopental and ketamine were used for rescue anesthesia. The authors concluded both PIVA techniques (IRK or isoflurane, guaifenesin, ketamine—IGK) were adequate to maintain surgical anesthesia in horses with an isoflurane-sparing effect, reduced need for rescue anesthetics, a more stable anesthetic depth, and without worsening recovery quality. (Nannarone *et al.* 2012)

For post-anesthesia sedation (extra-label): From a study to determine if in healthy horses romifidine would dose-dependently improve recovery quality from isoflurane anesthesia (>1 hour) more than postanesthetic sedation with xylazine. Authors concluded that the results of this study supported the use romifidine at 20 micrograms/kg IV (administered once the breathing circuit was disconnected and the patient was spontaneously breathing), rather than with lower romifidine doses or xylazine. (Woodhouse *et al.* 2013)

- **DOGS:**

For sedation (extra-label in USA): 40 – 120 micrograms/kg IV, IM or SQ. IV administration causes sedation within approximately 5 minutes. With SC or IM injection sedation is delayed until ≈ 30 minutes post-injection. Sedation depth is also lower than with IV injection. Atipamezole may be used to hasten recovery. An atipamezole dose of 200 micrograms/kg IM will reverse a dose of 120 micrograms/kg of romifidine. (Adapted from label; *Romydis*®—Virbac-Ireland)

As a preanesthetic (extra-label in USA): 40 – 120 micrograms/kg IV, IM or SQ. Induce anesthesia (with propofol or thiopental) approximately 10 minutes after IV injection and 10-15 minutes after IM or SC injection. Label states to maintain anesthesia with halothane. (Label information; *Romydis*®—Virbac-Ireland)

As an analgesic adjunct (extra-label in USA): 10 – 20 micrograms/kg IM, SQ. May combine with an anticholinergic agent in exercise-tolerant patients free from heart disease. (Lamont *et al.* 2002)

- **CATS:**

For sedation (extra-label in USA):

a) 200 – 400 micrograms/kg IV or IM. An IM injection of 200 micrograms/kg gives sedation in ≈ 10 minutes and persists for ≈ 60 minutes. IV administration gives a more rapid onset of action (5 minutes) and the duration is similar to IM. Atipamezole IM 30 minutes after IM romifidine injection may be used to hasten recovery. An atipamezole dose of 400 micrograms/kg IM will reverse a dose of 400 micrograms/kg of romifidine. (Label information; *Romydis*®—Virbac-Ireland)

b) In the study, doses as low as 80 micrograms/kg IM produced clinically useful sedation similar to that caused by 20 micrograms/kg of medetomidine. (Navarrete *et al.* 2011)

As a preanesthetic (extra-label in USA): 200 micrograms/kg IM 10-15 minutes prior to giving ketamine at 10 mg/kg IM will provide surgical anesthesia for up to 30 minutes. Increasing the dose of romifidine to 400 micrograms/kg will extend period of surgical anesthesia. A "top-up dose" of 50% of the initial doses of romifidine and ketamine can be used to prolong anesthesia. (Label information; *Romydis*®—Virbac-Ireland)

As an analgesic adjunct (extra-label in USA): 20 – 40 micrograms/kg IM, IV. May combine with an anticholinergic agent in exercise-tolerant patients free from heart disease. (Lamont *et al.* 2002)

- **CATTLE:**

Note: Romifidine is not FDA-approved for use in cattle or other food-producing animals in the USA. For guidance with determining withdrawal times, contact FARAD (see Phone Numbers & Websites in the appendix for contact information).

For epidural anesthesia for paralumbar analgesia or laparotomy: Romifidine 50 micrograms/kg plus morphine 0.1 mg/kg. Duration of analgesia is 12 hours maximum. (Anderson 2006)

Monitoring
- Level of sedation/analgesia.
- Respiratory rate.
- Heart rate/rhythm; blood pressure (during general anesthesia).
- Body temperature for longer procedures using higher dosages.

Client Information
- Veterinary professionals should only administer this medication.
- If clients are involved with handling horses after they are dosed with romifidine, they should be warned that although the horse looks fully sedated it may respond defensively (*e.g.,* kick) when stimulated.

Chemistry/Synonyms
Romifidine HCl is an alpha-2 adrenoreceptor agonist that is structurally related to clonidine. It has a molecular weight of 258.1 and occurs as a crystalline, white, odorless substance that is soluble in water.

Romifidine may also be known as: STH-2130, romifidiini, romifidin, romifidina, romifidinum, *Romidys*®, *Sedivet*®, and *Sedivan*®.

Storage/Stability
Romifidine HCl injection should be stored at controlled room temperature (15-30°C).

Compatibility/Compounding Considerations
No specific information noted.

Dosage Forms/Regulatory Status
VETERINARY-LABELED PRODUCTS:
Romifidine HCl 1% (10 mg/mL) Injection; *Sedivet*®; (Rx). In the USA: FDA-approved for use in horses not intended for human consumption. In the UK, slaughter withdrawal is 6 days for horses.

A small animal product, *Romidys*® containing 1 mg/mL is approved for use in dogs and cats in some European countries.

HUMAN-LABELED PRODUCTS: NONE.

Revisions/References
Monograph revised/updated August 2014.

Anderson, D. (2006). Urogenital surgery in cows. Proceedings: ACVIM 2006. accessed via Veterinary Information Network; vin.com

Lamont, L. & W. Tranquilli (2002). Alpha2-Agonists. *Handbook of Veterinary Pain Management.* J. Gaynor and W. Muir, Mosby: 199-220.

Lerche, P. (2013). Total Intravenous Anesthesia in Horses. Veterinary Clinics of North America-Equine Practice 29(1): 123-+.

Martin-Bouyer, V., et al. (2010). Cardiovascular effects following epidural injection of romifidine in isoflurane-anaesthetized dogs. Veterinary Anaesthesia and Analgesia 37(2): 87-96.

Nannarone, S. & C. Spadavecchia (2012). Evaluation of the clinical efficacy of two partial intravenous anesthetic protocols, compared with isoflurane alone, to maintain general anesthesia in horses. American Journal of Veterinary Research 73(7): 959-67.

Navarrete, R., et al. (2011). Sedative effects of three doses of romifidine in comparison with medetomidine in cats. Veterinary Anaesthesia and Analgesia 38(3): 178-85.

Wojtsiak-Wypart, M., et al. (2008). Pharmacokinetics and Pharmacodynamics of Romifidine Hydrochloride in the Horse. Peroceedings: IVECCS. accessed via Veterinary Information Network; vin.com

Woodhouse, K. J., et al. (2013). Effects of postanesthetic sedation with romifidine or xylazine on quality of recovery from isoflurane anesthesia in horses. Javma-Journal of the American Veterinary Medical Association 242(4): 533-9.

Ronidazole

(roe-nid-ah-zole)

Antiprotozoal

Prescriber Highlights

▶ Nitroimidazole antibiotic/antiparasitic drug that appears to be useful in treating *Tritrichomonas foetus* infections in cats; also used for treating trichomonas infections in non-food birds. Potentially useful as an alternative treatment for Giardia.

▶ Potentially carcinogenic; avoid human exposure.

▶ Neurotoxicity (reversible): more likely at higher doses (50 mg/kg twice daily), but can occur at lower dosages as well; GI effects possible.

▶ Many potential drug interactions.

▶ Must be compounded from bulk powder (100%) & ideally, put in gelatin capsules.

Uses/Indications

Ronidazole is a nitroimidazole antibiotic/antiparasitic drug that, at present, is considered the treatment of choice for *Tritrichomonas foetus* infections in cats. However a retrospective study concluded: "In most cats, ronidazole treatment at the currently recommended dosage (30 mg/kg PO q24h for 2 weeks) was efficacious in ameliorating clinical signs. However, in some cats clinical signs persisted despite use of ronidazole at the currently recommended dosages." (Xenoulis *et al.* 2013)

Ronidazole may also prove to be a viable alternative treatment for giardiasis in dogs and cats. The drug is also used for treating Trichomonas infections in non-food animal birds.

The drug is not commercially available in the USA and must be compounded from bulk powder by a compounding pharmacy.

Pharmacology/Actions

Ronidazole, like other 5-nitroimidazoles such as metronidazole is converted by hydrogenosomes (an organelle found in trichomonads) into polar autotoxic anion radicals. *T. foetus* infections in cats have been resistant to treatment by metronidazole and ronidazole appears to have greater activity against the organism, but ronidazole resistance has been documented (Gookin *et al.* 2010).

Pharmacokinetics

In cats, ronidazole is completely absorbed and bioavailable after oral dosing. Volume of distribution (steady state) is ≈ 0.7 L/kg and clearance ≈ 0.8 mL/kg/min. Elimination half-life is long at ≈ 10 hours (LeVine *et al.* 2008).

A guar gum-coated colon-targeted delayed-release tablet formulation had negligible release until 6 hours after administration. Peak plasma levels occurred at ≈ 14.5 hours, coinciding with colonic arrival. Repeated dosing did not appreciably affect bioavailability or other pharmacokinetic parameters (Papich *et al.* 2013).

Contraindications/Precautions/Warnings

Ronidazole should not be used in patients hypersensitive to it or other 5-nitroimidazoles (*e.g.*, metronidazole).

The compound has been demonstrated to be carcinogenic in mice but not rats. While humans should avoid contact with this compound or animal waste from treated patients, it can be safely compounded using a biological safety cabinet.

The FDA prohibits this drug for use in food animals.

Adverse Effects

Reversible neurotoxicity similar to that reported with metronidazole, has been reported in cats with ronidazole. Initial signs may include tremors, lethargy, anorexia, ataxia, nystagmus, seizures or behavior changes (agitation). Should neurotoxicity be diagnosed, discontinue ronidazole, treat supportively, and if necessary, consider administering a benzodiazepine such as diazepam to competitively inhibit GABA receptors in the CNS. Incidence of neurotoxicity appears to be higher when using the 50 mg/kg twice-daily dosage, but may occur at lower dosages as well. Potentially, gastrointestinal effects can occur (anorexia, vomiting). Ronidazole is very bitter and should be administered to cats in capsule form.

Ronidazole has been shown to increase the rate of benign mammary tumors in rats and benign and malignant pulmonary tumors in mice at dosages ≥ 20 mg/kg/day.

Dogs given 30 mg/kg per day for 2 years (40 mg/kg/day the first month) showed some testicular toxicity (type not specified), but no tumors.

Reproductive/Nursing Safety

Safety of this compound during pregnancy is not established. Teratology studies have been performed in mice, rats, and rabbits. In rabbits given 30 mg/kg/day, no embryotoxicity occurred, but fetal weights were significantly decreased. Mice demonstrated no teratogenic effects at dosages of up to 200 mg/kg/day. Rats given up to 150 mg/kg/day demonstrated no embryotoxic effects, but at dosages of 200 mg/kg/day both maternal and fetal weights were decreased.

If this compound is to be used in pregnant cats, weigh the potential benefits of treating with the potential for adverse effects in the offspring and queen.

It is not known if ronidazole is distributed into milk and safety cannot be assured. Consider using milk replacer if treating nursing queens.

Overdosage/Acute Toxicity

No specific information was located. Cats receiving doses of 50 mg/kg twice daily appear to have greater incidences of neurotoxicity (see Adverse Reactions). A case report of an overdose causing neurotoxicity, hemorrhage and death in society finches after consuming ronidazole in drinking water has been published (Woods *et al.* 2010). If overdoses cause neurotoxicity, discontinue further therapy and treat supportively. Consider administering a GABA inhibitor such as diazepam to competitively inhibit GABA receptors in the CNS.

Drug Interactions

In humans, the following drug interactions with metronidazole, a compound similar to ronidazole, have been reported or are theoretical and may be of significance in veterinary patients in patients receiving ronidazole. Unless otherwise noted, use together is not necessarily contraindicated, but weigh the potential risks and perform additional monitoring when appropriate.

- **ALCOHOL:** May induce a disulfiram-like (nausea, vomiting, cramps, etc.) reaction.
- **CIMETIDINE, KETOCONAZOLE:** May decrease the metabolism of ronidazole and increase the likelihood of dose-related side effects occurring.
- **CYCLOSPORINE, TACROLIMUS (systemic):** Ronidazole may increase the serum levels of cyclosporine or tacrolimus.
- **FLUOROURACIL (systemic):** Ronidazole may increase the serum levels of fluorouracil and risk for toxicity.
- **LITHIUM:** Ronidazole may increase lithium serum levels and risk for lithium toxicity.
- **OXYTETRACYCLINE:** Reportedly may antagonize the therapeutic effects of metronidazole (and presumably ronidazole).
- **PHENOBARBITAL, RIFAMPIN or PHENYTOIN:** May increase the metabolism of ronidazole thereby decreasing blood levels.
- **WARFARIN:** Metronidazole (and potentially ronidazole) may prolong INR/PT in patients taking coumarin anticoagulants; avoid concurrent use if possible; otherwise intensify monitoring.

Laboratory Considerations

- **AST, ALT, LDH (lactic dehydrogenase), Triglycerides, Hexokinase glucose:** A related compound, metronidazole can cause falsely decreased readings when determined using methods measuring decreases in ultraviolet absorbance when NADH is reduced to NAD. It is not known if ronidazole can also cause falsely decreased values.

Doses

- **DOGS;**

  For *Giardia* (extra-label): Study was in a kennel setting and combined strict hygiene control/disinfection, chlorhexidine shampoos and ronidazole at 30 – 50 mg PO twice daily for 7 days. Authors concluded this "was highly effective in reducing *Giardia* cyst excretion and may therefore constitute an alternative control strategy for canine giardiasis." (Fiechter *et al.* 2012)

- **CATS:**

  For treatment of *T. foetus* infections (extra-label): Recent studies investigating the pharmacokinetics of ronidazole in cats suggest that 30 mg/kg PO q24h for 14 days is likely to be most effective in resolving diarrhea and eradicating *T. foetus* infection. (Tolbert *et al.* 2009)

Monitoring

- Clinical efficacy (diarrhea improvement).
- Adverse effects (neurotoxicity, vomiting, anorexia).
- PCR testing (can be used to confirm infection, but negative results after treatment do not conclusively prove that infection has been eradicated).

Client Information

- Keep stored in the freezer.
- Give with food to avoid stomach or intestinal problems.
- Side effects in cats can include fever, loss of appetite, ataxia (*e.g.,* trouble keeping balance, trouble walking or climbing stairs, etc.), muscle twitching or weakness, seizures, lethargy (tiredness/lack of energy), nystagmus (eyes uncontrollably moving back and forth). Contact veterinarian immediately if any of these signs are seen.
- Has caused cancer at high doses in laboratory animals. Do not open or crush capsules; administer whole. Wear disposable gloves when handling and wash hands afterwards.
- Wear disposable gloves when cleaning the litter box, double bag feces and throw both gloves and feces in trash. Do not flush feces down toilet.
- Must not be used in any animals that will be consumed by humans.

Chemistry/Synonyms

Ronidazole is a 5-nitroimidazole compound that occurs as a white to yellowish-brown, odorless or almost odorless, bitter-tasting, powder. It is very slightly soluble in water or alcohol.

Ronidazole may also be known as ronidazol, ronidazolum, *Belga*®, *Ridsol-S*®, *Ronida*®, *Ronivet*®, *Ronizol*®, *Turbosol*®, *Tricho Plus*®, *Trichocure*®, or *Trichorex*®.

Storage/Stability

Compounded capsules should be stored in child-resistant, tight containers protected from light. Until further stability studies can be performed, capsules should be stored in the freezer.

Aqueous solutions are reportedly not very stable. It is recommended that fresh solutions using the 10% powder for addition to drinking water (used for pigeons) be freshly prepared every day.

Compatibility/Compounding Considerations

No specific information noted. See additional information in Dosage Form section.

Dosage Forms/Regulatory Status

VETERINARY-LABELED PRODUCTS:

None in the USA; a 10% ronidazole powder to be added to drinking water for treating Trichomonas infections in pigeons is available in some countries, but these products are unsuitable for use in cats due to the dosage required and the unpalatability (very bitter) of the powder and solution. Capsules prepared from 100% bulk powder for an individual feline patient should be obtained from a compounding pharmacy that can prepare the capsules in a bio-safety hood that will protect the compounder from drug exposure.

The FDA prohibits this drug for use in food animals.

HUMAN-LABELED PRODUCTS: NONE.

Revisions/References

Monograph revised/updated August 2014.

Fiechter, R., et al. (2012). Control of Giardia infections with ronidazole and intensive hygiene management in a dog kennel. Veterinary Parasitology 187(1-2): 93-8.

Gookin, J. L., et al. (2010). Documentation of In Vivo and In Vitro Aerobic Resistance of Feline Tritrichomonas foetus Isolates to Ronidazole. Journal of Veterinary Internal Medicine 24(4): 1003-7.

LeVine, D., et al. (2008). Ronidazole Pharmacokinetics in Cats After IV Administration and Oral Administration of an Immediate Release Capsule and a Colon-Targeted Delayed Release Tablet. Procedings: ACVIM. accessed via Veterinary Information Network; vin.com

Papich, M. G., et al. (2013). Ronidazole pharmacokinetics in cats following delivery of a delayed-release guar gum formulation. J. Vet. Pharmacol. Ther. 36(4): 399-407.

Tolbert, M. K. & J. L. Gookin (2009). Tritrichomonas foetus: A New Agent of Feline Diarrhea. Compendium-Continuing Education for Veterinarians 31(8): 374-+.

Woods, L. W., et al. (2010). Ronidazole Toxicosis in 3 Society Finches (Lonchura striata). Veterinary Pathology 47(2): 231-5.

Xenoulis, P. G., et al. (2013). Intestinal Tritrichomonas foetus infection in cats: a retrospective study of 104 cases. Journal of Feline Medicine and Surgery 15(12): 1098-103.

Rufinamide

(roo-fin-a-mide)   Banzel®, Inovelon®

Anticonvulsant

Prescriber Highlights

▶ Human-approved oral anticonvulsant that potentially could be useful in dogs; not enough data available at present to recommend clinical use in animals; should be considered 'investigational'.

▶ Most likely adverse effects are CNS (somnolence, fatigue, ataxia, etc.) and GI.

Uses/Indications

Rufinamide, a triazole-derivative antiepileptic drug is approved (USA) in humans for the management (in combination with other anticonvulsants) of seizures associated with Lennox-Gastaut syndrome in adults and children ≥4 years of age. It has shown some success in the adjunctive management of refractory or inadequately controlled partial seizures in adolescents and adults. The drug potentially could be useful in animal patients with seizure disorders.

Pharmacology/Actions

Rufinamide's exact mechanism of action as an anticonvulsant is not known. It appears to modulate sodium channel activity and prolong the inactive state of the channel. It does not appear to substantially affect cholinergic, histaminergic, GAB, glutamate, monoaminergic, or glycine receptors or systems.

Pharmacokinetics

In a six-dog pharmacokinetic study, a 20 mg/kg oral dose showed that, like humans, oral absorption is slow with peak plasma concentrations occurring ≈ 8-9 hours after dosing; peak concentrations averaged 19.6 mcg/mL and clearance was 1.41 L/kg. Mean half-life was 9.86 hours, but varied widely amongst the subjects (4.11-16.1 hours). The authors concluded that rufinamide's pharmacokinetics in dogs would be expected to allow twice-daily dosing in clinical practice, but that in some dogs every 8 hour dosing may be required. (Wright *et al.* 2012)

In humans, rufinamide is well absorbed after oral administration. However, the rate of absorption is relatively slow and absorption percentage is reduced as dosages increase. Food increases bioavailability. The oral bioavailability of the oral tablets and suspension are equivalent. Peak plasma levels occur ≈ 4-6 hours after dosing. Protein binding is low (34%) and drug interactions with highly protein-bound drugs are not likely. Elimination half-life is between 6-10 hours. Rufinamide is extensively metabolized predominantly by hydrolysis via carboxylesterase to the inactive metabolite GCP 47292. CYP enzymes or glutathione are not thought to be involved in metabolic pathways.

Most of the drug is eliminated in urine, primarily as metabolites with the majority being GCP 47292. Only ≈ 2% is excreted unchanged in urine.

Contraindications/Precautions/Warnings

No contraindications have been determined for dogs. In humans, rufinamide is contraindicated in people with Familial Short QT Syndrome. In patients with severe hepatic dysfunction rufinamide is not recommended.

When discontinuing the drug, gradual withdrawal is recommended.

Adverse Effects

The adverse profile for rufinamide in dogs is unknown. In humans, adverse effects are generally CNS related and fall into two general categories: 1) drowsiness/fatigue, and 2) ataxia, gait abnormalities, dizziness, blurred vision/diplopia. Gastrointestinal effects (nausea, vomiting) have also been reported, especially in children. Rufinamide can shorten QT interval but this is not likely to be of significance in animal patients. Multi-organ hypersensitivity reactions have been reported in human patients, but are very rare.

Reproductive/Nursing Safety

For humans, the FDA has classified this drug as Category C (*Animal studies have shown an adverse effect and there are no adequate studies in pregnant women; or no animal studies have been conducted and there are no adequate studies in pregnant women*). During laboratory animal studies, rufinamide was associated with increased fetal skeletal and visceral abnormalities. Decreased offspring weight, growth and survival were also noted.

Rufinamide is likely excreted into milk, and the manufacturer recommends that either rufinamide or nursing be discontinued.

Overdosage/Acute Toxicity

Specific toxic dosages have not been established. An adult human that received an overdose of 7.20 grams/day did not experience any major adverse effects. Management of rufinamide overdoses is generally supportive based upon clinical signs. GI decontamination is not recommended in human patients. In the event of a significant overdose in an animal, contact a veterinary poison control center for further advice.

Drug Interactions

Rufinamide is a weak inducer of CYP3A4 enzymes and a weak inhibitor of CYP2E1. The following drug interactions have either been reported or are theoretical in humans or animals receiving rufinamide and may be of significance in veterinary patients. Unless otherwise noted, use together is not necessarily contraindicated, but weigh the potential risks and perform additional monitoring when appropriate.

- **LAMOTRIGINE:** Levels can be decreased 7-13% in children receiving rufinamide.
- **PHENOBARBITAL:** Up to a 46% reduction in plasma rufinamide concentrations have been noted in humans receiving phenobarbital; likely due to phenobarbital inducing carboxylesterase activity in the liver. Phenobarbital levels can be slightly (10%) increased in humans receiving rufinamide.

Laboratory Considerations

No specific concerns noted.

Dosages

- **DOGS:**

  As an anticonvulsant: There is very little clinical experience using this drug in animal patients and nearly nothing published on its clinical usage; consider use at this time as experimental—use with caution. A single-dose pharmacokinetic study done in 6 dogs were dosed at 20 mg/kg PO in conjunction with a meal. No adverse effects were seen. Based upon this study, the authors concluded that a multiple-dosing study is warranted to confirm the drug's pharmacokinetics in dogs and that studies will be needed to investigate the drug's efficacy and safety with long-term use. (Wright *et al.* 2011; Wright *et al.* 2012)

Monitoring

- Clinical efficacy, adverse effects. In humans, monitoring plasma rufinamide levels or performing other lab tests are generally not recommended.

Client Information

- Because this drug is in its 'investigational' stage in veterinary medicine, informed consent should be obtained when prescribing.
- Give dosages with food. Tablets may be administered whole, as half tablets, or crushed; oral suspension should be shaken well before drawing into dosing syringe.
- Adverse effects are not well known in dogs; in humans CNS effects (drowsiness, ataxia-stumbling, dizziness) and gastrointestinal effects (nausea, vomiting) are most commonly reported.

Chemistry/Synonyms

Rufinamide (CAS Registry: 06308-44-5; ATC: N03AF03), a triazole derivative anticonvulsant, occurs a white, crystalline neutral powder. It is practically insoluble in water and very slightly soluble in alcohol.

Rufinamide may also be known as rufinamida, CGP 33101, E-2080, RUF-331, or 60231/4. Trade names include *Banzel*® and *Inovelon*®.

Storage/Stability

Rufinamide oral tablets or oral suspension should be stored at room temperature 25°C (77°F); excursions are permitted between 15-30°C (59-86°F). Tablets should be protected from moisture.

Compatibility/Compounding Considerations

No specific information noted.

Dosage Forms/Regulatory Status

VETERINARY-LABELED PRODUCTS: NONE.

HUMAN-LABELED PRODUCTS:

Oral Tablets (film-coated, scored): 200 mg, 400 mg; *Banzel*®; (Rx).

Oral Suspension: 40 mg/mL; *Banzel*®; (Rx)

Revisions/References

Monograph revised/updated August 2014.

Wright, H. M., et al. (2012). Pharmacokinetics of oral rufinamide in dogs. J. Vet. Pharmacol. Ther. 35(6): 529-33.

Wright, H. M., et al. (2011). Oral Rufinamide in Dogs: Pharmacokinetics and Safety. Journal of Veterinary Internal Medicine 25(3): 725-.

S-Adenosyl-Methionine

(ess-ah-den-oh-seel meth-ie-oh-neen)   SAMe, Ademetionine

Hepatoprotectant

Prescriber Highlights

▶ "Nutraceutical" that has been used in small animals as an adjunctive treatment for liver disease (chronic hepatitis), osteoarthritis, cognitive dysfunction, or treatment of hepatotoxicity, etc. Evidence is scant supporting clinical efficacy, but it is well tolerated.

▶ Not a regulated drug; choose products carefully.

Uses/Indications

In small animal medicine, S-adenosyl-methionine (SAMe; ademetionine) is most commonly used as an adjunctive treatment for liver disease (chronic hepatitis, hepatic lipidosis, cholangiohepatitis, feline triad disease, etc.). It potentially could be of benefit for osteoarthritis, age-related cognitive dysfunction, treatment of acute hepatotoxin-induced liver toxicity (*e.g.*, acetaminophen, xylitol toxicity, amatoxin), and in at-risk patients on long-term therapy using drugs with hepatotoxic potential; evidence is currently scant supporting its use for these. The authors in a 2013 review assessing the evidence for nutraceuticals for treating canine liver disease state: "Despite the lack of data supporting the use of SAMe as a hepatoprotectant, the compound is frequently recommended for dogs with hepatobiliary disease. Before veterinarians recommend use of SAMe, they should ensure that owners understand (informed consent) that data on its efficacy are lacking." (Vandeweerd *et al.* 2013)

A double-blinded, placebo-controlled, clinical trial (6 week) evaluating SAMe efficacy for the treatment of clinically inferred canine osteoarthritis (OA) did not find that it was an effective stand-alone treatment for reducing clinical signs of OA.

A proprietary combination (*Denamarin*®) of silymarin (silybin) and SAMe was found to minimize increased liver enzyme activity in dogs receiving lomustine (CCNU) chemotherapy and increased the likelihood of dogs completing a prescribed lomustine course of therapy (Skorupski *et al.* 2011), but this study had several weaknesses (low numbers of patients undergoing additional liver testing with bile acids, abdominal ultrasound examination and liver biopsies, low incidence of severe liver disease, lack of placebo in control group, non-blinded, occult preexisting liver disease in some dogs, combination of two agents, and author potential financial conflicts of interest) (Vandeweerd *et al.* 2013).

In humans, SAMe has been used as a treatment for depression, osteoarthritis, AIDS-related myopathy, intrahepatic cholestasis, liver disease, alcoholic liver cirrhosis, fibromyalgia, adult ADHD, Alzheimer's, migraines, etc.

Pharmacology/Actions

S-adenosyl-methionine (SAMe) is an endogenous molecule synthesized by cells throughout the body. It is formed from the amino acid methionine and ATP, in conjunction with SAMe synthetase enzyme (an enzyme manufactured in the liver; a rate-limiting step in the presence of liver compromise). SAMe is an essential part of three major biochemical pathways: transmethylation, transsulfuration, and aminopropylation. Normal function of these pathways is especially vital to the liver as many metabolic reactions occur there. In the transmethylation pathway, SAMe serves as a methyl donor (necessary for many substances and drugs to be activated and/or eliminated). Transmethylation is essential in phospholipid synthesis important to cell membrane structure, fluidity, and function. In aminopropylation, SAMe donates aminopropyl groups and is a source of polyamines. Aminopropylation is important in producing substances that have antiinflammatory effects, protein and DNA synthesis, and promoting cell replication and liver mass regeneration. In transsulfuration, SAMe generates sulfur-containing compounds important for conjugation reactions used in detoxification and as a precursor to glutathione (GSH). Glutathione is important in many metabolic processes and cell detoxification. The conversion of SAMe to glutathione requires the presence of folate, cyanocobalamin (B_{12}), and pyridoxine (B_6). Normally, the liver produces ample SAMe, but in liver disease or in the presence of hepatotoxic substances, endogenous conversion to glutathione may be deficient. Exogenous SAMe has been shown to increase liver and red cell glutathione levels and/or prevent its depletion. SAMe inhibits apoptosis secondary to alcohol or bile acids in hepatocytes.

In humans, the mechanism for its antidepressant effects are not well understood, but it apparently increases serotonin turnover and increases dopamine and norepinephrine levels. Neuro-imaging studies in humans show that SAMe affects the brain similarly to other antidepressant medications.

Pharmacokinetics

Oral bioavailability is dependent on the salt used to stabilize SAMe. Oral bioavailability of the tosylate salt is reportedly 1% whereas the 1,4-butanedisulfonate form has a bioavailability of 5%. Regardless of oral dosage form administered, presence of food in the gut can substantially reduce the amount of drug absorbed. Peak levels occur in 1-6 hours after oral dosing with the enteric-coated tablets. Once absorbed, SAMe enters the portal circulation and is primarily metabolized in the liver. In humans, 17% of a dose of radiolabeled SAMe was recovered in the urine within 48 hours of dosing; 27% in the feces.

In dogs, a chewable non-hygroscopic formulation of SAMe (*Denosyl*® Chewable) yielded similar areas under-the-curve when compared with the enteric-coated tablets (*Denosyl*®), but peak levels occurred sooner with the chewable tablets (Griffin *et al.* 2009).

Contraindications/Precautions/Warnings

There are no apparent contraindications to the use of SAMe.

Adverse Effects

Adverse effects appear to be minimal or non-existent in treated animals. Most studies in humans have shown adverse effects similar to that of placebo. There have been reports of immediate post-dose vomiting, anorexia, and anxiety. Oral SAMe in humans may cause anorexia, nausea, vomiting, diarrhea, flatulence, constipation, dry mouth, insomnia/nervousness, headache, sweating, and dizziness.

Reproductive/Nursing Safety

The safety of exogenous SAMe has not been proven in pregnancy; use with caution. Limited studies in laboratory animals and pregnant women with liver disease have not demonstrated any ill effects to mother or fetus.

It is unknown if SAMe enters maternal milk.

Overdosage/Acute Toxicity

SAMe appears to be quite safe. LD_{50} in rodents exceeds 4.65 grams/kg, and toxicity studies in dogs and cats at the usual prescribed dosages demonstrated no deleterious effects. In the case of an overdose, gastrointestinal effects may be observed, but unlikely to require treatment.

Drug Interactions

No interactions have been documented, but theoretically, concurrent use of SAMe with **tramadol, meperidine, dextromethorphan, pentazocine,** monoamine oxidase inhibitors (**MAOIs**) including **selegiline,** selective serotonin reuptake inhibitors (**SSRIs**) such as **fluoxetine,** or other antidepressants (*e.g.,* **amitriptyline, clomipramine**) could cause additive serotonergic effects.

Laboratory Considerations

- No specific laboratory interactions or considerations noted.

Doses

- **DOGS/CATS:**
  Daily dose for animals with body weights of:
  ≤12pounds (5.5 kg): one 90 mg tablet;
  12-25 pounds (5.5-11 kg): two 90 mg tablets (or one 225 mg tablet, if more convenient);
  25-35 pounds (11-16 kg): one 225 mg tablet;
  35-65 pounds (16-29.5 kg): two 225 mg tablets;
  65-90 pounds (29.5-41 kg): three 225 mg tablets;
  >90 pounds (41 kg+): four 225 mg tablets.

  Daily dosage may also be calculated based on 18 mg/kg of body weight and rounded to the closest tablet size or combination of sizes. Product should be given on an empty stomach, at least one hour before feeding. If giving more than one tablet, may divide total daily dosage and give twice daily. The number of tablets can be gradually reduced or may be increased at any time depending on the pet's needs. (Package information; *Denosyl*® —Nutramax)

  For adjunctive treatment of necro-inflammatory/cholestatic liver disease, vacuolar hepatopathy, or feline hepatic lipidosis (extra-label): 20 mg/kg PO once daily on an empty stomach; use a proven bioavailable product. (Center 2008)

Monitoring

- Clinical signs (appetite, activity, attitude).
- Liver enzymes, bilirubin, bile acids.

- Liver biopsies.
- Hepatic and erythrocyte glutathione levels (available at research institutions only at this time); may require 1-4 months before any changes in lab values are noted.

Client Information

- Keep tablets in original packaging until administration. Do not crush or split enteric-coated tablets.
- Very well tolerated, usually with no side effects.
- Give on an empty stomach, about an hour before feeding.
- SAMe is considered a nutritional supplement by the FDA, not a medication.

Chemistry/Synonyms

S-adenosyl-methionine (SAMe) is a naturally occurring molecule found throughout the body. Because pure SAMe is highly reactive and unstable, commercially available forms of SAMe are salt forms; sulfate, sulfate-p-toluenesulfonate (also known as tosylate), and butanedisulfonate salts can all be procured.

SAMe may also be known as: S-adenosyl-L-methionine, S-adenosylmethionine, SAM, SAM-e, ademetionine, adenosylmethionine, Sammy, methioninyl adenylate, *Donamet*®, *Gumbaral*®, *Isimet*®, *MoodLift*®, *S Amet*®, *Samyr*®, *Transmetil*®, and *Tunik*®.

Storage/Stability

Unless otherwise labeled, SAMe tablets should be stored at room temperature. Avoid conditions of high temperature or humidity. SAMe is inherently unstable in acidic or aqueous environments; store in tightly sealed, moisture-resistant containers.

Compatibility/Compounding Considerations

No specific information noted.

Dosage Forms/Regulatory Status

VETERINARY-LABELED PRODUCTS:

None as a pharmaceutical. The FDA considers SAMe a nutritional supplement. No standards have been accepted for potency, purity, safety, or efficacy by regulatory bodies. Supplements are available from a wide variety of sources and dosage forms include tablets in a variety of concentrations.

There are specific products marketed for use in animals, including:

Denosyl®, a 1, 4 –butanediolsulfonate salt in 90 mg, 225 mg, & 425 mg enteric-coated, blister-packed tablets and 225 mg chewable tablets.

Novifit® & *Zentonil*®, a tosylate salt in 100 mg, 200 mg and 400 mg tablets. Bioequivalence between SAMe products is not assured.

A combination product *Denamarin*®, containing SAMe and silybin (silymarin) is also labeled for use in dogs and cats.

HUMAN-LABELED PRODUCTS:

None as a pharmaceutical.

Revisions/References

Monograph revised/updated August 2014.

Center, S. (2008). Update on Canine & Feline Liver Disease. Proceedings: ECVIM. accessed via Veterinary Information Network; vin.com

Griffin, D., et al. (2009). Bioavailability of a Novel Formulation of S-Adenosylmethioine in Beagle Dogs. Preoceedings: ACVIM. accessed via Veterinary Information Network; vin. com

Skorupski, K. A., et al. (2011). Prospective Randomized Clinical Trial Assessing the Efficacy of Denamarin for Prevention of CCNU-Induced Hepatopathy in Tumor-Bearing Dogs. Journal of Veterinary Internal Medicine 25(4): 838-45.

Vandeweerd, J. M., et al. (2013). Nutraceuticals for Canine Liver Disease: Assessing the Evidence. Veterinary Clinics of North America-Small Animal Practice 43(5): 1171-+.

Saline Cathartics

Magnesium Oxide, Magnesium Sulfate, Magnesium Citrate, Sodium Sulfate

Laxative/Cathartic

Prescriber Highlights

▶ Saline/hyperosmotic agents for constipation or to increase elimination of GI toxins.
▶ Contraindications: Dehydrated patients or for long-term use. Used with extreme caution in patients with renal insufficiency, pre-existing water-balance or electrolyte abnormalities, or cardiac disease. Sodium sulfate contraindicated in patients with CHF or congenital megacolon.
▶ Adverse Effects: Cramping, nausea possible. Electrolyte disturbances possible, particularly with repeated use. If magnesium salts used chronically: hypermagnesemia (muscle weakness, ECG changes & CNS effects).
▶ Many drug interactions

Uses/Indications

Saline cathartics (laxatives) include: oral magnesium sulfate (epsom salts), magnesium oxide (milk of magnesia), magnesium citrate, and sodium sulfate (Glauber's salt). Saline cathartics can be used to relieve constipation or decrease intestinal transit time to reduce absorption of orally ingested toxicants. For small animals they are rarely recommended for treating constipation/obstipation.

Pharmacology/Actions

It is commonly believed that the hyperosmotic effect of poorly absorbed magnesium cations causes water retention, stimulates stretch receptors and enhances peristalsis in the small intestine and colon. Recent data, however, suggests that magnesium ions may directly decrease transit times and increase cholecystokinin release.

Pharmacokinetics

When magnesium salts are administered, up to 30% of the magnesium dose of magnesium can be absorbed.

Generally, the onset of action of saline cathartics (characterized by a loose, watery stool) occurs in 3-12 hours after dosing in monogastric animals and within 18 hours in ruminants.

Contraindications/Precautions/Warnings

Saline cathartics are contraindicated in dehydrated patients or for long-term use. Sodium containing laxatives are contraindicated in patients with congestive heart failure or congenital megacolon. Saline cathartics should be used with extreme caution in patients with significant diarrhea, renal insufficiency, pre-existing water-balance or electrolyte abnormalities, cardiac disease, or in severely depressed animals.

Adverse Effects

Except for possible cramping and nausea, adverse effects in otherwise healthy patients generally occur only with saline cathartics with chronic use or overdoses, but electrolyte disturbances (*e.g.,* hypernatremia, hypermagnesemia) can occur.

When magnesium salts are used, hypermagnesemia manifested by muscle weakness, ECG changes and CNS effects (depression) can occur.

Reproductive/Nursing Safety

In humans, the FDA categorizes magnesium sulfate as category *B* for use during pregnancy (*Animal studies have not yet demonstrated risk to the fetus, but there are no adequate studies in pregnant women; or animal studies have shown an adverse effect, but adequate studies in pregnant women have not demonstrated a risk to the fetus in the first trimester of pregnancy, and there is no evidence of risk in later trimesters.*) Other saline or hyperosmolar cathartics should be safe to use in pregnancy when used infrequently.

Magnesium emulsions administered orally did not affect the stools of nursing infants, although magnesium content in breast milk was slightly elevated compared with untreated patients. In veterinary patients, magnesium-containing cathartics should be safe to use during nursing if used infrequently.

Overdosage/Acute Toxicity

Clinical signs of overdosage of magnesium containing laxatives are described above. Treatment should consist of monitoring and correcting any fluid imbalances that occur with parenteral fluids.

If hypermagnesemia occurs, furosemide may be used to enhance the renal excretion of the excess magnesium. Calcium has been suggested to help antagonize the CNS effects of magnesium.

Drug Interactions

All orally administered saline laxatives may alter the rate and extent of absorption of **other orally administered drugs** by decreasing intestinal transit times. The extent of these effects has not been well characterized for individual drugs, however. The following drug interactions have either been reported or are theoretical in humans or animals receiving magnesium-containing oral products and may be of significance in veterinary patients. Unless otherwise noted, use together is not necessarily contraindicated, but weigh the potential risks and perform additional monitoring when appropriate.

- QUINIDINE: Increased risk for quinidine toxicity.
- SODIUM POLYSTYRENE SULFONATE: Increased risk for metabolic acidosis.

The following drugs or drug classes may have reduced oral bioavailability if administered with magnesium-containing cathartics; separate dosages by at least two hours if both drugs are needed:

- DIGOXIN
- FEXOFENADINE
- FLUOROQUINOLONES
- KETOCONAZOLE, ITRACONAZOLE
- LEVOTHYROXINE (Talcott 2012)
- MISOPROSTOL
- MYCOPHENOLATE
- PENICILLAMINE
- SOTALOL
- TETRACYCLINES

Laboratory Considerations

- No specific information noted.

Doses

- **DOGS/CATS:**

  As a cathartic (extra-label):

  Magnesium hydroxide (Milk of Magnesia) (extra-label): Rarely used in small animals as a laxative, but has been recommended as a cathartic for zinc phosphide ingestions at 5 – 15 mL per dog or cat PO. (Talcott 2012)

  Magnesium Sulfate or Sodium Sulfate (extra-label): Rarely used in small animals as a laxative, but can be used as a cathartic (although sodium sulfate is preferred) with or without activated charcoal to enhance toxin removal from the gut. Routine use is not recommended as sole treatment as there is a risk of volume depletion, hypotension, and electrolyte disturbances. 250 mg/kg as a 20% (or more dilute) solution in water. Activated charcoal (1 – 4 g/kg) combined with the cathartic (250 mg/kg) as a suspension in water (10X water) can also be used. In cases where repeated doses of activated charcoal are indicated and magnesium sulfate is used, the cathartic should be given with the initial dose of activated charcoal. If subsequent doses (up to two more times) of

magnesium sulfate are administered, use at ½ the amount used with charcoal. (Talcott 2012)

- **HORSES:**

  Magnesium Sulfate or Sodium Sulfate as a cathartic for plant intoxications (extra-label): Activated charcoal (AC) slurry dosage range of 1 – 5 grams/kg (≈1 gram of activated charcoal per 5 mL of water). Multi-dose activated charcoal is beneficial for a number of plant intoxications, including oleander. Administration of a cathartic mixed in the AC slurry helps to hasten elimination of contents from the gastrointestinal tract. Commonly used cathartics include sodium sulfate (Glauber's salts), magnesium sulfate (Epsom salts), and sorbitol. Sodium or magnesium sulfate can be administered at 250 – 500 mg/kg mixed in the AC slurry. Sorbitol (70%), also mixed in the AC slurry, can be administered at 3 mL/kg. There is little need to administer a cathartic if significant diarrhea is already present. (Puschner 2010)

  Magnesium Sulfate for cecal impactions (extra-label): 1 gram/kg dissolved in water and given via NG tube. Give with a balanced electrolyte solution IV to stimulate secretion into the dehydrated ingesta. (White 2005)

- **RUMINANTS:**

  Sodium sulfate as a cathartic (extra-label): Cattle: 500 – 750 grams PO as a 6% solution via stomach tube (Davis 1993). **Note:** When used in food animals, FARAD states that this salt is rapidly excreted and not considered a residue concern in animal tissues; therefore, a 24-hour preslaughter withdrawal interval (WDI) would be sufficient. (Haskell *et al.* 2005)

  Magnesium Sulfate or Sodium Sulfate as a cathartic for plant intoxications (extra-label): Activated charcoal (AC) slurry dosage range of 1 – 5 grams/kg (≈1 gram of activated charcoal per 5 mL of water). Multi-dose activated charcoal is beneficial for a number of plant intoxications, including oleander. Administration of a cathartic mixed in the AC slurry helps to hasten elimination of contents from the gastrointestinal tract. Commonly used cathartics include sodium sulfate (Glauber's salts), magnesium sulfate (Epsom salts), and sorbitol. Sodium or magnesium sulfate can be administered at 250 – 500 mg/kg mixed in the AC slurry. Sorbitol (70%), also mixed in the AC slurry, can be administered at 3 mL/kg. There is little need to administer a cathartic if significant diarrhea is already present. (Puschner 2010)

Monitoring

- Clinical efficacy.
- Fluid and electrolyte status in susceptible patients, especially with high or repeated doses.

Client Information

- Do not give dosages greater than, or for periods longer than, those recommended by veterinarian.
- Contact veterinarian if patient begins vomiting.

Chemistry/Synonyms

Magnesium cation containing solutions of magnesium citrate, magnesium hydroxide, or magnesium sulfate act as saline laxatives. Magnesium citrate solutions contain 4.71 mEq of magnesium per 5 mL. Magnesium hydroxide contains 34.3 mEq of magnesium per gram and milk of magnesia contains 13.66 mEq per 5 mL. One gram of magnesium sulfate (Epsom salt) contains approximately 8.1 mEq of magnesium.

Sodium sulfate (hexahydrate form) occurs as large, colorless, odorless, crystals or white crystalline powder. It will effloresce in dry air and partially dissolve in its own water of crystallization at about 33°C. 1 gram is soluble in about 2.5 mL of water. Sodium sulfate may also be known as E514, Glauber's Salt, natrii sulphas, natrio sulfata, or natrium sulfuricum.

Storage/Stability

Store milk of magnesia at temperatures less than 35°C, but do not freeze.

Compatibility/Compounding Considerations

No specific information noted.

Dosage Forms/Regulatory Status

VETERINARY-LABELED PRODUCTS:

Saline cathartic products have apparently not been formally FDA-approved for use in domestic animals. They are available without prescription (OTC).

HUMAN-LABELED PRODUCTS:

Saline Laxatives (not an inclusive list):

Magnesium Hydroxide Suspension (Milk of Magnesia): 400 mg/5mL (80 mg/mL); generic; (OTC)

Magnesium Hydroxide Suspension concentrated (Milk of Magnesia concentrated): 800 mg/5mL (160 mg/mL); generic; (OTC)

Magnesium Sulfate (Epsom Salt) Granules: in 120 g, 1 lb and 4 lbs; generic; (OTC)

Magnesium Citrate Solution 1.75 g/30 mL in 296 mL btls; generic; (OTC)

Sodium sulfate (hexahydrate) is available from chemical supply houses.

Revisions/References

Monograph revised/updated August 2014.

Davis, L. (1993). Drugs Affecting the Digestive System. *Current Veterinary Therapy 3: Food Animal Practice.* J. Howard. Philadelphia, W.B. Saunders Co.

Haskell, S., et al. (2005). Farad Digest: Antidotes in Food Animal Practice. JAVMA 226(6): 884-7.

Puschner, B. (2010). Diagnostic and therapeutic approach to plant poisonings in large animals. accessed via Veterinary Information Network; vin.com

Talcott, P. A. (2012). Decontamination Procedures in Poisoned Companion Animals - Facts & Fiction. Western Veterinary Conference. accessed via Veterinary Information Network; vin.com

White, N. (2005). Intestinal diseases. Western Veterinary Conference: Proceedings. accessed via Veterinary Information Network; vin.com

Saline, Hypertonic — see Hypertonic Saline

Selamectin

(sell-a-mek-tin)   Revolution®

Avermectin (Topical) Antiparasitic

Prescriber Highlights

▶ Topical avermectin antiparasiticide FDA-approved for multiple indications in dogs & cats.
▶ Applied monthly (usually; some indications one time dosing). More frequent dosing for some extra-label uses.
▶ Adverse effect profile appears minimal when used as labeled.

Uses/Indications

Topical selamectin (*Revolution®*) is indicated for flea infestations (*Ctenocephalides felis*), prevention of heartworm disease (*Dirofilaria immitis*), and ear mites (*Otodectes cynotis*) in both dogs and cats. Additionally in dogs, it is indicated for sarcoptic mange (*Sarcoptes scabeii*) and tick infestations (*Dermacentor variabilis*). In cats it is indicated for hookworms (*Ancylostoma tubaeforme*) and roundworms (*Toxocara cati*).

The product (*Revolution®*) is labeled as not effective against either adult heartworms or for clearing circulating microfilaria, but it possibly may have some efficacy with prolonged, continuous administration (Atkins 2007).

Topical selamectin has been used off-label successfully to treat a variety of ectoparasites in small animals, including notoedric mange (*Notoedres cati*), nasal mites in dogs (*Pneumonyssoides caninum*), cheyletiellosis in dogs, cats and rabbits, and cordyliobiolosis (cutaneous myiasis, *Cordylobia anthropophaga*) in dogs.

Selamectin has not been successful for treating generalized demodicosis; usually other treatments are preferred.

Pharmacology/Actions

Like other compounds in its class, selamectin is believed to act by enhancing chloride permeability or enhancing the release of gamma amino butyric acid (GABA) at presynaptic neurons. GABA acts as an inhibitory neurotransmitter and blocks the post-synaptic stimulation of the adjacent neuron in nematodes or the muscle fiber in arthropods. By stimulating the release of GABA, it causes paralysis and eventual death of the parasite. As liver flukes and tapeworms do not use GABA as a peripheral nerve transmitter, selamectin would probably be ineffective against these parasites.

Pharmacokinetics

After topical administration to dogs, ≈ 5% of the drug is bioavailable and peak plasma levels occur ≈ 3 days later. Selamectin bioavailability may be higher in female dogs. Elimination half-life after topical administration is ≈ 11 days.

After topical administration to cats, ≈ 75% of the drug is bioavailable and peak plasma levels occur ≈ 15 hours later. Elimination half-life after topical administration is ≈ 8 days. In cats, bioavailability is ≈ 75% and peak levels may be 64X those in dogs.

In rabbits, topical selamectin at 10 or 20 mg/kg had a mean terminal half-life of slightly less than one day. Maximum plasma concentrations of selamectin were 91.7 ng/mL (10 mg/kg) and 304.2 ng/mL (20 mg/kg) (Carpenter *et al.* 2012).

The persistence of the drug in the body is believed to be due to the drug forming reservoirs in skin sebaceous glands. It is secreted into the intestine to kill susceptible endoparasites in cats.

Contraindications/Precautions/Warnings

The manufacturer recommends caution when using in sick, underweight, or debilitated dogs or cats. It is not recommended for use in dogs under 6 weeks of age and in cats under 8 weeks of age.

At labeled doses of selamectin, dogs at risk for MDR1-allele mutation (Collies, Australian Shepherds, Shelties, Long-haired Whippets, etc.) should tolerate the medication, but use cautiously. Higher doses may cause neurological toxicity in these dogs.

Adverse Effects

In field trials (limited numbers of animals) adverse effects were rare. Approximately 1% of cats showed a transient, localized alopecia at the area of administration. Other effects reported (≤0.5% incidence) include diarrhea, vomiting, muscle tremors, anorexia, pruritus/urticaria, erythema, lethargy, salivation and tachypnea. Very rarely, seizures and ataxia have been reported in dogs.

Reproductive/Nursing Safety

Selamectin appears to be safe to use in pregnant or lactating dogs or cats.

Overdosage/Acute Toxicity

Dogs: Oral overdoses of up to 15 mg/kg did not cause adverse effects (except for ataxia in one avermectin sensitive collie). Topical overdoses (10X) to puppies caused no adverse effects; topical overdoses to avermectin-sensitive Collies caused salivation.

Cats: Oral ingestion may cause salivation and vomiting. Topical overdoses of up to 10X caused no observable adverse effects.

There were 97 exposures to selamectin reported to the ASPCA Animal Poison Control Center (APCC) during 2008-2009. In these cases 48 were dogs with 12 showing clinical signs and 53 cases were cats with 28 showing clinical signs. The remaining 3 cases consisted of 2 lagomorphs and 1 ferret none of which had clinical signs. Common findings in dogs recorded in decreasing frequency included hypersalivation and polydipsia. Common findings in cats recorded in decreasing frequency included hypersalivation, licking lips, vomiting, anorexia, depression, and lethargy.

Drug Interactions

None documented, but caution is advised if using other drugs that can inhibit **p-glycoprotein**. Those dogs at risk for MDR1-allele mutation (Collies, Australian Shepherds, Shelties, Long-haired Whippets, etc. "white feet") should probably not receive selamectin with the following drugs, unless tested "normal": Drugs and drug classes involved include:

- **AMIODARONE**
- **CARVEDILOL**
- **CLARITHROMYCIN**
- **CYCLOSPORINE**
- **DILTIAZEM**
- **ERYTHROMYCIN**
- **ITRACONAZOLE**
- **KETOCONAZOLE**
- **QUINIDINE**
- **SPIRONOLACTONE**
- **TAMOXIFEN**
- **VERAPAMIL**

Laboratory Considerations
- None reported.

Doses

- **DOGS:**

  For labeled indications (FDA-approved): For prophylaxis and treatment of dirofilariasis, it is suggested to review the guidelines published by the American Heartworm Society at www.heartwormsociety.org for more information: The recommended topical dose is 6 mg/kg. Dosing frequency: Heartworm prevention, flea control = monthly; Ticks = monthly (if heavy infestations, may repeat 2 weeks after the first dose); Ear Mites, Sarcoptes = once, repeat in one month if necessary. See the package for specific instructions on administration technique. (Adapted from label information; *Revolution®*—Pfizer)

  For sarcoptic mange (extra-label): Some dermatologists use a more aggressive approach (than labeled dose) using a protocol of 4-6 treatments at 2-week intervals. (Koch *et al.* 2011).

  For nasal mites in dogs (*Pneumonyssoides caninum*) (extra-label): In the study, dogs were dosed at 6 – 24 mg/kg for 3 times at 2-week intervals. (Gunnarsson *et al.* 2004)

  For cheyletiellosis (extra-label): 6 – 12 mg/kg topically every other week for a total of 4 treatments. (Mueller *et al.* 2002)

  For biting lice (extra-label): 6 mg/kg topically once. (Shanks *et al.* 2003)

- **CATS:**

  For labeled indications (FDA-approved): The recommended topical dose is 6 mg/kg. Dosing frequency: Heartworm prevention, flea control = monthly; Ear Mites = once, repeat in one month if necessary. Hookworms, Roundworms = once. See the package for specific instructions on administration technique. (Adapted from label information; *Revolution®*—Pfizer)

  For cheyletiellosis (extra-label): 6 – 12 mg/kg topically once monthly for a total of 3 treatments. (Koch *et al.* 2011)

  For notoedric (face/head) mange (*Notoedres cati*) (extra-label): 6 mg/kg topically once. (Arther 2009)

  For biting lice (extra-label): 6 mg/kg topically once. (Shanks *et al.* 2003)

- **FERRETS:**

  For heartworm prevention (extra-label): 18 mg/kg topically every 30 days. (Johnson 2006)

- **SMALL MAMMALS:**

  Rabbits; for ear mites (*P. cuniculi*) (extra-label): 6 – 18 mg/kg topically. (McTier *et al.* 2003)

  Rabbits; for fleas (*C. felis, C. canis*) (extra-label): Based on a safety, efficacy and pharmacokinetic study results suggested that topical administration at 20 mg/kg every 7 days is efficacious; further studies are needed to assess long-term safety in rabbits following repeated applications. (Carpenter *et al.* 2012)

  Guinea pigs; for *Trixacarus caviae* mange (extra-label): Results from the study suggested that a single topical application of selamectin at 15 mg/kg can eliminate *T. caviae mites* from guinea pigs within 30 days. (Eshar *et al.* 2012)

Monitoring
- Clinical efficacy.
- Owner compliance with treatment regimen.

Client Information
- Follow label directions for administration technique; do not massage into skin, and do not apply if hair coat is wet. Because the product contains alcohol, do not apply to broken skin.
- Avoid contact with animal while the application site is wet.
- Wait two hours or more after applying to bathe the animal (or allow to go swimming).
- Avoid getting the product on human skin; if contact occurs, wash off immediately. Dispose of tubes in regular household refuse.
- Do not expose to flame as the product is flammable.

Chemistry/Synonyms

A semi-synthetic avermectin, selamectin is commercially available as a colorless to yellow solution (flammable).

Selamectin may also be known as UK-124114, *Revolution®*, *Paradyne®* or *Stronghold®*.

Storage/Stability

The commercially available solution should be stored below 30°C (86°F). Keep away from flame or other igniters.

Compatibility/Compounding Considerations

No specific information noted.

Dosage Forms/Regulatory Status

VETERINARY-LABELED PRODUCTS:

Selamectin Topical Solution for Cats; *Revolution®*; (Rx):

Up to 5 lbs in wt, Pkg. Color: mauve. 15 mg/tube. Tube volume: 0.25 mL

5.1-15 lbs in wt, Pkg. Color: blue. 45 mg/tube. Tube volume: 0.75 mL

Selamectin Topical Solution for Dogs; *Revolution®*; (Rx)

Up to 5 lbs in wt, Pkg. Color: mauve. 15 mg/tube. Tube volume: 0.25 mL

5.1-10 lbs in wt, Pkg. Color: purple. 30 mg/tube. Tube volume: 0.25 mL

10.1-20 lbs in wt, Pkg. Color: brown. 60 mg/tube. Tube volume: 0.5 mL

20.1-40 lbs in wt, Pkg. Color: red. 120 mg/tube. Tube volume: 1 mL

40.1-85 lbs in wt, Pkg. Color: teal. 240 mg/tube. Tube volume: 2 mL

85.1-130 lbs in wt, Pkg. Color: plum. One 120 mg tube and one 240 mg tube. Total volume: 3 mL

There is also a re-labeled product called *Paradyne®*.

HUMAN-LABELED PRODUCTS: NONE.

Revisions/References

Monograph revised/updated August 2014.

Arther, R. (2009). Mites and Lice: Biology and Control. Vet Clin Small Anim **39**: 1159-71.

Atkins, C. (2007). What's new in heartworms. Proceedings: WVC. accessed via Veterinary Information Network; vin.com

Carpenter, J. W., et al. (2012). Pharmacokinetics, efficacy, and adverse effects of selamectin following topical administration in flea-infested rabbits. American Journal of Veterinary Research 73(4): 562-6.

Eshar, D. & T. Bdolah-Abram (2012). Comparison of efficacy, safety, and convenience of selamectin versus ivermectin for treatment of Trixacarus caviae mange in pet guinea pigs (Cavia porcellus). Javma-Journal of the American Veterinary Medical Association **241**(8): 1056-8.

Gunnarsson, L., et al. (2004). Efficacy of selamectin in the treatment of nasal mite (Pneumonyssoides caninum) infection in dogs. J. Am. Anim. Hosp. Assoc. **40**(5): 400-4.

Johnson, D. (2006). Ferrets: the other companion animal. Proceedings: ACVC. accessed via Veterinary Information Network; vin.com

Koch, S., et al. (2011). *Small Animal Dermatology Drug Handbook*, Wiley-Blackwell. Ames.

McTier, T., et al. (2003). Efficacy and safety of topical administration of selamectin for treatment of ear mite infestation in rabbits. J Am Vet Med Assoc 223(3): 322-4.

Mueller, R. S. & S. V. Bettenay (2002). Efficacy of selamectin in the treatment of canine cheyletiellosis. Veterinary Record 151(25): 773-.

Shanks, D. J., et al. (2003). Efficacy of selamectin against biting lice on dogs and cats. Veterinary Record 152(8): 234-+.

Selegiline HCl

(se-le-ji-leen)　l-deprenyl, Anipryl®, Eldepryl®

Monoamine Oxidase Inhibitor

Prescriber Highlights

▶ MAO-B inhibitor that may be useful for cognitive dysfunction syndrome (CDS) in dogs or cats or canine Cushing's (efficacy in doubt for Cushing's).

▶ May require 2-6 weeks of administration to show clinical improvement for CDS.

▶ Adverse Effects: Vomiting & diarrhea; CNS effects manifested by restlessness, repetitive movements, or lethargy; salivation & anorexia. Diminished hearing/deafness, pruritus, licking, shivers/trembles/shakes possible.

▶ Drug Interactions; some may be serious.

Uses/Indications

Selegiline is FDA-approved for use in dogs for the control of clinical signs associated with canine cognitive dysfunction syndrome (CDS; "old dog dementia") and control of clinical signs associated with uncomplicated canine pituitary dependent hyperadrenocorticism (PDH). While FDA-approved, its use for PDH is somewhat controversial as clinical studies evaluating its efficacy have shown disappointing results. In humans, selegiline's primary indication is for the adjunctive treatment of Parkinson's disease. Selegiline may have a role in treating dogs with chronic anxiety, particularly those that have high prolactin levels (Pageat *et al.* 2007). Combined with a benzodiazepine and a beta-blocker such as propranolol, selegiline may be particularly useful in treating social or noise phobias.

Selegiline may be of use in feline cognitive dysfunction syndrome.

Pharmacology/Actions

Selegiline's mechanism of action for treatment of Cushing's disease (pituitary dependent hyperadrenocorticism—PDH) is complex; a somewhat simplified explanation follows: In the hypothalamus, corticotropin-releasing hormone (CRH) acts to stimulate the production of ACTH in the pituitary and dopamine acts to inhibit the release of ACTH. As dogs age, there is a tendency for a decrease in dopamine production that can contribute to the development of PDH.

As dopamine is metabolized by monamino oxidase-B (MAO-B) and selegiline inhibits MAO-B, dopamine levels can be increased at receptor sites after selegiline administration. In theory, this allows the levels of dopamine and CRH to be in balance in the hypothal-

amus, thereby reducing the amount of ACTH produced and ultimately, cortisol.

While selegiline is labeled as a MAO-B inhibitor, at higher than labeled dosages, the drug loses its MAO-B specificity and also inhibits MAO-A. Two of three metabolites of selegiline are amphetamine and methamphetamine that may contribute to both the efficacy and the adverse effects of the drug.

Pharmacokinetics

There is only limited information on the pharmacokinetics of selegiline in dogs. A study done in 4 dogs showed that selegiline was absorbed rapidly and had an absolute bioavailability of ≈ 10%. The volume of distribution of the central compartment was measured at approximately 7 L/kg. Terminal half-life was ≈ 1 hour.

In humans, selegiline pharmacokinetics have wide interpatient variability. The drug has a high first pass effect where extensive metabolism to L-desmethylselegiline, methylamphetamine, and L-amphetamine occur. Each of these metabolites is active. While L-desmethylselegiline does inhibit MAO-B, the others do not, but they are CNS stimulants. The drug is excreted in the urine, primarily as conjugated and unconjugated metabolites.

Contraindications/Precautions/Warnings

Selegiline is contraindicated in patients known to be hypersensitive to it. In human patients, it is contraindicated in patients receiving meperidine or tramadol and possibly with other opioids as well.

The manufacturer cautions to perform appropriate diagnostic tests to confirm the diagnosis before starting therapy and not to attempt to treat hyperadrenocorticism not of pituitary origin.

Adverse Effects

Adverse reports in dogs include vomiting, diarrhea, CNS effects manifested by restlessness, repetitive movements or lethargy, salivation, and anorexia. Should GI effects be a problem, discontinue the drug for a few days and restart at a lower dose. Diminished hearing/deafness, pruritus, licking, shivers/trembles/shakes have also been reported. The manufacturer advises to observe animals carefully for atypical responses.

Adverse effects that have been reported in human patients include nausea (10%), hallucinations, confusion, depression, loss of balance, insomnia, and hypersexuality. These effects are noted because of their "subjective" nature and should they occur, they could help explain untoward behavioral changes in canine patients.

Because selegiline could potentially be abused by humans, veterinarians should be alert for drug "shoppers." Selegiline is classified by the Association of Racing Commissioners International (ARCI) as a class 2 agent (high abuse potential in racing horses).

Reproductive/Nursing Safety

Safety of selegiline in pregnant, breeding or lactating animals has not been established. Rat studies have not demonstrated overt teratogenicity. In humans, the FDA categorizes this drug as category C for use during pregnancy (*Animal studies have shown an adverse effect on the fetus, but there are no adequate studies in humans; or there are no animal reproduction studies and no adequate studies in humans.*)

It is not known whether selegiline is excreted in maternal milk.

Overdosage/Acute Toxicity

Oral LD_{50} in laboratory animals was ≈ 200 – 445 mg/kg. In limited data, dogs receiving 3X dosages showed signs of decreased weight, salivation, decreased pupillary response, panting, stereotypic behaviors and decreased skin elasticity (dehydration). Overdoses, if severe, should be treated with appropriate gut decontamination and supportive treatments.

Drug Interactions

Evaluating the potential for drug interactions for selegiline in dogs is problematic. There are a plethora of significant interactions with monamino oxidase inhibitors in humans for selegiline, but because there are significant species differences in quantities and locations of MOA-A and MOA-B, and the effect selegiline has at various dosages on these enzymes, these may not apply to dogs. However, the following are some of the more significant interactions reported (or are theoretical) in humans or animals; caution is advised particularly if using selegiline at higher than labeled dosages:

- **AMITRAZ:** The manufacturer recommends not using selegiline concurrently with amitraz (*Mitaban®*) in dogs.
- **BUPROPION:** Potential for serotonin syndrome.
- **EPHEDRINE:** The manufacturer recommends not using selegiline concurrently with ephedrine in dogs.
- **MEPERIDINE/OPIOIDS:** In humans, severe agitation, hallucinations and death have occurred in some patients receiving meperidine and an MAO inhibitor. Until the data can be clarified, it is recommended not to use selegiline and meperidine together. A separation of two weeks has been recommended. Other opioids (*e.g.,* **morphine**) should be safer, but use with extreme caution, if at all.
- **PHENYLPROPANOLAMINE, PSEUDOEPHEDRINE:** Possibility for increased risk for hypertension, hyperpyrexia.
- **SSRI'S** (*e.g.,* **fluoxetine**): Potentially, the so-called serotonin syndrome could occur if selegiline is used concurrently with selective serotonin reuptake inhibitors (SSRIs); several sources recommend a 5-week washout before administering selegiline in dogs after fluoxetine is discontinued and wait 2 weeks if switching from selegiline to an SSRI.
- **TRAMADOL:** Use together is contraindicated in humans; serotonin syndrome, nausea, vomiting, cardiovascular collapse.
- **TRICYCLIC & TETRACYCLIC ANTIDEPRESSANTS** (*e.g.,* **clomipramine, amitriptyline,** etc.): Potentially, the so-called serotonin syndrome could occur if selegiline is used concurrently with these agents and use together is not advised at this time; a 2-week separation between these compounds and selegiline is recommended.

Doses

- **DOGS:**

  For canine pituitary dependent hyperadrenocorticism (PDH; Canine Cushing's) (labeled dose; FDA-approved): 1 mg/kg PO in the AM (with food as needed). Reevaluate clinically over next 2 months; if no improvement, may increase to 2 mg/kg once daily; if no improvement or signs increase, reevaluate diagnosis or consider alternate treatment. Dogs should be monitored closely for possible adverse events associated with any increase in dose. (Adapted from label; *Anipryl®*).

  For canine cognitive dysfunction:

  Labeled-dose (FDA-approved): 0.5 – 1 mg/kg, PO once daily, preferably in the AM. Initially, dose to the nearest whole tablet; adjustments should then be made based upon response and tolerance to the drug. (Adapted from label; *Anipryl®*).

  Extra-label dose: 0.5 mg/kg PO q24h; if no response after 4 weeks give 1 mg/kg PO q24h. Also useful in some anxiety problems and sleep disorders. (Seksel 2008)

- **CATS:**

  For cognitive dysfunction syndrome (extra-label): 0.25 – 1 mg/kg PO once daily. There are no drugs licensed for the treatment of CDS in cats. However, a small open trial using selegiline showed a positive effect and the American Association

of Feline Practitioners supports the use of this drug for the treatment of CDS. (Gunn-Moore 2008)

Monitoring

- Clinical efficacy.
- Adverse effects. No correlation between low dose dexamethasone suppression test results and clinical efficacy of the drug. The manufacturer recommends physical exam and history as the primary methods to measure response to therapy.

Client Information

- May give with or without food. Dogs usually get the daily dose in the morning and cats in the evening.
- May take several weeks to see if the drug is working.
- Have veterinarian approve changes to diet/snacks and tick treatments (*e.g.,* collars, spot-ons) before using with selegiline.
- Side effects include gastrointestinal problems (*e.g.,* vomiting, diarrhea, lack of appetite, drooling, etc.) and behavioral changes.

Chemistry/Synonyms

Selegiline HCl, also commonly called l-deprenyl, occurs as a white to off-white crystalline powder that is freely soluble in water. It has a pKa of 7.5.

Selegiline HCl may also be known as: deprenyl, L-deprenyl, selegilini hydrochloridum; many trade names are available including *Anipryl®* and *Selgian®*.

Storage/Stability

Commercially available veterinary tablets should be stored at controlled room temperature 20-25°C (68-77°F). The commercially available human-labeled tablets and capsules are recommended to be stored from 15-30°C.

Compatibility/Compounding Considerations

No specific information noted.

Dosage Forms/Regulatory Status

VETERINARY-LABELED PRODUCTS:

Selegiline HCl Oral Tablets: 2 mg, 5 mg, 10 mg, 15 mg, 30 mg in blister-packs of 30 tablets; *Anipryl®*; (Rx). FDA-approved for use in dogs.

The ARCI (Racing Commissioners International) has designated this drug as a class 2 substance. See the appendix for more information.

HUMAN-LABELED PRODUCTS:

Selegiline HCl Tablets & Capsules 5 mg; *Eldepryl®*, generic; (Rx)

Selegiline Orally Dispersible Tablets 1.25 mg; *Zelapar®*; (Rx)

Selegiline HCl Transdermal Patch: 6 mg/24 hours (20 mg/20 cm²); 9 mg/24 hours (30 mg/30 cm²) & 12 mg/24 hours (40 mg/40 cm²); *Emsam®*; (Rx)

Revisions/References

Monograph revised/updated August 2014.

Gunn-Moore, D. (2008). Geriatric Cats and Cognitive Dysfunction Syndrome. Procedings: WSAVA. accessed via Veterinary Information Network; vin.com

Pageat, P., et al. (2007). An evaluation of serum prolactin in anxious dogs and response to treatment with selegiline or fluoxetine. Applied Animal Behaviour Science 105(4): 342-50.

Seksel, K. (2008). To medicate or not to medicate--That is the question! What to use, when and why. Proceedings: World Veterinary Congress. accessed via Veterinary Information Network; vin.com

Sertraline HCI

(sir-trah-leen)   Zoloft®

Selective Serotonin Reuptake Inhibitor (SSRI)

Prescriber Highlights

▶ Human-approved serotonin reuptake inhibitor that may be useful in treating a variety of behavior-related diagnoses in dogs & cats, including aggression, anxiety-related behaviors & other obsessive-compulsive behaviors.

▶ Caution: geriatric patients or those with severe hepatic disease; dosages may need to be adjusted.

▶ Adverse effect profile not well established. Potentially, **Dogs:** Anorexia, lethargy, GI effects, anxiety, irritability, insomnia/hyperactivity, or panting. Aggressive behavior in previously non-aggressive dogs possible. **Cats:** Sedation, decreased appetite/anorexia, vomiting, diarrhea, behavior changes (anxiety, irritability, sleep disturbances), & changes in elimination patterns.

▶ Drug-drug interactions.

Uses/Indications

Sertraline may be considered for use in treating a variety of behavior-related diagnoses in dogs and cats, including aggression, and anxiety-related or other obsessive-compulsive behaviors.

Pharmacology/Actions

Sertraline is a highly selective inhibitor of the reuptake of serotonin (5-hydroxytryptamine) in the CNS thus potentiating its pharmacologic activity. Sertraline apparently has little effect on dopamine or norepinephrine, and apparently no effect on other neurotransmitters.

Pharmacokinetics

In dogs, sertraline's volume of distribution is 25 L/kg and is 97% bound to plasma proteins. High first-pass metabolism occurs; clearance is >35 mL/min/kg. Bile is the major route of excretion in the dog.

In humans, sertraline peak levels occur 30-45 minutes after oral dosing. It is 98% bound to plasma proteins. Sertraline appears to be highly metabolized primarily to N-desmethylsertraline, which is active. Elimination half-lives for sertraline and desmethylsertraline average 26 and 80 hours respectively.

Contraindications/Precautions/Warnings

Sertraline is contraindicated in patients hypersensitive to it or any SSRI, or receiving a monoamine oxidase inhibitor (MAOI) or cisapride. Use with caution in geriatric patients and those with hepatic impairment; dosages may need to be decreased or dosing interval increased.

If using verbal orders, ascertain that sertraline is not confused with cetirizine.

Adverse Effects

Limited use of sertraline in dogs or cats makes it difficult to compare its adverse effect profile with other SSRIs (*e.g.*, fluoxetine, paroxetine, fluvoxamine). In dogs, SSRIs can cause lethargy, GI effects, anxiety, irritability, insomnia/hyperactivity, or panting. Anorexia is a common side effect in dogs (usually transient and may be negated by temporarily increasing the palatability of food and/or hand feeding). Some dogs have persistent anorexia that precludes further treatment. Aggressive behavior in previously non-aggressive dogs has been reported. SSRI's in cats can cause sedation, decreased appetite/anorexia, vomiting, diarrhea, behavior changes (anxiety, irritability, sleep disturbances), and changes in elimination patterns.

Reproductive/Nursing Safety

In humans, the FDA categorizes sertraline as a category *C* drug for use during pregnancy (*Animal studies have shown an adverse effect on the fetus, but there are no adequate studies in humans; or there are no animal reproduction studies and no adequate studies in humans.*) In rats and rabbits, sertraline was implicated in causing delayed ossification. Sertraline decreased pup survival in rats exposed *in utero*.

It is unknown if sertraline enters maternal milk.

Overdosage/Acute Toxicity

With overdoses, the SSRI's can cause vomiting, diarrhea, hypersalivation, and lethargy. Serotonin syndrome may occur with signs that include muscle tremors, rigidity, agitation, hyperthermia, vocalization, hypertension or hypotension, tachycardia, seizures, coma, and death. Most exposures below 20 mg/kg in dogs are not serious. The reported median lethal dosage for dogs following a single ingestion is 80 mg/kg of body weight (Fitzgerald *et al.* 2013). Human overdoses of as little of 2.5 grams have caused death, but one patient survived after taking 13.5 grams.

A retrospective review of sertraline ingestions reported to Pet Poison Helpline found approximately one-third of reports of ingestions in dogs had clinical signs, including CNS depression (60%), CNS stimulation (24%), cardiovascular signs (8%), respiratory signs (12%), GI signs (16%), and hyperthermia (8%). Median dose for causing clinical signs was 11.6 mg/kg, but the range was very wide (0.4 – 264 mg/kg). More severe signs such as tremoring and hyperthermia were not seen until the dose reached between 8 – 10 mg/kg of sertraline and seizure activity was not noted until the dose exceeded 25 mg/kg (Thomas *et al.* 2012). There were 814 single agent exposures to sertraline reported to the ASPCA Animal Poison Control Center (APCC) during 2009-2013. Of the 725 dogs, 160 were symptomatic with 33% being lethargic, 14% mydriatic and 13% vomiting. Of the 83 cats, 31 were symptomatic with hypersalivation (45%) and mydriasis (26%) being the most common.

Management of sertraline overdoses should be handled aggressively with supportive and symptomatic treatment. Intravenous lipid emulsions (ILE) have been successfully used to treat severe overdoses. Veterinarians are encouraged to contact an animal poison control center for further guidance.

Drug Interactions

The following drug interactions have either been reported or are theoretical in humans or animals receiving sertraline and may be of significance in veterinary patients. Unless otherwise noted, use together is not necessarily contraindicated, but weigh the potential risks and perform additional monitoring when appropriate.

- **BUSPIRONE:** Increased risk for serotonin syndrome.
- **CIMETIDINE:** May increase sertraline levels.
- **CYPROHEPTADINE:** May decrease or reverse the effects of SSRIs.
- **DIAZEPAM:** Sertraline may decrease diazepam clearance.
- **ISONIAZID:** Increased risk for serotonin syndrome.
- **MAO INHIBITORS** (including **amitraz** and **selegiline**): High risk for serotonin syndrome; use contraindicated; in humans, a 5 week washout period is required after discontinuing sertraline and a 2 week washout period is required if first discontinuing the MAO inhibitor.
- **PENTAZOCINE:** Serotonin syndrome-like adverse effects possible.
- **TRAMADOL:** SSRI's can inhibit the metabolism of tramadol to the active metabolites decreasing its efficacy and increasing the risk of toxicity (serotonin syndrome, seizures).
- **TRICYCLIC ANTIDEPRESSANTS** (*e.g.*, **clomipramine**, **am-**

itriptyline): Sertraline may increase TCA blood levels and the risk for serotonin syndrome.

- WARFARIN: Sertraline may increase the risk for bleeding.

Laboratory Considerations

- No significant laboratory interactions or considerations were located.

Doses

- **DOGS:**

For adjunctive treatment (with behavior modification) of behavior disorders (*e.g.*, obsessive/compulsive disorders, anxiety, etc.); (extra-label): Anecdotal dosage recommendations range from 1 – 4 mg/kg PO once daily (or divided twice daily). Most recommend starting at the low end of the dosing range. No specific studies supporting any one dosage were located. A minimum of a 6-8 week trial is usually recommended before assessing efficacy. If discontinuing treatment wean off over at least 2-3 weeks (or longer).

- **CATS:**

For adjunctive treatment (with behavior modification) of behavior disorders (*e.g.*, obsessive/compulsive disorders, anxiety, spraying, etc.); (extra-label): Anecdotal dosage recommendations range from 0.5 – 1.5 mg/kg PO once daily. Most recommend starting at the low end of the dosing range. No specific studies supporting any one dosage were located. A minimum of a 6-8 week trial is usually recommended before assessing efficacy. If discontinuing treatment wean off over at least 2-3 weeks (or longer).

Monitoring

- Efficacy.
- Adverse Effects; including appetite (weight).
- Consider doing baseline liver function tests and ECG; re-test as needed.

Client Information

- May take several days or weeks to determine if the drug is effective.
- Most common side effects are: drowsiness/sleepiness, reduced appetite.
- Rare side effects that can be serious (contact veterinarian immediately): seizures, aggression (threatening behavior/actions).
- Overdoses can be very serious; keep out of the reach of animals and children.
- If your animal wore a flea collar in the past two weeks, let your veterinarian know. Do not use one on your animal while it's getting this medicine without first talking to your veterinarian.

Chemistry/Synonyms

A selective serotonin reuptake inhibitor, sertraline hydrochloride is a white crystalline powder that is slightly soluble in water and isopropyl alcohol; sparingly soluble in ethanol. The commercially available oral solution contains 12% ethanol and has a menthol scent.

Sertraline may also be known as: CP-51974-01; *Altruline®, Anilar®, Aremis®, Atenix®, Besitran®, Bicromil®, Gladem®, Insertec®, Irradial®, Lustral®, Novativ®, Sealdin®, Serad®, Sercerin®, Serlain®, Serta®, Tatig®, Tolrest®, Tresleen®* or *Zoloft®.*

Storage/Stability

Store commercially available sertraline tablets and oral solution at controlled room temperature (25°C; 77°F); excursions permitted to 15-30°C (59-86°F).

Compatibility/Compounding Considerations

The manufacturer states to dilute the oral solution only in the following liquids: water, orange juice, ginger ale, lemonade or lemon/lime soda; use immediately after dilution.

Dosage Forms/Regulatory Status

VETERINARY-LABELED PRODUCTS: NONE.

The ARCI (Racing Commissioners International) has designated this drug as a class 2 substance. See the appendix for more information.

HUMAN-LABELED PRODUCTS:

Sertraline HCl Tablets: 25 mg, 50 mg & 100 mg (as base); *Zoloft®,* generic; (Rx)

Sertraline HCl Oral Solution Concentrate: 20 mg/mL in 60 mL; *Zoloft®,* generic; (Rx)

Revisions/References

Monograph revised/updated August 2014.

Fitzgerald, K. & A. C. Bronstein (2013). Topical Review: Selective Serotonin Reuptake Inhibitor Exposure. Topics in Companion Animal Medicine: 13-7.

Thomas, D. E., et al. (2012). Retrospective evaluation of toxicosis from selective serotonin reuptake inhibitor antidepressants: 313 dogs (2005-2010). J. Vet. Emerg. Crit. Care 22(6): 674-81.

Sevelamer

(se-vel-a-mer)   Renagel®

Phosphorus Binding Agent

Prescriber Highlights

▶ Phosphorus binding agent (in the gut) for hyperphosphatemia associated with chronic renal failure. Little veterinary experience.

▶ May be useful if patient cannot tolerate aluminum salts or aluminum salts are commercially unavailable.

▶ Expensive when compared to aluminum hydroxide or calcium carbonate products.

▶ Drug-drug interactions including nutrients.

Uses/Indications

Sevelamer may be useful for treating hyperphosphatemia associated with chronic renal failure, particularly when oral aluminum salts are not tolerated.

Pharmacology/Actions

Sevelamer binds phosphorus in the gut; when combined with decreased phosphorus in the diet it can substantially reduce serum phosphorus levels. It also reduces serum low-density lipoproteins and total cholesterol.

Pharmacokinetics

Sevelamer is administered orally, but is not absorbed systemically.

Contraindications/Precautions/Warnings

Sevelamer is contraindicated in patients with hypophosphatemia, or bowel obstruction and in patients hypersensitive to it.

Adverse Effects

Adverse effects in humans are reported to be the same as placebo. Potentially some GI effects occur.

As oral vitamin absorption may be reduced by sevelamer, consider the addition of vitamin supplementation during therapy.

Reproductive/Nursing Safety

Safety during pregnancy is not established; because of the potential for binding vitamins, additional vitamins (both fat and water soluble) may be necessary. In humans, the FDA categorizes this drug as category *C* for use during pregnancy (*Animal studies have shown an adverse effect on the fetus, but there are no adequate studies in hu-*

mans; or there are no animal reproduction studies and no adequate studies in humans.)

There are no adequate and well-controlled studies in nursing mothers.

Overdosage/Acute Toxicity

As sevelamer is not absorbed, acute toxicity potential appears to be negligible, but chronic overdoses may affect serum electrolytes and nutrient absorption.

Drug Interactions

The following drug interactions have either been reported or are theoretical in humans or animals receiving sevelamer and may be of significance in veterinary patients. Unless otherwise noted, use together is not necessarily contraindicated, but weigh the potential risks and perform additional monitoring when appropriate.

- **CIPROFLOXACIN:** Concurrent administration with sevelamer may decrease absorption by 50%; administer ciprofloxacin and other oral fluoroquinolones at least 1 hour before or 3 hours after sevelamer.
- **MYCOPHENOLATE:** Sevelamer may reduce absorption; administer 2 hours after mycophenolate.
- **ORAL MEDICATIONS:** There are only a few medications having documented reductions in oral absorption when administered with sevelamer; consider dosing other oral drugs separately, particularly for drugs with narrow therapeutic indexes.
- **THYROID HORMONES:** Sevelamer may reduce absorption; separate administering the two drugs by at least 4 hours.
- **VITAMINS:** Sevelamer may reduce vitamin absorption from food; consider administering vitamin supplements separately from sevelamer dose.

Doses

- **DOGS/CATS:**

  For adjunctive treatment of hyperphosphatemia in animals with chronic kidney disease (extra-label): No specific studies were noted that support any dosage. Practically, cats and small dogs would receive 200 – 400 mg per dose q8-12h with meals. Medium to large dogs would receive 400 – 1600 mg per dose q8-12h with meals. Monitor serum electrolytes and adjust as needed.

Monitoring

- Serum phosphorus (and other electrolytes calcium, bicarbonate, chloride).
- Consider a baseline coagulation-screening test before and after sevelamer therapy implementation as vitamin K absorption may be impacted.

Client Information

- Given with meals.
- Give separately (at least an hour apart) from other oral drugs or vitamins.
- Usually does not cause any side effects. Could cause reduced appetite, vomiting, constipation or diarrhea.
- Follow-up blood tests to measure phosphorous and other electrolytes are necessary.

Chemistry/Synonyms

A phosphorus binding agent, sevelamer HCl is a complex chemical that is hydrophilic, but insoluble in water. Sevelamer carbonate is also insoluble in water, but is hygroscopic.

Sevelamer may also be known as GT16-026A and *Renagel®* or *Renvela®*.

Storage/Stability

Sevelamer capsules should be stored at room temperature and protected from moisture.

Compatibility/Compounding Considerations

No specific information noted.

Dosage Forms/Regulatory Status

VETERINARY-LABELED PRODUCTS: NONE.

HUMAN-LABELED PRODUCTS:

Sevelamer HCl Oral Tablets: 400 mg & 800 mg; *Renagel®, Renvela®*; (Rx)

Sevelamer Carbonate Oral Tablets: 800 mg; *Renvela®*, generic; (Rx)

Sevelamer Carbonate Powder for Oral Suspension: 0.8 grams/packet & 2.4 grams/packet; *Renvela®*; (Rx)

Revisions/References

Monograph revised/updated August 2014.

Sevoflurane

(see-voe-floo-rane)   SevoFlo®, Ultane®

Inhalational Anesthetic

Prescriber Highlights

▶ Inhalational anesthetic similar to isoflurane, but with more rapid induction & recovery.
▶ Currently much more expensive than isoflurane.

Uses/Indications

While only FDA-approved for use in dogs and humans, sevoflurane may be useful in a variety of species (including cats, horses, small mammals and ruminants, birds, reptiles, etc.) when rapid induction and/or rapid recoveries are desired with an inhalational anesthetic. When mask inductions are necessary, sevoflurane is preferred over isoflurane or desflurane as it is better accepted and inductions are faster and smoother. Sevoflurane may be of particular usefulness in debilitated or geriatric patients as it is more easily dosed 'to effect' and may cause less hypotension than isoflurane.

Pharmacology/Actions

While the precise mechanisms how inhalant anesthetics produce their general anesthetic effects are not precisely known, they may interfere with functioning of nerve cells in the brain by acting at the lipid matrix of the membrane. Sevoflurane has a very low blood:gas partition coefficient (0.6) allowing very rapid anesthesia induction and recovery. Rapid mask induction is possible.

Pharmacologic effects of sevoflurane are similar to isoflurane and include: CNS depression, depression of body temperature regulating centers, increased cerebral blood flow, respiratory depression, hypotension, vasodilatation, myocardial depression (less so than with halothane), and muscular relaxation.

Approximate Minimal Alveolar Concentration (MAC; %) in oxygen reported for sevoflurane in various species: Dog = 2.09-2.4; Cat = 2.5-4; Horse = 2.31; Sheep = 3.3; Swine = 1.97-2.66; Human (adult) = 1.71-2.05. Several factors may alter MAC (acid/base status, temperature, other CNS depressants on board, age, ongoing acute disease, etc.).

Pharmacokinetics

Because of its low solubility in blood, only small concentrations of sevoflurane in the blood are required before alveolar partial pressures are in equilibrium with arterial partial pressures. This low solubility means that sevoflurane is rapidly removed from the lungs. It is unknown what percent sevoflurane is bound to plasma proteins. The majority of sevoflurane is excreted via the lungs, but ≈ 3% is metabolized in the liver via the cytochrome P450 2E1 isoenzyme system.

Contraindications/Precautions/Warnings

Sevoflurane is contraindicated in patients with a history or predilection towards malignant hyperthermia. It should be used with caution (benefits vs. risks) in patients with increased CSF or head injury, or renal insufficiency.

Because of its rapid action, use caution not to overdose during the induction phase. Because of the rapid recovery associated with sevoflurane use caution (and appropriate sedation during the recovery phase), particularly with large animals.

Geriatric animals may require less inhalation anesthetic.

In rabbits, sevoflurane (and isoflurane) can cause breath holding and struggling; premedication and close observation are required. Sevoflurane may have a low margin of safety in guinea pigs.

Sevoflurane can react with carbon dioxide absorbents to produce "compound A", a nephrotoxin. After extensive clinical use in humans and dogs nephrotoxicity has not been demonstrated to be of clinical concern. However sevoflurane should be used with good maintenance of the carbon dioxide absorbent (*i.e.*, should be changed regularly to prevent exhaustion or excessive drying) and should not be used with extremely low oxygen flows (*i.e.*, less than 500 mL/min) (Mathews 2008).

Adverse Effects

Sevoflurane seems to be well tolerated. Hypotension may occur and is considered dose related. Dose-dependent respiratory depression and GI effects (nausea, vomiting, ileus) have been reported. While cardiodepression generally is minimal at doses causing surgical planes of anesthesia, it may occur; bradycardia is possible. Chamber or facemask induction can significantly increase the risks for respiratory or cardiovascular depression.

Like other inhalational anesthetics, sevoflurane may rarely trigger malignant hyperthermia.

Sevoflurane should be used in precision, agent-specific, out of circuit vaporizers.

In ferrets, sevoflurane (and isoflurane) can cause temporary decreases in erythrocyte and white cell counts and total protein. Within 45 minutes after discontinuation of sevoflurane, this effect begins to revert to normal and is reversed within 2 hours.

Reproductive/Nursing Safety

No overt fetotoxicity or teratogenicity has been demonstrated in lab animal studies, but definite safety has not been established for use during pregnancy.

Overdosage/Acute Toxicity

In the event of an overdosage, discontinue sevoflurane; maintain airway and support respiratory and cardiac function as necessary.

Drug Interactions

The following drug interactions have either been reported or are theoretical in humans or animals receiving sevoflurane and may be of significance in veterinary patients. Unless otherwise noted, use together is not necessarily contraindicated, but weigh the potential risks and perform additional monitoring when appropriate.

- **AMINOGLYCOSIDES, LINCOSAMIDES:** May enhance neuromuscular blockade.
- **BARBITURATES (phenobarbital, pentobarbital,** etc.): May increase concentrations of inorganic fluoride.
- **ISONIAZID:** May increase concentrations of inorganic fluoride.
- **LIDOCAINE:** IV lidocaine can significantly reduce MAC in horses. (Rezende *et al.* 2011)
- **MIDAZOLAM:** May potentiate sevoflurane effects; decrease MAC.
- **NON-DEPOLARIZING NEUROMUSCULAR BLOCKING AGENTS (atracurium, pancuronium, vecuronium,** etc.): Additive neuromuscular blockade may occur.

- **OPIATES:** May potentiate sevoflurane effects; decrease MAC.
- **ST. JOHNS WORT:** Increased risk for anesthetic complications; recommend discontinuing St. John's Wort 5 days in advance of surgery.
- **SUCCINYLCHOLINE:** Sevoflurane may enhance effects.
- **SYMPATHOMIMETICS (dopamine, epinephrine, norepinephrine, ephedrine, metaraminol,** etc.): While sevoflurane sensitizes the myocardium to the effects of sympathomimetics less so than halothane, arrhythmias may still result; caution and monitoring is advised.
- **TRAMADOL:** May decrease MAC requirements.
- **VERAPAMIL:** May cause cardiodepression.

Laboratory Considerations

- Inhalational anesthetics may cause transient increases in **liver function tests, WBCs,** and **glucose.**

Doses

Minimal Alveolar Concentration (MAC; %) in oxygen reported for sevoflurane in various species: Dog = 2.09-2.4; Cat = 2.5-4; Horse = 2.31; Sheep = 3.3; Swine = 1.97-2.66; Human (adult) = 1.71-2.05. Several factors may alter MAC (acid/base status, temperature, other CNS depressants on board, age, ongoing acute disease, etc.)

- **DOGS/CATS:**

  Labeled-dose (FDA-approved): **Dogs:** Inspired Concentration: The delivered concentration of *SevoFlo®* (sevoflurane) should be known. Since the depth of anesthesia may be altered easily and rapidly, only vaporizers producing predictable percentage concentrations of sevoflurane should be used. Sevoflurane should be vaporized using a precision vaporizer specifically calibrated for sevoflurane. Sevoflurane contains no stabilizer. Nothing in the drug product alters calibration or operation of these vaporizers. The administration of general anesthesia must be individualized based on the patient's response. **When using sevoflurane, patients should be continuously monitored and facilities for maintenance of patient airway, artificial ventilation, and oxygen supplementation must be immediately available.**

  Replacement of Desiccated CO2 Absorbents: When a clinician suspects that the CO2 absorbent may be desiccated, it should be replaced. An exothermic reaction occurs when sevoflurane is exposed to CO2 absorbents. This reaction is increased when the CO2 absorbent becomes desiccated.

  Premedication: No specific premedication is either indicated or contraindicated with sevoflurane. The necessity for and choice of premedication is left to the discretion of the veterinarian. Preanesthetic doses for premedicants may be lower than the label directions for their use as a single medication.

  Induction: For mask induction using sevoflurane, inspired concentrations up to 7% sevoflurane with oxygen are employed to induce surgical anesthesia in the healthy dog. These concentrations can be expected to produce surgical anesthesia in 3-14 minutes. **Due to the rapid and dose dependent changes in anesthetic depth, care should be taken to prevent overdosing. Respiration must be monitored closely in the dog and supported when necessary with supplemental oxygen and/or assisted ventilation.**

  Maintenance: *SevoFlo®* may be used for maintenance anesthesia following mask induction using sevoflurane or following injectable induction agents. The concentration of vapor necessary to maintain anesthesia is much less than that required to induce it. Surgical levels of anesthesia in the healthy dog may be maintained with inhaled concentrations of 3.7 – 4% sevoflurane in oxygen in the absence of premedication and 3.3 – 3.6% in the presence of premedication. The use of injectable induction agents without premedication has little effect on the concentrations of sevoflurane required for maintenance. Anesthetic regimens that include opioid, alpha2-agonist benzodiazepine or phenothiazine premedication will allow the use of lower sevoflurane maintenance concentrations. (Label directions; *SevoFlo®*—Abbott Animal Health)

Extra-label doses:

a) **Dogs/Cats:** Where required, mask induction (particularly of cats) is achieved easily via a non-rebreathing system, usually starting at a concentration of around 4-4.5%. Maximum concentration (8%) is possible using the vaporizer and can be used for fresh gas flow for 'chamber' inductions as the concentrations in the box take time to reach high levels. However, concentrations administered must be reduced as soon as the animal loses consciousness (*i.e.*, take animal out of the box). For maintenance, vaporizer settings with non-rebreathing systems depend on the fresh gas flow rates as well as the residual effects of injectable drugs; a vaporizer setting of 3% for a circle system is a reasonable initial concentration. (Clarke 2008)

b) **Cats:** From a retrospective review of studies reporting sevoflurane MAC. Average MAC for sevoflurane in cats was 3.08 ± 0.4%, but ranged from 2.5 ± 0.2% to 3.95 ± 0.33%, reflecting a relatively wide range. Multiple variables and study methodology likely contributed to this wide range. (Shaughnessy *et al.* 2014)

■ **HORSES:**

For general anesthesia: (extra-label): Approximate MAC is 2.31-2.84.

■ **SHEEP/GOATS:**

For general anesthesia (extra-label): Small animal anesthetic circuits can be used to deliver inhalational anesthetics in small ruminants. Vaporizer should be set at 4% – 6% for induction; during maintenance vaporizer setting should be adjusted to 2.5-4%. Oxygen flow rate should be 2 – 4 L/min during induction and reduced to 0.5 – 1 L/min during maintenance. (Galatos 2011)

Monitoring

■ Respiratory and ventilatory status.

■ Cardiac rate/rhythm; blood pressure (particularly with "at risk" patients).

■ Level of anesthesia.

Chemistry/Synonyms

Sevoflurane is an isopropyl ether inhalational anesthetic with a molecular weight of 200, saturate vapor pressure at 20°C of 160 mmHg and a boiling pt. of 58.5°C. It is reported to have a pleasant odor and is not irritating to airways. It is non-flammable and non-explosive. Sevoflurane is a clear, colorless liquid that is miscible with ethanol or ether and slightly soluble in water. It does not possess an objectionable odor.

Sevoflurane may also be known as: BAX-3084, MR-654, *Sevocris®*, *SevoFlo®*, *Sevorane®*, *Petrem®*, or *Ultane®*.

Storage/Stability

Sevoflurane should be stored at room temperature. Sevoflurane does not react with metal but can react with Lewis acids to form hydrofluoric acid.

Compatibility/Compounding Considerations

No specific information noted.

Dosage Forms/Regulatory Status

VETERINARY-LABELED PRODUCTS:

Sevoflurane in 250 mL btls; *SevoFlo®*, *Petrem®*; (Rx). FDA-approved for use in dogs.

HUMAN-LABELED PRODUCTS:

Sevoflurane in 250 mL btls; *Ultane®*, *Sojourn®*, generic; (Rx)

Revisions/References

Monograph revised/updated August 2014.

Clarke, K. W. (2008). Options for inhalation anaesthesia. In Practice **30**(9): 513-8.
Galatos, A. D. (2011). Anesthesia and Analgesia in Sheep and Goats. Veterinary Clinics of North America-Food Animal Practice 27(1): 47-+.
Mathews, N. S. (2008). Newer Anesthetics: 2. Proceedings: ACVC. accessed via Veterinary Information Network; vin.com
Rezende, M. L., et al. (2011). Effects of intravenous administration of lidocaine on the minimum alveolar concentration of sevoflurane in horses. American Journal of Veterinary Research 72(4): 446-51.
Shaughnessy, M. R. & E. H. Hofmeister (2014). A systematic review of sevoflurane and isoflurane minimum alveolar concentration in domestic cats. Veterinary Anaesthesia and Analgesia 41(1): 1-13.

Sildenafil Citrate

(sil-**den**-ah-fil)   Viagra®, Revatio®

Vasodilator; Phosphodiesterase Type 5 Inhibitor

Prescriber Highlights

▶ Used in veterinary medicine for treating pulmonary hypertension.

▶ Contraindicated if patients receiving organic nitrates.

▶ Adverse effects not well known; inguinal flushing, possible GI effects reported.

▶ Treatment may be very expensive.

Uses/Indications

Sildenafil may be of benefit in the adjunctive treatment of pulmonary hypertension in small animals. An open label study in 5 dogs with Eisenmenger's syndrome found that sildenafil (0.5 mg/kg PO twice daily) improved clinical signs and secondary erythrocytosis (Nakamura *et al.* 2011).

In humans, sildenafil is indicated for erectile dysfunction or pulmonary hypertension.

Pharmacology/Actions

Sildenafil inhibits cyclic guanosine monophosphate (cGMP) specific phosphodiesterase type-5 (PDE5) found in the smooth muscle of the pulmonary vasculature, corpus cavernosum and elsewhere where PDE5 is responsible for degradation of cGMP. Sildenafil increases cGMP thereby resulting in nitric oxide mediated vasodilatation within pulmonary vascular smooth muscle cells.

In Thoroughbred horses, sildenafil (5 mg/kg) did not alleviate pulmonary hemorrhage or enhance performance-related indices (Colahan *et al.* 2010).

Pharmacokinetics

The pharmacokinetics of sildenafil has been reported in dogs (Walker *et al.* 1999). Oral bioavailability is ≈ 50% (approximately the same as in humans); volume of distribution is ≈ 5.2 L/kg (versus 1.2 L/kg in humans); elimination half-life ≈ 6 hours (significant interpatient variability; average human half life is ≈4 hours).

Contraindications/Precautions/Warnings

Sildenafil should not be used concurrently with nitrates (see drug interactions) or in patients documented as being hypersensitive to it.

Pulmonary vasodilators may significantly worsen the cardiovascular status of patients with pulmonary veno-occlusive disease (PVOD).

Use with extreme caution in patients with resting hypotension, fluid depletion, severe left ventricular outflow obstruction, or autonomic dysfunction.

Adverse Effects

Because of limited use in dogs, the adverse effect profile is not fully known. Cutaneous flushing of the inguinal region has been reported and GI effects are possible. In humans, headache, visual disturbances, dyspepsia, nasal congestion, myalgia, priapism, dizziness, and back pain have been reported.

Reproductive/Nursing Safety

No evidence of teratogenicity, embryotoxicity or fetotoxicity was observed in pregnant rats or rabbits, dosed at 200 mg/kg/day during organogenesis. In a rat pre- and postnatal development study, the no-observed-adverse-effect dose was 30 mg/kg/day. In humans, the FDA categorizes this drug as category *B* for use during pregnancy (*Animal studies have not yet demonstrated risk to the fetus, but there are no adequate studies in pregnant women; or animal studies have shown an adverse effect, but adequate studies in pregnant women have not demonstrated a risk to the fetus in the first trimester of pregnancy, and there is no evidence of risk in later trimesters.*)

It is not known if sildenafil or its metabolites are excreted in milk.

Overdosage/Acute Toxicity

Little information is available. An adult woman ingested 2000 mg and survived but developed tachycardia, nonspecific ST-T changes on ECG, headache, dizziness, and flushing.

It is expected that overdoses in animals would mirror the drugs adverse effect profile; treat supportively.

Drug Interactions

The following drug interactions have either been reported or are theoretical in humans or animals receiving sildenafil and may be of significance in veterinary patients. Unless otherwise noted, use together is not necessarily contraindicated, but weigh the potential risks and perform additional monitoring when appropriate.

- **ALPHA-ADRENERGIC BLOCKERS** (*e.g.,* **phentolamine, phenothiazines, phenoxybenzamine**): May increase hypotensive effects.
- **AMLODIPINE**: Potential to increase hypotensive effects.
- **ANTIHYPERTENSIVE, HYPOTENSIVE DRUGS**: Potentially could increase hypotensive effects.
- **AZOLE ANTIFUNGALS** (**ketoconazole, itraconazole,** etc.): May reduce sildenafil metabolism and increase AUC.
- **CIMETIDINE**: May reduce sildenafil metabolism and increase AUC.
- **ERYTHROMYCIN, CLARITHROMYCIN**: May reduce sildenafil metabolism and increase AUC.
- **HEPARIN**: May increase bleeding risks.
- **NITRATES** (*e.g.,* NTG, Isosorbide): Significant potentiation of vasodilatory effects; life-threatening hypotension possible.
- **NITROPRUSSIDE SODIUM**: Significant potentiation of vasodilatory effects; life-threatening hypotension possible.
- **PHENOBARBITAL**: May decrease sildenafil concentrations.
- **RIFAMPIN**: May decrease sildenafil concentrations.

Laboratory Considerations
- None noted.

Doses

- **DOGS/CATS:**

  For pulmonary hypertension (extra-label): Anecdotal dosage recommendations generally range from 0.5 – 3 mg/kg PO q8-12h. Start at the low end and titrate upwards as needed.

  a) Dogs: 1 mg/kg PO q8h. From a prospective short-term, randomized, placebo controlled, double blind, crossover study in 13 dogs. Authors concluded that sildenafil decreases systolic pressure gradients, increases exercise capacity, and improves quality of life in dogs with PAH and underlying cardiovascular disease. (Brown *et al.* 2010)

  b) Dogs: Median dose was 1.9 mg/kg (range from 0.5 – 2.7 mg/kg) q8-24h. From a retrospective study. Dogs may have been also treated with oxygen, ACE inhibitors, furosemide, amlodipine, diltiazem, theophylline, phenobarbital and/or antibiotics. (Bach *et al.* 2006)

  c) Dogs: 1 mg/kg PO q8-12h. From a retrospective study in 22 dogs. Treated dogs' clinical scores were significantly improved, but physical examination findings remained unchanged. (Kellum *et al.* 2007)

Monitoring
- Clinical efficacy (improved syncope, cough, respiratory effort).
- Pulmonary artery pressure, systemic blood pressure.
- Adverse effects.

Client Information
- May be given with or without food.
- Be sure to give exactly as prescribed.
- May cause flushing (redness) in groin area; gastrointestinal effects (*e.g.,* lack of appetite, vomiting, diarrhea, etc.) are possible.
- Not used often in veterinary medicine, so report any other side effects to veterinarian.

Chemistry/Synonyms

Sildenafil citrate occurs as a white to off-white crystalline powder with a solubility of 3.5 mg/mL in water and a molecular weight of 666.7.

Sildenafil may also be known as UK 92480, UK 92480-10, *Aphrodil*®, *Revatio*®, or *Viagra*®.

Storage/Stability

Sildenafil tablets should be stored at room temperature (25°C; 77°F); excursions permitted to 15-30°C (59-86°F).

Compatibility/Compounding Considerations

A stable 2.5 mg/mL sildenafil citrate oral suspension can be made with tablets and either a 1:1 mixture of methylcellulose 1% and simple syrup NF or a 1:1 mixture of *Ora-Sweet*® and *Ora-Plus*®. Crush thirty sildenafil 25 mg tablets in a mortar and reduce to a fine powder. Add small portions of chosen vehicle and mix to a uniform paste. Continue to add vehicle in incremental proportions to almost 300 mL and then transfer to a graduated cylinder, rinse mortar with vehicle, and add quantity of vehicle sufficient to make a total of 300 mL. Store in amber plastic bottles and label "shake well." Stable for 90 days at room temperature or when refrigerated. (Nahata *et al.* 2006)

Dosage Forms/Regulatory Status

VETERINARY-LABELED PRODUCTS: NONE.

HUMAN-LABELED PRODUCTS:

Sildenafil Citrate Oral Tablets: 20 mg, 25 mg, 50 mg & 100 mg (of sildenafil); *Revatio*® (20 mg only), *Viagra*®; (Rx)

Sildenafil Injection Solution: 10 mg/12.5 mL (dextrose 50.5 mg/mL) in 12.5 mL single-use vials; *Revatio*®; (Rx)

Revisions/References

Monograph revised/updated August 2014.

Bach, J., et al. (2006). Retrospective evaluation of sildenafil citrate as a therapy for pulmonary hypertension in dogs. J Vet Intern Med **20**: 1132-5.

Brown, A. J., et al. (2010). Clinical Efficacy of Sildenafil in Treatment of Pulmonary Arterial Hypertension in Dogs. Journal of Veterinary Internal Medicine **24**(4): 850-4.

Colahan, P. T., et al. (2010). The effect of sildenafil citrate administration on selected physiological parameters of exercising Thoroughbred horses. Equine Veterinary Journal **42**: 606-12.

Kellum, H. B. & R. L. Stepien (2007). Sildenafil citrate therapy in 22 dogs with pulmonary hypertension. Journal of Veterinary Internal Medicine **21**(6): 1258-64.

Nahata, M. C., et al. (2006). Extemporaneous sildenafil citrate oral suspensions for the treatment of pulmonary hypertension in children. Am J Health Syst Pharm **63**(3): 254-7.

Nakamura, K., et al. (2011). Effects of sildenafil citrate on five dogs with Eisenmenger's syndrome. Journal of Small Animal Practice **52**(11): 595-8.

Walker, D., et al. (1999). Pharmacokinetics and metabolism of sildenafil in mouse, rat, rabbit, dog and man. Xenobiotica **29**(3): 297-310.

Silymarin

(sill-e-mar-in)   Milk Thistle, Silybin, Marin®

Hepatoprotectant

Prescriber Highlights

▶ Nutraceutical that may be useful for treatment of chronic & acute liver disease, cirrhosis; as a hepato-protective agent when hepatotoxins (*e.g., Aminita phalloide*) ingested.

▶ Appears well tolerated; potentially could cause GI effects.

▶ Do not confuse Milk Thistle with Blessed Thistle.

▶ Potential drug interactions.

Uses/Indications

While controlled clinical studies demonstrating efficacy and a standardized form and concentration of silymarin are lacking, it is being used to treat a variety of liver diseases in humans and domestic companion animals (birds, dogs, cats, horses, rabbits). It is mostly of interest in treating chronic and acute liver disease, cirrhosis, and as a hepato-protective agent when hepatotoxic agents are ingested (*e.g., Aminita phalloide*; "Death Cap Mushrooms"). There is laboratory data that silymarin may be beneficial in preventing certain cancers and improving the efficacy and reducing the negative effects of chemotherapy for certain tumors. A study in dogs found evidence that silymarin and vitamin E provided some efficacy for preventing gentamicin-induced nephrotoxicity (Varzi *et al.* 2007) and another in cats showed some hepatoprotective effects in acetaminophen-induced hepatotoxicity (Avizeh *et al.* 2010). A proprietary combination (*Denamarin®*) of silymarin (silybin) and SAMe was found to minimize increased liver enzyme activity in dogs receiving lomustine (CCNU) chemotherapy and increased the likelihood of dogs completing a prescribed lomustine course of therapy (Skorupski *et al.* 2011), but this study had several weaknesses (low numbers of patients undergoing additional liver testing with bile acids, abdominal ultrasound examination, and liver biopsies, low incidence of severe liver disease, lack of placebo in control group, non-blinded, occult preexisting liver disease in some dogs, combination of two agents, and author potential financial conflicts of interest) (Vandeweerd *et al.* 2013).

Pharmacology/Actions

Silymarin has a variety of pharmacologic actions that may contribute to its apparent effects in treating liver disease. It inhibits lipid peroxidase and beta-glucoronidase and acts as an anti-oxidant and free radical scavenger. Silymarin also inhibits the cytotoxic, inflammatory, and apoptotic effects of tumor necrosis factor (TFN). It apparently can alter outer hepatocyte cell membranes that can prevent toxin penetration. Silymarin is thought to reduce hepatic collagen formation and increase hepatic glutathione content.

Pharmacokinetics

In humans, silymarin has an oral bioavailability of <50% and peak levels occur 2-4 hours post-dose. When silibinin (silybin, sylibin) is complexed with phosphatidylcholine, oral absorption can be increased. The drug undergoes extensive enterohepatic circulation and has significantly higher concentrations in liver cells and bile than in plasma. Elimination half-life in humans averages 6 hours. The majority of the drug is eliminated unchanged in the feces, but 20-40% is converted into glucuronide and sulfate conjugates which are eliminated in the feces; only ≈ 8% is excreted in the urine.

Contraindications/Precautions/Warnings

There are no reported absolute contraindications to silymarin in animals. Extracts from the plant parts of Milk Thistle (not the seeds which are used to make the extract silymarin), may possess estrogen-like activity and should not be used in patients where exogenous estrogens would be contraindicated.

Adverse Effects

Silymarin is apparently well tolerated when administered orally. In humans, GI disturbances have been reported on occasion (nausea to diarrhea). Patients who have allergies to other members of the Asteraceae/Compositae plant family (includes ragweed, marigolds, daisies, etc.) may exhibit allergic reactions to Milk Thistle derivatives. Do not confuse Milk Thistle with Blessed Thistle.

Reproductive/Nursing Safety

Data on the safety of silymarin use during pregnancy or nursing is not available; its potential benefit must be weighed against the uncertainty of its safety.

Overdosage/Acute Toxicity

Overdoses are unlikely to cause significant morbidity. Gastrointestinal effects may be seen and treated in a supportive manner.

Drug Interactions

Decreased efficacy of **antiviral drugs** is possible. Silymarin may inhibit cytochrome P450 isoenzyme 2C9 (CYP2C9). Drugs with narrow therapeutic indexes that are metabolized by this isoenzyme should be used with caution when using silymarin. Drugs that could be affected include: **warfarin, amitriptyline, verapamil**, etc.

Silymarin also may inhibit CYP3A4, but thus far this interaction does not appear to be clinically significant. Silymarin may increase the clearance of drugs that undergo hepatic glucuronidation (not cats), including: **acetaminophen, diazepam, morphine, and lamotrigine**.

Laboratory Considerations

- No interactions with laboratory tests are reported.

Doses

- **DOGS & CATS:**

  For hepatic dysfunction (extra-label): "Many oral formulations … are available. It is important to remember that silybin, the isomer of silymarin that comprises the majority of the flavonolignan in the milk thistle plant, is the most bioactive isomer but is found in varying concentrations in each product. There has been no consensus reached as to the proper dose of this compound in humans or veterinary patients." Proposed dosage range for *Marin®* is of 5 – 10 mg/kg daily in dogs and cats (McCord *et al.* 2011). Higher dosages have also been recommended: 20 – 50 mg/kg per day. (Center 2002), (Webb 2007)

Monitoring

- Clinical efficacy.

Client Information

- May be given with or without food.
- Not an approved drug; considered a nutritional agent.
- Seems to be very safe.
- Keep chewable tablets out of reach of children and animals.

Chemistry/Synonyms

Milk Thistle, the common name for *Silybum marianum*, has been used as a medicinal agent for at least 2000 years. The medicinal extract from the seeds of the plant is silymarin that contains the 4 flavolignans: silichristin (sylichristin), isosilibinin, silydianin (silidianin), and the most biological active component, silibinin (sylibin, silybin, silibide). Milk Thistle extract contains approximately 70% silymarin of which ≈ 70% is silibinin. Silymarin is reportedly fairly insoluble in water.

Silymarin or Milk thistle may also be known as *Carduus marianus*, Holy Thistle, Legalon, or Marian Thistle. Blessed Thistle is a different compound.

Storage/Stability

Unless otherwise labeled, commercially available products containing silymarin should be stored at room temperature in tight containers. Avoid storing the products in areas of high humidity.

Compatibility/Compounding Considerations

No specific information noted.

Dosage Forms/Regulatory Status

VETERINARY-LABELED PRODUCTS:

The FDA considers milk Thistle or silymarin a nutritional supplement. No standards have been accepted for potency, etc. by regulatory bodies. Supplements are available from a wide variety of sources and dosage forms include tablets and capsules in a variety of concentrations (150-1000 mg). When choosing a product it is recommended to purchase ones that state the concentration (usually 70-80%) of silymarin contained in the product.

Silybin A+B 9 mg (in a phosphatidylcholine complex) & Vitamin E 50 Units Tablets: *Marin® for Cats*.

Silybin A+B 24 mg (in a phosphatidylcholine complex), Vitamin E 105 Units, & Zinc 17 mg Chewable Tablets: *Marin® for Dogs*. Labeled for use in small to medium dogs.

Silybin A+B 70 mg (in a phosphatidylcholine complex), Vitamin E 300 Units, & Zinc 45 mg Chewable Tablets: *Marin® for Dogs*. Labeled for use in large dogs.

A combination product (*Denamarin®*) containing SAMe and silybin (silymarin) is also labeled for use in dogs and cats.

HUMAN-LABELED PRODUCTS:

None as a pharmaceutical.

Revisions/References

Monograph revised/updated August 2014.

Avizeh, R., et al. (2010). Evaluation of prophylactic and therapeutic effects of silymarin and N-acetylcysteine in acetaminophen-induced hepatotoxicity in cats. J. Vet. Pharmacol. Ther. 33(1): 95-9.

Center, S. (2002). Chronic hepatitis. Proceedings: Western Veterinary Conference. accessed via Veterinary Information Network; vin.com

McCord, K. W. & C. B. Webb (2011). Hepatic Dysfunction. Veterinary Clinics of North America-Small Animal Practice 41(4): 745-+.

Skorupski, K. A., et al. (2011). Prospective Randomized Clinical Trial Assessing the Efficacy of Denamarin for Prevention of CCNU-Induced Hepatopathy in Tumor-Bearing Dogs. Journal of Veterinary Internal Medicine 25(4): 838-45.

Vandeweerd, J. M., et al. (2013). Nutraceuticals for Canine Liver Disease: Assessing the Evidence. Veterinary Clinics of North America-Small Animal Practice 43(5): 1171-+.

Varzi, H. N., et al. (2007). Effect of silymarin and vitamin E on gentamicin-induced nephrotoxicity in dogs. J. Vet. Pharmacol. Ther. 30(5): 477-81.

Webb, C. (2007). Pushing the envelope in liver and pancreatic diseases. Proceedings: Western Vet Conference. accessed via Veterinary Information Network; vin.com

Sodium Bicarbonate

(soe-dee-um bye-kar-boe-nate)

Alkalinizer

Prescriber Highlights

▶ Alkalinizing agent used to treat metabolic acidosis & alkalinize urine; may be used adjunctively for hypercalcemic or hyperkalemic crises. Not commonly used secondary to potential complications/adverse effects.

▶ Contraindications: Parenteral bicarbonate is generally contraindicated in patients with metabolic or respiratory alkalosis, excessive chloride loss secondary to vomiting or GI suction, those at risk for development of diuretic-induced hypochloremic alkalosis, or with hypocalcemia where alkalosis may induce tetany.

▶ Extreme Caution: Hypocalcemia Caution: CHF, nephrotic syndrome, hypertension, oliguria or volume overload.

▶ Adverse Effects: Especially with parenteral (high dose): metabolic alkalosis, hypokalemia, hypocalcemia, "overshoot" alkalosis, hypernatremia, volume overload, congestive heart failure, shifts in the oxygen dissociation curve causing decreased tissue oxygenation, & paradoxical CNS acidosis leading to respiratory arrest. If used during CPR: hypercapnia, if the patient is not well ventilated; patients may be predisposed to ventricular fibrillation.

▶ Drug Interactions.

Uses/Indications

Sodium bicarbonate is sometimes used to treat severe metabolic acidosis. It is not a substitute for diagnosing and treating the underlying cause of the acid/base disturbance. In small animals acidosis that may be amenable to bicarbonate therapy include those as a result of cardiopulmonary arrest, renal failure, renal tubular acidosis, or toxins. Use of bicarbonate for metabolic acidosis secondary to diabetic crises is controversial.

Sodium bicarbonate can also be used as adjunctive therapy in treating hypercalcemic or hyperkalemia crises or to alkalinize the urine.

Pharmacology/Actions

Bicarbonate ion is the conjugate base component of bicarbonate:-carbonic acid buffer, the principal extracellular buffer in the body.

Contraindications/Precautions/Warnings

Parenterally administered sodium bicarbonate is considered generally contraindicated in patients with metabolic or respiratory alkalosis, excessive chloride loss secondary to vomiting or GI suction, those at risk for development of diuretic-induced hypochloremic alkalosis, or with hypocalcemia where alkalosis may induce tetany.

Use with extreme caution and give very slowly in patients with hypocalcemia. Ideally, low calcium or potassium serum concentrations should be corrected prior to administration. Bicarbonate therapy during a diabetic crisis (DKA) is rarely indicated. Administering bicarb before potassium replenishment can be detrimental and potentially life threatening as it can exacerbate hypokalemia.

Because of the potential sodium load, use with caution in patients with CHF, nephrotic syndrome, hypertension, oliguria, or volume overload.

Sodium bicarbonate is generally not effective for treating lactic acidosis. Fluid therapy remains the mainstay of treatment for lactic acidosis.

Adverse Effects

Sodium bicarbonate therapy (particularly high-dose parenteral use) can lead to metabolic alkalosis, hypokalemia, hypocalcemia, "overshoot" alkalosis, hypernatremia, volume overload, congestive heart failure, shifts in the oxygen dissociation curve causing decreased tissue oxygenation, and paradoxical CNS acidosis, leading to depression, stupor, coma, respiratory arrest and death.

When sodium bicarbonate is used during cardiopulmonary resuscitation, hypercapnia may result if the patient is not well ventilated; patients may be predisposed to ventricular fibrillation.

Oral and parenteral bicarbonate (especially at higher doses) may contribute significant amounts of sodium and result in hypernatremia and volume overload; use with caution in patients with CHF, or acute renal failure.

Reproductive/Nursing Safety

Reproductive safety studies have not been performed. Assess risk versus benefit before using.

Overdosage/Acute Toxicity

Sodium bicarbonate can cause severe alkalosis, with irritability or tetany if overdosed or given too rapidly. Dosages should be thoroughly checked and frequent monitoring of electrolyte and acid/base status performed.

Treatment may consist of simply discontinuing bicarbonate if alkalosis is mild or by using a rebreathing mask. Severe alkalosis may require intravenous calcium therapy. Sodium chloride or potassium chloride may be necessary if hypokalemia is present.

Drug Interactions

The following drug interactions have either been reported or are theoretical in humans or animals receiving sodium bicarbonate and may be of significance in veterinary patients. Unless otherwise noted, use together is not necessarily contraindicated, but weigh the potential risks and perform additional monitoring when appropriate.

- **ANTICHOLINERGIC AGENTS:** Concomitant oral sodium bicarbonate may reduce absorption; administer separately.
- **AZOLE ANTIFUNGALS** (*e.g.,* **ketoconazole, itraconazole,** etc.): Concomitant oral sodium bicarbonate may reduce absorption; administer separately.
- **CIPROFLOXACIN; ENROFLOXACIN:** The solubility of ciprofloxacin and enrofloxacin is decreased in an alkaline environment; patients with alkaline urine should be monitored for signs of crystalluria.
- **CORTICOSTEROIDS:** Patients receiving high dosages of sodium bicarbonate and ACTH or glucocorticoids may develop hypernatremia.
- **DIURETICS** (*e.g.,* **thiazides, furosemide,** etc.): Concurrent use of sodium bicarbonate in patients receiving potassium-wasting diuretics may cause hypochloremic alkalosis.
- **EPHEDRINE:** When urine is alkalinized by sodium bicarbonate, excretion may be decreased.
- **HISTAMINE$_2$ BLOCKING AGENTS** (*e.g.,* **cimetidine, ranitidine,** etc.): Concomitant oral sodium bicarbonate may reduce absorption; separate dosages by at least 2 hours.
- **IRON PRODUCTS:** Concomitant oral sodium bicarbonate may reduce absorption; separate dosages by at least 2 hours.
- **ORAL MEDICATIONS:** Because oral sodium bicarbonate can either increase or reduce the rate and/or extent of absorption of many orally administered drugs, it is recommended to avoid giving other drugs within 1-2 hours of sodium bicarbonate.
- **QUINIDINE:** When urine is alkalinized by sodium bicarbonate, excretion may be decreased.
- **SALICYLATES:** When urine is alkalinized by sodium bicarbonate, excretion of weakly acidic drugs may be increased.
- **SUCRALFATE:** Oral sodium bicarbonate may reduce the efficacy of sucralfate if administered concurrently; separate dosages by at least 2 hours.
- **TETRACYCLINES:** Concomitant oral sodium bicarbonate may reduce absorption; separate dosages by at least 2 hours.

Doses

- **DOGS & CATS:**

For severe metabolic acidosis (extra-label):

a) **Associated with cardiopulmonary arrest (CPA):** <u>RECOVER guidelines</u>: Given the evidence available, bicarbonate therapy after prolonged CPA of greater than 10-15 minutes with administration of 1 mEq/kg IV/IO of sodium bicarbonate may be considered. Contraindicated if patient is hypoventilating. (Fletcher *et al.* 2012)

b) <u>Main therapeutic goal</u> should be to eliminate the underlying cause of acidosis. If causes are not readily reversible, arterial pH is <7.2 (7.1 if diabetic ketoacidosis), and ventilatory procedures have not reduced acidemia, bicarbonate therapy should be considered. mEq of bicarbonate required = 0.5 x body weight in kg x (desired total CO_2 mEq/L minus measured total CO_2 mEq/L). Give 1/2 of the calculated dose slowly over 3-4 hours IV. Recheck blood gases and assess the clinical status of the patient. Avoid over-alkalinization. (Schaer 2006)

c) **For metabolic acidosis secondary to uremia:** In the majority of patients, definitive treatment of the urinary tract disorder and fluid diuresis is usually all that is required. In the unstable dog or cat with a pH <7.0 due to metabolic acidosis, sodium bicarb administration should be considered. The formula often recommended is 0.3 x body weight (kilograms) x the base deficit. This gives an approximation for the total bicarbonate deficit. Administration of one third of this dose slowly IV and the rest placed in the intravenous fluids will correct the metabolic acidosis over several hours. If measurement of blood gas is not possible and it is believed that the animal is severely acidemic, 1 – 2 mEq/kg of bicarbonate can be given as a slow IV bolus. Rapid intravenous boluses of sodium bicarbonate should be avoided because of the production of carbon dioxide and its diffusion into the central nervous system making CSF acidosis even worse. Other disadvantages of sodium bicarbonate administration include shifting of the oxygen/hemoglobin dissociation curve to the left and increasing osmolality. When monitoring the response to bicarbonate through the measurement of blood gases, remember that bicarbonate will increase initially in the intravascular space but then will be buffered by intracellular buffers. Immediate measurement of blood gases after bicarbonate administration may over-estimate the effect of the therapy. Diffusion and buffering of administered bicarbonate by intracellular buffers takes approximately 2-4 hours and a blood gas analysis should be performed after this time period as well. (Drobatz 2009)

For adjunctive therapy of diabetic ketoacidosis (extra-label): **Note:** Use of sodium bicarbonate for this indication is somewhat controversial and its use is falling out of favor. Bicarb therapy can be dangerous in DKA for several reasons. Like insulin, bicarbonate drives potassium intracellularly, potentially worsening hypokalemia. Bicarbonate shifts the oxyhemoglobin curve to the left decreasing oxygen release at the tissue level and can lead to paradoxical central nervous system acidosis, fluid overload, lactic acidosis, persistent ketosis, and cerebral edema (O'Brien 2010). Rarely needed as the acidemia corrects with fluid therapy and reversal of ketosis. Bicarbonate therapy is generally reserved for those patients with severe acidemia (pH <7.1, bicarbonate <8 mmol/L) and signs consistent with severe metabolic acidosis such as refractory hypotension, arrhythmias, and presence of stupor or coma. Slowly give 1/4 to 1/3 of the following: mEq of bicarbonate required = 0.3 x body weight in kg x (desired plasma bicarbonate mEq/L – measured plasma bicarbonate mEq/L). (Koenig 2013)

For adjunctive therapy for hyperkalemic crisis (extra-label): Must be used judiciously. Hyperkalemia associated with hypoadrenocorticism typically improves with fluid resuscitation alone (Koenig 2013). Dose is based on the base deficit, or an empirical dosage of 1–2 mEq/kg IV over 10-20 minutes can be used. (Monaghan *et al.* 2012)

To alkalinize the urine (extra-label): Rarely recommended today. Dosage must be individualized to the patient. Initially 650 mg – 5.85 grams PO per day depending on the size of the patient and the pretreatment urine pH value. Goal of therapy is to maintain a urine pH of ≈ 7; avoid pH >7.5. (Osborne *et al.* 1989)

- **HORSES:**
For metabolic acidosis associated with colic (extra-label): If pH is <7.3 and base deficit is >10 mEq/L estimate bicarbonate requirement using the formula: bicarbonate deficit (HCO^{-3} mEq) = base deficit (mEq/L) x 0.4 x body weight (kg). May administer as a 5% sodium bicarbonate solution. Each L of solution contains 600 mEq of bicarbonate (hypertonic) and should not be administered any faster than 1 – 2 L/hr. Because acidotic horses with colic tend also to be dehydrated, may be preferable to give as isotonic sodium bicarbonate (150 mEq/L). (Stover 1987)

- **RUMINANTS:**
For severely dehydrated (10-16% dehydrated) acidotic calves (usually comatose) (extra-label): Use isotonic sodium bicarbonate (156 mEq/L). Most calves require ≈ 2 liters of this solution given over 1-2 hours, then change to isotonic saline and sodium bicarbonate or a balanced electrolyte solution. Isotonic sodium bicarbonate may be made by dissolving 13 grams of sodium bicarbonate in 1 L of sterile water. Isotonic saline and sodium bicarbonate can be made by mixing 1 L of isotonic saline with 1 L of isotonic sodium bicarbonate. (Radostits 1986)

- **BIRDS:**
For metabolic acidosis (extra-label): 1 mEq/kg initially IV (then SC) for 15-30 minutes to a maximum of 4 mEq/kg. (Clubb 1986)

Monitoring
- Acid/base status.
- Serum electrolytes.
- Urine pH (if being used to alkalinize urine).

Chemistry/Synonyms
An alkalinizing agent, sodium bicarbonate occurs as a white, crystalline powder having a slightly saline or alkaline taste. It is soluble in water and insoluble in alcohol. One gram of sodium bicarbonate contains ≈ 12 mEq (mMol) each of sodium and bicarbonate; 84 mg of sodium bicarbonate contains 1 mEq each of sodium and bicarbonate. A 1.5% solution of sodium bicarbonate is approximately isotonic. An 8.4% solution of sodium bicarbonate can be made isotonic by diluting each mL with 4.6 mL of sterile water for injection.

Because converting volume measurements into weights is not very accurate for powders, it is recommended to actually weigh powders when using them for pharmaceutical purposes. However, if this is not possible, one (1) level teaspoon (5 mL) of commercially available baking soda contains approximately 4.8-5.9 grams of sodium bicarbonate.

Sodium Bicarbonate may also be known as: baking soda, E500, monosodium carbonate, natrii bicarbonas, natrii hydrogenocarbonas, sal de vichy, sodium acid carbonate, $NaHCO_3$, sodium hydrogen carbonate; many trade names are available.

Storage/Stability
Sodium bicarbonate tablets should be stored in tight containers, preferably at room temperature (15-30°C). Sodium bicarbonate injection should be stored at temperatures less than 40°C and preferably at room temperature; avoid freezing.

Sodium bicarbonate powder is stable in dry air, but will slowly decompose upon exposure to moist air.

Compatibility/Compounding Considerations
Sodium bicarbonate for injection is reportedly physically **compatible** with the following intravenous solutions and drugs: Dextrose in water, dextrose/saline combinations, dextrose-Ringer's combinations, sodium chloride injections, amikacin sulfate, aminophylline, amphotericin B, atropine sulfate, cefoxitin sodium, chloramphenicol sodium succinate, cimetidine HCl, clindamycin phosphate, erythromycin gluceptate/lactobionate, heparin sodium, hyaluronidase, hydrocortisone sodium succinate, lidocaine HCl, methotrexate sodium, oxytocin, phenobarbital sodium, phenylephrine HCl, phenytoin sodium, phytonadione, potassium chloride, prochlorperazine edisylate, and sodium iodide.

Sodium bicarbonate for injection **compatibility information conflicts** or is dependent on diluent or concentration factors with the following drugs or solutions: lactated Ringer's injection, Ringer's injection, sodium lactate 1/6 M, ampicillin sodium, calcium chloride/gluconate, penicillin G potassium, pentobarbital sodium, promazine HCl, thiopental sodium, vancomycin HCl, verapamil HCl, and vitamin B-complex with C. Consult specialized references or a hospital pharmacist for more specific information.

Sodium bicarbonate for injection is reportedly physically **incompatible** with the following solutions or drugs: alcohol 5%/dextrose 5%, D5-lactated Ringer's, ascorbic acid injection, carmustine, cisplatin, codeine phosphate, corticotropin, dobutamine HCl, epinephrine HCl, glycopyrrolate, hydromorphone HCl, imipenem-cilastatin, regular insulin, isoproterenol HCl, labetalol HCl, levorphanol bitartrate, magnesium sulfate, meperidine HCl, methadone HCl, metoclopramide HCl, norepinephrine bitartrate, oxytetracycline HCl, pentazocine lactate, and succinylcholine chloride.

Because converting volume measurements into weights is not very accurate for powders, it is recommended to actually weigh powders when using them for pharmaceutical purposes. However, if this is not possible, one (1) level teaspoon (5 mL) of commercially available baking soda contains approximately 4.8-5.9 grams of sodium bicarbonate.

Dosage Forms/Regulatory Status
VETERINARY-LABELED PRODUCTS:
Sodium Bicarbonate Injection: 8.4% (1 mEq/mL) in 50 mL (50 mEq/vial), 100 mL (100 mEq/vial) and 500 mL (500 mEq/vial) vials; available generically labeled; (Rx). FDA-approval status is uncertain.

HUMAN-LABELED PRODUCTS:
Injectable Products:
Sodium Bicarbonate Neutralizing Additive Solution: 4% (0.48 mEq/mL) in 5 mL (2.4 mEq) vials; 4.2% (0.5 mEq/mL) in 5 mL fill in 6 mL vials (2.5 mEq); *Neut*®, generic; (Rx)

Sodium Bicarbonate Injection: 4.2% (0.5 mEq/mL) in 10 mL (5 mEq) syringes, 10 mL (5 mEq) *Bristoject* syringes; generic; (Rx)

Sodium Bicarbonate Injection: 7.5% (0.9 mEq/mL) in 50 mL (44.6 mEq) amps, syringes, vials, *Bristoject* syringes and 200 mL (179 mEq) *MaxiVials*; generic; (Rx)

Sodium Bicarbonate Injection: 8.4% (1 mEq/mL) in 10 mL (10 mEq) and 50 mL (50 mEq) syringes and 50 mL vials (50 mEq/vial); generic; (Rx)

Oral Products:

Sodium Bicarbonate Tablets: 325 mg & 650 mg; generic; (OTC)

Sodium Bicarbonate Powder: 120 grams, 300 grams & 1 lb; generic; (OTC)

Omeprazole/Sodium Bicarbonate Capsules (immediate release): 20 mg or 40 mg omeprazole/1,100 mg sodium bicarbonate; *Zegerid*®, generic; (Rx)

Omeprazole/Sodium Bicarbonate Powder for Oral Suspension: 20 mg or 40 mg omeprazole/1,680 mg sodium bicarbonate in unit-dose packets; *Zegerid*®; (Rx)

Revisions/References

Monograph revised/updated August 2014.

Clubb, S. L. (1986). Therapeutics: Individual and Flock Treatment Regimens. *Clinical Avian Medicine and Surgery*. G. J. Harrison and L. R. Harrison. Philadelphia, W.B. Saunders: 327-55.

Drobatz, K. J. (2009). Emergencies of the urogenital tract. Proceedings: IVECCS. accessed via Veterinary Information Network; vin.com

Fletcher, D. J., et al. (2012). RECOVER evidence and knowledge gap analysis on veterinary CPR. Part 7: Clinical guidelines. J. Vet. Emerg. Crit. Care 22.

Koenig, A. (2013). Endocrine Emergencies in Dogs and Cats. Veterinary Clinics of North America: Small Animal Practice 43(4): 869-97.

Monaghan, K., et al. (2012). Feline Acute Kidney Injury: Approach to diagnosis, treatment and prognosis. Journal of Feline Medicine and Surgery 14(11): 785-93.

O'Brien, M. A. (2010). Diabetic Emergencies in Small Animals. Veterinary Clinics of North America-Small Animal Practice 40(2): 317-+.

Osborne, C. A., et al. (1989). Canine Urolithiasis. *Textbook of Veterinary Internal Medicine*. S. J. Ettinger. Philadelphia, WB Saunders: 2: 2083-107.

Radostits, O. M. (1986). Neonatal diarrhea in ruminants (calves, lambs and kids). *Current Veterinary Therapy 2: Food Animal Practice*. J. L. Howard. Philadelphia, WB Saunders: 105-13.

Schaer, M. (2006). Acute adrenocortical insufficiency. Proceedings: WSAVA World Congress. accessed via Veterinary Information Network; vin.com

Stover, S. M. (1987). Pre- and postoperative management of the colic patient. *Current Therapy in Equine Medicine: 2*. N. E. Robinson. Philadelphia, WB Saunders: 33- 8.

Sodium Bromide – see Bromides

Sodium Chloride Injections – see the Hypertonic Saline monograph or the Intravenous Fluids section in the appendix

Sodium Citrate – see Citrate Salts

Sodium Hyaluronate – see Hyaluronate Sodium

Sodium Iodide – see Iodide, Sodium

Sodium Nitroprusside – See Nitroprusside Sodium

Sodium Phosphate – see Phosphate, Parenteral

Sodium Polystyrene Sulfonate

(soe-dee-um pol-ee-stye-reen sulf-foe-nate) Kayexalate®, SPS

Cationic Exchange Resin (Hyperkalemia)

Prescriber Highlights

▶ Cation exchange resin used to treat hyperkalemia.

▶ Contraindications: Patients who cannot tolerate a large sodium load.

▶ Cause of hyperkalemia must be addressed.

▶ Adverse Effects: Constipation, anorexia, vomiting, or nausea. Sometimes mixed with sorbitol to prevent constipation. Overdosage/overuse may lead to hypokalemia, hypocalcemia & hypomagnesemia.

▶ If given PO, often mixed with sorbitol to expedite removal of resin (& potassium).

▶ Drug Interactions.

Uses/Indications

SPS is indicated as adjunctive treatment of hyperkalemia. The cause of hyperkalemia should be determined and corrected if possible.

Pharmacology/Actions

SPS is a resin that exchanges sodium for other cations. After being given orally, hydrogen ions will be exchanged for sodium (in an acidic environment). As the resin travels through the intestinal tract, the hydrogen ions will be exchanged with other more concentrated cations. Primary exchange with potassium occurs predominantly in the large intestine. When given as a retention enema, SPS generally exchanges sodium for potassium directly in the colorectum. While theoretically, up to 3.1 mEq of potassium could be exchanged per gram of SPS, it is unlikely that more than 1 mEq will be exchanged per gram of resin administered.

Pharmacokinetics

SPS is not absorbed from the GI tract. Its onset of action may be from hours to days; so severe hyperkalemia may require other treatments in the interim (*e.g.*, dialysis).

Contraindications/Precautions/Warnings

Because large quantities of sodium may be released and absorbed, patients on severely restricted sodium diets (severe CHF, hypertension, oliguria) may benefit from alternative methods of treatment. Overdosage/overuse may lead to hypokalemia, hypocalcemia and hypomagnesemia.

Adverse Effects

Large doses may cause constipation (fecal impactions have been reported rarely), anorexia, vomiting or nausea. Dose related hypocalcemia, hypokalemia and sodium retention have also been noted. To hasten the drug's action and prevent constipation, SPS is often mixed with 70% sorbitol (3 – 4 mL per 1 gram of resin) when dosed orally. Retention enemas with SPS and sorbitol have been implicated in some human cases of colonic necrosis, presumably secondary to sorbitol causing cellular dehydration.

Reproductive/Nursing Safety

While reproductive studies have apparently not been performed, it is unlikely the drug carries much teratogenic potential. In humans, the FDA categorizes this drug as category *C* for use during pregnancy (*Animal studies have shown an adverse effect on the fetus, but there are no adequate studies in humans; or there are no animal reproduction studies and no adequate studies in humans.*)

As SPS is not absorbed, it should be safe to use during nursing.

Overdosage/Acute Toxicity

Overdosage may cause the adverse effects noted (above); treat symptomatically.

Drug Interactions

The following drug interactions have either been reported or are theoretical in humans or animals receiving SPS and may be of significance in veterinary patients. Unless otherwise noted, use together is not necessarily contraindicated, but weigh the potential risks and perform additional monitoring when appropriate.

■ **ALUMINUM HYDROXIDE:** Increased risk for constipation.

■ **ANTACIDS, LAXATIVES (calcium- or magnesium-containing):** SPS may bind with magnesium or calcium found in laxatives (milk of magnesia, magnesium sulfate, etc.) or antacids which can prevent bicarbonate ion neutralization and lead to metabolic alkalosis. Concurrent use is not recommended during SPS therapy.

■ **LITHIUM:** May decrease lithium absorption; stagger doses if both drugs are needed.

■ **SORBITOL:** Use together (oral administration) is commonly employed in veterinary patients, but there is an increased risk for colon necrosis, especially if used as a retention enema.

Doses

- **DOGS:**

  For adjunctive treatment of hyperkalemia (extra-label): 2 g/kg of resin PO divided into 3-4 doses per day. Often mixed with 70% sorbitol to prevent constipation. Do not use a cathartic (*e.g.*, sorbitol) if using as a retention enema as it must be in the colon for at least 30 minutes. To prepare a retention enema from the powder add 15 grams per 100 mL of a 1% methylcellulose solution or 10% dextrose. If hyperkalemia is severe, 3-4 times the normal amount of resin may be given. Generally used for mild hyperkalemia; other treatments should be used for severe or life-threatening hyperkalemia. Adapted from: (Willard 1986), (Cowgill *et al.* 2005)

- **HORSES:**

  For life-threatening hyperkalemia in neonatal foals (extra-label):15 grams of resin in 100 mL of 10% dextrose via enema. Monitor serum potassium and sodium closely. (Madigan 2002)

Monitoring

- Serum electrolytes (sodium, potassium— at least once a day), calcium, magnesium.
- Acid/base status, ECG, if warranted.

Chemistry/Synonyms

A sulfonated cation exchange resin, sodium polystyrene sulfonate (SPS) occurs as a golden brown, fine powder. It is odorless and tasteless. Each gram contains 4.1 mEq of sodium and has an *in vitro* exchange capacity of ≈ 3.1 mEq of potassium (in actuality a maximum of 1 mEq is usually exchanged).

Sodium Polystyrene Sulfonate may also be known as: natrii polystyrenesulfonas, sodium polystyrene sulphonate, *Elutit-Natrium*®, *K-Exit*®, *Kayexalate*®, *Kexelate*®, *Kionex*®, *Resinsodio*®, *Resonium*®, *Resonium A*®, or *SPS*®.

Storage/Stability

Store products in well-closed containers at room temperature; do not heat. Suspensions made from powder should be freshly prepared and used within 24 hours.

Compatibility/Compounding Considerations

No specific information noted.

Dosage Forms/Regulatory Status

VETERINARY-LABELED PRODUCTS: NONE.
HUMAN-LABELED PRODUCTS:
Sodium Polystyrene Sulfonate Powder: Sodium content is approximately 100 mg (4.1 mEq) per g; in 1 lb. jars & 454 g; *Kayexalate*®, *Kionex*®; (Rx)

Sodium Polystyrene Sulfonate Suspension: 15 grams/60 mL (sodium 1.5 grams, 65 mEq) in 60 mL, 120 mL, 200 mL, 480 mL, 500 mL and UD 60 mL; *SPS*®, generic; (Rx)

Revisions/References

Monograph revised/updated August 2014.

Cowgill, L. & T. Francey (2005). Acute uremia. *Textbook of Veterinary Internal Medicine, 6th Ed.* S. Ettinger and E. Feldman, Elsevier: 1731-51.

Madigan, J. (2002). Renal and urinary disorders in equine neonates. Proceedings: Western Veterinary Conference. accessed via Veterinary Information Network; vin.com

Willard, M. D. (1986). Treatment of hyperkalemia. *Current Veterinary Therapy IX: Small Animal Practice.* R. W. Kirk. Phialdelphai, W.B. Saunders: 94-101.

Sodium Stibogluconate

(sti-boe-**gloo**-koe-nate)

Sodium Antimony Gluconate, Pentostam®

Antileishmanial

Prescriber Highlights

▶ Antimony compound for treatment of leishmaniasis in humans & dogs.

▶ Not commercially available in USA (CDC distributes).

▶ Contraindicated in renal failure, pre-existing arrhythmias.

▶ Many potential adverse effects, including some very serious.

Uses/Indications

Sodium stibogluconate has been used for the treatment of leishmaniasis in dogs. Availability issues and adverse effects limit usefulness.

Pharmacology/Actions

Sodium stibogluconate's exact mode of action is unknown. It is believed that it may reduce ATP and GTP synthesis in susceptible amistigotes.

Pharmacokinetics

In dogs, stibogluconate's volume of distribution (steady-state) was 0.25 L/kg, clearance 1.71 L/kg/hr, and terminal half-life ranged from 0.6-1.5 hours. The main route of excretion is via the kidneys; glomerular filtration rate determines excretion rate.

Contraindications/Precautions/Warnings

Stibogluconate is contraindicated in patients with pre-existing cardiac arrhythmias, or significantly impaired renal function. It should not be used in those that have had a serious adverse reaction to a previous dose.

Adverse Effects

Dogs given 40 mg/kg of stibogluconate developed increased AST levels. Other reported adverse effects (incidence unknown) include pain on injection, musculoskeletal pain, hemolytic anemia, leukopenia, vomiting, diarrhea, pancreatitis, myocardial injury and arrhythmias, renal toxicity, shock and sudden death. Intravenous administration can cause thrombophlebitis. Reportedly, the incidence of adverse effects increases if the drug is administered for longer than 2 months.

Reproductive/Nursing Safety

Sodium stibogluconate has not been shown to cause fetal harm, but the manufacturer states that the drug should be withheld during pregnancy unless the benefits outweigh the risks.

The use of this drug during nursing is controversial. Some (*e.g.*, The American Academy of Pediatrics) say that it is usually compatible with breast-feeding, but the manufacturer states that it should not be used in nursing mothers.

Overdosage/Acute Toxicity

In the unlikely event of a parenterally administered overdose, it is suggested to contact an animal poison control center. Potentially, antimony can be chelated with dimercaptosuccinic acid (DMSA) or d-penicillamine.

Drug Interactions

- No specific drug interactions were noted. Stibogluconate has reportedly been used with allopurinol, paromomycin, or pentamidine without problems.

Laboratory Considerations

- No specific laboratory interactions or considerations noted.

Doses

- **DOGS:**

    For treatment of cutaneous leishmaniasis: 30 – 50 mg/kg IV or SC daily for 3-4 weeks. Has severe side effects and may not be obtainable in the USA. If side effects occur, it can be administered every other day for longer periods. Intravenous administrations should be given over 5 minutes to prevent cardiac toxicity. The use of a fine needle or catheter is recommended to avoid thrombophlebitis. (Anon 2004; Brosey 2005), (Koch *et al.* 2011)

Monitoring

- Laboratory and clinical signs associated with adverse effects (CBC, liver enzymes, renal function tests, ECG, etc.).
- Bone marrow cultures for Leishmania.
- Clinical efficacy.

Client Information

- Clients should understand the potential public health implications of this disease in dogs (dependent on country), the guarded prognosis (even with treatment), risks of treatment and associated expenses.

Chemistry/Synonyms

Sodium stibogluconate is a pentavalent antimony compound that contains between 30-34% antimony and is a colorless, odorless or almost odorless, amorphous powder. Sodium stibogluconate is very soluble in water and practically insoluble in alcohol or ether. The commercially available (not in the USA) injection has a pH between 5-5.6.

Sodium stibogluconate may also be known as: sodium antimony gluconate, *stiboglucat-natrium*, natriumstibogluconat-9-wasser, solusurmin, stibogluconat, *sodio stibogluconato*, and *natrii stibogluconas*.

Storage/Stability

The commercially available injection (*Pentostam®*) should be stored at temperatures below 25°C (76°F) and protected from freezing and exposure to light. After removing the first dose, the vial should not be used after one month.

Compatibility/Compounding Considerations

No specific information noted.

Dosage Forms/Regulatory Status

VETERINARY-LABELED PRODUCTS: NONE.

HUMAN-LABELED PRODUCTS:

None in the USA. Sodium Stibogluconate (sodium antimony gluconate) 100 mg (of antimony)/mL for injection in 6 mL and 100 mL (*Pentostam®*) may be available from the Centers for Disease Control (CDC). It may or may not be released for use in domestic animals. Contact the CDC at 404-639-3670 from 8 AM-4:30 PM Eastern Time, Monday-Friday for more information or go to their website: www.cdc.gov/ncidod/srp/drugs/drug-service.html

Pentostam® is available commercially in several countries.

Revisions/References

Monograph revised/updated August 2014.

Anon (2004). Cutaneous Leishmaniasis. Associate Library, Veterinary Information Network. accessed via Veterinary Information Network; vin.com

Brosey, B. (2005). Leishmaniasis. Proceedings: ACVIM 2005. accessed via Veterinary Information Network; vin.com

Koch, S., et al. (2011). *Small Animal Dermatology Drug Handbook*, Wiley-Blackwell. Ames.

Sodium Thiosulfate

(soe-dee-um thye-oh-sul-fayte)   Sodium Hyposulfite

Antidote (Arsenic, Cyanide)

Prescriber Highlights

▶ Used for cyanide, arsenic, or copper poisoning; localized treatment for chemotherapy extravasation injuries.

▶ Contraindications: None.

▶ Adverse Effects: Large doses by mouth may cause profuse diarrhea.

▶ Injectable forms should be given slowly IV.

Uses/Indications

Sodium thiosulfate (alone or in combination with sodium nitrite) may be useful in the treatment of cyanide toxicity. It has been proposed for use in treating arsenic or other heavy metal poisonings but its efficacy is in question for these purposes. However, because sodium thiosulfate is relatively non-toxic and inexpensive, it may be tried to treat arsenic poisoning. When used in combination with sodium molybdate, sodium thiosulfate may be useful for the treatment of copper poisoning.

In humans, sodium thiosulfate has been used to reduce the nephrotoxicity of cisplatin therapy. A 3% or 4% solution has been used to infiltrate the site of extravasations of cisplatin, carboplatin, or dactinomycin. In combination with steroids, sodium thiosulfate may reduce the healing time associated with doxorubicin extravasation.

Topical sodium thiosulfate may be useful for treatment for some fungal infections (*Tinea* spp.).

Pharmacology/Actions

By administering thiosulfate, an exogenous source of sulfur is available to the body, thereby hastening the detoxification of cyanide using the enzyme rhodanese. Rhodanese (*thiosulfate cyanide sulfurtransferase*) converts cyanide to the relatively nontoxic thiocyanate ion; thiocyanate is then excreted in the urine.

Sodium thiosulfate has been used in humans to treat extravasation injuries secondary to carboplatin or cisplatin, for prophylaxis to prevent nephrotoxicity after cisplatin overdoses and ototoxicity with carboplatin overdoses.

Sodium thiosulfate's topical antifungal activity is probably due to its slow release of colloidal sulfur.

While sodium thiosulfate has been recommended for treating arsenic (and some other heavy metal) poisoning, the proposed mechanism of action is not known and its efficacy is in question. Presumably, the sulfate moiety may react with and chelate the metal allowing its removal.

Pharmacokinetics

Sodium thiosulfate is relatively poorly absorbed from the GI tract. When substantial doses are given PO, it acts a saline cathartic. When administered intravenously, it is distributed in the extracellular fluid and then rapidly excreted via the urine.

Contraindications/Precautions/Warnings

There are no absolute contraindications to the use of the drug.

Adverse Effects

The drug is relatively non-toxic. Large doses by mouth may cause profuse diarrhea. Injectable forms should be given slowly IV.

Reproductive/Nursing Safety

Safe use during pregnancy has not been established; use when benefits outweigh the potential risks. In humans, the FDA categorizes this drug as category C for use during pregnancy (*Animal studies have shown an adverse effect on the fetus, but there are no adequate studies in humans; or there are no animal reproduction studies and no adequate studies in humans.)*

No lactation information was found.

Drug Interactions/Laboratory Considerations

■ No specific drug or laboratory interactions or considerations were noted.

Doses

■ **DOGS, CATS:**

For cyanide toxicity (extra-label): Contact an animal poison control center for guidance.

For treating extravasation injuries secondary to doxorubicin, carboplatin, cisplatin infusions (extra-label): **Note:** These are recommendations for human patients.

Doxorubicin: Subcutaneous sodium thiosulfate 2% added to therapy with subcutaneous hydrocortisone and topical betamethasone decreased the healing time by half for cytotoxic drug extravasation (including doxorubicin and epirubicin) when compared to therapy without sodium thiosulfate.

Carboplatin: Prepare a 0.17 mole/L solution by mixing 4 mL sodium thiosulfate 10% w/v with 6 mL sterile water for injection. Inject 5 mL into extravasation site.

Cisplatin: For extravasation of large amounts (>20 mL) of highly concentrated (>0.5 mg/mL) solutions: Prepare a 0.17 mole/L solution by mixing 4 mL sodium thiosulfate 10% w/v with 6 mL sterile water for injection. Inject into extravasation site. (*Drugdex® Evaluations. Micromedex Healthcare Series; Thompson, 2007*)

■ **HORSES:**

For cyanide toxicity (extra-label): First give sodium nitrite in a 20% solution at a dose of 10 – 20 mg/kg IV followed with a 20% solution of sodium thiosulfate given at a dose of 30 – 40 mg/kg IV. (Osweiler 2003)

For arsenic toxicity (extra-label): Sodium thiosulfate at 20 – 30 grams in 300 mL of water orally with dimercaprol (BAL) 3 mg/kg IM q4h. (Jones 2004)

■ **RUMINANTS:**

Note: When used in food animals, FARAD states that this salt is rapidly excreted and not considered a residue concern in animal tissues; therefore a 24-hour preslaughter withdrawal interval (WDI) would be sufficient. (Haskell *et al.* 2005)

In combination with sodium molybdate for the treatment of copper poisoning (extra-label): In conjunction with fluid replacement therapy, 500 mg sodium thiosulfate in combination with 200 mg ammonium or sodium molybdate PO daily for up to 3 weeks will help decrease total body burden of copper. (Thompson *et al.* 1993)

For treatment of cyanide toxicity secondary to cyanogenic plants (extra-label): 660 mg/kg IV sodium thiosulfate in a 30% solution given rapidly using a 12 or 14 gauge needle. (Post *et al.* 2000)

For treatment of arsenic poisoning: (extra-label) In the meta-analysis, the most commonly administered antidote was sodium thiosulfate 20 – 40 mg/kg IV q8h and 80 mg/kg PO q24h, but one study using 40 mg/kg IV q8h and 80 mg/kg PO q24h reported better outcomes. Administration of oral or IV fluids was highly associated with survival. (Bertin *et al.* 2013)

Chemistry/Synonyms

Sodium thiosulfate occurs as large, colorless crystals or coarse, crystalline powder. It is very soluble in water, deliquescent in moist air and effloresces in dry air at temperatures >33°C.

Sodium thiosulfate may also be known as: natrii thiosulfas, na-

trium thiosulfuricum, sodium hyposulphite, sodium thiosulphate, *Consept Step 2®, Hiposul®, Hyposulfene®,* or *S-hydril®.*

Storage/Stability

Unless otherwise stated by the manufacturer, store at room temperature. Crystals should be stored in tight containers.

Compatibility/Compounding Considerations

Sodium thiosulfate is **not compatible** mixed with cyanocobalamin.

Dosage Forms/Regulatory Status

VETERINARY-LABELED PRODUCTS: NONE.

HUMAN-LABELED PRODUCTS:

Sodium Thiosulfate for Injection: 10% (100 mg/mL, as pentahydrate) & 25% (250 mg/mL as pentahydrate) preservative-free in 10 mL & 50 mL single-use vials; generic; (Rx)

Revisions/References

Monograph revised/updated August 2014.

Bertin, F. R., et al. (2013). Arsenic Toxicosis in Cattle: Meta-Analysis of 156 Cases. Journal of Veterinary Internal Medicine 27(4): 977-81.

Haskell, S., et al. (2005). Farad Digest: Antidotes in Food Animal Practice. JAVMA **226**(6): 884-7.

Jones, S. (2004). Inflammatory diseases of the gastrointestinal tract causing diarrhea. *Equine Internal Medicine 2nd Ed.* S. Reed, W. Bayly and D. Sellon. Philadelphia, Saunders: 884-912.

Osweiler, G. (2003). Toxicity of natural products in horses. Proceedings: Western Veterinary Conference. accessed via Veterinary Information Network; vin.com

Post, L. & W. Keller (2000). Current status of food animal antidotes. The Veterinary Clinics of North America: Food Animal Practice **16**:3(November).

Thompson, J. R. & W. B. Buck (1993). Copper-Molybdenum Toxicosis. *Current Veterinary Therapy 3: Food Animal Practice.* J. L. Howard. Philadelphia, W.B. Saunders: 396-8.

Somatotropin (Growth Hormone)

(soe-ma-toe-troe-pin)

Hormone

Prescriber Highlights

▶ Used for canine hypopituitary dwarfism or growth hormone-responsive dermatosis (in adult dogs).
▶ May cause diabetes mellitus.
▶ Availability & expense issues.

Uses/Indications

Somatotropin may be useful in treating hypopituitary dwarfism or growth hormone-responsive dermatosis (in adult dogs).

Pharmacology/Actions

Growth hormone (somatotropin) is responsible for, or contributes to, linear and skeletal growth, organ growth, and cell growth. It also is a factor in protein, carbohydrate, lipid, connective tissue, and mineral metabolism.

Pharmacokinetics

No canine information was located. Both the liver and kidney are major elimination organs for somatotropin.

Contraindications/Precautions/Warnings

Growth hormone derived from other species is contraindicated in patients hypersensitive to it.

Adverse Effects

Growth hormone may cause diabetes mellitus in dogs. This may be transient or permanent even after discontinuing treatment. Blood and urine glucose should be routinely monitored. If blood glucose exceeds 150 mg/dL, therapy should be stopped. Hypersensitivity reactions are possible, but less so if using porcine origin product. Long-term treatment at high doses may cause acromegaly. Acromegaly in dogs can cause increased size of paws and head, increased skin folds around head and neck area, prognathism, and inspiratory stridor.

Reproductive/Nursing Safety

In humans, the FDA categorizes this drug as category *C* for use during pregnancy (*Animal studies have shown an adverse effect on the fetus, but there are no adequate studies in humans; or there are no animal reproduction studies and no adequate studies in humans.*)

Overdosage/Acute Toxicity

Acute overdosage could cause hypoglycemia initially and then hyperglycemia. Blood glucose should be monitored and supportive treatment (glucose/insulin) performed.

Drug Interactions

The following drug interactions have either been reported or are theoretical in humans or animals receiving somatotropin and may be of significance in veterinary patients. Unless otherwise noted, use together is not necessarily contraindicated, but weigh the potential risks and perform additional monitoring when appropriate.

- **GLUCOCORTICOIDS:** May inhibit the growth promoting effect of somatotropin. When concurrent adrenal insufficiency is diagnosed, adjust glucocorticoid dose carefully to avoid negative effects on growth.

Doses

- **DOGS:**

  For treatment of hypopituitary dwarfism (extra-label):

  a) 0.1 Unit/kg (0.05 mg/kg) SC 3 times per week for 4-6 weeks. **Note:** May also require life-long thyroid hormone supplementation and if secondary adrenal insufficiency present, glucocorticoid treatment. If after successful treatment, dermatologic signs recur, may dose as above (0.1 Unit/kg 3 times weekly for one week). Repeat these weekly regimens at intervals determined by the time lapse between treatments and relapse. (Feldman *et al.* 1996)

  b) Porcine growth hormone 2 Units per dog SC every other day or 0.1 Unit/kg SC 3 times weekly for 4-6 weeks. Improvement of skin and hair coat signs can be seen within 6-8 weeks. Because growth plates close rapidly no significant change in stature is noted. Concurrent secondary adrenocortical insufficiency and hypothyroidism have to be treated appropriately. (Koch *et al.* 2011)

  For Alopecia X/Growth hormone responsive dermatosis (extra-label):

  a) 0.15 Units/kg of porcine growth hormone SC 2 times weekly for 6 weeks. (Hillier 2006)

  b) 2.5 Units for dogs weighting <14 kg and 5 Units for dogs >14 kg given SC every other day for 10 treatments. Other reported treatment regimens include 0.1 Units/kg 3 times weekly for 6 weeks or 0.015 Units/kg twice weekly for 6 weeks. Ovine growth hormone has not been shown to be effective. The majority of dogs previously diagnosed with adult-onset growth hormone responsive dermatosis fall into the category of alopecia X. Somatotropin should not be used as the first treatment choice for cases of Alopecia X because of potential for serious side effects and the infrequent and inconsistent response to this treatment modality. (Koch et al. 2011)

Monitoring

- Clinical efficacy.
- Blood glucose (weekly).
- Urine glucose (daily).
- Thyroid function, adrenal function (pituitary dwarfism pts.); initially and then periodically.

Client Information

- Clients should be instructed on the methods for SC injection and testing urine glucose.
- May be expensive to treat and diabetes (permanent) can occur.

Chemistry/Synonyms

Somatotropin may also be known as: CB-311, HGH, human growth hormone, LY-137998, somatropinum; many trade names are available.

Compatibility/Compounding Considerations

No specific information noted.

Dosage Forms/Regulatory Status

There are several manufacturers of human recombinant DNA origin somatotropin products, but these are expensive, can cause immunogenicity reactions in dogs, and not sold for veterinary use.

The bovine recombinant growth hormone product (*Posilac®*) is not suitable for canine use as it is a sustained release formulation and not easily diluted down to the smaller doses required for dogs.

Porcine growth hormone appears to have little immunogenicity in dogs and reportedly can be obtained via: Dr. A. F. Partlow at: 310-222-3537 E-Mail: Partlow@HUMC.edu WEBSITE: www.humc.edu/hormones

The ARCI (Racing Commissioners International) has designated this drug as a class 2 substance. See the appendix for more information.

Revisions/References

Monograph revised/updated August 2014.

Feldman, E. & R. Nelson (1996). *Canine and Feline Endocrinology and Reproduction*, Saunders. Philadelphia.
Hillier, A. (2006). Alopecia: is an endocrine disorder responsible? Proceedings: ACVC. accessed via Veterinary Information Network; vin.com
Koch, S., et al. (2011). *Small Animal Dermatology Drug Handbook*, Wiley-Blackwell. Ames.

Sorbitol

(sore-bit-ahl)

Laxative/Cathartic

Prescriber Highlights

▶ Orally administered cathartic that is generally not used alone in veterinary medicine; often used in combination with activated charcoal to accelerate expulsion of gut contents (toxins, poisons).

▶ Potential to cause fluid/electrolyte disturbances (*e.g.*, hypernatremia) and colonic necrosis.

Uses/Indications

Sorbitol is an osmotic laxative that can be used alone or in combination with activated charcoal for toxin/poison gut decontamination or with sodium polystyrene sulfonate (SPS) for treating mild hyperkalemia. Sorbitol is also used as a sweetener (1/2 the sweetening power of sucrose).

Pharmacology/Actions

Sorbitol is a non-absorbable sugar alcohol that acts as an osmotic laxative. Stool pH may be reduced in patients taking sorbitol, producing an "ammonia trap", which may be useful in patients with hepatic encephalopathy.

Pharmacokinetics

Depending on dose and additional fluid consumed, sorbitol can have a laxative effect within one hour of dosing.

Contraindications/Precautions/Warnings

Do not use sorbitol mixed with SPS as a retention enema. Retention enemas with SPS and sorbitol have been implicated in some human cases of colonic necrosis, presumably secondary to sorbitol causing cellular dehydration.

When used in combination with activated charcoal, generally only the first dose should contain sorbitol as multiple doses can increase the risks for hypernatremia and dehydration.

Adverse Effects

Products containing sorbitol may cause loose stools, diarrhea and vomiting. Fluid and electrolyte imbalances are possible.

There have been reports of hypernatremia occurring in small dogs and cats after activated charcoal and sorbitol administration, presumably due an osmotic effect pulling water into the GI tract. Reduced sodium fluids (*e.g.,* D5W, 1/2 normal saline/D2.5W) with warm water enemas can be administered to alleviate the condition.

Reproductive/Nursing Safety

In humans, the FDA categorizes this drug as category *C* for use during pregnancy (*Animal studies have shown an adverse effect on the fetus, but there are no adequate studies in humans; or there are no animal reproduction studies and no adequate studies in humans.*)

Safe use during nursing has not been established but it is unlikely to pose much risk to nursing offspring.

Overdosage/Acute Toxicity

Overdosage or multiple doses can cause fluid and electrolyte disorders including dehydration and hypernatremia.

Drug Interactions

The following drug interactions have either been reported or are theoretical in humans or animals receiving sorbitol and may be of significance in veterinary patients. Unless otherwise noted, use together is not necessarily contraindicated, but weigh the potential risks and perform additional monitoring when appropriate.

- **SODIUM POLYSTYRENE SULFONATE (SPS):** Use together (oral administration) is commonly employed in veterinary patients, but there is an increased risk for colon necrosis, especially if used as a retention enema.

Laboratory Considerations

- Sorbitol may cause false-positive **ethylene glycol test** results.

Doses

- **DOGS/CATS:**

  With activated charcoal as an adjunctive treatment for toxin ingestions (extra-label): **Note:** Depending on the toxin exposure, recommendations for using activated charcoal can vary. It is highly recommended to contact an animal poison control center for specific guidance on using activated charcoal in veterinary patients.

  Current recommended dosage for single-dose activated charcoal is 1 – 5 grams/kg PO. A "standard dose" is 2 g/kg PO. When a cathartic is not contraindicated, charcoal w/sorbitol is commonly employed to reduce GI transit time. For drugs/toxins that are enterohepatically recirculated (*e.g.,* caffeine, phenobarbital, theobromine, theophylline, bromethalin, pyrethrins, organophosphate insecticides, ivermectin, antidepressants), multiple doses of activated charcoal WITHOUT sorbitol at 1 – 2 grams/kg PO q4-8 hours for 24 hours is suggested. Dogs and cats with no clinical signs may freely drink the charcoal suspension if administered via syringe. A small amount of food may be added to the solution to enhance palatability. In animals exhibiting clinical signs, administration of activated charcoal slurries/suspensions may be administered via an orogastric tube with a cuffed endotracheal tube in place to help prevent aspiration. Administration via a nasogastric tube may be useful, particularly in cats. Adapted from: (Jutkowitz *et al.* 2009; Talcott 2012; Lee 2013)

  With sodium polystyrene sulfonate (SPS) for adjunctive treatment of hyperkalemia (extra-label): 2 g/kg of SPS resin PO divided into 3-4 doses per day. Often mixed with 70% sorbitol to prevent constipation. Do not use a cathartic (*e.g.,* sorbitol) if using as a retention enema as it must be in the colon for at least 30 minutes. To prepare a retention enema from the powder add 15 grams per 100 mL of a 1% methylcellulose solution or 10%

dextrose. If hyperkalemia is severe: 3-4X the normal amount of resin may be given. Generally used for mild hyperkalemia; other treatments should be used for severe or life-threatening hyperkalemia. Adapted from: (Willard 1986), (Cowgill *et al.* 2005)

- **HORSES:**

  With activated charcoal a cathartic for plant intoxications (extra-label): Activated charcoal (AC) slurry dosage range of 1 – 5 grams/kg (≈ 1 gram of activated charcoal per 5 mL of water). Multi-dose activated charcoal is beneficial for a number of plant intoxications, including oleander. Administration of a cathartic mixed in the AC slurry helps to hasten elimination of contents from the gastrointestinal tract. Commonly used cathartics include sodium sulfate (Glauber's salts), magnesium sulfate (Epsom salts), and sorbitol. Sodium or magnesium sulfate can be administered at 250 – 500 mg/kg mixed in the AC slurry. Sorbitol (70%), also mixed in the AC slurry, can be administered at 3 mL/kg. There is little need to administer a cathartic if significant diarrhea is already present. (Puschner 2010)

Monitoring

- Clinical efficacy.

Client Information

- Diarrhea, flatulence (excess gas), cramping and vomiting are possible.
- Sorbitol is available OTC (over-the-counter; without a prescription), but do not give sorbitol (or any other OTC medications) to your animal without first consulting a veterinarian.

Chemistry/Synonyms

Sorbitol is a sugar alcohol and occurs as a white, odorless, hygroscopic powder, granules, or crystalline masses having a sweet taste with a cold sensation. One gram is soluble in 0.45 mL of water; it is sparingly soluble in alcohol and practically insoluble in solvent ether.

Sorbitol may also be known as: D-glucitol, E420, D-sorbitol, sorbitoli, sorbitolis, sorbitolum, or szorbit.

Storage/Stability

Store the 70% oral solution at controlled room temperature (20-25°C; 68-77°F).

Compatibility/Compounding Considerations

No specific information noted.

Dosage Forms/Regulatory Status

VETERINARY-LABELED PRODUCTS:

None as the sole ingredient. In combination with: Activated charcoal 10%, Kaolin 6.25%, sorbitol 10% suspension in 240 mL bottles; *Toxiban*® *Suspension* with *Sorbitol*; (OTC). Labeled for use in small animals.

HUMAN-LABELED PRODUCTS:

Sorbitol 70% in pints; generic; (OTC). Sorbitol is also included in several activated charcoal products.

In combination with activated charcoal:

Activated Charcoal Oral Liquid/Suspension with sorbitol: 15 g & 30 g in 150 mL & 50 g in 240 mL; *CharcoAid*®; 25 g in 120 mL & 50 g in 240 mL; *Actidose*® with *Sorbitol*; (OTC)

Activated Charcoal Liquid/Suspension without sorbitol: 15 g & 50 g in 120 mL & 240 mL; *CharcoAid*® *2000*; (OTC); 208 mg/mL — 12.5 g in 60 mL & 25 g in 120 mL; 12.5 g in 60 mL, 15 g in 75 mL, 25 g in 120 mL, 30 g in 120 mL, 50 g in 240 mL; *Actidose-Aqua*®, generic; (OTC)

Revisions/References

Monograph written August 2014.

Cowgill, L. & T. Francey (2005). Acute uremia. *Textbook of Veterinary Internal Medicine, 6th Ed.* S. Ettinger and E. Feldman, Elsevier: 1731-51.

Jutkowitz, L. & J. Schildt (2009). Management of common household toxins. Proceedings: WVC. accessed via Veterinary Information Network; vin.com

Lee, J. A. (2013). Emergency Management and Treatment of the Poisoned Small Animal Patient. *Veterinary Clinics of North America: Small Animal Practice* **43**(4): 757-71.

Puschner, B. (2010). Diagnostic and therapeutic approach to plant poisonings in large animals. accessed via Veterinary Information Network; vin.com

Talcott, P. A. (2012). Decontamination Procedures in Poisoned Companion Animals - Facts & Fiction. Western Veterinary Conference. accessed via Veterinary Information Network; vin.com

Willard, M. D. (1986). Treatment of hyperkalemia. *Current Veterinary Therapy IX: Small Animal Practice.* R. W. Kirk. Phialdelphai, W.B. Saunders: 94-101.

Sotalol HCl

(soh-ta-lole)   Betapace®

Beta-Adrenergic Blocker

Prescriber Highlights

▶ Non-selective beta blocker/Class III antiarrhythmic for ventricular tachycardia.
▶ Adverse Effects: Most serious: negative inotropism & pro-arrhythmic but dyspnea/bronchospasm, fatigue/dizziness, & nausea/vomiting possible.
▶ Generic forms available, so cost is less of an issue than in the past.

Uses/Indications

Sotalol can be useful in the long-term treatment of ventricular tachycardias and, possibly, supraventricular tachycardias in dogs and cats. It is most often used in Boxers with arrhythmogenic cardiomyopathy and while research data support its efficacy to suppress ventricular ectopy it is unknown if it significantly impacts survival, particularly when compared with other therapies (mexiletine plus atenolol, or procainamide) (Caro-Vadillo *et al.* 2013). It is also used in dogs with ventricular tachycardia that are refractory to lidocaine and procainamide.

Pharmacology/Actions

Sotalol is a non-selective beta-blocker and Class III antiarrhythmic agent. The beta blocking activity of sotalol is ≈ 30% that of propranolol. The pharmacologic action is believed caused by selectively inhibiting potassium channels. Like other Class III drugs, it prolongs repolarization and refractoriness without affecting conduction. In animals with supraventricular tachycardias, sotalol may be more effective in preventing recurrence of the arrhythmia rather than terminating it.

Pharmacokinetics

Unlike propranolol, sotalol does not have any appreciable first pass effect after oral administration. Food may reduce the bioavailability of sotalol by ≈ 20% (human data) and, if given on an empty stomach, bioavailability is 90-100%. Peak plasma levels occur between 2-4 hours after a dose. The drug has relatively low lipid solubility and virtually no protein binding. Elimination is almost all via the kidney and most of the drug is excreted unchanged. In dogs, sotalol's elimination half-life is 5 hours; in humans ≈ 12 hours.

Contraindications/Precautions/Warnings

Sotalol is a rather weak non-specific beta-blocker, but it is still considered contraindicated in patients with asthma, sinus bradycardia, 2nd or 3rd degree heart block (unless artificially paced), long Q-T syndromes, cardiogenic shock or uncontrolled CHF. Because of the potential for negative inotropic effects, use with caution in CHF. Also, use with caution in patients with diabetes mellitus or hyperthyroidism (may mask signs). Use with caution in patients with renal dysfunction; dosage intervals may need to be extended.

Adverse Effects

Primary concerns with sotalol in dogs are the potential for negative inotropic, chronotropic and proarrhythmic effects. These generally are not clinically important if dosage is not excessive. Other potential adverse effects include dyspnea/bronchospasm, fatigue/dizziness, and nausea/vomiting. Sotalol's beta blocking effects can worsen syncope or cause lethargy, particularly if the ventricular tachyarrhythmia coexists with intermittent bradycardia (*e.g.*, AV block).

Reproductive/Nursing Safety

Sotalol did not cause any fetotoxicity or teratogenicity when given to pregnant lab animals at high dosages, but clear safety in pregnancy has not been established. Sotalol enters maternal milk in concentrations up to 5X found in the serum; consider using a milk replacer in nursing animals.

In humans, the FDA categorizes this drug as category *B* for use during pregnancy (*Animal studies have not yet demonstrated risk to the fetus, but there are no adequate studies in pregnant women; or animal studies have shown an adverse effect, but adequate studies in pregnant women have not demonstrated a risk to the fetus in the first trimester of pregnancy, and there is no evidence of risk in later trimesters.*)

Sotalol is excreted in milk; use with caution in nursing patients. It is not recommended for use in nursing humans.

Overdosage/Acute Toxicity

Overdoses may result in bradycardia, hypotension, CHF, bronchospasm, and hypoglycemia. Use gut decontamination (if not contraindicated) when significant risk of morbidity is possible. Treat adverse effects symptomatically and supportively. There were 110 single agent exposures to sotalol reported to the ASPCA Animal Poison Control Center (APCC) during 2009-2013. Of the 102 dogs, 17 were symptomatic with panting (24%), bradycardia (18%), lethargy (18%) and vomiting (18%) being the most common.

Drug Interactions

The following drug interactions have either been reported or are theoretical in humans or animals receiving sotalol and may be of significance in veterinary patients. Unless otherwise noted, use together is not necessarily contraindicated, but weigh the potential risks and perform additional monitoring when appropriate.

▪ **AMIODARONE:** May prolong refractory periods; concurrent use not recommended in human patients.
▪ **ANESTHETICS, GENERAL:** Additive myocardial depression may occur with the concurrent use of sotalol and myocardial depressant anesthetic agents.
▪ **ANTACIDS:** May reduce oral sotalol absorption; separate doses by at least 2 hours.
▪ **ANTIARRHYTHMICS, CLASS IA** (*e.g.*, **quinidine, procainamide, disopyramide,** etc.): May prolong refractory periods; concurrent use not recommended in human patients; may also prolong QT interval.
▪ **ANTIARRHYTHMICS, CLASS IB, 1C (lidocaine, mexiletine, phenytoin,** etc.): May prolong QT interval.
▪ **CALCIUM CHANNEL BLOCKERS** (*e.g.*, **verapamil, diltiazem,** etc.): Potential to increase hypotensive effects; may have additive effects on AV conduction or ventricular function; use with caution, particularly in patients with preexisting cardiomyopathy or CHF.
▪ **CISAPRIDE:** May prolong QT interval.
▪ **CLONIDINE:** If clonidine is discontinued after concomitant therapy with sotalol, there is an increased risk for rebound hypertension.
▪ **DIGOXIN:** Potential for increased risks for proarrhythmic events.

- ERYTHROMYCIN; CLARITHROMYCIN: May prolong QT interval.
- LIDOCAINE: Clearance may be impaired by sotalol.
- PHENOTHIAZINES: May prolong QT interval.
- RESERPINE: May have additive effects (hypotension, bradycardia) with sotalol.
- SYMPATHOMIMETICS, BETA 2 AGONISTS (*e.g.,* metaproterenol, terbutaline, albuterol, etc.): May have their actions blocked by sotalol.
- TRICYCLIC ANTIDEPRESSANTS: May prolong QT interval.

Laboratory Considerations

- Beta-blockers may produce hypoglycemia and interfere with **glucose** or insulin tolerance tests.
- Sotalol may falsely elevate urine **metanephrine** levels (pheochromocytoma screen) if using a fluorometric or photometric assay.

Doses

- **DOGS/CATS:**

For non-urgent control of ventricular tachyarrhythmias ± supraventricular tachycardia (extra-label): Most anecdotal dosage range recommendations are 1 – 2 mg/kg (some go up to 3 mg/kg) PO q12h. Initially, patients usually are started at the low end of the dosing range. Patients with significant renal dysfunction should receive reduced dosages or increased time between dosages.

For ventricular tachyarrhythmias in Boxers in combination with mexiletine (extra-label): Sotalol 1.5 – 3 mg/kg PO twice daily with mexiletine (5 – 7.5 mg/kg PO 3 times daily) (Prosek *et al.* 2006). Recent evidence (study done in normal dogs) suggests that when mexiletine is used with sotalol in dogs weighing >10 kg, mexiletine could be dosed at 8 – 10 mg/kg PO q12h. Additional confirmation in clinically affected dogs is needed. (Scollan *et al.* 2013)

For ventricular arrhythmias in German shepherds (GSD) with inherited arrhythmias (extra-label): Mexiletine (8 mg/kg PO q8h), and sotalol (2.5 mg/kg PO q12h) were more effective than either drug alone in suppressing ventricular premature complexes. Mexiletine levels were also higher when sotalol was added. (Gelzer *et al.* 2010)

Monitoring

- Efficacy (ECG).
- Adverse effects.

Client Information

- Best given on an empty stomach.
- Most common side effects include lethargy (tiredness/lack of energy) and weakness. Low blood pressure with fainting possible. A heartbeat that is too slow can occur if dose is too high and heart symptoms can get worse.
- When starting this drug, your veterinarian may start with a low dose and gradually increase the dose over time. Do not administer more at a time than your veterinarian prescribes.
- If the dose is too large for your animal, it may cause animal's condition to get worse. If animal loses its appetite, develops depression, or has trouble breathing, call your veterinarian immediately.

Chemistry/Synonyms

A non-selective beta-blocker and Class III antiarrhythmic agent, sotalol HCl is a racemic mixture of the d- and l- forms. Both isomers exhibit antiarrhythmic (Class II) activity, but only the levoform has beta blocking activity. Sotalol HCl occurs as white, crystalline solid that is soluble in water.

Sotalol may also be known as: MJ-1999, d,l-sotalol hydrochloride, or sotaloli hydrochloridum; many trade names are available.

Storage/Stability

Store tablets at room temperature.

Compatibility/Compounding Considerations

No specific information noted.

Dosage Forms/Approval

VETERINARY-LABELED PRODUCTS: NONE.

The ARCI (Racing Commissioners International) has designated this drug as a class 3 substance. See the appendix for more information.

HUMAN-LABELED PRODUCTS:

Sotalol HCl Tablets: 80 mg, 120 mg, 160 mg & 240 mg; *Betapace*®, generic; (Rx)

Revisions/References

Monograph revised/updated August 2014.

Caro-Vadillo, A., et al. (2013). Arrhythmogenic right ventricular cardiomyopathy in boxer dogs: a retrospective study of survival. Veterinary Record **172**(10).

Gelzer, A. R. M., et al. (2010). Combination therapy with mexiletine and sotalol suppresses inherited ventricular arrhythmias in German shepherd dogs better than mexiletine or sotalol monotherapy: A randomized cross-over study. Journal of Veterinary Cardiology **12**(2): 93-106.

Prosek, R., et al. (2006). Comparison of sotalol and mexiletine versus stand alone sotalol in treatment of Boxer dogs with ventricular arrhythmias. Proceedings: ACVIM. accessed via Veterinary Information Network; vin.com

Scollan, K. & D. Sisson (2013). Mexiletine Serum Levels with Twice-Daily Dosing in Combination with Sotalol in Healthy Dogs. Proceedings: 23rd ECVIM-CA Congress. accessed via Veterinary Information Network; vin.com

Spectinomycin

(spek-ti-noe-mye-sin)   Adspec®, Spectam®

Aminocyclitol Antibiotic

Prescriber Highlights

▶ Aminocyclitol antibiotic used primarily in food producing animals; relatively broad spectrum but minimal activity against anaerobes & most strains of Pseudomonas.

▶ Contraindications: Patients hypersensitive to it.

▶ Adverse Effects: Appears to have minimal adverse effects at labeled dosages; probably less nephrotoxicity/ototoxicity than other aminocyclitols. Can cause neuromuscular blockade. May cause swelling at SC injection sites.

Uses/Indications

Although occasionally used in dogs, cats, and horses for susceptible infections, Spectinomycin only has FDA-approved dosage forms for cattle, chickens, turkeys, and swine. Refer to the Dosage section below for more information on FDA-approved uses.

Pharmacology/Actions

Spectinomycin is primarily a bacteriostatic antibiotic that inhibits protein synthesis in susceptible bacteria by binding to the 30S ribosomal subunit.

Spectinomycin has activity against a wide variety of gram-positive and gram-negative bacteria, including *E. coli*, Klebsiella, Proteus, Enterobacter, Salmonella, Streptococci, Staphylococcus, and Mycoplasma. It has minimal activity against anaerobes, most strains of Pseudomonas, Chlamydia, or Treponema.

In human medicine, spectinomycin is used principally for its activity against *Neisseria gonorrhoeae*.

Pharmacokinetics

After oral administration only ≈ 7% of the dose is absorbed, but the drug that remains in the GI tract is active. When injected SC or IM, the drug is reportedly absorbed well with peak levels occurring in ≈ 1 hour.

Tissue levels of absorbed drug are lower than those found in the serum. Spectinomycin does not appreciably enter the CSF or the eye and is not bound significantly to plasma proteins. It is unknown whether spectinomycin crosses the placenta or enters milk.

Absorbed drug is excreted via glomerular filtration into the urine mostly unchanged. In cattle, terminal half-life is ≈ 2 hours.

Contraindications/Precautions/Warnings
Spectinomycin is contraindicated in patients hypersensitive to it.

Adverse Effects
When used as labeled, adverse effects are unlikely with this drug. It is reported that parenteral use of this drug is much safer than with other aminocyclitol antibiotics, but little is known regarding its prolonged use. It is probably safe to say that spectinomycin is significantly less ototoxic and nephrotoxic than other commonly used aminocyclitol antibiotics, but can cause neuromuscular blockade. Parenteral calcium administration will generally reverse the blockade.

Adverse effects that have been reported in human patients receiving the drug in single or multidose studies include soreness at injection site, increases in BUN, alkaline phosphatase and SGPT, and decreases in hemoglobin, hematocrit, and creatinine clearance. Although increases in BUN and decreases in creatinine clearance and urine output have been noted, overt renal toxicity has not been demonstrated with this drug.

Cattle receiving the sulfate form subcutaneously have developed swelling at the injection site.

Reproductive/Nursing Safety
In humans, the FDA categorizes this drug as category *B* for use during pregnancy (*Animal studies have not yet demonstrated risk to the fetus, but there are no adequate studies in pregnant women; or animal studies have shown an adverse effect, but adequate studies in pregnant women have not demonstrated a risk to the fetus in the first trimester of pregnancy, and there is no evidence of risk in later trimesters.*)

It is not known whether spectinomycin is excreted in milk; use caution when administering to nursing patients.

Overdosage/Acute Toxicity
No specific information was located on oral overdoses but because the drug is negligibly absorbed after oral administration, significant toxicity is unlikely via this route.

Injected doses of 90 mg produced transient ataxia in turkey poults.

Drug Interactions
- Antagonism has been reported when spectinomycin is used with **chloramphenicol** or **tetracycline**.

Doses
- **SMALL MAMMALS:**
  Rabbits; for susceptible infections (extra-label): 1 g/L in drinking water for 7 days in weanling rabbits; may cause diarrhea. (Donnelly 2012)
- **CATTLE:**
  For bovine respiratory disease (labeled dose; FDA-approved): 10 – 15 mg/kg SC (in the neck; not more than 50 mL per site) once daily (q24h) for 3-5 consecutive days. (Label directions; *Adspec*)
- **SWINE:**
  For bacterial enteritis (white scours) in baby pigs associated with *E. coli* susceptible to spectinomycin (labeled dose; FDA-approved): 50 mg/10 lbs of body weight PO twice daily for 3-5 days. (Label directions; *Spectam Scour-Halt*)

- **BIRDS:**
  For airsacculitis associated with *M. meleagridis* or chronic respiratory disease associated with *E. coli* in turkey poults (1-3 days old) (labeled dose; FDA-approved): Inject 0.1 mL (10 mg) SC in the base of the neck. (Label directions; *Spectam Injectable*)

  For control and to lessen mortality due to infections from *M. synoviae*, *S. typhimurium*, *S. infantis*, and *E. coli* in newly hatched chicks (labeled dose; FDA-approved): Dilute injection with normal saline to a concentration of 2.5 – 5 mg/0.2 mL and inject SC. (Label directions; *Spectam Injectable*)

  For prevention and control of chronic respiratory disease associated with *Mycoplasma gallisepticum* in broilers (labeled dose; FDA-approved): Add sufficient amount to drinking water to attain a final concentration of 2 grams/gallon. (Label directions; *Spectam Water-Soluble*)

  For infectious synovitis associated with *Mycoplasma synoviae* in broilers (labeled dose; FDA-approved): Add sufficient amount to drinking water to attain a final concentration of 1 gram/gallon. (Label directions; *Spectam Water-Soluble*)

  For improved weight gain/feed efficiency in floor-raised broilers (labeled dose; FDA-approved): Add sufficient amount to drinking water to attain a final concentration of 0.5 grams/gallon. (Label directions; *Spectam Water-Soluble*)

Monitoring
- Clinical efficacy.

Chemistry/Synonyms
An aminocyclitol antibiotic obtained from *Streptomyces spectabilis*, spectinomycin is available as the dihydrochloride pentahydrate and hexahydrate sulfate salts. It occurs as a white to pale buff, crystalline powder with pK$_a$s of 7 and 8.7. It is freely soluble in water and practically insoluble in alcohol.

Spectinomycin may also be known as: M-141, actinospectacin, spectinomycini, U-18409AE, *Adspec*, *Amtech Spectam*, *Kempi*, *Kirin*, *Spectoguard Scour-Chek*, *Stanilo*, *Togamycin*, *Trobicin*, *Trobicine*, or *Vabicin*.

Storage/Stability
Unless otherwise instructed by the manufacturer, spectinomycin products should be stored at room temperature (15-30°C). Protect from freezing.

Compatibility/Compounding Considerations
No specific information noted.

Dosage Forms/Regulatory Status
VETERINARY-LABELED PRODUCTS:
Spectinomycin Sulfate Injection: 100 mg/mL in 500 mL vials; *Adspec*; (Rx). When used as labeled, slaughter withdrawal in cattle = 11 days; not to be used in veal calves or in dairy cattle 20 months of age or older.

Spectinomycin Injection: 100 mg/mL in 500 mL vials; *Spectam Injectable*; (OTC). FDA-approved for use in 1-3 days old turkey poults and newly hatched chicks.

Spectinomycin Water Soluble Concentrate: 0.5 gram of spectinomycin per gram *Spectam Water Soluble*; (OTC). FDA-approved for use in chickens (not layers). Slaughter withdrawal (at labeled doses) = 5 days.

Spectinomycin Oral Solution: 50 mg/mL in 240 mL pump bottle and 500 and 1000 mL without pump; *Spectam Scour-Halt*, *Spectoguard Scour-Chek*, *Spectam Scour-Halt*; (OTC). FDA-approved for use in swine (Weighing less than 15 lbs and not older than 4 weeks of age). Slaughter withdrawal (at labeled doses) = 21 days.

Spectinomycin/Lincomycin in a 2:1 ratio; *LS 50 Water Soluble Powder*®, *Sepclinx-50*®, generic; in 2.65 oz packets. Each packet contains lincomycin 16.7 grams and spectinomycin 33.3 grams. FDA-approved for use in chickens up to 7 days of age.

Lincomycin 50 mg/Spectinomycin: 100 mg per mL in 20 mL vials; *Linco-Spectin*® *Sterile Solution*; (OTC). FDA-approved for use in semen extenders only.

HUMAN-LABELED PRODUCTS: NONE.

Revisions/References
Monograph revised/updated August 2014.
Donnelly, T. (2012). Rational Antimicrobial Therapeutics for Exotic Companion Mammals. ABVP Proceedings. accessed via Veterinary Information Network; vin.com

Spinosad

(spin-oh-sad)   Comfortis®

Oral Flea Adulticide

Prescriber Highlights
▶ Oral flea adulticide for dogs and cats; labeled for one month prevention/treatment. Combination product with milbemycin (*Trifexis*®) approved for dogs for heartworm prevention, fleas, hookworms, roundworms, & whipworms.
▶ Give with food. Rapid action. Appears very safe and well tolerated in dogs and cats.
▶ Potentially serious drug interaction with ivermectin (and possibly other drugs).

Uses/Indications

In dogs, oral spinosad is indicated for the prevention and treatment of flea (*Ctenocephalides felis*) infestations for one month in dogs 14 weeks of age and older (Label Information; *Comfortis*®). Advantages of this drug include: rapid response for a systemic once monthly product, killing adult fleas before egg laying is initiated, efficacy is not affected by bathing or swimming, and FDA-approved (not EPA-approved as are many topical flea products) (Ihrke 2009). A product combining spinosad and milbemycin (*Trifexis*®) is FDA-approved for the prevention of heartworm disease (*Dirofilaria immitis*), for the prevention and treatment of flea infestations (*Ctenocephalides felis*), and the treatment and control of adult hookworm (*Ancylostoma caninum*), adult roundworm (*Toxocara canis* and *Toxascaris leonina*) and adult whipworm (*Trichuris vulpis*) infections in dogs and puppies 8 weeks of age or older and 5 pounds of body weight or greater.

In cats, oral spinosad is approved to kill fleas and for the prevention and treatment of flea infestations (*Ctenocephalides felis*), for one month, on cats and kittens 14 weeks of age and older and two pounds of body weight or greater.

While spinosad is not labeled for use against ticks and it has been stated that it is not effective for this use, a pilot study evaluating the efficacy of spinosad dosed at 50 mg/kg (1.7X minimum flea dose) and 100 mg/kg (3.3X minimum flea dose) against adult brown dog tick (*R. sanguineus*) infestations in dogs, demonstrated high efficacy in killing ticks within 24 hours of dosing. The results suggested that some post-treatment residual tick control persisted up to 1 month. The authors concluded that the role of spinosad as a useful adjunct to currently marketed acaricidal products needs to be explored (Snyder *et al.* 2009).

In humans, spinosad as a topical suspension has been used to treat pediculosis capitis (head lice).

Pharmacology/Actions

Spinosad is a macrocyclic lactone containing two natural occurring macrocyclic lactones (spinosyn A and spinosyn D). Its primary mode of action in insects is as a nicotinic acetylcholine D-alpha receptor agonist causing involuntary muscle contractions and tremors secondary to motor neuron activation. Prolonged exposure causes paralysis and flea death. Flea death begins within 30 minutes of dosing and is complete in 4 hours. In insects, spinosad also opens chloride channels similarly to other macrocyclic lactones.

Pharmacokinetics

After oral administration of spinosad (with food) to dogs, peak plasma levels for spinosyn A and spinosyn D occur in ≈ 2 and 3 hours, respectively. Spinosyn D levels are ≈ 5 times greater than those of spinosyn A. Spinosyn A & D are extensively bound (≈ 99%) to canine plasma proteins. Spinosad is hepatically biotransformed with glutathione conjugates and 70-90% is eliminated in the feces via the bile. The plasma elimination half-life is ≈ 10 days.

Contraindications/Precautions/Warnings

No labeled contraindications. It has been recommended not to use spinosad with the high extra-label doses of ivermectin (Kuhl 2009; Jazic 2010).

The product label cautions use in breeding females and dogs with pre-existing epilepsy at higher than labeled dosages may decrease seizure threshold.

The chewable tablets are beef flavored and while they do not contain beef proteins, pork proteins and hydrolyzed soy are used. Dogs with pork or soy allergies may react (Rosenkrantz 2010).

A study evaluating the safety of spinosad (doses up to 5X) with or without milbemycin (doses up to 10X) in Collies homozygous and heterozygous for the *ABCB1* (MDR1) mutation did not cause signs of neuro-toxicosis (Sherman *et al.* 2010).

Adverse Effects

Spinosad appears to be very well tolerated in dogs and most animals will not show any adverse effects after dosing. The following adverse reactions are possible and based on post-approval adverse drug event reporting (listed in decreasing order of frequency): vomiting, depression/lethargy, anorexia, ataxia, diarrhea, pruritus, trembling, hypersalivation and seizures.

In cats, adverse effects are infrequent but vomiting, lethargy, reduced appetite, weight loss, and diarrhea have been reported.

Reproductive/Nursing Safety

The manufacturer states to use with caution in breeding females, but the drug appears to be relatively safe to use during pregnancy or lactation. In female Beagles dosed at 1.3X and 4.4X every 28 days prior to mating, during gestation, and during a six-week lactation period, no changes in dam conception rates or mortality, body temperature, necropsy, or histopathology were seen in dams or puppies. Treated dams experienced more vomiting, especially at one hour post-dose, than control dams. Puppies from dams treated at 1.3X had lower body weights; those from the 4.4X group experienced more lethargy, dehydration, weakness, and felt cold. Safe use in breeding males has not been evaluated.

The cat product label states: Safe use in breeding, pregnant, or lactating cats has not been evaluated.

In a pilot study in 3 dogs, spinosyns were excreted in milk at levels ≈ 2.5X of that found in the plasma. Puppy mortality and morbidity was highest in puppies from the dam with the highest spinosyn milk levels, but causal effect cannot be inferred due to the small sample size of the study.

Overdosage/Acute Toxicity

Spinosad appears to be very safe in mammals with the oral LD50 in mice >5000 mg/kg. Acute overdoses in dogs appear relatively innocuous. In a dose tolerance study, in adult Beagles dosed orally up to 100 mg/kg (16.7X) PO once daily for 10 consecutive days, vomiting was routinely seen after the dose was administered. No significant changes in hematology, blood coagulation or urinalysis parameters were noted, but phospholipidosis (vacuolation) of the lymphoid tissue and mild elevations in ALT occurred in all dogs.

There were 964 single agent exposures to spinosad reported to the ASPCA Animal Poison Control Center (APCC) during 2009-2013. Of the 851 dogs, 545 were symptomatic with 49% lethargic, 41% vomiting, 24% ataxic and 21% trembling. There were 114 cats, 39 of which were symptomatic (49% vomiting).

Drug Interactions

The following drug interactions have either been reported or are theoretical in humans or animals receiving spinosad and may be of significance in veterinary patients. Unless otherwise noted, use together is not necessarily contraindicated, but weigh the potential risks and perform additional monitoring when appropriate.

- **IVERMECTIN:** It has been recommended not to use with the high extra-label doses of ivermectin (Kuhl 2009), as spinosad can increase the plasma concentrations of ivermectin in dogs with the area under curve (AUC) increasing 3.6-fold (Dunn *et al.* 2011). When used with heartworm preventatives at their labeled doses, spinosad appears safe to use. No signs of signs of neuro-toxicosis were seen in Collies homozygous and heterozygous for the *ABCB1* (MDR1) mutation in a study evaluating the safety of spinosad (doses up to 5X) with or without milbemycin (doses up to 10X) (Sherman *et al.* 2010).

- **OTHER DRUGS AFFECTED BY P-GLYCOPROTEIN INHIBITORS:** Spinosad has been shown to be a substrate and potent inhibitor of canine p-glycoprotein, and other orally dosed drugs such as **cyclosporine**, **verapamil**, **ketoconazole**, or **loperamide** could potentially interact at the level of the intestinal tract. Because spinosad is so highly bound to plasma proteins, the risk for additional interactions at the blood-brain barrier appear to be to be limited (Schrickx 2014).

Laboratory Considerations

- No specific concerns noted.

Doses

- **DOGS:**

  Spinosad alone for prevention or treatment of flea infestations (labeled dose; FDA-approved): 30 – 60 mg/kg (minimum dosage of 30 mg/kg) PO once monthly with food. **Note:** Do not use the dosing table for cats as overdoses could occur. (Adapted from label information; *Comfortis*®)

  Spinosad/Milbemycin for the prevention of heartworm disease, for the prevention and treatment of flea infestations, and the treatment and control of adult hookworm, adult roundworm and adult whipworm infections in dogs and puppies 8 weeks of age or older and 5 pounds of body weight or greater (labeled-dose; FDA-approved): Given orally once a month at the minimum dosage of 30 mg/kg of spinosad and 0.5 mg/kg of milbemycin oxime. For heartworm prevention, give once monthly for at least 3 months after exposure to mosquitoes. See label information for a weight-based dosage table. (Adapted from label —*Trifexis*®)

- **CATS:**

  For prevention or treatment of flea infestations (labeled dose; FDA-approved): 50 mg/kg (minimum dosage) PO just prior to or after feeding once monthly. Alternatively, it may be offered in food or administered like other tablet medications. (Adapted from label information; *Comfortis*®)

Monitoring

- Efficacy.

Client Information

- Oral adult flea killer for dogs and cats; has rapid action.
- Give once a month with food. If vomiting occurs within an hour of administration, re-dose with another full dose.
- When used as directed on the label, it appears very safe.
- Can be harmful to wildlife so dispose of unused drug carefully. Keep chewable tablets well out of reach of children and animals.

Chemistry/Synonyms

Spinosad is a spinosyn class insecticide and contains two major factors, spinosyn A and spinosyn D that are derived from the naturally occurring bacterium, *Saccharopolyspora spinosa*. Spinosad may also be known as spinosyn A & B, DE-105, or XDE-105. Trade names include *Comfortis*® and *Natroba*® (human topical), or *Extinosad*®.

Storage/Stability

Chewable tablets should be stored at 20-25°C (68-77°F), excursions permitted between 15-30°C (59-86°F).

Compatibility/Compounding Considerations

No specific information noted.

Dosage Forms/Regulatory Status

VETERINARY-LABELED PRODUCTS:

Spinosad Chewable Tablets: 140 mg, 270 mg, 560 mg, 810 mg, 1620 mg; *Comfortis*®; (Rx). FDA-approved for use in dogs.

Spinosad Chewable Tablets: 90 mg, 140 mg, 270 mg, 560 mg; *Comfortis*® for Cats; (Rx). FDA-approved for cats.

Spinosad/Milbemycin Chewable Tablets: 140 mg/2.3 mg; 270 mg/4.5 mg; 560 mg/9.3 mg; 810 mg/13.5 mg; 1620 mg/27 mg; *Trifexis*®; (Rx). FDA-approved for use in dogs.

HUMAN-LABELED PRODUCTS:

None for systemic use. There is a topical product (for head lice) Spinosad 0.9% topical suspension in 120 mL: *Natroba*®; (Rx)

Revisions/References

Monograph revised/updated August 2014.

Dunn, S. T., et al. (2011). Pharmacokinetic Interaction of the Antiparasitic Agents Ivermectin and Spinosad in Dogs. Drug Metabolism and Disposition 39(5): 789-95.

Ihrke, P. (2009). Managing flea allergy- Where are we in 2009? Proceedings: WVC. accessed via Veterinary Information Network; vin.com

Jazic, E. (2010). Out With the Old, In With the New: New Approaches to the Management of Canine and Feline Demodicosis. Proceedings: WVC. accessed via Veterinary Information Network; vin.com

Kuhl, K. (2009). Integrated Parasite Control in Dogs. Proceedings: WVC. accessed via Veterinary Information Network; vin.com

Rosenkrantz, W. S. (2010). Flea Control Update. Proceedings: WVC. accessed via Veterinary Information Network; vin.com

Schrickx, J. A. (2014). Spinosad is a potent inhibitor of canine P-glycoprotein. Veterinary Journal 200(1): 195-6.

Sherman, J. G., et al. (2010). Evaluation of the safety of spinosad and milbemycin 5-oxime orally administered to Collies with the MDR1 gene mutation. American Journal of Veterinary Research 71(1): 115-9.

Snyder, D. E., et al. (2009). Preliminary study on the acaricidal efficacy of spinosad administered orally to dogs infested with the brown dog tick, Rhipicephalus sanguineus (Latreille, 1806) (Acari: Ixodidae). Veterinary Parasitology 166(1-2): 131-5.

Spironolactone

(speer-on-oh-lak-tone)   Aldactone®

Aldosterone Antagonist

Prescriber Highlights

▶ Aldosterone antagonist used as a potassium sparing diuretic or for adjunctive treatment for heart failure (use is controversial for heart failure in dogs); should not be substituted for furosemide in CHF.

▶ Contraindications: Hyperkalemia, Addison's disease, anuria, acute renal failure or significant renal impairment.

▶ Caution: Any renal impairment or hepatic disease.

▶ Adverse Effects: Facial dermatitis in cats. Hyperkalemia, hyponatremia, & dehydration possible; increased BUN & mild acidosis in patients with renal impairment. GI distress (vomiting, anorexia, etc.), CNS effects (lethargy, ataxia, etc.), & endocrine changes possible.

Uses/Indications

Spironolactone may be used in patients with congestive heart failure who do not adequately respond to furosemide and ACE inhibitors, who develop hypokalemia on other diuretics, and are unwilling or unable to supplement with exogenous potassium sources. In a study evaluating spironolactone's efficacy for improving survival in dogs with naturally occurring mitral regurgitation in myxomatous mitral valve disease (MMVD) the author's concluded that spironolactone added to conventional cardiac therapy decreased the risk of cardiac-related death, euthanasia, or severe worsening of the disease (Bernay *et al.* 2010). However the clinical relevance of these findings has been questioned due to the study design, event rate, patient withdrawals, and patient categorization with regard to heart failure (Kittleson *et al.* 2010). While efficacy remains in doubt, a randomized, double blinded, prospective study found that spironolactone added to conventional treatment (ACE-inhibitors, furosemide ± digoxin) did not increase risk for adverse effects, death caused by cardiac disease, renal disease, or both, hyperkalemia, or azotemia (Lefebvre *et al.* 2013).

Spironolactone may also be effective in treating ascites as it has less potential to increase ammonia levels than other diuretics.

It may find a (minor) role in treating renal disease. In rats, it has been shown to decrease proteinuria and glomerulosclerosis in experimental models of renal disease, but clinical effectiveness in dogs has been disappointing.

Pharmacology/Actions

Spironolactone is sometimes categorized as a potassium-sparing diuretic or a mineralocorticoid blocker. Aldosterone is competitively inhibited by spironolactone in the distal renal tubules with resultant increased excretion of sodium, chloride, and water, and decreased excretion of potassium, ammonium, phosphate, and titratable acid. Spironolactone has no effect on carbonic anhydrase or renal transport mechanisms and has its greatest effect in patients with hyperaldosteronism. When used alone in healthy dogs, spironolactone does not appear to cause significant diuresis (Jeunesse *et al.* 2004). As a diuretic, spironolactone is not commonly used alone as most sodium is reabsorbed at the proximal tubules. Combining it with a thiazide or loop diuretic maximize its diuretic effect.

In humans, spironolactone can have antifibrotic effects on cardiac muscle. Whether this occurs in veterinary patients with heart failure is controversial. One study in Maine Coon cats with hypertrophic cardiomyopathy but not in heart failure, showed that spironolactone did not cause significant changes in diastolic function or left ventricular mass after 4 months of treatment (MacDonald *et al.* 2008).

Pharmacokinetics

Because spironolactone is unstable if frozen and thawed, pharmacokinetic studies in animals are not readily performed. In fasted dogs, oral bioavailability of spironolactone (measured via its main metabolites) is ≈ 50%, but increases up to 90% when given with food. About 70% of a dose is found in the feces and 18% in the urine. In a recent pharmacodynamic study done in 15 Beagles, the dose required to inhibit the action of aldosterone by 50% was estimated to be ≈ 1.1 mg/kg and the authors suggest that the dose for spironolactone would be ≈ 2 mg/kg PO once daily to obtain concentrations effective at inhibiting the aldosterone levels associated with CHF in dogs (Guyonnet *et al.* 2010).

In humans, spironolactone is >90% bioavailable and peak levels are reached within 1-2 hours. The diuretic action of spironolactone (when used alone) is gradually attained and generally reaches its maximal effect on the third day of therapy.

Spironolactone and its active metabolite, canrenone, are both ≈ 98% bound to plasma proteins. Both spironolactone and its metabolites may cross the placenta. Canrenone has been detected in breast milk. Spironolactone is rapidly metabolized (half-life of 1-2 hours) to several metabolites, including canrenone, which has diuretic activity. Canrenone is more slowly eliminated, with an average half-life of ≈ 20 hours.

Contraindications/Precautions/Warnings

Spironolactone is contraindicated in patients with hyperkalemia, Addison's disease, anuria, acute renal failure or significant renal impairment. It should be used cautiously in patients with hepatic disease, but is often used to treat ascites.

The label for the canine product licensed in the U.K. states: Do not use in animals used for, or intended for use in breeding. Do not use the product in dogs suffering from hypoadrenocorticism, hyperkalemia or hyponatremia. Do not administer spironolactone in conjunction with NSAIDs to dogs with renal insufficiency.

Adverse Effects

Adverse effects are usually considered mild and reversible upon discontinuation of the drug. Gastrointestinal side effects, anorexia, and electrolyte (hyperkalemia, hyponatremia) and water balance (dehydration) abnormalities are the most likely adverse effects with spironolactone therapy. In dogs, electrolytes do not appear to be significantly affected. After cats received 2.7 mg/kg spironolactone twice daily for 7-9 days, the following serum values increased (on average) significantly: potassium 0.39 mEq/L, calcium 0.48 mg/dL, creatinine 0.22 mg/dL, phosphorus 0.63 mg/dL and total protein 0.51 mg/dL (Abbott *et al.* 2006).

A study in dogs found that spironolactone added to conventional treatment (ACE-inhibitors, furosemide ± digoxin) did not increase risk for adverse effects, death caused by cardiac disease, renal disease, or both, hyperkalemia, or azotemia (Lefebvre *et al.* 2013).

In cats, an interim report of a study using spironolactone (1.7 – 3.3 mg/kg PO once daily; n=16) with benazepril and furosemide reported no severe adverse events except worsening of heart failure (death, euthanasia, aortic thromboembolism and one case of severe anorexia). However, of the original 16 cats enrolled, 11 have died or been euthanized, 2 were withdrawn, 1 has completed 15 month follow-up and 2 cats remain in the study (James *et al.* 2013). In the study in Maine Coon cats, approximately 1/3 of treated subjects developed severe facial dermatitis.

Transient increases in BUN and mild acidosis may occur in patients with renal impairment. Use of spironolactone in patients with severe renal impairment may lead to hyperkalemia.

Spironolactone reportedly inhibits the synthesis of testosterone and may increase the peripheral conversion of testosterone to estradiol; gynecomastia has been reported in human males. Long-term toxicity studies in rats have demonstrated that spironolactone is tumorigenic in that species.

Reproductive/Nursing Safety

Spironolactone or its metabolites may cross the placental barrier. Feminization occurs in male rat fetuses. In humans, the FDA categorizes this drug as category *D* for use during pregnancy (*There is evidence of human fetal risk, but the potential benefits from the use of the drug in pregnant women may be acceptable despite its potential risks.*)

Canrenone, a metabolite of spironolactone, appears in maternal milk. In humans, the estimated maximum dose to the infant is ≈ 0.2% of the mother's daily dose. Use with caution in nursing patients, but it is unlikely of clinical significance in veterinary patients.

Overdosage/Acute Toxicity

Information on overdosage of spironolactone is apparently unavailable. Should an acute overdose occur, it is suggested to follow the guidelines outlined in the chlorothiazide and furosemide monographs. Contact an animal poison control center for further guidance.

Drug Interactions

The following drug interactions have either been reported or are theoretical in humans or animals receiving spironolactone and may be of significance in veterinary patients. Unless otherwise noted, use together is not necessarily contraindicated, but weigh the potential risks and perform additional monitoring when appropriate.

- **DIGOXIN**: Spironolactone may increase the half-life of digoxin; enhanced monitoring of digoxin serum levels and effects are warranted when spironolactone is used with these agents.
- **MITOTANE**: Spironolactone may mute the effects of mitotane if given concurrently, but very limited information is available on this potential interaction; monitor carefully.
- **NEUROMUSCULAR BLOCKERS, NON-DEPOLARIZING**: Increase in neuromuscular blockade effects possible.
- **POTASSIUM-SPARING DIURETICS, OTHER** (e.g., **triamterene**): Hyperkalemia possible.
- **POTASSIUM SUPPLEMENTS**: Hyperkalemia possible.
- **SALICYLATES**: Spironolactone's diuretic effects may be decreased if **aspirin** or other salicylates are administered concomitantly.

Laboratory Considerations

- Spironolactone may give falsely elevated **digoxin** values, if using a radioimmune assay (RIA) method.
- Fluorometric methods of determining plasma and urinary **17-hydroxycorticosteroids** (cortisol) may be interfered with by spironolactone.

Doses

- **DOGS:**

  For adjunctive treatment of heart failure (extra-label):
  a) U.K. labeled dose (extra-label in USA): 2 mg/kg PO once daily with food. (Adapted from label; *Prilactone®*)
  b) Extra-label doses: Most recommend using 1 – 2 mg/kg PO once daily, but dosing ranges of 0.5 – 4 mg/kg PO once daily have been noted. Whether any clinical benefit is derived from spironolactone is controversial.

  For treating ascites (extra-label): Attempt at treating underlying abnormality. When ascites is caused by right-sided heart failure: Be sure owner is administering medication properly and the prescription is correct. Increase furosemide to 4 – 6 mg/kg PO q8h (generally speaking dose should be increased until all the abnormal accumulated fluid is eliminated or unacceptable azo-

temia develops). Optimize ACE inhibitor dose. Restrict dietary sodium. Add spironolactone at 1 – 2 mg/kg PO q12h. Initially (3 times weekly) substitute one of the oral furosemide doses with a SC dose. Consider adding hydrochlorothiazide initially at 2 mg/kg PO every other day. (Connolly 2006)

  For adjunctive treatment of hypertension (extra-label): 1 – 2 mg/kg PO q12h. Not first-line therapy; effectiveness has been marginal when used as sole therapy for the management of hypertension. (Syme 2011)

- **CATS:**

  As a diuretic in heart failure (extra-label): No definitive studies documenting efficacy were located. Anecdotally, some may add spironolactone at dog dosages when furosemide and ACE inhibitors do not control fluid accumulation in refractory CHF.

  For adjunctive treatment of hypertension (extra-label): 1 – 2 mg/kg PO q12h. Not first-line therapy; effectiveness has been marginal when used as sole therapy for the management of hypertension, even in cats with aldosterone secreting tumors; cutaneous drug reactions may also limit usefulness. (Syme 2011)

Monitoring

- Serum electrolytes, BUN, creatinine. Initially, 5-14 days after starting therapy and q2 months thereafter (Rush 2013).
- Hydration status.
- Blood pressure, if indicated.
- Clinical signs of edema/ascites; patient weight, if indicated.

Client Information

- When beginning this medicine your animal may urinate more often than normal.
- May be given with or without food, but giving with food may help prevent vomiting or nausea.
- Because this drug can change electrolytes (salts) in the blood, more frequent testing may be required.
- If animal has sores or is scratching its face (cats), has severe or continuing vomiting or diarrhea, acts extremely tired, has trouble walking or keeping balance, or stops eating, drinking, or urinating, contact your veterinarian immediately.

Chemistry/Synonyms

A synthetically produced aldosterone antagonist, spironolactone occurs as a cream-colored to light tan, crystalline powder with a faint mercaptan-like odor. It has a melting range of 198°-207°, with decomposition. Spironolactone is practically insoluble in water and soluble in alcohol.

Spironolactone may also be known as: espironolactona, SC-9420, spirolactone, spironolactonum; many trade names are available.

Storage/Stability

Spironolactone tablets should be stored at room temperature in tight, light-resistant containers.

Compatibility/Compounding Considerations

An extemporaneously prepared oral suspension can be prepared by pulverizing commercially available tablets and adding cherry syrup. This preparation is reportedly stable for at least one month when refrigerated.

Dosage Forms/Regulatory Status

VETERINARY-LABELED PRODUCTS:
None in the USA; in the U.K. and elsewhere, the following may be available:

Spironolactone Tablets: 10 mg, 40 mg, 80 mg; *Prilactone®*; (POM-V). Licensed for use in dogs.

Spironolactone Chewable Tablets: 10 mg, 50 mg, 100 mg; *Tempora®*; (POM-V). Licensed for use in dogs.

Benazepril/Spironolactone Tablets: 2.5 mg/20 mg, 5 mg/40 mg, & 10 mg/80 mg; *Cardalis®*; (POM-V). Licensed for use in dogs.

The ARCI (Racing Commissioners International) has designated this drug as a class 4 substance. See the appendix for more information.

HUMAN-LABELED PRODUCTS:

Spironolactone Oral Tablets: 25 mg, 50 mg & 100 mg; *Aldactone®*, generic; (Rx)

Spironolactone/Hydrochlorothiazide Oral Tablets: 25 mg/25 mg & 50 mg/50 mg; *Aldactazide®*, generic; (Rx)

Revisions/References

Monograph revised/updated August 2014.

Abbott, J. & K. Saker (2006). Serum chemistry variables of healthy cats receiving spironolactone, Proceedings: ACVIM. accessed via Veterinary Information Network; vin.com

Bernay, F., et al. (2010). Efficacy of Spironolactone on Survival in Dogs with Naturally Occurring Mitral Regurgitation Caused by Myxomatous Mitral Valve Disease. Journal of Veterinary Internal Medicine 24(2): 331-41.

Connolly, D. (2006). The ascitic dog. Proceedings: BSAVA Congress. accessed via Veterinary Information Network; vin.com

Guyonnet, J., et al. (2010). A preclinical pharmacokinetic and pharmacodynamic approach to determine a dose of spironolactone for treatment of congestive heart failure in dog. J. Vet. Pharmacol. Ther. 33(3): 260-7.

James, R., et al. (2013). Safety of oral administration of spironolactone in cats with heart failure: Interim results of The SEISICAT Study. Journal of Veterinary Internal Medicine 27(3): 638-.

Jeunesse, E., et al. (2004). Spironolactone as a diuretic agent in the dog: Is the water becoming muddy? Proceedings: ACVIM Forum. accessed via Veterinary Information Network; vin.com

Kittleson, M. D. & J. Bonagura (2010). Letter to the Editor re: Efficacy of Spironolactone on Survival in Dogs with Naturally Occurring Mitral Regurgitation Caused by Myxomatous Mitral Valve Disease. J Vet Intern Med 24: 1245-6.

Lefebvre, H. P., et al. (2013). Safety of Spironolactone in Dogs with Chronic Heart Failure because of Degenerative Valvular Disease: A Population-Based, Longitudinal Study. Journal of Veterinary Internal Medicine 27(5): 1083-91.

MacDonald, K. A., et al. (2008). Effect of spironolactone on diastolic function and left ventricular mass in maine coon cats with familial hypertrophic cardiomyopathy. Journal of Veterinary Internal Medicine 22(2): 335-41.

Rush, J. E. (2013). Diuretics in the Management of Heart Failure. IVECCS. accessed via Veterinary Information Network; vin.com

Syme, H. (2011). Hypertension in Small Animal Kidney Disease. Veterinary Clinics of North America-Small Animal Practice 41(1): 63-+.

Stanozolol

(stah-no-zo-lahl)   Winstrol®-V

Anabolic Steroid

Prescriber Highlights

▶ Anabolic steroid; controlled substance in the USA. FDA-approved products no longer marketed in USA. Potentially useful in dogs for medical treatment of tracheal collapse.

▶ Contraindications: Pregnant animals, breeding stallions, food animals. Extreme Caution: Cats, hepatic dysfunction, hypercalcemia, history of myocardial infarction, pituitary insufficiency, prostate carcinoma, mammary carcinoma, benign prostatic hypertrophy, & during the nephrotic stage of nephritis. Caution: Cardiac & renal dysfunction with enhanced fluid & electrolyte monitoring.

▶ Adverse Effects: Potentially high incidence of hepatotoxicity in cats. Other possible effects: sodium, calcium, potassium, water, chloride, & phosphate retention; hepatotoxicity, behavioral (androgenic) changes, & reproductive abnormalities (oligospermia, estrus suppression).

▶ Category "X" for pregnancy; teratogenicity outweighs any possible benefit.

▶ Drug Interactions; lab interactions.

Uses/Indications

Labeled indications for the previously marketed veterinary stanozolol product *Winstrol®-V* (Winthrop/Upjohn) included "...to improve appetite, promote weight gain, and increase strength and vitality..." in dogs, cats and horses. The manufacturer also stated that: "Anabolic therapy is intended primarily as an adjunct to other specific and supportive therapy, including nutritional therapy." In a review of the evidence supporting anabolic steroid use in horses, the authors conclude: "Level 1 evidence for the efficacy of anabolic steroids in horses for therapeutic uses is not found in the biomedical literature. Evidence in other species exists for the efficacy of anabolic steroids in treating anemia and increasing muscle mass after illness or injury, but that evidence is not unequivocal, and the applicability to horses has not been demonstrated. There is little evidence in other species for the efficacy of anabolic steroids for increasing appetite." (Fajt *et al.* 2008)

A study in sheep using an experimental model of osteoarthritis, found that intra-articular stanozolol reduced osteophytes formation and subchondral bone reaction, and promoted articular cartilage regeneration (Spadari *et al.* 2013).

Like nandrolone, stanozolol has been used to treat anemia of chronic disease. Because stanozolol has been demonstrated to enhance fibrinolysis after parenteral injection it may be efficacious in the treatment of feline aortic thromboembolism or thrombosis in nephrotic syndrome, however clinical studies and/or experience are apparently lacking for this indication at present.

A controlled study in dogs using stanozolol as a conservative treatment for collapsing trachea (without bronchitis), reported that at the end of study (75 days), 93% of dogs in the stanozolol group had an improvement of the tracheal collapse grade. Eight of the 14 treated dogs were deemed 'cured' (Adamama-Moraitou *et al.* 2011).

Pharmacology/Actions

Stanozolol possesses the actions of other anabolic agents but it may be less androgenic than other anabolics that are used in veterinary medicine.

In the presence of adequate protein and calories, anabolic steroids promote body tissue building processes and can reverse catabolism. As these agents are either derived from or are closely related to testosterone, the anabolics have varying degrees of androgenic effects. Endogenous testosterone release may be suppressed by inhibiting luteinizing hormone (LH). Large doses can impede spermatogenesis by negative feedback inhibition of FSH.

Anabolic steroids can also stimulate erythropoiesis possibly by stimulation of erythropoietic stimulating factor. Anabolics can cause nitrogen, sodium, potassium and phosphorus retention and decrease the urinary excretion of calcium.

For medical treatment of tracheal collapse in dogs, it is postulated that stanozolol could increase tracheal wall strength via enhancing protein or collagen synthesis, increasing chondroitin sulfate content, increasing lean body mass, and decreasing inflammation.

Pharmacokinetics

In horses (n=26) following a 0.55 mg IM injection of compounded stanozolol suspension, peak levels occur at 7 days. Median half-life was 3-4 days, but ranged from 1.6-14.7 days (Moeller *et al.* 2013).

Contraindications/Precautions/Warnings

Stanozolol is contraindicated in pregnant animals and in breeding stallions and should not be administered to horses intended for food purposes.

Because of reported hepatotoxicity associated with stanozolol in cats, it should only be used in this species with extreme caution.

The manufacturer recommends using stanozolol cautiously in patients with cardiac and renal dysfunction with enhanced fluid and electrolyte monitoring.

In humans, anabolic agents are contraindicated in patients with hepatic dysfunction, hypercalcemia, patients with a history of myocardial infarction (can cause hypercholesterolemia), pituitary insufficiency, prostate carcinoma, benign prostatic hypertrophy, during the nephrotic stage of nephritis, and in selected patients with breast carcinoma.

Adverse Effects

The manufacturer lists only 'mild androgenic effects' in dogs, cats, and horses and then only when used with excessively high doses for a prolonged period of time.

One study in cats, demonstrated a very high incidence of hepatotoxicity associated with stanozolol use and the authors recommended that this drug not be used in cats until further toxicological studies are performed.

Potentially (from human data), adverse reactions of the anabolic agents in dogs and cats could include: sodium, calcium, potassium, water, chloride, and phosphate retention, hepatotoxicity, behavioral (androgenic) changes, and reproductive abnormalities (oligospermia, estrus suppression).

Reproductive/Nursing Safety

In humans, the FDA categorizes this drug as category *X* for use during pregnancy (*Studies in animals or humans demonstrate fetal abnormalities or adverse reaction; reports indicate evidence of fetal risk. The risk of use in pregnant women clearly outweighs any possible benefit.*) In a separate system evaluating the safety of drugs in canine and feline pregnancy (Papich 1989), this drug is categorized as in class: *D* (*Contraindicated. These drugs have been shown to cause congenital malformations or embryotoxicity.*)

It is not known whether anabolic steroids are excreted in maternal milk. Because of the potential for serious adverse reactions in nursing offspring, use with extreme caution in patients that are nursing.

Overdosage/Acute Toxicity

No information was located for this specific agent. In humans, sodium and water retention can occur after overdosage of anabolic steroids. It is suggested to treat supportively and monitor liver function should an inadvertent overdose be administered.

Drug Interactions

The following drug interactions have either been reported or are theoretical in humans or animals receiving stanozolol and may be of significance in veterinary patients. Unless otherwise noted, use together is not necessarily contraindicated, but weigh the potential risks and perform additional monitoring when appropriate.

- **ANTICOAGULANTS** (*e.g.,* **heparin, warfarin,** etc.): Anabolic agents as a class may potentiate the effects of anticoagulants; monitoring of INR/PT's and dosage adjustment, if necessary, of the anticoagulant are recommended.
- **CORTICOSTEROIDS:** Anabolics may enhance the edema that can be associated with ACTH or adrenal steroid therapy.
- **INSULIN:** Diabetic patients receiving insulin may need dosage adjustments if anabolic therapy is added or discontinued; anabolics may decrease blood glucose and decrease insulin requirements.

Laboratory Considerations

- Concentrations of protein bound iodine (PBI) can be decreased in patients receiving androgen/anabolic therapy, but the clinical significance of this is probably not important. Androgen/anabolic agents can decrease amounts of thyroxine-binding globulin and decrease **total T4** concentrations and increase resin uptake of **T3 and T4.** Free thyroid hormones are unaltered and there is no evidence of dysfunction.
- Both **creatinine** and **creatine** excretion can be decreased by anabolic steroids.
- Anabolic steroids can increase the urinary excretion of **17-keto-steroids.**

- Androgenic/anabolic steroids may alter **blood glucose** levels.
- Androgenic/anabolic steroids may suppress **clotting factors** II, V, VII, and X.
- Anabolic agents can affect **liver function tests** (BSP retention, SGOT, SGPT, bilirubin, and alkaline phosphatase).

Doses

- **DOGS:**

  As an anabolic agent per (formerly) labeled indications: Small Breeds: 1 – 2 mg PO twice daily; or 25 mg deep IM, may repeat weekly. Large Breeds: 2 – 4 mg PO twice daily; or 50 mg deep IM, may repeat weekly. Treatment should continue for several weeks, depending on response and condition of animal. (Package Insert; *Winstrol*-*V*)

  As a treatment for tracheal collapse: (extra-label): In the study, dogs in the treatment group received 0.15 mg/kg PO twice daily for 2 months then tapered for 15 days. (Adamama-Moraitou *et al.* 2011)

- **CATS:**

  Note: See warnings section above regarding hepatotoxicity in cats. Most do not recommend using in cats.

  As an anabolic agent per (formerly) labeled indications: 1 – 2 mg PO twice daily or 25 mg deep IM; may repeat weekly. Treatment should continue for several weeks depending on response and condition of animal. (Package Insert; *Winstrol*-*V*)

- **FERRETS:**

  As an anabolic (extra-label): 0.5 mg/kg PO or SC twice daily; use with caution in hepatic disease. (Williams 2000)

- **RABBITS, RODENTS, SMALL MAMMALS:**

  Rabbits; as an appetite stimulant (extra-label): 0.5 – 2 mg PO once. (Ivey *et al.* 2000)

- **HORSES:** (NOTE: ARCI UCGFS CLASS 4 DRUG)

  As an anabolic agent per (formerly) labeled indications: 0.55 mg/kg (25 mg/100 lb of body weight) IM deeply. May repeat weekly for up to and including 4 weeks. (Package Insert; *Winstrol*-*V*)

- **BIRDS:**

  As an anabolic agent to promote weight gain and recovery from disease (extra-label): 0.5 – 1 mL/kg (25 – 50 mg/kg) IM once or twice weekly. Use with caution in birds with renal disease. (Clubb 1986)

- **REPTILES:**

  For most species post-surgically and in very debilitated animals (extra-label): 5 mg/kg IM once a week as needed. (Gauvin 1993)

Monitoring

- Androgenic side effects.
- Fluid and electrolyte status, if indicated.
- Liver function tests if indicated.
- RBC count, indices, if indicated.
- Weight, appetite.

Client Information

- May give with or without food; give with food if vomiting or stomach upset occurs.
- Can cause behavior changes, including more sexual behaviors.
- Cats may be prone to developing liver problems while receiving this medication.
- Pregnant women should handle this drug with caution.
- Controlled substance in the USA. It is against federal law to use, give away or sell this medication to others than for whom it was prescribed.

Chemistry/Synonyms

An anabolic steroid, stanozolol occurs as an odorless, nearly colorless, crystalline powder that can exist in two forms: prisms that melt at approximately 235°C and needles that melt at ≈ 155°C. It is sparingly soluble in alcohol and insoluble in water.

Stanozolol may also be known as: androstanazole, estanozolol, methylstanazole, NSC-43193, stanozololum, win-14833, *Menabol*, *Neurabol*, *Stanol*, *Stromba*, *Strombaject* and *Winstrol*.

Storage/Stability

Stanozolol tablets should be stored in tight, light-resistant packaging, preferably at room temperature.

Compatibility/Compounding Considerations

No specific information noted.

Dosage Forms/Regulatory Status

VETERINARY-LABELED PRODUCTS: NONE.
Winstrol-V tablets and injection were previously marketed. Stanozolol may be available from compounding pharmacies.

The ARCI (Racing Commissioners International) has designated this drug as a class 4 substance. See the appendix for more information. A pharmacokinetic study concluded that following a single IM injection (0.55 mg/kg) of stanozolol suspension in exercise-conditioned Thoroughbred horses, a withdrawal guideline of 60 days is recommended (Moeller *et al.* 2013).

HUMAN-LABELED PRODUCTS: NONE.

Revisions/References

Monograph revised/updated August 2014.

Adamama-Moraitou, K. K., et al. (2011). Conservative management of canine tracheal collapse with stanozolol: A double blinded, placebo control clinical trial. International Journal of Immunopathology and Pharmacology 24(1): 111-8.

Clubb, S. L. (1986). Therapeutics: Individual and Flock Treatment Regimens. *Clinical Avian Medicine and Surgery*. G. J. Harrison and L. R. Harrison. Philadelphia, W.B. Saunders: 327-55.

Fajt, V. R. & C. McCook (2008). An evidence-based analysis of anabolic steroids as therapeutic agents in horses. Equine Veterinary Education 20(10): 542-4.

Gauvin, J. (1993). Drug therapy in reptiles. Seminars in Avian & Exotic Med 2(1): 48-59.

Ivey, E. & J. Morrisey (2000). Therapeutics for Rabbits. Vet Clin NA: Exotic Anim Pract 3:1(Jan): 183-216.

Moeller, B. C., et al. (2013). Pharmacokinetics of stanozolol in Thoroughbred horses following intramuscular administration. J. Vet. Pharmacol. Ther. 36(2): 201-4.

Papich, M. (1989). Effects of drugs on pregnancy. *Current Veterinary Therapy X: Small Animal Practice*. R. Kirk. Philadelphia, Saunders: 1291-9.

Spadari, A., et al. (2013). Effects of intraarticular treatment with stanozolol on synovial membrane and cartilage in an ovine model of osteoarthritis. Research in Veterinary Science 94(3): 379-87.

Williams, B. (2000). Therapeutics in Ferrets. Vet Clin NA: Exotic Anim Pract 3:1(Jan): 131-53.

Staphylococcal Phage Lysate

(staf-loe-kok-al faje lye-sate)   Staphage Lysate (SP)*, *SPL*

Immune Stimulant

Prescriber Highlights

▶ Injectable immune stimulant used to treat dogs with recurrent, idiopathic, staphylococcal pyodermas.

▶ May cause hypersensitivity (local or systemic).

Uses/Indications

Staphylococcal phage lysate (SPL) is labeled for treatment of canine pyoderma and related staphylococcal hypersensitivity, or polymicrobial skin infections with a staphylococcal component. Some veterinary dermatologists have used SPL most commonly to treat recurrent, idiopathic, staphylococcal pyodermas in combination (at least initially) with an appropriate antibiotic. There do not appear to be any controlled studies documenting efficacy, but anecdotally some state that it helps a subset of patients (up to 70%).

Pharmacology/Actions

SPL apparently enhances cell-mediated immunity increasing the capability of macrophages to inactivate staphylococci. It can stimulate production of tumor necrosis factor, interleukin-6, interleukin-γ, and γ-interferon.

Pharmacokinetics

No information was located.

Contraindications/Precautions/Warnings

The label states that "there are no known contraindications to the use of *SPL* except that in highly allergic patients, reduced desensitizing doses may be indicated." However, use with extreme caution, if at all, in patients with prior systemic hypersensitivity reactions to it or documented hypersensitivity reactions to beef products (contains unfiltered beef heart infusion broth).

Avoid administering subsequent doses at the same injection site.

The product contains no preservative so it must be handled aseptically. It is recommended to use the entire contents when the vial is opened.

Adverse Effects

Adverse effects reported for SPL include post vaccine-type reactions (fever, malaise, etc.) and injection site reactions (redness, itching, swelling) that may occur within 2-3 hours after injection and persist up to 3 days. If these effects are excessive, the manufacturer recommends dosage reduction.

Systemic hypersensitivity reactions are thought to occur rarely. Signs could include weakness, vomiting, diarrhea, severe itching, rapid breathing, and/or fatigue/lassitude. Should an anaphylactic-type reaction occur, treat supportively; the manufacturer recommends epinephrine and atropine as antidotes.

Reproductive/Nursing Safety

Studies performed in rats and rabbits demonstrated no impaired fertility or fetal harm.

No information was located on safety during nursing, but it is unlikely to be of concern.

Overdosage/Acute Toxicity

No specific information was located. Other than an increased risk for local or systemic hypersensitivity reactions, significant morbidity appears unlikely.

Drug Interactions

▪ **CELL-MEDIATED IMMUNOSUPPRESSIVE DRUGS** (*e.g., **corticosteroids, cyclosporine***): These drugs may reduce the efficacy of SPL.

Laboratory Considerations

▪ No significant concerns noted.

Doses

▪ **DOGS:**

For labeled indications (not an FDA-approved product): Highly allergic patients: Skin test with 0.05 – 0.1 mL intradermally. Therapy: Initially, 0.2 mL SC, then incremental increases of 0.2 mL once a week to 1 mL (a total of 5 injections). Then continue at 1 mL SC weekly for approximately 10-12 weeks.

For non-allergic patients: 0.5 mL SC twice weekly for 10-12 weeks, then 0.5 – 1 mL every 1-2 weeks.

Concomitant antibiotic therapy is recommended for an initial 4-6 week period.

Maximum dose should be decreased in small dogs and can be increased cautiously, if necessary, in large dogs to 1.5 mL. This dose is continued until improvement is demonstrated then the interval may be lengthened gradually to the longest interval that maintains adequate clinical control. (Label information; *Staphage Lysate (SPL)*)

For chronic recurrent idiopathic pyoderma (extra-label):

a) Pyoderma needs to be under control as this product is not a substitute for antibiotics. Injections are administered twice weekly (0.5 mL) and slowly reduced to 0.5 mL every 2 weeks. (Waisglass 2009)

b) 1 mL SC once per week or 0.5 mL twice weekly for 4-6 months. If no significant recurrence, decrease to every 2 weeks, then every 3 weeks, etc. Works best to keep pyoderma from recurring. Should be used with antibiotics initially to get pyoderma into remission. (Zabel 2011)

Monitoring

- Clinical efficacy.
- Local and systemic reactions (see adverse effects).

Client Information

- This medication should ideally be administered at a veterinary practice where suitable treatment can be instituted should a serious adverse effect (*e.g.*, anaphylaxis) occur.
- Report to veterinarian any adverse effects noted (*e.g.*, local effects at injection site, itching, change in behavior or activity level, difficulty or unexplained rapid breathing, vomiting, diarrhea).

Chemistry/Synonyms

SPL is prepared by lysing cultures of *Staphylococcal aureas* (Cowan serologic types I & III; human strains) by a staphylococcal bacteriophage. Pre-lysed cell counts (120 – 180 CFU/mL) are used to standardize the product; ultrafiltration achieves bacteriologic sterility. The prepared solution contains *Staphylococcal aureas* components (protein A extracts), bacteriophage, and unfiltered beef heart infusion.

Storage/Stability

SPL should be stored in the refrigerator (2-7°C); do not freeze.

Unopened, properly stored vials and ampules have an average expiration date of one year past the shipment date. The product contains no preservative and must be handled aseptically. It is recommended using the entire contents of the vial after opening. Do not use if contents are cloudy.

Compatibility/Compounding Considerations

Do not mix with other drugs or solutions prior to administration.

Dosage Forms/Regulatory Status

VETERINARY-LABELED PRODUCTS:

Staphylococcal Phage Lysate (serotypes I & III): in 1 mL ampules (box of 10) and 10 mL multi-dose vials (no preservative added and manufacturer recommends using entire contents when opened); *Staphage Lysate (SPL)*®; (Biologic OTC)

Note: This product is a USDA-licensed biologic and not an FDA-approved product.

HUMAN-LABELED PRODUCTS: NONE.

Revisions/References

Monograph revised/updated August 2014.

Waisglass, S. (2009). New Perspectives on Pyoderma--Something Old and Something New. Proceedings: WVC. accessed via Veterinary Information Network; vin.com

Zabel, S. (2011). Bacterial Pyoderma. World Small Animal Veterinary Association World Congress. accessed via Veterinary Information Network; vin.com

Streptozocin

(strep-toe-zoe-sin)   Streptozotocin, Zanosar®

Antineoplastic

Prescriber Highlights

▶ Antineoplastic used primarily for treating recurrent insulinoma in dogs.

▶ Severe vomiting after treatment may occur. May be nephrotoxic, myelotoxic, & hepatotoxic. Diabetes mellitus can occur.

▶ To reduce nephrotoxicity, must give saline diuresis during administration.

Uses/Indications

At present the primary purpose for streptozocin use in veterinary medicine is as a treatment for insulinomas in dogs, particularly those with refractory hypoglycemia and when tumors are non-resectable or have metastasized. Its use has been limited by high rates of nephrotoxicity and other serious adverse effects. Streptozocin potentially could be used for other oncologic conditions as well.

Pharmacology/Actions

While streptozocin has activity against gram-positive and gram-negative bacteria, its cytotoxicity prevents it from clinical usefulness for this purpose. While its antineoplastic activity is not well understood, streptozocin is considered an alkylating agent and it inhibits DNA synthesis, probably by inhibiting precursor incorporation into DNA.

Streptozocin also exhibits a species-specific (in dogs, not humans) diabetogenic effect by reducing nicotinamide adenine dinucleotide (NAD) concentration in pancreatic beta cells. This effect is usually irreversible in animals with preexisting normal beta cell function.

Pharmacokinetics

Streptozocin must be administered IV. Its distribution characteristics are not well known, but the drug does distribute to most tissues; concentrations in the pancreas are higher than those found in plasma. Streptozocin is metabolized, probably in the liver. Both unchanged and metabolized drug are excreted in the urine.

Contraindications/Precautions/Warnings

Should be used for recurrent insulinoma only in dogs that have undergone previous surgery in which all of the tumor could not be resected. Confirmed histologic diagnosis is mandatory.

Streptozocin must be used with extreme caution in patients with decreased renal, bone marrow, or hepatic function.

Adverse Effects

The primary concern when streptozocin is used for treating insulinomas in dogs is the potential for the development of serious, permanent renal toxicity. Aggressive saline diuresis during drug administration appears to reduce incidence of nephrotoxicity. GI effects (vomiting/nausea) often occur and can be severe or protracted; increased liver enzymes (ALT) are not uncommon. Acute, transient hypoglycemia (secondary to streptozocin-damaged tumor cells releasing intracellular insulin stores) and permanent diabetes mellitus have been reported. Less commonly, hematologic changes (mild myelosuppression) are seen. Injection site reactions (including severe necrosis) can occur if the drug extravasates.

In a study (n=19 dogs) using an every other week dosing schedule, all dogs developed at least one adverse effect that included: gastrointestinal signs (nausea, anorexia, vomiting, regurgitation, diarrhea, colitis, or some combination of these; n=12); diabetes mellitus (n=8); renal injury (n=2; 1 with Fanconi syndrome, 1 with probable nephrogenic diabetes insipidus); increased ALT (n=8); hypoglycemic collapse or seizure (n=2); no neutropenia or thrombocytopenia was observed (Northrup *et al.* 2013).

Reproductive/Nursing Safety

Streptozocin has been shown to be teratogenic in rats; use during pregnancy when the benefits outweigh the risks. In humans, the FDA categorizes this drug as category C for use during pregnancy (*Animal studies have shown an adverse effect on the fetus, but there are no adequate studies in humans; or there are no animal reproduction studies and no adequate studies in humans.*)

It is not known whether streptozocin is excreted in milk. Because of the potential for serious adverse reactions in nursing offspring, consider using milk replacer if used in nursing patients.

Overdosage/Acute Toxicity

Severe toxicity may result if acutely overdosed (see Adverse Effects); calculate dosages carefully.

Drug Interactions

The following drug interactions have either been reported or are theoretical in humans or animals receiving streptozocin and may be of significance in veterinary patients. Unless otherwise noted, use together is not necessarily contraindicated, but weigh the potential risks and perform additional monitoring when appropriate.

- **DOXORUBICIN:** Streptozocin may prolong the half-life of doxorubicin; dosage adjustment may be required.
- **MYELOSUPPRESSIVE DRUGS, OTHER:** When streptozocin is used with other myelosuppressive drugs (*e.g.,* **carmustine**) additive or synergistic myelosuppression may occur.
- **NEPHROTOXIC DRUGS, OTHER** (**aminoglycosides, amphotericin B, cisplatin,** etc.): May cause additive nephrotoxicity when used with streptozocin.
- **NIACINAMIDE** (**nicotinamide**): Can block the diabetogenic effects of streptozocin without altering its antineoplastic activity; this may be beneficial or detrimental depending on the reason for use.

Doses

- **DOGS:**

  Note: Because of the potential toxicity of this drug to patients, veterinary personnel and clients, and since chemotherapy indications, treatment protocols, monitoring and safety guidelines often change, the following dosages should be used only as a general guide. Consultation with a veterinary oncologist and referral to current veterinary oncology references [*e.g.,* (Withrow *et al.* 2012); (Dobson *et al.* 2011); (Henry *et al.* 2009); (North *et al.* 2009); (Argyle *et al.* 2008)] are strongly recommended.

  For treatment of insulinoma (extra-label):

  a) In the study, streptozocin at 500 mg/m^2 was diluted in 36.6 mL/kg of 0.9% NaCl and administered IV over 2 hours. Treatments were administered every 2 weeks for a total goal of 5 doses. A 7-hour diuresis protocol (18.3 mL/kg/h of 0.9% NaCl given IV for 3 hours before and 2 hours after streptozocin) and prophylactic antiemetic treatment was administered with each dose. Some patients with persistent hypoglycemia were given prednisone 0.5 – 1 mg/kg q24h or divided q12h PO. Authors concluded that streptozocin can be safely administered to dogs with insulinoma, but serious adverse effects are possible. Additional investigation is required to better define its role in managing dogs with insulinoma. (Northrup *et al.* 2013)

  b) Normal saline is given IV at 18.3 mL/kg/hr for 3 hours, then streptozocin is administered at 500 mg/m^2 over two hours with the saline diuresis continuing. After streptozocin infusion completed, continue saline diuresis for another 2 hours. Antiemetics are given. May repeat at 3-week intervals until evidence of tumor progression, recurrence of hypoglycemia,

or drug toxicity. Monitor for myelosuppression and nephrotoxicity. (Moore *et al.* 2002)

Monitoring

- Blood glucose (efficacy).
- Baseline renal function tests (including urinalyses) and after treatment.
- CBC.
- Baseline liver function tests and before retreatment.
- Hydration status (especially for the first few days after treatment or if vomiting a problem).

Client Information

- Streptozocin is a chemotherapy (cancer) drug. The drug and its byproducts can be hazardous to other animals and people that come in contact with it. On the day your animal gets the drug and then for a few days afterward, all bodily waste (urine, feces, litter), blood, or vomit should only be handled while wearing disposable gloves. Seal the waste in a plastic bag and then place both the bag and gloves in with the regular trash.

Chemistry/Synonyms

Streptozocin is an antineoplastic antibiotic produced by *Streptomyces achromogenes*, although the commercial product is prepared synthetically. It occurs as an ivory colored, crystalline powder. It is very soluble in water and has a pKa of 1.35.

Streptozocin may also be known as: NSC-85998, streptozotocin, U-9889 and *Zanosar*®.

Storage/Stability

The lyophilized powder for injection should be stored in the refrigerator and protected from light. It is stable for at least 3 years after manufacture. If stored at room temperature, it is stable for at least 1 year after manufacture.

After reconstitution, the lyophilized powder for injection has a pH of 3.5-4.5. Citric acid is added to buffer the solution at a concentration of 22 mg/mL. The solution is stable for 48 hours at room temperature and 96 hours if refrigerated, but as no preservative is added, the manufacturer recommends using the drug within 12 hours of mixing.

Compatibility/Compounding Considerations

Dextrose 5% or 0.9% sodium chloride are used to reconstitute the solution.

Dosage Forms/Regulatory Status

VETERINARY-LABELED PRODUCTS: NONE.

HUMAN-LABELED PRODUCTS:

Streptozocin Powder for Injection: 1 gram (100 mg/mL) in vials; *Zanosar*®; (Rx)

Revisions/References

Monograph revised/updated August 2014.

Argyle, D., et al. (2008). *Decision Making in Small Animal Oncology*, Wiley-Blackwell.

Dobson, J. & D. Lascelles (2011). *BSAVA Manual of Canine and Feline Oncology*, BSAVA.

Henry, C. & M. Higginbotham (2009). *Cancer Management in Small Animal Practice*, Saunders.

Moore, A., et al. (2002). Streptozocin for treatment of pancreatic islet cell tumors in dogs: 17 cases. JAVMA **221**: 811-18.

North, S. & T. Banks (2009). *Small Animal Oncology: An Introduction*, Saunders.

Northrup, N. C., et al. (2013). Prospective Evaluation of Biweekly Streptozotocin in 19 Dogs with Insulinoma. Journal of Veterinary Internal Medicine **27**(3): 483-90.

Withrow, S., et al. (2012). Withrow and MacEwen's Small Animal Clinical Oncology, 5th Ed., Saunders.

Succimer

(sux-i-mer)   Chemet®, DMSA, Dimercaptosuccinic acid

Antidote; Chelator

Prescriber Highlights

▶ Oral heavy metal chelator.

▶ Appears to be safe & effective despite limited experience.

▶ Most likely adverse effects noted are GI in nature; may also cause increased liver enzymes, rash.

▶ High doses may be fatal in birds.

▶ Unpleasant odor of capsules; may give feces, urine, saliva, etc. a very unpleasant odor.

▶ Cost is an issue.

Uses/Indications

In veterinary medicine, succimer may be useful for the oral treatment of lead poisoning in small animals (including birds). Potentially, it also may be of benefit for the treatment of other toxic heavy metals such as arsenic or mercury. Other advantages of succimer are that it is not nephrotoxic and does not increase elimination of other essential minerals.

Pharmacology/Actions

Succimer physically chelates heavy metals such as lead, mercury, and arsenic. These water-soluble chelates are then excreted via the kidneys.

Pharmacokinetics

No veterinary information was located. In humans, the drug is rapidly absorbed after oral ingestion, but only incompletely. Absorbed drug is excreted primarily through the kidneys into the urine. Half-life in humans is ≈ 2 days.

Contraindications/Precautions/Warnings

Succimer is contraindicated in patients hypersensitive to it. Chelation therapy should only be attempted if the source of lead is removed to prevent further exposure.

Adverse Effects

Most common adverse reactions reported in humans are GI related effects (vomiting, diarrhea, etc.) or "flu-like" symptoms (body aches, fatigue, etc.). Increases in liver enzymes and rashes have also been reported.

Reproductive/Nursing Safety

It is unknown if succimer is safe to use during pregnancy. At high doses it was fetotoxic and teratogenic in mice. Mothers are discouraged from nursing when taking succimer. In humans, the FDA categorizes this drug as category C for use during pregnancy (*Animal studies have shown an adverse effect on the fetus, but there are no adequate studies in humans; or there are no animal reproduction studies and no adequate studies in humans.*)

It is not known whether this drug is excreted in breast milk.

Overdosage/Acute Toxicity

In toxicology studies, doses of ≤ 200 mg/kg per day in dogs did not cause overt toxicity. Doses of 300 mg/day did cause fatalities in dogs; primarily kidney and GI tract lesions were seen. Doses of 80 mg/kg PO q12h did cause a significant number of fatalities in Cockatiels (but 40 mg/kg q12h did not). If an overdose situation is encountered, standardized gut evacuation with subsequent activated charcoal protocols are recommended.

Drug Interactions

The following drug interactions have either been reported or are theoretical in humans or animals receiving succimer and may be of significance in veterinary patients. Unless otherwise noted, use together is not necessarily contraindicated, but weigh the potential risks and perform additional monitoring when appropriate.

▪ **CHELATING AGENTS, OTHER (CaEDTA, dimercaprol, trientine, penicillamine,** etc.): Concomitant use with other chelating agents is not recommended in humans.

Laboratory Considerations

▪ False positive **urine ketones** can be reported when using nitroprusside reagent (*e.g.*, as in *Ketostix*®).

▪ Falsely low measurements of **CPK** or serum **uric acid** can be caused by succimer.

Doses

▪ **DOGS/CATS:**

For lead poisoning (extra-label): 10 mg/kg PO q8h for 10 days. Succimer has a good therapeutic index, few side effects, spares most other elements from being chelated and does not cause enhanced lead uptake from the gut. Blood lead levels should be rechecked a few days following the last dose of succimer; a second round of chelation therapy may be necessary to reduce the lead load (Talcott 2008). Another source recommends the same dosage for dogs and cats but adds: "the total length of treatment should be based on clinical improvement and determination of blood lead concentrations. In general, succimer (DMSA) is initially given for 5 days." (Puschner *et al.* 2010)

▪ **HORSES:**

For lead poisoning (extra-label): It is uncertain if succimer is absorbed and tolerated in horses and whether an extrapolated dose of 30 mg/kg per day (divided) PO is an alternative to edetate calcium (CaEDTA). (Puschner *et al.* 2010)

▪ **BIRDS:**

For lead poisoning (extra-label): 30 mg/kg PO twice daily for a minimum of 7 days. If severe neurologic signs, may supplement with one dose of CaEDTA (edetate calcium disodium; <50 mg/kg of body weight IM). (Hoogesteijn *et al.* 2003)

Monitoring

▪ Blood lead.

▪ GI adverse effects.

▪ Liver enzymes (AST, ALT).

Client Information

▪ Used to remove excess metals, particularly lead, from the body.

▪ Capsules may have an unpleasant odor; this is not a problem with the drug, but the odor may be transferred to saliva, urine, & feces.

▪ Animals should always have plenty of clean drinking water available to them while taking this medication.

▪ Can cause diarrhea and vomiting.

▪ Capsules can be opened and sprinkled on soft food.

Chemistry/Synonyms

A heavy metal chelating agent also known as meso-2,3 dimercaptosuccinic acid (DMSA), succimer is an analog of dimercaprol. It has an unpleasant odor.

Succimer may also be known as: meso-2,3 dimercaptosuccinic acid, dimercaptosuccinic acid, DIM-SA, DMSA, *Chemet*® or *Succicaptal*®.

Storage/Stability

Unless otherwise labeled, store succimer capsules in tight containers at room temperature. Protect from light.

Compatibility/Compounding Considerations

No specific information noted.

Dosage Forms/Regulatory Status

VETERINARY-LABELED PRODUCTS: NONE.

HUMAN-LABELED PRODUCTS:
Succimer Capsules: 100 mg; *Chemet*®; (Rx)

Revisions/References

Monograph revised/updated August 2014.

Hoogesteijn, A., et al. (2003). Oral treatment of avian lead intoxication with meso-2,3,dimercaptosuccinic acid. J Zoo Wildli Med **34**(1): 82-7.

Puschner, B. & M. Aleman (2010). Lead toxicosis in the horse: A review. Equine Veterinary Education **22**(10): 526-30.

Talcott, P. (2008). New and Used Topics in Toxicology. Proceedings: Western Veterinary Conference. accessed via Veterinary Information Network; vin.com

Succinylcholine Chloride

(suks-sin-i-nil-koe-leen)   Anectine®

Neuromuscular Blocking Agent

Prescriber Highlights

▶ Depolarizing neuromuscular blocking agent.

▶ Contraindications: Severe liver disease, chronic anemias, malnourishment, glaucoma or penetrating eye injuries, predisposition to malignant hyperthermia, & increased CPK values with resultant myopathies.

▶ Extreme Caution: Traumatic wounds or burns, receiving quinidine or digoxin therapy, hyperkalemia or electrolyte imbalances.

▶ Caution: Pulmonary, renal, cardiovascular, metabolic or hepatic dysfunction.

▶ Adverse Effects: Muscle soreness, histamine release, malignant hyperthermia, excessive salivation, hyperkalemia, rash, & myoglobinemia/myoglobinuria. Cardiovascular effects, (bradycardia, tachycardia, hypertension, hypotension, or arrhythmias).

▶ Specific recommendations for use in horses (see Contraindications below).

▶ No analgesic or anesthetic effects.

Uses/Indications

Succinylcholine chloride is indicated for short-term muscle relaxation needed for surgical or diagnostic procedures, to facilitate endotracheal intubation in some species, and reducing the intensity of muscle contractions associated with electro- or pharmacological-induced convulsions. Dogs, cats, and horses were the primary veterinary species where succinylcholine chloride was used. Newer non-depolarizing agents (*e.g.*, atracurium, vecuronium, rocuronium) with fewer adverse effects have largely replaced succinylcholine.

Pharmacology/Actions

An ultrashort-acting depolarizing skeletal muscle relaxant, succinylcholine bonds with motor endplate cholinergic receptors to produce depolarization (perceived as fasciculations). The neuromuscular block remains as long as sufficient quantities of succinylcholine remain and is characterized by a flaccid paralysis. Other pharmacologic effects are discussed in the precautions and adverse effects sections.

Pharmacokinetics

After IV administration, the onset of action with complete muscle relaxation, is usually within 30-60 seconds. In humans, this effect lasts for 2-3 minutes and then gradually diminishes within 10 minutes. The very short duration of action after a single IV dose is thought to occur because the drug diffuses away from the motor end plate. If multiple injections or a continuous infusion is performed, the brief activity is a result of rapid hydrolysis by pseudocholinesterases at the site of action. After IM injection, the onset of action is generally within 2-3 minutes and may persist for 10-30 minutes.

Dogs exhibit a prolonged duration of action ($\approx$ 20 minutes); this species appears unique in this idiosyncratic response.

Succinylcholine is metabolized by plasma pseudocholinesterases to succinylmonocholine and choline; 10% is excreted unchanged in the urine. Succinylmonocholine is partially excreted in the urine and may accumulate in patients with impaired renal function. Succinylmonocholine has approximately 1/20th the neuromuscular blocking activity of succinylcholine, but if it accumulates, prolonged periods of apnea may result.

Contraindications/Precautions/Warnings

Succinylcholine is contraindicated in patients with severe liver disease, chronic anemias, malnourishment (chronic), glaucoma or penetrating eye injuries, predisposition to malignant hyperthermia, and increased CPK values with resultant myopathies. As succinylcholine can exacerbate the effects of hyperkalemia, it should be used with extreme caution in patients who have suffered traumatic wounds or burns, are receiving quinidine or digoxin therapy, or have preexisting hyperkalemia or electrolyte imbalances as arrhythmias or cardiac arrest may occur. It should be used with caution in patients with pulmonary, renal, cardiovascular, metabolic, or hepatic dysfunction.

Succinylcholine should not be used if organophosphate agents have been given or applied recently.

Succinylcholine chloride does not have analgesic effects; and should be used with appropriate analgesic, sedative, and anesthetic agents.

Adverse Effects

Succinylcholine chloride can cause muscle soreness, histamine release, malignant hyperthermia, excessive salivation, hyperkalemia, rash, and myoglobinemia/myoglobinuria. Cardiovascular effects can include bradycardia, tachycardia, hypertension, hypotension, or arrhythmias.

Reproductive/Nursing Safety

It is unknown if succinylcholine can cause fetal harm. The drug does cross the placenta in low concentrations and a newly delivered neonate may show signs of neuromuscular blockade if the mother received high doses or prolonged administration of the drug prior to delivery. In humans, the FDA categorizes this drug as category *C* for use during pregnancy (*Animal studies have shown an adverse effect on the fetus, but there are no adequate studies in humans; or there are no animal reproduction studies and no adequate studies in humans.*) In a separate system evaluating the safety of drugs in canine and feline pregnancy (Papich 1989), this drug is categorized as in class: *B* (*Safe for use if used cautiously. Studies in laboratory animals may have uncovered some risk, but these drugs appear to be safe in dogs and cats or these drugs are safe if they are not administered when the animal is near term.*)

It is not known whether this drug is excreted into milk; exercise caution when succinylcholine is administered to a nursing patient.

Overdosage/Acute Toxicity

Inadvertent overdoses, or standard doses in patients deficient in pseudocholinesterase may result in prolonged apnea. Mechanical ventilation with O_2 should be used until recovery.

Repeated or prolonged high dosages may cause patients to convert from a phase I to a phase II block.

Drug Interactions

The following drug interactions have either been reported or are theoretical in humans or animals receiving succinylcholine and may be of significance in veterinary patients. Unless otherwise noted, use together is not necessarily contraindicated, but weigh the potential risks and perform additional monitoring when appropriate.

■ **AMPHOTERICIN B:** May increase succinylcholine's effects by causing electrolyte imbalances.

- **DIGOXIN:** Succinylcholine may cause a sudden outflux of potassium from muscle cells, thus causing arrhythmias in digitalized patients.
- **OPIATES:** Potential for increased incidences of bradycardia and sinus arrest.
- **THIAZIDE DIURETICS:** May increase succinylcholine's effects by causing electrolyte imbalances.

The following drugs/drug classes <u>may increase or prolong neuromuscular blockade</u> if used concurrently with succinylcholine:

- **AMINOGLYCOSIDES**
- **ANESTHETICS, INHALATION** (*e.g.,* **isoflurane, desflurane,** etc.)
- **ANTIARRHYTHMICS** (*e.g.,* **quinidine, lidocaine, procainamide,** etc.)
- **BETA-ADRENERGIC BLOCKERS**
- **CHLOROQUINE**
- **CLINDAMYCIN**
- **CORTICOSTEROIDS**
- **CYCLOPHOSPHAMIDE**
- **MAGNESIUM SALTS**
- **MAO INHIBITORS**
- **METOCLOPRAMIDE**
- **NEOSTIGMINE**
- **ORGANOPHOSPHATES**
- **OXYTOCIN**
- **PANCURONIUM**
- **PHENOTHIAZINES**
- **TERBUTALINE**
- **THIOTEPA**

Doses

- **DOGS/CATS:**

  As a neuromuscular blocker (extra-label): Rarely used today. Historically, anecdotal dosages of 0.07 – 0.11 mg/kg IV were generally recommended.

- **REPTILES:**

  As neuromuscular blocker (extra-label): Used predominately in Crocodilia, but also in chelonians and lizards. The recovery period is based upon the administered dose and the metabolic activity. Dosage is variable: 0.4 – 1 mg/kg IM with an induction of 5-30 minutes. Recovery is generally in 1 hour with these lower doses. Some species like large crocodiles need 2 – 5 mg/kg IM, but will have a recovery of 7-9 hours. Administration of an anxiolytic prior to induction is helpful. Again, the clinician should have a means to ventilate if the patient is severely apneic. Does not provide any analgesia. (Ferrell 2012)

Monitoring

- Level of muscle relaxation.
- Cardiac rate/rhythm.
- Respiratory depressant effect.

Client Information

- This drug should only be used by professionals familiar with its use.

Chemistry/Synonyms

A depolarizing neuromuscular blocking agent, succinylcholine chloride occurs as an odorless, white, crystalline powder. The dihydrate form melts at 190°C and the anhydrous form at 160°C. Aqueous solutions are acidic with a pH of approximately 4. One gram is soluble in ≈ 1 mL of water and ≈ 350 mL of alcohol. Commercially available injections have a pH from 3-4.5.

Succinylcholine chloride may also be known as: choline chloride succinate, succicurarium chloride, succinylcholine chloride, suxamethonii chloridum, suxametonklorid, suxamethonium chloride; many trade names are available.

Storage/Stability

Commercial injectable solutions should be stored refrigerated (2°-8°C). One manufacturer (*Anectine*®) states that multiple dose vials are stable up to 2 weeks at room temperature with no significant loss of potency.

The powder forms of the drug are stable indefinitely when stored unopened at room temperature. After reconstitution with either D$_5$W or normal saline, they are stable for 4 weeks at 5°C or 1 week at room temperature, but because they contain no preservative, it is recommended they be used within 24 hours.

Compatibility/Compounding Considerations

Succinylcholine chloride is physically **compatible** with all commonly used IV solutions, amikacin sulfate, isoproterenol HCl, meperidine HCl, norepinephrine bitartrate, and scopolamine HBr. It **may not be compatible** with pentobarbital sodium and is physically **incompatible** with sodium bicarbonate and thiopental sodium.

Dosage Forms/Regulatory Status

VETERINARY-LABELED PRODUCTS: NONE.

The ARCI (Racing Commissioners International) has designated this drug as a class 2 substance. See the appendix for more information.

HUMAN-LABELED PRODUCTS:

Succinylcholine Chloride Injection: 20 mg/mL; *Anectine*®, *Quelicin*®; (Rx)

Succinylcholine Chloride Injection, Solution: 100 mg/mL; *Quelicin-1000*®; (Rx)

Revisions/References

Monograph revised/updated August 2014.

Ferrell, S. T. (2012). Anesthesia & Analgesia in Reptiles & Amphibians. ABVP. accessed via Veterinary Information Network; vin.com

Papich, M. (1989). Effects of drugs on pregnancy. *Current Veterinary Therapy X: Small Animal Practice.* R. Kirk. Philadelphia, Saunders: 1291-9.

Sucralfate

(soo-kral-fate)   Carafate®

GI-mucosal Protectant

Prescriber Highlights

▶ Locally acting treatment for GI ulcers/esophagitis; may also protect somewhat against GI ulceration. Potentially could be useful for lowering serum phosphorus in renal patients.

▶ Contraindications: None, use with caution where decreased GI transit times may be harmful.

▶ Adverse Effects: Unlikely; constipation is possible. Vomiting reported in cats.

▶ Give on an empty stomach if possible.

▶ Drug Interactions.

Uses/Indications

Sucralfate has been used in the treatment of oral, esophageal, gastric, and duodenal ulcers. It has also been employed to prevent drug-induced (*e.g.,* aspirin) gastric erosions, but efficacy for this is not predictable.

Sucralfate has been used in human patients with hyperphosphatemia secondary to renal failure and potentially could be useful for this in animals as well. However in a study done in six healthy cats, sucralfate did not significantly change serum or urine phosphorus levels (Quimby *et al.* 2008).

Pharmacology/Actions

While the exact mechanism of action of sucralfate as an antiulcer agent is not known, the drug has a local effect rather than a systemic one. After oral administration, sucralfate reacts with hydrochloric acid in the stomach to form a paste-like complex that will bind to the proteinaceous exudates that generally are found at ulcer sites. This insoluble complex forms a barrier at the site and protects the ulcer from further damage caused by pepsin, acid, or bile. Sucralfate can inactivate pepsin and bind bile acids.

Sucralfate may have some cytoprotective effects, possibly by stimulation of prostaglandin E_2 and I_2. Sucralfate also has some antacid activity, but it is believed that this is not of clinical importance.

Sucralfate does not significantly affect gastric acid output, or trypsin or pancreatic amylase activity. It may decrease the rate of gastric emptying.

As an aluminum salt, sucralfate can bind to gastrointestinal phosphorus.

Pharmacokinetics

Animal studies have indicated that only 3-5% of an oral dose is absorbed which is excreted in the urine unchanged within 48 hours. By reacting with hydrochloric acid in the gut, the remainder of the drug is converted to sucrose sulfate, which is excreted in the feces within 48 hours. The duration of action (binding to ulcer site) may persist up to 6 hours after oral dosing.

Contraindications/Precautions/Warnings

There are no known contraindications to the use of sucralfate. Because it may cause constipation, it should be used with caution in animals where decreased intestinal transit times might be deleterious.

Adverse Effects

Adverse effects are uncommon with sucralfate therapy. Constipation is the most prominent adverse effect reported in humans (2%) and dogs receiving the drug. Vomiting has been reported in cats. Sucralfate can have an unpalatable taste and patient acceptance may be a problem.

Reproductive/Nursing Safety

It is unknown if sucralfate crosses the placenta and whether it may definitively be used safely during pregnancy. In rats, dosages up to 38X those used in humans caused no impaired fertility and doses up to 50X normal caused no symptoms of teratogenicity. In humans, the FDA categorizes this drug as category *B* for use during pregnancy (*Animal studies have not yet demonstrated risk to the fetus, but there are no adequate studies in pregnant women; or animal studies have shown an adverse effect, but adequate studies in pregnant women have not demonstrated a risk to the fetus in the first trimester of pregnancy, and there is no evidence of risk in later trimesters.*) In a separate system evaluating the safety of drugs in canine and feline pregnancy (Papich 1989), this drug is categorized as in class: *A* (*Probably safe. Although specific studies may not have proved he safety of all drugs in dogs and cats, there are no reports of adverse effects in laboratory animals or women.*)

It is not known whether this drug is excreted in milk, but it is unlikely to be of concern.

Overdosage/Acute Toxicity

Overdosage is unlikely to cause any significant problems. Laboratory animals receiving up to 12 grams/kg orally demonstrated no incidence of mortality.

Drug Interactions

The following drug interactions have either been reported or are theoretical in humans or animals receiving sucralfate and may be of significance in veterinary patients. Unless otherwise noted, use together is not necessarily contraindicated, but weigh the potential risks and perform additional monitoring when appropriate.

Sucralfate may impair the oral absorption of the following medications; separate dosing by at least 2 hours to minimize this effect:

- **AZITHROMYCIN**
- **CIPROFLOXACIN/ENROFLOXACIN** (assume other **oral fluoroquinolones** as well)
- **DICLOFENAC**
- **DIGOXIN**
- **DOXYCYCLINE**
- **ERYTHROMYCIN**
- **KETOCONAZOLE**
- **LEVOTHYROXINE**
- **MINOCYCLINE** (Hill *et al.* 2013; KuKanich *et al.* 2014)
- **PENICILLAMINE**
- **TETRACYCLINE**
- **THEOPHYLLINE**
- **VITAMINS (fat soluble)**
- **WARFARIN**

Doses

- **DOGS/CATS:**

  As a GI-mucosal protectant for conditions such esophagitis, gastric or duodenal ulcers, and uremic gastritis (extra-label): It is empirically dosed at ¼- ½ of a 1 gram tablet (250 – 500 mg) for toy breed dogs and cats to 1 gram per large dog PO 2-4 times a day. May be crushed and suspended in water or compounded into a suspension (see Compatibility/Compounding Considerations) and used within 14 days.

- **FERRETS:**

  As a GI-mucosal protectant (extra-label): 75 mg/kg PO q4-6h; give 10 minutes prior to feeding. (Williams 2000)

- **HORSES:**

  As a GI-mucosal protectant (extra-label):

  a) **For adjunctive treatment (used with acid suppressive drugs) for preventing stress-induced ulcers in foals**: 10 – 20 mg/kg PO q6-8h. (Sanchez 2004)

  b) Sucralfate alone may not be beneficial in **treatment of equine gastric ulcer syndrome**, but can be used in conjunction with acid-suppressive therapy and may be more suited for treatment of right dorsal colitis (colonic ulcers) at a dose of 22 mg/kg PO q6-8h. (Videla *et al.* 2009).

- **REPTILES:**

  For GI irritation in most species (extra-label): 500 – 1,000 mg/kg PO q6-8h. (Gauvin 1993)

Monitoring

- Clinical efficacy (dependent on reason for use); monitored by decrease in symptomatology, endoscopic examination, blood in feces, etc.

Client Information

- Best given on an empty stomach and not at the same time as other drugs (separate by two hours if possible).
- Must be given several times a day to be most effective.
- Shake liquids well before using. If using tablets (especially in horses), it is best to crush them and dissolve them in lukewarm water just before giving them.
- Usually tolerated very well; some animals may develop constipation. Some cats may vomit after a dose.

Chemistry/Synonyms

A basic, aluminum complex of sucrose sulfate, sucralfate occurs as a white, amorphous powder. It is practically insoluble in alcohol or water.

Sucralfate is structurally related to heparin, but does not possess any appreciable anticoagulant activity. It is also structurally related to sucrose, but is not utilized as a sugar by the body.

Sucralfate is also known as aluminum sucrose sulfate, basic and *Carafate*®.

Storage/Stability

Store sucralfate tablets in tight containers at room temperature.

Compatibility/Compounding Considerations

A sucralfate 200 mg/mL suspension can be extemporaneously prepared. To make 100 mL: crush twenty (20) sucralfate 1 gram tablets and add sufficient quantity of distilled water to bring the volume to 100 mL. Suspending agents such as acacia or tragacanth should not be used, as they can bind to sucralfate and make it inactive. Label "shake well" and "refrigerate". When refrigerated, it is stable for 14 days.

Dosage Forms/Regulatory Status

VETERINARY-LABELED PRODUCTS: NONE.

HUMAN-LABELED PRODUCTS:

Sucralfate Tablets: 1 gram; *Carafate*®, generic; (Rx)

Sucralfate Suspension: 1 gram/10 mL in 10 mL unit dose cups & 415 mL; *Carafate*®; (Rx)

Revisions/References

Monograph revised/updated August 2014.

Gauvin, J. (1993). Drug therapy in reptiles. Seminars in Avian & Exotic Med 2(1): 48-59.

Hill, T. L., et al. (2013). Sucralfate protects against acid-induced gastric mucosal barrier dysfunction (abstract). Journal of Veterinary Internal Medicine 27(3): 704-5.

KuKanich, K. S., et al. (2014). Effect of sucralfate on oral minocycline absorption in healthy dogs. J Vet Phamacol Ther **doi: 10.1111/jvp.12116.**

Papich, M. (1989). Effects of drugs on pregnancy. *Current Veterinary Therapy X: Small Animal Practice.* R. Kirk. Philadelphia, Saunders: 1291-9.

Quimby, J. & M. R. Lappin (2008). Effects of Sucralfate on the Serum Phosphorus Concentration and Urinary Fractional Excretion of Phosphorus in Healthy Cats. Proceedings: ACVIM. accessed via Veterinary Information Network; vin.com

Sanchez, L. (2004). Diseases of the stomach. *Equine Internal Medicine 2nd Ed.* S. Reed, W. Bayly and D. Sellon. Philadelphia, Saunders: 863-72.

Videla, R. & F. M. Andrews (2009). New Perspectives in Equine Gastric Ulcer Syndrome. Veterinary Clinics of North America-Equine Practice 25(2): 283-+.

Williams, B. (2000). Therapeutics in Ferrets. Vet Clin NA: Exotic Anim Pract 3:1(Jan): 131-53.

Sufentanil Citrate

(soo-fen-ta-nil)   *Sufenta*®

Opiate Agonist

Prescriber Highlights

▶ Injectable, extremely potent opiate that may be useful for adjunctive anesthesia or epidural analgesia.

▶ Marginal veterinary experience & little published data available to draw conclusions on appropriate usage in veterinary species.

▶ Dose-related respiratory & CNS depression most likely adverse effects.

▶ Class-II controlled substance; expensive when compared to fentanyl.

Uses/Indications

An opioid analgesic, sufentanil may be useful as an anesthesia adjunct or as an epidural analgesic. In humans, it has been used as the primary anesthetic in intubated patients with assisted ventilation, and as a post-operative analgesic.

Pharmacology/Actions

Sufentanil is a potent *mu* opioid with the expected sedative, analgesic, and anesthetic properties. When comparing analgesic potencies when injecting IM, 0.01 – 0.04 mg of sufentanil is equivalent to 0.4 – 0.8 mg of alfentanil, 0.1 – 0.2 mg of fentanyl, and ≈ 10 mg of morphine. Like fentanyl, sufentanil appears to have less circulatory effects than does morphine. Sufentanil has a rapid onset of action (1-3 minutes) and a faster recovery time than fentanyl.

Pharmacokinetics

In isoflurane-anesthetized cats a 1 mcg/kg IV bolus of sufentanil had a volume of distribution (steady-state) of ≈ 0.77 L/kg, clearance of ≈ 17.6 mL/min/kg and a terminal half-life ≈ 54 minutes. Disposition of sufentanil is expected to be more rapid than either fentanyl or alfentanil, due to a small volume of distribution and moderate clearance (Pypendop *et al.* 2014).

In humans, the drug has rapid onset of action (1-3 minutes) after intravenous injection. The drug is highly lipid soluble and has volume of distribution in the central compartment of 0.1 L/kg. Approximately 93% is bound to plasma proteins; plasma concentrations rapidly decline due to redistribution. Terminal elimination half-life is ≈ 2.5 hours. Plasma clearance has been reported to be 11.8 mL/min/kg. Sufentanil is metabolized primarily in the liver and small intestine via O-demethylation and N-dealkylation. The parent drug and these metabolites are excreted primarily in the urine. While the manufacturer states to use with caution in patients with impaired renal or hepatic function, limited pharmacokinetic studies in these patients rarely showed any drug accumulation.

Contraindications/Precautions/Warnings

Sufentanil is contraindicated in patients hypersensitive to it or other opioids. It should be used with caution in debilitated or geriatric patients and those with severely diminished renal or hepatic function.

Because of the drug's potency and potential for significant adverse effects, it should only be used in situations where patient vital signs can be continuously monitored. Initial dosage reduction may be required in geriatric or debilitated patients, particularly those with diminished cardiopulmonary function.

Do no not confuse sufentanil with fentanyl.

Adverse Effects

Adverse effects are generally dose related and consistent with other opiate agonists. Respiratory depression and/or CNS depression are most likely to be encountered.

In humans, bradycardia that is usually responsive to anticholinergic agents can occur. Dose-related skeletal muscle rigidity is not uncommon, and neuromuscular blockers are routinely used. Sufentanil has rarely been associated with asystole, hypercarbia and hypersensitivity reactions.

Respiratory or CNS depression may be exacerbated if sufentanil is given with other drugs that can cause those effects.

Reproductive/Nursing Safety

In humans, the FDA categorizes sufentanil as a category *C* drug for use during pregnancy (*Animal studies have shown an adverse effect on the fetus, but there are no adequate studies in humans; or there are no animal reproduction studies and no adequate studies in humans.*) While sufentanil is indicated for epidural use (mixed with bupivacaine ± epinephrine) in women for labor/delivery, it should not be administered systemically to a mother close to giving birth as offspring may show behavioral alterations (hypotonia, depression) associated with opioids.

The effects of sufentanil on lactation or its safety for nursing offspring is not well defined, but sufentanil milk levels approximate those found in serum. This coupled with its low oral bioavailability, make it unlikely to cause significant effects in nursing offspring.

Overdosage/Acute Toxicity

In dogs, the LD_{50} of intravenous sufentanil is 10.1-19.5 mg/kg. Intravenous severe overdoses may cause apnea, circulatory collapse, pulmonary edema, seizures, cardiac arrest and death. Treatment is a combination of supportive therapy and administration of an opiate antagonist such as naloxone. Although sufentanil has a fairly rapid half-life, multiple doses of naloxone may be necessary. Because of the drug's potency, the use of a tuberculin syringe to measure dosages less than 1 mL, with a dosage calculation and measurement double-check system is recommended.

Drug Interactions

The following drug interactions have either been reported or are theoretical in humans or animals receiving sufentanil and may be of significance in veterinary patients. Unless otherwise noted, use together is not necessarily contraindicated, but weigh the potential risks and perform additional monitoring when appropriate.

- **BETA-ADRENERGIC BLOCKERS:** May increase bradycardia and hypotension.
- **BUPRENORPHINE:** May reduce sufentanil's antinociceptive effects.
- **CALCIUM-CHANNEL BLOCKERS:** May increase bradycardia and hypotension.
- **CNS DEPRESSANTS, OTHER:** Additive effects can occur if sufentanil is used concurrently with other drugs that can depress CNS or respiratory function (*e.g.,* **barbiturates**, etc.).
- **NITROUS OXIDE:** Can cause cardiovascular depression if used with high dose sufentanil.

Laboratory Considerations

- Because opiates can increase biliary tract pressure and raise serum **amylase** and **lipase** values, these values may be unreliable for 24 hours after sufentanil is administered.

Doses

Note: In very obese patients, figure dosages based upon lean body weight.

- **DOGS/CATS:**

 As an opioid analgesic (IV); (extra-label): Dosages are not well defined and clinical experience is marginal. IV dosages of 2 – 3 micrograms/kg up to a maximum of 5 micrograms/kg have been noted. Dosage is titrated to effect.

 For epidural analgesia (extra-label): Dogs: 0.7 – 1 micrograms/kg diluted to a volume of 0.26 mL/kg with sterile saline. Onset of action in 10-15 minutes; duration 1-4 hours. (Otero 2006)

Monitoring

- Anesthetic and/or analgesic efficacy.
- Cardiac and respiratory rate.
- Pulse oximetry or other methods to measure blood oxygenation when used for anesthesia.

Client Information

- Sufentanil is a very potent opiate that should only be used by professionals in a setting where adequate patient monitoring is available.

Chemistry/Synonyms

A phenylpiperidine derivative opioid related to fentanyl, sufentanil citrate occurs as a white or almost white powder that is soluble in water, sparingly soluble in alcohol, acetone, or chloroform. The commercially available injection has a pH (adjusted with citric acid) of 3.5-6.

Sufentanil citrate may also be known as: R-33800, sufentanili citras, fentathienel citrate, sufentanyl citrate, sulfentanil citrate, *Fastfen®*, *Fentaientel®* and *Sufenta®*.

Storage/Stability

Unless otherwise labeled, sufentanil injection should be stored protected from light at room temperature. Sufentanil citrate is hydrolyzed in acidic solutions.

Compatibility/Compounding Considerations

Sufentanil citrate is reportedly **compatible** with D5W and bupivacaine. For Y-site injection it is **compatible** with solutions containing: atropine, dexamethasone sodium phosphate, diazepam, diphenhydramine, etomidate, metoclopramide, midazolam, phenobarbital, and propofol. It is **incompatible** with lorazepam, phenytoin and thiopental.

Dosage Forms/Regulatory Status

VETERINARY-LABELED PRODUCTS: NONE.

The ARCI (Racing Commissioners International) has designated this drug as a class 1 substance. See the appendix for more information.

HUMAN-LABELED PRODUCTS:

Sufentanil Citrate Injection: 50 micrograms/mL (as base) in 1 mL, 2 mL & 5 mL amps; *Sufenta®* (preservative free), generic; (Rx, C-II).

Revisions/References

Monograph revised/updated August 2014.

Otero, P. (2006). Epidural anesthesia and analgesia. Proceedings: WSAVA World Congress. accessed via Veterinary Information Network; vin.com

Pypendop, B. H., et al. (2014). Pharmacokinetics of fentanyl, alfentanil, and sufentanil in isoflurane-anesthetized cats. J. Vet. Pharmacol. Ther. 37(1): 13-7.

Sulfachlorpyridazine Sodium

(sul-fa-klor-pye-**rid**-a-zeen)   Vetisulid®

Sulfonamide Antimicrobial Agent

Prescriber Highlights

▶ Contraindications: Hypersensitivity to sulfas, thiazides, or sulfonylurea agents; severe renal or hepatic impairment.

▶ Caution: Diminished renal or hepatic function, or urinary obstruction.

▶ Adverse Effects: Can precipitate in the urine (especially with high dosages for prolonged periods, acidic urine or highly concentrated urine); **Dogs:** Keratoconjunctivitis sicca, bone marrow depression, hypersensitivity reactions (rashes, dermatitis), focal retinitis, fever, vomiting, & nonseptic polyarthritis possible.

▶ Potentially teratogenic; weigh risk vs. benefit.

▶ Too-rapid IV injection may cause muscle weakness, blindness, ataxia, & collapse; SC or IM injection may cause tissue irritation.

Uses/Indications

Sulfachlorpyridazine is indicated for the treatment of diarrhea caused or complicated by *E. coli* in calves <1 month of age or colibacillosis in swine. It is also used parenterally as a general-purpose sulfonamide in adult cattle and other species.

Pharmacology/Actions

Sulfonamides are usually bacteriostatic agents when used alone. They are thought to prevent bacterial replication by competing with para-aminobenzoic acid (PABA) in the biosynthesis of tetrahydrofolic acid in the pathway to form folic acid. Only microorganisms that synthesize their own folic acid are affected by sulfas.

Microorganisms that are usually affected by sulfonamides include some gram-positive bacteria, including some strains of streptococci, staphylococcus, *Bacillus anthracis*, *Clostridium tetani*, *C. perfringens*, and many strains of Nocardia. Sulfas have *in vitro* activity against some gram-negative species, including some strains of Shigella, Salmonella, *E. coli*, Klebsiella, Enterobacter, Pasteurella, and Proteus. Sulfas also have activity against some rickettsia and protozoa (Toxoplasma, Coccidia). Unfortunately, resistance to sulfas is a progressing phenomenon and many strains of bacteria that were once susceptible to this class of antibacterial are now resistant. The sulfas are less efficacious in pus, necrotic tissue, or in areas with extensive cellular debris.

Pharmacokinetics

Very limited information is available on the specific pharmacokinetics for this agent. In general, sulfonamides are readily absorbed from the GI tract of non-ruminants, but absorption can vary depending on the drug, species, disease process, etc. Food delays the rate, but usually not the extent of absorption. Peak levels occur within 1-2 hours in non-ruminant (and young pre-ruminant) animals. Adult ruminants may have significant delays before the drug is absorbed orally.

Sulfas are well distributed throughout the body and some reach significant levels in the CSF. Levels of the drugs tend to be highest in liver, kidney, and lung, and lower in muscle and bone. The sulfas can be highly bound to serum proteins, but the extent of binding is species and drug dependent. When bound to proteins the sulfa is not active.

Sulfonamides are both renally excreted and metabolized. Renal excretion of unchanged drug occurs via both tubular secretion and glomerular filtration. Protein bound drug is not filtered by the glomeruli. Metabolism is performed principally in the liver, but extra-hepatic metabolism is also involved. Mechanisms of metabolism are usually acetylation and glucuronidation. The acetylated metabolites may be less soluble and crystallization in the urine can occur with some sulfonamides, particularly at lower pH. The serum half-life of sulfachlorpyridazine is ≈ 1.2 hours in cattle.

Contraindications/Precautions/Warnings

Sulfonamides are contraindicated in patients hypersensitive to them, thiazides, or sulfonylurea agents. They are also considered contraindicated in patients with severe renal or hepatic impairment and should be used with caution in patients with diminished renal or hepatic function, or urinary obstruction.

Oral sulfonamides can depress the normal cellulytic function of the ruminoreticulum, but this effect is generally temporary and the animal adapts.

Adverse Effects

Sulfonamides (or their metabolites) can precipitate in the urine, particularly when given at high dosages for prolonged periods. Acidic or highly concentrated urine may also contribute to increased risk of crystalluria, hematuria, and renal tubule obstruction. Different sulfonamides have different solubilities at various pH. Alkalinization of the urine using sodium bicarbonate may prevent crystalluria, but it also decreases the amount available for tubular reabsorption. Crystalluria can usually be avoided with most of the commercially available sulfonamides by maintaining an adequate urine flow. Normal urine pH in herbivores is usually 8 or more, so crystalluria is not frequently a problem. Sulfonamides can also cause various hypersensitivity reactions or diarrhea by altering the normal gut flora.

Too rapid intravenous injection of the sulfas can cause muscle weakness, blindness, ataxia, and collapse.

In dogs, keratoconjunctivitis sicca has been reported with sulfonamide therapy. In addition, bone marrow depression, hypersensitivity reactions (rashes, dermatitis), focal retinitis, fever, vomiting and nonseptic polyarthritis have been reported in dogs.

Oral sulfonamides can depress the normal cellulytic function of the ruminoreticulum, but this effect is generally temporary and the animal adapts.

Because solutions of sulfonamides are usually alkaline, they can cause tissue irritation and necrosis if injected intramuscularly or subcutaneously.

Reproductive/Nursing Safety

Sulfas cross the placenta and may reach fetal levels of ≥50% than is found in maternal serum; teratogenicity has been reported in some laboratory animals when given at very high doses. They should be used in pregnant animals only when the benefits clearly outweigh the risks of therapy.

Sulfonamides are distributed into milk. Safe use during lactation cannot be assumed; use with caution.

Overdosage/Acute Toxicity

Acute toxicity secondary to overdoses apparently occurs only rarely in veterinary species. In addition to the adverse effects listed above, CNS stimulation and myelin degeneration have been noted after very high dosages.

Drug Interactions

The following drug interactions have either been reported or are theoretical in humans or animals receiving sulfachlorpyridazine and may be of significance in veterinary patients. Unless otherwise noted, use together is not necessarily contraindicated, but weigh the potential risks and perform additional monitoring when appropriate.

- **ANTACIDS:** May decrease the oral bioavailability of sulfonamides if administered concurrently.

Laboratory Considerations

- Sulfonamides may give false-positive results for **urine glucose** determinations when using the Benedict's method.

Doses

- **CATTLE:**

  In calves for labeled indications: 33 – 49.5 mg/kg PO, or IV twice daily for 1-5 days; suggest initiating therapy with intravenous preparation and then changing to oral if possible. (Package insert; *Vetisulid*®)

- **SWINE:**

  For labeled indications: 44 – 77 mg/kg PO per day (divide dose and give twice daily if treating individual animals) for 1-5 days. (Package insert; *Vetisulid*®)

- **BIRDS:**

  For enteric coccidial (*Atoxoplasma* spp.) or *E. coli* infections (extra-label):

  a) **For pigeons:** 1200 mg per gallon of drinking water. Very effective for *E. coli* and it is a good coccidiostat. (Harlin 2006)

  b) **For canaries, finches, and mynah birds** (especially in large groups of caged birds): *Atoxoplasma* spp. treatment is difficult. Sulfachlorpyridazine ¼ – ½ teaspoon (1.25 – 2.5 mL) per liter of drinking water for 5-10 days may be used. (Tully 2013)

Monitoring

- Clinical efficacy.
- Adverse effects.

Client Information

- To help reduce the possibility of crystalluria occurring, animals should have free access to water; avoid dehydration.

Chemistry/Synonyms

Sulfachlorpyridazine sodium is listed as a short to intermediate-acting, low lipid soluble sulfonamide antibacterial. It is reportedly very soluble in urine at usual pHs.

Sulfachlorpyridazine may also be known as cluricol, sulphachlorpyridazine, *Pyradan*®, *Prinzone*® or *Vetisulid*®.

Storage/Stability

The injection should be stored at room temperature and protected from light; avoid freezing. The oral suspension should be stored at room temperature; avoid freezing. The oral boluses and powder should be stored at room temperature; avoid excessive heat (above 40°; 104°F).

Dosage Forms/Regulatory Status

VETERINARY-LABELED PRODUCTS:

Sulfachlorpyridazine Sodium Oral powder: 54 grams per bottle; *Vetisulid® Powder*; (OTC). FDA-approved for use in calves < 1 month of age and swine. Slaughter withdrawal (at labeled doses) = 4 days for swine. When used orally in the milk or milk replacer for ruminating calves, treated calves must not be slaughtered for food during treatment and for 7 days after the last treatment.

An injectable solution, oral suspension, and oral tablets are still listed in FDA's Green Book.

HUMAN-LABELED PRODUCTS: NONE.

Revisions/References

Monograph revised/updated August 2014.

Harlin, R. (2006). Practical pigeon medicine. Proceedings: AAV 2006. accessed via Veterinary Information Network; vin.com

Tully, T. (2013). Avian Parasites. ABVP. accessed via Veterinary Information Network; vin.com

Sulfadiazine/Pyrimethamine – See Pyrimethamine/Sulfadiazine

Sulfadiazine/Trimethoprim
Sulfamethoxazole/Trimethoprim

(sul-fa-**dye**-a-zeen; sul-fa-meth-**ox**-a-zole/trye-**meth**-ohe-prim)

TMS, Co-trimoxazole, Tribrissen®

Potentiated Sulfonamide Antimicrobial

Note: In the USA, two separate combinations with trimethoprim are used clinically. There are trimethoprim/sulfadiazine products FDA-approved for use in dogs, cats, and horses in both parenteral and oral dosage forms. Many veterinarians also use the human FDA-approved, trimethoprim/sulfamethoxazole oral products. In Canada, sulfadoxine is available in combination with trimethoprim for veterinary use.

Prescriber Highlights

▶ Potentiated sulfonamide antimicrobial agent.

▶ Contraindications: Hypersensitivity to sulfas, thiazides, or sulfonylurea agents; severe renal or hepatic impairment; Doberman pinschers.

▶ Caution: Diminished renal or hepatic function, or urinary obstruction or urolithiasis.

▶ Adverse Effects: **Dogs:** Keratoconjunctivitis sicca, hypersensitivity (type 1 or type 3), acute neutrophilic hepatitis with icterus, vomiting, anorexia, diarrhea, fever, hemolytic anemia, urticaria, polyarthritis, facial swelling, polydipsia, crystalluria, hematuria, polyuria, cholestasis, hypothyroidism, anemias, agranulocytosis, idiosyncratic hepatic necrosis in dogs. **Cats:** Anorexia, crystalluria, hematuria, leukopenias & anemias. **Horses:** Transient pruritic (after IV injection). Oral: diarrhea, hypersensitivity reactions & hematologic effects (anemias, thrombocytopenia, or leukopenias).

▶ Local injection effects possible (check label for product recommendation for injection technique).

▶ Potentially teratogenic, weigh risk vs. benefit.

Uses/Indications

Although only FDA-approved for use in dogs and horses, trimethoprim/sulfadiazine etc. is used in many species to treat infections caused by susceptible organisms. See Dosage section for more information.

Trimethoprim/sulfa can be effective for some prostate infections.

Pharmacology/Actions

Alone, sulfonamides are bacteriostatic agents and trimethoprim is bactericidal, but when used in combination, the potentiated sulfas are bactericidal. Potentiated sulfas sequentially inhibit enzymes in the folic acid pathway, inhibiting bacterial thymidine synthesis. The sulfonamide blocks the conversion of para-aminobenzoic acid (PABA) to dihydrofolic acid (DFA), and trimethoprim blocks the conversion of DFA to tetrahydrofolic acid by inhibiting dihydrofolate reductase. Infected tissue and cellular debris can inhibit the activity of trimethoprim/sulfa by secreting PABA and thymidine.

The *in vitro* optimal ratio for most susceptible bacteria is approximately 1:20 (trimethoprim:sulfa), but synergistic activity can reportedly occur with ratios of 1:1-1:40. The serum concentration of the trimethoprim component is considered more important than the sulfa concentration. For most susceptible bacteria, the MIC's for TMP are generally above 0.5 micrograms/mL.

The potentiated sulfas have a fairly broad spectrum of activity. Gram-positive bacteria that are generally susceptible include most streptococci, many strains of staphylococcus (most veterinary strains of methicillin-resistant staphylococci are resistant), and Nocardia. In horses, ≈ 30% of strains tested of *Streptococcus zooepidemicus* are resistant to TMP/Sulfa. Many gram-negative organisms of the family Enterobacteriaceae are susceptible to the potentiated sulfas but not *Pseudomonas aeruginosa*. Some protozoa (*Pneumocystis carinii*, Coccidia, and Toxoplasma) are also inhibited by the combination. Potentiated sulfas reportedly have little activity against most anaerobes, but opinions on this vary.

Resistance development is thought to occur more slowly to the combination of drugs than to either one alone. In gram-negative organisms, resistance is usually plasmid-mediated. *E. coli* resistance development is an ongoing problem.

Pharmacokinetics

Trimethoprim/sulfa is relatively well absorbed after oral administration, with peak levels occurring ≈ 1-4 hours after dosing; the drug is more slowly absorbed after subcutaneous absorption, however. Oral bioavailability in fed horses after a single 30 mg/kg paste (*Norodine®*; Denmark) dose was 74% for sulfadiazine and 46% for trimethoprim (Winther *et al.* 2011). Food has no apparent effect on the absorption of sulfadiazine, but trimethoprim absorption is decreased.

In ruminants >8 weeks old, trimethoprim is apparently trapped in the ruminoreticulum after oral administration and undergoes some degradation limiting its usefulness.

Trimethoprim/sulfa is well distributed in the body, but in horses levels are lower in pulmonary epithelial lining fluid than in plasma (Winther *et al.* 2011). When meninges are inflamed, the drugs enter the CSF in levels of ≈ 50% those found in the serum. Both drugs cross the placenta and are distributed into milk. Trimethoprim/sulfa is relatively well distributed into the prostate. The volume of distribution for trimethoprim in various species are: 1.49 L/kg (dogs); 0.59-1.51 L/kg (horses). The volume of distribution for sulfadiazine in dogs is 1.02 L/kg. Sulfadiazine and trimethoprim are 20% and 35% bound to equine plasma proteins.

Trimethoprim/sulfa is both renally excreted unchanged via glomerular filtration and tubular secretion and metabolized by the liver. The sulfas are primarily acetylated and conjugated with glucuronic acid and trimethoprim is metabolized to oxide and hydroxylated metabolites. Trimethoprim may be more extensively metabolized in the liver in adult ruminants than in other species. The serum elimination half-lives for trimethoprim in various species are: 2.5 hours (dogs), 1.91-3 hours (horses), and 1.5 hours (cattle). The serum elimination half-lives for sulfadiazine in various species are: 9.84 hours (dogs), 2.71 hours (horses), and 2.5 hours (cattle). While trimethoprim is rapidly eliminated from the serum the drug may persist for a longer period of time in tissues.

Because of the number of variables involved, it is extremely difficult to apply pharmacokinetic values in making dosage recommendations with these combinations. Each drug (trimethoprim and the sulfa) has different pharmacokinetic parameters (absorption, distribution, elimination) in each species. Since different organisms have different MIC values and the optimal ratio of trimethoprim to sulfa differs from organism to organism, this problem is exacerbated.

There is considerable controversy regarding the frequency of administration of these combinations. The veterinary product, trimethoprim/sulfadiazine is labeled for once daily administration in dogs and horses, but many clinicians believe that the drug is more efficacious if given twice daily, regardless of which sulfa is used.

Contraindications/Precautions/Warnings
The manufacturer states that trimethoprim/sulfadiazine should not be used in dogs or horses showing marked liver parenchymal damage, blood dyscrasias, or those with a history of sulfonamide sensitivity. It is not for use in horses (or FDA-approved for other animals) intended for food.

Doberman pinschers appear to be very susceptible to sulfonamide-induced poly-systemic immune complex disease and most believe that these drugs are contraindicated in them.

This combination should be used with caution in patients with pre-existing hepatic or renal disease. In animals with moderate to severe renal dysfunction, consider dosage reduction; avoid products containing sulfadiazine.

Because of its potential for crystallization in the urine, it may be wise to avoid the use of sulfadiazine in dogs known to have uroliths, at increased risk for developing uroliths or known to have highly concentrated (dehydration) or acidic urine.

Adverse Effects
Adverse effects noted in dogs include: keratoconjunctivitis sicca (which may be irreversible), acute neutrophilic hepatitis with icterus, vomiting, anorexia, diarrhea, fever, hemolytic anemia, urticaria, polyarthritis, facial swelling, polydipsia, polyuria and cholestasis. Potentiated sulfonamides may cause hypothyroidism in dogs, particularly with extended therapy. Acute hypersensitivity reactions manifesting as Type I (anaphylaxis) or Type III reaction (serum sickness) can be seen. Hypersensitivity reactions appear to be more common in large breed dogs; Doberman Pinschers may possibly be more susceptible to this effect than other breeds. Other hematologic effects (anemias, agranulocytosis) are possible, but fairly rare. TMP/sulfa has rarely caused an idiosyncratic, moderate to massive hepatic necrosis in dogs. TMP/Sulfa may be a risk factor for developing acute pancreatitis, but cause and effect have not been definitively shown.

Adverse effects noted in cats may include anorexia, leukopenias and anemias.

In horses, transient pruritus has been noted after intravenous injection. Oral therapy has resulted in diarrhea in some horses, but incidence is relatively low. Previous administration of potentiated sulfas has been implicated in increasing the mortality rate associated with severe diarrhea. If the 48% injectable product is injected IM, SC, or extravasates after IV administration, swelling, pain and minor tissue damage may result. Hypersensitivity reactions, neu-

rologic effects (gait alterations and behavior changes), cutaneous vasculitis, and hematologic effects (anemias, thrombocytopenia, or leukopenias) may also be seen; long-term therapy should include periodic hematologic monitoring.

Sulfonamides (or their metabolites) can precipitate in the urine, particularly when given at high dosages for prolonged periods. Acidic urine or highly concentrated urine may also contribute to increased risk of crystalluria, hematuria, and renal tubule obstruction.

Trimethoprim/sulfa can significantly reduce tear production in rabbits (Shirani *et al.* 2010).

Reproductive/Nursing Safety
Safety of trimethoprim/sulfa has not been clearly established in pregnant animals. Reports of teratogenicity (cleft palate) have been reported. Studies thus far in male animals have not demonstrated any decreases in reproductive performance. In humans, the FDA categorizes this drug as category *C* for use during pregnancy (*Animal studies have shown an adverse effect on the fetus, but there are no adequate studies in humans; or there are no animal reproduction studies and no adequate studies in humans.*) In a separate system evaluating the safety of drugs in canine and feline pregnancy (Papich 1989), this drug is categorized as in class: *B* (*Safe for use if used cautiously. Studies in laboratory animals may have uncovered some risk, but these drugs appear to be safe in dogs and cats or these drugs are safe if they are not administered when the animal is near term.*)

Use TMP/sulfa products in nursing animals with caution. TMP-SMZ is not recommended for human use during the nursing period as sulfonamides are excreted in milk and may cause kernicterus. Premature infants and infants with hyperbilirubinemia or G-6-PD deficiency are also at risk for adverse effects.

Overdosage/Acute Toxicity
Manifestations of an acute overdosage can include clinical signs of GI distress (nausea, vomiting, diarrhea), CNS toxicity (depression, headache, and confusion), facial swelling, bone marrow depression and increases in serum aminotransferases. Oral overdoses can be treated by emptying the stomach, (following usual protocols), and initiating symptomatic and supportive therapy. Acidification of the urine may increase the renal elimination of trimethoprim, but could also cause sulfonamide crystalluria, particularly with sulfadiazine containing products. Complete blood counts (and other laboratory parameters) should be monitored as necessary. Bone marrow suppression associated with chronic overdoses may be treated with folinic acid (leucovorin) if severe. Peritoneal dialysis is not effective in removing TMP or sulfas from the circulation.

Drug Interactions
The following drug interactions have either been reported or are theoretical in humans or animals receiving trimethoprim/sulfa and may be of significance in veterinary patients. Unless otherwise noted, use together is not necessarily contraindicated, but weigh the potential risks and perform additional monitoring when appropriate.

- **AMANTADINE:** A human patient developed toxic delirium when receiving amantadine with TMP/sulfa.
- **ANTACIDS:** May decrease the bioavailability of sulfonamides if administered concurrently.
- **CYCLOSPORINE:** TMP/sulfa may increase the risk of nephrotoxicity.
- **DIGOXIN:** TMP/sulfa may increase digoxin levels.
- **DIURETICS, THIAZIDE:** May increase risk for thrombocytopenia.
- **HYPOGLYCEMIC AGENTS, ORAL:** TMP/sulfa may potentiate effects.

- **METHOTREXATE:** TMP/sulfa may displace from plasma proteins and increase risk for toxic effects; it can also interfere with MTX assays (competitive protein binding technique).
- **PHENYTOIN:** TMP/sulfa may increase half-life.
- **TRICYCLIC ANTIDEPRESSANTS:** TMP/sulfa may decrease efficacy.
- **WARFARIN:** TMP/sulfa may prolong INR/PT

Laboratory Considerations

- When using the Jaffe alkaline picrate reaction assay for **creatinine** determination, trimethoprim/sulfa may cause an overestimation of ≈ 10%.
- Sulfonamides may give false-positive results for **urine glucose** determinations when using the Benedict's method.

Doses

Note: There is significant controversy regarding the frequency of dosing these drugs. See the pharmacokinetic section above for more information. Unless otherwise noted, doses are for combined amounts of trimethoprim/sulfa.

- **DOGS:**

  For susceptible bacterial infections:

  For labeled indications (...for sensitive organisms alone or as an adjunct to surgery or debridement with associated infection; acute urinary tract infections; acute bacterial complications of distemper; acute respiratory tract infections; acute alimentary tract infections; wound infections; abscesses.); (FDA-approved): 30 mg/kg PO once daily. Alternatively, especially in severe infections, the initial dose may be followed by 15 mg/kg q12h. (Adapted from label —*Tribrissen*®)

  For superficial bacterial folliculitis (extra-label): 15 – 30 mg/kg PO twice daily. From the Antimicrobial Guidelines Working Group of the International Society for Companion Animal Infectious Diseases. Potentiated sulfas (trimethoprim/sulfa, ormetoprim/sulfa) are first tier drugs only if local regional susceptibility of *Staphylococcus pseudintermedius* is known. If prolonged (>7 day) therapy is anticipated, baseline Schirmer's tear testing is recommended, with periodic re-evaluation and owner monitoring for ocular discharge. Avoid in dogs that may be sensitive to potential adverse effects, such as keratoconjunctivitis sicca, hepatopathy, hypersensitivity and skin eruptions. (Hillier *et al.* 2014)

  For uncomplicated UTI while awaiting culture and susceptibility results; (extra-label): 15 mg/kg PO q12h. Can also be used as initial treatment for complicated UTI. From the Antimicrobial Guidelines Working Group of the International Society for Companion Animal Infectious Diseases. Same caveats as listed in the dosage (above) for superficial bacterial folliculitis. (Weese *et al.* 2011)

  For parasitic diseases (all are extra-label):

  For neosporosis: There is no approved or curative treatment for canine neosporosis. Arrestment of clinical disease is best achieved when treatment is initiated before the occurrence of contracture or paralysis. Dogs typically die without treatment, and some dogs die even with treatment. Trimethoprim/sulfadiazine 15 – 20 mg/kg PO q12h for 4 weeks in combination with pyrimethamine (1 mg/kg PO once daily for 4 weeks). If observable clinical improvement is slow, treatment should be extended beyond the recommended 4 weeks until 2 weeks after clinical signs have plateaued. All littermates of affected puppies should be treated regardless of clinical signs. Alternative treatment is clindamycin (12.5 – 25 mg/kg PO or IM q12h for 4 weeks). (CAPC 2014)

  For toxoplasmosis: There is no approved treatment for toxoplasmosis in cats or dogs. Trimethoprim/sulfa combination can be used at 15 mg/kg PO q12h for 4 weeks. Supportive care should be provided as needed. (CAPC 2014)

  For pneumocystosis (*Pneumocystis carinii*): 15 mg/kg PO q8h or 30 mg/kg PO q12h, both for 3 weeks. May be given with cimetidine and levamisole as potential immune stimulants. (Hawkins 2000)

  For American Canine Hepatozoonosis (*Hepatazoon americanum*): No treatment is effective in eliminating H. americanum in infected dogs. Treatment can increase survival time, improve the quality of life, and decrease the number and severity of clinical relapses. Supportive care can ensure hydration, and nonsteroidal anti-inflammatory drugs assist with pain control. Triple-combination therapy, referred to as TCP, consisting of trimethoprim-sulfadiazine (15 mg/kg PO q12h for 14 days), clindamycin (10 mg/kg PO q8h for 14 days), and pyrimethamine (0.25 mg/kg PO q24h for 14 days) OR ponazuril at a dose of 10 mg/kg PO q12h for 14 days. Prolonged therapy with decoquinate at 10 – 20 mg/kg mixed in the food twice daily; treatment continued for 2 years. If relapse occurs, either ponazuril or TCP should be administered again for 14 days followed by long-term decoquinate therapy. (CAPC 2014)

- **CATS:**

  For susceptible bacterial infections:

  For uncomplicated UTI while awaiting culture and susceptibility results; (extra-label): 15 mg/kg PO q12h. Can also be used as initial treatment for complicated UTI. From the Antimicrobial Guidelines Working Group of the International Society for Companion Animal Infectious Diseases. Same caveats as listed in the dosage (above) for superficial bacterial folliculitis. (Weese *et al.* 2011)

  For parasitic diseases (all are extra-label):

  For toxoplasmosis: There is no approved treatment for toxoplasmosis in cats or dogs. Trimethoprim/sulfa combination can be used at 15 mg/kg PO q12h for 4 weeks. Supportive care should be provided as needed. (CAPC 2014)

- **FERRETS:**

  For susceptible infections (all are extra-label):
  a) 30 mg/kg PO twice daily. (Williams 2000)
  b) For coccidiosis: 30 mg/kg PO once daily for 14 days. (Johnson 2006)

- **RABBITS, RODENTS, SMALL MAMMALS:**

  For susceptible infections (all are extra-label):
  a) **Rabbits:** 15 – 30 mg/kg, PO q12-24h; 30 – 48 mg/kg SC q12h. Sulfadiazine has a very short half-life (approx. 1 hour) in rabbits. (Ivey *et al.* 2000)
  b) **Chinchillas, Gerbils, Guinea Pigs, Hamsters, Mice, Rats:** 15 – 30 mg/kg PO q12h; or 30 mg/kg IM q12h. (Adamcak *et al.* 2000)
  c) **Chinchillas:** 30 mg/kg PO, SC or IM q12h. (Hayes 2000)

- **HORSES:**

  Labeled dose for susceptible infections (FDA-approved): 30 mg/kg PO once daily or 21.3 mg/kg IV once daily. (Package insert; *Tribrissen*®)

  For the treatment of lower respiratory tract infections by susceptible strains of *Streptococcus equi* **subsp.** *Zooepidemicus* (Labeled dose *Equisul-SDT*®; FDA-approved): 24 mg/kg (combined active ingredients) PO twice daily for 10 days. (Adapted from label; *Equisul-SDT*®)

  For respiratory infections (extra-label): A pharmacokinetic study using an oral paste (*Norodine®*; Denmark) concluded that clinically relevant drug concentrations (of mainly trimethoprim) are difficult to maintain in pulmonary epithelial lining fluid especially after oral administration. The use of potentiated sulfonamides for treatment against lower airway infections in horses should be restricted to treatment against highly susceptible pathogens if doses at 30 mg/kg PO or IV twice daily. (Winther *et al.* 2011)

For *Pneumocystis jiroveci* (formerly *P. carinii*) in foals: 30 mg/kg PO q12h.

- **BIRDS:**
  For susceptible infections (all are extra-label):
  a) **For respiratory and enteric infections in psittacines** using the 24% injectable suspension: 0.22 mL/kg IM once to twice daily.

     For coccidiosis in toucans and mynahs using TMP/SMX oral suspension (240 mg/5 mL): 2.2 mL/kg once daily for 5 days. May be added to feed.

     For respiratory and enteric infections in hand-fed baby psittacines using TMP/SMX oral suspension (240 mg/5 mL): 0.22 mL/30 grams 2-3 times daily for 5-7 days. (Clubb 1986)

  b) **For canaries, finches, and mynah birds:** *Atoxoplasma* spp. treatment is difficult. Trimethoprim/sulfa 100 mg/kg PO twice daily is the recommended treatment for avian coccidian parasitic diseases. (Tully 2013)

- **REPTILES:**
  For susceptible infections (extra-label):
  a) **For most species:** 30 mg/kg IM (upper part of body) once daily for 2 treatments, then every other day for 5-12 treatments. May be useful for enteric infections. (Gauvin 1993)

  b) **For all species:** 30 mg/kg IM, first two doses 24 hours apart and then every other day. (Jacobson 1999)

  c) 15 – 25 mg/kg/day IM for 7-14 days. (Lewbart 2001)

Monitoring

- Clinical efficacy.
- Adverse effects; with chronic therapy, periodic complete blood counts should be considered.
- In dogs if prolonged (>7 day) therapy is anticipated, baseline Schirmer's tear testing is recommended, with periodic (one suggestion is in 5 days and every 2-3 weeks) re-evaluation and owner monitoring for ocular discharge.
- Thyroid function tests should be considered (baseline and ongoing) particularly in dogs receiving long-term treatment. Some do not feel this is necessary.

Client Information

- If using oral suspension, shake well before using; does not need to be refrigerated.
- Animals must be allowed free access to water and must not become dehydrated while on therapy.
- If dog's eyes are dry or become irritated contact veterinarian.

Chemistry/Synonyms

Trimethoprim occurs as odorless, bitter-tasting, white to cream-colored crystals or crystalline powder. It is very slightly soluble in water and slightly soluble in alcohol.

Sulfadiazine occurs as an odorless or nearly odorless, white to slightly yellow powder. It is practically insoluble in water and sparingly soluble in alcohol.

Sulfamethoxazole occurs as a practically odorless, white to off-white, crystalline powder. Approximately 0.29 mg are soluble in 1 mL of water and 20 mg are soluble in 1 mL of alcohol.

In combination, these products may be known as: Co-trimoxazole, SMX-TMP, TMP-SMX, trimethoprim-sulfamethoxazole, sulfamethoxazole-trimethoprim, sulfadiazine-trimethoprim, trimethoprim-sulfadiazine, TMP-SDZ, SDZ-TMP, Co-trimazine or by their various trade names.

Storage/Stability

Unless otherwise instructed by the manufacturer, trimethoprim/sulfadiazine and co-trimoxazole products should be stored at room temperature (15-30°C) in tight containers. Shake suspensions well before use.

Compatibility/Compounding Considerations

No specific information noted.

Dosage Forms/Regulatory Status

VETERINARY-LABELED PRODUCTS:

Trimethoprim (TMP)/Sulfadiazine (SDZ) Oral Paste: Each gram contains 67 mg trimethoprim and 333 mg sulfadiazine. Available in 37.5 gram (total weight) syringes; *Tribrissen® 400 Oral Paste*; (Rx). FDA-approved for use in horses not intended for food.

Trimethoprim (TMP)/Sulfadiazine (SDZ) Oral Suspension: Each gram contains 67 mg trimethoprim and 333 mg sulfadiazine (proprietary formulation) in 150 mL, 135 mL, 625 mL, 560 mL, & 950 mL bottles; *Equisul-SDT®*; (Rx). FDA-approved (NADA 141-360) for horses.

Trimethoprim/Sulfadiazine Sterile Injection: 48% in 100 mL vials: *Di-Biotic® 48%*, *Tribrissen® 48% Injection*; (Rx) FDA-approved for use in horses not intended for food.

Trimethoprim/Sulfadiazine Powder: 67 mg trimethoprim and 333 mg sulfadiazine per gram: *Tucoprim® Powder* in 200 gram & 400 gram bottles and 2000 gram pails, *Uniprim® Powder* in 37.5 gram and 1,125 gram packets, 200 gram jar, and 12 kg box; (Rx). FDA-approved for use in horses not intended for food.

In Canada, trimethoprim and sulfadoxine are available for use in cattle and swine (*Trivetrin®*; *Borgal®*). Slaughter withdrawal = 10 days; milk withdrawal = 96 hours.

HUMAN-LABELED PRODUCTS:

Trimethoprim (alone) Tablets: 100 mg; generic; (Rx). A 50 mg/5 mL oral solution (trimethoprim HCl, *Primsol®*) is also available.

Trimethoprim & Sulfamethoxazole (Co-Trimoxazole; TMP-SMZ) Oral Tablets: 80 mg trimethoprim & 400 mg sulfamethoxazole; Double Strength Tablets: 160 mg trimethoprim & 800 mg sulfamethoxazole; *Bactrim®* & *Bactrim® DS*; generic; (Rx)

Trimethoprim 8 mg/mL and Sulfamethoxazole 40 mg/mL (labeled as 40 mg/5 mL & 200 mg/5mL) oral suspension; *Sulfatrim®*, generic; (Rx)

Trimethoprim & Sulfamethoxazole Injection: 80 mg sulfamethoxazole, 16 mg trimethoprim per mL in 5 mL single-use vials, 10 mL, or 30 mL multiple-dose vials; generic; (Rx)

Revisions/References

Monograph revised/updated August 2014.

Adamcak, A. & B. Otten (2000). Rodent Therapeutics. Vet Clin NA: Exotic Anim Pract 3:1(Jan): 221-40.

CAPC (2014). Companion Animal Parasite Council (CAPC) Recommendations, CAPCvet.org.

Clubb, S. L. (1986). Therapeutics: Individual and Flock Treatment Regimens. *Clinical Avian Medicine and Surgery*. G. J. Harrison and L. R. Harrison. Philadelphia, W.B. Saunders: 327-55.

Gauvin, J. (1993). Drug therapy in reptiles. Seminars in Avian & Exotic Med 2(1): 48-59.

Hawkins, E. (2000). Pulmonary Parenchymal Diseases. *Textbook of Veterinary Internal Medicine: Diseases of the Dog and Cat*. S. Ettinger and E. Feldman. Philadelphia, WB Saunders. 2: 1061-91.

Hayes, P. (2000). Diseases of Chinchillas. *Kirk's Current Veterinary Therapy: XIII Small Animal Practice*. J. Bonagura. Philadelphia, WB Saunders: 1152-7.

Hillier, A., et al. (2014). Guidelines for the diagnosis and antimicrobial therapy of canine superficial bacterial folliculitis (Antimicrobial Guidelines Working Group of the International Society for Companion Animal Infectious Diseases). Vet Derm.

Ivey, E. & J. Morrisey (2000). Therapeutics for Rabbits. Vet Clin NA: Exotic Anim Pract **3:1**(Jan): 183-216.

Jacobson, E. (1999). Bacterial infections and antimicrobial treatment in reptiles. The North American Veterinary Conference, Orlando. accessed via Veterinary Information Network; vin.com

Johnson, D. (2006). Ferrets: the other companion animal. Proceedings: ACVC. accessed via Veterinary Information Network; vin.com

Lewbart (2001). Reptile Formulary. Proceedings: Atlantic Coast Veterinary Conference. accessed via Veterinary Information Network; vin.com

Papich, M. (1989). Effects of drugs on pregnancy. *Current Veterinary Therapy X: Small Animal Practice.* R. Kirk. Philadelphia, Saunders: 1291-9.

Shirani, D., et al. (2010). Effects of short-term oral administration of trimethoprim-sulfamethoxazole on Schirmer II tear test results in clinically normal rabbits. Veterinary Record **166**(20): 623-5.

Tully, T. (2013). Avian Parasites. ABVP. accessed via Veterinary Information Network; vin.com

Weese, J. S., et al. (2011). Antimicrobial Use Guidelines for Treatment of Urinary Tract Disease in Dogs and Cats: Antimicrobial Guidelines Working Group of the International Society for Companion Animal Infectious Diseases. Veterinary Medicine International.

Williams, B. (2000). Therapeutics in Ferrets. Vet Clin NA: Exotic Anim Pract **3:1**(Jan): 131-53.

Winther, L., et al. (2011). Antimicrobial disposition in pulmonary epithelial lining fluid of horses. Part I. Sulfadiazine and trimethoprim. J. Vet. Pharmacol. Ther. **34**(3): 277-84.

Sulfadimethoxine

(sul-fa-dye-meth-ox-een)   Albon®

Sulfonamide Antimicrobial

Prescriber Highlights

▶ Sulfonamide antimicrobial agent. Usually used for coccidiosis.

▶ Contraindications: Hypersensitivity to sulfas, thiazides, or sulfonylurea agents; severe renal or hepatic impairment; Dobermans. Caution: Diminished renal or hepatic function, or urinary obstruction.

▶ Adverse Effects: Can precipitate in the urine (esp. with high dosages for prolonged periods, acidic urine or highly concentrated urine). **Dogs:** Keratoconjunctivitis sicca, bone marrow depression, hypersensitivity reactions (rashes, dermatitis), focal retinitis, fever, vomiting & nonseptic polyarthritis possible.

▶ Potentially teratogenic; weigh risk vs. benefit.

Uses/Indications

Sulfadimethoxine injection and tablets are FDA-approved for use in dogs and cats for respiratory, genitourinary, enteric and soft tissue infections caused by susceptible organisms. Sulfadimethoxine is used in the treatment of coccidiosis in dogs although not FDA-approved for this indication.

In horses, sulfadimethoxine injection is FDA-approved for the treatment of respiratory infections caused by *Streptococcus equi*.

In cattle, the drug is FDA-approved for treating shipping fever complex, calf diphtheria, bacterial pneumonia and foot rot caused by susceptible organisms.

In poultry, sulfadimethoxine is added to drinking water to treat coccidiosis, fowl cholera, and infectious coryza.

Pharmacology/Actions

Sulfonamides are usually bacteriostatic agents when used alone. They are thought to prevent bacterial replication by competing with para-aminobenzoic acid (PABA) in the biosynthesis of tetrahydrofolic acid in the pathway to form folic acid. Only microorganisms that synthesize their own folic acid are affected by sulfas.

Microorganisms that are usually affected by sulfonamides include some gram-positive bacteria, including some strains of streptococci, staphylococcus, *Bacillus anthracis*, *Clostridium tetani*, *C. perfringens*, and many strains of Nocardia. Sulfas also have *in vitro* activity against some gram-negative species, including some strains of Shigella, Salmonella, *E. coli*, Klebsiella, Enterobacter, Pasteurella, and Proteus. Sulfas have activity against some rickettsia and protozoa (Toxoplasma, Coccidia). Unfortunately, resistance to sulfas is a progressing phenomenon and many strains of bacteria that were once susceptible to this class of antibacterial are now resistant. The sulfas are less efficacious in pus, necrotic tissue, or in areas with extensive cellular debris.

Pharmacokinetics

In dogs, cats, swine, and sheep, sulfadimethoxine is reportedly readily absorbed and well distributed. Relative volumes of distribution range from 0.17 L/kg in sheep to 0.35 L/kg in cattle and horses. The drug is highly protein bound.

In most species, sulfadimethoxine is acetylated in the liver to acetylsulfadimethoxine and excreted unchanged in the liver. In dogs, the drug is not appreciably hepatically metabolized and renal excretion is the basis for the majority of elimination of the drug. Sulfadimethoxine's long elimination half-lives are a result of its appreciable reabsorption in the renal tubules. Serum half-lives reported in various species are: swine 14 hours; sheep 15 hours; and horses 11.3 hours.

Contraindications/Precautions/Warnings

Sulfonamides are contraindicated in patients hypersensitive to them, thiazides, or sulfonylurea agents. They are also considered contraindicated in patients with severe renal or hepatic impairment and should be used with caution in patients with diminished renal or hepatic function, or urinary obstruction.

Doberman pinschers appear to be very susceptible to sulfonamide-induced poly-systemic immune complex disease and most believe that these drugs are contraindicated in them.

Oral sulfonamides can depress the normal cellulytic function of the ruminoreticulum, but this effect is generally temporary and the animal adapts.

Adverse Effects

Sulfonamides (or their metabolites) can precipitate in the urine, particularly when given at high dosages for prolonged periods. Acidic urine or highly concentrated urine may also contribute to increased risk of crystalluria, hematuria, and renal tubule obstruction. Different sulfonamides have different solubilities at various pHs. Alkalinization of the urine using sodium bicarbonate may prevent crystalluria, but it also decreases the amount available for tubular reabsorption. Crystalluria can usually be avoided with most of the commercially available sulfonamides by maintaining an adequate urine flow. Normal urine pH in herbivores is usually 8 or more, so crystalluria is not frequently a problem. Sulfonamides can also cause various hypersensitivity reactions or diarrhea by altering the normal gut flora.

Too rapid intravenous injection of the sulfas can cause muscle weakness, blindness, ataxia, and collapse.

In dogs, keratoconjunctivitis sicca, bone marrow depression, hypersensitivity reactions (rashes, dermatitis), focal retinitis, fever, vomiting and nonseptic polyarthritis have been reported with sulfonamides.

Oral sulfonamides can depress the normal cellulytic function of the ruminoreticulum, but this effect is generally temporary and the animal adapts.

Because solutions of sulfonamides are usually alkaline, they can cause tissue irritation and necrosis if injected intramuscularly or subcutaneously.

Reproductive/Nursing Safety

Sulfas cross the placenta and may reach fetal levels of ≥50% than those found in maternal serum; teratogenicity has been reported in some laboratory animals when given at very high doses. They should be used in pregnant animals only when the benefits clearly outweigh the risks of therapy.

Sulfonamides are distributed into milk.

Overdosage/Acute Toxicity

Acute toxicity secondary to overdoses apparently occurs only rarely in veterinary species. In addition to the adverse effects listed above, CNS stimulation and myelin degeneration have been noted after very high dosages.

Drug Interactions

The following drug interactions have either been reported or are theoretical in humans or animals receiving sulfonamides and may be of significance in veterinary patients. Unless otherwise noted, use together is not necessarily contraindicated, but weigh the potential risks and perform additional monitoring when appropriate.

■ **ANTACIDS:** May decrease the oral bioavailability of sulfonamides if administered concurrently.

Laboratory Considerations

■ Sulfonamides may give false-positive results for **urine glucose** determinations when using the Benedict's method.

Doses

■ **DOGS/CATS:**

For coccidiosis (extra-label): 50 – 60 mg/kg PO once daily for 5-20 days. (CAPC 2014)

■ **FERRETS:**

For coccidiosis (extra-label): 50 mg/kg PO once, then 25 mg/kg q24h for 5-10 days. May not clear the organism.

■ **RABBITS, RODENTS, SMALL MAMMALS:**

a) Rabbits: 10 – 15 mg/kg PO q12h. (Ivey *et al.* 2000)

b) Rabbits: For coccidiosis: 25 mg/kg PO once daily. (Burke 1999)

c) Hedgehogs: 2 – 20 mg/kg/day IM, SC or PO. (Smith 2000)

d) Mice, Rats, Gerbils, Hamsters, Guinea pigs, Chinchillas: As a coccidiostat: 50 mg/kg PO once, then 25 mg/kg PO once daily for 10-20 days <u>or</u> 75 mg/kg PO for 7-14 days. (Adamcak *et al.* 2000)

■ **CATTLE:**

For susceptible infections: 55 mg/kg IV or PO initially, then 27.5 mg/kg q24h IV or PO for up to 5 days. If using sustained release boluses: 137.5 mg/kg PO every 4 days. (Package insert; *Albon*®)

■ **HORSES:**

For susceptible infections: 55 mg/kg IV or PO initially, then 27.5 mg/kg q24h IV. (Package insert; *Albon*®)

■ **CAMELIDS (NWC):**

a) For coccidiosis ("regular" coccidia: *E. alpacae, E. lamae, E. punoensis, E. peruviana*): 15 mg/kg PO twice daily for 5 days; monitor for signs of polioencephalomalacia. (Walker 2009)

b) **Treatment of Eimeria infection** is generally directed at clinically affected animals using sulfadimethoxine at 110 mg/kg PO q24h (or amprolium). Treatments are effective only against the immature stages and therefore may not have a significant impact on fecal oocyst count initially. Given the long prepatent period, it is prudent to treat *E. macusaniensis* infections for 10-15 days. Treatment should be directly administered to the animal rather than by medicating water supplies. (McKenzie 2008)

■ **REPTILES:**

For coccidia (extra-label): 90 mg/kg PO on day one and then 45 mg/kg PO on 5 successive days; may also be given IM or IV. Maintain adequate hydration. (Lewbart 2001)

Chemistry/Synonyms

A long-acting sulfonamide, sulfadimethoxine occurs as an odorless or almost odorless, creamy white powder. It is very slightly soluble in water and slightly soluble in alcohol.

Sulfadimethoxine may also be known as: solfadimetossina, solfadimetossipirimidina, sulphadimethoxine, *Albon*®, *Amtech*®, *Chemiosalfa*®, *Deltin*®, *Di-Methox*®, *Risulpir*®, *Ritarsulfa*®, *SDM*®, *Sulfadren*®, *Sulfastop*®, or *Sulfasol*®, and *Sulfathox*®.

Storage/Stability

Unless otherwise instructed by the manufacturer, store sulfadimethoxine products at room temperature and protect from light. If crystals form due to exposure to cold temperatures, either warm the vial or store at room temperature for several days to resolubolize the drug; efficacy is not impaired by this process.

Compatibility/Compounding Considerations

No specific information noted.

Dosage Forms/Regulatory Status

VETERINARY-LABELED PRODUCTS:

Sulfadimethoxine Injection: 400 mg/mL (40%) in 100 mL vials; *Albon*® *Injection 40%, Di-Methox*® *Injection 40%*, generic; (Rx) FDA-approved for use in dogs, cats, horses, swine and cattle. Not to be used in horses intended for food or calves to be processed for veal. Slaughter withdrawal (at labeled doses) = 5 days (cattle); milk withdrawal (at labeled doses) = 60 hours.

Sulfadimethoxine Oral Tablets: 125 mg, 250 mg, and 500 mg; *Albon*® *Tablets*; (Rx). FDA-approved for use in dogs and cats.

Sulfadimethoxine Oral Suspension: 50 mg/mL in 2 oz. and 16 oz. Bottles; *Albon*®; (Rx). FDA-approved for use in dogs and cats.

Sulfadimethoxine Oral Boluses: 5 grams, and 15 grams; *Albon*®; (OTC). FDA-approved for use in cattle. Not to be used in calves to be processed for veal. No withdrawal period has been established for this in preruminating calves. Slaughter withdrawal (at labeled doses) = 7 days (cattle); milk withdrawal (at labeled doses) = 60 hours.

Sulfadimethoxine Oral Boluses Sustained-Release: 12.5 g; *Albon*® *SR*; (Rx) FDA-approved for use in non-lactating cattle. Slaughter withdrawal (at labeled doses) = 21 days (cattle), a withdrawal period has not been established for pre-ruminating calves. Not for use in calves intended to be processed for veal.

Sulfadimethoxine Soluble Powder: 94.6 grams/packet (for addition to drinking water); *Albon*®, generic; FDA-approved for use in dairy calves, dairy heifers, beef cattle, broiler and replacement chickens only, and meat-producing turkeys. Slaughter withdrawal (at labeled doses) = 7 days (cattle); 5 days (poultry—do not use in chickens >16 weeks old or in turkeys >24 weeks old).

Sulfadimethoxine 12.5% Concentrated Solution (for addition to drinking water): *Albon*®, generic; (OTC). FDA-approved for use in chickens, turkeys and cattle. Slaughter withdrawal (at labeled doses) = 7 days (for dairy calves, dairy heifers and beef cattle only. Withdrawal for pre-ruminating calves has not been established. Not to be used in calves to be processed for veal; 5 days (poultry—do not use in chickens >16 weeks old or in turkeys >24 weeks old).

HUMAN-LABELED PRODUCTS: NONE.

Revisions/References

Monograph revised/updated August 2014.

Adamcak, A. & B. Otten (2000). Rodent Therapeutics. Vet Clin NA: Exotic Anim Pract 3:1(Jan): 221-40.

Burke, T. (1999). Husbandry and Medicine of Rodents and Lagomorphs. Proceedings: Central Veterinary Conference, Kansas City. accessed via Veterinary Information Network; vin.com

CAPC (2014). Companion Animal Parasite Council (CAPC) Recommendations, CAPCvet.org.

Ivey, E. & J. Morrisey (2000). Therapeutics for Rabbits. Vet Clin NA: Exotic Anim Pract 3:1(Jan): 183-216.

Lewbart (2001). Reptile Formulary. Proceedings: Atlantic Coast Veterinary Conference. accessed via Veterinary Information Network; vin.com

McKenzie, E. (2008). Diagnosis & Management of Diseases of Neonatal & Juvenile Camelids. Proceedings: ACVIM. accessed via Veterinary Information Network; vin.com

Smith, A. (2000). General husbandry and medical care of hedgehogs. *Kirk's Current Veterinary Therapy: XIII Small Animal Practice*. J. Bonagura. Philadelphia, WB Saunders: 1128-33.

Walker, P. (2009). Differential Diagnosis of Diarrhea in Camelid Crias. Proceedings: ACVIM. accessed via Veterinary Information Network; vin.com

Sulfadimethoxine/Ormetoprim

(or-me-toe-prim)   Primor ®

Potentiated Sulfonamide Antimicrobial

Prescriber Highlights

▶ Potentiated sulfa similar to trimethoprim/sulfa, but may have fewer adverse effects and is labeled for once daily dosing.

▶ Does not appear to be effective for prostate infections and is more expensive then generic trimethoprim/sulfa.

The following apply to TMP/Sulfa & may apply to this agent as well:

▶ Contraindications: Hypersensitive to sulfas, thiazides, or sulfonylurea agents; severe renal or hepatic impairment; Dobermans.

▶ Caution: Diminished renal or hepatic function, or urinary obstruction or urolithiasis.

▶ Adverse Effects: **Dogs:** Keratoconjunctivitis sicca, hypersensitivity (Type 1 or Type 3) acute neutrophilic hepatitis with icterus, vomiting, anorexia, diarrhea, fever, hemolytic anemia, urticaria, polyarthritis, facial swelling, polydipsia, crystalluria, hematuria, polyuria, cholestasis, hypothyroidism, anemias, agranulocytosis, idiosyncratic hepatic necrosis in dogs. **Cats:** Anorexia, crystalluria, hematuria, leukopenias & anemias.

▶ Potentially teratogenic, weigh risk vs. benefit.

Uses/Indications

Sulfadimethoxine/ormetoprim is FDA-approved for the treatment of skin and soft tissue infections in dogs caused by susceptible strains of *Staphylococcus aureus* and *E. coli*. Some feel that it has fewer adverse effects in dogs than trimethoprim/sulfa and can be dosed once daily. It is more expensive than trimethoprim/sulfa and does not appear to penetrate into the prostate as well.

Pharmacology/Actions

Sulfadimethoxine/ormetoprim shares mechanisms of action and probably the bacterial spectrum of activity with trimethoprim/sulfa. Alone, sulfonamides are bacteriostatic agents, but in combination with either ormetoprim or trimethoprim, the potentiated sulfas are bactericidal. Potentiated sulfas sequentially inhibit enzymes in the folic acid pathway, thereby inhibiting bacterial thymidine synthesis. The sulfonamide blocks the conversion of para-aminobenzoic acid (PABA) to dihydrofolic acid (DFA) and ormetoprim blocks the conversion of DFA to tetrahydrofolic acid by inhibiting dihydrofolate reductase.

The potentiated sulfas have a fairly broad spectrum of activity. Gram-positive bacteria that are generally susceptible include most streptococci, many strains of staphylococcus, and Nocardia. Many gram-negative organisms of the family Enterobacteriaceae are susceptible to the potentiated sulfas, but not *Pseudomonas aeruginosa*. Some protozoa (*Pneumocystis carinii*, Coccidia and Toxoplasma) are also inhibited by the combination. Potentiated sulfas reportedly have little activity against most anaerobes, but opinions on this vary.

Resistance will develop more slowly to the combination of drugs, than to either one alone. In gram-negative organisms, resistance is usually plasmid-mediated.

Pharmacokinetics

The pharmacokinetics of sulfadimethoxine are outlined in the previous monograph. Pharmacokinetic data for ormetoprim is not available at the time of this writing, but the manufacturer states that therapeutic levels are maintained over 24 hours at recommended doses. Unlike trimethoprim/sulfa, ormetoprim does not apparently attain clinically effective levels in the prostate for treating bacterial prostatic infections.

Contraindications/Precautions/Warnings

The manufacturer states that ormetoprim/sulfadimethoxine should not be used in dogs showing marked liver parenchymal damage, blood dyscrasias, or in those with a history of sulfonamide sensitivity.

Doberman pinschers appear to be very susceptible to sulfonamide-induced poly-systemic immune complex disease and most believe that these drugs are contraindicated in them.

This combination should be used with caution in patients with pre-existing hepatic or thyroid disease.

Adverse Effects

This combination would be expected to exhibit an adverse reaction profile in dogs similar to that seen with trimethoprim/sulfa, including: keratoconjunctivitis sicca (which may be irreversible), acute neutrophilic hepatitis with icterus, vomiting, anorexia, diarrhea, fever, hemolytic anemia, urticaria, polyarthritis, facial swelling, polydipsia, polyuria, and cholestasis. Acute hypersensitivity reactions manifesting as Type I, (anaphylaxis) or Type III reaction (serum sickness) can also be seen. Hypersensitivity reactions appear to be more common in large breed dogs; Doberman Pinschers may possibly be more susceptible to this effect than other breeds. Other hematologic effects (anemias, agranulocytosis) are possible, but fairly rare.

Long-term (8 weeks) therapy at recommended doses with ormetoprim/sulfadimethoxine (27.5 mg/kg once daily) resulted in elevated serum cholesterol, thyroid and liver weights, mild follicular thyroid hyperplasia, and enlarged basophilic cells in the pituitary. The manufacturer states that the principal treatment-related effect of extended or excessive usage is hypothyroidism.

Reproductive/Nursing Safety

Safety of ormetoprim/sulfadimethoxine has not been established in pregnant animals. Reports of teratogenicity (cleft palate) have been reported in some lab animals with trimethoprim/sulfa.

Overdosage/Acute Toxicity

In experimental studies in dogs, doses >80 mg/kg resulted in slight tremors and increased motor activity in some dogs. Higher doses may result in depression, anorexia, or seizures.

It is suggested that very high oral overdoses be handled by emptying the gut using standard precautions and protocols and by treating clinical signs supportively and symptomatically.

Drug Interactions; Laboratory Considerations

■ None have been noted for this combination, but it would be expected that the potential interactions outlined for the trimethoprim/sulfa monograph would also apply to this combination; refer to that monograph for more information.

Doses

■ **DOGS:**

Note: Unless otherwise noted, doses are for combined amounts of ormetoprim & sulfadimethoxine.

For labeled indications (skin and soft tissue infections in dogs caused by susceptible strains of *staphylococci* and *E. coli*);

(FDA-approved): Initially 55 mg/kg (combined drug) PO on the first day of therapy, then 27.5 mg/kg PO once daily for at least 2 days after remission of clinical signs. Not approved for treatment longer than 21 days. (Package insert; *Primor*®)

For superficial bacterial folliculitis (extra-label): 55 mg/kg on first day, then 27.5 mg/kg PO once daily. From the Antimicrobial Guidelines Working Group of the International Society for Companion Animal Infectious Diseases. Potentiated sulfas (trimethoprim/sulfa, ormetoprim/sulfa) are first tier drugs only if local regional susceptibility of *Staphylococcus pseudintermedius* is known. If prolonged (>7 day) therapy is anticipated, baseline Schirmer's tear testing is recommended, with periodic re-evaluation and owner monitoring for ocular discharge. Avoid in dogs that may be sensitive to potential adverse effects, such as keratoconjunctivitis sicca, hepatopathy, hypersensitivity and skin eruptions. (Hillier *et al.* 2014)

For coccidiosis (extra-label): 55 mg/kg for 7-23 days. (CAPC 2014)

Monitoring

- Clinical efficacy.
- Adverse effects.
- In dogs, monitor tear production (one suggestion is in 5 days after starting treatment and then every 2-3 weeks).

Client Information

- Animals must be allowed free access to water and must not become dehydrated while on therapy.

Chemistry/Synonyms

A diaminopyrimidine structurally related to trimethoprim, ormetoprim occurs as a white, almost tasteless powder. The chemistry of sulfadimethoxine is described in the previous monograph.

Sulfadimethoxine may also be known as: solfadimetossina, solfadimetossipirimidina, sulphadimethoxine, *Chemiosalfa*®, *Deltin*®, *Risulpir*®, *Ritarsulfa*®, *Sulfadren*®, *Sulfastop*®, or *Sulfathox*®.

Ormetoprim may also be known as NSC-95072, ormetoprima, ormétoprime, ormetoprimum, or Ro-5-9754.

Storage/Stability

Unless otherwise instructed by the manufacturer, store tablets in tight, light resistant containers at room temperature.

Compatibility/Compounding Considerations

No specific information noted.

Dosage Forms/Regulatory Status

VETERINARY-LABELED PRODUCTS:

Sulfadimethoxine/Ormetoprim Tablets (scored)

120's: 100 mg Sulfadimethoxine, 20 mg Ormetoprim

240's: 200 mg Sulfadimethoxine, 40 mg Ormetoprim

600's: 500 mg Sulfadimethoxine, 100 mg Ormetoprim

1200's: 1000 mg Sulfadimethoxine, 200 mg Ormetoprim; *Primor*®; (Rx). FDA-approved for use in dogs.

Sulfadimethoxine/Ormetoprim medicated premix: 113.5 grams sulfadimethoxine and 68.1 grams ormetoprim per pound in 50 lb bags. FDA-approved for use in chickens [broilers, replacements (breeders and layers)], turkeys, ducks, & Chukar partridges. Slaughter withdrawal (at labeled doses) = 5 days. Do not feed to chickens >6 weeks or age, turkeys or ducks producing eggs for food. *Rofenaid*® 40, *Romet*® 30; FDA-approved for use in salmonids (trout and salmon) and catfish. Slaughter or release as stocker fish = 42 days. (OTC)

HUMAN-LABELED PRODUCTS: NONE.

Revisions/References

Monograph revised/updated August 2014.

CAPC (2014). Companion Animal Parasite Council (CAPC) Recommendations, CAPCvet. org.

Hillier, A., et al. (2014). Guidelines for the diagnosis and antimicrobial therapy of canine superficial bacterial folliculitis (Antimicrobial Guidelines Working Group of the International Society for Companion Animal Infectious Diseases). Vet Derm.

Sulfasalazine

(sul-fa-**sal**-a-zeen)   Azulfidine®

Sulfonamide/Salicylate Antibacterial/Immunosuppressive

Prescriber Highlights

▶ Sulfa-analog that has GI antibacterial & antiinflammatory activity used for inflammatory bowel disease; has also been used for vasculitis.

▶ Contraindications: Hypersensitivity to it, sulfas or salicylates; intestinal or urinary obstructions; Dobermans.

▶ Caution: Liver, renal or hematologic diseases; cats.

▶ Adverse Effects: **Dogs:** Keratoconjunctivitis sicca, anorexia, vomiting, cholestatic jaundice, hemolytic anemia, leukopenia, vomiting, decreased sperm counts & an allergic dermatitis. **Cats:** Anorexia, vomiting, anemias.

Uses/Indications

Sulfasalazine is used for the treatment of inflammatory large bowel (colonic) disease in dogs and cats. It has also been suggested for adjunctive use in treating vasculitis in dogs. It is not effective for small intestinal inflammation as colonic bacteria are required to cleave the drug into mesalamine (5-ASA) and sulfapyridine.

Pharmacology/Actions

While the exact mechanism of action for its therapeutic effects in treating colitis in small animals has not been determined, it is believed that after sulfasalazine is cleaved into sulfapyridine and 5-aminosalicylic acid (5-ASA, mesalamine) by bacteria in the gut, the antibacterial (sulfapyridine) and/or antiinflammatory (mesalamine) activity alters the clinical signs/course of the disease. Levels of both drugs in the colon are higher then by giving them orally as separate agents.

Pharmacokinetics

No pharmacokinetic data for dogs or cats was located. In humans, only ≈ 10-33% of an orally administered dose of sulfasalazine is absorbed. Apparently, some of this absorbed drug is then excreted unchanged in the bile. Unabsorbed and biliary excreted drug is cleaved into 5-ASA and sulfapyridine in the colon by bacterial flora. The sulfapyridine component is rapidly absorbed, but only a small percentage of the 5-ASA is absorbed.

Absorbed sulfapyridine and 5-ASA are hepatically metabolized and then renally excreted.

Contraindications/Precautions/Warnings

Sulfasalazine is contraindicated in animals hypersensitive to it, sulfonamides or salicylates. It is also contraindicated in patients with intestinal or urinary obstructions. Doberman pinschers appear to be very susceptible to sulfonamide-induced polysystemic immune complex disease and most believe that these drugs are contraindicated in them.

It should be used with caution in animals with preexisting liver, renal or hematologic diseases. Because cats can be sensitive to salicylates (see the aspirin monograph), use caution when using this drug in this species.

Do not confuse sulfaSALAzine with sulfaDIAZINE.

Adverse Effects

Although adverse effects do occur in dogs, with keratoconjunctivitis sicca (KCS) reported most frequently, they are considered to occur relatively uncommonly. Other potential adverse effects include anorexia, vomiting, cholestatic jaundice, hemolytic anemia, leukopenia, vomiting, decreased sperm counts and an allergic dermatitis. Should decreased tear production be noted early, either reducing the dose or discontinuing the drug may prevent progression of KCS or increase tear production.

Cats can occasionally develop anorexia and vomiting which may be alleviated by use of the enteric-coated tablets. Anemias secondary to sulfasalazine are also potentially possible in cats.

Reproductive/Nursing Safety

Although sulfasalazine has not been proven harmful to use during pregnancy and incidences of neonatal kernicterus in infants born to women taking sulfasalazine are low, it should only be used when clearly indicated. In laboratory animal studies (rats, rabbits), doses of 6X normal (human) caused impairment of fertility in male animals; this effect is thought to be caused by the sulfapyridine component and was reversible upon discontinuation of the drug.

In humans, the FDA categorizes this drug as category *B* for use during pregnancy (*Animal studies have not yet demonstrated risk to the fetus, but there are no adequate studies in pregnant women; or animal studies have shown an adverse effect, but adequate studies in pregnant women have not demonstrated a risk to the fetus in the first trimester of pregnancy, and there is no evidence of risk in later trimesters.*) In a separate system evaluating the safety of drugs in canine and feline pregnancy (Papich 1989), this drug is categorized as in class: *B* (*Safe for use if used cautiously. Studies in laboratory animals may have uncovered some risk, but these drugs appear to be safe in dogs and cats or these drugs are safe if they are not administered when the animal is near term.*)

Sulfonamides are excreted in milk. In human newborns, they compete with bilirubin for binding sites on plasma proteins and may cause kernicterus. Use with caution in nursing patients.

Overdosage/Acute Toxicity

Little specific information is available regarding overdoses with this agent, but because massive overdoses could cause significant salicylate and/or sulfonamide toxicity, standard protocols (empty stomach, cathartics, etc.) should be considered. Urine alkalinization and forced diuresis may also be beneficial in selected cases.

Drug Interactions

The following drug interactions have either been reported or are theoretical in humans or animals receiving sulfasalazine and may be of significance in veterinary patients. Unless otherwise noted, use together is not necessarily contraindicated, but weigh the potential risks and perform additional monitoring when appropriate.

- **CHLORPROPAMIDE:** Hypoglycemic effects could be potentiated.
- **DIGOXIN:** Sulfasalazine may reduce absorption.
- **FERROUS SULFATE or other iron salts:** May decrease the blood levels of sulfasalazine if administered concurrently; clinical significance is unknown.
- **FOLIC ACID:** Oral absorption may be inhibited.
- **WARFARIN:** Potentially sulfasalazine could potentiate warfarin.

Doses

Note: Unless otherwise noted assume the following dosages are for the standard-release tablets.

- **DOGS:**
  For inflammatory large bowel disease (extra-label): Anecdotal dosage recommendations vary considerably and no definitive studies were located supporting any one dose. Initial dosages range from 20 – 50 mg/kg PO 2-3 times a day (most recommend 3 times daily). After 2-4 weeks (longer if at the low end of the dosing range) most taper off (reducing dosage every 2 weeks)

until eventual drug discontinuation while maintaining dietary treatment. Some dogs may require chronic therapy.
  For adjunctive treatment of vasculitis (extra-label): 20 – 40 mg/kg PO q8h. (Hillier 2006), (Griffin 2006)

- **CATS:**
  For inflammatory large bowel disease (extra-label): Use cautiously in cats because of their sensitivity to salicylates. Anecdotal dosage recommendations vary somewhat and no definitive studies were located supporting any one dose. Dosages range from 10 – 20 mg/kg PO 1-3 times a day (most recommend once daily). Some state to treat no longer than 10 days and others taper to the lowest effective dose.

- **FERRETS:**
  a) 10 – 20 mg/kg PO 2-3 times a day. (Williams 2000)
  b) 25 mg (total dose) PO twice daily. (Weiss 2002)

- **HORSES:**
  For chronic diarrhea (extra-label): From a case report. Sulfasalazine was used (with dietary adjustment) at 16 mg/kg PO once a day for 5 days, followed by 8 mg/kg PO once a day for 10 days. (Note: Although unconfirmed, the product used appears to be a delayed-release product; *Salazopyrin*® EN–Pfizer Italy). (Valle *et al.* 2013)

Monitoring

- Efficacy.
- Adverse effects, particularly KCS; Schirmer tear tests should be performed prior to therapy (and on rechecks), especially in middle-aged to older dogs.
- Occasional CBC, liver function tests are warranted with chronic therapy.

Client Information

- Give with food. Often dosage is raised until diarrhea is controlled and then it's reduced to the lowest effective dosage.
- Watch dogs for dry eye syndrome.
- Cats may be sensitive to the drug; report anything unusual to veterinarian.
- People allergic to sulfa drugs should handle this drug with caution.

Chemistry/Synonyms

Sulfasalazine is basically a molecule of sulfapyridine linked by a diazo bond to the diazonium salt of salicylic acid. It occurs as an odorless, bright yellow to brownish-yellow fine powder. Less than 0.1 mg is soluble in 1 mL of water and ≈ 0.34 mg is soluble in 1 mL of alcohol.

Sulfasalazine may also be known as: salazosulfapyridine, salicylazosulfapyridine, sulfasalazinum, sulphasalazine, *Sulfazine*® and *Azulfidine*®®®.

Storage/Stability

Sulfasalazine tablets (either plain or enteric-coated) should be stored at temperatures less than 40°C and preferably at room temperature (15-30°C, 59-86°F) in well-closed containers. The oral suspension should be stored at room temperature (15-30°C, 59-86°F); avoid freezing.

Compatibility/Compounding Considerations

No specific information noted.

Dosage Forms/Regulatory Status

VETERINARY-LABELED PRODUCTS: NONE.

HUMAN-LABELED PRODUCTS:

Sulfasalazine Tablets: 500 mg; *Azulfidine*®, *Sulfazine*®, generic; (Rx)

Sulfasalazine Delayed-Release Tablets: 500 mg (enteric coated); *Azulfidine*® EN-tabs®, *Sulfazine EC*®, generic; (Rx)

Revisions/References

Monograph revised/updated August 2014.

Griffin, C. (2006). Dermatologic diseases of the auricle. Proceedings: WSAVA Congress. accessed via Veterinary Information Network; vin.com

Hillier, A. (2006). Life threatening skin diseases. Proceedings: ACVC. accessed via Veterinary Information Network; vin.com

Papich, M. (1989). Effects of drugs on pregnancy. *Current Veterinary Therapy X: Small Animal Practice.* R. Kirk. Philadelphia, Saunders: 1291-9.

Valle, E., et al. (2013). Management of Chronic Diarrhea in an Adult Horse. Journal of Equine Veterinary Science 33(2): 130-5.

Weiss, C. (2002). Newly recognized diseases of ferrets. Proceedings: Atlantic Coast Veterinary Conference. accessed via Veterinary Information Network; vin.com

Williams, B. (2000). Therapeutics in Ferrets. Vet Clin NA: Exotic Anim Pract 3:1(Jan): 131-53.

Tadalafil

(ta-dal-a-fil)   Cialis®

Phosphodiesterase Type 5 Inhibitor

Prescriber Highlights

▶ PDP5 inhibitor that may be useful for treating pulmonary arterial hypertension in dogs.

▶ Very limited clinical experience or published data for use in dogs.

▶ Appears to have a longer duration action than sildenafil.

▶ Contraindicated if patients receiving organic nitrates.

▶ Adverse effects not well known for dogs; inguinal flushing, GI effects reported with sildenafil.

▶ Currently, very expensive.

Uses/Indications

Tadalafil is a phosphodiesterase-5 inhibitor similar to sildenafil and may be useful for treating pulmonary arterial hypertension (PAH) in dogs. A pilot study done in dogs with PAH, showed that tadalafil (1 mg/kg PO) caused modest, but significant decreases in diastolic pulmonary arterial pressure (PAP), mean PAP and tricuspid regurgitation suggesting that oral tadalafil, when added to conventional heart failure therapy, decreases PAP in dogs with PAH. Because of its longer duration of action, tadalafil has some advantages over sildenafil but it is currently very expensive.

In humans, tadalafil is approved for use in treating pulmonary artery hypertension (*Adcirca*®) and erectile dysfunction (*Cialis*®). Off-label uses include treating Raynaud's phenomenon.

Pharmacology/Actions

Tadalafil is a selective inhibitor of cyclic guanosine monophosphate (cGMP)–specific phosphodiesterase type 5 (PDE5). PDE5 is the enzyme responsible for the degradation of cGMP and is found (in humans) in the corpus cavernosum smooth muscle, pulmonary vascular and visceral smooth muscle, skeletal muscle, platelets, kidney, lung, cerebellum, and pancreas. In patients with PAH, vascular endothelium nitric oxide release is impaired with associated reduction of cGMP. PDE5 is the primary phosphodiesterase in pulmonary vasculature and tadalafil's PDE5 inhibition increases cGMP thereby relaxing pulmonary vascular smooth muscle with resultant vasodilation.

Pharmacokinetics

No pharmacokinetic data for tadalafil for dogs was located.

In humans, after oral administration maximum plasma concentrations occur ≈ 4 hours in patients with PAH. Food does not alter the rate or extent of absorption. Tadalafil is 94% bound to human plasma proteins. Tadalafil is metabolized by CYP3A4 to a catechol metabolite that then undergoes methylation and glucuronidation. These metabolites are not thought to be active. In PAH patients, mean terminal half-life is 35 hours. Excretion is primarily of the drug's metabolites via fecal routes (61%) with the majority of the remainder in the urine (≈ 36%).

Contraindications/Precautions/Warnings

Tadalafil is contraindicated in human patients using any form of organic nitrate (either regularly or intermittently), and in those with serious hypersensitivity to tadalafil. Dosage reductions may be required in patients with severe hepatic or renal impairment.

Adverse Effects

An adverse effect profile for dogs at suggested doses for PAH has not been determined. Cutaneous flushing of the inguinal region has been reported with sildenafil in dogs. GI effects are possible. In a 12-month tadalafil chronic toxicity study done in dogs, no disseminated arteritis was observed as was seen in rodent studies, but 2 dogs exhibited marked decreases in neutrophils and moderate decreases in platelets with inflammatory signs when dosed at ≈ 4-18X the equivalent human dose. These effects were reversible within 2 weeks after discontinuing the drug.

Most common adverse effects of tadalafil reported in humans with PAH, include dyspepsia, nausea, back pain, myalgia, nasal congestion, flushing and headache. Rare, but serious adverse effects include hypersensitivity, optic neuropathy, seizures, Stevens-Johnson syndrome and exfoliative dermatitis, and deafness.

Reproductive/Nursing Safety

Tadalafil animal reproduction studies in rats and mice demonstrated no evidence of teratogenicity, embryotoxicity, or fetotoxicity when tadalafil was given to pregnant rats or mice at exposures of up to 11X (human equivalent dose). The FDA categorizes tadalafil as category *B* for use during pregnancy (*Animal studies have not yet demonstrated risk to the fetus, but there are no adequate studies in pregnant women; or animal studies have shown an adverse effect, but adequate studies in pregnant women have not demonstrated a risk to the fetus in the first trimester of pregnancy, and there is no evidence of risk in later trimesters.*)

Tadalafil and/or its metabolites are secreted into the milk in lactating rats at concentrations ≈ 2.4-fold those found in the plasma. It is unlikely to pose much risk to nursing offspring.

Overdosage/Acute Toxicity

Little information is available. Single doses of up to 500 mg have been given to healthy men, and multiple daily doses of up to 100 mg have been given to men with erectile dysfunction; adverse reactions were similar to those seen at lower doses.

It is expected that overdoses in animals would mirror the drugs adverse effect profile; treat supportively. Contact an animal poison control center for guidance, if necessary.

Drug Interactions

The following drug interactions have either been reported or are theoretical in humans or animals receiving tadalafil and may be of significance in veterinary patients. Unless otherwise noted, use together is not necessarily contraindicated, but weigh the potential risks and perform additional monitoring when appropriate.

■ **ALPHA-ADRENERGIC BLOCKERS** (*e.g.,* **tamsulosin, prazosin, phenothiazines, phenoxybenzamine**): May increase hypotensive effects.

■ **AMLODIPINE**: Potential to increase hypotensive effects.

■ **ANTIHYPERTENSIVE, HYPOTENSIVE DRUGS**: Potentially could increase hypotensive effects.

■ **AZOLE ANTIFUNGALS** (*e.g.,* **ketoconazole, itraconazole**): May reduce tadalafil metabolism and increase AUC.

■ **CIMETIDINE**: May reduce tadalafil metabolism and increase AUC.

■ **ERYTHROMYCIN, CLARITHROMYCIN**: May reduce tadalafil metabolism and increase AUC.

■ **NITRATES** (*e.g.,* **NTG, isosorbide**): Significant potentiation of vasodilatory effects; life-threatening hypotension possible.

- **NITROPRUSSIDE SODIUM:** Significant potentiation of vasodilatory effects; life-threatening hypotension possible.
- **PHENOBARBITAL:** May decrease tadalafil concentrations.
- **RIFAMPIN:** May decrease tadalafil concentrations.

Laboratory Considerations
- None noted.

Doses
- **DOGS:**

  For pulmonary arterial hypertension (extra-label):

  a) From a case report in a Yorkshire terrier: 1 mg/kg PO q48h (every other day) was added to the background treatment (furosemide, spironolactone, benazepril, dexamethasone and oxygen). Dog's condition rapidly improved (<24 hours) and 7-day follow-up showed a decrease (up to 26 mmHg) in systolic pulmonary arterial pressure and disappearance of all respiratory and cardiac signs of PAH (cyanosis, syncope and tachypnea). Authors recommend long-term studies in more animals. (Serres *et al.* 2006)

  b) 1 mg/kg PO once daily. (Oyama 2009)

Monitoring
- Clinical efficacy (improved syncope, cough, respiratory effort).
- Pulmonary artery pressure, systemic blood pressure.
- Adverse effects.

Client Information
- May be given with or without food.
- Be sure to give exactly as prescribed.
- May cause flushing (redness) in groin area; gastrointestinal effects (*e.g.*, lack of appetite, vomiting, diarrhea, etc.) possible.
- Not used often in veterinary medicine, so report any other effects to veterinarian.

Chemistry/Synonyms
Tadalafil has a molecular weight of 389.41. It is insoluble in water and slightly soluble in ethanol.

Tadalafil may also be known as: GF-196960, IC-351, tadalafiili, tadalafilo, or tadalafilum. *Cialis®* and *Adcirca®* are trade names for tadalafil.

Storage/Stability
Tadalafil tablets should be stored at room temperature between 59°-86°F (15°-30°C).

Dosage Forms/Regulatory Status
VETERINARY-LABELED PRODUCTS: NONE.
HUMAN-LABELED PRODUCTS:
Tadalafil Oral Tablets: 2.5 mg, 5 mg, 10 mg, 20 mg: *Cialis®*, *Adcirca®* (20 mg only); (Rx)

Compatibility/Compounding Considerations
A method of preparing a stable 5 mg/mL oral suspension from tablets has been published. Crush fifteen 20 mg tadalafil tablets to a fine powder in a glass mortar. Mix together 30 mL of *Ora-Sweet®* and 30 mL of *Ora-Plus®*; stir vigorously. Add 30 mL of this solution in geometric proportions to the powder and mix to form a smooth suspension. Transfer the mixture to a 2 ounce (60 mL) amber plastic prescription bottle. Rinse mortar with a quantity of the vehicle sufficient to make a final volume of 60 mL. Label "shake well." Suspension is stable for 91 days when stored at room temperature in an amber plastic prescription bottle. (Pettit *et al.* 2012)

Revisions/References
Monograph revised/updated August 2014.

Oyama, M. (2009). Pulmonary Hypertension: What you can't see can kill you. Proceedings: ACVC. accessed via Veterinary Information Network; vin.com
Pettit, R., et al. (2012). Stability of an Extemporaneously Prepared Tadalafil Suspension. Am J Health Syst Pharm 7: 592-4.
Serres, F., et al. (2006). Efficacy of Oral Tadalafil, a New Long-acting Phosphodiesterase-5 Inhibitor, for the Short-term Treatment of Pulmonary Arterial Hypertension in a Dog. J Vet Med A 53: 129-33.

Tamsulosin
(tam-suh-low-sin)   Flomax®
Alpha-1 Adrenergic Antagonist

Prescriber Highlights
▶ Alpha-1 antagonist that causes selective blockade of smooth muscle in the ureters, urethra and prostate. Little clinical experience with this drug in dogs and cats, but could potentially be useful as a lower urinary tract (uretal/urethral) relaxant.
▶ Contraindications: Patients known to be hypersensitive to it. Hypersensitivity reactions (in humans) have included skin rash, urticaria, pruritus, angioedema and respiratory symptoms.
▶ Higher dosages could cause hypotension. Do not crush sustained-release pellets in capsules as rapid oral absorption may result in hypotension.
▶ Give on an empty stomach to increase bioavailability.

Uses/Indications
Tamsulosin is an alpha-1 adrenergic blocking agent similar to prazosin and phenoxybenzamine, but is longer acting. Although evidence for efficacy in animals is scant, it potentially could be useful to facilitate passage of nephroliths and ureteroliths, and for treating functional urinary obstruction, benign prostatic hypertrophy, or detrusor-urethral dyssynergia in dogs and cats.

In humans, tamsulosin is labeled for treatment of benign prostatic hyperplasia (BPH). It is also used off-label for ureteral relaxation to facilitate passage of urinary calculi. It has been shown to be superior to calcium channel blockers (*e.g.*, nifedipine) for this purpose.

Pharmacology/Actions
Tamsulosin blocks sympathetic nervous stimulation of alpha-1 adrenoreceptors, found in the prostate, prostatic capsule, prostatic urethra, and bladder neck. Blockade of these adrenoreceptors can cause smooth muscles in the bladder neck and prostate to relax resulting in improvement in urine flow rate and expulsion of urinary calculi. In conscious male dogs, tamsulosin caused a sustained inhibitory effect on phenylephrine-induced prostatic intraurethral pressure (IUP) response that was related to higher concentrations in the prostate and urethra, rather than in plasma and vascular tissues (Sato *et al.* 2007).

Pharmacokinetics
Tamsulosin exhibits significant interspecies variation in its pharmacokinetics. After oral dosing of a non-sustained release formulation in dogs, tamsulosin bioavailability is ≈ 30% and peak plasma levels occur ≈ 0.5 hours. Volume of distribution Vd_{ss} is 1.74 L/kg; protein binding is 90%; clearance is 4 L/hr/kg (estimated unbound clearance: 31-41 L/hr/kg) and elimination half-life ≈ 1.5 hours (Matsushima *et al.* 1998). Tamsulosin levels are significantly higher and retained longer in prostatic and urethral tissues than in plasma. At 6 hours post-dose (0.03 mg/kg), prostate/plasma and urethra/plasma ratios were 10.5 and 6.6 respectively (Sato *et al.* 2001), (Sato *et al.* 2007). Therefore despite a relatively fast plasma half-life, once or twice daily dosing may be possible in dogs, although pharmacokinetic/pharmacodynamic studies using the commercially available timed-release formulation are required to determine appropriate dosages. In dogs, cytochrome CYP3A4 is responsible for metabolism of tamsulosin to the M1 and AM-1 metabolites (Soeishi *et al.* 1996).

Pharmacokinetic data for cats was not located.

In humans, fasted state oral bioavailability is essentially complete

(> 90%). Tamsulosin exhibits linear kinetics following single and multiple dosing, with achievement of steady-state concentrations by the fifth day of once-a-day dosing. Plasma protein binding in humans is significant (98-99%). The terminal half-life of tamsulosin in humans is ≈ 6 hours (Matsushima *et al.* 1998).

Contraindications/Precautions/Warnings

Tamsulosin is contraindicated in patients known to be hypersensitive to it. Some humans with sulfonamide drug allergies reportedly have experienced hypersensitivity reactions (skin rash, urticaria, pruritus, angioedema and respiratory symptoms).

Tamsulosin capsules are manufactured in a sustained-release (beads) presentation to avoid rapid absorption and associated hypotensive effects; therefore they should not be crushed or compounded into an oral suspension.

Adverse Effects

The adverse effect profile in animals is not well documented, but hypotensive effects are possible. Hypotension may be more likely at very high doses or in older dogs (Kobayashi *et al.* 2009). When tamsulosin was administered to anesthetized female beagles at dosages from 0.003 – 0.01 mg/kg IV, urethral pressures were reduced in a dose-dependent fashion; almost no effect on mean arterial blood pressure was seen (Ohtake *et al.* 2006).

Reproductive/Nursing Safety

Safety in pregnancy has not been established; weigh any potential risks versus benefits in pregnant animals. However, tamsulosin given at 50X dosages to pregnant female rats and up to 50 mg/kg/day to pregnant rabbits revealed no evidence of harm to the fetus In humans, the FDA categorizes this drug as category *B* for use during pregnancy (*Animal studies have not yet demonstrated risk to the fetus, but there are no adequate studies in pregnant women; or animal studies have shown an adverse effect, but adequate studies in pregnant women have not demonstrated a risk to the fetus in the first trimester of pregnancy, and there is no evidence of risk in later trimesters.*)

For humans, infant risk cannot be ruled out if nursing. Use with caution in nursing veterinary patients.

Overdosage/Acute Toxicity

Moderate toxicity in humans generally occurs at 10X dosages. If hypotension occurs it is usually responsive to fluids. Severe hypotension may require norepinephrine or phenylephrine. Dialysis is unlikely to be of benefit.

There were 382 single agent exposures to tamsulosin reported to the ASPCA Animal Poison Control Center (APCC) during 2009-2013. Of the 324 dogs, 72 were symptomatic with 25% being lethargic, 19% tachycardic, 14% vomiting and 10% hypotensive. Of the 64 cats, 16 were symptomatic with lethargy (31%) and vomiting (25%) being the most common clinical signs.

Drug Interactions

The following drug interactions have either been reported or are theoretical in humans or animals receiving tamsulosin and may be of significance in veterinary patients. Unless otherwise noted, use together is not necessarily contraindicated, but weigh the potential risks and perform additional monitoring when appropriate:

- **ALPHA-1 ADRENERGIC BLOCKERS**, Others (*e.g.,* **prazosin, terazosin, doxazosin,** etc.): May have additive hypotensive effects.
- **CIMETIDINE:** May increase tamsulosin levels.
- **CLARITHROMYCIN & ERYTHROMYCIN:** May increase blood levels of tamsulosin.
- **KETOCONAZOLE:** May increase plasma levels of tamsulosin.
- **SILDENAFIL/TADALAFIL (PDE5 inhibitors):** May have additive hypotensive effects.
- **TERBINAFINE:** May increase plasma levels of tamsulosin.
- **WARFARIN:** Drug interaction studies with tamsulosin are inconclusive; use together with caution.

Laboratory Considerations

- No laboratory test interactions reported.

Doses

- **DOGS:**

  As an ureteral/urethral relaxant (extra-label): Safety, efficacy and dosages have not been determined and compounded capsules may be required for dosing. Anecdotal dosages of 0.1 mg per 10 kg (of weight) PO q24h or 0.4 mg total dose per dog PO once daily on an empty stomach initially; may increase frequency to q12h if no effects are seen at once daily dosing have been noted.

- **CATS:**

  As an ureteral/urethral relaxant (extra-label): Safety, efficacy and dosages have not been determined and compounded capsules are required. An anecdotal dosage of 0.004 – 0.006 mg/kg PO every 12-24 hours has been noted. May take up to 3 days for effects to occur.

Monitoring

- Clinical efficacy.
- Blood pressure if adverse effects occur.

Client Information

- Give on an empty stomach for best results.
- Do not crush or allow animal to chew beads found inside capsule.
- May take up to 3 days for the drug to work at its peak effect.

Chemistry/Synonyms

Tamsulosin hydrochloride is a white crystalline powder that melts with decomposition at ≈ 230°C. It is sparingly soluble in water or methanol, slightly soluble in glacial acetic acid or ethanol, and practically insoluble in ether.

Tamsulosin may also be known as LY253351, YM-12617-1, YM617, or *Flomax*®.

Storage/Stability

Do not store tablets above 25°C (77°F); protect from moisture.

Compatibility/Compounding Considerations

Tamsulosin capsules are manufactured in a sustained release presentation to avoid rapid absorption and associated hypotensive effects and should not be crushed or compounded into an oral suspension. Capsule contents are small timed-release beads and could be compounded into smaller sized capsules for use in dogs or cats.

Dosage Forms/Regulatory Status

VETERINARY-LABELED PRODUCTS: NONE.

HUMAN-LABELED PRODUCTS:

Tamsulosin HCl Capsules: 0.4 mg; *Flomax*®, generic; (Rx)

Revisions/References

Monograph written July 2014. Brittany Samples, PharmD (Wingate University) contributed to this monograph as part of a student project at NCSU.

Kobayashi, S., et al. (2009). Effects of silodosin and tamsulosin on the urethra and cardiovascular system in young and old dogs with benign prostatic hyperplasia. European Journal of Pharmacology 613(1-3): 135-40.

Matsushima, H., et al. (1998). Pharmacokinetics and plasma protein binding of tamsulosin hydrochloride in rats, dogs, and humans. Drug Metabolism and Disposition 26(3): 240-5.

Ohtake, A., et al. (2006). Effects of tamsulosin on resting urethral pressure and arterial blood pressure in anaesthetized female dogs. Journal of Pharmacy and Pharmacology 58(3): 345-50.

Sato, S., et al. (2007). Relationship between the functional effect of tamsulosin and its concentration in lower urinary tract tissues in dogs. Biological & Pharmaceutical Bulletin 30(3): 481-6.

Sato, S., et al. (2001). Pharmacological effect of tamsulosin in relation to dog plasma and tissue concentrations: Prostatic and urethral retention possibly contributes to uroselectivity of tamsulosin. Journal of Pharmacology and Experimental Therapeutics 296(3): 697-703.

Soeishi, Y., et al. (1996). Metabolism of tamsulosin in rat and dog. Xenobiotica 26(3): 355-65.

Taurine

(tor-een)

Amino Acid Nutritional

Prescriber Highlights

► Amino acid used primarily for the treatment of taurine deficiency cardiomyopathies in cats & dogs. Because of its low cost, low potential for toxicity, and the limitations of testing for taurine deficiency, routine taurine supplementation in cats with dilated cardiomyopathy is advised.

► May also be useful for many other conditions (*e.g.*, seizures, hepatic lipidosis), but little or no supporting data available.

► Laboratory considerations.

Uses/Indications

Taurine has proven beneficial in preventing retinal degeneration and the prevention and treatment of taurine-deficiency dilated cardiomyopathy in cats. Although modern commercial feline diets have added taurine, some cats still develop taurine-deficiency associated dilated cardiomyopathy. It may also be of benefit in taurine (± carnitine) deficient cardiomyopathy in American Cocker Spaniels and certain other breeds such as, Golden Retrievers, Labrador Retrievers, Newfoundlands, Dalmations, Portuguese Water Dogs, and English Bulldogs. Preliminary studies have shown evidence that it may be useful as adjunctive treatment for cardiac disease in animals even if taurine deficiency is not present. Because of its low toxicity, some have suggested it be tried for a multitude of conditions in humans and animals; unfortunately, little scientific evidence exists for these uses.

Pharmacology/Actions

While classically considered a "non-essential" nutrient, taurine has been found to play several "essential" roles in various mammalian species. Taurine is important for bile acid conjugation, especially in cats and dogs. *In vivo*, taurine is synthesized from methionine. Cysteinesulfinic acid decarboxylase (CSAD) and vitamin B_6 are involved with this synthesis. Deficiencies of either will depress taurine synthesis. Cats are particularly susceptible to taurine deficiency as they have low CSAD activity and use taurine almost exclusively for bile acid conjugation.

Additionally taurine is important in the modulation of calcium flux, thereby reducing platelet aggregation, stabilizing neuronal membranes, and affecting cardiac function. Taurine's effects on cardiac function include positive inotropic activity without affecting resting potential and modulating ionic currents across the cell membrane. Taurine is important for normal development of the CNS and it has a GABA-like effect that may make it useful for treating some seizure disorders.

Pharmacokinetics

No specific information was located. Excess taurine is rapidly excreted in the kidneys, but if a deficiency exists, urinary excretion is reduced via reabsorption.

Contraindications/Precautions/Warnings

While taurine is safe, it should not be used as a substitute for adequate diagnosis.

Adverse Effects

Taurine appears to be very well tolerated. Minor GI distress potentially could occur after oral dosing.

Overdosage/Acute Toxicity

No specific information was located, but toxic potential appears to be very low.

Drug Interactions

■ None noted.

Laboratory Considerations

■ To determine actual status of taurine in the body, whole blood taurine levels are preferred to plasma levels. Intracellular levels of taurine are much higher than in plasma and hemolysis or collection of the buffy coat will negate the results. However, whole blood assays may also yield false positive results in animals that are in a prolonged fasting state or anorectic; false negative results may be obtained after postprandial sampling, a recent dietary change, or recent thromboembolism (Hambrook *et al.* 2012).

Doses

■ **DOGS:**

For dilated cardiomyopathy (extra-label): Possible candidates are: 1) All American Cocker spaniels; 2) Consider in animals with dilated cardiomyopathy and cysteine or urate urolithiasis (*e.g.*, English Bulldogs and Dalmatians); 3) Consider in golden retrievers, Newfoundland dogs, Portuguese water dogs and any atypical breeds for dilated cardiomyopathy. The suggested taurine dose for dogs with dilated cardiomyopathy is 500 – 1000 mg PO q8-12h for dogs weighing <25 kg and 1 – 2 grams PO q8-12h for dogs weighing >25 kg. (Smith 2009)

As a complementary oral antiepileptic 400 mg/40 lbs. of body weight PO twice daily. "May" help decrease seizure activity. (Neer 2000)

■ **CATS:**

For taurine-deficiency related dilated cardiomyopathy (extra-label): No consensus regarding dosage, but usually 250 – 500 mg per cat PO q12h is noted. Taurine is safe and inexpensive.

As a complementary oral antiepileptic (extra-label): 100 – 400 mg per cat PO q24h. (Pakozdy *et al.* 2014)

For adjunctive treatment of hepatopathies (extra-label): No clinical studies document efficacy, but some *in vitro* data supports use. Consider 250 – 500 mg per cat PO twice daily.

Monitoring

■ Clinical efficacy. Clinical improvement in cats with taurine-responsive dilated cardiomyopathy is usually seen within 2 weeks; significant echocardiographic improvement may take 4 weeks or more (Hambrook et al. 2012).

■ Taurine levels (if possible and affordable; whole blood levels preferable to plasma/serum levels).

Client Information

■ Usually causes no side effects, but could cause vomiting.

■ Blood tests are often needed to check taurine levels in the blood.

■ If using a powder form, mix into food.

Chemistry/Synonyms

Taurine, an amino acid also known as 2-aminosulphonic acid, has a molecular weight of 125. Solubility in 100 mL of water at 20°C is 8.8 grams.

Storage/Stability

Unless otherwise labeled, store taurine tablets or capsules at room temperature. Protect from light and moisture.

Compatibility/Compounding Considerations
No specific information noted.

Dosage Forms/Regulatory Status
VETERINARY-LABELED PRODUCTS:
The following products are labeled (not FDA-approved drugs) for use in animals:

Taurine Tablets: 250 mg; *Formula V® Taurine Tablets*. Labeled for use in cats.

Taurine Liquid: 375 mg/4 mL (one pump); *Dyna-Taurine®*. Labeled for use in dogs and cats.

HUMAN-LABELED PRODUCTS:
There are several oral dosage form products available for taurine. Technically considered a "nutrient" they are all OTC and may need to be obtained from health food stores. Most dosage forms available range from 125 mg to 500 mg.

Revisions/References
Monograph revised/updated August 2014.

Hambrook, L. E. & P. F. Bennett (2012). Effect of pimobendan on the clinical outcome and survival of cats with non-taurine responsive dilated cardiomyopathy. Journal of Feline Medicine and Surgery 14(4): 233-9.

Neer, T. (2000). The refractory seizure patient: What should be my diagnostic and therapeutic approach? American Animal Hospital Assoc, Toronto. accessed via Veterinary Information Network; vin.com

Pakozdy, A., et al. (2014). Epilepsy in cats: Theory and practice. J Vet Intern Med.

Smith, F. (2009). Feline Cardiomyopathies: Diagnosis and treatment. Proceedings: WVC. accessed via Veterinary Information Network; vin.com

Telazol®—See Tiletamine/Zolazepam

Telmisartan
(tel- mi-sar-tan)   Semintra®, Micardis®

Angiotensin-II Receptor Blocker (ARB)

Prescriber Highlights
▶ ARB that potentially could be useful in dogs and cats for the adjunctive treatment of proteinuria, hypertension secondary to renal insufficiency, or congestive heart failure. An oral product (*Semintra®*), is at time of writing (2014) approved in EU for treatment of proteinuria associated with chronic kidney disease (CKD) in cats.

▶ Limited experience in veterinary medicine; little data on efficacy, safety, adverse effects, etc. especially in dogs.

▶ Adverse effects in cats: Hypotension and decreased red blood cell counts possible, but not common; rarely, GI effects (vomiting, diarrhea) and increases in liver enzyme values.

▶ Not safe during pregnancy.

Uses/Indications
Telmisartan is approved in the EU for the reduction of proteinuria associated with chronic kidney disease (CKD) in cats. It is an angiotensin-II AT1-receptor blocker that potentially could be useful for the adjunctive treatment of hypertension, proteinuria and cardiomyopathies in both dogs and cats, but there is little information published on its safety (in dogs) and clinical efficacy.

Pharmacology/Actions
Telmisartan is an angiotensin-II receptor blocker (ARB). By selectively blocking the AT1-receptor, aldosterone synthesis and secretion is reduced causing vasodilation and decreased potassium and increased sodium excretion. While plasma concentrations of renin and angiotensin-II are increased, this does not counteract the blood pressure lowering effects of telmisartan. Telmisartan does not interfere with substance P or bradykinin responses. The product label (U.K.) for cats states: "...telmisartan does not affect potassium excretion, as shown in the clinical field trial in cats."

A study in healthy cats (n=6) found that telmisartan (3 mg/kg PO) when compared to benazepril (2.5 mg/cat PO) significantly better attenuated blood pressure increases secondary to angiotensin I administration at 90 minutes and 24 hours (Coleman *et al.* 2013).

Pharmacokinetics
In cats, telmisartan oral solution bioavailability is ≈ 33% and peak levels occur in ≈ 30 minutes. Food does not affect overall absorption. Distribution data for cats was not located, but the drug is highly lipophilic and in other species (rats, dogs, humans) is highly bound (>99.5%) to plasma proteins. Absorbed drug is primarily metabolized via glucuronidation and the cat genetic defect UGT1A6 does not affect glucuronidation (Ebner *et al.* 2013). The major metabolite is telmisartan-O-acylglucuronide, which is not active. Elimination half-life is ≈ 8 hours.

No pharmacokinetic data for dogs was located.

In humans, oral bioavailability of telmisartan is dose dependent and ranges from 42% (40 mg) to 58% (160 mg). Food slightly reduces bioavailability. Absorbed drug is highly protein bound (>99.5%) and volume of distribution ≈ 500L. It is conjugated via glucuronidation to the pharmacologically inactive acylglucuronide. Elimination kinetics are bi-exponential and the terminal half-life is ≈ 1 day.

Contraindications/Precautions/Warnings
Telmisartan is contraindicated in patients that are allergic (hypersensitive) to it. It is not known if cross-reactivity occurs between other ARBs and telmisartan.

Hypotensive patients should not receive the drug. Patients that are volume or electrolyte depleted should not receive the drug until volume/electrolytes have been replenished/corrected.

The drug should not be used in pregnant animals. The human label has the following Black Box Warning: "Fetal toxicity: When pregnancy is detected, discontinue telmisartan as soon as possible. Drugs that act directly on the renin-angiotensin system can cause injury and even death to the developing fetus." See the Reproductive Safety section for more information.

Telmisartan should be used with caution in patients with moderate to severe hepatic impairment; dosage reduction may be warranted.

The label for the cat product (U.K.) reads: "The safety and efficacy of telmisartan has not been tested in cats under the age of 6 months."

Adverse Effects
Hypotension is potentially possible in cats, but has not been reported commonly at recommended dosages. Reduction in red blood cell counts could occur. Rarely, gastrointestinal effects (vomiting, diarrhea) and increases in liver enzyme values have been noted.

The adverse effect profile for this drug when used clinically in dogs is not known.

Reproductive/Nursing Safety
Telmisartan is not considered safe to use during pregnancy. The EU label for the cat product reads: "Do not use during pregnancy or lactation. The safety of *Semintra®* has not been established in breeding, pregnant or lactating cats."

Studies in pregnant rats given high doses of ARBs demonstrated a variety of fetal abnormalities (renal pelvic cavitation, hydroureter, absence of renal papilla). Smaller doses in rabbits caused increased maternal death and spontaneous abortion. In humans, the drug is considered teratogenic, particularly during the 2nd and 3rd trimesters. During this time, the FDA categorizes telmisartan as category D for use during pregnancy *(There is evidence of human fetal risk, but the potential benefits from the use of the drug in pregnant women may be acceptable despite its potential risks.)* If pregnancy is detected in patients receiving telmisartan, the drug should be discontinued as soon as possible.

It is not known if telmisartan is excreted into cat or dog milk and it is recommended to either halt nursing and use milk replacer or discontinue the drug in nursing animals.

Overdosage/Acute Toxicity

Limited information is available. Hypotension and tachycardia are possible; bradycardia could occur from parasympathetic (vagal) stimulation. Treat supportively. Telmisartan is not removed by hemodialysis.

In chronic toxicity studies done in cats of up to 5 mg/kg/day (5X) for 6 months, telmisartan did not cause lethality. Hypotension, decreased red blood cell counts, increase BUN and gastrointestinal effects are possible.

There were 89 single agent exposures to telmisartan reported to the ASPCA Animal Poison Control Center (APCC) during 2009-2013. Of the 85 exposed dogs, only 3 were symptomatic. Lethargy, anorexia, trembling and vomiting were reported.

Drug Interactions

The following drug interactions have either been reported or are theoretical in humans or animals receiving telmisartan and may be of significance in veterinary patients. Unless otherwise noted, use together is not necessarily contraindicated, but weigh the potential risks and perform additional monitoring when appropriate.

- **DIGOXIN:** Possible increased digoxin levels.

Laboratory Considerations

No specific information noted.

Dosages

- **DOGS:**

  Note: Published data supporting any safe and effective dosage for dogs is presently very limited. In a pre-clinical study done in dogs, telmisartan at 1 mg/kg PO once daily for 12 days significantly increased urine volume and renal excretion of sodium, chloride (Schierok *et al.* 2001).

- **CATS:**

  For reduction of proteinuria associated with chronic kidney disease (CKD); (extra-label in USA): Using the oral solution: 1 mg/kg PO (directly into mouth or with a small amount of food) once daily. (Adapted from *Semintra®* label— Boehringer Ingelheim U.K.)

Monitoring

- Depending on reason for use and patient's clinical condition: renal function, urine protein, blood pressure, volume status, and liver function tests.
- The label for cat product recommends monitoring red blood cell counts.

Client Information

- This medication may be given with or without food.
- Because this medication has not been frequently used in dogs or cats, side effects are not fully known; watch carefully for any side effects and report them to your veterinarian. Possible side effects could include: diarrhea, vomiting, lack of appetite, fatigue (reduced red blood cell count), and low blood pressure (fainting, weakness, inability to exercise, etc.).
- This drug has caused birth defects and should not be used in pregnant animals. If a human in the household is pregnant, they should be very careful not to ingest these tablets and should wear disposable gloves when administering doses and wash their hands after touching these tablets.

Chemistry/Synonyms

Telmisartan [CAS Registry: 144701-48-4; ATCvet code: QC-09CA07] occurs as a white or slightly yellowish, crystalline powder. It is practically insoluble in water, slightly soluble in methyl alcohol, sparingly soluble in dichloromethane, and dissolves in 1M sodium hydroxide.

The feline product (*Semintra®*) is a clear, colorless to yellowish viscous oral solution; excipients include: hydroxyethylcellulose, maltitol and benzalkonium chloride.

Telmisartan may also be known as: BIBR 277 SE. Trade names include *Micardis®* and *Semintra®*.

Storage/Stability

Telmisartan solution for cats may be stored at room temperature with the cap tightly closed. The label states that shelf life is 6 months after first opening bottle. Telmisartan tablets should be stored at room temperature (up to 30°C; 86F); do not remove from blisters until immediately before administration.

Compatibility/Compounding Considerations

The label (U.K.) for the cat product states: "In the absence of compatibility studies, this veterinary medicinal product must not be mixed with other veterinary products."

Dosage Forms/Regulatory Status

VETERINARY-LABELED PRODUCTS:
None in the USA; in the UK/EU: Oral Solution: 4 mg/mL in 30 mL bottle with oral measuring syringe; *Semintra®*; (POM-V; U.K.)

HUMAN-LABELED PRODUCTS:
Oral Tablets: 20 mg, 40 mg & 80 mg; *Micardis®*, generic; (Rx).

Revisions/References

Monograph revised/updated August 2014.

Coleman, A., et al. (2013). Attenuation of the Pressor Response to Exogenous Angiotensin by Angiotensin Receptor Blockers in Normal Cats (Abstract). ACVIM. accessed via Veterinary Information Network; vin.com

Ebner, T., et al. (2013). In vitro glucuronidation of the angiotensin II receptor antagonist telmisartan in the cat: a comparison with other species. J. Vet. Pharmacol. Ther. **36**(2): 154-60.

Schierok, H., et al. (2001). Effects of Telmisartan on Renal Excretory Function in Conscious Dogs. Journal of International Medical Research **29**: 131-9.

Tepoxalin

(te-pox-a-lin)   Zubrin®

Nonsteroidal Antiinflammatory Agent

Prescriber Highlights

▶ At time of writing (2014), no commercially products being marketed in USA.

▶ NSAID dual inhibitor of COX & LOX indicated for the treatment of pain & inflammation associated with osteoarthritis in dogs.

Uses/Indications

The formerly marketed product (*Zubrin®*) was indicated for the treatment of pain and inflammation associated with osteoarthritis in dogs.

Pharmacology/Actions

Tepoxalin is a dual inhibitor of both cyclooxygenase (COX) and 5-lipoxygenase (LOX). It inhibits both COX-1 and COX-2 enzymes, but it is not clear if it is COX-2 preferential in dogs (it is not COX-2 preferential in sheep uterine cells) or if its LOX inhibition reduces the adverse effects associated with COX-1 inhibition. LOX inhibition in dogs persists for only ≈ 6 hours after dosing. By inhibiting COX-2 enzymes, tepoxalin reduces the production of prostaglandins associated with pain, hyperpyrexia and inflammation. Its inhibition of LOX potentially reduces the production of leukotrienes, including leukotriene B_4. As leukotriene B_4 may contribute to increased GI tract inflammation by increasing cytokine production, neutrophil longevity and release of proteinases, inhibition may reduce the GI effects routinely seen in dogs with COX-1 inhibitors. Leukotrienes may also contribute to inflammatory responses seen in osteoarthritic conditions and their inhibition could reduce clinical signs seen with the condition.

Pharmacokinetics

After oral administration to dogs, tepoxalin is readily absorbed and peak levels occur between 2-3 hours post-dose. The presence of food in the gut increases bioavailability. Tepoxalin is rapidly metabolized to several metabolites, including one that it active (tepoxalin pyrazole acid). Tepoxalin and tepoxalin pyrazole acid are highly bound to plasma proteins (98-99%). Elimination half-lives for tepoxalin and tepoxalin pyrazole acid are ≈ 2 hours and 13 hours, respectively. Metabolites are eliminated in the feces; only 1% of the drug is eliminated in the urine.

In cats, tepoxalin elimination half-life is ≈ 5 hours; the active metabolite half-life is ≈ 4 hours.

Contraindications/Precautions/Warnings

Tepoxalin is contraindicated in dogs demonstrating prior hypersensitivity reactions to tepoxalin. It should be used with caution in patients with impaired hepatic, cardiovascular or renal function, or at risk for developing nephrotoxic affects associated with NSAIDs (*i.e.*, dehydrated or on concomitant diuretic therapy). Patients with active gastrointestinal ulcers should probably not receive this drug.

Dogs weighing <3 kg cannot be accurately dosed with available dosage forms. Safety in dogs <6 months old has not been established.

Adverse Effects

Adverse effects most likely seen in dogs include diarrhea, vomiting, anorexia/inappetence, enteritis, and lethargy. In one study where dogs received labeled doses for 4 weeks, 22% of dogs developed diarrhea and 20% vomited. It is unknown if giving the drug with food will decrease vomiting incidence. Other adverse effects reported (incidences <1%) include incoordination, incontinence, increased appetite, eating grass, flatulence, hair loss, and trembling. While all NSAIDs can potentially cause renal dysfunction, a study done in healthy dogs did not show that tepoxalin altered renal blood flow or renal function when used alone or with benazepril (for 7 days) or with enalapril (for 28 days) (Fusellier *et al.* 2005).

The manufacturer warns to discontinue the drug if signs such as inappetence, vomiting, fecal abnormalities, anemia, icterus, or lethargy are observed. Safety studies in dogs <6 months of age have not been completed.

Reproductive/Nursing Safety

Safety of this drug has not been determined in pregnant, breeding, or lactating dogs; use with caution and informed consent of client.

Overdosage/Acute Toxicity

Information on acute overdosage of tepoxalin was not located. Dogs receiving 300 mg/kg/day for 6 months showed decreases in total protein, albumin and calcium concentrations. At necropsy, all dogs showed gastric lesions. An acute overdose may cause significant GI distress and ulceration with GI bleeding. It is suggested to treat supportively and monitor CBC, hydration, renal function, and for evidence of GI bleeding. Contact an animal poison control center for more information.

Drug Interactions

A study in normal dogs showed no significant changes in renal function when **enalapril** was used with tepoxalin.

The following drug interactions have either been reported or are theoretical in humans or animals receiving tepoxalin and may be of significance in veterinary patients. Unless otherwise noted, use together is not necessarily contraindicated, but weigh the potential risks and perform additional monitoring when appropriate.

- **ASPIRIN**: May increase the risk of gastrointestinal toxicity (*e.g.*, ulceration, bleeding, vomiting, diarrhea).
- **CORTICOSTEROIDS**: As concomitant corticosteroid therapy may increase the occurrence of gastric ulceration, avoid the use of these drugs when also using tepoxalin.
- **DIGOXIN**: NSAIDS may increase serum levels.
- **FLUCONAZOLE**: Administration has increased plasma levels of celecoxib in humans, it is unknown if fluconazole affects tepoxalin levels in dogs.
- **FUROSEMIDE**: NSAIDs may reduce saluretic and diuretic effects.
- **METHOTREXATE**: Serious toxicity has occurred when NSAIDs have been used concomitantly with methotrexate; use together with extreme caution.
- **NEPHROTOXIC DRUGS** (*e.g.*, **furosemide, aminoglycosides, amphotericin B**, etc.): May enhance the risk of nephrotoxicity.
- **NSAIDS, OTHER**: May increase the risk of gastrointestinal toxicity (*e.g.*, ulceration, bleeding, vomiting, diarrhea).
- **WARFARIN**: The manufacturer cautions to closely monitor patients also receiving drugs that are highly bound to plasma proteins, as tepoxalin and its active metabolite are 98-99% protein bound in dogs.

Laboratory Considerations

- No specific laboratory interactions or considerations noted.

Doses

- **DOGS:**

  For pain and inflammation associated with osteoarthritis (labeled dose; FDA-approved): On first day of treatment give 20 mg/kg PO (or 10 mg/kg PO); subsequently give 10 mg/kg PO once daily. Duration of treatment should be based on clinical response and patient tolerance to therapy. (Package insert; *Zubrin*®)

Monitoring

- Clinical efficacy.
- Baseline and periodic CBC, chemistry panel (including bilirubin and serum creatinine).
- Signs associated with adverse effects (*e.g.*, GI effects, appetite, vomiting, diarrhea, etc.).

Client Information

- When dosing, the person administering the tablet should place it in dog's mouth and hold mouth closed for ≈ 4 seconds to assure tablet disintegration.
- Absorption may be enhanced (and vomiting reduced?) if given with food.
- Owners should be instructed to discontinue the drug and contact their veterinarian if diarrhea is severe or persists, or signs such as inappetence, vomiting, fecal abnormalities, anemia, icterus or lethargy are observed.
- Dogs should have access to water; dehydration should be avoided.
- The manufacturer provides a client information sheet and states to "Always provide client information sheet…".

Chemistry/Synonyms

A non-steroidal antiinflammatory agent (NSAID), tepoxalin occurs as a white, tasteless, crystalline material that is insoluble in water and soluble in alcohol and most organic solvents. The commercially available tablets contain a micronized form of the drug in a highly porous matrix that rapidly disintegrates in the mouth.

Drug particles are released into the saliva and swallowed by the dog where it is absorbed in the intestines.

Tepoxalin may also be known as ORF-20485, RWJ-20485 and *Zubrin®*.

Storage/Stability

Tablets should be kept in their foil blister packs until used and stored at temperatures between 2-30°C (36-86°F).

Compatibility/Compounding Considerations

No specific information noted.

Dosage Forms/Regulatory Status

VETERINARY-LABELED PRODUCTS:

At time of writing (2014) the following product has been discontinued: Tepoxalin Oral (rapidly-disintegrating) Tablets: 30 mg, 50 mg, 100 mg, 200 mg in foil blisters containing 10 tablets in boxes of 10 foil blisters; *Zubrin®*; (Rx). FDA-approved for use in dogs.

HUMAN-LABELED PRODUCTS: NONE.

Revisions/References

Monograph revised/updated August 2014.

Fuselier, M., et al. (2005). Effect of tepoxalin on renal function in healthy dogs receiving an angiotensin-converting enzyme inhibitor. J. Vet. Pharmacol. Ther. 28(6): 581-6.

Terbinafine HCl

(ter-bin-ah-fin)   Lamisil®

Antifungal

Prescriber Highlights

▶ Oral & topical antifungal; used primarily for dermatophytic infections, but may be useful for other systemic fungal infections.

▶ Comparatively (with azole antifungals) few drug interactions.

▶ Appears to be very well tolerated, but limited experience; vomiting most likely adverse effect.

▶ Caution if liver or renal disease.

▶ Treatment is relatively inexpensive at present (generics available).

Uses/Indications

Terbinafine may be useful for treating dermatophytic and other systemic fungal infections (blastomycosis, histoplasmosis, coccidioidomycosis, cryptococcosis, sporotrichosis, etc.) in dogs, cats, birds and other species.

Pharmacology/Actions

Terbinafine is an inhibitor of the synthesis of ergosterol, a component of fungal cell membranes. By blocking the enzyme squalene monooxygenase (squalene 2,3-epoxidase), terbinafine inhibits the conversion of squalene to sterols (especially ergosterol) and causes accumulation of squalene. Both these effects are thought to contribute to its antifungal action. Terbinafine's mechanism for inhibiting ergosterol is different from the azole antifungals.

Unlike the azole agents, terbinafine's actions are not mediated via the cytochrome P-450 enzyme system, and, therefore, do not have the concerns of drug interactions or altering testosterone or cortisol.

Terbinafine primarily has clinical activity (fungicidal) against dermatophytic organisms (*Microsporum* spp., *Trichophyton* spp., etc.). It may only be fungistatic against the yeasts (*Candida* spp.). Terbinafine has activity against Aspergillus, Blastomyces, Histoplasma, Sporothrix and Cryptococcus. It is not very effective for pythiosis.

Pharmacokinetics

In greyhound dogs, orally administered terbinafine (≈ 30 mg/kg) had a terminal half-life of ≈ 9 hours. A single dose study (30 – 35 mg/kg PO with food) in dogs (various breeds, ages) showed peak levels occurring ≈ 3 hours and peak plasma levels ≈ 2.7 mcg/mL (range from 1.3-4.9 mcg/mL) (Sakai *et al.* 2011).

Plasma protein binding of terbinafine is very high (>99%) in dogs, rabbits and humans. Measuring tissue or cellular (not plasma) concentrations of terbinafine would be more appropriate for determining the required kinetic parameters and dosage regimens for treating susceptible fungal organisms (Wang *et al.* 2012).

In cats, after an oral dose of 30 mg/kg, peak levels (≈ 3.2 mcg/mL) occur between 1-2 hours after dosing. Oral bioavailability is fairly low (≈ 30%). Elimination half-life is ≈ 8-10 hours. (Wang *et al.* 2012)

In cats dosed at 34 – 46 mg/kg PO once daily for 14 days, terbinafine persisted in hair above MIC for several weeks. (Foust *et al.* 2007)

In six horses, orally administered terbinafine pharmacokinetic values have been reported. The maximum plasma concentration was 0.31 (range: 0.21-0.61) mcg/mL and occurred at 1.7 (range: 0.75-4) hours after dosing. Mean half-life was ≈ 8 hours, but ranged widely (range: 3.9-11.6 hours); volume of distribution (Vd/F) was ≈ 131 L/kg (range: 50-266 L/kg); clearance was 187 mL/min/kg (range: 132-282 mL/min/kg). As intravenous terbinafine was not administered, volume of distribution and clearance are reported as per fraction of drug available (KuKanich *et al.* 2009). In horses, there was a large variability of terbinafine pharmacokinetic values; oral relative bioavailability was only 16% when compared to dogs (Williams *et al.* 2011).

In humans, terbinafine given orally is >70% absorbed; after first pass metabolism, bioavailability is ≈ 40%. Food may enhance absorption somewhat. Terbinafine is distributed to skin and into the sebum. Over 99% of drug in plasma is bound to plasma proteins. Drug in the circulation is metabolized in the liver and the effective elimination half-life is ≈ 36 hours. The drug may persist in adipose tissue and skin for very long periods.

Contraindications/Precautions/Warnings

Terbinafine is contraindicated in patients hypersensitive to it. The manufacturer does not recommend its use in patients with active or chronic liver disease or with significantly impaired renal function. If terbinafine is to be used in veterinary patents with markedly impaired liver or renal function, do so with extreme caution; dosage adjustments should be considered.

Adverse Effects

Because of limited usage in veterinary patients the adverse effect profile is not well defined, but the drug appears to be well tolerated. GI effects (vomiting, inappetence, diarrhea) are possible. In dogs, excessive panting and elevated liver enzymes have been noted (Berger *et al.* 2012). In a case report in two cats, one cat developed lethargy (Nuttall *et al.* 2008). Facial pruritus in some treated cats has also been reported.

Reportedly, the oral tablets can have an unpleasant taste and may contribute to GI or behavioral adverse effects or dosing avoidance. In a pharmacokinetic study in horses and dogs, one horse (and another in an earlier pilot study) exhibited behaviors (curling of lips, pawing at ground, opening/closing mouth) consistent with unpleasant taste or oral cavity irritation. Signs resolved, but the authors could not rule out that a transient colic developed. In dogs, whole tablets were used and did not cause GI or similar behaviors. (Williams *et al.* 2011)

Very rarely in humans, liver failure, neutropenia or serious skin reactions (*e.g.*, TEN, Stevens-Johnson syndrome) have occurred after terbinafine use.

Reproductive/Nursing Safety

High dose studies in pregnant rabbits and rats have not demonstrated overt fetotoxicity or teratogenicity, but definitive safety in pregnancy has not been determined. Use with caution (manufacturer recommends **NOT** using in pregnant women). In humans, the FDA categorizes this drug as category *B* for use during pregnancy (*Animal studies have not yet demonstrated risk to the fetus, but there are no adequate studies in pregnant women; or animal studies have shown an adverse effect, but adequate studies in pregnant women have not demonstrated a risk to the fetus in the first trimester of pregnancy, and there is no evidence of risk in later trimesters.*)

The drug enters maternal milk at levels 7X that found in plasma; the manufacturer recommends that mothers not nurse while taking this drug. Use with caution in nursing veterinary patients.

Overdosage/Acute Toxicity
Limited information; humans have taken doses of up to 5 grams without serious effects.

Drug Interactions
The following drug interactions have either been reported or are theoretical in humans or animals receiving terbinafine and may be of significance in veterinary patients. Unless otherwise noted, use together is not necessarily contraindicated, but weigh the potential risks and perform additional monitoring when appropriate.
- CYCLOSPORINE: Terbinafine may increase the elimination of cyclosporine.
- RIFAMPIN: May increase terbinafine clearance.

As it shares the same metabolic pathway (CYP2D6), terbinafine could affect the metabolism of:
- BETA-BLOCKERS
- MAO INHIBITORS (*e.g.*, **amitraz, selegiline**, etc.)
- SSRI'S (*e.g.*, **fluoxetine**, etc.)
- TRICYCLIC ANTIDEPRESSANTS

Laboratory Considerations
- No apparent issues.

Doses
- **DOGS**

  For systemic and subcutaneous mycoses (extra-label): Based upon a pharmacokinetic study and organism MIC's the following are proposed dosage regimens as an alternative to traditionally used systemic antifungals. **For the treatment of blastomycosis, histoplasmosis, and deep dermatophyte infections**: 30 – 35 mg/kg PO 2 times daily. **For coccidioidomycosis, or sporotrichosis**: administer 30 – 35 mg/kg PO 3 times daily. Expanded clinical trials should be performed in the future to document clinical efficacy and safety. Not recommended for *Pythium insidiosum*. (Sakai *et al.* 2011)

  For *Malassezia* dermatitis (extra-label): From a pilot study. Authors concluded that twice-weekly terbinafine administration (30 mg/kg PO once daily for 2 consecutive days, followed by no treatment for the next 5 consecutive days) may be an effective alternative treatment for canine *Malassezia* dermatitis and merits further investigation. (Berger *et al.* 2012)

  For cryptococcosis (extra-label): From a case report; after primary therapy with amphotericin B and fluconazole had failed. Dog received 30 mg/kg PO once daily. Insufficient data are currently available to recommend terbinafine as a first-line agent, but in cases where primary therapy has failed to yield a response, it may prove beneficial. (Olsen *et al.* 2012)

- **CATS:**

  For dermatophytic infections (extra-label):
  a) Using pulse therapy in cats: In the study, cats given 20 mg/kg PO once daily for 7 days and then 21 days off had clinical and mycological cures and terbinafine concentrations in hair were maintained above therapeutic concentrations. Cats given

higher doses (40 mg/kg) or continuous administration accumulated higher concentrations, but some developed emesis in the first week of therapy, and higher hepatic enzyme serum activities. There were no alterations in the values of ALT and FA in the pulse therapy group. (Balda *et al.* 2009)
  b) In the study (shelter cats), using 250 mg terbinafine tablets, cats <2.8 kg received 1/4 of a tablet (62.5 mg) per dose, cats 2.8-5.5 kg received 1/2 a tablet (125 mg) per dose, and cats >5.5 kg received 1 tablet (250 mg) per dose. Administered once daily with the morning feed for 21 days. Cats also received lime sulfur rinses twice weekly. Results (for 21 day course of treatment) were comparable to treatment trials using itraconazole. (Moriello *et al.* 2013)

  For sporotrichosis (extra-label): As an alternative for the treatment of cats that do not tolerate itraconazole, in cases that respond poorly, and/or if an azole resistance is suspected: 30 mg per cat PO once daily. May be used in combination with itraconazole. (Lloret *et al.* 2013)

  For adjunctive treatment (with topical therapy) of nasal Aspergillus infections if the cribriform pate is penetrated (extra-label): 5 – 10 mg/kg PO q12h for 3-6 months. (Kuehn 2007)

  For cryptococcal infections in cats that have become resistant to the azoles (extra-label): 10 mg/kg PO per day can rectify the clinical signs though cats with CNS Cryptococcus usually require treatment for life. (Legendre 2010)

- **BIRDS:**

  For aspergillosis (extra-label): A single oral dose pharmacokinetic study in red-tailed hawks concluded that a terbinafine dosage of 22 mg/kg PO q24h would result in steady-state trough plasma concentrations above the MIC and is recommended as a potential treatment option for aspergillosis in raptors. However, additional research is required to determine both treatment efficacy and safety (Bechert *et al.* 2010). A pharmacokinetic study using nebulized terbinafine (1 mg/mL solution nebulized for 15 minutes) in Hispaniolan Amazon parrots concluded that higher concentrations of nebulization solutions, nebulization times >15 minutes, or more frequent nebulization are likely needed to reach clinically relevant systemic terbinafine concentrations. The relationship between plasma concentrations and lung or air sac concentrations after nebulization of terbinafine still needs to be determined and further studies are warranted to determine the optimal technique for dissolving terbinafine in solution, as well as to determine the best concentration of terbinafine and particle size to nebulize. Additionally, pharmacodynamic studies are also necessary to determine therapeutic plasma concentrations.

Monitoring
- Clinical efficacy.
- Baseline liver enzymes and then as needed (especially if treating long-term).

Client Information
- Give with food, particularly if vomiting is a problem.
- Well tolerated; vomiting is the most common side effect.

Chemistry/Synonyms
A synthetic allylamine antifungal, terbinafine HCl occurs as a white to off-white, fine, crystalline powder. It is slightly soluble in water and soluble in ethanol.

Terbinafine HCl may also be known as: *Alamil®, Daskil®, Daskyl®, DesenexMax®, Finex®, Lamisil®, Maditez®, Micosil®,* or *Terekol®*.

Storage/Stability
Terbinafine tablets should be stored at room temperature, in tight containers; protect from light.

Compatibility/Compounding Considerations

In a pharmacokinetic study for terbinafine nebulization in parrots, one 250 mg tablet was crushed and dissolved into 250 mL sterile water to make a 1 mg/mL solution. Before nebulization, the solution was agitated before being mixed with a stir bar for 12 hours. Terbinafine concentrations of solutions made with a crushed tablet were significantly lower than those that made with raw powder, but plasma concentrations did not differ significantly. (Evans *et al.* 2013)

Dosage Forms/Regulatory Status

VETERINARY-LABELED PRODUCTS: NONE.

HUMAN-LABELED PRODUCTS:

Terbinafine HCl Oral Tablets: 250 mg; *Lamisil®*, generic; (Rx)

Terbinafine HCl Oral Granules (film-coated): 125 mg/packet & 187.5 mg/packet (as base); *Lamisil®*; (Rx)

A topical cream and spray (1%) are also available (Rx).

Revisions/References

Monograph revised/updated August 2014.

Balda, A. & C. Larsson (2009). Evaluation of Terbinafine Hair Concentration in Persian Cats with Dermatophytosis and Healthy Carriers of Microsporum canis Treated with Pulse or Continuous Therapy. Proceedings; WSAVA. accessed via Veterinary Information Network; vin.com

Bechert, U., et al. (2010). Pharmacokinetics of Terbinafine After Single Oral Dose Administration in Red-Tailed Hawks (Buteo jamaicensis). Journal of Avian Medicine and Surgery **24**(2): 122-30.

Berger, D. J., et al. (2012). Comparison of once-daily versus twice-weekly terbinafine administration for the treatment of canine Malassezia dermatitis - a pilot study. Veterinary Dermatology **23**(5).

Evans, E. E., et al. (2013). Pharmacokinetics of terbinafine after oral administration of a single dose to Hispaniolan Amazon parrots (Amazona ventralis). American Journal of Veterinary Research **74**(6): 835-8.

Foust, A., et al. (2007). Evaluation of persistence of terbinafine in the hair of normal cats after 14 days of daily therapy. Vet Derm **18**(4): 246-51.

Kuehn, N. (2007). Chronic rhinitis in dogs. Proceedings; ACVIM. accessed via Veterinary Information Network; vin.com

KuKanich, B., et al. (2009). Pharmacokinetics of Orally Administered Terbinafine in Horses. Proceedings: ACVIM. accessed via Veterinary Information Network; vin.com

Legendre, A. M. (2010). Novel Antifungal Drug Therapies for Deep Mycoses. Proceedings: ACVIM. accessed via Veterinary Information Network; vin.com

Lloret, A., et al. (2013). Sporotrichosis in cats: ABCD guidelines on prevention and management. Journal of Feline Medicine and Surgery **15**(7): 619-23.

Moriello, K., et al. (2013). Treatment of shelter cats with oral terbinafine and concurrent lime sulphur rinses. Veterinary Dermatology **24**(6): 618-+.

Nuttall, T. J., et al. (2008). Successful resolution of dermatophyte mycetoma following terbinafine treatment in two cats. Veterinary Dermatology **19**(6): 405-10.

Olsen, G. L., et al. (2012). Use of Terbinafine in the Treatment Protocol of Intestinal Cryptococcus neoformans in a Dog. J. Am. Anim. Hosp. Assoc. **48**(3): 216-20.

Sakai, M. R., et al. (2011). Terbinafine pharmacokinetics after single dose oral administration in the dog. Veterinary Dermatology **22**(6): 528-34.

Wang, A., et al. (2012). Single dose pharmacokinetics of terbinafine in cats. Journal of Feline Medicine and Surgery **14**(8): 540-4.

Williams, M. M., et al. (2011). Pharmacokinetics of oral terbinafine in horses and Greyhound dogs. J. Vet. Pharmacol. Ther. **34**(3): 232-7.

Terbutaline Sulfate

(ter-byoo-ta-leen)   Brethine®

Beta-Adrenergic Agonist

Prescriber Highlights

▶ Beta agonist used as a bronchodilator or tocolytic; sometimes used to treat bradyarrhythmias.

▶ Looks promising as a test to quantitate anhidrosis in horses.

▶ Caution: Diabetes, hyperthyroidism, hypertension, seizure disorders, or cardiac disease (especially with concurrent arrhythmias).

▶ Adverse Effects: Increased heart rate, tremors, CNS excitement (nervousness) & dizziness; after parenteral injection in horses, sweating & CNS excitation are possible.

Uses/Indications

Terbutaline is used as a bronchodilating agent in the adjunctive treatment of cardiopulmonary diseases (including tracheobronchitis, collapsing trachea, pulmonary edema, and allergic bronchitis) in small animals. It may be of some benefit in treating bradyarrhythmias in dogs and cats.

Terbutaline has been used occasionally in horses for its bronchodilating effects, but adverse effects, short duration of activity after IV administration and poor oral absorption have limited its use. It has been shown to be useful as a diagnostic agent to diagnose anhidrosis in horses after intradermal injection.

Oral and parenteral terbutaline has been used successfully in humans, dogs, and cats for the inhibition of premature labor (tocolytic).

Pharmacology/Actions

Terbutaline stimulates beta-adrenergic receptors found principally in bronchial, vascular, and uterine smooth muscles (beta2); bronchial and vascular smooth muscle relaxation occurs with resultant reduced airway resistance. At usual doses it has little effect on cardiac (beta1) receptors and usually does not cause direct cardiostimulatory effects. Occasionally, a tachycardia develops which may be a result of either direct beta stimulation or a reflex response secondary to peripheral vasodilation. Terbutaline has virtually no alpha-adrenergic activity.

Pharmacokinetics

The pharmacokinetics of this agent have apparently not been thoroughly studied in domestic animals. In humans, only ≈ 33-50% of an oral dose is absorbed; peak bronchial effects occur within 2-3 hours and activity persists up to 8 hours. Terbutaline is well-absorbed following SC administration with an onset of action occurring within 15 minutes, peak effects at 30-60 minutes, and duration of activity up to 4 hours.

In horses, terbutaline is very poorly absorbed after oral administration with a bioavailability <1%. When given IV, mean residence time is ≈ 30 minutes in horses and the drug probably needs to be given as a constant rate infusion if used therapeutically.

Terbutaline is distributed into milk at levels ≈ 1% of the oral dose given to the mother. Terbutaline is principally excreted unchanged in the urine (60%), but is also metabolized in the liver to an inactive sulfate conjugate.

Contraindications/Precautions/Warnings

Terbutaline is contraindicated in patients hypersensitive to it. One veterinary school formulary (Schultz 1986) states that terbutaline is contraindicated in dogs and cats with heart disease, especially with CHF or cardiomyopathy. It should be used with caution in patients with diabetes, hyperthyroidism, hypertension, seizure disorders, or cardiac disease (especially with concurrent arrhythmias).

Adverse Effects

Most adverse effects are dose-related and are those that would be expected with sympathomimetic agents including increased heart rate, tremors, CNS excitement (nervousness) and dizziness. These effects are generally transient, mild and do not require discontinuation of therapy. After parenteral injection in horses, sweating and CNS excitation have been reported.

Transient hypokalemia has been reported in humans receiving beta-adrenergic agents. If an animal is susceptible to developing hypokalemia, it is suggested that additional serum potassium monitoring be done early in therapy.

Reproductive/Nursing Safety

In humans, the FDA categorizes this drug as category *B* for use during pregnancy (*Animal studies have not yet demonstrated risk to the fetus, but there are no adequate studies in pregnant women; or animal studies have shown an adverse effect, but adequate studies in pregnant women have not demonstrated a risk to the fetus in the first trimester of pregnancy, and there is no evidence of risk in later trimesters.*)

Terbutaline is excreted in milk. In humans, nursing is not recommended with systemic terbutaline therapy.

Overdosage/Acute Toxicity

Clinical signs of significant overdose after systemic administration may include arrhythmias (bradycardia, tachycardia, heart block, extrasystoles), hyperkalemia, hypertension, fever, vomiting, mydriasis, and CNS stimulation. If a recent oral ingestion, it should be handled like other overdoses if the animal does not have significant cardiac or CNS effects (empty gut, give activated charcoal and a cathartic). If cardiac arrhythmias require treatment, a beta-blocking agent (*e.g.*, propranolol) can be used, but may precipitate bronchoconstriction.

Drug Interactions

The following drug interactions have either been reported or are theoretical in humans or animals receiving terbutaline and may be of significance in veterinary patients. Unless otherwise noted, use together is not necessarily contraindicated, but weigh the potential risks and perform additional monitoring when appropriate.

- **ANESTHETICS, INHALATION** (*e.g.*, **halothane, isoflurane, methoxyflurane**): Use with inhalation anesthetics may predispose the patient to ventricular arrhythmias, particularly in patients with preexisting cardiac disease—use cautiously.
- **BETA-ADRENERGIC BLOCKING AGENTS** (*e.g.*, **propranolol**): May antagonize the actions of terbutaline.
- **DIGOXIN**: Use with digitalis glycosides may increase the risk of cardiac arrhythmias.
- **MONOAMINE OXIDASE INHIBITORS**: May potentiate the vascular effects of terbutaline.
- **SYMPATHOMIMETICS, OTHER**: Use of terbutaline with other sympathomimetic amines may increase the risk of developing adverse cardiovascular effects.
- **TRICYCLIC ANTIDEPRESSANTS**: May potentiate the vascular effects of terbutaline.

Doses

- **DOGS:**

  For a trial to treat intrathoracic tracheal collapse, expiratory cough or dyspnea and marked exercise intolerance (extra-label): 1.25 – 5 mg (per dog) PO 2-3 times daily. (Johnson 2004)

  For bradyarrhythmias (extra-label): 0.2 mg/kg PO q8-12h; improvement usually partial and often temporary. (Rishniw *et al.* 2000)

  For adjunctive treatment of heart failure (extra-label): 0.2 mg/kg PO twice daily. While there is no data on bronchodilators in heart failure, the authors find them (theophylline or terbutaline) useful in patients with intractable cough, particularly when respiratory (airway collapse) disease complicates heart failure. Caution should be used as these drugs may produce tachycardia and predispose to arrhythmia. (Atkins *et al.* 2012)

  For treatment of premature labor as a tocolytic (extra-label): To suppress uterine contractility in bitches and queens with historical loss of otherwise normal pregnancies preterm, the initial dose is 0.03 mg/kg PO q8h. The dose is ideally titrated to effect using tocodynamometry. Terbutaline should be discontinued 48 hours prior to the calculated delivery date to permit normal labor and delivery to occur. Exogenous progesterone can be added if myometrial contractility cannot be controlled with tocolytics. (Davidson 2008), (Davidson *et al.* 2013)

- **CATS:**

  As a bronchodilator (extra-label):

  a) **For treatment (at home) for acute exacerbations of feline asthma**: 0.01 mg/kg SC or IM; Beneficial response (decrease of respiratory rate or effort by 50%) occurs in 15-30 minutes. A heart rate that approaches 240 BPM indicates that the drug has been absorbed. (Padrid 2000)

  b) **For acute bronchospasm** (initial crisis): 0.01 mg/kg IV, SC, IM. (Cohn 2007)

  c) **To prevent bronchospasm prior to trans-tracheal wash or bronchoalveolar lavage** (extra-label): 0.01 mg/kg SC q8h can be administered 12-24 hours before the procedure, with the final dose given 2-4 hours before anesthetic induction. (Finke 2013), (Venema *et al.* 2010)

  d) **To treat bronchospasm for non-bronchoscopic bronchoalveolar lavage** (extra-label): Have "on hand" in case of acute bronchoconstriction with the dose/amount pre-calculated (0.01 mg/kg). Can be given IV, IM, or SC, but until a full recovery, it is preferable to maintain IV catheter to enable IV dosing. (Foster *et al.* 2011)

  For bradyarrhythmias (extra-label): 0.625 mg per cat PO q8-12h; improvement usually partial and often temporary. (Rishniw *et al.* 2000)

- **HORSES:** (NOTE: ARCI UCGFS CLASS 3 DRUG)

  For use as a quantitative intradermal terbutaline sweat test (QITST) to identify anhidrosis (preliminary study); (extra-label): In the study a 6 cm wide strip of skin was clipped parallel with and 3 cm below the dorsal margin of the neck on the left side. Beginning at the caudal aspect of this strip, eight 0.1 mL intradermal injections of serial 10-fold dilutions of terbutaline sulfate in 0.9% saline were made through a 25 gauge needle at ≈ 5 cm intervals as follows: 0 (control), 0.001, 0.01, 0.1, 1, 10, 100 and 1000 mg/L. Individual sections of absorbent pad (3 x 3 cm; *Stayfree*® *Ultrathin* regular pads) were pre-weighed within plastic bags. Pads were then taped over each injection site. Thirty minutes later, they were removed, replaced in plastic bags and reweighed. Sweat weights at saline control sites were, in all cases, ≤8 mg. Sweat weights increased significantly at each successive terbutaline concentration up to a mean weight of 491 mg at the 1000 mg/L dose. The lower one-sided 95% confidence limits for sweat weights were 19, 57, 96, 195 and 267 mg for terbutaline concentrations of 0.1, 1, 10, 100 and 1000 mg/L, respectively. (MacKay 2008)

- **BIRDS:**

  For adjunctive treatment of respiratory distress (extra-label): Terbutaline at 0.01 mg/kg IM q6-8h, and butorphanol (1 – 2 mg/kg IM q2-3h) are usually given to birds in respiratory distress before placing in an oxygen-enriched incubator. Treatment can be continued via nebulizer. (Orosz *et al.* 2011)

- **REPTILES:**

  As a bronchodilator (extra-label): 0.01 – 0.02 mg/kg IM. (Schumacher 2011)

Monitoring

- Clinical symptom improvement; auscultation.
- Cardiac rate, rhythm (if indicated).
- Serum potassium, early in therapy if animal susceptible to hypokalemia.

Client Information

- Can increase heart rate (heartbeats) and cause excitement.
- Terbutaline can delay labor in pregnant animals.
- Contact veterinarian if animal's condition deteriorates or if it becomes acutely ill.
- Overdoses can be serious; keep well out of reach of children and animals.

Chemistry/Synonyms

A synthetic sympathomimetic amine, terbutaline sulfate occurs as a slightly bitter-tasting, white to gray-white, crystalline powder that may have a faint odor of acetic acid. One gram is soluble in 1.5 mL of water or 250 mL of alcohol. The commercially available injection has its pH adjusted to 3-5 with hydrochloric acid.

Terbutaline Sulfate may also be known as: KWD-2019, terbutaline sulphate, terbutalini sulfas. There are many trade names including, *Brethine*®.

Storage/Stability

Terbutaline tablets should be stored in tight containers at room temperature (15-30°C). Tablets have an expiration date of 3 years beyond the date of manufacture. Terbutaline injection should be stored at room temperature (15-30°C) and protected from light. The injection has an expiration date of 2 years after the date of manufacture.

Terbutaline injection is stable over a pH range of 1-7. Discolored solutions should not be used.

Compatibility/Compounding Considerations

Terbutaline injection is physically **compatible** with D5W and aminophylline.

Dosage Forms/Regulatory Status

VETERINARY-LABELED PRODUCTS: NONE.

The ARCI (Racing Commissioners International) has designated this drug as a class 3 substance. See the appendix for more information.

HUMAN-LABELED PRODUCTS:

Terbutaline Sulfate Tablets: 2.5 mg & 5 mg; generic; (Rx)

Terbutaline Injection: 1 mg/mL in 1 mL vials & 2 mL amps with 1 mL fill; generic; (Rx)

Revisions/References

Monograph revised/updated August 2014.

Atkins, C. E. & J. Haggstrom (2012). Pharmacologic management of myxomatous mitral valve disease in dogs. Journal of veterinary cardiology : the official journal of the European Society of Veterinary Cardiology **14**(1).

Cohn, L. (2007). Breathing easy: How to help cats with asthma. Proceedings: Western Vet Conf. accessed via Veterinary Information Network; vin.com

Davidson, A. (2008). Breeder Myths and the Veterinarian. Proceedings: WVC. accessed via Veterinary Information Network; vin.com

Davidson, A. P. & T. A. Baker (2013). Obstetrical Emergencies. 65th Convention of the Canadian Veterinary Medical Association. accessed via Veterinary Information Network; vin.com

Finke, M. D. (2013). Transtracheal Wash and Bronchoalveolar Lavage. Topics in Companion Animal Medicine **28**(3): 97-102.

Foster, S. F. & P. Martin (2011). Lower respiratory tract infections in cats: Reaching beyond empirical therapy. Journal of Feline Medicine & Surgery **13**(5): 313-32.

Johnson, L. (2004). Canine airway collapse. Proceedings: ACVIM Forum. accessed via Veterinary Information Network; vin.com

MacKay, R. J. (2008). Quantitative intradermal terbutaline sweat test in horses. Equine Veterinary Journal **40**(5): 518-20.

Orosz, S. & M. Lichtenberger (2011). Avian Respiratory Distress: Etiology, Diagnosis, and Treatment. Vet Clin Exot Anim **14**: 241-55.

Padrid, P. (2000). Feline bronchial disease: Therapeutic recommendations for the 21st Century. Proceedings: The North American Veterinary Conference, Orlando. accessed via Veterinary Information Network; vin.com

Rishniw, M. & W. Thomas (2000). Bradyarrhythmias. *Kirk's Current Veterinary Therapy: XIII Small Animal Practice*. J. Bonagura. Philadelphia, WB Saunders: 719-25.

Schumacher, J. (2011). Respiratory Medicine of Reptiles. Vet Clin Exot Anim **14**: 207-24.

Venema, C. M. & C. C. Patterson (2010). Feline asthma: What's new and where might clinical practice be heading? Journal of Feline Medicine & Surgery **12**(9): 681-92.

Testosterone

(tess-toss-ter-ohn)

Androgenic Hormone

Prescriber Highlights

► Principle endogenous androgen used primarily for the treatment of testosterone-responsive urinary incontinence in neutered male dogs/cats; in bovine medicine to produce an estrus-detector animal.

► Contraindications: Known hypersensitivity to the drug; prostate carcinoma. Caution: Renal, cardiac, or hepatic dysfunction.

► Adverse Effects: Uncommon (in males), but perianal adenomas, perineal hernias, prostatic disorders, & behavior changes possible.

► Testosterone products are controlled substances (C-III).

Uses/Indications

The use of injectable esters of testosterone in veterinary medicine is limited primarily to its use in dogs (and perhaps cats) for the treatment of testosterone-responsive urinary incontinence in neutered males. Testosterone has been used to treat a rare form of dermatitis (exhibited by bilateral alopecia) in neutered male dogs. These drugs are also used in bovine medicine to produce an estrus-detector (teaser) animal in cull cows, heifers, and steers.

The effectiveness of testosterone to increase libido, treat hypogonadism, aspermia, and infertility in domestic animals has been disappointing and is generally not recommended.

Theoretically, topically applied human transdermal products could be effective in animals, but no information was located on their efficacy or safety. Many older references list dosages using testosterone propionate (a shorter-acting injectable form), but commercially available products are no longer available in the USA.

Pharmacology/Actions

The principle endogenous androgenic steroid, testosterone is responsible for many secondary sex characteristic of the male as well as the maturation and growth of the male reproductive organs and increasing libido.

Testosterone has anabolic activity with resultant increased protein anabolism and decreased protein catabolism. Testosterone causes nitrogen, sodium, potassium and phosphorus retention and decreases the urinary excretion of calcium. Nitrogen balance is improved only when an adequate intake of both calories and protein occurs.

By stimulating erythropoietic stimulating factor, testosterone can stimulate the production of red blood cells. Large doses of exogenous testosterone can inhibit spermatogenesis through a negative feedback mechanism inhibiting luteinizing hormone (LH).

Testosterone may help maintain the normal urethral muscle tone and integrity of the urethral mucosa in male dogs. It may also be necessary to prevent some types of dermatoses.

Pharmacokinetics

Orally administered testosterone is rapidly metabolized by the GI mucosa and the liver (first-pass effect); very little reaches the systemic circulation. The esterified compounds, testosterone enanthate and cypionate, are less polar than testosterone and more slowly absorbed from lipid tissue after IM injection. The duration of action of these compounds may persist for 2-4 weeks after IM injection. Testosterone propionate reportedly has a much shorter duration of action than the enanthate or cypionate esters. Because absorption is dependent upon several factors (volume injected, perfusion, etc.), duration of action may be variable.

Testosterone is highly bound to a specific testosterone-estradiol globulin (98% in humans). The quantity of this globulin determines the amount of drug that is in the free or bound form. The free form concentration determines the plasma half-life of the hormone.

Testosterone is metabolized in the liver and is, with its metabolites, excreted in the urine ($\approx$ 90%) and feces ($\approx$ 6%). The plasma half-life of testosterone has been reported to be between 10-100 minutes in humans. The plasma half-life of testosterone cypionate has been reported to be 8 days.

Contraindications/Precautions/Warnings

Testosterone therapy is contraindicated in patients with known hypersensitivity to the drug or prostate carcinoma. It should be used with caution in patients with renal, cardiac or hepatic dysfunction.

Adverse Effects

Adverse effects are reportedly uncommon when injectable testosterone products are used in male dogs to treat hormone-responsive incontinence. Perianal adenomas, perineal hernias, prostatic disorders, and behavior changes (aggression) are all possible, however. In females (bitches), testosterone can cause clitoral hypertrophy/masculinization, and aggression. In cats, behavioral changes have been reported. High dosages or chronic usage may result in oligospermia or infertility in intact males.

Polycythemia has been reported in humans receiving high dosages of testosterone.

Reproductive/Nursing Safety

In humans, the FDA categorizes this drug as category *X* for use during pregnancy (*Studies in animals or humans demonstrate fetal abnormalities or adverse reaction; reports indicate evidence of fetal risk. The risk of use in pregnant women clearly outweighs any possible benefit.*) In a separate system evaluating the safety of drugs in canine and feline pregnancy (Papich 1989), this drug is categorized as in class: *D* (*Contraindicated. These drugs have been shown to cause congenital malformations or embryotoxicity.*)

It is not known whether androgens are excreted in milk; consider using milk replacer if using testosterone in nursing patients.

Overdosage/Acute Toxicity

No specific information was located; refer to the Adverse Effects section for further information.

Drug Interactions

The following drug interactions have either been reported or are theoretical in humans or animals receiving testosterone and may be of significance in veterinary patients. Unless otherwise noted, use together is not necessarily contraindicated, but weigh the potential risks and perform additional monitoring when appropriate.

- **CORTICOSTEROIDS:** Androgens may enhance the edema that can be associated with ACTH or adrenal steroid therapy.
- **INSULIN; ORAL ANTIDIABETIC AGENTS:** Testosterone may decrease serum glucose levels.
- **PROPRANOLOL:** Testosterone cypionate may increase propranolol clearance.
- **WARFARIN:** Testosterone may increase anticoagulant effects.

Laboratory Considerations

- Concentrations of **protein bound iodine (PBI)** can be decreased in patients receiving testosterone therapy, but the clinical significance of this is probably not important. Androgen agents can decrease amounts of **thyroxine-binding globulin** and decrease **total T4** concentrations and increase resin uptake of **T3 and T4**. Free thyroid hormones are unaltered and clinically, there is no evidence of dysfunction.
- Both **creatinine** and **creatine** excretion can be decreased by testosterone.

- Testosterone can increase the urinary excretion of **17-ketosteroids.**
- Androgenic/anabolic steroids may alter **blood glucose** levels.
- Androgenic/anabolic steroids may suppress **clotting factors II, V, VII, and X.**

Doses

- **DOGS:**

  For testosterone-responsive urinary incontinence (may be used with phenylpropanolamine) in males (extra-label): Testosterone cypionate 2.2 mg.kg IM once monthly.

  For estrus control (extra-label): **Note:** Rarely recommended. Side effects include masculinization, clitoral hypertrophy, and aggression. Concerns have been expressed about long-term suppression of estrous activity in bitches treated with testosterone. Research results disagree as to whether treatment with testosterone interferes with subsequent ability to induce estrus in bitches (Kustritz 2012). Testosterone enanthate or cypionate: 0.5 mg/kg IM once every 5 days or methyltestosterone tablets: 25 mg PO twice a week; these doses are for Greyhound-sized dogs. (Purswell 1999)

  To reduce mammary gland enlargement seen in pseudopregnancy (extra-label): **Note:** Rarely recommended. Testosterone enanthate or testosterone cypionate: 0.5 – 1 mg/kg IM once. (Purswell 1999)

- **CATTLE:**

  To produce an estrus-detector (teaser) animal (cull cows, heifers, steers); (extra-label): Testosterone enanthate 0.5 gram IM and 1.5 gram SC (divided in two separate locations). After 4 days attach chinball marker and put in with breeding herd. To maintain, give 0.5 – 0.75 gram SC every 10-14 days. (Wolfe 1986)

Monitoring

- Efficacy.
- Adverse effects.

Chemistry/Synonyms

The esterified compounds, testosterone cypionate, and enanthate are available commercially as injectable (in oil) products. Testosterone cypionate occurs as an odorless to having a faint odor, creamy white or white, crystalline powder. It is insoluble in water, soluble in vegetable oils, and freely soluble in alcohol. Testosterone cypionate has a melting range of 98°-104°C. It may also be known as testosterone cyclopentylpropionate.

Testosterone enanthate occurs as an odorless to having a faint odor, creamy white or white, crystalline powder. It is soluble in vegetable oils, insoluble in water and melts between 34-39°C.

Testosterone Cypionate may also be known as testosterone cyclopentylpropionate.

Storage/Stability

The commercially available injectable preparations of testosterone cypionate, enanthate and propionate should be stored at room temperature; avoid freezing or exposing to temperatures >40°C. If exposed to low temperatures a precipitate may form, but should redissolve with shaking and rewarming. If a wet needle or syringe is used to draw up the parenteral solutions, cloudy solutions may result but this will not affect the drug's potency.

Compatibility/Compounding Considerations

No specific information noted.

Dosage Forms/Regulatory Status

VETERINARY-LABELED PRODUCTS:

No known testosterone products (with the exception of combinations with estradiol as growth promotant implants) that are FDA-approved for use in veterinary species were located. Testosterone propionate (200 mg) is available in combination with estra-diol benzoate (20 mg) as a growth promotant. Trade names include *Component E-H*®; (OTC) and *Synovex-H*®; (OTC). For use in heifers weighing 400 or more pounds.

Testosterone propionate (200 mg) with estradiol benzoate (28 mg); *Synovex-Plus*®; (OTC). Approved for steers.

The ARCI (Racing Commissioners International) has designated this drug as a class 4 substance. See the appendix for more information.

HUMAN-LABELED PRODUCTS:
Testosterone Cypionate (in oil) Injection: 100 mg/mL & 200 mg/mL in 1 mL & 10 mL vials; *Depo-Testosterone*®, generic; (Rx, C-III)

Testosterone Enanthate (in oil) Injection: 200 mg/mL in 5 mL multi-dose vials; generic; (Rx, C-III)

Testosterone Undecanoate solution for injection: 750 mg/3 mL; *Aveed*®; (Rx; C-III)

Testosterone Pellets Implant for subcutaneous implantation: 75 mg in 1 pellet/vials; *Testopel*®; (Rx, C-III)

There are also testosterone transdermal patches and solutions, topical 1%, 1.6% & 2% gels, and buccal tablets available.

Revisions/References
Monograph revised/updated August 2014.

Kustritz, M. V. R. (2012). Managing the Reproductive Cycle in the Bitch. Veterinary Clinics of North America-Small Animal Practice **42**(3): 423-37.

Papich, M. (1989). Effects of drugs on pregnancy. *Current Veterinary Therapy X: Small Animal Practice*. R. Kirk. Philadelphia, Saunders: 1291-9.

Purswell, B. (1999). Pharmaceuticals used in canine theriogenology - Part 1 & 2. Proceedings: Central Veterinary Conference, Kansas City. accessed via Veterinary Information Network; vin.com

Wolfe, D. F. (1986). Surgical procedures of the reproductive system of the bull. *Current Therapy in Theriogenology 2: Diagnosis, treatment and prevention of reproductive diseases in small and large animals*. D. A. Morrow. Philadelphia, WB Saunders: 353-79.

Tetracycline HCl
(tet-ra-sye-kleen)

Tetracycline Antibiotic

Prescriber Highlights

▶ Prototype tetracycline antibiotic; many bacteria are now resistant, but still may be very useful to treat mycoplasma, rickettsia, spirochetes, & Chlamydia. Most common use is with niacinamide to help control sterile inflammatory skin conditions in dogs.

▶ Dosing frequency and adverse effects are issues; most prefer doxycycline or minocycline in small animals.

▶ Extreme Caution: Pregnancy. Caution: Liver or renal insufficiency.

▶ Adverse Effects: GI distress, staining of developing teeth & bones, superinfections, photosensitivity; long-term use may cause uroliths. Hepatopathy, especially if renal dysfunction, is possible. **Cats:** Do not tolerate very well. **Horses:** If stressed, may break with diarrheas (oral use). Ruminants: **High oral doses** can cause ruminal microflora depression & ruminoreticular stasis; **rapid IV** of undiluted propylene glycol-based products can cause intravascular hemolysis & cardiodepressant effects; **IM:** local reactions, yellow staining & necrosis may be seen at the injection site.

Uses/Indications
While tetracycline still is used as an antimicrobial, most small animal clinicians prefer doxycycline or minocycline and large animal clinicians prefer oxytetracycline when a tetracycline is indicated to treat susceptible infections. The most common use of tetracycline HCl today is in combination with niacinamide, which may be useful in controlling a variety of sterile inflammatory skin conditions in dogs including: discoid lupus erythematosus (DLE), sterile granulomatous/pyogranulomatous syndrome, sterile nodular panniculitis, cutaneous reactive histiocytosis, cutaneous vesicular lupus erythematosus, pemphigus erythematosus, pemphigus foliaceus, lupoid onychodystrophy/onychitis, German shepherd dog metatarsal fistulae, vasculitis, arteritis of the nasal philtrum, sebaceous adenitis and dermatomyositis (Koch *et al.* 2011). Controlled studies demonstrating clear efficacy are lacking, but anecdotally this combination appears effective in some patients, including up to 2/3 of dogs that are treated for DLE. Often used in conjunction with other immunomodulating drugs, especially in the initial treatment phase. Nicainamide/tetracycline may make take 1-2 months before efficacy is noted.

Pharmacology/Actions
Tetracyclines generally act as time-dependent antibiotics and inhibit protein synthesis by reversibly binding to 30S ribosomal subunits of susceptible organisms, thereby preventing binding to those ribosomes of aminoacyl transfer-RNA. Tetracyclines have been deemed bacteriostatic antibiotics but this nomenclature is more of historical importance than descriptive of their antibacterial actions. Tetracyclines are believed to reversibly bind to 50S ribosomes and additionally alter cytoplasmic membrane permeability in susceptible organisms. In high concentrations, tetracyclines can inhibit protein synthesis by mammalian cells.

As a class, the tetracyclines have activity against most mycoplasma, spirochetes (including the Lyme disease organism), Chlamydia, and Rickettsia. Against gram-positive bacteria, the tetracyclines have activity against some strains of staphylococcus and streptococci, but resistance of these organisms is increasing. Gram-positive bacteria that are usually covered by tetracyclines include *Actinomyces* spp., *Bacillus anthracis*, *Clostridium perfringens* and tetani, *Listeria monocytogenes*, and Nocardia. Among gram-negative bacteria that tetracyclines usually have *in vitro* and *in vivo* activity include *Bordetella* spp., Brucella, Bartonella, *Haemophilus* spp., *Pasteurella multocida*, Shigella, and Yersinia pestis. Many or most strains of *E. coli*, Klebsiella, Bacteroides, Enterobacter, Proteus and *Pseudomonas aeruginosa* are resistant to the tetracyclines. While most strains of Pseudomonas aeruginosa show *in vitro* resistance to tetracyclines, those compounds attaining high urine levels (*e.g.*, tetracycline, oxytetracycline) have been associated with clinical cures in dogs with UTI secondary to this organism. Hemoglobin at the site of the infection can reduce the antimicrobial activity of tetracycline.

Oxytetracycline and tetracycline share nearly identical spectrums of activity and patterns of cross-resistance and a tetracycline susceptibility disk is usually used for *in vitro* testing for oxytetracycline susceptibility.

Tetracyclines have antiinflammatory and immunomodulating effects. They can suppress antibody production and chemotaxis of neutrophils; inhibit lipases, collagenases, prostaglandin synthesis, and activation of complement component 3.

Pharmacokinetics
Both oxytetracycline and tetracycline are readily absorbed after oral administration to fasting animals. Bioavailabilities are ≈ 60-80%. The presence of food or dairy products can significantly reduce the amount of tetracycline absorbed, with reductions of 50% or more possible. After IM administration, tetracycline is erratically and poorly absorbed with serum levels usually lower than those attainable with oral therapy.

Tetracyclines as a class, are widely distributed to heart, kidney, lungs, muscle, pleural fluid, bronchial secretions, sputum, bile, saliva, urine, synovial fluid, ascitic fluid, and aqueous and vitreous humor. Only small quantities of tetracycline and oxytetracycline are distributed to the CSF, and therapeutic levels may not be achievable. While all tetracyclines distribute to the prostate and eye, doxycycline or minocycline penetrate better into these and most other tissues. Tetracyclines cross the placenta, enter fetal circulation and are distributed into milk. The volume of distribution of tetracycline is ≈ 1.2-1.3 L/kg in small animals. The amount of plasma protein binding is ≈ 20-67% for tetracycline. In cattle, the volume of distribution for oxytetracycline is between 1-2.5 L/kg. Milk to plasma ratios for oxytetracycline and tetracycline are 0.75 and 1.2-1.9, respectively.

Both oxytetracycline and tetracycline are eliminated unchanged primarily via glomerular filtration. Patients with impaired renal function can have prolonged elimination half-lives and accumulate the drug with repeated dosing. These drugs apparently are not metabolized, but are excreted into the GI tract via both biliary and nonbiliary routes and may become inactive after chelation with fecal materials. The elimination half-life of tetracycline is ≈ 5-6 hours in dogs and cats.

Contraindications/Precautions/Warnings

Tetracycline is contraindicated in patients hypersensitive to it or other tetracyclines. Because tetracyclines can retard fetal skeletal development and discolor deciduous teeth, they should only be used in the last half of pregnancy when the benefits outweigh the fetal risks. Oxytetracycline and tetracycline are considered more likely to cause these abnormalities than either doxycycline or minocycline.

In patients with renal insufficiency or hepatic impairment, tetracycline must be used cautiously; lower than normal dosages are recommended with enhanced monitoring of renal and hepatic function. Avoid concurrent administration of other nephrotoxic or hepatotoxic drugs if tetracyclines are administered to these patients. Monitoring of serum levels should be considered if long-term therapy is required.

Adverse Effects

Oxytetracycline and tetracycline given to young animals can cause discoloration (yellow, brown or gray color) of bones and teeth. High dosages or chronic administration may delay bone growth and healing.

Tetracyclines in high levels can exert an antianabolic effect that can cause an increase in BUN and/or hepatotoxicity, particularly in patients with preexisting renal dysfunction. As renal function deteriorates secondary to drug accumulation, this effect may be exacerbated.

In ruminants, high oral doses can cause ruminal microflora depression and ruminoreticular stasis. Rapid intravenous injection of undiluted propylene glycol-based products can cause intravascular hemolysis with resultant hemoglobinuria. Propylene glycol based products have also caused cardiodepressant effects when administered to calves. When administered IM, local reactions, yellow staining, and necrosis may be seen at the injection site.

In small animals, tetracyclines can cause nausea, vomiting, anorexia, and diarrhea. Cats do not tolerate oral tetracycline or oxytetracycline very well, and may present with clinical signs of colic, fever, hair loss, and depression. There are reports that long-term tetracycline use may cause urolith formation in dogs.

Horses that are stressed by surgery, anesthesia, trauma, etc., may break with severe diarrheas after receiving tetracyclines (especially with oral administration).

Tetracycline therapy (especially long-term) may result in overgrowth of non-susceptible bacteria or fungi (superinfections).

Tetracyclines have also been associated with photosensitivity reactions and, rarely, hepatotoxicity, formation of anti-nuclear antibodies, or blood dyscrasias.

Reproductive/Nursing Safety

In humans, the FDA categorizes this drug as category *D* for use during pregnancy (*There is evidence of human fetal risk, but the potential benefits from the use of the drug in pregnant women may be acceptable despite its potential risks.*) In a separate system evaluating the safety of drugs in canine and feline pregnancy (Papich 1989), this drug is categorized as in class: *D* (*Contraindicated. These drugs have been shown to cause congenital malformations or embryotoxicity.*)

Tetracyclines are excreted in milk but because much of the drug will be bound to calcium in milk, it is unlikely to be of significant risk to nursing animals.

Overdosage/Acute Toxicity

Tetracyclines are generally well tolerated after acute overdoses. Dogs given >400 mg/kg/day orally or 100 mg/kg/day IM of oxytetracycline did not demonstrate any toxicity. Oral overdoses would most likely be associated with GI disturbances (vomiting, anorexia, and/or diarrhea). Should the patient develop severe emesis or diarrhea, fluids and electrolytes should be monitored and replaced if necessary. Chronic overdoses may lead to drug accumulation and nephrotoxicity.

High oral doses given to ruminants, can cause ruminal microflora depression and ruminoreticular stasis. Rapid intravenous injection of undiluted propylene glycol-based products can cause intravascular hemolysis with resultant hemoglobinuria.

Rapid intravenous injection of tetracyclines has induced transient collapse and cardiac arrhythmias in several species, presumably due to chelation with intravascular calcium ions. Overdose quantities of drug could exacerbate this effect if given too rapidly IV. If the drug must be given rapidly IV (<5 minutes), some clinicians recommend pre-treating the animal with intravenous calcium gluconate.

Drug Interactions

The following drug interactions have either been reported or are theoretical in humans or animals receiving tetracyclines and may be of significance in veterinary patients. Unless otherwise noted, use together is not necessarily contraindicated, but weigh the potential risks and perform additional monitoring when appropriate.

- **ATOVAQUONE:** Tetracyclines have caused decreased atovaquone levels.
- **BETA-LACTAM OR AMINOGLYCOSIDE ANTIBIOTICS:** Bacteriostatic drugs, like the tetracyclines, have been historically thought to interfere with bactericidal activity of the penicillins, cephalosporins, and aminoglycosides but the actual clinical significance of this interaction is doubtful.
- **DIGOXIN:** Tetracyclines have increased the bioavailability of digoxin in a small percentage of human patients and caused digoxin toxicity. These effects may persist for months after discontinuation of the tetracycline.
- **DIVALENT OR TRIVALENT CATIONS (oral antacids, saline cathartics or other GI products containing aluminum, calcium, iron, magnesium, zinc, or bismuth cations):** When orally administered, tetracyclines can chelate divalent or trivalent cations that can decrease the absorption of the tetracycline or the other drug if it contains these cations; it is recommended that all oral tetracyclines be given at least 1-2 hours before or after the cation-containing products.
- **METHOXYFLURANE:** Fatal nephrotoxicity has occurred in humans when used with tetracycline; concomitant use with oxytetracycline not recommended.

- SUCRALFATE: Sucralfate may impair the oral absorption of tetracycline; separate dosing by at least 2 hours to minimize this effect.
- WARFARIN: Tetracyclines may depress plasma prothrombin activity and patients on anticoagulant therapy may need dosage adjustment.

Laboratory Considerations

- Tetracyclines (not minocycline) may cause falsely elevated values of **urine catecholamines** when using fluorometric methods of determination.
- Tetracyclines reportedly can cause false-positive **urine glucose results** if using the cupric sulfate method of determination (Benedict's reagent, *Clinitest®*), but this may be the result of ascorbic acid that is found in some parenteral formulations of tetracyclines. Tetracyclines have also reportedly caused false-negative results in determining urine glucose when using the glucose oxidase method (*Clinistix®*, *Tes-Tape®*).

Doses

- **DOGS:**

For adjunctive treatment of sterile inflammatory dermatoses (extra-label): Used with niacinamide. Recommended dosages are empirical and vary somewhat. Practically, for dogs weighing ≤5 kg: 100 mg niacinamide per dog PO 3 times a day; for dogs weighing 5-10 kg: 250 mg (1/2 of a 500 mg tablet) niacinamide per dog PO 3 times a day; for dogs weighing >10 kg: 500 mg niacinamide per dog PO 3 times a day. If efficacy/remission occurs, may reduce to twice daily administration and then tapered further over time when possible. If using tetracycline HCl, dose at the same amount of niacinamide PO 3 times daily. If using doxycycline consider 5 – 10 mg/kg PO twice daily. If using minocycline consider 7.5 mg/kg PO twice daily.

For susceptible infections (extra-label): 22 mg/kg PO q8h. Treatment duration recommendations generally range from 14-28 days.

- **CATS:**

For susceptible infections (extra-label): 15 – 22 mg/kg PO q8h. Treatment duration recommendations generally range from 14-28 days.

- **FERRETS:**

For susceptible infections (extra-label): 25 mg/kg PO 2-3 times daily. (Williams 2000)

- **RABBITS, RODENTS, SMALL MAMMALS:**
  a) Rabbits: 50 – 100 mg/kg PO q8-12h. (Ivey *et al.* 2000)
  b) Chinchillas: 50 mg/kg PO q8-12h. (Hayes 2000)
  c) Chinchillas, Guinea Pigs, Rats: 20 mg/kg PO q12h. Mice: 20 mg/kg PO q12h or 50 – 60 mg/L of drinking water Hamsters: 30 mg/kg PO q6h or 400 mg/L of drinking water. Gerbils: 20 mg/kg PO or IM q24h. (Adamcak *et al.* 2000)

- **CATTLE:**

For susceptible infections in calves (labeled dose): 11 mg/kg PO twice daily for up to 5 days. (Label directions; *Polyotic®*)

- **SHEEP:**

For susceptible infections (labeled dose): 11 mg/kg PO twice daily for up to 5 days. (Label directions; *Polyotic®*)

- **SWINE:**

For susceptible infections (labeled dose): 22 mg/kg PO for 3-5 days in drinking water. (Label directions; *Polyotic®*)

- **BIRDS:**

For susceptible infections (extra-label)
  a) **For treatment of psittacosis in conjunction with *LA-200®*** (see oxytetracycline doses) and/or medicated pellets and/or *Keet*

Life: Using 25 mg/mL oral suspension, mix 2 teaspoonsful to 1 cup of soft food. **For mild respiratory disease (especially flock treatment):** Mix 1 teaspoonful of 10 grams/6.4 oz. soluble powder per gallon of drinking water. Used as an adjunct for psittacosis with other tetracycline forms. Will not reach therapeutic levels by itself. Prepare fresh solution twice daily, as potency is rapidly lost. (McDonald 1989)
  b) Mix 1 teaspoonful of 10 grams/6.4 oz. soluble powder per gallon of drinking water and administer for 5-10 days. Prepare fresh solution 2-3 times daily, as potency is rapidly lost. For converting regimen to pelleted feeds administer oral suspension by gavage at 200 – 250 mg/kg once or twice daily until feeds are accepted. Is not an adequate therapy for long-term treatment of chlamydiosis (psittacosis). (Clubb 1986)

Monitoring

- Adverse effects.
- Clinical efficacy.
- Long-term use or in susceptible patients: periodic renal, hepatic, hematologic evaluations.

Client Information

- Avoid giving this drug orally within 1-2 hours of feeding, giving milk or other dairy products.
- If gastrointestinal upset occurs, giving with a small amount of food may help, but this may also reduce the amount of drug absorbed.

Chemistry/Synonyms

An antibiotic obtained from *Streptomyces aureofaciens* or derived semisynthetically from oxytetracycline, tetracycline HCl occurs as a moderately hygroscopic, yellow, crystalline powder. About 100 mg/mL is soluble in water and 10 mg/mL soluble in alcohol. Tetracycline base has a solubility of ≈ 0.4 mg per mL of water and 20 mg per mL of alcohol. Commercially available tetracycline HCl for IM injection also contains magnesium chloride, procaine HCl and ascorbic acid.

Tetracycline may also be known as: tetracyclini hydrochloridum; many trade names are available.

Storage/Stability

Unless otherwise instructed by the manufacturer, tetracycline oral tablets and capsules should be stored in tight, light resistant containers at room temperature (15-30°C). The oral suspension and powder for injection should be stored at room temperature; avoid freezing the oral suspension.

Compatibility/Compounding Considerations

No specific information noted.

Dosage Forms/Regulatory Status

VETERINARY-LABELED PRODUCTS:

There are a variety of Tetracycline HCl Soluble Powder (as a water additive) products available in various concentrations and sizes. Usual concentrations are either 25 grams/lb or 324 grams/lb and these products may be available in several sizes; may be FDA-approved for use in swine, cattle, or poultry. Withdrawal time may vary depending on age of animal and product.

HUMAN-LABELED PRODUCTS:

Tetracycline HCl Capsules: 250 mg & 500 mg; generic; (Rx)

Revisions/References

Monograph revised/updated August 2014.

Adamcak, A. & B. Otten (2000). Rodent Therapeutics. Vet Clin NA: Exotic Anim Pract 3:1(Jan): 221-40.
Clubb, S. L. (1986). Therapeutics: Individual and Flock Treatment Regimens. *Clinical Avian Medicine and Surgery.* G. J. Harrison and L. R. Harrison. Philadelphia, W.B. Saunders: 327-55.

Hayes, P. (2000). Diseases of Chinchillas. *Kirk's Current Veterinary Therapy: XIII Small Animal Practice*. J. Bonagura. Philadelphia, WB Saunders: 1152-7.

Ivey, E. & J. Morrisey (2000). Therapeutics for Rabbits. *Vet Clin NA: Exotic Anim Pract* **3:1**(Jan): 183-216.

Koch, S., et al. (2011). *Small Animal Dermatology Drug Handbook*, Wiley-Blackwell. Ames.

McDonald, S. E. (1989). Summary of medications for use in psittacine birds. *JAAV* 3(3): 120-7.

Papich, M. (1989). Effects of drugs on pregnancy. *Current Veterinary Therapy X: Small Animal Practice*. R. Kirk. Philadelphia, Saunders: 1291-9.

Williams, B. (2000). Therapeutics in Ferrets. *Vet Clin NA: Exotic Anim Pract* **3:1**(Jan): 131-53.

Theanine — See L-Theanine

Theophylline

(thee-off-i-lin)

Phosphodiesterase Inhibitor Bronchodilator

Prescriber Highlights

▶ Bronchodilator drug with mild diuretic activity. Used short-term for bronchospasm & cardiogenic pulmonary edema.

▶ Narrow therapeutic index in humans, but dogs appear to be less susceptible to toxic effects at higher plasma levels.

▶ Many drug interactions. Fluoroquinolones (*e.g.*, enrofloxacin) can increase theophylline levels substantially.

Uses/Indications

The theophyllines (aminophylline and theophylline) are used primarily for their bronchodilatory effects especially in animals with 'cough'. Theophylline could potentially be of benefit in dogs with pulmonary artery hypertension if the underlying cause is chronic obstructive pulmonary disease (COPD) (Kellihan *et al.* 2010).

Pharmacology/Actions

The theophyllines competitively inhibit phosphodiesterase thereby increasing amounts of cyclic AMP that then increase the release of endogenous epinephrine. The elevated levels of cAMP may also inhibit the release of histamine and slow reacting substance of anaphylaxis (SRS-A). The myocardial and neuromuscular transmission effects that the theophyllines possess may be a result of translocating intracellular ionized calcium.

The theophyllines directly relax smooth muscles in the bronchi and pulmonary vasculature, induce diuresis, increase gastric acid secretion and inhibit uterine contractions. They have weak chronotropic and inotropic action, stimulate the CNS and can cause respiratory stimulation (centrally-mediated).

Pharmacokinetics

Theophylline is distributed throughout the extracellular fluids and body tissues. It crosses the placenta and is distributed into milk (70% of serum levels). In dogs, at therapeutic serum levels only about 7-14% is bound to plasma proteins. The volume of distribution of theophylline for dogs has been reported to be 0.82 L/kg. After IV administration of aminophylline (= 7.88 mg/kg theophylline) to greyhounds, mean theophylline volume of distribution (steady state) was 0.72 L/kg, mean clearance 0.935 mL/min/kg; elimination half-life was ≈ 9 hours (KuKanich *et al.* 2012).

The volume of distribution in cats is reported to be 0.46 L/kg and in horses, 0.85-1.02 L/kg.

Because of the low volumes of distribution and theophylline's low lipid solubility, obese patients should be dosed on a lean body weight basis.

Theophylline is metabolized primarily in the liver (in humans) to 3-methylxanthine, which has weak bronchodilator activity. Renal clearance contributes only about 10% to the overall plasma clearance of theophylline. The reported elimination half-lives (mean values) in various studies include: dogs ≈ 5.7 hours; cats ≈ 7.8 hours; pigs ≈ 11 hours; and horses ≈ 11.9-17 hours. In humans, there are very wide interpatient variations in serum half-lives and resultant serum levels. It could be expected that similar variability exists in veterinary patients, particularly those with concurrent illnesses.

Contraindications/Precautions/Warnings

Theophylline is contraindicated in patients who are hypersensitive to any of the xanthines including aminophylline, theobromine or caffeine.

The theophyllines should be administered with caution in patients with severe cardiac disease, seizure disorders, gastric ulcers, hyperthyroidism, renal or hepatic disease, severe hypoxia, or severe hypertension. A 50% reduction in dosage has been suggested for patients in hepatic failure (Trepanier 2013). Because it may cause or worsen preexisting arrhythmias, patients with cardiac arrhythmias should receive theophylline only with caution and enhanced monitoring. Neonatal and geriatric patients may have decreased clearances of theophylline and be more sensitive to its toxic effects. Patients with CHF may have prolonged serum half-lives of theophylline.

Adverse Effects

The theophyllines can produce CNS stimulation and gastrointestinal irritation after administration by any route. Most adverse effects are related to the serum level of the drug and may be symptomatic of toxic blood levels; dogs appear to tolerate levels that may be very toxic to humans. Some mild CNS excitement and GI disturbances are not uncommon when starting therapy and generally resolve with chronic administration in conjunction with monitoring and dosage adjustments.

Dogs and cats can exhibit clinical signs of nausea and vomiting, insomnia, increased gastric acid secretion, diarrhea, polyphagia, polydipsia, and polyuria. Side effects in horses are generally dose related and may include nervousness, excitability (auditory, tactile, and visual), tremors, diaphoresis, tachycardia, and ataxia. Seizures or cardiac dysrhythmias may occur in severe intoxications.

Reproductive/Nursing Safety

In humans, the FDA categorizes this drug as category C for use during pregnancy (*Animal studies have shown an adverse effect on the fetus, but there are no adequate studies in humans; or there are no animal reproduction studies and no adequate studies in humans.*)

Overdosage/Acute Toxicity

Clinical signs of toxicity (see above) are usually associated with levels >20 micrograms/mL in humans and become more severe as the serum level exceeds that value. Tachycardias, arrhythmias, and CNS effects (seizures, hyperthermia) are considered the most life-threatening aspects of toxicity. Dogs appear to tolerate serum levels >20 micrograms/mL. There were 86 single agent exposures to theophylline reported to the ASPCA Animal Poison Control Center (APCC) during 2009-2013. Of the 75 dogs, 27 were symptomatic with tachycardia being the most commonly reported clinical sign (48%).

Treatment of theophylline toxicity is supportive. Patients suffering from seizures should have an adequate airway maintained and treated with IV diazepam. The patient should be constantly monitored for cardiac arrhythmias and tachycardia. Fluid and electrolytes should be monitored and corrected as necessary. Hyperthermia may be treated with phenothiazines and tachycardia treated with propranolol if either condition is considered life threatening.

Drug Interactions

The following drug interactions with aminophylline or theophylline have either been reported or are theoretical in humans or animals and may be of significance in veterinary patients. Unless otherwise noted, use together is not necessarily contraindicated, but weigh the potential risks and perform additional monitoring when appropriate.

The following drugs can <u>decrease</u> theophylline levels:
- **BARBITURATES** (*e.g.,* **phenobarbital**)
- **CARBAMAZEPINE**: May increase or decrease levels.
- **CHARCOAL**
- **HYDANTOINS** (*e.g.,* **phenytoin**)
- **ISONIAZID**: May increase or decrease levels.
- **KETOCONAZOLE**
- **LOOP DIURETICS** (*e.g.,* **furosemide**): May increase or decrease levels.
- **RIFAMPIN**
- **SYMPATHOMIMETICS** (*e.g.,* **beta-agonists**)

The following drugs can <u>increase</u> theophylline levels:
- **ALLOPURINOL**
- **BETA-BLOCKERS** (**non-selective such as propranolol**): May also antagonize theophylline's effects.
- **CALCIUM CHANNEL BLOCKERS** (*e.g.,* **diltiazem, verapamil**)
- **CIMETIDINE**
- **CORTICOSTEROIDS**
- **FLUOROQUINOLONES** (*e.g.,* **enrofloxacin, ciprofloxacin**): Consider reducing the dose of theophylline by 30%. Monitor for toxicity/efficacy. Marbofloxacin reduces clearance of theophylline in dogs, but not with clinical significance. In animals with renal impairment, marbofloxacin may interfere with theophylline metabolism in a clinically relevant manner.
- **MACROLIDES** (*e.g.,* **erythromycin; clindamycin, lincomycin**)
- **THIABENDAZOLE**
- **THYROID HORMONES** (in hypothyroid patients)

Theophylline may <u>decrease</u> the effects of following drugs:
- **BENZODIAZEPINES**
- **LITHIUM**
- **PANCURONIUM**
- **PROPOFOL**
- **EPHEDRINE, ISOPROTERENOL**: Toxic synergism (arrhythmias) can occur if theophylline is used concurrently with sympathomimetics (especially ephedrine) or possibly isoproterenol.
- **KETAMINE**: Theophylline with ketamine can cause an increased incidence of seizures.

Laboratory Considerations
- Theophylline can cause falsely elevated values of serum **uric acid** if measured by the Bittner or colorimetric methods. Values are not affected if using the uricase method.
- Immunoassays are specific for theophylline. If using a spectrophotometric method of assay, theophylline serum levels can be falsely elevated by **furosemide, phenylbutazone, probenecid, theobromine, caffeine, sulfathiazole, chocolate, or acetaminophen. Cefazolin** may interfere with HPLC assays. The Schack and Wexler method of determining theophylline concentrations may be interfered with by large doses of **thiamine**.

Doses
Note: Theophyllines have a relatively low therapeutic index; determine dosages carefully. Extended-release oral dosage forms are generally used, but bioavailability of currently marketed human products can be variable in veterinary species; attentive monitoring for adverse effects and efficacy are recommended. Contact a pharmacist for the current availability of products. Because of theophylline's pharmacokinetic characteristics, consider dosing using lean body weight in very obese patients. Dosage conversions between aminophylline and theophylline can be performed using the information found in the Chemistry section below.

- **DOGS:**
  As a bronchodilator (extra-label): Extended-release products are used, but pharmacokinetic data for currently marketed products was not located. Commonly, 10 mg/kg PO q12h initially is recommended; titrate dosage to balance efficacy and tolerability.
  For adjunctive treatment of heart failure (extra-label): Using a sustained-release product: 20 mg/kg PO once daily. While there is no data on bronchodilators in heart failure, the authors find them (theophylline or terbutaline) useful in patients with intractable cough, particularly when respiratory (airway collapse) disease complicates heart failure. Caution should be used as these drugs may produce tachycardia and predispose to arrhythmia (Atkins *et al.* 2012). **Note:** Consider using a 24-hour extended-release product for this dosage recommendation.

- **CATS:**
  As a bronchodilator (extra-label): Using a sustained-release (human) dosage form: 15 – 25 mg/kg (practically one 100 mg extended-release tablet/capsule) PO once daily in the evening has been suggested. Some cats may only require dosing every other day. **Note:** Consider using a 24-hour extended-release product for this dosage recommendation.

Monitoring
- Therapeutic efficacy and clinical signs of toxicity.
- Serum levels at steady state. The therapeutic serum levels of theophylline in humans are generally described to be between 10 – 20 mcg/mL. Dogs likely can tolerate higher peak levels. In small animals, one recommendation for monitoring serum levels is to measure trough concentration; level should be at least above 8-10 mcg/mL. If signs of toxicity are noted, monitoring peak levels should be considered. It is reported that sustained-release products peak 4-6 hours after dosing in dogs, and 8 hours post-dose in cats, but variable bioavailability occurs (Trepanier 2013). **Note:** Some recommend not exceeding 15 mcg/mL in horses.

Client Information
- Can give with or without food, but giving with some food may prevent stomach upset or vomiting.
- Do not crush or allow animals to chew extended release products.
- Keep out of reach of children and other pets; overdoses can be serious.

Chemistry/Synonyms
Xanthine derivatives, aminophylline and theophylline are considered to be respiratory smooth muscle relaxants but they also have other pharmacologic actions. Aminophylline differs from theophylline only by the addition of ethylenediamine to its structure and may have different amounts of molecules of water of hydration. 100 mg of aminophylline (hydrous) contains ≈ 79 mg of theophylline (anhydrous); 100 mg of aminophylline (anhydrous) contains ≈ 86 mg theophylline (anhydrous). Conversely, 100 mg of theophylline (anhydrous) is = 116 mg of anhydrous aminophylline and 127 mg of hydrous aminophylline.

Theophylline occurs as bitter-tasting, odorless, white, crystalline powder with a melting point between 270-274°C. It is sparingly soluble in alcohol and only slightly soluble in water at a pH of 7, but solubility increases with increasing pH.

Theophylline may also be known as: anhydrous theophylline, teofillina, or theophyllinum; many trade names are available.

Storage/Stability
Theophylline oral dosage forms should be stored at room temperature in tight containers. Theophylline injection should be stored at controlled room temperature and protected from freezing. Avoid excessive heat.

Compatibility/Compounding Considerations

Theophylline for injection is reportedly **compatible** when mixed with the following drugs: chlorpromazine, fluconazole, furosemide, lidocaine, methylprednisolone sodium succinate, and verapamil.

Theophylline for injection is reportedly **incompatible** (or data conflicts) with the following drugs:, ascorbic acid injection, ceftazidime, ceftriaxone, and phenytoin. Compatibility is dependent upon factors such as pH, concentration, temperature, and diluent used and it is suggested to consult specialized references for more specific information.

Dosage Forms/Regulatory Status

VETERINARY-LABELED PRODUCTS: NONE.

The ARCI (Racing Commissioners International) has designated this drug as a class 3 substance.

HUMAN-LABELED PRODUCTS:

Theophylline Time Released Capsules and Tablets: 100 mg, 125 mg 200 mg, 300 mg, 400 mg, 450 mg, & 600 mg (**Note:** Different products have different claimed release rates which may or may not correspond to actual times in veterinary patients); *Theo-24*®, *Theo-chron*®, generic; (Rx)

Theophylline Elixir: 80 mg/15 mL (26.7 mg/5 mL); *Elixophyllin*®, generic; (Rx)

Theophylline & Dextrose Injection: 200 mg/container in 50 mL (4 mg/mL) & 100 mL (2 mg/mL); 400 mg/container in 100 mL (4 mg/mL), 250 mL (1.6 mg/mL), 500 mL (0.8 mg/mL) & 1000 mL (0.4 mg/mL); 800 mg/container in 250 mL (3.2 mg/mL), 500 mL (1.6 mg/mL) & 1000 mL (0.8 mg/mL); generic; (Rx)

Revisions/References

Monograph revised/updated August 2014.

Atkins, C. E. & J. Haggstrom (2012). Pharmacologic management of myxomatous mitral valve disease in dogs. Journal of veterinary cardiology : the official journal of the European Society of Veterinary Cardiology 14(1).

Kellihan, H. B. & R. L. Stepien (2010). Pulmonary Hypertension in Dogs: Diagnosis and Therapy. Veterinary Clinics of North America-Small Animal Practice 40(4): 623-+.

KuKanich, B. & J. L. Nauss (2012). Pharmacokinetics of the cytochrome P-450 substrates phenytoin, theophylline, and diazepam in healthy Greyhound dogs. J. Vet. Pharmacol. Ther. 35(3): 275-81.

Trepanier, L. A. (2013). Applying Pharmacokinetics to Veterinary Clinical Practice. Veterinary Clinics of North America-Small Animal Practice 43(5): 1013-+.

Thiacetarsamide (no longer available) – See Melarsomine

Thiamine HCl

(thye-a-min)

Nutritional; B Vitamin   Thiamin, Vitamin B1

Prescriber Highlights

▶ A "B" vitamin used for treatment or prevention of thiamine deficiency. Possibly useful for adjunctive treatment of lead poisoning & ethylene glycol toxicity.

▶ Adverse Effects: hypersensitivity/anaphylactic reactions (rarely); tenderness, or muscle soreness after IM injection.

Uses/Indications

Thiamine is indicated in the treatment or prevention of thiamine deficiency states that may be secondary to either a lack of thiamine in the diet or the presence of thiamine destroying compounds in the diet (*e.g.*, bracken fern, raw fish, amprolium, thiaminase-producing bacteria in ruminants). Clinical signs of thiamine deficiency can manifest as gastrointestinal- (anorexia, salivation), neuromuscular/CNS- (ataxia, seizures, loss of reflexes), or cardiac- (brady- or tachyarrhythmias) related effects. Cats are more susceptible to thiamine deficiency than dogs as their daily requirements are 3X higher.

Thiamine may be supplemented in camelids and other species when long-term amprolium is used.

Thiamine has also been used in the adjunctive treatment of lead poisoning and ethylene glycol toxicity (to facilitate the conversion of glyoxylate to nontoxic metabolites).

Pharmacology/Actions

Thiamine combines with adenosine triphosphate (ATP) to form a compound (thiamine diphosphate/thiamine pyrophosphate) that is employed for carbohydrate metabolism, but it does not effect blood glucose concentrations.

Absence of thiamine results in decreased transketolase activity in red blood cells and increased pyruvic acid blood concentrations. Without thiamine triphosphate, pyruvic acid is not converted into acetyl-CoA; diminished NADH results with anaerobic glycolysis producing lactic acid. Lactic acid production is further increased secondary to pyruvic acid conversion; lactic acidosis may occur.

Pharmacokinetics

Thiamine is absorbed from the GI tract and is metabolized by the liver. Elimination is renal, the majority of the drug is eliminated as metabolites.

Contraindications/Precautions/Warnings

Thiamine injection is contraindicated in animals hypersensitive to it or to any component of it.

Adverse Effects

Hypersensitivity reactions have occurred after injecting this agent. Rarely, a vasovagal anaphylactic response (cardiac arrest or severe bradycardia, cardiac arrhythmias, apnea, hypotension, collapse, seizure, or protracted neuromuscular weakness) has been observed in a small number of cats when thiamine hydrochloride was administered subcutaneously. Some tenderness or muscle soreness may result after IM injection.

Reproductive/Nursing Safety

In humans, the FDA categorizes this drug as category *A* for use during pregnancy (*Adequate studies in pregnant women have not demonstrated a risk to the fetus in the first trimester of pregnancy, and there is no evidence of risk in later trimesters.*) If used in doses greater than the RDA, the FDA categorizes this drug as category *C* for use during pregnancy (*Animal studies have shown an adverse effect on the fetus, but there are no adequate studies in humans; or there are no animal reproduction studies and no adequate studies in humans.*)

It is not known whether this drug is excreted in milk, but it should not be of clinical concern.

Overdosage/Acute Toxicity

Very large doses of thiamine in laboratory animals have been associated with neuromuscular or ganglionic blockade but the clinical significance is unknown. Hypotension and respiratory depression may also occur with massive doses. A lethal dose of 350 mg/kg has been reported. Generally, no treatment should be required with most overdoses.

Drug Interactions

The following drug interactions have either been reported or are theoretical in humans or animals receiving thiamine and may be of significance in veterinary patients. Unless otherwise noted, use together is not necessarily contraindicated, but weigh the potential risks and perform additional monitoring when appropriate.

■ **NEUROMUSCULAR BLOCKING AGENTS:** Thiamine may enhance the activity of neuromuscular blocking agents; clinical significance is unknown.

Laboratory Considerations

■ Thiamine may cause false-positive **serum uric acid** results when using the phosphotungstate method of determination or urobilinogen urine spot tests using Ehrlich's reagent.

- The Schack and Wexler method of determining **theophylline concentrations** may be interfered with by large doses of thiamine.

Doses

- **DOGS/CATS:**

  For thiamine deficiency (extra-label): The ideal dose of thiamine is unknown and dosage recommendations vary widely. However thiamine has a relatively large margin for safety. One recommendation for cats is: 50 – 100 mg parenterally for 3-5 days, followed by PO administration for an additional 2-4 weeks (Markovich *et al.* 2013). Until further research determines optimal dosing recommendations, this could also be used in dogs.

  As adjunctive treatment of refeeding syndrome after critical illness (extra-label): 10 – 100 mg/day SC during the refeeding period. (Burns 2013)

- **CATTLE:**

  For thiamine deficiency (polioencephalomalacia) (extra-label): 10 mg/kg IV or IM q6h for 1-3 days, then daily. Prognosis is fair if the animals are still standing with some improvement within 24 hours; if still standing for up to a week, prognosis is good for a complete recovery. (Levy *et al.* 2013)

- **HORSES:**

  For thiamine deficiency (extra-label): 0.5 – 5 mg/kg IV, IM or PO (Robinson 1987); 100 – 1000 mg per horse IM, SC, or IV (depending on formulation) (Phillips 1988).

  For adjunctive treatment of perinatal asphyxia syndrome (hypoxic ischemic encephalopathy) (extra-label): Foals: 1 gram in one liter of fluids IV once a day. (Slovis 2003)

  As part of a parenteral nutrition (PN) formula (extra-label): B-complex vitamins (thiamine 12.5 mg/mL; niacinamide 12.5 mg/mL; pyridoxine 5 mg/mL; d-panthenol 5 mg/mL; riboflavin 2 mg/mL; cyanocobalamin 5 mg/mL) should be supplied at a rate of 1 – 2 mL/45 kg daily, diluted in fluids or PN. Vitamin C should be supplied at a rate of 20 mg/kg/day enterally whenever possible. (Magdesian 2010)

- **SWINE:**

  For thiamine deficiency (extra-label): 5 – 100 mg IM, SC, or IV (depending on formulation). (Phillips 1988)

- **SHEEP & GOATS:**

  For thiamine deficiency (polioencephalomalacia) (extra-label): 10 mg/kg IV initially, then 10 mg/kg q6h IV, IM, or SC for the first day. Dosing intervals may be tapered depending on the response to treatment; regaining appetite is a positive indicator. (Ermilio *et al.* 2011)

- **CAMELIDS (NWC):**

  For prophylaxis when animals with *E. macusaniensis* treated with amprolium for >5 days (extra-label): 10 mg/kg SC q24h after the 5th day of amprolium. From a retrospective study. (Cebra *et al.* 2007)

Monitoring

- Efficacy.

Client Information

- Reason for thiamine deficiency (diet, plants, raw fish, etc.) should be found with changes made to prevent recurrence.

Chemistry/Synonyms

A water-soluble "B" vitamin, thiamine HCl occurs as bitter-tasting, white, small hygroscopic crystals, or crystalline powder that has a characteristic yeast-like odor. Thiamine HCl is freely soluble in water, slightly soluble in alcohol and has pK_as of 4.8 and 9.0. The commercially available injection has a pH of 2.5-4.5.

Thiamine HCl may also be known as: aneurine hydrochloride, thiamin hydrochloride, thiamine chloride, thiamini hydrochloridum, thiaminii chloridum, vitamin B-1; many trade names available.

Storage/Stability

Thiamine HCl for injection should be protected from light and stored at temperatures <40°C and preferably between 15-30°C; avoid freezing.

Thiamine HCl is unstable in alkaline or neutral solutions or with oxidizing or reducing agents. It is most stable at a pH of 2.

Compatibility/Compounding Considerations

Thiamine HCl is reportedly physically **compatible** with all commonly used intravenous replacement fluids.

Do **not** mix thiamine with alkaline drugs or alkalinizing agents (barbiturates, citrates, carbonates, acetates, copper ions) or oxidizing/reducing agents (*e.g.*, sulfites).

Compatibility is dependent upon factors such as pH, concentration, temperature, and diluent used; consult specialized references or a hospital pharmacist for more specific information.

Dosage Forms/Regulatory Status

VETERINARY-LABELED PRODUCTS:

Thiamine HCl for Injection: 200 mg/mL & 500 mg/mL; generic; (Rx). Labeled for use in horses, dogs and cats.

Thiamine HCl Dietary Supplement: 8,200 mg/lb.; *Horse Care Durvit B-1 Crumbles*®; (OTC), Labeled for use in horses.

Thiamine HCl Supplement: 500 mg/oz in 1.5 lb, 4 lb and 20 lb containers; *Thia-Dex*®, *Vitamin B-1 Powder*®; (OTC). Labeled for use in dogs & horses.

There are several B-complex vitamin preparations available that may also have thiamine included.

HUMAN-LABELED PRODUCTS:

Thiamine Tablets: 50 mg, 100 mg & 250 mg; generic; (OTC)

Thiamine Enteric Coated Tablets: 20 mg; *Thiamilate*®; (OTC)

Thiamine HCl Injection: 100 mg/mL in 1 mL in 2 mL *Tubex*, 2 mL multi-dose vials; generic; (Rx)

Revisions/References

Monograph revised/updated August 2014.

Burns, K. (2013). Refeeding Syndrome After Critical Illness. Proceedings: Atlantic Coast Veterinary Conference. accessed via Veterinary Information Network; vin.com

Cebra, C. K., et al. (2007). Eimeria macusaniensis infection in 15 llamas and 34 alpacas. Javma-Journal of the American Veterinary Medical Association 230(1): 94-100.

Ermilio, E. M. & M. C. Smith (2011). Treatment of Emergency Conditions in Sheep and Goats. Veterinary Clinics of North America-Food Animal Practice 27(1): 33-+.

Levy, M. G. & C. Graham (2013). Diseases of the Brain and Brainstem of Feedlot Calves: From Videos to Histopathology. ACVIM. accessed via Veterinary Information Network; vin.com

Magdesian, K. G. (2010). Parenteral nutrition in the mature horse. Equine Veterinary Education 22(7): 364-71.

Markovich, J. E., et al. (2013). Timely Topics in Nutrition Thiamine deficiency in dogs and cats. Javma-Journal of the American Veterinary Medical Association 243(5): 649-56.

Phillips, R. W. (1988). Water-soluble Vitamins. Veterinary Pharmacology and Therapeutics - 6th Ed. N. H. Booth and L. E. McDonald. Ames, Iowa State University Press: 698-702.

Robinson, N. E. (1987). Table of Common Drugs: Approximate Doses. Current Therapy in Equine Medicine, 2. N. E. Robinson. Philadelphia, W.B. Saunders: 761.

Slovis, N. (2003). Perinatal asphyxia syndrome (Hypoxic ischemic encephalopathy). Proceedings: ACVIM Forum. accessed via Veterinary Information Network; vin.com

Thioguanine

(thye-oh-gwah-neen)

Antineoplastic

Prescriber Highlights

▶ Rarely used oral purine analog antineoplastic that may be useful as adjunctive treatment for acute lymphocytic or granulocytic leukemia in dogs or cats.

▶ Contraindications: Hypersensitivity to thioguanine. Caution: Hepatic dysfunction, bone marrow depression, infection, renal function impairment (adjust dosage), or history of urate urinary stones.

▶ Potentially mutagenic & teratogenic; use milk replacer if nursing.

▶ Adverse Effects: GI effects, bone marrow suppression, hepatotoxicity, pancreatitis, GI (including oral) ulceration, & dermatologic reactions.

▶ Cats may be more susceptible than dogs to adverse effects.

▶ Low therapeutic index; monitoring mandatory.

Uses/Indications

Thioguanine may be useful as adjunctive therapy for acute lymphocytic or granulocytic leukemia in dogs or cats. It is not commonly used in veterinary medicine.

Pharmacology/Actions

Intracellularly, thioguanine is converted to ribonucleotides that cause the synthesis and utilization of purine nucleotides to be blocked. The drug's cytotoxic effects are believed to occur when these substituted nucleotides are inserted into RNA and DNA. Thioguanine has limited immunosuppressive activity. Extensive cross-resistance usually occurs between thioguanine and mercaptopurine.

Pharmacokinetics

Thioguanine is administered orally, but absorption is variable. In humans, only ≈ 30% of a dose is absorbed. Thioguanine is distributed into the DNA and RNA of bone marrow, but several doses may be necessary for this to occur. It does not apparently enter the CNS, but does cross the placenta. It is unknown whether it enters maternal milk.

Thioguanine is rapidly metabolized primarily in the liver to a methylate derivative that is less active (and toxic) than the parent compound. This and other metabolites are eliminated in the urine.

Contraindications/Precautions/Warnings

Thioguanine is contraindicated in patients hypersensitive to it. The drug should be used cautiously (risk versus benefit) in patients with hepatic dysfunction, bone marrow depression, infection, renal function impairment (adjust dosage), or with a history of urate urinary stones. Thioguanine has a very low therapeutic index and should only be used by clinicians with experience in the use of cytotoxic agents and able to monitor therapy appropriately.

Adverse Effects

At usual doses, GI effects (nausea, anorexia, vomiting, diarrhea) may occur in small animals. However, bone marrow suppression, hepatotoxicity, pancreatitis, GI (including oral) ulceration, and dermatologic reactions are potentially possible. Cats may be particularly susceptible to the hematologic effects of thioguanine.

Reproductive/Nursing Safety

Thioguanine is potentially mutagenic and teratogenic and not recommended for use during pregnancy. In humans, the FDA categorizes this drug as category *D* for use during pregnancy (*There is evidence of human fetal risk, but the potential benefits from the use of the drug in pregnant women may be acceptable despite its potential risks.*)

Although it is unknown whether thioguanine enters milk, use of milk replacer is recommended for nursing bitches or queens.

Overdosage/Acute Toxicity

Toxicity may be acute (GI effects) or delayed (bone marrow depression, hepatotoxicity, gastroenteritis). It is suggested to use standard protocols to empty the GI tract if ingestion was recent and treat supportively.

Drug Interactions

The following drug interactions have either been reported or are theoretical in humans or animals receiving thioguanine and may be of significance in veterinary patients. Unless otherwise noted, use together is not necessarily contraindicated, but weigh the potential risks and perform additional monitoring when appropriate.

- **HEPATOTOXIC DRUGS** (*e.g.,* **halothane, ketoconazole, valproic acid, phenobarbital, primidone,** etc.): Thioguanine should be used cautiously with other drugs that can cause hepatotoxicity.

- **IMMUNOSUPPRESSIVE DRUGS** (*e.g.,* **azathioprine, cyclophosphamide, corticosteroids**): Use with other immunosuppressant drugs may increase the risk of infection.

- **MYELOSUPPRESSIVE DRUGS** (*e.g.,* **chloramphenicol, flucytosine, amphotericin B, or colchicine**): Use extreme caution when using concurrently with other drugs that are also myelosuppressive, including many of the other antineoplastics and other bone marrow depressant drugs; bone marrow depression may be additive.

- **VACCINES, LIVE:** Live virus vaccines should be used with caution during therapy, if at all.

Laboratory Considerations

- Thioguanine may increase serum **uric acid** levels in some patients.

Doses

- **DOGS:**

  Note: Because of the potential toxicity of this drug to patients, veterinary personnel and clients, and since chemotherapy indications, treatment protocols, monitoring and safety guidelines often change, the following dosages should be used only as a general guide. Consultation with a veterinary oncologist and referral to current veterinary oncology references [*e.g.,* (Withrow *et al.* 2012); (Dobson *et al.* 2011); (Henry *et al.* 2009); (North *et al.* 2009); (Argyle *et al.* 2008)] are strongly recommended.

  As part of protocols for treatment of acute myelogenous leukemias (extra-label): <u>Protocol 1</u>: Cytarabine 100 mg/m² SC daily for 2-6 days; Thioguanine 50 mg/m² PO q24-48h. <u>Protocol 2</u>: Cytarabine 100 mg/m² SC daily for 2-6 days; Thioguanine 50 mg/m² PO q24-48h; Doxorubicin 10 mg/m2 IV once a week. (Couto 2003)

- **CATS:**

  For acute lymphocytic and granulocytic leukemia (extra-label): 25 mg/m² PO once daily (q24 hours) for 1-5 days, then every 30 days thereafter as necessary. (Jacobs *et al.* 1992)

Monitoring

- Hemograms (including platelets) should be monitored closely; initially every 1-2 weeks and every 1-2 months once on maintenance therapy. It is recommended by some clinicians that if the WBC count drops to between 5,000-7,000 cells/mm³ the dose be reduced by 25%. If WBC count drops below 5,000 cells/mm³ treatment should be discontinued until leukopenia resolves.

- Liver function tests; serum amylase, if indicated.
- Efficacy.

Client Information

- Wear gloves when handling this medication and give it with food.
- Thioguanine is a chemotherapy (cancer) drug. The drug and its byproducts can be hazardous to other animals and people that come in contact with it. On the day your animal gets the drug and then for a few days afterward, all bodily waste (urine, feces, litter), blood, or vomit should only be handled while wearing disposable gloves. Seal the waste in a plastic bag and then place both the bag and gloves in with the regular trash.
- Most common side effect is GI toxicity (*e.g.*, vomiting, reduced appetite, diarrhea, etc.), but other serious side effects are possible.
- Contact veterinarian if animal exhibits clinical signs of abnormal bleeding, bruising, anorexia, vomiting, jaundice, or infection.

Chemistry/Synonyms

A purine analog antineoplastic agent, thioguanine occurs as a pale yellow, odorless or practically odorless, crystalline powder. It is insoluble in water or alcohol.

Thioguanine may also be known as: NSC-752, 6- thioguanine, TG, 6-TG, 2-Amino-6-mercaptopurine, WR-1141, *Lanvis*®, *Tabloid*®, or *Tioguanina*®.

Storage/Stability

Store tablets in tight containers at room temperature.

Compatibility/Compounding Considerations

No specific information noted.

Dosage Forms/Regulatory Status

VETERINARY-LABELED PRODUCTS: NONE.

HUMAN-LABELED PRODUCTS:

Thioguanine Tablets: 40 mg; *Tabloid*®; (Rx)

Revisions/References

Monograph revised/updated August 2014.

Argyle, D., et al. (2008). *Decision Making in Small Animal Oncology*, Wiley-Blackwell.

Couto, C. (2003). Oncology. *Small Animal Internal Medicine, 3rd Ed.* R. Nelson and C. Couto. St Louis, Mosby: 1093-155.

Dobson, J. & D. Lascelles (2011). *BSAVA Manual of Canine and Feline Oncology*, BSAVA.

Henry, C. & M. Higginbotham (2009). *Cancer Management in Small Animal Practice*, Saunders.

Jacobs, R., et al. (1992). Canine and Feline Reference Values. *Current Veterinary Therapy XI: Small Animal Practice*. R. Kirk and J. Bonagura. Philadelphia, W.B. Saunders Company: 1250-77.

North, S. & T. Banks (2009). *Small Animal Oncology: An Introduction*, Saunders.

Withrow, S., et al. (2012). Withrow and MacEwen's Small Animal Clinical Oncology, 5th Ed., Saunders.

Thiopental Sodium

(thye-oh-pen-tal)   Pentothal®

Ultra-Short Acting Thiobarbiturate

Prescriber Highlights

▶ Ultra-short acting thiobarbiturate used for anesthesia induction or anesthesia for very short procedures. Not available in USA or Canada. C-III controlled substance.

▶ **Absolute contraindications:** absence of suitable veins for IV administration, history of hypersensitivity reactions to barbiturates, status asthmaticus. **Relative contraindications:** severe cardiovascular disease or preexisting ventricular arrhythmias, shock, increased intracranial pressure, myasthenia gravis, asthma, & conditions where hypnotic effects may be prolonged (*e.g.*, severe hepatic disease, myxedema, severe anemia, excessive premedication, etc.). **Greyhounds (& other sight hounds)** metabolize thiobarbiturates much more slowly than other breeds; consider using methohexital instead. **Horses:** preexisting leukopenia; thiopental alone may cause excessive ataxia & excitement.

▶ Avoid: Extravasation, intra-carotid or intra-arterial injections, & use of concentrations of <2% in sterile water. Too rapid IV administration can cause significant vascular dilatation & hypoglycemia.

▶ Adverse Effects: **Dogs:** Ventricular bigeminy **Cats:** Apnea after injection, mild arterial hypotension. **Horses:** Excitement & severe ataxia (if used alone); transient leukopenias, hyperglycemia, apnea, moderate tachycardia, mild respiratory acidosis.

▶ Severe CNS toxicity & tissue damage has occurred in horses receiving intra-carotid injections of thiobarbiturates.

Uses/Indications

Because of its rapid action and short duration, in young, healthy animals, thiopental has been used as an induction agent (rapid IV bolus) for general anesthesia with other anesthetics or as the sole anesthetic agent for very short procedures. In sick or debilitated animals, thiopental may be used in a more cautious manner (IV, slowly to effect). Thiopental is no longer marketed in the USA or Canada.

Pharmacology/Actions

Because of their high lipid solubility, thiobarbiturates rapidly enter the CNS and produce profound hypnosis and anesthesia. They are also known as ultrashort-acting barbiturates. See the monograph: Barbiturates, Pharmacology of, for additional information.

Pharmacokinetics

Following IV injection of therapeutic doses, hypnosis and anesthesia occur within 1 minute and usually within 15-30 seconds. The drug rapidly enters the CNS and then redistributes to muscle and adipose tissue in the body. The short duration of action (10-30 minutes) after intravenous dosing of thiopental is due less to rapid metabolism than to this redistribution out of the CNS and into muscle and fat stores. Greyhounds and other sight hounds may exhibit longer recovery times than other breeds. This may be due to these breeds low body fat levels or differences in the metabolic handling of the thiobarbiturates. Although anesthesia is short, recovery periods may require several hours.

Thiopental is metabolized by the hepatic microsomal system and several metabolites have been isolated. The elimination half-life in dogs has been reported as being ≈ 7 hours and in sheep, 3-4 hours. Very little of the drug is excreted unchanged in the urine (0.3% in humans), so dosage adjustments are not necessary in patients with chronic renal failure.

Contraindications/Precautions/Warnings

The following are considered **absolute contraindications** to the use of thiopental: absence of suitable veins for IV administration, history of hypersensitivity reactions to the barbiturates, and status asthmaticus. **Relative contraindications** include: severe cardiovascular disease or preexisting ventricular arrhythmias, shock, increased intracranial pressure, myasthenia gravis, asthma, and conditions where hypnotic effects may be prolonged (*e.g.*, severe hepatic disease, myxedema, severe anemia, excessive premedication, etc.). These relative contraindications do not preclude the use of thiopental, but dosage adjustments must be considered and the drug must be given slowly and cautiously.

Patients with renal dysfunction or acidemia may show increased sensitivity to thiopental.

Because greyhounds (and other sight hounds) metabolize thiobarbiturates much more slowly than methohexital, many clinicians recommend using methohexital instead. In horses, thiopental should not be used if the patient has preexisting leukopenia. Some clinicians feel that thiopental should not be used alone in the horse as it may cause excessive ataxia and excitement.

Concentrations of <2% in sterile water should not be used as they may cause hemolysis. Extravasation and intra-arterial injections should be avoided because of the high alkalinity of the solution. Severe CNS toxicity and tissue damage has occurred in horses receiving intra-carotid injections of thiobarbiturates.

Adverse Effects

In dogs, thiopental has an arrhythmogenic incidence of ≈ 40%. Ventricular bigeminy is the most common arrhythmia seen; it is usually transient and generally responds to additional oxygen. Administration of catecholamines may augment the arrhythmogenic effects of the thiobarbiturates, while lidocaine may inhibit it. Cardiac output may also be reduced, but is probably only clinically significant in patients experiencing heart failure. Dose-related apnea and hypotension may be noted.

Cats are susceptible to developing apnea after injection and may develop a mild arterial hypotension.

Horses can exhibit clinical signs of excitement and severe ataxia during the recovery period if the drug is used alone. Horses can develop transient leukopenias and hyperglycemia after administration. A period of apnea and moderate tachycardia and a mild respiratory acidosis may also develop after dosing.

Too rapid IV administration can cause significant vascular dilatation and hypoglycemia. Repeated administration of thiopental is not advised as recovery times can become significantly prolonged. Parasympathetic side effects (*e.g.*, salivation, bradycardia) can be managed with the use of anticholinergic agents (atropine, glycopyrrolate).

Prolonged recoveries may occur when repeated dosages of thiopental are administered.

Thiopental's high pH (10-11) can cause significant tissue irritation and necrosis if administered perivascularly; administration through an IV catheter is advised.

Reproductive/Nursing Safety

Thiopental readily crosses the placental barrier and should be used with caution during pregnancy. In humans, the FDA categorizes this drug as category **C** for use during pregnancy (*Animal studies have shown an adverse effect on the fetus, but there are no adequate studies in humans; or there are no animal reproduction studies and no adequate studies in humans.*) In a separate system evaluating the safety of drugs in canine and feline pregnancy (Papich 1989), this drug is categorized as in class: **C** (*These drugs may have potential risks. Studies in people or laboratory animals have uncovered risks,*

and these drugs should be used cautiously as a last resort when the benefit of therapy clearly outweighs the risks.)

Small amounts of thiopental may appear in milk following administration of large doses, but is unlikely to be of clinical significance in nursing animals.

Overdosage/Acute Toxicity

Treatment of thiobarbiturate overdosage consists of supporting respirations (O_2, mechanical ventilation) and giving cardiovascular support (do not use catecholamines, *e.g.*, epinephrine, etc.).

Drug Interactions

A fatal interaction has been reported in a dog receiving the proprietary product, *Diathal®* (no longer marketed; contained procaine penicillin G, dihydrostreptomycin sulfate, diphemanil methylsulfate, and chlorpheniramine) and the related compound thiamylal.

The following drug interactions have either been reported or are theoretical in humans or animals receiving thiopental and may be of significance in veterinary patients. Unless otherwise noted, use together is not necessarily contraindicated, but weigh the potential risks and perform additional monitoring when appropriate.

- **CLONIDINE**: IV clonidine prior to induction may reduce thiopental dosage requirements by up to 37%.
- **CNS DEPRESSANTS, OTHER**: May enhance respiratory and CNS depressant effects.
- **DIAZOXIDE**: Potential for hypotension.
- **EPINEPHRINE, NOREPINEPHRINE**: The ventricular fibrillatory effects of epinephrine and norepinephrine may be potentiated when used with thiobarbiturates and halothane.
- **METOCLOPRAMIDE**: Given prior to induction may reduce thiopental dosage requirements.
- **MIDAZOLAM**: May potentiate hypnotic effects.
- **OPIATES**: Given prior to induction may reduce thiopental dosage requirements.
- **PHENOTHIAZINES**: May potentiate thiopental effects; hypotension possible.
- **PROBENECID**: May displace thiopental from plasma proteins.
- **SULFONAMIDES**: Thiopental and sulfas may displace one another from plasma proteins.

Doses

Note: Atropine sulfate (or glycopyrrolate) is often administered prior to thiobarbiturate anesthesia to prevent parasympathetic side effects; however, some clinicians question whether routine-administration of anticholinergic agents is necessary. Thiobarbiturates are administered strictly to effect; doses are guidelines only.

- **DOGS/CATS:**

    Labeled dose (No longer marketed in USA): 13.2 – 26.4 mg/kg IV depending on duration of anesthesia required. (Package insert; *Pentothal®*)

    Extra-label dose: Usually dosed at 12 – 15 mg/kg, with 1/3 of the drug administered rapidly and any additional amount administered to effect. Repeated doses will accumulate resulting in prolonged recoveries; residual effect may last several hours. (Hellyer 2005)

- **RABBITS, RODENTS, SMALL MAMMALS:**

    For chemical restraint (extra-label): **Mice:** 50 mg/kg IP; **Rats:** 40 mg/kg IP; **Hamsters/Gerbils:** 30 – 40 mg/kg IP; **Guinea pigs:** 15 – 30 mg/kg IV; **Rabbits:** 15 – 30 mg/kg IV. (Burke 1999)

- **CATTLE:**

    Labeled dose (No longer marketed in USA): 8.14 – 15.4 mg/kg IV; for unweaned calves from which food has been withheld for 6-12 hours: no more than 6.6 mg/kg IV for deep surgical anesthesia. (*Pentothal®* package insert)

- **HORSES:** (NOTE: ARCI UCGFS CLASS 2 DRUG)
  Labeled dose (No longer marketed in USA): With preanesthetic tranquilization: 6 – 12 mg/kg IV (an average of 8.25 mg/kg is recommended). Without preanesthetic tranquilization: 8.8 – 15.4 mg/kg IV (an average horse: 9.9 – 11 mg/kg IV). (Package insert; *Pentothal®*)

- **SWINE:**
  Labeled dose (No longer marketed in USA): 5.5 – 11 mg/kg IV. (Package insert; *Pentothal®*)

  Extra-label dose: For swine weighing 5-50 kg: 10 – 11 mg/kg IV. (Booth 1988)

- **SHEEP:**
  Labeled dose (No longer marketed in USA): 9.9 – 15 mg/kg IV depending on depth of anesthesia required. (Package insert; *Pentothal®*)

Monitoring

- Level of hypnosis/anesthesia.
- Respiratory status; cardiac status (rate/rhythm/blood pressure).

Client Information

This drug should only be used by professionals familiar with its effects in a setting where adequate respiratory support can be performed.

Chemistry/Synonyms

A thiobarbiturate, thiopental occurs as a bitter tasting, white to off-white, crystalline powder or a yellow-white hygroscopic powder. It is soluble in water (1 gram in 1.5 mL) and alcohol. Thiopental has a pK_a of 7.6 and is a weak organic acid. Thiopental solutions are very alkaline (pH>10).

Thiopental sodium may also be known as: thiopentone sodium, natrium isopentylaethylthiobarbituricum, penthiobarbital sodique, thiomebumalnatrium cum natrii carbonate, thiopentalum natricum, thiopentobarbitalum solubile, tiopentol sodico, *Anesthal®*, *Bensulf®*, *Farmotal®*, *Hipnopento®*, *Inductal®*, *Intraval®*, *Nesdonal®*, *Pensodital®*, *Pentothal®*, *Sandothal®*, *Sodipental®*, *Thionembutal®*, *Thiopentax®*, *Tiobarbital®*, or *Trapanal®*.

Storage/Stability

When stored in the dry form, thiopental sodium is stable indefinitely. Thiopental should be diluted with only sterile water for injection, sodium chloride injection, or D5W. Concentrations of <2% in sterile water should not be used as they may cause hemolysis. After reconstitution, solutions are stable for 3 days at room temperature and 7 days if refrigerated, however, as no preservative is present, it is recommended it be used within 24 hours after reconstitution. After 48 hours, the solution has been reported to attack the glass bottle in which it is stored. Thiopental may also adsorb to plastic IV tubing and bags. Do not administer any solution that has a visible precipitate.

Compatibility/Compounding Considerations

Preparation of Solution for Administration: Use only sterile water for injection, normal saline, or D5W to dilute. A 5 gram vial diluted with 100 mL will yield a 5% solution and diluted with 200 mL will yield a 2.5% solution. Discard reconstituted solutions after 24 hours

The following agents have been reported to be physically **compatible** when mixed with thiopental: aminophylline, chloramphenicol sodium succinate, hyaluronidase, hydrocortisone sodium succinate, neostigmine methylsulfate, oxytocin, pentobarbital sodium, phenobarbital sodium, potassium chloride, propofol (1:1 mixture), scopolamine HBr, sodium iodide, and tubocurarine chloride (recommendations **conflict** with regard to tubocurarine; some clinicians recommend not mixing with thiopental).

The following agents have been reported to be physically **incompatible** when mixed with thiopental: Ringer's injection, Ringer's in-

jection lactate, amikacin sulfate, atropine sulfate, chlorpromazine, codeine phosphate, dimenhydrinate, diphenhydramine, ephedrine sulfate, glycopyrrolate, hydromorphone, insulin (regular), meperidine, morphine sulfate, norepinephrine bitartrate, penicillin G potassium, prochlorperazine edisylate, promazine HCl, promethazine HCl, succinylcholine chloride, and tetracycline HCl. Compatibility is dependent upon factors such as pH, concentration, temperature, and diluent used; consult specialized references or a hospital pharmacist for more specific information.

Dosage Forms/Regulatory Status

VETERINARY-LABELED PRODUCTS:
None presently marketed in USA.

The ARCI (Racing Commissioners International) has designated this drug as a class 2 substance. See the appendix for more information.

HUMAN-LABELED PRODUCTS:
At the time of writing (June 2014), thiopental is not available for the US market.

Revisions/References

Monograph revised/updated August 2014.

Booth, N. H. (1988). Drugs Acting on the Central Nervous System. *Veterinary Pharmacology and Therapeutics - 6th Ed.* N. H. Booth and L. E. McDonald. Ames, Iowa State University Press: 153-408.

Burke, T. (1999). Husbandry and Medicine of Rodents and Lagomorphs. Proceedings: Central Veterinary Conference, Kansas City. accessed via Veterinary Information Network; vin.com

Hellyer, P. (2005). Anesthetic induction drugs. Proceedings: Western Vet Conf. accessed via Veterinary Information Network; vin.com

Papich, M. (1989). Effects of drugs on pregnancy. *Current Veterinary Therapy X: Small Animal Practice.* R. Kirk. Philadelphia, Saunders: 1291-9.

Thiotepa

(thye-oh-**tep**-ah)

Antineoplastic

Prescriber Highlights

▶ Rarely used antineoplastic for carcinomas (systemic administration), intracavitary for neoplastic effusions, & intravesical for transitional carcinomas.

▶ Contraindications: Hypersensitivity to thiotepa; Caution: Hepatic dysfunction, bone marrow depression, infection, tumor cell infiltration of bone marrow, renal dysfunction, or history of urate urinary stones.

▶ Adverse Effects: Leukopenia most likely adverse effect; other hematopoietic toxicity (thrombocytopenia, anemia, pancytopenia), GI toxicity possible. Intracavitary or intravesical instillation can also cause hematologic toxicity.

▶ Potentially teratogenic; use milk replacer if patient nursing.

▶ Monitor diligently.

Uses/Indications

Thiotepa is rarely used in veterinary medicine. Veterinary indications for thiotepa include: systemic use for adjunctive therapy against carcinomas, and intracavitary use for neoplastic effusions. In dogs with transitional cell bladder carcinoma, intravesical instillation of thiotepa had significantly less efficacy (mean survival time = 57 days) when compared to a systemic doxorubicin/cyclophosphamide protocol (mean survival time = 259 days).

Pharmacology/Actions

Thiotepa is an alkylating agent, thereby interfering with DNA replication and RNA transcription. It is cell cycle non-specific. Thiotepa has some immunosuppressive activity. When given via the intracavitary route, thiotepa is thought to control malignant effusions by a direct antineoplastic effect.

Pharmacokinetics

Thiotepa is poorly absorbed from the GI tract. Systemic absorption is variable from the pleural cavity, bladder, and after IM injection. Some studies in humans have shown that absorption from bladder mucosa ranges from 10-100% of an administered dose. Distribution characteristics are not well described; it is unknown if the drug enters maternal milk. Thiotepa is extensively metabolized and then excreted in the urine.

Contraindications/Precautions/Warnings

Thiotepa is contraindicated in patients hypersensitive to it. The drug should be used cautiously (weigh risk versus benefit) in patients with hepatic dysfunction, bone marrow depression, infection, tumor cell infiltration of bone marrow, renal function impairment (adjust dosage) or with a history of urate urinary stones. Thiotepa has a very low therapeutic index and should only be used by clinicians with experience in the use of cytotoxic agents and able to monitor therapy appropriately.

Adverse Effects

When used systemically, leukopenia is the most likely adverse effect seen in small animals. Other hematopoietic toxicity (thrombocytopenia, anemia, pancytopenia) may be noted. Intracavitary or intravesical instillation of thiotepa may cause hematologic toxicity. GI toxicity (vomiting, diarrhea, stomatitis, intestinal ulceration) may be noted and human patients have reported dizziness and headache as well.

Reproductive/Nursing Safety

Thiotepa is potentially mutagenic and teratogenic and is not recommended for use during pregnancy. In humans, the FDA categorizes this drug as category *D* for use during pregnancy (*There is evidence of human fetal risk, but the potential benefits from the use of the drug in pregnant women may be acceptable despite its potential risks.*)

Although it is unknown whether thiotepa enters milk, use of milk replacer is recommended for nursing bitches or queens.

Overdosage/Acute Toxicity

There is no specific antidote for thiotepa overdose. Supportive therapy, including transfusions of appropriate blood products, may be beneficial for treatment of hematologic toxicity.

Drug Interactions

The following drug interactions have either been reported or are theoretical in humans or animals receiving thiotepa and may be of significance in veterinary patients. Unless otherwise noted, use together is not necessarily contraindicated, but weigh the potential risks and perform additional monitoring when appropriate.

- IMMUNOSUPPRESSIVE DRUGS (*e.g.,* azathioprine, cyclophosphamide, corticosteroids): Use with other immunosuppressant drugs may increase the risk of infection.
- MYELOSUPPRESSIVE DRUGS (*e.g.,* chloramphenicol, flucytosine, amphotericin B, or colchicine): Use extreme caution when using concurrently with other drugs that are also myelosuppressive, including many of the other antineoplastics and other bone marrow depressant drugs; bone marrow depression may be additive.
- VACCINES, LIVE: Live virus vaccines should be used with caution during therapy, if at all.

Laboratory Considerations

- Thiotepa may increase serum **uric acid** levels in some patients.

Doses

- **DOGS:**

Note: Because of the potential toxicity of this drug to patients, veterinary personnel and clients, and since chemotherapy indications, treatment protocols, monitoring and safety guidelines often change,

the following dosages should be used only as a general guide. Consultation with a veterinary oncologist and referral to current veterinary oncology references [*e.g.,* (Withrow *et al.* 2012); (Dobson *et al.* 2011); (Henry *et al.* 2009); (North *et al.* 2009); (Argyle *et al.* 2008)] are strongly recommended.

For intracavitary use neoplastic effusions or systemically for adjunctive therapy of carcinomas (extra-label): 0.2 – 0.5 mg/m² intracavitary; IV. (Jacobs *et al.* 1992)

Monitoring

- Efficacy.
- CBC with platelets.

Client Information

- Thiotepa is a chemotherapy (cancer) drug. The drug and its by-products can be hazardous to other animals and people that come in contact with it. On the day your animal gets the drug and then for a few days afterward, all bodily waste (urine, feces, litter), blood, or vomit should only be handled while wearing disposable gloves. Seal the waste in a plastic bag and then place both the bag and gloves in with the regular trash.
- Contact veterinarian should animal exhibit clinical signs of abnormal bleeding, bruising, anorexia, vomiting, jaundice, or infection.

Chemistry/Synonyms

An ethylene derivative alkylating agent antineoplastic, thiotepa occurs as fine, white crystalline flakes. The drug has a faint odor and is freely soluble in water or alcohol.

Thiotepa may also be known as: NSC-6396, TESPA, thiophosphamide, triethylenethiophosphoramide, TSPA, WR-45312, *Ledertepa*®, *Onco Tiotepa*®, *Tespamin*®, or *Thioplex*®.

Storage/Stability

Store both the powder and the reconstituted solution refrigerated (2-8°C) and protected from light. Do not use solution that is grossly opaque (slightly opaque is OK) or if a precipitate is present. If refrigerated, reconstituted solutions are stable for up to 5 days.

Compatibility/Compounding Considerations

No specific information noted.

Dosage Forms/Regulatory Status

VETERINARY-LABELED PRODUCTS: NONE.

HUMAN-LABELED PRODUCTS:

Thiotepa Lyophilized Powder for Injection: 15 mg in vials; generic; (Rx).

Note: At time of writing (August 2014) thiotepa may not be available in the USA market. However, FDA is allowing temporary importation of *Tepadina*® (thiotepa) from Adienne Srl in Italy.

Revisions/References

Monograph revised/updated August 2014.

Argyle, D., et al. (2008). *Decision Making in Small Animal Oncology*, Wiley-Blackwell.

Dobson, J. & D. Lascelles (2011). *BSAVA Manual of Canine and Feline Oncology*, BSAVA.

Henry, C. & M. Higginbotham (2009). *Cancer Management in Small Animal Practice*, Saunders.

Jacobs, R., et al. (1992). Canine and Feline Reference Values. *Current Veterinary Therapy XI: Small Animal Practice*. R. Kirk and J. Bonagura. Philadelphia, W.B. Saunders Company: 1250-77.

North, S. & T. Banks (2009). *Small Animal Oncology: An Introduction*, Saunders.

Withrow, S., et al. (2012). Withrow and MacEwen's Small Animal Clinical Oncology, 5th Ed., Saunders.

Thyrotropin Alfa (RHTSH)

(thye-roe-troe-pin)   Thyroid Stimulating Hormone, TSH
Hormone

Prescriber Highlights

▶ Hormone used for thyroid stimulating hormone (TSH) test for thyroid function.
▶ Contraindications: Adrenocortical insufficiency, hyperthyroidism, coronary thrombosis, hypersensitivity to bovine thyrotropin. Cannot be used to evaluate thyroid function in patients receiving levothyroxine.
▶ Adverse Effects: Hypersensitivity (especially with repeated injections).
▶ Expense (human product) may be an issue.

Uses/Indications

The labeled indication for the formerly available bovine-source veterinary product *Dermathycin*® was for "the treatment of acanthosis nigrans and for temporary supportive therapy in hypothyroidism in dogs." In actuality however, TSH is used in veterinary medicine principally as a diagnostic agent in the TSH stimulation test to diagnose primary hypothyroidism. It can also be used for the diagnosis of congenital hypothyroidism. Commercially available TSH is supplied as a recombinant human product (rhTSH).

Pharmacology/Actions

Thyrotropin increases iodine uptake by the thyroid gland and increases the production and secretion of thyroid hormones. With prolonged use, hyperplasia of thyroid cells may occur.

Pharmacokinetics

No specific information was located; exogenously administered TSH apparently exerts maximal increases in circulating T4 ≈ 4-8 hours after IM or IV administration.

Contraindications/Precautions/Warnings

A previous veterinary manufacturer (Coopers), listed adrenocortical insufficiency and hyperthyroidism as contraindications to TSH use for treatment purposes in dogs. In humans, TSH is contraindicated in patients with coronary thrombosis, untreated Addison's disease, or hypersensitive to bovine thyrotropin.

Levothyroxine supplementation can cause thyroid atrophy and should be discontinued before thyroid testing with TSH. A washout period of 6-8 weeks after levothyroxine has been discontinued before testing has been proposed. (Campos *et al.* 2012)

Adverse Effects

Because the commercially available product is derived from human sources, hypersensitivity reactions are possible in patients sensitive to human proteins, particularly with repeated use. To date, no reports of anaphylaxis in animals receiving rhTSH have been reported.

Reproductive/Nursing Safety

In humans, the FDA categorizes this drug as category *C* for use during pregnancy (*Animal studies have shown an adverse effect on the fetus, but there are no adequate studies in humans; or there are no animal reproduction studies and no adequate studies in humans.*)

It is not known whether the drug is excreted in milk, but is unlikely to be clinically significant when used for diagnostic purposes.

Overdosage/Acute Toxicity

Chronic administration at high dosages can produce clinical signs of hyperthyroidism. Massive overdoses can cause clinical signs resembling thyroid storm. Refer to the levothyroxine monograph for more information on treatment.

Drug Interactions

No specific drug interactions reported, but see the information regarding levothyroxine (Contraindications section).

Laboratory Considerations

▪ Prior **levothyroxine** supplementation my negate results (see Contraindications section).

Doses

▪ **DOGS:**

For TSH stimulation test (extra-label):

a) From two studies where dogs received either 75 micrograms or 150 micrograms (per dog) IV of the human recombinant product. Blood samples were taken before and 6 hours after rhTSH administration for determination of total serum thyroxine (T4) concentration. The authors concluded: The TSH-stimulation test with rhTSH is a valuable diagnostic tool to assess thyroid function in selected dogs in which a diagnosis of hypothyroidism cannot be based on basal T4 and canine TSH concentrations alone. Using the higher dose of rhTSH resulted in a higher discriminatory power with regard to differentiating between primary hypothyroidism and non-thyroidal disease and the authors recommend the higher dose (150 micrograms) of rhTSH for performing a TSH stimulation test in a diseased animal or an animal on medication, especially if testing cannot be delayed. More well-controlled studies are needed to determine the optimal dosage and possibly also the optimal criteria for test interpretation in suspected hypothyroid dogs. (Boretti *et al.* 2006), (Boretti *et al.* 2009)

b) Using rhTSH : 50 – 100 micrograms (0.05 – 0.1 mg) IV. Measure serum T4 at 0 hours (pre-sample) and 4 hours post. Product may be frozen for at least 8 weeks with no loss of potency (see Storage/Stability). (Scott-Moncrieff 2006)

▪ **CATS:**

For TSH stimulation test (extra-label): 25 micrograms per cat IV. Draw post-TSH level at 6 hours. Can be useful for differentiating feline iatrogenic hypothyroidism from non-thyroidal illness. (Campos *et al.* 2012)

▪ **FERRETS:**

For TSH stimulation test (extra-label): In the study, 100 micrograms per ferret IM. Post-level (T4) drawn at 4 hours. Authors concluded that the results suggested that rhTSH can be used for TSH testing in ferrets when administered IM. Based on the results, a euthyroid ferret should have an increase of ≈ 30% in plasma T4 concentration 4 hours after rhTSH injection.

▪ **SMALL MAMMALS:**

Guinea pigs for TSH stimulation test (extra-label): In the study, 100 micrograms per guinea pig IM. Post-level (T4) drawn at 3-4 hours. Authors concluded that the results suggested that rhTSH can be used for TSH testing in guinea pigs when administered IM. Based on the results, authors suggest that the thyroxine concentration in a euthyroid guinea pig should at least double 3-4 hours after rhTSH injection. (Mayer *et al.* 2013)

▪ **BIRDS:**

For TSH stimulation test: Draw pre-dose baseline sample. Administer 1 Unit/kg IM. Collect sample for T4 6 hours after dose. (Greenacre 2009)

Chemistry/Synonyms

Commercially available thyrotropin (human; rhTSH) is now available only as a lyophilized powder for reconstitution obtained via DNA recombinant technology. Originally obtained from bovine anterior pituitary glands, thyrotropin is a highly purified preparation of thyroid-stimulating hormone (TSH). Thyrotropin is a glycoprotein and has a molecular weight of ≈ 28,000 – 30,000. Thyrotropin is measured in International Units (IU), which is abbreviated as Units in this reference. 7.5 micrograms of thyrotropin are ≈ equivalent to 0.037 Units.

Thyrotropin may also be known as: thyroid-stimulating hormone, thyrotrophic hormone, thyrotropin, TSH, *Ambinon®*, *Thyreostimulin®*, *Thyrogen®*, or *Thytropar®*.

Storage/Stability

Thyrotropin alfa (unreconstituted) should be stored between 2-8°C (36-46°F). If necessary, the reconstituted solution can be stored up to 24 hours at 2-8°C (36-46°F); avoid microbial contamination. However, it is reportedly stable if kept refrigerated (2-8°C) up to 4 weeks and up to 12 weeks if frozen (-20°C). Protect from light.

Compatibility/Compounding Considerations

After reconstitution visually inspect each vial for particulate matter or discoloration before use. Do not use any vial exhibiting particulate matter or discoloration. Do not use after the expiration date on the vial.

Dosage Forms/Regulatory Status

VETERINARY-LABELED PRODUCTS: NONE.

HUMAN-LABELED PRODUCTS:

Recombinant (human) Thyrotropin (Thyroid Stimulating Hormone) Powder for Injection, Lyophilized: 1.1 mg per vial; *Thyrogen®*; (Rx)

Revisions/References

Monograph revised/updated August 2014.

Boretti, F. S., et al. (2006). Evaluation of recombinant human thyroid-stimulating hormone to test thyroid function in dogs suspected of having hypothyroidism. American Journal of Veterinary Research 67(12): 2012-6.

Boretti, F. S., et al. (2009). Comparison of 2 Doses of Recombinant Human Thyrotropin for Thyroid Function Testing in Healthy and Suspected Hypothyroid Dogs. Journal of Veterinary Internal Medicine 23(4): 856-61.

Campos, M., et al. (2012). Recombinant Human Thyrotropin in Veterinary Medicine: Current Use and Future Perspectives. Journal of Veterinary Internal Medicine 26(4): 853-62.

Greenacre, C. (2009). Diagnostic Testing in the Field: The Researcher's Prospective on Thyroid Testing in Psittacine Birds. Proceedings: AAV. accessed via Veterinary Information Network; vin.com

Mayer, J., et al. (2013). Use of recombinant human thyroid-stimulating hormone for evaluation of thyroid function in guinea pigs (Cavia porcellus). Javma-Journal of the American Veterinary Medical Association 242(3): 346-9.

Scott-Moncrieff, J. (2006). Diagnosis and Treatment of Canine Hypothyroidism and Thyroiditis. Proceedings: ACVC. accessed via Veterinary Information Network; vin.com

Thyrotropin-Releasing Hormone

(thye-roe-troe-pin ree-lee-seen hor-mohn)   Protirelin, TRH
Hormone

Prescriber Highlights

▶ Most commonly used for diagnosing pituitary pars media dysfunction (PPID) in horses. Can also be used for some thyroid-related tests.

▶ May cause adverse effects after IV use; in horses: transient muscle trembling, yawning, lip smacking, flehmen and coughing.

▶ In USA, must be compounded.

Uses/Indications

Thyrotropin-releasing hormone (TRH; protirelin) is most commonly used in veterinary medicine as a diagnostic agent (TRH stimulation test) for diagnosing pituitary pars media dysfunction (PPID) in horses. While safe and fast, when measuring cortisol as the marker, false positive results are relatively common. Combining this test with a dexamethasone suppression test can improve diagnostic test sensitivity and specificity, but increases testing times and sampling requirements (McFarlane 2011). Measuring plasma corticotropin (ACTH) instead of cortisol after TRH now appears to offer the highest diagnostic sensitivity compared with other tests

for PPID and may allow for earlier detection (Beech *et al.* 2011).

In dogs, the TRH test can potentially be used to differentiate primary from secondary hypothyroidism. It is not a reliable test to diagnose primary hypothyroidism.

TRH or its analogs may improve function after acute intervertebral disk herniation.

Pharmacology/Actions

Thyrotropin-releasing hormone directly stimulates thyrotropin secretion by the pituitary gland thereby indirectly stimulating synthesis and secretion of thyroid hormones.

In horses, thyrotropin-releasing hormone (TRH) can stimulate the equine pars intermedia and appears to directly stimulate equine melanotropes. In healthy horses plasma alpha-melanocyte-stimulating hormones can be increased more than 400% after TRH. Normal horses will have slight increases in ACTH after TRH administration, subclinical PPID horses have a moderate increase in ACTH, while clinically ill PPID horses have dramatic increases in ACTH after TRH. Response to TRH is greater in autumn months than at other times of the year.

Pharmacokinetics

No specific information for veterinary species was noted. Onset of action after IV administration appears to be within minutes. In humans, buccal administration yielded statistically significant increases in thyrotropin levels above baseline at 30 and 60 minutes, although at 30 minutes both the thyrotrophic effect and adverse effects were less in some subjects. Deamidase, peptidase and imidopeptidase enzymes in the CNS and serum metabolize TRH to active and inactive metabolites. Elimination half-life is ≈ 5 minutes.

Contraindications/Precautions/Warnings

Contraindicated in patients that are hypersensitive to it. Use with caution in patients with seizure disorders as IV administration has rarely caused seizures in humans.

Adverse Effects

In horses, IV administration of TRH can cause transient muscle trembling, yawning, lip-smacking, flehmen and coughing.

In humans, TRH given by rapid IV injection or intranasally can cause nausea, a desire to urinate, flushing, dizziness, and a strange taste. Intranasal administration has rarely caused bronchospasm. Intravenous administration can cause transient increases in pulse rate, and changes in blood pressure; convulsions have rarely occurred.

Reproductive/Nursing Safety

In humans, the FDA categorizes this drug as category *C* for use during pregnancy (*Animal studies have shown an adverse effect on the fetus, but there are no adequate studies in humans; or there are no animal reproduction studies and no adequate studies in humans.*)

It is not known whether TRH is excreted in milk, but is unlikely to be clinically significant when used for diagnostic purposes.

Overdosage/Acute Toxicity

No specific information was located; determine dosages and drug volumes carefully.

Drug Interactions

The following drug interactions have either been reported or are theoretical in humans or animals receiving TRH and may be of significance in veterinary patients. Unless otherwise noted, use together is not necessarily contraindicated, but weigh the potential risks and perform additional monitoring when appropriate.

■ **CYPROHEPTADINE:** May cause decreased thyrotropin response to TRH.

■ **THYROID HORMONES** (*e.g.,* **levothyroxine**): May decrease thyrotropin response to TRH.

Laboratory Considerations
- Contact your laboratory for specific sampling guidelines, shipping requirements, etc.

Doses
- **DOGS:**

  To assess pituitary and thyroid gland function; primarily to differentiate primary from secondary hypothyroidism (extra-label): Collect a pre-TRH blood sample; administer 0.2 mg (200 mcg)/dog IV of TRH; collect a 4-hour post-TRH blood sample. Measure pre- and post-TRH serum T4 concentrations. **Note:** For measurement of thyrotropin (TSH) collect blood samples 30 minutes post-TRH administration. (Koch *et al.* 2011)

- **HORSES:**

  For the diagnosis of pituitary pars intermedia dysfunction (PPID) using the TRH stimulation test (extra-label):

  Using plasma ACTH as the marker:

  Protocol 1: Contact your diagnostic laboratory for specific sample requirements. Collect baseline (usually plasma) sample for ACTH analysis. Inject 1 mg TRH IV. Collect plasma sample at 10 minutes following TRH. A 10-minute post TRH ACTH level of 110 nanograms/L is the current diagnostic cut-off, but may differ depending on the laboratory used and additional research. Adapted from: (Beech *et al.* 2011), (Durham *et al.* 2014).

  Protocol 2: An alternative testing procedure is as above, but 0.5 mg is used for ponies and the post-TRH sample is drawn at 30 minutes. At Auburn Univ. Endocrine Diagnostic Laboratory: ACTH concentrations at T=0, 10 and 30 minutes should all be <35 picograms/mL, with even lower concentrations expected between December and June. **Note:** Can also be used to simultaneously "rule out" hypothyroidism by collecting samples for T3 and T4 at 0, 2, and 4 hours. Normal horse: a doubling of T4 after 4 hours and ≈ tripling of T3 after 2 hours is expected. A normal horse will have a small increase in ACTH concentration after 30 minutes (refer to seasonal reference ranges). PPID horse: T3 and T4 will increase the same as a normal horse, and the ACTH at T=0 will be elevated and at 30 minutes ACTH will be markedly elevated. Hypothyroid horse: No marked increase in T3 or T4. (Resting T3 and T4 concentrations are not very useful). (Stewart 2013)

  Combined dexamethasone suppression/TRH stimulation test using plasma cortisol as the marker: Collect plasma between 8-10 AM. Administer dexamethasone at 40 **micrograms**/kg IM. Three hours later administer 1 mg of TRH IV. Collect plasma 30 minutes after TRH was given and again 24 hours after the dexamethasone dose (21 hours post-TRH). Compared to baseline, a plasma cortisol >1 mcg/dL at 24h post-dexamethasone sample or a ≥66% increase for the 3-hour post TRH sample suggests PPID. **Note:** Some diagnostic laboratories prefer to use serum for measurement of cortisol levels. The effect of season on the combined test has not been assessed but would likely result in similar incidence of false-positive results as each of the component tests do.

Chemistry/Synonyms
TRH (protirelin) is a synthetic tri-peptide with the same sequence of amino acids as the natural hypothalamic neuro-hormone. It occurs as a white or yellowish-white hygroscopic powder that is very soluble in water and freely soluble in methyl alcohol.

Thyrotropin-releasing hormone may also be known as TRH, thyrotrophin-releasing hormone, lopremone, protirelin, thyroliberin, or thyrotropin-releasing factor (TRF).

Storage/Stability
TRH (protirelin) powder should be stored at 2-8°C and protected from light and moisture. If using a compounded preparation, store as instructed.

Compatibility/Compounding Considerations
No specific information noted.

Dosage Forms/Regulatory Status
VETERINARY-LABELED PRODUCTS: NONE.

HUMAN-LABELED PRODUCTS:

There are no commercially available products marketed in the USA at present, but TRH may be available from compounding pharmacies.

Revisions/References
Monograph revised/updated August 2014.

Beech, J., et al. (2011). Comparison of Cortisol and ACTH Responses after Administration of Thyrotropin Releasing Hormone in Normal Horses and Those with Pituitary Pars Intermedia Dysfunction. Journal of Veterinary Internal Medicine 25(6): 1431-8.

Durham, A. E., et al. (2014). Pituitary pars intermedia dysfunction: Diagnosis and treatment. Equine Veterinary Education 26(4): 216-23.

Koch, S., et al. (2011). *Small Animal Dermatology Drug Handbook*, Wiley-Blackwell. Ames.

McFarlane, D. (2011). Equine Pituitary Pars Intermedia Dysfunction. Vet Clin Equine 27: 93-113.

Stewart, A. (2013). Understanding Testing for Equine Endocrinopathies. ACVIM. accessed via Veterinary Information Network; vin.com

Thyroxine Sodium – See Levothyroxine Sodium

Tiamulin

(tye-am-myoo-lin)   Denagard®

Diterpine Pleuromutilin Antibiotic

Prescriber Highlights
- ▶ Antibiotic used primarily in swine.
- ▶ Contraindications: Access to feeds containing polyether ionophores (*e.g.*, monensin, lasalocid, narasin, or salinomycin); swine over 250 pounds.
- ▶ Adverse Effects are unlikely.
- ▶ Variable withdrawal times depending on dosage.

Uses/Indications
Tiamulin is FDA-approved for use in swine to treat pneumonia caused by susceptible strains of *Haemophilus pleuropneumoniae* and swine dysentery caused by *Treponema hyodysenteriae*. As a feed additive, it is used to cause increased weight gain in swine.

Pharmacology/Actions
Tiamulin is a pleuromutilin antibiotic that is usually bacteriostatic, but can be bactericidal in very high concentrations against susceptible organisms. The drug acts by binding to the 50S ribosomal subunit thereby inhibiting bacterial protein synthesis; it has good intracellular penetration.

Tiamulin has good activity against many gram-positive cocci, including most Staphylococci and Streptococci (not group D streptococci). It also has good activity against Mycoplasma and spirochetes. With the exceptions of *Haemophilus* spp., most isolates of *Lawsonia intracellularis*, and some *E. coli* and Klebsiella strains, tiamulin activity is quite poor against gram-negative organisms. Tiamulin does not have apparent efficacy against *Histomonas meleagridis*.

Pharmacokinetics
Tiamulin is well absorbed orally by swine. Approximately 85% of a dose is absorbed and peak levels occur between 2-4 hours after a single oral dose. Tiamulin is apparently well distributed, with highest levels found in the lungs.

Tiamulin is extensively metabolized to over 20 metabolites, some having antibacterial activity. Approximately 30% of these metabolites are excreted in the urine with the remainder excreted in the feces.

Contraindications/Precautions/Warnings

Tiamulin should not be administered to animals having access to feeds containing polyether ionophores (*e.g.*, monensin, lasalocid, narasin, or salinomycin) as adverse reactions may occur. Not for use in swine over 250 pounds.

Reproductive/Nursing Safety

Teratogenicity studies done in rodents demonstrated no teratogenic effects at doses up to 300 mg/kg. The manufacturer has concluded that the drug is not tumorigenic, carcinogenic, teratogenic, or mutagenic.

Adverse Effects

Adverse effects occurring with this drug at usual doses are considered unlikely. Rarely, redness of the skin, primarily over the ham and underline, has been observed. It is recommended to discontinue the medication, provide clean drinking water, and hose down the area or move affected animals to clean pens.

Overdosage/Acute Toxicity

Oral overdoses in pigs may cause transient salivation, vomiting, and CNS depression (calming effect). Discontinue drug and treat symptomatically and supportively if necessary.

Drug Interactions

- **POLYETHER IONOPHORES** (*e.g.*, **monensin, lasalocid, narasin**, or **salinomycin**): Tiamulin should not be administered to animals having access to feeds containing polyether ionophores as adverse reactions may occur.
- **LINCOSAMIDES, MACROLIDES** (*e.g.*, **clindamycin, lincomycin, erythromycin, tylosin**): Although not confirmed with this drug, concomitant use with other antibiotics that bind to the 50S ribosome could lead to decreased efficacy secondary to competition at the site of action.

Doses

- **SWINE:**

  For swine dysentery (labeled dose; FDA approved): 7.7 mg/kg PO daily in drinking water for 5 days. See package directions for dilution instructions. (Package insert; *Denagard® Liquid Concentrate*)

  For swine pneumonia (labeled dose; FDA approved): 23.1 mg/kg PO daily in drinking water for 5 days. See package directions for dilution instructions. (Package insert; *Denagard® Liquid Concentrate*)

  For use as a medicated premix see the label for the product.

Monitoring

- Clinical efficacy.

Client Information

- Prepare fresh medicated water daily.
- Avoid contact with skin or mucous membranes as irritation may occur.

Chemistry/Synonyms

A semisynthetic diterpene-class antibiotic derived from pleuromulin, tiamulin is available commercially for oral use as the hydrogen fumarate salt. It occurs as white to yellow, crystalline powder with a faint but characteristic odor. Approximately 60 mg of the drug are soluble in 1 mL of water.

Tiamulin may also be known as: 81723-hfu, SQ-14055, SQ-22947 (tiamulin fumarate), and *Denagard®*.

Storage/Stability

Protect from moisture; store in a dry place. In unopened packets, the powder is stable up to 5 years. Fresh solutions should be prepared daily when using clinically.

Compatibility/Compounding Considerations

No specific information noted.

Dosage Forms/Regulatory Status

VETERINARY APPROVED PRODUCTS:

Tiamulin Medicated Premix: 10 grams/1 lb in 35 lb bags; *Denagard® 10*; (OTC). FDA-approved for use in swine not weighing over 250 lbs. Slaughter withdrawal period at the 35 grams/ton use is 2 days; at the 200 grams/ton dose it is 7 days.

Tiamulin Solution: 12.3% tiamulin hydrogen fumarate in an aqueous base in 32 oz bottles; *Denagard® Liquid Concentrate, TiaGard®*; (OTC). FDA-approved for use in swine. Slaughter withdrawal: treatment at 3.5 mg/lb = 3 days, at 10.5 mg/lb = 7 days.

Tiamulin Soluble Powder: 45% in 2.28 oz packets (29.1 gram tiamulin per packet); *Denagard® Liquid Concentrate, TiaGard®*; (OTC). FDA-approved for use in swine. Slaughter withdrawal: treatment at 3.5 mg/lb = 3 days, at 10.5 mg/lb = 7 days.

There is also a chlortetracycline/tiamulin premix approved by the FDA.

HUMAN APPROVED PRODUCTS: NONE.

Revisions/References

Monograph revised/updated August 2014.

Ticarcillin Disodium + Clavulanate Potassium

(tye-kar-**sill**-in; klav-yoo-**lan**-ate)   Timentin®

Parenteral Extended Spectrum Penicillin +

Beta-Lactamase Inhibitor

Prescriber Highlights

▶ Parenteral, extended action penicillin with a beta lactamase inhibitor; has increased spectrum of activity when compared with ticarcillin alone.

▶ Used for serious systemic infections & as a compounded otic prep for Pseudomonas otitis.

▶ Limited experience or research in veterinary medicine, but appears quite safe.

▶ Patients with significantly impaired renal function or those receiving very high dosages may be more prone to develop platelet function abnormalities (bleeding) or CNS effects.

Uses/Indications

Ticarcillin/clavulanate is used systemically to treat serious infections such as sepsis or nosocomial pneumonias in dogs, cats and horses. By adding clavulanate, enhanced spectrum of activity against beta-lactamase producing bacteria can be obtained. This drug combination is sometimes used topically (otic) to treat Pseudomonas otitis in dogs.

Pharmacology/Actions

The extended-spectrum penicillins, sometimes called anti-pseudomonal penicillins, include both alpha-carboxypenicillins (carbenicillin and ticarcillin) and acylaminopenicillins (piperacillin). These agents have similar spectrums of activity as the aminopenicillins but with additional activity against several gram-negative organisms of the family Enterobacteriaceae, including many strains of *Pseudomonas aeruginosa*. Like the aminopenicillins, these agents are susceptible to inactivation by beta-lactamases.

By adding clavulanate, ticarcillin's efficacy can be extended against beta-lactamase-producing strains of otherwise resistant *E. coli, Pasteurella* spp., *Staphylococcus* spp., Klebsiella, and Proteus. Clavulanic acid acts by competitively and irreversibly binding to beta-lactamases, including types II, III, IV, and V, and penicillinases produced by Staphylococcus. Type I beta-lactamases that are often associated with *E. coli*, Enterobacter, and Pseudomonas are not generally inhibited by clavulanic acid.

Clavulanic acid has only weak antibacterial activity when used alone and, at present, is only available in fixed-dose combinations with either amoxicillin (oral) or ticarcillin (parenteral). Unlike sulbactam or tazobactam, clavulanic acid (clavulanate) can induce chromosomal beta-lactamases. A review of bacterial isolates cultured from canine and feline infections (Australia) found that ≈ 92% of *E. coli* (urine) and 82-90% of Pseudomonas isolates were susceptible; 12-23% of Pseudomonas isolates obtained from canine ear canal or tympanic bullae were resistant (Bennett *et al.* 2013). Another study (Croatia) found ≈ 90% of *P. aeruginosa* isolates obtained from canine ear canals susceptible to ticarcillin/clavulanate (Mekic *et al.* 2011).

Synergy against *Pseudomonas aeruginosa* can occur when used with an aminoglycoside, but the drugs cannot be physically mixed together (see Drug Interactions).

Pharmacokinetics

Ticarcillin is not appreciably absorbed after oral administration and must be given parenterally to achieve therapeutic serum levels. When given IM to humans, the drug is readily absorbed with peak levels occurring ≈ 30-60 minutes after dosing. The reported bioavailability in the horse after IM administration is ≈ 65%.

After parenteral injection, ticarcillin is distributed into pleural fluid, interstitial fluid, bile, sputum, and bone. Like other penicillins, CSF levels are low in patients with normal meninges (≈ 6% of serum levels), but increased (39% of serum levels) if meninges are inflamed. The volume of distribution is reportedly 0.34 L/kg in dogs and 0.22-0.25 L/kg in the horse. The drug is 45-65% bound to serum proteins (human). Ticarcillin is thought to cross the placenta and found in small quantities in milk. In cattle, mastitic milk levels of ticarcillin are ≈ 2X those found in normal milk, but are too low to treat most causal organisms.

Ticarcillin is eliminated primarily by the kidneys, via both tubular secretion and glomerular filtration. Concurrent probenecid administration can slow elimination and increase blood levels. In humans, ≈ 10-15% of the drug is metabolized by hydrolysis to inactive compounds. The half-life in dogs and cats is reportedly 45-80 minutes; ≈ 54 minutes in the horse. Clearance is 4.3 mL/kg/min in the dog and 2.8-3.2 mL/kg/min in the horse.

There is no evidence to suggest that the addition of clavulanic acid alters ticarcillin pharmacokinetics.

Clavulanic acid has an apparent volume of distribution of 0.32 L/kg in dogs and is distributed (with ticarcillin) into the lungs, pleural fluid and peritoneal fluid. Low concentrations of both drugs are found in the saliva, sputum and CSF (uninflamed meninges). Higher concentrations in the CSF are expected when meninges are inflamed, but it is questionable whether therapeutic levels are attainable. Clavulanic acid is 13% bound to proteins in dog serum.

Clavulanic acid is extensively metabolized in dogs (and rats) primarily to 1-amino-4-hydroxybutan-2-one. It is not known if this compound possesses any beta-lactamase inhibiting activity. Clavulanic acid is also excreted unchanged in the urine via glomerular filtration. In dogs, 34-52% of a dose is excreted in the urine as unchanged drug and metabolites, 25-27% in the feces, and 16-33% into respired air. The elimination half-life for clavulanic acid in dogs is faster than is ticarcillin.

Contraindications/Precautions/Warnings

Do not use this medication in patients with documented hypersensitivity reactions to penicillins or other beta-lactams.

Dosage adjustments should be made in patients with significantly impaired renal function.

Adverse Effects

Although clinical experience with this medication in veterinary patients is limited, it appears to be well tolerated; potentially, hypersensitivity reactions can occur. In humans, high dosages (particularly in patients with renal insufficiency) have caused platelet dysfunction and bleeding, and CNS effects (headache, giddiness, hallucinations, seizures). Intramuscular administration can cause pain, but reconstituting with 1% lidocaine (see Storage/Stability) can alleviate this effect. Local irritation to veins after IV administration is possible and best avoided by using dilute concentrations administered over not less than 30 minutes.

Antibiotic-associated diarrhea or colitis may occur.

Reproductive/Nursing Safety

Penicillins have been shown to cross the placenta and safe use during pregnancy has not been firmly established, but neither have there been any documented teratogenic problems associated with these drugs; however, use only when the potential benefits outweigh the risks. In humans, the FDA categorizes ticarcillin/clavulanate as category *B* for use during pregnancy (*Animal studies have not yet demonstrated risk to the fetus, but there are no adequate studies in pregnant women; or animal studies have shown an adverse effect, but adequate studies in pregnant women have not demonstrated a risk to the fetus in the first trimester of pregnancy, and there is no evidence of risk in later trimesters.*)

Although penicillins can be distributed into milk, it is unlikely that ticarcillin/clavulanate would be of significant clinical concern for nursing veterinary patients.

Overdosage/Acute Toxicity

A single inadvertent overdose is unlikely to cause significant morbidity. In humans, very high dosages of parenteral penicillins such as ticarcillin, especially in patients with renal disease, have induced CNS effects (hallucinations, headaches, seizures) and alterations in platelet function (bleeding).

Drug Interactions

The following drug interactions have either been reported or are theoretical in humans or animals receiving ticarcillin/clavulanate and may be of significance in veterinary patients. Unless otherwise noted, use together is not necessarily contraindicated, but weigh the potential risks and perform additional monitoring when appropriate.

- **AMINOGLYCOSIDES** (*e.g.*, **amikacin, gentamicin, tobramycin**): *In vitro* studies have demonstrated that penicillins can have synergistic or additive activity against certain bacteria when used with aminoglycosides. However, beta-lactam antibiotics can inactivate aminoglycosides *in vitro* and *in vivo* in patients in renal failure or when penicillins are used in massive dosages. Amikacin is considered the most resistant aminoglycoside to this inactivation. A study measuring amikacin in synovial fluid after regional limb perfusion with or without ticarcillin/clavulanate found significantly lower amikacin concentrations when ticarcillin/clavulanate was added (Zantingh *et al.* 2014).
- **PROBENECID**: Can reduce the renal tubular secretion of ticarcillin, thereby maintaining higher systemic levels for a longer period of time; it does not affect the elimination of clavulanate.
- **WARFARIN; HEPARIN**: As ticarcillin has been implicated in rarely causing bleeding, use with caution in patients receiving anticoagulant therapy.

Laboratory Considerations

- **Aminoglycoside serum quantitative analysis**: As penicillins and other beta-lactams can inactivate aminoglycosides *in vitro* (and *in vivo* in patients in renal failure or when penicillins are used in massive dosages), serum concentrations of aminoglycosides may be falsely decreased if the patient is also receiving beta-lactam antibiotics and the serum is stored prior to analysis. It is recommended that if the aminoglycoside assay is delayed, samples be frozen and, if possible, drawn at times when the beta-lactam antibiotic is at a trough.

- **Direct antiglobulin (Coombs') tests:** False-positive results may occur.
- **Urine protein:** May produce false-positive protein results with the sulfosalicylic acid and boiling test, nitric acid test, and acetic acid test. Strips using bromophenol blue reagent (*e.g., Multi-Stix*) do not appear to be affected by high levels of penicillins in the urine.

Doses

Note: Unless otherwise indicated, this drug combination is dosed on the basis of ticarcillin content.

- **DOGS/CATS:**

  For susceptible, serious systemic infections (extra-label): 15 – 25 mg/kg as an IV infusion over 15 minutes, followed by a CRI at 7.5 – 15 mg/kg/hour. (Trepanier 2012)

  For topical (otic) adjunctive treatment of Pseudomonas otitis in dogs (extra-label): Dilute the injection and store as detailed in Compatibility/Compounding Considerations; instill ≈ 0.25 – 0.5 mL into affected ear(s) 2 times a day.

- **HORSES:**

  For susceptible, serious infections in foals (extra-label): 50 mg/kg IV or IM (IM painful) q6h.

  For intrauterine infusion (extra-label): 3 – 6 grams with a minimum of 200 mL of saline. Mares need to be treated frequently (every 4-6 h) in order to maintain drug concentrations above MIC. (LeBlanc 2009)

Monitoring

- Efficacy for the infection treated (WBC, clinical signs, etc.)
- Serum levels and therapeutic drug monitoring are not routinely performed with this drug.

Client Information

- Limited experience in veterinary medicine when used systemically.
- Best suited for inpatient use.

Chemistry/Synonyms

An alpha-carboxypenicillin, ticarcillin disodium occurs as a white to pale yellow, hygroscopic powder or lyophilized cake with pK_as of 2.55 and 3.42. More than 600 mg is soluble in 1 mL of water. Potency of ticarcillin disodium is expressed in terms of ticarcillin and 1 gram of the disodium contains not less than 800 mg of ticarcillin anhydrous. One gram of the commercially available injection contains 5.2-6.5 mEq of sodium.

A beta-lactamase inhibitor, clavulanate potassium occurs as an off-white, crystalline powder that has a pK_a of 2.7 (as the acid) and is very soluble in water and slightly soluble in alcohol at room temperatures. Although available commercially as the potassium salt, potency is expressed in terms of clavulanic acid.

Ticarcillin Disodium may also be known as: BRL-2288, or ticarcillinum natricum. Clavulanate potassium may also be known by the following synonyms: clavulanic acid, BRL-14151K, or kalii clavulanas. International trade names for ticarcillin/clavulanate include *Timentin* and *Claventin*.

Storage/Stability

Unused vials should be stored at room temperature (below 24°C, 75°F).

A darkening of the sterile powder or solution indicates degradation and loss of potency of clavulanate.

When vials are reconstituted to 200 mg/mL for parenteral use, the resulting solution is stable for 6 hours at room temperature and 72 hours when refrigerated. Stability for solutions diluted for IV infusion (10-100 mg/mL):

Diluent	Room Temperature	Refrigerated	Frozen
NS	24 hrs.	7 days	30 days
D5W	24 hrs.	3 days	7 days
LRS	24 hrs.	7 days	30 days

All thawed solutions should be used within 8 hours and not refrozen.

Compatibility/Compounding Considerations

Ticarcillin/clavulanate should **not** be mixed with aminoglycosides (*e.g.,* gentamicin, amikacin) and **may not be compatible** when infused at a Y-site with solutions containing amphotericin B cholesteryl sulfate complex, azithromycin, or vancomycin. Y-site **compatible** drugs include (partial listing): propofol, dexmedetomidine, cefepime, diltiazem, doxorubicin HCl liposomes, etoposide, famotidine, fluconazole, heparin sodium, hetastarch, regular insulin, meperidine, morphine sulfate, and ondansetron.

For IM use, reconstitute vial with 2 mL of sterile water for injection, sodium chloride for injection, or 1% lidocaine (without epinephrine) per gram of ticarcillin. Each mL of the resulting solution will contain ≈ 385 mg/mL (1 gram per 2.6 mL) ticarcillin. For humans, IM injections are recommended to be given into a relatively large muscle and not to administer more than 1 gram (2.6 mL) IM per injection site.

For IV use, initially reconstitute 3.1 gram vials with 13 mL of sodium chloride injection, dextrose 5% or LRS. Resulting solution will contain ≈ 200 mg of ticarcillin per mL. If administered IV at this concentration, give as slowly as possible. Ideally, dilute further to a concentration of 10 – 100 mg (ticarcillin)/mL with a suitable diluent (*e.g.,* NS, LRS, D5W). Concentrations ≤50 mg/mL will cause less vein irritation; the solution should be administered as slowly as possible (over at least 30 minutes).

Otic Preparation Compounding:

An Australian study found that a 3.1 g vial of *Timentin* (for IV use) diluted in sterile water and then further diluted in the artificial tear product *Methopt* for otic use to be stable (determined by MIC/MBC against 4 different *Pseudomonas aeruginosa* isolates) when stored at various temperatures. Stock solutions diluted in 12.9 mL of sterile water and stored in 25 separate aliquots (tubes) at -20°C were stable for at least 12 months. Once an aliquot was thawed and further diluted 1:4 with sterile *Methopt* the solution was stable for 28 days when stored at either 4° or 24°C (Koch *et al.* 2011; Bateman *et al.* 2012). **Note:** *Methopt®* is a viscous, non-antigenic artificial tear product containing hydroxypropyl methylcellulose (hypromellose; 0.5%), and benzalkonium chloride as a preservative. In the USA, *Isopto Plain®* and *Isopto Tears®* appear to be equivalent products.

Another method using only sterile water: Reconstitute 3.1 g vial with 26 mL sterile water to make a 100 mg/mL solution. Draw up 0.5 mL into a 1 mL syringe; cap and freeze. Keep frozen and thaw individual syringe(s) on the day to be used. Instill 0.25 mL (1/2 of the amount) into ear, recap, and store in refrigerator until remainder used 12 hours later. (Cole 2013)

Dosage Forms/Regulatory Status

VETERINARY-LABELED PRODUCTS: NONE.

HUMAN-LABELED PRODUCTS:

Ticarcillin Disodium Powder for Injection (contains 4.75 mEq sodium/g) and Clavulanate Potassium (contains 0.15 mEq potassium/g): 3 grams ticarcillin and 0.1 gram clavulanic acid in 3.1 gram vials; *Timentin®*; (Rx)

Ticarcillin Powder for Injection (contains 18.7 mEq sodium/100 mL) and Clavulanate Potassium (contains 0.5 mEq potassium/100 mL): 3 grams ticarcillin and 0.1 gram clavulanic acid/100 mL; *Timentin®*; (Rx)

Ticarcillin (alone) has now been discontinued.

Revisions/References

Monograph revised/updated August 2014.

Bateman, F. L., et al. (2012). Biological efficacy and stability of diluted ticarcillin-clavulanic acid in the topical treatment of Pseudomonas aeruginosa infections. Veterinary Dermatology 23(2): 97-+.

Bennett, A. B., et al. (2013). In vitro susceptibilities of feline and canine Escherichia coli and Pseudomonas spp. isolates to ticarcillin and ticarcillin-clavulanic acid. Australian Veterinary Journal 91(5): 171-8.

Cole, L. K. (2013). Topical and Systemic Medications for Otitis Externa & Otitis Media. Proceedings: Western Veterinary Conference. accessed via Veterinary Information Network; vin.com

Koch, S., et al. (2011). *Small Animal Dermatology Drug Handbook*, Wiley-Blackwell. Ames.

LeBlanc, M. M. (2009). The current status of antibiotic use in equine reproduction. Equine Veterinary Education 21(3): 156-67.

Mekic, S., et al. (2011). Antimicrobial susceptibility of Pseudomonas aeruginosa isolates from dogs with otitis externa. Veterinary Record 169(5): 125-U46.

Trepanier, L. (2012). Antibiosis in Critical Care. Proceedings: WSAVA/FECAVA/BSAVA World Congress. accessed via Veterinary Information Network; vin.com

Zantingh, A. J., et al. (2014). Accumulation of Amikacin in Synovial Fluid After Regional Limb Perfusion of Amikacin Sulfate Alone and in Combination With Ticarcillin/Clavulanate in Horses. Veterinary Surgery 43(3): 282-8.

Tildipirosin

(til-di-pir-oh-sin)   Zuprevo®

Macrolide Antibiotic

Prescriber Highlights

▶ Injectable macrolide antibiotic used in cattle (see restrictions and withdrawal times) and swine (not approved for use in USA); given one-time SQ in cattle and IM in swine.

▶ Do not use cattle product in swine.

▶ Pain and swelling at injection site most common adverse effect.

Uses/Indications

Tildipirosin is an injectable macrolide antibiotic that is approved by the FDA for the treatment of bovine respiratory disease (BRD) associated with *Mannheimia haemolytica*, *Pasteurella multocida*, and *Histophilus somni* in beef and non-lactating dairy cattle, and for the control of respiratory disease in beef and non-lactating dairy cattle at high risk of developing BRD associated with *Mannheimia haemolytica*, *Pasteurella multocida*, and *Histophilus somni*. The U.K. cattle-product indications are similar (see Dosages). A study in heifers comparing metaphylactic antimicrobial administration of tildipirosin, tulathromycin, or placebo administered 10 days before experimental inoculation with *Mannheimia haemolytica* concluded that tildipirosin treated animals had less pulmonary damage and fewer clinical signs of illness when compared to the other groups (Amrine *et al.* 2014).

In the U.K, tildipirosin is also approved for the treatment of swine respiratory disease (SRD) associated with *Actinobacillus pleuropneumoniae*, *Pasteurella multocida*, *Bordetella bronchiseptica* and *Haemophilus parasuis* sensitive to tildipirosin.

Pharmacology/Actions

Similarly to other macrolides, the antimicrobial activity of tildipirosin is due to its binding to the ribosomal 50S subunit of bacterial cells and inhibiting bacterial protein synthesis. Tildipirosin is generally classified as a time-dependent antibiotic, although it may be concentration-dependent (AUC/MIC ratio) against some isolates of *M. haemolytica* and *P. multocida*.

Significant increases in MIC of *P. multocida* and *M. haemolytica* to tildipirosin can be conveyed by the presence of the *erm*(42) gene (Michael *et al.* 2012).

Pharmacokinetics

In cattle after a single, 4 mg/kg subcutaneous injection, bioavailability was 78%, and peak plasma levels of 0.7-0.8 mcg/mL occurred within 1 hour of dosing. Levels of tildipirosin in lung and bronchial fluid far exceed those in plasma. Lung:plasma ratios range from 28X at 4 hours to 214X at 240 hours. Bronchial fluid:plasma ratios are 5X at 4 hours; up to 72X at 240 hours. Elimination half-life was ≈ 9 days in plasma and 10-11 days in lung and bronchial fluid (Anon 2011; Menge *et al.* 2012).

In pigs, after a 4 mg/kg IM injection, peak plasma levels occurred within 23 minutes. Only ≈ 30% is bound to porcine plasma proteins. Mean terminal half-life was ≈ 4.4 days. Levels in the lung peaked about 1 day after dosing and lung half-life was ≈ 7 days (Anon 2012b; Rose *et al.* 2013).

Contraindications/Precautions/Warnings

Tildipirosin is contraindicated in animals hypersensitive (drug allergy) to it or other macrolide antibiotics. Tildipirosin is **NOT** for use in chickens or turkeys and the 18% product must **NOT** be used in swine. Tildipirosin must **NOT** be given intravenously.

Cross-resistance can occur with other macrolides and use with other macrolides or lincosamides is not advised. Subcutaneous injection in cattle may result in local tissue reactions that can persist beyond the slaughter withdrawal period and may result in trim loss of edible tissue at slaughter.

Care must be taken to avoid accidental injection in humans as toxicology studies in laboratory animals (including dogs) showed cardiovascular effects after IM administration. Do not use automatically powered syringes that do not have an additional protection system. In case of human injection, seek medical advice immediately and show the package insert or label to the physician. Avoid direct contact with skin and eyes. If accidental eye exposure occurs, rinse eyes with clean water. If accidental skin exposure occurs, wash the skin immediately with soap and water. Wash hands after use. Tildipirosin may cause sensitization by skin contact.

Adverse Effects

In cattle, pain and swelling at injection sites are the most commonly reported adverse effect with pain on palpation persisting for one day in most treated cattle. Swelling can last at the injection site for up to 21 days post treatment and tissue lesions have been be noted at 35 days post-injection (Anon 2011, 2012a).

In pigs, swelling at injection site after IM injection can persist up to 3 days, but in were not painful upon palpation. Injection site reactions resolved completely within 21 days of injection (Anon 2012b). Shock-like reactions with fatal outcomes can occur rarely (Anon 2012b).

Reproductive/Nursing Safety

The safety of the veterinary medicinal product has not been established during pregnancy and lactation, however no evidence for any selective developmental or reproductive effects was noted in any of the laboratory studies.

The product is not labeled for use in lactating dairy cattle.

Overdosage/Acute Toxicity

Limited information is available. In cattle, dosages up to 5X caused little demonstrable effects other than localized tissue reactions (Anon 2011).

Some piglets that were given 3X (12 mg/kg) & 5X (20 mg/kg) normal doses developed muscle tremors/weakness or showed subdued activity. One animal developed a shock-like syndrome after 20 mg/kg and was euthanized. Mortality was seen at dosages of 25 mg/kg or greater (Anon 2012b).

Dogs given IM doses of 20 mg/kg caused a slight, but significant decrease in blood pressure (Anon 2010a, 2012a).

Drug Interactions

No specific drug interactions were noted although the UK label states: "There is cross resistance with other macrolides. Do not administer with antimicrobials with a similar mode of action such as other macrolides or lincosamides." (Anon 2010b)

Laboratory Considerations

None noted.

Dosages

- **CATTLE:**

  Note: See restrictions and withdrawal times in the Dosage Forms/Regulatory Status section.

  Labeled dose (FDA-approved): **For the treatment of bovine respiratory disease (BRD) associated with *Mannheimia haemolytica*, *Pasteurella multocida*, and *Histophilus somni* in beef and non-lactating dairy cattle, and for the control of respiratory disease in beef and non-lactating dairy cattle at high risk of developing BRD associated with *Mannheimia haemolytica*, *Pasteurella multocida*, and *Histophilus somni*:** Inject subcutaneously as a single dose in the neck at a dosage of 4 mg/kg (1 mL/100 lb.) body weight (BW). Do not inject more than 10 mL per injection site. Do not puncture 50 & 100 mL vial stoppers more than 8 times or the 250 mL vial stopper more than 16 times. (Adapted from label information; *Zuprevo*®—MSD USA) (Anon 2011)

  Extra-label dose (USA); U.K. approved dose: **For the treatment and prevention of bovine respiratory disease (BRD) associated with *Mannheimia haemolytica*, *Pasteurella multocida* and *Histophilus somni* sensitive to tildipirosin:** Administer 4 mg/kg (equivalent to 1 mL/45 kg body weight) subcutaneously once only. For treatment of cattle over 450 kg body weight, divide the dose so that no more than 10 mL are injected at one site. The rubber stopper of the vial may be safely punctured up to 20 times. Otherwise, the use of a multiple-dose syringe is recommended. To ensure correct dosage, bodyweight should be determined as accurately as possible to avoid under-dosing. It is recommended to treat animals in the early stages of the disease and to evaluate the response to treatment within 2-3 days after injection. If clinical signs of respiratory disease persist or increase, treatment should be changed using another antibiotic, and continued until clinical signs have resolved. (Adapted from label information; *Zuprevo*®—MSD U.K.) (Anon 2010b)

- **SWINE:**

  Note: See restrictions and withdrawal times in the Dosage Forms/Regulatory Status section.

  Labeled dose (USA): None at time of writing (2014). The 18% cattle product states that it (tildipirosin 18%) should not be used in swine.

  Extra-label dose (USA); U.K. approved dose: **Note:** The swine product (U.K.) is 40 mg/mL (4%). **Treatment of swine respiratory disease (SRD) associated with *Actinobacillus pleuropneumoniae*, *Pasteurella multocida*, *Bordetella bronchiseptica* and *Haemophilus parasuis* sensitive to tildipirosin:** Administer 4 mg/kg IM (equivalent to 1 mL/10 kg body weight) once only. The injection volume should not exceed 5 mL per injection site. The rubber stopper of the vial may be safely punctured up to 20 times. Otherwise, the use of a multiple-dose syringe is recommended. To ensure correct dosage, body weight should be determined as accurately as possible to avoid under-dosing. It is recommended to treat animals in the early stages of the disease and to evaluate the response to treatment within 48 hours after injection. If clinical signs of respiratory disease persist or increase, or if relapse occurs, treatment should be changed using another antibiotic, and continued until clinical signs have resolved. (Adapted from label information; *Zuprevo*® for Pigs—MSD U.K.) (Anon 2012b)

Monitoring

Clinical efficacy. The product information for the UK products lists: In cattle, evaluate the response to treatment within 2-3 days after injection. If clinical signs of respiratory disease persist or increase, treatment should be changed using another antibiotic (Anon 2010b). In pigs, it is recommended to evaluate the response to treatment within 48 hours after injection. If clinical signs of respiratory disease persist, increase, or if relapse occurs, treatment should be changed using another antibiotic (Anon 2012b).

Client Information

- Understand and follow use restrictions and withdrawal times for food animals.
- Humans with known hypersensitivity (drug allergy) to macrolide antibiotics (*e.g.*, erythromycin, clarithromycin) should avoid contact with the medication.
- Do not use automatically powered syringes that do not have an additional protection system. If accidental self-injection, seek medical advice immediately and show the package leaflet or label to the physician. In case of skin or eye exposure, wash/flush with clean water.

Chemistry/Synonyms

Tildipirosin (CAS Registry: 328898-40-4; ATCvet code: QJ01FA96) is a 16-membered semi-synthetic macrolide antimicrobial agent.

The injectable solution is a clear, yellowish solution. Excipients in the injectable solution include citric acid monohydrate, propylene glycol and water for injection.

Tildipirosin may also be known as 20, 23-di-piperidynyl-mycaminosyl-tylonolide or "PMT". The trade name is *Zuprevo*®.

Storage/Stability

The injectable solution should be stored at temperatures at or below 30°C (86°F). Do not freeze. The U. K. label states not to store above 25°C.The maximum storage time after first puncture is 28 days at or below 25°C (77°F).

Compatibility/Compounding Considerations

No specific information noted. The UK label states: "In the absence of compatibility studies, this veterinary medicinal product must not be mixed with other veterinary medicinal products."

Dosage Forms/Regulatory Status

VETERINARY-LABELED PRODUCTS:
Tildipirosin Injection: 180 mg/mL (18%) in 50 mL, 100 mL & 250 mL multi-dose vials; *Zuprevo*®; (Rx). FDA-approved (NADA 141-334) for use in cattle (see below). There is a website (dailymed. nlm.nih.gov) with the FDA-approved veterinary product's label: *Zuprevo*®.

Withdrawal times/restrictions:

USA labeling: Cattle intended for human consumption must not be slaughtered within 21 days of the last treatment. Do not use in female dairy cattle 20 months of age or older. Use of this drug product in these cattle may cause milk residues. A withdrawal period has not been established in pre-ruminating calves. Do not use in calves to be processed for veal.

U.K. labeling: Cattle: (meat and offal): 47 days. Not authorised for use in lactating animals producing milk for human consumption. Do not use in pregnant animals, which are intended to produce milk for human consumption, within 2 months of expected parturition.

Pigs (meat and offal): 9 days.

Revisions/References

Monograph revised/updated August 2014.

Amrine, D. E., et al. (2014). Pulmonary lesions and clinical disease response to Mannheimia haemolytica challenge 10 days following administration of tildipirosin or tulathromycin. Journal of Animal Science **92**(1): 311-9.

Anon (2010a). Tildipirosin—European public MRL assessment report. Committee for Medicinal Products for Veterinary Use—European Medicines Agency.

Anon (2010b). Zuprevo® for Cattle—Product Leaflet. Milton Keynes, UK, MSD Animal Health.

Anon (2011). Zuprevo® (Tildipirosin 18%) - Product label. Summit, NJ, Merck Animal Health.

Anon (2012a). Freedom of Information Summary—Zuprevo (Tildiprisin 18%) NADA 141-334. FDA Database.

Anon (2012b). Zuprevo® (tildipirosin 40 mg/mL for pigs)—Product Leaflet. Milton Keynes UK, MSD Animal Health.

Menge, M., et al. (2012). Pharmacokinetics of tildipirosin in bovine plasma, lung tissue, and bronchial fluid (from live, nonanesthetized cattle). J. Vet. Pharmacol. Ther. **35**(6): 550-9.

Michael, G. B., et al. (2012). Increased MICs of gamithromycin and tildipirosin in the presence of the genes erm(42) and msr(E)-mph(E) for bovine Pasteurella multocida and Mannheimia haemolytica. Journal of Antimicrobial Chemotherapy **67**(6): 1555-7.

Rose, M., et al. (2013). Pharmacokinetics of tildipirosin in porcine plasma, lung tissue, and bronchial fluid and effects of test conditions on in vitro activity against reference strains and field isolates of Actinobacillus pleuropneumoniae. J. Vet. Pharmacol. Ther. **36**(2): 140-53.

Tiletamine HCl/Zolazepam HCl

(tye-let-a-meen and zoe-laze-a-pam)   Telazol®

Injectable Anesthetic/Tranquilizer

Prescriber Highlights

▶ Injectable anesthetic/tranquilizer combination similar to ketamine/diazepam.

▶ Contraindications: Pancreatic disease, rabbits, severe cardiac disease, use in cesarean section, or pulmonary disease. Caution: Renal disease, large exotic cats, especially tigers (use avoided).

▶ Protect patient's eyes after using.

▶ Dosages may need to be reduced in geriatric or debilitated animals, or animals with renal dysfunction.

▶ Adverse Effects: Respiratory depression, pain after IM injection, athetoid movements, tachycardia (esp. dogs), emesis during emergence, excessive salivation & bronchial/tracheal secretions, transient apnea, vocalization, erratic &/or prolonged recovery, involuntary muscular twitching, hypertonia, cyanosis, cardiac arrest, pulmonary edema, muscle rigidity, & either hypertension or hypotension.

▶ Monitor body temperature (may cause hypothermia).

▶ Class-III controlled substance.

Uses/Indications

Telazol® (tiletamine/zolazepam) is indicated for restraint or anesthesia combined with muscle relaxation in cats, and for restraint and minor procedures of short duration (≈ 30 minutes) which require mild to moderate analgesia in dogs. Although not FDA-approved for other species, it has been used in many domestic, exotic and wild species. A potential disadvantage of this product is that it is a fixed dose combination and the pharmacokinetics can vary significantly with each drug in a given species.

Pharmacology/Actions

In cats, tiletamine decreases cardiac rate and blood pressure after IM injections. Its effect on respiratory activity is controversial, and until these effects have been clarified, respiratory function should be closely monitored. The pharmacology of this drug combination is similar to that of ketamine and diazepam; for more information, refer to their monographs.

Pharmacokinetics

In cats, the onset of action is reported to be within 1-7 minutes after IM injection. Duration of anesthesia is dependent on dosage, but is usually about 21-60 minutes at peak effect. This is reported to be ≈ 3X the duration of ketamine anesthesia. The duration of effect of the zolazepam component is longer than that of the tiletamine, so there is a greater degree of tranquilization than anesthesia during the recovery period. The recovery times vary in length from ≈ 1-5.5 hours. Reported elimination half-life for tiletamine is 2.5 hours and 4.5 hours for zolazepam.

In dogs, the onset of action following IM injection averages 7.5 minutes. The mean duration of surgical anesthesia is ≈ 27 minutes, with recovery times averaging ≈ 4 hours. The duration of the tiletamine effect is longer than that of zolazepam, so there is a shorter duration of tranquilization than there is anesthesia. Less than 4% of the drugs are reported excreted unchanged in the urine in the dog. Reported elimination half-life for tiletamine is 2.5 hours and 1.5 hours for zolazepam.

In xylazine-sedated horses, tiletamine/zolazepam given 1.5 mg/kg IV (over 15 seconds) produced the following pharmacokinetic data (means reported): For tiletamine and zolazepam: clearance 96 mL/min/kg & 6.7 mL/min/kg; volume of distribution 0.79 L/kg & 0.76 L/kg; terminal half-life 29 minutes & 235 minutes. Tiletamine is cleared much more rapidly than zolazepam. At this dosage, recumbency lasted for 30-43 minutes, and the mean time to standing was 39 minutes. The authors judged recoveries to be excellent.

In pigs, higher concentrations of zolazepam were observed in pig plasma and it was cleared more slowly compared to tiletamine. Apparent clearance: 11 L/hour (zolazepam) versus 134 L/hour (tiletamine); half-life: 2.76 hours (zolazepam) versus 1.97 hours (tiletamine). Three metabolites of zolazepam and one metabolite of tiletamine were identified in pig urine, plasma and microsomal incubations. Authors concluded that the results collectively point to major pharmacokinetic and metabolic differences between the two components of this fixed-dose anesthetic combination (Kumar *et al.* 2014).

Contraindications/Precautions/Warnings

Telazol® is contraindicated in animals with severe cardiac, pulmonary or pancreatic disease. Animals with renal disease may have prolonged duration of anesthetic action or recovery times.

Because *Telazol®* may cause hypothermia, susceptible animals (small body surface area, low ambient temperatures) should be monitored carefully and supplemental heat applied if needed. Like ketamine, *Telazol®* does not abolish pinnal, palpebral, pedal, laryngeal, and pharyngeal reflexes and its use (alone) may not be adequate if surgery is to be performed on these areas.

It has been reported that this drug is contraindicated in rabbits due to renal toxicity.

Telazol® is generally avoided for use in large, exotic cats (contraindicated in tigers) as it may cause seizures, permanent neurologic abnormalities, or death.

Cats' eyes remain open after receiving *Telazol®*, and they should be protected from injury and an ophthalmic lubricant (*e.g., Lacrilube®*) should be applied to prevent excessive drying of the cornea. Cats reportedly do not tolerate endotracheal tubes well with this agent.

Dosages may need to be reduced in geriatric, debilitated, or animals with renal dysfunction.

Adverse Effects

Respiratory depression is a definite possibility, especially with higher dosages of this product. Apnea may occur; observe animal carefully. Pain after IM injection (especially in cats) has been noted which may be a result of the low pH of the solution. Athetoid movements (constant succession of slow, writhing, involuntary movements of flexion, extension, pronation, etc.) may occur; do not give additional *Telazol®* in the attempt to diminish these actions. Large doses given SC or IM, versus small doses given IV, may result in longer, rougher recoveries. Recoveries in dogs can be rougher than those usually seen in cats.

In dogs, tachycardia may be a common effect and last for 30 minutes. Insufficient anesthesia after recommended doses has been reported in dogs.

Telazol® has been implicated in causing nephrosis in lagamorphs (rabbits/hares) and is usually not recommended for use in these species.

Other adverse effects listed by the manufacturer include: emesis during emergence, excessive salivation and bronchial/tracheal secretions (if atropine not administered beforehand), transient apnea, vocalization, erratic and/or prolonged recovery, involuntary muscular twitching, hypertonia, cyanosis, cardiac arrest, pulmonary edema, muscle rigidity, and either hypertension or hypotension.

Reproductive/Nursing Safety

Telazol® crosses the placenta and may cause respiratory depression in newborns; the manufacturer lists its use in cesarean section as being contraindicated. The teratogenic potential of the drug is unknown, and it is not recommended for use during any stage of pregnancy.

Overdosage/Acute Toxicity

The manufacturer claims a 2X margin of safety in dogs, and a 4.5X margin of safety in cats. A preliminary study in dogs (Hatch et al. 1988) suggests that doxapram at 5.5 mg/kg will enhance respirations and arousal after *Telazol®*. In massive overdoses, it is suggested that mechanically assisted ventilation be performed if necessary and other clinical signs treated symptomatically and supportively.

High doses of tiletamine have caused acute tubular necrosis in New Zealand white rabbits.

Drug Interactions

Little specific information is available presently on drug interactions with this product. The following drug interactions have either been reported or are theoretical in animals receiving tiletamine/zolazepam and may be of significance in veterinary patients. Unless otherwise noted, use together is not necessarily contraindicated, but weigh the potential risks and perform additional monitoring when appropriate.

- **ANESTHETICS, INHALATIONAL**: Dosage may need to be reduced when used concomitantly with *Telazol®*.
- **BARBITURATES**: Dosage may need to be reduced when used concomitantly with *Telazol®*.
- **CHLORAMPHENICOL**: In dogs, chloramphenicol apparently has no effect on recovery times with *Telazol®*, but in cats, anesthesia is prolonged on average of 30 minutes by chloramphenicol.
- **PHENOTHIAZINES**: Can cause increased respiratory and cardiac depression.

For potential additional interactions from the related compounds, ketamine and midazolam:

Ketamine:

- **NEUROMUSCULAR BLOCKERS** (*e.g.,* **succinylcholine** and **tubocurarine**): May cause enhanced or prolonged respiratory depression.
- **THYROID HORMONES**: When given concomitantly with ketamine, thyroid hormones have induced hypertension and tachycardia in humans; beta-blockers (*e.g.,* **propranolol**) may be of benefit in treating these effects.

Midazolam:

- **ANESTHETICS, INHALATIONAL**: Midazolam may decrease the dosages required.
- **AZOLE ANTIFUNGALS** (*e.g.,* **ketoconazole, itraconazole, fluconazole,** etc.): May increase midazolam levels.

- **CALCIUM CHANNEL BLOCKERS** (*e.g.,* **diltiazem, verapamil,** etc.): May increase midazolam levels.
- **CIMETIDINE**: May increase midazolam levels.
- **CNS DEPRESSANTS, OTHER**: May increase the risk of respiratory depression.
- **MACROLIDES** (*e.g.,* **erythromycin, clarithromycin,** etc.): May increase midazolam levels.
- **OPIATES**: May increase the hypnotic effects of midazolam and hypotension has been reported when used with meperidine.
- **PHENOBARBITAL**: May decrease peak levels and AUC of midazolam.
- **RIFAMPIN**: May decrease peak levels and AUC of midazolam.
- **THIOPENTAL**: Midazolam may decrease the dosages required.

Doses

Note: Dosages are for the combined amounts of tiletamine/zolazepam.

- **DOGS:**

Labeled dose (FDA-approved): **For diagnostic purposes:** 6.6 – 9.9 mg/kg IM. **For minor procedures of short duration:** 9.9 – 13.2 mg/kg IM. If supplemental doses are necessary, give doses less than the initial dose and total dosage should not exceed 26.4 mg/kg. Atropine 0.04 mg/kg should be used concurrently to control hypersalivation. (Package Insert; *Telazol®*)

Extra-label dose: **For aggressive (difficult to handle) dogs:** Use only if there is insufficient sedation from opioid, higher dose medetomidine, and midazolam: 1 – 2 mg/kg IM. (Moffat 2008)

- **CATS:**

Labeled dose (FDA-approved): 9.7 – 11.9 mg/kg IM for procedures such as dentistry, abscess treatment, foreign body removal, etc. For procedures that require mild to moderate levels of analgesia (lacerations, castration, etc.) use 10.6 – 12.5 mg/kg IM. For ovariohysterectomy and onychectomy use 14.3 – 15.8 mg/kg IM. If supplemental doses are necessary, give doses less than the initial dose and the total dosage should not exceed 72 mg/kg. Atropine 0.04 mg/kg should be used concurrently to control hypersalivation. (Package Insert; *Telazol*)

Extra-label dose: 2 – 5 mg/kg IV or 5 – 10 mg/kg IM. Physiological effects are similar to those described for ketamine/valium. For procedures that will cause mild pain can reconstitute *Telazol®* vial with butorphanol (2.5 mL of 10 mg/mL) and dexmedetomidine (2.5 mL) & use IM in cats. Add an analgesic drug for moderate to severe pain.

- **RUMINANTS:**

For chemical restraint (extra-label):

In combination with ketamine and xylazine (TKX-Ru) for capturing intractable ruminant patients and large exotic hoof stock: Reconstitute a 500 mg vial of *Telazol®* with 250 mg of ketamine (2.5 mL) and 100 mg of large animal xylazine (1 mL) yielding a final volume of 4 mL. The dosing protocol for TKX-Ru is still evolving. Current recommendations are 1.25 – 1.5 mL/110-115 kg body weight for smaller ruminants patients, and 1 mL/110-115 kg body weight for larger ruminant patients. Typically administered via a dart gun or pole syringe. Patients generally become compliant and recumbent in 5-10 minutes. An excessive dose or accidental IV administration is assumed if onset of effects occur significantly earlier than 5 minutes after administration. If onset of effects has not occurred 20 minutes post-dose, may give another dose (25-50% of the original dose). There is wide interpatient variability with respect to the degree and duration of chemical restraint and analgesia. Ruminant double drip (ketamine, guaifenesin) or triple drip (ketamine, xylazine, guaifenesin) solutions may be used to enhance and/or extend systemic analgesia and patient cooperation. Generally, sternal recumbency occurs about 40-60 minutes after dosing and attempts to stand occur in another 20-40 minutes. Xylazine may be reversed if necessary. (Abrahamsen 2013)

In combination with ketamine and detomidine (TZDK) in free-range cattle: In the study the combination used contained detomidine 4.2 mg/mL, ketamine 52.6 mg/mL and tiletamine/zolazepam 52.6 mg/mL; 1 mL/100 kg body weight (BW estimated visually) was injected IM either by syringe or blowpipe, preferably in the back of the thigh. Animals whose procedures lasted longer than the expected duration of a single dose received that an additional dose (50% of the initial dose) when the first spontaneous pinna movement was observed. Atipamezole (0.02 – 0.06 mg/kg IV) was used to reverse effects. Respiratory depression was the most severe side effect and careful patient monitoring is recommended. (Re *et al.* 2013), (Re *et al.* 2011)

■ **SMALL MAMMALS:**

For chemical restraint in small rodents (extra-label): 6 – 10 mg/kg IM is adequate prior to inhalation anesthesia. Advantages over ketamine include better muscle relaxation, small volume of injection, rapid induction time and a wide margin of safety. Disadvantages of this drug combination are increased respiratory secretions, variability in recovery times, and short shelf-life after reconstitution (Bennett 2009). Not recommended for rabbits (Burke 1999).

■ **FERRETS:**

As a sedative/analgesic (extra-label): *Telazol®* alone: 22 mg/kg IM. *Telazol®* (1.5 mg/kg) plus xylazine (1.5 mg/kg) IM; may reverse xylazine with yohimbine (0.05 mg/kg IM). *Telazol®* (1.5 mg/kg) plus xylazine (1.5 mg/kg) plus butorphanol (0.2 mg/kg) IM; may reverse xylazine with yohimbine (0.05 mg/kg IM). (Williams 2000)

■ **HORSES:** (NOTE: ARCI UCGFS CLASS 2 DRUG)

For anesthesia (extra-label): Xylazine 1.1 mg/kg IV, 5 minutes prior to *Telazol®* at 1.65 – 2.2 mg/kg IV (Hubbell *et al.* 1989). A recent pharmacokinetics study, used xylazine 1 mg/kg IV followed by *Telazol®* 1.5 mg/kg (combined dose) administered IV over 15 seconds. Recumbency lasted 30-43 minutes and mean time to stand was 39 minutes. Both induction and recovery quality were subjectively evaluated as excellent. (Queiroz-Williams *et al.* 2013)

■ **CAMELIDS (NWC)**

As a sedative/analgesic (extra-label): Study was done in adult male llamas. Authors concluded that tiletamine-zolazepam alone (2 mg/kg IM) is only suitable for immobilization for non-painful procedures. Concurrent IM administration of xylazine at a dose of 0.2 or 0.4 mg/kg significantly increased the duration of antinociception induced by tiletamine-zolazepam, and there was a dose-dependent response for the antinociceptive effect of xylazine. Transient hypoxemia was associated with xylazine administration, but the authors did not consider this to be clinically important in healthy llamas. (Seddighi *et al.* 2013)

■ **REPTILES:**

a) Large Snakes: 3 mg/kg IM to facilitate handling and anesthesia. Administer 30-45 minutes prior to handling. Sedation may persist for up to 48 hours. May also be used in Crocodilians at 4 – 8 mg/kg. (Heard 1999)

b) 3 – 10 mg/kg IM. Lizards and snakes can generally be treated with lower end of dosage range and chelonians may require high end. If sedation is inadequate, may give incrementally up to the maximum dose. Monitor closely for apnea and ventilate if required. (Innis 2003)

c) Significant interspecies and interpatient differences in effectiveness. At lower doses of 4 – 10 mg/kg sedation may be sufficient for some procedures (venipuncture, gastric lavage, intubation for inhalation anesthesia). At higher doses (15 – 40 mg/kg), recovery may be greatly prolonged. Suggest starting out at 7 – 15 mg/kg the first few times this is used on reptiles in your practice (and to use on your own "in house" pets first!), and then use increasing dosages as needed. (Funk 2002)

d) Best used for sedation and tranquillization or to facilitate intubation, especially in large boids, crocodilians and venomous species. Author starts with a dose of 5 mg/kg IM and repeats if needed. Higher doses (6 mg/kg) are associated with very long recovery times, especially in chelonians (72 hours). (Mehler 2009)

■ **ZOO, EXOTIC, WILDLIFE SPECIES:**

For use in zoo, exotic and wildlife medicine refer to specific references, including:

a) *Zoo Animal and Wildlife Immobilization and Anesthesia.* West, G., Heard, D., Caulkett, N. (eds.). Blackwell Publishing, 2007.

b) Handbook of Wildlife Chemical Immobilization, 3rd Ed. Kreeger, T.J. and J.M. Arnemo. 2007.

c) Fowler's Zoo and Wild Animal Medicine Current Therapy, Volume 7, Miller, R.E., Fowler, M.E., Saunders. 2011.

d) *Exotic Animal Formulary, 4th Ed.* Carpenter, J.W., Saunders. 2012.

e) The 2009 American Association of Zoo Veterinarian Proceedings by D. K. Fontenot also has several dosages listed for restraint, anesthesia, and analgesia for a variety of drugs for carnivores and primates. VIN members can access them at: http://goo.gl/NNIWQ or http://goo.gl/9UJse

Monitoring

■ Level of anesthesia/analgesia.

■ Respiratory function; cardiovascular status (rate, rhythm, BP if possible).

■ Monitor eyes to prevent drying or injury.

■ Body temperature.

Client Information

Should only be administered by individuals familiar with its use.

Chemistry/Synonyms

Tiletamine is an injectable anesthetic agent chemically related to ketamine. Zolazepam is a diazepinone minor tranquilizer. The pH of the injectable product, after reconstitution, is 2.2-2.8.

Tiletamine HCl may also be known as: CI-634, CL-399, CN-54521-2, or *Telazol®*.

Zolazepam HCl may also be known as: CI-716.

Storage/Stability

After reconstitution, solutions may be stored for 4 days at room temperature and 14 days if refrigerated. Do not use solutions that contain a precipitate or are discolored.

Compatibility/Compounding Considerations

No specific information noted.

Dosage Forms/Regulatory Status

VETERINARY-LABELED PRODUCTS:

Tiletamine HCl (equivalent to 250 mg free base) and Zolazepam HCl (equivalent to 250 mg free base) as lyophilized powder/vial in 5 mL vials. When 5 mL of sterile diluent (sterile water) is added a concentration of 50 mg/mL of each drug (100 mg/mL combined) is produced; *Telazol®*; (Rx, C-III). FDA-approved for use in cats and dogs. *Telazol®* is a Class-III controlled substance.

No withdrawal guidelines for milk or meat withdrawal intervals are available (Smith 2013).

HUMAN-LABELED PRODUCTS: NONE.

Revisions/References

Monograph revised/updated August 2014.

Abrahamsen, E. J. (2013). Chemical Restraint and Injectable Anesthesia of Ruminants. Veterinary Clinics of North America-Food Animal Practice **29**(1): 209-+.
Bennett, R. (2009). Small Mammal Anesthesia--Rabbits and Rodents. Proceedings: ACVC. accessed via Veterinary Information Network; vin.com
Burke, T. (1999). Husbandry and Medicine of Rodents and Lagomorphs. Proceedings: Central Veterinary Conference, Kansas City. accessed via Veterinary Information Network; vin.com
Funk, R. (2002). Anesthesia in reptiles. Proceedings: Western Veterinary Conf. accessed via Veterinary Information Network; vin.com
Heard, D. (1999). Advances in Reptile Anesthesia. The North American Veterinary Conference, Orlando. accessed via Veterinary Information Network; vin.com
Hubbell, J. A. E., et al. (1989). Xylazine and tiletamine-zolazepam anesthesia in horses. Am J Vet Res **50**(5): 737-42.
Innis, C. (2003). Advances in anesthesia and analgesia in reptiles. Proceedings: Western Veterinary Conference. accessed via Veterinary Information Network; vin.com
Kumar, A., et al. (2014). Pharmacokinetic study in pigs and in vitro metabolic characterization in pig and human-liver microsomes reveal marked differences in disposition and metabolism of tiletamine and zolazepam (Telazol) [abstract]. Xenobiotica **44**(4): 379-90.
Mehler, S. (2009). Anaesthesia and care of the reptile. Proceedings: BSAVA. accessed via Veterinary Information Network; vin.com
Moffat, K. (2008). Addressing canine and feline aggression in the veterinary clinic. Vet Clin NA: Sm Anim Pract **38**: 983-1003.
Queiroz-Williams, P., et al. (2013). Pharmacokinetics of Intravenous Tiletamine and Zolazepam in Xylazine-Sedated Horses [abstract]. Proceedings: IVECCS. accessed via Veterinary Information Network; vin.com
Re, M., et al. (2011). Chemical restraint and anaesthetic effects of a tiletamine,Äìzolazepam/ketamine/detomidine combination in cattle. The Veterinary Journal **190**(1): 66-70.
Re, M., et al. (2013). Reversible chemical restraint of free-range cattle with a concentrated combination of tiletamine-zolazepam, ketamine, and detomidine. Canadian Journal of Veterinary Research-Revue Canadienne De Recherche Veterinaire **77**(4): 288-92.
Seddighi, R., et al. (2013). Physiologic and antinociceptive effects following intramuscular administration of xylazine hydrochloride in combination with tiletamine-zolazepam in llamas. American Journal of Veterinary Research **74**(4): 530-4.
Smith, G. (2013). Extralabel Use of Anesthetic and Analgesic Compounds in Cattle. Veterinary Clinics of North America-Food Animal Practice **29**(1): 29-+.
Williams, B. (2000). Therapeutics in Ferrets. Vet Clin NA: Exotic Anim Pract **3**:1(Jan): 131-53.

Tilmicosin

(til-mi-coe-sin)   Micotil®, Pulmotil®

Macrolide Antibiotic

Prescriber Highlights

► Macrolide antibiotic used in cattle, sheep, & sometimes rabbits; used in swine as a medicated feed article and in drinking water.

► Contraindications: Not to be used in automatically powered syringes or to be given IV; camelids(?).

► If injected may be fatal in swine, non-human primates, horses, and goats. May be fatal if injected IV in cattle and sheep.

► Adverse Effects: IM injections may cause a local tissue reaction resulting in trim loss; edema is possible at SC injection site.

► Avoid contact with eyes. In case of human injection, contact physician immediately.

Uses/Indications

Tilmicosin is indicated for the treatment of bovine respiratory disease (BRD) associated with *Mannheimia haemolytica*, *Pasteurella multocida* and *Histophilus somni* and the treatment of ovine respiratory disease (ORD) associated with *Mannheimia haemolytica*. It is also indicated for the control of respiratory disease in cattle at high risk of developing BRD associated with *Mannheimia haemolytica*. For oral use (in drinking water), tilmicosin is indicated for the control of swine respiratory disease associated with *Pasteurella multocida* and *Haemophilus parasuis* in groups of swine in buildings where a respiratory disease outbreak is diagnosed.

Pharmacology/Actions

Like other macrolides, tilmicosin has activity primarily against gram-positive bacteria, although some gram-negative bacteria are affected and the drug reportedly has some activity against mycoplasma. Preliminary studies have shown that 95% of studied isolates of *Pasteurella haemolytica* are sensitive. Bacterial isolates susceptible to tilmicosin at concentrations of ≤8 mcg/mL are reported as susceptible to tilmicosin. The MIC_{90} value reported for *M. haemolytica* and *P. multocida* in cattle with BRD is 32 mcg/mL. Oral tilmicosin does not have activity against *Cryptosporidium* spp. in goats (Paraud *et al.* 2010).

Pharmacokinetics

Tilmicosin apparently concentrates in lung tissue. At 3 days post injection, the lung:serum ratio is ≈ 60:1. MIC_{95} concentrations (3.12 mcg/mL) for *P. haemolytica* persist for a minimum of 3 days after a single injection.

Contraindications/Precautions/Warnings

Not to be used in automatically powered syringes or to be given intravenously as fatalities may result. Tilmicosin has been shown to be fatal in swine (when injected), non-human primates and potentially, in horses. Avoid contact with eyes.

There have been anecdotal reports of severe reactions in some camelids.

Accidental self-injection can be fatal in humans. Do not use in automatically powered syringes. Emergency treatment includes applying ice to injection site and contacting a physician immediately. Emergency medical telephone numbers are 1-800-722-0987 or 1-317-276-2000.

Adverse Effects

If administered IM, a local tissue reaction may occur resulting in trim loss. Edema may be noted at the site of subcutaneous injection.

Reproductive/Nursing Safety

Safe use in pregnant animals or animals to be used for breeding purposes has not been demonstrated.

Overdosage/Acute Toxicity

The cardiovascular system is apparently the target of toxicity in animals. In cattle, doses up to 50 mg/kg IM did not cause death, but SC doses of 150 mg/kg did cause fatalities, as well as IV doses of 5 mg/kg. Doses as low as 10 mg/kg in swine caused increased respiration, emesis and seizures; 20 mg/kg IM caused deaths in most animals tested. In monkeys, 10 mg/kg administered once caused no signs of toxicity, but 20 mg/kg caused vomiting; 30 mg/kg caused death.

In cases of human injection, contact physician immediately. The manufacturer has emergency telephone numbers to assist in dealing with exposure: 1-800-722-0987 or 1-317-276-2000.

Drug Interactions

In swine, **epinephrine** increased the mortality associated with tilmicosin. No other specific information was noted; refer to the erythromycin monograph for possible interactions.

Doses

- **CATTLE:**

  For labeled indications (FDA-approved): Administer a single SC dose of 10 – 20 mg/kg of body weight (1 – 2 mL/30 kg; 1.5 – 3 mL per 100 lbs.). Do not inject more than 10 mL per injection site. If no improvement is noted within 48-hours, the diagnosis should be reevaluated. Injection under the skin in the neck is suggested. If not accessible, inject under the skin behind the shoulders and over the ribs. (Adapted from label; *Micotil® 300*)

- **SHEEP:**

  For labeled indications (FDA-approved): In sheep >15 kg, administer a single SC dose of 10 mg/kg of body weight

(1 mL/30 kg; 1.5 mL per 100 lbs.). Do not inject more than 10 mL per injection site. If no improvement is noted within 48-hours, the diagnosis should be reevaluated. Injection under the skin in the neck is suggested. If not accessible, inject under the skin behind the shoulders and over the ribs. (Adapted from label; *Micotil® 300*)

- **SWINE:**

For labeled indications (FDA-approved): Must be diluted before administration to animals. Include in the drinking water to provide a concentration of 200 mg tilmicosin per liter (200 ppm). One 960 mL bottle is sufficient to medicate 1200 liters (320 gallons) of drinking water for pigs. The medicated water should be administered for 5 consecutive days. Use within 24 hours of mixing with water. Do not use rusty containers for medicated water as they may affect product integrity. When using a water medicating pump with a 1:128 inclusion rate, add 1 bottle (960 mL) of *Pulmotil AC®* per 2.5 gallons of stock solution. Swine intended for human consumption must not be slaughtered within 7 days of the last treatment with this product. Do not allow horses or other equines access to water containing tilmicosin. (Adapted from label: *Pulmotil® AC*—Elanco)

- **SMALL MAMMALS:**

Rabbits (extra-label): Two regimens: **1)** 25 mg/kg SC once; repeat in 3 days if necessary. **2)** 5 mg/kg SC on day 0, if no reaction, give 10 mg/kg SC on days 7 and 14. Can cause weakness, pallor, tachypnea and sudden death. May cause acute death if given IV. SC injections can cause local swelling and necrosis. (Ivey *et al.* 2000)

Monitoring

- Efficacy.
- Withdrawal times.

Client Information

- If clients are administering the drug, they should be warned about the potential toxicity to humans, swine, and horses if accidentally injected.
- Carefully instruct in proper injection techniques.
- Avoid contact with eyes.

Chemistry/Synonyms

A semi-synthetic macrolide antibiotic, tilmicosin phosphate is commercially available in a 300 mg/mL (of tilmicosin base) injection with 25% propylene glycol.

Tilmicosin may also be known as EL-870, LY-177370, *Micotil®* or *Pulmotil®*.

Storage/Stability

Store the injection at or below room temperature. Avoid exposure to direct sunlight. Store the oral liquid at or below 86° F (30° C). Protect from direct sunlight.

Compatibility/Compounding Considerations

No specific information noted.

Dosage Forms/Regulatory Status

VETERINARY-LABELED PRODUCTS:

Tilmicosin for Subcutaneous Injection: 300 mg/mL in 50 mL, 100 mL and 250 mL multi-dose vials; *Micotil® 300 Injection*; (Rx). FDA-approved for use in cattle and sheep. Not FDA-approved for use in female dairy cattle 20 months or older. Do not use in lactating ewes if milk is to be used for human consumption. Do not use in veal calves. Slaughter withdrawal (at labeled doses) = 28 days.

Tilmicosin Phosphate 250 mg/mL Aqueous Concentrate for oral use in drinking water in 960 mL bottles; *Pulmotil® AC*; (Rx). FDA-approved (NADA 141-361) for use in swine. Slaughter withdrawal is 7 days.

Tilmicosin Feed Medication: 90.7 grams/lb; *Pulmotil® 90, Tilmovet® 90*; (OTC). FDA-approved for veterinary use in swine and cattle (*Pulmotil® 90* only). Slaughter withdrawal (at labeled doses) = 7 days (swine); 28 days (cattle).

HUMAN-LABELED PRODUCTS: NONE.

Revisions/References

Monograph revised/updated August 2014.

Ivey, E. & J. Morrisey (2000). Therapeutics for Rabbits. Vet Clin NA: Exotic Anim Pract 3:1(Jan): 183-216.
Paraud, C., et al. (2010). Evaluation of oral tilmicosin efficacy against severe cryptosporidiosis in neonatal kids under field conditions. Veterinary Parasitology 170(1-2): 149-52.

Tiludronate Disodium

(til-yoo-droe-nate)   Tildren®, Tiludronic Acid

Bisphosphonate Bone Resorption Inhibitor

Prescriber Highlights

▶ Bisphosphonate bone resorption inhibitor for the intravenous treatment of navicular disease in horses.

▶ Must be given slowly and evenly as an IV infusion over 90 minutes.

▶ Adverse effects: Signs of colic, muscle tremor (hypocalcemia), fatigue/lassitude, sweating, injection site effects, salivation, tail hypertonia.

Uses/Indications

Tiludronate disodium (tiludronic acid) is a bisphosphonate bone resorption inhibitor that is indicated for the control of clinical signs associated with navicular syndrome in horses. It may be beneficial in managing lameness isolated to the navicular bone and distal tarsal osteoarthritis by decreasing bone resorption and inflammation (Kamm *et al.* 2008), (Gough *et al.* 2010). Treatment earlier in the course of the disease apparently results in greater efficacy.

For humans, there is an orally administered FDA-approved product for treating Paget's disease (osteitis deformans).

Pharmacology/Actions

Tiludronate, like other bisphosphonates, inhibit osteoclastic bone resorption by inhibiting osteoclast function after binding to bone hydroxyapatite thereby helping to regulate bone remodeling.

Pharmacokinetics

After intravenous injection in horses the drug is rapidly distributed to bone. Binding is greater to cancellous bone than cortical bone. Plasma protein binding is reported to be ≈ 85% and elimination half-life is ≈ 4.5 hours. Repeated daily doses do not result in accumulation in plasma. Tiludronate undergoes minimal metabolism. Unbound drug is eliminated unchanged in the urine. Approximately 25-50% of a single IV dose is eliminated in the urine over 96 hours. Quantifiable concentrations of tiludronate disodium in bone can still be detected at ≈ 6 months post-dose.

Contraindications/Precautions/Warnings

The product label states: "Do not use in horses with known hypersensitivity to tiludronate disodium or to mannitol. Do not use in horses with impaired renal function or with a history of renal disease. Bisphosphonates are excreted by the kidney; therefore, conditions causing renal impairment may increase plasma bisphosphonate concentrations resulting in an increased risk for adverse reactions. Do not use in horses intended for human consumption… not be used in pregnant or lactating mares, or mares intended for breeding."

Safe use has not been evaluated in horses <4 years of age.

Tiludronate affect can affect plasma concentrations of certain minerals and electrolytes, including calcium, magnesium and potassium, immediately post-treatment, with effects lasting up to several hours. Label states: "Caution should be used when administering *Tildren®* to horses with conditions affecting mineral or electrolyte homeostasis (*e.g.,* hyperkalemic periodic paralysis (HYPP), hypocalcemia, etc.) and conditions which may be exacerbated by hypocalcemia (*e.g.,* cardiac disease)."

Adverse Effects

Acute adverse effects reported in horses are most commonly seen during the infusion period or within 4 hours of beginning the infusion and include signs of abdominal pain or colic (pawing, evidence of pawing, getting up and down, pacing, restlessness, rolling, trying to roll, looking at or biting at side, stretching out/straining, kicking at belly/walls, and shifting weight), muscle tremors/fasciculation, fatigue/lassitude and sweating. The onset of colic signs appear within a few hours of treatment and generally resolve without treatment. Should they persist, conventional colic treatments are recommended. Muscle tremors may be treated with intravenous calcium if required. Adverse reactions occurring between 4-24 hours post treatment include: increased frequency of urination with or without increased drinking, reduced appetite, sore or stiff neck, fever, and uncomplicated colic.

Up to 9% of patients develop local reactions at the injection site (*e.g.,* phlebitis), particularly after the 4th injection.

Other adverse effects reported include salivation and tail hypertonia.

Reproductive/Nursing Safety

The product label states: "Bisphosphonates should not be used in pregnant or lactating mares, or mares intended for breeding…safe use has not been evaluated in pregnant or lactating mares, or in breeding horses; however, bisphosphonates are incorporated into the bone matrix, from where they are gradually released over periods of months to years. The extent of bisphosphonate incorporation into adult bone, and hence, the amount available for release back into the systemic circulation, is directly related to the total dose and duration of bisphosphonate use. Bisphosphonates have been shown to cause fetal developmental abnormalities in laboratory animals. The uptake of bisphosphonates into fetal bone may be greater than into maternal bone creating a possible risk for skeletal or other abnormalities in the fetus. Many drugs, including bisphosphonates, may be excreted in milk and may be absorbed by nursing animals."

Studies performed in male and female rats at dosages as high as 75 mg/kg/day demonstrated no effects on fertility. Studies in pregnant rabbits given 2X-5X human dosages showed no skeletal abnormalities. Pregnant mice given 7X human dosages showed some adverse effects (decreased litter size, malformed paws in 6 fetuses from one litter). Rat studies have shown decreased litter sizes, but no teratogenic effects. In humans, the FDA categorizes tiludronate as category *C* for use during pregnancy (Animal studies have shown an adverse effect on the fetus, but there are no adequate studies in humans; or there are no animal reproduction studies and no adequate studies in humans.)

Overdosage/Acute Toxicity

Limited information is available. The manufacturer reports that doses of 3X in horses caused an increased frequency of adverse effects, particularly signs of colic and muscle tremor. Intravenous calcium administration may be considered for signs associated with hypocalcemia.

Drug Interactions

- **AMINOGLYCOSIDES** (*e.g.,* **amikacin, gentamicin,** etc.): Product label warns that concurrent administration with other potentially nephrotoxic drugs should be approached with caution, and if administered, renal function should be monitored. Additionally, they warn other drugs that aminoglycoside toxicity may exacerbate a reduction in serum calcium.

- **CALCIUM-** or **MAGNESIUM-CONTAINING INTRAVENOUS FLUIDS**: May complex with tiludronate and reduce its availability; do not mix with fluids or administer with fluids such as **Lactated Ringer's, Ringer's,** *Plasma-Lyte®,* **Normosol®,** etc.

- **NSAIDS:** The product label warns that NSAIDs should not be used concurrently with tiludronate. Concurrent use may increase the risk of renal toxicity and acute renal failure. Acute renal failure has been reported in horses concurrently administered NSAIDs and tiludronate within a 48-hour period. Additionally, horses concurrently administered both drugs in field studies demonstrated a statistically significant increases in serum blood urea nitrogen (BUN) and creatinine concentrations, but were not always associated with clinical signs of renal dysfunction. Appropriate washout periods should be observed, and BUN and creatinine should be monitored. If treatment for discomfort is required after *Tildren®* administration, a non-NSAID treatment should be used.

- **TETRACYCLINES:** The product label warns to use with caution in horses receiving concurrent administration of other drugs that may reduce serum calcium (such as tetracyclines).

Laboratory Considerations

No specific concerns were noted.

Doses

- **HORSES:**

  For the control of clinical signs associated with navicular syndrome (labeled dose; FDA-approved): A single dose of 1 mg/kg as an intravenous infusion administered slowly and evenly over 90 minutes (to minimize adverse reactions) through a suitable IV catheter inserted into a jugular vein and connected to the infusion bag using sterile disposable infusion tubing. Maximum effect may not occur until 2 months post-treatment. (Adapted from label; *Tildren®*)

Monitoring

- Clinical Efficacy.
- Serum Calcium.
- Adverse Effects (particularly within first 4 hours after dosing).

Client Information

- This medication should be administered by a veterinary professional.
- Patient should be observed for up to 4 hours post-administration for signs of hypocalcemia (muscle tremors, etc.) or colic.

Chemistry/Synonyms

Tiludronate disodium is a bisphosphonate that occurs as a white powder having a molecular weight of 380.6. Commercially available products contain the disodium salt of tiludronic acid. 120 mg of tiludronate disodium is equivalent to 100 mg of tiludronic acid.

Tiludronate disodium or tiludronic acid may also be known as ME-3737, SR-41319, acidum tiludronicum, *Tildren®* or *Skelid®*.

Storage/Stability

Store unreconstituted powder at controlled room temperature 68-77°F (20-25°C). After preparation, the infusion should be administered either within 2 hours of preparation, or it can be stored for up to 24 hours under refrigeration at 36-46°F (2-8°C) and protected from light.

Shelf life of properly stored unreconstituted product is generally 3 years.

Compatibility/Compounding Considerations

Do **not** reconstitute or mix with calcium containing solutions or other solutions containing divalent cations such as LRS as it may form complexes with these ions.

For preparation of the reconstituted solution (20 mg/mL): Use strict aseptic technique. Remove 25 mL of solution from a 1 liter bag of sterile 0.9% Sodium Chloride Injection, USP and add to vial of *Tildren*®. Shake gently until the powder is completely dissolved. This reconstituted solution contains 20 mg of tiludronate disodium per mL. After reconstitution further dilution is required before administration.

Preparation of the solution for infusion: Using strict aseptic technique, withdraw the appropriate volume of the reconstituted solution based on the horse's body weight. Inject that volume back into the 1 liter bag of sterile 0.9% Sodium Chloride Injection, USP. Horses greater than 1,210 lbs. will require a second vial of reconstituted solution. Invert the infusion bag to mix the solution before infusion. Label the infusion bag to ensure proper use.

After preparation, the infusion should be administered either within 2 hours of preparation, or it can be stored for up to 24 hours under refrigeration at 36-46° F (2-8° C) and protected from light.

Administer for infusion through a suitable intravenous catheter inserted into a jugular vein and connected to the infusion bag using sterile disposable infusion tubing.

Dosage Forms/Regulatory Status

VETERINARY-LABELED PRODUCTS:

Tiludronic Acid: 500 mg (as tiludronate disodium) lyophilized powder for reconstitution per vial; *Tildren*®; (Rx). FDA-approved (NADA 141-420) for horses.

HUMAN-LABELED PRODUCTS:

Tiludronate Disodium Oral Tablets: 240 mg (equiv. to 200 mg tiludronic acid); *Skelid*®; (Rx)

Note: The information presented in this monograph pertains to the veterinary-labeled intravenous product only.

Revisions/References

Monograph revised/updated August 2014.

Gough, M. R., et al. (2010). Tiludronate infusion in the treatment of bone spavin: A double blind placebo-controlled trial. Equine Veterinary Journal 42(5): 381-7.

Kamm, L., et al. (2008). A review of the efficacy of tiludronate in the horse. Journal of Equine Veterinary Science 28(4): 209-14.

Tinidazole

(tye-ni-dah-zole)   Tindamax®

Nitroimidazole Antiprotozoal/Antibiotic

Prescriber Highlights

▶ Drug similar to metronidazole, used primarily as an alternative treatment for giardiasis. Potentially useful for treating anaerobic infections (especially in the mouth), trichomoniasis, amebiasis and balantidiasis.

▶ Little experience in veterinary medicine. Adverse effects most likely GI-related; like metronidazole and ronidazole, tinidazole could cause neurotoxicity.

▶ Many potential drug interactions.

Uses/Indications

Little information is presently available on the use of tinidazole in veterinary species. Because of its antiprotozoal effects, it has been used as an alternative for treating giardiasis in small animals. Tinidazole could have efficacy against amebiasis, trichomoniasis or balantidiasis, but documentation of efficacy is not available. Tinidazole potentially could be useful for treating anaerobic infections in small animals, particularly those associated with dental infections. Tinidazole has a longer duration of action than metronidazole in dogs and cats.

In a small study done in cats experimentally infected with *T. foetus*, tinidazole doses at 30 mg/kg PO once daily for 14 days, decreased fecal shedding of *T. foetus* but failed to eradicate the infec-

tion from 2 of 4 cats (Gookin *et al.* 2007). However, results from a pilot study indicated that tinidazole formulated in a gastro-resistant capsule coated with guar gum at 30 mg/kg PO once daily for 14 days resolved *T. foetus* infections and improved the clinical condition in 5 FIV-positive cats and was also effective against concomitant *Giardia duodenalis* infection in the 4 affected cats (Pennisi *et al.* 2012).

In humans, oral tinidazole is FDA-approved for treating extraintestinal and intestinal amebiasis, (*Entamoeba histolytica*), giardiasis (*Giardia duodenalis/lamblia*), and trichomoniasis (*T. vaginalis*).

Pharmacology/Actions

Tinidazole is a 5-nitroimidazole similar to metronidazole. It is bactericidal against susceptible bacteria. Its exact mechanism of action is not completely understood, but it is taken-up by anaerobic organisms where it is reduced to an unidentified polar compound. It is believed that this compound is responsible for the drug's antimicrobial activity by disrupting DNA and nucleic acid synthesis in the bacteria.

Tinidazole has activity against many obligate anaerobes and *H. pylori*. It has excellent activity against *Porphyromonas* spp. found in canine gingiva.

Tinidazole is also trichomonacidal and amebicidal. Its mechanism of action for its antiprotozoal activity is not well understood. It has therapeutic activity against *Entamoeba histolytica*, Trichomonas, and Giardia.

Pharmacokinetics

In dogs and cats, tinidazole is practically completely absorbed after oral administration. Apparent volumes of distribution are 0.66 L/kg in dogs and 0.54 L/kg in cats. Dogs clear the drug about twice as fast as cats; elimination half-lives are ≈ 4.4 hours in dogs, 8.4 hours in cats.

In horses, tinidazole is practically completely absorbed after oral administration. Apparent volume of distribution is 0.66 L/kg and elimination half-life is ≈ 5.2 hours.

Contraindications/Precautions/Warnings

Tinidazole should not be used in patients documented to be hypersensitive to it or other 5-nitroimidazoles (*e.g.*, metronidazole).

Tinidazole is metabolized by the liver; use with caution in patients with hepatic dysfunction.

As other 5-nitroimidazoles (*e.g.*, metronidazole, ronidazole) have been associated with neurotoxic signs in dogs and cats and seizures have been reported rarely with tinidazole use in humans, use with caution in animals susceptible to seizures.

The human labeling for tinidazole carries a "black box warning" stating: "Carcinogenicity has been seen in mice and rats treated chronically with another agent in the nitroimidazole class (metronidazole). Although such data has not been reported for tinidazole, avoid unnecessary use of tinidazole. Reserve its use for the conditions for which it is indicated."

Adverse Effects

The adverse effect profiles for dogs, cats or horses are not well described since clinical use of this medication has been limited. Gastrointestinal effects including vomiting, inappetence, and diarrhea are most likely. Giving the medication with food may help alleviate these effects. Other 5-nitroimidazoles (metronidazole, ronidazole) have been associated with neurotoxic signs in dogs and cats; seizures have been reported rarely with tinidazole use in humans.

Tinidazole reportedly is very bitter tasting. If using compounded products, consider using capsules or having a flavored suspension prepared.

Reproductive/Nursing Safety

In studies performed on male rats tinidazole decreased fertility and caused testicular histopathology.

Tinidazole crosses the placenta. While studies in mice and rats have not demonstrated significant fetal effects, because of its mutagenic potential, it is stated that it should **not be used in women during the first trimester** of pregnancy. In humans, the FDA categorizes tinidazole as category C for use during pregnancy (*Animal studies have shown an adverse effect on the fetus, but there are no adequate studies in humans; or there are no animal reproduction studies and no adequate studies in humans.*) If considering use of this product in a pregnant animal, weigh the potential benefits of treatment versus the risks.

Tinidazole is distributed into maternal milk at levels approximating those found in serum. It is suggested that milk replacer be used if tinidazole is necessary for treating a nursing dam.

Overdosage/Acute Toxicity

Very limited information is available. In studies done in rats and mice, the oral LD50 was >3.6 grams/kg for mice and >2 grams/kg for rats. Treatment of acute overdoses of tinidazole is symptomatic and supportive. Gastric lavage or induction of emesis may be helpful. Hemodialysis can remove ≈ 43% of the amount in the body (human) in a 6-hour session.

Drug Interactions

In humans, the following drug interactions with the related drug metronidazole have been reported or are theoretical and may be of significance in veterinary patients receiving tinidazole. Unless otherwise noted, use together is not necessarily contraindicated, but weigh the potential risks and perform additional monitoring when appropriate.

- **ALCOHOL:** May induce a disulfiram-like (nausea, vomiting, cramps, etc.) reaction.
- **BUSULFAN:** Tinidazole may increase the serum levels of busulfan.
- **CIMETIDINE, KETOCONAZOLE:** May decrease the metabolism of tinidazole and increase the likelihood of dose-related side effects occurring.
- **CISAPRIDE:** Tinidazole may increase the serum levels of cisapride; contraindicated in humans.
- **CYCLOSPORINE, TACROLIMUS (systemic):** Tinidazole may increase the serum levels of cyclosporine or tacrolimus.
- **FLUOROURACIL (systemic):** Tinidazole may increase the serum levels of fluorouracil and increase the risk of toxicity.
- **LITHIUM:** Tinidazole may increase lithium serum levels and increase the risk for lithium toxicity.
- **OXYTETRACYCLINE:** Reportedly, may antagonize the therapeutic effects of metronidazole (and presumably tinidazole).
- **PHENOBARBITAL, RIFAMPIN or PHENYTOIN:** May increase the metabolism of tinidazole thereby decreasing blood levels.
- **WARFARIN:** Metronidazole (and potentially tinidazole) may prolong the prothrombin time (PT) in patients taking warfarin or other coumarin anticoagulants. Avoid concurrent use if possible; otherwise, intensify monitoring.

Laboratory Considerations

- **AST, ALT, LDH, Triglycerides, Hexokinase glucose:** Tinidazole, like metronidazole may interfere with enzymatic coupling of the assay to oxidation-reduction of nicotinamide adenine. Falsely low values, including zero, may result.

Doses

- **DOGS:**

    For giardiasis (extra-label): 44 mg/kg PO q24h for 6 days. Potentially may be useful for treating trichomoniasis, amebiasis and balantidiasis, but efficacy data lacking for animals (Barr 2006).

Another source lists the same dosage, but treats for 3 days (Lappin 2012).

- **CATS:**

    For giardiasis (extra-label): 30 mg/kg PO for 7-10 days (Sherding 2013). Another source lists the same dosage, but treats for 3 days (Lappin 2012).

Monitoring

- Clinical efficacy in treating the infection.

Client Information

- Give this medication with food
- Animals should not have access to alcohol when receiving this medication.
- If gastrointestinal signs (*e.g.,* vomiting, lack of appetite, diarrhea) are severe or persist, contact veterinarian.
- Contact veterinarian immediately if animal shows signs of behavior changes, eyes moving back and forth (nystagmus), convulsions, or if it has difficulty walking, climbing stairs, etc. (ataxia); these could be signs that drug toxicity is occurring.

Chemistry/Synonyms

Tinidazole occurs as an almost white or pale yellow, crystalline powder. It is practically insoluble in water, soluble in acetone, and sparingly soluble in methyl alcohol.

Tinidazole may also be known as CP-12574 or tinidazolum. International trade names include: *Estovyn-T®, Fasigyn®, Tindamax®, Tiniba®, Tiniameb®,* or *Tinidazol®.*

Storage/Stability

Store tinidazole tablets at controlled room temperature (20-25°C) protected from light.

Compatibility/Compounding Considerations

No specific information noted.

Dosage Forms/Regulatory Status

VETERINARY-LABELED PRODUCTS: NONE.
As tinidazole is a nitroimidazole, its use is prohibited in animals to be used for food.

HUMAN-LABELED PRODUCTS:
Tinidazole Tablets (scored): 250 mg & 500 mg; *Tindamax®,* generic; (Rx)

Revisions/References

Monograph revised/updated August 2014.

Barr, S. (2006). Giardiasis. *Infectious Diseases of the Dog and Cat.* C. Greene, Elsevier: 736-42.
Gookin, J. L., et al. (2007). Efficacy of tinidazole for treatment of cats experimentally infected with Tritrichomonas foetus. American Journal of Veterinary Research **68**(10): 1085-8.
Lappin, M. R. (2012). Management of Giardiasis Infections in Dogs and Cats. Proceedings: Western Veterinary Conf. accessed via Veterinary Information Network; vin.com
Pennisi, M., et al. (2012). Pilot Study on Efficacy and Safety of Tinidazole Against Natural Tritrichomonas foetus Infection in Cats. Proceedings: International Society of Feline Medicine. accessed via Veterinary Information Network; vin.com
Sherding, R. G. (2013). Update on Intestinal Giardia and Tritrichomonas Infections. Proceedings: Atlantic Coast Veterinary Conf. accessed via Veterinary Information Network; vin.com

Tiopronin

(tye-oh-proe-nin)   Thiola®, 2-MPG

Antiurolithic (Cystine)

Prescriber Highlights

▶ For prevention (& treatment) of cystine urolithiasis in dogs.
▶ Avoid use in cats. Caution: Agranulocytosis, aplastic anemia, thrombocytopenia or other significant hematologic abnormality, impaired renal or hepatic function, or sensitivity to either tiopronin or penicillamine.
▶ Adverse Effects: Coombs'-positive regenerative spherocyte anemia, aggressiveness, proteinuria, thrombocytopenia, elevations in liver enzymes, dermatologic effects, & myopathy.
▶ Relatively expensive.

Uses/Indications

Tiopronin may be useful for the prevention of cystine urolithiasis in dogs where dietary therapy combined with urinary alkalinization is not completely effective. It may also be useful in combination with urine alkalinization and dietary (ultra-low protein diet) modification to dissolve stones.

Pharmacology/Actions

Tiopronin is considered an antiurolithic agent. It undergoes thiol-disulfide exchange with cystine (cysteine-cysteine disulfide) to form tiopronin-cystine disulfide. This complex is more water-soluble and readily excreted thereby preventing cystine calculi from forming.

Pharmacokinetics

Tiopronin has a rapid onset of action and in humans, up to 48% of a dose is found in the urine within 4 hours of dosing. Tiopronin has a relatively short duration of action and its effect in humans disappears in ≈ 10 hours. Elimination is primarily via renal routes.

Contraindications/Precautions/Warnings

Tiopronin's risks versus its benefits should be considered before using in patients with agranulocytosis, aplastic anemia, thrombocytopenia or other significant hematologic abnormalities, impaired renal or hepatic function, or sensitivity to either tiopronin or penicillamine.

Avoid use in cats; they reportedly do not tolerate the drug very well and dissolution of cystine uroliths has not been successful (Bartges 2011).

Adverse Effects

There is limited information available on the adverse effect profile of tiopronin in dogs. In a retrospective study evaluating tiopronin treatment for cystinuria in ≈ 16% of treated dogs, proteinuria, thrombocytopenia, anemia, increased liver enzymes and bile acids, lethargy, dermatologic effects (small pustules of the skin, dry crusty nose) aggressiveness, sulfur odor of the urine, or myopathy (noted as staggering and difficulty chewing) were noted (Hoppe *et al.* 2001). Tiopronin has been associated with Coombs'-positive regenerative spherocyte anemia in dogs. Should this effect occur, the drug should be discontinued and appropriate treatment started as needed (*e.g.*, corticosteroids, blood component therapy).

In cats, GI signs, liver disease, and anemia have been reported (Bartges 2011).

While tiopronin is thought to have fewer adverse effects than penicillamine in humans, adverse effects that occur more frequently include dermatologic effects (ecchymosis, itching, rashes, mouth ulcers, jaundice) and GI distress. Less frequently reported adverse effects include: allergic reactions (specifically adenopathy), arthralgias, dyspnea, fever, hematologic abnormalities, edema, and nephrotic syndrome.

Reproductive/Nursing Safety

There is limited information on the reproductive safety of tiopronin. Skeletal defects, cleft palates and increased resorptions were noted when rats were given 10X the human dose of penicillamine and, therefore, may also be of concern with tiopronin. Other animal studies have suggested that tiopronin may affect fetus viability at high doses. In humans, the FDA categorizes this drug as category *C* for use during pregnancy (*Animal studies have shown an adverse effect on the fetus, but there are no adequate studies in humans; or there are no animal reproduction studies and no adequate studies in humans.*)

Because tiopronin may be excreted in milk, at present it is not recommended for use in nursing animals.

Overdosage/Acute Toxicity

There is little information available. It is suggested to contact an animal poison control center for further information in the event of an overdose situation.

Drug Interactions

Potentially use of tiopronin with **other drugs causing nephrotoxicity, hepatotoxicity, or bone marrow depression** could cause additive toxic effects. Clinical significance is not clear.

Doses

- **DOGS:**

  For treatment or prevention of recurrence of cystine urinary calculi (extra-label):

  a) For dissolution: 15 mg/kg PO q12h. Feed a diet that is low protein, alkalinizing, and induces a diuresis. There are 2 commercially available diets formulated to be low in sulfur-containing amino acids: *Prescription Diet u/d*® (Hill's) and *UC Low Purine*® (Royal Canin). Canned diets may be better than dry diets. There are studies showing that administration of tiopronin without modifying diet may result in dissolution of cystine uroliths. (Bartges 2011)

  b) Prophylactic treatment: 30 mg/kg PO q12h. Increase water intake and urine diuresis. Alkalinize urine (pH 6.5-7.0) using potassium citrate. In cases with low cystine excretion and low urolith recurrence rate, tiopronin dose may be individually decreased (<30 mg/kg) or stopped.

  Dissolution of uroliths: Approximately 40 mg/kg PO q12h. Reevaluation of uroliths with ultrasound or radiography every 4th week. After urolith dissolution, give prophylactic dose of tiopronin. If urolith dissolution is not achieved after 2-3 months, surgery is recommended. Reexamination recommended 1, 3, 6, & 12 months after start of treatment and thereafter twice a year, including: physical examination, ultrasonography/radiography of the urinary tract, urinalyses (specific gravity, protein, pH, sediment, and cyanide nitroprusside reaction) using AM samples of urine, CBC (with platelets), liver enzymes (alkaline phos, ALT). Quantitative measurements of urinary cystine excretion related to the urinary creatinine excretion, AM urine samples, before start of treatment and once a year during treatment. If adverse reactions occur, stop treatment for 4 weeks. Blood and urine analysis every 1-2 weeks until remission of signs. When the adverse reactions disappear, start tiopronin again, gradually increasing the dose from 10 – 15 mg/kg q12h. If the adverse reactions reappear despite a lowered dose, tiopronin treatment has to be abandoned. (Hoppe *et al.* 2001)

Monitoring

- See the recommendations for monitoring in the dose section. (Hoppe et al. 2001)

Client Information

- Clients should be counseled on the importance of adequate compliance with this drug to maximize efficacy and detailed on the clinical signs to watch for regarding adverse effects.

Chemistry/Synonyms

A sulfhydryl compound related to penicillamine, tiopronin has a molecular weight of 163.2. It occurs as a white crystalline powder that is freely soluble in water.

Tiopronin may also be known as: SF 522, N-(2-Mercaptopropionyl)-glycine (MPG), 2-MPG, thiopronine, *Acadione®*, *Captimer®*, *Epatiol®*, *Mucolysin®*, *Mucosyt®*, *Sutilan®*, *Thiola®*, *Thiosol®*, or *Tioglis®*.

Storage/Stability

Store tablets at room temperature in tight containers.

Compatibility/Compounding Considerations

No specific information noted.

Dosage Forms/Regulatory Status

VETERINARY-LABELED PRODUCTS: NONE.

HUMAN-LABELED PRODUCTS:

Tiopronin Tablets: 100 mg; *Thiola®*; (Rx)

Revisions/References

Monograph revised/updated August 2014.

Bartges, J. (2011). Urine Heaven: Like a Rolling Stone - Uncommon Uroliths & Management. Proceedings: Western Veterinary Conference. accessed via Veterinary Information Network; vin.com

Hoppe, A. & T. Denneberg (2001). Cystinuria in the dog: Clinical studies during 14 years of medical treatment. Journal of Veterinary Internal Medicine 15(4): 361-7.

Tobramycin Sulfate

(toe-bra-mye-sin)   Nebcin®, TOBI®

Aminoglycoside Antibiotic

Prescriber Highlights

▶ Parenteral aminoglycoside antibiotic that has "good" activity against a variety of bacteria, predominantly gram-negative aerobic bacilli, also in ophthalmic preps.

▶ Because of potential adverse effects usually reserved for serious infections when given systemically, may be less nephrotoxic than gentamicin.

▶ Adverse Effects: Nephrotoxicity, ototoxicity, neuromuscular blockade.

▶ Cats may be more sensitive to toxic effects.

▶ Risk factors for nephrotoxicity: Preexisting renal disease, age (both neonatal & geriatric), fever, sepsis, & dehydration.

▶ At present, drug cost is more than gentamicin, but less than amikacin.

Uses/Indications

While there are no FDA-approved veterinary tobramycin products in the U.S., tobramycin can be useful clinically to treat serious gram-negative infections in most species. It is often used in settings where gentamicin-resistant bacteria are a clinical problem or when amikacin is unavailable. The inherent toxicity of the aminoglycosides limit their systemic use to serious infections when there is either a documented lack of susceptibility to other less potentially toxic antibiotics or when the clinical situation dictates immediate treatment of a presumed gram-negative infection before culture and susceptibility results are reported.

Whether tobramycin is less nephrotoxic than either gentamicin or amikacin when used clinically is somewhat controversial, but in controlled laboratory animal studies, it was less nephrotoxic.

Pharmacology/Actions

Tobramycin, like the other aminoglycoside antibiotics, acts on susceptible bacteria presumably by irreversibly binding to the 30S ribosomal subunit thereby inhibiting protein synthesis. It is considered a bactericidal antibiotic.

Tobramycin's spectrum of activity includes coverage against many aerobic gram-negative and some aerobic gram-positive bacteria, including most species of *E. coli*, Klebsiella, Proteus, *Pseudomonas, Salmonella*, Enterobacter, Serratia, Shigella, Mycoplasma, and Staphylococcus. Like amikacin, tobramycin may have more activity against Pseudomonas isolates than gentamicin.

Antimicrobial activity of the aminoglycosides is enhanced in an alkaline environment, but pus or cellular debris can reduce efficacy.

The aminoglycoside antibiotics are inactive against fungi, viruses and most anaerobic bacteria.

Pharmacokinetics

Tobramycin, like the other aminoglycosides, is not appreciably absorbed after oral or intrauterine administration, but it is absorbed from topical administration (not skin or urinary bladder) when used in irrigations during surgical procedures. Patients receiving oral aminoglycosides with hemorrhagic or necrotic enteritises may absorb appreciable quantities of the drug. Subcutaneous injection results in slightly delayed peak levels and more variability than after IM injection. Bioavailability from extravascular injection (IM or SC) is greater than 90%.

The pharmacokinetics of tobramycin in horses have been reported (Hubenov *et al.* 2007; Haritova *et al.* 2012; Newman *et al.* 2013). In a study where horses were given 4 mg/kg IV (Hubenov *et al.* 2007), the following approximate values were reported (**Note:** First value is a calculated value from a microbiologic assay and second is from an HPLC assay): volume of distribution (steady-state): 0.24-0.55 L/kg; clearance: 101-130 mL/kg/hr; elimination half-life: 2.5-4 hours. Another study where horses were administered 4 mg/kg IV, IM, or IV with concurrent IA (Newman *et al.* 2013), reported the following (means) after IV administration: volume of distribution 0.18 L/kg, clearance 1.18 mL/kg/min, and half-life 4.6 hours. IM mean bioavailability was 81% but there was wide variability (±44%). Concurrent IA administration did appear to alter IV pharmacokinetics.

After absorption, aminoglycosides are distributed primarily in the extracellular fluid. They are found in ascitic, pleural, pericardial, peritoneal, synovial and abscess fluids, and high levels are found in sputum, bronchial secretions and bile. Aminoglycosides (other than streptomycin) are minimally protein bound (<20%) to plasma proteins. Aminoglycosides do not readily cross the blood-brain barrier nor penetrate ocular tissue. CSF levels are unpredictable and range from 0-50% those found in the serum. Therapeutic levels are found in bone, heart, gallbladder and lung tissues after parenteral dosing. Aminoglycosides tend to accumulate in certain tissues such as the inner ear and kidneys, which may help explain their toxicity. Aminoglycosides cross the placenta and fetal concentrations range from 15-50% those found in maternal serum.

Elimination of aminoglycosides after parenteral administration occurs almost entirely by glomerular filtration. Patients with decreased renal function can have significantly prolonged half-lives. In humans with normal renal function, elimination rates can be highly variable with the aminoglycoside antibiotics.

Contraindications/Precautions/Warnings

Aminoglycosides are contraindicated in patients who are hypersensitive to them. Because these drugs are often the only effective agents in severe gram-negative infections, there are no other absolute contraindications to their use; however, they should be used with extreme caution in patients with preexisting renal disease with concomitant monitoring and dosage interval adjustments made. Other risk factors for the development of toxicity include age (both neonatal and geriatric patients), fever, sepsis, and dehydration. Refer to the Monitoring section to see The International Renal Interest

Society (www.iris-kidney.com) recommendations to prevent aminoglycoside-induced acute kidney injury in dogs and cats.

Because aminoglycosides can cause irreversible ototoxicity, they should be used with caution in "working" dogs (e.g., "seeing-eye", herding, dogs for the hearing impaired, etc.).

Aminoglycosides should be used with caution in patients with neuromuscular disorders (e.g., myasthenia gravis) due to their neuromuscular blocking activity.

Because aminoglycosides are eliminated primarily through renal mechanisms, they should be used cautiously, preferably with serum monitoring and dosage adjustment in neonatal or geriatric animals.

Aminoglycosides are generally considered contraindicated in rabbits/hares as they adversely affect the GI flora balance in these animals.

Adverse Effects

The aminoglycosides are notorious for their nephrotoxic and ototoxic effects. The nephrotoxic (tubular necrosis) mechanisms of these drugs are not completely understood, but are probably related to interference with phospholipid metabolism in the lysosomes of proximal renal tubular cells, resulting in leakage of proteolytic enzymes into the cytoplasm. Nephrotoxicity normally manifests by increases in BUN, creatinine, nonprotein nitrogen in the serum and decreases in urine specific gravity and creatinine clearance. Proteinuria and cells or casts may also be seen in the urine. Nephrotoxicity is usually reversible once the drug is discontinued. While gentamicin may be more nephrotoxic than the other aminoglycosides, the incidences of nephrotoxicity with all of these agents require equal caution and monitoring.

Ototoxicity (8th cranial nerve toxicity) of the aminoglycosides can manifest with either auditory and/or vestibular clinical signs and may be irreversible. Vestibular clinical signs are more frequent with streptomycin, gentamicin, or tobramycin. Auditory clinical signs are more frequent with amikacin, neomycin, or kanamycin, but either form can occur with any of the drugs. Cats are apparently very sensitive to the vestibular effects of the aminoglycosides.

The aminoglycosides can also cause neuromuscular blockade, facial edema, pain or inflammation at the injection site, peripheral neuropathy, and hypersensitivity reactions. Rarely, GI clinical signs, hematologic, and hepatic effects have been reported.

Reproductive/Nursing Safety

Tobramycin can cross the placenta and concentrate in fetal kidneys and, while rare, cause 8th cranial nerve toxicity or nephrotoxicity in fetuses. Total irreversible deafness has been reported in some human babies whose mothers received tobramycin during pregnancy. Because the drug should only be used in serious infections, the benefits of therapy may exceed the potential risks. In humans, the FDA categorizes this drug as category *D* for use during pregnancy (*There is evidence of human fetal risk, but the potential benefits from the use of the drug in pregnant women may be acceptable despite its potential risks.*) In a separate system evaluating the safety of drugs in canine and feline pregnancy (Papich 1989), this drug is categorized as in class: *C* (*These drugs may have potential risks. Studies in people or laboratory animals have uncovered risks, and these drugs should be used cautiously as a last resort when the benefit of therapy clearly outweighs the risks.*)

Small amounts of aminoglycoside antibiotics are excreted in milk, but are unlikely to cause clinically significant effects in nursing offspring.

Overdosage/Acute Toxicity

Should an inadvertent overdosage be administered, three treatment options have been suggested: 1) Hemodialysis is very effective in reducing serum levels of the drug, but is not a viable option for most veterinary patients; 2) Peritoneal dialysis also will reduce serum levels, but is much less efficacious; 3) Complexation of drug with ticarcillin (12 – 20 grams/day in humans) is reportedly nearly as effective as hemodialysis.

Drug Interactions

The following drug interactions have either been reported or are theoretical in humans or animals receiving tobramycin and may be of significance in veterinary patients. Unless otherwise noted, use together is not necessarily contraindicated, but weigh the potential risks and perform additional monitoring when appropriate.

- **BETA-LACTAM ANTIBIOTICS** (e.g., **penicillins**, **cephalosporins**): May have synergistic effects against some bacteria; some potential for inactivation of aminoglycosides *in vitro* (do not mix together) and *in vivo* (patients in renal failure).
- **CEPHALOSPORINS**: The concurrent use of aminoglycosides with cephalosporins is somewhat controversial. Potentially, cephalosporins could cause additive nephrotoxicity when used with aminoglycosides, but this interaction has only been well documented with cephaloridine and cephalothin (both no longer marketed).
- **DIURETICS, LOOP** (e.g., **furosemide**, **torsemide**) or **OSMOTIC** (e.g., **mannitol**): Concurrent use with loop or osmotic diuretics may increase the nephrotoxic or ototoxic potential of the aminoglycosides.
- **NEPHROTOXIC DRUGS, OTHER** (e.g., **cisplatin**, **amphotericin B**, **polymyxin B**, or **vancomycin**): Potential for increased risk for nephrotoxicity.
- **NEUROMUSCULAR BLOCKING AGENTS & ANESTHETICS, GENERAL**: Concomitant use with general anesthetics or neuromuscular blocking agents could potentiate neuromuscular blockade.

Laboratory Considerations

- Tobramycin serum concentrations may be falsely decreased if the patient is also receiving **beta-lactam antibiotics** and the serum is stored prior analysis. It is recommended that if assay is delayed, samples be frozen and, if possible, drawn at times when the beta-lactam antibiotic is at a trough level.

Doses

Note: There is significant inter-patient variability with aminoglycoside pharmacokinetic parameters. To insure therapeutic levels and minimize the risks for toxicity, consider monitoring serum levels. Like other aminoglycosides, most now recommend dosing mammals once daily.

In the Monitoring section refer to *The International Renal Interest Society* (www.iris-kidney.com) recommendations to prevent aminoglycoside-induced acute kidney injury.

- **DOGS & CATS:**

  For susceptible infections (extra-label): <u>Dogs</u>: 9 – 14 mg/kg IV, IM or SC once daily. <u>Cats</u>: 5 – 8 mg/kg IV, IM or SC once daily.

- **HORSES:**

  For susceptible infections (extra-label): Based upon a pharmacokinetic study and MIC data, the authors concluded: 4 mg/kg IV once daily would effectively treat 70% of *E. coli*, 67% of *K. pneumonia*, and 95% of *P. aeruginosa* isolates. If the IM route is used, only 67% of *E. coli* isolates would be effectively treated. All isolates of *S. aureus* would have been susceptible to either dosing regimen. (**Note:** There were only a low number of isolates for *K. pneumonia*, *P. aeruginosa*, and *S. aureus*.) Tobramycin provides an alternative choice of aminoglycoside antibiotic for use in horses and while IM administration appears to be safe, it may not be practical due to the large volume necessary for injection. (Newman *et al.* 2013)

- **LLAMAS:**
  For susceptible infections (extra-label): 4 mg/kg IV q24h. (Baird 2003)
- **BIRDS:**
  For susceptible infections (extra-label):
  a) 5 mg/kg IM every 12 hours. (Bauck *et al.* 1993)
  b) 2.5 – 5 mg/kg/day; must be given parenterally. (Flammer 2003)
- **REPTILES:**
  For susceptible infections (extra-label): 2.5 mg/kg once daily IM. (Gauvin 1993)

Monitoring

- Efficacy (cultures, clinical signs associated with infection).
- Gross monitoring of vestibular or auditory toxicity is recommended.
- Serum levels if possible (see below).
- Nephrotoxicity (see below).

The following recommendations are from *The International Renal Interest Society* (www.iris-kidney.com) to prevent aminoglycoside-induced acute kidney injury (in dogs and cats).

Prior to aminoglycoside treatment:

- Consider carefully the potential risk factors: dehydration, concomitant treatment with furosemide, use of other nephrotoxic drugs, arterial hypotension, hypokalemia, previous history of AKI, pre-existing chronic kidney disease (CKD). When such factors are identified, alternatives to aminoglycoside-treatment should be considered.
- Perform urinalysis (measure urine specific gravity, examine for glycosuria, proteinuria [measure UP / C], abnormal sediment]. If abnormalities are detected, investigate carefully to determine the underlying cause before deciding whether to prescribe aminoglycosides.
- Blood tests: determine blood creatinine concentration, referring to IRIS guidelines for CKD (www.iris-kidney.com). Consider avoiding use of aminoglycosides if the blood creatinine concentration is at the borderline between Stage I and Stage II or already in Stage II. In borderline cases, further investigations might be considered to evaluate renal risk.
- Imaging: abdominal radiograph and/or ultrasonographic examination.
- Measurement of arterial blood pressure (High risk hypertension: systolic >180 mm/ Hg is indicative of renal damage and risk).

During the treatment:

- Assess the hydration status of the patient (body weight, total plasma protein concentration and hematocrit) once weekly.
- If therapeutic drug monitoring is available, ensure the plasma concentration of gentamicin or tobramycin has decreased to below 1 mg/L (1 mcg/mL) before the next dose is administered.
- Re-assess carefully the pre-treatment urine and blood variables indicated above.
- Repeat these assessments every 3-4 days to detect any change. If any doubt of renal damage, perform the GGT:creatinine ratio in the urine (when available in the laboratory); an increase is an early indicator of nephrotoxicity.
- Continue monitoring for 1 week after discontinuing the treatment as AKI may occur later (aminoglycosides accumulate inside proximal tubular cells and persist for long periods after dosing).
- The risk of nephrotoxicity increases with the duration of the treatment, as aminoglycoside nephrotoxicity is cumulative.

- If findings suggest development of AKI (urine: presence of renal casts in the sediment, glycosuria; low specific gravity; blood:azotemia): Immediately stop aminoglycoside therapy. Hospitalize the patient and monitor urine production. Non-oliguric AKI occurs generally and is reversible. Oliguric AKI has a poor prognosis. Start adequate intravenous fluid therapy. Monitor: urea, creatinine and electrolytes (hypokalemia is frequent in nonoliguric AKI and should be corrected).
- If AKI is worsening, consider renal substitutive therapy (hemodialysis). After apparent recovery from aminoglycoside-induced AKI, some dogs may remain renally impaired.

Client Information

- Tobramycin must be injected if used for treating serious infections. It does not work if giving it by mouth.
- Can damage the nerves, hearing, and kidneys. Cats may be more likely to have damage to hearing.
- Given once daily either in the vein (by veterinarian) or under the skin (SC, subcutaneous).
- Can be used topically (in the eye or ear, on skin) for certain infections.

Chemistry/Synonyms

An aminoglycoside derived from Streptomyces tenebrarius, tobramycin occurs as a white to off-white, hygroscopic powder that is freely soluble in water and very slightly soluble in alcohol. The sulfate salt is formed during the manufacturing process. The commercial injection is a clear, colorless solution and the pH is adjusted to 6-8 with sulfuric acid and/or sodium hydroxide.

Tobramycin Sulfate may also be known as: tobramycin sulphate, *Nebcin®, Nebcine®, Tobra®, or TOBI®*.

Storage/Stability

Tobramycin sulfate for injection should be stored at room temperature (15-30°C); avoid freezing and temperatures above 40°C. Do not use the product if discolored.

Compatibility/Compounding Considerations

While the manufacturers state that tobramycin should not be mixed with other drugs, it is reportedly physically **compatible** and stable in most commonly used intravenous solutions (**NOT compatible** with dextrose and alcohol solutions, Polysal, Polysal M, or Isolyte E, M or P) and **compatible** with the following drugs: aztreonam, bleomycin sulfate, calcium gluconate, cefoxitin sodium, ciprofloxacin lactate, clindamycin phosphate (not in syringes), metronidazole (with or without sodium bicarbonate), ranitidine HCl, and verapamil HCl.

The following drugs or solutions are reportedly physically **incompatible** or only compatible in specific situations with tobramycin: furosemide and heparin sodium. Compatibility is dependent upon factors such as pH, concentration, temperature, and diluent used; consult specialized references or a hospital pharmacist for more specific information.

In vitro inactivation of aminoglycoside antibiotics by beta-lactam antibiotics is well documented; see the information in the Drug Interaction and Laboratory Consideration sections.

Dosage Forms/Regulatory Status

VETERINARY-LABELED PRODUCTS: NONE.

HUMAN-LABELED PRODUCTS:
Tobramycin Sulfate Injection: 0.8 mg/mL and 1.2 mg/mL (as sulfate) in 0.9% sodium chloride in 100 mL & 50 mL (respectively) single-dose containers; (Rx)

Tobramycin Solution for Injection: 10 mg/mL, 40 mg/mL & 80 mg/mL in vials; generic; (Rx)

Tobramycin Sulfate Powder for Injection: 1.2 grams (40 mg/mL after reconstitution), preservative free in 50 mL bulk package vial; generic; (Rx)

Tobramycin Solution for inhalation: 300 mg/4 mL or 5 mL; *TOBI®*, *Bethkis®*, generic; (Rx)

Also available in ophthalmic preparations and powder (capsule) for inhalation.

Revisions/References

Monograph revised/updated August 2014.

Baird, N. (2003). Antibiotic use in camelids. Proceedings: Western Veterinary Conference. accessed via Veterinary Information Network; vin.com

Bauck, L. & H. Hoefer (1993). Avian antimicrobial therapy. Seminars in Avian & Exotic Med 2(1): 17-22.

Flammer, K. (2003). Antimicrobic selection criteria in avian medicine. Proceedings: Western Veterinary Conf. accessed via Veterinary Information Network; vin.com

Gauvin, J. (1993). Drug therapy in reptiles. Seminars in Avian & Exotic Med 2(1): 48-59.

Haritova, A., et al. (2012). Population Pharmacokinetics of Tobramycin in Horses. Journal of Equine Veterinary Science 32(9): 531-5.

Hubenov, H., et al. (2007). Pharmacokinetic studies on tobramycin in horses. J. Vet. Pharmacol. Ther. 30(4): 353-7.

Newman, J. C., et al. (2013). Pharmacokinetics of tobramycin following intravenous, intramuscular, and intra-articular administration in healthy horses. J. Vet. Pharmacol. Ther. 36(6): 532-41.

Papich, M. (1989). Effects of drugs on pregnancy. *Current Veterinary Therapy X: Small Animal Practice.* R. Kirk. Philadelphia, Saunders: 1291-9.

Toceranib Phosphate

(toe-ser-a-nib)   Palladia®

Tyrosine Kinase Inhibitor Antineoplastic

Prescriber Highlights

▶ Tyrosine kinase inhibitor FDA-approved for grades II or III canine mast cell tumors.

▶ Most common adverse effects are: diarrhea, decreased/loss of appetite, lameness, weight loss and blood in the stool.

▶ Adverse effects can be serious and require treatment pause or dose reduction.

▶ Monitoring essential.

Uses/Indications

Toceranib is indicated for the treatment of Patnaik grade II or III, recurrent, cutaneous mast cell tumors with or without regional lymph node involvement in dogs.

Toceranib may prove useful for treating a variety of tumors in dogs, including sarcomas, carcinomas, melanomas, and myeloma. Toceranib as part of metronomic therapy (using low doses of chemotherapy) and/or combined with radiation therapy, and in combination with other anti-cancer agents such as vinblastine (Robat et al. 2012), cyclophosphamide (Mitchell et al. 2012), carboplatin (de Vos et al. 2012), lomustine (CCNU), piroxicam (Chon et al. 2012), prednisone, and calcitriol (Malone et al. 2010) are being investigated.

Preliminary data suggest that toceranib may have biological activity against feline squamous cell carcinomas, injection site sarcomas or mast cell tumors, and MCT. Additional clinical studies are necessary to define its safety in cast and efficacy.

Pharmacology/Actions

Toceranib is a small molecule tyrosine kinase inhibitor (TKIs) that selectively inhibits the tyrosine kinase activity of several split kinase receptor tyrosine kinases (RTK), including VEGFR-2 (vascular endothelial growth factor receptor-2), PDGFR-Beta (platelet-derived growth factor receptor-Beta), Kit (stem cell growth factor receptor), among others. These kinases are believed to be involved in growth, pathologic angiogenesis, and metastatic processes of certain tumors. By inhibiting TKIs, toceranib competitively inhibits ATP,

preventing receptor phosphorylation and subsequent downstream signal transduction. Toceranib exerts an antiproliferative effect on endothelial cells (*in vitro*) and can induce cell cycle arrest and subsequent apoptosis in tumor cell lines expressing activating mutations in Kit. As canine mast cell tumor growth can be enhanced by activating mutations in Kit, toceranib inhibition can reduce angiogenesis and subsequent growth of these cells.

Calcitriol may enhance the antiproliferative activity of toceranib in dogs with mast cell tumors and investigations exploring this potential are ongoing (Malone et al. 2010).

Pharmacokinetics

Oral bioavailability of toceranib phosphate in dogs is ≈ 77%. The presence of food does not significantly impact absorption. Binding to canine plasma proteins is ≈ 94% and the volume of distribution is very large (>20 L/kg). Terminal elimination half-life is ≈ 17 hours (after IV) and 31 hours (oral). While the metabolic fate of toceranib has not been completely determined, it appears that the drug is metabolized via cytochrome P450 and/or flavin monooxygenase to an N-oxide metabolite. (Yancey et al. 2010a; Yancey et al. 2010b)

A study evaluating toceranib peak plasma levels after lower doses (2.5 – 2.75 mg/kg PO every other day) resulted in an average 6-8 hour post-dose plasma concentration ranging from 100-120 ng/mL. These were significantly above the 40 ng/mL concentration that is associated with target inhibition, and the adverse event profile was substantially reduced from the one associated with the labeled dose (3.25 mg/kg every other day). The authors concluded that lower dose range of toceranib should be considered for future use in dogs with cancer (Bernabe et al. 2013).

Contraindications/Precautions/Warnings

The label lists toceranib contraindications as breeding, pregnant or lactating bitches. Safe use has not been evaluated in dogs less than 24 months of age or weighing <5 kg. Because toceranib can cause vascular dysfunction leading to edema and thromboembolism (including pulmonary emboli), wait at least 3 days after stopping the drug before performing surgery.

Use caution when handling this medication. See the product's *Client Information Sheet* for more details.

When toceranib is used in the presence of systemic mast cell tumors, significant mast cell degranulation with resultant adverse effects may result. The manufacturer states that attempts should be made to rule out systemic mastocytosis prior to starting toceranib.

Toceranib can cause clinical signs similar to those seen with aggressive mast cell tumors, when these occur, the drug should be stopped and the patient re-evaluated (Johannes 2010). The package insert has specific monitoring requirements with dosage adjustment or therapy pause guidelines when certain adverse effects (severe diarrhea, GI bleeding) occur or when laboratory monitoring indicates toxicity. Refer to the Monitoring section below, or the package insert for more information.

Adverse Effects

Most common adverse effects seen with toceranib in dogs include: diarrhea, decreased/loss of appetite, lameness, weight loss and blood in the stool. Severe diarrhea or GI bleeding require immediate treatment and dictate dose interruption or reduction (see monitoring below). Other potential adverse effects include muscle cramping/pain, neutropenia, hypoalbuminemia, thromboembolic disease, vasculitis, pancreatitis, nasal depigmentation, change in coat or skin color, epistaxis, seizures and pruritus. A recent retrospective study in 20 dogs found that the majority of toceranib-treated dogs had increases in systolic blood pressure (Markovic et al. 2013).

One source (London 2010) suggests starting certain drugs 4-7 days prior to staring toceranib to reduce the likelihood of toxicity, including antacids (*e.g.*, famotidine, omeprazole), an antihistamine (*e.g.*, diphenhydramine), prednisone (to reduce tumor inflammation and possibly decrease mast cell tumor mediators' effects), and sucralfate (if dog has a positive stool hemoccult). Additionally, in dogs that experience inappetence or vomiting after therapy has begun, administration of metoclopramide, ondansetron, or maropitant may be effective. Loperamide can be given on toceranib dosing days to help prevent or lessen diarrhea; others have found metronidazole useful. Another author states that prednisone can be continued after treatment has begun, but should only given on days when toceranib is not given and that NSAIDs and prednisone should never be used together (Garrett 2010).

In the small number of cats that have received toceranib, reported adverse effects include gastrointestinal toxicity, neutropenia and alopecia.

Reproductive/Nursing Safety

Toceranib is a likely teratogen and should not be used in pregnant females. It is labeled as contraindicated in breeding, pregnant, or lactating bitches.

Overdosage/Acute Toxicity

No acute toxicity data was located, but toceranib has a narrow margin of safety. In the event of an acute overdose, consider immediate gut decontamination; contact an animal poison center for further guidance.

Drug Interactions

The following drug interactions have either been reported or are theoretical in humans or animals receiving toceranib and may be of significance in veterinary patients. Unless otherwise noted, use together is not necessarily contraindicated, but weigh the potential risks and perform additional monitoring when appropriate.

- **CALCITRIOL:** An *in vitro* study found that calcitriol had synergist effects with toceranib against canine C2 mastocytoma cells. Authors concluded that calcitriol combination therapies might have significant clinical utility in the treatment of canine mast cell tumors but refinement of the calcitriol-dosing regimen must be carried out. (Malone *et al.* 2010)

- **NSAIDS:** The package insert states to use NSAIDs with caution in conjunction with toceranib due to an increased risk of gastrointestinal ulceration or perforation. While NSAIDs (*e.g.*, piroxicam) are sometimes used with toceranib as part of metronomic drug protocols, they should never be given on the same day as toceranib as GI toxicity can be exacerbated (London 2010).

- **CYP3A4 INHIBITORS** (*e.g.*, ketoconazole, fluconazole, itraconazole, grapefruit juice, clarithromycin, verapamil): May increase toceranib concentrations. This interaction with toceranib has not been documented in dogs to date and presently is speculative, however, use caution.

Laboratory Considerations

- None noted.

Doses

Note: There is a significant amount of ongoing research evaluating toceranib for use with other drugs, other species, and for extra-label indications and since chemotherapy indications, treatment protocols, monitoring and safety guidelines often change, the following dosages should be used only as a general guide. Consultation with a veterinary oncologist and referral to current veterinary oncology references [*e.g.*, (Withrow *et al.* 2012); (Dobson *et al.* 2011); (Henry *et al.* 2009); (North *et al.* 2009); (Argyle *et al.* 2008)] are strongly recommended.

- **DOGS:**

  For Patnaik grade II or III, recurrent, cutaneous mast cell tumors with or without regional lymph node involvement (labeled-dose; FDA-approved): Initial dose 3.25 mg/kg PO every other day (q48h). Dose reductions of 0.5 mg/kg (to a minimum dose of 2.2 mg/kg) every other day and dose interruptions (cessation of treatment) for up to 2 weeks may be utilized, if needed, to manage adverse reactions. May be administered with or without food. Do not split tablets. The package insert has a dosage table to determine the appropriate strength and number of tablets to use for a given dog's weight. (Adapted from label information; *Palladia®*)

  Extra-label Doses:

  a) **Lower than labeled dose:** Recent clinical experience with toceranib in dogs suggests that dosing at 2.5 - 2.75 mg/kg every other day is better tolerated than the higher dose, resulting in less toxicity, better owner compliance, and fewer drug holidays. Some dogs do not tolerate this dosing regimen even at the 2.5 mg/kg dose rate. The author and some other medical oncologists have found that a M/W/F schedule of dosing may be better tolerated by some dogs. This may be particularly useful when toceranib is combined with other drugs, such as cyclophosphamide or NSAIDs as part of a metronomic treatment protocol. When a dog cannot tolerate the M/W/F schedule, every third day dosing may be attempted, but this is not ideal and may result in sub-therapeutic drug exposure. (London 2010)

  b) **In combination with piroxicam:** A small, phase-I study concluded that toceranib at labeled dosage combined with piroxicam (0.3 mg/kg PO once daily) was generally safe, but that as with the labeled dosage, GI adverse effects may occasionally require treatment holidays and toceranib dosage reduction (Chon *et al.* 2012). However, at present, it is now recommended to administer piroxicam every other day (alternating with toceranib) to avoid GI effects (London 2013).

Monitoring

- CBC, Hematocrit, Serum Albumin, Creatinine, Serum Phosphate. Manufacturer recommends weekly (approximately) veterinary assessment for the first 6 weeks of therapy and approximately every 6 weeks thereafter. The package insert states: Temporarily discontinue drug if anemia, azotemia, hypoalbuminemia, and hyperphosphatemia occur simultaneously. Resume treatment at a dose reduction of 0.5 mg/kg after 1-2 weeks when values have improved and albumin is >2.5 g/dL. Temporary treatment interruptions may be needed if any one of these occurs alone: hematocrit <26%, creatinine ≥2 mg/dL or albumin <1.5 g/dL. Then resume treatment at a dose reduction of 0.5 mg/kg once the hematocrit is >30%, the creatinine is <2.0 mg/dL, and the albumin is >2.5 g/dL. Temporarily discontinue the use of toceranib if neutrophil count is ≤1000/microL. Resume treatment after 1-2 weeks at a dose reduction of 0.5 mg/kg, when neutrophil count has returned to >1000/microL. Further dose reductions may be needed if severe neutropenia reoccurs.

- Other laboratory tests that have been suggested for monitoring early (first 6 weeks) include urinalysis and full chemistry panels.

- Adverse Effects (Diarrhea): If ≥4 watery stools/day or diarrhea persists for 2 days, stop drug and institute supportive care until formed stools recur. When dosing is resumed, decrease dose by 0.5 mg/kg.

- Adverse Effects (GI-Bleeding): If fresh blood in stool or black tarry stool for >2 days or frank hemorrhage or blood clots in stool. Stop drug and institute supportive care until resolution of all clinical signs of blood in stool, then decrease dose by 0.5 mg/kg.

- Blood pressure. (Markovic *et al.* 2013)

- Tumor Size.

Client Information

- In the package insert, the manufacturer states to: "Always provide *Client Information Sheet* with prescription." In addition, it is highly recommended to verbally reiterate some of the key points found on the client information sheet, including the sections: "How do I give *Palladia*™ to my dog?"; "Stop *Palladia*™ immediately and contact your veterinarian if you notice any of the following changes in your dog"; and "Handling Instructions".

- May be given with or without food; do not split or crush tablets.

- Toceranib is a chemotherapy (cancer) drug. The drug and its byproducts can be hazardous to other animals and people that come in contact with it. On the day your animal gets the drug and then for a few days afterward, all bodily waste (urine, feces, litter), blood, or vomit should only be handled while wearing disposable gloves. Seal the waste in a plastic bag and then place both the bag and gloves in with the regular trash.

Chemistry/Synonyms

Toceranib phosphate is an idolinone with a molecular weight of 494.46. Toceranib may also be known as: PHA-291639, SU-11654, UNII-59L7Y0530C, toceranibum, or tocéranib.

Storage/Stability

Toceranib phosphate tablets should be stored at controlled room temperature 20-25°C (68-77°F).

Compatibility/Compounding Considerations

No specific information noted.

Dosage Forms/Regulatory Status

VETERINARY-LABELED PRODUCTS:

Toceranib Phosphate Oral Tablets: 10 mg, 15 mg, 50 mg; *Palladia*®; (Rx)

HUMAN-LABELED PRODUCTS: NONE.

Revisions/References

Monograph revised/updated August 2014.

Argyle, D., et al. (2008). *Decision Making in Small Animal Oncology*, Wiley-Blackwell.

Bernabe, L. F., et al. (2013). Evaluation of the adverse event profile and pharmacodynamics of toceranib phosphate administered to dogs with solid tumors at doses below the maximum tolerated dose. Bmc Veterinary Research **9**.

Chon, E., et al. (2012). Safety evaluation of combination toceranib phosphate (Palladia (R)) and piroxicam in tumour-bearing dogs (excluding mast cell tumours): a phase I dose-finding study. Veterinary and Comparative Oncology **10**(3): 184-93.

de Vos, J., et al. (2012). Primary frontal sinus squamous cell carcinoma in three dogs treated with piroxicam combined with carboplatin or toceranib. Veterinary and Comparative Oncology **10**(3): 206-13.

Dobson, J. & D. Lascelles (2011). *BSAVA Manual of Canine and Feline Oncology*, BSAVA.

Garrett, L. (2010). New Therapies for Cancer: The Role of Tyrosine Kinase Inhibitors in Practice. Proceedings: WVC. accessed via Veterinary Information Network; vin.com

Henry, C. & M. Higginbotham (2009). *Cancer Management in Small Animal Practice*, Saunders.

Johannes, C. (2010). Toceranib Phosphate (PalladiaTM): A New Treatment Option for Canine MCT. Proceedings: ACVIM. accessed via Veterinary Information Network; vin.com

London, C. A. (2010). Tyrosine Kinase Inhibitor (TKI) Therapy in Companion Animals: Year One. Proceedings: ACVIM. accessed via Veterinary Information Network; vin.com

London, C. A. (2013). Kinase dysfunction and kinase inhibitors. Veterinary Dermatology **24**(1): 181-+.

Malone, E. K., et al. (2010). Calcitriol (1,25-dihydroxycholecalciferol) enhances mast cell tumour chemotherapy and receptor tyrosine kinase inhibitor activity in vitro and has single-agent activity against spontaneously occurring canine mast cell tumours. Veterinary and Comparative Oncology **8**(3): 209-20.

Markovic, L. E. & R. L. Stepien (2013). Development of systemic hypertension after administration of toceranib phosphate (Palladia®) in dogs (2010-2012) [abstract]. Journal of Veterinary Internal Medicine **27**(3): 637-8.

Mitchell, L., et al. (2012). Clinical and Immunomodulatory Effects of Toceranib Combined with Low-Dose Cyclophosphamide in Dogs with Cancer. Journal of Veterinary Internal Medicine **26**(2): 355-62.

North, S. & T. Banks (2009). *Small Animal Oncology: An Introduction*, Saunders.

Robat, C., et al. (2012). Safety evaluation of combination vinblastine and toceranib phosphate (Palladia (R)) in dogs: a phase I dose-finding study. Veterinary and Comparative Oncology **10**(3): 174-83.

Withrow, S., et al. (2012). Withrow and MacEwen's Small Animal Clinical Oncology, 5th Ed., Saunders.

Yancey, M. F., et al. (2010a). Pharmacokinetic properties of toceranib phosphate (Palladia™, SU11654), a novel tyrosine kinase inhibitor, in laboratory dogs and dogs with mast cell tumors. J. Vet. Pharmacol. Ther. **33**(2): 162-71.

Yancey, M. F., et al. (2010b). Distribution, metabolism, and excretion of toceranib phosphate (Palladia (TM), SU11654), a novel tyrosine kinase inhibitor, in dogs. J. Vet. Pharmacol. Ther. **33**(2): 154-61.

Tolazoline HCl

(toe-laz-oh-leen)   Tolazine®

Alpha-Adrenergic Blocker

Prescriber Highlights

▶ Alpha-adrenergic blocker used primarily as a reversal agent for xylazine. Reversal effects may be partial and transitory.

▶ Contraindications: Horses exhibiting signs of stress, debilitation, cardiac disease, sympathetic blockage, hypovolemia or shock, hypersensitivity, or with coronary artery or cerebrovascular disease.

▶ Adverse Effects: **Horses:** Transient tachycardia; peripheral vasodilatation presenting as sweating & injected mucous membranes of the gingiva & conjunctiva; hyperalgesia of the lips (licking, flipping of lips); piloerection; clear lacrimal & nasal discharge; muscle fasciculations; apprehensiveness.

Uses/Indications

Tolazoline is FDA-approved and indicated for the reversal of effects associated with xylazine in horses. It has also been used for this purpose in a variety of other species as well, but less safety and efficacy data is available.

In humans, the primary uses for tolazoline are: treatment of persistent pulmonary hypertension in newborns, adjunctive treatment and diagnosis of peripheral vasospastic disorders, and as a provocative test for glaucoma after subconjunctival injection.

Pharmacology/Actions

By directly relaxing vascular smooth muscle, tolazoline has peripheral vasodilating effects and decreases total peripheral resistance. Tolazoline also is a competitive alpha$_1$ and alpha$_2$-adrenergic blocking agent helping explain its mechanism for reversing the effects of xylazine. Tolazoline is rapid acting (usually within 5 minutes of IV administration), but may not fully reverse effects on sedation, and heart rate and rhythm. It has a short duration of action; repeat doses may be required. A study in horses after SL detomidine, tolazoline's (4 mg/kg IV) effects on detomidine-induced changes in chin-to-ground distance were minimal and effects on detomidine-induced changes in heart rate and rhythm only persisted for 15-20 minutes (Knych *et al.* 2014).

After doses of 4 mg/kg IV in horses, average heart rate decreased beginning 2 minutes post-dose, with heart rate nadir at 45 minutes. No apparent effect on chin-to-ground distance was noted. PCV significantly increased in all horses throughout the times sampled with the maximal change at 15 minutes. Serum glucose concentrations increased significantly in all horses at the first time point measured through 1.5 hours post-dose. (Casbeer *et al.* 2013)

Pharmacokinetics

After a single IV injection (4 mg/kg) in 6 horses, tolazoline had a mean volume of distribution (steady-state) of 1.68 L/kg, a clearance (mean) of 0.757 L/hr/kg and an elimination half-life 2.08 hours (Casbeer *et al.* 2013). In a subsequent study after horses (n=9) were first given detomidine sublingually (0.04 mg/kg), then tolazoline (4 mg/kg IV 1-hour later), mean tolazoline pharmacokinetic values included: volume of distribution (steady-state) of 1.9 L/kg, a clearance of 11.2 mL/min/kg and an elimination half-life of 3.51 hours (Knych *et al.* 2014). An older pre-approval study done in ponies reported the elimination half-life as ≈ 1 hour (Anon 1996).

Animal studies have demonstrated that tolazoline is concentrated in the liver and kidneys.

Contraindications/Precautions/Warnings

The manufacturer does not recommend use in horses exhibiting signs of stress, debilitation, cardiac disease, sympathetic blockage, hypovolemia, or shock. Safe use for foals has not been established and some believe it should not be used in foals as adverse reactions and fatalities have been reported.

Tolazoline should be considered contraindicated in patients known to be hypersensitive to it, or with coronary artery or cerebrovascular disease. Humans having any of the above-contraindicated conditions should use extra caution when handling the agent.

Adverse Effects

In horses, adverse effects that may occur include: transient tachycardia; peripheral vasodilatation presenting as sweating and injected mucous membranes of the gingiva and conjunctiva; hyperalgesia of the lips (licking, flipping of lips); piloerection; clear lacrimal and nasal discharge; muscle fasciculations; apprehensiveness. Adverse effects should diminish with time and generally disappear within 2 hours of dosing. The potential for adverse effects increases if tolazoline is given at higher than recommended dosages or if xylazine has not be previously administered.

Ruminants and camelids appear to be more sensitive to tolazoline's effects than horses. In cattle, 1.5 mg/kg IV can cause coughing, increased frequency of defecation, and mild increases in breathing effort. At higher doses (2 – 10 mg/kg IV), bright red conjunctival mucous membranes, coughing, nasal discharge, salivation, labored breathing, CNS depression, signs of abdominal pain, straining, head pressing, restlessness, and severe diarrhea can be observed. Rapid IV injection has been reported to cause significant cardiac stimulation, tachycardia, increased cardiac output, vasodilation, and gastrointestinal distress.

Reproductive/Nursing Safety

Safety during pregnancy, in breeding or lactating animals has not been established. It is unknown if the drug enters maternal milk.

Overdosage/Acute Toxicity

In horses given tolazoline alone (no previous xylazine), doses of 5X recommended resulted in gastrointestinal hypermotility with resultant flatulence and defecation or attempt to defecate. Some horses exhibited mild colic and transient diarrhea. Intraventricular conduction may be slowed when horses are overdosed, with a prolongation of the QRS-complex noted. Ventricular arrhythmias may occur resulting in death with higher overdoses (5X). In humans, ephedrine (**NOT** epinephrine or norepinephrine) has been recommended to treat serious tolazoline-induced hypotension.

A llama that received 4.3 mg/kg IV and again 45 minutes later (≈ 5X overdose) developed signs of anxiety, hyperesthesia, profuse salivation, GI tract hypermotility, diarrhea, convulsions, hypotension, and tachypnea. Treatment including IV diazepam, phenylephrine, IV fluids, and oxygen was successful. (Reed *et al.* 2000).

8 mg/kg IV has reportedly caused a fatality in a sheep.

Drug Interactions

The following drug interactions have either been reported or are theoretical in humans or animals receiving tolazoline and may be of significance in veterinary patients. Unless otherwise noted, use together is not necessarily contraindicated, but weigh the potential risks and perform additional monitoring when appropriate.

- **ALCOHOL:** Accumulation of acetaldehyde can occur if tolazoline and alcohol are given simultaneously.
- **EPINEPHRINE, NOREPINEPHRINE:** If large doses of tolazoline are given with either norepinephrine or epinephrine, a paradoxical drop in blood pressure can occur followed by a precipitous increase in blood pressure.

Doses

- **HORSES:**

  For reversal of xylazine effects (labeled dose; FDA-approved): 4 mg/kg slow IV (4 mL/220 lb. of body weight); administration rate should approximate 1 mL/second. (Package Insert; *Tolazine*®)

- **DOGS/CATS:**

  For reversal of xylazine effects (extra label in USA): 4 mg/kg slow IV (4 mL/220 lb. of body weight); administration rate should approximate 1 mL/second. (Package Insert; *Tolazine*®—Lloyd Laboratories; New Zealand) **Warning:** If reversal is warranted, the high concentration (100 mg/mL) of the veterinary drug may make accurate dosing difficult. Tolazoline is not FDA-approved for use in dogs or cats and the US manufacturer does not recommend its use.

- **RUMINANTS:**

  Note: Not FDA-approved for cattle, sheep or goats. FARAD recommends a meat withdrawal interval of 8 days when tolazoline is given IV at doses between 2 – 4 mg/kg in cattle and a milk withdrawal in dairy cattle of 48 hours. (Smith 2013)

  For reversal of alpha-2 agonists (extra-label in USA): 0.5 – 1.5 mg/kg IV. Today, these lower dosages are now recommended for use in all ruminants including camelids. Others have suggested that IV administration of tolazoline should be avoided, except in emergency situations, to prevent adverse effects such as cardiac asystole. (Lin 2012)

- **CAMELIDS (NWC):**

  For reversal of alpha-2 agonists (extra-label):
  a) The preferred reversal agent for xylazine is tolazoline at 1 – 2 mg/kg IM or SC. IV administration (especially the labeled dose—4 mg/kg) should be avoided as adverse reactions have occurred. (Anderson 2013)
  b) 0.5 – 1.5 mg/kg IV. Today, these lower dosages are now recommended for use in all ruminants including camelids. Others have suggested that IV administration of tolazoline should be avoided, except in emergency situations, to prevent adverse effects such as cardiac asystole. (Lin 2012)

- **BIRDS:**

  As a reversal agent for alpha2-adrenergic agonists (*e.g.*, xylazine, detomidine, etc.); (extra-label): 15 mg/kg IV. (Clyde *et al.* 2000)

- **DEER:**

  Note: Not FDA-approved in the USA for use in food animals.

  For reversal of xylazine effects (extra-label in USA):
  a) 2 – 4 mg/kg slow IV; titrate to effect. Slaughter withdrawal: 30 days. (Label Directions; *Tolazine*®—Lloyd Laboratories; New Zealand)
  b) 2 – 4 mg/kg; 50% of dose given IV, 50% given IM. (Jensen 2011)

Monitoring

- Reversal effects (efficacy).
- Adverse effects (see above).

Client Information

- Because of the risks associated with the use of xylazine and reversal by tolazoline, these drugs should be administered and monitored by veterinary professionals only.

Chemistry/Synonyms

An alpha-adrenergic blocking agent, tolazoline HCl is structurally related to phentolamine. It occurs as a white to off-white, crystalline powder possessing a bitter taste and a slight aromatic odor. Tolazoline is freely soluble in ethanol or water. The commercially available (human) injection has pH between 3-4.

Tolazoline HCl may also be known as: benzazoline hydrochloride, tolazolinium chloratum, *Priscol®, Priscoline®, Tolazine®* or *Vaso-Dilatan®*.

Storage/Stability

Commercially available injection products should be stored between 15-30°C and protected from light.

Compatibility/Compounding Considerations

The drug is reportedly physically **compatible** with the commonly used IV solutions.

Dosage Forms/Regulatory Status

VETERINARY-LABELED PRODUCTS:

Tolazoline HCl Injection: 100 mg/mL in 100 mL multi-dose vials; *Tolazine®*; (Rx). FDA-approved for use in horses; not to be used in food-producing animals.

HUMAN-LABELED PRODUCTS: NONE.

Revisions/References

Monograph revised/updated August 2014.

Anderson, D. E. (2013). Handling, Restraint and Field Anesthesia of Camelids. Proceedings: Western Veterinary Conf. accessed via Veterinary Information Network; vin.com

Anon (1996). FOIA Drug Summary: NADA 140-994 Tolazine™Injection - original approval, FDA; Lloyd, Inc.

Casbeer, C. & H. K. Knych (2013). Pharmacokinetics and pharmacodynamic effects of tolazoline following intravenous administration to horses. Veterinary Journal **196**(3): 504-9.

Clyde, V. & J. Paul-Murphy (2000). Avian Analgesia. *Kirk's Current Veterinary Therapy: XIII Small Animal Practice*. J. Bonagura. Philadelphia, WB Saunders: 1126-8.

Jensen, J. (2011). Special Medical Considerations Related To Deer Production. Proceedings: ACVIM. accessed via Veterinary Information Network; vin.com

Knych, H. K. & S. D. Stanley (2014). Effects of three antagonists on selected pharmacodynamic effects of sublingually administered detomidine in the horse. Veterinary Anaesthesia and Analgesia **41**(1): 36-47.

Lin, H.-C. (2012). Large Ruminants Anesthesia: Review and Update. Western Veterinary Conference. accessed via Veterinary Information Network; vin.com

Reed, M., et al. (2000). Suspected tolazoline toxicosis in a llama. J AM Vet Med Assoc **216**: 227-9.

Smith, G. (2013). Extralabel Use of Anesthetic and Analgesic Compounds in Cattle. Veterinary Clinics of North America-Food Animal Practice **29**(1): 29-+.

Tolfenamic Acid

(tole-fen-a-mik)   Tolfedine®

Nonsteroidal Antiinflammatory Agent

Prescriber Highlights

▶ Oral and injectable NSAID approved in various countries for dogs, cats and cattle. No approved products in USA.

▶ Relatively safe for short-term use.

Uses/Indications

Tolfenamic acid may be useful for the treatment of acute or chronic pain and/or inflammation in dogs and acute pain/inflammation in cats. In some countries is also approved for use in cattle. Refer to the product label for approved products for further information.

Pharmacology/Actions

Tolfenamic acid exhibits pharmacologic actions similar to those of aspirin. It is a potent inhibitor of cyclooxygenase, thereby inhibiting the release of prostaglandins. It also has direct inhibition of prostaglandin receptors. Tolfenamic acid has significant anti-thromboxane activity and is not recommended for use pre-surgically because of its effects on platelet function.

Pharmacokinetics

Tolfenamic acid is absorbed after oral administration. In dogs, peak levels occur from 2-4 hours after dosing. Enterohepatic recirculation is increased if given with food. This can increase the bioavailability, but also creates more variability in bioavailability than when given to fasted dogs. The volume of distribution in

dogs is reported to be 1.2 L/kg and it has an elimination half-life of ≈ 6.5 hours. Duration of antiinflammatory effect is 24-36 hours. Dogs with experimentally induced renal failure had significantly increased clearances of the drug presumably via increasing hepatic metabolism or enterohepatic recycling of tolfenamic acid (Lefebvre et al. 1997).

Contraindications/Precautions/Warnings

Tolfenamic acid is contraindicated in animals hypersensitive to it or to other drugs in its class (*i.e.*, meclofenamic acid). Like other NSAIDs, it should not be used in animals with active GI bleeding or ulceration. Use with caution in patients with decreased renal or hepatic function.

Adverse Effects

Tolfenamic acid is relatively safe when given as recommended in dogs and cats. Vomiting and diarrhea have been reported after oral use. Experimental studies did not demonstrate significant renal or GI toxicity until doses were more than 10X labeled. Potentially, long-term use could cause renal failure, especially in cats. However one small (n=7) study where healthy cats received 4 mg/kg PO once daily for 14 days, did not find significant changes in renal scintigraphy or biochemical profiles when compared to baseline (Khwanjai et al. 2012).

Because of its anti-thromboxane activity and resultant effects on platelet function, tolfenamic acid is not recommended for use pre-surgically.

Reproductive/Nursing Safety

No specific information was located; like other NSAIDs, tolfenamic acid should be used with caution in pregnancy.

Overdosage/Acute Toxicity

No specific information was located. It is suggested that if an acute overdose occurs treatment follows standard overdose procedures (empty gut following oral ingestion, etc.). Supportive treatment should be instituted as necessary and IV diazepam used to help control seizures. Monitor for GI bleeding. Because tolfenamic acid may cause renal effects, monitor electrolyte and fluid balance carefully and manage renal failure using established guidelines.

Drug Interactions

The following drug interactions have either been reported or are theoretical in humans or animals receiving tolfenamic acid or other NSAIDs and may be of significance in veterinary patients. Unless otherwise noted, use together is not necessarily contraindicated, but weigh the potential risks and perform additional monitoring when appropriate.

- **ASPIRIN**: May increase the risk of gastrointestinal toxicity (*e.g.*, ulceration, bleeding, vomiting, diarrhea).
- **CORTICOSTEROIDS**: As concomitant corticosteroid therapy may increase the occurrence of gastric ulceration, avoid the use of these drugs when also using tolfenamic acid.
- **DIGOXIN**: NSAIDS may increase serum levels.
- **FLUCONAZOLE**: Administration has increased plasma levels of celecoxib in humans and potentially could also affect tolfenamic acid levels in dogs.
- **FUROSEMIDE**: NSAIDs may reduce saluretic and diuretic effects.
- **METHOTREXATE**: Serious toxicity has occurred when NSAIDs have been used concomitantly with methotrexate; use together with extreme caution.
- **NEPHROTOXIC DRUGS** (*e.g.*, **furosemide, aminoglycosides, amphotericin B**, etc.): May enhance the risk of nephrotoxicity.
- **NSAIDS, OTHER**: May increase the risk of gastrointestinal toxicity (*e.g.*, ulceration, bleeding, vomiting, diarrhea).
- **WARFARIN**: Closely monitor patients also receiving drugs that

are highly bound to plasma proteins (*e.g.,* warfarin), as tolfenamic acid and its active metabolite are 98-99% protein bound in the dog.

Doses

- **DOGS:**

  As an NSAID (extra-label in USA):

  a) For acute pain: 4 mg/kg once daily SC, IM or PO for 3-5 days. For chronic pain: 4 mg/kg, PO once daily for 3-5 consecutive days per week. The injectable is suggested for the first dose only. (Dowling 2000)

  b) First dose: 4 mg/kg SC or IM; follow with tablets at 4 mg/kg PO once daily for 2-4 days. The treatment may be repeated once a week as required, or as recommended by the veterinarian, PO once daily for 3-5 days. (Label information; *Tolfedine*®—Vetoquinol Canada)

- **CATS:**

  For acute pain (extra-label in USA): 4 mg/kg once daily SC, IM or PO for 3-5 days. The injectable is suggested for the first dose only. (Dowling 2000)

  For adjunctive treatment of upper respiratory disease in association with antimicrobial therapy (injectable) or for treatment of febrile syndromes (oral); (extra-label in USA): 4 mg/kg SC or PO (with food) once a day for 3 days. Injectable is labeled as a single injection or can be repeated one time. Tablets can follow inject up to a total maximum of 3 days treatment. (Adapted from label; *Tolfedine*®—Vetoquinol UK)

- **CATTLE:**

  As an aid in the treatment of pneumonia and acute mastitis in cattle (as registered for use in Australia); (extra-label in USA): Pneumonia: 2 mg/kg by IM injection high in the neck. Treatment may be repeated once only after 48 hours. Mastitis: 4 mg/kg as a single intravenous injection. **DO NOT** inject cattle other than into muscle tissues high on the side of the neck. Meat withdrawal = 10 days (IM), 4 days (IV); Milk withdrawal = 12 hours (1 milking) (Label Information; *Tolfejec*®—Troy Labs, Australia). **Note:** Other countries may have different withdrawal requirements; refer to product label. This drug is not approved in the United States and its administration would not be legal unless a veterinarian could provide justification for its use (Smith 2013).

- **SWINE:**

  As an aid in the treatment of metritis-mastitis-agalactia in pigs (as registered for use in Australia) extra-label in USA): 2 mg/kg IM once. Meat withdrawal = 6 days. (Label Information; *Tolfejec*®—Troy Labs, Australia). **Note:** Other countries may have different withdrawal requirements; refer to product label. This drug is not approved in the United States and its administration would not be legal unless a veterinarian could provide justification for its use (Smith 2013).

Monitoring

- Clinical efficacy.
- Adverse effects.

Client Information

- The weekly dosing regimen (3-5 consecutive days per week for dogs) is important to follow to minimize risks of adverse effects. Do not give longer to cats than the veterinarian prescribes.
- Give oral dosages should be given with food.
- Vomiting and diarrhea have been reported as side effects in dogs and cats.
- Report any changes in appetite, water consumption, or GI distress to veterinarian.

Chemistry/Synonyms

A non-steroidal antiinflammatory agent in the anthranilic acid (fenamate) category, tolfenamic acid is related chemically to meclofenamic acid.

Tolfenamic Acid may also be known as: acidum tolfenamicum, *Bifenac*®, *Clotam*®, *Clotan*®, *Fenamic*®, *Flocur*®, *Gantil*®, *Migea*®, *Polmonin*®, *Purfalox*®, *Rociclyn*®, *Tolfamic*®, *Tolfedine*®, *Tolfejec*® or *Turbaund*®.

Storage/Stability

Unless otherwise labeled, store tolfenamic acid tablets and solution at room temperature.

Compatibility/Compounding Considerations

No specific information noted.

Dosage Forms/Regulatory Status

VETERINARY-LABELED PRODUCTS:

None in the USA; in Canada, New Zealand, Australia and Europe: Tolfenamic Acid Tablets: 6 mg, 30 mg, 60 mg and Tolfenamic Acid Injection: 40 mg/mL are available. Common trade name is *Tolfedine*®.

HUMAN-LABELED PRODUCTS: NONE.

Revisions/References

Monograph revised/updated August 2014.

Dowling, P. (2000). Non-steroidal anti-inflammatory drugs for small animal practitioners. District of Columbia Academy of Veterinary Medicine, Fairfax VA. accessed via Veterinary Information Network; vin.com

Khwanjai, V., et al. (2012). Evaluating the effects of 14-day oral vedaprofen and tolfenamic acid treatment on renal function, hematological and biochemical profiles in healthy cats. J. Vet. Pharmacol. Ther. **35**(1): 13-8.

Lefebvre, H. P., et al. (1997). The effect of experimental renal failure on tolfenamic acid disposition in the dog. Biopharmaceutics & Drug Disposition **18**(1): 79-91.

Smith, G. (2013). Extralabel Use of Anesthetic and Analgesic Compounds in Cattle. Veterinary Clinics of North America-Food Animal Practice **29**(1): 29-+.

Toltrazuril

(tole-traz-yoo-ril)   Baycox®

Antiprotozoal/Anticoccidial

Prescriber Highlights

▶ Antiprotozoal approved in some countries (not USA) for treating coccidial infections in poultry, piglets, calves and lambs.

▶ May be considered as an alternative for treating coccidiosis in dogs, cats, rabbits, etc. and the oocyst shedding stage of toxoplasmosis in cats.

▶ Not commercially available in the USA, must be legally imported.

▶ Adverse effect profile not well described, but appears relatively safe.

Uses/Indications

Toltrazuril is an antiprotozoal agent that may be considered as an alternative treatment for coccidiosis in dogs, cats, calves, lambs, rabbits, mice, camelids and birds. Toltrazuril has been used for treating the oocyst shedding stage of toxoplasmosis in cats. It has also been used as a treatment for overwhelming parasitic loads in lizards (Bearded Dragons).

Toltrazuril has activity against parasites of the genus *Hepatozoon*, but other drugs (*e.g.,* imidocarb, primaquine, doxycycline) are generally used. Toltrazuril can induce initial excellent clinical responses in dogs with American canine hepatozoonosis (ACH), but cannot completely eliminate the parasites, and remission is transient in most dogs. A combination of toltrazuril/emodepside (*Procox*®) plus clindamycin while reducing infectivity, also did not completely clear the organism (De Tommasi *et al.* 2014).

While toltrazuril has been used to treat equine protozoal myeloencephalitis (EPM) caused by *Sarcocystis neurona*, use of FDA-approved products now available (*e.g.,* ponazuril, pyrimethamine/sulfadiazine) is preferred.

Toltrazuril is approved in some countries to treat *Isospora suis* in piglets and coccidiosis in lambs (*Eimeria crandallis* and *Eimeria ovinoidalis*) and calves (*Eimeria bovis* or *Eimeria zuernii*).

Pharmacology/Actions

Toltrazuril is the parent compound to ponazuril (toltrazuril sulfone). Its mechanism of action is not well understood, but it appears to inhibit protozoal enzyme systems.

Toltrazuril has activity against *Hepatozoon, Isospora, Sarcocystis, Toxoplasma*, and all intracellular stages of coccidia.

Pharmacokinetics

Little information is available. Toltrazuril is ≈ 50% absorbed after oral consumption in poultry. Highest concentrations are found in the liver; it is rapidly metabolized into the sulfone derivative (ponazuril).

In rabbits, the pharmacokinetics of toltrazuril were compared using a compounded toltrazuril formulation to improve solubility (prepared by solid dispersion technology using DMSO, PEG 400 and PEG 6000 as a carrier for drinking water) with a commercially available (China) 0.5% premix product. With the compounded preparation peak plasma levels were ≈ 3X greater and AUC was ≈ 2X greater. The authors concluded that using toltrazuril prepared with solid dispersion technology could provide better anticoccidial activity via attainment of higher blood concentrations (Hu *et al.* 2010).

Contraindications/Precautions/Warnings

Toltrazuril should not be used in patients who have had prior hypersensitivity reactions to it or other triazinone (triazine) antiprotozoals (*e.g.,* ponazuril, diclazuril).

The principle metabolite of toltrazuril reportedly persists in the environment and can contaminate groundwater, however there appears to be little risk for significant environmental contamination when toltrazuril is used in dogs, cats, horses, or other companion animals (pet birds, reptiles).

Do not confuse toltrazuril with toltrazuril sulfone (ponazuril).

Adverse Effects

Toltrazuril appears to be well tolerated in birds. An adverse effect profile in mammals is not well described. Potentially, GI signs could occur. Some horses receiving the related drug ponazuril developed blisters on their nose and mouth, and some, a rash or hives during field trials.

Reproductive/Nursing Safety

No reproductive or nursing safety information was located; weigh potential risks versus benefits of use during pregnancy or lactation.

Overdosage/Acute Toxicity

Very limited information is available. Doses of up to 10X in horses were tolerated without significant adverse effects. 5X overdoses in poultry have been tolerated without clinical signs noted. Decreased water intake has been seen if overdoses are greater than 5X.

Drug Interactions

- None reported.

Laboratory Considerations

- No issues were noted.

Doses

- **DOGS:**

  For coccidiosis (extra-label): No clear evidence for any dosage located. 15 – 20 mg/kg PO for 3 days can be considered, but noted anecdotal recommendations range from 10 – 30 mg/kg PO for 1-6 days.

- **CATS:**

  For enteroepithelial cycle of toxoplasmosis (oocyst shedding); (extra-label): 5 – 10 mg/kg PO once daily for 2 days. (Dubey *et al.* 2006)

  For coccidiosis (extra-label): No clear evidence for any dosage located. 20 mg/kg PO for 3 days can be considered, but noted anecdotal recommendations range from 20 – 30 mg/kg PO for 2-3 days.

- **SMALL MAMMALS:**

  For coccidiosis (extra-label):

  a) **Rabbits:** In the study a single oral dose of toltrazuril 2.5 mg/kg or 5 mg/kg PO reduced oocyte counts by 98.1% and 99.6%, respectively. Authors concluded that there appeared to be no advantage to using the higher dose and 2.5 mg/kg PO once is recommended. (Redrobe *et al.* 2010)

  b) **Mice:** Toltrazuril 0.5% at 10 – 20 mg/kg PO given for 3 days, pause for 5 days, and then repeat once more. (Huynh *et al.* 2013)

- **CATTLE:**

  In calves (extra-label in USA): **For the prevention of clinical signs of coccidiosis and reduction of coccidia shedding in housed calves replacing cows producing milk for human consumption (dairy cows) on farms with a confirmed history of coccidiosis caused by *Eimeria bovis* or *Eimeria zuernii*:** 15 mg/kg PO once for each animal. For the treatment of a group of animals of the same breed and same or similar age, the dosing should be done according to the heaviest animal of this group. To obtain maximum benefit, animals should be treated before the expected onset of clinical signs (i.e., in the prepatent period). Not for calves weighing >80 kg or in fattening units such as veal or beef calves. Not for dairy animals. Meat and offal withdrawal (U.K.) = 63 days. (Adapted from label *Baycox* 5%—Bayer U.K.)

- **SHEEP:**

  In lambs for the prevention of clinical signs of coccidiosis and reduction of coccidian shedding on farms with a confirmed history of coccidiosis (*Eimeria crandallis* and *Eimeria ovinoidalis*) (extra-label in USA): Each animal should be treated with a single dose of 20 mg/kg. To obtain maximum benefit, sheep should be treated in the prepatent period before the expected onset of clinical signs. The prepatent period of *Eimeria ovinoidalis* is 12-15 days and the prepatent period of *Eimeria crandalis* is 15-20 days. If animals are to be treated collectively rather than individually, they should be grouped according to their body weight and dosed accordingly. In order to maximize effectiveness it is important to time therapy according to individual farm management and lifecycle of the organism involved. Slaughter withdrawal time (Canada) = 48 days; not for use in dairy sheep. (Adapted from label *Baycox* 5%—Bayer Canada)

- **CAMELIDS:**

  For coccidiosis (*Eimeria* spp.) (extra-label): 5 – 20 mg/kg, PO once daily for up to 3 days. The higher doses and longer courses are for treatment of individuals; the lower doses may be used for control. (Cebra 2012)

- **SWINE:**

  For the treatment of preclinical coccidiosis due to *Isospora suis* in neonatal piglets (extra-label in USA): Weigh 3 representative litters at 3 days of age to determine an average piglet weight. The recommended dosage of toltrazuril is 20 mg/kg body weight PO once at 3-4 days of age. Slaughter withdrawal time (Canada) = 70 days; not for use in suckling or barbecue pigs. (Adapted from label *Baycox* 5%—Bayer Canada)

- **BIRDS:**
  For coccidiosis in raptors (extra-label): 7 mg/kg PO once daily for 2-3 days. (Jones 2004)
- **REPTILES:**
  For parasitism in Bearded Dragons (extra-label): 5 – 15 mg/kg PO once daily for 3 days. (Kramer 2006)

Monitoring
- Clinical efficacy.

Client Information
- Used to treat certain types of protozoa infections. Not currently available in the United States, but may be legally imported by a veterinarian.
- May be given either with food or on an empty stomach. If your animal vomits or acts sick after getting it on an empty stomach, give with food or small treat to see if this helps. If vomiting continues, contact your veterinarian.
- Avoid direct contact with the medication; wear disposable gloves and wash hands after giving medication.
- Appears to be well tolerated by many species of animals.

Chemistry/Synonyms
Related to other antiprotozoals such as ponazuril, toltrazuril is a triazinone (triazine) antiprotozoal (anticoccidial) agent. The commercially available (in Europe) 2.5% oral solution is an alkaline, clear, colorless to yellow brown solution that also contains triethanolamine 30 mg/mL and polyethylene glycol 80.7 mg/mL. Toltrazuril has a molecular weight of 425.4

Toltrazuril may also be known as Bay-Vi-9142, toltrazurilo, toltrazurilum and *Baycox*®.

Storage/Stability
The 2.5% solution should be stored at temperatures at 25°C or below.

Dilutions in drinking water more concentrated than 1:1000 (1 mL of the 2.5% solution to 1 liter of water) may precipitate. After dilution, the resulting solution is stable for 24 hours. It is recommended that medicated drinking water not consumed after 24 hours be discarded.

Compatibility/Compounding Considerations
No specific information noted.

Dosage Forms/Regulatory Status
VETERINARY-LABELED PRODUCTS:
None in the USA; in some countries: Toltrazuril 2.5% (25 mg/mL) solution for dilution in drinking water and/or 5% (50 mg/mL) Oral Suspension are available. Refer to the specific product label for withdrawal times or other restrictions for use.

A combination oral suspension for dogs and cats containing emodepside and toltrazuril (*Procox*®) is also available in some markets. (Petry *et al.* 2013)

HUMAN-LABELED PRODUCTS: NONE.

Revisions/References
Monograph revised/updated August 2014.
Cebra, C. (2012). Coccidiosis in New World Camelids. ACVIM. accessed via Veterinary Information Network; vin.com
De Tommasi, A. S., et al. (2014). Failure of imidocarb dipropionate and toltrazuril/emodepside plus clindamycin in treating Hepatozoon canis infection. Veterinary Parasitology **200**(3-4): 242-5.
Dubey, J. & M. Lappin (2006). Toxoplasmosis and Neosporosis. *Infectious Diseases of the Dogs and Cat, 3rd Ed.* C. Greene, Elsevier: 754-75.
Hu, L., et al. (2010). Pharmacokinetics and improved bioavailability of toltrazuril after oral administration to rabbits. J. Vet. Pharmacol. Ther. **33**(5): 503-6.
Huynh, M. & C. Pignon (2013). Gastrointestinal disease in exotic small mammals. Journal of Exotic Pet Medicine **22**(2): 118-31.
Jones, M. (2004). Update on infectious diseases of birds of prey. Proceedings: Western Veterinary Conference. accessed via Veterinary Information Network; vin.com
Kramer, M. (2006). Bearded Dragon Medicine. Proceedings: Western Veterinary Confernce. accessed via Veterinary Information Network; vin.com
Petry, G., et al. (2013). Efficacy of Emodepside plus Toltrazuril Oral Suspension for Dogs (Procox(A (R)), Bayer) against Trichuris vulpis in Naturally Infected Dogs. Parasitology Research **112**(1): 133-8.
Redrobe, S. P., et al. (2010). Comparison of toltrazuril and sulphadimethoxine in the treatment of intestinal coccidiosis in pet rabbits. Veterinary Record **167**(8): 287-90.

Topiramate
(toe-pie-rah-mate)   Topamax®
Anticonvulsant

Prescriber Highlights
- ▶ Antiseizure medication that may be useful for seizure disorders in dogs, particularly for partial seizure activity. May be of benefit in treating cats, but little information available.
- ▶ Very short half-life in dogs (2-4 hours), but therapeutic activity may persist secondary to high affinity for receptors in brain.
- ▶ Adverse effect profile may include GI distress, sedation, ataxia, inappetence, & irritability in dogs; in cats, sedation & inappetence have been noted.
- ▶ Expense may be an issue, but generics are now available.

Uses/Indications
Topiramate may be useful for treating seizures in dogs, particularly partial seizure activity. It may also be of benefit in treating cats, but little information is available. A case report of a cat with feline idiopathic ulcerative dermatitis treated with topiramate has been published (Grant *et al.* 2014).

Pharmacology/Actions
While the exact mechanism for its antiseizure action is not known, topiramate possesses three properties that probably play a role in its activity: Topiramate blocks in a time-dependent manner action potentials elicited repetitively by a sustained depolarization of neurons; it increases the frequency that GABA activates $GABA_A$ receptors; and it antagonizes the kainite/AMPA receptors without affecting the NMDA receptor subtype. Topiramate's actions are concentration-dependent; effects can first be seen at 1 microMole and maximize at 200 microMoles. Topiramate is a weak inhibitor of carbonic anhydrase isoenzymes CA-II and CA-IV, but it is believed that this effect does not contribute significantly to its antiepileptic actions.

Pharmacokinetics
In dogs, topiramate is rapidly absorbed after oral administration, but absolute bioavailability varies between 30-60%. Half-life ranges from 2-4 hours after multiple doses (Streeter *et al.* 1995). Comparatively, the half-life in humans is ≈ 21 hours in adults, but shorter in children. In humans, the drug is not extensively metabolized and ≈ 70% is excreted unchanged in the urine.

No information on sustained-release topiramate product (*e.g.*, 24-hour topiramate sprinkles) pharmacokinetics in dogs or cats was located.

Contraindications/Precautions/Warnings
Topiramate is contraindicated in patients hypersensitive to it. It should be used with caution (in humans) with impaired hepatic or renal function.

Adverse Effects
Because this drug has not commonly been used in veterinary patients, an accurate adverse effect profile is not well described. In dogs, the most prevalent adverse effects reported include GI distress, sedation, ataxia, inappetence, and irritability. In cats, sedation and inappetence have been noted.

In humans, the most likely adverse effects include somnolence, dizziness, nervousness, confusion, and ataxia. Very rarely, acute myopia with secondary angle closure glaucoma has been reported. Incidence of kidney stones is ≈ 2-4X higher in patients taking topiramate than in the general population. Topiramate can cause a hyperchloremic metabolic acidosis and reduce citrate excretion in the urine thus increasing urine pH leading to calcium phosphate renal calculi.

Reproductive/Nursing Safety

In humans, the FDA categorizes topiramate as a category **C** drug for use during pregnancy (*Animal studies have shown an adverse effect on the fetus, but there are no adequate studies in humans; or there are no animal reproduction studies and no adequate studies in humans.*) Teratogenic effects were noted in mice and rats given topiramate at dosages equivalent to those used in humans.

Topiramate enters maternal milk; use with caution in nursing patients.

Overdosage/Acute Toxicity

Overdoses in humans have caused convulsions, drowsiness/lethargy, slurred speech, blurred and double vision, impaired mentation/ stupor, ataxia, metabolic acidosis, hypotension, agitation, and abdominal pain.

There were 266 single agent exposures to topiramate reported to the ASPCA Animal Poison Control Center (APCC) during 2009-2013. Of the 248 dogs, 44 were symptomatic with 32% lethargic and 16% ataxic. Of the 22 cats, 4 were symptomatic with 75% vomiting.

Treatment consists of gut emptying protocols if the ingestion was recent, and supportive therapy. Hemodialysis is effective in enhancing the elimination of topiramate from the body.

Drug Interactions

The following drug interactions have either been reported or are theoretical in humans or animals receiving topiramate and may be of significance in veterinary patients. Unless otherwise noted, use together is not necessarily contraindicated, but weigh the potential risks and perform additional monitoring when appropriate.

- **AMITRIPTYLINE:** Topiramate may increase levels.
- **CARBONIC ANHYDRASE INHIBITORS** (*e.g.,* **acetazolamide, dichlorphenamide,** etc.): Used concomitantly with topiramate, may increase the risk of renal stone formation.
- **CNS DEPRESSANT DRUGS, OTHER:** Other CNS depressant drugs may exacerbate the CNS adverse effects of topiramate.
- **LAMOTRIGINE:** May increase topiramate levels.
- **PHENYTOIN:** May decrease topiramate levels; phenytoin levels may increase.
- **VALPROIC ACID:** May decrease topiramate and VPA levels.

Laboratory Considerations

- No specific laboratory interactions or considerations were noted. Plasma concentrations of topiramate are usually not monitored in human patients, but therapeutic levels are thought to range from 2-25 mg/L.

Doses

- **DOGS:**

  For refractory epilepsy (extra-label): No controlled clinical studies were noted that support clinical use or any dosage.

  a) **As an "add-on" drug** (to phenobarbital or bromides); (extra-label): From an open label, non-comparative trial in 10 dogs: Initially 2 mg/kg PO twice a day for the first 2 weeks. Then dosage increased to 5 mg/kg PO twice a day and continued for 2 months. If seizure frequency (SF) or seizure-day frequency (SDF) were not reduced by 50% or more (of those prior to topiramate) and no adverse effects occurred, the dosage was increased to 10 mg/kg PO twice a day and again continued for 2 months. At the end of that period and if the prior criteria were met, dosage was increased to 10 mg/kg PO 3 times a day. Some dogs had dosages increased sooner (than q2 months).

  Of the 5 (of 10) dogs that were responders, 3 responded with a dosage of 5 mg/kg twice a day, and two dogs with a dosage of 9 – 10 mg/kg twice a day. Seizure frequency was reduced by 66% in responding dogs. Authors concluded that topiramate may be effective as an add-on medication in treating canine idiopathic epilepsy. Apart from sedation and ataxia reported in some of the dogs, topiramate was well tolerated. (Kiviranta et al. 2013)

  b) Other anecdotal dosage recommendations range from 2 – 10 mg/kg PO q8-12h.

- **CATS:**

  For refractory epilepsy (extra-label): No controlled clinical studies were noted that support clinical use or any dosage. Anecdotally, 12.5 – 25 mg per cat (2.4 – 5 mg/kg) PO twice daily has been noted. To reduce adverse effects, dosage is usually started low and increased as tolerated. Inappetence can be dose limiting.

  For feline idiopathic ulcerative dermatitis (extra-label): 5 mg/kg PO twice daily. From a case report: remission occurred with 4 weeks and control has been maintained for 30 months. Two attempts to withdraw topiramate led to relapse within 24 hours. (Grant *et al.* 2014)

Monitoring

- Efficacy.
- Adverse effects.

Client Information

- Clients must understand that the clinical use of this agent is relatively "investigational" in veterinary patients, that it must be dosed often in dogs, and the potential costs.
- Caution clients not to stop therapy abruptly or "rebound" seizures may occur.
- Have clients maintain a seizure diary to help determine efficacy.

Chemistry/Synonyms

A sulfamate-substituted derivative of D-fructose antiepileptic, topiramate occurs as a white crystalline powder with a bitter taste. Its solubility in water is 9.8 mg/mL; it is freely soluble in alcohol.

Topiramate may also be known as: McN-4853, RWJ-17021, *Epitomax®, Topamac®, Topamax®,* or *Topimax®.*

Storage/Stability

Topiramate tablets should be stored in tight containers at room temperature (15-30°C; 59-86°F); protect from moisture. Topiramate sprinkle capsules should be stored in tight containers at temperatures below 25°C (76°F); protect from moisture.

Compatibility/Compounding Considerations

No specific information noted.

Dosage Forms/Regulatory Status

VETERINARY-LABELED PRODUCTS: NONE.

The ARCI (Racing Commissioners International) has designated this drug as a class 2 substance. See the appendix for more information.

HUMAN-LABELED PRODUCTS:

Topiramate Oral Tablets: 25 mg, 50 mg, 100 mg, & 200 mg; *Topamax®, Topiragen®,* generic; (Rx)

Topiramate Sprinkle Capsules: 15 mg & 25 mg; *Topamax® Sprinkle,* generic; (Rx)

Topiramate Sprinkle Capsules Extended-Release (24-hr for humans): 25 mg, 50 mg, 100 mg, 150 mg, 250 mg; *Qudexy XR®, Trokendi® XR;* (Rx)

Revisions/References

Monograph revised/updated August 2014.

Grant, D. & C. Rusbridge (2014). Topiramate in the management of feline idiopathic ulcerative dermatitis in a two-year-old cat. Veterinary Dermatology 25(3): 226-+.

Kiviranta, A. M., et al. (2013). Topiramate as an add-on antiepileptic drug in treating refractory canine idiopathic epilepsy. Journal of Small Animal Practice 54(10): 512-20.

Streeter, A. J., et al. (1995). Pharmacokinetics and bioavailability of topiramate in the beagle dog. Drug Metabolism and Disposition 23(1): 90-3.

Torsemide

(tor-se-myde) Demadex®, Torasemide

Loop Diuretic

Prescriber Highlights

▶ Potent loop diuretic potentially useful for adjunctive treatment of CHF in dogs & cats; marginal information available on clinical use in veterinary medicine.

▶ Approximately 10X more potent (dosed at 10% of furosemide dose), longer diuretic action, & more potassium-sparing (in dogs) than furosemide.

▶ May be more expensive than furosemide, but tablets are now available generically.

Uses/Indications

Torsemide is a loop diuretic similar to furosemide, but it is more potent, its diuretic effects can persist for a longer period, and it may not cause as much potassium excretion (in dogs). While clinical use in dogs and cats thus far has been minimal, it potentially may be a useful adjunctive treatment for congestive heart failure in dogs and cats, particularly in patients that have become refractory to furosemide or when furosemide is unavailable. The parenteral form has been discontinued in the USA, so use is limited to oral therapy.

Torsemide is ≈ 10X more potent than furosemide, so a starting dose of 10% of the furosemide dose could be considered. As torsemide has a more persistent diuretic effect (≈ 12 hours), dosing frequency may also be reduced. A study comparing furosemide (2 mg/kg PO twice daily) with torsemide (0.2 mg/kg PO twice daily) demonstrated that diuretic resistance developed after 14 days of furosemide, but not torsemide. But both drugs were associated with increased BUN and plasma creatinine concentrations when compared with values before treatment (Hori *et al.* 2007). A small (n=7), double-blinded, randomized, crossover design pilot study comparing oral furosemide vs. oral torsemide (dosed at 10% of the furosemide dose divided into twice daily dosages) concluded that torsemide is equivalent to furosemide at controlling clinical signs of CHF in dogs and is likely to achieve greater diuresis vs. furosemide. Larger clinical trials evaluating torsemide as a first or second-line loop diuretic for congestive heart failure in dogs are warranted (Peddle *et al.* 2012).

Pharmacology/Actions

Torsemide, like furosemide inhibits sodium and chloride reabsorption in the ascending loop of Henle via interference with the chloride-binding site of the 1Na+, 1K+, 2Cl- cotransport system.

Torsemide increases renal excretion of water, sodium, potassium, chloride, calcium, magnesium, hydrogen, ammonium, and bicarbonate.

In dogs, excretion of potassium is affected much less so than sodium (20:1); this is ≈ 2X the ratio of Na:K excreted than with furosemide. Diuretic activity begins within one hour of dosing, peaks at ≈ 2 hours and persists for ≈ 12 hours. In dogs, torsemide appears to have differing effects on aldosterone than furosemide. When compared to furosemide, torsemide increases plasma aldosterone levels and inhibits the amount of receptor-bound aldosterone, however, additional research must be performed to determine the clinical significance of these effects.

In cats, torsemide's effects on potassium excretion appear to be similar to that of furosemide. Peak diuresis occurs ≈ 4 hours post-dose and persists for 12 hours.

Pharmacokinetics

Limited information is available. Oral bioavailability has been reported to be between 80-100% in dogs and cats. Elimination half-life in dogs is ≈ 8 hours, which is longer than furosemide.

In humans, torsemide has high oral bioavailability; patients may be switched between IV and oral forms with no change in dose.

Contraindications/Precautions/Warnings

Torsemide should not be used in patients with known hypersensitivity to it or other sulfonylureas, or in anuric patients.

Use torsemide cautiously in patients with significant hepatic dysfunction, hyperuricemia (may increase serum uric acid), or diabetes mellitus (may increase serum glucose).

Adverse Effects

Adverse effect profiles for dogs and cats have not been fully established due to the limited use of this drug in veterinary medicine. Furosemide, a related drug, can induce fluid and electrolyte abnormalities. Patients should be monitored for hydration status and electrolyte imbalances (especially potassium, calcium, magnesium and sodium). Prerenal azotemia may result if moderate to severe dehydration occurs. Hyponatremia is probably the greatest concern, but hypocalcemia, hypokalemia, and hypomagnesemia may all occur. Animals with normal food and water intake are much less likely to develop water and electrolyte imbalances than those that do not.

Other potential adverse effects include gastrointestinal disturbances, hematologic effects (anemia, leukopenia), weakness, and restlessness. Torsemide, unlike furosemide, apparently only rarely causes significant ototoxic effects in humans; very high doses in laboratory animals have induced ototoxicity.

Reproductive/Nursing Safety

No effects on fertility were noted when female and male rats were administered up to 25 mg/kg/day.

No adverse teratogenic effects were seen when pregnant rats and rabbits were administered up to 15X (human dose) and 5X (human dose), respectively. Larger doses did increase fetal resorptions, decreased average body weight, and delayed fetal ossification. In humans, the FDA categorizes torsemide as category *B* for use during pregnancy (*Animal studies have not yet demonstrated risk to the fetus, but there are no adequate studies in pregnant women; or animal studies have shown an adverse effect, but adequate studies in pregnant women have not demonstrated a risk to the fetus in the first trimester of pregnancy, and there is no evidence of risk in later trimesters.*)

It is unknown if torsemide enters milk, but furosemide is distributed in milk. Clinical significance for nursing offspring is unknown.

Overdosage/Acute Toxicity

In dogs, the oral LD50 is >2 grams/kg. Fluid and electrolyte imbalance is the most likely risk associated with an overdose. Consider gut emptying protocols for very large or quantity unknown ingestions. Acute overdoses should generally be managed by observation with fluid, electrolyte and acid-base monitoring; supportive treatment should be initiated if required.

Drug Interactions

The following drug interactions have either been reported or are theoretical in humans or animals receiving torsemide and may be of significance in veterinary patients. Unless otherwise noted, use together is not necessarily contraindicated, but weigh the potential risks and perform additional monitoring when appropriate.

- **ACE INHIBITORS** (*e.g.,* enalapril, benazepril): Slight increased risk for hypotension, particularly in patients that are volume or sodium depleted secondary to diuretics.

- **AMINOGLYCOSIDES** (*e.g.,* gentamicin, amikacin, etc.): Other diuretics have been associated with increasing the ototoxic or nephrotoxic risks of aminoglycosides. It is unknown if torsemide can also have these effects and if so, what the clinical significance may be.

- **AMPHOTERICIN B**: Loop diuretics may increase the risk for nephrotoxicity development.

- **DIGOXIN**: Can increase the area under the curve of torsemide by 50%, but is unlikely to be of significance clinically; torsemide-induced hypokalemia may increase the potential for digoxin toxicity.

- **LITHIUM**: Torsemide may reduce lithium clearance.

- **NSAIDs**: Some NSAIDs may reduce the natriuretic effects of torsemide.

- **PROBENECID**: Can reduce the diuretic efficacy of torsemide.

- **SALICYLATES**: Torsemide can reduce the excretion of salicylates.

Laboratory Considerations

Torsemide can affect **serum electrolytes, glucose, uric acid,** and BUN concentrations.

Doses

- **DOGS/CATS:**

  As a diuretic for adjunctive treatment of heart failure (extra-label): Based on results from limited studies and clinical usage, a starting dose of 0.2 – 0.3 mg/kg PO q8-24h (usually twice a day) could be considered. Torsemide dosages are ≈ 1/10th (10%) of furosemide doses as torsemide is ≈ 10X more potent than furosemide. It may also have a more persistent diuretic effect (≈ 12 hours) and reduced dosing frequency may be possible. One reference states: "Use of doses that are, in terms of mg/kg, approximately 1/10th the daily furosemide dose typically requires halving or quartering the 5 mg tablet, and dosing of very small dogs can be difficult. The authors currently consider use of torsemide in dogs receiving doses of furosemide ≥4 mg/kg/day and that are experiencing recurrent episode of CHF." (Oyama *et al.* 2011)

Monitoring

- Serum electrolytes, BUN, creatinine, glucose (if diabetic).
- Hydration status.
- Blood pressure, if indicated.
- Clinical signs of edema, patient weight, if indicated.

Client Information

- Your animal may urinate more often than normal. This usually gets better after a while.
- May be given with or without food. Have water available at all times for your animal; encourage normal food intake.
- Because this drug can change electrolytes (salts) in the blood, your veterinarian will probably want to do more frequent testing.
- Contact veterinarian immediately if excessive thirst, weakness or collapsing/passing out, head tilt, lack of urination, or a racing heartbeat is noticed.

Chemistry/Synonyms

Torsemide is a pyridyl sulfonylurea loop diuretic that occurs as white to off-white, crystalline powder. It is practically insoluble in water and slightly soluble in alcohol. The injection has a pH >8.3.

Torsemide may also be known as torasemide, AC-3525, AC 4464, BM-02.015, JDL-464, and *Demadex*®. International trade names include *Torem*® and *Unat*®.

Storage/Stability

Torsemide tablets should be stored below 40°C; preferably between 15-30°C (59-86°F).

Compatibility/Compounding Considerations

No specific information noted.

Dosage Forms/Regulatory Status

VETERINARY-LABELED PRODUCTS: NONE.

The ARCI (Racing Commissioners International) has designated this drug as a class 3 substance.

HUMAN-LABELED PRODUCTS:

Torsemide Oral Tablets: 5 mg, 10 mg, 20 mg, & 100 mg; *Demadex*®, generic; (Rx)

Torsemide Injection: 10 mg/mL; generic; (Rx). Note: At time of writing (2014) not currently available.

Revisions/References

Monograph revised/updated August 2014.

Hori, Y., et al. (2007). Effects of oral administration of furosemide and torsemide in healthy dogs. American Journal of Veterinary Research 68(10): 1058-63.
Oyama, M. A., et al. (2011). Use of the loop diuretic torsemide in three dogs with advanced heart failure. Journal of veterinary cardiology : the official journal of the European Society of Veterinary Cardiology 13(4): 287-92.
Peddle, G. D., et al. (2012). Effect of torsemide and furosemide on clinical, laboratory, radiographic and quality of life variables in dogs with heart failure secondary to mitral valve disease. Journal of Veterinary Cardiology 14(1): 253-9.

Tramadol HCl

(tram-ah-doll)   Ultram®

Opiate-Like (mu-Receptor) Agonist

Prescriber Highlights

▶ Synthetic *mu*-receptor opiate-like agonist that also inhibits reuptake of serotonin & norepinephrine.

▶ May be useful as an analgesic or antitussive. May take up to two weeks for full analgesic activity in chronic pain states.

▶ Now a controlled drug (C-IV) in USA; has potential for human abuse.

▶ Appears well tolerated in dogs; sedation most likely adverse effect.

▶ Several potentially clinically significant drug interactions; avoid use with SSRIs (*e.g.,* fluoxetine, etc.) or MAOIs (*e.g.,* selegiline).

▶ Relatively inexpensive.

Uses/Indications

Tramadol may be a useful alternative or adjunct for the treatment of post-operative or chronic pain or cough in dogs, cats and potentially, other species. When used in combination with NSAIDs, or other analgesic drugs (*e.g.,* amantadine, gabapentin, alpha-2 agonists) it may be particularly useful for chronic pain conditions. A study in dogs evaluating the effects of perioperative oral administration of tramadol, firocoxib, and a tramadol-firocoxib combination on signs of pain and limb function after tibial plateau leveling osteotomy concluded that when used alone oral administration of tramadol may not provide sufficient analgesic efficacy to treat dogs with pain after orthopedic surgical procedures (Davila *et al.* 2013).

In horses, epidurally administered tramadol may also be useful as an analgesic but no appropriate commercial dosage forms are presently available in the USA. However a study evaluating the antinociceptive effects in horses after IV dosage found that at 2 mg/kg or 3 mg/kg, tramadol did not induce sedation or prolong hoof withdrawal reflex in conscious horses and that at 5 mg/kg tramadol caused produced excitement. The authors concluded that IV tramadol is apparently unsuitable for clinical use in horses (Milare *et al.* 2013).

Pharmacology/Actions

Tramadol is a centrally acting opiate-like agonist that has primarily *mu*-receptor activity, but also inhibits reuptake of serotonin and norepinephrine. These pharmacologic actions all contribute to its analgesic properties. At least one metabolite (O-desmethyltramadol; ODT; M1) has activity. When compared to tramadol in lab animal studies, M1 is 6X more potent an analgesic and has 20X more potency in binding to *mu*-receptors. Another metabolite (N-desmethyltramadol; M2) apparently also has pharmacologic activity. Naloxone only partially antagonizes the analgesic effects of tramadol; other partial antagonists include yohimbine and ondansetron.

Pharmacokinetics

In dogs after oral administration of immediate-release tablets, bioavailability is ≈ 65%, but there is significant interpatient variability. Rectal bioavailability is only ≈ 10%. Volume of distribution is ≈ 3.8 L/kg. Total body clearance and half-life are ≈ 55 mL/kg/min and 1.7 hours, respectively. Tramadol is extensively metabolized via several metabolic pathways to at least 20 metabolites. One metabolite (O-desmethyltramadol, M1) has agonist activity, but is a minor metabolite in dogs; M1 has a half-life of ≈ 2 hours after oral tramadol administration in dogs. Dogs appear to produce more substantial quantities of M2. A study in greyhounds reported a slightly shorter half-life (1.1 hours) for it than the parent compound (KuKanich *et al.* 2011).

One study in 8 cats using the immediate release oral tablet, showed high interpatient variability in absorption (with 2 cats there was not enough data to analyze). The elimination half-life for the parent compound was ≈ 2.5 hours; for the M1 metabolite, 4.5 hours. Neurologic effects (mydriasis, dysphoria) were seen in 25% of cats (2 of 4 females) in the study group and the drug was observed to be unpalatable to cats (Papich *et al.* 2007). Another study in 6 cats demonstrated approximate values of: oral bioavailability 60%; volume of distribution (steady-state) 2 L/kg; clearance 12 mL/min/kg; and terminal half-life 191 minutes. Terminal half-life for ODT after oral administration was ≈ 290 minutes (Pypendop *et al.* 2007).

In neonatal and weaned foals, tramadol has different pharmacokinetics. After oral administration, higher bioavailability (53% vs. 20%), shorter time to peak concentration (1 hr. vs. 1.25 hr.), and peak levels occurred with neonatal (2 week old) versus weaned foals (4 months old). Elimination half-life did not significantly differ (≈ 2 hours). The active metabolite (M1; ODT) remained above the reported therapeutic concentration for humans for 3 hours in neonatal foals and 8 hours in weaned foals (Stewart *et al.* 2006).

In adult horses, tramadol has relatively poor oral absorption (≈ 14%) and an elimination half-life has been reported to range from 2-10 hours, depending on the study. The active metabolite, (m1; ODT) half-life is reported as 4 hours in one study (Cox *et al.* 2010). Another study (Knych *et al.* 2013) reported elimination half-lives for tramadol, M1 and M2 of ≈ 1.5 – 2.5 hours for the parent compound and the two metabolites after dosages of tramadol at 3 mg/kg, 6 mg/kg and 9 mg/kg PO (Knych *et al.* 2013). At PO dosages of 3 mg/kg or 6 mg/kg tramadol and M1 plasma concentrations were within, but at the lower end of the analgesic range for humans and were only transiently maintained. The authors concluded that until effective analgesic plasma concentrations have been established, tramadol should be cautiously recommended for control of pain in horses. A follow-up study (Guedes *et al.* 2014) giving repeated oral dosages (5 mg/kg or 10 mg/kg PO q12h for 5 days) found wide interpatient variability in peak (C_{max}) and trough (C_{min}) plasma levels. Tramadol and M2 accumulated with repeated dosing, especially at the 10 mg/kg dose. The authors concluded: "Overall, tramadol was well tolerated, but the potential for gastrointestinal adverse effect exists in horses treated for longer periods of time, especially those

horses receiving higher dosage regimens. More restricted dosage regimens may be possible, if not necessary, in cases of long-term tramadol therapy."

In llamas, after IV dosing (2 mg/kg), tramadol & M1 pharmacokinetics values (approximate means) are: volume of distribution$_{(ss)}$ ≈ 4 L/kg & 26.5 L/kg; clearance ≈ 1.7 L/hr/kg & 2.03 L/hr/kg; half-life ≈ 2.1 hours & 10.4 hours. IM (2 mg/kg) bioavailability is high (Cox *et al.* 2011). In alpacas, oral bioavailability was poor (6-19%). After IV administration (3.4 – 4.4 mg/kg), volume of distribution was 5.50 ± 2.66 L/kg; total body clearance ≈ 4.6 L/hr/kg; and half-life ≈ 0.9 hours (Edmondson *et al.* 2012).

In red-tailed hawks, after an oral dose of 11 mg/kg, plasma levels of tramadol reached or exceeded concentrations associated with analgesia in humans for at least 4 hours after dosing. Elimination half-lives were 1.3 hours (tramadol) and 1.9 hours (M1) (Souza *et al.* 2011). Single dose IV doses to Hispaniolan Amazon parrots had half-lives of 1.54 hours (tramadol) and 2.55 hours (M2). Oral bioavailability was ≈ 24% (Souza *et al.* 2012).

Contraindications/Precautions/Warnings

Tramadol is contraindicated in patients hypersensitive to it or other opioids. The combination product containing acetaminophen is contraindicated in cats.

Use with caution in conjunction with other drugs that can cause CNS or respiratory depression. Because tramadol has caused seizures in humans, it should be used with caution in animals with preexisting seizure disorders or receiving other drugs that may reduce the seizure threshold. Like other opiate-like compounds, tramadol should be used with caution in geriatric or severely debilitated animals. Patients with impaired renal or hepatic function may need dosage adjustments.

While the risk of physical dependence occurring is less than that of several other opiates, it has been reported in humans. The drug should be withdrawn gradually in animals that have received it chronically. While not a controlled substance in the USA, humans can potentially abuse tramadol and significant diversion of the drug reportedly occurs. Veterinarians should be alert to "clients" seeking tramadol for their animals.

Extended-release tablets (generally not currently recommended or used in veterinary patients) must not be broken, crushed or chewed or toxicity could occur.

Do not confuse traMADol with traZODone.

Adverse Effects

Tramadol appears to be well tolerated in dogs. Potentially, it could cause a variety of adverse effects associated with its pharmacologic actions, including: CNS effects (excessive sedation, agitation, anxiety, tremor, dizziness), or GI effects (inappetence, vomiting, constipation to diarrhea).

Very limited information is available on the adverse effects in cats. Dose avoidance (unpalatability), vomiting, sedation, mydriasis, dysphoria or euphoria, and constipation have been reported.

Approximately 10% of humans receiving the drug develop pruritus. Injectable tramadol may cause respiratory and cardiac depression.

Reproductive/Nursing Safety

In humans, the FDA categorizes tramadol as a category *C* drug for use during pregnancy (*Animal studies have shown an adverse effect on the fetus, but there are no adequate studies in humans; or there are no animal reproduction studies and no adequate studies in humans.*) At dosages 3-15X usual, tramadol was embryotoxic and fetotoxic in laboratory animals.

Trazodone and its active metabolite enter maternal milk in very low levels, but the drug's safety in neonates has not been established.

Overdosage/Acute Toxicity

Acute oral overdoses may cause either CNS depressive signs or serotonin syndrome. Lethargy, mydriasis, ataxia and vomiting are most common, but stimulatory signs (tachycardia, tremors, vocalization) may also be seen.

There were 910 single agent exposures to tramadol reported to the ASPCA Animal Poison Control Center (APCC) during 2009-2013. Of the 749 dogs, 142 were symptomatic with 57% being sedated/lethargic, 12% vomiting, 10% tachycardic, 7% vocalizing or ataxic, and 6% agitated or tremoring. Of the 157 cats, 96 were symptomatic with 59% having mydriasis, 31% hypersalivating, 30% lethargic, 11% ataxic or tachycardic, and 8% vomiting.

Treatment is primarily supportive (maintaining respiration, treating seizures with benzodiazepines or barbiturates, etc.). Naloxone may NOT be useful in tramadol overdoses as it may only partially reverse some of the effects of the drug and may, in fact, increase the risk of seizures. Naloxone did not decrease the drug's lethality in tramadol overdoses given to mice. Cyproheptadine and phenothiazines can be used to treat the stimulatory signs.

Drug Interactions

The following drug interactions have either been reported or are theoretical in humans or animals receiving tramadol and may be of significance in veterinary patients. Unless otherwise noted, use together is not necessarily contraindicated, but weigh the potential risks and perform additional monitoring when appropriate.

- **CYPROHEPTADINE:** May decrease efficacy of tramadol.
- **DIGOXIN:** In humans, tramadol has been rarely linked to digoxin toxicity.
- **MAO INHIBITORS** (including **amitraz** and possibly, **selegiline**): Potential for serotonin syndrome; use together should be avoided.
- **ONDANSETRON:** In humans, use together may reduce the effectiveness of both drugs.
- **QUINIDINE:** May increase tramadol concentrations and decrease M1 (active metabolite) concentrations.
- **SAMe:** Theoretically, concurrent use of SAMe with tramadol could cause additive serotonergic effects.
- **SEVOFLURANE:** Pretreatment with tramadol reduced MAC values by ≈ 30% in dogs (Seddighi *et al.* 2009), and 40% in cats (Dirikolu *et al.* 2009).
- **SSRI ANTIDEPRESSANTS** (*e.g.,* **fluoxetine, sertraline, paroxetine**, etc.): Can inhibit the metabolism of tramadol to its active metabolites thereby decreasing its efficacy and increasing the risk of toxicity (serotonin syndrome, seizures).
- **TRICYCLIC ANTIDEPRESSANTS** (*e.g.,* **clomipramine, amitriptyline**, etc.): Increased risk for seizures; amitriptyline may inhibit tramadol metabolism.
- **YOHIMBINE:** May antagonize (partial) the pharmacologic effects of tramadol.
- **WARFARIN:** In humans, increased PT and INR in patients taking tramadol has been reported (relatively rare).

Laboratory Considerations

- No specific laboratory interactions or considerations were noted.

Doses

- **DOGS:**

  As an analgesic (extra-label): Dogs may benefit from tramadol administered 4 – 10 mg/kg PO 3 times a day. Maximum analgesic effects may not occur immediately and may be delayed up to 14 days for chronic pain conditions such as cancer and degenerative joint disease. Long-term efficacy of tramadol may decrease with time. Some data supports tramadol use in clinical veteri-

nary patients, but more studies need to be conducted to confirm its efficacy and safety. (KuKanich 2010), (KuKanich 2013)

- **CATS:**

  As an analgesic (extra-label): At present, there is no clear dosage for tramadol in cats based upon prospective studies. Most current recommendations for dosing in cats are 1 – 2 mg/kg PO q12h. Some suggest that some cats may only need once daily doses; others suggest going as high as 4 mg/kg. Has an unpleasant taste and dose avoidance may be an issue. Neurologic and opioid adverse effects can be seen, particularly at dosages higher than 2 mg/kg.

- **HORSES:**

  As an analgesic (extra-label): In a study of 10 horses with chronic laminitis pain: tramadol at 5 mg/kg PO twice daily for 7 days, alone or with ketamine at 0.6 mg/kg/hr IV during 6 hours each day for the first 3 days of treatment, pain relief was enhanced. (Guedes *et al.* 2009)

- **CATTLE:**

  For epidural analgesia (extra-label):

  a) From a study in 5 cattle: Authors concluded that tramadol at 2 – 3 mg/kg injected into the first intercoccygeal space provided sufficient analgesia in affected regions to allow common surgical procedures to be performed in standing cattle. Slight to mild sedation and ataxia were noted. (Baniadam *et al.* 2010)

  b) From a study in 5 cattle. A combination of lidocaine (0.11 mg/kg) and tramadol (0.5 mg/kg) injected into the first intercoccygeal space resulted in rapid onset time (≈ 5 minutes) and prolonged duration (≈ 175 minutes) of anesthesia in the regions of the tail and perineum in comparison with lidocaine and tramadol alone. (Bigham *et al.* 2010)

- **BIRDS:**

  As an analgesic (extra-label):

  a) From a pharmacokinetic study in red-tailed hawks: Authors concluded that an oral dose of 15 mg/kg PO q12h would be a reasonable starting point, additional pharmacodynamic and repeat dosing pharmacokinetic studies are needed. (Souza *et al.* 2011)

  b) From pharmacokinetic and antinociceptive studies in Hispaniolan Amazon parrots: 30 mg/kg PO q6-8h may provide clinical analgesia. Further studies are needed to fully evaluate the analgesic effects of tramadol in psittacines. (Guzman *et al.* 2012; Souza *et al.* 2012; Souza *et al.* 2013)

- **REPTILES:**

  As an analgesic (extra-label): A study in red-eared sliders concluded that the most clinically useful and safest dose range for tramadol in red-eared slider turtles is 5 –10 mg/kg PO (Baker *et al.* 2011). A review article on analgesia for reptiles suggests 5 – 10 mg/kg PO q48-72h. Good analgesic efficacy with relatively long duration when administered PO in chelonians; less respiratory depression than other opioids. (Sladky *et al.* 2012)

- **ZOO, EXOTIC, WILDLIFE SPECIES:**

  For use of tramadol in zoo, exotic and wildlife medicine refer to specific references, including: *Tramadol Use in Zoologic Medicine* by Souza, M. & Cox, S. in Vet Clin Exot Anim 14 (2011) 117–130.

Monitoring

- Clinical efficacy.
- Adverse effects.

Client Information

- May take up to 2 weeks to have an effect for chronic pain.
- May be given with or without food. If your animal vomits or acts sick after getting it on an empty stomach, give with food or small

treat to see if this helps. If vomiting continues, contact your veterinarian.

- May cause changes in alertness or behavior. Use with caution in working or service dogs.
- The combination product with acetaminophen (*Ultracet®*) must **NOT** be used in cats.
- Tramadol is a controlled substance in the USA. It is against the law to use, give away or sell this medication to others than for whom it was prescribed.

Chemistry/Synonyms

A *mu*-receptor opiate agonist, tramadol HCl occurs as a white crystalline powder that is freely soluble in water or alcohol, and very slightly soluble in acetone. Tramadol is not derived from opium nor is it a semi-synthetic opioid, but is entirely synthetically produced.

Tramadol HCl may also be known as: CG-315, CG-315E, tramadoli hydrochloridum, or U-26225A; many trade names are available.

Storage/Stability

Unless otherwise labeled, tramadol tablets should be stored at room temperature 25°C (77°F); excursions permitted to 15-30°C (59-86°F). Dispense in tight, light-resistant containers.

Compatibility/Compounding Considerations

Tramadol HCl injection 50 mg/mL (not available commercially in the USA) is reportedly **not compatible** when mixed in the same syringe with injectable diazepam, diclofenac sodium, indomethacin, midazolam, piroxicam, phenylbutazone, or lysine aspirin.

Dosage Forms/Regulatory Status

VETERINARY-LABELED PRODUCTS: NONE.
The ARCI (Racing Commissioners International) has designated this drug as a class 2 substance. See the appendix for more information.

HUMAN-LABELED PRODUCTS:
Note: As of August 18, 2014 all tramadol-containing products became controlled drugs (schedule C-IV) in the USA.

Tramadol HCl Oral Tablets (film-coated): 50 mg; *Ultram®*, generic; (Rx); (C-IV)

Tramadol HCl Extended-Release Tablets: 100 mg, 200 mg & 300 mg; *Ultram ER®*, *ConZip®*, generic; (Rx); (C-IV). **Note:** Dogs apparently do not absorb this product as well as humans, and potentially could "overdose" if the tablet is chewed.

Tramadol HCl Oral Disintegrating Tablets: 50 mg in UD 30s; *Rybix ODT®*; (Rx); (C-IV)

Tramadol is also available in a fixed dose combination of tramadol HCl 37.5 mg and acetaminophen 325 mg tablets. USA trade name is *Ultracet®*; (Rx); (C-IV). **Warning:** Be certain this combination product is **not** used in cats.

In several countries (but not the USA), tramadol injection is available commercially.

Revisions/References

Monograph revised/updated August 2014.

Baker, B. B., et al. (2011). Evaluation of the analgesic effects of oral and subcutaneous tramadol administration in red-eared slider turtles. Journal of the American Veterinary Medical Association 238(2): 220-7.
Baniadam, A., et al. (2010). Analgesic effects of tramadol hydrochloride administered via caudal epidural injection in healthy adult cattle. American Journal of Veterinary Research 71(7): 720-5.
Bigham, A. S., et al. (2010). Caudal epidural injection of lidocaine, tramadol, and lidocaine-tramadol for epidural anesthesia in cattle. J. Vet. Pharmacol. Ther. 33(5): 439-43.
Cox, S., et al. (2011). Pharmacokinetics of intravenous and intramuscular tramadol in llamas. J. Vet. Pharmacol. Ther. 34(3): 259-64.
Cox, S., et al. (2010). Determination of oral tramadol pharmacokinetics in horses. Research in Veterinary Science 89(2): 236-41.
Davila, D., et al. (2013). Comparison of the analgesic efficacy of perioperative firocoxib and tramadol administration in dogs undergoing tibial plateau leveling osteotomy. Javma-Journal of the American Veterinary Medical Association 243(2): 225-31.

Dirikolu, L., et al. (2009). Pyrilamine in the horse: detection and pharmacokinetics of pyrilamine and its major urinary metabolite O-desmethylpyrilamine. J. Vet. Pharmacol. Ther. 32(1): 66-78.
Edmondson, M. A., et al. (2012). Pharmacokinetics of tramadol and its major metabolites in alpacas following intravenous and oral administration. J. Vet. Pharmacol. Ther. 35(4): 389-96.
Guedes, A., et al. (2009). Analgesic Role of Tramadol and Ketamine in Horses with Laminitis-Associated Pain. Proceedings: IVECCS. accessed via Veterinary Information Network; vin.com
Guedes, A. G. P., et al. (2014). Pharmacokinetics and physiological effects of repeated oral administrations of tramadol in horses. J. Vet. Pharmacol. Ther. 37(3): 269-78.
Guzman, D. S. M., et al. (2012). Antinociceptive effects after oral administration of tramadol hydrochloride in Hispaniolan Amazon parrots (Amazona ventralis). American Journal of Veterinary Research 73(8): 1148-52.
Knych, H. K., et al. (2013). Pharmacokinetics and pharmacodynamics of tramadol in horses following oral administration. J. Vet. Pharmacol. Ther. 36(4): 389-98.
KuKanich, B. (2010). Managing Severe Chronic Pain: Maintaining Quality of Life in Dogs. Proceedings ACVIM. accessed via Veterinary Information Network; vin.com
KuKanich, B. (2013). Outpatient Oral Analgesics in Dogs and Cats Beyond Nonsteroidal Antiinflammatory Drugs: An Evidence-based Approach. Veterinary Clinics of North America-Small Animal Practice 43(5): 1109-+.
KuKanich, B. & M. G. Papich (2011). Pharmacokinetics and antinociceptive effects of oral tramadol hydrochloride administration in Greyhounds. American Journal of Veterinary Research 72(2): 256-62.
Milare, A. S., et al. (2013). Intravenous Tramadol Injection has no Antinociceptive Effect in Horses Undergoing Electrical and Thermal Stimuli. Journal of Equine Veterinary Science 33(10): 823-6.
Papich, M. & D. Bledsoe (2007). Tramadol pharmacokinetics in cats after oral administration of an immediate release product. Proceedings: ACVIM. accessed via Veterinary Information Network; vin.com
Pypendop, B. H. & J. E. Ilkiw (2007). Pharmacokinetics of Tramadol and O-Desmethyl-tramadol in Cats. Proceedings: IVECCS. accessed via Veterinary Information Network; vin.com
Seddighi, M. R., et al. (2009). Effects of tramadol on the minimum alveolar concentration of sevoflurane in dogs. Veterinary Anaesthesia and Analgesia 36(4): 334-40.
Sladky, K. K. & C. Mans (2012). Clinical analgesia in reptiles. Journal of Exotic Pet Medicine 21(2): 158-67.
Souza, M. J., et al. (2013). Pharmacokinetics of repeated oral administration of tramadol hydrochloride in Hispaniolan Amazon parrots (Amazona ventralis). American Journal of Veterinary Research 74(7): 957-62.
Souza, M. J., et al. (2012). Pharmacokinetics after oral and intravenous administration of a single dose of tramadol hydrochloride to Hispaniolan Amazon parrots (Amazona ventralis). American Journal of Veterinary Research 73(8): 1142-7.
Souza, M. J., et al. (2011). Pharmacokinetics of oral tramadol in red-tailed hawks (Buteo jamaicensis). J. Vet. Pharmacol. Ther. 34(1): 86-8.
Stewart, A., et al. (2006). Pharmacokinetics of tramadol in 2-week and 4-month-old foals. Proceedings: IVECC. accessed via Veterinary Information Network; vin.com

Trazodone HCl

(traz-oh-done) *Desyrel®*

Serotonin 2a Antagonist/Reuptake Inhibitor

Prescriber Highlights

▶ Antidepressant that may be useful for adjunctive treatment of behavioral disorders (esp. anxiety- or phobia-related) in dogs; not used in cats.

▶ Limited research or clinical experience available regarding appropriate veterinary use.

▶ Relatively inexpensive.

Uses/Indications

Trazodone may be useful in treating behavioral disorders in small animals, particularly as an adjunctive treatment in patients that do not adequately respond to conventional therapies.

It is commonly used in dogs as an antianxiety agent, particularly in intensive care situations. In a retrospective study of 56 dogs evaluating trazodone as an adjunctive treatment for anxiety disorders, it was found to be well tolerated over a wide dose range and enhanced behavioral calming. The authors concluded that further controlled studies are needed to more fully evaluate the pharmacokinetics, safety profile, and efficacy of this drug in dogs (Gruen *et al.* 2008).

Anecdotally, it has been used to decrease the hyperesthetic effects associated with strychnine toxicity.

In humans, trazodone is used for treating depression, aggressive behavior, alcohol or cocaine withdrawal, migraine prevention, and insomnia. It has fewer anticholinergic effects than the tricyclic antidepressants and is among the antidepressants with the lowest seizure risk.

Pharmacology/Actions

Trazodone is classified as a serotonin 2A antagonist/reuptake inhibitor (SARI) that primarily potentiates serotonin activity in the CNS. In laboratory animals, trazodone selectively inhibits serotonin uptake by brain synaptosomes and potentiates the behavioral changes induced by the serotonin precursor, 5-hydroxytryptophan. In dogs, trazodone exerts qualitatively different and less pronounced cardiac conduction effects than do the tricyclic antidepressants. Trazodone can antagonize alpha-1 adrenergic receptors and reduce blood pressure. As trazodone can antagonize 5-HT2 receptors and cause their down-regulation, it can augment the efficacy of SSRIs (Virga 2010).

Pharmacokinetics

In dogs after 8 mg/kg IV, volume of distribution was (all values are means) 2.53 L/kg, elimination half-life 169 minutes, and plasma total body clearance was 11.15 mL/min/kg. After 8 mg/kg PO, bioavailability was 85%, and elimination half-life was 166 minutes, peak plasma levels occurred at 445 minutes (mean), but there was wide inter-subject variation (± 271 minutes). IV administration was associated with transient tachycardia in all dogs and aggression in half the dogs (Jay *et al.* 2013).

In humans, oral bioavailability of trazodone (immediate-release tablets) is ≈ 65%; presence of food increases absorption (AUC is increased), but decreases Cmax (peak plasma level) and delays Tmax (time of peak level). It is ≈ 90-95% bound to plasma proteins. Volume of distribution ranges from 0.47 – 0.84 L/kg. Metabolism is extensive and occurs primarily in the liver. An active metabolite, m-chlorophenylpiperazine (mCCP) is formed via oxidative cleavage by CYP3A4 that is further metabolized to inactive compounds via CYP2D6. Excretion is mostly (70-75%) via renal mechanisms with only a very small amount (0.13%) excreted unchanged in the urine. About 21% of a dose is excreted in the feces. Elimination half-life of the parent compound is ≈ 7 hours (immediate-release tablets) and 10 hours (sustained-release tablets).

Contraindications/Precautions/Warnings

Trazodone is contraindicated in patients hypersensitive to it or those receiving MAO inhibitors (including amitraz and possibly, selegiline). It should be used with caution in patients with severe cardiac disease or hepatic or renal impairment.

Do not confuse traZODone with traMADol.

Adverse Effects

The adverse effect profile for trazodone in dogs is not well documented. Potential adverse effects include sedation, lethargy, ataxia, priapism, cardiac conduction disturbances, increased anxiety, and aggression. In a retrospective study in 56 dogs (Gruen *et al.* 2008), trazodone adverse effects were generally mild, and only 3 dogs had to have the drug discontinued. Approximately 80% of the dogs in the study had no reported adverse effects. Adverse effects that were reported included: vomiting/gagging (2), behavioral changes (within hours of a dose) such as getting onto counters (1), or into trash (1), increased excitement (2), sedation (2), increased appetite (2) and colitis (1). Should trazodone be used more extensively in dogs, a more defined adverse effect profile may be discerned.

Trazodone alone is unlikely to cause serotonin syndrome at clinically used dosages, but when used with other serotonergic drugs, it is possible. The most common clinical signs seen with serotonin syndrome in dogs include (in descending order): vomiting, diarrhea, seizures, hyperthermia, hyperesthesia, depression, mydriasis, vocalization, death, blindness, hypersalivation, dyspnea, ataxia/paresis, disorientation, hyperreflexia, and coma (Wismer 2006).

In humans, the most common adverse effects include blurred vision; confusion, dizziness, dry mouth, orthostatic hypotension, sweating, lethargy or somnolence. QT prolongation can occur, but is much less common in humans with trazodone than with the tricyclic antidepressants. Priapism has been reported rarely in men taking trazodone.

Reproductive/Nursing Safety

Trazodone appears to be relatively safe to use during pregnancy. At very high dosages (15-50X) in rats and rabbits, some increase in fetal death/resorption rates and congenital abnormalities were noted. For humans, the FDA categorizes trazodone as category **C** for use during pregnancy *(Animal studies have shown an adverse effect on the fetus, but there are no adequate studies in humans; or there are no animal reproduction studies and no adequate studies in humans.)* Tramadol is excreted into milk at very low levels and clinical effects in offspring seem unlikely. However, weigh the potential risks of using this medication versus the benefits in pregnant or nursing animals.

Overdosage/Acute Toxicity

No specific information was located regarding trazodone overdoses in veterinary patients. In humans, incidence of serious toxicity from trazodone overdose (alone) was low compared with tricyclic antidepressant overdoses. However, in the event of substantial overdose of trazodone, it is recommended to contact an animal poison control center for further guidance.

There were 418 single agent exposures to trazodone reported to the ASPCA Animal Poison Control Center (APCC) during 2009-2013. Of the 379 dogs, 104 were symptomatic with 43% sedated/lethargic, 16% ataxic and 14% vomiting. Of the 38 cats, 14 were symptomatic with lethargy (43%) and ataxia (36%) the most common.

Drug Interactions

The following drug interactions have either been reported or are theoretical in humans or animals receiving trazodone and may be of significance in veterinary patients. Unless otherwise noted, use together is not necessarily contraindicated, but weigh the potential risks and perform additional monitoring when appropriate.

- **ANTIHYPERTENSIVE DRUGS:** Trazodone may increase reductions in blood pressure and cause hypotension.
- **ASPIRIN:** Increase risk for GI bleeding; monitor.
- **AZOLE ANTIFUNGALS** (*e.g.*, **ketoconazole, fluconazole**): May increase trazodone blood levels.
- **CNS DEPRESSANTS:** Use with trazodone may cause additive CNS depressant effects.
- **DIGOXIN:** Trazodone may increase digoxin levels.
- **MACROLIDE ANTIBIOTICS:** (*e.g.*, **erythromycin, clarithromycin**): May increase trazodone blood levels.
- **METOCLOPRAMIDE:** Increased risk for serotonin syndrome.
- **NSAIDS:** Increased risk for GI bleeding; monitor.
- **PHENOTHIAZINES:** May increase trazodone blood levels; cause additive CNS effects.
- **SSRI ANTIDEPRESSANTS** (*e.g.*, **fluoxetine**): Increased risk for serotonin syndrome. Trazodone is commonly used together with SSRI's, but be alert for signs associated with serotonin syndrome (see adverse effects above).

Laboratory Considerations

- None noted.

Doses

- **DOGS:**
  Note: All dosages are for regular tablets (not extended-release) unless otherwise noted.

As an adjunctive treatment of anxiety-related disorders (extra-label):

a) From a retrospective study of 56 dogs. To allow dogs to become tolerant to the drug and avoid potential gastrointestinal adverse effects, trazodone was begun at an initial dose that was half of the target dose and administered for 3 days. Then the target dose was established as the lowest effective dose needed for behavioral calming. Additional dose increments were made empirically over time.

Weight (kg)	Initial Dosage (total; NOT mg/kg) Range	Target Dosage (total; NOT mg/kg) Range
<10 kg	≤ 25 mg q8-24h	≤ 50 mg q8-24h
≥10-20 kg	50 mg q12-24h	100 mg q8-24h
≥20-40 kg	100 mg q12-24h	200 mg q8-24h
>40 kg	100 mg q12-24h	200 – 300 mg q8-24h

In the study, the following minimum, maximum and mean daily dosages and dosing frequencies were used:

Daily medication only: 1.9 mg/kg/day to 16.2 mg/kg/day (mean = 7.3 mg/kg/day);

As needed only: 2.2 mg/kg/day to 14 mg/kg/day (mean 7.7 mg/kg/day);

Daily medication and as needed: 1.7 mg/kg/day to 19.5 mg/kg/day (mean 7.25 mg/kg/day). (Gruen *et al.* 2008)

b) **As an anxiolytic for short-term management of patients after surgery** (extra-label): A pharmacokinetic and hemodynamic study concluded that trazodone may be most useful in patients after surgery after complete recovery from anesthesia. In this study, dosages of 8 mg/kg PO were well tolerated but because of substantial variability in time to maximum plasma concentrations, individualized approaches in dosing intervals may be necessary. At the authors' institution trazodone treatment is instituted 12-24 hours after surgery for anxious patients and clinicians often prescribe trazodone for a treatment duration of weeks to months for surgical patients to facilitate cage rest and activity restriction, particularly following orthopedic procedures. Further studies are warranted.

c) In addition to the daily serotonin enhancing medication, trazodone can be used as an adjunctive drug to increase clinical control of anxiety related conditions. It is given about an hour prior to the onset of anxiety and with a typical starting dose between 2 – 5 mg/kg and adjusting upwards as necessary to get control (maximum dose 14 mg/kg/day). (Neilson 2010)

Monitoring
- Clinical efficacy and adverse effects.

Client Information
- Used in dogs for anxiety-related conditions, including thunderstorm or fireworks phobias, activity restrictions (cage rest) after surgery, etc. It is commonly used in combination with other drugs to help reduce anxiety.
- May give with food or on an empty stomach. If your animal vomits or acts sick after getting it on an empty stomach, try giving with food or small treat and see if this helps. If vomiting continues, contact your veterinarian.
- May take up to 2 weeks to achieve its calming effect, especially when used alone.
- Most common side effects are sleepiness and decreased activity. Use with caution in working/service dogs as they may be unable to perform their duties while on this medication.

Chemistry/Synonyms
Trazodone is a triazolopyridine antidepressant agent. It occurs as a white to off-white crystalline powder and is sparingly soluble in water, alcohol, or chloroform.

Trazodone may also be known as AF-1161, trazodona, trazodon, or "sleepeasy". A common trade name is *Desyrel*.

Storage/Stability
Store between 20-25°C (68-77°F); excursions are permitted to 15-30°C (59-86°F). Keep in an airtight container and protect from light.

Compatibility/Compounding Considerations
No specific information noted.

Dosage Forms/Regulatory Status
VETERINARY-LABELED PRODUCTS: NONE.
HUMAN-LABELED PRODUCTS:
Trazodone Oral Tablets: 50 mg, 100 mg, 150 mg, & 300 mg; generic; (Rx)

Trazodone Extended-Release (24-hour) Oral Tablets: 150 mg & 300 mg; *Oleptro*; (Rx)

Revisions/References
Monograph revised/updated August 2014.

Gruen, M. E. & B. L. Sherman (2008). Use of trazodone as an adjunctive agent in the treatment of canine anxiety disorders: 56 cases (1995-2007). Javma-Journal of the American Veterinary Medical Association 233(12): 1902-7.

Jay, A. R., et al. (2013). Pharmacokinetics, bioavailability, and hemodynamic effects of trazodone after intravenous and oral administration of a single dose to dogs. American Journal of Veterinary Research 74(11): 1450-6.

Neilson, J. (2010). Drug Therapy for Behavioral Problems. Proceedings: Western Veterinary Conference. accessed via Veterinary Information Network; vin.com

Virga, V. (2010). Case Files in Anxiety: Practical Management from the Trenches III, IV. Proceedings: WVC. accessed via Veterinary Information Network; vin.com

Wismer, T. (2006). Serotonin Syndrome. Proceedings: IVECC Symposium. accessed via Veterinary Information Network; vin.com

Triamcinolone Acetonide

(trye-am-sin-oh-lone)   Vetalog®

Glucocorticoid

Prescriber Highlights
- Oral, parenteral, topical & inhaled glucocorticoid that is 4-10X (some say up to 40X) more potent than hydrocortisone; no appreciable mineralocorticoid activity. Commonly used for intraarticular injection (especially in horses).
- Contraindications (relatively): Systemic fungal infections, manufacturer lists: "in viral infections, ...animals with arrested tuberculosis, peptic ulcer, acute psychoses, corneal ulcer, & Cushingoid syndrome. The presence of diabetes, osteoporosis, chronic psychotic reactions, predisposition to thrombophlebitis, hypertension, CHF, renal insufficiency, & active tuberculosis necessitates carefully controlled use."
- If using systemically for therapy, goal is to use as much as is required & as little as possible for as short an amount of time as possible.
- Primary adverse effects are "Cushingoid" in nature with sustained use.
- Many potential drug & lab interactions.

Uses/Indications
The systemic veterinary labeled product (*Vetalog® Injection*) is labeled as "indicated for the treatment of inflammation and related disorders in dogs, cats, and horses. It is also indicated for use in dogs and cats for the management and treatment of acute arthritis, allergic and dermatologic disorders."

In horses, intra-articular (IA) injection of triamcinolone acetonide (TA), particularly in high motion joints is often recommended as studies have demonstrated that IA injection can improve clinical lameness and reduce articular protein, inflammatory cell infiltration, intimal hyperplasia and subintimal fibrosis, and synovial levels of hyaluronan and glycosaminoglycan can be increased. Combining TA with a local anesthetic (*e.g.*, mepivacaine) has been shown not to alter the potency or duration of action of TA and may be useful to both confirm the joint causing lameness and to reduce synovitis (Kay *et al.* 2008). There is some evidence supporting the IA use of TA with hyaluronic acid. In clinically normal horses, IA triamcinolone acetonide diffused directly from the distal interphalangeal joint with or without hyaluronic acid and, after additional studies, may prove to be useful in treating navicular syndrome (Boyce *et al.* 2010).

Intralesional injection of triamcinolone into esophageal strictures has been done in dogs and cats prior to dilation (Richter 2009).

Glucocorticoids have been used in an attempt to treat practically every malady that afflicts man or animal, but there are three broad uses and dosage ranges for use of these agents. 1) Replacement of glucocorticoid activity in patients with adrenal insufficiency; 2) as an antiinflammatory agent; and 3) as an immunosuppressive. Among some of the uses for glucocorticoids include treatment of: endocrine conditions (*e.g.*, adrenal insufficiency), rheumatic diseases (*e.g.*, rheumatoid arthritis), collagen diseases (*e.g.*, systemic lupus), allergic states, respiratory diseases (*e.g.*, asthma), dermatologic diseases (*e.g.*, pemphigus, allergic dermatoses), hematologic disorders (*e.g.*, thrombocytopenias, autoimmune hemolytic anemias), neoplasias, nervous system disorders (increased CSF pressure), GI diseases (*e.g.*, ulcerative colitis exacerbations), and renal diseases (*e.g.*, nephrotic syndrome). Some glucocorticoids are used topically in the eye and skin for various conditions or are injected intra-articularly or intra-lesionally. The above listing is certainly not complete.

Pharmacology/Actions

Triamcinolone acetonide is considered an intermediate acting (metabolic activity of 24-48 hours when given orally) glucocorticoid that is ≈ 4-10X more potent than hydrocortisone. Triamcinolone has negligible mineralocorticoid effects. When injected IM, duration of activity may persist for 4-6 (and sometimes up to 8) weeks. A study in cats with allergic pruritus, found triamcinolone to be ≈ 7X more potent than methylprednisolone.

Glucocorticoids have effects on virtually every cell type and system in mammals. For more information, refer to the Glucocorticoid Agents, General Information monograph.

Pharmacokinetics

Like other corticosteroids, plasma levels are not a good indicator of biologic activity. A pharmacokinetic study to establish appropriate withdrawal times in Thoroughbred horses after IM or IA injection found: a plasma terminal elimination half-life of 11.4 (± 6.53) days for IM and 0.78 (±1) days for intra-articular administration. Levels below limit of detection after IM injection were by days 52 (plasma) and 60 (urine), and after intra-articular injection by day 7 (plasma) and day 8 (urine). Triamcinolone acetonide was also undetectable in any of the joints sampled following IM administration and remained above the limit of quantitation (LOQ) for 21 days following intra-articular administration. (Knych *et al.* 2013)

Contraindications/Precautions/Warnings

Systemic use of glucocorticoids is generally considered contraindicated in systemic fungal infections (unless used for replacement therapy in Addison's), when administered IM in patients with idiopathic thrombocytopenia or hypersensitive to a particular compound. Sustained-release injectable glucocorticoids use is considered contraindicated for chronic corticosteroid therapy of systemic diseases.

Animals that have received glucocorticoids systemically, other than with "burst" therapy, should be tapered off the drugs. Patients who have received the drugs chronically should be tapered off slowly as endogenous ACTH and corticosteroid function may return slowly. Should the animal undergo a "stressor" (*e.g.*, surgery, trauma, illness, etc.) during the tapering process or until normal adrenal and pituitary function resume, additional glucocorticoids should be administered.

Corticosteroid therapy may induce parturition in large animal species during the latter stages of pregnancy.

Adverse Effects

Adverse effects are generally associated with long-term administration of these drugs, especially if given at high dosages or not on an alternate day regimen. Effects generally are manifested as clinical signs of hyperadrenocorticism. When administered to young, growing animals, glucocorticoids can retard growth. Many of the potential effects, adverse and otherwise, are outlined above in the Pharmacology section.

In dogs, polydipsia (PD), polyphagia (PP) and polyuria (PU), may all be seen with short-term "burst" therapy as well as with alternate-day maintenance therapy on days when giving the drug. Adverse effects in dogs can include dull, dry haircoat, weight gain, panting, vomiting, diarrhea, elevated liver enzymes, pancreatitis, GI ulceration, lipidemias, activation or worsening of diabetes mellitus, muscle wasting and behavioral changes (depression, lethargy, viciousness). Discontinuation of the drug may be necessary; changing to an alternate steroid may also alleviate the problem. With the exception of PU/PD/PP, adverse effects associated with antiinflammatory therapy are relatively uncommon. Adverse effects associated with immunosuppressive doses are more common and potentially, more severe.

Cats generally require higher dosages than dogs for clinical effect, but tend to develop fewer adverse effects. Occasionally polydipsia, polyuria, polyphagia with weight gain, diarrhea, or depression can be seen. Long-term, high dose therapy can lead to "Cushingoid" effects, however.

In horses, the potential for dexamethasone or triamcinolone playing a contributory role in the development of laminitis has been a traditional concern, but good evidence linking laminitis to corticosteroid injection is lacking and current clinical evidence argues against generalizations of potential risk. Also there is no evidence that intra-articular corticosteroids cause harm to subchondral bone or promote catastrophic injury (McIlwraith 2010). Another review article on this subject states: "Although the association of laminitis with elevated serum cortisol in pituitary pars intermedia dysfunction suggests that chronic exposure to glucocorticoids may be part of laminitis pathogenesis, review of published reports and databases suggests that glucocorticoid-induced laminitis is a relatively rare occurrence...Generally, local glucocorticoid administration presents little risk as does systemic treatment of recurrent airway obstruction without concurrent disease. Caution should be used however in horses that are overweight and/or insulin resistant, or have had a recent bout of acute laminitis of alimentary or endotoxic origin." (Cornelisse *et al.* 2013).

Reproductive/Nursing Safety

Glucocorticoids are probably necessary for normal fetal development. They may be required for adequate surfactant production, myelin, retinal, pancreas and mammary development.

Excessive dosages early in pregnancy may lead to teratogenic effects. In horses and ruminants, exogenous steroid administration may induce parturition when administered in the latter stages of pregnancy. In humans, the FDA categorizes this drug as category C for use during pregnancy (*Animal studies have shown an adverse effect on the fetus, but there are no adequate studies in humans; or there are no animal reproduction studies and no adequate studies in humans.)*

Glucocorticoids unbound to plasma proteins will enter milk. High dosages or prolonged administration to mothers may potentially inhibit the growth of nursing newborns.

Overdosage/Acute Toxicity

Glucocorticoids when given short-term are unlikely to cause harmful effects, even in massive dosages. One incidence of a dog developing acute CNS effects after accidental ingestion of glucocorticoids has been reported. Should clinical signs occur, use supportive treatment if required.

Chronic usage of glucocorticoids can lead to serious adverse effects. Refer to Adverse Effects above for more information.

Drug Interactions

The following drug interactions have either been reported or are theoretical in humans or animals receiving triamcinolone and may be of significance in veterinary patients. Unless otherwise noted, use together is not necessarily contraindicated, but weigh the potential risks and perform additional monitoring when appropriate.

- **AMPHOTERICIN B:** Administered concomitantly with glucocorticoids may cause hypokalemia.
- **ANALGESICS, OPIATE** and/or **ANESTHETICS, LOCAL** (*e.g.*, **epidural injections**): Combination with glucocorticoids in epidurals has caused serious CNS injuries and death; do not use more volume than very small intrathecal test doses of these agents with glucocorticoids.
- **ANTICHOLINESTERASE AGENTS** (*e.g.*, **pyridostigmine, neostigmine,** etc.): In patients with myasthenia gravis, concomitant glucocorticoid and anticholinesterase agent administration may lead to profound muscle weakness. If possible, discontinue anticholinesterase medication at least 24 hours prior to corticosteroid administration.
- **ASPIRIN:** Glucocorticoids may reduce salicylate blood levels.
- **BARBITURATES:** May increase the metabolism of glucocorticoids and decrease blood levels.
- **CYCLOPHOSPHAMIDE:** Glucocorticoids may also inhibit the hepatic metabolism of cyclophosphamide; dosage adjustments may be required.
- **CYCLOSPORINE:** Concomitant administration of glucocorticoids and cyclosporine may increase the blood levels of each, by mutually inhibiting the hepatic metabolism of each other; the clinical significance of this interaction is not clear.
- **DIURETICS, POTASSIUM-DEPLETING** (*e.g.*, **spironolactone, triamterene**): Administered concomitantly with glucocorticoids may cause hypokalemia.
- **ERYTHROMYCIN, CLARITHROMYCIN:** May increase TMC levels.
- **ESTROGENS:** The effects of TMC, and possibly other glucocorticoids, may be potentiated by concomitant administration with estrogens.
- **INSULIN:** Insulin requirements may increase in patients receiving glucocorticoids.
- **ISONIAZID:** TMC may decrease isoniazid levels.
- **KETOCONAZOLE** and other **AZOLE ANTIFUNGALS:** May decrease the metabolism of glucocorticoids and increase TMC blood levels; ketoconazole may induce adrenal insufficiency when glucocorticoids are withdrawn by inhibiting adrenal corticosteroid synthesis.
- **MITOTANE:** May alter the metabolism of steroids; higher than usual doses of steroids may be necessary to treat mitotane-induced adrenal insufficiency.
- **NSAIDS:** Administration of ulcerogenic drugs with glucocorticoids may increase the risk of gastrointestinal ulceration.
- **PHENOBARBITAL:** May increase the metabolism of glucocorticoids and decrease TMC blood levels.
- **RIFAMPIN:** May increase the metabolism of glucocorticoids and decrease TMC blood levels.
- **VACCINES:** Patients receiving corticosteroids at immunosuppressive dosages should generally not receive live attenuated-virus vaccines as virus replication may be augmented; a diminished immune response may occur after vaccine, toxoid, or bacterin administration in patients receiving glucocorticoids.
- **WARFARIN:** TMC may affect INR's; monitor.

Laboratory Considerations

- Glucocorticoids may increase **serum cholesterol.**
- Glucocorticoids may increase **serum and urine glucose** levels.
- Glucocorticoids may decrease **serum potassium.**
- Glucocorticoids can suppress the release of thyroid stimulating hormone (TSH) and reduce T_3 & T_4 values. Thyroid gland atrophy has been reported after chronic glucocorticoid administration. Uptake of I^{131} by the thyroid may be decreased by glucocorticoids.
- Reactions to **skin tests** may be suppressed by glucocorticoids.
- False-negative results of the **nitroblue tetrazolium** test for systemic bacterial infections may be induced by glucocorticoids.
- Glucocorticoids may cause **neutrophilia** within 4-8 hours after dosing and return to baseline within 24-48 hours after drug discontinuation.
- Glucocorticoids can cause **lymphopenia,** which can persist for weeks after drug discontinuation in dogs.

Doses

Note: When used systemically (PO, IM or SC), initial doses of triamcinolone can be given at dosages that are ≈ 7-8X lower as the prednisone or prednisolone dose. For example: If the dosage of prednisone for the indication treated is 1 mg/kg PO, a corresponding dosage of triamcinolone acetonide would be ≈ 0.125 mg/kg PO. Triamcinolone has negligble mineralocorticoid effects and its biologic activity may persist for 36-48 hours. If given on a daily basis, therapy for longer than 1-2 weeks will suppress the HPA axis and recovery will take longer than 1 week. Therefore, if triamcinolone is used for longer than a few days, when discontinuing, dosage should be tapered off using alternate day, then every third day therapy.

- **DOGS/CATS:**

Labeled Doses (FDA-approved)

For glucocorticoid effects (labeled dose; FDA-approved): Using tablets: 0.11 mg/kg PO initially once a day, may increase to 0.22 mg/kg PO once daily if initial response is unsatisfactory. As soon as possible, but not later than 2 weeks, reduce dose gradually to 0.028 – 0.055 mg/kg/day. (Package insert; *Vetalog® Tablets*)

For injectable product: 0.11 – 0.22 mg/kg for inflammatory or allergic disorders, and 0.22 mg/kg for dermatological disorders. Effects generally persist for 7-15 days; if symptoms recur, may repeat or institute oral therapy.

For intralesional injection: Usual dose is 1.2 – 1.8 mg; inject around lesion at 0.5 – 2.5 cm intervals. Do not exceed 0.6 mg at any one site or 6 mg total dose. May repeat as necessary. (Package insert; *Vetalog® Injection*)

Extra-label Doses:

As an antiinflammatory agent:

a) Induction: 0.05 – 0.22 mg/kg PO q24h (manufacturer recommended dose). Maintenance: 0.05 – 0.1 mg/kg (or lower if possible) PO q48-72h. Taper off if discontinuing.

b) **For adjunctive treatment of pruritus in allergic cats** (extra-label): From a double-blinded, randomized, prospective study (n=16 in triamcinolone group). Initial induction dosage was 0.5 mg per cat PO once daily for cats weighing ≤5 kg, and 0.7 mg per cat PO once daily for cats >5 kg. Cats that did not achieve remission by day 7 had their once daily induction dose doubled for the next 7 days. Mean dosage required for induction of remission was 0.18 mg/kg (range 0.09 – 0.26 mg/kg) PO once daily; 94% of treated cats achieved remission by the end of the second week. Dosages used to achieve remission were then given every other day and tapered (from 100% to 25% of induction dose in 25% increments) to the lowest every other day dosage that maintained remission. Mean alternate day dosages were 0.08 mg/kg. (Ganz et al. 2012)

As an immunosuppressive:

a) **For autoimmune skin diseases:** Induction: 0.4 – 0.6 mg/kg PO q24h. Maintenance: 0.1 – 0.2 mg/kg PO q48-72h. (Koch *et al.* 2011)

b) **For feline pemphigus foliaceus** (extra-label): A retrospective study on feline pemphigus foliaceus reported an induction dose range for well-controlled cats of 0.6 – 2 mg/kg PO q24h and a maintenance dose range of 0.6 – 1 mg/kg PO every 2-7 days. Cats receiving triamcinolone had significantly fewer side effects than cats receiving prednisolone and chlorambucil. When used orally long-term, triamcinolone should be discontinued gradually.

For intralesional injection:

a) **To prevent re-stricture after esophageal dilation:** Using an endoscopically directed needle, inject 0.5 – 1 mL of *Vetalog®* (2 mg/mL) submucosally at time of dilation procedure. Infiltration is done circumferentially at four points around the site. (Marks 2004)

■ **HORSES:** (NOTE: ARCI UCGFS CLASS 4 DRUG)
For glucocorticoid effects (labeled dose; FDA-approved): 0.011 – 0.022 mg/kg PO twice daily; 0.011 – 0.022 mg/kg IM or SC; 6 – 18 mg intra-articularly or intrasynovially, may repeat after 3-4 days (Package inserts; *Vetalog® Powder* and I*njection*)

Monitoring

Monitoring of glucocorticoid therapy is dependent on its reason for use, dosage, agent used (amount of mineralocorticoid activity), dosage schedule (daily versus alternate day therapy), duration of therapy, and the animal's age and condition. The following list may not be appropriate or complete for all animals; use clinical assessment and judgment should adverse effects be noted:

■ Weight, appetite, signs of edema.
■ Serum and/or urine electrolytes.
■ Total plasma proteins, albumin.
■ Blood glucose.
■ Growth and development in young animals.
■ ACTH stimulation test if necessary.

Client Information

■ Give oral products with food.
■ Goal is to find the lowest dose possible and use it for the shortest period of time.
■ Many side effects are possible (see below), especially when it is used long term. Most common ones are: greater appetite, thirst, and need to urinate.
■ In dogs, stomach or intestinal ulcers, perforation or bleeding can occur. If your animal stops eating, or you notice a high fever, black tarry stools or bloody vomit, contact your veterinarian right away.

■ Do not stop therapy abruptly (cold turkey) without veterinarian's guidance as serious side effects could occur.

Chemistry/Synonyms

Triamcinolone acetonide, a synthetic glucocorticoid, occurs as slightly odorous, white to cream-colored, crystalline powder with a melting point between 290-294°C. It is practically insoluble in water, very soluble in dehydrated alcohol and slightly soluble in alcohol. The commercially available sterile suspensions have a pH range of 5-7.5.

Triamcinolone acetonide may also be known as: triamcinoloni acetonidum; many trade names are available.

Storage/Stability

Triamcinolone acetonide products should be stored at room temperature (15-30°C); the injection should be protected from light and protected from freezing.

Compatibility/Compounding Considerations

No specific information noted.

Dosage Forms/Regulatory Status

VETERINARY-LABELED PRODUCTS:

Triamcinolone Acetonide Tablets: 0.5 mg, 1.5 mg; *Cortalone®, Triamtabs®*, generic; (Rx). FDA-approved for use in dogs and cats.

Triamcinolone Acetonide Suspension for Injection: 2 mg/mL; 6 mg/mL; *Vetalog® Parenteral*; (Rx). FDA-approved for use in dogs, cats, and horses not intended for food.

The ARCI (Racing Commissioners International) has designated this drug as a class 4 substance. See the appendix for more information.

HUMAN-LABELED PRODUCTS:

Triamcinolone Acetonide Injection: 10 mg/mL & 40 mg/mL suspension in 1 mL, 5 mL and 10 mL vials; *Kenalog-10 & -40*; (Rx)

Triamcinolone Hexacetonide Injection: 5 mg/mL & 20 mg/mL suspension in 1 mL & 5 mL vials; *Aristospan Intralesional® & Intra-articular®*; (Rx)

Many topical preparations are available, alone and in combination with other agents. Oral mucosal paste & inhaled products are also FDA-approved. All are Rx.

Revisions/References

Monograph revised/updated August 2014.

Boyce, M., et al. (2010). Evaluation of diffusion of triamcinolone acetonide from the distal interphalangeal joint into the navicular bursa in horses. American Journal of Veterinary Research 71(2): 169-75.

Cornelisse, C. J. & N. E. Robinson (2013). Glucocorticoid therapy and the risk of equine laminitis. Equine Veterinary Education 25(1): 39-46.

Ganz, E. C., et al. (2012). Evaluation of methylprednisolone and triamcinolone for the induction and maintenance treatment of pruritus in allergic cats: a double-blinded, randomized, prospective study. Veterinary Dermatology 23(5).

Kay, A. T., et al. (2008). Anti-inflammatory and analgesic effects of intra-articular injection of triamcinolone acetonide, mepivacaine hydrochloride, or both on lipopolysaccharide-induced lameness in horses. American Journal of Veterinary Research 69(12): 1646-54.

Knych, H. K., et al. (2013). Pharmacokinetics of triamcinolone acetonide following intramuscular and intra-articular administration to exercised Thoroughbred horses. Equine Veterinary Journal 45(6): 715-20.

Koch, S., et al. (2011). *Small Animal Dermatology Drug Handbook*, Wiley-Blackwell. Ames.

Marks, S. (2004). What's new in veterinary endoscopy? Proceedings: ACVIM Forum. accessed via Veterinary Information Network; vin.com

McIlwraith, C. W. (2010). The use of intra-articular corticosteroids in the horse: What is known on a scientific basis? Equine Veterinary Journal 42(6): 563-71.

Richter, K. (2009). Esophageal Strictures--Update on Therapeutic Options. Proceedings: ACVIM. accessed via Veterinary Information Network; vin.com

Triamterene

(trye-am-the-reen)   Dyrenium®

Potassium-Sparing Diuretic

Prescriber Highlights

▶ Potassium-sparing diuretic that may be considered as an alternative to spironolactone for treating CHF in dogs; limited clinical experience with this drug in dogs/cats. Rarely used in veterinary medicine.

▶ Contraindications: Anuria, severe or progressive renal disease, severe hepatic disease, hypersensitivity to triamterene, preexisting hyperkalemia, concurrent therapy with another potassium-sparing agent (spironolactone, amiloride) or potassium supplementation.

▶ Hyperkalemia possible; must monitor serum K⁺.

Uses/Indications

Triamterene is a potassium-sparing diuretic that potentially could be an alternative to spironolactone for the adjunctive treatment of congestive heart failure in dogs, however, there is little experience associated with its use in dogs or cats and it is rarely recommended.

Pharmacology/Actions

By exerting a direct effect on the distal renal tubule, triamterene inhibits the reabsorption of sodium in exchange for hydrogen and potassium ions. Unlike spironolactone, it does not competitively inhibit aldosterone. Triamterene increases excretion of sodium, calcium, magnesium and bicarbonate; urinary pH may be slightly increased. Serum concentrations of potassium and chloride may be increased. When used alone, triamterene has little effect on blood pressure. Triamterene can reduce GFR slightly, probably by affecting renal blood flow. This effect is reversible when the medication is discontinued.

Pharmacokinetics

Pharmacokinetic data for dogs or cats was not located. In humans, triamterene is rapidly absorbed after oral administration and oral bioavailability is ≈ 85%. Onset of diuresis occurs in 2-4 hours, peaks at ≈ 6 hours and diuresis can persist up to 12-16 hours post-dose. Triamterene is metabolized in the liver to 6-p-hydroxytriamterine and its sulfate conjugate. These metabolites are eliminated in the bile/feces and urine; elimination half-life is ≈ 2 hours.

Contraindications/Precautions/Warnings

Triamterene is contraindicated for human patients (and presumably dogs and cats) with anuria, severe or progressive renal disease, severe hepatic disease, hypersensitivity to triamterene, preexisting hyperkalemia, history of triamterene-induced hyperkalemia, concurrent therapy with another potassium-sparing agent (spironolactone, amiloride) or potassium supplementation.

Adverse Effects

Because triamterene has been infrequently used in veterinary medicine, an accurate adverse effect profile for small animals is not known, however, hyperkalemia is a definite possibility and monitoring of electrolytes and renal function are necessary. In humans, hyperkalemia rarely occurs in patients with normal urine output and potassium intake.

Less common adverse effects reported in humans include headache/dizziness, GI effects, hyponatremia, and an increased sensitivity to sunlight. Rarely, hypersensitivity reactions have occurred in human patients taking triamterene. Other rare adverse effects include triamterene-nephrolithiasis, agranulocytosis, thrombocytopenia, or megaloblastosis.

Reproductive/Nursing Safety

Studies to determine triamterene's effects on fertility have not been performed.

Studies in pregnant rats given triamterene at 6-20X (human dose) did not show adverse effects to the fetuses. Triamterene crosses the placental barrier. For humans, triamterene is either in FDA category *B* or category *C*, depending on the reference. Category *C* for use during pregnancy states: *Animal studies have shown an adverse effect on the fetus, but there are no adequate studies in humans; or there are no animal reproduction studies and no adequate studies in humans.* If considering use of this product in a pregnant animal, weigh the potential benefits of treatment versus the risks.

Triamterene is distributed into milk. Although unlikely to pose much risk to nursing animals, safety during nursing cannot be assured.

Overdosage/Acute Toxicity

The oral LD50 for triamterene in mice is 380 mg/kg. Fluid and electrolyte imbalance is the most likely risk associated with an overdose. GI effects or hypotension are also possible. Consider gut emptying protocols for very large or quantity unknown ingestions. Acute overdoses should generally be managed by observation, with fluid, electrolyte (especially serum potassium) and acid-base monitoring. Supportive treatment should be initiated if required.

Drug Interactions

The following drug interactions have either been reported or are theoretical in humans or animals receiving triamterene and may be of significance in veterinary patients. Unless otherwise noted, use together is not necessarily contraindicated, but weigh the potential risks and perform additional monitoring when appropriate.

- **ACE INHIBITORS** (*e.g.,* **enalapril, benazepril**): Increased risks for hyperkalemia.
- **ANTIDIABETIC AGENTS** (*e.g.,* **insulin, oral hypoglycemic agents**): Triamterene may increase blood glucose.
- **ANTIHYPERTENSIVE AGENTS**: Possible potentiation of hypotensive effects.
- **DIURETICS, POTASSIUM-SPARING** (*e.g.,* **spironolactone, amiloride**): Increase risk of hyperkalemia; use of these drugs with triamterene in humans is contraindicated.
- **LITHIUM**: Triamterene may reduce lithium clearance.
- **NSAIDs**: Triamterene with NSAIDs (esp. **indomethacin**) may increase the risks of nephrotoxicity.
- **POTASSIUM SUPPLEMENTS** or **HIGH POTASSIUM FOODS**: Increased risk for hyperkalemia.

Laboratory Considerations

- **Quinidine**: Triamterene may interfere with fluorescent assay of quinidine.

Doses

- **DOGS:**

  For adjunctive treatment of heart failure: (extra-label): Scant published evidence to support use or any dosage; if a potassium-sparing diuretic is used, spironolactone is usually preferred. Anecdotal dosages of 1 – 2 mg/kg PO twice daily or 2 – 4 mg/kg per day have been noted.

Monitoring

- Serum electrolytes (especially potassium), BUN, creatinine.
- Hydration status.
- Blood pressure, if indicated.
- Signs of edema; patient weight, if indicated.

Client Information

- Give this medication with food to help prevent stomach upset.
- Urine may develop a bluish hue, this is normal.

- Because this medication has not been used very much in dogs or cats, report any unusual effects to the veterinarian.

Chemistry/Synonyms

Triamterene is structurally related to folic acid and occurs as a yellow, odorless, crystalline powder. It is practically insoluble in water and very slightly soluble in alcohol. At 50°C, it is slightly soluble in water. In acidified solutions, triamterene gives off a blue fluorescence.

Triamterene may also be known as NSC-77625, KF-8542, FI-6143, triamteren, trimaterenum, triamtereen, or *Dyrenium*®. International trade names include *Dytac*®, *Dyazide*®, *Maxzide-25*® and *Triteren*®. There are many international trade names for combination products with hydrochlorothiazide.

Storage/Stability

Triamterene capsules should be stored between 15-30°C (59-86°F) in tight, light-resistant containers.

Compatibility/Compounding Considerations

No specific information noted.

Dosage Forms/Regulatory Status

VETERINARY-LABELED PRODUCTS: NONE.
The ARCI (Racing Commissioners International) has designated this drug as a class 4 substance.

HUMAN-LABELED PRODUCTS:
Triamterene Capsules: 50 mg & 100 mg; *Dyrenium*®; (Rx)

In humans, triamterene is often prescribed as a fixed-dose combination with hydrochlorothiazide. Products include:

Triamterene 37.5 mg/Hydrochlorothiazide 25 mg Tablets and Capsules; *Dyazide*®, *Maxzide-25MG*®, generic; (Rx)

Triamterene 50 mg/Hydrochlorothiazide 25 mg Capsules; generic; (Rx)

Triamterene 75 mg/Hydrochlorothiazide 50 mg Tablets; *Maxzide*®, generic; (Rx)

Revisions/References

Monograph revised/updated August 2014.

Trientine HCl

(trye-en-teen)   2,2,2-tetramine, Syprine®
Chelating Agent

Prescriber Highlights

▶ Oral copper chelating agent for copper hepatopathy. Limited veterinary experience with this drug.

▶ Give on an empty stomach, about one hour prior to meals.

▶ Probably fewer adverse effects then penicillamine, but acute renal failure possible.

▶ More expensive than penicillamine; not readily available commercially and may need to be compounded into smaller dosages.

Uses/Indications

Trientine may be useful for the treatment of copper-associated hepatopathy in dogs, particularly when dogs cannot tolerate the adverse effects (*e.g.*, vomiting) associated with penicillamine.

Pharmacology/Actions

Trientine is an effective chelator of copper and increases its elimination via urinary excretion. It apparently has a greater affinity for copper in plasma than penicillamine, but penicillamine has a greater affinity for tissue copper.

Pharmacokinetics

No data was located.

Contraindications/Precautions/Warnings

Trientine is contraindicated in patients hypersensitive to it. It is not indicated for cystinuria, rheumatoid arthritis, or biliary cirrhosis.

Adverse Effects

Albeit with limited veterinary experience, trientine has had relatively minimal adverse effects in dogs treated for copper hepatotoxicity, but acute renal failure has been reported particularly when used in dogs with very high liver copper levels and at higher dosages. Human patients have developed iron deficiency anemia after taking trientine long-term. There is a chance for topical dermatitis developing if trientine gets on skin; wash off immediately. The drug should be given in a capsule (may need to be compounded) and not sprinkled on food.

Reproductive/Nursing Safety

Trientine is a potential teratogen. It was teratogenic in rats given doses similar to those for humans and should only be used in pregnancy when the benefits to the mother outweigh the risks to offspring. In humans, the FDA categorizes this drug as category *C* for use during pregnancy (*Animal studies have shown an adverse effect on the fetus, but there are no adequate studies in humans; or there are no animal reproduction studies and no adequate studies in humans.*)

It is not known whether this drug is excreted in breast milk. Exercise caution when administering to nursing patients.

Overdosage/Acute Toxicity

Little information is available; a case of a human ingesting 30 grams of trientine without significant morbidity has been reported.

Drug Interactions

The following drug interactions have either been reported or are theoretical in humans or animals receiving trientine and may be of significance in veterinary patients. Unless otherwise noted, use together is not necessarily contraindicated, but weigh the potential risks and perform additional monitoring when appropriate.

- **IRON:** Iron and trientine inhibit the absorption of one another; if iron therapy is needed, give doses at least 2 hours apart from one another.

- **ZINC:** Because trientine may also chelate zinc or other minerals, avoid concomitant therapy (most do not recommend using zinc for copper reduction until copper chelation therapy with penicillamine or trientine is completed) or separate dosages by at least 2 hours.

Doses

- **DOGS:**

  As a chelator for copper hepatotoxicity (extra-label): 10 – 15 mg/kg PO ≈ 1-2 hours prior to meals is usually recommended. However, one source (Center 2013) now recommends that initial dosages be lower, 5 – 7 mg/kg PO twice daily, 1-2 hours before meals to avoid acute renal injury in dogs with markedly increased hepatic copper.

Monitoring

- Periodic liver biopsies for quantitative hepatic copper levels and response to therapy.

- Baseline and periodic renal function tests.

Client Information

- It is best to give this medicine 1-2 hours before feeding. If your dog vomits after getting it, contact your veterinarian to see if giving it with a small amount of food is OK.

Chemistry/Synonyms

An oral copper chelator, trientine HCl occurs as a white to pale yellow crystalline powder. It is hygroscopic and freely soluble in water.

Trientine HCl may also be known as: MK-0681, 2,2,2-tetramine, trien hydrochloride, triethylenetetramine dihydrochloride, trientine hydrochloride or *Syprine*®.

Storage/Stability

Store trientine capsules in the refrigerator (2-8°C) in tightly closed containers.

Compatibility/Compounding Considerations

Trientine may need to be compounded into smaller capsules to give appropriate doses to dogs.

One sources states: "Modification of 2,2,2-tetramine (trientine) to 2,3,2-tetramine increases potency as a copper-chelating agent. Use of 2,3,2-tetramine in affected Bedlington terriers reduced liver copper concentrations significantly after 200 days of treatment at a dose of 15 mg/kg body weight. This drug is not commercially available, but can be obtained from chemical supply companies in the form of N,N'-bis(2-aminoethyl)-1,3-propanediamine and prepared as a salt for oral administration." (Marks 2013)

Dosage Forms/Regulatory Status

VETERINARY-LABELED PRODUCTS: NONE.

HUMAN-LABELED PRODUCTS:

Trientine HCl Oral Capsules: 250 mg; *Syprine*®; (Rx)

Revisions/References

Monograph revised/updated August 2014.

Center, S. (2013). Canine Copper-Associated Hepatopathy. Proceedings; 23rd ECVIM-CA Congress. accessed via Veterinary Information Network; vin.com

Marks, S. L. (2013). Advances in Dietary Management of GI Disorders. World Small Animal Veterinary Association World Congress Proceedings. accessed via Veterinary Information Network; vin.com

Trilostane

(try-low-stane)   Vetoryl®

Adrenal Steroid Synthesis Inhibitor

Prescriber Highlights

▶ Competitive inhibitor of 3-beta hydroxysteroid dehydrogenase thereby reducing the synthesis of cortisol, aldosterone, & adrenal androgens.

▶ May be useful in dogs for treatment of pituitary-dependent hyperadrenocorticism, adrenal dependent hyperadrenocorticism, Alopecia X in Pomeranians & Alaskan malamutes; in cats for treatment of feline pituitary dependent hyperadrenocorticism, & in horses for equine hyperadrenocorticism (HAC).

▶ Potential adverse effects in dogs include lethargy, inappetence, vomiting, electrolyte abnormalities, & diarrhea; there are case reports of hypoadrenocorticism & death. Lower dosage regimen (twice daily) appears to be effective and associated with fewer significant adverse effects.

▶ Expense of treatment (drug plus monitoring) may be an issue.

Uses/Indications

Trilostane may be useful for treating pituitary-dependent hyperadrenocorticism (HAC) or adrenal-dependent hyperadrenocorticism in dogs, feline pituitary-dependent hyperadrenocorticism, and equine hyperadrenocorticism (HAC). It is labeled as indicated for use in dogs for the treatment of pituitary-dependent hyperadrenocorticism or hyperadrenocorticism due to adrenocortical tumors.

While the mitotane versus trilostane debate for medical treatment of canine pituitary-dependent HAC continues, either treatment (drug) can be safe and effective, but both require diligent monitoring and client education (Reine 2012). One clinical study demonstrated that lower than labeled dosages given twice daily were both effective and safer than the labeled-dose (Feldman 2011). A second, smaller study in dogs weighing <5 kg reached the same conclusion (Cho *et al.* 2013).

Trilostane may also be useful in treating Pomeranians with Alopecia X and Alaskan malamutes with adult-onset alopecia.

In cats, one retrospective study (n=15) concluded that trilostane is a viable, well-tolerated, medical treatment option for management of cats with HAC (Mellet Keith *et al.* 2013).

Pharmacology/Actions

Trilostane is a competitive inhibitor of 3-beta hydroxysteroid dehydrogenase thereby reducing synthesis of cortisol, aldosterone, and adrenal androgens. Inhibition is reversible and apparently dose dependent.

After administration to dogs with pituitary-dependent HAC, cortisol concentrations decrease significantly 2-4 hours after trilostane administration. From baseline, significant increases occurred in endogenous ACTH concentrations between hours 3-12, significant increases in aldosterone concentrations occurred between hours 16-20 but were not deemed clinically significant, and significant increases in renin activity occurred between hours 6-20. Potassium concentrations decreased significantly between hours 0.5-2, but are not of clinical significance (Griebsch *et al.* 2014). Another study in dogs with pituitary-dependent hyperadrenocorticism assessed mitotane's and trilostane's effects on aldosterone secretory reserve and to see if aldosterone concentration correlates with electrolyte concentrations. They found that aldosterone concentrations in the mitotane- and trilostane-treated dogs at 30 and 60 minutes post-ACTH were significantly lower than in clinically healthy dogs and that treated dogs had a greater decrease in aldosterone secretory reserve at 30 minutes versus 60 minutes. There was no correlation between aldosterone and serum electrolyte concentrations (Reid *et al.* 2014).

Pharmacokinetics

In dogs, orally administered trilostane is rapidly, but erratically absorbed with peak levels occurring between 1.5-2 hours post dose. It is unknown whether the presence of food in the gut significantly alters absorption characteristics.

Trilostane is metabolized in the liver to several metabolites including ketotrilostane, which is active. An *ex vivo* study in canine adrenal glands found that ketotrilostane was 4.9X and 2.4X more potent than trilostane in inhibiting cortisol and corticosterone secretion (McGraw *et al.* 2011).

Contraindications/Precautions/Warnings

Trilostane is contraindicated in animals hypersensitive to it. It should be used with caution in patients with renal or hepatic impairment. Do not use in pregnant dogs.

When used for controlling clinical signs of Cushing's in dogs with adrenal tumors, trilostane will not shrink the tumor and adrenal glands may actually increase in size during treatment.

Adverse Effects

Trilostane appears to be relatively well tolerated in dogs, but up to 63% of treated dogs can develop lethargy, mild electrolyte abnormalities (hyponatremia, hyperkalemia), vomiting, diarrhea and inappetence during the first few days of therapy secondary to steroid withdrawal. These effects are usually relatively mild and self-limiting. Withholding the drug for a few days and then giving it every other day for a week may alleviate lethargy and vomiting. Although adrenal suppression caused by trilostane is reversible in most cases, rarely adrenal necrosis and death have occurred in dogs.

In cats with hyperadrenocorticism, adverse effects associated with trilostane therapy have included lethargy, anorexia and dulled mentation.

In one study of trilostane given to 20 horses with equine Cushing's, no adverse effects were noted (McGowan *et al.* 2003).

Reproductive/Nursing Safety

Because trilostane can significantly reduce the synthesis of progesterone *in vivo*, it should not be used in pregnancy. Trilostane reportedly (not confirmed) is classified by the FDA as a category *X* drug (*Contraindicated in pregnancy*).

Information on trilostane levels in maternal milk were not located; use with caution in lactating animals.

Overdosage/Acute Toxicity

Specific information on trilostane acute toxicity was not located. One source states that trilostane overdoses would be unlikely to threaten life and no clinical signs would be expected. However, blood pressure, hydration status, and electrolyte balance should be monitored. If the animal is stressed, consider giving exogenous corticosteroids short-term. Because the drug's effects are relatively short lived, monitoring of patients without complications should only be required for a few days post ingestion.

Drug Interactions

The following drug interactions have either been reported or are theoretical in humans or animals receiving trilostane and may be of significance in veterinary patients. Unless otherwise noted, use together is not necessarily contraindicated, but weigh the potential risks and perform additional monitoring when appropriate.

- **ACE INHIBITORS** (*e.g.,* **benazepril, enalapril**): Could increase risk for hyperkalemia.
- **AMINOGLUTETHIMIDE**: May potentiate the effects of trilostane and lead to hypoadrenocorticism.
- **KETOCONAZOLE**: May potentiate the effects of trilostane and lead to hypoadrenocorticism.
- **MITOTANE**: May potentiate the effects of trilostane and lead to hypoadrenocorticism.
- **POTASSIUM-SPARING DIURETICS** (*e.g.,* **spironolactone**): Could increase risk for hyperkalemia.
- **POTASSIUM-SUPPLEMENTS; HIGH POTASSIUM FOODS**: Could increase risk for hyperkalemia.

Laboratory Considerations

- No specific laboratory interactions or considerations were located.

Doses

- **DOGS:**

For treatment of canine hyperadrenocorticism (HAC):

a) Labeled dose; FDA approved: The starting dose for the treatment of hyperadrenocorticism in dogs is 2.2 – 6.7 mg/kg PO once a day with food based on body weight and capsule size. The package insert has a dosing table (Table 1) to help determine the appropriate size and number of capsules to administer.

After approximately 10-14 days at this dose, re-examine the dog and conduct a 4-6 hour post-dosing ACTH stimulation test. If physical examination is acceptable adjust dose according to Table 2 (found in the package insert). Individual dose adjustments and close monitoring are essential. Re-examine and conduct an ACTH stimulation test 10-14 days after every dose alteration. Care must be taken during dose increases to monitor the dog's clinical signs and serum electrolyte concentrations. Once daily administration is recommended. However, if clinical signs are not controlled for the full day, twice daily dosing may be needed. To switch from a once daily dose to a twice daily dose, increase the total daily dose by 1/3 to 1/2 and divide the total amount into two doses given 12 hours apart. (Label Information; *Vetoryl*®) **Note**: A prospective randomized study in 32 dogs with HAC comparing the efficacy of once daily (initial dosage 1 – 6.6 mg/kg; mean 2.9 mg/kg) vs. twice daily (initial dosage 2.5 – 5.5 mg/kg/day; mean 3.6 mg/kg/day) administration of trilostane found that more dogs in the twice daily group had complete clinical recovery, but there was no significant difference in the mean post-ACTH cortisol concentration between groups. At 6 months, once daily treated dogs had higher cortisol concentrations. There was no statistical difference in mean daily dosage in the 2 groups. Adverse effects were deemed "mild" and with no statistical difference between treatment groups. Authors concluded that giving trilostane twice daily might increase the number with good clinical response, but the results of adrenal function tests were similar in both groups. (Arenas *et al.* 2013). See also the dose (Feldman 2011) below.

b) Extra-label dose. Study done in dogs with naturally occurring HAC (n=47; 38 with pituitary dependent HAC, 9 with adrenocortical tumor): Initial treatment at 0.21 – 1.1 mg/kg PO q12h (mean: 0.86 mg/kg q12h). Slow adjustment of the treatment protocol to achieve clinical improvement may be needed on a case-by-case basis. Approximately 75% of the dogs in the study (35/47) never required more than 3 mg/kg per day to control their disease throughout the 1-year follow-up. Author concluded that the results of the present study indicated that trilostane is both potent and effective in dogs at doses less than those recommended by the manufacturer and that lower dose twice daily administration should be considered as it minimizes the incidence and severity of adverse effects and trilostane's effects have been shown to last less than 12 hours (Feldman 2011). There is some evidence that as body weight increases especially in dogs weighing >30 kg, the amount of trilostane (mg/kg/dose as well as mg/kg/daily dosage) required to control clinical signs decreases (Feldman *et al.* 2012).

For treatment of Alopecia X (extra-label):

a) In Alaskan Malamutes: 3 – 3.6 mg/kg PO twice a day for 4-6 months. From a case series (n=3); no adverse effects reported. (Leone *et al.* 2005)

b) In Miniature poodles and Pomeranians: Average dose was 10.85 mg/kg per day given either once a day or divided twice a day for 4-8 weeks. (Cerundolo *et al.* 2004)

- **CATS:**

For treatment of feline hyperadrenocorticism (extra-label):

a) From a retrospective study (n=15). Initial dosing frequency was once daily for 13/15 cats. The initial dosages in these cats were: 10 mg per cat PO once daily (n=8); and 30 mg per cat PO once daily (n=5). Dose adjustments were performed in 6 cases. Five were switched to twice daily dosing (Mellet Keith *et al.* 2013). Another retrospective study (n=9) trilostane dosages ranged from 0.5 – 12 mg/kg PO q24h or q12h (Valentin *et al.* 2014).

b) Treatment with trilostane may improve clinical signs, but cats typically remain diabetic. Effective doses range from 15 mg (per cat) PO once daily to 60 mg (per cat) PO q12h. ACTH stimulation tests should be used to titrate the dose, similar to the protocol for dogs. (Scott-Moncrieff 2010)

- **HORSES:**

For treatment of equine pituitary pars intermedia dysfunction (PPID; equine Cushing's syndrome) (extra-label): 0.4 – 1 mg/kg (total dose 120 – 240 mg) PO once daily (McGowan *et al.* 2003). **Note:** Trilostane may be beneficial to those horses with PPID with adrenal gland hyperplasia and hypercortisolemia, but it would have no effect on the excessive production of pituitary-derived hormones (McFarlane 2011).

Monitoring

- Clinical effects.
- Adverse effects.
- Serum electrolytes.
- Urinalysis including specific gravity, glucose and possibly urine cortisol:creatinine ratio (UCCR). **Note:** It appears that there is no advantage in performing the relatively expensive UCCR evaluation on each reevaluation, but urine specific gravity, glucose, protein or evidence for infection have potential in the assessment of dogs being treated long-term with trilostane (Feldman 2011).
- ACTH stimulation tests (see doses for recommendations). For long-term monitoring, the manufacturer recommends: Once an optimum dose has been reached, re-examine the dog at 30 days, 90 days and every 3 months thereafter. At a minimum, this monitoring should include a thorough history and physical examination, ACTH stimulation test conducted 4-6 hours after trilostane administration (**Note:** Results from one recent study suggests the optimal time point for an ACTH stimulation test to be performed is 2-4 hours after trilostane dosing), and serum biochemical tests (with particular attention to electrolytes, renal and hepatic function). A post-ACTH stimulation test resulting in a cortisol of <1.45 micrograms/dL (<40 nMol/L), with or without electrolyte abnormalities, may precede the development of clinical signs of hypoadrenocorticism. Good control is indicated by favorable clinical signs as well as post-ACTH serum cortisol of 1.45-9.1 micrograms/dL (40-250 nMol/L). If the ACTH stimulation test is <1.45 micrograms/dL (<40 nMol/L) and/or if electrolyte imbalances characteristic of hypoadrenocorticism (hyperkalemia and hyponatremia) are found, trilostane should be temporarily discontinued until recurrence of clinical signs consistent with hyperadrenocorticism and test results return to normal (1.45-9.1 micrograms/dL or 40-250 nMol/L). Trilostane may then be re-introduced at a lower dose. **Note:** One study concluded that a baseline cortisol concentration collected 4-6 hours after trilostane in dogs with HAC provided clinically useful information about control of adrenal gland function (Cook *et al.* 2010), but another study to see if baseline cortisol, endogenous ACTH and the cortisol/ACTH ratio could be used to monitor trilostane concluded that they cannot replace the ACTH stimulation test (Burkhardt *et al.* 2013).

Client Information

- Give exactly the way veterinarian has prescribed, don't give more or stop the drug unless you first talk to your veterinarian.
- Give in the morning with food, unless otherwise directed by veterinarian. If a dose is missed, give the prescribed dose at the regular dosing time the next day.
- Trilostane capsules do not require any special safety handling precautions. The manufacturer states: Wash hands after use. Do not empty capsule contents and do not attempt to divide the capsules. Do not handle the capsules if pregnant or if trying to conceive. Clients should report any adverse effects to the veterinarian. Contact veterinarian immediately if dog stops eating or drinking, or becomes ill.
- Keep out of reach of children and pets.
- Clients should understand that trilostane is a treatment for the condition and not a cure; improvements occur gradually and are difficult to see on a daily basis.

Chemistry/Synonyms

A synthetic steroid analog, trilostane has a molecular weight of 329.4 and its chemical name is 4-alpha, 5-alpha-Epoxy-17-beta-hydroxy-3-oxoandrostane-2-alpha-carbonitrile. It reportedly is relatively insoluble in water.

Trilostane may also be known as: WIN 24540, *Vetoryl®*, *Desopan®*, *Modrastane®* or *Modrenal®*.

Storage/Stability

Commercially available trilostane capsules should be stored at room temperature in tight, light-resistant containers.

Compatibility/Compounding Considerations

An evaluation of compounded trilostane capsules obtained from 8 compounding pharmacies found that 38% of compounded batches were outside the acceptance criteria for content (content ranged from 39%-152% of stated label) and 20% did not meet the established criteria for dissolution. Reformulation of the licensed trilostane product into a novel capsule size by a trained pharmacist did not affect dissolution characteristics and the target dose could be achieved. The authors concluded: "On the basis of these findings, compounded trilostane products should be used with caution as they may jeopardize the management of dogs with hyperadrenocorticism and potentially impact patient safety." (Cook *et al.* 2012)

Dosage Forms/Regulatory Status

VETERINARY-LABELED PRODUCTS:
Trilostane Oral Capsules: 10 mg, 30 mg, 60 mg & 120 mg packaged in aluminum foil blister cards of 10 capsules; *Vetoryl®*; (Rx).

HUMAN-LABELED PRODUCTS:
Modrastane® was withdrawn from the market in the USA in 1994.

Revisions/References

Monograph revised/updated August 2014.

Arenas, C., et al. (2013). Evaluation of 2 Trilostane Protocols for the Treatment of Canine Pituitary-Dependent Hyperadrenocorticism: Twice Daily versus Once Daily. Journal of Veterinary Internal Medicine 27(6): 1478-85.

Burkhardt, W. A., et al. (2013). Evaluation of Baseline Cortisol, Endogenous ACTH, and Cortisol/ACTH Ratio to Monitor Trilostane Treatment in Dogs with Pituitary-Dependent Hypercortisolism. Journal of Veterinary Internal Medicine 27(4): 919-23.

Cerundolo, R., et al. (2004). Treatment of Alopecia X with trilostane. Vet Derm 15: 285-93.

Cho, K. D., et al. (2013). Efficacy of Low- and High-Dose Trilostane Treatment in Dogs (< 5 kg) with Pituitary-Dependent Hyperadrenocorticism. Journal of Veterinary Internal Medicine 27(1): 91-8.

Cook, A. K. & K. G. Bond (2010). Evaluation of the use of baseline cortisol concentration as a monitoring tool for dogs receiving trilostane as a treatment for hyperadrenocorticism. Journal of the American Veterinary Medical Association 237(7): 801-5.

Cook, A. K., et al. (2012). Pharmaceutical Evaluation of Compounded Trilostane Products. J. Am. Anim. Hosp. Assoc. 48(4): 228-33.

Feldman, E. C. (2011). Evaluation of twice-daily lower-dose trilostane treatment administered orally in dogs with naturally occurring hyperadrenocorticism. Journal of the American Veterinary Medical Association 238(11): 1441-51.

Feldman, E. C. & P. H. Kass (2012). Trilostane Dose versus Body Weight in the Treatment of Naturally Occurring Pituitary-Dependent Hyperadrenocorticism in Dogs. Journal of Veterinary Internal Medicine 26(4): 1078-80.

Griebsch, C., et al. (2014). Effect of Trilostane on Hormone and Serum Electrolyte Concentrations in Dogs with Pituitary-Dependent Hyperadrenocorticism. Journal of Veterinary Internal Medicine 28(1): 160-5.

Leone, F., et al. (2005). The use of trilostane for the treatment of Alopecia X in Alaskan Malamutes. J Am Anim Hosp Assoc 41: 336-42.

McFarlane, D. (2011). Equine Pituitary Pars Intermedia Dysfunction. Vet Clin Equine 27: 93-113.

McGowan, C. & R. Neiger (2003). Efficacy of trilostane in the treatment of equine Cushing's syndrome. Equine Vet Jnl 35: 414-8.

McGraw, A., et al. (2011). Determination of the concentrations of trilostane and ketotrilostane that inhibit ex vivo canine adrenal gland synthesis of cortisol, corticosterone, and aldosterone. Am J Vet Res 72: 661-5.

Mellet Keith, A. M., et al. (2013). Trilostane Therapy for Treatment of Spontaneous Hyperadrenocorticism in Cats: 15 Cases (2004-2012). Journal of Veterinary Internal Medicine 27(6): 1471-7.

Reid, L. E., et al. (2014). Effect of Trilostane and Mitotane on Aldosterone Secretory Reserve in Dogs with Pituitary-Dependent Hyperadrenocorticism. Journal of Veterinary Internal Medicine 28(2): 443-50.

Reine, N. J. (2012). Medical Management of Pituitary-Dependent Hyperadrenocorticism: Mitotane versus Trilostane. Topics in Companion Animal Medicine 27(1): 25-30.

Scott-Moncrieff, J. C. (2010). Update on treatment of hyperadrenocorticism: What is the current recommendation? Proceedings: ACVIM Forum. accessed via Veterinary Information Network; vin.com

Valentin, S. Y., et al. (2014). Clinical Findings, Diagnostic Test Results, and Treatment Outcome in Cats with Spontaneous Hyperadrenocorticism: 30 Cases. Journal of Veterinary Internal Medicine 28(2): 481-7.

Trimeprazine Tartrate with Prednisolone

(trye-mep-ra-zeen)   Temaril-P®

Phenothiazine Antihistamine with Corticosteroid

Prescriber Highlights

► Combination phenothiazine antihistamine & corticosteroid used for pruritus & potentially as an antitussive.

► Relatively Contraindicated: Systemic fungal infections, hypovolemia, or shock & in patients with tetanus or strychnine intoxication. Caution: Hepatic dysfunction, cardiac disease, active bacterial or viral infections, peptic ulcer, acute psychoses, corneal ulcer, Cushingoid syndrome, diabetes, osteoporosis, chronic psychotic reactions, predisposition to thrombophlebitis, hypertension, CHF, renal insufficiency, general debilitation, very young animals.

► Primary adverse effects: Sedation, significant hypotension, cardiac rate abnormalities, hypo- or hyperthermia, "Cushingoid" effects with sustained use.

► Many potential drug & lab interactions.

Uses/Indications

Trimeprazine with prednisolone is used for the treatment of pruritic conditions, especially if induced by allergic conditions. There is reasonable evidence to support that when prednisolone is combined with trimeprazine (*Temaril-P®*), less prednisolone is required to control pruritus. The manufacturer suggests the drug is for use in dogs either for pruritic conditions or as an antitussive.

Pharmacology/Actions

Trimeprazine has antihistaminic, sedative, antitussive, and antipruritic qualities. The veterinary FDA-approved product also has prednisolone in its formulation that provides additional antiinflammatory effects.

Pharmacokinetics

The pharmacokinetics of trimeprazine have apparently not been studied.

Contraindications/Precautions/Warnings

The contraindications and precautions of this product follow those of the other phenothiazines and glucocorticoid agents. For more information, it is suggested to review the prochlorperazine and prednisone monographs.

Adverse Effects

For trimeprazine, possible adverse reactions include: sedation, depression, hypotension and extrapyramidal reactions (rigidity, tremors, weakness, restlessness, etc.).

Additional adverse effects, if using the product containing steroids include: elevated liver enzymes, weight loss, polyuria/polydipsia, vomiting, and diarrhea. If used chronically, therapy must be withdrawn gradually and Cushing's syndrome may develop.

The manufacturer of the veterinary combination product (*Temaril®-P*) includes the following adverse effects in its package insert: sodium retention and potassium loss, negative nitrogen balance, suppressed adrenocortical function, delayed wound healing, osteoporosis, possible increased susceptibility to and/or exacerbation of bacterial infections, sedation, protruding nictitating membrane, blood dyscrasias. In addition, intensification and prolongation of the action of sedatives, analgesics or anesthetics can be noted and potentiation of organophosphate toxicity and procaine HCl activity.

Reproductive/Nursing Safety

The manufacturer of the veterinary combination product (*Temaril®-P*) warns that corticosteroids can induce the first stages of parturition if administered during the last trimester of pregnancy.

Overdosage/Acute Toxicity

Acute overdosage should be handled as per the acepromazine monograph found at the beginning of the book.

Drug Interactions

The following drug interactions have either been reported or are theoretical in humans or animals receiving promethazine (a related phenothiazine antihistamine) or prednisolone and may be of significance in veterinary patients. Unless otherwise noted, use together is not necessarily contraindicated, but weigh the potential risks and perform additional monitoring when appropriate.

- **ACE INHIBITORS:** Phenothiazines may increase effects.
- **AMPHOTERICIN B:** When administered concomitantly with glucocorticoids may cause hypokalemia.
- **ANTACIDS:** May cause reduced GI absorption of oral phenothiazines.
- **ANTIDIARRHEAL MIXTURES** (*e.g.*, **Kaolin/pectin, bismuth subsalicylate mixtures**): May cause reduced GI absorption of oral phenothiazines.
- **ANTICHOLINESTERASE AGENTS** (*e.g.*, **pyridostigmine, neostigmine,** etc.): In patients with myasthenia gravis, concomitant glucocorticoid with these agents may lead to profound muscle weakness. If possible, discontinue anticholinesterase medication at least 24 hours prior to corticosteroid administration.
- **ASPIRIN** (**salicylates**): Glucocorticoids may reduce salicylate blood levels.
- **CISAPRIDE:** Increased risk for cardiac arrhythmias when used with phenothiazines.
- **CNS DEPRESSANT AGENTS** (*e.g.*, **barbiturates, narcotics, anesthetics,** etc.): May cause additive CNS depression if used with phenothiazines.
- **CYCLOPHOSPHAMIDE:** Glucocorticoids may also inhibit the hepatic metabolism of cyclophosphamide; dosage adjustments may be required.
- **CYCLOSPORINE:** Concomitant administration of may increase the blood levels of each, by mutually inhibiting the hepatic metabolism of each other; clinical significance of this interaction is not clear.
- **DIGOXIN:** Secondary to hypokalemia, increased risk for arrhythmias.
- **DIURETICS, POTASSIUM-DEPLETING** (*e.g.*, **furosemide, thiazides**): When administered concomitantly with glucocorticoids may cause hypokalemia
- **EPHEDRINE:** May increase metabolism
- **ESTROGENS:** The effects of hydrocortisone, and possibly other glucocorticoids, may be potentiated by concomitant administration with estrogens
- **INSULIN:** Requirements may increase in patients receiving glucocorticoids
- **KETOCONAZOLE:** May decrease metabolism.
- **MITOTANE:** May alter the metabolism of steroids; higher than usual doses of steroids may be necessary to treat mitotane-induced adrenal insufficiency
- **NSAIDS:** Administration of other ulcerogenic drugs with glucocorticoids may increase risk.
- **PAROXETINE:** May increase phenothiazine plasma levels.

- **PHENOBARBITAL:** May increase the metabolism of glucocorticoids.
- **PHENYTOIN:** May increase the metabolism of glucocorticoids.
- **RIFAMPIN:** May increase the metabolism of glucocorticoids.
- **VACCINES:** Patients receiving corticosteroids at immunosuppressive dosages should generally not receive live attenuated-virus vaccines as virus replication may be augmented; a diminished immune response may occur after vaccine, toxoid, or bacterin administration in patients receiving glucocorticoids.

Laboratory Considerations

- Glucocorticoids may increase serum **cholesterol** and **urine glucose** levels.
- Glucocorticoids may decrease serum **potassium**.
- Glucocorticoids can suppress the release of thyroid stimulating hormone (TSH) and reduce T_3 & T_4 values. Thyroid gland atrophy has been reported after chronic glucocorticoid administration. Uptake of I^{131} by the thyroid may be decreased by glucocorticoids.
- Reactions to **allergen tests** may be suppressed by glucocorticoids and/or trimeprazine. The actual effect of trimeprazine/prednisolone on allergen-specific intradermal tests (IDT) and allergen-specific IgE serological (ASIS) tests have not been reported (Olivry *et al.* 2013). A 4-week withdrawal time prior to IDT or ASIS is recommended in one veterinary dermatology reference (Koch *et al.* 2011).
- False-negative results of the **nitroblue tetrazolium test for systemic bacterial infections** may be induced by glucocorticoids.

Doses

- **DOGS:**

  For antipruritic and antitussive therapy (labeled dose; FDA-approved): Weight up to 10 lb = 1/2 tab PO twice daily; 11-20 lb = 1 tablet twice daily; 21-40 lb = 2 tablets twice daily; over 40 lb = 3 tablets twice daily. After 4 days reduce dose to 1/2 of initial dose or to an amount just sufficient to maintain remission of symptoms; adjust as necessary. (Package Insert; *Temaril*®*-P*)

  For adjunctive treatment of chronic pruritus (extra-label): 1 tablet/5 kg PO q12h for 4-7 days; then 1 tablet/5 kg PO once daily for 4-7 days, and finally 1 tablet/5 kg PO q24h every-other-day. This schedule may change according to each patient's needs; however, the ultimate goal for long-term glucocorticoid therapy is to give the lowest dosage that maintains control while administering the dosage every-other-day or less frequently if possible. However, since antihistamines should be administered daily for optimal effect, this complicates the use of this fixed dose combination product. (Koch *et al.* 2011)

- **CATS:**

  For pruritus (extra-label): The combination product (trimeprazine 5 mg with prednisolone 2 mg; *Temaril-P*®; *Vanectyl-P*®) has occasionally been used anecdotally in cats at 1 tablet per cat PO twice daily. (White 2012)

Monitoring

- Efficacy.
- Degree of sedation, and anticholinergic effects.
- Adverse effects associated with corticosteroids; consider serum chemistry profile, urinalysis and urine culture every 6-12 months if using long-term (Koch *et al.* 2011).

Client Information

- Follow veterinarian's dosage recommendations carefully. This is a combination of an antihistamine and a cortisone-like steroid used to reduce itching. It is sometimes used to treat cough.

- Can cause drowsiness, muscle tremors and rigidity; prednisolone can cause greater thirst, appetite and need to urinate.
- Long-term use can cause signs of Cushing's disease (*e.g.,* changes in hair coat, pot-belly, etc.)
- If side effects are worrisome, contact veterinarian.

Chemistry/Synonyms

A phenothiazine antihistamine related to promethazine, trimeprazine tartrate occurs as an odorless, white, to off-white crystalline powder with a melting range of 160-164°C. Approximately 0.5 gram is soluble in 1 mL water, and 0.05 gram is soluble in 1 mL of alcohol.

Trimeprazine Tartrate may also be known as: trimeprazine tartrate, alimemazine tartrate, or *Temaril*®.

Storage/Stability

Store trimeprazine products at room temperature (15-30°C); protect tablets from light.

Compatibility/Compounding Considerations

No specific information noted.

Dosage Forms/Regulatory Status

VETERINARY-LABELED PRODUCTS:

No single agent trimeprazine products are FDA-approved for veterinary medicine.

Trimeprazine Tartrate 5 mg with Prednisolone 2 mg Tablets; *Temaril-P*® Tablets; (Rx). FDA-approved for use in dogs. Trade name in Canada is *Vanectyl-P*®.

The ARCI (Racing Commissioners International) has designated this drug as a class 4 substance. See the appendix for more information.

HUMAN-LABELED PRODUCTS: NONE.

Revisions/References

Monograph revised/updated August 2014.

Koch, S., et al. (2011). *Small Animal Dermatology Drug Handbook*, Wiley-Blackwell. Ames.
Olivry, T., et al. (2013). Evidence-based guidelines for anti-allergic drug withdrawal times before allergen-specific intradermal and IgE serological tests in dogs. Veterinary Dermatology 24(2).
White, S. (2012). Feline Allergies: Atopic Dermatitis, Food & Fleas - Parts 1 & 2. Proceedings: AAFP. accessed via Veterinary Information Network; vin.com

Trimethoprim/Sulfa – See Sulfadiazine/Trimethoprim

Tripelennamine HCl

(tri-pel-ehn-a-meen)   Re-Covr®

Antihistamine

Prescriber Highlights

▶ Injectable antihistamine labeled for use in cattle and horses.
▶ Contraindications: Do not give IV to horses.
▶ Adverse Effects: CNS stimulation (if given IV to horses), sedation, depression, ataxia, GI effects (oral use).

Uses/Indications

Antihistamines are used in veterinary medicine to reduce or help prevent histamine mediated adverse effects. Tripelennamine has been used as a CNS stimulant in "Downer cows" when administered slow IV.

Pharmacology/Actions

Antihistamines (H_1-receptor antagonists) competitively inhibit histamine at H_1 receptor sites. They do not inactivate or prevent the release of histamine, but can prevent histamine's action on the cell. Besides their antihistaminic activity, these agents also have varying degrees of anticholinergic and CNS activity (sedation). Tripelennamine is considered to have moderate sedative activity and minimal anticholinergic activity when compared to other antihistamines.

Pharmacokinetics

The pharmacokinetics of tripelennamine have apparently not been thoroughly studied in domestic animals or humans. One study performed in horses and camels (Wasfi *et al.* 2000), showed that after IV administration similar pharmacokinetic profiles were obtained for both species. Terminal elimination half-lives were around 2+ hours; volumes of distribution steady-state ≈ 1.5-3 L/kg; protein binding was 80% and total body clearance ≈ 1 L/hour/kg.

Contraindications/Precautions/Warnings

Do not administer Tripelennamine IV in horses (see Adverse Effects).

Adverse Effects

CNS stimulation (hyperexcitability, nervousness, and muscle tremors) lasting up to 20 minutes, has been noted in horses after receiving tripelennamine intravenously. Other effects seen (in all species) include CNS depression, incoordination, and GI disturbances.

Overdosage/Acute Toxicity

Overdosage of tripelennamine reportedly can cause CNS excitation, seizures and ataxia. Treat symptomatically and supportively if clinical signs are severe. Phenytoin (IV) is recommended in the treatment of seizures caused by antihistamine overdose in humans; barbiturates and diazepam are generally avoided.

Drug Interactions

The following drug interactions have either been reported or are theoretical in humans or animals receiving tripelennamine and may be of significance in veterinary patients. Unless otherwise noted, use together is not necessarily contraindicated, but weigh the potential risks and perform additional monitoring when appropriate.

- **CNS DEPRESSANTS, OTHER**: Increased sedation can occur if tripelennamine is combined with other CNS depressant drugs.
- **HEPARIN, WARFARIN**: Antihistamines may partially counteract the anti-coagulation effects of heparin or warfarin.

Laboratory Considerations

- Antihistamines can decrease the wheal and flare response to **antigen skin testing**. In humans, it is suggested that antihistamines be discontinued at least 4 days prior to testing.

Doses

Note: It is recommended to warm the solution to near body temperature before injecting; give IM injections into large muscle areas.

- **CATTLE:**
  As an antihistamine (labeled dose; FDA-approved): 1.1 mg/kg (2.5 mL per 100 lbs. body weight) IV (for more immediate effect) or IM q6-12h as needed (Package Insert; *Re-Covr*®)

- **HORSES:** (NOTE: ARCI UCGFS CLASS 3 DRUG)
  As an antihistamine (labeled dose; FDA-approved): 1.1 mg/kg (2.5 mL per 100 lbs. body weight) IM (only) q6-12h as needed (Package Insert; *Re-Covr*®). **Note**: Do **NOT** administer IV to horses.

Monitoring

- Clinical efficacy.
- Adverse effects.

Chemistry/Synonyms

An ethylenediamine-derivative antihistamine, tripelennamine HCl occurs as a white, crystalline powder that will slowly darken upon exposure to light. It has a melting range of 188-192°C and pK_as of 3.9 and 9.0. One gram is soluble in 1 mL of water or 6 mL of alcohol.

Tripelennamine HCl may also be known as: tripelennaminium chloride, *Pyribenzamine*® or *Re-Covr*®.

Storage/Stability

Store the injection at room temperature and protect from light; avoid freezing or excessive heat.

Compatibility/Compounding Considerations

No specific information noted.

Dosage Forms/Regulatory Status

VETERINARY-LABELED PRODUCTS:

Tripelennamine HCl for Injection: 20 mg/mL in 20 mL, 100 mL, and 250 mL vials; *Re-Covr*®; (Rx). Tripelennamine HCl injection is FDA-approved for use in cattle and horses. Not for use in horses to be used for food purposes. Treated cattle must not be slaughtered for food purposes for 4 days following the last treatment. Milk must not be used for food for 24 hours (2 milkings) after treatment. No specific tolerance for residues has been published. Do not use in veal calves.

The ARCI (Racing Commissioners International) has designated this drug as a class 3 substance. See the appendix for more information.

HUMAN-LABELED PRODUCTS: NONE.

Revisions/References

Monograph revised/updated August 2014.

Wasfi, I. A., et al. (2000). Comparative disposition of tripelennamine in horses and camels after intravenous administration. J. Vet. Pharmacol. Ther. **23**(3): 145-52.

Trypan Blue

(trip-ann bloo)

Anti-Babesial Agent; Ophthalmologic Dye

Prescriber Highlights

▶ Uncommonly used alternative treatment for babesia (*B. canis*) in dogs that can rapidly alleviate clinical signs, but does not eliminate parasite.

▶ Must follow-up treatment with other anti-babesial drugs (*e.g.*, diminazene, imidocarb).

▶ Must be given IV.

▶ Will stain all body tissues and secretions for several weeks.

▶ Likely teratogen when used systemically.

Uses/Indications

Trypan blue was among the first agents used to treat Babesia. It may be useful as an adjunctive treatment for dogs with mild to moderate signs of infection with babesiosis (*B. canis*). Some have recommended its use in dogs with severe infections since it does not possess imidocarb's anticholinergic effects or the CNS toxic effects of some of the other diamidine drugs (*e.g.*, diminazene, pentamidine). Trypan blue suppresses parasitemia and can alleviate clinical signs, but it does not eliminate the infection and results can be variable. Other treatments (*e.g.*, imidocarb, diminazene) must be used within a month of trypan blue to be curative (Greene *et al.* 2006; Taboada *et al.* 2006). In a study comparing the effects of trypan blue and diminazene on hematocrit and parasitemia in dogs with clinically mild to moderate, uncomplicated babesiosis, there were no significant differences between diminazene and trypan blue on hematocrit or parasite clearance (Jacobson *et al.* 1996).

Trypan blue is also used as a dye in eye surgery to stain the anterior capsule of the lens and the epiretinal membranes.

Pharmacology/Actions

Trypan blue blocks the C3b receptor on both the erythrocyte membrane and the Babesia organism and likely prevents the parasite from entering the erythrocyte.

Pharmacokinetics

No information was located.

Contraindications/Precautions/Warnings

As trypan blue is a known teratogen it should be used during pregnancy in dogs only when the benefits to the dam outweigh the potential effects on puppies.

Adverse Effects

Trypan blue is well tolerated in dogs. The bluish-color change of secretions, urine, eyes and mucous membranes is most often the only adverse effect seen. This effect can persist for several weeks after treatment.

Reproductive/Nursing Safety

Trypan blue is teratogenic when used systemically in rats, mice, rabbits, hamsters, dogs, guinea pigs, and pigs. Systemically administered trypan blue to rats was teratogenic at 50 mg/kg (single dose) and 25 mg/kg/day (multiple doses). The FDA categorizes trypan blue used as a ophthalmologic dye as category C for use during pregnancy (*Animal studies have shown an adverse effect on the fetus, but there are no adequate studies in humans; or there are no animal reproduction studies and no adequate studies in humans.*)

Trypan blue can distribute into milk and cause it to have a bluish-tint. Safety in nursing offspring has not been established.

Overdosage/Acute Toxicity

No information located; figure dosages carefully.

Drug Interactions

- None noted.

Laboratory Considerations

- Trypan blue can tint plasma to a bluish color it may affect photometric-based test results or affect erythrocyte monitoring.

Doses

- **DOGS:**

  For *Babesia canis* (extra-label): 10 mg/kg IV as a 1% solution once. (Jacobson *et al.* 1996; Taboada *et al.* 2006) **Note:** Other treatments (*e.g.*, imidocarb, diminazene) must be used within a month of trypan blue to be curative (Greene *et al.* 2006; Taboada *et al.* 2006).

Monitoring

- Efficacy against babesia organism's effects on patient (bluish color change in plasma may make blood smear evaluation more difficult and affect erythrocyte counts and hematocrit determination).

Client Information

- This medication may cause a bluish color change in the dog's mucous membranes, eyes, urine, or secretions. This should diminish in a few weeks, but secretions may stain fabrics.

- Trypan blue does not completely eradicate the organism and additional treatments are required using other drugs.

Chemistry/Synonyms

Trypan blue is an azo-naphthalene dye derived from toluidine.

Trypan blue may also be known as azidione blue 3B, benzamine blue 3B, Niagara blue, Congo blue, diamine blue, CI Direct Blue 14, or trypanum caeruleum. Trade names include *VisionBlue®* and *MembranBlue®*.

Storage/Stability

Trypan blue powder or solutions should be stored at 15-25°C (59-77°F). Protect from direct sunlight.

Compatibility/Compounding Considerations

A 1% solution (10 mg/mL) is usually given intravenously. Trypan blue for injection that is compounded from powder should be administered through an in-line filter during intravenous administration.

Dosage Forms/Regulatory Status

VETERINARY-LABELED PRODUCTS: NONE.
Dosage forms may be available from compounding pharmacies.

HUMAN-LABELED PRODUCTS:
Trypan blue powder is available and it is also available as an ophthalmic stain in 0.06% and 0.15% solutions; *VisionBlue®*, *MembraneBlue®*; (Rx)

Revisions/References

Monograph revised/updated August 2014.

Greene, C. & S. Ewing (2006). Antiprotozoal Chemotherapy. *Infectious Diseases of the Dog and Cat, 3rd Ed.* C. Greene, Elsevier: 672-6.

Jacobson, L. S., et al. (1996). Changes in haematocrit after treatment of uncomplicated canine babesiosis: A comparison between diminazene and trypan blue, and an evaluation of the influence of parasitaemia. Journal of the South African Veterinary Association-Tydskrif Van Die Suid-Afrikaanse Veterinere Vereniging **67**(2): 77-82.

Taboada, J. & R. Lobetti (2006). Babesia. *Infectious Diseases of the Dog and Cat, 3rd Ed.* C. Greene, Elsevier: 722-36.

TSH – See Thyrotropin

Tulathromycin

(too-la-throe-mye-sin)   Draxxin®

Injectable Macrolide Antibiotic

Prescriber Highlights

▶ Injectable macrolide antibiotic labeled for cattle & swine.
▶ Very long tissue half-lives; one dose treatment.
▶ Not for lactating dairy cattle or veal calves.
▶ Local injection site reactions most likely adverse effect.

Uses/Indications

In beef and non-lactating dairy cattle, tulathromycin is indicated for the treatment of bovine respiratory disease (BRD) associated with *Mannheimia haemolytica*, *Pasteurella multocida*, *Histophilus somni* (*Haemophilus somnus*) and *Mycoplasma bovis*; and for the control of respiratory disease in cattle at high risk of developing BRD, associated with *Mannheimia haemolytica*, *Pasteurella multocida* and *Histophilus somni* (*Haemophilus somnus*). It is also FDA-approved for the treatment of bovine foot rot (interdigital necrobacillosis) associated with *Fusobacterium necrophorum* and *Porphyromonas levii* and for the treatment of infectious bovine keratoconjunctivitis (IBK) associated with *Moraxella bovis*. A study in heifers comparing metaphylactic antimicrobial administration of tildipirosin, tulathromycin, or placebo administered 10 days before experimental inoculation with *Mannheimia haemolytica* concluded that tildipirosin treated animals had less pulmonary damage and fewer clinical signs of illness when compared to the other groups (tulathromycin and placebo) (Amrine *et al.* 2014).

Tulathromycin is indicated for the treatment of swine respiratory disease (SRD) associated with *Actinobacillus pleuropneumoniae*, *Pasteurella multocida*, *Bordetella bronchiseptica*, *Haemophilus parasuis*, and *Mycoplasma hyopneumoniae* and for the control of SRD associated with *A. pleuropneumoniae*, *P. multocida*, and *M. hyopneumoniae* in groups of pigs where SRD has been diagnosed.

Tulathromycin may prove useful as a treatment of *Rhodococcus equi* infections in foals, but a study found the proportion of tulathromycin treated foals that recovered (27 of 30) was not significantly different from that of foals treated with a placebo.

Tulathromycin may be effective in treating various infections in small ruminants and rabbits.

Pharmacology/Actions

While tulathromycin is a macrolide antibiotic such as erythromycin or azithromycin, it is structurally unique in that it has three amine groups (tribasic), while erythromycin and azithromycin have one (monobasic) and two (dibasic) groups, respectively. The tribasic group of compounds are called triamilide macrolides.

It is believed that tulathromycin's tribasic structure allows it to better penetrate gram-negative pathogenic bacteria and its low affinity for bacterial efflux pumps may allow the drug to remain and accumulate within the bacteria.

The mechanism of action of tulathromycin is similar to other macrolides in that it inhibits protein synthesis by penetrating the cell wall and binding to the 50S ribosomal subunits in susceptible bacteria. It is considered a bacteriostatic antibiotic, but it possesses some bactericidal activity as well, particularly for *Mannheimia haemolytica* and *Pasteurella multocida*.

Tulathromycin's efficacy is enhanced by its ability to accumulate and persist in pulmonary epithelial lining fluid, macrophages and neutrophils. Neither time-dependent nor concentration-dependent models may accurately predict or describe the drug's efficacy. Some modern macrolides (*e.g.*, azithromycin) efficacy may be more predictive by assessing the total drug exposure to the pathogen; the AUC:MIC ratio may be helpful.

Bacterial isolates susceptible to tulathromycin at concentrations of 16 mcg/mL or less are reported as susceptible to tulathromycin. The MIC_{90} values reported for *M. haemolytica* and *P. multocida* in cattle with BRD are 2 mcg/mL and 1 mcg/mL, respectively. To date, resistance development to tulathromycin has not been a major problem.

Pharmacokinetics

In feeder calves given 2.5 mg/kg SC (in the neck), tulathromycin is rapidly and nearly completely absorbed (bioavailability >90%). Peak plasma concentrations generally occur within 15 minutes after dosing. Volume of distribution is very large ($\approx$ 11 L/kg) and total systemic clearance is $\approx$ 170 mL/hr/kg. This extensive volume of distribution is largely responsible for the long elimination half-life of this compound. In plasma, elimination half-life is $\approx$ 2.75 days, but in lung tissue it is $\approx$ 8.75 days. Tulathromycin is eliminated from the body primarily unchanged via biliary excretion.

Following intramuscular administration to feeder pigs at a dosage of 2.5 mg/kg, tulathromycin is readily and rapidly absorbed (bioavailability 88%) with peak levels occurring in $\approx$ 15 minutes. Tulathromycin rapidly distributes into body tissues, and the volume of distribution is 13-15 L/kg. Plasma half-life is $\approx$ 60-90 hours, but lung tissue half-life is $\approx$ 5.9 days. Tulathromycin is eliminated from the body primarily unchanged via the feces and urine.

Contraindications/Precautions/Warnings

Tulathromycin is contraindicated in animals with a prior hypersensitivity reaction to the drug.

Cattle intended for human consumption must not be slaughtered within 18 days from the last treatment. Do not use in female dairy cattle 20 months of age or older. A withdrawal period has not been established for this product in pre-ruminating calves. Do not use in calves to be processed for veal.

Swine intended for human consumption must not be slaughtered within 5 days from the last treatment.

Adverse Effects

At labeled doses, adverse effects appear to be minimal in cattle and swine. At therapeutic dosages, transient hypersalivation, head shaking, and pawing at the ground have been reported. One feeder calf in a field study developed transient dyspnea. Injection site reactions are most commonly reported and there have been some reports of anorexia in cattle to the FDA's Adverse Drug Reporting database. Subcutaneous or intramuscular injection can cause a transient local tissue reaction that may result in trim loss at slaughter.

In foals, self-limiting diarrhea, elevated temperature, and swelling at the injection site have been reported.

Hypersensitivity reactions are possible, but no reports were located.

Reproductive/Nursing Safety

Reproductive safety is not known, the product is labeled: "The effects of *Draxxin®* on bovine (and porcine) reproductive performance, pregnancy and lactation have not been determined."

Overdosage/Acute Toxicity

In cattle (feeder calves), single subcutaneous doses of up to 25 mg/kg caused transient indications of pain at the injection, including head shaking and pawing at the ground. Injection site swelling, discoloration of the subcutaneous tissues at the injection site and corresponding histopathologic changes were seen in animals in all dosage groups.

In swine, single IM doses of up to 25 mg/kg caused transient indications of pain at the injection site, restlessness, and excessive vocalization. Tremors occurred briefly in one animal receiving 7.5 mg/kg BW.

No systemic treatment for single overdoses should be necessary, localized treatment at the injection site (*e.g.*, ice pack) to reduce swelling and pain as well as FDA-approved analgesic medications can be considered.

Drug Interactions

- No drug interactions are noted in the manufacturer's label and none could be found in other references for tulathromycin.

Laboratory Considerations

- No concerns were noted.

Doses

- **CATTLE:**
  For labeled indications (FDA-approved): Inject subcutaneously as a single dose in the neck at a dosage of 2.5 mg/kg (1.1 mL/100 lb) body weight (BW). Do not inject more than 10 mL per injection site. (Label directions; *Draxxin®*)

- **SWINE:**
  For labeled indications (FDA-approved): Inject intramuscularly as a single dose in the neck at a dosage of 2.5 mg/kg (0.25 mL/22 lb) BW. Do not inject more than 2.5 mL per injection site. (Label directions; *Draxxin®*)

- **HORSES:**
  For foals with *R. equi* (extra-label): Anecdotally, 2.5 mg/kg IM every 5-7 days has been used successfully in milder clinical cases. (Divers 2009)

- **GOATS:**
  As an alternative for treatment of pneumonia associated with *Mannheimia haemolytica*, *Pasteurella multocida*, and *Mycoplasma* spp. (extra-label): 2.5 mg/kg SC; repeat in 7 days if necessary. Based on pharmacokinetic studies in meat and dairy goats, and FDA guidelines: a 34-day meat withdrawal interval and a 45 day milk withdrawal time are recommended (Romanet *et al.* 2012; Grismer *et al.* 2014).

Monitoring

- Clinical efficacy.

Client Information

- Follow dosing guidelines exactly; adhere to withdrawal times.
- Not for female dairy cattle (20 months or older) or veal calves.
- Cattle are dosed subcutaneously in the neck; not more than 10 mL per injection site.
- Swine are dosed intramuscularly in the neck; not more than 2.5 mL per injection site.

Chemistry/Synonyms

Tulathromycin is a semi-synthetic macrolide antibiotic of the subclass triamilide. It occurs as white to of-white-crystalline powder that is readily soluble in water at pH<8. At a pH of 7.4 (physiological pH), tulathromycin (a weak base) is ≈ 50X more soluble in hydrophilic than hydrophobic media.

The commercially available injection contains 100 mg/mL of tulathromycin in an equilibrated mixture of the two isomeric forms of tulathromycin in a 9:1 ratio. The injectable vehicle consists of 50% propylene glycol, monothioglycerol (5 mg/mL); citric and hydrochloric acids are added to adjust pH. It has a relatively low viscosity.

Tulathromycin may also be known as tulathromycine, tulathromycinum, CP-472295 (component A), CP-547272 (component B), or *Draxxin*.

Storage/Stability

Tulathromycin injection should be stored at, or below 25°C (77°F). The product is stable at room temperature for up to 36 months.

Compatibility/Compounding Considerations

No specific information noted.

Dosage Forms/Regulatory Status

VETERINARY-LABELED PRODUCTS:

Tulathromycin Injection: 100 mg/mL in 50, 100, 250, & 500 mL vials; *Draxxin*; (Rx). FDA-approved for use in cattle and swine. Cattle intended for human consumption must not be slaughtered within 18 days from the last treatment. Do not use in female dairy cattle 20 months of age or older. A withdrawal period has not been established for this product in pre-ruminating calves. Do not use in calves to be processed for veal.

Swine intended for human consumption must not be slaughtered within 5 days from the last treatment.

HUMAN-LABELED PRODUCTS: NONE.

Revisions/References

Monograph revised/updated August 2014.

Amrine, D. E., et al. (2014). Pulmonary lesions and clinical disease response to *Mannheimia haemolytica* challenge 10 days following administration of tildipirosin or tulathromycin. Journal of Animal Science 92(1): 311-9.

Divers, T. J. (2009). Diagnosing, treating and preventing Rhodococcus equi. Proceedings: WVC. accessed via Veterinary Information Network; vin.com

Grismer, B., et al. (2014). Pharmacokinetics of tulathromycin in plasma and milk samples after a single subcutaneous injection in lactating goats (*Capra hircus*). J. Vet. Pharmacol. Ther. 37(2): 205-8.

Romanet, J., et al. (2012). Pharmacokinetics and tissue elimination of tulathromycin following subcutaneous administration in meat goats. American Journal of Veterinary Research 73(10): 1634-40.

Venner, M., et al. (2013). Comparison of tulathromycin, azithromycin and azithromycin-rifampin for the treatment of mild pneumonia associated with Rhodococcus equi. Veterinary Record 173(16): 397-+.

Tylosin

(tye-loe-sin)   Tylan®

Macrolide Antibiotic

Prescriber Highlights

▶ Macrolide antibiotic related to erythromycin, used primarily in cattle & swine; sometimes used orally in cats/dogs for chronic colitis; has been used anecdotally in cats as an immunomodulating agent for treating FIP.

▶ Must be compounded for oral use in dogs and cats. Has a very unpleasant taste.

▶ Contraindications: hypersensitivity to it or other macrolide antibiotics; probably contraindicated in horses.

▶ Adverse Effects: Pain & local reactions after IM injection, GI upset (anorexia, & diarrhea) after PO administration. May cause severe diarrhea if administered PO to ruminants or by any route to horses. **Swine:** edema of rectal mucosa & mild anal protrusion with pruritus, erythema, & diarrhea.

Uses/Indications

Although the injectable form of tylosin was FDA-approved for use in dogs and cats, it is rarely used parenterally in those species. Oral tylosin is commonly recommended for the adjunctive treatment of inflammatory bowel disease (IBD; idiopathic antibiotic responsive diarrhea) in dogs, cats and some small mammals. A double-blinded prospective study, comparing tylosin to placebo in dogs with a history of chronic diarrhea that was thought to be responsive to tylosin in the past, showed that 85% of dogs receiving tylosin had perceived normal fecal consistency versus 29% of those receiving placebo (Kilpienn *et al.* 2009). A case-based review of the evidence for treatment of clinical signs (vomiting, diarrhea, weight loss) associated with mild lymphoplasmacytic, eosinophilic gastroenteritis, concluded that based upon current evidence, milder forms of IBD do not always require immunosuppression and can often be managed with a combination of diet change, antimicrobials (*e.g.,* tylosin), and time (Smee *et al.* 2011).

Tylosin has been used has been used anecdotally in cats as an immunomodulating agent for treating FIP. In dogs, tylosin has been anecdotally used orally to treat tear staining (epiphora).

Tylosin is also used clinically in cattle and swine for infections caused by susceptible organisms but newer, approved antibiotics are generally preferred for systemic therapy.

Pharmacology/Actions

Tylosin is thought to have the same mechanism of action as erythromycin (binds to 50S ribosome and inhibits protein synthesis) and exhibits a similar spectrum of activity. It is a bacteriostatic antibiotic. Tylosin may also have immunomodulatory effects on cell-mediated immunity. Over 50% of *Enterococcus faecalis* canine isolates from healthy dogs were resistant to tylosin in one study. Tylosin may increase concentrations of enterococci in the jejunum, which may have probiotic effects (Suchodolski *et al.* 2009).

Pharmacokinetics

Tylosin tartrate is well absorbed from the GI tract, primarily from the intestine. The phosphate salt is less well absorbed after oral administration. Tylosin base injected SC or IM is reportedly rapidly absorbed.

Like erythromycin, tylosin is well distributed in the body after systemic absorption, with the exception of penetration into the CSF. The volume of distribution of tylosin is reportedly 1.7 L/kg in small animals and 1-2.3 L/kg in cattle. In lactating dairy cattle, the milk to plasma ratio is reported to be between 1-5.4.

Tylosin is eliminated in the urine and bile apparently as unchanged drug. The elimination half-life of tylosin is reportedly 54 minutes in small animals, 139 minutes in newborn calves, and 64 minutes in calves 2 months of age or older.

Contraindications/Precautions/Warnings

Tylosin is contraindicated in patients hypersensitive to it or other macrolide antibiotics (*e.g.*, erythromycin). Most clinicians feel that tylosin is contraindicated in horses, as severe and sometimes fatal diarrheas may result from its use in that species.

Adverse Effects

Most likely adverse effects with tylosin are pain and local reactions at intramuscular injection sites, and mild GI upset (anorexia and diarrhea). Tylosin may induce severe diarrheas if administered orally to ruminants or by any route to horses. In swine, adverse effects reported include edema of rectal mucosa and mild anal protrusion with pruritus, erythema, and diarrhea.

Reproductive/Nursing Safety

In a system evaluating the safety of drugs in canine and feline pregnancy (Papich 1989), this drug is categorized as in class: *B* (*Safe for use if used cautiously. Studies in laboratory animals may have uncovered some risk, but these drugs appear to be safe in dogs and cats or these drugs are safe if they are not administered when the animal is near term.*)

Overdosage/Acute Toxicity

Tylosin is relatively safe in most overdose situations. The LD_{50} in pigs is greater than 5 grams/kg orally, and ≈ 1 gram/kg IM. Dogs are reported to tolerate oral doses of 800 mg/kg. Long-term (2 year) oral administration of up to 400 mg/kg produced no organ toxicity in dogs. Shock and death have been reported in baby pigs overdosed with tylosin, however.

Drug Interactions

Drug interactions with tylosin have not been well documented. It has been suggested that tylosin may increase **digoxin** blood levels with resultant toxicity. It is suggested to refer to the erythromycin monograph for more information on potential interactions.

- **BENTONITE**: Simultaneous administration of tylosin (in the drinking water or feed) and bentonite (mixed in the feed as a mycotoxin binder) should be avoided as it significantly reduced tylosin plasma levels and area-under-the-curve in chickens. (Devreese *et al.* 2012)

Laboratory Considerations

- Macrolide antibiotics may cause falsely elevated values of AST (SGOT), and **ALT** (SGPT) when using colorimetric assays.
- Fluorometric determinations of **urinary catecholamines** can be altered by concomitant macrolide administration.

Doses

- **DOGS/CATS:**

  Note: When using *Tylan® Soluble* (100 grams per bottle) powder: Using volumetric containers to measure powders is not necessarily accurate, but 1 level teaspoonful (5 mL) of powder contains ≈ 2.5-2.7 grams of tylosin; 1/8th of a teaspoonful contains ≈ 325 mg tylosin. Powder is very unpalatable.

  For adjunctive treatment of inflammatory bowel disease (IBD, idiopathic antibiotic responsive diarrhea); (extra-label):

  a) Dogs: 25 mg/kg PO once daily (in the study dogs were treated for 7 days, but the authors state that in dogs with tylosin-responsive diarrhea the stool remains normal as long as treatment continues, but diarrhea reappears within weeks after discontinuation). (Kilpienn *et al.* 2009)

  b) Other anecdotal dosage recommendations range from 10 – 40 mg/kg PO q8-12h. A recent review article suggested:

20 mg/kg PO q8-12h. There is no cure but signs may be controlled (Hall 2011). Milder cases with appropriate dietary change may eventually only require once daily dosing.

For campylobacteriosis (extra-label): 11 mg/kg PO q8h. (Weese 2011)

For *Clostridium perfringens*-associated diarrhea (extra-label): There is little objective information guiding decisions regarding when and how to treat, but tylosin at 10 – 20 mg/kg PO q12-24h is commonly recommended (Weese 2011). Animals with chronic clostridial colitis can often be controlled with one treatment every 2-3 days. (Willard 2006).

For *Cryptosporidium* spp. associated diarrhea in cats (extra-label): 10 – 15 mg/kg PO q12h will sometimes resolve diarrhea. Tylosin can be a GI irritant; if the cat is responding to the first 7 days of therapy and toxicity has not been noted, continue treatment for 1 week past clinical resolution of diarrhea. Some cats with *Cryptosporidium* spp. infection with or without *Giardia* co-infection require several weeks of treatment prior to resolution of diarrhea. (Lappin 2011)

- **FERRETS:**

  For susceptible enteric infections (extra-label): 10 mg/kg PO once to twice daily. (Williams 2000)

- **RABBITS, RODENTS, SMALL MAMMALS:**

  Rabbits: 10 mg/kg SC, IM q12-24h. (Ivey *et al.* 2000)

  Gerbils, Hamsters, Rats: 10 mg/kg SC q24h. (Adamcak *et al.* 2000)

- **CATTLE:**

  For susceptible infections (labeled dose; FDA-approved): 17.6 mg/kg IM once daily. Continue treatment for 24 hours after symptoms have stopped, not to exceed 5 days. Do not inject more than 10 mL per site. Use the 50 mg/mL formulation in calves weighing <200 pounds. (Package insert; *Tylosin® Injection*)

- **SWINE:**

  For susceptible infections (labeled dose; FDA-approved): 8.8 mg/kg IM twice daily. Continue treatment for 24 hours after symptoms have stopped, not to exceed 3 days. Do not inject more than 5 mL per site. (Package insert; *Tylosin® Injection*)

Monitoring

- Clinical efficacy.
- Adverse effects.

Client Information

- Most commonly used in dogs and cats to treat diarrhea and inflammation of intestines; may be used for respiratory infections in birds (including chickens) and reptiles.
- Do not give to horses or ponies.
- Oral doses may be given with or without food. Give with food if stomach upset or vomiting occurs.
- Powder has an extremely bitter taste. Placing the dose of powder in an empty gelatin capsule may be better accepted.
- When administered orally to small animals, tylosin is usually very well tolerated, but contact veterinarian if adverse effects are seen.

Chemistry/Synonyms

A macrolide antibiotic related structurally to erythromycin, tylosin is produced from *Streptomyces fradiae*. It occurs as an almost white to buff-colored powder with a pK_a of 7.1. It is slightly soluble in water and soluble in alcohol. Tylosin is considered highly lipid soluble. The tartrate salt is soluble in water. The injectable form of the drug (as the base) is in a 50% propylene glycol solution.

Tylosin may also be known as desmycosin, tilosina, tylozin, tylosiini, tylosinum, tylozyna or *Tylan®*.

Storage/Stability

Unless otherwise instructed by the manufacturer, injectable tylosin should be stored in well-closed containers at room temperature. Tylosin, like erythromycin, is unstable in acidic (pH <4) media. It is not recommended to mix the parenteral injection with other drugs.

Compatibility/Compounding Considerations

Because converting volume measurements into weights is not very accurate for powders, it is recommended to actually weigh powders when using them for pharmaceutical purposes. However, if this is not possible, one (1) level teaspoon (5 mL) of commercially available tylosin tartrate (*Tylan® Soluble*) contains ≈ 2.5-2.7 grams of tylosin; 1/8th of a teaspoonful contains ≈ 325 mg tylosin.

Tylan tartrate powder added to food can be very unpalatable for dogs or cats. Placing the proper dose in a gelatin capsule may be preferable to mixing it into food. Another suggestion for dogs or cats that absolutely won't eat food that has tylosin in it is to: Melt ≈ ¼ teaspoon of butter and place in one of the compartments in a mini-ice tray. Add the proper dose of tylosin powder, mix well and freeze. (**Note:** Stability information for this procedure has not been performed).

Dosage Forms/Regulatory Status

VETERINARY-LABELED PRODUCTS:

Note: The product *Tylan® Plus Vitamins* was used extensively orally in companion animals, but has been withdrawn from the market. *Tylan® Soluble* may be substituted, but is significantly more concentrated than *Tylan® Plus Vitamins* and dosage sizes (teaspoons are not equivalent) will be different.

Tylosin Injection: 50 mg/mL, 200 mg/mL; *Tylan®*, generic; (OTC). FDA-approved for use in nonlactating dairy cattle, beef cattle, swine, dogs, and cats. Slaughter withdrawal (at labeled doses): cattle = 21 days; swine = 14 days. **Note:** Although this author (Plumb) was unable to locate parenteral products FDA-approved for use in lactating dairy animals, one source (Huber 1988a) states that tylosin has a 72-hour milk withdrawal for dairy cattle, and 48 hour milk withdrawal in dairy goats and sheep. Contact FARAD for more information before using in lactating dairy animals.

Tylosin Tartrate Powder: (≈ 2.5-2.7 grams/level teaspoonful) in 100 gram bottles; *Tylan® Soluble, TyloMed®-WS*; (OTC). FDA-approved for use in turkeys (not layers), chickens (not layers) and swine. Slaughter withdrawal swine = 2 days; chickens = 1 day; turkeys = 5 days.

There are many FDA-approved tylosin products for addition to feed or water for use in beef cattle, swine, and poultry. Many of these products have other active ingredients included in their formulations.

HUMAN-LABELED PRODUCTS: NONE.

Revisions/References

Monograph revised/updated August 2014.
Adamcak, A. & B. Otten (2000). Rodent Therapeutics. Vet Clin NA: Exotic Anim Pract **3:1**(Jan): 221-40.
Devreese, M., et al. (2012). Interaction between tylosin and bentonite clay from a pharmacokinetic perspective. Veterinary Journal **194**(3): 437-9.
Hall, E. J. (2011). Antibiotic-Responsive Diarrhea in Small Animals. Veterinary Clinics of North America-Small Animal Practice **41**(2): 273-+.
Ivey, E. & J. Morrisey (2000). Therapeutics for Rabbits. Vet Clin NA: Exotic Anim Pract **3:1**(Jan): 183-216.
Kilpienn, S., et al. (2009). Effect of Tylosin on Dogs with Diarrhea: A Placebo-Controlled, Randomized, Double-Blinded, Prospective Clinical Trial. Proceedings: ECVIM. accessed via Veterinary Information Network; vin.com
Lappin, M. R. (2011). Diagnosis and Treatment of Cryptosporidium and Isospora in Cats. Proceedings: World Small Animal; Veterinary Association World Congress. accessed via Veterinary Information Network; vin.com
Papich, M. (1989). Effects of drugs on pregnancy. *Current Veterinary Therapy X: Small Animal Practice.* R. Kirk. Philadelphia, Saunders: 1291-9.
Smee, N. M. & T. L. Towell (2011). What Is the Evidence? Journal of the American Veterinary Medical Association **238**(9): 1111-3.
Suchodolski, J. S., et al. (2009). The Effect of Tylosin on Small Intestinal Microbiota in Healthy Dogs. Proceedings: ECVIM. accessed via Veterinary Information Network; vin.com
Weese, J. S. (2011). Bacterial Enteritis in Dogs and Cats: Diagnosis, Therapy, and Zoonotic Potential. Veterinary Clinics of North America-Small Animal Practice **41**(2): 287-+.
Willard, M. (2006). Chronic Diarrhea: Part 2. Proceedings: ACVC. accessed via Veterinary Information Network; vin.com
Williams, B. (2000). Therapeutics in Ferrets. Vet Clin NA: Exotic Anim Pract **3:1**(Jan): 131-53.

Ursodiol

(ur-soe-dye-ole)   Actigall®, Ursodeoxycholic acid

Bile Acid

Prescriber Highlights

► Bile acid that may be useful for adjunctive treatment of hepatobiliary disease in dogs/cats. May also be considered for medical treatment of mild cases of gall bladder mucocele.
► Contraindications: Rabbits & other hindgut fermenters. Caution: Complications associated with gallstones (*e.g.*, biliary obstruction, biliary fistulas, cholecystitis, pancreatitis, cholangitis).
► Adverse Effects: Appears to be well tolerated in dogs/cats.

Uses/Indications

In small animals, ursodiol may be useful as adjunctive therapy for the medical management of gallbladder mucocele ("sludge") and/or in patients with chronic liver disease, particularly where cholestasis (bile toxicity) plays an important role. Its use for the medical treatment of gallbladder mucocele is somewhat controversial as most recommend surgery for all, with the possible exception of very mild (asymptomatic or incidental discovery) cases. Ursodiol's benefit in treating canine or feline hepatobiliary disease in not known, but it may be of help in slowing the progression of inflammatory hepatic disorders, particularly autoimmune hepatitis and acute hepatotoxicity.

Pharmacology/Actions

After oral administration, ursodiol suppresses hepatic synthesis and secretion of cholesterol. Ursodiol also decreases intestinal absorption of cholesterol. By reducing cholesterol saturation in the bile, it is thought that ursodiol allows solubilization of cholesterol-containing gallstones. Ursodiol also increases bile flow and in patients with chronic liver disease, it apparently reduces the hepatocyte toxic effects of bile salts by decreasing their detergent action, and may protect hepatic cells from toxic bile acids (*e.g.*, lithocholate, deoxycholate, and chenodeoxycholate). In patients with chronic hepatitis, ursodiol may also reduce hepatocellular inflammatory changes and fibrosis.

Pharmacokinetics

Ursodiol is well absorbed from the small intestine after oral administration. In humans, up to 90% of dose is absorbed. After absorption, it enters the portal circulation. In the liver, it is extracted and combined (conjugated) with either taurine or glycine and secreted into the bile. Only very small quantities enter the systemic circulation and very little is detected in the urine. After each entero-hepatic cycle, some quantity of conjugated and free drug undergoes bacterial degradation; eventually most of the drug is eliminated in the feces after being oxidized or reduced to less soluble compounds. Ursodiol detected in the systemic circulation is highly bound to plasma proteins.

Contraindications/Precautions/Warnings

Ursodiol is contraindicated in rabbits and other hindgut fermenters as it is converted into lithocholic acid (toxic). Patients sensitive to other bile acid products may also be sensitive to ursodiol. The benefits of using ursodiol should be weighed against its risks in patients with complications associated with gallstones (*e.g.*, biliary obstruction, biliary fistulas, cholecystitis, pancreatitis, cholangitis). Some state that ursodiol should not be used unless bile duct obstruction has been ruled out and while it is not a substitute for surgery, others state that ursodiol does not have prokinetic effects, so it is not contraindicated.

Some patients with chronic liver disease may experience further impairment of bile acid metabolism.

Adverse Effects

Ursodiol use in animals has been limited, but it appears to be well tolerated in dogs and cats. Although hepatotoxicity has not been associated with ursodiol therapy, there are some human patients with an inability to sulfate lithocholic acid (a naturally occurring bile acid and also a metabolite of ursodiol). Lithocholic acid is a known hepatotoxin; veterinary significance is unclear. Diarrhea and other GI effects have rarely been noted in humans taking ursodiol. Ursodiol will not dissolve calcified radiopaque stones or radiolucent bile pigment stones.

Reproductive/Nursing Safety

In humans, the FDA categorizes this drug as category *B* for use during pregnancy (*Animal studies have not yet demonstrated risk to the fetus, but there are no adequate studies in pregnant women; or animal studies have shown an adverse effect, but adequate studies in pregnant women have not demonstrated a risk to the fetus in the first trimester of pregnancy, and there is no evidence of risk in later trimesters.*)

It is not known whether ursodiol is excreted in breast milk.

Overdosage/Acute Toxicity

Overdosage of ursodiol would most likely cause diarrhea. Treatment, if required, could include supportive therapy; oral administration of an aluminum-containing antacid (*e.g.*, aluminum hydroxide suspension); gastric emptying (if large overdose) with concurrent administration of activated charcoal or cholestyramine suspension.

Drug Interactions

The following drug interactions have either been reported or are theoretical in humans or animals receiving ursodiol and may be of significance in veterinary patients. Unless otherwise noted, use together is not necessarily contraindicated, but weigh the potential risks and perform additional monitoring when appropriate.

- **ALUMINUM-CONTAINING ANTACIDS:** May bind to ursodiol, thereby reducing its efficacy.
- **CHOLESTYRAMINE RESIN:** May bind to ursodiol, thereby reducing its efficacy.
- **TAURINE:** Although not documented, concern has been raised that chronic administration of ursodiol in cats may lead to taurine deficiency.

Laboratory Considerations

- As ursodiol is detected by many **serum bile acid** tests, bile acids may remain falsely elevated. One study in normal dogs did not show any effects. However if possible, stop ursodiol for 2-3 days before running test.

Doses

- **DOGS:**

  For adjunctive treatment of chronic hepatitis (extra-label): No prospective studies documenting efficacy or any one dosage were located, but anecdotal dosages of 10 – 15 mg/kg PO once per day or divided twice daily have been noted.

  For medical treatment with gall bladder mucoceles in dogs: of 5 – 7.5 mg/kg PO twice daily for medical treatment of cases with milder clinical signs.

- **CATS:**

  For adjunctive treatment of chronic hepatitis (extra-label): No prospective studies documenting efficacy or any one dosage were located, but anecdotal dosage of 10 – 15 mg/kg PO once per day or divided twice daily have been noted.

  For adjunctive treatment of feline triaditis (*e.g.*, **cholangitis, pancreatitis, inflammatory bowel disease**); (extra-label): 10 – 15 mg/kg per day is suggested. Fluid and electrolytes, antibiotics, analgesics, and antiemetics are also used. (Twedt 2012)

- **HORSES:**

  For medical treatment of cholangiohepatitis/colic, biliary "sludge" (extra-label): 15 mg/kg PO once daily; treatment is combined with antibiotics, fluid therapy, DMSO, and pentoxifylline. Treatment should be continued until GGT returns to normal range. (Divers 2013)

- **BIRDS:**

  For adjunctive treatment of liver disease (extra-label): 10 – 15 mg/kg PO once daily. (Oglesbee 2009)

Monitoring

- Efficacy (ultrasonography for gallstones; improved liver function tests for chronic hepatic disease).
- Monitoring of SGPT/SGOT (AST/ALT) on a routine basis (in humans these tests are recommended at the initiation of therapy and at 1 and 3 months after starting therapy; then every 6 months).

Client Information

- Ursodiol should be given with food.
- Usually well tolerated by dogs and cats.
- Used to help animals with cholesterol-containing gallstones and/or chronic liver disease.
- Do not give to rabbits, guinea pigs or rodents.

Chemistry/Synonyms

A naturally occurring bile acid, ursodiol, also known as ursodeoxycholic acid, has a molecular weight of 392.6.

Ursodiol may also be known as: acidum ursodeoxycholicum, UDCA, ursodesoxycholic acid; many trade names are available, including *Actigall*.

Storage/Stability

Unless otherwise specified by the manufacturer, ursodiol capsules should be stored at room temperature (15-30°C) in tight containers. Store tablets between 20°-25°C (68-77°F). Half tablets maintain acceptable quality up to 28 days when stored in the bottle at room temperature. Because of the bitter taste, segments should be stored separately from whole tablets.

Compatibility/Compounding Considerations

No specific information noted.

Dosage Forms/Regulatory Status

VETERINARY-LABELED PRODUCTS: NONE.

HUMAN-LABELED PRODUCTS:

Ursodiol Oral Capsules: 300 mg; *Actigall*, generic; (Rx)

Ursodiol Oral Tablets: 250 mg & 500 mg; *URSO* 250 & *-Forte*, generic; (Rx)

Revisions/References

Monograph revised/updated August 2014.

Divers, T. (2013). Diagnosis and Treatment of Acute Liver Disease and Renal Failure. Proceedings: IVECCS. accessed via Veterinary Information Network; vin.com

Oglesbee, B. (2009). Liver disease in pet birds. Proceedings: WVC. accessed via Veterinary Information Network; vin.com

Twedt, D. (2012). Managing Canine and Feline Liver Disease. Proceedings: Western Veterinary Conference. accessed via Veterinary Information Network; vin.com

Valproic Acid
Valproate Sodium
Divalproex Sodium

(val-**proe**-ik; val-**proe**-ayte; die-val-**proe**-ex)

Depakene®, Depakote®, Depacon®

Anticonvulsant

Prescriber Highlights

▶ 3rd to 4th line anticonvulsant that may be useful as adjunctive treatment in some dogs; most do not recommend its use in veterinary patients.

▶ Contraindications: Significant hepatic disease or dysfunction, previous hypersensitivity.

▶ Caution: Thrombocytopenia or altered platelet aggregation function.

▶ Adverse Effects: GI effects most likely (may be mitigated by giving with food), hepatotoxicity, CNS (sedation, ataxia, behavioral changes, etc.), dermatologic reactions, (alopecia, rash, etc.), hematologic reactions, (thrombocytopenia, reduced platelet aggregation, leukopenias, anemias, etc.), pancreatitis, & edema are possible.

▶ May be teratogenic.

Uses/Indications

Because of its cost, apparent unfavorable pharmacokinetic profile, and potential hepatotoxicity, valproic acid must be considered, at best, a third or fourth line drug in the treatment of seizures in the dog. Some clinicians feel it is of benefit when added to phenobarbital in patients not adequately controlled with that drug alone. Additionally, it is less protein bound in dogs than in humans, so the human serum therapeutic range of the drug (40-100 micrograms/mL) may be too high in dogs. The drug (free form) actually may concentrate in the CSF, and anticonvulsant effects may persist even after valproate levels are non-detectable in CSF, lending to the idea that serum levels do not accurately reflect clinical efficacy. Clearly, additional studies are needed to determine the clinical role, if any, for this drug.

Pharmacology/Actions

The mechanism of the anticonvulsant activity of valproic acid is not understood. Animal studies have demonstrated that valproic acid inhibits GABA transferase and succinic aldehyde dehydrogenase causing increased CNS levels of GABA. Additionally, one study has demonstrated that valproic acid inhibits neuronal activity by increasing potassium conductance.

Pharmacokinetics

Sodium valproate is rapidly converted to valproic acid in the acidic environment of the stomach where it is rapidly absorbed from the GI tract. The bioavailability reported in dogs following oral administration is ≈ 80%; peak levels occur in ≈ 1-hour. Food may delay absorption, but does not alter the extent of it. Divalproex in its enteric-coated form has an ≈ 1-hour delay in its oral absorption. Patients' who exhibit GI (nausea, vomiting) adverse effects may benefit from this dosage form.

Valproic acid is rapidly distributed throughout the extracellular water spaces and plasma. It is ≈ 80-95% plasma protein bound in humans, and 78-80% plasma protein bound in dogs. CSF levels are ≈ 10% those found in plasma. Milk levels are 1-10% those found in plasma; it readily crosses the placenta.

Valproic acid is metabolized in the liver and conjugated with glucuronide. These metabolic conjugates are excreted in the urine; only very small amounts of unchanged drug are excreted in the urine. The elimination half-life in humans ranges from 5-20 hours; in dogs from 1.5-2.8 hours. In cats, valproate is glucuronidated more slowly than other mammalian species so elimination half-life would be expected to be longer.

Contraindications/Precautions/Warnings

Valproic acid is contraindicated in patients with significant hepatic disease or dysfunction, or exhibiting previous hypersensitivity to the drug. It should be used with caution in patients with thrombocytopenia or altered platelet aggregation function.

Adverse Effects

Because of the limited experience with this agent, the following adverse effects may not be complete nor valid for dogs: Gastrointestinal effects consisting of nausea, vomiting, anorexia, and diarrhea are the most common adverse effects seen in people and also apparently, in dogs. GI effects may be diminished by administration with food. Hepatotoxicity is the most serious potential adverse (human) reaction reported and must be considered for canine patients also. Dose related increases in liver enzymes may be seen and, rarely, hepatic failure and death may occur. In humans, incidences of hepatotoxicity are greater in very young (<2 yr. old) patients, those on other anticonvulsants, or with multiple congenital abnormalities.

Other potential adverse effects include: CNS (sedation, ataxia, behavioral changes, etc.), dermatologic (alopecia, rash, etc.), hematologic (thrombocytopenia, reduced platelet aggregation, leukopenias, anemias, etc.), pancreatitis, and edema.

Reproductive/Nursing Safety

A 1-2% incidence of neural tube defects in children born of mothers taking valproic acid during the first trimester of pregnancy has been reported. Use in pregnant dogs only when the benefits outweigh the risks of therapy. In humans, the FDA categorizes this drug as category *D* for use during pregnancy (*There is evidence of human fetal risk, but the potential benefits from the use of the drug in pregnant women may be acceptable despite its potential risks.*) In a separate system evaluating the safety of drugs in canine and feline pregnancy (Papich 1989), this drug is categorized as in class: *C* (*These drugs may have potential risks. Studies in people or laboratory animals have uncovered risks, and these drugs should be used cautiously as a last resort when the benefit of therapy clearly outweighs the risks.*)

Concentrations of valproic acid in maternal milk are 1-10% of serum concentrations. It is unknown if this would have any detrimental effect on nursing offspring.

Overdosage/Acute Toxicity

Severe overdoses can cause profound CNS depression, asterixis, motor restlessness, hallucinations, and death. One human patient recovered after a serum level of 2000 micrograms/mL (20X over therapeutic) was measured. There were 48 single agent exposures to valproic acid reported to the ASPCA Animal Poison Control Center (APCC) during 2009-2013. Of the 43 exposed dogs, 5 were symptomatic and they all were ataxic.

Treatment consists of supportive measures and maintenance of adequate urine output is considered mandatory. Because the drug is rapidly absorbed, emesis or gastric lavage may be of limited value. Because of its delayed absorptive characteristics, the divalproex form may be removed by lavage or emesis if ingestion occurred recently. Naloxone is reported to be of benefit in reversing some of the CNS effects of valproic acid, but may also reverse the anticonvulsant properties of the drug.

Drug Interactions

The following drug interactions have either been reported or are theoretical in humans or animals receiving valproic acid and may be of significance in veterinary patients. Unless otherwise noted, use together is not necessarily contraindicated, but weigh the potential risks and perform additional monitoring when appropriate.

- **ANTICOAGULANTS:** Valproic acid may have effects on platelet aggregation; use with caution with other drugs that affect coagulation status.
- **ASPIRIN:** Salicylates may displace valproic acid from plasma protein sites, thus increasing valproic acid levels.
- **CLONAZEPAM:** The sedative effects of clonazepam may be enhanced by valproic acid and the anticonvulsant efficacy of both may be diminished.
- **CNS DEPRESSANTS, OTHER:** VPA may enhance the CNS depressant effects of other CNS active drugs.
- **PHENOBARBITAL, PRIMIDONE:** Valproic acid may increase serum levels of phenobarbital and primidone.

Laboratory Considerations
- A keto-metabolite of valproic acid is excreted into the urine and may yield false positive **urine ketone** tests.
- Altered **thyroid function tests** have been reported in humans with unknown clinical significance.

Doses
Note: Because of its very short half-life in dogs, most neurologists do not recommend using VPA in dogs.
- **DOGS:**
  For epilepsy (extra-label): Add on therapy with phenobarbital or bromide: 60 mg/kg PO q8h. (Thomas 2000)

Monitoring
- Anticonvulsant efficacy.
- If used chronically, routine CBC's and liver enzymes at least every 6 months.

Client Information
- Compliance with therapy must be stressed to clients for successful epilepsy treatment. Encourage administering daily doses at same time each day, preferably with food.
- Veterinarian should be contacted if animal develops significant adverse reactions (including clinical signs of anemia and/or liver disease) or if seizure control is unacceptable.

Chemistry/Synonyms
Structurally unrelated to other anticonvulsant agents; valproic acid, valproate sodium, divalproex sodium are derivatives of carboxylic acid. Valproic acid occurs as a colorless to pale yellow clear liquid. It is slightly viscous; has a characteristic odor, a pK_a of 4.8, is slightly soluble in water and freely soluble in alcohol. It is also known as Dipropylacetic acid, DPA, 2-propylpentanoic acid, and 2-propylvaleric acid.

Valproate sodium occurs as a white, crystalline, saline tasting, very hygroscopic powder. It is very soluble in water or alcohol. The commercially available oral solution has a pH of 7-8.

Divalproex sodium is a stable compound in a 1:1 molar ratio of valproic acid and valproate sodium. It occurs as a white powder with a characteristic odor. It is insoluble in water and very soluble in alcohol.

Valproate sodium may also be known as: Abbott-44090, natrii valproas; many trade names are available.

Storage/Stability
Valproic acid capsules should be stored at room temperature (15-30°C) and in tight containers; avoid freezing. Valproate sodium oral solution should be stored at room temperature and in tight containers; avoid freezing. Divalproex sodium enteric-coated tablets should be stored at room temperature in tight, light resistant containers.

Compatibility/Compounding Considerations
No specific information noted.

Dosage Forms/Regulatory Status
VETERINARY-LABELED PRODUCTS: NONE.
HUMAN-LABELED PRODUCTS:

Valproic Acid Oral Capsules: 250 mg; *Depakene*, generic; (Rx)

Valproate Sodium Syrup: 250 mg/5 mL in 473 mL; *Depakene*, generic; (Rx)

Divalproex Sodium Delayed/Extended Release Tablets/Capsules: 125 mg, 250 mg, 500 mg; *Depakote* & *Depakote ER*, *Stavzor*, generic; (Rx)

Divalproex Sodium Oral Capsules (Sprinkle): 125 mg; *Depakote*, generic; (Rx)

Valproate Sodium Injection Concentrate: 100 mg/mL in 5 mL single-dose vials (may be preservative free); *Depacon*, generic; (Rx)

Revisions/References
Monograph revised/updated August 2014.

Papich, M. (1989). Effects of drugs on pregnancy. *Current Veterinary Therapy X: Small Animal Practice*. R. Kirk. Philadelphia, Saunders: 1291-9.
Thomas, W. (2000). Idiopathic epilepsy in dogs. Vet Clin NA: Small Anim Pract **30:1**(Jan): 183-206.

Vanadium
Vanadyl Sulfate
(van-aye-dee-um; van-ah-dil)   Vanadyl Fuel®
Trace Metal

Prescriber Highlights
▶ Trace metal "nutraceutical" that may be useful as an adjunctive treatment for diabetes mellitus in cats.
▶ Efficacy questionable, but probably safe.

Uses/Indications
Vanadium supplementation may be useful in the adjunctive treatment of diabetes mellitus, particularly in cats with early type-2 diabetes mellitus. It is unknown whether vanadium has any benefit in cats with advanced type-2 or type-1 diabetes.

Pharmacology/Actions
In humans with non-insulin dependent diabetes mellitus (NIDDM; type-2), vanadium can reduce fasting blood glucose and glycosylated hemoglobin levels, reduce hepatic glucose release, and increase peripheral glucose disposal and uptake into skeletal muscle mediated by insulin. Vanadium does not influence blood glucose levels in normal patients. While the exact mechanism of action of vanadium is unknown, it apparently inhibits protein tyrosine phosphatase (PTP). PTP is important in signal transduction and allows vanadium to act via both insulin-dependent and insulin-independent pathways.

Pharmacokinetics
Little information on the pharmacokinetics of vanadium was located. Only ≈ 5% is absorbed from foodstuffs. *In vivo* it is converted to the vanadyl cation and forms complexes with ferritin and transferrin. Highest vanadium concentrations are found in the liver, bone and kidney. Vanadium is eliminated via renal routes. Effects on glucose in NIDDM humans may persist for weeks after discontinuation of therapy.

Contraindications/Precautions/Warnings
Vanadium supplements could potentially exacerbate renal insufficiency; use with caution in these patients.

Adverse Effects
Gastrointestinal effects have been reported in some cats receiving vanadium supplements; anorexia and vomiting is most commonly reported. It has been reported that cats initially unable to tolerate

vanadium, can have therapy re-instituted without ill effect. Vanadium in high dosages may have renal toxic effects.

Reproductive/Nursing Safety
It is unknown if supplemental vanadium is safe in pregnancy.

Vanadium is unlikely to have negative effects in nursing kittens.

Overdosage/Acute Toxicity
Vanadyl sulfate may be mildly toxic. The oral LD_{50} in rats is 450 mg/kg. Consider gut removal protocols if an acute overdose occurs. Contact an animal poison control center for further guidance. Chronic overdoses may cause kidney damage.

Drug Interactions
- No specific interactions of note were located. When used with other agents for diabetes management, effects may be additive.

Laboratory Considerations
- No specific laboratory interactions or considerations were noted.

Doses
Note: Because vanadium is given as a salt, do not confuse dosages for vanadium with vanadyl sulfate. Vanadyl sulfate reportedly contains 31% elemental vanadium, but labeled amounts of vanadium vary considerably.

- **CATS:**
  For adjunctive treatment of feline type-2 diabetes (extra-label): Vanadium (**Note:** *salt not specified, assume elemental vanadium*) 0.2 mg/kg PO once daily in food or water. (Greco 2002)

Monitoring
- As there is no reliable way to measure vanadium in the body, a clinical trial is the only way to determine whether vanadium is effective in helping to control blood glucose. Standard methods for monitoring efficacy of diabetes treatment should be followed (*e.g.*, fasting blood glucose, appetite, attitude, body condition, PU/PD resolution and, perhaps, serum fructosamine and/or glycosylated hemoglobin levels).

Client Information
- Clients should give the medication only as prescribed and not change brands without their veterinarian's guidance.
- Give with food.

Chemistry/Synonyms
A trace element, vanadium (V, atomic number 23) is usually given in the form of the inorganic salt, vanadyl sulfate. Vanadyl sulfate occurs as blue crystals and is very soluble in water. Vanadyl sulfate reportedly contains 31% elemental vanadium.

Vanadyl sulfate may also be known as: vanadium (IV) sulfate oxide; vanadium oxysulfate, oxo[sulfato(2-)-O]-vanadium, oxysulfato vanadium (IV); vanadyl (IV) sulfate, or vanadyl (IV)-sulfate hydrate.

Storage/Stability
While vanadyl sulfate is stable under ordinary conditions, refer to the label for each product used.

Compatibility/Compounding Considerations
No specific information noted.

Dosage Forms/Regulatory Status
VETERINARY-LABELED PRODUCTS: NONE.

HUMAN-LABELED PRODUCTS:
No oral products are FDA-approved as pharmaceuticals.

The FDA considers oral vanadyl sulfate products nutritional supplements. No standards have been accepted for potency, purity, safety or efficacy by regulatory bodies.

Supplements are available from a wide variety of sources. Common products include 7.5 mg and 10 mg tablets or 15 mg capsules.

One proprietary product that has been used in cats is *Super Vanadyl Fuel®*. This is a combination product that contains per capsule (among many other ingredients): 150 micrograms chromium (from chromium nicotinate and picolinate) and 1.25 mg of elemental vanadium (from BMOV [bi (maltolato) oxovanadium] and vanadyl sulfate). Bioequivalence between products cannot be assumed.

Revisions/References
Monograph revised/updated August 2014.
Greco, D. (2002). Feline Diabetes Mellitus II. Proceedings Western Vet Conf. accessed via Veterinary Information Network; vin.com

Vancomycin HCl
(van-koe-mye-sin)   Vancocin®
Glycopeptide Antibiotic

Prescriber Highlights
- ▶ Glycopeptide antibiotic reserved for IV use for life-threatening, multi-drug resistant Staph or Enterococcus infections; can also be used PO to treat *Clostridium difficile* diarrhea. Use in veterinary medicine is controversial.
- ▶ Oral vancomycin is not absorbed systemically and is only useful for treating GI *C. difficile* overgrowth.
- ▶ When used systemically, must be given IV; severe pain & tissue injury occurs with SC or IM injection.
- ▶ May be synergistic with aminoglycoside therapy, but increased risk of nephrotoxicity, ototoxicity & neutropenia also possible.
- ▶ If decreased renal dysfunction, adjust dosage.

Uses/Indications
Vancomycin should only be used to treat infections that are documented resistant to other antibiotics and susceptible to vancomycin, usually methicillin-resistant *Staphylococcus* spp. (MRSA) or multidrug-resistant *Enterococcus* spp. It potentially is useful for oral treatment of pseudomembranous colitis caused by *Clostridia difficile*.

Any use of this important human antibiotic in veterinary medicine is controversial. The BSAVA/SAMSoc PROTECT guidelines state: "There are very strong arguments that antimicrobials with restricted use in human medicine (*e.g.*, imipenem, linezolid, teicoplanin, vancomycin) should **not** be used in animals under any circumstances." The International Society for Companion Animal Infectious Diseases (ISCAID) guidelines state: "The use of drugs such as vancomycin, carbapenems and linezolid is **not** justified unless: 1) Infection must be documented on the basis of clinical, cytological abnormalities and culture. The use of these drugs for treatment of subclinical infections is not supported. 2) Resistance to all other reasonable options and susceptibility to the chosen antimicrobial must be documented. 3) The infection must be potentially treatable. The use of critical drugs in situations where the underlying cause cannot be managed or removed is not supported. 4) Consultation with someone with expertise in infectious diseases and antimicrobial treatment must be obtained to determine whether there are any other viable options and whether treatment is reasonable."

Pharmacology/Actions
Vancomycin inhibits cell-wall synthesis and bacterial cell-membrane permeability. It also affects bacterial RNA synthesis. It is only effective against gram-positive bacteria, including many strains of streptococci, staphylococci, and enterococci. Vancomycin is generally a bactericidal, time-dependent antibiotic, but is bacteriostatic against enterococci. Vancomycin also has activity against *Clostridium difficile*, *Rhodococcus equi*, *Listeria monocytogenes*, Corynebacterium, and *Actinomyces* spp. Vancomycin and aminoglycosides

can have synergistic action against susceptible bacteria. Pus and cellular debris may bind to vancomycin and reduce its efficacy.

Resistance to vancomycin by certain strains of enterococci and staphylococci is an increasing concern in human medicine and potentially, in veterinary patients.

Pharmacokinetics

When given orally, vancomycin is not appreciably absorbed. After intravenous administration, vancomycin is widely distributed. Therapeutic levels can be found in pleural, ascitic, pericardial, and synovial fluids. At usual serum levels, it does not readily distribute into the CSF.

The elimination half-life of vancomycin in patients with normal renal function is approximately 4-6 hours. Prolonged dosing can allow the drug to accumulate. The drug is eliminated primarily via glomerular filtration; small amounts are excreted into the bile.

Contraindications/Precautions/Warnings

Vancomycin is an important antibiotic for treating multi-drug resistant infections in humans. It should not be used in veterinary patients when other antibiotics can be used to successfully treat the infection; some believe that the drug should never be used in veterinary patients.

Intravenous vancomycin can be fatal in rabbits.

Patients with decreased renal function that require vancomycin should have dosages reduced or dosing interval increased. Serum levels should be monitored.

Adverse Effects

When given parenterally, nephrotoxicity and ototoxicity are the most serious potential adverse effects of vancomycin. Unlike aminoglycosides, these effects are believed to be uncommon. In humans, dermatologic reactions and hypersensitivity can occur; it is unknown if these effects are issues for veterinary patients. Reversible neutropenia has been reported in humans, particularly when dosage is high and prolonged.

Do not administer IV rapidly or as a bolus; thrombophlebitis, severe hypotension and cardiac arrest (rare) have been reported. Vancomycin must be given over at least 30 minutes as a dilute solution.

Do not give IM, SC, or IP. Severe tissue damage and pain may occur.

Oral therapy may cause GI effects (nausea, inappetence).

Reproductive/Nursing Safety

When used orally, vancomycin is relatively safe to use during pregnancy (FDA category *B*). When used IV, it is not known whether vancomycin can cause fetal harm. A limited study performed in humans did not detect fetal harm, but the numbers studied were small. In humans, the FDA categorizes IV vancomycin as a category *C* drug for use during pregnancy (*Animal studies have shown an adverse effect on the fetus, but there are no adequate studies in humans; or there are no animal reproduction studies and no adequate studies in humans.*) Because in veterinary patients vancomycin should only be used for serious infections, the potential benefits of therapy will probably outweigh the risks in most circumstances.

Vancomycin is excreted into milk. Because the drug is not appreciably absorbed, it is unlikely to pose significant harm to nursing animals, although diarrhea could occur.

Overdosage/Acute Toxicity

Patients with colitis associated with *Clostridia difficile* taking an oral overdose, could potentially absorb enough drug to cause adverse effects. The IV LD_{50} for vancomycin in mice and rats is 400 mg/kg and 319 mg/kg, respectively. Intravenous overdoses of vancomycin may cause an increased risk of adverse effects, particularly ototoxicity and nephrotoxicity. Supportive care is advised. Hemodialysis does not appear to remove the drug in significant amounts.

Drug Interactions

The following drug interactions have either been reported or are theoretical in humans or animals receiving vancomycin and may be of significance in veterinary patients. Unless otherwise noted, use together is not necessarily contraindicated, but weigh the potential risks and perform additional monitoring when appropriate.

- **AMINOGLYCOSIDES:** Vancomycin may increase the risk of aminoglycoside-related ototoxicity or nephrotoxicity. Because this combination of drugs may be medically required (there is evidence of synergy against staphylococci and enterococci), only enhanced monitoring is suggested.
- **ANESTHETIC AGENTS:** In children, vancomycin used with anesthetic agents has caused erythema and a histamine-like flushing.
- **NEPHROTOXIC DRUGS, OTHER** (*e.g.,* **amphotericin B, cisplatin**): Use with caution with other nephrotoxic drugs.

Laboratory Considerations

- No specific concerns were noted

Doses

- **DOGS/CATS:**

  For susceptible gram positive, systemic, life-threatening infections (extra-label): 15 mg/kg IV over 30-60 minutes q6-8h or give 3.5 mg/kg IV and follow with a constant rate infusion (CRI) of 1.5 mg/kg/hour. **Note:** Oral vancomycin is not appreciably absorbed and is only effective for susceptible enteric infections.

  For oral use to treat documented *C. difficile* enterocolitis (extra-label): 10 – 20 mg/kg PO q6h for 5-7 days.

- **HORSES:**

  For susceptible gram positive, systemic, life-threatening infections; IV (extra-label): From a retrospective study in 15 horses: Average dosage was 7.5 mg/kg IV over 30 minutes q8h. Authors recommend that the use of vancomycin in horses be limited to cases in which culture and susceptibility results clearly indicate that this agent is likely to be effective and in which there is no reasonable alternative. (Orsini *et al.* 2005)

  For susceptible gram positive, systemic, life-threatening infections; IV regional limb perfusion (IVRLP) or intraosseous regional limb perfusion (IORLP); (extra-label): In the studies: 300 mg vancomycin diluted in 60 mL 0.9% saline and infused IV (using an IV pump) or IO (administered manually) over 30 minutes. IVRLP or IORLP administration maintained their targeted trough drug concentration in synovial fluid. Authors concluded that IVRLP and IOPLP were safe and may be clinically useful in horses. IVRLP may be better for distal interphalangeal (DIP) joints and IORLP for metacarpophalangeal (MTCP) joints. Mean vancomycin concentration in the MTCP joint was 4 micrograms/mL for 24 hours after IORLP. (Rubio-Martinez *et al.* 2005a; Rubio-Martinez *et al.* 2005b; Rubio-Martinez *et al.* 2006)

Monitoring

When used parenterally:

- Renal function, baseline and periodic.
- Vancomycin levels, maintain trough level above 10 mcg/mL.
- Periodic CBC if therapy is prolonged.

Client Information

- Parenteral vancomycin is used in an inpatient setting and given IV.
- Oral vancomycin may be used for outpatient therapy; clients should be counseled to give as prescribed.
- May give oral dosage forms with a small amount of food.

Chemistry/Synonyms

A glycopeptide antibiotic, vancomycin HCl occurs as an odorless, tan to brown free-flowing powder. It is freely soluble in water. A 5% aqueous solution has a pH of 2.5-4.5.

Vancomycin may also be known as: vanco, vancomycini, or *Vancocin*®; there are many registered international trade names available.

Storage/Stability

Vancomycin should be stored at room temperature in tight containers that are protected from light. Once reconstituted (see directions in package insert or in the Doses section), the injectable or oral solutions are stable for 14 days if refrigerated. If diluted further with D5W or sodium chloride 0.9% for parenteral administration, solutions are stable for 24 hours at room temperature and 2 months if refrigerated.

Compatibility/Compounding Considerations

Vancomycin is **compatible** with D5W, 0.9% NaCl, and lactated Ringer's injection. To prepare parenteral solution using vancomycin 500 mg or 1 gram powder for injection: Reconstitute the 500 mg for injection vial by adding 10 mL of sterile water for injection; add 20 mL if using the 1 gram vial. Before administering to patient, further dilute reconstituted solutions with (at least 100 mL for 500 mg; 200 mL for 1 gram vial) a compatible diluent (*e.g.*, D5W, lactated Ringer's, 0.9% NaCl).

Dosage Forms/Regulatory Status

VETERINARY-LABELED PRODUCTS: NONE.

HUMAN-LABELED PRODUCTS:

Vancomycin HCl Powder for Injection (IV) Solution: 500 mg, 750 mg, 1 gram, & 5 grams; (some preservative free); generic; (Rx)

Vancomycin for IV Injection in dextrose: 500 mg/100, 750 mg/150 mL, & 1 gram/200 mL; generic; (Rx)

Vancomycin HCl Oral Capsules: 125 mg & 250 mg; *Vancocin*®, generic; (Rx). **Note:** Not for systemic infections; not appreciably absorbed.

Vancomycin Oral Solution: 25 mg/mL & 50 mg/mL; *First-Vancomycin*®-25, -50; (Rx). **Note:** Not for systemic infections; not appreciably absorbed.

Revisions/References

Monograph revised/updated August 2014.

Orsini, J. A., et al. (2005). Vancomycin for the treatment of methicillin-resistant staphylococcal and enterococcal infections in 15 horses. Can J Vet Res **69**: 278-86.

Rubio-Martinez, L., et al. (2005a). Medullary plasma pharmacokinetics of vancomycin after intravenous and Intraosseous perfusion of the proximal phalanx in horses. Veterinary Surgery **34**(6): 618-24.

Rubio-Martinez, L. M., et al. (2005b). Evaluation of safety and pharmacokinetics of vancomycin after intravenous regional limb perfusion in horses. American Journal of Veterinary Research **66**(12): 2107-13.

Rubio-Martinez, L. M., et al. (2006). Evaluation of safety and pharmacokinetics of vancomycin after intraosseous regional limb perfusion and comparison of results with those obtained after intravenous regional limb perfusion in horses. American Journal of Veterinary Research **67**(10): 1701-7.

Vasopressin

(vay-soe-**press**-in)

Pitressin®, Arginine Vasopressin, Antidiuretic hormone

Hormone; Pressor Agent

Prescriber Highlights

▶ Hormone used primarily as a diagnostic agent and for the adjunctive treatment of shock syndromes and cardiopulmonary-cerebral resuscitation (CPCR).

▶ Contraindications: Chronic nephritis until nitrogen retention is resolved to reasonable levels, or patients hypersensitive to it; Caution: Vascular disease, seizure disorders, heart failure, or asthma.

▶ Adverse Effects include: nausea, GI pain/cramping, local irritation at the injection site (including sterile abscesses), extravasation injuries, skin reactions, abdominal pain, hematuria, &, rarely, a hypersensitivity (urticarial) reaction.

▶ Overdosage can lead to exacerbation of adverse effects and possibly, water intoxication.

Uses/Indications

Vasopressin is used in veterinary medicine as a diagnostic agent (after water deprivation test), and in the past (as vasopressin tannate in oil is no longer commercially) as a treatment for, central diabetes insipidus (DI) in small animals. In recent years, there has been significant interest in using vasopressin for treating shock syndromes and for cardiopulmonary-cerebral resuscitation (CPCR) in humans and animals. In dogs and cats, evidence of vasopressin's efficacy when compared to epinephrine during CPCR is limited and one study in dogs (n=60) with naturally occurring cardiac arrest, found no difference in rates of return of spontaneous circulation (ROSC) (Buckley *et al.* 2011). However, in ventricular asystole or pulseless electrical activity, vasopressin has some potential advantages over epinephrine. Vasopressin can act as a vasoconstricting agent even when acidosis is present and it may cause less vasoconstriction of coronary and renal vasculature, thereby increasing myocardial perfusion. Also it does not have the arrhythmogenic or chronotropic effects that are associated with epinephrine.

In human medicine, vasopressin has been used to treat acute GI hemorrhage and stimulate GI peristalsis. Vasopressin CRI is also being used for treatment of hypotensive septic patients unresponsive to conventional vasopressor. Prior to radiographic procedures, it has been used to dispel interfering gas shadows or help concentrate contrast media.

Vasopressin has been documented to increase blood pressure in dogs with SIRS/sepsis-induced hypotension. A study reviewing the use of vasopressin in 5 dogs with dopamine-resistant, SIRS or sepsis-induced hypotension, found in all cases, mean arterial blood pressure increased within 15 minutes of adding vasopressin to the treatment regimen (Silverstein *et al.* 2007).

Pharmacology

Vasopressin or antidiuretic hormone (ADH) acts through at least 5 different receptors (three subtypes, V1, V2, V3, the oxytocin receptor, and the purinergic P2 receptor). It promotes the renal reabsorption of solute-free water in the distal convoluted tubules and collecting duct. ADH increases cyclic adenosine monophosphate (cAMP) at the tubule which increases water permeability at the luminal surface resulting in increased urine osmolality and decreased urine flow. Without vasopressin, urine flow can be increased up to 90% greater than normal.

At doses above those necessary for antidiuretic activity, vasopressin can cause smooth muscle contraction. Capillaries and small arterioles are most affected, with resultant decreased blood flow to several systems. Hepatic flow may actually be increased, however.

Vasopressin can cause contraction of smooth muscle of the bladder and gall bladder and increase intestinal peristalsis, particularly of the colon. Vasopressin may decrease gastric secretions and increase GI sphincter pressure; gastric acid concentration remains unchanged.

Vasopressin possesses minimal oxytocic effects, but at large doses may stimulate uterine contraction. Vasopressin also causes the release of corticotropin, growth hormone, and follicle-stimulating hormone (FSH).

Pharmacokinetics

Vasopressin is destroyed in the GI prior to being absorbed and therefore must be administered either intranasally or parenterally. After IM or SC administration in dogs, aqueous vasopressin has antidiuretic activity for 2-8 hours.

Vasopressin is distributed throughout the extracellular fluid. The hormone apparently is not bound to plasma proteins.

Vasopressin is rapidly destroyed in the liver and kidneys. The plasma half-life has been reported to be only 10-20 minutes in humans.

Contraindications/Precautions/Warnings

In humans, vasopressin is contraindicated in patients hypersensitive to it or with chronic nephritis until nitrogen retention is resolved to reasonable levels.

Because of its effects on other systems, particularly at high doses, vasopressin should be used with caution in patients with vascular disease, seizure disorders, heart failure, or asthma.

In human medicine, intravenous or intraosseous vasopressin is considered a "high alert" medication (medications that require special safeguards to reduce the risk of errors). Consider instituting practices such as redundant drug dosage and volume checking, special alert labels, etc.

Adverse Effects

Vasopressin adverse effects include: local irritation at the injection site (extravasation necrosis possible), bronchoconstriction, arrhythmias, skin reactions, platelet aggregation, hyperbilirubinemia, nausea, abdominal pain and cramping, hematuria, and, rarely, a hypersensitivity (urticarial) reaction. Overdosage can lead to water intoxication.

Reproductive/Nursing Safety

Although the drug has minimal effects on uterine contractions at usual doses, it should be used with caution in pregnant animals. In humans, the FDA categorizes this drug as category *C* for use during pregnancy (*Animal studies have shown an adverse effect on the fetus, but there are no adequate studies in humans; or there are no animal reproduction studies and no adequate studies in humans.*)

Overdosage/Acute Toxicity

Acute overdosages would likely exacerbate the adverse effects listed above. Heart rate rhythm and blood pressure should be monitored. Early clinical signs of overdose-induced water intoxication can include listlessness or depression. More severe intoxication clinical signs can include coma, seizures, and eventually, death. Treatment for mild intoxication is stopping vasopressin therapy and restricting water access until resolved. Severe intoxication may require the use of osmotic diuretics (mannitol, urea, or dextrose) with or without furosemide.

Drug Interactions

The following drugs may **inhibit** the antidiuretic activity of vasopressin:

- ALCOHOL
- EPINEPHRINE (large doses)
- HEPARIN
- NOREPINEPHRINE (large doses)

The following drugs may **potentiate** the antidiuretic effects of vasopressin:

- ANTIDEPRESSANTS, TRICYCLIC
- CARBAMAZEPINE
- CHLORPROPAMIDE
- FLUDROCORTISONE

Doses

- **DOGS/CATS:**

  As a diagnostic agent after the water deprivation test (WDT); (extra-label): Refer to a current small animal internal medicine text for further information on procedures, cautions and contraindications for WDT. After WDT if urine specific gravity is >1.025 (dogs) and >1.030 (cats), stop the test as patient does not have diabetes insipidus (DI). If urine specific gravity is not >1.025 (dogs) and >1.030 (cats), give 0.55 Units/kg (maximum dose of 5 Units) aqueous vasopressin IM. Empty the bladder and check urine specific gravity at 30, 60, and 120 minutes after vasopressin. If urine specific gravity increases <10%, nephrogenic DI is indicated; if urine S.G. increases 10-50%, partial central DI is indicated; if it increases 50-800%, complete central DI is indicated. (Tilley *et al.* 2004)

  For adjunctive treatment during CPCR (extra-label):

  a) From the RECOVER guidelines: Although further study is needed, the use of vasopressin (0.8 Units/kg IV or IO) as a substitute or in combination with epinephrine every 3-5 minutes may be considered. It is administered after every other basic life support cycle. If IV or IO access is not possible, intratracheal (IT) administration can be considered. Dilute in sterile saline or sterile water and administer via a catheter longer than the endotracheal tube. If giving IT, dosage has not been fully determined, but 1.2 Units/kg IT is currently recommended. (Fletcher *et al.* 2012)

  b) With pulseless electrical activity or ventricular asystole, vasopressin may be beneficial for myocardial and cerebral blood flow: 0.2 – 0.8 Units/kg, IV once. (Scroggin *et al.* 2009)

  For adjunctive treatment of hypotension/shock (extra-label):

  Warning: Do not confuse dosages listed as Units/kg/min; Units/kg/hour, milliUnits/kg/minute, etc. A dynamic drip rate table creation tool can be found at Global RPh: http://www. globalrph.com/drip.htm

  a) **For adjunctive post-CPCR treatment:** From the RECOVER guidelines: Vasopressin as a CRI at 0.5 – 5 milliUnits/kg/minute (0.003 – 0.03 Units/kg/hour) IV as a CRI. (Fletcher *et al.* 2012)

  b) **In patients with vasodilatory shock unresponsive to fluid resuscitation and catecholamine** (dobutamine, dopamine, and norepinephrine) administration: 0.01 – 0.04 Units/minute (not Units/kg/min) IV. (**Note:** This dose is not dependent upon patient weight). **DO NOT** exceed 0.04 Units/minutes as there is a risk for myocardial ischemia. **DO NOT** use in patients with cardiogenic shock. (Scroggin *et al.* 2009)

  c) **For adjunctive treatment of dogs with septic shock or severe SIRS** (extra-label): Goal is to raise the diastolic pressure to 70-90 mm Hg, which is usually associated with a mean pressure of 110-140 mm Hg and a systolic of 140-180 mm Hg. If norepinephrine at doses between 0.5 – 1 microgram/kg/min do not maintain goal, the author (Hansen) routinely adds an infusion a CRI of vasopressin at 1 – 4 milliUnits/kg/min. Infusion is begun at the low end of the range and titrated upwards in response to need. Supplementation with low doses of vasopressin can restore catecholamine and hemodynamic response. (Hansen 2013)

- **HORSES:**

  For refractory hypotension in critically neonatal foals (extra-label): From a retrospective study: Vasopressin dosages were titrated to the minimum infusion rate needed to achieve a mean arterial pressure (MAP) >65 mmHg and ranged from 0.1 – 2.5 milliUnits/kg/minute. All foals also received dobutamine and other supportive treatment. Vasopressin use was associated with a significant increase in MAP and urinary output, and a significant decrease in heart rate. (Dickey *et al.* 2010)

Monitoring

- Blood pressure; heart rhythm and rate; fluid and electrolyte status.
- For diagnostics (WDT): Urine output/frequency, specific gravity &/or osmolality, water consumption.

Chemistry/Synonyms

A hypothalamic hormone stored in the posterior pituitary, vasopressin is a 9-amino acid polypeptide with a disulfide bond. In most mammals (including dogs and humans), the natural hormone is arginine vasopressin, while in swine the arginine is replaced with lysine. Lysine vasopressin has only about 1/2 the antidiuretic activity of arginine vasopressin. The commercially available vasopressin products may be a combination of arginine or lysine vasopressin derived from natural sources or synthetically prepared. The products are standardized by their pressor activity in rats [USP posterior Pituitary (pressor) Units]; their antidiuretic activity can be variable. Commercially available vasopressin has little, if any, oxytocic activity at usual doses.

Vasopressin injection occurs as a clear, colorless or practically colorless liquid with a faint, characteristic odor. Vasopressin is soluble in water.

Vasopressin may also be known as: ADH, antidiuretic hormone, 8-arginine vasopressin, beta-hypophamine, *Neo-Lidocaton*, *Pitressin* or *Pressyn*.

Storage/Stability

Vasopressin (aqueous) injection should be stored at room temperature; avoid freezing.

Compatibility/Compounding Considerations

Vasopressin is **compatible** at Y-sites with the following: amiodarone, ciprofloxacin, diltiazem, dobutamine, dopamine, epinephrine, gentamicin, heparin, hydroxyethyl starch 130/0.4 in sodium chloride, imipenem-cilastatin, insulin (regular), lidocaine, meropenem, metronidazole, nitroglycerin, norepinephrine, pantoprazole, phenylephrine, piperacillin-tazobactam, procainamide, sodium bicarbonate, and voriconazole. It is **incompatible** with furosemide and phenytoin. Compatibility is dependent upon factors such as pH, concentration, temperature, and diluent used; consult specialized references or a hospital pharmacist for more specific information.

If the aqueous injection is to be administered as an intravenous or intra-arterial infusion, it may be diluted in either D5W or normal saline. For infusion use in humans, it is usually diluted to a concentration of 0.1 – 1 Unit/mL.

Dosage Forms/Regulatory Status

VETERINARY-LABELED PRODUCTS: NONE.

HUMAN-LABELED PRODUCTS:

Vasopressin Injection:: 20 pressor Units/mL in 0.5 mL, 1 mL & 10 mL vials; *Pitressin* Synthetic, generic; (Rx)

Vasopressin Tannate Sterile Suspension in oil is no longer commercially available.

Revisions/References

Monograph revised/updated August 2014.

Buckley, G. J., et al. (2011). Randomized, Blinded Comparison of Epinephrine and Vasopressin for Treatment of Naturally Occurring Cardiopulmonary Arrest in Dogs. Journal of Veterinary Internal Medicine 25(6): 1334-40.

Dickey, E. J., et al. (2010). Use of pressor therapy in 34 hypotensive critically ill neonatal foals. Australian Veterinary Journal 88(12): 472-7.

Fletcher, D. J., et al. (2012). RECOVER evidence and knowledge gap analysis on veterinary CPR. Part 7: Clinical guidelines. J. Vet. Emerg. Crit. Care 22.

Hansen, B. (2013). Cardiovascular System Support. Proceedings; Atlantic Coast Veterinary Conference. accessed via Veterinary Information Network; vin.com

Scroggin, R. D. & J. Quandt (2009). The use of vasopressin for treating vasodilatory shock and cardiopulmonary arrest. J. Vet. Emerg. Crit. Care 19(2): 145-57.

Silverstein, D. C., et al. (2007). Vasopressin therapy in dogs with dopamine-resistant hypotension and vasodilatory shock. J. Vet. Emerg. Crit. Care 17(4): 399-408.

Tilley, L. & F. Smith (2004). The 5-Minute Veterinary Consult: Canine and Feline 3rd Ed, Blackwell.

Vecuronium Bromide

(vek-yew-roe-nee-um)   Norcuron®

Nondepolarizing Neuromuscular Blocker

Prescriber Highlights

▶ Nondepolarizing neuromuscular blocking agent used primarily in dogs and cats.

▶ **Caution:** Severe renal dysfunction, myasthenia gravis hepatic, or biliary disease.

▶ Adverse Effects: None, other than pharmacologic actions.

▶ No analgesia or anesthetic effects.

Uses/Indications

Vecuronium is indicated as an adjunct to general anesthesia to produce muscle relaxation during surgical procedures or mechanical ventilation and facilitate endotracheal intubation. It causes very minimal cardiac effects and generally does not cause the release of histamine. Vecuronium has been used topically to cause mydriasis in birds.

Pharmacology/Actions

Vecuronium is a nondepolarizing neuromuscular blocking agent and acts by competitively binding at cholinergic receptor sites at the motor endplate thereby inhibiting the effects of acetylcholine. Vecuronium when compared to pancuronium (on a weight basis) has been described as being equipotent to up to 3X more potent.

The potency of vecuronium as a neuromuscular blocker appears to be lower in horses than other species and some horses appear to be relatively resistant to its effects (Martin-Flores *et al.* 2012), (Martin-Flores 2013).

Pharmacokinetics

The onset of neuromuscular blockade after IV injection is dependent upon the dose administered. Dogs given 50 mcg/kg IV (also receiving halothane anesthesia), experienced complete paralysis (Kariman *et al.* 2008). Duration of effect is ≈ 20-30 minutes when given as a bolus. Vecuronium has a shorter duration of action than pancuronium (≈ 1/3-1/2 as long), but duration of action is very similar to that of atracurium.

A study done in rats showed that vecuronium was absorbed after intratracheal administration with an onset of action that was slower than IV administration, but faster than after IM. Intratracheal administration resulted in a longer duration of action then after IV dosing (Sunaga *et al.* 2006).

Vecuronium is partially metabolized; it and its metabolites are excreted into the bile and urine. Prolonged recovery times may result in patients with significant renal or hepatic disease.

Contraindications/Precautions/Warnings

Vecuronium is contraindicated in patients hypersensitive to it. It should be used with caution in patients with severe renal dysfunction. Lower doses may be necessary in patients with hepatic or biliary disease. Vecuronium has no analgesic or sedative/anesthetic actions. In patients with myasthenia gravis, neuromuscular blocking agents (if needed) should be used with caution at dosages much lower than typical (15-20% of usual) and with continuous monitoring of neuromuscular transmission (Jones 2012).

Vecuronium's duration of action is shorter in dogs with diabetes mellitus (Clark *et al.* 2012).

In horses, vecuronium should be used with caution (Martin-Flores *et al.* 2011; Gurney *et al.* 2012; Martin-Flores *et al.* 2012).

In human medicine, vecuronium is considered a "high alert" medication (medications that require special safeguards to reduce the risk of errors). Consider instituting practices such as redundant drug dosage and volume checking, special alert labels, etc.

Adverse Effects

In human studies and one limited dog study, adverse effects other than what would be seen pharmacologically (skeletal muscle weakness to profound, prolonged musculoskeletal paralysis) have not been reported.

Reproductive/Nursing Safety

In humans, the FDA categorizes this drug as category *C* for use during pregnancy (*Animal studies have shown an adverse effect on the fetus, but there are no adequate studies in humans; or there are no animal reproduction studies and no adequate studies in humans.*)

Overdosage/Acute Toxicity

No cases of vecuronium overdosage have yet been reported (human or veterinary). Should an inadvertent overdose occur, treat conservatively (mechanical ventilation, O_2, fluids, etc.). Reversal of blockade might be accomplished by administering an anticholinesterase agent (*e.g.*, neostigmine) with an anticholinergic (atropine or glycopyrrolate). A suggested dose for neostigmine is 0.04 mg/kg IV. A case report of edrophonium failing to reverse prolonged vecuronium-induced neuromuscular blockade in a dog has been published (Martin-Flores *et al.* 2011).

Drug Interactions

The following drug interactions have either been reported or are theoretical in humans or animals receiving vecuronium and may be of significance in veterinary patients. Unless otherwise noted, use together is not necessarily contraindicated, but weigh the potential risks and perform additional monitoring when appropriate.

- **NON-DEPOLARIZING MUSCLE RELAXANT DRUGS, OTHER**: May have a synergistic effect or prolong duration of blockade if used with vecuronium.
- **SUCCINYLCHOLINE**: May speed the onset of action and enhance the neuromuscular blocking actions of vecuronium; do not give vecuronium until succinylcholine effects have subsided.

The following agents may enhance or prolong the neuromuscular blocking activity of vecuronium:

- **AMINOGLYCOSIDES**
- **ANESTHETICS** (*e.g.*, isoflurane, sevoflurane)
- **CLINDAMYCIN, LINCOMYCIN**
- **DANTROLENE**
- **MAGNESIUM SALTS**
- **PIPERACILLIN**
- **QUINIDINE**
- **TETRACYCLINES**
- **VERAPAMIL**

Doses

- **DOGS:**

  For neuromuscular relaxation/block (extra-label):

  a) From a study done in female Beagles: 25 micrograms/kg IV over 5 seconds. This dose of vecuronium was chosen after pi-

lot studies and was expected to produce partial block without causing apnea. In 9 of the 10 dogs, vecuronium at this dose produced a twitch reduction of >80%. Significant residual neuromuscular block could be measured at the hind limb with acceleromyography when ventilation spontaneously returned. In another study (Kariman *et al.* 2008) complete paralysis was induced at dosages of 50 micrograms/kg, suggesting that under inhalational anesthesia the ED_{90} of vecuronium in dogs is likely much lower than the previously reported 90 micrograms/kg. The authors concluded that monitoring spontaneous ventilation, including end-tidal CO_2, expired tidal volume, peak inspiratory flow or minute ventilation cannot be used as a surrogate for objective neuromuscular monitoring, and this practice may increase the risk of postoperative residual paralysis. (Martin-Flores *et al.* 2014)

  b) If using CRI propofol-fentanyl anesthesia: CRI maintenance infusion rate of vecuronium at 0.2 mg/kg/hour; If using CRI fentanyl-isoflurane or fentanyl-sevoflurane anesthesia: CRI maintenance infusion rate of vecuronium at 0.1 mg/kg/hour. (Nagahama *et al.* 2006)

- **CATS:**

  For neuromuscular relaxation/blockade (extra-label): 20 – 40 micrograms/kg (0.02 – 0.04 mg/kg) IV. (Morgan 2003)

Monitoring

- Level of neuromuscular block/relaxation. See Martin-Flores dose for dogs above for more information.

Client Information

- This drug should only be used by professionals familiar with its use.

Chemistry/Synonyms

Structurally similar to pancuronium, vecuronium bromide is a synthetic, nondepolarizing neuromuscular blocking agent. It contains the steroid (androstane) nucleus, but is devoid of steroid activity. It occurs as white to off-white, or slightly pink crystals or crystalline powder. In aqueous solution, it has a pK_a of 8.97, and the commercial injection has a pH of 4 after reconstitution. 9 mg are soluble in 1 mL of water; 23 mg are soluble in 1 mL of alcohol.

Vecuronium Bromide may also be known as: Org-NC-45, *Curlem*, *Norcuron*, *Rivecrum*, *Vecural*, or *Vecuron*.

Storage/Stability

The commercially available powder for injection should be stored at room temperature and protected from light. After reconstitution with sterile water for injection, vecuronium bromide is stable for 24 hours at either 2-8°C or at room temperature (<30°C) if stored in the original container. As it contains no preservative, unused portions should be discarded after reconstitution. The drug is stable for 48 hours at room temperature or refrigerated when stored in plastic or glass syringes, but the manufacturer recommends that it be used within 24 hours.

Compatibility/Compounding Considerations

Vecuronium bromide has been shown to be physically **compatible** with D5W, normal saline, D5 in normal saline, and lactated Ringer's.

It should not be mixed with alkaline solutions (*e.g.*, thiobarbiturates).

Dosage Forms/Regulatory Status

VETERINARY-LABELED PRODUCTS: NONE.

HUMAN-LABELED PRODUCTS:

Vecuronium Bromide Powder for Injection: 10 mg & 20 mg in 10 mL & 20 mL vials, with and without diluent; generic; (Rx)

Revisions/References

Monograph revised/updated August 2014.

Clark, L., et al. (2012). Diabetes mellitus affects the duration of action of vecuronium in dogs. Veterinary Anaesthesia and Analgesia 39(5): 472-9.

Gurney, M. & M. Mosing (2012). Prolonged neuromuscular blockade in a horse following concomitant use of vecuronium and atracurium. Veterinary Anaesthesia and Analgesia 39(1): 119-20.

Jones, R. (2012). Correspondence: The use of neuromuscular blocking agents for thymectomy in myasthenia gravis. Vet Anaesth Analg 39: 220.

Kariman, A. & R. Clutton (2008). The effects of medetomidine on the action of vecuronium in dogs anaesthetized with halothane and nitrous oxide. Vet Anaesth Analg 35: 400-8.

Martin-Flores, M. (2013). Neuromuscular Blocking Agents and Monitoring in the Equine Patient. Veterinary Clinics of North America-Equine Practice 29(1): 131-+.

Martin-Flores, M., et al. (2011). Failure to Reverse Prolonged Vecuronium-Induced Neuromuscular Blockade with Edrophonium in an Anesthetized Dog. J. Am. Anim. Hosp. Assoc. 47(4): 294-8.

Martin-Flores, M., et al. (2012). Observations of the potency and duration of vecuronium in isoflurane-anesthetized horses. Veterinary Anaesthesia and Analgesia 39(4): 385-9.

Martin-Flores, M., et al. (2014). Recovery from neuromuscular block in dogs: restoration of spontaneous ventilation does not exclude residual blockade. Veterinary Anaesthesia and Analgesia 41(3): 269-77.

Morgan, R. (2003). Appendix IV: Recommended Drug Dosages. *Handbook of Small Animal Practice 4th Ed.* R. Morgan, R. Bright and M. Swartout. Philadelphia, Saunders: 1279-308.

Nagahama, S., et al. (2006). The effects of propofol, isoflurane and sevoflurane on vecuronium infusion rates for surgical muscle relaxation in dogs. Vet Anaesth Analg 33(3): 169-74.

Sunaga, H., et al. (2006). The Efficacy of Intratracheal Administration of Vecuronium in Rats, Compared with Intravenous and Intramuscular Administration. Anesth Analg 103: 601-7.

Verapamil HCl

(ver-ap-a-mill)   Calan®, Isoptin®, Verelan®

Calcium-Channel Blocker

Prescriber Highlights

▶ Calcium channel blocking agent used for supraventricular tachycardias in dogs & cats.

▶ Contraindications: Cardiogenic shock or severe CHF (unless secondary to a supraventricular tachycardia), hypotension, sick sinus syndrome, 2nd or 3rd degree AV block, digoxin intoxication, or hypersensitive to verapamil. IV is contraindicated within a few hours of IV beta-adrenergic blockers.

▶ Caution: In herding dog breeds (*e.g.*, Collies) that may have the MDR1 gene mutation; patients with heart failure, hypertrophic cardiomyopathy, & hepatic or renal impairment. Use very cautiously in patients with atrial fibrillation & Wolff-Parkinson-White (WPW) syndrome.

▶ Adverse Effects: Hypotension, bradycardia, tachycardia, exacerbation of CHF, peripheral edema, AV block, pulmonary edema, nausea, constipation, dizziness, headache, or fatigue.

▶ Drug Interactions.

Uses/Indications

In dogs and cats, verapamil may be useful for supraventricular tachycardias and, possibly, treatment of atrial flutter or fibrillation. If systolic dysfunction is present, calcium channel blockers (diltiazem, verapamil) are often drugs of first choice for atrial or AV nodal tachycardia. When oral therapy is indicated, most prefer using diltiazem instead of verapamil.

Verapamil is being studied as an adjunctive treatment for pharmaco-resistant epilepsy, but results have thus far been disappointing.

Pharmacology/Actions

A slow-channel calcium blocking agent, verapamil is classified as a class IV antiarrhythmic drug. Verapamil exerts its actions by blocking the transmembrane influx of extracellular calcium ions across membranes of vascular smooth muscle cells and myocardial cells. The result of this blocking is inhibition of the contractile mechanisms of vascular and cardiac smooth muscle. Verapamil has inhibitory effects on the cardiac conduction system and these effects produce its antiarrhythmic properties. Electrophysiologic

effects include increased effective refractory period of the AV node, decreased automaticity and substantially decreased AV node conduction. On ECG, heart rate and RR intervals can be increased or decreased; PR and A-H intervals are increased. Verapamil has negative effects on myocardial contractility and it decreases peripheral vascular resistance.

Verapamil is an inhibitor of P-glycoprotein (Pgp), which potentially could increase toxicity risk for other substrate drugs, but also could be used for therapeutic advantage (*e.g.*, overcoming Pgp-mediated multi-drug resistance by blocking efflux of some chemo drugs).

Pharmacokinetics

In dogs, 90% of an oral dose is absorbed but due to a high first-pass effect bioavailability is only 10-23%. Verapamil's volume of distribution has been reported to be ≈ 4.5 L/kg in dogs. Serum half-lives of 1.8 hours and 2.5 hours have been reported in the dog, which appears to be significantly faster than in humans. Biotransformation occurs in the liver and like humans, several metabolites are formed including some that have activity. Elimination occurs primarily via the bile/feces in dogs.

No pharmacokinetic information was located for cats.

In humans, ≈ 90% of a dose of verapamil is rapidly absorbed after oral administration, but because of a high first-pass effect, only ≈ 20-30% is available to the systemic circulation. Patients with significant hepatic dysfunction may have considerably higher percentages of the drug systemically bioavailable. Food will decrease the rate and extent of absorption of the sustained-release tablets, but less so with the conventional tablets. Verapamil's volume of distribution is between 4.5-7 L/kg; ≈ 90% of the drug in the serum is bound to human plasma proteins. Verapamil crosses the placenta and milk levels may approach those in the plasma.

Verapamil is metabolized in the liver to at least 12 separate metabolites, with norverapamil being the most predominant. The majority of the amounts of these metabolites are excreted into the urine. Only 3-4% is excreted unchanged in the urine. In humans, the half-life of the drug is 2-8 hours after a single IV dose, but it can increase after 1-2 days of oral therapy (presumably due to a saturable process of the hepatic enzymes).

Contraindications/Precautions/Warnings

Verapamil is contraindicated in patients with cardiogenic shock or severe CHF (unless secondary to a supraventricular tachycardia amenable to verapamil therapy), hypotension (<90 mmHg systolic), sick sinus syndrome, 2nd or 3rd degree AV block, digoxin intoxication, or hypersensitive to verapamil.

IV verapamil is contraindicated within a few hours of IV beta-adrenergic blocking agents (*e.g.*, propranolol) as they both can depress myocardial contractility and AV node conduction. Use of this combination in patients with wide complex ventricular tachycardia (QRS >0.11 seconds) can cause rapid hemodynamic deterioration and ventricular fibrillation.

Verapamil should be used with caution in patients with heart failure, hypertrophic cardiomyopathy, and hepatic or renal impairment. Toxicity may be potentiated in patients with hepatic dysfunction. It should be used very cautiously in patients with atrial fibrillation and Wolff-Parkinson-White (WPW) syndrome as fatal arrhythmias may result.

Because verapamil may increase blood glucose in dogs, it should be used with caution in diabetic animals.

Verapamil is potentially a neurotoxic substrate of P-glycoprotein (Pgp); use with caution in those herding breeds (*e.g.*, Collies) that may have the gene mutation (MDR1; ABCB1) that causes a nonfunctional protein.

Adverse Effects

The following adverse reactions may occur: hypotension, bradycardia, tachycardia, exacerbation of CHF, peripheral edema, AV block, pulmonary edema, nausea, constipation, dizziness, headache or fatigue.

Reproductive/Nursing Safety

Oral verapamil in rats with doses 1.5-6X the human dose was embryocidal and retarded fetal growth and development, probably due to reduced weight gains in dams. Verapamil crosses the placenta and can be detected in umbilical vein blood at delivery. In humans, the FDA categorizes this drug as category *C* for use during pregnancy (*Animal studies have shown an adverse effect on the fetus, but there are no adequate studies in humans; or there are no animal reproduction studies and no adequate studies in humans.*)

Verapamil is excreted in milk. Consider discontinuing nursing if the dam requires verapamil therapy.

Overdosage/Acute Toxicity

Clinical signs of overdosage may include bradycardia, hypotension, QT interval prolongation, hyperglycemia, junctional rhythms, and 2nd or 3rd degree AV block. Sinus tachycardia is also possible presumably due to carotid sinus reflex stimulation. Other clinical signs that may be noted include: GI upset, hypothermia, CNS depression, non-cardiogenic pulmonary edema, hypokalemia, metabolic acidosis, and increased lactate production. Rarely, CNS stimulation (seizures, agitation, or tremors) occurs. (Hayes *et al.* 2012)

Because of the potential for severe toxic effects and the potentially complicated management for calcium-channel blocker overdoses, consider consulting with an animal poison control center for guidance. If overdose is secondary to a recent oral ingestion (<2 hours) and the patient is asymptomatic, GI decontamination (emesis, activated charcoal ± sorbitol) should be considered. Treatment is generally supportive in nature; vigorously monitor cardiac and respiratory functions. Intravenous calcium salts (1 mL of 10% solution per 10 kgs of body weight) have been suggested to treat the negative inotropic clinical signs, but may not adequately treat clinical signs of heart block. Use of fluids and pressor agents (*e.g.*, dopamine, norepinephrine, etc.) may be utilized to treat hypotensive clinical signs. The AV block and/or bradycardia can be treated with isoproterenol, norepinephrine, atropine, or cardiac pacing. Patients that develop a rapid ventricular rate after verapamil due to antegrade conduction in flutter/fibrillation with WPW syndrome, have been treated with D.C. cardioversion, lidocaine, or procainamide. Other therapies may include glucagon, insulin/glucose, and intravenous lipid emulsions.

Drug Interactions

The following drug interactions have either been reported or are theoretical in humans or animals receiving verapamil and may be of significance in veterinary patients. Unless otherwise noted, use together is not necessarily contraindicated, but weigh the potential risks and perform additional monitoring when appropriate.

- **ACE INHIBITORS**: May cause additive hypotensive effects.
- **ALPHA-ADRENERGIC BLOCKERS** (*e.g.*, **prazosin**): May cause additive hypotensive effects.
- **BETA-ADRENERGIC BLOCKERS** (*e.g.*, **propranolol**): May cause additive negative cardiac inotrope and chronotrope effects.
- **DOXORUBICIN**: Verapamil may increase concentrations.
- **COPP CHEMOTHERAPY** (**cyclophosphamide, vincristine, procarbazine, prednisone**): May decrease oral absorption of verapamil.
- **CYCLOSPORINE**: Verapamil may increase levels.
- **DANTROLENE**: Cardiovascular collapse reported in animals when used with verapamil.

- **DIGOXIN**: Verapamil may increase the blood levels of digoxin; monitoring of digoxin levels recommended.
- **DISOPYRAMIDE**: May cause additive effects; impair left ventricular function; use together within 24-48 hours not recommended.
- **DIURETICS**: May cause additive hypotensive effects.
- **ERYTHROMYCIN, CLARITHROMYCIN**: May increase verapamil levels.
- **NEUROMUSCULAR BLOCKERS**: Neuromuscular blocking effects of nondepolarizing muscle relaxants may be enhanced by verapamil.
- **PHENOBARBITAL**: May reduce verapamil levels.
- **QUINIDINE**: Additive alpha-adrenergic blocking activity; increased hypotensive effect; verapamil can block quinidine's AV conductive effects and increase quinidine levels.
- **RIFAMPIN**: May reduce verapamil levels.
- **THEOPHYLLINE**: Verapamil may increase serum levels of theophylline and lead to toxicity.
- **VINCRISTINE**: Calcium channel blockers may increase intracellular vincristine by inhibiting the drug's outflow from the cell.

Laboratory Considerations

- Verapamil may elevate blood glucose in dogs and confuse **blood glucose** determinations.

Doses

- **DOGS:**

  For treatment of supraventricular tachycardia (extra-label): Initially dosed 0.05 mg/kg IV (given over 1-2 minutes) while continuously monitoring ECG. If not effective, may repeat every 5-10 minutes until a total dose of 0.15 mg/kg has been administered. If effective, control may last only for 30 minutes (or less). A CRI of 2 – 10 micrograms/kg/minute can be administered for longer control. Adapted from: (Smith 2009), (Kittleson 2006)

- **CATS:**

  For treatment of supraventricular tachycardia (extra-label): Initially dosed 0.025 mg/kg IV (given over 1-2 minutes) while continuously monitoring ECG. If not effective, may repeat every 5-10 minutes until a total dose of 0.15 mg/kg has been administered. If effective, control may last only for 30 minutes (or less). A CRI of 2 – 10 micrograms/kg/minute can be administered for longer control. Adapted from: (Ware 2000)

- **HORSES:** (NOTE: ARCI UCGFS CLASS 4 DRUG)

  To control ventricular rate in atrial fibrillation (extra-label): 0.025 – 0.05 mg/kg IV q 30 minutes; give less than 0.2 mg/kg total dose. (Reimer 2002)

- **SMALL MAMMALS:**

  Hamsters: 0.25 – 0.5 mg (total dose per hamster) SC; **Rabbits:** 8 – 16 mg/kg PO plus 0.5 – 2 mg/kg SC once daily (q24h). (Heatley 2009)

Monitoring

- ECG.
- Clinical signs of toxicity (see Adverse Effects).
- Blood pressure, during acute IV therapy.
- Serum concentration, if efficacy or toxicity warrant (100 – 300 ng/mL is considered therapeutic).

Client Information

- Used in dogs and cats to treat heart rhythm problems (supraventricular tachycardias); being studied for use in the treatment of epilepsy that's resistant to drug therapy.
- Not very commonly used in veterinary medicine, so adverse effects are not well known in dogs or cats, but low blood pressure,

swelling (edema), too fast or too slow heartbeats, gastrointestinal effects (*e.g.*, vomiting, constipation, etc.) and drowsiness/tiredness/lack of energy are possible.

- Very important that animal gets all dosages that are prescribed or the heart rhythm problem can happen again.
- Animal will need to be seen regularly by veterinarian to check to see if the medication is working properly.

Chemistry/Synonyms

A calcium channel blocking agent, verapamil HCl occurs as a bitter-tasting, nearly white, crystalline powder. It is soluble in water and the injectable product has a pH of 4-6.5.

Verapamil HCl tablets should be stored at room temperature (15-30°C); the injectable product should be stored at room temperature (15-30°C) and protected from light and freezing.

Verapamil may also be known as: CP-16533-1, D-365, iproveratril hydrochloride, verapamili hydrochloridum; many trade names are available.

Compatibility/Compounding Considerations

Verapamil HCl for injection is physically **compatible** when mixed with all commonly used intravenous solutions. However, a crystalline precipitate may form if verapamil is added to an infusion line with 0.45% sodium chloride with sodium bicarbonate running. Verapamil is reported to be physically **compatible** with the following drugs: amikacin sulfate, aminophylline, ampicillin sodium, ascorbic acid, atropine sulfate, calcium chloride/gluconate, cefazolin sodium, cefotaxime sodium, cefoxitin sodium, chloramphenicol sodium succinate, cimetidine HCl, clindamycin phosphate, dexamethasone sodium phosphate, diazepam, digoxin, dobutamine HCl (slight discoloration due to dobutamine oxidation), dopamine HCl, epinephrine HCl, furosemide, gentamicin sulfate, heparin sodium, hydrocortisone sodium phosphate, hydromorphone HCl, insulin, isoproterenol, lidocaine HCl, magnesium sulfate, mannitol, meperidine HCl, methylprednisolone sodium succinate, metoclopramide HCl, morphine sulfate, multivitamin infusion, nitroglycerin, norepinephrine bitartrate, oxytocin, pancuronium Br, penicillin G potassium/sodium, pentobarbital sodium, phenobarbital sodium, phentolamine mesylate, phenytoin sodium, potassium chloride/phosphate, procainamide HCl, propranolol HCl, protamine sulfate, quinidine gluconate, sodium bicarbonate, sodium nitroprusside, tobramycin sulfate, vasopressin, and vitamin B complex with C.

The following drugs have been reported to be physically **incompatible** with verapamil: albumin injection, amphotericin B, hydralazine HCl, and trimethoprim/sulfamethoxazole. Compatibility is dependent upon factors such as pH, concentration, temperature, and diluent used; consult specialized references or a hospital pharmacist for more specific information.

Dosage Forms/Regulatory Status

VETERINARY-LABELED PRODUCTS: NONE.

The ARCI (Racing Commissioners International) has designated this drug as a class 4 substance. See the appendix for more information.

HUMAN-LABELED PRODUCTS:

Verapamil HCl Tablets: 40 mg, 80 mg, 120 mg; *Calan*®, generic; (Rx)

Verapamil HCl Sustained/Extended-Release Capsules: 100 mg, 120 mg, 180 mg, 200 mg, 240 mg, 300 mg, 360 mg; *Calan*® *SR*, *Isoptin*® *SR*, *Verelan*® *PM*, generic; (Rx)

Verapamil HCl for Injection: 2.5 mg/mL in 2 mL & 4 mL vials, amps and syringes; generic; (Rx)

Revisions/References

Monograph revised/updated August 2014.
Hayes, C. L. & M. Knight (2012). Calcium Channel Blocker Toxicity in Dogs and Cats. Veterinary Clinics of North America-Small Animal Practice 42(2): 263-+.
Heatley, J. (2009). Small Exotic Mammal Cardiovascular Disease. Proceedings: ABVP. accessed via Veterinary Information Network; vin.com
Kittleson, M. (2006). "Chapt 29: Drugs used in the treatment of cardiac arrhythmias." *Small Animal Cardiology, 2nd Ed* Veterinary Information Network.
Reimer, J. (2002). Treating life-threatening cardiac arrhythmias in the horse. Proceedings: ACVIM Forum. accessed via Veterinary Information Network; vin.com
Smith, F. (2009). Update on Antiarrhythmic Therapy. Proceedings: Western Veterinary Conference. accessed via Veterinary Information Network; vin.com
Ware, W. (2000). Therapy for Critical Arrhythmias: New Advances. Proceedings: The North American Veterinary Conference, Orlando. accessed via Veterinary Information Network; vin.com

Vinblastine Sulfate

(vin-blas-teen)   Velban®

Antineoplastic

Prescriber Highlights

▶ A Vinca alkaloid antineoplastic used for a variety of tumors in dogs & cats.
▶ Contraindications: Preexisting leukopenia or granulocytopenia (unless a result of the disease being treated) or active bacterial infection; reduce dose if hepatic disease. Use with caution in herding breeds (*e.g.*, Collies) that may have the gene mutation (MDR1; *ABCB1*).
▶ Adverse Effects: Gastroenterocolitis (nausea/vomiting), myelosuppression (more so than with vincristine); may also cause constipation, alopecia, stomatitis, ileus, inappropriate ADH secretion, jaw & muscle pain, & loss of deep tendon reflexes. Extravasation injury is possible.
▶ Cats can develop neurotoxicity causing constipation or paralytic ileus & aggravating anorexia; can also develop reversible axon swelling & paranodal demyelination.
▶ Potentially teratogenic.
▶ Wear gloves & protective clothing when preparing or administering.
▶ Drug Interactions.

Uses/Indications

Vinblastine may be employed in the treatment of lymphomas, carcinomas, mastocytomas, and splenic tumors in small animals. It is apparently more effective than vincristine in the treatment of canine mast cell tumors.

A prospective clinical trial in cats (n=40) to compare vincristine and vinblastine response rates, outcomes, and toxicity in a COP-based protocol for lymphoma, found that both arms had similar response rates, progression-free survival (PFS) times, lymphoma-specific survival (LSS) times, but vincristine treated cats had a higher incidence of gastrointestinal adverse effects (Krick *et al.* 2013).

A prospective clinical trial in dogs (n=28) using vinblastine to treat transitional cell bladder cancer, found 36% had a partial remission, 50% had stable disease, and 14% had disease progression. The majority of dogs (27 of 28) did not have clinically relevant adverse effects, but 61% required dosage reduction (from the initial 3 mg/m^2 IV q2 weeks) due to neutropenia. The authors concluded that vinblastine can be considered another treatment option (Arnold *et al.* 2011).

Pharmacology/Actions

Vinblastine apparently binds to microtubular proteins (tubulin) in the mitotic spindle, thereby preventing cell division during metaphase. It also interferes with amino acid metabolism by inhibiting glutamic acid utilization and preventing purine synthesis, citric acid cycle, and urea formation.

Pharmacokinetics

Vinblastine is administered IV. After injection, it is rapidly distributed to tissues. In humans, ≈ 75% is bound to tissue proteins and the drug does not appreciably enter the CNS.

Vinblastine is extensively metabolized by the liver and is primarily excreted in the bile/feces; lesser amounts are eliminated in the urine. CYP3A12 is the major cytochrome P450 isoform responsible for the metabolism of vinblastine in dogs (Achanta *et al.* 2014).

Contraindications/Precautions/Warnings

Vinblastine is contraindicated in patients with preexisting leukopenia or granulocytopenia (unless a result of the disease being treated), or active bacterial infection. One source states "Do not administer if neutrophil count is less than 3,000/mcL (Moore 2013).

Doses of vinblastine should be reduced in patients with hepatic disease. A 50% reduction in dose should be considered if serum bilirubin levels are >2 mg/dL.

Because vinblastine is potentially a neurotoxic substrate of P-glycoprotein, it should be used with caution in those herding breeds (*e.g.*, Collies) that may have the gene mutation (MDR1; *ABCB1*) that causes a nonfunctional protein. Bone marrow suppression (decreased blood cell counts, particularly neutrophils) and GI toxicity (anorexia, vomiting, diarrhea) are more likely to occur at normal doses in dogs with the A*BCB1* mutation. To reduce the likelihood of severe toxicity in these dogs (mutant/normal or mutant/mutant), the Veterinary Clinical Pharmacology Laboratory at Washington State University recommends reducing the dose by 25-30% and carefully monitoring these patients (Anon 2009).

As vinblastine may be a skin irritant, gloves and protective clothing should be worn when preparing or administering the medication. If skin/mucous membrane exposure occurs, thoroughly wash area with soap and water.

Adverse Effects

Vinblastine can cause gastroenterocolitis (nausea/vomiting), which generally lasts less than 24-hours. It can be myelosuppressive at usual dosages (nadir at 4-9 days after treatment; recovery at 7-14 days). Vinblastine is considered more myelosuppressive than is vincristine.

Vinblastine may not possess the degree of peripheral neurotoxic effects seen with vincristine, but at high doses, these effects may be seen. Additionally, vinblastine may cause constipation, alopecia, stomatitis, ileus, inappropriate ADH secretion, jaw and muscle pain, and loss of deep tendon reflexes.

Cats can develop neurotoxicity that can be associated with constipation or paralytic ileus thereby aggravating anorexia. They may develop reversible axon swelling and paranodal demyelination.

Extravasation of vinblastine may cause significant tissue irritation and cellulitis. Because of the vesicant action of this drug, it is recommended to use a different needle for injecting the drug than the one used to withdraw the drug from the vial. Should clinical signs of extravasation be noted, discontinue infusion immediately at that site and apply moderate heat to the area to help disperse the drug. Injections of hyaluronidase have also been suggested to help diffuse the drug.

Reproductive/Nursing Safety

Little is known about the effects of vinblastine on developing fetuses, but it is believed that the drug possesses some teratogenic and embryotoxic properties. It may also cause aspermia in males. In humans, the FDA categorizes this drug as category *D* for use during pregnancy (*There is evidence of human fetal risk, but the potential benefits from the use of the drug in pregnant women may be acceptable despite its potential risks.*)

It is not known whether vinblastine is excreted in milk. Because of the potential for serious adverse reactions in nursing offspring, consider using milk replacer if dams are being given this drug.

Overdosage/Acute Toxicity

In dogs, the lethal dose for vinblastine has been reported as 0.2 mg/kg. Effects of an overdosage of vinblastine are exacerbations of the adverse effects outlined above. Additionally, neurotoxic effects similar to those associated with vincristine may also be noted.

A case report of a cat receiving a 4X IV overdose has been published (Grant *et al.* 2010). The following were noted with this patient after the overdose: Within hours the cat developed depression and was unable to jump; days 1-11 anorexia; days 2-6 neutropenia with a fever on day 4; days 2-10 thrombocytopenia and anemia; days 4-10 vomiting and diarrhea, and on days 3-10 syndrome of inappropriate ADH (SIADH). Aggressive therapeutic interventions supporting the patient resulted in a positive outcome.

In humans, cardiovascular and hematologic monitoring are performed after an overdose. Treatment can include anticonvulsants, and prevention of ileus. Additionally, an attempt is made to prevent the effects associated with the syndrome of inappropriate antidiuretic hormone (SIADH) with fluid restriction and loop diuretics to maintain serum osmolality.

Do not confuse vinBLAStine with vinCRIStine; consider using "tall man lettering" when writing orders.

Drug Interactions

The following drug interactions have either been reported or are theoretical in humans or animals receiving vinblastine and may be of significance in veterinary patients. Unless otherwise noted, use together is not necessarily contraindicated, but weigh the potential risks and perform additional monitoring when appropriate.

- **OTOTOXIC DRUGS** (*e.g.*, **cisplatin, carboplatin**): May cause additive risk for ototoxicity

Caution is advised if using other drugs that can inhibit **p-glycoprotein** particularly in those dogs at risk for MDR1-allele mutation (Collies, Australian Shepherds, Shelties, Long-haired Whippet, etc. "white feet"), unless tested "normal". Drugs and drug classes involved include:

- **AMIODARONE**
- **AZOLE ANTIFUNGALS** (*e.g.*, **ketoconazole, itraconazole**)
- **CARVEDILOL**
- **CYCLOSPORINE**
- **DILTIAZEM**
- **ERYTHROMYCIN; CLARITHROMYCIN**
- **QUINIDINE**
- **SPIRONOLACTONE**
- **TAMOXIFEN**
- **VERAPAMIL**

Laboratory Considerations

- Vinblastine may significantly increase both blood and urine concentrations of **uric acid.**

Doses

Note: Because of the potential toxicity of this drug to patients, veterinary personnel and clients, and since chemotherapy indications, treatment protocols, monitoring and safety guidelines often change, the following dosages should be used only as a general guide. Consultation with a veterinary oncologist and referral to current veterinary oncology references [*e.g.*, (Withrow *et al.* 2012); (Dobson *et al.* 2011); (Henry *et al.* 2009); (North *et al.* 2009); (Argyle *et al.* 2008)] are strongly recommended.

- **DOGS/CATS:**

The following doses are general guidelines (see above). Depending on the protocol and the disease treated, vinblastine doses are usually 1.5 – 3 mg/m^2 (not mg/kg) IV every 1-2 weeks, often in combination with other chemo drugs (*e.g.,* in dogs, cyclophosphamide and prednisolone). There is one protocol for dogs (Woods 2010), where it is given on 4 subsequent days every 3 weeks.

Monitoring

- Efficacy.
- Toxicity (complete blood counts with platelets; liver function tests prior to therapy and repeated as necessary; serum uric acid).

Client Information

- Vinblastine is a chemotherapy (cancer) drug. The drug and its byproducts can be hazardous to other animals and people that come in contact with it. On the day your animal gets the drug and then for a few days afterward, all bodily waste (urine, feces, litter), blood, or vomit should only be handled while wearing disposable gloves. Seal the waste in a plastic bag and then place both the bag and gloves in with the regular trash.
- GI effects (*e.g.,* vomiting, reduced appetite, diarrhea, etc.) are common after a dose. If these become severe or bloody, contact your veterinarian.
- Can cause bone marrow suppression; if you notice bleeding, bruising, fever (indicating an infection), or if animal becomes very tired easily, contact veterinarian right away.
- Cats can develop nerve toxicity from vinblastine that results in severe constipation and loss of appetite.

Chemistry/Synonyms

Commonly referred to as a Vinca alkaloid, vinblastine sulfate is isolated from the plant Cantharanthus roseus (*Vinca rosea Linn*) and occurs as a white or slightly yellow, hygroscopic, amorphous or crystalline powder that is freely soluble in water. The commercially available injection has a pH of 3-5.5.

Vinblastine may also be known as: 29060-LE, NSC-49842, sulfato de vimblastina, vinblastini sulfas, vincaleukoblastine sulphate, VBL, *Alkaban®, Blastovin®, Cellblastin®, Cytoblastin®, Ifabla®, Lemblastine®, Periblastine®, Serovin®, Solblastin®, Velban®, Velbe®, Velsar®,* or *Xintoprost®.*

Storage/Stability

The sterile powder for injection, solution for injection and reconstituted powder for injection should all be protected from light. The powder for injection and injection liquid should be stored in the refrigerator (2-8°C). The intact powder for injection is stable at room temperature for at least 1 month. After reconstituting with bacteriostatic saline, the powder for injection is stable for 30 days if refrigerated.

Compatibility/Compounding Considerations

Vinblastine sulfate is reportedly physically **compatible** with the following intravenous solutions and drugs: D5W and bleomycin sulfate. In syringes or at Y-sites with: bleomycin sulfate, cisplatin, cyclophosphamide, droperidol, fluorouracil, leucovorin calcium, methotrexate sodium, metoclopramide HCl, mitomycin, and vincristine sulfate.

Vinblastine sulfate **compatibility information conflicts** or is dependent on diluent or concentration factors with the following drugs or solutions: doxorubicin HCl and heparin sodium (in syringes).

Vinblastine sulfate is reportedly physically **incompatible** with furosemide.

Compatibility is dependent upon factors such as pH, concentration, temperature and diluent used; consult specialized references or a hospital pharmacist for more specific information.

Dosage Forms/Regulatory Status

VETERINARY-LABELED PRODUCTS: NONE.

HUMAN-LABELED PRODUCTS:

Vinblastine Sulfate Injection: 1 mg/mL in 10 mL & 25 mL vials; generic; (Rx)

Vinblastine Powder for Injection: 10 mg in vials; *Velban®*, generic; (Rx)

Revisions/References

Monograph revised/updated August 2014.

Achanta, S. & L. K. Maxwell (2014). Reaction phenotyping of vinblastine in dogs [Abstract]. Vet Comp Oncol.

Anon (2009). Problem Drugs, Veterinary Clinical Pharmacology Lab, College of Vet Med, Washington State University.

Argyle, D., et al. (2008). *Decision Making in Small Animal Oncology*, Wiley-Blackwell.

Arnold, E. J., et al. (2011). Clinical Trial of Vinblastine in Dogs with Transitional Cell Carcinoma of the Urinary Bladder. Journal of Veterinary Internal Medicine 25(6): 1385-90.

Dobson, J. & D. Lascelles (2011). *BSAVA Manual of Canine and Feline Oncology*, BSAVA.

Grant, I. A., et al. (2010). Toxicities and salvage therapy following overdose of vinblastine in a cat. Journal of Small Animal Practice 51(2): 127-31.

Henry, C. & M. Higginbotham (2009). *Cancer Management in Small Animal Practice*, Saunders.

Krick, E. L., et al. (2013). Prospective Clinical Trial to Compare Vincristine and Vinblastine in a COP-Based Protocol for Lymphoma in Cats. Journal of Veterinary Internal Medicine 27(1): 134-40.

Moore, A. (2013). Chemotherapy Options for Carcinomas and Sarcomas in Pets. Porceedings: ACVIM. accessed via Veterinary Information Network; vin.com

North, S. & T. Banks (2009). *Small Animal Oncology: An Introduction*, Saunders.

Withrow, S., et al. (2012). Withrow and MacEwen's Small Animal Clinical Oncology, 5th Ed., Saunders.

Woods, J. (2010). Medical & Surgical Oncology: Diagnosis & Management of Mast Cell Tumors in Dogs & Cats. Proceedings: ACVIM. accessed via Veterinary Information Network; vin.com

Vincristine Sulfate

(vin-kris-teen)   Oncovin®

Antineoplastic

Prescriber Highlights

▶ A Vinca alkaloid antineoplastic used for a variety of tumors in dogs & cats (primarily lymphoid & hematopoietic neoplasms); also used for the treatment of immune-mediated thrombocytopenia.

▶ Caution: Hepatic disease, leukopenia, infection, or preexisting neuromuscular disease; reduce dose if hepatic disease. Use with caution in herding breeds (*e.g.,* Collies) that may have the gene mutation (MDR1; *ABCB1*).

▶ Adverse Effects: Much less myelosuppressive than vinblastine, but may cause more peripheral neurotoxic effects; neuropathic clinical signs can include proprioceptive deficits, spinal hyporeflexia, or paralytic ileus with resulting constipation; Cats can develop neurotoxicity causing constipation or paralytic ileus & aggravating anorexia; can also develop reversible axon swelling & paranodal demyelination.

▶ Potentially teratogenic.

▶ Avoid extravasation; wear gloves & protective clothing when preparing or administering.

▶ Drug Interactions.

Uses/Indications

Vincristine is used as an antineoplastic primarily in combination drug protocols in dogs and cats in the treatment of lymphoid and hematopoietic neoplasms. In dogs, it may be used alone in the therapy of transmissible venereal neoplasms.

A prospective clinical trial in cats (n=40) to compare vincristine and vinblastine response rates, outcomes, and toxicities in a COP-based protocol for lymphoma, found that both arms had similar response rates, progression-free survival (PFS) times, lymphoma-specific survival (LSS) times, but vincristine treated cats had a higher incidence of gastrointestinal adverse effects (Krick *et al.* 2013).

Because vincristine can induce thrombocytosis (at low doses) and has some immunosuppressant activity, it may also be employed in the treatment of immune-mediated thrombocytopenia (ITP). A prospective, randomized study in dogs (n=20) to compare the effect of hIVIG versus vincristine on platelet recovery in dogs with ITP found no significant differences in groups in platelet recovery time, hospitalization time, or survival at discharge, 6 months, and 1 year after entry into the study. The authors concluded that because of lower cost and ease of administration, vincristine should be the first-line adjunctive treatment for the acute management of canine ITP (Balog *et al.* 2013).

Pharmacology/Actions

Vincristine apparently binds to microtubular proteins (tubulin) in the mitotic spindle, thereby preventing cell division during metaphase. It also interferes with amino acid metabolism by inhibiting glutamic acid utilization and preventing purine synthesis, citric acid cycle and urea formation. Tumor resistance to one Vinca alkaloid does not imply resistance to another.

Vincristine can induce thrombocytosis (mechanism unknown) and has some immunosuppressant activity.

Pharmacokinetics

Vincristine is administered IV as it is unpredictably absorbed from the GI tract. After injection it is rapidly distributed to tissues. In humans, ≈ 75% is bound to tissue proteins and the drug does not appreciably enter the CNS.

In cats, vincristine and cyclophosphamide given intraperitoneally (IP) was considered safe and effective (Teske *et al.* 2014).

Vincristine is extensively metabolized, presumably by the liver and primarily excreted in the bile/feces; lesser amounts are eliminated in the urine. The elimination half-life in dogs is reportedly biphasic with an alpha half-life of 13 minutes and a beta half-life of 75 minutes.

Contraindications/Precautions/Warnings

Vincristine should be used with caution in patients with hepatic disease, leukopenia, infection, or preexisting neuromuscular disease.

Doses of vincristine should be reduced in patients with hepatic disease. A 50% reduction in dose should be considered if serum bilirubin levels are >2 mg/dL.

Because vincristine is potentially a neurotoxic substrate of P-glycoprotein, it should be used with caution in those herding breeds (*e.g.*, Collies) that may have the gene mutation (MDR1; ABCB1) that causes a nonfunctional protein. Bone marrow suppression (decreased blood cell counts, particularly neutrophils) and GI toxicity (anorexia, vomiting, diarrhea) are more likely to occur at normal doses in dogs with the *ABCB1* mutation. To reduce the likelihood of severe toxicity in these dogs (mutant/normal or mutant/mutant), the Veterinary Clinical Pharmacology Laboratory at Washington State University recommends reducing the dose by 25-30% and carefully monitoring these patients (Anon 2009).

Border Collies, unrelated to their *ABCB1* status, appear to be more susceptible than typical for developing vincristine-associated myelosuppression (Lind *et al.* 2013).

As vincristine may be a skin irritant, gloves and protective clothing should be worn when preparing or administering the medication. If skin/mucous membrane exposure occurs, thoroughly wash area with soap and water.

Do not confuse vinBLAStine with vinCRIStine; consider using "tall man lettering" when writing orders.

Adverse Effects

Although structurally related to and having a similar mechanism of action as vinblastine, vincristine has a different adverse reaction profile. Vincristine is much less myelosuppressive (mild leuko-penia) at usual doses than is vinblastine, but may cause more peripheral neurotoxic effects. Neuropathic clinical signs may include proprioceptive deficits, spinal hyporeflexia, or paralytic ileus with resulting constipation. In humans, vincristine commonly causes mild sensory impairment and peripheral paresthesias. These may also occur in animals, but are not usually noted due to difficulty in detection. Cats, however, can develop neurotoxicity that can be associated with constipation or paralytic ileus thereby aggravating anorexia. They can develop reversible axon swelling and paranodal demyelination.

Additionally, in small animals, vincristine may cause vomiting, diarrhea, anorexia, impaired platelet aggregation, increased liver enzymes, inappropriate ADH secretion, jaw pain, alopecia, stomatitis, or seizures.

A case report of cat developing pulmonary edema attributed to vincristine administration has been published (Polton *et al.* 2008).

While deemed not clinically significant, vincristine can cause erythrocyte dysplasia in dogs (Collicutt *et al.* 2013).

Extravasation injuries associated with perivascular injection of vincristine can range from irritation to necrosis and tissue sloughing. Because of the vesicant action of this drug, it is recommended to use a different needle for injecting the drug than the one used to withdraw it from the vial. Recommendations of therapy for extravasation include discontinuing the infusion immediately at that site and applying moderate heat to the area to help disperse the drug. Injections of hyaluronidase have been suggested to help diffuse the drug. Others have suggested applying ice to the area to limit the drug's diffusion and minimize the area affected. Topical dimethyl sulfoxide (DMSO) has also been recommended by some to treat the area involved.

Reproductive/Nursing Safety

Little is known about the effects of vincristine on developing fetuses, but it is believed that the drug possesses some teratogenic and embryotoxic properties. It may also cause aspermia in males. In humans, the FDA categorizes this drug as category *D* for use during pregnancy (*There is evidence of human fetal risk, but the potential benefits from the use of the drug in pregnant women may be acceptable despite its potential risks.*) In a separate system evaluating the safety of drugs in canine and feline pregnancy (Papich 1989), this drug is categorized as in class: *C* (*These drugs may have potential risks. Studies in people or laboratory animals have uncovered risks, and these drugs should be used cautiously as a last resort when the benefit of therapy clearly outweighs the risks.*)

It is not known whether this drug is excreted in milk. Because of the potential for serious adverse reactions in nursing offspring, consider using milk replacer if dams are being given this drug.

Overdosage/Acute Toxicity

In dogs, it is reported that the maximally tolerated dose of vincristine is 0.06 mg/kg every 7 days for 6 weeks. Animals receiving this dose showed signs of slight anemia, leukopenia, increased liver enzymes, and neuronal shrinkage in the peripheral and central nervous systems.

In cats, the lethal dose of vincristine is reportedly 0.1 mg/kg. Cats receiving toxic doses showed clinical signs of weight loss, seizures, leukopenia, and general debilitation. A case report of cat receiving a 5 mg/m^2 (10X) overdose has been published (Hughes *et al.* 2009). Despite intensive treatment including using calcium folinate, the cat died 72 hours after the overdose.

In humans, cardiovascular and hematologic monitoring are performed after an overdose. Treatment can include anticonvulsants, and prevention of ileus. Additionally, an attempt is made to prevent the effects associated with the syndrome of inappropriate antidiuretic hormone (SIADH) with fluid restriction and loop diuretics to maintain serum osmolality. There have been some reports of leucovorin calcium being used to treat vincristine overdoses in humans, but efficacy of this treatment has not yet been confirmed.

Drug Interactions

The following drug interactions have either been reported or are theoretical in humans or animals receiving vincristine and may be of significance in veterinary patients. Unless otherwise noted, use together is not necessarily contraindicated, but weigh the potential risks and perform additional monitoring when appropriate.

- **ASPARAGINASE:** Additive neurotoxicity may occur; is apparently less common when asparaginase is administered after vincristine.
- **MITOMYCIN:** In humans who have previously or simultaneously received mitomycin-C with Vinca alkaloids, severe bronchospasm has occurred.

Caution is advised if using other drugs that can inhibit **p-glycoprotein** particularly in those dogs at risk for MDR1-allele mutation (*e.g.*, Collies, Australian Shepherds, Shelties, Long-haired Whippet, etc. "white feet"), unless tested "normal". Drugs and drug classes involved include:

- **AMIODARONE**
- **AZOLE ANTIFUNGALS** (*e.g.*, **ketoconazole, itraconazole**)
- **CARVEDILOL**
- **CYCLOSPORINE**
- **DILTIAZEM**
- **ERYTHROMYCIN; CLARITHROMYCIN**
- **QUINIDINE**
- **SPIRONOLACTONE**
- **TAMOXIFEN**
- **VERAPAMIL**

Laboratory Considerations

- Vincristine may significantly increase both blood and urine concentrations of **uric acid.**

Doses

Note: Because of the potential toxicity of this drug to patients, veterinary personnel and clients, and since chemotherapy indications, treatment protocols, monitoring and safety guidelines often change, the following dosages should be used only as a general guide. Consultation with a veterinary oncologist and referral to current veterinary oncology references [*e.g.*, (Withrow *et al.* 2012); (Dobson *et al.* 2011); (Henry *et al.* 2009); (North *et al.* 2009); (Argyle *et al.* 2008)] are strongly recommended.

- **DOGS:**

For neoplastic diseases (extra-label): Usually used in combination protocols with other drugs; consultation with a veterinary oncologist is encouraged before use; see above. Vincristine is usually dosed in dogs at 0.5 – 0.75 mg/m² (**NOT** mg/kg) IV and administered every 1-2 weeks. When used for transmissible venereal tumor, vincristine is used as sole therapy usually at 0.5 mg/m² (maximum dose 1 mg) IV once weekly for 4-6 weeks of therapy.

For adjunctive treatment of immune-mediated thrombocytopenia (extra-label): In the study, dogs received vincristine at 0.02 mg/kg IV bolus once. Dogs also received glucocorticoids (usually prednisone at 1.5 – 2 mg/kg PO q12h) and doxycycline until results of serologic testing was confirmed negative. In dogs that did not have an increase in platelet count 7 days after treatment azathioprine (2 mg/kg PO q24h) was added. **Note:** At this dosage of vincristine, clinically significant myelosuppression has not been described. (Balog *et al.* 2013)

- **CATS:**

For neoplastic diseases (extra-label); (consultation with a veterinary oncologist is encouraged before use; see above): Vincristine is usually dosed in cats at 0.5 – 0.75 mg/m² (**NOT** mg/kg) IV and administered every 1-3 weeks.

- **HORSES:**

For neoplastic diseases (extra-label); consultation with a veterinary oncologist is encouraged before use: Usual doses used in horses are: 0.5 mg/m² (usually 2.5 – 3 mg total dose per horse) IV weekly. For generalized lymphoma the CAP protocol was used at the time of publication by one of the authors: cytarabine (cytosine arabinoside) at an average dose of 1 – 1.2 grams (total dose), SC or IM once every 1-2 weeks; cyclophosphamide at a dose of 1 gram (total dose) IV every 2 weeks (alternating with cytarabine); and prednisolone at a dose of 1 mg/kg PO every other day. Vincristine at 2.5 mg (total dose) IV is added on the weeks when the cytarabine is administered if there is no response. These are starting doses; the total doses can be increased by 20-30% without expecting complications. With remission, the starting doses are maintained for 2-3 months and then the horse is switched onto a maintenance protocol. The first cycle of maintenance therapy increases the treatment interval for each drug by one week (except prednisolone which is kept at the same frequency but with a reducing dose). If horse is still in remission after 2-3 months of the first cycle, the second cycle is begun by adding a further week to the treatment intervals of each drug. (Mair *et al.* 2006)

Monitoring

- Efficacy (tumor burden reduction or platelet count).
- Toxicity (peripheral neuropathic clinical signs; complete blood counts with platelets; liver function tests prior to therapy and repeated as necessary; serum uric acid).

Client Information

- Vincristine is a chemotherapy (cancer) drug. The drug and its byproducts can be hazardous to other animals and people that come in contact with it. On the day your animal gets the drug and then for a few days afterward, all bodily waste (urine, feces, litter), blood, or vomit should only be handled while wearing disposable gloves. Seal the waste in a plastic bag and then place both the bag and gloves in with the regular trash.
- Vincristine can be very toxic to Collie-like breeds that are positive for the MDR1 genetic mutation.
- Vincristine can cause a serious neurological toxicity that can result in weakness, severe constipation and loss of appetite.
- If leaked outside the vein, vincristine is very irritating and can cause severe damage to the affected limb.

Chemistry/Synonyms

Commonly referred to as a Vinca alkaloid, vincristine sulfate is isolated from the plant *Cantharanthus roseus* (*Vinca rosea Linn*) and occurs as a white or slightly yellow, hygroscopic, amorphous or crystalline powder that is freely soluble in water and slightly soluble in alcohol. The commercially available injection has a pH of 3-5.5. Vincristine sulfate has pK$_a$s of 5 and 7.4

Vincristine Sulfate may also be known as: leurocristine sulfate, VCR, LCR compound 37231, leurocristine sulphate, NSC-67574, 22-oxovincaleukoblastine sulphate, sulfato de vincristina, vincristini sulfas and *Oncovin*®; many other trade names are available.

Storage/Stability

Vincristine sulfate injection should be protected from light and stored in the refrigerator (2-8°C).

Compatibility/Compounding Considerations

Vincristine sulfate is reportedly physically **compatible** with the following intravenous solutions and drugs: D5W, bleomycin sulfate, cytarabine, fluorouracil, and methotrexate sodium. In syringes or at Y-sites with: bleomycin sulfate, cisplatin, cyclophosphamide, doxorubicin HCl, droperidol, fluorouracil, heparin sodium, leucovorin calcium, methotrexate sodium, metoclopramide HCl, mitomycin, and vinblastine sulfate.

Vincristine sulfate is reportedly physically **incompatible** with furosemide. Compatibility is dependent upon factors such as pH, concentration, temperature, and diluent used; consult specialized references or a hospital pharmacist for more specific information.

Dosage Forms/Regulatory Status

VETERINARY-LABELED PRODUCTS: NONE.

HUMAN-LABELED PRODUCTS:

Vincristine Sulfate Injection: 1 mg/mL in 1 mL, 2 mL & 5 mL vials and flip-top vials; *Vincasar*® *PFS*, generic; (Rx)

Revisions/References

Monograph revised/updated August 2014.

Anon (2009). Problem Drugs, Veterinary Clinical Pharmacology Lab, College of Vet Med, Washington State University.

Argyle, D., et al. (2008). *Decision Making in Small Animal Oncology*, Wiley-Blackwell.

Balog, K., et al. (2013). A Prospective Randomized Clinical Trial of Vincristine versus Human Intravenous Immunoglobulin for Acute Adjunctive Management of Presumptive Primary Immune-Mediated Thrombocytopenia in Dogs. Journal of Veterinary Internal Medicine 27(3): 536-41.

Collicutt, N. B. & B. Garner (2013). Erythrocyte dysplasia in peripheral blood smears from 5 thrombocytopenic dogs treated with vincristine sulfate. Veterinary Clinical Pathology 42(4): 458-64.

Dobson, J. & D. Lascelles (2011). *BSAVA Manual of Canine and Feline Oncology*, BSAVA.

Henry, C. & M. Higginbotham (2009). *Cancer Management in Small Animal Practice*, Saunders.

Hughes, K., et al. (2009). Vincristine overdose in a cat: clinical management, use of calcium folinate, and pathological lesions. Journal of Feline Medicine and Surgery 11(4): 322-5.

Krick, E. L., et al. (2013). Prospective Clinical Trial to Compare Vincristine and Vinblastine in a COP-Based Protocol for Lymphoma in Cats. Journal of Veterinary Internal Medicine 27(1): 134-40.

Lind, D. L., et al. (2013). Evaluation of vincristine-associated myelosuppression in Border Collies. American Journal of Veterinary Research 74(2): 257-61.

Mair, T. S. & C. G. Couto (2006). The use of cytotoxic drugs in equine practice. Equine Veterinary Education 18(3): 149-56.

North, S. & T. Banks (2009). *Small Animal Oncology: An Introduction*, Saunders.

Papich, M. (1989). Effects of drugs on pregnancy. *Current Veterinary Therapy X: Small Animal Practice*. R. Kirk. Philadelphia, Saunders: 1291-9.

Polton, G. A. & C. M. Elwood (2008). Pulmonary oedema as a suspected adverse drug reaction following vincristine administration to a cat: A case report. Veterinary Journal 177(1): 130-3.

Teske, E., et al. (2014). Intraperitoneal antineoplastic drug delivery: experience with a cyclophosphamide, vincristine and prednisolone protocol in cats with malignant lymphoma. Veterinary and Comparative Oncology 12(1): 37-46.

Withrow, S., et al. (2012). Withrow and MacEwen's Small Animal Clinical Oncology, 5th Ed., Saunders.

Vitamin A

Vitamin (Retinoid)

Prescriber Highlights

▶ Potentially useful for adjunctive treatment of some types of dermatoses in dogs. Evidence is weak to support use, but usually tolerated well.

▶ Give with food; may require 1-2 months before efficacy can be noted.

▶ Keratoconjunctivitis or increased liver enzymes possible.

Uses/Indications

In dogs, although evidence supporting its use is weak, exogenously administered (non-dietary) vitamin A may be useful for treating vitamin-A responsive dermatosis in cocker spaniels and other breeds, sebaceous adenitis, primary idiopathic seborrhea, and other primary keratinization disorders. It also can be used to treat hypovitaminosis A in other species, including chelonians and birds.

One retrospective study (n=24) using oral vitamin A (mean dosage was 1037 Units/kg/day) for a minimum of 1 month to treat sebaceous adenitis has been published (Lam *et al.* 2011). All but 2 dogs also received other treatments including systemic antibiotics, systemic antifungal medications, fatty acid supplementation or various topical treatments. At follow-up, approximately half of the owners were satisfied with the overall appearance of their dogs, reporting ≥25% improvement in clinical signs, but almost a third of owners reported no improvement. Authors concluded that no correlations could be made with vitamin A dosage and response to treatment; prognoses could not be made based on clinical and histopathologic findings.

Pharmacology/Actions

Vitamin A (and its derivatives) is necessary for growth, bone and dental development, vision, reproduction, cortisol synthesis, and the integrity of mucosal and epithelial surfaces. Vitamin A is a co-factor in various biochemical reactions including mucopolysaccharide synthesis, cholesterol synthesis, and hydroxysteroid metabolism. In the retina, retinol combines with the rod pigment opsin to form rhodopsin, which is necessary for visual dark adaptation.

Pharmacokinetics

Orally administered vitamin A (except retinoic acid) must be converted to retinol by pancreatic and mucosal hydrolases before it is absorbed in the small intestine and re-esterified in mucosal cells. These retinyl esters (primarily retinyl palmitate) enter the systemic circulation via the lymphatics after they are bound by chylomicrons and are then cleared from the circulation and stored by the liver. Retinoic acid is directly absorbed unchanged and then transported into systemic circulation via albumin.

Contraindications/Precautions/Warnings

Exogenously administered vitamin A is contraindicated in patients known to be hypersensitive to it or in patients with hypervitaminosis A. Vitamin A dosages in excess of recommended daily requirements are contraindicated during pregnancy.

To avoid hypervitaminosis A, consider all sources of vitamin A (dietary, other supplements, topicals, etc.).

Adverse Effects

Dogs appear to tolerate oral vitamin A well. Potential adverse effects in dogs can include GI effects, erythema, pruritus, and behavioral changes. Chronic over supplementation can cause hypervitaminosis A exhibited by localized or generalized papules (firm center), poor coat quality, alopecia, scaling, excessive bleeding, liver disease, and keratoconjunctivitis sicca. Adverse effects generally resolve after drug discontinuation.

Cats appear to be susceptible to chronic vitamin A toxicity. A case report of hypervitaminosis A in a cat fed raw liver that developed hepatic fibrosis and stellate cell lipidosis has been published (Guerra *et al.* 2014).

Reproductive/Nursing Safety

Exogenously administered vitamin A is contraindicated in pregnancy. In humans, the FDA categorizes this drug as category X for use during pregnancy (*Studies in animals or humans demonstrate fetal abnormalities or adverse reaction; reports indicate evidence of fetal risk.*)

Safety to nursing offspring is not known but vitamin A requirements in dams increase while nursing.

Overdosage/Acute Toxicity

Data on acute toxicity from oral vitamin A in dogs or cats was not located. In humans, acute toxic effects can include: GI effects (nausea, vomiting), drowsiness, headache, and vertigo. In adults blurred vision has been reported and in infants, bulging fontanels. Toxic (one time) doses reported are: 100,000 Units per dose for infants and children <6 years old, and >1,000,000 Units per dose for adults. Chronic overdosing appears to hold the greater risk for dogs (and cats); refer to the Adverse Effects section for more information.

Drug Interactions

The following drug interactions have either been reported or are theoretical in humans or animals receiving vitamin A and may be of significance in veterinary patients. Unless otherwise noted, use together is not necessarily contraindicated, but weigh the potential risks and perform additional monitoring when appropriate.

- **ACITRETIN; ISOTRETINOIN:** Increased risk for vitamin A toxicity.
- **CLOPIDOGREL:** High doses of vitamin A may increase risk for bleeding.
- **HEPARIN:** High doses of vitamin A may increase risk for bleeding.
- **MINERAL OIL:** May reduce the amount of vitamin A absorbed from the gut. Separate dosages by at least two hours if using concomitantly.
- **WARFARIN:** High doses of vitamin A may increase risk for bleeding.

Laboratory Considerations

- No specific information noted.

Doses

Note: Dosages are not well defined and little evidence exists to support any dosage regimen.

- **DOGS:**

  For adjunctive treatment of canine sebaceous adenitis (extra-label): Initially, 8,000 – 10,000 Units per dog PO twice a day; can increase to 20,000 – 30,000 Units per dog PO twice a day (Simpson *et al.* 2012). From a retrospective study (n=24): doses varied from 380 – 2667 Units/kg/day PO (mean dosage was 1037 Units/kg/day for a minimum of 1 month (Lam *et al.* 2011).

  For vitamin A-responsive dermatosis and primary idiopathic seborrhea (extra-label): 625 – 800 Units/kg PO q24h or 10,000 – 50,000 Units per dog PO q24h with a fatty meal. It may take 4-8 weeks before any improvement can be seen. (Koch *et al.* 2011)

- **REPTILES:**

  For adjunctive treatment of hypovitaminosis A in chelonians (extra-label): In addition to adding carrots and cod liver oil to the diet, vitamin A injection at 2000 Units/kg IM can be given. (Ward 2013)

Monitoring

- Efficacy.
- Schirmer tear test (STT) if using long-term. Recommendation for frequency for rechecking STT varies; every 3 weeks to every 6-12 months have been suggested.
- Liver enzymes; baseline and every 6-12 months.
- Other adverse effects as they arise.

Client Information

- Give with food (meals), preferably one that is high in fat.
- May take 1-2 months before it causes any improvement in condition.
- Do not give more than veterinarian prescribes. Vitamin A can be toxic, especially if given for a long time and dosages are too high.
- Watch for dry eyes.

Chemistry/Synonyms

Vitamin A may consist of retinol or its esters formed from edible fatty acids, principally acetic and palmitic acids. In liquid form, vitamin A is a light yellow to red oil that may solidify upon refrigeration. In solid form, it takes on the appearance of any diluent that has been added. Vitamin A can be practically odorless or it may have a mild fishy odor (but no rancid odor or taste). It is unstable in air and light. In liquid form, vitamin A is insoluble in water or glycerol; soluble in dehydrated alcohol or vegetable oils. In solid form, vitamin A may be dispersible in water.

Sources of vitamin A can be via retinols or provitamins. Retinols include retinol, retinal, and retinoic acid, and are found in foods such as milk, meat or eggs. Provitamins are plant derived and include alpha-, beta- and gamma-carotene, which are converted to vitamin A in the body. Food processing, such as freezing may reduce the amount of vitamin A in foods.

Formerly, vitamin A recommended daily allowances (for humans; RDA) were expressed in units, but now units has been replaced by retinol activity equivalents (RAE) where 1 RAE = retinol 1 mcg, beta-carotene (from supplements) 0.2 mcg, beta-carotene (from food) 12 mcg, alpha-carotene 24 mcg, or beta-cryptoxanthin 24 mcg.

Vitamin A may also be known as axerophthol, oleovitamin A, retinol or retinyl palmitate.

Storage/Stability

Store oral products in tight, light-resistant containers away from heat. Store the injection between 2-8°C; do not freeze. Protect from air and light.

Compatibility/Compounding Considerations

No specific information noted.

Dosage Forms/Regulatory Status

VETERINARY-LABELED PRODUCTS:

A liquid drop formulation is labeled for use in dogs and cats (supplement; not an FDA-approved drug product): *Liquid A Drops*® contains Vitamin A (as palmitate) 2000 Units/drop; also contains olive oil; (OTC)

HUMAN-LABELED PRODUCTS:

Vitamin A Oral Capsules: 7,500 Units, 8,000 Units, 10,000 Units & 25,000 Units; generic; (OTC)

Vitamin A Palmitate (Retinyl Palmitate) for IM Injection; 50,000 Units/mL; *Aquasol-A*®; (Rx). **Note:** IV administration is contraindicated.

Revisions/References

Monograph written August 2014.
Guerra, J. M., et al. (2014). Hypervitaminosis A-induced hepatic fibrosis in a cat. Journal of Feline Medicine and Surgery 16(3): 243-8.
Koch, S., et al. (2011). *Small Animal Dermatology Drug Handbook*, Wiley-Blackwell. Ames.
Lam, A. T. H., et al. (2011). Oral vitamin A as an adjunct treatment for canine sebaceous adenitis. Veterinary Dermatology 22(4): 305-11.
Simpson, A. & L. McKay (2012). Applied Dermatology: Sebaceous Adenitis in Dogs. Compendium 34(10).
Ward, D. A. (2013). Reptile and amphibian ophthalmology. Proceedings: . accessed via Veterinary Information Network; vin.com

Vitamin E ± Selenium

(vye-ta-min-ee; se-lee-nee-um)   Alpha-tocopherol

Nutritional; Vitamin

Prescriber Highlights

▶ Vitamin E (alone) has been used for various skin-related conditions (immune-mediated; ischemic dermatopathies); as an adjunctive treatment for hepatopathies; and vitamin E deficiency states caused by dietary deficiency, pancreatitis or genetics.

▶ Vitamin E with selenium is used for the treatment or prophylaxis of selenium-tocopherol deficiency (STD) syndromes in ewes and lambs (white muscle disease), sows, weanling and baby pigs (hepatic necrosis, mulberry heart disease, white muscle disease), calves and breeding cows (white muscle disease), and horses (myositis associated with STD).

▶ Contraindications: Vitamin E/selenium products should only be used in the species for which they are FDA-approved.

▶ Vitamin E/Selenium adverse effects: Anaphylactoid reactions; IM injections may cause transient muscle soreness. Selenium OD's can cause depression, ataxia, dyspnea, blindness, diarrhea, muscle weakness, & a "garlic" odor on the breath. Selenium overdoses can be extremely toxic.

Uses/Indications

Vitamin E may be useful as adjunctive treatment of discoid lupus erythematosus, canine demodicosis, and acanthosis nigricans in dogs. A review article on canine ischemic dermatopathies states: "The mainstay for pharmacologic management of ischemic dermatopathies is pentoxifylline in combination with vitamin E." (Morris 2013). Vitamin E may also be of benefit in the adjunctive treatment of hepatic fibrosis or adjunctive therapy of copper-associated hepatopathy in dogs. There is some evidence that vitamin E and silymarin have synergistic effects on hepatocytes and a study in dogs found evidence that silymarin and vitamin E provided some efficacy for preventing gentamicin-induced nephrotoxicity (Varzi *et al.* 2007). However, with respect to using vitamin E for canine liver disease, an article reviewing the evidence states: "…vitamin E supplements have been recommended for dermatologic and hepatobiliary diseases (cholestatic and necro-inflammatory hepatopathies) in which antioxidant activity may be of benefit. However, no scientific data support their use for any of these indications." (Vandeweerd *et al.* 2013)

Supplemental vitamin E appears useful for treating retinal pigment epithelial dystrophy (RPED) with neuroaxonal degeneration in English Cocker Spaniels (and presumably other breeds) (McLellan *et al.* 2012).

A double blinded and randomized pilot study (n=8 in treatment group) in a canine experimental osteoarthritis model found some evidence that dogs treated with vitamin E (≈ 400 Units per dog PO per day) showed a reduction in inflammation joint markers and histological expression, as well as a trend to improving signs of pain (Rhouma *et al.* 2013).

Some dogs and cats with dilated cardiomyopathy have low vitamin E levels, but it is unknown if vitamin E supplementation has any clinical effect.

Depending on the actual product and species, vitamin E with selenium is indicated for the treatment or prophylaxis of selenium-tocopherol deficiency (STD) syndromes in ewes and lambs (white muscle disease), sows, weanling and baby pigs (hepatic necrosis, mulberry heart disease, white muscle disease), calves and breeding cows (white muscle disease), and horses (myositis associated with STD). A small, non-controlled study indicated that vitamin E plus selenium may be useful as adjunct therapy to a miticide (ivermectin) for treating canine sarcoptic mange (Behera *et al.* 2011).

Pharmacology/Actions

Both vitamin E and selenium are involved with cellular metabolism of sulfur. Vitamin E has antioxidant properties and with selenium, protects against red blood cell hemolysis and prevents the action of peroxidase on unsaturated bonds in cell membranes.

Pharmacokinetics

After absorption, vitamin E is transported in the circulatory system via beta-lipoproteins. Water-soluble (water-dispersible) oral forms appear to be more bioavailable. It is distributed to all tissues and stored in adipose tissue. Vitamin E is only marginally transported across the placenta. Vitamin E is metabolized in the liver and excreted primarily into the bile. Absorption of vitamin E may be impaired in patients with severe cholestatic liver disease or in animals with fat malabsorption syndromes.

Pharmacokinetic parameters for selenium were not located.

Contraindications/Precautions/Warnings

Vitamin E (alone) should be used with caution in patients with coagulation disorders.

Vitamin E/selenium products should only be used in the species for which they are FDA-approved. Because selenium can be extremely toxic, the promiscuous use of these products cannot be condoned. Give slowly when administering intravenously to horses.

Adverse Effects

Anaphylactoid reactions have been reported. Intramuscular injections may be associated with transient muscle soreness. Other adverse effects are generally associated with overdoses of selenium (see below).

Overdosage/Acute Toxicity

Very large overdoses of vitamin E can cause coagulopathies.

Selenium is quite toxic in overdose quantities, but has a fairly wide safety margin. Cattle have tolerated chronic doses of 0.6 mg/kg/day with no adverse effects (approximate therapeutic dose is 0.06 mg/kg). Clinical signs of selenium toxicity include depression, ataxia, dyspnea, blindness, diarrhea, muscle weakness, and a "garlic" odor on the breath. Horses suffering from selenium toxicity may become blind, paralyzed, slough their hooves, and lose hair from the tail and mane. Dogs may exhibit clinical signs of anorexia, vomiting, and diarrhea at high dosages.

Drug Interactions

The following drug interactions have either been reported or are theoretical in humans or animals receiving vitamin E/selenium and may be of significance in veterinary patients. Unless otherwise noted, use together is not necessarily contraindicated, but weigh the potential risks and perform additional monitoring when appropriate.

- **IRON:** Large doses of vitamin E may delay the hematologic response to iron therapy in patients with iron deficiency anemia.
- **MINERAL OIL:** May reduce the absorption of orally administered vitamin E.
- **VITAMIN A:** Absorption, utilization and storage may be enhanced by vitamin E.
- **WARFARIN:** Vitamin E may increase the effects of warfarin.

Doses

The following are for **Vitamin E alone**, for doses of vitamin E/selenium veterinary-labeled products see the Dosage Form section.

- **DOGS:**

  For ischemic dermatopathies (extra-label): Vitamin E: 200 Units—small breeds, 400 units—medium breeds, 600 Units—large breeds PO every 12 hours. The ideal oral dosage of vitamin E for maximum cutaneous protection has not been elucidated, but it has a wide margin of safety for oral supplementation. Used in combination with pentoxifylline (15 mg/kg PO q8h to 30 mg/kg PO q12h). (Morris 2013)

For adjunctive treatment of immune-mediated skin diseases (*e.g.*, **discoid lupus erythematosus, canine demodicosis or dermatomyositis**) (extra-label): Used anecdotally as no controlled studies support use. 200 – 800 Units per dog PO twice daily.

For adjunctive treatment of hepatopathies or as an antioxidant hepatoprotective (extra-label): Dosage is anecdotal. 50 – 600 Units per dog PO once daily. Some recommend water-soluble (water-dispersible) dosage forms as oral bioavailability may be higher.

For treatment of tocopherol deficiency associated with exocrine pancreatic disease (extra-label): 100 – 400 Units PO once daily for 1 month then every 1-2 weeks as needed. (Williams 2000)

For treatment of retinal pigment epithelial dystrophy (RPED) (extra-label): Vitamin E at 600 – 900 Units per dog PO twice daily. Study was done in English Cocker Spaniels without diets deficient in vitamin E. Authors concluded that this dosage, vitamin E is absorbed enough to restore plasma vitamin E concentrations to the normal range in most affected dogs. (McLellan *et al.* 2012)

- **CATS:**
  For pansteatitis (extra-label): 10 – 15 Units/kg PO once daily.

- **HORSES:**
  For vitamin E deficiency (extra-label): Natural-source water-dispersible forms of vitamin E (*e.g.*, *Elevate W.S.* or *Nano•E*) at 10 Units/kg PO (*assume per day—Plumb*) seem like the obvious choice for optimal treatment as they are 5-6X more bioavailable than synthetic vitamin E acetate, and a 5000 Unit dose per horse (*assume per day—Plumb*) more than doubles serum vitamin E levels within 12 hours. Before implementing supplementation it is important to measure serum alpha-tocopherol concentrations in order to determine if there is an underlying deficiency and to monitor the efficacy of supplementation. (Finno *et al.* 2013)

  For adjunctive treatment of neurologic disease (extra-label): There are many recommendations for using high levels of vitamin E supplementation for horses with neurologic disease, ranging from 1,500 – 23,000 Units per 500 kg horse per day. The use of vitamin E for these conditions is empirical based on a belief that it could be neuroprotective in disorders not related to a deficiency of vitamin E. At this time (2012), there is no scientific evidence that supplementation with doses of vitamin E above the 2007 NRC-recommended dose will have a therapeutic effect in horses other than those associated with a vitamin E deficiency. Many of these dosage recommendations exceed the NRC upper safety recommendation of 20 IU/kg (10,000 Units/500 kg horse). Furthermore, many of these studies were performed before the development of natural forms of vitamin E in horses and these amounts could well be excessive if natural vitamin E is used therapeutically. (Finno *et al.* 2012)

Monitoring
- Clinical efficacy.
- Blood selenium levels (when using the combination product). Normal values for selenium have been reported as: >1.14 micromol/L in calves, >0.63 micromol/L in cattle, >1.26 micromol/L in sheep, and >0.6 micromol/L in pigs. Values indicating deficiency are: <0.40 micromol/L in cattle, <0.60 micromol/L in sheep, and <0.20 micromol/L in pigs. Intermediate values may result in suboptimal production.
- Optionally, glutathione peroxidase activity may be monitored.

Client Information
- Vitamin E is used to treat some skin, liver and eye conditions and is very safe when given as directed.
- Very large overdoses can cause bleeding.
- If using the vitamin E and selenium injection, do not give more than veterinarian recommends; selenium can be very toxic if overdosed.

Chemistry/Synonyms
Vitamin E is a lipid soluble vitamin that can be found in either liquid or solid forms. The liquid forms occur as clear, yellow to brownish red, viscous oils that are insoluble in water, soluble in alcohol and miscible with vegetable oils. Solid forms occur as white to tan-white granular powders that disperse in water to form cloudy suspensions. Vitamin E may also be known as alpha tocopherol.

Selenium in commercially available veterinary injections is found as sodium selenite. Each mg of sodium selenite contains ≈ 460 micrograms (46%) of selenium.

Compatibility/Compounding Considerations
No specific information noted.

Storage/Stability
Vitamin E/Selenium for injection should be stored at temperatures less than 25°C (77°F).

Dosage Forms/Regulatory Status
VETERINARY-LABELED PRODUCTS:
Vitamin E Oral Liquid

Many products may be labeled for use in animals and as they are considered supplements and not drugs, they are not necessarily "FDA-approved animal drugs". Two labeled products mentioned in the horse dosages are: *Elevate* W.S. 500 IU/mL (Kentucky Performance Products) and *Nano•E* 250 IU/mL (KERx); (OTC)

Vitamin E (Alone) Injection

Vitamin E Injection: 300 mg/mL in 250 mL vials; *Emulsivit* E-300, *Vital E*-300; (OTC or Rx)

Vitamin E/Selenium Oral

Equ-SeE (Vet-A-Mix) ;(one teaspoonful [5 mL] contains 1 mg selenium and 220 Units vitamin E) and *Equ-Se5E* (one teaspoonful [5 mL] contains 1 mg selenium and approximately 1100 Units vitamin E); (OTC). FDA-approved for oral use in horses.

Other top dress equine products containing Vitamin E and Selenium include: Vitamin E and Selenium Powder, *Vitamin E and Selenium Crumbles*; (OTC)

Vitamin E/Selenium Injection

Mu-Se; (Rx): Each mL contains: selenium 5 mg (as sodium selenite); Vitamin E 68 Units; 100 mL vial for injection. FDA-approved for use in non-lactating dairy cattle and beef cattle. Slaughter withdrawal (at labeled doses) = 30 days. Dose: For weanling calves: 1 mL per 200 lbs. body weight IM or SC. For breeding beef cows: 1 mL per 200 lbs. body weight during middle third of pregnancy and 30 days before calving IM or SC.

Bo-Se; (Rx): Each mL contains selenium 1 mg (as sodium selenite) and Vitamin E 68 Units; 100 mL vial for injection. FDA-approved for use in calves, swine and sheep. Slaughter withdrawal (at labeled doses) = 30 days (calves); 14 days (lambs, ewes, sows, and pigs). Dose: Calves: 2.5 – 3.75 mL/100 lbs. body weight (depending on severity of condition and geographical area) IM or SC. Lambs (2 weeks of age or older): 1 mL per 40 lbs. body weight IM or SC (1 mL minimum). Ewes: 2.5 mL/100 lbs. body weight IM or SC. Sows and weanling pigs: 1mL/40 lbs. body weight IM or SC (1 mL minimum). Do not use on newborn pigs.

L-Se®; (Rx): Each mL contains: selenium 0.25 mg (as sodium selenite) and Vitamin E 68 Units in 30 mL vials. FDA-approved for use in lambs and baby pigs. Slaughter withdrawal (at labeled doses) = 14 days. Lamb dose: 1 mL SC or IM in newborns and 4 mL SC or IM in lambs 2 weeks of age or older; Baby Pigs: 1 mL SC or IM.

E-Se®; (Rx): Each mL contains selenium 2.5 mg (as sodium selenite) and Vitamin E 68 Units in 100 mL vials. FDA-approved for use in horses. Equine dose: 1 mL/100 lbs. body weight slow IV or deep IM (in 2 or more sites; gluteal or cervical muscles). May be repeated at 5-10 day intervals.

Seletoc®; (Rx): Each mL contains selenium 1 mg (as sodium selenite) and Vitamin E 68 Units in 10 mL vials. FDA-approved for use in dogs. <u>Dog Dose</u>: Initially, 1 mL per 20 pounds of body weight (minimum 0.25 mL; maximum 5 mL) SC, or IM in divided doses in 2 or more sites. Repeat dose at 3-day intervals until satisfactory results then switch to maintenance dose. If no response in 14 days reevaluate. <u>Maintenance dose</u>: 1 mL per 40 lbs. body weight (minimum 0.25 mL) repeat at 3-7 day intervals (or longer) to maintain.

HUMAN-LABELED PRODUCTS:

Vitamin E Tablets: 100 Units, 200 Units, 400 Units, 500 Units & 800 Units; generic; (OTC)

Vitamin E Capsules: 100 Units, 200 Units, 400 Units & 1000 Units; *Mixed E 400 Softgels*® & *d'ALPHA E 1000 Softgels*®, *Vita-Plus E*®, generic; (OTC)

Vitamin E Drops: 15 Units/0.3 mL in 12 mL & 30 mL; *Aquasol E*®, *Aquavit-E*®; (OTC)

Vitamin E Liquid: 15 Units/30 mL in 30 mL, 60 mL & 120 mL; 798 Units/30 mL in 473 mL; (OTC)

Topicals are available. There are no FDA-approved vitamin E/selenium products, but there are many products that contain either vitamin E (alone, or in combination with other vitamins ± minerals) or selenium (as an injection alone or in combination with other trace elements) available.

Revisions/References

Monograph revised/updated August 2014.

Behera, S. K., et al. (2011). The curative and antioxidative efficiency of ivermectin and ivermectin plus vitamin E-selenium treatment on canine Sarcoptes scabiei infestation. Veterinary Research Communications 35(4): 237-44.

Finno, C. J. & S. J. Valberg (2012). A Comparative Review of Vitamin E and Associated Equine Disorders. Journal of Veterinary Internal Medicine 26(6): 1251-66.

Finno, C. J., et al. (2013). Vitamin E Supplementation in Horses with Neurologic Disorders. Proceedings: ACVIM. accessed via Veterinary Information Network; vin.com

McLellan, G. J. & P. G. C. Bedford (2012). Oral vitamin E absorption in English Cocker Spaniels with familial vitamin E deficiency and retinal pigment epithelial dystrophy. Vet. Ophthalmol. 15: 48-56.

Morris, D. O. (2013). Ischemic Dermatopathies. Veterinary Clinics of North America-Small Animal Practice 43(1): 99-+.

Rhouma, M., et al. (2013). Anti-inflammatory response of dietary vitamin E and its effects on pain and joint structures during early stages of surgically induced osteoarthritis in dogs. Canadian Journal of Veterinary Research-Revue Canadienne De Recherche Veterinaire 77(3): 191-8.

Vandeweerd, J. M., et al. (2013). Nutraceuticals for Canine Liver Disease: Assessing the Evidence. Veterinary Clinics of North America-Small Animal Practice 43(5): 1171-+.

Varzi, H. N., et al. (2007). Effect of silymarin and vitamin E on gentamicin-induced nephrotoxicity in dogs. J. Vet. Pharmacol. Ther. 30(5): 477-81.

Williams, D. (2000). Exocrine Pancreatic Disease. Textbook of Veterinary Internal Medicine: Diseases of the Dog and Cat. S. Ettinger and E. Feldman. Philadelphia, WB Saunders. 2: 1345-67.

Voriconazole

(vor-ih-koh-nah-zohl)   Vfend®

Second Generation Triazole Antifungal

Prescriber Highlights

▶ Broad-spectrum oral/parenteral triazole antifungal.

▶ Very little clinical experience thus far in veterinary medicine.

▶ Cats appear to be susceptible to adverse effects. Until further pharmacokinetic and safety studies can be done, it should only used in cats as a last resort.

▶ Like other compounds in this class, there are many potential drug interactions.

Uses/Indications

Voriconazole may be a useful treatment for a variety of fungal infections in veterinary patients, particularly against *Blastomyces*, *Cryptococcus*, and *Aspergillus*. It has high oral bioavailability in a variety of species and can cross into the CNS. Little clinical experience has occurred using voriconazole in veterinary patients. Because of adverse effects in cats, it is generally only recommended as "a last resort". Expense of the human dosages forms has been a significant issue, but now that generics are becoming available, prices may decrease. There is considerable interest in using voriconazole for treating aspergillosis in pet birds as their relative small size may allow the drug to be affordable; additional research must be performed before dosing regimens are available.

Pharmacology/Actions

Voriconazole a synthetic derivative of fluconazole, has broad-spectrum antifungal activity against a variety of organisms, including *Candida*, *Aspergillus*, *Trichosporon*, *Histoplasma*, *Cryptococcus*, *Blastomyces*, and *Fusarium* species. Like the other azole/triazole antifungals it inhibits cytochrome P-450-dependent 14-alpha-sterol demethylase that is required for ergosterol biosynthesis in fungal cell walls. Unlike fluconazole, voriconazole also inhibits 24-methylene dehydrolanosterol demethylation in molds such as *Aspergillus* giving it more activity against these fungi.

Pharmacokinetics

In dogs, voriconazole is rapidly and essentially completely absorbed after oral administration. Peak levels occur ≈ 3 hours after oral dosing. Voriconazole is only moderately (51%) bound to canine plasma proteins and volume of distribution is ≈ 1.3 L/kg. It is metabolized in the liver to a variety of metabolites with the N-oxide metabolite being the primary circulating metabolite. This metabolite has only weak (<100X as active as the parent) antifungal activity. The elimination pharmacokinetics of voriconazole in dogs is very complex. Both dose-dependent non-linear elimination and auto-induced metabolism after multiple dosages are seen complicating any dosage regimen scenarios; dosages may need to be increased over time. Auto-induction of metabolism apparently does not occur in humans, rabbits or guinea pigs.

In horses, voriconazole is well absorbed after oral administration with peak levels occurring at ≈ 1-3 hours post-dose. Voriconazole has low protein binding (31%); volume of distribution is ≈ 1.35-1.6 L/kg. The drug is distributed into the CSF, tears and synovial fluid. Elimination half-life is quite long ≈ 13 hours after oral dosing. It is not known if voriconazole self-induces hepatic metabolism after multiple doses in the horse. (Davis *et al.* 2006; Colitz *et al.* 2007)

After single oral doses to alpacas, voriconazole had a low bioavailability (≈ 24%), but IV doses of 4 mg/kg yielded plasma levels above 0.1 micrograms/mL for at least 24 hours. Elimination half-life is ≈ 8 hours (Chan *et al.* 2009).

In Hispaniolan Amazon parrots, oral voriconazole had a short half-life (≈ 1 hour). The authors concluded that the drug could be safely administered to this species at a dose of 18 mg/kg PO q8h for 11 days, but that further studies were necessary to determine safety and efficacy of long-term treatment (Guzman *et al.* 2010).

Contraindications/Precautions/Warnings

Voriconazole is contraindicated in patients hypersensitive to it or other azole antifungals.

It should be used with extreme caution in cats as they appear to be very prone to serious adverse effects. Voriconazole should be given with caution to patients with hepatic dysfunction, or proarrhythmic conditions.

The intravenous product contains 3200 mg of sulfobutyl ether beta-cyclodextrin sodium (SBECD) per vial. This compound can accumulate in patients with decreased renal function.

Adverse Effects

Accurate adverse effect profiles are unknown for veterinary species. Liver enlargement and up to a 2-3 fold increase in cytochrome P450 hepatic microsomal enzyme concentrations were noted in dogs orally dosed for 30 days. This may significantly impact the metabolism of other drugs that are hepatically metabolized (See Drug Interactions). A dog treated with an IV infusion of voriconazole developed significant pyrexia and tachypnea after the infusion.

Cats appear to be very susceptible to developing adverse effects from voriconazole. Two cats initially treated with 10 mg/kg PO once daily developed significant adverse reactions, including azotemia, inappetence, lethargy, and weight loss. One developed a presumed cutaneous drug reaction which resolved when voriconazole was discontinued and the other cat developed ataxia and hind limb paresis (Smith *et al.* 2010). In another published case report (Quimby *et al.* 2010), three cats receiving voriconazole at doses from 10 – 13 mg/kg PO once daily developed neurologic signs that included: ataxia in all subjects; 2 of the 3 cats developed paraplegia of hind limbs, 2 of the 3 cats had visual signs (mydriasis, decreased or absent pupillary light responses, and reduced menace response). One cat developed an arrhythmia and in one cat, hypokalemia was noted.

In humans, commonly encountered adverse effects include visual disturbances (blurring, spots, wavy lines) usually within 30 minutes of dosing or if higher drug concentrations are attained, and rashes (usually mild to moderate in severity). Less frequent adverse effects include gastrointestinal effects (nausea, vomiting, diarrhea), hepatotoxicity (jaundice, abnormal liver function tests), hypertension/hypotension, tachycardia, peripheral edema, hypokalemia, and hypomagnesemia. Rarely, eye hemorrhage, anemia, leukopenia, thrombocytopenia, pancytopenia, QT prolongation, torsade de pointes, and nephrotoxicity have been reported.

Reproductive/Nursing Safety

Voriconazole was teratogenic in rats at low dosages (10 mg/kg) and embryotoxic in rabbits at higher dosages (100 mg/kg). In humans, the FDA categorizes voriconazole as category *D* for use during pregnancy (*There is evidence of human fetal risk, but the potential benefits from the use of the drug in pregnant women may be acceptable despite its potential risks.*) Weigh the risks of treatment versus the benefits when considering use in pregnant patients.

It is unknown if voriconazole enters milk.

Overdosage/Acute Toxicity

The minimum lethal dose in rats and mice was 300 mg/kg (4-7X maintenance dose). Toxic effects included increased salivation, mydriasis, ataxia, depression, dyspnea, and seizures. Accidental single overdoses of up to 5X in human pediatric patients caused only brief photophobia. No antidote is known for voriconazole overdoses. Gut emptying should be considered for very large oral

overdoses, followed by close observation and supportive treatment if required.

Drug Interactions

There are many potential drug interactions involving voriconazole. The following partial listing includes reported or theoretical interactions in humans receiving voriconazole that may also be of significance in veterinary patients. Because, in dogs, voriconazole induces hepatic microsomal enzymes (in humans it does not) additional interactions and further clarification may be reported as clinical use increases in veterinary patients. Unless otherwise noted, use together is not necessarily contraindicated, but weigh the potential risks and perform additional monitoring when appropriate.

- **ANTIDIABETIC AGENTS (sulfonylureas):** Voriconazole may increase serum concentrations of these drugs and increase risk for hypoglycemia.
- **BARBITURATES** (*e.g.,* **phenobarbital,** etc.): Decreased voriconazole concentrations; use together contraindicated.
- **BENZODIAZEPINES:** Voriconazole may increase benzodiazepine concentrations.
- **CALCIUM-CHANNEL BLOCKERS** (*e.g.,* **amlodipine, diltiazem, verapamil**): Voriconazole may increase serum concentrations, dosage adjustment may be required.
- **CARBAMAZEPINE:** Decreased voriconazole concentrations; use together contraindicated.
- **CISAPRIDE:** Potential for serious cardiac arrhythmias; use is contraindicated.
- **CORTICOSTEROIDS** (*e.g.,* **prednisolone,** etc.): Potentially increased AUC for prednisolone.
- **IMMUNOSUPPRESSIVE AGENTS (systemic: cyclosporine, tacrolimus):** Increased cyclosporine and tacrolimus concentrations; decrease cyclosporine dosage by 50% when starting voriconazole; decrease tacrolimus dosage by 33% when starting voriconazole.
- **METHADONE:** Voriconazole may increase plasma concentrations of R-methadone; monitor for methadone toxicity and adjust dosage if necessary.
- **PHENYTOIN:** Can decrease voriconazole concentrations and voriconazole can increase phenytoin concentrations; monitoring and dosage adjustment may be required.
- **PIMOZIDE:** Potential for serious cardiac arrhythmias; use is contraindicated.
- **PROTON-PUMP INHIBITORS** (*e.g.,* **omeprazole**): Voriconazole may increase omeprazole (and potentially other PPI's) concentrations.
- **QUINIDINE:** Potential for serious cardiac arrhythmias; use is contraindicated.
- **RIFAMPIN, RIFABUTIN:** Decreased voriconazole concentrations; use together contraindicated.
- **VINCA ALKALOIDS** (*e.g.,* **vincristine, vinblastine**): Possible increased Vinca alkaloid concentrations; monitor for toxicity.
- **WARFARIN:** Voriconazole may potentiate warfarin's effects.

Laboratory Considerations

- No specific concerns were noted; see Monitoring for additional information.

Doses

- **DOGS:**

  For coccidioidomycosis (extra-label): 4 mg/kg PO q12h. (Graupmann-Kuzma *et al.* 2008)

  For systemic aspergillosis (extra-label): 4 – 5 mg/kg PO q12h; appears to be useful. (Sykes 2012)

- **CATS:**

    For aspergillosis (extra-label): From a published case report in 3 cats: Two of the cats were treated with oral voriconazole for orbital aspergillosis initially at 10 mg/kg PO once daily. Both responded to treatment, but significant systemic reactions were noted. Authors concluded that based on their experience, voriconazole should be used with caution as adverse side effects may be common (Smith *et al.* 2010). **Note:** Other anecdotal dosage recommendations range from 5 – 12 mg/kg PO once daily, but most suggest it be used as "a last resort".

- **HORSES:**

    For susceptible, systemic fungal diseases (extra-label): Based upon pharmacokinetic studies, doses of 3 mg/kg PO q24h should be sufficient to treat aspergillosis, but higher doses (4 – 5 mg/kg) are probably necessary to treat infections with *Fusarium* spp. However, clinical experience is lacking, and the drug is currently too expensive for practical use (Davis 2008). **Note:** Generically labeled products are now available.

- **BIRDS:**

    a) Based upon this pharmacokinetic study in Hispaniolan Amazon parrots the authors concluded that the drug could be safely administered to this species at a dose of 18 mg/kg PO q8h for 11 days, but that further studies were necessary to determine safety and efficacy of long-term treatment (Guzman *et al.* 2010).

    b) **For avian aspergillosis:** 12.5 mg/kg PO twice daily for 60-90 days or by nebulization as a 1 mg/mL solution for 60 minutes once daily. (Black 2008)

Monitoring

- Efficacy.
- Liver function tests, serum electrolytes.

Client Information

- Give at least 1 hour before or 1 hour after feeding.
- Because experience with this medication has been limited, report any possible adverse effects to the veterinarian immediately, including itching/rash, yellowing of whites of the eyes, reduced appetite, difficulty walking, vision problems, etc.

Chemistry/Synonyms

A triazole antifungal, voriconazole occurs as a white to light colored powder with a molecular weight of 349.3. Aqueous solubility is 0.7 mg/mL.

Voriconazole may also be known as UK-109496, voriconazol, voraconazolum, or *Vfend*®.

Storage/Stability

Voriconazole tablets should be stored at 15-30°C.

The unreconstituted powder for oral suspension should be stored in the refrigerator (2-8°C); it has a shelf life of ≈ 18 months. Once reconstituted, it should be stored in tightly closed containers at room temperature (15-30°C); do not refrigerate or freeze. After reconstitution, the suspension is stable for 14 days. The suspension should be shaken well for 10 seconds prior to each administered dose.

The powder for injection should be stored at room temperature (15-30°C). After reconstituting with 19 mL of sterile water for injection, the manufacturer recommends using immediately; however, chemical and physical stability remain for up to 24 hours if stored in the refrigerator (2-8°C). Discard solution if it is not clear or particles are visible.

Compatibility/Compounding Considerations

The injectable solution must be further diluted to a concentration of 5mg/mL or less for administration over 1-2 hours. Suitable diluents for IV infusion include (partial list): NS, LRS, D5LRS, and D5W.

Voriconazole is **not compatible** with simultaneous infusion with blood products.

Voriconazole tablets can be crushed and made into a 2.5 mg/mL oral suspension by mixing a crushed tablet with 25:75 *v/v* water:-*OraPlus*®. This suspension will pass through a 10-French feeding needle. To prepare, mix a crushed 200 mg tablet with 20 mL water and then add 60 mL *OraPlus*®. The suspension should be thoroughly vortex-mixed or shaken until no particles are visible (usually takes 2-3 minutes) and then for ≈ 30-60 seconds before each use. The suspension is stable under refrigeration for 14 days. (Guzman *et al.* 2010), (Flammer 2008)

Dosage Forms/Regulatory Status

VETERINARY-LABELED PRODUCTS: NONE.

HUMAN-LABELED PRODUCTS:

Voriconazole Tablets: 50 mg & 200 mg; *Vfend*®, generic; (Rx)

Voriconazole Powder for Oral Suspension: 45 grams (40 mg/mL after reconstitution) in 100 mL bottles; *Vfend*®, generic; (Rx)

Voriconazole Powder for Injection, Lyophilized: 200 mg in single-use vials; *Vfend I.V.*®, generic; (Rx). Also contains 3200 mg of sulfobutyl ether beta-cyclodextrin sodium (SBECD) per vial (See Warnings) to solubolize the drug for IV administration.

Revisions/References

Monograph revised/updated August 2014.

Black, D. (2008). Avian Aspergillosis. Proceedings: UEP. accessed via Veterinary Information Network; vin.com

Chan, H. M., et al. (2009). Pharmacokinetics of voriconazole after single dose intravenous and oral administration to alpacas. J. Vet. Pharmacol. Ther. 32(3): 235-40.

Colitz, C. M. H., et al. (2007). Pharmacokinetics of voriconazole following intravenous and oral administration and body fluid concentrations of voriconazole following repeated oral administration in horses. American Journal of Veterinary Research 68(10): 1115-21.

Davis, J. (2008). The use of antifungals. Comp Equine(April): 128-33.

Davis, J. L., et al. (2006). Pharmacokinetics of voriconazole after oral and intravenous administration to horses. American Journal of Veterinary Research 67(6): 1070-5.

Flammer, K. (2008). Avian Mycoses: Managing those difficult cases. Proceedings: AAV. accessed via Veterinary Information Network; vin.com

Graupmann-Kuzma, A., et al. (2008). Coccidioidomycosis in dogs and cats: A review. J. Am. Anim. Hosp. Assoc. 44(5): 226-35.

Guzman, D. S. M., et al. (2010). Pharmacokinetics of voriconazole after oral administration of single and multiple doses in Hispaniolan Amazon parrots (Amazona ventralis). American Journal of Veterinary Research 71(4): 460-7.

Quimby, J. M., et al. (2010). Adverse Neurologic Events Associated with Voriconazole Use in 3 Cats. Journal of Veterinary Internal Medicine 24(3): 647-9.

Smith, L. N. & S. B. Hoffman (2010). A case series of unilateral orbital aspergillosis in three cats and treatment with voriconazole. Vet. Ophthalmol. 13(3): 190-203.

Sykes, J. E. (2012). Recent Advances in Diagnosis and Treatment of Fungal Pneumonia in Dogs and Cats. Proceedings: 22nd ECVIM-CA Congress. accessed via Veterinary Information Network; vin.com

Warfarin Sodium

(war-far-in)   Coumadin®

Anticoagulant

Prescriber Highlights

▶ Coumarin derivative anticoagulant used primarily for long-term thromboprophylaxis, primarily in dogs. Requires careful monitoring and dosage adjustment.

▶ Contraindications: Cats (?); current evidence does not support use as risks appear to outweigh benefits of therapy. Preexistent hemorrhage, pregnancy, those undergoing or contemplating eye or CNS surgery, major regional lumbar block anesthesia, surgery of large, open surfaces, active bleeding from the GI, respiratory, or GU tract; aneurysm, acute nephritis, cerebrovascular hemorrhage, blood dyscrasias, uncontrolled or malignant hypertension, hepatic insufficiency, pericardial effusion, & visceral carcinomas.

▶ Adverse Effects: Dose-related hemorrhage; death is possible.

▶ Teratogenic; contraindicated in pregnancy.

▶ Many potentially significant drug interactions.

Uses/Indications

In veterinary medicine, warfarin has been used primarily for the oral, long-term treatment (or prevention of recurrence) of thrombotic conditions, primarily in dogs. Use of warfarin in veterinary species is somewhat controversial, especially in cats, due to unproven benefit in reducing mortality, increased expense associated with monitoring, and potential for serious effects (bleeding), many do not recommend its use.

Pharmacology/Actions

Warfarin acts indirectly as an anticoagulant (it has no direct anticoagulant effect) by interfering with the action of vitamin K_1 in the synthesis of the coagulation factors II, VII, IX, and X. Sufficient amounts of vitamin K_1 can override this effect. Warfarin is administered as a racemic mixture of S (+) and R (-) warfarin. The S (+) enantiomer is a significantly more potent vitamin K antagonist than the R (-) enantiomer in species studied.

Pharmacokinetics

Warfarin is administered as a racemic mixture of S (+) and R (-) warfarin. Warfarin is rapidly and completely absorbed in humans after oral administration. In cats, warfarin is also rapidly absorbed after oral administration.

After absorption, warfarin is highly bound to plasma proteins in humans, with ≈ 99% of the drug bound. In cats, >96% of the drug is protein bound. It is reported that there are wide species variations with regard to protein binding; horses have a higher free (unbound) fraction of the drug than do rats, sheep or swine. Only free (unbound) warfarin is active. While other coumarin and indanedione anticoagulants are distributed in human milk, warfarin does not enter milk.

Warfarin is principally metabolized in the liver to inactive metabolites that are excreted in urine and bile (and then reabsorbed and excreted in the urine). The plasma half-life of warfarin may be several hours to several days depending on the patient (and species?). In cats, the terminal half-life of the S enantiomer is approximately 23-28 hours and the R enantiomer approximately 11-18 hours.

Contraindications/Precautions/Warnings

Warfarin is contraindicated in patients with preexistent hemorrhagic tendencies or diseases, those undergoing or contemplating eye or CNS surgery, major regional lumbar block anesthesia, or surgery of large, open surfaces. It should not be used in patients with active bleeding from the GI, respiratory, or GU tract. Other contraindications include: aneurysm, acute nephritis, cerebrovascular hemorrhage, blood dyscrasias, uncontrolled or malignant hypertension, hepatic insufficiency, pericardial effusion, pregnancy, and visceral carcinomas.

Use with extreme caution in cats. Most no longer recommend use in cats as evidence does not support use and any benefit does not outweigh the risks of treatment (Smith 2012).

Adverse Effects

The principal adverse effect of warfarin use is dose-related hemorrhage, which may manifest with clinical signs of anemia, thrombocytopenia, weakness, hematomas and ecchymoses, epistaxis, hematemesis, hematuria, melena, hematochezia, hemathrosis, hemothorax, intracranial and/or pericardial hemorrhage, and death.

Reproductive/Nursing Safety

Warfarin is embryotoxic, can cause congenital malformations and is considered contraindicated during pregnancy. If anticoagulant therapy is required during pregnancy, most clinicians recommend using low-dose heparin. In humans, the FDA categorizes this drug as category *X* for use during pregnancy (*Studies in animals or humans demonstrate fetal abnormalities or adverse reactions; reports indicate evidence of fetal risk. The risk of use in pregnant women clearly outweighs any possible benefit.*) In a separate system evaluating the safety of drugs in canine and feline pregnancy (Papich 1989), this drug is categorized as in class: *D* (*Contraindicated. These drugs have been shown to cause congenital malformations or embryotoxicity.*)

Based on very limited published data, warfarin has not been detected in the breast milk of humans treated, but there are reports of some breast-fed infants whose mothers were treated having prolonged prothrombin times. Use with caution in nursing patients.

Overdosage/Acute Toxicity

Acute overdosages of warfarin may result in life-threatening hemorrhage. In dogs and cats, single doses of 5 – 50 mg/kg have been associated with toxicity. It must be remembered that a lag time of 2-5 days may occur before signs of toxicity occur, and animals must be monitored and treated accordingly.

Cumulative toxic doses of warfarin have been reported as 1 – 5 mg/kg for 5-15 days in dogs and 1 mg/kg for 7 days in cats. There were 204 single agent exposures to warfarin reported to the ASPCA Animal Poison Control Center (APCC) during 2009-2013. Of the 193 dogs, 20 were symptomatic with lethargy (50%) being the most common clinical sign. Of the 9 cats, 4 were symptomatic with 50% having anorexia, hematuria, lethargy, and vomiting.

If overdosage is detected early, prevent absorption from the gut using standard protocols. If clinical signs are noted, they should be treated with blood products and vitamin K_1 (phytonadione). Refer to the phytonadione monograph for more information.

Drug Interactions

Drug interactions with warfarin are perhaps the most important in human medicine. The following drug interactions have either been reported or are theoretical in humans or animals receiving warfarin and may be of significance in veterinary patients. Unless otherwise noted, use together is not necessarily contraindicated, but weigh the potential risks and perform additional monitoring when appropriate.

A multitude of drugs have been documented or theorized to interact with warfarin. The following drugs or drug classes may **increase the anticoagulant response** of warfarin (not necessarily a complete list):

■ **ACETAMINOPHEN**

■ **ALLOPURINOL**

- AMIODARONE
- ANABOLIC STEROIDS
- AZITHROMYCIN
- CHLORAMPHENICOL
- CIMETIDINE
- CISAPRIDE
- CO-TRIMOXAZOLE (trimethoprim/sulfa)
- DANAZOL
- DIAZOXIDE
- ERYTHROMYCIN
- FISH OIL
- FLUOROQUINOLONES
- FLUOXETINE
- HEPARIN
- METRONIDAZOLE
- NSAIDS
- PENTOXIFYLLINE
- PROPYLTHIOURACIL
- QUINIDINE
- SALICYLATES
- SERTRALINE
- SULFONAMIDES
- THYROID MEDICATIONS
- ZAFIRLUKAST

The following drugs or drug classes may **decrease the anticoagulant response** of warfarin (not necessarily a complete list):

- BARBITURATES (**phenobarbital**, etc.)
- CORTICOSTEROIDS
- ESTROGENS
- GRISEOFULVIN
- MERCAPTOPURINE
- RIFAMPIN
- SPIRONOLACTONE
- SUCRALFATE
- VITAMIN K

Should concurrent use of any of the above drugs with warfarin be necessary, enhanced monitoring is required. Refer to other references on drug interactions for more specific information.

Laboratory Considerations

- Warfarin may cause falsely decreased **theophylline** values if using the Schack and Waxler ultraviolet method of assay.

Doses

- **DOGS:**

For thromboprophylaxis (extra-label): No studies have prospectively evaluated the effectiveness of any warfarin regimen in animals. Initial doses of 0.22 mg/kg have been suggested, but a retrospective study described an initial dose of 0.05 – 0.2 mg/kg PO q24h (once daily), with dosage adjusted (see Monitoring) to achieve an INR of 2-3. The two most important principles in adjusting warfarin were to keep the dose adjustments small and to make adjustments to the total weekly dose rather than the total daily dose. Adapted from: (Smith 2012; Winter *et al.* 2012)

- **CATS:**

For thromboprophylaxis (extra-label): A recent review of the subject states: "Cats at risk for ATE receiving warfarin experience similar or shorter survival times than those receiving other agents or no thromboprophylaxis. Adverse event rates were high, with up to 1 in 6 experiencing fatal hemorrhage. Given the lack of demonstrable improvement in long-term survival, the need and expense of close monitoring, and the risk of fatal hemor-

rhage, the use of warfarin in cats is difficult to justify." (Smith 2012), (Smith *et al.* 2003)

- **HORSES:** (NOTE: ARCI UCGFS CLASS 5 DRUG)

As an anticoagulant (extra-label): Rarely recommended today. An anecdotal dose for adjunctive treatment of laminitis has been noted: 0.0198 mg/kg PO once daily; monitor OSPT (one-step prothrombin time) until prolonged 2-4 seconds beyond baseline. (Brumbaugh *et al.* 1999)

Monitoring

Note: The frequency of monitoring is controversial, and dependent on several factors including dose, patient's condition, concomitant problems, etc. See the Dosage section above for more information.

- While Prothrombin Times (PT) or International Normalized Ratio [INR; not validated for veterinary patients (Smith 2012)] are most commonly used to monitor warfarin, PIVKA (proteins induced by vitamin K antagonists) has been suggested as being more sensitive. PT's are usually recommended to be 1.5-2X normal and INR's to be between 2-3 (Smith 2012). A retrospective study in dogs used INR to adjust dosage. In that study, some dogs required weekly or biweekly dose adjustments based on the calculated INR value for the first 2-4 weeks. Based on concurrent disease processes or concomitant drug therapy, it is recommended that dogs (sensitive to diet changes or concomitant medications) have an INR value checked at least every 3 months (Winter *et al.* 2012).
- Platelet counts and hematocrit (PCV) should be done periodically.
- Occult blood in stool and urine; other observations for bleeding.
- Clinical efficacy.

Client Information

- Many drugs and foods can interact with warfarin and can either increase the risk for bleeding or reduce warfarin's anticoagulant effects. Before starting a new drug, including OTC (over the counter; without a prescription) drugs, or stopping drugs that your animal is currently taking, talk with your veterinarian or pharmacist.
- Do not allow your animal to be in situations where it might be injured or cut as serious bleeding could occur. If abnormal bleeding is seen, contact your veterinarian immediately.
- To assure that the dosage is correct, routine blood tests will be needed..

Chemistry/Synonyms

A coumarin derivative, warfarin sodium occurs as a slightly bitter tasting, white, amorphous or crystalline powder. It is very soluble in water and freely soluble in alcohol. The commercially available products contain a racemic mixture of the two optical isomers.

Warfarin Sodium may also be known as: sodium warfarin, warfarinum natricum, *Coumadin*®, *Jantoven*®, or *Panwarfin*®; there are many other trade names internationally.

Storage/Stability

Warfarin sodium tablets should be stored in tight, light-resistant containers at temperatures < 40°C, preferably at room temperature.

Compatibility/Compounding Considerations

A method of suspending warfarin tablets in an oral suspension has been described (Enos 1989). To make 30 mL of a 0.25 mg/mL suspension: Crush three 2.5 mg tablets with a mortar and pestle. Add 10 mL glycerin to form a paste; then add 10 mL of water; add sufficient amount of dark corn syrup (*Karo*®) to obtain a final volume of 30 mL. Warm gently; shake well and use within 30 days.

Dosage Forms/Regulatory Status

VETERINARY-LABELED PRODUCTS: NONE.

The ARCI (Racing Commissioners International) has designated this drug as a class 5 substance. See the appendix for more information.

HUMAN-LABELED PRODUCTS:

Warfarin Sodium Oral Tablets (scored): 1 mg, 2 mg, 2.5 mg, 3 mg, 4 mg, 5 mg, 6 mg, 7.5 mg & 10 mg; *Coumadin®*, *Jantoven®*, generic; (Rx)

Revisions/References

Monograph revised/updated August 2014.

Brumbaugh, G., et al. (1999). The pharmacologic basis for the treatment of laminitis. The Veterinary Clinics of North America: Equine Practice 15:2(August).

Enos, L. R. (1989). Personal Communication.

Papich, M. (1989). Effects of drugs on pregnancy. *Current Veterinary Therapy X: Small Animal Practice.* R. Kirk. Philadelphia, Saunders: 1291-9.

Smith, S., et al. (2003). Arterial thromboembolism in cats: acute crisis in 127 cases (1992-2001) and long-term management with low-dose aspirin in 24 cases. J Vet Intern Med **17**: 73-83.

Smith, S. A. (2012). Antithrombotic Therapy. Topics in Companion Animal Medicine 27(2): 88-94.

Winter, R. L., et al. (2012). Aortic thrombosis in dogs: presentation, therapy, and outcome in 26 cases. Journal of veterinary cardiology : the official journal of the European Society of Veterinary Cardiology **14**(2).

Xylazine HCl

(zye-la-zeen)   Rompun®

Alpha2-Adrenergic Agonist

Prescriber Highlights

▶ Alpha2-adrenergic agonist used for its sedative & analgesic in a variety of species; used as an emetic in cats.

▶ **Contraindications:** Animals receiving epinephrine or having active ventricular arrhythmias. **Extreme caution:** preexisting cardiac dysfunction, hypotension or shock, respiratory dysfunction, severe hepatic or renal insufficiency, preexisting seizure disorders, or if severely debilitated. Should generally not be used in the last trimester of pregnancy, particularly in cattle. Do not give to ruminants that are debilitated, dehydrated, or with urinary tract obstruction. Horses may kick after a stimulatory event (usually auditory); use caution. Avoid intra-arterial injection; may cause severe seizures & collapse. Caution in patients treated for intestinal impactions. Use cautiously in horses during the vasoconstrictive development phase of laminitis.

▶ **Adverse Effects: Cats:** emesis, muscle tremors, bradycardia with partial A-V block, reduced respiratory rate, movement in response to sharp auditory stimuli, & increased urination.

▶ **Adverse Effects: Dogs:** Muscle tremors, bradycardia with partial A-V block, reduced respiratory rate, movement in response to sharp auditory stimuli, emesis, bloat from aerophagia which may require decompression.

▶ **Adverse Effects: Horses:** Muscle tremors, bradycardia with partial A-V block, reduced respiratory rate, movement in response to sharp auditory stimuli, sweating, increased intracranial pressure, decreased GI motility, decreased mucociliary clearance.

▶ **Adverse Effects: Cattle:** Salivation, ruminal atony, bloating, regurgitation, hypothermia, diarrhea, bradycardia, premature parturition, & ataxia.

▶ Yohimbine, atipamezole, & tolazoline may be used alone or in combination to reverse effects or speed recovery times.

▶ Dosages between species can be very different; be certain of product concentration when drawing up into syringe, especially if treating ruminants.

▶ Drug Interactions.

Uses/Indications

Xylazine is FDA-approved for use in dogs, cats, horses, deer, and elk. It is indicated in dogs, cats, and horses to produce a state of sedation with a shorter period of analgesia, and as a preanesthetic before local or general anesthesia. Xylazine is often used in combination with other agents (opioids, ketamine, guaifenesin, etc.) for inducing anesthesia or perioperative sedation and analgesia in horses.

Xylazine use in small animals is somewhat controversial and because it can cause arrhythmias, reduce cardiac output, and increase risk for general anesthesia-related death, it is usually reserved for "healthy animals". Today, most prefer using newer alpha₂-agonists (*e.g.*, dexmedetomidine, etc.) that have a better adverse effect profile in dogs and cats.

Because of the emetic action of xylazine in cats, xylazine is used to induce vomiting after ingesting toxins or drug overdoses.

Pharmacology/Actions

A potent alpha₂-adrenergic agonist, xylazine is classified as a sedative/analgesic with muscle relaxant properties. Although xylazine possesses several of the same pharmacologic actions as morphine, it does not cause CNS excitation in cats, horses or cattle, but causes sedation and CNS depression. In horses, the visceral analgesia produced has been demonstrated to be superior to that produced by meperidine, butorphanol or pentazocine.

Xylazine can also have alpha₁-agonist activity and is less selective for alpha₂-receptors then detomidine, dexmedetomidine or romifidine.

Xylazine causes skeletal muscle relaxation through central mediated pathways. Emesis is often seen in cats, and occasionally in dogs receiving xylazine. While thought to be centrally mediated, neither dopaminergic blockers (*e.g.*, phenothiazines) nor alpha-blockers (*e.g.*, yohimbine, tolazoline) block the emetic effect. Xylazine does not cause emesis in horses, cattle, sheep or goats. Xylazine depresses thermoregulatory mechanisms and either hypo- or hyperthermia is a possibility depending on ambient air temperatures.

Effects on the cardiovascular system include an initial increase in total peripheral resistance with increased blood pressure followed by a longer period of lowered blood pressures (below baseline). A bradycardic effect can be seen with some animals developing a second-degree heart block or other arrhythmias. An overall decrease in cardiac output of up to 30% may be seen. Xylazine has been demonstrated to enhance the arrhythmogenic effects of epinephrine in dogs with or without concurrent halothane.

Xylazine's effects on respiratory function are usually clinically insignificant, but at high dosages it can cause respiratory depression with decreased tidal volumes and respiratory rates, and an overall decreased minute volume. Brachycephalic dogs and horses with upper airway disease may develop dyspnea.

Xylazine can increase blood glucose secondary to decreased serum levels of insulin; in non-diabetic animals, there appears to be little clinical significance associated with this effect.

In horses, sedatory signs include a lowering of the head with relaxed facial muscles and drooping of the lower lip. The retractor muscle is relaxed in male horses, but unlike acepromazine, no reports of permanent penile paralysis have been reported. Although, the animal may appear to be thoroughly sedated, auditory stimuli may provoke arousal with kicking and avoidance responses.

With regard to the sensitivity of species to xylazine, definite differences are seen. Ruminants are extremely sensitive to xylazine when compared with horses, dogs, or cats. Ruminants generally require ≈ 10% of the dosage that is required for horses to exhibit the same effect. In cattle (and occasionally cats and horses), polyuria is seen following xylazine administration, probably because of decreased production of vasopressin (antidiuretic hormone, ADH). Bradycardia and hypersalivation are also seen in cattle and diminished by pretreating with atropine. Because swine require 20-30X the ruminant dose, it is not routinely used.

Pharmacokinetics

Absorption is rapid following IM injection, but bioavailabilities are incomplete and variable. Bioavailabilities of 40-48% in horses, 17-73% in sheep, and 52-90% in dogs have been reported after IM administration.

In horses, the onset of action following IV dosage occurs within 1-2 minutes with a maximum effect 3-10 minutes after injection. The duration of effect is dose dependent but may last for ≈ 1.5 hours. The serum half-life after a single dose of xylazine is ≈ 50 minutes in the horse; recovery times generally take from 2-3 hours.

In dogs and cats, the onset of action following an IM or SC dose is ≈ 10-15 minutes, and 3-5 minutes following an IV dose. The analgesic effects may persist for only 15-30 minutes, but the sedative actions may last for 1-2 hours depending on the dose given. The serum half-live of xylazine in dogs has been reported as averaging 30 minutes. Complete recovery after dosing may take 2-4 hours in dogs and cats.

Xylazine is not detected in milk of lactating dairy cattle at 5 and 21 hours post-dose, but the FDA has not approved its use in dairy cattle and no meat or milk withdrawal times have been specified.

Contraindications/Precautions/Warnings

Xylazine is contraindicated in animals receiving epinephrine or having active ventricular arrhythmias. It should be used with extreme caution in animals with preexisting cardiac dysfunction, hypotension or shock, respiratory dysfunction, severe hepatic or renal insufficiency, preexisting seizure disorders, or if severely debilitated. Because it may induce premature parturition, it should generally not be used in the last trimester of pregnancy, particularly in cattle.

Be certain of product concentration when drawing up into syringe, especially if treating ruminants. Do not give to ruminants that are dehydrated, debilitated, or with urinary tract obstruction. It is not FDA-approved for any species to be consumed for food purposes.

Even though horses may appear sedated after xylazine, they have been known to kick after a stimulatory event (usually auditory); use caution. The addition of opioids (e.g., butorphanol) may help temper this effect, but may cause increased risks for hypotension or ileus development. Avoid intra-arterial injection; may cause severe seizures and collapse. The manufacturers warn against using xylazine in conjunction with other tranquilizers. Because this drug may inhibit gastrointestinal motility, use with caution in patients treated for intestinal impactions. Use cautiously in horses during the vasoconstrictive development phase of laminitis as xylazine has been shown to reduce digital flow of blood for about 8 hours after administration.

Adverse Effects

Emesis is generally seen within 3-5 minutes after xylazine administration in cats and occasionally in dogs. To prevent aspiration, do not induce further anesthesia until this time has lapsed. Other adverse effects listed in the package insert (*Gemini*®) for dogs and cats include: muscle tremors, bradycardia with partial A-V block, reduced respiratory rate, movement in response to sharp auditory stimuli, and increased urination in cats.

Xylazine can reduce tear production in cats and cause diuresis in dogs.

Dogs may develop bloat from aerophagia that may require decompression. Because of gaseous distention of the stomach, xylazine's use before radiography can make test interpretation difficult.

Adverse effects listed in the package insert (*AnaSed*®) for horses include: muscle tremors, bradycardia with partial A-V block, reduced respiratory rate, movement in response to sharp auditory stimuli, and sweating (rarely profuse). Additionally, horses receiving xylazine may develop transient hypertension, increased urine production, decreased gastric emptying, decreased motility of duodenum, jejunum and pelvic flexure, increased intrauterine pressure/contractions, and reduced mucociliary clearance rates.

Adverse reactions reported in cattle include: salivation, ruminal atony, bloating and regurgitation, hypothermia, diarrhea, and bradycardia. Hypersalivation and bradycardia may be alleviated by pretreating with atropine.

Large animals may become ataxic following dosing and caution should be observed.

Reproductive/Nursing Safety

Limited information was located on the safety of xylazine in pregnancy; apparently, there are no reports of teratogenicity in animals. Xylazine may induce premature parturition in cattle. For horses, one review concludes: "…alpha-2 agonists are safe in pregnant animals, but close monitoring is advised." (Valverde 2010)

Xylazine does not appear to be excreted in detectable quantities in cows' milk.

Overdosage/Acute Toxicity

In the event of an accidental overdosage, cardiac arrhythmias, hypotension, and profound CNS and respiratory depression may occur. Seizures have also been reported after overdoses. There has been much interest in using alpha-blocking agents as antidotes or reversal agents to xylazine. Yohimbine, atipamezole, and tolazoline have been suggested for use alone and in combination to reverse the effects of xylazine or speed recovery times. Refer to the monographs for atipamezole, tolazoline and yohimbine for more information.

To treat the respiratory depressant effects of xylazine toxicity, mechanical respiratory support with respiratory stimulants (*e.g.,* doxapram) have been recommended for use.

Drug Interactions

The manufacturers warn against using xylazine in conjunction with **other tranquilizers**. The following drug interactions have either been reported or are theoretical in humans or animals receiving xylazine and may be of significance in veterinary patients. Unless otherwise noted, use together is not necessarily contraindicated, but weigh the potential risks and perform additional monitoring when appropriate.

- **ACEPROMAZINE:** The combination use of acepromazine with xylazine is generally considered safe, but there is potential for additive hypotensive effects and this combination should be used cautiously in animals susceptible to hemodynamic complications.
- **CHLORAMPHENICOL:** Prolonged sedation and gastrointestinal stasis possible (Davis 2007).
- **CNS DEPRESSANT AGENTS, OTHER** (*e.g.,* **barbiturates, narcotics, anesthetics, phenothiazines,** etc.): May cause additive CNS depression if used with xylazine. Dosages of these agents may need to be reduced.
- **EPINEPHRINE:** The use of epinephrine with or without the concurrent use of halothane with xylazine may induce the development of ventricular arrhythmias.
- **RESERPINE:** A case of a horse developing colic-like clinical signs after reserpine and xylazine has been reported. Until more is known about this potential interaction, use of these two agents together should be avoided.

Doses

- **DOGS:**

  Note: Today, most prefer using newer alpha-2 agonists (*e.g.*, dexmedetomidine, etc.) that have a better adverse effect profile in dogs and cats.

  Labeled dose (FDA-approved): 1.1 mg/kg IV, 1.1 – 2.2 mg/kg IM or SC (Package Insert; *Rompun*®) **Note:** Many believe the labeled dosage is too high.

  As a preanesthetic (extra-label): Dosage range for xylazine 0.2 – 1 mg/kg IV, IM or SC is very broad, and dosages on the label are relatively high. Xylazine has depressant, sedative, analgesic, and muscle relaxing effects. It is very effective for restraint and analgesia, but does not produce immobilization and sedated animals can respond to noxious stimuli and noise. Xylazine is associated with significant cardiac rhythm disturbances when dosed according to the recommendations on the label, especially in dogs. In low doses, the benefits of xylazine can be realized while eliminating some of its detrimental side effects. (Hartsfield 2007)

  As an analgesic adjunct (extra-label): 0.05 – 0.5 mg/kg IV, IM or SC.

- **CATS:**

  Note: Except for its use as an emetic, most prefer using newer alpha-2 agonists (*e.g.*. dexmedetomidine, etc.) that have a better adverse effect profile in dogs and cats.

  Labeled Dose (FDA-approved): 1.1 mg/kg IV, 1.1 – 2.2 mg/kg IM or SC (Package Insert; *Rompun*®) **Note:** Many believe the labeled dosage is too high.

  As an emetic (extra-label):

  a) 1.1 mg/kg IM or SC. Side effects include CNS-mediated respiratory depression, bradycardia, and hypotension. Will not work with toxicants that target the CRTZ. To reverse adverse effects after emesis: Tolazoline (0.5 – 1 mg/kg IV) or yohimbine (0.1 mg/kg IV) can be considered. Tolazoline may be superior to yohimbine in the cat. (Talcott 2012)

  b) 0.44 mg/kg IM; reverse with yohimbine after emesis. (Lee 2013)

  As a preanesthetic (extra-label dose): Dosage range for xylazine 0.2 – 1 mg/kg IV, IM or SC is very broad, and dosages on the label are relatively high. Xylazine has depressant, sedative, analgesic, and muscle relaxing effects. It is very effective for restraint and analgesia, but does not produce immobilization and sedated animals can respond to noxious stimuli and noise. Xylazine is associated with significant cardiac rhythm disturbances when dosed according to the recommendations on the label, especially in dogs. In low doses, the benefits of xylazine can be realized while eliminating some of its detrimental side effects. (Hartsfield 2007)

  As an analgesic adjunct (extra-label): 0.05 – 0.5 mg/kg IV, IM or SC.

- **HORSES:** (NOTE: ARCI UCGFS CLASS 3 DRUG)

  Labeled Dose (FDA-approved) to produce a state of sedation with a shorter period of analgesia, and as a preanesthetic before local or general anesthesia: 1.1 mg/kg IV; 2.2 mg/kg IM. Allow animal to rest quietly until full effect is reached. (Package Insert; *Rompun*®)

  Extra-label Doses

  Note: There are a plethora of protocols published for use of xylazine in combination with other agents for equine anesthesia. A survey published in 2010 of American Association of Equine Practitioners (AAEP) found that the preferred agents for an induction protocol for short-term anesthesia (20 minutes or less) was xylazine administered as a sedative first and then followed by ketamine and diazepam. However, other alpha-2 agonists (detomidine, romifidine, etc.) or benzodiazepines (*e.g.*, midazolam) have been substituted. For longer procedures requiring anesthesia (>30 minute duration) protocols using guaifenesin, ketamine and xylazine (GKX), or isoflurane were used most commonly. The following are some examples of published protocols. A thorough discussion of balanced anesthesia, partial and total intravenous anesthesia for horses can be found in Vet Clin Equine 29 (2013) 89-122 (Valverde 2013), Vet Clin Equine 29 (2013) 123-129 (Lerche 2013) or other equine anesthesia references. The following are some examples of published recommended dosages and protocols:

  a) **For standing sedation and analgesia:** Full dose is 1 mg/kg IV; for intraoperative use IV dose is usually lower than the full dose or a CRI can be used. CRI dosages reported range from 2.1 – 4.2 mg/kg/hour. Epidural dosages range from 0.17 – 0.25 mg/kg (Valverde 2010). Alternately, 0.5 – 1.1 mg/kg IV (onset of peak action in 2-5 minutes; duration ≈ 30 minutes); 1 – 2 mg/kg IM (onset of peak action in 15 minutes; duration ≈ 30 minutes). For prolonged procedures: 0.5 mg/kg IV followed by a CRI of 0.65 mg/kg/hour (Michou *et al.* 2012).

  b) **For field anesthesia:** (extra-label): Sedate with xylazine (1 mg/kg IV; 2 mg/kg IM) given 5-10 minutes (longer for IM route) before induction of anesthesia with ketamine (2 mg/kg IV). Horse must be adequately sedated (head to the knees) before giving the ketamine (ketamine can cause muscle rigidity and seizures). If adequate sedation does not occur, either: **1)** Re-dose xylazine: up to half the original dose; or **2)** Add butorphanol (0.02 – 0.04 mg/kg IV). Butorphanol can be given with the original xylazine if you suspect that the horse will be difficult to tranquilize (*e.g.*, high-strung Thoroughbreds) or added before the ketamine. This combination will improve induction, increase analgesia and increase recumbency time by ≈ 5-10 minutes; or **3)** give diazepam (0.03 mg/kg IV). Mix the diazepam with the ketamine. This combination will improve induction when sedation is marginal, improve muscle relaxation during anesthesia and prolong anesthesia by ≈ 5-10 minutes; or **4)** Guaifenesin (5% solution administered IV to effect) can also be used to increase sedation and muscle relaxation. (Mathews 1999)

  c) **As part of induction protocols** (extra-label): **Note:** Must be used with caution; not recommended for field anesthesia.

  For normal healthy patients: Administer xylazine (0.44 – 0.66 mg/kg IV, or 200 – 300 mg/450 kg horse). Wait for sedation and muscle relaxation to occur (≈ 5 minutes). Guaifenesin (5% solution, or 50 mg/mL) is then rapidly infused using pressurization until marked sedation and muscle relaxation is achieved (generally a total dose of 30 – 50 mg/kg). Ketamine (2.2 mg/kg IV, 1000 mg/450 kg) should be administered at a point that allows for its slow onset to occur without the patient becoming excessively weak and collapsing from the effects of guaifenesin. Recumbency generally occurs ≈ 60 seconds following ketamine administration. The slow administration of guaifenesin described below can also be used in normal healthy patients in place of a supplemental dose of xylazine when the level of initial sedation is inadequate.

  For compromised patients: Try to use a very modest dose of xylazine (0.22 – 0.44 mg/kg IV, or 100 – 200 mg/450 kg horse) depending on status and demeanor to minimize its cardiovascular effects in compromised patients. Slow administration of guaifenesin (5% solution) can be used to gradually create the desired level of sedation. It is still important to allow adequate time for centralization of cardiac output to progress sufficiently prior to initiating the rapid phase of guaifenesin administration that precedes the induction bolus. Guaifenesin has a slow onset of action, when used to augment the level of pre-induction sedation. SLOW administration is important to avoid creating an overly weak and ataxic patient while waiting for centralization to progress sufficiently. Guaifenesin is then rapidly infused using pressurization until marked sedation and muscle relaxation is achieved (generally a total dose of 30 – 50 mg/kg IV). Ketamine (dose decreases as degree of compromise increases, 1.34 – 1.55 mg/kg IV, or 600 – 700 mg/450 kg) for extremely compromised patients should be administered at a point that allows for its slow onset to occur without the patient becoming excessively weak and collapsing from the growing effects of guaifenesin. Experience may be required to get the timing right. Recumbency takes even longer (up to a couple minutes) when ketamine dose is reduced in compromised patients. (Abrahamsen 2007)

d) **For long-term IV (>30 minutes) anesthesia using "GKX" or "triple-drip"** (extra-label): Guaifenesin (50 mg/mL), ketamine (1 – 2 mg/mL; 2 mg/mL concentration used for more painful or noxious procedures), and xylazine (0.5 mg/mL). Most practitioners prefer to induce with xylazine/ketamine or xylazine/diazepam/ketamine and then use GKX for maintenance. Typically the CRI runs at 1.5 – 2.2 mL/kg/hour depending on the procedure, patient response and ketamine concentration. (Wagner 2009)

- **CATTLE:**

Caution: Cattle are extremely sensitive to xylazine's effects; be certain of dose and dosage form. Use only the 20 mg/mL solution. Pretreatment with atropine can decrease bradycardia and hypersalivation. **Note:** Xylazine is approved for use in several countries, but not in the USA. Withdrawal times vary depending on labeling in each country. In the USA, when xylazine is used in an extra-label manner, FARAD recommends a meat withdrawal interval of 4 days and a milk withdrawal interval of 24 hours following xylazine administration in cattle. If xylazine sedation is reversed using tolazoline, both the meat and milk withdrawal intervals need to be increased (8 days meat; 48 hours milk); if yohimbine is used to reverse, meat withdrawal interval is 7 days and milk withdrawal interval is 72 hours. (Smith 2013)

For chemical restraint and injectable anesthesia (extra-label): The reader is encouraged to refer to the in depth review by (Abrahamsen 2013) where detailed discussions on the use of alpha-2 agonists alone and in combination with other anesthetic adjuncts (*e.g.,* "ketamine stun", etc.) for both standing and recumbent procedures can be found. An example of a combination (ketamine stun") from another reference follows: **For analgesia and restraint for standing procedures in cattle** (extra-label): A protocol for use of IM butorphanol/xylazine/ketamine (BXK; "ketamine stun") has been reported. It consists of butorphanol (0.01 – 0.025 mg/kg) + xylazine (0.02 – 0.05 mg/kg) + ketamine (0.04 – 0.1 mg/kg). For a 450 kg animal, 5 mg butorphanol, 10 mg xylazine, and 20 mg ketamine would constitute the low end of the dosing range. Up to an hour of cooperation was accomplished using this protocol, but more fractious patients may require increased doses. Suggested to give no more than 10 mg butorphanol or 20 mg of xylazine for the initial dose to an animal greater than 450 kg. (Coetzee 2010)

For standing sedation (extra-label): The following xylazine doses would be expected to produce standing sedation with a low incidence of recumbency for facilitating short diagnostic or therapeutic procedures. Patients will generally tolerate mildly uncomfortable stimuli, but these dosages should not be counted on to provide significant analgesia. Duration of effect generally lasts about 30-40 minutes.

Patient Type	IV	IM
Quiet Dairy Breeds	0.0075 – 0.01 mg/kg	0.015 – 0.02 mg/kg
Tractable Cattle	0.01 – 0.02 mg/kg	0.02 – 0.04 mg/kg
Anxious Cattle	0.02 – 0.03 mg/kg	0.04 – 0.06 mg/kg
Extremely Anxious or Unruly Cattle	0.025 – 0.05 mg/kg	0.05 – 0.1 mg/kg

Note: IV dosages given IM further reduces the chance for recumbency. (Abrahamsen 2013)

For sedation/analgesia: 0.1 – 0.3 mg/kg IM; 0.05 – 0.15 mg/kg IV; 0.05 – 0.07 mg/kg epidurally. When used IV/IM, analgesia can be very short-lived (1/2 hour). (Walz 2006)

- **SHEEP & GOATS:**

Note: Use xylazine with extreme caution in these species. Use only the 20 mg/mL solution. Consider using the FARAD meat and milk withdrawal recommendations for cattle when used in an extra-label manner. More information using xylazine as part of drug combinations for injectable sedation, anesthesia/analgesia protocols can be found in the following references: (Abrahamsen 2013), (Galatos 2011).

For light, standing sedation (extra-label): 0.01 mg/kg IV for light standing sedation to 0.2 mg/kg IM for recumbency of an hour's duration. Goats are bit more sensitive than sheep. When beginning to use these drugs, it is advisable to start with a conservative dose until one develops a feel for level of sedation provided. A reversal agent should always be on hand; reversal of sedative effects also reverses analgesic effects. (Snyder 2009)

- **CAMELIDS (NWC):**

Note: Use xylazine with extreme caution in these species. Use only the 20 mg/mL solution.

For procedural pain (*e.g.,* castrations) when recumbency (up to 30 minutes) is desired: Alpacas: butorphanol 0.046 mg/kg; xylazine 0.46 mg/kg; ketamine 4.6 mg/kg. Llamas: butorphanol 0.037 mg/kg; xylazine 0.37 mg/kg; ketamine 3.7 mg/kg. All drugs are combined in one syringe and given IM. May administer 50% of original dose of ketamine and xylazine during anesthesia to prolong effect up to 15 minutes. If doing mass castrations on 3 or more animals, can make up bottle of the "cocktail". Add 10 mg (1 mL) of butorphanol and 100 mg (1 mL) xylazine to a 1 gram (10 mL vial) of ketamine. This mixture is dosed at 1 mL/40 lbs. (18 kg) for alpacas, and 1 mL/50 lbs. (22 kg) for llamas. Handle quietly and allow plenty of time before starting procedure. Expect 20 minutes of surgical time; patient should stand 45-60 minutes after injection. (Miesner 2009)

As a sedative/analgesic with *Telazol®* (extra-label): Study was done in adult male llamas. Authors concluded that tiletamine-zolazepam alone (2 mg/kg IM) is only suitable for immobilization for non-painful procedures. Concurrent IM administration of xylazine at a dose of 0.2 or 0.4 mg/kg significantly increased the duration of antinociception induced by tiletamine-zolazepam, and there was a dose-dependent response for the antinociceptive effect of xylazine. Transient hypoxemia was associated with xylazine administration, but the authors did not consider this to be clinically important in healthy llamas. (Seddighi *et al.* 2013)

- **RABBITS, RODENTS, SMALL MAMMALS:**

As a sedative/analgesic (extra-label):

Rabbits: 1) Ketamine 35 mg/kg + xylazine 5 mg/kg IM; surgical anesthesia for 20-30 min, good relaxation, sleep time is 60-120 min, some effects reversible with atipamezole. 2) Ketamine 25 mg/kg + xylazine 5 mg/kg + butorphanol 0.1 mg/kg IM; surgical anesthesia for 60-90 min, good relaxation, sleep time is 120-180 min. 3) Ketamine 25 mg/kg + xylazine 5 mg/kg + acepromazine 1 mg/kg IM; surgical anesthesia for 45-75 min, good relaxation, sleep time is 100-150 min.

Gerbils: Ketamine 50 mg/kg + xylazine 2 mg/kg IP;

Guinea Pigs: Ketamine 40 mg/kg + xylazine 5 mg/kg IP;

Hamsters: Ketamine 200 mg/kg + xylazine 10 mg/kg IP;

Mice: Ketamine 80 mg/kg + xylazine 10 mg/kg IP;

Rats: Ketamine 75 mg/kg + xylazine 10 mg/kg IP.

Atipamezole 1 mg/kg SC, IM, IO or IV can be used to reverse xylazine. (Flecknell 2008)

- **FERRETS:**

  As a sedative/analgesic (extra-label):

  a) Xylazine: 0.5 – 2 mg/kg IM or SC. Usually combined with atropine (0.05 mg/kg) or glycopyrrolate (0.01 mg/kg IM); or butorphanol (0.2 mg/kg) plus xylazine (2 mg/kg) IM. (Finkler 1999)

  b) Xylazine (2 mg/kg) plus butorphanol (0.2 mg/kg) IM; *Telazol®* (1.5 mg/kg) plus xylazine (1.5 mg/kg) IM; may reverse xylazine with yohimbine (0.05 mg/kg IM); *Telazol®* (1.5 mg/kg) plus xylazine (1.5 mg/kg) plus butorphanol (0.2 mg/kg) IM; may reverse xylazine with yohimbine (0.05 mg/kg IM). (Williams 2000)

- **BIRDS:**

  As a sedative/analgesic (extra-label):

  a) 1 – 4 mg/kg IM; provides sedation for ketamine anesthesia. Has been used at dosages of up to 10 mg/kg in small psittacines. (Clyde *et al.* 2000)

  b) In combination with ketamine: Ketamine 10 – 30 mg/kg IM; Xylazine 2 – 6 mg/kg IM; birds <250 grams require a higher dosage (per kg) than birds weighing >250 g. Xylazine is not recommended for use in debilitated birds because of its cardiodepressant effects. (Wheler 1993)

- **ZOO, EXOTIC, WILDLIFE SPECIES:**

  For use in zoo, exotic and wildlife medicine refer to specific references, including:

  a) *Zoo Animal and Wildlife Immobilization and Anesthesia.* West, G., Heard, D., Caulkett, N. (eds.). Blackwell Publishing, 2007.

  b) Handbook of Wildlife Chemical Immobilization, 3rd Ed. Kreeger, T.J. and J.M. Arnemo. 2007.

  c) Fowler's Zoo and Wild Animal Medicine Current Therapy, Volume 7, Miller, R.E., Fowler, M.E., Saunders. 2011.

  d) *Exotic Animal Formulary, 4th Ed.* Carpenter, J.W., Saunders. 2012.

  e) The 2009 American Association of Zoo Veterinarian Proceedings by D. K. Fontenot also has several dosages listed for restraint, anesthesia, and analgesia for a variety of drugs for carnivores and primates. VIN members can access them at: http://goo.gl/NNIWQ or http://goo.gl/9UJse

Monitoring

- Level of anesthesia/analgesia.
- Respiratory function; cardiovascular status (rate, rhythm, BP if possible).
- Hydration status if polyuria present.

Client Information

- Xylazine should only be used by individuals familiar with its use.

Chemistry/Synonyms

Xylazine HCl is an alpha$_2$-adrenergic agonist structurally related to clonidine. The pH of the commercially prepared injections is ≈ 5.5. Dosages and bottle concentrations are expressed in terms of the base.

Xylazine HCl may also be known as Bay-Va-1470, *Rompun®*, *AnaSed®*, *Sedazine®*, *X-Ject®*, or *Xyla-Ject®*.

Storage/Stability

Do not store above 30°C (86°F).

Compatibility/Compounding Considerations

Xylazine is reportedly physically **compatible** in the same syringe with several compounds, including: acepromazine, buprenorphine, butorphanol, chloral hydrate, and meperidine.

A study (Taylor *et al.* 2009) evaluating the stability, sterility, pH, particulate formation and efficacy in laboratory rodents of compounded ketamine, acepromazine and xylazine ("KAX") supported the finding that the drugs are stable and efficacious for at least 180 days after mixing if stored at room temperature in the dark.

Dosage Forms/Regulatory Status
VETERINARY-LABELED PRODUCTS:

Xylazine Injection: 20 mg/mL in 20 mL vials or 100 mg/mL in 50 mL vials: *Rompun®*, *AnaSed®*, *Cervizine®* (300 mg/mL; for deer and elk), *Sedazine®*, *Chanazine®*, generic; (Rx). FDA-approved for use (depending on strength and product) in dogs, cats, horses, deer, and elk.

While xylazine is not FDA-approved for use in cattle in the USA, at labeled doses in Canada it reportedly has been assigned withdrawal times of 3 days for meat and 48 hours for milk. FARAD has reportedly suggested a withdrawal of 7 days for meat and 72 hours for milk for extra-label use.

The ARCI (Racing Commissioners International) has designated this drug as a class 3 substance. See the appendix for more information.

HUMAN-LABELED PRODUCTS: NONE.

Revisions/References

Monograph revised/updated August 2014.

Abrahamsen, E. (2007). Analgesia in equine practice. Proceedings: Western Vet Conference. accessed via Veterinary Information Network; vin.com

Abrahamsen, E. J. (2013). Chemical Restraint and Injectable Anesthesia of Ruminants. Veterinary Clinics of North America-Food Animal Practice 29(1): 209-+.

Clyde, V. & J. Paul-Murphy (2000). Avian Analgesia. *Kirk's Current Veterinary Therapy: XIII Small Animal Practice.* J. Bonagura. Philadelphia, WB Saunders: 1126-8.

Coetzee, H. (2010). How Do We Manage Pain in Cattle Effectively? Proceedings: WVC. accessed via Veterinary Information Network; vin.com

Davis, J. (2007). Potential Drug Interactions: What Every Technician Should Know. Proceedings: IVECCS. accessed via Veterinary Information Network; vin.com

Finkler, M. (1999). Anesthesia in Ferrets. Proceedings: Central Veterinary Conference, Kansas City. accessed via Veterinary Information Network; vin.com

Flecknell, P. (2008). Anaesthesia of Rodents, Rabbits and Ferrets. Proceedings: WVC. accessed via Veterinary Information Network; vin.com

Galatos, A. D. (2011). Anesthesia and Analgesia in Sheep and Goats. Veterinary Clinics of North America-Food Animal Practice 27(1): 47-+.

Hartsfield, S. (2007). Preanesthetic Drugs in Small Animal Anesthesia. Proceedings: ACVC. accessed via Veterinary Information Network; vin.com

Lee, J. A. (2013). Emergency Management and Treatment of the Poisoned Small Animal Patient. Veterinary Clinics of North America: Small Animal Practice 43(4): 757-71.

Lerche, P. (2013). Total Intravenous Anesthesia in Horses. Veterinary Clinics of North America-Equine Practice 29(1): 123-+.

Mathews, N. (1999). Anesthesia in large animals— Injectable (field) anesthesia: How to make it better. Proceedings: Central Veterinary Conference, Kansas City. accessed via Veterinary Information Network; vin.com

Michou, J. & E. Leece (2012). Sedation and analgesia in the standing horse 1. Drugs used for sedation and systemic analgesia. In Practice 34(9): 524-31.

Miesner, M. (2009). Field anesthesia techniques in camelids. Proceedings: WVC. accessed via Veterinary Information Network; vin.com

Seddighi, R., et al. (2013). Physiologic and antinociceptive effects following intramuscular administration of xylazine hydrochloride in combination with tiletamine-zolazepam in llamas. American Journal of Veterinary Research 74(4): 530-4.

Smith, G. (2013). Extralabel Use of Anesthetic and Analgesic Compounds in Cattle. Veterinary Clinics of North America-Food Animal Practice 29(1): 29-+.

Snyder, J. (2009). Anesthesia and pain management: Minor surgeries. Proceedings: WVC. accessed via Veterinary Information Network; vin.com

Talcott, P. A. (2012). Decontamination Procedures in Poisoned Companion Animals - Facts & Fiction. Western Veterinary Conference. accessed via Veterinary Information Network; vin.com

Taylor, B. J., et al. (2009). Beyond-Use Dating of Extemporaneously Compounded Ketamine, Acepromazine, and Xylazine: Safety, Stability, and Efficacy over Time. Journal of the American Association for Laboratory Animal Science 48(6): 718-26.

Valverde, A. (2010). Alpha-2 Agonists as Pain Therapy in Horses. Vet Clin Equine 26: 515-32.

Valverde, A. (2013). Balanced Anesthesia and Constant-Rate Infusions in Horses. Veterinary Clinics of North America-Equine Practice 29(1): 89-+.

Wagner, A. E. (2009). Injectable Field Anaesthesia in the Horse. Proceedings: AVA. accessed via Veterinary Information Network; vin.com

Walz, P. (2006). Practical management of pain in cattle. Proceedings: ABVP. accessed via Veterinary Information Network; vin.com

Wheler, C. (1993). Avian anesthetics, analgesics, and tranquilizers. Seminars in Avian & Exotic Med 2(1): 7-12.

Williams, B. (2000). Therapeutics in Ferrets. Vet Clin NA: Exotic Anim Pract 3:1(Jan): 131-53.

Yohimbine HCl

(yo-him-been)   Yobine®, Antagonil®

Alpha₂-Adrenergic Antagonist

Prescriber Highlights

► Alpha₂-adrenergic antagonist used to reverse xylazine, other alpha₂ agonists & potentially amitraz; may be used prophylactically before amitraz dips.

► Caution: Renal disease, seizure disorders. Possible that reversal effects will diminish before the agonist's effects dissipate.

► Adverse Effects: Transient apprehension or CNS excitement, muscle tremors, salivation, increased respiratory rates, & hyperemic mucous membranes; more likely in small animals and horses.

► Drug interactions.

Uses/Indications

Yohimbine is indicated to reverse the effects of xylazine in dogs, but it is being used clinically for other alpha₂ agonists and in several other species as well.

Yohimbine may be efficacious in reversing some of the toxic effects associated with other agents (*e.g.*, amitraz) and can be used prophylactically before amitraz dips.

Pharmacology/Actions

Yohimbine is an alpha₂-adrenergic antagonist that can antagonize the effects of xylazine and other alpha₂-adrenergic agonists. Alone, yohimbine increases heart rate, blood pressure, causes CNS stimulation and antidiuresis, and has hyperinsulinemic effects. A study in cats found that yohimbine can antagonize medetomidine-induced diuresis in healthy cats (Murahata *et al.* 2014).

A study in horses that received IV detomidine (0.03 mg/kg) followed 15 minutes later by IV yohimbine (0.2 mg/kg) found that yohimbine rapidly reversed the sedative effects of detomidine, effectively returned heart rate and the percent of atrio-ventricular conduction disturbances to pre-detomidine values, and effectively reduced detomidine-induced hyperglycemia (Knych *et al.* 2012b). Another study in horses after they received SL detomidine, showed yohimbine's (0.075 mg/kg IV) effects on detomidine-induced changes in chin-to-ground distance were minimal and effects on detomidine-induced changes in heart rate and rhythm only persisted for 15-20 minutes (Knych *et al.* 2014).

By blocking central alpha₂-receptors, yohimbine causes sympathetic outflow (norepinephrine) to be enhanced. Peripheral alpha₂-receptors are also found in the cardiovascular system, genitourinary system, GI tract, platelets, and adipose tissue.

Pharmacokinetics

When 0.12 mg/kg IV was administered to horses, a study found (using 2 compartment analysis) a large volume of distribution (mean 3.2 L/kg), a low clearance (mean 13.6 mL/kg/min) and long elimination half-life (4.4 hours). A separate study from the same group, using IV doses of 0.1, 0.2, and 0.4 mg/kg IV, reported similar results (DiMaio Knych *et al.* 2011b).

A study reported the pharmacokinetics yohimbine in steers and dogs (Jernigan et al. 1988). The apparent volume of distribution (steady-state) is ≈ 5 L/kg in steers and 4.5 L/kg in dogs. The total body clearance is ≈ 70 mL/min/kg in steers and 30 mL/min/kg in dogs. The half-life of the drug is ≈ 0.5-1 hours in steers and 1.5-2 hours in dogs.

Yohimbine is believed to penetrate the CNS quite readily and, when used to reverse the effects of xylazine, onset of action generally occurs within 3 minutes.

The metabolic fate of the drug is not fully understood, but in humans 90% of the drug is metabolized in the liver primarily by hydroxylation. In horses, at least 2 metabolites were detected in a pharmacokinetic study, both of which appeared to be hydroxylated metabolites (DiMaio Knych *et al.* 2011a). Whether any metabolites have activity is not known, but in humans there have been reports that the major metabolite, 11-hydroxy yohimbine may have pharmacologic activity.

Contraindications/Precautions/Warnings

Yohimbine is contraindicated in patients hypersensitive to it. In humans, yohimbine is contraindicated in patients with renal disease.

Yohimbine should be used cautiously in patients with seizure disorders. When used to reverse the effects xylazine, normal pain perception may result.

Yohimbine's alpha₂-adrenergic antagonist effects may diminish before the agonist's effects dissipate.

Prolonged withdrawal periods for horses in athletic events may be necessary. A pharmacokinetics study found in horses, yohimbine had a long half-life and they were able to detect the main metabolite, hydroxy-yohimbine in urine samples for as long as 96 hours post administration (DiMaio Knych *et al.* 2011a).

Adverse Effects

Yohimbine may cause transient apprehension or CNS excitement, muscle tremors, salivation, increased respiratory rates, and hyperemic mucous membranes. Adverse effects appear to be more probable in small animals and horses.

An *in vitro* study found that yohimbine inhibited collagen-induced aggregation of bovine and equine platelets (Yokota *et al.* 2013). Clinical significance is not known.

Reproductive/Nursing Safety

Safe use of yohimbine in pregnant animals has not been established. No information on safety during lactation was located.

Overdosage/Acute Toxicity

Dogs receiving 0.55 mg/kg (5X recommended dose) exhibited clinical signs of transient seizures and muscle tremors.

There were only 7 single agent exposures to yohimbine reported to the ASPCA Animal Poison Control Center (APCC) during 2009-2013. Yohimbine is commonly found in combination with other stimulants in over-the-counter medications. The most common signs are hyperactivity, tachycardia, anxiety, diarrhea, hind limb weakness, hyperthermia, injected sclera, and vocalization.

For more information on clinical effects and treatment for yohimbine toxicity see: (Volmer *et al.* 1994)

Drug Interactions

Little information is available, use with caution with **other alpha$_2$-adrenergic antagonists** or **other drugs that can cause CNS stimulation.**

- **DETOMIDINE:** In horses, a study found that giving yohimbine after prior administration of detomidine caused yohimbine clearance and volume of distribution to decrease with resultant increases in yohimbine peak plasma levels. The authors concluded that this increases the potential for untoward effects and warrants further study into the physiologic effects of this combination of drugs (Knych *et al.* 2012a).
- **TRICYCLIC ANTIDEPRESSANTS:** In humans, yohimbine is not recommended for use with antidepressants or other mood-altering agents; hypertension has been reported with tricyclics.

Doses

- **DOGS:**

  For alpha$_2$-adrenergic agonist (xylazine) reversal (labeled dose; FDA approved): For xylazine: 0.11 mg/kg IV slowly. (Package insert; *Yobine*®)

  For reversal or prevention of amitraz toxicity (extra-label): In cases of toxicity or to prevent a dog from having an acute episode of toxicity associated with demodicosis treatment: Yohimbine at 0.11 mg/kg IV or 0.25 mg/kg IM with atipamezole (50 micrograms/kg IM). (Torres 2007)

- **CATS:**

  As an antiemetic after xylazine-induced emesis (extra-label): Yohimbine at 0.1 mg/kg IV may reverse side effects. (Talcott 2012), (DeClementi *et al.* 2012)

- **RABBITS, RODENTS, SMALL MAMMALS:**

  To reverse the effects of xylazine and to partially antagonize the effects of ketamine and acepromazine (extra-label): **Rabbits:** 0.2 mg/kg IV as needed. **Mice/Rats:** 0.2 mg/kg IP as needed. (Huerkamp 1995)

- **BIRDS:**

  As a reversal agent for alpha$_2$-adrenergic agonists (*e.g.*, xylazine): 0.1 mg/kg IV. (Clyde *et al.* 2000)

- **CATTLE:**

  For alpha$_2$-adrenergic agonist (xylazine) reversal (extra-label): Yohimbine at a maximum dose of 0.125 mg/kg IM (or tolazoline) may be used to reverse the effects of xylazine to facilitate a quicker recovery at the end of a procedure and minimize the risks of gastrointestinal complications. The dose is reduced from the maximum to fit the circumstances. IM administration of the reversal agent is preferred in all but emergency situations as it decreases the risk of CNS excitement or cardiovascular complications. The amount of reversal agent used depends on the dose and time elapsed after administrating xylazine. Reversal of xylazine should not be attempted until sufficient time has elapsed (30-45 min. post IM and 15-30 min. post-IV administration) to allow ketamine or *Telazol*® used to reduce the chances of a rough recovery. When dosed properly the effects of reversal should start to become evident ≈ 10 minutes following IM administration. Emergency doses of yohimbine at 0.1 – 0.125 mg/kg can be administered IV, but the shorter duration of action when given IV can result in the return of the effects of IM administered xylazine. Adapted from: (Anderson *et al.* 2008), (Abrahamsen 2013)

- **HORSES:** (NOTE: ARCI UCGFS CLASS 2 DRUG)

  For alpha$_2$-adrenergic agonist reversal (extra-label): The less specific alpha-2 agonists— xylazine, detomidine, and romifidine—are typically reversed using yohimbine at 0.05 – 0.2 mg/kg administered IM or slowly IV (Brosnan 2013). A study where yohimbine was given at 0.2 mg/kg IV 15 minutes after IV detomidine, found that it effectively reversed detomidine-induced sedation, bradycardia, atrioventricular heart block and hyperglycemia (Knych *et al.* 2012b).

- **LLAMAS:**

  For xylazine reversal (extra-label): 0.25 mg/kg IV or IM. (Fowler 1989)

- **ZOO, EXOTIC, WILDLIFE SPECIES:**

  For use in zoo, exotic and wildlife medicine refer to specific references, including:

  a) *Zoo Animal and Wildlife Immobilization and Anesthesia.* West, G., Heard, D., Caulkett, N. (eds.). Blackwell Publishing, 2007.

  b) Handbook of Wildlife Chemical Immobilization, 3rd Ed. Kreeger, T.J. and J.M. Arnemo. 2007.

  c) Fowler's Zoo and Wild Animal Medicine Current Therapy, Volume 7, Miller, R.E., Fowler, M.E., Saunders. 2011.

  d) *Exotic Animal Formulary, 4th Ed.* Carpenter, J.W., Saunders. 2012.

  e) The 2009 American Association of Zoo Veterinarian Proceedings by D. K. Fontenot also has several dosages listed for restraint, anesthesia, and analgesia for a variety of drugs for carnivores and primates. VIN members can access them at: http://goo.gl/NNIWQ or http://goo.gl/9UJse

Monitoring

- CNS status (arousal level, etc.).
- Cardiac rate; rhythm (if indicated), blood pressure (if indicated and practical).
- Respiratory rate.

Client Information

- This agent should be used with direct professional supervision only.

Chemistry/Synonyms

A Rauwolfia or indolealkylamine alkaloid, yohimbine HCl has a molecular weight of 390.9. It is chemically related to reserpine.

Yohimbine may also be known as: aphrodine hydrochloride, chlorhydrate de quebrachine, corynine hydrochloride, *Aphrodyne*®, *Dayto Himbin*®, *Pluriviron mono*®, *Prowess Plain*®, *Urobine*®, *Virigen*®, *Yobine*®, *Yocon*®, *Yocoral*®, *Yohimex*®, *Yohydrol, Yomax*®, or *Zumba*®.

Storage/Stability

Yohimbine injection should be stored at room temperature (15-30°C) and protected from light and heat.

Compatibility/Compounding Considerations

No specific information noted.

Dosage Forms/Regulatory Status

VETERINARY-LABELED PRODUCTS:

Yohimbine Sterile Solution for Injection: 2 mg/mL in 20 mL vials; *Yobine*®; (Rx). FDA-approved for use in dogs.

HUMAN-LABELED PRODUCTS:

Oral 5.4 mg tablets are available, but would unlikely to be of veterinary benefit.

Revisions/References

Monograph revised/updated August 2014.

Abrahamsen, E. J. (2013). Chemical Restraint and Injectable Anesthesia of Ruminants. Veterinary Clinics of North America-Food Animal Practice 29(1): 209-+.

Anderson, D. & E. Abrahamsen (2008). Chemical Restraint in the Field--New Uses For Old Drugs. Proceedings: World Vet Congress. accessed via Veterinary Information Network; vin.com

Brosnan, R. J. (2013). Waking Up Is Hard To Do: Improving Anesthetic Recovery in Horses. Proceedings: Western Veterinary Conference. accessed via Veterinary Information Network; vin.com

Clyde, V. & J. Paul-Murphy (2000). Avian Analgesia. *Kirk's Current Veterinary Therapy: XIII Small Animal Practice.* J. Bonagura. Philadelphia, WB Saunders: 1126-8.

DeClementi, C. & B. R. Sobczak (2012). Common Rodenticide Toxicoses in Small Animals. Veterinary Clinics of North America-Small Animal Practice 42(2): 349-+.

DiMaio Knych, H. K., et al. (2011a). Pharmacokinetics of yohimbine following intravenous administration to horses. J. Vet. Pharmacol. Ther. 34(1): 58-63.

DiMaio Knych, H. K., et al. (2011b). Pharmacokinetics and pharmacodynamics of three intravenous doses of yohimbine in the horse. J. Vet. Pharmacol. Ther. 34(4): 359-66.

Fowler, M. E. (1989). *Medicine and Surgery of South American Camelids*, Iowa State University Press. Ames.

Huerkamp, M. (1995). Anesthesia and postoperative management of rabbits and pocket pets. *Kirk's Current Veterinary Therapy:XII*. J. Bonagura. Philadelphia, W.B. Saunders: 1322-7.

Knych, H. K. & S. D. Stanley (2014). Effects of three antagonists on selected pharmacodynamic effects of sublingually administered detomidine in the horse. Veterinary Anaesthesia and Analgesia 41(1): 36-47.

Knych, H. K., et al. (2012a). The effects of yohimbine on the pharmacokinetic parameters of detomidine in the horse. Veterinary Anaesthesia and Analgesia 39(3): 221-9.

Knych, H. K. D., et al. (2012b). Effect of yohimbine on detomidine induced changes in behavior, cardiac and blood parameters in the horse. Veterinary Anaesthesia and Analgesia 39(6): 574-83.

Murahata, Y., et al. (2014). Antagonistic Effects of Atipamezole, Yohimbine and Prazosin on Medetomidine-Induced Diuresis in Healthy Cats. Journal of Veterinary Medical Science 76(2): 173-82.

Talcott, P. A. (2012). Decontamination Procedures in Poisoned Companion Animals - Facts & Fiction. Western Veterinary Conference. accessed via Veterinary Information Network; vin.com

Torres, S. (2007). Diagnosis and treatment of canine and feline demodicosis. Proceedings: Western Vet Conf. accessed via Veterinary Information Network; vin.com

Volmer, P. A., et al. (1994). Acute Oral Yohimbine Toxicosis in a Dog. Canine Practice 19(2): 18-9.

Yokota, S., et al. (2013). Effects of imidazoline and nonimidazoline alpha-adrenergic agents, including xylazine, medetomidine, yohimbine, tolazoline, and atipamezole, on aggregation of bovine and equine platelets. American Journal of Veterinary Research 74(3): 395-402.

Zafirlukast

(zah-fur-luh-kast)   Accolate®

Leukotriene-Receptor Antagonist

Prescriber Highlights

▶ Leukotriene-receptor antagonist; potentially useful for canine atopic dermatitis, feline asthma, or inflammatory bowel disease, but efficacy has either been disappointing or not well studied in veterinary patients.

▶ Not for treatment of acute bronchospasm. Dose on an empty stomach.

▶ Well tolerated.

Uses/Indications

While zafirlukast potentially could be useful for treating a variety of conditions (*e.g.,* feline asthma, atopic dermatitis, inflammatory bowel disease) where leukotrienes are thought to contribute to morbidity, to date, efficacy has been shown to be disappointing, limited, or not fully studied. Zafirlukast failed to reduce airway eosinophilia or hyper-responsiveness in experimental feline asthma (Reinero *et al.* 2005). A study using zafirlukast to evaluate effects on pruritus (owner subjective evaluation) in dogs with atopic dermatitis, showed that only 11% of treated dogs had at least 50% reductions in pruritus (Senter *et al.* 2002).

Pharmacology/Actions

Zafirlukast selectively and competitively inhibits leukotriene receptors, specifically receptors for leukotriene D_4 and E_4 (LTD$_4$ and LTE$_4$). Additionally, it competes for receptors with some components of slow-reacting substance of anaphylaxis (SRS-A). These substances have all been implicated in the inflammatory and bronchoconstrictive aspects of bronchial asthma.

Pharmacokinetics

No specific veterinary data was located. In humans, zafirlukast is rapidly absorbed after oral administration. Food may impair the absorption of the drug, therefore, give on an empty stomach. Peak plasma levels occur ≈ 3 hours after dosing. Zafirlukast is highly bound to plasma proteins (>99%). The drug is extensively metab-

olized; <10% of a dose is excreted in the urine, the rest in the feces. Half lives in humans average ≈ 10 hours.

Contraindications/Precautions/Warnings

Zafirlukast is contraindicated in patients hypersensitive to it.

Zafirlukast is not indicated for, and is ineffective for treating bronchospasm associated with acute asthma attacks.

Patients with significantly decreased hepatic function may have reduced clearances (and increased plasma levels) of zafirlukast.

Adverse Effects

Veterinary experience is very limited, but some dogs reportedly have vomited after oral dosing. In humans, the adverse effect profile seems to be minimal; headache was noted most often, but incidence is not much different than placebo.

Reproductive/Nursing Safety

In humans, the FDA categorizes this drug as category *B* for use during pregnancy (*Animal studies have not yet demonstrated risk to the fetus, but there are no adequate studies in pregnant women; or animal studies have shown an adverse effect, but adequate studies in pregnant women have not demonstrated a risk to the fetus in the first trimester of pregnancy, and there is no evidence of risk in later trimesters.*)

Zafirlukast is excreted in milk, but it is probably safe to administer to nursing veterinary patients.

Overdosage/Acute Toxicity

In dogs, doses of up to 500 mg/kg were tolerated without mortality.

Drug Interactions

The following drug interactions have either been reported or are theoretical in humans or animals receiving zafirlukast and may be of significance in veterinary patients. Unless otherwise noted, use together is not necessarily contraindicated, but weigh the potential risks and perform additional monitoring when appropriate.

■ **ASPIRIN:** May significantly increase zafirlukast plasma levels.

■ **ERYTHROMYCIN:** May decrease the bioavailability of zafirlukast.

■ **THEOPHYLLINE:** May decrease plasma levels of zafirlukast.

■ **WARFARIN:** Zafirlukast may significantly increase the prothrombin time of patients taking warfarin.

Laboratory Considerations

■ None were noted.

Doses

■ **DOGS:**

For adjunctive treatment of atopic dermatitis (extra-label): In the study dogs received: 5 mg PO q12h, if the dog weighed less than 11.4 kg (25 lb); 10 mg PO q12h, if 11.4-22.3 kg (25-49 lb); 20 mg PO q12h, if 22.7-34.1 kg (50-75 lb); and 30 mg PO q12h, if greater than 34.1 kg (75 lb). Given on an empty stomach, 1 hour before, or 2 hours after meals. Only 11% of treated dogs had at least 50% reductions in pruritus. (Senter *et al.* 2002)

■ **CATS:**

For adjunctive treatment of feline bronchial "asthma" (extra-label): Anecdotal dosages 0.5 – 2 mg/kg (practically as 5 – 10 mg per cat) q12-24h have been suggested. A recent review of this subject deemed zafirlukast an "ineffective therapy" (Trzil *et al.* 2014).

For adjunctive treatment of mild inflammatory bowel disease (extra-label): 0.15 – 0.2 mg/kg PO once daily. Author has used a combination of zafirlukast (3 months), famotidine (4 weeks), and sucralfate (2 weeks) along with a low-allergen diet to successfully treat a case. (Boothe 2009)

Monitoring
- Clinical efficacy.

Client Information
- Best given on an empty stomach (1 hour before, or 2 hours after feeding), but if vomiting occurs after giving the medication, try giving it with a small amount of food to see if this helps.
- Zafirlukast has not been used in very many cats, but no significant side effects have been reported. Contact veterinarian if you see anything out of the ordinary for your animal

Chemistry/Synonyms
A leukotriene-receptor antagonist, zafirlukast occurs as a white to pale yellow, fine amorphous powder. It is practically insoluble in water.

Zafirlukast may also be known as: ICI-204219, *Accolate®*, *Accoleit®*, *Aeronix®*, *Azimax®*, *Olmoran®*, *Resma®*, *Vanticon®*, *Zafarismal®*, *Zafirst®*, or *Zuvair®*.

Storage/Stability
Zafirlukast tablets should be stored at room temperature and protected from light and moisture. The manufacturer states that the tablets should be dispensed only in the original, unopened container.

Compatibility/Compounding Considerations
No specific information noted.

Dosage Forms/Regulatory Status
VETERINARY-LABELED PRODUCTS: NONE.

The ARCI (Racing Commissioners International) has designated this drug as a class 4 substance. See the appendix for more information.

HUMAN-LABELED PRODUCTS:

Zafirlukast Tablets (film-coated): 10 mg & 20 mg; *Accolate®*, generic; (Rx)

Revisions/References
Monograph revised/updated August 2014.

Boothe, D. M. (2009). Control of Inflammatory Allergic Disease in Cats II. Proceedings; WVC. accessed via Veterinary Information Network; vin.com

Reinero, C. R., et al. (2005). Effects of drug treatment on inflammation and hyperreactivity of airways and on immune variables in cats with experimentally induced asthma. American Journal of Veterinary Research **66**(7): 1121-7.

Senter, D. A., et al. (2002). Treatment of canine atopic dermatitis with zafirlukast, a leukotriene-receptor antagonist: a single-blinded, placebo-controlled study. Canadian Veterinary Journal-Revue Veterinaire Canadienne **43**(3): 203-6.

Trzil, J. E. & C. R. Reinero (2014). Update on Feline Asthma. Veterinary Clinics of North America-Small Animal Practice **44**(1): 91-+.

Zidovudine

(zid-o-vew-den)   AZT, Retrovir®

Antiretroviral

Prescriber Highlights
▶ Antiretroviral agent that may be useful for adjunctive treatment of FeLV or FIV in cats.
▶ Use with caution if renal, hepatic, or bone marrow dysfunction present.
▶ Anemia (non-regenerative) most common adverse effect in cats.

Uses/Indications
In veterinary medicine, zidovudine may be useful for treating feline immunodeficiency virus (FIV) or feline leukemia virus (FeLV). While zidovudine can reduce the viral load in infected cats and improve clinical signs, it may not alter the natural course of the disease to a great extent. A placebo-controlled double-blinded trial assessing the efficacy of human interferon-alfa2a (10^5 IU/kg SC q24h),

zidovudine (5 mg/kg PO q12h), and a combination of both drugs in cats infected naturally with FeLV reported that although there was a trend for improved clinical status in treated cats they were unable to demonstrate measurable statistically significant efficacy of either drug alone or together when given for 6 weeks. However, no notable side effects were detected (Stuetzer *et al.* 2013). As drug resistance can be seen, one source recommends that zidovudine treatment is probably best reserved for those situations where symptomatic/supportive measures are not working (Sparkes 2011).

Pharmacology/Actions
Zidovudine is considered an antiretroviral agent. While its exact mechanism of action is not fully understood, zidovudine is converted *in vivo* to an active metabolite (triphosphate) that interferes with viral RNA-directed DNA polymerase (reverse transcriptase). This causes a virustatic effect in retroviruses.

Zidovudine has some activity against gram-negative bacteria and can be cytotoxic as well.

Pharmacokinetics
Zidovudine is well absorbed after oral administration. In cats, oral bioavailability is ≈ 95%. When administered with food, peak levels may be decreased, but total area under the curve may not be affected; peak levels occur ≈ 1 hour post-dosing in cats. The drug is widely distributed, including into the CSF. It is only marginally bound to plasma proteins. Zidovudine is rapidly metabolized and excreted in the urine. Half-life in cats is ≈ 1.5 hours.

Contraindications/Precautions/Warnings
Zidovudine is considered contraindicated in patients who have developed life threatening hypersensitivity reactions to it in the past.

Use zidovudine with caution in patients with bone marrow, renal or hepatic dysfunction. The European Advisory Board on Cat Diseases (ABCD) guidelines on prevention and management of feline immunodeficiency state that: Cats with bone marrow suppression should not be treated (with zidovudine; see monitoring guidelines, below). Dosage adjustment may be necessary in cats with renal or hepatic dysfunction.

Adverse Effects
In cats, reductions in RBC's, PCV and hemoglobin are the most common adverse effects reported. Anemia may be non-regenerative and is most commonly seen with the higher end of the dosage range (10 – 15 mg/kg). Diarrhea and weakness have also been reported. While there are many adverse effects reported in humans, granulocytopenia and GI effects appear to be the most likely to occur.

Reproductive/Nursing Safety
In humans, the FDA categorizes this drug as category C for use during pregnancy (*Animal studies have shown an adverse effect on the fetus, but there are no adequate studies in humans; or there are no animal reproduction studies and no adequate studies in humans.*)

Zidovudine is excreted in milk. Clinical significance is not clear for nursing offspring.

Overdosage/Acute Toxicity
Human adults and children have survived oral overdoses of up to 50 grams without permanent sequelae. Vomiting and transient hematologic effects are the most consistent adverse effects reported with overdoses.

Drug Interactions
The following drug interactions have either been reported or are theoretical in humans or animals receiving zidovudine and may be of significance in veterinary patients. Unless otherwise noted, use together is not necessarily contraindicated, but weigh the potential risks and perform additional monitoring when appropriate.

- **ANTIFUNGALS, AZOLE** (*e.g.,* **ketoconazole**, etc.): May increase zidovudine levels.

- ATOVAQUONE: May increase zidovudine levels.
- DOXORUBICIN: May antagonize each other's effects; avoid use together.
- INTERFERON ALFA: Increased risk for hematologic- and hepatotoxicity.
- MYELO-/CYTOTOXIC DRUGS (*e.g.*, **chloramphenicol, doxorubicin, flucytosine, vincristine, vinblastine**): Administered with zidovudine may increase the risk of hematologic toxicity.
- PROBENECID: May increase zidovudine levels.
- RIFAMPIN: May decrease blood levels (AUC) of zidovudine.

Laboratory Considerations
- None were noted.

Doses
- **CATS:**

  For adjunctive therapy of FeLV and FIV (extra-label):

  From the ABCB Guidelines: 5 – 10 mg/kg q12h PO or SC. The higher dose should be used carefully as side effects can develop. For SC injection, the lyophilized product should be diluted in isotonic sodium chloride solution to prevent local irritation. For PO dosing, syrup or gelatin capsules (dosage/weight calculated individually for each cat) can be given. See the ABCB monitoring guidelines below. (Hosie *et al.* 2009)

  From the AAFP feline retrovirus management guidelines: 5 – 10 mg PO or SC q12h. The higher dose should be carefully used in FeLV-infected cats because side effects, particularly non-regenerative anemia, can develop. (Levy *et al.* 2008)

Monitoring
- The European Advisory Board on Cat Diseases (ABCD) guidelines on prevention and management of feline immunodeficiency (Hosie *et al.* 2009) recommends: During treatment, a CBC should be performed weekly for the first month, because non-regenerative anemia is common, especially at higher doses. If the values are stable, monthly checks are sufficient. If hematocrit drops below 20%, treatment should be discontinued, and anemia then usually resolves within a few days.
- CD4/CD8 rates, if possible.
- Clinical efficacy.

Client Information
- Zidovudine must be administered as prescribed for it to work correctly.
- Side effects can include anemia, diarrhea and weakness. If your cat seems overly tired or has no energy, contact your veterinarian right away.
- Regular blood tests required.

Chemistry/Synonyms
A thymidine analog, zidovudine is synthetically produced and occurs as a white to beige-colored, odorless, crystalline solid. Approximately 20 mg are soluble in one mL of water.

Zidovudine may also be known as: ZDV,. azidodeoxythymidine, 3'-azido-2',3'-dideoxythymidine, azidothymidine, AZT, BW-A509U, BW-509U, compound-S, zidovudinum or *Retrovir*®; many other trade names are available.

Storage/Stability
Zidovudine oral tablets or capsules should be stored at room temperature. Protect from heat, light and moisture. The oral solution should be stored at room temperature. Zidovudine injection (for IV infusion) should be store at room temperature and protected from light.

Compatibility/Compounding Considerations
No specific information noted.

Dosage Forms/Regulatory Status
VETERINARY-LABELED PRODUCTS: NONE.
HUMAN-LABELED PRODUCTS:

Zidovudine Oral Tablets: 300 mg; *Retrovir*®, generic; (Rx)

Zidovudine Oral Capsules: 100 mg; *Retrovir*®, generic; (Rx)

Zidovudine Oral Syrup: 50 mg/5 mL in 240 mL; *Retrovir*®, generic; (Rx)

Zidovudine Injection Solution: 10 mg/mL in 20 mL single-use vials; *Retrovir*®; (Rx)

Revisions/References
Monograph revised/updated August 2014.

Hosie, M. J., et al. (2009). Feline Immunodeficiency: ABCD guidelines on prevention and management. Journal of Feline Medicine and Surgery 11(7): 575-84.

Levy, J., et al. (2008). 2008 American Association of Feline Practitioners' feline retrovirus management guidelines. Journal of Feline Medicine and Surgery 10(3): 300-16.

Sparkes, A. (2011). Let's Not Be Retro on Retroviruses. Proceedings: AAFP World Feline Congress in partnership with ISFM 2011. accessed via Veterinary Information Network; vin.com

Stuetzer, B., et al. (2013). A trial with 3'-azido-2',3'-dideoxythymidine and human interferon-alpha in cats naturally infected with feline leukaemia virus. Journal of Feline Medicine and Surgery 15(8): 667-71.

Zinc (Systemic)

(zink)

Nutritional; Trace Element

Prescriber Highlights
▶ Metal nutritional agent that may be used for zinc deficiency, to reduce copper toxicity in susceptible dog breeds (*e.g.*, Bedlington Terriers, West Highland White Terriers) with hepatic copper toxicosis, & treat hepatic fibrosis in dogs. Has astringent & antiseptic activity topically.

▶ Contraindications: None; consider obtaining zinc & copper levels before treating.

▶ Adverse Effects: Large doses may cause GI disturbances or hematologic abnormalities (usually hemolysis), particularly if a coexistent copper deficiency exists.

▶ Zinc overdoses (*e.g.*, U.S. pennies) can be serious.

Uses/Indications
Zinc sulfate is used systemically as a nutritional supplement in a variety of species. Oral zinc acetate has been shown to reduce copper toxicity in susceptible dog breeds (*e.g.*, Bedlington Terriers, West Highland White Terriers) with hepatic copper toxicosis. Zinc therapy may also be of benefit in the treatment of hepatic fibrosis and zinc-responsive dermatosis. In dogs and cats, zinc has been used for adjunctive therapy for superficial necrolytic dermatitis (metabolic epidermal necrosis; hepatocutaneous syndrome).

Zinc sulfate is used topically as an astringent and as a weak antiseptic both for dermatologic and ophthalmic conditions.

For more information, the reader is encouraged to refer to a thorough review of zinc physiology, pathophysiology, toxicity and deficiency in veterinary patients (Cummings *et al.* 2009).

Pharmacology/Actions
Zinc is a necessary nutritional supplement; it is required by over 200 metalloenzymes for proper function. Enzyme systems that require zinc include alkaline phosphatase, alcohol dehydrogenase, carbonic anhydrase, and RNA polymerase. Zinc is also necessary to maintain structural integrity of cell membranes and nucleic acids. Zinc dependent physiological processes include sexual maturation and reproduction, cell growth and division, vision, night vision, wound healing, immune response, and taste acuity.

When administered orally, large doses of zinc can inhibit the absorption of copper.

Pharmacokinetics

About 20-30% of dietary zinc is absorbed, principally from the duodenum and ileum. Bioavailability is dependent upon the food in which it is present. Phytates can chelate zinc and form insoluble complexes in an alkaline pH. Zinc is stored mostly in red and white blood cells, but is also found in the muscle, skin, bone, retina, pancreas, liver, kidney, and prostate gland. Elimination is primarily via the feces, but some is also excreted by the kidneys and in sweat. Zinc found in feces may be reabsorbed in the colon.

Contraindications/Precautions/Warnings

Zinc supplementation should be carefully considered before administering to patients with copper deficiency.

When dosing, do not confuse the concentrations of zinc salts with elemental zinc.

Adverse Effects

Large doses may cause GI disturbances. Hematologic abnormalities (usually hemolysis) may occur with large doses or serum levels >1000 micrograms/dL (1 mg/dL), particularly if a coexistent copper deficiency exists. Zinc acetate or methionine may be less irritating to the stomach. Mixing the contents of the capsule with a small amount of tuna or hamburger may minimize vomiting.

Reproductive/Nursing Safety

Although zinc deficiency during pregnancy has been associated with adverse perinatal outcomes, other studies report no such occurrences. In humans, since zinc deficiency is very rare, the routine use of zinc supplementation during pregnancy is not recommended. In humans, the FDA categorizes this drug as category C for use during pregnancy (*Animal studies have shown an adverse effect on the fetus, but there are no adequate studies in humans; or there are no animal reproduction studies and no adequate studies in humans.*)

Overdosage/Acute Toxicity

Signs associated with overdoses of zinc in mammals include hemolytic anemia, hypotension, acute pancreatitis, jaundice, vomiting, and pulmonary edema. There were 1248 single agent exposures to zinc acetate, zinc sulfate and zinc gluconate reported to the ASPCA Animal Poison Control Center (APCC) during 2009-2013. Of the 1200 dogs, 516 were symptomatic. Vomiting (75%), diarrhea (29%), polydipsia (21%), and lethargy (14%) were the most common clinical signs. Of the 47 cats, 18 were symptomatic with vomiting (89%), anorexia (50%), polydipsia (44%) and diarrhea (39%) being the most common.

Zinc intoxication in birds is relatively common, but clinical signs of intoxication in birds are varied and nonspecific. They include lethargy, anorexia, regurgitation, polyuria, polydipsia, hematuria, hematochezia, pallor, dark or bright green diarrhea, foul-smelling feces, paresis, seizures, and sudden death (Puschner *et al.* 2009). Treatment involves removing the source of zinc, chelation therapy (edetate calcium disodium or succimer), and supportive care.

Drug Interactions

The following drug interactions have either been reported or are theoretical in humans or animals receiving zinc and may be of significance in veterinary patients. Unless otherwise noted, use together is not necessarily contraindicated, but weigh the potential risks and perform additional monitoring when appropriate.

- **COPPER:** Large doses of zinc can inhibit copper absorption in the intestine; if this interaction is not desired, separate copper and zinc supplements by at least two hours.
- **FLUOROQUINOLONES** (*e.g.*, **enrofloxacin, ciprofloxacin**): Zinc salts may reduce the oral absorption of some fluoroquinolones.
- **PENICILLAMINE:** May potentially inhibit zinc absorption; clinical significance is not clear.

- **TETRACYCLINES:** Zinc salts may chelate oral tetracycline and reduce its absorption; separate doses by at least two hours.
- **URSODIOL:** May potentially inhibit zinc absorption; clinical significance is not clear.

Doses

Note: Zinc products may be labeled with concentrations expressed as the salt OR as elemental zinc. Assume the labeled concentration per tablet, capsule, etc. is elemental zinc unless the labeled ingredients and concentrations state otherwise. Dosages below are for elemental zinc unless otherwise noted.

- **DOGS:**

    For adjunctive treatment and prophylaxis of hepatic copper toxicosis (extra-label): 5 – 10 mg/kg elemental zinc q12h; use high end of dosage range initially for 3 months, then 50 mg PO q12h for maintenance. Separate dosage from meals by 1-2 hours. Zinc acetate or methionine may be less irritating to the GI than other salts. Mixing the contents of the capsule with a small amount of tuna or hamburger may also minimize vomiting. In dogs with active copper-induced hepatitis, do not use zinc alone, but in combination with a chelator (*e.g.*, D-penicillamine, trientine). Target zinc plasma levels >200 micrograms/dL but <400 micrograms/dL. Monitor levels every 2-3 months and adjust dosage as necessary. (Johnson 2000)

    For hepatic fibrosis (extra-label): Empirical dosage is 15 mg/kg of elemental zinc per day, (or 200 mg elemental zinc per medium sized dog per day, tapered to 50 – 100 mg per dog per day based on serum zinc levels). The goal is for serum zinc levels of 200-500 micrograms/dL (2-5 micrograms/mL). Zinc should ideally be given on an empty stomach (1 hour before or after a meal); mix with tuna oil if nausea noted. Author prefers to add zinc in as a single drug after stabilization of the patient with hepato-protective agents and glucocorticoids (if indicated). (Trepanier 2008)

    For adjunctive therapy for superficial necrolytic dermatitis or zinc-responsive dermatosis (extra-label): 2 mg/kg PO q24h of elemental zinc with food either once daily or divided q12h. Doses may need to be adjusted based on response to therapy. The addition of low-dose glucocorticoid therapy may benefit cases that do not respond solely to zinc supplementation. Syndrome I patients (fed balanced diets) that do not respond to oral zinc supplementation and low-dose glucocorticoid therapy, slow IV or IM injections with sterile zinc sulfate solutions at 10 – 15 mg/kg weekly (maximum of 600 mg/month) for at least one month have been recommended. Syndrome I patients require life-long therapy. Syndrome II patients (fed diets low in zinc or high in phytates [cereal grains, soy-based or corn-based diets], or with high levels of minerals [calcium, iron, or copper] that may bind dietary zinc), can have zinc supplementation discontinued after diet has been corrected and clinical signs resolve. Adapted from: (Koch *et al.* 2011)

- **CATS:**

    For adjunctive therapy of severe hepatic lipidosis (extra-label): 7 – 10 mg/kg PO once daily, in B-Complex mixture if possible. (Center 1994)

    For superficial necrolytic dermatitis (extra-label): Dosages are not well described; doses used in dogs could possibly be extrapolated for cats. (Koch *et al.* 2011)

Monitoring

- See information in individual doses above.
- There is poor correlation between serum zinc levels and zinc-deficient states in dogs, and zinc levels may have more value in de-

tection of potentially toxic intake or corroboration of a clinical diagnosis of toxicity or deficiency (Cummings *et al.* 2009).

Client Information

- Although it is best to give oral zinc acetate on an empty stomach if vomiting occurs, mix with hamburger or tuna fish to decrease this side effect.
- Do not give more than prescribed; zinc can be very toxic (especially in dogs).

Chemistry/Synonyms

Zinc acetate occurs as white crystals or granules. It has a faint acetous odor and effloresces slightly. One gram is soluble in 2.5 mL of water or 30 mL of alcohol. Zinc acetate contains 30% elemental zinc (100 mg zinc acetate = 30 mg elemental zinc).

Zinc sulfate occurs as a colorless granular powder, small needles, or transparent prisms. It is odorless but has an astringent metallic taste. 1.67 grams are soluble in 1 mL of water. Zinc sulfate is insoluble in alcohol and contains 23% zinc by weight (100 mg zinc sulfate = 23 mg elemental zinc).

Zinc gluconate occurs as white or practically white powder or granules. It is soluble in water; very slightly soluble in alcohol. Zinc gluconate contains 14.3% zinc (100 mg zinc gluconate = 14.3 mg elemental zinc).

Zinc methionine contains 18-21% elemental zinc. For very 5 mg of zinc methionine there is ≈ 1 mg of elemental zinc.

Zinc acetate may also be known as: E650, or zinci acetas dihydricus.

Zinc sulfate may also be known as: zinc sulphate; zinci sulfas, zincum sulfuricum; many trade names are available.

Storage/Stability

Store zinc acetate crystals in tight containers. Unless otherwise recommended by the manufacturer, store zinc sulfate products in tight containers at room temperature.

Compatibility/Compounding Considerations

If using bulk chemical powder: Zinc acetate contains 30% elemental zinc; zinc gluconate contains 14.3% elemental zinc; zinc sulfate contains 23% elemental zinc; zinc methionine contains 18-21% elemental zinc. 1 mg of elemental zinc is provided by the following: 2.8 mg zinc acetate, 2.09 mg zinc chloride, 7.14 mg zinc gluconate, and 4.4 mg zinc sulfate.

Dosage Forms/Regulatory Status

VETERINARY-LABELED PRODUCTS:

None as single-ingredient products for systemic use located; several vitamin/mineral supplements contain zinc, however. *NutriVed Chewable Zinpro*® Tablets contain 15 mg elemental zinc and 30 mg methionine; (OTC).

HUMAN-LABELED PRODUCTS:

Zinc Acetate is available from chemical supply houses.

Zinc Capsules: 25 mg & 50 mg elemental zinc (as zinc acetate); *Galzin*®; (Rx)

Zinc Injection: 1 mg/mL (as sulfate; as 4.39 mg heptahydrate or 2.46 mg anhydrous) in 10 mL & 30 mL vials; 5 mg/mL (as 21.95 mg sulfate) in 5 mL & 10 mL vials; 1 mg/mL (as 2.09 mg chloride) in 10 mL vials; *Zinca-Pak*®, generic; (Rx)

Zinc Tablets: 10 mg, 15 mg, 25 mg, 30 mg, & 50 mg elemental zinc (usually as zinc gluconate); generic; (OTC)

Zinc sulfate is also available in topical ophthalmic preparations.

Revisions/References

Monograph revised/updated August 2014.

Center, S. (1994). Hepatic lipidosis. *Consultations in Feline Internal Medicine: 2.* J. August. Philadelphia, W.B. Saunders Company: 87-101.
Cummings, J. E. & J. P. Kovacic (2009). The ubiquitous role of zinc in health and disease. J. Vet. Emerg. Crit. Care **19**(3): 215-40.
Johnson, S. (2000). Chronic Hepatic Disorders. *Textbook of Veterinary Internal Medicine: Diseases of the Dog and Cat.* S. Ettinger and E. Feldman. Philadelphia, WB Saunders. 2: 1298-325.
Koch, S., et al. (2011). *Small Animal Dermatology Drug Handbook*, Wiley-Blackwell. Ames.
Puschner, B. & A. Poppenga (2009). Lead and Zinc Intoxication in Companion Birds. Comp CE(January): E1- E12.
Trepanier, L. (2008). Choosing therapy for chronic liver disease. Proceedings: WSAVA. accessed via Veterinary Information Network; vin.com

Zinc Gluconate (Neutering Agent)

(zink gloo-koe-nayt)

Chemical Sterilant Zeuterin®

Prescriber Highlights

▶ Injectable (intra-testicular) chemical sterilant for male dogs.
▶ Contraindications: Undescended testicles (cryptorchid); disease or malformation of the testicle (including fibrosis of the testicles or epididymides); history of allergic reaction to any of the components of the drug; & pre-existing scrotal irritation or dermatitis, or transmissible venereal tumor (TVT).
▶ Specialized injection technique; requires training.
▶ Adverse Effects: Local reactions (scrotal; testicular) most common. Can cause vomiting; fasting for 12 hours prior is recommended.
▶ May be effective in male cats, but not approved for use.

Uses/Indications

Zeuterin® injectable is indicated for chemical sterilization in 3-10 month old male dogs.

Two studies have investigated zinc gluconate injection for use in male cats. At 120-days post-injection azoospermia occurred in 73% of treated cats (Oliveira *et al.* 2013), (Fagundes *et al.* 2014). The authors concluded that additional studies are warranted to determine if it could be used as a permanent contraceptive in cats.

Pharmacology/Actions

When injected into the testicle, zinc gluconate acts as a localized necrotizing agent that can result in: atrophy of testicles, epididymides, seminiferous tubules, and prostate gland, and/or testicular scar tissue formation thereby preventing movement of sperm from the seminiferous tubules to the epididymis.

Pharmacokinetics

No information noted.

Contraindications/Precautions/Warnings

Use is contraindicated in dogs with undescended testicles (cryptorchid), disease or malformation of the testicle (including fibrosis of the testicles or epididymides), history of allergic reaction to any of the components of the drug, and if there is pre-existing scrotal irritation or dermatitis, or transmissible venereal tumor (TVT). No more than 1 injection per testicle is to be performed. Do not use if the testicular width is <10 mm or >27 mm. Safety and effectiveness of *Zeuterin*® has not been established in dogs less than 3 months of age or in dogs greater than 10 months of age.

Withhold food for 12 hours before injection.

To avoid irritation to the scrotal skin, do not shave or clip the scrotal hair. Do not inject into scrotal sac or scrotal skin.

Do not allow dogs to bite or lick the scrotum after injection.

Adverse Effects

In field studies, local adverse effects were most commonly reported and included scrotal pain; some dogs (2.7%) reacted at the time of injection, but most dogs that exhibited signs of scrotal pain (6.3%) occurred within the first two days after injection. Other scrotal effects (irritation, selling, bruising, etc.) were also seen in some animals.

Systemic adverse affects include neutrophilia (6.3%), vomiting (4.4%), anorexia (4.1%), lethargy (2.2%), and diarrhea (1.9%) and were most commonly noted within the first 7 days after injection, but vomiting most often occurred between 1-4 hours post-injection.

Reproductive/Nursing Safety

Not for use in dogs to be used for breeding.

Overdosage/Acute Toxicity

Overdosages (up to 2X) increased likelihood of local reactions; determine dosages carefully.

Drug Interactions

- None noted.

Laboratory Considerations

- Nothing specific noted.

Doses

- **DOGS:**

  For chemical sterilization (labeled dose; FDA-approved): Dosage is determined by testicular width. Specialized injection techniques are used and the company requires training before it will authorize sales. Refer to the product (*Zeuterin®*) label for additional information.

Monitoring

- Local adverse effects.

Client Information

- Temporary swelling of the testicular area is expected.
- May not kill sperm present at the time of injection. Keep treated dogs away from females in heat for at least 60 days following the injection.
- Testosterone is not completely eliminated. Diseases that are related to testosterone (prostatic disease, testicular or perianal tumors) may not be prevented.
- Roaming, marking, aggression, or mounting may be displayed; contact your veterinarian if these get worse or are serious.

Chemistry/Synonyms

Zinc gluconate occurs as white or practically white powder or granules. It is soluble in water; very slightly soluble in alcohol. Zinc gluconate contains 14.3% zinc (100 mg zinc gluconate = 14.3 mg elemental zinc). The product *Zeuterin®* is an injectable aqueous solution containing 0.2 M zinc gluconate neutralized to pH 7.0 with 0.2 M L-arginine. Each mL contains 13.1 mg of elemental zinc and 34.8 mg of arginine.

Storage/Stability

Store the injection at controlled room temperature (15-30°C; 59-86°F).

Compatibility/Compounding Considerations

No specific information noted.

Dosage Forms/Regulatory Status

VETERINARY-LABELED PRODUCTS:

Zinc Gluconate (neutralized by arginine; 13.1 mg zinc/mL) Injectable Chemical Sterilant in 3.5 mL vials; *Zeuterin®*; (Rx). FDA-approved (NADA 141-217) for use in dogs.

HUMAN-LABELED PRODUCTS: NONE.

Revisions/References

Monograph written August 2014.

Fagundes, A. K. F., et al. (2014). Injection of a chemical castration agent, zinc gluconate, into the testes of cats results in the impairment of spermatogenesis: A potentially irreversible contraceptive approach for this species? Theriogenology 81(2): 230-6.

Oliveira, E. C. S., et al. (2013). Intratesticular injection of a zinc-based solution for contraception of domestic cats: A randomized clinical trial of efficacy and safety. Veterinary Journal 197(2): 307-10.

Zolazepam – see Tiletamine HCl/Zolazepam HCl

Zonisamide

(zoh-niss-a-mide)   Zonegran®

Anticonvulsant

Prescriber Highlights

▶ Antiseizure medication that may be useful as an "add-on" drug for refractory epilepsy. May be considered for initial treatment as monotherapy in dogs.

▶ Half-life of 15 hours makes twice daily dosing possible in dogs; 33-hour half-life in cats may allow once daily dosing.

▶ Adverse effect profile not fully elucidated for dogs; sedation, ataxia, inappetence, hepatopathy, urinary calculi, metabolic and acute tubular acidosis have been reported.

▶ Known teratogen in dogs.

▶ May need dosage adjustment when used with phenobarbital (see Drug Interactions).

Uses/Indications

Zonisamide may be useful as an "add-on" drug for refractory epilepsy in dogs. It has been suggested that it could be useful as monotherapy as the initial drug choice for dogs, particularly when the client wishes to avoid adverse effects associated with phenobarbital or bromides (Thomas 2010). No placebo-controlled prospective studies were located documenting efficacy in dogs or cats. Open label studies in dogs where zonisamide was used as monotherapy or as an add-on drug, reported response rates were 58-81% (Dewey *et al.* 2003), (von Klopmann *et al.* 2007), (Chung *et al.* 2012). Limited use in cats has occurred, but some report anecdotally to having success in controlling seizures.

Zonisamide administered rectally may be beneficial in treating status epilepticus.

Pharmacology/Actions

The exact mechanism of action for zonisamide is not known. It may produce its antiseizure activity by blocking sodium channels and reducing transient inward currents, thereby stabilizing neuronal membranes and suppressing neuronal hypersynchronization. It does not appear to potentiate GABA. Zonisamide has weak carbonic anhydrase inhibitory activity.

Pharmacokinetics

In dogs, zonisamide is well absorbed (bioavailability ≈ 70%) after oral administration and has low protein binding. Zonisamide has been demonstrated to be absorbed rectally in dogs. The elimination half-life in dogs is ≈ 15-17 hours. Most of the drug is excreted via the kidneys into the urine, but ≈ 20% is metabolized, primarily in the liver. Unlike in humans, zonisamide exhibits linear pharmacokinetics (dose to plasma trough concentrations) in dogs (at doses between 5 – 30 mg/kg PO twice daily) (Fukunaga *et al.* 2010).

An abstract (from a proceedings) reported that zonisamide 10 mg/mL in a polyethylene glycol solution (formulation not reported) that rectal bioavailability relative to oral dosing in dogs was 87%. The rectal solution in water had a relative bioavailability of 53%. The authors concluded: "With proportionately larger doses (based on relative bioavailability) of each rectal formulation, plasma zonisamide concentrations within the therapeutic range (10-40 mcg/mL) can probably be achieved clinically." (Brewer *et al.* 2008)

Zonisamide has a long half-life in cats of ≈ 33 hours (Hasegawa *et al.* 2008).

Contraindications/Precautions/Warnings

In humans, zonisamide is contraindicated in patients hypersensitive to it or to any of the sulfonamide drugs.

Adverse Effects

Because there has been limited use of this drug in veterinary patients the adverse effect profile is not fully known. Adverse effects that have been reported in dogs include sedation (usually transient), ataxia, and inappetence. Zonisamide is a sulfonamide, but not a sulfonylarylamine (the form of sulfonamide that generates toxic nitrosyl molecules that can cause direct tissue injury and act as allergens for hypersensitivity reactions), it is unlikely to cause KCS or other sulfonamide-related adverse effects in dogs or cats. Case reports of dogs developing zonisamide-associated apparent acute idiopathic hepatic necrosis, urinary calculi (Miller *et al.* 2011), hepatopathy (Schwartz *et al.* 2011) and acute tubular acidosis (Cook *et al.* 2011) have been published.

In a combined pharmacokinetic and toxicity study in cats, half of cats receiving 20 mg/kg per day developed adverse effects that included inappetence, diarrhea, vomiting, ataxia and somnolence (Hasegawa *et al.* 2008).

Tolerance to therapy is possible.

In humans, the most common adverse effects associated with zonisamide include anorexia, nausea, dizziness, somnolence, agitation and headache. Rarely, serious dermatologic reactions (Stevens-Johnson syndrome, TEN), blood dyscrasias, oligohidrosis, and hyperthermia have been reported in humans.

Reproductive/Nursing Safety

When zonisamide was administered to pregnant dogs at 10 or 30 mg/kg/day (approximate therapeutic dosages in dogs), ventricular septal defects, cardiomegaly and various valvular and arterial anomalies were seen at the higher dose. A plasma level of 25 micrograms/mL was the threshold level for malformation. If this drug is to be used in pregnant dogs, the owner must accept the significant risks associated with its use.

It is not known if zonisamide enters maternal milk; use with caution in nursing animals.

Overdosage/Acute Toxicity

The LD$_{50}$ of zonisamide in dogs is reportedly 1 gram/kg. In human overdoses, effects reported include coma, bradycardia, hypotension, and respiratory depression. In cats, toxic adverse effects (anorexia, vomiting, diarrhea, lethargy and ataxia) were noted in 50% of cats in one study (Hasegawa *et al.* 2008). There were 101 single agent exposures to zonisamide reported to the ASPCA Animal Poison Control Center (APCC) during 2009-2013. Eighty-eight of these were dogs, and 10 of them were symptomatic. The most common signs were sedation/lethargy (70%), and 20% with anxiety, ataxia and/or vomiting.

Treatment recommendations include GI decontamination if ingestion was recent, and supportive therapy. Because of the drug's long half-life, support may be required for several days.

Drug Interactions

The following drug interactions have either been reported or are theoretical in humans or animals receiving zonisamide and may be of significance in veterinary patients. Unless otherwise noted, use together is not necessarily contraindicated, but weigh the potential risks and perform additional monitoring when appropriate.

- **PHENOBARBITAL**: In dogs, phenobarbital may increase the clearance of zonisamide as repeated phenobarbital dosing decreased the bioavailability, peak concentrations, half-life, and area under the curve of zonisamide, but it did not affect the time to peak level or the volume of distribution of zonisamide. This effect persisted up to 10 weeks after phenobarbital discontinuation (Orito *et al.* 2008). If adding zonisamide to a dog already receiving phenobarbital, most recommend using zonisamide at the high end of the dosage range (10 mg/kg PO q12h) (Munana 2013), (Mariani 2010), (Thomas 2010), (Martin-Jimenez 2010), but one source recommends reducing phenobarbital dosage by 25% (Podell 2013).

Laboratory Considerations

- Zonisamide can decrease **total T4 levels**.
- While plasma concentrations of zonisamide are not routinely monitored in human patients, in dogs, the therapeutic range has been suggested to be from 10-40 mcg/mL.

Doses

- **DOGS:**

  For the treatment of seizures (extra-label): No placebo-controlled prospective studies were located. Most recommend an initial dosage of 5 mg/kg PO q12h, although recommendations when used as monotherapy range from 2 – 8 mg/kg PO q12h. If adding zonisamide to a dog already receiving phenobarbital, most recommend using zonisamide at the high end of the dosage range (10 mg/kg PO q12h) (Munana 2013), (Mariani 2010), (Thomas 2010), (Martin-Jimenez 2010), but one source recommends reducing phenobarbital dosage by 25% (Podell 2013).

- **CATS:**

  For treating seizure disorders in cats refractory to phenobarbital (extra-label): Because of its long half–life in cats, doses of 5 – 10 mg/kg PO once daily are likely to be appropriate although additional studies are needed to determine this. The authors report using the drug in 2 cats that were refractory to phenobarbital therapy; 1 developed anorexia and the drug had to be discontinued, but the other responded well. (Bailey *et al.* 2009)

Monitoring

- Efficacy.
- Monitoring zonisamide blood levels may be useful in veterinary patients, but this has not been confirmed nor have veterinary therapeutic blood concentrations been identified, but some feel that measurement of serum concentrations can be useful when seizures are not controlled. Therapeutic levels for humans are thought to be: 10-40 mcg/mL.
- Adverse effects.

Client Information

- May be given with or without food. If your animal vomits or acts sick after getting it on an empty stomach, give with food or small treat to see if this helps.
- Don't stop giving zonisamide suddenly ("cold turkey") or rebound seizures can occur.
- Keeping a seizure diary may help in determining how well this medication is working in your animal.
- If animal stops eating, has a lack of appetite, becomes overly lethargic (tired), or develops a yellowish tint to eyes or gums, contact veterinarian immediately.

Chemistry/Synonyms

A sulfonamide unrelated to other antiseizure drugs, zonisamide occurs as a white powder with a pKa of 10.2. It is moderately soluble in water (0.8 mg/mL).

Zonisamide may also be known as: AD-810, CI-912, PD-110843, *Excegran*®, or *Zonegran*®.

Storage/Stability

Zonisamide capsules should be stored at 25°C (76°F); excursions permitted to 15-30°C (59-86°F). Store in a dry place and protected from light.

Compatibility/Compounding Considerations

The preparation and stability of extemporaneously compounded (from 100 mg capsules) zonisamide 10 mg/mL suspensions in simple-syrup or methylcellulose (0.5%) has been published (Obobo *et al.* 2009). The simple-syrup suspension was stable for at least 28 days when stored at room temperature or under refrigeration and the methylcellulose (0.5%) suspension was stable for 28 days when stored under refrigeration and for 7 days when stored at room temperature.

Dosage Forms/Regulatory Status

VETERINARY-LABELED PRODUCTS: NONE.

HUMAN-LABELED PRODUCTS:

Zonisamide Capsules: 25 mg, 50 mg & 100 mg; *Zonegran*®, generic; (Rx)

Revisions/References

Monograph revised/updated August 2014.

Bailey, K. S. & C. W. Dewey (2009). The Seizuring Cat: Diagnostic work-up and therapy. Journal of Feline Medicine and Surgery **11**(5): 385-94.

Brewer, D., et al. (2008). Pharmacokinetics of Single-Dose Rectal Zonisamide Administration in Normal Dogs [Abstract]. Proceedings; IVECCS. accessed via Veterinary Information Network; vin.com

Chung, J. Y., et al. (2012). Zonisamide monotherapy for idiopathic epilepsy in dogs. New Zealand Veterinary Journal **60**(6): 357-9.

Cook, A. K., et al. (2011). Renal Tubular Acidosis Associated with Zonisamide Therapy in a Dog. Journal of Veterinary Internal Medicine **25**(6): 1454-7.

Dewey, C., et al. (2003). Zonisamide therapy for refractory idiopathic epilepsy in dogs. Proceedings: ACVIM Forum. accessed via Veterinary Information Network; vin.com

Fukunaga, K., et al. (2010). Steady-state pharmacokinetics of zonisamide in plasma, whole blood, and erythrocytes in dogs. J. Vet. Pharmacol. Ther. **33**(1): 103-6.

Hasegawa, D., et al. (2008). Pharmacokinetics and toxicity of zonisamide in cats. Journal of Feline Medicine and Surgery **10**(4): 418-21.

Mariani, C. (2010). Maintenance therapy for the routine & difficult to control epileptic patient. Proceedings: ACVIM Forum. accessed via Veterinary Information Network; vin.com

Martin-Jimenez, T. (2010). Newer agents for the treatment of epileptic disorders. Proceedings: WVC. accessed via Veterinary Information Network; vin.com

Miller, M. L., et al. (2011). Apparent Acute Idiosyncratic Hepatic Necrosis Associated with Zonisamide Administration in a Dog. Journal of Veterinary Internal Medicine **25**(5): 1156-60.

Munana, K. R. (2013). Update Seizure Management in Small Animal Practice. Veterinary Clinics of North America-Small Animal Practice **43**(5): 1127-+.

Obobo, C., et al. (2009). Stability of zonisamide in extemporaneously compounded oral suspensions. Am J Health-Syst Pharm **66**: 1105-9.

Orito, K., et al. (2008). Pharmacokinetics of zonisamide and drug interaction with phenobarbital in dogs. J. Vet. Pharmacol. Ther. **31**(3): 259-64.

Podell, M. (2013). Antiepileptic Drug Therapy and Monitoring. Topics in Companion Animal Medicine **28**(2): 59-66.

Schwartz, M., et al. (2011). Possible Drug-Induced Hepatopathy in a Dog Receiving Zonisamide Monotherapy for Treatment of Cryptogenic Epilepsy. Journal of Veterinary Medical Science **73**(11): 1505-8.

Thomas, W. B. (2010). Idiopathic Epilepsy in Dogs and Cats. Veterinary Clinics of North America-Small Animal Practice **40**(1): 161-+.

von Klopmann, T., et al. (2007). Prospective study of zonisamide therapy for refractory idiopathic epilepsy in dogs. Journal of Small Animal Practice **48**(3): 134-8.

Ophthalmic Products, Topical

The following section lists the majority of veterinary-labeled ophthalmic topical products and some of the more commonly used human-labeled products in veterinary medicine; written by Gigi Davidson, DICVP with input from Michael Davidson, DVM, DACVO. Drugs are listed in alphabetical order.

For additional information, an excellent review on veterinary ophthalmic pharmacology and therapeutics can be found in both of the following textbooks: *Slatter's Fundamentals of Veterinary Ophthalmology, 5th Edition*. Maggs, D.J., Miller, P.E., & Ofri, R., Eds. Saunders, 2012, 520 pp., and Veterinary Ophthalmology, 5th Edition; Gelatt, K.N., Gilger, B.C., Kern, T.J., Eds. Wiley-Blackwell, 2013. 2260 pp.

Routes of Administration For Ophthalmic Drugs

The route of administration selected to deliver therapy for an ocular condition is critical to successful therapy. The following table lists advantages and disadvantages of each route of administration for ocular medications.

Route	Tissues Reached	Dosage Forms	Advantages	Disadvantages	Comments
Topical	Conjunctiva; Cornea; Anterior uvea; Lids	Solutions Suspensions	Easier administration for small animals; minimal interference with vision; lower incidence of contact dermatitis; less toxic to interior of eye if penetrating wound	More difficult to administer to horses; less contact time with eye; requires more frequent application than ointment; diluted by tearing; generally more expensive than ointment; more systemic absorption	Doses >1 drop rarely indicated in small animals (maximum tear capacity is 10–20 ml, volume of a drop is 25–50 ml); allow 5 minutes between drops; instill in order of least viscous to most; instill in order of aqueous prior to oil base
		Ointments	Longer contact time; less frequent administration; protect cornea from drying; not diluted by tearing; generally less expensive than solutions/ suspensions	Contribute to volume of ocular discharge; temporary blurring of vision; more difficult for client administration; more contact dermatitis; should not be applied to penetrating corneal wounds as oils will cause a granulomatous uveitis; difficult to determine exact dose; metal tubes often fatigue and split before all medication is used	Owners should be counseled to avoid contact of application tube with eye; observe patient for short while after application due to temporarily blurred vision
Subconjunctival injection	Cornea; Anterior uvea	Sterile solutions and suspensions	Longer duration of action; higher anterior chamber concentrations than topical	Limited number of injections can be performed; may create scar tissue; cannot be removed once applied; temporary pain; drug vehicle residues	Indicated for poorly compliant owners, uncooperative patients; indicated for drugs with poor corneal penetration
Retrobulbar injection	Posterior segment; Optic nerve	Sterile solutions and suspensions			Primarily used for local anesthetic prior to enucleation of the eye
Intracameral injection	Anterior chamber; Posterior segment	Sterile solutions and suspensions	Allows very high drug concentrations for intraocular infections	Risk of hemorrhage, retinal detachment, cataract formation, and retinal degeneration	Rarely used except for severe intraocular infections or for administration of tPA to dissolve fibrin clots in the anterior chamber
Systemic Drugs	Lids; Posterior segment; Optic nerve; Anterior uvea (occasionally)	Oral Intramuscular Subcutaneous Intravenous	Allows drug penetration to areas where topical therapy will not reach	Systemic toxicity; Does not reach cornea; expense directly proportional to body weight in most cases	See monographs for use of systemic agents.

Ophthalmic Agents Listed by Class/Indication

Note: Some agents are listed in more than one category.

Analgesics (see also NSAIDs)
Morphine **1155**
Nalbuphine **1157**

Anesthetics, Ocular
Benoxinate **1124**
Proparacaine **1166**
Tetracaine **1174**

Antibacterials (single)
Amikacin **1117**
Azithromycin **1123**
Bacitracin **1123**
Besifloxacin **1125**
Chloramphenicol **1130**
Ciprofloxacin **1131**
Erythromycin **1140**
Gatifloxacin **1141**
Gentamicin **1145**
Levofloxacin **1151**
Moxifloxacin **1156**
Neomycin **1158, 1177**
Ofloxacin **1160**
Oxytetracycline **1161**
Polymyxin B **1117, 1161**
Povidone Iodine **1165**
Silver Sulfadiazine **1169**
Sulfacetamide **1171**
Tobramycin **1176**
Vancomycin **1179**

Antibiotic Combinations
Oxytetracycline/Polymyxin B **1161**
Triple Antibiotic **1177**

Antibiotic Corticosteroid Combinations
Gentamicin/Prednisolone **1145**
Tobramycin/Dexamethasone **1176**
Triple Antibiotic w/Hydrocortisone **1146, 1177**

Anticollagenase Agents
Acetylcysteine **1116**
Edetate Disodium **1138**
Polysulfated Glycosaminoglycan **1164**

Antifungals
Amphotericin B **1118**
Itraconazole **1148**
Miconazole **1154**
Natamycin **1157**
Silver Sulfadiazine **1169**
Voriconazole **1180**

Antihistamines (see also Mast Cell Inhibitors)
Alcaftadine **1117**
Azelastine **1122**
Bepotastine **1125**
Emedastine **1139**
Epinastine **1140**
Ketotifen **1150**
Olapatadine **1161**

Antineoplastics
Fluorouracil **1142**
Mitomycin **1154**

Antiseptics
Povidone Iodide **1165**
Silver Sulfadiazine **1169**

Antivirals
Acyclovir **1116**
Cidofovir **1130**
Ganciclovir **1144**
Idoxuridine **1147**
Trifluridine **1177**

Artificial Tears/Ocular Lubricants   1120

Chelating Agents
Edetate Disodium **1138**

Corticosteroids
Betamethasone **1126**
Dexamethasone **1135**
Difluprednate **1136**
Fluorometholone **1141**
Hydrocortisone **1146**
Loteprednol **1153**
Prednisolone **1165**
Rimexolone **1167**

Cycloplegic Mydriatics
Atropine **1121**
Cyclopentolate **1132**
Tropicamide **1178**

Mydriatic Combinations
Cyclopentolate/Phenylephrine **1132, 1162**

Hyperosmotic Agents
Sodium Chloride, Hypertonic **1170**

Glaucoma, Ocular Hypertension Agents
Miotics, Cholinesterase Inhibitors
Demecarium **1134**
Echothiophate **1138**

Miotics, Direct-Acting
Pilocarpine **1163**

Alpha-Adrenergic Agonists
Apraclonidine **1119**
Brimonidine **1127**

Beta-Blockers
Betaxolol **1126**
Carteolol **1129**
Levobunolol **1151**
Metipranolol **1153**
Timolol **1174**

Carbonic Anhydrase Inhibitors
Brinzolamide **1128**
Dorzolamide **1137**

Prostaglandin Analogs
Bimatoprost **1127**
Latanaprost **1150**
Tafluprost **1173**

Fixed Dose Combinations
Brimonidine/Timolol **1127, 1174**
Brinzolamide/Brimonidine **1127, 1128**
Dorzolamide/Timolol **1137, 1174**

Decongestants
Phenylephrine **1162**

Diagnostics
Fluorescein Sodium **1142**
Lissamine Green **1152**
Phenylephrine **1162**
Rose Bengal **1168**
Schirmer Tear Test **1169**

Fibrinolytics/Antifibrinolytics
Aminocaproic Acid **1118**
Tissue Plasminogen Activator (Alteplase) **1175**

Immunologics
Cyclosporine **1133**
Pimecrolimus **1163**
Tacrolimus **1172**

Irrigating Solutions   1147

Mast Cell Stabilizers
Cromolyn Sodium **1132**
Nedocromil **1158**

Nonsteroidal Antiinflammatory Drugs (NSAIDs)
Bromfenac **1129**
Diclofenac **1136**
Flurbiprofen **1143**
Ketorolac **1149**
Nepafenac **1159**
Suprofen **1172**

Surgical Adjuncts
Fluorouracil **1142**
Mitomycin **1154**

Acetylcysteine Ophthalmic

(a-see-tuhl-sis-teen)

Anticollagenase Agent

Prescriber Highlights

► Mucolytic agent used to stop melting effect of collagenases and proteases in the eye.

► Must be compounded. Solutions should be refrigerated.

► Foul odor is normal and does not affect drug activity.

Uses/Indications

In veterinary patients, acetylcysteine is used topically to treat corneal ulcers by preventing corneal melting caused by proteinases and collagenases.

Pharmacology/Actions

Acetylcysteine inhibits matrix metalloproteinase-9 (MMP-9) production by corneal epithelial cells. Although MMP's play a role in initial corneal wound healing, they must be down regulated to prevent corneal melting and allow for corneal wound healing.

Contraindications/Precautions/Warnings

Acetylcysteine is contraindicated in patients with a history of hypersensitivity to it or any component of the formulation. Acetylcysteine exposure to the pulmonary tree may result in severe bronchospasm and should be used with caution in asthmatic patients.

Adverse Effects

Adverse effects reported in humans or animals include irritation, redness, and tearing of the eyes. If inhaled, acetylcysteine can rarely cause bronchoconstriction and tracheal irritation. Concentrations of acetylcysteine >10% are irritating to the eye.

Doses

Corneal ulcers (extra-label): Acetylcysteine 5% or 10% Ophthalmic Solution (compounded), 1 drop in affected eye(s) every 1-2 hours for the first 24 hours, followed by 1 drop in affected eye(s) 3-4 times daily for 7-10 days.

Monitoring

■ Clinical efficacy; evidence of corneal wound healing.

Client Information

■ Used 3-4 times daily.

■ Wait 5 minutes after applying this medication before applying any other medications to the eye.

■ Foul, rotten-egg odor is normal and does not affect activity of the drug.

■ Store solutions in the refrigerator; do not freeze. Do not use if the color changes, becomes cloudy, or if particles are seen in the solution.

Storage/Stability

Store in refrigerator away from moisture and sunlight; do not freeze. Compounded 5% or 10% solutions of acetylcysteine are reported to be stable for 60 days in the refrigerator, protected from light.

Compatibility/Compounding Considerations

Acetylcysteine should not be mixed directly with any other drugs.

Dosage Forms/Regulatory Status

VETERINARY-LABELED PRODUCTS:
None; may be available from compounding pharmacies.

HUMAN-LABELED PRODUCTS: NONE.

Revisions/References

Monograph revised/updated September 2014.

Acyclovir Ophthalmic

(a-sye-klo-veer)

Antiviral

Prescriber Highlights

► Used as an ophthalmic ointment in cats with feline herpes virus-1 (FHV-1). Do not use systemically in cats; myelotoxic and poor efficacy against FHV-1.

► Ophthalmic dosage forms of acyclovir are approved in a few countries.

Uses/Indications

Acyclovir has been used topically as an ophthalmic ointment in cats with feline herpes virus-1 (FHV-1).

Pharmacology/Actions

Acyclovir is absorbed through the corneal epithelium and superficial ocular tissues and achieves significant concentrations in aqueous humor. Small quantities (2-16% of the applied dose) appear in urine. In animal studies, acyclovir can be detected in the blood after application of a topical dose. Acyclovir is selectively converted to thymidine kinase within herpes virus cells (not host cells) and inhibits viral replication through inhibition of herpes virus DNA polymerase.

Contraindications/Precautions/Warnings

Acyclovir is contraindicated in patients with a history of hypersensitivity to it or drugs like it (valacyclovir), or to any component of the formulation. Use of acyclovir systemically is contraindicated in cats. Cats receiving oral or parenteral acyclovir can suffer leukopenia and acute anemia. Acyclovir should be used cautiously in animals with dehydration, renal insufficiency, or neurological deficits.

Adverse Effects

Adverse effects reported in humans or animals include: bone marrow suppression, nephrotoxicity, and hepatotoxicity. Mild stinging and blepharitis may occur after application.

Doses

Feline Herpes Virus-1 (extra-label): Acyclovir 3% Ophthalmic Ointment (compounded), 1/8 in strip in the affected eye(s) 5 times daily.

Monitoring

■ Cats: renal function and CBC with prolonged topical therapy.

Client Information

■ Used 5 times daily.

■ Wait 5 minutes after applying this medication before applying any other medications to the eye.

■ Store at controlled room temperature away from moisture and sunlight; do not freeze. Discard if color change, or becomes cloudy.

■ Do not allow cats to lick this medication when grooming.

Storage/Stability

Store at controlled room temperature away from moisture and sunlight.

Compatibility/Compounding Considerations

Acyclovir should not be mixed directly with any other drugs.

Dosage Forms/Regulatory Status

VETERINARY-LABELED PRODUCTS: NONE.

HUMAN-LABELED PRODUCTS:
None in the USA; Acyclovir 3% Ophthalmic Ointment is available in Australia and Europe. It may be prepared (compounded) as an ophthalmic ointment by qualified compounding pharmacists in the absence of an approved product.

Revisions/References
Monograph revised/updated September 2014.

Alcaftadine Ophthalmic

(al-kaf-ta-deen)   Lastacaft®

Antihistamine

Prescriber Highlights

► Indicated for allergic conjunctivitis.
► May cause burning, stinging, and irritation.
► Very expensive.

Uses/Indications

Alcaftadine is approved for use in allergic conjunctivitis in humans and is used in animals to alleviate the clinical signs of allergic conjunctivitis.

Pharmacology/Actions

Alcaftadine is a histamine-1 receptor antagonist. It inhibits the release of mediators including histamine from cells (*e.g.*, mast cells) involved in hypersensitivity reactions and decreases chemotaxis and activation of eosinophils. It appears rapidly in systemic circulation following topical application to eye. Peak plasma concentrations of alcaftadine and its active metabolite occur at a median of 15 minutes and at 1 hour, respectively, after administration. Rapid onset of action with effect on ocular itching is apparent at 3 minutes after conjunctival antigen challenge. The half-life is about 2 hours with a duration of anti-pruritic effect lasting ≈ 16 hours in humans.

Contraindications/Precautions/Warnings

Alcaftadine is contraindicated in patients with a history of hypersensitivity to it or any component of the formulation.

Adverse Effects

Adverse effects reported in humans or animals include irritation, burning and stinging on application, redness, and pruritus. Nasopharyngitis and headache are experienced by humans and may be experienced by animals.

Doses

Allergic conjunctivitis (extra-label): 1 drop in affected eye(s) 1-2 times daily.

Monitoring

■ Clinical efficacy; resolution of ocular pruritus. If pruritus worsens, discontinue.

Client Information

■ Used 1-2 times daily.
■ Use proper administration techniques to avoid contamination of the solution. Keep dropper bottle tightly closed when not in use.
■ Wait 5 minutes after applying this medication before applying any other medications to the eye.
■ Store in the refrigerator or at controlled room temperature away from moisture and sunlight; do not freeze. Do not use if the color changes, becomes cloudy, or if particles are seen in the solution.

Storage/Stability

Store at controlled room temperature away from moisture and sunlight.

Compatibility/Compounding Considerations

Alcaftadine should not be mixed directly with any other drugs.

Dosage Forms/Regulatory Status

VETERINARY-LABELED PRODUCTS: NONE.

HUMAN-LABELED PRODUCTS:
Alcaftadine 0.25% Ophthalmic Solution (containing benzalkonium chloride 0.005%, edetate disodium; sodium phosphate, monobasic; purified water; NaCl; NaOH and/or HCl to adjust pH to 7, with osmolality of 290 mOsm/kg) in 3 mL ophthalmic dropper bottle; Lastacaft®; *(Rx)*

Revisions/References
Monograph revised/updated September 2014.

Amikacin Sulfate Ophthalmic

(am-uh-kay-sin sul-fate)

Aminoglycoside Antibiotic

Prescriber Highlights

► Aminoglycoside antibiotic for susceptible ocular infections that are resistant to other aminoglycoside antibiotics.
► Must be compounded.
► Cats may be more subject to toxic effects.

Uses/Indications

Amikacin sulfate is not manufactured in an ophthalmic dosage form, but it can be prepared (compounded) for use in ophthalmic infections caused by susceptible strains of Pseudomonas, E. coli, Proteus, Klebsiella and other gram-negative bacteria. Amikacin has activity against penicillinase and non-penicillinase-producing species of Staphylococcus, but it has a low order of activity against other gram-positive organisms. Amikacin is less toxic to the back of the eye than other aminoglycoside antibiotics and is sometimes used as an intravitreal injection to treat bacterial endophthalmitis.

Pharmacology/Actions

Amikacin sulfate binds irreversibly to the 30S subunit of the ribosome and inhibits bacterial protein synthesis. Amikacin solutions applied to the conjunctiva achieve therapeutic concentrations in the cornea and the aqueous humor.

Contraindications/Precautions/Warnings

Amikacin sulfate is contraindicated in patients with a history of hypersensitivity to it or any component of the formulation. Ophthalmic amikacin sulfate should be used carefully in animals with renal insufficiency. Cats appear to be more susceptible to the toxic effects of amikacin sulfate than other species.

Adverse Effects

When used systemically, amikacin sulfate can cause nephrotoxicity and neurotoxicity (ototoxicity and vestibular toxicity). Cats are more susceptible to the toxic effects of amikacin and it is recommended to monitor all patients receiving topical amikacin for systemic toxicity. Topical solutions of amikacin generally do not cause local adverse effects.

Doses

Ocular infections (extra-label): Amikacin sulfate 1% or 5% ophthalmic solution: 1 drop in the affected eye(s) or 0.2 mL in the SPL catheter for horses, every 1-2 hours for the first 24 hours, followed by 1 drop in the affected eye(s) or 0.2 mL in the SPL catheter every 4-6 hours.

Monitoring

■ Clinical efficacy: cultures and sensitivity to ensure continued susceptibility.
■ Adverse effects: gross monitoring for vestibular or auditory toxicity; monitor for signs of nephrotoxicity (*e.g.*, casts in the urine).

Client Information

■ Used 4-6 times daily.
■ Wait 5 minutes after applying this medication before applying any other medications to the eye.
■ Store in the refrigerator or at controlled room temperature away

from moisture and sunlight; do not freeze. Do not use if the color changes, becomes cloudy, or if particles are seen in the solution.

Storage/Stability

Store in refrigerator away from moisture and sunlight.

Compatibility/Compounding Considerations

Amikacin sulfate should not be mixed directly with any other drugs.

Dosage Forms/Regulatory Status

VETERINARY-LABELED PRODUCTS: NONE.

HUMAN-LABELED PRODUCTS: NONE.

Amikacin is not approved in an ophthalmic dosage form, but sterile solutions of amikacin 1% or 5% may be prepared (compounded) by qualified compounding pharmacists.

Revisions/References

Monograph revised/updated September 2014.

Aminocaproic Acid Ophthalmic

(a-mee-no-ka-pro-ik ass-id)   Caprogel®

Antifibrinolytic

Prescriber Highlights

▶ Available as an orphan drug (*Caprogel®*); may be submitted for FDA approval.

▶ Used to treat secondary ocular hemorrhage (hyphema) and to prevent intraocular re-bleeding episodes.

▶ May be useful in persistent corneal ulcerations by promoting re-epithelialization by maintaining fibronectin.

▶ Ophthalmic use may avoid severe systemic side effects such as nausea, dizziness, and hypotension.

Uses/Indications

In veterinary patients, aminocaproic acid is most commonly used topically for the treatment of persistent corneal ulceration. Aminocaproic acid maintains fibronectin in the wound to promote re-epithelialization (Regnier *et al.* 2005). Aminocaproic acid is also used topically in the eye to decrease or prevent intraocular re-bleeding episodes, and has been evaluated for treatment of traumatic hyphema in humans. Meta analyses of use of topical aminocaproic acid for resolution of traumatic hyphema in humans have been inconclusive. Topical aminocaproic acid is also used to promote healing in persistent corneal ulcerations by promoting re-epithelialization. In humans, it has been used topically to treat Rosacea.

Pharmacology/Actions

Aminocaproic acid inhibits fibrinolysis via inhibitory effects on plasminogen activator substances and antiplasmin action. It also promotes epithelialization by preserving fibronectin. Aminocaproic acid has been shown to reach antifibrinolytic concentrations in the aqueous humor of humans and rabbits.

Contraindications/Precautions/Warnings

Aminocaproic acid is contraindicated in patients with a history of hypersensitivity to it or any component of the formulation. Systemic aminocaproic acid is contraindicated in patients with active intravascular clotting, and extreme caution is warranted with topical use in these patients.

Adverse Effects

Adverse effects reported in humans or animals include nausea, vomiting, hypotension, and hyperkalemia following systemic administration. These effects are possible but not likely after topical administration.

Doses

Hyphema (extra-label): Clinical investigations applied 1-2 drops in the affected eye once daily for 5 days.

Monitoring

▪ Clinical efficacy. Prevention of re-bleeding. Resolution of hyphema.

Client Information

▪ Used 1 time daily.

▪ Use proper administration techniques to avoid contamination of the medication. Keep cap tightly closed when not in use.

▪ Wait 5 minutes after applying this medication before applying any other medications to the eye.

▪ Store in the refrigerator or at controlled room temperature away from moisture and sunlight; do not freeze. Do not use if the color changes, becomes cloudy, or if particles are seen in the gel.

Storage/Stability

Store in refrigerator or controlled room temperature away from moisture and sunlight; do not freeze.

Compatibility/Compounding Considerations

Aminocaproic acid topical gel should not be mixed directly with any other drugs.

Dosage Forms/Regulatory Status

VETERINARY-LABELED PRODUCTS: NONE.

HUMAN-LABELED PRODUCTS:

Aminocaproic Acid 25% topical gel in 2% carboxy polymethylene; *Caprogel®*; (Rx; Orphan Drug status). Available from: Eastern Virginia Medical School Department of Ophthalmology; 880 Kempsville Road, Suite 2500; Norfolk, VA 23502-3990.

Revisions/References

Monograph revised/updated September 2014.
Regnier, A., et al. (2005). Topical treatment of non-healing corneal epithelial ulcers in dogs with aminocaproic acid. Veterinary Record **157**(17): 510-3.

Amphotericin B Ophthalmic

(am-foe-ter-i-sin bee)

Antifungal

Prescriber Highlights

▶ Not commercially available in an ophthalmic dosage form. Must be compounded.

▶ Solutions may be used topically or injected subconjunctivally.

▶ Do not mix with saline-containing solutions; refrigerate and protect from light.

Uses/Indications

In veterinary patients, amphotericin B is used in the eye to treat fungal ophthalmic infections and fungal keratitis. It is effective against *Histoplasma, Coccidioides, Candida* spp. (except non-albicans), Blastomyces, Cryptococcus, Sporothrix, Mucor, and Aspergillus. Fusarium spp. are usually resistant.

Pharmacology/Actions

Amphotericin B acts by binding fungal sterols in cell membranes resulting in cell content leakage. Amphotericin B is usually fungistatic but can be fungicidal in higher concentrations. Amphotericin B is purported to have immunoadjuvant activity, but further investigation is necessary to confirm this effect.

Contraindications/Precautions/Warnings

Amphotericin B is contraindicated in patients with a history of hypersensitivity to it or any component of the formulation

Adverse Effects

Adverse effects reported in humans or animals include mild burning, stinging, irritation or redness.

Doses

- **AS AN ANTIFUNGAL (EXTRA-LABEL):**
  SPL Catheter: 0.2 mL of a 0.15 – 0.5% solution every 2-6 hours followed by air flush.

  Subconjunctival injection: 0.25 mL of a 0.5 mg/mL solution every 48 hours.

Monitoring

- Clinical efficacy. Corneal scraping to determine resolution of fungal infection.

Client Information

- Used 4-12 times daily.
- Use proper administration techniques to avoid contamination of the medication. Keep cap tightly closed when not in use.
- Wait 5 minutes after applying this medication before applying any other medications to the eye.
- Store in refrigerator protected from light. Discard if color change, or becomes cloudy, or if particles are observed in the solution.

Storage/Stability

Store in refrigerator away from moisture and sunlight; do not freeze.

Compatibility/Compounding Considerations

Amphotericin B should not be mixed with salt-containing solutions and should not be mixed directly with any other drugs. Amphotericin B is not available as an ophthalmic preparation but may be prepared as a topical solution (0.15 – 0.5% in dextrose 5% or sterile water) or as a subconjunctival injection (0.5 mg/mL in sterile water). Historically, only the non-liposomal injection was recommended for compounding topical solutions; however, recent studies demonstrate that liposomal amphotericin B ophthalmic solutions are equally effective and less irritating. Stability is concentration dependent, but most solutions are chemically stable for 7 days in the refrigerator protected from light and recent evidence suggests that ophthalmic solutions prepared from liposomal amphotericin B retain chemical potency for up to 6 months (Morand *et al.* 2007).

Dosage Forms/Regulatory Status

VETERINARY-LABELED PRODUCTS:
None it may be prepared (compounded) as an ophthalmic solution by qualified compounding pharmacists in the absence of an approved product.

HUMAN-LABELED PRODUCTS: NONE.

Revisions/References

Monograph revised/updated September 2014.

Morand, K., et al. (2007). Liposomal amphotericin B eye drops to treat fungal keratitis: Physico-chemical and formulation stability. International Journal of Pharmaceutics 344(1-2): 150-3.

Apraclonidine Ophthalmic

(a-pra-cloe-ni-deen)   Iopidine®

Alpha-Adrenergic Anti-Glaucoma Agent

Prescriber Highlights

▶ Do not use in cats.
▶ May cause dizziness or drowsiness.
▶ Tachyphylaxis may occur with chronic use. MAO inhibitors may inhibit effects.

Uses/Indications

In veterinary patients, apraclonidine is used as a short-term adjunct for patients that are maximally treated with other anti-glaucoma agents, but still require additional lowering of intraocular pressure.

Pharmacology/Actions

Apraclonidine is a relatively selective alpha-2-adrenergic agonist. By reducing the formation of aqueous humor, ocular apraclonidine has the action of reducing elevated, as well as normal, intraocular pressure (IOP), whether or not accompanied by glaucoma. Tachyphylaxis (loss of effect) may occur over time. In humans, tachyphylaxis usually occurs in <1 month.

Contraindications/Precautions/Warnings

Apraclonidine is contraindicated in patients with a history of hypersensitivity to it or any component of the formulation. Apraclonidine should not be used in patients that are receiving clonidine or MAO inhibitors. Do not use in cats as it can cause to bradycardia, hypersalivation, diarrhea, and vomiting. Apraclonidine should be used with caution, if at all, in animals with hepatic or renal insufficiency.

Adverse Effects

Adverse effects reported in humans or animals include conjunctival blanching, eyelid elevation, and mydriasis. Dogs may experience vomiting and diarrhea. Cats experience vomiting, diarrhea, hypersalivation, and bradycardia and apraclonidine should not be used in this species. Rarely, ophthalmic use of apraclonidine may cause dry mouth, dry eye, tachycardia, hypertension, and tachypnea.

Doses

Glaucoma (extra-label): 1 drop in the affected eye(s) every 8-12 hours.

Monitoring

- Clinical efficacy. Reduction of intraocular pressure.

Client Information

- Used 2-3 times daily.
- Use proper administration techniques to avoid contamination of the medication. Keep cap tightly closed when not in use.
- Wait 5 minutes after applying this medication before applying any other medications to the eye.
- Store in the refrigerator or at controlled room temperature away from moisture and sunlight; do not freeze. Do not use if the color changes, becomes cloudy, or if particles are seen in the solution.

Storage/Stability

Store in the refrigerator or at controlled room temperature away from moisture and sunlight; do not freeze.

Compatibility/Compounding Considerations

Apraclonidine should not be mixed directly with any other drugs.

Dosage Forms/Regulatory Status

VETERINARY-LABELED PRODUCTS: NONE.

HUMAN-LABELED PRODUCTS:
Apraclonidine 0.5% Ophthalmic Solution [containing benzalkonium chloride 0.01%, NaCl, sodium acetate, NaOH and/or HCl (pH 4.4-7.8) and purified water] in 5 mL and 10 mL dropper bottles; *Iopidine®; (Rx)*

Revisions/References

Monograph revised/updated September 2014.

Artificial Tears/Ocular Lubricants

Tear Replacement and Ocular Lubricating Agents

Prescriber Highlights

▶ Most human artificial tears and ocular lubricants are OTC.

▶ Preservative-free solutions are less likely to cause stinging or corneal damage with chronic use.

▶ Petroleum based ocular products should not be used in procedures where combustion may occur (*e.g.*, electrocautery, laser).

Uses/Indications

In veterinary patients, artificial tear solutions and ocular lubricants are used any time that tear production is decreased, tear loss through evaporation is increased, when corneal treatment with hydrophilic drugs is required, and when the tear film break up time is abnormal. Artificial tears and ocular lubricants are most commonly used for keratoconjunctivitis sicca (KCS), buphthalmos, lagophthalmos, during prolonged anesthesia to keep the cornea from drying, as a lubricant/cushion when performing gonioscopy, and as a vehicle when compounding water-soluble therapies to treat the cornea. The most commonly used solutions contain: polyvinylpyrrolidone, polyvinyl alcohol (PVA), cellulose solutions (hydroxypropyl methylcellulose (HMC), hydroxypropyl guar (HG), carboxy methylcellulose (CMC)), and hyaluronic acid (HA).

Polyvinyl alcohol (PVA) containing artificial tears work by lubricating the ocular surface. They are available in drops and gel formulations.

Carboxymethylcellulose (CMC) containing derivatives are widely used in artificial tear formulations. They increase the residence time of tears as well as increase the viscosity of tears. The refractive index of 1% methylcellulose is 1.336, which closely matches that of human tears. It has been shown that the mid-viscosity (1.0% CMC) solutions promote significant reduction in the signs and symptoms of dry eye compared to lower viscosity agents. CMC-based artificial tears may be indicated in patients that demonstrate ocular surface staining with vital dyes. Some CMC solutions are also hypotonic. Hyperosmolarity is a common feature of most forms of dry eye disease, and hypotonicity may provide comfort in dry eye patients.

Hydroxypropyl methylcellulose (HMC) containing artificial tears work on the simple principle of lubricating the ocular surface in order to promote the integrity of the surface.

Hydroxypropyl guar (HG) containing artificial tears are gel-forming and improve recovery of the ocular surface due to possible increased retention time of the artificial tear drop. Also, the increased retention time may be responsible for the increase in tear film break-up times observed with HP guar-based artificial tears compared to CMC-based tears. Tear evaporation may be reduced by the use of HP guar containing artificial tears. HP guar-based artificial tears may be helpful in patients with conditions causing evaporative dry eye as well as patients demonstrating ocular surface staining.

Hyaluronic Acid (HA) containing artificial tears are useful in improving subjective symptoms (as well as the ocular health) of dry eye patients, treating lipid tear-deficient patients and managing Sjogrens syndrome patients. Hyaluronic acid also seems to have protective effects on the corneal epithelium.

Petroleum based products (castor oil, petrolatum, and mineral oil) are useful in treating evaporative dry eye conditions and contribute to the re-formation of the lipid layer of the tear film which prevents evaporation of the existing tear film. Castor oil-based eye drops also improve tear stability and aid in the treatment of meibomian gland disease. Mineral oil containing products thicken the layer of the lipid film.

Pharmacology/Actions

Because purely aqueous solutions do not adhere to the lipophilic corneal epithelium they are not useful as tear replacers. To increase their utility in lubricating the eye or delivering drugs to the corneal epithelium, various mucopolysaccharide molecules such as polyvinylpyrrolidone, polyvinyl alcohol, cellulose polymers, and hyaluronic acid are added to aqueous solutions to increase their lipophilicity. Other agents are also added to increase viscosity and therefore retention time and include gelatin, glycerin, polyethylene glycol, pluronic gel, and polysorbate 80. Non-aqueous ocular lubricants such as white petrolatum and mineral oil are also formulated into ocular lubricant ointments to be used during anesthetic procedures where the animal's eyes may remain open without blinking for prolonged periods of time when tears are not produced. Petroleum based products pose potential risk of combustion, and should be used with caution in procedures where combustion is more likely: electrocautery, laser, etc.

Demulcents are included in an ophthalmic solution to provide proper consistency, viscosity, comfort and moisturization and include the following: cellulose derivatives: carboxymethylcellulose sodium 0.2-2.5%, hydroxyethyl cellulose 0.2-2.5%, hydroxypropyl methylcellulose 0.2-2.5%, methylcellulose 0.2-2.5%, dextran 70 0.1%, gelatin 0.01%, glycerin 0.2-1%, polyethylene glycol 300 0.2-1%, polyethylene glycol 400 0.2-1%, polysorbate 80 0.2-1%, polyvinyl alcohol 0.1-4%, and povidone 0.1-2%.

Emollients are lanolin preparations and oleaginous ingredients that provide lubrication and are intended to be soothing. Emollients include lanolin preparations (anhydrous lanolin 1-10% and lanolin 1-10%), oleaginous ingredients (light mineral oil ≤ 50%, Mineral oil ≤ 50%, paraffin ≤ 5%, petrolatum ≤ 100%, white petrolatum ≤ 100%, white wax ≤ 5%, and yellow wax ≤ 5%).

Contraindications/Precautions/Warnings

Artificial tear solutions are contraindicated in patients with a history of hypersensitivity to the mucopolysaccharide or any component of the formulation.

Adverse Effects

Adverse effects reported in humans or animals include eye pain, burning or stinging on instillation, and redness. Preservative-free solutions may decrease these adverse effects. Blurred vision is commonly reported in humans after application of ocular ointments. Sticky eyelashes and increased sensitivity to light are commonly reported with solutions containing hydroxypropyl cellulose.

Doses

Tear replacement (extra-label): 1-2 drops in the affected eye(s) every 2-3 hours or as often as possible.

Ocular lubrication during anesthetic procedures (extra-label): ¼ – ½ inch strip in each eye every 90 minutes. Do not use in procedures where combustion of petroleum based ocular lubricants may occur.

Monitoring

- Clinical efficacy. Chronic use of preserved solutions may cause corneal damage. Monitor corneal surface for any signs of disruption.

Client Information

- Place these drops in your pet's eye(s) as often as possible during the day. Longer acting ointments may be administered at bedtime.

- If you notice any increase in squinting or eye discharge, contact your veterinarian.

- Use proper administration techniques to avoid contamination of the medication. Keep cap tightly closed when not in use.

- Wait 5 minutes after applying this medication before applying any other medications to the eye.

- Store at controlled room temperature away from moisture and sunlight; do not freeze. Do not use if the color changes, becomes cloudy, or if particles are seen in the solution.

Storage/Stability

Store at controlled room temperature away from moisture and sunlight.

Compatibility/Compounding Considerations

Artificial tears and ocular lubricants are often used as vehicles when compounding topical ocular medications. Check to ensure compatibility of all ingredients and preservatives before compounding.

Dosage Forms/Regulatory Status

VETERINARY-LABELED PRODUCTS:
None are FDA approved.

Hyaluronic Acid Products:
Remend® Eye Lubricating Drops [hyaluronic acid 0.4 % (4 mg/mL) Hyasent-S cross-linked, modified hyaluronic acid (HA), in a preservative-free aqueous gel] in a 10 mL ophthalmic dropper bottle; (Rx). **Note:** There is also a 0.75% gel that is marketed as a corneal repair gel for superficial corneal ulcers: *Remend® Corneal Repair Gel*; (Rx)

HUMAN-LABELED PRODUCTS:
There are many products marketed; the following are representative:

Polyvinyl Alcohol Products:
HypoTears® (polyvinyl alcohol 1%, polyethylene glycol 400 1%, benzalkonium chloride 0.1 mg/mL, dextrose, edetate disodium, and purified water. May contain HCl and/or NaOH to adjust pH) in a 15 mL ophthalmic dropper bottle; (OTC)

Murine Tears® [polyvinyl alcohol 0.5%, benzalkonium chloride, dextrose, edetate disodium, potassium chloride, purified water, sodium bicarbonate, NaCl, sodium citrate, sodium phosphate (mono- and dibasic)] in a 15 mL ophthalmic dropper bottle; (OTC)

Polyvinylpyrrolidone Products:
Freshkote® [polyvinyl pyrrolidone 2%, polyvinyl alcohol 0.9% (87% hydrolyzed), polyvinyl alcohol 1.8% (99% hydrolyzed) boric acid, disodium edetate dihydrate, ethanol, glycerin, lecithin, polixetonium, polysorbate-80, potassium chloride, purified water, NaCl] in a 15 mL ophthalmic dropper bottle; (OTC)

Carboxymethylcellulose Products:
TheraTears® (carboxymethylcellulose sodium 1%, borate buffers, calcium chloride, magnesium chloride, potassium chloride, purified water, sodium bicarbonate, NaCl and sodium phosphate) in a 0.6 mL single use vial in containers of 4; (OTC)

Hydroxypropyl Methylcellulose Products:
Tears Naturale® (hypromellose 0.3%, dextran 70 0.1%, potassium chloride, purified water, sodium borate, NaCl, HCl and/or NaOH to adjust pH) in a 0.9 mL single dose vial in cartons of 60; (OTC)

Bion Tears® (hypromellose 0.3%, dextran 70 0.1%, calcium chloride, magnesium chloride, potassium chloride, purified water, sodium bicarbonate, NaCl, zinc chloride, HCl and/or NaOH and/or carbon dioxide to adjust pH) in 0.4 mL single use containers in cartons of 28; (OTC)

Genteal® (carboxymethylcellulose sodium 0.25%, hypromellose 0.3%, Boric acid, calcium chloride dihydrate, citric acid monohydrate, magnesium chloride hexahydrate, phosphonic acid, potassium chloride, purified water, NaCl and sodium perborate, HCl and/or NaOH to adjust pH) in a 15 mL ophthalmic dropper bottle; (OTC)

Visine Tears® (glycerin 0.2%, hypromellose 0.36%, polyethylene glycol 400 1%, ascorbic acid, benzalkonium chloride, boric acid, dextrose, glycine, magnesium chloride, potassium chloride, purified water, sodium borate, NaCl, sodium citrate, sodium lactate, sodium phosphate dibasic) in a 15 mL ophthalmic dropper bottle; (OTC)

Hydroxypropyl Guar Products:
Systane® (hypromellose 0.3%, carbopol 980, phosphonic acid, purified water, sodium perborate and sorbitol) in 10 gram ophthalmic dropper bottles; (OTC)

Hyaluronic Acid Products:
AQuify Comfort Drops® (sodium hyaluronate, NaCl, sodium phosphate and sodium perborate stabilized with phosphoric acid as a preservative) in 10 mL ophthalmic dropper bottles; (OTC)

Blink® [boric acid, calcium chloride, magnesium chloride, potassium chloride, purified water, sodium borate, NaCl, sodium chlorite (*Ocupure®* brand) as a preservative; sodium hyaluronate] in a 15 mL ophthalmic dropper bottle; (OTC)

Petroleum-Based Products:
Lacri-lube S.O.P.® (mineral oil 42.5% and petrolatum 56.8%) in 3.5 gram ophthalmic ointment tubes; (OTC)

Refresh Endura® [glycerin (1%), polysorbate 80 (1%); carbomer, castor oil, mannitol, purified water, and NaOH] in 0.3 mL x 20 single use containers; (OTC)

Soothe XP® (light mineral oil 1% and mineral oil 4.5%) in a 15 mL ophthalmic dropper bottle; (OTC)

Tears Again® (mineral oil 20% and white petrolatum 80%) in a 3.5 gram ophthalmic ointment tube; (OTC)

Revisions/References

Monograph revised/updated 01/2014.

Perry HD, Donnenfeld ED. Medications for dry eye syndrome: a drug-therapy review. Manag Care 2003; 12(12 Suppl): 26-32.

Murube J, Paterson A, Murube E. Classification of artificial tears. I: Composition and properties. Adv Exp Med Biol 1998; 438:693-704.

Simmons PA, Vehige JG. Clinical performance of a mid-viscosity artificial tear for dry eye treatment. Cornea 2007; 26(3): 294-302.

Atropine Sulfate Ophthalmic

(ah-troe-peen suhl-fate)

Mydriatic/Cycloplegic

Prescriber Highlights

▶ Do not use in primary glaucoma.

▶ Rarely can induce colic in horses when systemically absorbed.

▶ Ointment forms may avoid hypersalivation in dogs and cats.

▶ Use caution when handling to prevent cycloplegia/mydriasis in humans; wash hands after use.

Uses/Indications

In veterinary patients, atropine sulfate is used cycloplegic refraction, for pupillary dilation desired in inflammatory conditions of the iris and uveal tract. Atropine sulfate plays an important role in controlling pain secondary to corneal and uveal disease. It is also used perioperatively to maximally dilate the pupil during intraocular surgery. Atropine has also been used to break down synechiae in uveitis.

Pharmacology/Actions

Atropine causes anticholinergic effects by blocking the responses of the sphincter muscle of the iris and the accommodative muscle of the ciliary body to cholinergic stimulation, producing pupillary dilation (mydriasis) and paralysis of accommodation (cycloplegia).

It induces mydriasis in ≈ 1 hour and effects may persist up to 120 hours in dogs, 144 hours in cats, and for days to weeks in horses.

Contraindications/Precautions/Warnings

Atropine sulfate is contraindicated in patients with a history of hypersensitivity to it or any component of the formulation and should not be used in patients with primary glaucoma. Ophthalmic atropine may induce colic in horses secondary to systemic absorption, but this is rarely reported.

Adverse Effects

Adverse effects reported in humans or animals include sensitivity to bright light or sunlight, burning and irritation upon application, and in cats and dogs, decreased tear production and hypersalivation; ointment forms may avoid hypersalivation.

Doses

Mydriasis and Cycloplegia (extra-label): Solution: Initially, 1 drop in the affected eye(s) 2-3 times daily, and then once daily or every other day thereafter to achieve pupillary dilation. Ointment: Initially, 1/8th inch strip in the affected eye(s) 2-3 times daily, and then once daily or every other day thereafter to achieve pupillary dilation.

Monitoring

- Clinical efficacy. Confirm continued pupillary dilation.

Client Information

- Used 2-3 times daily initially and then once daily to once every other day to keep pupil dilated.
- Hypersalivation (drooling) can occur.
- Use proper administration techniques to avoid contamination of the medication. Keep cap tightly closed when not in use.
- Wait 5 minutes after applying atropine before applying any other medications to the eye.
- Wash hands after use to prevent it affecting your eyes.

Storage/Stability

Store at controlled room temperature away from moisture and sunlight; do not freeze.

Compatibility/Compounding Considerations

Atropine sulfate should not be mixed directly with any other drugs.

Dosage Forms/Regulatory Status

VETERINARY-LABELED PRODUCTS: NONE.

HUMAN-LABELED PRODUCTS: NONE.

Atropine Sulfate 1% Ophthalmic Ointment USP, (containing white petrolatum, mineral oil, lanolin oil and purified water) in 3.5 g ophthalmic tubes; *Isopto Atropine 1%*; (Rx)

Atropine Sulfate 1% Ophthalmic Solution, USP, [containing benzalkonium chloride 0.01%, boric acid, NaOH and/or HCl (to adjust pH), water for injection] in 2 mL, 5 mL and 15 mL dropper bottles; *Isopto Atropine®*; (Rx)

Revisions/References

Monograph revised/updated September 2014.

Azelastine Ophthalmic

(a-za-las-teen)   Optivar®

Antihistamine

Prescriber Highlights

▶ Selective H₁ receptor antagonist antihistamine. Rapid onset of action (3 minutes) and long duration of action (8 hours).

▶ Generics available.

Uses/Indications

In veterinary patients, azelastine is used to relieve pruritus caused by allergic conjunctivitis.

Pharmacology/Actions

Azelastine is a relatively selective histamine-1 antagonist and an inhibitor of the release of histamine and other mediators from cells (*e.g.*, mast cells) involved in the allergic response. Based on in-vitro studies using human cell lines, inhibition of other mediators involved in allergic reactions (*e.g.*, leukotrienes and PAF) has been demonstrated with azelastine. Decreased chemotaxis and activation of eosinophils has also been demonstrated. Azelastine has a rapid onset of action (3 minutes) and a long duration of antipruritic action (8 hours).

Contraindications/Precautions/Warnings

Azelastine is contraindicated in patients with a history of hypersensitivity to it or any component of the formulation.

Adverse Effects

Adverse effects reported in humans or animals include transient burning or stinging upon instillation in the eye. Humans experience headaches and a bad taste in the mouth; animals may also experience these side effects.

Doses

Allergic conjunctivitis (extra-label): 1 drop in the affected eye(s) 2 times daily.

Monitoring

- Clinical efficacy. Resolution of pruritus and conjunctivitis.

Client Information

- Used 2 times daily.
- Use proper administration techniques to avoid contamination of the medication. Keep lid tightly closed when not in use.
- Wait 5 minutes after applying this medication before applying any other medications to the eye.
- Store in the refrigerator or at controlled room temperature away from moisture and sunlight; do not freeze. Do not use if the color changes, becomes cloudy, or if particles are seen in the solution.

Storage/Stability

Store in refrigerator or at controlled room temperature away from moisture and sunlight.

Compatibility/Compounding Considerations

Azelastine should not be mixed directly with any other drugs.

Dosage Forms/Regulatory Status

VETERINARY-LABELED PRODUCTS: NONE.

HUMAN-LABELED PRODUCTS:

Azelastine HCl 0.05% Ophthalmic Solution (containing 0.01% benzalkonium chloride, disodium edetate dihydrate, hypromellose, sorbitol solution, NaOH and water for injection, pH of ≈ 5.0-6.5, osmolarity of ≈ 271-312 mOsm/kg) in a 6 mL dropper bottle; *Optivar®*; (Rx)

Revisions/References

Monograph revised/updated September 2014.

Azithromycin Ophthalmic

(uh-zith-roe-mye-sin)   Azasite®

Macrolide Antibiotic

Prescriber Highlights

▶ Used twice daily initially, then once daily.

▶ May cause reversible phospholipid accumulation in the cornea.

▶ Store in refrigerator. Discard 14 days after opening.

Uses/Indications

In veterinary patients, azithromycin ophthalmic solution is used to treat susceptible strains of Haemophilus, Streptococcus, and Staphylococcus.

Pharmacology/Actions

Azithromycin is a bacteriostatic macrolide antibiotic that acts by binding to the 50S ribosomal subunit of susceptible microorganisms and interfering with microbial protein synthesis.

Contraindications/Precautions/Warnings

Azithromycin is contraindicated in patients with a history of hypersensitivity to it or any component of the formulation. Azithromycin ophthalmic solution is indicated for topical ophthalmic use only, and should not be administered systemically, injected subconjunctivally, or introduced directly into the anterior chamber of the eye.

Adverse Effects

Adverse effects reported in humans or animals include burning, stinging and irritation upon application. Azithromycin ophthalmic solution has also caused phospholipidosis (intracellular phospholipid accumulation) causing cytoplasmic microvacuolation of the cornea that resolves upon discontinuation of the medication.

Doses

Bacterial conjunctivitis (extra-label): 1 drop in the affected eye(s) 2 times daily the first day, followed by once daily for 5 days.

Monitoring

▪ Clinical efficacy. Resolution of bacterial conjunctivitis.

Client Information

▪ Used 2 times daily the first day, then once daily for 5 more days.

▪ Wait 5 minutes after applying this medication before applying any other medications to the eye.

▪ Store in refrigerator and discard 14 days after opening or if solution color changes, becomes cloudy, or if particles are observed.

▪ Use proper administration techniques to avoid contamination of the medication. Keep cap tightly closed when not in use.

Storage/Stability

Store in refrigerator away from moisture and sunlight; do not freeze. Discard 14 days after opening.

Compatibility/Compounding Considerations

Azithromycin ophthalmic should not be mixed directly with any other drugs.

Dosage Forms/Regulatory Status

VETERINARY-LABELED PRODUCTS: NONE.

HUMAN-LABELED PRODUCTS:

Azithromycin 1% Ophthalmic Solution [containing *DuraSite®* (polycarbophil, edetate disodium, NaCl), 0.003% benzalkonium chloride. mannitol, citric acid, sodium citrate, poloxamer 407, polycarbophil, edetate disodium (EDTA), NaCl, water for injection, and NaOH to adjust pH to 6.3 with an osmolality of ≈ 290 mOsm/kg] in a 2.5 mL dropper bottle; *Azasite®*; (Rx)

Revisions/References

Monograph revised/updated September 2014.

Bacitracin Ophthalmic

(bas-i-tray-sin)

Polypeptide Antibiotic

Prescriber Highlights

▶ Typically one component of an antibiotic combination (*e.g.*, triple antibiotic); found only in ointment forms.

▶ Do not use OTC bacitracin dermatological ointment in the eye.

▶ Prolonged use of antibiotic preparations may result in overgrowth of non-susceptible organisms, including fungi.

Uses/Indications

Bacitracin ophthalmic products are used in combination primarily with neomycin and polymyxin B for topical treatment of superficial infections of the external eye and its adnexa caused by susceptible bacteria, including conjunctivitis, keratitis and keratoconjunctivitis, blepharitis, and blepharoconjunctivitis. Due to toxicity risks, systemic and irrigant uses of bacitracin should be limited to situations where less toxic alternatives would not be effective.

Pharmacology/Actions

Bacitracin is polypeptide antibiotic, produced by a strain of *Bacillus subtilis*. Bacitracin inhibits bacterial cell wall synthesis by preventing transfer of mucopeptides into the growing cell wall. It has a bactericidal activity *in vitro* against a variety of gram-positive organisms and a few gram-negative organisms. However, in practice, topical bacitracin is typically most useful for gram-positive bacillus infections. Bacitracin is minimally absorbed after oral administration and poorly penetrates the cornea. It is of limited value in deep corneal or intraocular infections.

Contraindications/Precautions/Warnings

Bacitracin combinations are contraindicated in patients with a history of hypersensitivity to any component of the formulation. Some cats are hypersensitive to the neomycin or polymyxin component of combination ointments. Prolonged use of antibiotic preparations may result in overgrowth of non-susceptible organisms, including fungi. Bacitracin is minimally absorbed after oral absorption, however severe gram-negative colitis may result if topical bacitracin is ingested through grooming.

Adverse Effects

Adverse effects reported in humans or animals include irritation and swelling upon instillation. Topically applied bacitracin has resulted in local sensitivity reactions in humans. Topical antibiotics, especially those containing neomycin sulfate and polymyxin B may cause cutaneous sensitization and anaphylaxis, particularly in cats. Clinical signs associated with sensitization to topical antibiotics can include itching, reddening, and edema of the conjunctiva and eyelid, but may progress to anaphylaxis. Symptoms usually subside quickly on withdrawing the medication.

Doses

Conjunctivitis or Keratitis: 1 drop of the triple antibiotic solution or ¼ inch strip of the triple antibiotic ointment in the affected eye(s) 3-4 times daily until resolution or microbial susceptibilities necessitate a change to another antimicrobial agent.

Monitoring

▪ Clinical efficacy. Resolution of conjunctivitis or keratitis as evidenced by cytology, cultures, or remission of symptoms.

Client Information

▪ Used 3-4 times daily.

▪ Cats can have a severe allergic reaction to one of the components of this medication. Contact your veterinarian immediately if your cat has difficulty breathing or facial swelling after receiving this medication.

- Use proper administration techniques to avoid contamination of the medication. Keep cap tightly closed when not in use.
- Wait 5 minutes after applying this medication before applying any other medications to the eye.
- Store at controlled room temperature; do not freeze. Do not use if the color changes.

Storage/Stability

Store at controlled room temperature away from moisture and sunlight.

Compatibility/Compounding Considerations

Bacitracin ophthalmic should not be mixed directly with any other drugs.

Dosage Forms/Regulatory Status

VETERINARY-LABELED PRODUCTS:

Triple Antibiotic Ophthalmic Ointment (containing: neomycin sulfate equivalent to 3.5 mg neomycin base, polymyxin B sulfate equivalent to 10,000 polymyxin B units, bacitracin zinc equivalent to 400 bacitracin units, and white petrolatum and mineral oil, q.s.) in a 3.5 g ophthalmic ointment tube; *TriOptic-P®*, *Vetropolycin®*; (Rx)

Triple Antibiotic with Hydrocortisone Ophthalmic Ointment; each gram contains: bacitracin zinc USP 400 units, neomycin sulfate 0.5% (equivalent to 3.5 mg neomycin base), polymyxin B sulfate USP 10,000 units, hydrocortisone acetate USP 1.0% in a base of white petrolatum and mineral oil; *TriOptic-S®*, *Vetropolycin HC®*; (Rx)

HUMAN-LABELED PRODUCTS:

Bacitracin 500 Units/g & Polymyxin B Sulfate 10,000 Units/g Ophthalmic Ointment in a 3.5 g tube; *Polysporin®*, *AK-Polybac®*, *Polycin®*, generic (Double Antibiotic Ophthalmic Ointment); (Rx)

Triple Antibiotic Ophthalmic Ointment (containing: neomycin sulfate equivalent to 3.5 mg neomycin base, polymyxin B sulfate equivalent to 5,000 or 10,000 polymyxin B units, bacitracin zinc equivalent to 400 bacitracin units, and white petrolatum, q.s) in a 3.5 gram ophthalmic ointment tube; *Neo-Polycin®*, generic; (Rx)

Revisions/References

Monograph revised/updated September 2014.

Benoxinate Ophthalmic

(bin-ak-sin-ate)   Oxybuprocaine, Altafluor®, Fluress®

Topical Ocular Anesthetic

Prescriber Highlights

▶ Less burning, stinging and chemosis than tetracaine.
▶ Only available in combinations with vital dyes.

Uses/Indications

In veterinary patients benoxinate has only recently been utilized. Benoxinate is only available in unapproved ophthalmic solutions combined with vital dyes such as fluorescein and is therefore most useful when determining the presence of corneal injury. Benoxinate causes fewer adverse reactions (burning, stinging, and chemosis) in dogs than tetracaine (Douet *et al.* 2013).

Pharmacology/Actions

Local anesthetics such as benoxinate stabilize the neuronal membrane by inhibiting the ionic fluxes required for the initiation and conduction of impulses thereby effecting local anesthetic action. Benoxinate appears to bind or antagonize the function of voltage gated sodium channels. The exact mechanism whereby local anesthetics influence the permeability of the cell membrane is unknown; however, several studies indicate that local anesthetics may limit sodium ion permeability through the lipid layer of the nerve cell membrane. Benoxinate may alter epithelial sodium channels through interaction with channel protein residues. This limitation prevents the fundamental change necessary for the generation of the action potential.

Contraindications/Precautions/Warnings

Benoxinate is contraindicated in patients with a history of hypersensitivity to it or any component of the formulation. Prolonged use of a topical ocular anesthetic may produce keratitis and permanent corneal opacification with accompanying loss of vision. Prolonged use results in retarded wound healing and causes corneal epithelial ulcers. The blink reflex is suppressed or absent after benoxinate administration, and the eye should be protected from external injury during use.

Adverse Effects

Adverse effects reported in humans or animals include transient stinging, burning, and conjunctival redness. Benoxinate is associated with less burning and chemosis than tetracaine. A rare, severe, immediate type allergic corneal reaction has been reported characterized by acute diffuse epithelial keratitis with filament formation and/or sloughing of large areas of necrotic epithelium, diffuse stromal edema, descemetitis and iritis.

Doses

Ophthalmic procedures requiring local anesthesia (extra-label): 1-2 drops in the target eye(s) prior to examination or procedure. Onset of action is in 6-20 seconds. Duration of corneal anesthesia is ≈ 15 minutes.

Monitoring

- **Diagnostic agent.** Chronic use will delay wound healing and cause loss of vision through corneal opacification.

Client Information

- Benoxinate is not administered by pet owners in the home. It is used for diagnostic procedures in the veterinary practice.

Storage/Stability

Store in refrigerator or at controlled room temperature (per product labeling) away from moisture and sunlight; do not freeze. Discard if color change, or becomes cloudy, or if particles are observed in the solution.

Compatibility/Compounding Considerations

Benoxinate should not be mixed directly with any other drugs.

Dosage Forms/Regulatory Status

VETERINARY-LABELED PRODUCTS: NONE.

HUMAN-LABELED PRODUCTS:

Benoxinate HCl 0.4% and Fluorescein Sodium 0.25% (containing: chlorobutanol 1%; povidone, boric acid; purified water; HCl may be added to adjust pH to 4.3-5.3) in 5 mL ophthalmic dropper bottles; *Altafluor®*, *Fluress®*; (Rx). No benoxinate ophthalmic products have been approved by the US FDA.

Revisions/References

Monograph revised/updated September 2014.

Douet, J. Y., et al. (2013). Degree and duration of corneal anesthesia after topical application of 0.4% oxybuprocaine hydrochloride ophthalmic solution in ophthalmically normal dogs. American Journal of Veterinary Research 74(10): 1321-6.

Bepotastine Ophthalmic

(be-po-tas-teen)   Bepreve®

Antihistamine

Prescriber Highlights

▶ H₁ receptor antagonist antihistamine.

▶ Used twice daily.

Uses/Indications

In veterinary patients, bepotastine is used to relieve pruritus caused by allergic conjunctivitis.

Pharmacology/Actions

Bepotastine acts a direct histamine (H1) antagonist. It also has mast cell stabilizing effects to prevent the release of histamine and other allergic reaction mediators.

Contraindications/Precautions/Warnings

Bepotastine is contraindicated in patients with a history of hypersensitivity to it or any component of the formulation.

Adverse Effects

Adverse effects reported in humans or animals include transient burning or stinging upon instillation in the eye. Humans experience headaches and a bad taste in the mouth; animals may also experience these side effects.

Doses

Allergic conjunctivitis (extra-label): 1 drop in the affected eye(s) 2 times daily.

Monitoring

▪ Clinical efficacy. Resolution of pruritus and conjunctivitis.

Client Information

▪ Used 2 times daily.

▪ Use proper administration techniques to avoid contamination of the medication. Keep cap tightly closed when not in use.

▪ Wait 5 minutes after applying this medication before applying any other medications to the eye.

▪ Store at controlled room temperature away from moisture and sunlight; do not freeze. Do not use if the color changes, becomes cloudy, or if particles are seen in the solution.

Storage/Stability

Store at controlled room temperature away from moisture and sunlight; do not freeze.

Compatibility/Compounding Considerations

Bepotastine should not be mixed directly with any other drugs.

Dosage Forms/Regulatory Status

VETERINARY-LABELED PRODUCTS: NONE.

HUMAN-LABELED PRODUCTS:

Bepotastine Besilate 1.5% Ophthalmic solution (containing benzalkonium chloride 0.005%, monobasic sodium phosphate dihydrate, NaCl, NaOH to adjust pH to 6.8, and water for injection, USP, with an osmolality of 290 mOsm/kg.) in 5 mL and 10 mL dropper bottles; *Bepreve®*; (Rx)

Revisions/References

Monograph revised/updated September 2014.

Besifloxacin Ophthalmic

(be-si-**flocks**-a sin)   Besivance®

Fluoroquinolone Antibiotic

Prescriber Highlights

▶ Fluoroquinolone antimicrobial used for bacterial conjunctivitis or keratitis.

▶ Physically incompatible with many drugs.

▶ Crystalline drug precipitates may be noted in the superficial portion of corneal defects during use.

Uses/Indications

In veterinary patients, besifloxacin ophthalmic may be useful for treating bacterial conjunctivitis caused by susceptible species/strains of staphylococci, streptococci, Corynebacteria, Haemophilus, and chlamydia. When administered via a subpalpebral lavage (SPL) catheter besifloxacin ophthalmic solution can be used for treating equine bacterial keratitis.

Pharmacology/Actions

Besifloxacin is a member of the fluoroquinolone class of anti-infective drugs. Its action results from inhibition of DNA gyrase, which is involved in replication, transcription and repair of bacterial DNA.

Contraindications/Precautions/Warnings

Besifloxacin is contraindicated in patients with a history of hypersensitivity to besifloxacin, to other fluoroquinolones, or any component of the formulation. For topical ophthalmic use only; not for injection subconjunctivally or into the anterior chamber of the eye. Fluoroquinolone-induced retinal toxicity in domestic cats has not been demonstrated with this product at time of writing (2014).

Adverse Effects

Adverse effects reported in humans or animals include blurred vision, tearing, eye pain, redness, itching, and a bad taste in the mouth. Crystalline drug precipitates may be noted in the superficial portion of corneal defects during use.

Doses

Conjunctivitis (extra-label): 1 drop affected eye(s) every 4-8 hours.

Keratitis (extra-label): 1 drop in the affected eye or 0.2 mL in the SPL catheter every 1-8 hours. May precipitate when mixed with other ophthalmic medications. Flush SPL catheter well with air between medications.

Monitoring

▪ Clinical efficacy. If blepharospasm, uveitis, or worsening of ulceration or no improvement in infection is noted in 7 days, reassess microbial susceptibility.

Client Information

▪ Used 3-12 times daily.

▪ Crystals may appear in the eyes for a few days after initiation of treatment.

▪ Wait 5 minutes after applying this medication before applying any other medications to the eye.

▪ Do not freeze. Dispose of unused medication in regular trash, do not put into sewer system.

Storage/Stability

Store at controlled room temperature away from moisture and sunlight; do not freeze.

Compatibility/Compounding Considerations

Fluoroquinolone antibiotics interact with many other drugs including those containing cations (*e.g.*, iron, aluminum, magnesium, calcium, etc.). Besifloxacin should not be mixed directly with any other drugs.

Dosage Forms/Regulatory Status

VETERINARY-LABELED PRODUCTS: NONE.

HUMAN-LABELED PRODUCTS:

Besifloxacin 0.6% (6 mg/mL) Ophthalmic Solution (containing benzalkonium chloride 0.01%, polycarbophil, mannitol, poloxamer 407, NaCl, edetate disodium dihydrate, NaOH and water for injection, with an osmolality of ≈ 290 mOsm/kg) in a 5 mL dropper bottle; *Besivance®*; (Rx).

Revisions/References

Monograph revised/updated September 2014.

Betamethasone Ophthalmic

(bate-uh-meth-uh-sown)

Corticosteroid Antiinflammatory Agent

Prescriber Highlights

► No longer commercially available; must be compounded.
► Do not use in feline herpes keratitis, fungal keratitis, or if corneal abrasion or ulceration are suspected.

Uses/Indications

In veterinary patients, betamethasone is used alone or in combination with aminoglycoside antibiotics for inflammatory conjunctivitis.

Pharmacology/Actions

A long-acting synthetic derivative of prednisolone, betamethasone has a 16β-methyl group that enhances the antiinflammatory action of the molecule and reduces the sodium- and water-retaining properties of prednisolone.

Contraindications/Precautions/Warnings

Betamethasone is contraindicated in patients with a history of hypersensitivity to it or any component of the formulation. Betamethasone should not be used if corneal abrasion or ulceration are suspected and should not be used to treat fungal or viral keratitis (*e.g.,* feline herpes keratitis). Ophthalmic steroids should be used with extreme caution in avian species due to increased risk for systemic adverse effects.

Adverse Effects

Adverse effects reported in humans or animals include burning, stinging and irritation upon application to the eye. Systemic absorption may result in suppression of the hypothalamus-pituitary-adrenal axis. Use of corticosteroids may produce posterior subcapsular cataracts, glaucoma with possible damage to the optic nerves, and may enhance the establishment of secondary ocular infections due to bacteria, fungi, or viruses. Intraocular pressure may increase in some animals with chronic use.

Doses

Inflammatory conjunctivitis (extra-label): 1 drop in the affected eye(s) up to 4 times daily.

Monitoring

▪ Clinical efficacy. Monitor for resolution of inflammatory signs; discontinue use if corneal abrasion or ulceration is present.

Client Information

▪ Used 4 times daily.
▪ Shake well before using.
▪ Use proper administration techniques to avoid contamination of the medication. Keep cap tightly closed when not in use.
▪ Wait 5 minutes after applying this medication before applying any other medications to the eye.
▪ Store in the refrigerator or at controlled room temperature away from moisture and sunlight; do not freeze.

Storage/Stability

Store in refrigerator or controlled room temperature away from moisture and sunlight; do not freeze.

Compatibility/Compounding Considerations

Betamethasone should not be mixed directly with any other drugs.

Dosage Forms/Regulatory Status

VETERINARY-LABELED PRODUCTS: NONE.

HUMAN-LABELED PRODUCTS: NONE.

Betamethasone 0.1% and gentamicin sulfate 0.3% ophthalmic suspension was formerly available as *Gentocin Durafilm®*. It is no longer commercially available but may be prepared (compounded) by appropriately qualified compounding pharmacists.

Revisions/References

Monograph revised/updated September 2014.

Betaxolol Ophthalmic

(be-tax-uh-lol)   Betoptic®

Beta-Adrenergic Blocker

Prescriber Highlights

► Must use 0.5% solution; 0.25% solutions are not effective in reducing intraocular pressure in veterinary patients.
► Delays onset of glaucoma in normal eye of dogs with unilateral glaucoma.

Uses/Indications

Betaxolol is used to reduce intraocular pressure in primary glaucoma and as prophylaxis to prevent glaucoma in the normal eye of animals with unilateral glaucoma.

Pharmacology/Actions

Betaxolol works through blockade of the ciliary body epithelium beta-receptors to reduce intraocular pressure. Several mechanisms have been postulated for this effect including beta-blockade of norepinephrine-induced tonic sympathetic stimulation, decreased activation of cAMP in the ciliary body leading to decreased aqueous humor production, inhibition of $Na^+K^+ATPase$ activity, or through vasoactive mechanisms. Betaxolol also inhibits glutamine-induced increases in intracellular calcium thereby providing a potential protective effect against ischemic insult to the retina.

Contraindications/Precautions/Warnings

Betaxolol is contraindicated in patients with a history of hypersensitivity to it or any component of the formulation. Betaxolol should be used carefully in patients with heart block, bradycardia, heart failure, asthma, chronic bronchitis, or other cardiopulmonary conditions, although systemic cardiopulmonary adverse effects are not likely with ocular use of betaxolol. Because beta-blockers can mask the signs of hypoglycemia, betaxolol should be used cautiously in diabetic patients.

Adverse Effects

Adverse effects reported in humans or animals include transient burning, stinging, and irritation upon application to the eye.

Doses

Glaucoma (extra-label): 1 drop in the affected eye(s) twice daily.

Monitoring

▪ Clinical efficacy. Monitor intraocular pressure.

Client Information

▪ Used 2 times daily.
▪ Shake well before using.
▪ Use proper administration techniques to avoid contamination of the medication. Keep cap tightly closed when not in use.

- Wait 5 minutes after applying this medication before applying any other medications to the eye.
- Store in the refrigerator or at controlled room temperature away from moisture and sunlight; do not freeze. Do not use if the color changes, becomes cloudy, or if particles are seen in the solution.

Storage/Stability

Store in refrigerator or controlled room temperature away from moisture and sunlight; do not freeze.

Compatibility/Compounding Considerations

Betaxolol should not be mixed directly with any other drugs.

Dosage Forms/Regulatory Status

VETERINARY-LABELED PRODUCTS: NONE.

HUMAN-LABELED PRODUCTS:

Betaxolol HCl 0.5% Ophthalmic Solution [containing benzalkonium chloride 0.01%, edetate disodium, NaCl, HCl and/or NaOH (to adjust pH), and purified water] in 2.5 mL, 5 mL, 10 mL and 15 mL ophthalmic dropper bottles; generic; (Rx)

Betaxolol 0.25% ophthalmic solution (*Betoptic-S*®) is generally not used by veterinary ophthalmologists as it is not effective in reducing intraocular pressure in animals.

Revisions/References

Monograph revised/updated September 2014.

Bartlett JR, Fiscella R. (2008) Ocular Hypotensive Drugs. *Clinical Ocular Pharmacology 5th ed.* J Bartlett and S Jaanus eds. St. Louis, Butterworth-Heinenmann: 139-174.

Bimatoprost Ophthalmic

(bi-mat-oh-prost)   Lumigan®

Prostaglandin Analog Ocular Hypotensive Agent

Prescriber Highlights

- ▶ Not effective for feline glaucoma.
- ▶ Not used if intraocular inflammation present; may worsen.
- ▶ Twice daily dosing results in less fluctuation of intraocular pressure. Lower concentration of benzalkonium chloride than latanoprost or travoprost; causes less ocular discomfort on administration.
- ▶ May increase brown pigment resulting in discoloration of light colored irises; increased eyelash growth.

Uses/Indications

In veterinary patients (not cats), bimatoprost is used to lower intraocular pressure in the management of glaucoma.

Pharmacology/Actions

Bimatoprost, a prostaglandin analog, is a synthetic structural analog of prostaglandin derived from a fatty acid precursor, anandamide. It selectively mimics the effects of naturally prostamides. Bimatoprost is believed to lower intraocular pressure (IOP) by increasing outflow of aqueous humor through both the trabecular meshwork and uveoscleral routes. The onset of action is in 4 hours with duration of action 8-12 hours.

Contraindications/Precautions/Warnings

Bimatoprost is contraindicated in patients with a history of hypersensitivity to it or any component of the formulation. Bimatoprost should not be used in the presence of intraocular inflammation (*e.g.*, uveitis) as it will worsen this condition.

Adverse Effects

Adverse effects reported in humans or animals include stinging, burning, erythema (conjunctival hyperemia) and irritation on administration. Macular edema has been reported in humans using bimatoprost. May cause darkening of the iris through direct stimulation of iris melanocytes. May cause increased eyelash growth.

May worsen intraocular inflammation through prostaglandin-mediated mechanisms.

Doses

Glaucoma (extra-label): Initially, 1 drop in the affected eye(s) once daily in the evening; increase to twice daily as glaucoma progresses.

Monitoring

- Clinical efficacy. Continued reduction of intraocular pressure.

Client Information

- Used 1 time daily initially but may be increased to 2 times daily as glaucoma progresses.
- Use proper administration techniques to avoid contamination of the medication. Keep cap tightly closed when not in use.
- Wait 5 minutes after applying this medication before applying any other medications to the eye.
- Store in the refrigerator or at controlled room temperature away from moisture and sunlight; do not freeze. Do not use if the color changes, becomes cloudy, or if particles are seen in the solution.

Storage/Stability

Store in the refrigerator or at controlled room temperature away from moisture and sunlight; do not freeze.

Compatibility/Compounding Considerations

Bimatoprost should not be mixed directly with any other drugs.

Dosage Forms/Regulatory Status

VETERINARY-LABELED PRODUCTS: NONE.

HUMAN-LABELED PRODUCTS:

Bimatoprost 0.01% Ophthalmic Solution (containing benzalkonium chloride 0.02%, NaCl; sodium phosphate, dibasic; citric acid; and purified water, NaOH and/or HCl to adjust pH to 6.8-7.8, with an osmolality of 290 mOsm/kg) in a 2.5 mL, 5 mL, and 7.5 mL dropper bottle; *Lumigan*®; (Rx).

Bimatoprost 0.03% Ophthalmic Solution (containing benzalkonium chloride 0.005%, NaCl; sodium phosphate, dibasic; citric acid; and purified water, NaOH and/or HCl to adjust pH to 6.8-7.8, with an osmolality of 290 mOsm/kg) in a 2.5 mL, 5 mL, and 7.5 mL dropper bottle; *Lumigan*®, *Latisse*®; (Rx). **Note:** *Latisse*® is approved for topical use only for inducing eyelash growth and should not be used in the eye.

Revisions/References

Monograph revised/updated September 2014.

Brimonidine Ophthalmic

(bri-moe-ni-deen)   Alphagan P®, Combigan®, Simbrinza®

Alpha-Adrenergic Anti-Glaucoma Agent

Prescriber Highlights

- ▶ Greenish-yellow color of solution is characteristic and not a sign of degradation or contamination.
- ▶ Longer duration of action than apraclonidine.
- ▶ Generics now available.

Uses/Indications

In veterinary patients, brimonidine (alone or in combination with timolol or brinzolamide) is used to treat elevated intraocular pressure (IOP) in patients with glaucoma or ocular hypertension.

Pharmacology/Actions

Brimonidine is a relatively selective alpha-2 adrenergic receptor agonist with a peak ocular hypotensive effect occurring at 2 hours post-dosing. Fluorophotometric studies in animals and humans suggest that brimonidine tartrate has a dual mechanism of action by reducing aqueous humor production and increasing uveoscleral outflow.

Contraindications/Precautions/Warnings

Brimonidine is contraindicated in patients with a history of hypersensitivity to it or any component of the formulation. Brimonidine should be used cautiously if at all in vascular insufficiency syndromes (*e.g.*, laminitis, cerebral or coronary vascular insufficiency). Concomitant use of MAO inhibitors may potentiate risk of systemic hypotension. Instruct pet owner to keep out of reach of household pets as ingestion of brimonidine ophthalmic solution has caused serious cardiovascular toxicities. Overdoses of brimonidine can be treated with atipamezole, yohimbine and other alpha-2 antagonists.

Adverse Effects

Adverse effects reported in humans or animals include allergic conjunctivitis, conjunctival hyperemia, ocular pruritus, burning, stinging and irritation.

Doses

Glaucoma (extra-label): 1 drop in the affected eye(s) 2-3 times daily.

Monitoring

- Clinical efficacy. Continued control of intraocular pressure.

Client Information

- Used 2-3 times daily.
- Keep out of reach of household pets as ingestion of brimonidine ophthalmic solution can cause serious heart problems.
- Use proper administration techniques to avoid contamination of the medication. Keep cap tightly closed when not in use.
- Wait 5 minutes after applying this medication before applying any other medications to the eye.
- Store in the refrigerator or at controlled room temperature away from moisture and sunlight; do not freeze. Do not use if the color changes, becomes cloudy, or if particles are seen in the solution.

Storage/Stability

Store at controlled room temperature away from moisture and sunlight; do not freeze.

Compatibility/Compounding Considerations

Brimonidine should not be mixed directly with any other drugs.

Dosage Forms/Regulatory Status

VETERINARY-LABELED PRODUCTS: NONE.

HUMAN-LABELED PRODUCTS:

Brimonidine Tartrate: 0.1%, 0.15%, or 0.2% Ophthalmic Solution (containing benzalkonium chloride 0.005%, citric acid, polyvinyl alcohol, NaCl, sodium citrate, purified water, HCl and/or NaOH added to adjust pH to 5.6-6.6, with an osmolality of 280-330 mOsm/kg) in a 5 mL, 10 mL and 15 mL dropper bottle; *Alphagan®*, generic; (Rx).

Brimonidine Tartrate 0.2% and Timolol Maleate 0.5% Ophthalmic Solution (containing benzalkonium chloride 0.005%, citric acid, polyvinyl alcohol, NaCl, sodium citrate, purified water, HCl and/or NaOH added to adjust pH to 5.6-6.6, with an osmolality of 280-330 mOsm/kg) in a 10 mL dropper bottle; *Combigan®*; (Rx).

Brimonidine Tartrate 0.2% and Brinzolamide 1% Ophthalmic Suspension; *Simbrinza®*; (Rx)

Revisions/References

Monograph revised/updated September 2014.

Brinzolamide Ophthalmic

(bryn-zoe-la-mide)   Azopt®, Simbrinza®

Carbonic Anhydrase Inhibitor Ocular Antihypertensive Agent

Prescriber Highlights

▶ May be better tolerated than dorzolamide; however, stinging upon application is likely.

▶ Sulfonamide derivative; caregivers with sulfa allergies should avoid direct contact.

▶ May be administered once daily in horses.

Uses/Indications

In veterinary patients, brinzolamide (alone or in combination with brimonidine) is used to decrease intraocular pressure in glaucoma and ocular hypertension.

Pharmacology/Actions

Carbonic anhydrase (CA) is an enzyme found in many tissues of the body including the eye. It catalyzes the reversible reaction involving the hydration of carbon dioxide and the dehydration of carbonic acid. In humans, carbonic anhydrase exists as a number of isoenzymes, the most active being carbonic anhydrase II (CA-II), found primarily in red blood cells (RBCs), but also in other tissues. Inhibition of carbonic anhydrase in the ciliary processes of the eye decreases aqueous humor secretion, presumably by slowing the formation of bicarbonate ions with subsequent reduction in sodium and fluid transport. The result is a reduction in intraocular pressure (IOP).

Contraindications/Precautions/Warnings

Brinzolamide is contraindicated in patients with a history of hypersensitivity to it or drugs like it such as sulfonamides, or any component of the formulation. Caregivers with sulfonamide allergies should use caution when applying brinzolamide.

Adverse Effects

Adverse effects reported in humans or animals include stinging, burning and irritation upon application. Cats are more susceptible to irritation from brinzolamide than other species. Corneal edema may occur in patients with low corneal endothelial cell counts. Humans experience headaches and a bitter taste in the mouth. It is possible that animals experience these side effects.

Doses

Glaucoma (extra-label):

Dogs and Cats: 1 drop in the affected eye(s) 2-3 times daily and adjusted according to effect on intraocular pressure.

Horses: 2 drops in the affected eye(s) once daily.

Monitoring

- Clinical efficacy. Confirm control of intraocular hypertension.

Client Information

- Used 2-3 times daily.
- Shake well before using.
- Use proper administration techniques to avoid contamination of the medication. Keep cap tightly closed when not in use.
- Wait 5 minutes after applying this medication before applying any other medications to the eye.
- Store in the refrigerator or at controlled room temperature away from moisture and sunlight; do not freeze. Do not use if the color changes or if particles are seen in the suspension.

Storage/Stability

Store in refrigerator or at controlled room temperature away from moisture and sunlight; do not freeze.

Compatibility/Compounding Considerations
Brinzolamide should not be mixed directly with any other drugs.

Dosage Forms/Regulatory Status
VETERINARY-LABELED PRODUCTS: NONE.
HUMAN-LABELED PRODUCTS:
Brinzolamide 1% Ophthalmic Suspension (containing, benzalkonium chloride 0.01%, mannitol, carbomer 974P, tyloxapol, edetate disodium, NaCl, purified water, HCl and/or NaOH to adjust pH to 7.5 and an osmolality of 300 mOsm/kg) in 10 mL and 15 mL dropper bottles; *Azopt®*; (Rx).

Brimonidine Tartrate: 0.2% and Brinzolamide: 1% Ophthalmic Suspension; *Simbrinza®*; (Rx)

Revisions/References
Monograph revised/updated September 2014.

Bromfenac Ophthalmic

(*brome-fen-ak*)   Bromday®, Xibrom®

NSAID

Prescriber Highlights
▶ Longer duration of action than diclofenac.
▶ May delay ocular wound healing and increase risk of intraocular bleeding.
▶ Available as drops; not available in an ointment form but may compounded.

Uses/Indications
Bromfenac is used for postoperative ocular analgesia in small animals and for treating equine recurrent uveitis.

Pharmacology/Actions
Bromfenac is a nonsteroidal antiinflammatory drug (NSAID) that has antiinflammatory activity. The mechanism of its action is thought to be due to its ability to block prostaglandin synthesis by inhibiting cyclooxygenase 1 and 2. Prostaglandins cause disruption of the blood-aqueous humor barrier, vasodilation, increased vascular permeability, leukocytosis, and increased intraocular pressure.

Contraindications/Precautions/Warnings
Bromfenac is contraindicated in patients with a history of hypersensitivity to it or any component of the formulation. Bromfenac contains sulfite; caregivers with sulfite allergies should avoid direct contact with bromfenac. Use of bromfenac and other NSAIDs may interfere with platelet aggregation and increase the risk of intraocular bleeding after surgery. Use bromfenac carefully in patients with bleeding tendencies or that are on systemic NSAIDs. Topical NSAID agents may also delay ocular healing.

Adverse Effects
Adverse effects reported in humans or animals include burning, stinging and irritation upon application, conjunctival hyperemia, risk of ocular bleeding, and delayed wound healing.

Doses
Equine Recurrent Uveitis (extra-label): 1 – 2 drops (0.09% solution) or 1/8th inch strip (compounded gel) in the affected eye(s) 3 times daily initially, then reduced to lowest effective dose.

Postoperative Ocular Analgesia (extra-label): 1 drop in the affected eye(s) every 6-8 hours as needed to control pain.

Monitoring
▪ Clinical efficacy. Evidence of effective analgesia. Control of intraocular inflammation.

Client Information
▪ Used 2-4 times daily.
▪ Use proper administration techniques to avoid contamination of the medication. Keep cap tightly closed when not in use.
▪ Wait 5 minutes after applying this medication before applying any other medications to the eye.
▪ Store in the refrigerator or at controlled room temperature away from moisture and sunlight; do not freeze. Do not use if the color changes, becomes cloudy, or if particles are seen in the solution. Discard compounded gels on the discard date indicated by the compounding pharmacist.

Storage/Stability
Store in refrigerator or at controlled room temperature away from moisture and sunlight; do not freeze.

Compatibility/Compounding Considerations
Bromfenac should not be mixed directly with any other drugs.

Dosage Forms/Regulatory Status
VETERINARY-LABELED PRODUCTS: NONE.
HUMAN-LABELED PRODUCTS:
Bromfenac 0.09% Ophthalmic Solution (containing with benzalkonium chloride, povidone, and sodium sulfite) in 2.5 mL ophthalmic dropper bottle; *Xibrom®, Bromday®*; (Rx)

Bromfenac is not available as an ophthalmic ointment. However, an ophthalmic gel can be prepared (compounded) by qualified compounding pharmacists.

Revisions/References
Monograph revised/updated September 2014.

Carteolol Ophthalmic

(*kar-tay-uh-lol*)   Ocupress®

Beta-Blocker

Prescriber Highlights
▶ Partial beta-agonist properties allow carteolol to be used in patients that suffer bradycardia from other beta-blockers.
▶ Effective for feline glaucoma (usually employed in addition to carbonic anhydrase inhibitors).

Uses/Indications
In veterinary patients, carteolol is used to reduce intraocular pressure in primary glaucoma and as prophylaxis to prevent glaucoma in the normal eye of animals with unilateral glaucoma.

Pharmacology/Actions
Carteolol is a nonselective beta-adrenergic blocking agent with associated intrinsic sympathomimetic activity and without significant membrane-stabilizing activity. The exact mechanism of the ocular hypotensive effect of beta-blockers has not been definitely demonstrated; however, several mechanisms have been postulated for this effect including beta-blockade of norepinephrine-induced tonic sympathetic stimulation, decreased activation of cAMP in the ciliary body leading to decreased aqueous humor production, inhibition of Na+K+ATPase activity, or through vasoactive mechanisms.

Contraindications/Precautions/Warnings
Carteolol is contraindicated in patients with a history of hypersensitivity to it or any component of the formulation. Carteolol should be used carefully in patients with heart block, bradycardia, heart failure, asthma, chronic bronchitis, or other cardiopulmonary conditions, although systemic cardiopulmonary adverse effects are not likely with ocular use of carteolol.

Adverse Effects

Adverse effects reported in humans or animals include transient burning, stinging, and irritation upon application to the eye.

Doses

Glaucoma (extra-label): 1 drop in the affected eye(s) 2 times daily.

Monitoring

- Clinical efficacy. Monitor intraocular pressure.

Client Information

- Used 2 times daily.
- Use proper administration techniques to avoid contamination of the medication. Keep cap tightly closed when not in use.
- Wait 5 minutes after applying this medication before applying any other medications to the eye.
- Store in the refrigerator or at controlled room temperature away from moisture and sunlight; do not freeze. Do not use if the color changes, becomes cloudy, or if particles are seen in the solution.

Storage/Stability

Store at controlled room temperature away from moisture and sunlight; do not freeze. Discard if color change, or becomes cloudy, or if particles are observed in the solution.

Compatibility/Compounding Considerations

Carteolol should not be mixed directly with any other drugs.

Dosage Forms/Regulatory Status

VETERINARY-LABELED PRODUCTS: NONE.

HUMAN-LABELED PRODUCTS:

Carteolol HCl 1% Ophthalmic Solution (containing NaCl, monobasic and dibasic sodium phosphate, purified water, benzalkonium chloride 0.005%, with a pH range of 6.2-7.2) in a 5 mL, 10 mL, and 15 mL dropper bottle; *Ocupress®*; (Rx).

Revisions/References

Monograph revised/updated September 2014.

Chloramphenicol Ophthalmic

(klor-am-fen-uh-kol)   Chloromycetin®

Broad-Spectrum Antibiotic

Prescriber Highlights

▶ Chloramphenicol has caused acute toxicity and death in humans; instruct caregiver to avoid contact with this drug.

▶ Chloramphenicol ophthalmic solutions are no longer commercially available but may be prepared (compounded) by a qualified compounding pharmacist.

▶ Useful to treat feline *Mycoplasma* or *Chlamydia* conjunctivitis.

Uses/Indications

In veterinary patients, chloramphenicol is used for the treatment of surface ocular infections involving the conjunctiva and/or cornea caused by chloramphenicol-susceptible organisms.

Pharmacology/Actions

Chloramphenicol acts by inhibition of protein synthesis by interfering with the transfer of activated amino acids from soluble RNA to ribosomes; chloramphenicol is a bacteriostatic antibiotic. Chloramphenicol is found in measurable amounts in the aqueous humor following local application to the eye. Development of resistance to chloramphenicol can be regarded as minimal for staphylococci and many other species of bacteria.

Contraindications/Precautions/Warnings

Chloramphenicol is contraindicated in patients with a history of hypersensitivity to it or any component of the formulation. Chloramphenicol is myelotoxic to approximately 1:10,000 humans, care-

givers should be instructed to wear gloves and wash hands after handling this drug. Chloramphenicol is banned for use in food producing animals.

Adverse Effects

Adverse effects reported in humans or animals include occasional burning or stinging on application. Bone marrow suppression and blood dyscrasias have been reported following

Doses

Bacterial conjunctivitis (extra-label): 1/8th inch strip (ointment) or 1 drop (solution) in the affected eye(s) every 6-8 hours.

Monitoring

- Clinical efficacy. Resolution of bacterial infection.
- Adverse effects: Monitor for bone marrow suppression.

Client Information

- Used 3-4 times daily.
- Wear gloves and wash hands after handling.
- Use proper administration techniques to avoid contamination of the medication. Keep cap tightly closed when not in use.
- Wait 5 minutes after applying this medication before applying any other medications to the eye.
- Store at controlled room temperature away from moisture and sunlight; do not freeze. Do not use if the color changes, becomes cloudy, or if particles are seen in the solution. Discard compounded preparations on the day the pharmacist indicates as the beyond-use-date.

Storage/Stability

Store at controlled room temperature away from moisture and sunlight; do not freeze.

Compatibility/Compounding Considerations

Chloramphenicol should not be mixed directly with any other drugs.

Dosage Forms/Regulatory Status

VETERINARY-LABELED PRODUCTS: NONE.

HUMAN-LABELED PRODUCTS: NONE.

Chloramphenicol was formerly available as a 0.5% ophthalmic solution or a 1% ointment, but are no longer commercially available. A qualified compounding pharmacists may prepare them if needed.

Revisions/References

Monograph revised/updated September 2014.

Cidofovir Ophthalmic

(sye-doe-fo-veer)   Vistide®

Antiviral

Prescriber Highlights

▶ Less frequent administration and shorter treatment duration when compared to other ophthalmic antiviral agents.

▶ Cidofovir is highly nephrotoxic in humans; irreversible kidney damage has occurred after exposure to a single dose; inform caregivers of exposure risks.

▶ Cidofovir has caused hypospermia and birth defects in humans and should not be used in animals intended for breeding.

▶ Not commercially available in an ophthalmic dosage form; can be compounded as a 0.5% ophthalmic solution.

▶ Must be refrigerated.

Uses/Indications

In veterinary patients, cidofovir is prepared (compounded) into a 0.5% ophthalmic solution for topical treatment of feline herpes virus-1 (FHV-1) keratitis. Cidofovir has a significant therapeutic advantage over other antiviral ophthalmic agents in treating FHV$_1$ as cidofovir is effective given twice daily for 10 days while other ophthalmic antiviral agents (trifluridine, vidarabine, and idoxuridine) must be given 4-6 times daily for 2-3 weeks. As feline herpes keratitis is induced and worsened by stress, less frequent administration for a shorter duration makes cidofovir a superior therapeutic choice for many veterinary ophthalmologists and cat owners.

Pharmacology/Actions

Cidofovir suppresses viral replication by selective inhibition of viral DNA synthesis. Biochemical data support selective inhibition of DNA polymerase by cidofovir diphosphate, the active intracellular metabolite of cidofovir. Cidofovir diphosphate inhibits herpes virus polymerases at concentrations that are 8- to 600-fold lower than those needed to inhibit human cellular DNA polymerases. Incorporation of cidofovir into the growing viral DNA chain results in reductions in the rate of viral DNA synthesis thereby exhibiting a virustatic effect.

Contraindications/Precautions/Warnings

Cidofovir is contraindicated in patients with a history of hypersensitivity to it or any component of the formulation. Do not use cidofovir in animals intended for breeding as cidofovir causes hypospermia and is mutagenic and teratogenic. Cidofovir has caused death by irreversible renal toxicity after single doses in humans; do not use in animals with existing renal impairment or concurrently with nephrotoxic drugs; warn human caregivers of risk of renal damage with exposure to cidofovir.

Adverse Effects

Adverse effects reported in humans or animals include burning or stinging on application. Severe adverse effects in humans include irreversible nephrotoxicity after one to two doses, hypospermia, birth defects from teratogenic effects, and neutropenia.

Doses

Feline Herpes Virus$_1$ Keratitis (extra-label): 1 drop in the affected eye(s) 2 times daily for 10 days.

Monitoring

- Clinical efficacy. Resolution of clinical signs of FHV1.

Client Information

- Used 2 times daily.
- Humans should avoid direct contact with this drug.
- Use proper administration techniques to avoid contamination of the medication. Keep cap tightly closed when not in use.
- Wait 5 minutes after applying this medication before applying any other medications to the eye.
- Store in the refrigerator or at controlled room temperature away from moisture and sunlight; do not freeze. Do not use if the color changes, becomes cloudy, or if particles are seen in the solution.

Storage/Stability

Store in refrigerator away from moisture and sunlight; do not freeze.

Reported chemical stability of this solution is 180 days stored in glass at 4°C, -20°C, and -80°C (Stiles *et al.* 2010). Sterility storage times are 14 days at 4°C in absence of additional sterility testing as required by USP <797> - Pharmaceutical Compounding—Sterile Preparations.

Compatibility/Compounding Considerations

Cidofovir should not be mixed directly with any other drugs.

Dosage Forms/Regulatory Status

VETERINARY-LABELED PRODUCTS: NONE.
HUMAN-LABELED PRODUCTS: NONE.
Cidofovir is not approved for use as an ophthalmic dosage form, but cidofovir 0.5% ophthalmic solution can be prepared by a qualified compounding pharmacist.

Revisions/References

Monograph revised/updated September 2014.
Stiles, J., et al. (2010). Stability of 0.5% cidofovir stored under various conditions for up to 6 months. Vet. Ophthalmol. 13(4): 275-7.

Ciprofloxacin Ophthalmic

(sip-rowe-**flocks**-a sin)   Cipro®

Fluoroquinolone Antibiotic

Prescriber Highlights

▶ Fluoroquinolone antimicrobial used for bacterial conjunctivitis or keratitis.
▶ Physically incompatible with many drugs.
▶ Crystalline drug precipitates may be noted in the superficial portion of corneal defects during use.
▶ Do not confuse pure fluoroquinolone eye medications with those that contain steroids.

Uses/Indications

In veterinary patients, ciprofloxacin ophthalmic may be useful for treating bacterial conjunctivitis caused by susceptible species/strains of staphylococci, streptococci, Corynebacterium, Haemophilus, and Chlamydia. When administered via a subpalpebral lavage (SPL) catheter ciprofloxacin ophthalmic solution can be used for treating equine bacterial keratitis.

Pharmacology/Actions

Ciprofloxacin is a member of the fluoroquinolone class of anti-infective drugs. Its action results from inhibition of DNA gyrase, which is involved in replication, transcription and repair of bacterial DNA.

Contraindications/Precautions/Warnings

Ciprofloxacin is contraindicated in patients with a history of hypersensitivity to it, other fluoroquinolones, or any component of the formulation. For topical ophthalmic use only; not for injection subconjunctivally or into the anterior chamber of the eye. Fluoroquinolone-induced retinal toxicity in domestic cats has not been demonstrated with this product at time of writing, but may be possible.

Adverse Effects

Adverse effects reported in humans or animals include blurred vision, tearing, eye pain, redness, itching, and a bad taste in the mouth. Crystalline drug precipitates may be noted in the superficial portion of corneal defects during use.

Doses

Conjunctivitis (extra-label): 1 drop affected eye(s) every 4-8 hours.

Keratitis (extra-label): 1 drop in the affected eye or 0.2 mL in the SPL catheter every 1-8 hours. May precipitate when mixed with other ophthalmic medications. Flush SPL catheter well with air between medications.

Monitoring

- Clinical efficacy. If blepharospasm, uveitis, or worsening of ulceration or no improvement in infection is noted in 7 days, reassess microbial susceptibility.

Client Information

- Used 3-6 times daily.
- Use proper administration techniques to avoid contamination of the medication. Keep cap tightly closed when not in use.
- Wait 5 minutes after applying this medication before applying any other medications to the eye.
- Store in the refrigerator or at controlled room temperature away from moisture and sunlight; do not freeze. Do not use if the color changes, becomes cloudy, or if particles are seen in the solution.

Storage/Stability

Store in refrigerator or at controlled room temperature away from moisture and sunlight; do not freeze.

Compatibility/Compounding Considerations

Ciprofloxacin should not be mixed directly with any other drugs.

Dosage Forms/Regulatory Status

VETERINARY-LABELED PRODUCTS: NONE.
HUMAN-LABELED PRODUCTS:

Ciprofloxacin 0.3% Ophthalmic Solution (containing benzalkonium chloride 0.006%, acetic acid, edetate disodium 0.05%, mannitol 4.6%, purified water, sodium acetate, HCl and/or NaOH may be used to adjust pH to 4.5 and the osmolality is 300 mOsm/kg) in 2.5 mL, 5 mL and 10 mL dropper bottles; *Cipro®*; (Rx)

Ciprofloxacin 0.3% Ophthalmic Ointment (containing mineral oil and white petrolatum) in 3.5 g ophthalmic ointment tubes; *Cipro®*; (Rx)

Revisions/References

Monograph revised/updated September 2014.

Cromolyn Sodium Ophthalmic

(kroe-mo-lin so-dee-um)   Opticrom®, Crolom®

Mast Cell Stabilizer

Prescriber Highlights

► Used for seasonal allergic conjunctivitis or atopic conjunctivitis.
► Administered 2-6 times daily.
► Mild transient stinging and burning upon application.

Uses/Indications

In veterinary patients, mast cell stabilizing ophthalmic agents are used to control the symptoms of allergic (seasonal) conjunctivitis and atopic conjunctivitis in dogs (usually in combination with topical corticosteroid ophthalmic agents). Symptomatic response to therapy (decreased itching, tearing, redness, and discharge) is usually evident within a few days, but longer treatment for up to six weeks is sometimes required. Once symptomatic improvement has been established, therapy should be continued for as long as needed to sustain improvement. If required, corticosteroids may be used concomitantly with cromolyn sodium ophthalmic solution.

Pharmacology/Actions

Cromolyn sodium inhibits the degranulation of sensitized mast cells and blocks the release of histamine and slow-releasing substance of anaphylaxis from mast cells following antigen recognition. Cromolyn sodium does not have intrinsic vasoconstrictor, antihistaminic, cyclooxygenase inhibition, or other antiinflammatory properties.

Contraindications/Precautions/Warnings

Cromolyn sodium is contraindicated in patients with a history of hypersensitivity to cromolyn sodium or any component of the formulation.

Adverse Effects

Adverse effects reported in humans or animals include a transient mild stinging and burning upon application.

Doses

Allergic Conjunctivitis (extra-label): 1 drop in each eye 2-6 times daily as needed to control symptoms of allergic conjunctivitis.

Monitoring

■ Clinical efficacy. Resolution of clinical signs of allergic conjunctivitis.

Client Information

■ Used 2-6 times daily.
■ Use proper administration techniques to avoid contamination of the medication. Keep cap tightly closed when not in use.
■ Wait 5 minutes after applying this medication before applying any other medications to the eye.
■ Store in the refrigerator or at controlled room temperature away from moisture and sunlight; do not freeze. Do not use if the color changes, becomes cloudy, or if particles are seen in the solution.

Storage/Stability

Store at controlled room temperature away from moisture and sunlight; do not freeze.

Compatibility/Compounding Considerations

Cromolyn sodium should not be mixed directly with any other drugs.

Dosage Forms/Regulatory Status

VETERINARY-LABELED PRODUCTS: NONE.
HUMAN-LABELED PRODUCTS:

Cromolyn Sodium 4% Ophthalmic Solution (containing benzalkonium chloride 0.01%. edetate disodium 0.1% and purified water, HCl and/or NaOH to adjust pH (4.0-7.0) in a 10 mL ophthalmic dropper bottle; *Opticrom®*, *Crolom®*; (Rx)

Revisions/References

Monograph revised/updated September 2014.

Cyclopentolate Ophthalmic

(sye-kloe-pen-toe-late)   Cyclogyl®, Cyclomydril®

Anticholinergic Cycloplegic/Mydriatic Agent

Prescriber Highlights

► Primarily used as a diagnostic agent to facilitate mydriasis and cycloplegia.
► Rapid and intense onset of mydriasis and cycloplegia in 15-60 minutes; longer duration of action in animals with darkly pigmented irises.
► Increases intraocular pressure, do not use in patients with glaucoma
► Higher concentrations (≥1%) cause stinging on application.
► Available as a combination product with phenylephrine (*Cyclomydril®*) to facilitate mydriasis with less cycloplegia.

Uses/Indications

In veterinary patients, cyclopentolate is primarily used to induce rapid mydriasis and cycloplegia for funduscopic examination and diagnostic purposes. It is also available as a combination with phenylephrine to accomplish greater mydriasis with a lesser degree of cycloplegia.

Pharmacology/Actions

Cyclopentolate blocks the responses of the sphincter muscle of the iris and the accommodative muscle of the ciliary body to cholinergic stimulation, producing papillary dilation (mydriasis) and paralysis of accommodation (cycloplegia). It acts rapidly, but has a shorter duration than atropine. Maximal cycloplegia occurs within 25-75 minutes after instillation. Complete recovery of accommodation usually takes 6-24 hours. Complete recovery from mydriasis in some individuals may require several days. Heavily pigmented irises may require more doses than lightly pigmented irises. When combined with phenylephrine, an adrenergic drug, synergistic mydriasis occurs with little accompanying cycloplegia.

Contraindications/Precautions/Warnings

Cyclopentolate is contraindicated in patients with a history of hypersensitivity to it or any component of the formulation. Cyclopentolate causes an increase in intraocular pressure and should not be used in patients with glaucoma. Cyclopentolate may interfere with the ocular anti-hypertensive action of pilocarpine or ophthalmic cholinesterase inhibitors.

Adverse Effects

Adverse effects reported in humans or animals include burning and stinging upon application. Increased intraocular pressure, photophobia, blurred vision, irritation, hyperemia, conjunctivitis, blepharoconjunctivitis, punctate keratitis, and synechiae have also been reported. Burning and stinging is usually associated with higher concentrations ($\geq$1%). CNS and cardiovascular disturbances are often noted in human pediatric patients and may occur when used in smaller animals. In smaller patients, the lacrimal sac should be compressed by digital pressure for 2-3 minutes after instillation to reduce excessive systemic absorption.

Doses

Mydriasis and Cycloplegia (extra-label): 1 drop in the desired eye(s) followed by a second drop 5 minutes later if necessary. **Note:** Use of a single drop may avoid adverse systemic effects in smaller patients. Administer 40-50 minutes prior to diagnostic procedure to ensure full effects.

Monitoring

- Clinical efficacy. Desired mydriasis and cycloplegia achieved. Full recovery in 24 hours. Advise caregiver to keep patient out of bright sunlight until pupils return to normal size.

Client Information

- This drug is rarely used at home.
- Wash hands after use to prevent accidently getting in your eyes (causes pupil dilation).
- Use to proper administration techniques to avoid contamination of the medication. Keep cap tightly closed when not in use.
- Wait 5 minutes after applying this medication before applying any other medications to the eye.
- Store in the refrigerator or at controlled room temperature away from moisture and sunlight; do not freeze. Do not use if the color changes, becomes cloudy, or if particles are seen in the solution.

Storage/Stability

Store at controlled room temperature away from moisture and sunlight; do not freeze.

Compatibility/Compounding Considerations

Cyclopentolate HCl should not be mixed directly with any other drugs.

Dosage Forms/Regulatory Status

VETERINARY-LABELED PRODUCTS: NONE.

HUMAN-LABELED PRODUCTS:

Cyclopentolate HCl 0.5%, 1% & 2% Ophthalmic Solution in a 2 mL, 5 mL, and 15 mL ophthalmic dropper bottle; *Cyclogyl*®, generic; (Rx)

Cyclopentolate HCl 0.2% and Phenylephrine HCl 1% Ophthalmic Solution in a 2 mL and 5 mL ophthalmic dropper bottle; *Cyclomydril*®; (Rx)

Revisions/References

Monograph revised/updated September 2014.

Cyclosporine Ophthalmic

(sye-klo-**spore**-in)   Cyclosporin A, Optimmune®, Restasis®

T-Cell Immunosuppressive Agent

Prescriber Highlights

▶ Approved as an ophthalmic ointment (*Optimmune*®) for treatment of keratoconjunctivitis sicca (KCS) in dogs. Cyclosporine also used to treat other ocular inflammatory diseases in animals.

▶ Human-approved cyclosporine 0.05% ophthalmic emulsion (*Restasis*®) does not appear to be effective in managing canine KCS.

▶ Animals not responding to the approved ophthalmic ointment (*Optimmune*®) may benefit from use of higher concentrations of cyclosporine ophthalmic solution.

▶ Normal tear production requires weeks of therapy with cyclosporine; however, cessation of therapy results in loss of tear production in days.

Uses/Indications

Cyclosporine is approved for treatment of keratoconjunctivitis sicca in dogs. In veterinary patients, cyclosporine is also used to treat ocular inflammatory disease such as canine pannus, equine uveitis and immune mediated keratitis. Intraocular implants (suprachoroidal disks and episcleral rods) are being used (investigationally) for treatment of equine recurrent uveitis and immune mediated keratitis (Gilger *et al.* 2006; Lee *et al.* 2007; Gilger *et al.* 2010; Weiner *et al.* 2010; Gilger *et al.* 2014).

Pharmacology/Actions

Cyclosporine is believed to act as a local immunomodulator (interferes with T-cell-mediated destruction of lacrimal glands) of diseases suspected to be immune-mediated such as keratoconjunctivitis sicca (KCS) and chronic superficial keratitis (CSK). In the management of KCS, the mechanism by which cyclosporine causes an increase in lacrimation is poorly understood. Cyclosporine stimulates tear production in healthy dogs (without KCS) and for this reason is thought to have direct stimulatory effects on the lacrimal gland. It may exert this effect by acting as a prolactin analog stimulating lacrimal prolactin receptors. Effective tear production after initiation of cyclosporine therapy takes several weeks; however, cessation of therapy results in return of symptoms in a matter of days. Clinical improvement in cases of KCS is not necessarily dependent on an increase in aqueous tear production (as measured by the Schirmer Tear Test [STT]). Cyclosporine ocular implants (episcleral or suprachoroidal) are sustained release implants aseptically inserted into the suprachoroid or episcleral space in horses suffering from uveitis or immune-mediated keratitis. The duration of effect for these implants is about 2 years. Cyclosporine has also been shown *in vitro* to have a direct inhibitory effect on the growth of leptospires, which have been implicated as a cause of equine uveitis.

Contraindications/Precautions/Warnings

Cyclosporine is contraindicated in patients with a history of hypersensitivity to it or any component of the formulation. Do not use in presence of ocular viral or fungal infections.

Cyclosporine is available as an ophthalmic solution for humans (*Restasis*® 0.05% ophthalmic solution), but this solution has not been shown to be effective in controlling KCS in dogs. More concentrated solutions of cyclosporine ophthalmic (1-2%) may be prepared (compounded) by qualified compounding pharmacists.

Do not administer cyclosporine ophthalmic ointment or solutions compounded in oil in a SPL catheter as they are likely to irreversibly obstruct the catheter necessitating replacement of the SPL system.

Adverse Effects

Adverse effects reported in humans or animals include local irritation, periocular erythema, and lid spasm, rubbing of the eye, alopecia, and epiphora.

Doses

For KCS or inflammatory conditions such as pannus: *Optimmune®:* ¼ inch strip to the affected eye(s) every 12 hours. Cyclosporine Solutions (1-2%) (extra-label): 1 drop in the affected eye(s) every 12 hours.

Monitoring

- Clinical efficacy. Test for adequate tear production (STT). Monitor for corneal abrasions or ulcerations from KCS. Prevent recurrent episodes of equine uveitis.

Client Information

- Used 2 times daily.
- Use proper administration techniques to avoid contamination of the medication. Keep cap tightly closed when not in use.
- Wait 5 minutes after applying this medication before applying any other medications to the eye.
- Cyclosporine ointment should be stored in the refrigerator or at controlled room temperature away from moisture and sunlight. Handle and squeeze the tube gently so the metal won't crack and leak.
- Cyclosporine solutions should be stored at room temperature and not refrigerated; do not freeze. Discard if color change, or becomes cloudy, or if particles are observed in the solution. Discard if color change, or becomes cloudy, or if particles are observed in the solution.

Storage/Stability

The ophthalmic ointment (*Optimmune®*) should be stored in the refrigerator or at controlled room temperature away from moisture and sunlight. Cyclosporine solutions should not be refrigerated; do not freeze.

Long-term stability of a 1% solution in corn oil has been established by USP to be 180 days; sterility storage times should be according to USP <797> defaults or per results of individual extended sterility testing.

Compatibility/Compounding Considerations

Cyclosporine should not be mixed directly with any other drugs. Do not administer cyclosporine ophthalmic ointment or solutions compounded in oil in the SPL catheter as they are likely to irreversibly obstruct the catheter necessitating replacement of the SPL system.

Dosage Forms/Regulatory Status

VETERINARY-LABELED PRODUCTS:

Cyclosporine 0.2% Ophthalmic Ointment (containing petrolatum, USP; corn oil, NF; petrolatum and lanolin alcohol) in a 3.5 g ophthalmic ointment tube; *Optimmune®*; (Rx). Approved for use in dogs.

Cyclosporine 1-2% Ophthalmic Solutions in fixed oils may be prepared (compounded) by qualified compounding pharmacists.

HUMAN-LABELED PRODUCTS:

Cyclosporine 0.05% Ophthalmic Emulsion; *Restasis®*; (Rx). **Note:** This solution has not been shown to be effective in controlling KCS in dogs.

Revisions/References

Monograph revised/updated September 2014.

Gilger, B. C., et al. (2006). A novel bioerodible deep scleral lamellar cyclosporine implant for uveitis. Investigative Ophthalmology & Visual Science 47(6): 2596-605.
Gilger, B. C., et al. (2014). Treatment of immune-mediated keratitis in horses with episcleral silicone matrix cyclosporine delivery devices. Vet. Ophthalmol. 17: 23-30.
Gilger, B. C., et al. (2010). Long-term outcome after implantation of a suprachoroidal cyclosporine drug delivery device in horses with recurrent uveitis. Vet. Ophthalmol. 13(5): 294-300.
Lee, S. S., et al. (2007). A pharmacokinetic and safety evaluation of an episcleral cyclosporine implant for potential use in high-risk keratoplasty rejection. Investigative Ophthalmology & Visual Science 48(5): 2023-9.
Weiner, A. L. & B. C. Gilger (2010). Advancements in ocular drug delivery. Vet. Ophthalmol. 13(6): 395-406.

Demecarium Bromide Ophthalmic

(deh-meh-kar-ee-um bro-mide)   Humorsol®

Anticholinesterase Ocular Anti-Hypertensive

Prescriber Highlights

- ▶ No longer commercially available; can be compounded.
- ▶ Used primarily for preventive management of glaucoma in the unaffected eye of canine patients diagnosed with primary glaucoma in one eye.
- ▶ Used 1-2 times daily.

Uses/Indications

In veterinary patients, demecarium bromide is used for preventive management of glaucoma in contralateral eye of canine patients diagnosed with primary glaucoma in the other eye.

Pharmacology/Actions

Demecarium bromide is a cholinesterase inhibitor or an anticholinesterase. Cholinesterase inhibitors prolong the effect of acetylcholine, which is released at the neuroeffector junction of parasympathetic postganglion nerves, by inactivating the cholinesterases that break it down. Demecarium inactivates both pseudocholinesterase and acetylcholinesterase. In the eye, this causes constriction of the iris sphincter muscle (causing miosis) and the ciliary muscle. The outflow of the aqueous humor is facilitated, which leads to a reduction in intraocular pressure. Demecarium is an organophosphate and may cause severe and even fatal dose-related systemic toxicity, especially in cats. Signs of systemic toxicity include vomiting, anorexia, diarrhea, lethargy and weakness.

Contraindications/Precautions/Warnings

Demecarium is contraindicated in patients with a history of hypersensitivity to it or any component of the formulation. Demecarium is contraindicated in pregnant animals; caregivers that are pregnant or intend to become pregnant should be warned to avoid contact with this medication.

Adverse Effects

Adverse effects reported in humans or animals include stinging, burning and ocular irritation. Demecarium is an organophosphate and can cause severe and even fatal dose-related systemic toxicity, especially in cats. Signs of systemic toxicity include vomiting, anorexia, diarrhea, lethargy and weakness.

Doses

Prophylaxis of glaucoma in normal eye (extra-label): 1 drop in the non-glaucomatous eye 1-2 times daily.

Monitoring

- Clinical efficacy. Maintenance of normal intraocular pressure in the contralateral eye of dogs with unilateral glaucoma.
- Toxicity: Monitor for signs of systemic toxicity: vomiting, anorexia, diarrhea, lethargy and weakness.

Client Information

- Used 1-2 times daily.
- Use proper administration techniques to avoid contamination of the medication. Keep cap tightly closed when not in use.
- Wait 5 minutes after applying this medication before applying any other medications to the eye.

- Store in the refrigerator or at controlled room temperature away from moisture and sunlight; do not freeze. Do not use if the color changes, becomes cloudy, or if particles are seen in the solution.

Storage/Stability

Store in refrigerator or at controlled room temperature away from moisture and sunlight; do not freeze.

Compatibility/Compounding Considerations

Demecarium bromide should not be mixed directly with any other drugs.

Dosage Forms/Regulatory Status

VETERINARY-LABELED PRODUCTS: NONE.

HUMAN-LABELED PRODUCTS: NONE.

Demecarium bromide is no longer commercially available but may be prepared (compounded) as a 0.25% ophthalmic solution by qualified compounding pharmacists.

Revisions/References

Monograph revised/updated September 2014.

Dexamethasone Ophthalmic

(decks-uh-**meth**-uh-sown)   Maxidex®

Corticosteroid

Prescriber Highlights

▶ Alcohol based dexamethasone solutions achieve better intra-ocular penetration than suspensions.

▶ Longer acting than prednisolone products, but less effective for treating equine uveitis than topical prednisolone.

▶ Do not use in feline herpes keratitis, fungal keratitis, or if corneal abrasion or ulceration are suspected.

Uses/Indications

In veterinary patients, dexamethasone ophthalmic is used for symptomatic relief of corticosteroid-responsive inflammatory conditions of the palpebral and bulbar conjunctiva, cornea, and anterior segment of the globe (*e.g.*, allergic conjunctivitis, acne rosacea, superficial punctate keratitis, iritis, and cyclitis). In horses it is used for treatment of uveitis. It may also be used to treat inflammation associated with corneal injury from chemical, radiation, or thermal burns or penetration of foreign bodies. Dexamethasone is also available in many combinations with antimicrobial agents for topical ophthalmic use.

Pharmacology/Actions

Corticosteroids work by inhibiting phospholipase A2 as well as cyclooxygenase (COX) and lipoxygenase (LOX) pathways. Corticosteroids can also penetrate the nucleus to interrupt specific DNA sequences that produce inflammatory mediators. In general, pro-inflammatory mediators are down-regulated and antiinflammatory mediators are up-regulated. Corticosteroids also reduce the migration of macrophages, decrease vascular permeability, and suppress lymphokines. They inhibit edema, cellular infiltration, capillary dilatation, fibroblastic proliferation, and deposition of collagen.

Contraindications/Precautions/Warnings

Dexamethasone is contraindicated in patients with a history of hypersensitivity to it or any component of the formulation. Topical corticosteroids are contraindicated in known or suspected corneal ulceration or corneal infection (fungal and viral). Use with caution in patients with diabetes mellitus or other endocrine diseases, infectious diseases, chronic renal failure, congestive heart failure, systemic hypertension, or gastric ulceration. When use is necessary in these conditions, the minimal effective dose should be administered for the shortest possible time.

Adverse Effects

Adverse effects reported in humans or animals include development of cataracts (via altered glucose or lenticular metabolic effects), increased intraocular pressure (via activation of glucocorticoid receptors in the trabecular meshwork), infection (via immunosuppression), decreased wound healing (via increased collagenolytic activity), mydriasis, and calcific keratopathy. Systemic effects are rare but include hepatopathy, suppression of endogenous glucocorticoid production, and focal alopecia. Concurrent use of systemic steroids increases risk of these adverse effects.

Doses

Conjunctivitis (extra-label): 1 drop or ¼ inch strip in affected eye(s) every 4-8 hours, then increase to longest dosing interval that still maintains efficacy.

Post Cataract Removal (extra-label): 1 drop in the affected eye(s) every 8-12 hours.

Monitoring

- Clinical efficacy. Absence of inflammation. Monitor intraocular pressure and observe for evidence of infection or delayed wound healing. Monitor for blood or urine glucose changes in diabetic animals.

Client Information

- Used 4-6 times daily.
- Shake suspensions well before using.
- Use proper administration techniques to avoid contamination of the medication. Keep cap tightly closed when not in use.
- Wait 5 minutes after applying this medication before applying any other medications to the eye.
- Store at controlled room temperature away from moisture and sunlight; do not freeze. Do not use if the color changes, becomes cloudy, or if particles are seen in the solution.

Storage/Stability

Store at controlled room temperature away from moisture and sunlight; do not freeze.

Compatibility/Compounding Considerations

Dexamethasone should not be mixed directly with any other drugs.

Dosage Forms/Regulatory Status

VETERINARY-LABELED PRODUCTS: NONE.

HUMAN-LABELED PRODUCTS:

Dexamethasone Sodium Phosphate 0.05% Ophthalmic Ointment (containing mineral oil and white petrolatum) in 3.5 g ophthalmic ointment tube; *Maxidex®*; (Rx)

Dexamethasone Sodium Phosphate 0.1% Ophthalmic Suspension [containing benzalkonium chloride 0.01%, hypromellose 0.5%, NaCl, dibasic sodium phosphate, polysorbate 80, edetate disodium, citric acid and/or NaOH (to adjust pH), purified water] in 5 mL and 15 mL ophthalmic dropper bottle; *Maxidex®*; (Rx).

Dexamethasone Sodium Phosphate 0.1% Ophthalmic Solution (containing sodium citrate, sodium borate, creatinine, polysorbate 80, edetate disodium dihydrate, purified Water, HCl to adjust pH to 6.6-7.8, sodium Bisulfite 0.1%, phenylethyl alcohol 0.25%, benzalkonium chloride 0.02%) in a 5 mL ophthalmic dropper bottle; generic; (Rx).

Revisions/References

Monograph revised/updated September 2014.

Diclofenac Ophthalmic

(dye-kloe-fen-ak)   Voltaren®

NSAID

Prescriber Highlights

▶ Diclofenac ophthalmic solution has a characteristic odor of castor oil.

▶ Ophthalmic ointment not commercially available, but may be prepared (compounded).

▶ Sulfite preservatives may trigger asthma attacks in susceptible patients.

Uses/Indications

In veterinary patients, nonsteroidal antiinflammatory agents (NSAIDs) are used to control inflammation and provide analgesia. Diclofenac Sodium Ophthalmic Solution, 0.1% is indicated for the treatment of postoperative inflammation in patients that have undergone cataract extraction. Diclofenac is also used topically in horses for uveitis. NSAIDs have also been used for treatment of allergic conjunctivitis.

Pharmacology/Actions

NSAIDs work by decreasing prostaglandin formation through inhibition of cyclooxygenase and also decrease neutrophil chemotaxis and migration, decrease expression of inflammatory cytokines, decrease mast cell degranulation, and scavenge free radicals. NSAIDs are organic acids and therefore accumulate at inflammation sites increasing their overall antiinflammatory effect. Diclofenac is also used to induce mydriasis during cataract surgery.

Contraindications/Precautions/Warnings

Diclofenac is contraindicated in patients with a history of hypersensitivity to it or any component of the formulation.

Adverse Effects

Adverse effects reported in humans or animals include burning or stinging on administration. Superficial punctate keratitis has been reported with chronic use. NSAIDs may also cause direct cellular damage causing delayed wound healing. Although unlikely, systemic side effects have occurred with use of topical NSAIDs and include gastric ulceration, decreased platelet aggregation, bronchial asthma attacks (due to shunting to lipoxygenase pathways), and renal damage. Concurrent use of systemic NSAIDs increases the risk of systemic adverse effects.

Doses

Peri and post-operative Cataract Surgery (extra-label): 1 drop in the affected eye(s) every 8-12 hours.

Equine Uveitis (extra-label): 2 drops or ½ inch strip in the affected eye(s) every 12 hours.

Allergic Conjunctivitis (extra-label): 1 drop in the affected eye 2-4 times daily.

Monitoring

■ Clinical efficacy: Decreased or absent inflammation. Monitor for delayed wound healing.

Client Information

■ Used 2-4 times daily.

■ May cause burning or stinging on administration.

■ May increase risk of bleeding.

■ Use proper administration techniques to avoid contamination of the medication. Keep cap tightly closed when not in use.

■ Wait 5 minutes after applying this medication before applying any other medications to the eye.

■ Store at controlled room temperature away from moisture and sunlight; do not freeze. Do not use if the color changes, becomes cloudy, or if particles are seen in the solution.

Storage/Stability

Store at controlled room temperature away from moisture and sunlight; do not freeze. Discard if color change, or becomes cloudy, or if particles are observed in the solution.

Compatibility/Compounding Considerations

Diclofenac should not be mixed directly with any other drugs.

Dosage Forms/Regulatory Status

VETERINARY-LABELED PRODUCTS: NONE.

HUMAN-LABELED PRODUCTS:

Diclofenac Sodium 0.1% Ophthalmic Solution [containing boric acid, edetate disodium (1 mg/mL), polyoxyl 35 castor oil, purified water, sorbic acid (2 mg/mL), tromethamine with buffers added to achieve a pH of 7.2, osmolality 300 mOsm/kg] in a 2.5 mL or 5 mL ophthalmic dropper bottle; generic; (Rx)

Revisions/References

Monograph revised/updated September 2014.

Difluprednate Ophthalmic

(dye-floo-pred-nate)   Durezol®

Corticosteroid

Prescriber Highlights

▶ Shortens duration of inflammation of anterior uveitis compared to prednisolone.

▶ Superior to prednisolone in protecting the cornea and reducing macular thickening after cataract surgery.

▶ Do not use in viral or fungal keratitis.

Uses/Indications

In veterinary patients, difluprednate is used to treat inflammation following ocular injury or cataract surgery. It may also be used to treat anterior uveitis. Difluprednate has been shown to be more effective in preventing corneal edema and retinal thickening after cataract surgery and to shorten the duration of anterior uveitis compared to prednisolone (Foster *et al.* 2010), (Donnenfeld *et al.* 2011).

Pharmacology/Actions

Corticosteroids work by inhibiting phospholipase A2 as well as cyclooxygenase (COX) and lipoxygenase (LOX) pathways. Corticosteroids can also penetrate the nucleus to interrupt specific DNA sequences that produce inflammatory mediators. In general, pro-inflammatory mediators are down-regulated and antiinflammatory mediators are up-regulated. Corticosteroids also reduce the migration of macrophages, decrease vascular permeability, and suppress lymphokines. They inhibit edema, cellular infiltration, capillary dilatation, fibroblastic proliferation, and deposition of collagen.

Contraindications/Precautions/Warnings

Difluprednate is contraindicated in patients with a history of hypersensitivity to it or any component of the formulation. Topical corticosteroids are contraindicated in known or suspected corneal ulceration or corneal infection (fungal and viral). Use with caution in patients with diabetes mellitus or other endocrine diseases, infectious diseases, chronic renal failure, congestive heart failure, systemic hypertension, or gastric ulceration. When use is necessary in these conditions, the minimal effective dose should be administered for the shortest possible time.

Adverse Effects

Adverse effects reported in humans or animals include development of cataracts (via altered glucose or lenticular metabolic effects), increased intraocular pressure (via activation of glucocorticoid receptors in the trabecular meshwork), infection (via immunosuppression), decreased wound healing (via increased collagenolytic activity), mydriasis, and calcific keratopathy. Systemic effects are rare but include hepatopathy, suppression of endogenous glucocorticoid production, and focal alopecia. Concurrent use of systemic steroids increases risk of these adverse effects.

Doses

Conjunctivitis (extra-label): 1 drop in affected eye(s) every 4-8 hours, then increase to longest dosing interval that still maintains efficacy.

Post Cataract Removal (extra-label): 1 drop in the affected eye(s) every 8-12 hours.

Monitoring

- Clinical efficacy. Absence of inflammation. Monitor intraocular pressure and observe for evidence of infection or delayed wound healing. Monitor for blood or urine glucose changes in diabetic animals.

Client Information

- Used 2-4 times daily.
- Use proper administration techniques to avoid contamination of the medication. Keep cap tightly closed when not in use.
- Wait 5 minutes after applying this medication before applying any other medications to the eye.
- Store at controlled room temperature away from moisture and sunlight; do not freeze.

Storage/Stability

Store at controlled room temperature away from moisture and sunlight; do not freeze.

Compatibility/Compounding Considerations

Difluprednate should not be mixed directly with any other drugs. Difluprednate is not available as an ophthalmic ointment.

Dosage Forms/Regulatory Status

VETERINARY-LABELED PRODUCTS: NONE.

HUMAN-LABELED PRODUCTS:

Difluprednate 0.05% Ophthalmic Emulsion (containing sorbic acid 0.1%, boric acid, castor oil, glycerin, polysorbate 80, water for injection, sodium acetate, sodium EDTA, NaOH to adjust the pH to 5.2-5.8, with tonicity of 304-411 mOsm/kg) in 5 mL ophthalmic dropper bottle; *Durezol®*; (Rx)

Revisions/References

Monograph revised/updated September 2014.

Donnenfeld, E. D., et al. (2011). A Multicenter Randomized Controlled Fellow Eye Trial of Pulse-Dosed Difluprednate 0.05% Versus Prednisolone Acetate 1% in Cataract Surgery. American Journal of Ophthalmology 152(4): 609-17.

Foster, C. S., et al. (2010). Durezol (R) (Difluprednate Ophthalmic Emulsion 0.05%) Compared with Pred Forte (R) 1% Ophthalmic Suspension in the Treatment of Endogenous Anterior Uveitis. Journal of Ocular Pharmacology and Therapeutics 26(5): 475-83.

Dorzolamide Ophthalmic

(dor-zoe-la-mide)   Trusopt®, Cosopt®

Carbonic Anhydrase Inhibitor Anti-Glaucoma Agent

Prescriber Highlights

- ▶ 3 times a day dosing recommended over twice daily dosing.
- ▶ More stinging on application compared to brinzolamide.
- ▶ Sulfonamide derivative, inform clients with sulfa allergies.
- ▶ Available as a single agent or in combination with timolol maleate; generics now available.

Uses/Indications

In veterinary patients, dorzolamide (alone or in combination with timolol) is used to reduce intraocular pressure in patients with glaucoma.

Pharmacology/Actions

Dorzolamide is an inhibitor of carbonic anhydrase II. Inhibition of carbonic anhydrase in the ciliary processes of the eye decreases aqueous humor secretion, presumably by slowing the formation of bicarbonate ions with subsequent reduction in sodium and fluid transport. The result is a reduction in intraocular pressure (IOP). It equilibrates between acidic and basic forms allowing for both lipid and water solubility and greater corneal and scleral penetration.

Contraindications/Precautions/Warnings

Dorzolamide is contraindicated in patients with a history of hypersensitivity to it or sulfonamides or any component of the formulation.

Adverse Effects

Adverse effects reported in humans or animals include burning and stinging upon application (due to low pH), superficial punctate keratitis, local hypersensitivity reactions, and corneal edema. Systemic adverse effects are not usually observed with topical application.

Doses

Glaucoma (extra-label): 1 drop in the affected eye(s) every 8-12 hours.

Monitoring

- Clinical efficacy. Measure intraocular pressure. Monitor for corneal edema.

Client Information

- Used 2-3 times daily.
- Use proper administration techniques to avoid contamination of the medication. Keep cap tightly closed when not in use.
- Wait 5 minutes after applying this medication before applying any other medications to the eye.
- Store at controlled room temperature away from moisture and sunlight; do not freeze.

Storage/Stability

Store at controlled room temperature away from moisture and sunlight.

Compatibility/Compounding Considerations

Dorzolamide should not be mixed directly with any other drugs.

Dosage Forms/Regulatory Status

VETERINARY-LABELED PRODUCTS: NONE.

HUMAN-LABELED PRODUCTS:

Dorzolamide HCl 2% Ophthalmic Solution [containing benzalkonium chloride 0.0075%, hydroxyethyl cellulose, mannitol, sodium citrate dihydrate, NaOH (to adjust pH) and water for injection] in 5 mL and 10 mL ophthalmic dropper bottles; *Trusopt®*, generic; (Rx)

Dorzolamide 2% and Timolol 0.5% Ophthalmic Solution (containing benzalkonium chloride 0.0075%, sodium citrate, hydroxyethyl cellulose, NaOH, mannitol, and water for injection, with a pH of 5.65 and an osmolality of 242-323 mOsm/kg) in 10 mL ophthalmic dispenser bottles. *Cosopt*®, generic; (Rx)

Revisions/References
Monograph revised/updated September 2014.

Echothiophate Iodide Ophthalmic

(ek-oh-thye-oh-fate eye-oh-dide)   Phospholine Iodide®

Acetylcholinesterase Inhibitor Anti-Glaucoma Agent

Prescriber Highlights
▶ Risk for systemic organophosphate toxicity; may cause acute pancreatitis in dogs.
▶ Do not combine with pilocarpine or organophosphate/carbamate parasiticides.
▶ Do not use in patients with myasthenia gravis (drug interactions).
▶ Long duration of activity may be optimal for non-adherent owners.

Uses/Indications
Echothiophate iodide is very rarely used to treat glaucoma in animals due to risks for severe adverse effects. Because of the long duration of activity, echothiophate iodide remains an option for non-adherent pet owners. Use in humans to treat and diagnose accommodative esotropia continues, so the product remains commercially available.

Pharmacology/Actions
Echothiophate iodide for ophthalmic solution is a long-acting cholinesterase inhibitor for topical use that enhances the effect of endogenously liberated acetylcholine in iris, ciliary muscle, and other parasympathetically innervated structures of the eye. It thereby causes miosis, increase in facility of outflow of aqueous humor, fall in intraocular pressure, and potentiation of accommodation. Echothiophate iodide for ophthalmic solution will depress both plasma and erythrocyte cholinesterase levels in most patients after a few weeks of eye drop therapy. The effect on acetylcholinesterase is irreversible.

Contraindications/Precautions/Warnings
Echothiophate iodide is contraindicated in patients with a history of hypersensitivity to it or any component of the formulation. Use is contraindicated in uveitis. Echothiophate should be used cautiously if at all in patients with a history of pancreatitis. Do not use in patients being treated for myasthenia gravis. Paralytic agents (succinylcholine and atracurium) should not be used in animals being treated with echothiophate iodide.

Adverse Effects
Adverse effects reported in humans or animals include retinal detachment, which has been reported in a few cases during the use of echothiophate iodide for ophthalmic solution in adult human patients without a previous history of this disorder. Stinging, burning, lacrimation, lid muscle twitching, conjunctival and ciliary redness, browache, induced myopia with visual blurring may occur. Activation of latent iritis or uveitis may occur. Iris cysts may form, and if treatment is continued, may enlarge and obscure vision. The cysts usually shrink upon discontinuance of the medication, reduction in strength of the drops or frequency of instillation. Prolonged use may cause conjunctival thickening and obstruction of nasolacrimal canals. Lens opacities occurring in patients under treatment for glaucoma with echothiophate iodide for ophthalmic solution have

been reported and similar changes have been produced experimentally in normal monkeys. Routine examinations should accompany clinical use of the drug.

Paradoxical increase in intraocular pressure may follow anticholinesterase instillation. This may be alleviated by prescribing a sympathomimetic mydriatic such as phenylephrine. Cardiac irregularities have been reported.

Doses
Glaucoma (extra-label): 1 drop of the lowest concentration (0.03%) initially every 24 hours, then reduce dosing frequency to the longest interval that maintains reduced intraocular pressure.

Monitoring
- Clinical efficacy. Monitor intraocular pressure. Observe for signs of systemic organophosphate toxicity (ataxia, urinary incontinence, dyspnea, and tachycardia).

Client Information
- Used once daily then as directed.
- Do not use flea and tick preparations or collars without consulting your veterinarian.
- Use proper administration techniques to avoid contamination of the medication. Keep cap tightly closed when not in use.
- Wait 5 minutes after applying this medication before applying any other medications to the eye.
- Store in refrigerator prior to mixing. Once mixed, store at controlled room temperature away from moisture and sunlight; do not freeze. Discard 28 days after mixing or if color changes, becomes cloudy, or if particles are observed in the solution.

Storage/Stability
Store in refrigerator prior to mixing. Once mixed, store at controlled room temperature away from moisture and sunlight; do not freeze. Discard 28 days after mixing.

Compatibility/Compounding Considerations
Echothiophate iodide should not be mixed directly with any other drugs.

Dosage Forms/Regulatory Status
VETERINARY-LABELED PRODUCTS: NONE.
HUMAN-LABELED PRODUCTS:
Each package contains materials for dispensing 5 mL of eye drops: (1) Bottle containing sterile echothiophate iodide for ophthalmic solution in one of four potencies [1.5 mg (0.03%), 3 mg (0.06%), 6.25 mg (0.125%), or 12.5 mg (0.25%)] as indicated on the label, with 40 mg potassium acetate in each case. NaOH or acetic acid may have been incorporated to adjust pH during manufacturing. (2) A 5 mL bottle of sterile diluent containing chlorobutanol (chloral derivative), 0.55%; mannitol, 1.2%; boric acid, 0.06%; and sodium phosphate, 0.026%. (3) Sterilized dropper; *Phospholine Iodide*®; (Rx)

Revisions/References
Monograph revised/updated September 2014.

Edetate Disodium Ophthalmic

(ed-uh-tayt dye-so-dee-um)   EDTA

Chelating Agent

Prescriber Highlights
▶ No longer commercially available, must be compounded.
▶ Used 4-6 times daily for dissolution of corneal calcium deposits.
▶ Must use within 2 minutes of exposure for zinc chloride eye injury to achieve efficacy.
▶ Do not mix with other calcium-containing drugs.

Uses/Indications

In veterinary patients, edetate disodium is used topically to remove exogenous or endogenous calcific corneal deposits occur in the superficial cornea in band keratopathy that may cause pain or impair vision. Removal of superficial calcium deposits may improve vision, unless scarring and vascularization have occurred. Edetate disodium has been used as emergency treatment to decontaminate the eye after injury by zinc chloride and for emergency management and follow-up treatment of calcium hydroxide burns in the eye.

Pharmacology/Actions

Edetate disodium forms a soluble complex with calcium ions. Deposits from band keratopathy and other corneal calcium deposits associated with chronic uveitis, advanced interstitial keratitis, or hypercalcemia are dissolved from the conjunctiva, corneal epithelium, and anterior layers of the stroma. Calcium deposits in the deep stroma are not affected. Edetate disodium is lipid-insoluble and does not penetrate the corneal epithelium. Therefore, the epithelium must be completely removed before application, unless the deposit extends to the surface.

Contraindications/Precautions/Warnings

Edetate disodium ophthalmic should not be used in patients that are hypersensitive to it or to any component of the formulation.

Adverse Effects

Adverse effects reported in humans or animals include swelling of the stroma, usually following application of concentrations >1%, stinging on application, and swelling of the eyelids.

Doses

Calcium chelation (extra-label): 1 drop of the solution (0.35-1.85%, but most commonly 1%) to the affected eye(s) initially 4-6 times daily and then 3-4 times daily as indicated.

Zinc chloride injury (extra-label): Topical, to the cornea, as a 1.7% (0.046 M) solution as irrigation for 15 minutes; more likely to be effective if started within 2 minutes of exposure.

Monitoring

- Clinical efficacy. Monitor mineral deposits in cornea.

Client Information

- Used 4-6 times daily then as directed.
- Must be prepared (compounded) by a qualified compounding pharmacist. Give ample notice for refills.
- Use proper administration techniques to avoid contamination of the medication. Keep cap tightly closed when not in use.
- Wait 5 minutes after applying this medication before applying any other medications to the eye.
- Store in the refrigerator; do not freeze. Do not use if the color changes, it becomes cloudy, or if particles are seen in solutions. Discard by date indicated on label.

Storage/Stability

Store in refrigerator; do not freeze.

Compatibility/Compounding Considerations

Edetate disodium should not be mixed directly with any other drugs, especially those that contain calcium.

Dosage Forms/Regulatory Status

VETERINARY-LABELED PRODUCTS: NONE.
HUMAN-LABELED PRODUCTS: NONE.
Edetate disodium ophthalmic solution must be prepared (compounded) by a qualified compounding pharmacist. It is usually prepared as a 1% solution in an artificial tear solution that does not contain calcium.

Revisions/References

Monograph revised/updated September 2014.

Emedastine Ophthalmic

(em-uh-dast-teen)   Emadine®
Antihistamine

Prescriber Highlights

► Relatively selective H-1 blocker for treatment of allergic conjunctivitis.
► Used up to 4 times daily.

Uses/Indications

In veterinary patients, emedastine is used for the temporary relief of the signs and symptoms of allergic conjunctivitis.

Pharmacology/Actions

Emedastine is a relatively selective, histamine-1 antagonist.

Contraindications/Precautions/Warnings

Emedastine is contraindicated in patients with a history of hypersensitivity to it or any component of the formulation.

Adverse Effects

Adverse effects reported in humans include headache and abnormal dreams. It is not known if this adverse effect occurs in animals. The following adverse experiences have also been reported: asthenia, bad taste, blurred vision, burning or stinging, corneal infiltrates, corneal staining, dermatitis, discomfort, dry eye, foreign body sensation, hyperemia, keratitis, pruritus, rhinitis, sinusitis, and tearing. Some of these events may be similar to the underlying disease being treated.

Doses

Allergic conjunctivitis (extra-label): 1 drop in the affected eye(s) 4 times daily.

Monitoring

- Clinical efficacy. Resolution or relief of signs and symptoms of allergic conjunctivitis (pruritus, tearing, squinting, erythema).

Client Information

- Used 4 times daily.
- Use proper administration techniques to avoid contamination of the medication. Keep cap tightly closed when not in use.
- Wait 5 minutes after applying this medication before applying any other medications to the eye.
- Store in the refrigerator or at controlled room temperature away from moisture and sunlight; do not freeze. Do not use if the color changes, it becomes cloudy, or if particles are seen in solutions.

Storage/Stability

Store in refrigerator or at controlled room temperature away from moisture and sunlight; do not freeze. Discard if color change, or becomes cloudy, or if particles are observed in the solution.

Compatibility/Compounding Considerations

Emedastine should not be mixed directly with any other drugs.

Dosage Forms/Regulatory Status

VETERINARY-LABELED PRODUCTS: NONE.
HUMAN-LABELED PRODUCTS:
Emedastine Difumarate 0.05% Ophthalmic Solution [containing 0.884 mg emedastine difumarate equivalent to 0.5 mg Emedastine, benzalkonium chloride 0.01%, tromethamine; NaCl; hydroxypropyl methylcellulose; HCl/NaOH (adjust pH); and purified water. It has a pH of ≈7.4 and an osmolality of ≈300 mOsm/kg] in a 5 mL ophthalmic dropper bottle; *Emadine®*; (Rx)

Revisions/References

Monograph revised/updated September 2014.

Epinastine Ophthalmic

(ep-i-nas-teen)   Elestat®

Antihistamine

Prescriber Highlights

▶ Used to relieve symptoms and prevent pruritus associated with allergic conjunctivitis.

▶ Longer duration of action (8 hours) allows for twice daily dosing.

Uses/Indications

In veterinary patients, epinastine is used to treat and prevent pruritus associated with allergic conjunctivitis.

Pharmacology/Actions

Epinastine is a topically active, direct H1-receptor antagonist and an inhibitor of the release of histamine from the mast cell. Epinastine is selective for the histamine H1-receptor and has affinity for the histamine H2-receptor. Epinastine also possesses affinity for the α1-, α2-, and 5-HT2–receptors. The duration of action is ≈ 8 hours making this antihistamine suitable for twice daily administration.

Contraindications/Precautions/Warnings

Epinastine is contraindicated in patients with a history of hypersensitivity to it or any component of the formulation.

Adverse Effects

Adverse effects reported in humans or animals include were burning sensation in the eye, folliculitis, hyperemia, and pruritus. The most frequently reported non-ocular adverse reactions include cold symptoms and upper respiratory infections, seen in ≈ 10% of human patients, and headache, rhinitis, sinusitis, increased cough, and pharyngitis, seen in ≈ 3% of human patients. Some of these adverse effects may be related to the underlying disease being treated.

Doses

Allergic conjunctivitis (extra-label): 1 drop in the affected eye(s) every 12 hours.

Monitoring

▪ Clinical efficacy. Relief of symptoms associated with allergic conjunctivitis (pruritus, tearing, squinting).

Client Information

▪ Used 2 times daily.

▪ Use proper administration techniques to avoid contamination of the medication. Keep cap tightly closed when not in use.

▪ Wait 5 minutes after applying this medication before applying any other medications to the eye.

▪ Store at controlled room temperature away from moisture and sunlight; do not freeze. Do not use if the color changes, it becomes cloudy, or if particles are seen in solutions.

Storage/Stability

Store at controlled room temperature away from moisture and sunlight; do not freeze.

Compatibility/Compounding Considerations

Epinastine should not be mixed directly with any other drugs.

Dosage Forms/Regulatory Status

VETERINARY-LABELED PRODUCTS: NONE.

HUMAN-LABELED PRODUCTS:

Epinastine HCl 0.05% Ophthalmic Solution [containing epinastine 0.5 mg/mL, benzalkonium chloride 0.01%, edetate disodium; purified water; NaCl; sodium phosphate, monobasic; and NaOH and/or HCl (to adjust pH to 7) and an osmolality range of 250 to 310 mOsm/kg] in a 5 mL ophthalmic dropper bottle; *Elestat*®; (Rx)

Revisions/References

Monograph revised/updated September 2014.

Erythromycin Ophthalmic

(eh-rith-rowe-mye-sin

Macrolide Antibiotic

Prescriber Highlights

▶ For treatment of susceptible superficial ocular infections (*e.g.,* *Mycoplasma* and *Chlamydia* in cats).

▶ Not available in an ophthalmic solution; only ointment.

▶ Used up to 6 times daily.

▶ Use with caution in pocket pets that may ingest the drug via grooming.

Uses/Indications

In veterinary patients, erythromycin ophthalmic ointment is used for the treatment of superficial ocular infections involving the conjunctiva and/or cornea caused by organisms susceptible to erythromycin.

Pharmacology/Actions

Erythromycin inhibits protein synthesis without affecting nucleic acid synthesis. Erythromycin is usually active against *Streptococcus* and *Staphylococcus* spp., Mycoplasma, and Chlamydia.

Contraindications/Precautions/Warnings

Erythromycin is contraindicated in patients with a history of hypersensitivity to it or any component of the formulation. Topical macrolides should be used carefully if at all in pocket pets (*e.g.,* rabbits, hamsters, chinchillas) that may ingest macrolides while grooming.

Adverse Effects

Adverse effects reported in humans or animals include mild stinging, burning, irritation and redness. Pocket pets ingesting macrolides may suffer from an acute and potentially fatal diarrhea.

Doses

Susceptible ocular infections (extra-label): ¼ – ½ inch strip in the affected eye(s) up to 6 times daily depending on severity of infection.

Monitoring

▪ Clinical efficacy. Resolution of ocular infection. Discontinue if diarrhea occurs following use on pocket pets.

Client Information

▪ Used up to 6 times daily.

▪ Do not administer to pocket pets without supervision of veterinarian.

▪ Use proper administration techniques to avoid contamination of the medication. Keep cap tightly closed when not in use.

▪ Wait 5 minutes after applying this medication before applying any other medications to the eye.

▪ Store at controlled room temperature; do not freeze. Do not use if the color or consistency changes.

Storage/Stability

Store at controlled room temperature; do not freeze.

Compatibility/Compounding Considerations

Erythromycin should not be mixed directly with any other drugs. Erythromycin is not available as an ophthalmic solution.

Dosage Forms/Regulatory Status

VETERINARY-LABELED PRODUCTS: NONE.

HUMAN-LABELED PRODUCTS:

Erythromycin 0.5% Ophthalmic Ointment (containing erythromycin 5 mg/g in a sterile ophthalmic base of mineral oil and white petrolatum) in a 3.5 g ointment tube; generic; (Rx)

Revisions/References

Monograph revised/updated September 2014.

Fluorometholone Ophthalmic

(flew-roe-meth-oh-lone)   Flarex®, FML®

Corticosteroid

Prescriber Highlights

▶ Do not use for existing or suspected viral or fungal ocular infections.

▶ Prolonged use may elevate intraocular pressure; use with caution in glaucoma. Onset of elevated intraocular pressured is delayed when compared to dexamethasone.

▶ Use with caution in avian species as systemic adrenal suppression may result.

▶ Shake suspension well before using.

Uses/Indications

In veterinary patients, fluorometholone ophthalmic is used for the treatment of corticosteroid-responsive inflammation of the palpebral and bulbar conjunctiva, cornea and anterior segment of the globe.

Pharmacology/Actions

Ocular corticosteroids are thought to act by the induction of phospholipase A2 inhibitory proteins, collectively called lipocortins. It is postulated that these proteins control the biosynthesis of potent inflammatory mediators such as prostaglandins and leukotrienes by inhibiting the release of their common precursor, arachidonic acid. Arachidonic acid is released from membrane phospholipids by phospholipase A2.

Contraindications/Precautions/Warnings

Fluorometholone is contraindicated in patients with a history of hypersensitivity to it or any component of the formulation. Ocular corticosteroids should not be used in animals with concurrent fungal or viral infections or if corneal ulcerations are present.

Adverse Effects

Adverse reactions experienced by humans and animals include, in decreasing order of frequency, elevation of intraocular pressure (IOP) with possible development of glaucoma (following prolonged use) and infrequent optic nerve damage, posterior subcapsular cataract formation, and delayed wound healing. Although systemic effects are extremely uncommon, avian species may suffer systemic adrenocortical suppression following topical administration of corticosteroids. Corticosteroid-containing preparations have also been reported to cause acute anterior uveitis and perforation of the globe. Keratitis, conjunctivitis, corneal ulcers, mydriasis, conjunctival hyperemia, loss of accommodation and ptosis have occasionally been reported following local use of corticosteroids. The development of secondary ocular infection (bacterial, fungal and viral) has occurred. Fungal and viral infections of the cornea are particularly prone to develop or worsen coincidentally with long-term applications of steroids. Transient burning and stinging upon instillation and other minor symptoms of ocular irritation have been reported with the use of fluorometholone suspension. Other adverse events reported with the use of fluorometholone include: allergic reactions; foreign body sensation; erythema of eyelid; eyelid edema/eye swelling; eye discharge; eye pain; eye pruritus; lacrimation increased; rash; taste perversion; visual disturbance; and visual field defect.

Doses

Antiinflammatory (extra-label): 1 drop in the affected eye(s) every 4 hours for 24-48 hours and then reduce to every 6-12 hours as indicated.

Monitoring

- Clinical efficacy. Monitor intraocular pressure and discontinue use if elevated. Observe/culture for secondary bacterial, fungal or viral infections.

Client Information

- Used 2-6 times daily.
- Shake suspension well before using.
- Use proper administration techniques to avoid contamination of the medication. Keep cap tightly closed when not in use.
- Wait 5 minutes after applying this medication before applying any other medications to the eye.
- Store in the refrigerator or at controlled room temperature away from moisture and sunlight; do not freeze. Do not use if the color changes or if particles are seen in the suspension.

Storage/Stability

Store in refrigerator or at controlled room temperature away from moisture and sunlight; do not freeze.

Compatibility/Compounding Considerations

Fluorometholone ophthalmic should not be mixed directly with any other drugs. Instruct caregivers to wait 5 minutes after applying this medication before applying any other medications to the eye.

Dosage Forms/Regulatory Status

VETERINARY-LABELED PRODUCTS: NONE.

HUMAN-LABELED PRODUCTS:

Fluorometholone 0.1% Ophthalmic Suspension (containing fluorometholone 1mg/mL; benzalkonium chloride 0.004%; edetate disodium; polysorbate 80; polyvinyl alcohol 1.4%; purified water; NaCl; sodium phosphate, dibasic; sodium phosphate, monobasic; and NaOH to adjust pH from 6.2-7.5 and an osmolality range of 290-350 mOsm/kg) in 5 mL, 10 mL and 15 mL ophthalmic dropper bottles; *FML®*; (Rx)

Fluorometholone 0.25% Ophthalmic Suspension (containing fluorometholone 2.5 mg/mL; benzalkonium chloride 0.005%; edetate disodium; polysorbate 80; polyvinyl alcohol 1.4%; purified water; NaCl; sodium phosphate, dibasic; sodium phosphate, monobasic; and NaOH to adjust the pH from 6.2-7.5) in 5 mL, 10 mL and 15 mL ophthalmic dropper bottles; *FML Forte®*; (Rx)

Fluorometholone 0.1% Ophthalmic Ointment [containing fluorometholone 1 mg/mL; phenylmercuric acetate (0.0008%); mineral oil; petrolatum (and) lanolin alcohol; and white petrolatum] in 3.5 gram ophthalmic ointment tubes; *FML S.O.P.®*; (Rx)

Revisions/References

Monograph revised/updated September 2014.

Fluorouracil Ophthalmic

(flewr-oh-your-uh-sil)   5-fluorouracil, 5-FU

Antineoplastic Agent

Prescriber Highlights

▶ Antineoplastic used for susceptible tumors.

▶ Do **NOT** use on cats or patients with bone marrow suppression or serious infections.

▶ Known teratogen.

▶ Adverse effects include dose-dependent myelosuppression, gastrointestinal toxicity, and neurotoxicity.

Uses/Indications

Because of its ability to reduce fibroblastic proliferation and prevent subsequent scarring, fluorouracil (5-fluorouracil; 5-FU) is used as an adjunct in ocular and periorbital surgeries. It is also used to treat ocular surface neoplasia such as squamous cell carcinoma and periorbital tumors such as neoplasia and sarcoids.

Pharmacology/Actions

5-FU is a pyrimidine analog that is converted through intracellular mechanisms into an active metabolite, fluorouridine monophosphate (FUMP) and fluorouridine triphosphate (FUTP) that intercalate into DNA and RNA and disrupt cellular function.

Contraindications/Precautions/Warnings

5-FU is contraindicated in patients hypersensitive to it or any component of the formulation. 5-FU is absolutely contraindicated in cats by any route of administration including topical administration. Cats develop a severe, potentially fatal neurotoxicity when exposed to 5-FU by any route. Although systemic adverse effects are less likely after topical application in other species, they can occur. Do not use in patients with myelosuppression, with concurrent serious infections, or that are hypersensitive to 5-FU.

Adverse Effects

Although less likely after topical administration, adverse effects reported in humans or animals include bone marrow suppression, GI toxicity (*e.g.,* diarrhea, gastrointestinal ulceration, sloughing, stomatitis), and neurotoxicity (seizures). The most frequent adverse reactions to topical 5-FU occur locally and are often related to an extension of the pharmacological activity of the drug. These include burning, crusting, allergic contact dermatitis, erosions, erythema, hyperpigmentation, irritation, pain, photosensitivity, pruritus, scarring, rash, soreness and ulceration. Periorbital alopecia is also reported after topical ocular use in horses.

Doses

Ocular surface neoplasia (extra-label): 5-FU 1% ophthalmic solution (compounded) 1 drop in affected eye(s) q6h.

Monitoring

▪ Clinical efficacy. Morphological smears for cell cytology or biopsy to confirm remission of neoplasia.

Client Information

▪ Used 4 times daily.

▪ This is a chemotherapy drug. Pregnant women should avoid contact.

▪ Wear protective gloves and mask when administering.

▪ Loss of hair around the eyes may occur after use.

▪ Wait 5 minutes after applying this medication before applying any other medications to the eye.

▪ Store at controlled room temperature away from moisture and sunlight; do not freeze. Do not use if the color changes, it becomes cloudy, or if particles are seen in solutions.

▪ Dispose of unused medication in regular trash, do not put into sewer system.

Storage/Stability

Store at controlled room temperature away from moisture and sunlight; do not freeze.

Compatibility/Compounding Considerations

Fluorouracil should not be mixed directly with any other drugs. Fluorouracil (5-FU) ophthalmic solution is not commercially available but may be prepared by qualified compounding pharmacists by utilizing the 50 mg/mL injectable solution, *Adrucil®*. Fluorouracil 1% ophthalmic solution prepared this way is reported to be stable for 3 weeks (Midena *et al.* 2000).

Dosage Forms/Regulatory Status

VETERINARY-LABELED PRODUCTS: NONE.

HUMAN-LABELED PRODUCTS: NONE.

Revisions/References

Monograph revised/updated September 2014.
Midena, E., et al. (2000). Treatment of conjunctival squamous cell carcinoma with topical 5-fluorouracil. British Journal of Ophthalmology **84**(3): 268-72.

Fluorescein Sodium Ophthalmic

(flur-e-seen)

Ocular Diagnostic Agent

Prescriber Highlights

▶ Yellow-green dye that binds to corneal stroma to delineate full thickness loss of corneal epithelium (corneal injury).

▶ Used to evaluate tear film breakup time and patency of nasolacrimal outflow system.

▶ Fluorescein binds only to corneal stroma and not to corneal epithelium or Descemet's membrane.

▶ Fluorescein should **not** be used during intraocular surgery.

Uses/Indications

In veterinary patients, fluorescein is used to delineate corneal injury, to evaluate tear film break up time, and to determine the patency of the nasolacrimal outflow system. While fluorescein solutions have been prepared, they are easily contaminated, so individually wrapped fluorescein strips are preferred. Fluorescein injection is also used in fluorescein angiography.

Pharmacology/Actions

Fluorescein is a water-soluble dye that does not stain normal cornea because it does not pass through the hydrophobic epithelium. If the epithelium is damaged, fluorescein penetrates the hydrophilic corneal stroma and stains it bright yellow-green. The green color is best excited with blue light from a cobalt filter attached to a penlight or transilluminator. A Wood's Lamp may also be used. Intravenous fluorescein is also used in fluorescein angiography to investigate retinal and choroidal vascular patency, vessel-wall permeability, and pigmentary abnormalities of the fundus. Vessels in active areas of inflammation and neovascularization show increased permeability to the dye. Fluorescein fluoresces in light with a wavelength between 485-500 nm with maximal emission between 520-530 nm.

Contraindications/Precautions/Warnings

Fluorescein is contraindicated in patients with a history of hypersensitivity to it or any component of the formulation. Fluorescein should not be used during intraocular surgery.

Adverse Effects

Adverse effects reported in humans or animals following application of the strips include local hypersensitivity reactions. Temporary staining of the skin and fur may result after use. Adverse events following intravenous administration can be severe and include nausea, vomiting, gastrointestinal distress, headache, syncope, hypotension, and symptoms and signs of hypersensitivity have occurred. Cardiac arrest, basilar artery ischemia, severe shock, convulsions, thrombophlebitis at the injection site, and rare cases of death have been reported in humans. Extravasation of the solution at the injection site causes intense pain at the site and a dull aching pain in the injected limb.

Doses

Determination of Corneal Injury: Wet the surface of the fluorescein strip with 1-2 drops of normal saline solution. Apply moistened tip to conjunctiva or fornix as required. It is recommended that the patient blink several times after application. Wait 60 seconds, rinse the eye with sterile irrigating solution, and examine the eye with a light source. Defects in the corneal epithelium appear as bright green. In deep corneal lesions the center of the lesion may fail to take up stain and appears black, indicating that a descemetocele is present.

Tear Film Breakup: Wet the surface of the fluorescein strip with 1-2 drops of normal saline solution. Apply moistened tip to conjunctiva or fornix as required. It is recommended that the patient blink several times after application. Conduct tear film break up time measurements immediately. Normal values are considered to be <19 seconds.

Nasolacrimal Outflow Patency: Wet the surface of the fluorescein strip with 1-2 drops of normal saline solution. Apply moistened tip to conjunctiva or fornix as required. It is recommended that the patient blink several times after application. Normal wait times are 2-5 minutes in dogs and up to 10 minutes in cats for fluorescein stain to show up at the nose.

Fluorescein Angiography: 2 – 5 mL of fluorescein 100 mg/mL injection is rapidly administered intravenously (~1 ml/second), usually in the antecubital vein. Luminescence usually appears in the retina and choroidal vessels in 7-14 seconds and can be observed by standard viewing equipment.

Note: No fluorescein products are FDA-approved and all use is extra-label.

Monitoring
- Diagnostic product. No monitoring is required.

Client Information
- Fluorescein strips are not used by pet owners at home.

Storage/Stability
Store at controlled room temperature away from moisture and sunlight; do not freeze.

Compatibility/Compounding Considerations
Fluorescein should not be mixed directly with any other drugs.

Dosage Forms/Regulatory Status
VETERINARY-LABELED PRODUCTS: NONE.
HUMAN-LABELED PRODUCTS:
No fluorescein products have been approved by the US Food and Drug Administration, although several are marketed, including:

Fluorescein Sodium 10% Injection (containing: fluorescein 100 mg/mL and sterile water for injection; NaOH and/or HCl to adjust pH) in 5 mL ampules; *Fluorescite®*; (Rx)

Fluorescein Sodium 0.25% and Benoxinate HCl 0.4% (containing: chlorobutanol 1%; povidone, boric acid; purified water; HCl may be added to adjust pH to 4.3-5.3) in 5 mL ophthalmic dropper bottles; *Altafluor®, Fluress®*; (Rx)

Fluorescein Sodium Ophthalmic Strips U.S.P. 1 mg per strip individually wrapped strips in cartons of 50, 100, or 300; *Glostrips®, Fluor-I-Strips®, SoftGlo®, Dry Eye Test®, Ful-Glo®*; (Rx)

Revisions/References
Monograph revised/updated September 2014.

Flurbiprofen Ophthalmic
(flur-bi-proe-fin)   Ocufen®
NSAID

Prescriber Highlights
▶ May cause transient increases in intraocular pressure.
▶ Immunosuppressive activity may worsen infected corneal ulcers.
▶ May delay wound healing.

Uses/Indications
In veterinary patients, flurbiprofen is used to treat a variety of inflammatory conditions of the eye including uveitis, iritis, and pre-and postoperative cataract surgery. It is a nonsteroidal antiinflammatory agent (NSAID) and avoids the adverse effects associated with chronic use of corticosteroids. Flurbiprofen also inhibits miosis and is sometimes used to prevent miosis during intraocular surgery. However, since prostaglandin blockade may result in increase in intraocular pressure, the use of preoperative flurbiprofen has become obsolete. Inhibition of miosis by flurbiprofen is, however, useful in the management of uveal inflammation.

Pharmacology/Actions
Flurbiprofen sodium is one of a series of phenylalkanoic acids that have shown analgesic, antipyretic, and antiinflammatory activity in animal inflammatory diseases. Its mechanism of action is believed to be through inhibition of the cyclooxygenase enzyme that is essential in the biosynthesis of prostaglandins known to be mediators of certain kinds of intraocular inflammation. In studies performed on animal eyes, prostaglandins have been shown to produce disruption of the blood-aqueous humor barrier, vasodilatation, increased vascular permeability, leukocytosis, and increased intraocular pressure.

Prostaglandins also appear to play a role in the miotic response produced during ocular surgery by constricting the iris sphincter independently of cholinergic mechanisms. In human clinical studies, flurbiprofen sodium ophthalmic solution 0.03% has been shown to inhibit the miosis induced during the course of cataract surgery. Results from clinical studies indicate that flurbiprofen sodium has no significant effect upon intraocular pressure.

Contraindications/Precautions/Warnings
Flurbiprofen is contraindicated in patients with a history of hypersensitivity to it or any component of the formulation. Cross-sensitivity with other NSAIDs has occurred in humans and may occur in animals. Flurbiprofen may be as immunosuppressive as topical steroids, so it should be used with caution in patients with infected corneal ulcers. NSAIDs inhibit thrombocyte aggregation and may prolong bleeding; use during intraocular surgery may promote intraocular bleeding. Although clinical studies with acetylcholine chloride and animal studies with acetylcholine chloride or carbachol revealed no interference and there is no known pharmacological basis for an interaction, there have been reports that acetylcholine chloride and carbachol have been ineffective when used in patients treated with flurbiprofen sodium ophthalmic solution 0.03%.

Adverse Effects
Adverse effects reported in humans or animals include transient burning and stinging upon instillation and other minor symptoms of ocular irritation. Other adverse reactions reported with the use of flurbiprofen sodium include: fibrosis, miosis, and mydriasis. In-

creased bleeding tendency of ocular tissues in conjunction with ocular surgery has also been reported.

Doses

Pre-surgery (extra-label): 1 drop every 20 minutes for 4 applications.

Antiinflammatory (keratitis, uveitis) (extra-label): 1 drop in affected eye(s) every 8 hours, may be reduced to once daily after resolution of initial episodes.

Monitoring

- Clinical efficacy. Effective blockade of miosis during intraocular surgery; resolution of inflammation associated with keratitis or uveitis.

Client Information

- Used 3-4 times daily.
- Use proper administration techniques to avoid contamination of the medication. Keep cap tightly closed when not in use.
- Wait 5 minutes after applying this medication before applying any other medications to the eye.
- Store in the refrigerator or at controlled room temperature away from moisture and sunlight; do not freeze. Do not use if the color changes, it becomes cloudy, or if particles are seen in solutions.

Storage/Stability

Store in refrigerator or at controlled room temperature away from moisture and sunlight; do not freeze.

Compatibility/Compounding Considerations

Flurbiprofen should not be mixed directly with any other drugs. Flurbiprofen is not available as an ophthalmic ointment.

Dosage Forms/Regulatory Status

VETERINARY-LABELED PRODUCTS: NONE.

HUMAN-LABELED PRODUCTS:

Flurbiprofen sodium 0.03% Ophthalmic Solution (containing flurbiprofen 0.3 mg/mL; thimerosal 0.005%; citric acid; edetate disodium; polyvinyl alcohol 1.4%; potassium chloride; purified water; NaCl; and sodium citrate; HCl and/or NaOH to adjust pH to 6.0-7.0; osmolality of 260-330 mOsm/kg) in 2.5 mL ophthalmic dropper bottles; *Ocufen®*; (Rx)

Revisions/References

Monograph revised/updated September 2014.

Ganciclovir Ophthalmic

(gan-**sye**-kloe-veer)   Zirgan®

Antiviral Agent

Prescriber Highlights

▶ Used 4-6 times daily.

▶ May cause myelosuppression and nephrotoxicity in cats if ingested.

▶ *In vitro* efficacy double against FHV-1 as compared to cidofovir and penciclovir, and 10-fold higher than acyclovir.

Uses/Indications

In veterinary patients, ganciclovir is used to treat acute herpes keratitis in cats and horses.

Pharmacology/Actions

Ganciclovir is a guanosine derivative that, upon phosphorylation, inhibits DNA replication by herpes simplex viruses (HSV). Ganciclovir is transformed by viral and cellular thymidine kinases (TK) to ganciclovir triphosphate, which works as an antiviral agent by inhibiting the synthesis of viral DNA in 2 ways: competitive inhibition of viral DNA-polymerase and direct incorporation into viral primer strand DNA, resulting in DNA chain termination and prevention of replication.

Contraindications/Precautions/Warnings

Ganciclovir is contraindicated in patients with a history of hypersensitivity to it or any component of the formulation. Myelosuppression and nephrotoxicity occur in cats after systemic treatment; warn caregiver to not allow cats to groom ganciclovir from the eye area.

Adverse Effects

Adverse effects reported in humans or animals include blurred vision, eye irritation, punctate keratitis, and conjunctival hyperemia. Myelosuppression and nephrotoxicity are possible in cats after ingestion by grooming.

Doses

Herpes Keratitis (extra-label): 1 drop in each eye every 4-6 hours for 21 days.

Monitoring

- Clinical efficacy. Resolution of signs of herpes keratitis.
- Safety: CBC and chemistry panel for cats to detect myelosuppression and nephrotoxicity.

Client Information

- Used 4-6 times daily.
- Wipe your cat's face after applying; do not let cats lick this medication.
- Use proper administration techniques to avoid contamination of the medication. Keep cap tightly closed when not in use.
- Wait 5 minutes after applying this medication before applying any other medications to the eye.
- Store at controlled room temperature away from moisture and sunlight; do not freeze. Do not use if the color changes, it becomes cloudy, or if particles are seen in the gel.

Storage/Stability

Store at controlled room temperature away from moisture and sunlight.

Compatibility/Compounding Considerations

Ganciclovir should not be mixed directly with any other drugs. Ganciclovir is not available as an ophthalmic solution.

Dosage Forms/Regulatory Status

VETERINARY-LABELED PRODUCTS: NONE.

HUMAN-LABELED PRODUCTS:

Ganciclovir 0.15% Ophthalmic Gel [containing ganciclovir 1.5 mg/mL; carbopol, water for injection, NaOH (to adjust the pH to 7.4), mannitol; benzalkonium chloride 0.075 mg] in a 5 g ophthalmic gel tube; *Zirgan®*; (Rx)

Revisions/References

Monograph revised/updated September 2014.

Gatifloxacin Ophthalmic

(gat-i-**flocks**-a sin)   Zymaxid®, Zymar®

Fluoroquinolone Antibiotic

Prescriber Highlights

▶ Fluoroquinolone antimicrobial used for bacterial conjunctivitis or keratitis.

▶ Physically incompatible with many drugs.

▶ Crystalline drug precipitates may be noted in the superficial portion of corneal defects during use.

Uses/Indications

In veterinary patients, gatifloxacin ophthalmic may be useful for treating bacterial conjunctivitis caused by susceptible species/strains of staphylococci, streptococci, Corynebacterium, Haemophilus, and Chlamydia. When administered via a subpalpebral lavage (SPL) catheter it can be used for treating keratitis in horses.

Pharmacology/Actions

Gatifloxacin is a member of the fluoroquinolone class of anti-infective drugs. Its action results from inhibition of DNA gyrase, which is involved in replication, transcription and repair of bacterial DNA. The mechanism of action of fluoroquinolones including gatifloxacin is different from that of aminoglycoside, macrolide, and tetracycline antibiotics. Therefore, gatifloxacin may be active against pathogens that are resistant to these antibiotics and these antibiotics may be active against pathogens that are resistant to gatifloxacin. There is no cross-resistance between gatifloxacin and the aforementioned classes of antibiotics. Cross-resistance has been observed between systemic gatifloxacin and some other fluoroquinolones.

Contraindications/Precautions/Warnings

Gatifloxacin is contraindicated in patients with a history of hypersensitivity to it, other fluoroquinolones, or any component of the formulation. For topical ophthalmic use only. Not for injection subconjunctivally or into the anterior chamber of the eye. Fluoroquinolone-induced retinal toxicity in domestic cats has not been demonstrated with this product at time of writing, but may be possible.

Adverse Effects

Adverse effects reported in humans or animals include blurred vision, tearing, eye pain, redness, itching, and a bad taste in the mouth. Crystalline drug precipitates may be noted in the superficial portion of corneal defects during use.

Doses

Conjunctivitis (extra-label): 1 drop in affected eye(s) every 4-8 hours.

Keratitis (extra-label): 1 drop in the affected eye or 0.2 mL in the SPL catheter every 1-8 hours. May precipitate when mixed with other ophthalmic medications. Flush SPL catheter well with air between medications.

Monitoring

- Clinical efficacy. If blepharospasm, uveitis, or worsening of ulceration or no improvement in infection is noted in 7 days, reassess microbial susceptibility.

Client Information

- Used 3-12 times daily. Use proper administration techniques to avoid contamination of the medication. Keep cap tightly closed when not in use.
- Crystals may appear in the eyes for a few days after initiation of treatment.
- Wait 5 minutes after applying this medication before applying any other medications to the eye.
- Store at controlled room temperature away from moisture and sunlight; do not freeze. Dispose of unused medication in regular trash, do not put into sewer system.

Storage/Stability

Store at controlled room temperature away from moisture and sunlight; do not freeze.

Compatibility/Compounding Considerations

Gatifloxacin should not be mixed directly with any other drugs. Gatifloxacin is not available as an ophthalmic ointment.

Dosage Forms/Regulatory Status

VETERINARY-LABELED PRODUCTS: NONE.

HUMAN-LABELED PRODUCTS:

Gatifloxacin 0.3% Ophthalmic Solution (containing: gatifloxacin 3 mg/mL; benzalkonium chloride 0.005%; edetate disodium; purified water and NaCl; HCl and/or NaOH to adjust pH to ≈ 6; osmolality of 260-330 mOsm/kg) in 2.5 and 5 mL ophthalmic dropper bottles; *Zymar*®; (Rx)

Gatifloxacin 0.5% Ophthalmic Solution (containing: gatifloxacin 5 mg/mL; benzalkonium chloride 0.005%; edetate disodium; purified water and NaCl; HCl and/or NaOH to adjust pH to ≈ 6; osmolality of 260-330 mOsm/kg) in a 2.5 mL ophthalmic dropper bottle; *Zymaxid*®; (Rx)

Revisions/References

Monograph revised/updated September 2014.

Gentamicin Sulfate Ophthalmic

(jen-ta-mye-sin sul-fate)   Gentocin®, Genoptic®, Gentak®

Aminoglycoside Antibiotic

Prescriber Highlights

▶ Do not use if cornea penetrated; gentamicin is toxic to the interior of the eye.

▶ Do not confuse pure gentamicin sulfate ophthalmic preparations with those containing combination with steroids.

▶ Fortified solutions of gentamicin sulfate up to 13.6 mg/mL may be compounded for use in susceptible infections of equine bacterial keratitis.

Uses/Indications

In veterinary patients, gentamicin sulfate ophthalmic is primarily used for patients with ocular infections of *Pseudomonas aeruginosa*. Due to the intraocular toxicity of gentamicin sulfate, it is also injected into the eye to perform chemical enucleation in end-stage glaucoma or other conditions that cause loss of vision.

Pharmacology/Actions

Gentamicin sulfate, an aminoglycoside, is actively transported across the bacterial cell membrane and binds to a specific receptor protein on the 30 S subunit of bacterial ribosomes. It consequently interferes with an initiation complex between mRNA (messenger RNA) and the 30 S subunit, inhibiting protein synthesis. DNA may be misread, thus producing nonfunctional proteins; polyribosomes are split apart and are unable to synthesize protein. Aminoglycosides are bactericidal, while most other antibiotics that interfere with protein synthesis are bacteriostatic.

Contraindications/Precautions/Warnings

Gentamicin sulfate is contraindicated in patients with a history of hypersensitivity to it or any component of the formulation. Gentamicin sulfate should not be used if the cornea is penetrated, as gentamicin is extremely toxic to the interior of the eye.

Adverse Effects

Adverse effects reported in humans or animals include are ocular burning and irritation upon drug instillation, nonspecific conjunctivitis, conjunctival epithelial defects, and conjunctival hyperemia. Other adverse reactions that have occurred rarely are allergic reactions, thrombocytopenic purpura, and hallucinations (humans).

Doses

Susceptible Ocular Infections (extra-label): 1 drop of the solution or ¼ – ½ inch strip in the affected eye(s) 2-3 times daily. Frequency may be increased to every 30-60 minutes for treating equine corneal ulcers.

Chemical Enucleation (extra-label): 0.25 mL of gentamicin sulfate 100 mg/mL injection into the vitreous.

Monitoring

- Clinical efficacy. Resolution of bacterial infection.

Client Information

- Used 3-4 times daily.
- Use proper administration techniques to avoid contamination of the medication. Keep cap tightly closed when not in use.
- Wait 5 minutes after applying this medication before applying any other medications to the eye.
- Store in the refrigerator or at controlled room temperature away from moisture and sunlight; do not freeze. Do not use if the color changes, it becomes cloudy, or if particles are seen in solutions.

Storage/Stability

Store in refrigerator or at controlled room temperature away from moisture and sunlight; do not freeze.

Compatibility/Compounding Considerations

Gentamicin sulfate should not be mixed directly with any other drugs.

Dosage Forms/Regulatory Status

VETERINARY-LABELED PRODUCTS: NONE.
Gentamicin Sulfate 0.3% Ophthalmic Ointment (containing gentamicin sulfate equivalent to 3 mg/mL of gentamicin in a base of white petrolatum and mineral oil, with methylparaben and propylparaben as preservatives) in a 3.5 g ophthalmic ointment tube; *Gentocin®*; (Rx)

HUMAN-LABELED PRODUCTS:
Gentamicin 0.3% Ophthalmic Solution (containing gentamicin sulfate equivalent to 3 mg/mL gentamicin base; benzalkonium chloride; edetate disodium, polyvinyl alcohol 1.4%; purified water; NaCl; sodium phosphate, dibasic; and HCl and/or NaOH to adjust the pH in an aqueous, buffered solution with a pH of 6.5-7.5) in 5 mL ophthalmic dropper bottles; *Genoptic®*; (Rx)

Gentamicin 0.3% Ophthalmic Ointment (containing gentamicin sulfate equivalent to 3 mg/mL of gentamicin in a base of white petrolatum and mineral oil, with methylparaben and propylparaben as preservatives) in a 3.5 g ophthalmic ointment tube; *Gentak®*; (Rx)

Combination Products:

Prednisolone Acetate 0.6% and Gentamicin 0.3% Ophthalmic Ointment in 3.5 g; *Pred-G®*; (Rx)

Prednisolone Acetate 1% and Gentamicin 0.3% Ophthalmic Suspension in 5 & 10 mL; *Pred-G®*; (Rx)

Revisions/References

Monograph revised/updated September 2014.

Hydrocortisone Ophthalmic

(hye-dro-kort-uh-sown)

Corticosteroid Antiinflammatory Agent

Prescriber Highlights

▶ Usually combined with double or triple antibiotic.
▶ Do not use in feline herpes keratitis, fungal keratitis, or if corneal abrasion or ulceration are suspected.
▶ Use with caution in avian species due to risk of systemic corticosteroid effects.

Uses/Indications

In veterinary patients, hydrocortisone is used alone or in combination with triple antibiotic (neomycin, polymyxin, ± bacitracin) for inflammatory conjunctivitis.

Pharmacology/Actions

Hydrocortisone is a naturally occurring corticosteroid produced by the adrenal glands. It decreases inflammation by stabilizing leukocyte lysosomal membranes, preventing release of destructive acid hydrolases from leukocytes, and inhibiting macrophage accumulation in inflamed areas. Corticosteroids also reduce leukocyte adhesion to capillary endothelium, and reduces capillary wall permeability and edema formation. Corticosteroids decrease complement components. Corticosteroids antagonize histamine activity and release of kinin from substrates.

Contraindications/Precautions/Warnings

Hydrocortisone is contraindicated in patients with a history of hypersensitivity to it or any component of the formulation. Hydrocortisone should not be used if corneal abrasion or ulceration are suspected and should not be used to treat fungal or viral keratitis (*e.g.*, feline herpes keratitis). Ophthalmic steroids should be used with extreme caution in avian species due to increased risk for systemic adverse effects.

Adverse Effects

Adverse effects reported in humans or animals include burning, stinging and irritation upon application to the eye. Systemic absorption may result in suppression of the hypothalamus-pituitary-adrenal axis. Use of corticosteroids may produce posterior subcapsular cataracts, glaucoma with possible damage to the optic nerves, and may enhance the establishment of secondary ocular infections due to bacteria, fungi, or viruses. Intraocular pressure may increase in some animals with chronic use.

Doses

Inflammatory conjunctivitis (extra-label): 1 drop in the affected eye(s) up to 4 times daily.

Monitoring

- Clinical efficacy. Monitor for resolution of inflammatory signs; discontinue use if corneal abrasion or ulceration is present.

Client Information

- Used up to 4 times daily.
- Shake drops well before using.
- Use proper administration techniques to avoid contamination of the medication. Keep cap tightly closed when not in use.
- Wait 5 minutes after applying this medication before applying any other medications to the eye.
- Store at controlled room temperature away from moisture and sunlight; do not freeze. Discard if color change occurs.

Storage/Stability

Store at controlled room temperature away from moisture and sunlight.

Compatibility/Compounding Considerations

Hydrocortisone ophthalmic should not be mixed directly with any other drugs. Instruct caregivers to wait 5 minutes after applying this medication before applying any other medications to the eye.

Dosage Forms/Regulatory Status

VETERINARY-LABELED PRODUCTS:
No ophthalmic products containing only hydrocortisone are available; available commercially in combination with antimicrobial agents.

Neomycin/Bacitracin/Polymyxin/Hydrocortisone Ophthalmic Ointment (containing: neomycin sulfate equivalent to 3.5 mg neomycin base, polymyxin B sulfate equivalent to 10,000 polymyxin B units, bacitracin zinc equivalent to 400 bacitracin units, hydrocortisone 10 mg per gram, and white petrolatum) in a 3.5 gram ophthalmic ointment tube; *Vetropolycin HC®*, *Trioptic-S®*; (Rx)

HUMAN-LABELED PRODUCTS: NONE.

Revisions/References
Monograph revised/updated September 2014.

Hypertonic Sodium Chloride Ophthalmic — See Sodium Chloride, Hypertonic Ophthalmic

---

Idoxuridine Ophthalmic

(eye-docks-yoor-uh-deen)   Stoxil®, Herplex®, Dendrid®

Antiviral

Prescriber Highlights
▶ Must be used 4-5 times daily.
▶ Less stinging compared to other antiviral drugs (except cidofovir).
▶ No longer commercially available, must be compounded.

Uses/Indications
In veterinary patients, idoxuridine is used for topical treatment of feline herpes virus-1 (FHV-1) keratitis.

Pharmacology/Actions
Idoxuridine is chemically similar to thymidine and its substitution into viral DNA causes misreading of the viral genetic code thereby inhibiting viral replication. Because idoxuridine is a non-specific inhibitor of DNA synthesis, it affects any cellular function requiring thymidine and is not suitable for systemic use. Even with topical therapy corneal toxicity can occur. Idoxuridine is virustatic, not virucidal.

Contraindications/Precautions/Warnings
Idoxuridine is contraindicated in patients with a history of hypersensitivity to it or any component of the formulation.

Adverse Effects
Adverse effects reported in humans or animals include acute ocular irritation including burning, corneal stippling, vascularization, and clouding has been reported. Following prolonged use of idoxuridine, ocular irritation characterized by follicular conjunctivitis, blepharitis with punctal swelling, bulbar conjunctival hyperemia, and corneal epithelial staining has also been reported. In either case, the drug should be discontinued.

Doses
Feline herpes virus-1 keratitis (extra-label): 1 drop in the affected eye(s) every 2-3 hours for 48 hours then 4-5 times daily for a week beyond resolution of clinical signs.

Monitoring
■ Clinical efficacy. Resolution of clinical signs of FHV-1.

Client Information
■ Used every 2-3 hours for 2 days then 4-5 times daily.
■ Use proper administration techniques to avoid contamination of the medication. Keep cap tightly closed when not in use.
■ Wait 5 minutes after applying this medication before applying any other medications to the eye.
■ Store in the refrigerator or at controlled room temperature away from moisture and sunlight; do not freeze. Do not use if the color changes, it becomes cloudy, or if particles are seen in solutions.

Storage/Stability
Store in refrigerator or at controlled room temperature away from moisture and sunlight; do not freeze.

Compatibility/Compounding Considerations
Idoxuridine should not be mixed directly with any other drugs.

Dosage Forms/Regulatory Status
VETERINARY-LABELED PRODUCTS: NONE.
HUMAN-LABELED PRODUCTS: NONE.
Idoxuridine is no longer approved for use as an ophthalmic dosage form, but idoxuridine 0.1% ophthalmic solution or 0.5% ophthalmic ointment can be prepared by a qualified compounding pharmacist.

Revisions/References
Monograph revised/updated September 2014.

Irrigating Solutions, Ophthalmic

BSS, Collyrium®, OCuSOFT®

Irrigants

Prescriber Highlights
▶ Two categories of irrigants: intraocular and extraocular (eyewashes); extraocular (eyewashes) products should **not** be used for intraocular procedures.
▶ BSS Plus® solutions must be mixed (parts 1 & 2) before use.

Uses/Indications
The primary use of intraocular irrigation solutions (*e.g.*, BSS, *BSS Plus®*) is during intraocular surgery (cataract removal). Ocular irrigating solutions maintain the shape of the anterior chamber during surgery, cool phacoemulsification handpieces, and lavage emulsified lens and surgical byproducts from the eye. A study evaluating cooled versus room temperature irrigating solutions have demonstrated no significant adverse effects between the two temperatures (Praveen *et al.* 2009). They are also used for flushing the nasolacrimal system, for removing debris from the eye, and to remove excess stain after diagnostic staining of the cornea.

OTC eyewash products are used to flush eyes to remove loose foreign material, or help relieve eye irritation caused by air pollutants (smog or pollen) or chlorinated water.

Pharmacology/Actions
Intraocular sterile irrigating solution (BSS, *BSS Plus®*) are sterile, preservative-free physiological balanced salt solutions that are isotonic to ocular tissue and contain electrolytes required for normal cellular metabolic functions. The ideal ocular irrigation solution mimics the composition of the aqueous humor in terms of physiologic pH, osmolality and ion composition. Some intraocular irrigating solutions (*e.g.*, *BSS Plus®*) contain glutathione, which is responsible for stabilizing endothelial cell junctions and intraocular pumping functions.

OTC eye wash products are sterile isotonic solutions containing preservatives for general ophthalmic use. As they have short contact time with the eye, they do not need to provide nutrients to cells.

Contraindications/Precautions/Warnings
Adding other medications to intraocular irrigating solutions may result in damage to intraocular tissue. In humans with diabetes undergoing vitrectomy, it is recommended to use intraocular irrigating solutions with caution as intraoperative lens changes have been noted in some patients.

Extraocular solution (eyewashes) are contraindicated during intraocular surgery or if the patient is hypersensitive to any component of the formulation. Preservative components are very toxic to corneal endothelium.

Adverse Effects
BSS solutions have caused corneal clouding and edema in some patients.

Doses

For intraocular use (extra-label): Using a sterile, preservative-free balanced salt solution (not an OTC eyewash) use according to the established practices for each surgical procedure.

As an eyewash (extra-label): Flush affected eye(s) as needed; control rate of flow by exerting pressure on bottle.

Monitoring

- No specific recommendations.

Client Information

- Pet owners do not use intraocular BSS solutions.
- If using an OTC eyewash use proper administration techniques to avoid eye injury or contamination of the medication. Keep cap tightly closed when not in use.
- Wait 5 minutes after use before applying any other medications to the eye.
- Store at controlled room temperature away from moisture and sunlight; do not freeze. Discard if color changes or the solution becomes cloudy.

Storage/Stability

Store BSS solutions at 8-30°C (46-86°F); avoid excessive heat and do not freeze. Discard solution after 6 hours.

Store *BSS Plus*® solutions at 2-25°C (36-77°F); do not freeze. Discard prepared solution after 6 hours.

Store OTC eyewash products as labeled, usually at controlled room temperature away from moisture and sunlight; do not freeze.

Compatibility/Compounding Considerations

It is not recommended to add any other medication to intraocular or extraocular irrigating solutions, but off-label additives in some protocols have included heparin, epinephrine, antibiotics or local anesthetics.

For reconstituting *BSS Plus*® solutions: Reconstitute solution just prior to use in surgery. Follow the same strict aseptic reconstitution procedures as is used for intravenous additives. Remove the blue flip-off seal from the Part 1 (240 mL) bottle. Remove the blue flip-off seal from the Part 2 (10 mL) vial. Clean and disinfect the rubber stoppers on both containers by using sterile alcohol wipes. Transfer the contents of the Part 2 vial to the Part 1 bottle using the vacuum transfer device (provided). An alternative method of solution transfer may be accomplished by using a 10 mL syringe to remove the Part 2 solution from the vial and transferring exactly 10 mL to the Part 1 container through the outer target area of the rubber stopper. An excess volume of Part 2 solution is provided in each vial. Gently agitate the contents to mix the solution. Place a sterile cap on the bottle. Remove the tear-off portion of the label. Record the time and date of reconstitution and the patient's name on the bottle label.

Dosage Forms/Regulatory Status

VETERINARY-LABELED PRODUCTS:

There are several products marketed as eye washes or rinses for animal patients including: *Clear Eyes*®, *Clear Oph*®, *Conquer Hy-Optic*®, *Eye Rinse*®, *Opticlear*®, & *Vetericyn*®. Ingredients vary and some are labeled only as tear stain removers. None of these products appear to be FDA-approved and they should **NOT** be used for intraocular procedures.

HUMAN-LABELED PRODUCTS:

Irrigating Solutions, Intraocular

Balanced Salt Solution Irrigating Solution in 15 mL, 18 mL, 30 mL 250 mL or 500 mL; preservative-free containing 0.64% NaCl, 0.075% KCl, 0.03% magnesium chloride, 0.048% calcium chloride, 0.39% sodium acetate, 0.17% sodium citrate and NaOH or HCl; *BSS*®, generic; (Rx)

Balanced Salt Solution Plus; in 2 parts in 10 ml (part 1) and 240 mL (part 2) in a 250 mL bottle; preservative-free containing 0.0154% calcium chloride, 0.714% sodium chloride, 0.038% potassium chloride, 0.02% magnesium chloride, 0.42% sodium phosphate, 0.2% sodium bicarbonate, 0.092% dextrose, 0.0184% glutathione disulfide; *BSS Plus*®; (Rx)

Irrigating Solutions, Extraocular (Eyewash)

Collyrium for Fresh Eyes Wash® (containing: boric acid, sodium borate, benzalkonium Cl) in a 120 mL bottle; (OTC)

Eye Stream® (containing: 0.64% NaCl, 0.075% KCl, 0.03% magnesium Cl hexahydrate, 0.048% calcium Cl dihydrate, 0.39% sodium acetate trihydrate, 0.17% sodium citrate dihydrate, 0.013% benzalkonium Cl) in 30 mL & 118 mL bottles; (OTC)

Eye Wash® (containing: boric acid, KCl, EDTA, anhydrous sodium carbonate, 0.01% benzalkonium Cl) in a 118 mL bottle; (OTC)

Eye Irrigating Solution® (containing: NaCl, mono- and dibasic sodium phosphate, benzalkonium Cl, EDTA) in a 118 mL bottle; (OTC)

OCuSOFT® (containing: benzalkonium chloride, edetate disodium, NaCl, sodium phosphate dibasic, sodium phosphate monobasic) in a 30 mL bottle; (OTC)

Revisions/References

Monograph revised/updated September 2014.

Itraconazole Ophthalmic

(it-ruh-kon-uh-zohl)   Sporanox®

Azole Antifungal Agent

Prescriber Highlights

▶ Not commercially available; must be compounded.

▶ Compounded forms contain 30% DMSO, which may be irritating to horses.

▶ Warn caregivers to wear nitrile gloves when applying this medication to protect from DMSO exposure.

Uses/Indications

In veterinary patients, itraconazole ophthalmic ointment is used to treat fungal keratitis in horses.

Pharmacology/Actions

Itraconazole interacts with 14-demethylase, a cytochrome P-450 enzyme necessary to convert lanosterol to ergosterol. As ergosterol is an essential component of the fungal cell membrane, inhibition of its synthesis results in increased cellular permeability causing leakage of cellular contents. Itraconazole may also inhibit endogenous respiration, interact with membrane phospholipids, inhibit the transformation of yeasts to mycelial forms, inhibit purine uptake, and impair triglyceride and/or phospholipid biosynthesis. Because itraconazole specifically targets oxidative enzymes of fungal species, it has higher efficacy and lower host toxicity. Itraconazole is usually effective against *Aspergillus* and *Candida* spp., but it is not effective against *Fusarium* spp. Identification of fungal species prior to treatment is critical to success of treatment.

Contraindications/Precautions/Warnings

Itraconazole is contraindicated in patients with a history of hypersensitivity to it or any component of the formulation. Compounded itraconazole 1% in DMSO 30% ointment may cause irritation to the cornea. A solution of DMSO 1% is commonly used as a control for corneal irritation in ophthalmic drug studies (Pintor *et al.* 2014).

Adverse Effects

Adverse effects reported in humans or animals include stinging and corneal irritation from the DMSO component. Although systemic absorption of topically applied ointments is unlikely, systemic exposure to itraconazole has resulted in hepatotoxicity and hearing loss in humans.

Doses

Equine Fungal Keratitis (extra-label): ½ inch strip to the affected eye(s) every 2-3 hours initially followed by tapering of frequency based on clinical response.

Monitoring

- Clinical efficacy. Corneal scrapings to determine efficacy; monitor for corneal irritation from DMSO.

Client Information

- Used up to 8 times daily initially and then as directed.
- A garlic-like odor is normal (from the DMSO solvent).
- Wear nitrile gloves when applying to prevent absorption of DMSO solvent.
- Use proper administration techniques to avoid contamination of the medication. Keep cap tightly closed when not in use.
- Wait 5 minutes after applying this medication before applying any other medications to the eye.
- Store at controlled room temperature away from moisture and sunlight; do not freeze. Discard if color or consistency changes.

Storage/Stability

Store at controlled room temperature away from moisture and sunlight; do not freeze.

Compatibility/Compounding Considerations

Itraconazole should not be mixed directly with any other drugs, although a compounded preparation containing 30% DMSO has been described (Ball *et al.* 1997a; Ball *et al.* 1997b).

Dosage Forms/Regulatory Status

VETERINARY-LABELED PRODUCTS: NONE.

HUMAN-LABELED PRODUCTS: NONE.

Itraconazole ophthalmic products are not commercially available and must be prepared (compounded) by a qualified compounding pharmacist. It has been compounded into a 1% ophthalmic ointment in a base containing DMSO 30%. (Ball *et al.* 1997a; Ball *et al.* 1997b)

Revisions/References

Monograph revised/updated September 2014.

Ball, M. A., et al. (1997a). Evaluation of itraconazole dimethyl sulfoxide ointment for treatment of keratomycosis in nine horses. Journal of the American Veterinary Medical Association 211(2): 199-&.

Ball, M. A., et al. (1997b). Corneal concentrations and preliminary toxicological evaluation of an itraconazole/dimethyl sulphoxide ophthalmic ointment. J. Vet. Pharmacol. Ther. 20(2): 100-4.

Pintor, J., et al. (2014). Cytotoxic Effect on Corneal Surface of Multipurpose Soft Contact Lens Solution Which Contains Aloe Vera. Biochem Pharmacol 3: 128.

Ketorolac Ophthalmic

(kee-toe-role-ak)   Acular®

Nonsteroidal Antiinflammatory Drug (NSAID)

Prescriber Highlights

► Usually used 4 times daily to decrease inflammation.
► May increase risk of ocular bleeding.
► May delay wound healing.
► Cross sensitivity with allergies to other NSAIDs has occurred in humans.

Uses/Indications

In veterinary patients, ketorolac is primarily used to control surgical or non-surgical uveitis particularly in cases with concurrent bacterial infection or ulceration where corticosteroids are contraindicated. Ketorolac is also used to treat the symptoms of allergic conjunctivitis. It is also used before cataract surgery to prevent miosis during intraocular surgery. Ketorolac has also been used to treat postoperative cystoid macular edema and ocular surface inflammation. In diabetic patients, ketorolac may be useful to avoid the systemic effects of topically applied corticosteroids.

Pharmacology/Actions

Like other NSAIDs, ketorolac is presumed to possess antiinflammatory properties via prostaglandin synthetase inhibition. The biological activity of ketorolac tromethamine is associated with the S enantiomer.

Contraindications/Precautions/Warnings

Ketorolac is contraindicated in patients with a history of hypersensitivity to it or any component of the formulation. Potential for cross-sensitivity to acetylsalicylic acid, phenylacetic acid derivatives, and other NSAIDs exists. There have been reports of bronchospasm or exacerbation of asthma associated with the use of ketorolac tromethamine ophthalmic solution in patients that have either a known hypersensitivity to aspirin or NSAIDs or a past medical history of asthma. Therefore, caution should be used when treating individuals that have previously exhibited sensitivities to these drugs. Topical nonsteroidal antiinflammatory drugs (NSAIDs) may slow or delay healing. Topical corticosteroids are also known to slow or delay healing. Concomitant use of topical NSAIDs and topical steroids may increase the potential for healing problems. Due to interference with thrombocyte aggregation, ocular applied nonsteroidal antiinflammatory drugs may cause increased bleeding of ocular tissues (including hyphema) in conjunction with ocular surgery. It is recommended that ketorolac ophthalmic solution be used with caution in patients with known bleeding tendencies or that are receiving other medications, which may prolong bleeding time.

Adverse Effects

Adverse effects reported in humans or animals include transient stinging and burning on instillation, corneal edema, iritis, ocular inflammation, ocular irritation, superficial keratitis, and superficial ocular infections. Ocular bleeding may occur due to interference with thrombocyte aggregation. Use of topical NSAIDs may result in keratitis. In some susceptible patients, continued use of topical NSAIDs may result in epithelial breakdown, corneal thinning, corneal erosion, corneal ulceration, or corneal perforation. Other adverse effects that have rarely occurred in humans include corneal infiltrates, corneal ulcer, eye dryness, headaches, and visual disturbance (blurry vision).

Doses

Allergic conjunctivitis (extra-label): 1 drop in the affected eye(s) 4 times daily.

Monitoring

- Clinical efficacy. Resolution of signs and symptoms of allergic conjunctivitis.

Client Information

- Used 4 times daily.
- Use proper administration techniques to avoid contamination of the medication. Keep cap tightly closed when not in use.
- Wait 5 minutes after applying this medication before applying any other medications to the eye.
- Store in the refrigerator or at controlled room temperature away from moisture and sunlight; do not freeze. Do not use if the color changes, it becomes cloudy, or if particles are seen in solutions.

Storage/Stability
Store at controlled room temperature away from moisture and sunlight; do not freeze.

Compatibility/Compounding Considerations
Ketorolac should not be mixed directly with any other drugs. Ketorolac is not available as an ophthalmic ointment.

Dosage Forms/Regulatory Status
VETERINARY-LABELED PRODUCTS: NONE.
HUMAN-LABELED PRODUCTS:
Ketorolac Tromethamine 0.5% Ophthalmic Solution (containing ketorolac tromethamine 5 mg/mL; benzalkonium chloride 0.01%; edetate disodium 0.1%; octoxynol 40; purified water; NaCl; HCl and/or NaOH to adjust the pH to 7.4 and osmolality of 290 mOsm/kg) in a 5 mL ophthalmic dropper bottle; *Acular®*; (Rx)

Revisions/References
Monograph revised/updated September 2014.

Ketotifen Ophthalmic
(kee-toe-tye-fin)   Alaway®, Zaditor®

Antihistamine Agent

Prescriber Highlights
▶ Relatively selective H-1 blocker for treatment of allergic conjunctivitis.
▶ Used up to 2 times daily.

Uses/Indications
In veterinary patients, ketotifen is used for the temporary relief of the signs and symptoms of allergic conjunctivitis.

Pharmacology/Actions
Ketotifen is a relatively selective, non-competitive histamine antagonist (H1-receptor) and mast cell stabilizer. Ketotifen inhibits the release of mediators from mast cells such as histamine, leukotrienes C4 and D4 (SRS-A) and Platelet Activating Factor that are involved in hypersensitivity reactions. Decreased chemotaxis and activation of eosinophils have also been demonstrated.

Contraindications/Precautions/Warnings
Ketotifen is contraindicated in patients with a history of hypersensitivity to it or any component of the formulation.

Adverse Effects
Adverse effects reported in humans or animals include conjunctival injection, rhinitis, and ocular allergic reactions, burning or stinging of eye, conjunctivitis, eye discharge, dry eye, eye pain, eyelid disorder, itching eye, keratitis, lacrimation disorder, mydriasis, photophobia, rash, and pharyngitis.

Doses
Allergic conjunctivitis (extra-label): 1 drop in the affected eye(s) 2 times daily.

Monitoring
- Clinical efficacy. Resolution or relief of signs and symptoms of allergic conjunctivitis (pruritus, tearing, squinting, erythema).

Client Information
- Used 2 times daily.
- Use proper administration techniques to avoid contamination of the medication. Keep cap tightly closed when not in use.
- Wait 5 minutes after applying this medication before applying any other medications to the eye.
- Store in the refrigerator or at controlled room temperature away from moisture and sunlight; do not freeze. Do not use if the color changes, it becomes cloudy, or if particles are seen in solutions.

Storage/Stability
Store in refrigerator or at controlled room temperature away from moisture and sunlight; do not freeze.

Compatibility/Compounding Considerations
Ketotifen should not be mixed directly with any other drugs. Ketotifen is not available as an ophthalmic ointment.

Dosage Forms/Regulatory Status
VETERINARY-LABELED PRODUCTS: NONE.
HUMAN-LABELED PRODUCTS:
Ketotifen Fumarate 0.025% Ophthalmic Solution (containing: ketotifen fumarate equivalent to 0.25 mg ketotifen per milliliter; benzalkonium chloride 0.015, glycerol; NaOH/ HCl to adjust pH to 4.4 -5.8 and purified water; with an osmolality of 210-300 mOsm/kg) in a 5 mL ophthalmic dropper bottle; *Zaditor®*, *Alaway®*, many other trade names available, generic; (OTC)

Revisions/References
Monograph revised/updated September 2014.

Latanoprost Ophthalmic
(la-ta-noe-prost)   Xalatan®

Prostaglandin Analog Anti-Glaucoma Agent

Prescriber Highlights
▶ Not effective for feline glaucoma.
▶ Twice daily dosing results in less fluctuation of intraocular pressure.
▶ Preservative systems may cause ocular irritation/discomfort.
▶ May increase brown pigment resulting in discoloration of light colored irises and increase eyelash growth.
▶ May worsen intraocular inflammation through prostaglandin-mediated mechanisms

Uses/Indications
In veterinary patients, latanoprost is used to reduce intraocular pressure to manage canine glaucoma. It is not effective for treating feline glaucoma (Studer *et al.* 2000). Use in horses is not effective and is associated with a high incidence of adverse effects including ocular discomfort (Davidson *et al.* 2002).

Pharmacology/Actions
Prostaglandin analogs are chemically modified versions of prostaglandin F2-alpha, and endogenous inflammatory mediator that causes ocular hypotensive effects. Latanoprost is believed to lower intraocular pressure (IOP) by increasing outflow of aqueous humor through both the trabecular meshwork and uveoscleral routes.

Contraindications/Precautions/Warnings
Latanoprost is contraindicated in patients with a history of hypersensitivity to it or any component of the formulation. Latanoprost should not be used in the presence of intraocular inflammation (*e.g.*, uveitis) as it will worsen this condition.

Adverse Effects
Adverse effects reported in humans or animals include blurred vision, burning and stinging, conjunctival hyperemia, foreign body sensation, itching, increased pigmentation of the iris, and punctate epithelial keratopathy. May cause darkening of the iris through direct stimulation of iris melanocytes. May cause increased eyelash growth. May worsen intraocular inflammation. Eyelash changes (increased length, thickness, pigmentation, and number of lashes); eyelid skin darkening; intraocular inflammation (iritis/uveitis); iris pigmentation changes; and macular edema, including cystoid macular edema, have all been reported after use of latanoprost in humans.

Doses

Glaucoma (extra-label): 1 drop in the affected eye(s) twice daily.

Monitoring

- Clinical efficacy. Continued reduction of intraocular pressure.

Client Information

- Used 2 times daily.
- Use proper administration techniques to avoid contamination of the medication. Keep cap tightly closed when not in use.
- Protect from light. Store unopened bottle(s) under refrigeration at 2-8°C (36-46°F); do not freeze. Once a bottle is opened for use, it may be stored at room temperature up to 25°C (77°F) for 6 weeks. Do not use if the color changes, it becomes cloudy, or if particles are seen in solutions.
- Wait 5 minutes after applying this medication before applying any other medications to the eye.

Storage/Stability

Protect from light. Store unopened bottle(s) under refrigeration at 2-8°C (36-46°F); do not freeze. During shipment to the patient, the bottle may be maintained at temperatures up to 40°C (104°F) for a period not exceeding 8 days. Once a bottle is opened for use, it may be stored at room temperature up to 25°C (77°F) for 6 weeks.

Compatibility/Compounding Considerations

Latanoprost should not be mixed directly with any other drugs. Latanoprost is not available as an ophthalmic ointment.

Dosage Forms/Regulatory Status

VETERINARY-LABELED PRODUCTS: NONE.

HUMAN-LABELED PRODUCTS:

Latanoprost 0.005% Ophthalmic Solution (containing 50 micrograms of latanoprost per milliliter; benzalkonium chloride 0.02%, NaCl, sodium dihydrogen phosphate monohydrate, disodium hydrogen phosphate anhydrous, and water for injection, with a pH of ≈ 6.7 and an osmolality of ≈ 267 mOsm/kg) in 2.5 mL ophthalmic dropper bottles. One drop contains ≈ 1.5 μg of latanoprost; *Xalatan®*; (Rx)

Revisions/References

Monograph revised/updated September 2014.

Davidson, H., et al. (2002). Effect of topical ophthalmic latanoprost on intraocular pressure in normal horses. Vet Therapeutics 3: 1220-4.

Studer, M. E., et al. (2000). Effects of 0.005% latanoprost solution on intraocular pressure in healthy dogs and cats. American Journal of Veterinary Research **61**(10): 1220-4.

Levobunolol Ophthalmic

(lee-voe-byoon-uh-lol)   Betagan®

Beta-Adrenergic Blocker

Prescriber Highlights

▶ Partial beta-agonist properties allow it to be used in patients that suffer bradycardia from other beta-blockers.

▶ Effective for feline glaucoma (usually employed in addition to carbonic anhydrase inhibitors)

Uses/Indications

In veterinary patients, levobunolol is used to reduce intraocular pressure in primary glaucoma and as prophylaxis to prevent glaucoma in the normal eye of animals with unilateral glaucoma.

Pharmacology/Actions

Levobunolol is a nonselective beta-adrenergic blocking agent with associated intrinsic sympathomimetic activity but it does not have significant membrane-stabilizing activity. The exact mechanism of the ocular hypotensive effect of beta-blockers is not clear, but may involve vasoactive mechanisms, beta-blockade of norepineph-rine-induced tonic sympathetic stimulation, decreased activation of cAMP in the ciliary body leading to decreased aqueous humor production, and/or inhibition of $Na^+K^+ATPase$ activity.

Contraindications/Precautions/Warnings

Levobunolol is contraindicated in patients with a history of hypersensitivity to it or any component of the formulation. Levobunolol should be used carefully in patients with heart block, bradycardia, heart failure, asthma, chronic bronchitis, or other cardiopulmonary conditions, although systemic cardiopulmonary adverse effects are not likely with ocular use of levobunolol.

Adverse Effects

Adverse effects reported in humans or animals include transient burning, stinging, and irritation upon application to the eye.

Doses

Glaucoma (extra-label): 1 drop in the affected eye(s) twice daily.

Monitoring

- Clinical efficacy. Monitor intraocular pressure.

Client Information

- Used 2 times daily.
- Use proper administration techniques to avoid contamination of the medication. Keep cap tightly closed when not in use.
- Wait 5 minutes after applying this medication before applying any other medications to the eye.
- Store in the refrigerator or at controlled room temperature away from moisture and sunlight; do not freeze. Do not use if the color changes, it becomes cloudy, or if particles are seen in solutions.

Storage/Stability

Store in refrigerator or at controlled room temperature away from moisture and sunlight; do not freeze.

Compatibility/Compounding Considerations

Levobunolol should not be mixed directly with any other drugs. Levobunolol is not available as an ophthalmic ointment.

Dosage Forms/Regulatory Status

VETERINARY-LABELED PRODUCTS: NONE.

HUMAN-LABELED PRODUCTS:

Levobunolol 0.25% or 0.5% Ophthalmic Solution [containing: benzalkonium chloride (0.004%), polyvinyl alcohol 1.4%, edetate disodium, sodium metabisulfite, sodium phosphate, dibasic; potassium phosphate, monobasic; NaCl; HCl or NaOH to adjust the pH; and purified water] in 2, 5, 10, & 15 mL ophthalmic dropper bottles; *Betagan®*; (Rx)

Revisions/References

Monograph revised/updated September 2014.

Levofloxacin Ophthalmic

(lev-oh-flocks-a sin)   Quixin®

Fluoroquinolone Antibiotic

Prescriber Highlights

▶ Fluoroquinolone antimicrobial used for bacterial conjunctivitis or keratitis.

▶ Physically incompatible with many drugs.

▶ Crystalline drug precipitates may be noted in the superficial portion of corneal defects during use.

Uses/Indications

In veterinary patients, ophthalmic may be useful for treating bacterial conjunctivitis caused by susceptible species/strains of staphylococci, streptococci, Corynebacterium, Haemophilus, and Chlamydia. When administered via a subpalpebral lavage (SPL) catheter it can be used for treating equine bacterial keratitis.

Pharmacology/Actions

Levofloxacin is a member of the fluoroquinolone class of anti-infective drugs. Its action results from inhibition of DNA gyrase, which is involved in replication, transcription and repair of bacterial DNA.

Contraindications/Precautions/Warnings

Levofloxacin is contraindicated in patients with a history of hypersensitivity to it, other fluoroquinolones, or any component of the formulation. For topical ophthalmic use only. Not for injection subconjunctivally or into the anterior chamber of the eye. Fluoroquinolone-induced retinal toxicity in domestic cats has not been demonstrated with this product at time of writing, but may be possible.

Adverse Effects

Adverse effects reported in humans or animals include blurred vision, tearing, eye pain, redness, itching, and a bad taste in the mouth. Crystalline drug precipitates may be noted in the superficial portion of corneal defects during use.

Doses

Conjunctivitis (extra-label): 1 drop affected eye(s) every 4-8 hours.

Keratitis (extra-label): 1 drop in the affected eye or 0.2 mL in the SPL catheter every 1-8 hours. May precipitate when mixed with other ophthalmic medications. Flush SPL catheter well with air between medications.

Monitoring

- Clinical efficacy: If blepharospasm, uveitis, or worsening of ulceration or no improvement in infection is noted in 7 days, reassess microbial susceptibility.

Client Information

- Used 3-12 times daily.
- Crystals may appear in the eyes for a few days after initiation of treatment.
- Wait 5 minutes after applying this medication before applying any other medications to the eye.
- Use proper administration techniques to avoid contamination of the medication. Keep cap tightly closed when not in use.
- Store in refrigerator; do not freeze. Dispose of unused medication in regular trash, do not put into sewer system.

Storage/Stability

Store in refrigerator or at controlled room temperature away from moisture and sunlight; do not freeze.

Compatibility/Compounding Considerations

Fluoroquinolone antibiotics interact with many other drugs including those containing cations (*e.g.*, iron, aluminum, magnesium, calcium, etc.). Levofloxacin should not be mixed directly with any other drugs. Levofloxacin is not available as an ophthalmic ointment.

Dosage Forms/Regulatory Status

VETERINARY-LABELED PRODUCTS: NONE.

HUMAN-LABELED PRODUCTS:

Levofloxacin 0.5% ophthalmic solution (containing levofloxacin 5 mg/mL, benzalkonium chloride 0.005%, NaCl and water. May also contain HCl and/or NaOH to adjust pH to 6.5 with an osmolality of ≈ 300 mOsm/kg) in a 5 ml ophthalmic dropper bottle; *Quixin®*; (Rx)

Revisions/References

Monograph revised/updated September 2014.

Lissamine Green Ophthalmic

(lis-ah-meen)

Ocular Diagnostic Agent

Prescriber Highlights

▶ Less stinging than with Rose Bengal.

▶ Requires broader interpretive experience than fluorescein staining.

▶ Unapproved drug and periodically backordered in the market.

Uses/Indications

In veterinary patients, lissamine green is used as a diagnostic agent when superficial corneal or conjunctival tissue change is suspected. Lissamine green does not sting like Rose Bengal does, but interpretation of results requires broader evaluative experience than that for Rose Bengal and fluorescein.

Pharmacology/Actions

Lissamine green works by staining the cornea blue upon instillation, resulting in a speckling of the cornea if any corneal ulcerations or dry patches from muco-deficient or damaged corneal cells.

Contraindications/Precautions/Warnings

Lissamine green is contraindicated in patients with a history of hypersensitivity to it or any component of the formulation.

Adverse Effects

Adverse effects reported in humans or animals include stinging upon instillation but not as much as with Rose Bengal.

Doses

Detection of corneal change: Wet the surface of the lissamine green strip with 1-2 drops of normal saline solution. Apply moistened tip to conjunctiva or fornix as required. It is recommended that the patient blink several times after application. Wait 60 seconds, and then read with a white light source. Blue speckling will be evident for areas of damaged or muco-deficient cornea. **Note:** No dosage forms of lissamine green are approved by US FDA.

Monitoring

- Diagnostic agent. Monitoring not required.

Client Information

- Lissamine green is not used at home by pet caregivers.

Storage/Stability

Store in refrigerator or at controlled room temperature away from moisture and sunlight; do not freeze.

Compatibility/Compounding Considerations

Lissamine green should not be mixed directly with any other drugs.

Dosage Forms/Regulatory Status

VETERINARY-LABELED PRODUCTS: NONE.

HUMAN-LABELED PRODUCTS:

Lissamine Green 1.5 mg Strips (containing 1.5 mg of lissamine green per strip) in individually wrapped strips in containers of 100 strips; *GreenGlo®*; (Rx). There are no FDA-approved forms of lissamine strips.

Revisions/References

Monograph revised/updated September 2014.

Loteprednol Ophthalmic

(lote-uh-pred-nole)   Lotemax®, Alrex®, Zylet®

Corticosteroid Antiinflammatory Agent

Prescriber Highlights

▶ Do not use in fungal keratitis, feline herpes keratitis, or if corneal abrasion or ulceration are suspected.

▶ Use with caution in avian species due to risk of systemic corticosteroid effects.

Uses/Indications

In veterinary patients, loteprednol ophthalmic is used for symptomatic relief of corticosteroid-responsive inflammatory conditions of the palpebral and bulbar conjunctiva, cornea, and anterior segment of the globe (*e.g.*, allergic conjunctivitis, acne rosacea, superficial punctate keratitis, iritis, and cyclitis). In horses it is used for treatment of uveitis. It may also be used to treat inflammation associated with corneal injury from chemical, radiation, or thermal burns or penetration of foreign bodies.

Pharmacology/Actions

Corticosteroids work by inhibiting phospholipase A2 as well as cyclooxygenase (COX) and lipoxygenase (LOX) pathways. Corticosteroids can also penetrate the nucleus to interrupt specific DNA sequences that produce inflammatory mediators. In general, pro-inflammatory mediators are down-regulated and antiinflammatory mediators are up-regulated. Corticosteroids also reduce the migration of macrophages, decrease vascular permeability, and suppress lymphokines. They inhibit edema, cellular infiltration, capillary dilatation, fibroblastic proliferation, and deposition of collagen.

Contraindications/Precautions/Warnings

Loteprednol is contraindicated in patients with a history of hypersensitivity to it or any component of the formulation. Topical corticosteroids are contraindicated in known or suspected corneal ulceration or corneal infection (fungal and viral). Use with caution in patients with diabetes mellitus or other endocrine diseases, infectious diseases, chronic renal failure, congestive heart failure, systemic hypertension, or gastric ulceration. When use is necessary in these conditions, the minimal effective dose should be administered for the shortest possible time.

Adverse Effects

Adverse effects reported in humans or animals include development of cataracts (via altered glucose or lenticular metabolic effects), increased intraocular pressure (via activation of glucocorticoid receptors in the trabecular meshwork), infection (via immunosuppression), decreased wound healing (via increased collagenolytic activity), mydriasis, and calcific keratopathy. Systemic effects are rare but include hepatopathy, suppression of endogenous glucocorticoid production, and focal alopecia. Concurrent use of systemic steroids increases risk of these adverse effects.

Doses

Conjunctivitis (extra-label): 1 drop or ¼ inch strip in affected eye(s) every 4-8 hours, then increase to longest dosing interval that still maintains efficacy.

Post Cataract Removal (extra-label): 1 drop in the affected eye(s) every 8-12 hours.

Monitoring

▪ Clinical efficacy. Absence of inflammation. Monitor intraocular pressure and observe for evidence of infection or delayed wound healing. Monitor for blood or urine glucose changes in diabetic animals.

Client Information

▪ Used 4-6 times daily.

▪ Shake suspensions well before using.

▪ Use proper administration techniques to avoid contamination of the medication. Keep cap tightly closed when not in use.

▪ Wait 5 minutes after applying this medication before applying any other medications to the eye.

▪ Store in the refrigerator or at controlled room temperature away from moisture and sunlight; do not freeze. Do not use if the color changes, or if particles are seen in solutions.

Storage/Stability

Store in refrigerator or at controlled room temperature away from moisture and sunlight.

Compatibility/Compounding Considerations

Loteprednol should not be mixed directly with any other drugs.

Dosage Forms/Regulatory Status

VETERINARY-LABELED PRODUCTS: NONE.

HUMAN-LABELED PRODUCTS:

Loteprednol etabonate 0.5% Ophthalmic Suspension in 2.5 mL, 5 mL, 10 mL, and 15 mL ophthalmic dropper bottles; *Lotemax®*; (Rx)

Loteprednol etabonate 0.5% and Tobramycin 0.3% Ophthalmic Suspension in 2.5 mL, 5 mL, & 10 mL; *Zylet®*; (Rx)

Revisions/References

Monograph revised/updated September 2014.

Metipranolol Ophthalmic

(meh-tee-pran-uh-lol)   OptiPranolol®

Beta-Adrenergic Blocker

Prescriber Highlights

▶ Partial beta-agonist properties allow it to be used in patients that suffer bradycardia from other beta-blockers.

▶ May be associated with more ocular burning, stinging, and granulomatous anterior uveitis than other beta-blocking agents.

▶ Effective for feline glaucoma (usually employed in addition to carbonic anhydrase inhibitors)

Uses/Indications

In veterinary patients, metipranolol is used to reduce intraocular pressure in primary glaucoma and as prophylaxis to prevent glaucoma in the normal eye of animals with unilateral glaucoma. Although metipranolol is cost effective for treating glaucoma, it is associated with more adverse effects as compared to other beta-blocking agents (Sorensen *et al.* 1996).

Pharmacology/Actions

Metipranolol is a nonselective beta-adrenergic blocking agent with associated intrinsic sympathomimetic activity and without significant membrane-stabilizing activity. The exact mechanism of the ocular hypotensive effect of beta-blockers has not been definitely demonstrated; however, several mechanisms have been postulated for this effect including beta-blockade of norepinephrine-induced tonic sympathetic stimulation, decreased activation of cAMP in the ciliary body leading to decreased aqueous humor production, inhibition of Na+K+ATPase activity, or through vasoactive mechanisms.

Contraindications/Precautions/Warnings

Metipranolol is contraindicated in patients with a history of hypersensitivity to it or any component of the formulation. Metipranolol should be used carefully in patients with heart block, bradycardia, heart failure, asthma, chronic bronchitis, or other cardiopulmonary conditions, although systemic cardiopulmonary adverse effects are not likely with ocular use of metipranolol.

Adverse Effects

Adverse effects reported in humans or animals include transient burning, stinging, and irritation upon application to the eye.

Doses

Glaucoma (extra-label): 1 drop in the affected eye(s) twice daily.

Monitoring

- Clinical efficacy. Monitor intraocular pressure.

Client Information

- Used 2 times daily.
- Use proper administration techniques to avoid contamination of the medication. Keep cap tightly closed when not in use.
- Wait 5 minutes after applying this medication before applying any other medications to the eye.
- Store at controlled room temperature away from moisture and sunlight; do not freeze. Do not use if the color changes, it becomes cloudy, or if particles are seen in solutions.

Storage/Stability

Store at controlled room temperature away from moisture and sunlight.

Compatibility/Compounding Considerations

Metipranolol should not be mixed directly with any other drugs. Metipranolol is not available as an ophthalmic ointment.

Dosage Forms/Regulatory Status

VETERINARY-LABELED PRODUCTS: NONE.

HUMAN-LABELED PRODUCTS:

Metipranolol 0.3% Ophthalmic Solution (containing: metipranolol 3 mg per milliliter, benzalkonium chloride 0.004%, povidone, glycerin, HCl, NaCl, edetate disodium, and purified water, NaOH and/or HCl may be added to adjust pH to 5.0-5.8 with an osmolality of 265-330 mOsm/kg) in 5 mL and 10 mL ophthalmic dropper bottles; *OptiPranolol*®; (Rx)

Revisions/References

Monograph revised/updated September 2014.

Sorensen, S. J. & S. R. Abel (1996). Comparison of the ocular beta-blockers. Annals of Pharmacotherapy **30**(1): 43-54.

Miconazole Ophthalmic

(mye-kon-uh-zohl)

Azole Antifungal Agent

Prescriber Highlights

▶ Not commercially available, must be compounded, give ample notice for prescription preparation.

▶ Penetrates cornea more efficiently than natamycin.

Uses/Indications

In veterinary patients, miconazole ophthalmic solution is used to treat fungal keratitis in horses.

Pharmacology/Actions

Miconazole interacts with 14-demethylase, a cytochrome P-450 enzyme necessary to convert lanosterol to ergosterol. As ergosterol is an essential component of the fungal cell membrane, inhibition of its synthesis results in increased cellular permeability causing leakage of cellular contents. Miconazole may also inhibit endogenous respiration, interact with membrane phospholipids, inhibit the transformation of yeasts to mycelial forms, inhibit purine uptake, and impair triglyceride and/or phospholipid biosynthesis. Miconazole has a wide antifungal spectrum against most fungi and yeasts of veterinary interest. Sensitive organisms include *Blastomyces dermatitidis*, *Paracoccidioides brasiliensis*, *Histoplasma capsulatum*, *Candida* spp., *Coccidioides immitis*, *Cryptococcus neoformans*, and *Aspergillus fumigatus*. Some *Aspergillus* and *Madurella* spp. are only marginally sensitive.

Contraindications/Precautions/Warnings

Miconazole is contraindicated in patients with a history of hypersensitivity to it or any component of the formulation.

Adverse Effects

Adverse effects reported in humans or animals include transient burning or stinging on application. Miconazole may cause local irritation if injected subconjunctivally. Although systemic absorption of topically applied solutions is unlikely, systemic exposure to miconazole has resulted in hepatotoxicity and hearing loss in humans.

Doses

Equine Fungal Keratitis (extra-label): 1-2 drops or 0.2 mL through the SPL catheter to the affected eye(s) every 2-3 hours initially followed by tapering of frequency based on clinical response.

Monitoring

- Clinical efficacy. Corneal scrapings to determine efficacy.

Client Information

- Used up to 8 times daily.
- Use proper administration techniques to avoid contamination of the medication. Keep cap tightly closed when not in use.
- Wait 5 minutes after applying this medication before applying any other medications to the eye.
- Store in the refrigerator or at controlled room temperature away from moisture and sunlight; do not freeze. Do not use if the color changes, it becomes cloudy, or if particles are seen in solutions.

Storage/Stability

Store in refrigerator or at controlled room temperature away from moisture and sunlight.

Compatibility/Compounding Considerations

Miconazole should not be mixed directly with any other drugs.

Dosage Forms/Regulatory Status

VETERINARY-LABELED PRODUCTS: NONE.

HUMAN-LABELED PRODUCTS: NONE.

Miconazole has been compounded into a 1% ophthalmic solution that mimics the formerly commercially available *Monistat IV*®. Miconazole topical creams and ointments for dermatological use should **NOT** be used in the eye.

Revisions/References

Monograph revised/updated September 2014.

Mitomycin Ophthalmic

(mye-toe-mye-sin see)   Mitomycin C, Mitosol®

Cytotoxic Anti-tumor Agent

Prescriber Highlights

▶ Chemotherapy agent. Mix using appropriate hazardous drug standards, instruct caregivers in appropriate personal protection and waste disposal.

▶ Mitomycin is normally blue in color.

▶ May cause orbital and facial alopecia in treated horses.

Uses/Indications

Mitomycin (mitomycin C) is used for topical therapy of equine limbal and eyelid squamous cell carcinoma. It is also used as an antimetabolite to limit fibrosis over the body of gonioimplant devices used to artificially shunt aqueous humor out of the eye in glaucoma as well as improve long-term performance of the implant.

Pharmacology/Actions

Mitomycin selectively inhibits the synthesis of deoxyribonucleic acid (DNA). The guanine and cytosine content correlates with the degree of mitomycin-induced cross-linking. At high concentrations of the drug, cellular RNA and protein synthesis are also suppressed.

Contraindications/Precautions/Warnings

Mitomycin is contraindicated in patients with a history of hypersensitivity to it or any component of the formulation. Mitomycin is contraindicated in patients with thrombocytopenia, coagulation disorder, or an increase in bleeding tendency due to other causes.

Pregnant women or women attempting to become pregnant should avoid contact with this drug.

Adverse Effects

Adverse effects reported in humans or animals include burning and stinging upon application and corneal irritation. Some horses have experienced orbital and facial alopecia after application. Although unlikely with topical therapy, systemic use of mitomycin C has been associated with bone marrow suppression, particularly thrombocytopenia and leukopenia, and nephrotoxicity.

Doses

Equine Squamous Cell Carcinoma (extra-label): Apply 0.2 mL of a 0.04% solution to the affected site 3 times daily for 21 days in a cycle of 7 days of drug application followed by a 7 day drug vacation.

Monitoring

- Clinical efficacy. Resolution of squamous cells at surgical margins.

Client Information

- Used 3 times daily.
- Chemotherapy agent. Wear gloves, wash hands, and avoid handling if pregnant or attempting to become pregnant.
- Use proper administration techniques to avoid contamination of the medication. Keep cap tightly closed when not in use.
- Wait 5 minutes after applying this medication before applying any other medications to the eye.
- Store in the refrigerator; do not freeze. Do not use if the color changes (it is normally blue), it becomes cloudy, or if particles are seen in solutions.
- Dispose of any waste in a doubled plastic bag.

Storage/Stability

Store in refrigerator away from moisture and sunlight.

Compatibility/Compounding Considerations

Mitomycin should not be mixed directly with any other drugs. Mitomycin ophthalmic solution is not commercially available, but mitomycin lyophilized powder for injection can be compounded into appropriate ophthalmic solutions as follows:

If using the 5 mg vial: Reconstitute vial with 12.5 mL sterile 0.9% NaCl injection to make a 0.4 mg/mL (0.04%) solution.

If using the 20 mg vial: Reconstitute with 50 mL sterile 0.9% NaCl injection to make a 0.4 mg/mL (0.04%) solution. **Note:** Commercially available mitomycin 20 mg vials may not contain 50 mL volume. Use caution when reconstituting and aseptically transfer contents to 50 mL empty sterile vial when volume restrictions require.

Dosage Forms/Regulatory Status

VETERINARY-LABELED PRODUCTS: NONE.
HUMAN-LABELED PRODUCTS:

Mitomycin ophthalmic topical solution for multi-use is not commercially available, but mitomycin lyophilized powder for injection (5 mg or 20 mg/vial) can be compounded into a suitable ophthalmic. A commercially available kit for mitomycin ophthalmic topical (single-use) as an adjunct to ab externo glaucoma surgery is available; *Mitosol*®; (Rx).

Revisions/References

Monograph revised/updated September 2014.

Morphine Sulfate Ophthalmic

(mor-feen suhl-fate)
Opioid Analgesic Agent

Prescriber Highlights

- ▶ Opioid analgesic for corneal ulcers.
- ▶ Schedule II Controlled Substance: Requires a new prescription each time; medication cannot be refilled.
- ▶ Must be prepared (compounded) by a qualified pharmacist since no dosage forms suitable for the eye are manufactured.
- ▶ Do not use in animals receiving naloxone, nalbuphine or nalorphine as these drugs have opioid antagonist properties.

Uses/Indications

In veterinary patients, morphine sulfate ophthalmic solution is used to manage the pain associated with corneal ulcers.

Pharmacology/Actions

Morphine interacts predominantly with the opioid *mu*-receptor. These *mu*-binding sites are discretely distributed in the brain, with high densities in the posterior amygdala, hypothalamus, thalamus, nucleus caudatus, putamen, and certain cortical areas. They are also found on the terminal axons of primary afferents within laminae I and II (substantia gelatinosa) of the spinal cord and in the spinal nucleus of the trigeminal nerve. They are present in the cornea although in smaller numbers than delta receptors in canine cornea (Stiles *et al.* 2003). Its primary actions of therapeutic value are analgesia and sedation. Morphine appears to increase tolerance for pain and decrease discomfort, although the presence of the pain itself may still be recognized. In addition to analgesia, alterations in mood, euphoria and dysphoria, and drowsiness commonly occur. Opioids also produce respiratory depression by direct action on brain stem respiratory centers when administered systemically.

Contraindications/Precautions/Warnings

Morphine sulfate is contraindicated in patients with a history of hypersensitivity to it or any component of the formulation. Although unlikely with topical administration, adverse effects following concomitant use with MAO inhibitors (*e.g.*, amitraz) or within 14 days of such treatment may occur.

Adverse Effects

Adverse effects reported in humans or animals include stinging and burning on application. Although unlikely with topical administration, the following effects have been reported after systemic administration: respiratory insufficiency or depression; severe CNS depression; attack of bronchial asthma; heart failure secondary to chronic lung disease; cardiac arrhythmias; increased intracranial or cerebrospinal pressure; head injuries; brain tumor; convulsive disorders; after biliary tract surgery; suspected surgical abdomen; surgical anastomosis; concomitantly with MAO inhibitors (*e.g.*, amitraz) or within 14 days of such treatment.

Doses

Corneal ulcers: 1 drop of a morphine 1% solution in the affected eye(s) every 8 hours.

Monitoring

- Clinical efficacy. Adequate ocular analgesia.

Client Information

- Used 3 times daily.
- This is a controlled substance and may not be refilled. Your pet will require a new prescription each time.
- Use proper administration techniques to avoid contamination of the medication. Keep cap tightly closed when not in use.
- Wait 5 minutes after applying this medication before applying any other medications to the eye.
- Store in the refrigerator or at controlled room temperature away from moisture and sunlight; do not freeze. Do not use if the color changes, it becomes cloudy, or if particles are seen in solutions.

Storage/Stability

Store in the refrigerator or at controlled room temperature away from moisture and sunlight; do not freeze.

Compatibility/Compounding Considerations

Morphine sulfate should not be mixed directly with any other drugs.

Dosage Forms/Regulatory Status

VETERINARY-LABELED PRODUCTS: NONE.

HUMAN-LABELED PRODUCTS: NONE.

Morphine sulfate ophthalmic solution is not commercially available. It must be compounded. Ideally, the preservative-free morphine sulfate injection may be aseptically diluted with sterile 0.9% NaCl injection to achieve a 1% (10 mg/mL) sterile ophthalmic solution.

Revisions/References

Monograph revised/updated September 2014.

Stiles, J., et al. (2003). Effect of topical administration of 1% morphine sulfate solution on signs of pain and corneal wound healing in dogs. American Journal of Veterinary Research **64**(7): 813-8.

Moxifloxacin Ophthalmic

(mox-ih-**flox**-uh-sin) Vigamox®, Moxeza®

Fluoroquinolone Antimicrobial

Prescriber Highlights

- ▶ Fluoroquinolone antimicrobial used for bacterial conjunctivitis or keratitis.
- ▶ Physically incompatible with many drugs.
- ▶ Crystalline drug precipitates may be noted in the superficial portion of corneal defects during use.
- ▶ *Moxeza®* gel is very viscous and will obstruct subpalpebral lavage (SPL) catheters; solutions should be used.

Uses/Indications

In veterinary patients, moxifloxacin ophthalmic may be useful for treating bacterial conjunctivitis caused by susceptible species/strains of staphylococci, streptococci, *Corynebacterium, Haemophilus,* and chlamydia. When administered via a subpalpebral lavage (SPL) catheter it can be used for treating keratitis.

Pharmacology/Actions

Moxifloxacin is a member of the fluoroquinolone class of anti-infective drugs. Its action results from inhibition of DNA gyrase, which is involved in replication, transcription and repair of bacterial DNA.

Contraindications/Precautions/Warnings

Moxifloxacin is contraindicated in patients with a history of hypersensitivity to moxifloxacin, to other fluoroquinolones, or to any of the components of this medication. For topical ophthalmic use only; not for injection subconjunctivally or into the anterior chamber of the eye.

Moxeza® should not be used in SPL catheters (too viscous) for treating equine keratitis.

Fluoroquinolone-induced retinal toxicity in domestic cats has not been demonstrated with this product at time of writing, but may be possible.

Adverse Effects

Adverse effects reported in humans or animals include blurred vision, tearing, eye pain, redness, itching, and a bad taste in the mouth. Crystalline drug precipitates may be noted in the superficial portion of corneal defects during use.

Doses

Conjunctivitis (extra-label): 1 drop in the affected eye(s) every 4-8 hours.

Keratitis (extra-label): 1 drop in the affected eye or 0.2 mL in the SPL catheter every 1-8 hours. May precipitate when mixed with other ophthalmic medications. Flush SPL catheter well with air between medications.

Monitoring

- Clinical efficacy. If blepharospasm, uveitis, or worsening of ulceration or no improvement in infection is noted in 7 days, reassess microbial susceptibility.

Client Information

- Used 3-12 times daily.
- Crystals may appear in the eyes for a few days after initiation of treatment.
- Wait 5 minutes after applying this medication before applying any other medications to the eye.
- Store in the refrigerator or at controlled room temperature away from moisture and sunlight; do not freeze. Do not use if the color changes, it becomes cloudy, or if particles are seen in solutions.
- Dispose of unused medication in regular trash, do not put into sewer system.

Storage/Stability

Store in refrigerator or controlled room temperature away from moisture and sunlight; do not freeze.

Compatibility/Compounding Considerations

Fluoroquinolone antibiotics interact with many other drugs including those containing cations (*e.g.*, iron, aluminum, magnesium, calcium, etc.). Moxifloxacin should not be mixed directly with any other drugs. Moxifloxacin is not available as an ophthalmic ointment, but *Moxeza®* gel may be used in place of an ophthalmic ointment.

Dosage Forms/Regulatory Status

VETERINARY-LABELED PRODUCTS: NONE.

HUMAN-LABELED PRODUCTS:

Moxifloxacin 0.5% Ophthalmic Solution (containing boric acid, NaCl and purified water) in 3 mL ophthalmic dropper bottle; *Vigamox®*; (Rx)

Moxifloxacin 0.5% Ophthalmic Gel (containing NaCl, xanthan gum, boric acid, sorbitol tyloxapol, purified water and HCl and/or NaOH to adjust pH) in 3 mL ophthalmic dropper bottle; *Moxeza®*; (Rx)

Revisions/References

Monograph revised/updated September 2014.

Nalbuphine Ophthalmic

(nal-byoo-feen)   Nubain®

Opioid Agonist-Antagonist Analgesic Agent

Prescriber Highlights

▶ Decrease in corneal sensitivity in rabbits, dogs and horses not supported by evidence.

▶ Do not use in combination with other opioid ocular analgesics (*e.g.*, morphine sulfate).

Uses/Indications

In veterinary patients, nalbuphine ophthalmic solution use is controversial; it has been used as a corneal analgesic, but investigations have showed that corneal sensitivity is not decreased in horses, rabbits, or dogs (Wotman *et al.* 2010; Clark *et al.* 2011; Silva *et al.* 2012).

Pharmacology/Actions

Nalbuphine is a synthetic opioid agonist-antagonist analgesic of the phenanthrene series. Nalbuphine's analgesic potency is essentially equivalent to that of morphine on a milligram basis. The opioid antagonist activity of nalbuphine is 1/4th as potent as nalorphine and 10X that of pentazocine. Nalbuphine by itself has potent opioid antagonist activity at doses equal to or lower than its analgesic dose. When administered following or concurrent with *mu* agonist opioid analgesics (*e.g.*, morphine, oxymorphone, fentanyl), nalbuphine may partially reverse or block opioid-induced respiratory depression from the *mu*-agonist analgesic.

Contraindications/Precautions/Warnings

Nalbuphine is contraindicated in patients with a history of hypersensitivity to it or any component of the formulation. Nalbuphine is a partial opioid antagonist and should not be used in patients receiving other opioid agents as analgesia may be reversed by nalbuphine. Nalbuphine used systemically has potential to depress respiratory and cardiac systems; although it is not likely to have these effects when used topically.

Adverse Effects

Adverse effects reported in humans or animals include burning, stinging and irritation on application. Systemic adverse effects, although unlikely following topical use include respiratory and cardiovascular depression, somnolence, and ataxia.

Doses

Corneal analgesia (extra-label): 1 drop in the affected eye(s) every 8 hours.

Monitoring

- Clinical efficacy. Evaluate pain and blepharospasm to determine adequate analgesia.

Client Information

- Used 3 times daily.
- Use proper administration techniques to avoid contamination of the medication. Keep cap tightly closed when not in use.
- Wait 5 minutes after applying this medication before applying any other medications to the eye.
- Store in the refrigerator or at controlled room temperature away from moisture and sunlight; do not freeze. Do not use if the color changes, it becomes cloudy, or if particles are seen in solutions.

Storage/Stability

Store in refrigerator or at controlled room temperature away from moisture and sunlight; do not freeze.

Compatibility/Compounding Considerations

Nalbuphine should not be mixed directly with any other drugs. Nalbuphine is not commercially available and must be compounded by a qualified compounding pharmacist.

Dosage Forms/Regulatory Status

VETERINARY-LABELED PRODUCTS: NONE.

HUMAN-LABELED PRODUCTS: NONE.

Nalbuphine is not commercially available as an ophthalmic preparation, but may be compounded by qualified compounding pharmacists into a 1% or 1.2% ophthalmic solution. Evidence to support long-term stability of this solution could not be located at time of writing (2014).

Revisions/References

Monograph revised/updated September 2014.

Clark, J. S., et al. (2011). Evaluation of topical nalbuphine or oral tramadol as analgesics for corneal pain in dogs: a pilot study. Vet. Ophthalmol. **14**(6): 358-64.

Silva, M. L., et al. (2012). Topical 1% Nalbuphine on corneal sensivity and epitheilization after experimental lamellar keratectomy in rabbits. Ciencia Rural **42**(4): 679-84.

Wotman, K. L. & M. E. Utter (2010). Effect of treatment with a topical ophthalmic preparation of 1% nalbuphine solution on corneal sensitivity in clinically normal horses. American Journal of Veterinary Research **71**(2): 223-8.

Natamycin Ophthalmic

(nat-uh-mye-sin)   Natacyn®, Pimaracin

Antifungal

Prescriber Highlights

▶ Poorly soluble and does not efficiently penetrate corneal epithelium, used primarily for *Fusarium* infections.

▶ Well-tolerated; fewer adverse effects than amphotericin B.

▶ Natamycin suspensions may block SPL catheters; ensure catheter patency by flushing the line with air after each dose.

▶ Extravasation from SPL catheter can cause severe swelling and pain in eyelid area.

▶ Expensive.

Uses/Indications

In veterinary patients, natamycin is primarily used to treat superficial equine fungal keratitis caused by *Fusarium*.

Pharmacology/Actions

Natamycin is a tetraene polyene antibiotic derived from *Streptomyces natalensis*. It possesses in vitro activity against a variety of yeast and filamentous fungi, including Candida, Aspergillus, Cephalosporium, *Fusarium* and Penicillium. The mechanism of action appears to be through binding of the molecule to the sterol moiety of the fungal cell membrane. The polyenesterol complex alters the permeability of the membrane to produce depletion of essential cellular constituents. Although the activity against fungi is dose-related, natamycin is predominantly fungicidal.

Contraindications/Precautions/Warnings

Natamycin is contraindicated in patients with a history of hypersensitivity to it or any component of the formulation.

Adverse Effects

Adverse effects reported in humans or animals include corneal opacity, dyspnea, eye discomfort, eye edema, eye hyperemia, eye irritation, eye pain, foreign body sensation, paresthesia, and tearing. In horses, extravasation from SPL catheter into local tissues can cause severe irritation and swelling.

Doses

Equine Fungal Keratitis (extra-label): 0.1 mL in the SPL catheter every 30-60 minutes for 1-3 days, then every 6 hours for 4-6 weeks or until resolution of fungal keratitis. Ensure catheter patency by flushing the line with air after each dose.

Monitoring

- Clinical efficacy. Corneal scrapings to detect fungal organisms.

Client Information

- Used every 30-60 minutes for the first day then every 6 hours.
- Use proper administration techniques to avoid contamination of the medication. Keep cap tightly closed when not in use.
- Wait 5 minutes after applying this medication before applying any other medications to the eye.
- Store at controlled room temperature away from moisture and sunlight; do not freeze. Do not use if the color changes.

Storage/Stability

Store at controlled room temperature away from moisture and sunlight; do not freeze.

Compatibility/Compounding Considerations

Natamycin should not be mixed directly with any other drugs. Natamycin is not available as an ophthalmic ointment.

Dosage Forms/Regulatory Status

VETERINARY-LABELED PRODUCTS: NONE.

HUMAN-LABELED PRODUCTS:

Natamycin 5% Ophthalmic Suspension (containing: Natamycin 50 mg/mL, benzalkonium chloride 0.02%, NaOH and/or HCl to adjust the pH to 5-7.5, and purified water) in a 15 mL amber glass dropper bottle; *Natacyn®*; (Rx)

Revisions/References

Monograph revised/updated September 2014.

Nedocromil Ophthalmic

(ne-doe-krow-mill)   Alocril®

Mast Cell Stabilizing Ophthalmic Agent

Prescriber Highlights

▶ Used primarily for allergic conjunctivitis.

▶ May not be as well tolerated or as effective as ketotifen for allergic conjunctivitis (Greiner *et al.* 2003).

Uses/Indications

In veterinary patients, nedocromil is used for the treatment of itching associated with allergic conjunctivitis.

Pharmacology/Actions

Nedocromil is a mast cell stabilizer and inhibits histamine release from mast cells. Decreased chemotaxis and decreased activation of eosinophils (antiinflammatory effects) have also been demonstrated following administration of nedocromil (Corin 2000).

Contraindications/Precautions/Warnings

Nedocromil is contraindicated in patients with a history of hypersensitivity to it or any component of the formulation.

Adverse Effects

Adverse effects reported in humans or animals include ocular burning, irritation and stinging, unpleasant taste, and nasal congestion. Approximately 40% of humans report headaches and a bad taste in their mouths after use. Other less common adverse events include asthma, conjunctivitis, eye redness, photophobia, and rhinitis.

Doses

Allergic Conjunctivitis (extra-label): 1 drop in the affected eye(s) twice daily. Treatment should be continued throughout the period of exposure (*i.e.,* until exposure to the offending allergen is terminated), even when symptoms are absent.

Monitoring

- Clinical efficacy. Resolution of signs of allergic conjunctivitis.

Client Information

- Used 2 times daily.
- Use proper administration techniques to avoid contamination of the medication. Keep cap tightly closed when not in use.
- Wait 5 minutes after applying this medication before applying any other medications to the eye.
- Store in the refrigerator or at controlled room temperature away from moisture and sunlight; do not freeze. Do not use if the color changes, becomes cloudy, or if particles are seen in the solution.

Storage/Stability

Store in refrigerator or at controlled room temperature away from moisture and sunlight; do not freeze.

Compatibility/Compounding Considerations

Nedocromil should not be mixed directly with any other drugs. Nedocromil is not available as an ophthalmic ointment.

Dosage Forms/Regulatory Status

VETERINARY-LABELED PRODUCTS: NONE.

HUMAN-LABELED PRODUCTS:

Nedocromil 2% Ophthalmic Solution (containing nedocromil 20 mg/mL; benzalkonium chloride 0.01%; edetate disodium 0.05%; purified water; NaCl 0.5%, buffered to a pH of 4.0-5.54 with an osmolality range of 270-330 mOsm/kg) in a 5 mL ophthalmic dropper bottle; *Alocril®*; (Rx)

Revisions/References

Monograph revised/updated September 2014.

Corin, R. E. (2000). Nedocromil sodium: a review of the evidence for a dual mechanism of action. Clinical and Experimental Allergy **30**(4): 461-8.

Greiner, J. V. & G. Minno (2003). A placebo-controlled comparison of ketotifen fumarate and nedocromil sodium ophthalmic solutions for the prevention of ocular itching with the conjunctival allergen challenge model. Clinical Therapeutics **25**(7): 1988-2005.

Neomycin Sulfate Ophthalmic

(nee-oh-mye-sin suhl-fate)

Aminoglycoside Antibiotic

Prescriber Highlights

▶ Typically one component of an antibiotic combination (*e.g.,* triple antibiotic). Multiple approved ophthalmic products containing neomycin sulfate exist; many contain corticosteroids.

▶ Cats may experience hypersensitivity/anaphylaxis when exposed to topical neomycin.

▶ Prolonged use of antibiotic preparations may result in overgrowth of non-susceptible organisms, including fungi.

Uses/Indications

In veterinary patients, neomycin sulfate ophthalmic products are used in combination primarily with bacitracin and polymyxin B for topical treatment of superficial infections of the external eye and its adnexa caused by susceptible bacteria. Neomycin sulfate contributes activity against gram-negative organisms. Such infections encompass conjunctivitis, keratitis and keratoconjunctivitis, blepharitis and blepharoconjunctivitis. Due to toxicity risks, systemic and irrigant uses of neomycin sulfate are rare in treating ocular disorders and should be limited to situations where less toxic alternatives would not be effective.

Pharmacology/Actions

Neomycin sulfate is an aminoglycoside antibiotic. Aminoglycosides work by binding to the bacterial 30S ribosomal subunit, causing misreading of t-RNA, leaving the bacterium unable to synthesize proteins vital to its growth. Aminoglycosides are useful primarily in infections involving aerobic, gram-negative bacteria, such as *Pseudomonas*, *Acinetobacter*, and *Enterobacter*. In addition, some mycobacteria, including the bacteria that cause tuberculosis, are susceptible to aminoglycosides. Infections caused by gram-positive bacteria can also be treated with aminoglycosides, but other types of antibiotics are more potent and less damaging to the host. Aminoglycosides are mostly ineffective against anaerobic bacteria, fungi and viruses.

Contraindications/Precautions/Warnings

Neomycin sulfate combinations are contraindicated in patients with a history of hypersensitivity to any component of the formulation. Some cats are hypersensitive to the neomycin or polymyxin component of triple antibiotic ointments. This hypersensitivity has not been associated with steroid-containing neomycin sulfate products. Prolonged use of antibiotic preparations may result in overgrowth of non-susceptible organisms, including fungi. Neomycin sulfate is minimally absorbed after oral absorption; however, renal damage and ototoxicity may result if topical neomycin sulfate is ingested through grooming.

Adverse Effects

Adverse effects reported in humans or animals include irritation and swelling upon instillation. Topical antibiotics, especially neomycin sulfate and polymyxin B, may cause cutaneous sensitization and anaphylaxis, particularly in cats. Clinical signs of cutaneous sensitization to topical antibiotics usually include itching, reddening, and edema of the conjunctiva and eyelid, but may progress to anaphylaxis. Effects usually subside quickly after withdrawing the medication.

Doses

Conjunctivitis or Keratitis: 1 drop of the triple antibiotic solution or ¼ inch strip of the triple antibiotic ointment in the affected eye(s) 3-4 times daily until resolution or microbial susceptibilities necessitate a change to another antimicrobial agent.

Monitoring

- Clinical efficacy. Resolution of conjunctivitis or keratitis as evidenced by cytology, cultures, or remission of symptoms.

Client Information

- Used 3-4 times daily.
- Cats may have a severe allergic reaction to one of the components of this medication. Contact your veterinarian immediately if your cat has difficulty breathing or facial swelling after receiving this medication.
- Use proper administration techniques to avoid contamination of the medication. Keep cap tightly closed when not in use.
- Wait 5 minutes after applying this medication before applying any other medications to the eye.
- Store in the refrigerator or at controlled room temperature away from moisture and sunlight; do not freeze. Do not use if the color changes, becomes cloudy, or if particles are seen in the solution.

Storage/Stability

Store at controlled room temperature away from moisture and sunlight; do not freeze.

Compatibility/Compounding Considerations

Neomycin sulfate ophthalmic should not be mixed directly with any other drugs.

Dosage Forms/Regulatory Status

VETERINARY-LABELED PRODUCTS:

Triple Antibiotic Ophthalmic Ointment (containing: neomycin sulfate equivalent to 3.5 mg neomycin base, polymyxin B sulfate equivalent to 10,000 polymyxin B units, bacitracin zinc equivalent to 400 bacitracin units, and white petrolatum and mineral oil, q.s.) in a 3.5 g ophthalmic ointment tube; *TriOptic-P®, Vetropolycin®*; (Rx)

Triple Antibiotic with Hydrocortisone Ophthalmic Ointment; each gram contains: bacitracin zinc USP 400 units, neomycin sulfate 0.5% (equivalent to 3.5 mg neomycin base), polymyxin B sulfate USP 10,000 units, hydrocortisone acetate USP 1.0% in a base of white petrolatum and mineral oil; *TriOptic-S®, Vetropolycin HC®*; (Rx)

HUMAN-LABELED PRODUCTS:

Triple Antibiotic Ophthalmic Ointment (containing: neomycin sulfate equivalent to 3.5 mg neomycin base, polymyxin B sulfate equivalent to 5,000 or 10,000 polymyxin B units, bacitracin zinc equivalent to 400 bacitracin units, and white petrolatum, q.s) in a 3.5 gram ophthalmic ointment tube; *Neo-Polycin®*, generic; (Rx)

Neomycin-Polymyxin-Gramicidin Ophthalmic Solution (containing: polymyxin B equivalent to 1.75 mg polymyxin B base, polymyxin B sulfate equivalent 10,000 polymyxin B units, and gramicidin 0.025 mg per mL; alcohol 0.5%; thimerosal 0.001%; propylene glycol; polyoxyethylene polyoxypropylene compound; NaCl; and Water for Injection) in a 10 mL ophthalmic dropper bottle; *Neosporin®*, generic; (Rx)

Revisions/References

Monograph revised/updated September 2014.

Nepafenac Ophthalmic

(ne-paf-en-ak)   Nevanac®

Nonsteroidal Antiinflammatory Drug (NSAID)

Prescriber Highlights

▶ Prodrug to amfenac, which is bioavailable to the posterior segment.

▶ May be useful in ocular anti-angiogenic therapies.

▶ May increase risk of intraocular bleeding, retard corneal wound healing and promote corneal melting.

▶ Very expensive.

Uses/Indications

In veterinary patients, nepafenac is used to decrease inflammation following cataract surgery. It may be administered in conjunction with other topical ophthalmic medications such as beta-blockers, carbonic anhydrase inhibitors, alpha-agonists, cycloplegics, and mydriatics.

Pharmacology/Actions

Nepafenac is a nonsteroidal antiinflammatory and analgesic prodrug. After topical ocular dosing, nepafenac penetrates the cornea where it is converted by ocular tissue hydrolases to amfenac. Amfenac is thought to inhibit the action of prostaglandin H synthase (cyclooxygenase), an enzyme required for prostaglandin production.

Contraindications/Precautions/Warnings

Nepafenac is contraindicated in patients with a history of hypersensitivity to it or any component of the formulation or to other NSAIDs. Caution should be exercised when utilizing nepafenac in patients that have previously exhibited sensitivity to other NSAID drugs as there is potential for cross-sensitivity. Nepafenac should be used cautiously in patients concomitantly receiving systemic anticoagulants (*e.g.,* aspirin, clopidogrel, warfarin, and heparin) as concomitant use may increase risk of intraocular bleeding.

Nepafenac has been associated with increased bleeding of ocular tissues (including hyphema) in conjunction with ocular surgery due to interference with platelet aggregation. All topical NSAIDs may slow or delay healing. Concomitant use with topical steroidal agents may increase the potential for delayed healing.

Use of topical NSAIDs may result in keratitis due to epithelial breakdown, corneal thinning, corneal erosion, corneal ulceration, or corneal perforation and it should be discontinued immediately in patients exhibiting evidence of corneal epithelial breakdown.

Post-marketing experience with topical NSAIDs suggests that use more than 24 hours prior to surgery or use beyond 14 days after surgery may increase patient risk for the occurrence of corneal adverse events.

Adverse Effects

Adverse effects reported in humans or animals include capsular opacity, decreased visual acuity, foreign body sensation, increased intraocular pressure, and sticky sensation. Other ocular adverse events include conjunctival edema, corneal edema, dry eye, lid margin crusting, ocular discomfort, ocular hyperemia, ocular pain, ocular pruritus, and photophobia, tearing and vitreous detachment. Some of these events may be the consequence of the cataract surgical procedure. Non-ocular adverse events reported by humans include headache, hypertension, nausea/vomiting, and sinusitis.

Doses

Post cataract surgery (extra-label): 1 drop in the affected eye(s) 3 times daily for up to 2 weeks following cataract surgery.

Equine Uveitis (extra-label): 2 drops in the affected eye(s) every 8 hours.

Allergic Conjunctivitis (extra-label): 1 drop in the affected eye 2-4 times daily.

Monitoring

- Clinical efficacy. Decreased or absent inflammation. Monitor for delayed wound healing.

Client Information

- Used 3-4 times daily.
- Shake well before using.
- Use proper administration techniques to avoid contamination of the medication. Keep cap tightly closed when not in use.
- Wait 5 minutes after applying this medication before applying any other medications to the eye.
- Store in the refrigerator or at controlled room temperature away from moisture and sunlight; do not freeze. Do not use if the color changes.

Storage/Stability

Store in refrigerator or at controlled room temperature away from moisture and sunlight; do not freeze.

Compatibility/Compounding Considerations

Nepafenac should not be mixed directly with any other drugs. Nepafenac is not available as an ophthalmic ointment.

Dosage Forms/Regulatory Status

VETERINARY-LABELED PRODUCTS: NONE.

HUMAN-LABELED PRODUCTS:

Nepafenac 0.1% Ophthalmic Solution (containing: nepafenac 1 mg/mL; mannitol; carbomer 974P; NaCl; tyloxapol; edetate disodium; benzalkonium chloride 0.005%; NaOH and/or HCl to adjust pH to 7.4; and purified water, USP, with an osmolality of 305 mOsm/kg) in a 3 mL ophthalmic dropper bottle; *Nevanac®*; (Rx)

Revisions/References

Monograph revised/updated September 2014.

Ofloxacin Ophthalmic

(o-flocks-uh-sin)   Ocuflox®

Fluoroquinolone Antimicrobial

Prescriber Highlights

▶ Fluoroquinolone antimicrobial used for bacterial conjunctivitis or keratitis.

▶ May be considerably less expensive than ciprofloxacin or moxifloxacin ophthalmic solutions.

▶ Physically incompatible with many drugs.

▶ Crystalline drug precipitates may be noted in the superficial portion of corneal defects during use.

Uses/Indications

In veterinary patients, ofloxacin ophthalmic may be useful for treating bacterial conjunctivitis caused by susceptible species/strains of staphylococci, streptococci, Corynebacterium, Haemophilus, and chlamydia. When administered via a subpalpebral lavage (SPL) catheter it can be used for treating keratitis.

Pharmacology/Actions

Ofloxacin is a member of the fluoroquinolone class of anti-infective drugs. Its action results from inhibition of DNA gyrase, which is involved in replication, transcription and repair of bacterial DNA.

Contraindications/Precautions/Warnings

Ofloxacin is contraindicated in patients with a history of hypersensitivity to ofloxacin, to other fluoroquinolones, or to any of the components of this medication. For topical ophthalmic use only; not for injection subconjunctivally or into the anterior chamber of the eye. Fluoroquinolone-induced retinal toxicity in domestic cats has not been demonstrated with this product at time of writing, but may be possible.

Adverse Effects

Adverse effects reported in humans or animals include blurred vision, tearing, eye pain, redness, itching, and a bad taste in the mouth. Crystalline drug precipitates may be noted in the superficial portion of corneal defects during use.

Doses

Conjunctivitis (extra-label): Days 1 and 2: 1 drop in the affected eye(s) every two to four hours; Days 3 through 7: 1 drop in the affected eye(s) 4 times daily.

Keratitis (extra-label): 1 drop in the affected eye or 0.2 mL in the SPL catheter every 1-8 hours. May precipitate when mixed with other ophthalmic medications. Flush SPL catheter well with air between medications.

Monitoring

- Clinical efficacy. If blepharospasm, uveitis, or worsening of ulceration or no improvement in infection is noted in 7 days, reassess microbial susceptibility.

Client Information

- Used 3-12 times daily.
- Crystals may appear in the eyes for a few days after initiation of treatment.
- Wait 5 minutes after applying this medication before applying any other medications to the eye.
- Store in the refrigerator or at controlled room temperature away from moisture and sunlight; do not freeze. Do not use if the color changes, it becomes cloudy, or if particles are seen in solutions.
- Dispose of unused medication in regular trash, do not put into sewer system.

Storage/Stability

Store in refrigerator or controlled room temperature away from moisture and sunlight; do not freeze.

Compatibility/Compounding Considerations

Fluoroquinolone antibiotics interact with many other drugs including those containing cations (*e.g.*, iron, aluminum, magnesium, calcium, etc.). Ofloxacin should not be mixed directly with any other drugs. Ofloxacin is not available as an ophthalmic ointment.

Dosage Forms/Regulatory Status

VETERINARY-LABELED PRODUCTS: NONE.

HUMAN-LABELED PRODUCTS:

Ofloxacin 0.3% Ophthalmic Solution (containing ofloxacin 3 mg/mL; benzalkonium chloride 0.005%; NaCl; HCl and/or NaOH to adjust pH to a range of 6.0-6.8; and purified water; with an osmolality of 300 mOsm/kg.) in a 5 mL and 10 mL ophthalmic dropper bottle; *Ocuflox®*; (Rx)

Revisions/References

Monograph revised/updated September 2014.

Olopatadine Ophthalmic

(o-la-pat-a-deen)   Pataday®, Patanol®

H1 Receptor Antagonist Antihistamine Agent

Prescriber Highlights

▶ Selective H₁ receptor antagonist antihistamine.

▶ Longer duration of action allows once to twice daily dosing.

▶ Relatively expensive.

Uses/Indications

In veterinary patients, olopatadine is used to relieve pruritus caused by allergic conjunctivitis.

Pharmacology/Actions

Olopatadine is a mast cell stabilizer and a histamine H1 antagonist. Decreased chemotaxis and inhibition of eosinophil activation has also been demonstrated.

Contraindications/Precautions/Warnings

Olopatadine is contraindicated in patients with a history of hypersensitivity to it or any component of the formulation.

Adverse Effects

Adverse effects reported in humans or animals include transient burning or stinging upon instillation in the eye. Humans experience headaches and a bad taste in the mouth; animals may also experience these side effects.

Doses

Allergic conjunctivitis (extra-label): 1 drop in the affected eye(s) once daily (*Pataday®*) or twice daily (*Patanol®*).

Monitoring

▪ Clinical efficacy. Resolution of pruritus and conjunctivitis.

Client Information

▪ Used once daily (*Pataday®*) or twice daily (*Patanol®*).

▪ Use proper administration techniques to avoid contamination of the medication. Keep lid tightly closed when not in use.

▪ Wait 5 minutes after applying this medication before applying any other medications to the eye.

▪ Store at controlled room temperature away from moisture and sunlight; do not freeze. Do not use if the color changes, it becomes cloudy, or if particles are seen in solutions.

Storage/Stability

Store at controlled room temperature away from moisture and sunlight; do not freeze.

Compatibility/Compounding Considerations

Olopatadine should not be mixed directly with any other drugs.

Dosage Forms/Regulatory Status

VETERINARY-LABELED PRODUCTS: NONE.

HUMAN-LABELED PRODUCTS:

Olopatadine 0.1% Ophthalmic Solution (containing 1.11 mg olopatadine HCl equivalent to 1 mg Olopatadine per mL; povidone; dibasic sodium phosphate; NaCl; edentate disodium; benzalkonium chloride 0.01%; HCl/NaOH to adjust pH to ≈ 7; and purified water; with an osmolality of ≈ 300 mOsm/kg) in 2.5 mL ophthalmic dropper bottles; *Patanol®*; (Rx)

Olopatadine 0.2% Ophthalmic Solution (containing 2.22 mg olopatadine HCl equivalent to 2 mg Olopatadine per mL; povidone; dibasic sodium phosphate; NaCl; edentate disodium; benzalkonium chloride 0.01%; HCl/NaOH to adjust pH to ≈ 7; and purified water; with an osmolality of ≈ 300 mOsm/kg) in 2.5 mL ophthalmic dropper bottles; *Pataday®*; (Rx)

Revisions/References

Monograph revised/updated September 2014.

Oxytetracycline/Polymyxin B Ophthalmic

(ocks-ih-tet-rih-sye-kleen; pol-lee-mix-in)   Terramycin®

Combination Antibiotic

Prescriber Highlights

▶ Frequently unavailable, but may be prepared by qualified compounding pharmacists during shortages.

▶ Useful for treating *Chlamydial* and *Mycoplasma* conjunctivitis in cats.

▶ Treat *Chlamydia* infections for 3-4 weeks beyond resolution of symptoms to disrupt *Chlamydia* reproductive cycle.

▶ Some cats have severe allergic reactions to the polymyxin B component.

Uses/Indications

In veterinary patients, oxytetracycline is used to treat for the treatment of superficial ocular infections involving the conjunctiva and/or cornea caused by oxytetracycline and polymyxin B sulfate-susceptible organisms, including gram-positive and gram-negative bacteria, rickettsiae, spirochetes, large viruses, and certain protozoa. It is most commonly used to treat known or suspected Chlamydia and Mycoplasma conjunctivitis in cats. Polymyxin B Sulfate, one of a group of related antibiotics derived from *Bacillus polymyxa*, is rapidly bactericidal. This action is exclusively against gram-negative organisms. It is particularly effective against *Pseudomonas aeruginosa* (*B. pyocyaneus*), and Koch-Weeks bacillus.

Pharmacology/Actions

Tetracyclines bind irreversibly to the 30S ribosomal subunits of susceptible organisms disrupting RNA synthesis, and to the 50S subunits of ribosomes altering cytoplasmic membrane permeability. Oxytetracycline is also a potent inhibitor of matrix metalloproteinase-9 and a moderate inhibitor of matrix metalloproteinase-2. Polymyxin B sulfate has a bactericidal action against almost all gram-negative bacilli except the Proteus group. Polymyxin B sulfate interacts with the lipopolysaccharide of the cytoplasmic outer membrane of gram-negative bacteria, altering membrane permeability and causing cell death. It does not need to enter the cell. It is not absorbed orally so systemic toxicity is not a concern.

Contraindications/Precautions/Warnings

Oxytetracycline and polymyxin are contraindicated in patients with a history of hypersensitivity to it, drugs like it, or any component of the formulation.

Adverse Effects

Adverse effects reported in humans or animals are rare. Oxytetracycline with polymyxin B sulfate is well tolerated by the epithelial membranes and other tissues of the eye. Allergic or inflammatory reactions due to individual hypersensitivity are rare; however, some cats are allergic to the polymyxin B component.

Doses

Conjunctivitis: ¼ inch strip in the affected eye(s) 2-4 times daily until resolution of conjunctivitis.

Monitoring

- Clinical efficacy. Resolution of conjunctivitis.

Client Information

- Used 2-4 times daily.
- Use proper administration techniques to avoid contamination of the medication. Keep cap tightly closed when not in use.
- Wait 5 minutes after applying this medication before applying any other medications to the eye.
- Store in the refrigerator or at controlled room temperature away from moisture and sunlight; do not freeze. Do not use if the color changes.

Storage/Stability

Store at controlled room temperature away from moisture and sunlight; do not freeze.

Compatibility/Compounding Considerations

Oxytetracycline should not be mixed directly with any other drugs.

Dosage Forms/Regulatory Status

VETERINARY-LABELED PRODUCTS:

Oxytetracycline HCl and Polymyxin B Ophthalmic Ointment (containing oxytetracycline 5mg/g; polymyxin B sulfate 10,000 units/g; white petrolatum, and liquid petrolatum.) in 3.5 g ointment tubes; *Terramycin®*; (Rx)

HUMAN-LABELED PRODUCTS: NONE.

Revisions/References

Monograph revised/updated September 2014.

Phenylephrine Ophthalmic

(fen-il-ef-rin)   Altafrin®, Neofrin®, Cyclomydril®

Alpha Agonist Vasoconstrictor

Prescriber Highlights

▶ Used to differentiate 2nd from 3rd order Horner's syndrome.
▶ Not an effective mydriatic in cats or horses when used alone and should be combined with atropine sulfate.
▶ Used to limit bleeding during minor ocular surface procedures.
▶ Local discomfort may occur after application.
▶ Cardiovascular adverse effects are more likely in small dogs and cats and following use of 10% concentrations.

Uses/Indications

In veterinary patients, phenylephrine is most commonly used to induce mydriasis prior to phacoemulsification for cataract removal. It may also be used prior to minor ocular surface procedures to limit bleeding. Phenylephrine can also be used to diagnose 2nd and 3rd order Horner's syndrome.

Pharmacology/Actions

Phenylephrine is an alpha-1 adrenergic receptor agonist used for dilation of the pupil due to its vasoconstrictor and mydriatic action. Phenylephrine possesses predominantly α-adrenergic effects. In the eye, phenylephrine acts locally as a potent vasoconstrictor and mydriatic, by constricting ophthalmic blood vessels and the radial muscle of the iris.

Contraindications/Precautions/Warnings

Phenylephrine is contraindicated in patients with a history of hypersensitivity to it or any component of the formulation. Phenylephrine should be used cautiously in patients with thyrotoxicosis or hypertension as cardiovascular adverse effects may occur.

Adverse Effects

Adverse effects reported in humans or animals include eye pain and stinging on instillation, temporary blurred vision and photophobia, and conjunctival sensitization. Systemic absorption of phenylephrine may result in cardiovascular adverse effects such as marked increase in blood pressure, syncope, myocardial infarction, tachycardia, and arrhythmia. Cardiovascular reactions are more likely following use of phenylephrine 10% solutions.

Doses

Diagnosis of Horner's syndrome (extra-label): 1 drop of a 0.25% phenylephrine solution in each eye. Patients suffering from third order Horner's syndrome will experience mydriasis from this low concentration while normal patients will not. If no response in 20-30 minutes, apply 1 drop of a 2.5% solution to each eye. If mydriasis occurs, 2nd order Horner's syndrome is likely.

Preoperative cataract removal (extra-label): 1 drop of 2.5% or 10% in the affected eye(s) every 15 minutes for 2 hours. Severe cardiovascular adverse effects are more likely with small dogs and cats and following use of the 10% solution.

Monitoring

- Clinical efficacy. Monitor heart rate.

Client Information

- Use exactly as your veterinarian has prescribed; watch your pet for signs of rapid heartbeat or dizziness.
- Use proper administration techniques to avoid contamination of the medication. Keep cap tightly closed when not in use.
- Wait 5 minutes after applying this medication before applying any other medications to the eye.
- Store in the refrigerator or at controlled room temperature away from moisture and sunlight; do not freeze. Do not use if the color changes, it becomes cloudy, or if particles are seen in solutions.

Storage/Stability

Store in refrigerator; do not freeze.

Compatibility/Compounding Considerations

Phenylephrine should not be mixed directly with any other drugs.

Dosage Forms/Regulatory Status

VETERINARY-LABELED PRODUCTS: NONE.

HUMAN-LABELED PRODUCTS:

Phenylephrine HCl 2.5% & 10% Ophthalmic Solution in 15 mL ophthalmic dropper bottles; *Altafrin®*, *Neofrin®*, generic; (Rx)

Phenylephrine HCL 1% & Cyclopentolate HCl 0.2% Ophthalmic Solution; *Cyclomydril®*; (Rx)

Revisions/References

Monograph revised/updated September 2014.

Pilocarpine Ophthalmic

(pye-loe-kar-peen)   Isopto-Carpine®

Cholinergic Miotic Agent

Prescriber Highlights

▶ Do not use in secondary glaucoma (*e.g.*, caused by uveitis); rarely used to treat primary glaucoma in dogs.

▶ Given orally in food to stimulate salivation to treat neurogenic keratoconjunctivitis sicca.

▶ Do not use in cases of lens luxation or subluxation due to risk of papillary block.

▶ Monitor for systemic toxicity (vomiting, diarrhea, bradycardia, hypersalivation, bronchiolar spasm, pulmonary edema).

Uses/Indications

In veterinary patients, pilocarpine is primarily used to diagnose localization of parasympathetic denervation of the iris sphincter caused by lesions or trauma to Cranial Nerve III. Prior to the approval of cyclosporine for treating keratoconjunctivitis sicca, pilocarpine was used orally (in food) to induce salivation to treat neurogenic keratoconjunctivitis sicca. Historically, pilocarpine was used to treat primary glaucoma in dogs, but has largely been replaced by beta-blockers and prostaglandin agents.

Pharmacology/Actions

Pilocarpine stimulates cholinergic receptors to cause the ciliary body muscle to constrict placing posteriorly directed tension on the base of the iris to mechanically pull open the iridocorneal angle structures resulting in miosis and reducing uveoscleral outflow. Pilocarpine does not reduce intraocular pressure in horses.

Contraindications/Precautions/Warnings

Pilocarpine is contraindicated in patients with a history of hypersensitivity to it or any component of the formulation. Avoid use in dogs with glaucoma secondary to uveitis. Do not use in cases of lens luxation or subluxation due to risk of papillary block.

Adverse Effects

Adverse effects reported in humans or animals include irritation (due to the low pH) upon application, which may result in inflammation of the uveal tract. Local irritation is reported to resolve after 3 days of therapy in humans. Chronic use may result in an irreversible miosis due to dilator muscle atrophy and sphincter muscle fibrosis. Systemic absorption of pilocarpine may result in vomiting, diarrhea, increased salivation, bronchiolar spasm, and pulmonary edema.

Doses

Diagnosis of parasympathetic denervation/Cranial Nerve III lesions (extra-label): 1 drop of 0.2% solution applied to the affected eye(s).

Neurogenic keratoconjunctivitis sicca (extra-label): 2 drops/20 lbs. of a 2% solution in food to be consumed orally twice daily. The dose is increased weekly until signs of toxicity occur or until symptoms are controlled.

Primary glaucoma (extra-label): 1 drop in the affected eye(s) 3 times daily.

Monitoring

- Clinical efficacy. Adequate salivation from oral pilocarpine for neurogenic keratoconjunctivitis sicca.
- Toxicity: Observe for signs of systemic toxicosis including vomiting, diarrhea, increased salivation, bronchiolar spasm (coughing) and pulmonary edema.

Client Information

- Used in food 2 times daily. Follow veterinarian's instructions exactly.
- Observe for signs of toxicity; including: vomiting, diarrhea, increased salivation, and coughing.
- Use proper administration techniques to avoid contamination of the medication. Keep cap tightly closed when not in use.
- Wait 5 minutes after applying this medication before applying any other medications to the eye.
- Store at controlled room temperature away from moisture and sunlight; do not freeze. Do not use if the color changes, it becomes cloudy, or if particles are seen in solutions.

Storage/Stability

Store at controlled room temperature away from moisture and sunlight; do not freeze.

Compatibility/Compounding Considerations

Pilocarpine should not be mixed directly with any other drugs.

Dosage Forms/Regulatory Status

VETERINARY-LABELED PRODUCTS: NONE.

HUMAN-LABELED PRODUCTS:

Pilocarpine HCl 1%, 2%, or 4% Ophthalmic Solution (containing: pilocarpine 10 mg/mL, 20 mg/mL, or 40 mg/mL respectively; benzalkonium chloride 0.01%; monobasic sodium phosphate; hypromellose; edetate disodium; dibasic sodium phosphate, purified water; NaOH and/or HCl may be added to adjust pH to 3.5-5.5) in a 15 mL ophthalmic dropper bottle; *Isopto Carpine*®, generic; (Rx)

Revisions/References

Monograph revised/updated September 2014.

Pimecrolimus Ophthalmic

(pi-mek-kroe-li-mus)

Immunosuppressive Lacrimimetic Agent

Prescriber Highlights

▶ Similar action as tacrolimus but has fewer systemic adverse effects; may be useful for cyclosporine-resistant cases of keratoconjunctivitis sicca.

▶ Not commercially available, must be compounded. *Elidel*® topical (skin) pimecrolimus ointment should **NOT** be used in the eye.

▶ Advise caregivers to wear gloves when handling pimecrolimus.

Uses/Indications

In veterinary patients, pimecrolimus is used to stimulate tear production in dogs that do not respond to cyclosporine. Pimecrolimus 1% administered 3 times daily to keratoconjunctivitis sicca patients demonstrated a favorable response (Nell *et al.* 2005). An investigation comparing pimecrolimus 1% to cyclosporine 0.2% demonstrated favorable improvement for both drugs over an 8 week period (Ofri *et al.* 2009).

Pharmacology/Actions

Pimecrolimus is a macrolide antibiotic that has a similar immunopharmacological profile as cyclosporine but is ≈ 100X more potent than cyclosporine. Both cyclosporin and pimecrolimus are calcineurin inhibitors that reversibly inhibit T-cell proliferation and prevent the release of pro-inflammatory cytokines. Calcineurin inhibitors bind to intracellular immunophilins and form complexes that subsequently bind to and inhibit calcineurin. In blocking calcineurin, translocation of the cytoplasmic component of the nuclear factor of activated T cells to the nucleus is prevented. This prevention of translocation impairs transcription of the genes encoding

IL-2 and other cytokines, thereby suppressing T-cell proliferation and normal immune function. In addition to increasing tear production by inhibiting T-helper lymphocyte proliferation and infiltration of lacrimal gland acini, pimecrolimus restores conjunctival goblet cell mucin production.

Contraindications/Precautions/Warnings

Pimecrolimus is contraindicated in patients with a history of hypersensitivity to it or any component of the formulation. Caregivers should be advised to avoid contact with pimecrolimus as skin contact with pimecrolimus has been associated with the development of cancer in humans.

Adverse Effects

Adverse effects to ocular use of pimecrolimus are rare but include orbital alopecia, which may be related to oil vehicles used to compound pimecrolimus solutions.

Doses

Keratoconjunctivitis Sicca (extra-label): 1 drop of a pimecrolimus 1% solution in each eye 2 times daily.

Monitoring

- Clinical efficacy. Schirmer Tear Test to determine adequate tear production.

Client Information

- Used 2 times daily.
- This is a lifelong medication and must be given daily. Missed doses may cause return of dry eye.
- Wear gloves when handling pimecrolimus. Use proper administration techniques to avoid contamination of the medication. Keep cap tightly closed when not in use.
- Wait 5 minutes after applying this medication before applying any other medications to the eye.
- Store at controlled room temperature away from moisture and sunlight; do not freeze. Do not use if the color changes, it becomes cloudy, or if particles are seen in solutions.

Storage/Stability

Store at controlled room temperature away from moisture and sunlight.

Compatibility/Compounding Considerations

Pimecrolimus should not be mixed directly with any other drugs.

Dosage Forms/Regulatory Status

VETERINARY-LABELED PRODUCTS: NONE.

HUMAN-LABELED PRODUCTS: NONE.

Pimecrolimus has been prepared (compounded) by qualified compounding pharmacists in 1% solutions in oil vehicles including olive oil, corn oil, and medium chain triglyceride oil.

Revisions/References

Monograph revised/updated September 2014.

Nell, B., et al. (2005). The effect of topical pimecrolimus on keratoconjunctivitis sicca and chronic superficial keratitis in dogs: results from an exploratory study. Vet. Ophthalmol. 8(1): 39-46.

Ofri, R., et al. (2009). Clinical evaluation of pimecrolimus eye drops for treatment of canine keratoconjunctivitis sicca: A comparison with cyclosporine A. Veterinary Journal 179(1): 70-7.

Polysulfated Glycosaminoglycan Ophthalmic

(pol-ee-sulf-ate-id glye-kos-uh-meen-oh-glye-kan)
  PSGAG, Adequan®

Collagen Enhancing Agent

Prescriber Highlights

▶ Used to manage indolent corneal ulcers in dogs and horses.
▶ Not commercially available, ophthalmic dosage form must be prepared from the commercially available injectable solution
▶ Superiority to keratectomy has not been demonstrated.

Uses/Indications

In veterinary patients, polysulfated glycosaminoglycan is used to manage corneal ulcers. The efficacy of PSGAG in inhibiting gelatinase in the tear film of dogs was found to be inferior to EDTA and other gelatinase inhibitors (Couture *et al.* 2006).

Pharmacology/Actions

Polysulfated glycosaminoglycan inhibits a number of enzymes (gelatinase, lysozyme, hyaluronidase, and plasmin), decreases prostaglandin E2 synthesis, reduces production of toxic superoxide radicals, and increases synthesis of collagen proteoglycans and hyaluronic acid. The effect on healing of corneal ulcers by PSGAG does not appear to be due to inhibition of lacrimal protease (Willeford *et al.* 1998).

Contraindications/Precautions/Warnings

Polysulfated glycosaminoglycan is contraindicated in patients with a history of hypersensitivity to it or any component of the formulation.

Adverse Effects

Adverse effects reported in humans or animals include inflammation or cellulitis at the injection site; however, these adverse effects are not usually observed after topical ophthalmic use.

Doses

Indolent corneal ulcer (extra-label): 1 drop in the affected eye(s) 3 times daily for up to 2 weeks.

Monitoring

- Clinical efficacy. If no significant response in 2 weeks, consider keratectomy.

Client Information

- Used 3 times daily.
- Use proper administration techniques to avoid contamination of the medication. Keep cap tightly closed when not in use.
- Wait 5 minutes after applying this medication before applying any other medications to the eye.
- Store in the refrigerator or at controlled room temperature away from moisture and sunlight; do not freeze. Do not use if the color changes, it becomes cloudy, or if particles are seen in solutions.

Storage/Stability

Store in refrigerator or at controlled room temperature away from moisture and sunlight; do not freeze.

Compatibility/Compounding Considerations

Polysulfated glycosaminoglycan should not be mixed directly with any other drugs. PSGAG is not available as an ophthalmic dosage form but may be prepared aseptically combining the commercially available 100 mg/ml injection 1:1 with sterile artificial tear solutions.

Dosage Forms/Regulatory Status

VETERINARY-LABELED PRODUCTS: NONE.

A 100 mg/mL injection is approved for use in horses and dogs, but no dosage forms appropriate for the eye are currently manufactured. Approved injections can be diluted to 5% with artificial tear solutions for use in the eye.

HUMAN-LABELED PRODUCTS: NONE.

Revisions/References

Monograph revised/updated September 2014.

Couture, S., et al. (2006). Topical effect of various agents on gelatinase activity in the tear film of normal dogs. Vet. Ophthalmol. **9**(3): 157-64.

Willeford, K., et al. (1998). Modulation of proteolytic activity associated with persistent corneal ulcers in dogs. Vet. Ophthalmol. **1**(1): 508.

Povidone Iodine Ophthalmic

(poe-veh-done eye-oh-dyne)   Betadine®

Ocular Disinfectant

Prescriber Highlights

▶ Inexpensive alternative to traditional anti-fungal or anti-viral ophthalmic agents.

▶ May be used to debride non-vital corneal epithelium from indolent ulcers.

▶ Solutions >1% must be thoroughly lavaged from the eye within 5 minutes of administration to avoid corneal toxicity.

Uses/Indications

In veterinary patients, povidone iodine ophthalmic solutions (1-5%) are used to chemically debride loose epithelium in canine indolent ulcers. Povidone iodine 5% solutions have been used once daily as inexpensive antifungal therapy for fungal keratitis, but due to corneal epithelial toxicity must be lavaged from the eye within 5 minutes after administration. Povidone iodine 0.5-1% solution is also sometimes used topically in the eye as an inexpensive option to treat feline herpes virus (FHV-1). Solutions with concentrations >1% used for any indication should always be lavaged from the eye within 5 minutes after administration to avoid corneal damage.

Pharmacology/Actions

Povidone iodine is an iodophor that penetrates the cell wall of microorganisms quickly, and lethal effects are believed to result from disruption of protein and nucleic acid structure and synthesis. Iodines are bactericidal and virucidal and may also be fungicidal and sporicidal depending on organism and contact time.

Contraindications/Precautions/Warnings

Povidone iodine is contraindicated in patients with a history of hypersensitivity to it or any component of the formulation.

Adverse Effects

Adverse effects reported in humans or animals include local burning and stinging upon application; however, concentrations of 0.5-1% seem to be well tolerated. Some patients may experience a local hypersensitivity reaction. Solutions of >1% are toxic to the corneal epithelium if left in contact for more than 5 minutes.

Doses

Fungal keratitis (extra-label): 1 – 2 drops of a 5% solution to the affected eye(s) once every 24 hours. Treated eye(s) must be thoroughly lavaged no more than 5 minutes after administration to avoid corneal damage.

Feline herpes keratitis (extra-label): 1 drop of a 0.5-1% solution to the affected eye(s) 3-4 times daily.

Debridement of non-vital epithelium in indolent ulcers (extra-label): 1 – 2 drops of a 5% solution to the affected eye(s) once. Irrigate

thoroughly to remove all povidone iodine not more than 5 minutes after application to avoid damage to healthy corneal epithelium.

Monitoring

- **Clinical efficacy.** Ensure that solutions >1% are thoroughly lavaged from treated eyes not more than 5 minutes after application.

Client Information

- Used 1-3 times daily.
- Rinse your animal's eyes thoroughly with eyewash within 5 minutes of application if instructed by your veterinarian.
- Use proper administration techniques to avoid contamination of the medication. Keep cap tightly closed when not in use.
- Store at controlled room temperature away from moisture and sunlight; do not freeze. Do not use if the color changes, becomes cloudy, or if particles are seen in the solution.

Storage/Stability

Store at controlled room temperature away from moisture and sunlight; do not freeze.

Compatibility/Compounding Considerations

Povidone iodine should not be mixed directly with any other drugs. Sterile povidone iodine ophthalmic preparation is available as a 5% solution intended for application to the eyes, but solutions of 0.5-1% may be prepared by diluting this solution with normal saline. Non-sterile povidone iodine solutions should not be administered to the eye.

Dosage Forms/Regulatory Status

VETERINARY-LABELED PRODUCTS: NONE.

HUMAN-LABELED PRODUCTS:

Povidone Iodine 5% Ophthalmic Prep (containing: povidone-iodine 5 mg/mL as a sterile dark brown solution; citric acid; glycerin; nonoxynol-9; NaCl; NaOH; and dibasic sodium phosphate) in a 30 mL bottle; *Betadine Sterile Ophthalmic Prep®*; (Rx)

Revisions/References

Monograph revised/updated September 2014.

Prednisolone Ophthalmic

(pred-niss-oh-lone)   Pred Forte®, Omnipred®

Corticosteroid Antiinflammatory Agent

Prescriber Highlights

▶ Superior penetration into anterior segment compared to other topical corticosteroids. Acetate salts achieve better penetration than phosphate salts.

▶ Use cautiously in small diabetic patients to avoid deregulation.

▶ Do not use in fungal keratitis, feline herpes keratitis, or if corneal abrasion or ulceration are suspected.

Uses/Indications

In veterinary patients, prednisolone ophthalmic is used for symptomatic relief of corticosteroid-responsive inflammatory conditions of the palpebral and bulbar conjunctiva, cornea, and anterior segment of the globe (*e.g.*, allergic conjunctivitis, acne rosacea, superficial punctate keratitis, iritis, and cyclitis). In horses it is used for treatment of uveitis. It may also be used to treat inflammation associated with corneal injury from chemical, radiation, or thermal burns or penetration of foreign bodies. Prednisolone is also available in many combinations with antimicrobial agents for topical ophthalmic use.

Pharmacology/Actions

Corticosteroids work by inhibiting phospholipase A2 as well as cyclooxygenase (COX) and lipoxygenase (LOX) pathways. Corticosteroids can also penetrate the nucleus to interrupt specific DNA sequences that produce inflammatory mediators. In general, pro-inflammatory mediators are down-regulated and antiinflammatory mediators are up-regulated. Corticosteroids also reduce the migration of macrophages, decrease vascular permeability, and suppress lymphokines. They inhibit edema, cellular infiltration, capillary dilatation, fibroblastic proliferation, and deposition of collagen. Prednisolone is a synthetic corticosteroid with ≈ 3-5X the potency of hydrocortisone.

Contraindications/Precautions/Warnings

Prednisolone is contraindicated in patients with a history of hypersensitivity to it or any component of the formulation. Topical corticosteroids are contraindicated in known or suspected corneal ulceration or corneal infection (fungal and viral). Use with caution in patients with diabetes mellitus or other endocrine diseases, infectious diseases, chronic renal failure, congestive heart failure, systemic hypertension, or gastric ulceration. When use is necessary in these conditions, the minimal effective dose should be administered for the shortest possible time.

Adverse Effects

Adverse effects reported in humans or animals include development of cataracts (via altered glucose or lenticular metabolic effects), increased intraocular pressure (via activation of glucocorticoid receptors in the trabecular meshwork), infection (via immunosuppression), decreased wound healing (via increased collagenolytic activity), mydriasis, and calcific keratopathy. Systemic effects are rare but include hepatopathy, suppression of endogenous glucocorticoid production, and focal alopecia. Concurrent use of systemic steroids increases risk of these adverse effects.

Doses

Anterior Uveitis (extra-label): 1 drop in the affected eye(s) 4 times daily initially and then taper depending on clinical response.

Conjunctivitis (extra-label): 1 drop or ¼ inch strip in affected eye(s) every 4-8 hours, then increase to longest dosing interval that still maintains efficacy.

Post Cataract Removal (extra-label): 1 drop in the affected eye(s) every 8-12 hours.

Monitoring

- Clinical efficacy. Resolution of inflammation. Monitor intraocular pressure and observe for evidence of infection or delayed wound healing. Monitor for blood or urine glucose changes in diabetic animals.

Client Information

- Used 4-6 times daily.
- Shake well before using.
- Use proper administration techniques to avoid contamination of the medication. Keep cap tightly closed when not in use.
- Wait 5 minutes after applying this medication before applying any other medications to the eye.
- Store at controlled room temperature away from moisture and sunlight; do not freeze. Do not use if the color changes.

Storage/Stability

Store at controlled room temperature away from moisture and sunlight; do not freeze.

Compatibility/Compounding Considerations

Prednisolone should not be mixed directly with any other drugs.

Dosage Forms/Regulatory Status

VETERINARY-LABELED PRODUCTS: NONE.
HUMAN-LABELED PRODUCTS:

Prednisolone Acetate 1% Ophthalmic Suspension (containing: prednisolone acetate 10 mg/mL; benzalkonium chloride; boric acid; edetate disodium; hypromellose; polysorbate 80; purified water; sodium bisulfite; NaCl; and sodium citrate, with a pH of 5-6) in 1 mL, 5 mL, 10 mL, and 15 mL ophthalmic dropper bottles; *Pred Forte 1%, Omnipred®*; (Rx)

Prednisolone Sodium Phosphate 1% Ophthalmic Suspension [containing prednisolone sodium phosphate 10 mg/mL (equivalent to 9.1 mg/mL prednisolone); hypromellose; monobasic and dibasic sodium phosphate; NaCl, edetate disodium and purified water; NaOH and/or HCl may be added to adjust the pH to 6.2-8.2] in 5 mL, 10 mL, and 15 mL ophthalmic dropper bottles; generic; (Rx)

Combination Products:

Prednisolone Acetate 0.6% and Gentamicin 0.3% Ophthalmic Ointment in 3.5 g; *Pred-G®*; (Rx)

Prednisolone Acetate 1% and Gentamicin 0.3% Ophthalmic Suspension in 5 mL & 10 mL; *Pred-G®*; (Rx)

Prednisolone Acetate 0.2% and Sulfacetamide Sodium 10% Ophthalmic Suspension in 2.5 mL, 5 mL, & 10 mL; *Blephamide®*; (Rx)

Prednisolone Sodium Phosphate 0.25% and Sodium 10% Ophthalmic Suspension in 5 mL & 10 mL; generic; (Rx)

Prednisolone Acetate 0.2% and Sulfacetamide Sodium 10% Ophthalmic Ointment in 3.5 g tubes; *Blephamide®*; (Rx)

Revisions/References

Monograph revised/updated September 2014.

Proparacaine Ophthalmic

(proe-pare-a-kane)   Alcaine®, Flucaine®

Topical Ocular Anesthetic

Prescriber Highlights

▶ Rapid-acting topical anesthetic for ocular diagnostic procedures.

▶ 5-10 minute duration.

▶ Chronic use results in corneal opacification and vision loss.

▶ Some products must be stored in the refrigerator; consult labeling.

Uses/Indications

In veterinary patients, proparacaine is indicated for topical anesthesia in ophthalmic practice. Representative ophthalmic procedures in which the preparation provides good local anesthesia include measurement of intraocular pressure (tonometry), removal of foreign bodies and sutures from the cornea, conjunctival scraping in diagnosis and gonioscopic examination; it is also indicated for use as a topical anesthetic prior to surgical operations such as cataract extraction.

Pharmacology/Actions

Proparacaine stabilizes the neuronal membrane by inhibiting the ionic fluxes required for the initiation and conduction of impulses thereby effecting local anesthetic action. More specifically, proparacaine appears to bind or antagonize the function of voltage gated sodium channels. The exact mechanism whereby proparacaine and other local anesthetics influence the permeability of the cell membrane is unknown; however, several studies indicate that local anesthetics may limit sodium ion permeability through the lipid layer of the nerve cell membrane. Proparacaine may alter epithelial sodium channels through interaction with channel protein residues. This limitation prevents the fundamental change necessary for the generation of the action potential.

Contraindications/Precautions/Warnings

Proparacaine is contraindicated in patients with a history of hypersensitivity to it or any component of the formulation. Prolonged use of a topical ocular anesthetic may produce permanent corneal opacification with accompanying loss of vision.

Adverse Effects

Adverse effects reported in humans or animals include pupillary dilatation or cycloplegic effects. The drug appears to be safe for use in patients sensitive to other local anesthetics, but local or systemic sensitivity occasionally occurs. Instillation of proparacaine in the eye at recommended concentration and dosage usually produces little or no initial irritation, stinging, burning, conjunctival redness, lacrimation or squinting. However, some local irritation and stinging may occur several hours after the instillation. Rarely, a severe, immediate hypersensitivity may occur, manifested by intense and diffuse epithelial keratitis; a gray, ground-glass appearance; sloughing of large areas of necrotic epithelium; corneal filaments and, sometimes, iritis with descemetitis. Softening and erosion of the corneal epithelium and conjunctival congestion and hemorrhage have been reported.

Doses

Ophthalmic procedures requiring local anesthesia (extra-label): 1 – 2 drops in the target eye(s) prior to examination or procedure. May repeat 1 drop every 5-10 minutes for 5-7 times. Duration of corneal anesthesia is ≈ 5-10 minutes per application.

Monitoring

- Diagnostic agent. Chronic use will delay wound healing and cause loss of vision through corneal opacification.

Client Information

- Proparacaine is not administered by pet owners in the home. It is reserved for diagnostic procedures in the veterinary practice.

Storage/Stability

Store in refrigerator or at controlled room temperature (depending on product labeling) away from moisture and sunlight; do not freeze. Discard if color change, or becomes cloudy, or if particles are observed in the solution.

Compatibility/Compounding Considerations

Proparacaine should not be mixed directly with any other drugs.

Dosage Forms/Regulatory Status

VETERINARY-LABELED PRODUCTS: NONE.
HUMAN-LABELED PRODUCTS:
Proparacaine HCl 0.5% Ophthalmic Solution (containing: proparacaine 5 mg/mL; benzalkonium chloride 0.1 mg/mL; glycerin as a stabilizer; water for injection; HCl and/or NaOH may be added to adjust pH to 3.5-6) in 15 mL ophthalmic dropper bottles; *Alcaine®*, *Flucaine®*; (Rx)

Revisions/References

Monograph revised/updated September 2014.

Rimexolone Ophthalmic

(rye-mecks-uh-lone) Vexol®
Corticosteroid Antiinflammatory Agent

Prescriber Highlights

- ► "Soft" steroid similar in action to prednisolone acetate, but steroid response more similar to fluorometholone.
- ► May be safer for use in diabetic patients due to rapid inactivation to non-toxic metabolites.
- ► Administered in pulse doses for mild to moderate keratitis.
- ► Do not use in fungal keratitis, feline herpes keratitis, or if corneal abrasion or ulceration are suspected.

Uses/Indications

In veterinary patients, rimexolone ophthalmic is used for symptomatic relief of corticosteroid-responsive inflammatory conditions of the palpebral and bulbar conjunctiva, cornea, and anterior segment of the globe (*e.g.*, allergic conjunctivitis, acne rosacea, superficial punctate keratitis, iritis, and cyclitis). In horses it is used for treatment of uveitis. It may also be used to treat inflammation associated with corneal injury from chemical, radiation, or thermal burns or penetration of foreign bodies. Rimexolone is also available in many combinations with antimicrobial agents for topical ophthalmic use.

Pharmacology/Actions

Corticosteroids work by inhibiting phospholipase A2 as well as cyclooxygenase (COX) and lipoxygenase (LOX) pathways. Corticosteroids can also penetrate the nucleus to interrupt specific DNA sequences that produce inflammatory mediators. In general, pro-inflammatory mediators are down-regulated and antiinflammatory mediators are up-regulated. Corticosteroids also reduce the migration of macrophages, decrease vascular permeability, and suppress lymphokines. They inhibit edema, cellular infiltration, capillary dilatation, fibroblastic proliferation, and deposition of collagen. Rimexolone is a synthetic corticosteroid with ≈ 3-5X the potency of hydrocortisone. Rimexolone is a "soft" steroid that is a biologically active compound with a predictable inactivation to a nontoxic substance after achieving its therapeutic purpose. The aim of this type of drug is to lower toxicity and increase more specific actions at a target organ. For this reason, rimexolone may be a safer choice for use in diabetic animals. Rimexolone was also found to cause less of an increase in IOP compared to prednisolone acetate in patients with uveitis (Foster *et al.* 1996).

Contraindications/Precautions/Warnings

Rimexolone is contraindicated in patients with a history of hypersensitivity to it or any component of the formulation. Topical corticosteroids are contraindicated in known or suspected corneal ulceration or corneal infection (fungal and viral). Use with caution in patients with diabetes mellitus or other endocrine diseases, infectious diseases, chronic renal failure, congestive heart failure, systemic hypertension, or gastric ulceration. When use is necessary in these conditions, the minimal effective dose should be administered for the shortest possible time.

Adverse Effects

Adverse effects reported in humans or animals include development of cataracts (via altered glucose or lenticular metabolic effects), increased intraocular pressure (via activation of glucocorticoid receptors in the trabecular meshwork—but to a lesser degree than with prednisolone), infection (via immunosuppression), decreased wound healing (via increased collagenolytic activity), mydriasis, and calcific keratopathy. Systemic effects are rare but include hepatopathy, suppression of endogenous glucocorticoid production, and focal alopecia. Concurrent use of systemic steroids increases risk of these adverse effects.

Doses

Anterior uveitis (extra-label): 1 drop in the affected eye(s) 4 times daily initially and then taper depending on clinical response.

Conjunctivitis (extra-label): 1 drop or ¼ inch strip in affected eye(s) every 4-8 hours, then increase to longest dosing interval that still maintains efficacy.

Post cataract removal (extra-label): 1 drop in the affected eye(s) every 8-12 hours.

Monitoring

- Clinical efficacy. Absence of inflammation. Monitor intraocular pressure and observe for evidence of infection or delayed wound healing. Monitor for blood or urine glucose changes in diabetic animals.

Client Information

- Used 4 times daily.
- Shake suspensions well before using.
- Use proper administration techniques to avoid contamination of the medication. Keep cap tightly closed when not in use.
- Wait 5 minutes after applying this medication before applying any other medications to the eye.
- Store at controlled room temperature away from moisture and sunlight; do not freeze. Do not use if the color changes.

Storage/Stability

Store at controlled room temperature away from moisture and sunlight; do not freeze.

Compatibility/Compounding Considerations

Rimexolone should not be mixed directly with any other drugs.

Dosage Forms/Regulatory Status

VETERINARY-LABELED PRODUCTS: NONE.

HUMAN-LABELED PRODUCTS:

Rimexolone Acetate 1% Ophthalmic Suspension (containing: rimexolone 10 mg/mL; benzalkonium chloride 0.01%; carbomer 974P; polysorbate 80; NaCl; edetate disodium; NaOH and/or HCl to adjust pH to 6-8; purified water, with a tonicity of 260-320 mOsm/kg.) in 5 mL and 10 mL ophthalmic dropper bottles; *Vexol®*; (Rx)

Revisions/References

Monograph revised/updated September 2014.

Foster, C. S., et al. (1996). Efficacy and safety of rimexolone 1% ophthalmic suspension vs 1% prednisolone acetate in the treatment of uveitis. American Journal of Ophthalmology 122(2): 171-82.

Rose Bengal Ophthalmic

(rose ben-gall)   Glostrips®, Rosets®

Ocular Diagnostic Agent

Prescriber Highlights

▶ Diagnostic method of choice to delineate dendritic corneal ulcers. Full thickness loss of corneal epithelium is not necessary (only dead epithelial cells) to detect corneal epithelium deficits with Rose Bengal.

▶ Used to determine damage to corneal epithelium in early keratoconjunctivitis sicca.

▶ Very toxic to cornea; irrigate eye(s) well after use.

▶ Stings upon application.

Uses/Indications

In veterinary patients, Rose Bengal stain is used to detect viral keratitis in cats. Feline herpes virus tends to infect one cell and moves to an adjacent cell causing dendritic tracts in the cornea. Because Rose Bengal binds to dead corneal epithelial cells without full thickness loss of corneal epithelium, Rose Bengal is an ideal diagnostic agent to detect dendritic corneal damage. Rose Bengal can also be used to detect early damage in undiagnosed or newly diagnosed keratoconjunctivitis sicca.

Pharmacology/Actions

Rose Bengal stains both the nuclei and cell walls of dead or degenerated epithelial cells of the cornea and conjunctiva. Rose Bengal will also stain the mucus of the precorneal tear film and does not require full thickness loss of corneal epithelium to indicate damage to the cornea.

Contraindications/Precautions/Warnings

Rose Bengal is contraindicated in patients with a history of hypersensitivity to it or any component of the formulation. Rose Bengal is very toxic to the cornea and treated eye(s) should be thoroughly irrigated after exposure. Rose Bengal is virucidal and may confound results of diagnostics for viral keratitis.

Adverse Effects

Adverse effects reported in humans or animals include burning and stinging upon application. Rose Bengal is very toxic to the cornea and treated eye(s) should be thoroughly irrigated after exposure.

Doses

Detection of Corneal and Conjunctival Cell Damage: Wet the surface of the Rose Bengal strip with 1-2 drops of normal saline solution. Apply moistened tip of strip or instill 1 drop of Rose Bengal 1% solution to conjunctiva or fornix as required. It is recommended that the patient blink several times after application. Wait 60 seconds, rinse the eye with sterile irrigating solution, and examine the eye with a light source. Degenerated or dead epithelial cells will appear red in color. **Note:** Rose Bengal is not FDA-approved.

Monitoring

- Diagnostic agent. Topical anesthetic agents may be indicated to prevent stinging upon application. Flush exposed eye(s) thoroughly with ophthalmic irrigation solutions following procedure to prevent corneal toxicity.

Client Information

- Rose Bengal should only be administered in the veterinary practice.

Storage/Stability

Store in refrigerator or at controlled room temperature away from moisture and sunlight as directed on packaging or by compounding pharmacist; do not freeze. Unpreserved solutions of Rose Bengal carry a high risk of contamination with bacteria. Store as directed and observe all assigned beyond-use dates.

Compatibility/Compounding Considerations

Rose Bengal should not be mixed directly with any other drugs. Rose Bengal solution is no longer commercially available but may be compounded as a 1% solution either with or without preservatives; however, preservation systems are strongly recommended to prevent microbial and fungal contamination (McElhiney 2012).

Dosage Forms/Regulatory Status

VETERINARY-LABELED PRODUCTS: NONE.

HUMAN-LABELED PRODUCTS: NONE.

Rose Bengal 0.13% & 0.15% Strips (containing: Rose Bengal 1.3 mg or 1.5 mg per strip) as individually wrapped strips in containers of 100 sterile strips; *Rose Glo®*, generic; (Rx). No FDA-approved dosage forms of Rose Bengal are currently available.

Rose Bengal may be prepared (compounded) by qualified compounding pharmacists into a 1% sterile solution in sterile water for injection.

Revisions/References
Monograph revised/updated September 2014.
McElhiney, L. (2012). I see colors: Using vital dyes in diagnosing ophthalmic disease. Int Journal Pharmaceut Comp 6(3): 190-5.

Schirmer Tear Test Ophthalmic

(shir-mer teer test)

Ocular Diagnostic Agent

Prescriber Highlights

► Used to quantitatively measure aqueous aspect of tear production to diagnose lacrimal disorders such as keratoconjunctivitis sicca.

► Does not cause burning or stinging upon application.

► Bend strip at right angle at notch to facilitate retention in conjunctival sac.

► Do not use sedation, atropine, or local anesthetics prior to testing.

Uses/Indications

In veterinary patients, Schirmer tear test strips are used to quantitatively measure the aqueous aspect of basal and reflexive tear production. Reflexive tear production describes the quantity of tears produced in response to an irritant. Quantitative tear production is an important diagnostic factor when deficiency of the lacrimal system is suspected. Canine tear production measured as <10 mm/min is associated with keratoconjunctivitis (KCS), but only in the context of other signs of quantitative tear deficiency (such as conjunctival hyperemia, mucopurulent discharge, corneal vascularization, corneal fibrosis, corneal pigmentation, and/or blepharospasm). Additional testing (tear film breakup time and conjunctival goblet cell density) may reveal qualitative differences in the tears produced.

Pharmacology/Actions

Schirmer tear tests are strips of 5 mm x 35 mm Whatman no. 41 filter paper impregnated with a blue dye and marked with 1 mm gradations. A strip within a plastic sleeve is first bent at a notch 5 mm below a rounded tip and placed in the conjunctival sac. The test strips remain in place for exactly 1 minute. Tear production is visualized by dye migration down the strip (distance in mm) and recorded in units of mm/min.

Contraindications/Precautions/Warnings

Schirmer tear test strips are contraindicated in patients with a history of hypersensitivity to the blue dye component or any component of the formulation. In order to maximize test result validity, do not excessively manipulate the eyelids prior testing and do not administer topical anesthesia or systemic tranquilizers. Do not administer atropine prior to testing.

Adverse Effects

Adverse effects reported in humans or animals include mild irritation during the insertion period.

Doses

Tear production: Open the Schirmer tear test packet and bend the strip at a right angle at the notch above the rounded tip. Place the short end of the strip in the conjunctival sac with the calibrated end facing out of the eye. Leave the strip in place for 1 minute. Remove and read calibrations quickly to avoid false migration of dye (higher than actual result) or drying of the strip (lower than actual result). The normal rate of canine lacrimation established by Schirmer tear testing is in the range of 18.64 ± 4.47 mm/min to 23.90 ± 5.73 mm/min. The normal value for cats is 20.2 ± 4.5 mm wetting per minute. The normal value for rabbits is 5.3 ± 2.9 mm wetting per minute.

Monitoring

■ Ocular Diagnostic Product. No monitoring is required.

Client Information

■ Schirmer Tear Tests are used in the veterinary practice and not at the caregiver's home.

Storage/Stability

Store at controlled room temperature away from moisture and sunlight; do not freeze.

Compatibility/Compounding Considerations

Do not mix with other agents.

Dosage Forms/Regulatory Status

VETERINARY-LABELED PRODUCTS: NONE.

HUMAN-LABELED PRODUCTS:

Schirmer Tear Tests Strips are 5 mm x 35 mm Whatman no. 41 filter paper impregnated with a blue dye and marked with 1 mm gradations conveniently marked for right and left eyes. Supplied in individually wrapped strips or pairs in containers of 50 pairs per box, or 300 strips per box; generic; (Rx)

Revisions/References
Monograph revised/updated September 2014.

Silver Sulfadiazine Ophthalmic

(sil-ver sul-fa-dye-a zeen)   Silvadene®, SSD

Broad Spectrum Antibacterial/Antifungal Agent

Prescriber Highlights

► Inexpensive antimicrobial/antifungal topical cream alternative to traditional therapies for fungal keratitis in horses.

► Chronic use may result in discoloration of the sclera due to argyrism.

► Do not use in SPL catheters as occlusion will likely result.

► Best dispensed in 1 mL sterile tuberculin syringes with sterile tip caps for administration in the conjunctival sac.

Uses/Indications

In veterinary patients, silver sulfadiazine (SSD) is used as a broad spectrum antibacterial and antifungal ophthalmic agent. It is used most commonly as a less expensive alternative to conventional therapy for fungal keratitis in horses. It has been demonstrated to be effective in treating fungal keratitis in humans (Mohan *et al.* 1988). Silver sulfadiazine was found to be superior to natamycin in antifungal sensitivity testing for fungal isolates in horses with fungal keratitis (Betbeze *et al.* 2006).

Pharmacology/Actions

Studies utilizing radioactive micronized silver sulfadiazine, electron microscopy, and biochemical techniques have revealed that the mechanism of action of silver sulfadiazine on bacteria differs from silver nitrate and sodium sulfadiazine. Silver sulfadiazine acts only on the cell membrane and cell wall to produce its bactericidal effect. A specific mechanism of action has not been determined, but silver sulfadiazine's effectiveness may possibly be from a synergistic interaction, or the action of each component. Silver is a biocide, which binds to a broad range of targets. Silver ions bind to nucleophilic amino acids, as well as sulfhydryl, amino, imidazole, phosphate, and carboxyl groups in proteins, causing protein denaturation and enzyme inhibition. Silver binds to surface membranes and proteins, causing proton leaks in the membrane, leading to cell death. Sulfadiazine is a competitive inhibitor of bacterial para-aminobenzoic acid (PABA), a substrate of the enzyme dihydropteroate synthetase. The inhibited reaction is necessary in these organisms for the synthesis of folic acid.

Contraindications/Precautions/Warnings

Silver sulfadiazine is contraindicated in patients with a history of hypersensitivity to it or any component of the formulation.

SSD should not be administered through SPL catheters as occlusion will result.

Adverse Effects

Adverse effects reported in humans or animals include argyrism (bluish discoloration of the skin and sclera due to silver accumulation). Pain, burning and itching may occur after application.

Doses

Note: All dosages are extra-label, and the package insert of the topical cream clearly states that it is **NOT** for use in the eye. It is recommended to obtain informed consent from client before prescribing.

Bacterial or fungal keratitis: 0.2 mL in the conjunctival sac every 30-60 minutes initially, then tapered to every 4 hours and then per clinical response. Avoid chronic use; risks argyrism.

Monitoring

- Clinical efficacy. Resolution of keratitis as evidenced by cytology and cultures. Discontinue use if sclera becomes blue or gray in color (argyrism).

Client Information

- Used 4-6 times daily.
- Do not use in SPL catheters.
- Use proper administration techniques to avoid contamination of the medication. Keep cap tightly closed when not in use.
- Wait 5 minutes after applying this medication before applying any other medications to the eye.
- Store at controlled room temperature away from moisture and sunlight; do not freeze. Do not use if the color changes.

Storage/Stability

Store at controlled room temperature away from moisture and sunlight; do not freeze.

Compatibility/Compounding Considerations

Silver sulfadiazine should not be mixed directly with any other drugs.

Dosage Forms/Regulatory Status

VETERINARY-LABELED PRODUCTS: NONE.

HUMAN-LABELED PRODUCTS: NONE.

Silver sulfadiazine is **not** approved for ophthalmic use. It is available as a topical cream, silver sulfadiazine 10 mg/g in a water miscible base in 20 g, 50 g, 400 g, and 1000 g containers. It is optimally dispensed in sterile, single use tuberculin syringes tipped with a sterile tip cap (needle removed) for administration in the conjunctival sac.

Note: The package insert of all brands of silver sulfadiazine topical creams warns against use in the eye.

Revisions/References

Monograph revised/updated September 2014.

Betbeze, C. M., et al. (2006). In vitro fungistatic and fungicidal activities of silver sulfadiazine and natamycin on pathogenic fungi isolated from horses with keratomycosis. American Journal of Veterinary Research 67(10): 1788-93.

Mohan, M., et al. (1988). Topical silver sulphadiazine - A new drug for ocular keratomycosis. British Journal of Ophthalmology 72(3): 192-5.

Sodium Chloride (Hypertonic) Ophthalmic

Muro 128®, Altachlore®, Sochlor®

Hyperosmotic Corneal Diuretic

Prescriber Highlights

▶ Short acting corneal diuretic used for temporary relief of corneal edema.

▶ Ointment forms have longer contact time and are preferred.

▶ Available without prescription.

▶ Efficacy reduced in presence of corneal ulceration due to loss of concentration gradient across intact corneal epithelium.

Uses/Indications

In veterinary patients, hypertonic sodium chloride is used for the temporary relief of corneal edema caused by bullous keratopathy, superficial corneal erosions, and chronic corneal edema due to endothelial dysfunction. Corneal diuresis is short-lived, only lasting about 90 seconds after application.

Pharmacology/Actions

Ocular fluid continuously seeps into the corneal stroma from tear film and aqueous humor. When removal of this fluid is disrupted, fluid accumulates in pockets (bullae) and migrates to the surface of the cornea causing discoloration, disruption of the corneal surface, and visual impairment.

Contraindications/Precautions/Warnings

Hypertonic sodium chloride is contraindicated in patients with a history of hypersensitivity to any component of the formulation. It should not be used in the presence of corneal ulceration, as intact corneal epithelium is required to create the concentration gradient by which fluid is drawn from the bullae. Application of hypertonic sodium chloride will only further increase irritation caused by ulcerative keratitis.

Adverse Effects

Adverse effects reported in humans or animals include temporary burning and stinging upon application.

Doses

Corneal Edema (extra-label): 1 – 2 drops or ¼ – ½ inch strip in the affected eye(s) every 3-4 hours.

Monitoring

- Clinical efficacy. Observe for resolution of corneal edema. Discontinue use if corneal ulceration present and employ antimicrobials and mydriatics until ulcer is healed.

Client Information

- Used 3-4 times daily.
- Available without a prescription but should be used only as directed by your veterinarian.
- Use proper administration techniques to avoid contamination of the medication. Keep cap tightly closed when not in use.
- Wait 5 minutes after applying this medication before applying any other medications to the eye.
- Store at controlled room temperature away from moisture and sunlight; do not freeze. Do not use if the color changes, it becomes cloudy, or if particles are seen in solutions.

Storage/Stability

Store at controlled room temperature away from moisture and sunlight; do not freeze. Discard if color changes, becomes cloudy, or if particles are observed in the solution.

Compatibility/Compounding Considerations

Hypertonic sodium chloride should not be mixed directly with any other drugs to avoid dilution of the active ingredient.

Dosage Forms/Regulatory Status

VETERINARY-LABELED PRODUCTS: NONE.

HUMAN-LABELED PRODUCTS:

Sodium Chloride 5% Ophthalmic Ointment (containing: sodium chloride 50 mg/mL, lanolin oil, mineral oil, water for injection and white petrolatum) in a 3.5 g ophthalmic ointment tube; *Muro 128®*, *Altachlore®*, *Sochlor®*; (OTC)

Sodium Chloride 2% or 5% Ophthalmic Solution (containing: sodium chloride 20 mg/mL or 50 mg/mL, methylparaben 0.023%, propylparaben 0.01% boric acid, hypromellose, propylene glycol, purified water, sodium borate, NaOH ad/or HCl to adjust pH) in a 15 mL ophthalmic dropper bottle; *Muro 128®*, *Altachlore*; (OTC)

Revisions/References

Monograph revised/updated 01/2014.

Sulfacetamide Ophthalmic

(sul-fa-seet-uh-mide)   Bleph-10®

Sulfonamide Antimicrobial Agent

Prescriber Highlights

▶ 15-25% of dogs treated with sulfonamides develop keratoconjunctivitis sicca.

▶ Warn caregivers with sulfonamide allergies to avoid contact with this medication.

▶ Some sulfacetamide ophthalmic products are combined with prednisolone; do not use in viral or fungal keratitis.

Uses/Indications

In veterinary patients, sulfacetamide is used to treat conjunctivitis and other superficial ocular infections due to susceptible microorganisms. Topical sulfacetamide is also used concurrently with systemic sulfonamides for ocular manifestations of trachoma. Sulfacetamide is considered active against *E. coli*, *Staphylococcus aureus*, *Streptococcus pneumoniae*, and *Streptococcus viridans* spp., Haemophilus, Klebsiella, and Enterobacter. Sulfacetamide has no activity when applied topically for Neisseria, *Serratia marcescens*, or *Pseudomonas aeruginosa*. A significant percentage of staphylococcal isolates are completely resistant to sulfa drugs. It is also found in combination products with prednisolone (*e.g.*, *Blephamide®*).

Pharmacology/Actions

The sulfonamides are bacteriostatic agents and the spectrum of activity is similar for all. Sulfonamides inhibit bacterial synthesis of dihydrofolic acid by preventing the condensation of the pteridine with aminobenzoic acid through competitive inhibition of the enzyme dihydropteroate synthetase. Resistant strains have altered dihydropteroate synthetase with reduced affinity for sulfonamides or produce increased quantities of aminobenzoic acid.

Contraindications/Precautions/Warnings

Sulfacetamide is contraindicated in patients with a history of hypersensitivity to it or any component of the formulation. Use cautiously in patients with blood dyscrasias. Patients with ocular infections due to viral or fungal organisms should not receive corticosteroid-containing sulfacetamide products.

Adverse Effects

Adverse effects reported in humans or animals include gastrointestinal disturbances, allergic skin reactions, renal damage, and blood dyscrasias. In dogs, sulfonamides are known to cause keratoconjunctivitis sicca (KCS) due to a direct toxicity to the lacrimal acinar cells. This effect is caused by the nitrogen-containing pyridine and pyrimidine rings in sulfonamides and is dose-related. The estimated incidence is 1525% in dogs treated with sulfonamides and may be latent in onset. Dogs exhibiting squinting or excess ocular mucus discharge should be evaluated for KCS. This condition may be reversible if sulfonamide use is discontinued in time.

Doses

Conjunctivitis and susceptible ocular infections (extra-label): 1 drop in the conjunctival sac every 2-3 hours initially and then tapered according to clinical response. Duration of therapy is usually 7-10 days.

Monitoring

- Clinical efficacy. Resolution of bacterial conjunctivitis as evidenced by cytology and cultures. Dogs should be observed for signs of keratoconjunctivitis sicca.

Client Information

- Used 3-12 times daily.
- Caregivers with sulfa allergies should avoid contact with this medication.
- Observe dogs for signs of dry eye (squinting, excessive mucus eye discharge) and consult veterinarian if this occurs.
- Use proper administration techniques to avoid contamination of the medication. Keep cap tightly closed when not in use.
- Wait 5 minutes after applying this medication before applying any other medications to the eye.
- Store in the refrigerator or at controlled room temperature away from moisture and sunlight; do not freeze. Do not use if it becomes cloudy, or if particles are seen in solutions. Sulfacetamide solutions will darken over time; throw it out if this occurs.

Storage/Stability

Store in refrigerator or at controlled room temperature away from moisture and sunlight; do not freeze.

Compatibility/Compounding Considerations

Sulfacetamide should not be mixed directly with any other drugs.

Dosage Forms/Regulatory Status

VETERINARY-LABELED PRODUCTS: NONE.

HUMAN-LABELED PRODUCTS:

Sulfacetamide Sodium 10% Ophthalmic Solution in 15 mL ophthalmic dropper bottles; *Bleph-10®*, generic; (Rx)

Sulfacetamide Sodium 10% Ophthalmic Ointment in 3.5 g tubes; generic; (Rx)

Sulfacetamide Sodium 10% and Prednisolone Acetate 0.2% Ophthalmic Suspension in 2.5 mL, 5 mL, & 10 mL; *Blephamide®*; (Rx)

Sulfacetamide Sodium 10% and Prednisolone Sodium Phosphate 0.25% Ophthalmic Suspension in 5 mL & 10 mL; generic; (Rx)

Sulfacetamide Sodium 10% and Prednisolone Acetate 0.2% Ophthalmic Ointment in 3.5 g tubes; *Blephamide®*; (Rx)

Revisions/References

Monograph revised/updated September 2014.

Suprofen Ophthalmic

(soo-proe-fin)   Profenal®

NSAID

Prescriber Highlights

▶ May cause transient increases in intraocular pressure but these are not usually significant.

▶ Immunosuppressive activity may worsen infected corneal ulcers.

▶ May delay wound healing.

Uses/Indications

Suprofen is a nonsteroidal antiinflammatory agent (NSAID) that is used to treat a variety of inflammatory conditions of the eye including uveitis, iritis, and pre- and postoperative cataract surgery. Suprofen also inhibits miosis and is sometimes used to prevent miosis during intraocular surgery. However, since prostaglandin blockade may result in increase in intraocular pressure, the use of preoperative suprofen has become obsolete. Inhibition of miosis by suprofen is, however, useful in the management of uveal inflammation.

Pharmacology/Actions

Suprofen sodium is one of a series of phenylalkanoic acids that have shown analgesic, antipyretic, and antiinflammatory activity in animal inflammatory diseases. Its mechanism of action is believed to be through inhibition of the cyclooxygenase enzyme that is essential in the biosynthesis of prostaglandins known to be mediators of certain kinds of intraocular inflammation. In studies performed on animal eyes, prostaglandins have been shown to produce disruption of the blood-aqueous humor barrier, vasodilatation, increased vascular permeability, leukocytosis, and increased intraocular pressure.

Prostaglandins also appear to play a role in the miotic response produced during ocular surgery by constricting the iris sphincter independently of cholinergic mechanisms. Suprofen sodium has no significant effect upon intraocular pressure.

Contraindications/Precautions/Warnings

Suprofen is contraindicated in patients with a history of hypersensitivity to it or any component of the formulation. Cross-sensitivity with other NSAIDs has occurred in humans and may occur in animals. Suprofen may be as immunosuppressive as topical steroids, so it should be used with caution in patients with infected corneal ulcers. NSAIDs inhibit thrombocyte aggregation and may prolong bleeding; use during intraocular surgery may promote intraocular bleeding.

Adverse Effects

Adverse effects reported in humans or animals include transient burning and stinging upon instillation and other minor symptoms of ocular irritation. Other adverse reactions reported with the use of suprofen sodium include fibrosis, miosis, and mydriasis. Increased bleeding tendency of ocular tissues in conjunction with ocular surgery has also been reported.

Doses

Pre-surgery (extra-label): 1 drop in affected eye(s) every 20 minutes for 4 applications.

Antiinflammatory (keratitis, uveitis); (extra-label): 1 drop in affected eye(s) every 8 hours; may be reduced to once daily after resolution of initial episodes.

Monitoring

▪ Clinical efficacy. Effective blockade of miosis during intraocular surgery; resolution of inflammation associated with keratitis or uveitis.

Client Information

▪ Used 3-4 times daily.

▪ Use proper administration techniques to avoid contamination of the medication. Keep cap tightly closed when not in use.

▪ Wait 5 minutes after applying this medication before applying any other medications to the eye.

▪ Store at controlled room temperature away from moisture and sunlight; do not freeze. Do not use if the color changes, it becomes cloudy, or if particles are seen in solutions.

Storage/Stability

Store at controlled room temperature away from moisture and sunlight; do not freeze.

Compatibility/Compounding Considerations

Suprofen should not be mixed directly with any other drugs. Suprofen is not available as an ophthalmic ointment.

Dosage Forms/Regulatory Status

VETERINARY-LABELED PRODUCTS: NONE.

HUMAN-LABELED PRODUCTS:

Suprofen sodium 1% Ophthalmic Solution (containing: suprofen 10 mg/mL; thimerosal 0.05 mg/mL; caffeine 20 mg/mL; edetate disodium; dibasic sodium phosphate; monobasic sodium phosphate; NaCl; NaOH and/or HCl to adjust pH to 7.4; and purified water) in a 2.5 mL ophthalmic dropper bottle; *Profenal*®; (Rx)

Revisions/References

Monograph revised/updated September 2014.

Tacrolimus Ophthalmic

(ta-kroe-li-mus)

Immunosuppressive Lacromimetic Agent

Prescriber Highlights

▶ May be useful for cyclosporine-resistant cases of keratoconjunctivitis sicca.

▶ Not commercially available, must be compounded. *Protopic*® topical tacrolimus ointment should not be used in the eye.

▶ Advise caregivers to wear gloves when handling tacrolimus.

Uses/Indications

In veterinary patients, tacrolimus is used to stimulate tear production in dogs that do not respond to cyclosporine. An investigation comparing cyclosporine 2% to tacrolimus 0.03% demonstrated that tacrolimus is equally efficacious as cyclosporine 2% for canine keratoconjunctivitis sicca (Hendricks *et al.* 2011). Concentrations of 0.01-0.03% have been successful in controlling canine keratoconjunctivitis sicca.

Pharmacology/Actions

Tacrolimus is a macrolide antibiotic that has a similar immunopharmacological profile as cyclosporine, but is ≈ 100X more potent than cyclosporine. Both cyclosporine and tacrolimus are calcineurin inhibitors that reversibly inhibit T-cell proliferation and prevent the release of proinflammatory cytokines. Calcineurin inhibitors bind to intracellular immunophilins and form complexes that subsequently bind to and inhibit calcineurin. In blocking calcineurin, translocation of the cytoplasmic component of the nuclear factor of activated T cells to the nucleus is prevented. This prevention of translocation impairs transcription of the genes encoding IL-2 and other cytokines, thereby suppressing T-cell proliferation and normal immune function. In addition to increasing tear production by inhibiting T-helper lymphocyte proliferation and infiltration of lacrimal gland acini, tacrolimus restores conjunctival goblet cell mucin production.

Contraindications/Precautions/Warnings

Tacrolimus is contraindicated in patients with a history of hypersensitivity to it or any component of the formulation. Caregivers should be advised to avoid contact with tacrolimus as skin contact with tacrolimus has been associated with the development of cancer in humans. Systemic use of tacrolimus is nephrotoxic in dogs.

Adverse Effects

Adverse effects to ocular use of tacrolimus are rare but include orbital alopecia, which may be related to oil vehicles used to compound tacrolimus solutions.

Doses

Keratoconjunctivitis Sicca (extra-label): 1 drop of a tacrolimus 0.03% solution in each eye 2 times daily.

Monitoring

- Clinical efficacy. Schirmer Tear Test to determine adequate tear production.

Client Information

- Used 2 times daily.
- This is a lifelong medication and must be given daily. Missed doses may cause return of dry eye.
- Use proper administration techniques to avoid contamination of the medication. Keep cap tightly closed when not in use.
- Wait 5 minutes after applying this medication before applying any other medications to the eye.
- Store at controlled room temperature away from moisture and sunlight; do not freeze. Do not use if the color changes, it becomes cloudy, or if particles are seen in solutions.

Storage/Stability

Store at controlled room temperature away from moisture and sunlight; do not freeze.

Compatibility/Compounding Considerations

Tacrolimus should not be mixed directly with any other drugs. It is not commercially available and must be prepared (compounded) by a qualified compounding pharmacist.

Dosage Forms/Regulatory Status

VETERINARY-LABELED PRODUCTS: NONE.

HUMAN-LABELED PRODUCTS: NONE.

Tacrolimus has been prepared (compounded) in concentrations varying from 0.01-0.03% in oil vehicles including olive oil, corn oil, and medium chain triglyceride oil.

Revisions/References

Monograph revised/updated September 2014.

Hendricks, D., et al. (2011). An Investigation Comparing the Efficacy of Topical Ocular Application of Tacrolimus and Cyclosporine in Dogs. Vet Med Intl(ID 487592).

Tafluprost Ophthalmic

(ta-floo-prost)   Zioptan®

Prostaglandin Analog

Prescriber Highlights

▶ For glaucoma in dogs; not effective for feline glaucoma.

▶ Twice daily dosing results in less fluctuation of intraocular pressure.

▶ Preservative free and may be better tolerated than preservative-containing prostaglandin analogs.

▶ May increase brown pigment resulting in discoloration of light colored irises. Causes increased eyelash growth.

▶ May worsen intraocular inflammation through prostaglandin-mediated mechanisms.

Uses/Indications

In veterinary patients, tafluprost is used to reduce intraocular pressure to manage canine glaucoma. It is not effective for feline glaucoma. Use in horses is not effective and is associated with a high incidence of adverse effects including ocular discomfort.

Pharmacology/Actions

Prostaglandin analogs are chemically modified versions of prostaglandin F2-alpha, and endogenous inflammatory mediator that causes ocular hypotensive effects. Tafluprost is believed to lower intraocular pressure (IOP) by increasing outflow of aqueous humor through both the trabecular meshwork and uveoscleral routes.

Contraindications/Precautions/Warnings

Tafluprost is contraindicated in patients with a history of hypersensitivity to it or any component of the formulation. It should not be used in the presence of intraocular inflammation (*e.g.*, uveitis), as it will worsen this condition.

Adverse Effects

Adverse effects reported in humans or animals include blurred vision, burning and stinging, conjunctival hyperemia, foreign body sensation, itching, increased pigmentation of the iris, and punctate epithelial keratopathy. May cause darkening of the iris through direct stimulation of iris melanocytes. May cause increased eyelash growth. May worsen intraocular inflammation. Eyelash changes (increased length, thickness, pigmentation, and number of lashes); eyelid skin darkening; intraocular inflammation (iritis/uveitis); iris pigmentation changes; and macular edema, including cystoid macular edema, have all been reported after use of tafluprost in humans.

Doses

Glaucoma (extra-label): 1 drop in the affected eye(s) 2 times daily.

Monitoring

- Clinical efficacy. Continued reduction of intraocular pressure.

Client Information

- Used 2 times daily.
- Use proper administration techniques to avoid contamination of the medication. Keep cap tightly closed when not in use.
- Wait 5 minutes after applying this medication before applying any other medications to the eye.
- Store in the original pouch in the refrigerator at 2-8°C (36-46°F). After the pouch is opened, the single-use containers may be stored in the opened foil pouch for up to 28 days at room temperature: 20-25°C (68-77°F). Protect from light and moisture. Discard any unused containers 28 days after first opening the pouch. Do not use if the color changes, it becomes cloudy, or if particles are seen in solutions.

Storage/Stability

Store in the original pouch in the refrigerator at 2-8°C (36-46°F). After the pouch is opened, the single-use containers may be stored in the opened foil pouch for up to 28 days at room temperature: 20-25°C (68-77°F). Protect from light and moisture. Discard any unused containers 28 days after first opening the pouch.

Compatibility/Compounding Considerations

Tafluprost should not be mixed directly with any other drugs. Tafluprost is not available as an ophthalmic ointment.

Dosage Forms/Regulatory Status

VETERINARY-LABELED PRODUCTS: NONE.

HUMAN-LABELED PRODUCTS:

Tafluprost 0.0015% Ophthalmic Solution (containing: tafluprost 0.015 mg/mL; glycerol; sodium dihydrogen phosphate dihydrate; disodium edetate; polysorbate 80; water for injection; and HCl and/or NaOH to adjust pH to 5.5-6.75 and an osmolality of

260-300 mOsm/kg) in 0.3 mL single use containers in boxes of 30 or 90 pouches; *Zioptan®*; (Rx)

Revisions/References
Monograph revised/updated September 2014.

Tetracaine Ophthalmic

(teh-trah-kane)   Altacaine®, Tetravisc®

Topical Ocular Anesthetic

Prescriber Highlights

▶ Faster onset of action, but more burning, stinging and chemosis than with proparacaine.

▶ Viscous forms have longer duration of action (30 minutes).

Uses/Indications
In veterinary patients, tetracaine is used when a more rapid and deeper plane of local anesthesia is required. Tetracaine causes more adverse reactions (burning, stinging, and chemosis) in dogs than proparacaine (Parchen *et al.* 2011). A formulation of viscous tetracaine (*Tetravisc®*) decreases corneal sensitivity and has a longer duration of action in horses compared to proparacaine or non-viscous tetracaine (Sharrow-Reabe *et al.* 2012).

Pharmacology/Actions
Local anesthetics such as tetracaine, stabilize the neuronal membrane by inhibiting the ionic fluxes required for the initiation and conduction of impulses thereby effecting local anesthetic action. Tetracaine appears to bind or antagonize the function of voltage gated sodium channels. The exact mechanism whereby local anesthetics influence the permeability of the cell membrane is unknown; however, several studies indicate that local anesthetics may limit sodium ion permeability through the lipid layer of the nerve cell membrane. Tetracaine may alter epithelial sodium channels through interaction with channel protein residues. This limitation prevents the fundamental change necessary for the generation of the action potential.

Contraindications/Precautions/Warnings
Tetracaine is contraindicated in patients with a history of hypersensitivity to it or any component of the formulation. Prolonged use of a topical ocular anesthetic may produce keratitis and permanent corneal opacification with accompanying loss of vision. Prolonged use results in retarded wound healing and causes corneal epithelial ulcers. The blink reflex is suppressed or absent after tetracaine administration, and the eye should be protected from external injury during use.

Adverse Effects
Adverse effects reported in humans or animals include transient stinging, burning, and conjunctival redness. Tetracaine is associated with more burning and chemosis than proparacaine. A rare, severe, immediate type allergic corneal reaction has been reported characterized by acute diffuse epithelial keratitis with filament formation and/or sloughing of large areas of necrotic epithelium, diffuse stromal edema, descemetitis and iritis.

Doses
Ophthalmic procedures requiring local anesthesia (extra-label): 1-2 drops in the target eye(s) prior to examination or procedure. Onset of action is in 15 seconds. May repeat 1 drop every 5-10 minutes for 5-7 times. Duration of corneal anesthesia is ≈ 5 minutes with aqueous formulations and up to 30 minutes with viscous formulations.

Monitoring
▪ Diagnostic agent. Chronic use will delay wound healing and cause loss of vision through corneal opacification.

Client Information
▪ Tetracaine is not administered by pet owners in the home. It is reserved for diagnostic procedures in the veterinary practice.

Storage/Stability
Store at controlled room temperature away from moisture and sunlight; do not freeze. Discard if color change, or becomes cloudy, or if particles are observed in the solution.

Compatibility/Compounding Considerations
Tetracaine should not be mixed directly with any other drugs.

Dosage Forms/Regulatory Status
VETERINARY-LABELED PRODUCTS: NONE.

HUMAN-LABELED PRODUCTS:

Tetracaine HCl 0.5% Ophthalmic Solution (containing: tetracaine 5 mg/mL; benzalkonium chloride; boric acid; edetate disodium; hypromellose; potassium chloride; sodium borate; NaCl; and water for injection) in 0.6 mL and 5 mL ophthalmic dropper bottles; *Tetravisc®*; (Rx)

Tetracaine HCl 0.5% Ophthalmic Solution (containing: tetracaine 5 mg/mL; chlorobutanol; boric acid; edetate disodium; potassium chloride; water for injection; USP; HCl and/or NaOH to adjust pH) in 15 mL ophthalmic dropper bottles; *Altacaine®*, generic; (Rx)

Revisions/References
Monograph revised/updated September 2014.

Parchen, H. D., et al. (2011). Ophthalmic and anesthetic evaluation of topical 1% tetracaine and 0.5% proparacaine in dogs. Arquivo Brasileiro De Medicina Veterinaria E Zootecnia 63(6): 1337-44.

Sharrow-Reabe, K. L. & W. M. Townsend (2012). Effects of action of proparacaine and tetracaine topical ophthalmic formulations on corneal sensitivity in horses. Javma-Journal of the American Veterinary Medical Association 241(12): 1645-9.

Timolol Maleate Ophthalmic

(teh-moe-lol) or (tye-moe-lol)   Timoptic®

Beta Blocker

Prescriber Highlights

▶ 0.25% concentrations are minimally effective; 0.5% concentrations are preferentially used.

▶ Effective for feline glaucoma (usually employed in addition to carbonic anhydrase inhibitors).

▶ Use with caution in asthmatic patients (bronchospasm) and diabetic patients (may mask signs of acute hypoglycemia).

Uses/Indications
In veterinary patients, timolol maleate is primarily used as prophylaxis to prevent glaucoma in the normal eye of animals with unilateral glaucoma. The 0.25% concentration has minimal ocular hypotensive effects in animals and the 0.5% concentration is preferentially employed. It rarely used to treat glaucoma as a sole agent (except for prophylaxis of the normal eye) and is most commonly used in combination with dorzolamide (*Cosopt®*) in cats (Dietrich *et al.* 2007). Gel-forming 0.5% solutions of timolol (accomplished by interaction of xanthum gum with tears) reduce intraocular pressure by a mean of 5.3 mmHg in dogs (Takiyama *et al.* 2006). Timolol 0.5% either alone or in combination with dorzolamide 2% can be used twice daily in horses to effectively reduce intraocular pressure (van der Woerdt *et al.* 2000; Willis *et al.* 2001). Timolol may also be combined with alpha-adrenergic agonists (*e.g.*, brimonidine) to potentiate ocular hypotensive effects through increased outflow of aqueous humor in addition to decreased aqueous humor production.

Pharmacology/Actions

Timolol maleate is a nonselective beta-adrenergic blocking agent with associated intrinsic sympathomimetic activity and without significant membrane-stabilizing activity. The exact mechanism of the ocular hypotensive effect of beta-blockers has not been definitely demonstrated; however, several mechanisms have been postulated for this effect including beta-blockade of norepinephrine-induced tonic sympathetic stimulation, decreased activation of cAMP in the ciliary body leading to decreased aqueous humor production, inhibition of Na$^+$K$^+$ATPase activity, or through vasoactive mechanisms.

Contraindications/Precautions/Warnings

Timolol maleate is contraindicated in patients with a history of hypersensitivity to it or any component of the formulation. Timolol maleate should be used carefully in patients with heart block, bradycardia, heart failure, asthma, chronic bronchitis, or other cardiopulmonary conditions, although systemic cardiopulmonary adverse effects are not likely with ocular use of timolol maleate. Use with caution in diabetic patients as beta-blockers may mask the signs of acute hypoglycemia in these patients.

Adverse Effects

Adverse effects reported in humans or animals include transient burning, stinging, and irritation upon application to the eye. Timolol may cause slight miosis in dogs, cats and horses. Timolol maleate may trigger attacks in cats with asthma.

Doses

Glaucoma or prophylaxis in the normal eye of unilateral glaucoma (extra-label): 1 drop in the affected eye(s) twice daily.

Monitoring

- Clinical efficacy. Monitor intraocular pressure. Observe asthmatic and diabetic pets for respiratory difficulty or acute hypoglycemia, respectively.

Client Information

- Used 2 times daily.
- May delay onset of glaucoma in the normal eye of dogs with glaucoma in the other eye.
- The 0.5% concentration is more commonly used for treating glaucoma in animals.
- Use carefully in pets with asthma or diabetes.
- Adhere to proper administration techniques to avoid contamination of the medication. Keep cap tightly closed when not in use.

Storage/Stability

Store at controlled room temperature away from moisture and sunlight; do not freeze. Discard if color change, or becomes cloudy, or if particles are observed in the solution.

Compatibility/Compounding Considerations

Timolol maleate should not be mixed directly with any other drugs. Timolol maleate is not available as an ophthalmic ointment. Instruct caregivers to wait 5 minutes after applying this medication before applying any other medications to the eye.

Dosage Forms/Regulatory Status

VETERINARY-LABELED PRODUCTS: NONE.

HUMAN-LABELED PRODUCTS:

Timolol 0.25% or 0.5% Ophthalmic Solution [containing: timolol maleate 2.5 mg/mL of timolol (3.4 mg of timolol maleate) and 5 mg/mL of timolol (6.8 mg of timolol maleate), respectively; benzalkonium chloride 0.01%; monobasic and dibasic sodium phosphate; purified water; and NaOH to adjust pH to 6.5-7.5] in a 2 mL, 5 mL, 10 mL, and 15 mL ophthalmic dropper bottle; *Timoptic*, *Betimol*; (Rx)

Timolol 0.25% or 0.5% Gel-Forming Solution [containing: 2.5 mg/mL of timolol (3.4 mg of timolol maleate) or 5 mg/mL of timolol (6.8 mg of timolol maleate); benzododecinium bromide 0.012%; xanthan gum; tromethamine; boric acid; mannitol; polysorbate-80; and purified water with a pH of ≈ 6.9 and an osmolality of ≈290 mOsm/kg] in 2.5 mL and 5 mL ophthalmic dropper bottles; *Timoptic-XE*, generic; (Rx)

Timolol 0.5% and Dorzolamide 2% Ophthalmic Solution [containing: 20 mg/mL dorzolamide (22.26 mg of dorzolamide HCl) and 5 mg/mL timolol (6.83 mg timolol maleate); benzalkonium chloride 0.0075%; sodium citrate; hydroxyethyl cellulose; NaOH; mannitol; and water for injection with a pH of ≈5.65; and an osmolarity of 242-323 mOsm/kg] in 10 mL ophthalmic dropper bottles; *Cosopt*; (Rx)

Brimonidine Tartrate: 0.2% and Timolol Maleate 0.5% Ophthalmic Solution (containing benzalkonium chloride 0.005%, citric acid, polyvinyl alcohol, NaCl, sodium citrate, purified water, HCl and/or NaOH added to adjust pH to 5.6-6.6, with an osmolality of 280-330 mOsm/kg) in a 10 mL dropper bottle; *Combigan*; (Rx).

Revisions/References

Monograph revised/updated September 2014.

Dietrich, U. M., et al. (2007). Effects of topical 2% dorzolamide hydrochloride alone and in combination with 0.5% timolol maleate on intraocular pressure in normal feline eyes. Vet. Ophthalmol. **10**: 95-100.

Takiyama, N., et al. (2006). The effects of a timolol maleate gel-forming solution on normotensive beagle dogs. Journal of Veterinary Medical Science **68**(6): 631-3.

van der Woerdt, A., et al. (2000). Effect of single- and multiple-dose 0.5% timolol maleate on intraocular pressure and pupil size in female horses. Vet. Ophthalmol. **3**: 165-8.

Willis, A. M., et al. (2001). Effect of topical administration of 2% dorzolamide hydrochloride or 2% dorzolamide hydrochloride-0.5% timolol maleate on intraocular pressure in clinically normal horses. American Journal of Veterinary Research **62**(5): 709-13.

Tissue Plasminogen Activator (Alteplase) Ophthalmic

(tiss-you plaz-min-uh-gin ak-ti-vate-er)   t-PA, Activase®

Fibrinolytic

Prescriber Highlights

- For intracameral injection to achieve fibrinolysis of intraocular blood clots; not effective for fibrinolysis by the topical route.
- Toxic to the cornea in intracameral doses >50 mcg.
- Not approved for intraocular injection; must be prepared from the injection intended for intracatheter administration.
- Very expensive.

Uses/Indications

In veterinary patients, tissue plasminogen factor (alteplase; t-PA) is most commonly used for lysis of intraocular blood clots. Intracameral injection of alteplase in humans following cataract surgery dissolves fibrin clots, reduces posterior synechiae, and does not result in re-bleeding (Heiligenhaus *et al.* 1998). Topical application of alteplase does not result in therapeutic aqueous humor concentrations and are of little value in lysing intraocular clots (Gerding *et al.* 1992). In dogs and cats, intracameral injection of 25 mcg of alteplase results in fibrinolysis without corneal toxicity, while doses of 50 mcg lead to corneal endothelial toxicity (Gerding *et al.* 1992), (Hrach *et al.* 2000).

Pharmacology/Actions

Alteplase (t-PA) is an enzyme (serine protease) that has the property of fibrin-enhanced conversion of plasminogen to plasmin. It produces limited conversion of plasminogen in the absence of fibrin. Alteplase binds to fibrin in a thrombus and converts the entrapped plasminogen to plasmin, thereby initiating local fibrinolysis.

Contraindications/Precautions/Warnings

Tissue plasminogen activator is contraindicated in patients with a history of hypersensitivity to it or any component of the formulation. The most frequent adverse reaction associated with all thrombolytics in all approved indications is bleeding. Caution should be exercised with patients that have thrombocytopenia, other hemostatic defects (including those secondary to severe hepatic or renal disease), or any condition for which bleeding constitutes a significant hazard. Intracameral doses of 50 mcg have resulted in toxicity to the corneal epithelium in dogs and cats.[3, 4]

Adverse Effects

Adverse effects reported in humans or animals include increased risk of bleeding following administration. Corneal toxicity is likely with intracameral doses of 50 mcg but do not occur with doses of 25 mcg.

Doses

Intraocular fibrinolysis (extra-label): Intracameral injection of 0.1 mL of a 0.25 mg/mL sterile solution.

Monitoring

- Clinical efficacy. Resolution of intraocular clot. Observe for signs of re-bleeding.

Client Information

- This medication is not administered outside of the veterinary practice.

Storage/Stability

Store unreconstituted alteplase in the refrigerator, protected from light until use. Tissue plasminogen activator contains no preservatives. Aliquots of reconstituted and further diluted solutions should be stored in a refrigerator or at controlled room temperature and used within 8 hours or stored in an ultralow (-80 C) freezer for 45 days unless extended stability and sterility testing has been conducted. Frozen aliquots should not be re-frozen once thawed. Discard if color change, or becomes cloudy, or if particles are observed in the solution.

Compatibility/Compounding Considerations

Tissue plasminogen activator should not be mixed directly with any other drugs. It is not available as an ophthalmic injection. For intraocular injection, *Cathflo Activase®* is further diluted with normal saline to a final concentration of 0.25 mg/mL.

Dosage Forms/Regulatory Status

VETERINARY-LABELED PRODUCTS: NONE.

HUMAN-LABELED PRODUCTS: NONE.

Tissue Plasminogen Activator (Alteplase) is not approved for ophthalmic use. *Cathflo Activase®* is available (containing: 2.2 mg of alteplase [which includes a 10% overfill], 77 mg of L-arginine, 0.2 mg of polysorbate 80, and phosphoric acid for pH adjustment. Each reconstituted vial will deliver 1 mg/mL of alteplase, at a pH of ≈7.3). For intraocular injection, this solution is further diluted with normal saline to a final concentration of 0.25 mg/mL.

Revisions/References

Monograph revised/updated September 2014.

Gerding, P. A., et al. (1992). Use of tissue plasminogen-activator for intraocular fibrinolysis in dogs. American Journal of Veterinary Research 53(6): 894-6.

Heiligenhaus, A., et al. (1998). Recombinant tissue plasminogen activator in cases with fibrin formation after cataract surgery: a prospective randomised multicentre study. British Journal of Ophthalmology 82(7): 810-5.

Hrach, C. J., et al. (2000). Retinal toxicity of commercial intravitreal tissue plasminogen activator solution in cat eyes. Archives of Ophthalmology 118(5): 659-63.

Tobramycin Sulfate Ophthalmic

(tobe-ra-mye-sin sul-fayt)   Tobrex®

Aminoglycoside Antimicrobial Agent

Prescriber Highlights

▶ Subconjunctival injections of tobramycin sulfate may increase ocular concentrations of tobramycin if not achieved with topical application.

▶ Do not confuse pure tobramycin sulfate ophthalmic preparations with those containing combination with steroids.

▶ Fortified solutions of tobramycin sulfate >13.5 mg/mL may be compounded for use in susceptible infections where commercially available products are not concentrated enough to achieve inhibitory concentrations.

Uses/Indications

In veterinary patients tobramycin sulfate ophthalmic is primarily used for patients with ocular infections of *Pseudomonas aeruginosa*. Commercially available tobramycin solutions and ointments may not achieve inhibitory concentrations in the eye and must be either compounded in fortified concentrations (≥13.5 mg/mL) or injected subconjunctivally (Gorden *et al.* 1982; Allen 2011).

Pharmacology/Actions

Tobramycin, like the other aminoglycoside antibiotics, acts on susceptible bacteria presumably by irreversibly binding to the 30S ribosomal subunit thereby inhibiting protein synthesis. It is considered a bactericidal antibiotic.

Tobramycin's spectrum of activity includes coverage against many aerobic gram-negative and some aerobic gram-positive bacteria, including most species of *E. coli*, Klebsiella, Proteus, Pseudomonas, Salmonella, Enterobacter, Serratia, Shigella, Mycoplasma, and Staphylococcus. Like amikacin, tobramycin may have more activity against Pseudomonas isolates than gentamicin.

Antimicrobial activity of the aminoglycosides is enhanced in an alkaline environment, but pus or cellular debris can reduce efficacy.

The aminoglycoside antibiotics are inactive against fungi, viruses and most anaerobic bacteria.

Contraindications/Precautions/Warnings

Tobramycin sulfate is contraindicated in patients with a history of hypersensitivity to it or any component of the formulation. Cross sensitivity with other aminoglycosides has been known to occur.

Adverse Effects

Adverse effects reported in humans or animals include are ocular burning and irritation upon drug instillation, nonspecific conjunctivitis, conjunctival epithelial defects, and conjunctival hyperemia.

Doses

Susceptible Ocular Infections (extra-label): 1 drop of the solution or ¼ - ½ inch strip in the affected eye(s) 2-3 times daily. Frequency may be increased to every 30-60 minutes for treating equine corneal ulcers.

Subconjunctival Injection (extra-label): 10 mg of tobramycin injection once.

Monitoring

- Clinical efficacy. Resolution of bacterial infection as evidenced by cytology and bacterial cultures.

Client Information

- Used 3-4 times daily.
- Adhere to proper administration techniques to avoid contamination of the medication. Keep cap tightly closed when not in use.

- Wait 5 minutes after applying this medication before applying any other medications to the eye.
- Store in the refrigerator or at controlled room temperature away from moisture and sunlight; do not freeze. Do not use if the color changes, becomes cloudy, or if particles are seen in the solution.

Storage/Stability
Store in refrigerator or at controlled room temperature as directed in product labeling away from moisture and sunlight; do not freeze.

Compatibility/Compounding Considerations
Tobramycin sulfate should not be mixed directly with any other drugs. Tobramycin may be compounded into a fortified ophthalmic solution in concentrations of ≥13.5mg/mL by aseptically adding tobramycin injection in appropriate amounts to commercially available tobramycin ophthalmic solution.

Dosage Forms/Regulatory Status
VETERINARY-LABELED PRODUCTS: NONE.
HUMAN-LABELED PRODUCTS:
Tobramycin 0.3% Ophthalmic Solution; *Tobrex®*; (Rx)

Tobramycin 0.3% Ophthalmic Ointment; *Tobrex®*; (Rx)

Tobramycin 0.3% and Dexamethasone 0.1% Ophthalmic Suspension; *Tobradex®, Tobradex ST®*, generic; (Rx)

Tobramycin 0.3% and Loteprednol 0.5% Ophthalmic Suspension in 2.5 mL, 5 mL, & 10 mL; *Zylet®*; (Rx)

Revisions/References
Monograph revised/updated September 2014.
Allen, L. (2011). Tobramycin 13.5 mg/mL fortified Ophthalmic Solution. Int Journal Pharmaceut Comp 15(6): 507.
Gorden, T. & R. Cunningham (1982). Tobramycin levels in aqueous humor after subconjunctival injection in humans. Am J Ophthalmol 93(1): 107-10.

Trifluridine Ophthalmic
(try-floor-ih-deen)   trifluorothymidine, F3TdR, F3T, Viroptic®
Antiviral

Prescriber Highlights
▶ Must be used 4-5 times daily.
▶ Rarely used due to irritation and pain upon administration.
▶ Trifluridine is a corneal toxin. Use should not exceed 3 weeks duration per episode.

Uses/Indications
In veterinary patients, trifluridine is occasionally used for topical treatment of feline herpes virus-1 (FHV-1) keratitis and has also been used for equine herpes virus (EHV-2) infection of the cornea.

Pharmacology/Actions
Trifluridine interferes with DNA synthesis in cultured mammalian cells. However, its antiviral mechanism of action is not completely known. Trifluridine is virustatic, not virucidal.

Contraindications/Precautions/Warnings
Trifluridine is contraindicated in patients with a history of hypersensitivity to it or any component of the formulation.

Adverse Effects
Adverse effects reported in humans or animals include acute ocular irritation including burning, corneal stippling, vascularization, and clouding has been reported. The irritation associated with administration of trifluridine may be more intense than the inflammation caused by FHV-1. Following prolonged use of trifluridine, ocular irritation characterized by follicular conjunctivitis, blepharitis with punctal swelling, bulbar conjunctival hyperemia, and corneal epithelial staining has also been reported. In either case, the drug should be discontinued.

Doses
Feline Herpes Virus-1 or Equine Herpes Virus-2 Keratitis (extra-label): 1 drop in the affected eye(s) every 2-3 hours for 48-hours then 4-5 times daily for a week beyond resolution of clinical signs. Trifluridine is a corneal toxin and should not be used for more than 3 consecutive weeks per episode.

Monitoring
- Clinical efficacy. Resolution of clinical signs of FHV1.

Client Information
- Used every 2-3 hours for 2 days then 4-5 times daily.
- Do not use for more than 3 consecutive weeks.
- May cause stinging upon administration.
- Use proper administration techniques to avoid contamination of the medication. Keep cap tightly closed when not in use.
- Wait 5 minutes after applying this medication before applying any other medications to the eye.
- Store in the refrigerator away from moisture and sunlight; do not freeze. Do not use if the color changes, it becomes cloudy, or if particles are seen in solutions.

Storage/Stability
Store in refrigerator away from moisture and sunlight; do not freeze.

Compatibility/Compounding Considerations
Trifluridine should not be mixed directly with any other drugs. Trifluridine is not available as an ophthalmic ointment.

Dosage Forms/Regulatory Status
VETERINARY-LABELED PRODUCTS: NONE.
HUMAN-LABELED PRODUCTS: NONE.
Trifluridine aqueous 1% Ophthalmic Solution (containing: NaCl; thimerosal 0.001%; acetic acid and sodium acetate to adjust the pH to 5.5-6 with an osmolality of ≈ 283 mOsm/kg) in a 7.5 mL ophthalmic dropper bottle; *Viroptic®*; (Rx)

Revisions/References
Monograph revised/updated September 2014.

Triple Antibiotic Ophthalmic
Broad Spectrum Antimicrobial Combination Agent

Prescriber Highlights
▶ First choice for antimicrobial prophylaxis of conjunctivitis and keratitis until cytology and sensitivities are available.
▶ Some animals, particularly cats, may be hypersensitive to neomycin or polymyxin components in ointments.
▶ Do not confuse hydrocortisone-containing triple antibiotic ophthalmic ointment with those that lack corticosteroids.
▶ Prolonged use of antibiotic preparations may result in overgrowth of non-susceptible organisms, including fungi.

Uses/Indications
In veterinary patients, triple antibiotic ophthalmic products are used for topical treatment of superficial infections of the external eye and its adnexa caused by susceptible bacteria. Such infections encompass conjunctivitis, keratitis and keratoconjunctivitis, blepharitis and blepharoconjunctivitis. Triple antibiotic is often used as the first choice for symptomatic treatment of conjunctivitis in dogs and for prophylactic antimicrobial treatment prior to and following ophthalmic surgery. Triple antibiotic ophthalmic is also used for antimicrobial prophylaxis of corneal injuries and wounds. Triple antibiotic ophthalmic ointments may also contain hydrocortisone. Triple antibiotic ophthalmic solutions substitute gramicidin for bacitracin.

Pharmacology/Actions

A wide range of antibacterial action is provided by the overlapping spectra of neomycin, polymyxin B sulfate, and bacitracin or gramicidin. Neomycin is bactericidal for many gram-positive and gram-negative organisms. It is an aminoglycoside antibiotic, which inhibits protein synthesis by binding with ribosomal RNA and causing misreading of the bacterial genetic code. Polymyxin B is bactericidal for a variety of gram-negative organisms. It increases the permeability of the bacterial cell membrane by interacting with the phospholipid components of the membrane. Bacitracin is bactericidal for a variety of gram-positive and gram-negative organisms. It interferes with bacterial cell wall synthesis by inhibition of the regeneration of phospholipid receptors involved in peptidoglycan synthesis. Neomycin sulfate, polymyxin B sulfate, and bacitracin zinc together are considered active against the following microorganisms: *Staphylococcus aureus*, streptococci including *Streptococcus pneumoniae*, *Escherichia coli*, *Haemophilus influenzae*, *Klebsiella/Enterobacter* species, *Neisseria* species, and *Pseudomonas aeruginosa*. The product does not provide adequate coverage against *Serratia marcescens*.

Contraindications/Precautions/Warnings

Triple antibiotic combinations are contraindicated in patients with a history of hypersensitivity to any component of the formulation. Some cats are hypersensitive to the neomycin or polymyxin component of triple antibiotic ointments. This hypersensitivity has not been associated with steroid-containing triple antibiotic products. Prolonged use of antibiotic preparations may result in overgrowth of non-susceptible organisms, including fungi.

Adverse Effects

Adverse effects reported in humans or animals include irritation and swelling upon instillation. Topical antibiotics, especially neomycin sulfate and polymyxin B, may cause cutaneous sensitization and anaphylaxis, particularly in cats. The manifestations of sensitization to topical antibiotics are usually itching, reddening, and edema of the conjunctiva and eyelid, but may progress to anaphylaxis. Symptoms usually subside quickly on withdrawing the medication.

Doses

Conjunctivitis or Keratitis (extra-label): 1 drop of the solution or ¼ inch strip of the ointment in the affected eye(s) 3-4 times daily until resolution or microbial susceptibilities necessitate a change to another antimicrobial agent.

Monitoring

- Clinical efficacy. Resolution of conjunctivitis or keratitis as evidenced by cytology, cultures, or remission of symptoms.

Client Information

- Used 3-4 times daily.
- Cats may have a severe allergic reaction to one of the components of this medication. Contact your veterinarian immediately if your cat has difficulty breathing or facial swelling after receiving this medication.
- Use proper administration techniques to avoid contamination of the medication. Keep cap tightly closed when not in use.
- Wait 5 minutes after applying this medication before applying any other medications to the eye.
- Store at controlled room temperature away from moisture and sunlight; do not freeze. Do not use if the color changes, or it becomes cloudy.

Storage/Stability

Store at controlled room temperature away from moisture and sunlight; do not freeze.

Compatibility/Compounding Considerations

Triple antibiotic Ointment or should not be mixed directly with any other drugs.

Dosage Forms/Regulatory Status

VETERINARY-LABELED PRODUCTS:

Triple Antibiotic Ophthalmic Ointment (containing: neomycin sulfate equivalent to 3.5 mg neomycin base, polymyxin B sulfate equivalent to 10,000 polymyxin B units, bacitracin zinc equivalent to 400 bacitracin units, and white petrolatum and mineral oil, q.s.) in a 3.5 g ophthalmic ointment tube; *TriOptic-P®*, *Vetropolycin®*; (Rx)

Triple Antibiotic with Hydrocortisone Ophthalmic Ointment; each gram contains: bacitracin zinc USP 400 units, neomycin sulfate 0.5% (equivalent to 3.5 mg neomycin base), polymyxin B sulfate USP 10,000 units, hydrocortisone acetate USP 1.0% in a base of white petrolatum and mineral oil; *TriOptic-S®*, *Vetropolycin HC®*; (Rx)

HUMAN-LABELED PRODUCTS:

Triple Antibiotic Ophthalmic Ointment (containing: neomycin sulfate equivalent to 3.5 mg neomycin base, polymyxin B sulfate equivalent to 5,000 or 10,000 polymyxin B units, bacitracin zinc equivalent to 400 bacitracin units, and white petrolatum, q.s) in a 3.5 gram ophthalmic ointment tube; *Neo-Polycin®*, generic; (Rx)

Neomycin-Polymyxin-Gramicidin Ophthalmic Solution (containing: polymyxin B equivalent to 1.75 mg polymyxin B base, polymyxin B sulfate equivalent 10,000 polymyxin B units, and gramicidin 0.025 mg per mL; alcohol 0.5%; thimerosal 0.001%; propylene glycol; polyoxyethylene polyoxypropylene compound; NaCl; and water for injection) in a 10 mL ophthalmic dropper bottle; *Neosporin®*, generic; (Rx)

Revisions/References

Monograph revised/updated September 2014.

Tropicamide Ophthalmic

(troe-pik-uh-myde)   Mydriacyl®

Anticholinergic Mydriatic/Cycloplegic Agent

Prescriber Highlights

▶ Used for funduscopic examination or to induce prevent synechiae formation following cataract surgery.

▶ More rapid onset and shorter duration of action compared to atropine. Poor cycloplegic compared to atropine and is a poor analgesic for ciliary spasm.

▶ Good corneal penetration due to lack of ionization at physiological pH.

▶ Do not apply prior to Schirmer Tear Test; tropicamide decreases tear production for several hours following administration.

Uses/Indications

In veterinary patients, tropicamide is used to produce rapid and short acting mydriasis for funduscopic evaluation. Tropicamide has also been used to break down synechiae in uveitis and to prevent synechiae formation following cataract surgery. It is not as effective as atropine in inducing cycloplegia and is consequently a poor choice for controlling ocular pain caused by ciliary spasm.

Pharmacology/Actions

Tropicamide causes anticholinergic effects by blocking the responses of the sphincter muscle of the iris and the accommodative muscle of the ciliary body to cholinergic stimulation, producing pupillary dilation (mydriasis) and, to a lesser degree, paralysis of accommodation (cycloplegia). Tropicamide induces mydriasis in about 15-30 minutes, and pupil returns to normal in 6-12 hours.

Contraindications/Precautions/Warnings

Tropicamide is contraindicated in patients with a history of hypersensitivity to it or any component of the formulation. It should not be used in patients with primary glaucoma.

Adverse Effects

Adverse effects reported in humans or animals include sensitivity to bright light or sunlight, burning and irritation upon application, and hypersalivation in cats and dogs. May decrease tear production for several hours after application in dogs and cats.

Doses

Mydriasis: (extra-label) 1 drop in the affected eye(s) 2-3 times daily to achieve pupillary dilation.

Monitoring

- Clinical efficacy. Confirm continued pupillary dilation.

Client Information

- Used 2-3 times daily to keep pupil dilated following cataract surgery.
- Dogs and cats may drool excessively after administration.
- Use proper administration techniques to avoid contamination of the medication. Keep cap tightly closed when not in use.
- Wash hands after application to prevent accidentally getting the drug into your eyes, which can cause pupil dilation.
- Wait 5 minutes after applying this medication before applying any other medications to the eye.
- Store at controlled room temperature away from moisture and sunlight; do not freeze. Do not use if the color changes, it becomes cloudy, or if particles are seen in solutions.

Storage/Stability

Store at controlled room temperature away from moisture and sunlight; do not freeze.

Compatibility/Compounding Considerations

Tropicamide should not be mixed directly with any other drugs.

Dosage Forms/Regulatory Status

VETERINARY-LABELED PRODUCTS: NONE.

HUMAN-LABELED PRODUCTS: NONE.

Tropicamide 0.5% and 1% Ophthalmic Solution, USP, (containing tropicamide 5 mg/mL and 10 mg/mL, respectively; benzalkonium chloride 0.01%; NaCl; edetate disodium; purified water; and HCl and/or NaOH to adjust pH to 4-5.8) in 3 mL and 15 mL dropper bottles; *Mydriacyl®*, *Mydral®*, generic; (Rx)

Revisions/References

Monograph revised/updated September 2014.

Vancomycin Sulfate Ophthalmic

(van-kohe-mye-sin sul-fate)

Glycopeptide Antimicrobial Agent

Prescriber Highlights

▶ Reserved for treatment of infections by methicillin-resistant gram-positive organisms.

▶ Is not effective against gram-negative bacteria.

▶ Not approved in an ophthalmic dosage form in the United States, although ocular dosage forms are approved in other countries.

Uses/Indications

In veterinary patients, vancomycin ophthalmic is used for cases of methicillin-resistant microorganisms such as methicillin-resistant *Staphylococcus aureus* (MRSA) or *Staphylococcus pseudintermedius* (MRSP). Vancomycin 0.3-1% ophthalmic ointments have been shown to be effective in treating methicillin-resistant *Staphylococcus* keratitis in rabbits (Eguchi *et al.* 2009). Vancomycin is also administered intravitreally for severe cases of methicillin-resistant endophthalmitis. Intracameral injection of vancomycin nanoparticles has also demonstrated good prophylactic activity against MRSA in rabbits with minimal adverse effects (Kodjikian *et al.* 2010).

Pharmacology/Actions

The bactericidal action of vancomycin results primarily from inhibition of cell-wall biosynthesis. In addition, it alters cell membrane permeability and RNA synthesis. There is no cross-resistance between vancomycin and other antibiotics. Vancomycin is not active *in vitro* against gram-negative bacilli, mycobacteria, or fungi.

Contraindications/Precautions/Warnings

Vancomycin is contraindicated in patients with a history of hypersensitivity to it or any component of the formulation. Vancomycin is extremely ototoxic and should not be used in the ear.

Adverse Effects

Adverse effects reported in humans or animals include burning or stinging upon application. Renal damage and severe gram-negative colitis have been associated with systemic use of vancomycin; risk of these adverse effects are not likely following ophthalmic use.

Doses

Methicillin-resistant bacterial conjunctivitis or keratitis (extra-label): 1 drop of solution or ¼ inch strip of ointment applied to the affected eye(s) 5 times daily.

Monitoring

- Clinical efficacy. Resolution of conjunctivitis or keratitis as evidenced by cytology and cultures.

Client Information

- Used 5 times daily.
- Use proper administration techniques to avoid contamination of the medication. Keep cap tightly closed when not in use.
- Wait 5 minutes after applying this medication before applying any other medications to the eye.
- Store in the refrigerator; do not freeze. Do not use if the color changes, it becomes cloudy, or if particles are seen in solutions.

Storage/Stability

Store solutions in refrigerator away from moisture and sunlight; do not freeze.

Compatibility/Compounding Considerations

Vancomycin should not be mixed directly with any other drugs.

Dosage Forms/Regulatory Status

VETERINARY-LABELED PRODUCTS: NONE.

HUMAN-LABELED PRODUCTS: NONE.

Vancomycin ophthalmic dosage forms are not approved in the USA but are approved in other countries. Vancomycin ointments and ophthalmic solutions may be prepared (compounded) by an appropriately qualified compounding pharmacist.

Revisions/References

Monograph revised/updated September 2014.

Eguchi, H., et al. (2009). The inhibitory effect of vancomycin ointment on the manifestation of MRSA keratitis in rabbits. Journal of Infection and Chemotherapy 15(5): 279-83.
Kodjikian, L., et al. (2010). Experimental Intracameral Injection of Vancomycin Microparticles in Rabbits. Investigative Ophthalmology & Visual Science 51(8): 4125-32.

Voriconazole Ophthalmic

(vohr-uh-kon-uh-zohl)   VFend®

Azole Antifungal

Prescriber Highlights

► Not commercially available, must be compounded, give ample notice for prescription preparation.

► Penetrates cornea more efficiently than natamycin and achieves effective concentrations in the aqueous humor.

► Considerably more effective against filamentous fungal organisms than amphotericin B.

► Relatively expensive.

Uses/Indications

In veterinary patients, voriconazole ophthalmic solution is used topically to treat fungal keratitis in horses. It has also been administered by intrastromal injection to humans with recalcitrant deep fungal keratitis (Sharma *et al.* 2011). Voriconazole is not available as an ophthalmic dosage form but voriconazole 1% compounded solution has been shown to achieve effective antifungal concentrations in the aqueous humor (Clode *et al.* 2006). A case report of successful treatment using topical and subconjunctival voriconazole 1% in a horse with *Fusarium* keratitis has been published (Gilmour 2012).

Pharmacology/Actions

Voriconazole is a triazole antifungal agent. The primary mode of action of voriconazole is the inhibition of fungal cytochrome P-450-mediated 14 alpha-lanosterol demethylation, an essential step in fungal ergosterol biosynthesis. The accumulation of 14 alpha-methyl sterols correlates with the subsequent loss of ergosterol in the fungal cell wall and may be responsible for the antifungal activity of voriconazole. Voriconazole has a wide antifungal spectrum against most fungi and yeasts of veterinary interest. Sensitive organisms include *Aspergillus* spp., *Candida* spp., *Fusarium* spp., and *Aspergillus* spp.

Contraindications/Precautions/Warnings

Voriconazole is contraindicated in patients with a history of hypersensitivity to it or any component of the formulation.

Adverse Effects

Adverse effects reported in humans or animals include transient burning or stinging on application.

Doses

Equine Fungal Keratitis (extra-label): 1-2 drops or 0.2 mL through the SPL catheter to the affected eye(s) every 2-3 hours initially followed by tapering of frequency based on clinical response.

Monitoring

■ Clinical efficacy. Corneal scrapings with cytology and cultures to determine efficacy.

Client Information

■ Used up to 8 times daily.

■ Use proper administration techniques to avoid contamination of the medication. Keep cap tightly closed when not in use.

■ Wait 5 minutes after applying this medication before applying any other medications to the eye.

■ Store in the refrigerator; do not freeze. Do not use if the color changes, it becomes cloudy, or if particles are seen in solutions.

Storage/Stability

Store in refrigerator; do not freeze. Compounded solutions (see below) are stable for 28 days when refrigerated.

Compatibility/Compounding Considerations

Voriconazole should not be mixed directly with any other drugs.

Voriconazole is not approved in an ophthalmic dosage form, but has been compounded into a 1% ophthalmic solution by aseptically reconstituting the *VFend®* 200 mg vial for injection with 19 mL of either sterile water for injection or normal saline. This solution is stable for 28 days at controlled cold (refrigerated) temperature (Clode *et al.* 2006).

Dosage Forms/Regulatory Status

VETERINARY-LABELED PRODUCTS: NONE.

HUMAN-LABELED PRODUCTS: NONE.

Revisions/References

Monograph revised/updated September 2014.

Clode, A. B., et al. (2006). Evaluation of concentration of voriconazole in aqueous humor after topical and oral administration in horses. American Journal of Veterinary Research 67(2): 296-301.

Gilmour, M. A. (2012). Subconjunctival voriconazole for the treatment of mycotic keratitis in a horse. Equine Veterinary Education 24(10): 489-92.

Sharma, N., et al. (2011). Evaluation of intrastromal voriconazole injection in recalcitrant deep fungal keratitis: case series. British Journal of Ophthalmology 95(12): 1735-7.

Principles of Compounding Ophthalmic Products

GIGI DAVIDSON, DICVP

Physiochemical Considerations for Compounding Ophthalmic Preparations

The availability of suitable commercially available products for every veterinary ophthalmic indication is highly unlikely. Many agents used in veterinary ophthalmology are no longer or never were commercially available. Examples of agents that are commonly used by veterinarians but are no longer commercially available currently include oxytetracycline ophthalmic ointment, idoxuridine ophthalmic solution and ointment, miconazole solution, vidarabine ophthalmic solution, trifluridine ophthalmic solution, tetracycline ophthalmic solution, rose bengal solution, and chloramphenicol ophthalmic ointment. Even if commercially available, products may be of inappropriate concentration to achieve a therapeutic effect in a given patient (*e.g.*, cyclosporine) or may have agents and excipients that have adverse effects in animal patients (*e.g.*, neomycin sulfate in cats). In other cases, no product is commercially available and must be compounded from other non-ophthalmic drugs or from bulk chemicals (*e.g.*, acetylcysteine ophthalmic solution and disodium edetate ophthalmic solution). For these reasons, pharmacists are frequently called upon to compound products to be used in the animal eye. These products may be administered topically in the form of solutions, suspensions or ointments, by periocular or intraocular injection, by drug-implanted collagen shields, or by drug-impregnated disposable contact lens delivery systems. The quality and sterility of these products is critical. To ensure adequate stability, uniformity, and sterility, both the American Society of Health-Systems Pharmacists and the United States Pharmacopoeial (USP) Convention have published guidelines for pharmacy-prepared ophthalmic products. These guidelines address the following areas of concern.

Validation of Formulation

Before compounding any product for ophthalmic use, the pharmacist should obtain documentation that substantiates the stability, safety and benefit of the requested formulation. Pharmacists may call the manufacturer of the drug, refer to primary literature, call regional eye centers, or call professional compounding organizations to obtain such information. If no such documentation is available, the pharmacist must employ professional judgment in determining a suitable formulation for ophthalmic administration. Factors to consider when making this judgment include: sterility, tonicity, pH and buffering, toxicity of the drug, need for preservatives, solubility, stability in the chosen vehicle, viscosity, packaging, and any precautions necessary to keep drug residues from occurring in any food-producing animals.

Documentation

A written procedure for each ophthalmic product compounded should be recorded and kept in a readily retrievable place. This master formulation sheet should indicate the name of the product, the dosage form, the specifications and source of each ingredient used, the weights and measures of each ingredient used, the equipment required, a complete description of each step in the compounding process with special notation of aseptic techniques utilized and which method of terminal sterilization is appropriate, beyond-use dating, storage requirements, specific packaging requirements, sample label and auxiliary labeling, quality control testing performed, and references for formula. Production records for each batch should include the date of compounding, lot or batch number assigned, the manufacturer and lot number and expiration date of each ingredient used, a sign-off provision for compounder and checker, the amount compounded, and the projected beyond-use date for the batch compounded.

Sterility

Ophthalmic dosage forms must be compounded in aseptic conditions. Sterile Compounding Guidelines should be consulted in the United States Pharmacopeia General Chapter <797>. Sterility is the most important consideration for ophthalmic products. Contaminated ophthalmic products can result in eye infections leading to blindness or even loss of the eye, especially if pathogens such as Pseudomonas are present. Eye infections from contamination can also lead to systemic infections requiring hospitalization and may even result in death. All ophthalmics should be compounded in a laminar flow hood that has undergone annual checkups and certification of acceptable performance. It is also important to note that the laminar flow hood does not guarantee sterility. The compounding pharmacist must also use impeccable aseptic technique when handling products intended for use in the eye. All products must be rendered sterile after formulation in the laminar flow hood.

Sterilization of the final product is most easily achieved through filtration through 0.2μ filters, which also remove particulate matter. This method is obviously only suitable for ophthalmic solutions. Ophthalmic suspensions and ointments must be sterilized by other means to avoid filtering out active drug. Other methods of sterilization available to the pharmacist include dry heat, autoclaving, and ethylene oxide gas sterilization. Gamma radiation is also commercially available for bulk sterilization, but is very expensive. Preservatives may also be added to prevent bacterial growth, especially if the container is intended for multiple use. The preservative selected must be compatible with the active drug and excipients as well as non-toxic to the eye or to the patient. A description of commonly used ophthalmic preservatives and maximal concentrations in provided in Table 1.

Table 1. Agents used for preserving ophthalmic products.

Agent	Maximum concentration (%)*
Benzalkonium chloride	0.01
Benzethonium chloride	0.01
Phenylmercuric acetate	0.004
Phenylmercuric nitrate	0.004
Methylparaben	0.2
Propylparaben	0.04
Thimerosal	0.01
Chlorobutanol	0.5

*As recommended by FDA Advisory Review Panel on OTC Ophthalmic Drug Products

Clarity

Drugs prepared as ophthalmic solutions should be free from foreign particles. This can be accomplished through filtration with a 0.45μ filter needle attached to a sterile syringe, or through the use of clarifying agents such as polysorbate 20 (maximum of 1%) and polysorbate 80 (maximum of 1%). Drugs prepared as ophthalmic suspensions, obviously cannot be filtered, but must be of a particle size that does not irritate or scratch the cornea. A micronized form of the drug is required. The use of an ointment mill is highly recommended to decrease particle size for ophthalmic ointments.

Tonicity

Ophthalmic products do not need to be isotonic if the contact time with the cornea is only for a few minutes. The eye can tolerate a range of 200-600 mOsm/L for short periods of time. For ointments, irrigations and products that will remain in contact with the eye longer than a few minutes, isotonic products should be used. Hypotonic agents may cause corneal edema and hypertonic agents may dehydrate the cornea and cause pain. Tear fluid and normal saline have identical osmotic pressures making 0.9% sodium chloride an excellent vehicle for ophthalmic products. For products that are hypotonic, sodium chloride equivalencies can be used to determine how much sodium chloride to render the product isotonic.

Buffering and pH

Ophthalmic preparations are generally buffered in a range from 4.5-11.5. Buffering is necessary to provide maximal stability of the drug or for comfort and safety of the patient. Alkaloids such as atropine and pilocarpine are usually buffered. If the activity and stability of the drug are not pH dependent, and the pH of the product is not irritating, then buffers may be omitted from the formulation. Commonly used buffers for ophthalmic preparations include Palitzsch buffer, boric acid buffer, boric acid/sodium borate buffer, sodium acetate/boric acid buffer, Sorensen's modified phosphate buffer, Atkins and Pantin buffer solution, Feldman buffer, and Gilford ophthalmic buffer. Formulations for these solutions and ratios required to achieve a desired pH are referenced in the International Journal of Pharmaceutical Compounding, Vol. 2, No. 3 May/June 1998.

Viscosity Enhancers

Because tears and blinking reflexes reduce the total amount of drug available for penetration, an increase in residence time in the eye will increase drug absorption. Increasing the viscosity of the drug is the most common way to prolong contact time. Methylcellulose is the most commonly used agent and is generally formulated at a concentration of 0.25%. Hydroxypropylmethylcellulose is used in concentrations of 0.5-1%. Polyvinyl alcohol has also been used in concentrations of 0.5-1% w/v. Agents used to increase the viscosity of ophthalmic products are shown in Table 2.

Table 2. Agents used to increase viscosity of ophthalmic solutions and suspensions.

Agent	Maximum Concentration (%)
Hydroxyethylcellulose	0.8
Hydroxypropylmethylcellulose	1
Methylcellulose	2
Polyvinyl alcohol	1.5
Polyvinylpyrrolidone	1.7

Quality Control

Finished products should be thoroughly inspected visually for clarity and uniformity of suspension. The pH of the final product should always be checked and the value recorded on the master formula record for that batch. Most compounded products should have a pH of 5-7 unless otherwise indicated for stability or penetration of ocular tissue. Practitioners compounding large volumes of ophthalmic products should periodically perform testing to ensure sterility. Various agencies provide this service. The nearest college of pharmacy can be consulted for a list of providers of this service.

Packaging

Ophthalmic preparations should be packaged in sterile dropper bottles (glass or plastic), or individual doses can be placed in sterile syringes with sterile tip caps. Ointments should be packaged in sterile ointment tubes and heat-sealed.

Beyond Use Dating

The USP/NF standards for preparation of ophthalmic medications indicate that, unless otherwise documented, the beyond-use date for water containing formulations is 14 days. For non-aqueous liquids, the recommendation is not more than 25% of the time remaining until the expiration date of the starting product or 6 months, whichever is earlier. For all other products, the expiration dating should be the duration of therapy or 30 days whichever is shorter. These beyond-use recommendations can be extended in the face of supporting, valid, scientifically conducted stability information.

Considerations for use of ophthalmics in veterinary patients:

Veterinary patients experience many of the same ophthalmic diseases and conditions as humans, and treatments are often based on human therapy. Animals, however, have a variety of species-related characteristics that might cause human-designed therapies to fail or be toxic. Behavioral characteristics such as grooming may significantly reduce the contact time of ophthalmic agents with the eye, and increase systemic exposure through ingestion. Anatomical differences such as size must be considered. Horses and other large animals may simply elevate their eyes out of a caregiver's reach if ophthalmic treatments are objectionable. Specialized delivery devices have been created to treat these patients. Subcutaneous palpebral lavage systems are tunneled under the skin over the animal's brow and allow for passage of medication through long catheters that are easily reachable by caregivers. Food-producing animals require special consideration. Systemic absorption of ophthalmic agents in food-producing animals could result in violative drug residues in food intended for human consumption.

General Principles of Ocular Penetration

Corneal penetration

Drugs must generally be administered topically to treat corneal and intraocular conditions. While the eye would appear to be an easy target for topical administration, the eye has several anatomical barriers to prevent penetration by foreign substances. Instantaneous tear production, strong blinking reflexes, and alternating layers of lipophilic and hydrophilic tissue all work in conjunction to prevent entry of foreign substances. The clear tissue known as the cornea covers the visible outer surface of the eye between the lids. The cornea must be clear in order to allow for vision, and nature has accomplished this by omitting blood vessels in the cornea. Because of this lack of vascular tissue, systemically administered drugs do not penetrate into the cornea. The cornea is composed of several layers of lipophilic (outer layers) and hydrophilic (inner layer) tissue. For a topically administered drug to fully penetrate the cornea, the drug must be able to exist in ready equilibrium between both ionized and non-ionized forms (*e.g.*, chloramphenicol, atropine, and pilocarpine). Most antibiotics are water-soluble and will not penetrate the lipophilic outer layer of the cornea unless ulcers are present. Small molecular weight (<350) and high local concentration of drugs will also increase penetration even if the drugs are ionized and hydrophilic. Topical administration is ideal as it allows for very high local concentrations of drug on the cornea. For a topically administered drug to reach the anterior chamber and bind to intraocular structures (*e.g.*, ciliary body, iris, aqueous humor), the drug must pass through the cornea. Drugs may also reach the anterior chamber to some extent by passive absorption through the conjunctiva.

Key points for corneal penetration of drugs:
- lipophilic
- equilibrium between ionized and non-ionized forms
- small molecular weight (<350)
- high local concentrations

Intravitreal Penetration

Topically administered drugs reach the vitreous only in very small concentrations. To treat severe conditions of the anterior chamber (uveitis) as well as intravitreal conditions, drugs must be administered by periocular or intraocular injection. The periocular routes include subconjunctival injection and sub-Tenon's membrane injection while the intraocular routes are intracameral injection (directly into the aqueous humor) or intravitreal injection (directly into the vitreous humor). Periocular injections can be administered under sedation and topical anesthesia. Intraocular injections are usually only performed in the operating room while the patient is completely anesthetized. These routes bypass the outermost chemical and physical ocular defenses and allow for better concentration of drug in the vitreous. The volume of administration for these routes is relatively small. Periocular injections should not exceed 0.5 – 1 mL in small animals and 2 mL in large animals. Intraocular injections should not exceed 0.1 mL in small animals and 0.25 mL in large animals due to the risk in increasing intraocular pressure. Drugs injected into the eye should be free of preservatives and buffers.

Route of Therapy for Given Ocular Target:

Tissue	Routes of Administration
Eyelids	Topical, systemic
Corneal surface	Topical
Anterior segment	Topical if good penetration or mild disease
	Systemic if poor penetration or severe disease
Posterior segment	Systemic or intraocular injection (rarely)
Any site where multiple dosing is impractical	Subconjunctival depot injection

Questions to Ponder Prior to Compounding Ophthalmic Products:

1. Where is the target of therapy? (eyelids, corneal surface, cornea, anterior segment, posterior segment)
2. What is the character of the drug?
   - Lipophilic? Hydrophilic?
   - What is the molecular weight?
   - What is the inherent toxicity of the drug to the eye (gentamicin)? To the caregiver (chloramphenicol); to the patient (neomycin sulfate in cats)?
   - Is there data to support what concentration is necessary for corneal penetration?
   - Is the drug soluble in a vehicle that is not toxic to the eye?
   - If not soluble, will the particle size of the suspension or the ointment scratch the corneal or conjunctiva?
   - What is the pH of the final product? Is this in an acceptable range to avoid irritation (4.5-11.5)?
   - What is the tonicity of the final product? Hypertonic? Hypotonic? How long will the product be in contact with the cornea if not isotonic?
   - Will the viscosity need to be enhanced in order to prolong contact with the eye? Which agent is compatible?
   - What is the duration of therapy? Will the product require preservation if long term multiple use? Which preservative is compatible?

Dermatological Agents, Topical

The following section lists many of the active ingredients and examples of corresponding preparations used topically for their local action in veterinary medicine. It includes both veterinary-labeled dermatological products and some potentially useful human-labeled products. The drug sponsor, availability and formulation of these products tend to change rapidly in the marketplace so this listing should be used as a basic guide; always refer to actual label. Active ingredients are listed by therapeutic class. Products that are applied topically, but are absorbed systemically and used primarily for their systemic effects are found in the general monograph section. For veterinary products, refer to the complete label for additional information. **Note**: While many of these products do not legally require a prescription (OTC), they are often marketed as "Sold only through licensed veterinarians" or "Sold by professionals only."

Portions of this section are adapted from: Koch, Torres, & Plumb. (2012) *Canine and Feline Dermatology Drug Handbook.* Wiley-Blackwell. This reference provides additional detail on these and other compounds and products.

Antipruritics/Antiinflammatories, Topical

Non-Corticosteroids

Aluminum Acetate Solution (Burow's Solution)

(ah-**loo**-mi-num **ass**-ih-tate)

For otic use, refer to the Otics section

Indications/Actions

An astringent antipruritic agent, aluminum acetate solution (Burows or Burow's solution, modified Burow's solution) can be useful for adjunctive treatment of minor skin irritations such as insect bites, and localized inflamed and exudative skin conditions, including acute moist dermatitis, fold dermatitis (intertrigo) and contact dermatitis. It can also be used for the treatment of otitis externa (see Otics section).

In addition to Burow's solution's astringent and antipruritic actions, it also has acidifying effects and it mildly antiseptic. The exact mechanisms of action for these effects are not fully understood.

Suggested Dosages/Use

Topical use of Burow's solution (alone) is usually as a wet compress, dressing or soak. Application for 15-30 minutes is generally recommended and the affected area is air-dried between applications. Use can be as often as necessary, but every 4-6 hours is often employed. The veterinary-labeled products containing hydrocortisone may be directly applied. As Burow's solution products come in various dosage forms (powder or tablets for dissolving, liquid); refer to package directions for proper dilutions. Dilutions of 1:40, 1:20, or 1:10 are commonly used.

Precautions/Adverse Effects

Do not use plastic or any occlusive dressing material to prevent evaporation. Use room temperature water for dissolving and application. Avoid contact with eyes. Clients should wash hands after application or wear gloves when applying.

Burows solution may cause dry skin or skin irritation on some patients.

Veterinary-Labeled Products

Product (Company)	Form: Concentration All contain: Hydrocortisone 1%; Aluminum Acetate 2%	Label Status	Other Ingredients; Comments; Size(s)
Cort/Astrin Solution® (Vedco)	Solution	OTC	1 oz. dropper btl, 16 oz.
Corti-Derm Solution® (First Priority)	Solution	OTC	1 oz.
Bur-O-Cort 2:1® (Q.A. Labs)	Solution	OTC	1, 16 oz.
Hydro-B 1020® (Schein)	Solution	Rx	1, 2, 16 oz.
Hydro-Plus® (Clipper)	Solution	Rx	1, 2, 16 oz.

Human-Labeled Products

Product (Company)	Form: Concentration	Label Status	Other Ingredients; Size(s)
Aluminum Acetate Topical Solution (Burows Solution) (Humco)	Solution	OTC	480 mL btls.
A-Mantle® (Pharmaderm)	Cream: Aluminum acetate (Burow's)	OTC	30 g, 120 g, 480 g

Colloidal Oatmeal

(ko-loyd-al ote-meel)

Indications/Actions

Colloidal oatmeal is used topically as an antiinflammatory and antipruritic, but an exact mechanism for this effect is not known. It is thought that as the concentration of oatmeal increases, both its drying and antipruritic effects increase; it has been suggested that it may inhibit prostaglandin synthesis.

Suggested Dosages/Use

Spray can be used 2-3 times per day as needed for itching or pain. Shampoo or conditioner is usually used once a day to once a week. Shampoo should be in contact with skin for at least 10 minutes and then rinsed well. Refer to each product's label for further details.

Precautions/Adverse Effects

Other than the potential for increased drying of already dry skin, colloidal oatmeal is very safe. In humans, there are some reports of contact dermatitis associated with its use.

Veterinary-Labeled Products

Note: Products listed are representative of those containing only colloidal oatmeal as the principle active ingredient. For other products that contain colloidal oatmeal, see Diphenhydramine, Pramoxine, Hydrocortisone, Permethrin, or Pyrethrins listings.

Product (Company)	Form: Concentration	Label Status	Other Ingredients; Comments; Size(s)
Dermallay® Oatmeal Spray Conditioner (Dechra)	Leave-On Spray	OTC	12 oz; 1 gal.
ResiSoothe® Leave-On Lotion (Virbac)	**Lotion**: % not listed	OTC	Sunflower oil (omega 6 FA's), vitamin E. 8 oz. Shake well.
Aloe & Oatmeal Skin and Coat Conditioner® (Vetoquinol)	**Conditioner**: % not listed	OTC	Aloe vera gel, vitamins A, D & E, chamomile. 16 oz; 1 gal.
Dermallay® Oatmeal Shampoo (Dechra)	**Shampoo**: 2%	OTC	12 oz; 1 gal.
Moisturizing Oatmeal Shampoo (Schuyler)	Shampoo	OTC	12 oz
Soothe Oatmeal Shampoo (Pet Naturals)	Shampoo	OTC	16 oz, 1 gal.
Simply Pure Oatmeal & Aloe Shampoo® (Davis)	**Shampoo**: % not listed	OTC	Aloe vera, panthenol, Vitamin E.; 1 gal.

Human- Products

Note: There are several human products available containing colloidal oatmeal, including creams, lotions and products to be added to the bath. Common trade names include: *Aveeno®*, *Geri Silk®*, and *Actibath®*.

Essential Fatty Acids, Topical

For systemic use of essential fatty acids, refer to the Fatty Acids, Essential monograph found in the main section.

Indications/Actions

Essential fatty acids are indicated primarily for pruritic and inflammatory conditions such as atopic dermatitis and sebaceous adenitis, and keratinization disorders such as seborrhea. They may also be used to improve coat quality and ameliorate dry skin. Some of these products may contain other active ingredients, including other natural oils, which may have other adjunctive indications.

The exact mechanism of action of essential fatty acids is not well understood. However, essential fatty acids affect the arachadonic acid levels in plasma lipids and platelet membranes. They affect production of inflammatory prostaglandins in the body, thereby reducing inflammation and pruritus. Essential oils may also play a role in restoring the skin barrier.

Suggested Uses/Dosages

If using spray: up to 2-3 times applications a day or as needed. If spot-on: treatment may vary from weekly to every 2 weeks or monthly. If shampoo or conditioner: daily to weekly baths/after baths; leave shampoo in contact with the skin for at least 10 minutes prior to rinsing well. Refer to product label for details on individual use.

Precautions/Adverse Effects

No specific precautions or adverse effects are described for these products.

Veterinary-Labeled Products

Product (Company)	Form: Concentration	Label Status	Ingredients; Comments; Size(s)
HyLyt® Shampoo (Teva)	Shampoo	OTC	Omega 6 fatty acids. Soap free. Labeled for dogs and cats. 8, 12 (spray) oz; 1 gal.
Dermallay® Oatmeal Shampoo and Spray (Dechra)	Shampoo, Spray	OTC	Solubilized oatmeal, linoleic acid, ceramide complex in 8, 12 oz; 1 gal
DermaLyte® Shampoo (Dechra)	Shampoo	OTC	Omega 6 fatty acids, Vitamin E, Coconut oil. Soap free. 1 oz pouch, 12 oz; 1 gal.

Product (Company)	Form: Concentration	Label Status	Ingredients; Comments; Size(s)
Hyliderm® Shampoo +PS (Sogeval)	Shampoo	OTC	Omega 6 fatty acids. Soap free. Labeled for dogs and cats. 2, 8, 16 oz; 1 gal.
Allermyl® Shampoo (Virbac)	Shampoo	OTC	Omega 6 fatty acids (linoleic acid), Ceramides 1, 3 and 6, Cholesterol, L-rhamnose, D-mannose, D-galactose; polysaccharide: alkyl polyglucoside. Fragrance free. Indicated for control of pruritus, specifically labeled for management of allergic skin conditions in dogs and cats. Also has skin barrier restoring properties. 8, 16 oz
HyLyt® Crème Rinse (Teva)	Crème Rinse	OTC	Labeled for dogs and cats. 8 oz; 1 gal.

Human-Labeled Products

Note: Several human over-the-counter products are available in the USA but may contain other ingredients. They are generally not used in dogs and cats.

Diphenhydramine HCl, Topical

(dye-fen-hye-dra-meen)   Benadryl®

For systemic use, see the monograph found in the main section

Indications/Actions

A first generation antihistamine, diphenhydramine has some local anesthetic activity that probably is its main antipruritic mechanism of action. Diphenhydramine may be absorbed in small amounts transdermally, but should not cause systemic side effects.

Suggested Dosages/Use

Topical creams, gels, lotion or sprays are usually applied 2-3 times a day. The shampoos and conditioners are generally used once a day to once a week after bathing. Shampoos should remain in contact with skin for at least 10 minutes prior to rinsing.

Precautions/Adverse Effects

Avoid contact with eyes or mucous membranes. Do not apply to blistered or oozing areas of skin. Clients should wash hands after application or wear gloves when applying.

Prolonged use could potentially cause local irritation and/or hypersensitization. Residual activity may affect intradermal or allergy serum tests; it has been suggested to stop use 2 weeks prior to allergy testing.

Veterinary-Labeled Products

Product (Company)	Form: Concentration	Label Status	Other Ingredients; Comments; Size(s)
Atopicream® (VetriMax)	Cream: 2%	Rx	Aloe Vera, Maltodextrin, Conjugated Linoleic Acid, Lactic Acid, Butyrospermum Parkii Butter Extract, Sodium Starch Octenylsuccinate, Isomerized Safflower Acid, Hydroxypropyl Bispalmitamide MEA, Tocopheryl Acetate, Phytosterols. 2 oz.
Benasoothe® Conditioner (Schuyler)	Conditioner: Diphenhydramine 1%; Pramoxine 1%	OTC	Ceramides, glycerin, lanolin, fragrance. 8 oz.
Benasoothe® Shampoo (Schuyler)	Conditioner: Diphenhydramine 1%; Pramoxine 1%	OTC	Ceramides, cocamidopropyl betaine, coconut oil, lauramide DEA, fragrance. 12 oz.

Human-Labeled Products

Product (Company)	Forms: Concentration	Label Status	Other Ingredients; Comments; Size(s)
Products include: *Benadryl®*, *Derma-Pax®*, *Dermarest®*; (various manufacturers and additional trade name modifiers such as Maximum Strength, etc. may be found)	Lotion: 0.5% Gel: 2% Cream: 2% Stick: 2% Strip: 12.5 mg	OTC	These products may also contain astringents (calamine, zinc oxide or acetate), other antihistamines (pyrilamine, tripelennamine), and/or counter irritants (menthol, camphor)

Lidocaine, Topical
Lidocaine/Prilocaine (EMLA Cream)

(lye-doe-kane; prye-loe-kane)

For systemic use of lidocaine, see the monograph found in the main section

Indications/Actions

Lidocaine is used topically as a dermal anesthetic or antipruritic and is included in several products used for acute moist dermatitis, pruritic lesions, or painful skin conditions. When combined with prilocaine (commonly called EMLA cream), it may be useful for dermal anesthesia prior to painful or invasive procedures (*e.g.*, catheter placement, etc).

Lidocaine exerts its anesthetic properties via alteration of cell membrane ion permeability, thereby inhibiting conduction from sensory nerves.

Suggested Dosages/Use
Thin layers can be applied every 3-4 hours as needed.

Precautions/Adverse Effects
Topical lidocaine may be absorbed systemically, but systemic toxicity is unlikely to occur unless used on a significant percentage of body area, for prolonged times or at high concentrations. Be extra vigilant in patients also receiving Class-I antiarrhythmics (*e.g.*, lidocaine, mexiletine). Avoid contact with eyes and do not use in ears, unless specifically labeled for such. Clients should wash hands after application or wear gloves when applying.

Hypersensitivity reactions or skin irritation (burning, tenderness, etc) are possible, but apparently do not occur commonly. Products containing prilocaine (EMLA) may be more likely to cause methemoglobinemia or systemic toxicity, but these occur rarely.

Veterinary-Labeled Products

Product (Company)	Form: Concentration	Label Status	Other Ingredients; Comments; Size(s)
Allercaine® w/*Bittran*® II for *Dogs* (Tomlyn)	Spray: 2.4%	OTC	Denatonium benzoate (bittering agent), Benzalkonium Chloride 0.1%. Do not apply to entire body or to large areas of broken skin. 4, 12 oz.
Barrier® Wound Care Spray (Aurora)	Spray: Lidocaine 2.4%; Povidone Iodine 2%	OTC	Denatonium benzoate (bittering agent), ethyl alcohol; isopropyl alcohol. 16 oz, 1 gal.
Barrier® II Wound Care Spray (Aurora)	Spray: Lidocaine 2.4%; Povidone Iodine 2%	OTC	Ethyl alcohol; isopropyl alcohol. 16 oz, 1 gal.
Dermacool w/ *Lidocaine Spray*® (Virbac)	Spray: 1.5%	OTC	Hamamelis extract, lactic acid, colloidal oatmeal, PCMX. 4 oz
Hexa-Caine® (PRN)	Spray: 2.4%	OTC	Denatonium benzoate (bittering agent), Benzalkonium Chloride 0.1%, aloe vera gel, allantoin, lanolin. 4, 8, 16 oz.

Human-Labeled Products

Product	Form: Concentration	Label Status	Other Ingredients; Size(s)
EMLA®; Lidocaine/Prilocaine Cream (generic various)	Cream: Lidocaine 2.5%; Prilocaine 2.5% Kit: Lidocaine 2.5%; Prilocaine 2.5%	Rx	Depending on manufacturer: 5, 15, 30 g.
Lidocaine (alone) includes: *Topic-aine*®, Lidoderm®, various.	Ointment: 5%; Cream: 2%, 5%; Gel: 4%; Jelly: 2%; Patch: 5%	Rx and OTC	Depending on manufacturer: 10, 15, 30, 35, 45, 50, 113 g; jelly – 5, 30 mL, UD 5, 10, 20 mL

Phytosphingosine
(fye-tos-fin-joe-seen)   DOUXO®

Indications/Actions
The *Douxo*® *Calm* products containing phytosphingosine are labeled as indicated for localized and generalized inflammatory conditions that may be associated with pruritus including allergic diseases such as atopic dermatitis. *Douxo Gel*® is also indicated as a liquid wound dressing for localized inflammation and after surgery (can be sprayed on sutures). There are also products marketed for seborrheic conditions and an otic cleanser.

Phytosphingosine is a modified pro-ceramide with salicylic acid and a key molecule in the natural defense mechanism of the skin. Ceramides comprise 40-50% of the main lipids responsible for maintaining the cohesion of the stratum corneum, therefore; restoring the skin lipid barrier, controlling local flora (antibacterial and antifungal effects), and maintaining the correct moisture balance. It is also anti-inflammatory as it has anti-IL-1 activity, impairing the production of PGE2 and inhibits kinase protein C.

Suggested Dosages/Use
If using spray or gel: up to 2-3 times a day as needed for itching/pain relief. If shampoo or conditioner: daily to weekly baths/after baths; leave shampoo in contact with the skin for at least 10 minutes prior to rinsing well. Refer to product label for details on individual use.

Precautions/Adverse Effects
Skin redness or irritation may occur.

Veterinary-Labeled Products

Product (Company)	Form: Concentration	Label Status	Other Ingredients; Comments; Size(s)
DOUXO® Calm Gel (Sogeval)	Gel: 0.1%	OTC	Hinokitiol 0.2%, Raspberry seed oil, natural to-copherol, extract of creosote bush. 2 oz.
DOUXO® Calm Micro-emulsion Spray (Sogeval)	Spray: 0.05%	OTC	Hinokitiol 0.1%, Raspberry seed oil. 6.8 oz.

Product (Company)	Form: Concentration	Label Status	Other Ingredients; Comments; Size(s)
DOUXO® Calm Shampoo (Sogeval)	Shampoo: 0.05%	OTC	Hinokitiol 0.1%, Raspberry seed oil, allantoin, lipidure C. 6.8, 16.9 oz, 3L.
DOUXO® Seborrhea Shampoo (Sogeval)	Shampoo: 0.1%	OTC	Fomblin (stabilizer), cationic conditioners; 6.8 oz
DOUXO® Chlorhexidine PS (Sogeval)	Shampoo: Chlorhexidine 3%, Phytosphingosine 0.05%	OTC	*Lipicid®* C8G; 6.8 oz
DOUXO® Seborrhea MicroEmulsion Spray (Sogeval)	Spray: 0.2%	OTC	*Boswellia serrata* extract, glycerin; 6.8 oz
DOUXO® Seborrhea Spot-on (Sogeval)	Spot-on Solution: 1%	OTC	Transcutol (surface diffuser)

Human-Labeled Products

Note: There are several over-the-counter human cosmetic products containing phytosphingosine in the USA. These products target mostly lipid barrier restoration and are generally not used in dogs and cats.

Pramoxine HCl

(pra-moks-een)

Indications/Actions

Pramoxine is a surface and local anesthetic affecting peripheral nerves. It is not related structurally to procaine-type anesthetics. Pramoxine is often combined with other topical medications to reduce pain and/or itching. Precise mechanism of action is not known.

Suggested Dosages/Use

Depending on the product labeling, pramoxine 1% may be applied every 3-4 hours. Peak local anesthetic effects occur within 3-5 minutes of application. It provides only temporary effects. Shampoos are used once daily to once weekly and should remain in contact with the skin for at least 10 minutes prior to rinsing well.

Precautions/Adverse Effects

Avoid contact with eyes; pramoxine is too irritating for ophthalmic use. Depending on product labeling, clients should wash hands after application or wear gloves when applying. Adverse effects are unlikely, but localized dermatitis is possible.

Veterinary-Labeled Products

Product (Company)	Form: Concentration	Label Status	Other Ingredients; Comments; Size(s)
Benasoothe® Conditioner (Schuyler)	Conditioner: Diphenhydramine 1%, Pramoxine 1%	OTC	Ceramides, glycerin, lanolin, fragrance. 8 oz.
Benasoothe® Shampoo (Schuyler)	Conditioner: Diphenhydramine 1%, Pramoxine 1%	OTC	Ceramides, cocamidopropyl betaine, coconut oil, lauramide DEA, fragrance. 12 oz.
Micro-Pearls Advantage Dermal-Soothe® Anti-Itch Spray (Vetoquinol)	Spray: 1%	OTC	Lactamide monoethanolamine and *Novasome®* micro-vesicles. 12 oz. Shake well and repeat as necessary.
Relief® Spray (Bayer)	Spray: 1%	OTC	Colloidal oatmeal. 8 oz. For dogs or cats.
Pramoderm® HC Spray (Schein)	Spray: Hydrocortisone 1%, Pramoxine 1%	OTC	Colloidal oatmeal; EFA's. 8 oz.
Pramoxine Anti-Itch® Spray (Davis)	Spray: 1%	OTC	8 oz. For dogs or cats. Labeled for daily use or as directed by DVM
Pramosoothe® HC Spray (Sogeval)	Spray: Hydrocortisone 1%, Pramoxine1%	OTC	Colloidal oatmeal, essential fatty acids. 8 oz.
Micro-Pearls Advantage Dermal-Soothe® Anti-Itch Shampoo (Vetoquinol)	Shampoo: 1%	OTC	Colloidal Oatmeal, *Novasome®* microvesicles, Skin respiratory factor. 12 oz, 1 gal. Labeled for dogs, cats, and horses.
Pramoxine Anti-Itch® Shampoo (Davis)	Shampoo: 1%	OTC	Colloidal oatmeal, emollients. 12 oz, 1 gal. Labeled for dogs, cats, puppies, kittens
Relief® Shampoo (Bayer)	Shampoo: 1%	OTC	Colloidal oatmeal, Omega-6 FA's. 8, 12 oz, 1 gal.
Micro-Pearls Advantage Dermal-Soothe® Anti-Itch Cream Rinse (Vetoquinol)	Rinse: 1%	OTC	Colloidal Oatmeal, *Novasome®* microvesicles, Skin respiratory factor. 12 oz, 1 gal. Labeled for dogs, cats, & horses.
Pramoxine Anti-Itch® Crème Rinse (Davis)	Rinse: 1%	OTC	Colloidal oatmeal, emollients, Omega-6 FA's. 12 oz, 1 gal. Labeled for dogs, cats, puppies, kittens
Relief® Crème Rinse (Bayer)	Rinse: 1%	OTC	Colloidal oatmeal, emollients, Omega-6 FA's. 8, 12 oz, 1 gal.
Phytovet P Cream Rinse® (Schein)	Rinse: 1.5%	OTC	Colloidal Oatmeal, Phytosphingosine-salicyloyl 0.05%. 237 mL

Human-Labeled Products

Product (Company)	Form: Concentration	Label Status	Other Ingredients; Comments; Size(s)
Tronothane® HCl (Abbott)	Cream: 1%	OTC	Usually used for extremely dry, painful or itchy skin in humans. 28.4 g
Prax® (Sebela)	Lotion: 1%	OTC	Mineral oil, cetyl alcohol, glycerin, lanolin, 0.1% potassium sorbate, 0.1% sorbic acid. 120, 240 mL
Sarna Sensitive Anti-Itch® (Stiefel)	Lotion: 1%	OTC	Usually used for extremely dry, painful or itchy skin in humans. Benzyl alcohol, cetyl alcohol, petrolatum. 220 mL
Itch-X® (Ascher)	Spray: 1%	OTC	Benzyl alcohol 10%, aloe vera gel. 60 mL
Itch-X® (Ascher)	Gel: 1%	OTC	Benzyl alcohol 10%, aloe vera gel. 35.4 g.
PrameGel® (Bioglan)	Gel: 1%	OTC	0.5% menthol, emollient base, benzyl alcohol. 118 g.

Phenol/Menthol/Camphor

(fee-nol; men-thol; kam-for)

Indications/Actions

When used in low concentrations, these agents can be used as counterirritants and may be added to proprietary or compounded products primarily as antipruritics. Camphor and phenol may also have some antiseptic properties.

Precautions/Adverse Effects

These compounds may cause local irritation and should not be used around, or in eyes. Products containing phenol should **not** be used on cats.

Veterinary-Labeled Products

Note: There are also several over the counter products not listed containing menthol, phenol or camphor used primarily on equine patients for overexertion, soreness, or stiffness. These include a variety of liniments (*e.g.,* white liniment, Choate's liniment) or gels (*e.g., Cool Gel®, Ice-O-Gel®, Shin-O-Gel®,* etc.).

Product (Company)	Form/Concentration	Label Status	Other Ingredients; Size(s)
Scarlet Oil Pump Spray (various)	Spray: Menthol, Phenol, Oil of Camphor, Oil of Eucalyptus & Oil of Pine each at 7.5mg/mL; Oil of Thyme 2.8mg/mL; Peru Balsam 1.5mg/mL; Biebrich Scarlet Red 100 ppm.	OTC	Labeled for superficial cuts, wounds, burns, etc for horses and mules. Shake well. 500 mL

Zinc Gluconate (Neutralized), Topical

For otic use, refer to the Otics section.

Indications/Actions

Can be used alone for mild itching or as an adjunctive treatment for more pruritic conditions, mild bacterial infections, or dry skin. It can be used for minor skin irritations such as insect bite reactions, acute moist dermatitis, acral lick dermatitis, fold dermatitis (intertrigo), feline acne and post surgery wounds.

Exact mechanism of action is unknown. Zinc plays a role in extra-cellular matrix remodeling, wound healing, connective tissue repair, inflammation, and cell proliferation. Zinc also has antiseptic and astringent properties.

Suggested Dosages/Use

May be applied to affected areas 2 times a day or as needed to relief itching and soothe the skin. Refer to product label for details on individual use.

Precautions/Adverse Effects

Avoid contact with eyes.

Veterinary-Labeled Products

Product (Company)	Form: Concentration	Label Status	Other Ingredients; Comments; Size(s);
Maxi/Guard® ZN7 Derm (Addison)	Solution and Spray: Zinc gluconate 0.9-1.1%	OTC	Taurine, L-lysine, glycerin. 2 oz btl.

Human-Labeled Products

There are several OTC zinc gluconate or zinc oxide products available for use in humans, and many of the products contain other ingredients. A common trade name is *Calamine lotion*, which contains zinc oxide and 0.5% iron(III) oxide.

Corticosteroids, Topical

Note: There are at least 20 chemical entities (plus a variety of salts) used in humans for topical corticosteroid therapy. The following section includes many veterinary topical products and some human products that may be of use in veterinary medicine. Also, see the *Otics section* for more products.

Betamethasone Dipropionate, Topical

(bet-ah-meth-ah-zone)

For systemic use, see the monograph found in the main section

Indications/Actions

Considered a high potency topical corticosteroid, betamethasone may useful for adjunctive treatment of localized pruritic or inflammatory conditions. Because risks associated with betamethasone (HPA axis suppression, systemic corticosteroid effects, skin atrophy) are greater than with hydrocortisone, betamethasone products are generally reserved for more serious localized pruritic conditions or when hydrocortisone is not effective. All veterinary-labeled products are in combination with gentamicin and labeled indications are for treatment of infected superficial lesions caused by bacteria sensitive to gentamicin. Additional otic products are available that contain gentamicin and clotrimazole, but these can be used in an extra-label manner for treating mixed bacterial and yeast infections when strong antiinflammatory activity is desired. Sole ingredient betamethasone topical forms are available with human labeling.

Corticosteroids are non-specific anti-inflammatory agents. They probably act by inducing phospholipase A2 inhibitory proteins (lipocortins) in cells, thereby reducing the formation, activity, and release of endogenous inflammatory mediators (*e.g.*, histamine, prostaglandins, kinins, etc). Corticosteroids also reduce DNA synthesis via an anti-mitotic effect on epidermal cells. Topically applied corticosteroids also inhibit the migration of leukocytes and macrophages to the area reducing erythema, pruritus and edema.

Suggested Dosages/Use

Betamethasone formulations are best suited for focal (*e.g.*, pedal) or multifocal lesions for relatively short durations (*e.g.*, <2 months). Initially, topical corticosteroids are usually used sparingly 1-4 times per day and then frequency is tapered when control is achieved. Long term, frequent use can cause HPA axis suppression; risk can be reduced by treating for only as long as necessary on as small an area as possible. Refer to individual product labeling for actual dosing recommendations for veterinary products.

Precautions/Adverse Effects

Several veterinary topical products list tuberculosis of the skin or pregnancy as a contraindication. Systemic corticosteroids can be teratogenic or induce parturition during the third trimester of pregnancy in animals. If considering use during pregnancy, weigh the respective risks with treating versus potential benefits. Clients should wash hands after application or wear gloves when applying. Avoid contact with eyes. Do not allow animal to lick or chew at affected sites for at least 20-30 minutes after application.

Residual activity may affect intradermal or allergy serum tests; it has been suggested to stop use 2 weeks prior to allergy testing.

Use care when treating large areas, or when used on smaller patients. Increased risks of HPA axis suppression, systemic corticosteroid effects (polydipsia/polyuria, Cushing's, gastrointestinal effects) and skin atrophy (skin fragility, alopecia, localized pyoderma and comedones are other possible complications) occur as product concentration and duration of use increases. Betamethasone may delay wound healing particularly if used longer than 7 days in duration. Vomiting and diarrhea have been reported with use of the products containing betamethasone. Local skin reactions (burning, itching, redness) are possible, but unlikely to occur.

Veterinary-Labeled Products

Note: At time of writing there are no veterinary-labeled sole active ingredient betamethasone products in the USA.

Product (Company)	Form: Concentration	Label Status	Other Ingredients; Comments; Size(s)
Gentocin Topical Spray® (Merck) *Gentacalm® Topical Spray* (Dechra) *GentaSpray®* (Schein) *Betagen Topical Spray®* (Med-Pharmex) *Gentamicin Topical Spray®* (RXV) *Gentaved Topical Spray®* (Vedco) *GenOne Spray®* (VetOne) *Relifor®* (Schuyler)	Spray (all products listed): Gentamicin 0.57 mg/mL; Betamethasone (as valerate) 0.284 mg/mL	All are Rx	Depending on product: 15 & 30 g, 60, 72, 120, 240 mL
Otomax® (Merck) *Gentizol®* (VetOne) *Vetromax®* (Dechra) *MalOtic®* (Vedco) *Otibiotic®* (Schein)	Ointment (otic): All Products contain: Gentamicin 3 mg/g; Betamethasone (as valerate) 1 mg/g; Clotrimazole 10 mg/g	Rx	Mineral oil base. Approved for otic use in dogs; used in extra-label manner for bacterial skin lesions or Malassezia dermatitis; 7.5, 10, 15, 20 and 215 g bottles or tubes
Fuciderm Gel® (Dechra)	Gel: Betamethasone valerate 0.1%, Fusidic acid 0.5%	Rx (not in USA); available in EU and Canada	Labeled for dogs. Can be used extra-label in cats. 15, 30 g tubes.

Human-Labeled Products

Note: Partial listing; there are also topical branded products (two common trade names are *Diprosone®* and *Maxivate®*) available with betamethasone dipropionate. Do not confuse products containing *augmented* betamethasone dipropionate (*Diprolene®*, etc.) with betamethasone dipropionate. Augmented betamethasone dipropionate is not equivalent with betamethasone dipropionate as it is more potent. For more information on human-labeled betamethasone products, refer to a comprehensive human drug reference (*e.g., Facts and Comparisons*) or contact a pharmacist.

Product	Form: Concentration	Label Status	Size(s); Comments
Betamethasone Dipropionate Ointment	Ointment: 0.05%	Rx	15, 45 g.
Betamethasone Dipropionate Cream	Cream: 0.05%	Rx	15, 45 g.
Betamethasone Dipropionate Lotion	Lotion: 0.05%	Rx	60 mL
Clotrimazole & Betamethasone Diprop. Lotion (various)	Lotion: Clotrimazole 1%, Betamethasone dip. 0.05%	Rx	30 mL
Clotrimazole & Betamethasone Diprop. Cream (various); *Lotrisone*® (Schering)	Cream: Clotrimazole 1%, Betamethasone dip. 0.05%	Rx	15, 45 g.

Hydrocortisone, Topical
(hye-droe-kor-ti-zone)

Indications/Actions
Considered a low potency topical corticosteroid, hydrocortisone may useful for adjunctive treatment of localized pruritic and/or inflammatory conditions. Because risks associated with hydrocortisone are significantly less when compared to higher potency corticosteroids, hydrocortisone is a reasonable first choice, particularly when treating large areas, or when used on smaller patients. Some products also contain the astringent Burow's solution, which may have additional antipruritic effects.

Corticosteroids are non-specific anti-inflammatory agents. They probably act by inducing phospholipase A2 inhibitory proteins (lipocortins) in cells, thereby reducing the formation, activity, and release of endogenous inflammatory mediators (*e.g.*, histamine, prostaglandins, kinins, etc). Corticosteroids also reduce DNA synthesis via an anti-mitotic effect on epidermal cells. Topically applied corticosteroids also inhibit the migration of leukocytes and macrophages to the area reducing erythema, pruritus and edema.

Suggested Dosages/Use
Hydrocortisone formulations are best suited for focal (*e.g.*, pedal) or multifocal lesions for relatively short durations (*e.g.*, <2 months). Initially, topical corticosteroids are usually used sparingly 1-4 times per day and then frequency is tapered when control is achieved. In contrast to some of the more potent topical corticosteroids, hydrocortisone can be applied more frequently and over a greater surface area without undue risk for local or systemic adverse effects. Long-term, frequent use can cause HPA axis suppression; risk can be reduced by treating for only as long as necessary on as small an area as possible.

Shampoos containing hydrocortisone are generally used once a day to once a week. They should remain in contact with skin for at least 10 minutes prior to rinsing. Refer to individual product labeling for actual dosing recommendations for veterinary products.

Precautions/Adverse Effects
Several veterinary topical products list tuberculosis of the skin or pregnancy as contraindications. Clients should wash hands after application or wear gloves when applying. Avoid contact with eyes. Do not allow animal to lick or chew at affected sites for at least 20-30 minutes after application.

Local skin reactions are possible, but unlikely to occur. Atrophy associated with skin fragility, superficial follicular cysts (milia) and comedones may be seen with long term, frequent use, but this occurs more commonly when using more potent, topical corticosteroids. Although systemic absorption is rare with hydrocortisone, long-term use may lead to HPA axis suppression.

Residual activity may affect intradermal or allergy serum tests; it has been suggested to stop use 2 weeks prior to allergy testing.

Veterinary-Labeled Products

Product (Company)	Form: Concentration	Label Status	Other Ingredients; Comments; Size(s)
Resicort Leave-On Lotion® (Virbac)	Lotion: 1%	Rx	8, 16 oz.
Zymox Topical Cream® with HC (PKB)	Cream: 1%	OTC	Lactoperoxidase, lysozyme, lactoferrin. 1 oz.
MalAcetic HC Wipes® (Dechra)	Wipes: Hydrocortisone 1%, Acetic Acid 1%, Boric Acid 1%	OTC	25 count jar.
Pramosoothe® HC Spray (Sogeval)	Spray: Hydrocortisone 1%, Pramoxine 1%	OTC	Colloidal oatmeal, essential fatty acids. 8 oz.
Dermacool HC Spray® (Virbac)	Spray: 1%	Rx	Colloidal oatmeal, hamamelis extract, lactic acid, menthol, propylene glycol. 2, 4 oz.
Hartz Advanced Care Hydrocortisone Spray w/Aloe® (Hartz)	Spray: 0.5%	OTC	Aloe. 5 oz.
Zymox Topical Spray® with HC Shampoo (PKB)	Spray: 1%	Rx	Lactoperoxidase, lysozyme, lactoferrin. 2 oz.
MalAcetic Ultra Spray® (Dechra)	Spray: Hydrocortisone 1%, Ketoconazole 0.15%	Rx	Acetic Acid 1%, Boric Acid 2%; 8 oz.

Product (Company)	Form: Concentration	Label Status	Other Ingredients; Comments; Size(s)
Cort/Astrin Solution® (Vedco) *Corti-Derm Solution®* (First Priority) *Bur-O-Cort 2:1®* (Q.A. Labs) *Hydro-B 1020®* (Schein) *Hydro-Plus®* (Clipper)	Solution: Hydrocortisone 1%, Burow's Solution 2%	OTC or Rx	Depending on product: 1, 2, 16 oz btl
Cortisoothe Shampoo® (Virbac)	Shampoo: Hydrocortisone 1%, Colloidal oatmeal 1%	Rx	Labeled for dogs and cats. 8, 16 oz.
Chlorhexidine 4% HC Shampoo (Sogeval)	Shampoo: Chlorhexidine 4%, Hydrocortisone 1%	OTC	Labeled for dogs and cats. 8, 16 oz.
MalAcetic Ultra Shampoo® (Dechra)	Shampoo: Hydrocortisone 1%, Ketoconazole 0.15%, Acetic Acid 1%, Boric Acid 2%	OTC	Labeled for dogs and cats. 8 oz.

Human-Labeled Products

Note: Partial listing; there are many branded products available with hydrocortisone. For more information on human-labeled hydrocortisone products, refer to a comprehensive human drug reference (*e.g., Facts and Comparisons*) or contact a pharmacist.

Product	Form: Concentration	Label Status	Size(s)
Hydrocortisone Ointment	Ointment: 0.5, 1%	OTC/Rx. Status determined by labeling.	25, 28, 28.35, 28.4, 30, 56, 110, 430, 454 g.
Hydrocortisone Ointment	Ointment: 2.5%	Rx	20, 28.35, 435.6, 454 g
Hydrocortisone Cream	Cream: 0.5, 1%	OTC/Rx. Status determined by labeling.	1, 1.5 g pkts, 14, 14.2, 15, 20, 26, 28, 28.3, 28.35, 28.4, 30, 42, 56,120, 454 g.
Hydrocortisone Cream	Cream: 2.5%	Rx	15, 20, 28, 28.35, 30, 454 g
Hydrocortisone Lotion	Lotion: 1%	OTC/Rx. Status determined by labeling	30, 59, 60, 88.7, 99, 113, 114, 118, 120 mL
Hydrocortisone Lotion *Ala Scalp®* (2%, Crown Labs), *Scalacort®* (2%, Avidas Pharm.); generic (2.5%)	Lotion: 2 & 2.5%	Rx	29.6 mL (2% only); 59, 118 mL (2.5% only)
Hydrocortisone Gel (various)	Gel: 1%	OTC	28, 30, 42.53, 56 g
Hydrocortisone Gel	Gel: 2.5%	Rx	43 g
Hydrocortisone Gel Kit, *First-Hydrocortisone®* (Cutis Pharma)	Gel: 10%	Rx	Propylene glycol, simethicone, compounding kit. 60 g jar.
Hydrocortisone Solution; Liquid	Solution: 1%, 2.5%	OTC/Rx	30, 44, 59, 120 mL
Itch-X® (B.F. Ascher)	Foam: 1%	OTC	88.7 mL

Isoflupredone Acetate, Topical

(eye-soe-flue-pre-done **ass**-i-tate)

Indications/Actions

Considered a high potency topical corticosteroid, isoflupredone in combination with neomycin and tetracaine may be useful for adjunctive treatment of otic or topical localized pruritic or inflammatory conditions that may be associated with a bacterial skin infection and pain. Because risks associated with isoflupredone (HPA axis suppression, systemic corticosteroid effects, skin atrophy) are greater than with hydrocortisone, these products are generally reserved for more serious localized pruritic conditions or when hydrocortisone is not effective. All veterinary-labeled products (*Tritop® Ointment* and *Neo-Predef w/Tetracaine Powder®*) have labeled indications for conditions associated with neomycin-susceptible organisms and/or allergy with anesthetic properties due to tetracaine, or as a superficial dressing applied to minor cuts, wounds, lacerations, and abrasions, and for post-surgical pain application where reduction in pain and inflammatory response is deemed desirable. In addition, *Tritop® Ointment* is also labeled for acute (and possibly chronic) otitis externa, acute moist dermatitis and anal sac inflammation/infection, and *Neo-Predef w/Tetracaine Powder®* for acute otitis externa, acute moist dermatitis and interdigital dermatitis in dogs and cats.

Corticosteroids are non-specific anti-inflammatory agents. They probably act by inducing phospholipase A2 inhibitory proteins (lipocortins) in cells, thereby reducing the formation, activity, and release of endogenous inflammatory mediators (*e.g.,* histamine, prostaglandins, kinins, etc). Corticosteroids also reduce DNA synthesis via an anti-mitotic effect on epidermal cells. Topically applied corticosteroids also inhibit the migration of leukocytes and macrophages to the area reducing erythema, pruritus and edema.

Suggested Dosages/Use

Labeled dose for *Tritop®* when used on skin or mucous membranes: Cleanse area, apply a small amount and spread and rub in gently. Involved area may be treated 1-3 times daily and continued in accordance with clinical response.

Labeled dose for *Neo-Predef w/Tetracaine Powder®*: Cleanse area, apply by compressing bottle with short, sharp squeezes; once daily application usually sufficient, but may use 1-3 times as required.

Precautions/Adverse Effects

Several veterinary topical products containing corticosteroids list tuberculosis of the skin or pregnancy as a contraindication. Systemic corticosteroids can be teratogenic or induce parturition during the third trimester of pregnancy in animals. If considering use during pregnancy, weigh the respective risks with treating versus potential benefits. Residual activity may affect intradermal or allergy serum tests; it has been suggested to stop use 2 weeks prior to allergy testing.

Clients should wash hands after application or wear gloves when applying. Avoid contact with eyes. Do not allow the animal to lick or chew at affected sites for at least 20-30 minutes after application. Isoflupredone may delay wound healing particularly if used longer than 7 days in duration.

Use care when treating large areas, or when used on smaller patients. Treat for only as long as necessary on as small an area as possible. Risk for HPA axis suppression, systemic corticosteroid effects (polydipsia/polyuria, Cushing's, gastrointestinal effects) and skin atrophy increase with prolonged duration of use. Local skin reactions (burning, itching, redness) are possible, but unlikely to occur. Hypersensitivity reactions to neomycin and/or tetracaine are possible.

Veterinary-Labeled Products

Note: At time of writing there are no veterinary-labeled sole active ingredient isoflupredone products in the USA.

Product (Company)	Form: Concentration	Label Status	Other Ingredients; Comments; Size(s)
Tritop® (Zoetis)	Ointment: Isoflupredone acetate 0.1%; Neomycin sulfate 0.5%; Tetracaine HCl 0.5%	Rx	10 g. tube. Labeled for dogs and cats.
Neo-Predef w/ Tetracaine Powder® (Zoetis)	Powder: Isoflupredone acetate 1mg/g; Neomycin Sulf. 5 mg/g; Tetracaine HCl 5 mg/g	Rx	Myristyl-gamma-picolinium Cl (germicidal surfactant) 0.2 mg/g. 15 g. insufflator bottle. Store in dry place, do not allow tip of bottle to contact moisture. Labeled for use on dogs and cats.

Human-Labeled Products

None.

Mometasone Furoate
(moe-met-a-zone fyur-oh-ate)

For otic use, refer to the Otics section.

Indications

Considered a highly potent topical corticosteroid, mometasone furoate may be useful for adjunctive treatment of pruritic and/or inflammatory conditions that may be associated with bacterial and/or yeast skin infections. Because risks associated with mometasone (HPA axis suppression, skin atrophy) are greater than with hydrocortisone, mometasone products are generally reserved for more serious pruritic conditions or when hydrocortisone is not effective. Mometasone is found in a veterinary-labeled suspension (*MoMetaMax®*) in combination with gentamicin and clotrimazole indicated for otic use. It can also be used extra-label for yeast and/or bacterial skin infections sensitive to clotrimazole and gentamicin, when a strong anti-inflammatory effect is also needed.

Corticosteroids are non-specific anti-inflammatory agents. They probably act by inducing phospholipase A2 inhibitory proteins (lipocortins) in cells, thereby reducing the formation, activity, and release of endogenous inflammatory mediators (*e.g.,* histamine, prostaglandins, kinins, etc). Corticosteroids also reduce DNA synthesis via an anti-mitotic effect on epidermal cells. Topically applied corticosteroids also inhibit the migration of leukocytes and macrophages to the area reducing erythema, pruritus and edema.

Suggested Dosages/Use

Initially, topical corticosteroids are usually used sparingly 1-2 times per day, then tapered to less frequent use. Mometasone formulations are best suited for focal (*e.g.* pedal) or multifocal lesions and for relatively short durations (*e.g.,* <2 months). However, clinicians must tailor the frequency and duration of application to the severity of clinical signs. Refer to the actual product labeling for additional usage information.

Precautions/Adverse Effects

Several veterinary topical products list tuberculosis of the skin or pregnancy as a contraindication. Use care when treating large areas, or when used on smaller patients. Risks can be reduced by treating for only as long as necessary on as small an area as possible. Increased risks of HPA axis suppression, systemic corticosteroid effects (polydipsia/polyuria, Cushing's, gastrointestinal effects) and cutaneous atrophy associated with skin fragility, alopecia, localized pyoderma, superficial follicular cysts (milia) and comedones occur as product concentration and duration of use increases. Local skin reactions (burning, itching, redness) are possible, but unlikely to occur. Mometasone may delay wound healing particularly if used longer than 7 days in duration.

Residual activity may affect intradermal or allergy serum tests; it has been suggested to stop use 2 weeks prior to allergy testing.

Clients should wash hands after application or wear gloves when applying. Avoid contact with eyes. Do no let animal lick or chew at affected areas for at least 20-30 minutes after application.

Veterinary-Labeled Products

Product (Company)	Form: Concentration	Label Status	Other Ingredients; Comments; Size(s)
MoMetaMax Otic Suspension® (Merck)	Suspension (otic): Per gram: Mometasone 1 mg; Gentamicin 3 mg; Clotrimazole 10 mg	Rx	Mineral-oil base. Approved for otic use in dogs, but used extra-label (see above). In 7.5, 15, 30, 215 g tubes

Human-Labeled Products

Note: Partial listing; for more information on human-labeled mometasone products (nasal, etc), refer to a comprehensive human drug reference (*e.g., Facts and Comparisons*) or contact a pharmacist.

Product (Company)	Form: Concentration	Label Status	Other Ingredients; Comments; Size(s)
Elocon® (Schering- Plough); generic	Cream, Ointment, Lotion, Solution (external): 0.1%	Rx	Cream: stearyl alcohol. 15, 45, 50 g. Ointment: 15, 45, 50 g. Lotion: Propylene glycol, isopropyl alcohol. 30, 60 mL Solution: 30, 60 mL

Triamcinolone Acetonide, Topical

(trye-am-sin-ohe-lone ass-si-toe-nide)

For systemic use, see the monograph found in the main section.

Indications/Actions

Considered a medium potency topical corticosteroid when used at concentrations <0.5% (high potency), triamcinolone acetonide may useful for adjunctive treatment of pruritic conditions. Because risks associated with triamcinolone (HPA axis suppression, skin atrophy) are greater than with hydrocortisone, triamcinolone acetonide products are generally reserved for more serious pruritic conditions or when hydrocortisone is not effective. Triamcinolone can be found in a veterinary-labeled sole agent cream (*Medalone®*) or spray (*Genesis®*). It is also an ingredient in combination with antibiotics and anti-yeast ingredients in several veterinary products (*e.g., Panalog®*) that are labeled for otic use. However, these products can be used in an extra-label manner to treat bacterial and yeast skin infections sensitive to gentamicin and nystatin, including pododermatitis and anal sac disease, when a strong anti-inflammatory effect is needed.

Corticosteroids are non-specific anti-inflammatory agents. They probably act by inducing phospholipase A2 inhibitory proteins (lipocortins) in cells, thereby reducing the formation, activity, and release of endogenous inflammatory mediators (*e.g.*, histamine, prostaglandins, kinins, etc). Corticosteroids also reduce DNA synthesis via an anti-mitotic effect on epidermal cells. Topically applied corticosteroids also inhibit the migration of leukocytes and macrophages to the area reducing erythema, pruritus and edema.

Suggested Dosages/Use

Triamcinolone formulations are best suited for focal (*e.g.*, pedal) or multifocal lesions for relatively short durations (*e.g.*, <2 months). Initially, topical corticosteroids are usually used sparingly 1-4 times per day and then frequency is tapered when control is achieved. Long term, frequent use can cause HPA axis suppression; risk can be reduced by treating for only as long as necessary on as small an area as possible. Refer to individual product labeling for actual dosing recommendations for veterinary products.

Precautions/Adverse Effects

Several veterinary topical products list tuberculosis of the skin or pregnancy as a contraindication. Systemic corticosteroids can be teratogenic or induce parturition during the third trimester of pregnancy in animals. If considering use during pregnancy, weigh the respective risks with treating versus potential benefits. Clients should wash hands after application or wear gloves when applying. Avoid contact with eyes. Do not allow animal to lick or chew at affected sites for at least 20-30 minutes after application.

Residual activity may affect intradermal or allergy serum tests; it has been suggested to stop use 2 weeks prior to allergy testing.

Use care when treating large areas, or when used on smaller patients. Increased risks of HPA axis suppression, systemic corticosteroid effects (polydipsia/polyuria, Cushing's, gastrointestinal effects) and skin atrophy (skin fragility, alopecia, localized pyoderma and comedones are other possible complications) occur as product concentration and duration of use increases. Local skin reactions (burning, itching, redness) are possible, but unlikely to occur.

Veterinary-Labeled Products

Product	Form: Concentration	Label Status	Other Ingredients; Comments; Size(s)
Genesis Spray®	Spray: 0.015%	Rx	16 oz spray bottle. Approved for dogs. Indication is for control of pruritus associated with allergic dermatitis. Bacterial skin infection needs to be resolved prior to use. Strongly recommend referring to the package insert information for maximum allowable dosages, treatment durations, etc.
Medalone Cream®	Cream: 0.1%	Rx	Labeled for topical treatment of allergic dermatitis and summer eczema in dogs. 7.5, 15 g.
Panolog Cream® *Animax Cream®* *Derma-Vet Cream®*	Cream: Nystatin 100,000 Units/g Triamcinolone Acet. 1 mg Neomycin Sulf. 2.5 mg Thiostrepton 2,500 Units	Rx	Aqueous vanishing cream. 7.5, 15 g.

Product	Form: Concentration	Label Status	Other Ingredients; Comments; Size(s)
Panolog Ointment® *Animax Ointment®* *Quadritop Ointment®* *Derma-Vet Ointment®* *Dermalog Ointment®* *Dermalone Ointment®* *EnteDerm Ointment®* *Resortin®*	Ointment: Nystatin 100,000 Units/g Triamcinolone Acet. 1 mg Neomycin Sulf. 2.5 mg Thiostrepton 2,500 Units	Rx	7.5, 15, 30, 240 mL

Human-Labeled Products

Note: Partial listing; there are several topical branded products (two common trade names are *Aristocort®* and *Kenalog®*) available with triamcinolone. For more information on human-labeled triamcinolone products, refer to a comprehensive human drug reference (*e.g., Facts and Comparisons*) or contact a pharmacist.

Product	Form: Concentration	Label Status	Size(s); Comments
Triamcinolone Acetonide Ointment	Ointment: 0.025, 0.1, 0.5%	Rx	15, 17, 80, 85, 453.6, 454 g.
Triamcinolone Acetonide Cream	Cream: 0.025, 0.1, 0.5%	Rx	15, 30, 80, 453.6, 454 g.
Triamcinolone Acetonide Lotion	Lotion: 0.025, 0.1%	Rx	60 mL
Kenalog® Spray	Aerosol Spray: 0.1%	Rx	63 g, 100 g. 10.3% alcohol.
Nystatin-Triamcinolone Acetonide Cream	Cream: Nystatin 100,000 units/g, Triamcinolone Acet. 0.1%	Rx	Depending on product: 15, 30, 60 g.
Nystatin-Triamcinolone Acetonide Ointment	Ointment: Nystatin: 0.1 Million Units/g, Triamcinolone Acet.: 0.1%	Rx	15, 30, 60 g

Antimicrobials, Topical

Antibacterial Agents

See also the Sulfur listing the keratolytic section

Bacitracin, Topical
(bass-ih-trase-in)

Indications/Actions

Bacitracin is used topically to prevent infection after dermal lacerations, scrapes or minor burns. Bacitracin acts by inhibiting cell wall synthesis of susceptible bacteria and is either bactericidal or bacteriostatic depending on drug concentration and bacterial susceptibility. Bacitracin is primarily active against gram-positive bacteria, but *Staphylococci* spp. are becoming increasingly resistant. Bacitracin activity is not impaired by blood, pus, necrotic tissue or large inocula. Bacitracin is not recommended in the treatment of ulcerated and chronic canine dermatoses (sensitization may occur).

Suggested Dosages/Use

May be applied up to 3 times daily and be covered by a suitable dressing. Use is usually not recommended to continue more than 1 week.

Precautions/Adverse Effects

Bacitracin topical ointment should not be used in or around eyes, for the treatment of ulcerated lesions, or in patients known to be hypersensitive to it. There have been anecdotal reports of cats developing fatal anaphylactic reactions after administered ophthalmic "triple" antibiotic ointment. Deep puncture wounds, animal bites or deep cutaneous infections may require systemic antibiotic therapy. While topical administration generally results in negligible systemic levels, if used over large areas of the body or on serious burns or puncture wounds, measurable absorption and potential toxicity may occur. Do no let animal lick or chew at affected areas for at least 20-30 minutes after application. Clients should wash hands after application or wear gloves when applying.

Veterinary-Labeled Products

Veterinary-labeled bacitracin formulations for topical use are not available. However, ophthalmic preparations containing bacitracin in combination with other antibiotics w/ or w/o hydrocortisone could be used in an extra-label manner.

Human-Labeled Products

Bacitracin ointment is available alone as 500 Units/g in various tube sizes. There are many OTC human products available with formulas equivalent to the formally available veterinary-labeled triple antibiotic preparations that contained neomycin, polymyxin B, and bacitracin. A well-known trade name is *Neosporin®* or it is available generically as Triple Antibiotic Ointment. When combined with only polymyxin B, a common trade name is *Polysporin®*.

Product (Company)	Form: Concentration	Label Status	Other Ingredients; Size(s)
Bacitracin (various generic)	Ointment: 500 Units/gram	OTC	Depending of manufacturer: white petrolatum, mineral oil. 14, 14.2, 28, 28.4, 120 g tubes, 454 g jar

Benzoyl Peroxide

(ben-zoyl per-oks-ide)

Indications/Actions

Benzoyl peroxide products are used topically either as gels or in shampoos. Shampoos are generally used for oily and scaly skin (seborrhea oleosa), superficial and deep pyodermas, crusty pyodermas (such as seborrheic dermatitis/pyoderma commonly seen in Cocker Spaniels), furunculosis, and as adjunctive therapy for generalized demodicosis and Schnauzer comedo syndrome. Gels may be useful for treating localized superficial and deep pyodermas, chin acne, fold pyodermas, and localized Demodex lesions.

Benzoyl peroxide possesses antimicrobial (especially antibacterial), comedolytic ("follicular flushing"), keratolytic and antiseborrheic actions. It also is It has some mild antipruritic activity and wound healing effects, and is thought to increase follicular flushing. Benzoyl peroxide's antimicrobial activity is due to the oxidative benzoyl peroxy radicals formed that disrupt cell membranes.

Suggested Dosages/Use

Gels are usually recommended for use once to twice daily and shampoos up to once daily. Shampoos should remain in contact with skin for at least 10 minutes before rinsing. For veterinary products, refer to product label for details on use.

Precautions/Adverse Effects

Avoid contact with eyes or mucous membranes. Clients should wash hands after application or wear gloves when applying. Benzoyl peroxide will bleach colored fabrics, jewelry, clothing or carpets and may bleach the patient's fur. Clients should be advised to keep treated animals away from fabrics during treatment. Do no let animal lick or chew at affected areas for a few minutes after application.

Benzoyl peroxide can be drying or irritating (erythema, pruritus, pain) in some patients particularly at higher (>5%) concentrations. Reducing frequency of use, application of emollients after bathing, or using shampoos with moisturizing microvesicles may alleviate or prevent this problem. Benzoyl peroxide shampoos do not lather well.

Veterinary-Labeled Products

Product (Company)	Form: Active Ingredients; Concentration	Label Status	Other Ingredients; Comments; Size(s)
Pyoben Gel® (Virbac)	Gel: 5%	Rx	Labeled for dogs and cats and for use once or twice daily after cleaning. 30 g
Micro-Pearls Advantage Benzoyl-Plus® (Vetoquinol)	Shampoo: 2.5%	OTC	*Novasome*® microvesicles. Labeled for dogs & cats. Shake well; wear gloves. May be used up to once daily as directed. 12 oz, 1 gal
Benzoyl Peroxide Shampoo® (Davis)	Shampoo: 2.5%	OTC	Labeled for OTC use. 12 oz, 1 gal
glycoBenz® *Shampoo* (Dermazoo)	Shampoo: 2.5%	OTC	1% glycolic acid. 8 oz.
Pyoben Medicated Shampoo® (Virbac)	Shampoo: 3%	Rx	*Spherulites*® microcapsules, chitosanide. Labeled for dogs and cats. Use initially 2-3 times/week, then once a week or as directed by DVM. 8, 16 oz.
BPO-3® *Shampoo* (Vetoquinol)	Shampoo: 3%	OTC	Labeled for dogs and cats. 16 oz; 1 gal.
Oxibenz-3 Shampoo® (Clipper) *Peroxiderm S Shampoo*® (Schein)	Shampoo: Benzoyl peroxide 3%, Sulfur 2%, Salicylic acid 2%	OTC	8, 12, 16 oz
Oxiderm® *+PS Shampoo* (Sogeval) *PhytoVet PSS Shampoo*® (Schein)	Shampoo: Benzoyl peroxide 3%, Sulfur 2%, Salicylic acid 2%, Phytosphingosine	OTC	8, 16 oz.
Dermabens$_s$ *Shampoo*® (Dechra)	Shampoo: Benzoyl peroxide 2.5%, sodium thiosulfate 1%, Salicylic Acid 1%	OTC	Moisturizing factors, Vitamin E. 8 oz, 1 gal
Peroxiderm Shampoo® (Schuyler) *Sulfur Benz Shampoo*® (Davis)	Shampoo: Benzoyl peroxide 2.5%, Sulfur 1%, Salicylic Acid 1%	OTC	12 oz., 1 gal.

Human-Labeled Products

There are many human products available containing benzoyl peroxide (2.5-10%), but with the possible exception of the 5% gel products, the veterinary formulations would be more suitable for use on dogs or cats. Benzoyl peroxide 5% gel can be labeled as either Rx or OTC depending on product and are available as generics or with the following trade names: *Benzac*®, *Desquam-X*®, or *PanOxyl*®.

Clindamycin, Topical

(klin-da-mye-sin) Cleocin®

For systemic use, see the monograph found in the systemic drug section.

Indications/Actions

Topical clindamycin may be used for the treatment of feline acne or other localized skin infections caused by bacteria susceptible to it. It has been recommended by some veterinary dermatologists that topical clindamycin only be used when other topical antibiotics such as gentamicin have failed. Ideally, treatment should be based on culture and susceptibility results.

Clindamycin inhibits bacterial protein synthesis by binding to the 50S ribosome; primary activity is against anaerobic and gram-positive aerobic bacteria. For more information on the pharmacology of clindamycin, refer to the monograph for systemic use found in the main section.

Suggested Dosages/Use

When used for feline acne, topical clindamycin is generally applied in a thin film once to twice daily.

Precautions/Adverse Effects

Topical clindamycin should not be used in patients with a history of hypersensitivity to clindamycin or lincomycin. Avoid contact with eyes. Clients should wash hands after application or wear gloves when applying.

Contact reactions (pain, burning erythema, itching, drying, peeling) are possible. Clindamycin lotions and gels may cause less burning than the topical solutions or foams. As clindamycin can be absorbed through the skin, systemic adverse effects are possible. Antibiotic associated diarrheas are potentially possible, but severe, life-threatening diarrheas (so-called Pseudomembranous colitis) are thought to occur very rarely in animal patients when clindamycin is used systemically.

Veterinary-Labeled Products

None as a topical.

Human-Labeled Products

Product	Form: Concentration	Label Status	Other Ingredients; Comments; Size(s)
Clindamycin Phosphate Lotion (various generic); *Cleocin T®*; *Clindamax®*	Lotion: 1%	Rx	60 mL
Clindamycin Phosphate Gel (various generic); *Cleocin T®*; *Clindagel®*; *Clindamax®*	Gel: 1%	Rx	30, 60 g; 40, 79 mL
Clindamycin Phosphate Solution (various generic); *Cleocin T®*	Solution: 1%	Rx	30, 60 mL
Evoclin®	Aerosol Foam: 1%	Rx	Cetyl alcohol, ethanol 58%, stearyl alcohol, propylene glycol. 50, 100 g.
Clindamycin Phosphate Swabs (various generic); *Cleocin T®*; *Clindacin-ETZ*; *Clindacin-P®*	Swabs: 1%	Rx	60 per box/jar

Gentamicin Sulfate, Topical

(jen-ta-**mye**-sin **sul**-fate)

For systemic use, see the monograph found in the systemic drug section.

Indications/Actions

Topical gentamicin can be useful for treating both primary and secondary superficial bacterial skin infections caused by bacteria susceptible to it. It can also be used prophylactically after lacerations/abrasions or after minor surgery. In small animal medicine, topical gentamicin is usually used in combination with the corticosteroid betamethasone to treat superficial lesions, including "hot spots" (acute moist dermatitis, pruritic lesions).

The products containing betamethasone or mometasone and clotrimazole are labeled for otic use, but can also be used in an extra-label manner for yeast and/or bacterial skin infections sensitive to gentamicin and clotrimazole, when an anti-inflammatory effect is also desired. Formulations containing betamethasone ore mometasone are best suited for focal (*e.g.*, pedal) or multifocal lesions for relatively short durations (*e.g.*, <2 months). Initially, topical corticosteroids are usually used sparingly 1-4 times per day and then frequency is tapered when control is achieved. Sole ingredient gentamicin sulfate topical forms are available with human labeling.

Gentamicin has activity against many Streptococci, Staphylococci (coagulase negative/positive and some penicillinase-producing strains) and gram-negative bacteria including many Klebsiella, *E. coli*, and some strains of Pseudomonas. Gentamicin-resistant strains of Pseudomonas are an ongoing issue.

Suggested Dosages/Use

Topical gentamicin/betamethasone sprays are labeled for use 2-4 times day for up to 7 days. Topical gentamicin creams and ointments are generally applied to affected areas up to 4 times daily. Creams are generally used for secondary or greasy infections; ointments on dry skin infections.

Precautions/Adverse Effects

Topical gentamicin may be absorbed systemically if used on ulcers, burned or denuded skin. Creams are more likely to be absorbed than are ointments. Systemic toxicity is unlikely to occur unless used on a significant percentage of body area or for prolonged times. Do not let animal lick or chew at affected areas for at least 20-30 minutes after application.

With products containing betamethasone or mometasone, long-term or frequent use can cause HPA axis suppression. Risk can be reduced by treating for only as long as necessary on as small an area as possible. Residual activity may affect intradermal or allergy serum tests; it has been suggested to stop use 2 weeks prior to allergy testing.

Avoid contact with eyes. Clients should wash hands after application or wear gloves when applying.

Refer to individual product labeling for actual dosing recommendations for veterinary products.

Veterinary-Labeled Products

Note: There are no topical gentamicin-only labeled veterinary products in the USA.

Product (Company)	Form: Concentration	Label Status	Other Ingredients; Size(s)
MoMetaMax Otic Suspension® (Merck)	Suspension (otic): Gentamicin 3 mg/g Mometasone 1 mg/g Clotrimazole 10 mg/g	Rx	Mineral oil based. Approved for otic use in dogs. Extra label use in dogs and cats with localized inflamed or infected cutaneous lesions (e.g., bacterial skin lesions or Malassezia dermatitis.) 7.5, 15, 30, 215 g tubes.
Gentocin Topical Spray® (Merck) Gentacalm® Topical Spray (Dechra) GentaSpray® (Schein) Betagen Topical Spray® (Med-Pharmex) Gentamicin Topical Spray® (RXV) Gentaved Topical Spray® (Vedco) GenOne Spray® (VetOne) Relifor® (Schuyler)	Spray (all products listed): Gentamicin 0.57 mg/mL; Betamethasone (as valerate) 0.284 mg/mL	All are Rx	Depending on product: 15 & 30 g, 60, 72, 120, 240 mL
Otomax® (Merck) Gentizol® (VetOne) Vetromax® (Dechra) MalOtic® (Vedco) Otibiotic® (Schein)	Ointment (otic): All Products contain: Gentamicin 3 mg/g; Betamethasone (as valerate) 1 mg/g; Clotrimazole 10 mg/g	Rx	Mineral oil base. Approved for otic use in dogs; used in extra-label manner for bacterial skin lesions or Malassezia dermatitis; 7.5, 10, 15, 20 and 215 g bottles or tubes

Human-Labeled Products

Product (Company)	Form: Concentration	Label Status	Other Ingredients; Comments; Size(s)
Gentamicin (various generic)	Cream: 0.1% (as base) Ointment: 0.1% (as base)	Rx	Cream may contain propylene glycol and parabens. 15, 30 g tubes Ointment may contain white petrolatum and parabens. 15, 30 g. tubes

Mupirocin (Pseudomonic Acid A)

(myoo-pye-roe-sin)   Bactroban®, Muricin®

Indications/Actions

Mupirocin is FDA-approved for treating infections in dogs (e.g., superficial pyoderma, fold pyoderma, interdigital cysts/draining tracts, acne, pressure point pyodermas, etc.) caused by susceptible strains of Staphylococcus aureus or Staphylococcus pseudintermedius, including beta-lactamase producing and methicillin-resistant strains. It may also be of use in other species and conditions (e.g., feline acne, equine pyoderma, superficial pyoderma, interdigital abscesses, pressure point pyodermas, etc). It may also be of use in feline acne. It also shows activity against other gram-positive pathogens, including strains of Corynebacterium, Clostridium, Proteus and Actinomyces.

Mupirocin is not related structurally to other commercially available antibiotics and acts by inhibiting bacterial protein synthesis by binding to bacterial isoleucyl transfer-RNA synthetase. While bacterial resistance is rare, resistant strains of Staphylococcal aureus have been identified and resistance transference is thought to be plasmid-mediated. It is thought that resistance occurs more frequently when mupirocin is used over a prolonged period and over larger areas of skin, therefore; it may be best to use mupirocin for short-term treatment and on small, localized areas. Cross-resistance with other antimicrobials has not been identified. Mupirocin also has activity against some gram-negative bacteria, but it is not used clinically for gram-negative infections. Pseudomonas is particularly resistant to mupirocin.

Mupirocin is not significantly absorbed through the skin into the systemic circulation, but does penetrate well into granulomatous deep pyoderma lesions. It is not suitable for application to burns.

Suggested Dosages/Use

Mupirocin is labeled for twice daily application on dogs. It requires 10 minutes of contact time to be active. In cats with feline acne, once a course of once to twice-daily mupirocin therapy has been completed (control attained), some cats can be maintained with 1-2 applications per week.

Precautions/Adverse Effects

Mupirocin is contraindicated in patients with a history of hypersensitive reactions it or other ointments containing polyethylene glycol. Because the ointment has a polyethylene glycol base, the manufacturer warns that nephrotoxicity may potentially develop if used on extensive deep lesions. Avoid contact with eyes.

Mupirocin appears to be very well tolerated; contact reactions (pain, erythema, itching) are possible, but thought to occur rarely. Overgrowth of non-susceptible organisms (superinfection) is also possible with prolonged use. Anecdotally, very rare renal toxicity has been reported.

Veterinary-Labeled Products

Product (Company)	Form: Concentration	Label Status	Other Ingredients; Size(s)
Muricin® (Dechra), generic (Putney)	Ointment: 2%	Rx	Labeled for use on dogs; Polyethylene glycol base. 15 g.

Human-Labeled Products

Product (Company)	Form: Concentration	Label Status	Other Ingredients; Size(s)
Mupirocin (various generic); *Bactroban*® (GlaxoSmithKline)	Ointment: 2%	Rx	Polyethylene glycol base. 1, 22, 30 g.
Centany® and *Centany AT*® Kit (Medimetriks)	Ointment: 2%	Rx	Castor oil, hard fat base. 30 g tube; 1 kit/box
Mupirocin Calcium (generic); *Bactroban*® Cream (GlaxoSmithKline)	Cream: 2%	Rx	Oil/water base. 15, 30 g

Nitrofurazone, Topical
(nye-troe-fur-ah-zone)   Furazone®

Indications/Actions
Nitrofurazone is a nitrofuran antibacterial that can be used topically as an antibacterial for treating or preventing superficial infections. It is bactericidal for many bacteria, including *E. coli, S. aureus*, etc. Clinical efficacy demonstrating efficacy for the treatment of minor burns or surface bacterial infections is apparently unavailable.

Nitrofurazone's mechanism of action is thought to be associated with inhibiting bacterial enzymes that primarily degrade glucose and pyruvate.

Suggested Dosages/Use
Apply once daily until lesions resolve or as directed by the veterinarian. For veterinary products, refer to product label for details on individual use.

Precautions/Adverse Effects
As nitrofurazone has been shown to cause mammary tumors when fed in high doses to rats and ovarian tumors in mice, U.S.A. **federal law prohibits the use of nitrofurazone products in (or on) food animals, including horses to be used for food**.

The soluble dressing contains polyethylene glycols and if used on large areas of denuded skin significant amounts of polyethylene glycol could be absorbed and cause nephrotoxicity.

Avoid ointment contact with eyes or mucous membranes. Clients should wash hands after application or wear gloves when applying. Do not allow animal to lick or chew treated area for at least 30 minutes. Avoid exposure to sunlight, strong fluorescent lighting, excessive heat, or alkaline materials.

Topical nitrofurazone appears to be well tolerated; hypersensitivity or skin reactions (pain, erythema, itching) are possible, but thought to occur rarely. Overgrowth of non-susceptible organisms (superinfection) is also possible with prolonged use.

Veterinary-Labeled Products

Product (Company)	Form: Concentration	Label Status	Other Ingredients; Comments; Size(s)
Nitrofurazone Soluble Dressing (generic). Also available under a variety of trade names.	Ointment (soluble): 0.2%	OTC	Water-soluble or polyethylene glycol base. 1 lb. jars.
NFZ Puffer (various)	Soluble Powder: 0.2%	OTC	Labeled for eye and ear infections, surface wounds, cuts and abrasions in dogs and cats. Shake or rotate to loosen powder. Restricted drug in California. 45 g.

Human-Labeled Products
None. Nitrofurazone products are no longer available with human labeling in the USA.

Silver Sulfadiazine (SSD)
(sil-ver sul-fa-dye-ah-zeen)   Silvadene®

Indications/Actions
Topical silver sulfadiazine (SSD) is labeled for topical prophylaxis and treatment of 2nd and 3rd degree burns. In veterinary medicine, it is can be useful in treating localized bacterial skin infections, particularly those caused by *Pseudomonas* spp.

SSD has extensive antimicrobial activity and is bactericidal for yeasts and many gram-negative and gram-positive bacteria. SSD acts by disrupting microbial cell membranes and cell walls; this differs from the antibacterial actions of silver nitrate or sodium sulfadiazine. It can enhance epithelization, but can retard granulation.

Suggested Dosages/Use
When used for burns SSD is applied once to twice daily at a thickness of approx. 1/16th of an inch (1-2 mm). Dressings may be applied over the cream. When used for localized bacterial infections once to twice daily treatment with the cream rubbed in is suggested.

Precautions/Adverse Effects
Patients hypersensitive to sulfonamides may also react to SSD. Risks of continued treatment must be weighed against the risks of not treating with SSD. Patients with significant hepatic or renal dysfunction may accumulate drug, particularly when used over large areas. Because SSD can retard granulation, avoid use in non-granulated wounds. Avoid contact with eyes. Clients should wash hands after application or wear gloves when applying.

Adverse effects associated with sulfonamides (*e.g.*, KCS in dogs, blood dyscrasias in dogs/cats, etc) are possible particularly when used over large areas or for extended periods. Refer to the Sulfadiazine/Trimethoprim monograph in the main section of the reference for more information.

Veterinary-Labeled Products

There are no topical products labeled for veterinary patients. An otic preparation (*Baytril Otic*®) contains SSD. See the Otics section for more information.

Human-Labeled Products

Product	Form: Concentration	Label Status	Other Ingredients; Size(s)
Silvadene®; *Thermazene*®; *SSD Cream*®	Cream: 1% (10 mg/gm)	Rx	Water-miscible base containing white petrolatum, stearyl alcohol, methylparaben. 20, 25, 50, 85, 400 & 1000 g.

Antiseptics

Acetic Acid/Boric Acid
(ah-see-tik ass-id; bor-ik assi-id)

Indications/Actions

Indicated for the treatment of skin infections caused by bacteria including *Staphylococcus* spp., *Pseudomonas* spp. and yeast such as *Malassezia* spp. Also indicated for fold dermatitis, acute moist dermatitis, pododermatitis, and seborrhea oleosa. Some products contain other antimicrobials such as chlorhexidine and ketoconazole or antiinflammatory agents such as hydrocortisone for anti-pruritic effects.

Acetic and boric acids are potent antibacterial and antifungal agents with a rapid killing effect. They also possess ceruminolytic, keratolytic, keratoplastic, and astringent.

Suggested Uses/Dosages

If using spray or wipes: up to 2-3 times a day. If shampoo or conditioner: daily to weekly baths/after baths according to the veterinarian's recommendations. Leave shampoos in contact with the skin for at least 10 minutes prior to rinsing. Refer to the product for individual label directions.

Precautions/Adverse Effects

Skin redness and irritation may occur. Do no let animal lick or chew at affected areas for at least 20-30 minutes after application.

Veterinary-Labeled Products

Product (Company)	Form: Concentration	Label Status	Other Ingredients; Comments; Size(s);
Malacetic Ultra Spray® (Dechra)	Spray: Acetic Acid 1%, Boric Acid 2%, Ketoconazole 0.15%, Hydrocortisone 1%	OTC	Labeled for dogs and cats. 8 oz.
HexaChlor-K Spray® (Schuyler)	Spray: Acetic Acid 2%, Chlorhexidine 2%, Ketoconazole 1%	OTC	8 oz.
Malacetic Spray® Conditioner (Dechra)	Spray: Acetic Acid 2%, Boric Acid 2%	OTC	Labeled for dogs and cats. 8, 16 oz.
Mal-A-Ket Wipes® (Dechra) *HexaChlor-K Wipes*® (Schuyler)	Wipes: Acetic Acid 2%, Chlorhexidine 2%, Ketoconazole 1%	OTC	Labeled for dogs and cats. 50 count jar.
Malacetic HC Wipes® (Dechra)	Wipes: Acetic Acid 1%, Boric Acid 1%, Hydrocortisone 1%	OTC	Labeled for dogs and cats. 25 count jar.
Malacetic Wet Wipes® (Dechra)	Wipes: Acetic Acid 1%, Boric Acid 1%	OTC	Labeled for dogs and cats. Indicated for anal sac expression, skin folds and cleaning of ears. 25 and 100 count jars and 25-count brick pack.
Malacetic Shampoo® (Dechra)	Shampoo: Acetic Acid 2%, Boric Acid 2%	OTC	Labeled for dogs and cats. 12, 16 oz; 1 gal.
Malacetic Ultra Shampoo® (Dechra)	Shampoo: Ketoconazole 0.15%, Hydrocortisone 1%, Acetic Acid 1%, Boric Acid 2%.	OTC	Labeled for dogs and cats. 8 oz.
Mal-A-Ket® Shampoo (Dechra)	Shampoo: Ketoconazole 2%, Acetic Acid 2%, Chlorhexidine 2%	OTC	Labeled for dogs and cats. 1 oz pouch, 8 oz; 1 gal.
HexaChlor-K Shampoo® (Schuyler)	Shampoo: Ketoconazole 1%, Acetic Acid 2%, Chlorhexidine 2%	OTC	12 oz.

Human-Labeled Products

There are several OTC human products available containing acetic acid or boric acid (alone or containing other ingredients). For more information on human-labeled acetic acid or boric acid products, refer to a comprehensive human drug reference (*e.g.*, *Facts and Comparisons*) or contact a pharmacist.

Chlorhexidine

(klor-heks-ih-deen)   Nolvasan®

Indications/Actions

A topical antiseptic, chlorhexidine has activity against many bacteria, but apparently, it is not predictably active against *Pseudomonas* or *Serratia* spp. It is available with veterinary labels in many different forms (solutions, shampoos, scrubs, ointments, sprays, etc).

Because it causes less drying and is usually less irritating than benzoyl peroxide, it is sometimes used in patients that cannot tolerate benzoyl peroxide. However, it does not have the keratolytic, comedolytic or degreasing effects of benzoyl peroxide. Chlorhexidine possesses some residual effects and can remain active on skin after rinsing. Chlorhexidine products may also contain other ingredients such as antifungals (ketoconazole and miconazole), salicylic acid, phytosphingosine, etc.

At usual concentrations, chlorhexidine acts by damaging bacterial cytoplasmic membranes. Antifungal activity can be obtained with 2% or higher concentrations.

Suggested Dosages/Use

For wound irrigation or foot soaking, 0.05-0.1% dilution in water is recommended. If using spray or wipes/pads: 1-2 times a day. If using shampoo or conditioner: daily to weekly baths/after baths; leave shampoo in contact with the skin for at least 10 minutes prior to rinsing. For veterinary products, refer to product label for details on individual use.

Precautions/Adverse Effects

Keep away from eyes as chlorhexidine products can damage eyes. Clients should wash hands after application or wear gloves when applying. Chlorhexidine is safe used on cats, although irritation and corneal ulcers have been reported.

Hypersensitivity and local skin irritant reactions are possible. Likelihood of irritation increases with increased concentrations. Chlorhexidine may retard wound healing; not recommended for long-term use particularly on granulating lesions.

Veterinary-Labeled Products

There are also a several teat dip and udder wash products, a lubricant, and oral rinses are available. There are several trade names used for chlorhexidine products, including *Nolvasan®, Chlorhexiderm®*, Dermachlor®, Chlorasan®, Chloradine®, Privasan®, and *Chlorhex®*.

Product (Company)	Form: Concentration	Label Status	Other Ingredients; Comments; Size(s)
Chlorhexidine Ointment (*Nolvasan®, Chlorhex®*)	Ointment: 1%	OTC	7 oz, 16 oz
Chlorhexidine Spray (various manufacturers and trade names)	Spray: 4%	OTC	Aloe. 8 oz. Shake well. Labeled for dogs, cats, & horses
TrizChlor 4® Spray Conditioner (Dechra)	Spray: Chlorhexidine 4%, TrizEDTA	OTC	Labeled for dogs and cats. 8 oz, 1 gal.
Mal-A-Ket Plus TrizEDTA Spray Conditioner® (Dechra)	Spray: Chlorhexidine 2%, Ketoconazole 1%, TrizEDTA	OTC	Labeled for dogs and cats. 8 oz.
DOUXO® Chlorhexidine PS Micro-emulsion Spray (Sogeval)	Spray: Chlorhexidine 3%, Phytosphingosine 0.05%	OTC	Labeled for dogs and cats. 6.8 oz.
Chlorhex 2X 4%® Spray (Vedco)	Spray: 4%	OTC	4% Isopropyl alcohol. Labeled for dogs and cats. 8 oz.
ChlorhexiDerm Spray® (DVM)	Spray: 4%	OTC	Labeled for dogs and cats. 8 oz.
Ketoseb-D® Spray (Sogeval)	Spray: Chlorhexidine 2%, Ketoconazole 1%	OTC	Labeled for dogs and cats. 8 oz.
Chlorhexidine Shampoo *Chloradine 4%®* (RXV) *Chlorhex 2X 4%®* (Vedco)	Shampoo: Chlorhexidine 4%	OTC	8 oz, 1 gal.
TrizCHLOR® 4 Shampoo (Dechra)	Shampoo: 4%, TrizEDTA	OTC	8oz, 1 gal.
Chlorhexidine Shampoo 2% (various manufacturers and trade names)	Shampoo: 2%	OTC	8, 16 oz, 1 gal
Chlorhex Shampoo® (Vedco)	Shampoo: Chlorhexidine 1%	OTC	8 oz, 1 gal.
DOUXO® Chlorhexidine PS+- Climbazole Shampoo	Shampoo: Chlorhexidine 3%, Climbazole 0.5%, Phytosphingosine 0.05%	OTC	200, 500 mL, 3 L
Mal-A-Ket® Shampoo (Dechra)	Shampoo: Ketoconazole 1%, Chlorhexidine 2%, Acetic acid 2%	OTC	8 oz, 1 gal
Ketochlor Shampoo® (Virbac)	Shampoo: Chlorhexidine 2.3%, Ketoconazole 1%	Rx	*Spherulites®* Microcapsules. Glycotechnology (monosaccharides: L-rhamnose, D-mannose, D-galactose; polysaccharide: alkyl polyglucoside), chitosanide. Labeled for dogs and cats. 8, 16 oz, 1 gal.

Product (Company)	Form: Concentration	Label Status	Other Ingredients; Comments; Size(s)
KetoHex Shampoo® (VetOne)	Shampoo: Ketoconazole 1%, Chlorhexidine 2%	OTC	8, 16 oz, 1 gal.
HexaChlor-K Shampoo® (Schuyler)	Shampoo: Ketoconazole 1%, Acetic Acid 2%, Chlorhexidine 2%	OTC	12 oz.
Malaseb Shampoo® (Bayer)	Shampoo: Miconazole nitrate 2%, Chlorhexidine 2%	OTC	8, 12 oz, 1 gal.
Chlorhexidine Solution (various manufacturers and trade names)	Solution: 2%	OTC	As the gluconate. 16 oz, 1 gal. May be labeled for use on dogs, horses, cattle and swine.
Chlorhexidine Concentrate (Davis)	Solution for dilution: 20%	OTC	For 1%: Dilute 6 oz into 1 gal water or shampoo. For 2%: 12 oz into one gal.
DOUXO® Chlorhexidine 3% PS pads (Sogeval)	Medicated pads: Chlorhexidine 3%, Climbazole 0.5%, Phytosphingosine 0.05%	OTC	Alcohol free. Labeled for dogs and cats. 30 count jar.
Ketoseb-D® Wipes + PS (Sogeval) *PhytoVet CK®* Wipes (Schein)	Wipes: Chlorhexidine 20 mg, Ketoconazole 17 mg, Phytosphingosine 0.4 mg	OTC	Labeled for dogs and cats (*Ketoseb-D®*) + horses (*Phytovet CK®*). 50 count jar.
KetoHex® Wipes (VetOne)	Wipes: Chlorhexidine 20 mg, Ketoconazole 17 mg	OTC	Labeled for dogs, cats, and horses. 50 count jar.
Mal-A-Ket® Wipes (Dechra)	Wipes: Chlorhexidine 2%, Ketoconazole 1%, Acetic Acid 2%	OTC	Labeled for dogs and cats. 50 count jar.
TrizChlor® 4 Wipes (Dechra)	Wipes: Chlorhexidine 4%, TrizEDTA	OTC	Labeled for dogs and cats. 50 count jar.
Chlorhexidine Flush (various manufacturers and trade names)	Flush: Depending on product concentration may not be not listed	OTC	4, 12 oz
TrizChlor® Flush (Dechra)	Flush: Chlorhexidine 0.15%, TrizEDTA	OTC	Labeled for dogs and cats. 4 oz.
Mal-A-Ket Plus TrizEDTA® Flush (Dechra)	Flush: Chlorhexidine 0.15%, Ketoconazole 0.15%, TrizEDTA	OTC	A multicleanse flush to aid in the treatment of bacterial and fungal (dermatophytosis and Malassezia) infections. Labeled for dogs and cats. 4, 12 oz.
Dermachlor Flush Plus® (Schein)	Flush: Lidocaine 0.5%, Chlorhexidine 0.2%	OTC	Propylene glycol, malic acid, benzoic acid, salicylic acid, glycerin. 4 oz.
Hexadene Flush® (Virbac)	Flush: Chlorhexidine 0.25%, Triclosan	OTC	*Spherulites®* Microcapsules. Labeled for dogs and cats. 12 oz.
Malaseb® Flush (Bayer)	Flush: Chlorhexidine 2%, Miconazole 2%	OTC	Labeled for dogs and cats. 4, 12 oz.
Chlorhexidine 0.2% Solution	Flush: Chlorhexidine 2%	OTC	4, 8, 16 oz.
Ketoseb Flush +PS® (Sogeval)	Flush: Chlorhexidine 2%, Ketoconazole 1%, Phytosphingosine 0.02%	OTC	Labeled for dogs and cats. 4, 16 oz.
ResiKetoChlor Leave-On Lotion® (Virbac)	Lotion: Chlorhexidine 2.3%, Ketoconazole 1%	Rx	*Spherulites®* Microcapsules. Glycotechnology (monosaccharides: L-rhamnose, D-mannose, D-galactose; polysaccharide: alkyl polyglucoside), chitosanide. Labeled for dogs and cats. 8 oz.
Chlorhexidine Scrub (various)	Scrub: 2%, 4%	OTC	1 gal.

Human-Labeled Products

There are several topical skin cleansers available in the 2-4% range. Trade names include: *Hibiclens®*, *Hibistat®*, *Betasept®*, *Exidine®*, *Dyna-Hex®* and *BactoShield®*.

Chloroxylenol (PCMX)

(kloro-zye-len-ol)

For otic use, refer to the Otics section

Indications/Actions

Chloroxylenol is an antimicrobial disinfectant with demonstrated efficacy against gram-negative and gram-positive bacteria, in addition to a wide variety of fungal organisms, and against RNA and DNA viruses. It can be used in pre-surgical preparation of skin, cleaning wounds and in the treatment of bacterial, fungal and yeast skin infections.

Chloroxylenol, also known as PCMX, is a chlorinated phenolytic antiseptic. Its antibacterial action is due to disruption of bacterial cytoplasmic membranes by blocking production of adenosine triphosphate.

Suggested Uses/Dosages
If using shampoo, leave shampoo in contact with the skin for at least 10 minutes prior to rinsing. Refer to product label for details on individual use.

Precautions/Adverse Effects
May cause skin irritation.

Veterinary-Labeled Products
This list represents only products where chloroxylenol is one of the main active ingredients.

Product (Company)	Form: Concentration	Label Status	Other Ingredients; Comments; Size(s)
Surgical Scrub and Handwash (Vetoquinol)	Scrub: 2%	OTC	Deionized Water, Sodium Laureth Sulfate, Propylene Glycol, Sodium Lauryl Sulfate, Polyquaternium-7, Hydroxyethylcellulose, Polysorbate-20. 16 oz, 1 gal
Medicated Shampoo® (Sogeval; VetOne) *Universal Medicated Shampoo®* (Vetoquinol)	Shampoo: Chloroxylenol 2%, Salicylic acid 2%, Sodium thiosulfate 2%	OTC	Propylene glycol, citric acid. Also has antiseborrheic effect. Labeled for dogs and cats. 16 oz; 1 gal.
Vet Solutions Sebozole Shampoo® (Vetoquinol)	Solution: Chloroxylenol 1%, Miconazole nitrate 1%	OTC	Also has antimycotic effect. Labeled for dogs and cats. 8, 16 oz; 1 gal.

Human-Labeled Products
There are several topical products available containing chloroxylenol usually combined with other ingredients such as hydrocortisone, menthol, pramoxine, and benzocaine. They are presented in different forms (creams, ointments, lotions and shampoos), but are not commonly used in dogs and cats. Trade names include: *Aurinol®*, *Calamycin®*, *Cortamox®*, *Cortane-B®*, *Dermacoat®* and *Foille®*.

Enzymes, Topical (Lactoperoxidase, Lysozyme, Lactoferrin)
For otic use, refer to the Otics section

Indications/Actions
These products may be useful for bacterial and fungal skin infections and are reported to be effective against *Staphylococcus* spp., *Pseudomonas* spp., *Malassezia* spp., *Candida albicans*, and *Microsporum* spp. The can be used alone, or especially with products containing hydrocortisone, for mild itching or as an adjunctive treatment for more pruritic conditions such as atopic dermatitis.

The veterinary products contain the milk-derived enzymes lactoperoxidase, lysozyme and lactoferrin. These enzymes are reported to be effective against bacterial, fungal and viral microorganisms. Lactoperoxidase combined with hydrogen peroxide, thiocyanate, and/or iodide produce hypothiocyanate or hypoiodite ions that are bactericidal by oxidizing components of bacterial cell walls. Hypoiodite also is fungicidal. Lactoferrin acts as a bacteriostatic agent against many bacteria by depriving them of iron.

Suggested Uses/Dosages
If using spray, cream or wipes: 1-2 times a day applications. If shampoo or rinse: daily to weekly baths/after baths; leave shampoo in contact with the skin for at least 10 minutes prior to rinsing well. May be applied to affected areas 2 times a day or as needed to relief itching and soothe the skin. Refer to product label for details on individual use.

Precautions/Adverse Effects
Overall appears to be safe. No reported side effects, but skin irritation is possible.

Veterinary-Labeled Products

Product (Company)	Form: Concentration	Label Status	Ingredients; Comments; Size(s)
Zymox Topical Spray® w/ and w/o Hydrocortisone (PKB)	Spray	OTC	Lactoperoxidase, lysozyme, lactoferrin. Available with and without Hydrocortisone 1%. 2 oz.
Zymox Topical Cream® w/ and w/o Hydrocortisone (PKB)	Cream	OTC	Lactoperoxidase, lysozyme, lactoferrin. Available with and without Hydrocortisone 1%. 1 oz.
Zymox Shampoo® (PKB)	Shampoo	OTC	Lactoperoxidase, lysozyme, lactoferrin. 12 oz.
Zymox Rinse® (PKB)	Rinse	OTC	Lactoperoxidase, lysozyme, lactoferrin. 12 oz.

Human-Labeled Products
None.

Ethyl Lactate
(eth-il lak-tate) Etiderm®

Indications/Actions
Ethyl lactate shampoos can be used for bacterial skin infections, including surface and superficial pyodermas. It also has a keratoplastic effect, which provides anti-seborrheic activity.

A lipid soluble compound, ethyl lactate rapidly penetrates hair follicles and sebaceous glands where bacterial lipases convert it into lactic acid and ethanol, which are responsible for its antibacterial action. Ethanol helps solubolize fats and reduces sebaceous secretions. It is not as active as benzoyl peroxide against staphylococcal organisms, but it is less irritating and drying.

Suggested Dosages/Use
Daily to 2-3 weekly baths. Shampoo should remain in contact with the skin for at least 10 minutes prior to rinsing well. Refer to product label for details on individual use.

Precautions/Adverse Effects
Ethyl lactate shampoos are often used in conjunction with oral antibiotics and are usually used 2-3 times per week initially; frequency of use may be reduced when pyoderma is under control.

Avoid contact with eyes. Clients should wash hands after application or wear gloves when applying.

Adverse effects are unlikely, but local effects (erythema, pain, itching) are possible.

Veterinary-Labeled Products

Product (Company)	Form: Concentration	Label Status	Other Ingredients; Comments; Size(s)
Etiderm Shampoo® (Virbac)	Shampoo: 10% (in Spherulite® and free form)	OTC	Chitosanide (in Spherulite® and free form), benzalkonium chloride (in encapsulated form), lactic acid, propylene glycol in a shampoo base. Labeled for dogs & cats. Shake well. 8, 16 oz, 1 gal.

Human-Labeled Products
None.

Hypochlorous Acid
(hye-poe-klor-us ass-id)

Indications/Actions
The proprietary products, *Vetericyn®* and *Microcyn®* contain hypochlorous acid and sodium hypochlorite and are labeled for the management of wounds, abscesses, cuts, abrasions, skin irritations, ulcers, post surgical incision sites, burns and wound odors and to accelerate healing. It may be used for prevention of bacterial skin infections or as an adjunctive topical therapy for bacterial skin infections, including Methicillin-Resistant *Staphylococcus* spp. and *Pseudomonas* spp. Hypochlorous acid also has anti-fungal and antiviral properties and is reported to reduce inflammation, pain and itching.

These products are a proprietary formulation and have broad-spectrum antimicrobial activity and act rapidly against gram-positive and gram-negative bacteria and fungal/yeast organisms. They may also be effective against viruses. The products *Vetericyn®* and *Microcyn®* contain oxychlorine (bleach-like) compounds and have a neutral pH. Mode of action is to disrupt the cellular membrane of single cell organisms. Because mode of action is primarily chemical in nature, resistance does not appear to be an issue.

Suggested Dosages/Use
Clip hair if necessary and apply spray or gel to affected areas up to 3 times a day; may be used with dressing applications on wounds. Refer to product label for details on individual use. No rinsing is required. Labeled as safe to use around eyes, nose and mouth.

Precautions/Adverse Effects
No precautions or adverse effects reported. Reported as non-toxic; does not sting or irritate the skin, however treated area may become reddened secondary to increased blood flow.

Veterinary-Labeled Products

Product (Company)	Form: Concentration	Label Status	Other Ingredients; Comments; Size(s)
Vetericyn® VF (Innovacyn)	Spray/liquid: Hypochlorous Acid 0.011%	OTC	Sodium Hypochlorite. Labeled for dogs and cats, including puppies and kittens. 4, 8, 16 oz.
Vetericyn Utility Gel® (Innovacyn)	Gel: Hypochlorous Acid 0.01%	OTC	Boric Acid, Sodium Hypochlorite. Labeled for all animal species. 4, 8, 16 oz
Vetericyn® VF Hydrogel (Innovacyn)	Spray: Hypochlorous Acid 0.08%	OTC	Boric Acid, Sodium Hypochlorite. Labeled for all animal species. 4, 8, 16 oz. Also a product labeled for cats.
Vetericyn® Wound & Infection Treatment Spray Vetericyn® Hot Spot Spray Vetericyn® Reptile Wound & Skin Care Treatment (Innovacyn)	Spray/liquid: (all products contain the same formula): Hypochlorous Acid 0.04%	OTC	Sodium Hypochlorite. Depending on product, labeled for dogs, cats, horses, reptiles, or all animals. 4, 8, 16 oz.

Human-Labeled Products

Product	Form: Concentration	Label Status	Other Ingredients; Comments; Size(s)
Microcyn® Skin & Wound HydroGel *Microcyn® Dermatology HydroGel Micro-* *cyn® Dermatology Spray* *Microcyn® Solution w/Preservatives* *Microcyn® Skin and Wound Care* *Microcyn® Negative-Pressure Wound* *Therapy Solution* All products are by: Oculus Innovative	All products contain: Hypochlorous Acid 0.008%, Sodium Hypochlorite 0.002%	Depending on labeling either OTC or Rx	Product sizes range from 1.5 oz to 990 mL
Myclyns® Spray (Union Spring)	Spray: Hypochlorous Acid 0.00025%, Sodium Hypochlorite 0.0036%	OTC	pH: 6.2-7.8. 2 oz.

Povidone Iodine

(poe-vi-done eye-oh-dine)   Betadine®

Indications/Actions

Povidone iodine can be used as a topical pre-surgical skin cleanser/antiseptic and may be used for superficial pyoderma and Malassezia dermatitis, however; it is infrequently used in small animal dermatology due to its drying, irritating and staining effects.

An iodophore antiseptic, povidone iodine is rapidly bactericidal (against gram-positive and –negative bacteria) at low concentration. It is also fungicidal and sporicidal (as a 1% aqueous solution). Povidone acts by slowly releasing iodine to tissues. It has prolonged activity (4-6 hours), but not as long as chlorhexidine. Povidone iodine also has mild degreasing and debriding activity.

Suggested Dosages/Use

For veterinary products, refer to product label for details on individual use.

Precautions/Adverse Effects

Povidone may be drying, irritating and staining to skin, hair and fabrics. Can be extremely irritating to the scrotal skin and external ears. Use with emollients may alleviate the drying effects. Avoid contact with eyes. Clients should wash hands after application or wear gloves when applying. Systemic absorption can result in renal and thyroid dysfunction.

Veterinary-Labeled Products

There are several trade names used for povidone iodine products, including *Poviderm®*, *Prodine®*, *Vetadine®*, *Betadine®*, *Lanodine®*, *Viodine®* and *Povidine®*. There are also hoof dressings, teat dips, and udder washes available (not listed) that contain povidone iodine.

Note: 10% povidone iodine yields 1% titratable iodine and so forth. Labels may be confusing.

Product (Company)	Form: Concentration	Label Status	Other Ingredients; Comments; Size(s)
Povidone Iodine Shampoo (various manufacturers and trade names)	Shampoo: 5%	OTC	Depending on manufacturer: 8 & 32 oz, 1 gal.
Povidone Iodine Solution (various manufacturers and trade names)	Solution: 10%	OTC	1 qt, 1 gal
Povidone Iodine Ointment (various manufacturers and trade names)	Ointment: 10%	OTC	1 lb.
Povidone Iodine Surgical Scrub (various manufacturers and trade names)	Scrub: 7.5%	OTC	1 gal

Human-Labeled Products

There are several trade names used for povidone iodine products, including *Betadine®*, *Betagen®*, *Biodine®*, *Etodine®*, *Mallisol®*, *Minidyne®*, *Polydine®* and *Povidine®*. There are also vaginal gels, swabs, sponges, and foaming skin cleansers available (not listed).

Product	Form: Concentration	Label Status	Other Ingredients; Size(s)
Povidone Iodine Solution (various manufacturers and trade names)	Solution: 1%, 5%, 10%	OTC	15, 59, 118, 237, 472, 473, 946, 3780, 3800 mL, 1 pt, 1 qt, 1 gal
Betadine® Spray	Aerosol: 5%	OTC	88.7 mL
Povidone Iodine Skin Cleanser & Surgical Scrub (various manufacturers and trade names)	Scrub: 0.75%, 1%, 7.5%	OTC	5 mL packet (5% only); 59, 89, 118, 237, 473, 946, 3780, 3800 mL
Povidone Iodine Ointment (various manufacturers and trade names)	Ointment: 10%	OTC	1 g pkts, 28.35, 28.4 gm tubes

Triclosan

(trye-klose-san)   Irgasan

Indications/Actions

Found in several products, often with other active ingredients, triclosan's antibacterial effects may be useful in treating superficial pyodermas. Veterinary products labeled for small animals containing triclosan as the sole active ingredient are all shampoos.

Triclosan is a bis-phenol disinfectant/antiseptic. It has activity against a wide range of organisms, including both gram-positive and gram-negative bacteria and acts via inhibiting bacterial fatty acid synthesis leading to disruption of cell membrane integrity. Triclosan reportedly is not effective against *Pseudomonas* spp. and may be less effective against staphylococci than either chlorhexidine or ethyl lactate.

Suggested Dosages/Use

Daily to weekly baths; leave shampoo in contact with the skin for at least 10 minutes prior to rinsing. For veterinary products, refer to product label for details on individual use.

Precautions/Adverse Effects

Triclosan should not be used on burned or denuded skin, or mucous membranes. Avoid contact with eyes.

Triclosan is not recommended as a surgical scrub. Clients should wash hands after application or wear gloves when applying. Allergic contact reactions may occur.

Veterinary-Labeled Products

There are also triclosan products labeled for use as topical creams, hand soaps, sprays and cattle teat sealants (*Uddergold Dry®*).

Product (Company)	Form: Concentration	Label Status	Other Ingredients; Comments; Size(s)
Equine America Fungazol Shampoo® (WF Young)	Shampoo: Triclosan 0.65%	OTC	Aloe. Labeled for animals. 32 oz.
Sulfodene Shampoo (Farnam)	Shampoo: Coal tar, Sulfur, Triclosan %'s not listed	OTC	Labeled for dogs; do not use on cats. 8, 12 oz.
Triclosan Deodorizing® Shampoo (Davis)	Shampoo: % not listed	OTC	12 oz, 1 gal.

Human-Labeled Products

There are several human triclosan products labeled as hand, face or body washes for acne treatment. Trade names include *Septisoft®*, *Clearasil Antibacterial®*, *Clearasil Daily Face Wash®*, *Stri-Dex®*, *Oxy Medicated Soap®*, and *ASC®*. However, due to environmental concerns many products are phasing out triclosan as an ingredient.

Antifungals

Clotrimazole, Topical

(kloe-trye-ma-zole)   Lotrimin®

Indications/Actions

Topical clotrimazole has activity against dermatophytes and yeasts; it may be useful for localized lesions associated with *Malassezia*. It is not very effective in treating dermatophytosis in cats. Most veterinary products contain gentamicin and either, betamethasone or mometasone, and are labeled for otic use. However, these products may be used in an extra-label manner for bacterial and yeast skin infections with concurrent inflamed/pruritic skin.

Clotrimazole inhibits the biosynthesis of ergosterol, a component of fungal cell membranes leading to increased membrane permeability and probable disruption of membrane enzyme systems.

Suggested Dosages/Use

If sprays, twice daily applications are usually recommended. Ointments are generally applied to affected areas up to 4 times daily. For veterinary products, refer to product label for details on individual use.

Precautions/Adverse Effects

Products with clotrimazole alone:

Avoid contact with eyes and mucous membranes. Clients should wash hands after application or wear gloves when applying. Skin irritation is possible, but unlikely to occur with products containing only clotrimazole.

If using products containing betamethasone or mometasone:

Several veterinary topical products list tuberculosis of the skin or pregnancy as a contraindication. Systemic corticosteroids can be teratogenic or induce parturition during the third trimester of pregnancy in animals. If considering use during pregnancy, weigh the respective risks with treating versus potential benefits. Clients should wash hands after application or wear gloves when applying. Avoid contact with eyes. Do not allow animal to lick or chew at affected sites for at least 20-30 minutes after application. Residual activity may affect intradermal or allergy serum tests; it has been suggested to stop use 2 weeks prior to allergy testing.

Use care when treating large areas, or when used on smaller patients. Risks can be reduced by treating for only as long as necessary on as small an area as possible. Increased risks of HPA axis suppression, systemic corticosteroid effects (polydipsia/polyuria, Cushing's, gastrointestinal effects) and skin atrophy (skin fragility, alopecia, localized pyoderma and comedones are other possible complications) occur as product concentration and duration of use increases. Betamethasone may delay wound healing particularly if used longer than 7 days in duration. Vomiting and diarrhea have been reported with use of the products containing betamethasone. Local skin reactions (burning, itching, redness) are possible, but unlikely to occur.

Veterinary-Labeled Products
Note: There are several products containing clotrimazole for otic use; refer to that section for more information.

Product (Company)	Form: Concentration	Label Status	Other Ingredients; Size(s)
Clotrimazole Solution (various) *ClotrimaTop®* (Schein)	Solution: 1%	OTC or Rx	30 mL
Otomax® (Merck) *Gentizol®* (VetOne) *Vetromax®* (Dechra) *MalOtic®* (Vedco) *Otibiotic®* (Schein)	Ointment (otic): All products contain: Gentamicin 3 mg/g; Betamethasone (as valerate) 1 mg/g; Clotrimazole 10 mg/g	Rx	Mineral oil base. Approved for otic use in dogs; used in extra-label manner for bacterial skin lesions or Malassezia dermatitis; 7.5, 10, 15, 20 and 215 g bottles or tubes
MoMetaMax Otic Suspension® (Merck)	Suspension (otic): Per gram: Mometasone 1 mg; Gentamicin 3 mg; Clotrimazole 10 mg	Rx	Mineral-oil base. Approved for otic use in dogs, but used extra-label (see above). In 7.5, 15, 30, 215 g tubes.

Human-Labeled Products
In addition to the products listed below, there vaginal creams and suppositories, and oral 10 mg troches.

Product	Form: Concentration	Label Status	Other Ingredients; Size(s)
Clotrimazole (various); *FungiCure® Intensive/NailGuard*	Solution: 1%	OTC/Rx. Status determined by labeling	Depending on product: 10, 30 mL
Clotrimazole (various); *Lotrimin AF®* *Desenex®*	Cream: 1%	OTC/Rx. Status determined by labeling	Depending on product: 10, 30 mL
Alevazol®	Ointment: 1%	OTC	56.7 g tube
Clotrimazole & Betamethasone Diprop. (various)	Lotion: Clotrimazole 1% Betamethasone dip. 0.05%	Rx	30 mL
Clotrimazole & Betamethasone Diprop. (generic) *Lotrisone®*	Cream: Clotrimazole 1% Betamethasone dip. 0.05%	Rx	15, 45 g.

Enilconazole
(ee-nil-kon-a-zole)

Indications/Actions
Although no dosage forms are currently commercially available for topical use in the USA, enilconazole is used topically for treating dermatophytosis in small animals and horses using compounded products. A commercially available topical rinse *Imaverol®* (Janssen) 10% is available with canine, bovine and equine use labeling in many countries. Intranasal instillation of enilconazole after plaque debridement has also been shown useful in treating nasal aspergillosis in small animals.

Use of topical enilconazole on cats with dermatophytosis is somewhat controversial as there are apparently no products with feline labeling available in Europe or Canada. There are reports of safely and successfully using enilconazole on dermatophytic cats alone, or in combination with oral itraconazole.

A topical product and a poultry environmental disinfectant product (*Clinafarm EC®*) are available in the USA. This formulation has been used off-label to treat dermatophytosis at a dilution of 55.6 mL per gallon water as a topical antifungal. However, it is technically illegal to use this product other than it is labeled, as it is an EPA-licensed product in the USA.

Suggested Dosages/Use
Using *Imaverol®*: 10% concentrate is diluted in 50 parts of lukewarm water, which yields a 0.2% emulsion. Remove crusts with a hard brush, which has been soaked in the diluted emulsion. It is highly recommended that the animal be sprayed entirely at the first treatment so as to reach subclinical lesions as well. **Horses:** The lesions and surrounding skin are to be washed with the diluted emulsion 4 times at 3-4 day intervals. **Dogs:** Clip longhaired dogs prior to treatment and wash with the diluted emulsion 4 times at 3-4 day intervals. While doing this, one should rub thoroughly in the direction opposite to the hair growth to make sure that the skin is thoroughly wet. Dispose of all unused diluted solutions. Refer to product label for details on individual use.

Precautions/Adverse Effects
Avoid contact with eyes. Clients should wear gloves when applying and use eye protection.

When used topically in cats, hypersalivation, vomiting, anorexia/weight loss, muscle weakness, and a slight increase in serum ALT levels have been reported.

Veterinary-Labeled Products

Product (Company)	Form: Concentration	Label Status	Other Ingredients; Comments; Size(s)
Imaverol® (Janssen)	Concentrate: 10%	Not available in USA	May also use as a dip. Not labeled for use on cats. 100 mL
Clinafarm EC® (Schering Plough)	Emulsifiable Concentrate: 13.8%	OTC-EPA Pesticide	Labeled for the control of *Aspergillus fumigates* contamination in poultry hatchery equipment. It is a violation of US Federal Law to use this product in a manner inconsistent with its labeling. Corrosive; may cause irreversible eye damage. Labeling includes several warnings on ingestion or exposure. 750 mL

Human-Labeled Products

None.

Ketoconazole, Topical

(kee-toe-kah-na-zole)   Nizoral®, Ketochlor®

For systemic use, see the monograph found in the main section.

For otic use, see the Otics section.

Indications/Actions

Topical ketoconazole has activity against dermatophytes and yeasts and ketoconazole shampoos can be effective treatment for *Malassezia* dermatitis. Patients with severe, generalized infections may require additional systemic therapy. Topical ketoconazole shampoos are generally ineffective (or minimally effective) when used alone for dermatophytosis.

Suggested Dosages/Use

If using spray or wipes/pads: 1-2 times a day. If shampoo or conditioner: daily to weekly baths/after baths; leave shampoo in contact with skin for at least 10 minutes prior to rinsing. For veterinary products, refer to product label for details on individual use.

Precautions/Adverse Effects

Avoid contact with eyes. Clients should wash hands after application or wear gloves when applying. Skin irritation is possible.

Veterinary-Labeled Products

Product (Company)	Form: Concentration	Label Status	Other Ingredients; Comments; Size(s)
Mal-A-Ket Plus TrizEDTA Spray Conditioner® (Dechra)	Spray: Chlorhexidine 2%, Ketoconazole 1%, TrizEDTA	OTC	Labeled for dogs and cats. 8 oz.
Ketoseb-D® Spray (Sogeval)	Spray: Chlorhexidine 2%, Ketoconazole 1%	OTC	Labeled for dogs and cats. 8 oz.
Malacetic Ultra Spray® (Dechra)	Spray: Ketoconazole 0.15%, Hydrocortisone 1%, Acetic Acid 1%, Boric Acid 2%	Rx	Labeled for dogs and cats. 8 oz.
Mal-A-Ket® Shampoo (Dechra)	Shampoo: Ketoconazole 1%, Chlorhexidine 2%, Acetic acid 2%	OTC	8 oz, 1 gal
Ketochlor Shampoo® (Virbac)	Shampoo: Chlorhexidine 2.3%, Ketoconazole 1%	Rx	*Spherulites®* Microcapsules. Glycotechnology (monosaccharides), chitosanide. Labeled for dogs and cats. 8, 16 oz, 1 gal.
KetoHex Shampoo® (VetOne)	Shampoo: Ketoconazole 1%, Chlorhexidine 2%	OTC	8, 16 oz, 1 gal.
HexaChlor-K Shampoo® (Schuyler)	Shampoo: Ketoconazole 1%, Acetic Acid 2%, Chlorhexidine 2%	OTC	12 oz.
Ketoseb-D® Wipes + PS (Sogeval) *PhytoVet CK® Wipes* (Schein)	Wipes: Chlorhexidine 20 mg, Ketoconazole 17 mg, Phytosphingosine 0.4 mg	OTC	Labeled for dogs and cats (*Ketoseb-D®*) + horses (*Phytovet CK®*). 50 count jar.
KetoHex® Wipes (VetOne)	Wipes: Chlorhexidine 20 mg, Ketoconazole 17 mg	OTC	Labeled for dogs, cats, and horses. 50 count jar.
Mal-A-Ket® Wipes (Dechra)	Wipes: Chlorhexidine 2%, Ketoconazole 1%, Acetic Acid 2%	OTC	Labeled for dogs and cats. 50 count jar.
T8 Keto Flush (Teva)	Flush: 0.1%	OTC	4, 12 oz.
Mal-A-Ket Plus TrizEDTA® Flush (Dechra)	Flush: Chlorhexidine 0.15%, Ketoconazole 0.15%, TrizEDTA	OTC	A multicleanse flush to aid in the treatment of bacterial and fungal (dermatophytosis and Malassezia) infections. Labeled for dogs and cats. 4, 12 oz.
TrizULTRA® + KETO Flush (Dechra)	Flush: 0.15% ketoconazole, USP tris-EDTA	OTC	4, 12 oz

Product (Company)	Form: Concentration	Label Status	Other Ingredients; Comments; Size(s)
Dermachlor® Flush (Schein) *KetoHex® Flush* (VetOne)	Flush: Chlorhexidine 0.2%, Ketoconazole 0.1%	OTC	8 oz.
Ketoseb Flush +PS® (Sogeval)	Flush: Chlorhexidine 2%, Ketoconazole 1%, Phytosphingosine 0.02%	OTC	Labeled for dogs and cats. 4, 16 oz.
ResiKetoChlor Leave-On Lotion® (Virbac)	Lotion: Chlorhexidine 2.3%, Ketoconazole 1%	Rx	*Spherulites®* Microcapsules. Glycotechnology (mono-saccharides), chitosanide. Labeled for dogs and cats. 8 oz.

Human-Labeled Products

Product	Form: Concentration	Label Status	Other Ingredients; Size(s)
Nizoral A-D®	Shampoo: 1%	OTC	125, 200 mL
Nizoral®, generic	Shampoo: 2%	Rx	Aqueous suspension. 120 mL
Ketoconazole Cream (generic)	Cream: 2%	Rx	Aqueous vehicle containing cetyl alcohol, stearyl alcohol, sodium sulfite. 15, 30 60 g.
Ketoconazole Foam (generic)	Foam: 2%	Rx	50, 100 g cans
Xolegel®	Gel: 2%	Rx	45 g tube

Lime Sulfur (Sulfurated Lime Solution)
(lyme sul-fur)

Indications/Actions
Lime sulfur applications are very effective and relatively inexpensive as a generalized topical treatment for dermatophytosis. Both lime sulfur and enilconazole are thought to have the most topical activity against *M. canis* of commercially available compounds. In addition, it is the most efficacious treatment of surface demodicosis (*Demodex gatoi*) in cats. Lime sulfur can also be useful in the adjunctive treatment of Malassezia dermatitis, Cheyletiellosis, Chiggers, Sarcoptic and Notoedric mange, fur mites, lice, canine demodicosis and sarcoptic mange.

Lime sulfur has antibacterial and antifungal (and some anti-yeast) properties secondary to the formation of pentathionic acid and hydrogen sulfide after application. Both lime sulfur and enilconazole are thought to have the most topical activity against *M. canis*. Lime sulfur may also have keratolytic, keratoplastic, antiparasitic, and antipruritic effects.

Suggested Dosages/Use
Labeled dose for *Lime Sulfur Dip®* (Vetoquinol): Shake concentrate well. Add 4 oz. of concentrate to 1 gallon of water. After adding concentrate to water, mix well. For chronic or resistant cases, concentrate may be diluted at 8 oz. per gallon of water. Wear Gloves. Carefully pour dilute dip over the animal making sure to reach affected areas. Re-apply every 5-7 days or as directed by your veterinarian. Do not rinse or blow-dry animal. Do not allow animal to ingest. Apply a protective collar until dry if necessary to prevent ingestion.

When used for dermatophytosis, once to twice-weekly treatments have been recommended, if patients can tolerate the treatment's irritating effects, until 2 consecutive negative cultures are obtained. When used for confirmed cases of feline surface demodicosis, applications are recommended every 5-7 days for a total of 6 treatments. If using lime sulfur as a treatment trial for surface demodicosis, 3 applications should be performed and if there is significant improvement in clinical signs, 3 more applications should be performed to complete treatment. If no significant improvement is seen after 3 applications, demodicosis should be ruled out and other diagnosis should be considered.

Precautions/Adverse Effects
Avoid contact with eyes and mucous membranes. Can stain porous surface (*e.g.*, concrete, porcelain) or permanently discolor jewelry. Clients should wear gloves and protect skin and eyes from solution. Because of its very unpleasant odor, application should be performed in a well-ventilated area or clients should wear a protective (respirator-type) mask.

While reasonably non-toxic, lime sulfur may cause skin irritation or drying. Adding mineral oil to the solution may reduce its drying effects. Lime sulfur can stain (temporarily) light colored fur and rarely cause hair loss on the pinnae in cats. Lime sulfur's odor may persist on treated animals, but generally is tolerable once the patient dries. Oral ingestion can rarely cause nausea and oral ulcers, mainly in cats; an Elizabethan collar may help prevent this from occurring.

Veterinary-Labeled Products

Product (Company)	Form: Concentration	Label Status	Other Ingredients; Comments; Size(s)
LimePlus Dip® (Dechra)	Concentrate: 97.8%	OTC	Labeled for dogs, puppies, kittens and cats. Shake well and dilute before use (see dosages above). 4, 16 oz., 1 gal.
Lime Sulfur Dip® (Vetoquinol)	Concentrate: 97.8%	OTC	Labeled for dogs, puppies, kittens and cats. Shake well and dilute before use (see dosages above). 4 oz.
Lime Sulfur Dip® (Davis)	Concentrate: 97.8%	OTC	Labeled for dogs, puppies, kittens and cats. Shake well and dilute before use (see dosages above). 16 oz, 1 gal.

Human-Labeled Products
None.

Miconazole, Topical

(mye-kah-nah-zole)

For otic use, see the Otics section.

Indications/Actions

Topical miconazole has activity against dermatophytes and yeast. It is especially effective for the treatment of Malassezia dermatitis. Patients with severe, generalized infections may require systemic therapy. Lotions, sprays and creams are generally used for localized lesions associated with *Malassezia* sp. or dermatophytes. Topical miconazole products are generally ineffective (or minimally effective) when used alone for dermatophytosis; adjunctive systemic treatment is usually required.

Miconazole's actions are a result of altering permeability of fungal cellular membranes and interfering with peroxisomal and mitochondrial enzymes, leading to intracellular necrosis. Miconazole products are fungicidal with repeated application.

Suggested Dosages/Use

If using spray, creams, lotions or wipes/pads: 1-2 times a day applications. If using a shampoo or conditioner: daily to weekly baths; leave in contact with skin for at least 10 minutes prior to rinsing. For veterinary products, refer to product label for details on individual use.

Precautions/Adverse Effects

Avoid contact with eyes. Clients should wash hands after application or wear gloves when applying. Do not allow animal lick or chew at affected areas for at least 20-30 minutes after application.

Skin irritation is possible, but unlikely to occur, but in very inflamed, eroded to ulcerated skin, the pledgets, wipes, towelettes, and spray containing alcohol (*Malaseb®*) can be severely irritating.

Veterinary-Labeled Products

Note: Miconazole nitrate is the salt generally used in pharmaceutical products. While technically, a 1% concentration of miconazole nitrate contains <1% miconazole, the following products are rounded to the closest full percent regardless of how much miconazole base is actually in each product.

Product (Company)	Form: Concentration	Label Status	Other Ingredients; Comments; Size(s)
Micro-Pearls Advantage Miconazole 1% Spray® (Vetoquinol)	Spray: 1%	Rx	Labeled for dogs, cats, & horses. 4 oz.
Miconazole Spray *Conofite Spray® 1%* (Merck) *MicaVed Spray® 1%* (Vedco) *Micazole Spray®* (Schein) *Priconazole Spray®* (First Priority)	Spray: 1%	Rx	Labeled for dogs and cats. 60, 120, 240 mL
Malaseb® Flush (Bayer)	Flush: Miconazole nitrate 2%, Chlorhexidine 2%	OTC	Labeled for use on dogs and cats. 4, 12 oz.
Conofite Cream® 2% (Merck)	Cream: 2%	Rx	Labeled for use on dogs and cats. 15 g
Miconazole Lotion 1% *Conofite®* (Merck) *Conzol®* (VetOne) *Priconazole®* (First Priority) *MicaVed®* (Vedco) *Miconosol®* (Med-Pharmex) *Micazole®* (Schein)	Lotion: 1%	Rx	Labeled for dogs and cats. 30, 60 mL
Sebazole® Shampoo (Vetoquinol)	Shampoo: Miconazole 2%, Chloroxylenol 1%	OTC	Salicylic acid, sodium thiosulfate. Labeled for dogs, cats, and horses. 8, 12 oz, 1 gal.
Malaseb Shampoo® (Bayer)	Shampoo: Miconazole 2%, Chlorhexidine 2%	OTC	Labeled for dogs, cats, and horses. 8, 12 oz, 1 gal.
Miconazole Shampoo (Schuyler)	Shampoo: Miconazole 2%	OTC	12 oz
Miconazole Shampoo (Davis)	Shampoo: Miconazole 2%, Colloidal Oatmeal 2%	OTC	12 oz, 1 gal.

Human-Labeled Products

In addition to the products listed below, there are 2% topical vaginal creams, vaginal suppositories, 2% powders and spray powders available. Most human-labeled products are OTC.

Product	Form: Concentration	Label Status	Other Ingredients; Size(s)
Miconazole Nitrate Ointment (various; many proprietary named products)	Ointment: 2%	OTC	Depending on product: 4 gm package; 30, 57, 56.7, 113, 142 g
Miconazole Nitrate Spray (various; many proprietary named products)	Aerosol Spray or Powder: 2%	OTC	30, 43, 85, 85, 90, 113, 133 g cans

Product	Form: Concentration	Label Status	Other Ingredients; Size(s)
Miconazole Nitrate Cream (various; many proprietary named products)	Cream: 2%	OTC	Depending on product: 14, 28, 35, 45, 56.7, 57, 92 g; 118 mL

Nystatin & Nystatin Combinations

(nye-sta-tin)

For oral use, see the monograph found in the main section.

Indications/Actions

Because of limited dosage forms and other alternative anti-yeast medications readily available, nystatin is not usually used alone in small animal medicine. The combination products (*e.g., Panalog®,* etc.) can be useful for topical lesions caused by yeasts or yeast-like organisms; they have been used for mixed otitis infections for many years.

Nystatin has efficacy against many yeasts and yeast-like organisms (Malassezia). Its mechanism of action is believed secondary to binding to sterols in the fungal cell membranes thereby increasing membrane permeability with leakage of intracellular components. Nystatin does not have activity against bacteria and is ineffective against other fungi.

Suggested Dosages/Use

Nystatin (topical) is rarely used alone in veterinary medicine. In humans, the cream is usually used instead of the ointment in treating candidal-infections involving intertriginous areas; nystatin topical powder is best used for very moist lesions.

Nystatin products that contain triamcinolone are best suited for focal (*e.g.,* pedal) or multifocal lesions for relatively short durations (*e.g.,* <2 months). Initially, topical corticosteroids are usually used sparingly 1-4 times per day and then frequency is tapered when control is achieved.

Precautions/Adverse Effects

Avoid contact with eyes. Clients should wash hands after application or wear gloves when applying

Nystatin alone is very safe, although hypersensitivity reactions are possible. The combination veterinary products are usually well tolerated when used on skin. Neomycin can cause localized sensitivity and those containing glucocorticoids can potentially cause cutaneous atrophy HPA-axis suppression.

Veterinary-Labeled Topical Products

Product	Form: Concentration	Label Status	Other Ingredients; Comments; Size(s)
Panolog Cream® *Cortalone Cream®* *Animax Cream®* *Derma-Vet Cream®*	Cream: Nystatin 100,000 Units/g Triamcinolone Acet. 1 mg Neomycin Sulf. 2.5 mg Thiostrepton 2,500 Units	Rx	Aqueous vanishing cream. 7.5, 15 g.
Panolog Ointment® *Animax Ointment®* *Quadritop Ointment®* *Derma-Vet Ointment®* *Dermalog Ointment®* *Dermalone Ointment®* *EnteDerm Ointment®* *Resortin®*	Ointment: Nystatin 100,000 Units/g Triamcinolone Acet. 1 mg Neomycin Sulf. 2.5 mg Thiostrepton 2,500 Units	Rx	7.5, 15, 30, 240 mL

Human-Labeled Products

In addition to the products listed below, there are vaginal tablets and oral products. Oral products are found in the main section.

Product	Form: Concentration	Label Status	Other Ingredients; Size(s)
Nystatin (various); *Nyamyc®*; *Nystop®*; *Pedi-Dri®*	Powder: 100,000 Units/g (0.1 million Units/gm)	Rx	Depending on product: 15, 30, 56.7, 60 g.
Nystatin (various)	Ointment: 100,000 Units/g (0.1 million units/gm)	Rx	Depending on product: 15, 30 g.
Nystatin (various)	Cream: 100,000 Units/g (0.1 million Units/gm)	Rx	Depending on product: 15, 30 g.
Nystatin-Triamcinolone Acetonide (various)	Ointment: Nystatin 100,000 Units/g (0.1 million Units/gm) Triamcinolone Acet. 0.1%	Rx	Depending on product: 15, 30, 60 g.
Nystatin-Triamcinolone Acetonide (various)	Cream: Nystatin 100,000 Units/g (0.1 million Units/gm) Triamcinolone Acet. 0.1%, 1 mg/gm	Rx	Depending on product: 1.5 g. pkts, 15, 30, 60 g.

Selenium Sulfide

(si-leen-ee-um sul-fide)

Indications/Actions

Selenium sulfide may be useful in seborrheic disorders (mainly for seborrhea oleosa) and for adjunctive treatment of Malassezia dermatitis, particularly in dogs exhibiting signs of waxy, greasy or scaly (seborrheic) dermatitis. There may be some residual activity on the skin.

Selenium sulfide possesses antifungal (including sporicidal activity), keratolytic, keratoplastic and degreasing properties. It affects cells of the epidermis and follicular epithelium (alters the epidermal turnover) and interferes with hydrogen bond formation of keratin thereby reducing corneocyte production. Selenium sulfide's antifungal mechanism of action is not well understood.

Suggested Dosages/Use

Frequency of shampooing will vary according to the patient's needs. When using a medicated shampoo allow 10 minutes contact time. Another acceptable regimen is to allow the shampoo act for 3-5 minutes, rinse it thoroughly and thereafter repeat the procedure. Completely rinse to prevent skin irritation and/or excessive drying.

Precautions/Adverse Effects

Selenium sulfide products should **not be used on cats**. Avoid contact with eyes. Selenium sulfide can discolor jewelry. Clients should wear gloves when using these products.

Selenium sulfide can be irritating, cause excessive drying and hair-coat staining. Mucous membranes and scrotal areas may be particularly sensitive to the irritating effects of the drug.

After discontinuation, a rebound seborrhea can occur where signs could be worse than prior to treatment. Gastrointestinal effects (nausea, vomiting, diarrhea) may occur selenium sulfide is ingested orally. Neurologic signs are possible if large quantities are ingested. Contact an animal poison center if a substantial oral ingestion occurs.

Veterinary-Labeled Products

There apparently are no labeled veterinary products containing selenium sulfide currently available in the USA; *Seleen®* may be available in other countries.

Human-Labeled Products

Product (Company)	Form: Concentration	Label Status	Other Ingredients; Size(s)
Selenium Sulfide (various); *Selsun Blue®*; *Dandrex®*	Shampoo/Lotion: 1%	OTC	Depending on product: 207, 240 mL
Selenium Sulfide (various); *Selsun®*; *Tersi®*	Lotion: 2.5%	Rx	Depending on product: 70, 118, 120 mL

Terbinafine HCl, Topical

(ter-bin-a-feen)   Lamisil®

For systemic use, see the monograph found in the main section

Indications/Actions

An allylamine antifungal agent, terbinafine may be useful for localized lesions associated with *Malassezia*. With its current topical dosage forms, it does not appear to be very useful for treating dermatophytosis in cats.

Terbinafine inhibits the biosynthesis of ergosterol, but its mechanism for inhibiting ergosterol is different from the azole antifungals. Terbinafine inhibits the fungal squalene epoxidase enzyme. The resultant depletion of ergosterol within the fungal cell membrane and the intracellular accumulation of squalene are believed to be responsible for the fungicidal effect of terbinafine. It is fungicidal against dermatophytes, but may only be fungistatic against yeasts.

Suggested Dosages/Use

Topical terbinafine is not commonly used in veterinary medicine at present, but it could be used topically to affected areas once to twice a day.

Precautions/Adverse Effects

Avoid contact with eyes and mucous membranes. Clients should wash hands after application or wear gloves when applying. Skin irritation is possible, but unlikely to occur.

Veterinary-Labeled Products

None.

Human-Labeled Products

Product	Form: Concentration	Label Status	Other Ingredients; Size(s)
LamiSIL AT®, various generic	Cream: 1%	OTC	12, 15, 24, 30, 36, 42 g
LamiSIL® Spray	Solution: 1%	Rx	Alcohol. 30 mL
Lamisil Advanced®	Gel: 1%	OTC	Ethanol, propylene glycol. 12 g

Keratolytic Agents

Also see the:

- **Benzoyl Peroxide** monograph in the Antibacterials section
- **Phytosphingosine** monograph in the Non-Corticosteroid Antipruritic/Antiinflammatories section
- **Selenium Sulfide** monograph in the Antifungals section

Salicylic Acid
(sal-i-sil-ic ass-id)

Indications/Actions

Often combined with sulfur, salicylic acid shampoos are employed to treat patients with seborrheic disorders (seborrhea sicca and oleosa) exhibiting mild to moderate scaling, with mild waxy and keratinous debris. When combined with benzoyl peroxide, salicylic acid and sulfur containing shampoos can also be used to manage seborrhea oleosa. In higher concentrations, topicals such as *Solva-Ker®* Gel (6.6% salicylic acid) can be used to remove localized excessive tissues associated with hyperkeratotic disorders, such as calluses and idiopathic thickening of the planum nasale and footpads.

Salicylic acid has mildly antipruritic, antibacterial (bacteriostatic), keratoplastic and keratolytic actions. Lower concentrations are primarily keratoplastic and higher concentrations, keratolytic. Salicylic acid lowers skin pH, increases corneocyte hydration and dissolves the intercellular binder between corneocytes. Salicylic acid and sulfur are thought to be synergistic in their keratolytic actions.

Suggested Dosages/Use

Frequency of shampooing will vary according to the patient's needs. When using a medicated shampoo allow 10 minutes contact time. Another acceptable regimen is to allow the shampoo act for 3-5 minutes, rinse it thoroughly and thereafter repeat the procedure. Completely rinse to prevent skin irritation and/or excessive drying.

Precautions/Adverse Effects

Avoid contact with eyes, mucous membranes and open sores/cuts. Clients should wash hands after application or wear gloves when applying.

Skin irritation is possible. Burning, itching, pain, erythema, swelling can occur from salicylic acid, particularly when used in higher concentrations (>2%). A rebound seborrheic effect can occur.

Veterinary-Labeled Products

Product (Company)	Form: Concentration	Label Status	Other Ingredients; Size(s)
Solva-Ker Gel® (VetriMax)	Gel: 6.6%	Rx	Labeled for use on dogs, cats, & horses. Rub in well. Usually used once daily initially, may reduced to 2-3 times per week once remission occurs. Often requires life-long treatment. 30 mL
Derma-Clens® Cream (Zoetis)	Cream: Salicylic acid, Benzoic acid, Malic acid. Concentrations not listed (proprietary).	OTC	Labeled as an acidic cleansing cream for use on wounds, abrasions, burns, and other dermatological conditions. 1oz, 14 oz.
Stanisol® Spray (QA Labs)	Spray: Salicylic acid 1%, tannic acid 5.7%, boric acid 2.6%	OTC	Labeled for moist dermatitis. 4 oz.
Dermazole Shampoo® (Virbac)	Shampoo: Miconazole 2%, Salicylic Acid 2%	Rx	6, 16 oz.
Sebolux Shampoo® (Virbac)	Shampoo: Salicylic Acid 2%, Sulfur 2%	Rx	Chitosanide, urea, glycerin. Ingredients in free form and in Spherulites®. Shake well; wear gloves. 8, 16 oz; 1 gal
Sebosal-T® Shampoo (Clipper)	Shampoo: Salicylic acid 3%, Coal Tar 2%, Menthol 1%	Rx	Labeled for dogs; do not use on cats. 12 oz.
Dermabenss® Shampoo® (Dechra)	Shampoo: Benzoyl peroxide 2.5%, sodium thiosulfate 1%, Salicylic Acid 1%	OTC	Moisturizing factors, Vitamin E. 8 oz, 1 gal
Micro Pearls Advantage Seba-Hex Shampoo® (Vetoquinol)	Shampoo: Chlorhexidine 2%, Salicylic Acid 2%, Sulfur 2%	OTC	*Novasome®* microvesicles. Labeled for dogs, cats and horses. Shake well; wear gloves. 12 oz, 1 gal.
Keraseb® Shampoo (Schuyler)	Shampoo: Salicylic Acid 2%, Sulfur 2%	OTC	12 oz.
Gentleseb Shampoo +PS® (Sogeval) *PhytoVet S Shampoo* (Schein)	Shampoo: Salicylic Acid 2%, Sulfur 2%, Phytosphingosine	OTC	8, 16 oz, 1 gal.
Oxibenz-3 Shampoo® (Clipper) *Peroxiderm S Shampoo®* (Schein)	Shampoo: Benzoyl peroxide 3%, Sulfur 2%, Salicylic acid 2%	OTC	8, 12, 16 oz

Product (Company)	Form: Concentration	Label Status	Other Ingredients; Size(s)
Oxiderm® +PS Shampoo (Sogeval) *PhytoVet PSS Shampoo®* (Schein)	Shampoo: Benzoyl peroxide 3%, Sulfur 2%, Salicylic acid 2%, Phytosphingosine	OTC	8, 16 oz.
Peroxiderm Shampoo® (Schuyler) *Sulfur Benz Shampoo®* (Davis)	Shampoo: Benzoyl peroxide 2.5%, Sulfur 1%, Salicylic Acid 1%	OTC	12 oz., 1 gal.

Human-Labeled Products

Note: There are many topical salicylic acid products labeled for human use, including topical creams, ointments, transdermal patches, liquids and gels that are principally labeled for wart removal. Except for one product (*Salex®*; 6% cream), they are available OTC. There are also many OTC skin cleansers and shampoos containing salicylic acid and usually sulfur (sometimes coal tar or menthol). As there are several similar products formulated and labeled for animal use, human products will not be listed. For more information on these products, refer to a comprehensive human drug reference or contact a pharmacist.

Sulfur, Precipitated
(sul-fer)

Indications/Actions

Often combined with salicylic acid, sulfur-containing shampoos are often employed to treat patients with seborrheic disorders exhibiting mild to moderate scaling, with mild waxiness and keratinous debris.

Sulfur has keratoplastic and keratolytic actions. Lower concentrations of sulfur are primarily keratoplastic secondary to assisting conversion of cysteine to cystine, thought an important factor in the maturation of corneocytes. Like salicylic acid, sulfur's keratolytic effects increase with concentration. Salicylic acid and sulfur are believed synergistic in their keratolytic actions. Sulfur also has mild degreasing effects and can be mildly antipruritic.

Sulfur also has antibacterial, antifungal, and antiparasitic effects secondary to sulfur conversion to hydrogen sulfide and pentathionic acid by bacteria and keratocytes.

Suggested Dosages/Use

Frequency of shampooing will vary according to the patient's needs. When using a medicated shampoo allow 10 minutes contact time. Another acceptable regimen is to allow the shampoo act for 3-5 minutes, rinse it thoroughly and thereafter repeat the procedure. Completely rinse to prevent skin irritation and/or excessive drying.

Precautions/Adverse Effects

Avoid contact with eyes, mucous membranes and open sores/cuts. Clients should wash hands after application or wear gloves when applying.

Skin irritation is possible. Sulfur can be drying, cause pruritus and be irritating. Residual odor is often bothersome to clients. Sulfur may stain fabrics and hair. A rebound seborrheic effect can occur when using shampoo products containing sulfur.

Veterinary-Labeled Products

Product (Company)	Form: Concentration	Label Status	Other Ingredients; Size(s)
Sebolux Shampoo® (Virbac)	Shampoo: Salicylic Acid 2%, Sulfur 2%	Rx	Chitosanide, urea, glycerin. Ingredients in free form and in Spherulites®. Shake well; wear gloves. 8, 16 oz; 1 gal
Dermabenss® Shampoo® (Dechra)	Shampoo: Benzoyl peroxide 2.5%, sodium thiosulfate 1%, Salicylic Acid 1%	OTC	Moisturizing factors, Vitamin E. 8 oz, 1 gal
Micro Pearls Advantage Seba-Hex Shampoo® (Vetoquinol)	Shampoo: Chlorhexidine 2%, Salicylic Acid 2%, Sulfur 2%	OTC	*Novasome®* microvesicles. Labeled for dogs, cats and horses. Shake well; wear gloves. 12 oz, 1 gal.
Keraseb® Shampoo (Schuyler)	Shampoo: Salicylic Acid 2%, Sulfur 2%	OTC	12 oz.
Gentleseb Shampoo +PS® (Sogeval) *PhytoVet S® Shampoo* (Schein)	Shampoo: Salicylic Acid 2%, Sulfur 2%, Phytosphingosine	OTC	8, 16 oz, 1 gal.
Oxibenz-3 Shampoo® (Clipper) *Peroxiderm S Shampoo®* (Schein)	Shampoo: Benzoyl peroxide 3%, Sulfur 2%, Salicylic acid 2%	OTC	8, 12, 16 oz
Oxiderm® +PS Shampoo (Sogeval) *PhytoVet PSS Shampoo®* (Schein)	Shampoo: Benzoyl peroxide 3%, Sulfur 2%, Salicylic acid 2%, Phytosphingosine	OTC	8, 16 oz.
Peroxiderm Shampoo® (Schuyler) *Sulfur Benz Shampoo®* (Davis)	Shampoo: Benzoyl peroxide 2.5%, Sulfur 1%, Salicylic Acid 1%	OTC	12 oz., 1 gal.
Paraguard Shampoo® (RXV)	Shampoo: Captan 2%, Sulfur 1%	OTC	Labeled as an anti-ringworm, antifungal, antibacterial shampoo for dogs, cats & horses. 32 oz.

Human-Labeled Products

Note: There are several topical products containing sulfur labeled for human use, including topical creams, lotions, shampoos, soaps and masks that are principally labeled for acne or dandruff. For more information on these products, refer to a comprehensive human drug reference (*e.g.*, *Facts and Comparisons*) or contact a pharmacist.

Coal Tar & Coal Tar Combinations

(kole tar)

Indications/Actions

Use of coal tar containing shampoos in veterinary medicine is somewhat controversial, particularly since almost all veterinary-labeled products have been withdrawn from the market. However, coal tar shampoos have been used in dogs for treating greasy dermatoses (seborrhea oleosa) for many years.

Coal tar possesses keratoplastic, keratolytic, vasoconstrictive, antipruritic, and degreasing actions. Coal tar's mechanism of keratoplastic (keratoregulating) action is probably secondary to decreasing mitosis and DNA synthesis of basal epidermal cells.

Suggested Dosages/Use

Frequency of shampooing will vary according to the patient's needs. When using a medicated shampoo allow 10 minutes contact time. Another acceptable regimen is to allow the shampoo act for 3-5 minutes, rinse it thoroughly and thereafter repeat the procedure. Completely rinse to prevent skin irritation and/or excessive drying.

Precautions/Adverse Effects

The carcinogenic risks associated with coal tar products are hotly debated. At present, most (including the FDA) believe that coal tar products with concentrations of 5% or less are safe for human use. However, should they be used on animals, clients should wear gloves when applying and wash off any product that contacts their skin. Carcinogenic risk assessment for dogs using coal tar products was not located.

Coal tar products should **not be used on cats**, patients who have prior sensitivity reactions to tar products or have dry scaling dermatoses.

Be careful in comparing coal tar concentrations on labels. Coal tar solution contains approximately 20% coal tar extract or refined tar. For example, a 10% coal tar solution contains approximately 2% coal tar (refined).

Photosensitization, skin drying and skin irritation are possible with tar therapy. Adverse effects are more likely with tar concentrations >3%. Residual odor is often bothersome to clients. Tar may stain fabrics or haircoats and discolor jewelry.

Veterinary-Labeled Products

Product (Company)	Form: Concentration	Label Status	Other Ingredients; Comments; Size(s)
Sebosal-T® Shampoo (Clipper)	Shampoo: Salicylic acid 3%, Coal Tar 2%, Menthol 1%	Rx	Labeled for dogs; do not use on cats. 12 oz.
Imrex Tar and Sulphur Shampoo® (Imrex)	Shampoo: Salicylic acid 2%, Sulfur 2%, Coal Tar 3%, Chloroxylenol 0.6%	OTC	Labeled for dogs; do not use on cats. 8 oz.
Sulfodene Shampoo® (Farnam)	Shampoo: Coal tar, Sulfur, Triclosan; %'s not listed	OTC	Labeled for dogs; do not use on cats. 8, 12 oz.
Sulfur and Tar Shampoo® (Davis)	Shampoo: Sulfur, Coal Tar, Salicylic Acid, Zinc Oxide, Menthol and Aloe Vera; %'s not listed	OTC	Labeled for dogs; do not use on cats. 12 oz, 1 gal.

Human-Labeled Products

There are also several products labeled for human use containing coal tar, including ointments, lotions, and creams, available in concentrations ranging from 0.5-5% coal tar (not coal tar extract).

Product	Form: Concentration (Concentrations listed as refined tar or extract)	Label Status	Other Ingredients; Size(s)
DHS Tar®, Tera-Gel®, Polytar®	Shampoo: Coal Tar 0.5%	OTC	120, 177, 240, 355, 480 mL
Ionil T®, PC-Tar, Zetar®	Shampoo: Coal Tar 1%	OTC	180, 473 mL
Neutrogena T/Gel Original®	Shampoo: Coal Tar 2%	OTC	132,255, 480 mL
MG 217 Medicated Tar®	Shampoo: Coal Tar 3%	OTC	120, 240 mL

Antiseborrheic Products

See the:

- **Benzoyl Peroxide** monograph in the Antibacterials section
- **Essential Fatty Acids, Topical** monograph in the Non-Corticosteroid Antipruritic/Antiinflammatories section
- **Phytosphingosine** monograph in the Non-Corticosteroid Antipruritic/Antiinflammatories section
- **Selenium Sulfide** monograph in the Antifungals section
- **Salicylic Acid**, **Sulfur** and **Coal Tar** monographs in the Keratolytics section

Immunomodulators, Topical

Imiquimod, Topical
(imi-i-kwi-mod)   Aldara®

Indications/Actions

An immune response modifier, imiquimod may be useful in the treatment of a variety of topical conditions in animals. It is labeled for use on humans as a treatment for genital or perianal warts, superficial basal cell carcinomas and actinic keratoses of the face and scalp. In dogs and cats, imiquimod potentially may be of benefit in treating feline herpes virus dermatitis, actinic keratosis, squamous cell carcinoma and Bowen's disease, papillomas virus lesions, and localized solar dermatitis or solar carcinoma *in situ*. Many of these indications are based upon anecdotal evidence, as there are very few studies published for veterinary use. In horses, imiquimod has been anecdotally used with success in treating sarcoids.

Imiquimod stimulates the patient's own immune system to release a variety of cytokines including interferon-alpha and interleukin-12. This locally generated cytokine milieu induces a Th1-immune response with the generation of cytotoxic effectors Imiquimod itself does not have in vitro activity against wart viruses, but stimulates monocytes and macrophages to release cytokines that induce a regression in viral protein production.

Suggested Dosages/Use

Use in animals is still rather limited and ongoing research on this agent is being performed. Doses and treatment regimens will vary depending on the disease treated and tolerance to the drug. At present, dosing ranges from applying a thin film once daily to 2-3 times weekly or every-other-week. Treatment duration and frequency may need to be adjusted depending on patient response and adverse reactions.

Precautions/Adverse Effects

Clients administering the drug should wear gloves when handling or applying the cream. It is advised to avoid getting in eyes or on mucous membranes; but dogs with oral mucosal papillomas have been treated without significant problems. While there are low chances the drug would be absorbed systemically, do not allow animal to groom/lick the applied site; occlusive dressings should not be used over the treatment site. Application site should not be touched after application. Avoid exposure of the site to sunlight; there is concern that there may be an increased risk for sunburn after use (not proven).

Local skin reactions are common with imiquimod therapy and include application site reactions: erythema, burning, tenderness, pain, irritation, oozing/exudate and erosion. Treatment duration and frequency may need to be adjusted depending on response and irritant reactions. Depigmentation and hair loss may occur at application sites as post-treatment sequelae.

Veterinary-Labeled Products
None.

Human-Labeled Products

Product	Form: Concentration	Label Status	Other Ingredients; Size(s)
Aldara®, generic	Cream: 5%	Rx	Cetyl alcohol, stearyl alcohol, white petrolatum, benzyl alcohol, parabens. Single use 250 mg packets in boxes of 1, 12 or 24.
Zyclara®	Cream: 2.5, 3.75%	Rx	7.5 g pump bottles, ingle use 250 mg packets in boxes of 28.

Pimecrolimus, Topical
(pim-e-kroe-li-mus)   Elidel®

Indications/Actions

A relatively new addition to the human topical armamentarium, pimecrolimus cream may be of benefit in veterinary patients in the adjunctive treatment of atopic dermatitis, discoid lupus erythematosus, pemphigus erythematosus or foliaceous, pinnal vascular disease or other cutaneous vasculopathies, alopecia areata, vitiligo, perianal fistulas (terminal phase or maintenance treatment after cyclosporine therapy), and for feline proliferative and necrotizing otitis externa. Unlike topical corticosteroids, pimecrolimus does not have atrophogenic or metabolic effects associated with long-term or large area treatment.

Pimecrolimus acts similarly as cyclosporine and tacrolimus, namely inhibiting T-lymphocyte activation primarily by inhibiting the phosphatase activity of calcineurin. It also inhibits the release of inflammatory cytokines and mediators from mast cells and basophils. Pimecrolimus may not have identical mechanisms of action as tacrolimus, as it did not impair the primary immune response (as did tacrolimus) in mice after a contact sensitizer was applied. Both drugs did impair the secondary response however. Any clinical significance associated with this difference is not yet clear.

Suggested Dosages/Use
Only limited experience has occurred with this drug in veterinary patients. Most dosing recommendations are to use the product twice daily until signs are controlled, then reduce application frequency to the fewest times that allow control of the disease.

Precautions/Adverse Effects
Both tacrolimus and pimecrolimus have FDA-mandated "black box" warnings that use may increase risks for skin cancer and lymphomas in humans, although a causal relationship has not been established. Because of the rarity of these occurrences in humans, these drugs are probably relatively safe to use in veterinary patients. However, clients should be informed and instructed to wear gloves or use an applicator (*e.g.*, a Q-tip) when applying the cream. The long-term adverse effects of topical pimecrolimus are currently unknown; therefore, it is prudent to avoid using this medication on a continuous maintenance basis. When long-term treatment is required, the ultimate goal should be to achieve the lowest possible dose that keeps the disease under control.

Topical pimecrolimus appears well tolerated in dogs, but localized irritation and pruritus have been reported in humans and dogs using the drug. Early anecdotal reports state that pimecrolimus may be less irritating than tacrolimus in dogs, but that it also may not be as effective. The cost of the medication may be prohibitive for some clients.

Veterinary-Labeled Products
None.

Human-Labeled Products

Product (Company)	Form: Concentration	Label Status	Other Ingredients; Size(s)
Elidel® (Valeant)	Cream: 1%	Rx	30, 60, 100 g.

Tacrolimus, Topical
(ta-kroe-li-mus)   Protopic®

Indications/Actions
Tacrolimus ointment may be of benefit in veterinary patients in the adjunctive treatment of atopic dermatitis, discoid lupus erythematosus, pemphigus erythematosus or foliaceous, pinnal vascular disease, alopecia areata, vitiligo and for perianal fistulas (terminal phase or maintenance treatment after cyclosporine therapy). Unlike topical corticosteroids, tacrolimus or pimecrolimus do not have atrophogenic or metabolic effects associated with long-term or large area treatment.

Tacrolimus acts similarly as cyclosporine, namely inhibiting T-lymphocyte activation primarily by inhibiting the phosphatase activity of calcineurin. It also inhibits the release of inflammatory cytokines and mediators from mast cells and basophils.

Suggested Dosages/Use
Only limited experience has occurred with this drug in veterinary patients. Most dosing recommendations are to use the product twice daily until signs are controlled, then reduce application frequency to the fewest times that allow control of the disease.

Precautions/Adverse Effects
Both tacrolimus and pimecrolimus have FDA-mandated "black box" warnings that use may increase risks for skin cancer and lymphomas in humans, although a causal relationship has not been established. Because of the rarity of these occurrences in humans, these drugs are probably relatively safe to use in veterinary patients. However, clients should be informed and instructed to wear gloves or use an applicator (*e.g.*, a Q-tip) when applying the ointment. The long-term adverse effects of topical tacrolimus are currently unknown; therefore, it is prudent to avoid using this medication on a continuous maintenance basis. When long-term treatment is required, the ultimate goal should be to achieve the lowest possible dose that keeps the disease under control.

The commercially available ointment should not be used as, or compounded into an ophthalmic preparation for treating KCS in dogs as it contains propylene carbonate, a known ocular toxin.

Thus far, topical tacrolimus is appears to be well tolerated in dogs, but localized irritation and pruritus have been reported in humans and dogs using the drug. Early anecdotal reports state that pimecrolimus may be less irritating than tacrolimus in dogs, but that it may also not be as effective. The cost of the medication may be cost prohibitive for some clients.

Veterinary-Labeled Products
None.

Human-Labeled Products

Product (Company)	Form: Concentration	Label Status	Other Ingredients; Size(s)
Protopic® (Astellas)	Ointment: 0.03, 0.1%	Rx	30, 60, 100 g.

Retinoids, Topical

Tretinoin (trans-Retinoic Acid; Vitamin A Acid)
(tret-in-oyn)   Retin-A®

Indications/Actions

Topical tretinoin may be useful in treating localized follicular or hyperkeratotic disorders such as acanthosis nigrans, idiopathic nasal and footpad hyperkeratosis, callous pyodermas, or chin acne.

Tretinoin's exact mechanism of action is not well understood, but it stimulates cellular mitotic activity, increases cell turnover, and decreases the cohesiveness of follicular epithelial cells.

Suggested Dosages/Use

In small animals, topical tretinoin gel is usually used initially at a concentration of 0.05% and is applied once daily. Treatment continues as long as the animal tolerates the treatment or until controlled. Once controlled, usage is then reduced to as needed. In animals unable to tolerate therapy, concentration may be reduced to 0.025-0.01% in an attempt to balance efficacy with adverse effects.

Precautions/Adverse Effects

Avoid sun exposure during treatment with tretinoin. Avoid contact with eyes, nostrils, inner ears, or mouth. Clients should wear gloves when applying the product.

Adverse effects can include hypersensitivity reactions or local irritation (erythema, dryness, peeling, pruritus).

Veterinary-Labeled Products

None.

Human-Labeled Products

Product	Form: Concentration	Label Status	Other Ingredients; Size(s)
Tretinoin Cream (various); *Retin-A®, Renova®, Avita®, Altinac®, Tretin-X®, Refissa®*	Cream: 0.02, 0.025, 0.038, 0.05, 0.1%	Rx	40, 44, 45, 60 g.
Tretinoin Gel (various); *Retin-A®, Retin-A Micro®, Atralin®, Avita®*	Gel: 0.01, 0.025, 0.04, 0.05%	Rx	15, 45 g. *Retin-A Micro®* is in microspheres. 20, 45, 50 g.

Antiparasitic Agents, Topical

For agents such as **eprinomectin, ivermectin, levamisole, moxidectin** and **selamectin** that may be administered topically, but absorbed through the skin to treat internal parasites as well as external parasites, refer to the monographs in the main (systemic drugs) section of the reference. Also see monographs in the main section for those products administered orally for their external parasitic actions, including **lufenuron, nitenpyram, milbemycin,** and **spinosad.**

Amitraz & Amitraz Combinations
(a-mi-traz)   Mitaban®

Indications/Actions

In dogs, amitraz solution is used topically primarily in the treatment of generalized demodicosis. A topical spot-on solution (*Certifect®* for Dogs) and a collar (*Preventic®*) are available for treatment and prevention of flea and tick infestation. It is also used as a general insecticidal/miticidal agent in several other species (see label information). The pharmacologic action of amitraz is not well understood, but it is a monoamine oxidase (MAO) inhibitor (in mites) and may have effects on the CNS of susceptible organisms. It apparently also possesses alpha-2 adrenergic activity and inhibits prostaglandin synthesis. Amitraz can cause a significant increase in plasma glucose levels, presumably by inhibiting insulin release via its alpha2-adrenergic activity. Yohimbine (alpha2 blocker) or atipamezole can antagonize this effect.

Suggested Dosages/Use

- **DOGS:**

  For treatment of generalized demodicosis: Note: The general <u>rule of thumb</u> for therapy duration independent of the protocol chosen involves treating for 30 days past two consecutive negative skin scrapings.

  <u>Labeled Dose Protocol:</u> Long and medium haired dogs should be clipped closely and given a shampoo with mild soap and water prior to first treatment. Topically treat at a concentration of 250 ppm (one 10.6 mL bottle of *Mitaban®* in 2 gallons of warm water), by applying to entire animal and allowing to air dry. DO NOT rinse or towel dry. Use a freshly prepared dilution for additional dogs or additional treatments. Repeat every 14 days for 3-6 treatments (continue until 6 treatments done or 2 successive skin scrapings demonstrate no live mites). Chronic cases may require additional courses of therapy. (Package Insert; *Mitaban®*—Upjohn)

  <u>Extra-label Protocols:</u>

  1) For dogs whose owners accept the risk of using the drug in an "unlicensed" manner with the goal of increasing efficacy, first try the 250 ppm solution (as above) <u>once weekly</u> for 4 weeks. If positive response is seen, continue treatment for an additional 30 days after

obtaining two consecutive negative skin scrapings (rule of thumb). If weekly 250-ppm application fails, a 500-ppm solution may be tried (1 bottle in 1 gallon of water) weekly as above. In dogs failing 500 ppm, 1000 ppm may also be attempted, but likelihood of toxicity increases and the authors have no experience using this high concentration. If these methods fail, the dog is unlikely to be cured using amitraz.

2) Prepare a 0.125% solution by diluting 1 mL of the 12.5% commercially available large animal product (*Taktic®*) in 100 mL of water. Using a sponge rub the diluted solution (0.125%) <u>daily onto one-half of the dog's body and alternate sides on a daily basis</u>. Air dry. During the first week of therapy, keep dog hospitalized and observe for adverse effects.

Follow rule of thumb above for duration of therapy. Dogs with severe pododemodicosis should be also treated with daily foot soaks of the 0.125% solution. Dogs with otic demodicosis can be treated with a diluted solution of amitraz (1 mL of Tactic in 8.5 mL of mineral oil) every 3-7 days unless irritation develops. Owners accepting the extra-label therapy, must be carefully screened and trained to carefully handle the amitraz solutions.

- **CATS:**
  For follicular demodicosis (*Demodex cati*) (extra-label): Dilute amitraz to 0.0125% (125 ppm) and apply every 7-14 days. Monitor cats very closely for potential side effects. Place an Elizabethan-collar until the solution is completely dry.

  For surface demodicosis (*Demodex gatoi*) (extra-label): Dilute amitraz to 0.0125% (125 ppm) and apply every 7 days for 12 weeks. Monitor cats very closely for potential side effects. Place an Elizabethan-collar until the solution is completely dry. (Saari S. AM. et al. Acta Veterinaria Scandinavica; 51:40, 2009).

- **SMALL MAMMALS**
  Mice, Rats, Gerbils, Hamsters, Guinea pigs, Chinchillas (extra-label): 1.4 mL per liter topically every 2 weeks (q14 days) for 3-6 treatments. Caution: Not recommended in young animals or rabbits. (Adamcak, A. & B. Otten (2000). Rodent Therapeutics. Vet Clin NA: Exotic Anim Pract 3:1(Jan): 221-240)

Precautions/Adverse Effects/Drug Interactions

Amitraz liquid concentrates are flammable until diluted with water. Do not stress animals for at least 24 hours after application of *Mitaban®*. When mixing with water, protect exposed skin with rubber gloves, etc. After application to anima, wash hands and arms well. Dispose of unused diluted solution by flushing down the drain. Rinse *Mitaban®* container with water and dispose; do not re-use. Do not re-use collar or container; wrap in newspaper and throw in trash. Avoid inhalation of vapors. Animals treated may exhibit signs of sedation; if animal cannot be aroused or sedation persists for longer than 72 hours, contact your veterinarian.

Safety has not been demonstrated in dogs <4 months of age. The manufacturer of *Mitaban®* does not recommend use in these animals. Toy breeds may be more susceptible to CNS effects (transient sedation); lower dose rates (1/2 of recommended) have been recommended in these breeds. Because of the drug's effects on plasma glucose, use with caution in brittle diabetic patients. Reproductive safety has not been established. Use only when benefits outweigh potential risks of therapy

The most commonly reported adverse effect after amitraz topical administration is transient sedation that may persist for up to 72 hours (24 hours is usual). If treating around eyes, use an ophthalmic protectant (*e.g.*, petrolatum ophthalmic ointment) before treating. Do not use if dog has deep pyodermas with drainage tracts; postpone application until lesions improve after treating with antibiotic and shampoo therapy. Other adverse effects include: ataxia, bradycardia, vomiting, diarrhea, hypothermia and a transient hyperglycemia. Rarely, seizures have been reported. Topical effects can include edema, erythema and pruritus. Adverse effects are more likely to be seen in debilitated, geriatric, or very small breed dogs.

Amitraz can be toxic to cats and rabbits and it is probably best to avoid its use in these species, although amitraz has been used safely in cats in diluted form for the treatment of demodicosis.

Amitraz may be toxic if swallowed (by either animals or humans). Beagles receiving 4 mg/kg PO daily for 90 days, demonstrated transient ataxia, CNS depression, hyperglycemia, decreased pulse rates and lowered body temperature. No animals died.

Amitraz toxicity can be significant if amitraz-containing insecticide collars are ingested. Treatment should consist of emesis, retrieval of the collar using endoscopy if possible and administration of activated charcoal and a cathartic to remove any remaining collar fragments. Because of the risk of an increased chance of gastric dilatation, gastrotomy may not be a viable option. Yohimbine at a dose of 0.11 – 0.2 mg/kg IV (start with low dosage) may be of benefit for overdose effects. Because yohimbine has a short half-life it may need to be repeated, particularly if the animal has ingested an amitraz-containing collar that has not been retrieved from the GI tract. Atipamezole has also been used to treat amitraz toxicity; refer to that monograph for more information. Contact a poison center for more information, if necessary.

Because of their immunosuppressive effects, **corticosteroids** and **other immunosuppressant drugs** (*e.g.*, **azathioprine, cyclophosphamide**, etc.) should not be used in animals with demodicosis.

Amitraz may interact with other MAO inhibitors (including **selegiline**) or tricyclic antidepressants (**amitriptyline, clomipramine**). Concomitant use is not recommended.

Clients should wear gloves when applying and wash off any product that contacts their skin.

Veterinary-Labeled Products

Product (Company)	Form: Concentration	Label Status	Other Ingredients; Comments; Size(s)
Mitaban® (Zoetis)	Solution for Dilution: 19.9%	Rx	10.6 mL btls. FDA labeled and approved for use on dogs. Note: Liquid is flammable until diluted.
Taktic® EC (Merck)	Solution (emulsifiable concentrate) for Dilution: 12.5%	OTC-EPA	760 mL cans. EPA labeled for use on swine, dairy or beef cattle. Label states not to use on dogs or horses.

Product (Company)	Form: Concentration	Label Status	Other Ingredients; Comments; Size(s)
Certifect® for Dogs (Merial)	Spot-On Solution: Side A: fipronil 9.8%, (S)-methoprene 8.8%; Side B: Amitraz 22.1%	OTC-EPA	For dogs and puppies 8 weeks of age or older and at least 5 lbs. body weight. Not for cats. 1.7, 2.14, 4.28 & 6.42 mL/applicator.
Preventic® (Virbac)	Collar: 9% Amitraz; 25 inch	OTC-EPA	18 & 25 in. adjustable (cut off excess). EPA labeled for dogs 12 weeks and older only. Effective for 3 months.

Human-Labeled Products
None.

Crotamiton
(kroe-ta-mye-ton) Eurax®

Indications/Actions
Crotamiton is a topical miticide/scabicide and has been used primarily for adjunctive treatment (with ivermectin) for treating mite infections (*e.g.*, *Knemidopkoptes*) in birds. Crotamiton has both miticidal and antipruritic actions, but the mechanism for each is not known.

Suggested Dosages/Use
Once to twice daily applications are usually recommended.

Precautions/Adverse Effects
Do not apply around eyes or mouth. Little is known of the compound's safety profile; irritation or hypersensitivity reactions are possible.

Veterinary-Labeled Products
None.

Human-Labeled Topical Products

Product (Company)	Form: Concentration	Label Status	Other Ingredients; Size(s)
Eurax® (Ranbaxy)	Cream: 10%	Rx	Cetyl alcohol, vanishing base. 60 g.
Eurax® (Ranbaxy)	Lotion: 10%	Rx	Cetyl alcohol, emollient base. 60, 454 g.

Deltamethrin
(del-ta-meeth-rin)

Indications/Actions
In the United States, deltamethrin-impregnated collars are labeled for killing fleas and ticks on dogs. In countries where leishmaniasis is a problem, deltamethrin-impregnated collars are also indicated for repelling and killing the phlebotomine sandfly vectors.

Deltamethrin is a synthetic pyrethroid and acts by disrupting the sodium channel current in arthropod nerve cell membranes, resulting in paralysis and death.

Suggested Dosages/Use
The manufacturer recommends applying a new collar every 6 months and claims that maximum effect may not occur before 2-3 weeks after collar placement. Follow label for specific use instructions.

Precautions/Adverse Effects
Collars containing deltamethrin should not be used in dogs younger than 12 weeks of age. Avoid contact with eyes, skin or clothing. Consult a veterinarian before using on debilitated, pregnant, nursing, old or medicated animals. Skin reactions at the application site may occur. Mammalian exposure to deltamethrin is classified as safe; however, it should be used very carefully around water because deltamethrin is highly toxic to aquatic animals, especially fish.

Veterinary-Labeled Products

Product (Company)	Form: Concentration	Label Status	Other Ingredients; Size(s)
Scalibor® Protector Band for Dogs (Merck)	Collar: Deltamethrin 4%	OTC-EPA	One size fits all. 0.9 oz

Human-Labeled Products
None.

Dinotefuran + Pyriproxyfen (± Permethrin)

Indications/Actions
The product containing dinotefuran and pyriproxyfen (*Vectra®*) labeled for dogs and cats is used for control of adult and all immature flea stages including eggs, larvae and pupae. The exclusive dog product contains in addition to dinotefuran and pyriproxyfen, permethrin (*Vectra 3D®*), which kills and repels adult and immature fleas, ticks and mosquitoes.

Dinotefuran is a nitroguanidine, neonicotinoid insecticide with a structure similar to acetylcholine. It permanently binds to the same insect receptor sites as acetylcholine and activates the nerve impulse at the synapse causing stimulation, which results in tremors, incoordination and insect death. Dinotefuran does not bind to mammalian acetylcholine receptor sites.

The commercially available products also contain pyriproxyfen (a second-generation insect growth regulator) and, in the case of *Vectra 3D®* (for dogs only), permethrin.

Suggested Dosages/Use

Refer to the package information for specific instructions on application and dosages of dinotefuran-containing products. Monthly applications are recommended for dogs and cats. It is labeled for cats and kittens 8 weeks of age or older and dogs or puppies 7 weeks of age or older. Apparently bathing or swimming does not interfere with efficacy; however, the authors do not recommend bathing the pet until two days after application.

Precautions/Adverse Effects

The dog product containing permethrin (*Vectra 3D®*) **must not be used on cats or on dogs that cohabit with a cat.** The manufacturer recommends not using *Vectra 3D®* or *Vectra®* on debilitated, aged, medicated, pregnant or nursing animals and animals known to be sensitive to pesticide products. Mild transitory skin erythema may occur at the application site. Avoid eye and oral contact since Dinotefuran can cause substantial, but temporary eye irritation.

Veterinary-Labeled Products

Product (Company)	Form: Concentration	Label Status	Comments; Size(s)
Vectra® for Cats and Kittens (Ceva)	Topical Solution: Dinotefuran 22%, Pyriproxyfen 3%	EPA-OTC	For cats and kittens under 9 lbs. and over 8 weeks of age.
Vectra® for Cats (Ceva) *First Shield®* (Schuyler)	Topical Solution: Dinotefuran 22%, Pyriproxyfen 3%	EPA-OTC	For cats weighting 9 lbs. or over.
Vectra for Dogs & Puppies® (Ceva)	Topical Solution: Dinotefuran 22%, Pyriproxyfen 3%	EPA-OTC	Can be used on dogs and puppies 8 weeks of age or older. For dogs and puppies 2.5-10 lbs.– dose volume 1.3mL For dogs and puppies 11-20 lbs. – dose volume 2 mL For dogs 21-55 lbs. – dose volume 4 mL For dogs 56-100 lbs. – dose volume 6 mL
Vectra 3D® (Ceva) *First Shield Trio®* (Schuyler)	Topical Solution: Dinotefuran 4.95%, Pyriproxyfen 0.44%, Permethrin 36.08%	EPA-OTC	Must not be used on cats or on dogs that cohabit with a cat. For dogs and puppies 2.5-20 lbs., 7 weeks of age or over – dose volume 1.6 mL. For dogs and puppies 21-55 lbs., 7 weeks of age or over – dose volume 3.6 mL For dogs 56-95 lbs. – dose volume 4.7 mL For dogs over 95 lbs. – dose volume 8 mL

Human-Labeled Products

None.

Fipronil & Fipronil Combinations

(fip-roe-nil; meth-oh-preen)   Frontline®

Indications/Actions

In the USA, fipronil is indicated for the treatment of fleas, ticks and chewing lice infestations in dogs and cats. It has also been used successfully for *Trombicula autumnalis* (chigger) infestation, sarcoptic mange, cheyletiellosis, chewing lice and otoacariosis.

Fipronil is a phenylpyrazole antiparasitic agent that in invertebrates interferes with the passage of chloride ions in GABA regulated chloride channels, thereby disrupting CNS activity causing death of the flea or tick. The manufacturer states that fipronil collects in the oils of the skin and hair follicles and continues to be released over a period a time resulting in long residual activity. Topically applied, the drug apparently spreads over the body in approximately 24 hours via translocation.

When fipronil is combined with the insect growth regulator (S)-methoprene (*Frontline® Plus*), additionally flea eggs and flea larvae are killed. (S)-methoprene mimics flea juvenile growth hormone, halting development during metamorphosis and larval development. It also concentrates in female flea ovaries, causing non-viable eggs to be produced. Additional combination products with etofenprox, cyphenothrin or amitraz are available.

Suggested Dosages/Use

For fleas, ticks or chewing lice: Monthly treatments are usually recommended when used for fleas, ticks or chewing lice. See product labels for specific directions on administration and recommendations on bathing/swimming, etc. after administration.

For *Trombicula autumnalis* infestation: Fipronil spray (0.25%) is recommended Monthly applications throughout the trombiculid season at the dose of 3 – 6 mL/kg. It is important to thoroughly wet the coat with special emphasis on the areas typically affected (feet, ears, face, perineum and tail). In some cases, the interval between applications needs to be shortened to every 14 days.

For otoacariosis: Apply 0.05 mL of fipronil solution inside each ear canal and 0.4 mL between the shoulder blades. Resolution of clinical signs can be seen as early as seven days post-treatment. Additional applications may be needed. Fipronil needs to be applied in the ear canals to be effective.

Precautions/Adverse Effects

Do not use on puppies or kittens <8 weeks of age. This product is reportedly to be contraindicated in rabbits as deaths have occurred with the spray. Do not apply or spray in eyes. While temporary irritation may occur at the site of administration, animals that have demonstrated sensitivity reactions to fipronil or any of the ingredients in the product should probably not be retreated.

The manufacturer recommends consulting a veterinarian before using on debilitated, aged, or medicated patients.

Do not contaminate food or water and dispose of container properly. Avoid human contact with skin, eyes or clothing and wear gloves when applying/spraying. If using spray, do so in a well ventilated area. Avoid contact with animal until dry. Wash well with soap and water if contact occurs.

Product is labeled as remaining effective after bathing (but do not shampoo within 48 hours of application), water immersion, or exposure to sunlight. Spotted areas may appear wet or oily for up to 24 hours after application.

Temporary irritation may occur at the site of administration. Rarely, hypersensitivity has been reported.

Veterinary-Labeled Products

Product (Company)	Form: Concentration	Label Status	Other Ingredients; Comments; Size(s)
Frontline® Spray Treatment (Merial) *Martin's Flee®* (Control Solutions) *Spectra Sure®* (Durvet) *Sentry Fiproguard®* or *Pronyl OTC®* (Sergeant's)	Spray: 0.29% fipronil	OTC-EPA	Labeled for use on dogs, cats, puppies, kittens 8 weeks of age or older. 8.5, 17 oz.
Frontline® Top Spot for Cats and Kittens (Merial) *Barricade®* or *Fortress® Spot On* (Farnam) *Easyspot®* (Novartis) *Spectra Sure®* (Durvet) *Effipro®* (Virbac) *Hartz First Defense®* (Hartz Mountain) *Martin's Prefurred® One* (Control Solutions) *PetArmor®* or *Sentry Fiproguard®* or *Pronyl OTC®* (Sergeant's)	Solution: 9.7% fipronil; (*Effipro®*: 9.61% fipronil)	OTC-EPA	Labeled for use on cats or kittens 8 weeks of age or older. Single dose applicators 0.5 mL in 3's & 6's.
Frontline® Plus for Cats and Kittens (Merial)	Solution: 9.8% fipronil, (s)-methoprene 11.8%	OTC-EPA	Labeled for use on cats or kittens 8 weeks of age or older. Single dose applicators 0.5 mL in 3's & 6's.
Martin's Prefurred® Plus for Cats (Control Solutions) *Sentry Fiproguard® Max* (Sergeant's) *Spectra Sure® Plus* (Durvet)	Solution: 9.8% fipronil, 15% etofenprox	OTC-EPA	Single dose applicators in 3's; Labeled for 12 weeks of age or older. Single dose applicators 0.5 mL in 3's.
Frontline® Tritak for Cats and Kittens (Merial)	Solution: 9.8% fipronil, etofenprox 15%, (s)-methoprene 11.8%	OTC-EPA	Labeled for use on cats or kittens 12 weeks of age or older. Single dose applicators 0.5 mL in 3's.
Parastar® (Novartis) *PetArmor®* or *Sentry Fiproguard®* or *Pronyl OTC®* (Sergeant's) *Spectra Sure®* (Durvet)	Solution: 9.7% fipronil	OTC-EPA	For dogs and puppies 8 weeks or older.
Frontline® Plus for Dogs & Puppies (Merial)	Solution: 9.8% fipronil, (s)-methoprene 8.8%	OTC-EPA	Single dose applicators in 3's and 6's; Labeled for dogs or puppies 8 weeks of age or older. For dogs weighing 11-22 lb.: 0.67 mL For dogs weighing 23-44 lb.: 1.34 mL For dogs weighing 45-88 lb.: 2.68 mL For dogs weighing 89-132 lb.: 4.02 mL
Parastar Plus® (Novartis) *Martin's Prefurred® Plus for Dogs* (Control Solutions) *Spectra Sure® Plus* (Durvet) *Sentry Fiproguard® Max* or *Pronyl OTC Max® for Dogs* (Sergeant's)	Solution: 9.8% fipronil, 5.2% cyphenothrin	OTC-EPA	Single dose applicators in 3's; Labeled for dogs or puppies 12 weeks of age or older. Not for cats. For dogs weighing up to 22 lb.: 0.67 mL For dogs weighing 23-44 lb.: 1.34 mL For dogs weighing 45-88 lb.: 2.68 mL For dogs weighing 89-132 lb.: 4.02 mL
Frontline® Tritak for Dogs (Merial)	Solution: 9.8% fipronil, cyphenothren 5.2% (s)-methoprene 8.8%	OTC-EPA	Labeled for use dogs 12 weeks of age or older and at least 4 lbs. Single dose applicators in 4 sizes in 3's. For dogs weighing up to 22 lb.: 0.67 mL For dogs weighing 23-44 lb.: 1.34 mL For dogs weighing 45-88 lb.: 2.68 mL For dogs weighing 89-132 lb.: 4.02 mL
Certifect® for Dogs (Merial)	Spot-On Solution: Side A: fipronil 9.8%, (S)-methoprene 8.8%; Side B: Amitraz 22.1%	OTC-EPA	For dogs and puppies 8 weeks of age or older and at least 5 lbs. body weight. Not for cats. 1.7, 2.14, 4.28 & 6.42 mL/applicator.

Human-Labeled Products

None.

Imidacloprid & Imidacloprid Combinations

(eye-mi-da-kloe-prid)   Seresto®

Indications/Actions

Imidacloprid topical solution (*Advantage®*) is indicated for the treatment of adult and larval stage fleas in dogs and cats. The combination product with permethrin (*K9 Advantix®*) is indicated for adulticide/larvicide for fleas, to repel and kill ticks, and mosquitoes in dogs only. The canine combination product with moxidectin (*Advantage® Multi for Dogs* in USA and *Advocate®* in Europe) is indicated for the prevention of heartworm disease, adult fleas, adult and immature hookworms, adult roundworms, and adult whipworms. It has been also used successfully for the treatment of sarcoptic mange, cheyletiellosis and mild cases of demodicosis.

The feline combination product (*Advantage® Multi for Cats*) is indicated for the prevention of heartworm disease, adult fleas, ear mites, adult and immature hookworms, and adult roundworms. It is also approved for use in ferrets.

Imidacloprid's mechanism of action as an insecticide is to act on nicotinic acetylcholine receptors on the postsynaptic membrane causing CNS impairment and death. Certain insect species are more sensitive to these agents than are mammalian receptors. This is a different mechanism of action than other insecticidal agents (organophosphates, pyrethrins, carbamates, insect growth regulators (IGR's) and insect development inhibitors (IDI's). The manufacturer states that imidacloprid is non-teratogenic, non-hypersensitizing, non-mutagenic, non-allergenic, non-carcinogenic, and non-photosensitizing. The manufacturer states that when applied topically the compound is not absorbed into the bloodstream or internal organs. One combination product for dogs (*K9 Advantix®*) also contains permethrin, a pyrethroid (synthetic pyrethrin) that will kill and repel ticks and mosquitoes. Permethrin's insecticidal activity is as a neurotoxin in susceptible species by slowing sodium ions through sodium channels in neuron membranes. Moxidectin is found in combination products (*Advantage® Multi for Dogs* and *Cats*) with imidacloprid. Moxidectin is a macrocyclic lactone that binds to the glutamate-gated ion channels specific to parasites thereby increasing the influx of chloride ions resulting in hyperpolarization of neuronal cells causing paralysis and death.

Suggested Dosages/Use

Refer to the package information for specific instructions on application of imidacloprid products. They are generally administered once monthly. While swimming, bathing, and rain do not apparently significantly affect the duration of action, repeated shampooing may require additional treatment(s) before the monthly dosing interval is completed. Do not reapply more often than once weekly for these animals.

Precautions/Adverse Effects

The manufacturer lists the following contraindications for imidacloprid and pyripoxyfen: Do not use in puppies <7 weeks old, dogs weighing <3 lbs. or kittens <8 weeks old. The manufacturer recommends consulting a veterinarian before using on debilitated, aged, pregnant, or nursing animals or those on medication.

The combination product with permethrin (*K9 Advantix II®*) **must not be used on cats.** Use with caution in households with both dogs and cats, particularly if cats are in close contact or will groom dogs in the household.

When used as directed, adverse effects are unlikely. Because the drug is bitter tasting, oral contact may cause excessive salivation. Do not get product in eyes. If eye contact occurs (human or animal), flush well with ophthalmic irrigation solution or water. While gloving is not mandated it should be encouraged, as contact with skin should be avoided. Wash hands with soap and water after handling. Keep out of reach of children and do not contaminate feed or food. Dispose of product carefully (in the trash); the permethrin-containing product is extremely toxic to fish.

Imidacloprid topical solutions are usually very well tolerated. Dermal irritation has been reported at the site of application. Hypersalivation, tremors, vomiting and reduced appetite may occur in cats after oral exposure to *Advantage Multi®*. Uncommon to rare adverse reactions reported in dogs treated with *Advantage Multi®* in a field study included pruritus, lethargy, reduced appetite and hyperactivity.

Overdoses/Acute Toxicity

Most problems are seen following oral dosing of topical products. Signs include hypersalivation and vomiting, oral ulcers have been rarely reported in cats. There were 119 exposures to imidacloprid reported to the ASPCA Animal Poison Control Center (APCC) during 2008-2009. In these cases 57 were dogs with 25 showing clinical signs, 60 cases were cats in which 42 showed clinical signs, 1 case was a turtle that showed clinical signs and the remaining case was a lagomorph that showed no clinical signs. Common findings in dogs recorded in decreasing frequency included vomiting, hypersalivation, and trembling. Common findings in cats recorded in decreasing frequency included hypersalivation, vomiting, lethargy, and hiding.

Veterinary-Labeled Products

Product (Company)	Form: Concentration	Label Status	Other Ingredients; Comments; Size(s)
Advantage® For Dogs (Bayer)	Topical Solution: imidacloprid 9.1%	OTC-EPA	Flea adulticide/larvicide for use on dogs and puppies 7 weeks of age and older. In cards of 4 or 6 tubes: Under 10 lb. = 0.4 mL (small dog) 11-20 lb. = 1 mL (medium dog) 21-55 lb. = 2.5 mL (large dog) Over 55 lb. = 4 mL (extra-large dog)
Advantage® II For Dogs (Bayer)	Topical Solution: imidacloprid 9.1%, pyripoxyfen 0.46%	OTC-EPA	Flea adulticide/larvicide for use on dogs and puppies 7 weeks of age and older. In cards of 4 or 6 tubes: Under 10 lb. = 0.4 mL (small dog) 11-20 lb. = 1 mL (medium dog) 21-55 lb. = 2.5 mL (large dog) Over 55 lb. = 4 mL (extra-large dog)

Product (Company)	Form: Concentration	Label Status	Other Ingredients; Comments; Size(s)
Advantage® *for Cats* (Bayer)	Topical Solution: imidacloprid 9.1%	OTC-EPA	Flea adulticide/larvicide for use on cats and kittens 8 weeks of age and older. In cards of 4 or 6 tubes: 9 lb and under = 0.4 mL (small cat) Over 9 lb. = 0.8 mL (large cat)
Advantage® *II for Cats* (Bayer)	Topical Solution: imidacloprid 9.1%, pyripoxyfen 0.46%	OTC-EPA	Flea adulticide/larvicide for use on cats and kittens 8 weeks of age and older. In cards of 4 or 6 tubes: 9 lb and under = 0.4 mL (small cat) Over 9 lb. = 0.8 mL (large cat)
K9 Advantix® (Bayer)	Topical Solution: imidacloprid 8.8%, permethrin 44%	OTC-EPA	Flea adulticide/larvicide, tick and mosquito repellant and treatment. For use on dogs and puppies 7 weeks of age. **NOT** for cats. In cards of 4 or 6 tubes: Under 10 lb. = 0.4 mL (small dog) 11-20 lb. = 1 mL (medium dog) 21-55 lb. = 2.5 mL (large dog) Over 55 lb. = 4 mL (extra large dog)
K9 Advantix II® (Bayer)	Topical Solution: imidacloprid 8.8%, permethrin 44%, pyripoxyfen 0.44%	OTC-EPA	Flea adulticide/larvicide, tick and mosquito repellant and treatment. For use on dogs and puppies 7 weeks of age. **NOT** for cats. In cards of 4 or 6 tubes: Under 10 lb. = 0.4 mL (small dog) 11-20 lb. = 1 mL (medium dog) 21-55 lb. = 2.5 mL (large dog) Over 55 lb. = 4 mL (extra large dog)
Advantage Multi® *for Dogs* (Bayer)	Topical Solution: imidacloprid 10%, moxidectin 2.5%	Rx	Approved for use on dogs 7 weeks of age or greater, and more than 3 lb body weight. 0.4 mL tubes x 6 1 mL tubes x 6 2.5 mL tubes x 6 4 mL tubes x 6 5 mL tubes x 6
Advantage Multi® *for Cats* (Bayer)	Topical Solution: imidacloprid 10%, moxidectin 1%	Rx	Approved for use on cats 9 weeks of age or greater, and more than 2 lb body weight and ferrets. 0.23 mL tubes x 3 0.4 mL tubes x 6 0.8 mL tubes x 6
Seresto® *Small* or *Large Dog* (Bayer)	Collar: imidacloprid 10%, flumethrin 4.5%	OTC-EPA	For 8-month prevention and treatment of ticks and fleas on dogs and puppies 7 weeks of age and older.
Seresto® *Cat* (Bayer)	Collar: imidacloprid 10%, flumethrin 4.5%	OTC-EPA	For 8-month prevention and treatment of ticks and fleas on cats or kittens 10 weeks of age and older.

Human-Labeled Products
None.

Indoxacarb ± Permethrin

(in-**dox**-ah-carb)   Activyl®

Indications/Actions

Indoxacarb products (*Activyl*®) are labeled for once a month topical application for treatment of fleas in dogs and cats. For dogs, the combination product containing permethrin (*Activyl*® *Tickplus*) is also indicated for ticks.

Indoxacarb is an oxadiazine insecticide. It is considered a pro-insecticide as it requires bio-activation in insects via esterification to a de-carbomethoxylated form of the drug. This process does not occur in mammals. After bioactivation it induces irreversible hyperpolarization of insect nerve cell membranes and blocks sodium current amplitude in neurons differently than pyrethroids. In susceptible insects, nerve function is impaired with resultant feeding cessation, paralysis and death.

Suggested Dosages/Use

These products are used monthly in dogs and cats for flea (*Activyl*®) and tick (*Activyl*® *Tickplus*; only in dogs) control.

Precautions/Adverse Effects

Appears to have a relatively high safety margin.

The combination product with permethrin (*Activyl Tickplus*®) **must not be used on cats**. Use with caution in households with both dogs and cats, particularly if cats are in close contact or will groom dogs in the household. Do not have contact or allow children to have contact with treated area until it is completely dry.

Veterinary-Labeled Products

Product (Company)	Form: Concentration	Label Status	Other Ingredients; Comments; Size(s)
Activyl® Spot-On for Cats (Merck)	Topical Solution: indoxacarb 19.53%	OTC-EPA	For use on cats and kittens at least 2 lbs. Product comes in two sizes: for cats <9 lbs., and for those over 9 lbs.
Activyl® Spot-On for Dogs (Merck)	Topical Solution: indoxacarb 19.53%	OTC-EPA	Once-A-Month Topical Flea Spot-On for dogs and puppies 8 weeks and older and weighing over 4 lb. Packaged in 5 different sizes according to dog's weight.
Activyl TickPlus® for Dogs (Merck)	Topical Solution: indoxacarb 13.01%; permethrin 42.5% mg/mL	OTC-EPA	Once-A-Month Topical Flea and Tick Treatment for dogs and puppies 8 weeks and older and weighing over 11 lb. **Must not be used on cats.** See the product label for more information. Packaged in 5 different sizes according to dog's weight.

Human-Labeled Products
None.

Isopropyl Myristate
(eye-so-proe-pil meer-is-tate)   Resultix®

Indications/Actions
Resultix® (50% isopropyl myristate solution) is a non-insecticidal product labeled for the removal and killing of attached and crawling ticks on dogs and cats. It acts by dissolving the outer wax layer covering the hard shell (cuticle) of the tick resulting in uncontrollable water loss and death. Ticks die and fall off generally within 3 hours.

Suggested Dosages/Use
Direct nozzle at tick and spray until tick is covered with solution (2 sprays). The tick will be dead within 3 hours; it will fall off of the dog or cat or will be immobile when removed. After 3 hours, if the tick has not fallen off, remove carefully with gloves or tweezers and dispose of tick. Wash hands after accidental exposure to any ticks.

Precautions/Adverse Effects
Do not use near dog's or cat's eyes. Do not use on irritated skin. Stop treatment with this product and consult a veterinarian if skin irritation or skin infection develops during use of product.

Do not discharge this product into lakes, streams, pond, estuaries, oceans, or other waters where aquatic invertebrates or fish may be found.

Veterinary-Labeled Products

Product (Company)	Form: Concentration	Label Status	Other Ingredients; Comments; Size(s)
Resultix® (Bayer)	Topical Spray: Isopropyl myristate 50%.	OTC-EPA	Labeled for dogs and cats. 20 mL.

Human-Labeled Products
None.

(s)-Methoprene Combinations
(meth-oh-preen)

Indications/Actions
Methoprene is added to premise sprays and topical products to eliminate insects (usually fleas) via its ability prevent maturation of eggs or larva.

(s)-methoprene mimics insect juvenile growth hormone, halting development during metamorphosis and larval development. It also concentrates in female flea ovaries, causing non-viable eggs to be produced. When combined with an adulticide (*e.g.,* permethrin, fipronil, phenothrin) all stages of the parasite are killed and re-infestation is less likely.

Suggested Dosages/Use
For specific use and dosage recommendations, refer to the actual product's label.

Precautions/Adverse Effects
Methoprene may be found in products also containing **permethrin, cyphenothren or phenothrin, which can be toxic to cats**, particularly small kittens. **Only use on cats those products containing permethrin or other pyrethroids labeled specifically for use on cats.** Hypersensitivity can occur to these compounds. Do not use in eyes or on mucous membranes.

Methoprene (used alone) has low toxicity in mammals. Potentially, skin irritation or hypersensitivity reactions could occur. As methoprene is broken down by UV light, protect unused product from light.

Veterinary-Labeled Products

Note: There are many products marketed, including collars, topical sprays, foggers, and spot-ons; the following are representative:

Product (Company)	Form: Concentration	Label Status	Other Ingredients; Comments; Size(s)
Adams Spot On® Flea & Tick Control (Farnam)	Topical Solution: (s)-Methoprene: 3%, Permethrin: 45%	OTC-EPA	Kills and repels adult fleas, ticks and mosquitoes. It also prevents flea eggs from developing into adult fleas. For dogs 6 months of age or older. **Must not be used on cats or on dogs that cohabit with a cat.** Packaged and labeled by the dog's weight in tubes of 3: <15-30 lbs. = 0.034 oz; 31-60 lbs. = 0.068 oz; >60 lbs. = 0.101 oz
Bio Spot On® Flea & Tick Control For Dogs (Farnam)	Topical Solution: (s)-Methoprene: 3%, Permethrin: 45%	OTC-EPA	Kills and repels adult fleas, ticks and mosquitoes. It also prevents flea eggs from developing into adult fleas. For dogs 6 months of age or older **Must not be used on cats or on dogs that cohabit with a cat.** Packaged and labeled by the dog's weight in tubes of 3: <15-30 lbs. = 0.034 oz; 31-60 lbs. = 0.068 oz; >60 lbs. = 0.101 oz
Certifect® for Dogs (Merial)	Spot-On Solution: Side A: fipronil 9.8%, (S)-methoprene 8.8%; Side B: Amitraz 22.1%	OTC-EPA	For dogs and puppies 8 weeks of age or older and at least 5 lbs. body weight. Not for cats. 1.7, 2.14, 4.28 & 6.42 mL/applicator.
Hartz UltraGuard Plus® Flea & Tick Drops for Dogs and Puppies®; Hartz UltraGuard Pro® (Hartz Mountain)	Topical Solution: (s)-Methoprene: 2.3%, Phenothrin: 85.7%	OTC-EPA	Note: Phenothrin is a pyrethroid similar to permethrin; refer to the permethrin monograph for more information. For dogs 12 weeks of age and older or weighting more than 4 pounds. Kills fleas, ticks, mosquitoes and flea eggs for 30 days; repels fleas and ticks. **Must not be used on cats or on dogs that cohabit with a cat.** Packaged and labeled by dogs weight in tubes of 3: 4-15 lb. = 1.1 mL; 16-30 lb. = 1.3 mL; 31-60 lb. = 4.1 mL; >60 lb. = 5.9 mL
Hartz UltraGuard One Spot® Treatment for Cats and Kittens® (Hartz Mountain)	Topical Solution: (s)-Methoprene: 2.9%	OTC-EPA	For kittens 12 weeks of age and older. Kills and prevents flea eggs and larvae for up to 30 days. 1 mL
Hartz UltraGuard Plus® Drops for Cats; Hartz UltraGuard Pro® (Hartz Mountain)	Topical Solution: (s)-Methoprene: 3.6%, Etofenprox: 40%	OTC-EPA	For kittens 12 weeks of age and older. Kills fleas, flea eggs and deer ticks; kills and repels mosquitoes. 1.8 mL applicators.
Bio-Spot® Flea & Tick Spray for Dogs and Puppies (Farnam)	Topical Spray: (s)-Methoprene: 0.27%, Pyrethrins: 0.2%, Piperonyl Butoxide: 0.37%	OTC-EPA	Kills and repels fleas, ticks and mosquitoes. Prevents flea eggs from hatching. For dogs 12 weeks of age or older. 24 oz.
Frontline® Plus for Cats and Kittens (Merial)	Solution: 9.8% fipronil, (s)-methoprene 11.8%	OTC-EPA	Labeled for use on cats or kittens 8 weeks of age or older. Single dose applicators 0.5 mL in 3's & 6's.
Frontline® Tritak for Cats and Kittens (Merial)	Solution: 9.8% fipronil, etofenprox 15%, (s)-Methoprene 11.8%	OTC-EPA	Labeled for use on cats or kittens 12 weeks of age or older. Single dose applicators 0.5 mL in 3's.
Frontline® Plus for Dogs & Puppies (Merial)	Solution: 9.8% fipronil, (s)-Methoprene 8.8%	OTC-EPA	Single dose applicators in 3's and 6's; Labeled for dogs or puppies 8 weeks of age or older. For dogs weighing 11-22 lb.: 0.67 mL For dogs weighing 23-44 lb.: 1.34 mL For dogs weighing 45-88 lb.: 2.68 mL For dogs weighing 89-132 lb.: 4.02 mL
Frontline® Tritak for Dogs (Merial)	Solution: 9.8% fipronil, cyphenothren 5.2%, (s)-methoprene 8.8%	OTC-EPA	Labeled for use dogs 12 weeks of age or older and at least 4 lbs. Single dose applicators in 4 sizes in 3's. For dogs weighing up to 22 lb.: 0.67 mL For dogs weighing 23-44 lb.: 1.34 mL For dogs weighing 45-88 lb.: 2.68 mL For dogs weighing 89-132 lb.: 4.02 mL

Human-Labeled Products

None.

Permethrin & Permethrin Combinations
(per-meth-rin)

Indications/Actions
Permethrin is synthetic pyrethroid that acts as an adulticide insecticide/miticide. It has knockdown activity against fleas, lice, ticks, and certain mites (*e.g.*, Cheyletiella, *Sarcoptes scabiei*). Permethrin also has repellant activity. In small animal medicine, it is used primarily for fleas and ticks on dogs. In large animal and food animal medicine, there are many products (not listed below) available for pour-on, dusting, and spray use for flies, lice, mites, mosquitoes, ticks and keds.

Permethrin acts by disrupting the sodium channel current in arthropod nerve cell membranes, resulting in paralysis and death.

Suggested Dosages/Use
Refer to each product's label.

Precautions/Adverse Effects
Permethrin and other synthetic pyrethroids can be toxic to cats, particularly small kittens. **Only use products containing pyrethroids labeled for use on cats on this species.** Hypersensitivity can occur to these compounds. Do not use in eyes or on mucous membranes. Clients should wear gloves when applying and wash off any product that contacts their skin.

Pruritus or mild skin irritation can occur at application site, but occur uncommonly.

Veterinary-Labeled Products
Not an inclusive list; many shampoos, pour-ons, sprays, foggers, dusts are available.

Product (Company)	Form: Concentration	Label Status	Other Ingredients; Comments; Size(s)
Bansect® Squeeze-On Flea & Tick Control for Dogs® (Sergeant's)	Topical Solution: Permethrin 45%	OTC-EPA	Kills and repels fleas and ticks. For dogs, older than 6 months old. **Must not be used on cats or on dogs that cohabit with a cat.** Individual packaging for dog's weighing: <33 lb. = 1.5 mL; >33 lb. = 3 mL; 3 per package.
Bio Spot On® Flea & Tick Control For Dogs (Farnam)	Topical Solution: Permethrin 45%, (s)-Methoprene: 3%	OTC-EPA	Kills and repels adult fleas, ticks and mosquitoes. It also prevents flea eggs from developing into adult fleas. For dogs 6 months of age or older. **Must not be used on cats or on dogs that cohabit with a cat.** Packaged and labeled by the dog's weight in tubes of 3: <15-30 lbs. = 0.034 oz; 31-60 lbs. = 0.068 oz; >60 lbs. = 0.101 oz
Flea Halt® Flea and Tick Spray for Dogs (Farnam)	Topical Spray: Permethrin 0.1%, Pyrethrins 0.05%, Piperonyl Butoxide 0.5%	OTC-EPA	Kills and repels fleas, ticks, flies, mosquitoes, gnats, chiggers and lice. For dogs older than 3 months of age. **Must not be used on cats or on dogs that cohabit with a cat.** 32 oz bottle.
K9 Advantix® (Bayer)	Topical Solution: imidacloprid 8.8%, permethrin 44%	OTC-EPA	Flea adulticide/larvicide, tick and mosquito repellant and treatment. For use on dogs and puppies 7 weeks of age. **NOT** for cats. In cards of 4 or 6 tubes: Under 10 lb. = 0.4 mL (small dog) 11-20 lb. = 1 mL (medium dog) 21-55 lb. = 2.5 mL (large dog) Over 55 lb. = 4 mL (extra large dog)
K9 Advantix II® (Bayer)	Topical Solution: imidacloprid 8.8%, permethrin 44%, pyripoxyfen 0.44%	OTC-EPA	Flea adulticide/larvicide, tick and mosquito repellant and treatment. For use on dogs and puppies 7 weeks of age. **NOT** for cats. In cards of 4 or 6 tubes: Under 10 lb. = 0.4 mL (small dog) 11-20 lb. = 1 mL (medium dog) 21-55 lb. = 2.5 mL (large dog) Over 55 lb. = 4 mL (extra large dog)
Scratchex® Flea & Tick Spray For Dogs and Cats (Farnam)	Topical Spray: Permethrin 0.05%, Pyrethrins 0.056%, Related compounds 0.004%	OTC-EPA	Kills and ticks. For dogs and cats 12 weeks of age or older. 7 oz bottle.
Vectra 3D® (Ceva)	Topical Solution: Permethrin 36.08%, Pyripoxyfen 0.44%, Dinotefuran, 4.95%	OTC-EPA	For use on dogs over 7 weeks old only. **Must not be used on cats or on dogs that cohabit with a cat.** In 4 different package sizes for dogs weighing >2.5. lb.
Activyl TickPlus® for Dogs (Merck)	Topical Solution: indoxacarb 13.01%; permethrin 42.5% mg/mL	OTC-EPA	Once-A-Month Topical Flea and Tick Treatment for dogs and puppies 8 weeks and older and weighing over 11 lb. **Must not be used on cats.** See the product label for more information. Packaged in 5 different sizes according to dog's weight.

Human-Labeled Products

Product (Company)	Form: Concentration	Label Status	Other Ingredients; Comments; Size(s)
Generic (various), *Elimite*® (Prestium Pharma), *Acticin*® (Mylan)	Cream: Permethrin 5%	Rx	Used for treating scabies in humans. 60 g.
Generic (various)	Lotion/Cream Rinse: Permethrin 1%	OTC	Used for treating head lice in humans. 59 mL

Pyrethrins & Pyrethrin Combinations

(pye-ree-thrins)

For otic use, refer to the Otics section

Indications/Actions

Pyrethrins are naturally derived insecticides that act as adulticide insecticides/miticides. They have knockdown activity against fleas, lice, ticks, and Cheyletiella. In small animal medicine, pyrethrins are used primarily for fleas and ticks on dogs and cats. In large animal and food animal medicine, there are many products (not listed below) available for pour-on, dusting, and spray use.

Pyrethrins act by disrupting the sodium channel current in arthropod nerve cell membranes, resulting in paralysis and death. Pyrethrins are often found in combination with the insect growth regulators, methoprene or pyriproxyfen and with the synergist piperonyl butoxide. Piperonyl butoxide inhibits insect metabolic enzymes (P450 system) allowing a lower dose of primary insecticide to be used.

Suggested Dosages/Use

For specific dosage recommendations, refer to the actual product's label.

Precautions/Adverse Effects

Pyrethrins are among the safest insecticidal products available, but cats should not be allowed to groom wet product after using dips or sprays. Hypersensitivity can occur to these compounds. Do not use in eyes or on mucous membranes. Avoid hypothermia when using liquid products (sprays, dips, etc), particularly in small animals and when ambient temperatures are low.

Pruritus or mild skin irritation can occur at application site, but occur uncommonly.

Clients should wear gloves when applying and wash off any product that contacts their skin.

Veterinary-Labeled Products

Not an inclusive list, but representative of the types of products available; many shampoos, pour-ons, sprays, dusts, ointments are available.

Product (Company)	Form: Concentration	Label Status	Other Ingredients; Comments; Size(s)
Adams Flea & Tick Mist with IGR® (Farnam) *Adams Flea & Tick Mist for Cats*® (Farnam)	Topical Spray: Pyrethrins 0.18%, Pyriproxyfen 0.125%	OTC-EPA	N-octyl bicycloheptane dicarboxamide 1% (insecticide synergist). For dogs and cats. 16, 32 oz.
Vet-Kem Ovitrol Plus Flea, Tick & Bot Spray® (VPL)	Topical Spray: (s)-Methoprene: 0.27%, Pyrethrins: 0.2%, Piperonyl Butoxide 0.37%	OTC-EPA	N-octyl bicycloheptene dicarboximide: 0.62%. 16 oz., 1 gal. Labeled for use on dogs, cats, puppies, kittens, horses, and ponies. Not for puppies or kittens <12 weeks old.
Bio-Spot® *Flea & Tick Spray for Dogs and Puppies* (Farnam)	Topical Spray: Pyrethrins: 0.2%, Piperonyl Butoxide: 0.37%, (s)-Methoprene: 0.27%	OTC-EPA	Kills and repels fleas, ticks and mosquitoes. Prevents flea eggs from hatching. For dogs 12 weeks of age or older. 24 oz.
Flea Halt® *Flea and Tick Spray for Dogs* (Farnam)	Topical Spray: Pyrethrins 0.05%, Permethrin 0.1%, Piperonyl Butoxide 0.5%	OTC-EPA	Kills and repels fleas, ticks, flies, mosquitoes, gnats, chiggers and lice. For dogs older than 3 months of age. Must not be used on cats or on dogs that cohabit with a cat. 32 oz bottle.
Scratchex® *Flea & Tick Mist For Dogs and Cats* (Farnam)	Topical Spray: Pyrethrins 0.056%, Permethrin 0.05%	OTC-EPA	Kills fleas and ticks. For dogs and cats 12 weeks of age or older. 7 oz bottle.
Bio Spot Shampoo® *for Dogs and Puppies* (Farnam)	Shampoo: Pyrethrins 0.15%, (s)-methoprene 0.1%, Piperonyl butoxide 1.5%	OTC-EPA	For dogs and cats 12 weeks of age or older. 12 oz.
Adams® *Plus Flea & Tick Shampoo with Insect Growth Regulator (IGR)* (Farnam)	Shampoo: Pyrethrins 0.075%, Pyriproxyfen 0.086%, Piperonyl butoxide 0.75%	OTC-EPA	Kills fleas, ticks and lice. Prevent flea eggs from hatching. For dogs and cats. 12 oz.
Vet-Kem Ovitrol Plus Flea & Tick Shampoo® (VPL)	Shampoo: (s)-Methoprene: 1.1%, Pyrethrins: 0.15%, Piperonyl butoxide:1.05%	OTC-EPA	12 oz. Not for puppies or kittens <12 weeks old.
Ecto-Soothe® *3X Shampoo* (Virbac)	Shampoo: Pyrethrins 0.15%, Piperonyl butoxide 1.5%, *Spherulite*® microcapsules	OTC-EPA	N-octyl bicycloheptane dicarboxamide (MGK 264) 0.5%. Kills ticks, fleas, and lice. For dogs and cats 12 weeks of age or older. 8 oz, 16 oz, 1 gal.

Product (Company)	Form: Concentration	Label Status	Other Ingredients; Comments; Size(s)
Vet-Kem Ovitrol Plus Flea & Tick Shampoo® (VPL)	Shampoo: Pyrethrins: 0.15%, Piperonyl butoxide:1.05%, (s)-Methoprene: 1.1%	OTC-EPA	Kills adult fleas, ticks and lice and prevents flea larvae from hatching. Not for puppies or kittens <12 weeks old. 12 oz.
Adams Pyrethrin Dip® (VPL)	Dip: Pyrethrins: 0.97%,Piperonyl butoxide: 3.74%	OTC-EPA	N-octyl bicycloheptene dicarboxamide 5.7% Di-n-propyl isocinchomerate 1.94%. Kills and repels fleas, ticks, lice, gnats, mosquitoes and flies. Not for puppies or kittens <12 weeks old. Must be diluted before use. 4 oz.
Pyrethrin Dip® (Virbac)	Dip: Pyrethrins 1%, Piperonyl butoxide 4%, N-Octyl Bicycloheptene Dicarboximide 6%, Di-n-Propyl Isocinchomeronate 4%	OTC-EPA	For puppies or kittens over 12 weeks old. Shake well. May be flammable. Must be diluted: ½ oz makes one gallon. Keep away from open flame. 4 oz, 1 gal.

Human-Labeled Products
None.

Pyriproxyfen & Pyriproxyfen Combinations
(pye-ri-proks-i-fen)   Nylar®

Also see to the Dinotefuran and Imidacloprid listings

Indications/Actions
Pyriproxyfen is a second-generation insect growth regulator and is added to premise sprays and topical products to eliminate insects (usually fleas) via its ability to prevent maturation of eggs or larva.

Pyriproxyfen mimics insect juvenile growth hormone, halting development during metamorphosis and larval development. It also concentrates in female flea ovaries, causing non-viable eggs to be produced. When combined with an adulticide (*e.g.*, permethrin, fipronil) all stages of the parasite are killed and re-infestation is less likely. It is more resistant to UV light than is methoprene.

Suggested Dosages/Use
For specific dosage recommendations, refer to the actual product's label.

Precautions/Adverse Effects
Pyriproxyfen may be found in products also containing **permethrin, which can be toxic to cats**, particularly small kittens. **Only use on cats those products containing permethrin or other pyrethroids labeled specifically for use on cats.**

Pyriproxyfen (used alone) has low toxicity in mammals. Potentially, skin irritation or hypersensitivity reactions could occur.

Clients should wear gloves when applying products containing permethrin or other insecticides and wash off any product that contacts their skin.

Veterinary-Labeled Products
Not necessarily inclusive, there are premise sprays and other topical products containing pyriproxyfen.

Product (Company)	Form: Concentration	Label Status	Other Ingredients; Comments; Size(s)
Adams® Plus Flea & Tick Mist with Insect Growth Regulator (IGR) (Farnam)	Topical Spray: Pyriproxyfen 0.125%, Pyrethrins 0.18%	OTC-EPA	Kills and repels fleas, ticks and mosquitoes. Also kills flea eggs and larvae. For dogs and cats. N-octyl bicycloheptane dicarboxamide 1% (insecticide synergist). 16, 32 oz.
Adams® Flea & Tick Mist for Cats (Farnam)	Topical Spray: Pyriproxyfen 0.125%, Pyrethrins 0.18%	OTC-EPA	Kills and repels fleas, ticks and mosquitoes. Also kills flea eggs and larvae. For cats. N-octyl bicycloheptane dicarboxamide 1% (insecticide synergist). 16 oz.
Adams® Plus Flea & Tick Shampoo with Insect Growth Regulator (IGR) (Farnam)	Shampoo: Pyriproxyfen 0.086%, Pyrethrins 0.075%, Piperonyl butoxide 0.75%	OTC-EPA	Kills fleas, ticks and lice. Prevent flea eggs from hatching. For dogs and cats. 12 oz.
Bio Spot® Shampoo (Farnam)	Shampoo: Pyriproxyfen 0.01%, Pyrethrins 0.1%, Piperonyl butoxide 0.5%	OTC-EPA	Kills adult and larval fleas, and ticks. For dogs only. 12 oz.
Advantage® II For Dogs (Bayer)	Topical Solution: imidacloprid 9.1%, pyripoxyfen 0.46%	OTC-EPA	Flea adulticide/larvicide for use on dogs and puppies 7 weeks of age and older. In cards of 4 or 6 tubes: Under 10 lb. = 0.4 mL (small dog); 11-20 lb. = 1 mL (medium dog); 21-55 lb. = 2.5 mL (large dog); Over 55 lb. = 4 mL (extra-large dog)
Advantage® II for Cats (Bayer)	Topical Solution: imidacloprid 9.1%, pyripoxyfen 0.46%	OTC-EPA	Flea adulticide/larvicide for use on cats and kittens 8 weeks of age and older. In cards of 4 or 6 tubes: 9 lb and under = 0.4 mL (small cat) Over 9 lb. = 0.8 mL (large cat)

Product (Company)	Form: Concentration	Label Status	Other Ingredients; Comments; Size(s)
K9 Advantix II® (Bayer)	Topical Solution: imidacloprid 8.8%, permethrin 44%, pyripoxyfen 0.44%	OTC-EPA	Flea adulticide/larvicide, tick and mosquito repellant and treatment. For use on dogs and puppies 7 weeks of age. NOT for cats. In cards of 4 or 6 tubes: Under 10 lb. = 0.4 mL (small dog) 11-20 lb. = 1 mL (medium dog) 21-55 lb. = 2.5 mL (large dog) Over 55 lb. = 4 mL (extra large dog)

Human-Labeled Topical Products
None.

Spinetoram

(spin-et-oh-ram)   Cheristin®

Topical Flea Insecticide

Indications/Actions

Spinetoram (*Cheristin*®) is an EPA-registered product once-a-month topical solution for the prevention and treatment of flea infestations for cats and kittens 8 weeks and older. The currently marketed product for cats (*Cheristin*®) is an 11.2% solution of spinetoram. The formerly marketed product (*Assurity*®) was 39.4% spinetoram, but was discontinued primarily due to alopecia at the site of application (Credille *et al.* 2013).

Spinetoram is a semi-synthetic second-generation derivative of spinosad. It acts on both GABA and nicotinic acetylcholine receptors in the CNS of insects, leading to CNS hyperexcitation followed by paralysis and death. Product label states that once applied fleas begin to die in 30 minutes.

Spinetoram is a semi-synthetic derivative of <u>spinosad</u>, a natural insecticide extracted from cultures of *Saccharopolyspora spinosa*, a soil bacterium. It is a combination of 3'-O-ethyl-5,6-dihydro Spinosyn J (XDE-175-J) and 3'-O-ethyl Spinosyn L (XDE-175-L). Trade names include: *Delegate*® WG, *Radiant*® SC, *Exalt*® SC, *Assurity*® and *Cheristin*®.

Suggested Dosages/Use

- **CATS:**

   For the prevention and treatment of flea infestations for cats and kittens 8 weeks and older and weighing at least 1.8 lbs.: Apply one applicatorful (regardless of cat's weight) monthly. Part the hair on the neck at the base of the head until the skin is visible. Place the tip of the tube directly above the skin and squeeze the tube 2-4 times to expel the contents of the tube directly on the skin. For best results, apply at the base of the head, not between shoulder blades. Avoid getting the product in pet's eyes or mouth. Treatment at the base of the head will minimize the opportunity for the cat to directly lick the product. Do not allow cat to ingest this product. (There may be a small residual remaining in the tube after a full dose is expelled.) (Adapted from label; *Cheristin*®)

Precautions/Adverse Effects

Label states: "Do not use on kittens less than eight (8) weeks of age or weighing less than 1.8 lb. Do not allow cat to ingest product. Use only a single dose on cats weighing more than 20 lbs. As with any product, consult your veterinarian before using this product on debilitated, aged, pregnant or nursing animals or animals known to be sensitive to pesticides."

The product is not labeled for use in dogs. Of dogs, mice, and rats, dogs appear to be the most toxicologically sensitive species to spinetoram exposure (Anon 2009).

Adverse effects on the product label include: application site reactions such as application site hair loss, hair change (greasy, clumping or matting) or redness, inflammation and itching. Other side effects such as inactivity, vomiting and inappetence have also been reported.

EPA's Fact Sheet states: "Spinetoram was shown to produce reproductive effects in parental female rats. The effects were characterized by treatment-related depletion of primordial and/or "growing" ovarian follicles, dystocia and other parturition abnormalities, late resorptions/retained fetuses and increased post-implantation loss. However, no adverse effects were observed on the offspring at dose levels that produced parental toxicity. The developmental toxicity and reproduction studies indicated no evidence of increased susceptibility of the offspring with pre and/or postnatal exposures." (Anon 2009)

Data was not located with respect to safe use while nursing.

Store in original package in a cool dry place.

Veterinary-Labeled Products

Product (Company)	Ingredients	Label Status	Size
Cheristin® (Elanco)	Spinetoram 11.2%	OTC-EPA; EPA Reg. No. 72642-10.	Do not use on kittens less than eight (8) weeks of age. One applicator tube contains 0.019 oz (0.57 mL). Single-dose and six-dose dispensing packs.

Human-Labeled Products
None.

Revisions/References
Monograph revised/updated August 2014.

Anon (2009). Spinetoram; EPA Pesticide Fact Sheet, United States Environmental Protection Agency: Office of Prevention, Pesticides and Toxic Substances
Credille, K. M., et al. (2013). Evaluation of hair loss in cats occurring after treatment with a topical flea control product. Veterinary Dermatology 24(6): 602-+.

Otic Preparations

While not a complete list, the following examples are representative of the types of topical otic preparations available to veterinarians. Included are both veterinary-labeled and human-labeled products that may be of use in veterinary medicine. Much of this section is adapted from: Koch, Torres, & Plumb. (2012). _**Canine and Feline Dermatology Drug Handbook**_. Wiley-Blackwell. This reference provides additional detail on these, and other related compounds and products.

Ceruminolytic Agents

Ceruminolytic products emulsify and remove ceruminous and purulent exudate by providing a surfactant, detergent and bubbling activity. They work best if applied 10-15 minutes prior to cleaning. Ceruminolytic agents should not be used with ruptured tympanic membrane because of potential for ototoxicity (be especially careful in cats with ruptured tympanum). If they are needed during in-hospital ear flushing procedures, their use should be followed by multiple flushes with warm sterile isotonic saline. Docusate sodium (DSS), calcium sulfosuccinate, and urea (carbamide) peroxide are considered potent ceruminolytic agents. Squalene, triethanolamine polypeptide elite condensate and hexamethyltetracosane are less potent agents. Propylene glycol, glycerin and oil are considered very mild ceruminolytic agents. Urea peroxide containing products will release oxygen when activated and produce a foaming action that helps breakdown down cerumen. This product however, can be irritating to already inflamed ears. If mild ceruminolytic products will be used at home by the client (intact tympanic membrane), demonstrate proper cleaning technique in the examination room. Advise the client to discontinue product application and contact the veterinarian if the ears become redder or more inflamed at any time during the course of cleaning. The frequency of cleaning varies according to the needs of the individual patient.

Trade Name (Manufacturer)	Ingredients	Sizes
Cerumene® (Vetoquinol)	25% squalene in isopropyl myristate liquid, petrolatum base	4 oz
Cerumotic® Ear Cleanser (Schuyler)	22% squalene, isopropyl myristate, mineral oil.	4 oz
Corium-20® Ear Cleaner (Virbac)	Water, specially denatured alcohol, glyceride mixture, polysorbate 80, fragrance, BHT.	8, 16 oz
Douxo® Micellar Solution (Sogeval)	Phytosphingosine, polysorbate, propylene glycol, poloxamer 184, imidazolidin urea, polidocanol, polysaccharides, alcohol, light fragrance	4.2, 8.4 oz
Earoxide® Pet Ear Cleanser (Tomlyn)	Carbamide peroxide 6.5% in a glycerin base	4 oz
Epiklean® Ear Cleanser (Dechra)	Propylene glycol, glycerin, salicylic acid	8, 12 oz
KlearOtic® Ear Cleanser (Dechra)	Squalene 22%	4 oz

Cleaning/Drying Agents

Cleaning and drying agents are typically used after debris or exudate has been removed from the ear canals with a ceruminolytic agent. Their primary ingredient is usually an acid (_e.g.,_ boric acid) or isopropyl alcohol. Cleaning and drying ear solutions can be used on a maintenance regimen to help prevent ear infections and after bathing or swimming to keep the external ear canals water free. It is important to demonstrate the cleaning technique in the examination room. Advise the client to discontinue application and contact the veterinarian if the ears become more red or more inflamed at any time during the course of cleaning. The frequency of cleaning varies according to the needs of the individual patient.

There are an overwhelming number of these products marketed and the following are representative. They do not appear to be FDA-approved products. Many products also contain ceruminolytic ingredients.

Trade Name (Manufacturer)	Ingredients	Sizes
Aller 911® Ear Wash (Naturvet)	Deionized Water, Dioctyl Sodium Sulfosuccinate, Grapefruit Seed Extract, Calcium Disodium EDTA (Chelating Agent), Calendula Extract, Mullein Extract, St. John's Wort Extract, Olive Leaf Extract, Lavender Extract and Citric Acid	8 oz
Aloeclens® Ear Cleanser (Schein)	Deionized Water, Propylene Glycol, Aloe Vera Gel, SD Alcohol 40-2, Lactic Acid, Glycerin, Dioctyl Sodium Sulfosuccinate, Salicylic Acid, Fragrance, Benzoic Acid, Benzyl Alcohol.	8 oz
Aurocin® Ear Cleanser (Vet One)	Deionized water, Propylene Glycol, Aloe Vera Gel, SD Alcohol 40, Lactic Acid, Glycerin, Dioctyl Sodium Sulfosuccinate, Salicylic Acid, Fragrance, Benzoic Acid, Benzyl Alcohol.	4, 8 oz
Corium-20® Ear Cleaner (Virbac)	Water, specially denatured alcohol, glyceride mixture, polysorbate 80, fragrance, BHT.	8, 16 oz

Trade Name (Manufacturer)	Ingredients	Sizes
Ceruclean Ear Cleanser (Schuyler)	Water, propylene glycol, lactic acid, microcapsules, docusate sodium, salicylic acid, PCMX, dimethicone, fragrance and FD&C blue #1. Lactic acid and salicylic acid are present in encapsulated microcapsules and free forms. Chitosanide is present in encapsulated form.	8, 12 oz
Clean Ear with Aloe Vera (Vedco)	Deionized Water, Propylene Glycol, Aloe Vera Gel, SD Alcohol 40-2, Lactic Acid, Glycerin, Dioctyl Sodium Sulfosuccinate, Salicylic Acid, Fragrance, Benzoic Acid, Benzyl Alcohol.	8 oz, 1 gallon
Conquer® Hy-Otic (Kinetic)	Deionized water, propylene glycol, aloe vera gel, SD alcohol 40, lactic acid, glycerin, dioctyl sodium sulfosuccinate, sodium hyaluronate, salicylic acid, fragrance, benzoic acid, benzyl alcohol.	4, 8 oz
Ear Cleansing Pads (Nutri-Vet)	Deionized Water, Isopropyl Alcohol, Polysorbate 20, Glycerin USP, Propylene Glycol, Salicylic Acid, Benzoic Acid, FD&C Blue #1, Fragrance.	90 pads
Ear Cleansing Solution (RXV)	Deionized Water, Propylene Glycol, Aloe Vera Gel, SD Alcohol 40-2, Lactic Acid, Glycerin, Dioctyl Sodium Sulfosuccinate, Salicylic Acid, Fragrance, Benzoic Acid, Benzyl Alcohol.	4, 8 oz, 1 gallon
Ear Cleansing Solution (Vetoquinol)	SD-Alcohol 40-2, 10%; Lactic Acid, 1.76%; Benzoic Acid, 0.15%; Salicylic Acid, 0.1%.	4, 8, 16 oz, 1 gallon
Ear Flushing Drying Lotion (ADL)	Deionized water, isopropyl alcohol, acetamide mea, propylene glycol, polysorbate 80, eucalyptol, polyethylene glycol, glycerin	4, 6, 8, 12, 32 oz, 1 gallon
EarMed® Boracetic® Flush (Davis)	Odor Neutralizing Agents, Boric Acid, Acetic Acid, Aloe Vera, Lan-Aqua-Sol, Propylene Glycol, Cosmetic Grade Dye, Phospholipid Complex, Ethanol, Purified Water	12 oz, 1 gallon
EarMed® Cleansing Solution & Wash (Davis)	Odor Neutralizing Agents, Lan-Aqua-Sol, Propylene Glycol, Cosmetic Grade Dye, Phospholipid Complex, Ethanol, Purified	12 oz, 1 gallon
EarMed® Wipes (Davis)	Colalipid, SDA40 Ethanol, Lan-Aqua-Sol, Propylene Glycol, Odor Neutralizing Agents, Peppermint Oil, Fragrance	40 Wipes 5 x 6 160 Wipes 6 x 7
EpiKlean® Ear Cleanser (Dechra)	SD alcohol #40, propylene glycol, nonoxynol-9, glycerin, salicylic acid, fragrance	8 oz
Epi-Otic® Advanced (Virbac)	Salicylic Acid 0.2%, in a mild citrus aroma cleansing solution with patented anti-odor technology, containing disodium EDTA, docusate sodium, PCMX, a monosaccharide complex (l-rhamnose, d-galactose, d-mannose), and FD&C Blue #1.	4, 8 oz
Epi-Otic® Ear Cleanser (Virbac)	Water, propylene glycol, lactic acid, Spherulites, docusate sodium, salicylic acid, PCMX, dimethicone, fragrance and FD&C blue #1. Lactic acid and salicylic acid are present in encapsulated and free forms. Chitosanide is present in encapsulated form.	4, 8, 16 oz
Euclens Otic Cleanser (Schein)	Propylene Glycol, Malic Acid, Benzoic Acid, Salicylic Acid, Eucalyptus Oil, FD&C Yellow #6, in a water base.	4, 16 oz
ExpertCare® Ear Cleansing Rinse (Bayer)	Contains wax-dissolving agents and aloe vera	4 oz
Fresh-Ear® (Q.A. Labs)	De-ionized water, isopropyl alcohol, propylene glycol, glycerine, fragrance, salicylic acid, PEG 75 lanolin oil, lidocaine hydrochloride, boric acid, acetic acid, FD & C blue #1.	4 oz, 1 gallon
Gent-L-Clens® (Merck)	Water, propylene glycol, lactic acid, salicylic acid, chloroxylenol, and fragrance.	4 oz
glycoZoo® Otic (DermaZoo)	2% Glycolic Acid, 2% Boric Acid with surfactants.	4, 16 oz
MalAcetic Otic® Cleanser (Dechra)	2% acetic acid, 2% boric acid, glycerin, polysorbate, triethanolamine, fragrance.	4, 8, 16 oz
MalAcetic® Ultra Otic (Dechra)	Acetic acid 1%, boric acid 1%, ketoconazole 0.15%, Hydrocortisone 1%	2, 8 oz
MAX Ear Cleanser® (ADL)	Deionized water, cocamidopropyl betaine: a mild non-irritating foaming surfactant, peg almond glycerides (mildness additive), eucalyptol.	2, 4, 8, 16 oz
Maxi/Guard® Zn 4.5 Otic® (Addison)	Deionized Water, Zinc Gluconate, Boric Acid, Taurine, L-lysine, Propylene Glycol, Methylparaben, Propylparaben.	2, 4 oz
Nolva-Cleanse® (Zoetis)	Propylene glycol	4, 8 oz
Nolvasan® Otic (Zoetis)	Otic solvent, surfactant(s)	4, 16 oz
Otic Clear® (Schein)	Deionized water, isopropyl alcohol, propylene glycol, glycerine, fragrance, salicylic acid, PEG 75 lanolin oil, lidocaine hydrochloride, boric acid, acetic acid, FD&C blue #1.	4, 8 oz, 1 gallon
Oticetic Flush® (Schuyler)	2% acetic acid, 2% boric acid, glycerin, polysorbate, triethanolamine, apple fragrance.	4, 12 oz

Trade Name (Manufacturer)	Ingredients	Sizes
Oti-Clens® (Zoetis)	Propylene glycol, malic acid, benzoic acid, salicylic acid	4 oz
OtiRinse® Ear Solution (Bayer)	Water, benzyl alcohol, propylene glycol, fragrance, dioctyl sodium sulfosuccinate, DM-DM hydantoin, glycerin, nonoxynol-12, salicylic acid, benzoic acid, lactic acid, aloe vera	8 oz
Oti-Soothe®+PS Ear Cleansing Solution (Sogeval)	Deionized water, Propylene Glycol, Aloe Vera Gel, SD Alcohol 40, Lactic Acid, Glycerin, Dioctyl Sodium Sulfosuccinate, Salicylic Acid, Fragrance, Benzoic Acid, Benzyl Alcohol, Phytosphingosine-HCl 0.01%.	4, 8, 16 oz & 1 gallon
Oti-Soothe® Ear Cleansing Solution (Sogeval)	Deionized water, Propylene Glycol, Aloe Vera Gel, SD Alcohol 40, Lactic Acid, Glycerin, Docusate sodium, Salicylic Acid, Fragrance, Benzoic Acid, Benzyl Alcohol.	4, 8, 16 oz & 1 gallon
Oti-Tris Flush (Schuyler)	TrizEDTA (tromethamine USP, disodium EDTA dehydrate), deionized water.	4 oz
Otocetic Solution® (Vedco)	2% Boric acid and 2% acetic acid with surfactants	4, 16 oz
PhytoVet Ear Cleansing Solution (Schein)	Phytosphingosine HCl 0.01%, Lactic Acid, Salicylic Acid, Benzoic Acid, Aloe Vera Gel.	4, 8, 16 oz
SENTRY® 2-in-1 Ear Cleaner For Dogs (Sergeant's)	Purified Water, Isopropyl Alcohol, Propylene Glycol, Glycerin, Docusate Sodium, FD&C Blue #1, Lanolin, Sodium Benzoate, Aloe Vera, Sodium Hydroxide.	4 oz
Soothables® Crystal-Ear (A.A.H.)	Purified Water, Polyethylene Glycol, Isopropyl Alcohol, Lactic Acid, Polyoxyethylene 20-Sorbitan Monolaurate, Tea Tree Oil and Aloe Vera.	8 oz
Sulfodene® Ear Cleaner (Farnam)	USP purified water, alcohol, acetic acid, nonoxynol 12, methyl paraben, fragrance, dm hydantoin, aloe vera gel.	4 oz
Swimmer's Ear® Astringent (Vedco)	SD-Alcohol 40, Deionized Water, Butylene Glycol, Carbomer, Chloroxylenol, AMP, Fragrance, FD&C Blue No. 1.	4 oz
TrizEDTA® Aqueous and Crystals Flush (Dechra)	Tromethamine (tris-EDTA) USP	4, 16 oz
Vetericyn® Ear Rinse (Innovacyn)	Hypochlorous Acid (HOCl) (0.004%) **Inactive:** Electrolyzed Water (H2O), Sodium Chloride (NaCl), Sodium Hypochlorite (NaOCl)	4 oz
Vetericyn® VF Otic Rinse (Innovacyn)	Hypochlorous Acid (HOCl) (0.011%) **Inactive:** Electrolyzed Water (H2O) (99.816%), Sodium Chloride (NaCl) (0.023%), Sodium Phosphate (NaH2PO4/Na2HPO4) (0.15%)	4 oz
Zymox® Otic with Hydrocortisone (PKB)	Glycerin, Deionized Water, Hydroxy Propyl Cellulose, Benzyl Alcohol, Potassium Iodide, Hydrocortisone, Dextrose, Propylene Glycol, Glucose Oxidase, Lysozyme, Lactoperoxidase, Lactoferrin.	1.25, 4, 8 oz
Zymox® Ear Cleanser (PKB)	Purified Water, Glycerin, Propylene Glycol, Benzyl Alcohol, Sodium Lauryl Sarcosinate, Fragrance, Zinc Gluconate, Glucose Oxidase, Lactoperoxidase, Lactoferrin, Lysozyme.	4 oz
Zymox® Otic Hydrocortisone Free (PKB)	Glycerin, Deionized Water, Hydroxy Propyl Cellulose, Benzyl Alcohol, Potassium Iodide, Dextrose, Propylene Glycol, Glucose Oxidase, Lysozyme, Lactoperoxidase, Lactoferrin.	1.25, 4, 8 oz

Antiseptic Agents

Topical antiseptic ear flushes include acetic acid, chlorhexidine and ketoconazole containing products. These products are typically used as adjunctive therapy for ear infections (*e.g.*, bacterial and/or yeast) but can also be used as sole treatment in mild, first time infections. Acetic acid works as an acidifying and antimicrobial agent. Chlorhexidine has activity against gram-positive and gram-negative bacteria and fungi. Chlorhexidine containing products should be used cautiously in ear canals with ruptured tympanic membranes because of potential for ototoxicity. Ketoconazole is a fungistatic antifungal. When recommending ear flushing as part of the treatment regimen, it is important to demonstrate the cleaning technique in the examination room and advise the client to discontinue application and contact the veterinarian if the ears become more red or more inflamed at any time during the course of cleaning. The frequency of cleaning varies according to the needs of the individual patient.

Trade Name (Manufacturer)	Active Ingredients	Sizes
MalAcetic Otic® *MalAcetic Otic® AP* (Dechra)	Acetic acid 2%, boric acid 2%; *MalAcetic® Otic AP* contains apple fragrance	4, 8, 16 oz
MalAcetic® Ultra Otic (Dechra)	Acetic acid 1%, boric acid 1%, ketoconazole 0.15%, Hydrocortisone 1%	2, 8 oz
Mal-A-Ket Plus TrizEDTA Flush® (Dechra)	Ketoconazole (0.15%), chlorhexidine 0.15%, tris-EDTA	4, 12 oz
Otocetic Solution® (Vedco)	2% Boric acid and 2% acetic acid with surfactants.	4, 16 oz

Trade Name (Manufacturer)	Active Ingredients	Sizes
Vetericyn® Ear Rinse (Innovacyn)	Hypochlorous Acid (HOCl) (0.004%) **Inactive:** Electrolyzed Water (H2O), Sodium Chloride (NaCl), Sodium Hypochlorite (NaOCl)	4 oz
Vetericyn® VF Otic Rinse (Innovacyn)	Hypochlorous Acid (HOCl) (0.011%) **Inactive:** Electrolyzed Water (H2O) (99.816%), Sodium Chloride (NaCl) (0.023%), Sodium Phosphate (NaH2PO4/Na2HPO4) (0.15%)	4 oz

Corticosteroid Preparations

Refer also to the Corticosteroid + Antimicrobial section

Corticosteroid-containing ear medications are used in cases of acute or chronic otitis with the goal of reducing inflammation, edema, tissue hyperplasia, pain and pruritus. In addition, they are helpful in decreasing secretions from sebaceous and apocrine glands thereby reducing the build up of debris in ear canals. Ear cleaning solutions that contain glucocorticoids without an antibiotic can be used as maintenance therapy in cases of allergic otitis, but use the least potent glucocorticoid at the lowest possible frequency to balance efficacy and prevent undesirable side effects.

Trade Name (manufacturer)	Active Ingredients	Sizes
Cort/Astrin Solution® (Vedco)	Hydrocortisone 1% (10 mg), Burow's solution (20 mg)	1, 16 oz
Fluocinolone Otic (various) *DermOtic®* (Royal)	Fluocinolone Acetonide 0.01%	20 mL; human product (Rx)
Synotic Otic Solution® (Zoetis)	Fluocinolone 0.01%; DMSO 60%	8, 60 mL
Zymox® Plus Otic-HC (PKB)	Hydrocortisone 1%	1.25 oz

Antibacterials

Refer also to the Corticosteroid + Antimicrobial section

Antibacterial ear preparations are commonly used to treat infections caused by *Staphylococcus* spp. or *Pseudomonas* spp. Very few otic products containing solely an antibiotic are commercially available to treat bacterial otitis; therefore, the clinician often must use ophthalmic products or injectable antibiotics directly into the ear canals to treat these infections. When using acidifying ear cleansers and with an aminoglycoside- or fluoroquinolone-containing agent, it is recommended to use these products about one hour apart since low pH can decrease the activity of aminoglycosides and fluoroquinolones. When treating a Pseudomonas ear infection, culture and susceptibility should be performed to select the appropriate antibiotic as resistance is a major concern.

These products should be used 2-3 times daily in adequate amounts to coat the entire ear canal. Advise the client to discontinue the medication and contact the veterinarian if the ears become more red or more inflamed at any time during treatment. Patients should be rechecked before discontinuing treatment.

Trade Name (Manufacturer)	Active Ingredients	Sizes; Label Status
Baytril® Otic (Bayer)	Enrofloxacin 0.5%, Silver sulfadiazine (SSD)1%.	15 mL, 30 mL; (Rx)
Ofloxacin Otic (various)	Ofloxacin 0.3%	5, 10 mL; Human-labeled product (Rx)
Tobramycin Ophthalmic Solution (various) *Tobrex®*	Tobramycin 0.3%	5 mL; Human-labeled ophtho product (Rx)

Antibiotic Potentiating Agents

Tromethamine-ethylenediaminetetraacetic acid (tris-EDTA) has antimicrobial and antibiotic potentiating activity. It is alkalinizing (pH8), blocks the *Pseudomonas* efflux pump, potentiates antibiotics such as enrofloxacin and aminoglycosides, disrupts the bacterial cell wall by chelating metal ions and making it more porous, inhibits the effects of ulcerating bacterial enzymes. Tris-EDTA is non-ototoxic and safe to use in the middle ear. Tris-EDTA containing products are most effective when applied 15-30 minutes before the topical antibiotic.

Products containing tris-EDTA are available as a sole ingredient or combined with chlorhexidine or ketoconazole. When recommending ear flushing as part of the treatment regimen, it is important to demonstrate the cleaning technique in the examination room and advise the client to discontinue application and contact the veterinarian if the ears become redder or more inflamed at any time during the course of cleaning. The frequency of cleaning varies according to the needs of the individual patient.

Trade Name (Manufacturer)	Active Ingredients	Sizes
Mal-A-Ket Plus TrizEDTA Flush® (Dechra)	Ketoconazole 0.15%, chlorhexidine 0.15%, tris-EDTA	4, 12 oz
KetoTris Flush + PS (Sogeval)	Ketoconazole 0.1%, Phytosphingosine-HCl 0.01%, Tromethamine (Tris), Ethylenediaminetetraacetic acid (EDTA) in a pH 8 buffered solution.	4, 16 oz

Trade Name (Manufacturer)	Active Ingredients	Sizes
KetoTris Flush (Sogeval)	Ketoconazole 0.1%, Tromethamine (Tris), Ethylenediaminetetraacetic acid (EDTA) in a pH 8 buffered solution.	4, 16 oz
TrizCHLOR® (Dechra)	tris-EDTA, chlorhexidine 0.15%	4 oz
TrizEDTA®, Aqueous or *Crystals Flush* (Dechra)	tris-EDTA	4, 16 oz
TrizULTRA + Keto® (Dechra)	tris-EDTA, ketoconazole 0.15%	4, 12 oz

Antifungals

Refer also to the Corticosteroid + Antimicrobial section

Antifungal ear preparations are used to treat Malassezia otitis and rarely otic candidiasis. Most of the commercially available products also contain an antibiotic and/or a glucocorticoid. Listed here are exclusively the products without an antibiotic agent. These products are not labeled as otics, but have commonly been used in veterinary patients.

These products should be used 2-3 times daily in adequate amounts to coat the entire ear canal. Advise the client to discontinue the medication and contact the veterinarian if the ears become more red or more inflamed at any time during treatment. Patients should be rechecked before discontinuing treatment.

Trade Name (Manufacturer)	Active Ingredients	Sizes
Clotrimazole Solution (various, several brand names)	Clotrimazole 1%	30, 60 mL
Miconazole Lotion (various; several brand names)	1.15% miconazole nitrate (equivalent to 1% miconazole base by weight), polyethylene glycol 400 and ethyl alcohol 55%.	60 mL

Corticosteroid + Antimicrobial Preparations

Refer also to the Corticosteroid + Antimicrobial section

Most of these products should be used 2-3 times daily in adequate amounts to coat the entire ear canal. Advise the client to discontinue the medication and contact the veterinarian if the ears become more red or more inflamed at any time during treatment. Patients should be rechecked before discontinuing treatment.

Trade Name (Manufacturer)	Active Ingredients	Size(s): Label Status
Ciprodex® (Alcon)	Ciprofloxacin 0.3%, Dexamethasone 0.1%	7.5 mL; human product (Rx)
Cipro HC Otic® (Alcon)	Ciprofloxacin 0.2%, Hydrocortisone 1%	10 mL; human product (Rx)
Clotrimazole, Gentamicin and Betamethasone Ointment *Gentizol®* (Vet One) *Malotic®* (Vedco) *Otibiotic®* (Schein) *Otomax®* (Merck); *Remicin®* (Schuler) *Tri-Otic®* (Med-Pharmex) *Vetromax®* (Dechra)	Clotrimazole 1%, Gentamicin sulfate 0.3%, Betamethasone valerate 0.1%	Depending on brand: 7.5, 10, 15, 20, 25, 30 & 215 g
Coly-Mycin S® Otic (JHP) *Cortisporin-TC® Otic* (Monarch)	Neomycin 3.3 mg/mL; Colistin 3 mg/mL, Thonzonium Br 0.5 mg/mL, Hydrocortisone 1%	10 mL; human product (Rx)
Easotic® Otic Suspension (Virbac)	Hydrocortisone aceponate 1.11 mg/mL, miconazole nitrate 15.1 mg/mL and gentamicin sulfate 1.5 mg/mL.	10 - 1mL doses; (Rx)
Gentamicin and Betamethasone Otic Solution *Vet Beta-Gen®* (Med-Pharmex) *GenOne Otic Solution®* (VetOne) *Gentaotic®* (Schein) *GentaVed Otic Solution®* (Vedco)	Gentamicin sulfate 3 mg/mL, Betamethasone valerate 1 mg/mL	Depending on brand: 7.5, 15, & 240 mL
KC-Oto Pak® (Dermazoo)	Ketoconazole 0.15% Hydrocortisone 1 %	54 mL (OTC)
MalAcetic® Ultra Otic Cleanser (Dechra)	Acetic acid 1%, boric acid 1%, ketoconazole 0.15%, Hydrocortisone 1%	2, 8 oz
MoMetaMax® Otic Suspension (Merck)	Gentamicin 3 mg/g, Mometasone 1 mg/g, Clotrimazole 10 mg/g	15, 30 g

Trade Name (Manufacturer)	Active Ingredients	Size(s): Label Status
Neomycin, Polymyxin B, Hydrocortisone Otic Solution and Suspension (various; several brand name products)	Neomycin 3.5 mg/mL, Polymyxin B 10,000 Units/mL, Hydrocortisone 10 mg/mL	7.5 mL or 10 mL depending on brand. Both veterinary and human-labeled products available; (Rx)
Nystatin, Neomycin, Thiostrepton Ointment *Animax®* (Dechra) *Derma Vet®* (Med-Pharmex; Clipper) *Dermalog®* (RXV) *Dermalone®* (Vedco) *Quadritop®* (Schein) *Panolog®* (Zoetis)	Nystatin 100,000 Units/mL, Neomycin sulfate 0.25%, Thiostrepton 2,500 Units, Triamcinolone acetonide 0.1%	Depending on brand: 7.5, 15, 30, & 240 mL
Posatex® Otic Suspension (Merck)	Orbifloxacin 10 mg/g; Mometasone Furoate 0.1%, Posaconazole 0.1%	7.5, 15, & 30 g btls; (Rx). Dosed once daily.
Surolan® Otic Suspension (Elanco)	Miconazole 23 mg/mL, Polymyxin B 0.5293 mg/mL, Prednisolone acetate 5 mg/mL	15 & 30 mL
Tresaderm® (Merial)	Neomycin 0.25%, Dexamethasone 0.1%, Thiabendazole 4%	7.5 mL, 15 mL
Tritop® (Zoetis)	Neomycin sulfate 0.5%, Isoflupredone acetate 0.1%, Tetracaine hydrochloride 0.5%	10 g

Antiparasitic Preparations

Refer also to the Selamectin and Fipronil monographs.

Included are only preparations labeled to be applied directly into the ear canals for the treatment of otoacariosis. However, parasiticides with systemic or more generalized effect such as, selamectin or fipronil are preferred because *Otodectes cynotis* mites are known to also live outside ear canals and can re-infest the ears.

Trade Name (manufacturer)	Active Ingredients	Dose/Use	Comments; Size(s)
Acarexx® Otic Suspension (BIVI)	0.01% Ivermectin	Clean ear and apply 0.5 mL in each ear; repeat one time if necessary	For ear mite infestation in cats or kittens four weeks of age or older. 12 foil pouches with 2 ampules per foil pouch containing 0.5 mL.
Adams Ear-Mite Treatment® (Farnam)	Pyrethrins 0.05% Piperonyl butoxide 0.5%	Clean ears. May be applied daily for 7-10 days. Repeat in 2 weeks if necessary.	Recommended for dogs and cats 12 weeks of age or older. 0.5 oz
Cooper's Best® Ear Mite Lotion (Aspen)	Oil of pennyroyal, Oil of lemongrass, Oil of lavender	Clean ear and apply daily for 7-10 days. Repeat the procedure in 2 weeks if needed.	Aloe. For ear mite infestation on dogs and cats. 6 oz
EarMed® Mite Lotion (Davis)	Oil of pennyroyal, Oil of lemongrass, Oil of lavender	Clean ear and apply once daily for 7-10 days.	Aloe. For ear mite infestation on dogs and cats. 2 oz
Ear Mite Killer® (AgriLabs)	Pyrethrins 0.15%, piperonyl butoxide 1%, N-Octyl bicyclopoheptene dicarboximede 0.5%, di-n-propyl isocinchomeronate 1%	Clean ears. Apply daily for 7-10 days. Do not repeat treatment for 3-5 days if using as a repellent. Horses treated daily for 2-3 days then every 3-5 days as needed for controlling ticks, gnats, etc.	Not for use in horses/foals intended for slaughter. Not for use on puppies or kittens under 12 weeks old; consult veterinarian before using on debilitated, medicated, aged, pregnant or nursing animals. 6 oz
Ear Mite Lotion® (First Companion)	Essential oils, Lavender, Lemongrass and Pennyroyal	Clean ears. Apply daily for 7-10 days.	6 oz
Ear-Rite® Insecticidal Ear Wash (Lambert Kay)	Pyrethrins 0.15%, piperonyl butoxide 1%, N-Octyl bicyclopoheptene dicarboximede 0.5%, di-n-propyl isocinchomeronate 1%	Clean ears. Apply daily for 7-10 days. Do not repeat treatment for 3-5 days if using as a repellent.	Not for use on puppies or kittens under 12 weeks old; consult veterinarian before using on debilitated, medicated, aged, pregnant or nursing animals. 4 oz
Ear-Rite® Miticide for Cats & Kittens (Lambert Kay)	Pyrethrins 0.15%, Piperonyl butoxide 1.5%	Single dose. May repeat every 2 days until condition has cleared up. As a preventative treatment, apply every 15 days.	Not for use on cats <12 weeks of age; consult veterinarian before using on debilitated, medicated, aged, pregnant or nursing animals. 1 oz

Trade Name (manufacturer)	Active Ingredients	Dose/Use	Comments; Size(s)
Eradimite® (Zoetis)	Pyrethrins 0.15%, Piperonyl butoxide 1.5%	Clean ear and apply once. Repeat every 2 days until resolution of infestation. As a preventative treatment, apply every 15 days.	For ear mite and spinose ear tick infestation on dogs and cats. Not for use on dogs, cats or rabbits under 12 weeks of age; consult veterinarian before using on debilitated, medicated, aged, pregnant or nursing animals. 1 oz
Happy Jack Mitex® (Happy Jack)	Pyrethrins 0.05% Piperonyl butoxide 0.5%	Clean ear and apply once daily for 7-10 days. Repeat in 2 weeks if needed.	For ear mite infestation in dogs and cats. 0.5, 1 oz
Hartz® UltraGuard® Ear Mite Treatment for Cats; for Dogs (Hartz)	Pyrethrins 0.05% Piperonyl butoxide 0.5%	Apply once daily for 7-10 days. Repeat in 2 weeks if needed.	For ear mite infestation in cats or puppies <12 weeks old; consult veterinarian before using on debilitated, medicated, aged, pregnant or nursing animals. 3 & 9 mL
MilbeMite® Otic Solution (Novartis)	Milbemycin oxime 0.1%	Clean ear and apply entire contents of tube in external ear canal; one tube per ear. Repeat in 30 days if recommended by the veterinarian.	For ear mite infestation on cats or kittens 4 weeks of age or older; safe use in cats used for breeding purposes, pregnant or lactating has not been evaluated. Box of 10 pouches of 2 tubes of 0.25 mL each
Mita-Clear® (Zoetis)	Pyrethrins 0.15%, Technical piperonyl butoxide 1.5%, N-Octyl bicyclopoheptene dicarboximede 0.5%, di-n-propyl isocinchomeronate 1%	Clean ear; instill enough to wet ear canal and massage. Do not reapply for 7 days.	For ear mite infestation on dogs and cats over 12 weeks of age; consult veterinarian before using on debilitated, medicated, aged, pregnant or nursing animals. 12 mL, 22 mL
No-Bite® Ear Mite Control (Durvet)	Pyrethrins 0.06%, Technical piperonyl butoxide 0.60%,	Apply 2 times a day until ticks/mites are eliminated.	For use on dogs and cats over 12 weeks of age. Consult veterinarian before using on debilitated, medicated, aged, pregnant or nursing animals. 4 oz
Otomite® Plus (Virbac)	Pyrethrins 0.15%, Technical piperonyl butoxide 1.5%, N-octyl bicyclopheptene dicarboximide 0.5%, di-n-propyl isocinchomeronate 1%	Clean ear and instill enough to wet ear canal and massage. Retreat in 7 days.	For ear mite infestation on dogs, cats, puppies and kittens. 15 mL
Sentry HC EARMITEfree® Ear Miticide (Sergeant)	Pyrethrins 0.06%, Piperonyl butoxide 0.6%	Clean ears and apply twice daily until the infestation is resolved.	For mite and tick ear infestation on dogs and cats 12 weeks of age or older; consult veterinarian before using on debilitated, medicated, aged, pregnant or nursing animals. 1 oz
Sergeant's® Vetscription® MITEaway® Ear Mite & Tick Treatment (Sergeant)	Pyrethrins 0.06%, Piperonyl butoxide 0.6%	Clean ears and apply twice daily until the infestation is resolved.	For use on cats and dogs 12 weeks of age or older; consult veterinarian before using on debilitated, medicated, aged, pregnant or nursing animals. 3 oz

Appendix
Multidrug Sensitivity in Dogs

Editor's Note: The following information is adapted, with permission from Washington State University, College of Veterinary Medicine Clinical Pharmacology Laboratory's (VCPL) website: http://www.vetmed.wsu.edu/vcpl/

Reviewed by: Katrina L. Mealey, DVM, PhD, DACVIM, DACVCP; College of Veterinary Medicine, Washington State University, Pullman, WA

Introduction:

Many herding breed dogs—but not exclusively so—have a gene mutation (MDR1; ABCB1) that affects P-glycoprotein, a drug transport pump that plays an important role in limiting drug absorption and distribution (particularly to the brain), as well as enhancing the excretion of many drugs. Dogs with this mutation can have a defective ability to limit drug absorption and distribution, and drugs that are normally transported by P-glycoprotein can have excretion delayed. These effects can lead to potentially serious toxicity.

Affected Breeds:

Approximately 3 of 4 Collies in the United States have the mutant MDR1 gene. The frequency is about the same in France and Australia, so it is likely that most Collies worldwide have the mutation. The MDR1 mutation has also been found in Shetland Sheepdogs (Shelties). Australian Shepherds, Old English Sheepdogs, English Shepherds, German Shepherds, Long-haired Whippets, Silken Windhounds, and a variety of mixed breed dogs. As more dogs are tested, more breeds will likely be added and these frequencies may be change.

Breed	Frequency (approx.)
Australian Shepherd	50%
Australian Shepherd, Mini	50%
Border Collie	< 5%
Collie	70%
English Shepherd	15%
German Shepherd	10%
Herding Breed Cross	10%
Long-haired Whippet	65%
McNab	30%
Mixed Breed	5%
Old English Sheepdog	5%
Shetland Sheepdog	15%
Silken Windhound	30%

Problem Drugs:

Many different drugs and drug classes have been reported to cause problems in dogs that carry the MDR1 mutation. The following drugs have been documented to cause problems in dogs with the MDR1 mutation:

- **ACEPROMAZINE** (tranquilizer and pre-anesthetic agent). In dogs with the MDR1 mutation, acepromazine tends to cause more profound and prolonged sedation. We recommend reducing the dose by 25% in dogs heterozygous for the MDR1 mutation (mutant/normal) and by 30-50% in dogs homozygous for the MDR1 mutation (mutant/mutant).

- **BUTORPHANOL** (analgesic and pre-anesthetic agent). Similar to acepromazine, butorphanol tends to cause more profound and prolonged sedation in dogs with the MDR1 mutation. We recommend reducing the dose by 25% in dogs heterozygous for the MDR1 mutation (mutant/normal) and by 30-50% in dogs homozygous for the MDR1 mutation (mutant/mutant).

- **EMODEPSIDE** (*Profender®*) is a deworming drug approved for use in cats only in the U.S., but is approved for use in dogs in some other countries. Use of this drug in dogs with the MDR1 mutation has resulted in neurological toxicity.

- **ERYTHROMYCIN**. Erythromycin may cause neurological signs in dogs with the MDR1 mutation. A mutant/mutant collie exhibited signs of neurological toxicity after receiving erythromycin. After withdrawal of the drug, the dog's neurological signs resolved. There were no other potential causes of neurological toxicity identified in the dog.

- **IVERMECTIN** (antiparasitic agent). While the dose of ivermectin used to prevent heartworm infection is SAFE in dogs with the mutation (6 micrograms per kilogram), higher doses, such as those used for treating mange (300-600 micrograms per kilogram) will cause neurological toxicity in dogs that are homozygous for the MDR1 mutation (mutant/mutant) and can cause toxicity in dogs that are heterozygous for the mutation (mutant/normal).

- **LOPERAMIDE** (*Imodium®*; antidiarrheal agent). At doses used to treat diarrhea, this drug will cause neurological toxicity in dogs with the MDR1 mutation. This drug should be avoided in all dogs with the MDR1 mutation.

- **SELAMECTIN, MILBEMYCIN,** and **MOXIDECTIN** (antiparasitic agents). Similar to ivermectin, these drugs are safe in dogs with the mutation if used for heartworm prevention at the manufacturer's recommended dose. Higher doses (generally 10-20 times higher than the heartworm prevention dose) have been documented to cause neurological toxicity in dogs with the MDR1 mutation.

- **VINCRISTINE, VINBLASTINE, DOXORUBICIN** (chemotherapy agents). Based on some published and ongoing research, it appears that dogs with the MDR1 mutation are more sensitive to these drugs with regard to their likelihood of having an adverse drug reaction. Bone marrow suppression (decreased blood cell counts, particularly neutrophils) and GI toxicity (anorexia, vomiting, diarrhea) are more likely to occur at normal doses in dogs with the MDR1 mutation. To reduce the likelihood of severe toxicity in these dogs, MDR1 mutant/normal dogs should have their dose reduced by 25% while MDR1 mutant/mutant dogs should have their dose reduced by a full 50%. These patients should be closely monitored for adverse effects.

The following drugs appear to be safely tolerated by dogs with the MDR1 mutation:

- **CYCLOSPORINE** (immunosuppressive agent). While we know that cyclosporin is pumped by P-glycoprotein (the protein encoded by the MDR1 gene), we have not documented any increased sensitivity to this drug in dogs with the MDR1 mutation compared to "normal" dogs. Therefore, we do not recommend altering the dose of cyclosporin for dogs with the MDR1 mutation, but we do recommend therapeutic drug monitoring.

- **DIGOXIN** (cardiac drug). While we know that digoxin is pumped by P-glycoprotein (the protein encoded by the MDR1 gene), we have not documented any increased sensitivity to this drug in dogs with the MDR1 mutation compared to "normal" dogs. Therefore, we do not recommend altering the dose of digoxin for dogs with the MDR1 mutation, but do recommend therapeutic drug monitoring.

- **DOXYCYCLINE** (antibacterial drug). While we know that doxycycline is pumped by P-glycoprotein (the protein encoded by the MDR1 gene), we have not documented any increased sensitivity to this drug in dogs with the MDR1 mutation compared to "normal" dogs. Therefore, we do not recommend altering the dose of doxycycline for dogs with the MDR1 mutation.

- **MORPHINE, BUPRENORPHINE, FENTANYL** (opioid analgesics or pain medications). We suspect that these drugs are pumped by P-glycoprotein (the protein encoded by the MDR1 gene) in dogs because they have been reported to be pumped by P-glycoprotein in people, but we are not aware of any reports of toxicity caused by these drugs in dogs with the MDR1 mutation. We do not have specific dose recommendations for these drugs for dogs with the MDR1 mutation.

Use caution. The following drugs have been reported to be pumped by P-glycoprotein in humans, but there is currently no data stating whether they are or are not pumped by canine P-glycoprotein:

- **DOMPERIDONE**
- **ETOPOSIDE**
- **MITOXANTRONE**
- **ONDANSETRON**
- **PACLITAXEL**
- **RIFAMPICIN**

There are many additional drugs pumped by human P-glycoprotein (the protein encoded by the MDR1 gene), but data is not yet available with regard to their effect in dogs with the MDR1 mutation.

Testing:

While certain breeds have a predilection for the mutation, only PCR testing can identify normal dogs (normal/normal), heterozygote dogs (normal/mutant, mutant/normal), or homozygote mutant dogs (mutant/mutant). The test is patented and available in the USA, Europe and Australia/New Zealand.

- In the USA (or any country **except** Australia & New Zealand): More information and testing kit ordering information can be obtained by contacting the Veterinary Clinical Pharmacology Laboratory at Washington State University: www.vetmed.wsu.edu/vcpl by phone at 509-335-3745 or email at VCPL@vetmed.wsu.edu

- In Australia/New Zealand: Contact Gribbles Veterinary Pathology 1868 Dandenong Road Clayton VIC 3168 Australia. Phone: +61 3 9538 2241 Fax: +61 3 9538 6778 email: rick.mccoy@healthscope.com.au web: http://www.gribblesvets.com.au/

Overdose and Toxin Exposure Decontamination Guidelines

Camille DeClementi, VMD, DABT, DABVT
ASPCA Animal Poison Control Center

All patients should be stabilized prior to attempts at decontamination. Once stabilization has been accomplished, decontamination should be considered to prevent systemic absorption of the toxicant.

The specific method of decontamination chosen in each case must be guided by the species exposed and the exposure circumstances. When a patient has ingested a potentially toxic dose of a substance, the clinician has many options for decontamination including dilution, induction of emesis, gastric lavage, the use of adsorbents, cathartics, and administration of enemas. In many cases, the best treatment plan will include more than one of these methods.

Dilution using a small amount of milk or water is recommended in cases where irritant or corrosive materials have been ingested. A dose of 2-6 mL/kg is suggested (Mathews, 2006), which for an average-sized cat, would be approximately only 1 – 2 teaspoons. Giving only a small amount is important since using excessive amounts could lead to vomiting and re-exposure of the esophagus to the damaging material (Rosendale, 2002). Juicy fruits and vegetables can be fed to accomplish dilution in some patients, especially birds and reptiles. Dilution is not appropriate in patients who are at an increased risk for aspiration, including those who are actively seizing or obtunded (Rosendale, 2002). Dilution with milk, yogurt and cottage cheese has been useful in cases of oral irritation following ingestion of plants containing insoluble calcium oxalate crystals (Philodendron species, for example) (Means, 2004).

Emetics are usually most effective if used within 2-3 hours after the ingestion (Rosendale, 2002) but in some cases, emesis may be effective even after that time frame. If the substance ingested could coalesce to form a bezoar in the stomach or a timed-released medication was ingested, emesis may be effective later than 3 hours after the ingestion. Chocolate (Albretsen, 2004) and chewable medications are examples of products, which may form bezoars. Emetics generally empty 40-60% of the stomach contents (Beasley and Dorman, 1990). Feeding a small moist meal before inducing vomiting can increase the chances of an adequate emesis.

Animals that are able to vomit safely include dogs, cats, ferrets, and potbelly pigs. Emetics should not be used in birds, rodents, rabbits, horses or ruminants. Rodents are unable to vomit. Rabbits have a thin-walled stomach putting them at risk for gastric rupture if they vomit (Donnelly, 2004).

Induction of emesis is **contraindicated** with ingestion of corrosive agents including alkalis and acids. The protective epithelial lining of the esophagus may be damaged initially when one of these products is swallowed. The muscular layer of the esophagus may be exposed and at risk for ulceration, perforation and scarring if vomiting does occur (Beasley and Dorman, 1990). Emesis is also not recommended after petroleum distillate ingestion due to the risk of aspiration. The clinician must also take into account when deciding whether to induce emesis, any pre-existing conditions of the patient that can cause vomiting to be hazardous including severe cardiac disease or seizure disorder. In all instances the attending veterinarian must carefully weigh the benefits of emesis against the risks. Emesis may not be needed if the animal has already vomited and is not appropriate if the animal is already exhibiting clinical signs such as coma, seizures or recumbency, which make emesis hazardous. Additionally, if the patient has ingested a CNS stimulant and is already agitated, the additional stimulation of vomiting could lead to seizures (Rosendale, 2002).

Hydrogen peroxide, apomorphine hydrochloride and xylazine hydrochloride are commonly used emetics in the veterinary clinical setting. Preliminary data obtained from the ASPCA Animal Poison Control's toxicology database indicate that hydrogen peroxide and apomorphine are effective emetics in dogs. Emesis was successful in ninety-two percent of dogs when administered either 3% hydrogen peroxide or apomorphine. No significant adverse effects were reported in dogs after emetic use. Apomorphine was poorly effective as an emetic in cats and using it in cats is controversial. Xylazine was an effective emetic in only fifty-seven percent of cats. When emesis was successfully induced, sixty-eight percent of patients vomited some portion of the ingested toxicant (Khan, 2009). Some clinicians are also using dexmedetomidine as an emetic in cats. Please see the monographs in the text for additional information on using these as emetics.

Several other agents have been suggested by various sources as emetics. These include table salt, liquid dishwashing liquid, syrup of ipecac and powdered mustard. They are not as effective as those mentioned, and salt and syrup of ipecac may cause significant adverse effects. Table salt (sodium chloride) has been associated with hypernatremia and CNS dysfunction (Beasley and Dorman, 1990) and there are concerns that syrup of ipecac can be cardiotoxic (Rosendale, 2002). Human pediatricians no longer routinely recommend syrup of ipecac for home use and The American Association of Poison Control Centers reported in 2001 that the use of ipecac in human exposures has fallen by more than 95% over a 15-year period (Shannon, 2003).

An October 12, 2010 bulletin by the American Society of Health-System Pharmacists indicates that syrup of ipecac has been discontinued (http://goo.gl/dwbY2).

Gastric lavage can be considered in cases where emesis is contraindicated, not possible or has been unsuccessful. For example, lavage is an option if the patient is agitated, seizing or recumbent or has other health concerns, such as recent abdominal surgery, that increase the risks associated with induction of emesis. Gastric lavage should be considered in rabbits and rodents, which are unable to vomit safely. Lavage is unlikely to be as effective as emesis (Beasley and Dorman, 1990) and is associated with significant potential risks (Rosendale, 2002). For these reasons, it should not be chosen routinely as a decontamination method over emesis. Lavage should also not be used to remove caustic materials or volatile hydrocarbons for the same reasons emesis is contraindicated in such cases (Rosendale, 2002).

The patient should be under general anesthesia when performing gastric lavage unless the patient is comatose. In all instances, a cuffed endotracheal tube should be in place to prevent aspiration. If the patient is a species with cheek pouches, the cheek pouches should be emptied gently with a finger or swab prior to the lavage. Risks associated with gastric lavage include esophageal or stomach damage or perforation, electrolyte abnormalities, hypothermia and the accidental placement of the tube in the trachea and the instillation of fluid into the patient's lungs (Rosendale, 2002).

Adsorbents may be utilized instead of or in addition to using an emetic or performing gastric lavage to prevent further systemic absorption of a toxicant. These agents act by adsorbing to a chemical or toxicant in the gastrointestinal tract and facilitating its excretion in the feces. Activated charcoal is the most commonly used adsorbent.

Activated charcoal is composed of large porous particles that adsorb to and therefore trap a wide range of organic compounds within the gastrointestinal tract. It is created from materials such as coal, wood, rye starch and coconut shells through a process using acid and steam treatments. The surface binding area of activated charcoal is large, in the range of 900 – 1500 m²/g (Rosendale, 2002). Charcoal tablets and capsules available over the counter, which are used to control flatulence, and bloating are not likely to be as effective adsorbents as the commercially prepared products (Buck and Bratich, 1986). The concentration of charcoal in the capsules is often low and the binding area much smaller.

Repeated doses of activated charcoal should be considered in some instances where toxicants are known to undergo enterohepatic recirculation. In enterohepatic recirculation, the toxicant is first carried to the liver by either the portal vein after absorption from the gastrointestinal tract or via the systemic circulation. Once in the liver, the toxicant enters the bile and is excreted into the gastrointestinal tract where it is again available for absorption. Examples of toxicants known to undergo this type of recycling include most NSAIDs, marijuana and digoxin.

Another instance where multiple doses of activated charcoal are appropriate is in the treatment of ivermectin toxicosis. Ivermectin is a substrate for the P-glycoprotein pump that transports drugs across cell membranes. This pump is found in various cells including intestinal epithelial cells and brain capillary endothelial cells. In the intestine, ivermectin is absorbed into the enterocyte. However, once in the cell, the P-glycoprotein pump moves the ivermectin back into the gastrointestinal lumen. This cycling allows the ivermectin molecules to have multiple opportunities to bind with the repeated doses of activated charcoal (DeClementi, 2007). Other P-glycoprotein substrates include loperamide, diltiazem and doxorubicin (Mealey, 2006).

When repeated doses are indicated, half the original dose should be given at 4 to 8 hour intervals (Peterson, 2006). It is important to mention that if medications are excreted in the bile, activated charcoal can be beneficial regardless of the route the medication was administered. Thus if a patient received an overdose of injectable ivermectin subcutaneously, use of activated charcoal will still be a very useful (DeClementi, 2007).

Administration of activated charcoal does carry some risks and it does not bind all compounds equally. Some chemicals that are not bound effectively include: ethanol, methanol, fertilizer, fluoride, petroleum distillates, most heavy metals, iodides, nitrates, nitrites, sodium chloride, and chlorate. Activated charcoal should not be given to animals that have ingested caustic materials. It is unlikely to bind them, can be additionally irritating to the mucosal surfaces, and make visualization of oral and esophageal burns difficult (Buck and Bratich, 1986). Activated charcoal can cause a false positive on an ethylene glycol test since propylene glycol is found in many formulations. Additionally, the timing of the activated charcoal administration should be taken into account when deciding on dosing of other oral medications since the charcoal can also bind them.

Activated charcoal administration carries a significant risk of aspiration. If a patient does aspirate the charcoal, the prognosis is poor, hence proper placement of the stomach tube and a protected airway are required in symptomatic patients. Constipation and black bowel movements are possible making it difficult to determine if melena is present. If the activated charcoal resides within the gastrointestinal tract for a significant period, it may release the compound it has adsorbed. It is for this reason that activated charcoal is frequently administered with a cathartic. Many commercially available preparations do contain a cathartic such as sorbitol.

Hypernatremia is another possible adverse effect of activated charcoal administration. In humans, hypernatremia has been reported primarily in children when multiple doses of a charcoal-sorbitol mixture were administered. The mechanism for hypernatremia is attributed to a water shift from the intracellular and extracellular spaces into the gastrointestinal tract as a result of the osmotic pull of the sorbitol cathartic (Allerton and Strom, 1991). The ASPCA Animal Poison Control Center (APCC) has also received reports of elevated serum sodium following activated charcoal administration in dogs. Hypernatremia appears to be reported more often in small dogs receiving multiple doses of activated charcoal, but it has also been reported in large dogs and in cases receiving only a single dose. Furthermore, unlike the human reports, elevated serum sodium has also been noted in cases where no cathartic was present in the charcoal (Ball, 2014). In hypernatremia cases, the APCC has found that administration of a warm water enema is effective at lowering the serum sodium and controlling the resultant central nervous system effects (DeClementi, 2007).

<u>Cathartics</u> enhance elimination of substances, including administered activated charcoal, by promoting their movement through the gastrointestinal tract. Activated charcoal only binds to toxicants by weak chemical forces, so without cathartics the bound toxicant can eventually be released and reabsorbed (Rosendale, 2002). When used with activated charcoal, the cathartic is given immediately following or mixed with the charcoal. Cathartics are contraindicated if the animal is dehydrated, has diarrhea, if ileus is present, or if intestinal obstruction or perforation are possible (Peterson, 2006).

There are bulk, osmotic, and lubricant cathartics. The most commonly used bulk cathartic is psyllium hydrophilic mucilloid (*e.g.*, *Metamucil*®). Another bulking cathartic that can be used in dogs and cats is unspiced canned pumpkin. In birds and reptiles, dilute peanut butter, fruit or vegetables can also be used as bulking agents. Timothy hay can be utilized in rabbits. Osmotic cathartics have limited absorption from the gastrointestinal tract so they are able to pull water into the gastrointestinal tract, thereby increasing the fluid volume and stimulating motility to hasten expulsion in the feces.

There are saline and saccharide osmotic cathartics. Sorbitol is the most commonly used saccharide osmotic cathartic; it is the cathartic of choice and is frequently combined with activated charcoal in commercially prepared charcoal products. The saline cathartics include sodium sulfate (Glauber's salts) and magnesium sulfate (Epsom salts). Saline cathartics should not be used in patients with renal insufficiency or in birds or reptiles.

Of the lubricant cathartics, mineral oil is the most often used. Mineral oil is not recommended following activated charcoal administration as the mineral oil may render the charcoal less effective (Buck and Bratich, 1986; Galey, 1992). Since all cathartics alter the water balance in the gastrointestinal tract, electrolyte abnormalities, especially hypernatremia, are a potential risk to their use. Hydration status should be monitored frequently and fluids administered, intravenously or via an enema as needed.

<u>Enemas</u> may be indicated when elimination of toxicants from the lower gastrointestinal tract is desired (Beasley and Dorman, 1990). Medications formulated as extended-release or controlled-release are absorbed from the entire gastrointestinal tract, including the colon (Buckley et al., 1995). An enema can be used to move those medications through the colon quickly and lessen additional systemic effects. The general technique is to use plain warm water or warm soapy water. Phosphate enema solutions should be avoided due to the risk of electrolyte and acid-base disturbances (Beasley and Dorman, 1990). In reptiles, enemas may be useful since ingested materials often lag for prolonged periods in the colon. Enemas are not recommended for birds since they already have a rapid gastrointestinal transit time.

Resources/References:
Animal Poison Centers: The following are known 24-hour poison control centers in the USA that specialize in providing information specific for veterinary patients. Fees listed are those at the time of writing (August 2014).

- <u>ASPCA Animal Poison Control Center</u>: Phone: **888-426-4435**; $65 consultation fee. http://www.aspca.org/pet-care/animal-poison-control

- <u>Pet Poison Helpline</u>: Phone: **800-213-6680**; $39 consultation fee. http://www.petpoisonhelpline.com

Albretsen, J.C. (2004). Methylxanthines. In "Clinical Veterinary Toxicology" (K.H. Plumlee, Ed.), pp. 322-326. Mosby, St. Louis.

Allerton, J.P., and Strom, J.A. (1991). Hypernatremia due to repeated doses of charcoal-sorbitol. Am J Kidney Dis 17, 581-584.

Ball, A. (2014). Toxicology case: Managing hypernatremia after activated charcoal administration. http://veterinarymedicine.dvm360.com/vetmed/Toxicology/Toxicology-case-Managing-hypernatremia-after-activ/ArticleStandard/Article/detail/839410

Beasley, V.R., and Dorman, D.C. (1990). Management of Toxicoses. Vet Clin North Am Small Anim Pract 20, 307-337.

Buck, W.B., and Bratich, P.M. (1986). Activated charcoal: preventing unnecessary death by poisoning. Vet Med 81, 73-77.

Buckley, N.A., Dawson, A.H., and Reith, D.A. (1995). Controlled release drugs in overdose Clinical considerations. Drug Safety 12, 73-84.

DeClementi, C. (2007). Prevention and treatment of poisoning. In "Veterinary Toxicology Basic and Clinical Principles" (R.C. Gupta, Ed.), pp. 1143 – 1147. Elsevier, Amsterdam.

Donnelly, T.M. (2004). Rabbits. Basic Anatomy, Physiology, and Husbandry. In "Ferrets, Rabbits, and Rodents Clinical Medicine and Surgery" (K.E. Quesenberry and J.W. Carpenter, Eds.), 2nd Ed, pp. 136-139. Saunders, St. Louis.

Galey, F.D. (1992). Diagnostic Toxicology. In "Current Therapy in Equine Medicine 3" (N.E. Robinson, Ed.), pp. 337-340. W.B. Saunders Company, Philadelphia.

Khan, S., McLean, M.K., Hansen, S., Luchinski, D., and Zawistowski, S. (2009) ASPCA Animal Poison Control Center uses its databases to study the efficacy and safety of three different emetics in dogs and cats utilizing 3R principles. Poster presented at 7th World Congress on Alternatives and Animal Use in the Life Sciences. Rome, Italy.

Mathews, K.A. (2006). "Veterinary Emergency and Critical Care Manual." Lifelearn Inc., Guelph. pp. 4-8, 12-17, 85, 630-640, 655-659.

Mealey, K.L. (2006). Adverse drug reactions in herding-breed dogs: the role of P-glycoprotein. Compend Contin Educ Pract Vet 28, 23-33.

Means, C. (2004). Insoluble Calcium Oxalates. In "Clinical Veterinary Toxicology" (K.H. Plumlee, Ed.), pp. 340-341. Mosby, St. Louis.

Peterson, M.E. (2006). Toxicological Decontamination. In "Small Animal Toxicology" (M.E. Peterson and P.A. Talcott, Eds.), 2nd Ed, pp. 127-141. Elsevier Inc., St. Louis.

Rosendale, M.E. (2002). Decontamination strategies. Vet Clin North Am Small Anm Prac 32, 311-321.

Shannon, M. (2003). The demise of ipecac. J Pediatr Vol. 112, 1180-1181.

"Drug Store" Toxins in Small Animals

Trishna Patel, PharmD
Resident in Veterinary Pharmacy
University of California-Davis

Ahna Brutlag, DVM, MS, DABT, DABVT
Associate Director of Veterinary Services
Pet Poison Helpline & SafetyCall International, PLLC

The following is a list of products or compounds that may be found in retail settings, pharmacies, or in 'human' drugs, that may be potentially toxic to dogs, cats, or other pets. It is a <u>partial list only</u> and is not meant to be inclusive of all potentially toxic items. In addition, there are many human prescription drugs with significant toxic potential for small animals. Refer to the systemic monograph section; if the drug is not listed consult with an animal poison center for more information (see listing at the end of this section).

Over-the-Counter (OTC) Medications

- **5-HYDROXYTRYPTOPHAN** (5-HTP or *Griffonia* seed extract): Human dietary supplement; serotonin precursor. Toxic to dogs and cats as it induces serotonin syndrome. Clinical signs include sedation at low doses. High doses cause agitation, tremors, seizures, hyperthermia, GI upset, ataxia, abdominal pain, hyperesthesia, and transient blindness. The minimum oral toxic dose for dogs is 24 mg/kg; the minimum oral lethal dose for dogs is 128 mg/kg. (Peterson *et al.* 2013)

- **ACETAMINOPHEN** (*e.g.*, *Tylenol*®; APAP): Human analgesic/antipyretic. Contraindicated in cats at any dosage and not recommended for ferrets. In cats, can cause methemoglobinemia, hepatic necrosis, and death. Clinical signs include shock, brown mucous membranes, respiratory distress, cyanosis, lethargy, depression, coma, and edema of face and paws. In dogs, hepatotoxicity and methemoglobinemia can also occur and dosages above 100 mg/kg are considered toxic. Clinical signs include anorexia, nausea, vomiting, lethargy, abdominal pain, icterus, hepatic encephalopathy, and coma. (Osweiler *et al.* 2011)

- **ALPHA LIPOIC ACID** (thioctic acid, ALA): Dietary supplement used to manage diabetes. Dose dependent toxicity in dogs and cats; cats are more sensitive. Clinical signs develop in 30 minutes to several hours with acute hypoglycemia as the primary concern. Other clinical signs include hypersalivation, vomiting, ataxia, tremors and seizures. Anecdotal therapeutic dose in cats is 1 – 5 mg/kg daily; the minimum toxic dose is 13 mg/kg. ALA is considered 10 times more toxic to cats than dogs. In dogs, the experimental minimum tolerated dose is 126 mg/kg but suspicious deaths have been reported at 100 mg/kg.

- **ASPIRIN** (ASA): Toxicity is dose dependent—see Aspirin monograph for more information. Used therapeutically in dogs and cats but at very different doses. Cats are very sensitive to salicylates and have half-lives of 38-45 hours at 25 mg/kg. Severe intoxication occurs at 80+ mg/kg in cats and 100 – 500 mg/kg in dogs. Clinical signs: vomiting, GI ulceration, hematemesis, melena, Heinz body anemia (cats), metabolic acidosis, hyperthermia, renal and liver damage.

- **CAFFEINE** (*e.g., No-Doze*®, also found in analgesics, coffee, energy drinks & gums, foods such as chocolate): Toxic to dogs and cats. Clinical signs include vomiting, diarrhea, polyuria, polydipsia, hyperactivity, ataxia, tachycardia, tachypnea, hypertension, weakness, cardiac arrhythmias, tremors, seizures, and coma. Death can result from cardiac arrhythmia or respiratory failure. Clinical signs begin at 15 mg/kg. The oral LD_{50} in dogs is 140 mg/kg and 80 – 150 mg/kg in cats. (Osweiler *et al.* 2011)

- **DEXTROMETHORPHAN** (*e.g., Delsym*®; *Robitussin-DM*®): Human cough suppressant. Toxicity is dose dependent. Has been used anecdotally in dogs at 2 mg/kg PO twice daily to treat repetitive behavioral disorders. Clinical signs of toxicity include agitation, hallucination, nervousness, mydriasis, shaking, vomiting, or diarrhea. Some clinical signs may be similar to serotonin syndrome such as tremors, seizures, hyperesthesia, hyperthermia, hypersalivation, and death. (Osweiler *et al.* 2011)

- **IBUPROFEN** (*e.g., Advil*®, *Motrin*®): Human NSAID. Toxic to dogs, cats, and ferrets; not recommended for veterinary use. Gastrointestinal ulceration may occur as evidenced by hematemesis, diarrhea, melena (black-tarry stool), weakness, pale mucus membranes, abdominal pain, lethargy, and inappetence. With larger ingestions acute renal failure, liver failure and neurological signs such as tremors or seizures can develop. In ferrets, toxicity affects gastrointestinal, renal, and central nervous systems. (Dunayer 2004)

- **IMIDAZOLINES** (*e.g.,* oxymetazoline [*Afrin*®], tetrahydrozoline [*Visine*®], naphazoline, tolazoline): Toxic to all pets. Not recommended for veterinary use. Poisoning occurs most commonly after pets chew open product vials. Clinical signs of intoxication may include vomiting, bradycardia, cardiac arrhythmias, poor capillary refill time, hypotension or hypertension, panting, depression, weakness, nervousness, hyperactivity, or shaking. These signs appear within 30 minutes to 4 hours post-exposure. In general, imidazoline decongestant exposure may affect the GI, cardiopulmonary, and nervous systems. Veterinary alpha$_2$ adrenergic antagonists such as atipamezole (*Domitor*®) or yohimbine may be antidotal.

- **IRON** (Fe): Found in over-the-counter iron supplements (see the Ferrous Sulfate monograph), multivitamins, prenatal vitamins, fertilizers, pesticides, one-time use hand warmers or heating pads such as *ThermaCare*®, and oxygen absorber sachets in food packaging (*e.g.,* beef jerky). Toxicity in dogs observed at doses greater than 20 mg/kg of elemental iron. Clinical signs include vomiting, bloody diarrhea, lethargy, abdominal pain, and gastrointestinal ulcerations. More severe signs such as metabolic acidosis, shock, hypotension, hypovolemia, tachycardia, coagulation deficits, hepatic necrosis, tremors, seizures, and coma can occur. Amount of elemental iron ingested should be determined to assess toxicity. Oxygen absorbers used in food packaging are commonly mistaken for silica gel packets, which are non-toxic. (Albertson 2006)

- **NAPROXEN** (*Aleve*®): Human NSAID. Highly toxic to dogs, cats, and ferrets. No longer recommended for veterinary use in small animals. See the Naproxen monograph for more information. In dogs, doses of 5 mg/kg may result in gastrointestinal irritation or ulceration, and doses greater than 10 – 20 mg/kg may result in acute renal failure. Stomach ulcers, bloody vomiting, diarrhea, black-tarry stool, weakness, pale gums, abdominal pain, lethargy, and inappetence may occur.

- **PERMETHRIN**: Topical insecticide. Toxic to cats in concentrated formulas (typically greater than 5-7%). Over-the-counter lice treatment products typically contain 1% permethrin or pyrethrins/piperonyl butoxide and are not usually of concern. Cats are highly sensitive to pyrethrins and pyrethroids, application of concentrated products could be fatal. The most common clinical signs observed are nervous system effects such as hyperesthesia, generalized tremors, muscle fasciculation, hyperthermia, and seizures. Clinical signs can develop within hours or may be delayed up to 72 hours and generally last 2-3 days. (Richardson 2000)

- **PHENAZOPYRIDINE** (*Pyridium*®; PAP): Human urinary analgesic. May be toxic to dogs and cats; not recommended for veterinary use. Cyanosis, methemoglobinemia, rhabdomyolysis and hepatotoxicity possible. (Holahan *et al.* 2010)

- **PHENYLEPHRINE** (*Sudafed-PE*®): Human oral decongestant. May be toxic to dogs and cats at high doses. Ingestion can result in hyperactivity, agitation, vomiting, mydriasis, tachycardia, hypertension, hyperthermia, cyanosis, arrhythmias, tremors, and seizures. Pet owners purchasing antihistamines for their pets may unwittingly select a combination product. (Osweiler *et al.* 2011)

- **PSEUDOEPHEDRINE** (*Sudafed*®): Human oral decongestant with sympathomimetic properties. Can be highly toxic to dogs and cats. In dogs, 5 – 6 mg/kg results in moderate to severe clinical signs with death possible at 10 – 12 mg/kg. Ingestion can result in hyperactivity, agitation, vomiting, mydriasis, tachycardia, hypertension, hyperthermia, cyanosis, arrhythmias, tremors, and seizures. Pet owners purchasing antihistamines for their pets may unwittingly select a combination product. See the Pseudoephedrine monograph for additional information. (Osweiler *et al.* 2011)

- **VITAMIN D** (D2, D3; cholecalciferol): Found in rodenticides, multivitamins and flavored chewable vitamins, such as *Viactiv*®. Ingestion of cholecalciferol-rodenticides carries a greater risk of toxicosis than ingestion of over the counter supplements. Intoxication results from hypercalcemia and hyperphosphatemia followed by metastatic mineralization, typically presenting as acute renal failure. Clinical signs are observed within the first 48 hours of overdose and can include vomiting, lethargy, muscle weakness, bloody diarrhea, depression, polyuria and polydipsia. With high doses, death from acute renal failure can result. (Morrow 2001)

Medicinal Oils, Solvents or Excipients

- **BENZYL ALCOHOL:** Preservative. Commonly found in injectable drug products. Cats may be very susceptible to toxic effects. Clinical signs associated benzyl alcohol toxicity include ataxia, hyperesthesia, muscle fasciculation, depression, coma, respiratory failure, and death. (Wilcke 1984)
- **PEPPERMINT OIL** (menthol): Toxic to cats. Ingested peppermint oil may cause gastrointestinal upset, CNS depression, and hepatotoxicity. Inhalation may cause aspiration pneumonia. Caution: Some formulations (i.e., wintergreen oil) contain aspirin derivatives with additional toxic potential.
- **PROPYLENE GLYCOL:** Commonly found in 'safer' alternative antifreeze ('pet-safe' antifreeze, RV antifreeze, etc.), hair dyes, disinfectants, and paints/varnish. The canine oral LD_{50} is 9 mL/kg of undiluted propylene glycol. Initial clinical signs can include depression, weakness, ataxia, polyuria, and polydipsia. Lactic acidosis occurs later. Heinz body anemia occurs in cats. Hypotension, cardiovascular collapse and seizures can occur. (Osweiler et al. 2011)
- **TEA TREE OIL** (melaleuca oil): Topical antibacterial agent. Toxicosis is common following exposure to 100% oil (oral or dermal exposure). As little as 7 drops of oil have caused poisoning in pets. Cats are more susceptible to toxicosis than dogs. Clinical signs observed include ataxia, hypothermia, dehydration, muscle tremors and coma. May be hepatotoxic to cats. (Bischoff et al. 1998)
- **XYLITOL:** Natural sweetener with a low glycemic index. Commonly found in many sugar-free foods and chewing gum, breath mints, nicotine gum, baked goods, oral care products, nasal sprays, chewable vitamins and some prescription medications, including gabapentin (Neurontin®) oral liquid, and some oral dispersing tablet (ODT) formulations. Can be toxic to dogs; hypoglycemia, lethargy, vomiting, ataxia, collapse, and seizures can occur. Acute liver failure possible. Dogs ingesting greater than 0.1 g/kg of xylitol are considered at risk for developing hypoglycemia; doses greater than 0.5 g/kg may be hepatotoxic. (Murphy et al. 2012)

Foods

- **ALLIUM-CONTAINING FOODS** (garlic, onion, leeks, chives): May be toxic to dogs and cats. Oral consumption can lead to toxicosis. Clinical signs result from hemolytic anemia and often include depression, hemoglobinuria, icterus, tachypnea, tachycardia, weakness, and exercise intolerance. Inappetence, abdominal pain, and diarrhea may also occur. Development of clinical signs is delayed; they may not be observed until several days after ingestion. (Cope 2005)
- **CHOCOLATE:** Toxic to dogs and cats. Primary toxic component is theobromine. Clinical signs occur 6-12 hours after ingestion. Initial signs include polydipsia, vomiting, diarrhea, and restlessness, followed by hyperactivity, polyuria, ataxia, tremors, and seizures. Other effects include tachycardia, premature ventricular contractions, tachypnea, cyanosis, hypertension, hyperthermia, and coma. Pancreatitis can occur 24-72 hours after ingestion, due to the high fat content in chocolate. Death can result from cardiac arrhythmias or respiratory failure. Dogs can easily ingest a toxic dose of chocolate. (Gwaltney-Brant 2001)
- **GRAPES/RAISINS/ZANTE CURRANTS** (Vitis spp.): Toxic to dogs. Clinical signs can appear within hours and include vomiting, diarrhea, lethargy, and polydipsia. Acute renal failure may develop within 24 hours to several days after exposure. No toxic dose has been established and all exposures are concerning. (McKnight 2005)

- **MACADAMIA NUTS:** Toxic to dogs. Common clinical signs of macadamia nut ingestion include weakness, depression, vomiting, ataxia, tremors, joint pain, lameness, hind limb weakness, hyperthermia, recumbency, and abdominal pain. Clinical signs are typically seen at doses greater than 2 g/kg. Reports of clinical signs seen at doses as low as 0.7 mg/kg. (Osweiler et al. 2011)
- **XYLITOL:** See above in "Medicinal Oils, Solvents or Excipients" section.

Household Products/Solvents

- **ACIDS** (found in drain/toilet bowl cleaners, hair wave neutralizers, metal cleaners, rust removers and vinegar): Tissue damage is related to pH and concentration. Products with a pH of 2-4 can cause mild to moderate tissue irritation. Products with a pH <2 are corrosive; some examples include acetic acid (>50%), aluminum sulfate (>20%), HCl (>10%), and sulfuric acid (>10%). Clinical signs include oral/dermal/GI ulcerations, dysphagia, vomiting, hematemesis, abdominal pain, stridor, and coughing. Inducing emesis is not recommended. (Osweiler et al. 2011)
- **ALKALIS/BASES** (found in drain cleaners, dry cell batteries, hair relaxers, lye, non-chlorine bleach, oven cleaners): Tissue damage is related to pH and concentration. Products with a pH of 10-11 can cause mild tissue irritation. Products with a pH of 11-12 may cause corrosive tissue injury; examples include sodium hypochlorite (>10%), sodium carbonate (>15%), NaOH (>2%), and sodium silicate (>20%). Clinical signs include ulcerations, dysphagia, vomiting, hematemesis, abdominal pain, stridor, and coughing. Inducing emesis is not recommended. (Osweiler et al. 2011)
- **RODENTICIDES, ANTICOAGULANTS** (e.g., d-Con®): Toxic to all mammals and birds; dogs are more sensitive than cats. Active ingredients can include brodifacoum, bromadiolone, chlorphacinone, difethialone, diphacinone, and warfarin. Clinical signs typically develop 3-5 days after ingestion. Most common clinical signs following ingestion can include dyspnea, coughing, lethargy, exercise intolerance and hemoptysis. Nonspecific signs can include lethargy, anorexia, or lameness. Signs of bleeding can occur such as hematuria, hematemesis, melena, hyphema, and epistaxis. Phytonadione (Vitamin K_1) is antidotal and dosed at 2.5 – 5 mg/kg orally in dogs and cats. See the Phytonadione monograph for more information. **Note:** As of April 2015 retail stores in the USA will no longer be allowed to legally carry residential use rodenticide products that contain brodifacoum, bromadiolone, or difethialone.
- **RODENTICIDES, BROMETHALIN:** Toxic to all species; cats more sensitive than dogs. Intoxication is due to cerebral edema (white matter vacuolization). No antidote is available. The minimum lethal dose in dogs is 2.5 mg/kg active ingredient; in cats it is 0.45 mg/kg. Dogs may exhibit ataxia, weakness, paralysis, tremors, seizures and coma. Cats are more prone to paralytic signs. (Osweiler et al. 2011)
- **DEET** (e.g., Off®; N,N-diethyl-meta-toluamide): Found in insect repellants. Neurological signs (tremors, hyperexcitation, ataxia, and seizures), skin irritation, hypersalivation and vomiting, can result. Up to 13% of DEET is absorbed through the skin in dogs.
- **ETHANOL** (alcohol, Purell® and other hand sanitizers): Ingesting large amounts may cause hypoglycemia, hypothermia, and hypotension. Clinical signs include weakness, lethargy, vomiting, collapse, hypothermia, weak respirations, and coma. The minimum oral lethal dose in dogs is 5.55 grams/kg. See the Ethanol monograph for additional information.
- **ETHYLENE GLYCOL** (found in automotive antifreeze): The minimum lethal dose of undiluted ethylene glycol antifreeze is 4.2 – 6.6 mL/kg in dogs and 1.5 mL/kg in cats. Toxicity typically

occurs in three stages. The first stage occurs within 30 minutes to 12 hours and clinical signs include nausea, vomiting, polyuria, polydipsia, ataxia, and metabolic acidosis. The second stage occurs 12-24 hours after ingestion, and is characterized by dehydration, tachypnea, and tachycardia. The third stage occurs 12-24 hours after ingestion in cats and 36-72 hours in dogs and clinical signs include renal failure, anorexia, depression, lethargy, oral ulcers, hypersalivation, coma, and seizures. Products such as wall paint, printer ink, etc., that contain < 5% ethylene glycol rarely cause problems. See the Fomepizole and Ethanol monographs for additional information. (Osweiler *et al.* 2011)

- **ICE MELTS CONTAINING CALCIUM CHLORIDE:** Exposure may cause severe skin, gastrointestinal tract irritation and electrolyte imbalance. Clinical signs associated with exposure include salivation, depression, disorientation, polydipsia, diarrhea, vomiting, and anorexia. (Foss 2002)

- **METALDEHYDE** (commonly found in snail and slug baits): Concentrations of active ingredient range from 3.25-4% and are toxic to pets. Clinical signs are similar in dogs and cats and may appear minutes to hours after ingestion. Typical signs include anxiety, tachycardia, nystagmus, mydriasis, hyperpnea, panting, hypersalivation, and ataxia. Vomiting, diarrhea, tremors, hyperesthesia, continuous seizures, metabolic acidosis, rigidity, opisthotonos, and severe hyperthermia may also be seen. Delayed signs that may develop are depression, coma, and liver failure. Death from respiratory failure can occur within a few hours of exposure. (Dolder 2003)

- **METHANOL** (organic solvent found in windshield washer fluid, paint thinners, household cleaning products): Toxic to dogs and cats. The canine oral LD_{50} of undiluted methanol is 5 – 11.25 mL/kg. Clinical signs in cats and dogs are similar to ethanol intoxication and include ataxia, depression, lethargy, sedation, hypothermia, and metabolic acidosis. Does not cause blindness as it does in humans. (Osweiler *et al.* 2011)

- **MOTHBALLS** (naphthalene or paradichlorobenzene [PDB]): Toxic to all species via ingestion, inhalation or dermal contact. Ingestion may cause severe GI upset, neurological stimulation followed by depression, hemolytic anemia, liver and kidney damage. Dogs ingesting 1.5 g/kg of naphthalene mothballs resulted in hemolytic anima. PDB is approximately 50% less toxic than naphthalene. Mothballs typically weigh 2.7-4 g. (Osweiler *et al.* 2011)

- **POLYURETHANE GLUES** (*e.g., Gorilla*® glue, *Elmer's Pro-Bond*®): Expanding adhesive glues that contain diisocyanate. Although not poisonous, the glue expands significantly once ingested to create a firm, foam-like foreign body that can cause gastric or esophageal obstructions. Clinical signs can be seen 15 minutes to 20 hours after ingestion and include vomiting, abdominal distension, stomach pain, inappetence, and lethargy. Surgical removal is almost always necessary. Inducing emesis is not often recommended.

Miscellaneous Items

- **GLOW JEWELRY & TOYS** (liquid filled plastic necklaces, earrings, plastic wands, safety sticks): Mildly toxic to cats and dogs. Contains dibutyl phthalate, a chemical with a bitter taste capable of causing immediate eye, skin and mucus membrane irritation. Most commonly, cats are exposed after piercing jewelry with their teeth. Significant but self-limiting hypersalivation results but is of little toxicological concern.

- **LILIES** (plants in the *Lilium* and *Hemerocallis* spp.): Highly toxic to cats. *Lilium spp.* are frequently sold as cut flowers in retail settings as they are inexpensive, fragrant and long lasting.

Specific *Lilium* plants include the Easter lily, stargazer lily, tiger lily, and other Asiatic hybrid lilies. *Hemerocallis*, day lilies, are more often sold in pots for outdoor planting. Small ingestions of leaves, petals, pollen or vase water can cause acute renal failure in cats within 1-2 days. If untreated, the prognosis is grave.

- **LIQUID POTPOURRI** (simmer pot potpourri): Cats are more susceptible to toxicosis than dogs. Products may contain cationic detergents and essential oils. Ingestion of cationic detergents can result in ulceration or severe inflammation of the mouth and upper gastrointestinal tract. Essential oils are absorbed across the skin and mucus membranes and result in tissue irritation, gastrointestinal upset, CNS depression and dermal hypersensitivity. Inducing emesis is not recommended. (Peterson *et al.* 2013)

- **LITHIUM ION DISC BATTERIES:** Ingestion can be toxic to dogs and cats. Toxicity caused by electrical current flow in the gastrointestinal tract, which leads to tissue necrosis. The greatest concern is for esophageal necrosis followed by perforation, potential aortic fistula and fatal hemorrhage. Clinical signs include ulceration of the gums, teeth discoloration, hypersalivation, food/water refusal, abdominal pain, shock and pallor, and abdominal distension. (Osweiler *et al.* 2011)

- **U.S. PENNIES** (1¢): Pennies minted after 1982 are toxic to dogs and cats due to high (97%) zinc content. Ingestion can cause oxidative damage to red blood cells (hemolytic anemia) and acute gastrointestinal distress. Additionally, damage to the kidneys, liver, gastrointestinal tract, pancreas, and red blood cells can occur. (Richardson 2002)

Resources/References

Animal Poison Centers: The following are known 24-hour poison control centers in the USA that specialize in providing information specific for veterinary patients. Fees listed are those at the time of writing (August 2014).

- Pet Poison Helpline: Phone: **800-213-6680;** $39 consultation fee. http://www.petpoisonhelpline.com

- ASPCA Animal Poison Control Center: Phone: **888-426-4435;** $65 consultation fee. http://www.aspca.org/pet-care/animal-poison-control

Albertson, J. (2006). The toxicity of iron, an essential element. Veterinary Medicine(February).

Bischoff, K. & F. Guale (1998). Australian tea tree (*Melaleuca alternifolia*) oil poisoning in three purebred cats. Journal of Veterinary Diagnostic Investigation 10(2): 208-10.

Cope, R. B. (2005). *Allium* species poisoniong in dogs and cats. Veterinary Medicine(August).

Dolder, L. (2003). Metaldehyde toxicosis. Veterinary Medicine(March): 213-5.

Dunayer, E. (2004). Ibuprofen toxicosis in dogs, cats, and ferrets. Veterinary Medicine(July).

Foss, T. (2002). The Hazards of Ice Melt. Veterinary Technician(February): 94-104.

Gwaltney-Brant, S. (2001). Chocolate intoxication. Veterinary Medicine(February): 108-11.

Holahan, M. L., et al. (2010). Presumptive hepatotoxicity and rhabdomyolysis secondary to phenazopyridine toxicity in a dog. J. Vet. Emerg. Crit. Care 20(3): 352-8.

McKnight, K. (2005). Grape and Raisin Toxicity in Dogs. Veterinary Technician(February).

Morrow, C. (2001). Cholecalciferol Poisoning. Veterinary Medicine(December): 905-11.

Murphy, L. A. & A. E. Coleman (2012). Xylitol Toxicosis in Dogs. Veterinary Clinics of North America-Small Animal Practice 42(2): 307-+.

Osweiler, G. D., et al. (2011). Blackwell's Five-Minute Veterinary Consult Clinical Companion: Small Animal Toxicology, Wiley-Blackwell. Ames.

Peterson, M. E. & P. A. Talcott (2013). Small Animal Toxicology, 3rd Ed., Saunders. St. Louis.

Richardson, J. A. (2000). Permethrin Spot-On Toxicosis in Cats. J. Vet. Emerg. Crit. Care 10(June): 103-6.

Richardson, J. A. (2002). Zinc Toxicosis from penny ingestions in dogs. Veterinary Medicine(February): 96-9.

Wilcke, J. R. (1984). Idiosyncracies of drug metabolism in cats: Effects on pharmacotherapeutics in feline practice. Vet Clin North Am Small Anim Pract 14(6): 1345-54.

Importation of Unapproved New Animal Drugs into the USA

As of October 2009, the Food and Drug Administration's Center for Veterinary Medicine is no longer accepting requests nor issuing "no-objection" letters facilitating veterinarians' personal importation of foreign animal drugs that are not approved for use in the United States. FDA previously allowed licensed veterinarians to apply for permission to import small amounts of unapproved animal drugs under the Medically Necessary Personal Import Policy (a 13 step letter detailing the intended use for a specific patient under specific circumstances, such as when the drug posed no threat to human or animal health and there were no adequate drug substitutes available.) The burden of importation now appears to rest upon the exporter in completing necessary Customs and Border Patrol (CBP) documents that will allow the drugs to clear US Customs upon entry into the United States. It is important to note that drug shipments may still be seized by US Customs and returned to the exporter in spite of efforts to provide necessary documentation.

Veterinarians seeking to import these types of foreign animal drugs are now directed to FDA's guidance on the Coverage of Personal Importation, which is available at: http://goo.gl/GiWys

This supplier from the U.K. has been recommended to the author and may be able to assist U.S. veterinarians in obtaining medically necessary products from abroad:

Manor Veterinary Exports
Telephone (from USA): 01144-1993-830-278
Email: johngrippervet@compuserve.com
www.manorveterinaryexports.com

ARCI UCGFS Classifications

The Association of Racing Commissioners International, Inc. is a non-profit corporation whose mission and vision is: To protect and uphold the integrity of the pari-mutuel sports of horse racing, dog racing and jai-alai through an informed membership, by encouraging forceful and uniform regulation, by promoting the health and welfare of the industry through various programs and projects.

The organization's website has the most current information of the: Uniform Classification Guidelines for Foreign Substances and Recommended Penalties and Model Rule. It can be accessed at: arcicom.businesscatalyst.com/index.html

Conversion Tables for Weight in Kilograms to Body Surface Area (m²)

The following tables are derived from the equation:
Approximate surface area in m² = $\dfrac{10.1 \ (10 \ for \ cats) \times (weight \ in \ grams)^{2/3}}{10000}$

Dogs

Weight in Kg	m²	Weight in Kg	m²	Weight in Kg	m²
0.5	0.06	17	0.66	38	1.13
1	0.1	18	0.69	40	1.17
2	0.15	19	0.71	42	1.21
3	0.2	20	0.74	44	1.25
4	0.25	21	0.76	46	1.28
5	0.29	22	0.78	50	1.36
6	0.33	23	0.81	54	1.44
7	0.36	24	0.83	58	1.51
8	0.4	25	0.85	62	1.58
9	0.43	26	0.88	66	1.65
10	0.46	27	0.9	70	1.72
11	0.49	28	0.92	74	1.78
12	0.52	29	0.94	80	1.88
13	0.55	30	0.96		
14	0.58	32	1.01		
15	0.6	34	1.05		
16	0.63	36	1.09		

Cats

Weight in Kg	m²
2	0.159
2.5	0.184
3	0.208
3.5	0.231
4	0.252
4.5	0.273
5	0.292
5.5	0.311
6	0.33
6.5	0.348
7	0.366
7.5	0.383
8	0.4
8.5	0.416
9	0.432
9.5	0.449
10	0.464

Tables of Parenteral Fluids

(Not a complete listing; includes both human- and veterinary-approved products)

Sodium Chloride Solutions	Sodium (mEq/L)	Chloride (mEq/L)	Osmolality (mOsm/L)	Available as:
Sodium Chloride 0.2%	34	34	69	3 mL
Sodium Chloride 0.45% ; (Half-Normal Saline)	77	77	155	3, 5, 500, and 1000 mL
Sodium Chloride 0.9% (Normal Saline)	154	154	310	1, 2, 2.5. 3, 4, 5, 10, 20, 25, 30, 50, 100, 130, 150, 250, 500, & 1000 mL
Sodium Chloride 3%	513	513	1030	500 mL
Sodium Chloride 5%	855	855	1710	500 mL

Dextrose Solutions	Dextrose (g/L)	Calories (kCal/L)	Osmolality (mOsm/L)	Available as:
Dextrose 2.5%	25	85	126	250, 500, & 1000 mL
Dextrose 5%	50	170	253	10, 25, 50, 100, 130, 150, 250, 400, 500, 1000 mL
Dextrose 10%	100	340	505	250, 500, & 1000 mL
Dextrose 20%	200	680	1010	500 & 1000 mL
Dextrose 25%	250	850	1330	in 10 mL syringes
Dextrose 30%	300	1020	1515	500 & 1000 mL
Dextrose 38.5%	385	1310	1945	1000 mL
Dextrose 40%	400	1360	2020	500 & 1000 mL
Dextrose 50%	500	1700	2525	50, 250, 500, & 1000 mL
Dextrose 60%	600	2040	3030	500 & 1000 mL
Dextrose 70%	700	2380	3535	250, 500, & 1000 mL

Dextrose & Saline Solutions	Sodium (mEq/L)	Chloride (mEq/L)	Dextrose (g/L)	Calories (kCal/L)	Osmolality (mOsm/L)	Available as:
$D_{2.5}$ & 0.45% NaCl	77	77	25	85	280	250, 500, & 1000 mL
D_5 & 0.11% NaCl	19	19	50	170	290	500 & 1000 mL
D_5 & 0.2% NaCl	34	34	50	170	320	250, 500, & 1000 mL
D_5 & 0.33% NaCl	56	56	50	170	365	250, 500, & 1000 mL
D_5 & 0.45% NaCl	77	77	50	170	405	250, 500, & 1000 mL
D_5 & 0.9% NaCl	154	154	100	170	560	250, 500, & 1000 mL
D_{10} & 0.45% NaCl	77	77	100	340	660	1000 mL
D_{10} & 0.9% NaCl	154	154	100	340	815	500 & 1000 mL

Electrolyte Solutions	Na^+ (mEq/L)	K^+ (mEq/L)	Ca^{++} (mEq/L)	Mg^{++} (mEq/L)	Cl^- (mEq/L)	Gluconate (mEq/L).4;	Lactate (mEq/L)	Acetate (mEq/L)	Osmolarity (mOsm/L)	Available as:
Ringer's Injection	147	4	4		156				310	250, 500, 1000 mL
Lactated Ringer's Injection (LRS)	130	4	4		109		28		272	250, 500, 1000, 5000 mL
Plasma-Lyte® 56	40	13		3	40			16	111	500 & 1000 mL
Plasma-Lyte® R	140	10	5	3	103		8	47	312	1000 mL
Plasma-Lyte A; Normosol®-R pH 7.4	140	5		3	98	23		27	294	500, 1000, & 5000 mL
Isolyte® S pH 7.4	141	5		3	98	23		29	295	500 & 1000 mL

Dextrose & Electrolyte Solutions	D5 in Ringer's	D2.5 in Half-strength lactated Ringer's	D5 in lactated Ringer's	Normosol®-M w/D5; Plasma-Lyte 56 w/D5	Plasma-Lyte® 148 and D5	Normosol®-R and D5
Dextrose (g/L)	50	25	50	50	50	50
Calories (kCal/L)	170	89	179	170	190	185
Na+ (mEq/L)	147	65.5	130	40	140	140
K+ (mEq/L)	4	2	4	13	5	5
Ca++ (mEq/L)	4.5	1.4	2.7			
Mg++ (mEq/L)				3	3	3
Cl- (mEq/L)	156	54	109	40	98	98
Gluconate (mEq/L)					23	23
Lactate (mEq/L)		14	28			
Acetate (mEq/L)				16	27	27
Osmolarity (mOsm/L)	562	263	527	368 (363)	547	552
Available as:	500 & 1000 mL	250, 500 & 1000 mL	250, 500 & 1000 mL	500 & 1000 mL	500 & 1000 mL	500 & 1000 mL

Abbreviations Used in Prescription Writing

A warning and the strange case of S.I.D.: Although prescription abbreviations are used throughout many references and they are generally fairly well recognized, they do increase the potential for mistakes to occur. When writing a prescription, this author recommends writing out the directions in plain English and avoiding the use of abbreviations entirely. If abbreviations are to be used, definitely avoid q.d., q.o.d., q.i.d. and s.i.d. because they can be easily confused with other abbreviations.

S.I.D. is an abbreviation virtually unknown to health professionals outside of veterinary medicine and the vast majority of pharmacists have never seen it. **S.I.D. should be eliminated from all veterinary usage and replaced with "once a day".** The additional time to write out "once a day" versus "SID" is approximately 3 seconds, but by doing so, a potentially serious, avoidable error could be prevented.

a.c.	before meals
a.d.	right ear
a.s.	left ear
a.u.	both ears
amp.	ampule
b.i.d.	twice a day
c.	with
cap.	capsule
cc	cubic centimeter
disp.	dispense
g or gm	gram
gtt(s).	drop(s)
h.	hour
h.s.	at bedtime
IM	intramuscular
IO	intraosseous
IP	intraperitoneal
IV	intravenous
lb.	pound
m2	meter squared
mg.	milligram
ml. or mL	milliliter
o.d.	right eye

o.s.	left eye
o.u	both eyes
p.c.	after meals
p.o	by mouth
p.r.n.	as needed
q.	every
q4h, etc	every 4 hours
q.i.d.	four times a day
q.o.d.	every other day
q.s.	a sufficient quantity
q4h	every 4 hours, etc.
s.i.d.	once a day
Sig:	directions to pt.
stat	immediately
SubQ, SQ, SC, Subcut	subcutaneous
susp.	suspension
t.i.d.	three times a day
tab	tablet
Tbsp., T	tablespoon (15 mL)
tsp., t	teaspoon (5 mL)
Ut dict	as directed

Solubility Definitions

The following definitions are used throughout the book in the chemistry section for each agent:

Descriptive Term	Parts of Solvent for 1 Part of Solute
Very Soluble	Less than 1
Freely Soluble	From 1 to 10
Soluble	From 10 to 30
Sparingly Soluble	From 30 to 100
Slightly Soluble	From 100 to 1000
Very Slightly Soluble	From 1000 to 10,000
Practically Insoluble, or Insoluble	More than 10,000

Conversion: Weights; Temperature; Liquids

Weights

1 pound (lb) = 0.454 kg = 454 grams = 16 ounces
1 kilogram (kg) = 2.2 pounds = 1000 grams
1 grain (gr.) = 64.8 mg (often rounded to 60 or 65 mg)
1 gram = 15.43 grains = 1000 mg
1 ounce = 28.4 grams
1 gram = 1000 mg
1 milligram (mg) = 1000 mcg (µg)
1 microgram (mcg or µg) = 1000 nanograms (ng)

Temperatures

$9 \times (°C) = (5 \times °F) - 160$
°C to °F = (°C x 1.8) + 32 = °F
°F to °C = (°F – 32) x 0.555 = °C

Liquids

1 gallon (gal.) = 4 qts. = 8 pts. = 128 fl. oz. = 3.785 liters = 3785 mL
1 quart (qt) = 2 pints = 32 fl. oz. = 946 mL
1 pint = 2 cups = 16 fl. oz. = 473 mL
1 cup = 8 fl. oz = 237 mL = 16 tablespoons
1 tablespoon = 15 mL = 3 teaspoons
1 teaspoon = 5 mL
4 liters = 1.057 gals.
1 liter = 1000 mL = 10 deciliters
1 deciliter (dl) = 100 mL
1 milliliter (mL) = 1 cubic centimeter (cc) = 1000 microliters (µl; mcl)

Milliequivalents & Molecular Weights

Milliequivalents: The term milliequivalents (mEq) is usually used to express the quantities of electrolytes administered to patients. A mEq is 1/1000 of an equivalent (Eq). For pharmaceutical purposes an equivalent may be thought of as equal to the equivalent weight of a given substance. This, in practical terms, is the molecular weight of the substance divided by the valence or the radical. For example:

How many milligrams are equivalent to 1 mEq of potassium chloride (KCl)?

1. Determine the equivalent weight = gram atomic weight ÷ valence; Molecular weight of KCl = 74.5; Valence = 1 (K⁺; Cl⁻); Equivalent weight = 74.5 ÷ 1 = 74.5 grams

2. Determine the mEq weight: Equivalent weight ÷ 1000; 74.5 ÷ 1000 = 74.5 mg = 1 mEq of KCl = 1 mEq of K⁺ & 1 mEq of Cl⁻

If the substance would have been $CaCl_2$, the process would be identical using the gram molecular weight of $CaCl_2$ (MW 111 if anhydrous; 147 if dihydrate) and a valence of 2.

Listed below are several commonly used electrolytes with their molecular weights and valences in parentheses:

Electrolyte	Molecular Weight (valence)
Sodium Chloride	58.44 (1)
Sodium Bicarbonate	84 (1)
Sodium Acetate, anhydrous	82 (1)
Sodium Acetate, trihydrate	136 (1)
Sodium Lactate	112 (1)
Potassium Chloride	74.55 (1)
Potassium Gluconate	234.25 (1)
Calcium Gluconate	430.4 (2)
Calcium Lactate, anhydrous	218.22 (2)
Calcium Chloride, anhydrous	111 (2)
Calcium Chloride, dihydrate	147 (2)
Magnesium Sulfate, heptahydrate	246.5 (2)
Magnesium Sulfate, anhydrous	120.4 (2)
Magnesium Chloride, anhydrous	95.21 (2)
Magnesium Chloride, hexahydrate	203.3 (2)

"Normal" Vital Signs

Temperature	Celsius (°C)	Fahrenheit (°F)
Dog	37.5–39.2	99.5–102.5
Cat	37.8–39.5	100–102.5
Ferret	37.8–39.2	100–102.5
Cattle, up to one year old	38.6–39.4	101.5–103.5
Cattle, over one year old	37.8–39.2	100–102.5
Horse, adult	37.2–38.5	99–101.3
Horse, foal	37.5–39.3	99.5–102.7
Goat	38.5–40.2	101.3–104.5
Sheep	38.5–40	101.3–104
Swine, piglet	38.9–40	102–104
Swine, adult	37.8–38.9	100–102
Rabbit	38.5–39.3	100.4–105

Temperature (Rectal): Temperatures will normally fluctuate over the course of the day. The following may increase body temperature: Time of day (evening), food intake, muscular activity, approaching estrus, during gestation, high external temperatures. The following may decrease body temperature: intake of large quantities of cool fluids, time of day (morning), and low atmospheric temperature. Small breed dogs tend to have higher normal temperatures than large breeds.

Pulse Rate	BPM
Cattle, calves	100–120
Cattle, adults	55–80
Cat, young	130–140
Cat, old	100–120
Dog, young	110–120
Dog, adult large breed	80–120
Ferret	300
Goat	70–120
Horse, adult	28–40
Horse, 3 months–2 years	40–80
Horse, foals–3 months	64–128
Rabbit	120–150
Sheep	66–115
Swine, young	100–130
Swine, adult	60–90

Pulse Rates (resting and healthy) in beats per minute (BPM). Pulse rates for very young animals are usually in the higher ranges and older animals in the lower ranges of those values listed.

Respiratory Rates	RPM
Cattle, young	15–40
Cattle, adults	10–30
Cats	20–30
Dog	15–30
Ferret	33–36
Horse	10–14
Swine	8–18
Rabbit	50–60
Sheep, Goat	10–30

Respiratory Rates (resting & healthy) respirations per minute.

Estrus and Gestation Periods: Dogs & Cats

	Dog	Cat
Appearance of first estrus at the age of:	7–9 months	4–12 months
Estrous cycle in animals not served:	Mean = 7 months Range = every 5–8 months	Every 4–30 days (14–19 day model) if constant photoperiod
Duration of estrus period:	7–42 days (proestrus plus estrus)	2–19 days
First occurrences after parturition:	Pregnancy does not alter interval	7–9 days
Gestation Period	Mean = 63 days; Range 58–71 days	Mean = 63 days; Range 58–70 days
Number of Young	8–12 Large Breeds 6–10 Medium Breeds 2–4 Small Breeds	4–6
Suckling Period	3–6 weeks	3–6 weeks

Conversion of Conventional Chemistry Units to SI Units

The Système Internationale d'Unites (SI), or the International System of Units was recommended for use in the health professions by the World Health Assembly in 1977. It is slowly being adopted in the United States and many journals now require its use. The following is an abbreviated table of conversion values for some of the more commonly encountered tests that may now be reported in SI Units.

	Chemistry Units to SI Units
Albumin	g/dL x 10 = g/L
Ammonia	mg/dL x 0.5872 = mmol/L
Bilirubin	mg/dL x 17.10 = mmol/L
Calcium	mg/dL x 0.2495 = mmol/L
Cholesterol	mg/dL x 0.02586 = mmol/L
CO_2 pressure, pCO_2	mmHg x 0.1333 = kPa
Creatinine	mg/dL x 88.4 = mmol/L
Glucose	mg/dL x 0.05551 = mmol/L
Lactate	mg/dL x 0.111 = mmol/L
Magnesium	mg/dL x 0.4114 = mmol/L
O_2 pressure, pO_2	mmHg x 0.1333 = kPa
Phosphorus	mg/dL x 0.3229 = mmol/L
Protein	g/dL x 10 = g/L
Urea Nitrogen	mg/dL x 0.7140 = mmol/L
Amylase	IU/L = Units/L
AST (SGOT)	IU/L = Units/L
ALT (SGPT)	IU/L = Units/L
Lipase	IU/L = Units/L
ALP	IU/L = Units/L
SDH (Sorbitol)	IU/L = Units/L

Bicarbonate, Chloride, CO_2 (total), Potassium, & Sodium do not require conversion from conventional to SI units.

Reference Laboratory Ranges

Note: The following reference ranges are as a general reference only; for clinical use refer to the "normals" for your laboratory.

Values are from: **Marshfield Clinic Laboratories, Veterinary Diagnostic Service;** http://www.marshfieldlabs.org/veterinary/ Data accessed: 2014.

Ferret values adapted from: **Biology and Diseases of the Ferret 3rd ed.** (2014); edited by Fox, JG and Marini, RP; Wiley-Blackwell.

Rabbit values adapted from: **Animal Models in Toxicology, 3rd ed.** (2013); edited by Gad, SC; CRC Press.

Rat hematology values adapted from: **Schalm's Veterinary Hematology, 6th ed.** (2010) edited by Weiss, DJ and Wardrop, KJ; Wiley-Blackwell.

Chemistry: Companion/Small Animals

Values are from: Marshfield Clinic Laboratories, Veterinary Diagnostic Service; http://www.marshfieldlabs.org/veterinary/ Data accessed: 2014.

Test	Units	Canine	Feline	Ferret	Rat	Rabbit
Albumin	gm/dL	2.6 – 4.0	2.3 – 3.9	3.5 – 4.2	3.2 – 3.7	3.5 – 5.5
Alkaline phosphatase	Units/L	13 – 289	8 – 115	9 – 84	232 – 632	40 – 140
Alanine Amino Transferase (ALT)	Units/L	14 – 151	23 – 145	78 – 149	59 – 166	15 – 50
Amylase	Units/L	268 – 1653	627 – 1572	**	545 – 847	**
Anion Gap		17 – 28	17 – 32	**	24 – 39	**
Aspartate Amino Transferase	Units/L	18 – 86	14 – 68	28 – 120	90 – 345	15 – 45
Betahydroxybutyrate	mg/dL	0.2 – 0.8	0.3 – 1.9	**	2.2 – 5.1	**
Bicarbonate	mmol/L	16 – 31	11 – 21	20 – 28	18 – 27	**
Bile acids, fasting	umol/L	0.0 – 12.0	0.0 – 5.0	**	NA	**
Bile acids, post prandial (or non-fasting)	umol/L	5.0 – 25.0	5.0 – 15.0	**	2.2 – 5.1	**
Bilirubin - Direct	mg/dL	0.0 – 0.2	0.0 – 0.2	**	0.0 – 0.0	**
Bilirubin - Total	mg/dL	0.1 – 0.5	0.0 – 0.4	0.0 – 0.1	0.0 – 0.1	0.1 – 0.5
Blood Urea Nitrogen	mg/dL	8 – 30	13 - 36	11 – 25	13 – 19	11 – 25
Calcium	mg/dL	8.7 – 12.0	8.1 – 11.8	8.7 – 9.4	9.5 – 13.9	12.5 – 15.5
Chloride	mmol/L	100 – 121	114 – 130	118 – 126	98 – 104	96 - 106
Cholesterol	mg/dL	98 – 300	81 – 275	119 – 201	50 – 92	30 – 100
Corticosterid-induced	Units/L	0 – 50	NA	**	NA	**
Creatine Kinase	Units/L	50 – 554	52 – 462		113 - 692	**
Creatinine	mg/dL	0.4 – 2.0	0.5 – 2.5	0.4 – 0.9	0.3 – 0.5	0.9 – 1.7
Iron	ug/dL	46 – 214	43 – 226	**	184 – 497	**
Fructosamine (for non-diabetic animals)	micromol/L	180 – 330	164 – 356	**	139 – 176	**
Gamma Glutamyl Transferase	Units/L	3 – 19	0 – 2	1 – 8	0 – 0	0 – 10
Globulin	g/dL	2.2 – 4.1	2.8 – 5.4	**	2.6 – 3.5	**
Glucose	mg/dL	74 – 145	65 – 155	107 – 138	70 – 308	100 – 190
Haptoglobin	mg/mL	1.0 – 5.0	0.5 – 3.8	**	0.9 – 2.1	**
Insulin	microU/mL	5.0 – 65.0	NA	4.9 – 34.8	NA	**
Lactate	mmol/L	0.99 – 4.77	0.83 – 4.95		1.60 – 17.29	**
Lactate Dehydrogenase	Units/L	19 – 162	35 – 325	241 – 752	364 – 1706	**
Lipase	Units/L	109 – 750	15 – 246	**	14 – 41	**
Magnesium	mg/dL	1.6 – 2.3	1.7 – 2.6	**	3.8 – 5.5	**
Phosphorus	mg/dL	2.5 – 7.9	2.7 – 7.3	5.2 – 7.6	5.6 – 16.8	2.0 – 9.0
Potassium	mmol/L	3.4 – 5.6	3.4 – 5.4	4.3 – 5.3	3.8 – 5.6	3.5 – 6.0
Sorbitol Dehydrogenase	Units/L	0.7 – 20.0	1.8 – 22.1	**	27.3 – 118.5	**
TSH	ng/mL	0.03 – 0.32	NA	NA	NA	NA

Test	Units	Canine	Feline	Ferret	Rat	Rabbit
Free T4-MEIA	ng/mL	0.42 – 2.19	0.63 – 1.92	NA	NA	NA
Sodium	mmol/L	141 – 159	151 – 164	146 – 160	146 – 151	133 – 150
Total T4	ug/dL	0.4 – 3.7	0.6 – 3.6	0.7 – 8.3	0.6 – 3.9	**
Total protein	gm/dL	5.0 – 8.3	5.7 – 8.6	6.2 – 7.1	5.8 – 7.1	5.2 – 7.5
Triglycerides	mg/dL	36 – 240	24 – 169	10 – 32	101 – 369	30 – 180
Uric acid	ng/dL	0.2 – 0.7	0.0 – 0.4	0.8 – 3.1	3.7 – 9.1	**

**no normal range established in this laboratory

Hematology: Companion/Small Animals

Values are from: Marshfield Clinic Laboratories, Veterinary Diagnostic Service; http://www.marshfieldlabs.org/veterinary/ Accessed: 2014

Test	Units	Canine	Feline	Ferret	Rat	Rabbit
Red Blood count (RBC)	x 10⁶/microL	4.48 – 8.53	5.80 – 11.00	7.30 – 12.18	5.00 – 7.20	7.00 – 9.00
Hemoglobin	g/dL	10.5 – 20.1	8.6 – 16.0	12.0 – 17.4	10.5 – 15.0	13.7 – 16.8
Hemtocrit	%	33.0 – 58.7	28.0 – 47.0	36.0 – 61.0	32.0 – 45.0	37.9 – 49.9
Mean corp. volume (MCV)	fL	63.0 – 78.3	37.7 – 50.0	42.6 – 51.0	55.0 – 70.0	49.9 – 58.3
Mean corp. HGB (MCH)	pg	21.0 – 27.0	12.3 – 17.2	13.7 – 16.0	19.0 – 23.0	17.8 – 29.0
Mean corp. HGB conc. (MCHC)	f/dL	30.8 – 35.9	31.1 – 36.0	30.3 – 34.9	30.0 – 35.0	33.2 – 37.9
Red cell dis. Width (RDW)	%	11.9 – 18.1	17.0 – 24.0	7.3 – 12.2	**	10.5 – 14.9
Platelet count	x 10³/microL	140 – 540	160 – 660	297 – 910	300 – 750	680 – 1280
White blood count (WBC)	x 10³/microL	4.0 – 18.2	3.7 – 20.5	4.4 – 19.1	4.0 – 13.0	1.1 – 7.5
Segmented neutrophil absolute #	x 10³/microL	2.50 – 15.70	1.3 – 15.7	1.3 – 3.7	1.00 – 6.00	0.20 – 1.50
Band neutrophil absolute #	x 10³/microL	0.00 – 0.20	0.00 – 0.50	0.00 – 0.10	0.00 – 0.10	0.00 – 0.10
Lymphocyte absolute #	x 10³/microL	0.30 – 3.90	1.00 – 7.90	1.50 – 6.70	2.00 – 9.00	0.80 – 5.70
Monocyte absolute #	x 10³/microL	0.00 – 1.40	0.00 – 1.00	0.10 – 0.80	0.00 – 0.50	0.00 – 0.20
Eosinophil absolute #	x 10³/microL	0.00 – 1.30	0.10 – 2.00	0.10 – 0.90	0.00 – 0.40	0.00 – 0.20
Basophil absolute #	x 10³/microL	0.00 – 0.10	0.00 – 0.10	0.00 – 0.10	0.00 – 1.00	0.00 – 0.30

Chemistry: Equine, Food, & Fiber Animals

Values are from: Marshfield Clinic Laboratories, Veterinary Diagnostic Service; http://www.marshfieldlabs.org/veterinary/ Data accessed: 2014

Test	Units	Alpaca	Bovine	Camelid (Llama)	Caprine	Equine	Ovine	Porcine
Albumin	gm/dL	2.7 – 4.4	3.1 – 4.3	1.9 – 4.9	2.3 – 3.4	2.4 – 3.7	2.8 – 3.7	3.2 – 4.2
Alkaline phosphaase	Units/L	17 – 232	12 – 154	15 – 115	18 – 220	96 – 385	47 – 681	61 – 147
Alanaine Amino Transferase	Units/L	5 – 21	10 – 33	5 – 18	11 – 28	5 – 13	11 – 26	30 – 53
Amylase	Units/L	561 – 1211	11 – 21	**	10 – 73	1 – 5	5 – 40	744 – 2330
Anion Gap		11 – 22	10 – 25	**	12 – 20	10 – 24	14 – 21	13 – 30
Aspartate Amino Transferase	Units/L	73 – 282	48 – 204	98 – 256	60 – 118	204 – 390	52 – 122	17 – 63
Betahydroxybutyrate	mg/dL	0.4 – 0.9	1.9 – 14.8	0.3 – 1.2	2.3 – 4.9	1.2 – 4.4	0.6 – 5.4	0.2 – 1.2
Bicarbonate	mmol/L	20 – 32	22 – 29	13 – 38	23 – 3 2	21 – 33	21 – 32	18 – 32
Bile acids, fasting	micromol/L	NA	NA	**	NA	NA	NA	NA
Bile acids, post prandial (or non-fasting)	micromol/L	11.0 – 82.0	1.9 – 14.8	**	5.0 – 69.0	1.2 – 4.4	3 – 86	1.0 – 31.0
Bilirubin – Direct	mg/dL	0.0 – 0.0	0.0 – 0.2	**	0.0 – 0.7	0.0 – 0.4	0.0 – 0.0	0.0 – 0.2
Bilirubin – Total	mg/dL	0.0 – 0.1	0.0 – 0.2	0.1 – 0.2	0.0 – 0.1	0.2 – 2.2	0.0 – 0.1	0.0 – 0.1

Test	Units	Alpaca	Bovine	Camelid (Llama)	Caprine	Equine	Ovine	Porcine
Blood Urea Nitrogen	mg/dL	13 – 30	8 – 22	8 – 34	7 – 22	9 – 27	13 – 28	10 – 24
Calcium	mg/dL	8.5 – 10.1	7.9 – 10.5	7.8 – 10.7	8.2 – 10.3	10.2 – 13.4	9.4 – 11.0	10.1 – 11.8
Chloride	mmol/L	107 – 116	100 – 109	106 – 129	101 – 109	92 – 107	100 – 112	91 – 109
Cholesterol	mg/dL	15 – 63	112 – 331	16 – 57	52 – 120	59 – 125	31 – 85	41 – 89
Corticosteriod-induced	Units/L	NA	NA	NA	NA	NA	NA	NA
Creatine Kinase	Units/L	31 – 232	50 – 271	**	98 – 267	131 – 548	47 – 273	136 – 1609
Creatinine	mg/dL	0.8 – 2.0	0.3 – 0.8	0.4 – 3.1	0.4 – 0.9	0.4 – 1.9	0.5 – 0.9	0.8 – 1.7
Iron	mcg/dL	53 – 206	97 – 261		13 – 215	98 – 213	90 – 310	109 – 222
Fructosamine (for non-diabetic animals)	umol/L	222 – 386	186 – 243	**	187 – 273	227 – 347	182 – 278	217 – 299
Gamma Glutamyl Transferase	Units/L	12 – 29	4 – 41	9 – 41	31 – 58	6 – 32	26 – 75	34 – 82
Globulin	g/dL	1.4 – 5.5	2.0 – 4.0	0.8 – 4.5	3.5 – 5.3	2.3 – 5.3	2.5 – 4.5	5.3 – 6.4
Glucose	mg/dL	93 – 137	44 – 75	61 – 173	40 – 76	54 – 118	45 – 85	44 – 91
Haptoglobin	mg/mL	0.3 – 1.6	0.1 – 1.7	**	0.0 – 4.9	0.9 – 5.0	0.1 – 1.8	0.0 – 1.8
Insulin	uU/mL	NA	NA	**	NA	0.5 – 10.0	NA	NA
Lactate	mmol/L	0.31 – 5.06	0.38 – 1.83	**	0.67 – 4.43	0.60 – 7.97	8.18 – 15.14	1.43 – 5.52
Lactate Dehydrogenase	Units/L	171 – 445	744 – 1592	**	172 – 441	244 – 802	280 – 597	328 – 782
Lipase	Units/L	2 – 130	1 – 10	**	11 – 42	10 – 32	10 – 38	2 – 12
Magnesium	mg/dL	1.8 – 2.5	1.8 – 2.9	**	2.1 – 3.2	1.5 – 2.4	1.9 – 2.7	1.9 – 3.1
Phosphorus	mg/dL	2.8 – 9.0	4.1 – 8.3	1.5 – 8.9	3.8 – 9.6	1.4 – 5.9	4.5 – 9.2	6.0 – 9.3
Potassium	mmol/L	4.0 – 5.8	3.7 – 5.6	3.7 – 5.8	4.4 – 6.5	3.2 – 5.5	4.1 – 5.9	4.5 – 7.6
Sorbitol Dehydrogenase	Units/L	1.5 – 16.0	6.6 – 37.8	**	19.7 – 71.9	3.3 – 15.5	10.2 – 54.3	4.7 – 18.8
TSH	ng/mL	NA	NA	NA	NA	NA	NA	NA
Free T4-MEIA	ng/mL	NA	NA	NA	NA	0.35 – 1.25	NA	NA
Sodium	mmol/L	145 – 153	135 – 145	145 – 166	139 – 147	130 – 140	139 – 150	128 - 151
Total T4	mcg/dL	5.5 – 12.0	1.5 – 5.3	5.5 – 12.0	4.1 – 8.9	0.5 – 3.1	4.2 – 9.6	2.4 – 7.1
Total protein	gm/dL	4.8 – 8.7	5.6 – 7.8	3.3 – 8.8	6.3 – 8.2	5.2 – 8.2	5.7 – 7.7	5.8 – 8.1
Triglycerides	mg/dL	11 – 55	4 – 26	6 – 41	11 – 66	10 – 61	10 – 32	34 – 165
Uric Acid	mg/dL	0.0 – 0.1	0.5 – 1.6	**	0.0 – 0.2	0.1 – 0.6	0.0 – 0.2	0.0 - 02

**no normal range established in this laboratory

Hematology: Equine, Food, & Fiber Animals

Values are from: Marshfield Clinic Laboratories, Veterinary Diagnostic Service; http://www.marshfieldlabs.org/veterinary/ Data accessed: 2014

Test	Units	Alpaca	Bovine	Camelid (Llama)	Caprine	Equine	Ovine	Porcine
Red blood count (RBC)	x 10⁶/microL	8.60 – 15.90	5.00 – 10.00	9.33 – 17.06	12.20 – 20.00	5.63 – 12.09	9.90 – 14.50	6.40 – 8.00
Hemoglobin	g/dL	8.6 – 16.5	8.0 – 15.0	10.6 – 17.3	7.0 – 12.0	9.8 – 17.1	10.2 – 14.3	12.9 – 15.9
Hematocrit	%	21.1 – 41.8	24.0 – 46.0	25.8 – 45.6	19.2 – 33.0	27.0 – 47.5	32.3 – 47.4	38.3 – 47.8
Mean corp. volume (MCV)	fL	21.6 – 29.9	40.0 – 60.0	23.3 – 31.0	13.2 – 19.7	33.5 – 55.8	28.6 – 36.7	55.1 – 65.1
Mean corp. HGB (MCH)	pg	8.6 – 11.7	11.0 – 17.0	9.2 – 12.1	5.1 – 6.7	12.2 – 19.3	8.9 – 11.2	18.2 – 22.0
Mean corp. HGB conc. (MCHC)	f/dL	38.1 – 41.1	30.0 – 36.0	36.3 – 41.9	33.1 – 40.0	32.4 – 37.4	29.3 – 32.3	31.4 – 35.1
Red cell dis. Width (RDW)	%	18.8 – 31.4	14.0 – 31.0	20.3 – 29.6	24.9 – 41.2	20.6 – 29.0	19.9 – 26.4	14.2 – 17.7
Platelet count	x 10³/microL	269 – 912	230 – 690	185 – 1007	300 – 600	95 – 385	78 – 1309	157 – 618

Test	Units	Alpaca	Bovine	Camelid (Llama)	Caprine	Equine	Ovine	Porcine
Whte blood count (WBC)	x 10³/microL	4.7 – 28.6	4.0 – 12.0	5.9 – 18.9	9.5 – 30.5	4.1 – 14.3	3.7 – 11.7	10.9 – 21.8
Segmented neutrophil absolute #	x 10³/microL	1.30 – 12.00	0.60 – 4.00	2.60 – 13.10	4.20 – 17.50	1.7 – 10.4	0.8 – 3.6	3.2 – 13.1
Band neutrophil absolute #	x 10³/microL	0.00 – 0.100	0.00 – 0.10	0.00 – 0.05	0.00 – 0.10	0.00 – 0.10	0.00 – 0.10	0.00 – 0.10
Lymphocyte absolute #	x 10³/microL	0.60 – 11.00	2.50 – 7.50	0.73 – 6.90	1.60 – 9.60	0.60 – 6.70	0.80 – 7.40	3.30 – 11.50
Monocyte absolute #	x 10³/microL	0.00 – 4.70	0.00 – 0.80	0.00 – 0.61	0.10 – 1.50	0.00 – 0.90	0.00 – 0.40	0.00 – 1.90
Eosinophil absolute #	x 10³/microL	0.30 – 6.40	0.00 – 2.40	0.00 – 4.32	0.00 – 3.50	0.00 – 0.50	0.00 – 1.10	0.00 – 1.50
Basophil absolute #	x 10³/microL	0.00 – 3.60	0.00 – 0.20	0.00 – 0.27	0.00 – 0.60	0.00 – 0.20	0.00 – 0.40	0.00 – 0.20

Coagulation: Bovine, Canine, Equine, Feline

Values are from: Marshfield Clinic Laboratories, Veterinary Diagnostic Service; http://www.marshfieldlabs.org/veterinary/ Accessed: 2014

Test	Units	Bovine	Canine	Equine	Feline
Antithrombin III	%	10 – 1000	75 – 108	10 – 1000	87 – 143
APTT (Activated Partial Thromboplastin Time)	seconds	21.3 – 35.8	9.1 – 15.6	33.0 – 55.0	9.9 – 23.4
Fibrinogen (quantitative)	mg/dL	300 – 700	200 – 400	100 – 400	50 – 300
Fibrinogen, Semi-quantitative	mg/dL	300 – 700	100 – 500	100 – 400	50 – 300
PT (Prothrombin time)	seconds	16.8 – 20.7	5.4 – 8.8	9.1 – 12.6	7.2 – 12.5

Urinalysis: Canine, Feline

Test	Units	Canine	Feline
Specific Gravity		1.001–1.070	1.001–1.080
pH		5.5–7.5	5.5–7.5
Volume	mL/kg/day	24–41	22–30
Osmolality		500–1200 50 min; 2400 max.	50 min; 3000 max.
Sediment: erythrocytes (per HPF)		0–5	0–5
Sediment: leukocytes (per HPF)		0–5	0–5
Sediment: casts (per HPF)		0	0
Glucose/Ketones		0	0
Bilirubin		0–trace	0
Calcium	mEq/L	2–10	
Creatinine	mg/dL	100–300	110–280
Chloride	mEq/L	0–400	
Magnesium	mg/kg/24h	1.7–3.0	3
Phosphorus	mEq/L	50–180	
Potassium	mEq/L	20–120	
Sodium	mEq/L	20–165	
Urea Nitrogen	mg/kg/24h	140–2302	374–1872

Cerebral Spinal Fluid: Canine, Feline

Test	Units	Canine	Feline
Pressure	mm of Water	<170	<100
Specific gravity		1.005–1.007	1.005–1.007
Lymphocytes	per mcl	<5	<5
Pandy's		neg.–trace	neg.
Protein	mg/dL	<25	<25
CK	Units/L	9–28	
K	mEq/L	3.5–6.0	
CL	mEq/L	96–106	
Trig	mg/dL	30–180	
GGT	Units/L	0–10	

Phone Numbers & Websites

Governmental Veterinary Drug-Related Websites

Food and Drug Administration Center for Veterinary Medicine (FDA-CVM)

Call to report an adverse effect for a pharmaceutical, etc. 888-463-6332 (888-INFO-FDA); Emergency: 866-300-4374. After hours call and leave a recorded message. May also file a report on-line www.fda.gov/cvm/

U.S. Department of Agriculture (USDA)

For adverse effect reporting on biologics: 800-752-6255. May also file a report on-line at: http://goo.gl/5hoCO

U.S. Environmental Protection Agency (EPA)

Most of the products used topically for the control of ectoparasites and insects on animals are regulated by the Environmental Protection Agency (EPA) under the Federal Insecticide Fungicide and Rodenticide Act. The EPA may be reached at 800-858-7378.

The National Pesticide Information Center has a hotline and an online site for veterinarians or their staff to report adverse effects of topical pesticides: 800-858-7378; http://pi.ace.orst.edu/vetrep/

Food Animal Residue Avoidance & Depletion Program (FARAD)

1-888-USFARAD (1-888-873-2723) http://www.farad.org/

Drug Enforcement Administration (DEA)

800-882-9539 Toll-free number for registration information. www.deadiversion.usdoj.gov/

Outside of USA:

Australia: APVMA Website: http://www.apvma.gov.au/
Canada: Health Canada website with many veterinary links: http://goo.gl/cGDua
New Zealand: NZFSA Ag Compounds and Vet Medicines website: http://goo.gl/UvHLa
United Kingdom: Veterinary Medicines Directorate website: http://www.vmd.gov.uk/

The Animal Health & Production Compendium

CABI maintains a listing of global and country/region specific websites and databases pertaining to veterinary drug products. It can be accessed at:
http://www.cabi.org/ahpc/more-resources/drug-databases/

Drug Shortage Websites

The Food and Drug Administration (FDA) maintains a drug shortage web page. E-mail notification service is available:
http://goo.gl/16ICZ

The American Society of Health-System Pharmacists (ASHP) has a website for drug shortages (human drugs):
http://www.ashp.org/shortages

Animal Poison Control Centers

The following are known 24-hour poison control centers in the USA that specialize in providing information specific for veterinary patients. Fees listed are those at the time of writing (August 2014).

ASPCA Animal Poison Control Center: 888-426-4435; $65 consultation fee. http://www.aspca.org/pet-care/animal-poison-control

Pet Poison Helpline: 800-213-6680; $39 consultation fee. http://www.petpoisonhelpline.com

There are many regional poison centers that may be of assistance with animal poisonings; refer to your local poison center for more information.

In the UK:

Veterinary Poisons Information Center: 020 7188 0200; Subscription service. http://www.vpisuk.co.uk

Animal Blood Banks

The following list are some known animal blood banks or companies that sell blood products. There are many University-affiliated or emergency clinic blood bank programs as well; contact your local veterinary school or emergency clinic for more information. **Note:** Primary location(s) are listed in parentheses.

Animal Blood Resources (MI, CA)

1-800-243-5759
http://www.abrint.net

Blue Ridge Veterinary Blood Bank (VA)

800-949-3822
http://www.brvbb.com

Buddies for Life Canine Blood Bank (MI)

248-334-6877
www.ovrs.com/canine_blood_bank/index.php

Canadian Animal Blood Bank Inc. (Canada; MB)

http://www.rrc.mb.ca/abb/

Hemopet (CA)

714-891-2022, Ext 114
www.hemopet.com

HemoSolutions (CO)

800-791-2507
www.hemosolutions.com

LifeStream Animal Blood Bank Inc. (Canada; ON)

www.animalbloodbank.ca

Northwest Veterinary Blood Bank (WA)

360-752-5554
www.northwestbloodbank.com/

Rocky Mountain Blood Services (CO)
719-522-3227
www.rockymountainbloodservices.com

Sun States Animal Blood Bank (AZ)
844-430-4300
www.sunstates.org/

The Animal Blood Bank at The Ohio State University (OH)
614-688-8460
http://vet.osu.edu/vmc/animal-blood-bank

The Pet Blood Bank (TX)
Tel: 800-906-7059
www.pettransfusion.com

The Veterinarians' Blood Bank (IN)
877-838-8533
www.vetbloodbank.com

Dog/Cat Food Companies

The following are links to some of the major canine and feline dog food companies in the USA.

Blue Buffalo
www.bluebuffalo.com

Eukanuba/Iams
www.iams.com
www.eukanuba.com

Hill's/Science Diet
www.hillspet.com

Mars Petcare
Includes: *Pedigree, Royal Canin, Nutro, Whiskas*
www.marspetcare.com

PetAg
www.petag.com

Nestle Purina
www.purinaveterinarydiets.com/

Veterinary Pharmaceutical Manufacturers & Suppliers

The following lists customer service phone numbers and website URLs for several companies that provide veterinary drug-related products for the USA market.

Abbott Animal Health
888-299-7416
www.abbottanimalhealth.com

Agri Laboratories LTD
800-542-8916
www.agrilabs.com

Aspen Veterinary Resources Ltd.
816-415-4324
www.aspenveterinaryresources.com

Bayer HealthCare LLC, Animal Health Division
General Inquiries: 800-255-6517
www.bayer-ah.com

Bimeda, Inc., Div. Cross Vetpharm Group, Ltd.
888-524-6332
www.bimeda.com

Bioniche Animal Health USA, Inc.
800-265-5464
www.bioniche.com

Boehringer Ingelheim Vetmedica, Inc.
800-325-9167
www.bi-vetmedica.com

Colorado Serum Company
800-525-2065
www.colorado-serum.com

Davis Mfg.
800-292-2424
www.davismfg.com

Dechra Veterinary Products
913-327-0015
www.pharmadermah.com

Delmont Laboratories, Inc.
800-562-5541
www.delmont.com

Durvet, Inc.
800-821-5570
www.durvet.com

DVM Formula (Vets Plus, Inc)
715-231-1234
www.dvmformula.com

Elanco Animal Health
A Division of Eli Lilly & Co.
800-428-4441
www.elanco.com
www.elancopet.com

Farnam
800-234-2269
www.farnam.com

Figuerola Laboratories
800-219-1147
http://www.figuerola-labs.com/

First Priority, Inc.
800-650-4899
www.prioritycare.com

Ford Dodge Labs
—See Zoetis

Greer Laboratories, Inc.
877-777-1080
www.greerlabs.com

Halocarbon Products Corporation
201-262-8899
www.halocarbon.com

Hanford Pharmaceuticals
800-234-4263
www.hanford.com

Happy Jack, Incorporated
800-326-5225
www.happyjackinc.com

The Hartz Mountain Corporation
800-275-1414
www.hartz.com

Henry Schein Animal Health
855-724-3461
www.henryscheinvet.com

Heska Corporation
800-464-3752 (800-GO HESKA)
www.heska.com

I-Med Pharma Inc.
800-463-1008
www.imedanimalhealth.com

Innovacyn, Inc
866-318-3116
www.vetericyn.com

Lloyd Laboratories
800-831-0004
www.lloydinc.com

Luitpold Pharmaceuticals, Inc.
800-458-0163
www.luitpoldanimalhealth.com/

MVP Laboratories, Inc
800-856-4648
www.mvplabs.com

Macleod Pharmaceuticals, Inc.
800-850-5432
www.macleodpharma.com

Med-Pharmex, Inc.
www.med-pharmex.com

Merial Ltd.
678-638-3000
www.merial.com

Merck Animal Health
800-224-5318 Companion Animals
800-211-3573 Livestock
866-349-3497 Equine
www.merck-animal-health-usa.com

Modern Veterinary Therapeutics, LLC
305-669-4150
www.modernveterinarytherapeutics.com

Neogen Corporation
800-525-2022
www.neogen.com

Norbrook Inc.
913-599-5777
www.norbrookinc.com

Novartis Animal Health USA, Inc.
800-637-0281
www.ah.novartis.com

Nutramax Laboratories, Inc.
888-886-6442
www.nutramaxlabs.com

Nutri-Vet
877-729-8668
www.nutri-vet.com

OPK Biotech
866-933-2472
www.opkbiotech.com

Paladin Labs Inc.
514-340-1112
www.paladin-labs.com/index.asp

Pala-Tech Laboratories, Inc.
888-337-2446
www.palatech.com

PetAg, Inc.
800-323-6878
www.petag.com

Pfizer Animal Health
—see Zoetis

Pharmacia & Upjohn Company
—see Zoetis

Phibro Animal Health
888-403-0074
www.phibroah.com

PRN Pharmacal
800-874-9764
www.prnpharmacal.com

Putney Inc.
866-683-0660
www.putneyvet.com

Purica
866-334-2463
http://www.purica.com/

RXV
817-859-3000

Schering
—see Merck

Sergeant's Pet Care Products, Inc.
800-224-7387 (800-224-PETS)
www.sergeants.com

Sogeval Laboratories, Inc.
866-866-8896
www.sogevalus.com

Sparhawk Laboratories, Inc.
800-255-6368
www.sparhawklabs.com

The Hartz Mountain Corporation
800-275-1414
www.hartz.com

Tomlyn Products
877-580-7729
www.tomlyn.com

Van Beek Natural Science
800-346-5311
www.vanbeeknaturalscience.com/

Vedco, Inc.
816-238-8840
www.vedco.com

Veterinary Products Laboratories
www.vpl.com

Vet One
www.vetone.net

Vet Tek, Inc.
800-821-5570
www.durvet.com

Vetoquinol USA, Inc.
800-267-5707
www.vetoquinolusa.com

Virbac Corporation
817-831-5030 (US)
www.virbac.com

Vortech Pharmaceuticals, Ltd.
800-521-4686

Wildlife Pharmaceuticals, Inc.
866-823-9314
www.wildpharm.com

Zinpro Corporation
952-983-4000
www.zinpro.com

Zoetis
888-963-8471
www.zoetis.com

Systemic Drugs Sorted by Therapeutic Class or Major Indication

The following lists systemic drugs by their therapeutic class or major indication. Classifications are based upon the American Society of Health-System Pharmacists (ASHP) drug classification system. If a dosage for a given species is listed, the following species codes are used in parentheses after the drug name:

A   = Avian; Pet Bird
B   = Bovine, Cattle
C   = Cat, Feline
D   = Dog, Canine
Fer = Ferret
Fi = Fish
H   = Horse, Equine
L   = Llama, Alpacas, Camelids
Po = Pocket Pets, Rabbits, Small Lab Animals
R   = Reptiles/Amphibians
Ru = Ruminants
Sh = Sheep/Goats; Ovine/Caprine; Small Ruminants
SA = Small Animals
Sw = Swine, Pigs
Z   = Wildlife/Zoo Animals

Note: As some drugs have multiple indications, there may not be a specific dosage listed for that indication for every species noted.

Antihistamines

Cetirizine (D, C, H) 200
Chlorpheniramine (D, C, Fer, A) 213
Clemastine Fumarate (D, C) 234
Cyproheptadine (D, C, H) 273
Diphenhydramine (D, C, Fer, Po, A, H, B) 342
Doxepin (D, C, H, A) 361
Fexofenadine (D, C) 440
Hydroxyzine (D, C, Fer, H, A) 534
Loratadine (D, C) 638
Meclizine (D, C, Po) 662
Promethazine (D, C, H) 899
Pyrilamine (H) 919
Trimeprazine (D, C) 1066
Tripelennamine (B, H) 1067

Central Nervous System Drugs

(including antiinflammatories, analgesics, muscle relaxants)

CNS/Respiratory Stimulants

Doxapram (D, C, Fer, Po, B, Sw, H, A, R) 359

Analgesics, Opioid Agonists

Alfentanil (D, C) 30
Codeine (D, C, Po) 256
Fentanyl Injection (D, C, Fer, Po, H) 430
Fentanyl Transdermal Patch (D, C, H, Sw, Po, Sh) 432
Fentanyl Transdermal Solution (D) 436
Hydrocodone (D, C) 521
Hydromorphone (D, C, Fer, Po, R) 526
Meperidine (D, C, Fer, Po, Sw, B, H) 680
Methadone (D, C) 688
Morphine (D, C, Po, H, L, Z) 743
Oxymorphone (D, C, Fer, H, A, Po, Z) 799
Sufentanil (D, C) 985
Tramadol (D, C, H, B, A, R, Z) 1052

Analgesics, Opioid Agonist/Antagonists

Buprenorphine (D, C, Po, Fer, H, Z) 127
Butorphanol (D, C, Fer, Po, B, H, A, L, Z) 135
Nalbuphine (D, C, Po) 756
Pentazocine (D, C, Po, Fer, H) 830

Analgesics, Other

Amantadine (D, C) 38
Clonidine (D, C, B) 247
Gabapentin (D, C) 478
Ketamine (D, C, Po, Fer, B, H, Sw, L, R, A, Z) 592
Pregabalin (D, C) 887

Nonsteroidal Antiinflammatory/Analgesic Agents

Acetaminophen (D, Po) 6
Aspirin (D, C, Po, Fer, H) 83
Carprofen (D, C, Po, H, B, Fer, A, R) 161
Colchicine (D, A) 258
Deracoxib (D) 291
Diclofenac (H) 321
Dimethyl Sulfoxide (D, H) 335
Etodolac (D) 412
Firocoxib (D, C, H) 444
Flunixin (D, C, Fer, Po, B, H, Sh, Sw, Z) 458
Ketoprofen (D, C, Fer, Po, H, Sw, A, Z) 603
Ketorolac Tromethamine (D, Po) 605
Mavacoxib (D) 658
Meloxicam (D, C, H, B, Sh, Sw, L, Fer, Po, A, R, Z) 675
Naproxen (D, Po, H) 762
Phenylbutazone (D, H, Ru) 845
Piroxicam (D, C, H, Po) 865
Robenacoxib (D, C) 935
Tepoxalin (D) 1002
Tolfenamic Acid (D, C, B, Sw) 1046

Behavior-Modifying Agents

Amitriptyline (D, C, A) 50
Buspirone (D, C) 131
Clomipramine HCl (D, C, A) 243
Clorazepate (D, C) 253
Diazepam (D, C, Po, Fer, A, H, Z) 312
Fluoxetine (D, C) 462
Fluvoxamine (D, C) 467
Imipramine (D, C, H)
Lorazepam (D, C) 639
Methylphenidate (D) 704

Paroxetine HCl (D, C, A) 820
Pheromones (D, C, H) 852
SAMe (D, C) 945
Sertraline (D, C) 953
Trazodone (D) 1055

Tranquilizers/Sedatives

Acepromazine (D, C, Fe, PO, B, H, Sw, Sh, Z) 2
Alprazolam (D, C) 33
Azaperone (Sw, Z) 97
Chlordiazepoxide (D, C) 209
Detomidine (D, H, B, Sh, L, A) 299
Dexmedetomidine (D, C) 306
Diazepam (D, C, Po, Fer, A, H, Z) 312
Doxepin (D, C, H, A) 361
L-Theanine (D, C) 607
Lorazepam (D, C) 639
Medetomidine (D, C, Fer, A, R, Z) 663
Midazolam (D, C, Po, A, H, Z) 722
Romifidine (D, C, H, B) 940
Tiletamine/Zolazepam (D, C, Po, Fer, H, Ru, L, R, Z) 1030
Xylazine (D, C, H, B, Sh, L, Po, Fer, A, Z) 1099

Anesthetic Agents, Barbiturates

Methohexital Sodium (D, C) 698
Pentobarbital (D, C, Po, H) 832
Thiopental (D, C, Po, B, H, Sw, Sh) 1018

Anesthetic Agents, Inhalants

Desflurane 293
Isoflurane (D, C, Po, H, Sh, R, A) 573
Sevoflurane (D, C, H, Sh) 955

Anesthetic Agents, Miscellaneous

Alfaxalone (D, C) 26
Alfentanil (D, C) 30
Etomidate (D, C, Fe, Po) 414
Fentanyl Injection (D, C, Fer, Po, H) 430
Fentanyl Transdermal Patch (D, C, H, Sw, Po, Sh) 432
Fentanyl Transdermal Solution (D) 436
Ketamine (D, C, Po, Fer, B, H, Sw, Sh, L, R, A, Z)
Propofol (D, C, H, Sh, Po, R, Z) 904
Remifentanil (D, C, H) 931
Sufentanil (D, C) 985
Tiletamine/Zolazepam (D, C, Po, Fer, H, Ru, L, R, Z) 1030
Xylazine (D, C, H, B, Sh, L, Po, Fer, A, Z) 1099

Reversal Agents

Atipamezole D, C, Po, H, B, L, A, R, Z) 86
Flumazenil (D, C, Z) 454
Naloxone (D, C, Po, H) 757
Naltrexone (D, C, Z) 759
Neostigmine (D, C, B, H, Sw, Sh) 766
Tolazoline (D, C, H, Ru, L, A) 1044
Yohimbine (D, C, Po, A, B, H, L, Z) 1104

Anticonvulsants
Imepitoin (D) 541
Bromides (D, C) 120
Carbamazepine (D, H) 154
Clonazepam (D, C) 246
Clorazepate (D, C) 253
Diazepam (D, C, Po, Fer, A, H, Z) 312
Felbamate (D) 424
Gabapentin (D, C) 489
Levetiracetam (D, C) 617
Lorazepam (D, C) 639
Phenobarbital (D, C, Fer, B, H) 840
Phenytoin (D, C, H) 850
Pregabalin (D, C) 887
Primidone (D) 890
Rufinamide (D) 944
Topiramate (D, C) 1049
Valproic Acid (D) 1075
Zonisamide (D, C) 1111

Muscle Relaxants, Skeletal
Atracurium (D, C, Po, H) 91
Baclofen (D) 106
Dantrolene (D, C, H) 283
Guaifenesin (H, Sh, L) 507
Methocarbamol (D, C, H) 697
Pancuronium (D, C) 813
Rocuronium (D, C, H) 938
Succinylcholine (D, C, R) 982
Vecuronium (D, C) 1081

Euthanasia Agents
Pentobarbital/Phenytoin (D, C, Ru, H) 415

Cardiovascular Agents
Inotropic Agents
Digoxin (D, C, Fer, H) 325
Dobutamine (D, C, H, A) 349
Pimobendan (D, C) 858

Antiarrhythmic Drugs
Amiodarone (D, H) 48
Disopyramide (D) 347
Lidocaine (D, C, H) 623
Mexiletine (D) 720
Procainamide (D, H) 894
Quinidine (D, H) 925
Verapamil (D, C, H, Po) 1083

Anticholinergics (Parasympatholytics)
Atropine (D, C, B, H, Po, Fer, Sw, Sh, A, R) 93
Glycopyrrolate (D, C, Fer, Po, H, R) 500
Hyoscyamine (D) 536

ACE Inhibitors
Benazepril (D, C) 107
Captopril (D, C) 152
Enalapril (D, C, Fer, A) 374
Imidapril (D) 543
Lisinopril (D, C) 630
Ramipril (D, C) 927

Calcium Channel Blocking Agents
Amlodipine (D, C) 52
Diltiazem (D, C, Fer) 330
Verapamil (D, C, H, Po)

Vasodilating Agents
Hydralazine (D, C, H) 516
Isosorbide (D, C) 579
Isoxsuprine (H, D) 582
Nitroglycerine (D, C, Fer) 773
Nitroprusside (D, C) 774
Sildenafil (D, C) 957
Tadalafil (D) 997

Agents Used in Treatment of Shock
Dobutamine (D, C, H, A) 349
Dopamine (D, C) 355
Epinephrine (D, C, Po, A, H, Ru, Sw) 385
Isoproterenol HCl (D, C) 577
Norepinephrine (D, C, H) 777
Phenylephrine (D, C, H) 847
Vasopressin (D, C, H) 1079

Alpha-Adrenergic Blocking Agents
Phenoxybenzamine (D, C, H) 843
Prazosin (D, C) 882

Beta-Adrenergic Blocking Agents
Atenolol (D, C, Fer) 86
Carvedilol (D) 163
Esmolol (D, C) 400
Metoprolol (D, C) 713
Propranolol (D, C, Fer, H) 908
Sotalol HCl (D, C) 969

Angiotensin Receptor Blockers (ARBs)
Candesartan (D) 151
Irbesartan (D, C) 568
Losartan (D) 641
Telmisartan (D, C) 1001

Miscellaneous Antihypertensive Agents
Fenoldopam (D, C) 428
Nitroprusside (D, C)

Other Cardiovascular Agents
Carnitine (D, C) 159
Taurine (D, C) 1000

Respiratory Drugs
Sympathomimetics
Albuterol (D, C, H) 23
Clenbuterol (H) 236
Ephedrine (D, C) 383
Epinephrine (D, C, Po, A, H, B, Sh, Sw) 385
Isoproterenol HCl (D, C) 577
Pseudoephedrine HCl (D, C) 911
Terbutaline (D, C, H, A, R) 1006

Xanthines
Aminophylline (D, C, H) 46
Theophylline (D, C) 1013

Antitussives
Benzonatate (D) 109
Butorphanol (D, C, Fer, Po, B, H, A, L, Z) 135
Codeine (D, C, Po) 256
Hydrocodone (D, C) 521

Mucolytics
Acetylcysteine (D, C, H) 11

Other Respiratory Agents
Cromolyn Sodium (H) 264
Ipratropium Br (Po H) 567
Montelukast (C) 741
Zafirlukast (D, C) 1106

Renal & Urinary Tract Agents
Diuretics, Carbonic Anhydrase Inhibitors
Acetazolamide (D, C, H) 7
Dichlorphenamide (D, C) 317
Methazolamide (D, C) 690

Diuretics, Thiazides
Chlorothiazide (D, C) 211
Hydrochlorothiazide (D, C, H) 518

Diuretics, Loop
Bumetanide (D, C) 125
Furosemide (D, C, Fer, Po, B, H, A, R) 475
Torsemide (D, C) 1051

Diuretics, Potassium Sparing
Spironolactone (D, C) 974
Triamterene (D) 1061

Diuretics, Osmotic
Glycerin, Oral (D, C) 499
Mannitol (D, C, B, Sw, Sh, H) 650

Agents for Urinary Incontinence/Retention
Baclofen (D) 106
Bethanechol (D, C, H, B) 112
Ephedrine (D, C) 383
Flavoxate (D) 447
Imipramine (D, C, H) 548
Oxybutynin (D, C) 798
Phenoxybenzamine (D, C, H) 483
Phenylpropanolamine (D, C) 849
Pseudoephedrine HCl (D, C) 911
Tamsulosin (D, C) 998

Urinary Alkalinizers
Sodium Bicarbonate (D, C, H, Ru, A) 960

Urinary Acidifiers
Ammonium Chloride (D, C, H, Sh) 54
Methionine (D, C, Sh) 695

Agents for Urolithiasis
Acetohydroxamic Acid (D) 10
Allopurinol (D, A, R) 31
Ammonium Chloride (D, C, H, Sh) 54
Citrate, Potassium (D, C) 230
Methionine (D, C, Sh) 695
Tiopronin (D) 1038

Miscellaneous Renal/Urinary Agents
Amitriptyline (D, C, A) 50
Pentosan (D, C, H) 835
Probenecid (R) 892

Gastrointestinal Agents

Antiemetic Agents
Chlorpromazine (D, C, B, H, Sw, Sh) 215
Dimenhydrinate (D, C) 332
Diphenhydramine (D, C, Fer, Po, A, H, B) 342
Dolasetron (D, C) 352
Granisetron (D, C) 505
Maropitant (D, C) 654
Meclizine (D, C, Po) 662
Metoclopramide (D, C, Po, H) 710
Mirtazapine (D, C) 732
Ondansetron (D, C) 787
Prochlorperazine (D, C) 898
Promethazine (D, C, H) 899

Antacids
Aluminum Hydroxide (D, C, Po, B, H) 37
Calcium Acetate (D, C) 145
Calcium Carbonate (D, C) 146
Sodium Bicarbonate (D, C, H, Ru, A) 960

H-2 Antagonists
Cimetidine (D, C, Fer, Po, H) 222
Famotidine (D, Fer, Po, H) 418
Nizatidine (D, C) 776
Ranitidine (D, C, Fer, H, Po) 929

Gastromucosal Protectants
Sucralfate (D, C, Fer, H, R) 983

Prostaglandin E Analogs
Misoprostol (D, C, H) 734

Proton Pump Inhibitors
Esomeprazole (D, C, H) 402
Omeprazole (D, C, Fer, H, Sw) 785
Pantoprazole (D, C, H, L) 815

Appetite Stimulants
Cyproheptadine (D, C, H) 273
Diazepam (D, C, Po, Fer, A, H, Z) 312
Mirtazapine (D, C) 732
Oxazepam (D, C) 795

GI Antispasmodics-Anticholinergics
Aminopentamide (D, C) 45
Hyoscyamine (D) 536
N-Butylscopolammonium Br (H) 754
Propantheline (D, C, H) 901

GI Stimulants
Cisapride (D, C, Po, H) 226
Dexpanthenol (D, C, H) 308
Domperidone (D, C, H) 353
Metoclopramide (D, C, Po, H) 710
Neostigmine (D, C, B, H, Sw, Sh) 766

Digestive Enzymes
Pancrelipase (D, C, Po, A) 812

Laxatives
Bisacodyl (D, C) 114
Docusate (D, C, H) 351
Lactulose (D, C, A, R) 608
Mineral Oil (D, C, Po, B, H, Sw, Sh, A) 728
Polyethylene Glycol (PEG) 3350 (D, C) 867
Psyllium (D, C, H) 913
Saline Cathartics (D, C, H, B) 947
Sorbitol (D, C, H) 967

Antidiarrheals
Bismuth Subsalicylate (D, C, Fer, B, H, Sw) 115
Clonidine (D, C, B) 247
Diphenoxylate/Atropine (D, C) 344
Kaolin/Pectin (D, C, Fer, Po, B, H, Sw, A) 591
Loperamide (D, C, Po) 636
Paregoric (D, C) 817

Emetics
Apomorphine (D) 77
Hydrogen Peroxide 3% (D) 525
Xylazine (D, C, H, B, Sh, L, Po, Fer, A, Z) 1099

Miscellaneous GI Drugs
Bismuth Subsalicylate (D, C, Fer, B, H, Sw) 115
Budesonide (D, C) 124
Dirlotapide (D) 345
Glutamine (D, C) 497
Olsalazine Sodium (D) 784
SAMe (D, C) 945
Silymarin (D, C) 959
Sulfasalazine (D, C, Fer, H) 995
Ursodiol (D, C, H, A) 1073

Hormones/Endocrine/ Reproductive Agents

Sex Hormones, Estrogens
Diethylstilbestrol (DES) (D) 323
Estradiol (D, C, B, H) 404
Estriol (D) 406

Sex Hormones, Progestins
Altrenogest (D, H, Sw) 35
Medroxyprogesterone (D, C, H) 666
Megestrol Acetate (D, C) 668

Sex Hormones, Androgens
Danazol (D, C) 281
Methyltestosterone (D) 709
Mibolerone (D, C) 721
Testosterone (D, B) 1008

Anabolic steroids
Boldenone (H) 118
Nandrolone (D, C, R) 761
Stanozolol (D, C, Fer, Po, H, A, R) 976

Posterior Pituitary Hormones
Desmopressin (D, C, H) 295
Vasopressin (D, C, H) 1079

Oxytocics
Oxytocin (D, C, Po, B, H, Sw, Sh, A, L, R) 806

Adrenal Cortical Steroids
Corticotropin-ACTH (D, C, H, A) 260
Cortisone Acetate (D) 261
Cosyntropin (D, C, H) 263

Mineralocorticoids
Desoxycorticosterone (D, C) 297
Fludrocortisone (D, C, Fer) 453

Glucocorticoids
Betamethasone (D, H) 110
Dexamethasone (D, C, Po, B, H) 301
Flumethasone (D, C, H) 455
Fluticasone (D, C, H) 465
Hydrocortisone (D, C) 522
Isoflupredone (B, H, Sw) 571
Methylprednisolone (D, C, H) 705
Prednisolone (D, C, Po, B, H, L, A, R) 883
Prednisone (D, C, Po, B, H, L, A, R) 883
Triamcinolone (D, C, H) 1057

Adrenal Steroid Inhibitors
Ketoconazole (D, C, H, Po, A, R) 599
Metyrapone (C) 718
Mitotane (D, Fer) 737
Selegiline (D, C) 951
Trilostane (D, C, H) 1063

Antidiabetic Agents
Acarbose (D, C) 1
Chlorpropamide (D, C) 217
Chromium (C) 221
Glimepiride (C) 488
Glipizide (C) 490
Glyburide (C) 498
Insulin (D, C, Fer, Po, B, H, L, A) 552
Metformin (C, H) 686
Vanadium (C) 1076

Glucose Elevating Agents
Diazoxide, Oral (D, C, Fer, Po) 316
Glucagon (D, C, B) 491
Octreotide Acetate (D, Fer) 783

Thyroid Hormones
Levothyroxine (D, C, H, A, R) 619
Liothyronine (D, C) 628
Thyrotropin (D, C, Fer, Po, A) 1022

Antithyroid Drugs
Carbimazole (C) 156
Ipodate Sodium (C) 566
Methimazole (C, Po) 693

Prostaglandins
Cloprostenol (D, B, H, Sw, Sh, L) 251
Dinoprost (D, C, H, Sw, Sh) 339

Misc. Endocrine/Reproductive Drugs
Aglepristone (D, C) 17
Bromocriptine (D, C, H) 122
Cabergoline (D, C, A) 140
Chorionic Gonadotropin-HCG (D, C, A, B, Sw) 220
Deslorelin (D, Fer, H) 294
Finasteride (D, Fer) 443
Gonadorelin (D, C, B) 503
Leuprolide (Fer, A) 613
Melatonin (D, C, Fer, H) 673
Metergoline (D, C) 685
Mibolerone (D, C) 721
Octreotide Acetate (D, Fer) 783
Osaterone Acetate (D) 790
Pergolide (H) 838
Somatotropin (D) 966
Thyrotropin-Releasing Hormone (D, H) 1023
Zinc Gluconate (neutering agent) (D) 1110

Anti-infective Drugs
Antiparasitics
Afoxolaner (D) 16
Albendazole (D, C, Po, B, Sh) 19
Atovaquone (D, C) 90
Clorsulon (B, Sh, L) 254
Dichlorvos (Po, Sw) 318
Diclazuril (D, C, H, B, Sh) 319
Diminazene (D, H, B, Sh) 337
Doramectin (D, C, B, Sw, Po) 357
Emodepside + Praziquantel (C, D, R) 373
Eprinomectin (C, H) 392

Epsiprantel (D, C) 394
Fenbendazole (D, C, Po, Fer, B, H, Sw, Sh, L, A, R, Z) 425
Fluralaner (D) 464
Furazolidone (C) 474
Imidocarb (D, C, H) 544
Ivermectin (D, C, B, Fer, Po, H, Sw, Sh, L, A, R) 586
Levamisole (D, H, B, Sh, R) 615
Lufenuron (D, C, Po) 643
Meglumine Antimoniate (D) 670
Melarsomine (D) 671
Metronidazole (D, C, Fer, Po, H, A, R) 715
Milbemycin Oxime (D, C) 726
Miltefosine (D) 727
Morantel (B, Sh) 742
Moxidectin (D, C, Fer, Sh, L, H, B) 747
Nitazoxanide (C, H) 769
Nitenpyram (D, C, R) 770
Oxfendazole (H, B, Sw) 796
Oxibendazole (H, Po) 797
Paromomycin (D, C, L, R) 819
Piperazine (D, C, Po, A, R) 863
Ponazuril (D, C, Po, H, L, A, R) 869
Praziquantel (D, C, Po, Sh, H, L, A, R) 879
Primaquine (C) 889
Pyrantel (D, C, Po, H, L, A) 914
Pyrimethamine (D, C, H, A) 920
Pyrimethamine + Sulfadiazine (H) 922
Quinacrine (D, C, R) 923
Ronidazole (D, C) 942
Selamectin (D, C, Fer, Po) 949
Sodium Stibogluconate (D) 964
Spinosad (D, C) 972
Tinidazole (D, C) 1036
Trypan Blue (D) 1068

Anticoccidial Agents
Amprolium (D, C, Fer, Po, B, Sw, Sh, L, A) 71
Decoquinate (D, B, Sh, L) 288
Diclazuril (D, C, H, B, Sh) 319
Toltrazuril (D, C, Po, B, Sh, L, Sw, A, R) 1047

Antibiotics, Aminocyclitols
Amikacin (D, C, Fer, Po, H, A, R, Fi) 40
Apramycin (B, Sw, A) 78
Gentamicin (D, C, Fer, Po, H, Sw, A, R) 485
Neomycin (D, C, Po, Fer, B, H, Sh, A, R) 764
Spectinomycin (Po, B, Sw, A) 970
Tobramycin (D, C, H, L, A, R) 1039

Antibiotics, Carbapenems
Ertapenem (D, C) 396
Imipenem-Cilastatin (D, C, H) 546
Meropenem (D, C) 684

Antibiotics, Cephalosporins
Cefaclor (D, C) 167
Cefadroxil (D, C, Fer) 168
Cefazolin (D, C, H, R) 170
Cefepime (D, C, H) 172
Cefixime (D, C) 173
Cefotaxime (D, C, H, A, R) 174
Cefotetan Disodium (D, C) 176
Cefovecin (D, C) 178
Cefoxitin (D, C, H) 180
Cefpodoxime Proxetil (D, C, H) 182
Ceftazidime (D, C, R) 183
Ceftiofur HCl (B, Sw) 188
Ceftiofur Crystalline Free Acid (B, Sw, H) 185
Ceftiofur Sodium (B, Sw, Sh, H, D, C, A, R) 190
Ceftriaxone (D, C, H) 193
Cefuroxime (D, C, Sh) 195
Cephalexin (D, C, Po, Fer, H, R, A) 196
Cephapirin (B) 199

Antibiotics, Macrolides
Azithromycin (D, C, H, Po, A) 102
Clarithromycin (D, C, Fer, H) 232
Erythromycin (D, C, Fer, A, B, H) 397
Gamithromycin (B) 481
Tildipirosin (B, Sw) 1028
Tulathromycin (B, Sw, H, Sh) 1069
Tylosin (D, C, Fer, Po, B, Sw) 1071

Antibiotics, Penicillins
Amoxicillin (D, C, Po, Fer, A, R) 56
Amoxicillin/Clavulanate (D, C, Fer, A) 59
Ampicillin (D, C, B, H, Fer, Po, R) 67
Ampicillin/Sulbactam (D, C) 69
Cloxacillin (B) 255
Dicloxacillin (D, C) 322
Oxacillin (D, C, H) 793
Penicillin G (D, C, Fer, Po, B, H, Sw, A) 825
Penicillin V (D, C, H) 829
Piperacillin/Tazobactam (D, C, A, R) 861
Ticarcillin/Clavulanate (D, C, H) 1025

Antibiotics, Tetracyclines
Chlortetracycline (C, Po, A) 218
Doxycycline (D, C, Po, H, A, R) 365
Minocycline HCl (D, C, H) 730
Oxytetracycline (D, C, B, H, Sw, Sh, A, R) 802
Tetracycline (D, C, Fer, Po, B, Sh, Sw, A) 1010

Antibiotics, Lincosamides
Clindamycin (D, C, Fer, A, R) 237
Lincomycin (D, C, Fer, Sw) 626
Pirlimycin (B) 864
Tilmicosin (B, Sh, Sw, Po) 1033

Antibiotics, Quinolones

Ciprofloxacin (D, C, Fer, Po, A) 224
Danofloxacin (B, R) 282
Enrofloxacin (D, C, H, B, Sw, Fer, Po, R, A, L) 379
Marbofloxacin (D, C, R) 652
Orbifloxacin (D, C, H, A) 788
Pradofloxacin (D, C) 875

Antibiotics, Sulfonamides

Sulfachlorpyridazine (B, Sw, A) 986
Sulfadiazine/Trimethoprim (D, C, Fer, Po, B, H, A, R) 988
Sulfamethoxazole/Trimethoprim (D, C, Fer, Po, B, H, A, R) 988
Sulfadimethoxine (D, C, Fer, Po, B, H, L, R) 992
Sulfadimethoxine/Ormetoprim (D) 994

Miscellaneous Antibiotics, Antibacterials

Aztreonam (D, H, Fi) 104
Chloramphenicol (D, C, Po, Fer, H, A, R) 206
Clofazimine (D, C, A) 242
Dapsone (D, C, H) 285
Ethambutol (D, C, A) 407
Florfenicol (D, C, B, Sh, Sw) 447
Fosfomycin (D, H) 472
Isoniazid (D, C, B) 575
Methenamine (D, C) 692
Metronidazole (D, C, Fer, Po, H, A, R) 715
Nitrofurantoin (D, C) 771
Novobiocin (D, B) 779
Rifampin (D, C, H) 933
Ronidazole (D, C) 942
Sodium Iodide (D, C, B, Sh, H) 561
Tiamulin (Sw) 1024
Tinidazole (D, C, H)
Vancomycin (D, C, H) 1077

Antifungal Agents

Amphotericin B (D, C, H, Po, L, A, R) 62
Caspofungin (D, C) 165
Fluconazole (D, C, H, Po, A, R) 449
Flucytosine (D, C) 451
Griseofulvin (D, C, Po, H) 506
Itraconazole (D, C, Po, A, H, R) 583
Ketoconazole (D, C, H, Po, A, R) 599
Nystatin (D, C, H, A, R) 780
Posaconazole (D, C) 871
Terbinafine HCl (D, C, A) 1004
Voriconazole (D, C, H, A) 1094

Antiviral Agents

Acyclovir (A, H) 14
Amantadine (D, C) 38
Famciclovir (C) 416
Interferon Alfa (D, C) 558
Interferon Omega (D, C) 560
Lysine (C) 644
Oseltamivir (D, H) 791
Zidovudine (AZT) (C) 1107

Blood Modifying Agents

Anticoagulants/Antithrombotics

Aspirin (D, C, Po, Fer, H) 83
Clopidogrel (D, C) 249
Dalteparin (D, C, H) 279
Enoxaparin (D, C, H) 377
Heparin (D, C, H) 512
Warfarin (D, C, H) 1097

Erythropoietic Agents

Cyanocobalamin (D, C, H, Sw, B, Sh) 265
Darbepoetin (D, C) 287
Epoetin Alfa (Erythropoietin) (D, C, Fer, Po) 390
Ferrous Sulfate (D, C) 438
Folic Acid (D, C, H) 469
Iron Dextran (D, C, Fer, Sw, A) 570

Misc. Blood Modifying Agents

Aminocaproic Acid (D, H) 43
Filgrastim (D, C, H) 442
Gemfibrozil (D, C) 484
Hemoglobin Glutamer (D, C) 510
Lithium (D) 632
Pentoxifylline (D, C, H) 836
Phytonadione (SA, B, Sh, H, A) 857
Protamine Sulfate (D, C, B) 910

Fluid & Electrolyte Modifiers

Albumin (D, C) 20
Aluminum Hydroxide (D, C, Po, B, H) 37
Butaphosphan (H, B, Sw, A) 134
Calcitonin (D, R) 141
Calcitriol (D, C) 143
Calcium Acetate (D, C) 145
Calcium Carbonate (D, C) 146
Calcium, Injectable (D, C) 147
Dextran 70 (D, C, B) 311
Dihydrotachysterol (D, C) 328
Ergocalciferol (D, C) 394
Etidronate (D, C) 411
Glycerin, Oral (D, C) 499
Hydroxyethyl Starch (D, C, H, A, L) 530
Hypertonic saline (7% - 7.5%) (D, C, H, B, A) 537
Lanthanum Carbonate (C) 609
Magnesium/Aluminum Oral (D, C, B, H, Sh, Sw) 645
Magnesium Intravenous (D, C, H, B, Sw) 647
Mannitol (D, C, B, Sw, Sh, H) 650
Pamidronate (D, C) 811
Phosphate (D, C) 854
Potassium (D, C, H, Ru) 872
Sevelamer HCl (D, C) 954
Sodium Polystyrene Sulfonate (D, H) 963

Antineoplastics

Antineoplastics, Alkylating Agents

Busulfan (D, C) 132
Carboplatin (D, C, Po) 158
Chlorambucil (D, C, H) 204
Cisplatin (D, H) 228
Cyclophosphamide (D, C, H, Po) 266
Dacarbazine (D) 276
Ifosfamide (D, C) 539
Lomustine (D, C) 634
Mechlorethamine (D, C) 660
Melphalan (D, C) 678
Procarbazine (D, C) 896
Thiotepa (D) 1020

Antineoplastics, Antimetabolites

Cytarabine (D, C, H) 274
Fluorouracil (5-FU) (D, C, H) 461
Mercaptopurine (D) 682
Methotrexate (D, C) 700
Thioguanine (D, C) 1017

Antineoplastics, Antibiotics

Bleomycin (D, C) 117
Dactinomycin (D) 278
Doxorubicin (D, C, Fer) 362
Epirubicin (D) 388
Streptozocin (D) 979

Antineoplastics, Mitotic Inhibitors

Vinblastine (D, C) 1085
Vincristine (D, C, H) 1087

Antineoplastics, Miscellaneous

Asparaginase (D, C) 81
Gemcitabine (D, C) 482
Hydroxyurea (D, C) 533
Masitinib (D) 656
Mitoxantrone (D, C) 739
Paclitaxel (D) 809
Piroxicam (D, C, H, Po) 865
Toceranib (D) 1042

Immunomodulators

Immunosuppressive Drugs

Azathioprine (D, C, Fer, H) 99
Cyclophosphamide (D, C, H, Po) 266
Cyclosporine (D, C) 269
Dexamethasone (D, C, Po, B, H) 301
Flumethasone (D, C, H) 455
Hydroxychloroquine (D) 529
Immune Globulin (Human), Intravenous (D) 550
Leflunomide (D, C) 610
Mercaptopurine (D) 682
Methotrexate (D, C) 700
Methylprednisolone (D, C, H) 705
Mycophenolate (D, C) 752
Oclacitinib (D) 782
Prednisolone (D, C, Po, B, H, L, A, R) 883
Prednisone (D, C, Po, B, H, L, A, R) 883
Triamcinolone (D, C, B, H)

Gold Compounds
Auranofin (D, C) 96

Immunostimulants
Mycobacterial Cell Wall Fraction Immuno-
modulator (D, H) 751
Parapox Ovis Virus Immunomodulator (H)
816
Propionibacterium acnes Inj. (D, C, H) 903
Staphylococcal Phage Lysate (D) 978

Antidotes
Acetylcysteine (D, C, H) 11
Ammonium Molybdate (Sh) 56
Ammonium Tetrathiomolybdate (Sh) 56
Antivenin Black Widow Spider (D, C) 76
Antivenin Coral Snake (D, C, H) 75
Antivenin Crotalidae (D, C, H) 73
Atipamezole (D, C, Po, H, B, L, A, R, Z) 86
Charcoal, Activated (D, C, H, B, Ru) 202
Deferoxamine (D, C, H) 289
Dexrazoxane (D) 309
Dimercaprol (D, C, H, B) 334
Edetate Calcium Disodium (D, C, Po, H, A,
Ru, Sw) 370
Ethanol (D, C, H) 409
Fat Emulsion, Intravenous 420
Fomepizole (D, C) 471
Leucovorin Calcium (D, C, H) 612
Methylene Blue (D, C, Ru, H) 702
Naloxone (D, C, Po, H) 757
Penicillamine (D, C, Ru, A) 822

Physostigmine (D, H, B) 855
Phytonadione (SA, B, Sh, H, A) 857
Pralidoxime (D, C, Ru, H, A) 877
Protamine Sulfate (D, C, B) 910
Pyridoxine (D, C) 918
SAMe (D, C) 945
Silymarin (D, C) 959
Sodium Polystyrene Sulfonate (D, H) 963
Sodium Sulfate (B, Sh, Sw) 947
Sodium Thiosulfate (D, C, H, Ru) 965
Succimer (D, C, H, A) 981
Thiamine (D, C, B, H, Sw, Sh, L) 1015
Trientine HCl (D) 1062
Zinc (systemic) (D, C) 1108

Bone/Joint Agents
Alendronate Sodium (D, C) 25
Allopurinol (D, A, R) 31
Clodronate (H) 240
Glucosamine ± Chondroitin (D, C) 495
Hyaluronate (D, H) 515
Etidronate (D, C) 411
Pentosan (D, C, H) 835
Polysulfated Glycosaminoglycan (H, D, C,
Po) 868
Tiludronate Disodium (H) 1034

Dermatologic Agents (Systemic)
Acitretin (D, C) 13
Fatty Acids, Essential (D, C) 422
Isotretinoin (D, C) 580
Pentoxifylline (D, C, H) 836

Vitamins & Minerals/Nutrients
Ascorbic Acid (D,C, Po, H, B) 79
Carnitine (D, C) 159
Cyanocobalamin (D, C, H, Sw, B, Sh) 265
Fat Emulsion, Intravenous 420
Fatty Acids, Essential (D, C) 422
Folic Acid (D, C, H) 6
Medium Chain Triglycerides (D) 665
Niacinamide (D) 768
Pyridoxine (D, C) 918
Thiamine (D, C, B, H, Sw, Sh, L) 1015
Vitamin A (D, R) 1090
Vitamin E ± Selenium (D, C, H) 1092
Zinc (systemic) (D, C) 1108

Cholinergic Muscle Stimulants
Edrophonium Chloride (D, C, H) 371
Pyridostigmine (D, C) 916

Systemic Acidifiers
Acetazolamide (D, C, H) 7
Acetic Acid (B, H) 9

Systemic Alkalinizers
Sodium Bicarbonate (D, C, H, Ru, A) 960

Unclassified
Aminocaproic Acid (D, H) 43
Colchicine (D, A) 258
Iodixanol 563
Iohexol (D, C, A) 564

Index

Note: Trade names are not italicized or indicated by ® or ™.

(s)-Methoprene Combinations, Topical, 1225
1-beta-D-Arabinofuranosylcytosine, 276
2,2,2-tetramine, 1063
2,2,-dichlorovinyl dimethyl phosphate, 319
2-Bromergocriptine, 123
2-MPG, 1038, 1039
2-PAM, 877, 878
2-propylpentanoic acid, 1076
2-propylvaleric acid, 1076
3'-azido-2',3'-dideoxythymidine, 1108
4-epidoxorubicin, 390
4-Methylpyrazole, 471
4-MP, 471
5-fluorocytosine, 453
5-fluorouracil, 1142
5-FU, 461, 1142
5-HTP, 1241
5-Hydroxytryptophan, 1241
6-thioguanine, 1018
6-alpha-methylprednisolone, 708
6-aminohexanoic acid, 44
6-mercaptopurine, 683
6-TG, 1018
6% Hetastarch, 532
9-alpha fluorohydrocortisone acetate, 454

A180, 282
A-ase, 82
ABCD, 65
Abelcet, 62, 65, 66
ABL, 65
ABLC, 65
Abraxane, 810
Acarbose, 1
Acarexx, 1236
Accolate, 1106, 1107
AccuNeb, 24
Accutane, 580, 581
Aceproject, 5
Acepromazine Maleate, 2
Acetadote, 13
Acetaminophen, 6, 1241
Acetazolamide, 7
Acetic Acid, 9
Acetic acid oxime, 11
Acetic Acid/Boric Acid, 1200
Acetohydroxamic Acid, 10, 11
Acetoxymethylprogesterone, 667
Acetylcysteine, 11
Acetylcysteine Ophthalmic, 1116
Acetylpromazine, 5
Acetylsalicylic Acid, 83, 85
Acitretin, 13, 14
ACP, 5
ACTH, 260, 261
ACTH gel, 261
ACTHAR, 260
Acticin, 1228
Actidose with Sorbitol, 203, 968
Actidose-Aqua, 203, 968

Actigall, 1073, 1074
Actinomycin D, 278, 279
Activase, 1175
Activated carbon, 203
Activated charcoal, 203
Active Carbon, 203
Activyl TickPlus, 1225, 1227
Activyl Spot-On, 1225
Acular, 1149
ACV, 15
Acycloguanosine, 15
Acyclovir, 14
Acyclovir Ophthalmic, 1116
Adams Pyrethrin Dip, 1229
Adams Spot On, 1226
Adams Flea & Tick Mist, 1228, 1229
Adaptil, 853
Adcirca, 998
Ademetionine, 945, 947
Adequan, 868, 1164
Adequan I.A., 869
Adequan I.M., 869
Adrenaclick, 387
Adrenalin, 385, 387
Adrenocorticotropic Hormone, 261
Adriamycin, 362
Adriamycin PFS, 365
Adriamycin RDF, 364, 365
Adrucil, 461, 462
Adsorbent charcoal, 203
Adspec, 970, 971
Advantage Multi, 749, 750, 1224
Advantage, 1223, 1224
Advantage II, 1223, 1224, 1229
Advil, 1242
Advocate, 751, 1223
Advocin, 282
AeroHippus, 24, 467
Aeropulmin, 237
Afrin, 1242
Aglepristone, 17
AHA, 10, 11
A-HydroCort, 525
Alavert, 639
Alaway, 1150
Albadry Plus, 780
Albaplex, 779, 780
Albaplex, 779
Albendazole, 19
Albenza, 19, 20
Albon, 992, 993
Albumin, Canine, 20
Albumin, Human, 20
Albuterol Sulfate, 23
Alcaftadine Ophthalmic, 1117
Alcaine, 1166
Alcohol, Ethyl, 409
Aldactazide, 520, 976
Aldactone, 974, 976
Aldara, 1216
Alendronate Sodium, 25
Alevazol, 1207
Aleve, 762, 1242
Alfast, 31
Alfaxalone, 26
Alfaxan, 29

Alfenta, 30, 31
Alfentanil HCl, 30
Alfentanyl, 31
Alinia, 770
Alizin, 17
Alizine, 17
Alka-Seltzer, 85
Alkeran, 678, 679
Allegra, 440, 441, 442
Aller 911 Ear Wash, 1231
Allercaine, 1187
Allermyl Shampoo, 1186
Allopurinol, 31
Alloxanthine, 33
Alocril, 1158
Aloe & Oatmeal, 1185
Aloeclens, 1231
Aloprim, 31
Alpha Lipoic Acid, 1242
Alpha Tocopherol, 1093
Alphagan P, 1127
Alpha-Tocopherol, 1092
Alprazolam, 33
Alrex, 1153
Altacaine, 1174
Altace, 927
Altafluor, 1124, 1143
Altafrin, 1162
Alteplase, 1176
Alteplase Ophthalmic, 1175
Altinac, 1218
Altrenogest, 35, 36
Aluminium Hydroxide, 37
Aluminum Hydroxide, 37
Aluminum Sucrose Sulfate, Basic, 985
Amantadine HCl, 38
A-Mantle, 1184
Amaryl, 488, 489
Ambien, 455
Ambisome, 65, 66
A-Methapred, 709
Amethopterin, 700
Amicar, 43, 44
Amidate, 414, 415
Amidine HCl, 690
Amiglyde-V, 40
Amikacin Sulfate, 40
Amikacin Sulfate Ophthalmic, 1117
Amikin, 40
Aminobenzylpenicillin, 69
Aminocaproic Acid, 43
Aminocaproic Acid Ophthalmic, 1118
Aminopentamide Hydrogen Sulfate, 45
Aminophylline, 46
Aminosidine, 819
Aminoxin, 919
Amiodarone HCl, 48
Amitraz, 1218
Amitriptyline HCl, 50
Amlodipine Besylate, 52
Ammonil Tablets, 696
Ammonium Chloride, 54
Ammonium Molybdate, 56
Ammonium Tetrathiomolybdate, 56
Amnesteem, 582
Amoxicillin, 56

Amoxicillin/Clavulanate Potassium, 59
Amoxi-Drop, 59
Amoxil, 56, 59
Amoxi-Tabs, 56
Amoxycillin, 59, 62
Amphogel, 37
Amphotec, 65, 66
Amphotericin B Cholesteryl Sulfate Complex, 65
Amphotericin B Colloidal Dispersion, 65
Amphotericin B lipid complex, 65
Amphotericin B liposomal, 65
Amphotericin B Ophthalmic, 1118
Ampicillin, 67
Ampicillin Sodium, 69
Ampicillin sodium/Sulbactam sodium, 69
Amprolium Hydrochloride, 71
AmproMed, 71, 72
Amtech Prostamate, 341
Am-Vet Renakare, 874
Anafen, 603
Anafranil, 243, 245
AnaSed, 1099, 1103
Anaspaz, 537
Ancef, 170
Ancobon, 451, 453
Android, 709
Anectine, 983
Anihist, 920
Animax Ointment, 1195, 1211, 1236
Anipryl, 951, 952
Anipsyll Powder, 914
Antagonil, 1104
Anthelcide EQ, 797, 798
Antidiuretic Hormone, 297, 1079
Antihistamine Granules, 920
Antilirium, 855
Antirobe, 237, 240
Antisedan, 89
Antivenin (Crotalidae) Polyvalent, 74
Antivenin (Latrodectus Mactans) Black Widow Spider, 76, 77
Antivenin (Micrurus Fulvias) Coral Snake, 75, 76
Antivert, 662, 663
Antizol, 472
Antizol-Vet, 471
Antizol-Vet, 472
Anxitane, 607
Anzemet, 352, 353
APAP, 6
Apokyn, 77, 78
Apomorphine HCl, 77
Apoquel, 782, 783
Apraclonidine Ophthalmic, 1119
Apralan, 78, 79
Apramycin Sulfate, 78
Apresoline, 516, 518
Aquasol E, 1094
Aquasol-A, 1091
Aquavit-E, 1094
AQuify Comfort Drops, 1121
Arabinosylcytosine, 276
ara-C, 276
Aranesp, 287, 288
Arava, 610, 612

Aredia, 811
Arestin, 732
Arginine Vasopressin, 1081
ASA, 83, 85
Ascorbic Acid, 79
ASN-ase, 82
Asparaginase, 81
Aspirin, 83, 1242
Astramorph PF, 747
Atacand, 151, 152
Atarax, 534
Atenolol, 86
Atgard, 318, 319
Atipamezole HCl, 88
Ativan, 639, 641
Atopica, 272
Atovaquone, 90
Atracurium Besilate, 93
Atracurium Besylate, 91
Atralin, 1218
Atridox, 369
Atropine Sulfate, 93
Atropine Sulfate Ophthalmic, 1121
Atrovent, 567
Atrovent HFA, 568
Augmentin, 59, 62
AUPEN5000, 836
Auranofin, 96
Aureomycin, 218, 219
Aurocin, 1231
Auvi-Q, 387
Avalide, 570
Avapro, 568, 570
Aveed, 1010
Avinza, 747
Avita, 1218
Axid, 776, 777
Azactam, 104, 105
Azaperone, 97
Azasan, 101
Azasite, 1123
Azathioprine, 99, 101
Azelastine Ophthalmic, 1122
Azidodeoxythymidine, 1108
Azidothymidine, 1108
Azithromycin, 102
Azithromycin Ophthalmic, 1123
Azium, 301, 305
Azopt, 1128
AZT, 1107
Aztreonam, 104
Azulfidine, 995, 996

Bacitracin, Topical, 1195
Baclofen, 106, 454
Bactocill, 794
Bactrim, 991
Bactroban, 1199
BAL in Oil, 334, 335
Banamine, 458, 460
Banophen, 343
Bansect Squeeze-On Flea & Tick Control for Dogs, 1227
Banzel, 944, 945
Barricade, 1222
Barrier II Wound Care, 1187

Barrier Wound Care, 1187
Baycox, 1047, 1049
Baytril, 379, 382, 383
Baytril 100, 383
Baytril Otic, 1234
Benadryl, 342, 343, 1186
Benasoothe, 1186, 1188
Benazepril HCl, 107
Benemid, 892
Benoxinate Ophthalmic, 1124
Benuryl, 892
Benzac, 1196
Benzonatate, 109
Benzoyl Peroxide, 1196
Benzoyl Peroxide Shampoo, 1196
Benzyl alcohol, 1243
Bepotastine Ophthalmic, 1125
Bepreve, 1125
Berenil, 337
Besifloxacin Ophthalmic, 1125
Besivance, 1125
Betadine, 1165, 1205
Betagan, 1151
Betagen Topical Spray, 1190, 1198
Beta-Gen Otic Solution, 1235
Betamethasone, 110, 112
Betamethasone Ophthalmic, 1126
Betamethasone, Topical, 1190, 1191
Betapace, 969, 970
Betasone, 112
Betaxolol Ophthalmic, 1126
Bethanechol Chloride, 112
Bethkis, 1042
Betimol, 1175
Betoptic, 1126
Beuthanasia -D Special, 416
Biaxin, 232, 234
Bicillin L-A, 828
Biltricide, 881
Bimatoprost Ophthalmic, 1127
Bio Spot On, 1226, 1227
Bio Spot Shampoo, 1228, 1229
Biocyl, 805
Biodry, 780
Biomycin, 805
Bion Tears, 1121
Biosol, 764
Bio-Spot Flea & Tick Spray, 1228
Bio-Statin, 781
Bisacodyl, 114
Bismuth Subsalicylate, 115, 117
Blenoxane, 117, 118
Bleomycin Sulfate, 117
Bleph-10, 1171
Blephamide, 1166, 1171
Blink, 1121
Boldenone Undecenoate, 119
Boldenone Undecylenate, 118, 119
Bonine, 662, 663
Borgal, 991
Bo-Se, 1093
Bravecto, 464, 465
Brethine, 1006, 1008
Brevibloc, 400, 402
Brevital, 698, 699
Brimonidine Ophthalmic, 1127

Brinzolamide Ophthalmic, 1128
British Anti-Lewisite, 335
Brodifacoum, 1243
Bromadiolone, 1243
Bromday, 1129
Brom-ergocryptine, 123
Bromethalin, 1243
Bromfenac Ophthalmic, 1129
Bromides, 120
Bromocriptine Mesylate, 122
Bromocryptine, 123
BSS, 115, 1148
BSS Plus, 1148
Budesonide, 124
Bumetanide, 125
Bumex, 125
Buprenex, 127, 130
Buprenorphine Hcl, 127
Burinex, 125
Bur-O-Cort 2:1, 1184, 1192
Burow's Solution, 1184
Buscapina, 756
Buscoban, 754
Buscopan, 754, 755
Buscopan Compositum, 755
BuSpar, 1031, 1032
Buspirone HCl, 131
Busulfan, 132
Busulfex, 132, 133
Butaphosphan w/Cyanocobalamin, 134
Butazolidin, 845
Bute, 845
Butorphanol Tartrate, 135
Butorphic, 139
Butylscopolamine Bromide, 755

Cabergoline, 140
Caduet, 53
CaEDTA, 371
Caffeine, 1242
Calamine lotion, 1189
Calan, 1083, 1085
Calcidol, 396
Calciferol, 394, 396
Calcijex, 143
Calcimar, 141
Calcitonin Salmon, 141
Calcitriol, 143
Calcium Carbonate, 146
Calcium Chloride, 1244
Calcium Chloride Injection, 150
Calcium Disodium Versenate, 370, 371
Calcium EDTA, 370
Calcium Folinate, 612
Calcium Gluconate Injection, 150
Calcium Salts, Parenteral, 147
Cal-Dextro, 150
Cal-Dextro Special, 650, 855
Cal-Phos #2, 650
Camphor, 1189
Camphorated Tincture of Opium, 817, 818
Cancidas, 165, 166
Candesartan Cilexetil, 151
Caninsulin, 557
Capoten, 152, 153
Caprogel, 1118

Capstar, 644, 770, 771
Captan, 1214
Carafate, 983, 985
Carbamazepine, 154
Carbazole, 156, 157
Carbimazole, 156
Carboplatin, 158
Cardalis, 976
Cardizem, 330, 332
Carimune NF, 551
Carisoprodol, 454
Carmilax, 647
Carnitine, 159
Carnitor, 159, 160
Carprofen, 161
Carteolol Ophthalmic, 1129
Cartia XT, 332
Cartrophen-Vet, 835, 836
Carvedilol, 163
Caspofungin Acetate, 165
Cataflam, 322
Catapres, 247, 249
Catapres-TTS, 249
Cathflo Activase, 1176
Catosal, 134
Cayston, 106
CCNU, 634
CDDP, 230
Ceclor, 167
Cecon, 81
CeeNu, 634, 635
Cefaceptin, 199
Cefaclor, 167
Cefa-Dri, 199, 200
Cefadroxil, 168
Cefa-Lak, 199, 200
Cefazolin Sodium, 170, 171
Cefepime HCl, 172
Cefixime, 173
Cefotan, 176
Cefotaxime Sodium, 174, 176
Cefotetan Disodium, 176
Cefovecin Sodium, 178
Cefoxitin Sodium, 180, 181
Cefpodoxime Proxetil, 182
Ceftazidime, 183
Ceftiflex, 193
Ceftin, 195
Ceftiofur Crystalline Free Acid, 185
Ceftiofur HCl, 188
Ceftiofur Sodium, 190
Ceftriaxone Sodium, 193
Cefuroxime, 195
Celestone, 110
Celestone Soluspan, 112
CellCept, 752, 754
Centany, 1199
Centrine, 45
Cephalexin, 196
Cephapirin, 199
Cephorum, 199
Cephulac, 608, 609
Ceporex, 199
Ceptaz, 183
Cerebyx, 852
Cerenia, 654, 656

Certifect, 1220, 1222, 1226
Ceruclean, 1232
Cerumene, 1231
Cerumotic, 1231
Cervizine, 1103
Cestex, 394
Cetirizine HCl, 200
Chanazine, 1103
CharcoAid, 203, 968
CharcoAid 2000, 203, 968
Charcoal, Activated, 202
Chemet, 981, 982
Cheque Drops, 721, 722
Cheristin, 1230
Chloradine, 1201
Chlorambucil, 204
Chloramphenicol, 206
Chloramphenicol Ophthalmic, 1130
Chloramphenicol Sodium Succinate, 206
Chlorasan, 1201
Chlordiazepoxide, 209
Chlorhex, 1201
Chlorhex 2X 4% Spray, 1201
Chlorhexiderm, 1201
ChlorhexiDerm Spray, 1201
Chlorhexidine, 1201, 1202
Chloromycetin, 206, 1130
Chlorothiazide, 211
Chlorphacinone, 1243
Chlorpheniramine Maleate, 213
Chlorpromazine Hcl, 215
Chlorpropamide, 217
Chlortetracycline, 218
Chlor-Trimeton, 214
Chlorxylenol, 1202
Chocolate, 1243
Cholecalciferol, 1242
Chondroitin Sulfate, 496
Chondroprotec, 868, 869
Chorionic Gonadotropin, 220, 221
Chorulon, 220, 221
Chromium, 221
Chromium Picolinate, 221
Cialis, 997, 998
Ciclosporin, 269
Cidofovir Ophthalmic, 1130
Cimetidine, 222
Cipro, 224, 226 1131
Cipro HC Otic, 1235
Ciprodex, 1235
Ciprofloxacin, 224
Ciprofloxacin Ophthalmic, 1131
Cisapride, 226
cis-DDP, 230
cis-diamminedichloroplatinum, 230
Cisplatin, 228, 230
cis-Platinum II, 230
Citrolith, 232
Claforan, 174, 176
Claravis, 582
Clarithromycin, 232
Claritin, 639
Clavamox, 59, 62
Clavulanate Potassium, 62, 1027
Clavulanic Acid, 62, 1027

Clean Ear with Aloe Vera, 1232
Clear Eyes, 1148
Clemastine Fumarate, 234, 235
Clenbuterol HCl, 236
Cleocin, 237, 240
Cleocin T, 1197
Clidinium Bromide, 209
Clinafarm EC, 1208
Clindacin-ETZ, 1197
Clindacin-P, 1197
Clindagel, 1197
Clindamax, 1197
Clindamycin, 237, 240
Clindamycin, Topical, 1196
Clinicox, 319, 320
Clinsol, 240
Clintabs, 240
Clodronate, 240
Clodronic Acid, 240
Clofazimine, 242
Clomicalm, 243, 245
Clomipramine HCl, 243
Clonazepam, 246
Clonazepam, 247
Clonidine, 247
Clopidogrel Bisulfate, 249
Cloprostenol Sodium, 251, 252
Clorazepate Dipotassium, 253
Clorsulon, 254, 590
ClotrimaTop, 1207
Clotrimazole, 1190, 1191, 1194, 1198, 1206,
    1207, 1235
Clotrimazole & Betamethasone, 1207
Clotrimazole, Gentamicin & Betamethasone
    Ointment, 1235
Cloxacillin, 255
CMPK, 650, 855
Coal Tar, 1215
Colace, 351
Colchicine, 258
Colcrys, 259
Colloidal Oatmeal, 1185
Collyrium for Fresh Eyes Wash, 1148
Coloaspase, 82
Coly-Mycin S Otic, 1235
CoLyte, 868
Combigan, 1127, 1175
Combivent, 24
ComboCare, 750, 881
Comforion Vet, 604
Comfortis, 972, 973
Compazine, 898, 899
Composure, 607, 608
Compound F, 524
Compro, 898
Concerta, 705
Conofite, 1210
Conquer, 516
Conquer Hy-Optic, 1148
Conquer Hy-Otic, 1232
Constulose, 609
Contralac, 685
Convenia, 179
ConZip, 1055
Cooper's Best Ear Mite Lotion, 1236
Co-phenotrope, 345

Cordarone, 48
Coreg, 163, 165
Coreg CR, 165
Corid, 71, 72
Corium-20, 1231
Corlopam, 428, 429, 430
Cort/Astrin Solution, 1184, 1192, 1234
Cortalone Cream, 1211
Cortef, 522, 525
Corticotropin, 260, 261
Corti-Derm Solution, 1184, 1192
Cortisol, 524
Cortisone Acetate, 261
Cortisoothe Shampoo, 1192
Cortisporin-TC Otic, 1235
Cortrosyn, 263, 264
Cosequin, 495, 497
Cosmegen, 278, 279
Cosopt, 1137, 1175
Cosyntropin, 263
Co-trimazine, 991
Co-trimoxazole, 988, 991
Coumadin, 1097, 1099
Cozaar, 641, 642
CPM, 269
CroFab, 73, 74
Crolom, 1132
Cromolyn Sodium, 264
Cromolyn Sodium Ophthalmic, 1132
Crotamiton, 1220
Crystamine, 266
Crysti, 266
CTX, 269
Cuprimine, 822, 823
Curatrem, 254, 255
Cyanocobalamin, 265
Cyanoject, 266
Cyclogyl, 1132
Cyclomydril, 1132, 1133, 1162
Cyclopentolate Ophthalmic, 1132
Cyclophosphamide, 266, 269
Cyclosporine, 269
Cyclosporine A, 269
Cyclosporine Ophthalmic, 1133
Cydectin, 747, 750
Cyproheptadine HCl, 273
Cystolamine, 850
Cystorelin, 504
Cystospaz, 537
CYT, 269
Cytarabine, 274, 276
Cytomel, 628, 630
Cytosar-U, 274
Cytosine Arabinoside, 274
Cytotec, 734, 736
Cytoxan, 266, 269

D.A.P., 852, 853
Dextrose & Sodium Chloride IV Fluids, 1246
Dacarbazine, 276
Dactinomycin, 278
Dalteparin Sodium, 279
Danazol, 281
Dandrex, 1212
Danocrine, 281
Danofloxacin Mesylate, 282

Dantrium, 283, 285
Dantrium Intravenous, 285
Dantrolene Sodium, 283
DAP, 853
Dapsone, 285
Daranide, 317
Daraprim, 920, 922
Darbazine, 898
Darbepoetin Alfa, 287
Dari-Clox, 256
Dayhist-1, 235
Dazamide, 7
d-Con, 1243
DDAVP, 295, 297
DDP, 230
DDS, 285
Decadron, 305
Deca-Durabolin, 761
Deccox, 288, 289
Decolorizing Carbon, 203
Decoquinate, 288
Dectomax, 357, 358
DEET, 1243
Deferoxamine, 289, 439
Delestrogen, 405
Delsym, 1242
Delta Albaplex, 780
Deltahydrocortisone, 886
Deltamethrin, 1220
Demadex, 1051, 1052
Demecarium Bromide Ophthalmic, 1134
Demerol, 680, 682
Denagard, 1024, 1025
Denamarin, 947, 960
Dendrid, 1147
Denosyl, 947
Depacon, 1075, 1076
Depakene, 1075, 1076
Depakote, 1075, 1076
Depen, 822, 823
DepoCyt, 276
DepoDur, 747
Depo-Estradiol Cypionate, 405
Depo-Medrol, 705, 708
Depo-Provera, 667
Depo-Testosterone, 1010
Deracoxib, 291
Deramaxx, 291, 292
Derma Vet, 1236
Dermabenss Shampoo, 1196, 1213, 1214
Dermachlor, 1201, 1209
Dermachlor Flush Plus, 1202
Derma-Clens, 1213
Dermacool HC Spray, 1191
Dermacool w/ Lidocaine Spray, 1187
Dermallay Oatmeal, 1185
Dermalog, 1195, 1211, 1236
Dermalone, 1195, 1211, 1236
DermaLyte Shampoo, 1185
Derma-Pax, 1186
Dermapet Eicosderm, 424
Dermapet OFA plus EZ-C Caps, 424
Dermarest, 1186
Dermathycin, 1022
Dermatonin, 674
Derma-Vet Ointment, 1195, 1211

Dermazole Shampoo, 1213
DermOtic, 1234
Desenex, 1207
Desferal, 289, 290
Desferoxamine Mesylate, 290
Desflurane, 293
Deslorelin Acetate, 294
Desmopressin Acetate, 295
Desoxycorticosterone Pivalate, 297
Desquam-X, 1196
Desyrel, 1055
Detomidine HCl, 299
Detomidine HCl for Injection, 301
Dexamethasone, 301
Dexamethasone Ophthalmic, 1135
Dexamethasone Sodium Phosphate, 301
Dexasone, 301
Dexdomitor, 306
DexFerrum, 571
Dexmedetomidine, 306
Dexpanthenol, 308
Dexpanthenol Injection, 309
Dexrazoxane, 309
Dextran 70, 311
Dextromethorphan, 1242
Dextrose 10%-70%, 1246
DFO, 290
DHS Tar, 1215
DHT, 328, 329
Diabenese, 217, 218
DiaBeta, 499
Diamox, 7
Diastat, 312, 315
Diazepam, 312
Diazoxide, Oral, 316
Dibenzyline, 843, 845
Di-Biotic, 991
Dichlorphenamide, 317
Dichlorvos, 318
Dichysterol, 329
Diclazuril, 319
Diclofenac Ophthalmic, 1136
Diclofenac Sodium, 321
Dicloxacillin, 322
Didronel, 411
Diethylstilbestrol, 323, 324
Difethialone, 1243
Diflucan, 449, 451
Difluprednate Ophthalmic, 1136
Digitalis glycosides, 325
Digoxin, 325
Dihydrotachysterol, 328, 329
Dilacor, 330, 332
Dilantin, 850, 852
Dilatrate-SR, 580
Dilaudid, 526, 528
Dilt-CD, 332
Diltia, 332
Diltiazem HCl, 330
Dimenhydrinate, 332, 333
Dimercaprol, 334
Dimercaptopropanol, 335
Dimercaptosuccinic acid, 981
Di-Methox, 993
Dimethyl Sulfoxide, 335
Dimethyl-nortestosterone., 722

Diminazene Aceturate, 337
Dinoprost Tromethamine, 339, 341
Dinotofuran, 1220
Dio, 797
Dioctyl Sodium Succinate, 351, 352
Dioctynate, 352
Dipentum, 784, 785
Diphacinone, 1243
Diphenhist, 343
Diphenhydramine, 342, 343
Diphenhydramine HCl, Topical, 1186
Diphenoxylate HCl, 345
Diphenoxylate HCl/Atropine Sulfate, 344
Diphenylhydantoin, 852
Diprivan, 904, 907, 908
Diprolene, 1190
Dipropylacetic acid, 1076
Diprosone, 1190
Dirlotapide, 345
Disal, 478
Disodium Cromoglycate, 264
Disopyramide Phosphate, 347
Ditropan, 798, 799
Diuril, 211, 212
Divalproex Sodium, 1075
dl-Hyoscyamine, 95
dl-Methionine, 695
DMSA, 981
DMSO, 335
Dobutamine HCl, 349
Dobutrex, 349
DOCP, 297, 298
Docusate, 351, 352
Docu-Soft, 352
Dog Appeasing Pheromone, 853
Dolasetron Mesylate, 352
Dolophine, 688, 690
Dolorex, 139
Domitor, 663, 664
Domoso, 335, 337
Domperidone, 353
Dopamine HCl, 355
Dopram, 361
Dopram-V, 359, 360
Doramectin, 357
Dorbene, 664
Dormilan, 664
Dormosedan, 299, 301
Doryx, 369
Dorzolamide Ophthalmic, 1137
DOSS, 351
Dostinex, 140
DOUXO Calm, 1187
DOUXO Chlorhexidine PS, 1188, 1202
DOUXO Chlorhexidine PS Micro-emulsion, 1201
Douxo Micellar Solution, 1231
DOUXO Seborrhea MicroEmulsion Spray, 1188
DOUXO Seborrhea, 1188
Doxapram HCl, 359
Doxepin HCl, 361
Doxil, 362, 365
Doxirobe, 365, 369
Doxorubicin HCl, 362, 365
Doxy, 369

DPA, 1076
D-Panthenol, 308
D-Penicillamine, 823
DPH, 852
Dramamine, 332, 333
Draxxin, 1069, 1071
Dried ferrous sulfate, 440
Drisdol, 394, 396
Droncit, 879, 881
Drontal, 881, 916
Drontal Plus, 881, 916
Droxia, 533, 534
Dry Eye Test, 1143
Dry-Clox, 256
DSS, 351, 352
DTIC, 276
DTIC-Dome, 277
Dulcolax, 114, 115
Duoneb, 24, 568
Duraclon, 247, 249
Duragesic, 432
Duragesic-, 435
Durezol, 1136
D-Worm, 914
Dyazide, 1062
Dynapen, 322
Dyna-Taurine, 1001
Dyrenium, 1061, 1062

E.E.S., 400
EAP, 853
Ear Mite Killer, 1236
Ear Mite Lotion, 1236
EarMed Mite Lotion, 1236
EarMed Boracetic Flush, 1232
EarMed Cleansing Solution & Wash, 1232
EarMed Wipes, 1232
Earoxide Ear Cleanser, 1231
Ear-Rite Insecticidal Ear Wash, 1236
Ear-Rite Miticide for Cats & Kittens, 1236
Easotic Otic Suspension, 1235
Easyspot, 1222
Echothiophate Iodide Ophthalmic, 1138
ECP, 404, 405
Ecto-Soothe 3X, 1229
Edetate Calcium Disodium, 370, 371
Edetate Disodium Ophthalmic, 1138
Edrophonium Chloride, 371
ED-SPAZ, 537
EDTA, 1138
Effipro, 1222
EHDP, 412
Elavil, 50
Eldepryl, 951, 952
Elestat, 1140
Elevate W.S., 1093
Elidel, 1216, 1217
Eligard, 614
Elimite, 1228
Elixophyllin, 1015
Ellence, 388, 390
Elmer's ProBond, 1244
Elmiron, 835, 836
Elocon, 1194
Elspar, 81, 82
Emadine, 1139

Emedastine Ophthalmic, 1139
EMLA Cream, 1186
EMLA, 1187
Emodepside + Praziquantel, 373
Emsam, 952
Emulsivit E-300, 1093
Enacard, 374, 376, 377
Enalapril, 374
Enilconazole, 1207
Enisyl, 645
Enlon, 371, 373
Enlon-Plus, 373
Enoxaparin Sodium, 377
Enroflox, 383
Enrofloxacin, 379
EnteDerm, 1211
EnteDerm Ointment, 1195
Entocort EC, 124, 125
Enulose, 609
Enzymes, Topical, 1203
Epakitin, 147
Ephedrine Sulfate, 383, 385
Epiklean, 1231
EpiKlean Ear Cleanser, 1232
Epinastine Ophthalmic, 1140
Epinephrine, 385
Epi-Otic Advanced, 1232
Epi-Otic Ear Cleanser, 1232
Epirubicin HCl, 388, 390
Epizyme Powder, 813
EPO, 390
Epoetin, 390
Epoetin Alfa, Recombinant, 392
Epogen, 390, 392
Eprinomectin, 392
Epsilon Aminocaproic Acid, 43
Epsiprantel, 394
Epsom Salt, 949
Eqstim, 903, 904
Equa Aid Psyllium, 914
Equidin, 797
Equidone, 353, 355
Equimectrin, 590
Equimune, 751
Equimune I.V., 752
Equine Appeasing Pheromone, 853
Equine Enteric Colloid, 914
Equine Haler, 24
Equine Thyroid Supplement, 622
Equine-haler, 467
Equioxx, 444, 446
Equi-Phar, 116
Equi-Phar Equi-Hist 1200 Granules, 920
Equi-Phar, 914
Equiphed, 911, 919, 920
Equipoise, 118, 119
Equisul-SDT, 991
Equitac, 797
Equron, 515
Equ-Se5E, 1093
Equ-SeE, 1093
Eqvalan, 590
Eqvalan, 590
Eradimite, 1237
Ergamisol, 617
Ergocalciferol, 394

Ertapenem Sodium, 396
Ery-Tab, 400
Erythromycin, 397
Erythromycin Gluceptate, 397
Erythromycin Ophthalmic, 1140
Erythropoietin, 390
E-Se, 1094
Eserine, 855
Esmeron, 938, 939
Esmolol HCl, 400
Esomeprazole, 402
Essential Fatty Acids, Topical, 1185
Estrace, 405
Estradiol Cypionate, 404, 405
Estriol, 406
estroPLAN, 252
Estrumate, 251, 252
Ethambutol HCl, 407, 409
Ethanol, 409, 1243
Ethyl Alcohol, 409
Ethyl Lactate, 1204
Ethylene Glycol, 1243
Ethylenediamine Dihydroiodide, 563
Etiderm, 1204
Etiderm Shampoo, 1204
Etidronate Disodium, 411, 412
Etodolac, 412
EtoGesic, 412, 414
Etomidate, 414, 415
Euclens Otic Cleanser, 1232
Eudemine, 317
Eudolat, 682
Eurax, 1220
Euthanasia Agents w/Pentobarbital, 415
Euthanasia-6 GR, 416
Euthanasia-III Solution, 416
Euthasol, 416
Evoclin, 1197
Excede, 185, 187
Excenel, 188
Excenel RTU, 190
ExpertCare Ear Cleansing Rinse, 1232
Extraocular Irrigating Solutions, 1148
Eye Irrigating Solution, 1148
Eye Rinse, 1148
Eye Stream, 1148
Eye Wash, 1148
Eythrocin, 400

F.A. Caps, 424
F.A. Caps ES, 424
F3T, 1177
F3TdR, 1177
Factrel, 504
Factrel, 504
Famciclovir, 416
Famotidine, 418
Famvir, 416, 417
Fansidar, 923
Fat Emulsion, Intravenous, 420
Fatal-Plus, 416
Fatty Acids, Essential/Omega, 422
Felbamate, 424
Felbatol, 424, 425
Feldene, 865, 866
FeliFriend, 853

Felimazole, 695
Feline Facial Pheromone, 853
Feliway, 852, 853
Fenbendazole, 425
Fenoldopam, 428
Fentanyl, 432, 436
Fentanyl Citrate, 430, 432, 435
Feosol, 438, 440
Fer-In-Sol, 438, 440
FeroSul, 440
Ferretonin, 674
Ferrous Sulfate, 438
Fertagyl, 504
Fertalin, 504
Fexofenadine HCl, 440
FFP-F3 fraction, 853
Filgrastim, 442
Finadyne, 460
Finasteride, 443
Fiproguard, 1222
Fipronil, 1221
Fipronil ± (S)-Methoprene, Topical, 1221
Firocoxib, 444
First Shield, 1221
First Shield Trio, 1221
Fish Oil, 422
Flagyl, 715, 718
Flarex, 1141
Flavoxate HCl, 447
Flea Halt, 1227, 1228
Flebogamma, 551
Flomax, 998, 999
Flo-Pred, 887
Florfenicol, 447
Florinef, 453
Florvio, 449
Flovent, 465, 467
Flucaine, 1166
Fluconazole, 449
Flucort, 455
Flucytosine, 451
Fludrocortisone Acetate, 453, 454
Flumazenil, 454
Flumeglumine, 460
Flumethasone, 455
Flumethrin, 1224
Flu-Nix, 460
Flunixamine, 460
Flunixin Meglumine, 458
Fluocinolone Otic, 1234
Fluohydrisone Acetate, 454
Fluohydrocortisone Acetate, 454
Fluorescite, 1143
Fluor-I-Strips, 1143
Fluorometholone Ophthalmic, 1141
Fluorouracil, 461
Fluorouracil Ophthalmic, 1142
Fluoxetine, 462
Flurbiprofen Ophthalmic, 1143
Fluress, 1124, 1143
Fluticasone Propionate, 465
Fluvoxamine, 469
Fluvoxamine Maleate, 467
FML, 1141
FML Forte, 1141
FML S.O.P., 1141

Folacin, 469
Folate, 469
Folic Acid, 469
Folinic Acid, 612
Follicular Hormone Hydrate, 407
Folvite, 470
Fomepizole, 471
Forane, 575
Formula V Taurine Tablets, 1001
Fortaz, 183
Fortekor, 107
Fortical, 142
Fortress, 1222
Fosamax, 26
Fosfomycin Trometamol, 473
Fosfomycin Tromethamine, 472
Fosphenytoin Sodium, 852
Fosrenol, 609, 610
Fragmin, 279, 281
Fresh-Ear, 1232
Freshkote, 1121
Frontline Plus, 1222, 1226
Frontline Spray, 1222
Frontline Tritak, 1222, 1226
Frusemide, 477
Fuciderm, 1190
Ful-Glo, 1143
Fulvicin, 506
Fungazol Shampoo, 1206
FungiCure, 1207
Fungizone, 62
Furadantin, 772, 773
Furazolidone, 474
Furazone, 1199
Furosemide, 475
Furoxone, 474

Gabapentin, 478
Gabapentin oral liquid, 1243
Galastop, 141
Galastop, 140
Gallimycin, 397
Galzin, 1110
Gamithromycin, 481
Gammagard, 551
Gammaked, 551
Gammaplex, 551
Gamunex, 551
Ganciclovir Ophthalmic, 1144
Garacin, 488
Garamycin, 485
Garasol, 488
Gastrocrom, 265
Gastrogard, 786
Gatifloxacin Ophthalmic, 1144
GCSF, 442
Gelnique, 799
Gemcitabine HCl, 482
Gemfibrozil, 484
Gemzar, 482, 483
Generlac, 609
Genesis Spray, 1194
Gen-Gard, 488
Gengraf, 272
Gen-L-Clens, 1232
GenOne Otic Solution, 1235

GenOne Spray, 1190, 1198
Genoptic, 1145
Gentacalm, 1190, 1198
Gentak, 1145
Gentamicin & Betamethasone Otic Solution, 1235
Gentamicin Sulfate, 485
Gentamicin Sulfate Ophthalmic, 1145
Gentamicin Topical, 1190, 1197, 1198
Gentaotic, 1235
Gentaspray, 1190, 1198
Gentaved Topical Spray, 1190, 1198
Genteal, 1121
Gentizol, 1190, 1198, 1207, 1235
Gentleseb, 1213, 1214
Gentocin, 485
Gentocin Durafilm, 1126
Gentocin Topical Spray, 1190, 1198
Gentoved, 1235
Gentran, 312
Gen-Xene, 253
GG, 509
Glauber's Salt, 948
GlaucTabs, 691
Glimepiride, 488
Glipizide, 490
Glostrips, 1143, 1168
Glow jewelry, 1244
Glucagon, 491
Glucantim, 671
Glucantime, 671
Glucantime, 670
Glucocorticoid Agents, General Information, 493
GlucoGen, 491, 492, 493
Glucophage, 686, 688
Glucosamine, 496
Glucosamine/Chondroitin Sulfate, 495
Glucotrol XL, 491
Glucotrol, 490, 491
Glutamine, 497
Gly Chon, 497
Glyburide, 498
Glycerine, 499, 500
Glycerol, 499
Glyceryl Guaiacolate, 509
glycoBenz Shampoo, 1196
GlycoLax, 868
Glycopyrrolate, 500
glycoZoo Otic, 1232
Glydiazinamide, 491
Goat Care-2X, 743
GoLYTELY, 868
GONABreed, 504
Gonadorelin, 503, 504
Gorilla glue, 1244
Granisetron HCl, 505
Granulocyte Colony Stimulating Factor, 442
Grapes, 1243
Gravol, 332
GreenGlo, 1152
Griffonia seed extract, 1241
Griseofulvin, 506, 507
Gris-PEG, 507
Growth Hormone, 966
Guaifenesin, 507

Guailaxin, 507
Guaiphenesin, 509
Gulcantim, 670
Gynodiol, 405

H.P. Acthar Gel, 261
Half-Normal Saline, 1246
Happy Jack Mitex, 1237
Hartz Advanced Care Ear Mite Treatment, 1237
Hartz Advanced Care Hydrocortisone Spray w/Aloe, 1191
Hartz First Defense, 1222
Hartz UltraGuard One Spot, 1226
Hartz UltraGuard Plus, 1226
Hartz UltraGuard Pro, 1226
HBOC-301, 510
HCG, 220, 221
Heartgard, 586, 590
Heartgard for Cats, 590
Heartgard Plus Chewables, 590, 916
Hemerocallis spp., 1244
Hemoglobin Glutamer-200 (Bovine), 510
Heparin Sodium, 512-514
Herplex, 1147
Hespan, 532
Hexa-Caine, 1187
HexaChlor-K, 1200, 1208
Hexadene Flush, 1202
Hexadrol, 306
Hexasol, 805
Hextend, 532
Hiprex, 692, 693
Histagranules, 920
Histall, 919, 920
hIVIG, 550
HN2, 661
Homatropine MBr, 521
Horizant, 480
Horse Care Durvit B-1 Crumbles, 1016
Humalog, 557
Humatin, 819
Humorsol, 1134
Humulin, 557
Humulin 50/50, 558
Humulin 70/30, 558
Humulin N, 557
Hyalovet, 515
Hyaluronan, 515
Hyaluronate Sodium, 515
Hyaluronic Acid, 515
Hycodan, 521
Hycodan, 521
Hydralazine HCl, 516
Hydrallazine, 518
Hydrea, 533, 534
Hydro-B 1020, 1184, 1192
Hydrochlorothiazide, 518
Hydrocodone Bitartrate, 521
Hydrocortisone, 522
Hydrocortisone Topical, 1192
Hydrocortisone Ophthalmic, 1146
Hydrocortisone sodium succinate, 524
Hydrocortisone, Topical, 1191
HydroDIURIL, 518, 520
Hydrogen Peroxide 3% (oral), 525

Hydromet, 522
Hydromorphone, 526
Hydro-Plus, 1184
Hydroxychloroquine Sulfate, 529
Hydroxyurea, 533
Hydroxyzine, 534
Hydroxyzine Pamoate, 534
Hylartin V, 515
Hyliderm +PS Shampoo, 1186
HyLyt EFA Rinse, 1186
HyLyt Shampoo, 1185
Hyoscine Butylbromide, 754
Hyoscyamine Sulfate, 536
Hyperstat IV, 316
Hypochlorous Acid, 1204
HypoTears, 1121
Hysocine Butylbromide, 755
Hytakerol, 328
Hyvisc, 515

IB-Stat, 537
Ibuprofen, 1242
Ice melts, 1244
Idoxuridine Ophthalmic, 1147
IFE, 420
Ifex, 539, 541
Ifosfamide, 539
IGIV, 550
ILE, 420
Ilopan, 308
Imaverol, 1207, 1208
Imdur, 580
Imepitoin, 541
Imidacloprid, 1223
Imidocarb Dipropinate, 544
Imipenem-Cilastatin Sodium, 546
Imipramine, 548
Imipramine Pamoate, 548
Imiquimod, Topical, 1216
Imizol, 544, 546
Immiticide, 673
Immune Globulin (Human), Intravenous, 550
Immunoregulin, 903, 904
Imodium, 636
Imodium A-D, 637
Impavido, 728
Imrex Tar and Sulphur Shampoo, 1215
Imuran, 99
Incurin, 406, 407
Inderal, 908
Inderal LA, 910
InFeD, 571
Infumorph, 747
INH, 575
Inovelon, 944, 945
Instamag, 647
In-Synch, 341
Intal, 264
Interceptor, 727
Interferon Alfa-2a, Human Recombinant, 558
Interferon-ω, 560
Intrafungol, 583
Intralipid, 422
Intraocular Irrigating Solution, 1148

Intravenous Lipid Emulsion, 420
Intron A, 560
Intron-A, 558
Intropin, 355
Invanz, 397
Iodide, Potassium, 561
Iodide, Sodium, 561
Iodixanol, 563
Iodoject, 561
Iohexol, 564
Ionsys, 435
Iopidine, 1119
Ipodate, 566
Ipratropium Bromide, 567, 568
Irbesartan, 568, 570
Iron, 1242
Iron Dextran, 570, 571
Irrigating Solutions, Ophthalmic, 1147
Ismo, 580
Isochron, 580
Isoflo, 573, 575
Isoflupredone Acetate, 571, 573
Isoflupredone Acetate, Topical, 1192
Isoflurane, 573
Isolyte S, 1246
Isoniazid, 577
Isoniazide, 575
Isonicotinic acid hydrazide, 575
Isoprenoline, 577
Isoproterenol HCl, 577, 579
Isoptin SR, 1085
Isopto Atropine, 1122
Isopto Carpine, 1163
Isordil, 579, 580
Isosorbide Dinitrate, 579, 580
Isosorbide Mononitrate, 579, 580
Iso-Thesia, 573, 575
Isotretinoin, 580
Isoxsuprine HCl, 582
Istin, 52
Isuprel, 577
Itch-X, 1189, 1192
Itraconazole, 583
Itraconazole Ophthalmic, 1148
Iverhart Max, 881, 916
Ivermectin, 586
IVIG, 550
Ivomec, 586, 590
Ivomec Plus, 254
Ivomec, 590
Ivomec Eprinex, 392, 393
Ivomec Plus, 255, 590

Jantoven, 1099

K9 Advantix, 1224
K9 Advantix II, 1224, 1227, 1230
Kadian, 747
Kaolin/Pectin, 591
Kao-Pec, 592
Kao-Pect, 592
Kaopectolin, 591
Kayexalate, 963, 964
K-Caps, 858
KC-Oto Pak, 1235
Keflex, 196, 199

Kefzol, 170
Kenalog, 1060, 1195
Keppra, 617, 619
Keraseb, 1213, 1214
Ketaflo, 592
Ketaject, 598
Ketalar, 598
Ketamine HCl, 592
Ketaset, 592, 598
Keta-sthetic, 598
Ketochlor, 1201, 1208
Ketoconazole, 599
Ketoconazole, Topical, 1208
Ketofen, 603, 605
KetoHex, 1208, 1209
Ketoprofen, 603
Ketorolac Ophthalmic, 1149
Ketorolac Tromethamine, 605
Ketoseb Flush +PS, 1202
Ketoseb-D, 1201, 1208, 1209
Ketotifen Ophthalmic, 1150
KetoTris Flush, 1234
KetoTris Flush + PS, 1234
Kinavet CA-1, 656, 658
Kionex, 964
K-Ject, 858
KlearOtic Ear Cleanser, 1231
Klonopin, 246, 247
Kondremul Plain, 730
Kristalose, 609
Kytril, 505

L- Asparaginase, 81
Lacri-lube S.O.P., 1121
Lactated, 1246
Lactoperoxidase, Lysozyme, Lactoferrin Topical, 1203
Lactulose, 608, 609
L-AMB, 65
Lamisil, 1004, 1005, 1006, 1212
Lamisil Advanced, 1212
Lamisil AT, 1212
Lamprene, 242, 243
Lanodine, 1205
Lanoxin, 325-328
Lanthanum Carbonate, 609
Lantharenol, 609
Lantus, 558
Lasix, 475-478
Lastacaft, 1117
Latanoprost Ophthalmic, 1150
Latisse, 1127
Laurabolin, 762
Laxade, 647
Laxatone, 728
L-Carnitine, 159
L-deprenyl, 951
Leflunomide, 610, 612
Legend, 515
Leucovorin Calcium, 612, 613
Leukeran, 204, 205
Leuprolide, 613
Leurocristine Sulfate, 1089
Levamisole, 615
Levamisole hydrochloride, 617
Levamisole phosphate, 617

Levarterenol, 777
Levasole, 615
Levbid, 537
Levemir, 558
Levetiracetam, 617, 619
Levobunolol Ophthalmic, 1151
Levocarnitine, 159
Levofloxacin Ophthalmic, 1151
Levophed, 777
Levotabs, 622
Levothyroxine Sodium, 619-622
Levoxine, 622
Levoxyl, 622
Levsin, 536, 537
Levsinex, 537
Levsin-SL, 537
Librax, 209, 211
Librium, 209
Lidocaine HCl, 623, 626
Lidocaine, Topical, 1186
Lidocaine/Prilocaine, 1186
Lidocaine/Prilocaine Cream, 1187
Lidoderm, 1187
Lilies, 1244
Lilium spp., 1244
Lime Sulfur, 1209
Lime Sulfur Dip, 1209
LimePlus Dip, 1209
Lincocin, 626, 628
Lincomix, 626, 628
Lincomycin, 626, 628
Linco-Spectin, 972
Lioresal, 106, 107
Liothyronine Sodium, 628
Liposyn, 422
Liquamycin, 805
Liquamycin LA-200, 805
Liqui-Char-Vet, 203
Liquid A Drops, 1091
Liquid paraffin, 729
Liquid petrolatum, 729
Liserdol, 685
Lisinopril, 630
Lithium ion disc batteries, 1244
Lithostat, 10, 11
L-Lysine, 644, 645
Lodine, 412
Loditac, 797
Lofene, 345
Lomotil, 344, 345
Lomustine, 634, 636
LongRange, 393
Lonox, 345
Loperamide HCl, 636
Lopid, 484, 485
Lopremone, 1024
Lopressor, 713, 715
Lorazepam, 639, 641
Lortabs, 522
Losartan Potassium, 641
Losec, 787
Lotemax, 1153
Lotensin HCT, 109
Lotensin, 107, 109
Loteprednol Ophthalmic, 1153
Lotrel, 53, 109

Lotrimin, 1206, 1235
Lotrisone, 1191, 1207
Lovenox, 377, 378
L-PAM, 679
L-Phenylalanine Mustard, 679
LRS, 1246
LS 50, 972
L-Se, 1094
L-triiodothyronine, 630
Lufenuron, 643
Lumigan, 1127
Luminal, 843
Lupron, 613, 614
Lupron Depot, 614
Lutalyse, 339, 341
Luvox, 467
Lyrica, 887, 889
Lysine, 644
Lysine vasopressin, 1081
Lysodren, 737, 739

MA, 669
Maalox, 647
Macadamia Nuts, 1243
Macrobid, 771, 772, 773
Macrodantin, 771, 772, 773
Magnadex, 855
Magnalax, 647
Magnesium Chloride, 650
Magnesium Citrate, 947
Magnesium Hydroxide, 645, 647, 949
Magnesium Oxide, 947
Magnesium Sulfate, 650, 947, 949
Magnesium/Aluminum Antacids, 645
Malacetic, 1200
Malacetic HC Wipes, 1191, 1200
MalAcetic Otic, 1232, 1233
MalAcetic Otic AP, 1233
Malacetic, 1200
Malacetic Ultra Shampoo, 1191, 1192, 1200,
    1208, 1232, 1233, 1235
Mal-A-Ket, 1200,1202, 1208
Mal-A-Ket Plus TrizEDTA Flush, 1201, 1202,
    1208, 1233, 1234
Malanil, 91
Malarone, 91
Malaseb Shampoo, 1202, 1210
Malaseb Flush, 1202, 1210
MalOtic, 1190, 1198, 1207, 1235
Mannitol, 650
MAP, 667
Marbofloxacin, 652
Marin, 959, 960
Maropitant Citrate, 654
Marquis, 869, 870
Mar-Spas, 537
Martin's Flee, 1222
Martin's Prefurred One, 1222
Martin's Prefurred Plus, 1222
Masitinib Mesylate, 656
Masivet, 656, 658
Matrix, 36
Matulane, 896, 897
Mavacoxib, 658
MAX Ear Cleanser, 1232
Maxi/Guard Zn 4.5 Otic, 1232

Maxi/Guard ZN7, 1189
Maxidex, 1135
Maxipime, 172, 173
Maxivate, 1190
Maxzide, 1062
MCT Oil, 665
Mechlorethamine HCl, 660
Meclastine Fumarate, 235
Meclizine HCl, 662
Mecloprodin Fumarate, 235
Medalone Cream, 1194
Medamycin, 805
Medetomidine HCl, 663
Medicated Shampoo, 1203
Medicinal Charcoal, 203
Medium Chain Triglycerides, 665
Medrol, 705, 708, 709
Medroxyprogesterone Acetate, 666, 667
Mefoxin, 180, 181
Megace, 668, 669
Megestrol Acetate, 668, 669
Meglumine Antimoniate, 670
Melaleuca oil, 1243
Melarsomine, 671
Melatonin, 673
Meloxicam, 675
Melphalan, 678
MembraneBlue, 1069
Menthol, 1189, 1243
Mepacrine HCl, 924
Meperidine HCl, 680, 682
Mephyton, 857, 858
Mepron, 90, 91
Mercaptopurine, 682, 684
Meropenem, 684
Merrem I.V., 684, 685
Mesna, 540
Mestinon, 916, 917
Metacam, 675, 678
Metacortandralone, 886
Metadate, 705
Metaglip, 491
Metaldehyde, 1244
Metamucil, 913
Metergoline, 685
Metformin HCl, 686
Methadone HCl, 688
Methadose, 690
Methanol, 1244
Methazolamide, 690
Methenamine, 692
Methigel, 696
Methimazole, 693, 695
Methio-Form, 696
Methionine, 695
Methitest, 709, 710
Methitest, 709
Methocarbamol, 697
Methohexital Sodium, 698
Methoprene Combinations, Topical, 1225
Methotrexate, 700
Methotrexate LPF, 702
Methylene Blue, 702, 703
Methylin, 705
Methylphenidate, 704
Methylphenyl Isoxazolyl Penicillin, 794

Methylprednisolone, 705
Methylprednisolone Acetate, 705
Methylprednisolone Sodium Succinate, 705
Methyltestosterone, 709
Metipranolol Ophthalmic, 1153
Metoclopramide HCl, 710, 712
Metopirone, 718
Metoprolol, 713
Metronidazole, 715, 718
Metyrapone, 718
Mexiletine HCl, 720
Mexitil, 720
MG 217 Medicated Tar, 1215
Miacalcin, 141
Mibolerone, 721, 722
Micalcin, 142
Micardis, 1001, 1002
MicaVed, 1210, 1235
Micazole, 1210, 1235
Miconazole Ophthalmic, 1154
Miconazole, Topical, 1210, 1235
Miconosol, 1210, 1235
Micotil, 1033
Micotil 300 Injection, 1034
Micro Pearls Advantage Seba-Hex Shampoo, 1213, 1214
Microcyn, 1205
Micronase, 498
Micro-Pearls Advantage Benzoyl-Plus, 1196
Micro-Pearls Advantage Dermal-Soothe, 1188, 1210
Microzide, 520
Midazolam HCl, 722
Milbemite, 727, 1237
Milbemycin Oxime, 726
Milk of Magnesia, 949
Milk Thistle, 959
Millipred, 887
Milteforan, 727, 728
Miltefosine, 727
Miltex, 728
Mineral Oil, 728
Minipress, 883
Minitran, 773, 774
Minocin, 730, 732
Minocycline HCl, 730
MiraLax, 868
Mirtazapine, 732
Misoprostol, 734
Mitaban, 1218, 1219
Mitaban, 1219
Mita-Clear, 1237
Mitomycin C, 1154
Mitomycin Ophthalmic, 1154
Mitosol, 1154, 1155
Mitotane, 737
Mitoxantrone Hcl, 739
Mobic, 678
Mobicox, 677, 678
Modified Burow's Solution, 1184
Modipher EQ, 853
Modrastane, 1065
Molybdate, 56
Molypen, 56
MometaMax Otic, 1194, 1198, 1207, 1235
Mometasone Furoate, 1193

Monodox, 369
Monoket, 580
Montelukast Sodium, 741
Monurol, 473
Morantel Tartrate, 742
Morphine Sulfate, 743
Morphine Sulfate Ophthalmic, 1155
Mothballs, 1244
Motilium, 353, 355
Motrin, 1242
MoviPrep, 868
Moxeza, 1156
Moxidectin, 747
Moxifloxacin Ophthalmic, 1156
MPA, 667
MS Contin, 747
MTX, 700
Mucomyst, 11
Mupirocin, 1198, 1199
Muriate of Ammonia, 55
Muricin, 1198
Murine Tears, 1121
Mu-Se, 1093
Mustargen, 660
Mustargen, 661
Mustine, 661
Myambutol, 407, 409
Myclyns, 1205
Mycobacterial Cell Wall Fraction Immuno-modulator, 751
Mycophenolate Mofetil, 752
Mycostatin, 781
Mydral, 1179
Mydriacyl, 1178
Myfortic, 754
Mylepsin, 892
Myleran, 132, 133
Mylocel, 533
Myotonachol, 112
Mysoline, 890, 892

Na2EHDP, 412
N-acetylcysteine, 11, 12
N-Acetylhydroxylamide, 11
N-Acetyl-L-cysteine, 12
N-acetyl-p-aminophenol, 6
Nalbuphine HCl, 756
Nalbuphine Ophthalmic, 1157
Naloxone HCl, 757
Naltrexone HCl, 759
Nandrolone Decanoate, 761, 762
Nandrolone Laurate, 762
Nano•E, 1093
Naphazoline, 1242
Naphthalene, 1244
Naprelan, 763, 764
Naprosyn, 762, 763, 764
Naproxen, 762, 1242
Naquasone Bolus, 305
Narcan, 757, 759
Nasalcrom, 265
Natacyn, 1157
Natamycin Ophthalmic, 1157
Natroba, 973
Natulan, 897
Navigator, 770

Naxcel, 190, 193
n-butylscopolammonium Bromide, 754
Nebcin, 1039
Nedocromil Ophthalmic, 1158
Nembutal, 832
Nemex, 914, 915
Nemex-2, 915
Neo Mercazole, 157
Neo-Carbimazole, 156, 157
Neo-Darbazine, 898
Neo-fradin, 766
Neofrin, 1162
Neomix, 764
Neomycin Sulfate, 764
Neomycin, Polymyxin B, Hydrocortisone Otic Solution and Suspension, 1236
Neo-Predef w/ Tetracaine Powder, 1193
Neoral, 269, 273
Neosar, 266
Neosol, 537
Neosporin, 1195
Neostigmine, 766
Neostigmine Methylsulfate, 766
Neo-Synephrine, 847, 848
Neovet, 766
Nepafenac Ophthalmic, 1159
Neptazane, 690
Neupogen, 442, 443
Neurontin, 478, 480, 1243
Neurosyn, 890, 892
Neut, 962
Neutrogena T/Gel Original, 1215
Nevanac, 1159
NexHA, 515
NexIUM, 404
NFZ Puffer, 1199
N-Hydroxyacetamide, 11
Nicotinamide, 769
Nilstat, 781
Niravam, 35
Nitazoxanide, 769
Nitenpyram, 770
Nitro-BID, 773, 774
Nitro-Dur, 774
Nitrofurantoin, 771
Nitrofurazone, Topical, 1199
Nitrogen Mustard, 661
Nitroglycerin, 773
Nitropress, 774, 776
Nitroprusside Sodium, 774
Nizatidine, 776
Nizoral, 1208
Nizoral A-D, 1209
Nizoral, 599, 602, 1209
N-methyl-glucamine antimoniate, 670
No-Bite Ear Mite Control, 1237
No-Doze, 1242
Nolva-Cleanse, 1232
Nolvasan, 1201
Nolvasan Otic, 1232
Noradrenaline, 777
Norcalciphos, 150, 649, 855
Norco, 522
Norcuron, 1081, 1082
Norepinephrine Bitartrate, 777
Normal Saline, 1246

Normosol-M w/D5, 1247
Normosol-R pH 7.4, 1246
Norocarp, 163
Norodine, 990
Noromycin, 805
Norpace, 347, 349
Norpace CR, 349
North American Pit Viper Antivenin, 73
Notensil, 5
Novantrone, 739, 741
Novobiocin Sodium, 779
Novocox, 163
Novolin, 557
Noxafil, 871, 872
NTG, 773
Nubain, 756, 757
Nuflor Gold, 449
NuFlor, 447, 449
NuLev, 537
NuLytely, 868
Numorphan, 799, 801
NutreStore, 498
Nutrived, 232, 622
NutriVed Chewable Zinpro, 1110
Nyamyc, 1211
Nylar, 1229
Nystatin, 780, 1211
Nystatin, Neomycin, Thiostrepton Ointment, 1236
Nystatin-Triamcinolone Acetonide, 1195
Nystatin-Triamcinolone Acetonide Ointment, 1195
Nystop, 1211

o, p' – DDD, 737
OCL Solution, 868
Oclacitinib, 782
Octreotide Acetate, 783
Ocufen, 1143
Ocuflox, 1160
Ocupress, 1129
OCuSOFT, 1148
Oestriol, 406
OFA Gel Capsules Extra Strength, 424
Off, 1243
Ofloxacin Ophthalmic, 1160
Ofloxacin Otic, 1234
Oleptro, 1057
Olopatadine Ophthalmic, 1161
Olsalazine Sodium, 784
Omedga, 424
Omega EFA Capsules, 424
Omeprazole, 785
Omnipaque, 564, 566
Omnipred, 1165
Oncovin, 1087
Ondansetron, 787
Onmel, 585
Onsior, 935, 938
Opana, 801
Opticlear, 1148
Opticrom, 1132
Optimmune, 1133
OptiPranolol, 1153
Optivar, 1122
Oramorph SR, 747

Orapred, 887
Orapred ODT, 887
Orbax, 788, 790
Orbenin-DC, 256
Orbifloxacin, 788
Ormetoprim, 994
Osaterone Acetate, 790
Oseltamivir Phosphate, 791
Osmoglyn, 499
OSPHOS, 240
Otibiotic, 1190, 1198, 1207, 1235
Otic Clear, 1232
Oticetic Flush, 1232
Oti-Clens, 1233
OtiRinse Ear Solution, 1233
Oti-Soothe Ear Cleansing Solution, 1233
Oti-Soothe+PS Ear Cleansing Solution, 1233
Oti-Tris Flush, 1233
Otocetic Solution, 1233
Otomax, 1190, 1198, 1207
Otomax, 1235
Otomite Plus, 1237
Otrexup, 702
Ovaban, 668, 669
Ovacyst, 504
Ovuplant, 295
Oxacillin Sodium, 793
Oxazepam, 795
Oxfendazole, 796
Oxibendazole, 797
Oxibenz-3, 1196, 1213, 1214
Oxipurinol, 33
Oxybuprocaine, 1124
Oxybutinyn HCl, 799
Oxybutynin Chloride, 798
Oxyderm Shampoo, 1196, 1214
Oxyglobin, 510
Oxyglobin, 512
Oxyject, 805
Oxymetazoline, 1242
Oxymorphone HCl, 799
Oxypurinol, 33
Oxytet, 805
Oxytetracycline, 802
Oxytetracycline Ophthalmic, 1161
Oxytocin, 806.808
Oxytrol, 798, 799

P.G. 600 Estrus Control, 221
Paccal-Vet, 810
Pacccal-Vet-CA1, 809
Pacerone, 48
Palabis, 116
Palladia, 1042, 1044
Pamidronate Disodium, 811
Panacur, 425, 427
Panakare Plus Powder, 813
Pancrelipase, 812
Pancrepowder Plus, 813
Pancreved Powder, 813
Pancrezyme Powder, 813
Pancuronium Bromide, 813
Panolog, 1194, 1211, 1236
PanOxyl, 1196
Pantoloc, 815
Pantoprazole, 815

Paracetamol, 6
Paradichlorobenzene, 1244
Paradyne, 950
Paraguard Shampoo, 1214
Paraplatin, 158
Parapox Ovis Virus Immunomodulator, 816
Parastar, 1222
Parastar Plus, 1222
Paregoric, 817, 818
Parlodel, 122, 123
Paromomycin Sulfate, 819
Paroxetine HCl, 820
Pataday, 1161
Patanol, 1161
Paxil, 820, 821
Paxil CR, 821
PCMX, 1202
Pediapred, 887
Pedi-Dri, 1211
Penicillamine, 822
Penicillin G, 825
Penicillin G (aqueous) Procaine, 828
Penicillin G Benzathine, 828
Penicillin G Procaine, 828
Penicillin V Potassium, 829, 830
Penicillins, General Information, 823
Pennies (U.S.), 1244
Pentasol, 416
Pentaspan, 533
Pentastarch, 530, 533
Pentazocine HCL, 830
Pentobarbital Sodium, 832
Pentosan Polysulfate Sodium, 835
Pentostam, 964, 965
Pentothal, 1018, 1020
Pentoxifylline, 836
Pepcid, 418, 419
Peppermint oil, 1243
Pepto-Bismol, 115, 716
Percorten-V, 297, 298
Performer, 424
Pergolide Mesylate, 838
Periactin, 273
Periostat, 369
Permethrin, 1227, 1242
Peroxiderm, 1214
Peroxiderm S, 1213, 1214
Peroxiderm Shampoo, 1196, 1214
Pet Care Liquid Wormer, 915, 916
PetArmor, 1222
Pethidine, 680
Pethidine HCl, 682
Petrem, 957
Petrolatum, 729
'Pet-safe' antifreeze, 1243
Pexeva, 821
Pexion, 541
Phenadoz, 901
Phenazopyridine, 1242
Phenergan, 899, 901
Phenobarbital, 840
Phenobarbitone, 840, 843
Phenol, 1189
Phenoxybenzamine HCL, 843
Phenoxymethylpenicillin, 829
Phentolamine, 848

Phenylbutazone, 845
Phenylbute, 847
Phenylephrine HCl, 847,1242
Phenylephrine Ophthalmic, 1162
Phenylpropanolamine HCl, 849
Phenytek, 852
Phenytoin Sodium, 850
Pheromones, 852
PhosLo, 145, 146
Phosphate, Parenteral, 854
Phospholine Iodide, 1138
p-Hydroxyampicillin, 59, 62
Physostigmine Salicylate, 855
Phytonadione, 857, 858, 1243
Phytosphingosine Salicylol, 1187
PhytoVet Ear Cleansing Solution, 1233
Phytovet P Cream Rinse, 1188
PhytoVet PSS, 1214
PhytoVet PSS Shampoo, 1196, 1214
PhytoVet S, 1214
Pilocarpine Ophthalmic, 1163
Pima, 563
Pimaracin, 1157
Pimecrolimus Ophthalmic, 1163
Pimecrolimus, Topical, 1216
Pimobendan, 858
Pin-X, 916
Pipa-Tabs, 864
Piperacillin Sodium + Tazobactam, 861
Piperazine, 863, 864
Piperazine Dihydrochloride, 864
Pirlimycin HCl, 864
Piroxicam, 865
Pirsue, 864, 865
Pit Viper Antivenin, 73
Pitocin, 806, 808
Pitressin, 1079
Plaquenil, 530
Plasma-Lyte A, 1246
Plasma-Lyte 56, 1246
Plasma-Lyte R, 1246
Platinol-AQ, 228
Plavix, 249, 251
Plegicil, 5
Polycitra, 232
Polyflex, 67, 69
Polymag, 647
Polyotic, 1012
Polyox II, 647
Polysporin, 1195
Polysulfated Glycosaminoglycan, 868
Polysulfated Glycosaminoglycan Ophthalmic, 1164
Polytar, 1215
Polyurethane Glues, 1244
Ponazuril, 869
Posaconazole, 871
Posatex Otic Suspension, 1236
Posilac, 967
Potassiject, 874
Potassium Acetate, 872
Potassium Bromide, 120
Potassium Chloride, 872
Potassium Citrate, 230
Potassium Gluconate, 872
Potassium Iodide, 561, 563

Potassium Phosphate, 854, 855
Potpourri, liquid, 1244
Poviderm, 1205
Povidine, 1205
Povidone Iodine, Topical 1205
Povidone Iodine Ophthalmic, 1165
PPA, 849
PPS, 835
Pradofloxacin, 875
Pralidoxime Chloride, 877
PrameGel, 1189
Pramosoothe HC, 1188, 1191
Pramoxine, 1188
Prascend, 838, 839
Prax, 1189
Praziquantel, 879
Prazosin HCl, 882
Precedex, 308
Precose, 1
Pred Forte, 1165
Predef 2x, 571, 573
Pred-G, 1146, 1166
Prednisolone, 883-886
Prednisolone Acetate, 886
Prednisolone Ophthalmic, 1165
Prednisolone Sodium Succinate, 883
Prednisone, 883-886
Prednis-Tab, 887
Pregabalin, 887
Preventic, 1220
Previcox, 444-446
Prevpak, 234
Priconazole, 1210, 1235
Prilactone, 975
Prilium, 543, 544
Prilosec, 785, 787
Primaquine Phosphate, 889, 890
Primaxin, 546, 548
Primidone, 890
Primor, 994, 995
Primsol, 991
Prinivil, 630, 631
Priscoline, 1046
Privasan, 1201
Privigen, 551
ProAir HFA, 24
Probanthine, 902
Pro-Banthine, 901
Probenecid, 892
Procainamide HCl, 894
Procanbid, 894, 896
Procarbazine HCl, 896
Prochlorperazine, 898, 899
Procox, 1049
Procrit, 390, 392
Prodine, 1205
Profenal, 1172
Profender, 373, 374, 881
Proglycem, 316
Program, 643, 644, 771
ProHeart6, 750
Prohibit, 617
Proin, 849, 850
PromAce, 2, 5
Promethazine HCl, 899
Promethegan, 901

Pronestyl, 894, 896
Pronyl OTC, 1222
Pronyl OTC Max, 1222
Propalin, 850
Propan B, 902
Propantheline Bromide, 901, 902
Proparacaine Ophthalmic, 1166
Propecia, 443, 444
Propionibacterium Acnes Injection, 903
PropoClear, 908
PropoFlo, 904, 907, 908
Propranolol HCl, 908
Propylene Glycol, 1243
Proscar, 443, 444
Prostaglandin F2a Tromethamine, 339
Prostaglandin F2alpha, 341
Prostigmin, 766, 767, 768
Protamine Sulfate, 910, 911
Protazil, 319, 320
Protirelin, 1023, 1024
Protonix, 815, 816
Protopam Chloride, 877, 878
Protopic, 1217
Proventil, 23
Provera, 666, 667
Prozac, 462-464
ProZinc, 557
Pseudoephedrine, 911, 1242
Pseudomonic Acid A, 1198
PSGAG, 868, 869, 1164
Psyllium Hydrophilic Mucilloid, 913
PTX, 836
Pulmotil, 1033, 1034
Pulmotil AC, 1034
Purell, 1243
Purepsyll Powder, 914
Purinethol, 682, 683, 684
Pyoben Gel, 1196
Pyoben Shampoo, 1196
Pyrantel, 914
Pyrantel Tartrate, 914
Pyrethrin Dip, 1229
Pyrethrins and Pyrethrin Combinations, Topical, 1228
Pyridium, 1242
Pyridostigmine Bromide, 916
Pyridoxine HCl, 918
Pyrilamine Maleate, 919
Pyrimethamine, 920
Pyrimethamine + Sulfadiazine, 922
Pyriproxyfen & Pyriproxyfen Combinations, Topical, 1229

Quadratop Ointment, 1195, 1211, 1236
Qudexy XR, 1050
Quelicin, 983
quellin, 163
Quest, 750
Quest Plus, 751, 881
Quinacrine HCl, 923
Quinidine, 925
Quinidinium, 927
Quixin, 1151

Racemethionine, 695
Ramipril, 927

Ranitidine HCl, 931
Rapinovet, 904, 907
Ravap E.C., 319
ReBalance, 922, 923
Recombinant Omega Interferon (Feline), 560
Reconcile, 462, 464
Re-Covr, 1067, 1068
Recuvyra, 438
Reese's Pinworm, 915
Refresh Endura, 1121
Reglan, 710
Regonol, 917
Regressin-V, 751, 752
Regulin, 673, 674
Regu-Mate, 35, 36
Relief Creme Rinse, 1188
Relief HC Spray, 1188
Relief Shampoo, 1188
Relief Spray, 1188
Relifor, 1190, 1198
Remend, 1121
Remeron, 732
Remicin, 1235
Remicit, 932
Remifentanil HCl, 931
Renagel, 954, 955
Renakare, 874
Renalzin, 610
Renova, 1218
Renvela, 955
Resflor Gold, 449, 460
Resichlor Leave-On Conditioner, 1202, 1209
Resicort Lotion, 1191
ResiKetoChlor Leave-On, 1209
Resisoothe Leave-On Lotion, 1185
Resortin, 1195, 1211
Respiram, 360
Restasis, 1133
Restor-A-Flex, 497
Resultix, 1225
Retin-A, 1218
Retin-A Micro, 1218
Retin-A, 1218
Retrovir, 1107, 1108
Revatio, 957, 958
ReVia, 759, 760
Revolution, 949, 950
rFeIFN-ω, 560
RHTSH, 1022
RHuEPO, 390
Ridaura, 96, 97
Rifadin, 935
Rifamate, 577
Rifampicin, 933
Rifampin, 933
Rifater, 577
Rilexine, 196, 199
Rimadyl, 161, 163
Rimexolone Ophthalmic, 1167
Rimso-50, 337
Ringer's, 1246
Ritalin, 704, 705
RMS, 747
Robaxin, 698
Robaxin-V, 697, 698
Robenacoxib, 935

Robinul, 500
Robinul Forte, 503
Robinul, 503
Robitussin-DM, 1242
Rocaltrol, 143, 144
Rocephin, 193, 194
Rocuronium Bromide, 938
Rofenaid, 995
Romazicon, 454, 455
Romet, 994, 995
Romidys, 942
Romifidine HCl, 940
Rompun, 1099
Ronidazole, 942
Rose Glo, 1168
Rosets, 1168
Roxanol, 747
Rubesol, 266
Rufinamide, 944
Rumatel, 742, 743
Rumen Bolus, 647
RV antifreeze, 1243
Rybix ODT, 1055

(s)-Methoprene Combinations, Topical, 1225
S-Adenosyl-Methionine, 945
Safe-Guard, 425, 427
Safeguard, 427
sal ammoniac, 55
Salazopyrin EN, 996
Salbutamol, 23
Salex, 1214
Salicylic Acid, 1213
Saline Cathartics, 947
Salix, 478
Sal-Tropine, 96
SAMe, 945
Sandclear 99, 914
Sandimmune, 269, 272, 273
Sandostatin, 783, 784
Sarafem, 464
Sarna Sensitive Anti-Itch, 1189
Scalibor Protector, 1220
Scarlet Oil Pump Spray, 1189
Scratchex, 1227
Scratchex Flea & Tick, 1228
SDZ-TMP, 991
Sebazole Shampoo, 1210
Sebolux Shampoo, 1213, 1214
Sebosal-T, 1213, 1215
Sebozole, 1203
Sedanorm, 664
Sedazine, 1103
Sedivet, 940-942
Selamectin, 949
Selegiline HCl, 951
Selenium, 1093
Selenium Sulfide, 1212
Seletoc, 1094
Selgian, 952
Selsun, 1212
Selsun Blue, 1212
Semintra, 1001, 1002
Sentinel, 643, 644, 727, 771
Sentinel Flavor Tabs, 644, 727
Sentinel Spectrum, 644, 727, 881

Sentry Fiproguard, 1222
Sentry Fiproguard Max, 1222
Sentry HC EARMITEfree, 1237
Sentry 2-in-1 Ear Cleaner, 1233
Sepclinx-50, 972
Serax, 795, 796
Seresto, 1224
Sergeant's MITEaway, 1237
Sertraline HCl, 953
Sevelamer, 954
SevoFlo, 955, 957
Sevoflurane, 955
Shohl's solution, 231
Sildenafil Citrate, 957
Silibinin, 959
Silvadene, 1169, 1200
Silver Sulfadiazine (SSD), Topical, 1199
Silver Sulfadiazine Ophthalmic, 1169
Silybin, 959
Silymarin, 959
Simbadol, 127
Simbrinza, 1127, 1128
Simplicef, 182, 183
Sinequan, 361-362
Singulair, 741, 742
Skelid, 1035, 1036
Sleepaway, 416
Slentrol, 345, 47
SMX-TMP, 991
Socumb-6gr, 416
Sodium Antimony Gluconate, 964
Sodium Bicarbonate, 960, 962
Sodium Bromide, 120
Sodium Calcium edetate, 371
Sodium Chloride 0.2%, 1246
Sodium Chloride 0.45%, 1246
Sodium Chloride 3%, 1246
Sodium Chloride 5%, 1246
Sodium Cloxacillin, 256
Sodium Cromoglicate, 264
Sodium Etidronate, 412
Sodium Hyaluronate, 515
Sodium Hypochlorite, 1204
Sodium Hyposulfite, 965
Sodium Iodide, 561, 563
Sodium Oxacillin, 794
Sodium Phosphate, 854
Sodium Phosphate Injection, 855
Sodium Polystyrene Sulfonate, 963, 964
Sodium Selenite, 1093
Sodium Sulfate, 947
Sodium Thiosulfate, 965
SoftGlo, 1143
Sojourn, 957
Solfoton, 843
Solodyn, 732
Soloxine, 619, 622
Solu-Cortef, 522, 525
Solu-Delta-Cortef, 887
Solu-Medrol, 709
Solva-Ker Gel, 1213
Somatotropin, 966
Somlethol, 416
Somnasol, 416
Soothables Crystal-Ear, 1233
Soothe Oatmeal Shampoo, 1185

Soothe XP, 1121
Sorbitol, 967
Soriatane, 13, 14
Sotalol HCl, 969
Sotret, 582
SP5, 416
Spect-Aid, 55
Spectam, 970, 971
Spectinomycin, 970
Spectoguard Scour-Chek, 971
Spectra Sure, 1222
Spectra Sure Plus, 1222
Spectramast, 188
Spectramast DC, 190
Spectramast LC, 190
Spinetoram, 1230
Spinosad, 972
Spironolactone, 974
SPL, 978
Sporanox, 583, 585
Spriafil, 872
SPS, 963, 964
SSD, 1169, 1199
SSD Cream, 1200
SSKI, 561
Stadol, 135, 139
Stanisol, 1213
Stanozolol, 976, 978
Staphage Lysate (SPL), 978, 979
Staphylococcal Phage Lysate, 978
Stiglyn, 766, 767, 768
Stimate, 295, 297
Stoxil, 1147
Streptozocin, 979
Streptozotocin, 980
Stresnil, 97
Stromectol, 590
Stronghold, 950
Strongid C, 916
Strongid T, 914, 916
Strongid, 916
Sublimaze, 430, 432
Subutex, 130
Succimer, 981
Succinylcholine Chloride, 982
Sucralfate, 983, 985
SucroMate Equine, 295
Sudafed, 911, 912, 1242
Sudafed-PE, 1242
Sufenta, 985, 986
Sufentanil Citrate, 985
Suicalm, 98
Sulbactam Sodium, 69
Sulfacetamide Ophthalmic, 1171
Sulfachlorpyridazine Sodium, 986
Sulfadiazine-Trimethoprim, 988, 991
Sulfadimethoxine, 992
Sulfadimethoxine-Ormetoprim, 994
Sulfamethoxazole-Trimethoprim, 988, 991
Sulfasalazine, 995
Sulfasol, 993
Sulfatrim, 991
Sulfazine, 996
Sulfazine EC, 996
Sulfodene Shampoo, 1206, 1215
Sulfodene Ear Cleaner, 1233

Sulfur and Tar Shampoo, 1215
Sulfur Benz, 1196, 1214
Sulfur, Precipitated, 1214
Sulfurated Lime Solution, 1209
Suntheanine, 607
Super Vanadyl Fuel, 1077
Suprane, 293, 294
Suprax, 173
Suprofen Ophthalmic, 1172
Surolan, 1236
Surpass, 321, 322
Swimmer's Ear Astringent, 1233
Symax FasTab, 537
Symax-SR, 537
Symmetrel, 38
Synacid, 515
Synanthic, 796, 797
Synotic, 337, 1234
Synovex-H, 1010
Synovex-Plus, 1010
Synthroid, 619, 622
Syprine, 1062, 1063
Systane, 1121

T3, 630
T3 thyronine sodium, 630
T4, 622
T8 Keto Flush, 1208
Tabloid, 1018
Tacrolimus Ophthalmic, 1172
Tacrolimus, Topical, 1217
Tadalafil, 997
Tafluprost Ophthalmic, 1173
Tagamet, 222, 224
Taktic EC, 1219
Talwin, 830, 832
Tamiflu, 791, 793
Tamsulosin, 998
Tanatril, 544
Tapazole, 693, 695
Taurine, 1000
Tavist, 234, 235
Taxol, 810
Tazicef, 183
Taztia XT, 332
Tea Tree oil, 1243
Tears Again, 1121
Tears Naturale, 1121
Tegretol, 154
Telazol, 1030, 1032
Telfast, 440, 441
Telmisartan, 1001
Temaril-P, 887, 1066, 1067
Tempora, 975
Tenormin, 86
Tensilon, 371
Tepadina, 1021
Tepoxalin, 1002
Tera-Gel, 1215
Terbinafine HCl, 1004
Terbinafine HCl, Topical, 1212
Terbutaline Sulfate, 1006
Terramycin, 802, 805, 1161
Terramycin Scours Tablets, 805
Terrell, 575
Tersi, 1212

Tessalon, 109, 110
Testopel, 1010
Testosterone, 1008
Testosterone Cyclopentylpropionate, 1009
Testosterone Cypionate, 1009
Testosterone Enanthate, 1009
Testred, 710
Tetracaine Ophthalmic, 1174
Tetracosactide, 263
Tetracycline HCl, 1010
Tetrahydrozoline, 1242
Tetramine, 1062
Tetrastarch, 530
Tetrathiomolybdate, 56
Tetravisc, 1174
TG, 1018
Theelol, 407
Theo-24, 1015
Theochron, 1015
Theophylline, 1013
TheraTears, 1121
Therios, 199
ThermaCare, 1242
Thermazene, 1200
Thiacetarsamide, 1015
Thia-Dex, 1016
Thiamilate, 1016
Thiamin, 1015
Thiamine HCl, 1015, 1016
Thioctic acid, 1242
Thioguanine, 1017
Thiola, 1038, 1039
Thiopental Sodium, 1018
Thiopentone sodium, 1020
Thiopronine, 1039
Thiotepa, 1020
Thorazine, 215
Throxine-L Powder, 622
Thyrogen, 1023
Thyroid Stimulating Hormone, 1022
Thyrokare Powder, 622
Thyro-L, 622
Thyroliberin, 1024
Thyrotropin, 1022, 1023
Thyrotropin Alfa (RHTSH), 1022
Thyrotropin-Releasing factor, 1024
Thyrotropin-Releasing Hormone, 1023
Thyrozine, 622
TiaGard, 1025
Tiamulin, 1024
Tiazac, 332
Ticarcillin Disodium + Clavulanate
   Potassium, 1025
Tildipirosin, 1028
Tildren, 1034-1036
Tiletamine, 1032
Tiletamine HCl/Zolazepam HCl, 1030
Tilmicosin, 1033
Tilmovet 90, 1034
Tiludronate Disodium, 1034
Timentin, 1025, 1028
Timolol GFS, 1175
Timolol Maleate Ophthalmic, 1174
Timoptic, 1174
Timoptic-XE, 1175
Tindamax, 1036, 1037

Tinidazole, 1036
Tiopronin, 1038
Tiptone, 333
Tissue Plasminogen Activator Ophthalmic, 1175
TMP-SDZ, 991
TMP-SMX, 991
Tobi, 1039, 1041
Tobradex, 1177
Tobramycin Sulfate, 1039
Tobramycin Sulfate Ophthalmic, 1176, 1234
Tobrex, 1177, 1234
Toceranib Phosphate, 1042
Today, 200
Tofranil, 548, 549
Tofranil-PM, 549
Tolazine, 1044, 1046
Tolazoline HCl, 1044
Tolfedine, 1046, 1047
Tolfejec, 1047
Tolfenamic Acid, 1046
Toltrazuril, 1047
Toltrazuril Sulfone, 869
Tomorrow, 200
Topamax, 1049, 1050
Topicaine, 1187
Topiragen, 1050
Topiramate, 1049
Toprol XL, 713, 715
Toradol, 605
Torasemide, 1051
Torbugesic, 135, 139
Torbugesic-SA, 139
Torbutrol, 135, 139
Torsemide, 1051
Toxiban, 203
Toxiban Suspension with Sorbitol, 203, 968
t-PA, 1175
Tracrium, 91, 93
Tramadol HCl, 1052
Tramisol, 615
trans-Retinoic Acid, 1218
Tranxene, 253
Tranxene T-tab, 254
Tranxene-SD, 253
Trazodone, 1055
Trental, 836, 838
Tresaderm, 1236
Tretinoin, 1218
Trexan, 759
TRH, 1023, 1024
Triamcinolone Acetonide, 1057
Triamcinolone Acetonide Cream, 1195
Triamcinolone Acetonide Lotion, 1195
Triamcinolone Acetonide Ointment, 1195
Triamcinolone Acetonide, Topical, 1194
Triamterene, 1061
Tribrissen, 988, 991
Triclosan, 1206
Trientine HCl, 1062
Trifexis, 727, 973
Trifluorothymidine, 1177
Trifluridine Ophthalmic, 1177
Tri-Hist Granules, 920
Trilostane, 1063
Trimeprazine, 1066

Trimeprazine Tartrate w/Prednisolone, 1066
Trimethoprim-Sulfadiazine, 988, 991
Trimethoprim-Sulfamethoxazole, 988, 991
Trimox, 59
Trioptic-S, 1147
Triostat, 628, 630
Tri-Otic, 1235
Tripelennamine HCl, 1067
Triple Antibiotic Ophthalmic, 1177
Tritop, 1193, 1236
Trivetrin, 991
TrizChlor 4 Spray, 1201
TrizCHLOR, 1235
TrizChlor 4 Wipes, 1202
TrizChlor Flush, 1202
TrizEDTA Aqueous and Crystals Flush, 1233
TrizEDTA, 1235
TrizULTRA + Keto, 1235
TrizULTRA + KETO Flush, 1208
Trocoxil, 658, 660
Trokendi XR, 1050
Tronothane, 1189
Tropicamide Ophthalmic, 1178
Trusopt, 1137
Trypan Blue, 1068
TSH, 1022
TTM, 56
Tucoprim, 991
Tulathromycin, 1069
Tumil-K, 874
Tussigon, 521, 522
Tylan, 1071, 1073
Tylan Soluble, 1073
Tylenol, 6, 7, 1241
Tylenol with Codeine, 258
TyloMed-WS, 1073
Tylosin, 1071

UAA (Universal Animal Antidote) Gel, 203
Ulcergard, 787
Ultane, 955, 957
Ultiva, 931, 932, 933
Ultracet, 1055
Ultram, 1052, 1055
Ultram ER, 1055
Unasyn, 69, 71
Uniferon, 571
Uniprim, 991
Unithroid, 622
Universal Medicated Shampoo, 1203
Urecholine, 112, 114
Urex, 692, 693
UriKare, 55
Urispas, 447
Urocit-K, 230, 232
Uroeze, 54, 55
Urolene Blue, 703
Urso, 1073, 1074
Ursodeoxycholic acid, 1073, 1074
Ursodiol, 1073

Valbazen, 19
Valium, 312, 315
Valproate Sodium, 1075
Valproic Acid, 1075
Vanadium, 1076

Vanadyl Fuel, 1076
Vanadyl Sulfate, 1076
Vancocin, 1077, 1079
Vancomycin HCl, 1077
Vancomycin Sulfate Ophthalmic, 1179
Vanectyl-P, 1067
Vantin, 182, 183
Vasodilan, 582
Vasodilan, 582, 1081
Vasopressin, 1081
Vasopressin Tannate, 1081
Vasotec, 374, 376, 377
Vasotop, 927
VCR, 1089
Vebonol, 119
Vectra, 1221
Vectra 3D, 1221, 1227
Vecuronium Bromide, 1081
Veetids, 830
Vegetable Oil Dietary Supplements, 422
Velban, 1085-1087
Ventipulmin, 236, 237
Ventolin, 23
Veraflox, 875, 876, 877
Verapamil HCl, 1083
Verelan, 1083, 1085
Veripred, 887
Versed, 722, 725
Vet Solutions BPO-3, 1196
Vetadine, 1205
VetaKet, 598
Vetalar, 592, 598
Vetalog, 1057, 1060
Vetalog Parenteral, 1060
Vetamine, 598
Vetasyl, 914
Vetericyn, 1148, 1204
Vetericyn VF, 1204, 1233, 1234
Vetisulid, 986, 988
Vet-Kem Ovitrol Plus, 1228, 1229
Vetmedin, 858, 860
Vetoryl, 1063, 1065
Vetprofen, 163
Vetromax, 1190, 1198, 1207, 1235
Vetropolycin HC, 1147
Vetsulin, 554, 557
Vexol, 1167
Vfend, 1094-1096, 1180
Viactiv, 1242
Viagra, 957, 958
Vibramycin, 365-359
Vibra-Tabs, 369
Vicodin, 522
Vidalta, 157
Vigamox, 1156
Vinblastine Sulfate, 1085, 1087
Vincasar PFS, 1090
Vincristine Sulfate, 1087, 1090
Vinegar, 9
Viodine, 1205
Viokase, 812
Viokase-V Powder, 813
Viralys Gel, 645
Virbagen Omega, 560, 561
Viroptic, 1177
Visine, 1242

Visine Tears, 1121
VisionBlue, 1069
Visipaque, 563, 564
Vistaril, 534
Vistide, 1130
Vita-Flex Sand Relief, 914
Vita-Jec, 858
Vital E, 1093
Vitamin A, 1090
Vitamin A Acid, 1218
Vitamin A Palmitate, 1091
Vitamin B1, 1015
Vitamin B12, 265
Vitamin B6, 918
Vitamin BT, 160
Vitamin C, 79
Vitamin D, 1242
Vitamin D2, 394
Vitamin E, 1092, 1093
Vitamin E/Selenium, 1092
Vitamin K1, 857, 1243
Vivitrol, 760
VLB, 1087
Voltaren Ophthalmic, 1136
Voltaren-XR, 322
Voluven, 533
Voriconazole, 1094
Voriconazole Ophthalmic, 1180

Warfarin Sodium, 1097, 1243
Wellvone, 91
White Mineral Oil, 729
White Petrolatum, 728
Winstrol-V, 976

Xalatan, 1150
Xanax, 33, 35
X-Ject, 1103
Xolegel, 1209
Xyla-Ject, 1103
Xylazine HCl, 1099
Xylitol, 479, 1243
Xylocaine, 623, 625

Yobine, 1104, 1105
Yohimbine HCl, 1104
Ypozane, 790, 791

Zactran, 481, 482
Zaditor, 1150
Zafirlukast, 1106
Zanosar, 979, 980
Zantac, 929-931
ZDV, 1108
Zegerid, 787, 963
Zelapar, 952
Zemuron, 938, 939, 940
Zeniquin, 652, 654
Zentonil, 947
Zestril, 630, 631
Zetar, 1215
Zeuterin, 1110, 1111
Zidovudine (AZT), 1107
Zimecterin Gold, 590, 881
Zimectrin, 590
Zinacef, 195-196
Zinc (Systemic, 1108
Zinc Acetate, 1110
Zinc Gluconate, 1110
Zinc Gluconate (Neutering Agent), 1110
Zinc Gluconate (Neutralized), Topical, 1189

Zinc Sulfate, 1108, 1110
Zinca-Pak, 1110
Zinecard, 309, 310
Zioptan, 1173, 1174
Zirgan, 1144
Zithromax, 102, 104
Zofran, 787, 788
Zolazepam, 1030-1032
Zolicef, 170
Zoloft, 953, 954
Zolpidem, 454
Zonatuss, 109
Zonegran, 1111-1113
Zonisamide, 1111
Zosyn, 861-863
Zovirax, 14, 15, 16
Zubrin, 1002, 1003, 1004
Zuplenz, 788
Zuprevo, 1028, 1029
Zyclara, 1216
Zydax, 836
Zylet, 1153, 1177
Zylexis, 816, 817
Zyloprim, 31, 33
Zymar, 1144
Zymaxid, 1144, 1145
Zymox Spray, 1191
Zymox Topical, 1203
Zymox Cream, 1191
Zymox Ear Cleanser, 1233
Zymox Otic Hydrocortisone Free, 1233
Zymox Otic with Hydrocortisone, 1233
Zymox Plus Otic-HC, 1234
Zyrtec, 200, 201

Plumb's Veterinary Drug Handbook, Eighth Edition

offers an update to the most extensive and comprehensive source of drug information relevant to veterinary medicine. Easy to use and packed with detailed information encompassing monitoring, chemistry, storage, compounding, and dosages, this bestselling book provides reliable information on the use of an exhaustive list of drugs in a wide variety of species, including dogs, cats, exotic animals, and farm animals. Designed for fast access, the Eighth Edition has been revised to significantly reduce the number of dosage entries for a given indication, providing clearer guidance for selecting the correct dosage.

The Eighth Edition adds 43 new systemic drug monographs, and listed dosages have been extensively revised to address FDA status, current clinical use, and supporting evidence. New appendices cover multidrug sensitivity in dogs and provide a list of compounds and ingredients found in common household items and over-the-counter drugs that are potentially toxic to animals.

Plumb's Veterinary Drug Handbook is available as both an 8½ x 11-inch desk size, offering enhanced readability and ease of use, and in the convenient 5- by 8-inch pocket size. Plumb's exhaustive one-volume coverage of drugs approved for veterinary species and non-approved (human) drugs that are used in veterinary practices today make this book an essential reference for veterinarians, veterinary technicians, veterinary pharmacologists, pharmacists with veterinary patients, animal research or zoological facilities, and libraries that serve these groups.

Key Features

› Fully updated edition of the classic veterinary drug handbook, now with fewer dosages per indication for clearer guidance on selecting a dose
› Features 43 new drugs, as well as updated dosages and information for existing monographs and new appendices covering multidrug sensitivity in dogs and compounds potentially toxic to animals
› Offers an authoritative, complete reference for detailed information about animal medication
› Designed to be used every day in the fast-paced veterinary setting
› Includes dosages for a wide range of species, including dogs, cats, exotic animals, and farm animals
› Provides a must-have reference for veterinarians and veterinary students

The Author

DONALD PLUMB was formerly Director of Pharmacy Services and Hospital Director at the University of Minnesota's Veterinary Medical Center. Now retired from the University of Minnesota, he focuses full-time on providing veterinary drug information to veterinarians, other health professionals, and animal caretakers.